Schmidek & Sweet

# *Operative Neurosurgical Techniques*

## Indications, Methods, and Results

*Henry H. Schmidek, MD, FACS*

*Marion, Massachusetts*

### Fourth Edition
#### Volume 1

**W.B. SAUNDERS COMPANY**
A Harcourt Health Sciences Company
Philadelphia London New York St. Louis Sydney Toronto

**W.B. SAUNDERS COMPANY**
*A Harcourt Health Sciences Company*

The Curtis Center
Independence Square West
Philadelphia, Pennsylvania 19106

**Library of Congress Cataloging-in-Publication Data**

Schmidek & Sweet operative neurosurgical techniques: indications, methods, and results / edited by Henry H. Schmidek—4th ed.

p.    cm.

Includes bibliographical references and index.

ISBN 0–7216–7813–0 (set). ISBN 0–7216–7814–9 (vol. 1).
ISBN 0–7216–7815–7 (vol. 2).
1. Nervous system—Surgery.   I. Schmidek, Henry H.   II. Sweet, William Herbert.
   III. Operative neurosurgical techniques. IV. Title: Schmidek and Sweet operative
   neurosurgical techniques.   V. Title: Operative neurosurgical techniques.
   [DNLM: 1. Neurosurgery—methods.     WL 368 S348 2000]

RD 593.063   2000     617.4′8—dc21

DNLM/DLC                                                                99-38473

*Acquisitions Editor:* Richard Zorab
*Developmental Editor:* Catherine Carroll
*Manuscript Editor:* Marjory I. Fraser
*Production Manager:* Paul Nigel Harris
*Illustration Specialist:* Walter Verbitski

SCHMIDEK & SWEET OPERATIVE NEUROSURGICAL TECHNIQUES:
Indications, Methods, and Results

ISBN 0–7216–7813–0 (set)
ISBN 0–7216–7814–9 (vol. 1)
ISBN 0–7216–7815–7 (vol. 2)

Printed in the United States of America.

Last digit is the print number:     9    8    7    6    5    4    3    2    1

*Time present and time past*
*Are both perhaps present in time future*
*And time future contained in time past*

*—T.S. Eliot*


*Dedicated to*

*Alexandra Schmidek, MD*
*and*
*William H. Sweet, MD*

# Contributors

**DIANA ABSON-KRAEMER, M.D.**
Department of Neurosurgery, Swedish Medical Center, Seattle, Washington
*Diagnostic Techniques in Surgical Management of Epilepsy: Strip Electrodes, Grids, and Depth Electrodes*

**CHRIS B. T. ADAMS, M.Chir., F.R.C.S.**
Lecturer in Neurosurgery, University of Oxford; Consultant Neurosurgeon, Radcliffe Infirmary, Oxford, United Kingdom
*Transcranial Surgery for Pituitary Macroadenomas; Management of Craniopharyngiomas: Additional Comment*

**MAHMOUD AL-YAMANY**
Academic and Educational Organizer and Acting Head, Department of Neurosurgery, Riyadh Medical Complex, Riyadh, Saudi Arabia
*Surgical Management of Cranial Dural Arteriovenous Fistulas*

**JEAN-YVES ALNOT**
Professor and Surgeon, Groupe Hospitalier Bichat—Claude Bernard; Chief of Department of Orthopedics–Traumatology, Paris, France
*Surgical Management of Lesions of the Adult Brachial Plexus*

**MELVIN G. ALPER, M.D.**
Attending Physician, Washington Hospital Center, Washington, D.C.
*Anterior and Lateral Approaches to the Orbit and Orbital Apex*

**ARUN PAUL AMAR, M.D.**
Clinical Instructor, Department of Neurosurgery, University of Southern California School of Medicine, Los Angeles, California
*Surgical Management of Growth Hormone–Secreting and Prolactin-Secreting Pituitary Adenomas; Transcallosal Approach to the Third Ventricle*

**SEPIDEH AMIN-HANJANI, M.D.**
Clinical Fellow in Surgery, Harvard Medical School; Resident in Neurosurgery, Massachusetts General Hospital, Boston, Massachusetts
*Surgical Management of Cavernous Malformations of the Nervous System*

**OLEH M. ANTONYSHYN, M.D., F.R.C.S.C.**
Associate Professor, University of Toronto Faculty of Medicine; Chief of Plastic Surgery, Division of Plastic Surgery, Department of Surgery, Sunnybrook Health Science Centre, Toronto, Ontario, Canada
*Cranioplasty: Indications, Techniques, and Results*

**RONALD I. APFELBAUM, M.D.**
Professor of Neurosurgery, University of Utah School of Medicine; Neurosurgeon, University of Utah Hospital; Primary Children's Medical Center, Salt Lake VA Medical Center, Salt Lake City, Utah
*Neurovascular Decompression in Surgical Disorders of Cranial Nerves V, VII, IX, and X*

**MICHAEL L. J. APUZZO, M.D.**
Edwin M. Todd/Trent H. Wells, Jr., Professor of Neurological Surgery and Professor of Radiation Oncology, Biology, and Physics, University of Southern California School of Medicine, Los Angeles, California
*Transcallosal Approach to the Third Ventricle*

**MARK ARGINTEANU, M.D.**
Clinical Assistant Attending Physician, Mount Sinai–New York University Medical Center; Associate Attending Physician, Mt. Sinai Hospital, New York, New York
*Surgical Management of Primary and Metastatic Tumors of the Spine*

**PAUL M. ARNOLD, M.D.**
Associate Professor of Surgery (Neurosurgery), University of Kansas Medical School, Kansas City, Kansas
*Surgical Management of Spinal Infections*

**ANDREW W. ARTENSTEIN, M.D., F.A.C.P.**
Clinical Assistant Professor of Medicine, Brown University School of Medicine, Providence, Rhode Island; Consultant, Infectious Diseases, Hawthorn Medical Associates, New Bedford, Massachusetts
*Suppurative Intracranial Infections*

**ADAM S. ARTHUR, M.D.**
Department of Neurosurgery, University of Utah School of Medicine and University of Utah Hospital; Primary Children's Medical Center, Salt Lake VA Medical Center, Salt Lake City, Utah
*Neurovascular Decompression in Surgical Disorders of Cranial Nerves V, VII, IX, and X*

TAKAO ASANO, M.D., D.M.Sc.
Department of Neurosurgery, Saitama Medical Center/
School, Kawagoe, Saitama, Japan
*Surgical Management of Ossification of the Posterior
Longitudinal Ligament*

PETER WOLF ASCHER, M.D.
Professor and Chairman of the Neurosurgical Department
and Surgical Clinics, University of Rostock, Rostock, Germany
*Percutaneous Lumbar Disk Excision*

ERIK-OLOF BACKLUND, M.D., Ph.D.
Emeritus Professor of Neurosurgery, Department of Clinical Neurosciences, University Hospital, Linköping, Sweden
*Stereotactic Radiosurgery for Pituitary Adenomas and
Craniopharyngiomas*

ROY A. E. BAKAY, M.D.
Department of Neurological Surgery, Emory University
School of Medicine and Hospital; Crawford Long Hospital;
Grady Memorial Hospital; VA Medical Center, Atlanta,
Georgia
*Transplantation in the Human Nervous System in
Parkinson's Disease*

JONATHAN J. BASKIN, M.D.
Neurosurgical Group of Chatham, Chatham, New Jersey
*Surgical Techniques for the Stabilization of the Subaxial
Cervical Spine*

ARMANDO BASSO, M.D., Ph.D.
Professor and Chairman, Neurosurgical Department, University of Buenos Aires School of Medicine and Hospital,
Buenos Aires, Argentina
*Transcranial Approach to Lesions of the Orbit; Sphenoid
Ridge Meningiomas*

JAMES S. BATH, B.S.
Radionics, Inc., Burlington, Massachusetts
*Image-Guided Neurosurgery*

ULRICH BATZDORF, M.D.
Professor, Department of Neurosurgery, UCLA Medical
Center, Los Angeles; Medical Staff, Santa Monica UCLA
Medical Center, Santa Monica, California
*Microsurgery of Syringomyelia and Syringomyelic Cord
Syndrome*

BERNHARD L. BAUER, M.D.
Professor Emeritus, Nordstadt-Krankenhaus, Department of
Neurosurgery, Hannover, Germany
*Surgical Management of Arachnoid, Suprasellar, and
Rathke's Cleft Cysts*

JANET W. BAY, M.D.
Department of Surgery, Riverside Methodist Hospitals; Columbus Children's Hospital; Mt. Carmel Medical Center;
Doctors Hospital West; University Hospital, Columbus,
Ohio
*Surgery of the Sympathetic Nervous System*

P. BEAUCHESNE, M.D.
Medical Doctor, Service de Neurochirurgie, Hôpital Bellevue, Saint Etienne, France
*Lumboperitoneal Shunting*

CARTER E. BECK, M.D.
Chief Resident, Department of Neurosurgery, Stanford University Medical Center, Stanford, California
*Surgical Approaches to the Cervicothoracic Junction;
Surgical Management of Lumbar Spinal Stenosis*

DONALD P. BECKER, M.D.
Professor and Chairman, Division of Neurosurgery, School
of Medicine, University of California, Los Angeles; UCLA
Health Sciences Center, Los Angeles, California
*Surgical Management of Severe Closed Head Injury in
Adults*

JOSHUA BEDERSON, M.D.
Associate Professor of Neurosurgery, Mount Sinai School
of Medicine, New York, New York
*Surgical Management of Spinal Cord Tumors and
Arteriovenous Malformations*

A. L. BENABID, M.D., Ph.D.
J. Fourier University; Hospital of Grenoble, Grenoble,
France
*Multilobar Resections for the Control of Epilepsy*

VALLO BENJAMIN, M.D.
Professor of Neurosurgery, New York University School of
Medicine; Attending in Neurosurgery, Institute of Neurology-Neurosurgery, Beth Israel North Hospital, New York,
New York
*Surgical Management of Tuberculum Sellae and Sphenoid
Ridge Meningiomas*

RAVI BHATIA, M.S., M.Ch.
Professor of Neurosurgery, Department of Neurosurgery,
Indraprastha Apollo Hospital, New Delhi, India
*Surgical Management of Tuberculous Infections of the
Nervous System*

ROLFE BIRCH, M.Chir., F.R.C.S.
Honorary Visiting Professor in Neurology, Royal London
Hospital; Honorary Surgeon, National Hospital for Nervous
Diseases; Hospitals for Sick Children and Royal Postgraduate Medical School, London; Consultant Orthopaedic Surgeon, Royal National Orthopaedic Hospital, Middlesex,
United Kingdom
*Surgical Management of Spinal Nerve Root Injuries*

PERRY BLACK, M.D.
Professor of Neurosurgery, MCP Hahnemann University,
Philadelphia, Pennsylvania
*Surgical and Radiotherapeutic Management of Brain
Metastasis*

NIKOLAS BLEVINS, M.D.
Assistant Professor, Tufts University School of Medicine,
Boston, Massachusetts
*Surgical Management of Glomus Jugulare Tumors*

**GÖRAN C. BLOMSTEDT, M.D., Ph.D.**
Assistant Professor, Helsinki University; Consultant, Helsinki University Central Hospital, Helsinki, Finland
*Considerations of Infections After Craniotomy*

**WARREN BOLING, Jr., M.D., F.R.C.S.(C.)**
Neurosurgeon, Montreal Neurological Hospital, Montreal, Canada
*Stereotactic Intracranial Recording
(Stereoelectroencephalography)*

**SVEND ERIK BØRGESEN, M.D.**
Associate Professor and Chief Surgeon, University Clinic of Neurosurgery, The Neuroscience Center, University of Copenhagen and Rigshospitalet, Copenhagen, Denmark
*Translabyrinthine Approaches to Vestibular Schwannomas*

**JAMES M. BORTHWICK, B.Sc., M.B., Ch.B., F.R.C.A.**
Honorary Clinical Senior Lecturer, University of Glasgow; Consultant Anaesthetist, Institute of Neurological Sciences, Southern General Hospital, Glasgow, Scotland
*Surgical Management of the Rheumatoid Cervical Spine*

**ROBERT E. BREEZE, M.D.**
Division of Neurosurgery and Neural Transplantation Program for Parkinson's Disease, University of Colorado School of Medicine; Division of Neurosurgery, Denver General Hospital; St. Anthony Hospital Central; The Children's Hospital; University Hospital; VA Medical Center, Denver, Colorado
*Transplantation in the Human Nervous System in Parkinson's Disease*

**ALBINO BRICOLO, M.D.**
Professor of Neurosurgery, University of Verona Medical School; Chairman, Section of Neurosurgery, Department of Neurological Sciences and Vision, University Hospital of Verona, Verona, Italy
*Petroclival Meningiomas*

**GAVIN W. BRITZ, M.D.**
Acting Instructor in Neurological Surgery, Department of Neurological Surgery, University of Washington, Seattle, Washington
*Craniofacial Resection for Anterior Skull Base Tumors*

**JASON A. BRODKEY, M.D.**
Neurosurgeon, Michigan Brain and Spine Institute, Ann Arbor, Michigan
*Transtemporal Approaches to the Posterior Cranial Fossa*

**JEFFREY A. BROWN, M.D.**
Medical College of Ohio, Toledo, Ohio
*Percutaneous Trigeminal Nerve Compression*

**JEFFREY N. BRUCE, M.D.**
Associate Professor of Neurological Surgery, College of Physicians and Surgeons of Columbia University; Associate Attending in Neurological Surgery, New York Presbyterian Hospital, New York, New York
*Surgical Management of Intraorbital Tumors;
Supracerebellar Approach to Pineal Region Neoplasms*

**FRANZ XAVER BRUNNER, M.D., D.D.S.**
Professor and Director, Department of Otorhinolaryngology, Zentralklinikum, Augsburg, Germany
*Surgical Management of Trauma Involving the Skull Base and Paranasal Sinuses*

**JACQUES BRUNON, M.D.**
Professor of Neurosurgery, University of Saint Etienne; Head of the Neurosurgical Department, University Hospital (Bellevue), Saint Etienne, France
*Lumboperitoneal Shunting*

**JOHN C. M. BRUST, M.D.**
Professor of Clinical Neurology, College of Physicians and Surgeons of Columbia University; Director of Neurology, Harlem Hospital Center, New York, New York
*Surgical Management of Intracranial Aneurysms Caused by Infection*

**MICHAEL BUCHFELDER, M.D.**
Associate Professor, Department of Neurosurgery, University of Erlangen-Nürnberg, Erlangen, Germany
*Transsphenoidal Microsurgery of Craniopharyngioma*

**JAMES A. BURNS, M.D.**
Assistant Professor, Wright State University School of Medicine; Medical Director, Otolaryngology–Head and Neck Surgery, Wright-Patterson Air Force Base Medical Center, Dayton, Ohio
*Transnasal Endoscopic Repair of Cranionasal Fistulas*

**RICHARD W. BYRNE, M.D.**
Assistant Professor of Neurosurgery, Rush Medical College; Attending Neurosurgeon, Rush–Presbyterian Medical Center, Chicago, Illinois
*Multiple Subpial Transection for Epilepsy*

**JACQUES CAEMAERT, M.D.**
Professor, Department of Neurosurgery, University Hospital of Ghent, Ghent, Belgium
*Endoscopic Neurosurgery*

**GIAMPAOLO CANTORE, M.D.**
Professor of Neurosurgery and Chairman, Department of Neurological Sciences, State University of Rome Medical School, La Sapienza; Chief, Neurosurgical Service, Hospital Policlinico Umberto I, Rome, Italy
*Surgical Management of Tumors of the Cervical Spine and Spinal Cord*

**PAOLA CAPPABIANCA, M.D.**
Department of Systematic Pathology, Federico II University School of Medicine, Naples, Italy
*Repair of the Sella Turcica After Transsphenoidal Surgery*

**JOHN CARBONE, M.D.**
Assistant Professor of Surgery–Orthopaedics and Chief, Division of Spine Surgery, Johns Hopkins Bayview Medical Center and Johns Hopkins University School of Medicine; University of Maryland, R. Adam Crowley Shock Trauma, Baltimore, Maryland
*Surgical Management of Injuries of the Cervical Spine and Spinal Cord*

**THOMAS P. CARLSTEDT, M.D., Ph.D.**
Associate Professor, Karolinska Institute, Stockholm, Sweden; Senior Lecturer, University College of London, London, United Kingdom; Consultant Orthopaedic Surgeon, The Royal National Orthopaedic Hospital, Stanmore, United Kingdom
*Surgical Management of Spinal Nerve Root Injuries*

**ANTONIO G. CARRIZO, M.D.**
Assistant Professor of Neurosurgery, School of Medicine, Buenos Aires National University; Chief of the Neurosurgical Unit, Santa Lucia Hospital, Buenos Aires, Argentina
*Transcranial Approach to Lesions of the Orbit; Sphenoid Ridge Meningiomas*

**BENJAMIN S. CARSON, M.D.**
Professor and Director, Pediatric Neurosurgery, Johns Hopkins School of Medicine, Baltimore, Maryland
*Surgical Management of Achondroplasia and Its Neurosurgical Complications*

**C. MICHAEL CAWLEY, M.D.**
Professor, Emory University School of Medicine, Atlanta, Georgia
*Surgical Management of Aneurysms and Fistulas of the Cavernous Sinus*

**CECIL GUANG-SHIUNG CHANG, M.D.**
Associate Professor of Neurosurgery, Stanford University School of Medicine; Neurosurgeon, Stanford University Hospital, Palo Alto, California
*Failed Microvascular Decompression for Trigeminal Neuralgia*

**PAUL H. CHAPMAN, M.D.**
Neurosurgeon, Department of Neurological Surgery, Massachusetts General Hospital; Professor of Surgery, Harvard Medical School, Boston, Massachusetts
*Surgical Management of Occult Spinal Dysraphism*

**E. THOMAS CHAPPELL, M.D.**
Department of Surgery, Division of Neurosurgery, University of California, Davis, East Bay; Almeda County Medical Center, Oakland, California
*Neurosurgical Management of HIV-Related Brain Lesions*

**DER-YANG CHO, M.D.**
Associate Professor, Neurosurgery, and Chairman, Department of Neurosurgery, China Medical College Hospital, Taichung, Taiwan R.O.C.
*Failed Microvascular Decompression for Trigeminal Neuralgia*

**PASQUALE CIAPPETTA, M.D.**
Professor of Neurosurgery, University of Perugia; Chief, Neurosurgical Service, Hospital S. Maria, Terni, Italy
*Surgical Management of Tumors of the Cervical Spine and Spinal Cord*

**JAMES C. COLLIAS, M.D.**
Assistant Clinical Professor, University of Connecticut School of Medicine, Farmington; Honorary Staff, Department of Neurosurgery, Hartford Hospital, Hartford, Connecticut
*Posterior Surgical Approaches in Cervical Disk Herniation and Spondylotic Myelopathy*

**SCHLOMO CONSTANTINI, M.D., M.Sc.**
Professor of Neurosurgery, Tel-Aviv University; Chief, Division of Pediatric Neurosurgery, Dana Children's Hospital, Tel-Aviv, Israel
*Surgical Management of Intramedullary Spinal Cord Tumors*

**G. REES COSGROVE, M.D., F.R.C.S.(C.)**
Associate Professor of Surgery, Harvard Medical School; Associate Visiting Neurosurgeon, Massachusetts General Hospital, Boston, Massachusetts
*Stereotactic Interstitial Radiosurgery in the Management of Brain Tumors; Cingulotomy for Intractable Psychiatric Illness*

**PAUL R. COSYNS, M.D.**
Professor of Psychiatry, University of Antwerp, Faculty of Medicine; Head of Department of Psychiatry, University Hospital, Antwerp, Belgiuim
*Cerebral Lesions for Psychiatric Disorders and Pain*

**WILLIAM T. COULDWELL, M.D., Ph.D.**
Professor and Chairman, Department of Neurosurgery, New York Medical College, Valhalla, New York
*Surgical Management of Growth Hormone–Secreting and Prolactin-Secreting Pituitary Adenomas*

**T. FORCHT DAGI, M.D., M.P.H., F.A.C.S.**
Department of Surgery, The Uniformed Services University of the Health Sciences; Department of Neurosurgery, St. Joseph's Hospital; Scottish Rite Children's Medical Center; Northside Hospital, Atlanta, Georgia
*Surgical Management of Penetrating Missile Injuries of the Head; Management of Cerebrospinal Fluid Leaks; Vascular Tumors of the Spine*

**RONAN M. DARDIS, M.B., M.Med.Sc., F.R.S.C.I.**
Specialist Registrar in Neurosurgery, King's College Hospital, London, United Kingdom
*Carbon Fiber Implants in Anterior Cervical Disk Surgery*

**ARTHUR L. DAY, M.D.**
Professor, James and Newton Eblen Eminent Scholar in Cerebrovascular Surgery, University of Florida, Gainesville, Florida
*Surgical Management of Aneurysms and Fistulas of the Cavernous Sinus*

**J. DIAZ DAY, M.D.**
Clinical Assistant Professor, Department of Neurological Surgery, University of Southern California; Director, Neurological Surgery, Hoase Ear Clinic, Los Angeles, California
*Surgical Management of Tumors Involving the Cavernous Sinus; Surgical Management of Vertebro–Posterior Inferior Cerebellar Artery Aneurysms*

**ENRICO de DIVITIIS, M.D.**
Department of Systematic Pathology, Federico II University School of Medicine, Naples, Italy
*Repair of the Sella Turcica After Transsphenoidal Surgery*

**PATRICK J. DeROME, M.D.**
University of Paris VIII; Chief of Neurosurgery (Emeritus), Hospital Foch, Suresnes, France
*Transbasal Approach to Tumors Invading the Skull Base; Surgical Management of Endocrinologically Silent Pituitary Tumors*

**ROBERT DERUTY, M.D.**
Professor, School of Medicine; Head of Department of Neurosurgery, Neurological Hospital, Lyon, France
*Surgical Management of Cerebral Arteriovenous Malformations*

**ANAND P. DESAI, M.D.**
Professor of Neuropathology and Head, Department of Pathology, Seth G. S. Medical College; Professor of Neuropathology, K. E. M. Hospital, Parel, Mumbai, Maharashtra State, India
*Surgical Management of Fungal Infections of the Nervous System*

**JACQUEZ CHARL de VILLIERS, M.D., F.R.C.S. (Eng.), F.R.C.S. (Edin.)**
Emeritus Professor of Neurosurgery, Department of Neurosurgery, Groote Schuur Hospital, University of Cape Town, Cape Town, South Africa
*Surgical Management of Arteriovenous Malformations of the Scalp*

**P. C. TAYLOR DICKINSON, M.D.**
Assistant Clinical Professor of Medicine, Columbia University College of Physicians and Surgeons, New York; Attending Physician in Medicine, Nyack Hospital, Nyack, New York
*Surgical Management of Intracranial Aneurysms Caused by Infection*

**CURTIS A. DICKMAN, M.D.**
Associate Chief, Spine Section, and Director, Spinal Research, Division of Neurological Surgery, Barrow Neurological Institute, Phoenix, Arizona
*Surgical Techniques for Stabilization of the Subaxial Cervical Spine*

**JÜRGEN DIETRICH, M.D., Ph.D.**
Department of Radiology, University of Leipzig, Leipzig, Germany
*Open Magnetic Resonance Imaging–Guided Neurosurgery Focusing on Intracranial Gliomas*

**DONALD D. DIETZE, Jr., M.D.**
Assistant Professor of Neurosurgery, Tulane University, Department of Neurosurgery; Tulane Hospital and Clinics; Medical Center of Louisiana–Charity Hospital; Veterans Administration Medical Center, New Orleans, Louisiana
*Primary Reconstruction for Spinal Infections; Surgical Approaches to the Cervicothoracic Junction*

**CONCEZIO Di ROCCO, M.D.**
Professor of Pediatric Neurosurgery, Catholic University Medical School; Head of Pediatric Neurosurgery, Policlinico Gemelli, Rome, Italy
*Surgical Management of Craniosynostosis and Craniofacial Deformities*

**ZAYNE DOMINGO, M.B.Ch.B. (Natal), M.Med. (U.C.T.), D.Phil. (Oxon.), F.C.S. (S.A.)**
Specialist Neurosurgeon, Constantia Medi-clinic, Cape Town, South Africa
*Surgical Management of Arteriovenous Malformations of the Scalp*

**NICHOLAS W. C. DORSCH, M.B.B.S., F.R.C.S., F.R.A.C.S.**
Clinical Associate Professor, Department of Surgery, University of Sydney; Staff Neurosurgeon, Westmead Hospital, Sydney, New South Wales, Australia
*Perioperative Care After an Aneurysmal Subarachnoid Hemorrhage*

**CHARLES G. DRAKE, M.D., F.A.C.S., F.R.C.S.(C.) (deceased)**
Division of Neurosurgery, University of Western Ontario Faculty of Medicine and Hospital, London, Ontario, Canada
*Surgical Management of Terminal Basilar Artery and Posterior Cerebral Artery Aneurysms*

**JAMES M. DRAKE, M.B., B.Ch., F.R.C.S.C.**
Associate Professor, University of Toronto; Staff Neurosurgeon, Hospital for Sick Children, Toronto, Ontario, Canada
*Current Systems for Cerebrospinal Fluid Shunting and Management of Pediatric Hydrocephalus: Endoscopic and Image-Guided Surgery in Hydrocephalus*

**THOMAS B. DUCKER, M.D.**
Professor of Neurosurgery, Johns Hopkins University School of Medicine and Hospital; University of Maryland, Baltimore, Maryland
*Circumferential Spinal Fusion (Cervical)*

**CHRISTOPHER DUMA, M.D.**
Medical Director, HOAG/UCI Gamma Knife Center; Director, Movement Disorder Clinic, Hoag Memorial Hospital Presbyterian, Newport Beach, California
*Sphenoid Ridge Meningiomas*

**JOHN A. DUNCAN III, M.D., Ph.D.**
Assistant Professor, Department of Clinical Neurosciences, Program in Neurosurgery, and Department of Pediatrics, Brown University School of Medicine; Chief, Pediatric Neurosurgery, Rhode Island Hospital/Hasbro Children's Hospital, Providence, Rhode Island
*Surgical Management of Hydrocephalus in Adults*

**STEWART B. DUNSKER, M.D.**
Department of Neurosurgery, University of Cincinnati College of Medicine; Mayfield Neurological Institute, Cincinnati, Ohio
*Surgical Management of Thoracic Disk Herniations*

**ROBERT DUTHEL, M.D.**
Adjunct Professor, University of St. Etienne; Hospital Practitioner, Hôpital Bellevue, Neurosurgical Service, St. Etienne, France
*Lumboperitoneal Shunting*

**W. JEFFREY ELIAS, M.D.**
Resident Neurosurgeon, University of Virginia, Charlottesville, Virginia
*Transsphenoidal Approaches to Lesions of the Sella*

**FRED J. EPSTEIN, M.D., F.A.C.S.**
Professor, Albert Einstein College of Medicine; Chief of Pediatric Neurosurgery and Director, Neurosurgery, Institute of Neurology and Neurosurgery, Beth Israel Medical Center, New York, New York
*Surgical Management of Intramedullary Spinal Cord Tumors*

**MEL H. EPSTEIN, M.D.**
Professor and Co-Chairman, Department of Clinical Neurosciences, Brown University School of Medicine; Neurosurgeon-in-Chief, Rhode Island Hospital, Providence, Rhode Island
*Surgical Management of Hydrocephalus in Adults; Surgical Management of Segmental Spinal Instability*

**NANCY E. EPSTEIN, M.D., F.A.C.S., F.I.C.S.**
Associate Clinical Professor of Neurosurgery, Cornell University Medical College, New York; Chief, Division of Neurosurgery, North Shore University Hospital, Manhasset, New York
*Surgical Management of Far Lateral Lumbar Disks*

**CALVIN B. ERNST, M.D.**
Clinical Professor of Surgery, University of Michigan Medical School, Ann Arbor, Michigan
*Surgical Exposure of the Distal Internal Carotid Artery*

**R. FRANCISCO ESCOBEDO, M.D.**
Professor of Neurology and Neurosurgery, School of Medicine, National University; Chairman of Clinical Research Division, National Institute of Neurology and Neurosurgery, Mexico City, Mexico
*Neurosurgical Aspects of Neurocysticercosis*

**RUDOLF FAHLBUSCH, M.D.**
Chairman, Department of Neurosurgery, University of Erlangen-Nürnberg, Erlangen, Germany
*Transsphenoidal Microsurgery for Craniopharyngioma*

**MAHMOOD FAZL, M.D., F.R.C.S.C.**
Assistant Professor, University of Toronto; Attending Neurosurgeon, Division of Neurosurgery, Department of Surgery, Sunnybrook Health Science Centre, Toronto, Ontario, Canada
*Cranioplasty: Indications, Techniques, and Results*

**RICHARD G. FESSLER, M.D., Ph.D.**
Dunspaugh-Dalton Professor of Brain and Spinal Surgery, Department of Neurological Surgery, University of Florida Brain Institute; Shands Hospital of the University of Florida; Veterans Administration Medical Center, Gainesville, Florida
*Primary Reconstruction for Spinal Infections; Surgical Approaches to the Cervicothoracic Junction*

**BERNARD E. FINNESON, M.D., F.A.C.S.**
Emeritus Director, Low Back Pain Center; Former Chief of Neurosurgery, Crozer-Chester Medical Center, Upland, Pennsylvania
*Lumbar Disk Excision*

**NORMAN D. FISHER-JEFFES, M.B.Ch.B., F.C.S. (S.A.)**
Senior Specialist, Department of Neurosurgery, University of Cape Town; Specialist Neurosurgeon, Panorama Mediclinic, Cape Town, South Africa
*Surgical Management of Arteriovenous Malformations of the Scalp*

**KEVIN T. FOLEY, M.D.**
Director, Complex Spine Service, Semmes-Murphey Clinic; Medical Director, Medical Education and Research Institute; Medical Director, Image Guided Surgery Research Center, Memphis, Tennessee; Clinical Assistant Professor of Surgery, Uniformed Services University of the Health Sciences, Bethesda, Maryland; Associate Professor of Neurosurgery and Biomedical Engineering, University of Tennessee; Attending Physician at Baptist Memorial Hospital, Bowld Hospital, Regional Medical Center, and Methodist Hospitals of Memphis, Memphis, Tennessee
*Microendoscopic Diskectomy*

**ROBERT D. FOSTER, M.D.**
Plastic Surgery Fellow, Division of Plastic Surgery, University of California at San Francisco and San Francisco General Hospital, San Francisco, California
*Cranioplasty: Indications, Techniques, and Results*

**M. J. FOTSO, M.D.**
Medical Doctor, Service de Neurochirurgie, Hôpital Bellevue, Saint Etienne, France
*Lumboperitoneal Shunting*

**RICHARD S. FOX, M.D.**
Assistant Director, Plastic and Reconstructive Surgery, St. Luke's Hospital, New Bedford, Massachusetts
*Surgical Repair of Major Defects of the Scalp and Skull*

**NATALE FRANCAVIGLIA**
Neurosurgical Clinic, St. Martin Hospital, University of Genoa, Genoa, Italy
*Anterolateral Techniques for Stabilization in the Thoracic Spine*

**S. FRANCIONE, M.D.**
Department of Neurology, University of Genoa, Genoa, Italy
*Multilobar Resections for the Control of Epilepsy*

**CLAIR FRANCOMANO, M.D.**
Departments of Medicine and Pediatrics, The Johns Hopkins School of Medicine and Hospital, Baltimore; Medical Genetics Branch, National Center for Human Genome Research, National Institutes of Health, Bethesda, Maryland
*Management of Achondroplasia and Its Neurosurgical Complications*

**CURT R. FREED**
Division of Clinical Pharmacology and Toxicology, University of Colorado School of Medicine; Neurotransplantation Program for Parkinson's Disease, University of Colorado Hospital, Denver, Colorado
*Transplantation in the Human Nervous System in Parkinson's Disease*

**STEPHEN R. FREIDBERG, M.D.**
Department of Neurosurgery, Lahey Clinic, Burlington;
Courtesy Staff, New England Deaconess Hospital, Boston;
Atlanticare Medical Center, Lynn, Massachusetts
*Surgical Management of Cerebrospinal Fluid Leakage
After Spinal Surgery*

**GERHARD FRIEHS, M.D.**
Assistant Professor of Neurosurgery, Brown University
School of Medicine; Rhode Island Hospital, Providence,
Rhode Island
*Surgical Management of Segmental Spinal Instability*

**TAKANORI FUKUSHIMA, M.D., D.M.Sc.**
Department of Neurosurgery, Medical College of Pennsyl-
vania and Allegheny General Hospital, Pittsburgh; Univer-
sity of Southern California, Los Angeles; Karolinska Insti-
tute, Stockholm, Sweden; Komonji Hospital, Kitakyushu;
St. Mary's Hospital, Kurume; Nagasaki Morinoki Hospital,
Nagasaki; Kagoshima Acsuchi Hospital, Kagoshima;
Nishikasai Moriyama Hospital, Tokyo, Japan; Kaiser Per-
manente Hospital, Honolulu, Hawaii
*Surgical Management of Tumors Involving the Cavernous
Sinus*

**MICHAEL R. GAAB, M.D., Ph.D.**
Professor and Chairman, Ernst Moritz Arndt University
Medical School and Hospital, Department of Neurosurgery,
Greifswald, Germany
*Neuroendoscopic Approach to Intraventricular Tumors*

**STÉPHANE GAILLARD, M.D.**
Assistant Neurosurgeon, AIHL–ACCA, University of Paris
VIII; and Foch Hospital, Suresnes, France
*Transbasal Approach to Tumors Invading the Skull Base;
Surgical Management of Endocrinologically Silent
Pituitary Tumors*

**GALE GARDNER, M.D.**
Clinical Professor, Department of Otolaryngology, Univer-
sity of Tennessee College of Medicine, Memphis, Tennes-
see
*Transtemporal Approaches to the Posterior Cranial
Fossa; Surgical Management of Glomus Jugulare Tumors*

**BERNARD GEORGE, M.D.**
Professor of Neurosurgery, University of Paris; Head, De-
partment of Neurosurgery, Lariboisiere Hospital, Paris,
France
*Meningiomas of the Foramen Magnum*

**STEVEN L. GIANNOTTA, M.D.**
Professor, Department of Neurological Surgery, University
of Southern California, Los Angeles, California
*Surgical Management of Vertebro–Posterior-Inferior
Cerebellar Artery Aneurysms*

**RENATO GIUFFRÈ, M.D.**
Professor and Chairman, Institute of Neurosurgery, Depart-
ment of Neurosciences, Tor Vergata University of Rome
Medical School, Rome, Italy
*Surgical Management of Low-Grade Gliomas*

**KEITH Y. C. GOH, M.B.B.S., F.R.C.S., F.H.K.A.M.**
Clinical Tutor, National University of Singapore; Associate
Consultant, Specialist Neurosurgeon, Department of Neuro-
surgery, Singapore General Hospital and Department of
Pediatric Neurosurgery, KK Women's and Children's Hos-
pital, Singapore
*Surgical Management of Intramedullary Spinal Cord
Tumors*

**ALFREDO GÓMEZ-AVIÑA, M.D.**
Professor of Neurology and Neurosurgery, University of
Guadalajara School of Medicine, Jalisco; Medical Division
Director, National Institute of Neurology and Neurosurgery,
Mexico City, Mexico
*Neurosurgical Aspects of Neurocysticercosis*

**TODD A. GOODGLICK, M.D.**
Assistant Clinical Professor, Georgetown University De-
partment of Ophthalmology; Attending Physician, Wash-
ington Hospital Center; Washington, D.C.; Clinical Faculty,
National Eye Institute, National Institutes of Health,
Bethesda, Maryland
*Anterior and Lateral Approaches to the Orbit and Orbital
Apex*

**SERGEY K. GORELYSHEV, M.D.**
Chief, Neurosurgeon and Pediatric Department, Burdenko
Neurosurgical Institute, Moscow, Russia
*Surgical Management of Diencephalic and Brain Stem
Tumors*

**CHARLES W. GROSS, M.D.**
Professor, University of Virginia School of Medicine, Char-
lottesville, Virginia; President, Triologic Society of the
American Academy of Otolaryngology–Head and Neck
Surgery, Alexandria, Virginia
*Transnasal Endoscopic Repair of Cranionasal Fistulas*

**ROBERT G. GROSSMAN, M.D.**
Professor and Chairman, Department of Neurosurgery,
Baylor College of Medicine; Chief of Neurosurgery Ser-
vice, The Methodist Hospital, Houston, Texas
*Temporal Lobe Operations for Drug-Resistant Epilepsy*

**RICHARD W. GULLAN, M.B., B.Sc., M.R.C.P., F.R.C.S.**
Consultant Neurosurgeon, King's College Hospital, Lon-
don, United Kingdom
*Carbon Fiber Implants in Anterior Cervical Disk Surgery*

**BJÖRN GUNTERBERG, M.D., Ph.D.**
Associate Professor of Orthopaedic Surgery, Department
of Surgical Sciences, Gothenburg University; Consultant,
Department of Orthopaedics, Sahlgrenska University Hos-
pital, Gothenburg, Sweden
*Technique of High Sacral Amputation*

**BARTON L. GUTHRIE, M.D.**
Associate Professor, University of Alabama at Birmingham,
Birmingham, Alabama
*Neurosurgical Management of HIV-Related Brain Lesions*

## JAN M. GYBELS, M.D., Ph.D.
Professor Emeritus of Neurosurgery, Department of Neurosciences and Psychiatry, University of Leuven School of Medicine and Hospital, Leuven, Belgium; Member of the Royal Academy of Medicine of Belgium
*Brain Stimulation in the Management of Persistent Pain; Cerebral Lesions for Psychiatric Disorders and Pain*

## MICHAEL M. HAGLUND, M.D., Ph.D.
Assistant Professor of Neurosurgery and Neurobiology, Duke University Medical Center, Durham, North Carolina
*Optical Imaging in Epilepsy Surgery*

## MICHAEL V. HAJJAR, M.D.
Resident, Department of Neurosurgery, University of South Florida College of Medicine, Tampa, Florida
*Surgical Management of Tumors of the Nerve Sheath Involving the Spine*

## STEN HÅKANSON, M.D., Ph.D.
Associate Professor and Consultant, Tawam Hospital, Abu Dhabi, United Arab Emirates
*Retrogasserian Glycerol Rhizolysis in Trigeminal Neuralgia*

## AKIRA HAKUBA, M.D., D.M.Sc.
Professor and Chairman, Department of Neurosurgery, Osaka City University, Osaka, Japan
*Orbitozygomatic Infratemporal Approach to Parasellar Meningiomas*

## MARK G. HAMILTON, M.D.C.M., F.R.C.S.(C.)
Department of Neurosurgery, University of Calgary, Faculty of Medicine; Alberta Children's Hospital; Foothills Hospital; Tom Baker Cancer Center, Calgary, Alberta, Canada
*Surgical Management of Midbasilar and Lower Basilar Aneurysms*

## WINIFRED J. HAMILTON, Ph.D.
Department of Neurosurgery, Baylor College of Medicine, Houston, Texas
*Temporal Lobe Operations for Drug-Resistant Epilepsy*

## RUSSELL W. HARDY, Jr., M.D.
Professor, Department of Neurological Surgery, University Hospital, Case Western Reserve University, Cleveland, Ohio
*Surgery of the Sympathetic Nervous System*

## J. FREDERICK HARRINGTON, Jr., M.D.
Assistant Professor of Neurosurgery, Brown University School of Medicine; Surgeon-in-Charge, Spinal Neurosurgery, Rhode Island Hospital, Providence, Rhode Island
*Surgical Management of Segmental Spinal Instability*

## GRIFFITH R. HARSH, M.D.
Professor, Stanford University Medical School; Director, Brain Tumor Center, Stanford Medical Center, Stanford, California
*Surgical Management of Recurrent Gliomas*

## CARL B. HEILMAN, M.D.
Assistant Professor, Tufts University School of Medicine; Tufts New England Medical Center, Boston, Massachusetts
*Surgical Management of Glomus Jugulare Tumors; Distal Anterior Cerebral Artery Aneurysms*

## OLAVI HEISKANEN, M.D., Ph.D.
Chief of Service (Emeritus), Department of Neurosurgery, Helsinki University Central Hospital, Helsinki, Finland
*Surgical Management of Unruptured Cerebral Aneurysms*

## DIETER HELLWIG, M.D.
Associate Professor, Department of Neurosurgery, Philipps-University of Marburg, Marburg, Germany
*Surgical Management of Arachnoid, Suprasellar, and Rathke's Cleft Cysts*

## SANDRA L. HELMERS, M.D.
Assistant Professor in Neurology, Harvard Medical School; Assistant in Neurology and Director, Evoked Potential Laboratory, Harvard Medical School and Children's Hospital, Boston, Massachusetts
*Treatment of Intractable Epilepsy by Electrical Stimulation of the Vagal Nerve*

## JUHA A. HERNESNIEMI, M.D., Ph.D.
Professor, Department of Neurosurgery, School of Medicine, University of Helsinki; Chairman, Department of Neurosurgery, University Central Hospital of Helsinki, Helsinki, Finland
*Surgical Management of Aneurysms of the Middle Cerebral Artery; Surgical Management of Terminal Basilar Artery and Posterior Cerebral Artery Aneurysms*

## ROBERTO C. HEROS, M.D.
Professor, Co-Chairman, and Program Director, Department of Neurosurgery, University of Miami School of Medicine, Miami, Florida
*Surgical Management of Unclippable Intracranial Aneurysms*

## D. HOFFMANN, M.D.
Hospital of Grenoble, Grenoble, France
*Multilobar Resections for the Control of Epilepsy*

## MARTIN HOLLAND, M.D.
Assistant Professor, University of California at San Francisco; Attending Neurosurgeon, Department of Neurosurgery, San Francisco General Hospital, San Francisco, California
*Cranioplasty: Indications, Techniques, and Results*

## ROBERT N. N. HOLTZMAN, M.D.
Associate Clinical Professor of Neurological Surgery, Columbia University College of Physicians and Surgeons; Associate Attending in Neurosurgery, New York Presbyterian Hospital, New York, New York
*Surgical Management of Intracranial Aneurysms Caused by Infection*

## JÜRGEN HONEGGER, M.D.
Assistant Professor, Department of Neurosurgery, University of Freiburg, Freiburg, Germany
*Transsphenoidal Microsurgery of Craniopharyngioma*

**JOHN H. HONEYCUTT, Jr., M.D.**
Neurosurgery Resident, University of Oklahoma, Department of Neurosurgery, Oklahoma City, Oklahoma
*Surgical Management of Extracranial Carotid Artery Disease*

**MICHAEL B. HOROWITZ, M.D.**
Associate Professor of Neurosurgery and Radiology, Department of Neurological Surgery, University of Pittsburgh School of Medicine and Medical Center, Pittsburgh, Pennsylvania
*Surgical Management of Intraoperative Aneurysm Rupture*

**MOHAMMED HOSBAN, M.B., B.S., F.R.C.S.**
Consultant Neurosurgeon, King Hussein Medical Centre, Amman, Jordan
*Carbon Fiber Implants in Anterior Cervical Disk Surgery*

**EDGAR M. HOUSEPIAN, M.D.**
Professor Emeritus of Neurological Surgery, Columbia University College of Physicians and Surgeons; Attending in Neurological Surgery, Columbia–Presbyterian Medical Center, New York, New York
*Surgical Management of Intraorbital Tumors*

**ALAN R. HUDSON, M.B., Ch.B., F.R.C.S.(C.)**
Professor of Neurosurgery, University of Toronto, Faculty of Medicine; President and CEO, The Toronto Hospital, Toronto, Ontario, Canada
*Surgical Management of Peripheral Nerve Tumors*

**JAMES E. O. HUGHES, M.D.**
Assistant Clinical Professor of Neurological Surgery, College of Physicians and Surgeons of Columbia University; Chief, Division of Neurosurgery, Harlem Hospital Center, New York, New York
*Surgical Management of Intracranial Aneurysms Caused by Infection*

**OREST HURKO, M.D.**
Departments of Neurology and Medicine, Johns Hopkins University School of Medicine; Division of Neurogenetics, Johns Hopkins Hospital, Baltimore, Maryland
*Management of Achondroplasia and Its Neurosurgical Complications*

**MARK R. IANTOSCA, M.D.**
Clinical Assistant Professor, Department of Neurosurgery, University of Connecticut, Farmington; Director, Division of Pediatric Neurosurgery, Connecticut Children's Medical Center, Hartford, Connecticut
*Current Systems for Cerebrospinal Fluid Shunting and Management of Pediatric Hydrocephalus: Endoscopic and Image-Guided Surgery in Hydrocephalus*

**HAE-DONG JHO, M.D., Ph.D.**
Professor of Neurosurgery, University of Pittsburgh Medical Center, Pittsburgh, Pennsylvania
*Endoscopic Transsphenoidal Surgery*

**J. PATRICK JOHNSON, M.D.**
Associate Professor, University of California, Los Angeles School of Medicine; Co-Director, UCLA Comprehensive Spine Program, Division of Neurosurgery, UCLA Medical Center, Los Angeles, California
*Thoracoscopic Sympathectomy*

**FRANCIS JOHNSTON, F.R.C.S.**
Consultant Neurosurgeon, Atkinson Morely Hospital, London, England, United Kingdom
*Craniofacial Resection for Anterior Skull Base Tumors*

**R. A. JOHNSTON, M.D., F.R.C.S.**
Honorary Clinical Senior Lecturer, University of Glasgow; Consultant Neurosurgeon, Institute of Neurological Sciences and Queen Elizabeth National Spinal Injuries Unit, Southern General Hospital NHS Trust, Glasgow, Scotland
*Surgical Management of the Rheumatoid Cervical Spine*

**P. KAHANE, M.D.**
J. Fourier University; Hospital of Grenoble, Grenoble, France
*Multilobar Resections for the Control of Epilepsy*

**ANDREW KAM, M.B.B.S., F.R.A.C.S.**
Neurosurgical Registrar, Royal Alexandra Hospital for Children, Sydney, New South Wales, Australia
*Perioperative Care After an Aneurysmal Subarachnoid Hemorrhage*

**MICHAEL KAZIM, M.D.**
Assistant Professor of Ophthalmology, College of Physicians and Surgeons of Columbia University; Attending in Neurological Surgery, New York Presbyterian Hospital, New York, New York
*Surgical Management of Intraorbital Tumors*

**DANIEL F. KELLY, M.D.**
Division of Neurosurgery, University of California, Los Angeles, School of Medicine and Health Sciences Center, Los Angeles; Harbor-UCLA Medical Center, Torrance, California
*Surgical Management of Severe Closed Head Injury in Adults*

**PATRICK J. KELLY, M.D.**
Professor and Chairman of Neurosurgery, Department of Neurosurgery, New York University School of Medicine; Attending Neurosurgeon, Tisch Hospital–NYU Medical Center, New York, New York
*CT/MRI-Based Computer-Assisted Volumetric Stereotactic Resection of Intracranial Lesions*

**SANFORD KEMPIN, M.D.**
Associate Professor of Clinical Medicine, Cornell University Medical College; Associate Attending Physician and Acting Chief, Hematology Service, Memorial Sloan-Kettering Cancer Center, New York, New York
*Disorders of the Spine Related to Plasma Cell Dyscrasias*

**ELENA A. KHUHLAEVA, M.D.**
Pediatric Neurologist, Bukenko Neurosurgical Institute, Pediatric Department, Moscow, Russia
*Surgical Management of Diencephalic and Brain Stem Tumors*

**DANIEL H. KIM, M.D.**
Assistant Professor, Department of Neurosurgery, and Director of Spinal Neurosurgery and Reconstructive Peripheral Nerve Surgery, Stanford University Medical Center, Stanford, California
*Surgical Approaches to the Cervicothoracic Junction; Surgical Management of Peripheral Nerve Tumors*

**JEROME H. KIM, M.D., F.A.C.P.**
Clinical Assistant Professor of Medicine, University of Maryland School of Medicine, Baltimore; Chief, Section of Virology, Henry M. Jackson Foundation, Rockville, Maryland
*Suppurative Intracranial Infections*

**RICHARD KIM, M.D., M.S.**
Assistant Clinical Professor, Department of Neurological Surgery, University of California, Irvine, Orange, California
*Surgery for Mesial Temporal Sclerosis*

**HIROYUKI KINOUCHI, M.D., Ph.D.**
Assistant Professor, Department of Neurosurgery, Akita University School of Medicine, Akita, Japan
*Intraoperative Endovascular Techniques in the Management of Intracranial Aneurysms*

**DAVID L. KIRSCHMAN, M.D.**
Resident, Department of Neurosurgery, University of Kansas Medical School, Kansas City, Kansas
*Surgical Management of Spinal Infections*

**RIKU KIVISAARI, M.D.**
Resident, Department of Neurosurgery, University Central Hospital of Helsinki, Helsinki, Finland
*Surgical Management of Aneurysms of the Middle Cerebral Artery*

**DAVID G. KLINE, M.D.**
Boyd Professor and Chairman, Department of Neurosurgery, Louisiana State University Medical Center; Visiting Staff, Charity Hospital and University Hospital; Academic Staff, Ochsner Hospital; Senior Staff, Memorial Hospital and Touro; Consultant, New Orleans Veterans Affairs and Kessler AFB Hospitals, New Orleans, Louisiana
*Surgical Management of Peripheral Nerve Tumors*

**SHIGEAKI KOBAYASHI, M.D., Ph.D.**
Professor, Shinshu University School of Medicine, Matsumoto, Japan
*Surgical Management of Paraclinoid Aneurysms*

**ALEXANDER N. KONOVALOV, M.D.**
Director, Burdenko Neurosurgical Institute, Moscow, Russia
*Surgical Management of Diencephalic and Brain Stem Tumors*

**THOMAS A. KOPITNIK, Jr., M.D.**
Associate Professor of Neurological Surgery, Southwestern Medical School, University of Texas, Dallas, Texas
*Surgical Management of Intraoperative Aneurysm Rupture*

**JOHN P. KOSTUIK, M.D.**
Professor, Johns Hopkins University School of Medicine, Baltimore, Maryland
*Surgical Management of Injuries of the Cervical Spine and Spinal Cord*

**MARK D. KRIEGER, M.D.**
Clinical Instructor, Department of Neurological Surgery, University of Southern California School of Medicine, Los Angeles, California
*Surgical Management of Growth Hormone–Secreting and Prolactin-Secreting Pituitary Adenomas*

**RAKESH KUMAR, M.D., F.R.C.S.(E.)**
Department of Neurosurgery, University of Cincinnati College of Medicine and Hospital, Cincinnati, Ohio
*Surgical Management of Thoracic Disk Herniations*

**RON C. KUPERS, Ph.D.**
Assistant Professor, Positron Emission Tomography Center, Aarhus University Hospital, Aarhus, Denmark
*Brain Stimulation in the Management of Persistent Pain*

**KAZUHIKO KYOSHIMA, M.D., Ph.D.**
Associate Professor, Shinshu University School of Medicine, Matsumoto, Japan
*Surgical Management of Paraclinoid Aneurysms*

**SANTOSH D. LAD, M.B.B.S., M.S.**
Undergraduate and Postgraduate Clinical Tutor in Neurosurgery and Accident and Emergency Surgery, Sultan Quaboos University; Oman Medical Specialty Board; Senior Consultant Neurosurgeon and Head, Department of Neurosurgery, National Neurosurgical Centre, Khoula Hospital, Muscat, Oman
*Surgical Management of Fungal Infections of the Nervous System*

**ALEX M. LANDOLT, M.D.**
Professor of Neurosurgery, University of Zurich; Consultant Neurosurgeon, Klinik im Park, Zurich, Switzerland
*Surgical Management of Recurrent Pituitary Tumors*

**EDWARD R. LAWS, Jr., M.D.**
Professor of Internal Medicine and Neurosurgery, University of Virginia School of Medicine, Charlottesville, Virginia
*Transsphenoidal Approaches to Lesions of the Sella*

**CHEN LEE, M.D., F.R.C.S.C., F.A.C.S.**
Assistant Professor, University of California at San Francisco; Attending Plastic Surgeon, Division of Plastic Surgery, Department of Surgery, San Francisco General Hospital, San Francisco, California
*Cranioplasty: Indications, Techniques, and Results*

**ADAM I. LEWIS, M.D.**
Neurosurgeon, St. Dominic's Neuroscience Center; Jackson Neurosurgery Clinic, Jackson, Mississippi
*Surgical Management of Giant Aneurysms of the Anterior Circulation; Surgical Management of Thalamic-Basal Ganglia Vascular Malformations; Surgical Management of Brain Stem Vascular Malformations*

**BENGT LINDEROTH, M.D., Ph.D.**
Associate Professor, Department of Clinical Neuroscience, Section of Neurosurgery, Karolinska Institute; Head, Section of Functional Neurosurgery, Department of Neurosurgery, Karolinska Hospital, Stockholm, Sweden
*Retrogasserian Glycerol Rhizolysis in Trigeminal Neuralgia; Spinal Cord Stimulation for Chronic Pain*

**CHRISTER LINDQUIST, M.D., Ph.D.**
Professor and Consultant Neurosurgeon, Cromwell Hospital, London, United Kingdom
*Gamma Surgery in Cerebral Vascular Lesions, Malformations, Tumors, and Functional Disorders*

**MICHAEL J. LINK, M.D.**
Senior Associate Consultant, Neurologic Surgery, Mayo Clinic, Rochester, Minnesota
*Surgical Management of Thalamic-Basal Ganglia Vascular Malformations; Surgical Management of Brain Stem Vascular Malformations*

**ALI LIU, M.D.**
Professor, Capital University of Medical Science; Director of Gamma-Knife Center, Beijing Neurosurgery Institute, Beijing, China
*Surgical Management of Nonglomus Tumors of the Jugular Foramen*

**JAY S. LOEFFLER, M.D.**
Professor of Radiation Oncology, Harvard Medical School; Director, Northeast Proton Therapy Center, Massachusetts General Hospital, Boston, Massachusetts
*Stereotactic Interstitial Radiosurgery in the Management of Brain Tumors*

**CHRISTOPHER M. LOFTUS, M.D.**
Esther and Ted Greenberg Professor and Chair, Department of Neurosurgery, University of Oklahoma College of Medicine Health Sciences Center, Oklahoma City, Oklahoma
*Surgical Management of Extracranial Carotid Artery Disease*

**DONLIN M. LONG, M.D., Ph.D.**
Professor and Director, Department of Neurosurgery, Johns Hopkins University School of Medicine; Neurosurgeon-in-Chief, Johns Hopkins Hospital, Baltimore, Maryland
*Management of Persistent Symptoms After Lumbar Disk Surgery*

**RUSSEL R. LONSER, M.D.**
Resident, Department of Neurosurgery, University of Utah School of Medicine and Hospital; Primary Children's Medical Center; Salt Lake VA Medical Center, Salt Lake City, Utah
*Neurovascular Decompression in Surgical Disorders of Cranial Nerves V, VII, IX, and X*

**G. Lo RUSSO, M.D.**
Department of Neurosurgery, Epilepsy Surgery Regional Center, Niguarda Hospital, Milan, Italy
*Multilobar Resections for the Control of Epilepsy*

**DARREN S. LOVICK, M.D.**
Neurosurgery Resident, University of Minnesota Medical School, Minneapolis, Minnesota
*Parasagittal and Falcine Meningioma Surgery; Convexity Meningioma Surgery; Posterior Fossa Meningiomas*

**PATRICK G. LYNCH, F.R.C.(Path.)**
Consultant Neuropathologist, Royal Preston Hospital, Preston, United Kingdom
*Surgical Management of Fungal Infections of the Nervous System*

**JOSEPH R. MADSEN, M.D.**
Assistant Professor of Surgery, Harvard Medical School; Associate in Neurosurgery, Children's Hospital and Brigham and Women's Hospital, Boston, Massachusetts
*Treatment of Intractable Epilepsy by Electrical Stimulation of the Vagal Nerve*

**MARCO MAIELLO, M.D.**
Neurosurgical Clinic, St. Martin Hospital, University of Genoa, Genoa, Italy
*Anterolateral Techniques for Stabilization in the Thoracic Spine*

**GIULIO MAIRA, M.D.**
Professor of Neurosurgery, Catholic University School of Medicine; Head of Department of Neurosurgery, A. Gemelli Polyclinic, Rome, Italy
*Surgical Management of Lesions of the Clivus*

**PAOLO MANGIONE, M.D.**
Centre Aquitain du Dos, Clinique Saint Martin, Pessac, France
*Endoscopic Approach to the Thoracic Spine for Removal of Thoracic Disk Herniation*

**ROBERT E. MAXWELL, M.D., Ph.D.**
Professor and Head, Department of Neurosurgery, University of Minnesota Medical School, Minneapolis, Minnesota
*Parasagittal and Falcine Meningioma Surgery; Convexity Meningioma Surgery; Posterior Fossa Meningiomas*

**DUNCAN Q. McBRIDE, M.D.**
Division of Neurosurgery, School of Medicine, University of California, Los Angeles; Harbor-UCLA Medical Center, Torrance, California
*Surgical Management of Severe Closed Head Injury in Adults*

**BRUCE McCORMACK, M.D.**
Department of Neurosurgery, University of California, San Francisco, School of Medicine; Moffit-Long Hospital; Mount Zion Hospital and Medical Center; Veterans Affairs Medical Center, San Francisco, California
*Surgical Management of Tuberculum Sellae and Sphenoid Ridge Meningiomas; Surgical Management of Lumbar Spinal Stenosis*

**PAUL C. McCORMICK, M.D., M.P.H.**
Associate Professor of Clinical Neurosurgery, Columbia University College of Physicians and Surgeons; Associate Attending Physician in Neurosurgery, New York Presbyterian Hospital, New York, New York
*Surgical Management of Pelvic Tumors with Intraspinal Extension*

**ARNOLD H. MENEZES, M.D., F.A.C.S.**
Professor of Neurosurgery, Department of Neurosurgery, University of Iowa College of Medicine and Hospital, Iowa City, Iowa
*Craniovertebral Abnormalities and Their Neurosurgical Management*

**PATRICK MERTENS, M.D., M.Sc.**
Privat Docent, University of Lyon; Neurosurgeon, Pierre Wertheimer Neurological Hospital, Lyon, France
*Neurosurgical Management of Spasticity*

**BJÖRN A. MEYERSON, M.D., Ph.D.**
Department of Neurosurgery, Karolinska Institute and Hospital, Stockholm, Sweden
*Anterior Capsulotomy for Intractable Anxiety Disorders*

**J. DOUGLAS MILLER, M.D., Ph.D., F.R.C.S.(Edin.), F.R.C.S.(E.)**
Department of Clinical Neurosciences, University of Edinburgh; Western General Hospital, Edinburgh, Scotland
*Surgical Management of Traumatic Intracranial Hematomas*

**H. MILLESI, M.D.**
Department of Plastic and Reconstructive Surgery, University of Vienna Medical School, Vienna, Austria
*Surgical Management of Lesions of the Peripheral Nerves and Brachial Plexus*

**PER MINDUS, M.D., Ph.D.**
Department of Psychiatry, Karolinska Hospital, Stockholm, Sweden; University of Trondheim, Trondheim, Norway
*Anterior Capsulotomy for Intractable Anxiety Disorders*

**VERONICA D. MITCHELL, M.D.**
Department of Anesthesia, Georgetown University Medical Center, Washington, D.C.
*Current Concepts in the Neurosurgical Management of Persistent Pain*

**KAZUO MIZOI, M.D.**
Professor and Chairman, Department of Neurosurgery, Akita University School of Medicine, Akita, Japan
*Intraoperative Endovascular Techniques in the Management of Intracranial Aneurysms*

**FRANK MOORE, M.D.**
Assistant Clinical Professor of Neurosurgery, Mount Sinai-New York University Medical Center; Associate Attending Physician, Mount Sinai Hospital, New York, New York
*Surgical Management of Primary and Metastatic Tumors of the Spine*

**MICHAEL K. MORGAN, M.D., F.R.A.C.S.**
Professor of Neurosurgery, University of Sydney; Consultant Neurosurgeon, Royal North Shore Hospital, Sydney, New South Wales, Australia
*Perioperative Care After an Aneurysmal Subarachnoid Hemorrhage*

**JOHN F. MULLAN, M.D., D.Sc., F.R.C.S.**
University of Chicago, Pritzker School of Medicine; University of Chicago Medical Center, Chicago, Illinois
*Percutaneous Trigeminal Nerve Compression*

**CLAUDIO MUNARI, M.D.**
Department of Neurosurgery, University of Genoa, Genoa, Italy; Hospital of Grenoble, Grenoble, France
*Multilobar Resections for the Control of Epilepsy*

**CHERYL A. MUSZYNSKI, M.D.**
Assistant Professor of Neurosurgery, Albert Einstein College of Medicine, Bronx; Attending Neurosurgeon, Beth Israel Medical Center, New York, New York
*Surgical Management of Penetrating Injuries to the Spine*

**RAJ K. NARAYAN, M.D., F.A.C.S.**
Professor and Chairman, Department of Neurosurgery, Temple University School of Medicine, Philadelphia, Pennsylvania
*Surgical Management of Penetrating Injuries to the Spine*

**RICHARD B. NORTH, M.D.**
Professor of Neurosurgery, Anesthesiology and Critical Care Medicine, Johns Hopkins University School of Medicine; Director, Functional Neurosurgery, and Director, Neurosurgery Spine Service, Department of Neurosurgery, Johns Hopkins Hospital, Baltimore, Maryland
*Current Concepts in the Neurosurgical Management of Persistent Pain; Spinal Cord Stimulation for Chronic Pain*

**CHRISTOPHE NUTI, M.D.**
Assistant Neurosurgeon, School of Medicine, University of Saint Etienne; Bellevue Hospital, Department of Neurosurgery, Saint Etienne, France
*Lumboperitoneal Shunting*

**CHRISTOPHER S. OGILVY, M.D.**
Associate Professor of Surgery, Harvard Medical School; Director, Cerebrovascular Surgery, and Associate Visiting Neurosurgeon, Brain Aneurysm/AVM Center; Neurosurgical Service, Massachusetts General Hospital, Boston, Massachusetts
*Management of Dissections of the Carotid and Vertebral Arteries; Surgical Management of Cavernous Malformations of the Nervous System*

**KENJI OHATA, M.D., D.M.Sc.**
Associate Professor, Department of Neurosurgery, Osaka City University, Osaka, Japan
*Orbitozygomatic Infratemporal Approach to Parasellar Meningiomas*

**ROBERT G. OJEMANN, M.D.**
Professor, Department of Surgery, Harvard Medical School; Visiting Neurosurgeon and Vice Chairman, Neurosurgical Service, Massachusetts General Hospital, Boston, Massachusetts
*Surgical Management of Olfactory Groove Meningiomas; Suboccipital Transmedial Transmeatal Approach to Vestibular Schwannoma; Surgical Management of Cavernous Malformations of the Nervous System*

**ANDRÉ OLIVIER, M.D., Ph.D.**
W. Cone Professor and Chairman, Division of Neurosurgery, McGill University; Chief, Department of Neurosurgery, McGill University Health Centre, Montreal, Quebec, Canada
*Stereotactic Intracranial Recording (Stereoelectroencephalography)*

**TY I. OLSON, M.D.**
Resident, Department of Neurological Surgery, The Neurological Institute of New York, Columbia-Presbyterian Medical Center, New York, New York
*Optical Imaging in Epilepsy Surgery*

**DWIGHT PARKINSON, M.D.**
Professor of Neurosurgery, Faculty of Medicine, Department of Anatomy, University of Manitoba, Winnipeg, Manitoba, Canada
*Anatomy of the Lateral Sellar Compartment (Cavernous Sinus); Surgical Management of Traumatic Intracranial Aneurysms*

**FRANCESCO S. PASTORE, M.D.**
Assistant Professor, Institute of Neurosurgery, Department of Neurosciences, School of Medicine, Tor Vergata University of Rome, Italy
*Surgical Management of Low-Grade Gliomas*

**RANA PATIR, M.S., M.Ch.(Neurosurg.)**
Senior Consultant, Sir Ganga Ram Hospital, New Delhi, India
*Surgical Management of Tuberculous Infections of the Nervous System*

**BRYAN RANKIN PAYNE, M.D.**
Lars Leksell Fellow, University of Virginia School of Medicine, Charlottesville, Virginia
*Gamma Surgery in Cerebral Vascular Lesions, Malformations, Tumors, and Functional Disorders*

**SIDNEY J. PEERLESS, M.D.**
Department of Neurosurgery, University of Miami School of Medicine; Jackson Memorial Hospital; Neuroscience Institute, Mercy Hospital, Miami, Florida
*Surgical Management of Terminal Basilar Artery and Posterior Cerebral Artery*

**ISABELLE PELISSOU-GUYOTAT, M.D., Ph.D.**
Head, Department of Emergency Neurosurgery, Neurological Hospital, Lyon, France
*Surgical Management of Cerebral Arteriovenous Malformations*

**NOEL PERIN, M.D.**
Associate Professor of Neurosurgery, Mount Sinai School of Medicine and Hospital, New York, New York
*Surgical Management of Spinal Cord Tumors and Arteriovenous Malformations*

**JOSEPH PIEPMEIER, M.D.**
Professor, Department of Neurosurgery, Yale University, New Haven, Connecticut
*Approaches to Lateral and Third Ventricular Tumors*

**CHARLES E. POLETTI, M.D.**
Hartford Hospital, Hartford, Connecticut
*Complications of Percutaneous Rhizotomy and Microvascular Decompression; Open Cordotomy and Medullary Tractotomy*

**CHARLES E. POLKEY, M.D., F.R.C.S.**
Professor of Functional Neurosurgery, Division of Clinical Neurosciences, Guys King's and St. Thomas' School of Medicine, King's College Hospital, London, England
*Temporal Lobe Resection—Amygdalohippocampectomy*

**MATTI PORRAS, M.D., Ph.D.**
Neuroradiologist, Department of Radiology, Helsinki University Central Hospital, Helsinki, Finland
*Surgical Management of Unruptured Cerebral Aneurysms*

**KALMON D. POST, M.D.**
Professor and Chairman of Neurosurgery, Mount Sinai School of Medicine; Director of Neurosurgery, Mount Sinai Hospital, New York, New York
*Surgical Management of Spinal Cord Tumors and Arteriovenous Malformations; Surgical Management of Pelvic Tumors with Intraspinal Extension*

**LARS POULSGAARD, M.D.**
Associate Professor, University Clinic of Neurosurgery, The Neuroscience Center, University of Copenhagen; Chief Surgeon, University Clinic of Neurosurgery, The Neuroscience Center, Rigshospitalet, Copenhagen, Denmark
*Translabyrinthine Approaches to Vestibular Schwannomas*

**DHEERENDRA PRASAD, M.D.**
Assistant Professor of Neurosurgery, University of Virginia School of Medicine, Charlottesville, Virginia
*Technique of Gamma Surgery; Gamma Surgery in Cerebral Vascular Lesions, Malformations, Tumors, and Functional Disorders*

**ANTONIO RACO, M.D.**
Assistant Professor of Neurosurgery, University of Rome, La Sapienza; Director, Medico I Fascia, Policlinico Umberto I, Rome, Italy
*Surgical Management of Cerebellar Infarction and Cerebellar Hemorrhage*

**Y. RAJA RAMPERSAUD, M.D.**
Department of Neurosurgery, University of Tennessee, Memphis, Tennessee
*Microendoscopic Diskectomy*

**ALBERT L. RHOTON, Jr., M.D.**
Professor of Neurosurgery, Department of Neurological Surgery, University of Florida, Gainesville, Florida
*Microsurgery of Syringomyelia and the Syringomyelia-Chiari Complex*

**THOMAS RIEGEL, M.D.**
Department of Neurosurgery, Philipps-University Marburg, Marburg, Germany
*Surgical Management of Arachnoid, Suprasellar, and Rathke's Cleft Cysts*

**DANIELE RIGAMONTI, M.D., F.A.C.S.**
Professor of Neurosurgery and Professor of Radiology, Johns Hopkins University School of Medicine, Baltimore, Maryland
*Management of Achondroplasia and Its Neurosurgical Complications; Surgical Management of Injuries of the Cervical Spine and Spinal Cord*

**JAAKKO RINNE, M.D., Ph.D.**
Assistant Professor, Department of Neurosurgery, School of Medicine, University of Kuopio; Associate Chief Physician, Department of Neurosurgery, Kuopio University Hospital, Kuopio, Finland
*Surgical Management of Aneurysms of the Middle Cerebral Artery*

**DAVID W. ROBERTS, M.D.**
Professor of Surgery (Neurosurgery), Dartmouth Medical School, Hanover; Chief, Section of Neurosurgery, Dartmouth-Hitchcock Medical Center, Lebanon, New Hampshire
*Callosotomy in the Management of Epilepsy*

**MELVILLE P. ROBERTS, M.D.**
Emeritus Professor, Department of Neurosurgery, University of Connecticut School of Medicine and Health Center, Farmington, Connecticut
*Posterior Surgical Approaches in Cervical Disk Herniation and Spondylotic Myelopathy*

**JON H. ROBERTSON, M.D.**
Professor and Chairman, Department of Neurosurgery, University of Tennessee College of Medicine, Memphis, Tennessee
*Transtemporal Approaches to the Posterior Cranial Fossa; Surgical Management of Glomus Jugulare Tumors*

**SETH I. ROSENBERG, M.D.**
Clinical Assistant Professor, University of Pennsylvania School of Medicine, Philadelphia, Pennsylvania; Vice-President, Ear Research Foundation, Sarasota, Florida
*Vestibular Nerve Section in the Management of Intractable Vertigo*

**J. PETER RUBIN, M.D.**
Clinical Fellow in Plastic Surgery, Harvard Medical School, Boston, Massachusetts
*Surgical Repair of Major Defects of the Scalp and Skull*

**SALVADOR RUIZ-GONZÁLEZ, M.D.**
Professor of Neurosurgical Technics, National School of Obstetrics and Nurses, National University of Mexico City, Mexico City, Mexico
*Neurosurgical Aspects of Neurocysticercosis*

**MAURICE I. SABA, M.D.**
Division of Neurosurgery, School of Medicine and Medical Center, American University of Beirut, Beirut, Lebanon
*Surgical Management of Missile Injuries of the Head*

**AMIR SAMII, M.D., Ph.D.**
Hannover Medical School, Department of Neurosurgery; Nordstadt Medical Center, Department of Neurosurgery, Hannover, Germany
*Surgical Management of Craniopharyngiomas*

**MADJID SAMII, M.D., Ph.D.**
Professor and Chairman, Department of Neurosurgery, Hannover Medical School; Director, Nordstadt Medical Center, Department of Neurosurgery, Hannover, Germany
*Surgical Management of Craniopharyngiomas*

**PRAKASH SAMPATH, M.D.**
Assistant Professor and Director, Neurosurgical Oncology, Brown University School of Medicine, Providence, Rhode Island
*Surgical Management of Injuries of the Cervical Spine and Spinal Cord*

**DUKE S. SAMSON, M.D.**
Professor and Chairman, Department of Neurological Surgery, University of Texas Southwestern Medical School, Dallas, Texas
*Surgical Management of Intraoperative Aneurysm Rupture*

**KEIJI SANO, M.D., Ph.D., Dr.H.C.**
Emeritus Professor, Faculty of Medicine, University of Tokyo; Director, Fuji Brain Institute, Fujinomiya, Japan
*Alternate Surgical Approaches to Pineal Region Neoplasms*

**PAUL D. SAWIN, M.D.**
Winter Memorial Hospital, Winter Park; Florida Hospital, Orlando, Florida
*Surgical Techniques for Stabilization of the Subaxial Cervical Spine*

**DAVID SCALZO, M.D.**
St. Dominic's Neuroscience Center, Jackson, Mississippi
*Surgical Management of Giant Aneurysms of the Anterior Circulation*

**HENRY H. SCHMIDEK, M.D.**
Marion, Massachusetts
*Surgical Management of Arachnoid, Suprasellar, and Rathke's Cleft Cysts; Surgical Management of Supratentorial Hemispheric Gliomas in Adults; Management of Pineal Region Neoplasms; Surgical Management of Cerebellar Tumors in Adults; Surgical Management of Posterior Communicating, Anterior Choroidal, and Carotid Bifurcation Aneurysms; Suppurative Intracranial Infections; Surgical Management of Tumors of the Nerve Sheath Involving the Spine; Vascular Tumors of the Spine; Anterior Cervical Diskectomy and Fusion in Cervical Spondylosis; Lumbar Disk Excision*

**JENS-PETER SCHNEIDER, M.D.**
Department of Radiology, University of Leipzig, Leipzig, Germany
*Open Magnetic Resonance Imaging–Guided Neurosurgery Focusing on Intracranial Gliomas*

**HENRY W. S. SCHROEDER, M.D.**
Assistant Professor, Ernst Moritz Arndt University Medical School and Hospital, Department of Neurosurgery, Greifswald, Germany
*Neuroendoscopic Approach to Intraventricular Tumors*

**KURT SCHÜRMANN, M.D.**
University Professor Emeritus; Formerly, Chairman of the Neurosurgical Department, Johannes Gutenberg University, Mainz, Germany
*Surgical Management of Meningiomas of the Orbit: A Personal Series*

**LUIS SCHUT, M.D.**
Department of Neurosurgery and Pediatrics, University of Pennsylvania School of Medicine; Neurosurgical Services, Children's Hospital, Philadelphia, Pennsylvania
*Surgical Management of Encephaloceles*

**VOLKER SEIFERT, M.D., Ph.D.**
Professor and Chairman, Department of Neurosurgery, Johann Wolfgang Goethe University, Frankfurt/Main, Germany
*Open Magnetic Resonance Imaging–Guided Neurosurgery Focusing on Intracranial Gliomas; Anterior Approaches in Multisegmental Cervical Spondylosis*

**R. P. SENGUPTA, M.Sc., F.R.C.S., F.R.C.S.E.**
Honorary Lecturer in Neurosurgery, University of Newcastle Upon Tyne; Senior Consultant Neurosurgeon and Head of the Department of Neurosurgery, Regional Neurosciences Centre, Newcastle General Hospital, Newcastle Upon Tyne, United Kingdom
*Surgical Management of Anterior Cerebral and Anterior Communicating Artery Aneurysms*

**REWATI RAMAN SHARMA, M.B.B.S., M.S.(Neurosurg.), D.N.B.(Neurosurg.)**
Clinical Tutor, Neurosurgery, Sultan Qaboos University; Senior Specialist Neurosurgeon, National Neurosurgical Centre, Khoula Hospital, Muscat, Sultanate of Oman
*Surgical Management of Fungal Infections of the Nervous System*

**BASSEM SHEIKH, M.D., F.R.C.S., F.K.F.U.(NS)**
Assistant Professor, Neurosurgery, King Faisal University, Dammam; Consultant Neurosurgeon and Acting Chairman, Department of Neurosurgery, King Fahd Teaching Hospital, Al-Khobar, Saudi Arabia
*Orbitozygomatic Infratemporal Approach to Parasellar Meningiomas*

**HU SHEN, M.D.**
Associate Chief Neurosurgeon, Department of Neurosurgery, North Hospital, Shenyang, Liaoning, China
*Surgical Management of Aneurysms of the Middle Cerebral Artery*

**MASATO SHIBUYA, M.D., Ph.D.**
Director, Chukyo Hospital, Nagoya, Japan
*Surgical Management of Paraclinoid Aneurysms*

**WILLIAM A. SHUCART, M.D.**
Professor and Chair, Department of Neurosurgery, Tufts Medical School; Chief, Department of Neurosurgery, Tufts New England Medical Center, Boston, Massachusetts
*Distal Anterior Cerebral Artery Aneurysms*

**TALI SIEGAL, M.D.**
Professor of Oncology and Neurology, Medical Faculty, Hebrew University; Director, Neuro-Oncology Center, Hadassah Hebrew University Hospital, Jerusalem, Israel
*Surgical Management of Malignant Epidural Tumors Compressing the Spinal Cord*

**TZONY SIEGAL, M.D., D.M.D.**
Director, Chosen Specialties Clinics; Attending Spinal Surgeon, Assuta Hospital, Tel Aviv, Israel
*Surgical Management of Malignant Epidural Tumors Compressing the Spinal Cord*

**ADRIAN M. SIEGEL, M.D.**
Epilepsy Fellow, Dartmouth Medical School, Hanover; Dartmouth-Hitchcock Medical Center, Lebanon, New Hampshire
*Callosotomy in the Management of Epilepsy*

**HERBERT SILVERSTEIN, M.D.**
Clinical Professor, University of Pennsylvania School of Medicine, Philadelphia, Pennsylvania; President, Ear Research Foundation, Sarasota, Florida
*Vestibular Nerve Section in the Management of Intractable Vertigo*

**MARC P. SINDOU, M.D., D.Sc.**
Professor of Neurosurgery, University of Lyon; Chairman of Neurosurgical Department, Pierre Wertheimer Neurological Hospital, Lyon, France
*Microsurgical DREZotomy; Neurosurgical Management of Spasticity*

**ROBERT J. SINGER, M.D.**
Neurosurgeon, Neurological Surgeons, P.C., Nashville, Tennessee
*Management of Dissections of the Carotid and Vertebral Arteries*

**DONALD A. SMITH, M.D.**
Assistant Professor, Department of Neurosurgery, College of Medicine, University of South Florida, Tampa, Florida
*Surgical Management of Tumors of the Nerve Sheath Involving the Spine*

**MAURICE M. SMITH, M.D.**
Image-Guided Surgery Research Center, Memphis, Tennessee
*Microendoscopic Diskectomy*

**ROBERT R. SMITH, M.D.**
Professor of Neurosurgery (Emeritus), University of Mississippi Medical Center; St. Dominic's Neuroscience Center, Jackson, Mississippi
*Surgical Management of Giant Aneurysms of the Anterior Circulation*

**VOLKER K. H. SONNTAG, M.D., F.A.C.S.**
Vice Chairman; Director, Residency Program; Chairman, BNI Spine Section, Division of Neurological Surgery, Barrow Neurological Institute, Phoenix, Arizona
*Surgical Techniques for Stabilization of the Subaxial Cervical Spine*

**RENATO SPAZIANTE, M.D.**
Department of Systematic Pathology, Federico II University School of Medicine, Naples, Italy
*Repair of the Sella Turcica After Transsphenoidal Surgery*

**DENNIS SPENCER, M.D.**
Harvey and Kate Cushing Professor and Chair, Department of Neurosurgery, Yale University School of Medicine, New Haven, Connecticut
*Surgery for Mesial Temporal Sclerosis*

**ROBERT F. SPETZLER, M.D., F.A.C.S.**
Division of Neurosurgery, University of Arizona College of Medicine, Tucson; St. Joseph's Hospital and Barrow Neurological Institute, Phoenix, Arizona
*Surgical Management of Midbasilar and Lower Basilar Aneurysms*

**PATRICK F. X. STATHAM, M.B., F.R.C.S.(Eng.), F.R.C.S.(SN)**
Department of Clinical Neurosciences, University of Edinburgh; Western General Hospital, Edinburgh, Scotland
*Surgical Management of Traumatic Intracranial Hematomas*

**STEPHEN N. STEEN, Sc.D., M.D.**
Professor of Anesthesiology and Director of Research/Anesthesiology, University of Southern California School of Medicine; Professor of Anesthesiology, Charles R. Drew University of Medicine and Science; Director of Research/Anesthesiology, Martin Luther King, Jr. Hospital/Charles R. Drew Medical Center, Los Angeles, California
*Anesthetic Management of the Patient After Aneurysmal Subarachnoid Hemorrhage*

**BENNETT M. STEIN, M.D.**
Byron Stookey Professor Emeritus, College of Physicians and Surgeons of Columbia University, New York, New York
*Supracerebellar Approach to Pineal Region Neoplasms; Surgical Management of Spinal Cord Tumors and Arteriovenous Malformations*

**DAVID R. STEINBERG, M.D.**
Assistant Professor, Department of Orthopaedic Surgery, University of Pennsylvania School of Medicine, Philadelphia, Pennsylvania
*Open Carpal Tunnel Release*

**GARY K. STEINBERG, M.D., Ph.D.**
Lacroute-Hearst Professor and Chairman, Department of Neurosurgery, Stanford University School of Medicine; Co-Director, Stanford Stroke Center, Stanford, California
*Surgical Management of Intracranial Arteriovenous Malformations*

**ALFRED A. STEINBERGER, M.D.**
Assistant Clinical Professor of Neurosurgery, Mount Sinai School of Medicine, New York, New York; Chief of Neurosurgery, Englewood Hospital Medical Center, Englewood, New Jersey
*Surgical Management of Primary and Metastatic Tumors of the Spine*

**LADISLAU STEINER, M.D., Ph.D.**
Alumni Professor of Neurosurgery and Radiology, University of Virginia School of Medicine, Charlottesville, Virginia
*Technique of Gamma Surgery; Gamma Surgery in Cerebral Vascular Lesions, Malformations, Tumors, and Functional Disorders*

**MELITA STEINER, M.D.**
Research Professor of Neurosurgery, University of Virginia School of Medicine, Charlottesville, Virginia
*Gamma Surgery in Cerebral Vascular Lesions, Malformations, Tumors, and Functional Disorders*

**BERTIL STENER, M.D., Ph.D.**
Professor Emeritus of Orthopaedic Surgery, Gothenburg University, Gothenburg, Sweden
*Technique of Complete Spondylectomy in the Thoracic and Lumbar Spine; Technique of High Sacral Amputation*

**MARCUS A. STOODLEY, Ph.D., F.R.A.C.S.**
Cerebrovascular Surgery Fellow, Department of Neurosurgery, Stanford University School of Medicine; Stanford Stroke Center, Stanford, California
*Surgical Management of Intracranial Arteriovenous Malformations*

**JOHN STRUGAR, M.D.**
Assistant Professor, Department of Neurosurgery, Yale University School of Medicine, New Haven, Connecticut
*Approaches to Lateral and Third Ventricular Tumors*

**NARAYAN SUNDARESAN, M.D.**
Clinical Professor of Neurosurgery, Mount Sinai School of Medicine; Attending Neurosurgeon, Mount Sinai Hospital, New York, New York
*Disorders of the Spine Related to Plasma Cell Dyscrasias; Surgical Management of Primary and Metastatic Tumors of the Spine*

**BROOKE SWEARINGEN, M.D.**
Department of Neurosurgery, Harvard Medical School; Massachusetts General Hospital, Boston, Massachusetts
*Surgical Management of Cushing's Disease*

**WILLIAM H. SWEET, M.D., D.Sc.**
Department of Neurosurgery, Harvard Medical School; Massachusetts General Hospital, Boston, Massachusetts
*Optic Gliomas: Their Diagnosis, Capacity for Spontaneous Regression, and Radical Surgical Treatment; Craniopharyngiomas: A Summary of Data; Surgical Management of Arachnoid, Suprasellar, and Rathke's Cleft Cysts; Complications of Percutaneous Rhizotomy and Microvascular Decompression Operations for Facial Pain; Cervicothoracic Ankylosing Spondylitis*

**JAMAL M. TAHA, M.D.**
Assistant Professor, Department of Neurosurgery, University of Cincinnati College of Medicine, Cincinnati, Ohio
*Percutaneous Rhizotomy in the Treatment of Intractable Facial Pain*

**AKIRA TAKAHASHI, M.D.**
Professor and Chairman, Department of Neuroendovascular Therapy, Tohoku University School of Medicine, Sendai, Japan
*Intraoperative Endovascular Techniques in the Management of Intracranial Aneurysms*

**TOSHIHIRO TAKAMI, M.D., D.M.Sc.**
Lecturer, Department of Neurosurgery, Osaka City University, Osaka, Japan
*Orbitozygomatic Infratemporal Approach to Parasellar Meningiomas*

**PRAKASH NARAIN TANDON, M.D., M.S., F.R.C.S.**
Emeritus Professor, All India Institute of Medical Sciences, New Delhi, India
*Surgical Management of Tuberculous Infections of the Nervous System*

**R. R. TASKER, M.D., M.A., F.R.C.S.(C.)**
Professor Emeritus, Department of Surgery, University of Toronto; Senior Neurosurgeon, Toronto Western Hospital, University Health Network, Toronto, Ontario, Canada
*Surgical Treatment of the Dyskinesias; Percutaneous Cordotomy*

**L. TASSI, M.D.**
Department of Neurology, Epilepsy Surgery Regional Center, Niguarda Hospital, Milan, Italy
*Multilobar Resections for the Control of Epilepsy*

**JUAN M. TAVERAS**
Harvard Medical School; Department of Radiology, Massachusetts General Hospital, Boston, Massachusetts
*Optic Gliomas: Their Diagnosis, Capacity for Spontaneous Regression, and Radical Surgical Treatment*

**JOHN M. TEW, Jr., M.D.**
Frank H. Mayfield Professor and Chair, Department of Neurosurgery, University of Cincinnati College of Medicine, Cincinnati, Ohio
*Surgical Management of Giant Aneurysms of the Anterior Circulation; Surgical Management of Thalamic-Basal Ganglia Vascular Malformations; Surgical Management of Brain Stem Vascular Malformations; Percutaneous Rhizotomy in the Treatment of Intractable Facial Pain*

**SUZIE C. TINDALL, M.D.**
Professor of Neurological Surgery, Emory University School of Medicine, Atlanta, Georgia
*Surgical Management of Thoracic Outlet Syndrome and Peripheral Entrapment Neuropathies*

**GIUSTINO TOMEI, M.D.**
Director, Institute of Neurosurgery, Hospital Maggiore Policlinico—IRCCS, Milan, Italy
*Transcallosal Approach to Tumors of the Third Ventricle*

**CHRISTOS TRANTAKIS, M.D.**
Neurosurgical Clinic, Leipzig, Germany
*Open Magnetic Resonance Imaging–Guided Neurosurgery Focusing on Intracranial Gliomas*

**NOBUYUKI TSUZUKI, M.D., D.M.Sc.**
Department of Orthopedics, Saitama Medical Center/School, Kawagoe, Saitama, Japan
*Surgical Management of Ossification of the Posterior Longitudinal Ligament*

**SONYA D. TUERFF, M.D.**
Research Fellow, Division of Vascular Surgery, Hahnemann University School of Medicine, Philadelphia, Pennsylvania
*Surgical Exposure of the Distal Internal Carotid Artery*

**SERGIO TURAZZI, M.D.**
Chief, Division of Neurosurgery, Department of Neurosurgery, City Hospital, Verona, Italy
*Petroclival Meningiomas*

**FRANCIS TURJMAN, M.D., Ph.D.**
Professor, School of Medicine, University of Lyon; Head, Interventional Neuroradiology, Department of Radiology, Neurological Hospital, Lyon, France
*Surgical Management of Cerebral Arteriovenous Malformations*

**JOHN C. VanGILDER, M.D.**
Professor and Chairman, Department of Neurosurgery, University of Iowa School of Medicine; University of Iowa Hospitals and Clinics, Iowa City, Iowa
*Craniovertebral Abnormalities and Their Neurosurgical Management*

**ROBERTO M. VILLANI, M.D.**
Professor of Neurosurgery, Institute of Neurosurgery, University of Milan; Head, Institute of Neurosurgery, Ospedale Maggiore Policlinico, IRCCS, Milan, Italy
*Transcallosal Approach to Tumors of the Third Ventricle*

**JEAN-GUY VILLEMURE, M.D., F.R.C.S.C.**
Professor, University of Lausanne; Head of Neurosurgery, University Centre Hospital Vandois, Lausanne, Switzerland
*Cerebral Hemispherectomy for Epilepsy*

**ANDRÉ VISOT, M.D.**
University of Paris VIII; Chief of Neurosurgical Department, Hospital Foch, Suresnes, France
*Transbasal Approach to Tumors Invading the Skull Base; Surgical Management of Endocrinologically Silent Pituitary Tumors*

**KLAUS R. H. Von WILD, M.D.**
Professor, Medical Faculty, Westfalien Wilhelms University; Professor and Head, Department of Neurosurgery and Division of Early Neurological-Neurotraumatological Rehabilitation, Clemens Hospital, Münster, Germany
*Perioperative Management of Severe Head Injuries in Adults*

**FRANK D. VRIONIS, M.D., Ph.D.**
Assistant Professor and Director of Skull Base Surgery, Department of Neurosurgery, University of South Florida College of Medicine; Chief of Neurosurgery, James A. Haley Veterans Administration Hospital, Tampa, Florida
*Transtemporal Approaches to the Posterior Cranial Fossa*

**M. CHRISTOPHER WALLACE, M.D.**
Professor, Department of Surgery and Fondation Baxter et Alma Ricard Chair in Cerebrovascular Neurosurgery, University of Toronto; Attending Physician, Toronto Western Hospital, University Health Network, Toronto, Canada
*Surgical Management of Cranial Dural Arteriovenous Fistulas*

**CHUNG-CHENG WANG, M.D.**
Professor, Capital University of Medical Science; Director, Beijing Neurosurgery Institute, Beijing, China
*Surgical Management of Nonglomus Tumors of the Jugular Foramen*

**LYNDELL V. WANG, M.D.**
Resident in Neurosurgery, Tufts New England Medical Center, Boston, Massachusetts
*Distal Anterior Cerebral Artery Aneurysms*

**YEOU-CHIH WANG, M.D.**
Associate Professor, Neurosurgery, National Defense Medical Center, Taipei; National Yang-Ming University, Taipei; Chung Shan Medical and Dental College, Taichung; Chairman, Department of Neurosurgery, Taichung Veterans General Hospital, Taichung, Taiwan, R.O.C.
*Failed Microvascular Decompression for Trigeminal Neuralgia*

**RONALD E. WARNICK, M.D.**
Associate Professor of Neurosurgery and Director of Surgical Neuro-Oncology, University of Cincinnati School of Medicine, Cincinnati, Ohio
*Image-Guided Neurosurgery*

**HOWARD L. WEINER, M.D.**
Assistant Professor of Neurosurgery, Department of Neurosurgery, New York University School of Medicine; Attending Neurosurgeon, Tisch Hospital–NYU Medical Center, New York, New York
*CT/MRI-Based Computer-Assisted Volumetric Stereotactic Resection of Intracranial Lesions*

**PHILIP R. WEINSTEIN, M.D.**
Department of Neurological Surgery, University of California, San Francisco, School of Medicine and Hospitals, San Francisco, California
*Surgical Management of Lumbar Spinal Stenosis*

**MARTIN H. WEISS, M.D.**
Professor and Chairman, Department of Neurological Surgery, University of Southern California School of Medicine, Los Angeles, California
*Surgical Management of Growth Hormone–Secreting and Prolactin-Secreting Pituitary Adenomas*

**WALTER W. WHISLER, M.D., Ph.D.**
Professor and Chairman Emeritus, Rush Medical College; Attending Neurosurgeon, Rush-Presbyterian Medical Center, Chicago, Illinois
*Multiple Subpial Transection for Epilepsy*

**ALLEN R. WYLER, M.D.**
Medical Director, Neuroscience Institute, Swedish Medical Center, Seattle, Washington
*Diagnostic Techniques in Surgical Management of Epilepsy: Strip Electrodes, Grids, and Depth Electrodes*

**MICHAEL J. YAREMCHUK, M.D.**
Clinical Associate Professor of Surgery, Harvard Medical School; Chief of Craniofacial Surgery, Massachusetts General Hospital, Boston, Massachusetts
*Surgical Repair of Major Defects of the Scalp and Skull*

**TAKASHI YOSHIMOTO, M.D.**
Professor and Chairman, Department of Neurosurgery, Tohoku University School of Medicine, Sendai, Japan
*Intraoperative Endovascular Techniques in the Management of Intracranial Aneurysms*

**CHUN-JIANG YU, M.D.**
Professor, Capital University of Medical Science; Vice-Chairman of Department of Neurosurgery, Beijing Tiantan Hospital, Beijing, China
*Surgical Management of Nonglomus Tumors of the Jugular Foramen*

**SETH M. ZEIDMAN, M.D.**
Assistant Professor of Neurological Surgery and Neurology, University of Rochester Medical Center; Chief, Complex Spinal Surgery, Department of Neurological Surgery, University of Rochester Medical Center, Rochester, New York; Uniformed Services University of the Health Sciences, Bethesda, Maryland
*Circumferential Spinal Fusion (Cervical)*

**VLADIMIR ZELMAN, M.D., Ph.D.**
Professor of Anesthesiology, Neurological Surgery, and Neurology, University of Southern California School of Medicine; Co-Chairman of Clinical Affairs, Department of Anesthesiology, and Director of Neuroanesthesia, Los Angeles County–University of Southern California Medical Center, Los Angeles, California
*Anesthetic Management of the Patient After Aneurysmal Subarachnoid Hemorrhage*

**NICHOLAS T. ZERVAS, M.D.**
Professor of Surgery, Harvard Medical School; Chief, Neurosurgical Service, Massachusetts General Hospital, Boston, Massachusetts
*Surgical Management of Cushing's Disease; Stereotactic Interstitial Radiosurgery in the Management of Brain Tumors*

**MICHAEL ZIMMERMAN, M.D.**
Neurosurgical Clinic, University of Leipzig, Leipzig, Germany
*Open Magnetic Resonance Imaging–Guided Neurosurgery Focusing on Intracranial Gliomas*

# Preface

In 1977, Dr Sweet and I coedited a single volume entitled *Current Techniques in Operative Neurosurgery,* which reflected our own interests not only in the day-to-day topics of clinical importance but also in topics at the forefront of contemporary neurosurgical practice. In the intervening years, we edited three editions of *Operative Neurosurgical Techniques: Indications, Methods, and Results*—a first edition in 1982, a second edition in 1988, and a third edition in 1995. The overwhelming positive response by the neurosurgical community to these volumes, as reflected both by their worldwide sales and by the clones that they have generated, has encouraged the publisher, W.B. Saunders, to "memorialize" this and subsequent editions of the book with the ongoing appellation of "Schmidek & Sweet." Dr Sweet retired from his editorial duties in 1996.

Conceptually, we have attempted in these volumes to provide the "working neurosurgeon" with the information that he or she would find particularly useful when taking an adult patient with a particular brain, spinal, or peripheral nerve problem to the operating room. When grappling with the decision-making process, the surgeon does not require an encyclopedic coverage but rather one that provides an overview of the topic followed by a discussion of the available options and experiences by which the problem can be treated. In many cases, alternative and reasonable surgical and nonsurgical options are available for dealing with a particular clinical situation. This book supplies chapters by contributors who describe the different choices in detail. Often, there is overlap in these presentations, which reiterates that which is common ground and highlights differences. In the daily routine of the busy clinician, it is extremely useful to have the information in a single source, available immediately, while planning a patient's care, and that is what I have again attempted to provide in this edition.

The fourth edition reflects the continuing technologic and social changes in neurosurgery that have evolved from the 517-page, 33-chapter volume in 1977 to the current two-volume, 2200-page, 188-chapter, and 275-contributor set in 2000. Operating under constraints imposed by the publisher, this material is presented without exceeding the size of the third edition in order to keep down the cost of the book. This edition also reflects the quality and diversity of contributions made to neurosurgical advances from around the world. Approximately 40% of the chapters are from neurosurgical centers located in 26 different countries outside of the United States. This book is among the first surgical texts of international scope and participation.

In 1973, a colleague wrote in the May 17th issue of the *New England Journal of Medicine* that "Neurosurgery has stopped evolving. Although it is unlikely that the specialty will follow the dinosaur's path to extinction, for many it is becoming lifeless and uninteresting. The promise and excitement that once permeated neurosurgery have yielded too often to an easy acceptance of the status quo." The intervening quarter century has belied this viewpoint with spectacular innovations of computed tomography, magnetic resonance imaging, image-guided surgery, endoscopic neurosurgery, endovascular techniques, and techniques in management of medically intractable epilepsy, as well as techniques that have revolutionized the surgical management of spinal disorders. Each of these areas is presented in this edition. In addition, chapters have been added on preoperative management of head injury, aneurysmal subarachnoid hemorrhage, and the anesthetic management of aneurysmal subarachnoid hemorrhage, along with new chapters on cranioplasty, hydrocephalus, management of low-grade and recurrent gliomas, and management of dissections of the carotid and vertebral arteries and of intracranial and intraspinal infections, as well as management of spinal nerve root injuries. Of the remaining chapters, all have been carefully evaluated and often extensively rewritten and updated.

I want to express to each of the contributors my sincerest thanks for the time and effort that have been devoted to preparing their chapters and also to the staff of W.B. Saunders. In particular I wish to thank Mr. Richard Zorab and Ms. Cathy Carroll for having done everything possible to justify the contributors' participation in producing a work of editorial excellence.

*Henry H. Schmidek, MD*

# Contents

xxviii   Contents

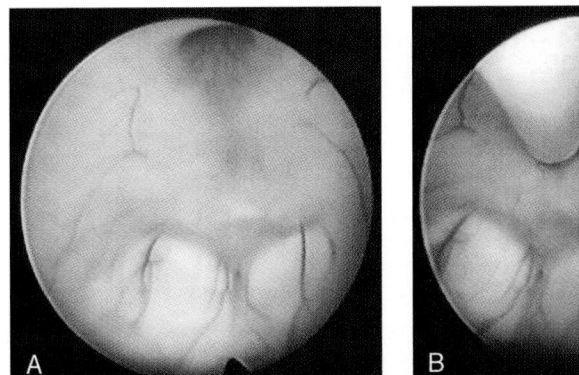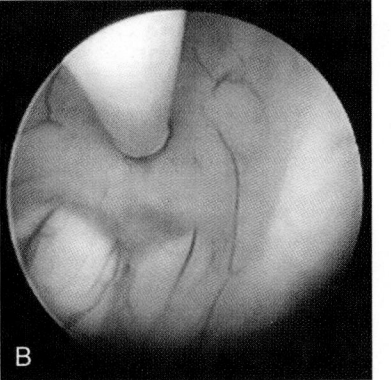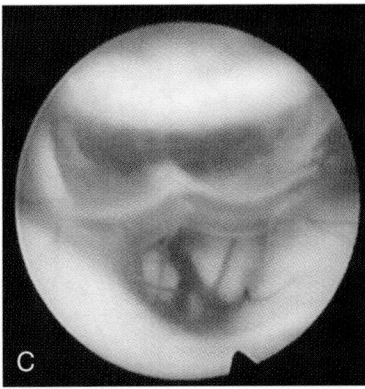

FIGURE 42–18 ■ *A,* Exact site of perforation for third ventriculostomy. *B,* Bipolar coagulation of the floor of the third ventricle. *C,* Splitting of the basilar artery into both posterior cerebral arteries and interpeduncular perforant branches shining through the thinned floor of the third ventricle.

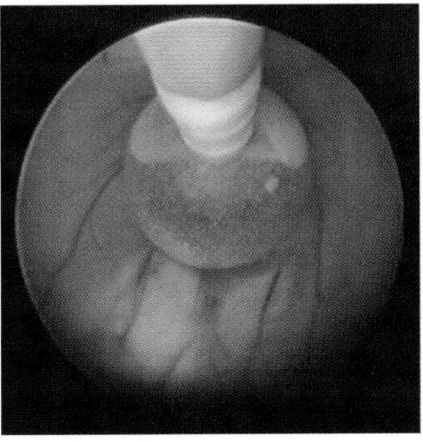

FIGURE 42–19 ■ Balloon dilatation of the perforation in third ventriculostomy.

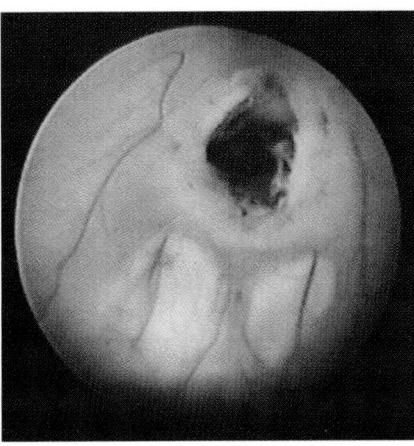

FIGURE 42–20 ■ Correct third ventriculostomy opening.

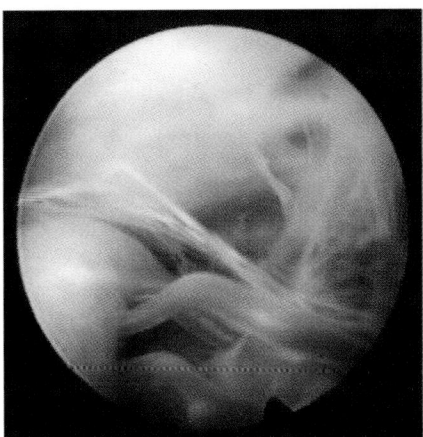

FIGURE 42–21 ■ Image of the subarachnoid space with the basilar artery and perforate pontine branches seen through third ventriculostomy.

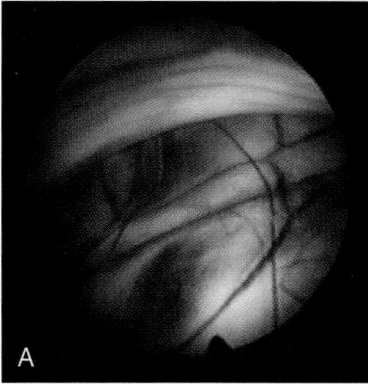 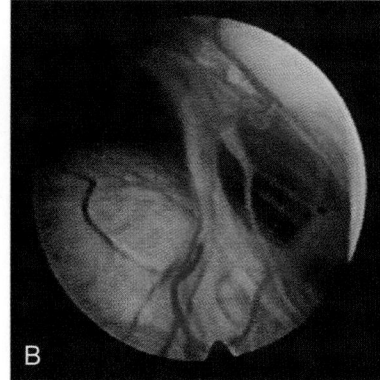

**FIGURE 42–23** ■ *A*, Typical bluish dome crossed by small vessels. *B*, Blood vessels between the ventricular wall and the dome of a suprasellar arachnoid cyst.

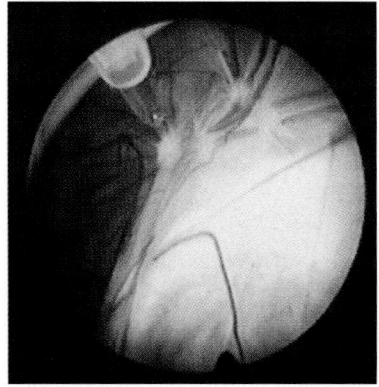

**FIGURE 42–24** ■ Coagulation of a circle in the dome of a suprasellar arachnoid cyst.

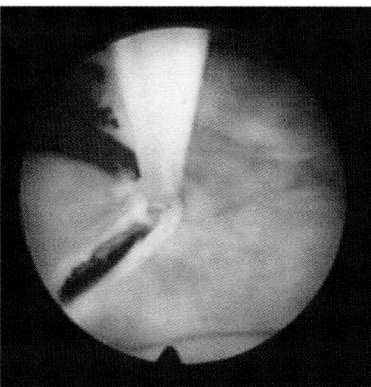

**FIGURE 42–25** ■ Cutting out of a roundel in the dome of an arachnoid cyst.

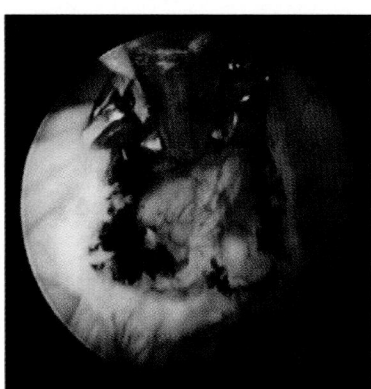

**FIGURE 42–26** ■ Grasping of the cut-out part of the membrane in a suprasellar arachnoid cyst.

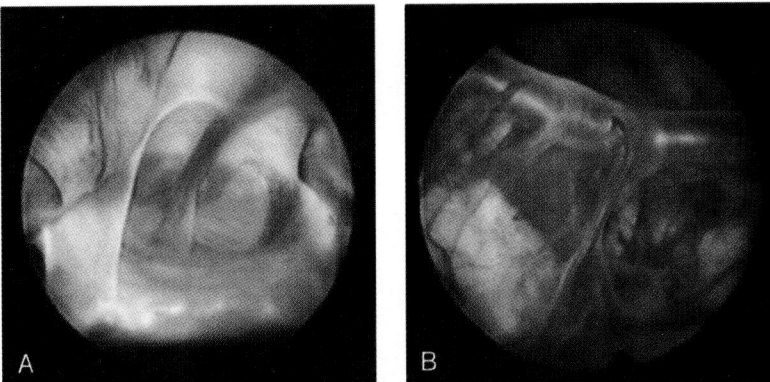

FIGURE 42–30 ■ *A,* The pituitary gland, pituitary stalk, and dorsum sellae in a suprasellar arachnoid cyst. *B,* Interpeduncular perforate branches in the splitting of the basilar artery in the depth of a suprasellar arachnoid cyst. Dorsum sellae, posterior clinoid processes, oculomotor nerve, posterior communicating artery, and posterior cerebral artery in the depth of a suprasellar arachnoid cyst.

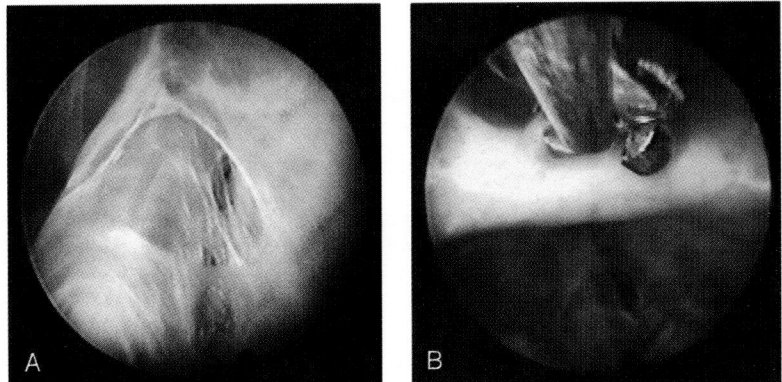

FIGURE 42–31 ■ *A,* Slit valve in the arachnoid membrane around the basilar artery. *B,* Grasping of the arachnoid membrane over the dorsum sellae.

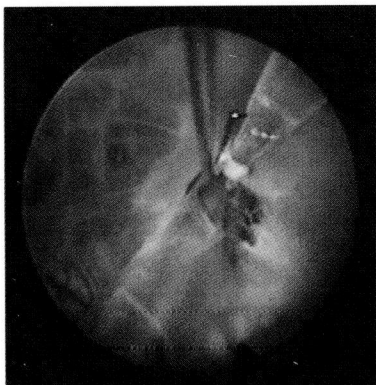

FIGURE 42–32 ■ Cutting by laser in the contact mode of an arachnoid membrane stretched by means of a hooklet to destroy the slit valve around the basilar artery.

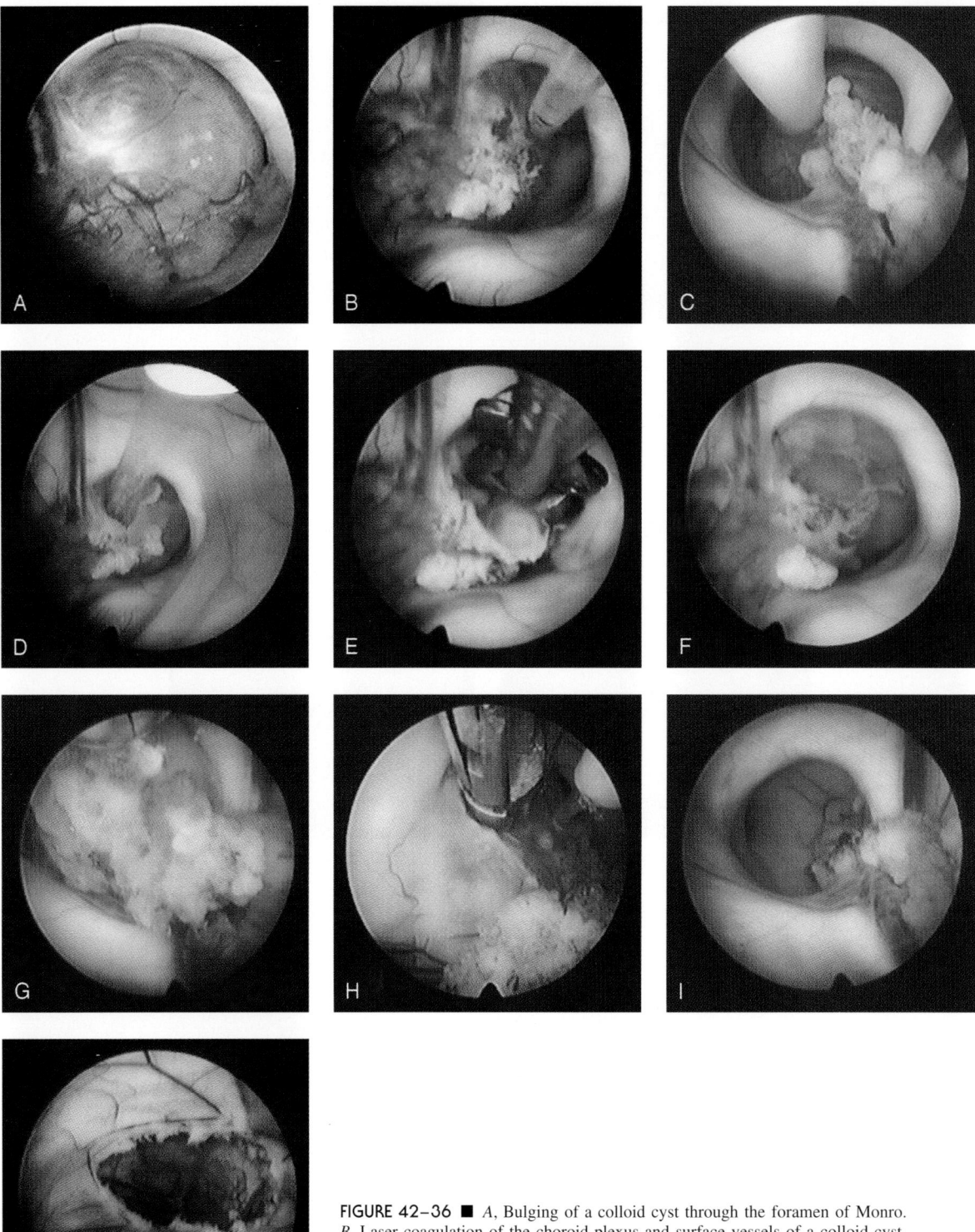

FIGURE 42–36 ■ *A*, Bulging of a colloid cyst through the foramen of Monro.
*B*, Laser coagulation of the choroid plexus and surface vessels of a colloid cyst.
*C*, Aspiration catheter to remove semisolid contents. *D*, Aspiration of blubbery
contents in colloid cysts. *E*, Grasping forceps to remove the solid parts of colloid
cysts. *F*, Flaccid capsula after the removal of the contents of a colloid cyst.
*G*, Pulling out of a cyst capsula through the foramina of Monro. *H*, Simultaneous
use of two instruments. *I*, Final result: a wide-open foramen of Monro. *J*, Septostomy after the removal of a colloid cyst.

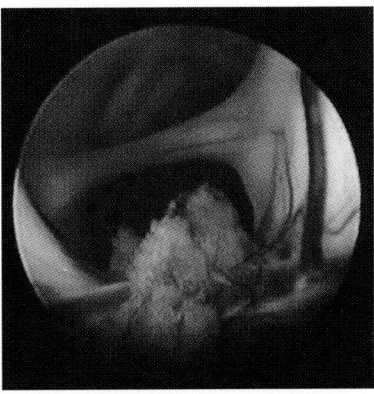

**FIGURE 42–42** ■ Foramen of Monro, approaching a pineal gland tumor with the fornix caudate vein, thalamostriate vein, choroid plexus, septal vein, and interthalamic commissure in the depth.

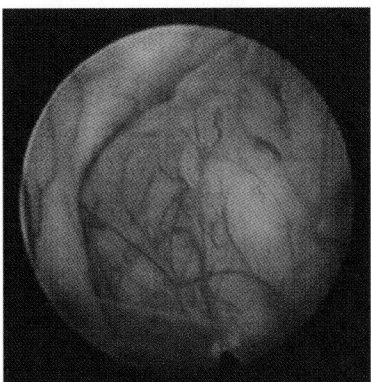

**FIGURE 42–46** ■ An endoscopic image of a pinealoblastoma.

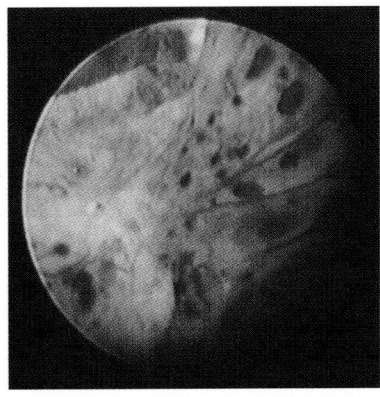

**FIGURE 42–47** ■ An endoscopic image of a pineal germinoma.

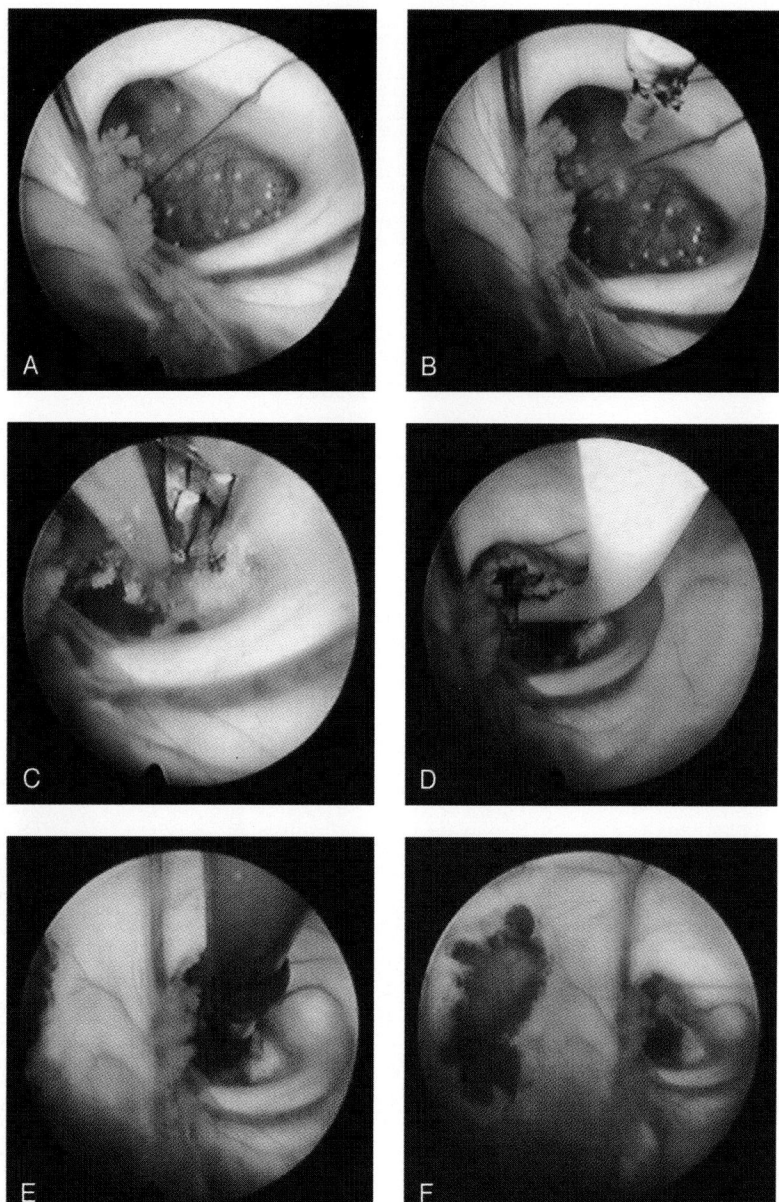

**FIGURE 42–49** ■ *A,* Solid craniopharyngioma, with cystic parts and calcifications, bulging through the foramina of Monro. *B,* Laser coagulation of surface vessels in a craniopharyngioma capsula. *C,* Simultaneous use of grasping forceps and a cutting laser. *D,* Aspiration of the contents of a craniopharyngioma with a catheter with a pre-bent tip to work around the corner. *E,* Inspection of the third ventricle with the flexible endoscope through the working channel of the rigid endoscope after the removal of a craniopharyngioma. *F,* Final results after the removal of a craniopharyngioma and septostomy (left in the image).

# Trauma to the Scalp, Skull, and Brain

# Surgical Repair of Major Defects of the Scalp and Skull

■ MICHAEL J. YAREMCHUK and J. PETER RUBIN

Major defects of the scalp and skull are most often the result of trauma or extirpation for tumor. Although a careful physical examination is paramount in the preoperative evaluation, computed tomography (CT) or magnetic resonance imaging (MRI) is performed in most cases to provide optimal definition of the real or anticipated defect and the status of the adjacent structures.

This chapter presents plastic surgical concepts and techniques used to reconstruct major defects of the scalp and skull. The first section addresses the reconstruction of the scalp; the second section covers the reconstruction of the skull.

## THE SCALP

### Anatomy of the Scalp

The scalp consists of five distinct anatomic layers. Listed from the most superficial to the deepest, these layers include: (1) the skin with its characteristic thick dermis; (2) the subcutaneous tissue; (3) the relatively rigid galea aponeurotica, which is continuous with the superficial musculoaponeurotic system, frontalis, occipitalis, and superficial temporal fascia; (4) underlying areolar tissue; and (5) skull periosteum. The rich vascular supply of the subcutaneous layer, in which there is an abundant communication of vessels, can result in significant blood loss when the scalp is lacerated. The relatively poor fixation of the galea to the underlying periosteum of the skull provides little resistance to shear injuries, resulting in large flaps or "scalping" injuries. This layer's resultant potential space also provides little resistance to hematoma or abscess formation. As a result, extensive fluid collections related to scalp injury tend to accumulate in the subgaleal plane.

### Lacerations of the Scalp

The scalp wound should always be inspected for fractures. Because the scalp has a rich vascular supply, lacerations may result in significant blood loss, particularly in children. The large diameter of the scalp vessels often requires that they be individually clamped and ligated for control. Bleeding from a scalp wound can be controlled emergently until definitive care is provided with temporary pressure dressings, Raney clip placement of the wound edges, or an over-and-over continuous stitch with large sutures.

The rich intercommunicating blood supply of the scalp is such that one set of superficial temporal vessels alone may nourish the entire scalp. This rich vascularity allows the survival of large, narrow-pedicled avulsion flaps that would never survive anywhere else on the body. For that reason, almost all traumatic scalp flaps should be appropriately cleansed, minimally débrided, and anatomically replaced. Only the hair adjacent to the lacerated edges needs to be shaved to allow easier suture placement and removal. The subgaleal space is drained with a closed suction drainage system before the scalp is closed in layers. In general, the galea and the dermis are closed with 2–0 or 3–0 polyglycolic acid sutures before the skin is closed with running or interrupted 3–0 or 4–0 nylon sutures.

### Wounds with Tissue Loss

The management of scalp wounds with soft tissue loss is determined by the amount of soft tissue lost and the type of tissue exposed.

#### Local Advancement (Galeal Scoring)

The surface area of the scalp adjacent to the defect can be enlarged considerably by galeal scoring to allow closure by advancement of the wound edge. Each cut, which is made at 1-cm intervals in a parallel or cross-hatch fashion, allows the scalp to be stretched approximately 4 to 6 mm. This scoring maneuver requires a complete division of the substantial galeal layer (Fig. 1–1). Tissue loss of more than 1 to 2 cm may require extension of the laceration to allow greater undermining and scoring. Defects that are 3 cm in diameter can be routinely closed with this technique.

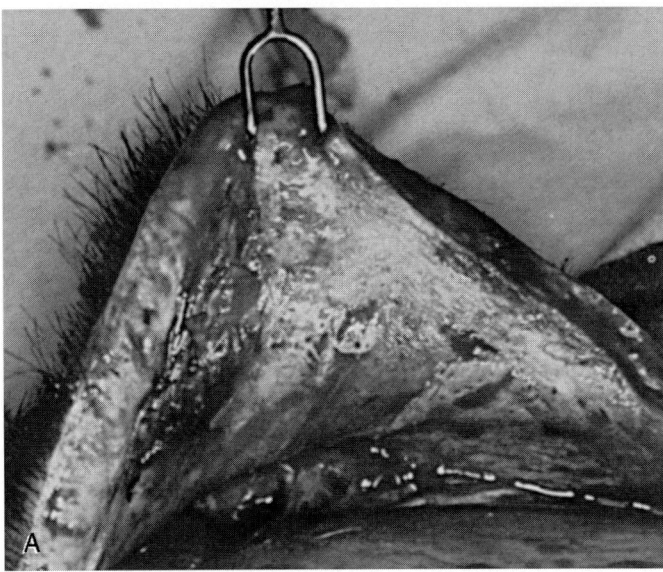
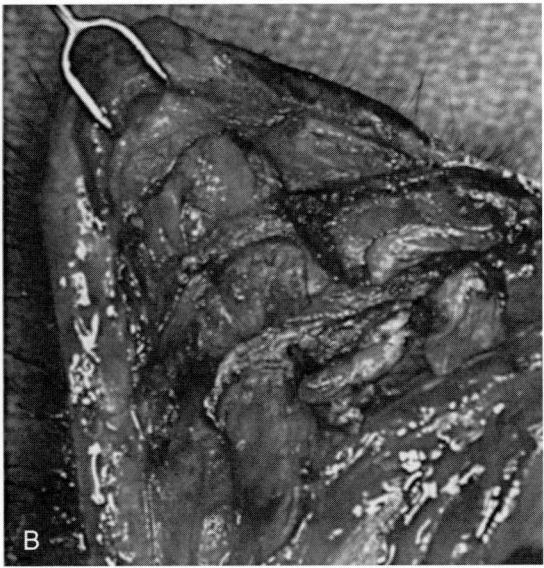

FIGURE 1–1 ■ Scalp flaps can be enlarged considerably by galeal scoring. The galea is completely divided at 1-cm intervals. *A,* The appearance of galea before scoring. *B,* The appearance of galea after scoring. Note the increase in surface area.

## Skin Grafts

Wounds in which soft tissue loss is so extensive that the skin edges cannot be approximated are closed with either skin grafts or flaps. Full-thickness skin grafts contain the epidermis and the complete thickness of dermis from the recipient area. Split-thickness grafts contain the epidermis and a variable thickness of the dermis. Grafts with a greater thickness of dermis contract less on the wound bed and provide more durable coverage. Thin grafts have the advantage of more rapid revascularization, so that they are more likely to be successful. Thin grafts, however, tend to provide less durable coverage.

A skin graft may cover any scalp wound that has capillary circulation, which will ultimately provide a source of vascular ingrowth for that graft. For that reason, skull periosteum or any more superficial scalp layer will support a skin graft. Most scalp defects are closed with thin (0.010- to 0.014-inch thickness) "meshed" skin grafts.

Meshed grafts are those that are mechanically perforated in a grid pattern, which allows them to be expanded and to conform to irregular surfaces. The perforations also provide egress for wound drainage. The resultant improved graft bed contact optimizes conditions for graft take (Fig. 1–2). For scalp defects, meshed grafts should not be perforated and expanded more than 1.5 times their normal size, unless donor skin is in short supply. A widely expanded graft is less desirable, because larger open areas take longer to epithelialize and provide poorer protective coverage.

Skin grafts are most easily harvested with an electric dermatome. The upper lateral thigh has skin of sufficient thickness to allow uncomplicated healing of the donor site. Donor site scarring in this area is usually covered with clothing.

To ensure optimal graft-bed interface for graft take, the graft should be immobilized to the scalp recipient site. A tie-over stent dressing or a quilt dressing in which the overlying dressing is sutured to the intact wound edges is most often used to achieve this immobilization.

Several flap designs allow closure of scalp wounds with significant soft tissue loss.[1, 2] However, the wound should not be enlarged considerably to close a large traumatic wound emergently; rather, if the periosteum remains, a split-thickness skin graft should be applied. When scalp with periosteum is lost, a closed wound is obtained most expeditiously if, at the time of presentation, the outer table is drilled down to find bleeding points that can provide a bed for a split-thickness skin graft take. A meshed, nonexpanded, split-thickness skin graft is placed immediately at the time of the drilling. An older, well-proved technique involves removing the outer table of the skull to expose the diploë and treating the wound with wet dressings for 5 to 7 days, at which time luxuriant granulation tissue usually forms. This granulation tissue readily accepts a skin graft.

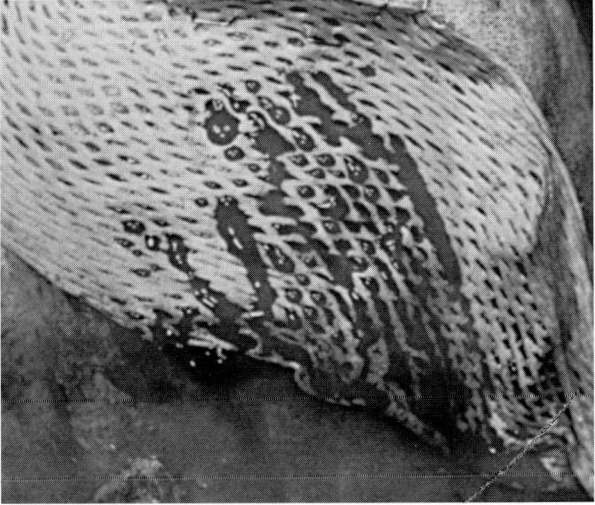

FIGURE 1–2 ■ A meshed skin graft placed minimally expanded over a scalp wound. Note how perforations in the graft allow egress for drainage from the wound bed.

Another method involves making small drill holes 1 cm apart through the outer table down into the diploë space. Usually, granulation tissue arises from these holes and grows over the exposed calvarium to coalesce and form a suitable bed for skin grafting.

Skin grafting directly onto bone is susceptible to breakdown after minimal trauma and leaves an area with alopecia and significant contour deformity. This problem can be corrected as a delayed reconstruction with advancement or rotational flaps after galeal scoring or with tissue expanders.

## Flaps

Wounds with exposed vital structures or wounds that do not have exposed capillary circulation require flap coverage. Whereas skin grafts provide only thin coverage and depend on the wound bed for their revascularization and survival, flaps carry their own blood supply and provide soft tissue bulk to the wound.

The basic principles of flap coverage are: (1) to move available tissue with its intact circulation from an area of relative excess to the area of deficiency, and (2) to optimize vascularity of the flap. In the scalp, the lateral and posterior aspects are usually used as donor sites to avoid distortion of the forehead or frontal hairline. The flaps are designed to include axial vessels in their base. Usually, the superficial temporal artery or the occipital artery provides the basic blood supply to these flaps. The flaps should be designed with respect to previous incisions, which may block vascular inflow to the flap. Although many types of rotation flaps are possible, their design requires considerable expertise and extensive mobilization of the scalp tissues. Usually, most of the scalp must be degloved, and the galea should be scored to allow primary closure of the secondary defect.

Full-thickness skin coverage for the skull can usually be provided by galeal scoring and direct advancement or by the creation of a bipedicle flap. As noted earlier, galeal scoring and advancement of wound edges usually close defects up to 3 or 4 cm in diameter. Defects greater than this can be closed by creating a bipedicle flap and by closing the secondary defect with a split-thickness skin graft on the skull periosteum. This can be considered equivalent to the situation of local advancement and placement of a relaxing incision (Fig. 1–3; see Case Report 1). Wounds too large to allow bipedicle flap coverage usually require coverage with a free tissue transfer (free flap).

### FREE FLAPS

A free flap is one that is completely detached from the donor area and moved to another site on the body. After this movement, circulation to the flap is restored by the microsurgical anastomosis of flap and available recipient site vasculature. The superficial temporal artery or other branches of the external carotid system in the neck most often provide donor site vasculature for free tissue transfers used to reconstruct the scalp. The addition of free flaps to the reconstructive surgeon's armamentarium makes almost any size of wound reconstructable (Fig. 1–4; see Case Report 2).

## Tissue Expansion

Tissue expansion makes use of the long-observed principle that skin expands to accommodate itself to gradual stretching. In 1978, Radovan was the first to report successful clinical applications of this observation and to demonstrate prototypes of the expanders in clinical use today.[3–5] The expanders that are currently in use are silicone bags with self-sealing valves placed beneath the areas to be expanded.

Tissue expansion has become a preferred technique of scalp reconstruction, because it provides hair-bearing skin for reconstruction. The distance between hair follicles does not increase to a clinically noticeable amount, and, unlike many rotation flaps, the resultant advancement flap created by the expansion process does not appreciably change the orientation of the hair follicles.

Tissue expanders are placed adjacent to the defect in a subgaleal pocket. Saline may be injected percutaneously through a one-way valve into the expander once or twice per week to increase the volume. The duration required to inflate the expander varies with each clinical situation, but it is usually between 4 and 8 weeks. At a second operation, the expander is removed, and the resultant scalp flap is used to close the defect.

Disadvantages of tissue expansion include the need for two or more operations, the interim deformity, and usually, the fact that the expander cannot be placed in the acute setting. Tissue expanders are usually placed after the wound has been closed temporarily by simpler but less definitive techniques (Fig. 1–5; see Case Report 3).

### ■ Case Report 1 (see Fig. 1–3)

A 65-year-old woman was referred for treatment of a recurrent meningioma arising in the right parietal area. This patient had undergone high-dose radiation treatment for the lesion as well as extirpative surgery. Complications led to loss of the bone flap in this area. On preoperative examination, the patient was found to have extremely atrophic skin in the area of her previous surgery and radiation and a large parietal skull defect beneath it.

The patient's previous craniotomy scars were reopened; the recurrent tumor was removed; and a dural repair was performed. A separate bone flap in the occipital area was harvested, and the inner table removed using the Midas Rex drill. The outer table of the occipital bone was returned to its anatomic position. The right parietal defect was repaired with the bone harvested from this flap, and fixation was provided with microplates and screws. At the time of closure, the unstable skin was excised and replaced with a sagittally oriented bipedicle flap, which was harvested in a supraperiosteal plane. The resultant defect located in the left parietal area was skin grafted with a meshed, split-thickness skin graft that was harvested from the left lateral thigh. This graft was meshed 1 to 1.5 times and placed nonexpanded on the secondary skull defect.

The patient's postoperative course was unremarkable. Two years later, another meningioma was found in an adjacent area. The anterior aspect of the previ-

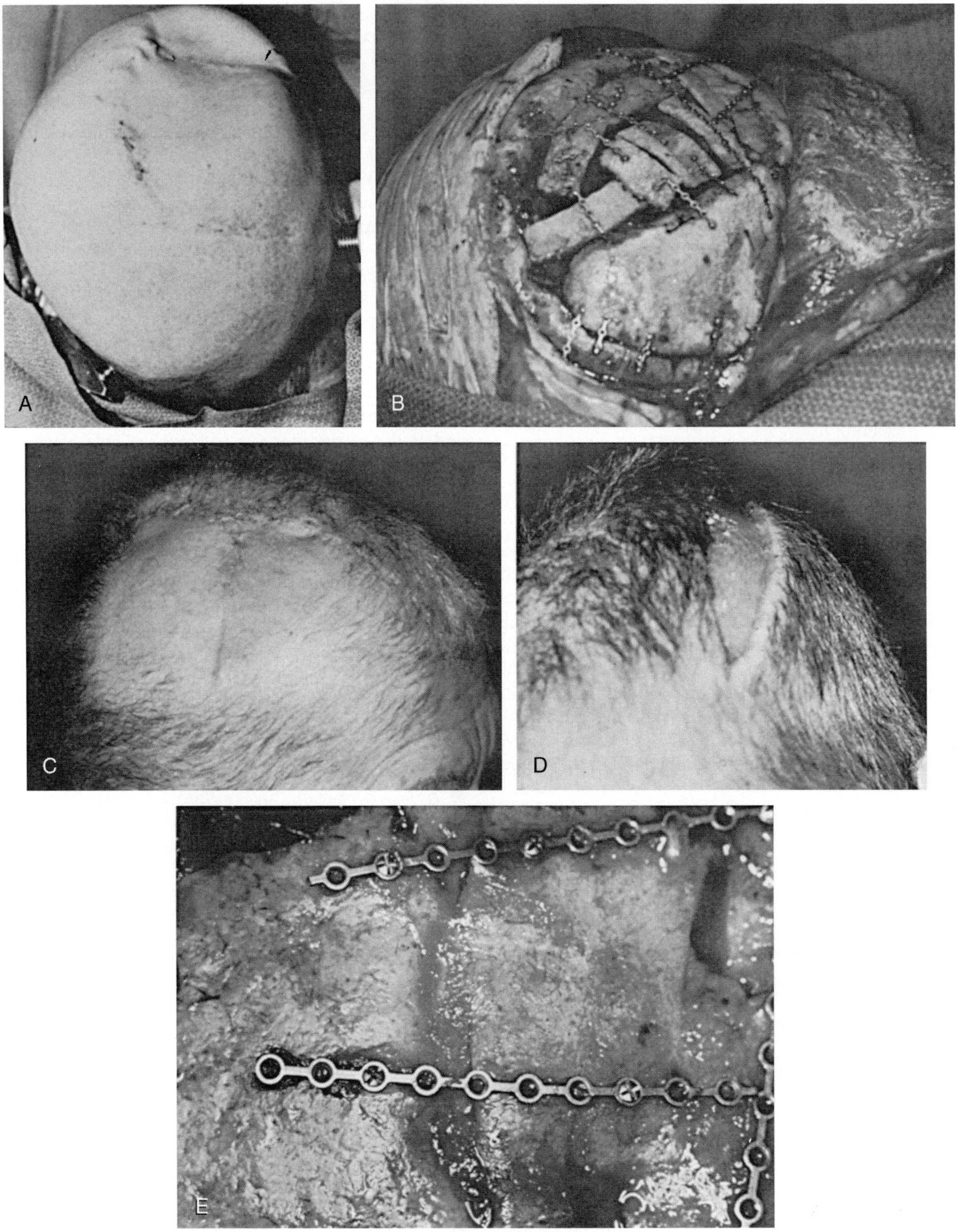

**FIGURE 1–3** ■ Scalp reconstruction and split cranial bone cranioplasty after removal of a recurrent meningioma that had been previously irradiated. A bipedicle flap was advanced to replace the unstable skin. The secondary defect was resurfaced with a skin graft. *A,* Intraoperative appearance from behind and above. Note that positioning allows access to and exposure of as much skull as possible. *B,* Reconstruction of a right temporoparietal defect from behind, with split cranial bone stabilized with microplates and screws. *C,* Postoperative appearance from the right side of the reconstruction site. *D,* Frontal postoperative appearance of a skin-grafted secondary defect after rotation of the bipedicle flap. *E,* Appearance of skull reconstruction at the time of reoperation 2 years later.

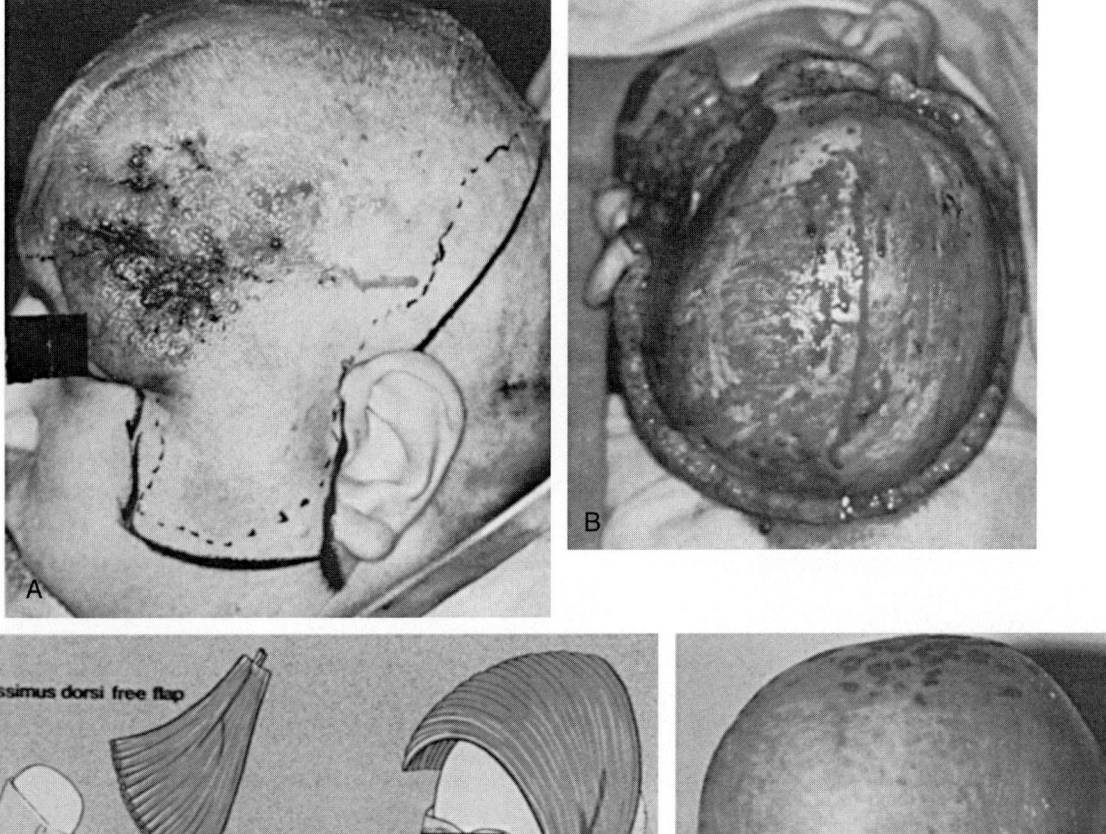

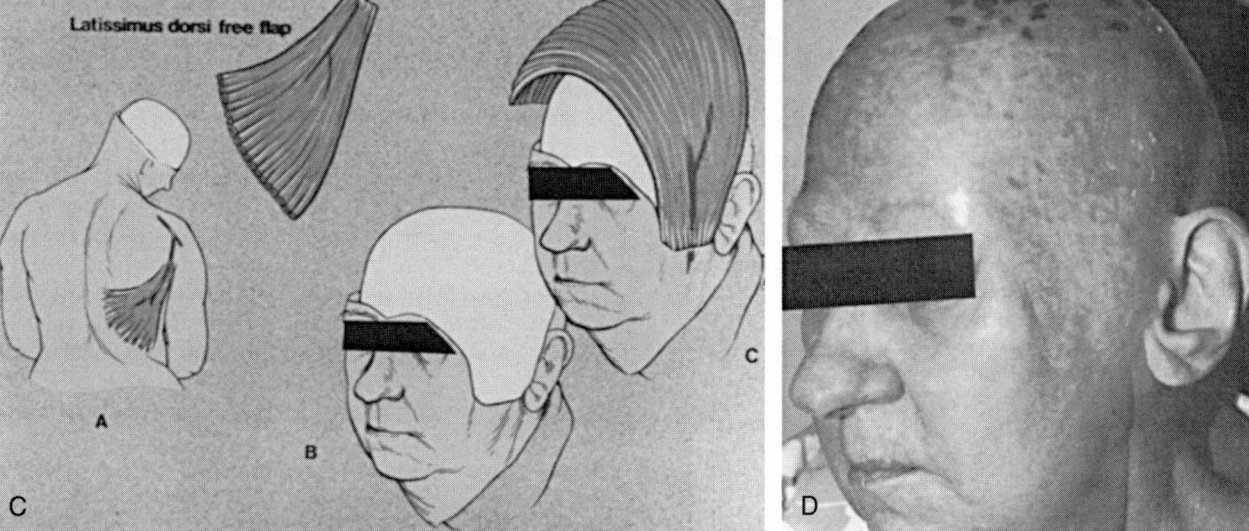

FIGURE 1–4 ■ *A,* Preoperative lateral view of a scalp tumor. *B,* Intraoperative view of the defect from above and behind. *C,* A diagrammatic representation of the procedure. *D,* The postoperative result.

ous operative site was exposed during this surgery to reveal complete healing of the previous reconstruction of the skull vault.

### Case Report 2 (see Fig. 1–4)

A 58-year-old previously healthy woman was referred with a 6-month history of a rapidly growing scalp tumor. The preoperative evaluation revealed no evidence of tumor spread beyond the scalp. A biopsy revealed that the tumor was an angiosarcoma.

The entire tumor, along with a 2-cm margin of grossly normal-appearing skin, was removed down to the outer table of the skull. In addition, a left-sided parotidectomy was performed. The defect was reconstructed with a latissimus dorsi muscle free tissue transfer. The muscle was then covered with a split-

thickness skin graft that was harvested from the left thigh.

The patient's postoperative course was unremarkable. Chemotherapy was administered postoperatively. The patient died of metastatic disease approximately 2.5 years after surgery.

### Case Report 3 (see Fig. 1–5)

A 47-year-old man was referred with a massive dermatofibrosarcoma protuberans carcinoma of the scalp, which had been treated 8 years previously with a topical solution. A preoperative evaluation revealed clinical and CT evidence that the tumor focally involved the outer table of the skull.

The lesion was excised together with a 2-cm margin of grossly normal-appearing tissue. Removal re-

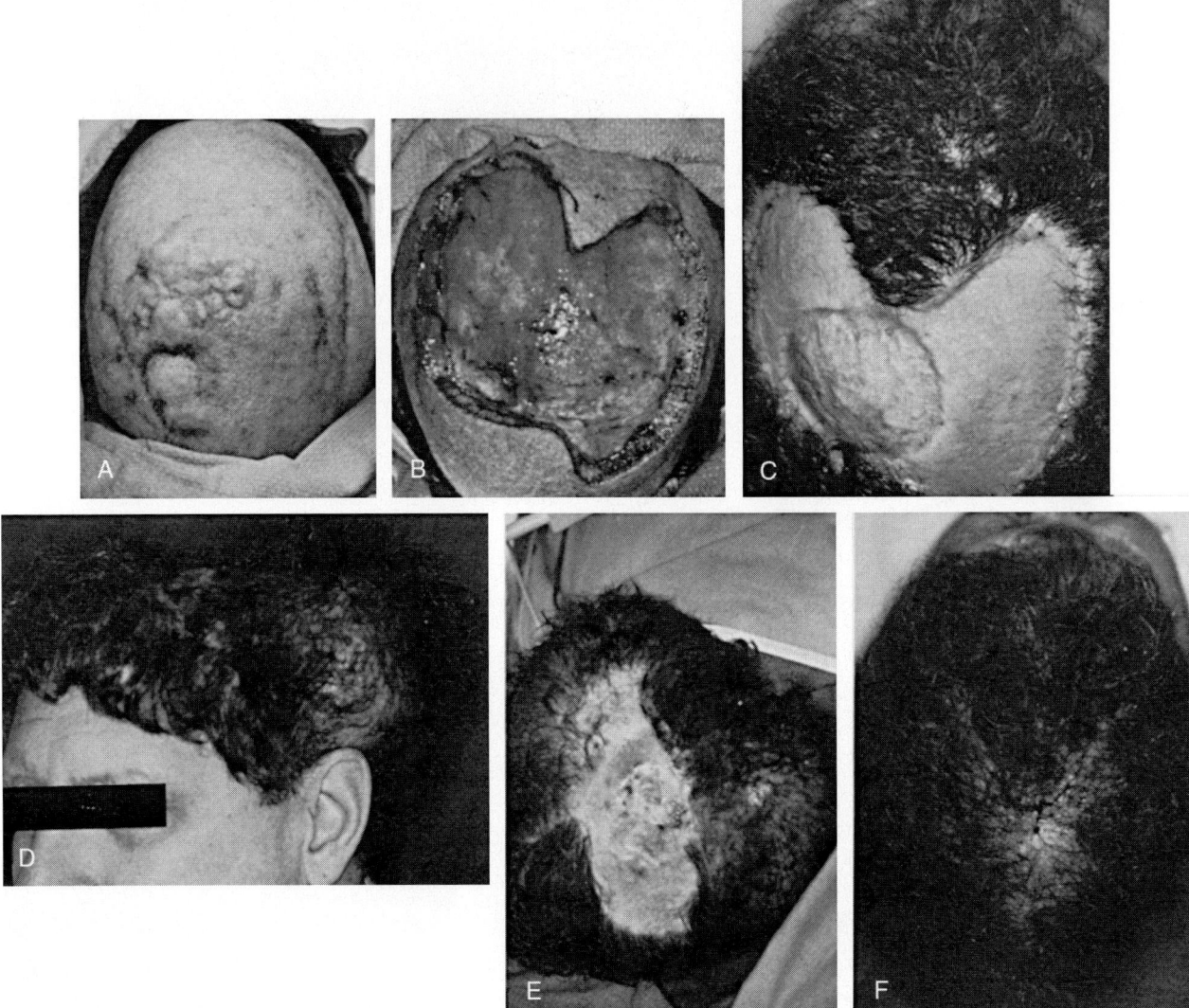

**FIGURE 1–5** ■ This patient underwent radical excision of a scalp cancer and staged reconstruction using tissue expansion. *A,* Preoperative appearance of a scalp tumor. *B,* An intraoperative view of the resultant scalp defect. *C,* Postoperative appearance after placement of a meshed split-thickness skin graft. The central area is where the outer table was removed and the split graft was placed on the diploë. *D,* Appearance with tissue expander in place. Scalp expansion and advancement were performed twice to close the defect. *E,* Intraoperative appearance during removal of a second set of expanders. *F,* Postoperative appearance after removal of the second set of expanders, flap advancement, and closure.

sulted in a defect down to the periosteum of 17 × 12 cm. Where the tumor was adjacent to the outer table, the outer table was excised to an area 8 cm². The wound was immediately closed by the placement of a meshed, split-thickness skin graft of approximately 0.014-inch thickness on the patient's periosteum and drilled-down outer table. This recipient site was dressed with Adaptic and saline-soaked gauze, which was immobilized by sewing the dressing to the intact scalp. The dressing was removed after 7 days, at which time the graft had almost completely taken. The area was observed for a recurrence for 1 year, but none occurred. During this time, small areas of skin graft breakdown occurred; these areas were managed with local dressing care. Approximately 1.5 years after radical removal of the tumor, two large tissue expanders were placed in the hair-bearing skin in the occipital and temporal areas. These expanders

were gradually filled over the next 10 weeks, after which the expanders were removed, and the resultant scalp flap was advanced. This action resulted in a remaining defect of approximately 8 × 10 cm. Two more tissue expanders were placed, and the expansion process was repeated. At the time of removal of the second set of expanders, the entire area of skin-grafted skull was resurfaced with hair-bearing skin.

## SKULL

### Anatomy of the Skull

The calvaria has three distinct layers in the adult: the hard internal and external laminae and the cancellous middle layer, or diploë. The bony vault has an average thickness of about 5 mm but varies considerably across areas and among individuals. Skull thickness lessens considerably in the elderly. The thickest area is usually the occipital and the thinnest, the temporal.

The calvaria is covered with periosteum on both the outer and inner surfaces. On the inner surface, it fuses with the dura to become the dura's outer layer. Unlike other areas of the skeleton, and perhaps because of the lack of functional stresses on the skull, the periosteum of the skull seems to have little osteogenic potential in the adult. Therefore, the loss or removal of the calvaria requires its replacement if its location is important from a protective or esthetic standpoint.

Esthetically, the frontal bone is the most important calvaria, because only a small portion of it is concealed by hair-bearing scalp. In addition, it forms the roof and portions of the medial and lateral walls of the orbit. Displaced frontal fractures may, therefore, cause a visible deformity or globe malposition. The frontal bone also includes the frontal sinuses, which are paired structures that lie between the inner and outer lamellae of the frontal bone. The lesser thickness of the anterior wall of the frontal sinus makes this area more susceptible to fracture than the adjacent temporo-orbital areas.

## Fractures of the Skull

Skull fractures should be considered after any craniofacial trauma. Bruises, lacerations, ocular injuries, brain impairment, or adjacent facial fractures should alert the physician to the possibility of skull fracture.

The radiographic examination is essential for the diagnosis. Plain films are limited by artifact secondary to suture lines, density overlap, and vessel grooves. For that reason, a CT scan has become the gold standard when evaluating injuries to the craniofacial skeleton and the intracranial structures.

### Indications for Surgery on Fractures of the Skull

Surgery for skull fracture is indicated for three main reasons: (1) to address a dural tear or an associated brain injury, (2) to avoid early or late sinus dysfunction, or (3) to avoid deformity.

#### SURGICAL TECHNIQUE FOR FRONTOBASILAR FRACTURES

**Exposure.** The bicoronal incision provides ideal exposure to the frontobasilar region for both the neurosurgeon and the craniofacial surgeon. Neurosurgical exploration, if necessary, is usually conducted through this access under the control provided by a craniotomy and bone flap. The dural repair should provide a watertight seal. In addition to allowing a panoramic view to compare for symmetry, the coronal incision provides easy access to cranial bone grafts. The resultant scalp scar is usually hidden inconspicuously within the hair. Unless they are very extensive or preclude the use of a bicoronal approach, pre-existing lacerations are rarely used for access to this area. The access provided by lacerations is often limited and usually requires their significant enlargement; the resultant long scar is often

the most deforming sequela of the injury. We have been disappointed with the postoperative appearance of the eyebrow incision and, therefore, avoid its use.

**Management of Frontal Sinus Injuries.** Management of frontal sinus injuries has long been controversial for several reasons. Because injuries are relatively infrequent, very few surgeons have extensive experience with this injury. Their care tends to be fragmented by different specialties, which also limits the experience by any one surgeon or surgical group. This fragmentation by specialization also results in varied criteria for evaluating the results of surgery. In addition, the infectious complications that may arise after treatment of these injuries do so many years later. Finally, the evaluation of esthetic results is quite arbitrary.

Our treatment algorithm is determined by the extent of the injury. Because the skeletal injury can be well documented by a preoperative CT scan, this imaging modality is important in the preoperative assessment. In any frontal sinus injury, the status of the brain, the anterior and posterior frontal walls of the sinus, the nasofrontal ducts, and the sinus mucosa must be considered. Injuries isolated to the anterior wall of the frontal sinus have a very low incidence of nasofrontal duct dysfunction[6]; therefore, if the anterior wall displacement does not constitute an objectionable contour deformity, these injuries are observed but are not necessarily treated operatively. If a significant contour deformity exists, surgery can be undertaken to correct it. During the surgery, any devitalized sinus mucosa is removed, the nasofrontal ducts are examined for patency, and fracture segments are replaced anatomically and stabilized in position.

Injuries extending into the adjacent supraorbital area have a much greater likelihood of nasofrontal duct injury and subsequent dysfunction.[6] These injuries are explored, and the frontal sinus is defunctionalized. To avoid frontal sinus mucocele formation, the walls of the sinus are drilled with a high-speed drill under constant irrigation to remove any sinus invaginations along venous channels that might later allow mucus formation.[7] The frontal sinus is further defunctionalized and isolated from the nasal cavity by obstruction of the nasofrontal ducts with contour-fit bone graft plugs. Finally, the sinus is obliterated with autogenous material. Craniofacial surgeons tend to obliterate the sinus with cancellous bone, whereas otolaryngologic surgeons usually employ autogenous fat.[8, 9] Alloplastic materials, such as hydroxyapatite, have also been used.[10] The superiority of any one material has not been documented.

Injuries that include the posterior wall have the greatest potential for intracranial contamination with sinus contents. When the posterior wall is badly disrupted, it is removed, thus "cranializing" the frontal sinus. When cranialization is performed, care is taken to effectively seal the expanded intracranial cavity from the nasal cavity. This process may require reconstruction of the cranial base with bone grafts. Pericranial and galeal frontalis flaps may be particularly useful in providing a well-vascularized seal.[11]

Note that no attempts are made to restore nasofrontal duct or sinus function once concern exists for its compromise; rather, the sinus is defunctionalized by mucosal exenteration and sinus obliteration or cranialization.

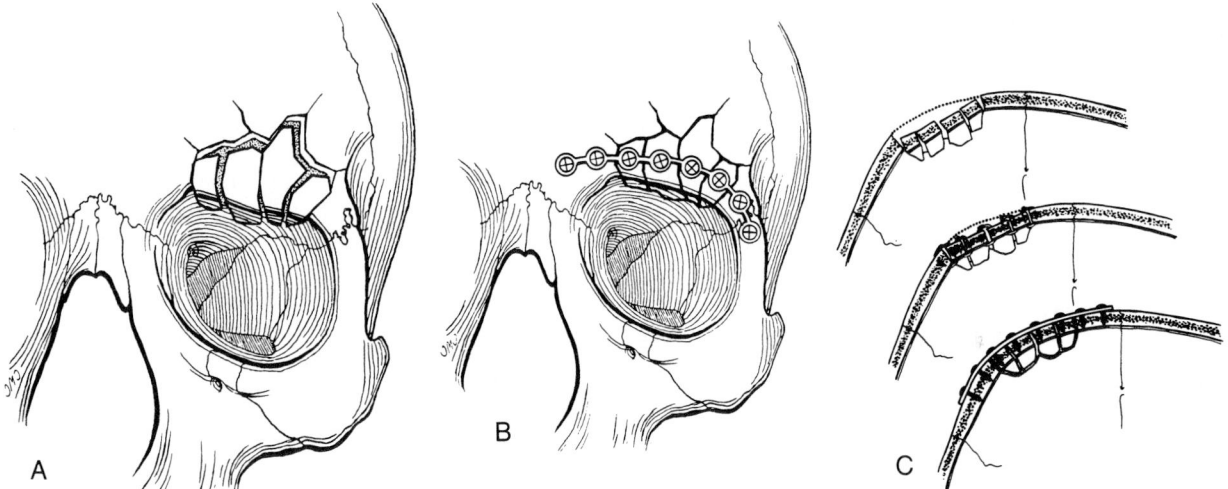

FIGURE 1–6 ■ Miniaturized plates and screws are used to maintain three-dimensional anatomic reduction of the fronto-orbital area. *A,* A comminuted supraorbital rim fracture. *B,* Fracture segments are anatomically reduced and stabilized with plates and screws. *C,* Axial view *(top)* of a supraorbital rim fracture showing resultant loss of projection *(dotted lines).* Fixation with interfragmentary wires *(middle)* does not restore the projection. Fixation with plates and screws *(bottom)* restores the projection. (From Yaremchuk MJ, Gruss JS, Manson PN [eds]: Rigid Fixation of the Craniofacial Skeleton. Boston: Butterworth Publishers, 1992.)

**Frontal Bone Reconstruction.** The reconstructive goal in frontal bone reconstruction is to restore the fronto-orbital contour. In most cases, this can be performed in the acute setting. The creation of a surgically clean wound allows replacement of frontal bone fragments and acute bone grafting in most injuries. This process may require débridement of devitalized soft tissue edges to allow primary wound healing and effective management of the sinuses as noted earlier.

The key to restoring fronto-orbital contour is the anatomic replacement of fracture segments in three dimensions. Interfragmentary wiring of fracture segments alone is usually inadequate, because wiring allows bone fragments to sink posteriorly and inferiorly, thus losing projection. Bone loss at multiple sites and particularly along craniotomy cuts tends to aggravate this problem. In fact, surgical restoration of preinjury contour often requires fracture segment replacement without bone-to-bone contact. Such replacement can be accomplished only by stabilizing bone segments with plates and screws. The plates are bent to the appropriate shape and are fixed to a stable anatomic point. The fracture segments or bone grafts are then attached to the plates with screws (Fig. 1–6). Titanium has become a popular material for craniofacial plates because of its high strength and decreased artifact on CT and MRI studies compared with stainless steel or cobalt chromium (Vitallium).[12, 13]

When autogenous bone grafts are required for replacement or augmentation, they are often harvested from the inner table of the bone flaps used to obtain neurosurgical access (Fig. 1–7) (see Case Report 4 and Fig. 1–10).

**Cranioplasty.** Cranioplasty may become necessary when primary repair or bone replacement was not possible at the time of injury. Eradication of infection may require removal of bone flaps used in elective procedures or bone fragments replaced immediately after trauma. The resultant deformity is reconstructed after the clinical infection has been treated, and the area remains clinically free of infection.

As is true of acute craniomaxillofacial reconstruction, the reconstructive goal in cranioplasty is to provide protection for the brain and restore the preinjury appearance. The two major indications for cranioplasty are protection and esthetics. In addition, speech problems and hemiparesis may improve by cranial reconstruction, but the more vague symptoms related to the "syndrome of the trephined" are less reliably improved.[14–17] Skull defects larger than 2 or 3 cm should be considered for repair. However, this decision varies with location of the defect. Even small defects in the frontal area can be disturbing to the patient and can, therefore, be considered for repair. Defects of the temporal

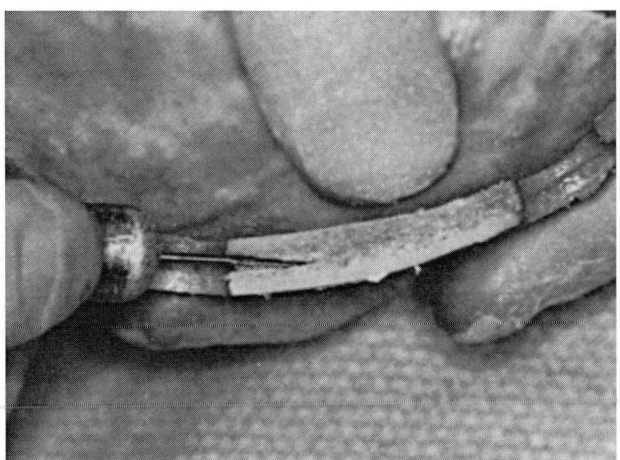

FIGURE 1–7 ■ The bone flap is being split with a Midas Rex drill (Midas Rex Pneumatic Tools, Fort Worth, TX) using a C-1 bit.

and occipital areas, which are covered by thick muscle, are usually not reconstructed.

## TIMING OF SURGERY

The incidence of infection is influenced by the timing of cranioplasty. A significant reduction in incidence of infection has been shown when 1 year is allowed to elapse between the initial injury or infection and the subsequent reconstruction.[18–20]

Bone cranioplasty has been advocated when the reconstruction is performed adjacent to sinus cavities or in areas in which previous infection occurred, despite objective evidence to support this contention.[17, 21, 22]

A recent review of the literature shows that a history of infection increases the incidence of infection after cranioplasty an average of 14% and that cranioplasty in the frontal area causes twice the incidence of infection noted for all other areas (5%).[22, 23] In reviewing their experience of 42 post-traumatic reconstructions of frontal defects in which both bone and acrylic were used, Manson and colleagues found that the material employed was not as important as the timing of reconstruction (more than 1 year after infection), eradication of communication between the cranial vault reconstruction and the nasal and frontal sinus cavities, and absence of any ethmoidal or frontal sinus inflammatory disease.[18] These data are consistent with our clinical observations. We prefer to delay cranioplasty for ideally 1 year after control of infection, to treat all sinus disease before reconstruction, and to eradicate communication between the sinus cavities and the reconstruction. Bone is used when potential for sinus communication or a history of recurrent infection exists; otherwise, most reconstructions are performed with acrylic.

## TECHNIQUE OF CRANIOPLASTY

Before cranioplasty, poorly vascularized skin areas are revised, and residual frontal or ethmoidal sinus disease is eliminated. At surgery, the patient is positioned so that a panoramic view of the skull is possible and, if appropriate, the upper face can be draped into the field. This position allows the surgeon to compare the contralateral anatomy and to avoid unnatural transitions. Preinjury photographs may be helpful in certain situations. A skull model should be available to aid in the creation of complex curvatures and landmarks.

Old scars are usually incised for exposure, and the skull flap is removed carefully from the underlying dura and brain. Any dural tears are repaired. Resection of the bone edge to identify normal dura and establishment of a plane of dissection may be necessary.

The freed bone edge is saucerized by removal of the outer table with rongeurs or a high-speed bur. This lip prevents the implant from slipping into the defect and provides a ledge for subsequent fixation.

## CHOICE OF MATERIAL FOR CRANIOPLASTY

Today, the most commonly used materials for cranioplasty are acrylic and bone.

Bone is preferred by many plastic surgeons, because it is believed to be "natural" and less susceptible to infection and late complications. It has the disadvantages of requiring a donor site, being technically demanding to perform, and exhibiting variable resorption and therefore being prone to irregular contour.

Methyl methacrylate reconstruction has the advantages of ease of reconstruction and avoidance of donor site morbidity. The contour of this substance is stable. It is radiolucent and, therefore, does not affect postoperative radiologic imaging. It is not affected by temperature and is very strong. Methyl methacrylate is believed by some to be more susceptible to infection and late complications.[18, 24]

**Methyl Methacrylate.** Cranioplasty kits are available that contain a single dose of 30 g of powdered polymer and 17 ml of liquid monomer. The elements are mixed with a spatula in a bowl. The mixing should be conducted under ventilation so that the person who is mixing the substance is not overcome by fumes. The mixing process takes about 30 seconds. The bowl is then covered to avoid evaporation of the monomer. Doughing time varies with the temperature and takes approximately 5 minutes at 72° F.

Shaping of the plastic implant is usually performed by placing the doughy mixture in a plastic sleeve provided in the cranioplasty kit. The sleeve containing the still pliable implant mixture is placed onto the skull defect and molded by digital compression. The molding process occurs under continuous irrigation to avoid thermal damage to the dura and brain. The molding time usually takes 6 to 8 minutes. The very exothermic polymerization process is allowed to take place away from the surgical field.

Some surgeons place a wire mesh into the skull defect. Methyl methacrylate is then cured directly on the mesh. This technique allows more risk for burn damage to the dura during the exothermic reaction. However, data from Manson and colleagues show that temperature rises less than 3° C when the implant is continuously irrigated.[18]

Complex curvatures, particularly in the supraorbital area, are created by adding material to an initial construct. Final adjustments can be made with a contouring bur on a high-speed drill. The implants may be secured with wires or, more simply and rapidly, with microscrews. The plate may be perforated to allow the dura to be tented up to it. This method reduces the potential for epidural collection. Perforations in the implant also allow for drainage and for soft tissue ingrowth, which also aids in implant fixation (see Case Study 5).

**Bone Cranioplasty.** Bone cranioplasty is technically more challenging than alloplastic cranioplasty. Bone donor sites include the ribs, the calvaria, and less frequently, the iliac crest.

Split ribs are useful when large defects are to be reconstructed and calvarial bone is in short supply. Split ribs are usually fitted into a shelf created in the adjacent intact skull. In the past, an interlocking "chain link" technique was used for fixation, but most craniofacial surgeons now use a combination of plates and screws (Fig. 1–8).

Calvarial bone is the preferred donor site of most craniofacial surgeons. Clinical experience and several animal studies have shown that calvarial bone maintains its volume better than split rib or iliac crest. The calvarial bone is harvested in two ways. The outer table may be harvested

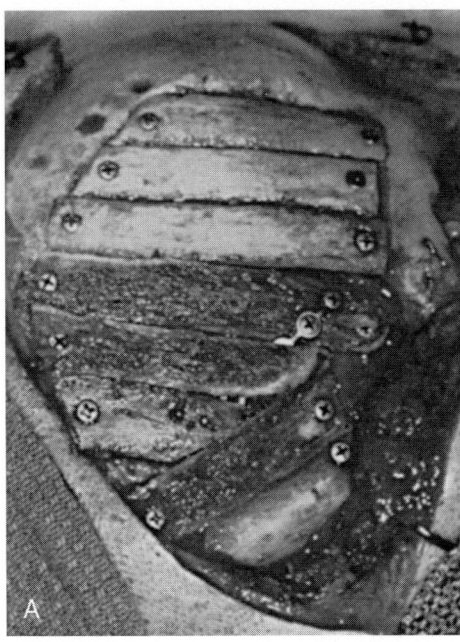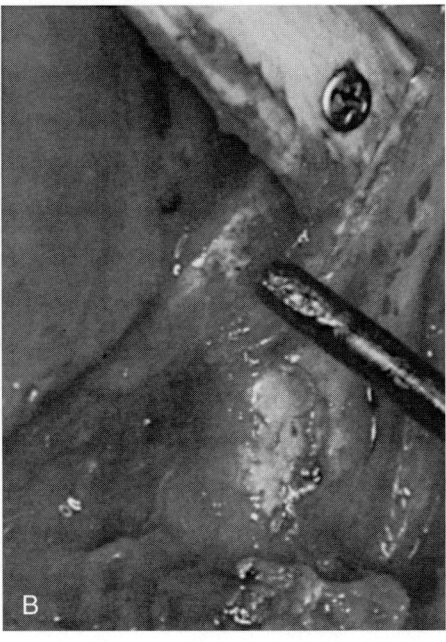

FIGURE 1–8 ■ *A*, An example of a split-rib cranioplasty stabilized with plates and screws on the right frontotemporal area. *B*, A close-up view shows a ledge created by removing the outer table at the edge of the defect. This allows a ledge for the rib graft and ease of screw fixation.

from the intact skull. The parietal area usually serves as the donor site, because this area is usually accessible and the donor site contour deformity is hidden by the patient's hair (see Case Report 6 and Fig. 1–12).

Another technique for harvesting cranial bone is to perform a craniotomy and harvest a full-thickness piece of skull of appropriate size and curvature. The inner table is split from the outer table. A simple way to do this is with the aid of the Midas Rex drill and the C-1 bit (see Fig. 1–7). This thin bit is placed in the diploë between the two skull cortices. The outer cortex can be replaced, and the inner cortex is used for reconstruction of the defect. Most often, microplates and screws are used to stabilize this reconstruction.

**Other Materials.** Porous polyethylene (Medpor) has been used for the reconstruction of small defects. This substance has the advantages of easy contourability, potential for adjacent soft tissue ingrowth, and ease of fixation with miniaturized plates and screws. Various-sized implants are available (Fig. 1–9).

Hydroxyapatite is a ceramic biomaterial that consists of calcium phosphate. It can be manufactured synthetically or formed by chemically converting the naturally porous calcium carbonate skeleton of marine coral. Absorption is minimal, and the material allows bony ingrowth when used as an onlay or interpositional graft.[25] Hydroxyapatite granules can also be mixed with autologous blood and fibrillar collagen to form a moldable paste, but osseointegration does not occur with this method.[26]

**Computer-Aided Design/Computer-Aided Manufacture (CAD/CAM).** CT imaging of skull defects provides digitized information that can be transferred to design software. Data describing the contour along the edge of the defect and the surface characteristics of the normal cranium surrounding the defect can be used to design a custom-fit implant. The electronic data describing the newly designed prosthesis are then used by a computer-controlled manufac-turing system to create a wax model, which is then cast, or to directly mill raw material into the finished implant (Fig. 1–10).[27–29]

## Case Report 4

A 38-year-old man was referred with a frontal fracture 1 week after being involved in a motor vehicle accident (Fig. 1–11*A–D*). The patient had no neurologic symptoms, and a preoperative axial CT scan showed the fracture to be confined to the anterior wall of the frontal sinus. Surgery was performed through a bicoronal incision. The fracture segments were elevated, and the frontal sinus was explored. No injury to the nasofrontal ducts was found. The devitalized mucosa was removed, and the fracture segments were replaced anatomically and fixed in position with microplates and screws. The patient was discharged on the fourth postoperative day. His postoperative course has been unremarkable over the past 2 years.

## Case Report 5

A 65-year-old man was referred for cranioplasty (Fig. 1–12*A–C*). The patient had undergone tumor resection in the parietal area 1 year before and postoperative infection required removal of the bone flap. The patient's previous surgical scar was incised. The scalp flap was dissected off to the dura, and an acrylic cranioplasty with methyl methacrylate was performed. The patient's postoperative course was unremarkable.

## Case Report 6

A 10-year-old girl was referred from Armenia after having had an open skull fracture in an earthquake (Fig. 1–13). Emergency treatment consisted of dé-bridement of bone fragments and soft tissue closure. The patient had no neurologic abnormalities. The physical examination and CT scan revealed a large

*Text continued on page 18*

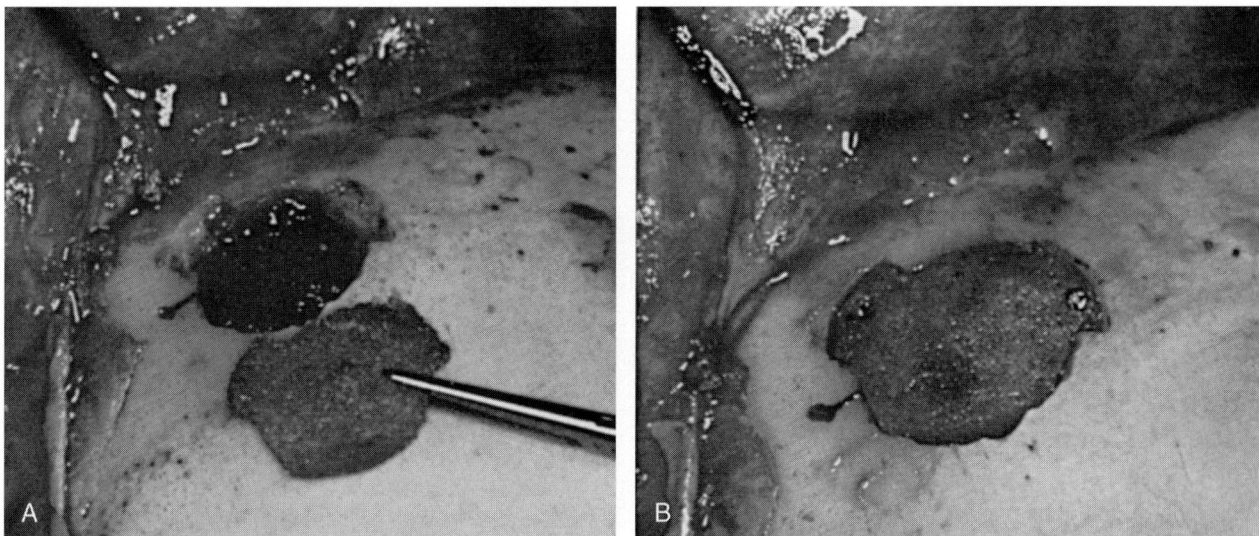

FIGURE 1–9 ■ A 3-cm left frontal defect after removal of a benign bone tumor was reconstructed with a Medpor implant. *A,* An intraoperative view showing the defect and the implant. *B,* The implant is in place. A ledge was created in the frontal bone by removing the outer table in two places. A flange of Medpor was affixed to this ledge with microscrews.

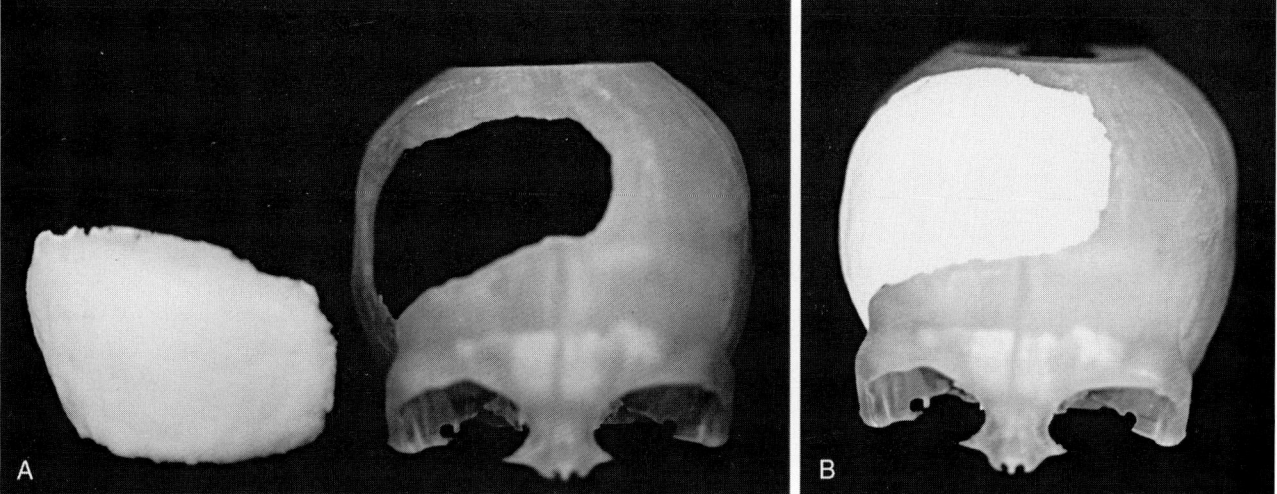

FIGURE 1–10 ■ A three-dimensional model of a skull defect with a CAD/CAM–generated polyethylene implant adjacent to the skull *(A),* and fitted into the defect *(B).*

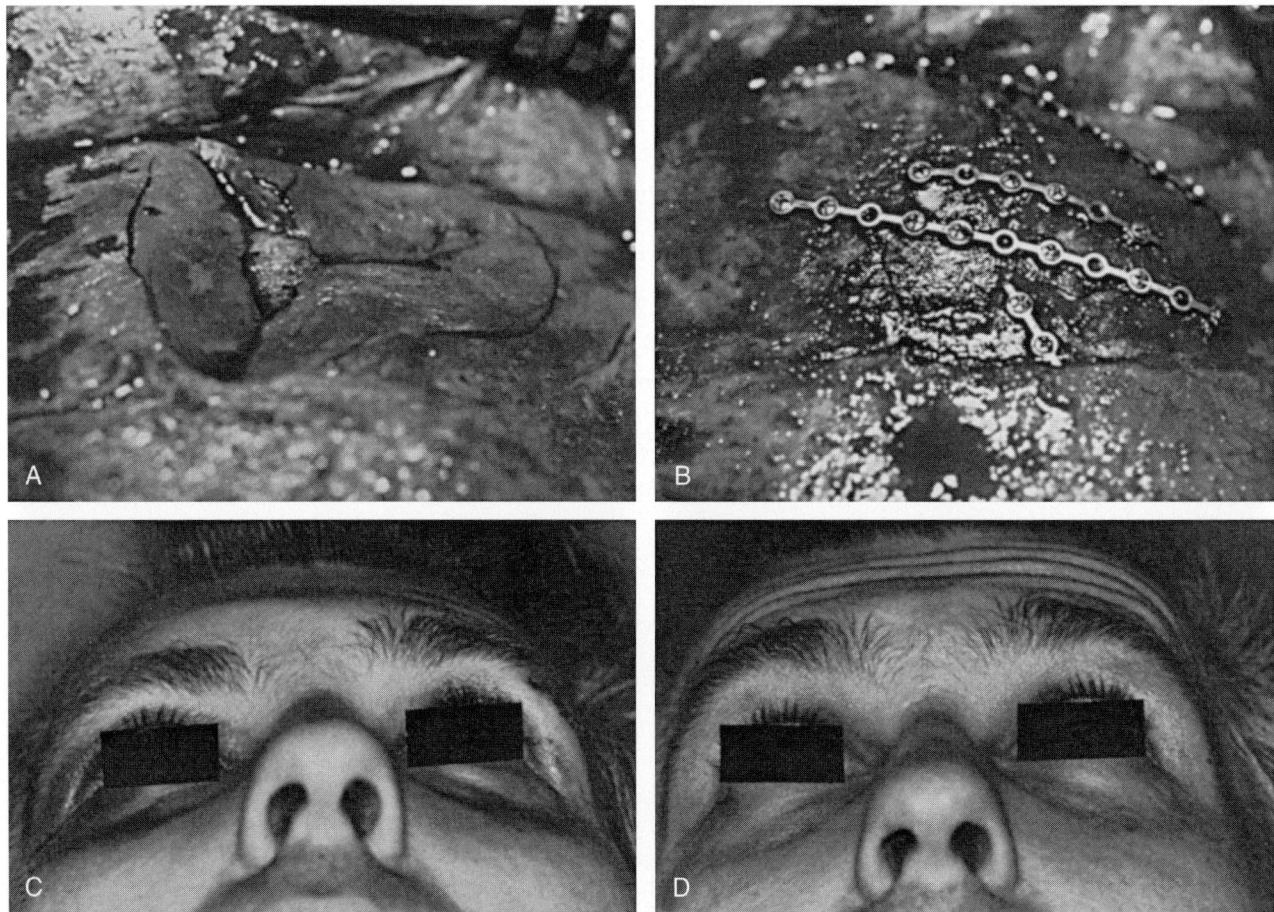

FIGURE 1–11 ■ A patient with a frontal sinus fracture managed by open reduction and internal fixation. *A*, Intraoperative appearance of a fracture as seen from above through the coronal approach. *B*, After reduction and fixation. Miniplates and screws were used for fixation. *C*, A preoperative worm's eye view. *D*, A postoperative worm's eye view.

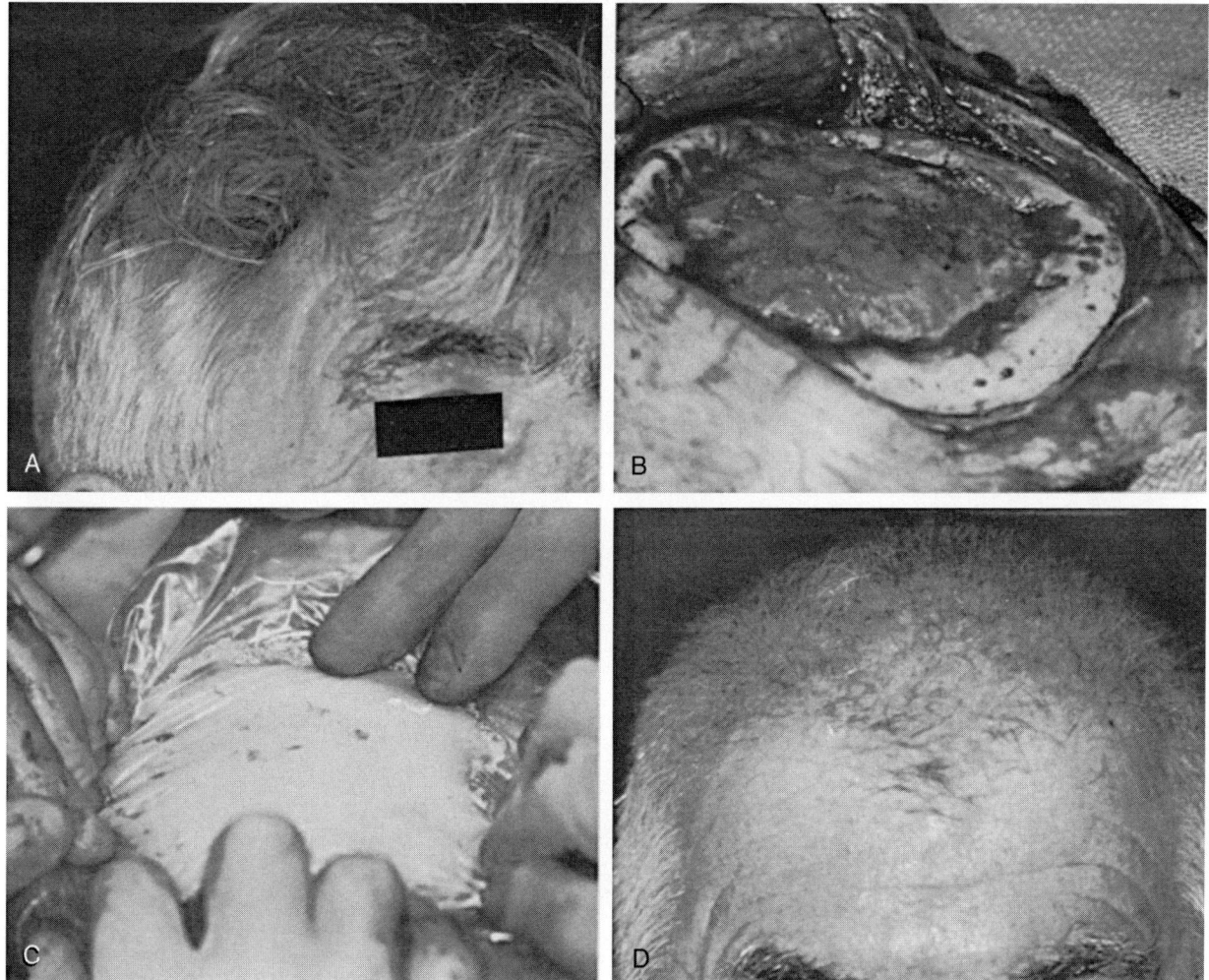

**FIGURE 1–12** ■ Acrylic cranioplasty. *A,* The preoperative appearance. *B,* An intraoperative view of the right frontoparietal defect. *C,* Molding of methyl methacrylate to the defect. *D,* The postoperative result.

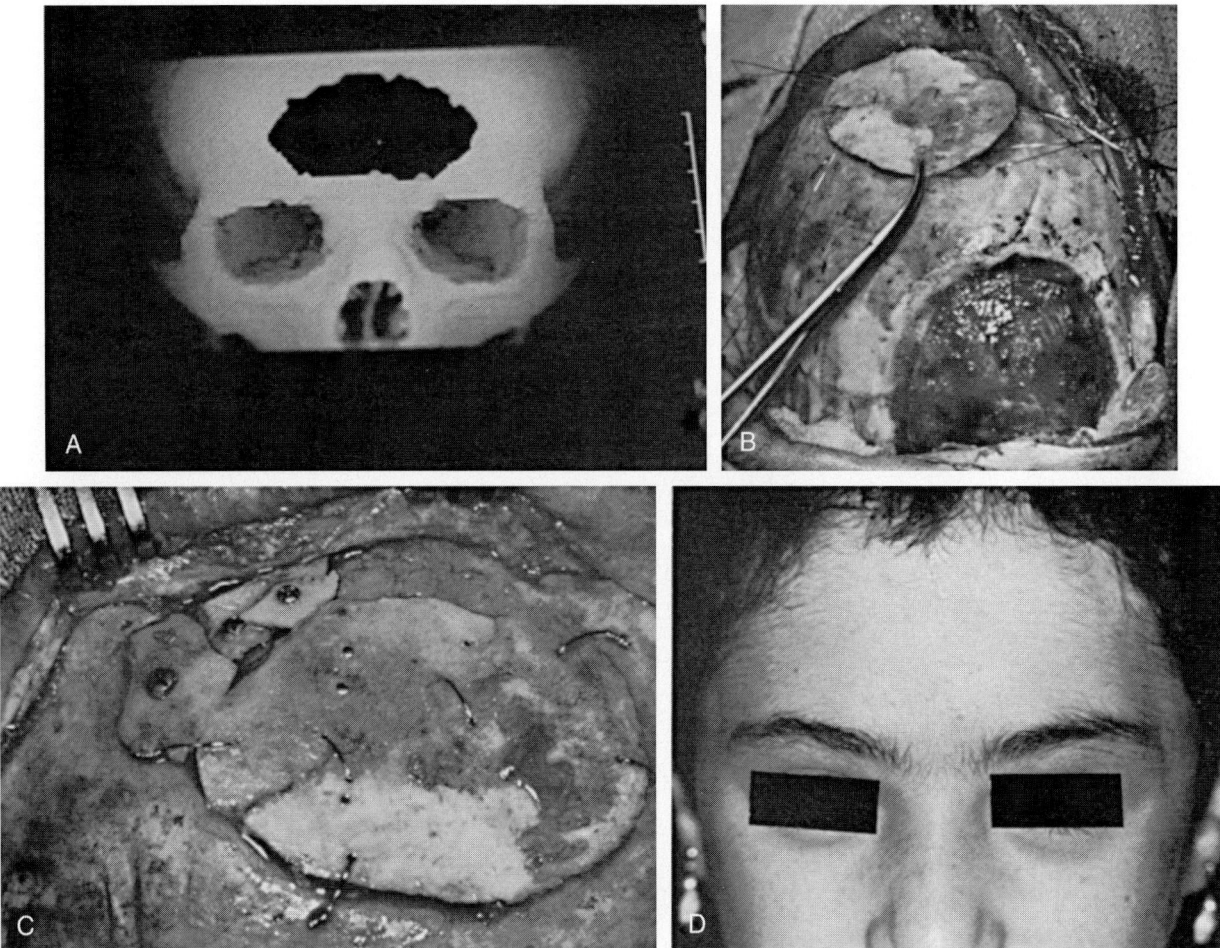

**FIGURE 1–13** ■ A frontal cranioplasty is performed with an outer table cranial bone. *A,* A preoperative three-dimensional computed tomography scan shows the frontal defect. *B,* An intraoperative view shows the donor site and the graft in position. *C,* A close up view of the graft, which is stabilized with screws. The supraorbital rim was augmented with onlay grafts. *D,* The postoperative appearance.

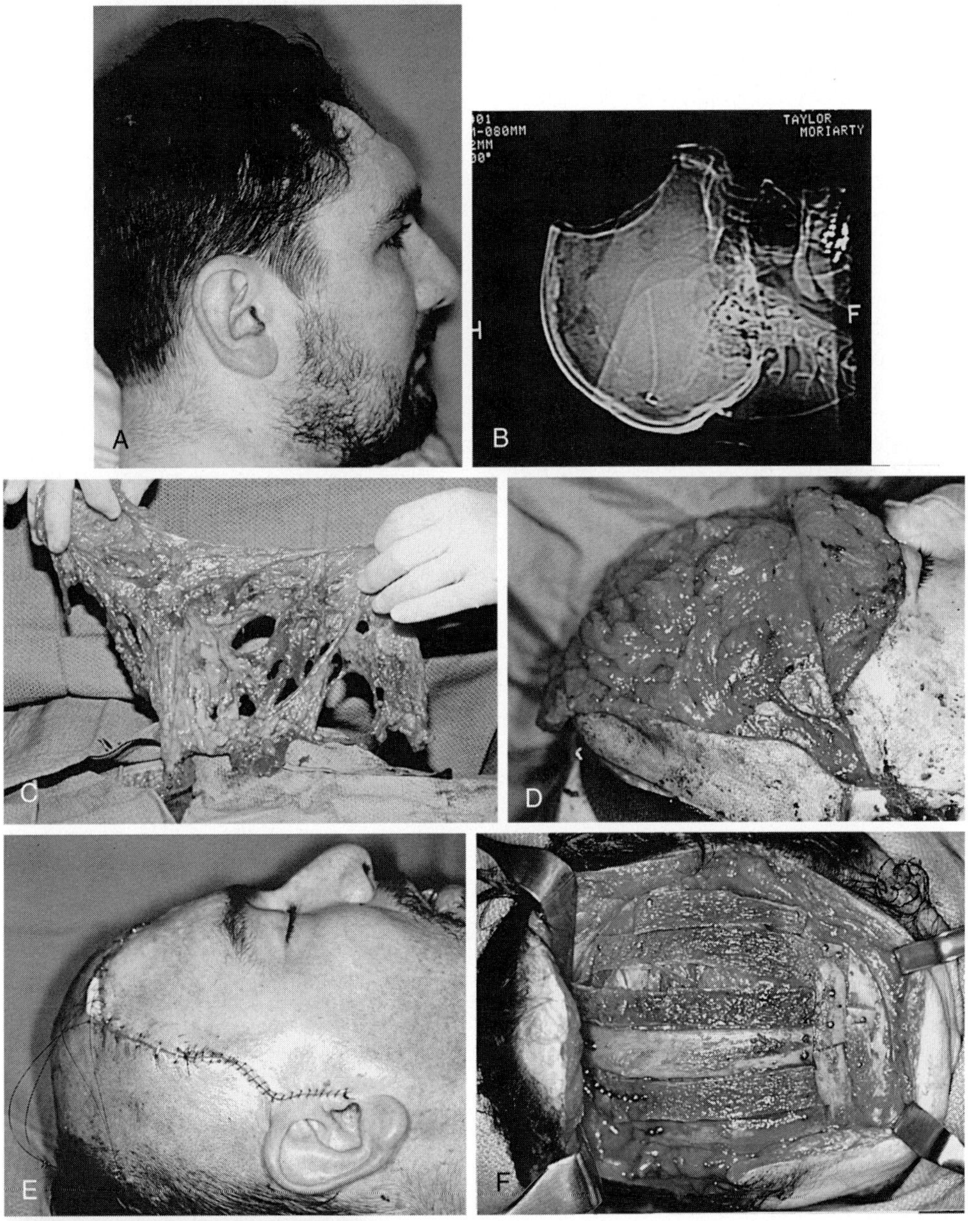

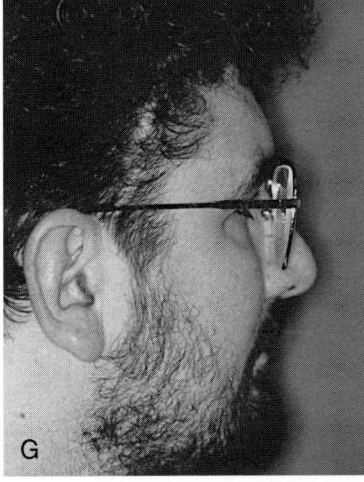

**FIGURE 1–14** ■ Repair of the traumatic frontal defect is complicated by a cerebrospinal fluid fistula and infection. *A,* The preoperative profile. *B,* Sagittal plane computed tomography (CT) scan image of the defect. *C,* Harvest of an omental flap; *D,* placement in defect. *E,* Postoperative view from the omental flap. *F,* Split rib grafts are in place. *G,* A late postoperative photograph showing restoration of the normal contour.

frontal defect. In addition, there were unrepaired fractures of the supraorbital rim, resulting in supraorbital depression on the left side. Surgery was performed though a bicoronal incision. The scalp flap was dissected away from the dura. A template of the defect was placed over the parietal area, and bone from the outer table of the skull was removed. This bone was transferred to the central frontal area to reconstruct the defect and was stabilized with microplates and screws. In addition, left supraorbital contour was restored by the placement of onlay grafts of outer table cranial bone. These grafts were fixed with microscrews and contoured in situ. The patient was discharged on the fifth postoperative day, and her postoperative course was unremarkable.

## Case Report 7

A 32-year-old man sustained an open frontal injury in a high-speed motor vehicle accident (Fig. 1–14A–G). He developed a cerebrospinal spinal fluid fistula and meningitis, necessitating lumbar drainage and intravenous antibiotics. The skull deformity persisted, and the overlying skin remained unstable. An omental free flap was used to cover the dura and fill dead space. Six months later, split rib grafts were used to restore the bone contour.

## REFERENCES

1. Juri J, Juri C, Aurfe HN: Use of rotation scalp flaps for treatment of occipital baldness. Plast Reconstr Surg 61:23–26, 1978.
2. Ortichchea M: New three flap reconstruction technique. Br J Plast Surg 24:184–188, 1971.
3. Nordstrom REA, Devine JW: Scalp stretching with a tissue expander for closure of scalp defects. Plast Reconstr Surg 75:578–581, 1985.
4. Radovan C: Breast reconstruction after mastectomy using the temporary expander. Plast Reconstr Surg 69:195–206, 1982.
5. Radovan C: Tissue expansion in soft tissue reconstruction. Plast Reconstr Surg 74:482–490, 1984.
6. Stanley RB Jr: Fractures of the frontal sinus. Clin Plast Surg 16:115–123, 1989.
7. Donald PJ: The tenacity of frontal sinus mucosa. Otolaryngol Head Neck Surg 87:557–566, 1979.
8. Donald PJ, Ettin M: The safety of frontal sinus fat obliteration when sinus walls are missing. Laryngoscope 96:190–198, 1986.
9. Wolfe SA, Johnson P: Frontal sinus injuries: Primary care and management of late complications. Plast Reconstr Surg 82:781–789, 1988.
10. Rosen G, Nachtigal D: The use of hydroxyapatite for obliteration of the human frontal sinus. Laryngoscope 105:553–555, 1995.
11. Gruss JS, Pollock RA, Phillips JH, Antonyshyn O: Combined injuries of the cranium and face. Br J Plast Surg 42:385–398, 1989.
12. Fiala TGS, Paige KT, Davis TL, et al: Comparison of artifact from craniomaxillofacial internal fixation devices: Magnetic resonance imaging. Plast Reconstr Surg 93:725–731, 1994.
13. Saxe AW, Doppman JL, Brennan MF: Use of titanium surgical clips to avoid artifacts seen on computed tomography. Arch Surg 117:978–979, 1982.
14. Grantham EG, Landis HP: Cranioplasty and posttraumatic syndrome. J Neurosurg 5:19–26, 1948.
15. Carmichael FA: The reduction of hernia cerebri by tantalum cranioplasty: A preliminary report. J Neurosurg 2:379–384, 1945.
16. Tabaddor K, LaMorgese J: Complication of a large cranial defect: Case report. J Neurosurg 44:506–512, 1976.
17. Stula D: The problem of "sinking skin-flap syndrome" in cranioplasty. J Craniomaxillofac Surg 10:142–146, 1982.
18. Manson PN, Crawley WA, Hoopes JE: Frontal cranioplasty: Risk factors and choice of cranial vault reconstructive material. Plast Reconstr Surg 77:888–900, 1986.
19. Hammon WM, Kempe LG: Methyl methacrylate cranioplasty; 13 years experience with 417 patients. Acta Neurochir 25:69–76, 1971.
20. Rish BL, Dillon JD, Meirowsky AM, et al: Cranioplasty: A review of 1030 cases of penetrating head injury. Neurosurgery 4:381–386, 1979.
21. Munro IR, Guyuron B: Split-rib cranioplasty. Ann Plast Surg 7:341–346, 1981.
22. White JC: Late complications following cranioplasty with alloplastic plates. Ann Surg 128:743–751, 1948.
23. Woolf JI, Walker AE: Cranioplasty. Int J Surg 81:1–9, 1945.
24. Wofle SA: In discussion: Manson PN, Crawley WA, Hoopes JE: Frontal cranioplasty: Risk factors and choice of cranial vault reconstructive material. Plast Reconstr Surg 77:901–904, 1986.
25. Holmes R, Hagler H: Porous hydroxyapatite as a bone graft substitute in cranial reconstruction: A histometric study. Plast Reconstr Surg 81:662, 1988.
26. Byrd HS, Hobar PC, Shewmake K: Augmentation of the craniofacial skeleton with porous hydroxyapatite granules. Plast Recontr Surg 91:15–26, 1993.
27. Wehmoller MW, Eufinger H, Kruse D, Massberg W: CAD by processing of computed tomography data and CAM of individually designed prostheses. Int J Oral Maxillofac Surg 24:90–97, 1995.
28. Eufinger H, Wehmoller MW, Machtens E, et al: Reconstruction of craniofacial bone defects with individual alloplastic implants based on CAD/CAM manipulated CT data. J Craniomaxillofac Surg 23:175–181, 1995.
29. Ono I, Gunji H, Kaneko F, et al: Treatment of extensive cranial bone defects using computer-designed hydroxyapatite ceramics and periosteal flaps. Plast Reconstr Surg 92:819–830, 1993.

# CHAPTER 2

# Surgical Repair of the Major Defects of the Scalp and Skull

■ RICHARD S. FOX

Since America's first encounters with scalping, and even back to 2000 BC, surgeons and shaman have been both astonished and confounded with large defects of the scalp and skull.[1, 2] It was not until the latter part of the 19th century that skin grafting was found to be effective in treating some of these large open defects.[3, 4] Subsequently, in the early part of the 20th century and particularly since the 1970s, there have been significant technical achievements allowing for successful treatment of these injuries. Indeed, there is a plethora of different approaches and techniques, and this chapter is designed to allow the surgeon to select the technique most appropriate for the defect at hand.

## ANATOMY

The scalp constitutes the soft tissue coverage of this area and is divided into five layers (Fig. 2–1):

1. Skin (epidermis and dermis)
2. Subcutaneous tissue
3. Galea aponeurotica
4. Loose areolar connective tissue
5. Periosteum

The essential element for any successful repair is epidermis, to prevent desiccation and infection.

The bony skull has four major components:

1. Outer cortex
2. Diploë
3. Inner cortex
4. Dura

With respect to defects greater than 1 cm, the skin and dura are indispensable as the absolute minimal requirements.

The scalp has an extensive blood supply with a thick network of collateralization. There are six principal arteries on each side (Fig. 2–2). These are invaluable when considering the design of axial pattern flaps or planning a microvascular anastomosis.

## DEFECT ASSESSMENT AND PLANNING

### Acute Defects

The appropriate initial treatment and surgical plan is fundamental to ultimate success or failure. For example, in a complete avulsion of the scalp, the residual soft tissues must be protected from desiccation. Similarly, an amputated scalp must be cooled and protected from desiccation and unnecessary trauma. Finally, this surgery must occur in the shortest time frame possible. All tissue must be handled gently, and topical cytotoxic agents are to be avoided.

When life-threatening, brain, cardiovascular, or pulmonary injury takes precedence, efforts should be made to protect the soft tissue and bone for subsequent repair. Because of the extensive collateralization of the blood supply, scalp tissue in situ will survive despite extraordinary injury. Débridement should be carefully considered before being carried out. Such tissues may be protected with sponges and moistened with topical antibiotic solution

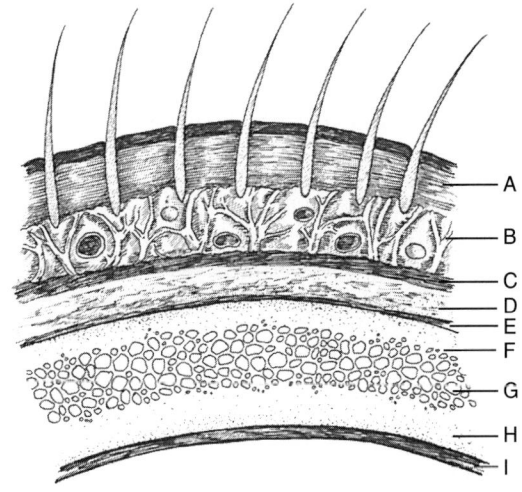

FIGURE 2–1 ■ Anatomy of the scalp. *A,* Skin (epidermis/dermis). *B,* Subcutaneous tissue. *C,* Galeal aponeurotica. *D,* Loose areolar connective tissue. *E,* Periosteum. *F,* Outer cortex. *G,* Diploe. *H,* Inner cortex. *I,* Dura.

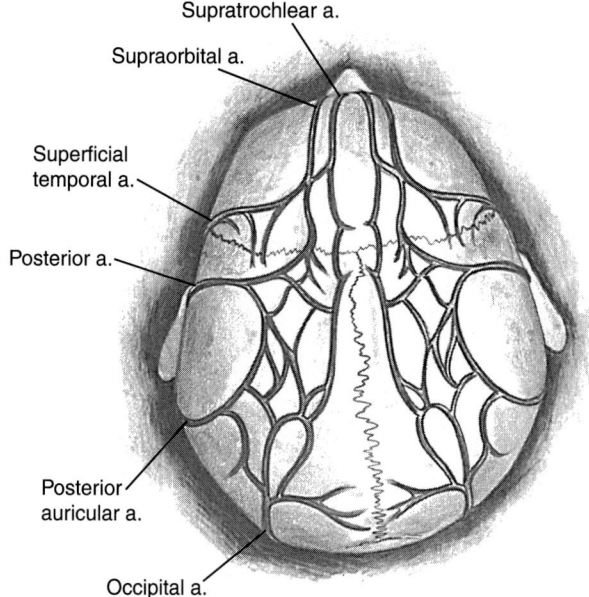

FIGURE 2–2 ■ Blood supply to the scalp. Note the six major vessels on each side and the extensive collateralization.

or one-quarter-strength povidone-iodine (Betadine). If repair is to be delayed more than 24 hours, silver sulfadiazine (Silvadene) may be applied topically every 12 to 24 hours. Infection control is excellent and desiccation minimal. At the time of repair, the gelatinous coating is easily removed with a gauze sponge.

## Chronic Defects

Long-standing defects characteristically harbor chronic, low-grade infection. Before closure, this must be addressed with surgical débridement, systemic antibiotics, and occasionally topical antibiotics. If the wound is ischemic (i.e., radiation injury or cicatrix), nonsalvageable tissue clearly must be débrided. If the chronic infection or ischemia is not addressed definitively at the outset, any reconstruction will fail as a result of infection or wound breakdown. When assessing and planning to treat any defect, one must recognize that plans sometimes fail; tumors recur, a flap may die. Thus, inherent in any plan *A* is plan *B* and avoidance of any procedures that might destroy options for future treatment.

For either acute or chronic defects, metabolic factors must be recognized, dealt with, and considered in the surgery plan. Diabetes, malnutrition, and immunosuppressants are to be optimally corrected and surgical plans kept simple and straightforward, strongly entertaining the possibility of secondary or delayed reconstruction when physiologic conditions are optimal.

## INJURIES

### Lacerations

Lacerations of any length or complexity (stellate) are appropriately and safely closed with monofilament suture

(4–0 nylon or 4–0 Prolene) or staples. Efforts should be made to include the galea in such repairs as a separate layer with absorbable sutures.

Before closure, the wounds must be visually and palpably examined for any underlying fractures. Radiographs are not necessary in all scalp injuries.

Bleeding is often prolific. In an emergency setting, pressure dressings, if quickly applied, can effectively control such hemorrhage. It is important that 4 × 4s be folded and put directly over an area of bleeding and compressed snugly. A large, all-encompassing, thick layer of soft dressings is not effective and leads to unnecessary blood loss. When repair is undertaken, large vessels are controlled with electrocautery or ties. Smaller skin bleeding is controlled with skin sutures.

It is not necessary to shave the hair when repairing almost any scalp injury. The hair can be washed with Hibiclens (antiseptic/antimicrobial skin cleanser) preoperatively in elective settings. At the time of surgery, it can be parted to either side of the wound with petroleum-based ointment or water-soluble jelly.

In any injury in which the subgaleal space has been extensively opened, it is wise to consider a closed suction drain for 24 to 48 hours and occasionally longer.

## Defects Up to 10 cm²

If such defects contain viable periosteum, they can be closed quickly with a retroauricular full-thickness skin graft or a split-thickness skin graft. A tie-over dressing is necessary for 5 to 7 days. Such a repair leaves a bald, hairless patch.

To avoid this, galeal release or cross-hatching permits an approximately 20% increase in soft tissue available for coverage. Cross-hatching must be perpendicular to the desired axis of extension and must be completely through the galea, without damaging the underlying vessels. Wounds may require extension to allow exposure of the galea for its adequate release (Fig. 2–3). Alternatively, a

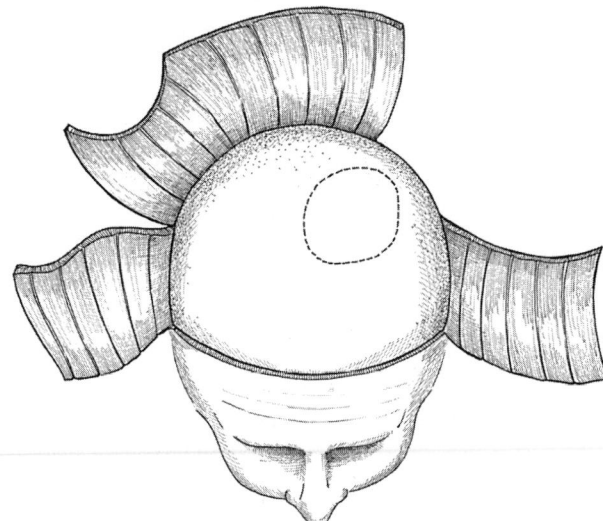

FIGURE 2–3 ■ Elevation of multiple skin flaps at the subgaleal level. Cross-hatching must carefully avoid the underlying axial blood vessels. Each elevated flap should be based on the course of an axial vessel.

limited rotation flap with galeal release closes the defect without the need for skin grafting of the donor site.

It is argued that in acute injuries, extensive undermining or flap elevation should be avoided. Skin grafting over intact periosteum or decorticated bone with skin grafting is safe; secondary reconstruction of the subsequent defect may be performed in the future.

In my experience, many acute wounds can be treated safely with topical care (topical antibiotics, silver sulfadiazine) and systemic antibiotics until conditions are optimal for extended repair. This avoids potential infection in the initial procedure and avoids the need for a secondary procedure itself. It also significantly reduces the total surgical manipulation of the soft tissue.

In the instance of bone loss, replacement can be safely carried out with harvest of outer table cortical bone from the adjacent skull.[5, 6] Bone from the iliac crest or split rib should be considered when it is inappropriate to use split skull. Edges of the defect should be sculpted to create a ridge for support of the bone graft or methyl methacrylate. It is my preference to fix bone grafts with microplates and screws. In acute wounds with a high potential for infection and those wounds characterized by suboptimal metabolic conditions, bone is preferred over methyl methacrylate. Comments on the techniques of harvesting split calvarial bone graft are appropriate at this time. This is a procedure that is conceptually simple and straightforward, but in fact has significant risks and requires precision and focus. Alloplastic materials such as methyl methacrylate molded to the defect or titanium mesh cut to fit the defect are alternatives to bone autografts.

It is recommended that the outer cortex be burred down into the diploë circumferentially around the piece of bone to be harvested. Great care must be taken throughout the course of the procedure to prevent penetration of the inner table. This outer cortex should then be harvested with curved osteotomes that have been recently sharpened and are in excellent condition. An osteotome that requires unusual force with the mallet to force its way through the diploë carries with it a risk of penetrating the inner table.

In isolated situations, it is not unreasonable for a segment of full-thickness bone to be removed from the skull and split on a back table with a Midas Rex drill or osteotome. The inner cortex then can be returned to its original location and anchored there, and a graft can be placed in the defect as desired. When a two-team approach is being used, this may be of great value.

## Defects Less Than 20 cm²

In many situations, skin grafts are the best choice of treatment. This is particularly true if the periosteum is viable. Patients suffering from other life-threatening injuries that take precedence can be quickly closed with minimal surgical trauma and time. No bridges are burned, and the appropriate secondary reconstruction can be carried out to achieve a more stable closure with improved esthetics.

Several helpful tips make skin grafting reliable and expeditious. High on the lateral thigh is the ideal donor site. Its scar is easily concealed with clothing. It is distant from the operative site on the scalp, permitting a two-team approach. A subcutaneous injection of 0.5%, 1:200,000 epinephrine subdermally, 10 minutes before harvesting, virtually eliminates donor-site bleeding. Donor sites are dressed with transparent dressing (Opsite) anchored with liquid adhesive (Mastisol) at the margins. Such dressings provide biologic protection of the raw wound and are remarkably comfortable for the patient. Opsite is removed in 5 to 7 days, and the donor site exposed to air. Topical antibiotic ointment is occasionally helpful for painful cracking or desiccation. Should cellulitis develop, silver sulfadiazine for 24 hours generally eliminates the problem.

Harvested grafts should be 0.01 to 0.014 inches in thickness. Meshing of such grafts, in a 1.5 to 1.0 ratio, has several advantages. There is a small donor defect: The perforations in the graft permit serous drainage and significantly increase the probability of "graft take." I find that topical mesh Silastic dressings with tie-over stents provide excellent protection and appear to be associated with a greater and more satisfactory take. When measuring the defect to determine the size of the graft, it is important that the vertical height of the wound margins be included. If not, the graft when anchored will tend to tent from the base of the wound. A combination of staples to quickly affix the graft followed by tie-over sutures (4–0 nylon) with a stent provides stable fixation of the graft at the margins. Defects in this size range are minimal to flap coverage.

The choice of flaps ranges from a single rotation flap with skin grafting of the donor site to multiple flaps as described by Orticochea (Fig. 2–4).[7, 8] There are three points to be made. First, flaps on the scalp are hardy and reliable if designed to include one of the axial blood vessels to its tip. Second, great care must be given when designing such flaps to prevent arbitrary destruction of an axial vessel or tissues, which would significantly compromise future treatment options. Third, release of the galea makes such flaps easily manipulated and extends their coverage. However, excess tension must be avoided. Generally, as a rule of thumb, if 4–0 nylon cannot tolerate tensile strength at the tip, tension is too great. The major advantage of flap closure for defects of this size is the ability to achieve a stable, esthetically satisfactory closure in a single surgical procedure. Disadvantages include that it is not a reasonable procedure in an acute, significantly contaminated wound. Patients with significant medical problems or life-threatening injuries are not good candidates. There is more residual scarring that may limit any future treatment options.

Calvarial bone is the first choice for replacement of bony defects. There is some increased risk in that the graft lies under the apex of the flaps. This is inherently a relatively ischemic area. Chances of infection are higher with the bone graft in such places. Certainly, if there is necrosis of a distal flap, the bone graft will be lost with a resultant difficult wound.

Secondary bone grafting is to be considered in these wounds. A second procedure through scar tissue (particularly over the dura), however, makes this a delicate procedure.

## Wounds Greater Than 20 cm² (Up to 60% of the Scalp)

Evolution of tissue expansion has been the single most important technologic achievement in managing wounds of

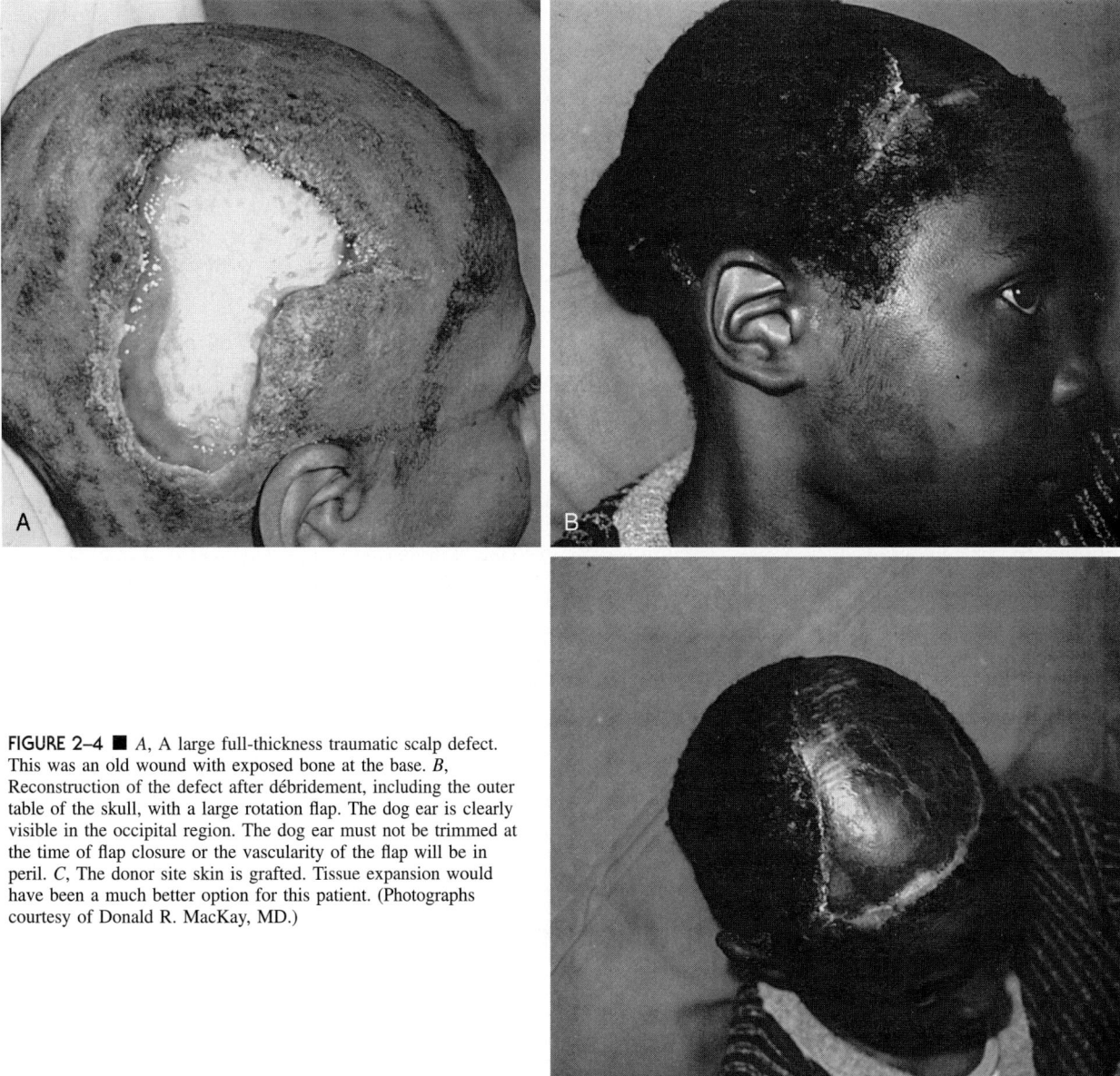

**FIGURE 2–4** ■ *A*, A large full-thickness traumatic scalp defect. This was an old wound with exposed bone at the base. *B*, Reconstruction of the defect after débridement, including the outer table of the skull, with a large rotation flap. The dog ear is clearly visible in the occipital region. The dog ear must not be trimmed at the time of flap closure or the vascularity of the flap will be in peril. *C*, The donor site skin is grafted. Tissue expansion would have been a much better option for this patient. (Photographs courtesy of Donald R. MacKay, MD.)

this size. It should not always be considered in acute settings but certainly is invaluable for secondary reconstruction. As discussed earlier, temporary coverage of such wounds can be achieved with skin grafting.

When conditions are appropriate, the initial defect can be closed with either rotation flaps or bipedicle flaps. The donor sites will require skin grafting. Fundamental principles of flap design and elevation still apply.

The esthetic result of such reconstruction is poor. The donor sites are relatively unstable wounds. Secondary reconstruction for an improved final result can be difficult. However, in selected patients who would not tolerate any extended surgical procedure (i.e., free-flap-staged procedure with tissue expansion), this may be the most appropriate treatment. Examples of such patients are those with significant debility or immunosuppression.

When there is a stable, closed wound with a substantial scalp defect, tissue expansion is an ideal choice (Fig. 2–5).[9–11] Detailed planning is essential. In general, more than one expander is required. The shape and the size of the expander are selected to give maximum expansion for the tissue available. As a rule, 20% of the increased surface area is lost with removal of the inflated expander. Galeal cross-hatching is to be avoided; evidence suggests that a significant percentage of the blood flow to the flap travels through the capsule of the expander.[12]

The expander should be placed at least 3 cm from the margin defect. For scalp reconstruction, the injection ports are best self-contained. Care must be taken to avoid the potential for extrusion. A slow, weekly rate of expansion may be necessary to prevent such extrusion. The expansion process takes between 2 and 6 months. It has been recommended that expanders not be used in children younger than 3 years when the calvarial sutures have not been closed. Lidocaine/prilocaine (Emla) cream, 1 hour prior to expansion, is suggested, particularly in children.

Bony replacement is generally undertaken as a secondary procedure with defects of this size. Stable soft tissue reconstruction should have been placed for a minimum of 1 year before reconstruction of the skull. Infection is of the greatest concern. The rate of infection has been shown to be significantly reduced in a wound that has been stable and infection-free for at least 1 year.[13, 14] Cranioplasty in frontal bone or areas of previous sinus infection are particularly treacherous.

Cranial bone grafts are the first choice. Iliac crest and split ribs are also options. Data suggest that membranous bone has a lower resorption rate.[15] The focus of cranioplasty is to restore protection to the brain and to improve esthetic appearance. In general, defects in the occipital and temporal areas do not require restoration because of their thick muscular coverage.

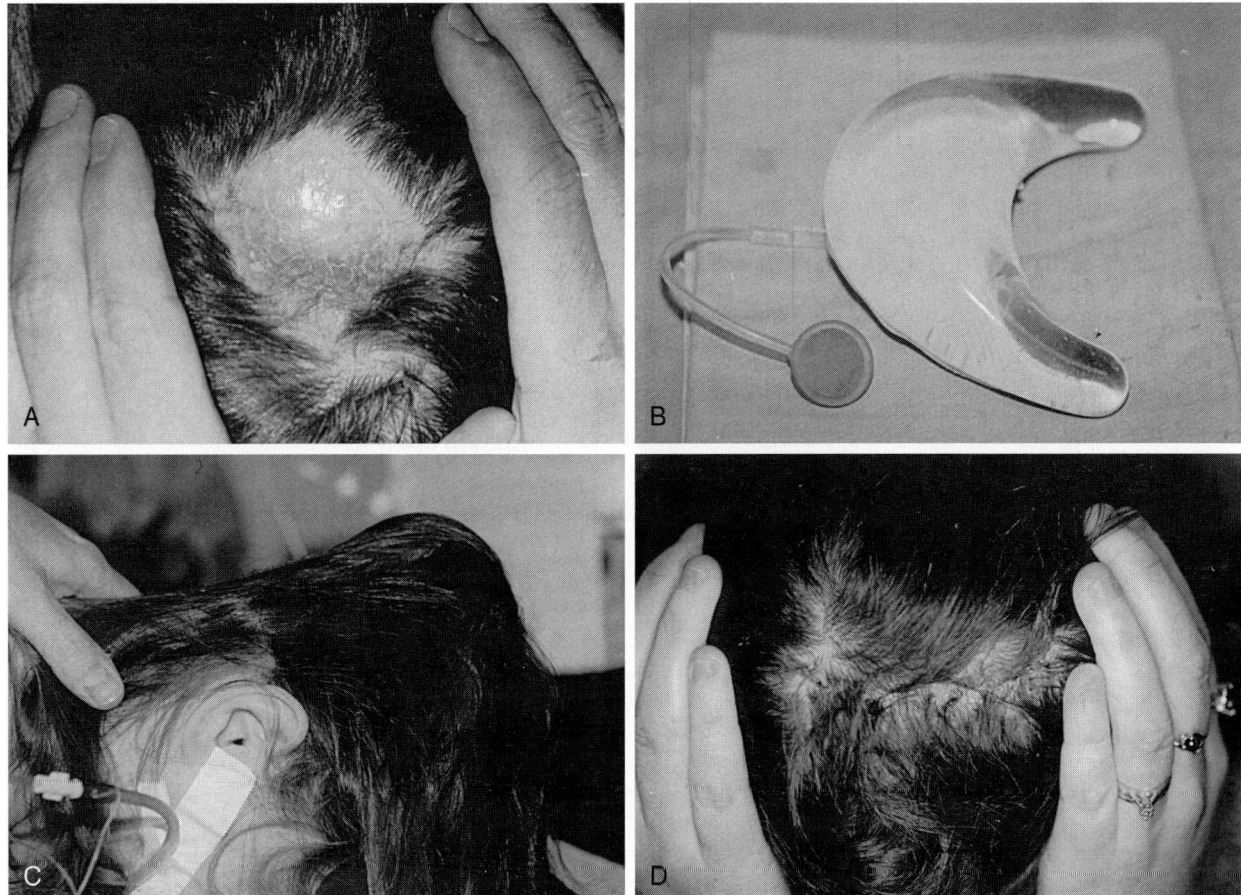

**FIGURE 2–5** ■ *A*, Scalp defect approximately 15 × 8 cm. *B*, "Croissant" tissue expander. *C*, Expander in place with a modified external inflation tube. *D*, The final result after removal of the expander and closure. (Photographs courtesy of Donald R. MacKay, MD.)

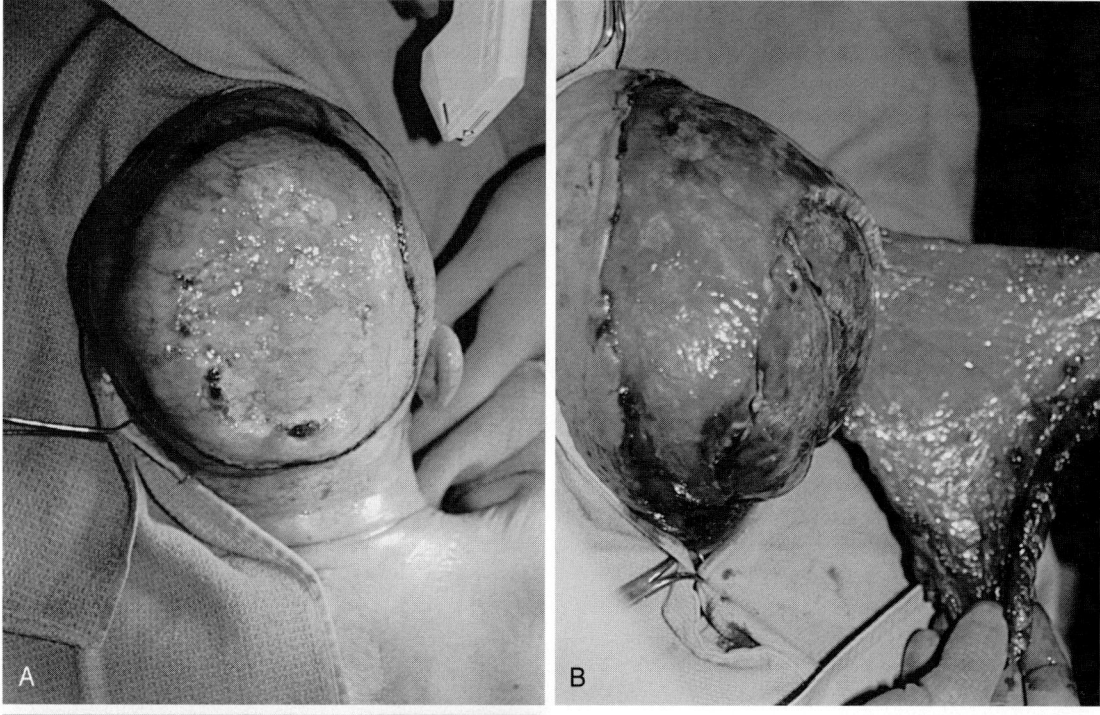

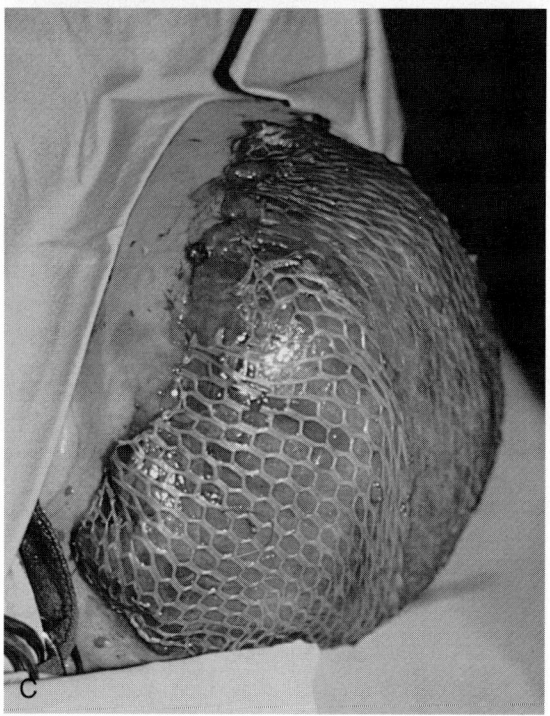

FIGURE 2–6 ■ *A,* A large basal cell carcinoma covering the posterior scalp. *B,* A large defect of the scalp and a smaller skull defect after resection of the tumor. A free latissimus dorsi muscle flap is used to cover the defect. *C,* The latissimus dorsi muscle flap is covered with a meshed split-thickness skin graft. (Photographs courtesy of Donald R. MacKay, MD.)

## Defects of 50% or Greater

Free tissue transfers have been the greatest technologic achievement for defects of this size. In 1972, McLean and Buncke reported successful coverage of a large scalp defect with free omentum.[16] Immediate, reliable coverage was achieved. The omentum readily accepted a split-thickness skin graft and conformed to the necessary contours of the defect. Multiple vessels are available for microanastomosis, as located throughout the face and cervical region (Fig. 2–6). Disadvantages were clearly the bulkiness of the free graft, limited esthetic function, and the necessity for an intra-abdominal surgical procedure.

The first successful replantation of a completely avulsed scalp was reported by Miller and associates in 1976.[17] This was the first time in history a problem that had both astonished and confounded surgeons, from 2000 BC up through the Industrial Revolution, was solved in a satisfactory, successful, and dramatic fashion (Fig. 2–7).

Despite these advancements, persistent osteomyelitis, patients who had no scalp to replant, and those who had undergone previous abdominal procedures remained a problem. Maxwell and colleagues reported the first successful use of latissimus dorsi myocutaneous flap in 1978.[18] Distinct advantages included a safe, reliable free flap with a predictable satisfactory pedicle, relative ease of harvesting with minimal donor site morbidity and deformity, and a flap that was relatively thin with excellent blood supply from the muscle to underlying tissues. This is a distinct advantage in wounds with a history of infection or osteomyelitis and in wounds compromised by multiple previous surgical procedures or radiation.

At this juncture, the latissimus dorsi muscle, either as a free muscle or myocutaneous free flap, is the ideal choice for reconstruction of these large defects. Other options include a free scapular flap or radial forearm flap. These provide for satisfactory coverage but they do lack muscle, which can provide increased blood supply to underlying bone and its protection. Radial forearm flaps have the additional disadvantage of leaving a substantial donor defect. Free temporalis fascia or free omentum with skin grafting is the second echelon of choice with free tissue transfer (Fig. 2–8).

## CONCLUSIONS

The treatment options available, coupled with their anatomic principles, advantages, and disadvantages for a variety of defects of the scalp have been presented. It is hoped that these will provide reliable guideline for reconstruction of defects of the scalp and skull, given their size.

Future technologic advances are expected. Such advances will include more appropriate materials for bone grafting. Ultimately, perhaps, xenografts will prove to be both esthetically pleasing and highly functional.

Future problems certainly exist as well. In our current milieu, cost concessions are a major concern, making it mandatory that the appropriate procedures be undertaken at the outset. The tolerance level for haphazard treatment programs and morbidity will be significantly reduced and penalized.

The emergence of VIRSA (vancomycin intermediate-resistant *Staphylococcus aureus*) presages greater difficulty in the management of patients with these defects. Minimization of surgical treatment and hospitalizations, coupled with reinforcement of fundamental principles of surgical asepsis, will be all the more important.

Technologically, what looms brightest in the future is the development of a satisfactory bone substitute. This is one that will have adequate biomechanical properties to absorb stress without increasing the risk of infection and one that can be procured easily from the shelf or pharmacy

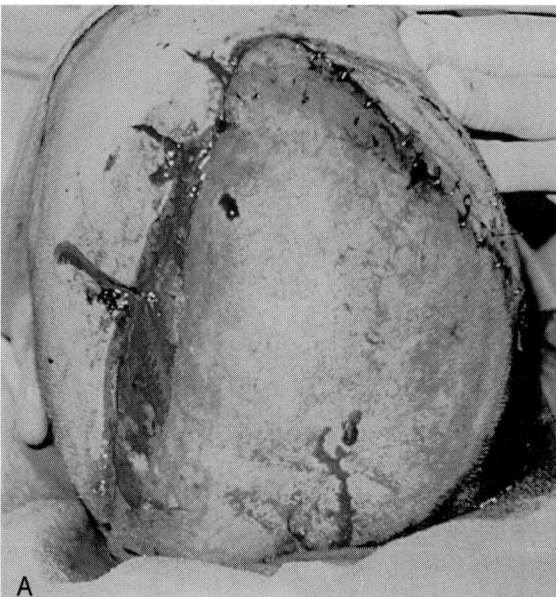
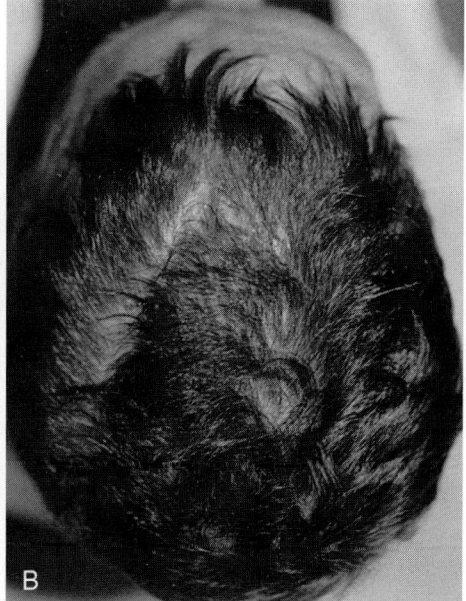

FIGURE 2–7 ■ *A*, Large traumatic scalp avulsion salvaged by carrying out an immediate replantation with microsurgical anastomosis of veins and arteries. *B*, Late result of replanted scalp. (Photographs courtesy of Donald R. MacKay, MD.)

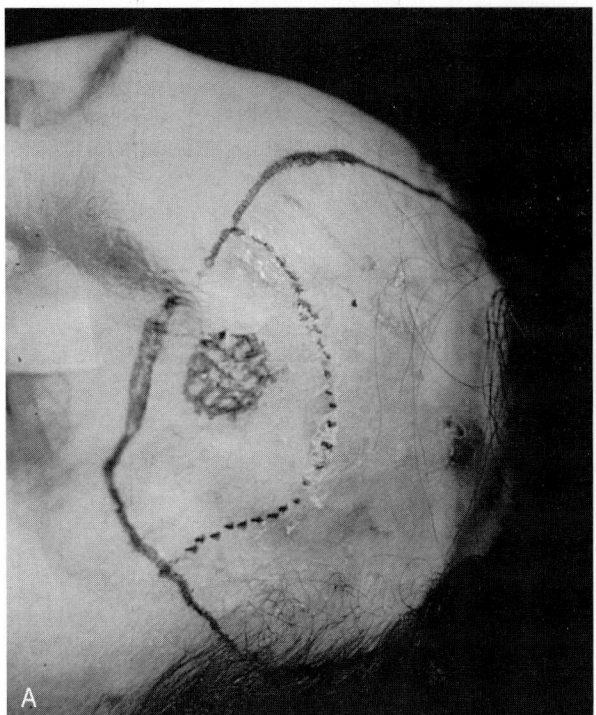

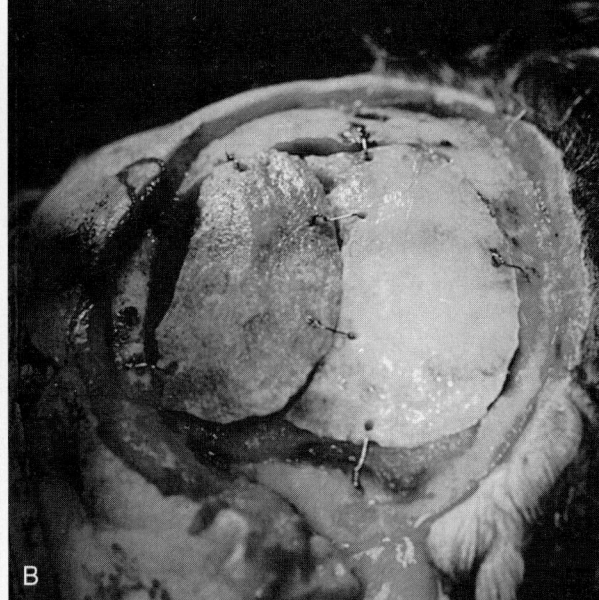

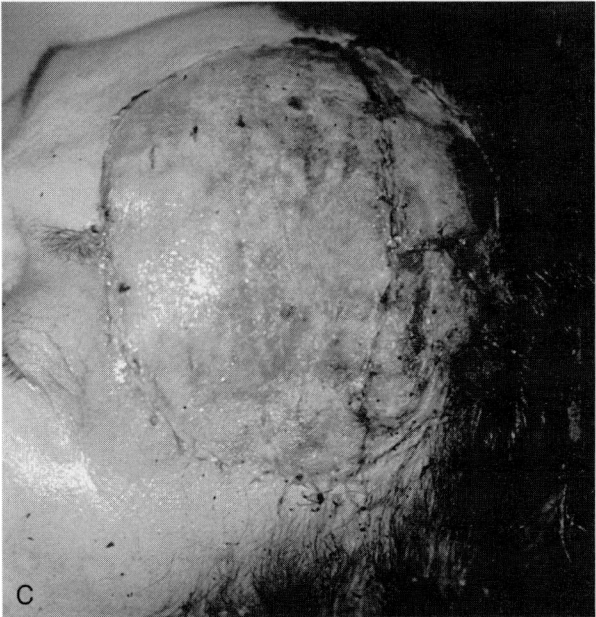

FIGURE 2–8   ■   *A*, Recurrent basal cell carcinoma of the scalp involving the underlying skull. Outline of the resection marked on the scalp. *B*, Large full-thickness defect of the scalp and skull following invasive basal cell carcinoma resection. The bone defect is reconstructed with a split calvarium. The split donor bone and graft are seen wired in place. Microplates and screws are a preferable fixation system currently. *C*, A soft tissue defect covered with a free temporoparietal flap and a skin graft. (Photographs courtesy of Donald R. MacKay, MD.)

in the hospital and used immediately. Certainly, with the development of such a bone substitute, donor-site morbidity will drop to zero. The ideal bone substitute will ultimately be integrated and resorbed into the skeletal structure such that it leaves no detectable sequelae. Current work with hydroxyapatite is promising, and there should be development in this area in the near future.

The range of available reconstructive options and the defects with which they can be used have been outlined. There should be no scalping injury, of any size or complexity, that presents today that cannot be repaired by adhering to the principles outlined in this chapter.

## REFERENCES

1. Dieck VA: Archaologische belege fur den brauch des skalpierens in Europa. Neue Ausgrabungen und Forschungen in Niedersachsen 4:359, 1969.
2. McGrath MH: Scalping: The savage and the surgeon. Clin Plast Surg 10:679, 1983.
3. Abbe R: Thiersch's method of skin grafting a great step in surgical progress. Postgrad Med 7:295, 1892.
4. Bartlett SC: Removal of the entire scalp: Wound healed by skin grafting. Am J Med Sci 64:573, 1872.
5. McCarthy J, Zide B: The spectrum of bone grafting: Introduction of the vascularized calvarial bone flap. Plast Reconstr Surg 74:10, 1984.
6. Tessier P: Autogenous bone grafts taken from the calvaria for facial and cranial applications. Clin Plast Surg 9:531, 1982.
7. Orticochea M: Four-flap scalp reconstruction technique. Br J Plast Surg 20:159, 1967.
8. Orticochea M: New three-flap scalp reconstruction technique. Br J Plast Surg 24:184, 1971.
9. Argenta LC, Watanabe MJ, Grabb WC: The use of tissue expansion in head and neck reconstruction. Ann Plast Surg 11:31, 1983.
10. Manders EK, et al: Skin expansion to eliminate large scalp defects. Ann Plast Surg 12:305, 1984.
11. Argenta LC: Control tissue expansion in reconstructive surgery. Br J Plast Surg 37:520, 1984.
12. Sasaki CH, Pang GY: Pathophysiology of skin flaps raised on expanded skin. Plast Reconstr Surg 74:59, 1984.

13. Manson PN, Crawley WH, Hoopes JE: Frontal cranioplasty: Risk factors and choice of cranial vault reconstruction material. Plast Reconstr Surg 77:888–900, 1986.
14. Rish BL, Dillon JD, Meirowsky AM, et al: Cranioplasty: A review of 1030 cases of penetrating head injury. Neurosurgery 4:381–386, 1979.
15. Zins JE, Whitaker LA: Membranes versus endochondral bone implications for craniofacial reconstruction. Plast Reconstr Surg 72:778, 1983.
16. McLean DH, Buncke HJ Jr: Autotransplant of omentum to a large scalp defect with microsurgical revascularization. Plast Reconstr Surg 49:268, 1972.
17. Miller GDH, Anstec EJ, Snell JA: Successful replantation of an avulsed scalp by microvascular anastomoses. Plast Reconstr Surg 58:133, 1976.
18. Maxwell GP, Stuber K, Hoopes JE: A free latissimus dorsi myocutaneous flap. Plast Reconstr Surg 62:462, 1978.

# Cranioplasty: Indications, Techniques, and Results

■ ROBERT D. FOSTER, OLEH M. ANTONYSHYN, CHEN LEE, MARTIN HOLLAND, and MAHMOOD FAZL

Historically, the reconstruction of cranial vault defects is considered by some to be the earliest operation performed on humans, dating back to prehistoric times. The Inca culture, around 3000 BC, is credited with using gold plates to cover cranial defects resulting from trauma or to ward off spirits.[1] Since that time, various materials have been advocated for coverage including autogenous bone, methyl methacrylate, and titanium mesh.[2–4] Although the choice of implant material remains somewhat controversial, the reconstructive goals, to protect the underlying brain and restore the preinjury appearance, have remained essentially the same.

## ETIOLOGY OF CRANIAL DEFECTS

The majority of cranial defects are acquired, most commonly as a result of traumatic injury. Young adults and children are affected most frequently, either from depressed skull fractures or penetrating injuries. Other causes include ablative tumor resections, bone flap infections, and decompression craniectomies.

Neoplasms invading the skull can be benign or malignant. Benign tumors requiring cranioplasty include pediatric eosinophilic granulomas, osteomas, fibrous bone dysplasia of the anterior skull, and juvenile nasopharyngeal angiofibromas. Malignant tumors include carcinomas of the ethmoid and frontal sinuses extending to bone, sarcomas or meningiomas, and less commonly metastases from melanomas or hypernephromas, which can result in significant surgical defects.

Congenital defects involve mainly dysraphic disorders including encephaloceles, meningoencephaloceles, large parietal foramina, aplasia cutis congenita, cranium bifidum, and sphenoid wing defects. In addition, defects following the surgical correction of craniosynostosis may persist subsequently requiring cranioplasty.[5]

## INDICATIONS

In their landmark review, in 1939, of more than 1300 cranioplasties, Grant and Norcross[6] outlined indications for

cranioplasty that remained standards of care for many years: (1) severe headache and other symptoms of the syndrome of the trephined, such as dizziness, vague discomfort at the site of the defect, and intolerance to vibration; (2) epilepsy, when assumed to be the result of the defect; (3) those cases in which there is danger of trauma at the site of the defect; (4) cases that have an unsightly defect; and (5) defects that pulsate unduly or that are painful. Although some authors have reported good results following cranioplasty for the syndrome of the trephined[7] (dizziness, nausea, headache, motion intolerance), most of these complaints are not reliably altered by cranioplasty.

The relationship between epilepsy and cranial defects and their repair remains controversial. In 1939, Grant reported clinical improvement in 18 of 27 patients with cranial defects and epilepsy who underwent cranioplasty.[6] This was followed up by Weiford and Gardner's study in 1949 in which 6 of 10 patients were seizure-free for a period of 10 to 48 months following cranioplasty.[8] Three of those six patients, however, also had cortical excisions during the cranioplasty. Since then, multiple studies have found no beneficial effect of cranioplasty for post-traumatic seizures. Currently, cranioplasty cannot be recommended to reliably treat seizures. The accepted major indications for cranioplasty remain the protection of the cerebrum and improved cosmetic appearance.

Because most cranial defects are associated with dirty or contaminated wounds, cranioplasty is rarely performed in the acute setting of the injury. In such a case, bone fragments should be removed, the wound débrided, and the intracranial pathology treated before any reconstruction is attempted. Following trauma, extensive cerebral edema and increased intracranial pressure would also be contraindications to any definitive coverage. Therefore, typically cranioplasty is not attempted before several months after the initial injury.

## TECHNIQUES

Successful clinical outcome following cranioplasty depends on the selection of an implant material to reproduce the rigid framework of the skull and preparation of the recipient bed to optimize implant stability and vascularity. The choice of implant material has been controversial.[9] Alloplastic materials have the advantage of abundant supply without any donor site morbidity and as a result have been popular in uncomplicated primary cranioplasties.[10, 11] Alloplasts, however, remain inert, avascular foreign bodies and, therefore, are contraindicated in problem recipient beds where external erosion of the soft tissues or internal paranasal sinus exposure may lead eventually to implant infection or exposure. Furthermore, late exposure and failure of alloplastic cranioplasties have been reported repeatedly in the literature.[12, 13] For these purposes, autogenous bone reconstruction has been advocated because of its ability to become incorporated as living tissue with reparative capabilities. Skull bone of appropriate contour is available in abundant supply directly within the operation site and, therefore, donor site morbidity and scarring are minimal.[14, 15]

A cranioplasty failure is manifested by a poor esthetic result (Fig. 3–1) and inadequate cerebral protection (Fig. 3–2). Implant infection is the most common cause (Fig. 3–3). The risk can be minimized by securing a well-vascularized soft tissue cover, sealing any internal paranasal sinus communication (see Fig. 3–2), using principles of rigid internal fixation to stabilize grafts, and deferring the definitive cranial reconstruction in a previously infected bed until the recipient wound has matured, confirming clearance of all bacterial foci.

Patients with a history of infection causing failure of a previous cranial reconstruction have up to an 8-fold increased risk of reinfection with subsequent cranioplasties.[16] When the surgery is delayed, however, longer than one year, the incidence of infection approaches that of routine cranioplasty. In our experience, definitive autogenous bone cranioplasty should not be attempted before a minimum of 6 months following removal of a failed infected alloplast or bone flap (see Fig. 3–3). Preoperative computed tomography (CT) scans with three-dimensional reconstructions can be useful in determining the integrity of the paranasal sinuses and their proximity to the defect as well as visualizing the location, shape, and size of the cranial defect (Fig. 3–4).

Prior to definitive cranial vault reconstruction, it is essential to verify that adequate scalp and skin cover are available to resurface the expanded reconstructed skull. A deficiency in the external coverage is anticipated when the measured sagittal length of skin overlying the defect is less than that of the external convex surface of the planned cranial reconstruction (Fig. 3–5). If insufficient tissue exists, then surgical planning must include a consideration of techniques to provide increased external soft tissue. Tissue expansion is helpful for this purpose. In cases with extreme soft tissue deficiencies, microsurgical-free tissue transfer should be considered[17] (Fig. 3–6).

Dissection of the cranial defect is commonly performed in conjunction with a neurosurgical team. Extradural exposure of the defect is attempted in all cases. Pericranial flaps are routinely elevated during exposure when paranasal sinus exposure is anticipated. Exposed sinuses are treated by stripping the mucosal lining followed by bone graft (iliac crest cancellous) obliteration[18] (see Fig. 3–2D). Sealing the sinus with either the pericranial flap or a galeal frontalis flap further augments the barrier. The bony cranial defect margins are débrided until healthy margins of bleeding bone are identified.

## AUTOGENOUS BONE

**Split Skull Cranioplasty.** To optimize the fit and contour match of the donor bone to the recipient site, a malleable lead template is fashioned from the cranial defect. The template is then transposed to a site of healthy normal skull. The selection site for the donor bone is based on availability and desired contour match. With extremely large defects, a better recipient site match can be achieved by dividing the lead template into two halves to isolate separate but well-matched smaller skull donor sites (Fig. 3–7).

Several principles are strictly adhered to when choosing a skull donor site. In most cases, the parietal regions are the preferred donor sites, providing a reasonable match for the contour of the frontal bone. Under no circumstance is bone harvested from the frontal region, where iatrogenically produced contour irregularities would be readily observed. A 4-cm sagittal bar is maintained intact to protect the sagittal sinus and provide a stable skeletal reference for subsequent skull donor site reconstruction. A similar bone bar is maintained over the coronal suture, providing a stable index to normal skull width and height (Fig. 3–8).

Following delineation of an appropriate donor site, a

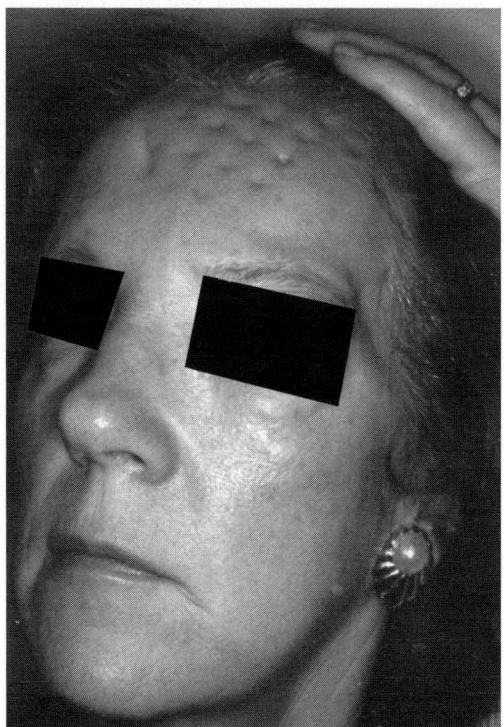

FIGURE 3–1 ■ Poor esthetic result from perforated metal plate cranioplasty. There is lack of recognition of the normal skull shape and the presence of a temporal hollow. The perforations of the metallic implant are accentuated by the contracted capsule with adhesions between scalp and dura through the implant perforations.

*Text continued on page 35*

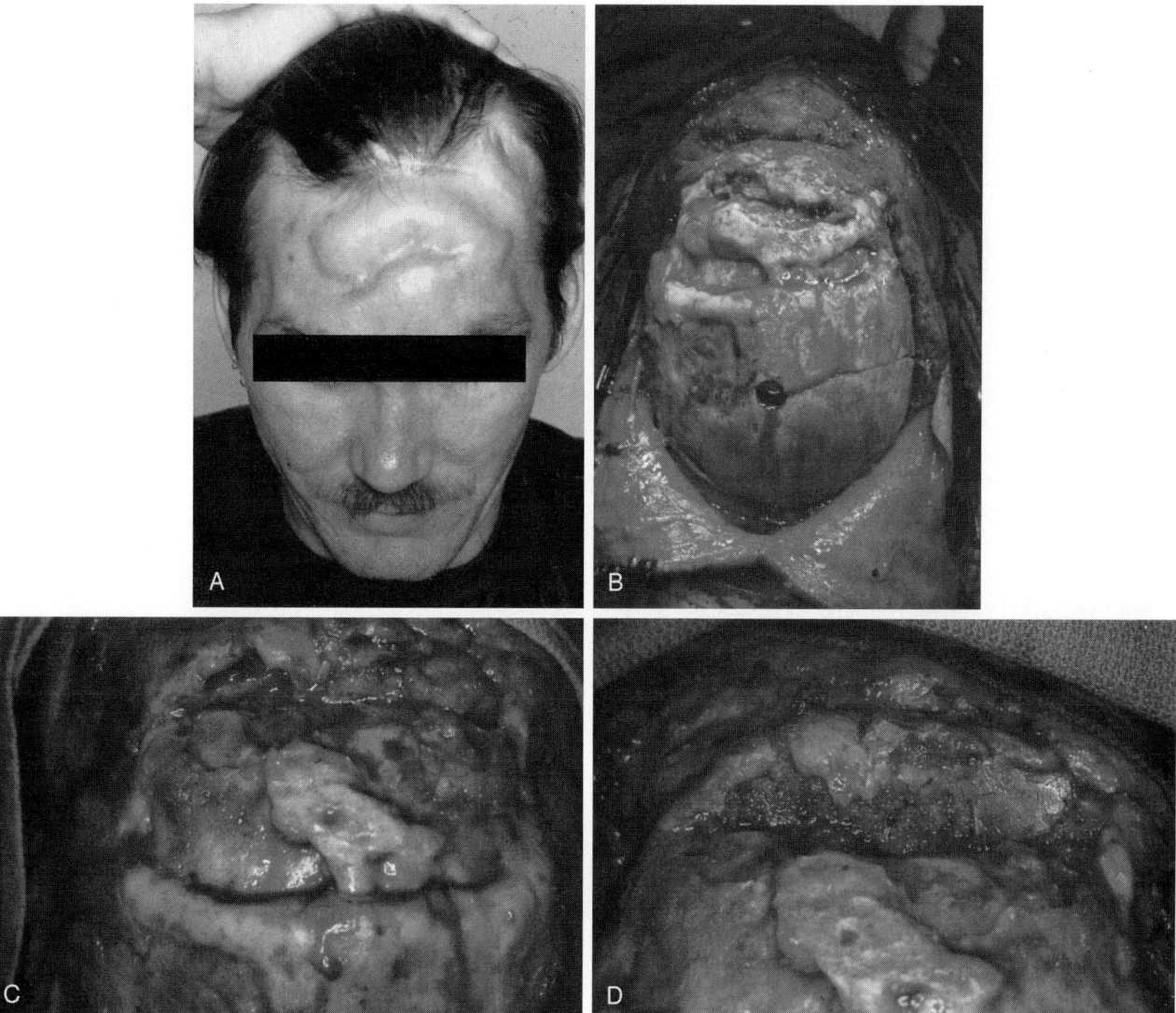

**FIGURE 3–2** ■ *A,* Significant bone resorption with loss of cranial protection following open reduction internal fixation of a frontal bone fracture. *B,* Intraoperative views demonstrate full thickness defects of the frontal bone. *C,* Close-up views of the frontal sinus demonstrate cranial defects to be in communication with the frontal sinus. *D,* Operative treatment rendered included frontal sinus obliteration with iliac crest cancellous bone.

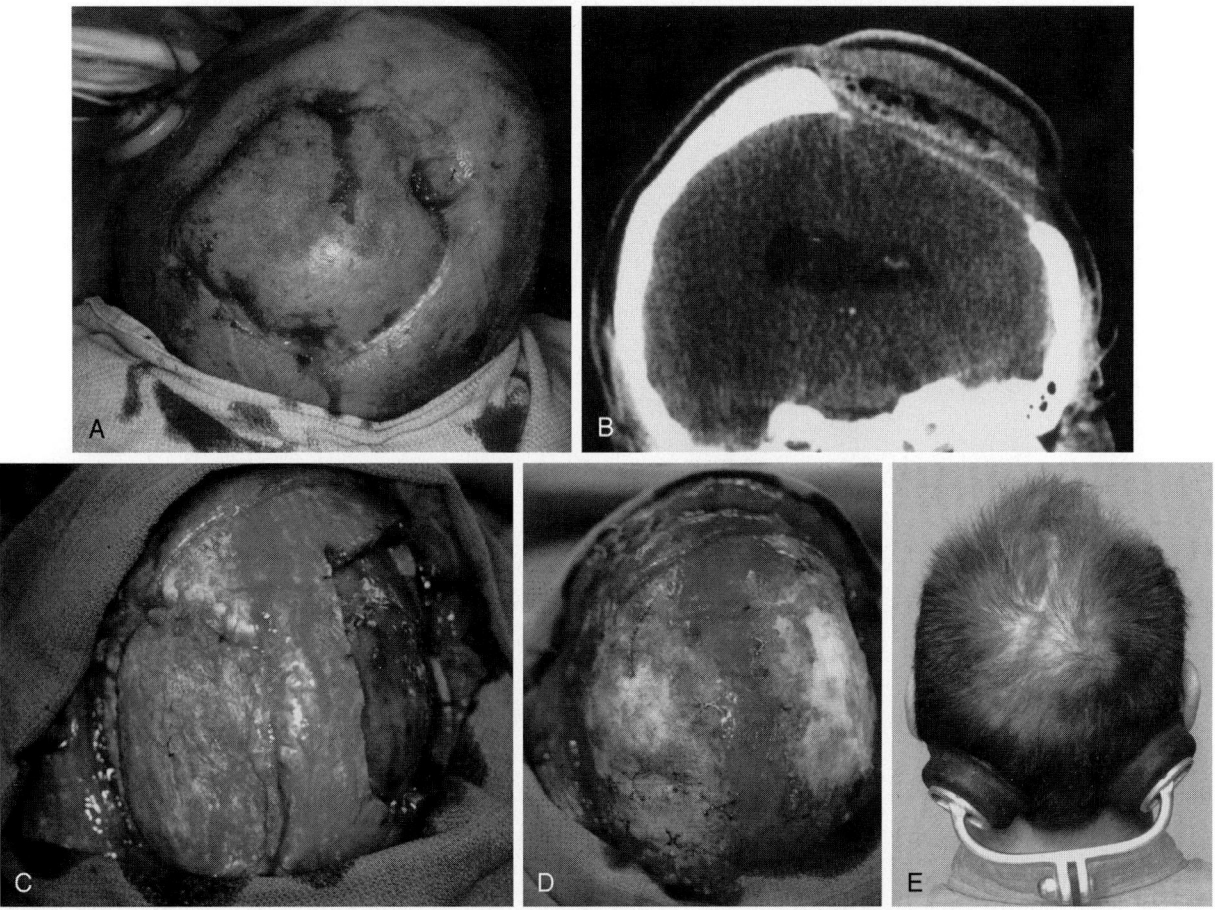

**FIGURE 3–3  ■** *A,* Infected and exposed acrylic cranioplasty. *B,* Computed tomography (CT) scans infected space deep to the acrylic implant. *C,* The infected acrylic implant was removed, and the definitive reconstruction was deferred for 6 months to permit maturation of the wound. The intraoperative view demonstrates the 6-month-old left parietal cranial defect formally being reconstructed with split skull bone harvested from the contralateral normal skull. *D,* Autogenous reconstruction was rigidly fixated with micro/mini titanium plates and screws. *E,* The split skull cranioplasty demonstrated excellent restoration of the cranial shape.

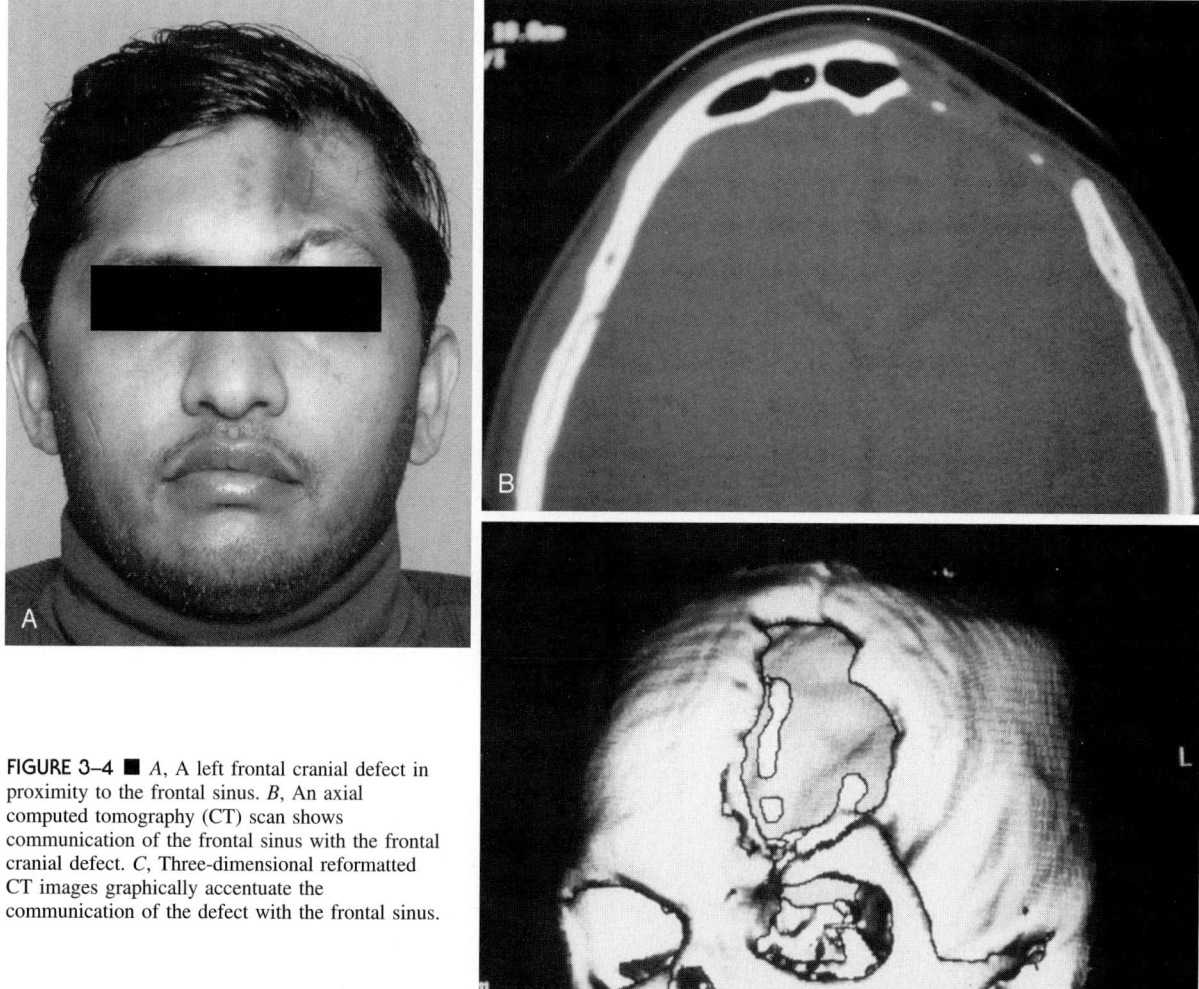

FIGURE 3–4 ■ *A*, A left frontal cranial defect in proximity to the frontal sinus. *B*, An axial computed tomography (CT) scan shows communication of the frontal sinus with the frontal cranial defect. *C*, Three-dimensional reformatted CT images graphically accentuate the communication of the defect with the frontal sinus.

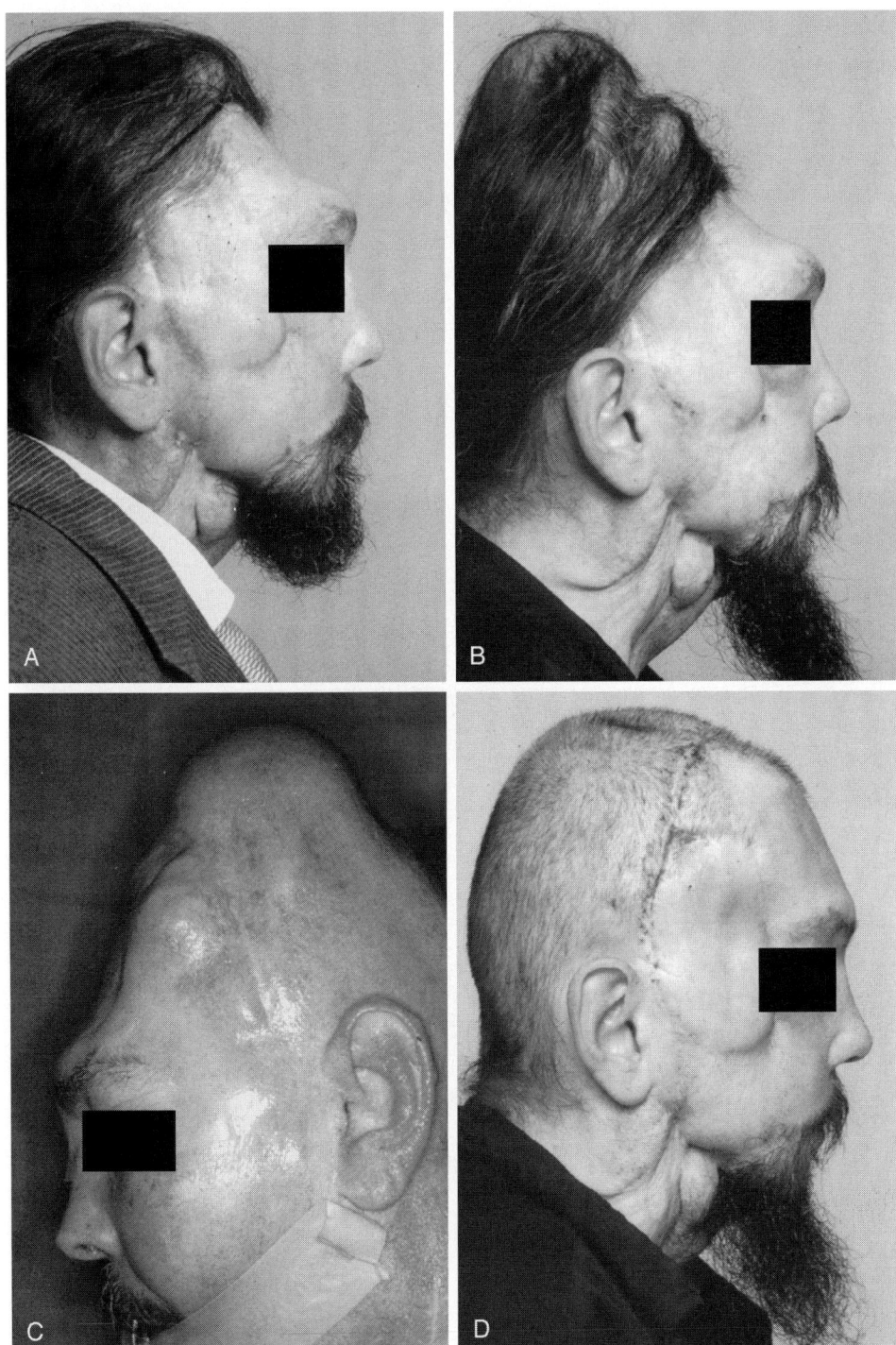

**FIGURE 3–5** ■ *A,* A preoperative lateral view demonstrates insufficient soft tissue in the sagittal plane to externally resurface a cranioplasty. *B* and *C,* Tissue expansion has increased the volume of tissue in the sagittal plane. *D,* The split skull cranioplasty was successfully covered with tissue-expanded scalp.

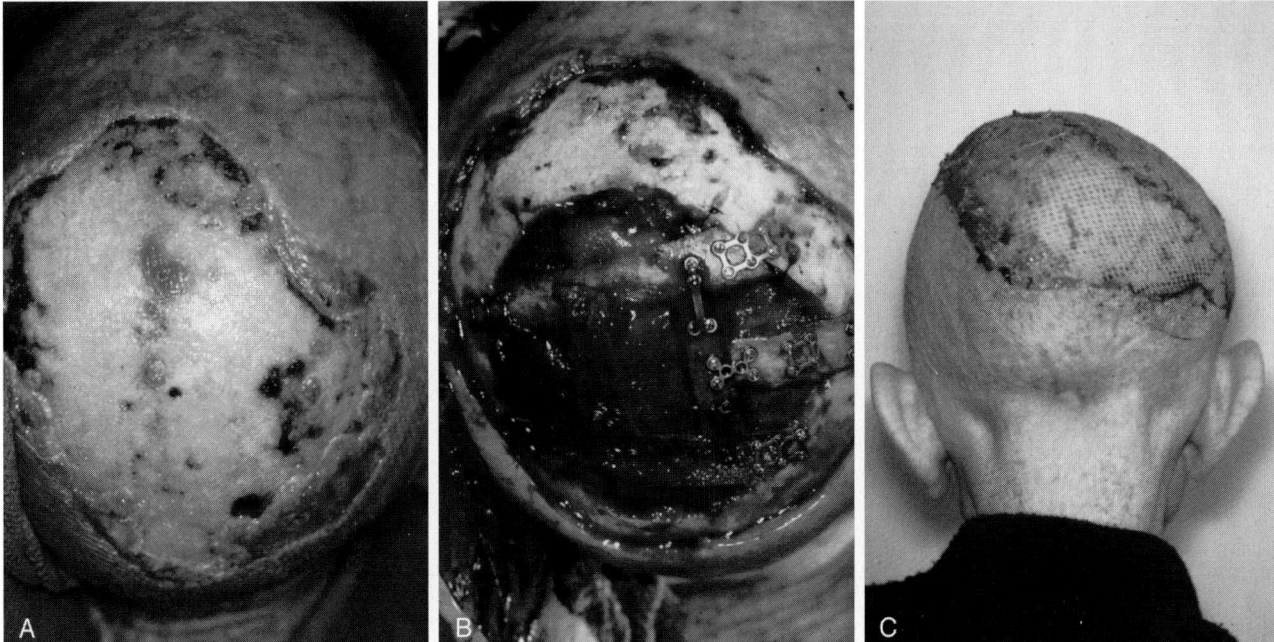

**FIGURE 3–6** ■ *A*, This 80-year-old man suffered from squamous cell carcinoma of the scalp and skull following teenage radiation for tinea capitis. Adequate treatment demands tumor ablation, reconstruction of the resected cranium, and soft tissue coverage. *B*, The skull was thin with no diploë, precluding its use for cranioplasty. Thus, a split rib was used to build a structural framework. *C*, Soft tissue coverage was achieved with a latissimus dorsi muscle microsurgical-free transfer and split-thickness skin grafts.

full-thickness bone flap is harvested. The skull bone is then split along the diploic interface between the inner and outer tables using a water-cooled reciprocating saw and fine osteotomes. The continuity of the skull donor site is restored by replacing the inner table while the outer table is used to reconstruct the cranial defect.

Although the lead templates allow reasonable contour approximation, there are still minor mismatches. The contour mismatches are easily corrected by a technique of controlled bending of the cranial bone.[19] Micro- or mini-fixation plates are first applied to the site to be contoured. Bone cuts are then made perpendicular to the plate to allow unopposed bending of the plate at the site of the osteotomies (see Fig. 3–8*D*). Once the donor bone is properly contoured, the cranioplasty is completed by rigidly fixating the bone grafts to the recipient site with titanium micro- or miniplates (see Fig. 3–8).

In addition to membranous (calvarial) bone grafts, endochondral bone can be used in the form of rib or iliac bone grafts. Calvarial bone is still preferred because of decreased donor site morbidity and the membranous bone of the skull withstands resorption better than rib or iliac bone. Studies in rabbits and monkeys show that endochondral bone harvested from rib or ileum resorbs 3- to 4-fold more rapidly than calvarial bone grafts.[20] If rib is chosen, the entire rib can be resected from the transverse process to the costochondral junction by subperiosteal dissection. With the periosteum intact, the rib will regenerate; this process usually takes several months. The rib can then be split, providing a graft of cortical bone on one side and cancellous bone on the other[21, 22] (see Fig. 3–6). Subperiosteal removal of two adjacent ribs or three or more alternate ribs can be performed without any pulmonary compromise. Rib grafts, though, can lead to significant contour deformities

because of the shape of the bone. In fact, Korlof and coworkers found that cranioplasty with split-thickness rib grafts produced an uneven skull surface contour in 50% of their patients.[23] Stabilization of the rib segments can also be a problem, and the hardware necessary for fixation can often be palpated through the skin.[24]

Iliac crest can provide a significant amount of bone for grafting.[25] Pieces as large as 10 to 20 cm² can be harvested in adults. As with rib grafts, the ileum can be split to provide increased bone coverage. Disadvantages include marked postoperative pain, use of a second operative site, and differences in contour between the cranial vault and iliac graft.

## ALLOPLASTIC GRAFTS

In the modern era of cranial vault reconstruction, the initial metals used, such as tantalum,[26] posed problems with thermoconductivity and were radiopaque, heavy, and expensive. Currently, many surgeons favor acrylic (methyl methacrylate) (Fig. 3–9) or metal (titanium) (Fig. 3–10), which provides radiolucency, cosmesis, and strength in addition to being relatively inexpensive. More recently, bioresorbable bone substitutes (hydroxyapatite paste) have been introduced into clinical practice (Fig. 3–11).

**Methyl Methacrylate.** Methyl methacrylate is inert, causing minimal tissue reaction, adhering tightly to bone, and is not thermoconductive. It does not create paramagnetic artifacts on magnetic resonance imaging (MRI), and on CT scans it is hyperdense, creating only a minor amount of scatter. Methyl methacrylate is prepared intraoperatively by

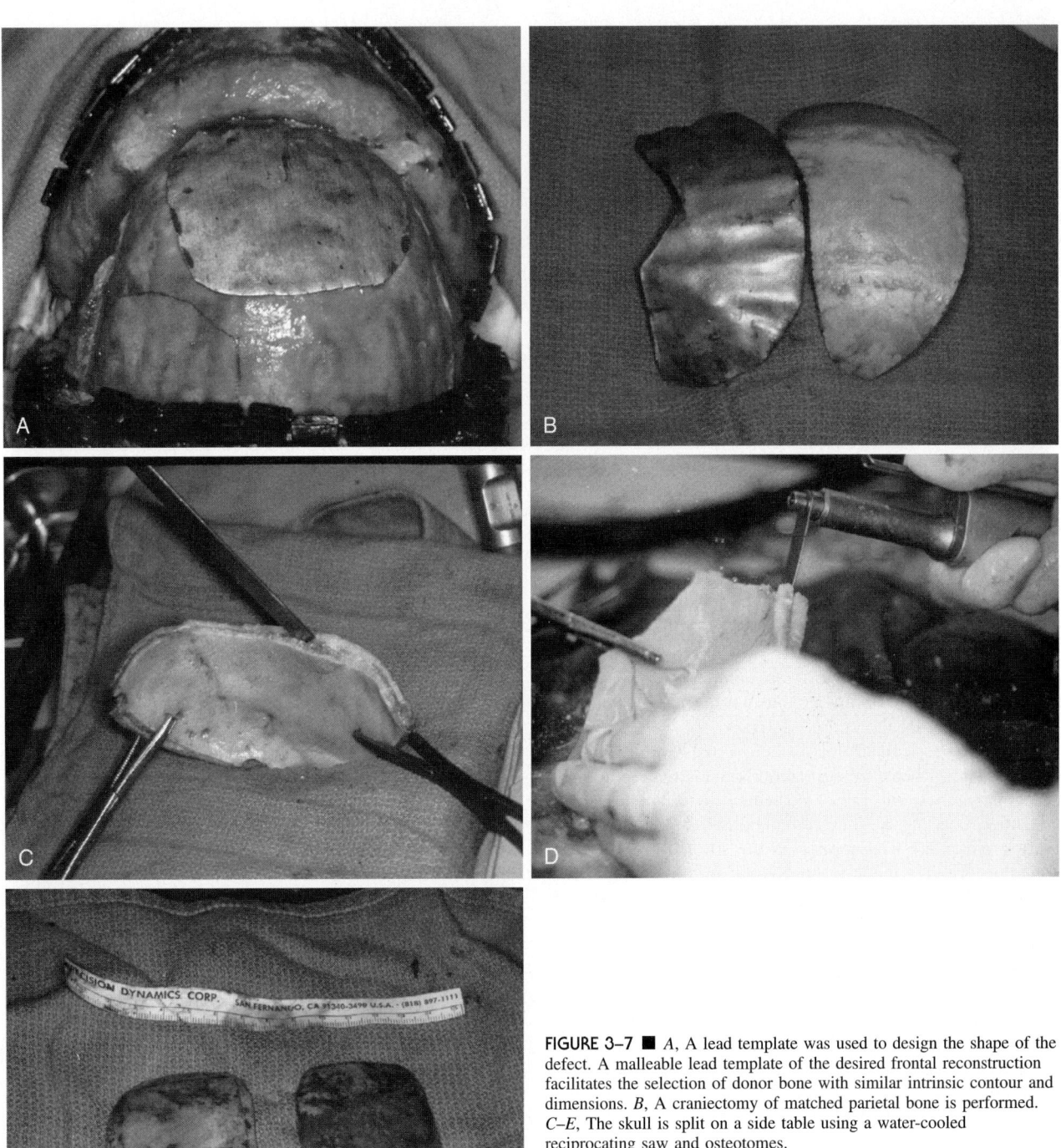

**FIGURE 3–7** ■ *A*, A lead template was used to design the shape of the defect. A malleable lead template of the desired frontal reconstruction facilitates the selection of donor bone with similar intrinsic contour and dimensions. *B*, A craniectomy of matched parietal bone is performed. *C–E*, The skull is split on a side table using a water-cooled reciprocating saw and osteotomes.

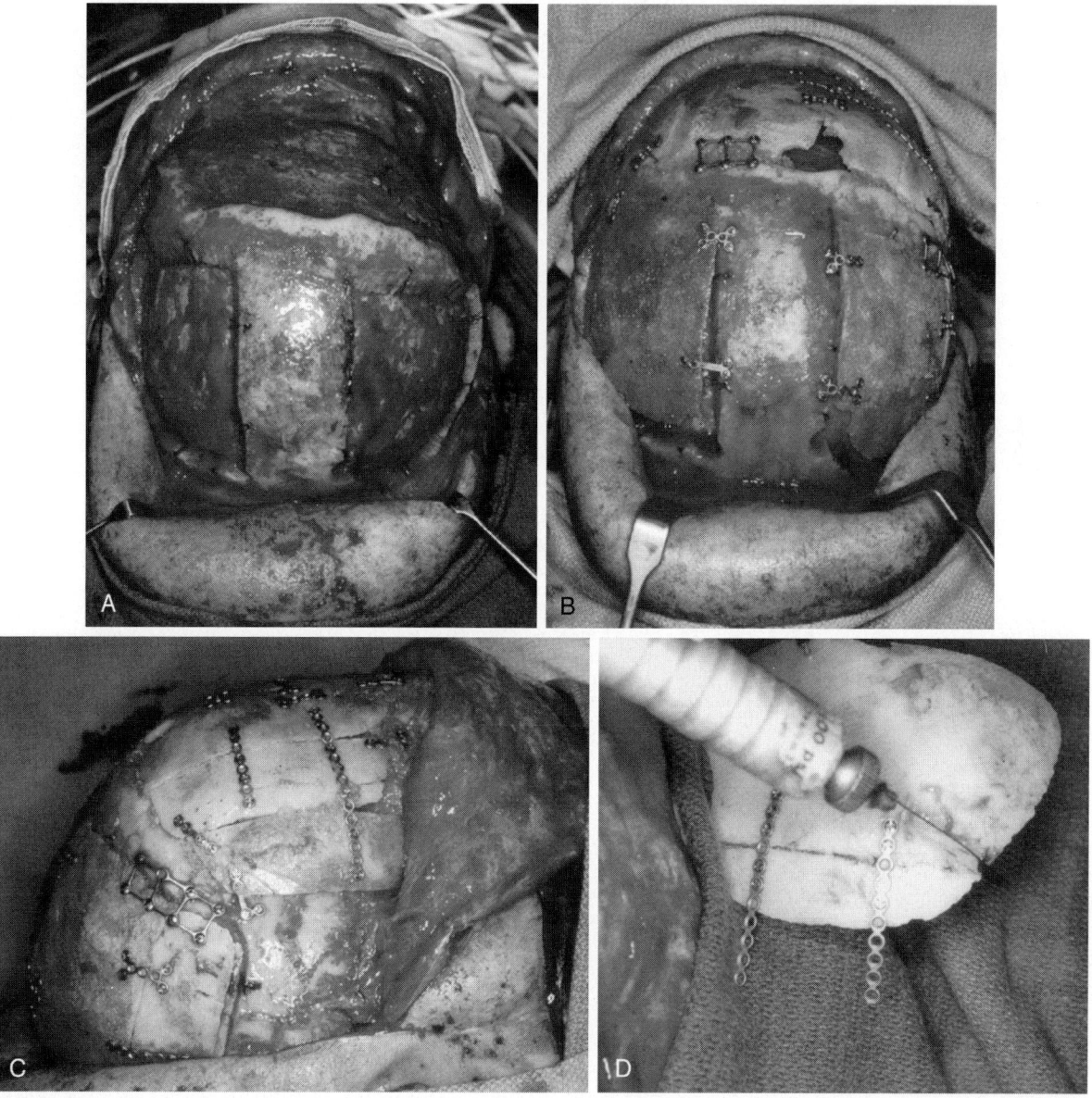

**FIGURE 3–8** ■ *A*, The transverse and sagittal planes are preserved as means of protecting the sagittal sinus in order to provide a stable point for fixation and to be a stable skeletal reference for the reconstruction. *B*, The large frontal defect is reconstructed with split skull harvested from bilateral parietal regions. *C*, The lateral operative view demonstrates the restoration of anatomic contours to the forehead. *D*, Minor adjustments to bone contour are made by "controlled bending" of the bone.

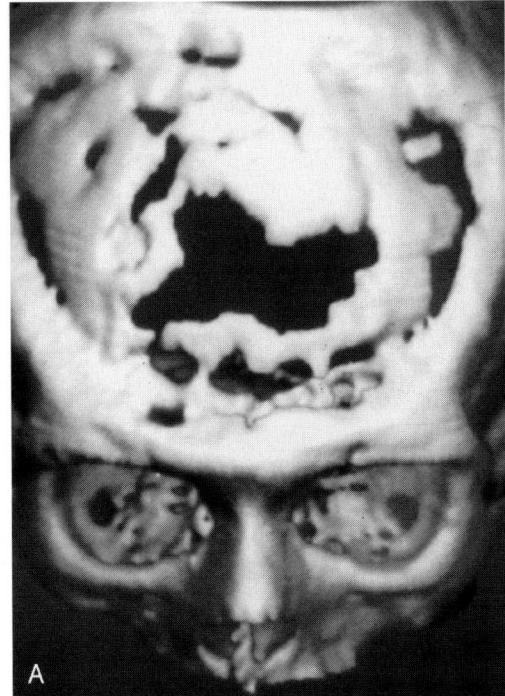

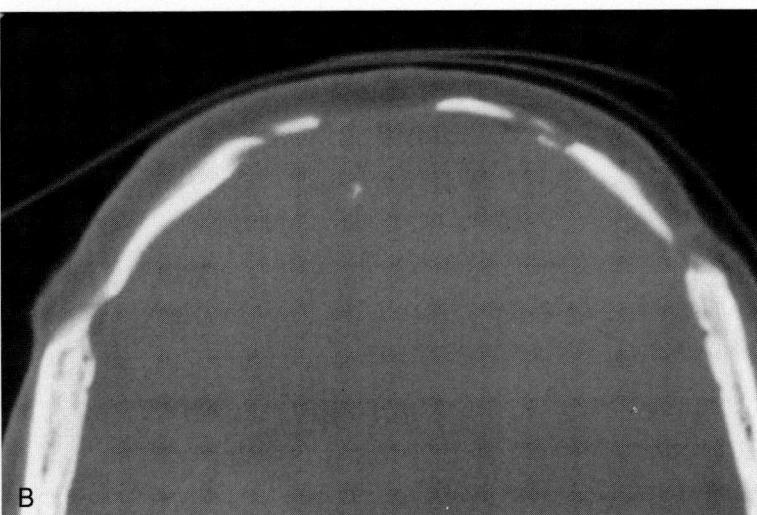

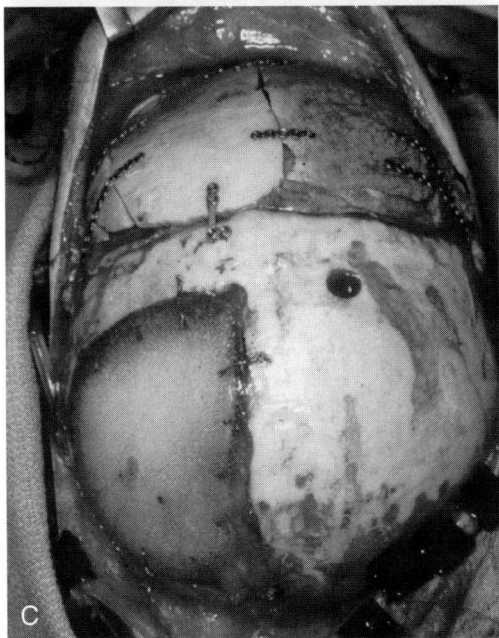

FIGURE 3–9 ■ *A* and *B*, A large frontal defect with dural calcifications communicates with the frontal sinus on three-dimensional and axial computed tomography (CT) scans. *C*, Reconstruction of the frontal region was achieved using split skull harvested from the left parietal bone. Intraoperatively, this patient became medically unstable. To reduce the physiologic stress and shorten the operative time, the donor parietal defect was reconstructed with methyl methacrylate. Intraoperative view with methyl methacrylate left parietal cranioplasty. A standard split skull frontal reconstruction was performed.

a polymerization process, mixing a powder polymer with a liquid monomer in a 2:1 ratio. The polymerization process is an exothermic reaction that reaches temperatures in excess of 1000°C. The material, once mixed, is placed in a plastic bag to facilitate the molding of the doughy substance precisely to the defect while simultaneously irrigating with copious amounts of saline to mitigate the local effects of the rise in temperature. It is important to thoroughly blend in the monomer, because it has been associated with cardiovascular collapse when injected into the marrow cavity of long bones in orthopedic procedures.[27] The polymer hardens in approximately 20 minutes, while the polymerization continues for several days. Final, subtle

contouring can be achieved with the use of a sharp polishing bur (see Fig. 3–9C).

**Titanium.** Titanium was first developed commercially in 1946 and is currently available as an alloy with aluminum, which stabilizes and strengthens it. It is corrosive resistant and light, yet twice as strong with double the fatigue resistance as stainless steel, and highly biocompatible. It possesses a thermal expansion comparable to bone; it is also well tolerated by soft tissue and bone and has minimal fibrous encapsulation.[28] Titanium is relatively inexpensive and does not cause hypersensitivity reactions. It is fairly radiolucent, although less so than acrylics.[10] In the past, its

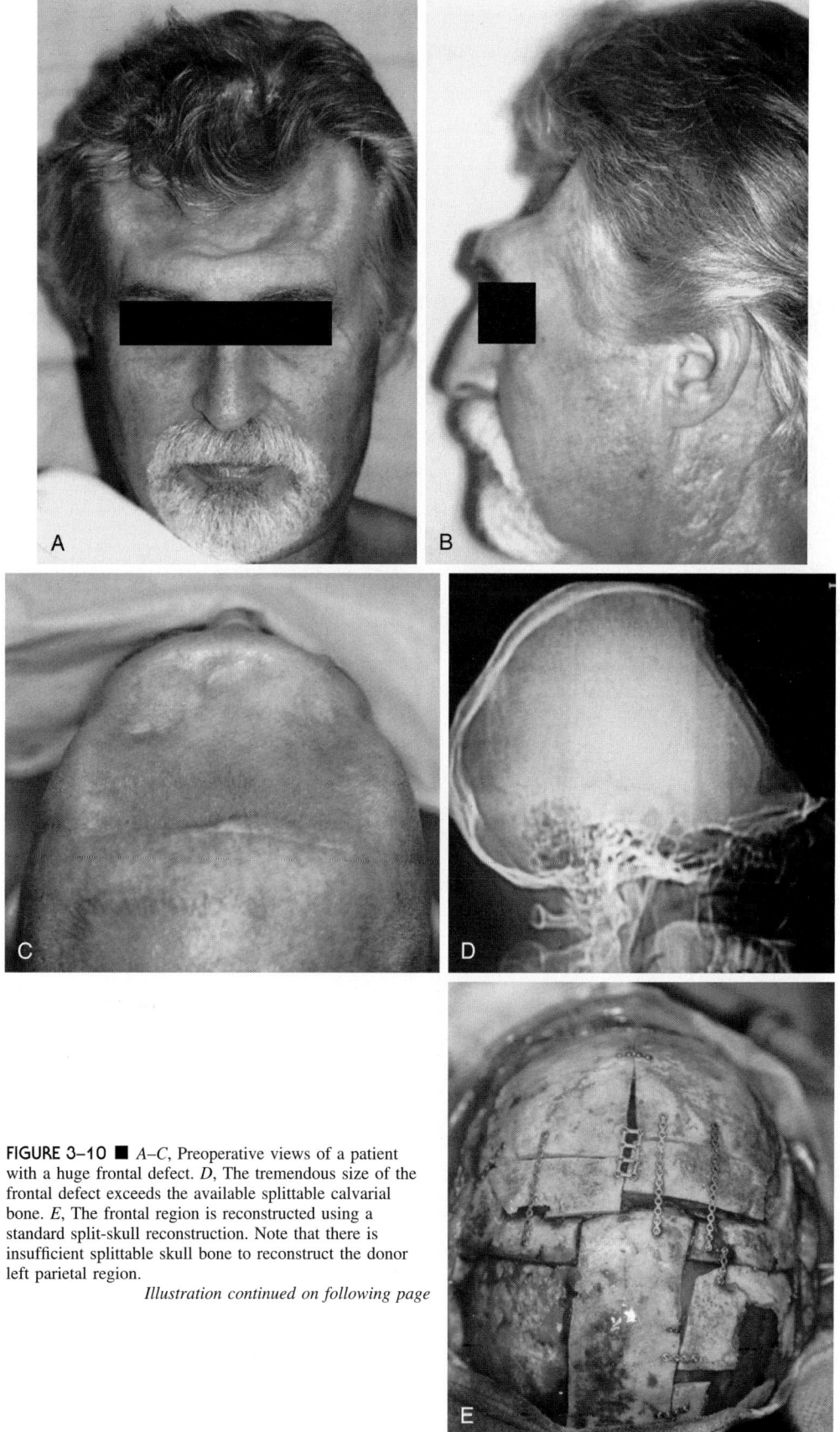

**FIGURE 3–10** ■ *A–C*, Preoperative views of a patient with a huge frontal defect. *D*, The tremendous size of the frontal defect exceeds the available splittable calvarial bone. *E*, The frontal region is reconstructed using a standard split-skull reconstruction. Note that there is insufficient splittable skull bone to reconstruct the donor left parietal region.

*Illustration continued on following page*

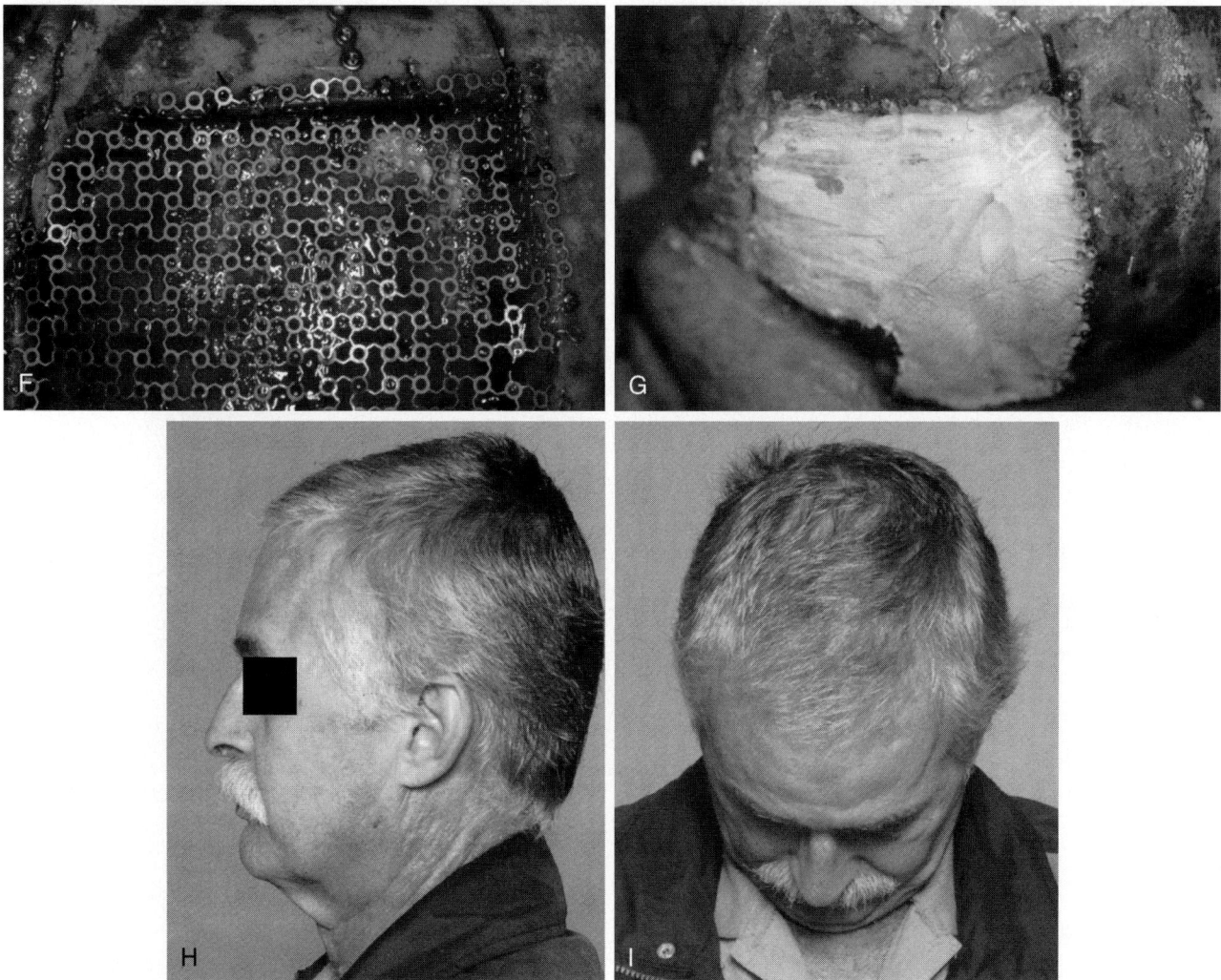

**FIGURE 3–10  ■**  *Continued. F,* The left parietal donor region was reconstructed using titanium mesh and hydroxyapatite paste. The titanium mesh was recessed into the defect and rigidly fixed to the surrounding bone margins with screws. *G,* This provided the recessed supportive framework from which to layer and sculpt the hydroxyapatite paste. *H* and *I,* Postoperative results demonstrate an anatomic restoration of the skull.

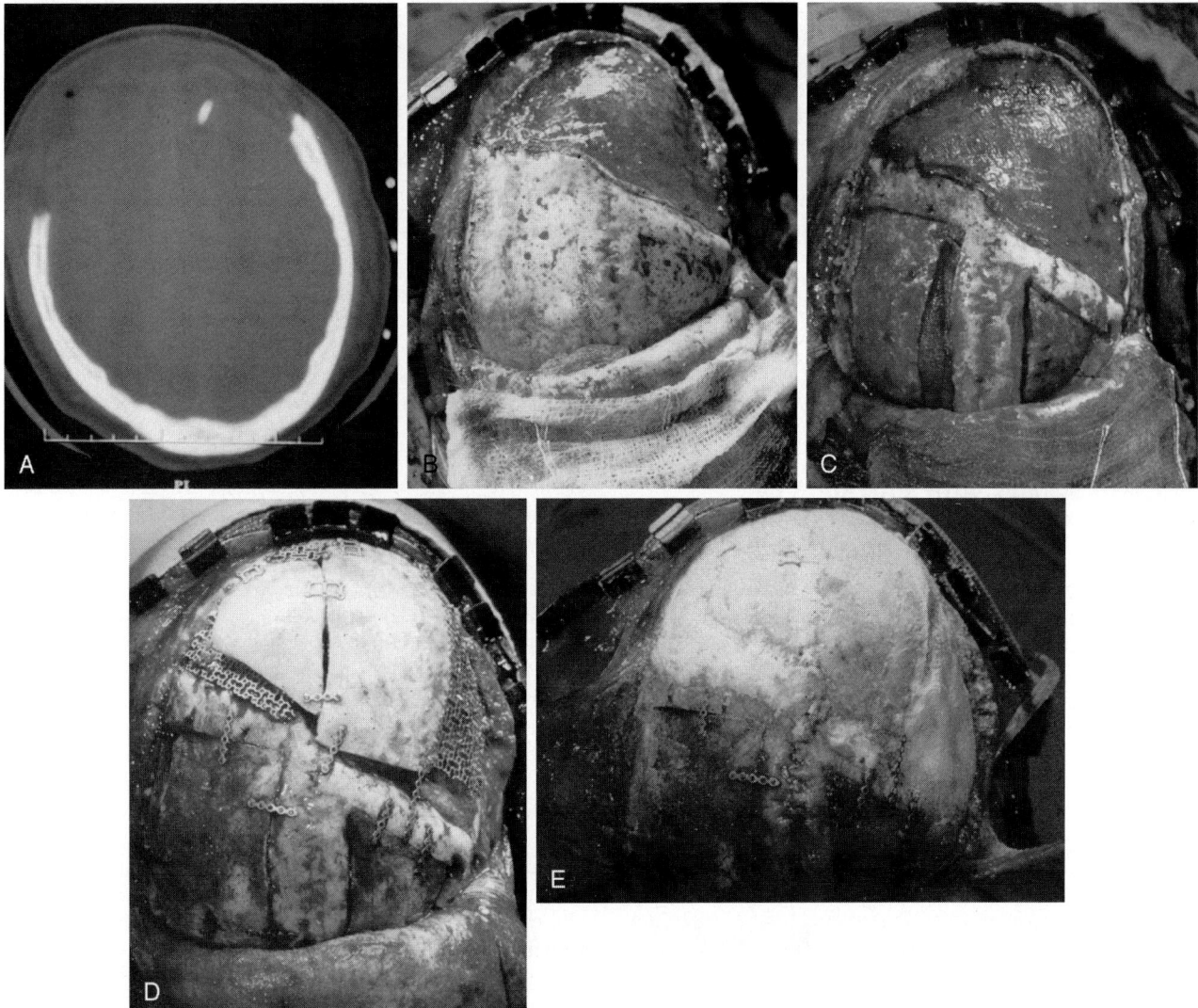

**FIGURE 3–11** ■ *A–E*, This massive frontal defect was treated with a combination of a split skull for the frontal reconstruction and titanium mesh with hydroxyapatite paste for the remaining donor site deficiencies.

major disadvantage was the difficulty molding it to fit the contour of the skull; however, the current complex mesh patterns available allow it to be shaped without difficulty while maintaining its strength in the final formed position (see Fig. 3–10F).

**Bioresorbable Bone Substitutes.** Hydroxyapatite cement is a calcium phosphate–based material that, when mixed with water, forms a dense paste that sets isothermically and converts in vivo to a microporous hydroxyapatite implant. The "putty-like" physical characteristics during the curing of the hydroxyapatite cement facilitate accurate three-dimensional reconstruction of the bony cranium[29, 30] (see Fig. 3–10G). Compressive strength, compliance, and setting time for this bone substitute can be adjusted by chemically altering the aqueous liquid with which the calcium phosphate–based material is mixed.[31–34] Once implanted, there is steadfast adherence to the adjacent bone, thus preventing micromotion and migration of the implant. Typically, bone ingrowth takes place at the surface of the hydroxyapatite implant in contact with the native bone. Replacement of the hydroxyapatite cement implants by new bone is postulated to occur by osteoconduction.[29, 30] Radiographically,[35] hydroxyapatite cement is homogeneously radiopaque on CT scans and plain radiographs. On an MRI scan, the hydroxyapatite cement is a signal void.

## RECONSTRUCTION WITH MATERIALS OF DISSIMILAR COMPOSITION

Autogenous split skull reconstruction is especially advantageous for cranial defects involving the visible fronto-orbital region of the cranium and for defects juxtaposed to paranasal sinuses. Occasionally, the recipient cranial defect may be too large to permit complete split skull cranioplasty (see Figs. 3–10 and 3–11). Under such circumstances, priority is given to split skull reconstruction of the esthetically sensitive frontal region. Donor bone graft is still harvested from the parietal skull; however, remaining parietal cranial donor deficiencies are then reconstructed with alloplastic implants. Combined materials of differing composition facilitate accurate and stable reconstruction of the remaining parietal cranial donor sites. Preferential use of titanium mesh, anatomically sculpted with a layer of hydroxyapatite paste, should be considered. This novel combined application of titanium mesh and hydroxyapatite paste permits rigid stabilization and provides a construct on which to use hydroxyapatite paste to sculpt the anatomic contours of an osteoconductive cranial construct (Fig. 3–12).

## RESULTS

The debate over the most appropriate material for cranial defect reconstruction remains somewhat unresolved. Historically, autogenous bone has been advocated when the reconstruction is performed adjacent to sinus cavities or in areas with a previous history of infection because of the subsequent increased risk of infection. Despite their advantages, methyl methacrylate and metallic cranioplasty implants are foreign bodies with a significant risk of complications. Abscess formation, draining sinus tracts, local skin breakdown, epidural granulomas, and pneumatoceles have all been reported as complications of methyl methacrylate and metallic cranioplasties.[36, 37] The incidence of these complications has been reported to be as high as 14%[2, 7] compared with less than 5% in most autogenous bone reconstructions. Manson and associates challenged that notion in their review of 42 frontal cranioplasties in 1986.[38] They found that the material used was not as important as the timing of the reconstruction (waiting at least 1 year after the initial injury), communication between the cranial vault reconstruction and the nasal and frontal sinuses, and residual ethmoidal or frontal sinus inflammatory disease. They found no infections in those patients reconstructed with methyl methacrylate compared with a 23% incidence of infection in patients treated with autogenous bone. However, other studies find a much lower rate of infection using bone under similar conditions. Wolfe[39] reported no infections in 73 autogenous bone cranioplasties; half of those patients were operated on for fronto-orbital defects similar to those described by Manson, eight of which were successfully reconstructed with autogenous bone after previous failures with alloplastic materials. In 1994, Wong and Manson[40] described a technique of incorporating titanium mesh within acrylic cranioplasties to facilitate rigid screw stabilization of the alloplastic construct to the native skull. The absence of complications in their six treated patients was ascribed to the rigid stability and avoidance of micromotion at the alloplastic-bone interface.

**Dead Space Morbidity.** The presence of a dead space posterior to the planned cranioplasty deserves special consideration. Posnick and associates demonstrated that intracranial dead space arising after cranial vault expansion in children is obliterated spontaneously by brain expansion in the early postoperative period.[41] The natural history of the dead space arising after restoration of a normal cranial vault in an adult patient with an acquired defect has not been delineated. Patients with acquired cranial defects may have reduced brain substance from traumatic or ablative loss, a contracted fibrotic dura from a long-standing deformity, or a calcified dura that can restrict brain re-expansion and maintain the dead space. In such cases, the dead space becomes fluid-filled and postoperative CT scans performed as late as 1 year following cranioplasty demonstrate persistence of the dead space.[42]

Classically, the healing of bone grafts has been thought to necessitate complete enclosure within a well-vascularized soft tissue pocket.[43] Problems with vascularity on the internal surface of a bone graft cranioplasty have prompted some authors to alter their surgical treatment by importing well-vascularized tissue.[17, 44] This surgical strategy has been most commonly employed when there is an intracranial dead space associated with the autogenous bone graft cranioplasty. Advocates have used microvascular-free tissue transfer to obliterate the intracranial dead space.[44] Arguments against such a procedure include a potential intracranial mass effect from early flap edema, prolonged surgery, and morbidity of the flap donor site.[45] Clinically, the dead space does not alter either the external

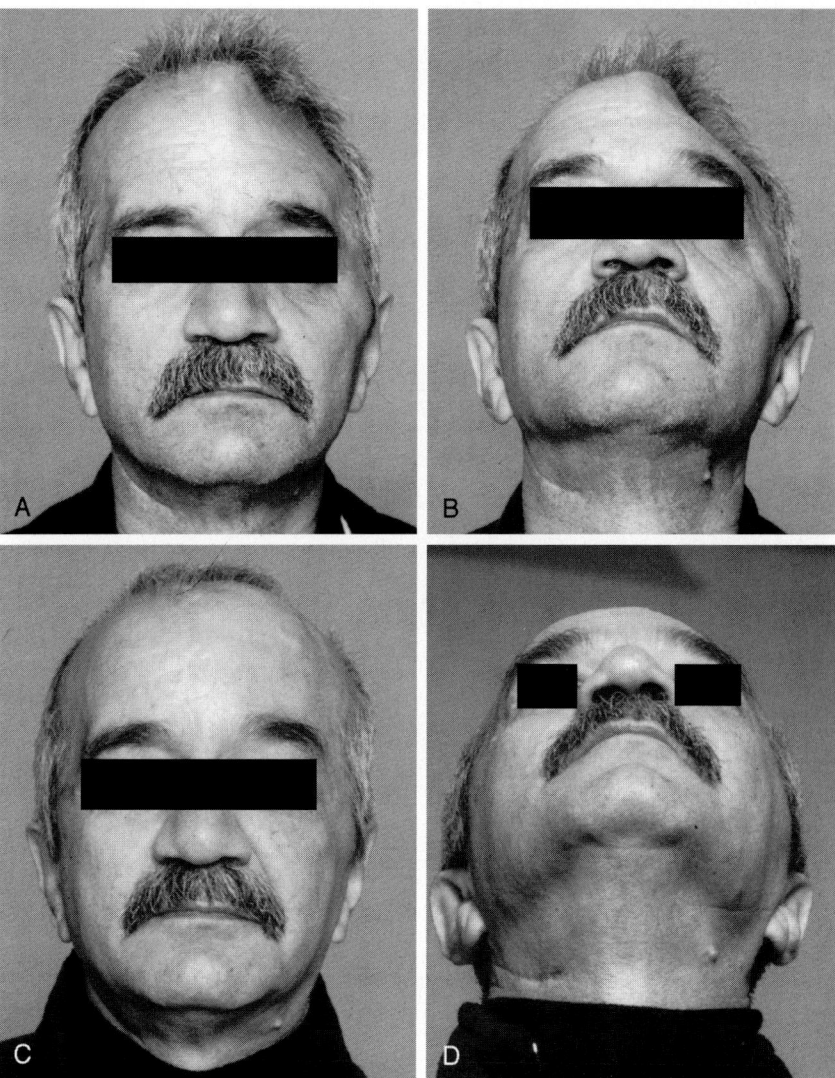

FIGURE 3-12 ■ A combination of titanium mesh and layered hydroxyapatite paste was used in this patient. The frontal sinus was not involved. The left enophthalmos and depressed malar bone were treated with a zygomatic osteotomy. *A* and *B*, Preoperative views. *C* and *D*, Postoperative views.

contour or the protective function achieved. Late infection of the fluid-filled dead space is a known complication, most commonly as a result of inadequate débridement at the time of the primary reconstruction. Usually, though, these infections can be treated with simple drainage without systemic complications and without any adverse effect on the cranial reconstruction.[42]

## PEDIATRIC CRANIOPLASTY

The goals of cranioplasty in children are similar to those in adults, primarily to provide protection and cosmesis. Unlike adults, young children (younger than 36 to 48 months) can regenerate calvarial bone, particularly in acquired defects with the dura and pericranium intact. In such cases, cranioplasty is considered only after a period of conservative management (approximately 1 year) to allow calvarial bone to form.

The qualities of an ideal material for pediatric cranioplasty are similar to those for adults. In general, autogenous bone is preferred over alloplastic materials because the rapid growth of the skull in childhood makes an artificial material unsuitable. We would not consider placement of alloplastic material in children younger than 7 to 8 years, because until that age the cranium continues to develop significantly. Either full-thickness calvarial grafts in infants or split skull grafts in older children are preferred.

## FUTURE DEVELOPMENTS

Hydroxyapatite paste bone substitutes have been available since 1995. In this brief time, we have seen innovative and imaginative uses develop for these materials. At present the handling characteristics and limited capacity for osteoconduction with existing substances fall short of an ideal bone replacement. Nevertheless, it has positively impacted on our ability to manage osseous cranial defects and is rapidly becoming the "ideal" implant. With continued advances in bioresorbable technology and tissue engineering, there remains a glimmer of hope that one day we will cease to have controversies regarding the "ideal" bone replacement.

## REFERENCES

1. Kunz Z: Neurochirurgi. Prague: Statni Zdravotnicke Nakladatelsti, 1968, pp 11–14.
2. Hammon WM, Kempe LG: Methyl methacrylate cranioplasty: Thirteen years' experience with 417 patients. Acta Neurochir 25:69–77, 1971.
3. Jackson IT, Pellett C, Smith JM: The skull as a bone graft donor site. Ann Plast Surg 11:527–532, 1963.
4. Simpson D: Titanium in cranioplasty. J Neurosurg 22:292–293, 1965.
5. Delashaw JB, Persing JA, Jane JA: Cranial deformation in craniosynostosis. Neurosurg Clin North Am 2:611–620, 1991.
6. Grant FC, Norcross NC: Repair of cranial defects by cranioplasty. Ann Surg 110:488–512, 1939.
7. Stula D: Cranioplasty. Berlin: Springer-Verlag, 1984.
8. Weiford EC, Gardner WJ: Tantalum cranioplasty: Review of 106 cases in civilian practice. J Neurosurg 6:13–32, 1949.
9. Prolo DJ, Oklund SA: The use of bone grafts and alloplastic materials in cranioplasty. Clin Orthop 268:270–278, 1993.
10. Blake GB, MacFarlane MR, Hinton JW: Titanium in reconstructive surgery of the skull and face. Br J Plast Surg 43:528–535, 1990.
11. Cabanela ME, Coventry MB, Maccarty CS, et al: The fate of patients with methyl methacrylate cranioplasty. J Bone Joint Surg 54A:278–281, 1972.
12. Psillakis JM, Nocchi VLB, Zanini SA: Repair of large defect of the frontal bone with free graft of outer table of parietal bones. Plast Reconstr Surg 64:827–830, 1979.
13. Thompson HG, Munro IR, Birch JR: Exposed cranial implants—a salvage operation. Plast Reconstr Surg 59:395–397, 1977.
14. Edwards MSB, Ousterhout DK: Autogeneic skull bone grafts to reconstruct large or complex skull defects in children and adolescents. Neurosurg 20:273–280, 1987.
15. Habal MB: Repair of a skull defect by a split cranial bone graft. J Craniofac Surg 3:230–234, 1992.
16. Rish BL, Dillon JD, Meirowsky AM, et al.: Cranioplasty: A review of 1030 cases of penetrating head injury. Neurosurgery 4:381–385, 1979.
17. Stueber K, Salcman M, Spence RJ: The combined use of the latissimus dorsi musculocutaneous free flap and split-rib grafts for cranial vault reconstruction. Ann Plast Surg 15:155–160, 1985.
18. Cabbabe EB, Shively RE, Malik P: Cranioplasty for traumatic deformities of the fronto-orbital area. Ann Plast Surg 13:175–184, 1984.
19. Antonyshyn O, Caputy G: Controlled bending of cranial bone grafts: A simple surgical technique. J Craniomaxillofac Surg 21:82–85, 1993.
20. Zins JE, Whitaker LA: Membranous versus endochondral bone: Implications for craniofacial reconstruction. Plast Reconstr Surg 72:778–785, 1983.
21. Nickell WB, Jurkiewicz MJ, Salyer KE: Repair of skull defects with autogenous bone. Ann Surg 105:431–433, 1972.
22. Longacre JJ, Stefano GA: Reconstruction of extensive defects of the skull with split rib grafts. Plast Reconstr Surg 19:186–200, 1957.
23. Korlof B, Nylen B, Rietz K: Bone grafting of skull defects. Plast Reconstr Surg 52:378–382, 1973.
24. Munro IR, Guyuron B: Split-rib cranioplasty. Ann Plast Surg 7:341–346, 1981.
25. McClintock HG, Dingman RO: The repair of cranial defects with iliac bone. Surgery 30:955–963, 1951.
26. Mayfield JF, Levitch LA: Repair of cranial defects with tantalum. Am J Surg 67:319–332, 1945.
27. Leininger RI, Bigg DM: Polymers. In Von Recum AF (ed): Handbook of Biomaterials Evaluation. New York: Macmillan, 1986, pp 25–37.
28. Linder I, Albreklsson T, Branemark P, et al: Electron microscopic analysis of the bone-titanium interface. Acta Orthop 54:45–52, 1983.
29. Stelnicki EJ, Ousterhout DK: Hydroxyapatite paste (BoneSource) used as an onlay implant for supraorbital and malar augmentation. J Craniofac Surg 8:367–372, 1997.
30. Costantino PD, Friedman CD, Jones K, et al: Experimental hydroxyapatite cement cranioplasty. Plast Reconstr Surg 90:174–185, 1992.
31. Ishikawa K, Miyamoto Y, Takechi M, et al: Non-decay type fast-setting calcium phosphate cement: Hydroxyapatite putty containing an increased amount of sodium alginate. J Biomed Mater Res 36:393–399, 1997.
32. Kurashina K, Kurita H, Hirano M, et al: In vivo study of calcium phosphate cements: Implantation of an alpha-tricalcium phosphate/dicalcium phosphate dibasic/tetracalcium phosphate monoxide cement paste. Biomaterials 18:539–543, 1997.
33. Maruyama M, Ito M: In vitro properties of a chitosan-bonded self-hardening paste with hydroxyapatite granules. J Biomed Mater Res 32:527–532, 1996.
34. Ito M, Yamagishi T, Yagasaki H, Kafrawy AH: In vitro properties of a chitosan-bonded bone-filling paste: Studies on solubility of calcium phosphate compounds. J Biomed Mater Res 32:95–98, 1996.
35. Weissman JL, Snyderman CH, Hirsch BE: Hydroxyapatite cement to repair skull base defects: radiologic appearance. AJNR Am J Neuroradiol 17:1569–1574, 1996.
36. Meirowski AM, Hazouri LA, Freiner DJ: Epidural granulomata in the presence of tantalum plates. J Neurosurg 7:485–491, 1950.
37. Woodhall B, Cramer FJ: Extradural pneumatocele following tantalum cranioplasty. J Neurosurg 2:524–529, 1945.
38. Manson PN, Crawley WA, Hoopes JE: Frontal cranioplasty: Risk factors and choice of cranial vault reconstructive material. Plast Reconstr Surg 77:888–900, 1986.
39. Wolfe SA: In discussion: Manson PN, Crawley WA, Hoopes JE: Frontal cranioplasty: Risk factors and choice of cranial vault reconstructive material. Plast Reconstr Surg 77:901–904, 1986.
40. Wong L, Manson PN: Rigid mesh fixation for alloplastic cranioplasty. J Craniofac Surg 5:265–269, 1994.
41. Posnick JC, Al Qattan MM, Armstrong D: Extradural dead space following monoblock and facial bipartition osteotomies for reconstruction of craniofacial malformations. Presented at the 62nd Annual Meeting of the American Society of Plastic and Reconstructive Surgery, New Orleans, Louisiana, September, 1993.
42. Lee C, Antonyshyn OM, Forrest CR: Cranioplasty: Indications, technique, and early results of autogenous split skull cranial vault reconstruction. J Craniomaxillofac Surg 23:133–142, 1995.
43. Lukash FN, Zingaro EA, Salig J: The survival of free non-vascularized bone grafts in irradiated areas by wrapping in muscle flaps. Plast Reconstr Surg 74:783–786, 1984.
44. Netscher DT, Stal S, Shenaq S: Management of residual cranial vault deformities. Clin Plast Surg 19:301–313, 1992.
45. Moore MH, Tan E, Reilly PL, David DJ: Frontofacial advancement with a free flap: Deadspace versus drainage. J Craniofac Surg 2:33–37, 1991.

# Perioperative Management of Severe Head Injuries in Adults

■ KLAUS R. H. VON WILD

The last 4 decades has seen advances and approaches in the perioperative management strategies of patients with severe traumatic brain injury (TBI).[1–29] This is especially true concerning the avoidance or minimization of hypotensive insults and the attitudes regarding monitoring during treatment.[30–46] In 1960, Lundberg published his paper on the "continuous recording and control of ventricular fluid pressure in neurosurgical practice."[42] This paper has proved to be important for current neurointensive care management. In 1965, Ruf (Professor of Neurosurgery at the University Clinic in Frankfurt, Germany) realized the life-saving opportunities provided by proper perioperative management of neurosurgical patients and opened the first neurosurgical intensive care unit (ICU). This unit consisted of 22 beds adjacent to the neurosurgical operating rooms. His philosophy held that the neurosurgeon has to be trained in the physiology of brain injury, in neurointensive care medicine, and in early rehabilitation medicine.[20, 30, 33, 39, 47–56]

An increasing number of evidence-based guidelines have been published for the management of patients with TBI who have severe (GCS 3 to 8) moderate (GCS 9 to 12) and minor (GCS 13 to 15) Glasgow Coma Scale (GCS) scores.[1, 13–15, 17, 27, 57–59] These management guidelines reflect a degree of consensus among different medical specialists based on evidence and literature searches of topics important for diagnosis, medical treatment, and technique.[1, 13, 14] There is wide variation in clinical management in the United States (US) among centers treating severe TBI. The variation is not only in terms of trauma level designation (level I, II, or III) and the number of patients with severe TBI who are routinely treated but also within such categories at a time when most treatment strategies were not based on published literature.[25] In Germany, we were able to demonstrate the variation in management of patients with mild head injury in neurosurgical departments when using the European Federation of Neurological Societies (EFNS) survey questionnaire published by Twijnstra (1997).[60]

## EPIDEMIOLOGY

In western industrialized countries, it is estimated that approximately 300 per 100,000 inhabitants are at the risk of suffering a head injury (HI) every year and that HI is responsible for a disproportionate number of critically injured patients.[1, 13, 47] One third of these critical cases die, making HI the main contributor to trauma-related mortality and disability.[61] Furthermore, 70% of patients with multiple injuries have associated head injuries including long bone fracture (60%), thoracic injury (40%), abdominal injury (20%), and spinal trauma (5% to 15%).[20, 36, 62–70]

## GRADING

In order to assess management versus outcome in HI, a reliable criteria for grading the severity of the injury patterns is essential.[1, 15, 27, 57, 62, 63, 68, 71–74] Tools used for the classification of injury severity include the Revised Trauma Score (RTS),[75, 76] the Abbreviated Injury Score (AIS),[77, 78] and the GCS.[58, 103, 130] The RTS is based on physiologic variables, whereas the AIS is based on the relative severity of the anatomic injury of the head or neck, face, chest, abdominal or pelvic contents, extremities, or pelvic girdle and external tissue. The AIS is rated on a scale of 1 (minor) to 6 (major) in terms of severity. It is useful when estimating the risk for patients with multiple lesions before operative treatment, especially when used in combination with the Index Injury Severity Score (ISS)[79] (calculated by squaring the AIS scores of the three most seriously injured organ systems and summing up the squares.) Although the RTS correlates almost linearly with the lethality in TBI, the ISS shows a steep lethality peak for the 16- to 25-year age bracket by considering only three regions of the most severe body injuries, a feature that is insufficient. With multiple injuries, the severity of the injuries determines the chronologic sequence and the extent of the necessary surgical therapy with regard to the proven risk of secondary brain damage (graduated therapy plan).[1, 15, 17, 62–66]

The Coma Remission Scale (CRS) is based on the GCS and incorporates the neurologic impairment and neurobehavioral disturbances and their functional recovery over time. The latter is done by testing the patient's neuropsychological response intensity to different stimuli, using algebraic points on the total score (Table 4–1). The CRS

TABLE 4–1  ■  **COMA REMISSION SCALE (CRS)**

**German Task Force on Neurologic-Neurosurgical Early Rehabilitation, 1993 (Lit. No. 7, pp 118–119)**

**Patient name:**

| Name of institution: | **Date:** | |
|---|---|---|
| Date of brain injury: | **Investigator (initials):** | |

**1. Arousability/attention** (to any stimulus)

| | | |
|---|---|---|
| Attention span for 1 minute or longer | 5 | |
| Attention remains on a stimulus (longer than 5 sec) | 4 | |
| Turning towards a stimulus | 3 | |
| Spontaneous eye opening | 2 | |
| Eye opening in response to pain | 1 | |
| None | 0 | |

**2. Motoric response** (minus 6 points from max. attainable sum if tetraplegic)

| | | |
|---|---|---|
| Spontaneous grasping (also from prone position) | 6 | |
| Localized movement in response to pain | 5 | |
| Body posture recognizable | 4 | |
| Unspecific movement in response to pain (vegetative or spastic pattern) | 3 | |
| Flexion in response to pain | 2 | |
| Extension in response to pain | 1 | |
| None | 0 | |

**3. Response to acoustic stimuli (e.g., clicker)** (minus 3 points from max. attainable sum if deaf)

| | | |
|---|---|---|
| Recognizes a well-acquainted voice, music, etc. | 3 | |
| Eye opening, turning of head, perhaps smiling | 2 | |
| Vegetative reaction (startle) | 1 | |
| None | 0 | |

**4. Response to visual stimuli** (minus 4 points from max. attainable sum if blind)

| | | |
|---|---|---|
| Recognizes pictures, persons, objects | 4 | |
| Follows pictures, persons, objects | 3 | |
| Fixates on pictures, persons, objects | 2 | |
| Occasional, random eye movements | 1 | |
| None | 0 | |

**5. Response to tactile stimuli**

| | | |
|---|---|---|
| Recognizes by touching/feeling | 3 | |
| Spontaneous, targeted grasping (if blind), albeit without comprehension of sense | 2 | |
| Only vegetative response to passive touching | 1 | |
| None | 0 | |

---

TABLE 4–1 ■ **COMA REMISSION SCALE (CRS)** *Continued*

---

**6. Auditory response** (tracheostoma = 3 if lips can be heard to utter guttural sounds/seen to mime "letters")

| | | |
|---|---|---|
| At least one understandably articulated word | 3 | |
| Unintelligible (unarticulated) sounds | 2 | |
| Groaning, screaming, coughing (emotional, vegetatively tinged) | 1 | |
| No phonetics/articulation audible/recognizable | 0 | |

| | | |
|---|---|---|
| **Sum score:** | | |
| Max. attainable score (of 24) for this patient | | |

1. **Arousability/attention**
   5 pts: The patient can direct his/her attention toward an interesting stimulus for at least 1 minute (e.g., perceivable by vision, hearing, or touching; stimulus: persons, objects, noises, music, voices) without being diverted by secondary stimuli.
   4 pts: Attention fixed to a stimulus for a discernible moment (fixation with the eyes, grasping, and feeling or "pricking up of ears"); the patient is, however, easily diverted or "switches off."
   3 pts: The patient turns to a source of stimulus by moving the eyes, head, or body; the patient follows moving objects. Vegetative reactions should also be observed (the patient is capable only of vegetative reaction).
   2 pts: Spontaneous opening of the eyes without any external stimulis, e.g., in connection with a sleep-waking state rhythm.

2. **Motor response**
   6 pts: The patient spontaneously grasps held-out everyday objects (only if the patient's vision function is intact, otherwise lay the object on the back of the patient's hand) or the patient is able to respond to such gestures with an invitational character only with a delay or inconsistently yet adequately, due to paralysis or contraction.
   *Note regarding the following items (use of pain stimuli):*
      The pain stimuli must be applied to the various limbs and to the body trunk, because there may be regional stimulus-perception impairment; pain stimuli can take the form, e.g., of a gentle twisting pinch of a fold of skin, pressure applied to a fingernail fold, tickling of the nose.
   5 pts: The patient responds to painful stimuli defensively after localization by a targeted and adequate measure, e.g., pushing away, sweeping motions of the hand, etc.
   4 pts: The patient should be seated upright: tests for the sense of balance and/or posture by slight pushes applied to the body (corrective movements of trunk or extremities).
   3 pts: Untargeted withdrawal from a pain stimulus or merely vegetative reactions (tachycardia, tachypnea, agitation) or an increase of spastic pattern.
   2 pts: Strong, hardly resolvable flexion, especially in the arms/elbows. The legs may stretch out.
   1 pt:  Typical "decerebrate rigidity" with spastic extension of all extremities, in many cases opisthotonus (dorsal overextension/hyperlordosis).

3. **Response to acoustic stimuli (tests as a rule to be carried out beyond the patient's field of vision!)**
   3 pts: The patient can recognize voices or music, i.e, he/she is able either to name the stimulus or to react in a differentiated manner (e.g., to certain pieces of music or persons with pleasure or defensively).
   2 pts: The patient only opens his/her eyes, fixates or turns to the source of the stimulus with his/her head, in some cases accompanied by emotional expressions such as smiling or crying.
   1 pt:  Rise in pulse and/or blood pressure, perspiration or agitation, excessive twitching of the body, slight triggering of eye blinking.
   *Note:* Similar to the procedures applied when testing the motor responsiveness by the application of pain stimuli, the use of a clicker held directly next to each of the patient's ears (bilateral testing) suggests itself as the relatively strongest non–pain-involving stimulus for items 1 and 2; if the response is positive, the patient can be assumed to still be in possession of his/her hearing and the stimuli can be made more manifold.

4. **Response to visual stimuli (must be presented without speaking or any other form of comment)**
   4 pts: The patient recognizes pictures, objects, portraits of familiar persons.
   3 pts: Follows pictures, etc., with the eyes without any sign of recognition or questioning, inconsistent recognition.
   2 pts: Fixates on moving pictures or objects without being able to follow them properly, or when the picture/object moves outside the patient's field of vision the patient makes no attempt to keep track.

5 **Response to tactile stimuli**
   3 pts: The patient is capable of feeling and recognizing objects, the hands of other persons, etc., even if his/her sense of vision is absent and the objects must be placed on the skin or in the hands; adequate response to stimuli in the area of the mouth/face (edible/inedible, e.g., response to a kiss).
   2 pts: Touches, feels, and grasps aiming at or targeting but without an adequate reaction.
   1 pt:  Unspecific response to stroking and touch (vegetative signs, e.g., agitation, raised pulse).

6. **Auditory response**
   3 pts: The patient is capable of expressing an intelligible word, even if this is not related to the context or situation. Names also count as words here.
   2 pts: The patient utters unintelligible sounds (e.g., slurred sounds), also repetition of syllables or similar sounds ("ma-ma," "oh," . . .).

**Total score:** In the event that certain channels of sense or motor systems are completely absent ("blind," "deaf," "plegic"), the point scores of the respective category must be subtracted from the maximum attainable score, e.g., 12/21 points instead of 12/24 points.

---

TABLE 4–2 ■ **GLASCOW COMA SCALE***

| | | |
|---|---|---|
| **Eyes Open** | Spontaneously (eyes open, does not imply awareness) | 4 |
| | To speech (any speech, not necessarily a command) | 3 |
| | To pain (should not use supraorbital pressure for pain stimulus) | 2 |
| | Never | 1 |
| **Best Verbal Response** | Oriented (to time, person, place) | 5 |
| | Confused speech (disoriented) | 4 |
| | Inappropriate (swearing, yelling) | 3 |
| | Incomprehensible sounds (moaning, groaning) | 2 |
| | None | 1 |
| **Best Motor Response** | Obeys commands | 6 |
| | Localizes pain (deliberate or purposeful movement) | 5 |
| | Withdrawal (moves away from stimulus) | 4 |
| | Abnormal flexion (decortication) | 3 |
| | Extension (decerebration) | 2 |
| | None (flaccidity) | 1 |
| **Total Score** | | |

*The Glasgow Coma Scale is a practical means of monitoring changes in the level of consciousness based on eye opening and verbal and motor responses. The responsiveness of the patient can be expressed by summation of the figures. The lowest score is 3; the highest is 15.

was developed by specialists from the fields of neurointensive care and early neurologic-neurosurgical rehabilitation.[6] This was an attempt to render the complex lesions and their functional regression under therapy measurable and comparable nationally and internationally.[71] Like the Glasgow Outcome Score (GOS), it is easy to apply and permits a good, graduated functional assessment for each item of interest and in the sum of the item scores in the most critically brain-injured patients.[72] Table 4–2 depicts the criteria used in the GCS.

## MONITORING

Although no clear guidelines are yet available for a graduated surgical emergency protocol, definitive surgical therapy of non–life-threatening injuries associated with severe HI should be postponed until the patient's condition is stabilized to avoid hypotension, hypovolemia, and secondary cerebral hypoxemia due to blood loss and stress reactions.[62–67] In a prospective study of 33 patients with severe TBI, subjected to multimodal monitoring in the ICU, it was possible to show that cerebral hypoxia may be present even though ICP and cerebral perfusion pressure (CPP) were adequately treated.[80] Moreover, and in contrast to former reports,[67] it was also demonstrated in a prospective multicenter study in 172 patients with TBI (GCS <12) and multiple fractures (extremities 38%, pelvis 12%) that the operative stabilization did not significantly influence the early outcome when the patients were monitored and treated according to European Brain Injury Criteria (EBIC) guidelines.[64, 65] Miller[11, 12, 33] and coworkers who demonstrated the high frequency of secondary silent insults that occurred in patients in the ICU and in patients studied during transportation within the hospital.[27–32, 36, 37, 39, 45, 46, 51, 54–56, 80–83] However, the continuous measurement of jugular venous oxygen saturation and brain tissue $Po_2$ in patients with severe TBI is still restricted to a few centers.[51, 84–86] The same is true for microdialysis for monitoring brain tissue metabolism[87] in local and global cerebral ischemia

and neuroprotection. By contrast, intracranial pressure (ICP) monitoring has been universally accepted as indicated in patients with a GCS less than 8 and perioperatively when elevated ICP or an expanding mass lesion is suspected.[88] In addition to the routinely monitored parameters (electrocardiogram [ECG], $Sao_2$, invasive arterial blood pressure, temperature, and end-tidal $CO_2$ in ventilated patients) as recommended in the EBIC guidelines,[15] neuromonitoring is helpful in both the continuous evaluation of neurologic functions in comatose patients during intensive care treatment as well as in treatment controls.[38, 57] Noninvasive continuous cortical electroencephalogram (EEG) recording with computerized analysis and intermittently recorded evoked potentials (EPs) provides information regarding the functional status in terms of the depth of coma and recovery as well as the localization of functional blocks along the peripheral and central pathways (Fig. 4–1).[28, 89–92]

Electrophysiologic monitoring may demonstrate central effects of neuroprotective and stimulating drugs (phar-

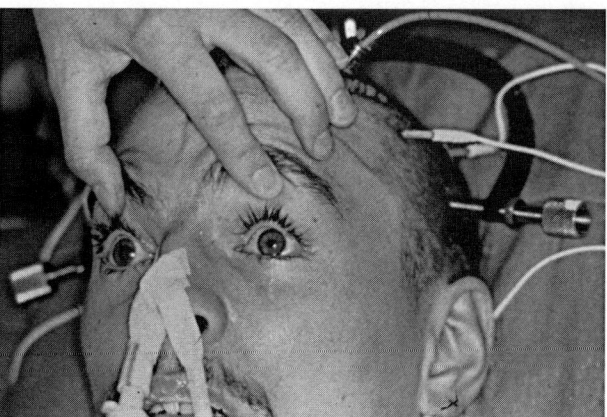

**FIGURE 4–1** ■ Gardner-Wells cervical spine distraction owing to a vertebral body fracture C4-C5 in connection with traumatic brain injury (GCS 3). Intensive care unit treatment, multimodal monitoring with an electroencephalogram, and evoked potentials. Onset of herniation with mydriatic pupil on the right. The outcome is fatal.

maco-EEG)[93–96] and the response to coma-stimulating measures.[81, 82] For ICP monitoring, ventricular pressure measurement is the reference standard owing to the accuracy, reliability, therapeutic potential with CSF drainage (Fig. 4–2), and the relatively low cost.[13–15, 17, 30–33, 41, 42] Parenchymal catheter tip pressure-transducer devices do not always correlate well with intraventricular ICP and tend to drift from baseline measurements over time.[1] However, the acceptance of ICP monitoring is still remarkably low proportional to the number of patients treated for severe TBI.[12, 20, 46, 50, 55, 83] The reluctance may be due to concern about complications such as cerebrospinal fluid (CSF) infection, which is the most common problem associated with the ventricular catheter.[20] However, in our 20-year experience employing percutaneous needle trepanation in approxi-

mately 800 patients in the ICU,[81] the infection rate is less than 0.3%.

Because varying cerebral perfusion pressure (CPP) produces specific changes in cerebral blood flow (CBF) velocity as measured by transcranial Doppler (TCD) ultrasonography,[98] autoregulation vasoreactivity can easily be measured with the noninvasive TCD. CBF and TCD vasoreactivity vary by the same magnitude ($\sim$ 3% change) per millimeter of mercury of $Pa_{CO_2}$.[99–101] However, single TCD of the basal arteries can yield only very limited information about CBF. Moreover, in the case of TCD, many patients have been shown to have raised ICP values but do not have a markedly increased pulse index or systolic/diastolic flow ratio.[99–101] This well-known correlation between flow velocity and $P_{CO_2}$ may cause signal misinterpretation in

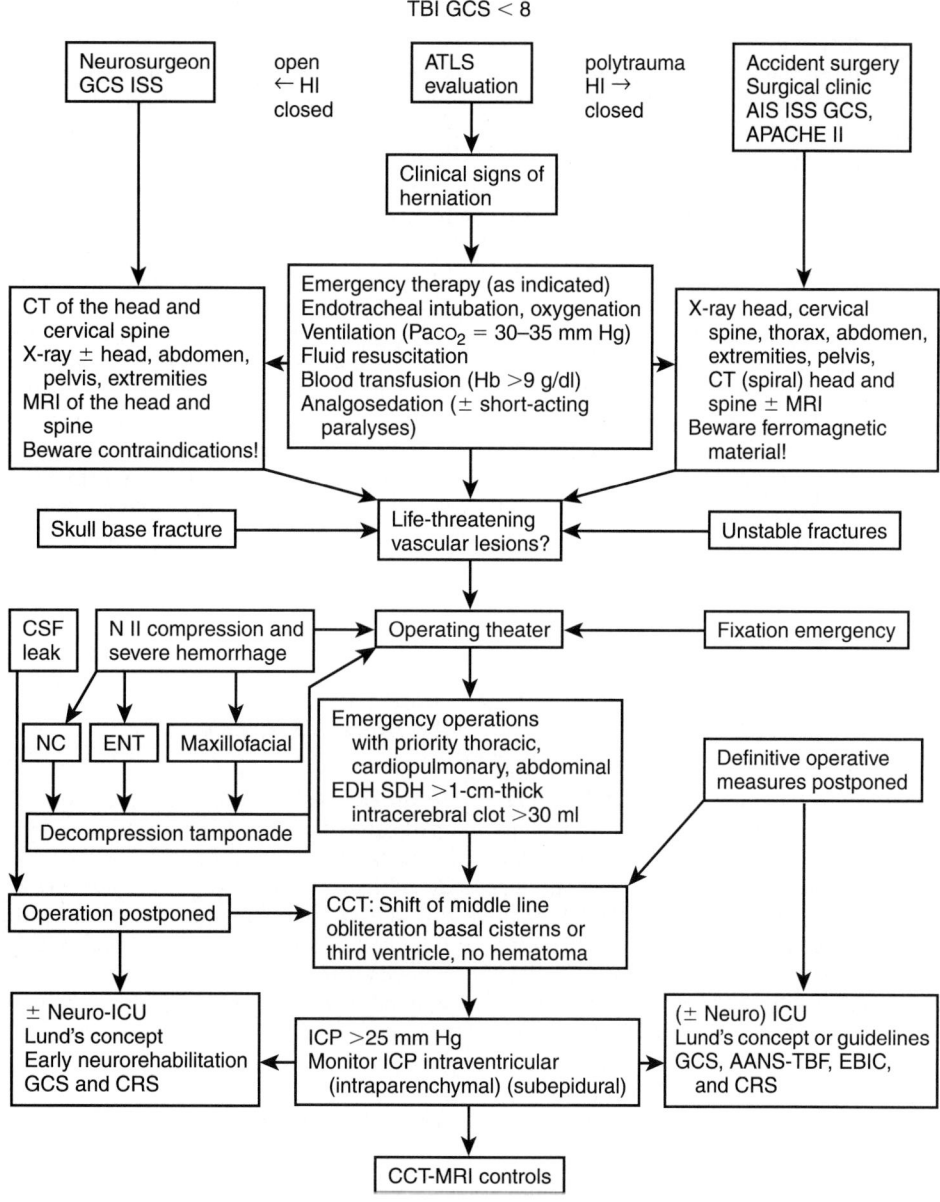

**FIGURE 4–2** ■ Management algorithm in patients with severe traumatic brain injury in the acute phase. Evidence-based treatment options are founded on the consensus of experts.[1, 15, 17, 129–138] (ATLS, advanced trauma life support; APACHE II, acute physiology and chronic health evaluation; CT, computed tomography; MRI, magnetic resonance imaging; ICP, intracranial pressure; GCS, Glasgow Coma Score; AIS, Abbreviated Injury Score; ISS, Injury Severity Score.)

ventilated patients.[43, 85] One may, therefore, conclude that the estimation of CPP using the noninvasive TCD method might only have limited value in severe TBI without ICP monitoring when measurement of relative changes in CPP is required.

## GUIDELINES

The American Association of Neurological Surgeons (AANS) and Brain Trauma Foundation (BTF) guidelines for the management of severe TBI (1995) are empirical and evidence-based in respect to a carefully reviewed and classified literature research.[1, 13, 14] The recommendations are ranked as *standards* (class I); representing principles of a high degree of clinical certainty and based on prospective, randomized, placebo-controlled trials; *guidelines* (class II), representing principles that reflect a moderate degree of clinical certainty; and *options* (class III), representing principles of unclear clinical certainty. There are only three class I studies to support standards in the areas of hyperventilation, steroid usage, and anticonvulsant treatment. Most recommendations use class II or class III as guidelines or options.[15, 17, 27, 32, 41] The main target and most important task in the management of patients with severe TBI is the diagnosis, prevention, and treatment of hypotension, hypoxia, elevated ICP, and intracranial mass lesions.[25, 30, 31, 33, 44–46, 102] Rapid and effective resuscitation and stabilization of physiologic conditions are recommended. Resuscitation includes an assessment of the patient's level of consciousness, depth of coma, airway protection in a patient with a GCS less than 9 or with severe bleeding from skull-based fractures, and sufficient fluid volume substitution. The stabilization of the spine has to be performed whenever a fracture is suspected in HI with extracranial injuries before further diagnostic procedures and transportation can be performed (see Fig. 4–2).[1, 15, 17, 41]

## IMAGING (Figs. 4–3 to 4–6)

For a general survey and assessment of major extracranial injuries and life-threatening vascular lesions such as cardiac tamponade, major thoracic or abdominal vascular injuries, tension pneumothorax, and cervical spine fractures, radiologic examination must be performed.[1, 15, 17] In the event that computed tomography (CT) is unavailable, initial radiologic studies should include three-plane skull radiographs in anterior posterior and sagittal views, including one additional sagittal view with the head turned about 15 degrees with the nose to the side of the film, so that temporoparietal skull fracture lines are better visualized as they move with the turned head, and the sharp line indicating the fracture at the side of the film. One mandatory aspect is the three-view cervical spine series plus chest and pelvic films during the initial radiographic studies. Cranial CT[103] must be performed in patients with a GCS score of less than 9 and is recommended in patients with a GCS score of less than 13 in association with skull fractures.[104, 105] However, acute epidural and subdural hematomas may be missed in emergency cranial computed tomography (CCT) so that CCT controls are indicated according to the neurologic findings. Currently, spiral CT of the head and body is the fastest and most efficient diagnostic emergency radiographic procedure.[106]

Coronal CCT thin-slide sections of the anterior skull base are superior to all other radiologic examinations in demonstrating primary and secondary lesions of the bulb, nerve structures, major vessels, and fractures with CSF fistula. MRI is superior to CCT in demonstrating diffuse axonal injury (DAI) and cortical and subcortical contusions.[106–109] However, the long examination time and ferromagnetic material (e.g., bullets or ventilators, cardiac pacemakers, artificial valves) are contraindications.

## SURGICAL TREATMENT

In an algorithim on emergency trauma care, the emergency life-saving operative procedures (see Fig. 4–2) involve the treatment of major thoracic vascular lesions, abdominal lesions causing severe blood loss, and epidural hematoma producing compression of the brain and brain stem with herniation.[15, 17, 62–67] When primary optic nerve lesions are suspected because of bone fracture or intraorbital hematoma emergency, ophthalmologic examination is mandatory and, if indicated, immediate decompression of the optic nerve performed as an emergency procedure (preferably via the minimal noninvasive transethmoidal route or by the subfrontal transorbital approach depending on the location of bone fragments). Facial reconstruction and revision and closure of CSF fistulas should be postponed until after the patient's condition has stabilized (to normal ICP and CPP values) to prevent secondary brain damage by local operative manipulation and hypotension during the operation. Invasive reconstruction of bone fractures must also be postponed in respect to blood loss and additional secondary trauma to the HI.

## MEDICAL TREATMENT

In patients with severe TBI, the most important target of medical treatment is the prevention of hypotension (defined at <90 mm Hg) and of intracranial hypertension (defined at >20 to 25 mm Hg). Any imbalance of the electrolytes and serum osmolality must be treated and controlled. Sedation and analgesia play an important role in ventilated patients with TBI.[14, 15, 17, 33, 54–56, 102] Anticonvulsant treatment may be indicated. The clinical role of neuroprotective substances in human TBI remains uncertain.[47, 48, 52, 111]

### Intravenous Fluid Resuscitation

From a CNS viewpoint, therapeutic aim in fluid resuscitation is to maintain sufficient CPP (CPP >60 mm Hg). Hemodynamic volume support is mandatory in hypotensive patients, especially in those displaying signs of hemorrhagic shock, noting that aggressive replacement therapy

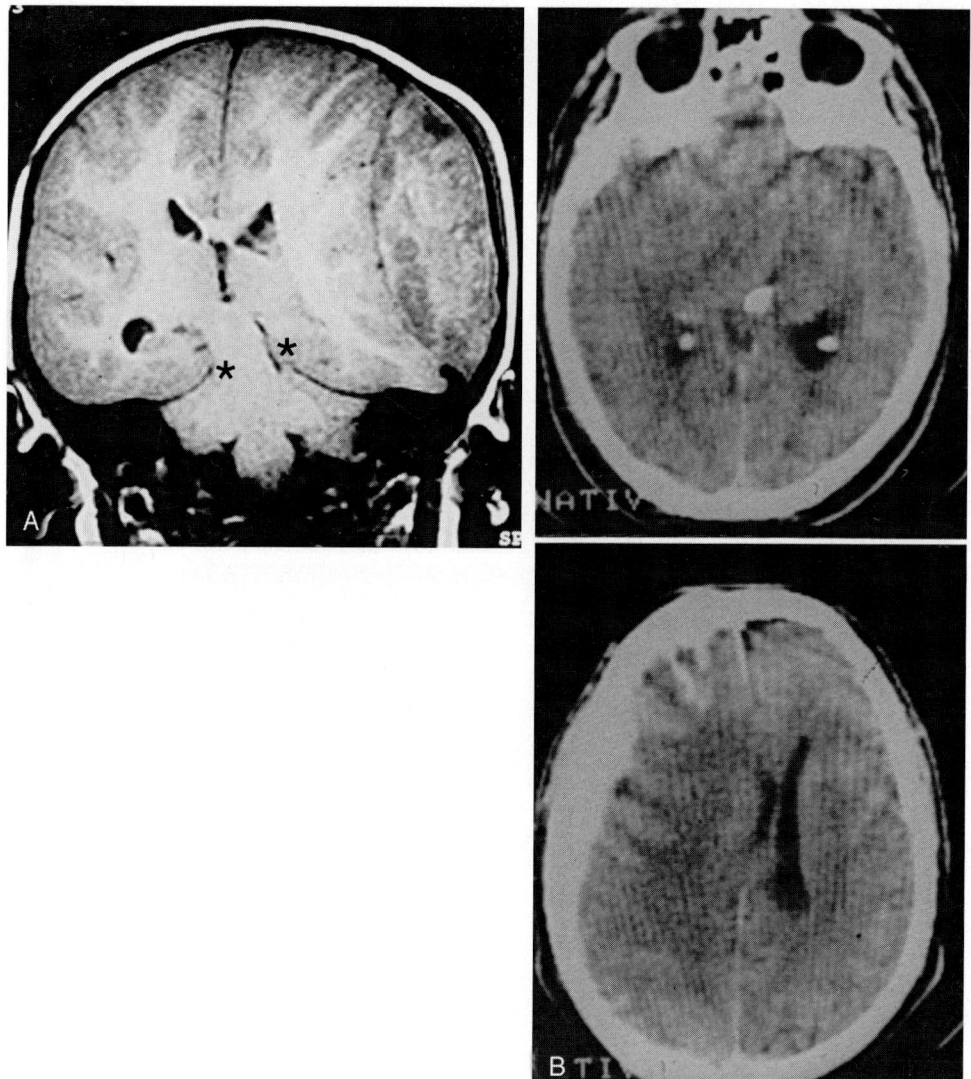

FIGURE 4–3 ■ *A–D,* Cranial computed tomography (CCT) best demonstrates intracranial mass lesions as an indication for immediate operative treatment, and today CCT is regarded as a standard emergency diagnostic procedure in head injury (HI), especially in acute unstable severe traumatic brain injury (TBI). Magnetic resonance imaging (MRI) often provides additional important information; however, several contraindications must be observed, such as the relatively long duration of the investigative procedure, ferromagnetic materials, indwelling ventilators, pressure bolts, and cardiac pacemakers. *A,* MRI (T₁, TR 730 TE 17) demonstrates typical, biconvex acute epidural hematoma (EDH) (Glasgow Coma Score 5) over the left hemisphere, partly hypointense and partly isointense and hyperintense to brain tissue, with compression of the brain and brain stem *(asterisk:* herniation of the medial temporal lobe); CT was not available at the time. After an emergency evacuation, the patient's postoperative course was uneventful. *B,* This CCT image demonstrates a typical, acute convex-concave–shaped SDH >1 cm over the right hemisphere of the brain (GCS score of 4). With the shift of the middle line, compression of the cerebral subdural hematoma (SDH) and interpeduncular cisterns is not visible. The outcome was fatal.

*Illustration continued on following page*

can aggravate hemorrhage from a systemic injury. When the loss of blood is substantial, transfusion with blood and blood products should be enacted as soon as possible, even though this may result in a coagulopathy and an increased risk of hemorrhage.[31, 36, 37] Isotonic solutions (e.g., Ringer's, NaCl 0.9%) and colloidal infusions are the first-choice agents, whereas hypotonic crystalloid solutions (e.g., glucose 5%, lactated Ringer's solution) are not recommended for neurosurgery patients because they increase brain edema.[1, 15, 112] If volume replacement alone does not produce a sufficient mean arterial blood pressure, the use of vasoactive substances is indicated; however, none of these agents is superior to others. Serum electrolyte abnormalities have not been shown to be statistically associated with the

outcome; however, these should be monitored carefully. Salt depletion of central origin, which may induce severe hyponatremia and seizures, frequently occurs secondary to traumatic hypothalmic lesions and diffuse axonal injury.[113]

Numerous experimental studies support the usefulness of hypertonic saline in improving the resuscitation of brain-injured animals; however, it is unclear why the administration of hypertonic saline solution has not become a standard practice in the resuscitation of severe TBI in humans.[55] Vassar et al. compared the use of 250 ml of lactated Ringer's solution with 7.5% saline solution in 6% dextran 70 (HSD) during the prehospital resuscitation of patients in whom systolic blood pressure was ≤100 mm Hg.[114] Although there was no overall difference in mortality, in

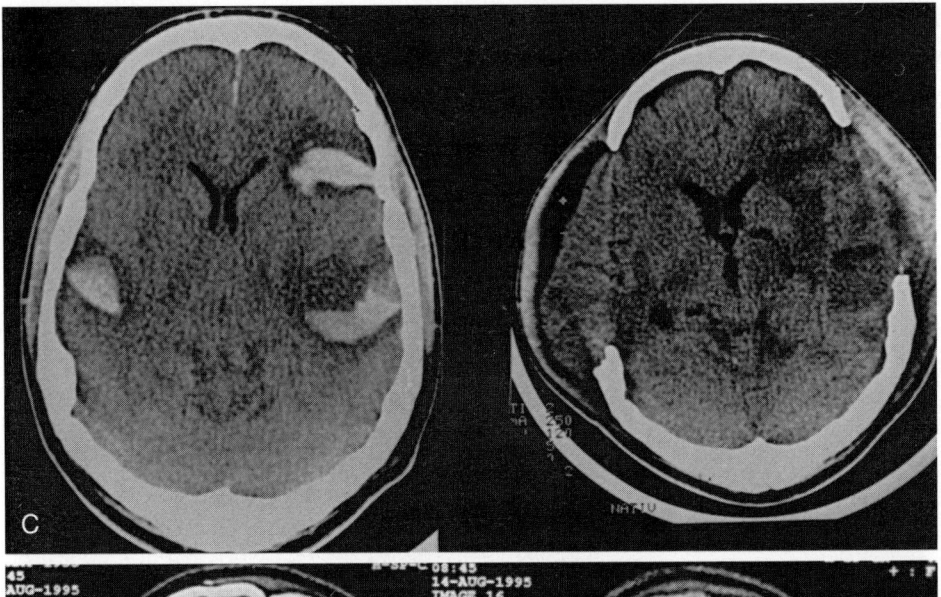

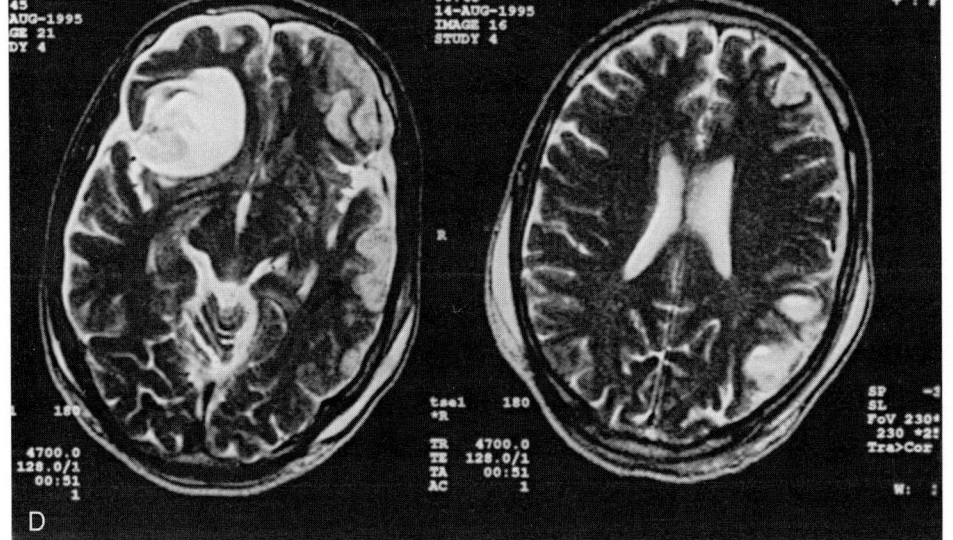

FIGURE 4–3 ■ *Continued C,* CCT in severe TBI shows bilateral hemorrhagic brain contusions (causing elevated intracranial pressure [ICP] with transtentorial herniation). The GCS score is 4. A major bilateral decompressive craniotomy was done with evacuation of clots greater than 30 ml bilaterally. The patient recovered over weeks. *D,* An MRI (T₂, TR4700, TE 128), which was performed on the second day after the patient's admission because of increased ICP (>25 mm Hg) and a deterioration in condition from a GCS score of 9 to that of 7, showed a right frontobasal contusional hemorrhage and left cortical contusion. A soft tissue hemorrhage is seen on the right (the region of primary impact). Immediate evacuation of the intracerebral clot was followed by normal ICP.

the subset of patients with severe HI (53 of 186 patients), 32% in the HSD group survived compared with 16% of the patients who received lactated Ringer's solution (*P* = .04). Furthermore, Vassar et al. compared the effects of 250 ml of 7.5% sodium chloride with and without 6% and 12% dextran 70 with those of 250 ml of lactated Ringer's solution for the prehospital resuscitation of hypotensive trauma patients.[115] The subgroup with severe HI and without severe anatomic injury seemed to benefit most from resuscitation with 7.5% saline solution. The salutary effects of hypertonic resuscitation might be caused by the rapid increase in systolic arterial pressure compared with a comparable volume of isotonic solution and probably also with a reduction in ICP.

## Sedation and Analgesia

An adequate degree of sedation and analgesia is recommended in intubated and ventilated patients and in combative patients. Benzodiazepines, morphine derivatives, phenothiazines, and propofol should be used as needed. Because

severe TBI results in stress and a rise in the serum catecholamines with a rise in heart rate, blood pressure, muscular tone, and raised bronchial secretions, clonidine and β-sympatholytic agents are particularly useful.[1, 7, 15, 17, 28, 29, 31, 56, 93, 116]

## Neuroprotective (Cerebroprotective) Medication[47, 111]

In contrast to a great deal of experimental evidence concerning the benefit of a various glutamate antagonists in models of focal cerebral ischemia, randomized double-blind clinical studies in humans with severe TBI have not revealed a significant benefit. Moreover, clinical studies employing antagonists or agonists to cholinergic or monoaminergic systems have also not been able to demonstrate the anticipated effectiveness.

Pyritinol is reported to activate cerebral glucose and protein metabolism, an effect attributed to the synaptic release of acetylcholine in the brain's cholinergic system in addition to effects on binding free radicals.[94–96]

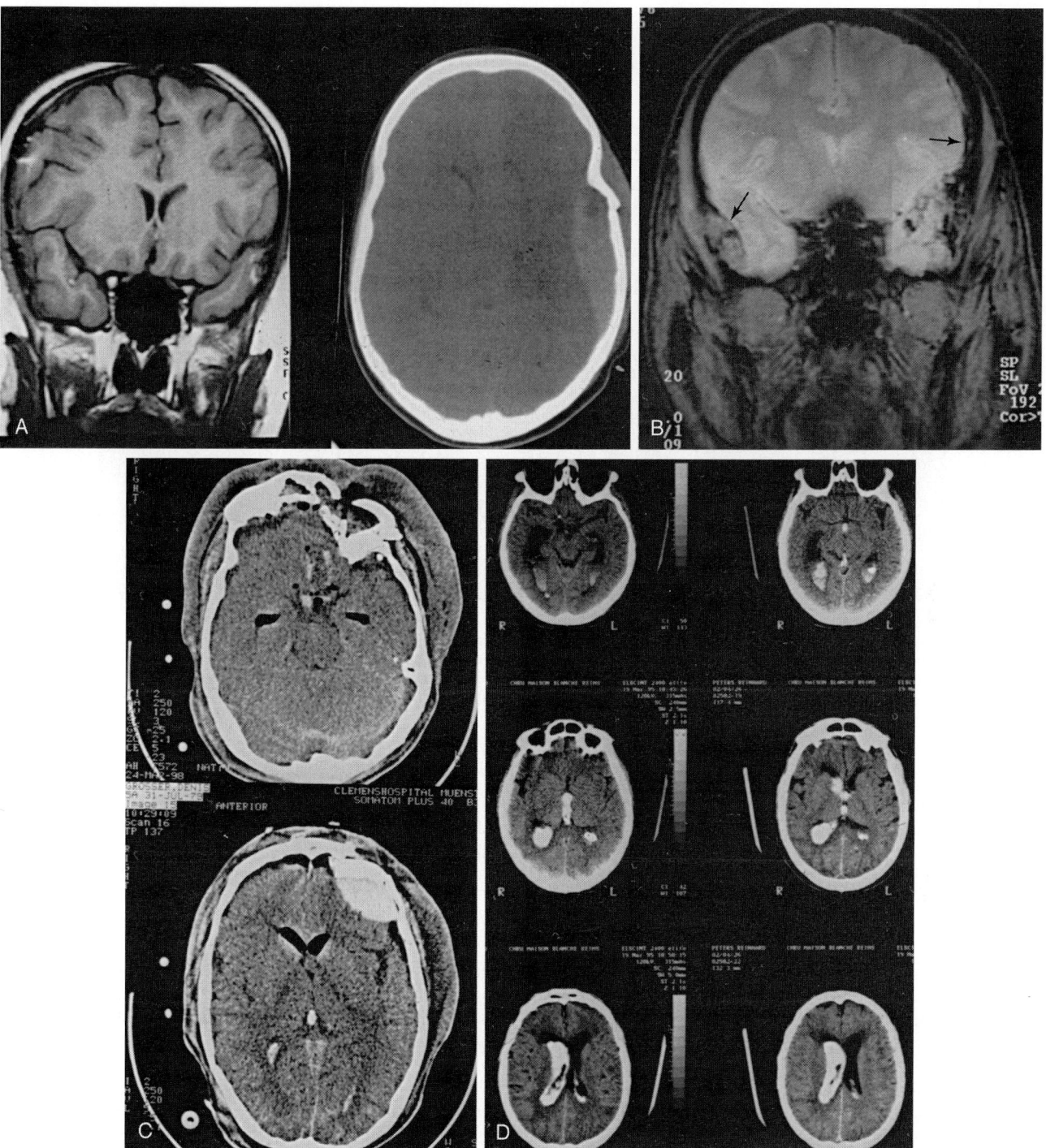

FIGURE 4–4 ■ Cranial computed tomography (CCT) and magnetic resonance imaging (MRI) controls are indicated in traumatic brain injury (TBI) in the event of progressive neurologic impairment (e.g., loss of consciousness and in conservatively treated intracranial hematomas and mass lesions as well as postoperatively). *A,* CCT (right) demonstrates a temporal fracture and EDH on the left side (GCS score of 12). An evacuation was done. Postoperative MRI control (T$_1$, coronal) *(left)* shows a left temporocortical contusion (left). *B,* An MRI (T$_1$, TR 800/TE 26) with an acute epidural hematoma (EDH) (temporobasal right side). Conservative treatment after an initial GSC of 7 *(closed arrow)* and subdural hematoma (SDH) *(open arrow)* over a left temporoparietal hemorrhagic contusion (contrecoup); the latter is much less evident in T$_1$-weighted images than on T$_2$-weighted images. The MRI scan was taken 5 days after TBI (GCS score of 12) because of deterioration to a GCS score of 8. Conservative treatment was given and ICP monitoring was maintained. The patient had a good recovery. *C,* CCT in TBI with brain contusion and a frontobasal skull fracture (left) on admission (GCS score of 6) (same patient as in Fig. 4–6 *B*). ICU and ICP monitoring were maintained. A CT control image, which was taken on the following day, shows an acute left frontobasal EDH. The ICP is higher than 25 mm Hg. Evacuation and decompression were performed. Reconstruction was postponed after the patient made a partial recovery (GCS score of 12). The patient's postoperative course was uneventful. *D,* The initial CCT (95.03.19) demonstrates an intraventricular hemorrhage in a 69-year-old orchestra conductor with a high-level paraplegic syndrome, 2 hours after a highway accident that involved his car overturning three times due to aquaplaning.

*Illustration continued on following page*

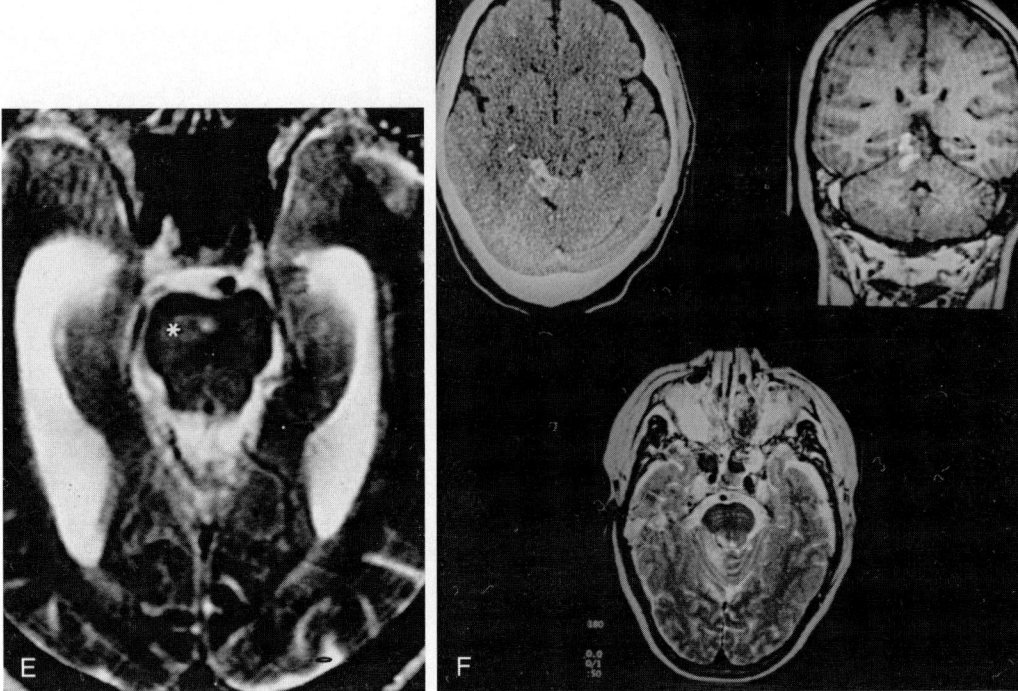

FIGURE 4–4 ■ *Continued E,* An MRI (95.06.25, TR 4700, TE 120) demonstrates a DAI lesion in the upper brain stem (*) after 3 months of conservative treatment because of neurologic and neuropsychological impairments secondary to traumatic diffuse axonal injury (DAI). After 2 weeks in a neurologic intensive care unit and 5 months' early rehabilitation, the patient recovered almost completely after 3 years (the conductor returned to the concert stage). *F,* CCT (axial, upper left) and MRI (T₁ coronal, upper right; T₂ axial, lower figure) show contusion hemorrhage with traumatic SAH and clots within the quadrigeminal cistern and the peduncle in a 63-year-old woman in the acute post-traumatic stage (GCS score of 6). The patient recovered completely after ICU and early rehabilitation treatment.

In the clinical trials with calcium antagonists in HI, there appears to be a trend toward a more favorable outcome in the subgroup of patients with traumatic subarachnoid hemorrhage (SAH) when treated with nimodipine.[47, 110, 117] Trials using other, newer calcium antagonists are currently in progress.

The free radical scavengers have not proved to be beneficial in clinical trials involving patients with severe TBI. Steroids, which were introduced 25 years ago in the medical management of TBI, have not shown a significant beneficial effect[47]; however, steroids are still used in two thirds of US centers for the treatment of TBI and new prospective clinical studies are on the way in all parts of the world despite numerous studies showing their lack of efficacy.[60] We stopped using steroids in TBI in 1979. The exception to this experience is one double-blind prospective randomized multicenter clinical trial,[118] which noted the efficacy of triamcinolone acetonide (Volon A soluble) administered within 4 hours of the trauma as producing a better outcome in patients with a GCS less than 9. In this group, a good recovery resulted in 34.8% compared with 21.3% of the placebo group and a mortality of 19.6% in the treated group compared with 38.3% in the control group.

Recent results of a prospective, randomized, multicenter trial in TBI involving 957 patients with a GCS score less than 9 (85%) and 163 patients with a GCS in the range of 9 to 12 to assess the efficacy of tirilazad mesylate, a novel aminosteroid, in HI does not show any differences in good recovery when this agent is used except (39% compared with 42%) and death (26% compared with 25% in the placebo group, respectively) in the subgroup of HI patients with SAH.[119]

## Antiseizure Prophylaxis

Seizures may cause an elevation of blood pressure, CPP, and ICP, with changes in oxygen delivery and neurotransmitter release. Following TBI, seizures may occur either immediately (within seconds and minutes after impact, i.e., *immediate fits*); within hours until the end of the first week *(early fits)* with most of them occurring in the first 24 hours (one third within the first hour, one third during the first day, one third during the first week after injury), or after the first week *(late fits).*

In patients with TBI, early fits occur more often in the first hours after injury, especially among patients with depressed and open frontotemporobasal skull fractures and loss of consciousness lasting for more than 24 hours and in those with GCS less than 10 and hemorrhagic brain contusion, often postoperatively. The incidence of seizures is 12 times higher than that of the general population within the first year after trauma.[120, 121]

During the acute phase of treatment of HI patients with a GCS higher than 10 at the risk of post-traumatic seizures (PTS), prophylactic anticonvulsants (phenobarbital, phenytoin, carbamazepine or sodium valproate) are indicated.[121] Anticonvulsant medicine has not been shown to prevent

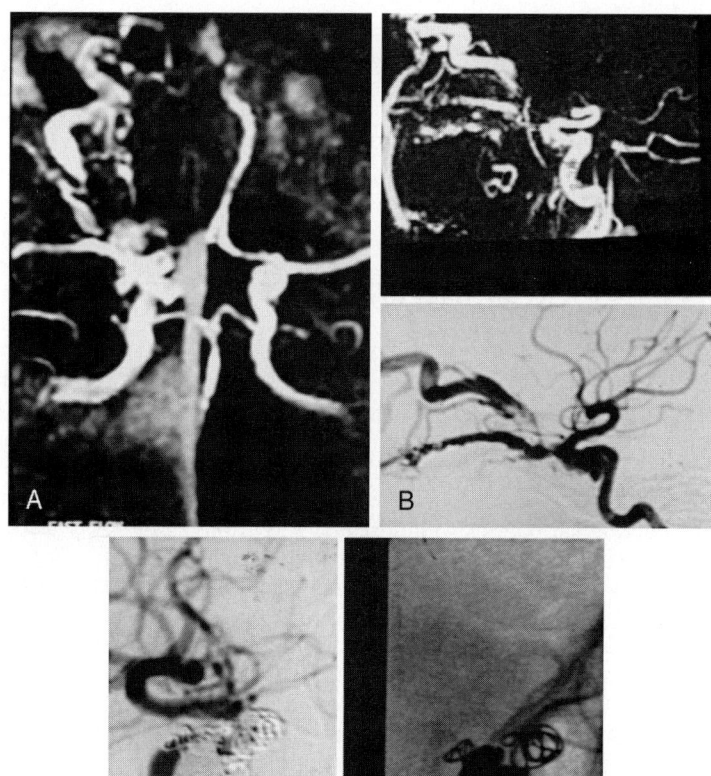

**FIGURE 4–5** ■ Magnetic resonance angiography has proved to be the most effective method of screening patients for vascular intracranial lesions in traumatic brain injury. Corresponding to the clinical syndrome of cavernous sinus, at the right side in a 51-year-old man after head trauma with skull-base fracture magnetic resonance imaging (MRI) (96.02.03) demonstrates the post-traumatic arteriovenous fistula in the cavernous sinus with increased flow in the right ophthalmic artery and ophthalmic vein. This is demonstrated in the axial *(A)* and sagittal MRI sections *(B)* and the sagittal conventional digital right ACI angiography *(C)*. Please note the complete occlusion after interventional endovascular occlusions of the fistula. (Courtesy of Prof. Dr. Kühne, Neuroradiologist, A.-Krupp-Hospital, Essen, Germany.) The recovery was uneventful.

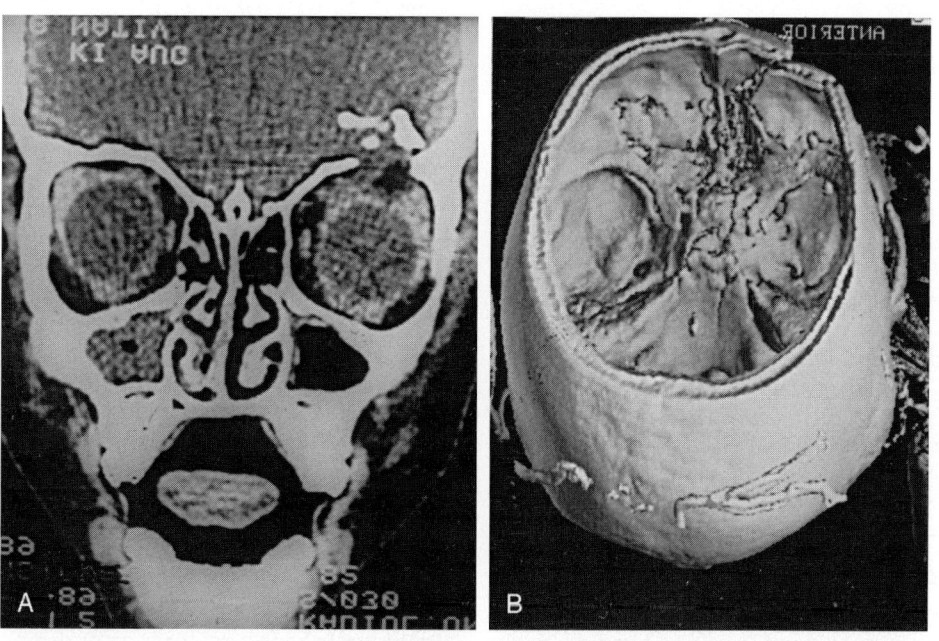

**FIGURE 4–6** ■ Thin-layer coronal images best demonstrate frontobasal skull fractures for the assessment of the extent and the severity of head injuries with regard to the most sparing and most effective operative interdisciplinary method of treatment. Spiral computed tomography also provides a spatial image for the reconstruction of dislocated structures (e.g., in injuries in the middle of the face and frontobasal injuries). *A,* Coronal computed tomography (CT) image in traumatic brain injury taken on admission demonstrating an orbital roof fracture with an intracerebral bone fragment (GCS score of 11). Neurosurgical removal and plastic covering of the repair after 1 week (GCS score of 14). The patient recovered completely. *B,* A spiral CT demonstrates best the three-dimensional situation of dislocated bone fragments in skull base fractures as shown (the same patient as shown in Fig. 4–4 *C*).

late PTS in severe TBI patients.[1] For acute treatment of PTS, we administer 10 to 40 mg/70 kg diazepam intravenously followed by clonazepam 1 to 3 ml slowly IV until the seizures are controlled and then carbamazepine or phenytoin are used for the following weeks, depending on the respective patient's neurologic and neuropsychological recovery (CRS 71) (see Table 4–1).

## MEDICAL MANAGEMENT OF RAISED INTRACRANIAL PRESSURE

There are insufficient data to support a standard treatment for ICP; however, mannitol and furosemide are recommended as diuretics that are effective in controlling elevated ICP after severe head injury. Limited data suggest that intermittent boluses with doses ranging from 0.25 g to 1 g/kg body weight may be more effective than the continuous infusion of mannitol. Hypovolemia should be avoided by fluid replacement, and serum osmolarity should be kept below 320 mOsm when there is concern for renal failure as recommended as options; furosemide (Lasix) 0.4 mg/kg or 10 mg IV has an additional potentiating effect. Glycerol and sorbitol are no longer recommended.[1, 15, 17, 57]

The use of barbiturates in the control of intracranial hypertension[19] may be considered in hemodynamically stable, salvageable patients with severe HI refractory to maximal medical and surgical ICP–lowering therapy. Pentobarbital, with a loading dose of 10 mg/kg over 30 minutes, 5 mg/kg every hour in 3 doses, followed by a maintenance infusion at 1 mg/kg/hr is used. Maximum reduction of cerebral metabolism and cerebral blood flow occurs when EEG burst suppression is induced.[122, 123]

### Antithrombotic Medication

Patients with severe head injuries are at high risk of deep vein thrombosis and pulmonary embolism as a result of the long-term immobilization in combination with trauma-induced pathologic changes in coagulation. For 4 years, all severe TBI patients at our clinic receive low-molecular-weight heparin (Inoxaparin 0.4 ml/day) with Clexane 40 to prevent deep vein thrombosis. We have not seen any increase in intracranial hemorrhage. There are no prospective randomized studies regarding these agents in TBI patients. Concerning the rare allergic reactions on low-molecular-weight heparin and in high-risk patients in Europe the recombinant hirudin (Desidurin INN 15 mg/day) may be preferable.[123, 124]

## HYPERVENTILATION

Current data suggest that routine and especially aggressive hyperventilation ($Pa_{CO_2}$ of 25 or lower), at one time a central principle of ICP management, should not be a first-line therapy,[43, 125] because in the first 24 hours after TBI the CBF is less than half that of normal individuals.[14, 51, 53, 55] Occasionally, hyperventilation may result in a local, paradoxical increase in CBF and inversal steal. However, hyperventilation remains the most rapid method to reduce increased ICP in patients in whom the cerebral vasculature is reactive by causing cerebral vasoconstriction with a subsequent reduction in CBF.[1, 17] In a prospective randomized study, Muizelaar (1991) found an improved outcome at 3 and 6 months when prophylactic hyperventilation was not used for 5 days after injury compared with when it was used.[40] Ventilatory parameters while on intermittent positive-pressure ventilation (IPPV) adjust ventilation to maintain $Pa_{O_2}$ less than 13 kPa (100 mm Hg) and $Pa_{CO_2}$ at 4 to 4.5 kPa (30 to 35 mm Hg). However, more intensive hyperventilation ($Pa_{CO_2} < 30$ mm Hg) may be indicated only in selected cases of elevated ICP refractory to mannitol and furosemide (Lasix).[1, 15, 41, 43, 45, 116, 122]

If we detect one or more hemorrhagic contusions in connection with deterioration in the patient's state of consciousness, or the neurologic findings, or deepening of coma stages, with a persistently raised ICP higher than 25 mm Hg despite therapy, these lesions are surgically removed immediately. The ICP values often drop by 20 mm Hg following measures. With extreme, bilateral swelling of the brain, consideration is given to the generous decompressive craniotomy over both halves of the brain down to the skull base (see Fig. 4–3C). However, these results require a prospective critical analysis.[117]

## HYPOTHERMIA

Moderate hypothermia of 32°C, which has been reported to limit postishemic neuronal damage, is used increasingly in connection with severe TBI.[19–22, 92] A controlled trial is now being undertaken in the US. With the aid of a venovenous extracorporeal heat exchanger, cooling of the brain is achieved within 6 hours and is maintained for 2 days without complications.

Over the years the classic management of elevated ICP[1, 9, 11, 12, 20] involved the head raised to 30 degrees, normotension, resuscitation, sedation, intubation, hyperventilation, if necessary paralyzed, and drug administration based on ICP values. This policy has now been switched to CPP therapy[1, 13, 14, 28–30, 44–46, 50, 55] with the head kept flat, normocapnia, CPP higher than 60 mm Hg, hypervolemia, vasopressors, and inotropism, and the avoidance of cardiovascular depressants. Finally, the "Lund concept" therapy,[31, 32, 116] focused at minimizing hydrostatic brain edema by physiologic conditions, has been introduced into clinical practice, albeit very slowly, and is now being used increasingly by us and by other centers.[5, 37] Guidelines for the Lund therapy of post-traumatic brain edema with raised ICP (not for patients with large traumatic SAH)[117, 122] are given in Table 4–3.

## NUTRITIONAL AND METABOLIC MANAGEMENT

The systemic response to severe TBI includes hypermetabolism, hypercatabolism, altered vascular permeability, increased hormone and cytokine release (shock reaction)

## TABLE 4–3 ■ "LUND CONCEPT"[113, 117] GUIDELINES FOR THE TREATMENT OF POST-TRAUMATIC BRAIN EDEMA WITH ICP >20 mm Hg

1. Surgical evacuation of hematomas and space occupying contusions
2. No extra head elevation (<15 degrees)
3. Ventilation to a $PaCO_2$ 30–33 mm Hg, $PaCO_2$ >98 mm Hg
4. Avoid hypothermia 38 degrees; accept hypothermia (34 degrees)
5. Avoid hypoglycemia (blood glucose <7 mmol/L)
6. Avoid hyponatremia; accept hypernatremia up to 150 mmol/L
7. Low-dose continuous thiopental (1–3 mg/kg/hr IV) best when cortical EEG pattern of burst suppression
8. Reduction of arterial hypertension (lowest CPP 50 mm Hg) $\beta_1$-antagonist (metoprolol 0.2–0.3 mg/kg/24hr IV) $\beta_2$-agonist (clonidine 0.5–1 µg/kg × 8 IV)
9. Aim at a dry and normovolemic patient. Negative fluid balance (furosemide), no antidiuretics
   Red blood cell transfusions (Hb >11g/dl)
   Albumin infusions (alb/s >40 g/L)
10. If ICP >25 mm Hg start a continuous dihydroergotamine infusion with maximum doses per day (d): d1:0.8; d2:0.6; d3:0.4; d4:0.2; d5:0.1 µg/kg/hr
11. Drainage of CSF via the intraventricular catheter
12. When life-threatening ICP values despite the measures 1–11 large decompressive bilateral craniotomy indicated

IV, intravenous; ICP, intracranial pressure; EEG, electroencephalogram; CPP, cerebral perfusion pressure.

with altered gastric voiding, mineral metabolism, glucose metabolism, and immune status. Nutritional support is targeted at providing an optimal environment for recovery with prevention of secondary systemic and brain lesions. Although the optimal route of nutrient supplementation is unknown, we prefer early jejunal or gastric enteral tube feeding, depending on the extent of gastric and intestinal atony, starting within 48 hours. This helps to prevent gastric ulcers, which may occur despite routine administration of cimetidine 200 to 400 mg/75 kg/day. Because of skull-base fractures and possible occlusion of the paranasal sinus, with secondary infections, enteral access is best established by the oral route instead of the nasal route. Feeding starts at 50 ml/hr and increases to 125 ml/hr of 25 to 35 kcal/kg/day (15% of calories as protein by the seventh day) in most critical TBI patients. In the event of hyperglycemia, which is not uncommon in severe TBI, insulin is administered to maintain the serum glucose below 200 mg/dl. During the acute post-traumatic phase when enteral feeding cannot be initiated, we start with parenteral nutrition bearing the risk of IV line infection. After two 2 to 3 weeks, critically ill patients are fed by way of a percutaneously positioned jejunal feeding tube, which they will continue as required for weeks or months, because swallowing disorders are common in these patients and they are at the risk of aspiration and pneumonia.[5, 8, 129]

## ACKNOWLEDGMENTS

*I want to express my gratitude to Mrs. Gabriele Kühling for her patience in preparing this manuscript and to Mr. Guy Jeffries for translating this paper.*

## REFERENCES

1. American Association of Neurological Surgeons and Brain Trauma Foundation: Guidelines for the Management of Severe Head Injury. New York: The Brain Trauma Foundation, 1995.
2. Ciba Foundation: Outcome of Severe Damage to the Central Nervous System. New York: Elsevier, 1975.
3. Narayan K, Wilberger JR Jr, Povlishock JT(eds): Neurotrauma. New York: McGraw-Hill, 1996.
4. Diemath HE, Sommerauer J, Wild KRH von (eds): Brain protection in severe head injury: Accident prevention, rescue systems and primary care. Proceedings of the Euroacademy for Multidisciplinary Neurotraumatology. Munich: W. Zuckschwerdt Verlag, 1996.
5. Wild KRH von: Pathophysiological principles and controversies in neurointensive care: Minimizing mortality in head injured patients by "The Lund Concept"? Proceedings of the Euroacademy for Multidisciplinary Neurotraumatology. Munich: W. Zuckschwerdt Verlag, 1997.
6. Wild K von, Janzik HH (eds): Neurologische Frührehabilitation. Munich: W. Zuckschwerdt Verlag, 1990.
7. Wild K von (ed): Spektrum der Neurorehabilitation. Munich: W. Zuckschwerdt Verlag, 1993.
8. Horn LJ, Zasler ND (eds): Medical Rehabilitation of Traumatic Brain Injury. Philadelphia: Hanley & Belfus, 1996.
9. Lawrence F, Marshall MD, Randall W, et al: The outcome with aggressive treatment in severe head injuries. J Neurosurg 50: 26, 1979.
10. Sharon A, Bowers BSN, Lawrence F, et al: Outcome in 200 consecutive cases of severe head injury treated in San Diego County: A prospective analysis. Neurosurgery 6: 237, 1980.
11. Jennett WB: Douglas Miller Memorial Lecture: Half a century of head injury care. In Diemath HE, Sommerauer J, Wild KRH von (eds): Brain Protection in Severe Head Injury. Munich: W. Zuckschwerdt Verlag, 1996, pp 1–7.
12. Bricolo A: Past, present and the future of neurotraumatology. J. Douglas Miller Memorial Lecture. In Wild KRH von (ed): Pathophysiological Principles and Controversies in Neurointensive Care. Munich: W. Zuckschwerdt Verlag, 1997, pp IX–XV.
13. Bullock R, Chesnut R, Clifton G, et al: Guidelines for the management of severe head injury. J Neurotrauma 13: 639, 1996.
14. Chesnut RM: Guidelines for the management of severe head injury: What we know and what we think we know. J Trauma 5:19, 1997.
15. Maas AIR, Dearden M, Teasdale GM, et al: EBIC: Guidelines for management of severe head injury in adults. Acta Neurochir (Wien) 139: 286, 1997.
16. Holbrook TL, Anderson JP, Sieber WJ, et al: Outcome after major trauma: Discharge and 6-month follow-up results from the trauma recovery project. J Trauma 45: 315, 1998.
17. Fernandez R, Firsching R, Lobato R, et al: Guidelines for treatment of head injury in adults. Zentralbl Neurochir 58: 72, 1997.
18. Ragnarrsson KT, Thomas JP, Zasler ND: Model systems of care for individuals with traumatic brain injury. J Head Trauma Rehabil 8:1 1993.
19. Spiss CK, Illievich UM: Hypothermie bei erhöhtem intrakraniellen Druck—Was ist gesichert? Zentralbl Neurochir 58: 133, 1997.
20. Marshall LF, Gautilley T, Klauber MR, et al: The outcome of severe closed head injury. J Neurosurg 75(Suppl): 528, 1991.
21. Shiozaki T, Sugimoto H, Taneda M, et al: Selection of severely head injured patients for mild hypothermia therapy. J Neurosurg 89: 206, 1998.
22. Piepgras A, Roth H, Schürer L, et al: Rapid active internal core cooling for induction of moderate hypothermia in head injury by use of an extracorporeal heat exchanger. Neurosurgery 42:311, 1998.
23. Servadei F: Prognostic factors in severely head injured adult patients with epidural haematomas. Acta Neurochir (Wien) 139:273, 1997.
24. Servadei F: Prognostic factors in severely head injured adult patients with acute subdural hematomas. Acta Neurochir (Wien) 139:279, 1997.
25. Ghajar J, Hariri RJ, Narayan RK, et al: Survey of critical care management of comatose, head-injured patients in the United States. Crit Care Med 23:560, 1995.
26. Guirguis EM, Hong C, Lin D, et al: Trauma outcome analysis of two Canadian centers using the TRISS method. J Trauma 30:426, 1990.
27. Prough DS, Lang J: Therapy of patients with head injuries: Key parameters for management. J Trauma 42:10, 1997.
28. Stocker R, Bernays R, Imhof HG: Monitoring and treatment of acute head injury. In Goris RJA, Trentz O (eds): The integrated approach to trauma care and emergency medicine 22. Berlin: Springer, 1995, pp 196–210.
29. Keidel M, Miller JD: Head trauma. In Neurological disorders:

Course and Treatment. Intensive Care in Neurology, Chapter 48. Academic Press, 1995, pp 1–14.

30. Rosner MJ: Pathophysiology and management of increased intracranial pressure. In Andrews BT (ed): Neurosurgical Intensive Care. New York: McGraw-Hill, 1993, pp 57–112.

31. Nordström CH, Messeter K, Sundbarg G, et al: Severe traumatic brain lesions in Sweden. 1: Aspects on management in non-neurosurgical clinics. Brain Injury 3:247, 1989.

32. Asgeirsson B, Grände PO, Nordström CH: A new therapy of posttrauma brain edema based on hemodynamic principles for brain volume regulation. Intensive Care Med 20:260, 1994.

33. Miller JD: Head injured and brain ischemia: Implications for therapy. Br J Anaesth 57:120, 1985.

34. Werner C: Hyperventilation bei erhöhtem intrakraniellen Druck-Möglichkeiten und Grenzen. Zentralbl Neurochir 58:118, 1997.

35. Prange HW, Nau R: Pharmakodynamik und Pharmakokinetik der Osmotherapeutika bei erhöhtem intrakraniellen Druck. Zentralbl Neurochir 58:127, 1997.

36. Dick W, Heene DL, Schuster HP (eds): Aktuelle Entwicklungen der Intensivmedizin Monitoring, Transfusion. Intensivmedizin und Notfallmedizin. 35 (Suppl 1), 1998.

37. Naredi S, Edén E, Zäll S, et al: A standardized neurosurgical/neurointensive therapy directed toward vasogenic edema after severe traumatic brain injury: Clinical results. Intensive Care Med 24:446, 1998.

38. Burchardi H, Wöbker G, Engelhardt W, et al: Beatmung. Zentralbl Neurochir 58:76, 1997.

39. Chesnut, RM, Marshall SB, Piek J, et al: Early and late systemic hypotension as frequent and fundamental source of cerebral ischemia following severe brain injury in the Traumatic Coma Data Bank. Acta Neurochir 59 (Suppl):121, 1993.

40. Muizelaar JP, Marmarou A, Ward JD, et al: Adverse effects of prolonged hyperventilation in patients with severe head injury: A randomized clinical trial. J Neurosurg 75:731, 1991.

41. Piek J, Jantzen JP, et al: Leitlinien zur Primärversorgung von Patienten mit Schädel-Hirntrauma. Arbeitsgemeinschaft Intensivmedizin und Neurotraumatology der DGNC, Wissenschaftlicher Arbeitskreis Neuroanästhesie der DGAI. Zentralbl Neurochir 58:13, 1997.

42. Lundberg N: Continuous recording and control of ventricular fluid pressure in neurosurgical practice. Thesis. Munksgaard, Copenhagen, 1960.

43. Marion, DW, Firlik A, McLaughlin MR: Hyperventilation therapy for severe traumatic brain injury. New Horiz 3:439, 1995.

44. Andrews PJD: What is optimal perfusion pressure after brain injury: A review of evidence with an emphasis on arterial pressure. Acta Anaesth Scand 39:112, 1995.

45. Rosner MJ, Rosner SD, Johnson AH: Cerebral perfusion pressure: Management protocol and clinical results. J Neurosurg 83:949, 1995.

46. Marmarou A, Bullock R, Young HF, et al: The contribution of raised ICP and hypotension to reduced cerebral perfusion pressure in severe brain injury. In Nagai H, Kamiya K, Ishii S (eds): Intracranial Pressure IX. Berlin: Springer, 1994, pp 302–304.

47. Teasdale GM, Graham DI: Craniocerebral trauma: Protection and retrieval of the neuronal population after injury. Neurosurgery 43:723, 1998.

48. Stein DG: Brain damage and recovery. In Bloom F (ed): Progress in Brain Research. New York: Elsevier Science, 1994, pp 203–211.

49. Baethman A, Jantzen JP, Piek J, et al: Physiologie und Pathophysiologie des intrakraniellen Drucks. Anasthesiol Intensivmed Notfallmed Schmerzther 7/8:357, 1997.

50. Marmarou A, Bandoh K, Yoshihara M, et al: Measurement of vascular reactivity in head injured patients. Acta Neurochir 59 (Suppl):18, 1993.

51. Unterberg AW, Schneider GH, Lanksch WR (eds): Monitoring of cerebral blood flow and metabolism in intensive care. Acta Neurochir Suppl 59, 1993.

52. Boyeson MG, Jones JL: Theoretical mechanisms of brain plasticity and therapeutic implication. In Horn LJ, Zasler ND (eds): Medical Rehabilitation of Traumatic Brain Injury. Philadelphia: Hanley & Belfus, 1996, pp 77–102.

53. Bouma GJ, Muizelaar JP, Bandoh K, et al: Blood pressure and intracranial pressure volume dynamics in severe head injury: Relationship with cerebral blood flow. J Neurosurg 77:15, 1992.

54. Chesnut RM: Secondary brain insults after head injury: Clinical perspectives. New Horiz 3:366, 1995.

55. Chesnut RM: Avoidance of hypotension: Condition sine qua non of successful severe head-injured management. J Trauma 42:4, 1997.

56. Piek J, Chesnut RM, Marshall LF, et al: Extracranial complications of severe head injury. J Neurosurg 77:901, 1992.

57. Brooks DN, Truelle JL, et al: EBIS Document: Evaluation of traumatic brain injury. Document réalisé avec la collaboration du groupe de travail EBIS et le concours de la Direction Générale de la Science, de la Recherche et du Développement—DG XII—de la Commission de L'Union Européenne (Contrat M.R. 4 10201), Vol 1, 30 pp.

58. Teasdale G, Jennett WB: Assessment of coma and impaired consciousness: A practical scale. Lancet ii;81, 1974.

59. Miller JD: Minor, moderate and severe head injury. Neurosurg Rev 9:135, 1986.

60. Wild KRH von, Terwey S: Is mild traumatic brain injury (MTBI) a mistakable diagnosis? Lessons from clinical practice and a European Federation of Neurological Societies (EFNS) inquiry. Eur J Neurol 5 (Suppl 3): 235, 1998.

61. Janzik HH, Wild KRH von, Hömberg V: Gutachten zu den Standards der neurologischen Rehabilitation unter besonderer Berücksichtigung der Frührehabilitation und der Nachsorge und Verwirklichungsmöglichkeiten im bestehenden Versicherungssystem. In Ministerium für Arbeit, Gesundheit und Soziales des Landes NRW (eds): Hilfen zur Versorgung Schädel-Hirnverletzter. Ahlen: Partner Druck, 1992.

62. Kossmann T, Stover JF, Trentz O: Brain injury with multiple trauma. In Diemath HE, Sommerauer J, Wild KRH von (eds): Brain Protection in Severe Brain Injury. Munich: W. Zuckschwerdt Verlag, 1996, pp 52–59.

63. Firsching W, Woischneck D: Cooperative study: Multiple injuries. Zentralbl Neurochir 59:195, 1998.

64. Pakos P, Terhag D, Ernestus RI, et al: Management of multiple injuries with fractures of pelvis and extremities. Zentralbl Neurochir 59:195, 1998.

65. Moskopp D, Cortbus F, Terhaag D, et al: Thoracoabdominal injuries: Their influence on the early outcome in multiple injuries. Zentralbl Neurochir 59:196, 1998.

66. Pagni CA, Massaro F: Concomitant craniocerebral and vertebromedullary injuries: Analysis of 121 cases. Acta Neurochir 111:1, 1991.

67. Karimi-Nejad A, Wenzel SC: Timing of extracranial surgery in severely head injured patients. In Diemath HE, Sommerauer J, Wild KRH von (eds): Brain Protection in Severe Head Injury. Munich: Zuckschwerdt Verlag, 1996, pp 86–94.

68. Neugebauer E, Bouillon B: Scoring systems: To what purpose? Unfallchirurg 97:172, 1994.

69. Regel G, Pape HC, Pohlemann T, et al: Score systems—an instrument of decision making in trauma care. Unfallchirurg 97:211, 1994.

70. Baker SP, O'Neill B, Haddon W, et al: The Injury Serverity Score: A method for describing patients with multiple injuries and evaluating emergency care. J Trauma 15:187, 1994.

71. Voss A, Blumenthal W, Wild KRH von, et al: Standards der neurologisch-neurochirurgischen Frührehabilitation. In Wild K von (ed): Spektrum der Neurorehabilitation. Munich: W. Zuckschwerdt Verlag, 1993, pp 112–120.

72. Spittler JF, Langenstein H, Calabrese P: Die Quantifizierung krankhafter Bewußtseinsstörungen. Anasthesiol Intensivmed Notfallmed Schmerzther 28:213, 1993.

73. Oestern HJ, Kabus K: Comparison of different trauma scoring systems: A review. Unfallchirurg 97:177, 1994.

74. Varney M, Gross-Weege W, Becker H: Followup of severely injured patients with scoring systems on the intensive care unit. Unfallchirurg 97:205, 1994.

75. Champion HR, Sacco WJ, Copes, WS, et al: A revision of trauma score. J Trauma 29:632, 1989.

76. Copes WS, Champion HR, Sacci WJ, et al: Progress in characterizing anatomic injury. J Trauma 30:1200, 1990.

77. Committee of Medical Aspects of Automotive Safety: Rating the severity of tissue damage. I: The Abbreviated Scale. JAMA 215:277, 1971.

78. Committee on Injury Scaling: Abbreviated Injury Scale 1990 Revision. Des Plaines, IL: Association for the Advancement of Automovement Medicine, 1990.

79. Baker SP, O'Neill B, Haddon W, et al: The Injury Severity Score: A method for describing patients with multiple injuries and evaluating emergency care. J Trauma 14:187, 1974.

80. Bardt TF, Sarrafzadeh AS, Schneider GH, et al: Monitoring of patients with traumatic brain injury: Cerebral hypoxia is frequent despite sufficient ICP and CPP therapy. Zentralbl Neurochir 59:189, 1998.

81. Wild K von, et al: Zur Indikation, Technik und praktischer Bedeutung des Monitoring bei Patienten mit Schädelhirntraumen. In Wieck HH (ed): Neurotraumatologie. Stuttgart: Thieme Verlag, 1980, pp 193–196.

82. Sabel H, Simons P, Wild K von: Neuromonitoring unter intensivmedizinischen Bedingungen. In Wild K von, Janzik HH (eds): Neurologische Frührehabilitation. Munich: W. Zuckschwerdt-Verlag, 1990, pp 110–114.

83. Chan KH, Dearden NM, Miller JD: Multimodality monitoring as a guide to treatment of intracranial hypertension after severe brain injury. Neurosurgery 32:547, 1993.

84. Santbrink H van, Maas AIR, Avezaat CJJ: Continuous monitoring of partial pressure of brain tissue oxygen in patients with severe head injury. Neurosurgery 38:21, 1996.

85. Dings J, Meixensberger J, Amschler B, et al: Brain tissue $pO_2$ in relation to cerebral perfusion pressure, TCD findings and TDC-$CO_2$ reactivity after severe head injury. Acta Neurochir (Wien) 138:425, 1996.

86. Unterberg A, Kiening K, Barth T, et al: Monitoring of cerebral oxygenation. In Diemath HE, Sommerauer J, Wild KRH von (eds): Brain protection in severe brain injury. Munich: W. Zuckschwerdt Verlag, 1996, pp 125–129.

87. Ungerstedt U, Nordström CH: Microdialysis monitoring of brain biochemistry during neurointensive care. In Wild K von (ed): Pathophysiological Principles and Controversies in Neurointensive Care. Munich: W. Zuckschwerdt Verlag, 1997, pp 83–90.

88. Miller JD: ICP monitoring: Current status and future directions. Acta Neurochir (Wien) 85:80, 1997.

89. Nuwer MR: Electroencephalograms and evoked potentials: Monitoring cerebral function in the neurosurgical intensive care unit. Neurosurg Clin N Am 5:647, 1994.

90. Greenberg RP, Becker DM, Miller JD, et al: Evaluation of brain function in severe head trauma with multimodality evoked potentials. II: Localization of brain dysfunction and correlation with posttraumatic neurologic conditions. J Neurosurg 47:163, 1977.

91. Gütling E, Gonser A, Imhof HG, et al: EEG reactivity in the prognosis of severe head injury. Neurology 45:915, 1995.

92. Kochs E: Electrophysiological monitoring and mild hyperthermia. J Neurosurg Anesthesiol 7:222, 1995.

93. Wöbker G, Bock WJ: Stellenwert der Barbiturate bei erhöhtem intrakraniellen Druck. Zentralbl Neurochir 58:122, 1997.

94. Wild K von: Encephalotropic drugs in neurology and neurosurgery. In Herrmann WM (ed): Higher Nervous Functions. Wiesbaden; Vieweg, 1988, pp 131–160.

95. Wild K von, Dolce C: Pathophysiological aspects concerning the treatment of apallic syndrome. J Neurol 213:143, 1976.

96. Wild K von, Simons P, Schoeppner H: Effect of pyritinol on EEG and SSEP in comatose patients in the acute phase of intensive care therapy. Pharmopsychiatry 25:157, 1992.

97. Overgaard J, Christensen S, Hvid-Hansen O, et al: Prognosis after head injury based on early clinical examination. Lancet ii:631, 1973.

98. Aaslid R, Huber P, Nornes H: Evaluation of cerebrovascular spasm with transcranial Doppler ultrasound. J Neurosurg 60:37, 1984.

99. Markwalder ThM, Grolimund P, Seiler R, et al: Depency of blood flow velocity in the middle cerebral artery on end-tidal carbon dioxide partial pressure: A transcranial ultrasound Doppler study. J Cereb Blood Flow Metab 4:368, 1984.

100. Czosnyka M, Matta BF, Smielewski P, et al: Cerebral perfusion pressure in head-injured patients: A noninvasive assessment using transcranial Doppler ultrasonography. J Neurosurg 88:802, 1998.

101. Smielewski P, Kirkpatrick P, Minhas P, et al: Can cerebrovascular reactivity be measured with near-infrared spectroscopy? Stroke 26 26:2285, 1995.

102. Lang EW: Target therapy for posttraumatic brain swelling with induced hypertension. In Wild K von (ed): Pathophysiological principles and Controversies in Neurointensive Care. Munich: W. Zuckschwerdt Verlag, 1997, pp 114–122.

103. Marshall LF, Marshall SB, Klauber MR, et al: A new classification of head injury based on computerized tomography. The Trauma Coma Data Bank. J Neurosurg (Suppl) 75:S14, 1991.

104. Mendelow AD, Teasdale G, Jennett B, et al: Risks of intracranial haematomas in head injured adults. BMJ 287(6400):1173, 1983.

105. Lobato RD, Rivas JJ, Gomez PA: Head-injured patients who talk and deteriorate into coma: Analysis of 211 cases studied with computed tomography. J Neurosurg 75:256, 1991.

106. Lindell RG: Imaging of closed head injury. Radiology 191:1, 1994.

107. Wild KRH von: Magnetic resonance imaging (MRI) in acute traumatic brain injury (TBI). In Diemath HE, Sommerauer J, Wild KRH von (eds): Brain Protection in Severe Head Injury. Munich: W. Zuckschwerdt Verlag, 1996, pp 74–85.

108. Cecil KM, Hills EC, Sandel ME, et al: Proton magnetic resonance spectroscopy for detection of axonal injury in the splenium of the corpus callosum of brain-injured patients. J Neurosurg 88:795, 1998.

109. Firsching R, Woischneck D, Diedrich M, et al: Early magnetic resonance imaging of brain stem lesion after severe head injury. J Neurosurg 89:707, 1998.

110. Harders A, Kakarieka A, Braakman R, the German SHT Study Group: Traumatic subarachnoid hemorrhage and its treatment with nimodipine. J Neurosurg 85: 82, 1996.

111. Bollock R: Opportunities for neuroprotective drugs in clinical management of head injury. J Emerg Med 11: 23, 1993.

112. Berger S, Schürer L, Härtl R, et al: Reduction of posttraumatic intracranial hypertension by hypertonic/hyperoncotic saline/dextran and hypertonic mannitol. Neurosurgery 37: 98, 1995.

113. Berendes E, Walter M, Cullen P, et al: Secretion of brain natriuretic peptide in patients with aneurysmal subarachnoid haemorrhage. Lancet 349: 245, 1997.

114. Vassar MJ, Perry CA, Gannaway WL, et al: 7.5% sodium chloride/dextran for resuscitation of trauma patients undergoing helicopter transport. Arch Surg 126: 1065, 1991.

115. Vassar MJ, Fischer RP, O'Brian PE, et al: A multicenter trial for resuscitation of injured patients with 7.5% sodium chloride: The effect of added dextran 70. The multicenter Group for Study of Hypertonic Saline in Trauma Patients. Arch Surg 128: 1003, 1993.

116. Nordström CH, Grände PO: The "Lund concept" in neurointensive care—clinical results. In Wild KRH von (ed): Pathophysiological Principles and Controversies in Neurointensive Care. Munich: W. Zuckschwerdt Verlag, 1997, pp 67–74.

117. Kakarieka A (ed): Traumatic Subarachnoid Haemorrhage. Berlin: Springer Verlag, 1997.

118. Grumme T, Baethmann A, Kolodziejczyk D, et al: Treatment of patients with severe head injury by triamcinolone: A prospective, controlled multicenter clinical trial of 396 cases. Res Exp Med (Berl) 2995: 217, 1995.

119. Marshall LF, Maas AIR, Bowers Marshall S, et al: A multicenter trial on the efficacy of using tirilazad mesylate in cases of head injury. J Neurosurg 89: 519, 1998.

120. Pagni CA, Lo Russo GM, Bana P, et al: Posttraumatic epilepsy. In Wild K von (ed): Spektrum der Neuro-rehabilitation. Munich: W. Zuckschwerdt Verlag, 1993, pp 71–78.

121. Wild K von: Entstehungsbedingungen und Möglichkeiten antikonvulsiver Prophylaxe der post-traumatischen Epilepsie aus neurochirurgischer Sicht. In Ritz A (ed): Forum der Epilepsien. medicin + pharmacie. Hamburg: Dr. Werner Rudat & Co, 1993, pp 45–59.

122. Grände PO, Nordström CH: Treatment of increased ICP in severe head-injured patients. In Wild KRH von (ed): Pathophysiological Principle and Controversies in Neurointensive Care. Munich: W. Zuckschwerdt Verlag, 1997, pp 123–128.

123. Erikson BL, Wille-Jorgensen P, Kälebo P, et al: A comparison of recombinant hirudin with a low-molecular-weight heparin to prevent thromboembolic complications after total hip replacement. N Engl J Med 337: 1329, 1997.

124. Erikson BL, Ekman S, Lindbratt S, et al: Prevention of thromboembolism with use of recombinant hirudin: Results of a double-blind study, multicenter trial comparing the efficacy of desirudin (REVASC) with that of unfractionated heparin in patients having a total hip replacement. J Bone Joint Surg 79-A: 326, 1997.

125. Werner C: Hyperventilation bei erhöhtem intrakraniellen Druck - Möglichkeiten und Grenzen. Zentralbl Neurochir 58: 118, 1997.

126. Hadley MN: Hypermetabolism following head trauma: Nutritional conservations. In Barrow DL (ed): Complications and Sequelae of Head Injury. Park Ridge, IL: AANS Publications Committee, 1992, pp 151–168.

127. Young B, Ott L: Nutritional and metabolic management of head injured patient. In Narayan RK, Wilberger JE Jr, Povlishock JT (eds): Neurotrauma. New York: McGraw-Hill, 1996, pp 345–363.

128. Heylen R, De Deyne C, De Jongh R, et al: Legal aspects of the

withdrawal of support in the ventilated unconscious patient in an intensive care unit. Eur J Anaesthesiol 15 (Suppl 17): 105, 1998.

129. Wild KRH von, Hoffmann B: Early neurological-neurosurgical rehabilitation after coma. Eur J Anaesthesiol 15 (Suppl 17): 97, 1998.

130. Teasdale G, Murray G, Parker L, et al: Adding up the Glasgow coma scale. Acta Neurochir 28 (Suppl): 13, 1979.

131. Stoll W: Operative Versorgung frontobasaler Verletzungen (inklusive Orbita) durch den HNO-Chirurgen. Otorhinolaryngol (Suppl): 287, 1993.

132. Wild K von: Fronto basale Verletzungen—Eine Einführung in das Thema. In Hausamen JE, Schmelzeisen R (eds): Traumatologie der Schädelbasis. Reinbeck: Einhorn Presse Verlag, 1996, pp 16–26.

133. Katayama Y, Tsubokawa T, Kinoshita K, et al: Intraparenchymal blood-fluid levels in traumatic intracerebral haematomas. Neuroradiology 34: 381, 1992.

134. Wild K von, Samii M, Moringlane JR, et al: Zur Indikation, Technik und praktischer Bedeutung des Monitoring bei Patienten mit Schädelhirntraumen. In Wieck HH (ed): Neurotraumatologie. Stuttgart: Thieme Verlag, 1980, pp 193–196.

135. Knaus WA, Draper EA, Wagner DP, et al: APACHE II: A severity of disease classification system. Crit Care Med 13: 818, 1985.

136. Waydhas D, Nast-Kolb S, Ruchholtz S, et al: Praktische und theorethische Grenzen von Score-systemen. Unfallchirurg 97: 185, 1994.

137. Wild K von: Neurotraumatologische Frührehabilitation. In Frommelt P, Grötzbach H (eds): Neurorehabilitation. Berlin: Blackwell Wissenschafts-Verlag, 1998, pp 419–433.

138. Kemper B, Wild K von: Neurpsychologische Aspekte in der Frührehabilitation schädelhirnverletzter Patientin. In Frommelt P, Grötzbach H (eds): Neurorehabilitation. Berlin: Blackwell Wissenschafts-Verlag, 1998, pp 434–439.

# Surgical Management of Severe Closed Head Injury in Adults

■ DANIEL F. KELLY, DUNCAN Q. McBRIDE, and DONALD P. BECKER

Closed head injury, broadly defined, encompasses all nonmissile head injuries, including those associated with simple or compound skull fractures. *Severe head injury* usually refers to an initial postresuscitation Glasgow Coma Scale (GCS) of 8 or less or a subsequent deterioration to a GCS of 8 or less.[31, 103] Patients with a GCS of 7 or less are in coma, defined by the International Coma Data Bank as an inability to obey commands, utter words, or open eyes; only a portion of patients with a GCS of 8 fulfill these criteria for coma.[51]

Fewer than half of patients who sustain a severe nonpenetrating head injury require craniotomy for evacuation of a mass lesion.[1, 5, 74] In the Traumatic Coma Data Bank (TCDB), comprising 746 severe head injury victims, 37% of patients underwent surgery for removal of an epidural (EDH), subdural (SDH), or intracerebral hematoma (ICH).[64] Diffuse brain injury often accompanies focal mass lesions in the severely brain-injured patient and has a significant impact on outcome. Secondary insults such as hypotension, hypoxia, raised intracranial pressure (ICP), seizures, and hyperthermia can further hinder recovery of the injured brain. Consequently, aggressive medical intervention aimed at preventing secondary injury and optimizing conditions for brain recovery plays a major role in managing patients with severe head injury. This chapter focuses on both surgical and perioperative critical care aspects of managing such patients.

## EPIDEMIOLOGY

In the United States, trauma is the leading cause of death in people younger than 45 years of age. In older age groups, it is also a major cause of death and disability, accounting for approximately 30,000 deaths annually in people aged 65 years or older.[4] It is estimated that approximately half of the 148,000 injury-related deaths that occurred in the United States in 1990 involved a serious brain injury, which was primarily responsible for the patient's death.[54] Gennarelli and associates,[36] in assessing over 49,000 trauma victims from 95 trauma centers in the United States, found that the overall mortality rate was three times

higher in patients with head injury compared with those who did not sustain cranial trauma. In the head-injured patients, the cause of death was attributed to the brain injury in 67.8% of patients, to extracranial injuries in 6.6% of patients, and to both cranial and extracranial trauma in 25.6% of patients.

Approximately 500,000 head injuries requiring admission to a hospital occur annually in the United States; 50,000 of these patients die before reaching a medical facility. Of the 450,000 initial survivors, approximately 80% sustain minor injuries (GCS 13 to 15), 10% have moderate injuries (GCS 9 to 12), and 10% have severe brain injuries (GCS 3 to 8).[54] Given current survival and outcome data, another 15,000 to 20,000 of these patients will die after reaching the hospital, and approximately 50,000 will have some form of permanent disability.[64, 89]

Although men and women of all ages are affected, severe closed head injury is predominantly a disease of young adult men. The peak incidence in the United States is in the age range of 15 to 24 years.[54] In the TCDB cohort, 77% of patients were male, with a mean age of approximately 30 years.[64] The most common mechanism of closed head injury in the United States is motor vehicle accidents, followed by falls, pedestrian-vehicular accidents, and assaults. Concomitant extracranial trauma, including facial, thoracic, abdominal, and orthopedic injuries, compounds up to 70% of severe closed head injuries; 5% to 10% of patients also sustain a cervical spine injury.[38, 74, 110] Alcohol intoxication is another compounding factor in up to 72% of traumatic brain injuries.[54]

## INITIAL PATIENT ASSESSMENT AND STABILIZATION

Stabilization of the head injury victim ideally begins at the site of the accident by emergency medical personnel. Their tasks are numerous and vital; they include securing the patient's airway, providing adequate oxygenation, initiating fluid resuscitation, stabilizing the cervical and thoracolumbar spine, assessing the patient's level of consciousness, obtaining an account of the accident, and providing safe and rapid transport to a qualified medical facility.

Once in hospital, the initial evaluation and care of the patient should proceed in an expedient and systematic manner, with diagnostic and therapeutic maneuvers proceeding simultaneously. This approach is best facilitated by a designated trauma team, which has become the standard of care for acute management of the trauma victim. Given that many severely brain-injured patients have sustained multiple injuries, a thorough but brief general examination is mandatory. Life-threatening insults, such as tension pneumothorax, cardiac tamponade, or major vascular injuries with hypovolemic shock, take precedence over neurologic injury and are addressed immediately.

## Airway Management

Hypoxia during resuscitation was documented in approximately 46% of patients in the TCDB cohort and was significantly associated with poor outcome.[17] Early establishment of a patent airway in the patient with severe head injury is a primary means of preventing cerebral ischemia. All patients with a GCS of 8 or less require intubation and assisted ventilation as a result of their depressed level of consciousness. Some patients have sustained additional injuries that further impair oxygenation, such as flail chest, hemothorax or pneumothorax, upper airway trauma, and cervical spinal cord injury. Intoxication with alcohol or other central nervous system depressants also diminishes protective airway reflexes. The establishment of a secure airway is especially important when patients leave the emergency department for diagnostic procedures such as computed tomography (CT), or when they are transported to the operating room.

Most head injury victims can be safely intubated by the orotracheal route with in-line stabilization of the cervical spine. This method of intubation with strict maintenance of a neutral head position and slight or no axial traction causes minimal movement of the potentially unstable cervical spine and has not been associated with new neurologic deficit.[58, 88, 102] Oral endotracheal intubation in the head-injured patient is best facilitated by rapid-sequence induction, using thiopental, 3 to 5 mg/kg, and succinylcholine, 1 to 2 mg/kg.[22, 102] Despite the risk of transiently aggravating intracranial hypertension with the use of succinylcholine, this method of intubation appears to be the safest for most acutely brain-injured patients.[22, 63] In patients with major facial or upper airway trauma, cricothyroidotomy may be required, although the complication rate in the emergency setting may be as high as 32%.[22] The nasotracheal route of intubation is contraindicated in patients with possible anterior cranial base fractures, requires considerably more experience and time, and has a lower success rate and a higher complication rate than orotracheal intubation.[22] Once the patient is intubated, providing adequate sedation and paralysis is essential; "bucking" by the patient on the endotracheal tube and excessive motor activity are to be strictly prevented. Narcotic sedation with morphine or fentanyl is effective in averting this activity; muscle paralysis with vecuronium or pancuronium can be added if motor activity persists.

## Neurologic Assessment

The initial neurologic examination in the severely brain-injured patient is necessarily abbreviated and should focus on the level of consciousness, using the GCS and evaluation of the patient's pupillary light reflexes, extraocular eye movements, lower brain stem reflexes, when appropriate, and asymmetries of the motor examination.[103] This initial neurologic survey, along with examination of the head, neck, and thoracolumbar spine, should take no longer than 5 to 10 minutes. A depressed or deteriorating level of consciousness, pupillary abnormalities, and hemiparesis with or without abnormal posturing are the findings most frequently associated with a traumatic hematoma and, when noted, should heighten the urgency of evaluation. Although such signs are highly suggestive of a traumatic mass lesion, they can be falsely localizing and are seen in patients with diffuse brain injuries as well.[111] Alcohol intoxication is another factor that frequently confounds early diagnostic efforts in the head injury victim. In most people, however, a blood alcohol level of less than 200 mg/dL is insufficient to explain a significantly impaired level of consciousness.[34, 48]

Because of factors such as ethanol and falsely localizing signs, the neurologic examination is often misleading and unreliable in accurately predicting an intracranial lesion. Hence, a definitive diagnostic procedure is always warranted. As discussed later, noncontrast axial CT is the imaging modality of choice. Additional signs that severe cranial trauma has occurred are manifestations of a basilar skull fracture, including hemotympanum, cerebrospinal fluid (CSF) otorrhea or rhinorrhea, ecchymosis over the mastoid area, or bilateral periorbital ecchymosis. In comatose patients, cranial base fractures are often associated with an intracranial hematoma and, when detected, should hasten the patient's trek to the CT scanner.

Given the aggressive prehospital and emergency care that is common today, many critically ill trauma patients are intubated, sedated, and pharmacologically paralyzed before being seen by a neurosurgeon. Close cooperation and communication with the trauma or emergency physicians is essential to obtain information on the patient's initial neurologic status and to plan a coherent sequence of diagnostic and therapeutic procedures, especially in the patient who has sustained multiple injuries.

## Radiographic Spine Evaluation

Before the patient leaves the emergency department, the cervical spine is evaluated radiographically with a lateral view that includes the cervicothoracic junction, plus anteroposterior and open-mouth views. If the C7 to T1 junction is not visualized on the lateral view despite arm traction or a swimmer's view, then a CT scan through the level with 3-mm cuts suffices. An important but often overlooked consideration in the severe head injury patient is that a normal three-view cervical spine radiography series does not rule out a ligamentous injury. The finding of posterior cervical spine tenderness in an alert and cooperative patient, without fracture or subluxation on the initial radiographic studies, warrants lateral flexion/extension views.

Because of the risk of missing a significant ligamentous injury in a comatose patient, the neurosurgical team should perform gentle flexion and extension views of the cervical spine of 20 to 30 degrees when the initial three views are normal. If instability is demonstrated on flexion/extension radiographs, the collar is left in place or appropriate traction is applied. Experience indicates this is a low-risk, yet reliable maneuver in demonstrating ligamentous injury. These additional flexion/extension views are particularly important in patients injured in a motor vehicle accident or a fall, in whom the risk of sustaining a cervical spine injury is high. Patients who demonstrate a paucity of extremity movement during initial evaluation, however, may have already sustained a cervical spinal cord injury; flexion/extension radiographs are not recommended in these patients unless performed under fluoroscopic guidance. This policy of early flexion/extension views is certainly safer than removing the collar after the initial series of radiographs, whereby the patient may then go to the operating room and considerable head rotation be used for positioning. Flexion and extension of the cervical spine in a controlled fashion also poses less risk to the patient than the unpredictable movement of the head and neck that frequently occurs in comatose and often agitated patients during transport and in the intensive care unit, even when a rigid collar is in place. When time or other circumstances do not permit these additional views to be obtained in the emergency department, the collar should be left on until such radiographs are performed or until the patient is awake enough to detect cervical spine tenderness.

Radiographic studies of the thoracic and lumbar spine are also obtained when indicated, especially in patients injured in a motor vehicle accident or in a fall of more than several feet. These views of the lower spine are preferably performed early in the evaluation process to minimize the time the patient spends on a spine board, where pressure sores can develop rapidly in a comatose person. Given the high incidence of traumatic intracranial hematomas in severe head injury victims, however, an urgent head CT is usually warranted before radiographic evaluation of the thoracolumbar spine.

## DIAGNOSTIC PROCEDURES

The noncontrast axial CT scan is the imaging modality of choice for evaluation of a head-injured patient. It is performed in less than 10 minutes and clearly defines the location, extent, and type of intracranial lesion. With the lateral scout view and CT bone windows, skull fractures usually are well visualized, thus obviating the need for skull radiographic studies.

The presence of a skull fracture on skull radiography, although highly suggestive of a traumatic hematoma, does not identify the type of intracranial injury. Skull fractures are seen in 66% to 100% of patients with EDH, with a lower incidence of fracture occurring in younger patients. In patients with SDH, skull fractures are seen 18% to 60% of the time and most frequently are contralateral to the side of the hematoma. With ICH and cerebral contusions, skull fractures have been noted in 40% to 80% of cases.[20] The

lack of specificity and time required to obtain skull films make them a wasteful endeavor when CT is readily available.

In situations in which CT is unavailable, emergency cerebral angiography can adequately demonstrate most traumatic hematomas and a midline shift. If both CT and angiography are unobtainable, a rapidly deteriorating patient can undergo twist drill ventriculostomy followed by air ventriculography in the emergency department. A ventricular shift indicative of a mass lesion usually can be demonstrated.

### Newer Imaging Modalities

Magnetic resonance imaging (MRI) can clearly demonstrate traumatic hematomas, especially those that are subacute and appear isodense on CT. However, MRI does not demonstrate acute blood as clearly as CT does, takes significantly longer than CT, and requires a ventilator with nonferromagnetic components for intubated patients. These factors make MRI impractical for initial evaluation of the severely head-injured patient.[20, 43]

Transcranial near-infrared spectroscopy has been shown by Gopinath and associates[40] accurately to detect the presence of an acute intracranial hematoma in head-injured patients. In a study of 40 patients with EDH, SDH, or ICH confirmed by CT, a significant difference in optical density was noted between the hemisphere with the hematoma and the contralateral hemisphere. This rapidly performed, noninvasive technique for detecting acute traumatic hematomas may have its greatest utility in the hemodynamically unstable trauma patient who must be taken immediately to the operating room for management of an extracranial injury, before obtaining a head CT. Near-infrared spectroscopy may also obviate the need for performing exploratory bur holes in the rapidly deteriorating head-injured patient. The major limitation of this technique is the possible inability to detect bilateral hematomas. It is hoped that further studies with near-infrared spectroscopy are forthcoming.

### Exploratory Bur Holes

Fortunately, there are increasingly rare situations in which a patient is deteriorating so rapidly that diagnostic studies are unobtainable and placement of exploratory bur holes is indicated. Nonetheless, it is a procedure with which all neurosurgeons should be familiar. It is of value only if the surgeon is prepared to proceed with a formal craniotomy, because acute traumatic hematomas cannot be dealt with adequately through bur holes.

The patient is placed supine with the brow up to provide access to both sides of the head (Fig. 5–1). The first bur hole should be made in the temporal region, immediately above the zygomatic arch, according to the following scheme based on the relative localizing value of neurologic findings: (1) ipsilateral to a dilated pupil, (2) contralateral to the most abnormal motor response, and (3) ipsilateral to the side of a skull fracture. Subsequent trephinations are then made in the parietal and frontal regions. The scalp incisions and bur holes should be placed to permit their

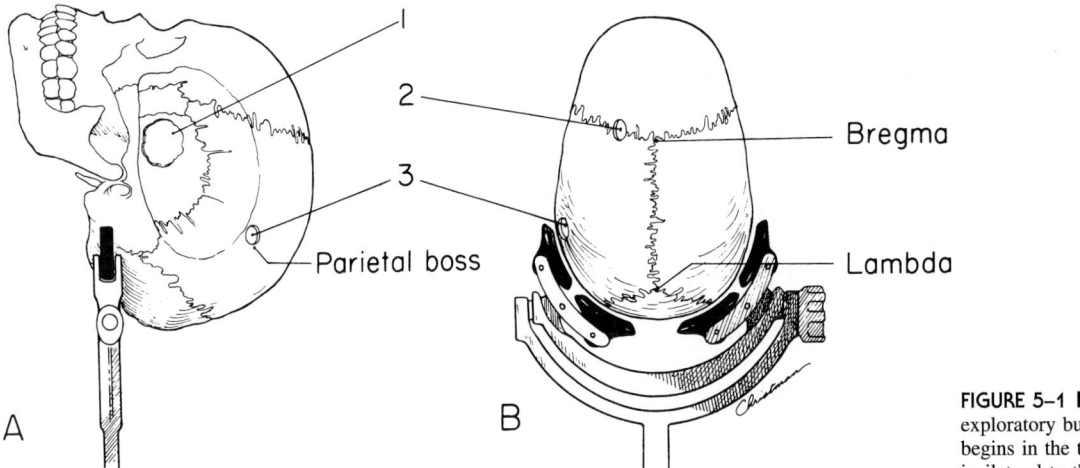

FIGURE 5–1 ■ Positioning of exploratory bur holes. Placement begins in the temporal fossa, ipsilateral to the suspected lesion.

incorporation into a formal craniotomy if a hematoma is encountered. When the procedure is completed on one side of the head, it should be repeated on the other side.

Intraoperative ultrasound studies have been shown to improve the diagnostic accuracy of exploratory bur holes.[3] This technique also may be of use in patients who, after evacuation of a hematoma, still have a tense brain during surgery. The possibility of an evolving ipsilateral ICH or expansion of a contralateral hematoma can be evaluated in the operating room, without the need for a repeat CT. However, given the possibility of not detecting some lesions by this technique, an immediate repeat CT scan is always indicated if the intraoperative ultrasound is negative but brain swelling persists.

## SURGICAL MANAGEMENT OF TRAUMATIC INTRACRANIAL HEMATOMAS

### Indications for Surgery

The most important factors in deciding whether to proceed with surgery are the patient's overall clinical condition, his or her neurologic status, and the imaging findings. There is little debate in the surgical management of a rapidly deteriorating patient with focal neurologic deficit harboring an expanding intracranial hematoma associated with significant mass effect and midline shift. For less obvious situations controversy persists, but several reasonable statements can be made. In general, an SDH or EDH of over 5 mm in thickness with a commensurate midline shift, in a comatose patient (GCS of 8 or less), should be evacuated urgently. On the other hand, surgical decompression of a thin-rim SDH of 3 mm or less, associated with marked hemispheric swelling and a large midline shift, is unlikely to improve the patient's condition or reduce intracranial pressure.[2, 20, 72] Such patients are best managed medically. A CT scan should be repeated, especially if the first scan was obtained within a few hours of injury or if there are other associated lesions, such as contusions, on the original CT that may have progressed in the interim.

Perhaps the most controversy exists over when to evacu-

ate ICHs and hemorrhagic contusions, and whether such removal is helpful in controlling ICP and improving outcome.[72] Miller and colleagues,[74] in their experience with over 200 severely head-injured patients, found that despite removing such lesions, patients with contusions or ICHs had the highest incidence of poor ICP control of all subgroups in the study. On that basis, they recommend an initial nonoperative course in most cases, resorting to surgery if medical management of ICP has failed. Others, such as Cooper,[20] believe that early surgical removal of larger ICHs and cerebral contusions provides early control of ICP and helps prevent the cascade of secondary events leading to later ICP problems. Despite such debate, there is general agreement that the decision to remove an ICH or cerebral contusion should be based on several key factors, including the size of the lesion, its depth and exact location from the cortical surface, the presence of associated lesions, and the ICP.[20, 72] Cortical contusions of over 2 cm in diameter usually should be removed if there is significant mass effect and treatment intensity for ICP is high. Frontal pole and temporal lobe hematomas or contusions of 2 cm or more in diameter, when associated with significant mass effect and shift of over 5 mm, should also be removed if ICP is poorly controlled. An initial conservative approach is warranted, however, when eloquent cortex is involved, such as dominant temporal lobe lesions or lesions near the central sulcus. In general, an expectant course is indicated in all comatose but neurologically stable patients with small lesions associated with a less than 5-mm midline shift and open basilar cisterns on CT. Similarly, lesions confined to the deep white matter or basal ganglia are best managed without surgery. ICP should be carefully monitored and controlled by medical means. If such measures fail, the patient can be reconsidered for surgery.

Finally, there are situations in which the dismal clinical status of the patient warrants a nonoperative course despite the presence of a radiographic surgical lesion. Such cases include the adult patient who is moribund and flaccid with a GCS of 3, nonreactive and dilated pupils, and no spontaneous respirations. Similarly, in patients older than 75 years of age with a GCS of 5 or less, a nonoperative course usually should be taken given their consistently poor outcome with or without surgery.[47, 110] All other patients with surgical mass lesions, even those with a postre-suscitation GCS of 3, warrant emergency operative intervention. A significant albeit small portion of such patients will make a satisfactory recovery. In addition, in some patients a low GCS may in part be due to intoxication.[48]

## Potential Operative Mass Lesions and Early Repeat Computed Tomography Scan

In patients with potential surgical lesions on the initial CT scan, it is best to repeat the study sooner rather than later, when the scan may then be prompted by irreversible neurologic deterioration. McBride and associates,[69] based on a review of 154 consecutive closed head injury patients requiring surgical intervention, recommend a repeat CT scan within 4 to 8 hours of the initial scan in all patients with abnormal initial scans, given that 47.5% of patients received surgical intervention based on the findings of the follow-up CT scan. Patients receiving craniotomy after the second CT scan comprised 53% of the operated cerebral contusions, 25% of the SDHs, and 23% of the EDHs. In another study by Stein and coworkers,[99] 44.5% of 337 consecutive patients sustaining a closed head injury had delayed or progressive brain injury, defined as new or progressive lesions seen on a follow-up CT scan. Highly significant indicators for the development of delayed cerebral insults included increasing severity of the initial head injury, as defined by GCS; the need for cardiopulmonary resuscitation at the accident site; the presence of SDH on the first CT scan; and the presence of coagulopathy on admission.

Addressing further the issue of coagulopathy after closed head injury in another report, the same investigators found elevated prothrombin time (PT), partial thromboplastin time (PTT), or low platelet count in 37.5% of 253 patients on admission.[100] Of those patients with delayed brain injury, as defined earlier, 55% had an abnormal PT, PTT, or platelet count, whereas, of those patients whose follow-up CT scans did not worsen, only 9% had abnormal coagulation studies. The risk for development of a delayed insult on CT was 85% in those with at least one abnormal clotting study and only 31% for those without such abnormalities. When coagulopathy is present on hospital admission, Stein and colleagues[99] advocate early repeat CT scanning. This concept of timely follow-up evaluation is particularly relevant in many of today's trauma centers, where patients are routinely scanned within 1 to 2 hours of injury, when the hemorrhagic process may still be evolving.

## Preoperative Preparation

In preparing a severe head injury victim for emergency craniotomy, the most important goals are avoiding hypotension and hypoxia, gaining early control of ICP, preventing seizures, and assessing for coagulopathy. The risk of hypoxia and hypotension is minimized with supplemental oxygen and aggressive fluid resuscitation using crystalloid and colloid, and type-specific blood, if indicated. Preemptive measures against intracranial hypertension include use of additional sedation and paralyzing agents, assisted ventilation to maintain the $PaCO_2$ at 32 to 35 mm Hg, and mannitol. A 1 g/kg bolus of intravenous (IV) mannitol should be given without delay when the CT scan has demonstrated an intracranial hematoma with signs of raised intracranial pressure, such as midline shift, compressed basilar cisterns, or diffuse swelling. Any patient who demonstrates a precipitous decline in his or her level of consciousness, pupillary abnormalities, or hemiparesis can be given a mannitol bolus even before imaging in the likelihood that a traumatic hematoma and raised ICP are responsible for the patient's condition. Mannitol boluses larger than 1 g/kg are not significantly more effective in lowering ICP and run the risk of intravascular depletion and hypotension, especially if adequate fluid replacement is not provided. Because generalized seizures in the setting of raised ICP can have devastating consequences, all patients should be given a preoperative 18 mg/kg loading dose of IV phenytoin as early as possible. Rapid infusion of phenytoin of over 50 mg/min is to be avoided because significant hypotension or arrhythmias may result.

When coagulopathy is present with a significantly elevated PT or PTT, fresh frozen plasma or cryoprecipitate should be available in the operating room and transfused if hemostasis is problematic.[2] A platelet count of less than 50,000 or a significantly prolonged bleeding time (> 10 minutes) should be treated with platelet transfusion. Disseminated intravascular coagulopathy (DIC) is often associated with severe traumatic brain injury.[84] If coagulopathy is suggested by excessive bleeding or by abnormalities of PT, PTT, or platelet count, a complete screen for DIC should be undertaken.[84] If DIC is confirmed by low fibrinogen level, elevated levels of fibrin degradation products, and prolonged thrombin time, then transfusion of platelets, cryoprecipitate, and fresh frozen plasma is indicated.[39] Surgery should not be delayed, however, while waiting for blood products, especially in the neurologically deteriorating patient.

## Surgical Evacuation of Traumatic Hematomas

### Basic Trauma Craniotomy

Relatively small, localized EDHs or contusions of the temporal pole occasionally can be evacuated through a vertical scalp incision and limited temporal craniotomy (Fig. 5–2). However, most traumatic injuries are best addressed through a generous frontotemporal parietal craniotomy that provides access to the frontal and temporal poles and the area along the vertex. Hemorrhage from bridging veins and from draining veins to the sagittal sinus can be seen and controlled, and fractures, dural lacerations, and vascular injuries at the skull base can be visualized and treated.

The patient should be positioned with the head turned almost 90 degrees to the side, supported on a donut or a similar headrest, with the head slightly elevated above the level of the heart. A bolster placed under the ipsilateral shoulder helps prevent positional obstruction of cranial venous outflow. If the cervical spine has not been radiographically cleared and a collar is still in place, the patient should be put in the lateral position to maintain the head and neck in neutral alignment.

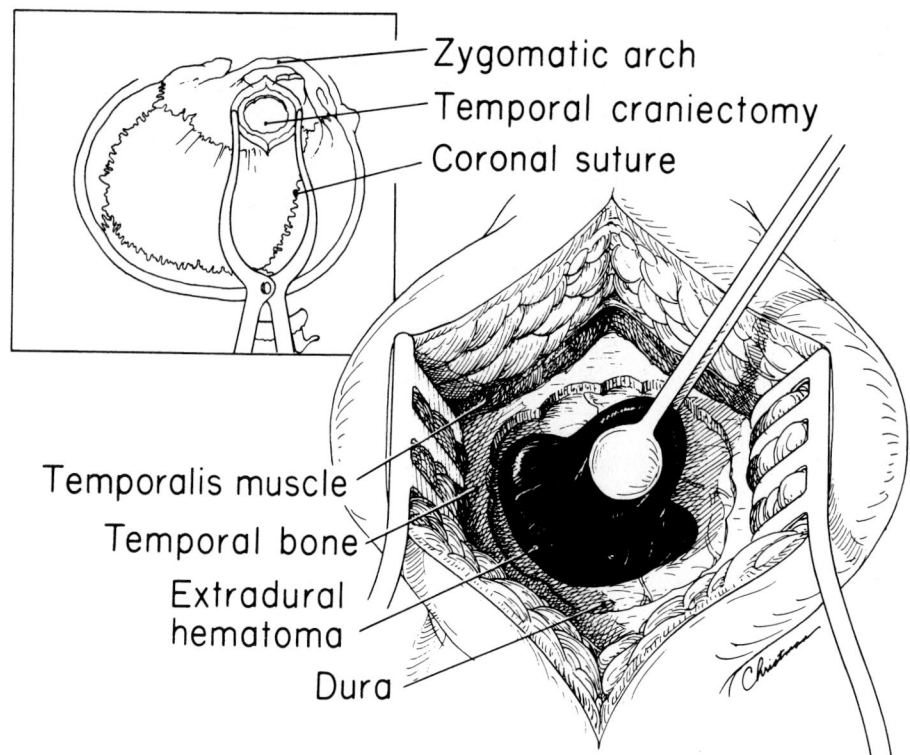

Zygomatic arch
Temporal craniectomy
Coronal suture

Temporalis muscle
Temporal bone
Extradural
hematoma
Dura

**FIGURE 5–2** ■ A limited craniectomy for a small epidural hematoma. The same exposure provides access to localized contusion of the temporal pole.

The scalp incision is begun directly in front of the tragus, curved posteriorly above the helix of the ear, and continued in a question mark fashion from the parietal area toward the frontal midline, ending, if possible, behind the hairline (Fig. 5–3). In a patient who is deteriorating and has a known temporal fossa lesion, the temporal end of the incision should be opened and a limited temporal craniectomy performed immediately. The dura is opened and hematoma and contused brain are removed, thereby achieving prompt decompression and relief of raised ICP. The scalp incision then can be completed, and a large free or osteoplastic bone flap, which extends to within 2 or 3 cm of the midline and curves low over the frontal region, can be elevated. Taking the medial craniotomy cut any closer to the midline gains little in exposure and increases the risk of transgressing large venous tributaries near the sagittal sinus. If necessary, additional bone can be removed medially more safely with a rongeur under direct vision after the initial craniotomy flap has been removed. In cases in which fractures cross the sagittal sinus, the surgeon and anesthesiologist should be prepared for major blood loss at the time the bone flap is elevated. Resection of the lateral sphenoid wing often is necessary to provide adequate exposure of the middle fossa.

With a relatively thin SDH and underlying swollen brain, great care must be taken in opening the dura and avoiding a cortical laceration. In such cases, performing only slit openings in the dura should be considered. Otherwise, the dural opening should begin over the area of maximal clot thickness, or in the anterior temporal region, because if brain begins to herniate through the exposure here, relatively silent cortex is affected (Fig. 5–4). Hematoma and

cerebral contusions are evacuated, and the subdural space is explored (Fig. 5–5). A severely contused or pulped frontal or temporal pole should be resected. Gentle handling of the injured brain is critical because further trauma from rough instrumentation and forceful retraction is poorly tolerated. Meticulous hemostasis with use of bipolar and hemostatic agents such as Avitene, Surgicel, or Gelfoam is essential in avoiding recurrent hematoma formation.

After the intradural portion of the procedure is completed, the dura is closed in a watertight fashion, either primarily or with a pericranial or fascia lata graft, if necessary. If dural closure is difficult secondary to swelling and significant intracranial hypertension is anticipated, a generous subtemporal decompression can be performed. Multiple dural tacking sutures are placed around the craniotomy margin and one or two are placed in the bone flap to prevent a postoperative EDH. The bone flap is secured with nonabsorbable suture or with cranial miniplates. A subgaleal drain may be placed and brought out through a separate incision and left in place for 12 to 24 hours. The scalp is closed in two layers. Prophylactic antibiotics, such as nafcillin, 1 g every 6 hours, and gentamicin, 80 mg every 8 hours, are given until the drain is removed, unless a ventriculostomy is in place, in which case they are continued.

In the less common situations in which parietal, occipital, or interhemispheric posterior fossa lesions are present, the approach is modified accordingly.

Before leaving the operating room, all patients with severe head injury should have an ICP monitor placed because intracranial hypertension develops in 50% to 75%

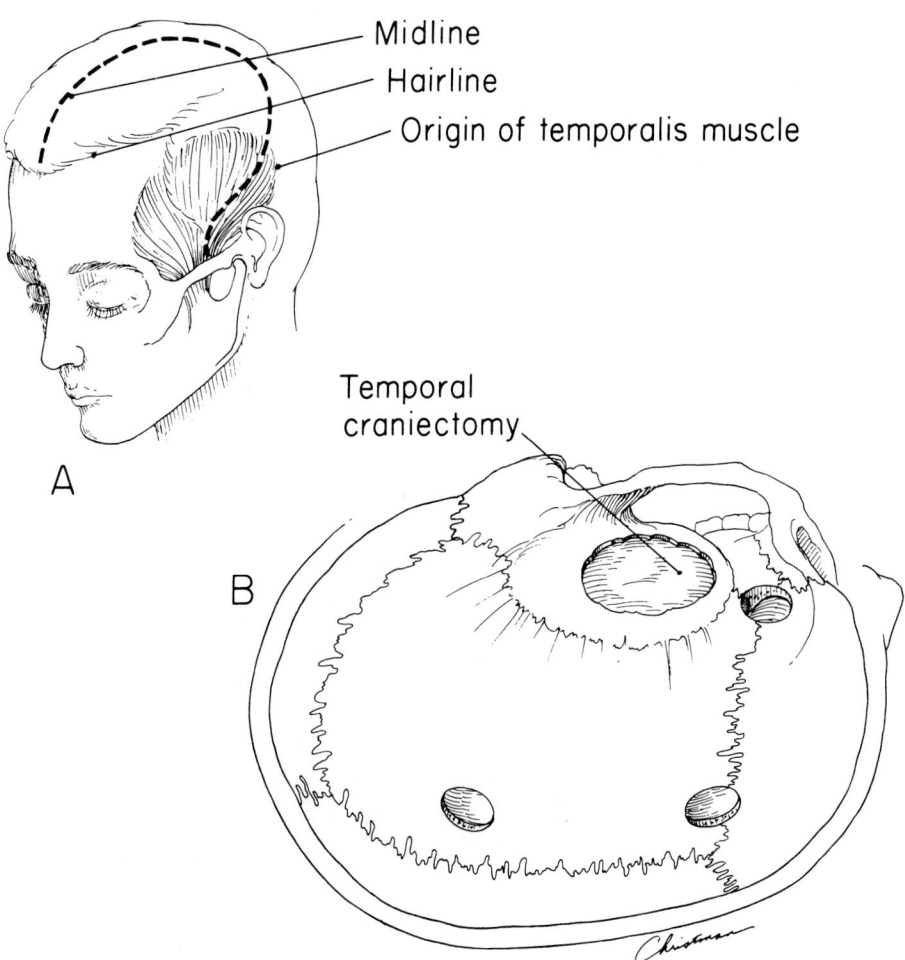

FIGURE 5–3 ■ Scalp incision and bur hole placement for a standard trauma craniotomy. Note the temporal craniectomy for the initial decompression.

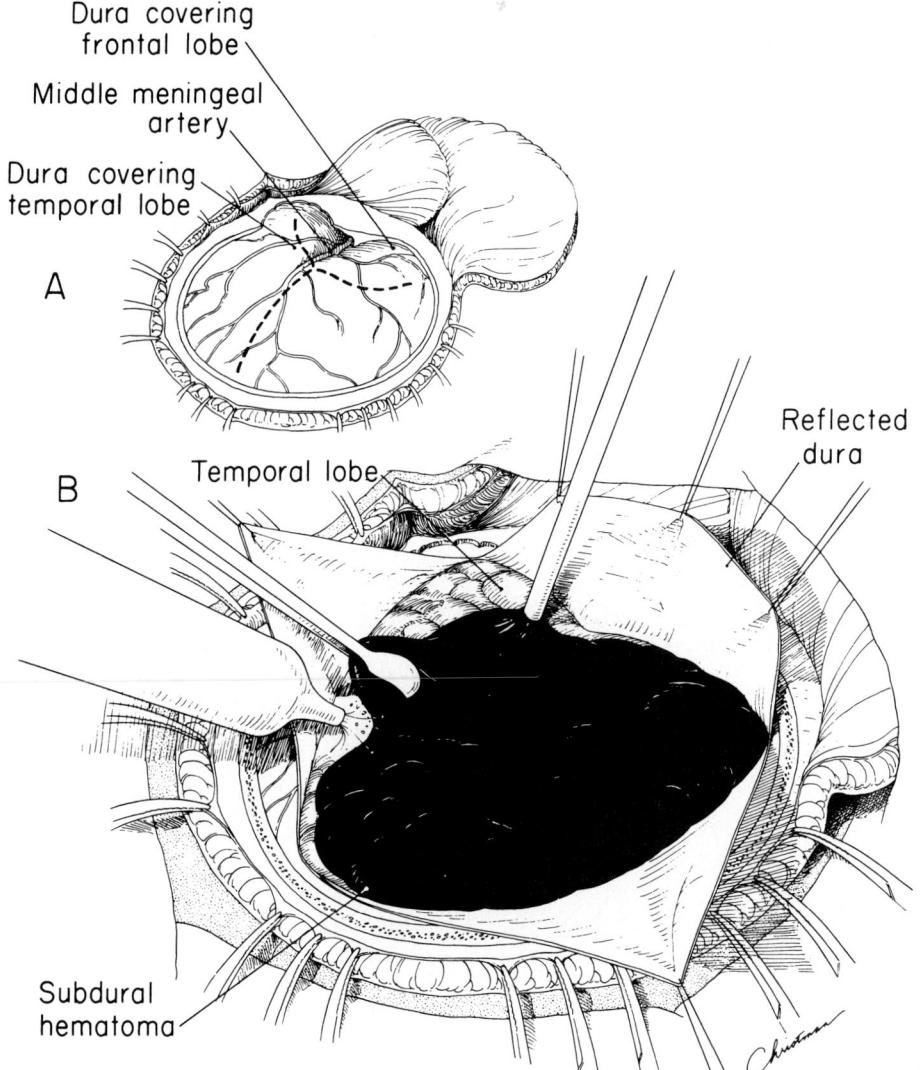

Dura covering
frontal lobe

Middle meningeal
artery

Dura covering
temporal lobe

A

B

Temporal lobe

Reflected
dura

Subdural
hematoma

**FIGURE 5–4** ■ *A*, The dural opening for evacuation of a subdural hematoma. The incision begins over the temporal lobe. *B*, Removal of clot.

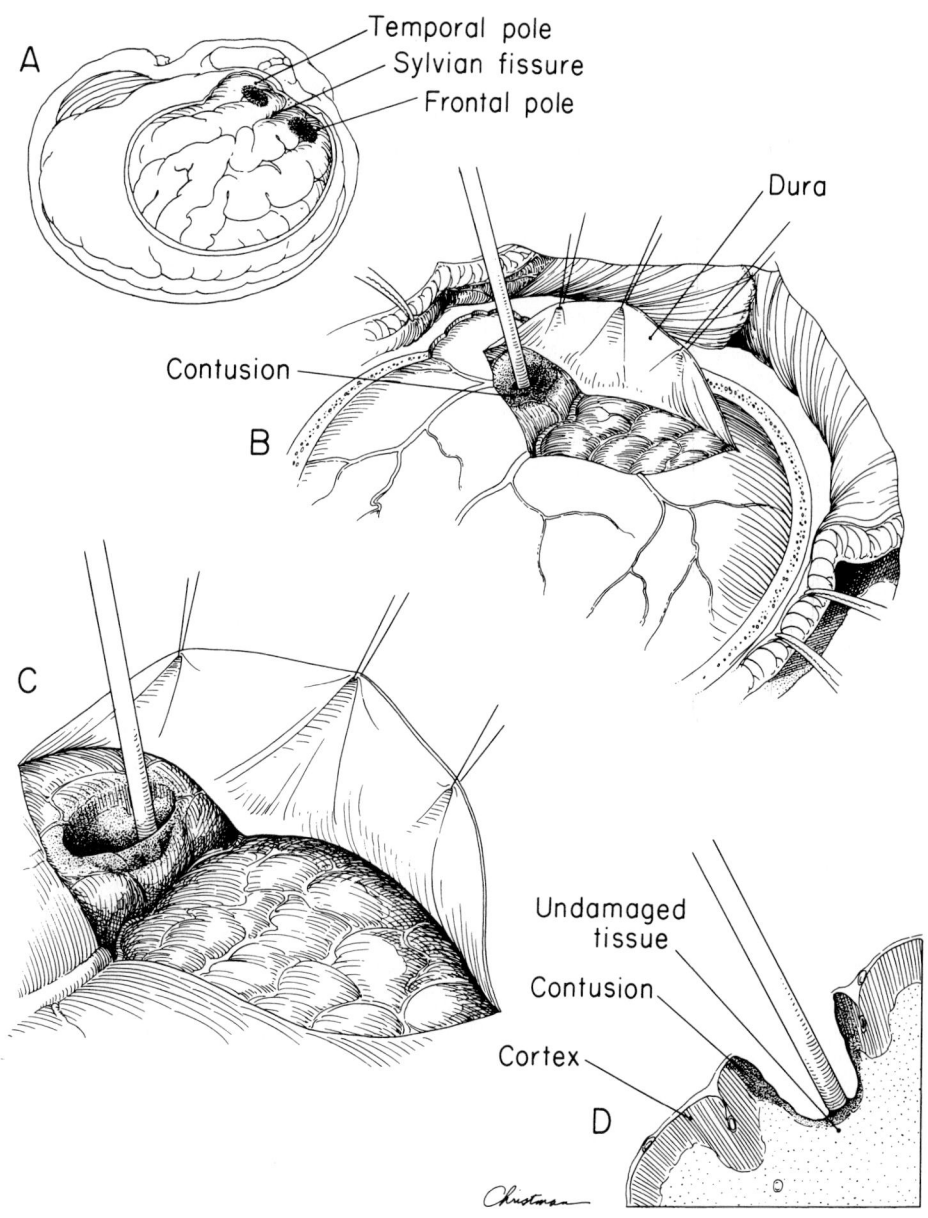

FIGURE 5–5 ■ *A,* The usual location of contusions. *B,* The dural opening for access to contusions. *C* and *D,* Resection of contusion limited to the damaged brain.

of them.[61, 75] A ventriculostomy is preferable over other monitoring devices because it permits drainage of CSF as an additional and effective means of treating raised ICP. Typically, the catheter is placed through the nondominant frontal lobe into the frontal horn of the lateral ventricle from an entry point 1 to 2 cm anterior to the coronal suture and 2 to 3 cm lateral to the midline. However, if the trauma occurs over the dominant side, it is reasonable to place the catheter through the injured hemisphere, provided there is no effacement of the ventricle from swelling or residual mass effect. Intraoperative ultrasound can be helpful in guiding placement and limiting the number of passes made. If the operative site was contaminated by an open depressed fracture or an ipsilateral slit ventricle is present, the contralateral ventricle is used. After placement, the catheter is tunneled at least 4 or 5 cm in the subgaleal space and externalized through a separate stab incision. When a ventricle cannot be cannulated, a fiberoptic subarachnoid or parenchymal monitor should be placed.

## Intraoperative Brain Swelling

Despite thorough clot removal, some patients have severe intraoperative brain swelling. A systematic approach to finding the cause and controlling it is critical. The endotracheal tube position is assessed. The head of the operating table is elevated, and rotation of the head and neck is minimized. Marked arterial hypertension should be controlled, but even modest hypotension is to be avoided. As these maneuvers are carried out, further sedation, paralyzing agents, and mannitol are given and a ventriculostomy should be attempted for drainage of CSF. The possibility of occult bleeding must be investigated, including an evolving ipsilateral ICH or a contralateral hematoma. An intraoperative ultrasound study, if available, should be obtained, and contralateral bur holes can be placed.[3] In extremely recalcitrant cases, provided the patient is normovolemic and normotensive, pentobarbital coma can be initiated with a 10 mg/kg IV bolus, given over 20 to 30 minutes.[17] At this juncture, if brain swelling remains relentless and without apparent cause, a decision must be made to proceed with further surgical decompression or to repeat a CT scan. If the surgeon is relatively confident that no other mass lesion exists based on the first CT and intraoperative ultrasound, an anterior temporal lobectomy and elevation of herniated medial temporal lobe can be performed. In one series of 10 patients treated in this manner for severe unilateral hemispheric swelling, 7 of the patients recovered satisfactorily.[81] Leaving the entire bone flap out as an external decompression is another option. The utility of this tactic as a means of improving ICP remains controversial, and earlier studies did not support its use.[20, 21] More recently, however, both Miller[72] and Gaab and colleagues[33] have stated that this option is a reasonable approach in selected patients younger than 40 years of age with uncontrollable brain swelling. In 34 such patients treated with wide frontotemporal parietal craniectomy and dural enlargement, Gaab and colleagues[33] reported that 68% of patients made a satisfactory recovery, whereas 15% of patients died. ICP control was improved after craniectomy.[33] When brain swelling does preclude replacement of the bone flap, it can be temporarily placed in an abdominal subcutaneous pocket

for later insertion, avoiding a large and often problematic cranioplasty.[94] After such an intraoperative crisis, a repeat CT scan immediately after closure is mandatory, especially when no obvious cause for swelling was identified.

## Epidural Hematoma

The mortality rate for patients with acute EDH is directly related to the level of consciousness before surgery. In patients who present comatose with an acute EDH, the mortality rate is approximately 40%, whereas in those who are awake and alert without focal deficit before surgery, the mortality rate approaches zero. Associated intracranial injuries, such as cerebral contusions, SDH, and brain lacerations, also have an adverse impact on the patient's outcome. Such injuries are seen in 50% to 75% of patients who present in coma with EDH, but they are seen in only 25% to 40% of patients with acute EDH overall.[97] Rapid diagnosis and urgent evacuation are the keys to optimizing outcome in patients with an acute EDH.

The scalp incision and craniotomy flap should be fashioned to provide complete exposure of the hematoma. Because most epidural clots are located in the middle or frontal fossa, or both, a standard frontotemporal craniotomy, as described earlier, is typically most appropriate. The initial bur hole should be placed over or near the area of maximal clot thickness, which is usually in the low temporal area. After rapidly widening this opening to a small craniectomy, the hematoma is removed to provide prompt ICP reduction (Fig. 5–6). A formal craniotomy is then completed, and the hematoma is removed with irrigation, suction, and cup forceps. It is crucial to achieve adequate exposure through the craniotomy so that all of the clot can be easily removed without retracting the brain. Such exposure is also necessary to visualize and control the epidural bleeding source, which, in most cases, is a branch of the middle meningeal artery. With petrous bone fractures, exposure of the main trunk of the middle meningeal artery at or near the foramen spinosum is often necessary. This bleeding usually is easily controlled with bipolar coagulation, but packing the foramen spinosum with bone wax occasionally may be necessary. After removal of the hematoma, if the dura remains tense or has a bluish color suggestive of subdural blood, or if there is a significant underlying cerebral contusion seen on CT, the subdural space is inspected. This exposure can be initiated through a small linear incision and expanded as necessary. A watertight dural closure should follow. After achieving meticulous hemostasis in the epidural space with bipolar coagulation and hemostatic agents, circumferential and bone flap dural tacking stitches are placed followed by routine scalp closure (Fig. 5–7).

## Subdural Hematoma

Rates of mortality and morbidity after an acute SDH are the highest of all traumatic mass lesions. This poor outcome results largely from associated parenchymal injuries and subsequent intracranial hypertension. Approximately 50% of patients have associated lesions, including intracerebral contusions, hematomas, and cortical lacerations, most being located in the frontal and temporal lobes.[47, 49]

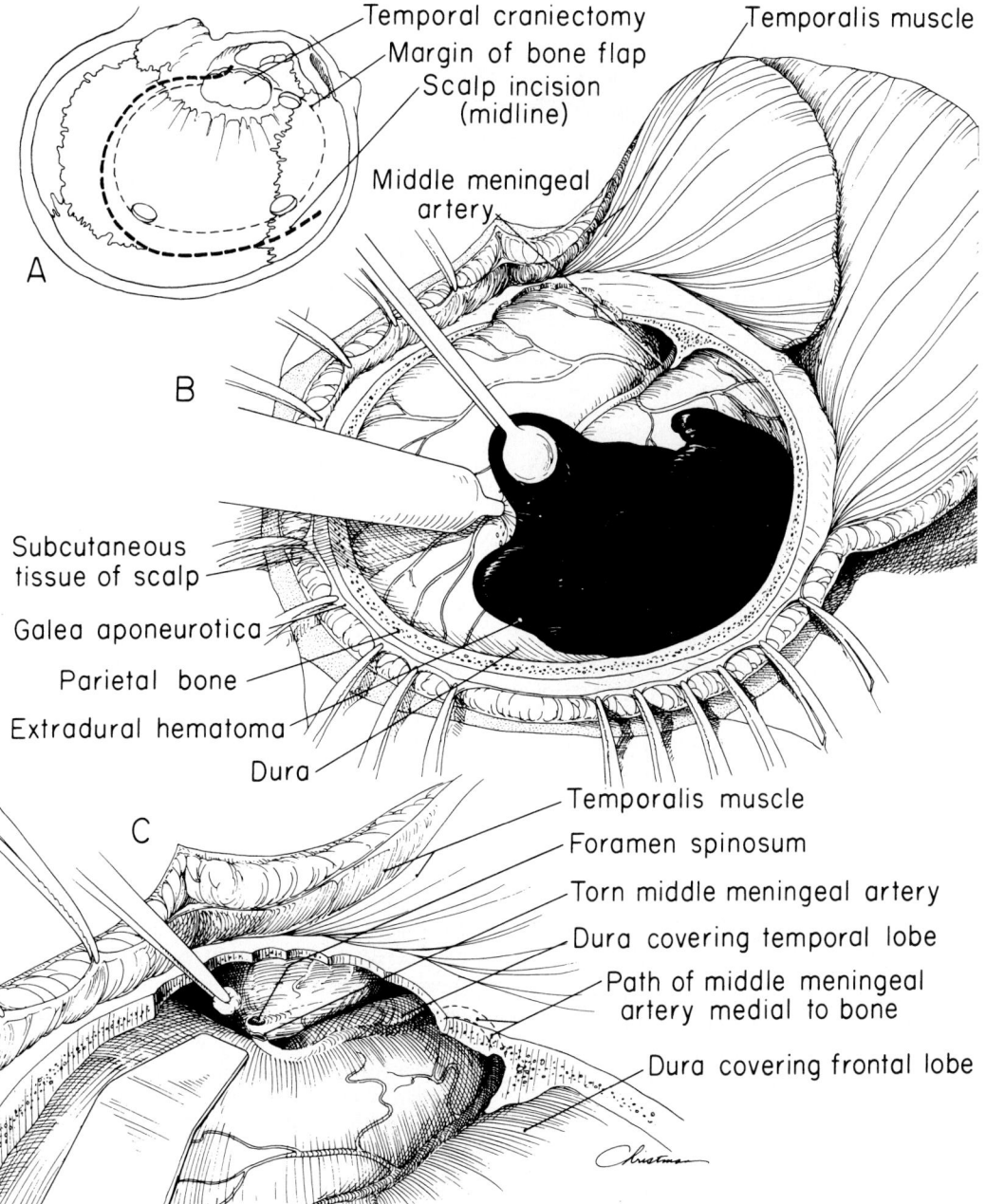

**FIGURE 5-6** ■ *A*, The scalp incision and bone flap for removal of a large extradural hematoma. *B*, Removal of the clot. *C*, Packing of the foramen spinosum.

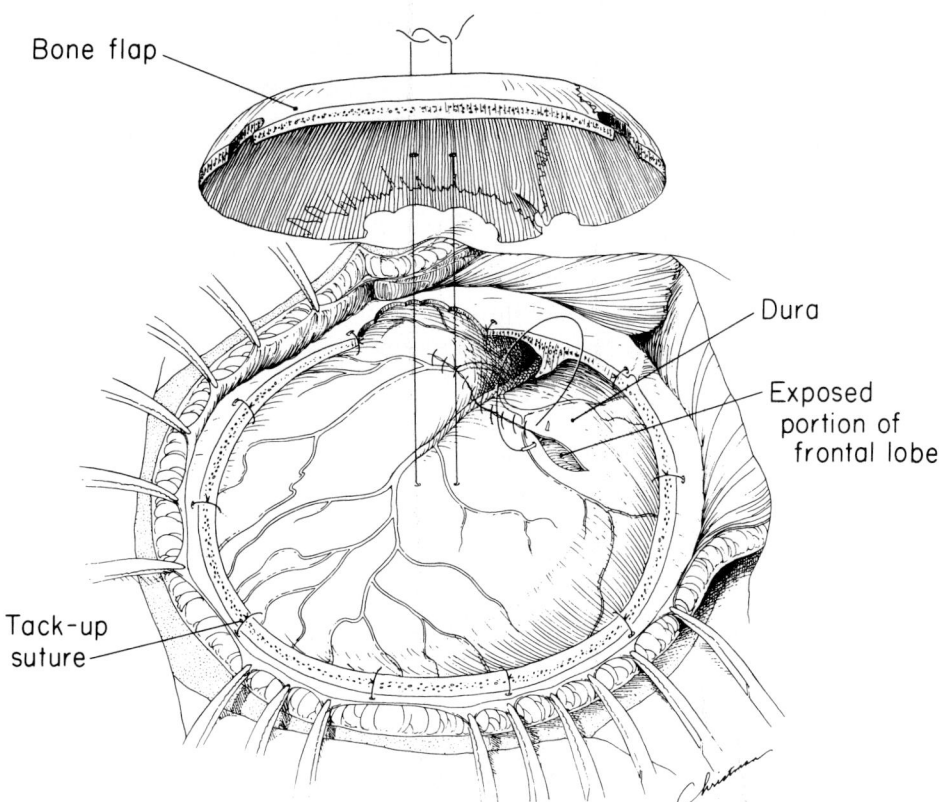

Bone flap

Dura

Exposed
portion of
frontal lobe

Tack-up
suture

**FIGURE 5–7** ■ Closure of an
exploratory dural incision and
tacking up of the dura to the bone
flap and craniotomy edges.

In the TCDB cohort and in previous series, the mortality rate for severe head injury patients with an acute SDH requiring evacuation has ranged from 42% to 65%.[5, 64, 74]

A large frontotemporal parietal craniotomy, as described earlier, usually is required adequately to remove an acute SDH and to treat associated parenchymal injuries. Exposure of the frontal and temporal poles is especially important, as is visualization along the sagittal sinus if the hematoma extends that far medially. Again, in the comatose patient with evidence of raised ICP, an immediate temporal craniectomy and partial clot removal should initiate the procedure before a craniotomy is performed.

After a generous dural opening, the clot is carefully removed with irrigation, suction, and cup forceps (see Fig. 5–4). The subdural space and cortical surface should be widely inspected for additional hematoma, bleeding, and surface contusions. Bleeding points on the cortical surface are coagulated with the bipolar, whereas more troublesome, diffuse ooze can often be controlled with hemostatic agents. Areas of cerebral contusion over 1 to 2 cm in size with irreparably damaged brain, appearing purplish and mottled, should be removed with gentle aspiration (see Fig. 5–5). In eloquent areas, such as along the dominant superior temporal gyrus and the central sulcus, a more limited removal of such contusions is prudent. Hemorrhage from draining veins along the sagittal sinus can be troublesome. If cautious bipolar coagulation is ineffective, tamponade with Gelfoam is used. Small amounts of clot that cannot be visualized adequately, that require undue brain retraction for exposure, or that are adjacent to bleeding points along the sagittal sinus should be left undisturbed. After hematoma removal, disimpaction of a herniated medial temporal lobe from the tentorial hiatus can be attempted with great care. Effective reduction usually is accompanied by a flow of CSF as the tentorial edge is visualized.[46] If reversal of herniation is unsuccessful with gentle elevation, no further efforts are warranted. A watertight dural closure should be attempted, followed by routine closure of the craniotomy.

## Intracerebral Hematoma

Intracerebral hematomas occur most frequently in the frontal and temporal lobes but are usually more deeply situated than cerebral contusions. The diagnosis of these well defined collections of parenchymal blood has become common with the routine use of CT scanning. Because they frequently are associated with other traumatic lesions, the standard trauma craniotomy usually is indicated. The approach is by a limited cortical incision through already traumatized or otherwise noneloquent brain. If the hematoma is a considerable depth from the cortical surface according to the CT scan, ultrasound can be helpful for precise localization. After thorough clot removal, adjacent contused brain should be resected. In eloquent areas, less aggressive removal of injured parenchyma should be performed. After bipolar coagulation of obvious bleeding vessels, placement of cotton balls soaked in half-strength hydrogen peroxide into the hematoma cavity is effective in achieving hemostasis. This tactic is not recommended, however, if the ventricle has been entered. After removal of the cotton balls, the hematoma bed is lined with Surgicel, followed by routine closure.

## POSTOPERATIVE CRITICAL CARE

After removal of an intracranial hematoma in the severely head-injured patient, intensive postoperative care is essential to optimize recovery. The major focus of therapy is aimed at maintaining an adequate cerebral perfusion pressure (CPP) and normalizing ICP. Prompt recognition and treatment of secondary insults, including hypotension, hypoxia, seizures, hyperthermia, electrolyte disturbances, and infection, is also crucial in achieving the best possible outcome. Described in the following sections is a management regimen that incorporates the most recent findings concerning CPP, the modified use of hyperventilation, and other data that appear to have a significant impact on recovery after traumatic brain injury. A critical aspect of any such treatment plan is maintaining close communication with the nursing staff using clearly defined goals and unambiguous orders.

## Treatment Rationale

### Cerebral Ischemia

Cerebral ischemia as documented by direct measurements of blood flow, inferred by the presence of hypotension or hypoxia, or confirmed by postmortem brain examination, is a common and ominous event after severe head injury.[9, 17, 41] Bouma and colleagues[9, 10] have documented global ischemia, defined as a cerebral blood flow (CBF) of 18 ml/100 g/min or less, by the [133]Xe method or by stable xenon CT in approximately one third of severe head injury patients who underwent CBF measurements within 6 to 8 hours of injury. Hypotension or hypoxia was documented in 57% of the severe head injury patients in the TCDB cohort. A single episode of hypotension was associated with an 85% increase in mortality.[17] In a postmortem study of 112 head injury fatalities, Graham and associates[41] documented histopathologic evidence of ischemic brain damage in 88% of subjects. As the devastating effects of cerebral ischemia have become increasingly recognized as a major contributor to poor outcome, greater emphasis has been placed on identifying and correcting factors that diminish CBF.[9, 72] Two of the most significant and easily manipulated factors that appear to have a direct impact on CBF are the CPP and the use of hyperventilation to lower ICP.

### Cerebral Perfusion Pressure

Cerebral perfusion pressure is defined as the difference between the mean arterial pressure and the ICP. In normal subjects, the mean arterial pressure ranges from 80 to 100 mm Hg and the ICP is 5 to 10 mm Hg, resulting in a normal CPP range of 70 to 95 mm Hg. Cerebral autoregulation normally has a lower CPP limit of approximately 40 mm Hg and an upper limit of 140 mm Hg. Below a perfusion pressure of 40 mm Hg, compensatory cerebral vasodilatation that augments cerebral blood flow is exhausted and cerebral ischemia results. Above a perfusion pressure of 140 mm Hg, cerebral vasoconstriction is overcome and hyperemia or even hemorrhage ensues.[15, 85]

After traumatic brain injury, impairment of pressure autoregulation is relatively common, occurring in approximately one third to one half of patients as reported in several investigations by Bouma and associates[7, 8] and Muizelaar and colleagues.[78] Equally important, however, is the concept that the lower limit at which autoregulatory mechanisms will function appears to be significantly elevated in the injured brain.[28, 42] Previous studies of head-injured patients indicated that a CPP of 50 to 60 mm Hg was adequate for maintaining relatively normal CBF and autoregulatory function.[73, 80, 106] However, several investigations now suggest that a perfusion pressure of 60 mm Hg is probably the absolute lowest acceptable level and that maintaining a perfusion pressure at 70 mm Hg or higher is optimal. When perfusion pressure is sustained at 60 to 70 mm Hg or higher, autoregulatory mechanisms are more likely to function, secondary ischemic insults appear to be minimized, and long-term outcome is substantially improved.[13, 19, 60, 70, 90, 91]

A concern in maintaining relatively high perfusion pressures has been the possibility of exacerbating intracranial hypertension through passive increases in CBF, especially in patients with impaired autoregulation.[82] This issue of hyperemia-induced intracranial hypertension is important, given that autoregulatory dysfunction may persist in a significant proportion of patients even when CPP is maintained above 70 mm Hg.[7, 8] Studies suggest, however, that systemic blood pressure elevations do not worsen intracranial hypertension in most severe head injury victims even though CBF may be substantially improved. In two reports by Bouma and associates,[7, 8] autoregulation was tested and changes in CBF and ICP were assessed in response to alterations in blood pressure. In the first report, in patients with impaired autoregulation, induced hypertension resulted in an increase of CPP from an average of 74 to 107 mm Hg and a decrease of ICP from an average of 18 mm Hg to 16 mm Hg.[7] In the second report, in patients with impaired autoregulation, induced hypertension resulted in an average increase of CPP from 73 to 106 mm Hg and an ICP increase from 16 to 20 mm Hg.[8] In both series, CBF increased with induced hypertension by approximately 50% and in the second series flows were in the hyperemic range.[82] These data suggest that for most patients with impaired autoregulation, induced hypertension results in a significant improvement in CBF with minimal or no increase in ICP. Equally important was the finding that in patients with intact autoregulation, induced hypertension did not cause significant changes in CBF or ICP; however, a reduction of blood pressure resulted in significant intracranial hypertension, presumably because of reflex vasodilatation and increased cerebral blood volume. When patients with impaired autoregulation were subjected to induced hypotension, a reduction in both ICP and CBF occurred.

Thus, the rationale for maintaining CPP at 70 mm Hg or higher is to improve CBF in patients with impaired autoregulation and to prevent reflex vasodilatation and a subsequent exacerbation of intracranial hypertension in those with intact autoregulation. By optimizing CBF after severe head injury, outcome appears to be improved.[9, 95] In a report by Sheinberg and colleagues,[95] the highest survival occurred in patients with normal and high blood flows, that is, in patients with either relative or absolute hyperemia, as defined by Obrist and associates,[82] compared with those patients with low blood flows.

At the time of this writing, randomized trials in severe head injury patients using different CPP goals have not been performed. A retrospective study of over 180 closed head injury patients by McGraw,[70] however, demonstrated significantly better outcome by Glasgow Outcome Scale and significantly less mortality when CPP was maintained above 80 mm Hg, compared with when CPP was below 80 mm Hg during the first 48 hours after injury. Two other reports by Rosner[90] and Marion and coworkers[60] document outcome after severe closed head injury when CPP was maintained at 70 mm Hg or greater and $PaCO_2$ was kept in the range of 35 mm Hg. Rosner[90] reported on 120 patients with a GCS of 7 or less. A favorable outcome was seen in 55% of patients, defined as good outcome or moderate disability by Glasgow Outcome Scale; the mortality rate was 31%. Likewise, Marion and colleagues[60] have treated 94 severely head-injured adults (GCS 7 or less), with 84 patients evaluated at 6 months after injury. A favorable outcome was achieved in 51% of the patients and the mortality rate was 20%.[60] These two reports compare favorably with the TCDB cohort, which is one of the largest and most extensive reports of severe closed head injury available. In the TCDB centers, a specific CPP goal was not established and hyperventilation to a $PaCO_2$ of 25 to 30 mm Hg was used routinely. If considering only TCDB patients with an initial GCS of 7 or less, the outcome was favorable in 37% of patients (good recovery or moderate disability), whereas the mortality rate was 40% at a mean follow-up of 674 days after injury[64] (Table 5-1). Even more relevant to this discussion is a comparison of those patients with traumatic hematomas requiring surgery treated with these two different management strategies. In Rosner's[90] report of the use of CPP therapy and minimal hyperventilation, a favorable outcome was achieved in 60% of operated patients, versus a favorable outcome in 23% of patients in the TCDB cohort who underwent surgery and were managed with more liberal use of hyperventilation and without stringent CPP goals.

In summary, it is recommended that CPP be maintained at 70 mm Hg or above in patients after severe head injury.

**TABLE 5-1  ■  OUTCOME AFTER SEVERE CLOSED HEAD INJURY (GLASGOW COMA SCALE 7 OR LESS) COMPARING CEREBRAL PERFUSION PRESSURE THERAPY AND MINIMAL HYPERVENTILATION REGIMEN\* VERSUS TRADITIONAL MANAGEMENT (TCDB COHORT)**

| | Favorable (%) | Unfavorable (%) | Mortality (%) |
|---|---|---|---|
| Rosner\*[90] | 55 | 45 | (31) |
| Marion and colleagues\*[60] | 51 | 49 | (20) |
| TCDB[64] | 37 | 63 | (40) |

\*Outcome as defined by Glasgow Outcome Scale: favorable outcome includes good recovery and moderate disability; unfavorable outcome includes severe disability, vegetative, and dead.
TCDB, Traumatic Coma Data Bank.

A perfusion pressure at this level minimizes the risk of cerebral ischemia and may represent a critical threshold for cerebral autoregulatory mechanisms to function. This goal is ideally achieved by maintaining the patient in a euvolemic state with a mean arterial pressure of at least 90 mm Hg, and an ICP of less than 20 mm Hg.

### Hyperventilation

Despite its effectiveness, the use of hyperventilation as a primary means of controlling ICP has been tempered substantially. This change is based on evidence that maintaining $PaCO_2$ in the range of 25 to 30 mm Hg can result in significant cerebral vasoconstriction, leading to ischemia.[77, 108] Such levels of hypocapnia, which previously had been considered moderate, have been associated with worse outcome compared with the use of milder degrees of hypocapnia after severe head injury.[77] In addition, in most patients, significant hyperventilation is not essential for control of ICP.[60, 77, 90] In studies of patients with severe head injury, the lowest CBFs consistently occurred within the first 6 to 12 hours after injury and then progressively increased over the ensuing hours and days.[9, 10, 83] These findings suggest that hyperventilation may have its most deleterious effect during the first day after injury when relative or absolute cerebral ischemia may already exist. Maintaining $PaCO_2$ at approximately 35 mm Hg during the initial 24 hours after injury appears warranted. Thereafter, maintaining $PaCO_2$ in the range of 30 to 35 mm Hg is recommended in that a modest degree of ICP control is provided without a significant risk of hyperventilation-induced ischemia.

## Management of Neurologic Injury

### Physiologic Monitoring

Essential monitoring equipment for the patient with severe head injury includes an ICP monitor, central venous pressure (CVP) line, an arterial line, pulse oximetry, and end-tidal $CO_2$ monitoring. A Foley catheter and nasogastric or orogastric tube also are placed.

Additional modalities that provide further information on regional and global CBF and metabolism are being used increasingly in the neurosurgical intensive care unit. Jugular bulb catheterization allows continuous recording of cerebral venous oxygen saturation ($SJO_2$), which is reflective of global CBF.[13, 72, 95] CBF measurements by the $^{133}Xe$ technique (or by stable xenon CT) can also aid in the detection of ischemia and can be used with $SJO_2$ values to optimize CPP and $PaCO_2$, particularly when ischemia is suspected.[9, 10, 60, 72, 83] Transcranial Doppler measurements of middle cerebral artery flow velocity, when combined with cervical internal carotid flow velocity or CBF measurements, appear to allow differentiation between traumatic arterial spasm with ischemia versus hyperemia. Given that up to 40% of patients with severe head injury have post-traumatic spasm, the use of serial transcranial Doppler measurements appears warranted in such patients.[14, 66, 67, 93] The ultimate utility of these technologies in the management of severe traumatic brain injury remains to be proved, but initial experiences indicate such information helps further optimize therapy.

## Cerebral Perfusion Pressure Management

To maintain CPP at or above 70 mm Hg, normovolemia is essential. Full maintenance IV fluids are given at a rate of 1.5 ml/kg/hr of 5% dextrose in half-normal or normal saline. A CVP line or a Swan-Ganz catheter is placed to optimize fluid management. A Swan-Ganz catheter is recommended in patients older than 55 years of age; in those with known cardiac disease, or chest or visceral injury; or when pressor agents or high-dose barbiturates are used. The CVP is maintained from 5 to 10 mm Hg or the pulmonary artery wedge pressure (PAWP) is kept at 10 to 14 mm Hg.

A maximal wedge pressure of 14 mm Hg is chosen because this level has been associated with maximal cardiac performance in previously healthy patients with subarachnoid hemorrhage without cardiac disease; raising wedge pressure above 14 mm Hg did not improve cardiac or stroke volume indices.[56] In some patients, especially the elderly and those with cardiac disease or hypertension, higher filling pressures may be needed to achieve optimal cardiac output.

Additional fluids in the form of colloid (250 ml of 5% albumin) are given as needed when the CVP drops below 5 mm Hg or the PAWP is less than 10 mm Hg. If the goal of maintaining CPP at 70 mm Hg is not being met with the CVP or PAWP in the desired range, then additional albumin is given. Once CVP is over 10 mm Hg or PAWP is over 14 and CPP is still less than 70 mm Hg, a pressor agent such as norepinephrine (Levophed) is recommended to achieve the CPP goal. Levophed infusion should not exceed 0.2 μg/kg/min. If urine output falls below 0.5 ml/kg/hr, dopamine should be started and Levophed discontinued or decreased. When the cardiac index is less than 3.0 L/min/m², the cardiac inotropic agent dobutamine is highly effective in improving CPP.[57] Some patients occasionally require more than one pressor to achieve adequate cerebral perfusion. In patients with acute intraparenchymal blood on CT scan, an upper limit for systolic blood pressure of 180 to 200 mm Hg is probably prudent, given the risk of worsening such hemorrhage with excessive hypertension. Chronic hypertensive patients, however, are likely to tolerate and, in fact, require higher systemic pressures to maintain adequate cerebral perfusion.[90] Further measures to reduce ICP, which are outlined in the next section, also improve CPP.

Strict and frequent monitoring of total intake (crystalloid, colloid, blood products, parenteral nutrition and tube feedings) and output (urine, nasogastric, CSF) are essential in maintaining a euvolemic state. Negative fluid balance is corrected by replacement of the fluid deficit every 2 hours. With intensive fluid management as described, the risk of pulmonary edema is significant. Careful clinical assessment and daily chest radiographs are mandatory, especially in elderly patients and in those with multiple injuries.

## Intracranial Hypertension Management

Intracranial hypertension is defined as an ICP of over 15 mm Hg; an ICP of over 20 mm Hg sustained for more than 5 minutes should be treated. In patients with temporal lobe or deep frontal lobe lesions in whom the risk of uncal herniation is greater, an ICP treatment threshold of 15 mm Hg may be warranted.[17]

The treatment of intracranial hypertension should proceed in a stepwise manner. Routine pre-emptive measures exercised in all patients with severe head injury include maintenance of normothermia, head elevation to 30 degrees, and mild hyperventilation to a Paco₂ of 30 to 35 mm Hg.[30] Seizure prophylaxis should be used for at least the first week after injury or for longer if intracranial hypertension persists. Phenytoin with serum levels maintained in the high therapeutic range (15 to 20 μg/L) appears most effective.[104] Additional therapies to control ICP are used as needed, starting with narcotic sedation, muscle relaxants, and ventricular drainage, followed by bolus mannitol administration and finally, in some select patients, induction of pentobarbital coma. When acute and sustained rises in ICP occur, rapid manual hyperventilation of the patient should be avoided because the Paco₂ may drop dramatically, resulting in critical cerebral vasoconstriction and ischemia. Instead, the maneuvers outlined in the following paragraphs should be done in an expedient and, if necessary, simultaneous manner.

Sedation can be initiated with a 10-mg bolus of IV morphine, which may be repeated once. If it is effective in lowering ICP, a continuous morphine infusion starting at 5 mg/hr is begun. The rate can be increased by 5-mg increments up to 20 mg/hr as needed for agitation or excess motor activity. When intracranial hypertension persists despite narcotic sedation, and the patient is agitated, has increased motor tone, is shivering, or is resisting the ventilator, a neuromuscular blocking agent is added to help control ICP. Vecuronium, 10 mg every 30 minutes, is given as needed. Alcohol withdrawal also may contribute to agitation and intracranial hypertension, and is typically poorly controlled with narcotics. If withdrawal is suspected, lorazepam (Ativan), 5 mg IV every 6 hours, is administered empirically for 48 to 72 hours. Chlordiazepoxide (Librium) is an effective alternative.

When these initial measures are inadequate to control ICP or achieve an adequate CPP, ventricular drainage is used. In patients without significant agitation or motor activity, ventricular drainage can be used as the initial intervention to reduce ICP before narcotic administration. The ventriculostomy drip chamber is placed at 5 cm above the level of the ventricle, with the stopcock turned to the transducer only. This arrangement provides a continuous ICP reading for the nursing staff and allows for relatively rapid but not excessive CSF drainage when needed. The ventriculostomy is opened for drainage only when ICP exceeds the treatment threshold. Continuous ventricular drainage is not recommended because significant ICP spikes may be missed when the ICP is monitored only intermittently. If the transduced waveform is lost, the catheter should be checked for patency.

If ventricular drainage is inadequate or a functioning ventriculostomy is not in place, bolus mannitol therapy is the next line of treatment for intracranial hypertension or low CPP. Mannitol not only removes extravascular water from the brain, but acts as a fluid bolus to improve CPP, and is thought to reduce blood viscosity and thus improve cerebral oxygen delivery.[90] Because boluses of 0.25 g/kg have been shown to be equally effective in lowering ICP as have larger doses, it is recommended that smaller doses be used first.[65] For most adults, a 25-g bolus is effective in lowering ICP and for improving CPP and can be repeated as necessary. Serum osmolality should not be allowed to rise above 310 mOsm/kg. If total input and output are regularly matched, a hyperosmolar state rarely develops. Given that excessive mannitol use may result in acute oliguric renal failure, total daily doses of mannitol should not exceed 200 g; in patients with renal insufficiency, substantially lower doses are recommended.[24]

When ICP remains elevated and CPP is 70 mm Hg or less, despite use of the aforementioned maneuvers, an attempt to raise CPP further to the range of 80 to 100 mm Hg can be made before resorting to barbiturate therapy. Rosner[90] notes numerous patients who require a CPP considerably above 70 mm Hg before adequate ICP control is achieved. A corollary to the concept of a minimally acceptable perfusion pressure is that at an adequate CPP, modest intracranial hypertension appears to be well tolerated if clinical status and CT findings do not suggest impending herniation. The studies of Miller[72] and Rosner[90] support this idea. The precise level and duration of raised ICP that does not adversely affect outcome at a given perfusion pressure, however, remains to be defined. Given the strong correlation between elevated ICP and poor outcome in the TCDB and numerous other reports, an aggressive attempt to maintain ICP below 20 mm Hg should still be made.[1, 61, 62, 74] Twenty-four hours after injury, mild hyperventilation to a $PaCO_2$ of 30 mm Hg can be used if there is no evidence of cerebral ischemia.

## Barbiturate Coma

When all previously outlined measures fail to control ICP, barbiturate therapy can be considered in select patients, provided it is not begun too late in the course of treatment.[17, 72] Only one randomized study, performed by Eisenberg and associates,[27] has demonstrated some benefit from the use of barbiturate coma in the severely head-injured patient. Indications for initiating barbiturate treatment have not been rigidly defined. However, it appears a favorable outcome is most likely to occur in young patients who do not have evidence of brain stem injury and who have a Glasgow motor score of 4 or greater before sedation and paralysis. Reasonable indications to begin high-dose barbiturates include 30 minutes of ICP over 30 mm Hg with CPP less than 70 mm Hg, or ICP over 40 mm Hg despite a CPP of 70 mm Hg, after all previously outlined measures to control ICP have been exhausted. Given the high rate of complications with barbiturate coma, these patients must be monitored extremely closely. The patient should be in a normovolemic state before onset of therapy and should have a Swan-Ganz catheter inserted if it is not already in place. Pentobarbital administration begins with a 10-mg/kg loading dose over 30 minutes followed by 5 mg/kg/hr over the next 3 hours. An adverse hemodynamic response to high-dose barbiturates is more likely to occur in older patients and in those with previous cardiac instability. In such patients, initiating therapy with lower doses is prudent. Ideally, CPP should be maintained above

70 mm Hg and vasopressors instituted rapidly if blood pressure falls. A maintenance infusion of 1 to 3 mg/kg/hr is usually sufficient to maintain burst suppression on electroencephalogram and reasonable control of ICP. Serum pentobarbital levels should be monitored; ICP control usually is achieved with serum levels of 30 to 50 mg/100 ml. Gradual withdrawal of barbiturate therapy over several days can begin after ICP control has been achieved for 24 to 48 hours. Patients in barbiturate coma are at increased risk for pneumonia and sepsis and should be carefully monitored for such complications. For a more in-depth discussion of the use of barbiturate coma, the reader is referred to the work by Chesnut and colleagues.[17]

## Delayed Neurologic Deficit, Refractory Intracranial Hypertension, and Recurrent Hematoma Formation

If control of intracranial hypertension becomes increasingly problematic in a given patient, or if the patient otherwise worsens neurologically, the possibility of a new or reaccumulating intracranial hematoma must be investigated by a repeat CT scan. As discussed earlier, this procedure is especially important in patients who receive a CT scan within a few hours of injury and in those patients with coagulopathy on admission. In a report by Bullock and associates,[12] recurrent hematoma requiring reoperation developed at the operative site in almost 7% of 850 patients who underwent craniotomy for evacuation of a traumatic intracranial lesion. EDHs comprised 69% of these secondary lesions, but subdural and intracerebral accumulations were also seen. Patients with postoperative hematoma had a significantly worse outcome and a higher incidence of alcohol intoxication, and were more likely to have received preoperative mannitol. Coagulopathy was also more common in patients requiring reoperation. Delayed ICHs are also relatively common after severe closed head injury, occurring in 1.5% to 7% of patients.[20] As reported by Gentleman and associates,[37] development of a delayed ICH was almost always associated with persistent intracranial hypertension, clinical worsening, or failure to improve neurologically. Approximately 80% of delayed ICHs become evident within 48 hours of injury.[98]

Two other causes of delayed neurologic deterioration that may be associated with raised ICP are traumatic cervical internal carotid dissection and traumatic vasospasm. Carotid dissection typically occurs after severe blunt head and neck trauma, and is usually manifested in a subacute manner within hours to days of injury.[76] It is often heralded by a new hemiparesis in the absence of associated CT findings.

Significantly more common than carotid dissection, traumatic arterial spasm has a time course similar to that seen in patients with aneurysmal subarachnoid hemorrhage, usually occurring at least 3 days after injury. The development of spasm is most likely to occur in patients with CT evidence of subdural, subarachnoid, intraventricular, or intraparenchymal hemorrhage.[66, 67] When a repeat CT scan does not provide an explanation for the patient's neurologic deterioration, transcranial and cervical Doppler studies are indicated, followed by angiography in some cases. Ideally, transcranial Doppler studies are performed on a daily basis in patients with severe head injury to allow detection of increased flow velocities before the development of a delayed ischemic deficit.

## Neurologic Assessment During the Postoperative Period

When narcotics and neuromuscular blocking agents are routinely used for ICP control, neurologic assessment is limited until such medications are withheld. After surgery, in patients whose ICP is easily controlled, narcotics and paralytics are suspended early to permit clinical evaluation. However, in patients with problematic ICP, diffuse swelling, or poorly visualized cisterns on CT, little is to be gained by reversing such therapy shortly after surgery.[72] In fact, a marked and often dangerous spike in ICP may develop. In such cases, no attempt should be made neurologically to assess the patient other than evaluating his or her pupillary response for at least 24 to 48 hours after surgery, and then only if the ICP treatment intensity significantly lessens.

## Duration of Intracranial Pressure Monitoring

The criteria for how long to monitor ICP are not firmly established. Post-traumatic swelling, edema, and progression of hemorrhagic lesions typically are maximal within 48 to 96 hours of injury. However, delayed increases in ICP are not uncommon. In a series of 53 patients with severe head injury, 15 (31%) had a secondary rise in ICP occurring 3 to 10 days after injury.[107] In 6 of the 15 patients, the delayed rise in ICP was uncontrollable, resulting in death; only 2 patients had a good outcome. The most frequent initial diagnoses in these 15 patients were multiple contusions (7 patients) and acute SDH (5 patients). Possible explanations for the secondary rise in ICP were available in only seven patients and included delayed ICH in three patients, vasospasm detected by transcranial Doppler in two patients, and hypoxia or hyponatremia in two others.

Discontinuation of ICP monitoring is reasonable in patients who maintain normal ICP without specific therapy or with only minimal sedation for at least 24 hours. Such patients should also show significant and steady clinical improvement to a GCS of 9 or greater (unless a primary brain stem injury is evident) and demonstrate resolving lesions on follow-up CT scans, including visible cisterns. Even if these criteria are met, a longer period of observation may be warranted when the initial diagnosis is acute SDH or multiple contusions, in patients with significant vasospasm by transcranial Doppler, and in those patients with major systemic derangements. In addition, intraoperative ICP monitoring is strongly recommended in patients with severe head injury who require general anesthesia within 7 to 10 days of injury for an extracranial operation that cannot otherwise be delayed.

## Ventriculostomy-Related Complications

Ventriculostomy placement is certainly not without risk, the most damaging complications being parenchymal injury, hemorrhage, and infection. The incidence of ventriculostomy-related hemorrhage was 1.4% in the series by Narayan and colleagues[79] and was related to presence of coagulopathy and the number of passes made during catheter placement. In patients with clotting abnormalities, placement of an ICP monitor should be deferred until such deficiencies are at least temporarily corrected.

Ventriculitis in association with ventricular catheter placement is a more frequent problem, being seen in 11% of general neurosurgical patients in the series by Mayhall and coworkers.[68] From this study, the risk of infection was thought to be related largely to the length of time the catheter was in place. Ventriculitis developed in only 6% of patients if the catheter was removed within 5 days, whereas this complication developed in 18% of patients when the catheter was in place longer. However, a new series of 205 neurosurgical patients, including 76 with head injuries, reported by Winfield and associates[114] demonstrated no relationship between the duration of ICP monitoring and incidence of infection with up to 2 weeks of monitoring. The overall infection rate was 7%, with an average monitoring time of 7 days. From their data and a review of the literature, they conclude that the duration of monitoring should be dictated by the clinical need to follow ICP, not the concern of infection. They also stress the need for prophylactic antibiotics and minimal manipulation and irrigation of the catheter system. This report is a welcome addition to the ventriculostomy literature given the significant time, cost, and risk to the patient that accompany catheter replacement, especially in those with small ventricles. Thus, it appears reasonable to leave a ventriculostomy in place for up to 2 weeks, provided prophylactic antibiotics are used, the catheter is tunneled several centimeters away from the insertion site, and CSF samples taken every 2 or 3 days show no evidence of incipient infection. If ventriculitis does develop, removal or changing of the catheter to another site is mandatory and the patient is placed on appropriate antibiotics. Prophylactic antibiotics are not routinely used for fiberoptic ICP monitors, which are not placed in the ventricle.

## Postoperative Intracranial Infections

Osteomyelitis, subdural empyema, meningitis, and brain abscess are seen in 2% to 10% of patients after craniotomy for traumatic intracranial hematoma, with the highest incidence reported in patients with an associated open depressed fracture.[92, 101] Perioperative prophylactic antibiotics and meticulous operative débridement and wound closure are essential to minimize this risk. Once infection is diagnosed, broad-spectrum antibiotics are begun without delay, followed by more targeted therapy when cultures are available. In all cases of osteomyelitis and subdural empyema and in most cases of brain abscess, surgery is also indicated.[55]

## Post-Traumatic Seizures

Early post-traumatic seizures, occurring in the first week after injury, are seen in approximately 25% of patients with traumatic intracranial hematomas.[50] Temkin and colleagues,[104] in a well designed randomized study of head-injured patients with intracranial injury on CT scan or a GCS of 10 or less, demonstrated a significant beneficial effect with the use of prophylactic phenytoin during the first week after injury. If early seizures do occur despite high therapeutic levels of phenytoin and an underlying cause, including electrolyte derangements, hypoglycemia, hypoxemia, or a new lesion on CT scan has been excluded, administration of phenobarbital should be started.

Late post-traumatic epilepsy with onset after the first week of injury occurs in up to 15% of severely head-injured patients and in approximately 35% of patients with intracranial hematomas. Early seizures also significantly increase the risk of late seizures.[50] No randomized studies have shown a beneficial effect from prophylactic anticonvulsant therapy in controlling late seizures.[104] However, given the high risk of late seizures in patients with severe head injury with intracranial hematomas, especially in those with early seizures, prophylactic anticonvulsant therapy for at least 6 months appears reasonable in this subset of patients, despite the lack of definitive evidence to support such a practice.

## Management of Systemic and Extracranial Complications

### Hyperthermia

Hyperthermia, a general metabolic stimulant, has been associated with worse outcome after severe head injury.[52] Conversely, the use of mild systemic hypothermia of 30°C to 34°C (86°F to 93.2°F) in the treatment of severe head injury has yielded promising results in four preliminary clinical studies, prompting a randomized, multicenter study of its use in severe traumatic brain injury.[18, 59, 96, 109] For the present, an aggressive attempt to maintain normothermia (core temperature <37.5°C) appears warranted. A regimen using a combination of acetaminophen, cooling blankets, craniocervical ice packs, and ice water lavage usually is effective. If shivering is noted, a muscle relaxant such as vecuronium should be added.

### Hematologic, Electrolyte, and Nutritional Concerns

In the acute postoperative period, a complete blood count should be obtained at least once daily and packed red blood cells transfused if the hematocrit falls below 30% to optimize cerebral oxygen delivery.[90] Serum electrolytes, including calcium and magnesium, should be checked at least twice daily.

Hyponatremia lowers the seizure threshold and can exacerbate cerebral edema.[23, 87] Low serum sodium is relatively common after head injury, occurring in 8% of patients with moderate or severe injuries in one study.[23] If serum sodium falls below 135 mmol/L, the maintenance IV infusion should be changed to normal saline. For hyponatremia below 130 mmol/L, which typically begins several days after injury, intravenous urea has proved safe and rapidly effective in correcting this problem, whether it is attributed to the syndrome of inappropriate antidiuretic hormone or to cerebral salt wasting.[53, 87] Urea is effective because it is a potent osmotic diuretic and has the unique property of significantly increasing sodium resorption at the kidney.

Forty grams of urea in 150 ml of normal saline is given over 2 hours and repeated every 8 hours. A significant rise in serum sodium is typically seen after two or three doses. Infusion of hypertonic saline is also an effective method of correcting significant hyponatremia but usually takes longer than urea and requires close monitoring of urine electrolytes. Most important, marked fluid restriction is not an option in these patients, in whom maintaining normovolemia is essential.

Magnesium levels should be carefully followed in severely brain-injured patients because low serum and low brain magnesium levels are frequently seen in these patients.[35] Hypomagnesemia lowers the seizure threshold, frequently complicates alcohol withdrawal, and in experimental traumatic brain injury, hinders neurologic recovery.[71] Conversely, administration of intravenous magnesium after injury in a rat head injury model was shown significantly to improve motor function compared with saline-treated animals.[71] A randomized trial of magnesium in the treatment of severe head injury is under way, and early outcome data suggest that there is a therapeutic benefit from its use.[35] It appears reasonable and safe to maintain serum levels in the upper range of normal (1.8 to 2.2 mEq/L) with IV supplementation. Magnesium sulfate, 2 g every 4 hours, can be given as needed, provided renal function is normal.

Hyperglycemia is another common metabolic derangement seen early after both experimental and human traumatic brain injury and is a significant predictor of poor outcome.[112] It is thought that high glucose levels enhance ischemia-mediated cell damage, probably through lactate accumulation.[112, 113] Based on these data, hyperglycemia of over 200 mg/dl should be treated with an insulin drip or sliding scale coverage, and enteral or parental nutrition withheld until 48 hours after injury to minimize early elevations in serum glucose.[16] Dextrose should also be limited to 5% or less in IV fluids during this early postinjury phase.

### Pneumonia

Pneumonia is a frequent and often serious complication after severe head injury, occurring in 41% of the TCDB patients.[86] Aspiration at the scene of injury, impaired airway reflexes, prolonged intubation, and treatment with barbiturates make the severe head injury victim highly predisposed to the development of pneumonia. A high index of suspicion must be maintained. In febrile patients who show new infiltrates on chest radiographs, an evolving leukocytosis, and sputum analysis showing copious white blood cells, empiric antibiotic treatment is indicated. Aggressive chest physiotherapy is an important adjunct to antimicrobial therapy. In patients with problematic ICP, chest percussion and nasotracheal suctioning should be preceded by IV lidocaine, up to 100 mg/hr, to blunt the stimulation that may result in ICP spikes.[16]

An important contributing factor in the development of pneumonia in intubated neurosurgical patients appears to be the use of antacids or histamine type 2 ($H_2$) antagonists (cimetidine or ranitidine) for stress ulcer prophylaxis. In three randomized trials composed of over 250 ventilator-dependent intensive care unit patients, including neurosurgical patients, the incidence of pneumonia averaged 31% in the patients treated with antacids, $H_2$ blockers, or both, whereas in patients treated with sucralfate, the incidence of pneumonia averaged 10%.[25, 26, 105] The frequency of clinically significant gastrointestinal hemorrhage using either method of ulcer prophylaxis was low in both groups, approximately 1% for the patients treated with an antacid and an $H_2$ antagonist and 2% for those patients treated with sucralfate. The higher rate of pneumonia in the patients treated with an $H_2$ antagonist or antacids is thought to be related to a higher gastric pH, which allows gastric colonization of aerobic gram-negative bacilli and subsequent oropharyngeal and tracheal colonization. Thus, sucralfate is recommended as the initial ulcer prophylactic agent in the intubated brain-injured patient. When sucralfate is used, however, absorption of enterally administered medications may be impaired. In particular, this problem has been noted with anticonvulsants; consequently, the IV route of administration for such medication is preferable.

## Thromboembolic Events

Deep vein thrombosis (DVT) and pulmonary embolism (PE) are both relatively frequent and often devastating complications in head-injured patients. The incidence of these complications is reduced by the use of pneumatic compression stockings. In a study of both neurologic and neurosurgical patients treated with compression stockings, the incidence of clinically evident DVT was 2.3%, and for PE, the incidence was 1.8%.[6] More recently, Frim and associates[32] administered low-dose subcutaneous heparin to 138 consecutive neurosurgical patients requiring operation, including 58 patients with head injuries. The patients were treated with a regimen using perioperative compression stockings and subcutaneous heparin, 5000 units twice daily, starting on the first day after surgery. In these patients, there were no thromboembolic events and no postoperative hemorrhages. In the control group of 473 patients treated with only compression stockings during and after surgery, thromboembolic complications developed in 3.2% of patients, including eight patients with DVT and seven with PE. From this study, low-dose subcutaneous heparin in conjunction with compression stockings appears to be a safe and effective measure against thromboembolic events in the postoperative head-injured population. However, in patients with abnormal coagulation studies or in those whose hemorrhagic lesions have not stabilized on CT scan, a delay in use of low-dose heparin is warranted.

A high degree of suspicion for DVT and PE must be maintained in the severe head injury victim. If a PE is suspected, a ventilation-perfusion ($\dot{V}/\dot{Q}$) scan should be obtained. In patients with intermediate probability or indeterminate scans in whom the clinical suspicion of PE is high, a pulmonary angiogram is indicated. If a PE is detected by a high-probability $\dot{V}/\dot{Q}$ scan or by angiography, an inferior vena cava filter is placed without delay. A DVT occurring above the level of the knee also warrants filter placement.[16] The unacceptable risk of intracranial hemorrhage with full anticoagulation precludes such treatment in the acutely head-injured patient for at least 10 days to 2 weeks after injury. The ideal timing for safe anticoagulation after head injury remains unclear, however.[16]

## Gastrointestinal Hemorrhage

Erosive gastrointestinal lesions are remarkably common after severe head injury. In one endoscopic study, 91% of such patients had gastritis within 24 hours of injury.[11] Significant gastrointestinal bleeding requiring transfusion or other intervention has been reported in 2% to 11% of severely head-injured patients.[29, 45] Routine ulcer prophylaxis in all patients with severe head injury is warranted. Use of sucralfate is recommended because of the significantly lower incidence of associated pneumonia and equivalent ulcer prophylaxis compared with $H_2$ antagonists or antacids.[25, 26, 105]

## OUTCOME AND FUTURE EFFORTS

The strongest predictors of poor outcome after severe closed head injury, as documented by the TCDB cohort and largely confirmed by earlier studies, include patient age, postresuscitation GCS, pupil reactivity, proportion of time ICP is over 20 mm Hg, presence of hypotension, and initial CT findings.[1, 5, 61, 64, 74] There is mounting evidence that maintaining CPP at 60 to 70 mm Hg or higher is also associated with an improved outcome.[19, 60, 70, 90, 91]

Regarding the effect of age in the TCDB, no patient older than 55 years of age made a good recovery, whereas 91% of such patients were severely disabled, vegetative, or dead at 6 months after injury. In patients aged 16 to 35 years, good recovery at 6 months after injury was seen in approximately 30%. Concerning the postresuscitation GCS, the percentage of patients reaching an outcome of good or moderate disability at last contact ranged from 7% of those with a GCS of 3 to 77% of patients with a GCS of 8. In patients with normal pupils after resuscitation and throughout their hospital course, 8.5% were left vegetative or dead compared with 74% to 80% vegetative or dead in those with both pupils abnormal at some point after injury.[64] Hypotension, defined as a systolic blood pressure of 90 mm Hg or less, occurred in almost 35% of TCDB patients and was associated with an 85% increase in mortality compared with those who did not sustain a hypotensive episode.[17]

Finally, in patients undergoing evacuation of a traumatic hematoma in the TCDB group, a favorable outcome was seen in 23% of patients (47% of patients with EDH, 27% with ICH, and 14% with SDH), whereas the mortality rate was 39%.[64] Compared with perioperative treatment focused on CPP, Rosner[90] reported a favorable outcome in 60% of operated patients and a mortality rate of 29% in patients with a GCS 7 or less. These favorable results, which are being replicated by others, appear to result largely from aggressive prevention of cerebral ischemia.[60]

Further improvement in recovery after severe traumatic brain injury will be forthcoming with greater understanding of secondary injury phenomena, more refined physiologic and metabolic monitoring, and an even greater reduction of cerebral ischemia. The addition of cerebral protectants currently under investigation, including the antioxidant 21-aminosteroids, calcium channel blockers, N-methyl-D-aspartate (NMDA) antagonists, buffering agents such as tromethamine (THAM), mild hypothermia, and magnesium supplementation, also holds promise in reducing the devastating personal and societal impact of head injury.[18, 35, 44, 52, 71, 72, 96, 109]

## REFERENCES

1. Alberico AM, Ward JD, Choi SC, et al: Outcome after severe head injury, relationship to mass lesions, diffuse injury, and ICP course in pediatric and adult patients. J Neurosurg 67:648–656, 1987.
2. Aldrich EF, Eisenberg HM: Acute subdural hematoma. In Apuzzo MLJ (ed): Brain Surgery Complication Avoidance and Management. New York: Churchill Livingstone, 1993, pp 1283–1298.
3. Andrews BT, Bederson JB, Pitts LH: Use of intraoperative ultrasonography to improve the diagnostic accuracy of exploratory burr holes in patients with traumatic tentorial herniation. Neurosurgery 24:345–347, 1989.
4. Baker SP, O'Neill B, Ginsburg MJ, et al: Injuries in relation to other health problems. In The Injury Fact Book, 2nd ed. New York: Oxford University Press, 1992, pp 8–16.
5. Becker DP, Miller JD, Ward JD, et al: The outcome from severe head injury with early diagnosis and intensive management. J Neurosurg 47:491–502, 1977.
6. Black PM, Baker MF, Snook CP: Experience with external pneumatic calf compression in neurology and neurosurgery. Neurosurgery 18:440–444, 1986.
7. Bouma GJ, Muizelaar JP: Relationship between cardiac output and cerebral blood flow in patients with intact and with impaired autoregulation. J Neurosurg 73:368–374, 1990.
8. Bouma GJ, Muizelaar JP, Bandoh K, et al: Blood pressure and intracranial pressure-volume dynamics in severe head injury: Relationship with cerebral blood flow. J Neurosurg 77:15–19, 1992.
9. Bouma GJ, Muizelaar JP, Choi SC, et al: Cerebral circulation and metabolism after severe traumatic brain injury: The elusive role of ischemia. J Neurosurg 75:685–693, 1991.
10. Bouma GJ, Muizelaar JP, Stringer WA, et al: Ultra-early evaluation of regional cerebral blood flow in severely head-injured patients using xenon-enhanced computerized tomography. J Neurosurg 77:360–369, 1992.
11. Brown TH, Davidson PF, Larson GM: Acute gastritis occurring within 24 hours of severe head injury. Gastrointest Endosc 35:37–40, 1989.
12. Bullock R, Hannemann CO, Murray L, et al: Recurrent hematomas following craniotomy for traumatic intracranial mass. J Neurosurg 72:9–14, 1990.
13. Chan K, Dearden NM, Miller JD, et al: Multimodality monitoring as a guide to treatment of intracranial hypertension after severe brain injury. Neurosurgery 32:547–553, 1993.
14. Chan K, Dearden NM, Miller JD, et al: Transcranial Doppler waveform differences in hyperemic and nonhyperemic patients after severe head injury. Surg Neurol 38:433–436, 1992.
15. Chan K, Miller JD, Dearden NM, et al: The effect of changes in cerebral perfusion pressure upon middle cerebral artery blood flow velocity and jugular bulb venous oxygen saturation after severe brain injury. J Neurosurg 77:55–61, 1992.
16. Chesnut RM: Medical complications of the head-injured patient. In Cooper PR (ed): Head Injury, 3rd ed. Baltimore: Williams & Wilkins, 1993, pp 459–501.
17. Chesnut RM, Marshall LF, Marshall SB: Medical management of intracranial pressure. In Cooper PR (ed): Head Injury, 3rd ed. Baltimore: Williams & Wilkins, 1993, pp 225–246.
18. Clifton GL, Steven A, Plenger PM, et al: A phase II study of systemic hypothermia in severe brain injury (Abstract). 61st Annual Meeting of the American Association of Neurological Surgeons, Boston, April, 1993.
19. Contant CF, Robertson CF, Gopinath SP, et al: Determination of clinically important thresholds in continuously monitored patients with head injury (Abstract). 2nd International Neurotrauma Symposium, Glasgow, July, 1993.
20. Cooper PR: Post-traumatic intracranial mass lesions. In Cooper PR (ed): Head Injury, 3rd ed. Baltimore: Williams & Wilkins, 1993, pp 275–329.
21. Cooper PR, Rovit RL, Ransohoff J: Hemicraniectomy in the treatment of acute subdural hematoma: A re-appraisal. Surg Neurol 5:25–29, 1976.
22. Delaney KA, Goldfrank LR: Initial management of the multiply injured or intoxicated patient. In Cooper PR (ed): Head Injury, 3rd ed. Baltimore: Williams & Wilkins, 1993, pp 43–63.
23. Doczi T. Tarjanyi J, Huszka E, et al: Syndrome of inappropriate secretion of antidiuretic hormone (SIADH) after head injury. Neurosurgery 10:685–688, 1982.
24. Dorman HR, Sondheimer JH, Cadnapaphornchai P: Mannitol-induced acute renal failure. Medicine (Baltimore) 69:153–159, 1990.
25. Driks MR, Craven DE, Celli BR, et al: Nosocomial pneumonia in intubated patients given sucralfate as compared with antacids or histamine type 2 blockers, the role of gastric colonization. N Engl J Med 317:1376–1382, 1987.
26. Eddleston JM, Vohra A, Scott P, et al: A comparison of the frequency of stress ulceration and secondary pneumonia in sucralfate- or ranitidine-treated intensive care unit patients. Crit Care Med 19:1491-1496, 1991.
27. Eisenberg HM, Frankowski RF, Contant CF, et al: High-dose barbiturate control of elevated intracranial pressure in patients with severe head injury. J Neurosurg 69:15–23, 1988.
28. El Adawy Y, Rosner MJ: Cerebral perfusion pressure, autoregulation and the PVI reflection point: Pathological ICP. In Hoff JT, Betz AL (eds): Intracranial Pressure VII. New York: Springer-Verlag, 1988, pp 829–833.
29. Epstein FM, Ward JD, Becker DP: Medical complications of head injury. In Cooper PR (ed): Head Injury, 2nd ed. Baltimore: Williams & Wilkins, 1987, pp 390–421.
30. Feldman Z, Kanter MJ, Robertson CS, et al: Effect of head elevation on intracranial pressure, cerebral perfusion pressure, and cerebral blood flow in head-injured patients. J Neurosurg 76:207–211, 1992.
31. Foulkes MA, Eisenberg HM, Jane JA, et al: The traumatic coma data bank: Design, methods, and baseline characteristics. J Neurosurg 75 (Suppl):S8–S13, 1991.
32. Frim DM, Barker FG, Poletti CE: Postoperative low-dose heparin decreases thromboembolic complications in neurosurgical patients. Neurosurgery 30:830–833, 1992.
33. Gaab MR, Rittierodt M, Lorenz M, et al: Traumatic brain swelling and operative decompression: A prospective investigation. Acta Neurochir Suppl (Wien) 51:326–328, 1990.
34. Galbraith S, Murray WR, Patel AR, et al: The relationship between alcohol and head injury and its effect on the conscious level. Br J Surg 63:128–130, 1976.
35. Gennarelli TA. Personal communication, 1993.
36. Gennarelli TA, Champion HR, Sacco WJ, et al: Mortality of patients with head injury and extracranial injury treated in trauma centers. J Trauma 29:1193–1202, 1989.
37. Gentleman D, Nath F, MacPherson P: Diagnosis and management of delayed traumatic intracerebral hematoma. Br J Neurosurg 3:367–372, 1989.
38. Gentleman D, Teasdale G, Murray L: Cause of severe head injury and risk of complications. BMJ 292:449, 1986.
39. Goodnight SH, Kenoyer G, Rapaport SI, et al: Defibrination after brain tissue destruction: A serious complication of head injury. N Engl J Med 290:1043–1047, 1974.
40. Gopinath SP, Robertson CS, Grossman RG, et al: Near-infrared spectroscopic localization of intracranial hematomas. J Neurosurg 79:43–47, 1993.
41. Graham DI, Ford I, Hume-Adams J, et al: Ischaemic brain damage is still common in fatal non-missile head injury. J Neurol Neurosurg Psychiatry 52:346–350, 1989.
42. Gray WJ, Rosner MJ: Pressure-volume index II: The effects of low cerebral perfusion pressure and autoregulation. J Neurosurg 67:377–380, 1987.
43. Grossman CB: Magnetic Resonance Imaging and Computed Tomography of the Head and Spine. Baltimore: Williams & Wilkins, 1990, pp 184–201.
44. Hall ED, Braughler JM, McCall JM: Antioxidant effects in brain and spinal cord injury. J Neurotrauma 9 (Suppl 1):S165–172, 1992.
45. Halloran LG, Zfass AM, Gayle WE, et al: Prevention of acute gastrointestinal complications after severe head injury: A controlled trial of cimetidine prophylaxis. Am J Surg 139:44–48, 1980.
46. Horwitz NH: Comment of: Nussbaum ES, Wolf AL, Sebring L, et al: Complete temporal lobectomy for surgical resuscitation of patients with transtentorial herniation secondary to unilateral hemispheric swelling. Neurosurgery 29:62–66, 1991.
47. Howard MA, Gross AS, Dacey RG, et al: Acute subdural hemato-

mas: An age-dependent clinical entity. J Neurosurg 71:858–863, 1989.

48. Jagger J, Fife D, Venberg K, et al: Effect of alcohol intoxication on the diagnosis and apparent severity of brain injury. Neurosurgery 15:303–306, 1984.

49. Jamieson KG, Yelland JDN: Surgically treated traumatic subdural hematomas. J Neurosurg 37:137–149, 1972.

50. Jennett B: Epilepsy After Nonmissile Injuries, 2nd ed. Chicago: Year Book, 1975.

51. Jennett B, Teasdale G, Galbraith S, et al: Severe head injury in three countries. J Neurol Neurosurg Psychiatry 40:291–298, 1977.

52. Jones PA, Piper IR, Corrie J, et al: Microcomputer based detection of secondary insults and 12 month outcome after head injury (Abstract). 2nd International Neurotrauma Symposium, Glasgow, July, 1993.

53. Kelly DF, Laws ER, Fossett DT: Fluid and sodium abnormalities after transsphenoidal surgery for pituitary adenomas with emphasis on delayed hyponatremia: A review of 99 patients (Abstract). Congress of Neurological Surgeons Annual Meeting, Vancouver, October, 1993.

54. Kraus JF: Epidemiology of head injury. In Cooper PR (ed): Head Injury, 3rd ed. Baltimore: Williams & Wilkins, 1993, pp 1–25.

55. Landesman S, Cooper PR: Infectious complications of head injury. In Cooper PR (ed): Head Injury, 3rd ed. Baltimore: Williams & Wilkins, 1993, pp 503–523.

56. Levy ML, Giannotta SL: Cardiac performance indices during hypervolemic therapy for cerebral vasospasm. J Neurosurg 75:27–31, 1991.

57. Levy ML, Rabb CH, Zelman V, et al: Cardiac performance enhancement from dobutamine in patients refractory to hypervolemic therapy for cerebral vasospasm. J Neurosurg 79:494–499, 1993.

58. Majernick TG, Bieniek R, Houston JB, et al: Cervical spine movement during orotracheal intubation. Ann Emerg Med 15:417–420, 1986.

59. Marion D, Obrist WD, Carlier PM, et al: The use of moderate therapeutic hypothermia for patients with severe head injuries: A preliminary report. J Neurosurg 79:354–362, 1993.

60. Marion D, Obrist WD, Penrod LE, et al: Treatment of cerebral ischemia improves outcome following severe traumatic brain injury (Abstract). The 61st Annual Meeting of the American Association of Neurological Surgeons, Boston, April, 1993; and personal communication.

61. Marmarou A, Anderson RL, Ward JD, et al: NINDS traumatic coma data bank: Intracranial pressure monitoring methodology. J Neurosurg 75:S21–S27, 1991.

62. Marmarou A, Anderson RL, Ward JD, et al: Impact of ICP instability and hypotension on outcome in patients with severe head trauma. J Neurosurg 75:S59–S66, 1991.

63. Marsh ML, Dunlop BJ, Shapiro HM, et al: Succinylcholine: Intracranial pressure effects in neurosurgical patients. Anesth Analg 59:550–551, 1980.

64. Marshall LF, Gautille, T, Klauber MR, et al: The outcome of severe closed head injury. J Neurosurg 75 (Suppl):S28–S36, 1991.

65. Marshall LF, Smith R, Rauscher L, et al: Mannitol dose requirements in brain-injured patients. J Neurosurg 48:169–172, 1978.

66. Martin NA, Doberstein C, Khanna R, et al: Post-traumatic cerebral arterial spasm (Abstract). 2nd International Neurotrauma Symposium, Glasgow, July, 1993.

67. Martin NA, Doberstein C, Zane C, et al: Posttraumatic cerebral arterial spasm: Transcranial Doppler ultrasound, cerebral blood flow, and angiographic findings. J Neurosurg 77:575–583, 1992.

68. Mayhall CG, Archer NH, Lamb VA, et al: Ventriculostomy-related infection: A prospective epidemiologic study. N Engl J Med 310:553–559, 1984.

69. McBride DQ, Patel AB, Caron M: Early repeat CT scan: Importance in detecting surgical lesions after closed head injury (Abstract). 2nd International Neurotrauma Symposium, Glasgow, July, 1993.

70. McGraw CP: A cerebral perfusion pressure greater than 80 mm Hg is more beneficial. In Hoff JT, Betz AL (eds): Intracranial Pressure, Vol VII. Berlin: Springer-Verlag, 1989, pp 839–841.

71. McIntosh TK. Pharmacologic strategies in the treatment of experimental brain injury. J Neurotrauma 9 (Suppl 1):S201–S209, 1992.

72. Miller JD: Evaluation and treatment of head injury in adults. Neurosurg Q 2:28–43, 1992.

73. Miller JD: Head injury and brain ischemia. Br J Anaesth 57:120–129, 1985.

74. Miller JD, Butterworth JF, Gudeman SK, et al: Further experience in the management of severe head injury. J Neurosurg 54:289–299, 1981.

75. Miller JD, Dearden NM, Piper IR, et al: Control of intracranial pressure in patients with severe head injury. J Neurotrauma 9 (Suppl 1):S317–S326, 1992.

76. Mokri B, Piepgras DG, Houser OW: Traumatic dissections of the extracranial internal carotid artery. J Neurosurg 68:189–197, 1988.

77. Muizelaar JP, Marmarou A, Ward JD, et al: Adverse effects of prolonged hyperventilation in patients with severe head injury: A randomized clinical trial. J Neurosurg 75:731–739, 1991.

78. Muizelaar JP, Ward JD, Marmarou A, et al: Cerebral blood flow and metabolism in severely head-injured children. Part 2: Autoregulation. J Neurosurg 71:72–76, 1989.

79. Narayan RK, Kishore PRS, Becker DP, et al: Intracranial pressure: To monitor or not to monitor? A review of our experience with severe head injury. J Neurosurg 56:650–659, 1982.

80. Nordstrom CH, Messeter K, Sundbarg G, et al: Cerebral blood flow, vasoreactivity, and oxygen consumption during barbiturate therapy in severe traumatic brain lesions. J Neurosurg 68:424–431, 1988.

81. Nussbaum ES, Wolf AL, Sebring L, et al: Complete temporal lobectomy for surgical resuscitation of patients with transtentorial herniation secondary to unilateral hemispheric swelling. Neurosurgery 29:62–66, 1991.

82. Obrist WD, Langfitt TW, Jaggi JL, et al: Cerebral blood flow and metabolism in comatose patients with acute head injury: Relationship to intracranial hypertension. J Neurosurg 61:241–253, 1984.

83. Obrist WD, Marion DW, Aggarwal S: Time course of cerebral blood flow and metabolic changes following severe head injury (Abstract). 61st Annual Meeting of the American Association of Neurological Surgeons, Boston, April, 1993.

84. Olson JD, Kaufman HH, Moake J, et al: The incidence and significance of hemostatic abnormalities with head injuries. Neurosurgery 24:825–832, 1989.

85. Paulson OB, Strandgaard S, Edvinsson L: Cerebral autoregulation. Cerebrovasc Brain Metab Rev 2:161–192, 1990.

86. Piek J, Chesnut RM, Marshall LF, et al: Extracranial complications of severe head injury. J Neurosurg 77:901–907, 1992.

87. Reeder RF, Harbaugh RE: Administration of intravenous urea and normal saline for treatment of hyponatremia in neurosurgical patients. J Neurosurg 70:201–206, 1989.

88. Rhee KJ, Green W, Holcroft JW, et al: Oral intubation in the multiply injured patient: The risk of exacerbating spinal cord damage. Ann Emerg Med 19:511–514, 1990.

89. Rimel RW, Giordani B, Barth JT: Moderate head injury: Completing the clinical spectrum of brain trauma. Neurosurgery 11:344–351, 1982.

90. Rosner MJ: Pathophysiology and management of increased intracranial pressure. In Andrews BT (ed): Neurosurgical Intensive Care. New York: McGraw-Hill, 1993, pp 57–112.

91. Rosner MJ, Daughton S: Cerebral perfusion pressure management in head injury. J Trauma 30:933–941, 1990.

92. Sande GM, Galbraith SL, McLatchie G: Infection after depressed fracture in the west of Scotland. Scott Med J 25:227–229, 1980.

93. Seiler RW, Groge U, Steiger HJ, et al: Detection and monitoring of traumatic vasospasm (Abstract). 2nd International Neurotrauma Symposium, Glasgow, July, 1993.

94. Sekhar L: Personal communication, 1993.

95. Sheinberg M, Kanter MJ, Robertson CS, et al: Continuous monitoring of jugular venous oxygen saturation in head-injured patients. J Neurosurg 76:212–217, 1992.

96. Shiozaki T, Sugimoto H, Taneda M, et al: Effect of mild hypothermia on uncontrollable intracranial hypertension after severe head injury. J Neurosurg 79:363–368, 1993.

97. Smith MM, Young HF: Acute epidural hematoma. In Apuzz MLJ (ed): Brain Surgery Complication Avoidance and Management. New York: Churchill Livingstone, 1993, pp 1323–1334.

98. Sprick C, Bettag M, Bock WJ: Delayed traumatic intracranial hematomas: Clinical study of seven years. Neurosurg Rev 12 (Suppl 1):228–230, 1989.

99. Stein SC, Spettell C, Young G, et al: Delayed and progressive brain injury in closed-head trauma: Radiological demonstration. Neurosurgery 32:25–31, 1993.

100. Stein SC, Young GS, Talucci RC, et al: Delayed brain injury after head trauma: Significance of coagulopathy. Neurosurgery 30:160–165, 1992.

101. Stone JL, Rifai MHS, Sugar O, et al: Subdural hematomas. I: Acute subdural hematoma: Progress in definition, clinical pathology, and therapy. Surg Neurol 19:216–231, 1983.
102. Talucci RC, Shaikh KA, Schwab CW: Rapid sequence induction with oral endotracheal intubation in the multiply injured patient. Am Surg 54:185–187, 1988.
103. Teasdale G, Jennett B: Assessment of coma and impaired consciousness: A practical scale. Lancet 2:81–84, 1974.
104. Temkin NR, Dikmen SS, Wilensky AJ, et al: A randomized, double-blind study of phenytoin for the prevention of post-traumatic seizures. N Engl J Med 323:497–502, 1990.
105. Tryba M: Risk of acute stress bleeding and nosocomial pneumonia in ventilated intensive care unit patients: Sucralfate versus antacids. Am J Med 83 (Suppl 3B):117–124, 1987.
106. Tsutsumi H, Ide K, Mizutani T, et al: The relationship between intracranial pressure, cerebral perfusion pressure and outcome in head-injured patients: The critical level of cerebral perfusion pressure. In Miller JD, Teasdale GM, Rowan JO, et al (eds): Intracranial Pressure, Vol VI. Berlin: Springer-Verlag, 1986, pp 661–666.
107. Unterberg A, Kiening K, Schmidek P, et al: Long-term observations of intracranial pressure after severe head injury: The phenomenon of secondary rise of intracranial pressure. Neurosurgery 32:17–24, 1993.
108. van Helden A, Schneider GH, Unterberg A, et al: Monitoring of jugular venous oxygen saturation as a guide to therapy of severe head injury (Abstract). 2nd International Neurotrauma Symposium, Glasgow, July, 1993.
109. Vice MV: A metabolic approach to the management of neurological trauma: Hypothermic hypokalemic coma (Abstract). 61st Annual Meeting of the American Association of Neurological Surgeons, Boston, April, 1993.
110. Vollmer DG, Torner JC, Jane JA: Age and outcome following traumatic coma: Why do older patients fare worse? J Neurosurg 75:S37–S49, 1991.
111. Wilberger JE, Rothfus WE, Tabas J, et al: Acute tissue tear hemorrhages of the brain: Computed tomography and clinicopathological correlations. Neurosurgery 27:208–213, 1990.
112. Young B, Ott L, Dempsey R, et al: Relationship between admission hyperglycemia and neurological outcome of severely brain-injured patients. Ann Surg 210:466–473, 1989.
113. Young B, Ott L, Yingling B, et al: Nutrition and brain injury. J Neurotrauma 9 (Suppl 1):S375–S383, 1992.
114. Winfield JA, Rosenthal P, Kanter RK, et al: Duration of intracranial pressure monitoring does not predict daily risk of infectious complications. Neurosurgery 33:424–431, 1993.

# Surgical Management of Traumatic Intracranial Hematomas

■ J. DOUGLAS MILLER and PATRICK F. X. STATHAM

## DEFINING THE THERAPEUTIC PROBLEM

The formation of intracranial hematomas after a head injury is a common occurrence; exactly how common this situation is has become clear only since the application of computed tomographic (CT) imaging in large consecutive series of head-injured patients of all degrees of severity. One of the first such reports, which showed a 40% incidence of intracranial hematomas requiring surgical evacuation in comatose, head-injured patients, was by Becker and colleagues in 1977.[1] Since then, many reports have confirmed this high frequency and have allowed definition of risk factors for hematoma formation after head injury (see later).[2–6]

Post-traumatic intracranial hematomas take several forms in terms of size, location, and speed of development and also the effects that they exert on patients. These effects depend on the characteristics of the hematoma and those of the brain on which the hematoma presses, whether it is swollen, tight and noncompliant, or atrophic with ample compensatory cerebrospinal fluid (CSF) space. The effects also depend on whether the brain has previously been injured, diseased, or affected by degenerative disorders.

Not all intracranial hematomas need to be surgically removed, but failing to detect a hematoma that does need to be removed or making a wrong decision to treat such a hematoma conservatively is a catastrophe that could result in death or disability for the patient. Such decisions are a measure of poor clinical judgment on the part of the treating surgeon and are a potential source of medical litigation.

Many patients show evidence of deterioration of neurologic function and level of consciousness as the hematoma develops in size. In the patient who is already comatose or becomes comatose, brain failure exists, and intervention must begin immediately because the prospects for independent survival ebb away minute by minute. All efforts should be directed toward obtaining brain decompression. To detect hematomas at an early stage, a pre-emptive approach is essential, and this depends on the identification of risk factors that increase the chances that a given patient will be harboring an intracranial hematoma. These risk factors are simple, consisting of the presence of a skull fracture on radiograph or by clinical inference and a decrease in the level of consciousness. The factors are additive and apply both to adults and to children.[7] All patients with skull fracture must have a CT scan, as should head-injured patients with any neurologic dysfunction, depression of level of consciousness that lasts for more than a few hours, a seizure, or severe headaches and vomiting.

## CLASSIFICATION AND CLINICAL FEATURES

Traumatic intracranial hematomas are conventionally divided into extradural or epidural hematoma, subdural hematoma, and intracerebral hematoma. Traumatic subarachnoid hemorrhage is more common than any of these but never constitutes a surgical problem in itself, although it may be followed by hydrocephalus requiring CSF shunting at a later stage. Each of the principal types of surgical intracranial hematoma has subtypes according to the location and timing of their development. The clinical features of hematoma are general features of elevated intracranial pressure and signs of focal brain dysfunction, depending on the site of the hematoma; however, both of these sets of clinical features may be overshadowed and totally obscured by the neurologic consequences of the primary trauma. It is, therefore, unwise to depend on the detection of "characteristic" clinical signs or temporal patterns, and it is important to obtain CT imaging regardless of whether the patient is in a static clinical state, deteriorating, or even apparently improving.

### Epidural Hematoma

Epidural hematomas, which lie between the inner surface of the skull and the stripped-off dural membrane, are almost always caused by, and located near, a skull fracture.[8, 9] The association of hematoma and skull fracture is somewhat less strong in patients younger than 30 years of age. Seventy percent of hematomas are located in the temporoparietal area, because skull fractures in this area cross the path of the middle meningeal artery and its dural branches. Frontal and occipital epidural hematomas occur less frequently (10% each), and the latter sometimes extend both above and below the tentorium or, rarely, lie entirely in the posterior cranial fossa.

In the past, too much emphasis has been laid on the so-called typical presentation of an epidural hematoma, referring to the sequence of events in which a patient has a relatively minor head injury, which may cause a brief loss of consciousness. The patient regains consciousness, then deteriorates once again into coma, with a fixed dilated pupil ipsilateral to a skull fracture and a contralateral hemiparesis or extensor motor response. This type of presentation accounts for fewer than 20% of epidural hematomas detected in the modern series of head injuries. Epidural hematomas usually form within a matter of hours from the time of injury but sometimes run a more chronic course, being detected only days after injury. CT removes most of the mysteries from diagnosis and, most important, shows precisely the location of the hematoma, thus guiding the surgeon to the location and extent of craniotomy that will be required to evacuate the hematoma.

In rare circumstances in which neurologic deterioration is extremely rapid and CT is either unavailable or will take too long to obtain, and in which epidural hematoma is strongly suspected, the surgeon may need to initiate treatment without CT. In that rare event, the exploratory bur hole should be located close to, but not over, the fracture because this is where the hematoma will be found, if it is epidural. However, prompt intubation, ventilation, and intravenous mannitol administration usually provide sufficient time to obtain a CT scan. In some cases, the initial CT may be performed too soon in a patient in whom an epidural hematoma is still in the process of forming. In circumstances in which CT is obtained within the first 6 hours of injury and the patient shows subsequent deterioration, a second CT scan must be obtained. In a few cases, repeat CT reveals a sizeable epidural hematoma that was not shown on the first films.[10]

There are no typical clinical features of posterior fossa epidural hematoma, but the surgeon should be aware that clinical deterioration can be dramatic. The patient may literally be conscious and speaking one minute and apneic the next.

## Subdural Hematoma

Subdural hematomas, which form between the inner surface of the dura mater and the pial surface of the brain, are more stereotypical in location. In most cases, the collection lies over the lateral surface of the anterior temporal lobe and adjacent frontal and parietal areas. The collections are not always locally associated with skull fracture, although, like epidural hematoma, they are causally associated. In many cases, the hematoma is on the opposite side of the brain to a unilateral skull fracture. In a few cases, the hematoma may lie in an unusual location, for example, in the interhemispheric fissure.

Acute subdural hematomas, which form within minutes or hours of injury, may be one or more of three distinct types. The first is a hematoma associated with laceration of the brain, usually at the temporal pole, in which there is a mixture of intracerebral contusion and hemorrhage and an acute subdural hematoma, a condition known by some neurosurgeons as "burst temporal lobe." The second variety is an acute subdural hematoma that results from tearing of a bridging vein between the surface of the brain and one of the main draining venous sinuses, either the sagittal sinus or the lateral sinus. In these cases, the hematoma forms remarkably quickly. Patients often say a few words after a blow to the head, only to lapse into coma within a matter of minutes, entirely as a result of brain compression. When the hematoma is removed and the bleeding point is located and sealed, the brain looks completely intact. The third type of hematoma also forms extremely quickly after the injury, but in this type, the bleeding vessel is a small artery on the surface of the brain that may have been injured by an overlying fracture of the skull, or in some cases, because the vessels are arteriosclerotic. The hematoma forms concentrically around the site of the hemorrhage, and on CT, the image of clotted blood of increased radiodensity may show a lucent area within the clot that represents fresh areas of as yet unclotted blood, the so-called hyperacute subdural hematoma.

Acute subdural (and epidural) hematomas form against a broad spectrum of primary brain injury of diffuse axonal type. Thus, patients who develop hematomas may be in widely varying states of consciousness (from fully awake to deeply comatose) before the onset of the additional problems of brain compression.

In the past, a condition of subacute subdural hematoma was defined, in which patients who showed some deterioration 2 to 3 days after a head injury and were at that time discovered to be harboring a subdural hematoma (usually of the burst temporal lobe variety).[11] Most of these patients probably had the hematoma within 12 hours of injury, and the cause of the later deterioration was swelling and edema of the brain around the area of the temporal lobe laceration and contusion rather than formation of fresh hematoma.

Chronic subdural hematoma is, however, an entirely separate and distinct entity consisting of a collection of liquid blood or blood product over the surface of the brain. This collection may, in long-standing cases, be contained by a membrane of fibrin adherent to the inner aspect of the dura and the pial surface of the brain. In some patients, there is a history of a minor or moderate head injury several weeks before presentation. In other patients, no history of trauma is ever obtained. Patients show a general pattern of deterioration of level of consciousness and the appearance of focal neurologic signs consisting of hemiparesis and hemisensory neglect. Although the overall pattern is one of neurologic deterioration, over shorter periods of time, patients' level of consciousness may fluctuate, which can be confusing for both the family and the medical observer. Visual field impairment is rare, but neglect of one side is not. In some cases, these unilateral signs may be ipsilateral to the hematoma and are caused by the massive midline shift of the brain structures that often accompanies these lesions and compression of the contralateral cerebral peduncle against the edge of the tentorium, sometimes known as Kernohan's notch.[12] If unilateral pupillary dilatation occurs, however, it is always on the side of the hematoma. Skull fracture is most often absent. This form of subdural collection is seen in the elderly and in very young children. If chronic subdural hematomas occur in the intervening age period, they are mainly associated with prior brain atrophy and are often associated with alcohol abuse.

Sudden neurologic deterioration may occur in patients with chronic subdural hematoma. In some cases, this deterioration is a reflection of the exponential relationship between added intracranial volume and intracranial pressure (ICP); a steep rise in pressure results in tentorial herniation. In other cases, however, the slowly enlarging hematoma tears loose a small pial artery, producing fresh arterial hemorrhage that rapidly results in severe headache and progressive loss of consciousness. CT shows the combination of acute (radiodense) and chronic (radiolucent) hematoma, but the patient must be treated with all of the urgency demanded by the acute subdural bleeding and by craniotomy rather than by multiple bur holes.

## Intracerebral Hematoma

Before the advent of CT, intracerebral hematomas diagnosed during life were limited to large collections that were associated with mass effect and could, therefore, be detected by angiography or ventriculography. In contrast, the pathologist has long been aware that patients dying of head injury commonly show a wide range of intracerebral bleeding, ranging from petechial hemorrhages to substantial collections, usually in the temporal or frontal lobes, but also occurring less commonly in the occipital lobe and cerebellum. CT now permits such lesions to be observed during life. This development has created therapeutic dilemmas for the surgeon faced with an acutely ill head-injured patient in whom CT reveals a sizeable frontal and temporal hematoma but no collection over the surface of the brain. Some such lesions are pure hematomas; others are hemorrhagic contusions. In the early stage after head injury, seldom do such hematomas contribute to the coma, which relates to the primary brain injury; however, in some cases, continued expansion of the hematoma or reaction of the surrounding brain to the products of the hematoma may lead to delayed deterioration and subsequent need to evacuate the collection. Hemorrhagic contusions or hematomas in the basal ganglia area after severe, blunt, deceleration head injury represent an extreme end of the spectrum of diffuse axonal injury, and surgical evacuation is not indicated for these lesions.[13]

In a few patients, intracerebral hemorrhage that was not present at first may appear in later CT examinations ("delayed intracerebral hematoma").[14] The appearance of these lesions is often unheralded by a change in ICP. The hemorrhage may form in an area where vascular damage occurred previously, and in at least one report the frequency of the condition was higher in patients who had been hypoxic after the head injury. These hemorrhagic areas seldom need to be evacuated, and successful medical management and follow-up CT often reveal resolution of the hemorrhagic process. However, the prognosis in such patients is more often poor.

**Preoperative Evaluation and Indications for Surgery.** Through the use of the Glasgow Coma Scale, head-injured patients may be triaged into three groups: (1) severe head injury, in which patients are in a coma and score eight or less on the Glasgow Coma Scale with no eye opening; (2) moderate head injury, in which patients score 9 to 12 points on the Glasgow Coma Scale; and (3) minor injury, in which patients score 13 to 15 points.[3] Severely head-injured patients must have CT scanning as soon as it is safely possible; that is, once the airway and hemodynamic circumstances of the patient are stable. This is the case regardless of whether or not a skull fracture is demonstrated. Comatose patients have a one in two to one in four risk of harboring intracranial hematoma.[7] Patients with moderate head injury should have CT within 6 hours of the injury and sooner if a skull fracture, abnormal neurologic signs, or seizures are present. Patients with minor head injury should have CT within 24 hours of admission or sooner if skull fracture, focal neurologic signs, or any indication of neurologic deterioration is present.

When an extracerebral hematoma is disclosed (epidural or subdural), the decision on whether or not surgical evacuation is to be carried out depends on many factors, including the thickness of the hematoma, its volume as shown by the number of CT sections on which it appears, and the degree of associated shift of brain structures. A midline shift of more than 5 mm is generally an indication for surgical evacuation. A thick hematoma with little midline shift suggests the possibility of an isodense hematoma on the other side. A thin hematoma with a disproportionately large shift may suggest infarction and swelling of the brain underlying the hematoma, or it may suggest that part of the hematoma is isodense with brain on CT. The use of ICP monitoring to select patients who will require decompression has not been very helpful.[15] The time elapsed after injury is also very important. In comatose patients, every effort should be made to evacuate an acute subdural hematoma or an epidural hematoma within 4 hours of the onset of coma. Evacuation of a clot later than this causes much poorer results.[16]

The clinical status of the patient is also important. Severe headache, repeated vomiting, and any impairment of the level of consciousness all suggest the need for surgical evacuation of a hematoma disclosed on CT in a noncomatose patient. Clinical and radiologic features suggesting raised ICP, such as obliteration of all subarachnoid CSF spaces, dilatation of the lateral ventricle contralateral to the hematoma, oculomotor paresis ipsilateral to a sizeable hematoma, bradycardia, and arterial hypertension, all indicate an urgent need for surgical decompression.[17] The sooner the decompression is achieved the better.[16]

Children are more likely to need to have moderate or small hematomas removed than are adults because of a generally lower level of craniospinal compliance than is found in older patients, who have a degree of brain atrophy and a larger amount of displaceable CSF that can compensate for the formation of an extracerebral hematoma. Patients with drug-induced or other blood coagulation disorders should be observed particularly carefully for progressive enlargement of hematomas, and the clotting disorders must be vigorously treated.

## REGIONAL SURGICAL ANATOMY

In patients with scalp lacerations, the planning of suitable scalp incision for craniotomy to remove an intracranial

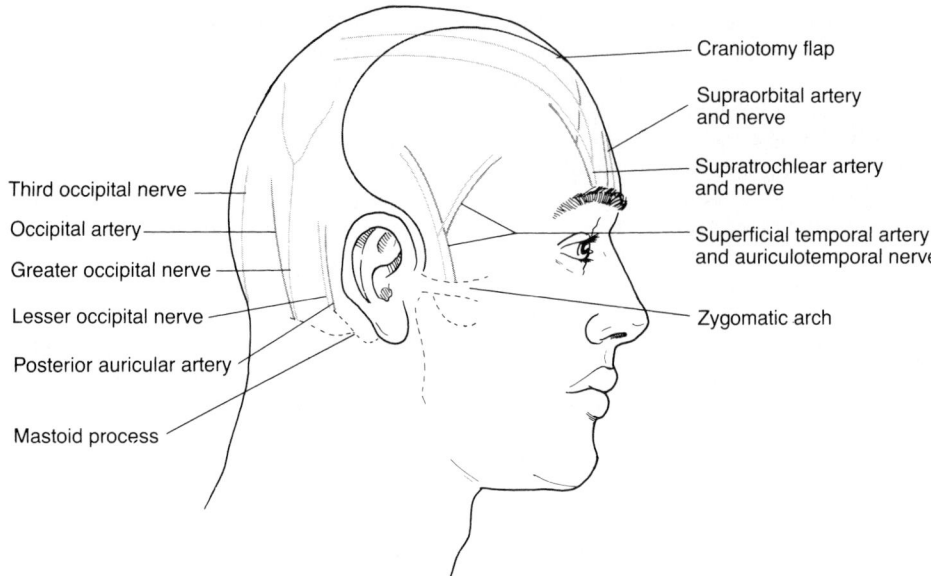

FIGURE 6–1 ■ Course of major vessels and nerves of the scalp.

hematoma can pose problems. If a decision is made to contain the laceration within the bounds of a craniotomy flap, the location of the blood and nerve supply to that area of scalp must be recognized, and steps must be taken to ensure that scalp distal to the traumatic laceration does not become ischemic. The surgeon should be aware of the location and course of the major vessels and nerves that supply the scalp (Fig. 6–1). For hematomas in the temporal region, including almost all acute subdural hematomas and most epidural hematomas, the temporal bur hole for the craniotomy should be low and parallel with the floor of the middle cranial fossa. When the bone flap is being turned, the surgeon should be aware of the location of the middle meningeal artery and be prepared to rapidly arrest bleeding from it (Fig. 6–2). The bone flap should be beveled to avoid the poor cosmetic effect that results from the flap sinking in. After the bone flap is turned and the dura

opened, the surgeon should be aware of the location of the principal frontal and temporal gyri; the sylvian veins; the branches of the middle cerebral artery within the sylvian fissure; the anastomotic veins of Trolard, running upward to the superior sagittal sinus; and the veins of Labbé, running across the temporal lobe of the sigmoid sinus.

## ANESTHESIA FOR CRANIOTOMY

Operations are usually carried out with the patient under general anesthesia, and all patients should have an intra-arterial line and a central venous line placed in situ. Patients are moderately hyperventilated with intravenous anesthesia and are placed in 10 to 15 degrees of head-up tilt on the operating table. At the point at which the skull is

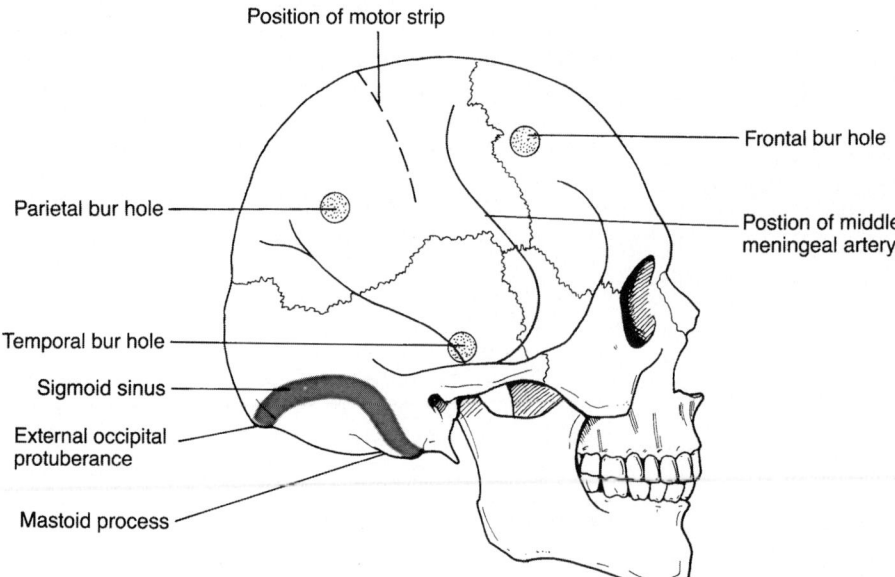

FIGURE 6–2 ■ Position of bur holes with respect to the middle meningeal artery.

opened and epidural or subdural hematoma begins to be removed, thus effecting cranial decompression, the surgeon should warn the anesthetist that a drop in blood pressure may occur, because in many cases, the blood pressure is being held up by a vasopressor response consequent on the brain compression.

In a patient who has deteriorated rapidly despite ventilation and intravenous mannitol administration, urgent partial surgical decompression through a bur hole may be required before insertion of all intravascular lines. In epidural hematomas, this initial bur hole should be close to the fracture but not in the line of the proposed craniotomy. In acute subdural hematomas, the initial bur hole should be low down on the temporal bone, with the skin incision extending vertically down in front of the ear to the level of the zygomatic arch, splitting the temporalis muscle. This method puts the bur hole close to the floor of the middle fossa and ensures that the dural opening is well below the level of the sylvian veins.

## SURGICAL APPROACHES

### Epidural Hematoma

If the hematoma has been clearly demarcated by preoperative CT, the patient should be placed on the operating table with the head positioned with the hematoma uppermost, and a skin and bone flap should be fashioned that encloses the area of the hematoma as much as possible. In hematomas that extend to the floor of the temporal fossa, the surgeon must ensure that there is visual access across the floor of the middle fossa as far as the foramen spinosum. Epidural hematomas, which are almost always clotted and may be adherent to the dura surface, should be removed by suction and dissection as rapidly as possible so that the principal bleeding point can be identified and secured. In most cases, this point will be the middle meningeal artery or one of its main branches lying in the dura mater, and secure coagulation can be easily obtained with bipolar diathermy. In some patients, the bleeding may originate directly from the foramen spinosum, with no visible artery available to coagulate. In such cases, the hemorrhage can be arrested by plugging the foramen spinosum with a mixture of cotton wool and bone wax packed in with a blunt hook. In some cases, brisk arterial bleeding may emanate from a wide fracture running across the temporal bone, and the surgeon should be careful with any exploration in case the carotid artery is itself damaged and bleeding. Any suspicion of this should be confirmed through either carotid angiography followed by an endovascular approach to occlude the bleeding point or exposure of the carotid bifurcation in the neck and temporary occlusion of the internal carotid artery.

After the hematoma has been evacuated, some surgeons like to make a very small opening in the dura to ensure that no underlying subdural hematoma exists; however, if at the end of the hematoma evacuation the dura is lying slack, then this maneuver is unnecessary. Injection of saline into the subdural space is helpful to float the dura away from the brain and to reduce the epidural space left after removal of the clot. This procedure should be reinforced by tacking the dura up to the edge of the bone flap to eliminate as much as possible the epidural space that has formed with the stripping off of the dura mater by the formation of the hematoma. The separation of dura from brain by saline reduces the risk of hemorrhage from the brain surface that is produced by the needle carrying the "tack-up" suture. At this stage, considerable oozing of blood from the dural surface is often present, and time must be taken to ensure that this area is dry before closure. A combination of bipolar diathermy and oxidized cellulose usually suffices for this purpose. If the bone flap is large, then a tacking suture can be put through the dura and taken through two holes drilled in the center of the bone flap to tent up the dura centrally as well as around the edges of the craniotomy. This action minimizes the dead space left at the end of the operation. If bleeding persists, a clotting screen should be performed immediately because platelet malfunction or more severe disturbances of coagulation are common. Drainage of the epidural space should not be necessary and is not generally very effective, except in a patient with a clotting disorder.

### Subdural Hematoma

#### Acute

Because subdural hematomas are generally more extensive than epidural hematomas, and because the bleeding points may be variously located close to the sagittal sinus or under the frontal lobes, at the anterior tip or posterior aspect of the temporal lobe, the bone flap needs to be larger. The skin incision is usually made in the form of a question mark, with the medial limb running up the midline and the posterior limb sweeping downward, then forward over the top of the ear and ending at the zygomatic arch. If the patient was in a coma before the operation, the procedure should begin with a limited skin incision in the line of the skin flap in the anterior temporal area. Rapid formation of a bur hole and small craniectomy, cruciate incision in the dura, and evacuation of some of the hematoma should be performed so that surgical decompression begins as rapidly as possible. Once pulsation of the brain is seen, the remainder of the skin incision is made; the bone flap is turned back; and the dura is opened more widely.

Because of the size of the bone flap, the surgeon must be confident at the start of the operation that obtaining sufficient surgical decompression for the flap to be safely replaced will be possible. A problem may arise if the preoperative CT scan suggests that the subdural hematoma is thin and it is uncertain whether swelling of subjacent brain or a thicker, but isodense, subdural collection exists. In this case, the surgeon should start the operation with a small craniectomy in the anterior temporal area. If, indeed, only a few millimeters depth of acute subdural hematoma exists, this may be verified by a frontal bur hole (using a skin incision that will still permit craniotomy) and a further check of hematoma depth at this site. If the hematoma is uniformly thin and the brain is very swollen, it is better not to proceed with the full craniotomy but to insert a pressure-monitoring device and to try to control the brain swelling and intracranial hypertension by medical means. To perform a large bone decompression under these circumstances is to invite progressive extrusion of brain tissue through the margins of the craniotomy, and venous obstruction around its margins, leading to extensive brain infarction.

When a craniotomy has been completed in a patient with a large acute subdural hematoma, the dura mater should be opened gradually but extensively so that obtaining wide access over the lateral surface of the cerebral hemisphere is possible. If the clot is found to be thin and underlying brain swollen after the large bone flap has been fashioned, multiple short dural openings should be made to evacuate clot, and the dura should not be widely opened until ICP is reduced. Clotted blood should be removed by irrigation, gentle suction, and dissection until the brain surface is clear and the location of the bleeding point can be ascertained. This point may be a vein or an artery on the surface of the brain that can be coagulated with the bipolar forceps, or the hemorrhage may be coming from the margins of a ragged brain laceration, which would necessitate removing a small amount of necrotic brain tissue and accessible intracerebral clot before the margins of the laceration are sealed with bipolar diathermy and a layer of hemostatic gauze over the raw surface of brain.

In some cases, the source of bleeding is an anastomotic vein between the cortex and the superior sagittal sinus. This source necessitates a large craniotomy, close to the midline, so that the bleeding point can be directly visualized and sealed by bipolar diathermy. If the vein has torn out from the dura, leaving a bleeding hole in the dura, a muscle plug can be secured onto it.

The advantage of taking the craniotomy low in the temporal fossa, if necessary by piecemeal removal of some of the temporal bone, is that this method enables the surgeon to see across the floor of the middle cranial fossa and over the superior surface of the tentorium. In patients who have already suffered temporal lobe herniation with production of an oculomotor palsy, gentle upward retraction or irrigation on the undersurface of the temporal lobe may help to ease the herniated brain out of the tentorial hiatus. Successful completion of this maneuver is signaled by free flow of CSF up through the hiatus. If the brain is swollen and tense and difficult to retract, then this maneuver should not be attempted forcibly because it is likely only to produce more brain distortion.

When the hematoma has been evacuated and hemostasis attained, the dura should be closed, although watertight closure is not essential. Tacking sutures around the margins of the craniotomy is important if dura has been stripped away from the margins. The bone flap should be replaced and attached superiorly such that the inferior edge can ride up a little, if necessary.

## Chronic

Chronic subdural hematomas are always liquid and can be removed through a bur hole or twist drill hole in the skull. When the patient is lying supine, layering tends to occur within the hematoma such that the thicker material lies posteriorly. To drain the usual extensive collection, two bur holes are advisable, one over the parietal eminence and the other in the lateral frontal position. If the collection extends down into the temporal fossa, a third, low anterior temporal bur hole is also advisable. The advantage of using two bur holes rather than a single one is that more effective irrigation of the cavity can be obtained by irrigating first into one cavity, then removing effluent from the other. A soft catheter should be used to try to remove thick oily hematoma fluid from the posterior aspects of the collection. Excessive suction should not be applied so that stimulation of fresh bleeding is avoided, and the principle of siphon drainage can be used. Although some hematomas are associated with formation of a thick membrane over the surface of the brain, an attempt to remove this membrane surgically is not advisable.

At the end of hematoma evacuation, the brain may be left lying some distance away from the inner aspect of the skull, and attempts should be made to reduce this space as much as possible before wound closure. Reduction may be accomplished by reversing any head-up tilt that has been used and putting the patient in a slight Trendelenberg position. If an extensive subdural space is still present, then when the wounds are closed, a soft drainage tube connected to a simple drainage bag should be left in the space for 24 hours. After surgery, patients should be positioned flat or with the head slightly down for 24 to 48 hours. Mobilization should occur gradually over 2 or 3 days.

In the postoperative period, the clinician should be guided by the clinical status of the patient rather than the results of repeat CT scanning, because CT usually shows a fairly extensive amount of residual hematoma. Occasionally, however, repeat evacuation is required, and in some young children, a chronic subdural hygroma develops that requires permanent drainage from a subdural to peritoneal shunt.

## Intracerebral Hematoma

Emergency operations on hematomas within the brain substance should be avoided, if possible; however, when the hematoma is large and near to the surface of the brain, and the shift of midline structures is great, immediate surgical decompression is necessary. The location of the flap to be used depends on the location of the hematoma. The craniotomy can be much smaller than that used for evacuation of acute subdural hematoma. Access should normally be available to the anterior part of the temporal lobe and to the undersurface of the frontal lobe, because hematomas frequently point in these areas. Limited cortical excision and the gentlest suction should be employed lest fresh hemorrhage be caused. For this reason, trying to manage such patients conservatively is preferable at first. If it is necessary to remove the hematoma surgically because of increasing shift of persistent intracranial hypertension, this should be a delayed maneuver performed when fresh bleeding is less likely to result from clot removal. Deeply located hematomas in the basal ganglia are not suitable for surgical evacuation.

## Insertion of an Intracranial Pressure Monitoring Device

The prevalence of postoperative intracranial hypertension is extremely high (>75%)[18] in patients who were in a coma before removal of an intracranial hematoma. In all such patients, therefore, an ICP monitoring device should be inserted at the end of the procedure. This device should be inserted through a bur hole and skin incision separate from the craniotomy. In most cases, this area will be on the opposite side from the surgery site. The bur hole is usually made just anterior to the coronal suture in line with the pupil. A small dural slit is then made. The device may be an intraventricular cannula, which is inserted by directing the point of the cannula along a line 2 cm anterior to the external auditory meatus toward the inner canthus of the ipsilateral eye or, if this is not successful, to the bridge of the nose. The device may also be a subdural catheter or transducer, which is inserted by gently depressing the brain and sliding the device over the surface. Another alternative is an intraparenchymal pressure monitor, which may be inserted simply by pushing it approximately 2 cm into the brain and then withdrawing it by 2 to 3 mm. The tubing from the device should be securely attached to the skin to minimize the risk of it being pulled out when patients are moved during routine nursing care maneuvers.

## INTRAOPERATIVE COMPLICATIONS

Intraoperative complications mainly comprise difficulties in arresting the hemorrhage and in controlling severe brain swelling. Although arterial hemorrhage may occur as a result of in-driven bone fragments or foreign bodies in patients with traumatic intracranial hematoma, the most common source of hemorrhage during operation is the venous system. Because intracranial venous pressure rises in parallel with the ICP, such venous bleeding may be profuse and difficult to control. The most important principle in controlling such hemorrhage is to reduce the ICP. For this purpose, close cooperation between the surgeon and the anesthetist is paramount. When venous bleeding is becoming difficult to control, the surgeon should apply a cotton pack over the area and wait while ICP is reduced by increased hyperventilation, intravenous mannitol, or administration of a bolus of barbiturate. The anesthetist should check that the airway is free and that the head position has not changed to cause obstruction of one of the jugular veins. As the brain becomes more slack, venous bleeding diminishes, and identifying the bleeding point and controlling it with bipolar coagulation or hemostatic gauze becomes easier.

Similar principles apply to the management of acute intraoperative brain swelling, but the surgeon should also be aware that a hematoma could be forming on the opposite side. If brain swelling remains problematic throughout the procedure despite the employment of adequate maneuvers in the operating room, an immediate postoperative CT scan should be obtained.

A dural laceration that extends into one of the dural venous sinuses or the venous lakes that may lie beside them can pose a major problem for the surgeon. Two pairs of hands are essential. In these cases, the assistant puts pressure over the sinus close to the breach and applies suction to allow the other surgeon to see the tear, which can be either sutured or closed by oversewing a muscle plug.

## POSTOPERATIVE MANAGEMENT AND OUTCOME

The intensity of care and monitoring applied to the postoperative patient after evacuation of an intracranial hematoma and the anticipated outcome both depend on the patient's level of consciousness before induction of anesthesia. If the patient was comatose, then intermittent positive-pressure ventilation should be continued after the operation, and the patient should be transferred to the intensive care unit. The indwelling arterial line should be left in situ together with a long central venous line. Arterial pressure should be monitored continuously, and arterial oxygen saturation should also be monitored, through pulse oximetry. An ICP monitoring device should be inserted, and continuous monitoring of ICP should be instituted.

It has been the experience of several groups that these patients suffer a high rate of intracranial hypertension in the postoperative phase. If repeated or protracted treatment for intracranial hypertension is envisaged, then insertion of an oxygen-saturation monitoring catheter into the jugular bulb may be advisable if such devices and the expertise to manage them are available.[19]

Such patients may lie flat or with a modest degree of head-up tilt (depending on other injuries) and should be given adequate intravenous fluids, including colloids when indicated, to avoid arterial hypotension. The ventilation is adjusted to provide moderate hypocapnia, and the arterial $Pco_2$ should be around 30 mm Hg. Core and peripheral temperatures should be monitored. Arterial oxygen saturation is kept as close to 100% as possible by meticulous airway management, frequent chest physiotheraphy, and modest degrees of positive end-expiratory pressure and increased $Fio_2$ if required.

When ICP is increased beyond 25 mm Hg, and particularly if it is associated with neurologic deterioration, measures are required to reduce ICP and optimize cerebral perfusion pressure. Ideally, in the severely head injured patient, cerebral perfusion pressure should be kept at 70 mm Hg or above.[20, 21] The choice of therapy for reduction of raised ICP lies between treatments that act on the cerebral vascular and metabolic systems (e.g., increased hyperventilation and barbiturates and other sedative drugs) and osmotic agents (intravenous mannitol solution).[22, 23] Patients who develop intracranial hypertension following evacuation of a hematoma generally respond best to mannitol solution. If sedative drugs are used, the clinician must ensure that arterial pressure does not fall. To optimize the effect of mannitol and to avoid rebound rises in pressure and hypovolemia, mannitol infusion can be accompanied by furosemide and followed by intravenous plasma protein solution. If ICP therapy is used, jugular venous oxygen saturation should be monitored because a reduction in saturation below 50% indicates that cerebral ischemia is occurring as a complication of therapy.[24]

In the noncomatose patient whose hematoma is evacuated, it is the practice in most centers to allow the patient to awaken after the operation. In such cases, it is important that the anesthetic used will permit this to happen. Thereafter, monitoring in the intensive care unit or high-dependency unit consists of measurement of arterial pressure and arterial oxygen saturation by pulse oximetry. These events are monitored, together with frequent assessments of level of consciousness, by use of a neurosurgical nursing chart that incorporates the Glasgow Coma Scale and assessment of pupil size and limb strength.

The principal factor regulating outcome after evacuation of an intracranial hematoma is the patient's level of consciousness before the operation. Comatose patients have a mortality rate 5 to 10 times higher than that of noncomatose patients undergoing evacuation of hematomas (30% to 60% versus 0% to 5%). For this reason, strong advocacy exists for a pre-emptive approach in diagnosing and evacuating intracranial hematomas at a stage at which the patient remains conscious. Other factors that adversely affect outcome are a delay of more than 4 hours in instituting decompression and the numbers and duration as well as the severity of secondary insults in the postoperative period. Such insults include periods of arterial hypotension, raised ICP with reduced cerebral perfusion pressure, hypoxemia, and elevated body temperature.

## REFERENCES

1. Becker DP, Miller JD, Ward JD, et al: The outcome from severe head injury with early diagnosis and intensive management. J Neurosurg 47:491–502, 1977.
2. Miller JD, Butterworth JF, Gudeman SK, et al: Further experience in the management of severe head injury. J Neurosurg 54:289–299, 1981.
3. Miller JD: Minor, moderate and severe head injury. Neurosurg Rev 9:135–139, 1986.
4. Marshall LF, Toole BM, Bowers SA: The National Traumatic Coma Data Bank. II: Patients who talk and deteriorate: Implications for treatment. J Neurosurg 59:285–288, 1983.
5. Miller JD, Jones PA: The work of regional head injury unit. Lancet i:1141–1144, 1985.
6. Miller JD, Jones PA, Dearden NM, Tocher JL: Progress in the management of head injury. Br J Surg 79:60–64, 1992.
7. Teasdale GM, Murray G, Anderson E, et al: Risks of acute traumatic intracranial haematoma in children and adults: Implications for managing head injuries. BMJ 300:363–367, 1990.
8. Servadei F, Piazza A, Seracchioli A, et al: Extradural haematomas: An analysis of the changing characteristics of patients admitted from 1980 to 1986. Diagnostic and therapeutic implications in 158 cases. Brain Inj 2:87–100, 1988.
9. Bricolo AP, Pasut LM: Extradural haematoma: Toward zero mortality. Neurosurgery 14:8–12, 1984.
10. Knuckey NW, Gelbard S, Epstein MH: The management of asymptomatic epidural hematomas: A prospective study. J Neurosurg 70:392–393, 1989.
11. McKissock W, Richardson A, Bloom WH: Subdural haematoma: A review of 389 cases. Lancet i:1365–1369, 1960.
12. Miller JD, Adams JH: The pathophysiology of raised intracranial pressure. In Adams JH, Duchen LW (eds): Greenfield's Neuropathology, 5th ed. London: Arnold, 1992, pp 69–105.
13. Adams JH: Head injury. In Adams JH, Duchen LW (eds): Greenfield's Neuropathology, 5th ed. London: Arnold, 1992, pp 106–152.
14. Gudeman SK, Kishore PRS, Miller JD, et al: The genesis and significance of delayed traumatic intracerebral hematoma. Neurosurgery 5:309–311, 1979.
15. Bullock R, Golek J, Blake G: Traumatic intracerebral haematoma–which patients should undergo surgical evacuation? CT scan features and ICP monitoring as a basis for decision making. Surg Neurol 32:181–187, 1989.
16. Seelig JM, Becker DP, Miller JD, et al: Traumatic acute subdural haematoma: Major mortality reduction in comatose patients treated in under four hours. N Engl J Med 304:1511–1518, 1981.
17. Teasdale E, Cardoso E, Galbraith S, Teasdale G: CT scan in severe diffuse head injury: Physiological and clinical correlations. J Neurol Neurosurg Psychiatry 47:600–603, 1984.
18. Miller JD, Becker DP, Ward JD, et al: Significance of intracranial hypertension in severe head injury. J Neurosurg 47:503–516, 1977.
19. Andrews PJD, Dearden NM, Miller JD: Jugular bulb cannulation: Description of a cannulation technique and validation of a new continuous monitor. Br J Anaesth 67:553–558, 1991.
20. Chan KH, Miller JD, Dearden NM, et al: The effect of changes in cerebral perfusion pressure upon middle cerebral artery blood flow velocity and jugular venous oxygen saturation after severe brain injury. J Neurosurg 77:55–61, 1992.
21. Chan KH, Dearden NM, Miller JD, et al: Multimodality monitoring as a guide to treatment of intracranial hypertension after severe brain injury. Neurosurgery 32:547–553, 1993.
22. Miller JD, Dearden NM, Piper IR, Chan KH: Control of intracranial pressure in patients with severe head injury. J Neurotrauma 9: (Suppl 1):S317–S326, 1992.
23. Miller JD, Piper IR, Dearden NM: Management of intracranial hypertension in head injury: Matching treatment with cause. Acta Neurochir (Wien) 57 (Suppl):152–159, 1993.
24. Dearden NM: Jugular bulb venous oxygen saturation in the management of severe head injury. Curr Opin Anaesthesiol 4:279–286, 1991.

# Surgical Management of Penetrating Missile Injuries of the Head

■ T. FORCHT DAGI

Until the turn of the 20th century, penetrating missile injuries of the brain were almost universally fatal. During World War I, Harvey Cushing, Geoffrey Jefferson, and others demonstrated that the mortality rate could be reduced by early débridement with meticulous attention to neurosurgical technique. Since then, the expectations of neurosurgical intervention have shifted from simple survival to the improvement of ultimate functional outcome. This chapter addresses the techniques that have proven best suited to this purpose.

Gunshot wounds of the head are usually sustained in warfare. In many parts of the world, however, urban strife has changed this injury from one almost uniquely military to a broadly civilian concern. Although military and civilian penetrating injuries often do differ significantly, the principles of managing such injuries are identical. It is the nature of the injury that differs, primarily with respect to the penetrating missile, its energy level on impact, the conditions under which treatment must be rendered, and collateral factors affecting survival.

Each war has taught the surgeon different lessons. World War I, for example, proved the efficacy of vigorous surgical intervention and its importance in improving patient survival. The Spanish Civil War demonstrated that blast effect was a significant component of craniofacial injury after aerial bombardment. During World War II, the importance of initial dural repair and antibiotic medication was debated, and ultimately universally accepted.[1–3] The Korean War confirmed the effectiveness of early evacuation of the wounded and of initial definitive surgery in improving survival and reducing infection.[2, 4] The civil disturbances in Belfast took place so close to the neurosurgical center that the natural history of penetrating injury could be studied virtually from the moment of injury.[5] In the course of the Israeli expedition into Lebanon, all head-injured patients were brought to a single institution, and, for the first time, the place of computed tomography (CT) in combat neurosurgery could be evaluated. In the wake of the Vietnam conflict, the Vietnam Head Injury Study (VHIS), a unique cooperative effort funded by the Veterans Administration and involving the U.S. Army, Navy, and Air Force,

the American Red Cross, and the National Institutes of Health, was established to register and study outcome after penetrating head injury. For approximately 18 years, the VHIS has followed a large population using sophisticated epidemiologic, radiologic, and neuropsychological techniques, successfully eliciting data that were often lost in the past, when injured veterans were not aggressively followed once they returned to their communities.[6] Finally, reports and casualty analyses from the Iran-Iraq conflict, from Afghanistan, and from Bosnia-Herzegovina and the Baltics confirm the commonality of experience across many fields of battle.[7–13]

Regardless of venue or circumstance of injury, a small number of subjects is responsible for the most heated debate whenever gunshot wounds of the head and neck are discussed. These topics stake out the most important controversies in the management of these injuries. They are:

1. The practical significance of distinguishing between high-velocity and low-velocity wounds
2. The importance of early transport and treatment of the wounded, as opposed to delaying treatment until optimal specialist attention can be provided
3. The definition of what constitutes adequate surgical débridement
4. Specific methods of dealing with complex wounds involving the orbit, the air sinuses, and major vascular structures
5. The management of cerebrospinal fluid (CSF) fistulas
6. The prevention and diagnosis of acute infection, and of delayed abscess and hematoma
7. The epidemiology of post-traumatic seizure disorders

Maurice Saba, in his excellent chapter in this book, has provided an overview and general approach to the problem of penetrating missile injuries. Our companion chapter is directed at some specific areas of pathophysiology and their management. We draw heavily, but certainly not exclusively, on lessons learned from military neurosurgery. We have also sought to reflect the evolution of ideas concerning the treatment of open and closed head injury in nonmilitary settings.

## BALLISTICS AND THEIR CLINICAL SIGNIFICANCE

Injury to the brain is a function of energy release over time, and of the volume and location of tissue disruption. A brief consideration of ballistics provides a useful vocabulary and conceptual framework through which to analyze penetrating injuries.

The simplest useful classification divides penetrating missile injuries into high-velocity and low-velocity categories. Although the severity of wounds is clearly associated with the muzzle or initial velocity and energy content of the missile, it is the terminal or striking velocity that determines the energy at impact and that correlates more exactly with the extent of trauma.[14, 15] Nevertheless, by convention, the initial or muzzle velocity of bullets and aimed missiles is used as a shorthand to describe the *potential* for injury. Thus, all things being equal, a high-velocity missile would be assumed to strike with more energy, and therefore to create greater havoc, than its low-velocity counterpart.

By convention, high-velocity missiles exceed 2000 feet per second. This velocity is commonly achieved by rifle bullets. Most modern high-velocity rifle ammunition surpasses a velocity of 2500 ft/sec at the muzzle. Most handgun ammunition, however, leaves the barrel with a velocity somewhere between 800 and 1400 ft/sec. Penetrating fragments or shrapnel, however, typically have a velocity on the order of 600 ft/sec. Most survivable injuries in wartime are ascribable to shrapnel injuries.

The energy (E) released during the terminal ballistic events (terminal ballistic events are those that ensue when the free path of a missile is disrupted by impact with anything in its path) in tissue depend on the missile mass (M) and velocity (V). The greater the energy release, the greater the potential for damage. This is a key concept: all things being equal, it is the quantity of energy transferred or energy *released,* not the level of energy per se, that determines the potential for injury. In addition, the shorter the time span over which release occurs, the more violent the injury. As the time span approaches 0, the energy release resembles an explosion more and more closely, and can be effectively modeled as an explosion with localized, and sometimes contained, blast effect. The relationship between E, M, and V can be modeled in a number of ways: *momentum* (MV), *kinetic energy* ($\frac{1}{2}$ MV$^2$), and *power* (MV$^3$). Each of these models places a different emphasis on velocity. The models were developed, and justified, because of the need to justify radically different concepts of ammunition and armament design.

At the turn of the century, for example, the chamber pressures attainable in military weapons were limited by metallurgic considerations, and ballistic design was focused on massive bullets with relatively low velocity, similar to those used for hunting big game. Steel technology quickly progressed to the point where high chamber pressures could be achieved without difficulty, and ammunition after World War I was no longer limited in any practical sense by the

design of the weapon. As a result, modern ammunition is designed to attain very high velocity through tremendous chamber pressures. There are secondary advantages of this design; weapons, for example, tend to cycle more easily. Because high-velocity ammunition requires light bullets, the foot soldier can carry a larger quantity of ammunition for the same weight.

Light bullets are easily deflected, however. They also lose energy rapidly over distance (hence the importance of distinguishing between muzzle velocity and striking velocity or energy). For this reason, there is continued worldwide reliance on slower and more massive bullets, particularly for sniper and long-distance operations. As a result, in most NATO and former Warsaw Pact armies, low-mass, small-caliber, high-velocity bullets such as the 55-grain .223 fired in the American M-16 assault rifle or its Soviet equivalent are supplemented by slower, more massive rounds—such as the 150-grain .308 or 7.62-caliber bullet—for sniper use. Neurosurgeons must be aware of this point because sniper tactics emphasize aiming at the head, and terrorists who have been trained as snipers are taught to target prominent people in positions of leadership. Despite the deadliness of sniper rounds, some sniper wounds are survived because of the distances at which most such injuries are delivered.

Terrorist incidents are increasingly likely to affect the innocent public throughout the world. The neurosurgeon may be called on to deal with the consequences of such acts. The injuries created are very likely to differ from those to which she or he may be accustomed. It is wise to shed any preconceived ideas. Many weapons and rounds can be modified to deposit far more energy than usual. Standard handgun ammunition, for example, can be hand-loaded to attain 1600 ft/sec. "Hot" ammunition designed for submachine gun use can be discharged in most 9-mm pistols. Cast bronze, Teflon-clad bullets, heavy metal–derived, and expanding or exploding bullets produce unusual cavitation. Moreover, blast effects from exploding bullets, grenades, plastic explosive, and incendiary devices in closed spaces create wounds that combine the worst characteristics of closed and penetrating head injury.[16]

A missile's energy is greatest at the moment at which it is launched, and decays with time and distance. A .30/30-caliber, 170-grain bullet can be discharged with a muzzle velocity of 2220 ft/sec, for example, but at 100 yards, the velocity drops to 1350 ft/sec, and at 200 yards, to 1000 ft/sec, well in the range of handgun ammunition. Most survivable injuries occur at low impact velocity. From a practical standpoint, and as already noted, the terminal ballistic events, the striking velocity, the quantity of energy released, and the explosive force developed, are more important than muzzle velocity or bullet mass. What counts is the *striking,* or *impact* energy, rather than the muzzle velocity.

The degree of tissue injury is proportional to the quantity of energy delivered. The amount of energy imparted to tissue when a projectile strikes is limited by the energy at impact. As a rule, more energy is imparted by penetrating injuries than by perforating (through-and-through) injuries. Penetrating missiles release all their energy in the tissue, whereas in perforating injuries, the difference between the energy at impact and the residual energy at exit determines the energy delivered.

The "perfect" bullet from a ballistician's standpoint would release all of its energy instantaneously: $dE/dt$ (t = time) would be infinite. Thus, ballistic design is calculated to create smooth, friction-free flight in air, but infinite resistance to passage in tissue. This goal is achieved by physical changes that affect the shape or ballistic characteristics of the bullet by expansion, tumbling, yaw, or fragmentation. The sudden loss of spin, for example, causes energy to be released in two ways: first, a significant quantity of angular energy is released; then, the bullet destabilizes, slows, tumbles, and sometimes fragments. Even a glancing, tangential injury can generate significant injury because of the energy transmitted to adjacent structures.[17, 18]

Although many wartime injuries are sustained at considerable distance, in civilian life most injuries occur at less than 50 yards, and impact velocity is effectively equal to muzzle velocity. The distance at which a soldier in wartime is shot is usually an unknown variable that helps account for survival after ostensibly high-energy bullet wounds.

## PATHOPHYSIOLOGY

What happens when a missile strikes determines the limits of successful surgical intervention after penetrating injury. Harvey and colleagues[19] provided the classic description of the five principal events that accompany bullet penetration:

1. Shock waves at an angle to the bullet path
2. A temporary cavity lasting approximately 20 msec that develops pari passu as energy is transferred to the tissue
3. Pulsation of the temporary cavity before it collapses, sending pressure waves through adjacent tissue, and causing remote injury and herniation of the brain
4. Collapse of the temporary cavity, leaving a residual permanent cavity, the bullet track, with an area of surrounding tissue damage
5. Extravasation of blood around the missile track, occupying a space larger than but fundamentally concentric with the temporary cavity

### Nature of the Bullet Track

At close ranges, the permanent cavity bears little relationship to the muzzle velocity of the missile, At greater distances, however, a high-velocity bullet creates a beet-shaped cavity, and a low-velocity bullet creates a carrot-shaped cavity. With long-range perforating injuries, the exit wound is always larger than the entrance wound; this rule does not hold after injuries at short range.

The cavitary effect of low-velocity missiles is inconsistent. The extent of cavitation is determined both by the direction of travel and extent of yaw. High-velocity missiles, in general, create a more consistent cavity.

When bullets fragment, however, the nature of the cavitary events cannot be reliably predicted. The configuration of the cavity remains a function of the complexities of energy transfer.[20]

### Bone Chips

Bone chips invariably accompany penetration of the skull, and may be thrown off by tangential injuries as well.[21] The path of a missile wound can often be determined on plain skull films by the track of bone chips. Bone chips occasionally form a secondary track different from that of the bullet, but the volume of this tract is usually small, and bone chips that take on the role of secondary missiles rarely assume ballistic significance. The volume of residual chips on plain skull films after surgery has been traditionally regarded as a measure of the adequacy of débridement, but this point of view is no longer uncritically promoted[22] (see later).

### Acute Bursts of Intracranial Pressure

Signs of acute bursts of intracranial pressure (ICP) are seen in over 90% of fatal head injuries. These acute bursts are to be distinguished from the rise in ICP that parallels the brain swelling that may take place within the first 12 to 36 hours, particularly with high-energy wounds. The significance of these pressure marks is controversial.[23–25] The degree of acute ICP change does not correlate directly with missile velocity, cavity size, or duration of survival. Low-velocity wounds observed in civilian practice have not been consistently associated with cerebral edema unless the brain stem is traversed.

### Contusions and Hematomas

Cortical contusions are present at the site of entry in 50% of cases, and elsewhere in another 50%. Regardless of bullet path, subfrontal contusions occur in 25%. Other remote contusions are also commonly found.[17] CT scan data from the VHIS substantiates the long-standing clinical impression that the degree of actual injury usually far surpasses the surgeon's estimate.

During the Korean war, 46.2% of patients seen within 8 hours of injury had intracranial hematomas; this figure dropped to 27% after 12 to 35 hours, and 7% after 48 to 72 hours.[26] In civilian practice, hematomas were found in 44% of patients seen within 5.5 hours of injury.[18] The decline in prevalence with time most probably reflects the early death of patients with significant mass effect or intracranial hematomas. The early mortality rate in Croatia in front-line hospitals is uncannily close to the incidence of hematomas in the Korean war: 46.4%.[12]

In a study of 316 cases seen within 8 hours of wounding, 3% had extradural clots, 21% subdural clots, 23% intracerebral clots, and 0.2% had intraventricular clots. Two or more hematomas were not uncommon.[20] It is quite likely that the incidence of both early and late hematomas will be recalculated when CT scans are used to evaluate patients acutely close to the front. In military practice, hematomas at the site of exit can be more significant than those elsewhere.[27]

## Fractures and Fracture Lines

Fracture lines that accompany gunshot wounds to the brain tend to pass from the point of impact to the opposite pole, sparing or shifting directions at buttress lines. Shock waves within the skull cause fractures of the orbital roofs and cribriform plate even when the missile proceeds elsewhere.[17] This helps to explain why CSF leaks after penetrating missile injuries can be so difficult to define and treat: there are many widely separated areas where the leptomeninges could be lacerated by fracture lines.

## Tangential Injuries

Tangential injuries are common and carry the best prognosis of all types of missile injuries, despite carrying a significant morbidity. In the pre-CT era, it was estimated that 75% would have significant cortical contusions, subcortical hematomas, subdural hematomas, or venous sinus disruption. Comparable data using modern diagnostic techniques have not been elicited, but there is nothing in the aggregate experience of managing penetrating missile wounds to contradict this expectation.

## Blast Injuries

In the urban setting, blast injuries complicate penetrating trauma with diffuse acceleration-deceleration forces akin to those encountered in closed head injury. This type of injury was characteristic in patients who were evacuated from the Lebanon conflict. The major pathophysiologic finding is a rapid and diffuse increase in intracranial pressure, out of keeping with the extent of actual penetration. The term *blast* is invoked to express the idea that, as in an explosion, the time course of energy deposition (corresponding to $dt$ in the energy transfer equation, $dE/dt$) may be vanishingly small. As a result, the value of the energy transfer equation can be immense.

## OPERATIVE CONSIDERATIONS

### General Principles

The approach to penetrating missile injuries in the military does not differ significantly from that in civilian practice, although specific concerns and limitations inherent to combat medicine in the military setting may affect certain details of operative management. The overall expectations of surgery must be restricted because of the surgically irreparable damage resulting from the pathophysiologic events that accompany missile penetration of the brain. Thus, the goals of surgery are both defined and specific: (1) to remove space-occupying lesions; (2) to prevent infec-

tion; (3) to ensure hemostasis; and (4) to repair and restore anatomic integrity to injured structures.

The guiding principles of operative management were enunciated by Cushing and Jefferson, and reiterated by Cairns, Lewin, and Matson, among others. The original literature bears review. In brief, vigorous operative débridement of the missile track is recommended to prevent abscess formation. The need for satisfactory dural closure and scalp reconstruction has become axiomatic. The dura should be closed in watertight fashion, with an autologous or, if necessary, an allographic graft to prevent tension. Vascularized, and therefore vital grafts are in theory preferable. In practice, however, dural grafts revascularize quickly, even though they are technically nonvital. Potential donor sites include temporalis fascia, pericranium, fascia lata, and transversalis fascia, in order of accessibility and preference. Galea is usually needed to close the scalp, and is not recommended for use as a dural substitute. All foreign bodies should be avoided; synthetic dural substitutes are contraindicated. Lyophilized human dural, pericranial, fascial, and amniotic material, however, seems to act like true autogenic dura despite having been processed and preserved.

Finally, a meticulous reconstruction and closure of the scalp is effected. Tension should be avoided in repair of skin and subcutaneous tissues. Flaps can be rotated immediately, even over contaminated wounds, and may, in fact, facilitate healing of locally infected areas. If absolutely necessary, the closed dura can be dressed and left uncovered by skin, allowing a flap to be rotated once granulation has set in with healing by secondary intention. The older literature advocated this technique, but it is probably unnecessary when antibiotics are available. Absorbable suture material should be placed in the galea. Monofilament thread or stainless steel staples can be used for the skin. Single-layer skin closures have been advocated for grossly contaminated wounds: the correct technique requires the use of interrupted vertically mattressed monofilament sutures spaced at 1- to 1.5-cm intervals. Because scalp closure is a major barrier to CSF leak, the two-layer closure is preferable. The use of drains for 48 to 72 hours does not seem to increase the risk of wound infections.

### Steroids and Alimentation

There is no evidence to support the use of steroids in head-injured patients. Similarly, aggressive dehydration has not been shown to be effective in controlling diffuse cerebral edema, and may be harmful. Caloric intake, on the other hand, is highly correlated with improvements in outcome. The increased metabolic demands of head-injured patients make hyperalimentation and careful nutritional support an integral part of the medical management.

### Anticonvulsants

Anticonvulsant prophylaxis is required. Although a number of factors have been shown to influence the likelihood of seizures developing,[25, 26] it is becoming apparent that many patients who do not have seizures immediately after injury will do so within 5 to 15 years. There is no evidence, however, to suggest that the ultimate seizure history is affected by phenytoin, the anticonvulsant most commonly used for routine prophylaxis and treatment.[28] The correlation of hematomas with seizure disorders is well defined. Retained bone fragments do not seem to exert a deleterious effect on seizure prevalence, but whether the same holds true for retained metal fragments remains to be seen. Whenever the onset of seizures is other than immediately after injury, CT should be performed to exclude late hematoma and abscess formation even as anticonvulsant treatment is begun.

## Antibiotics

Antibiotics should be given prophylactically as soon as feasible. This holds regardless of whether proposed management includes surgery, and has proved useful in both the civilian and the military experience.

It is necessary to determine in each situation what antibiotics are the most appropriate. For a start, skin flora should be covered. The use of antibiotics in this setting is *therapeutic*, and not prophylactic; antibiotics should be prescribed in meningeal doses.[11, 29–32]

## Intracranial Pressure Monitoring

The role of ICP monitoring has yet to be defined. It was rarely used in Vietnam. In Northern Ireland, other parameters proved more useful in patient evaluation and management.[33] In contrast, ICP monitoring proved to be one of the cornerstones of therapy in Haifa, between 1982 and 1985, and has become one of the parameters used in monitoring patients when less invasive management is advocated.

The disparity among these views may be accounted for in part by differences in the venue of injury—combat environment or civilian injury, urban setting or long-range shooting. ICP monitoring can be especially useful where blast injury constitutes a significant component of the overall problem. In most patients who survive penetrating missile injuries, however, initial increases of ICP are due to mass effect surrounding hematomas and collections of debris, and late increases are due to delayed hematoma or abscess formation.[36] These lesions can be visualized on CT and should be treated surgically, in accordance with the usual indications for relief of mass lesions. Although angiography is not called for routinely, it should be considered as part of the evaluation and management of delayed or recurring hematoma to rule out the possibility of traumatic aneurysm or other vascular injury. Magnetic resonance angiography has not been evaluated as a diagnostic method in this setting. The use of spiral CT and three-dimensional arterial reconstruction has been shown to be quite promising, however.[35–37]

## Evolving Techniques and Ongoing Controversies

### Débridement and Management of Bone Fragments

With the advent of CT, the existence of modern antibiotics, and the availability of ICP monitoring and neurosurgical intensive care, some serious questions have been raised concerning the extent of necessary débridement: must *all* fragments of bone be removed to minimize the risk of abscess, even to the point of threatening relatively normal brain and performing secondary and tertiary operations, or can a more conservative approach be justified?

The reasons for pursuing this issue are several. First, from a number of sources, including the VHIS, the military experience on the neurosurgical service of the Walter Reed Army Medical Center, and the follow-up experience with head trauma in a more general sense, it is becoming evident that there is no such thing as a truly "silent" area of brain and that there is a definable risk to reoperation in enthusiastic pursuit of retained fragments.[38] An impressive body of evidence emanating from the Iran-Iraq war reinforces these impressions and underscores the absence of correlation, all other factors held equal, between retained bone fragments and late infection.[11] Second, civilian institutions have reported satisfactory outcomes with limited débridement under an antibiotic umbrella. Third, the extensive availability of CT scanning allows patients at risk for delayed abscess to be restudied serially.[39] Fourth, by using CT rather than relying simply on plain skull films, the VHIS has demonstrated that "complete" débridement of all foreign material and bony fragments is achieved in any event much less often than previously believed, or than memorialized as an impression in the operative note by the operating neurosurgeon.[40] Finally, experience in Israel suggests that many patients can be treated with relatively limited cerebral débridement, dural repair, and scalp closure without imperiling the eventual outcome, followed by ICP monitoring and serial CT.[41]

Present levels of experience do not warrant a dogmatic approach. Even so, with the evidence at hand, it appears reasonable to withhold secondary reoperation for retained fragments in the event that three critical conditions are met:

1. Adequate initial débridement in qualified neurosurgical hands
2. Availability of serial CT scanning for long-term follow-up
3. Ready availability of satisfactory continuing neurosurgical care

Should any of these conditions *not* be satisfied, the level of bony débridement required may have to be re-evaluated. A secondary operation may be indicated. This decision is undertaken by the neurosurgeons primarily responsible for operative management. Their sense of the conditions under which neurosurgical treatment can be provided serves as the basis for tailoring decisions in time of war, or when external circumstances limit the extent to which optimal neurosurgical care can be delivered. No part of this discussion is intended to negate the importance of initial vigorous débridement of injured tissue. This discussion is directed only at the practice of *uncritical* secondary or tertiary operation to débride residual bone fragments, an approach that was once mandated in American military hospitals but now seems outdated—so long as serial sectional images and satisfactory neurosurgical follow-up can be obtained when needed.

## Metallic and Migrating Fragments

Although the possible epileptogenic effects of retained metal fragments—especially copper—have been mentioned,[42, 43] there is no definite indication to pursue metallic fragments beyond those that are readily accessible. An exception to this rule is the migrating metallic fragment. There are two categories of migrating fragments, those in the ventricle, and those in the parenchyma of the brain. Intraventricular fragments have been implicated anecdotally in hydrocephalus, ventriculitis, and hypothalamic syndromes characterized by central disturbances of temperature control (central neurogenic hyperthermia) and obtundation. By judicious positioning of the patient, it is possible to guide the fragment in the occipital horn of the lateral ventricle, where it can be reached relatively easily. Intraoperative radiography is necessary to confirm that the fragment is attainably lodged. Intraventricular metallic fragments associated with infection or obstructive hydrocephalus should also be removed, even if they do not appear migratory at the time. Endoscopic and stereotactic techniques may be useful in retrieving intraventricular fragments.

Inaccessible fragments deep in the parenchyma of the brain do not migrate as a rule, but when they do, the patient should be positioned in such a manner as to allow gravity to bring the fragment to the surface in an innocuous area. Fragments that spontaneously migrate to the cortex pose no particular technical difficulty and should be removed.

## Exploding Bullets

Explosive bullets that detonate on impact or shortly after are formally prohibited by the rules of war, but have been available on the civilian market and are used by terrorist groups. When the bullet explodes, the surgeon encounters a combination of blast effect and penetrating missile injury. When the bullet has failed to detonate, the surgeon faces a certain risk of personal injury in removing or manipulating the missile. Some explosive bullets have a characteristic radiologic appearance: a central cavity filled with explosive, sometimes sealed with a ball bearing, a pellet, or a BB. Hollow-nosed and dum-dum (blunt-tipped) bullets are not explosive. It is recommended that long-handled instruments be used, that electrocautery not be used in the vicinity of such missiles, that they be grasped gently from the base rather than from the nose of the bullet, and that, at all costs, the nose of the bullet not be crushed. The surgeon should wear goggles to protect his or her eyes.

Although it has been suggested on theoretical grounds that ultrasound and microwaves could cause explosive bullets to detonate, we know of no published data on this point. (It may be of some small comfort to note that explosive bullets have a high failure rate.)

## Dural Sinus Repair

Lacerations of the dural sinuses are common in wartime. Techniques for the repair of the dural sinuses have been well described.[44] In most respects, the classic approaches have not been outdated. The application of modern micro-vascular techniques to trauma surgery, however, makes it possible to contemplate the functional repair of dural sinus injuries that in the past would have been treated by packing only.

A full complement of vascular instruments and clips should be available when undertaking sinus repair. The first step in repair involves hemostasis. Temporary hemostasis can usually be achieved by compressing the lacerated sinus with cottonoid over Gelfoam while elevating the head (reverse Trendelenburg's position). Because of the risks of air embolus during sinus repair, the cottonoids covering the laceration and the wound edges should be soaking wet. A central line in the right atrium and Doppler echocardiography monitoring are mandatory. The use of positive end-expiratory pressure (PEEP) helps prevent air from entering the venous system, but may be limited by cardiopulmonary constraints. Although PEEP may increase the amount of active bleeding, it is easier to contend with the bleeding than with massive air embolus.

Repair of the dural sinuses is done to restore patency, rather than simply to staunch hemorrhage. Hemorrhage can be stopped without attempting to repair the sinus.

The surgery of penetrating missile injuries thus requires a familiarity with microvascular techniques and a psychological preparedness to use these techniques even under relatively primitive circumstances. For example, although commercial shunts or Silastic T-tubes may not be available at all times, a workable alternative can be improvised from a floppy pediatric endotracheal tube to which a second balloon cuff has been affixed.

## Cerebrospinal Fluid Leaks

At the time of initial débridement, a search should be made for potential sites of CSF fistulas, particularly when the air sinuses, skull base, and orbit have been violated. The complex craniofacial wounds are always treated more vigorously than other penetrating injuries because CSF fistulas are almost inevitable, and infection usually sets in if contaminated nasopharyngeal bone and mucosa are implanted within the brain. If a CSF leak has been detected, the entire frontal floor, as far posteriorly as the optic foramina and the limbus sphenoidale, must be inspected.

Neither bone nor polymethyl methacrylate is needed to close a dural fistula leaking CSF from the skull base*; indeed, this can be accomplished simply by patching or reinforcing the dura with pericranium, temporalis fascia, or an adjacent dural flap. The patch is tacked down with several 4–0 or 5–0 sutures intradurally. The pressure of CSF and the brain holds the graft in place until after it vascularizes and fuses to the dura. Sometimes, fat must be used to plug a particularly large fistula, with the dural graft or dural reflection used to hold the fat in place. Acrylic tissue adhesives for attaching the dural graft have been used with some initial success, but have significant toxicity to neural elements. Furthermore, the seal produced by this type of tissue adhesive is not watertight; the cement sepa-

---

*Despite an initial enthusiasm for early repair of cosmetic and structural skull defects with polymethyl methacrylate, the infectious complications resulting from this practice make it inadvisable. Polymethyl methacrylate is also not a satisfactory substance for obtaining a watertight seal because it shrinks and can become porous with time.

rates the tissues, impeding contact, fibroblastic ingrowth, and eventual healing.

Many of these problems may be solved by fibrin glues. No glue, however, will repair a leak that is caused by a local or generalized disturbance of CSF circulation rather than a simple anatomic defect.

Cerebrospinal fluid fistula can develop years after injury, and can recur even after careful repair.

## Hydrocephalus

There are a number of circumstances that predispose to the development of hydrocephalus after penetrating missile injury. The most obvious case is disruption or occlusion of the ventricular system by bone fragments (rarely) or metal. When possible, these should be removed (see Metallic and Migrating Fragments). Ventriculitis and subarachnoid and intraventricular hemorrhage are known to cause both communicating and obstructive hydrocephalus. Lumbar puncture may be used as a temporizing measure in communicating hydrocephalus.

Ventriculostomy (in contaminated or infected cases) and ventriculoperitoneal shunting can be used in both communicating and obstructive hydrocephalus. In diffuse intracerebral edema, the ventricles may be so small that they cannot be cannulated, but if a successful ventriculostomy can be placed, intracranial pressure should be measured at the same time. The cause of any delayed rise in ICP, as well as the onset of hydrocephalus, needs to be understood before it is treated.

## Replacement of Bone Fragments

Should bone fragments be replaced at time of initial débridement to achieve immediate reconstruction of the calvaria? In fresh injuries, large pieces of bone with aesthetically important functions, such as the forehead or the orbital ridge, can be replaced after scrubbing and soaking with antibiotic solution, or even sterilization, and fixation with plates and screws. Moreover, most neurosurgeons have had reasonable success at treating smaller open skull fractures by immediate repositioning of bone fragments. Nonetheless, there is an inevitable risk of infection and osteomyelitis. Close neurosurgical observation must be available before primary reconstruction is undertaken. If, because of a long evacuation path from the field of battle, with multiple stations or other special circumstances, adequate follow-up cannot be provided, it is preferable to leave out the bone, and perform a cranioplasty at 9 to 12 months after injury. Delayed reconstruction is almost always preferable when an injury is not seen acutely. Under no circumstances should synthetics or plastics be incorporated into an initial bony repair. Infection is almost certain to supervene.

## Strategic Considerations

In most mass casualty situations, international conflicts, terrorist incidents, or natural disasters, definitive care will probably be available at a site removed from the epicenter of the incident. Transportation is all important, particularly to reduce the interval between wounding and definitive care. In Vietnam, the interval between wounding and arrival at a treatment facility was frequently 1 hour or less, and rarely more than 6 hours.[45] During the Lebanon conflict, in Israel, the average interval between wounding and CT was less than 1 hour, with a physician-manned helicopter on the scene within 15 to 30 minutes. Resuscitation can be begun during transportation, and the neurosurgeon can expect to be close to the scene of injury in time, if not in actual distance. This should help minimize secondary hypoxic damage after injury, and limit the number of untreated cases of acutely increased ICP. If the Vietnam experience holds true, most patients will be conscious when they arrive.

It can reasonably be anticipated that a CT scan will be available wherever the neurosurgeon operates. Ideally, a senior neurosurgeon would review the scan and be responsible for triage decisions in mass casualty situations. This arrangement proved quite satisfactory in Haifa, where the senior neurosurgeon was available to the emergency room and could accompany a patient to CT. Although it would be preferable to have at least two neurosurgeons at every location where neurosurgery is to be carried out, a partially trained neurosurgeon, or even a general surgeon, could be called to assist a single, fully qualified neurosurgeon working alone.

Patients can be moved as soon as they are stable, using the ordinary neurosurgical criteria. At times, it may be necessary to relax these criteria under mass casualty conditions. If necessary, patients can be transferred intubated or under anesthesia.

## SUMMARY

We have entered an era of less aggressive surgery in the management of penetrating missile injuries. The VHIS has demonstrated that there are no silent areas of the brain when it comes to débridement after penetrating trauma. Regardless of how well patients seem to recover, very complex psychobehavioral and cognitive functions are adversely affected. Community adjustment can be severely affected. Whatever brain tissue can be saved, should be saved. With modern imaging techniques and dependable follow-up, multiple operations to achieve a "perfect" débridement of penetrating missile tracks are no longer indicated, provided the initial débridement sufficed.

## REFERENCES

1. Meirowsky AM (ed): Neurological Surgery of Trauma. 1964. Office of the Surgeon General, Washington, DC.
2. Matson DD: The Treatment of Acute Craniocerebral Injuries Due to Missiles. Charles C. Thomas, Springfield, IL 1948.
3. War Surgery Supplement. Br J Surg 1947.
4. Lewin W, Gibon MR: Missile head wounds in the Korean campaign: A survey of British casualties. Br J Surg 43:628–632, 1956.
5. Byrnes DP, Crockard HA, Gordon DS, et al: Penetrating craniocerebral missile injuries in the civil disturbances in Northern Ireland. Br J Surg 61:169–176, 1971.
6. Meyers PW, Salazar AM: Vietnam Head Injury Study: Combat-caused penetrating head wounds—assessment 14 years after injury. Annual Meeting, American Academy of Neurology, Course #104, April 27, 1986.
7. Danic D, Prgomet D, Milicic D, et al: War injuries to the head and neck. Mil Med 163:117–119, 1998.

8. Prgomet D, Danic D, Milicic D, et al: Mortality caused by war wounds to the head and neck encountered at the Slavonski Brod Hospital during the 1991–1992 war in Croatia. Mil Med 163:482–485, 1998.
9. Al-Harby SW: The evolving pattern of war-related injuries from the Afghanistan conflict. Mil Med 161:163–164, 1996.
10. Tudor M: Prediction of outcome in patients with missile craniocerebral injuries during the Croatian War. Mil Med 163:486–489, 1998.
11. Aarabi B, Taghipour M, Alibaii E, Kamgarpour A: Central nervous system infections after military missile head wounds. Neurosurgery 42:500–507; Discussion 507–509, 1998.
12. Vrankovic D, Splavski B, Hecimovic I, et al: Analysis of 127 war inflicted brain missile injuries sustained in north-eastern Croatia. J Neurosurg Sci 40:107–114, 1996.
13. Porteous MH, Edwards SA, Groom AF: Inner city gunshot wounds. Injury 28:385–387, 1997.
14. Demuth WE Jr: Bullet velocity as applied to military rifle wounding capacity. J Trauma 9:27–32, 1969.
15. Demuth WE Jr: Bullet velocity and design as determinants of wounding capability: An experimental study. J Trauma 6:222–232, 1966.
16. Dobbyn RC, Bruckly WL Jr, Shubin LD: An evaluation of police handgun ammunition: Summary report. Washington, D.C:, U.S. Department of Justice, 1975.
17. Dodge PR, Meirowsky AM: Tangential wounds of the scalp and skull. J Neurosurg 9:472–483, 1952.
18. Adelola A, Odehu EL: A syndrome characteristic of tangential bullet wounds of the vertex of the skull. J Neurosurg 34:155–158, 1971.
19. Harvey EW, Butler EG, McMillen JH, et al: Mechanisms of wounding. War Med 8:91–104, 1945.
20. Kirpatrick JB, DiMaio VD: Civilian gunshot wounds of the brain. J Neurosurg 49: 185–198, 1978.
21. Meirowsky AM: Secondary removal of retained bone fragments in missile wounds of the brain. J Neurosurg 57:617–621, 1982.
22. Hammon WM: Retained intracranial bone fragments: analysis of 42 patients. J Neurosurg 34:142–154, 1971.
23. Freytag E:Autopsy findings in head injuries from firearms: Statistical evaluation of 254 cases. Arch Pathol 76:215–225, 1963.
24. Raimondi AS, Samuelson GH: Craniocerebral gunshot wounds in civilian practice. J Neurosurg 32:647–653, 1970.
25. Crockard HA. Bullet injuries of the brain. Ann R Coll Surg Eng 55:111–123, 1974.
26. Barnett JC, Meirowsky AM: Intracranial hematoma associated with penetrating wounds of the brain. J Neurosurg 12:34–48, 1955.
27. Matson DD, Wolkin J: Hematoma associated with penetrating wounds of the brain. J Neurosurg 3:46–53, 1946.
28. Young B, Rapp R, Norton A: Failure of prophylactically administered phenytoin to prevent early posttraumatic seizures. J Neurosurg 58:231–241, 1983.
29. Webster JE, Schneider RC, Loftram JE: Observations on early types of brain abscess following penetrating wounds of the brain. J Neurosurg 3:7–14, 1946.
30. Ecker AD: A bacteriologic study of penetrating wounds of the brain from a surgical point of view. J Neurosurg 3:1–6, 1946.
31. Carey ME, Young, H, Mathis JL, et al: A bacteriological study of craniocerebral missile wounds from Vietnam. J Neurosurg 34:145–154, 1971.
32. Hagan RE: Early complications following penetrating wounds of the brain. J Neurosurg 34:127–131, 1971.
33. Crockard HA: Early intracranial pressure studies in gunshot wounds of the brain. J Trauma 15:339–347, 1975.
34. Morin MA, Pitts, FW: Delayed apoplexy following head injury ("traumatische Spaet-Apoplexie"). J Neurosurg 33:542–547, 1970.
35. Gaskill-Shipley MF, Tomsick TA: Angiography in the evaluation of head and neck trauma. Neuroimaging Clin N Am 6:607–624, 1996.
36. Patel MR, Edelman RR: MR angiography of the head and neck. Top Magn Reson Imaging 8:345–365, 1996.
37. Rieger J, Hosten N, Neumann K, et al: Initial clinical experience with spiral CT and 3D arterial reconstruction in intracranial aneurysms and arteriovenous malformations. Neuroradiology 38:245–251, 1996.
38. Carey ME, Tutton RH, Strub RL, et al: The correlation between surgical and CT estimates of brain damage following missile wounds. J Neurosurg 60:947–954, 1984.
39. Rappaport ZH, Sahar A, Shaked I, et al. Computerized tomography in combat-related craniocerebral penetrating missile injuries. Isr J Med Sci 20:668–671, 1984.
40. Meyers PW, Salazar AM, Dillon JD, et al: The significance of retained intracranial bone fragments in penetrating combat head wounds. A preliminary report from the Vietnam Head Injury Study. Abstract presented at the American Congress of Neurosurgeons, Chicago, Illinois, November, 1983.
41. Feinsod M: The Israeli experience with penetrating missile injuries in Lebanon. Presented at the Army-Navy Neurosurgical Conference, Walter Reed Army Medical Center, Bethesda, Maryland, October, 1985.
42. Caveness WF, Meirowsky, AM, Rish BL, et al: The nature of post traumatic epilepsy. J Neurosurg 50:545–553, 1979.
43. Weiss GH, Feeney DM, Caveness WF, et al. Prognostic factors for the occurrence of posttraumatic epilepsy. Arch Neurol 40:7–10, 1983.
44. Meirowsky AM: Wounds of the dural sinuses. J Neurosurg 10:496–514, 1953.
45. Hammon WM: Missile wounds. In Vinken PJ, Bruyn GW, Braakman R, (eds): Handbook of Clinical Neurology: Injuries of the Brain and Skull, Part I. New York: American Elsevier, pp 505–526.

# Surgical Management of Missile Injuries of the Head

■ MAURICE I. SABA

Gunshot wounds of the head are on the increase. The easy availability of handguns, revolvers, shotguns, and rifles and the continued and increasing armed struggle in various parts of the world demand a renewed and serious interest in and a better understanding of both the ballistic characteristics of missiles and the surgical pathology of missile wounds. Simple adherence to the general surgical principles of wound care leaves much to be desired when the neurosurgeon is confronted with a missile or gunshot wound of the brain. Gurdjian[1] has reviewed the stages through which the treatment of penetrating wounds of the brain sustained in warfare has evolved. Reports from the great wars of the 20th century detailed some of the early work on missile and gunshot wounds to the head.[2–7] An analysis of penetrating brain wounds from Vietnam by Hammon[8, 9] has familiarized neurosurgeons with the difficult and multifaceted problems facing the surgeon who must deal with these types of wounds on a day-to-day basis. The high rate of complications,[10, 11] the problems associated with bacterial contamination of these wounds,[12, 13] and the increased rates of morbidity and mortality from reoperation will be improved only when the surgeon becomes familiar with certain specific surgical principles based on vast experiences in the care of such wounds. Meirowsky[7] has described some of the basic principles involved in the surgical care of such patients drawn from the Korean War experience. More recently, Hammon,[8] Saba and colleagues,[14, 15] and Brandvold and associates[16] outlined some basic principles in the surgical management of these patients drawn from the Vietnam and Middle East conflicts. Adherence to these basic surgical principles and a thorough understanding of the ballistic characteristics of the wounding agents and the mechanisms of wounding and tissue damage should be the prerequisites to a carefully executed and definitive surgical management, when possible. Management should begin as early as possible after wounding. This approach ensures that more lives will be saved and more neurologic function preserved.

## BALLISTIC DATA

A voluminous literature offers ballistic data from a number of institutions and authors.[17–27] Ballistic data related to civilian and military injuries are summarized here. Most handguns and revolvers use heavy bullets weighing approximately 0.5 oz and have muzzle velocities ranging from 550 to 900 ft/sec. These are referred to as *low-velocity missiles*. In contrast, most current rifles use very light bullets (<10 g) and have muzzle velocities averaging 3000 ft/sec, with a range of 2300 to 6000 ft/sec.

In our practice at the American University of Beirut Medical Center, in which an large number of patients have been seen between 1975 and 1990, we have encountered and become familiar with three basic types of missiles that cause penetrating wounds to the brain:

1. The 7.62-mm bullet fired from the Russian AK-47 assault rifle. This is an expanding-type bullet that weighs 150 g and has a diameter of 0.311 in and a length of 1.08 in. It has a muzzle velocity of 2329 ft/sec and is used for close-range and street fighting.[17]
2. The 5.56-mm (0.223-in diameter) bullet fired from the M-16 rifle. This soft-point, jacketed bullet weighs 55 g and has a muzzle velocity of 3250 ft/sec.[18] This bullet is commonly used for long-range combat and for sniping.
3. Fragments of high-explosive devices. These are of various shapes and sizes and can weigh as much as 100 g. These should be regarded as high-velocity missiles because initially they travel at speeds of over 3000 ft/sec, although they rapidly lose speed because of their volume, irregular shape, and aerodynamic instability, becoming low-velocity missiles after having traveled as little as 10 m.

Although rifle and machine gun fire causes only 15% to 20% of such wounds in modern warfare, they are encountered with greater frequency in civil strife, guerrilla warfare, and civilian injuries, in which wounding usually occurs at very close range.

The ballistic analysis of shotgun and pellet injuries has been discussed by Sights,[28] who analyzed 24 shotgun injuries to the central nervous system and indicated 4 types of injuries in which wound production was a feature of pellet skull penetration requiring a unit per cross-sectional area energy in excess of $6.5 \times 10^4$ ft-lb/in².

## SURGICAL PATHOLOGY

The behavior of a missile depends on several variables such as its size, shape, aerodynamic stability, and velocity. Tissue density and elasticity greatly modify both the stability and the velocity of the missile. This factor, to a great degree, determines the extent of tissue damage produced by the passage of the missile.

Because the center of gravity is behind the center of mass, bullets are aerodynamically unstable. This instability is usually overcome by the rifling of the barrel, which gives the bullet a spinning action and more stability. Stability is lost as the bullet hits the tissue, however, because the high density of the tissue retards the bullet as a result of the phenomenon of yaw. On average, human tissue is approximately 800 times denser than air. The human brain is similar to a gelatin foam preparation in its density and response to missile penetration.

The extent of tissue damage depends on the amount of energy expended by the missile at the point of tissue penetration. Although the physics of missile energy is beyond the scope of this discussion, in general, tissue injury manifests in three different patterns (Fackler[29] has shed some light on some of the common misconceptions regarding tissue injury):

1. *Laceration and crushing of tissues*: In this type of injury, there is no significant energy transmitted to the tissues. This frequently occurs with low-velocity missile wounds. There is no cavitation except for the limited track produced by the passage of the missile, a pathologic picture similar to that produced by hand weapons and sharp objects. The wound is equal in size at the entry and exit points.
2. *Shock waves*: As the missile hits and enters the tissue, it compresses the tissue medium ahead of it, which momentarily spreads in the form of a spherical shock wave of very short duration but of considerable energy and produces damage distant from the missile track. According to Owen-Smith,[30] this energy can be in excess of 1000 lb/in².
3. *Temporary cavitation*: On entry of a high-velocity missile into tissue, the tissue moves both forward and sideways, producing what is referred to as *temporary cavitation*. The area affected may be as large as 30 times the diameter of the actual track of the missile. With the outward movement of the tissue, a sudden drop of pressure to subatmospheric levels occurs; this produces a sucking action that introduces debris, foreign material, and bacteria from the air into the cavity. This temporary cavitation is similar to a shock wave and is of very short duration. It immediately collapses and forms the permanent cavity, which is invariably larger than the actual track of the missile. This mechanism of injury is exclusively produced by high-velocity missiles.

The extent of tissue damage in penetrating and perforating wounds of the head is modified by the existence of two distinct physical properties of the tissues involved. First, the brain is a semisolid medium (closer to a liquid system), and second, it is encased in a rigid skull that has

the physical property of being able to stretch. This ability of the skull to stretch, in addition to the low density of the brain, perhaps accounts for the occurrence of limited cavitation in the brain. In contrast, because the skull is filled with the semisolid brain tissue, extensive fracturing of the skull occurs when the energy expended by the missile is great, such as with a high-velocity missile. Owen-Smith[30] studied this phenomenon by firing bullets into empty skulls. The entry and exit wounds produced were small and neat. He then filled the skulls with a gelatin medium and placed a pressure transducer in them. He noted that extensive fracturing of the skull occurred with pressure recordings in excess of 400 lb/in² when bullets were fired into the gelatin-filled skulls. He suggested that it is difficult to attain pressures high enough extensively to fracture an empty skull, whereas a gelatin-filled skull extensively fractures with much lower pressures. Therefore, the brain may actually aid in cracking the skull from within.

In summary, the surgeon should keep in mind the following:

1. High-velocity missiles traveling at speeds greater than 3000 ft/sec produce extensive tissue damage by shock waves and temporary cavitation.
2. The cavitary necrosis is much larger than the actual track of the missile.
3. The suction effect of temporary cavitation actively draws large volumes of bone, dirt, hair, skin fragments, clothing, and bacteria into the track, which also contains devitalized brain tissue.
4. Bacterial contamination of these wounds occurs as a result of the temporary cavitation and suction effect, and it is uniformly distributed throughout the wound.
5. Low-velocity missiles produce limited tissue damage consisting mainly of tissue laceration and crushing.
6. Larger wounds at exit sites are the result of the phenomenon of bullet deformation and yaw, occurring most commonly with high-velocity bullets. The degree of yaw angle is greatest at 10 cm or more of tissue penetration.

Wound ballistics have been detailed by Weiner and Barrett[18] and others,[20–27] and the reader is referred to their work for details.

## SURGICAL MANAGEMENT

To some extent, in the straightforward case, knowledge of the type of missile and the circumstances of injury dictates the operative approach and the technical details. The presence of signs of increased intracranial pressure caused by an expanding hematoma or the presence of gross sepsis with meningitis or brain fungus may alter the timing and the type of operative management used.

### Preoperative Evaluation

If such information is available, a detailed history of the time, place, and circumstances of wounding, as well as the type of weapon and the bullet used, is essential. A careful neurologic evaluation should be made in terms of any neurologic deficit secondary either to the primary injury or to the effects of expanding intracranial hematomas. The picture of impending herniation and brain stem compression must be recognized immediately. Plain roentgenograms of the skull in three projections (anteroposterior, lateral, and Towne) should be obtained to determine the following:

1. The entry and exit points of the missile
2. The extent of bony fractures
3. The volume of any bone that has been driven intracranially
4. The presence of any metallic fragments
5. The trajectory of the bullet, which may suggest the areas of penetration and bullet fragmentation and the extent of radial fragment scatter such as occurs with soft-point and copper-jacketed military bullets, to predict the expected neurologic deficit
6. The type, caliber, shape, and size of the missile
7. The location of the missile and its accessibility for removal at the time of definitive surgery

Computed tomography (CT) of the brain should be obtained in every case when feasible. The findings should be correlated with the plain roentgenograms (mainly for foreign material, bone, and metal) and the clinical picture. CT scans can be obtained within 15 to 20 minutes and should be obtained even in patients with rapidly deteriorating clinical pictures. We have routinely used CT for gunshot wounds to the head at the American University of Beirut Medical Center since 1982. In addition to the information obtained from the plain roentgenograms, CT scans help assess the following:

1. The extent of brain injury
2. Size and location of hematomas along the track of injury
3. The presence of subdural or epidural hematomas close to or distant from the site of the injury
4. The extent of cerebral injury in tangential wounds
5. The trajectory of the missile, predictive of outcome, such as in transventricular wounds, tracks through deep gray matter, or diagonal injury with crossover from one hemisphere to another
6. Cerebral injury distant from the surgical field, such as intracerebral hematoma or brain infarction, secondary to vascular injury
7. The volume of in-driven bone as well as postdébridement retained bone (best seen on CT scans)

Computed tomography scanning not only helps tailor the definitive operative procedure after wounding but is a valuable tool in assessing the true extent of brain damage after missile wounds. Carey and colleagues[31] have clearly demonstrated the value of CT imaging in the estimate of true brain damage after such wounds.

Cerebral angiography was used before the advent of CT imaging and is now used only if CT imaging is not available, and mainly to determine the presence of distant hematomas, extradural and subdural hematomas, and major vascular injury. Postoperative cerebral angiography has been used in patients who have had subarachnoid hemorrhage to determine the presence of traumatic aneurysms,[32, 33] which seem to occur more frequently with shell fragments than with bullets. Cerebral angiography is most valuable in the postoperative period if a subarachnoid hemorrhage develops in the patient.

Preoperative osmotic diuretics are used sparingly and only when an expanding intracranial lesion is suspected. In contrast, corticosteroids are used routinely in a dosage range of 24 to 36 mg/day given in six divided doses. We resort to higher dosages when CT imaging reveals severe hemispheric swelling. All patients are started on anticonvulsants immediately; diphenylhydantoin is the drug most commonly used, with a loading dose of 500 to 1000 mg given intravenously by slow infusion. Antibiotics are started only after all cultures are taken. We routinely take cultures from the entry and exit wounds, cerebral debris, bone fragments driven into the wound, and foreign matter. Because this procedure is feasible only at the time of surgery, antibiotics are started either during or immediately after surgery. Specimens must be cultured in both aerobic and anaerobic media.

The entire scalp is shaved in the emergency ward, the wounds are dressed with sterile gauze soaked with a solution of 1% povidone-iodine (Betadine), and a heavy sterile dressing is applied.

## Operative Technique

Accurate assessment of tissue loss can be performed only in the operating room. The most crucial factor in successful closure of the wound is the amount of scalp loss. The primary aim of the surgical intervention is to save the patient's life and preserve his or her neurologic function. The most opportune time for cranial exploration after gunshot wounds of the head is within the first 2 to 3 hours after injury. Every effort should be made to make this early exploration the definitive one, because reoperations carry a higher rate of mortality and morbidity.

The guidelines to follow for such an operation are as follows:

1. Adequate débridement and excision of the edges of the scalp wound
2. Adequate débridement of all bone edges
3. Exposure of the entire edge of the torn dura, and débridement of the shredded dural edge
4. Thorough débridement of all necrotic brain tissue, hair, soil, skin fragments, and blood clots from the cavity in the brain
5. Hemostasis of the cerebral wound and torn dural venous sinuses
6. Removal of all bone fragments driven into the wound: injuries associated with bone fragments have the highest incidence of bacterial infection, and their retention in the depth of the cerebral wound predisposes the patient to the development of cerebritis or brain abscess, or both
7. Watertight closure of the dura, preferably with a graft and a tight skin closure without tension to prevent cerebrospinal fluid (CSF) leakage (which is associated with an increased rate of morbidity from postoperative infection)

We prepare the entire scalp and drape it to facilitate either the extension of scalp wounds across the midline or bilateral exploration of both entry and exit wounds. Betadine solution is used for skin antisepsis. In the presence of entry and exit wounds, we prefer to débride the entry wound first because of the smaller amount of tissue damage and the larger volume of foreign matter that is usually driven in. The entry wound, which is usually small, is excised and sent for culture. The wound is enlarged by Z extensions or flaps, and the bony defect is enlarged with rongeurs to expose a clean and intact dural edge. The dura is opened with a cruciate incision, and the cerebral wound is inspected. The cortical wound is usually much smaller than the track of the missile in the cerebral white matter. The track is then gently explored for debris and hematoma. For this maneuver, we prefer to introduce a blunted tip of an Asepto syringe (Becton Dickinson & Co., Rutherford, NJ) into the wound and wash the debris out by steady and gentle irrigation of the track with saline under moderate constant pressure while the syringe tip is withdrawn slowly. Care is taken to avoid blocking the cerebral entry wound with the irrigating syringe because this allows water to dissect into the brain with undesirable consequences, instead of allowing back drainage of debris and necrotic, hemorrhagic brain tissue. This maneuver is repeated several times and effects a thorough débridement of the track because foreign matter usually is floated out with the irrigation. We avoid using the metal-tipped suction because it can induce deep bleeding that results in further neurologic deficit. Metal suction tips tend to suck up swollen brain from the wall of the track, brain that is not necessarily necrotic. We attempt to save as much viable brain tissue as possible and débride only necrotic brain in the center of the track. We sometimes use diluted hydrogen peroxide solution, which also stops capillary oozing from the walls of the cerebral cavitary track. After this irrigation débridement, attention is directed toward removing all bone fragments embedded in the cerebral wound. Large fragments can be picked up easily with fine forceps; small, lightweight chips float out with irrigation. We have occasionally encountered large buttons of bone driven deep into the center of the hemisphere as a bullet hit the skull and ricocheted tangentially after it had separated the bone button and driven it in as a secondary missile. In such cases, the track created by the bone is small and not cavitary. Such fragments are found easily by sounding the track with a long brain needle, and the fragment can be picked up with a fine bayonet forceps. The track is then irrigated with saline. Hemostasis of the brain wound should be complete to avoid the use of hemostatic material. No attempt should be made to remove small metallic shrapnel fragments at the expense of further injury to brain tissue. These fragments are not associated with bacterial infection, as bone fragments often are, and it is unlikely that such metallic fragments left in place form a nidus for cerebral infection provided that all necrotic brain in the vicinity has been débrided. The dural defect is patched with a pericranial graft and sutured with fine monofilament nylon to achieve watertight closure. The bone edge is waxed, and the skin edge is approximated with a continuous 2–0 nylon suture. There should be no tension on the skin edge because of possible skin edge necrosis. A Hemovac drain is left in the subgaleal space in the craniectomy defect for 24 hours.

Attention then is directed to the exit wound, where a larger amount of tissue loss, particularly of the scalp, poses a challenge to closure. More skin exposure is necessary here, and extension of the skin is carried out with easier closure in mind. The bone, which is usually extensively fractured, can be removed easily. Brisk and active bleeding may be encountered after fractured bone fragments are elevated, particularly over the high convexity or close to the dural sinuses. Bleeding may occur from the torn surface of the dura or from lacerated brain, where the bleeding points were tamponaded as the swollen brain pushed against the calvarium. The surgeon must alert the anesthesiologist to the possibility of brisk bleeding, especially when working close to the dural sinuses. The surgeon also must be equipped to control bleeding quickly with Gelfoam, Oxycel, and cottonoid patties. Sometimes, several hundred milliliters of blood can be lost quickly from these sites. When torn sinuses are anticipated, it is important that generous bone removal be performed before removing the impacted bone fragment. After the bone has been removed, the diploë are waxed; we do not hesitate to coagulate the dural surface for hemostasis because we rely on grafting for closure. At times, tears of the sinuses have been repaired with a patch of dura. More often, the tear is so irregular and extensive, with massive cerebral laceration in the vicinity, that packing with muscle and Gelfoam is necessary. The torn dural edge is excised completely, and the dura is tacked up to the bone with interrupted 4–0 nylon sutures. The cerebral wound is then explored. Usually, there is very little foreign material in the wound; in particular, there are no bone fragments. The volume of necrotic brain tissue, however, is much larger than that in the entry wound. Both hemorrhagic brain and hematomas usually are found; these can be removed with copious saline irrigation. Care should be taken not to produce fresh bleeding from the adjacent swollen brain that may be difficult to control. Hemostasis of the edge of the lacerated cortex is secured by coagulation of the pia-arachnoid around the entire edge with bipolar coagulation. Again, we emphasize the débridement only of necrotic brain tissue; swollen brain should not be débrided because it will function after the edema has subsided. Brain débridement should be thorough but gentle. Exploration of the bottom of the cerebral wound for hematoma is mandatory. If a persistently high degree of brain swelling is present, the surgeon should suspect the development of a deep hematoma until it has been searched for and not found. Unless there is a deep hematoma, the bulk of the brain responds to mannitol with a rapid decrease in volume. In our experience, when brain swelling could not be satisfactorily explained, we have found a deep intracerebral hematoma in every instance. Occasionally, the brain swells and no hematoma is found; this situation can be addressed by placing gentle, even pressure on the surface of the brain by the surgeon's hands for 10 to 15 minutes, after which the brain may settle back to its normal size. This could be caused by the phenomenon of reactive hyperemia. After the hematoma is evacuated, the cerebral wound is copiously irrigated with a diluted solution of hydrogen peroxide (half-strength with saline, 1:1/volume), and then with saline.

This approach ensures the removal of large amounts of devitalized brain and hemostasis. We sometimes also use a diluted solution of 1% Betadine (100 ml diluted in 1000 ml of saline). No untoward effects have been seen with the use of either solution.

Dural closure is routinely performed with a graft. Pericranium or temporalis fascia usually suffices and is easy to handle. Pericranium is more accessible and has been used routinely. We do not recommend the use of fascia lata because it does not withstand infection as well as pericranium. Watertight closure of the dura is recommended, and the patch is sutured with a running locked-stitch suture of 4–0 monofilament nylon. We share the opinion with many that dura is a good barrier to intracranial extension of infection should the superficial wound become infected. The dural patch is not stretched and is left redundant to accommodate postoperative brain swelling. The devitalized edges of the scalp are excised, and with Z extensions, rotation flaps, or gridiron incisions into the galea, closure of the wound becomes feasible. Tension on the edge produces necrosis and predisposes the wound to infection. After closure of the dura, the skin wound is irrigated with copious amounts of diluted Betadine solution and saline. Subgaleal Hemovac drains are used routinely for 24 hours. The skin edges are approximated with 2–0 nylon sutures in one layer.

# CASE REPORTS

Unusual problems occasionally can be encountered that may require some modification of the recommended technique. Unusual circumstances of wounding and delayed referral to a specialized center may require a change in strategy toward definitive treatment.

## Case Report 1

A 35-year-old woman was hit with a sniper's high-velocity 5.56-mm bullet and was immediately rendered unconscious. She was brought to the hospital 1 hour after injury. She had a 0.8-cm entry wound in the left frontal area, a larger exit wound in the right frontal area, and extensive fractures of the frontal bone (Figs. 8–1 and 8–2). She had no clinical evidence of expanding hematoma, but hemorrhagic, necrotic brain was oozing out of both wounds. She underwent a large bifrontal craniotomy, débridement of brain, removal of all bone fragments, dural repair, and wiring of the extensive fractures of the frontal bone (Figs. 8–3 and 8–4). After surgery, the wound healed without infection and within 3 weeks she was neurologically intact except for a slight blunting of affect, and was discharged on anticonvulsants. Five years after injury, this patient was doing well and had returned to her job as a factory worker and was subsequently lost to follow-up.

This case illustrates the extensive fracturing of the skull and the damage to brain produced by high-velocity bullets, as was mentioned in the section on Surgical Pathology. Prompt, definitive, meticulous surgery along the lines of the recommended technique saved the life and neurologic function of this patient.

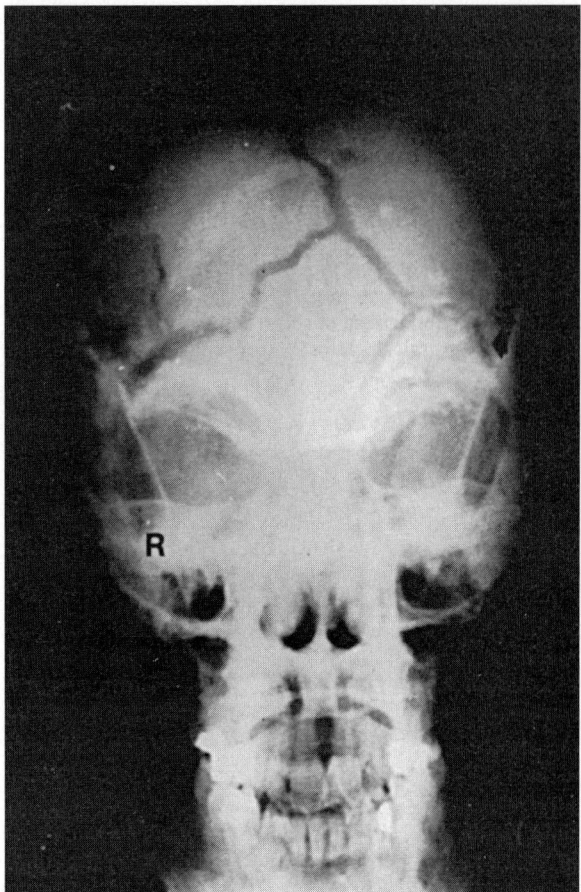

FIGURE 8–1 ■ Case report 1. An anteroposterior radiograph of the skull showing the entry wound (*short arrow*), the exit wound (*curved arrow*), and the blowout and comminuted fracture of the entire frontal bone. Note the increased density medial to the entry wound representing the bone fragments that were driven into the brain and embedded deep in the left frontal lobe.

## Case Report 2

A 20-year-old man was hit by a 7.62-mm bullet at close range. The injury produced a large scalp wound in the right frontal area with loss of skin, bone, and dura (Fig. 8–5). When he was examined 48 hours after injury, the patient had necrotic and hemorrhagic brain coming out of his wound, producing a cerebral fungus. He had a fever of 40°C (104°F), a stiff neck, and left hemiplegia, and was somnolent. A smear from the wound revealed gram-negative rods, and the CSF as well as the wound subsequently grew *Proteus vulgaris*, which was sensitive to gentamicin. Because of his general condition, surgery was postponed. The patient's head was shaved, the wound edge débrided, the depth of the wound packed with gauze soaked with 1% Betadine solution, and an occlusive external dressing applied. He was given 80 mg of gentamicin intravenously every 8 hours and 5 mg of gentamicin intrathecally every other day, along with 30 million units of crystalline penicillin G intravenously daily. On the sixth day after injury, the fever was reduced, the neck was less stiff, and the patient was

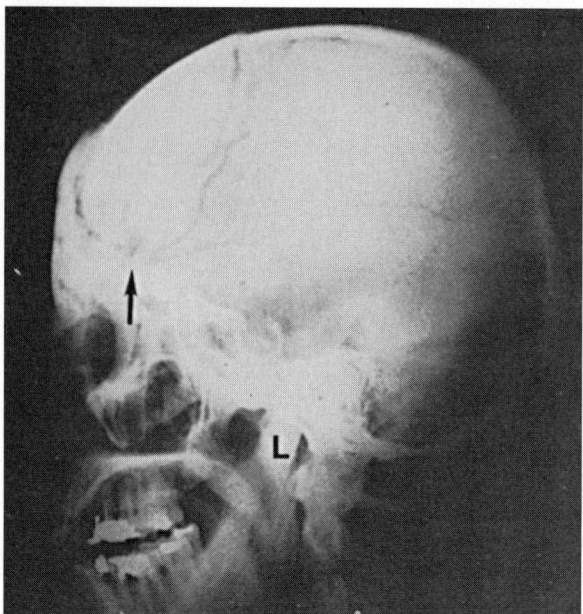

FIGURE 8–2 ■ Case report 1. This lateral radiograph of the skull shows the extensive frontal bone fractures. A frontoparietal linear fracture line is also visible. The bullet entered just above the roof of the orbit (*straight arrow*).

in controlling both the CSF and wound infections. Soaking these wounds with Betadine works both as a débriding agent for the necrotic brain fungus and as a local antiseptic. Continued use of Betadine locally is an acceptable alternative to early surgical débridement of an infected cerebral fungus. We seldom encountered a deep, persistent infection in such patients and believe that delayed débridement of such wounds is a less traumatic and effective surgical approach. In terms of neurologic function, the postoperative result has been satisfactory. This method is not recommended for routine use, but it can be a good alternative to early surgical intervention in a patient with a heavily infected wound with meningitis and an infected cerebral fungus due to delayed referral.

## Case Report 3

A 7-year-old boy was struck by a bullet as it descended vertically. The bullet was 7.62 mm in caliber, and it entered the head in the right frontoparietal area just posterior to the coronal suture (Fig. 8–7) and 6 cm lateral to the midline. It made an 8-mm linear scalp wound, traversed the hemisphere after piercing

more alert. Since admission, the head wound had been dressed with Betadine twice daily, with some débridement of the brain wound with each dressing change. The wound looked clean on the sixth day. The previously swollen brain had shrunk back into the confines of the bony defect and was pulsating gently, and clear CSF welled up from around the brain wound. It appeared that the cerebral wound had been effectively débrided of necrotic brain with the daily dressings. On the seventh day, the wound was explored. All bone fragments were removed, the brain débrided with irrigation, the dura closed with a patch and stainless steel wire sutures (Fig. 8–6), a clean craniectomy performed, and excision of the skin wound and its closure with relaxing and gridiron galeal incisions was conducted. The skin was closed in one layer with 2–0 nylon over catheter drains that were used to irrigate the wound for 1 week with 2 mg of gentamicin diluted in 10 ml of saline. The wound healed without infection, and within 3 weeks after débridement the patient was fully conscious and his left hemiplegia had cleared completely. The patient was followed regularly and showed no evidence of skull infection. Eighteen months later, a cranioplasty was performed. Twenty years later, he is still well, on anticonvulsants without seizures, and has not experienced a delayed cerebral infection.

Delayed definitive surgical débridement has been performed on some patients who came to hospital 36 hours or more from the time of injury. As this case illustrates, these patients have grossly infected wounds and most have a gram-negative rod as the infective organism. *Proteus* and *Escherichia coli* are the most common organisms cultured from these wounds. Treatment with aminoglycosides is effective

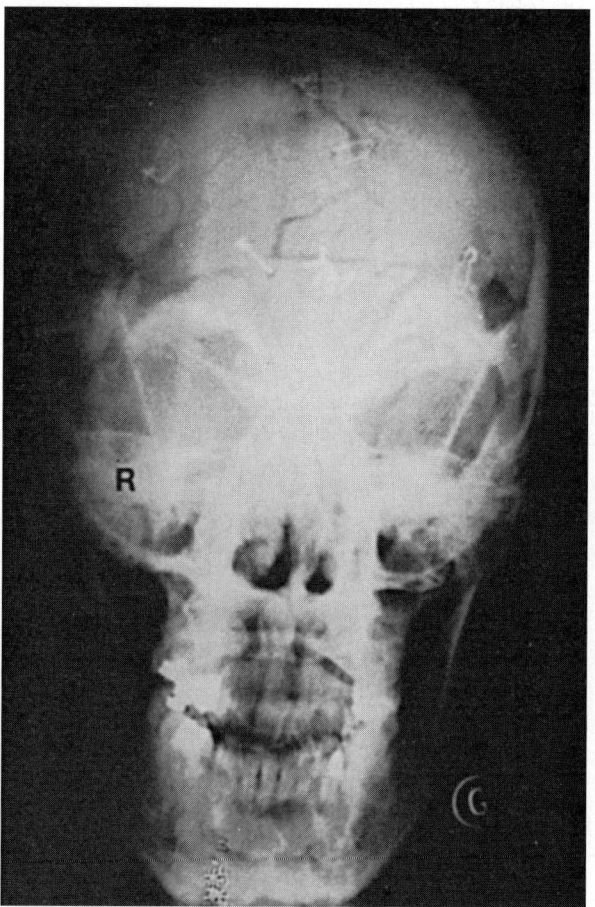

FIGURE 8–3 ■ Case report 1. An anteroposterior radiograph of the skull after débridement of the bone, dura, and brain. The bone fragments driven into the brain have been removed, and the frontal fractures have been wired to reconstitute the normal contour of the forehead. The midline metallic clips were used to stop bleeding from a tear of the dural venous sinus.

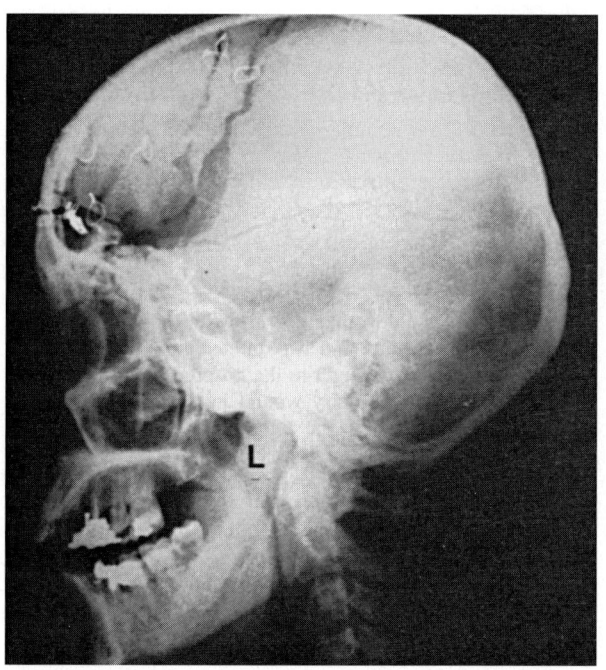

FIGURE 8–4 ■ Case report 1. A postoperative lateral view of the skull with the fractured frontal bone wired in place. A bifrontal craniotomy had been performed.

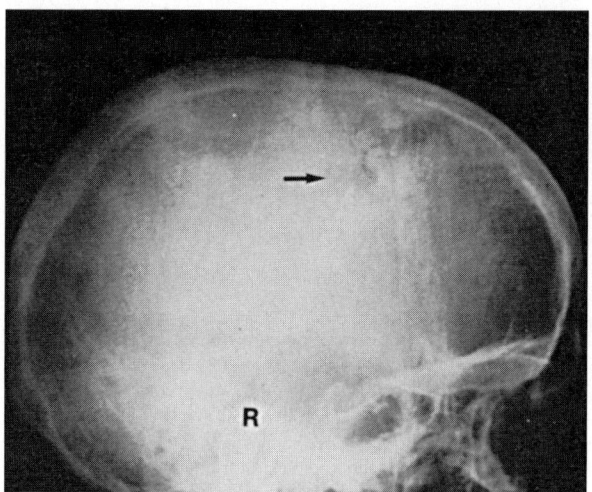

FIGURE 8–5 ■ Case report 2. A lateral view of the skull demonstrating the bony defect produced by the entry of the bullet in the right frontal area. The bullet drove several large fragments of bone intracranially, ricocheted, and exited 5 cm posterolaterally at the level of the coronal suture (*arrow*).

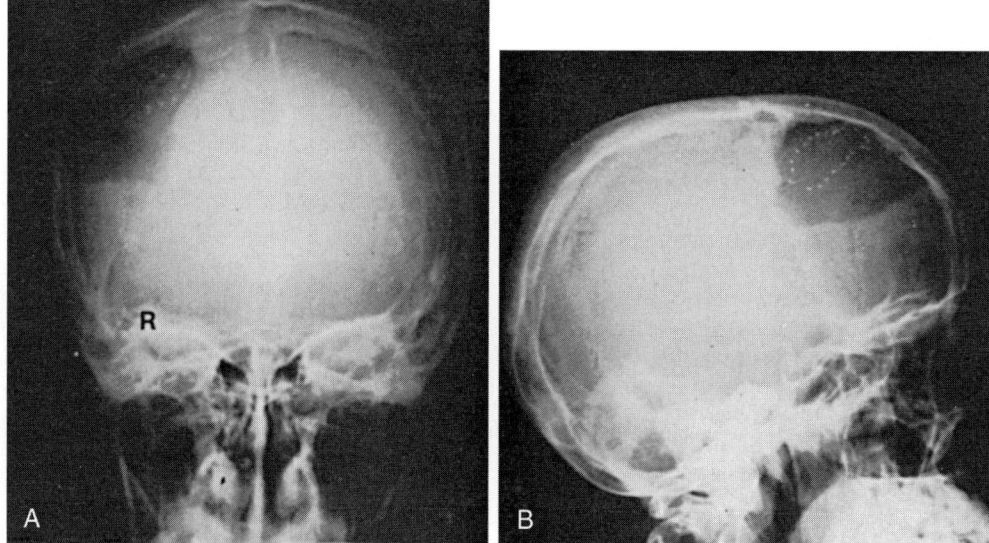

FIGURE 8–6 ■ Case report 2. Anteroposterior (*A*) and lateral (*B*) views of the skull demonstrating the extent of the craniectomy, the absence of any retained bone fragments, and the stainless steel wire suture outlining the pericranial dural patch.

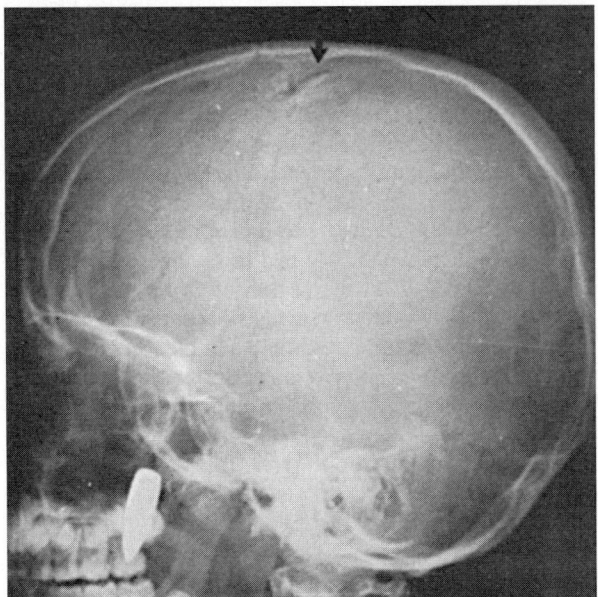

FIGURE 8–7 ■ Case report 3. The spent bullet, which was descending vertically, entered the skull just behind the coronal suture over the convexity (*arrow*), traveled through the white matter of the right hemisphere, and lodged in the facial bones just anterior and inferior to the zygoma. No bone fragments were driven intracranially. The scalp wound was less than 1 cm in diameter.

the calvarium, produced a small depressed fracture (Fig. 8–8), and lodged in the maxilla just anterior and inferior to the zygoma. The boy was dazed, fell to the ground, but soon got up and was able to walk. Results of a neurologic examination were normal except for a mild left facial weakness. There were no bone fragments driven into the wound on plain skull radiography. The scalp wound was excised and closed, and the patient was treated with corticosteroids and intravenous mannitol drip (15 ml/hr of 20% mannitol solution), anticonvulsants, and antibiotics. On the fourth day, his facial weakness had cleared and a right frontoparietal craniotomy centered on the wound was performed. The surface of the brain was hemorrhagic, and the cortical wound was covered with necrotic cerebral tissue. The cerebral track was irrigated with saline. All loose brain tissue separated easily with the water jet, and there was no need for débridement with metal-tipped suction. There were no bone fragments and no foreign material. The dura was closed with a pericranial patch and sutured with fine nylon. The bone flap was anchored in place, and the scalp flap was closed with 2–0 nylon. The bullet was then removed transorally through a mucosal incision above the last molar tooth. The patient's postoperative course was smooth, and he was discharged on anticonvulsants on the sixth postoperative day, neurologically intact and without wound sepsis.

## SPENT BULLETS

Patients who are injured by a spent bullet present a totally different pathologic picture from patients injured by a gun-

shot or shrapnel at a close range. These bullets descend vertically and have sufficient energy to penetrate the scalp, the calvarium, and the dura and descend through cerebral tissue to varying distances. They sometimes traverse the whole brain to come to lie on the bone of the base of the skull. The wound they produce is similar to a simple laceration of the brain, with a small track without cavitary necrosis along their trajectory. They neither produce cavitation nor drive bone fragments into the cerebral depth. Necrotic brain is limited to the passage track, and the level of bacterial contamination is extremely low. When the patient is neurologically intact at the time of admission, only the external wound is débrided, and delayed operation for brain débridement is performed toward the end of the first week, when all brain edema has subsided and necrotic brain along the wall of the track has separated from the adjacent swollen brain. In this setting, the operation is simple and bloodless, and effective cerebral débridement can be performed without any risk of added neurologic deficit. We attempt to remove these bullets unless they are located deep in the brain. These bullets move in the brain substance as a result of their weight and smooth surface. This happens more often in children and infants. It is, therefore, important to obtain repeat radiographs of the skull on the morning of the operation to locate their position. The craniotomy is a routine one, and we prefer small flaps because of the limited cerebral pathologic process and the small passage track. Probing of the track with

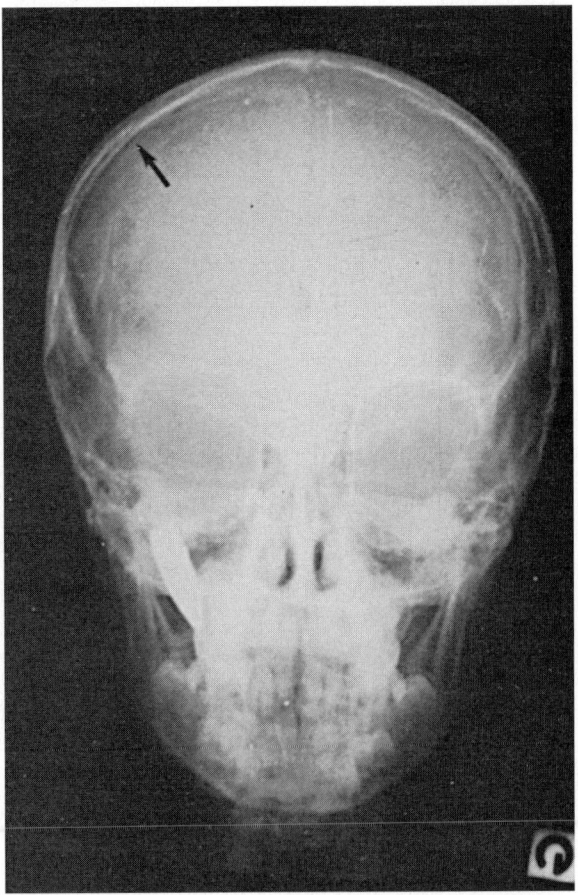

FIGURE 8–8 ■ Case report 3. An anteroposterior view of the skull showing the entry point of the bullet (*arrow*) and its position anterior to the zygoma.

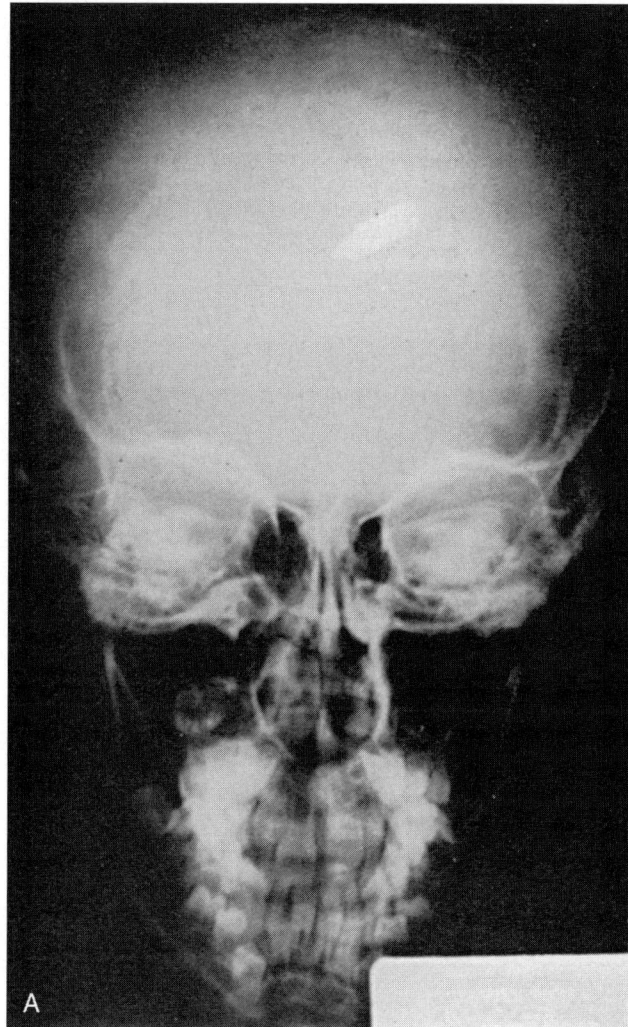

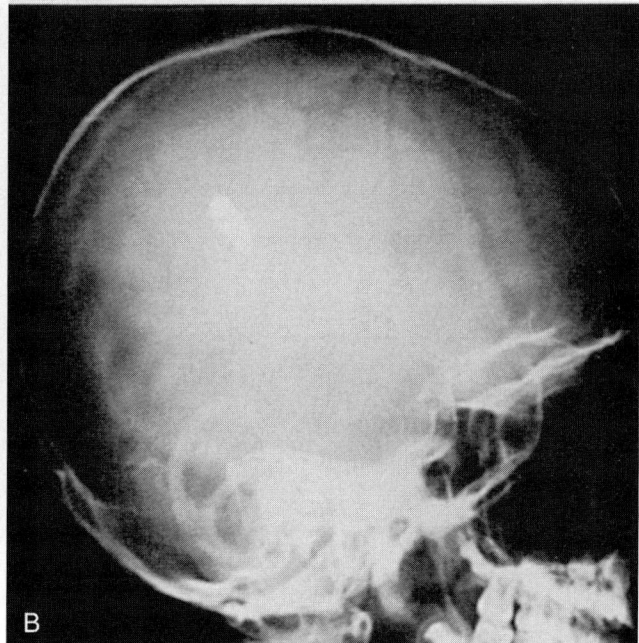

**FIGURE 8–9** ■ Posteroanterior (*A*) and lateral (*B*) projections showing a spent bullet in the center of the skull to the right of the midline.

instruments often is not necessary, and necrotic brain is washed out of the cerebral wound with saline. If the brain is unduly swollen 1 week after the injury, an intracerebral hematoma, usually deep in the track, must be sought. No foreign hemostatic material is to be left in the wound.

Most of these injuries occur during the vertical descent of the bullet. The relative benignity of these injuries, unless penetration of deep structures with deep hemorrhage into the ventricles occurs, has been established from the cases reported by Hanieh,[34] and our experience concurs with his. Although they behave like low-velocity missiles, they travel a distance into the skull and sometimes exit. Removal of these bullets may require a small additional craniotomy over the location of the bullet. Spent bullets in the depths of the brain that were inaccessible initially may change location by gravity and move with time to more accessible areas, where they can be easily removed. This is common in children injured with heavy, smooth bullets (Figs. 8–9 and 8–10).

## SPECIAL CONSIDERATIONS

From the experience of 15 years of continued military operations and civil war in Lebanon and the Middle East,

during which more than 2000 civilian and military gunshot wounds and missile injuries to the head were treated at the American University of Beirut Medical Center, we have come to recognize specific types of cerebral injury and special circumstances of ballistic wounds that are closely related to the extent of the injury and trajectory of the wounding agent, and that carry with them a high risk of complications and a grave prognosis for neurologic function and for life. I have briefly summarized these in the following patient categories: deep injuries, diagonal injuries, transventricular wounds, tangential injuries, CSF leak complicating missile injury to the head, retained bone fragments and infection, and traumatic intracranial aneurysms with penetrating head injuries.

## Deep Injuries

Bullets and shrapnel penetrating to the depths of the brain and traversing areas of deep gray matter carry with them a mortality rate of higher than 50%. Our observations concur with the physiologic study and experimental model presented by Gerber and Moody.[35] Many of these patients have a concomitant ventricular injury and hematoma, and the patient model is not as neat as the experimental one. Nonetheless, the mortality rate seems to be very high.

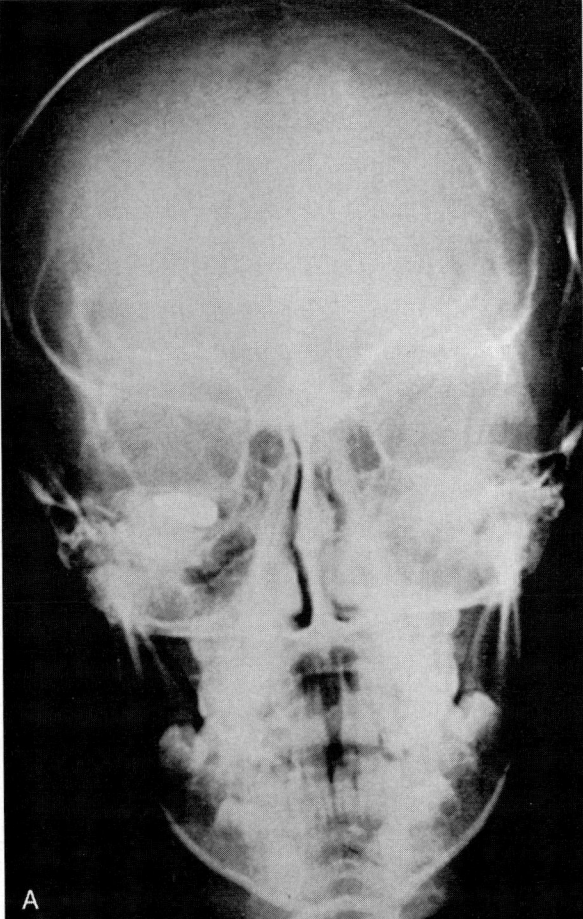

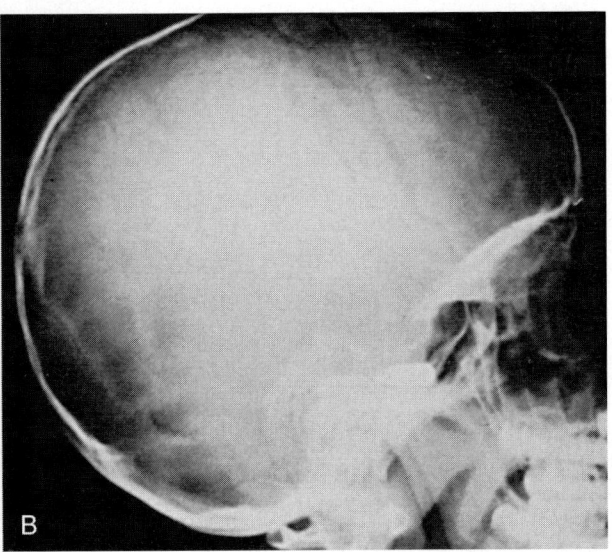

FIGURE 8–10 ■ Posteroanterior (*A*) and lateral (*B*) views of the skull of the same patient (as in Fig. 8–9) 7 months after the initial injury illustrating the descent of the bullet through the brain substance to lie on the bone of the middle fossa. No clinical deficits occurred with the migration of the bullet.

Many of these patients are comatose, and their clinical presentation is often associated with death. Rish and colleagues[36] have alluded to this finding from the Vietnam Head Injury Registry.

## Diagonal Injuries

Diagonal or crossover injuries from one hemisphere to another carry a poor prognosis in terms of residual cerebral function, with a devastating fixed neurologic deficit. The deficit is usually bilateral, and the patient is incapacitated, should he or she survive. The mortality rate has also been high, although a little better than with injuries of the deep gray matter. The overall mortality rate is approximately 25% to 30%. Diagonal injuries usually are associated with large hematomas at the exit site, and if the wounding agent is an expanding or fragmenting bullet, the damage from one hemisphere to the other by the fragmented metallic jacket is tremendous. Figures 8–11 and 8–12 illustrate this kind of injury with its usual sequelae.

## Transventricular Wounds

Whether they lodge in the ventricular system or traverse both walls of the ventricle, penetrating objects, such as

bullets and shrapnel, carry with them a mortality rate approximating 40%. This high mortality rate is due largely to deep gray matter injury and the effects of meningitis, ventriculitis, and brain abscess. There seems to be a high incidence of associated CSF leak in this type of wound, and there is a high risk of infection as well as a high rate of morbidity and mortality. Figure 8–13 illustrates a transventricular injury with the development of both an intracerebral and intraventricular hemorrhage.

## Tangential Injuries

Although tangential injuries look relatively benign, they are frequently associated with areas of local cerebral tissue damage that are larger than expected and produce devastating focal neurologic deficits. They occur with high-velocity bullets and shell fragments, and the cerebral cavitary necrosis, with or without extensive skull fracturing, is substantial and involves the white matter sometimes down to the ventricular surface. Vertex and convexity injuries produce a trough in the scalp and the calvarium with a torn dura. Bone fractures are the result of cavitary necrosis in the calvarium, and a large volume of bone fragments is driven through torn dura into the cortex and underlying white matter. In most instances, the volume of the in-driven bone is large and the adjacent cerebral injury is

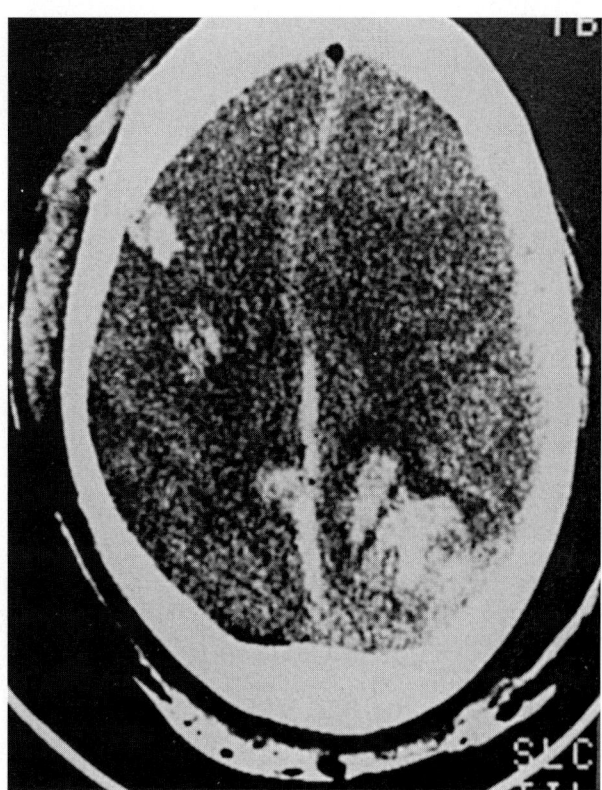

**FIGURE 8–11** ■ A computed tomography scan of a patient with a diagonal crossover of a bullet from the right hemisphere into the left. Note the larger hematoma toward the exit side.

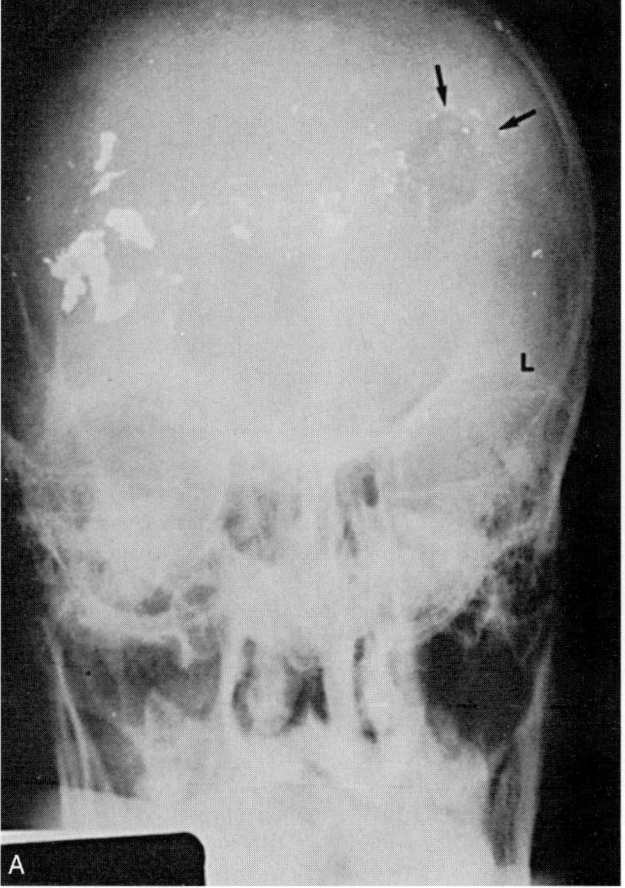

**FIGURE 8–12** ■ Anteroposterior (A) and lateral (B) views of the skull of a patient with a diagonal injury from the right hemisphere into the left. Note the larger bony wound at the exit site in the left parietal area (arrows). The track of the bullet is clearly outlined by the fragmentation of the soft jacket of the bullet.

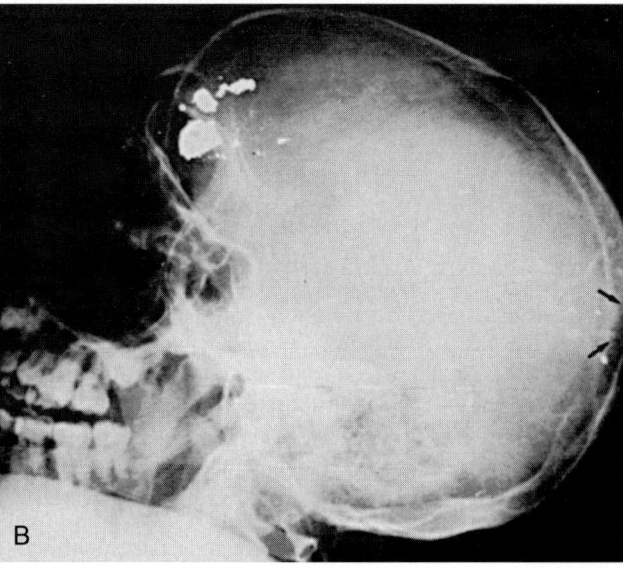

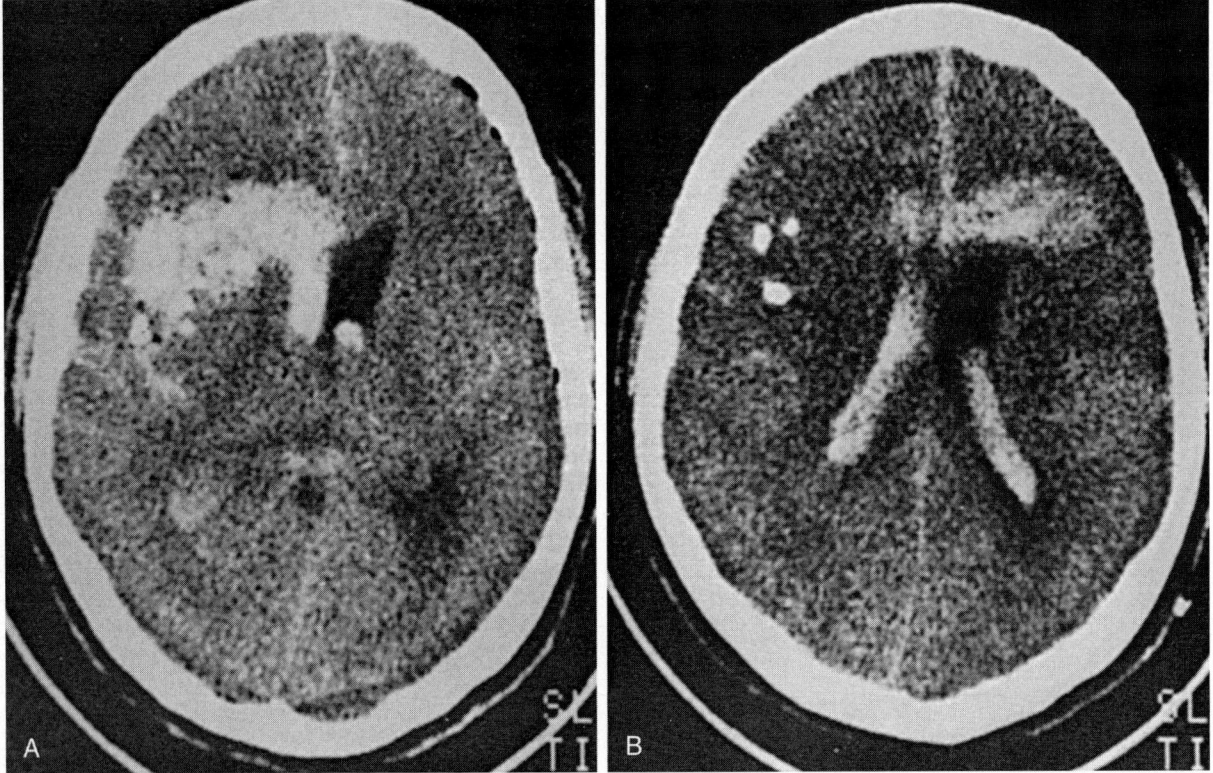

FIGURE 8–13 ■ Two computed tomography scans in sequence illustrating a gunshot wound with a transventricular track. Note the in-driven bone in the right frontotemporal area at the entry and the track going through both frontal horns with a large hematoma along the track and intraventricular hemorrhage.

tremendous, leading to a marked focal neurologic deficit. Although tangential injuries are often limited to one hemisphere, vertex tangential injuries as well as paramedian injuries can affect both hemispheres with a bilateral neurologic problem. This is not necessarily related to sagittal sinus injury, and in the presence of an intact sinus, bilateral cavitary necrosis and cerebral infarction have been observed in patients who had vertex injuries. CT imaging clarifies the neurologic problem in what seems to be a superficial and simple injury. We have seen such injuries associated with high-velocity missiles in which the cerebral injury is due to bone that has been driven bilaterally. However, there have been occasional instances in which large shell fragments weighing over 100 g have descended and struck the bone of the vertex without driving the bone in, and the patient still had a major bilateral lower extremity neurologic deficit, with CT imaging revealing extensive necrosis and infarction in the high convexity and both medial cortices. Figure 8–14 illustrates a tangential gunshot wound to the left frontoparietal area with minimal bony injury and extensive cerebral injury with hemorrhage. Figure 8–15 illustrates a high-convexity tangential wound with extensive fracturing, torn dura and sagittal sinus, and extensive underlying cerebral injury. Figure 8–16 illustrates the large amount of in-driven bone in such injuries. Although the mortality rate is low in such injuries, the neurologic deficit is profound and often permanent. Such injuries are extremely serious, and if CT imaging reveals a large volume of bone and cerebral injury, thorough primary débridement of the brain is mandatory.

## Cerebrospinal Fluid Leak Complicating Missile Injury to the Head

A CSF leak complicating missile injury is not an uncommon problem and frequently occurs in gunshot and missile wounds through the base of the skull, that is, in the anterior cranial fossa with involvement of the paranasal sinuses. In such cases, thorough débridement and closure of the craniofacial wound allows the use of fascia lata for watertight closure of the dura. This method is not difficult or fraught with a substantially increased risk of graft infection. Much greater difficulties, however, arise in wounds through the orbit that produce extensive damage to the globe and bony injury to the roof of the orbit or its posterior wall into the middle cranial fossa. CSF leaks are almost invariable after orbital exenteration or evisceration, especially if the orbital contents become infected. Hence, the use of fascia lata or a pericranial patch over the cranial defect in the floor of the anterior fossa is mandatory at the time of initial craniocerebral débridement, despite the high risk of infection of the graft from an extension of the orbital infection. CSF may not leak until after the globe has been exenterated. If the defect has not been patched at the initial operation and the globe is exenterated later, the patient certainly will require a secondary cranial operation for repair of the leak. In general, the surgeon is advised to try to patch the defect of the cranial floor at the time of the first operation, provided that the injured and massively swollen brain allows both good visualization and access. Although this may not be difficult in defects of the orbital

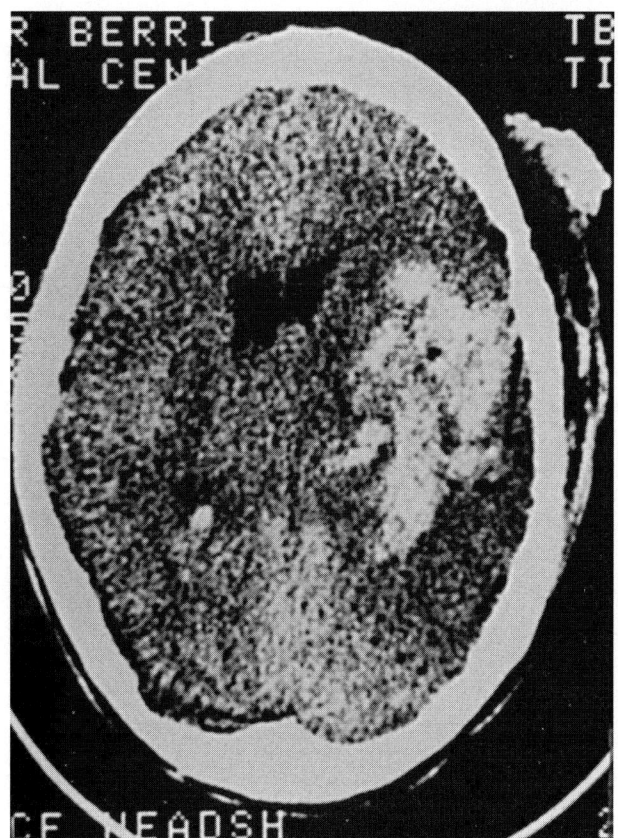

FIGURE 8–14 ■ A computed tomography scan of a tangential gunshot wound to the left temporoparietal area with minimal bone injury and extensive cerebral injury with intracerebral hemorrhage and mass effect at the midline.

risk of brain infection (cerebritis, abscess, ventriculitis, or meningoencephalitis) associated with such retained bone. Bone has a higher yield of positive cultures than metal fragments,[12] and this factor is the basis for the dictum to débride all bone driven into the brain. In principle, we concur with this dictum and strongly recommend the removal of all *accessible* bone at the primary débridement operation. The issue becomes more difficult when a substantial amount of bone is inaccessible or when a considerable volume of retained bone is discovered on a postoperative CT scan after a primary débridement operation has been performed. Meirowsky,[7] reporting on the Korean experience, stated that "whenever postoperative roentgenograms reveal a residual bone fragment, secondary craniotomy should be carried out for purpose of removal of that fragment even though the patient may be doing well clinically. We are convinced that rigid adherence to that policy has played a considerable part in the reduction of meningocerebral infections in Korean casualties from 41% initially to less than 1% ultimately." The idea that bone fragments were the main cause of deep infection came out of the study of Carey and associates in 1971,[12] reporting on the bacteriologic data of such wounds from the Vietnam conflict. They found that between 45% and 83% of retained bone at the time of primary or secondary exploration was

roof or the frontal bone with extension into the sinuses, it may prove unattainable in the middle fossa and particularly below the sphenoid wing in the posterior wall of the orbit. Leaks from these locations and into the orbit do not heal spontaneously. Caution must be taken to explore the fracture site well and to cover the fracture site with the graft beyond its limit.

CSF leaks through calvarial wounds over the convexity and the temporal region can occur in transventricular missile wounds or when meningitis or ventriculitis develops with breakdown of the wound secondary to infection. Closure of all the dural defects must be watertight to prevent the occurrence of CSF leaks. CSF leaks not only predispose the defect to reoperation and wound débridement, but they also are associated with a high incidence of infection. Our experience relates well to that of Meirowsky and colleagues,[11] who found that not only was the incidence of infection high (4.6% in patients without CSF leak versus 49.5% in patients with CSF leak), but the mortality rate was also greater from missile wounds of the brain in patients with CSF leak (22.8% in patients with CSF leak versus 5.1% when CSF leak did not occur).

## Retained Bone Fragments and Infection

The problem of retained intracranial in-driven bone remains of paramount importance in view of the increased

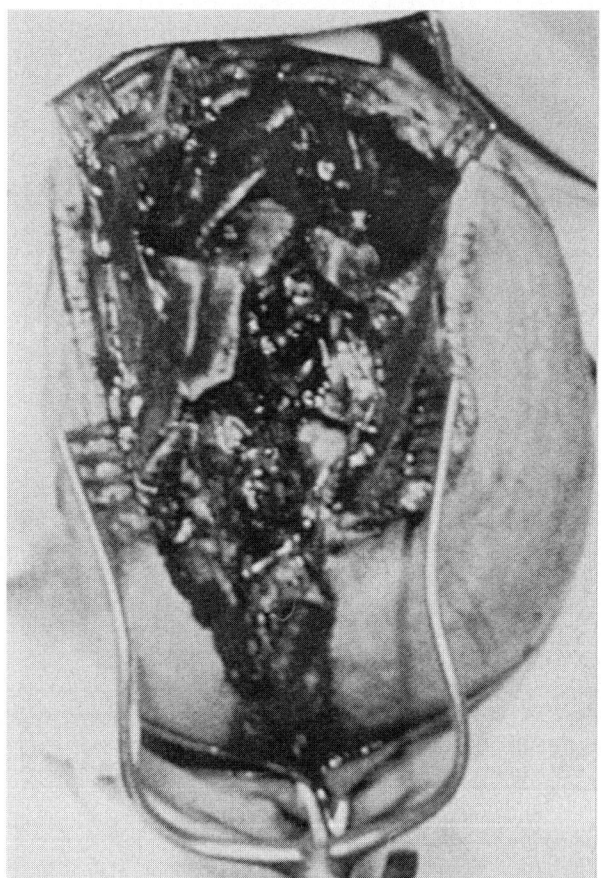

FIGURE 8–15 ■ The extent of a tangential gunshot wound to the left hemisphere convexity as seen at exploration. Note the extensive bone fracturing and the tearing of the dura to involve the sagittal sinus medially. Extensive cerebral injury is seen in the bottom of the wound into the depth of the white matter and hemorrhagic brain.

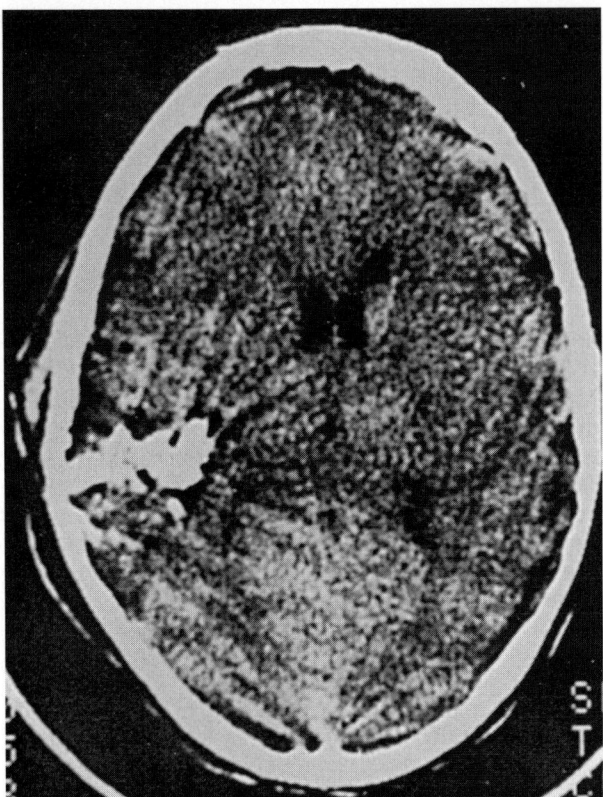

**FIGURE 8–16** ■ A computed tomography scan at the level of a tangential gunshot wound to the right temporoparietal area. Note the remarkable absence of significant cerebral injury and the large volume of in-driven bone in the hemisphere.

contaminated. This high incidence of bone contamination should have resulted in serious deep cerebral infection in a large number of patients. However, this was not the case as reported by Aarabi,[13] who followed up 102 patients from the Iraq-Iran war. On the other hand, many authors reported that an abscess developed around a cluster of bone fragments within 6 to 8 weeks from the occurrence of the injury. The extreme opinion was that bone fragments can stay in place with impunity.[37] In 1970, Pitlyk[38] reported on the experimental significance of retained intracranial bone fragments. His work indicated that bone fragments, regardless of their bacteriologic contamination, carried up to a 7% chance of abscess formation in the dog brain. However, this chance of abscess formation increased to 60% when retained bone was contaminated with animal fur and scalp.

In an attempt to resolve this issue and draw some conclusions from our experience at the American University of Beirut Medical Center, we analyzed the records of 403 patients seen between 1979 and 1986.[39] The analysis was directed toward the issue of retained bone as a possible cause of meningocerebral infection. All patients were followed up between 2 weeks and 84 months, with a mean of 30 months, and were divided into two main groups: those who had a primary cerebral débridement (349 patients), and those who had no cerebral débridement and had their external wound débrided and closed in the emergency unit (54 patients). Of the 349 débrided patients, 286 had no radiologically demonstrable retained bone after surgery, and 63 patients (18.1%) had postoperative retained bone by CT scan. Of the 54 patients whose wounds were closed in the emergency unit, 32 patients had no retained bone and 22 had retained bone on CT imaging. When all patient groups were analyzed for the actual risk and incidence of meningocerebral infection, we noted that

1. There was no relationship between the contaminating wound bacteria and the infective agent after débridement, as reported elsewhere.[13]
2. In the well-débrided group without retained bone, the incidence of infection was 3.1%, versus 28.6% in the group with retained bone. In the nondébrided group with retained bone, the incidence was 13.6%, and no infection occurred in patients when bone was not retained.
3. The volume of retained bone correlated well with the incidence of infection. The overall incidence of 50% with volumes of bone greater than 1 cm$^3$ dropped to 20% when the volume of bone was smaller than 1 cm$^3$.
4. When all patient groups were analyzed for infection in the presence of CSF leak from the wound, there was a marked increase in the incidence of infection when retained bone was associated with CSF leak as opposed to those with retained bone without CSF leak (Table 8–1).

Our analysis led us to conclude that minor cerebral injury, smaller volumes of retained bone, and the absence of CSF leak place a patient with retained bone at low risk for infection. A case can be made for this particular group of patients that observation, prophylactic antibiotic coverage, and external wound closure is a viable alternative to extensive débridement, although patients who have large volumes of retained bone and a CSF leak are at high risk

**TABLE 8–1** ■ **INCIDENCE OF MENINGOCEREBRAL INFECTION IN THE ABSENCE OR PRESENCE OF A CEREBROSPINAL FLUID LEAK: REVIEW OF 403 CASES**

| Patient Category | Total No. of Patients | Patients Without a CSF Leak | No. of Infections and Percentage | Patients with a CSF Leak | No. of Infections and Percentage |
|---|---|---|---|---|---|
| Débrided primarily (no retained bone) | 286 | 276 | 6/276 (2.1%) | 10 | 3/10 (30%) |
| Débrided primarily (postoperative retained bone) | 63 | 50 | 9/50 (18%) | 13 | 11/13 (84.6%) |
| Nondébrided (no retained bone) | 32 | 32 | 0/32 (0%) | 0 | 0 (0%) |
| Nondébrided (retained bone) | 22 | 19 | 0/19 (0%) | 3 | 3/3 (100%) |

CSF, cerebrospinal fluid.

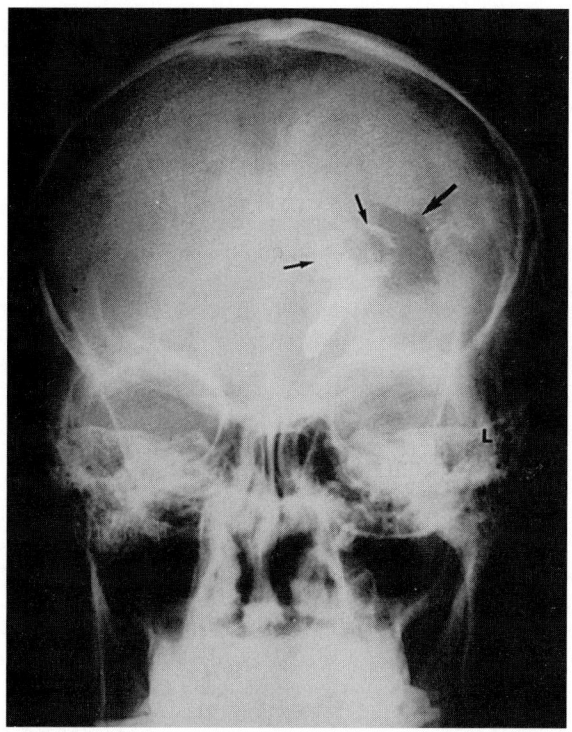

**FIGURE 8-17** ■ Posteroanterior view of plain skull radiograph to show the extent of the injury.

retrospective study by Aarabi and colleagues[40] is in agreement with Meirowsky and coworkers'[11] and our experience at the American University of Beirut Medical Center.[39] Although every attempt should be made to remove all bone at the primary débridement operation, in some instances in which bone is retained deep in the cerebral wound, making its removal particularly hazardous, it is advisable to leave it behind, provided watertight closure of the dura and external wound is performed to prevent CSF leak. This method is very important in patients with large volumes of bone close to the ventricular system. Figures 8–17 and 8–18 are of a young man who was shot through his left occiput with large volume of in-driven bone and metallic shrapnel. He had a profound left parieto-occipital neurologic deficit. He was débrided gently—postoperative plain radiographs and CT revealed a fairly sizable retained piece of bone. Because of previous adequate cerebral débridement (seen on a CT scan) and his profound neurologic deficit, we elected to observe him. Since 1981, he has been regularly checked neurologically and by CT and has had no evidence of infection. When mass casualties occur, however, the surgeon may resort to minor external débridement and heavy antibiotic coverage in a group of patients who may or may not have retained bone intracranially and who have a small area of cerebral injury, provided that wound closure obviates CSF leakage. This approach has been summarized by a protocol drawn from our experience.[15]

## Traumatic Intracranial Aneurysms with Penetrating Head Injuries[41]

A systematic study by Aarabi[32] has put the incidence of traumatic aneurysms after penetrating wounds at 4%; patients with intracerebral hematoma are a high-risk group who require cerebral angiography after surgery. The incidental discovery of these aneurysms and their exclusion

for infection. We have proposed a protocol for patients who do not need intracranial débridement at the time of injury.[15] These 32 patients (20 with retained bone and 12 without) had no CSF leakage from their wounds. The incidence of infection (1/32) is significantly less than in those complicated by CSF leakage[11] (see Table 8–1). CSF leak seems to be the single most important factor in the increased risk for infection, and not the volume of bone as an isolated variable without CSF leak. A more recent,

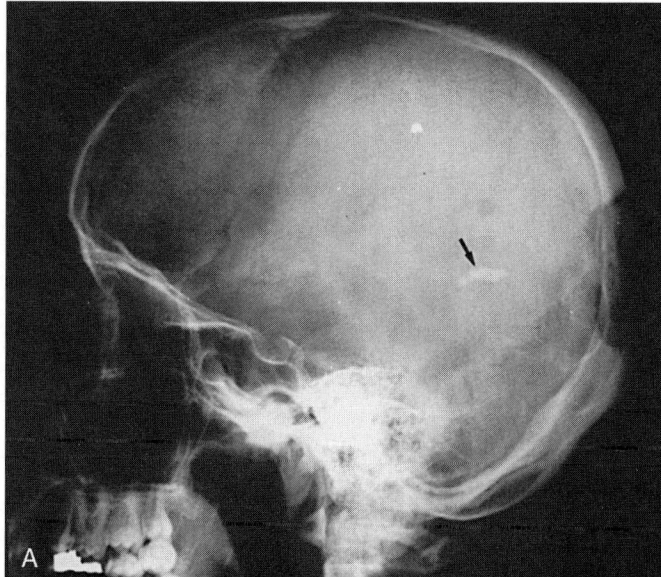
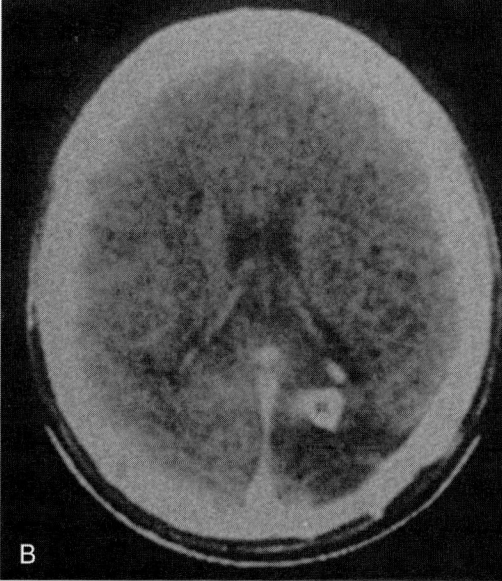

**FIGURE 8-18** ■ *A,* Lateral plain skull radiograph to show retained bone in-driven deep into the parietal lobe. *B,* A computed tomography scan is done postoperatively to show the exact location of the bone in a well-débrided parietal lobe.

from the circulation by surgery decreases the mortality rate from their subsequent rupture. Experience at the American University of Beirut Medical Center has been reported by Haddad and colleagues,[33] who discovered 19 traumatic aneurysms in 15 patients. An accompanying hematoma was frequently found, which indicates that angiography should be used when intracerebral and subdural hematomas complicate missile brain injury.

## POSTOPERATIVE CARE

Postoperative care of patients with penetrating head injuries is the same as that of patients with other forms of severe head injury. They require general supportive care in an intensive care unit and specific therapy for their increased intracranial pressure. Cerebral edema resulting from injury and surgery is combated with large doses of corticosteroids for 5 to 7 days. Repeated small boluses of osmotic diuretics or a continuous intravenous infusion of 20% mannitol solution for 3 to 5 days may be necessary to keep brain bulk down. Adequate monitoring of serum osmolarity is essential. It may be necessary to resort to ventilatory care and hyperventilation. Anticonvulsant therapy is started and maintained for a long period in view of the high risk of post-traumatic epilepsy associated with penetrating brain wounds. If the patient has a postoperative CSF leak, it should be repaired as soon as the patient's condition permits to prevent the development of infection. Leaks that are repaired within a week of onset are associated with a low incidence of infection. The high yield of positive cultures from these wounds, with both gram-positive cocci and gram-negative bacilli, requires prophylactic and therapeutic antibiotics. The prophylactic use of antibiotics is not meant to replace thorough wound débridement in these cases, because it has been shown that well-débrided wounds have a low incidence of infection. The clinician may face the problem of resistant *Staphylococcus* infections, as well as resistant gram-negative infections. In heavily contaminated wounds, third-generation cephalosporins may be used either prophylactically, before the onset of infection, or therapeutically, after infection is present. Postoperative CT imaging is performed, when the patient's condition permits, to determine whether foreign matter has been retained and the extent of local and distant cerebral injury. CT imaging also shows delayed postoperative hematoma, infection, post-traumatic hydrocephalus, and cerebral infarction. We have not encountered increased bone flap infection, although most débrided patients had their bone flaps replaced at the initial operation. Brain fungal infection remains a difficult problem, but its incidence has been greatly reduced with prompt initial definitive débridement and the use of meticulous technique and antibiotic coverage. We have occasionally dealt with brain fungal infection in patients whose transfer to our facility was delayed for 3 to 5 days after wounding when primary treatment was inadequate.

## SUMMARY

Gunshot and missile wounds of the head can present with different clinical pictures, which are based mainly on the different types of damage inflicted on the brain and the area involved. The clinical presentation depends on the size, shape, stability, and velocity of the missile. Low-velocity missiles may present a relatively benign clinical picture; high-velocity missiles produce large areas of cavitary necrosis with extensive skull fracturing, and such injuries are often incompatible with survival. A thorough knowledge of the pathologic process of missile wounds and wound ballistics is essential in the execution of an early definitive cranial operation, which consists of thoroughly débriding the cavitary track of all necrotic tissue, foreign bodies, and bone and metal fragments. This approach lessens the chance of deep cerebral wound infection with cerebritis or abscess. Watertight closure of the dura is mandatory and is easier with a graft. The scalp wound should be débrided, and the edges should be excised and closed without tension using relaxing sutures or rotating flaps. Unusual circumstances may present, and these problems should be dealt with as they arise by modification of the recommended technique. Every effort should be made to prevent CSF leak or infection secondary to leakage or retained bone. In the well-executed primary débridement operation and proper wound closure, a large number of patients have their lives saved and more of their neurologic function preserved.

## REFERENCES

1. Gurdjian ES: The treatment of penetrating wounds of the brain sustained in warfare: A historical review. J Neurosurg 40:157–167, 1974.
2. Ascroft PB: Treatment of head wounds due to missiles: Analysis of 500 cases. Lancet 2:211–218, 1943.
3. Cushing H: A study of various wounds involving the brain and its enveloping structure. Br J Surg 5:558–684, 1918.
4. Haynes WG: Penetrating brain wounds: Analysis of 342 cases. J Neurosurg 2:365–378, 1945.
5. Jefferson G: The physiological pathology of gunshot wounds of the head. Br J Surg 7:262–289, 1919.
6. Matson DD: The management of acute craniocerebral injuries due to missiles. In Surgery in World War II. Neurosurgery, Vol I. Washington, DC: Office of the Surgeon General, 1958.
7. Meirowsky AM: Penetrating wounds of the brain. In Meirowsky AM (ed): Neurological Surgery of Trauma. Washington, DC: U.S. Government Printing Office, 1965.
8. Hammon WM: Analysis of 2178 consecutive penetrating wounds of the brain from Vietnam. J Neurosurg 32:127, 1971.
9. Hammon WM: Retained intracranial bone fragments: Analysis of 42 patients. J Neurosurg 32:142, 1971.
10. Hagan RE: Early complications following penetrating wounds of the brain. J Neurosurg 34:132, 1971.
11. Meirowsky AM, Caveness WF, Dillon JD, et al: Cerebrospinal fluid fistulas complicating missile wounds of the brain. J Neurosurg 54:44–48, 1981.
12. Carey ME, Young H, Mathis JL, et al: A bacteriological study of craniocerebral missile wounds from Vietnam. J Neurosurg 34:145, 1971.
13. Aarabi B: Comparative study of bacteriological contamination between primary and secondary exploration of missile head wounds. Neurosurgery 20:610, 1987.
14. Saba MI: Surgical management of gunshot wounds of the head. In Schmidek HH, Sweet WH (eds): Operative Neurosurgical Techniques: Indications, Methods, and Results, 2nd ed. Philadelphia: WB Saunders, 1988.
15. Taha JM, Saba MI, Brown JA: Missile injuries to the brain treated by simple wound closure: Results of a protocol during the Lebanese conflict. Neurosurgery 29:380–384, 1991.
16. Brandvold B, Levi L, Feinsod M, et al: Penetrating craniocerebral injuries in the Israeli involvement in the Lebanese conflict, 1982–1985. J Neurosurg 72:15–21, 1990.

17. Smith WHB, Smith JE: The Book of Rifles, 4th ed. Harrisburg, PA: Stackpole, 1972, pp 400, 434.
18. Weiner SL, Barrett J: Trauma Management. Philadelphia: WB Saunders, 1986, pp 1–12.
19. Bowen TE, Bellamy RF: Emergency War Surgery: Second United States Revision of the Emergency War Surgery NATO Handbook. Washington, DC: United States Department of Defense.
20. McSwain NE, Kerstein MD (eds): Evaluation and Management of Trauma. Norwalk, CT: Appleton-Century-Crofts, 1987, pp 25–41.
21. Engel J, Kessler I (eds): The War Injuries of the Upper Extremity (Review). Prog Surg 16:53–67, 1979.
22. Fackler ML: Ballistic injury. Ann Emerg Med 15:1451–1455, 1986.
23. Fackler ML, Bellamy RF, Malinowski JA, et al: Wounding mechanism of projectiles striking at more than 1.5 km/sec. J Trauma 26:250–254, 1986.
24. Fackler ML, Bellamy RF, Malinowski JA, et al: A reconsideration of the wounding mechanisms of very high projectiles: Importance of projectile shape. J Trauma 28:563–567, 1988.
25. Fackler ML, Bellamy RF, Malinowski JA, et al: The wound profile: Illustration of the missile-tissue interaction. J Trauma 28(Suppl 1):S21–S29, 1988.
26. Fackler ML: Wounding patterns of military rifle bullets. International Defense Review l:9–64, 1989.
27. Adams DB, Fackler ML: Grenade fragmentation injuries. J Trauma (China) 6(Suppl):48–52, 1990.
28. Sights WO Jr: Ballistic analysis of shotgun injuries to the central nervous system. J Neurosurg 31:25, 1969.
29. Fackler ML: Wound ballistics: A review of common misconceptions. JAMA 259:2730–2736, 1988.
30. Owen-Smith: Surgical Pathology of Missile Injuries. Graves Medical Audiovisual Library 77.38. Chelmsford, United Kingdom: Medical Recording Service Foundation, 1980.
31. Carey ME, Tutton RH, Strub RL, et al: The correlation between surgical and CT estimates of brain damage following missile wounds. J Neurosurg 60:947–954, 1984.
32. Aarabi B: Traumatic aneurysms of brain due to high velocity missile head injuries. Neurosurgery 22:1056–1062, 1988.
33. Haddad FS, Haddad GF, Taha J: Traumatic intracranial aneurysms caused by missiles: Their presentation and management. Neurosurgery 28:1–7, 1991.
34. Hanieh A: Brain injury from a spent bullet descending vertically. J Neurosurg 34:222, 1971.
35. Gerber A, Moody R: Craniocerebral missile injuries in the monkey: An experimental physiological model. J Neurosurg 36:43, 1972.
36. Rish BL, Dillon JD, Weiss GH: Mortality following penetrating craniocerebral injuries: An analysis of the deaths in the Vietnam Head Injury Registry population. J Neurosurg 59:775–780, 1983.
37. Haddad FS: Nature and management of penetrating head injuries during the civil war in Lebanon. Can J Surg 21:233–240, 1978.
38. Pitlyk PJ: The experimental significance of retained intracranial bone fragment. J Neurosurg 33:19–24, 1970.
39. Saba MI: Retained intracranial bone following gunshot and missile injuries of the head: Correlation of risk of infection with the volume of bone. Presented at the 19th Congress of the Middle East Neurosurgical Society, Beirut, Lebanon, May 1992.
40. Aarabi B, Taghipour M, Alibaii E, et al: Central nervous system infections after military missile head wounds. Neurosurgery 42:500–509, 1998.
41. Achram M, Rizk G, Haddad FS, et al: Angiographic aspects of traumatic intracranial aneurysms following war injuries. Br J Radiol 53:1144–1149, 1980.

# Craniofacial Lesions

# Surgical Management of Craniosynostosis and Craniofacial Deformities

■ CONCEZIO DI ROCCO

C raniosynostosis is the premature fusion of one or more cranial sutures with secondary changes in the shape or volume of the skull, or both. The term *fusion* means the partial or total ossification of the strips of connective tissue interposed between the adjacent vault bones that permit bone movements and prevent separation. The abnormal fusion of the cranial sutures interferes with their main function of allowing the molding of the skull during its passage through the birth channel and, subsequently, its enlargement to accommodate the physiologic growth of the neural mass.[1, 2]

The ossification of the cranial sutures is a normal event at a certain age, and the pathologic process of craniosynostosis is related to the prematurity of the phenomenon and to its effects on the development of the skull and brain. The goal of surgery is to re-establish an intracranial volume adequate for physiologic cerebral expansion, which takes place in early postnatal life, and to correct as much as possible the cosmetic defect resulting from the diminished or unbalanced growth of the skull. In most cases, premature fusion of the cranial sutures in craniosynostosis leads to a narrowing of the sutural space between the adjacent margins of the calvarial bones rather than to its actual closure. In general, only the area near the center of the fused segment exhibits complete obliteration because of lamellar bony deposition, whereas the adjacent areas may show only partial bony union or minimal histologic changes. However, because the fused suture cannot stretch, there is diminished addition of new bone at the sutural edges. This results in insufficient growth of the cranial bones that, combined with their reduced capacity to separate, produces insufficient enlargement of the skull volume in response to brain expansion.

Overwhelming evidence indicates that calvarial and skull base growth influence each other reciprocally, although they depend on different mechanisms. Under normal conditions, calvarial growth is directly determined by the "growth effect" of the neural mass, the expansion of which molds the inner (meningeal) and outer (cutaneous) periosteal layers, within which each flat bone of the vault is suspended.

As these bones are drawn apart, new bony tissue forms at their perimeter (sutural interface), the amount of which corresponds to the amount of the displacement. Conversely, skull base growth is relatively independent from that of the brain, as demonstrated by the normal development of the sphenoid, clivus, and occipital bones in anencephalic subjects. However, because it is a borderline structure, the cranial base adapts its growth to that of the calvaria and the facial complex.

In the mid-1970s, Moss[3, 4] and other researchers investigated the role of the cranial base in craniosynostosis. They suggested that a primary malformation of this structure, probably occurring during embryonic life and depending on alterations of the bilateral prosencephalic organization center in the forehead, could impede normal chondrocranial growth and result in early synostosis of the frontosphenoidal and frontoethmoidal sutures. The authors elaborated a morphogenetic theory to explain the growth of the cranial base and that of the calvaria. According to this theory, the expansion of the neurocranial capsule, formed by the neural mass, the dura, and its external coverings, acts as a "functional matrix" for the development of the supporting "skeleton unit." The growth of the last structure would then be a rather passive phenomenon, which carries adjacent bones away from each other and determines the secondary and compensatory deposition of new bone at the sutural borders to accommodate the centrifugal expansion of intracranial content.[5] The growth of the neurocapsule is directed by bundles of the dura mater that are connected to the skull base at five main points (the crista galli, the two lesser sphenoidal wings, and the two petrous crests) and then run upward, following the major calvarial sutures.[6] Without these dural fiber tracts, which guide the vectors of the growing neural mass in specific directions, the neurocranium would assume a hemispheric shape.

If Moss' theory were tenable, in primary craniosynostosis, premature fusion of the cranial sutures would represent a secondary manifestation of a developmental alteration of the skull base, where the dura fiber bundles are attached. Supporting this hypothesis are: (1) observations made in experimental animals; (2) the occurrence of

119

craniosynostosis and anomalies of the skull base in complex malformations, such as faciocraniostenosis, and in the so-called simple, or primary, craniosynostosis, in which only the neurocranium should be involved; (3) the obliteration of the cranial sutures when tensile forces transmitted by the dura mater are attenuated (secondary craniosynostosis in shunted hydrocephalic subjects); and (4) the possibility that the various forms of craniosynostosis can be explained in terms of altered genetic information encoded in the cells of the functional matrix rather than by a direct genetic determination.[5, 7]

Moss' hypothesis has the advantage of conceptually unifying the various forms of craniosynostosis. In fact, the theory also can be applied to cases in which the pathologic activity of the suture seems to be the main factor responsible for its early fusion. In such cases, congenital or acquired causes (dysmetabolic, hormonal, teratogenic, or genetic), acting on the functional matrix as a whole or directly on the neurocranial capsule, result in early fusion of the cranial sutures. The alterations of the chondrocranium are the consequence rather than the cause of the synostotic process.

Although craniosynostosis appears to be pathogenetically heterogeneous, and although the only common factor seems to be failure of bony growth, depending on the suture stretch, enough evidence exists to support the role of primitive changes in the osteoconnective structure that envelops the brain. First, investigators have reported on newborns with craniosynostosis provoked by abnormal intrauterine pressure,[8–10] as well as early fusion of the cranial sutures in animals that was caused by cranial constraints that directed the cerebral and cranial growth along abnormal vectors.[11, 12] In addition, numerous clinical forms exist in which craniosynostosis depends on metabolic disorders (calcium metabolism alterations, hyperthyroidism, mucopolysaccharidosis, and mucolipidosis) or on the abnormal position or insertion of the dura mater (linear sebaceous nevus syndrome), or is part of teratogenically induced syndromes characterized by abnormal growth of the neural mass (aminopterin syndrome or fetal hydantoin syndrome).[13, 14] The genetic etiology of many forms of craniosynostosis is indicated by numerous examples of well-determined chromosomal or monogenic syndromes characterized by the early fusion of one or more cranial sutures.[13, 14] In simple, or primary, craniosynostosis, genetic causality is again supported by the geographic and racial variations in its incidence and by the general male and particular female prevalence of bicoronal craniosynostosis. Other support is offered by examples of familial disposition and the occurrence of the same type of craniosynostosis in twins.[15–30] The modes of transmission have not been completely determined, but they are probably different for the different types of craniosynostosis.

The precocious fusion of one or more cranial sutures is followed by a cranial deformity due to the growth of the neural mass along abnormal vectors. An obvious relationship exists between the type of suture involved in the synostotic process, the precocity and extent of the process, and the resulting modification in shape of the skull—the cranial growth perpendicular to the fused suture is inhibited, while compensatory growth occurs parallel to the suture itself. Four of the five major sutures in the calvaria,

two single (sagittal, metopic) and three paired (coronal, lambdoid, and squamosal), have major roles in craniosynostosis. The early fusion of these sutures results in a specific anomaly of calvarial shape. The anterior sutures (sphenofrontal, frontoethmoidal, and frontonasal) are the most commonly involved sutures of the cranial base.

Besides the cosmetic defect, various clinical manifestations, such as mental retardation, focal neurologic deficits, epilepsy, increased intracranial pressure, and hydrocephalus, have been described in older children with craniosynostosis. These manifestations could result from the distorted brain growth that occurs secondary to the cranial deformity and, possibly, from a chronic state of increased intracranial pressure, thus suggesting the need for early surgical treatment.

Psychomotor retardation is relatively common in craniosynostosis and has three main causes, acting alone or in combination: impaired growth of the brain and increased intracranial pressure, both of which depend on the abnormally shaped skull, and primary brain malformation. The incidence of mental retardation is, however, very low in patients with isolated single-suture fusion and no other congenital anomalies. Indeed, mental retardation is practically absent in cases of metopic synostosis, provided that underlying brain malformations, such as arhinencephaly, are excluded, in cases of anterior or posterior plagiocephaly, and in cases of sagittal synostosis. In fact, in the last condition, subjects with superior ability have been described.[21, 25, 30–32]

Conversely, bilateral involvement of both coronal sutures and craniosynostosis with early fusion of more than one cranial suture are frequently accompanied by mental retardation, occurring in up to 33% to 50% in cases of oxycephaly and 70% to 80% in cases of Apert's syndrome.[16, 26, 27, 33] Mental retardation is commonly associated with cloverleaf skull anomaly, which is also characterized by multiple fusion of the cranial sutures.[34] However, results obtained in patients with Apert's syndrome indicate that a high percentage of them may reach normal or borderline intelligence when treated at an early age.[30, 35, 36] Psychomotor retardation has been reported in approximately 10% to 20% of patients with Crouzon's syndrome. However, in both Apert's and Crouzon's syndromes, as well as in the cloverleaf skull malformation, the frequently associated hydrocephalus, when unrecognized and untreated, may contribute significantly to the delay in psychomotor development.[16, 27, 37, 38]

With regard to focal neurologic deficits, most of the early reports on craniosynostosis are on optic nerve damage, and investigators stress the risk of blindness in untreated cases or cases treated too late. The same factors influence focal neurologic deficits that influence mental retardation; decreased visual acuity is practically absent in patients with fusion of a single cranial suture, whereas it occurs in approximately one third of older children and young adults with oxycephaly, bilateral coronal synostosis, and Crouzon's syndrome who did not receive appropriate treatment.[16, 27, 39–42] Again, associated hydrocephalus and chronically increased intracranial pressure may contribute substantially to the genesis of focal neurologic deficits. Nevertheless, some authors have identified as possible causes direct compression of the optic fibers in a narrowed optic canal, compression of the vascular supply to the optic nerve, or stretching or kinking of the third nerve or its mechanical compression by the carotid artery, secondary to the deformation of the skull base.[16, 43–51]

Alteration of the anterior skull base has a direct role in determining ophthalmologic manifestations of craniosynostosis, such as proptosis, enophthalmos, hypertelorism, hypotelorism, and strabismus. Therefore, anomalies in the position of the ocular globe and disturbances in ocular mobility are also surgical indications. Exophthalmos is common because of characteristic anatomic changes induced by premature synostosis of the cranial and midface sutures, which modify the shape and reduce the volume of the orbit. Exorbitism is related to the degree of forward displacement of the greater wing of the sphenoid bone, shortening of the anterior cranial base, hypoplasia of the maxillary bone, and changes of the planum sphenoidale. Proptosis is almost constant and is usually severe in patients with Crouzon's syndrome, and it is very common in Apert's syndrome; in these conditions, intracranial hypertension may also be a cause, possibly because of the associated increase in orbital vein pressure, which leads to orbital congestion.[4, 14] The incidence of exophthalmos progressively diminishes in patients with multiple cranial suture and bicoronal synostosis and becomes rare in patients with early fusion of the metopic and sagittal sutures.

Hypertelorism may be associated with exophthalmos, especially in patients with Crouzon's and Apert's syndromes; hypotelorism is uncommon in patients with craniosynostosis except in those with early fusion of the metopic suture, in whom it is a typical finding. Strabismus is relatively common although differently estimated in various series; it is typically convergent in patients with metopic synostosis and unilateral in those with anterior plagiocephaly, because of the vertical canthal displacement. Besides the optic and the oculomotor nerves, damage to the first, fifth, sixth, seventh, and eighth cranial nerves has been described in craniosynostosis. Anosmia has been related to anomalies of the cribriform plate resulting from the synostotic process or to chronically increased intracranial pressure.[16] Primary anomalies of the temporal bone and stretching or compression of the eighth nerve in the auditory canal have been implicated as causes of hearing loss, which occurs in approximately 10% of patients with craniosynostosis.[16, 27, 32, 52]

Epilepsy has also been associated with craniosynostosis. Its incidence was high in papers published in the mid-20th century, when approximately one fourth of patients appeared to be affected by a seizure disorder[16]—hence the justification for the definition of *turricephalic epilepsy*. However, epilepsy is rarely described in most recent series of patients with craniosynostosis, in which its incidence ranges between 0% and 8%. This difference is probably related to the younger age of patients at treatment and the more accurate diagnosis of their condition.[27, 28, 30, 37]

Increased intracranial pressure, which results from restriction in skull growth related to the precocious closure of the cranial sutures, is considered the most important indicator for surgical treatment in craniosynostosis.[53] Indeed, in early descriptions of craniosynostosis, optical atrophy and blindness, presumably resulting from chronic intracranial hypertension, were regarded as typical events of the condition's natural history.[16] The postulate that intracranial volume is decreased in craniosynostosis and, consequently, that intracranial pressure is increased has been widely accepted in medical literature in spite of the surprisingly scarce direct demonstration of this phenomenon. In fact, clinical signs and symptoms of increased intracranial pressure are uncommon in cases of craniosynostosis, except in those associated with hydrocephalus. Only in some patients, especially those with multiple premature fusion of the cranial sutures or those with craniofacial stenosis, does the skull volume appear to be clearly reduced at physical inspection. Actually, in many craniosynostotic patients, intracranial volume is normal or only minimally decreased when evaluated by indirect intracranial volume measurements using computed tomographic (CT) scanning.[54] In these cases, normal intracranial volume may be maintained in spite of the cranial deformity because of the local compensatory cranial growth in areas where function of the sutures is still preserved or because of the absorption of bone from the inner surface of the skull.

Direct recording of intracranial pressure very rarely demonstrates chronically elevated intracranial pressure values; in some patients, abnormally increased intracranial pressures do not necessarily correlate with reduced intracranial volumes and, conversely, patients with decreased cranial volume may not show evidence of chronic intracranial hypertension.[55] Consequently, critical attention should be paid when evaluating reports of craniosynostosis series in which 5% to 31% of patients have intracranial hypertension, although clinical evidence consists only of occasional headache.[27, 37] In most cases, laboratory findings thought to suggest chronically increased intracranial pressure are limited to the radiologic demonstration of a "copper-beaten" or "fingerprinting" pattern of the skull, a finding that is inconstant, occurs relatively late, and is mainly related to specific forms of craniosynostosis. Nevertheless, even though mean intracranial pressure remains within normal limits, the cumulative experience shows a significant percentage of children with intermittently elevated intracranial pressure. In fact, prolonged pressure recordings may demonstrate abnormal cerebrospinal fluid (CSF) dynamics in approximately one third of children with craniosynostosis by showing transitory abnormal increases during the rapid eye movement phases of sleep.[56] Further evidence of reduced intracranial compliance, especially in patients with multiple-suture involvement, is provided by the results of examinations (e.g., spinal subarachnoid infusion test) that indicate a reduced ability to accommodate for rapidly induced increases in intracranial volume, even in patients with apparently normal baseline intracranial pressure.[57–59]

Investigators have noted focal dilatations of the subarachnoid spaces that seem to occur with a pattern specific to the various types of craniosynostosis corresponding to areas of compensatory focal cranial enlargement.[60] These focal dilatations may play a role in the determination of compensatory deformities of the skull through a hydrodynamic mechanism that can be identified in the augmented transmission of CSF pulsations traveling through these dilated subarachnoid spaces.[60] Such a pathogenetic mechanism does not, however, always imply a chronically increased mean intracranial pressure.

The association of hydrocephalus and craniosynostosis

is relatively common in patients with multiple-suture involvement, those with craniofaciostenosis (i.e., Apert's and Crouzon's syndromes), or those with the so-called cloverleaf anomaly.[61–63] There is no single explanation for the ventricular dilatation in craniosynostosis because both communicating and noncommunicating types of hydrocephalus have been described.[64] The more widely accepted pathogenetic interpretations are an impairment in CSF flow (compression of the subarachnoid spaces and cisterns, compression of the infratentorial structures, or aqueductal stenosis) or an obstruction of the venous drainage of the brain (narrowing of the venous sinuses, narrowing of the jugular foramens), both of which depend on deformation of the vault or involvement of the cranial base in the stenotic process.[64] In the past, hydrocephalus sometimes remained long undetected and contributed to mental retardation because of the limited ability of the skull to expand in patients with craniosynostosis. Today, ventricular dilatation is usually recognized by CT examination simultaneously with the diagnosis of craniosynostosis; therefore, the hydrocephalus can be treated in the first months of life, with a clear advantage for psychomotor development. However, such surgical management requires procedures designed to prevent the risk that excessive reduction in pressure and volume of the CSF will limit the expansion of the skull, which is expected to follow the opening of the precociously fused cranial sutures. Furthermore, the cephalic end of the CSF shunting device should be placed in a region of the calvaria that does not interfere with the operation for the correction of the craniosynostosis.

## PREOPERATIVE EVALUATION AND CLASSIFICATION

The diagnosis of craniosynostosis is based on morphologic features. However, clinical, genetic, and radiologic evaluation is required in nearly all cases to differentiate the various clinical forms and syndromes. A good basic classification of craniosynostosis is proposed in Table 9–1.[13] More detailed classifications are available in the literature, but these may be redundant for surgical purposes.[14]

The primary, idiopathic, or true craniosynostosis group I includes all forms that can be treated satisfactorily in the first year of life by the neurosurgeon. The choice of surgical procedure—cranial or orbitocranial, when the deformity affects the orbits and the nasoethmoidal complex—is determined by the specific suture or sutures that have undergone precocious fusion. Groups II and III consist mostly of all forms of craniosynostosis that, in addition to surgical treatment required in early life for fostering brain development, require further operations later to treat the associated malformation of the face (e.g., in Crouzon's and Apert's syndromes). These patients need more extensive and reconstructive operations that demand a team approach with various specialists. In some syndromes, however, the associated malformations can be so severe and the psychomotor retardation so significant that any surgical treatment is precluded. The surgical indication is also disputable in many cases of group IV craniosynostosis, which includes

### TABLE 9–1 ■ CLASSIFICATION OF CRANIOSYNOSTOSIS

I. Idiopathic craniosynostosis
   A. Scaphocephaly or dolichocephaly (boat head)—premature fusion of the sagittal suture
   B. Brachycephaly, acrobrachycephaly, or turricephaly (short head)—premature fusion of both coronal sutures
   C. Plagiocephaly (oblique head)—unilateral premature fusion of one coronal or lambdoid suture
   D. Trigonocephaly (triangular head)—premature fusion of the metopic suture
   E. Pachycephalus (flat head)—premature fusion of both lambdoid sutures
   F. Oxycephaly (pointed head)—premature fusion of all cranial sutures
II. Craniosynostosis as part of other known malformative syndromes
   A. Chromosomal syndromes
   B. Monogenic syndromes
   C. Teratogenically induced syndromes
   D. Syndromes of unknown genesis
III. Craniosynostosis in association with other conditions
   A. Hematologic disorders
   B. Metabolic disorders
   C. Iatrogenic disorders
IV. Craniosynostosis induced by mechanical compression

forms resulting from fetal constraint, posture, and intentional deformations.

## SURGICAL CLASSIFICATION

Goals for the surgical treatment of craniosynostosis are to reduce the potential for further cranial or craniofacial deformity, to ensure the growth of the skull and the underlying cerebrovascular structures along normal vectors, and to correct the cosmetic defect. In many cases, the immediate re-expansion of the skull and the relief of compression on the underlying subarachnoid spaces and nervous tissue caused by the surgical correction account for the normalization of eventually impaired CSF dynamics.

Operations performed early in life carry the best surgical prognosis, and younger children tolerate even extensive surgical procedures surprisingly well, once adequate anesthesiologic and postoperative care is provided (Table 9–2). In younger children, surgical correction of simple craniosynostosis can be performed with relatively unsophisticated anesthesia and basic surgical instrumentation. The limited cranial bone resistance in this age group, the typically limited involvement of the cranial sutures, and the greater potential for cranial reshaping, depending on the rapid cerebral growth, all contribute to a better postoperative outcome. However, more refined surgical instrumentation and techniques are required when the craniosynostosis is treated in older children or adolescents who need radical bone reconstruction and simultaneous correction of the soft tissue defects.

The main purpose of surgical treatment varies according to the patient's age at operation, the type and the number of the sutures involved, and whether the operation is prophylactic, functional, or cosmetic. However, a clear-cut distinction between craniosynostoses that require treatment

## TABLE 9–2 ■ ANESTHESIOLOGY IN CRANIOSYNOSTOSIS

| | | |
|---|---|---|
| Clinical evaluation | Craniofacial deformities<br>Intracranial hypertension<br>Focal neurologic deficits<br>Mental retardation<br>Epilepsy | |
| Anesthesiologic management | Induction:<br>Myoresolution:<br><br><br>Maintenance:<br>Intravenous access: | Halothane in facial mask<br>Vecuronium bromide (0.1 mg/kg) or suxamethonium<br>    (1 mg/kg)<br>Isoflurane or halothane<br>1. 22-gauge cannula (first choice, vena saphena) for<br>    hemotransfusion<br>2. 22–24-gauge cannula for balanced glucose<br>    solution infusion |
| Intraoperative monitoring | Cardiocirculatory:<br><br><br>Respiratory:<br><br><br><br><br>Temperature: | Heart rate<br>Electrocardiogram<br>Noninvasive blood pressure measurement<br>Tidal volume<br>Bronchomanometry<br>$Sao_2$<br>$Fio_2$<br>End-tidal $CO_2$ and anesthetic agents<br>Central (rectal) and peripheral temperatures<br>    (Thermadrape, humidified and warmed gases,<br>    warmed hematic and saline infusions) |
| Postoperative monitoring (6, 12,<br>    24, and 48 hours after the<br>    operation) | Blood pressure<br>Heart rate<br>Hematocrit and hemoglobin levels<br>Diuresis<br>Blood glucose level<br>Water and electrolyte balance<br>Neurologic status | |

Data from Zanghi F, Petrini D: Institute of Anesthesiology, Catholic University Medical School, Rome, Italy.

for cosmetic reasons and those that require correction to re-establish a normal space relationship between the brain and the skull is not always possible in clinical practice. In fact, some forms of craniosynostoses (e.g., multiple cranial suture synostosis) that are accompanied by clinical signs of cerebral disturbance suggesting the need for functional correction may also need cosmetic treatment. In the same way, some types of craniosynostoses—for example, the sagittal and the metopic synostoses, for which correction appears to be cosmetic—may be associated with alterations of the cephalic skeleton or impaired CSF dynamics that demand prophylactic or functional therapy.

Consequently, for practical purposes, the subdivision of craniosynostoses based on the recognition of an anatomofunctional lesion seems to be more convenient. From this point of view, it is possible to distinguish two main groups of craniosynostoses: a first group, in which the lesion is centered mainly on the sagittal suture, and a second group, in which the pathologic process involves the coronal, frontosphenoidal, and sphenoethmoidal sutures. The first group may be approached satisfactorily through linear craniectomy techniques directed at restoring the function of the sagittal suture. Additional craniectomies along the remaining principal sutures may also be necessary, but only to improve the immediate cosmetic result. In the first group, the skull base anomalies are secondary and can be corrected by early surgical treatment of the vault deformity.

The second group of craniosynostoses can be defined as anterior craniosynostoses; examples of the simple forms include the unilateral and the bilateral coronal synostoses, and the complex and syndromic forms are the craniofaciostenoses. However, the metopic craniosynostoses could also be regarded as belonging to this group because of the nearly constant functional involvement of the coronal and anterior cranial base sutures. In all affected patients, the failure of the skull to expand at the level of the anatomofunctional ring formed by the continuation of the coronal, sphenoethmoidal, and frontoethmoidal sutures causes a shortening of the anteroposterior diameter of the anterior cranial fossa and of the orbits very early in life. Consequently, surgical treatment cannot be limited to the opening of the prematurely fused coronal suture but should also be extended to the cranial base to achieve an immediate increase in volume of the anterior part of the skull.

Less important groups of craniosynostosis exist, one of which is characterized by contemporary involvement of the coronal-sphenoethmoidal ring and the sagittal suture. Because of its rarity in infancy and childhood, the clinical impact of this form, usually classified under the generic term of *oxycephaly*, is rather limited. The surgical treatment, which meets functional, cosmetic, and prophylactic criteria, must be tailored according to the specific anatomofunctional lesion encountered. Another group—posterior plagiocephaly and pachycephaly—is characterized by the early fusion of one or both lambdoid sutures. The surgical indication is disputed because of the limited cosmetic and functional impairment associated with the condition.

## SAGITTAL CRANIOSYNOSTOSIS

The premature fusion of the sagittal suture is the most common congenital deformity of the head in an otherwise normal child. Its relative incidence among craniosynostoses cases is approximately 5%; its estimated general incidence is 0.4 cases per 1000 live births. Boys outnumber girls with a ratio of 3 to 3.5 to 1.[64] Familial cases, although rare, have been reported.[25, 26]

The head is typically elongated, narrow, and keel or boat shaped, often already at birth. A ridge is commonly palpable along the sagittal suture, often more prominent in its posterior half. Frequently, the value of the ratio between the transverse vault diameter and the interaural skull diameter is below 1. In most children, the forehead becomes prominent and, frequently, wedge shaped when seen from above. In most cases, a disproportion between the anterior region, which is enlarged transversely, and the narrowed parietal and occipital regions is created by the relative expansion of the skull allowed by the anterior fontanelle and metopic suture. In a relatively high percentage of infants, only limited segments of the suture undergo precocious closure. Early fusion of one or both coronal sutures may be an associated finding in less than 10% of cases; the association with fusion of other sutures is considerably less common. Facial bones are rarely involved, but a wide range of accompanying malformations has been described in children with sagittal synostosis, such as congenital heart defects, syndactyly, club feet, hypospadias, and communicating or obstructive hydrocephalus.

### Surgical Indications

The surgical indications in sagittal craniosynostosis are still debated. The usual absence of clinical signs of intracranial hypertension and the rarity of mental or neurologic deficits have led many to emphasize the purpose of surgical treatment as mainly cosmetic because the skull deformity could be a cause of relevant psychosocial disturbance for many patients. However, studies on CSF dynamics have challenged such a concept. Indeed, CT scan examination demonstrates obvious changes in the configuration and distribution of CSF pathways: the basal cisterns appear compressed, the cortical sulci are barely discernible over the cerebral hemispheres, and CSF collections are visible at both the anterior and posterior cerebral poles and within the interhemispheric fissure. In some cases, the ventricular system is initially enlarged. Prolonged intracranial pressure recording as well as a spinal subarachnoid infusion test may reveal reduced intracranial compliance in a significantly high percentage of patients.[56, 58]

In infants younger than 6 months of age, almost all methods devised for surgical correction of the malformation, including simple sagittal synostectomy or strip craniectomies running parallel to the fused sagittal suture, may

suffice for obtaining normal head shape. The main advantage of these simple procedures is that they reduce the need for blood transfusion, whereas their principal limitation is the relatively frequent early reclosure. Of all the techniques proposed to reduce the incidence of this complication, such as the application of caustic agents on the dura mater, the excision of the external dural layer, or the use of biologic or foreign interpositioned material, only the insertion of silicone sheets (Silastic; Dow-Corning) on the bone edges of the craniectomies is still used in some centers. Because of the greater risk of infection or allergic reaction from the last methodology, most authors prefer to rely both on more extensive craniectomies to prevent premature refusion and on reconstructive procedures aimed at the immediate reshaping of the head (transposition technique by Marchac and Renier[65] and the squeeze procedure by Jane and coworkers[66]). However, sagittal synostosis is usually a simple condition to cure, so that procedures such as radical osteoclastic craniectomies or extended cranial morcellation, which involve excessive blood loss, appear to be relatively unjustified in most of cases. The technique the author uses—a wide craniectomy involving the sagittal suture, with extensions both anteriorly along the coronal sutures and posteriorly along the lambdoid sutures—is similar to that proposed by Stein and Schut.[67] The procedure has been satisfactorily applied on 270 children younger than 1 year of age. No interpositional material has been used in any of these patients; four children, all of them operated on in the first 2 months of life, required a second operation because of premature reclosure.

### Surgical Technique

After induction of anesthesia, the child is placed in a supine position, with the head at the top of the table and flexed resting on a soft roll placed underneath the nape of the neck. This position provides access to the entire extension of the skull, from the frontal to the occipital region. In cases in which early fusion involves mainly the posterior two thirds of the sagittal suture and the narrowing of the skull prevails in the posterior region with a noticeable occipital prominence, the prone position is preferred, with the child's head positioned on a well padded headrest in a way that avoids pressure on the eyes. Good access to the entire skull is also offered by Park's modified prone position, with the child's head hyperextended and resting on the cheeks and the chin.[68]

Two large-bore peripheral intravenous lines are placed and the main physiologic parameters are monitored (see Table 9–2). A thermal mattress ensures temperature control. After sterile preparation of the head, a biparietal incision is made across the vertex, the edges of which end at the tragus or turn posteriorly, parallel to the base of the skull, for 2 to 3 cm above the ear pavilion to give easier access to the posterior half of the skull and to avoid visible scars (Fig. 9–1). A zig-zag skin incision offers the advantage that the resulting scar is more easily hidden by the hair than conventional linear incisions of the scalp. Subcutaneous infiltrations with epinephrine solution are never used, and stitches preventively placed at the border of the incision line to limit blood loss are used only in cases

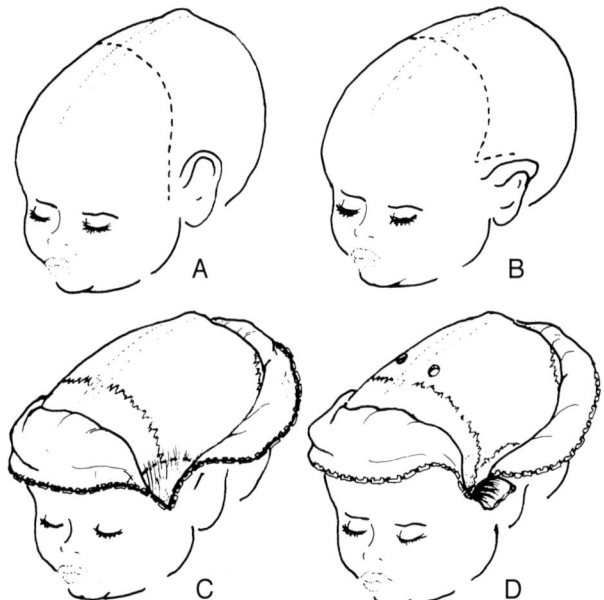

FIGURE 9–1 ■ Sagittal synostosis. The calvaria is exposed by a coronal scalp incision that ends at the tragus *(A)* or runs for 2 cm parallel to the base of the skull above the ear pavilion *(B)*. The temporal muscle is cut at its cranial insertion and retracted laterally in order to expose the pterional region *(C and D)*.

A further curvilinear incision of the pericranium is performed to detach the temporal muscle from the basolateral aspect of the frontal bone and the anterior temporal squama. Four bur holes are then made bilaterally at the anterosuperior and posterosuperior angles of the parietal bones; in infants, small nibbles at the coronal and lambdoid sutures may suffice for insertion of the foot plate of the craniotome. Linear craniectomies with a high-speed craniotome or rongeur are then performed along each side of the sagittal suture, followed by strip craniectomies (2 cm wide), which include both coronal and lambdoid sutures (Fig. 9–2). The bone bridges connecting the two anterior bur holes at the posterior border of the anterior fontanelle and the two posterior bur holes at the inion are removed with a rongeur to avoid accidental damage of the underlying venous channel. Frequent saline irrigations and bone wax on the edges of the craniectomies allow a clear exposure of the surgical field, reducing blood loss that would ensue from the generous use of suction. The bone at the pterion is also removed with a rongeur; in the author's experience, this maneuver corrects the depression that often narrows the basolateral frontal and temporal regions in children with such craniosynostoses. The inferior ends of the coronal and lambdoid craniectomies are then extended, parallel to the base and across the temporal squama, leaving a bone bridge (3 to 4 cm wide) to facilitate the lateral mobilization of the parietal bone flap at the end of the procedure.

The dura mater and the superior sagittal sinus are separated from beneath the strip of bone that contains the fused sagittal suture. Such separation can usually be done easily, although some difficulty can be encountered in cases in which the superior sagittal sinus is encased in a sulcus in the bone. Minimal dural tears above the venous sinus and the interruptions of small perforating veins, mainly posteriorly, may result in some oozing of blood, which is easily controlled by cautious bipolar coagulation or local application of Surgicel. Once the strip of bone containing

with marked engorgement of the scalp veins. Hemostasis is obtained with Children's Hospital clips (Codman-Shurtleff, Randolph, MA) or, more simply, using a microtip needle high-frequency electrocautery. The scalp flaps are reflected by means of a subgaleal dissection anteriorly at the level of the midfrontal region and below the occipital shelf posteriorly. To reduce bone bleeding, the pericranium is incised only along the craniectomy lines, which run approximately 1.5 to 2 cm on either side of the sagittal suture and 1 cm on either side of the coronal and lambdoid sutures.

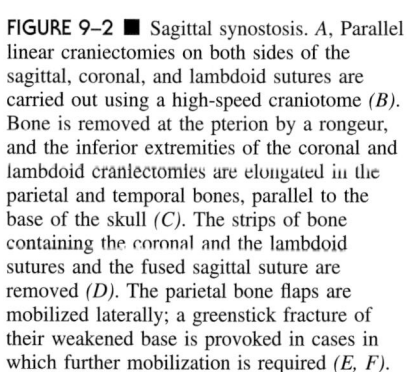

FIGURE 9–2 ■ Sagittal synostosis. *A,* Parallel linear craniectomies on both sides of the sagittal, coronal, and lambdoid sutures are carried out using a high-speed craniotome *(B)*. Bone is removed at the pterion by a rongeur, and the inferior extremities of the coronal and lambdoid craniectomies are elongated in the parietal and temporal bones, parallel to the base of the skull *(C)*. The strips of bone containing the coronal and the lambdoid sutures and the fused sagittal suture are removed *(D)*. The parietal bone flaps are mobilized laterally; a greenstick fracture of their weakened base is provoked in cases in which further mobilization is required *(E, F)*.

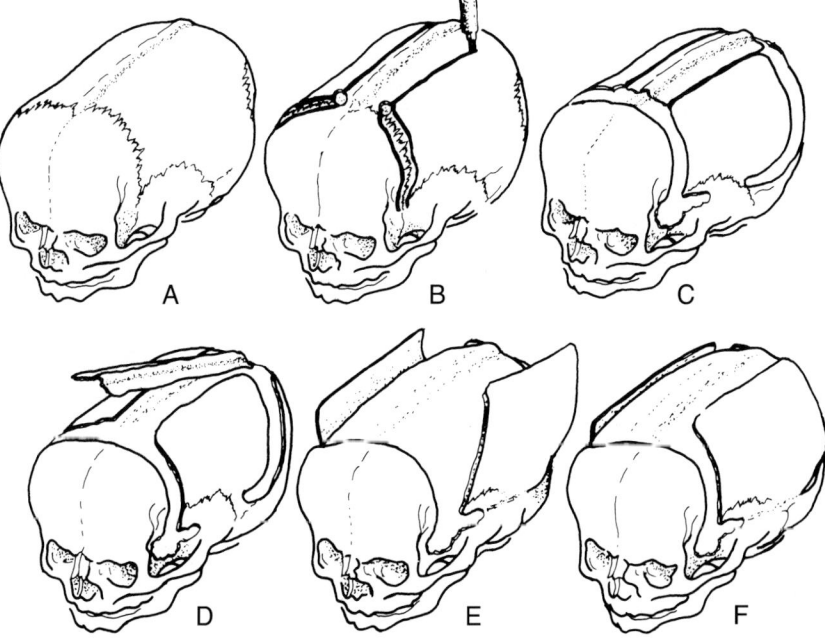

the fused sagittal suture is removed, the dura is separated from the inner surface of the parietal bone flaps; these bone structures are forced laterally, pivoting on their artificially weakened base. A greenstick fracture provoked at the base of the parietal bone flaps ensures maximal mobility in cases in which the transverse diameter of the skull is particularly reduced. The galea is approximated in a single layer with absorbable sutures, and the skin is closed with monofilament nylon. A subgaleal drain is used during the first 24 to 48 hours after the operation to reduce the pooling of blood and serum under the scalp and to have better control of possible postoperative bleeding. The hematocrit level is checked regularly during the first 48 postoperative hours.

In older children, a total skull reshaping can be performed by cutting the frontal and parietal bones in several transverse segments and by eventually replacing the various pieces of bone, after having modified their curvature with other cuts or greenstick fractures. The frontal bossing, which appears to be the most disturbing feature of the condition, is treated by removal of the malformed frontal bone 1 cm above the supraorbital bar. The bone is replaced with a "new" forehead using the most convenient piece of bone, usually a transverse segment of the parietal bone. The new forehead is placed in a more posterior and vertical position to correct the abnormal frontonasal angle. The lateral ends of the new forehead overlap the temporal areas, compensating for the narrowed transverse temporal diameter of the skull (Fig. 9–3).

## ANTERIOR CRANIOSYNOSTOSES

### Bicoronal Craniosynostosis

The relative incidence of bicoronal craniosynostosis is difficult to calculate because of its frequent association with premature fusion of other cranial sutures; indeed, the coronal suture is involved in approximately 13% of craniosynostoses.[64] Familial inheritance and a higher incidence among girls have been noted. Frequently, the condition is associated with some degree of mental retardation.

The abnormal flattening of the anterior part of the head is often noticed at birth. Characteristically, the head is broad, with a reduced anteroposterior diameter that results in two main morphologic patterns, brachycephaly and acrocephaly, according to the type of compensatory skull growth. The first pattern is characterized by a rounded

aspect of the superior part of the head and depends on compensatory growth at the sagittal suture. In acrocephaly, which is more common, the anterior fontanelle closes later and accommodates most of the compensatory growth, thus accounting for the typical pointy vertex. The combination of the two patterns is termed *acrobrachycephaly.* The facies in this craniosynostosis is typical: the forehead is uniformly flattened, the orbits are shallow, and proptosis may be evident because of the poorly formed orbital ridges. Mild hypertelorism is common, as are cleft palate, uvula bifida, hypospadias, hydrocephalus, and congenital heart diseases.

### Unicoronal Craniosynostosis

Unilateral flattening of the frontal bone, which is the main feature of anterior plagiocephaly, results from the defective growth of the frontal bone along one coronal suture. However, the first step of the process leading to this condition is the early fusion of the frontosphenoidal suture in the anterior skull base. The relative incidence of anterior plagiocephaly is approximately 12%[64]; no sex predominates, and both sutures are equally affected. Psychomotor development is normal.

In affected patients, the forehead is characteristically flattened on the pathologic side with a poorly formed supraorbital ridge. The eyebrow is retracted laterally and is elevated. The orbit is hypoplastic because of the elevated and steep lesser wing of the sphenoid, resulting in an apparent eye protrusion. Some ocular malalignment can be noticed, as well as a specific vertical strabismus. The nose is frequently deviated opposite the affected side; the maxillary and mandibular bones may be asymmetric and deviated (facial scoliosis). The ear pavilion is displaced anteriorly on the pathologic side. Compensatory growth of the skull can be observed at the level of the contralateral anterior cranial fossa or the homolateral temporal region. The head is typically tilted because of the obliquity of the cervicospinal junction caused by the asymmetric development of the occipital condyles and the lateral masses of the atlas. The various combinations of abnormalities of the nasal pyramid and the vomer, sphenobasilar, and petrous bones determine the severity of the condition and its associated surgical prognosis.[31] Associated malformations are absent or very rare.

### Craniofacial Dysostosis

Although several forms of craniofacial dysostosis have been classified according to clinical variants and genetic

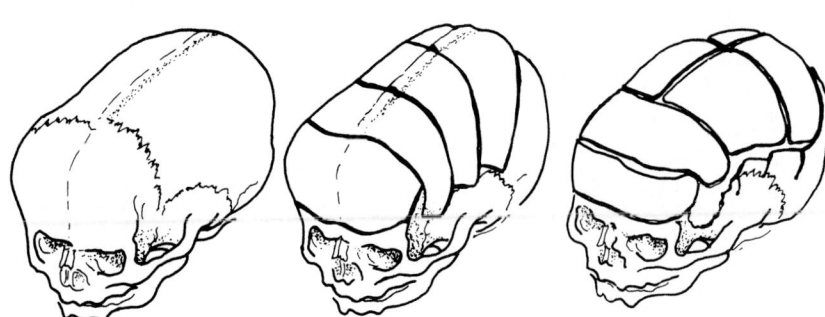

FIGURE 9–3 ■ Sagittal synostosis. The transposition technique is used for older children.

patterns, Crouzon's and Apert's craniofacial dysostoses have attracted interest because of their higher incidence. The approximate incidence of Apert's syndrome is 1 per 100,000 to 160,000 live births, and the incidence of Crouzon's syndrome is 1 per 20,000 live births.[64] The relative incidence in clinical series of craniosynostosis varies significantly with the accessibility of specialized centers for multidisciplinary treatment, which can attract large percentages of patients. Crouzon's syndrome is now regarded as an autosomal dominant trait inherited by both sexes. A similar mode of transmission has also been described in Apert's syndrome. In both syndromes, however, most cases are sporadic occurrences resulting from fresh gene mutation.

The phenotype of both syndromes is similar, but the most distinguishing feature is the syndactyly, or digital fusion, of the four extremities typical of Apert's syndrome. The shortening of the anteroposterior diameter of the skull depends on the recession of the frontal bone and supraorbital bar, which can be masked by the simultaneous retrusion of the facial skeleton. The orbits are severely hypoplastic secondary to the verticalization of the orbital roof, the frontalization of the great wing of the sphenoid, and the ballooning of the ethmoid. Consequently, exophthalmos is a constant feature, accentuated by the contemporary hypoplasia of the infraorbital rim. The orbital axis may be altered and directed downward and outward. The parrot's-beak shape of the nose results from the retrusion and vertical shortness of the middle third of the face. The retrusion of the upper face is accentuated by the protrusion of the mandible; the maxillary bone is hypoplastic with secondary deformity of the alveolar arch and the palate. Associated malformations, such as otologic anomalies, vertebral deformities, polycystic kidney, and syringomyelia, are common in both Apert's and Crouzon's syndromes.

The ocular and facial abnormalities described earlier also can be found in a particularly severe form of craniosynostosis, the cloverleaf skull deformity, in which the head assumes a characteristic trilobar configuration. Hydrocephalus is almost always associated with this craniosynostosis. The condition has been specifically described, although some investigators have proposed including it in Crouzon's syndrome.

## Metopic Craniosynostosis

The early fusion of the metopic suture causes a typical triangular deformity of the head—trigonocephaly—when viewed from above. Because the process occurs in utero, the condition can be noticed at birth; consequently, its relative incidence increases in series mainly dealing with infants.[64] In mild cases, metopic craniosynostosis should be distinguished from alterations of the skull secondary to forebrain morphogenetic anomalies or frontal lobe atrophy. Besides the hypoplastic anterior cranial fossa with abnormally angulated frontal bones, the hypoplastic flat or anteriorly concave supraorbital margins, and the relatively shallow orbits with antimongoloid slant of the palpebral fissure, the most typical feature of the condition is the presence of a prominent midline ridge of the frontal bone. The interocular distance is decreased because of the underdevelopment

of the ethmoid bone. An increase in the biparietal diameter or parietal height may result from compensatory cranial growth. Epicanthic folds, cleft palate, and cardiac anomalies are the most commonly associated malformations.

## Surgical Indications

The first goal of surgical treatment of craniosynostoses resulting from early fusion of the sutures of the anterior part of the skull is to provide adequate room for cerebral growth, which can be achieved through cranial expansion operations, nearly always carried out exclusively by the neurosurgeon and performed in the first months of life. A second goal of surgical treatment is to ensure a normal relationship between the various components of the craniofacial skeleton. Although early operations that enlarge the anterior segment of the skull may have a positive influence on the development of the facial skeleton, more complex malformations due to the precocious fusion of the coronal and anterior skull base sutures usually require several staged operations performed from childhood to adolescence. Even though the neurosurgeon may still maintain an important role even in this late phase of treatment, in nearly all cases the final correction requires the intervention of the maxillofacial and plastic surgeon to treat the midface retrusion by a Le Fort III or monoblock advancement.

Coronal synostosis results in a decreased volume of the anterior cranial fossa because of the restricted growth of the frontal vault and the secondary alteration of the angle along which this structure joins the cranial base. Both anomalies can be corrected by the simple release of the prematurely fused suture. Indeed, in patients in whom the synostotic process concerns the coronal suture exclusively or principally, wide linear craniectomy along the coronal sutures extended laterally and inferiorly to bisect the upper margin of the sphenoid bone is followed, when carried out early in life, by an immediate, long-lasting modification of skull shape and a relative normalization of the basocranial angle.

Simple strip craniectomies, however, are not sufficient to obtain satisfactory functional and cosmetic results in patients with associated involvement of the frontoethmoidal, frontosphenoidal, and frontozygomatic sutures because of the secondary development impairment of the anterior cranial base. In such cases, creating "neosutures" at the base of the skull is necessary. The restriction of anteroposterior growth of the skull base takes place during the first 2 months of life and results in an abnormal faciocranial relationship; consequently, surgical correction must be performed at a very early age to have prophylactic value.

During the 1970s, several surgical procedures were propounded to correct more complex forms of coronal synostosis by extending the craniectomy into the base of the skull.[69–73] In particular, the opening of the frontosphenoidal segment of the coronal suture produced an increase in the sagittal diameter of the anterior cranial fossa in infants with Apert's or Crouzon's syndromes.[73] Anterior displacement of the supraorbital margin, after the supraorbital plate is opened from the crista galli to the pterion and the osteotomy is extended through the frontozygomatic process, appeared to ensure better functional and cosmetic results than previous operations. Such procedures consisted of simple overimposition of a 180-degree rotated frontal flap on the hypoplastic supraorbital ridge left in place.[70–72]

Advancement of the supraorbital ridge is also an essential step in surgical procedures used to treat metopic synostosis. In fact, the maneuver provides room for immediate re-expansion of the frontal lobes constricted within the hypoplastic anterior cranial fossa, consequently overcoming the limits of previous procedures based on the simple opening of the fused suture and the removal of the midline frontal bone ridge.

## Surgical Technique

After the same general preparation described for sagittal synostosis, the child is placed in the supine position; the head is slightly rotated toward the normal side in case of anterior plagiocephaly. A bicoronal skin incision is made from one antitragus to the symmetric opposite region. The scalp flap is elevated by blunt separation of the galea from the periosteum. Blood transfusion is started in this phase. The scalp is reflected anteriorly, and the coronal suture is exposed. The pterion is visualized by detachment and lateral retraction of the temporal muscle from the infratemporal fossa to the level of the zygomatic arch, after its insertion is cut at the level of the superior temporal line with a Bovie knife.

In patients with simple bilateral coronal synostosis, a coronal synostectomy, 2 cm wide, may be sufficient to release the frontal cranial vault. A subtemporal decompression may be associated with the coronal synostectomy in patients whose pterional region is depressed. In infants and young children, strip coronal craniectomies are easily performed with a bone rongeur, starting from the lateral aspect of the anterior fontanelle, continuing along the entire coronal sutures to encompass the sphenozygomatic sutures, and ending at the level of the inferior orbital fissures.

During the procedure, the lateral aspect of the overgrown sphenoid bone should be removed, with careful preservation of the orbit's contents.

Strip coronal craniectomies are not sufficient, however, to achieve a satisfactory functional and cosmetic correction in patients with more severe forms of bicoronal synostosis and for those with contemporary involvement of the sutures of the anterior cranial base. In such cases, it is necessary to obtain a wider exposure of the frontal bone by turning the scalp flap further forward to perform orbital decompression and advance the retrocessed supraorbital ridge (Fig. 9–4). The periosteum is then incised parallel to the skull base, approximately 2 cm above the superior orbital rim. The supraorbital portion of the periosteum is carefully dissected and reflected anteriorly to expose the anterosuperior orbital margin; during the maneuver, the surgeon should avoid damaging the supraorbital nerve, which usually is lodged in a groove on the inferior surface of the superior orbital ridge. More rarely, the nerve runs in a channel that goes through the frontal bone and must be freed with a high-speed drill.

It is important to preserve the continuity of the pericranium with the periorbita and to avoid entering the latter structure. Once this part of the procedure is finished, a synostectomy is carried out along the metopic suture down to the nasion. Small-caliber and fragile veins entering the superior sagittal sinus at its origin may be torn during this phase; the bleeding, however, is easily controlled by bipolar coagulation or local absorbable gelatin sponge (Gelfoam) application. A linear craniectomy, running approximately 1 cm above and parallel to the orbital rim, is then carried out to join the coronal and metopic craniectomies and to obtain unilateral (unicoronal synostosis) or bilateral (bicoronal synostosis, craniofacial dysostosis, or metopic synostosis) free frontal bone flaps. The frontal lobe is retracted extradurally, and the orbital roof is exposed, incised up to its mesial margin, and partially removed to-

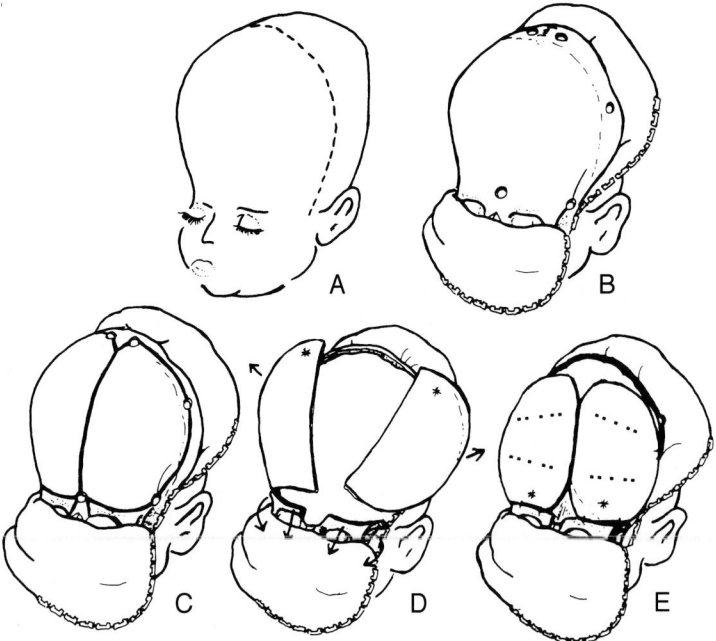

FIGURE 9–4 ■ Anterior craniosynostosis. The anterior part of the calvaria is exposed by a bicoronal scalp incision (A). Burr holes are made, and two frontal bone flaps, which contain a segment of the fused coronal suture, are freed (B and C). The superior orbital rims are advanced, especially at their lateral canthi, after cutting their lateral and mesial extremities and removing the upper half of the nasal bones (D). The frontal flaps are rotated and replaced after their curvature (E) has been modified appropriately.

gether with the lateral third of the lesser wing of the sphenoid.

The superior orbital ridge is cut free at its most lateral and mesial extremities and is detached from the thin underlying capsule, which borders the orbital content. It is then placed in a more advanced position. Alternatively, advancement of the structure may be obtained by angling its freed lateral canthus anteriorly and pivoting it on its superomesial border, while its resistance is lessened by a greenstick fracture. The new position of the superior orbital ridge may be maintained by use of a buttress of bone obtained from the calvaria and placed between the lateral canthus and the temporal border of the coronal craniectomy (Fig. 9–5). In older children, rigid microplates and screws can be used. The free frontal flaps are remodeled with Tessier's rib benders, then rotated to provide the most appropriate contour and replaced over the advanced superior orbital ridges, thereby further stabilizing their advanced position.

Alternatively, the frontal flaps can be laid over the superior orbital ridge, contributing to a more prominent new orbital rim. The frontal flaps are secured with silk stitches or microscrews inferolaterally and posteriorly, but they are left "floating" on the midline. The continuity of the periosteum is reconstituted as much as possible. In cases

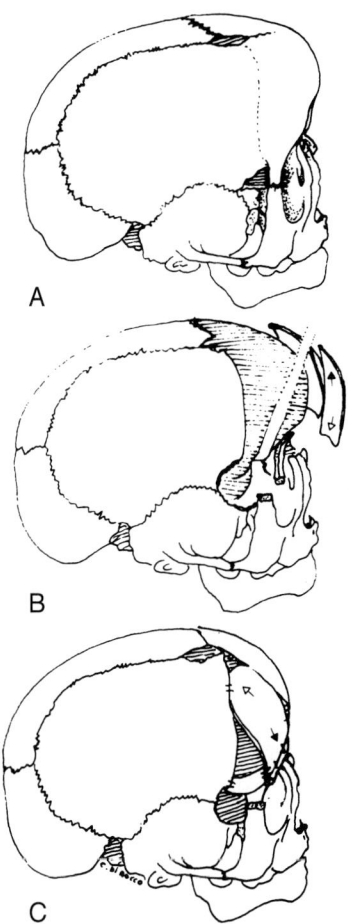

FIGURE 9–5 ■ A–C, Anterior plagiocephaly (bilateral approach): the advanced freed superior orbital margins are maintained in the new position by the rotated frontal flaps and by bone bridges interposed between the anterior border of the parietal bone and the lateral orbital canthus.

in which the anterior aspect of the superior orbital ridge is excessively concave and its remodeling cannot be achieved, the structure can be completely removed. In these cases, the frontal bone can be turned and its posterior border remodeled to form a new orbital rim (Fig. 9–6). This type of procedure is indicated particularly in older children with severe bilateral coronal synostosis and in some children with trigonocephaly.

In patients with unilateral coronal craniosynostosis, the hypoplastic superior orbital ridge must be advanced to a more anterior position than that of the normal contralateral orbital rim. In fact, the malformed orbital ridge usually tends to retrocede from the artificially created new position. Furthermore, it may appear to be relatively hypoplastic late in life because of the frequent failure of the frontal sinus to develop on the side of the operation.[74] To avoid this complication, a bilateral approach can be used, especially when it is necessary to correct a contralateral compensatory frontal bossing. A sinus-sparing osteotomy, with the basal frontal craniectomy line angled upward at its mesial border in the vicinity of the future frontal sinus, has been suggested as a possible alternative.[75]

In children with trigonocephaly, extension of the metopic craniectomy by removal of the upper part of the nasal bones is a simple but effective measure that counteracts the hypotelorism. In these children as well as in patients with severe frontal hypoplasia treated with the technique described earlier, the frontal flaps may leave an uncovered median triangular area above the glabella when they are replaced after a 180-degree rotation, which in rare cases may fail to ossify. In the author's experience, the best method to avoid this complication is to leave a mosaic of minute bone fragments, such as those that can be obtained from the midline craniectomy, and to let them lie freely above the dura mater and fill the artificially created gap in the calvaria. Alternatively, the frontal bone can be removed en bloc to be replaced, rotated 180 degrees when necessary, after reshaping its curvature by means of multiple radial cuts and drilling of the bone ridge of the prematurely fused metopic suture—the so-called *shell operation*[76] (Fig. 9–7). With this simpler and shorter technique compared with the more traditional operations for metopic synostosis, the resulting craniolacunia is in the upper aspect of the operative field, that is, in the area of the bregmatic fontanelle. The reossification of this area is more rapid than that of the supraglabellar region, and the patient's parents are reassured because the postoperative craniolacunia seems to represent only the reopening of the prematurely closed anterior fontanelle.

## MULTIPLE-SUTURE CRANIOSYNOSTOSES

Different patterns of craniosynostosis originate from the various combinations of fusion of the major cranial sutures, and all of the patterns share the morphologic characteristics of a small cranial vault. In the most typical instance, early fusion of all cranial sutures produces a typical tower-shaped or pointed-head oxycephaly, which results from the growth of the skull toward the vertex in the direction where resistance is less. Besides oxycephaly, two other common

FIGURE 9-6 ■ Anterior craniosynostosis: alternative methods for frontal bone advancement. A bilateral tongue-in-groove procedure is carried out for frontal bar advancement *(A)*. A new frontal visor is created by using a rotated frontal bone flap. The hypoplastic superior orbital ridges have been completely removed *(B)*.

morphologic patterns may be recognized. The first, acrocephaly, recalls bicoronal craniosynostosis because it depends predominantly on the failure of this suture. The facial skeleton anomalies are also similar, such as hypoplastic orbits with a reduced anteroposterior diameter and the gothic arch palate. The second pattern, microcephaly, is characterized by global reduction of skull volume.

The actual incidence of multiple-suture craniosynostoses is difficult to evaluate. However, the impressively low relative incidence in series dealing with younger children compared with those considering subjects of all ages suggests that the condition may represent the late evolution of craniosynostoses that, in the first months of life, are characterized only by the fusion of one major cranial suture and by the incomplete fusion of the other sutures. Consequently, the current policy of early correction of craniosynostosis could account for the apparent decrease in the incidence of oxycephaly in most of the more recent clinical reports.

## Surgical Indications

The main goal of the surgical correction of multiple-suture craniosynostosis is to eliminate the compression effect on the brain that occurs early in life. When the diagnosis is obtained in late childhood, the main rationale for operative treatment is cosmetic. Several surgical procedures have been proposed, varying from linear craniectomies along the fused sutures to King's morcellation technique or the creation of multiple bone flaps.[21, 33, 39, 44] The extensive subperiosteal resection of the skull vault and base introduced by Powiertowski[77] is very rarely performed today. In fact, most surgeons prefer to leave a mosaic of bone to be possibly molded by an external device[78] or to use for various bone transposition techniques (Fig. 9–8).[65] According to some authors, in these forms of craniosynostosis, and especially in the cloverleaf skull syndrome, a posterior release of the skull performed before 3 months of age may dramatically improve the cranial shape and allow the neurosurgeon to postpone or even avoid the need for a fronto-orbital advancement.[79]

## LAMBDOID CRANIOSYNOSTOSIS

The early fusion of one or both lambdoid sutures is relatively unusual; in most cases, the bilateral or unilateral

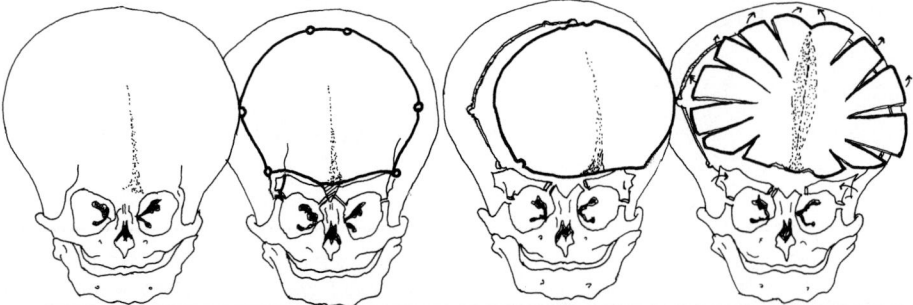

FIGURE 9-7 ■ "Shell" operation for metopic synostosis. The curvature of the en bloc frontal bone flap is modified by drilling the thick bone ridge along the metopic suture in order to bend the two hemifrontal segments anteriorly. Further increase in volume of the anterior cranial fossa is obtained by appropriate bending of the bone segments resulting from radial cuts of the frontal bone flap. The modified frontal bone flap is then replaced maintaining its normal orientation or after a 180-degree rotation, as required for functional and cosmetic purposes.

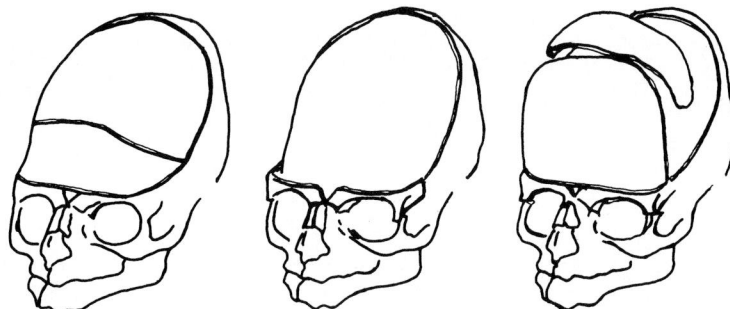

FIGURE 9–8 ■ Multiple suture synostosis. A transposition technique is used for cranial remodeling and expansion.

flattening of the posterior aspect of the head is only a transitory deformity, which can disappear spontaneously or be corrected by external molding of the skull.[80] Most of the discussion concerning the surgical indication in children presenting with a flattening of the posterior aspect of the head derives from the difficulties in differentiating the rare cases of posterior plagiocephaly resulting from an intrinsic disorder of the lambdoid suture, which leads to its early fusion (true craniosynostosis), from the more frequent posterior skull asymmetries secondary to the action of external forces (skull molding).[81–86] Unlike the coronal and sagittal sutures, which exhibit clear radiologic or intraoperative evidence of early fusion in their respective forms of craniosynostosis, the lambdoid suture fuses only in exceptional instances. However, because asymmetry or deformation of the occipital bone from unilateral or bilateral posterior flattening of the skull is relatively common, several attempts have been made to identify radiologic or functional criteria that could allow the diagnosis of lambdoid synostosis even in the absence of the typical appearance of a prematurely fused cranial suture. In children with posterior flattening of the skull, various radiologic changes of the lambdoid suture have been proposed, including "incomplete fusion," "partial fusion," "sclerosis of the sutural borders," "bony bridges," "bony spiculae," "spot-welding pattern," "inward prominence" of the inner calvarial table, and so on. Correspondingly, the search for some pathogenetic explanation of impaired skull growth at the level of a suture that is still apparently open at radiologic examination has resulted in "pathogenetic" definitions such as "lazy" or "blocked" suture or "functional lambdoid synostosis."[80]

The high incidence of cases of "false" lambdoid synostosis is related to the recent increase in the relative incidence of posterior plagiocephaly among the various forms of craniosynostosis, which in turn is due to changes in infants' sleeping positions resulting from the formal actions undertaken in several European countries in the early 1990s to encourage parents to avoid placing their child in a prone position. These actions followed a variety of reports supporting a possible relationship between the prone position and the sudden infant death syndrome, and received strong support from the 1992 report of the American Academy of Pediatrics Task Force on Infant Positioning. Infants placed in either the supine or prone position usually remain in that position throughout sleep, at least during the first months of life. By the end of the 1970s, several investigations already had suggested the possible role of the supine position in inducing molding of the posterior aspect of the head because of an easily compressible occipital bone, and emphasized the risk of performing unnecessary operations on patients whose molded skull could be treated by physical measures.

## Surgical Indications and Techniques

Most children with a molded skull may be treated by nonsurgical methods such as changing the sleep position, neck muscle stretching, or wearing corrective helmets for a certain period of time. Only a small proportion of subjects with posterior plagiocephaly (i.e., one of six or seven cases) continue to show progression of their deformity in spite of aggressive early positioning and helmet remodeling.[87] In such cases, the modifications of the skull resemble, although they are less severe, those of unilateral coronal synostosis, with a unilateral posterior flattening associated with a contralateral occipital bulging and, possibly, with opposite changes of the frontal bone as well as shifting of the ears, facial scoliosis, and mandibular malalignment.

Techniques for treatment include simple excision of the fused suture, release of a parieto-occipital bone flap, which contains the pathologic suture, and creation of free unilateral or bilateral bone flaps that are replaced after adequate remolding and rotation (Fig. 9–9).

More aggressive surgical techniques (Fig. 9–10) offer the advantage of a more complete and immediate correction of the skull anomaly than with linear strip craniectomies of the lambdoid suture or the creation of a free bone flap of limited size, the effect of which relies on the expanding forces of the underlying brain.

## COMPLICATIONS

Blood loss during and after surgical correction is the most important risk of surgical treatment of craniosynostosis. The main role of the anesthetist in this type of procedure is the careful evaluation and adequate replacement of blood volume lost during the operation. However, in spite of accurate efforts to weigh sponges and repeated controls of hemoglobin concentration, assessment of blood loss may remain difficult. Fortunately, the experience of the anesthetist who is familiar with the surgical treatment of craniosynostosis in empirical transfusion practice proves to be sufficient in most cases, thereby challenging the need for the routine use of invasive monitoring.[79]

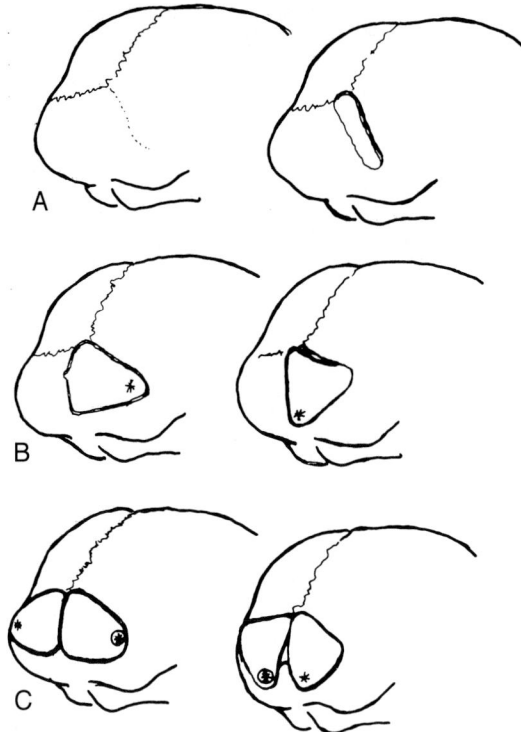

**FIGURE 9–9** ■ Lambdoid synostosis: alternative methods for correction. A strip craniectomy is shown to contain the fused suture *(A)*. Unilateral *(B)* or bilateral *(C)* creation of free bone flaps to be reversed or transposed (or both) before replacement.

The use of hypotensive anesthesia in infants has had little effect in reducing blood loss during craniectomy. The efficacy of scalp infiltrations with local anesthetic solutions in diminishing blood loss is also disputable because most of the blood volume during the surgical procedure is lost at the periosteal and bone levels. Hemostatic scalp sutures or clamps adequately control hemorrhage from the skin incision. Their use, however, may be avoided in cases in which a microtip needle high-frequency electrocautery is used for the skin incision. The use of high-speed craniotomes significantly diminishes blood loss related to the craniotomy; when bone rongeurs are used, frequent irrigation with saline is preferred to the constant use of suction to maintain a clean surgical field. Blood loss increases according to the number of sutures involved and the severity of the surgical procedure, varying from 20% to 40% to 60% of the total estimated blood volume.[88] Repeated hematocrit controls are necessary during the first 24 to 48 postoperative hours because in some cases further blood

replacement may be required to compensate for postoperative blood loss. Subgaleal drainages are particularly useful in the evaluation of the amount of blood lost locally after the operation and in the reduction of postoperative accumulation of fluids beneath the scalp.

In the 1990s, the risk of post-transfusion infections has been drastically reduced; for example, the risk for hepatitis dropped from 1:25 to 1:100,000, and for human immunodeficiency virus infection, from 1:5000 in 1982 to the current 1:600,000. However, allogeneic blood transfusions still represent a major concern for the family of children undergoing surgical correction of craniosynostosis, and continue to constitute a cause of theoretically avoidable postoperative infective and immunologic reactions. No definitive information is available yet for the more recently identified hepatitis viruses, non-A, non-B virus and hepatitis C virus. Some kind of immunosuppression attributable to blood transfusion has been advocated to explain an increased susceptibility of the recipient to infection by a virus possibly present in one of the blood units transfused. Furthermore, there is some evidence that repeated blood transfusions, as required in cases of staged surgical correction of complex faciocraniostenotic syndromes, might determine a nonlinear increase in the predisposition of the patient to immunologic reactions. The significant attention paid to this type of complication, as well as (to a lesser extent) the necessity of respecting the convictions of those people who might oppose blood transfusion because of religious beliefs, have resulted in protocols that diminish or even avoid the use of allogeneic blood transfusions in the surgical correction of craniosynostosis.[89] These protocols are based on a complex group of techniques that include predeposited autologous blood donation, acute preoperative normovolemic hemodilution, and intraoperative blood salvage (Table 9–3). The application of these protocols requires an experienced team comprising the neurosurgeon familiar with blood-sparing craniosynostosis repair techniques, the pediatric neuroanesthesiologist, the hematologist, the hemapheresis and intraoperative blood salvage technician, the pediatrician, and the pediatric intensivist.

Major and potentially life-threatening complications are very rare during the surgical correction of simple craniosynostoses. They are essentially related to systemic hypotension and usually result from excessive blood loss, such as in cases of generalized bleeding or accidental tearing of the venous sinuses. Accidental dural tearing during the operation can be easily repaired with silk sutures or local application of fibrin glue. Major complications are also very rare during the immediate postoperative period; they include CSF leak and infection, blood loss, and shock.

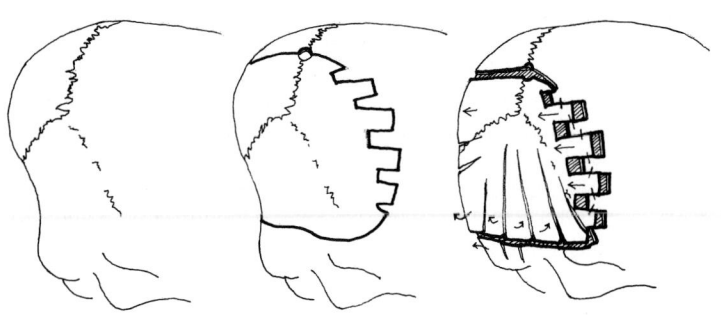

**FIGURE 9–10** ■ En bloc posterior displacement of the posterior part of the parietal and occipital bones. The bone flap is replaced after modification of its shape and curvature by appropriately bending the bone segments created with radial cuts. The "new" more posterior position is maintained using the "ad hoc" designed craniotomy lines as a guide.

## TABLE 9–3 ■ NO ALLOGENEIC BLOOD TRANSFUSION (NABT) PROTOCOL, CATHOLIC UNIVERSITY MEDICAL SCHOOL, ROME, ITALY

**Preoperative Phase**

*Exclusionary Criteria*
Age, clinical condition *(e.g, infants younger than 4 months of age, subjects with hematologic or cardiorespiratory disorders)*

*Age for the Operation*
4–6 Months *(85% of fetal hemoglobin [Hb] substituted by adult-type Hb)*

*Optimal Hematologic Condition*
97th Percentile for Hb concentration and hematocrit (Ht) (Hb ~13g/dl, Ht = 35%)
- *Possibly obtained with recombinant human erythropoietin, 3 times/week for 21 days before performing the autotransfusion, plus iron administration*
- *High values of Hb concentration and Ht should be avoided to exclude a possible increase in blood viscosity*

*Predeposited Autologous Blood Donation (PABD)*
Deposited 20 days before the planned surgical procedure in patients in optimal hematologic condition
- *Blood donation volumes calculated according to the equation for acceptable blood loss:*
$$PABD\ volume = EBV\ Ht1 - Ht2/Ht1$$
   *where EBV (estimated blood volume) = body weight (kg) × 80; Ht1 = actual Ht; and Ht2 = Ht targeted after PABD (under no circumstances should it be <27)*
   *For safety purposes (Ht1 − Ht2) ≤ 5*
   *The storage limit for predeposited autologous blood is 28 days.*

*Actual Preoperative Normovolemic Hemodilution*
Children older than 10 months of age or weighing 12 kg or more in optimal hematologic condition
- *Blood autodonation replaced by simultaneous administration of colloids*
- *Crystalloid solutions to be avoided to minimize hemodilution*

**Intraoperative Phase**

*Anesthesiologic Monitoring*
- *Inhalatory induction of anesthesia with halothane (no barbiturates, propofol, sedatives, fentanyl, muscle relaxant drugs)*
- *Anesthesia maintained with isoflurane or sevoflurane MAC1-2*
- *Anesthesiologic monitoring (electrocardiogram, invasive arterial blood pressure, central venous pressure, body temperature [rectal or tympanic plus cutaneous], urinary output, end-tidal carbon dioxide, end-tidal anesthetic agents, oxygen and nitrous oxide, pulse oxymetry, airway pressure, preoperative and sequential intraoperative Hb and Ht values, blood loss volume)*

*Blood Salvage*
- *Continuous autotransfusion system for intraoperative blood salvage (IOBS apparatus): the shed blood of the patient is continuously processed and retransfused as soon as the separation chamber of the IOBS apparatus is full of red blood cells (current systems: 25–40 ml)*
- *Avoid contamination of the operative field by:*
   *Iodine or hydrogen peroxide (risk of massive hemolysis)*
   *Colloid fibrin microparticles, fibrin glue (risk for microembolism because the microparticles with a molecular weight similar to that of red blood cells migrate and are reinfused together with the erythrocytes)*

**Postoperative Phase**

Patient Extubated if Presents with
- *Rapid recovery*
- *Hemodynamic stability*
- *Spontaneous ventilation*
- *Normothermia*
- *No continuous bleeding in the surgical drain*

*Intensive Care*
Evaluation of blood volumes collected in the surgical drain
Sequential monitoring of Hb and Ht
Patient transfused with autologous blood if still available
Patient transfused with allogeneic blood if Hb <7.5 g/dl plus two of the following:
- *Systolic arterial pressure <10th percentile for age and sex*
- *Heart rate at rest >75th percentile for age*
- *Respiratory rate at rest >mean + 2 SD, with no signs of pulmonary engorgement*
- *Central venous pressure <2 cm $H_2O$*
- *Right atrium blood oxygen saturation <58% at $FIO_2 = 0.21$, without pulmonary engorgement*
- *Metabolic acidosis (standard bicarbonates <21 mmol/L, pH <7.35, $PaCO_2$ <38 mm Hg)*

Although postoperative CSF fistulas may require surgical closure of the dural defect, in most cases lumbar CSF drainage is sufficient. Infections are practically absent in simple craniosynostosis cases, and prophylactic antibiotic therapy consequently is unnecessary. However, infection can represent an important risk in faciocraniostenosis, especially in patients undergoing frontofacial monoblock advancement in whom the nasal mucosa can be breached, or in patients with tracheostomies.[90] Postoperative hemorrhagic complications are infrequent; nevertheless, one of the two deaths recorded in the author's series of 540 patients resulted from disseminated intravascular coagulation that occurred 1 hour after an apparently uneventful correction of a sagittal craniosynostosis.

Additional postoperative complications, usually transient, have been reported, such as deficits of the cranial nerves, inappropriate antidiuretic hormone secretion, and chemosis.[80] When this last complication is expected, Frost sutures can be applied and secured with adhesive tape.

Late complications are essentially due to inadequate correction of the malformation, with refusion of previously operated sutures or fusion of other cranial sutures. The recurrence of craniosynostosis, which was common after linear craniectomy, has become a relatively less important problem in modern series in which reconstructive procedures are adopted in most cases. Consequently, the methods used in the past to interfere with regrowth of bone across the craniectomy, such as creating barriers against bone regrowth or acting on the osteogenic power of the dura mater, have been mostly abandoned.

## REFERENCES

1. Holland E: Cranial stress in the foetus during labour and on the effects of excessive stress on the intracranial content, with an analysis of 81 cases of torn tentorium cerebelli and subdural hemorrhage. J Obstet Gynaecol Br Emp 29:549–571, 1922.
2. McPherson GU, Kriewall TJ: The elastic modulus of fetal cranial bone: A first step towards an understanding of the biomechanics of fetal head molding. J Biomech 13:9–16, 1980.
3. Moss ML: Functional anatomy of cranial synostosis. Childs Nerv Syst 1:22–23, 1975.
4. Moss ML: New studies of cranial growth. Birth Defects 11:283–295, 1975.
5. Moss ML: Growth of the calvaria in the rat. Am J Anat 94:333–362, 1954.
6. Popa GT: Mechanostruktur und Mechanofunktion der Dura Mater des Menschen. Gegenbaurs Morphol Jahrb 78:85–187, 1936.
7. Moss ML: Functional analysis and the functional matrix. Speech Hear Assoc Rep 6:5–18, 1971.
8. Graham JM, Badura RJ, Smith DW: Sagittal craniostenosis: Fetal head constraint as one possible cause. J Pediatr 95:747–750, 1979.
9. Graham JM, Badura RJ, Smith DW: Coronal craniostenosis: Fetal head constraint as one possible cause. Pediatrics 65:995–999, 1980.
10. Graham JM, Smith DW: Metopic craniostenosis as a consequence of fetal head constraint: Two interesting experiments of nature. Pediatrics 65:1000–1002, 1980.
11. Persson KM, Roy WA, Persing JA, et al: Craniofacial growth following experimental craniosynostosis and craniectomy in rabbits. J Neurosurg 50:187–197, 1979.
12. Persing JA, Babler W, Winn HR, et al: Age as a critical factor in the success of surgical correction of craniosynostosis. J Neurosurg 54:601–606, 1981.
13. Di Rocco C, Velardi F: Classification, forms and varieties; classification tables. In Galli G (ed): Craniosynostosis. Boca Raton, FL: CRC Press, 1984, pp 76–107.
14. Cohen MM Jr: Syndromes with craniosynostosis. In Cohen MM Jr (ed): Craniosynostosis. New York: Raven Press, 1986, pp 413–590.
15. Franceschetti A, Klein D: Oxicéphalie chéz trois paires de jumeaux univitellins, assoc iée dans un des cas à une cutis frontis gyrata. Acta Genet Med Gemellol (Roma) 1:48–65, 1952.
16. Bertelsen TI: The premature synostosis of the cranial sutures. Acta Ophthalmol Suppl (Copenh) 51:1–174, 1958.
17. Bell HS, Clare FB, Wentworth AR: Familiar scaphocephaly. J Neurosurg 18:239–241, 1961.
18. Acquaviva R, Tamie PM, Lebascle J, et al: Les craniosténoses en milieu marocain: A propos des 140 observations. Neurochirurgie 12:561–566, 1966.
19. Keith J, Datta Bonik NN, Falkner F: Identical twins with craniosynostosis of the sagittal suture. Indian J Pediatr 35:229–231, 1968.
20. Pereira W-C, De Barras GN, De Almeida M, Saldanha PH: Craniostenose em gemeos: Estudio genetico. Arch Neuropsiquiatr S Paulo 26:236–239, 1968.
21. Shillito J, Matson DD: Craniosynostosis: A review of 519 surgical patients. Pediatrics 41:829–853, 1968.
22. Armendares S: On the inheritance of craniostenosis: Study of thirteen families. J Hum Genet 18:121–134, 1970.
23. El Sharif H, Khalita AS, Abou-Jenna AM, Ghaly AF: Craniosynostosis in Egypt. J Neurosurg 33:29–34, 1970.
24. Gooding CA: Cranial sutures and fontanelles. In Newton TH, Potts DH (eds): Radiology of the Skull and Brain, Vol 1. St. Louis: CV Mosby, 1971, pp 216–237.
25. Hunter AGW, Rudd NL: Craniosynostosis. I: Sagittal synostosis: Its genetics and associated clinical findings in 214 patients who lacked involvement of the coronal suture(s). Teratology 14:185–193, 1976.
26. Hunter AGW, Rudd NL: Craniosynostosis. II: Coronal synostosis: Its familial characteristics and associated clinical findings in 109 patients lacking bilateral polysyndactyly or syndactyly. Teratology 15:301–310, 1977.
27. Montaut J, Stricker M: Dysmorphie crânio-faciales: Les synostoses prématurées (craniosténoses et faciosténoses). Neurochirurgie 23 (Suppl 2):1–299, 1977.
28. Giuffré R, Vagnozzi R, Savino S: Infantile craniosynostosis: Clinical, radiological, and surgical considerations based on 100 surgically treated cases. Acta Neurochir (Wien) 44:49–67, 1978.
29. Mohr G, Hoffman HJ, Munro IR, et al: Surgical management of unilateral and bilateral coronal craniosynostosis: 21 years of experience. Neurosurgery 2:83–92, 1978.
30. Di Rocco C, Marchese E, Velardi F: Craniosynostosis: Surgical treatment during the first year of life. J Neurosurg Sci 36:129–137, 1992.
31. Di Rocco C, Velardi F: Nosographic identification and classification of plagiocephaly. Childs Nerv Syst 4:9–15, 1988.
32. Freeman JM, Borkowf S: Craniosynostosis: Review of the literature and report of thirty-four cases. Pediatrics 30:57–70, 1962.
33. Anderson FM, Geiger L: Craniosynostosis. J Neurosurg 22:229–240, 1965.
34. Kokich VG, Moffet BC, Cohen MM Jr: The cloverleaf skull anomaly: An anatomic and histologic study of two specimens. Cleft Palate Craniofac J 19:89–99, 1982.
35. Galli ML: Apert syndrome does not equal mental retardation (Letter). J Pediatr 89:691, 1976.
36. Camfield PR, Camfield CS: Neurologic aspects of craniosynostosis. In Cohen MM Jr (ed): Craniosynostosis. New York: Raven Press, 1986, pp 215–226.
37. David DJ, Poswillo D, Simpson D: The Craniosynostoses: Causes, Natural History, and Management. Berlin: Springer-Verlag, 1982.
38. De Castro P, Pascual-Castroviejo I: Evolucion mental de 108 casos con craneosinostosis. An Esp Pediatr 15:443–448, 1981.
39. Ingraham FD, Alexander E Jr, Matson DD: Clinical studies in craniosynostosis. Surgery 24:518–541, 1948.
40. McLaurin RL, Matson DD: Importance of early surgical treatment in craniosynostosis: Review of thirty-six cases treated during the first six months of life. Pediatrics 10:637–652, 1952.
41. Laitinen L, Miettinin P, Sulamaa M: Ophthalmological observations in craniosynostosis. Acta Ophthalmol (Copenh) 34 (Suppl 44–45):121–132, 1956.
42. Blodi FC: Developmental anomalies of the skull affecting the eye. Acta Ophthalmol (Copenh) 57:593–610, 1957.
43. Lecuire J, Lapras C: A propos des craniosténoses et de leur traitement chirurgical. Neurochirurgie 7:35–42, 1961.
44. Pemberton JW, Freeman JM: Craniosynostosis. Am J Ophthalmol 54:641–650, 1962.
45. Vigouroux R, Choux M, Baurand C: Les craniosténoses: A propos de 11 cas. Pediatrie 20:409–412, 1965.

46. Farnarier G, Mouly A, Liechstenteger J, Djiane D: Les signes ophthal-mologiques des craniosynostoses (à propos de 219 cas). Bull Soc Ophthalmol Fr 77:853–856, 1977.
47. Loffredo A, Sammartino A, De Crecchio G: Crouzon disease in twins. Ophthalmologica 175:297–304, 1977.
48. Greig DM: Oxycephaly. Edinb Med J 33:189–218, 280–302, 357–376, 1926.
49. Cayotte JL: Les Troubles Oculaires dans L'Oxycéphalie. Nancy: These Med, 1927.
50. Lindenberger R, Walsh FP: Vascular compression involving intracran-ial visual pathways. Trans Am Acad Ophthalmol Otolaryngol 68:677–694, 1964.
51. Wood-Smith D, Epstein F, Marello D: Transcranial decompression of the optic nerve in the osseous canal in Crouzon's disease. Clin Plast Surg 3:621–623, 1976.
52. Bergstrom L, Nesblett L, Hemenway W: Otologic manifestations of acrocephalosyndactyly. Arch Otolaryngol Head Neck Surg 96:117–123, 1972.
53. Di Rocco C: Intracranial volume and intracranial pressure in cranio-synostosis. Crit Rev Neurosurg 3:235–240, 1993.
54. Posnick JC, Bite U, Nakano P, et al: Indirect intracranial volume measurements using CT scans: Clinical application for cranio-synostosis. Plast Reconstr Surg 89:34–35, 1992.
55. Fox H, Jones BB, Gault DG, et al: Relationship between intracranial pressure and intracranial volume in craniosynostosis. Br J Plast Surg 45:394–397, 1992.
56. Renier D, Sainte-Rose C, Marchac D, Hirsch JF: Intracranial pressure in craniostenosis. J Neurosurg 57:370–377, 1982.
57. Caldarelli M, Di Rocco C, Rossi GF: Lumbar subarachnoid infusion test in pediatric neurosurgery. Dev Med Child Neurol 21:71–82, 1979.
58. Di Rocco C, Iannelli A, Velardi F: Early diagnosis and surgical indication in craniosynostosis. Childs Nerv Syst 6:176–188, 1980.
59. Lundar T, Norne SH: Steady-state lumbar infusion tests in the man-agement of children with craniosynostosis. Childs Nerv Syst 7:31–33, 1991.
60. Chadduck WM, Chadduck JB, Boop FA: The subarachnoid spaces in craniosynostosis. Neurosurgery 30:867–871, 1992.
61. Hogan G, Bauman M: Hydrocephalus in Apert's syndrome. J Pediatr 79:782–787, 1971.
62. Hoffman HJ, Hendrick EB: Early neurosurgical repair in craniofacial dysmorphism. J Neurosurg 51:796–803, 1979.
63. Holtermuller K, Wiedemann HR: Kleeblattschädel-syndrome. Med Monatsschr 14:439–446, 1960.
64. Shiroyama Y, Ito H, Yamashita T, et al: The relationship of cloverleaf skull syndrome to hydrocephalus. Childs Nerv Syst 7:382–385, 1991.
65. Marchac D, Renier D: Craniofacial Surgery for Craniosynostosis. Boston: Little, Brown, 1982.
66. Jane JA, Edgerton MT, Futrell JW, Park TS: Immediate correction of sagittal synostosis. J Neurosurg 11:537–542, 1978.
67. Stein SC, Schut L: Management of scaphocephaly. Surg Neurol 7:153–155, 1977.
68. Park TS, Haworth CS, Jane JA, et al: A modified prone position for cranial remodeling procedures in children with craniofacial dys-morphism: A technical note. Neurosurgery 16:212–214, 1985.
69. Seeger JF, Gabrielsen TO: Premature closure of the frontosphenoidal suture in synostosis of the coronal suture. Radiology 101:631–635, 1971.
70. Hoffmann HJ, Mohr G: Lateral canthal advancement of the supraor-bital margin. J Neurosurg 45:376–381, 1976.
71. Raimondi AJ, Gutierrez FA: A new surgical approach to the treatment of coronal synostosis. J Neurosurg 46:210–214, 1977.
72. Marchac D, Cophignon J, Hirsch JF, Renier D: Remodelage fronto-cranien des craniosténoses avec mobilisation du bandeau frontal. Neurochirurgie 24:23–27, 1978.
73. Epstein F, McCarthy JG, Coccaro PJ: Prophylactic craniofacial sur-gery. Childs Nerv Syst 5:204–215, 1979.
74. McCarthy JG, Karp NS, Lo Trenta GS, Thorne CHM: The effect of early fronto-orbital advancement on frontal sinus development and forehead aesthetics. Plast Reconstr Surg 86:1078–1084, 1990.
75. Cohen SR, Kawamoto HK, Burstein F, Peacock WJ: Advancement-onlay: An improved technique of fronto-orbital remodeling in cranio-synostosis. Childs Nerv Syst 7:264–271, 1991.
76. Di Rocco C, Velardi F, Ferrario A, Marchese E: Metopic synostosis: In favour of a "simplified" surgical treatment. Childs Nerv Syst 12:654–663, 1996.
77. Powiertowski H: Surgery of craniostenosis in advanced cases. In Krayenbuhl H (ed): Advances and Technical Standards in Neurosur-gery, Vol 1. New York: Springer-Verlag, 1974, pp 93–119.
78. Persing JA, Jane JA, Delashaw JB: Treatment of bilateral coronal synostosis in infancy: A holistic approach. J Neurosurg 72:171–175, 1990.
79. Goldin JH: The timing of surgical treatment for severe cranio-synostosis. In Caronni EP (ed): Craniofacial Surgery, Vol 3. Bologna: Moduzzi Editore, 1991, pp 307–309.
80. Di Rocco C, Scogna A, Velardi F, Zambelli HJL: Posterior plagio-cephaly: Craniosynostosis or molding? Crit Rev Neurosurg 8:122–130, 1998.
81. Dias MS, Klein DM, Backstrom JW: Occipital plagiocephaly: Defor-mation or lambdoid synostosis? I. Morphometric analysis and results of unilateral lambdoid craniectomy. Pediatr Neurosurg 24:61–68, 1996.
82. Dias MS, Klein DM: Occipital plagiocephaly: Deformation or lamb-doid synostosis? II. A unifying theory regarding pathogenesis. Pediatr Neurosurg 24:69–73, 1996.
83. Huang MHS, Gruss JS, Clarren SK, et al: The differential diagnosis of posterior plagiocephaly: true lambdoid synostosis versus positional molding. Plast Reconstr Surg 98:765–774, 1996.
84. Lo LJ, Marsh JL, Pilgram TK, Vannier MW: Plagiocephaly: Differen-tial diagnosis based on endocranial morphology. Plast Reconstr Surg 97:282–291, 1996.
85. Pople IK, Sanford RA, Muhlbauer MS: Clinical presentation and management of 100 infants with occipital plagiocephaly. Pediatr Neu-rosurg 25:1–6, 1996.
86. Sawin PD, Muhonen MG, Menezes AH: Quantitative analysis of cerebrospinal fluid spaces in children with occipital plagiocephaly. J Neurosurg 85:428–434, 1996.
87. Goodrich JT, Argamaso R: Lambdoid stenosis (posterior plagioceph-aly) and craniofacial asymmetry: Long-term outcomes. Childs Nerv Syst 12:720–726, 1996.
88. Kearney RA, Rosales JK, Howes WJ: Craniosynostosis: An assess-ment of blood loss and transfusion practices. Can J Anaesth 36:473–477, 1989.
89. Velardi F, Di Chirico A, Di Rocco C, et al: "No allogeneic blood transfusion" protocol for the surgical correction of craniosynostosis: I. Rationale. Childs Nerv Syst 14:722–731, 1998.
90. Jones BM, Jani P, Bingham RM, et al: Complications in paediatric craniofacial surgery: An initial four year experience. Br J Plast Surg 45:225–231, 1992.

# CHAPTER 10

# Surgical Management of Encephaloceles

■ LUIS SCHUT

Among the less common of the congenital malformations of the central nervous system (CNS), hernias of the cerebral contents through an opening in the cranium have long been recognized. The presence of a cranial opening (cranium bifidum) is similar to the more common problem of spina bifida occulta and, as in the latter entity, does not by itself presuppose the presence of cerebral hernia. However, when a mass extrudes through the defect, it can be composed entirely of meninges and cerebrospinal fluid (CSF) (meningocele), can be accompanied by a variable amount of CNS tissue (encephalocele), or can be a combination of these—myeloencephalocele or, in the most severe cases, a true herniation of the brain, the meninges, and the ventricular system (hydroencephalomeningocele). The incidence of this congenital malformation is between 5% and 15% of all dysraphic states.

The true incidence of this malformation changes with the geographic location[1] of the patient and has been reported as one in 3000 live births in portions of the Far East to one in 10,000 live births in the Western Hemisphere.[2] The location of the encephalocele could be in the occipital region, frontoethmoidal area, or at the base of the cranium. Other reported sites for these hernias are in the interparietal region and, much less commonly, lateral to the midline in the region of the pterion or asterion. The pathophysiology of encephaloceles is still obscure and has generated many theories. One of the theories is the failure of the anterior neuropore at the cephalic end of the neural tube to close, an event that normally occurs on the 24th day of development at the level of the foramen cecum in the frontal bone. The resultant malformation is usually severe and is often incompatible with life, in the form of anencephaly or exencephaly (Fig. 10–1). Other pathophysiologic possibilities include the often quoted ideas of Dr. James Gardner,[3] who postulated that the single origin for many of the congenital malformations is the failure of the rhombic roof to perforate, producing hydrocephalus and secondary rupture of the neural tube at different levels. This theory could explain different pathologic variations from myelomeningocele to encephalocele. Another possible explanation is the production of blebs or ruptures of the neural tube with secondary adhesions between the neuroectoderm and ectoderm and defects in the mesoderm. Finally, defects in the membra-

nous cranium and shortening of the cranial base with mesodermal insufficiency could be the etiologic factor.

## CLINICAL FEATURES

A visible and palpable mass exists in cranial vault encephaloceles, more commonly in the occipital region just below or above the expected location of the torcula. The defect is sometimes covered completely with skin or a tenuous membrane. The defect is usually accompanied by other cutaneous signs, such as hemangioma or hypertrichosis. Characteristically, the hair at the base of the encephalocele is much coarser and thicker. In unusual cases, there is complete absence of cutaneous coverage and exposed neural tissue. In anterior encephaloceles, hypertelorism fre-

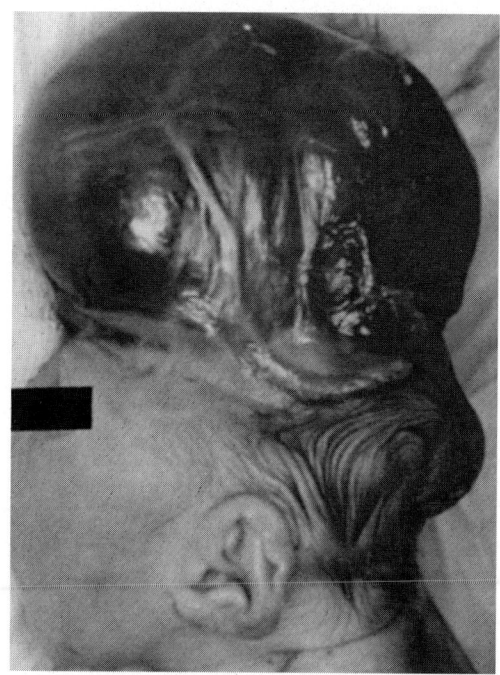

FIGURE 10–1 ■ An encephalic newborn.

quently exists, sometimes accompanied by clefts and ocular problems (e.g., coloboma). On basal encephaloceles, the patient frequently presents with respiratory or swallowing difficulties because of masses in the region of the nose or anterior pharynx and the volume of the encephalocele.

## PREOPERATIVE EVALUATION

The patient presenting with encephalocele must be evaluated by a team that includes the neonatologist, neuroanesthesiologist, intensive care specialist, and neurosurgeon. The neurosurgeon decides if the patient should be operated on as an emergency, such as when tissue is either exposed or leaking CSF or when correction can be delayed if the area is covered by good skin.

## PATIENT SELECTION AND DECISION MANAGEMENT

The family must be thoroughly informed of the problems likely to be encountered during the surgical management of the encephalocele and the prognosis. They should also be told what the experience has been with similar cases in a long-term follow-up. The pediatric consultant and neonatologist should ensure that no other congenital defects exist that would alter the prognosis. Obviously, in cases in which another major anomaly exists (e.g., congenital heart disease or trisomy), the viability of the patient may come into question. In these cases, proceeding with repair of the encephalocele until the total health of the child is considered makes little sense. Even in cases in which large portions of nonviable cerebral tissue extrude from the defect and there are gross indications of cerebral damage by the presence of either microcephaly or marked hydrocephalus, it is still important to make the family aware of problems that will occur in the future. Most of these children do not die rapidly unless there is an infection or severe respiratory involvement. We have encountered problems with placement of such patients in nursing facilities simply because of the mechanical problems of dealing with large encephaloceles. Surgical repair is commonly forced on the neurosurgeon by the practical necessities of daily nursing care of the infant.

## CHOICE OF SURGICAL APPROACH

The surgical approach depends entirely on the location of the encephalocele and the results of the assessment of the contents of the mass. With the advent of modern neuroimaging techniques, it is now imperative that the neurosurgeon have a clear idea of the anatomic variations involved and be aware of the possibility of other congenital malformations of the CNS in the patient being treated. Computed tomography (CT) scan, particularly with bone windows or three-dimensional reconstruction, allows the location to be determined and, in most cases, permits assessment of the contents of the encephalocele sac. Magnetic resonance imaging (MRI) is invaluable in identifying more complicated associated anomalies, and we have been using nuclear magnetic angiography to study the vasculature of the herniated portions of the CNS, particularly in relation to the large venous sinuses.

## ANESTHESIA CONSIDERATIONS

The neuroanesthesiologist familiar with the treatment of children with congenital abnormalities is an integral part of the team that evaluates these patients. Because of the variations in location of the masses and the difficult problems that may arise during intubation, operative procedure, and postoperative management, the necessity of having the patients under the care of well-trained personnel is self-evident. All of these operations are done with the patient under general endotracheal anesthesia, and this procedure could become quite difficult if the patient has a large nasopharyngeal mass. Because of the unexpected locations of the major venous sinuses, provisions should be made for transfusion that, in unusual cases, could equal or surpass the circulating blood volume. The possibility of raised intracranial pressure (ICP) due to pre-existing hydrocephalus is also a consideration, as is the position of the patient on the operating table, which is dictated by the location of the mass.

## CASE REPORTS

Figure 10–2 shows the intrauterine diagnosis of a nasoethmoidal encephalocele. In this case, it was possible to discuss with the parents the implications of the malformation as well as to make arrangements to have the child delivered by cesarean section because of the large volume of the encephalocele.

Figure 10–3 reveals a child born with an occipital encephalocele, which was found to be mostly CSF and meninges with very little neural tissue.

Figure 10–4 shows the surgical exposure and demonstrates the communication of the large encephalocele with the ventricular system as well as the extruded choroid plexus through the cranial opening. Surgical correction in this case is relatively simple, necessitating only the preparation of the false dura mater by preservation of the inner layer of the sac. The sac is then imbricated and sutured in a watertight fashion, with secondary closure of the scalp itself. In most cases, a cranioplasty is unnecessary because if the ICP is under control, secondary ossification of the defect will occur.

Figure 10–5 shows an enormous occipital encephalocele that consists mainly of CSF, but MRI (Fig. 10–6) clearly demonstrates that portions of the CNS are herniating through and a well-demarcated hernia of the occipital pole exists that could be dissected free from the rest of the encephalocele and returned to the cranial cavity. Care should be taken in similar cases to ascertain the location

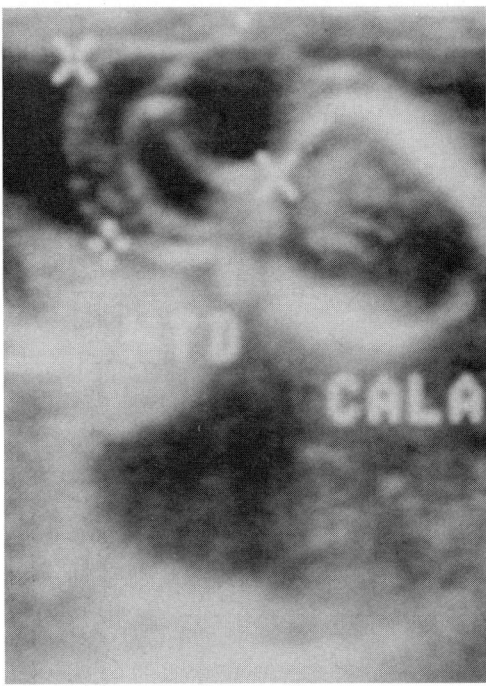

FIGURE 10–2 ■ Encephalocele in utero.

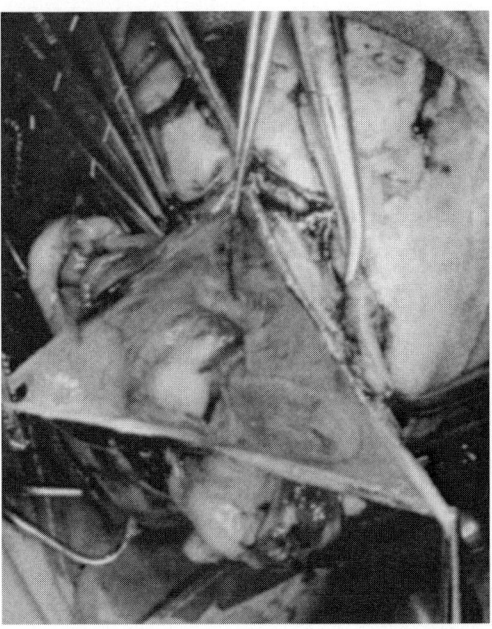

FIGURE 10–4 ■ Operative view demonstrating communication with the ventricle.

of the torcula and, obviously, preserve the vascular anatomy and reintegrate it into the cranial cavity.

Figure 10–7 shows a newborn baby with occipital encephalocele, but in this case, the contents are mainly herniated neural tissue with very little CSF. This presents a surgical dilemma to the neurosurgeon. If the examination, both radiologic and at the time of surgery, shows that the mass has extruded through a very small opening and does not have the cytoarchitecture of normal brain, the tissue can be amputated and then repair can be performed. However, if assessment reveals viable brain in the mass, every effort should be made to preserve the tissue. The opening

in the cranium must be enlarged to ameliorate the compression of the brain. The dura mater should be closed either with the inner layer of the sac or, if not available, with artificial dura, such as fascia lata, pericrania, or lyophilized cadaveric dura. Although this method will not correct the large defect, a secondary operation can be done later to reconstruct the bone defect.

Figures 10–8 and 10–9 show two examples of encephaloceles not covered with skin. In both cases, the tissue was necrotic and nonviable and could be safely removed.

Figure 10–10 is an example of a nasoethmoidal encephalocele, in this case a pedunculated one, that can clearly be seen from the intracranial exposure. This encephalocele has a small tract that can be easily divided and repaired.

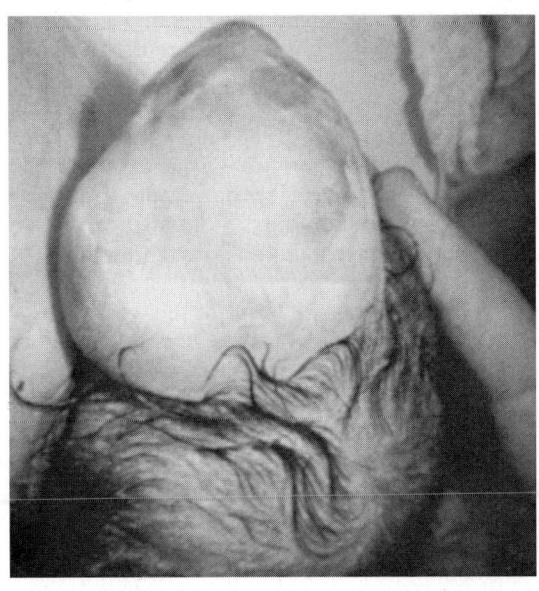

FIGURE 10–3 ■ Occipital encephalocele.

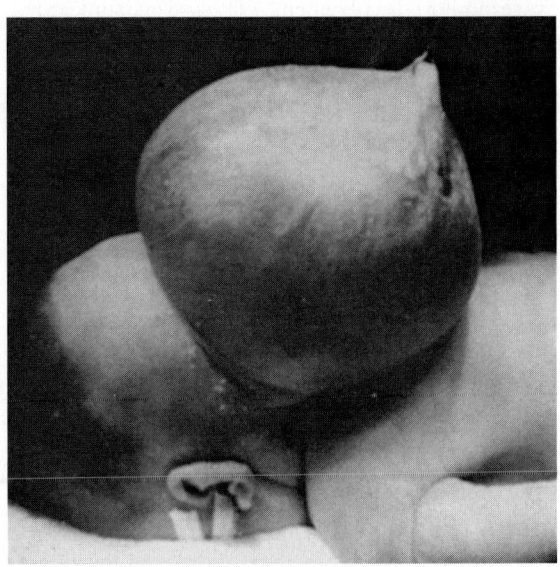

FIGURE 10–5 ■ A large occipital encephalocele.

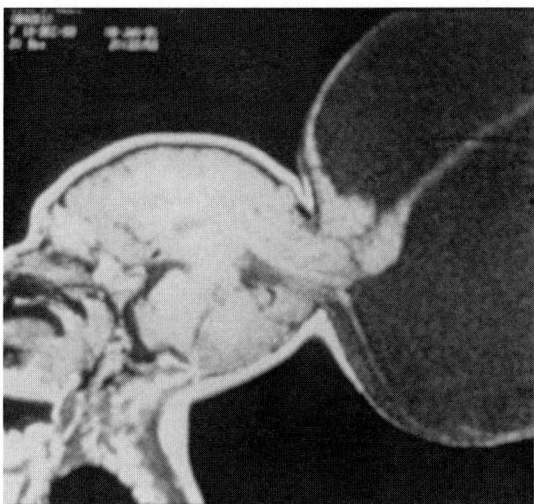

FIGURE 10–6 ■ A magnetic resonance imaging scan of the same patient as in Figure 10–5.

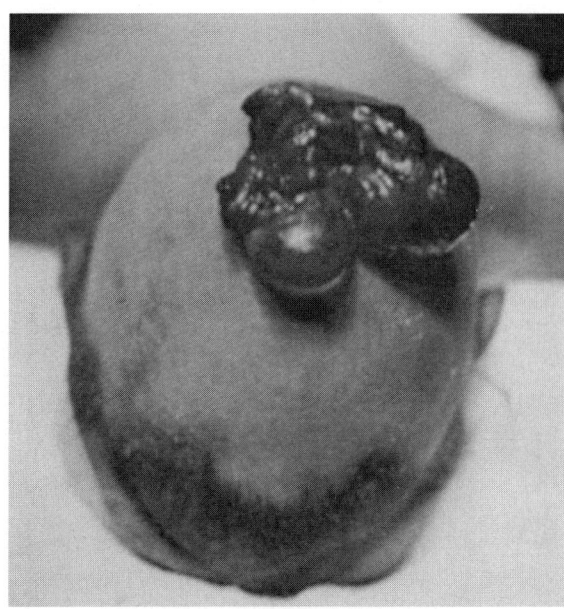

FIGURE 10–8 ■ Cerebral hernia.

The defect in the skull was closed in this case (Fig. 10–11) by a small portion of bone obtained from the squamous portion of the temporal bone underneath the temporalis muscle. The bone will regenerate quickly.

Figures 10–12 and 10–13 show a patient with a more complicated naso-orbital encephalocele who presented at birth with a large interocular mass, herniation of the meninges through the inner canthus of the eye, and hypertelorism. In such cases, the experienced craniofacial reconstruction team should be able to repair the encephalocele, close the cranial defect, and treat the hypertelorism in the same operation.

In the newborn, it is very easy to approximate the orbital walls after removal of the medial portion of bone, and this should be done at an early stage, if possible, to prevent more severe deformities and a much more complicated repair later in life (Figs. 10–14 and 10–15).

Figures 10–16 and 10–17 represent a very large nasoencephalocele composed exclusively of meninges and

CSF. The surgical correction is straightforward, but in our experience, this defect always requires an intracranial approach. In practically all cases, intradural exploration is necessary as well to identify the posterior aspect of the herniated sac and prepare it for further imbrication and surgical closure.

Figures 10–18 and 10–19 show a patient with a nasoethmoidal encephalocele with a broader base. Both the CT scan (Fig. 10–20) and three-dimensional reconstruction of the skull (Fig. 10–21) allowed an intelligent assessment of the surgical approach before the actual operation. In this case, a bifrontal craniotomy with intradural exploration allowed return of the contents of the sac to the cranial cavity and closure of the dura mater. The craniofacial reconstruction team was able to correct the hypertelorism at the same time.

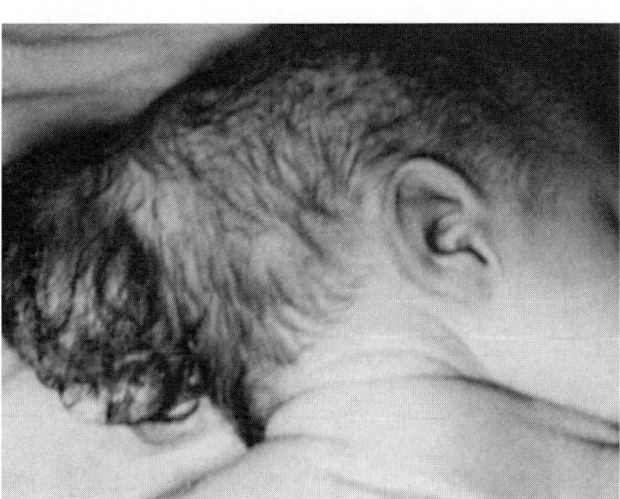

FIGURE 10–7 ■ An occipital encephalocele with neural tissue.

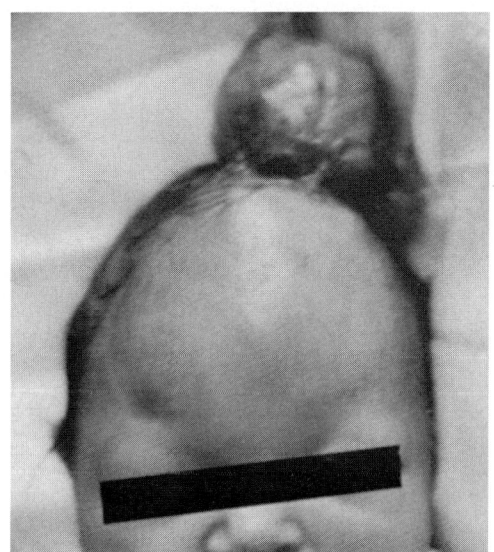

FIGURE 10–9 ■ Cerebral hernia.

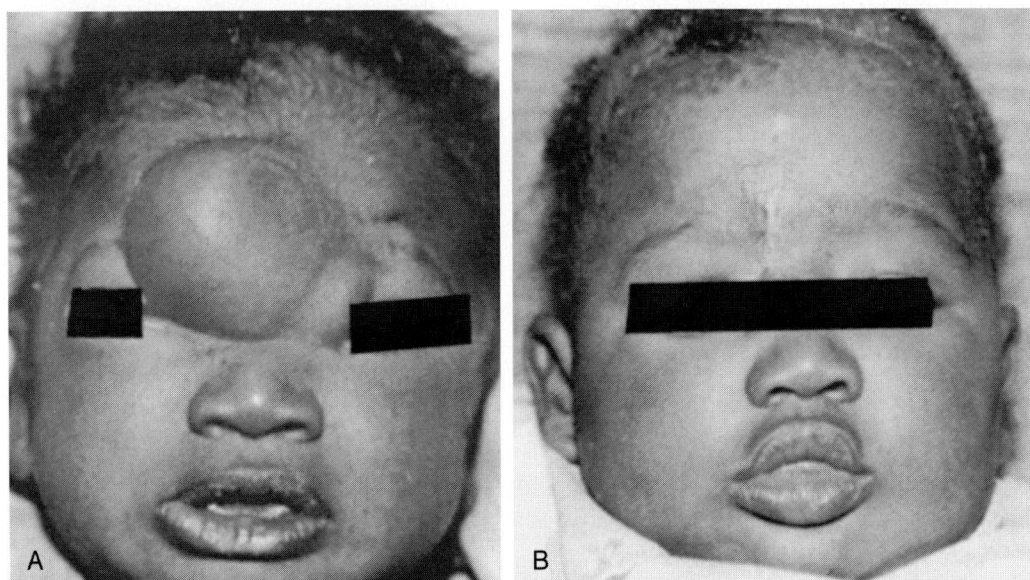

**FIGURE 10–10** ■ *A*, Preoperative nasoethmoidal encephalocele. *B*, Postoperative nasoethmoidal encephalocele.

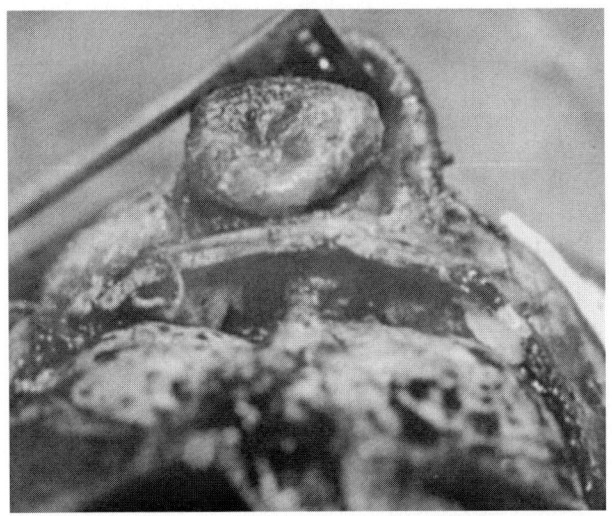

**FIGURE 10–11** ■ Operative view of the same patient as in Figure 10–10.

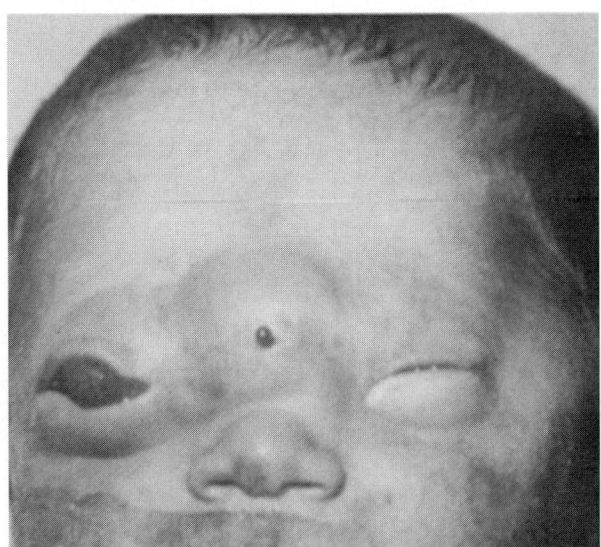

**FIGURE 10–12** ■ Complicated naso-orbital encephalocele.

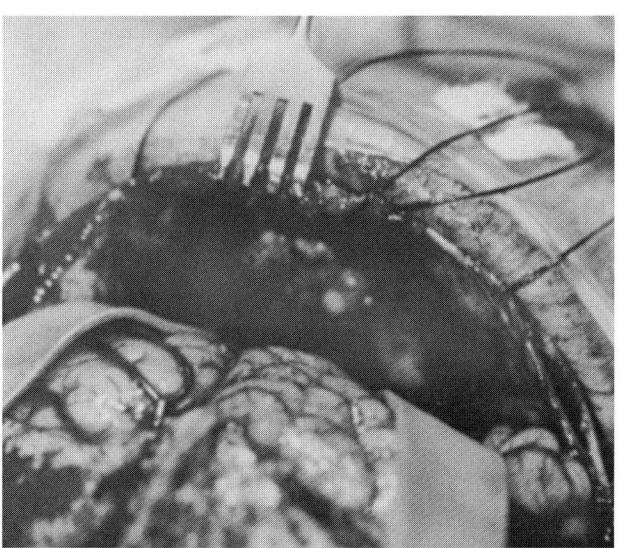

**FIGURE 10–13** ■ Operative view of the same patient as in Figure 10–12.

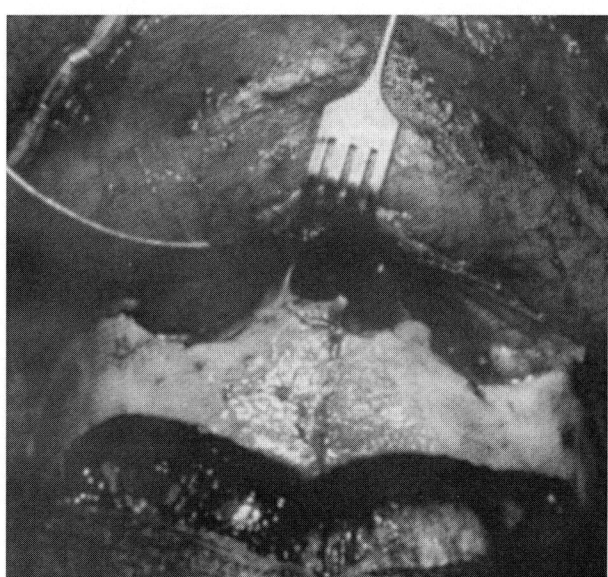

**FIGURE 10–14** ■ Repair of the hypertelorism found in the same patient as in Figure 10–12.

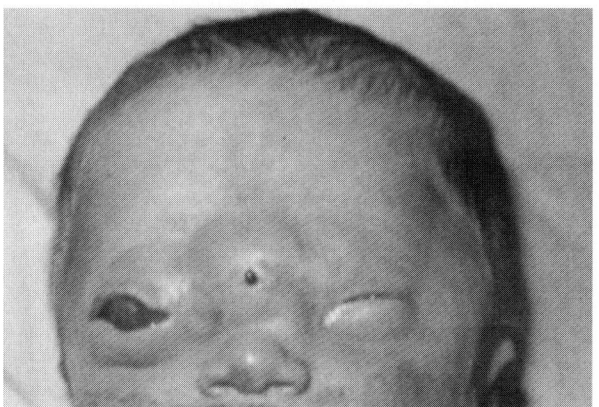

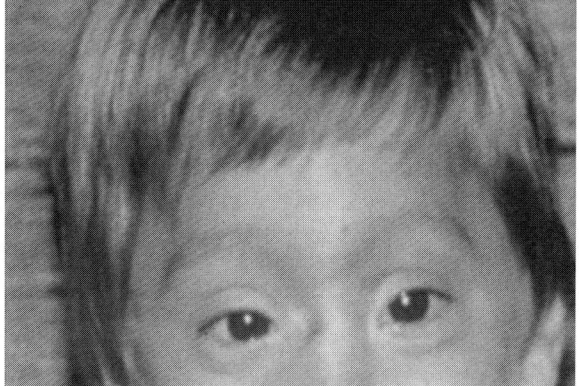

**FIGURE 10–15** ■ The end result of surgery in the same patient as in Figure 10–12.

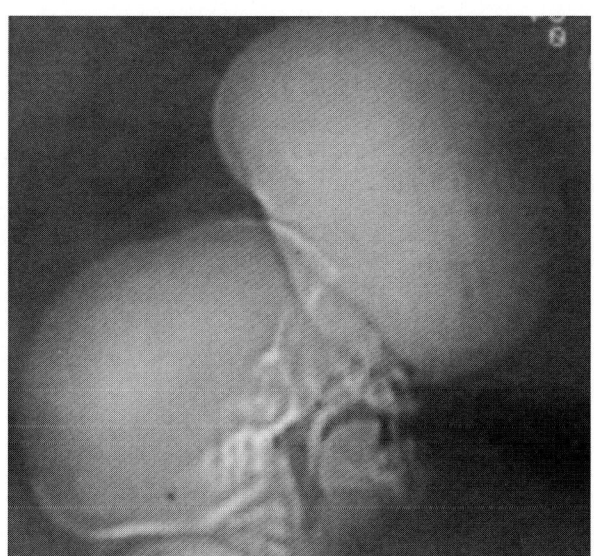

**FIGURE 10–16** ■ A computed tomography scan of a patient with a large nasal encephalocele.

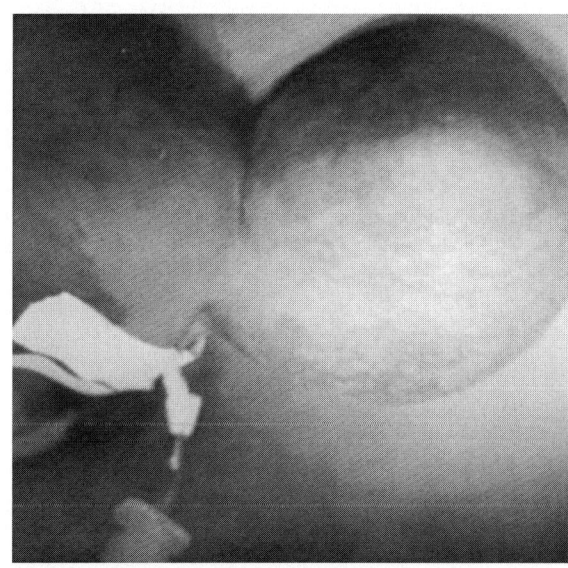

**FIGURE 10–17** ■ A preoperative view of the same patient as in Figure 10–16.

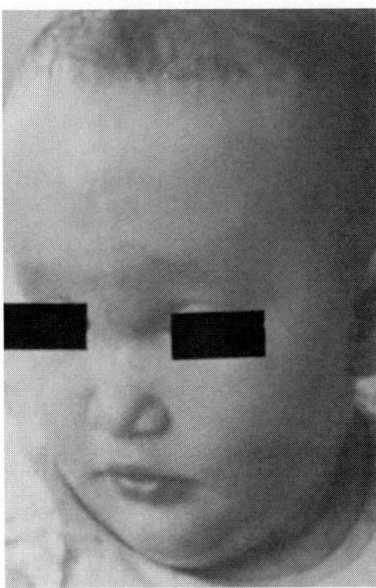

**FIGURE 10–18** ■ A postoperative view of the same patient as in Figure 10–16.

Figures 10–22 and 10–23 show one of the most complicated dilemmas confronting the neurosurgeon dealing with encephaloceles. This child presented with respiratory distress and inability to swallow. Examination of the nasopharynx demonstrated a large mass protruding at the base of the skull. This mass was diagnosed initially as a nasal polyp, but it is important to remember that infants do not commonly have this disorder, and masses of this type are much more likely to represent encephaloceles. We have seen past attempts at biopsy that resulted in CSF leakage and secondary meningitis. In this child, MRI revealed a

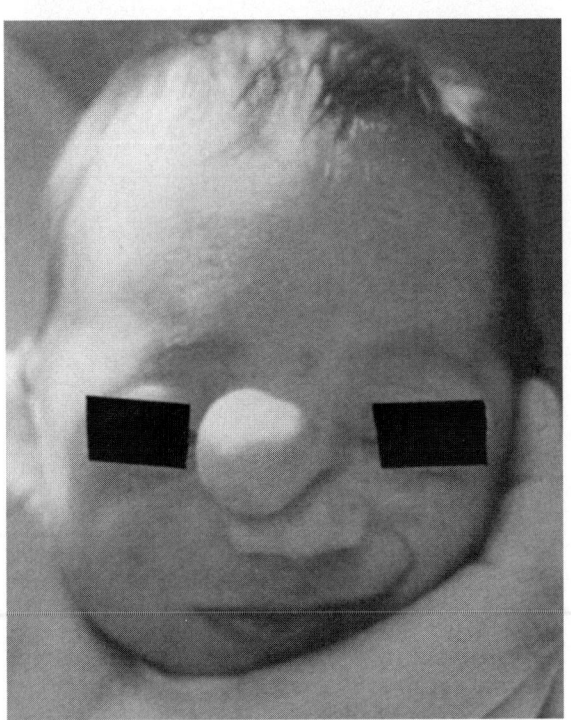

**FIGURE 10–19** ■ A patient with a broad-based nasal encephalocele.

herniation not only of the meninges but also of the anterior third ventricle, portions of the chiasm, and much of the hypothalamus. The neurosurgeon should be extremely cautious in these cases. Obviously, any attempts at amputating the extruded mass will result in a catastrophe. In this particular case, a shunt was inserted 1 week before the operation, which allowed enough relaxation of the intracranial contents to be able to bring back to the cranial cavity all of the herniated material. Both an extradural and an intradural approach were used to the encephalocele, which was then repaired, and, with portions of autologous bone, the floor of the cranium was closed, preventing further herniation through the region of the sphenoid sinus.

Figure 10–24 represents a lateral cleft syndrome with nasoencephalocele and colobomas of the eye. The encephalocele was repaired through a bicoronal craniotomy with both intradural and extradural dissection and return of the hernia to the cranial cavity. The cleft lip and palate were subsequently treated surgically.

Figure 10–25 illustrates a bilateral cleft syndrome with hydrocephalus and cerebral hernia, which on CT scan (Fig. 10–26) was found to result from a ruptured ventricular system that had herniated through the anterior fontanelle. The treatment would be the insertion of a ventriculoperitoneal shunt as a first step to reduce the ICP, secondary repair of the cranial hernia, and, later, plastic repair of the facial clefts.

Figure 10–27 is an illustration of the so-called nasal glioma, which consists of small portions of brain tissue that have extruded, usually through the foramen cecum. Subsequently, during development, there is complete closure of the cranial bones as well as the meninges. Thus, the CNS tissue becomes trapped outside the cranium. Although these do not represent true gliomas, the term has become ingrained in the literature. These masses are better taken care of through an external approach after ensuring through CT with bone windows that no communication with the intracranial cavity exists.

## MAJOR INTRAOPERATIVE COMPLICATIONS

Major intraoperative complications are usually related to blood loss secondary to inadvertent opening of the venous sinuses, which can be displaced and can sometimes be extracranial in position. In rare cases, the complication results from removal of tissue at the time of surgery that involves vital structures of the brain, such as the hypothalamus or brain stem in occipital encephaloceles. In the postoperative period, the patient should be watched carefully for the onset of hydrocephalus, which should be treated accordingly. Many of these children remain in follow-up for years for treatment of their other malformations and may require multiple procedures, both by the neurosurgical team and by plastic surgeons.

The end result is not usually dictated by the neurosurgical procedure per se but by the involvement of the brain in the encephalocele and the presence of other congenital anomalies. In long-term follow-up, cases with an anterior defect have a better prognosis for function: More than half of the children have normal intelligence,[4] and another 20% are mildly affected. In large posterior defects, the prognosis is more severe. In children with hydrocephalus, fewer than 20% will have normal intelligence, and in those without

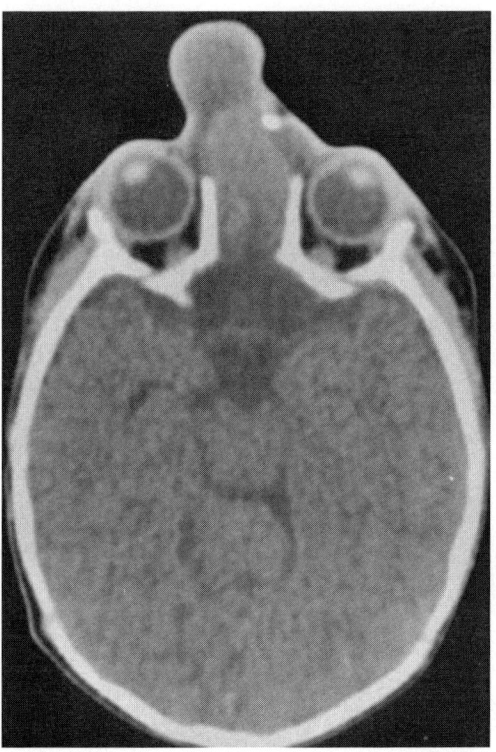

FIGURE 10–20 ■ A computed tomography scan of the same patient as in Figure 10–19.

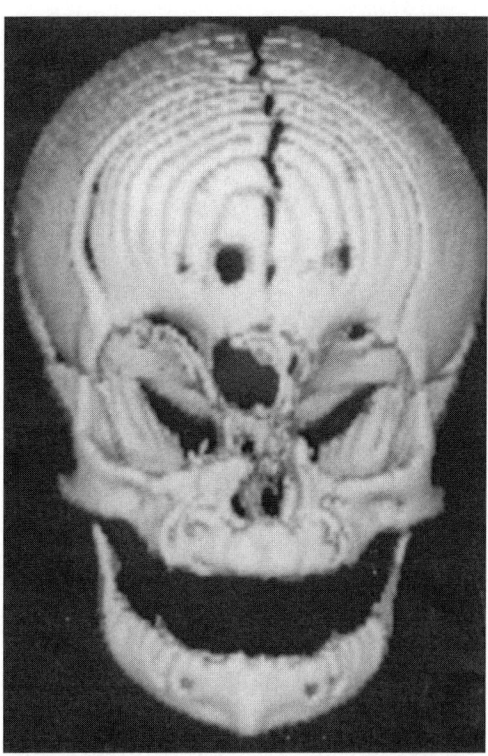

FIGURE 10–21 ■ Three-dimensional computed tomography reconstruction of the same patient as in Figure 10–20, demonstrating a cranial defect.

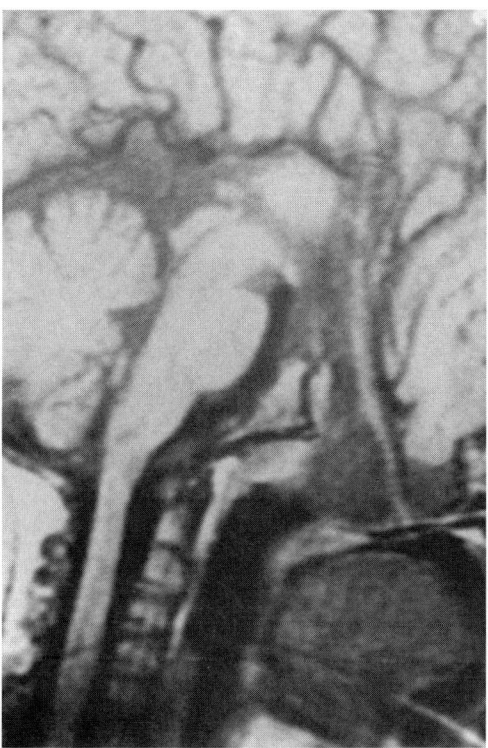

FIGURE 10–22 ■ A magnetic resonance imaging scan of a sphenoid encephalocele (lateral view).

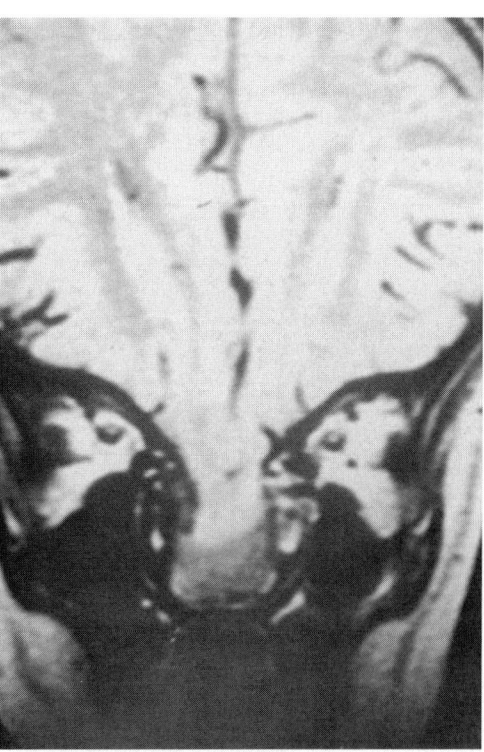

FIGURE 10–23 ■ A magnetic resonance imaging scan of a sphenoid encephalocele (coronal view).

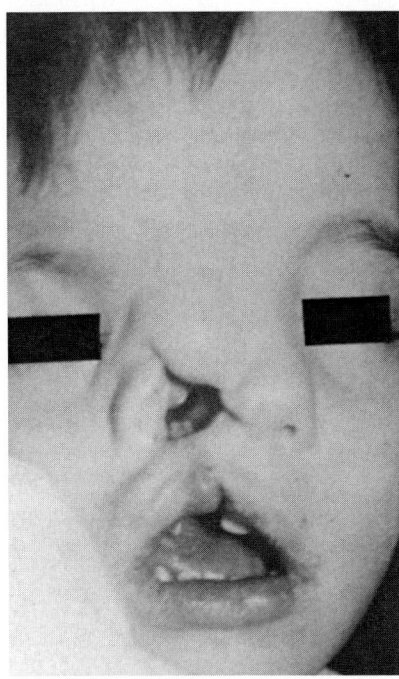

FIGURE 10–24 ■ Lateral cleft syndrome.

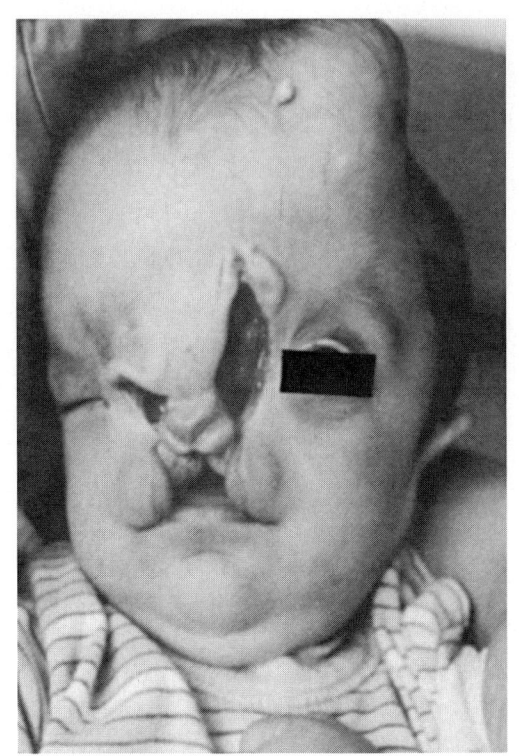

FIGURE 10–25 ■ Bilateral cleft syndrome with hydrocephalus.

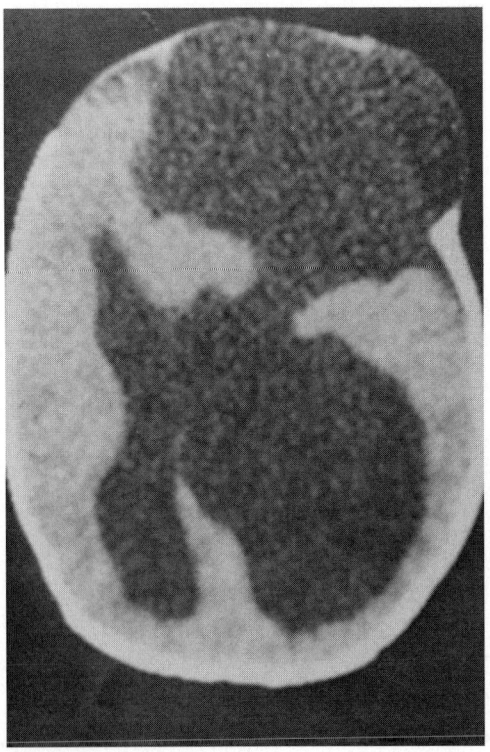

FIGURE 10–26 ■ A computed tomography scan of the patient with bilateral cleft syndrome as in Figure 10–25.

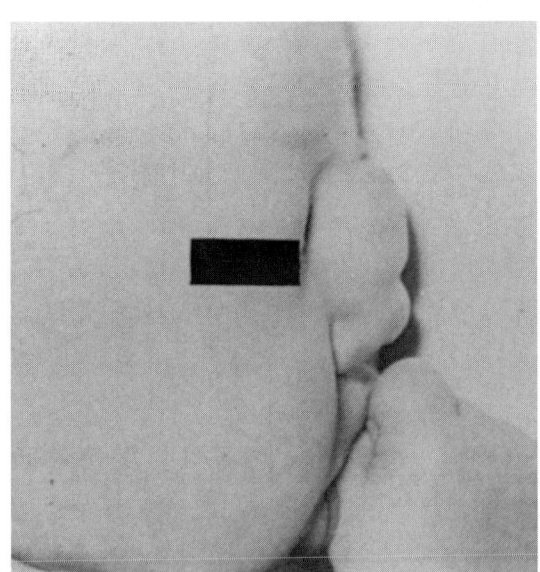

FIGURE 10–27 ■ Nasal glioma.

hydrocephalus, 50% either will have normal intelligence or will be in the mildly retarded range.

## REFERENCES

1. Suwanwela C, Chaturaporn H: Frontoethmoidal encephalocele. J Neurosurg 25:172, 1966.
2. James H: Encephaloceles, dermoid sinus and arachnoid cyst. In McLaurin L, Schut L, Venes L, Epstein F (eds): Pediatric Neurosurgery, 2nd ed. Philadelphia: WB Saunders, 1989, pp 97–106.
3. Gardner WJ: The dysraphic states from syringomyelia to anencephaly. Amsterdam: Excerpta Medica, 1973.
4. Brown M, Sheridan-Pereira M: Outlook for the child with a cephalocele. Pediatrics 90:914–919, 1992.

## CHAPTER 11

# Surgical Management of Trauma Involving the Skull Base and Paranasal Sinuses

■ FRANZ XAVER BRUNNER

Traffic accidents frequently cause trauma to the midface and frontal skull base. In many cases, there are post-traumatic functional deficits, deformities, and stressful psychosocial problems accompanying facial distortions. The availability of microsurgical reconstruction techniques, using tissue adhesive, preserved dura, resorbable materials, and thin rigid titanium plates for osteosynthesis, puts more demands on the quality of surgery in maxillofacial and skull base trauma. By means of miniplate and microplate osteosynthesis, secure stabilization of the midface can be achieved after even extensive fractures of the midface or the floor of the anterior cranial fossa. This procedure is considered a satisfactory operative treatment in terms of cosmetic and functional results. As a rule, sealing of the frontal skull base should be performed before repairing the fractures of the midface. The postoperative results depend on the extent of the primary bone or soft tissue lesions. To achieve satisfactory results in operative treatment, a team approach is necessary.

## MECHANISMS OF INJURY

Most midfacial fractures occur in men and are related to high-impact forces usually sustained in motor vehicle accidents, industrial accidents, fist fights, aggravated assaults, sports injuries, and falls. Direct injuries lead to skull base and Le Fort maxillary fractures. In many cases, isolated depressed pieces of bone occur in addition to multiple fractures of the glabellar area and the anterior walls of frontal sinuses combined with skull base fractures.

Head-on collisions account for approximately one half of all motorist injuries. For drivers who fail to use lap and shoulder seat belts, such a collision is likely to throw them face on into the windshield. In a broadside collision on the driver's side, bony injuries to the temporal skull area and zygomatic and nasal bones may occur, whereas midfacial fractures are less likely.

## ANATOMIC AND PATHOPHYSIOLOGIC ASPECTS AND FRACTURE CLASSIFICATIONS

The maxillary bones consist of a body and four processes: frontal, zygomatic, palatine, and alveolar. The body contains the maxillary sinus. All paranasal sinuses are air-filled extensions of the nasal cavity, which is developed in the bones of the skull.

The anterior group comprises the frontal sinus, the maxillary sinus, and the anterior ethmoidal cells. The posterior group comprises the posterior ethmoidal cells and the sphenoidal sinus. The sinuses are classified according to drainage rather than to the actual anatomic distribution. The sinuses vary widely in their positions during development so that the distinction between anterior and posterior may be misleading. The anterior group of sinuses drains into the middle meatus, whereas the posterior group drains into the superior meatus and the sphenoethmoidal recess.

The fully developed maxillary sinus usually extends from the first premolar to the third molar tooth. The sinus reaches up to the floor of the orbit, occupying practically the whole body of the maxillary bone. The ostium lies in the medial wall. Additionally, a small accessory ostium may be anterior and inferior to it.

The frontal sinus occupies the space in the frontal bones between the inner and the outer tables. The sinus is not present at birth. It develops until the age of 5 years, when the air cells extend above the level of the supraorbital ridge. The fully developed frontal sinus may extend to the outer orbital angle, cranially into the frontal bone for a distance of several centimeters, and posteriorly above the roof of the orbit. The frontal sinuses are rarely symmetric and usually are separated from each other by a thin bony plate. The roof of the orbit forms the floor of the frontal sinus, containing the supraorbital nerve running toward the inner orbital angle and having attached to it, more medially, the trochlea of the superior oblique muscle.

The ethmoidal cells, although divided into two groups, must be regarded as one cell system from the point of view of development and treatment. In contrast to the other

147

sinuses, the ethmoidal cells consist of many small air-filled cells that do not have a regular symmetry or fixed number. They lie in the upper part of the lateral wall of the nose. Located laterally is the orbital periosteum, located inferiorly is a part of the maxillary air sinus, and superiorly the cells meet at the apex, although in the anterior part, the frontal sinus may be considered to be a superior anatomic structure.

The two sphenoidal sinuses occupy the body of the sphenoid bone. The sphenoidal sinuses may vary widely in shape and position. The ostium is high on the anterior wall of the sinus. In most skulls, pneumatization extends inferiorly below the pituitary fossa, which bulges into the sinus. At the outer anterior angle where the roof and the lateral wall meet, the optic foramen, which contains the optic nerve, is in close relation to the sphenoidal sinus. The lateral wall is in contact with the cavernous sinus and the carotid artery.

All sinuses are lined by ciliated mucous membranes, richly provided with glands, which are found mainly around the ostium. The cilia are constantly beating to reach the openings.

The bony structures of the midface are connected to the skull base by four vertical bony buttresses. The nasomaxillary or anterior buttress consists of the anterior part of the alveolus, the pyriform aperture, and the nasal process of the maxilla through the anterior lacrimal crest to the superior orbital rim and frontocranial attachment. The lateral buttress extends from a bony crest of the maxilla above the anterior molar teeth to the zygomatic process of the frontal bone superiorly and the zygomatic arch laterally. Posteriorly, the pterygomaxillary buttress joins the maxillary tuberosity to the cranial base through the pyramidal process of the palatine bone and the medial pterygoid plate of the sphenoid. Finally, there is an important median buttress or frontoethmoidal vomerine pillar connecting the frontal bone to the median palatine suture containing thinner and thicker parts of the bony nasal septum.

Fractures of the frontal sinuses are mainly fissures of the anterior walls, but in severe cases, they may involve the inner table and the dura. Serious effects may be expected if the fracture extends into the cribriform area with tearing of the dura. Maxillary fractures involve the middle third of the face, in which both maxillae are pushed backward. Initially, swelling obscures the displacement. If this swelling is not recognized quickly and reduced, an ugly "dish-face" deformity occurs.

Zygomatic fractures result from a blow or kick to the cheekbone. This type of fracture generally leads to an inward and downward displacement, which is commonly combined with a fracture of the orbital floor. Usually, there is an immediate diplopia, periorbital swelling, and enophthalmos. The affected eye lies at a lower level when compared with the contralateral one.

The Le Fort classifications (Fig. 11–1A) of midfacial fractures are still evolving and may continue to do so. Although midfacial fractures occur only infrequently in a pure Le Fort form and often present as comminuted fractures, the classification system provides useful means for analysis and communication (see Fig. 11–1B). In approximately 50% of all cases, the so-called Le Fort maxillary fractures are combined with fractures of the frontal skull

base. The Le Fort I fracture is a transverse low maxillary fracture involving a traumatic separation of the palate from the body of the maxilla. Le Fort II or pyramidal fractures are the most common of the three types; the fracture line passes through the nasal bones across the frontal process of the maxilla and the lacrimal bones descending through the infraorbital rim and through the lateral inferior wall of the maxillary sinus. Le Fort III fractures represent the most severe form of maxillary and craniofacial injury and result in a separation of the facial skeleton from the skull base. These fractures occur in approximately 20% of cases. In Le Fort III injuries, the fracture line originates high on the nasal bones, crosses the upper part of the frontal processes of the maxilla and lacrimal bones, and passes through the lamina papyracea and ethmoid sinuses. In the orbit, the fracture line passes posterior to the inferior orbital fissure. Combination fractures refer to Le Fort fractures on the same side of the face, such as Le Fort I and Le Fort III fractures. These fractures are uncommon and are often confused with nasal, nasomaxillary, and zygomatic fractures.

Isolated crush fractures within the nasal area or anterior wall of the frontal sinus, so-called central midfacial fractures (see Fig. 11–1C) without malocclusion, are often caused by impact forces (horse kick, foreign body) and are associated with fractures of the anterior skull base. The varieties of the different fractures of the anterior skull base or the *rhinobase* have been classified by Escher[1] (Fig. 11–2) as follows:

Type 1, the extended rhinobase fracture, a frontal crush fracture, is normally treated by both neurosurgeons and rhinosurgeons.
Type 2, the localized fracture, normally is a small fracture, often a microgap or a dura tear. The areas of predilection are the lamina cribrosa, crista galli, posterior area of the ethmoidal walls, and roof of sphenoid sinus.
Type 3 typically comprises the rhinobasal fractures with posterior displacement of the viscerocranium. Consequent on the depression and compression of the viscerocranium accompanying this posterior shift, a crush fracture of the rhinobase is often caused as well, particularly within the roof of the ethmoidal cell system.
Type 4 fractures are fronto-orbital within the rhinobase. The fracture gap runs from the lateral frontal area to the roof of the orbit. Dural tears and brain prolapse are often difficult to diagnose because of the natural packing caused by the orbital contents.

## DIAGNOSIS AND INDICATIONS FOR SURGERY

The diagnosis and treatment of frontobasal injuries require an interdisciplinary approach and should take into account potential lesions of the midfacial region, orbit, paranasal sinuses, and intracranial cavity. The upper paranasal sinuses, the posterior wall of the frontal sinus, the roof of the ethmoidal cells, and the sphenoid sinus are directly adjacent to the frontal skull base. Even without soft tissue lesions of the face, fractures of the frontal skull base have to be considered indirect open wounds. Lacerations of

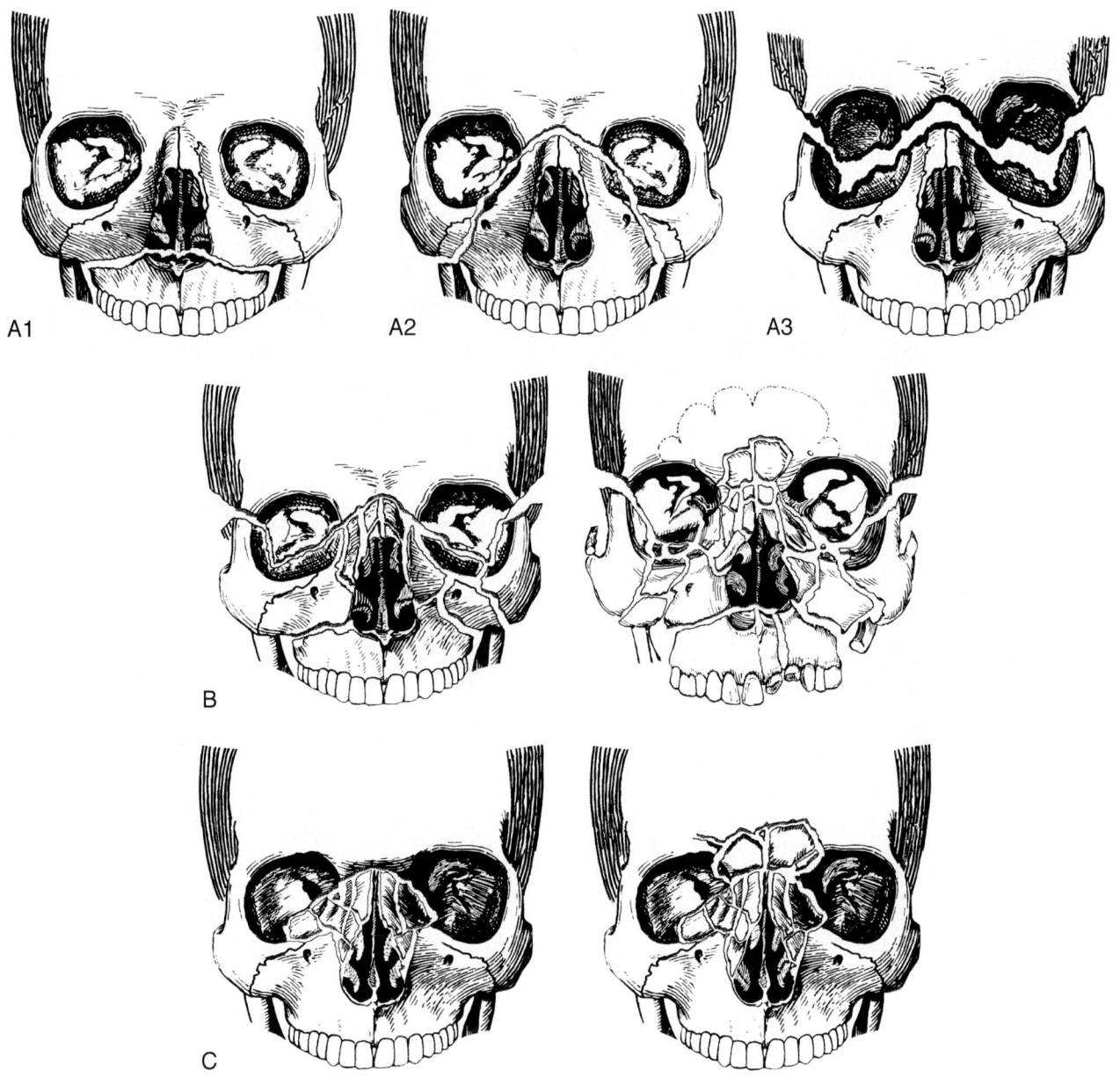

FIGURE 11–1 ■ *A*, Le Fort fractures. *B*, Comminuted Le Fort fractures. *C*, Central midfacial fractures without malocclusion.

nasal mucosa and the mucous membranes of the paranasal sinuses are always present in these cases, and a high risk exists for ascending infection to lead to involvement of the endocranium. Cerebrospinal fluid (CSF) leakage from the nose or nasopharynx demands localization of the site of the leak and subsequent surgical repair, even if the leak stops spontaneously. The cicatricial healing of dural lesions in areas of the skull base that are in contact with the nose or paranasal sinuses—the rhinobase—does not adequately seal the cranial cavity. Because bacterial flora normally exist in the nose and paranasal sinuses at all times, intracranial complications, such as meningitis, encephalitis, and brain abscess, can develop years after the trauma. Therefore, the leak has to be definitively sealed by an appropriate duraplasty, a conclusion enunciated during World War II.

As a consequence, nearly every case of frontal skull base fracture requires some form of operative intervention.

Current concepts for treatment of midface and frontal skull base injuries have evolved since 1927, based on the work of various surgeons.[2-9] These principles remain valid:

1. Closure of open or indirectly open fractures is necessary; fractures of the frontal skull base must be sealed to avoid endocranial complications.
2. The management of soft tissue lesions and facial bone fractures should take into account all esthetic and functional aspects during primary treatment.

Spinal fluid leakage may remain clinically undetected for some time before complications occur. Diagnostic procedures include head-down positioning and jugular vein compression, the use of glucose test strips, and the measurement of $\beta_2$-transferrin and the albumin-to-prealbumin ratio. For the diagnosis of CSF leak, $\beta_2$-transferrin is a highly sensitive parameter, but the procedure used to meas-

**Type 1**                                    **Type 2**

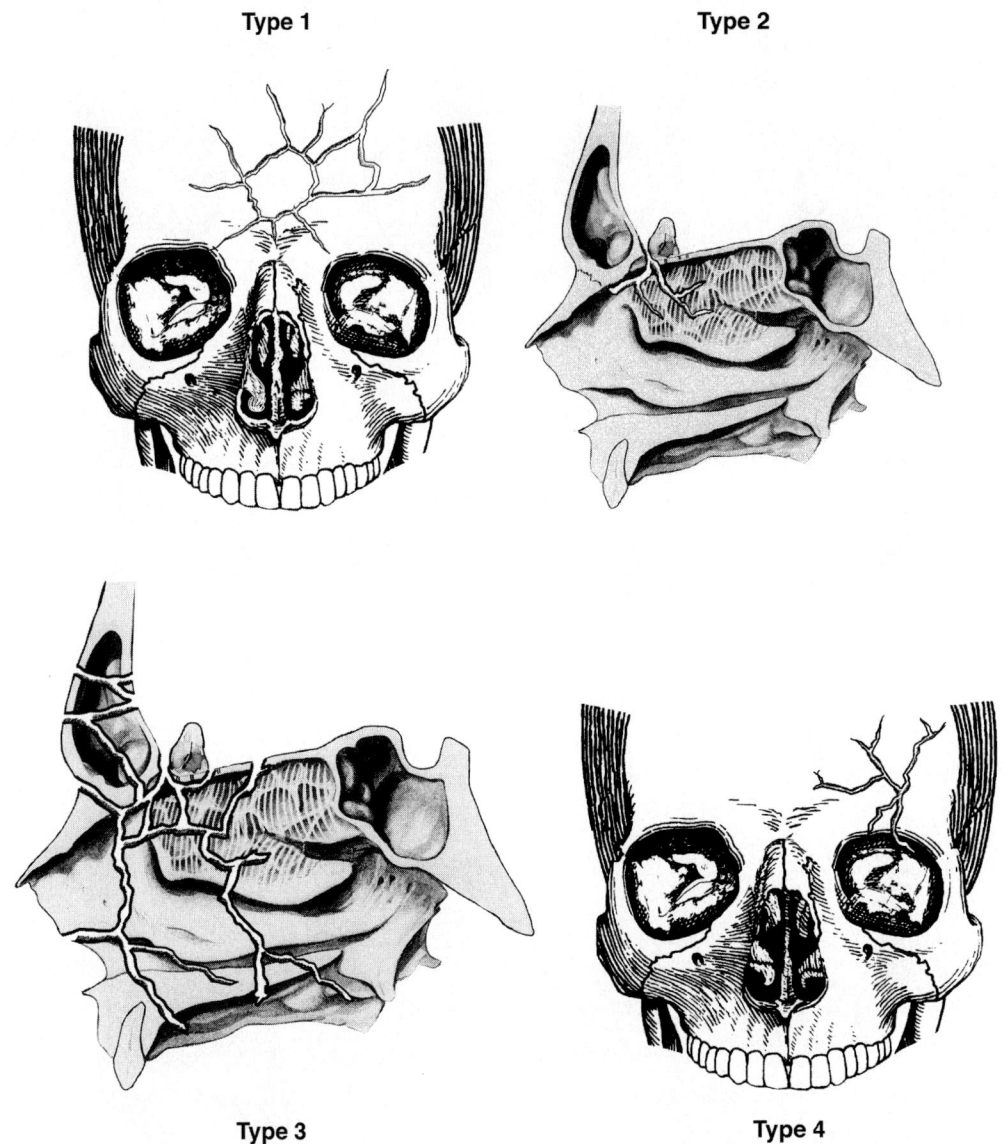

**Type 3**                                    **Type 4**

FIGURE 11–2 ■ Escher classification of frontal skull base fractures.

ure this element is time-consuming and needs at least 1.5 ml of fluid and a lot of experience on the part of the examiner. In particularly difficult cases, the leak can be localized by injecting fluorescin into the lumbar canal. The yellow-stained CSF can be detected endoscopically with a special blue filter.[10] Methods using intralumbar injections of [131]I albumin, [169]Y, or [111]In do not produce reliable results.

Radiologic examinations with coronal computed tomography (CT) scans are of major importance. Although ordinary x-ray studies of the skull in the anteroposterior, lateral, semiaxial, and basal projections sufficiently demonstrate the extent of the fractures and possibly existing pneumatoceles, modern CT scans provide improved resolution of even tiny fractures without increased exposure to radiation. Using a shoulder device and a gantry deviation of 20 degrees enables coronal scans even in cases in which overstretching of the head would cause a dangerous increase of intracranial pressure.

Most CSF leaks (Fig. 11–3) result from dural injury at the ethmoidal roof. The second most common cause of CSF leakage is fractures of the posterior wall of the frontal sinus. Only rarely is the dural defect located at the sphenoid area in the region of the tuberculum sellae, the anterior wall of the sella, or the planum sphenoidale. With extensive comminuted injuries of the anterior skull base, the frontal sinus, the roof of the ethmoidal cells, and the sphenoid sinus may all be involved concurrently. The absence of intracranial air does not prove that the dura is intact. In my experience, in 75% of all cases, air is resorbed after 48 hours, even after a large bony fracture gap.

Among the 58 patients suffering from an anterior skull base fracture that were treated in the ear, nose, and throat clinic of Würzburg from 1986 to 1988 (Table 11–1), the most common defect was located in the area of the ethmoidal roof and at the junction between the posterior wall of the frontal sinus and the ethmoidal roof (Fig. 11–4A and B). Thirty-one patients showed defects only in the form of bony gaps, and 27 patients had a bony defect greater than

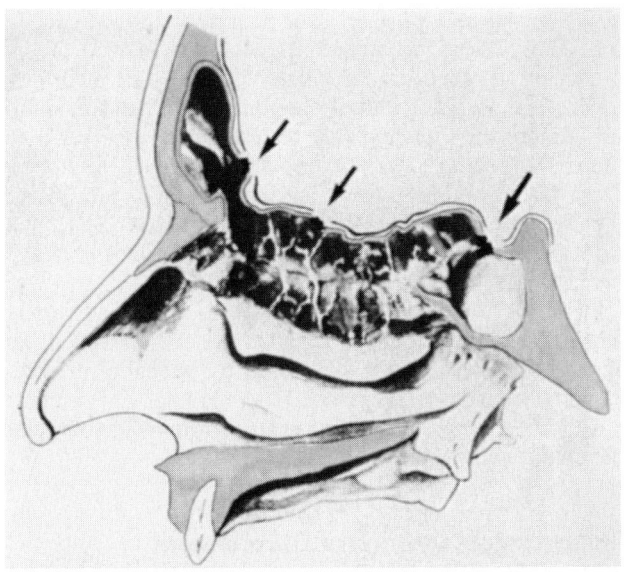

FIGURE 11–3 ■ Common sites of frontal skull base fractures.

| Localization of Anterior Skull Base Fractures | Size of Defect (No. = 58) (%) | (%) |
|---|---|---|
| Posterior wall of frontal sinus | 6 (10, 3) gap | 31 (53) |
| Posterior wall of frontal sinus + roof of ethmoid cells | 21 (36, 2) >0, 5 cm² | 27 (47) |
| Roof of ethmoid cells | 24 (41, 4) | |
| Roof of ethmoid cells + sphenoid sinus | 7 (12, 1) | |

0.5 cm². The size of the defect of the skull base, as revealed in coronal CT scans, was compared with the lesion found during surgery. A dural lesion existed in 92.4% of the cases in which the CT scan had shown a gap greater than 2 mm and in all cases with a gap greater than 4 mm.

## OPERATIVE TREATMENT

The timing of surgical treatment depends on the patient's general condition, the type of injury involved, and the requirements of the specialties involved. Serious bleeding demands emergency surgery, even without complete preoperative diagnostic evaluation. If the patient is in a poor general condition, the definitive treatment of the fractures may be delayed for hours, days, or weeks. In these cases, emergency procedures can be of only short duration. Bleeding is stopped by nasal and pharyngeal packing, and soft tissue lesions are closed adequately by suturing mucosa, subcutaneous tissue, and skin wounds. In most of these cases, tracheostomy cannot be avoided. Soft tissue lesions of the face should be closed within 12 hours, however. Nasal fractures should be treated within the first 5 days. Midfacial fractures should be reduced and stabilized within the first 2 to 3 weeks. Duraplasty should be performed as soon as possible in cases of comminuted fractures of the posterior wall of the frontal sinus, combined with extensive CSF rhinorrhea. Duraplasty of localized fractures in the area of the ethmoidal roof and sphenoid sinus roof can be performed as a delayed second procedure. In these cases,

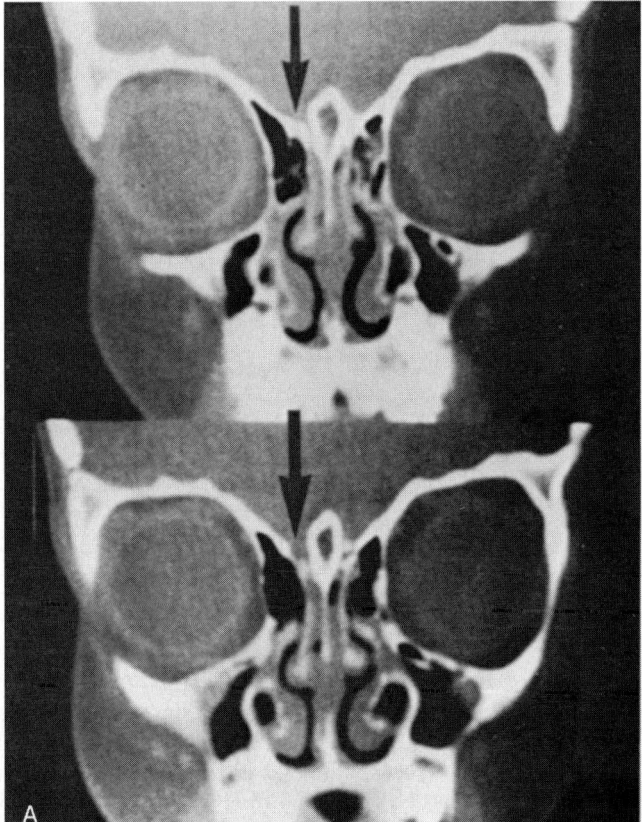

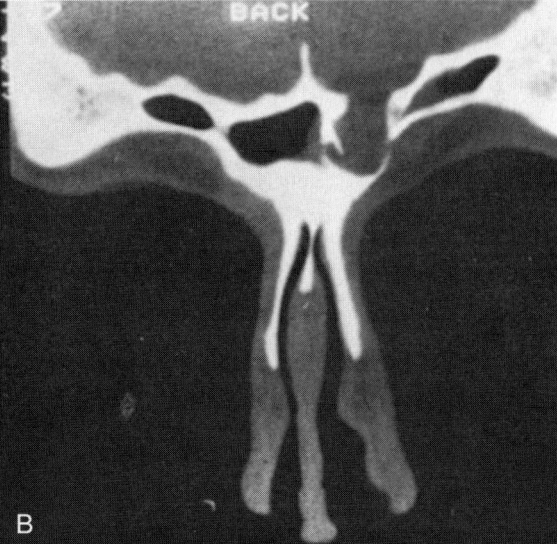

FIGURE 11–4 ■ A, Coronary computed tomography (CT) scan: localized fracture of the ethmoid roof. B, Coronary CT scan: large fracture of the posterior wall of the frontal sinus.

high-dose antibiotic coverage should be given over at least 1 week, and a constant follow-up of the trauma patient has to be maintained. After having completed clinical and radiologic examinations, surgical approaches and techniques should be discussed in a joint meeting with all relevant disciplines to plan surgery in which neurosurgeons, rhinosurgeons, and maxillofacial surgeons cooperate.

## Rhinosurgical Approach to the Frontal Skull Base

The classic epidurotransethmoidal rhinosurgical approach for the closure of CSF leaks localized in the median and paramedian frontal skull base and sphenoidal region has been favored by various specialists. Using this approach, via a Killian (eyebrow) or bilateral Killian incision (Fig. 11–5A), defects of the ethmoidal roof and the sella-sphenoidal planes can be closed. Fractures of the posterior wall of the frontal sinus can be sealed using an osteoplastic approach involving temporary removal of the anterior wall of the frontal sinus (Fig. 11–5B). The area is cut out earlier

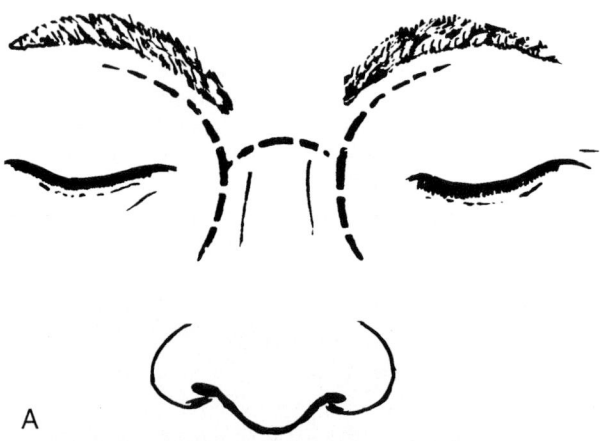

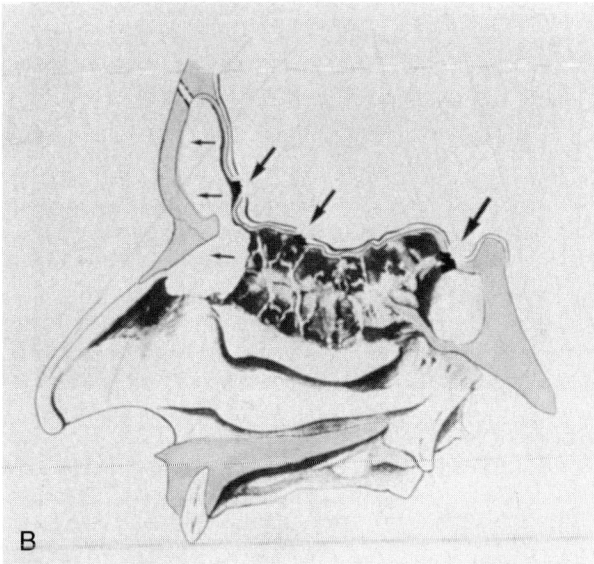

FIGURE 11–5 ■ A, Rhinosurgical exposure of the frontal skull base via the bilateral eyebrow (Killian) incision. B, Osteoplastic rhinosurgical approach.

as a cone-shaped lid, then later, it is repositioned exactly by osteosynthesis. A disadvantage of this method of approaching the skull base in cases of laterally situated fractures of the posterior wall of the frontal sinus can be painful irritation of the supratrochlear and supraorbital nerves over months and years after surgery. This approach cannot be recommended for extensive and comminuted fractures of the posterior wall of the frontal sinus and the whole frontal skull base with brain herniation, intracranial bleeding, and hematoma.

If the only problems are pre-existing facial and frontal wounds and the patient is in good general condition, an approach to the anterior skull base by widening the pre-existing wounds, if necessary, is preferable. The wounds have to be cleaned and closed exactly from inside out after beginning with repair of the dural defect.

## Rhinosurgical Closure of Dura Lesions

As just noted, the first step consists of closing the defect within the anterior skull base. In a rhinosurgical approach, the patient's fascia lata, fascia of the temporalis muscle, or preserved dura or fascia lata is used. A generously sized graft undermines the defect, allowing the surgeon to close it without tension. A double layer of fascia transplants attached with fibrin glue is even more efficient (Fig. 11–6). Sealing CSF leaks tightly within the area of the roof or posterior wall of the sphenoid sinus often presents a major problem. Draf and Samii[6, 9] describe the sealing technique of Kley, which uses a "tobacco-pouch" consisting of fascia lata filled with gelatin sponges. It can be recommended to cover the tobacco-pouch packing with fibrin glue and glue it in (Fig. 11–7). Provided that a small leak within the roof or posterior wall of the sphenoid sinus can be totally visualized under the microscope, merely a cover of fascia lata coated with fibrin glue is sufficient. In cases without malocclusion and an intact lateral bone frame, the easiest way to induce osteosynthesis is by putting back the conic bone lid, which was removed earlier, using resorbable sutures.

## Combined Neurosurgical and Rhinosurgical Procedures

The management of major intracranial fragment dislocations and multiple dural tears should incorporate a combined intracranial and extracranial transfrontal approach. According to Samii and Draf,[9] this procedure was described first by Unterberger and involved division of the olfactory fibers in cases requiring bilateral exposure of the cribriform plate because of the necessity of elevating the dura. This technique, however, can be modified by stopping the intracranial approach before reaching the olfactory fibers. Exposure and sealing of posteriorly situated dural lesions can be performed without dissection by subcranial preparations similar to the techniques developed by Tessier[11, 12] for craniofacial surgery. After coronal incision, periosteal flaps based frontally or laterally are created, if necessary (Fig. 11–8A). The supraorbital nerves are then exposed if a bony supraorbital canal exists. The next step provides laterally

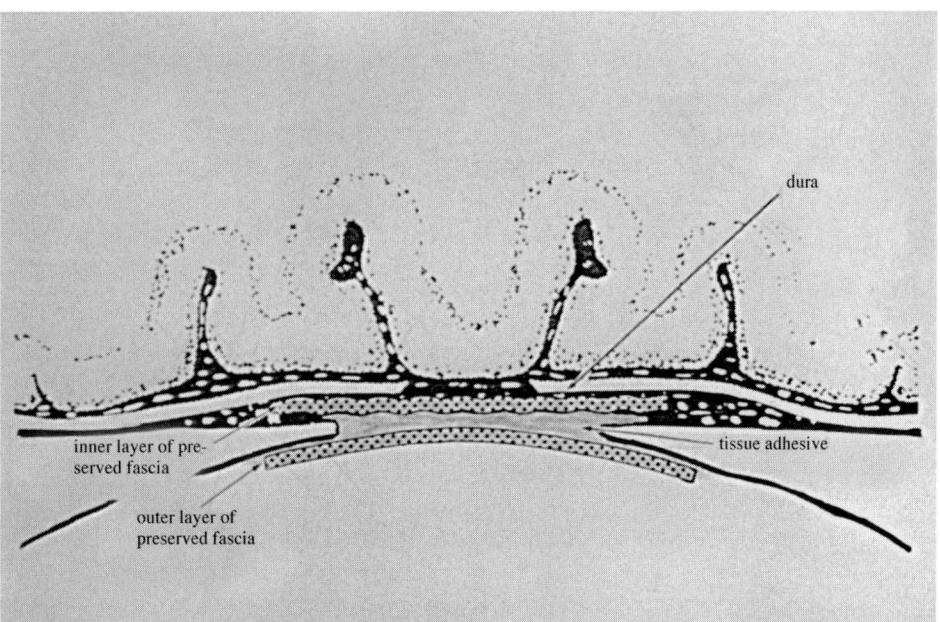

**FIGURE 11–6** ■ Rhinosurgical closure of dural leaks. This technique uses two layers of fascia and tissue adhesive.

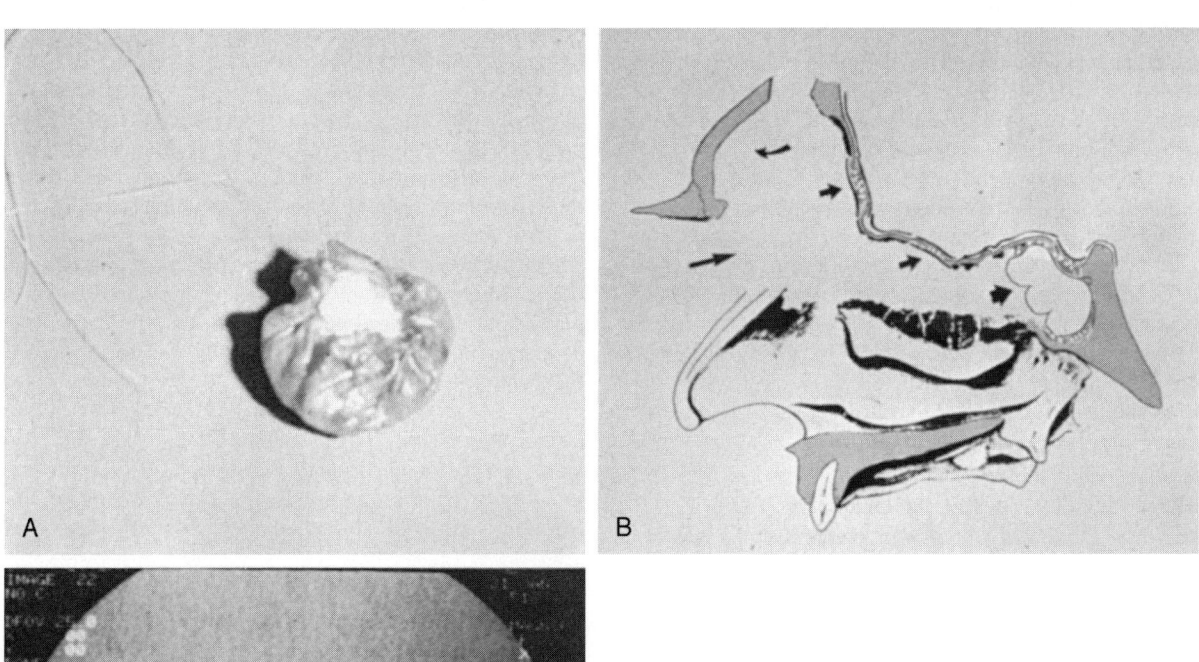

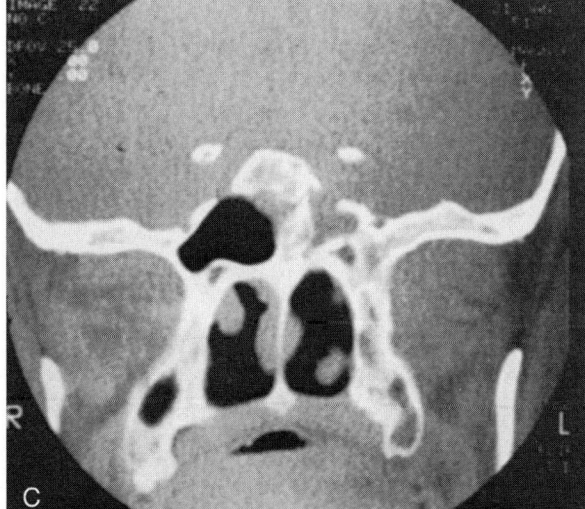

**FIGURE 11–7** ■ *A*, Tobacco-pouch technique, according to Kley. *B*, Osteoplastic approach. The tobacco pouch is fixed with fibrin glue. *C*, X-ray control study 1 year after surgery showing tight seal of the sphenoidal roof.

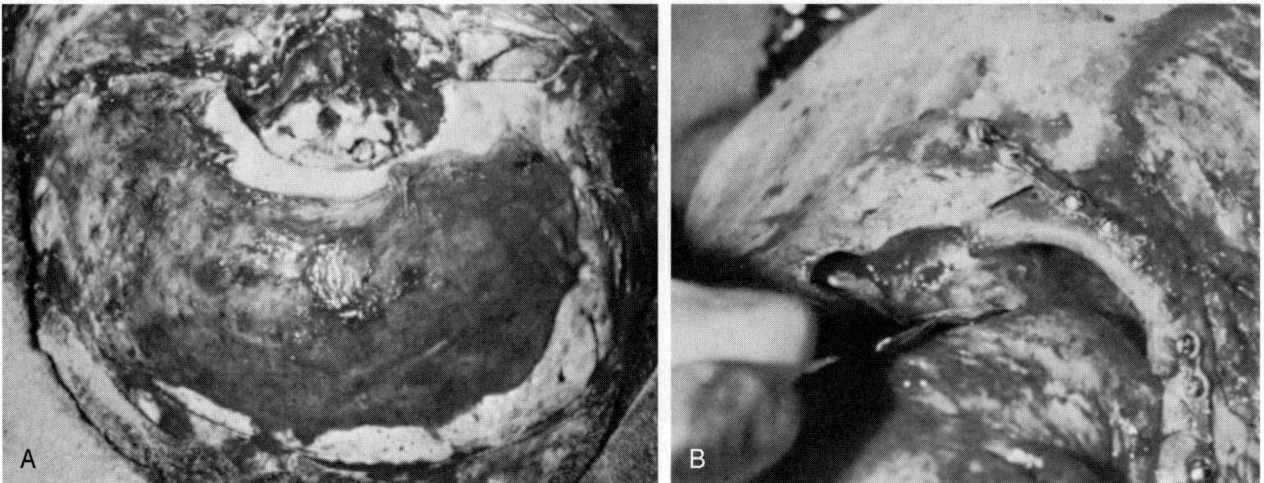

FIGURE 11–8 ■ *A*, Rhinosurgical approach to the frontal skull base using a coronary incision; the anterior wall of the frontal sinus is sawn out, and a laterally based periosteal flap is created. *B*, Exposure of the orbital roof.

an exposure of the frontozygomatic junction by moving exactly frontally and inferiorly along the fascia of the temporal muscle. The bony supraorbital rims are then identified. The bony orbital roofs (Fig. 11–8*B*) are stripped subperiosteally, and this process is continued to the complete medial and lateral wall of the orbit. Then the nasal bones and the fracture lines of the lamina papyracea are identified. After removal of the fragments of the anterior areas of the lamina papyracea and coagulation of the anterior ethmoidal artery, the anterior and medial parts of the ethmoidal roof can be identified. By removing bony fragments in this area by an extradural rhinosurgical approach, the areas of the posterior ethmoid roof and sphenoidal sinus usually can be surveyed carefully and dural tears can be sealed.

In severe craniofacial injuries and midfacial fractures, the incidence of involvement of the skull base with concomitant major dural tears is significantly high. Regarding functional and esthetic results, treatment consisting of primary urgent neurosurgical exploration, combined with rhinosurgical and maxillofacial reconstruction, produces the best results. The major advantage of this method is the

possibility of an early one-stage craniofacial reconstruction, avoiding extreme frontal lobe retraction and damage to the olfactory fibers. Reduction of telecanthus, decompression of the optic nerve, and meticulous reconstruction of the bony structures of the midface and frontal skull base can be performed in a one-session procedure.

Extensive fractures and depressions within the area of the frontal bone are often associated with vast crush fractures of the posterior wall of the frontal sinus. In these cases, dura lesions and subdural hematomas are common; these problems require primary or secondary interdisciplinary involvement of a neurosurgeon.

The surgical approach chosen in these cases is a frontal or frontotemporal bone lid type of craniotomy. An intradural or an extradural approach may also be used. In cases of excessively large crush defects of the posterior wall of the frontal sinus, the reconstruction is no longer possible. Partial or total cranialization of the frontal sinus may then be necessary (Fig. 11–9*A*). Tears of the dura are mended using sutures or fibrin glue. Bony edges at the transition of the former frontal sinus with the tabula interna of the os frontale have to be smoothed down to avoid a bony over-

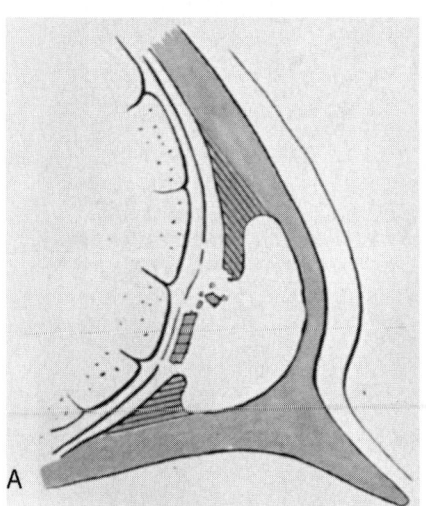

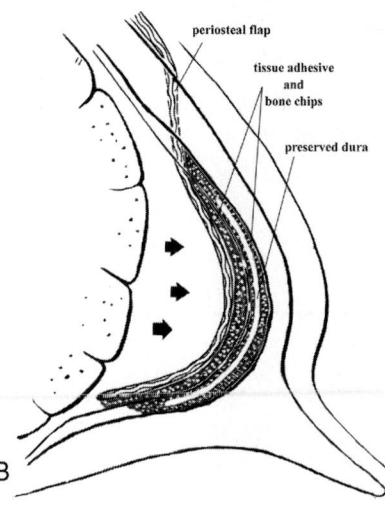

periosteal flap

tissue adhesive
and
bone chips

preserved dura

FIGURE 11–9 ■ *A*, Extensive fracture of the posterior wall of the frontal sinus. *B*, Situation after complete cranialization.

hang and to give the brain and the dura the chance to use up the newly gained space completely. The mucosa of the frontal sinus must be entirely removed. For sealing the area toward the nose and the ethmoid roof, a pedicle flap consisting of periosteum and muscle and periosteum, fibrin glue, bone meal, and bone chips of the wall of the former frontal sinus, minus all mucosa, is used (see Fig. 11–9*B*).

If fracture lines involve only the superior parts of a large frontal sinus, partial cranialization is performed by removing the upper fragments only and pushing the mucosa downward (Fig. 11–10). If the parietotemporofrontal bone of one side is markedly involved and the posterior wall of the frontal sinus of only one side is crushed, it suffices merely to conceal the injured frontal sinus, approaching it laterally. This technique, combining rhinosurgical and neurosurgical treatment, has been used successfully in the head clinic of Würzburg.

## Drainage of the Frontal Sinus and the Ethmoidal Cell System

In most cases of midfacial and anterior skull base fractures, the frontal sinus and ethmoidal cell system remains pneumatized. To avoid the development of mucoceles or inflammation, a wide, fully epithelialized access to the frontal sinus, the ethmoidal cells, and the nose has to be created.

In cases of a primary crush fracture of the upper bony septum associated with corresponding lesions of the mucosa, the construction of a median drainage route by resection of the upper parts of the bony nasal septum can be suggested. In cases without major fractures in the upper parts of the septum, this method should not be applied to

avoid further instability in the area of the forehead-nose pillar, which has to be reconstructed. Because there is a bony crush within the area of the nose and glabella already, any further bony destabilization should be avoided.

In these cases, I prefer a local mucosal flap. This rotating flap (Fig. 11–11) is created, using the mucosa of the middle parts of the middle concha, which is tipped sideways and cranially, thereby epithelializing the access to the frontal sinus and ethmoidal cells before one carries out the osteosynthesis of the forehead-nose pillar. Because of the anatomically narrow passages, bone must be reduced in the area of the nasofrontal junction. Nevertheless, it is important to avoid extensive thinning to achieve a stable bony union. Fibrin glue is used for the attachment of the mucosaperiosteal flap of the frontal parts of the middle turbinate.

## DEVELOPMENT OF OSTEOSYNTHESIS

In the past, the treatment of fractures of the frontomaxillary area—the so-called interorbital space[4]—and the sealing of fractures of the frontal skull base were commonly osteoclastic procedures. Loss of bony structures created visible and disturbing facial defects, however.

Secondary correction required considerable effort, for example, using the implantation of bone or cartilage or individually prepared plates of tantalum. These types of correction were possible only in a few cases. Wiring has been the standard procedure for stabilizing fractured facial bones, but it has not always given satisfactory results. Wiring promotes readaptation of bony fragments but cannot

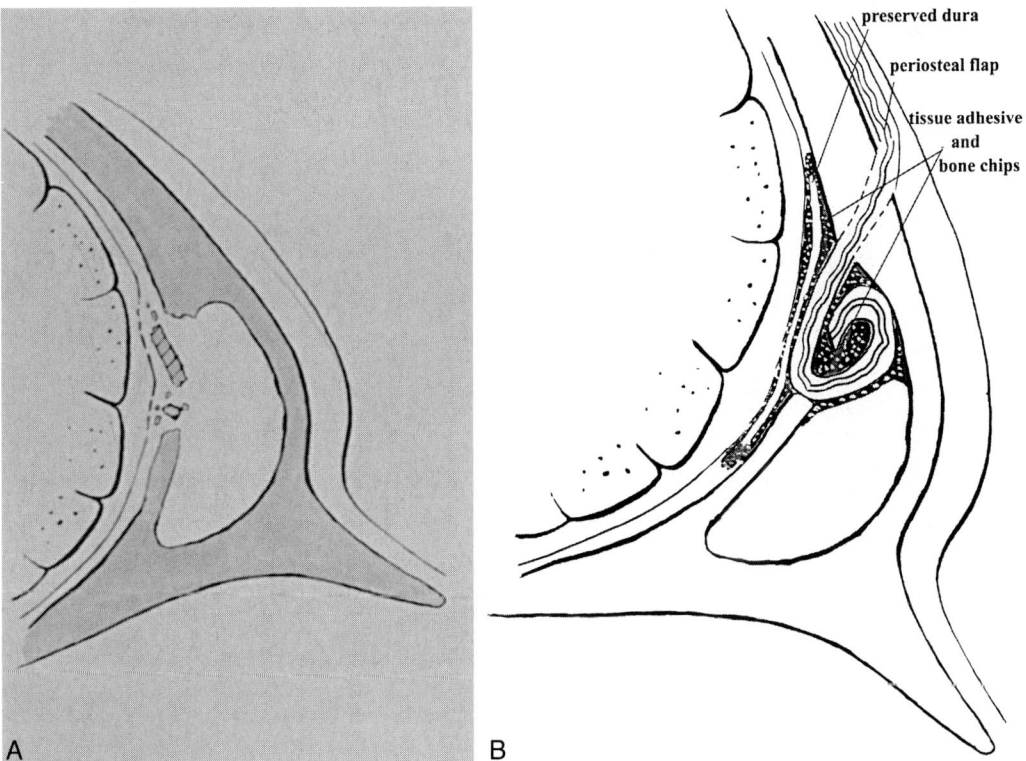

FIGURE 11–10 ■ *A*, Fractures within the superior or lateral parts of the posterior wall of the frontal sinus. *B*, Situation after partial cranialization.

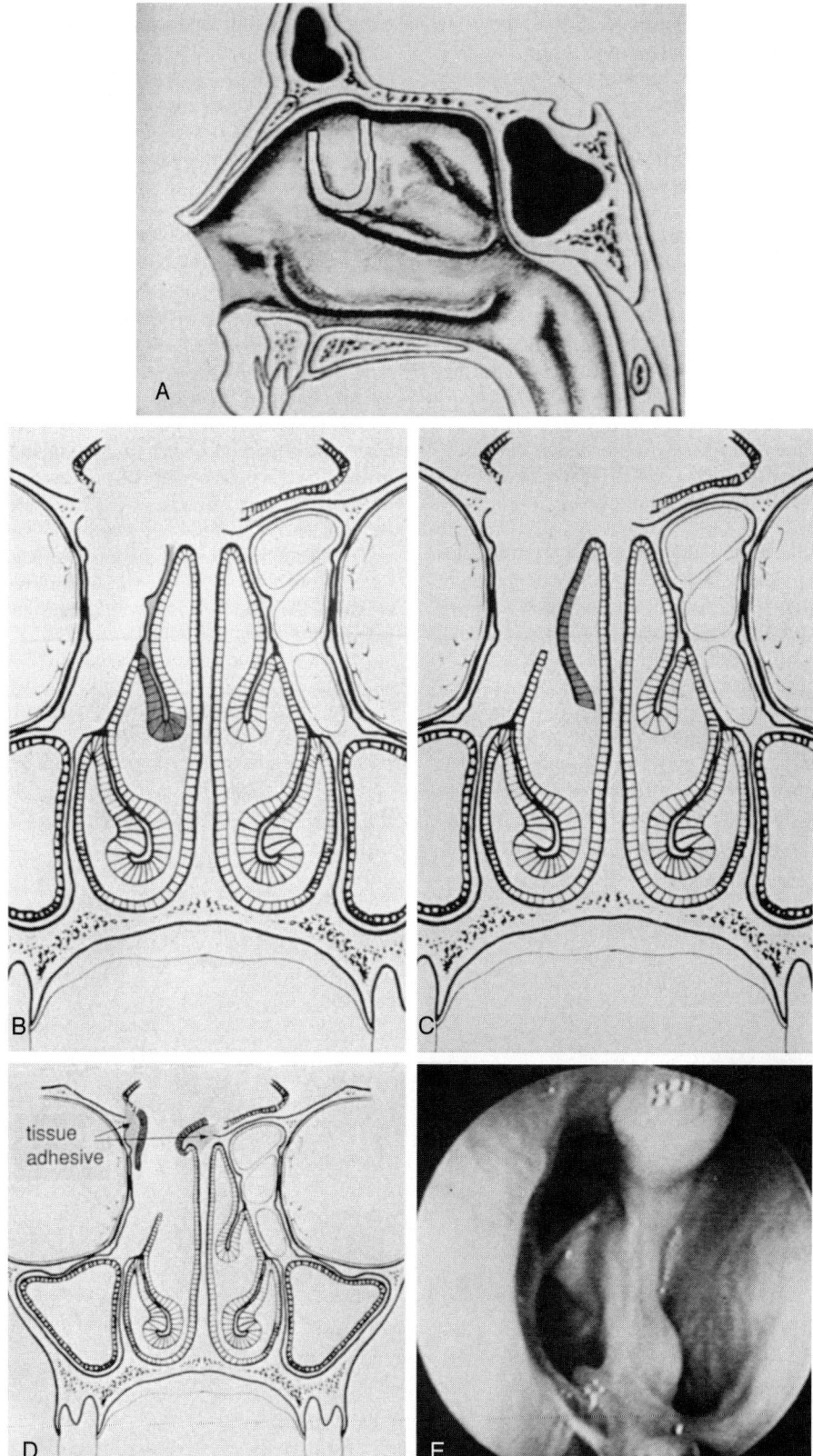

**FIGURE 11–11** ■ Operative technique creating a rotating flap using the middle turbinate. *A*, Superiorly based mucosal flap. *B* and *C*, Bony lamella and inferior and lateral parts of the mucosa are removed. *D*, The mucosal flap is turned upward. The flap and free mucosal transplant are fixed with fibrin glue. *E*, Endoscopic control 8 weeks after surgery. Wide and fully epithelialized frontal sinus and ethmoid cavity openings.

achieve a stable three-dimensional reconstruction of the frontomaxillary area in cases of multiple fractures.

Clinical observations made it obvious that wiring of the frontomaxillary area could not prevent secondary dislocations of the affected bones by the forces present at the time of the repair and during the period of any intermaxillary fixation. Repositioning the maxilla and its wire suspension to the zygomatic process of the frontal bone also creates pressure on the rebuilt osseous nasal or frontomaxillary complex. In the case of the frontomaxillary complex, deforming pressure is exerted toward the back and the side. Despite intermaxillary fixation, pressure transferred by the masticatory muscles acts in the same manner. In general, in these cases, wiring of the osseous fragments of the interorbital space cannot prevent traumatic bony telecanthus and a traumatic saddle-nose deformity.

Based on the investigations of Michelet and associates[13] and Champy and colleagues,[14] various bone plates were developed in many clinics, such as those created by Luhr.[15] Developing bone plate osteosynthesis for facial bone was continued in the basic investigations of Perren and coworkers[16] in the surgical treatment of fractures of the extremities. Thin bone plates were used primarily for osteosynthesis of the zygomatic bone.

To create a bone plate fixation able to withstand any normal functional loads, an anatomic and clinical study[2] was initiated in 1979 in the ear, nose, and throat clinic of the University of Würzburg. These investigations first tried to define which sizes and forms of the plates and screws might be ideal for use in the frontomaxillary area. The thickness of the bone in the areas to be considered for plate osteosynthesis were measured on adult skulls and skull pieces, using the skull collections of the Department of Anatomy of the Universities of Würzburg and Innsbruck. Measuring instruments used were dental calipers, which are normally used in maxillofacial orthopedics and orthodontic techniques. With these instruments, the deep-seated and usually inaccessible bone in the area of the nasal roof could be measured with a precision 0.1 mm.

As in most of the skulls, the calvaria had already been separated, permitting the thickness of the anterior walls of the frontal sinuses and of the skull caps also to be measured. Forty-five skulls and 21 right or left halves or skull pieces were studied. Significant differences between the right and the left sides were not found.

In the medial part of the nasal bone and up to the roof of the nose, the bone has a mean thickness of 1.5 to 4.2 mm. The thickness of the bony wall of the frontal process of the maxilla increases similarly to its upper areas. Mean values of 2.1 mm were found inferiorly, whereas mean values of 3.2 mm were found superiorly. Consequently, the superior parts of the osseous base of the bony nose seem to be thick enough to allow fixation of bone plates with screws 5 to 7 mm long (Miniplate system).

The mean thickness of the anterior wall of the frontal sinus varies from 1.75 to 2.42 mm. The differences are due to bone crests at the back of the bone, which usually arise from the interfrontal septum.

The mean thickness of the calvarial bone was 5.5 mm in each of the specimens studied, making it suitable for bone plate fixation in every case. The bone of the anterior wall of the frontal sinus also seems to be generally suitable for bone plate osteosynthesis, although sites less than 2 mm thick are too thin to allow satisfactory miniplate osteosynthesis, and therefore in these areas, microplate osteosynthesis is preferable. Elsewhere, all bones of the supraorbital and infraorbital rims with a mean thickness of more than 5 mm were found to allow miniplate fixation.

Figure 11–12A and B shows all sites of the upper cranial and facial skeleton at which miniplate or microplate bone fixation might be considered. In essence, bony walls that are at least 2 mm thick should provide sufficient retention only for microscrews. Miniplate osteosynthesis, however, requires bone at least 3 mm thick.

## CLINICAL EXPERIENCES

Most midfacial fractures are associated with frontal skull base fractures. Cases of maxillary fractures with malocclusion (Le Fort II or III fractures) in the Head Clinic of the University of Würzburg were treated in cooperation with colleagues from the Department of Maxillofacial Surgery. The first step of the operation is the removal of any debris of the sinuses and the sealing of the frontal skull base, as needed. After this step is completed, reconstruction of the osseous base of the nose follows, with stable osteosynthesis performed by the ear, nose, and throat surgeon.

In contrast to Champy's vitallium miniplates, handling with titanium minisystems and microsystems is easier. Their versatility is due to their better design and construction. This design is also more variable and allows anatomic reconstruction to be carried out even in those cases having spatially irregular points of fixation. Further, because the quality of the titanium material is excellent, it allows the surgeon to bend the material over edges much more easily than with Champy's vitallium plates. The titanium plate can be formed quickly and without difficulty, so that it is even possible to reconstruct a previously prominent and angular nose. The osseous infraorbital rim can be readily joined to a bone plate framing the osseous nose. Repositioning the maxilla to the frontal bone with its wire fixation to the zygomatic process cannot damage an initially performed stable reconstruction of the nose using plates (Fig. 11–13). The stability provided by such plates is a real improvement in comparison to the former wiring technique.

If the bone of the anterior wall of the frontal sinus is thick enough in cases of single-piece fractures in the glabellar area, two or three 5-mm-long screws give sufficient stability to hold the reconstructed osseous frame of the nose in place. The fragments of superior parts of the osseous nose can usually be fixed with 7- or 5-mm screws.

It is more difficult to reconstruct multiple fractures of the glabellar area because they are often associated with multiple fractures of the anterior wall of the frontal sinus. Solid osseous structures are needed for a stable reconstruction of the osseous base of the nasofrontal area, but they are generally located beyond the frontal sinus in the lateral or superior frontal bone. Such repairs require superior fixation in the calvaria (Fig. 11–14). In these cases, reconstruction of the anterior wall of the frontal sinus is best performed as a combination osteosynthesis. First, the fragments of the anterior wall of the frontal sinus are

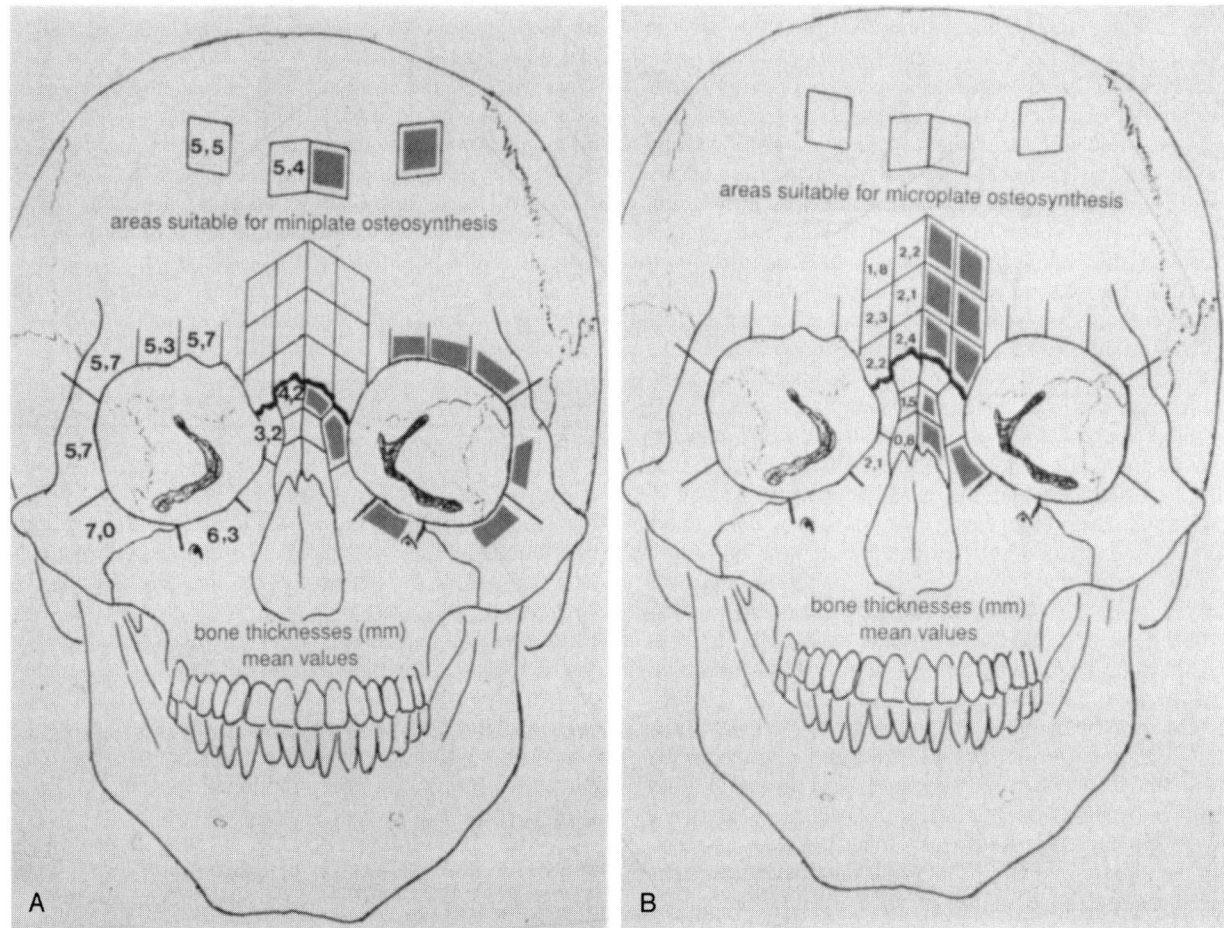

FIGURE 11–12 ■ *A* and *B*, Average values of bone thicknesses of areas important for miniplate and microplate osteosynthesis.

readapted with wires or microplates and microscrews before they are elevated so that they act as a lid. Following this step, definite fixation and stabilization can be performed by miniplate osteosynthesis.

Therefore, the methods of osteoplastic treatment of fractures of the osseous nasofrontomaxillary area with miniplate and microplate osteosynthesis allow: (1) a stable medial fixation of the maxilla to the frontal bone, (2) an effective treatment for traumatic telecanthus, and (3) prevention of a bony saddle-nose deformity.

With a stable bone plate osteosynthesis of the osseous nasofrontomaxillary complex, the osseous base of the nose is restructured as a well-fixed medial osseous block. This block acts as a solid foundation against any lateral traction arising from the more laterally situated suspension of the maxilla to the zygomatic process of the frontal bone. Similarly, this solid medial osseous block prevents redislocation produced by the masticatory muscles. The advantage of this step is that it prevents the occurrence of a dish-face deformity, as was commonly seen in the past. Thus, a good esthetic result is achieved, and satisfactory functional conditions are also possible. In patients with these conditions, tracheotomy often can be avoided. The osseous base of the nose that has been reconstructed by bone plates is usually so stable that nasal intubation is generally possible after rhinosurgical treatment. If nasal intubation is per-

formed, it is preferable that the procedure be completed by the ear, nose, and throat surgeon.

The advantage of bone plate maxillofacial osteosynthesis is the stable fixation of bony fragments. This method allows better healing of the overlying soft tissues and especially prevents excessive tissue shrinkage and scar formation. My experience has also shown that tiny fragments of the anterior wall of the frontal sinus with a bone thickness less than 1 mm do not heal and were completely resorbed when the bone plates were removed. To avoid inflammatory complications, it is preferable in these cases to use the biggest bone pieces only (having at least a wall thickness of 2.5 mm) to reconstruct the anterior wall of the frontal sinus. For fixation of the fragments, micro-osteosynthetic material is preferable.

As long as good frontal sinus drainage is gained, it is not necessary to remove the mucosa of the back part of the big bone pieces used for osteosynthesis. Remaining gaps can be closed by using adapted bone transplants from the skull (Fig. 11–15). The free bone transplants are adjusted using wires or micro-osteosynthetic material. The edges of the transplants are formed in a way as to create broad bony contact areas. Gaps are filled with bone meal and fibrin glue. This reconstruction technique is performed only after a primary coronal incision has been selected.

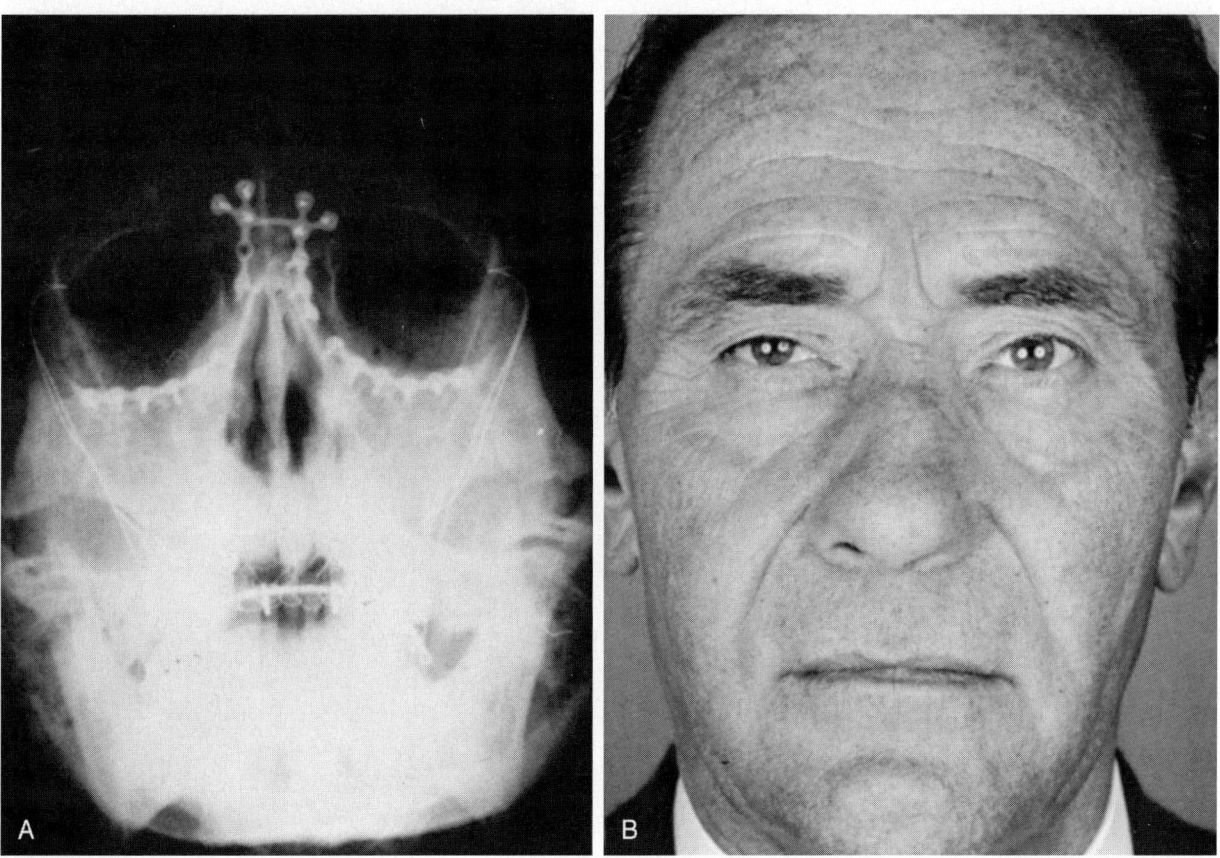

**FIGURE 11–13** ■ Radiologic and clinical example of miniplate osteosynthesis after Le Fort III fracture combined with a localized fracture of the ethmoidal roof; strong fixation of the medial bony midfacial fractures to the anterior wall of the frontal sinus.

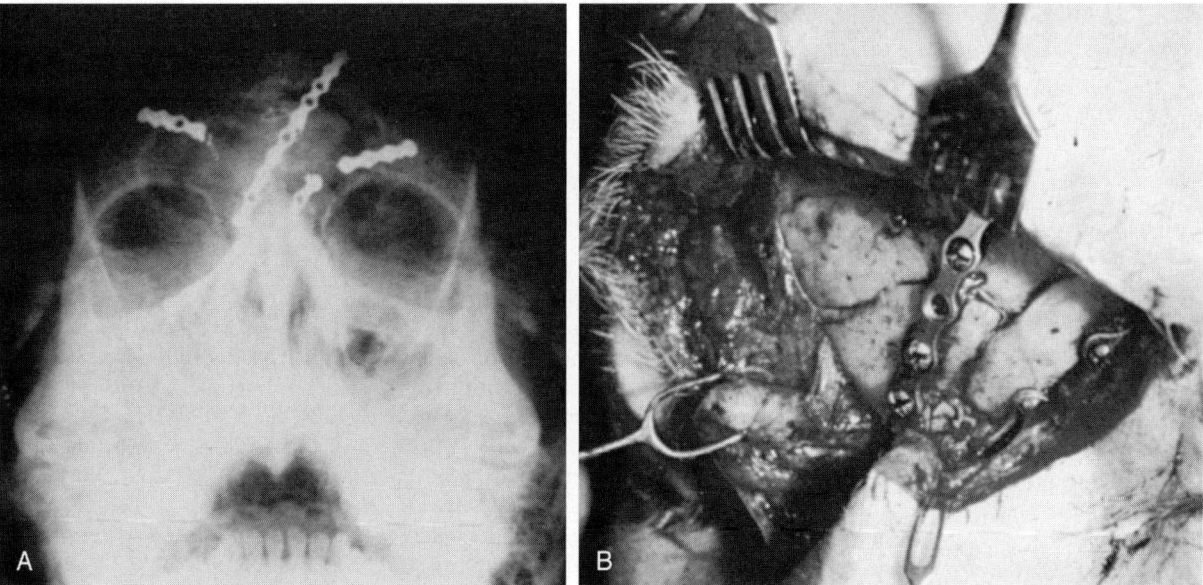

**FIGURE 11–14** ■ Radiologic and clinical example of a central midfacial and comminuted frontal sinus wall fracture. *A*, Osteosynthesis using wires and miniplates, with fixation to the calvarium. *B*, Situation 9 months later. Bony healing is complete, and the material used for osteosynthesis can be removed.

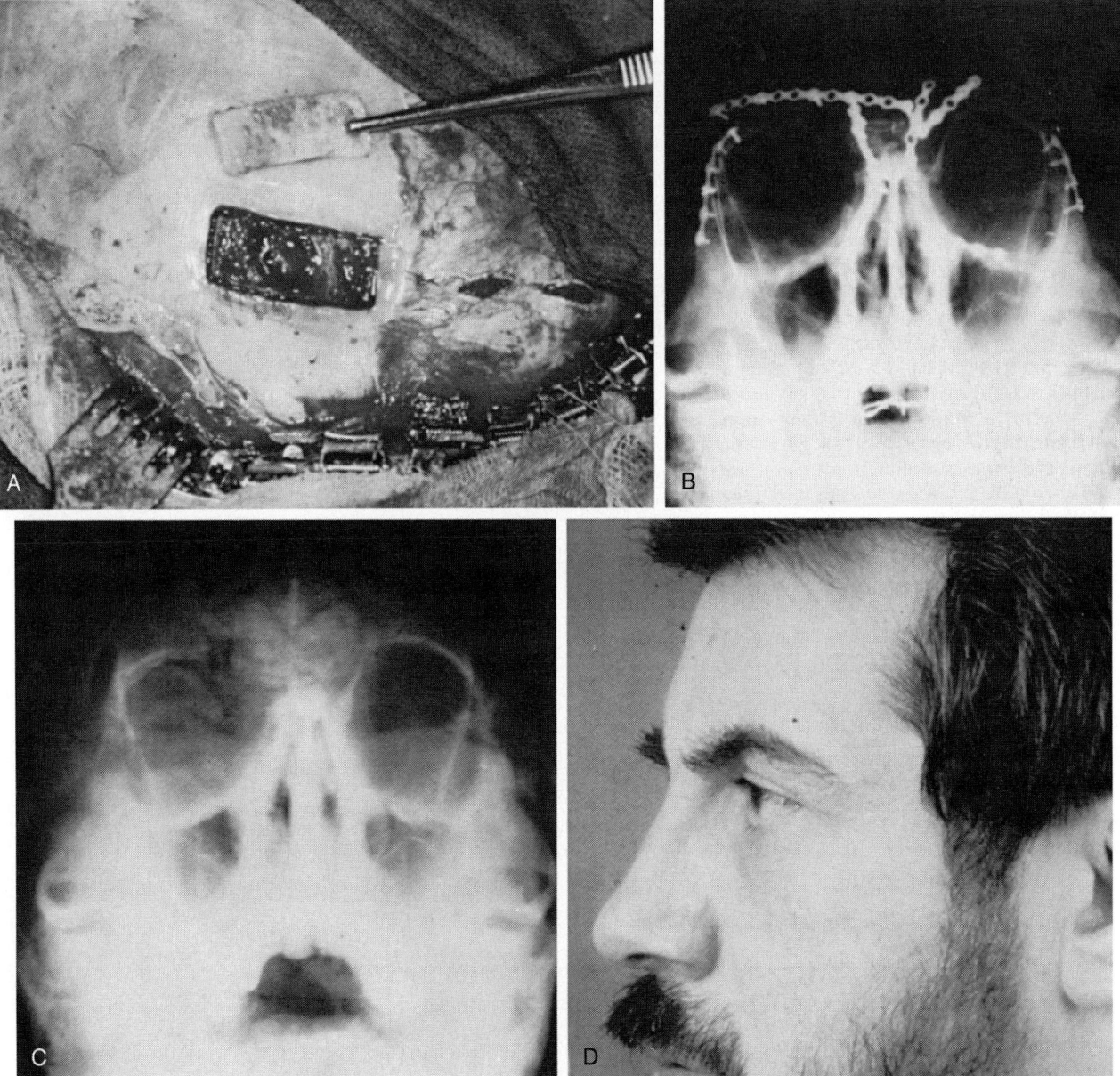

FIGURE 11–15 ■ Radiologic and clinical example of adapted bone transplants from the skull. *A*, Removal of a piece of split skull from the parietotemporal area. *B*, Reconstruction using miniplates and wires. *C*, Radiologic control 10 months after surgery; free bone transplant completely healed. *D*, Clinical situation 1 year after surgery.

## POSTOPERATIVE PROGRESS, PROBLEMS, AND COMPLICATIONS AND SECONDARY RECONSTRUCTIVE TECHNIQUES

Even with the extensive experience with osteosynthesis, it is not possible to prevent screws from having contact with the mucosa of the upper paranasal sinuses, thus allowing infection to spread from the mucosa to the bone. Therefore, it seems to be important to carry out careful management of the nasal region, including frequent suctioning of the nose and inhalation with cortisol and other aerosols to reduce inflammation of the soft tissues.

The osteosynthetic material should be removed immediately after bony consolidation has taken place. Before dis-

charge from the hospital, the patient and his or her family are instructed to attend follow-up examinations on a regular basis and to be certain that osteosynthetic material is removed at a later date. In addition, all patients with paranasal sinus surgery, especially those with osteosynthetic material above the frontal or ethmoidal sinus, are registered in an osteosynthesis chart and are asked to attend follow-up examinations.

Important diagnostic procedures in these follow-up examinations at 1 week, then 3 weeks, and later yearly periods are endoscopy of the nose and paranasal sinuses using various items of optical equipment, including a flexible endoscope; ultrasound; and the conventional x-ray study, CT scan, or magnetic resonance imaging study.

From 1980 to 1983, 73 patients with fractures of the

central and lateral viscerocranium and of the rhinobase were treated in the ear, nose, and throat clinic of Würzburg using miniplate osteosynthesis. The results using this method are satisfying in both the esthetic and the functional aspects. Postoperative follow-up studies showed that an astonishingly high percentage of patients remained without any complaints, even those who suffered from extensive crush fractures and the loss of precious mucosa. Fifteen patients were found to have rhinitis sicca, and 13 showed recurrent mucopurulent sinusitis. Accompanying edema of the upper and lower eyelids, which is a sign of a threatening orbital complication, was found in 6.8% of all cases. To date, only two patients had a true complication of menacing pyesis.

Early complications usually are due to penetration of ascending infection from the nasal and sinus mucosa along the screws reaching the frontal bone, thus creating frontal sinus empyema, a subperiosteal abscess, or osteitis within the frontal area. Late complications are caused by scar formation in the area of the newly created frontal sinus opening. Following blocking of the drainage, mucoceles and secondary inflammatory reactions may develop months or even years later; if one fails to diagnose and treat them at an early stage, meningitis, frontal bone osteitis, or subdural or brain abscess can occur (Fig. 11–16).

Different opinions exist as to whether osteosynthetic material may remain permanently or always must be removed. In Germany, because there are still serious disadvantages, nearly all metal implants are removed after bony consolidation takes place. This approach creates additional costs, however. Reasons for removal of the material are at first cosmetic. Usually after a few months, because of a thin cover of soft tissue, plates and screws within the face and the skull can be palpated by the patient and become disturbing foreign bodies. Chromium, nickel, cobalt, and a few other alloys have proved to be potential causes of

cancer in animal studies. It cannot be denied that leaving metallic (or other) foreign material within the human body may cause cancer.

Because even the so-called Titan alloys may be corroded in vivo, and because frequently high concentrations of titanium oxide (up to 2000 parts per million) were found in the localized areas of Titan implants, especially those within soft tissue, all kinds of Titan material should be removed, as far as possible, even if a few manufacturers have claimed that the removal of the so-called pure Titan is not absolutely necessary. Exceptions have to be considered concerning the elderly or patients with tumors. Metallic implants covering nasal sinuses should always be removed 6 to 9 months after bony consolidation because at least one of the screws has contact with the mucosa of the nasal sinus. Thus, an infection within the nasal sinus may easily reach a screw and cause an acute large osteolytic infection of the frontal bone and adjacent skull bone or even initiate an endocranial complication as well.

In the case of allergic reactions, the metallic implants have to be removed immediately. In my practice two such cases were observed: one 4 months after a midfacial osteosynthesis with titanium plates (Fig. 11–17) and another one 6 months after refixation of a frontonasal osteotomy lid with a chromium-cobalt plate. In both cases, punctiform, itching, pimple-like skin irritations occurred, starting in the face within the area covering the osteosynthesis material, causing severe itching, foreign body sensation, and malaise. In both cases, shortly after that time, pruritic skin eruptions could be found on the entire body as well and even on the extremities. After removal of the osteosynthetic material, the skin irritations disappeared completely. In both cases, an epicutaneous skin test showed the specific sensitization.

Ionomer cement proved to be a good material for secondary reconstructive surgery, such as for the reconstruction of the frontonasal or supraorbital bone defects as well

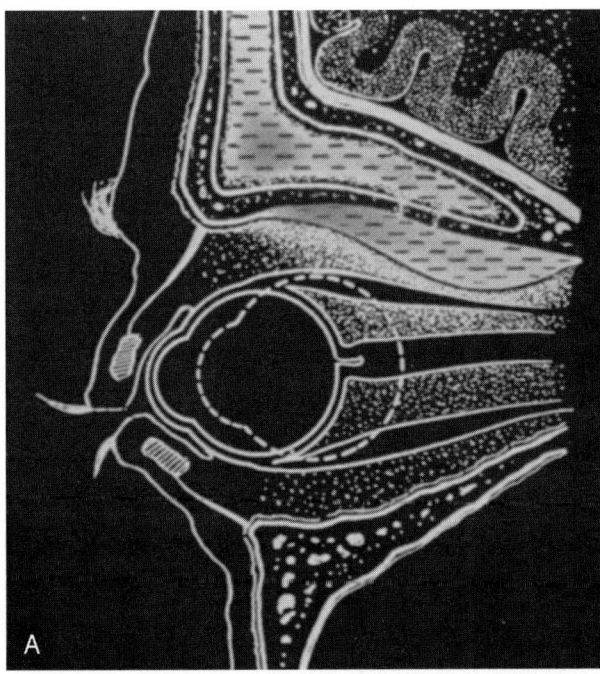 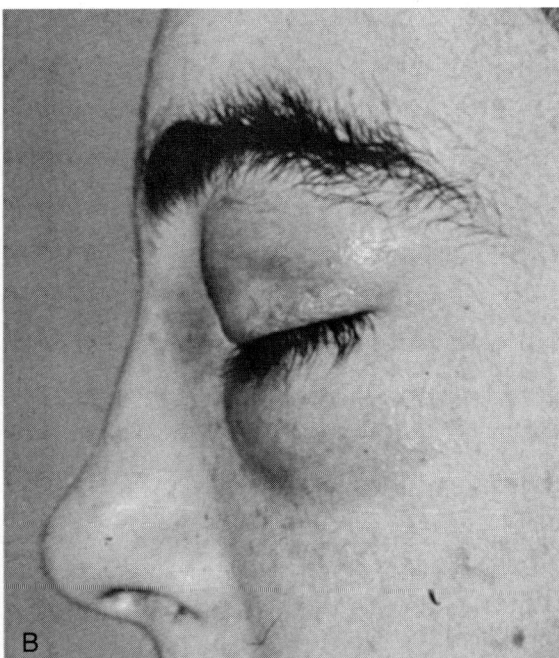

FIGURE 11–16 ■ *A* and *B*, Orbital complication due to ascending inflammation.

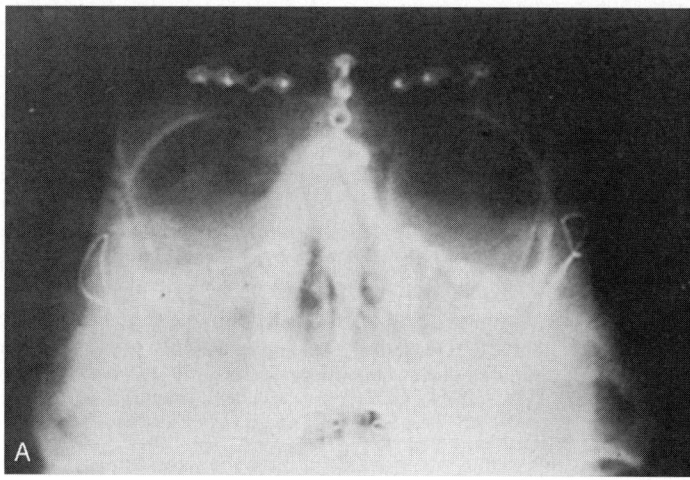
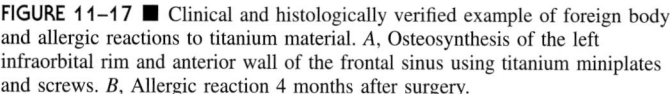
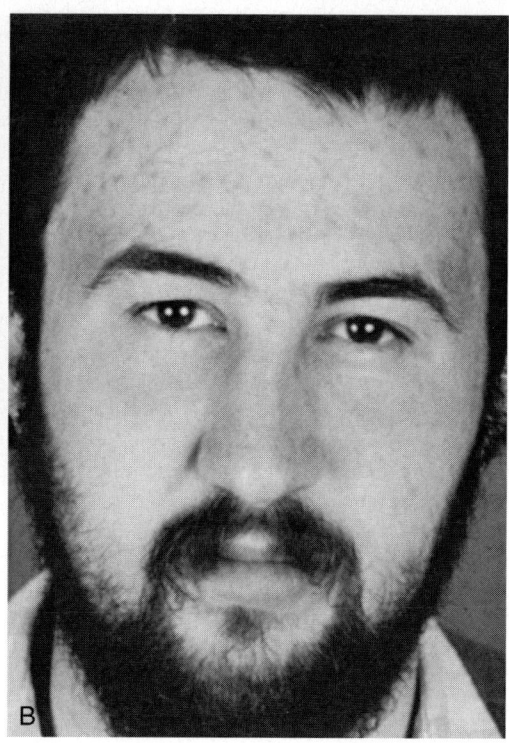

**FIGURE 11-17** ■ Clinical and histologically verified example of foreign body and allergic reactions to titanium material. *A*, Osteosynthesis of the left infraorbital rim and anterior wall of the frontal sinus using titanium miniplates and screws. *B*, Allergic reaction 4 months after surgery.

as for the roof of the skull. Although pure acrylates have the disadvantage of producing heat during polymerization, ionomer cement remains at an almost constant temperature. Because ionomer cement is sensitive to water, it has to be applied in almost perfectly dry areas. If all of these items are considered, this material attaches well to the bone, and the bone itself is not altered at all, especially not in its vitality. Since 1989, this material proved to be useful in the ear, nose, and throat clinic of Würzburg for reconstruction of defects within the frontal and lateral skull base and for the skull itself as well. Ionomer cement is especially suited for skull defects in the form of a paste, which can be formed individually. It is also available in the form of premanufactured parts, which are put in place using only a little freshly prepared cement.[17]

## SUMMARY

Surgical experience in Europe and my personal work in the area of anterior skull base and midfacial trauma proves that closing dural tears offers protection against primary and secondary meningitis resulting from ascending infection. The use of the operative microscope, well-tolerated implants, fibrin glue, miniosteosynthesis and micro-osteosynthesis, and cooperation among all participant specialists guarantee a high quality of functional and esthetic results in most cases. The result of the surgery, however, depends on the extent of bone and soft tissue destruction. Therefore, in cases in which only emergency treatment is possible, insufficient functional and esthetic results may occur and require secondary treatment. In several of these cases,

ionomer cement proves to be a good solution for filling skull defects.

## ACKNOWLEDGMENTS

*Thanks are due to all colleagues and staff members of the Head Clinic of the University of Würzburg, especially to Professor Roosen, Department of Neurosurgery; Professor Reuther, Department of Maxillofacial Surgery; and Professor Kampik, Department of Ophthalmology, and to Professor Nadjmi and colleagues, Department of Neuroradiology, for preparing the x-ray studies and CT scans.*

## REFERENCES

1. Escher F: Clinical classification and treatment of frontobasal fractures. In Hamberger CA, Wersäll J (eds): Disorders of the Skull Base Region. Proceedings of the Tenth Nobel Symposium Stockholm, August 1968. Stockholm: Almquist & Wiksell; New York: Wiley, 1969, pp 343–352.
2. Teachenor FR: Intracranial complications of fracture of skull involving frontal sinus. JAMA 88:987–989, 1927.
3. Cairns H: Injuries of the frontal and ethmoidal sinuses with special reference to cerebrospinal rhinorrhoea and aeroceles. J Laryngol 52:589, 1937.
4. Converse JM, Smith B, Wood-Smith D: Orbital and naso-orbital fractures. In Converse JM (ed): Reconstructive Plastic Surgery, Philadelphia: WB Saunders, 1977, pp 748–793.
5. Dingman RO, Converse JM: The clinical management of facial injuries and fractures of the facial bones. In Converse JM (ed): Reconstructive Plastic Surgery. Philadelphia: WB Saunders, 1977, pp 599–747.
6. Draf W, Samii M: Fronto-basal injuries—principles in diagnosis and treatment. In Samii M, Brihaye J (eds): Traumatology of the Skull Base. Berlin: Springer, 1983, pp 61–69.

7. Brunner FX, Kley W, Plinkert K: Anatomical studies and a correlative management of facial skeleton and skull base injuries with bone plate fixation. Arch Otorhinolaryngol 245:61–68, 1988.
8. Raveh J, Vuillemin T: The surgical one-stage management of combined cranio-maxillo-facial and frontobasal fractures. J Craniomaxillofac Surg 16:160–172, 1988.
9. Samii M, Draf W: Surgery of the Skull Base. Berlin: Springer, 1989, pp 114–158.
10. Oberascher G: Cerebrospinal fluid otorrhoea-rhinorrhea. The Salzburg concept of cerebrospinal fluid diagnosis. Laryngol Rhinol Otol (Stuttg) 67:375–381, 1988.
11. Tessier P: Relationship of craniostenoses to craniofacial dysostoses, and to faciostenoses: A study with therapeutic implications. Plast Reconstr Surg 48:224–237, 1971.
12. Tessier P: Definitive plastic surgical treatment of the severe facial deformities of craniofacial dysostosis: Crouzon's and Apert's diseases. Plast Reconstr Surg 48:419–442, 1971.
13. Michelet FX, Deymes J, Dessus B: Osteosynthesis with miniaturized screwed plates in maxillo-facial surgery. J Maxillofac Surg 1:79–84, 1973.
14. Champy M, Loddé JP, Schmitt R, et al: Mandibular osteosynthesis by miniature screwed plates via a buccal approach. J Craniomaxillofac Surg 6:14–21, 1978.
15. Luhr HG: Indications for use of a microsystem for internal fixation in craniofacial surgery. J Craniomaxillofac Surg 1:35–52, 1990.
16. Perren SM, Russenberger M, Steinemann S, et al: A dynamic compression plate. Acta Orthop Scand 125(Suppl):29–41, 1969.
17. Helms J, Geyer G: Alloplastic materials in skull base reconstruction. In Sekhar LN, Janecka IP (eds): Surgery of Cranial Base Tumors: A Color Atlas. New York: Raven Press, 1993, pp 461–469.

# CHAPTER 1 2

# Management of Cerebrospinal Fluid Leaks

■ T. FORCHT DAGI

Cerebrospinal fluid (CSF) fistula is a serious, frustrating, and potentially fatal condition whose successful management requires a fundamental understanding of the anatomy and pathophysiology of the problem. The evolution of the current operative approaches is best understood from a historical perspective.

## HISTORICAL OVERVIEW

The correlation of post-traumatic rhinorrhea with leakage of CSF was made in the 17th century by a Dutch surgeon, Bidloo the Elder.[1, 2] Cases in which nontraumatic CSF rhinorrhea resulted from increased intracranial pressure were then reported by Miller in 1826[3] and King in 1834.[4] The full significance of CSF fistulas was not appreciated, however, until 1884, when Chiari[5] demonstrated a fistulous connection between a pneumatocele in the frontal lobes and the ethmoid sinuses of a patient who died of meningitis following rhinorrhea. The introduction of roentgenography enabled the diagnosis of a fistula to be made in vivo through the detection of intracranial air,[6] ultimately leading to the development of pneumoencephalography as a diagnostic procedure[7] and, less directly, to the refinement of surgical techniques for the repair of CSF fistulas.[8, 9] Despite a number of early attempts, successful repair was not consistently achieved until the mid-1930s. In 1937, Cairns[10] published a series of cases demonstrating that CSF leaks could be repaired by the extradural application of fascia lata. The need for such intervention was not, however, universally acknowledged. World War II heightened interest in this problem. By 1944, Dandy[11] advocated surgical repair of any CSF leak within 2 weeks of onset to prevent meningitis. Lewin's review of the British combat experience and of a large series of basilar skull fractures.[12, 13] strongly influenced the adoption of aggressive operative management as the standard of care. The cessation of a leak, he argued, did not eliminate the risk of meningitis. By the mid-1950s, it became virtually axiomatic to operate on all CSF fistulas that did not close within several days.

There has never been a consensus regarding which operative route is most successful: intracranial or extracranial. Although the extradural repair described by Cairns and

Dandy was initially supplanted, among neurosurgeons, by an intradural approach to the fistula,[14] the extradural technique has enjoyed a resurgence of respect in both otolaryngologic and neurosurgical circles.[15–17] The introduction of minimally invasive approaches to CSF fistulas—the use of endoscopic procedures, for example—has simultaneously facilitated the extradural approach and blurred the distinction between truly extradural and intradural repair. For purposes of this discussion, endoscopic repair is considered extradural when it is intended to patch or plug a fistula from outside in and intradural when it is intended to facilitate the location or repair of a fistula intradurally.[18, 19]

The danger of CSF leakage has been framed in terms of the potential for meningitis, and the indication for treatment has been driven by the rarity of spontaneous and permanent cessation of the leak. Recent years have witnessed an increasing appreciation for the inherent complexity of this problem. Why should some leaks stop and others not? Why should some recur? Why should 20% or more of repairs that are done come to failure? With these questions in mind, the principle promoted by Lewin,[12] the idea that *all* cranial CSF fistulas, without exception, be repaired surgically unless they resolve spontaneously within 5 days or a week, has come under increasing scrutiny. The observations that have led to this situation are as follows:

1. Some fistulas seem to heal spontaneously with time, especially if external CSF drainage is used as an adjunctive maneuver.
2. A recurrence rate of 6% to 25% and a not inconsequential operative morbidity and mortality accompany the various forms of reparative surgery.
3. The incidence and severity of meningitis in otherwise uncomplicated CSF leaks may be diminished by treatment with antibiotics.[2, 20–28]

## CONVENTIONS AND DEFINITIONS

The term *rhinorrhea* is used to describe fluid dripping from the nose. *Otorrhea* is used to describe fluid dripping from the ear. These terms must be understood to reflect the site of the drip, rather than the site of the leak. CSF leaking

164

through temporal bone fractures, for example, can easily reach the nasopharynx through the eustachian tube and mimic a leak through the cribriform plate. There is no specific term to describe leaks from the spinal subarachnoid space.

Transcranial CSF leaks fall into two major categories: *traumatic* leaks and the so-called *spontaneous,* or nontraumatic, leaks. The traumatic group, in turn, is divided into two groups: *acute or early* leaks that present within 1 week of injury and *delayed* leaks that occur months or years later. The nontraumatic group is also divided into subsets, including leaks associated with intracranial mass lesions; leaks associated with congenital defects of the skull base; leaks associated with osteomyelitis and other causes of bony erosion; leaks associated with focal cerebral atrophy[4]; and leaks associated with an ill-defined group of acquired hernias, meningoceles, and meningeal diverticula perforating pneumatized bone in the anteromedial middle fossa.[29] Nontraumatic fistulas are divided again into high-pressure and low-pressure categories.[4, 30] There is good reason to attempt to apply this nosology to the traumatic group as well.[24] Iatrogenic or postoperative leaks are usually included in the category of traumatic fistulas.

Spinal CSF leaks are classified analogously. Most spinal CSF leaks are postoperative and therefore traumatic. A number of rare congenital anomalies can give rise to meningopleural or meningoperitoneal fistulas.[31] The distinction between high-pressure and low-pressure fistulas is particularly important in the management of spinal leaks. In children with spinal dysraphism or other anomalies, the leak may be the first expression of hydrocephalus or shunt failure.[32, 33]

## CAUSE AND EPIDEMIOLOGY

### Traumatic Leaks

The most common cause of CSF leaks is head trauma, particularly basilar skull fracture.[34] In Lewin's series[12] of 100 patients with head injury, 7% had basal skull fractures, and 2% had CSF leaks. A CSF leak was detected in 2.8% of 1250 head injuries and 11.5% of the basilar fractures studied by Brawley.[14] In another study of 1077 skull fractures, including a particularly large proportion of high-speed road traffic accidents, 20.8% of 168 basilar skull fractures had an acute CSF leak.[35] The incidence in cases of penetrating missile injuries is comparable: In 1133 cases, 101 (8.9%) developed a CSF fistula. The proportion is somewhat higher with transventricular penetration.[36] Thus, CSF leaks occur in approximately 3% of all head injuries, 9% of high-energy penetrating injuries, and 12% to 30% of basilar skull fractures, depending on the accelerative forces involved.

In childhood, the incidence of traumatic CSF leaks is far lower: 1% or less of closed head injuries.[37] This disparity may be due to differences in fragility between the adult and the pediatric skull as well as to the lack of development of the air sinuses in children. As a rule, the frontal sinuses become visible between the 4th and 12th year and are always detected by age 15. They are often asymmetric until age 20. The ethmoids are present at birth, enlarge by age 3, and are fully formed by age 16 or 17. The cavity of the sphenoid sinus is usually recognizable by age 4 and fully developed by puberty. In the pediatric age range, the interpretation of sinus x-ray studies is often difficult because of small size, variations in development, and normal calcification and clouding.[32]

### Spontaneous Leaks

The term *spontaneous leak* is a 19th century misnomer that has entered into common use. The term ideally should be restricted to refer to leaks explained neither by trauma nor by any other cause if it is to have any useful meaning. The literature allows the term a far broader license. In any event, there have been few series of nontraumatic leaks collected. There are insufficient data to extrapolate quantitative estimates of incidence or cause.[28] Anecdotal series suggest that pituitary tumors are the most common cause of spontaneous CSF leaks when the underlying cause is an intracranial mass lesion, with or without excessive CSF pressures. Because of the structures eroded by sellar masses, such leaks generally present as rhinorrhea.[30, 38, 39] Other presentations—including a serous otitis media—have also been reported.[40, 41]

### Postoperative Leaks

Large, annoying, and potentially dangerous subgaleal collections of CSF were common before the modern era of neurosurgery. In retrospect, they generally represented the visible manifestations of altered postoperative CSF flow characteristics, increases in intracranial pressure, unrecognized or untreated hydrocephalus, or some combination of these conditions. These collections often leaked through the incision. In consequence, postoperative incisional CSF leaks were understood to be common neurosurgical complications. Attempts to prevent this complication were focused on careful dural closure, buttressing the suture line, multiple-layer incisional repair, and other techniques for reconstruction and reinforcement of violated tissue planes. All of these technical details were important, but none was as important as control of intracranial pressure and CSF dynamics postoperatively and the contributions to postoperative management rendered through serial sectional imaging techniques.

More radical approaches to cerebellopontine angle lesions and tumors straddling the nasopharynx and the anterior and middle fossas as well as the skull base more generally have created problems of a different sort. The true overall incidence of incisional CSF leaks is difficult to estimate, even though the factors responsible are not difficult to outline. After transfrontal surgery, the most common cause is failure to seal an opened frontal sinus. Rhinorrhea and otorrhea after cerebellopontine angle tumor resection are recorded in 2% to 22% of large series.[42] The incidence has been reduced by waxing and plugging mastoid air cells as they are opened and placing a graft of adipose tissue in the opened porus acusticus.[43, 44] The use of endoscopy to inspect the craniectomy site for unsealed air sinuses has been reported to reduce the incidence of otorrhea even further.[45] Rhinorrhea in this setting is a false localizing sign. In the trans-sphenoidal approach to the pituitary, leaks occur in 1.4% to 6.4%.[46–48]

## PNEUMOCEPHALUS

Intracranial air, a pathognomonic sign of CSF fistula after trauma or spontaneous rhinorrhea (but not after surgery), is demonstrable in approximately 20% of patients with CSF leaks.[49] Pneumocephalus is post-traumatic in 75% and spontaneous, or otherwise unexplained, in 10%.[50]

## MENINGITIS

Meningitis occurs in approximately 20% of acute post-traumatic leaks and 57% of delayed leaks.[34] Although these figures vary in different series, meningitis occurs more frequently in the delayed post-traumatic group. The incidence of meningitis in nontraumatic CSF leaks has not been well documented. Anecdotally, copious, continuous leakage of the high-pressure type is less likely to be associated with meningitis than intermittent leakage.[30] The overall risk of meningitis from traumatic CSF leaks of all types is on the order of 25%.[13, 51-54] In postoperative leaks, the incidence of meningitis can be calculated to be on the order of 20%, but this figure is admittedly complicated by the problem of distinguishing aseptic from bacterial meningitis, by factors such as immunosuppression that might, because of an association with poor wound healing, precipitate both the leak and the meningitis.

## DEFINING AND LOCALIZING A FISTULA

The management of CSF leaks involves three steps: (1) confirming that the leaking fluid is really CSF, (2) delineating the site of the fistula, and (3) defining its mechanism.

### Clinical Evidence to Confirm the Presence of Cerebrospinal Fluid

#### Glucose

The presence of glucose in clear leaking fluid has been used historically to differentiate CSF from nasal secretions and other sources of serous or serosanguineous drainage. The concentration of glucose in CSF equals or exceeds 50% of the serum concentration except as follows: (1) during meningitis, (2) after subarachnoid hemorrhage, or (3) under other unusual circumstances. The glucose concentration in nasal secretions, in contrast, is 10 mg/dl or less.[55] Quantitative measurements of glucose concentration are diagnostic. *Qualitative* spot tests, such as those provided by chemical testing strips (e.g., Clinistix, Dextrostix, Uristix, or Tes-Tape), are *not* definitive for two reasons: (1) The glucose oxidase test on which they are based is too sensitive, turning positive at values less than 20 mg/100 ml of glucose. (2) Normal nasopharyngeal secretions often elicit false-positive reactions even in the absence of glucose.[56, 57] Thus, although a *negative* glucose oxidase reaction effectively eliminates the possibility of CSF rhinorrhea, a positive result does not.

### Reservoir Sign

It is widely held that true CSF leaks produce quantities of fluid sufficient for collection and quantitative analysis at some time in their course. The reservoir sign, the ability of a patient to produce CSF at will by positioning the head in a certain way, is generally taken to be quite specific for a fistula with pooling in the sphenoid sinus.[29] Although Dandy[11] believed that this sign would differentiate leakage through the frontal sinus from ethmoidal and sphenoidal leaks, it is not reliably localizing.

### Target Sign

The target sign refers to the differential, pseudochromatographic diffusion of CSF admixed with blood or other serosanguineous fluid on filter paper or bedclothes. CSF migrates further, creating a bull's-eye stain with blood in the center. This is a convenient but unreliable sign because whenever watery nasal secretions and blood are mixed, the same phenomenon occurs.

### Headache

CSF leaks can be accompanied by high-pressure or low-pressure headaches. Intermittent high-pressure leaks are characterized by *high* CSF pressure headaches that are relieved by the sudden discharge of fluid and build up again over time. Normal-pressure leaks, in contrast, are characterized by postural *low* CSF pressure headaches, relieved by reclining or otherwise allowing pressure in the subarachnoid space to rise to normal levels.

### Other Confirmatory Evidence

The finding of unusually low opening pressure in the lumbar subarachnoid space is corroborating evidence for CSF leak. Unilateral or bilateral *anosmia* is associated with defects or leaks in the region of the cribriform plate and the fovea ethmoidalis. Olfaction may be preserved, however, in cases of spontaneous CSF rhinorrhea with congenital defects of the cribriform fossa.[30, 51] *Optic nerve* lesions point to the tuberculum sella, the sphenoid sinus, and the posterior ethmoids. Impaired *vestibular function, facial nerve palsy,* and *cochlear damage* accompany fractures in the temporal bone.

## Imaging Techniques

Imaging techniques are used to detect intracranial air, fractures and defects in the skull base, mass lesions, and hydrocephalus and to demonstrate flow through fistulas or skull defects.[58] Plain films, multiplanar tomography, computed tomography (CT), and magnetic resonance imaging (MRI) delineate the anatomy and pathology of the skull base, sinuses, and calvaria. Stains, contrast agents, and radioactive tracers are injected into the ventricular or lumbar subarachnoid space to prove that leaking fluid is CSF and to show, directly or by inference, the location of the leak.

Radiographic data must be interpreted in accordance with the clinical setting. As a general rule, *positive* data obtained from radiography are helpful, but *negative* data are often meaningless.

## Plain Radiography and Computed Tomography

Plain films and CT are examined for evidence of fracture; air/fluid levels in the frontal, ethmoidal, and sphenoid sinuses; intracranial air; chronic increased intracranial pressure; erosion of bone by tumor or infection; congenital anomalies; and penetrating objects. Although multiplanar tomography provides exquisite detail of bony anatomy, it has been supplanted in most centers by high-accuracy CT with overlapping 2-mm cuts.[59] Contrast cisternography in conjunction with CT provides dynamic information about flow patterns of CSF.[60] MRI also provides superb detail of soft tissue pathology at the skull base and in the nasopharynx.

## Tracers

The ultimate proof of CSF fistula is the ability to retrieve extracranially a tracer substance injected into the CSF. Historically the nonradioactive subtances injected into the CSF have included methylene blue, phenolsulfonphthalein, indigo carmine, and fluorescein.[61, 62] Only indigo carmine and fluorescein remain in common use. The others proved toxic.[4]

In the presence of an active leak, cotton pledgets placed along the anterior roof of the nose, the posterior roof and the sphenoethmoid recess, and the middle meatus and below the posterior end of the inferior turbinate can be used to confirm that a leak exists. When differentially stained or contaminated by radioactive isotopes, they indicate the location of the leak.[28] The following procedure has been recommended to localize a leak with fluorescein:

1. A spinal tap is performed.
2. Ten milliliters of spinal fluid are withdrawn after measuring the opening pressure.
3. The fluid is mixed with 0.5 ml of 5% fluorescein.
4. The mixture is slowly reinjected intrathecally.
5. The patient assumes a recumbent position for about 30 minutes, depending on the size of the leak.
6. The pledgets are removed and examined under ultraviolet illumination.

The findings are interpreted in Table 12–1. The use of fluorescein in the CSF is controversial. Similar techniques, however, can be adapted to other tracers.

Staining behind the tympanic membrane indicates a leak into the middle ear. In the presence of an active leak, tracer methods are sensitive and reasonably specific. With slow, low-volume, or intermittent leaks, tracer methods may give false-negative results.

There is an important controversy regarding the use of fluorescein intrathecally. Although the ear, nose and throat community uses fluorescein tracer almost routinely, neurosurgeons have become wary of its use because of reports of transverse myelitis and other serious reactions.[63] Indigo carmine is the tracer stain preferred by most neurosurgeons. Indigo carmine is more visible than fluorescein to the unaided eye. This characteristic makes it useful to check for the presence of CSF fistulas intraoperatively, when ultraviolet illumination may not be readily available.[29]

Because it is easier to detect minute amounts of radioactivity than to distinguish faint color on pledgets stained by bloody fluid or mucus, radioactive tracers are more sensitive than stains. [131]I (RISA) was widely used for cisternography in the past. It has been replaced by [111]In DTPA, an isobaric tracer that combines improved physical properties, fewer adverse reactions, better imaging quality, and shorter half-life (2.8 days). [169]Yb DTPA and [99m]Tc albumin have also been approved for CSF imaging, but these tracers suffer from inferior imaging characteristics and from inconvenient half-lives (32 days and 6 hours).

Isotope cisternography is an excellent method by which to prove the existence of a CSF leak. It provides inaccurate localization, however. An active leak of any magnitude quickly oversaturates the pledgets and surrounding tissues, so that differential localization becomes impossible.[34, 64, 65]

Many radiologists and neurosurgeons fail to appreciate the importance of the timing of radioactive contamination. Active leaks contaminate accurately placed pledgets within 0.5 to 2 hours. Slow or intermittent leaks can be detected by leaving the pledgets in place or replacing them continuously over 6 to 48 hours. Over the extended time span, however, the isotope can be absorbed into the bloodstream from the CSF and undergo secondary secretion into the nasopharynx. These events cause a false-positive test result.[66]

An alternate pathway for isotope contamination of nasopharyngeal secretions was first recognized in normal dogs. It may result from active transport from the CSF, passage via the olfactory nerves, or passive lymphatic drainage.[67] The same type of contamination has been documented in normal human volunteers. In short, low-level radioactivity in pledgets exposed to the nasal mucosa over many hours should be viewed with suspicion. This finding may just as easily represent spurious secondary contamination as a slow leak.

The accuracy of faintly positive tests can be improved slightly by calculating a radioactivity index ratio. This ratio compares the radioactivity (RI) in counts per minute of an exposed pledget with that of 1 ml of blood, as follows:

$$\text{RI ratio} = \frac{\text{RI}_{\text{pledget}}}{\text{RI}_{\text{1 ml blood}}}$$

An RI ratio less than 0.3 is normal. Canine studies suggest that the ratio in the presence of a leak is at least five times greater. In the canine model, the RI ratio of nasal activity to CSF is 1:14, 2 to 5 hours after cisternal injection of radiosotope. The RI ratio of nasal activity to blood is 1:2 to 3, 2 to 5 hours after intravenous injection of radioisotope. Thus, the RI ratio of CSF to blood is 4.6:7. Thus, the

TABLE 12–1 ■ **INTERPRETATION OF NASAL PLEDGET STAINS IN CEREBROSPINAL FLUID FISTULAS**

| Location of Stain | Probable Site of Fistula |
| --- | --- |
| Anterior nasal | Cribriform plate or anterior ethmoidal roof |
| Posterior nasal or sphenoethmoidal | Posterior ethmoid or sphenoid sinus |
| Middle meatus | Frontal sinus |
| Below posterior end of inferior turbinate | Eustachian tube (middle fossa) |

significance of tracer substances appearing in low concentrations more than 5 hours after injection should be carefully evaluated.

It has been suggested that tracer injected into the cervical subarachnoid cistern can be forced through a slow, intermittent, or low-pressure leak by raising the CSF pressure with saline or artificial CSF delivered via a constant infusion pump.[68] Delayed scans carried out 24 and 48 hours after injection of isotopes can help define the mechanism of a leak by detecting defects in CSF absorption and circulation.

## Contrast Enhancement

Early attempts at demonstrating CSF leaks by injecting air or iophendylate (Pantopaque) into the subarachnoid space failed to produce consistently satisfactory images. The combination of CT and metrizamide cisternography has come to yield excellent visualization of *active* leaks. Smaller fistulas have been demonstrated by having the patient cough or carry out a Valsalva maneuver.[34] For maximal contrast enhancement, cisternal injections can be performed via C1-C2 punctures. Overlapping views in both the coronal and the axial planes are required.[59] Direct coronal studies are preferable to reconstructed images. The risk of provoking seizures and aseptic or chemical meningitis with metrizamide cisternography should be kept in mind.

## Immunologic Methods

Irjala and colleagues[69] have described the use of an immunofixation technique for the identification of microaliquots (<100 μl) of CSF by demonstrating two electrophoretically characteristic bands of transferrin. The B1 fraction consists of normal transferrin and sometimes two variant fractions. The B2 fraction characteristic of CSF contains smaller amounts of neuraminic acid. This method is not subject to contamination from other body fluids (tears, nasal secretions). The immunofixation method could theoretically be used for localization of the leak by differential suction techniques in the nasopharynx, but large-scale clinical trials of this method have yet to be reported.

# ANATOMIC CONSIDERATIONS: SITES OF LEAKAGE

## Trauma

CSF leak can occur wherever the dura is lacerated during an injury. It is more likely to persist or recur, rather than close spontaneously, where a meningeal hiatus is maintained by bony spicules, by dura entrapped in the edges of a fracture, or by herniating brain and leptomeninges. Avulsion of the olfactory fibrils can cause a dural fistula through the cribriform plate even without a fracture. Post-traumatic fistulas are frequently complex and multiple.

## Spontaneous

Nontraumatic leaks are usually confined to one region where an anatomic defect is demonstrable. It is usually

easier to demonstrate the defect than the leak. High-pressure leaks that act as safety valves for hydrocephalus occur where the skull is thinnest, usually the cribriform fossa and the sellar region. This is the case, for example, in Crouzon's disease and osteopetrosis (Albers-Schoenberg disease).

The middle fossa can be the site of CSF leaks that are direct in that they do not cross the inner ear. Such fistulas have been described mainly in conjunction with a pneumatized temporal fossa. Pulsatile CSF forces induce additional thinning of the bone and enlargement of pits and small bony defects that are normally present. The leptomeninges and brain herniate, thinning the dura and leading to rupture of the arachnoid. The leak may be constant or intermittent, depending on several factors: the underlying intracranial pressure, whether an arachnoid diverticulum is created, and whether brain tissue temporarily obliterates the leak. A similar sequence of events has been postulated to explain CSF leaks in the empty sella syndrome[29] and in focal atrophy.[30]

Indirect fistulas through the temporal bone are the most elusive. In *extralabyrinthine fistulas* the defect occurs in the *middle fossa,* in the region of the tegmen tympani. In *intralabyrinthine fistulas,* CSF escapes into the labyrinth through the subarachnoid space of the *posterior fossa.* In either case, the leak can present as otorrhea or, when the tympanic membrane is intact, as rhinorrhea.[49] The possibility of temporal bone dysplasia should be investigated whenever a patient with severe hearing loss develops unexplained or recurrent meningitis.[29, 34, 70] In the Mondini malformation, for example (unreactive ear with a shortened cochlear coil, dilated semicircular canal system, and widened inner ear vestibule), it is hypothesized that a widened, patent cochlear aqueduct allows CSF to pass from the subarachnoid space to the inner ear via a leak in the oval window. Other proposed routes include defects of the scala tympani, the footplate of the stapes, or thin bony plate separating the internal auditory canal and the inner ear vestibule and perforated by nerve fibers innervating the utricular and saccular macula.[70–73]

# HIGH-PRESSURE VERSUS LOW-PRESSURE LEAKS

When a CSF leak is the manifestation of increased intracranial pressure from mass effect or hydrocephalus, the underlying cause must be treated before the leak can be effectively repaired. The existence of increased intracranial pressure can be inferred from several sources. Skull films and CT scans disclose signs of pressure, mass effect, and tumors. Radiographic signs suggestive of defective circulation and absorption of CSF include periventricular lucencies, enlarged temporal horns, disproportionately plump third ventricle narrowed at the massa intermedia, and an empty sella. Extracerebral collections of CSF can represent the so-called fifth ventricle phenomenon, a hydrocephalus variant. Other concomitants of high-pressure leakage include papilledema and optic atrophy; pallor of the optic disk; enlarged central scotoma or subtle binasal visual field cuts; a history of headaches worse in the morning or while recumbent, relieved by a gush of fluid; variable or intermittent diplopia; intermittent clonus or pyramidal tract signs reversing spontaneously after leakage; and a history of granulomatous meningitis, subarachnoid hemorrhage, head trauma, or some other event that might adversely affect the circulation of CSF.

Infants with incisional leaks after fresh meningomyelocele repair can be assumed to have hydrocephalus, especially if there is an accompanying Dandy-Walker malformation. In contrast to other cases of postoperative leak, in which the temporizing maneuvers discussed subsequently are frequently effective, CSF shunting is generally required.

## INITIAL MANAGEMENT

The initial management of CSF leaks is intended to slow or stop the leak and prevent meningitis. Usually, both these ends are satisfied simultaneously.

### Antibiotics

Antibiotics have not been proven effective in changing the incidence of meningitis in post-traumatic or postoperative CSF leaks. In traumatic leaks, they are no longer prescribed routinely.[14–16, 20, 35, 74] For postoperative leaks, however, prophylactic antibiotics are commonly, if not universally, employed. There is some theoretical justification for distinguishing between the two situations. When antibiotics are administered, several principles should be kept in mind:[75]

1. Patients should not be kept on antibiotics indefinitely in the hope that a leak will seal; a trial of conservative therapy is reasonable, but the end point should be decided a priori.
2. Wide-spectrum antibiotics are not desirable for prophylaxis; the most specific antibiotic capable of eliminating the potential pathogens should be used.
3. Patients of different ages and in different locations harbor different vulnerabilities because of changes in nasopharyngeal and environmental flora; thus, *Haemophilus influenzae* is a common cause of meningitis in children and in the elderly, whereas diplococcus is more common in healthy adults.
4. Patients can develop meningitis even while on prophylactic antibiotics; after the usual investigations are carried out, the antibiotics are changed to cover the appropriate organisms and sensitivities.
5. Bactericidal antibiotics should be chosen when possible.

### Intensive Care

The admission of patients with CSF leak to intensive care units was universally advocated by the older literature. This admission may certainly be warranted in some cases of trauma or spontaneous high-pressure leaks but is not always needed for recurrent or postoperative leak. A great deal depends on nursing and house staff coverage in a

given institution and on any unique aspects of nursing policy. One consideration to keep in mind is that opportunistic infections arising in intensive care units are usually due to resistant organisms and are often highly recalcitrant to treatment with the usual antibiotics.

### Position

The preferred position for patients with cranial leaks is between 45 and 70 degrees. Patients with a spinal leak should be kept flat if at all possible.

## EXTERNAL DRAINAGE OF CEREBROSPINAL FLUID

External drainage of CSF has been used in various forms for many years. External ventricular drainage[76, 77] has been replaced in most centers by continuous lumbar drainage, first described in 1963.[78] Since then, lumbar drainage has been found useful in controlling and sometimes curing CSF leak of every cause.[22–24] McCoy[79] provided theoretical justification for the initial management of CSF fistulas with CSF diversion by demonstrating that granulation can seal the fistulas, provided that the leakage has stopped. Lumbar drainage should be considered therefore whenever positioning alone does not eliminate, or at least significantly diminish, a leak within 24 hours.

### Technique

A 19-gauge catheter is threaded percutaneously through a 17-gauge Touhy needle inserted into the lumbar subarachnoid space between L4-L5 and L2-L3. Aside from increased attention to sterile technique, there is no difference from standard lumbar puncture procedure. After 10 to 20 cm have been threaded rostrally, the needle is removed over the catheter. If there is any significant resistance to passage, the needle and the catheter should be removed as a unit. *Under no circumstances should the catheter be withdrawn through the needle once the tip has protruded:* The needle tip may shear the catheter, leaving the tip irretrievably lost in the subarachnoid space or the subcutaneous tissue. The proximal end of the catheter is connected, via the appropriate adapters, to a closed, sterile drainage system. Prepackaged kits for epidural anesthesia generally provide all the necessary catheters, needles, and fittings. Specialized drainage kits for lumbar CSF drainage have also been marketed commercially. In their absence, a blood transfusion pack connected to the catheter with intravenous tubing can be used for collection. Antibiotic ointment may be placed at the skin entry site. A waterproof, occlusive dressing should be applied, with the catheter coiled and taped to relieve strain and prevent disconnection.

### Prevention of Infection

The infection rate with indwelling catheters can be prohibitive, ranging, in some series, as high as 10% or more.[80]

The risk is lower with lumbar catheters.[25] Infection can be controlled by prophylactic antibiotics, potentially capable of reducing infection by two thirds,[80] and by externalization of the catheter through an extended subcutaneous tunnel.[81] *Staphylococcus* species and other skin flora are the major threat: Antibiotics should be chosen to reflect the sensitivities of local pathogens. Prophylaxis is continued for 8 to 24 hours after the catheter is withdrawn. Daily samples of CSF are obtained, cultured, and examined by Gram stain and analyzed for cell count and differential, glucose, and protein. The presence of a catheter does not, of its own accord, lower the CSF glucose or evoke a major leukocytotic reaction; the cell count and glucose concentration remain quite stable in uninfected CSF over 4 to 9 days. Any persisting variation of 2 standard deviations or more from the cumulative average cell count and glucose concentration over several days is cause for concern and careful re-examination of the CSF for signs of opportunistic infection.[82]

External drainage has been maintained in large series for 10 days without infection. Longer durations have been reported in exceptional cases.[23] By analogy with central venous access lines, it may be wise to change catheters if drainage is continued beyond 7 days.

## How Long to Drain

Drainage should be continued for 3 to 5 days after stoppage of the leak to allow healing. If leakage recurs, operative repair is indicated. If the underlying problem is increased intracranial pressure or hydrocephalus, implantation of a drain acts purely as a temporizing maneuver: No "cure" is effected. Similarly, patients whose leak is not controlled by external drainage should be considered for early operation. In Findler's series of 50 patients,[28] drainage of 350 to 420 ml daily was continued for an average of 10 days, with a leak recurrence rate of 14%. There was an additional 8% incidence of delayed leak at the site of lumbar puncture.

As a rule, acute post-traumatic and postoperative normal-pressure leaks respond to external drainage. Transitory high-pressure leaks also respond, so long as the pressure elevation recedes over the duration of the drainage. Delayed and recurring leaks cannot be definitively managed by drainage.

## Pharmacologic Adjuvants

Pharmacologic agents such as acetazolamide (Diamox) that retard the production of CSF may be helpful in reducing CSF pressure after the drain has been removed. These agents are not effective as a primary mode of therapy.

## Complications

High CSF protein concentrations predispose against a successful drainage. If, for technical reasons, patency of the drainage catheter cannot be maintained, the same effect can be achieved with repetitive lumbar punctures through a large needle.

Calcaterra[17] records one case of fatal postoperative suboccipital hemorrhage in an elderly patient attributed to overdrainage of CSF. Similar complications have followed spinal anesthesia.[83–85] Overdrainage of CSF can also cause life-threatening pneumocephalus.[51, 86–88] The CSF pressure should be lowered substantially but not reduced to less than zero. The acute reduction of CSF pressure can also precipitate headache, nausea, and vomiting. This reaction can be prevented, according to Findler,[28] by gradually lowering the pressure and increasing the drainage over several days. An accidental siphon effect can be avoided by relating the height of the drainage valve or the drainage bag to the level of the ventricular system rather than the bed. In this way, the pressure column remains constant as the bed is raised and lowered or as the patient is moved. Most commercial systems incorporate a micropore filtered air port to prevent siphonage. Improvised systems are generally unable to include such a port, and positioning becomes critical.

There has been long-standing concern regarding the possibility of inducing meningitis by retrograde migration of bacteria into an open fistula under the influence of negative CSF pressure induced by an external drain.[4] This situation has not occurred in practice, however, and seems avoidable by maintaining a low but steady positive pressure in the CSF.

Catheters should not be removed forcibly. If a catheter resists withdrawal, serious consideration should be given to whether it ought to be removed in the operating room under direct vision. As the catheter is removed, the tip is examined to ensure that no part of it has been left behind. An unused catheter should be available for comparison because the indwelling catheter may be distorted or elongated during withdrawal.

If the catheter is not intact, an effort should be made to locate and identify the retained segment. Although most catheters are intended to be radiopaque, they are easily missed on plain x-ray studies and are better visualized on CT. There are two strong indications for retrieval of a broken catheter tip: infection in the region of the tip and radicular pain or paresis associated with juxtaposition of the retained catheter to an appropriate root. In most cases, the retained fragment can be ignored safely. If symptoms in the region point to possible catheter involvement at some future time, sectional imaging studies should be obtained and the matter reviewed anew.

Dural cutaneous fistulas can occur at the site of catheter insertion, particularly in the setting of a high-pressure leak. Most such fistulas stop spontaneously or seal with a single stitch. Low-pressure or normal-pressure leaks can also be sealed by an injection of 10 to 20 ml of autologous blood as an epidural blood patch. This technique is favored by anesthetists and obstetricians for the treatment of low-pressure "spinal" headaches. It has been shown by a number of studies to improve over natural history[89–93] with a success rate of 93%.[94] Epidural blood patching has resulted in symptomatic mass effect, hemorrhagic complications,[95] and infection. Surgical repair of the dura may still be needed. External lumbar drainage is contraindicated when the source of increased intracranial pressure can be related to posterior fossa masses.

## OPERATIVE MANAGEMENT

### Timing of Surgery

The debate regarding the timing of surgery centers on three issues:

1. Most CSF leaks stop spontaneously and do not recur.
2. Surgery is neither universally successful nor without hazard.
3. Modern antibiotics have significantly reduced the morbidity from any infection that may develop while waiting for the leak to stop or that may ensue should the leak recur.

There are some leaks that should always be given the opportunity to stop spontaneously. Most acute post-traumatic leaks stop within 10 days of injury; in Mincy's series[2] of 54 cases of rhinorrhea in frontal fossa injury, 35% had stopped within 24 hours, 68% within 48 hours, and 85% within 1 week. The use of lumbar drainage may further increase the rate of sealing.

There are three classic criteria for surgical intervention: a bout of meningitis, pneumocephalus, or active leak (persistent or recurring). Lewin's insistence on surgery for virtually all leaks was based on a fear of meningitis rather than on accurate figures for recurrence. It has yet to be shown that operation offers a real improvement over natural history in patients with acute post-traumatic leaks that have stopped within the first week.

Most leaks or dural tears associated with midface fractures stop permanently when the facial fractures are reduced.[96] Meningitis is relatively uncommon in dural tears associated with facial fractures, despite the fact that the incidence of dural laceration in facial fractures (43%) is higher than in closed head injury (7%) and CSF leak occurs far more commonly (36%).[96]

Most postoperative incisional leaks also stop spontaneously or with lumbar drainage, particularly if the incision is reinforced or oversewn and any underlying abnormality of intracranial pressure is properly treated. Postoperative rhinorrhea and otorrhea are less likely to seal. If position and lumbar drainage do not stop the leak within 48 hours or if the leak stops then recurs, most authors favor re-exploration of the wound and direct repair of the fistula. The air sinuses in these cases have usually been violated. In the series by Spaziante and colleagues[47] of 140 transsphenoidal operations, four of six leaks stopped with lumbar drainage alone; Ciric[48] estimates that 2% of transsphenoidal cases require reoperation for CSF leak.

Surgical intervention may be indicated without further delay in the following circumstances:

1. Acute traumatic or postoperative leaks that recur or persist after 10 to 13 days of conservative management, including external drainage
2. Proven intermittent or delayed leaks
3. High-pressure leaks acting as a "safety valve" for hydrocephalus
4. Leaks associated with erosion, destruction, or severe comminution of the skull base or the paranasal sinuses
5. Leaks associated with congenital dysplasias of the brain, skull base, orbit, or ear, particularly after a bout of meningitis
6. Leaks caused by high-energy missile wounds
7. Postoperative rhinorrhea and otorrhea that cannot be controlled by position and drainage, especially when the air sinuses have been violated as part of the operative route

High-volume leaks through the petrous bone and the sella are particularly recalcitrant to conservative management.

### Operative Techniques

There are three major operative approaches currently in use. Often combined, they are as follows: (1) craniotomy, including intradural and extradural techniques; (2) extracranial extradural, endoscopic or not, with degrees of complexity ranging from simple packing to complicated mucoperiosteal grafts; and (3) CSF shunting procedures. Table 12–2 summarizes current techniques and their applications.

### Craniotomy

#### Anterior Fossa

In the anterior fossa, the two techniques that are most used are *intracranial extradural* and *intracranial intradural*. The intracranial extradural approach has several substantial limitations: (1) Dural tears are virtually inevitable in the course of dissection, (2) areas of cerebral tissue herniation into bony defects cannot be easily visualized, and (3) permanent dural repair is not reliably achieved. For these reasons, the intracranial intradural route is preferred when craniotomy is indicated.

Preoperatively, steroids, anticonvulsants, and prophylactic antibiotics are given. The patient is positioned supine in a three-point or four-point frame or on a cerebellar head rest, body flexed, knees bent, nose at the midline, head hyperextended with the malar eminences uppermost. A Doppler probe monitors for air emboli during the procedure; arterial and central venous access is obtained. A bicoronal scalp flap is turned. A bone flap is elevated ipsilateral to the leak for a unilateral exposure, bilaterally otherwise. Although in some situations, satisfactory access can be obtained from a unilateral exposure, a full exploration of the anterior fossa generally requires a bifrontal flap. Should the frontal air sinus be entered, the mucosa is stripped from both the flap and the sinus, the sinus is packed with bacitracin-soaked Gelfoam sponge, and a pericranial flap reflected from the scalp is sutured over open sinus to the dura. Instruments used to close the sinus are considered contaminated and replaced.

The intracranial intradural approach allows a full exposure of the anterior fossa. A satisfactory exposure results in the demonstration of both sphenoid wings, both cribriform fossas, and both orbital roofs. The middle fossa is usually out of reach. The exposure should always extend as far posteriorly as possible. The anterior clinoids should be visualized. If the leak is to be repaired in conjunction with the definitive resection of an intracranial mass, other

**TABLE 12–2 ■ OPERATIVE PROCEDURES FOR MANAGEMENT OF CEREBROSPINAL FLUID LEAKS AND THEIR INDICATIONS**

| Procedure | Indications |
|---|---|
| Intracranial, intradural exploration | Acute or delayed traumatic leak from anterior or middle fossas |
| | Anterior fossa leak with extrasellar intracranial mass |
| | Congenital anomaly of brain |
| | Definable dysplasia of the anterior or middle fossas |
| | Postoperative leak after anterior or middle fossa surgery |
| | Complex penetrating or through-and-through injuries involving cerebral tissue as well as extracranial structures |
| | Whenever a craniotomy is indicated for other reasons |
| | Whenever a significant dural hiatus is demonstrable |
| Extracranial, extradural approach: *open* (trans-septal, trans-sphenoidal, or transethmoidal with mucoperiosteal flap) or *endoscopic* (tissue transfer, placement of fat plug or muscle pledget, injection of fibrin glue) | Clearly defined spontaneous leaks from the anterior fossa, including the cribriform fossa and fovea ethmoidalis |
| | Postoperative leaks after treatment of sellar and parasellar lesions |
| Extracranial, extradural approach: dural repair and simple packing | Leaks associated with temporal bone dysplasia and ear anomalies |
| | Leaks through the mastoid air cells, not originating in the middle fossa |
| Primary repair of facial fractures: sinus repair and ablation as necessary | Le Fort type II or type III fracture with dural tear or cerebrospinal fluid leak but without evidence of gross bony disruption of the skull base, or significant cerebral contusion |
| | Complex facial fractures involving orbit or air sinuses in which the initial leak has spontaneously sealed, without evidence of gross bony disruption of the skull base or significant cerebral contusion |
| Osteoplastic sinusotomy: repair of posterior sinus wall or cranialization of sinus and packing | Leaks associated with simple fractures through the posterior wall of the frontal sinus without evidence of comminution of the skull base or significant cerebral contusion |
| Ventricular or lumboperitoneal shunting | Carried out in conjunction with anatomic repair of a fistula or resection of a space-occupying mass in the face of hydrocephalus |
| | Small leaks that cannot be identified |

considerations may govern the exposure conjointly. Dehydrating agents and drainage of CSF facilitate retraction.

The fistula is often betrayed by a palpable or visible dural defect or by a contusion, adhesion, or herniation of cerebral tissue. An obvious fistula is sealed by inserting a plug of abdominal fat and covering the defect with a free or reflected flap of dura. The dura can be obtained from the adjacent bone or from the falx cerebri, depending on the location of the fistula. Alternatively a free patch of pericranium, temporalis fascia, fascia lata, or lyophilized dura can be sutured to the surrounding dura and, if needed, used to reinforce a plug of fat. Fat forms a more durable plug than muscle. Muscle fibroses and shrinks, whereas fat remains viable by recruiting a blood supply from adjacent tissues. Simple dural laceration can often be sutured primarily. A dural patch graft may be inserted when necessary. Dural grafts should be harvested from autologous tissue (temporalis fascia, pericranium, fascia lata, transversalis fascia) or from commerically prepared cadaver tissue (dura, pericardium, amniotic sac) but not from synthetic material, for fear of infection or secondary leak at the suture site.

If no discrete fistula is visualized, the entire floor of the frontal fossa, including both cribriform plates, and the limbus sphenoidale are invested with a large free pericranial graft. Sutures are placed to maintain approximation rather than obtain a watertight seal. The vector of CSF pressure tends to approximate the graft to the dura and stop the leak. Although dural substitutes have been used to repair dural defects, there is usually enough pericranium available for this purpose to obviate the need for synthetic grafts.

## Middle Fossa

For leaks from the middle fossa, the temporal floor must be thoroughly inspected. This is most efficiently done with an intradural approach. An extradural dissection runs an additional risk of damaging the facial nerve by inadvertent traction on the geniculate ganglion during exposure and dissection.

The principles of repair are identical to those in the anterior fossa. Free pericranial grafts are easier to manipulate than dural flaps in the middle fossa. Additionally, because the middle fossa is bounded by venous sinuses, reflecting a flap of any substantial size is impossible. Because only a unilateral exposure can be obtained in the middle fossa, it is particularly important to identify the site of the leak preoperatively. Craniotomy is the preferred route to the floor of middle fossa because of the anatomic consideration noted earlier. Leaks involving the petrous bone and the posterior margins of the temporal fossa are often better approached from an extradural approach or a combined exposure.

Air can be insufflated through specially designed tubes that seal the nares and occlude the posterior pharynx during surgery. By flooding the field with saline, it is sometimes possible to identify, by the bubbles, a fistula that would not otherwise be evident.[53] As a rule, it is simpler and more prudent to cover the entire anterior or middle fossa with a graft than to count on this technique.

## Posterior Fossa

CSF does not leak from the posterior fossa except in fractures extending through the petrous bone, after surgery, and in conjunction with some rare congenital anomalies. Otorrhea from petrous fractures rarely presents a problem because it usually stops spontaneously or with external CSF drainage. The same holds true for rhinorrhea emanating in the posterior fossa and presenting as a false localizing sign.

Postoperative CSF leaks can also trickle through the suture line. This trickling is a recognized complication of cerebellopontine angle surgery. Postoperative leaks through the mastoid or through the temporal bone can be quite challenging. It is standard technique to wax or otherwise seal any opened mastoid air cells. This task can be facilitated endoscopically.[53] Some surgeons also recommend plugging the porus acusticus with fat when it has been enlarged for tumor removal. Watertight closure of the dura is achieved using a dural graft.[42–44]

In the event of a leak, re-exploration of the incision is indicated. Some surgeons prefer an extradural approach via mastoidectomy, particularly for recalcitrant cases. When the ear is nonfunctional, this approach, combined with an obliteration of the inner and middle ear, ensures the maximal likelihood of detection and obliteration of the site of leakage. It does not address the problem of altered CSF dynamics, however.

For "spontaneous" leaks, such as those associated with the Mondini malformation, the extradural approach is generally adopted. These are complex cases, and multiple layer closures may be required.[97]

Most incisional leaks after posterior fossa surgery can be repaired by oversewing the wound and draining CSF. As a rule, incisional leaks reflect increased intracranial pressure. If the leak recurs or the wound bulges with subgaleal CSF after drainage is discontinued, permanent CSF diversion should be considered. In children particularly, but also in adults, increasing the dose of corticosteroids, or slowing a taper, may reduce the pressure and allow tissue barriers to re-establish.

## Closure

A routine craniotomy closure is carried out. The patient is nursed in the head-up position for 3 to 5 days postoperatively and treated with laxatives and stool softeners to prevent straining. All heavy labor and lifting are prohibited for 3 months.

## Combined Craniotomy and Reduction of Facial Fractures

Most CSF leaks associated with fractures of the midface can be managed definitively by reducing the facial fracture. Complex fractures impacted into the skull base often require reduction via craniotomy before realignment of the facial fracture. No definitive rules can be given for these injuries; treatment must be carefully individualized and often requires a team approach using ear, nose, and throat; dental surgery; ophthalmology; plastic surgery; and neurosurgery.

## Extracranial Approaches

Aside from the classic trans-sphenoidal operations, the extracranial approaches to the skull base are generally performed by or in conjunction with otolaryngologists. Both neurosurgeons and otolaryngologists have begun to explore the limits of endoscopic approaches. This minimally invasive approach is promising but depends on one's ability to find with certainty the source of the leak. Even so, remarkably complex procedures have been carried out with endoscopic visualization only.[20, 21, 98] The broad principles of extracranial techniques are reviewed.

## Indications

There are four situations for which the extracranial approach is particularly suited:

1. Discrete and definable normal pressure leaks through the cribriform plate or adjacent ethmoid labyrinth
2. Fractures that abut on an air sinus, particularly when the bony defect is limited to the cranial wall of that sinus
3. Postoperative leaks after trans-sphenoidal surgery
4. Leaks through the oval window, petrous bone, or other parts of the ear

## Special Techniques

Intrathecal dye injected at the beginning of the procedure helps to visualize the leak intraoperatively. Indwelling catheters are often used: saline or artificial CSF can be injected intrathecally to distend the subarachnoid space and provoke an intermittent leak, and CSF can be drained postoperatively to encourage approximation of the flap and dural packing.

When CSF fistulas traverse an air sinus, the sinus is ablated with fat or muscle. The packing acts as a seal in its own right and serves to hold mucoperiosteal, periosteal, or free fascia lata grafts against the dura. To inhibit the formation of a mucocele, the mucosa of the sinus must be stripped before packing.

Transfrontal extradural procedures can be carried out either through a forehead incision or via a bicoronal incision. There is one important advantage to the bicoronal incision: Should it be necessary to obtain a more generous view of the frontal fossa, a craniotomy can be carried out without difficulty. This eventuality should be considered and discussed with the patient before surgery. The anterior wall of the frontal sinus is removed with a Stryker saw or the Midas Rex with the C1 attachment, following a template obtained from a 72-inch sinus film. The posterior wall is fully exposed: The mucosa is resected, and enough bone is removed to display the dural defect. The dura can be patched or sutured primarily. Depending on the extent of damage, the fragments of the posterior wall can be replaced or totally removed, thereby cranializing the frontal sinus. In either case, the sinus is ablated with fat, and the frontal wall is restored.

Endoscopic techniques have been adapted to each of these approaches. The learning curve is high for endoscopic manipulation. In the event that a leak can be pinpointed and the necessary tissue manipulation achieved, endoscopic procedures have the advantage of reduced hospitalization and, quite often, better visualization. With rare exceptions currently entering the market, three-dimensional visualization is lost, and the field of view is extremely limited.[99]

Depending on the angle required, the width of the desired window, the site of the leak, and the surgeon's preference, the sphenoid sinus and the sella can be approached trans-septally, via a sublabial or a transnasal route, or transethmoidally, via an external rhinotomy incision. The first is more familiar to neurosurgeons, but the second is shorter, gives a wider exposure, and permits complete resection of the sphenoid septae. This is an important consideration in reoperation for CSF leak after trans-sphenoidal surgery and reconstruction of the sellar floor. The leak is sealed by a flap of mucoperiosteum elevated with or without the underlying cartilage and folded over the dural defect. Sometimes a free graft of fascia lata is interposed. The ethmoid or sphenoid sinus is packed to hold the graft in place. Lumbar drainage is implemented for 5 days.

Endoscopic endonasal surgery has been used to operate in the parasellar area and to seal CSF leaks.[100, 101] Mucoperiosteum from the inferior turbinate serves as a convenient source of tissue. Dural defects up to $10 \times 10$ mm have been successfully treated. Parasellar leaks have also been treated by injecting fibrin glue transmucosally under CT guidance.[102]

If an open extracranial approach to the cribriform fossa and fovea ethmoidalis is preferred, these structures are best approached through a curved naso-orbital incision and a complete ethmoidectomy. A flap rotated from the middle turbinate or the septum is used to cover the cribriform plate and the ethmoid roof from below. The posterior ethmoidal artery is a landmark situated directly anterior to the optic nerve.

Extracranial techniques, whether open or endoscopic, carry a lower morbidity than craniotomy and avoid anosmia. They are sometimes successful in situations in which multiple craniotomies have failed. They do not permit a wide visual inspection of the orbitofrontal cortex or of the floor of the anterior fossa.

## Other Technical Considerations

### Methyl Methacrylate

When methyl methacrylate first became available, it was hailed as the paean for CSF leaks.[49, 103] Experience has not justified the initial round of enthusiasm. With time, methacrylate shrinks with the result that leaks recur. If infection sets in, the plug becomes a septic nidus. More importantly, it has become evident that the concept behind the use of methacrylate was faulty: It is the dura, not the bone, that requires repair. Leaks seal when the dural fistula is closed. Except in rare instances, the bony structures do not require reinforcement. When they do, however, autologous bone or cartilage is preferable to foreign material. Should the underlying problem be hydrocephalus or increased intracranial pressure, control of the intracranial pressure should be carried out before, or in conjunction with the exploration.

### Lumbar Drainage

Lumbar drainage is not generally carried out after craniotomy, because it is hoped that the CSF pressure will com-

press the graft onto the dura surrounding the fistula and create a seal. In extracranial extradural approaches, drainage of CSF helps create a seal and promotes healing.

### Tissue Adhesives

The availability of tissue adhesives was heralded with great initial enthusiasm. Similar to the methyl methacrylate to which they were chemically related, the cyanoacrylates seemed particularly suited to the management of CSF fistulas. It was hoped that adhesives might overcome some of the problems associated with obtaining a durable seal, especially in relatively inaccessible areas. The first generation of acrylic tissue adhesives has proved disappointing. In addition to carrying a risk of meningitis and of neural toxicity, particularly to the optic apparatus, they form a barrier between layers of tissue, inhibiting granulation and preventing fibroblastic proliferation from fusing one layer to the next. With time, tissue adhesives become porous and can result in recurring leaks.[104–107] More recently, the use of autogenous or prepackaged fibrin clot adhesives has prompted a reconsideration of the role of these agents.

## Use of Cerebrospinal Fluid Shunts

High-pressure leaks cannot be sealed without reducing the intracranial pressure. The primary pathology must be treated first, either by resection of the space-occupying lesion or by reduction of CSF volume and flow in hydrocephalus. Nonetheless, several types of recalcitrant fistulas have been successfully treated with lumboperitoneal shunts.[108, 109]

CSF shunting can be attempted in normal-pressure leaks when other means of repair have failed or when, after exhaustive investigation, the site of the leak cannot be delineated. Lumboperitoneal shunting has been advocated as the only treatment needed for small leaks that cannot be visualized.[68, 110] This empirical approach assumes that the resistance to flow through the shunt will be less than the resistance to passage through the fistula. With shunt malfunction, the leak may recur. Moreover, tension pneumocephalus can occur when air is aspirated intracranially through an open fistula under negative pressure.[49, 86, 87] The treatment for this complication is ligation of the shunt initially and replacement of the valve with a higher pressure unit once the mass effect has been treated and the air resorbed.

## Treatment of Spinal Cerebrospinal Fluid Leaks

Spontaneous spinal CSF leaks rarely occur outside the setting of spinal dysraphism or unusual spinal anomalies except that some rare leaks have been attributed to bone spurs at the skull base or cervical spine.[111] Traumatic leaks occur after penetrating injury, after surgery, after lumbar puncture, and after spinal anesthesia. Leaks that are less explicable as truly *traumatic*, at least in the sense that penetration of the dura cannot always be demonstrated convincingly, occur after multiple epidural injections with steroid preparations. Intraoperative observations by the author suggest that the dura both thickens and thins after multiple injections. The dura is sometimes gossamer-thin and almost porous. The CSF that leaks from this location more accurately *seeps* than *leaks*. Epidural fat grafts seem to contain this seepage without too much difficulty. The dura is easily torn in these locations, however.

Prevention of postoperative leaks is far more preferable to cure. Dural defects should be closed in a watertight fashion whenever possible. The dura should not be closed under tension; a graft, taken from the lumbodorsal fascia, can be inserted if necessary. Dural flaps should be studiously avoided. They embody the potential to become ball valves. Closure of the fascial and superficial layers should not be left to inexperienced surgeons.

Much has been said regarding the importance of intraoperative Valsalva maneuvers in detecting small meningeal tears and proving the adequacy of dural repair. Although the emergence of CSF obviously implies that satisfactory repair has not been achieved, the absence of CSF with increase in intrathoracic pressure does not eliminate the possibility of a delayed leak.

For patients undergoing elective repair of spinal anomalies, such as spinal lipomas associated with dysraphism, or in other situations in which the skin or subcutaneous tissue is defective, consideration should be given to rotating a generous myocutaneous flap. This technique is also useful when there is a recurrence of CSF leak with breakdown of the wound edges, when difficulty with wound healing can be anticipated, and in the face of infection. Despite the dictum that infection should be cleared before a graft is applied, the myocutaneous flaps seem to survive rotation onto a clean but infected base and even to facilitate healing in chronically infected wounds.

Other principles of management are analogous to those already described for transcranial leaks. In meningomyeloceles and other dysraphic states, the repair of the leak becomes part of the repair of the anomaly. Increased intracranial pressure must be controlled before the leak stops. Except in open injuries, transcutaneous leaks, and obvious anomalies, the site of the leak may be quite difficult to determine.[94] Isotope cisternography and contrast CT are usually accurate in active leaks.[112] Most uncomplicated traumatic leaks seal within several days so long as there is no ball-valve dural defect to resist healing. Certain maneuvers may be helpful: Incisional leaks should be initially repaired by resuturing the wound and applying an abdominal binder over a pressure pad to increase resistance to CSF flow. External CSF drainage from the cervical subarachnoid space via C1-C2 puncture has been used on several occasions to good effect at the Walter Reed Army Medical Center. The Touhy needle and drainage catheter must be inserted under fluoroscopy. Although the cervical subarachnoid catheters are more likely to kink, no other major difficulties have been encountered. If the leak persists over 10 days and if the intracranial pressure is normal, re-exploration of the wound is generally indicated.

A number of other techniques have been reported. Three are mentioned as additions to the surgeon's armamentarium, although they cannot be recommended as a routine: (1) an infusion of 100 ml of 20% mannitol every 4 hours for 7 days and positioning in a head-down attitude for 1 week,[113] (2) insertion of a fat plug through a limited midline

durotomy for small rents of the anterior and lateral thecal walls,[114] and (3) the use of tissue adhesives to seal the dura.[115] It is particularly important not to confuse an infected serous exudate with a delayed spinal CSF leak. It is necessary to re-explore a recalcitrant postoperative leak to determine what tissue layers need to be repaired for the leak to be contained.

## CONCLUSIONS

The large number of solutions to the problem of CSF leak attests to the difficulty of the problem. CSF leaks can be managed only after the mechanism of causation, the anatomic origin, and the pathophysiology have been understood. Both extradural and intradural approaches are effective in the appropriate setting. A team approach may well be desirable. Leaks that decompress increased intracranial pressure do not stop until the pressure is reduced. The usefulness of CSF diversion should be kept in mind. A long duration of follow-up is necessary before the possibility of recurrence can be dismissed absolutely.

## REFERENCES

1. Bidloo the Elder, quoted in Morgagni: De Sedibus et Causis Morborum, 1, 15, art 21. Cited in Lewin W: Cerebrospinal fluid rhinorrhea in nonmissile head injuries. Clin Neurosurg 12:237–252, 1966.
2. Mincy JE: Post traumatic cerebrospinal fluid fistula of the frontal fossa. J Trauma 6:618–622, 1966.
3. Miller C: Case of hydrocephalus chronicus with some unusual symptoms and appearances on dissection. Trans Med Chir Soc Edinb 2:243–248, 1826.
4. Ommaya AK: Spinal fluid fistulae. Clin Neurosurg 23:363–392, 1975.
5. Chiari H: Ueber einem Fall von Luftansammlung in den Ventrikeln des menchichen Gehirns. Z Heilkd 5:383–390, 1884.
6. Luckett WH: Air in the ventricles of the brain, following a fracture of the skull: Report of a case. Surg Gynecol Obstet 17:237–240, 1913.
7. Wilkins RH: Neurosurgical Classics. New York and London: Johnson Reprint Corporation, 1965, pp 242–256.
8. Grant FC: Intracranial aerocele following fracture of the skull: Report of a case with review of the literature. Surg Gynecol Obstet 36:251–255, 1923.
9. Dandy WE: Pneumocephalus (intracranial pneumatocele or aerocele). Arch Surg 12:949–982, 1926.
10. Cairns H: Injuries of the frontal and ethmoidal sinuses with special reference to cerebrospinal fluid rhinorrhea and aeroceles. J Laryngol Otol 52:589–623, 1937.
11. Dandy WE: Treatment of rhinorrhea and otorrhea. Arch Surg 49:75–85, 1944.
12. Lewin W: Cerebrospinal fluid rhinorrhea in closed head injuries. Br J Surg 42:1–18, 1954.
13. Lewin W: Cerebrospinal fluid rhinorrhea in nonmissile head injuries. Clin Neurosurg 12:237–252, 1966.
14. Eden K: Traumatic cerebrospinal rhinorrhoea: Repair of a fistula by a transfrontal intradural operation. Br J Surg 29:299–303, 1941.
15. Dohlman G: Spontaneous cerebrospinal rhinorrhoea: Case operated by rhinologic methods. Acta Otolaryngol (Stockh) 67 (Suppl):20–23, 1948.
16. McCabe NF: The osteo-mucoperiosteal flap in repair of cerebrospinal fluid rhinorrhea. Laryngoscope 86:537–539, 1976.
17. Calcaterra TC: Extracranial surgical repair of cerebrospinal rhinorrhea. Ann Otol 89:108–116, 1980.
18. Wormald PJ, McDonogh M: 'Bath-plug' technique for the endoscopic management of cerebrospinal fluid leaks. J Laryngol Otol 111:1042–1046, 1997.
19. Sethi DS, Chan C, Pillay PK: Endoscopic management of cerebro-

spinal fluid fistulae and traumatic cephalocoele. Ann Acad Med Singapore 25:724–727, 1996.
20. Appelbaum E: Meningitis following trauma to the head and face. JAMA 173:116–120, 1968.
21. Brawley B, Kelly W: Treatment of skull fractures with and without cerebrospinal fluid fistula. J Neurosurg 26:57–61, 1967.
22. Einhorn A, Mizrahia EM: Basilar skull fractures in children: Incidence of CNS infection and the use of antibiotics. Am J Dis Child 132:1121–1124, 1978.
23. Krayenbuhl HA: Questions and answers. Clin Neurosurg 14:23–24, 1967.
24. Leech PJ, Patterson R: Conservative and operative management for cerebrospinal leakage after closed head injury. Lancet 1:1013–1016, 1973.
25. Vourc'h G: Continuous cerebrospinal fluid drainage by indwelling spinal catheter. Br J Anaesth 35:118–120, 1963.
26. Aitken RR, Drake CG: Continuous spinal drainage in the treatment of postoperative cerebrospinal-fluid fistulae. J Neurosurg 21:275–277, 1964.
27. McCallum J, Maroon JC, Janetta PJ: Treatment of postoperative cerebrospinal fluid fistulas by subarachnoid drainage. J Neurosurg 42:434–437, 1975.
28. Findler G, Sahar A, Beller AJ: Continuous lumbar drainage of cerebrospinal fluid in neurosurgical patients. Surg Neurol 8:455–457, 1977.
29. Kaufman B, Nulsen FE, Weiss MH, et al: Acquired spontaneous nontraumatic normal-pressure cerebrospinal fluid fistulas originating from the middle fossa. Radiology 122:379–387, 1977.
30. Ommaya AK, Di Chiro G, Baldwain M, Pennybacker JB: Nontraumatic cerebrospinal fluid rhinorrhoea. J Neurol Neurosurg Psychiatry 31:214–225, 1968.
31. Scievink WI, Meyer FB, Atkinson JJ, Mokri B: Spontaneous spinal cerebrospinal fluid leaks and intracranial hypotension. J Neurosurg 84:598–605, 1996.
32. Droste DW, Krauss JK: Oscillations of cerebrospinal fluid in nonhydrocephalic persons. Neurol Res 19:135–138, 1997.
33. Schievink WI, Morreale VM, Atkinson JL, et al: Surgical treatment of spontaneous spinal cerebrospinal fluid leaks. J Neurosurg 88:2430–2436, 1998.
34. Park JI, Strelzow VV, Friedman WH: Current management of cerebrospinal fluid rhinorrhea. Laryngoscope 93:1294–1300, 1983.
35. Dagi TF, Meyer FB, Poletti CA: The incidence and prevention of meningitis after basilar skull fracture. Am J Emerg Med 3:295–298, 1983.
36. Meirowsky AM, Caveness WF, Dillon JD, et al: Cerebrospinal fluid fistulas complicating missile wounds of the brain. J Neurosurg 54:44–48, 1981.
37. Shulman K: Later complications of head injuries in children. Clin Neurosurg 19:371–380, 1971.
38. Nutkiewicz A, DeFeo DR, Kohut RI, Fierstien S: Cerebrospinal fluid rhinorrhea as a presentation of pituitary adenoma. Neurosurgery 6.195–197, 1980.
39. Haran RP, Chandy MJ: Symptomatic pneumocephalus after transsphenoidal surgery. Surg Neurol 48:575–578, 1997.
40. Landy LB, Graham MD, Kartush JM, LaRouere MJ: Temporal bone encephalocele and cerebrospinal fluid leaks. Am J Otol 17:461–469, 1996.
41. Piziak VK, Gilliland PF, Boyd G, et al: Pituitary tumor initially seen as serous otitis media. JAMA 251:3131–3132, 1984.
42. Horowitz NH, Rizzoli HV: Postoperative Complications of Intracranial Surgery. Baltimore: Williams & Wilkins, 1982, p 76.
43. Montgomery WW: Surgery for acoustic neurinoma. Ann Otolaryngol 82:428–444, 1973.
44. Ojemann RG: Microsurgical suboccipital approach to cerebellopontine angle tumors. Clin Neurosurg 25:461–479, 1978.
45. Valtonen HJ, Poe DS, Heilman CB, Tarlov EC: Endoscopically assisted prevention of cerebrospinal fluid leak in suboccipital acoustic neuroma surgery. Am J Otol 18:381–385, 1997.
46. Horowitz NH, Rizzoli HV: Postoperative Complications of Intracranial Surgery. Baltimore: Williams & Wilkins, 1982, pp 123–124.
47. Spaziante R, de Divitiis E, Cappabianca P: Reconstruction of the pituitary fossa in transsphenoidal surgery: An experience of 140 cases. Neurosurgery 17:453–458, 1985.
48. Ciric I: Comment on Spaziante et al. Neurosurgery 17:458, 1985.
49. Bakay L, Glasauer FE: Head Injury. Boston: Little, Brown, 1980, p 280.
50. Markham JW: The clinical features of pneumocephalus based upon a survey of 284 cases with report of 11 additional cases. Acta Neurochir 16:1–78, 1967.
51. Hubbard JL, Thomas JM, Pearson BW, Laws ER: Spontaneous cerebrospinal fluid rhinorrhea: Evolving concepts in diagnosis and surgical management based on the Mayo Clinic experience from 1970 through 1981. Neurosurgery 16:314–321, 1985.
52. Flanagan JC, McLachlan DL, Shannon GM: Orbital roof fractures: Neurologic and neurosurgical considerations. Ophthalmology 87:325–329, 1980.
53. Ray BS, Bergland RM: Cerebrospinal fluid fistula: Clinical aspects, techniques of localization, and methods of closure. J Neurosurg 30:399–405, 1969.
54. Jamieson KG, Yelland JDN: Surgical repair of the anterior fossa because of rhinorrhea, aerocele, or meningitis. J Neurosurg 39:328–331, 1973.
55. Kosoy J, Trieff N, Winkelmann P, et al: Glucose in nasal secretions. Arch Otolaryngol 95:225–229, 1975.
56. Healy CE: Significance of a positive reaction for glucose in rhinorrhea. Clin Pediatr 8:239, 1969.
57. Kirsch AP: Diagnosis of cerebrospinal fluid rhinorrhea: Lack of specificity of the glucose oxidase Tes-Tape. J Pediatr 71:718, 1967.
58. Ghoshhajra K: Radiologic techniques for identification and localization of cerebrospinal fluid fistulae. Semin Neurol 2:115–125, 1982.
59. Levy JM, Christensen FK, Nykamp PW: Detection of a cerebrospinal fluid fistula by computed tomography. AJR 131:344–345, 1978.
60. Ahmadi J, Weiss MH, Segali HD, et al: Evaluation of cerebrospinal fluid rhinorrhea by metrizamide computed tomographic cisternography. Neurosurgery 16:54–60, 1985.
61. Strauss H: Fluorescein als Indikator fuer die Nierenfunktion. Berliner Klin Wchschr 50:2226–2227, 1913.
62. Fox N: Cure in a case of cerebrospinal rhinorrhea. Arch Otolaryngol 17:85–86, 1933.
63. Mahaley MS, Odom GL: Complications following intrathecal injections of fluorescein. J Neurosurg 25:298, 1966.
64. Staab EV, Shirkhoda A: Cerebrospinal fluid scanning. Clin Nucl Med 6:103–109, 1981.
65. Coletti PM, Siegel ME: Posttraumatic lumbar cerebrospinal fluid leak: Detection by retrograde In-111-DTPA myeloscintigraphy. Clin Nucl Med 6:403–404, 1981.
66. Hasegawa M, Watanabe I, Hiratsuka H, et al: Transfer of radioisotope from CSF to nasal secretion. Acta Otolaryngol (Stockh) 95:359–364, 1983.
67. Di Chiro G, Stein SC, Harrington T: Spontaneous cerebrospinal fluid rhinorrhea in normal dogs: Radioisotope studies of an alternate pathway of CSF drainage. J Neuropathol Exp Neurol 31:447–453, 1972.
68. Spetzler RF, Wilson CB: Management of reucrrent CSF rhinorrhea of the middle and posterior fossa. J Neurosurg 49:393–397, 1978.
69. Irjala K, Suonpaa J, Laurent B: Identification of CSF leakage by immunofixation. Arch Otolaryngol 105:447–448, 1979.
70. Parisier SC, Briken EA: Recurrent meningitis secondary to idiopathic oval window CSF leak. Laryngoscope 86:1503–1515, 1976.
71. Nenzelius C: On spontaneous cerebrospinal otorrhea due to congenital malformations. Acta Otolaryngol (Stockh) 39:314–328, 1951.
72. Bottema T: Spontaneous cerebrospinal fluid otorrhea. Arch Otolaryngol 101:693–694, 1975.
73. Rice WJ, Waggoner LG: Congenital cerebrospinal fluid otorrhea via defect in the stapes footplate. Laryngoscope 77:341–349, 1967.
74. Ignelzi RJ, VanderArk GD: Analysis of the treatment of basilar skull fractures with and without antibiotics. J Neurosurg 43:75–78, 1975.
75. Dagi TF, Ojemann RG, Zervas NT: Incidence and prevention of infection after neurosurgical operations. In Thompson RA, Green JR (eds): Infectious Diseases of the Central Nervous System. Jamaica, NY: Spectrum Publications, 1984, pp 155–173.
76. Ingraham FD, Campbell JB: An apparatus for closed drainage of the ventricular system. Ann Surg 114:1096–1098, 1941.
77. White RJ, Dakters JG, Yashon D, et al: Temporary control of cerebrospinal fluid volume and pressure by means of an externalized valve-drainage system. J Neurosurg 30:264–269, 1969.
78. Vourc'h G: Continuous cerebrospinal fluid drainage by indwelling spinal catheter. Br J Anaesth 35:118–120, 1963.
79. McCoy G: Cerebrospinal rhinorrhea: A comprehensive review and a definition of the responsibility of the rhinologist in the diagnosis and treatment. Laryngoscope 73:1125–1157, 1963.

80. Wyler AR, Kelly WA: Use of antibiotics with external ventriculostomies. J Neurosurg 37:185–187, 1972.

81. Friedman WA, Vries JK: Percutanous tunnel ventriculostomy: Summary of 100 procedures. J Neurosurg 53:662–665, 1980.

82. Dagi TF, Ondra SL: The role of artificial intelligence systems in neurosurgical intensive care. International Congress on Trends in Neurosurgery, Diagnostic and Surgical Perspectives, Vienna, Austria, May 14–17, May, 1986.

83. Brownridge P: Spinal anesthesia revisited: An evaluation of subarachnoid block in obstetrics. Anaesth Intensive Care 12:334–342, 1984.

84. Rudehill A, Gordon E, Rahn T: Subdural haematoma: A rare but life-threatening complication after spinal anaesthesia. Acta Anaesthesiol Scand 27:376–377, 1983.

85. Benzon HT: Intracerebral hemorrhage after dural puncture and epidural blood patch: Nonpostural and noncontinuous headache. Anesthesiology 60:258–259, 1984.

86. Ikeda K, Nakano M, Tani E: Tension pneumocephalus complicating ventriculoperitoneal shunt for cerebrospinal fluid rhinorrhea: Case report. J Neurol Neurosurg Psychiatry 41:319–322, 1978.

87. Little JR, McCarty CS: Tension pneumocephalus after insertion of ventriculoperitoneal shunt for aqueductal stenosis. J Neurosurg 44:383–385, 1976.

88. Jooma R, Grant DN: Cerebrospinal fluid rhinorrhea and intraventricular pneumocephalus due to intermittent shunt obstruction. Surg Neurol 20:231–124, 1983.

89. Katz J: Treatment of a subarachnoid-cutaneous fistula with an epidural blood patch. Anesthesiology 60:603–604, 1984.

90. Digiovanni AJ, Galbert MW, Wahle WM: Epidural injection of autologous blood for postlumbar-puncture headache: I. Additional clinical experiences and laboratory investigation. Anesth Analg 51:226–228, 1972.

91. Crawford JS: Experiences with epidural blood patch. Anaesthesia 35:513–515, 1980.

92. Casement BA, Danielson DR: The epidural blood patch: Are more than two ever necessary? Anesth Analg 63:1033–1035, 1984.

93. Rosenberg PH, Heavner JE: In vitro study of the effect of epidural blood patch on leakage through a dural puncture. Anesth Analg 64:501–504, 1985.

94. Harrington H, Tyler HR, Welch K: Surgical treatment of post-lumbar puncture dural CSF leak causing chronic headache. J Neurosurg 57:703–707, 1982.

95. Reynolds AF, Hameroff SR, Blitt CD, et al: Spinal subdural epiarachnoid hematoma: A complication of a novel epidural blood patch technique. Anesth Analg 59:702–703, 1980.

96. O'Brien MD, Reade PC: The management of dural tear resulting from mid-facial fracture. Head Neck Surg 6:810–818, 1984.

97. da Cruz MJ, Ahmed SM, Moffat DA: An alternative method for dealing with cerebrospinal fluid fistulae in inner ear deformities. Am J Otol 19:288–291, 1998.

98. Kelley TF, Stankiewicz JA, Chow JM, et al: Endoscopic closure of postsurgical anterior cranial fossa cerebrospinal fluid leaks. Neurosurgery 39:743–746, 1996.

99. Hughes RG, Jone NS, Robertson IJ: The endoscopic treatment of cerebrospinal fluid rhinorrhoea: The Nottingham experience. J Laryngol Otol 111:125–128, 1997.

100. Jho HD, Carrau RL, Ko Y, Daly MA: Endoscopic pituitary surgery: An early experience. Surg Neurol 47:213–223, 1997.

101. Gjuric M, Goede U, Keimer H, Wigand ME: Endonasal endoscopic closure of cerebrospinal fluid fistulas at the anterior cranial base. Ann Otol Rhinol Laryngol 105:620–623, 1996.

102. Fraioli B, Pastore FS, Floris R, et al: Computed tomography-guided transsphenoidal closure of postsurgical cerebrospinal fluid fistula: A transmucosal needle technique. Surg Neurol 48:409–413, 1997.

103. Jakoby RK: The use of a methylmethacrylate seal in spinal fluid otorrhea and rhinorrhea. J Neurosurg 18:614–615, 1961.

104. Lehman RAW, Hayes GJ, Martins AN: The use of adhesive and lyophilized dura in the treatment of cerebrospinal rhinorrhea. J Neurosurg 26:92–95, 1967.

105. VanderArk GD, Pitkethly DT, Ducker TB, et al: Repair of cerebrospinal fluid fistulas using a tissue adhesive. J Neurosurg 33:151–155, 1970.

106. Maxwell JA, Goldware SI: Use of tissue adhesive in the surgical treatment of cerebrospinal fluid leaks: Experience with isobutyl-2 cyanoacrylate in 12 cases. J Neurosurg 39:332–336, 1973.

107. Mickey BE, Samson D: Neurosurgical applications of the cyanoacrylate adhesives. Clin Neurosurg 29:429–444, 1982.

108. Greenblatt SH, Wilson DH: Persistent cerebrospinal fluid rhinorrhea treated by lumboperitoneal shunt: Technical note. J Neurosurg 38:524–526, 1973.

109. Bret P, Hor F, Huppert J, et al: Treatment of cerebrospinal fluid rhinorrhea by percutaneous lumboperitoneal shunting: Review of 15 cases. Neurosurgery 16:44–47, 1985.

110. Spetzler RF: Commentary on Bret P, et al. Neurosurgery 16:47, 1985.

111. Vishteh AG, Scievink WI, Baskin JJ, Sonntag VK: Cervical bone spur presenting with spontaneous intracranial hypotension: Case report. J Neurosurg 89:483–484, 1998.

112. Gass H, Goldstein AS, Ruskin R, et al: Chronic postmyelogram headache: Isotopic demonstration of dural leak and surgical cure. Arch Neurol 25:108–170, 1971.

113. Rosenthal JD, Hahn JF, Martinez GJ: A technique for closure of leak of spinal fluid. Surg Gynecol Obstet 140:948–950, 1975.

114. Mayfield FH, Kurokawa K: Watertight closure of the spinal dura mater: Technical note. J Neurosurg 43:639–640, 1975.

115. Papadakis N, Mark VH: Repair of spinal cerebrospinal fluid fistula with the use of a tissue adhesive: Technical note. Neurosurgery 6:63–65, 1980.

# Transnasal Endoscopic Repair of Cranionasal Fistulas

■ JAMES A. BURNS and CHARLES W. GROSS

Cerebrospinal fluid (CSF) rhinorrhea presents a major challenge for otolaryngologists and skull base surgeons. Difficulties in diagnosis and localization add to the complexity of the problem, and management varies with etiology and site. Immediate measures must be taken to repair the defect because the risk of intracranial infection and its sequelae is high. Since its first report by Dohlman in 1948,[1] repair of CSF rhinorrhea has evolved considerably. Several recent reports describe various endoscopic techniques used to manage CSF rhinorrhea.[2–8] Increasing incidences of CSF leaks from neurosurgical and otolaryngologic procedures, as well as from noniatrogenic trauma, have led to refinements in endoscopic techniques. Because endoscopic repair may involve defects that do not present with CSF rhinorrhea (e.g., cephaloceles), we now refer to these defects as *cranionasal fistulas*.

This chapter describes the pertinent anatomy, pathophysiology, and manifestations of cranionasal fistulas, as well as current methods of diagnosis and localization. The endoscopic repair of cranionasal fistulas is detailed.

## PATHOPHYSIOLOGY

Leakage of CSF occurs when arachnoid, dura, bone, and mucosal epithelium are violated. Etiologies of CSF rhinorrhea can be divided into traumatic and nontraumatic causes (Table 13–1).[9]

### Traumatic Cerebrospinal Fluid Rhinorrhea

The roof of the ethmoid and the cribriform plate are the most frequent sites of CSF rhinorrhea because dura is tightly adherent to bone in this area.[10] Also, the lateral cribriform plate is easily fractured where the anterior ethmoid artery creates a natural dehiscence. Fractures through the frontal sinus, ethmoid roof, and sphenoid roof drain into the posterosuperior aspects of the nasal vault. CSF may also enter the nasal vault by way of the eustachian tube and middle ear through dural defects surrounding the petrous portion of the temporal bone[4] (Fig. 13–1). CSF

may appear immediately after trauma or days to weeks later. Delayed leaks may be caused by delayed increases in intracranial pressure after trauma, lysis of clot in an area of bone and dural dehiscence, resolution of soft tissue edema, or loss of vascularity and necrosis of soft tissue and bone around the wound. Also, dura may herniate and, with continued pulsations and physiologic changes in CSF pressure, the herniation may progress with eventual dehiscence and CSF leak.[11, 12]

CSF rhinorrhea secondary to intracranial and extracranial surgery can often be avoided with proper technique. Postoperative rhinorrhea is present in 3% to 6% of cases after trans-sphenoidal hypophysectomy, ethmoidectomy, and anterior skull base tumor ablation.[13] Today, advances in skull base surgery and the introduction of functional endoscopic sinus surgery (FESS) for inflammatory paranasal sinus disease have led to an increase in the incidence of postsurgical cranionasal fistulas.

### Nontraumatic Cerebrospinal Fluid Rhinorrhea

Rhinorrhea from tumors or hydrocephalus occurs as a result of elevated intracranial pressure leading to continued erosion and weakening of bone with the eventual development of a cranionasal fistula.[14] Again, the ethmoid roof and cribriform plate are the most common sites because they are the thinnest areas of the anterior skull base. Tumors

**TABLE 13–1 ■ CEREBROSPINAL FLUID RHINORRHEA**

| Traumatic | Atraumatic |
|---|---|
| **Nonsurgical** | **High-Pressure Flow** |
| Blunt trauma | Intracranial tumors |
| Projectile trauma | Hydrocephalus |
| **Surgical** | **Low-Pressure Flow** |
| Craniotomy | Bony erosion |
| Paranasal sinus surgery | Sellar atrophy |
| Tumor ablation | Olfactory atrophy |
| | Congenital anomalies |
| | Idiopathic |

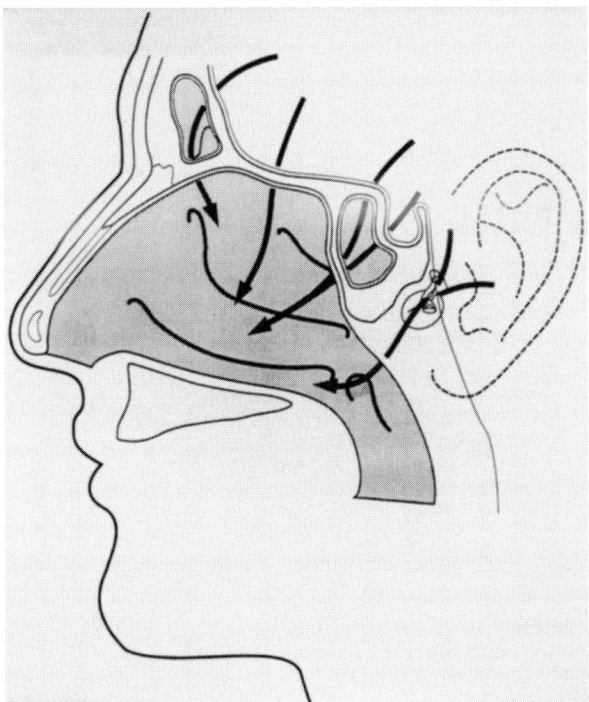

FIGURE 13–1 ■ Common pathways of cerebrospinal fluid (CSF) drainage presenting as CSF rhinorrhea. (From Papay FA, Maggiano H, Dominquez S, et al: Rigid endoscopic repair of paranasal sinus cerebrospinal fluid fistulas. Laryngoscope 99:1195–1201, 1989.)

may also cause CSF rhinorrhea through direct erosion of bone.

Low-pressure–flow rhinorrhea likely results from normal physiologic elevations of CSF pressure. Pressure elevations of up to 80 mm H$_2$O normally occur spontaneously every few seconds.[15] This increase in CSF pressure in general is not able to erode or fracture bone. However, the presence of sudden, short-lived, marked increases in intracranial pressure due to coughing or straining may be an important precipitating factor in the development of spontaneous CSF rhinorrhea.[11] There is commonly a history of remote head trauma years before.

Differentiating between CSF rhinorrhea caused by a congenitally dehiscent area and that which occurs spontaneously may be difficult. Because management of these entities is identical, this difficulty is not clinically relevant. Similarly, the empty sella syndrome can be classified as either congenital or spontaneous. The empty sella syndrome occurring because of an absent portion of the diaphragma sellae is classified as congenital, whereas that occurring because of pituitary gland atrophy is classified as spontaneous.[11]

## DIAGNOSIS

Symptoms of cranionasal fistula include clear, watery rhinorrhea, anosmia due to olfactory nerve damage at the cribriform plate, and headaches due to the presence of a pneumocephalus. Cephaloceles may not produce CSF rhinorrhea and present with nasal obstruction. As much as

20% of patients with CSF rhinorrhea have meningitis as their initial manifestation, and the risk for development of meningitis in the first 3 weeks after trauma is 3% to 11%.[13]

Paramount in the diagnosis of cranionasal fistula is the clear demonstration that extracranial CSF exists. In cases where the rhinorrhea is profuse, the diagnosis is obvious. However, diagnosis is more difficult when the drainage is minimal or intermittent. When CSF rhinorrhea is a direct result of FESS procedures, the intraoperative presence of a clear fluid draining from the roof of the nasal cavity and washing away blood is pathognomonic of a CSF leak. Testing the fluid for β$_2$-transferrin is a highly accurate way of determining the presence of CSF.[7, 8]

Radiographic studies can confirm the presence of a CSF leak, determine its precise site, identify the underlying cause, and precisely measure the size of cranionasal fistulas. The definitive test is computed tomographic (CT) cisternography. High-resolution CT scans are performed after the administration of intrathecal iohexal (Omnipaque 300; Winthrop Pharmaceuticals, New York, NY) or other low-osmolar, nonionic iodine contrast media.[8] CT shows extravasation of the dye through the cranionasal fistula, thus demonstrating the leak and localizing the site (Fig. 13–2). Magnetic resonance imaging is helpful for delineating the defect and identifying potentially treatable causes of CSF rhinorrhea, like cephaloceles (Fig. 13–3).

Along with advances in imaging techniques, clinical localization of cranionasal fistulas has improved dramatically with the use of endoscopes. One of the main advantages of the endoscopic repair of cranionasal fistulas is the excellent field of vision, allowing exact localization of the

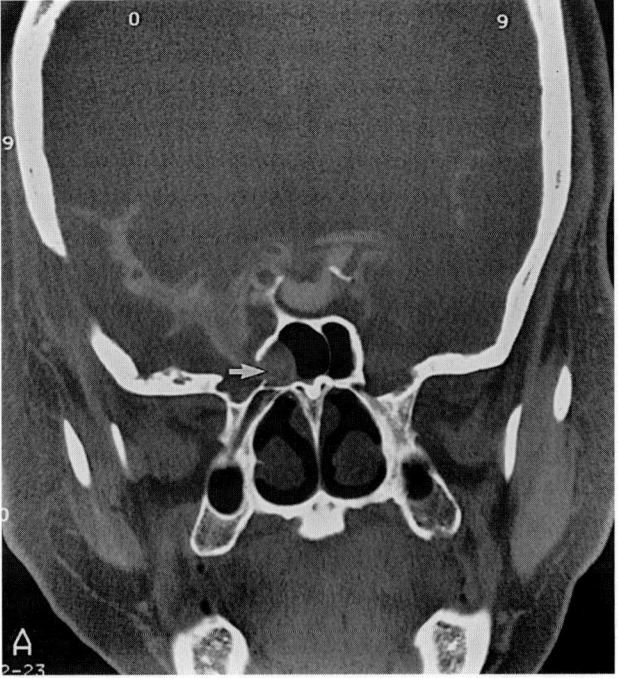

FIGURE 13–2 ■ A coronal computed tomography scan showing cranionasal fistula in the sphenoid sinus with Iohexal dye collecting in the sphenoid sinus (arrow). (From Burns JA, Dodson EE, Gross GW: Transnasal endoscopic repair of cranio-nasal fistulae—a refined technique with long term follow-up. Laryngoscope 106:1080–1083, 1996.)

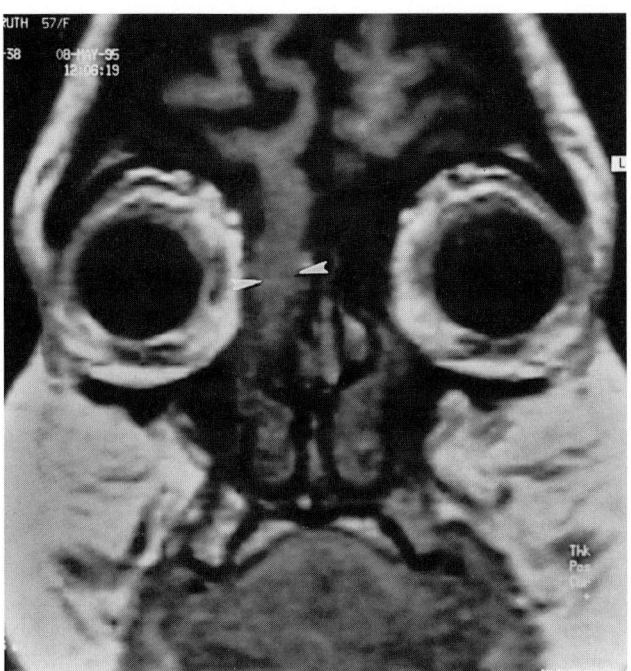

FIGURE 13–3 ■ Coronal $T_2$-weighted magnetic resonance imaging scan showing a cephalocele presenting through the ethmoid roof defect. The cranionasal fistula measured 2.2 × 1 cm. (From Burns JA, Dodson, EE, Gross GW: Transnasal endoscopic repair of cranio-nasal fistulae—a refined technique with long term follow-up. Laryngoscope 106:1080–1083, 1996.)

leak.[3, 7, 8] Fluorescein is routinely used to aid in the clinical localization of CSF leaks. Intrathecal fluorescein is administered through a lumbar puncture. Ten milliliters of CSF is withdrawn, mixed with 0.5 ml of 5% fluorescein (injectable, not ophthalmic preparation), and slowly reinjected into the lumbar subarachnoid space. After allowing 20 to 30 minutes for diffusion throughout the CSF, the bright yellow-green fluorescein dye can be seen readily with the rigid nasal endoscope. No special light source is needed. A Valsalva maneuver given by the anesthetist can enhance flow of CSF through a defect for better visualization. Because iohexal and fluorescein can be given simultaneously, CT cisternography and rigid nasal endoscopy can work in a complementary fashion precisely to localize cranionasal defects.[16–18] Although complications ranging from lower extremity weakness to seizures and cranial nerve deficits have been described with the use of intrathecal fluorescein,[19] several large series of endoscopic repairs using fluorescein for localization did not experience these complications.[3–5, 8] Most adverse reactions were associated with much higher doses of fluorescein, and even those complications rarely produced permanent neurologic sequelae.

## MANAGEMENT

Intracranial repairs of cranionasal fistulas were initially described by Dandy in 1926.[20] Although still the preferred route by many neurosurgeons, disadvantages include permanent anosmia, intracerebral hemorrhage, and brain edema due to retraction during exposure. Despite the mag-

nitude of the procedure, closure is not guaranteed after a craniotomy approach, with success reported to be as low as 60% after the first attempt.[14]

Several studies report success rates of 86% to 100% for closure of CSF fistulas and cranionasal defects using the endoscopic approach.[3, 7, 8, 21] Nasal endoscopy aids in diagnosis and diminishes the need for surgical trauma to the external skin and intervening bone.[21] Also, permanent anosmia and direct manipulation of the brain are avoided. Using the endoscopic approach, intraoperative leaks can and should be treated as soon as the problem is recognized.

## REPAIR OF SPECIFIC SITES

### Sphenoid Sinus

With the patient under general anesthesia, the nasal cavities and sphenoid sinus are injected with a solution of 2% lidocaine with 1:50,000 epinephrine. A third-generation cephalosporin is given before surgery. Diagnostic nasal endoscopy is performed with or without intrathecal injection of the intravenous form of 5% fluorescein (0.5 ml diluted in 10 ml of CSF).

An endoscopic sphenoidotomy is then accomplished medial to the middle turbinate. This opening is enlarged only to the point of adequate exposure, to provide maximal support for the graft anteriorly. It is important to preserve as much of the face of the sphenoid sinus as possible to prevent extrusion of the graft. The bony defect is exposed, and all mucosa are removed from the sinus (Fig. 13–4).

A fat graft is harvested from the abdomen with either attached dermis or rectus abdominis fascia. The graft is then trimmed to the appropriate size and placed into the sphenoid, after application of fibrinogen and topical throm-

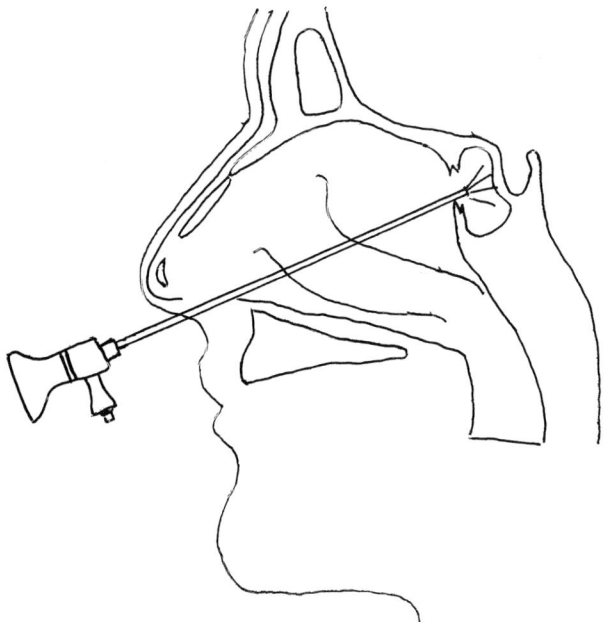

FIGURE 13–4 ■ Sagittal view showing the sphenoidotomy opening viewed with an endoscope for a sphenoid sinus fistula.

bin (fibrin glue). Great care is taken to place the dermal or fascial surface over the defect. Additional fibrin glue is then used to seal the graft, and the face of the sphenoid and ethmoid recess is packed firmly with Surgicel (Johnson & Johnson Medical, Arlington, TX) or Gelfoam (The Upjohn Company, Kalamazoo, MI). A nasal trumpet airway or nasal balloon is usually placed in the posterior nasal cavity for support.

## Ethmoid Roof and Cribriform Plate

The repair of fistulas in the ethmoid roof and cribriform area is identical to repair of sphenoid fistulas in the use of general anesthesia, local anesthetic/vasoconstrictor, perioperative antibiotics, and diagnostic nasal endoscopy.

If not previously accomplished, a partial or complete ethmoidectomy is performed to expose defects in the skull base for lesions less then 0.5 cm² in diameter. The site of the fistula is identified and any remaining adjacent mucosa removed to expose the bone as a graft recipient site (Fig. 13–5). It is important to remove mucosa surrounding the defect because residual mucosa prevents adhesion of the mucosal graft. A turbinate graft is harvested from the opposite nasal cavity and prepared on a back table. The mucosa is carefully removed from the underlying turbinate bone, trimmed to the appropriate size, and placed over the defect after application of fibrin glue. For defects larger than 0.5 cm² in diameter, composite grafts (consisting of turbinate bone, submucosal tissue, and mucosa) are prepared by removing the mucosa and submucosa from one side of the resected turbinate. The denuded side of the composite graft is placed against the defect and held in place with fibrin glue. The free graft can also be placed on the intracranial side of larger defects positioned between the dura and the skull base. In this case, a neuro-otologic

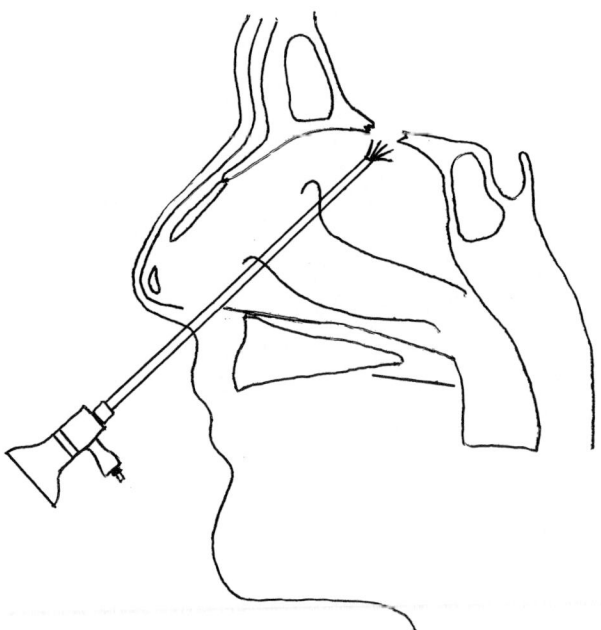

**FIGURE 13–5** ■ Sagittal view showing an ethmoid roof defect as viewed by an endoscope after performing a standard total ethmoidectomy.

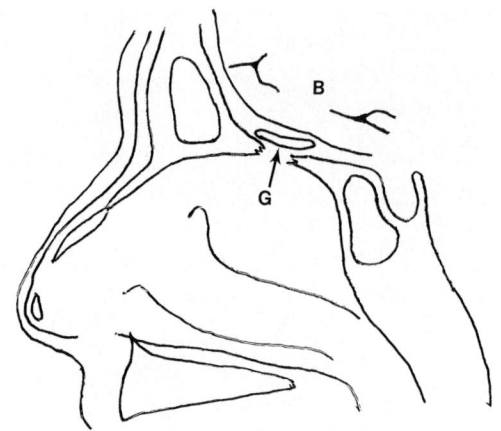

**FIGURE 13–6** ■ Schematic representation of placement of a free composite graft through an ethmoid roof defect. The graft lies in the epidural space. (B, brain; G, graft.)

elevator is used to elevate the dura off the skull, thereby creating an epidural space. The graft is then carefully inserted through the skull defect to lie in the epidural space (Fig. 13–6). Additional support is established with Surgicel or Gelfoam, followed by petroleum jelly–impregnated gauze, a nasal balloon, or both.

Repair of ethmoid roof and cribriform fistulas varies based on the size of the defect. In general, we favor free tissue grafts as opposed to pedicled grafts. This approach is favored by Mattox and Kennedy,[3] but Yessenow and McCabe[22] have achieved good results using pedicled grafts. For defects less than 0.5 cm², a free mucosa graft is used. For defects larger than 0.5 cm², a composite graft with rigid support from turbinate bone or septal cartilage is used. As additional support, we use a pedicled turbinate graft in those cases where the composite graft provides the main repair in larger defects.

## Cephaloceles

Sphenoid and ethmoid roof cephaloceles are managed by removing the mucosa from the mass and reducing the mass through the bony defect. This is accomplished by direct manipulation or by using bipolar cautery. Dissection is meticulous and slow to avoid intracranial hemorrhage. The mass is resected if its size precludes easy manipulation or there is incomplete mucosa removal. After closure of the dura, if possible, composite grafts are used as previously described. Figure 13–7 shows the endoscopic view of a large ethmoid roof encephalocele. Excision of this lesion created a cranionasal fistula measuring 2.2 × 1 cm. The fistula was successfully repaired endoscopically with use of a free composite turbinate graft, showing that even very large skull base defects can be managed endoscopically.

## POSTOPERATIVE CARE

After the procedure, patients are kept at bed rest with the head of the bed elevated. Intravenous antibiotics are

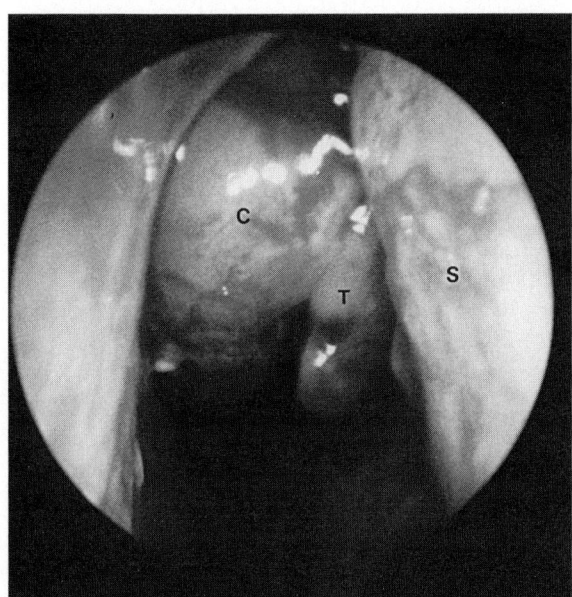

**FIGURE 13–7** ■ Endoscopic view of large cephalocele originating through an ethmoid roof cranio-nasal fistula. (S, septum; T, middle turbinate; C, cephalocele.) The resultant defect measured 2.2 × 1 cm. (From Burns JA, Dodson EE, Gross GW: Transnasal endoscopic repair of cranio-nasal fistulae—a refined technique with long term follow-up. Laryngoscope 106:1080–1083, 1996.)

continued for 24 to 48 hours and stool softeners are prescribed to reduce straining. If used, the lumbar drain is removed on the second postoperative day. The nasal packing is commonly removed after 48 hours, and the patient is discharged from the hospital after an additional 24 hours if there are no other medical problems. The average hospital stay ranges from 2 to 4 days. Patients are then required to avoid heavy lifting or strenuous activity for 4 to 6 weeks.

## CONCLUSION

The growing number of patients with cranionasal defects has provided ample experience with this endoscopic algorithm. By using a consistent technique for each location and defect size, the success rate for closure is optimized. Precise localization afforded by the rigid nasal endoscope avoids the use of huge grafts or flaps and preserves normal nasal structure and function. The transnasal endoscopic approach effectively repairs cranionasal fistulas with excellent long-term results.

## REFERENCES

1. Dohlman G: Spontaneous cerebrospinal rhinorrhea. Acta Otolaryngol 67 (Suppl):20–23, 1948.
2. Levine HL: Endoscopic diagnosis and management of cerebrospinal fluid rhinorrhea. Oper Tech Otolaryngol Head Neck Surg 2:282–284, 1991.
3. Mattox DE, Kennedy DW: Endoscopic management of cerebrospinal fluid leads and cephaloceles. Laryngoscope 100:857–862, 1990.
4. Papay FA, Maggiano H, Dominquez S, et al: Rigid endoscopic repair of paranasal sinus cerebrospinal fluid fistulas. Laryngoscope 99:1195–1201, 1989.
5. Papay FA, Benninger MS, Levine HL, et al: Transnasal transseptal endoscopic repair of sphenoidal cerebral spinal fluid fistula. Otolaryngol Head Neck Surg 101:595–597, 1989.
6. Stankiewicz JA: Cerebrospinal fluid fistula and endoscopic sinus surgery. Laryngoscope 101:250–256, 1991.
7. Dodson EE, Gross CW, Swerdloff JL, Gustafson LM: Transnasal endoscopic repair of cerebrospinal fluid rhinorrhea and skull base defects: A review of 29 cases. Otolaryngol Head Neck Surg 111:600–605, 1994.
8. Burns JA, Dodson EE, Gross GW: Transnasal endoscopic repair of cranio-nasal fistulae: A refined technique with long term follow-up. Laryngoscope 106:1080–1083, 1996.
9. Ommaya AK, Dichuro G, Baldwin M, et al: Non-traumatic cerebrospinal fluid rhinorrhea. J Neurol Neurosurg Psychiatry 31:214–225, 1968.
10. Calcaterra TC: Diagnosis and management of ethmoid cerebrospinal rhinorrhea. Otolaryngol Clin North Am 18:99–117, 1985.
11. Applebaum EL, Chow JE: CSF leaks. In Cummings CW (ed): Otolaryngology: Head and Neck Surgery, 2nd ed. St. Louis: CV Mosby, 1993, pp 965–974.
12. McCormack B, Hunt CE, Sofer S: Extracranial repair of cerebrospinal fluid fistulae: Techniques and results in 37 patients. Neurosurgery 27:412–417, 1998.
13. Loew F, Loh KK: Traumatic, spontaneous and postoperative CSF rhinorrhea. Adv Tech Stand Neurosurg 11:169–171, 1984.
14. Park JI, Strelzow VV, Friedman WH: Current management of cerebrospinal fluid rhinorrhea. Laryngoscope 93:1294–1300, 1983.
15. VonHaeke NP, Craft CB: Cerebrospinal fluid rhinorrhea and otorrhea: Extracranial repair. Clin Otolaryngol 8:317–345, 1983.
16. Chow JM, Goodman D, Mafee MF: Evaluation of CSF rhinorrhea by computerized tomography with metrizamide. Otolaryngol Head Neck Surg 100:99–105, 1989.
17. Luotonen J, Jokinen K, Laitinen J: Localization of a CSF fistula by metrizamide CT cisternography. J Laryngol Otol 100:955–958, 1986.
18. Schaefer SD, Briggs WH: The diagnosis of CSF rhinorrhea by metrizamide CT scanning. Laryngoscope 90:871–875, 1980.
19. Moseley JI, Carton CA, Stern WE: Spectrum of complications in the use of intrathecal fluorescein. J Neurosurg 48:765–767, 1978.
20. Dandy WE: Pneumocephalus (intracranial pneumatocele or aerocele). Arch Surg 12:949–982, 1926.
21. Lanza DC, O'Brien DA, Kennedy DW: Endoscopic repair of cerebrospinal fluid fistulae and encephaloceles. Laryngoscope 106:1119–1125, 1996.
22. Yessenow RS, McCabe BF: The osteo-cutaneous flap in repair of cerebrospinal fluid rhinorrhea: A 20-year experience. Otolaryngol Head Neck Surg 101:555–558, 1989.

# SECTION III

# Orbit

CHAPTER 14

# Surgical Management of Intraorbital Tumors

■ JEFFREY N. BRUCE, MICHAEL KAZIM, and EDGAR M. HOUSEPIAN

To appreciate the details of a surgical technique, the objectives of the operation must be clearly understood. These objectives are derived from a clear understanding of the nature of the pathologic process and the details of the regional anatomy. Once this is achieved, the objectives, advantages, and limitations of a given surgical approach can be understood and a rational choice of technique can be made. The transcranial neurosurgical approach to the orbit is of greater advantage when dealing with disease processes that span the orbital and intracranial spaces. It also affords superior access to the apical portion of the optic nerve and to the medial and lateral superior quadrants of the orbital apex.

The great variety of tumors and other mass lesions that occur behind the eye and cause proptosis are of interest to several surgical disciplines, and access to a multidisciplinary team can be valuable when contemplating surgical management. Ophthalmic surgeons can deal with many of these problems by one of a number of direct orbital approaches. The otolaryngologist can gain access to pathologic conditions arising within sinuses bordering the superior, medial, and inferior margins of the orbit. The neurologic surgeon has access to those tumors that involve both the intracranial and the intraorbital space. With the advent of modern neurosurgery, which allows safe access to the orbit by the cranial route, the neurosurgical literature began to reflect an increasing application of the transcranial orbital exploration to a large number of orbital problems.[1-5]

As one might expect, this encroachment on a traditionally ophthalmologic field led to a period of justifiable controversy regarding the proper approach to orbital problems.[6-10] Fortunately, the rapid development of diagnostic radiologic procedures has provided a means of more precisely defining the nature and extent of a lesion and has brought a rational basis to the surgical approach to orbital surgery.

## SURGICAL ANATOMY

The purpose of surgical anatomy is to describe and define significant anatomic interrelationships and to correlate the anatomy with clinical and surgical considerations.[11-16]

## The Orbit

The surgeon must be oriented to the medial obliquity of the apex of the orbit (Fig. 14–1).

The 5- to 10-mm-long optic canal enters the intracranial cavity medial to the anterior clinoid process, beneath which lies one of the two roots of the lesser wing of the sphenoid bone. This root forms the lateral wall of the optic canal and the medial margin of the superior orbital fissure. The lateral margin of the superior orbital fissure is bordered by the greater wing of the sphenoid bone, and together with the frontosphenoid process of the zygomatic bone, it forms the lateral wall of the orbit. The roof of the orbit and the floor of the anterior cranial fossa are, of course, one and the same, and the orbital plate of the maxillary bone forms both the floor of the orbit and the roof of the maxillary sinus. The medial wall of the orbit is formed by the

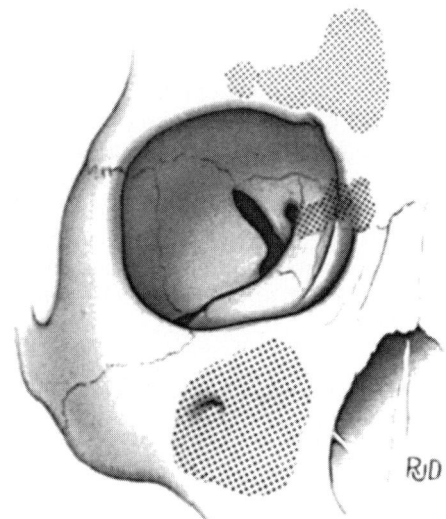

FIGURE 14–1 ■ The integrity of the bone orbit and the size and shape of its fissures and foramina can be defined by plain skull radiographs and computed tomography (CT) bone windows. The frontal, ethmoidal, and maxillary sinuses are shown in diagrammatic fashion. Attention is directed to one of the two roots of the lesser wing of the sphenoid, which lies beneath the anterior clinoid and forms the lateral margin of the optic canal in the medial margin of the superior orbital fissure.

lacrimal bone and the fragile lamina papyracea, which covers the ethmoid sinuses, and closer to the apex, the sphenoid sinus. The frontal sinus, to a variable extent, fills that portion of the frontal bone forming the supraorbital rim.

## Optic Nerve

Starting at the chiasmal end, the optic nerve has a flattened horizontal oval shape and measures approximately 4 × 6 mm (Fig. 14–2).

After it enters the cranial end of the optic canal, it is circular and 5 mm in diameter and continues to the globe as a 6 × 4 mm vertically oval structure. A pial membrane, carrying the blood supply, accompanies the nerve from the chiasm throughout its entire course to the sclera. The intracranial arachnoid, in like fashion, continues as a discrete structure through the optic canal and fuses with the pia at the globe. There are loose trabeculations in the subarachnoid space. At the apical orbital portion of the nerve, however, the pia and arachnoid are fused dorsomedially and ventrally with the dura and the fibrous annulus of Zinn, tethering the optic nerve and partially occluding the subarachnoid space but not obliterating its continuity. Normally, the intraocular pressure is slightly higher than the intracranial pressure; therefore, it is most likely that the papilledema found in conditions producing increased intracranial pressure is directly related to this continuity of the subarachnoid space from the cranial cavity to its termination at the lamina cribrosa.

## Periorbita

The intracranial dura extends into and lines the optic canal, and at the orbital exit of the canal, it splits into an outer periosteal (or periorbital) layer and an inner layer that accompanies the optic nerve to the globe, where it fuses with the arachnoid, pia, and sclera (Fig. 14–3).

To remove the optic nerve from the globe to the chiasm, as in cases of optic nerve glioma and meningioma, it is therefore necessary to section the annulus of Zinn and its fibrous attachment to the nerve. The periorbital dura is also continuous with the intracranial dura at the superior orbital fissure and, of course, lines the inferior orbital fissure as well as the other foramina, becoming continuous with the

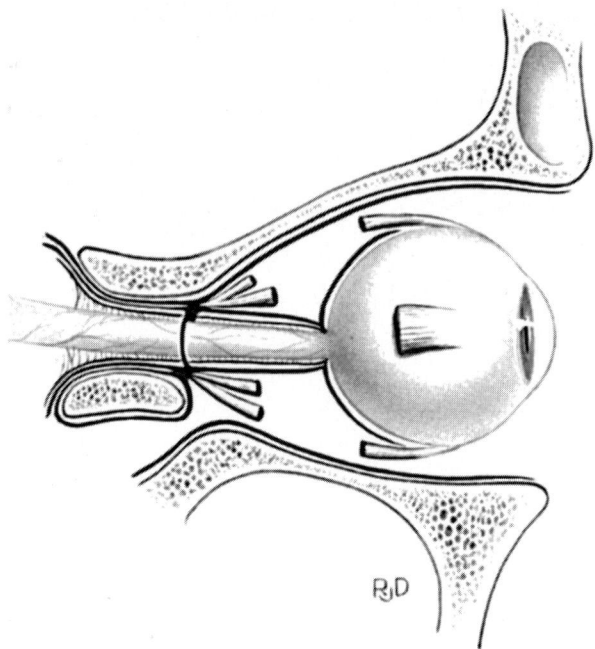

FIGURE 14–3 ■ The membranes investing the optic nerve and lining the intracranial cavity, optic canal, and orbit are shown. A double-layered intracranial dura is seen extending through the optic canal and superior orbital fissure. The inner layer continues in the orbit as the dural sheath of Schwann. The outer layer forms the periorbita beyond the annulus of Zinn. There is a continuous subarachnoid space that extends from the intracranial space to the junction of the pia, arachnoid, and dura at the scleral margin. This space is partially obliterated at the annulus of Zinn.

periosteum of the skull at these sites. Anteriorly, the periorbita is continuous with the periosteum at the orbital margin; structural modifications in the periorbita enclose the lacrimal gland and fix the pulley of the superior oblique tendon.

This confluence of the periorbita with the intracranial dura at the superior orbital fissure may serve as a route of entry of en plaque meningioma. Arachnoidal rests at this border zone may be the source of intraorbital meningiomas that appear to arise from the periorbita. Resection of a meningioma invading the superior fissure cannot be achieved without a risk of injury to the oculomotor nerves passing therein. Primary optic nerve sheath meningiomas can be defined preoperatively and safely removed by the transcranial approach. When these tumors occur at the extreme apex, where the dural sheath of the optic nerve is fused with the origins of the extraocular muscles at the annulus of Zinn, total excision can be achieved without injury to these structures if they have not been invaded by the tumor.

Meningiomas may have a propensity for more rapid growth in children; therefore, exenteration may be advisable in children if there is microscopic residual tissue at the annulus of Zinn or the superior orbital fissure. In older patients, microscopic residual tissue within the muscle cone may be acceptable because the tumors grow more slowly. The annulus of Zinn provides no barrier against extension of a tumor through the optic nerve (Fig. 14–4), and routine monitoring of the canal for hyperostosis, together with computed tomography (CT) or magnetic resonance imaging

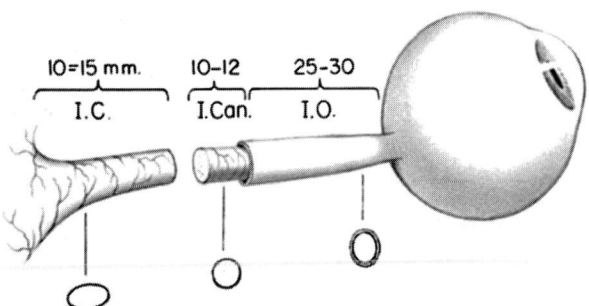

FIGURE 14–2 ■ The dimensions and contours of the intracranial, intracanalicular, and intraorbital portions of the optic nerve.

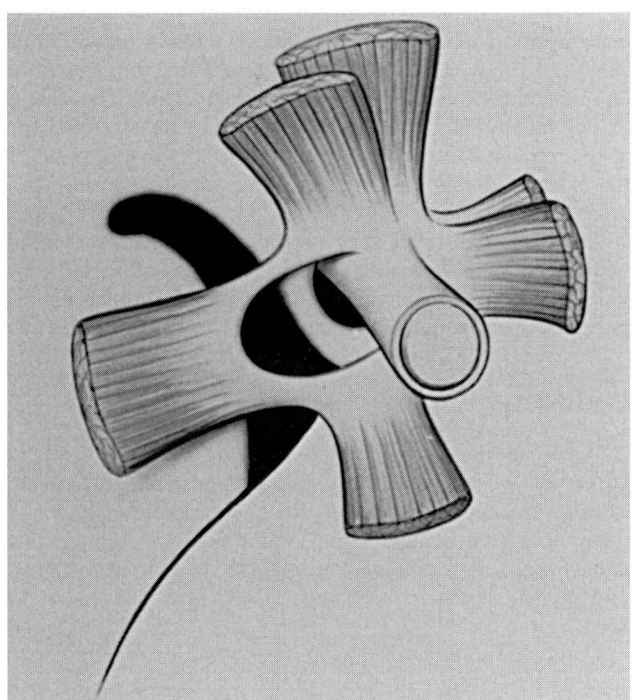

**FIGURE 14-4 ■** The annulus of Zinn is a fibrous band giving rise to the origins of six of the seven extraocular muscles. This fibrous tissue is in continuity with the dural sheath of the optic nerve. The two heads of the lateral rectus loop around that portion of the superior orbital fissure are known as the oculomotor foramen.

(MRI) scans, must be performed to detect the presence of intracanalicular tumors.

## Muscle Cone and Annulus of Zinn

The fibrous annulus tendineus (annulus of Zinn), previously described, serves as the origin of six of the seven extraocular muscles (see Fig. 14-4).

Superiorly, the superior rectus muscle arises from the annulus, which, at this point, is fused with the leptomeninges and dura of the optic nerve. The origin of the levator palpebrae is medial and superior to that of the superior rectus muscle. More medial and inferior to this are the origins of the medial rectus and superior oblique muscles. Although it is firmly fused to the optic nerve dorsally, the annulus of Zinn loops widely around the nerve, laterally and inferiorly, giving rise to the lateral rectus muscle, which has its origin from two heads; the inferior rectus derives its origin from the inferior head; the space between the two heads of the lateral rectus muscle is known as the oculomotor foramen. Thus, it is evident that this arrangement separates the portal of entry of the nerves, arteries, and veins into essentially three spaces: the optic foramen, the superior orbital fissure, and the oculomotor foramen.

## Arterial Supply and Venous Drainage

The ophthalmic artery arises from the internal carotid artery at its emergence from the cavernous sinus, passes on the medial side of the anterior clinoid, and runs in a split layer of dura beneath the optic nerve as it enters the orbital cavity through the optic foramen. On entering the orbit, it curves over the lateral margin of the optic nerve, gives off the central retinal branch, which perforates the dural sheath approximately 10 mm from the optic foramen, and then, within several millimeters, enters the nerve obliquely about 1 cm behind the globe. After giving off the central retinal branch, the ophthalmic artery crosses medially forward, giving off two long posterior ciliary arteries and six or eight short posterior ciliary arteries, and then anastomoses freely with the external carotid circulation. Two small branches of the ophthalmic artery supply the ocular muscles at their origin near the annulus.

Although obstruction of the central retinal artery results in loss of vision, obstruction of the ophthalmic artery may not if the arterial anastomoses are sufficient to preserve blood flow to the retina and choroidal circulation.

The orbital cavity is drained principally by the superior and inferior ophthalmic veins. Both of these valveless channels have extensive anastomoses with each other as well as with external tributaries. The superior ophthalmic vein passes through the superior orbital fissure to drain into the cavernous sinus. The inferior ophthalmic vein, which primarily drains a network of channels on the medial wall and floor of the orbit, divides; one branch drains the pterygoid plexus through the inferior orbital fissure, and the other joins the superior ophthalmic vein before it enters the superior orbital fissure. These extensive communications between the pterygoid plexus and the angular and deep facial veins accommodate minor alterations in venous drainage; however, occlusion of the superior ophthalmic vein may result in severe orbital venous congestion, chemosis, and proptosis.

## Orbital Nerves

When the orbit is unroofed from above, the frontalis nerve is usually visible through the thin periorbita. Once the periorbita is opened, the surgeon finds the frontalis nerve overlying the levator and superior rectus muscles. In the same plane but closer to the apex lies the fine trochlear nerve. The trochlear nerve, the frontalis branch of the fifth nerve, and its lacrimal branch pass through the superior orbital fissure in that order and lie within the periorbita but over the extraocular muscles (Fig. 14-5).

The remaining nerves traversing the superior orbital fissure enter the orbit and the muscle cone through the so-called oculomotor foramen between the two heads of the lateral rectus muscle in the following order: the superior division of the oculomotor nerve, which supplies the superior rectus and levator muscles; the nasociliary branch of the ophthalmic nerve; the sixth nerve; and the inferior division of the third nerve. The nasociliary nerve crosses over the optic nerve to reach the medial wall of the orbit. The ciliary ganglion lies lateral to the optic nerve. The inferior division of the oculomotor nerve crosses beneath the optic nerve to reach the medial and inferior rectus muscles.

Because of this arrangement, it is clear that the optic nerve can be approached directly through the medial com-

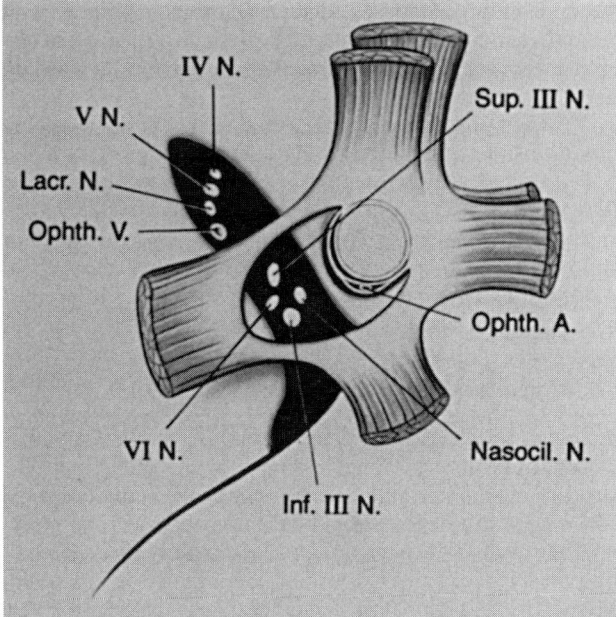

FIGURE 14–5 ■ Partial obliteration of the subarachnoid space of the optic nerve at the annulus of Zinn is shown, and the medial origin of the levator muscle is evident. The ophthalmic artery enters the orbit through the optic canal. The trochlear, frontalis, and lacrimal nerves and the ophthalmic vein enter through the superior orbital fissure and thus lie within the periorbita but outside the muscle cone, whereas the superior division of the oculomotor nerve, the abducens nerve, nasociliary nerve, and the inferior division of the oculomotor nerve enter the muscle cone through the oculomotor foramen and lie within the muscle cone.

partment, between the medial rectus and the levator muscles, without fear of injury to the nerve supply of any extraocular muscle (Fig. 14–6).

The trochlear nerve rarely can be spared. When optic nerve resection is the objective, however, there is little functional or cosmetic consequence of fourth nerve section.

Careful dissection through the lateral compartment, between the lateral and superior rectus and levator muscles, allows access to solitary neurofibromas, which most frequently arise from branches of the long ciliary nerves lying lateral to the optic nerve.

Tumors or mass lesions that arise external to the muscle cone are most likely to cause proptosis without limitation of extraocular movements or loss of vision. Some tumors within the muscle cone cause proptosis without causing neurologic or ophthalmologic deficits; however, tumors that crowd the apex are most likely to lead to dysfunction of one or more of the extraocular muscles or their nerve supply, causing specific deficits.

A clear understanding of orbital apical anatomy should help the surgeon approach the apical region safely and provides a basis for understanding the surgical limitations imposed by specific pathologic conditions.

## DIAGNOSIS

When an orbital pathologic entity is suspected and, in particular, when unilateral exophthalmos exists, a logical sequential work-up should follow the clinical examination.

Computed tomography (CT) has effectively supplanted the use of skull and orbital roentgenograms. Because of the contrast with orbital fat, CT is useful in defining orbital pathologic processes and is best used to image bony anatomy.[17] A well-performed study shows normal orbital anatomy, including the size and position of the globe, optic nerve, and extraocular muscles. The size and extent of a meningioma, optic glioma, or neurofibroma can be defined preoperatively. Most of these tumors enhance with contrast. CT scanning with bone windows offers the best definition of destructive or invasive pathology of the bone margins of the orbit and is also available with three-dimensional reconstructions.

MRI with fat suppression is now widely available and provides excellent definition of orbital pathology.[18–20] Fat suppression eliminates $T_1$-associated bright signals that can obscure intraorbital pathology. Gadolinium-enhanced MRI is superior to CT for resolution of soft tissue structures and is the best modality for demonstrating orbital apex lesions as well as the intracranial extension of gliomas and meningiomas.

Orbital angiography has a limited place in defining vascular lesions in the orbit and is required with less frequency now that a combination of noninvasive studies are available. Angiography can be useful when highly vascular tumors are suspected or to identify tumors that might benefit from embolization.

## CASE SELECTION

When a thoughtful sequential diagnostic work-up has been completed, the location and extent of the pathologic

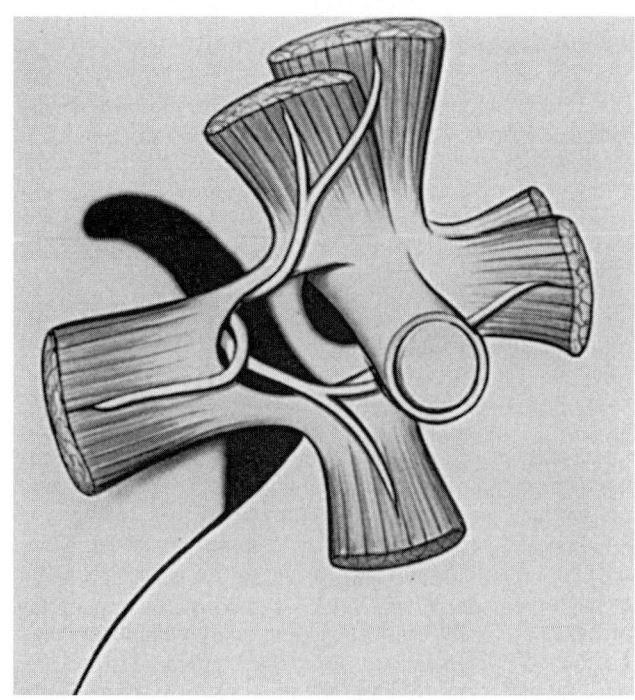

FIGURE 14–6 ■ The nerve supply to the extraocular muscles is shown entering through the oculomotor foramen. A medial superior approach to the optic nerve between the lateral and medial rectus muscles provides direct access, with minimal chance of injury to this nerve supply to the extraocular muscles.

process can be defined. Is a tumor present at all? If so, is it confined within the muscle cone? Does it arise from the optic nerve, or is it medial to or lateral to the optic nerve? Is the optic canal enlarged or hyperostotic? Is the bone integrity of the orbit violated? Are the fissures normal? Is the process erosive or destructive? Does the pathologic process extend to or from a sinus or arise from or enter the cranial cavity?

The clinical diagnosis of optic nerve glioma can be made with a high degree of accuracy. For optic nerve glioma confined to a single optic nerve, primary treatment is excision via the transcranial approach.[21] The ideal surgical candidate is a patient with a glioma of a single optic nerve who has disfiguring proptosis and poor vision in the involved eye. The rationale for the transcranial orbital approach is based on the conclusion that a wide excision, from the globe to the chiasm, is necessary to ensure total removal. A simple orbital resection too often leaves residual tumor in the apical stump of the transected, tumor-bearing nerve thus risking chiasmal extension.

Surgical indications are more complicated for tumors extending beyond a single nerve. Surgical resection would not be considered for multicentric optic glioma but exophytic chiasmal glioma should be excised. The role of radiotherapy is controversial; however, there is convincing evidence from our own large series of cases that astrocytoma of the optic nerve is a benign but often progressive process, similar to pilocystic astrocytoma of childhood in other locations. Our experience suggests that, in many cases, radiotherapy effectively arrests the course and improves proptosis and vision.[22]

The risks of radiation therapy to growth and maturation in infants and young children under the age of 5 years are more problematic. Initial treatment with chemotherapy, allowing for the deferral of radiotherapy in these cases, is recommended although long-term results await further analysis.

Primary meningiomas of the optic nerve most often produce visual impairment with minimal proptosis. When a meningioma of the optic nerve or orbit is responsible for nonfunctional vision, transcranial exploration is the preferred approach. Meningiomas also frequently arise between the optic nerve and carotid artery and involve both the cranial and orbital cavities. The transcranial approach allows direct and safe access to the apical and intracanalicular part of the optic nerve.[23] Tumors occurring distal to the orbital apex and close to the globe may be explored by a direct approach.[24]

Tumors involving the lateral periorbita from arachnoidal rests near the superior orbital fissure are frequently associated with multicentric or en plaque lesions on the cranial side of the superior orbital fissure. Pterional and skull base approaches are desirable in these circumstances both for exposure and to facilitate radical resection of tumor and involved bone.

A microsurgical technique is essential for the successful removal of solitary neurofibromas, which are usually found lateral to the optic nerve. Although the transcranial approach provides better access to the most apical lesions, more anteriorly located lesions can also be accessed via lateral canthotomy (Krönlein operation). In view of the

relative difficulty in making this diagnosis clinically, the latter approach may be advantageous.

Osteomas and other bony lesions arising from the posterior ethmoid region can be defined and the transcranial approach selected for primary removal because of their medial epiperiorbital location. Reconstruction is important for these patients to prevent a cerebrospinal fluid (CSF) leak and encephaloceles.

Obviously, encephaloceles must be treated by a neurosurgical approach, and some dermoid cysts and hemangiomas of the orbit can also be treated neurosurgically. Lesions such as ossifying fibromas and aneurysmal bone cysts that border both the orbit and the cranial cavity can be best approached transcranially.

Most problems arising within the orbit can be dealt with more simply by a direct approach, including the most common mucoceles and most hemangiomas and lymphangiomas. Similarly, malignant processes of the orbit may require extensive skull base approaches for en bloc resection and orbital exenteration. Finally, the surgeon dealing with proptosis must be aware of the very common nonsurgical causes, such as pseudotumor and thyrotoxicosis which are generally diagnosed by preoperative noninvasive imaging.

Under certain conditions in which clinical parameters have not firmly established the surgical indications, and particularly when a lymphoid lesion is suspected, a fine-needle aspiration biopsy can be useful for directing management decisions.[25] This technique is limited by sampling error and cytologic misinterpretation and can be complicated by orbital hemorrhage or globe perforation.

## PREOPERATIVE MANAGEMENT AND ANESTHESIA

General anesthesia is used in all cases of transcranial orbital exploration. The principles of neuroanesthesia are adhered to, and there are no special anesthetic requirements for exploring the orbit. Dexamethasone is used as an intraoperative and postoperative adjunct to reduce postoperative edema. Mannitol is used intraoperatively to reduce intraocular tension as well as intracranial tension so that a suitable surgical field is obtained without unnecessary retraction. Placement of a lumbar spinal drain for CSF removal can be useful for brain relaxation.

## AIDS TO SURGERY

Besides deserving credit for systematizing the preoperative work-up in patients with orbital tumors, neurosurgery can also claim contributions to improved instrumentation and techniques for operating within the orbit. Maroon and Kennerdell[26] have described the advantages of neurosurgical techniques in an ophthalmologic lateral approach to the orbit. Magnification with a microscope is mandatory when operating on the fine and attenuated structures within the orbit. Similarly, cottonoids and controlled suction are indispensable, as is the use of malleable retractors. Bipolar coagulation has materially added to the safety of operating within the orbit by either the cranial or the direct orbital approach. The $CO_2$ and neodymium:yttrium aluminum garnet (Nd:YAG) lasers can be valuable adjuncts for tumor removal.[20] The $CO_2$ laser can be mounted on surgical microscope and targeted with a micromanipulator. The shallow depth of energy penetration facilitates vaporization of tumor tissue while sparing deeper normal anatomic structures.

## OPERATIVE PROCEDURE[20, 26–28]

It is not necessary to resect and replace the orbital rim to gain access to the apex of the orbit. It is most important, however, to plan a flap that is medial in order to allow a medial orbital approach to the optic nerve when dealing with primary tumors of the optic nerve. The frontotemporal approach, which is so useful for most invasive tumors of the lateral orbit, such as sphenoid wing meningiomas, does not provide sufficient medial exposure for surgery on optic nerve tumors.

### Exposure

The patient is placed supine on the operating table and a Mayfield three-point headholder or a similar device is used to secure the head. The head is extended to allow the frontal lobe to fall away from the orbital roof. A bicoronal incision is made 1 to 2 cm behind the hairline extending from the tragus on the ipsilateral side to the superior temporal line on the contralateral side. A smaller incision extending to the midline can be used if the orbital rim is not going to be removed and if medial exposure is not needed. The incision is carried down to the pericranium but the temporalis muscle and fascia are allowed to remain intact. It is preferable to leave the pericranium attached to the scalp to preserve its blood supply during the course of the operation. It can be easily dissected free and left attached to its vascularized pedicle at the end of the operation when it is needed for reconstruction. If the lateral orbital rim and zygoma are to be removed or exposed, the temporalis fascia should be brought forward with the scalp flap to ensure that the frontal branches of the seventh nerve are preserved. The scalp flap is brought forward far enough to expose the frontal bone so that the inferior portion of the craniotomy provides exposure of the floor of the anterior fossa. The extent of the craniotomy should be anticipated to decide whether or not the galeal dissection must extend to the orbital rim since it will be associated with considerable postoperative ecchymosis and swelling. In addition, there may be injury to the supraorbital vessels and nerve. However, if the supraorbital rim is to be removed, the scalp flap should be brought lower to expose the supraorbital rim so that the periorbital fascia, which is continuous with the pericranium, can be freed up from the orbital roof. This dissection must avoid damage to the supraorbital nerve as it exits through the supraorbital foramen. A fine osteotome or rongeur may be needed to unroof the foramen if the nerve is completely enclosed by bone.

Following placement of a small bur hole in the postero-lateral portion of the frontal bone, a craniotome is used to turn a craniotomy flap extending to the floor of the anterior fossa and just ipsilateral to the sagittal sinus (Fig. 14–7). A simple median frontal craniotomy is sufficient for most exposures that are required in the orbit.

For lesions extending beyond the orbit itself, modifications of the simple frontal craniotomy can be made depending on the required degree of exposure. If the orbital lesion extends anteriorly, the supraorbital rim may be removed. When removing the orbital rim, it is desirable to include as much of the orbital roof with it as possible to minimize the orbital defect to be repaired at the conclusion of the operation. This can be done by drilling an opening in the orbital roof and using an oscillating saw or Gigli saw threaded through the opening to make a cut through the orbital rim both medially and laterally. For cosmetic purposes, the width of the cut should be small so that a noticeable gap is not left when the rim is replaced at the end of the operation. If the lesion extends laterally in the orbit, or into the cavernous sinus or parasellar area through the optic foramen or superior orbital fissure, then a frontotemporal exposure is necessary. This is done by incising the temporalis muscle and bringing it forward with the scalp flap to expose the inferior temporal area. The craniotomy should include the temporal bone and pterion. When the cavernous sinus is involved, the lateral wing of the sphenoid bone is drilled off, thus unroofing the optic foramen and superior orbital fissure and removing the anterior clinoid process.

If the lesion extends medially into the ethmoid sinus and a wide exposure is needed, an orbitoethmoidal osteotomy can be utilized by making cuts through the supraorbital rim, frontonasal suture, and the contralateral, medial orbital rim. The frontal craniotomy in this situation must extend across the midline, exposing the sagittal sinus. Although this opening invariably sacrifices the ipsilateral olfactory nerve, the contralateral olfactory nerve should be preserved if possible. When the olfactory nerve is cut at its sheath

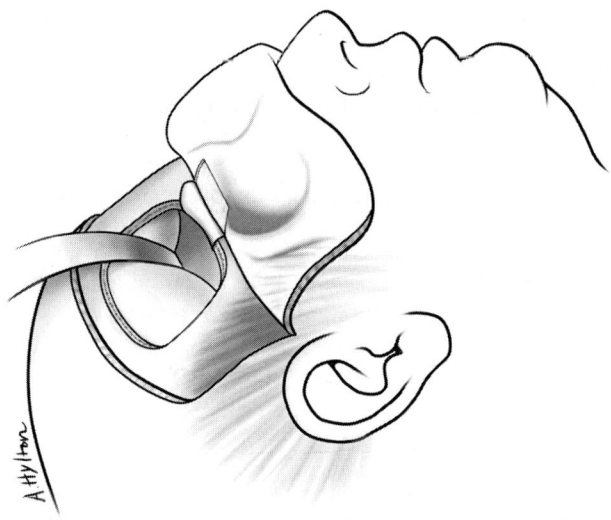

**FIGURE 14–7 ■** The coronal incision and low medial frontal craniotomy flap are used in exposing the floor of the anterior fossa. Drainage of cerebrospinal fluid from a spinal drain before beginning the epidural approach to the orbital roof minimizes the need for frontal retraction.

the ensuing dural opening must be repaired primarily. To complete the orbitoethmoidal osteotomy, additional cuts are made through the cribriform plate and orbital roof. An osteotome is used to release the final attachment through the ethmoidal bone.

If the frontal sinus is opened with the craniotomy, which is often the case, the mucosa is exenterated and the sinus obliterated with either a fat graft from the patient's abdomen or with portions of pericranium, temporalis muscle or temporalis fascia. At the end of the procedure, a flap of vascularized pericranium is brought over the frontal sinus defect and sutured to the dura, cordoning off the sinus.

Following the craniotomy, the orbital roof is exposed extradurally with careful preservation of the dura to minimize the possibility of CSF leaks and infection. The frontal lobe is gently retracted extradurally, and the orbit is unroofed with a high-speed cutting drill. Depending on the location of the lesion, it may be necessary to drill out the optic foramen. In this case, a diamond drill bit is used under copious irrigation to avoid heat injury to the nerve. Once the orbit is exposed, the lesion may be removed using microsurgical techniques.

If the orbit is being explored for optic glioma, it is advisable to open the dura and inspect the intracranial optic nerve before proceeding with the orbital unroofing. In so doing, the removal of CSF from the chiasmatic cistern aids in the development of an excellent operative field without the need for spinal drainage or excessive retraction. If the tumor is found to extend into the chiasm, indicating that gross total resection cannot be achieved, the procedure can be discontinued after a biopsy specimen is obtained. Once the tumor is identified within the nerve but not extending to the chiasm, the optic nerve is cut perpendicular to its direction at the chiasm. Hemostasis of the fine pial circulation is achieved with Surgicel or other hemostatic material. If the tumor is not seen in the intracranial space, the optic nerve should not be sectioned until pathology is identified within the orbit.

An epidural approach is desirable for orbital exploration, because the underlying brain remains protected during gentle retraction. In addition, it protects the olfactory nerve and bulb from avulsion. Because the dura inserts at the cribriform fossa lateral to the olfactory nerve, epidural retraction avoids injury in this location. Malleable self-retaining retractors are shaped and curved to expose the entire anterior fossa up to the clinoid. Moist cottonoids are placed at the lateral margins of the exposure to advance the epidural dissection, allow irrigation, and facilitate suctioning.

The orbital unroofing is begun with a chisel or a high-speed bur. Once a small opening is made in the midportion of the floor of the anterior fossa, the remainder of the resection is facilitated by the use of fine double-action mastoid or infant Leksell rongeurs (Fig. 14–8). The canal can be unroofed, if required, with a drill. The orbital unroofing does not need to come closer than 1 cm to the orbital rim anteriorly; it should extend approximately 1.5 cm from the medial margin and should be extended laterally to within 0.5 cm of the lateral orbital margin. This unroofing must be carried through the optic canal.

The periorbita is usually thin and transparent. When there is a significant orbital mass, the intraorbital structures

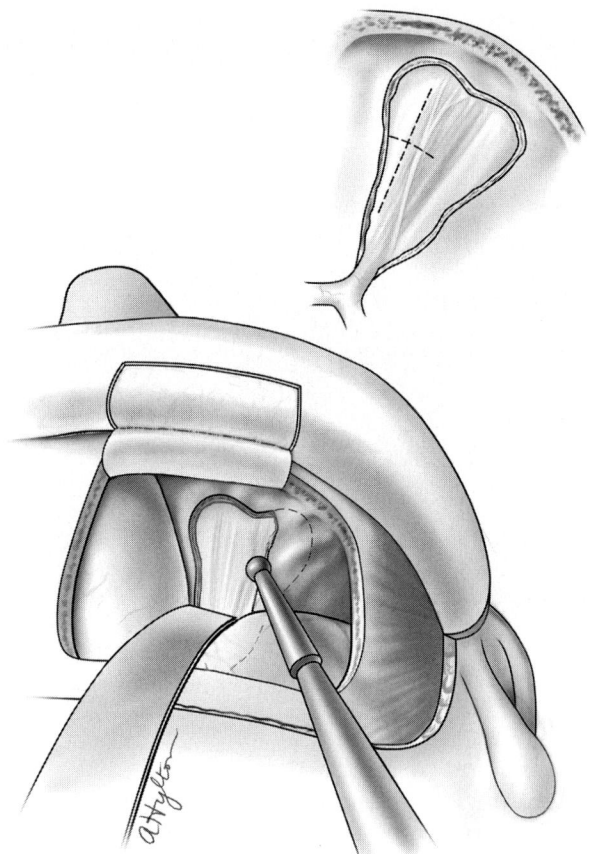

FIGURE 14–8 ■ The thin orbital roof is entered with a chisel or bur. The extent of orbital unroofing is outlined. The unroofing is completed with fine double-action and Leksell rongeurs. The optic canal is opened as illustrated. The frontalis nerve can be seen through the thin periosteum and is a landmark indicating the course of the levator and superior rectus muscles, otherwise seen with difficulty. The dura is incised medial or lateral to these structures as indicated.

are attenuated and blanched and may be difficult to see. The periorbita is incised in a cruciate fashion with a No. 11 blade. The vertical limb is placed lateral or medial to the levator and superior rectus muscles, depending on whether a lateral or medial approach to the orbit is planned. The frontalis nerve is usually visible through the periorbita, because it lies over these muscles. It serves to approximate their location. The trochlear nerve lies beneath the periorbita but outside of the muscle cone. It lies close to the apex, is extremely fine, and cannot be easily spared if the optic nerve is to be resected. There is, of course, no functional or cosmetic consequence to fourth nerve section in a blind eye.

## Approach to the Medial Orbit

A medial approach to the optic nerve is preferred when dealing with meningioma or optic glioma (Fig. 14–9). The primary advantage of this approach relates to preservation of the nerve supply to extraocular muscles. The third (oculomotor) nerve, after it enters the orbit through the superior orbital fissure and oculomotor foramen lateral to the optic nerve, sends branches *over* the nerve to supply the under-

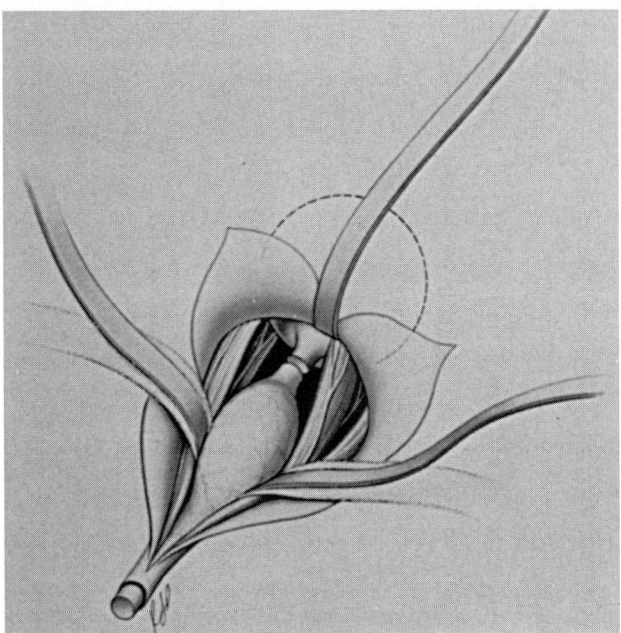

**FIGURE 14–9 ■** Narrow malleable retractors and cottonoid pledgets are used to gently retract the orbital structures. The preferred approach to the optic nerve is shown.

belly of the levator and superior rectus muscles and *beneath* the nerve to the inferior and medial rectus muscles. A medial approach to the optic nerve thus can be made without traversing the course of these nerves to the extraocular muscles. Small malleable retractors are individually bent to retract the levator and superior rectus complex laterally and anteriorly. The tumor is approached by blunt dissection through residual orbital fat. Magnification and gentle handling of tissues are essential to this portion of the procedure. Both optic gliomas and primary optic nerve sheath meningiomas are fairly firm encapsulated tumors, and a plane of dissection is started directly on the tumor capsule. Gentle retraction and the placement of moist cottonoids allow the development of a plane entirely around the tumor capsule, which is not adherent to the surrounding residual areolar tissue. This tissue separates and protects the normal neurovascular structures, which therefore can be spared during tumor removal.

The junction of the tumor and the posterior margin of the globe is readily found. At this point, the nerve is transected between two fine mosquito forceps, which are used to clamp the tumor-bearing optic nerve. Use of this technique avoids injury to the posterior margin of the globe and the sclera. After the nerve is sectioned, the distal clamp is removed and any bleeding from the cut margin is carefully electrocoagulated with bipolar cautery. The proximal clamp can be used as a handle for further tumor dissection toward the apex.

In the case of optic nerve glioma, in order to remove the tumor in one piece from the globe to the chiasm (Fig. 14–10), the origin of the levator muscle, which inserts at the annulus of Zinn medial to the superior rectus, must be sectioned. Only in this way can the annulus of Zinn be opened from above to remove the canalicular portion of the optic nerve tethered at the orbital end of the canal. The

origin of the levator muscle can then be resutured after the tumor is removed. This maneuver is difficult, and in young infants, the structures are small and the exposure limited, making the procedure more difficult. The optic nerve can be sectioned with curved scissors at the extreme apex and the orbital specimen removed. At this juncture, the ophthalmic artery is sometimes severed, but the bleeding can be controlled with bipolar electrocautery. The intracranial portion of the nerve then can be removed as a second specimen. In order to accomplish this, the epidural retractors must be removed and placed intradurally again, re-exposing the intracranial optic nerve so that it can be pulled through the canal. If the surgeon believes that there may be a small amount of residual glioma at the canalicular face of the annulus, brief electrocoagulation on an angled nerve hook can be used safely and may limit recurrence. A small pledget of temporalis muscle placed within the canal will prevent the flow of CSF into the orbital space in the immediate postoperative period.

When dealing with a primary optic nerve sheath meningioma, however, it is *mandatory* to unroof the optic canal, open the intracanalicular dura, section the origin of the levator at the annulus of Zinn, and open the annulus. This approach permits inspection at high magnification and gross total removal of the entire intracanalicular tumor with the optic nerve from the orbit close to the globe, back to the cranial end of the optic nerve near the chiasm. The annulus and levator origin should then be resutured with fine atraumatic silk or synthetic suture. Unlike the situation with optic nerve gliomas, electrocoagulation of residual meningioma at the orbital apex or in the canal is *not* an acceptable technique and *will lead to recurrence.*

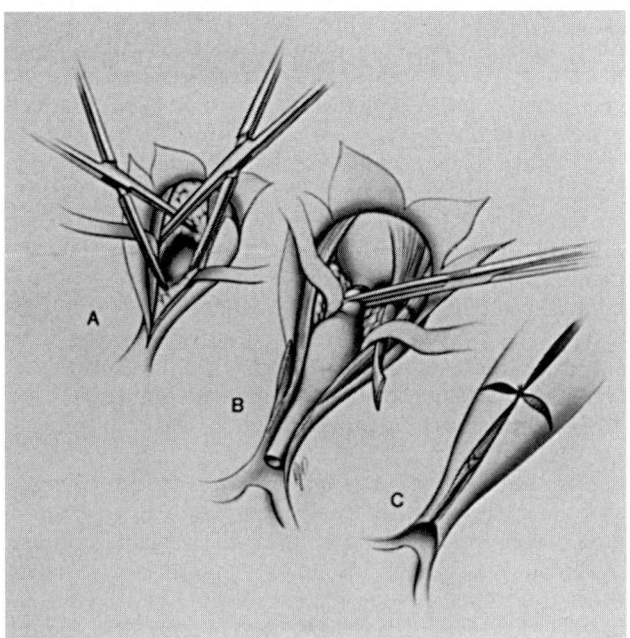

**FIGURE 14–10 ■** The technique of sectioning the levator. The annulus of Zinn cannot be opened without performing this maneuver. After resecting a tumor-bearing optic nerve from the globe to the chiasm, the origin of the levator muscle is resutured. This maneuver is useful in some cases of optic glioma and meningioma. (From Housepian EM, Marquardt MD, Behrens M: Orbital tumors. In Wilkins RH, Renganchary SS [eds]: Neurosurgery, Vol 1. New York: McGraw-Hill, 1985.)

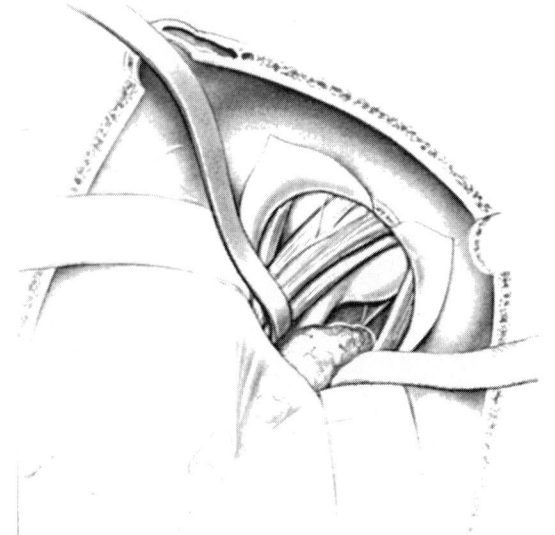

FIGURE 14–11 ■ The lateral transcranial orbital approach to an apical neurofibroma. Dissection in the areolar tissue is avoided, and cottonoid pledgets and narrow, shaped, malleable retractors are used to define a plane directly on the tumor capsule. Injury to the extraocular nerve supply is avoided in this way.

There is ample histopathologic evidence for the primary intraorbital origin of optic nerve meningiomas. Cushing and Eisenhardt[1] described a psammomatous meningioma arising at the sheath of Schwann and growing into the optic nerve. Although it is not clearly defined, it may represent the origin of some nerve sheath meningiomas. These tumors have been shown to traverse the optic canal by microscopic spread along the subarachnoid space or within the nerve, without producing enlargement or hyperostosis of the optic canal.

## Lateral Orbital Approach

The transcranial orbital approach to the lateral superior quadrant of the orbit can be used for some cases of suspected solitary neurofibroma believed to arise from the long ciliary nerves. They are thus found in a position lateral to the optic nerve. In these cases, the periorbital opening is made lateral to the superior rectus insertion (Fig. 14–11), and using the techniques described for orbital exploration with malleable retractors and cottonoids, a plane is developed directly on the tumor capsule. Efforts are made to separate the loose areolar tissue from the tumor itself and minimize dissection within this tissue. To achieve exposure of the lateral quadrant, the superior rectus muscle is retracted medially. If the tumor is large, it can be broken into several pieces for removal. Efforts should be made to avoid the extreme apex in the lateral approach in order to minimize the chance of injury to the third and sixth cranial nerves.

The Berke modification of the Krönlein operation[6] may provide good access to pathologic processes in the lateral quadrant of the orbit. The application of neurosurgical techniques, as described by Maroon and Kennerdell,[26] and adherence to strict microsurgical technique should allow safe access to the lateral apex and minimize the possibility

of injury to the sixth nerve. This approach is not recommended for primary optic nerve tumors, however, because of the anatomic configuration of the nerve supply to the extraocular muscles, as described previously.

## Closure and Reconstruction

Once removal of the tumor is complete and before retraction is released, cottonoids are carefully removed and the apical bed is inspected for hemostasis. Bipolar electrocoagulation should be used sparingly to achieve this. Extensive electrocauterization behind the globe should be avoided, because it can injure the retinal blood supply as well as the autonomic nerves and result in pupillary dilatation and corneal anesthesia. When the field is dry, all retractors and cottonoids are removed; the origin of the levator is resutured, if it has been sectioned; and the periorbita is closed loosely by approximating the four corners.

With small orbital roof defects, the vascularized pericranium flap is usually sufficient to provide support, and no further reconstruction is needed. If the orbital defect is large, reconstruction is needed to avoid enophthalmos or pulsating exophthalmos. We generally prefer to reconstruct the orbital defect with a piece of bone from the inner table of the craniotomy flap plated to the orbital rim (Fig. 14–12). If the defect is large, a cancellous bone graft may be taken from the iliac crest. Although defects may be repaired with titanium mesh, autologous bone is generally preferred

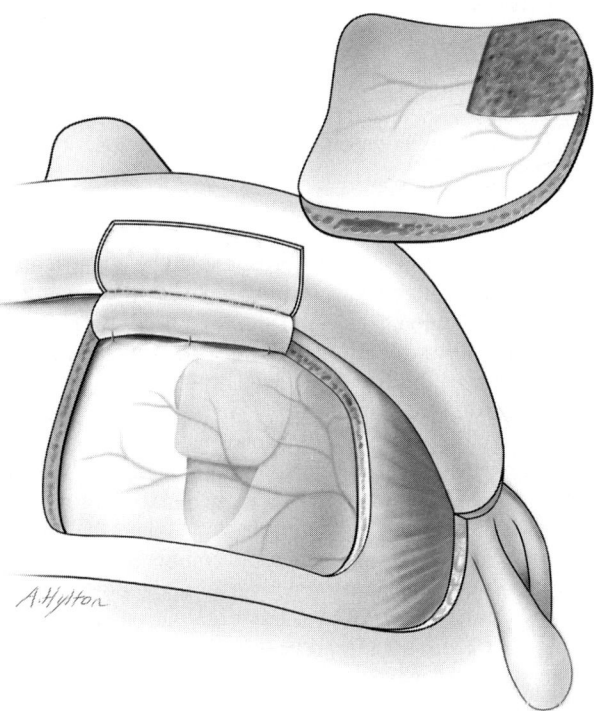

FIGURE 14–12 ■ On completion of tumor removal, the periorbita is closed with one or several fine atraumatic sutures. A bridge formed from a split thickness of bone taken from the craniotomy flap is placed at the orbital roof defect to avoid postoperative pulsation of the globe. Dural tenting sutures are then placed, and any defect in the frontal sinus repaired and a flap of pericranium sutured to the dura to cover the bone defect.

because there is decreased risk of infection and less interference with postoperative radiographic imagining.

If the ethmoid sinus is entered during the exposure, it must be covered with vascularized tissue. A pericranium flap is most convenient for this purposes, and should be developed and separated from the scalp, while preserving its blood supply anteriorly. If the olfactory nerve has been sacrificed, the pericranium should be sutured back behind the area of the closure of dural sleeve, completely covering it. If the dura has been torn or has been purposely opened to remove an intradural lesion, a watertight dural repair is needed to prevent CSF leakage. If the dural opening is small this can be accomplished primarily, but a larger opening must be covered with a patch taken from either the pericranium or temporalis fascia.

The craniotomy flap is replaced with wires or titanium plates. The orbital rim is replaced first and is secured with plates or wire. The galea and skin are closed as separate layers. A subgaleal hemovac is placed and brought out through a separate stab incision to remain in place for 24 hours. A snug head wrap will discourage the accumulation of any subcutaneous or subgaleal fluid collection. If the spinal drain has been used, it is removed immediately unless there has been a significant dural repair with potential for CSF leakage postoperatively in which case it may be left on continuous drainage (5 to 10 ml/hr) for up to 5 days to allow the leaks to seal.

## Tarsorrhaphy

Before extubation and after the head dressing has been applied, temporary tarsorrhaphy should be performed in all cases of orbital exploration when optic nerve function has been sacrificed. In other cases, the lids are not closed to allow for monitoring of vision. The procedure is simple and atraumatic (Fig. 14–13). The lids are washed with a cotton ball, and the cornea and conjunctiva are irrigated with saline. Sterile towels are placed to keep the sutures sterile. A double-ended 6–0 suture is used to place a horizontal mattress with two rubber band bumper guards. The thin skin of the lid is protected with the bumpers and makes removal of the tarsorrhaphy simple. In principle, the suture should pass through the tarsal plate posterior to the anterior extension of the orbicularis muscle (gray line) of both lids. Care should be taken to see that there are no inverted lashes before the suture is tied. When the tarsorrhaphy is completed, an ophthalmic ointment is used to lubricate the cornea and conjunctiva. A pledget of nonstick gauze is placed over the eye; fluffy cotton balls then are used to gently diffuse the pressure when taped to the head dressing. It is important for the surgeon to remove the tarsorrhaphy dressing daily to inspect the eye for signs of irritation and to reapply ophthalmic ointment. The tarsorrhaphy is left in place until the peak edema period has passed. It is advisable to remove the pressure dressing 1 day before the tarsorrhaphy suture is removed. In this way, if pressure has been removed prematurely and the eye begins to bulge, the cornea will be protected.

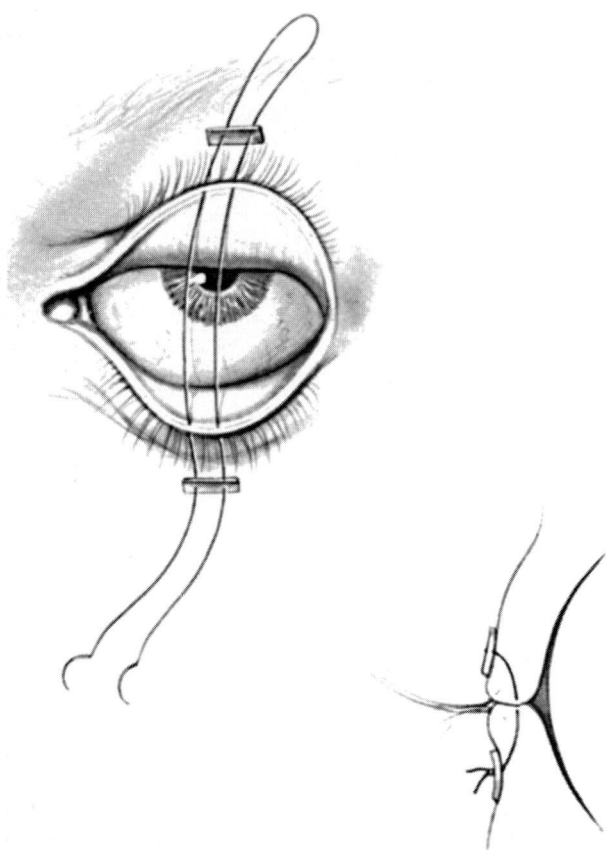

**FIGURE 14–13** ■ The technique for temporary tarsorrhaphy. A fine double-ended atraumatic suture is placed through the tarsal plate of each lid. Small rubber bumpers prevent maceration of the thin skin of the lid.

## POSTOPERATIVE CARE

Intraoperative antibiotics are used routinely, and dexamethasone is administered in high doses through the fourth postoperative day and then tapered over the ensuing week. With care in hemostasis, blood transfusion should not be required. Anticonvulsant therapy can be used, although there is usually little retraction injury to the orbital brain surface.

## Complications

Transcranial orbital exploration should be a relatively benign procedure; however, transient levator and superior rectus palsy occurs in almost all cases of optic nerve tumor resection by this route; it may be complete or partial. Improvement is seen from several days to 3 to 6 weeks and recovery is usually complete by 3 months. Ptosis and limitation of extraocular movements may infrequently be a permanent accompaniment to removal of orbital tumors by any approach. Loss of vision may occur in orbital exploration for the optic nerve tumor, even when the optic nerve is preserved; and a potential complication of blindness may accompany resection of tumors at the chiasm. Late postoperative vitreous hemorrhage, uveitis, and avascular necrosis are also infrequent but recognized complications that can lead to enucleation. Infection is a potential complication in any operative procedure. Recurrence of glioma within the orbit occurred in only one case in which the tumor was seeded by earlier Krönlein exploration. Serious arterial hemorrhage is rare but occurred in 1 of 76 patients operated on for resection of primary optic nerve tumor.

## SUMMARY

The diagnostic techniques that are currently available have vastly improved our ability to predict the nature, precise location, and extent of tumors of the orbit. Familiarity with the variety of diseases that occur in the orbit and that can produce proptosis is essential for the neurosurgeon involved in the management of patients with orbital disease. A clear understanding of the regional anatomy will allow the surgeon to plan his or her surgical approach based on rational surgical objectives. The availability of a multidisciplinary team comprised of surgeons experienced in ophthalmology and neurosurgery provides the best opportunity for successful management of these tumors.

## REFERENCES

1. Cushing H, Eisenhardt L: Meningiomas. Springfield, IL: Charles C Thomas, 1938.
2. Dandy WE: Results following transcranial attack on orbital tumors. Arch Ophthalmol 25:191, 1941.
3. Love JG, Benedict WL: Transcranial removal of intraorbital tumors. JAMA 121:777, 1945.
4. Matson DD: Unilateral exophthalmos in childhood. Clin Neurosurg 5:116, 1958.
5. Van Buren JM, Poppen JL, Horax G: Unilateral exophthalmos: A consideration of symptom pathogenesis. Brain 80:139, 1957.
6. Berke RN: A modified Krönlein operation. Trans Am Ophthalmol Soc 51:193, 1953.
7. Davis FA: Primary tumors of the optic nerves. Arch Ophthalmol 23:735, 957, 1940.
8. Jackson H: Orbital tumors. Proc Soc Med 38:587, 1945.
9. Reese AB: Expanding lesions of the orbit. Trans Ophthalmol Soc UK 91:85, 1971.
10. Spencer WH: Primary neoplasms of the optic nerve and its sheaths: Clinical features and current concepted pathogenetic mechanisms. J Am Ophthalmol Soc 70:490, 1972.
11. Pernkopf E: Fernen H (ed): Atlas of Topographical and Applied Human Anatomy, Vol 1. Philadelphia: WB Saunders, 1963.
12. Last RJ: Wolff's Anatomy of the Eye and Orbit, 6th ed. Philadelphia: WB Saunders, 1968.
13. Doxanas MT, Anderson RL: Clinical Orbital Anatomy. Baltimore: Williams & Wilkins, 1984.
14. Zide BM, Jelks GW: Surgical Anatomy of the Orbit. New York: Raven Press, 1985.
15. Natori Y, Rhoton AL. Transcranial approach to the orbit: Microsurgical anatomy. J Neurosurg 81:78, 1994.
16. Housepian EM: Microsurgical anatomy of the orbital apex and principles of transcranial orbital exploration. In Keener EB (ed): Clinical Neurosurgery, Vol 25. Baltimore: Williams & Wilkins, 1978, pp 556–573.
17. Jakobiec FA, Depot MJ, Kennerdell JS, et al: Combined clinical and computed tomographic diagnosis of orbital glioma and meningioma. Ophthalmology 91:137, 1984.
18. Bilaniuk LT, Schenck JF, Zimmerman RA, et al: Ocular and orbital lesions: Surface coil MR imaging. Radiology 156:669–674, 1985.
19. Haik BG, et al: Magnetic resonance imaging in the evaluation of optic nerve gliomas. Ophthalmology 94:709, 1987.
20. Kazim M, Bruce J: Neurogenic tumors. In Bosniak S (ed): Ophthalmic Plastic and Reconstructive Surgery. Philadelphia: WB Saunders, 1996, pp 983–993.
21. Housepian EM: Surgical treatment of unilateral optic nerve gliomas. J Neurosurg 31:604, 1969
22. Housepian EM, Bruce JN, Habif D Jr: Current concepts in the diagnosis and treatment of optic gliomas. In Tindall G (ed): Contemporary Neurosurgery, Vol 14. Baltimore: Williams & Wilkins, 1992, pp 1–5.
23. Housepian EM: The surgical treatment of optic nerve sheath meningiomas. In Ransohoff JR (ed): Modern Techniques in Surgery: Neurosurgery. Mt Kisco, NY: Futura, 1981, pp 1–4.
24. Mark LE, Kennerdell JS, Maroon JC, et al: Microsurgical removal of a primary intraorbital meningioma. Am J Ophthalmol 86:704–709, 1978.
25. Kennerdell JS, Dekker A, Johnson BL, et al: Fine-needle aspiration biopsy. Its use in orbital tumors. Arch Ophthalmol 97:1315, 1979.
26. Maroon JC, Kennerdell JS: Surgical approaches to the orbit. J Neurosurg 60:1226, 1984.
27. Jane JA, Park TS, Doberskin LH, et al: The supraorbital approach. Neurosurgery 11:537, 1982.
28. Housepian EM: Optic gliomas. Rangenchary SS (ed): In AANS Color Atlas of Neurosurgical Techniques, Vol 1. Baltimore: Williams & Wilkins, 1991, pp 1–13.

# Anterior and Lateral Approaches to the Orbit and Orbital Apex

■ TODD A. GOODGLICK and MELVIN G. ALPER

The surgical removal of retrobulbar tumors with retention of the globe was first devised by Krönlein in 1888.[1] Using a lateral approach with a curvilinear incision parallel to the orbital rim and lateral lid creases, this approach remains, although modified, in use today. Before World War II, relatively few such operations were performed by ophthalmic surgeons because most orbitotomies were performed through a transcranial approach by neurosurgeons. Dandy[2] believed that 75% of orbital tumors arose within the cranial cavity and that the only proper surgical approach for them was a transcranial route. All surgically treatable orbital diseases, however, involve the highly complex visual apparatus. With this realization, orbital surgery came to lie properly within the province of ophthalmic surgery as a subspecialty of its own. The most successful approaches to such skull-based surgery have developed from interacting teams of neurosurgeons, otolaryngologists, plastic surgeons, maxillofacial specialists, and orbital surgeons, each contributing their specific expertise regarding this complex anatomic territory.

The transition from intracranial to intraorbital procedures requires a paradigm change in approach. The orbit is a mechanical device, in contrast to the "solid state" configuration of the brain. Injury to any of its components is likely to interfere with the overall function of the whole mechanism rather than producing focal deficits seen in neurologic procedures. With multiple structures running in all directions and surrounded and supported by a cushion of orbital fat, the concept of distinct surgical tissue planes and wide excisional margins requires revision.

As a hybrid of ophthalmic; plastic; ear, nose, and throat; and neurosurgical techniques, orbital surgery has advanced over the last 2 decades, particularly with the advent of computed tomography (CT) scanning, magnetic resonance imaging (MRI), angiography, ultrasonography, and endoscopic techniques. A combination of various ophthalmic and neurosurgical instruments is used as well as loupe and microscope magnification. Except for anterior and superficial procedures, cases are performed most safely and comfortably under general anesthesia. Even with these techniques, the primary challenge confronting surgery in the orbit remains the difficulties in manipulating the complex and often microscopic orbital structures without disturbing the mechanical precision that is required for sight.

## FUNCTIONAL ORBITAL ANATOMY

The orbit, cranium, and sinuses function as an integrated anatomic system despite the fact that the medical specialties that deal with these often work with vastly different perspectives. Relational anatomy becomes critical as the surgeon passes across distinct anatomic subspecialty boundaries.

The orbital cavity is a 30-ml four-walled, pear-shaped structure oriented anterior and laterally such that the lateral walls form a 90-degree angle with each other, and the medial walls are parallel. The central axis of the orbit and the visual axis of the globe are separated by 23 degrees (Figs. 15–1 to 15–5). The floor of the orbit slopes upward posteriorly.

In addition to sharing common boundaries with the sinuses, the orbital walls lie adjacent to the intracranial space. The orbital roof is the floor of the anterior fossa, the greater sphenoid wing is both the posterior lateral orbital wall and the medial wall of the middle fossa, and the superior third of the medial orbital wall lies above the level of the cribriform plate. The apex is formed by the greater and lesser wings of the sphenoid bone with the gap between these creating the superior and inferior orbital fissures. A continuous leptomeningeal sheath extends from the intracranial space through the optic canal of the lesser sphenoid wing and along the optic nerve to its insertion into the globe. The blood supply to the intraorbital optic nerve traverses this sheath, explaining why resection of meningiomas in this location poses a risk to the nerve itself.[3, 4] The annulus of Zinn forms the tendinous insertion of the extraocular muscle cone at the apex. It spans the superior orbital fissure creating an intraconal and extraconal compartment of the fissure dividing the structures that run through it. Through the former, the optic nerve, ophthalmic artery, cranial nerve III (both superior and inferior branches) and cranial nerve VI, nasociliary branch of cranial nerve V, and the sympathetic fibers enter the orbit from the arachnoid space and cavernous sinus. Through the extraconal aspect of the fissure courses cranial nerve IV, the frontal and lacrimal branches of cranial nerve V, and the venous drainage back to the cavernous sinus. These

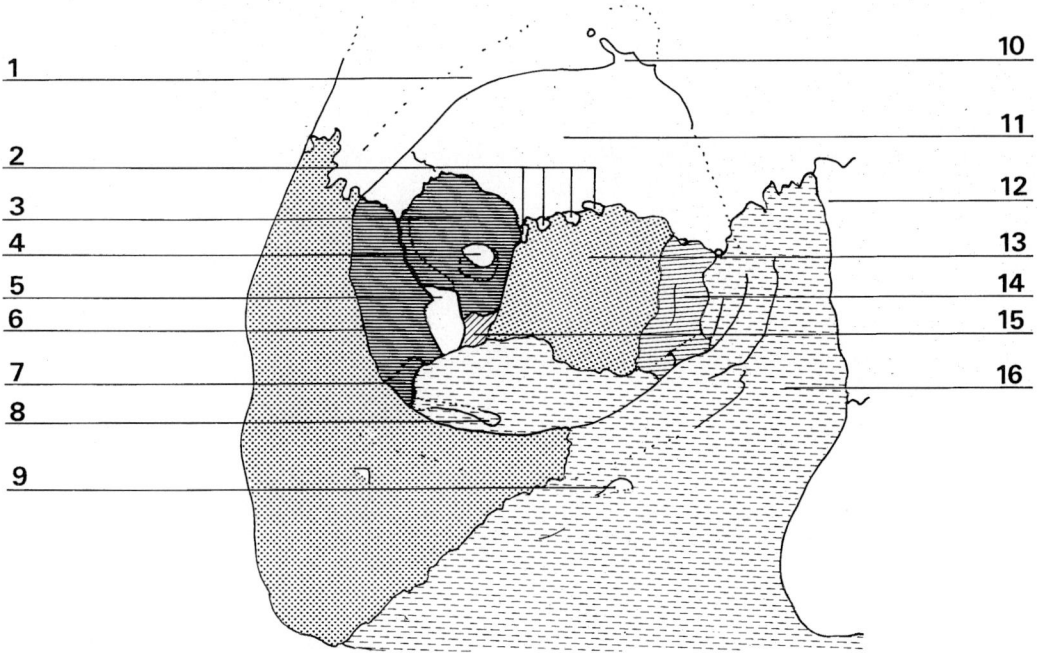

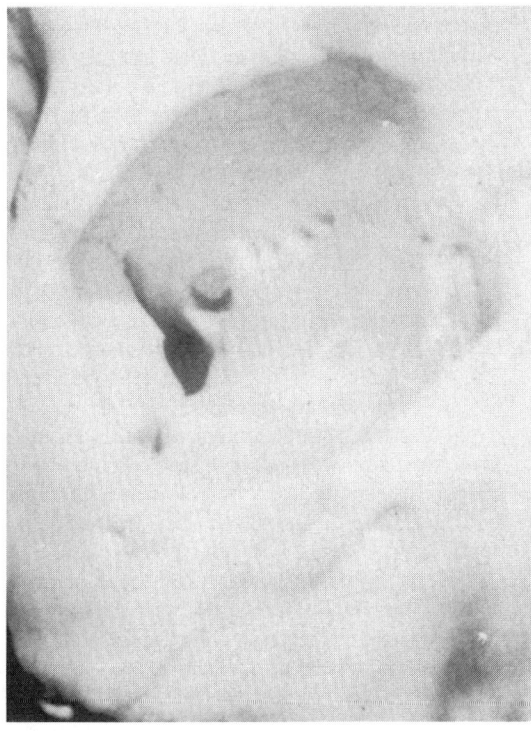

FIGURE 15–1 ■ A frontal view of the orbit with the optic foramen, the medial orbital wall, and the roof visible. (1, supraorbital ridge; 2, ethmoid foramina; 3, lesser wing of the sphenoid bone; 4, optic foramen; 5, superior orbital fissure; 6, greater wing of the sphenoid bone; 7, inferior orbital fissure; 8, infraorbital groove; 9, intraorbital foramen; 10, supraorbital notch; 11, orbital roof (frontal); 12, nasal bone; 13, orbital plate of the ethmoid bone; 14, lacrimal bone; 15, orbital process of the palatine bone; 16, maxilla.) (From Waddington MA: Atlas of the Human Skull. Rutland, VT: Academy Books, 1981. With permission of Academy Books.)

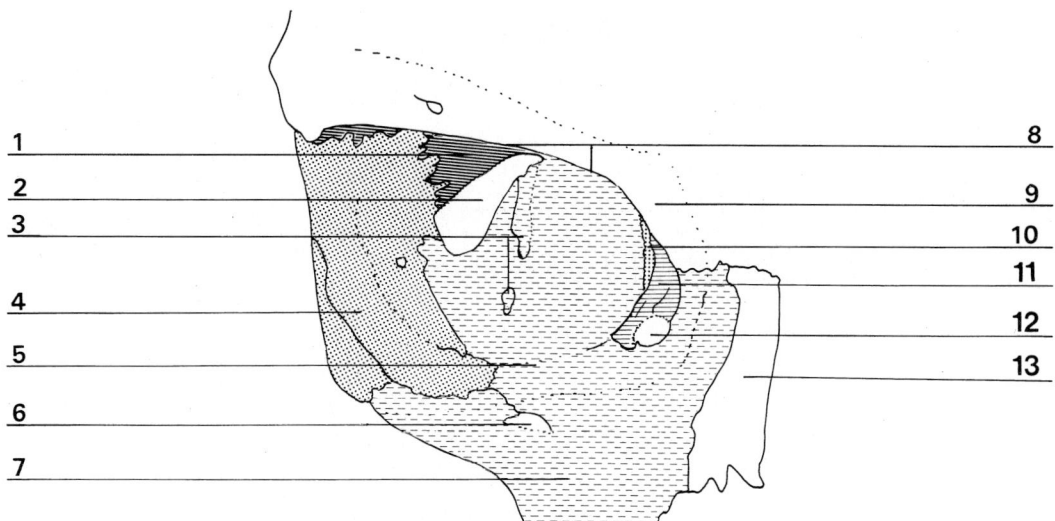

**FIGURE 15–2** ■ A view of the inferior orbital surface and the medial wall of the orbit. (1, greater wing of the sphenoid bone; 2, inferior orbital fissure; 3, infraorbital groove; 4, zygomatic bone; 5, inferior orbital margin; 6, infraorbital foramen; 7, maxilla; 8, superior orbital margin; 9, frontal bone; 10, ethmoid bone; 11, lacrimal gland; 12, lacrimal canal; 13, nasal bone.) (From Waddington MA: Atlas of the Human Skull. Rutland, VT: Academy Books, 1981. With permission of Academy Books.)

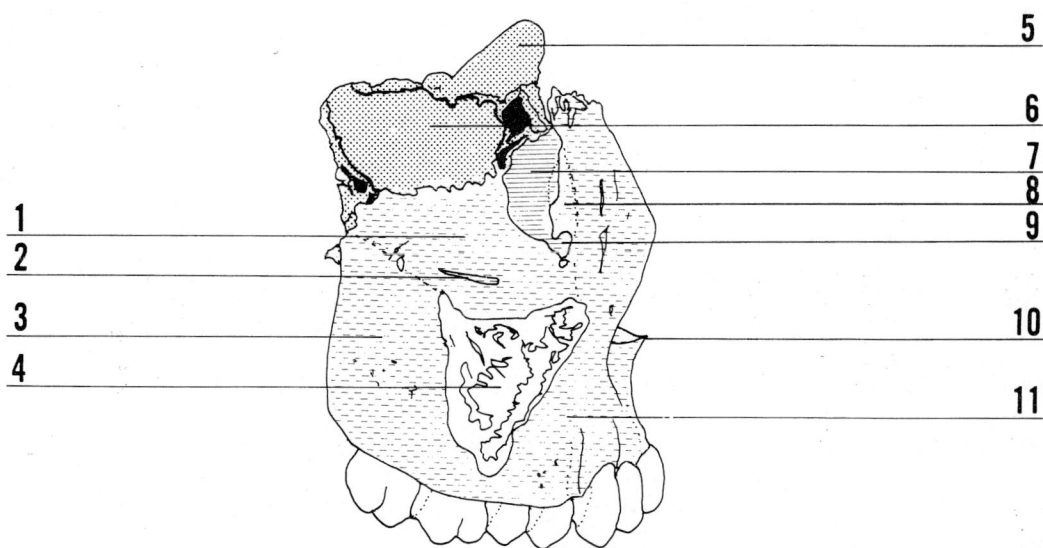

**FIGURE 15–3** ■ A composite view of the floor of the orbit with the maxillary sinus exposed. (1, orbital floor of the maxilla; 2, infraorbital groove; 3, infraorbital surface of the maxilla; 4, articular surface for zygomatic bone; 5, crista galli; 6, orbital plate of the ethmoid bone; 7, lacrimal gland; 8, lacrimal fossa; 9, lacrimal hamulus; 10, anterior nasal spine; 11, maxilla.) (From Waddington MA: Atlas of the Human Skull. Rutland, VT: Academy Books, 1981. With permission of Academy Books.)

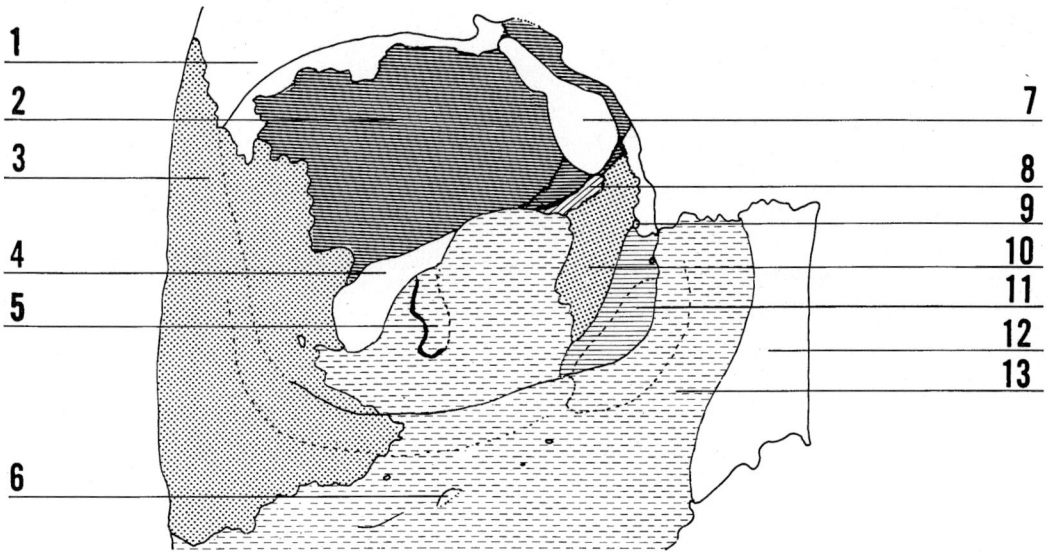

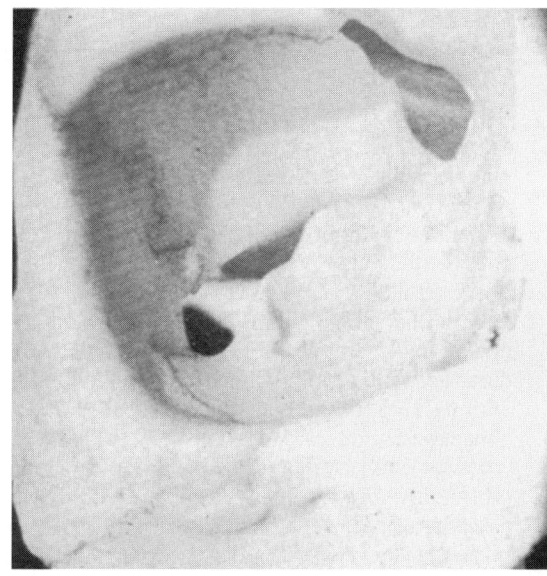

**FIGURE 15–4** ■ View of the orbital floor and the orbital fissures near the apex. (1, frontal bone; 2, greater wing of the sphenoid bone; 3, zygomatic bone; 4, inferior orbital fissure; 5, infraorbital groove; 6, infraorbital foramen; 7, superior orbital fissure; 8, orbital process of the palatine bone; 9, anterior ethmoid foramen; 10, orbital plate of the ethmoid bone; 11, lacrimal fossa; 12, maxilla.) (From Waddington MA: Atlas of the Human Skull. Rutland, VT: Academy Books, 1981. With permission of Academy Books.)

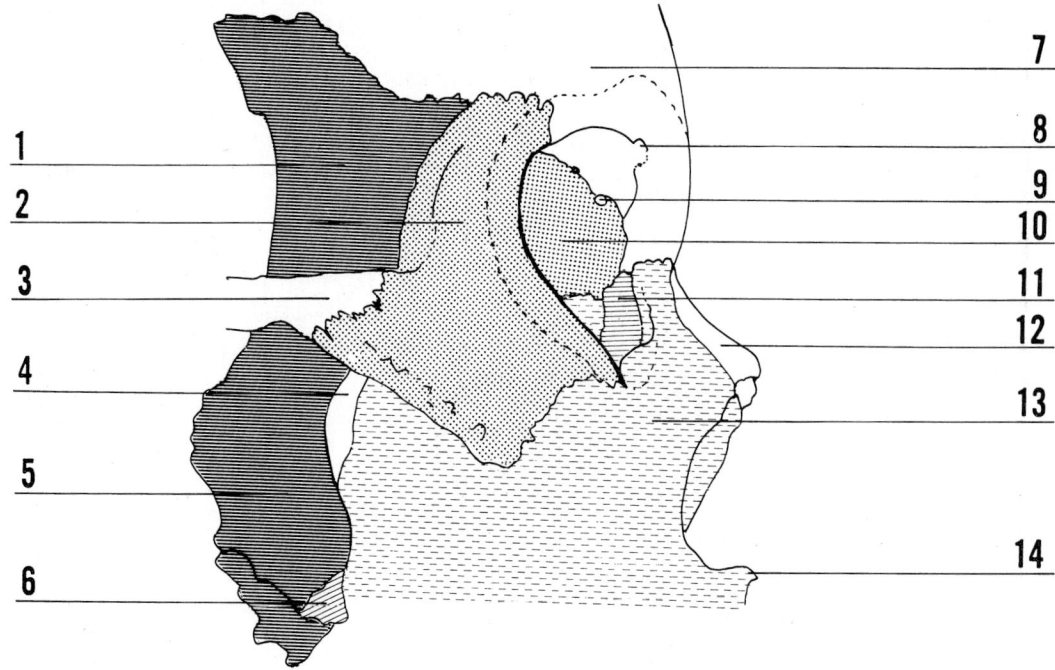

FIGURE 15-5 ■ Lateral external view of the orbital wall. (1, greater wing of the sphenoid bone; 2, zygomatic bone; 3, temporal bone [zygomatic arch]; 4, pterygopalatine fissure; 5, lateral pterygoid process of the sphenoid bone; 6, pyramidal process of the palatine bone; 7, frontal bone; 8, supraorbital notch; 9, ethmoid foramen; 10, orbital process of the ethmoid bone; 11, lacrimal gland; 12, nasal bone; 13, maxilla; 14, anterior nasal spine.) (From Waddington MA: Atlas of the Human Skull. Rutland, VT: Academy Books, 1981. With permission of Academy Books.)

structures lie below the orbital roof in a superficial plane immediately observable during a transcranial approach to the superior orbit.

Modern CT and MRI have revolutionized the ability to localize and characterize disease processes preoperatively. Each technique offers advantages over the other in evaluating orbital diseases. Both are frequently required on the same patient and should not be considered unnecessary duplication of testing. CT scans, particularly when fine cuts of the orbit are specified, allow the details of the bony walls and the surrounding sinuses to be viewed. Soft tissues, such as extraocular muscles, the globe, and the optic nerve, are also seen well. MRI, specifically with fat-suppression techniques, provides superior imaging of orbital soft tissues, particularly of their pathology. MRI with various intravenous enhancing agents is the most sensitive method presently available for detecting inflammatory lesions and some tumors, such as meningiomas.[5] With the availability of CT and MRI, plain films can no longer be considered adequate in ruling out an abnormality of the orbit or sinuses.

Orbital ultrasound is used at some centers as a diagnostic modality and can reveal information about the consistency of lesions.[6, 7] It requires significant technical skill, particularly in interpreting the images, and for this reason has not found widespread use. When available, however, it offers a rapid, noninvasive adjunct to the other radiologic methods and can be useful in obtaining precise measurements of extraocular muscle size and the subarachnoid fluid of the optic nerve sheath, which are useful in diagnostic considerations regarding thyroid orbitopathy and optic nerve swelling. Color Doppler imaging can aid in the assessment of orbital arterial and venous blood flow in cases regarding ocular ischemic syndrome or dural sinus fistulas.[8]

## COMPLICATIONS OF ORBITAL SURGERY

Structures peripheral in the orbit, such as the lacrimal gland, trochlea, lacrimal sac, and inferior oblique muscle, are easily damaged when dissection of the periorbita is performed without caution. Cerebrospinal fluid leaks can occur with overaggressive bone removal of the roof, posterior lateral wall, or superior lateral rim. Long-standing tumors and inflammation can erode orbital bone creating unexpectedly fragile barriers between the orbital fat and dura. Persistent cerebrospinal fluid leaks need to be closed with packing, fibrin glue, and a lumbar drain to avoid fluid collections in the orbit.

Ptosis can occur after an anterior, superior, or lateral orbitotomy, but it usually resolves within weeks. Severe damage to the levator muscle or its innervation can result in permanent ptosis. Similarly, prolonged or excessive retraction of extraocular muscles can lead to paresis and diplopia, and retraction of the globe can induce ischemia and subsequent blindness. This latter complication is thought to be a result of occlusion of the short posterior ciliary arteries or the central retinal artery. Eyes with a history of glaucoma, optic neuropathy, or retinal disease may be more susceptible to injury. When such retraction is necessary, pupillary size and function should be monitored closely. One of the more dreaded intraoperative complications during orbital surgery is hemorrhage. Careful blunt dissection through orbital fat and the use of bipolar cautery are helpful in avoiding excessive bleeding that can be difficult to control. Postoperative infection is unusual, even when orbital contents are placed in direct contact with the sinus cavities.

The ophthalmic complications of neurosurgical and orbital procedures can ultimately prove more devastating than many other neurologic sequelae. These complications include vision and visual field loss, diplopia, eye pain and irritation, pupil abnormalities, secondary glaucoma, ocular inflammation as well as cosmetic deformity. Damage to the ciliary ganglion can result in permanent iridoplegia. Injury to the ophthalmic branch of the trigeminal nerve during cavernous sinus and orbital apex procedures results in corneal anesthesia leading to corneal ulceration (neurogenic keratitis) frequently requiring permanent tarsorrhaphy. Despite these cautions, orbital procedures are now routinely performed, with large series recording fairly low rates of complications.[9, 10]

## SURGICAL APPROACHES TO THE ORBIT

The four surgical areas of the orbit are the subperiosteal, extraconal, intraconal, and Tenon's (including intraocular) spaces. The subperiosteal space harbors bony tumors, abscesses, and dermoid cysts. Cavernous hemangiomas, fibrous histiocytomas, hemangiopericytomas, and lacrimal gland tumors are found in the extraconal space. The intraconal space can also be a common site for cavernous hemangiomas as well as optic nerve tumors (gliomas, meningiomas) and neurilemomas. Malignant tumors, such as rhabdomyosarcomas, metastases, and inflammatory lesions, can be found in all of these locations as well as in Tenon's space, which is also the area where intraocular tumors extend as they breach the scleral boundary.

In general, lesions of the apex are best approached transcranially or laterally, and the intraconal space is approached through either a lateral orbitotomy or a medial-transconjunctival orbitotomy route. The medial extraconal space can be entered transnasally, through the medial orbital wall or through a medial conjunctival or lid skin incision (Table 15–1).[29]

## LATERAL ORBITOTOMY

Lateral orbitotomy involves removal of the lateral bony wall, usually from the frontal zygomatic suture to the

TABLE 15–1 ■ ROUTE OF CHOICE FOR SURGERY OF ORBITAL TUMORS

| Location of Orbital Tumor | Surgical Route |
|---|---|
| Intracranial extension | Superior |
| Apex and canal | Superior |
| Apex only | Lateral |
| Superior extraconal | Anterior |
| Superonasal | Anterior and lateral |
| Superotemporal | Lateral and anterior |
| Inferior | Lateral and anterior |
| Medial | Anterior and medial |
| All others | Lateral |

zygomatic arch and posteriorly to the junction of the temporal and sphenoid bones. This approach includes the classic Krönlein procedure and subsequent modifications (Figs. 15–6 to 15–18) and can be combined with a superior or anterior approach for maximal exposure or with a medial approach, including disinsertion of the medial rectus muscle to displace the globe laterally to access the medial intraconal space.[11]

Exposure of the lateral orbital rim is achieved with a lateral canthotomy or with an anterolateral skin incision lateral to the lateral canthus over the bony rim as advocated by Wright.[12] The lateral rectus muscle is tagged at its insertion. This suture exerts traction on the globe and the lateral rectus muscle to aid in dissection when the muscle cone is opened.

For lesions in the upper orbit, an S-type skin incision beginning in the outer third of the lateral supraorbital area is made, extending along Langer's skin lines into the preauricular area for a distance of 30 to 40 mm. Alternatively, if the tumor is located in the lower part of the orbit, we perform an inverted S-type skin incision beginning in the outer third of the lateral infraorbital area and extending along Langer's skin lines. Dissection is rapidly carried down to the periorbita of the lateral orbital rim. With the anterolateral skin incisions described, it is unnecessary to remove the lateral canthal ligament from the periorbita as is the case with a lateral canthotomy incision. The orbicularis muscle insertions are then freed from the lateral orbital rim to an area above the zygomaticofrontal suture line and below the zygomaticomaxillary suture line by elevating the periosteum. The temporalis muscle can be dissected off the bone if the deep posterior third of the orbit is to be explored, or it can be left intact on the posterior aspect of the lateral bony wall if more extensive exposure is not necessary. Cutting maneuvers on the muscle can be performed with electrocautery instruments. This practice achieves hemostasis at the same time as cutting and is a much faster technique than cutting and clamping bleeders.

An incision is made into the periorbita parallel to the lateral orbital rim 4 mm behind the bony edge. It is then extended up and down the zygomatic arch, the suture lines already described being used to delimit the superior and inferior aspects of the incision. The periosteum then is stripped forward to the orbital rim and around into the orbital cavity. In the orbit, it is easily separated from the lateral wall posteriorly. Bleeding can be encountered in the subperiosteal space, and one may identify the zygomatic artery anteriorly and the meningeal branch of the lacrimal artery posteriorly. These are usually eliminated with bipolar coagulation causing no problems. Attention is once again turned to the temporalis muscle, which is reflected posteriorly by blunt dissection to expose the posterolateral aspect of the orbital wall and the temporalis fossa. Marks are now made with the Stryker saw in the bony lateral wall just above the zygomaticofrontal suture line and at the zygomatic arch. The orbital contents must be protected during this maneuver by means of malleable ribbon retractors placed in the subperiosteal space. If the temporalis muscle has been disinserted, two drill holes are made so that the bone can be wired or plated back into place at the completion of the operation. If the temporalis muscle has been left intact, it acts as a hinge for the bony lateral wall,

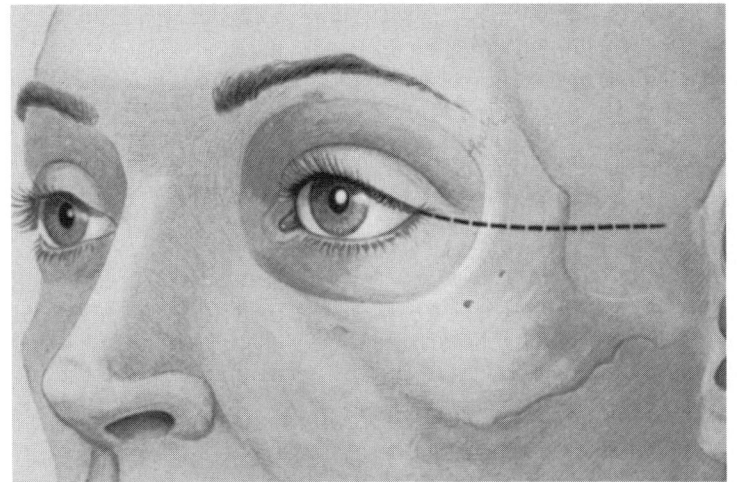

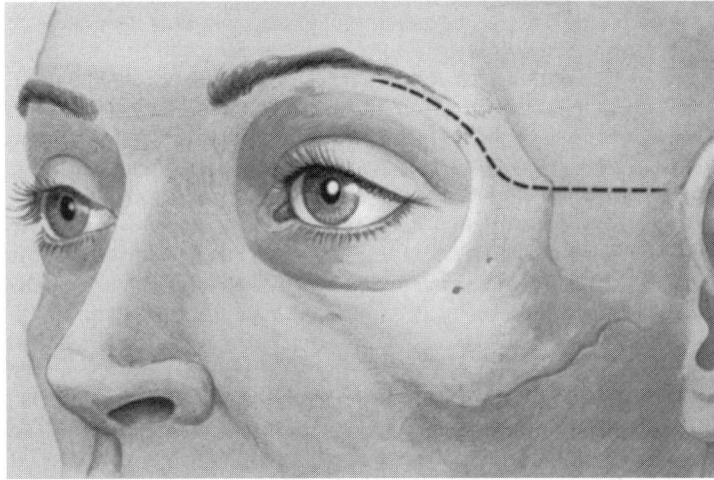

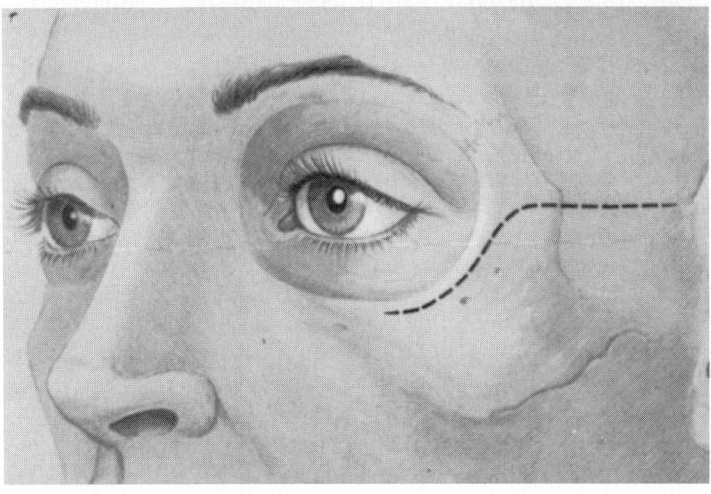

FIGURES 15–6, 15–7, and 15–8 ■ The lateral surgical approach may offer several options depending on the area of needed exposure and anatomic variations.

which can be reflected laterally to expose the temporalis fossa. Once the bone cuts have been made above the zygomaticofrontal suture and at the zygomatic arch, the lateral bony wall is removed. If the temporalis muscle has been left intact, one can merely break back the bone with a Coker clamp. Alternatively, if the muscle has been disinserted, the Stryker saw can be used to join the upper and lower bone cuts by incising bone at the junction of the zygoma with the greater wing of the sphenoid. The bone becomes thin at the sphenozygomatic suture, and in some patients it has been noted to be almost membranous in character, so that great care must be taken in joining the superior and inferior bone cuts with the Stryker saw. More bone can be removed from the greater wing of the sphenoid with a rongeur until the thicker temporal bone is exposed. With this technique, adequate exposure of the middle third of the orbit can be obtained.

Hemostasis is of the utmost importance as an orbital case progresses. Bipolar cautery is preferred to protect the optic nerve from potentially damaging electrical current.

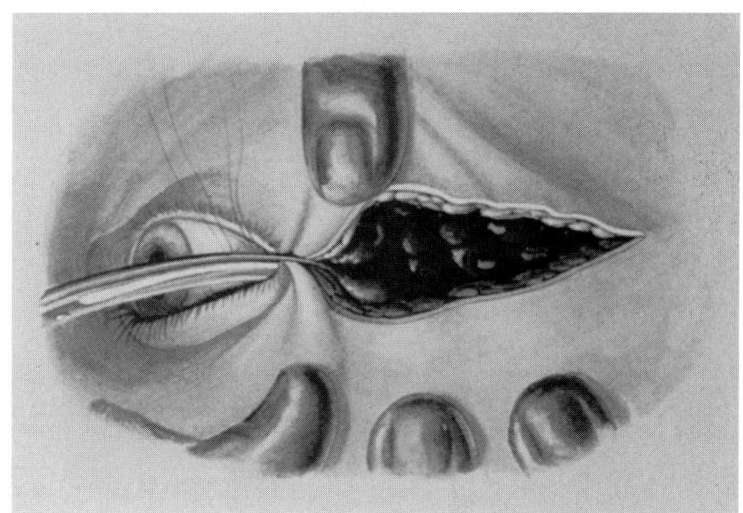

**FIGURE 15–9** ■ The lateral approach to the orbit requires that the soft tissue be retracted before the zygomatic bone is exposed.

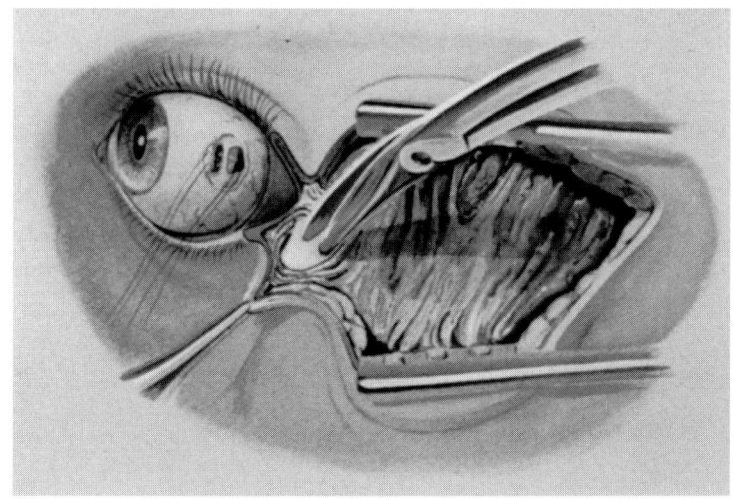

**FIGURE 15–10** ■ The zygomatic bone is identified as the soft tissue is divided, exposing the periosteum of the orbital wall. A lateral canthotomy has been carried out with disinsertion of the lateral canthal tendon.

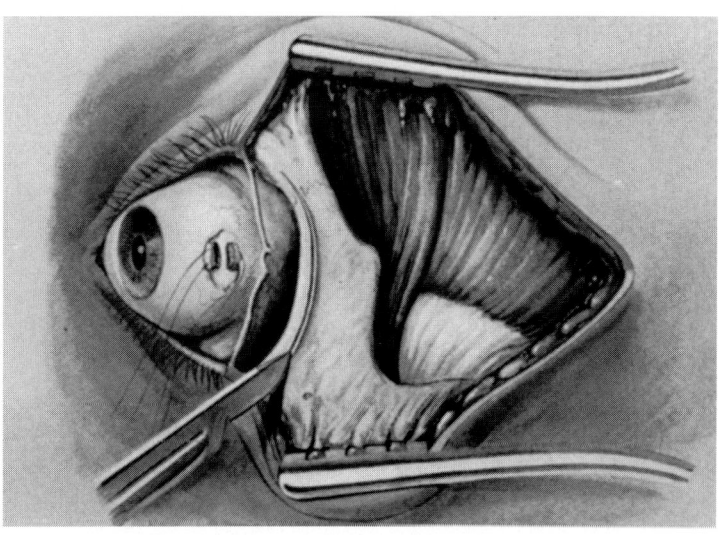

**FIGURE 15–11** ■ After the lateral bone structures of the orbit have been exposed, the periosteum is incised on the surface. The lateral rectus is identified.

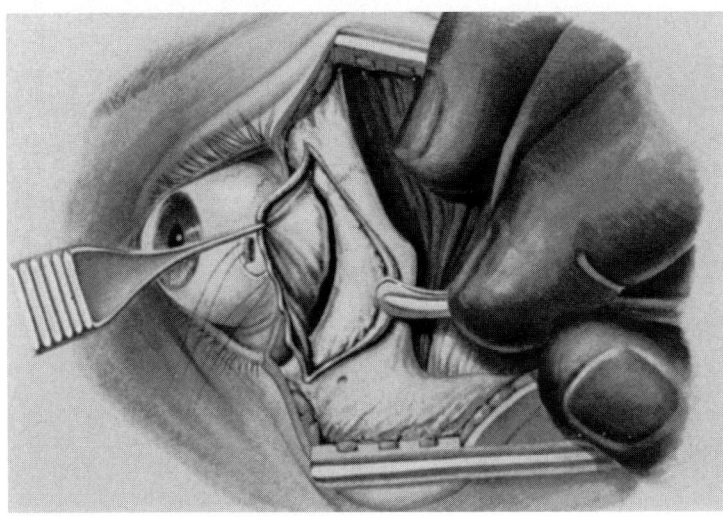

FIGURE 15–12 ■ The periosteum is divided and elevated using a periosteal elevator.

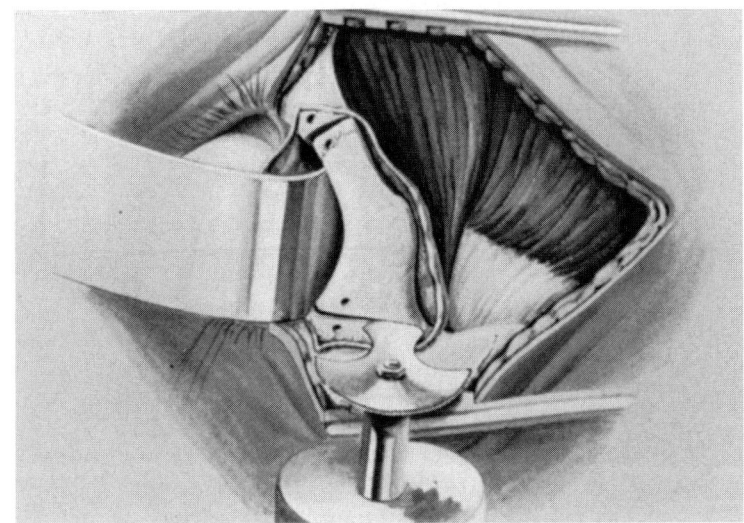

FIGURE 15–13 ■ The zygomatic bone is divided using a bone saw, and care is taken to protect the globe. Holes for plating at the completion of surgery are prepared for better placement.

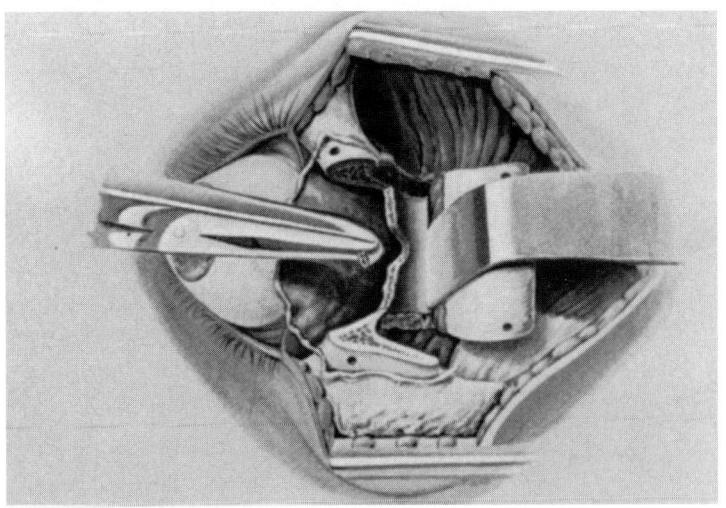

FIGURE 15–14 ■ Additional exposure is obtained by removing the lateral wall of the orbit using the rongeur.

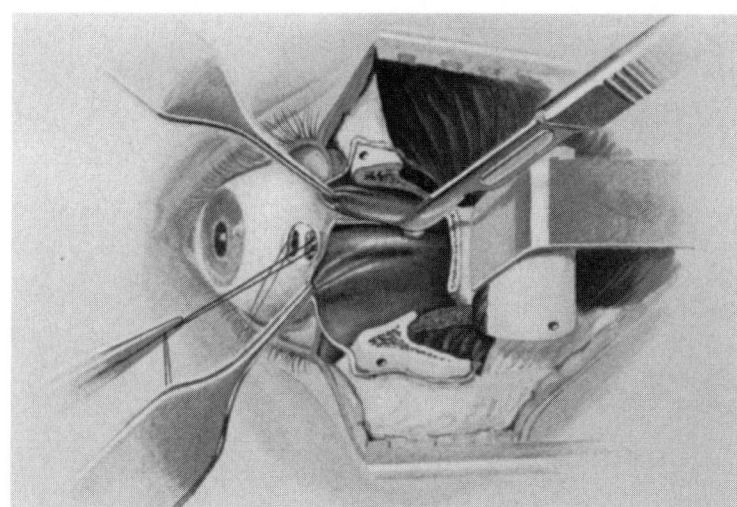

**FIGURE 15–15** ■ The bony lateral wall has been removed, and the periorbita is divided to provide exposure to the orbital contents.

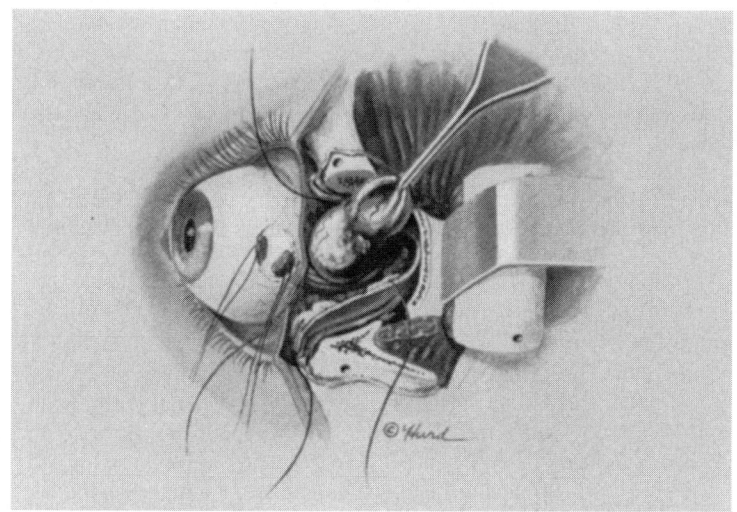

**FIGURE 15–16** ■ A tumor can be removed via the exposed site in the lateral orbital wall and the periorbita.

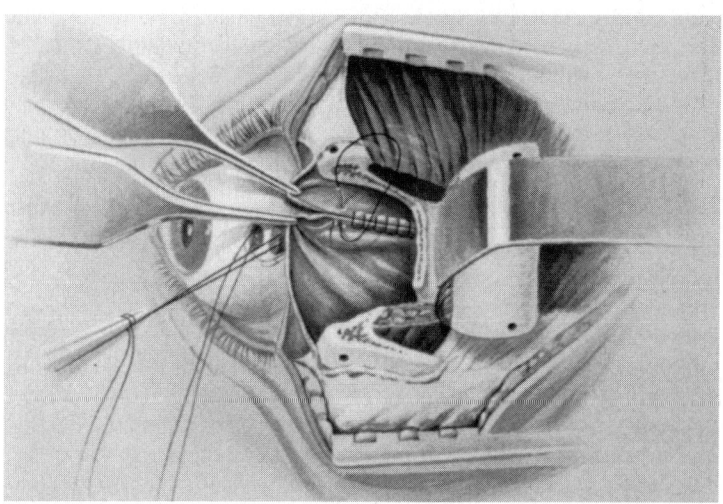

**FIGURE 15–17** ■ The periorbita is closed with sutures as the first step in the repair of the lateral orbitotomy.

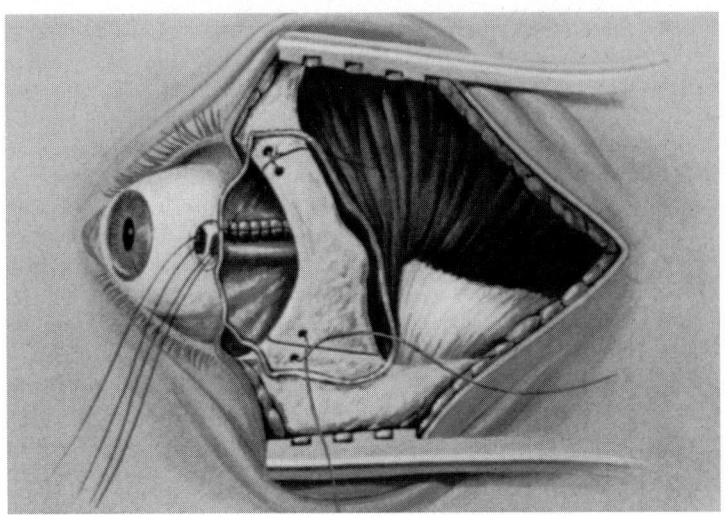

FIGURE 15–18  ■  Plates or wire are used to fix the bone segment of the zygoma in place using the predrilled holes. The periosteum, soft tissue, and skin are closed in layers. This approach allows exposure to at least two thirds of the lateral orbit.

Bleeding risks compression and inflammatory injury post-operatively and reduces visibility already compromised by orbital fat and the reduced operating field. Orbital fat is laced with fine septae in which run vascular bundles, so that rough handling can precipitate additional bleeding that has to be contained.

Once the bone has been removed, the retrobulbar contents are accessible through the subperiosteal space. Gentle digital palpation of a tumor now can be carried out. Periodic careful observation of the pupil for dilation must be made when palpating the optic nerve; pressure in the orbit should be immediately removed if this occurs. Some authors have reported continuously monitoring the visual evoked response during intraorbital surgery for more sensitive observation of adverse effects.[13] Tugging on the suture applied to the lateral rectus muscle aids in orientation before incising the periorbita.

An incision next is made into the outer layer of Tenon's fascia just above or below the lateral rectus muscle. It is advisable not to strip the fascia from the muscle because doing so would promote scarring of the muscle itself or adhesions of the muscle to the canthotomy scar. The intraconal space is now available for surgical intervention. Exploration of the intraconal space must be done with uninhibited visibility. Magnification is useful at this stage to avoid neurovascular structures. The lateral rectus muscle is retracted upward or downward, depending on the location of the mass within the muscle cone.

Cystic lesions can be removed intact with the aid of a cryoprobe, but if such a mass is large, it is safer to open the cyst wall and aspirate the contents before removing the capsule to avoid inadvertent rupture of its inflammatory contents. Infiltrative lesions sometimes are difficult to separate from the surrounding structures without causing serious injury. In such situations, surgical judgment is important. If, on clinical grounds, the surgeon believes that intraorbital surgery may not be the definitive treatment, removing an adequate biopsy specimen that debulks the orbit suffices. Lesions such as inflammatory pseudotumors, lymphomas, metastatic tumors, and rhabdomyosarcomas fall into this category. Before performing any radical surgery, it is prudent to await review of permanent sections and consultation with pathologists who are familiar with orbital pathologic conditions. Debulking, with incomplete surgical removal, is useful in dealing with a number of incurable tumors that have invaded from adjacent structures. Lesions such as inverting papillomas from the nasal and paranasal cavities, chondrosarcomas, and sphenoid ridge meningiomas have been treated in this fashion. In some patients, vision has been restored or binocularity regained by such debulking.

For evaluation of the area behind the globe, gentle traction can be exerted on the suture placed around the scleral insertion of the lateral rectus muscle. This maneuver pulls the optic nerve into view without direct pressure by the surgeon. The short posterior ciliary arteries are readily seen and should not be torn.

The optic nerve courses nasally, so that dissection in the intraconal space should be performed cautiously with adequate exposure. The central retinal artery enters the dural sheath inferolaterally 10 to 15 mm posterior to the globe.

If the bone has been left hinged to the temporalis muscle, there is no need to reattach it back into place because merely suturing the overlying periosteum accomplishes repositioning of the bone flap. In the event that the muscle has been stripped off the bone, plating is necessary if the bone is to be replaced. The lateral canthal ligament is reattached by closing the periosteum with 5–0 polyglycolic acid suture (Vicryl). Subcutaneous tissue is closed in layers, using 5–0 Vicryl for the fascia of the temporalis and orbicularis muscles. The skin is closed with a continuous running suture.

## SURGERY OF LACRIMAL GLAND TUMORS

Special consideration should be given to tumors of the lacrimal gland. Wright and coworkers,[14, 15] Stewart and colleagues,[16] Henderson and associates,[17, 18] and Font and Gamel[19, 20] have published excellent papers on this subject.

As Wright and coworkers[14] point out, if there is a history of a mass in the lacrimal fossa with a duration of less than 6 months, the lesion should be regarded as malignant until proved otherwise by an adequate biopsy specimen.

Adenoid cystic carcinoma of the lacrimal gland carries such a poor prognosis that radical surgery is necessary to attempt a cure. The decision for such a procedure should not be made on the basis of frozen sections but should await histopathologic diagnosis of permanent sections. Death usually results from intracranial extension and bony invasion, although lymph node metastases can occur.[21]

It is important to obtain a satisfactory amount of representative lacrimal gland tissue for histopathologic examination. The surgical approach for biopsy must be adequate to achieve this goal. Reese and Jones[11] have stressed the importance of making a lateral approach without removing bone for this purpose. This approach uses a modified anterolateral skin incision. The upper part of the lateral canthal ligament is disinserted from the bone and the skin undermined upward over the brow to expose the lateral portion of the superior orbital rim in the lateral aspect of the roof. The lateral horn of the levator aponeurosis crosses the gland but is reflected upward with the detached lateral canthal ligament when the tumor of the lacrimal gland is exposed.

If the biopsy specimen proves to be adenoid cystic carcinoma of the lacrimal gland, exenteration with radical removal of bone must be considered. Wright and coworkers[14-16] advocate a radical combined neurosurgical and orbital procedure that removes the bony lateral wall and roof of the orbit together with exenteration of the orbital contents. Craniotomy is performed to remove the roof. Closure is accomplished with split-thickness skin grafts. If the duration of the mass is longer than 1 year, the entire mass is removed in the initial procedure because benign mixed (pleomorphic) adenoma of the lacrimal gland is the most likely diagnosis, and there is a risk of recurrence and malignant transformation if resection is incomplete.

## ANTERIOR ORBITOTOMY

The anterior approach involves an incision either beneath the superior orbital rim through the lid crease or a subciliary incision through the lower lid (Figs. 15–19 to 15–21). It affords entrance into the subperiosteal space and the anterior two thirds of the extraconal area. This approach was devised by Knapp[22] in 1874 and later popularized by Benedict.[23]

An incision is made superiorly along the inferior margin of the eyebrow from the medial canthus to the lateral canthus or through the upper lid crease. If it is necessary to explore the superonasal quadrant as well, the skin incision is carried across halfway between the medial canthus and the anterior aspect of the nasal bone. With the subbrow approach, the supraorbital notch is encountered with its neurovascular bundle. It is sometimes necessary to sacrifice this neurovascular bundle, and anesthesia in that dermatome results. The supratrochlear and dorsal nasal arteries also pierce the septum and must be coagulated at this time. To access the subperiosteal space, an opening is made into the periosteum along the entire length of the incision. This space is entered as the periosteum is elevated from the overlying bone. Medially the anterior and posterior ethmoid arteries are encountered at the frontoethmoid suture line. Bleeding from these vessels can be quite brisk but can be readily controlled by cautery.

The levator muscle runs below the orbital roof and is separated from it by the periorbita, a thin layer of fat, and the frontal nerve. The levator is loosely suspended from the periorbita by connective tissue but joins with the orbital septum anteriorly as the levator aponeurosis approaches the tarsus. Injury to these anatomic relationships can result in a permanent ptosis. There often is some degree of postoperative ptosis, which resolves after 2 to 3 weeks in most cases.

As exploration of the superior subperiosteal space continues, care must be taken in palpating the roof or in passing a periosteal elevator in this area because the bone can be quite thin. Penetration at this point may tear the dura underlying the anterior cranial cavity and unnecessarily complicate the operation. Exploration medially may result in contact with the trochlea. Damage to this structure results in postoperative diplopia from malfunction of the superior oblique muscle. Elevation of the trochlea with the periosteum, however, can preserve its function when the periorbita is repositioned during closing. Laterally the lacrimal gland and nerve are encountered just behind the rim. Closure is accomplished by suturing the periorbita with

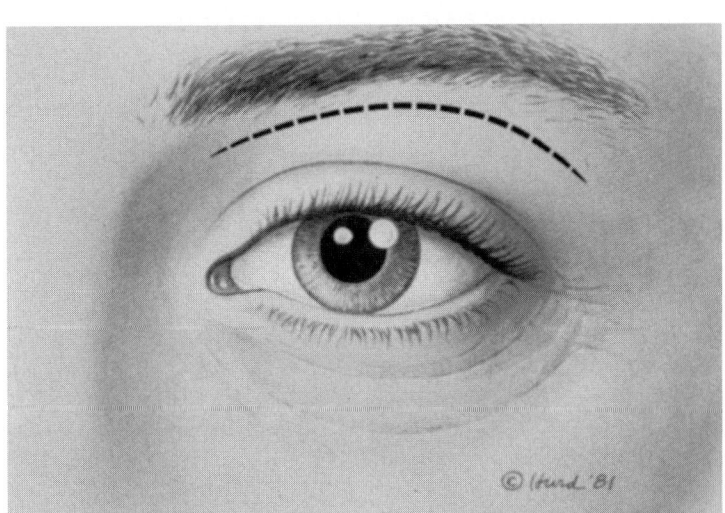

FIGURE 15–19 ■ The approach to the superior aspect of the orbit utilizes the lid crease or an initial incision above or below the brow. The area of the orbit to be approached determines the exact placement of the initial incision. (Copyright © 1981, Hurd.)

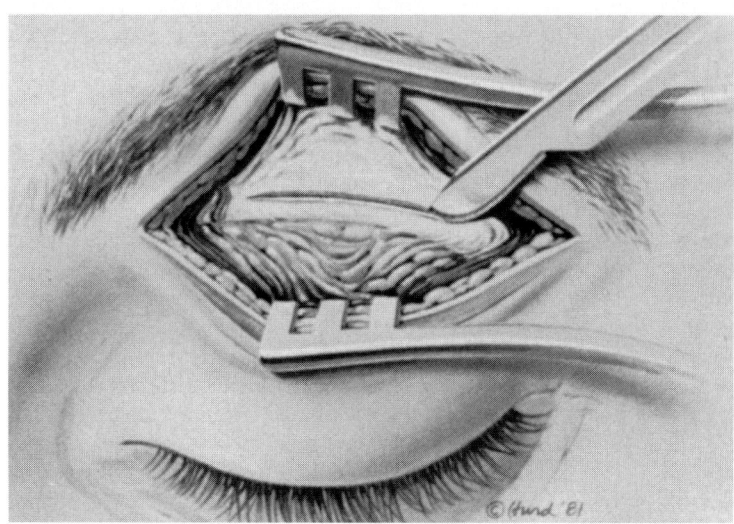

FIGURE 15–20 ■ The orbital rim and periosteum are exposed after separating the soft tissue and muscle. The periosteum is cleanly elevated, and a periosteal elevator is used to follow the roof of the orbit to the area of interest. (Copyright © 1981, Hurd.)

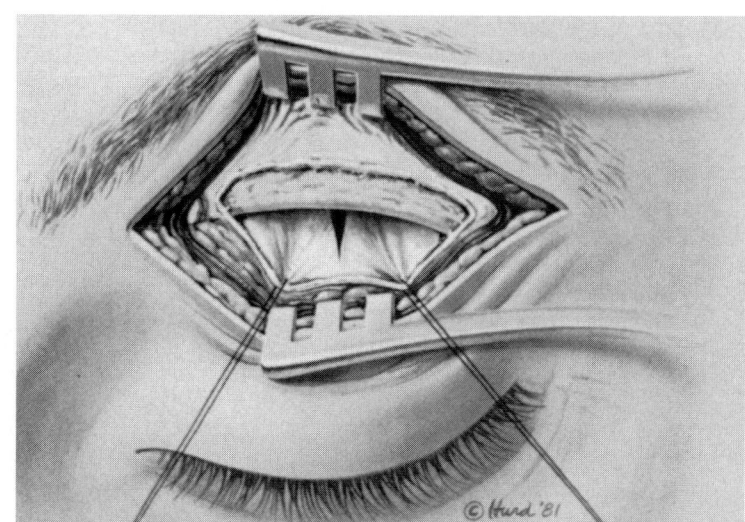

FIGURE 15–21 ■ The periorbita is divided and the orbital contents are exposed. Layer-by-layer closure is required. (Copyright © 1981, Hurd.)

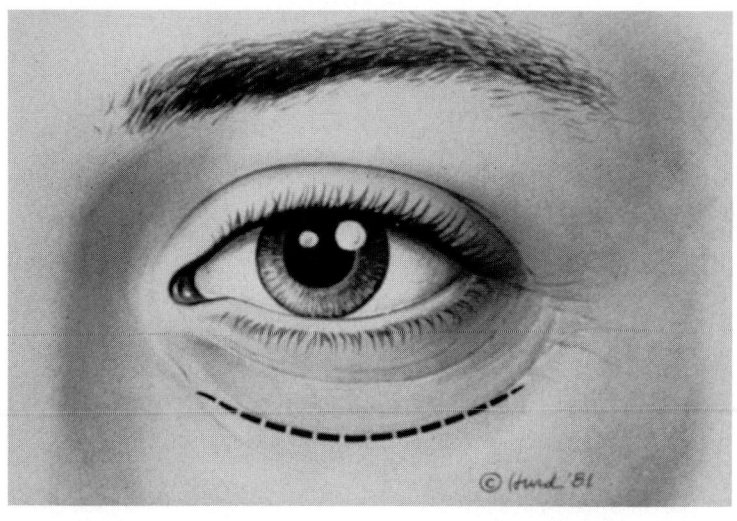

FIGURE 15–22 ■ The inferior approach to the orbit requires selection of an incision line along normal subciliary skin folds.

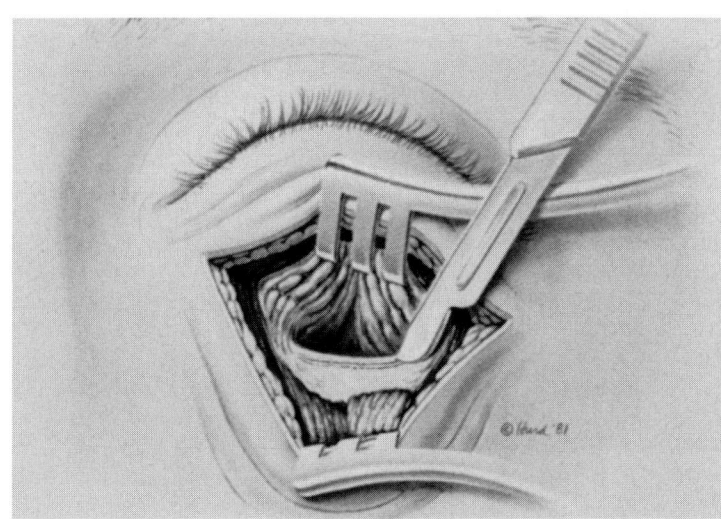

**FIGURE 15–23** ■ The orbital rim is identified, and the muscle and soft tissue are divided. (Copyright © 1981, Hurd.)

5–0 absorbable suture. It is most important to reattach the periosteum to the orbital rim carefully to support the upper lid. Drains are not usually inserted, but if drainage is deemed necessary, a Penrose drain can be brought out through the skin incision and anchored laterally or passed through the ethmoid air cells into the nasal cavity medially. This anterior approach is used to gain access to the superior ophthalmic vein for canalization and embolization to treat dural sinus fistulas.[24]

Incisions at the inferior rim are somewhat less common than those at the superior margin. This surgical approach (Figs. 15–22 to 15–24) is used commonly to decompress the orbit into the maxillary antrum in cases of Graves' orbitopathy. A transconjunctival approach through the lower lid retractors achieves similar exposure without a skin incision. The incision is made through the skin 2 to 3 mm below the lower lid lash line. A skin muscle flap can be dissected inferiorly to the orbital rim. The septum can be avoided because the periosteum is incised below the rim. The periorbita is elevated, and the subperiosteal space is entered. The infraorbital nerve and vessels are visible lying in the infraorbital canal and can usually be avoided. The patient should have been warned of postoperative

anesthesia of the lip. The periosteum is stripped from the floor up toward the apex, then is opened vertically in an anteroposterior direction to gain access to the peripheral surgical space. The origins of the inferior oblique muscle and tear sac lie medially and should be avoided or elevated carefully.

Closure is accomplished with 5–0 interrupted absorbable sutures to reattach the periosteum to the orbital rim. Drains can be brought out at the temporal aspect of the wound or through a separate stab wound, especially if the inferior incision is combined with a lateral approach.

## MEDIAL ORBITOTOMY

Lesions of the medial orbit can be approached through an anteronasal incision, such as a modified Lynch incision, or through a transconjunctival dissection (Figs. 15–25 to 15–28). The latter can be directed medially into the extraconal space or, when combined with disinsertion of the medial rectus muscle, into the intraconal space behind the globe. Optic nerve sheath fenestration, to decompress the anterior

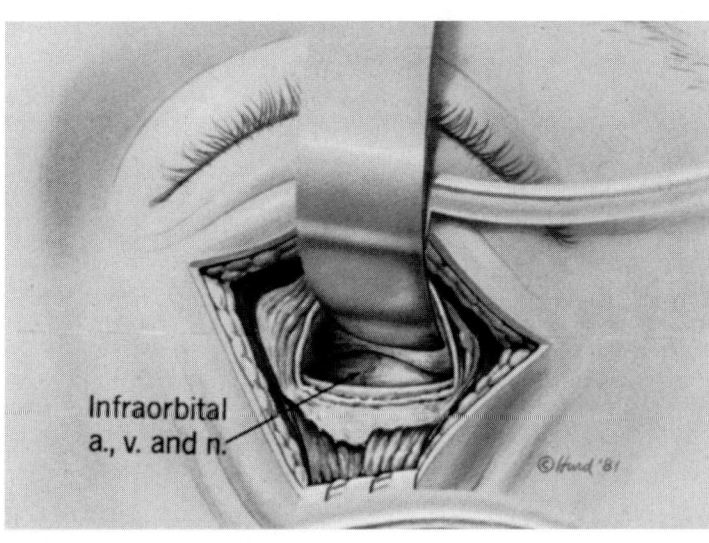

**FIGURE 15–24** ■ The periosteum is divided using a sharp blade. The periosteal elevator allows exposure back along the inferior aspect of the orbit. On completion of the operation, the incisions are closed layer by layer, and the periosteum is closed. The infraorbital artery, nerve, and vein are visible as the floor is exposed. (Copyright © 1981, Hurd.)

Infraorbital a., v. and n.

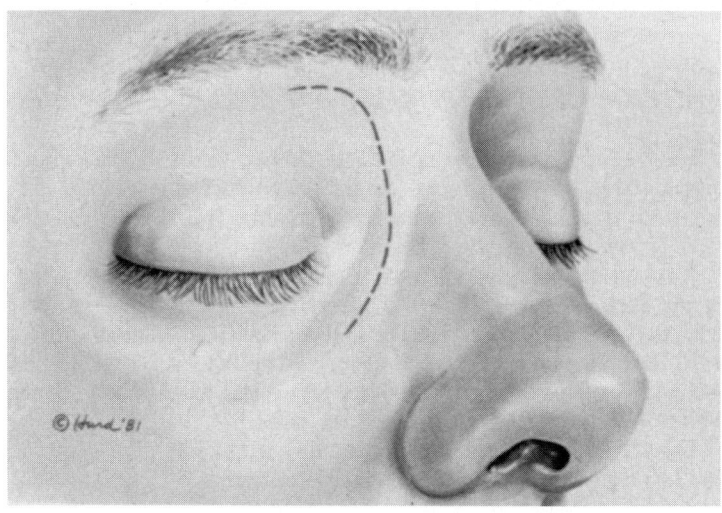

FIGURE 15–25 ■ The approach to the medial side of the orbit and the lacrimal fossa. The angular artery and vein may be encountered. (Copyright © 1981, Hurd.)

optic nerve when indicated in pseudotumor cerebri or chronic papilledema, is performed through either this medial or analogous lateral approach.[25, 26] The optic nerve can be directly visualized as it enters the sclera, and the posterior ciliary vessels can be gently retracted to incise two or three small windows into the dural sheath and produce drainage of the subarachnoid fluid.

The medial orbital wall contains the attachment of the medial canthus into the periosteum. Elevating this tendon with its periosteal attachment and reflecting it laterally carries the tear sac off of the lacrimal bone and exposes the medial wall. Posteriorly along the medial wall, one encounters the anterior and posterior ethmoidal arteries in the subperiosteal space. Most posterior along the medial wall is the optic foramen at the apex. Here, one encounters the optic nerve if the subperiosteal dissection is carried out in too vigorous a fashion.

The ethmoid sinus lies medial to the ethmoid bone. This bone is quite thin, as can be the lacrimal bone. Dissection that is too aggressive with pressure on these structures can result in penetration into the nasal cavity anteriorly through the lacrimal bone or into the ethmoid sinus through the ethmoid bone.

Access to the medial orbit and particularly the medial orbital wall can also be achieved with an incision through the caruncle. The incision leads to the periosteum posterior to the medial canthus attachments and the lacrimal sac.[27] This approach has the advantage of avoiding a skin incision in the area of the medial canthus, which frequently causes webbing as healing occurs across the concave area. It also maintains preservation of the medial canthal tendon attachments whose disruption can result in telecanthus and lid laxity.

Nasal and sinus endoscopy is now routinely used to view and remove the medial and inferior orbital walls without external incisions during decompression surgery. Posterior ethmoidectomy with entrance into the sphenoid sinus enables bony decompression as far back as the optic canal.[28]

## SUPERIOR TRANSCRANIAL ORBITOTOMY

The superior orbitotomy, which was first devised and popularized by Dandy,[2] involves a transcranial approach to the

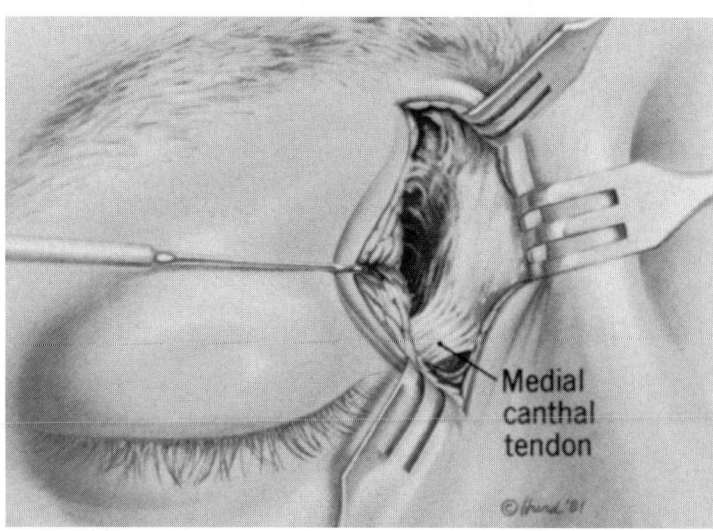

FIGURE 15–26 ■ The tissue is reflected until the medial canthal tendon is identified. (Copyright © 1981, Hurd.)

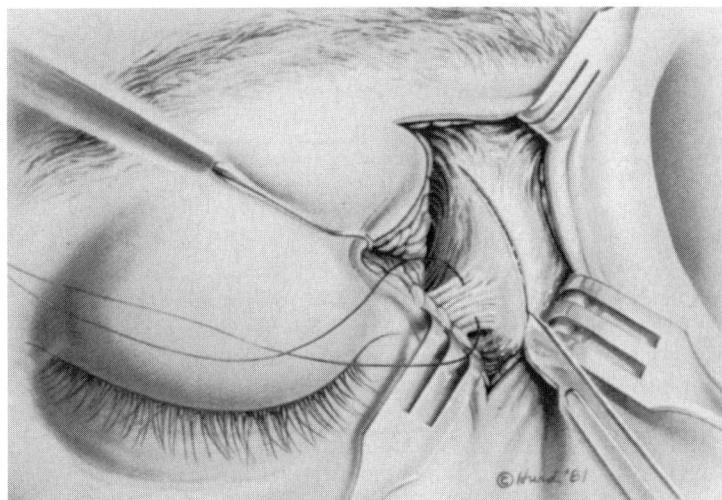

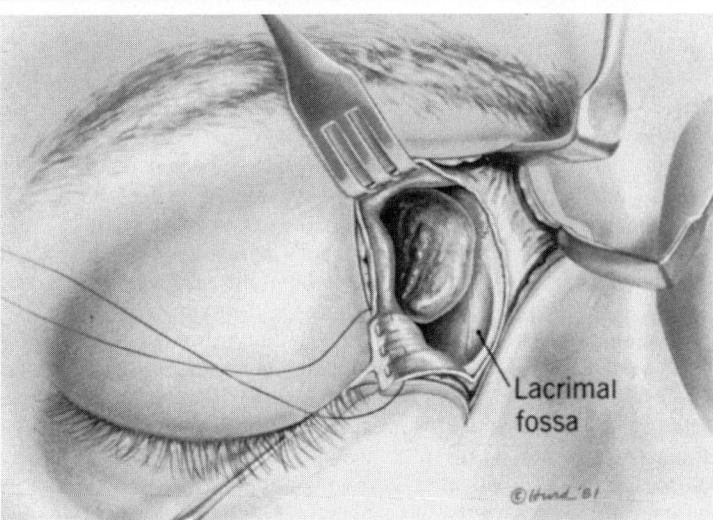

**FIGURES 15–27 and 15–28** ■ The periosteum is divided anterior to the medial canthal tendon, and the tissue is reflected laterally to expose the lacrimal sac and fossa. Further exploration can be made with periosteal elevation. The ethmoidal vessels can be identified. (Copyright © 1981, Hurd.)

orbit, which is then unroofed often with the optic canal as well. It is indicated for lesions arising in the orbital apex with or without extension into the optic canal or intracranial compartment tumors extending anteriorly into the orbit. The orbital roof may be quite thin or may have eroded creating a passage into the anterior fossa.

Approaching the orbit through the roof requires a shared approach between the neurosurgeon for the craniotomy and the orbital surgeon for the unroofing and orbitotomy. The roof can be accessed with a coronal incision and anterior craniotomy through the frontal bone. Alternatively a pterional approach reveals an optimal view of the sphenoid wing and apex.[30] The frontal and temporal lobes are then retracted as an extradural procedure that can be performed with relatively low risk. This approach enables excellent exposure and is thus preferred for lesions in the deep orbit. In such cases, maximal exposure and visualization are essential for successful treatment and minimizing iatrogenic injury to adjacent orbital structures.

On incising the periorbita, the frontal and lacrimal nerves are identified in the superior orbital fat. The supraorbital nerve and vessels exit through the supraorbital notch or foramen at the juncture of the inner and middle thirds of the superior orbital rim. Directly inferiorly courses the levator palpebrae muscle with the superior rectus below it.

Innervation of the extraocular muscles comes from the intraconal surface. Exploration through the orbital fat is best accomplished with blunt dissection using cottonoids and small malleable retractors and Penfield dissectors. The annulus can most safely be incised medially between the superior oblique and the levator–superior rectus insertions. The intraconal space can then be entered with cautious lateral retraction of the superior rectus. The periorbita is closed with absorbable suture to prevent orbital fat from forming adhesions to the dura. The orbital roof does not require replacement after this dissection because the periorbita and dura form adequate support that usually prevents pulsatile proptosis postoperatively.

## FINE-NEEDLE ASPIRATION BIOPSY

Fine-needle aspiration biopsy of the orbit was introduced by Schyberg in 1975.[31] A 22-gauge needle under local or topical anesthesia can be used to obtain a sufficient specimen for a skilled cytopathologist to interpret, thereby avoiding an orbitotomy biopsy procedure. The technique is limited to circumstances in which particular pathologic lesions are suspected by clinical presentation.[31, 32]

## CONCLUSION

Surgery at the skull base is best performed by a team of subspecialists because each anatomic area involves its own particular subtleties in approach and clinical follow-up. Orbital surgery exemplifies this principle. Even more so, careful ophthalmic and neuro-ophthalmic examination, both preoperatively and postoperatively, is essential for evaluating patients who have undergone such procedures. Detailed assessment of vision, assessment of pupillary function, measurements of eye motility, and indirect ophthalmoscopy provide essential information in determining the indications and approaches for surgical intervention and assessing their efficacy.

## REFERENCES

1. Krönlein RU: Zur pathologie und operativen behandlung der dermoidcysten der orbita. Beitr Klin Chir 4:149, 1888.
2. Dandy WE: Results following transcranial operative attack on orbital tumors. Arch Ophthalmol 25:191, 1941.
3. Wright JE, McNab A, McDonald W: Primary optic nerve sheath meningioma. Br J Ophthalmol 73:960, 1989.
4. Dailey RA: Optic nerve sheath meningioma. Ophthalmol Clin North Am 4:519, 1991.
5. Zimmerman C, Schatz N, Glaser J: Magnetic resonance imaging of optic nerve meningiomas: Enhancement with gadolinium-DPTA. Ophthalmology 97:585, 1990.
6. Byrne SF: Standardized echography of the eye and orbit. Neuroradiology 28:618, 1986.
7. Galetta S, Byrne SF, Smith JL: Echographic correlation of optic nerve sheath size and cerebrospinal fluid pressure. J Clin Neuro-Ophthalmol 9:79, 1989.
8. Erickson SJ, Hendrix LE, Massaro BM, et al: Color doppler flow imaging of the normal and abnormal orbit. Radiology 172:511, 1989.
9. Wright JE: Surgery in the orbit. In Miller S (ed): Operative Surgery, 3rd ed. London: Butterworths, 1976.
10. Kennerdell JS, Maroon JC: Lateral microsurgical approach to intraorbital tumors. J Neurosurg 44:556, 1976.
11. Reese AB, Jones IS: Bone resection in the excision of epithelial tumors of the lacrimal gland. Arch Ophthalmol 71:382, 1964.
12. Wright JE: The role of surgery in the management of orbital tumors. Mod Probl Ophthalmol 14:553, 1975.
13. Wright JE, Arden G, Jones BR: Continuous monitoring of the visual evoked response during intraorbital surgery. Trans Ophthalmol Soc UK 93:311, 1973.
14. Wright JE, Stewart WB, Krohel GB: Clinical presentation and management of lacrimal gland tumors. Br J Ophthalmol 63:600, 1979.
15. Wright JE: Factors affecting the survival of patients with lacrimal gland tumors. Can J Ophthalmol 17:3, 1982.
16. Stewart WB, Krohel G, Wright JE: Lacrimal gland and fossa lesions: An approach to diagnosis and management. Ophthalmology 86:886, 1979.
17. Henderon JW, Neult RW: En bloc removal of intrinsic neoplasms of the lacrimal gland. Am J Ophthalmol 82:905, 1976.
18. Henderson WJ, Farrow GM: Primary malignant mixed tumors of the lacrimal gland. Ophthalmology 87:466, 1980.
19. Font RL, Gamel JW: Epithelial tumors of the lacrimal gland: An analysis of 265 cases. In Jakobiec FA (ed): Ocular and Adnexal Tumors. Birmingham, AL: Aesculapius, 1978.
20. Font RL, Gamel JW: Adenoid cystic carcinoma of the lacrimal gland: A clinicopathologic study of 79 cases. In Nicholson DH (ed): Ocular Pathology Update. New York: Masson, 1980.
21. Spencer WH: Lacrimal gland tumors. In Ophthalmic Pathology, 3rd ed. Philadelphia: WB Saunders, 1986, pp 2496–2525.
22. Knapp H: A case of carcinoma of the outer sheath of the optic nerve, removed with preservation of the eyeball. Arch Ophthalmol 4:323, 1874.
23. Benedict WL: Surgical treatment and tumors and cysts of the orbit. Am J Ophthalmol 32:763, 1949.
24. Hanneken AM, Milles NR, Debrum GM, et al: Treatment of carotid-cavernous fistulas using a detachable balloon catheter through the superior ophthalmic vein. Arch Ophthalmol 107:87, 1989.
25. Corbett JJ, Nerad JA, Tse DT, et al: Results of optic nerve sheath fenestration for pseudotumor cerebri: The lateral orbitotomy approach. Arch Ophthalmol 106:1391, 1988.
26. Spoor TC, McHenry JG: Long-term effectiveness of optic nerve sheath decompression for pseudotumor cerebri. Arch Ophthalmol 111:632, 1993.
27. Shorr N, Baylis H: Transcaruncular approach to the medial orbit and orbital apex. Oral presentation, American Society of Ophthalmic Plastic and Reconstructive Surgeons, 24th Annual Scientific Symposium, Chicago, November 13, 1993.
28. Hobson SR: Endoscopic surgery for lacrimal and orbital disease. Curr Opin Ophthalmol 5:32, 1994.
29. Kennerdell JS, Maroon JC, Malton ML: Surgical approaches to orbital tumors. Clin Plast Surg 15:273, 1988.
30. Maroon JC, Kennerdell JS: Surgical approaches to the orbit. J Neurosurg 60:1225, 1984.
31. Kennerdell JS, Slamovits TL, Dekker A: Orbital fine needle aspiration biopsy. Am J Ophthalmol 99:547, 1985.
32. Midena E, Segato T, Piermarocchi S, et al: Fine needle aspiration biopsy in ophthalmology. Surv Ophthalmol 29:410, 1985.

# Transcranial Approach to Lesions of the Orbit

■ ANTONIO G. CARRIZO and ARMANDO BASSO

The orbit is an anatomic region located between the facial structures, paranasal sinuses, and the skull base that is occupied by the organs of sight and their adnexa. From the surgical viewpoint, it represents a field shared by ophthalmology, neurosurgery, maxillofacial surgery, and ear-nose-throat surgery—each with its own techniques for orbital approach.[1]

The orbit can be considered as a quadrangular pyramid that may be approached by its open base or by one of its four walls resected in a transient or permanent way. In the anteroposterior direction, three sections may be discerned: one anterior, ample and superficial with regard to the base; another intermediate; and the last posterior, deep and narrow with many vascular, nervous, and muscular structures, making access to this section the most complex of the three.[1, 2]

The anatomic structure of the orbital contents encompasses three areas: the periosteal, located between the periorbita and the bone; the muscular cone, which encloses the intricate components of the apex; and the area limited by the preceding two, mainly occupied by orbital fat. Primary space-occupying lesions that develop in these divisions tend to remain confined within them, requiring a different access for each compartment.[1, 3]

Selecting the most suitable surgical treatment for orbital tumors requires a thorough knowledge of the diverse surgical approaches as well as their advantages, indications, limitations, and contraindications. The main considerations are the location and size of the lesion, its apparent site of origin, its routes of propagation, and its probable histologic status. Such features are gleaned from clinical evaluation and complementary examinations. Current technologies allow accurate anatomic localization and earlier, more reliable diagnosis than former methods, resulting in improved treatment planning.[1, 3]

## SURGICAL APPROACHES TO THE ORBIT

Historically, the earliest approaches were anterior orbitotomies. One of the pioneers of this technique was the German ophthalmologist Bartisch, who described a kind of subtotal exenteration with preservation of eyelids in 1583. In 1744, Thomas Hope reported one of the first orbital interventions that spared the eyeball. Herman Knapp described the transconjunctival approach through the upper eyelid in 1874.[4]

The so-called "transpalpebral" access was reported by Rollet (1907, 1924), Elschnig (1927), Golovine (1930),[3, 4] and Benedict[2] (1949). In fact, the skin incision is performed on the superior orbital rim. This technique remains virtually unchanged.[3, 4]

In 1940, Davis[5] described the removal of optic nerve gliomas through an incision along the inferior orbital rim. Callahan[6] adapted this approach in 1948 to other tumor types.

Philip Gustav Passavant in Frankfurt was the first to use a lateral approach to the orbit for a vascular malformation in 1866, the same year that Wagner described its application to the removal of foreign bodies. However, this technique is associated with Krönlein's name on the basis of his complete description in 1888 for the excision of a dermoid cyst. Later, multiple modifications were advanced, mainly concerning the cutaneous incision. The most widely adopted is Berke's[7] (1954), which uses Swift's horizontal incision.

The earliest craniotomy to remove an intracranial tumor causing exophthalmos was carried out by Durante in Rome in 1887.[3] In 1941, Walter Dandy[8] published his landmark paper advancing the transcranial approach to the orbit as the procedure of choice, which he regarded as superior to "that performed by ophthalmologists." This route was used during the same decade by Naffziger for decompressive purposes, as well as by Poppen[9] (1943) and Love and Benedict[10] (1945) for tumor removal.

In 1913, Frazier[11] described an approach to the hypophyseal region by means of frontal craniotomy and resection of the superior orbital rim at the anterior portion of the roof, with later replacement. This technique, which allows minimal cerebral retraction, fell into disuse with improvement in anesthetic techniques, but later proved extremely valuable for gaining access to the orbital apex after the work of Johnson and Tym (1961), Bachs (1962),[3] and, more recently, that of Jane and colleagues,[12] Maroon and Kennerdell,[13] and Leone and Wissinger.[14]

## REGIONAL SURGICAL ANATOMY OF THE ORBIT

The orbital cavity is generally visualized as a quadrangular pyramid in its anterior part and a cone in its posterior. The inner wall is formed by the lacrimal and ethmoid bones, along with the body of the sphenoid bone; the zygomatic bone and the greater wing of the sphenoid form the lateral wall; the floor consists of the zygomatic, the maxillary, and the palatine bones; the roof, finally, is formed by the horizontal portion of the frontal bone and by the lesser wing of the sphenoid bone.[15] The depth of the orbital cavity ranges from 42 to 50 mm, with a maximum base width of roughly 40 mm and a height of 35 mm.[16]

The optic canal, actually a tubular cavity lying in the deepest portion of the orbit, is sculpted in the base of the minor sphenoid wing at an angle of roughly 37 degrees with regard to the sagittal axis. It measures on average 5 to 10 mm long, 4.5 mm wide, and 5 mm high. The thickness of the roof varies from 1 to 3 mm, and it merges backward into the falciform process, a sheet of dura mater covering the optic nerve.[13, 17]

The superior orbital fissure, through which the intracranial dura mater joins the periorbita, is delimited by the minor sphenoid wing along its superointernal margin and by the major wing along its inferolateral border. It allows passage of the oculomotor and ophthalmic nerves, as well as exit of the ophthalmic vein, which drains into the medial sector of the cavernous sinus.[16, 17]

The intracranial portion of the optic nerve, whose cross-section is $4 \times 6$ mm and whose length is 10 to 15 mm, is flattened in the horizontal direction. The intracanalicular portion of the nerve is 10 to 12 mm long, and its section is circular, almost 5 mm in diameter. The intraorbital segment extends from 25 to 30 mm and presents an oval section, measuring $6 \times 4$ mm, whose major vertical axis lies at the exit from the optic foramen.[13, 17]

The meninges and subarachnoid space accompany the optic nerve up to the sclera. At the orbital apex, the pia mater and the arachnoid fuse in the dorsal, medial, and ventral portions with the dura mater and the annulus of Zinn, partially occluding the subarachnoid space. The annulus of Zinn, a fibrous band that attaches the optic nerve at the orbital apex, receives the insertion of the levator palpebralis and extraocular muscles, with the exception of the minor oblique. The annulus is in close contact with the optic nerve dorsally, but separates from it in its lateral and inferior portions, creating a space between the two heads of the lateral rectus muscle, forward to the basal sector of the superior orbital fissure. This opening is termed the *oculomotor foramen*, and is traversed by the superior division of the oculomotor nerve innervating the superior rectus and levator palpebralis, the nasociliary branch of the ophthalmic nerve, the abducens, and the inferior division of the oculomotor nerve.[13, 18]

Through the superior orbital fissure, but outward from the oculomotor foramen, the frontal and lacrimal branches of the ophthalmic nerve, as well the sympathetic nerves, are directed inward, just below the periorbita, to gain entry into the orbit. The ciliary ganglion is located external to the optic nerve, emerging from the nasociliary branch of the ophthalmic nerve, which crosses the optic nerve superiorly to proceed toward the medial orbital wall.[19]

The ophthalmic artery arises from the anteromedial or superomedial surface of the internal carotid artery at its exit from the cavernous sinus (occasionally emerging from the intracavernous portion) and crosses the optic canal laterally and inferiorly with respect to the optic nerve. In turn, the central retinal artery arises from the ophthalmic artery and crosses the dura mater of the nerve 5 to 20 mm behind the eyeball. The ophthalmic artery then crosses above (in 82.5% of cases) or below (in 17.5%) the optic nerve, according to Rengachary and Kishore,[20] proceeding forward parallel to the internal orbital wall to reach the trochlea, where it divides into its two terminal branches, frontal (or supratrochlear) and nasal. Its collateral branches comprise the ocular (central retinal, short and long posterior ciliary, and collaterals to the optic nerve), orbital (lacrimal, superior and inferior muscular, and branches to the orbital periosteum and areolar tissue), and extraorbital (anterior and posterior ethmoidal, supraorbital, and medial palpebral) branches.[17, 21]

The superior and inferior ophthalmic veins drain the orbit. These veins lack valves and anastomose several times with one another and with external tributaries. The much more developed superior ophthalmic vein passes over the lateral rectus muscle and drains into the cavernous sinus. The inferior ophthalmic vein receives the veins from the medial wall and from the floor of the orbit and divides into two branches, one draining toward the pterygoid plexus through the inferior orbital fissure and the other reaching the superior ophthalmic vein just before traversing the superior orbital fissure.[17, 22]

## DIAGNOSIS OF ORBITAL LESIONS

Before the widespread availability of computed tomography (CT), orbital lesions were studied by means of plain radiography, orbitography with positive contrast, orbital phlebography, and echography. Data provided by these methods were indirect and poorly characteristic, so that a thorough knowledge of the patient's clinical history and physical examination was crucial for a presumptive diagnosis and for determination of the surgical indication— usually exploration, decompression, or biopsy.

Computed tomography scanning had a great impact on the diagnosis of orbital disease, greater perhaps than that on the field of neurologic diagnosis, and led to earlier diagnosis, more accurate lesion localization, closer delineation of lesion extension, and determination of the status of the orbital walls and neighboring areas.[1, 23] In tomographic imaging, the bone structure of orbital walls, the eyeball, the optic nerve, and the extraocular muscles are clearly outlined in contrast to the low-density backdrop of the orbital fat. As a rule, space-occupying lesions also are depicted sharply against adjacent structures and may enhance with endovenous contrast.[23]

An optic nerve glioma is commonly observed at CT scanning as a spindle-shaped thickening of the optic nerve, with a rounded, enlarged section on coronal views (Fig. 16–1).[24] Meningiomas involving the optic nerve sheath

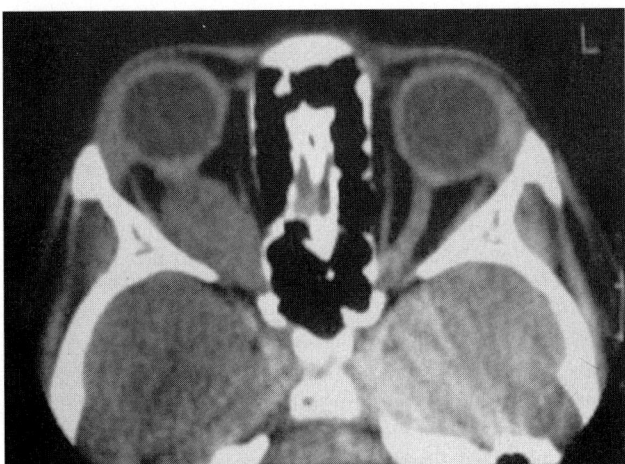

FIGURE 16–1 ■ A computed tomography scan. An axial view of an optic nerve glioma.

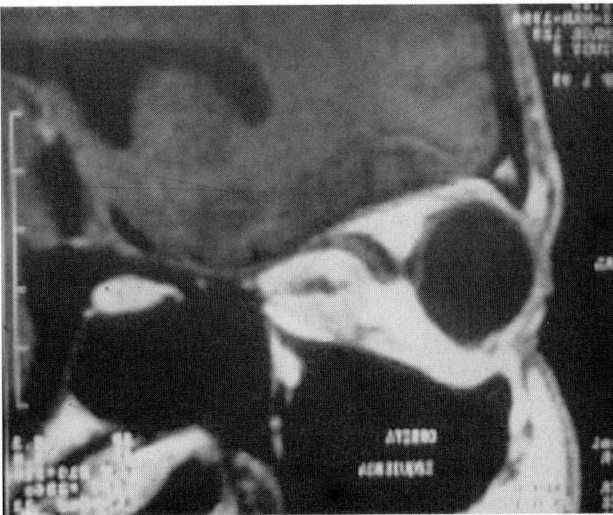

FIGURE 16–3 ■ A T₁-weighted magnetic resonance imaging scan with an oblique view along the optic nerve course showing an infraoptic neurinoma.

present diverse tomographic features, such as diffuse thickening of the optic nerve image that expands toward the apex, occasionally accompanied by a negative shadow of the optic nerve in its interior or, at other times, by calcification of the enlarged sheath. Another image typical of meningioma is that of an extensive lesion surrounding the optic nerve and presenting irregular borders.[24, 25] Cavernous hemangiomas are characterized by well defined, rounded images that enhance with contrast. These must be distinguished from neurinomas, which are similar in aspect and location, but more elongated and heterogeneous in structure.[1, 23] Orbital roof lesions include osteomas, dysplasias, aneurysmal bone cysts, and osteolytic lesions such as cholesteatomas, mucoceles, histiocytosis X, and metastases, all of which are clearly visualized in bone algorithm images.[1, 24]

More recently, the incorporation of magnetic resonance imaging (MRI) has enriched orbital diagnosis by allowing lateral incidence, parasagittal oblique views in the direction of the optic nerve, weighting at different times, and fat saturation techniques, in addition to axial and coronal sections. MRI provides greater anatomic detail of normal structures as well as better comparative delineation of the pathologic process (Figs. 16–2 and 16–3).[23]

Magnetic resonance imaging is of special interest in the study of optic nerve disease, often distinguishing whether the lesion is attached to the nerve or arises from the nerve itself or from its meningeal sheath. Gadolinium enhancement commonly and accurately delineates tumoral extension, mainly toward the endocranium. In the case of meningiomas, this spreading is observed more frequently than expected (Fig. 16–4). Another finding in perioptic meningiomas is that of perioptic arachnoid cyst anterior to the tumoral obstruction.[23, 26]

Digital subtraction angiography is mainly indicated in vascular lesions or highly vascularized tumors. It has been increasingly replaced by CT and MR angiography.

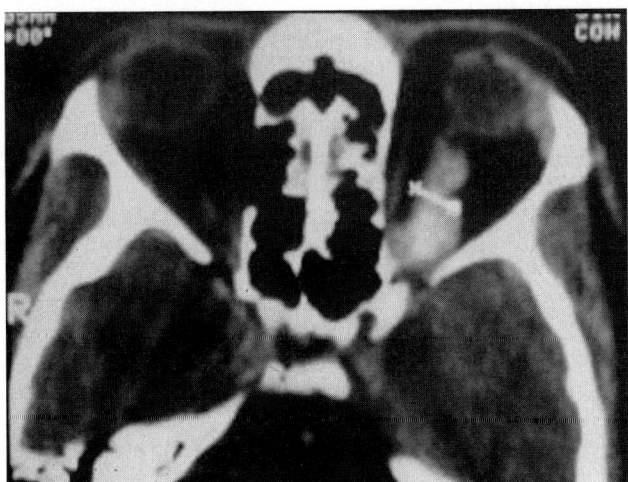

FIGURE 16–2 ■ A T₁-weighted magnetic resonance imaging scan with an axial view of an optic nerve sheath meningioma.

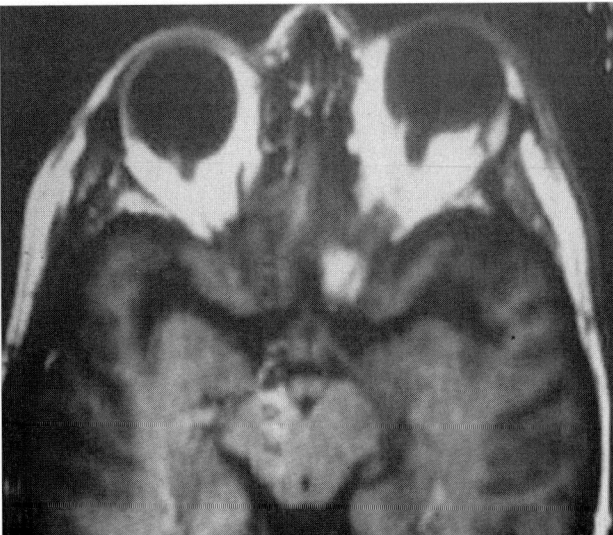

FIGURE 16–4 ■ A T₁-weighted magnetic resonance imaging scan with gadolinium enhancement of the intracranial extension of an optic nerve sheath meningioma.

## SURGICAL TECHNIQUE

### Transcranial Approach to the Orbit

Orbital approach by means of craniotomy is the most complex and demanding route. It is reliably indicated in cranio-orbital disease, including sphenoid wing or anterior fossa meningiomas with orbital extension, fronto-orbital fibrous dysplasia, chondromas, chondrosarcomas, and large epidermoid cysts, as well as in bone lesions arising from the orbital roof, most commonly osteomas and aneurysmal bone cysts. In such cases, frontal or frontotemporal craniotomy is performed according to lesion extension, with tumor resection including the roof and, occasionally, the lateral wall of the orbit, followed by plastic reconstruction of invaded orbital walls, and, if necessary, of compromised dura mater.[1]

The primary types of intraorbital tumors that should be approached by the transcranial route are those arising in the orbital apex or in the superointernal quadrant of the orbit. In our experience, optic nerve sheath meningiomas, optic nerve gliomas, neurinomas, intraconal cavernous hemangiomas, inflammatory pseudotumors, perioptic metastases, vascular malformations, and lymphangiomas represent most of such lesions (Fig. 16–5).[1]

Since 1985, we have performed supraorbital craniotomy for primary tumors of the orbital apex. In sheath meningiomas, optic gliomas, and other tumors types extending toward the intracranial cavity, this procedure is followed by extradural decompression of the optic canal and exploration of the optic nerve by the intradural route. In meningiomas, an annular or cuff-like tumoral growth may be observed extending from the orbit and surrounding the intracranial segment of the optic nerve. In optic nerve gliomas, it is advisable to carry out prechiasmatic section of the nerve to avoid tumor extension toward the optic chiasm. Such combined extradural and intracranial procedures can be performed only by the transcranial route because the other approaches to the orbit prove insufficient.[24–26]

### Supraorbital Craniotomy

Under general anesthesia and with endotracheal intubation, the patient is placed supine, with the head slightly extended to allow separation of the frontal lobe from the orbital roof by the effect of gravity. The sagittal axis of the skull is rotated 10 degrees toward the contralateral side. A strip of scalp is shaved along the line of incision.

Bearing cosmesis in mind, we use a hemicoronal incision behind the hairline, starting in front of the tragus and extending upward and forward, crossing the midline. The cutaneous flap is raised and dissected from the pericranium and from the temporal muscle aponeurosis, including the superior branch of the facial nerve in the folded planes.

A sickle-shaped incision with a lower concavity is made in the periosteum. The incision continues toward the lateral orbital rim, dissects the flap up to the superior orbital rim, and then proceeds toward the periorbita. The supraorbital nerve is released from the notch and, if a bony bridge exists, it is sectioned with a fine chisel.

The most anterior portion of the temporal muscle is dissected and a bur hole is made in the temporal fossa, behind the zygomatic process of the frontal bone, exposing the dura mater of the anterior fossa in its upper portion and the periorbita in its lower portion, both separated by the orbital roof. A second opening is made immediately above the orbital rim in the superointernal angle, outside the glabella. Because this opening usually crosses the frontal sinus, standard precautions are required. Both openings may be connected with a craniotome. Otherwise, a third frontal bur hole is made, equidistant from the first two and approximately 4 to 5 cm from the orbital rim. This opening is connected to the former two with a Gigli saw.[1, 12]

From the lateral bur hole first described, a Gigli saw or an oscillating saw is passed toward the lateral rim, which is then sectioned. From this same opening, while the dura mater and the periorbita are protected with small spatulas, the orbital roof is sectioned with a fine chisel directed toward the midline. From the medial frontal opening, the superior orbital rim and the orbital roof are sectioned with the chisel directed laterally and posteriorly toward the osteotomy previously performed. The frontal bone flap is then easily raised, together with the superior orbital rim and the anterior and wider sector of the orbital roof, exposing the frontal dura mater and the periorbita (Fig. 16–6).[1, 12, 13]

In apical tumors, it is necessary to complete bone resection of the orbital roof and the upper margin of the optic canal using a high-speed drill with a diamond bit.[1, 13]

The surgical microscope and self-retaining retractors are placed with only minimal frontal displacement. The use of spatulas on the meninges is avoided. The periorbita frequently opens during osteotomy and flap elevation maneuvers; should the periorbita remain intact, an anteroposterior incision is made medially to the levator palpebralis muscle.[13, 21]

Next, the inner and superior rectus muscles are explored by microsurgical technique until the optic nerve is located.

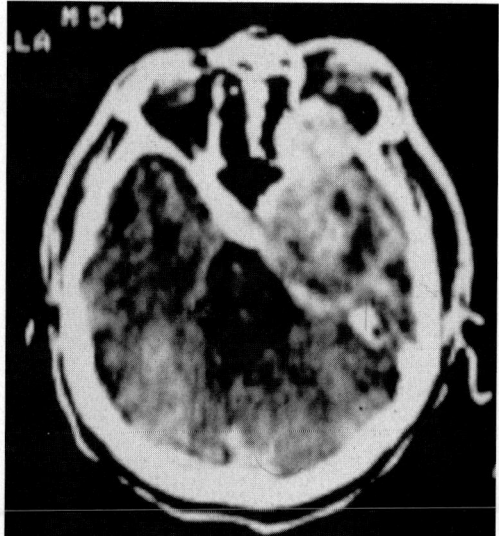

**FIGURE 16–5** ■ A computed tomography scan with an axial view demonstrating a dumb-bell neurinoma occuping the orbital apex and the middle cranial fossa, trespassing an enlarged superior orbital fissure.

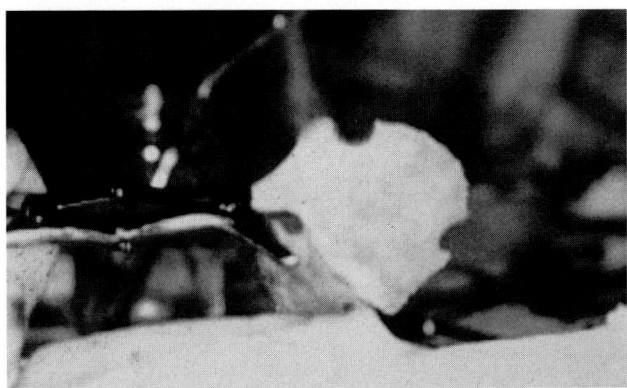

**FIGURE 16–6** ■ Surgical photograph of a supraorbital bone flap, including the superior orbital rim and the anterior part of the orbital roof.

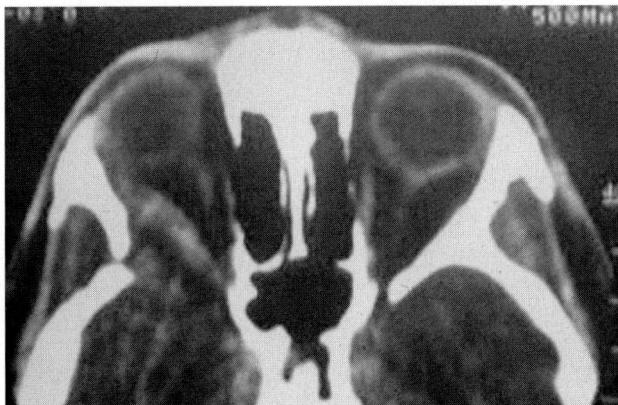

**FIGURE 16–7** ■ A preoperative axial computed tomography scan of an eosinophilic granuloma of the lateral orbital wall.

This method carries the least risk of causing irreversible ophthalmoplegia.[21, 22]

In optic nerve gliomas, the nerve is often extremely thickened in its distended meningeal coverings, showing regular contours. In these cases, the lesion is dissected laterally, the anterior portion from behind the eyeball and the posterior one at the level of the annulus of Zinn, followed by opening of the frontobasal dura mater to explore the optic nerve along its intracranial course. The nerve is then resected from the prechiasmatic level toward the optic canal, including the foraminal portion.[1, 13, 21]

In sheath meningiomas presenting as diffuse thickening, the dural sheath may be opened anteroposteriorly, and the tumor may be dissected jointly with the invaded sheath by following the subarachnoid space. Exceptionally, particularly in lesions located anteriorly, sight preservation may be achieved, provided that careful dissection is carried out and vascularization is spared in the nerve and retina. When the tumoral mass is larger, is not clearly restricted to the nerve course, and exhibits micronodular infiltration of the muscles at the apex, the eye is most likely amaurotic. Thus, it is advisable to resect this type of mass with the nerve, because the latter cannot be spared from the former. In such cases, it is essential to perform intracranial exploration of the optic nerve, which may be surrounded by tumor extending through the optic canal.[1]

In neurinomas and cavernous hemangiomas, the procedure is often simpler. Once the lesion has been located, it is dissected by microsurgical technique and may be removed in toto because attachment to critical structures is unusual. In rare cases, we have found hourglass neurinomas extending toward the middle cerebral fossa through a markedly enlarged superior orbital fissure that required resection by a combined intracranial and intraorbital procedure.[1, 22]

## Transcranial Approach with Resection of the Orbital Roof

Tumors invading or arising from the orbital roof demand a technique differing from the one used for purely intraorbital lesions. We resort to a frontal or frontotemporal craniotomy, according to lesion extension. When marked hyperostosis is present, as in pterional meningioma, fibrous dyspla-

sia, or osteoma, the procedure begins with a gradual resection of the pathologic bone with burs, drills, and gouges before the bone flap is raised, so that the dura mater is protected by that bony sector during such maneuvers. It often is necessary to continue bone resection toward the roof and lateral orbital wall, leaving the orbital contents amply exposed. In purely osseous lesions, this stage ends with total removal of the lesion (Figs. 16–7 and 16–8).[27]

In sphenoid wing meningiomas, it is essential to proceed with dural opening and resection of invaded dura mater, as well as the attached meningioma en plaque. Occasionally, in a large intradural tumor with temporal or frontotemporal extension that projects toward the sylvian fissure, tumoral dissection proceeds from the cerebral cortex and along the internal carotid and middle cerebral arteries using microsurgical technique.[27]

The final step is to perform plastic reconstruction of the resected dura mater with pericranium. Lyophilized dura mater produced good results in some of our earlier patients, but was abandoned after some cases of Creutzfeldt-Jakob disease associated with its use were reported in the literature.[27] The roof and, at times, the lateral wall of the orbit are reconstructed with methyl methacrylate. Initially, we carried out plastic reconstruction with costal autografts, but

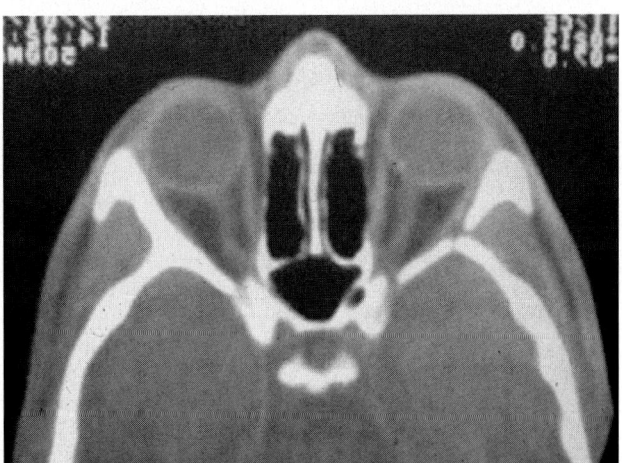

**FIGURE 16–8** ■ A postoperative computed tomography scan of the same patient showing remodelling of the lateral orbital wall.

the procedure proved protracted and tedious because graft modeling was highly complex and the cosmetic results were suboptimal.[27]

## Complications

In primary intraorbital tumors lacking intracranial extension operated on by the diverse methods described, no mortality or neurologic complications, such as seizures, hemipareses, or sensory disorders, occurred. Infrequently, signs of intracranial hypotension or pneumocephalus may be detected during the first 48 postoperative hours in patients operated on transcranially.

In tumors extending toward the apex, mainly optic nerve gliomas and sheath meningiomas, most patients presented with subtotal ophthalmoplegia and ptosis immediately after surgery, followed by nearly entire remission within 2 to 3 months. Although amaurosis of the corresponding eye is the rule in gliomas and most meningiomas, in a few cases of spared sight, preservation of useful sight was achieved with the technique described. In other histologic forms, the cosmetic and functional results were most satisfactory, barring transient inflammatory pseudoptosis in the upper eyelid. Neither cerebrospinal fluid collection nor leaks were observed; no infectious processes occurred.[27]

With sphenoid wing meningiomas, the most crucial complications occurred in the earlier cases of the series, mainly in the internal third of the wing. They consisted mostly of contralateral hemiparesis or hemiplegia in 4%, seizures in 3%, and transient disorders of consciousness in 4% of the cases. The mortality rate in these cases was 2%. Almost invariably, such complications resulted from damage to the internal carotid or middle cerebral arteries in the course of dissection. However, these undesirable effects have been avoided during the last two decades owing to improvements in microsurgical technique and instruments, such as the ultrasonic aspirator.[27]

Our experience is based on a series of 553 operative cases of orbital disease from 1974 to the present (Table 16–1). The surgical techniques used are presented in Table 16–2. Most cases were resolved by superior orbitotomy, although the transcranial approach was necessary in 24.4% of patients with primary intraorbital disease. Including tumors extending secondarily to the orbit increased the incidence of craniotomies to 37.7% of all interventions.

In primary intraorbital tumors, Berke lateral orbitotomy was used in 11.4% and inferior orbitotomy in 4.5% of patients. Eight cases had a superolateral approach by means of a Kocher incision, and 17 had an inferolateral transmalar access, 9 with large primary tumors and 8 with tumors extending to the orbit, mostly pterional meningiomas from the start of our series. Exenteration was required in 13 patients from early in the series with advanced malignant tumors. Eight cases of paranasal sinus tumor with orbital invasion received a transantral approach.[1] Revision surgery, using the initial or an alternative route, was necessary in 18 patients.

The diversity of procedures used in our series is the result of a systematic and thorough evaluation of the patient's clinical history and of complementary examinations

### TABLE 16–1 ■ SURGICAL EXPERIENCE WITH ORBITAL TUMORS (1974–1998)

| Tumor Type | No. |
| --- | --- |
| **Primary Orbital Tumors** | |
| Mucoceles | 108 |
| Cholesteatomas | 61 |
| Neurinomas | 33 |
| Meningiomas | 33 |
| Lacrimal gland tumors | 30 |
| Cavernous hemangiomas | 27 |
| Lymphomas | 21 |
| Metastases | 18 |
| Inflammatory pseudotumors | 16 |
| Sarcomas | 15 |
| Optic nerve gliomas | 14 |
| Localized bone lesions | 12 |
| Hydatid cysts | 12 |
| Miscellaneous | 28 |
| Subtotal | 428 |
| **Propagated Orbital Tumors** | |
| Sphenoid ridge meningiomas | 102 |
| Paranasal sinus carcinomas | 7 |
| Fibrous dysplasias | 6 |
| Chondromas, chondrosarcomas | 4 |
| Miscellaneous (e.g., reticulosarcoma, Ewing's sarcoma, metastases) | 6 |
| Total | 553 |

to select the most suitable treatment for each particular case.[1, 13, 21]

## SUMMARY

The choice of the most suitable surgical treatment for space-occupying orbital lesions is made on the basis of tumor location, size, apparent site of origin, propagation routes, and probable histologic type.

Superior orbitotomy, the technique most frequently used, is mainly indicated in frontoethmoidal mucoceles, dermoid cysts, and lacrimal gland tumors. Lateral orbitotomy allows access to the lateral quadrants of the orbital cavity, where cavernous hemangiomas, neurinomas, inflammatory pseudotumors, and metastases may develop.

### TABLE 16–2 ■ SURGICAL APPROACHES TO ORBITAL TUMORS

| | Primary Tumors | | Propagated Tumors | | Total | |
| --- | --- | --- | --- | --- | --- | --- |
| | *No.* | *%* | *No.* | *%* | *No.* | *%* |
| Superior orbitotomy | 218 | 50.93 | | | 218 | 39.42 |
| Transcranial approach | 104 | 24.29 | 102 | 81.6 | 206 | 37.25 |
| Lateral orbitotomy | 48 | 11.21 | 4 | 3.2 | 52 | 9.40 |
| Inferior orbitotomy | 19 | 4.43 | | | 19 | 3.43 |
| Exenteration | 13 | 3.03 | | | 13 | 2.35 |
| Superolateral | 10 | 2.33 | | | 10 | 1.80 |
| Inferolateral | 8 | 1.86 | 14 | 11.2 | 22 | 3.97 |
| Transantral approach | 8 | 1.86 | 5 | 4 | 13 | 2.35 |
| Total | 428 | 100 | 125 | 100 | 553 | 100 |

We found fewer indications for inferior orbitotomy, which is used in rare lesions, such as some lymphomas and metastases. For tumors originating in ethmoid cells or the maxillary sinus, a transantral approach is indicated.

Less frequently, larger lesions require extended approaches (e.g., superolateral or inferolateral) according to tumor topography. Such techniques are used mainly for removal of hydatid cysts or huge cavernous hemangiomas or neurinomas.

The transcranial approach to the orbit is indicated for cranio-orbital meningioma of the sphenoid wing, and with anterior cranial fossa disease with orbital extension—fronto-orbital fibrous dysplasia, chondroma, chondrosarcoma, aneurysmal bone cyst, osteoma, and large epidermoid cysts. Primary intraorbital tumors requiring a transcranial approach are those located in the apex or in the superointernal quadrant that are large or extend posteriorly. The most common lesions are optic nerve sheath meningioma, optic nerve glioma, cavernous hemangioma, neurinoma, inflammatory pseudotumor, vascular malformation, lymphangioma, hemangiopericytoma, and perioptic metastases. The transcranial route is the only one that allows decompression of the optic canal and intracranial exploration of the optic nerve along its prechiasmatic course.

## REFERENCES

1. Basso A, Carrizo A, Kreutel A: Transcranial approach to lesions of the orbit. In Schmidek H, Sweet W (eds): Operative Neurosurgical Techniques. Philadelphia: WB Saunders, 1995, pp 205–212.
2. Benedict W: Surgical treatment of tumors and cysts of the orbit. Am J Ophthalmol 32:765–773, 1949.
3. Brihaye J: Neurosurgical approaches to orbital tumors. In Krayenbuhl H (ed): Advances and Technical Standards in Neurosurgery, Vol 3. Wien/New York: Springer-Verlag, 1976, pp 103–121.
4. Duke-Elder S: Systems of Ophthalmology, Vol 13, part II. London: Henry Kimpton, 1974, pp 774–1230.
5. Davis F: Primary tumors of the optic nerve. Arch Ophthalmol 23:735–821, 1940.
6. Vergez A: Les voies temporales d'abord de l'orbite. Arch Ophthal (Paris) 18:294–343, 1958.
7. Berke R: A modified Kronlein operation. Arch Ophthalmol 51:609–632, 1954.
8. Dandy W: Orbital tumors. New York: Oskar Piest, 1941, pp 154–160.
9. Poppen J: Exophthalmos. Am J Surg 64:64–79, 1943.
10. Love J, Benedict W: Transcranial removal of intraorbital tumors. JAMA 129:777–784, 1945.
11. Frazier C: An approach to the hypophysis through the anterior cranial fossa. Ann Surg 57:145–152, 1913.
12. Jane J, Park T, Pobereskin L, et al: The supraorbital approach: Technical note. Neurosurgery 11:537–542, 1982.
13. Maroon J, Kennerdell J: Surgical approaches to the orbit. J Neurosurg 60:1226–1235, 1984.
14. Leone C, Wissinger J: Surgical approaches to diseases of the orbital apex. Ophthalmology 95:391–397, 1988.
15. Reese A: Tumors of the eye. New York: Hoeber Medical Division, 1963, pp 562–570.
16. Casper D, Linda Chi T, Trokel S: Orbital Disease: Imaging and Analysis. New York: Thieme, 1993, pp 64–79.
17. Doxanas M, Anderson R: Clinical orbital anatomy. Baltimore: Williams & Wilkins, 1984, pp 153–169.
18. Shields J: Diagnosis and Management of Orbital Tumors. Philadelphia: WB Saunders, 1989, pp 8–10.
19. Towsend D: Orbital surgical techniques. In Albert D, Jakobiec F (eds): Principles and Practice of Ophthalmology, Vol 3. Philadelphia: WB Saunders, 1994, pp 1890–1895.
20. Rengachary S, Kishore P: Intraorbital ophthalmic aneurysms and arteriovenous fistulae. Surg Neurol 9:35–40, 1978.
21. Housepian E: Microsurgical anatomy of the orbital apex and principles of transcranial orbital exploration. Clin Neurosurg 25:556–573, 1977.
22. Housepian E, Trokel S: Tumors of the orbit. In Youmans J (ed): Neurological Surgery, Vol 3. Philadelphia: WB Saunders, 1973, pp 1275–1296.
23. Lindblom B, Truwit C, Hoyt W: Optic nerve sheath meningioma: Definition of intraorbital, intracanalicular and intracranial components with magnetic resonance imaging. Ophthalmology 99:560–566, 1992.
24. Jakobiec F, Depot M, Kennerdell J: Combined clinical and computed tomographic diagnosis of orbital glioma and meningioma. Ophthalmology 91:137–155, 1984.
25. Wright J, Call N, Liaricos S: Primary optic nerve meningioma. Br J Ophthalmol 64:553–558, 1980.
26. Basso A, Carrizo A, Kreutel A, Tomecek F: Primary intraorbital meningiomas. In Schmidek H (ed): Meningiomas and Their Surgical Management. Philadelphia: WB Saunders, 1991, pp 311–323.
27. Basso A, Carrizo A: Sphenoid ridge meningiomas. In Schmidek H (ed): Meningiomas and Their Surgical Management. Philadelphia: WB Saunders, 1991, pp 233–241.

# Surgical Management of Meningiomas of the Orbit: A Personal Series*

■ KURT SCHÜRMANN

Between 1955 and 1988, 436 space-occupying lesions of the orbit were treated surgically at the Neurosurgical Department of Johannes Gutenberg University in Mainz, West Germany (Table 17–1). Of these masses, 17% were intraorbital meningiomas. Excluded from this series were meningiomas of the sphenoid wing, sphenoidal plane, orbital plate, and other intracranial meningiomas that secondarily invaded the orbit; however, tumors diagnosed by arteriography and orbitophlebography and those that antedated computed tomography (CT) were included (Fig. 17–1; Tables 17–2 and 17–3). Since 1975, CT, particularly high-resolution CT, has been used to deter-

*This chapter has been adapted from Schmidek H: Meningiomas and Their Surgical Management. Philadelphia: WB Saunders, 1991.

mine the site and size of an orbital tumor and to define its relation to the optic nerve, the globe, and the optic canal (Fig. 17–2). Included in this series of cases were the tumors whose surgical treatment antedated the routine use of microsurgical technique. In this chapter, I report my experience in treating these complex lesions. (Fig. 17–3).

Based on my observations, I differentiate between two types of intraorbital meningiomas: (1) tumors that are global meningiomas and are unrelated to the optic nerve sheath and (2) tumors that are meningiomas of the optic nerve sheath. This distinction is important in deciding the indications for operation, the choice of approach, the prognosis for subsequent visual function, and the probability of recurrence of tumor.

*Global meningiomas* are spherical tumors with a usually sharp demarcation from the surrounding tissue, which renders them similar to cavernous hemangiomas. In general, they displace rather than invade important intraorbital structures. These tumors can be removed in most cases without producing additional iatrogenic damage. Global intraorbital meningiomas are usually located within the anterior and middle part of the orbit and are rarely located within the retrobulbar muscle cone. Nevertheless, the more posteriorly the tumor is situated within the orbit, the more primary damage and secondary surgical deficits are to be expected because the functionally important structures of the orbit are closest together within the tight space of the dorsal cone. I have 52 such tumors in my series (Table 17–4). For total removal of these tumors, limited osteoplastic craniotomy that is specific to tumor site is preferable

## TABLE 17–1 ■ SPACE-OCCUPYING LESIONS OF THE ORBIT (JANUARY 1955 TO MARCH 1988)

| Lesion | n |
|---|---|
| Meningiomas | 74 |
| Cavernous hemangiomas | 62 |
| Hemangiopericytoma | 1 |
| Optic nerve gliomas | 21 |
| Hematoma | 1 |
| Lacrimal gland tumors (mixed tumors, cylindromas, carcinomas) | 35 |
| Mesenchymal tumors (fibromas, myxomas, lipomas) | 33 |
| Neurofibromas | 12 |
| Lymphomas (including 9 primary low-grade non-Hodgkin's B-cell lymphomas after Kieler classification) | 21 |
| Dermoids and epidermoids | 20 |
| Osteomas | 7 |
| Rhabdomyosarcomas (children) | 9 |
| Malignant neoplasms (carcinomas, sarcomas, metastases, melanomas) | 34 |
| Granulomas | 12 |
| Chronic inflammatory fibrous pseudotumors | 45 |
| Fibrous dysplasia | 2 |
| Aneurysmal bone cyst | 1 |
| Leukemic or leukoblastic tumors | 2 |
| Unclassified tumors | 30 |
| Inflammatory processes and mucoceles | 14 |
| *Total* | 436 |

## TABLE 17–2 ■ CLINICAL SYMPTOMS OF INTRAORBITAL LESIONS

Unilateral exophthalmos and bulbar protrusion with conjunctival hyperemia, chemosis, or both
Dislocation of the globe, laterally, medially, inferiorly, or superiorly, according to the site of the lesion
Diplopia due to dislocation of the globe or paresis of cranial nerves III, IV, VI
Palpable intraorbital resistance
Diminished vision

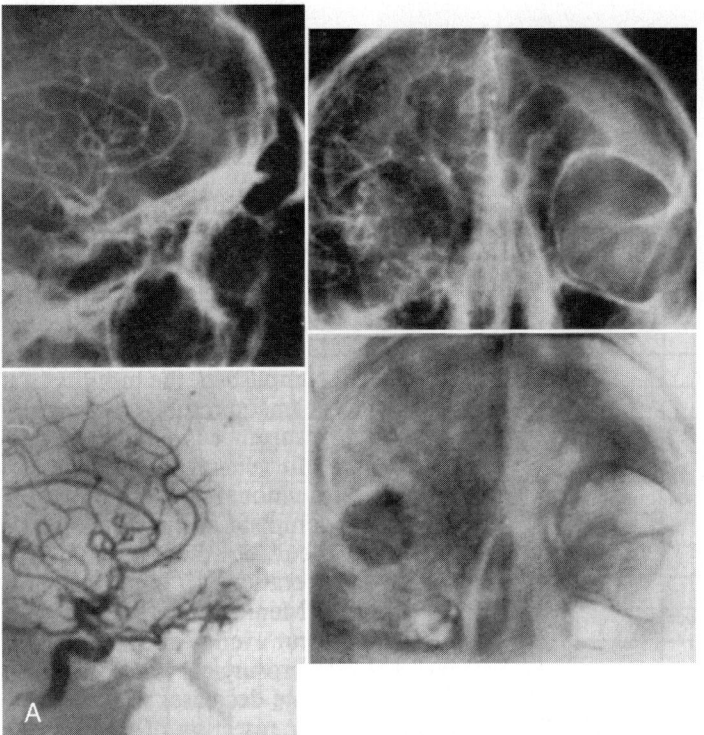

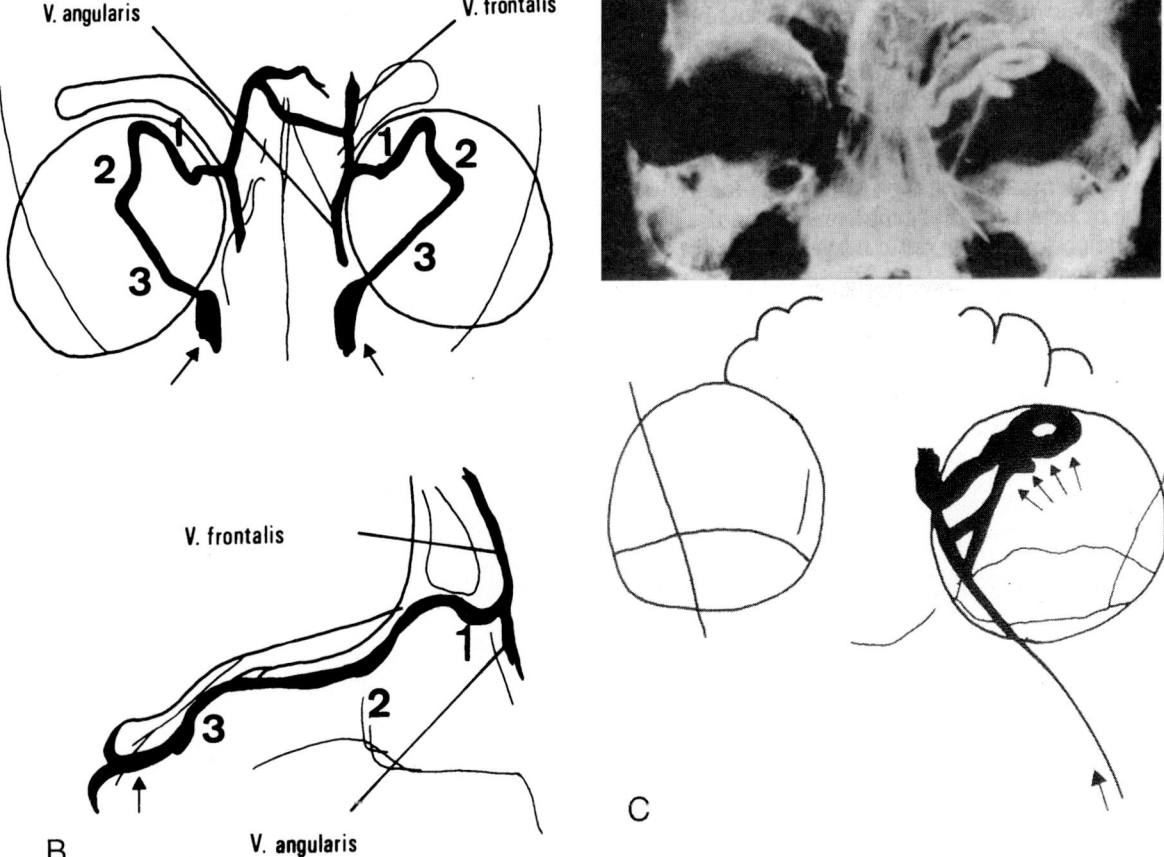

FIGURE 17–1 ■ *A*, Retrobulbar meningioma of the right superior lateral orbit. Hypertrophic ophthalmic artery and global enhancement in the capillary phase are shown. Complete removal by osteoplastic craniotomy was accomplished without functional deficits and with no recurrence since 1969. *B*, Diagram of the normal course of the superior orbital vein as visualized by orbitophlebography. (*Top*, Anteroposterior view; *bottom*, lateral view.) *C*, orbitophlebography reveals a big retrobulbar meningioma within the dorsal tip of the left orbit, causing compression, dislocation, and increasing dilatation of the posterior part of the vein, near the entry zone of the cavernous sinus. (*B* and *C*, From Schürmann K: The development of orbital surgery from a neurosurgeon's viewpoint [Fedor Krause Memorial Lecture]. Adv Neurosurg 17:1, 1989.)

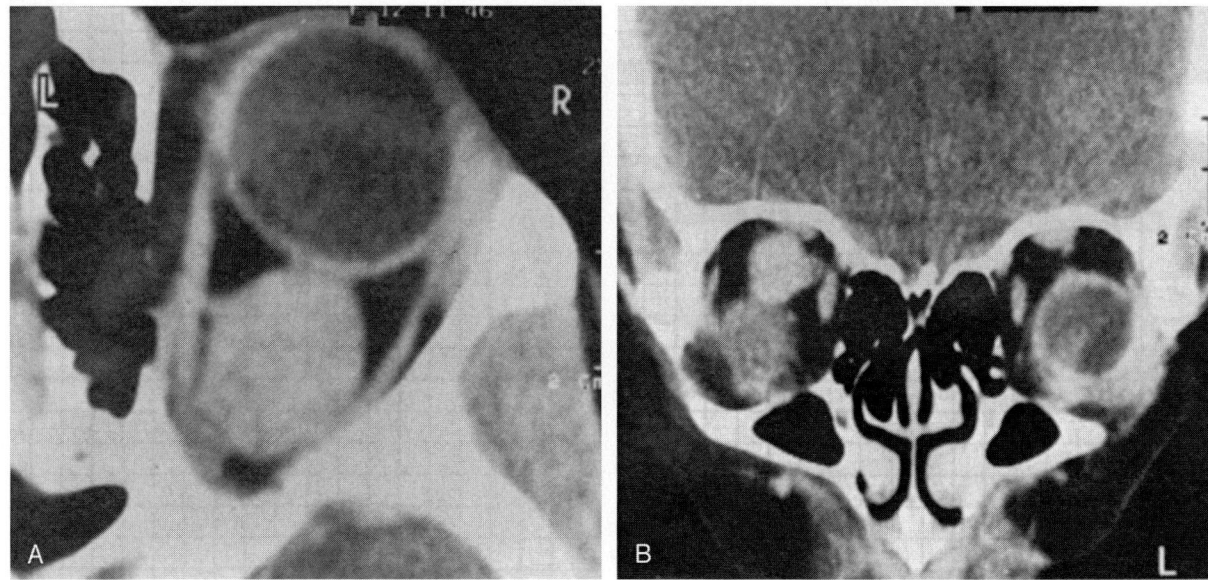

FIGURE 17–2  ■  A sharply demarcated right-sided retrobulbar global tumor within the middle and upper parts of the muscle cone. A 41-year-old woman underwent an operation through a frontal osteoplastic craniotomy in 1987. No postoperative visual or motor damage occurred.

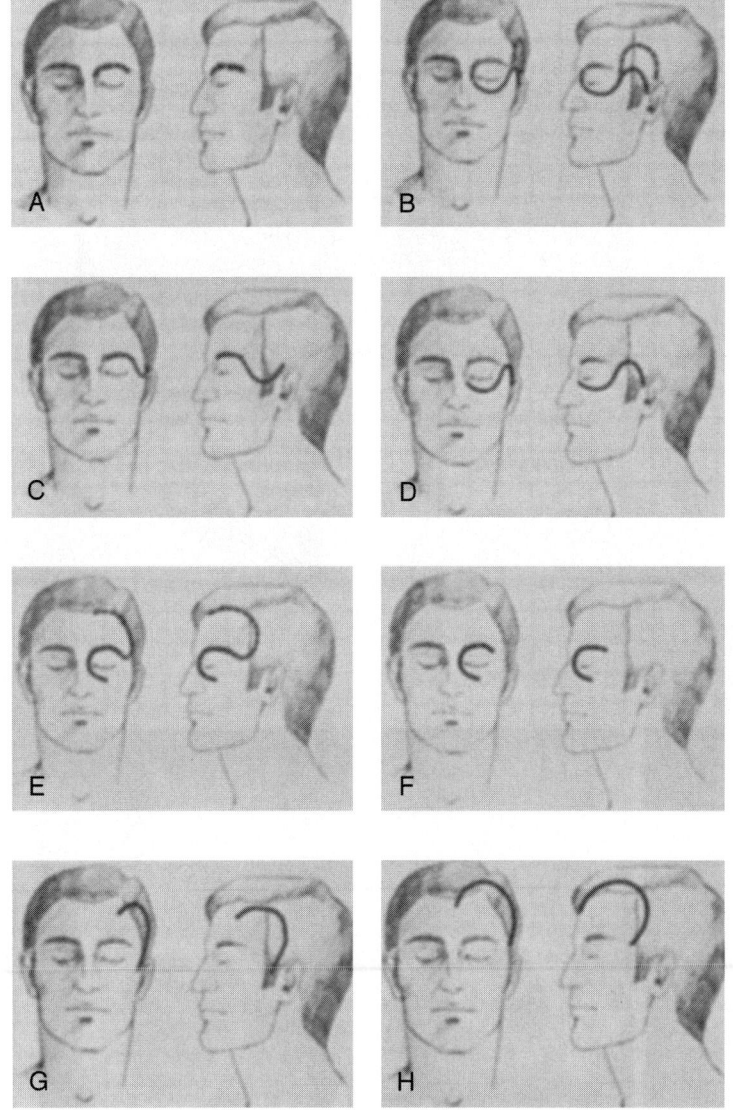

FIGURE 17–3  ■  Surgical approaches to the orbit. *A*, Simple superior orbitotomy. (Lateral or medial extension is possible.) *B*, Simple inferior (basal) orbitotomy, extended to a lateral osteoplastic orbitotomy or lateral craniotomy, or both. *C*, Simple superior orbitotomy, extended to lateral osteoplastic orbitotomy. *D*, Simple inferior (basal) orbitotomy, extended to lateral osteoplastic orbitotomy. *E*, Superior medial orbitotomy, extended to lateral osteoplastic orbitotomy or craniotomy, or both. *F*, Simple medial orbitotomy, extended superiorly. *G*, Transfrontal lateral orbitotomy. *H*, Transfrontal medial orbitotomy. (From Schürmann K: The development of orbital surgery from a neurosurgeon's viewpoint [Fedor Krause Memorial Lecture]. Adv Neurosurg 17:1, 1989.)

## TABLE 17–3 ■ NEURORADIOLOGIC INVESTIGATION OF ORBITAL LESIONS

| Investigative Technique | Application |
| --- | --- |
| Plain x-ray film | Detects soft tissue mass, erosion and destruction of bone walls, bone sclerosis or atrophy, and dilatation of the optic canal |
| Computed tomography | Provides information about site, size, nature, and relation to neighboring structures of the lesions (standard 400 HU). Bone window (3200 HU) gives precise information on bone lesions |
| Carotid arteriography | Used in vascular lesions (AVM) and in suspected intracranial lesions |
| Orbitophlebography | Used in vascular lesions of the venous system |
| Ultrasonography | Determines site, size, and nature of lesions |
| Magnetic resonance imaging | Particularly effective for soft tissue imaging |

HU, Hounsfield unit; AVM, arteriovenous malformation.

(see Fig. 17–3*G*). Only when the lesion is located in the lateral third of the orbit is a modified lateral osteoplastic (Krönlein) orbitotomy used to advantage (Figs. 17–4 and 17–5). Some anatomic and clinical examples further clarify the particular situation of global meningiomas of the orbit (Figs. 17–6 to 17–12).

Two types of expansion are exhibited by *optic nerve sheath meningiomas*. Each of these types requires a different surgical strategy. Fungoid optic nerve sheath meningiomas arise from a limited part of the optic nerve sheath and tend to grow outside of the optic nerve sheath. This type of meningioma is treated in a manner that is similar to treatment of global meningiomas. Total removal of these tumors may be possible if the surgeon succeeds in their microsurgical isolation from the optic nerve and optic nerve sheath. In these cases, the surgeon has a chance of preventing impairment of visual function, especially if the tumor has compressed and not invaded the optic nerve.

In my patients, this type of tumor was located near the globe or near the optic canal and not in the middle part of the course of the optic nerve. I differentiated between the growth of these tumors in the anterior and in the posterior parts of the optic nerve. The prognosis for preservation of

## TABLE 17–4 ■ INTRAORBITAL MENINGIOMAS*

| Tumor Type | *n* |
| --- | --- |
| Meningiomas without relation to the optic nerve sheath (mainly within the anterior middle part of the orbit) | 52 |
| Meningiomas of the optic nerve sheath | 17 |
| Hemangiopericytomas | 2 |
| Malignant meningiomas | 2 |
| Micromeningioma of the optic nerve sheath combined with a fibrous pseudotumor | 1 |
| *Total* | 74 |

*Neurosurgical clinic of the Johannes Gutenberg University of Mainz, West Germany, 1955 through 1988.

## TABLE 17–5 ■ POSTOPERATIVE VISUAL FUNCTION ASSOCIATED WITH PRIMARY OPTIC NERVE SHEATH MENINGIOMAS

| Results After Tumor Removal* | No. Tumors |
| --- | --- |
| Improved visual function | 0 |
| Unchanged visual function | 2 |
| Worsened visual function | 3 |
| Complete resection of tumor-bearing optic nerve | 12 |
| *Total* | 17 |

*Severely diminished visual function was found in every case preoperatively.

visual function is better for anteriorly situated tumors. I have not seen an improvement in visual function among the posteriorly situated tumors, even after their successful removal (Table 17–5).

The second type of optic nerve sheath meningioma is a tumor that grows around and along the length of the optic nerve sheath from the globe to the optic canal, compromises the blood supply to the optic nerve, and compresses the optic nerve. Most patients with these tumors exhibit only slight exophthalmos and demonstrate intact ocular motility and no diplopia. The main symptom is a decrease of visual acuity that slowly progresses to blindness; such progression may occur over 3 to 5 years or more. The diagnosis is established by CT examination. Operation is indicated if no useful vision remains or if there is tumor extension along the optic canal or intracranially. The last case is an absolute indication for surgical intervention.

Based on my experience with 17 cases of optic nerve sheath meningiomas, limited lateral frontal osteoplastic craniotomy is the surgical approach of choice (see Fig. 17–3*G*). In a few cases, microsurgical separation of the optic nerve from the enveloping tumor has been attempted. Useful vision was not successfully preserved in any of these cases, however. In addition, within 2 to 3 years after total tumor removal, tumor usually recurred. The preferable plan involves total removal of the tumorous optic nerve between globe and optic canal at the time of the first operation, when the optic nerve is surrounded by tumors. When total removal of the optic nerve has been accomplished, the motility of the eyeball is preserved, the cosmetic result is satisfactory, and the chance of tumor recurrence is significantly reduced.

In general, meningiomas of the orbit have a good functional and life prognosis, if one succeeds in their complete removal. Meningiomas may recur; however, most of them are cured by reoperation if it is radical enough.

Meningiomas within the posterior orbital tip tend to recur even if one succeeds in their seemingly complete microsurgical removal. The risk of recurrence decreases if one directly performs a complete en bloc resection of the tumor mass with its surrounding tissue, such as nerves, muscles, and bone. In my opinion, such a radical and mutilating primary intervention is not absolutely indicated; it can be postponed until the second operation for the tumor recurrence or until the patient demonstrates total blindness of the afflicted eye.

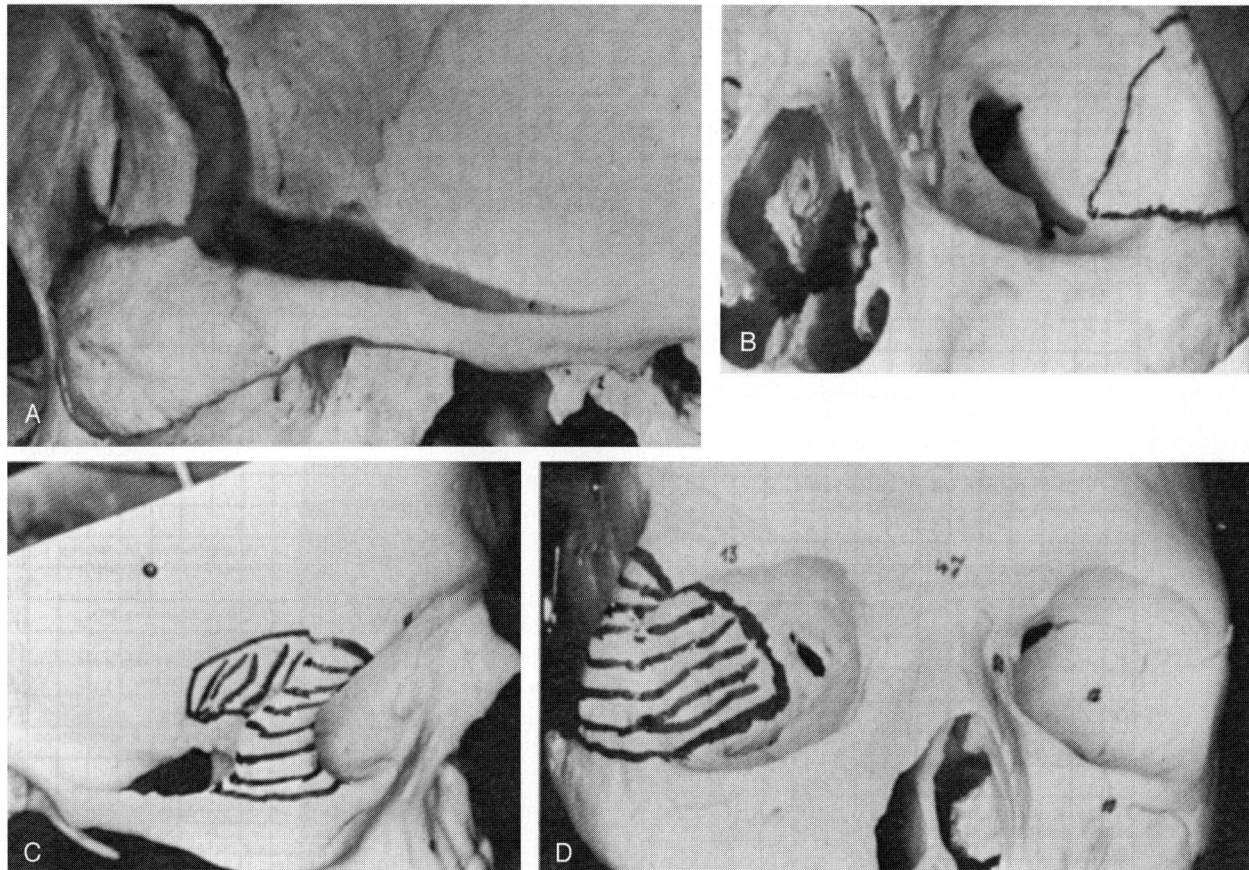

**FIGURE 17–4** ■ Lateral osteoplastic orbitotomy. *A*, Extension of the original Krönlein operation in 1886 (left side). *B*, Anteroposterior view of an extension of the original Krönlein operation (left side). *C*, Lateral view of a more extensive lateral orbitotomy (right side). *D*, Anteroposterior view of a more extensive lateral orbitotomy.

## SURGICAL APPROACHES TO THE ORBIT IN ORBITAL MENINGIOMAS

In most global meningiomas of the orbit, limited frontal osteoplastic craniotomy provides an excellent exposure of the orbital contents, which allows total removal of the tumor and protection of important structures. In meningiomas of the anteromedial quadrant of the orbit, medial craniotomy is advantageous (see Fig. 17–3*H*), whereas in retrobulbar meningiomas within the muscle cone or within the dorsal tip of the orbit, craniotomy that is more laterally localized is preferred (see Fig. 17–3*G*). I recommend an exposure involving resection of the orbital roof and the lateral orbital wall, along with opening of the superior orbital fissure and, if necessary, unroofing of the optic canal. In this way, the surgeon obtains good exposure of the elements of the dorsal orbital apex (see Fig. 17–8). As a rule, the orbit is approached extradurally after the craniotomy is performed. The dura is usually easy to detach from the bone in the region of the lower sphenoid wing, the superior orbital fissure, and the optic canal.

When the tumor site is in the anterolateral quadrant of the orbit, it is approached through a modified lateral orbitotomy (see Fig. 17–5*A*). In the case of anterolateral-to-posterolateral tumor extension, an extended lateral or-

bitotomy may be sufficient (see Fig. 17–5*B*). If the tumor extends within the dorsal muscle cone in the posterior orbital apex, the preferred method consists of a limited lateral osteoplastic orbitotomy or widening of the lateral orbitotomy to a limited frontal craniotomy, in which an extended Krönlein exposure is combined with a frontal orbitotomy (see Fig. 17–3*C*).

These modified lateral approaches are usually also practicable by using the extradural route. Only if the tumor extends into the intracranial space is opening of the dura necessary. Subsequently the dural defect is repaired by a flap of the inner layer of galea-periosteum, fascia lata, or lyophilized dura mater fixed by sutures and fibrin glue.

When the orbital contents are approached after resection of the orbital roof, the lateral wall of the orbit, and the lesser sphenoid wing, the periorbita is opened by a longitudinal, ventral-to-dorsal incision just behind the bulb toward the opened superior orbital fissure. The incision of the periorbita is placed between the levator muscle of the upper eyelid and the lateral straight muscle of the eyeball. The lips of this incision are carefully retracted, and the orbital fat is handled carefully. The superior orbital vein and the first branch of the trigeminal nerve (nervus frontalis) must be identified and separated. The vein can be ligated and divided, if necessary. The origins of the extracular muscles, which are fused at the annulus, should be identified

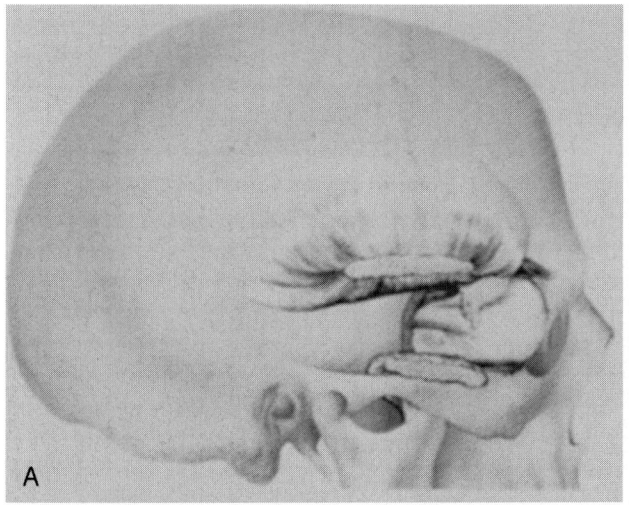
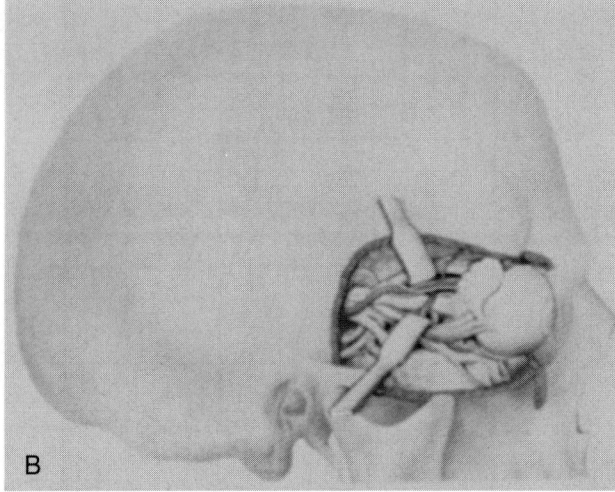

FIGURE 17–5 ■ Operative sketch of a lateral osteoplastic orbitotomy. *A,* Limited approach for an anterolateral tumor site, particularly of the lacrimal gland. *B,* More extensive lateral approach with complete removal of the lateral orbital wall to the superior orbital fissure, subtotal resection of the orbital roof, and temporary removal of the zygomatic arch for reaching the dorsal orbital cone. Extradural resection of a large part of the sphenoid wing is also possible, if needed. This extended lateral approach is sometimes preferred in elderly patients, because it involves fewer risks than craniotomy. (*B,* From Schürmann K: The development of orbital surgery from a neurosurgeon's viewpoint [Fedor Krause Memorial Lecture]. Adv Neurosurg 17:1, 1989.)

and isolated. The surgeon should now identify the nerves and, if possible, the ophthalmic artery situated below the optic nerve (see Figs. 17–6 and 17–7).

After the optic canal is dorsally and laterally unroofed, the regional anatomy is clearer. If the optic nerve is followed ventrally after the dural and subarachnoid sheaths are split, exposure over the orbital apex is optimized. The optic canal, the optic nerve, the ophthalmic artery, and the more laterally located oculomotor nerves are visible. The lacrimal, trochlear, and ophthalmic division of the trigeminal nerve enter the superior orbital fissure, and the ophthalmic vein leaves the orbit through this opening. These structures lie within the periorbita, outside of the muscle cone (see Fig. 17–7A). The two divisions of the third and the sixth cranial nerves and the nasociliary nerves enter through the superior orbital fissure and fall directly within the muscle cone.

In treating primary optic nerve sheath meningiomas, the surgeon should plan to perform a frontal osteoplastic craniotomy with an extradural approach to the orbit. After the optic canal is unroofed, a longitudinal split is made in the dural and subarachnoid sheaths of the optic nerve within the optic canal, and the optic nerve is transected as far proximally as possible (in its tumor-free part). The unaffected part of the optic nerve can then be held by a mosquito clamp and be carefully extracted from the optic canal. The ophthalmic artery can now be seen; this vessel should be clipped or occluded by bipolar coagulation, then divided. This extraction of the optic nerve from the optic canal and the isolation of the ophthalmic artery must be done carefully to avoid tearing this vessel from the internal carotid artery. After the ophthalmic artery is protected, the optic nerve is followed to the posterior aspect of the globe, and the nerve is cut close to the sclera to accomplish a total removal of the tumor along with the strangled optic nerve. If the meningioma has invaded the intracranial cavity through the optic canal, the operation should be extended to include an intradural exploration. The intradural

operation is the same as any approach to the optic chiasm involving the pterion.

## RECONSTRUCTIVE MEASURES

When extensive bone resections are performed, various materials may be used for reconstruction. For extensive bone removal (see Fig. 17–8), a plastic repair of the defect is carried out. A resected anterolateral orbital wall can also be reconstructed with the use of plastic materials. In the case of extreme preoperative exophthalmos, modeling of the plastic in a larger curve may be useful to enlarge the orbital cavity and produce a more symmetric appearance. If one has used another material, it should be placed to achieve the same effect. If possible, orbital fat should not be resected to reduce the degree of exophthalmos because the orbital fat protects the fine internal neurovascular structures that are necessary for synchronized eye movements.

If ethmoidal cells or paranasal sinuses are opened, the preferred method of closure involves use of a pedicled flap of galea-periosteum. This flap must have a vascularized pedicle to promote rapid, safe healing. The same applies to a flap of the temporal muscle and its fascia. The strip or flap should be fixed by a few sutures to the dura mater of the anterior skull base and by human fibrin glue. In exceptional cases, one must use fascia lata or lyophilized dura mater to achieve a watertight closure.

The approach to the orbit to remove meningiomas should be adapted to the individual case and necessitates adequate bone resection to provide optimal exposure of the orbital contents, especially in the region of the dorsal orbital muscle cone.

## RESULTS

The extradural approach to the orbit is the preferable route because of its lower risk. Before 1963, the transfrontal

*Text continued on page 233*

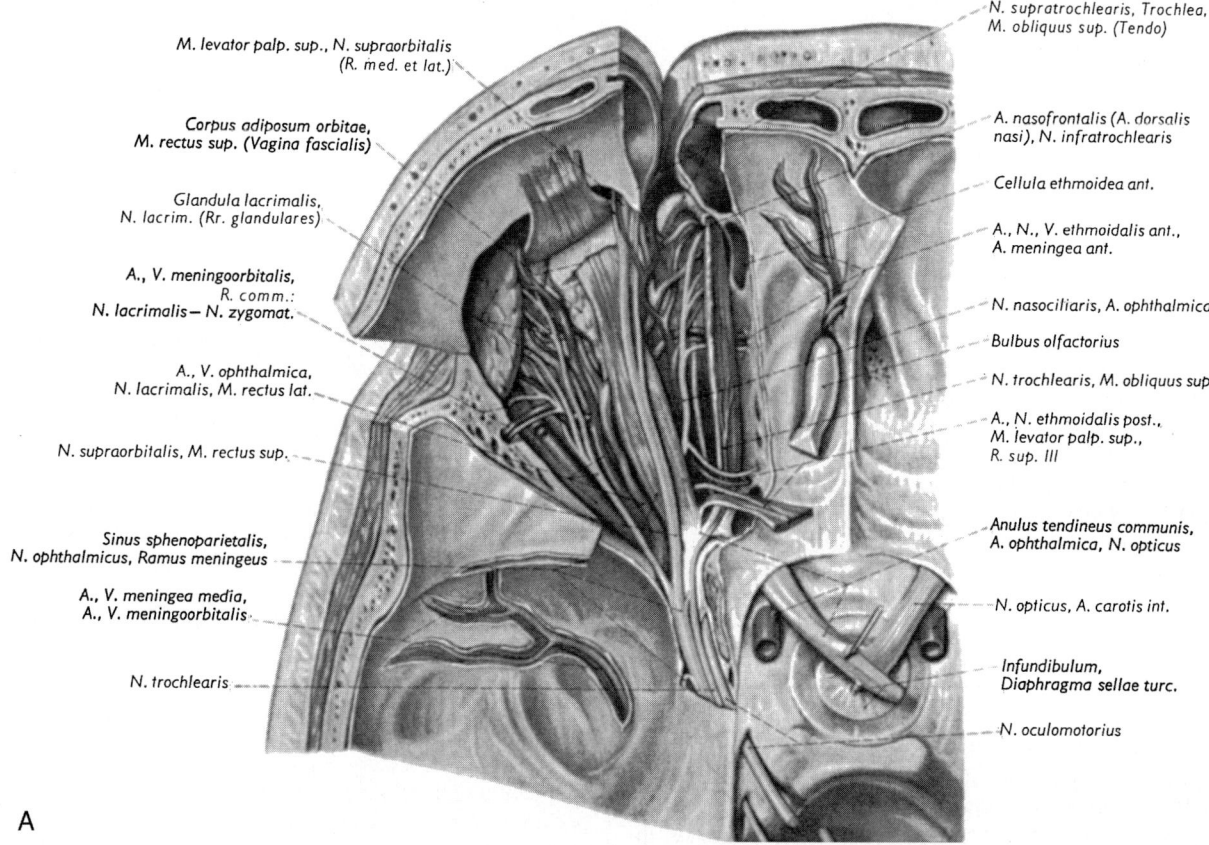

*M. levator palp. sup., N. supraorbitalis
(R. med. et lat.)*

*Corpus adiposum orbitae,
M. rectus sup. (Vagina fascialis)*

*Glandula lacrimalis,
N. lacrim. (Rr. glandulares)*

*A., V. meningoorbitalis,
R. comm.:
N. lacrimalis – N. zygomat.*

*A., V. ophthalmica,
N. lacrimalis, M. rectus lat.*

*N. supraorbitalis, M. rectus sup.*

*Sinus sphenoparietalis,
N. ophthalmicus, Ramus meningeus*

*A., V. meningea media,
A., V. meningoorbitalis*

*N. trochlearis*

*N. supratrochlearis, Trochlea,
M. obliquus sup. (Tendo)*

*A. nasofrontalis (A. dorsalis
nasi), N. infratrochlearis*

*Cellula ethmoidea ant.*

*A., N., V. ethmoidalis ant.,
A. meningea ant.*

*N. nasociliaris, A. ophthalmica*

*Bulbus olfactorius*

*N. trochlearis, M. obliquus sup.*

*A., N. ethmoidalis post.,
M. levator palp. sup.,
R. sup. III*

*Anulus tendineus communis,
A. ophthalmica, N. opticus*

*N. opticus, A. carotis int.*

*Infundibulum,
Diaphragma sellae turc.*

*N. oculomotorius*

A

**FIGURE 17–6 ■** *A,* Anatomic view of the orbital contents viewed from above. The tight space in the dorsal orbital cone is shown, with nerves, vessels, and tendinous muscle origins in close relationship. The superior orbital fissure is opened.

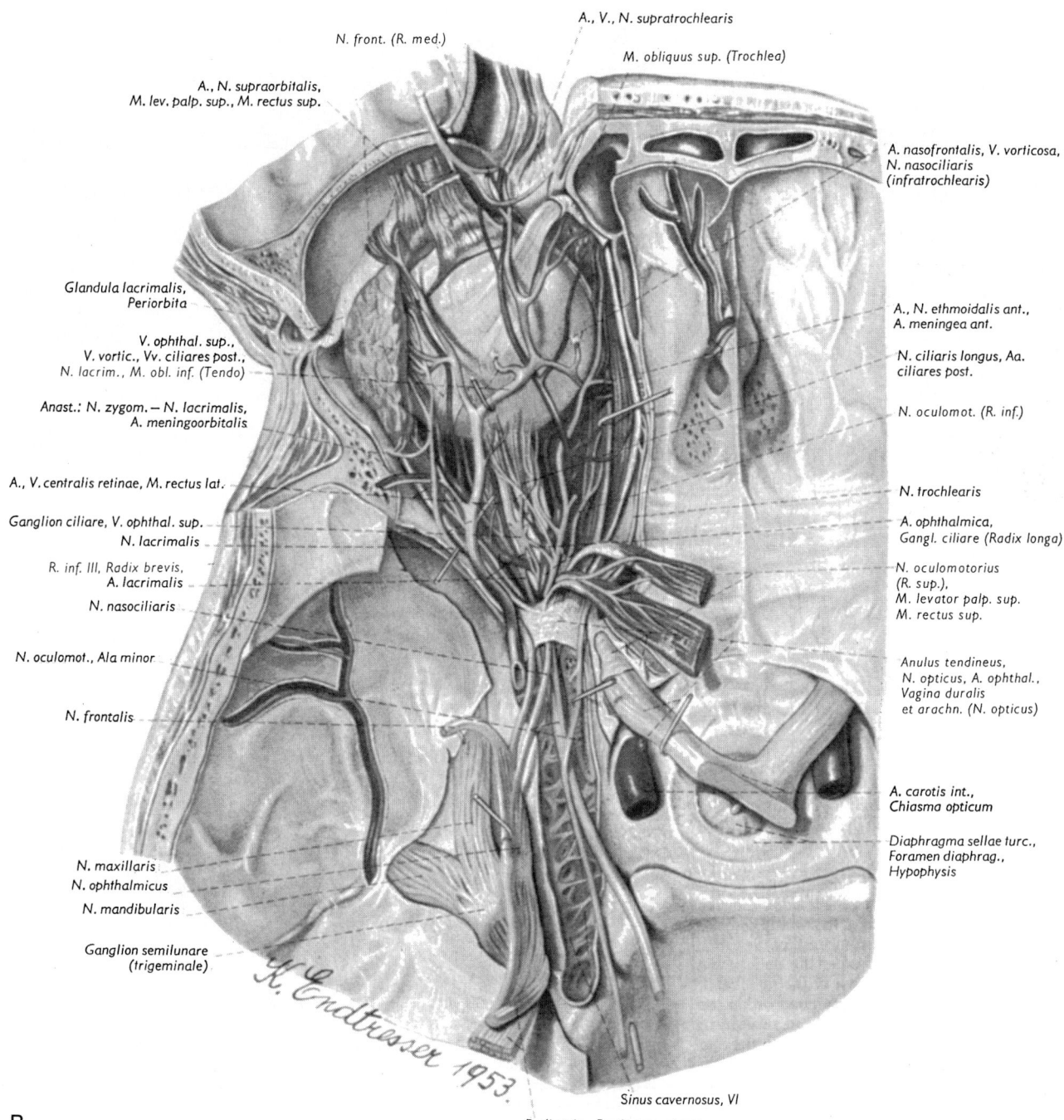

N. front. (R. med.)

A., V., N. supratrochlearis

M. obliquus sup. (Trochlea)

A., N. supraorbitalis,
M. lev. palp. sup., M. rectus sup.

A. nasofrontalis, V. vorticosa,
N. nasociliaris
(infratrochlearis)

Glandula lacrimalis,
Periorbita

A., N. ethmoidalis ant.,
A. meningea ant.

V. ophthal. sup.,
V. vortic., Vv. ciliares post.,
N. lacrim., M. obl. inf. (Tendo)

N. ciliaris longus, Aa.
ciliares post.

Anast.: N. zygom. – N. lacrimalis,
A. meningoorbitalis

N. oculomot. (R. inf.)

A., V. centralis retinae, M. rectus lat.

N. trochlearis

Ganglion ciliare, V. ophthal. sup.,
N. lacrimalis

A. ophthalmica,
Gangl. ciliare (Radix longa)

R. inf. III, Radix brevis,
A. lacrimalis

N. oculomotorius
(R. sup.),
M. levator palp. sup.
M. rectus sup.

N. nasociliaris

N. oculomot., Ala minor

Anulus tendineus,
N. opticus, A. ophthal.,
Vagina duralis
et arachn. (N. opticus)

N. frontalis

A. carotis int.,
Chiasma opticum

Diaphragma sellae turc.,
Foramen diaphrag.,
Hypophysis

N. maxillaris
N. ophthalmicus

N. mandibularis

Ganglion semilunare
(trigeminale)

Sinus cavernosus, VI

Radix trig., Portio sens. et mot.

B

**Figure 17–6 ■** *Continued. B,* The same anatomic view at a deeper level and with retraction of the levator palpebrae and superior rectus muscles (see also Fig. 17 8). (From Pernkopf E, et al: Atlas of Topographical and Applied Human Anatomy, 2nd ed. I: Head and Neck. Munich: Urban & Schwarzenberg, 1980.)

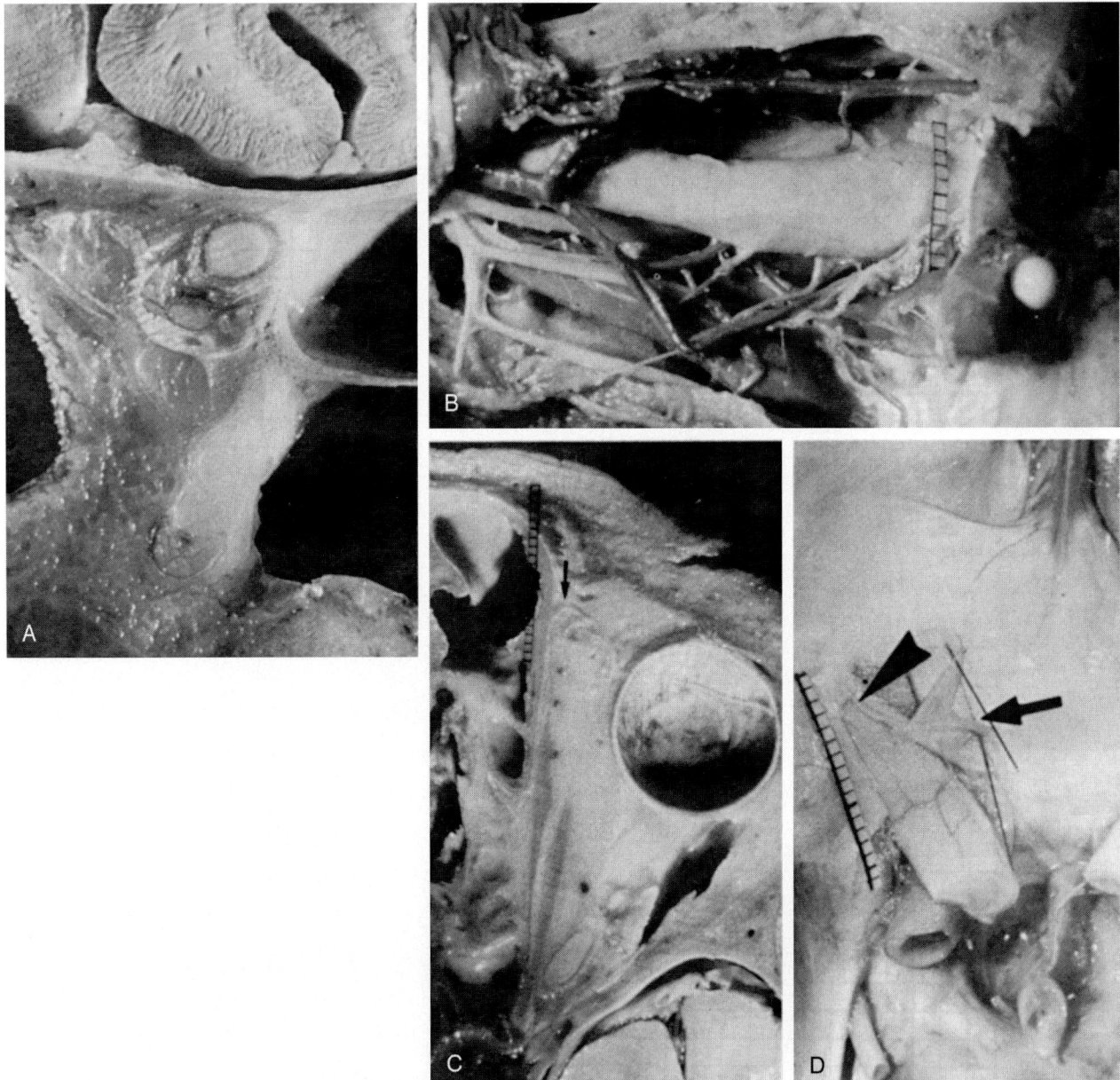

**FIGURE 17–7** ■ Anatomic dissections by Professor Johannes Lang, Head of the Anatomical Institute of the University of Würzburg. *A,* Coronal cut through the dorsal tip of the right orbit, which shows the optic nerve (above), the ophthalmic artery (middle), the oculomotor nerve (below), the trochlear nerve (middle), and the muscles. *B,* Lateral view of the optic nerve (right side), showing Krönlein's lateral approach to the orbit. From the left, the ophthalmic artery comes out of the canal, and some of its branches enter the optic nerve from below. *C,* Horizontal cut of the right orbit, the optic nerve, and the muscle cone within the dorsal orbital tip. Ventromedially in relation to the globe, the trochlea *(arrow)* is seen. In the case of simple superior medial orbitotomy, the trochlea is temporarily detached and refixed after tumor removal. (*A–C,* From Schürmann K: The development of orbital surgery from a neurosurgeon's viewpoint [Fedor Krause Memorial Lecture]. Adv Neurosurg 17:1, 1989.) *D,* Proximal view of partial unroofing of the left optic canal. *Arrow,* Dura mater of the anterior skull base. *Arrowhead,* Dura mater of the optic nerve.

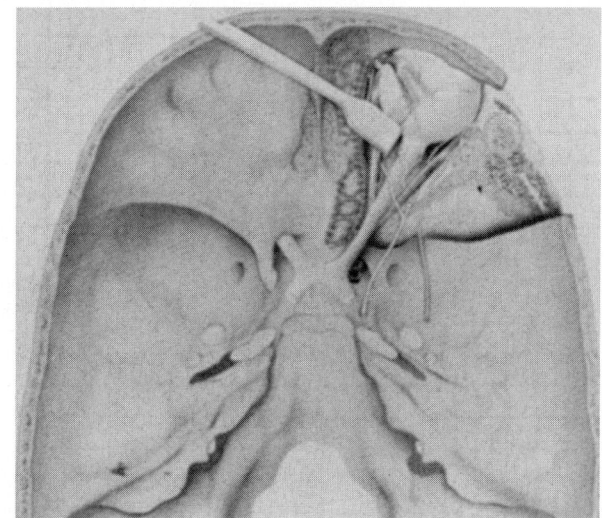

**FIGURE 17-8** ■ Bone resection provides an excellent view over the orbit and its contents. (From Schürmann K: The development of orbital surgery from a neurosurgeon's viewpoint [Fedor Krause Memorial Lecture]. Adv Neurosurg 17:1, 1989.)

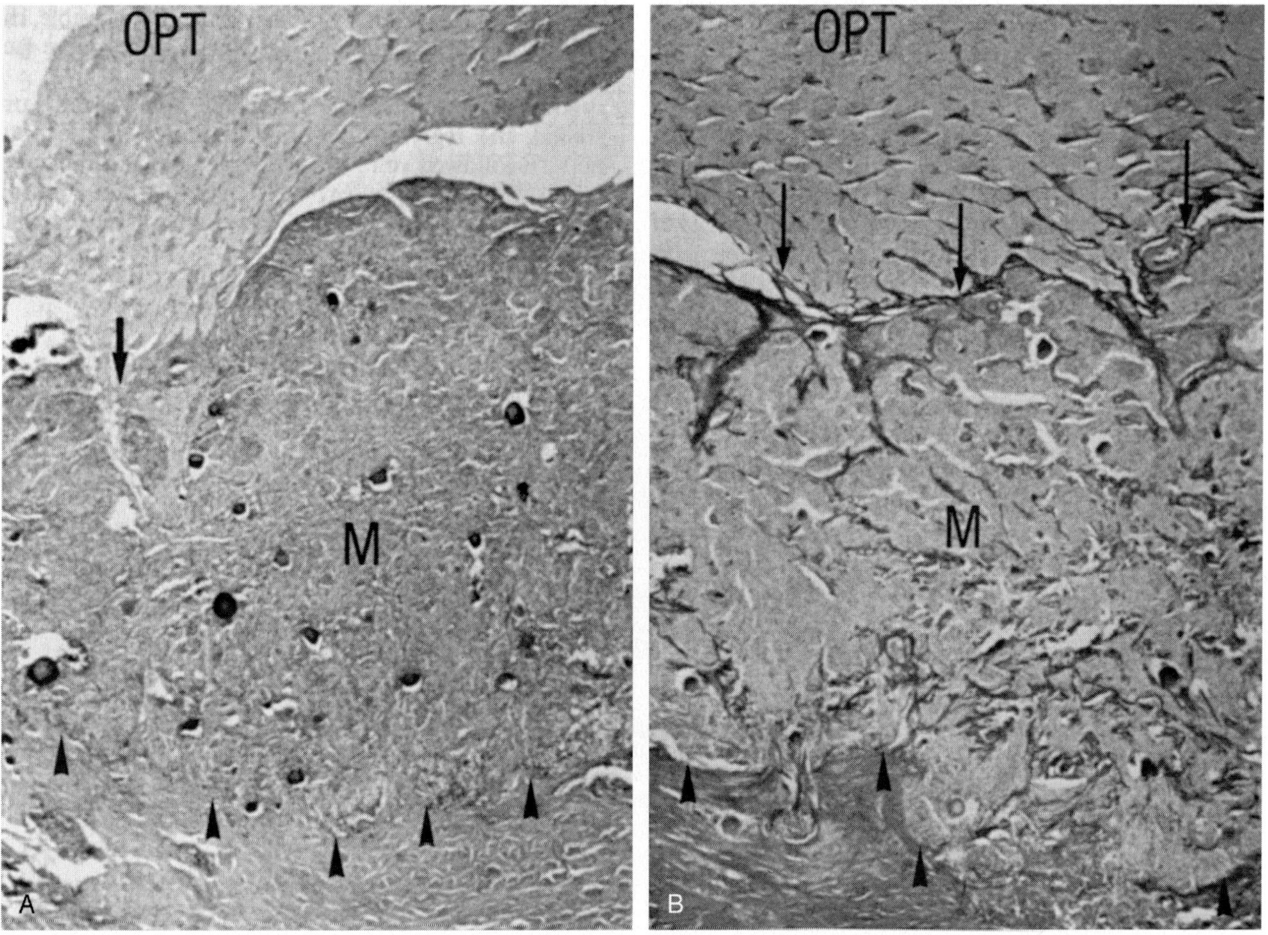

**FIGURE 17-9** ■ Primary optic nerve sheath meningioma, (endotheliomatous type). *A,* The tumor (M) compresses optic nerve (OPT) and begins to invade the nervous tissue *(arrow). B,* The tumor is tightly fixed to the dura mater *(arrowheads)* and to the optic nerve on the other side *(arrows).*

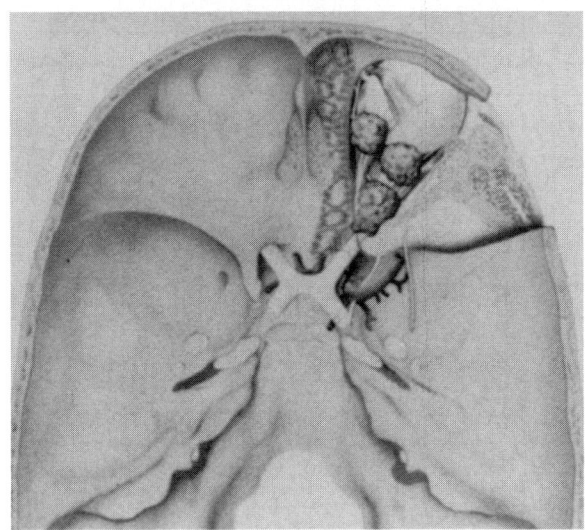

FIGURE 17–10 ■ Surgical sketch of an anterior and dorsal fungoid optic nerve sheath meningioma and a ventromedially located global meningioma. A surgical approach to the tumor within the dorsal tip of the orbit requires extensive bone resection to obtain adequate exposure. Such a procedure helps to prevent damage to functionally important elements.

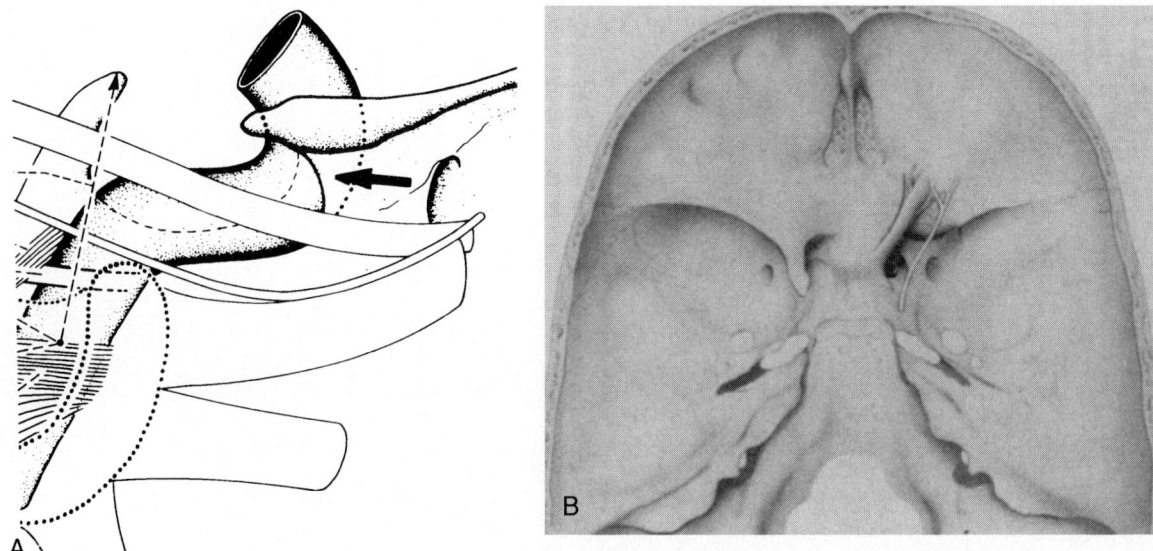

FIGURE 17–11 ■ A, Anatomic diagram of the right carotid artery in its intracavernous and supraclinoid course. The infraclinoid structure *(arrow)* is the anterior siphon knee, which is outside of the cavernous sinus between the clinoid process and the circular line. (From Perneczky A, et al: Direct surgical approach to infraclinoidal aneurysms. Acta Neurochir (Wien) 76:36, 1985, with permission. After Professor Johannes Lang, Head of the Anatomical Institute of the University of Würzburg.) B, Operative sketch shows the approach to the anterior siphon knee after resection of the anterior clinoid process and opening of the optic canal.

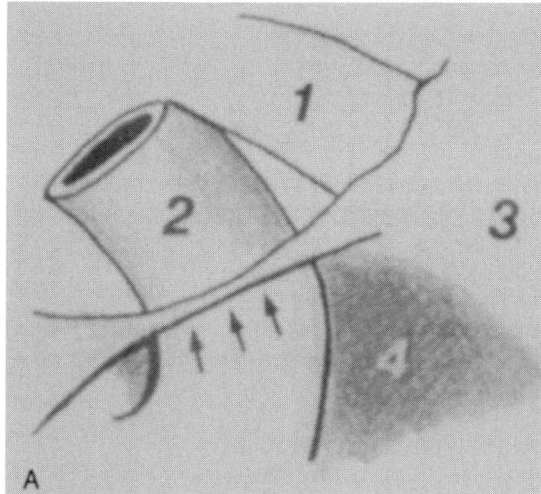

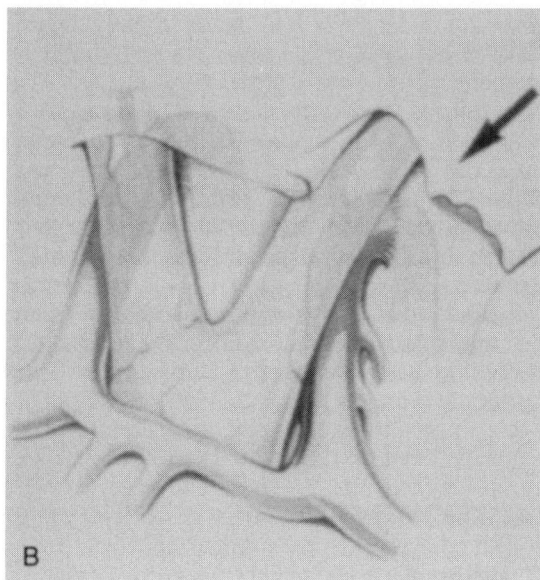

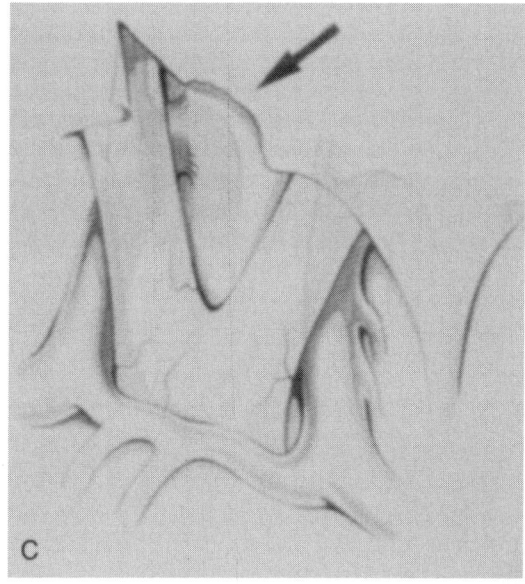

FIGURE 17–12 ■ Operative approach to the anterior part of the cavernous sinus and to the anterior knee of the carotid artery after resection of the anterior clinoid process on the right side. *A, 1,* Opening of the ipsilateral optic canal for mobilization of the optic nerve after splitting of its dural sheath. *2,* Removal of the anterior clinoid process. *3,* Identification of the upper wall of the cavernous sinus. *4,* Dissection of the fibrous ring around the carotid artery up to the anterior siphon knee. *B,* Ipsilateral approach. Space of 3 to 4 mm is usually present. *C,* Contralateral approach. Space of 3 to 4 mm is usually present. (From Perneczky A, et al: Direct surgical approach to infraclinoidal aneurysms. Acta Neurochir [Wien] 76:36, 1985.)

intradural approach was usually used to explore the orbit; on the average, this method required patients to have hospital stays of 3 weeks. After the switch to using the extradural approach to explore the orbit, the hospital stay was reduced to 8 to 10 days.

In my series of 436 cases of surgically treated space-occupying lesions of the orbit, craniotomy was used in 69%, lateral orbitotomy (Krönlein) in 19%, and simple orbitotomy in 12% of cases. Three postoperative deaths occurred among the cases from 1955 to 1963, when the intradural route was preferred. In two of these cases, the patients were elderly and had extensive malignant tumors. These patients were severely hypertensive and arteriosclerotic and suffered severe postoperative intracerebral hemorrhage, which was related to retraction of the frontal lobe.

One patient died on the third postoperative day, and one died on the fifth postoperative day. The third postoperative death was that of a 24-year-old man who had an extremely large spheno-orbital encephalocele, which caused marked anterior displacement of the internal carotid artery. This vessel was injured during the transfrontal craniotomy, which was performed to replace the brain that had prolapsed into the orbit back into the intracranial cavity. The injury to the internal carotid artery required immediate occlusion of this vessel and caused the patient's death several days later. Modification of the transcranial approach and use of the extradural approach to the orbit, combined with the improvements in anesthesia and in surgical techniques, resulted in no postoperative deaths in my series since 1963.

# CHAPTER 18

# Optic Gliomas: Their Diagnosis, Capacity for Spontaneous Regression, and Radical Surgical Treatment

■ WILLIAM H. SWEET and JUAN M. TAVERAS

The operative techniques for removal of the anteriormost tumor of the anterior visual pathways—optic nerve glioma—have been well established, following Dandy's pioneering efforts.[1, 2] His usual superb artist's drawings show why his transcranial approach to the orbit is the best, even for a purely orbital tumor requiring exposure from the globe to the optic canal. The 31 lesions whose treatments were reported in Dandy's two accounts were all neoplasms except for one inflammatory mass. Four gliomas arose in the anterior visual pathways—all large—and all patients died shortly after a partial tumor removal. One of these tumors, which extended from the orbit via the optic tract into the temporal, parietal, and occipital lobes, would have been recognized as inoperable today. The patients with the other three gliomas would probably have easily survived a biopsy or partial removal by today's vastly improved methods, especially for parasellar lesions requiring endocrine replacement during and after operation.

Evidence is steadily accumulating that indicates that gliomas of the optic nerve that arise in the orbit have enough potential for growth back into the chiasm that if they are to be removed, the posterior transection of the nerve should occur just in front of the chiasm, necessitating exposure of the suprasellar area, as emphasized by Dandy.

The growth rate of these tumors is one of the most variable of any in the human body, ranging from that of great malignancy to extremely sluggish growth, with the attainment of a steady state of little or no growth in a significant number of tumors arising in childhood. One or more episodes of substantial growth may punctuate these indolent growths, whereas others may become frankly malignant. Even a spontaneous decrease in the size of a few of these tumors has been unequivocally demonstrated. Those with a torpid course have led many observers to classify them as entering into a hamartomatous or nonneoplastic phase, in which they are presumed to persist, growing only at the rate of normal tissues. These phenomena are considered later. Extreme variations in advice for treating them have arisen, with the sole exception of those producing hydrocephalus; in these cases, all agree on the use of a shunt.

Gliomas of the anterior visual pathways are rare, occurring in 1 in 10,000 to 1 in 100,000 ophthalmic patients.[3] They occur so infrequently at any age that it was not until 1955 that Henschen[4] collected 180 cases from the literature and found that 39% arose before the age of 5 years and 60% before the age of 10. As diagnostic methods have improved, an even greater percentage in the young has become evident. Of Matson's[5] 23 patients younger than 17 years of age, 21 (91%) were younger than 9 years old—an important fact that sharply limits the dosage of radiation therapy, if used.

This chapter discusses (1) special diagnostic considerations, (2) decisive evidence against classifying any of the tumors as hamartomas, (3) evidence for an antitumor mechanism that may partially or even completely destroy the tumor spontaneously, (4) indications for radiotherapy, and (5) indications for radical surgery and methods for achieving it. A massive amount of literature on optic gliomas has developed that reflects the difficulty of predicting the course of this disorder and of generalizing from small numbers of cases.

## SPECIAL DIAGNOSTIC CONSIDERATIONS

### Calcification

Although the parasellar tumors most commonly showing calcification are craniopharyngiomas, calcification can also occur in optic gliomas. Schuster and Westberg[6] noted this in 5 of 25 operatively verified cases; Fletcher and colleagues,[7] in 3 of 22 cases (11 histologically verified); Bynke and colleagues,[8] in 1 of 10 histologically proven cases; Myles and Murphy,[9] in 2 of 20 cases; Kahn and colleagues,[10] in 1 case; and Weiss and colleagues,[11] in intrasellar and suprasellar areas in 1 of 16 cases. Calcification was present in 9 of 21 of our verified cases and was often identifiable only with computed tomography (CT) scans. A common misdiagnosis was craniopharyngioma. More surprising to us was perineoplastic calcification in extra-cerebral intradural fibrous tissue in two patients (cases 5 and 9, to be discussed later). Its presence was not associated with recurrence of tumor. In 16 patients whose tumors were irradiated by Fletcher and colleagues,[7] three of the tumors, all involving the optic tract, contained calcium. In two of these, the calcification was progressive in the lenticular nuclei and thalamus after radiation of 74 and 49.5 Gy. The clinical significance of this postirradiation calcification in the basal ganglia and elsewhere is uncertain. Such calcification was noted also in one of our patients and in one of three children treated by Beyer and associates.[12] Hypothalamic and frontal lobe calcification accompanied by a progressive memory and learning deficit developed in a 4-year-old child with a craniopharyngioma after exposure to more than 5000 rads.[13]

## Computed Tomography and Magnetic Resonance Imaging

The development of the third generation of CT scans around 1988 revolutionized diagnosis for many disorders, including intracranial tumors, as was documented in the second edition of this book. Representative ophthalmologists from six major units in the United States defined the CT differences between the two major intraorbital nerve tumors after study of 22 gliomas and 47 meningiomas.[14] The gliomas had a markedly fusiform shape (tapering toward each end) extending from the sclera to the orbital apex. They had a well-demarcated margin in 17 instances because they tend not to invade the dura. The meningiomas have a somewhat reversed shape, with a diffuse swelling of the nerve and an expansion posteriorly in 16 cases or anteriorly in 2 cases. Psammoma bodies gave rise to visible calcification in 10 of the meningiomas, whereas the calcospherites in gliomas are usually not so conspicuous as to create radiodensities. The intracranial optic gliomas present far greater diversity in size and shape, as illustrated in 22 patients, aged newborn to 12 years, seen by Fletcher and associates.[7] The commonest appearance seen in 10 patients was a globular expanded suprasellar mass that did not involve the intraorbital optic nerves, but any symmetric or, more often, asymmetric expansion of nerves, chiasm, or tracts may occur. All but 4 of the 22 tumors enhanced with contrast material; 2 of the 4 produced tubular expansion of both nerves and the chiasm, and the other 2 tumors were accompanied by optic tract calcification. Enhancement occurred in 6 of 10 cases reported by Byrd and coworkers.[15]

The fundamental concept of nuclear magnetic resonance was recognized by Gorter,[16] 40 years after Roentgen discovered the existence of the radiation named for him. Within less than a year, these emanations, soon called *x-rays*, swept into clinical medical uses and many other uses throughout the Western world. For example, a live demonstration of skeletal imaging was presented to a Bos-

ton medical society in April 1896.[17] The vastly greater complexity of using magnetic resonance resulted in a 40-year delay, until several groups produced the first images of human anatomy by magnetic resonance imaging (MRI) in 1976. A succession of steadily more superior instruments followed that used detailed conceptions of intricate subatomic behavior, including that of the enormous magnetic fields and the superconducting magnets required to produce them.

The development of MRI has mainly used the behavior of the hydrogen atom in its manifold relations to the other atoms of the body. MRI has the potential for imaging any odd-numbered isotope in the entire table of isotopes. Present devices have barely scratched the surface of what the biologic imaging center of the future may do. A fundamental feature of MRI behavior is the enormous inherent contrast that can be several hundred percent for two soft tissues. In an x-ray image, however, including that generated by CT, contrast is contingent on differences in the attenuation coefficients for two adjacent structures and is, at best, a few percent. Attenuation coefficients, which are related to electron densities, are roughly proportional to the atomic numbers of elements in biologic compounds. Fat, rich in carbon (atomic number 6), is more transparent to x-rays and is darker on CT scans than is water, richer in oxygen (atomic number 8).

As MRI techniques have continued to improve, their margin of superiority over CT has steadily increased. A rapid succession of technical MRI improvements and interpretive skills have made obsolete most articles published more than 10 years ago on CT and within an even shorter time on MRI. MRI has several specific advantages over CT in depicting gliomas of the visual pathways. Because MRI does not image bone, it presents no marked density to distort the registration of various grades of soft tissues, as occurs with CT. MRI tends not to induce artifacts at the orbital apex and demonstrates better the intracanalicular portion of optic nerve gliomas than does CT.[18]

MRI delineates the intraorbital and intracranial extent of tumor with excellent contrast and spatial resolution without the need for ionizing radiation. For example, in two of the optic nerve gliomas reported by Wright and colleagues,[19] both CT and visual evoked potential results were normal, and only MRI showed the chiasmal involvement. The absence of radiation hazards with MRI is particularly important in these tumors because of their predominance in the young and the frequent need to observe them serially. The rare, highly malignant optic glioma seen mainly in adults[20] may have a gelatinous interior and may present on CT scan as a low-density suprasellar mass with ring enhancement, leading to the mistaken diagnosis of cystic pituitary adenoma or craniopharyngioma.[21] MRI provides better visualization of the chiasm and is more sensitive to posterior optic pathway (optic tract, lateral geniculate body, and optic radiation) involvement than is CT.[22, 23] The multiplanar capability of MRI also permits excellent visualization of tumors and aids in the demonstration of the relationship of the mass to normal structures.[11, 24] This flexibility has eliminated the need for reformatting coronal and sagittal images in section CT, a process that entailed some loss of resolution.

Supplementary vascular imaging with magnetic resonance angiography can provide useful additional information on the status of the major intracranial vessels. Pulse sequences that allow for intraorbital fat saturation (fat-suppression technique) improve the detection of intratumoral contrast enhancement.[25]

The MRI appearance of intraorbital optic nerve glioma shows a peculiar feature of its histopathology, first described by Stern and coworkers.[26] In 18 patients whose optic nerve gliomas were accompanied by stigmata of neurofibromatosis type 1, 17 showed perineural arachnoidal gliomatosis surrounding the optic nerve. This condition results in a characteristic fusiform enlargement of an intraorbital optic nerve glioma. By contrast, in 14 of 16 patients without neurofibromatosis, the tumor grew exclusively intraneurally. In the series by Wright and associates,[19] however, this intraneural arachnoid hyperplasia was correlated more with active growth of the tumor, and no relationship existed between neurofibromatosis and pattern or grade of glioma. Typically the tumor is isodense to hypodense relative to white matter on $T_1$-weighted images.[27, 28] $T_2$-weighted sequences demonstrate a peripheral hyperintense signal surrounding a core of hypointensity.[28, 29] Enhancement of the intraorbital tumor is described as inconsistent, but the enhancement of pilocytic astrocytomas is generally intense, despite their being low-grade malignancies.[30, 31] Based on the work of Stern and coworkers,[26] the tumor would be expected to show more uniform signal changes on $T_2$-weighted images if most of the dilated optic nerve sheath is occupied by the expanded optic nerve without an associated perineural process.

Brown and colleagues[23] found MRI abnormalities of the posterior optic pathways in 10 of 21 patients; contrast-enhanced CT detected none of the lesions. In the absence of enhancement to indicate tumor involvement, the significance of these abnormal signal regions is uncertain, especially because pathologic correlation of posterior pathway abnormalities is rare. Chiasmal tumors tend to present as a hypointense mass lesion on $T_1$-weighted images and have an increased signal relative to brain parenchyma on proton density and $T_2$-weighted sequences. Enhancement with gadolinium chelated with diethylenetriamine penta-acetic acid (Gd-DTPA) increases contrast in certain pathologic tissues by speeding up hydrogen-proton spin-lattice relaxation, causing shortening of $T_1$. In one study, Gd-DTPA defined brain tumor margins better in 14 of 17 cases and depicted intraneoplastic vessels, necrosis, and cysts better than enhanced CT or unenhanced MRI.[32] One of the three optic gliomas in this study showed large vessels in the tumor only with Gd-DTPA enhancement, and the other two, chiasmatic gliomas, showed enhancement of residual tumor after surgery. Gd-DTPA does not cross the intact blood-brain barrier but leaks into any brain tissue in which the barrier is impaired with the shortening of $T_1$.[32]

Vascular encasement is not a feature of these tumors. Stenoses of branch vessels of the circle of Willis may be present in patients with neurofibromatosis type 1, however. Magnetic resonance angiography can be useful in determining the tumor relationship to vessels and in documenting vascular occlusive disease.

## Hemorrhage into Glioma of Optic Pathway

Four hemorrhages into an anterior optic pathway glioma had been reported by 1989.[33–36] CT scans showed them as high-density chiasmal or intraorbital masses. The lesions were: (1) bilateral optic nerve tumors with neurofibromatosis,[33] (2) glioma of one optic nerve and chiasm,[34] (3) glioma of the optic chiasm and both optic nerves,[35] and (4) cystic glioma of the optic nerve.[36] The case of the glioma of the optic chiasm and both optic nerves is of special interest because the patient's bilateral tumors had blinded her before an acute spontaneous hemorrhage occurred in one optic nerve. The chemical changes within an enclosed intracranial hematoma have been studied by MRI and indicate that the potential of the method has yet to be fully realized. The bleeding into this intraorbital retrobulbar glioma could be analyzed sequentially because no indication for surgical evacuation existed, and the complex evolution of the images during the chemical degradation of the hematoma could be observed by MRI. The right globe had been pushed forward by the large right retrobulbar nonhemorrhagic glioma, which had a predominantly medium signal intensity. The superiority of MRI over an immediately preceding CT scan was at once evident when the CT scan showed a linear streak of increased density across the mass that was diagnosed as a streak artifact from the density of adjoining bony orbit. MRI, not being affected by bone, is not beset by such distortions. Three days after an abrupt intraneoplastic hemorrhage, all but the center of the lesion was markedly hyperdense as a result of methemoglobin on MRI on both $T_1$-weighted and $T_2$-weighted images. MRI changes early after intracerebral or intraneoplastic hemorrhage included a central isointensity or mild hypointensity on $T_1$-weighted images and marked hypointensity in $T_2$-weighted images as a result of deoxyhemoglobin in still-intact red blood cells. There was also a fine, low-intensity black rim around the hematoma, especially on $T_2$-weighted images, that reflects early deposition of hemosiderin.[37] Six months later, the MRI scan of the high-signal methemoglobin area early after the bleed had reverted to the prebleed intensity. In addition, scattered, ring-shaped areas of low signal intensity existed—probably residual deposits of hemosiderin.

MRI is also a uniquely sensitive imager of the peculiar cerebral lesions associated with neurofibromatosis type 1 because it demonstrates high signal abnormalities on $T_2$-weighted studies not only in the optic nerve and chiasm, but also at times into both optic tracts and even both optic radiations.[22, 23, 38–40] Hyperdense areas similar to those seen in neurofibromatosis type 1 may be seen in a bewildering number of other cerebral sites—in basal ganglia, brain stem, and cerebellar peduncles[40] and in one or both sides of the optic chiasm, optic tracts, globus pallidus, cerebellar white matter, thalamus, and genu of internal capsule.[41] Several of these sites in each of four children aged 5 to 7 years were affected. In the absence of contrast enhancement, the significance of these widespread abnormalities outside optic pathways is uncertain. Cohen and coworkers[40] and Hurst and coworkers[41] believe that hamartomas and glial scars cannot be reliably differentiated from tumor, and no pathologic correlation with the widespread hyperdense zones exists. MRI is also the diagnostic imaging procedure of choice in neurofibromatosis type 1 for the investigation of seizures and mental retardation.

Stenoses of branch vessels of the circle of Willis may be present in patients with neurofibromatosis type 1, but vascular encasement is not a feature of these tumors. Magnetic resonance angiography can be useful in determining the tumor relationship to vessels and in identifying vascular occlusive disease.

The technical advances of MRI have been dramatic. The importance of communication between the referring physician and radiologist cannot be overemphasized, however, to ensure that an optimal examination is obtained.

## Visual Evoked Potentials

Visual evoked potentials is a valuable method for determining visual function in patients who cannot cooperate for studies such as testing of visual fields and needs wider usage, especially in children. The procedure consists of placement of occipital scalp electrodes as follows: two on each side, 2.5 and 5 cm from midline, and three in midline posteriorly—one at the inion, one 2.5 or 5 cm above, and one 5 cm below the inion. A reference electrode is placed 12 mm above the nasion.[42] Responses are measured to bright flashes (one 106 cd/m²) at a rate of 1 second and to a more complicated pattern reversal consisting of a black-and-white checkerboard whose squares have luminances of 8 and 227 cd/m². Pattern reversal stimulation is effected by rapid lateral displacement of the checkerboard through one square at a frequency of 10 msec per displacement. Flash responses are better preserved than pattern responses and are widely distributed across the occipital scalp; they are of no value in determining whether the chiasm is involved when standard tests show a lesion in only one eye.

Groswasser and coworkers[42] studied 25 patients aged 2 to 25 years who had optic gliomas and were followed 52 months. They illustrated many response patterns. In one patient, who was blind in one eye and whose visual evoked potential response pattern was initially normal in the fellow eye, abnormalities in this response preceded deterioration in all other parameters of visual function. A 6-year-old girl showed the following unusual sequence: On removal of the entire glioma-laden right optic nerve, its posterior end showed tumor cells but only on microscopic examination. She was followed for 5 years with 10 visual evoked potential studies. The first, 5 months before the tumor excision, yielded normal results in the left eye, but the next, which was performed 1.5 years later, and the seven studies thereafter during a 3-year interval all revealed electrical abnormalities in the left temporal field. A dramatic return to normal was seen at the final study 6 months later, indicating spontaneous recovery. Another 6-year-old girl exhibited a similar sequence of events but with somewhat less recovery.

The sensitivity of the method to detect progression of abnormality is illustrated by two patients seen by Wright and coworkers.[19] In their primary optic nerve gliomas, visual evoked potential evidence of chiasmal involvement preceded a succession of other signs. Likewise, Flickinger and associates[43] recorded visual evoked potential worsening in a 19-month-old child that led to a decision to treat rather than wait for the child to become older and more tolerant of radiation. Sensitive detection of improvement is also a feature of visual evoked potentials: Williams and colleagues,[44] using the visual evoked potential flash response

in a 13-month-old totally blind girl, demonstrated recovery. This response returned 6 weeks after the end of radiotherapy and before pupillary response to light and reaching for objects recovered. Majorchik and coworkers[45] found that the more caudad the spread of tumor, the more abnormal were the visual evoked potential components: prolongation of peak latencies, decrease in amplitude, and change of signal-to-noise ratio. These data also help distinguish glioma of optic pathways from other suprasellar tumors and inflammatory disorders.

## CONTROVERSIAL POINTS

### Optic Gliomas—Neoplasms or Hamartomas?

Do optic gliomas, which often start in early childhood, continue to grow, or do they "tend to enlarge, cause symptoms early in life, and remain static thereafter" so that "[e]xcision of the tumor is justified only for the relief of severe proptosis of a blind eye" because "[t]he tumor is non-neoplastic, self-limiting, and has a good prognosis for life"?[46] The quotations are from Hoyt and Baghdassarian's[46] study regarding 36 patients with chiasmal or optic nerve tumors (proved by biopsy in only 58%). As one of their examples, they cite the clinical course of three patients whose tumors in one optic nerve were present in the chiasm, causing no visual loss in the remaining eye (duration of follow-up not stated). The bases for this view have been augmented by Glaser and colleagues.[47] Miller and coworkers,[48] from the Wilmer Eye Institute of Johns Hopkins, studied 40 biopsy-proven optic gliomas, 11 of an optic nerve and 29 of the chiasm. They "agree that this type of tumor probably represents a congenital hamartoma of low potential morbidity."[48] Borit and Richardson,[49] of the Massachusetts General Hospital, also said with respect to all gliomas of the optic pathways, "our findings. . .are in general agreement. . .that the mortality and morbidity are much the same regardless of whether the patients have been treated surgically or by irradiation, or have received no treatment directed against the tumors." Wong and Lubow[50] reached similar conclusions after follow-up of 42 cases for 1 to 20 years. The prestige of these groups and the documentation they provided have given their views widespread credence. Three of our cases, with some of the longest follow-ups on record, present divergent answers about the self-limiting nature of these lesions.

### Case Report 1

The patient, a 3-year-old girl, underwent enucleation of the left eye and excision of some *glioma of optic nerve* (Fig. 18–1). Fifteen months later, further growth of the tumor extruded the glass eyeball implant. She underwent orbital exenteration of a glioma of optic nerve. Despite requests, the patient and her mother did not return until 22 years later. She came to her ophthalmic surgeon with a mass "slightly smaller than a tennis ball" protruding from the left orbit. Donahue[51] reported that the patient was leading a comparatively normal life 22 years after orbitotomy. She had gone

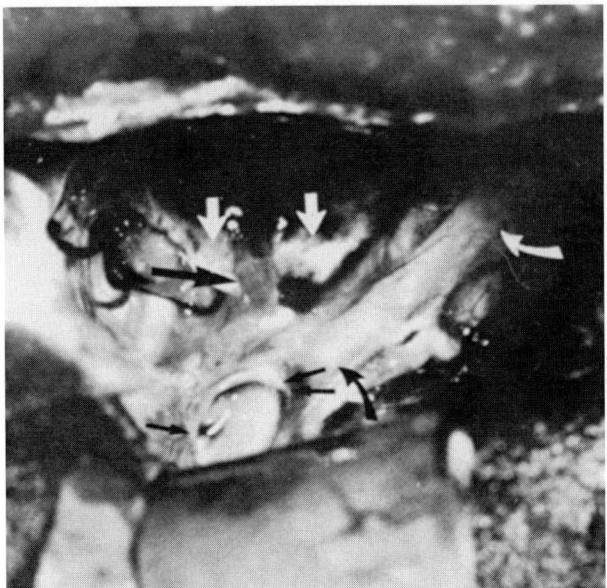

**FIGURE 18–1** ■ This intraoperative photograph shows the parasellar field after removal of the tumor in Case Report 1. An ovoid erosion in the lamina terminalis that discloses the interior of the third ventricle lies just posterior to the narrow strip of chiasm, the left side of which was virtually compressed out of existence and not attached to the tumor. All these structures are displaced markedly backward. (*Straight white arrows,* dorsum sellae; *large black arrow,* pituitary stalk; *small black arrows,* inferior rim of the hole in the lamina terminalis; *curved black arrow,* junction of the right optic nerve and chiasm; *curved white arrow,* anterior end of the intracranial portion of the right optic nerve.) Intact arachnoid covers the posterior communicating, posterior cerebral, and basilar arteries. The tumor capsule is separated easily from the normal structures, including, to our amazement, the chiasm.

through high school and secretarial school and was working in an office. She declined surgery. Sweet first saw her at age 32, when she inquired about a cosmetic procedure for her extruding orbital mass, mentioning as symptoms only occasional dizziness and loss of taste of food for 2 years. She declined study but returned at age 35, describing brief temporal lobe seizures, only about one per month for the previous 5 years, and consenting to hospitalization.

Examination showed a visual acuity of 20/40 in the right eye, with relative temporal hemianopia to dim light but full field to bright light. Calcification on skull films and a pneumoencephalogram outlined an additional subfrontal intracranial tumor the size of a grapefruit, 9 cm in transverse diameter. Sweet removed the intracranial tumor in one stage on September 3, 1965, and the posterior segment of the intraorbital mass 1 month later. He then placed a ventriculoatrial shunt on January 19, 1966. Casten, an ophthalmic surgeon, removed the remaining 5- × 6- × 6.5-cm anterior orbital part of the glioma on May 25, 1966. Removal of the intracranial tumor left the patient with a temporal hemianopia that precisely split the macula and a corrected visual acuity of 20/30. Six years after these operations, she was no longer experiencing seizures, was functioning well, and was supported by cortisone, levothyroxine (Synthroid), and phenytoin (Dilantin). She was lost to follow-up, and it was later learned

she had died from an infected shunt and ventriculitis on June 20, 1980, at age 50.

### Summary

A glioma initially of one optic nerve apparently grew steadily for 32 years until totally removed.

## Case Report 2

A 6-month-old boy underwent exploratory surgery by Mixter, assisted by Sweet, on February 18, 1941. A reddened right optic nerve was found, the pencil-sized enlargement of which extended back into the right side of the chiasm and optic tract. Examination of the biopsy specimen revealed a low-grade glioma. The boy was seen again 6 years later, having gradually lost vision in the right eye, with a sudden increase of the proptosis to an extreme degree for the previous 6 to 8 months. The ophthalmic surgeon removed the right eyeball and the orbital portion of the tumor on July 9, 1947. At that time, the patient's visual acuity was 20/200 in the left eye, and optic atrophy was present. He was followed up assiduously every few years by his ophthalmologist. The visual field and acuity remained stable for 34 years until 1981. A new superior altitudinal defect and a decline in visual acuity to 20/400 were then found, but these changes were not accompanied by certain changes on CT scans obtained in February 1982 and September 1983 or on an MRI scan obtained in February 1986. Greater resolution of the involved structures was provided by the MRI, however. Enlargements of the intraorbital parts of both optic nerves and of the slightly calcified chiasm were found (Fig. 18–2). The patient continues to work full-time and, with an almost stable intracranial status for 43 years, without treatment. Slight tumor growth may have occurred in the mid-1980s but did not further increase by the last follow-up in December 1992, 46 years after the last operation—exactly as predicted by the Hoyt group.

### Summary

A glioma initially of one optic nerve grew sporadically for 6 years, then remained virtually stationary with a visual acuity of only 20/200 in the remaining eye.

## Case Report 3

At age 4 years, the patient's grade I astrocytoma of one optic nerve that slightly invaded the chiasm was almost totally removed on March 17, 1947. Removal commenced from in front of the chiasm up to and including the globe, and the patient was given a tumor dose of 40 Gy of radiation. In the 26 days from April 8 to May 13, 1947, the patient had 30 fractions each of about 1.33 Gy given through five 4- × 5-cm portals: right and left lateral chiasms, anterior forehead, left orbit, and occiput. Radiation was given at 200 kV, 20 mA, Filteri 0.5 mm Cu, 1 mm Al, and at a tube-skin distance of 50 cm. Six years later, the tumor, now a grade II astrocytoma, completely refilled the orbit and extended on the left side as a gray carpet from beneath the left frontal lobe back to the

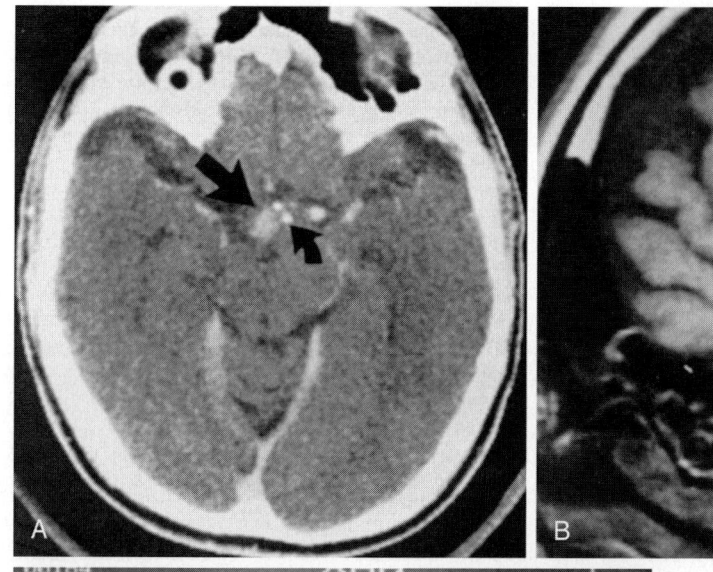
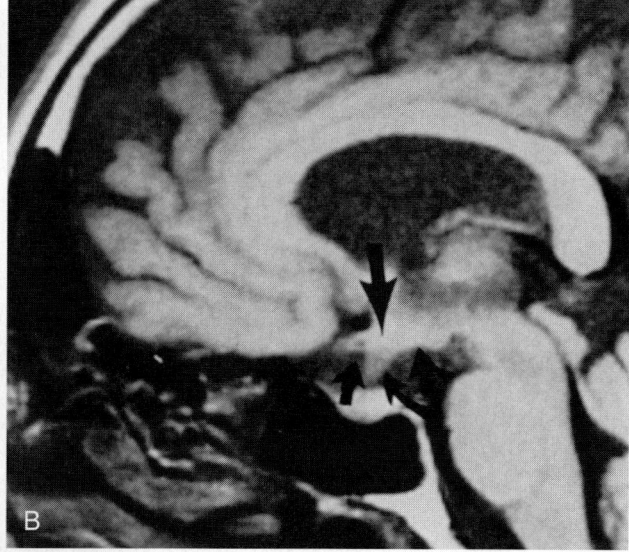
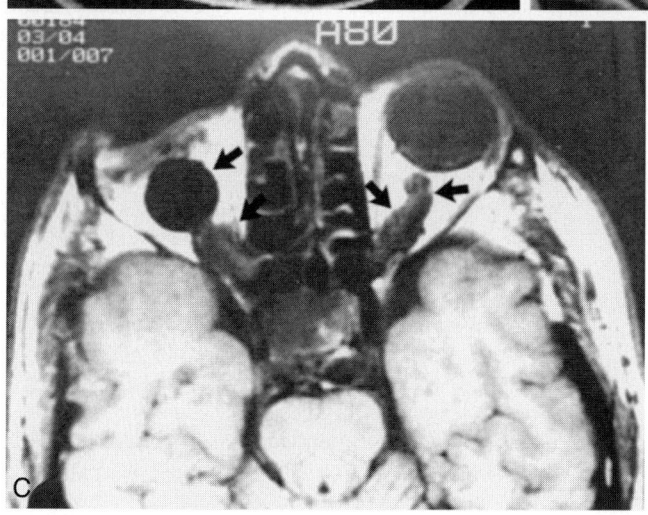

FIGURE 18–2 ■ Case Report 2. *A*, A Computed tomography scan, which was obtained on February 21, 1982, shows an enhancing tumor of the chiasm *(large straight arrow)* with two calcified globules *(small curved arrow)*. *B*, A magnetic resonance imaging scan that was obtained on March 31, 1986, shows a dense chiasmal tumor (three *large arrows*) and the less dense enlarged pituitary stalk *(arrowhead)*. Note the much less dense neighboring cerebrospinal fluid. *C*, A negative image of gliomas of each optic nerve is enclosed by dense images of periorbital fat.

hypothalamus, covering the internal carotid artery. The intraorbital portion only was removed on August 21, 1953, and the anterior intracranial portion was removed on November 4, 1953. Further radiation therapy was thought useless.

In the 40 years since then, the patient has remained nearly normal, including a normal visual field and acuity in the remaining eye. Her menses, sleep patterns, temperature regulation, and fluid intake and output were normal, but she has always been obese and now weighs 245 pounds, which is the only evidence of her hypothalamopituitary disorder. Closely spaced CT scans and MRI scans in 1987 showed no definite intracranial tumor. Its previous site, the suprasellar fossas, most of the intrasellar fossa, and the left subfrontal area were filled with cerebrospinal fluid. The left posterior orbital and intraorbital canalicular spaces contained tissue that was presumably non-neoplastic. Figure 18–3 shows an axial CT scan at the horizontal level of the proximal parts of the anterior and middle cerebral arteries as they appeared in January 1987. Figures 18–4*A* and *B* and 18–5*A* and *B* show comparable MRI sections from January 30, 1987, and September 18, 1993, and the

five parts of Figure 18–6 of essentially the same axial view displayed by five different techniques show remarkable preservation of normal structures in the otherwise empty basal cerebrospinal fluid cisterns of the middle cranial fossa.

### Summary

A glioma, initially of one optic nerve and slightly involving the chiasm, recurred massively despite removal of the nerve and 4000 rads of radiation at age 4. Extensive intracranial tumor was seen at operation 6 years later, then spontaneously disappeared almost completely for the next 34 years.

## Evidence for the Variable Growth Rate of Optic Gliomas

In 1912, Hudson[52] presented one of the first comprehensive discussions of collations of gliomas of the optic nerve that included 118 cases. His conclusion was that about 80% of optic nerve tumors were gliomas, and 20% were *endothelial tumors* (i.e., meningiomas of the nerve sheath). His statement is widely quoted, "in no single instance has a

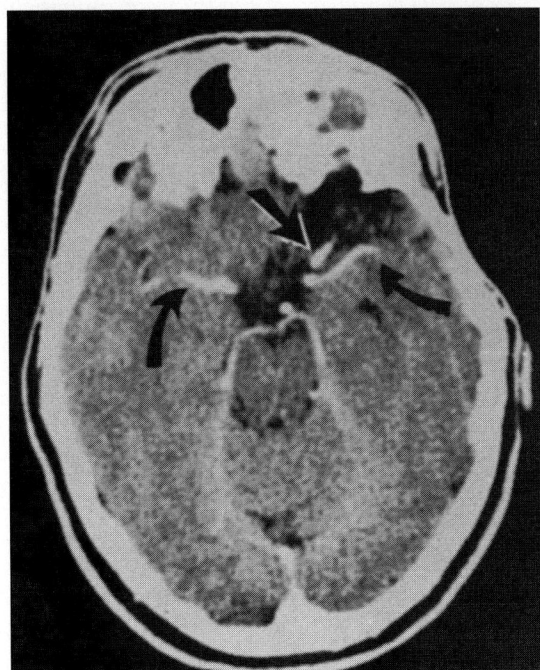

**FIGURE 18–3** ■ Case Report 3. A computed tomography axial scan with contrast taken on January 30, 1987, at the level of proximal portions of the middle cerebral and posterior cerebral arteries. In the suprasellar cistern and extending forward and to the left, note an empty space filled with cerebrospinal fluid at the previous site of a large tumor mass biopsied by Dr. J.C. White on November 4, 1953. This is about the same section as that of Figure 18–6, which was taken on September 18, 1993. (*Straight arrow*, anterior cerebral artery; *curved arrows*, middle cerebral arteries.)

recurrence of new growth in the orbit after removal of one of these tumors been recorded."[52] The tumors were incompletely removed in 51 cases; freedom from recurrence was noted in 13 cases from 3 to 24 years later. This result led Hudson to suggest that the process is a *degenerative gliomatosis* rather than a true neoplasm. Not as widely quoted but recognized by Dandy[53] were the findings in 23 autopsies reported by Byers[54] between 1901 and 1903 and by Hudson[52] on patients with intraorbital optic nerve gliomas. "In only one instance did the cranial cavity contain no tumor."[52] Fourteen of the patients died of meningitis a few days after removal of the orbital tumor, three died later of increased intracranial pressure, and five died of intercurrent disease.[52, 54] In Hudson's 15 autopsied cases, the intracranial growth affected one or both optic nerves with or without the chiasm and included neighboring brain in 5 cases. Recurrence of tumor caused death in six patients, and probable recurrence occurred in five others. Although 34 patients had a 1-year *cure*, follow-up reports at 6 years existed for only 6 patients. Fifty-seven of the patients had been followed up for less than 1 year. Hudson[52] stated, "The large size attained by the cerebral new formations without the production of severe symptoms has in several cases been very remarkable, and is to be attributed to the very slow rate of increase."

At the other end of the spectrum of growth rate are the relatively few malignant gliomas of the anterior visual pathways. Hoyt and associates[20] discussed 15 adult patients: 5 of their own and 10 more from the literature. The

patients were 23 to 59 years of age at onset, with an average age of 42 years. Since the publication of that article, at least 19 other articles have described malignant astrocytomas of the anterior visual pathways. Although most lesions have appeared in adults, Reese[55] described a grade IV and Brand and Hoover[56] a grade III optic glioma in infants. Helcl and Petraskova[57] had one anaplastic glioma in their 18 otherwise pilocytic optic astrocytomas in children. In addition, two Japanese reports were published of an aggressively growing type of optic glioma in infants.[58, 59] Of Kanamori and coworkers'[59] six patients 3 years old or younger at onset, three soon died, and a fourth was bedridden. These four tumors were histologically malignant and gave rise to severe hypothalamic dysfunction. Hoyt and Baghdassarian[46] also described two anaplastic astrocytomas as giant tumors in infants and five more *moderately anaplastic* gliomas in 12 children with chiasmal gliomas. Borit and Richardson[49] described a 9-month-old infant with neurofibromatosis whose bilateral tumor of both optic nerves and chiasm at surgery was hypercellular with many mitoses, killing the patient 2 years later. Heiskanen and colleagues[60] reported on two children whose initially benign optic gliomas underwent malignant transformation with extensive invasion of the frontal lobes. One had had early hypothalamic signs; the first signs in the other child were visual. Wilson and associates[61] reported on the case of a 7-year-old girl given 56.7 Gy in 6 weeks for her tumor. The patient died at age 27 with benign gliomatous areas in her visual pathways that became anaplastic in the massive basal spread of the lesion. At postmortem, no features of radiation effect were identified. These reports further emphasize the potential for erratic and dangerous growth of these lesions at all ages.

A *hamartoma*, as defined in *Stedman's Medical Dictionary*, 21st edition, is a "malformation resembling a neoplasm but developing and growing at virtually the same rate as normal components and not likely to result in compression of adjacent tissue." Similar definitions are given in other dictionaries. This definition simply does not fit the tumors in question, which at some phase all grow faster than does the child, similar to true neoplasms, for a long or a short time, compressing or invading the optic pathways. By 1902, five publications described the recurrence of a glioma of one optic nerve after intraorbital excision (see Table 18–6).[54, 62–65]

We see no justification from that era or thereafter for referring to gliomas as *hamartomas*, a term that lulls the physician into a false sense of security with regard to the growth potential of the lesion. Hoyt's colleagues, Anderson and Spencer,[66] described three "mechanisms for enlargement of the tumor": (1) proliferation of tumor cells, (2) hyperplasia of surrounding tissues, and (3) accumulation of mucin within the tumor.

In the past 6 years, further crushing refutations have arisen about the hamartoma concept, with the conclusions that neither radiation nor surgery is of value in the slowly growing or nonchanging optic gliomas seen principally in childhood. These refutations apply also to nearly all of the slowly growing subgroup described by Wright and colleagues.[19] The most comprehensive of these rebuttals is that of Alvord and Lofton,[67] who subjected to statistical analysis[68, 69] the results in 425 chiasmal tumors and 198

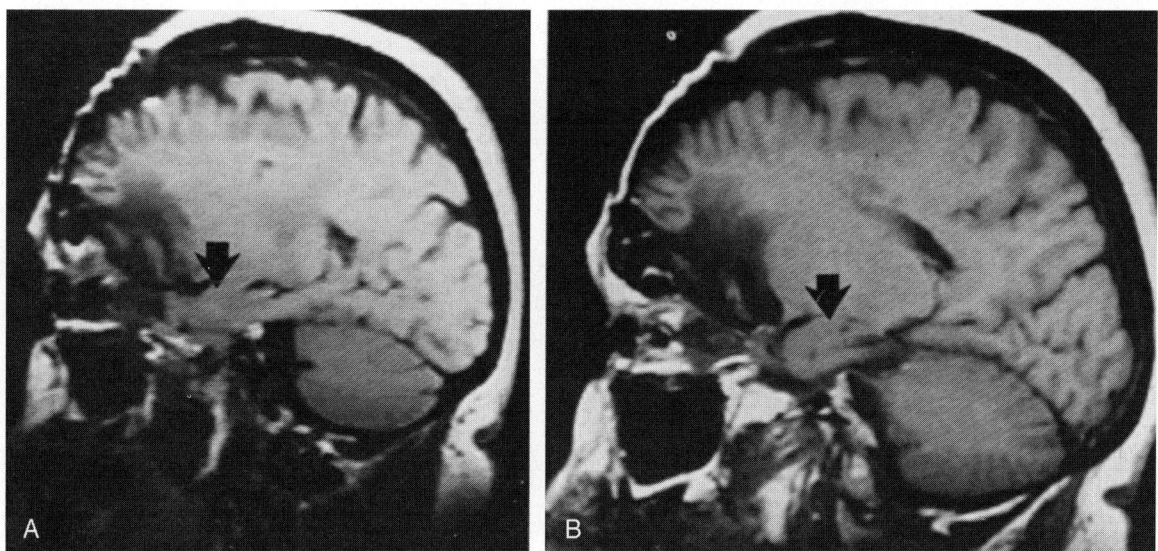

**FIGURE 18–4** ■ *A*, A magnetic resonance imaging (MRI) scan, 0.3 Tesla, taken January 30, 1987, T1, TR 575, TE 30, 4 mm thick through the temporal horn of the left ventricle. *B*, An MRI scan, 1.5 Tesla, taken September 18, 1993, T1, TR 600, TE 16, 3 mm thick through the temporal horn of the left ventricle. The huge left subfrontal area, which is filled almost completely with cerebrospinal fluid, now replaces in its posterior portion the large tumor that had grown forward from the left optic nerve and chiasm (according to the operative note of Dr. White, dated November 4, 1953). The temporal lobe is indicated by *closed arrows*.

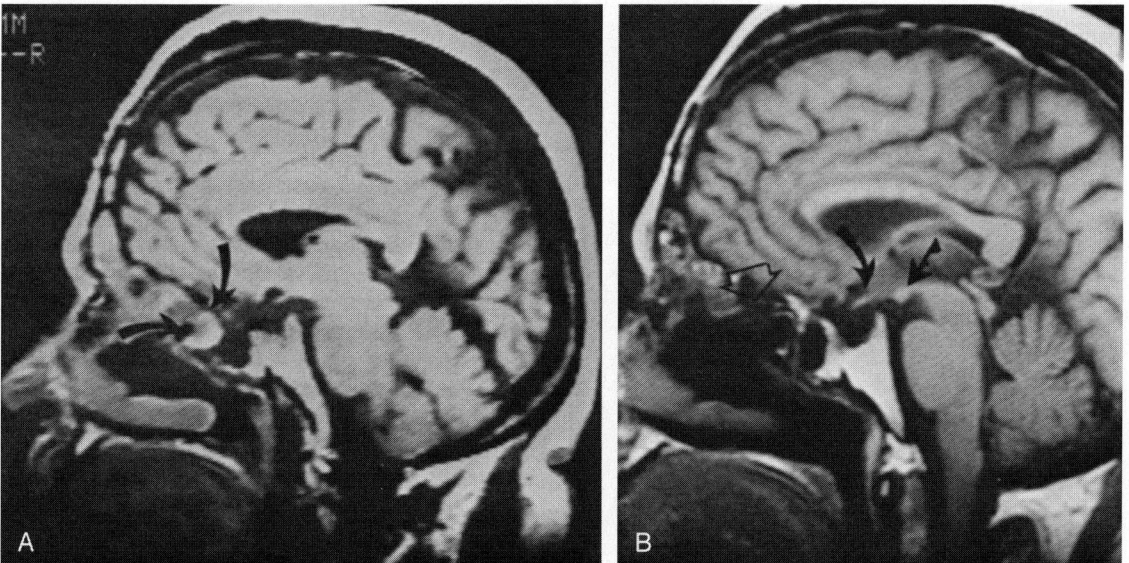

**FIGURE 18–5** ■ *A*, A magnetic resonance imaging (MRI) 0.3 Tesla magnet, taken on January 30, 1987, T1, TR 575, TE 30, slice 4 mm thick. *B*, MRI 1.5 Tesla magnet, taken on September 18, 1993, T1, TR 600, TE 16, slice 3 mm thick.

These virtually identical sections were taken 6.7 years apart. The most dramatic difference is the complete absence in *B* of the hyperintense concavoconvex mass beneath the frontal lobe outlined by the *curved arrows* in *A*. The corresponding empty space in *B* is indicated by the *closed arrowhead*. In front of the mass in *A*, one sees the ethmoid sinus and, further anterior, the frontal sinus filled with mucus. An ethmoidectomy had been carried out a few months before *B*, which shows the sinuses. (*Small straight arrow*, mammillary body dipping into the prepeduncular cistern; *small curved arrow*, optic chiasm and tract dipping into the suprasellar cistern; *open arrowhead*, site of a tumor 80 months earlier.)

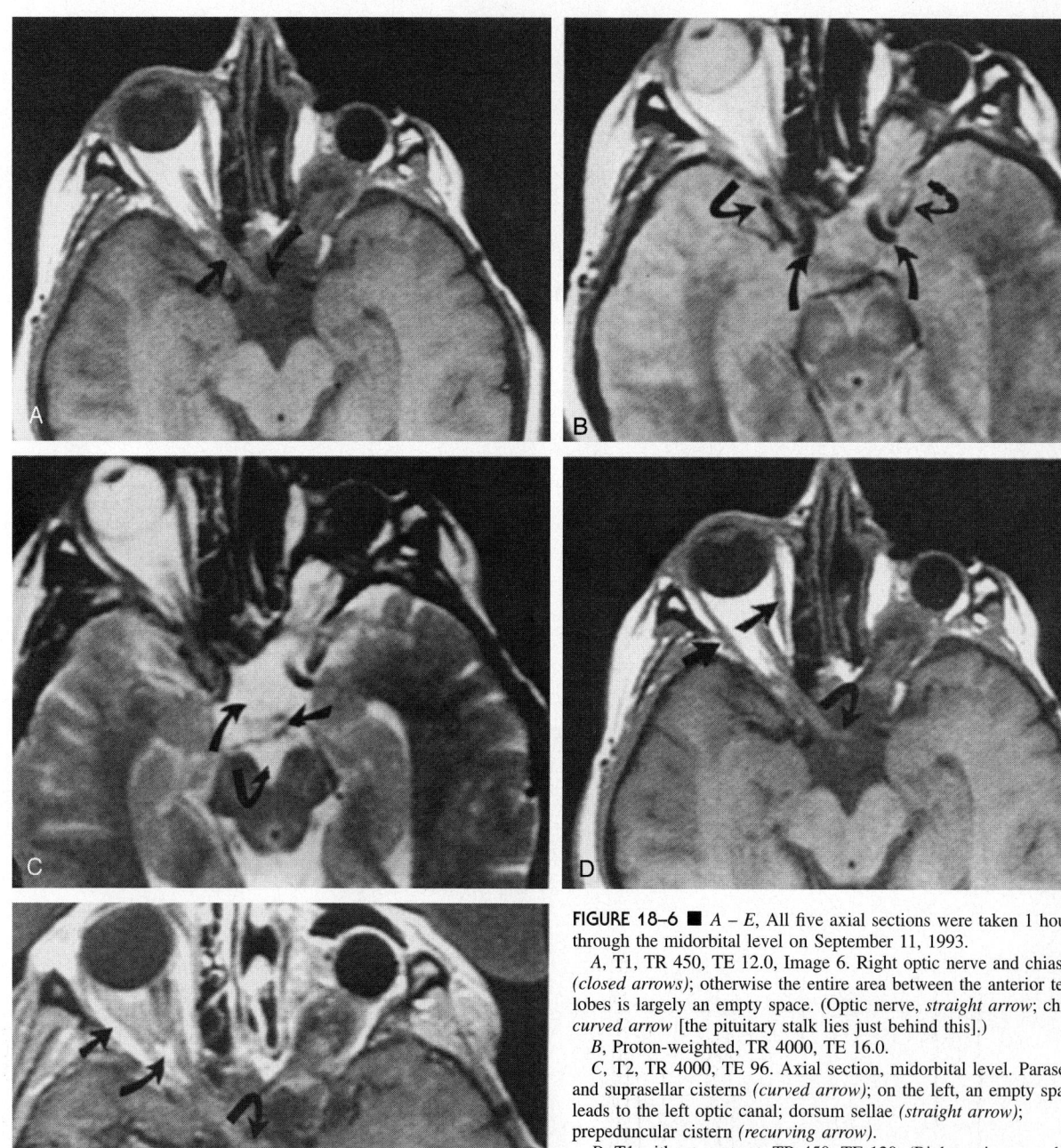

**FIGURE 18–6** ■ *A – E,* All five axial sections were taken 1 hour through the midorbital level on September 11, 1993.

*A,* T1, TR 450, TE 12.0, Image 6. Right optic nerve and chiasm *(closed arrows);* otherwise the entire area between the anterior temporal lobes is largely an empty space. (Optic nerve, *straight arrow;* chiasm, *curved arrow* [the pituitary stalk lies just behind this].)

*B,* Proton-weighted, TR 4000, TE 16.0.

*C,* T2, TR 4000, TE 96. Axial section, midorbital level. Parasellar and suprasellar cisterns *(curved arrow);* on the left, an empty space leads to the left optic canal; dorsum sellae *(straight arrow);* prepeduncular cistern *(recurving arrow).*

*D,* T1 without contrast, TR 450, TE 120. (Right optic nerve, hilt of the *recurving arrow;* right optic chiasm, point of the *recurving arrow;* right intraorbital white, *black arrow;* right retrobulbar group lateral streaks, muscle; central streak, optic nerve.)

*E,* T1 with gadolinium diethylenetriaminepentaacetic acid (Gd-DTPA) contrast. Right optic nerve, hilt of the *recurving arrow;* chiasm, point of the *recurving arrow.* Note that chiasm and nerve are larger in Gd-DTPA images than in noncontrast images. (Pituitary stalk, *arrowhead;* peripheral intraorbital, *long white streaks;* lateral and medial rectus muscles, *straight arrows* [muscles take up contrast]; apical stump remainder of extraocular muscles, *curved arrow.*) Note that there is no intracranial increased uptake anywhere.

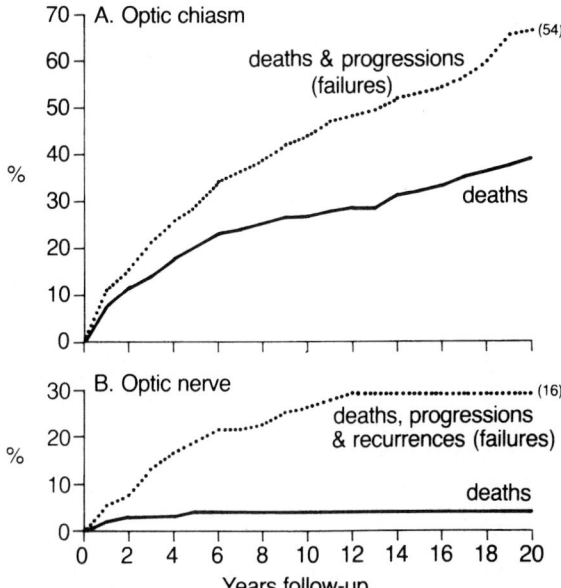

FIGURE 18–7 ■ Actuarial data showing the percentage of deaths, recurrences and progressions of gliomas, almost all astrocytomas of the anterior visual pathways. The numbers at the end of the failure lines indicate the percentage of deaths among the failures. All tumors involving the chiasm (468) are included in this figure. There were 155 gliomas of the optic nerve only when the patient was first seen. (From Alvord EC, Lofton S: Gliomas of the optic nerve or chiasm: Outcome of patients' age, tumor site, and treatment. J Neurosurg 68:85–95, 1988.)

The top of Figure 18–9 compares actuarial survival and the bottom of Figure 18–9 compares actuarial relapse-free survival in patients with tumors of the optic nerve with survival in patients with tumors of the chiasm. Alvord and Lofton[67] also found that complete surgical excision of optic nerve gliomas was better than irradiation. No recurrence is on record in any patient in whom no tumor was seen microscopically in the posterior face of the nerve cut just in front of the chiasm.

In the study by Flickinger and colleagues,[43] actuarial survival for 25 patients whose tumors were confined to the optic nerve was 100% at 5, 10, and 15 years and for tumors involving the chiasm was 93%, 88%, and 88% at 5, 10, and 15 years. Actuarial survival in 25 patients irradiated for biopsy-proven chiasmal gliomas was 96%, 90%, and 90% at 5, 10, and 15 years. Actuarial progression-free survival in this same group of 25 was 87% at 5, 10, and 15 years, and stabilization or improvement in vision occurred in almost the same 86% of patients. In patients with chiasmal tumors, 100% of those radiated with more than 4500 cGy enjoyed actuarial progression-free survival, whereas only 62% of those given less than 4500 cGY had progression-free survival. The value of radiation was shown more explicitly by Wong and colleagues[70] because they had an unradiated control group. Of their 27 patients with chiasmal tumors, 7 were not irradiated, and 6 of them

tumors with clinical involvement of the intraorbital portion of the optic nerve. They included in the chiasmal group 43 *dumbbell* tumors also involving the optic nerve, the entire lot culled from 107 publications. Figure 18–7 shows a continuing, although decelerating, growth rate in both groups. Figure 18–8 compares actuarial relapse-free survival rates in patients with chiasmal gliomas whose tumors were irradiated with the rates in patients whose tumors were not. The radiation is valuable to promote survival.

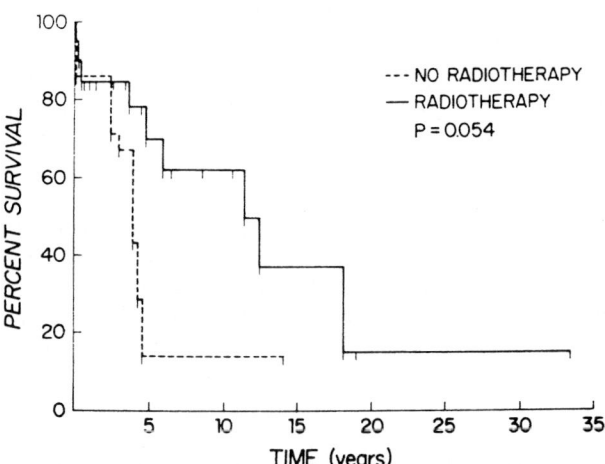

FIGURE 18–8 ■ Actuarial relapse-free survival with and without therapy for patients with chiasmal glioma. (From Wong JYC, Uhl V, Wora WM, et al: Optic gliomas: A reanalysis of the University of California, San Francisco experience. Cancer 60:1853, 1987. Copyright © 1987 American Cancer Society. Reprinted by permission of Wiley-Liss, Inc., a subsidiary of John Wiley & Sons, Inc.)

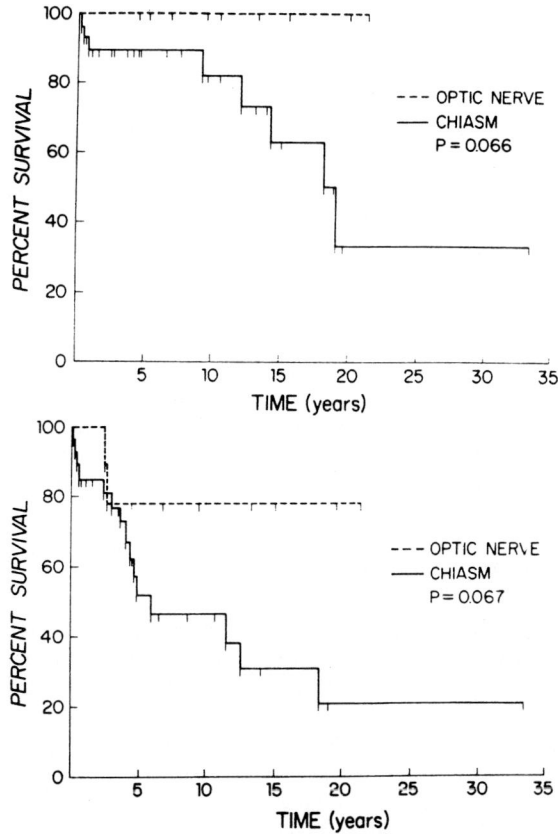

FIGURE 18–9 ■ *Top*, Actuarial survival versus tumor location. *Bottom*, Actuarial relapse-free survival versus tumor location. (From Wong JYC, Uhl V, Wora WM, et al: Optic gliomas: A reanalysis of the University of California, San Francisco experience. Cancer 60:1852, 1987. Copyright © 1987 American Cancer Society. Reprinted by permission of Wiley-Liss, Inc., a subsidiary of John Wiley & Sons, Inc.)

did not respond to therapy. Only 9 of 20 patients in the irradiated group did not respond to therapy. This article includes the work of the late distinguished radiation oncologist Sheline and comes from the same institution as that of the Hoyt group, the University of California at San Francisco. Its cases overlap those of Hoyt and colleagues, and the authors point out that orthovoltage radiation was used for the earlier Hoyt cases in the 1940s, whereas in the Wong series, the use of megavoltage levels probably accounts for the discrepant results.

The specific question of whether or not the slowly changing optic gliomas are tumors has been addressed by a new technique derived from the concept that in the nucleolus, a specialized area called the *organizer region* exists whose proteins may be impregnated with colloidal silver for histologic quantification. The features of the silver impregnation of the nucleolar organizing regions (AgNORs) permit assessment of growth potential by their size, number, and morphology. Cell proliferation rate measured with $^3$H-thymidine has shown a linear relationship with the amount of AgNOR proteins in 12 different types of human tumor cell lines from various parts of the body.[71]

A report on AgNOR counts per nucleus in 305 surgical specimens of meningiomas divided them into two atypical faster-growing types and two more numerous slow-growing types. The mean AgNOR counts in the former group were 2.73 0.12 and 2.91 0.18; in the latter two groups they were 1.41 0.34 and 1.38 0.31. These substantial differences permit one to predict which tumors require more vigilance.

In an article by Burnstine and colleagues,[73] AgNOR was counted in 31 optic gliomas, 14 optic nerve meningiomas, and 1 giant cell glioblastoma of the optic chiasm. The optic gliomas contained 2.0 0.09 AgNOR per nucleus, and the optic nerve meningiomas 2.15 0.15 per nucleus, counts similar to those reported (2.22 0.1) in 12 diffuse grade II fibrillary astrocytomas.[74] The counts in all three groups were significantly higher than the 1.15 0.02 counts in 14 cases of reactive astrocytes. The glioblastoma count in these cases was 2.91. In a group of cerebellar and hypothalamic pilocytic astrocytomas, there were 2.00 0.40 AgNOR counts per nucleus. Burnstine and colleagues[73] concluded that these data "suggest that optic gliomas may be true neoplasms." The presence of compound AgNORs also distinguishes benign from various malignant processes.[74]

## Neurofibromatosis

The abnormal cells in neurofibromatosis type 1 differ in several ways from those in pure gliomas. With respect to excessive glial non-neoplastic growth in the anterior visual pathways, there are a few reported cases of neurofibromatosis in which one or both optic nerves became diffusely thickened as a consequence of proliferation of astrocytic, arachnoidal, and other connective tissue elements.[75] Such an unusual patient typically has neurofibromatosis, enlarged optic canals, and pallor of the optic disks but no visual complaints or visual field loss.[76] Two patients described by Pfeiffer[77] and Reese[78] were 44 and 40 years of age; the disorder had presumably been present for decades. Both authors described enlarged optic foramens without loss of vision in the presence of neurofibromatosis.

We describe here the case of patient in whom the diagnosis of probable tumor rather than hyperplasia in the visual pathways was made, even though she had no visual complaints.

### Case Report 4*

The patient, aged 14, with the cutaneous stigmata of neurofibromatosis, had a similarly affected mother in whom a glioma of one optic nerve had been removed 10 years previously. The patient's visual fields showed the scotomas illustrated in Figure 18–10, of which the asymptomatic patient was unaware. CT (Fig. 18–10A–C) demonstrated a tumor in the chiasm and at least one optic nerve. By August 1986, the scotoma in the left eye was larger and denser than in July 1985. This loss receded, however, and a succession of five visual field analyses on the sensitive Humphrey automated perimeter from February 1985 to August 1987 showed no statistically significant change in the visual fields.

Careful follow-up was also the course of action chosen by Horwich and Bloom[79] for a similar patient with von Recklinghausen's disease, a tumor in one optic nerve, and no evidence of progression of disease.

### Case Report 5

In a patient with neurofibromatosis, the right optic nerve, which contained a glioma, was removed from the chiasm to the globe when the patient was 34 months old in 1971. The visual field and acuity of the left eye were normal in 1975. Although he was totally asymptomatic and free of all neurologic deficits except those in his visual system, follow-up studies at age 17 revealed a quadrantic temporal field defect in the left eye, and CT scans and MRI showed three large tumors in the third ventricle and right and left cerebellar hemispheres (Fig. 18–11A–C). In addition, MRI revealed at least seven tiny nodules of indeterminate (astroglial?) nature scattered bilaterally in the frontal lobe white matter (Fig. 18–11C shows two of these). Martuza removed the large left cerebellar astrocytoma, and radiation therapy was given to the chiasmal region.

Horwich and Bloom[79] described another patient with von Recklinghausen's disease whose bilateral optic nerve gliomas were treated by radiation. Thirty-one years later, the patient had developed four other intracranial tumors, including a large grade III astrocytoma of the thalamus. Lewis and coworkers,[80] in radiologic studies including CT scans on 207 patients diagnosed as having von Recklinghausen's neurofibromatosis, found tumors of the anterior visual pathways in 15%. In two thirds, such lesions were not suspected either from the patient's history or from ophthalmologic examination. Aron and coworkers[39] reported on two more unsuspected chiasmal lesions detected on CT scans in such patients.

---

*Case provided by Robert Martuza, M.D.

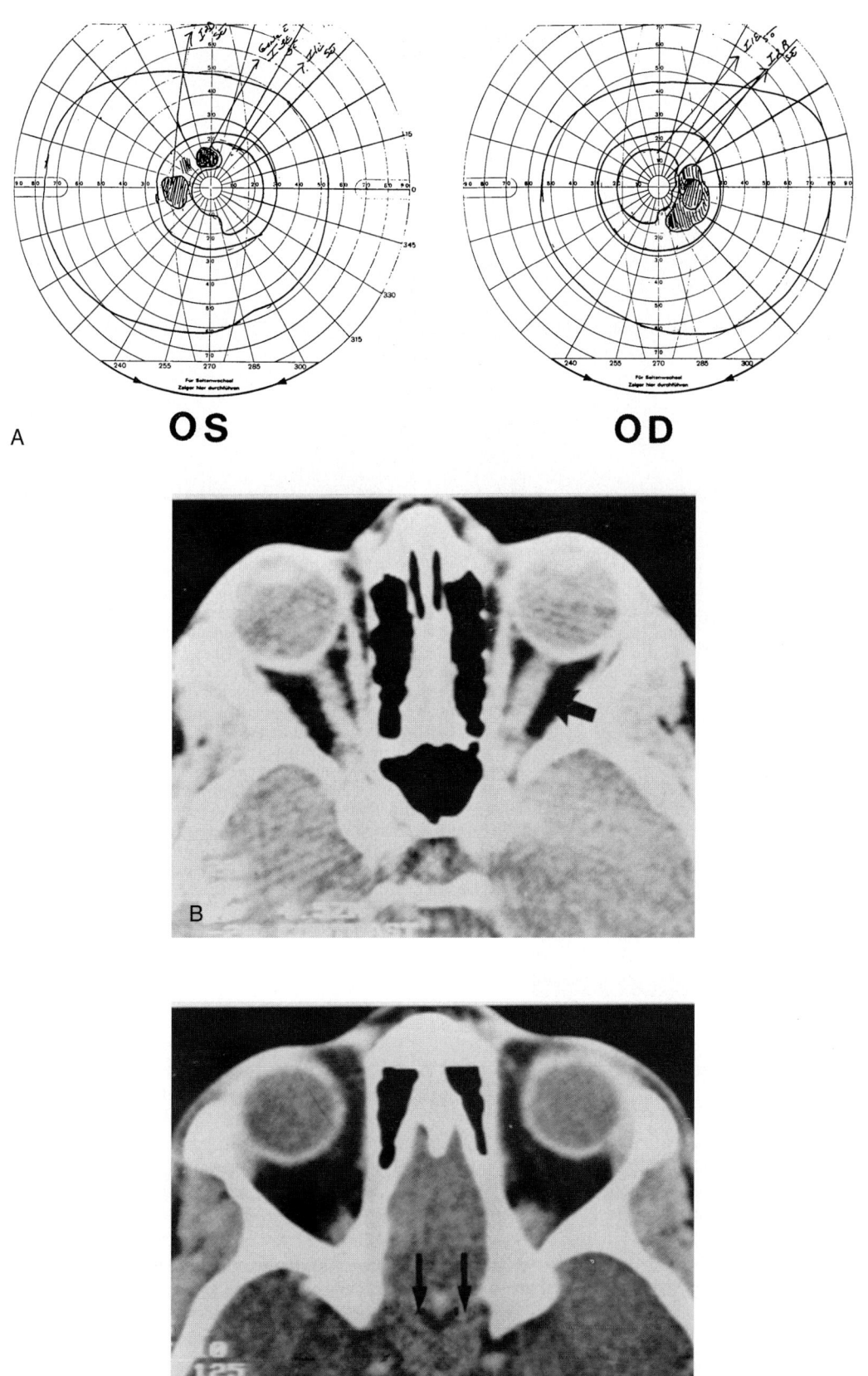

**FIGURE 18–10** ■ This 14-year-old patient was asymptomatic and had subjectively normal vision. *A*, The visual fields showed these scotomas. Those of the left eye worsened 13 months later. *B*, A Computed tomography (CT) scan through the orbit shows a greatly enlarged left optic nerve *(black arrow)*. *C*, A CT scan through the chiasm shows substantial enlargement; the estimated diameter is 1.5 cm *(arrows)*.

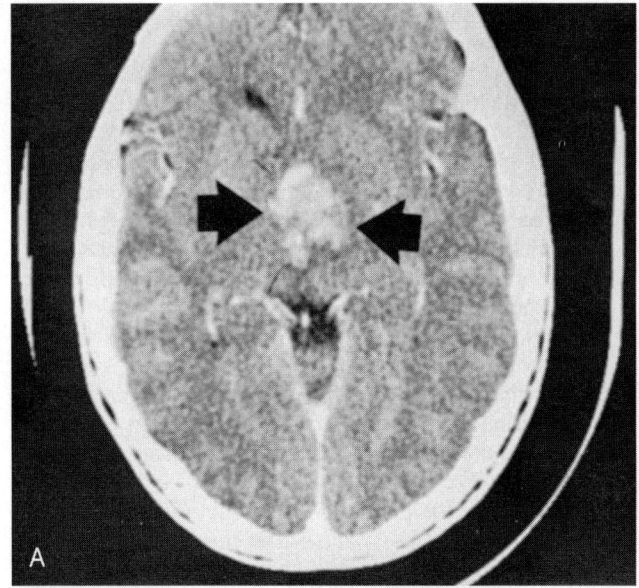

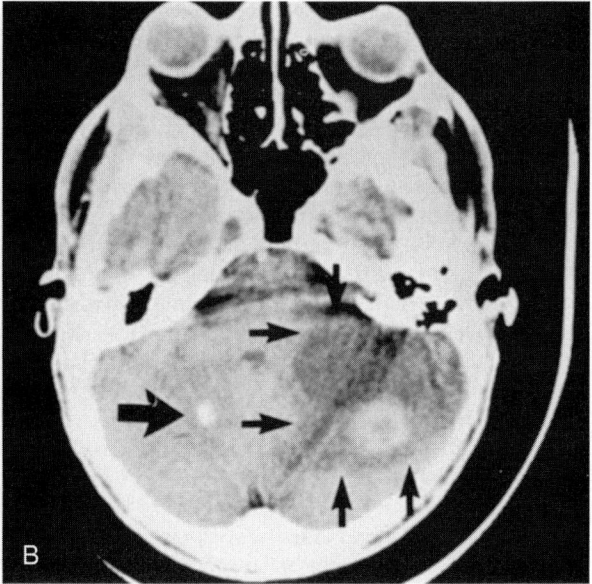

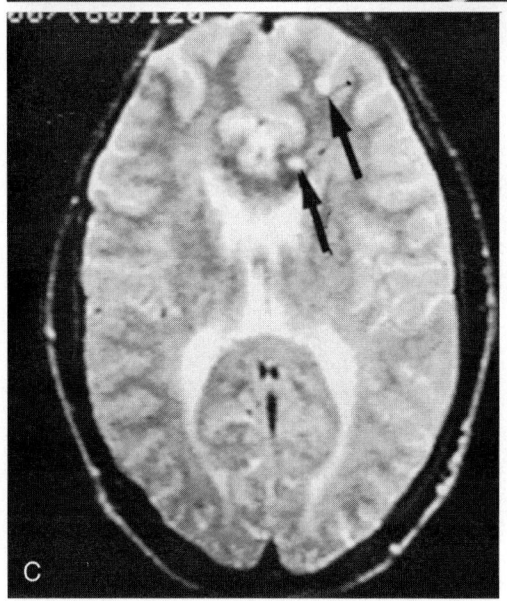

**FIGURE 18–11** ■ Case Report 5. These computed tomography (CT) scans were obtained on August 1, 1986. At 34 months of age, the boy had numerous café au lait spots and right optic nerve glioma. In August 1971, removal back to chiasm. Fifteen years later on a routine check-up, the patient's only symptom is that he sleeps from 3:00 to 5:00 PM three times per week; the only sign is blindness. Magnetic resonance imaging (MRI) technology offered increased clarity. *A,* Contrast-enhanced tumor *(arrows)* in the region of the upper third ventricle. *B,* The *small arrows* outline the huge cyst with a contrast-enhanced solid component near the surface of this left cerebellar cystic astrocytoma. (*Large arrow;* small tumor nodule in the center of the right cerebellar hemisphere.) *C,* One of a series of MRI scans shows a total of seven small nodules of indeterminate nature. The two in this image are indicated by the *arrows.* The larger left cerebellar cystic grade 1 astrocytoma was removed, and the patient had a briskly normal convalescence. On May 17, 1987, the patient had a hemorrhage into the right temporoparietal glioblastoma. Five months later, the patient developed a third ventricle grade 1 astrocytoma, $2 \times 3 \times 4$ cm, that involved the thalamus and hypothalamus and spared the chiasm; thus, it was independent of the original optic glioma as well as the glioblastoma. The sequence suggests three different stages of evolution of three adverse gene mutations.

All patients with neurofibromatosis with or without pallor of an optic disk probably should be studied for optic and other gliomas and for smaller lesions, so that early diagnosis can be made and the natural history more fully documented. This group requires conservative but assiduous follow-up, including visual evoked potentials, with subsequent surgery or radiation therapy when advisable.

## Spontaneous Regression of Optic Gliomas

In addition to the patient in Case Report 3, who experienced the spectacular disappearance of her tumor, we have identified other cases in the literature of significant, although often modest spontaneous improvement in symptoms and objective findings in optic gliomas. The report of Hoyt and Baghdassarian[46] describes spontaneous improvement in 4 of 23 eyes in untreated patients—nearly all

without surgical verification of the diagnosis. The largest series of patients with verified diagnoses and protracted stationary status (three cases) or actual regression (two cases) is that of Tym.[81] It includes a patient followed for 39 years whose chiasmal tumor had reduced visual acuity to less than J20 in each eye after 25 years of worsening. Vision then recovered to J6 and J18 over the next 14 years. In a 2-year-old child, the optic nerves at transfrontal exploration "were swollen like spring onions in contact with each other"; the massively proptotic eyeball and the nerve on one side were removed.[81] Eight years later, the patient was developing normally, with J2 vision in the remaining cyc. In three other cases, despite a swollen chiasm, one eye in each case had conserved normal visual acuity and field for 16, 8, and 6 years. Other convincing reports include two cases from Borit and Richardson,[49] in which residual tumor remained at surgery, but none was found at autopsy in each case 13 years later with no radiation therapy. In the first case, a 14-year-old girl, the eyeball and entire orbital and intracranial optic nerve had been resected, leaving only microscopic remnants in the chiasm, but in the second case, a 3-month-old boy, only a biopsy specimen had been taken. The case reported on by Kahn and colleagues,[10] consisted of a biopsy-proven glioma of the nerves and chiasm extending into and filling the third ventricle that had caused papilledema. A bilateral Torkildsen procedure was followed by complete recovery, despite the fact that the planned radiation treatment was never given. On re-examination 9 years later, the patient was perfectly well, with 20/20 vision in both eyes and normal optic fundi. This patient probably represents a more dramatic spontaneous disappearance of huge optic glioma than our Case 3 because of the sparing of virtually the entire normal visual system during the selective destruction of massive tumor.

With the advent of high-resolution CT, at least one visual demonstration exists of a marked decrease in tumor size. A large suprasellar astrocytoma (grade II), of which only the exophytic component was surgically removed, was far smaller in scans made 10 months after surgery than in those made 3 months after surgery; there also was some recovery of visual acuity,[82] changes that may, however, have been radiation induced. As already noted, the visual evoked potential responses to pattern stimulation improved spontaneously in two patients with optic nerve gliomas.[42] Berke[83] reported on two patients in whom bilaterally enlarged optic canals decreased in size after unilateral removal of a tumor via one-sided lateral orbitotomy. Wright and colleagues[19] noted spontaneous improvement in visual acuity in 3 of 31 patients with gliomas of the nerve; the most marked change was from 6/24 to 6/6 in 7 years. In one of these patients, proptosis receded by 2 mm and in another by 3 mm.

Two patients were reported whose abrupt, mysterious, sustained improvements after steady major deterioration are perhaps explicable on the basis of spontaneous regression of the tumor or regression triggered by the craniotomy. A 51-year-old woman reported on by Hird[84] had had headaches for 2 years and failing vision for 2 months. She had a blind right eye with no pupillary reaction to light, plus markedly blurred vision on the left and bilateral papilledema with hemorrhage and exudates. Stammer's small biopsy of the swollen right optic nerve and chiasm confirmed the diagnosis of glioma. After this minor surgical procedure, the headaches ceased, and the papilledema and the left eye's visual field and acuity gradually recovered completely, to the astonishment of her physicians.

Wulc and associates[85] reported on a 31-year-old woman with neurofibromatosis type 1 who was blind in the left eye when biopsy of the swollen left optic nerve and chiasm revealed a grade I astrocytoma. After radiotherapy, she remained free of new symptoms for 7 years. Then a rapidly developing left proptosis led to exenteration of the left orbit and another course of radiotherapy. One year later, left temporal hemianopia and increased intracranial pressure led to subtotal resection involving a left frontal lobectomy of a now malignant astrocytoma. At this cheerless juncture, the patient amazed all by recovering with good vision and no change in the visual field of the right eye.

The range of spontaneous behavior of these anterior visual pathway gliomas varies from complete disappearance of a large growing mass to minor degree of regression just cited, then to cessation of growth with maintenance of the same tumor size for years, to resumption of slow growth in grade I, and, finally, to more rapid growth in one of the higher grades. This behavior is consonant with evolving concepts of neoplastic and non-neoplastic growth and suppression related to genes that promote normal growth, genes that promote one or more steps in development of neoplasia, and oppositely oriented suppressor genes or those whose activity promotes a bizarre growth. Such growth may be seen in neurofibromatosis type 1 patients, who have large areas in the brain that appear hyperintense on $T_2$-weighted MRI scans and whose pathologic features have yet to be fully described.

Molecular geneticists have introduced a complex world of bewildering genetic changeability, with the final result in any cell group depending on different genes or groups of genes at each of several steps in cellular growth, retardation, or dissolution. The tumor-suppressor genes, of which eight have been identified, are prone to develop nonsuppressing mutants that permit tumor development.[86] Jacoby[87] notes that point mutations in the P53 tumor-suppressor gene are generally useful for the study of the nervous system tumors in general and astrocytomas in particular. Of interest to the neurosurgeon is the fact that P53 RNA and that of some other genes can be identified in tiny liquid nitrogen–cooled biopsy specimens, readily secured by the neurosurgeon by stereotactic open operative methods. The neurosurgeon can search for the known suppressor genes, using this knowledge to guide therapy in conservative or radical paths. The presence of this or another appropriate suppressor gene would then warn the surgeon that radical excision might not be needed. The same P53 mutation as that in astrocytomas that had progressed to a higher grade was found in a primary astrocytoma. Initiation of astrocytoma is less well understood at present, but it is known that in humans, astrocytoma-altered genes are at 17p, 13p, 9p, and 10p.

This mechanism, rather than vascular changes promoting ischemia, is the preferable hypothesis to explain regression of these tumors. In particular, the astounding complete wipeout of tumor in Case Report 3 requires a highly specific modus operandi similar to that of antigen-antibody reactions. All of the tumors except that reported by Venes and colleagues[82] showed slow or no change or somewhat faster steady growth and were classified as grade I astrocytomas. Standard microscopy is of no help for selecting only the clinically significant tumor growers for surgery.

The patient in Case Report 3 and that of Kahn and coworkers[10] demonstrated three remarkable capacities: Not only can they keep the tumor at bay, as first pointed out by Imes and Hoyt,[29] but also they can destroy it in a highly selective fashion, while sparing completely enough of the immediately adjoining structures so that they function normally. The patients apparently did this at a pace that did not outrun the capacity of the body's scavenger mechanisms to prevent the accumulation or the persistence of a noxious mass of debris, as may occur in radiation therapy of some intracranial tumors. A mechanism that can do these remarkable things while the patient notes only a feeling of progressive well-being is worth further study.

## Gliomas Initially of One Optic Nerve

Most patients suffer from significant enlargement of neoplasm at some stage in the course of the disease. These cases are analyzed here in two groups: those with a tumor confined at least initially to one optic nerve and those with more extensive tumors. A survey of the literature on gliomas confined to one optic nerve and including our own cases is given in Tables 18–1 to 18–6.*

Wright and colleagues,[19, 107] in two important papers covering 31 patients with glioma of one optic nerve, confirmed their earlier finding that the patients fell into two groups: one with a relatively static, *slow indolent course* and the other with a more rapid progression of symptoms. Fifteen patients were in the rapidly growing group and 16 in the slow-growing group, of whom 11 had neurofibromatosis. Of the latter group, four were lost to follow-up, illustrating one major hazard of the tactic of following the patient without treatment until signs and symptoms worsen. The largest increase in proptosis in the slow-growing group was from 3 to 6 mm over 6 years. We would now favor early operation for the patient with a 3 mm protrusion when first seen.

As seen in Table 18–1, in most services, if the glioma was thought to be confined to one optic nerve when the patient was first seen, a macroscopically complete excision was carried out from variable distances in front of the chiasm to the globe. Of the 237 patients in this group of grossly total removal, there were 15 recurrences in 10 patients. A recurrence from the stump of the nerve at the globe took place in two patients, one of whom also had recurrence posteriorly. We do not know how many of these patients had tumor in the cut posterior end of the excised nerve. In our only presumed recurrence, the patient's autopsy revealed that the chiasm was not invaded by the patient's later development of a huge hypothalamothalamic glioma. He did not have a recurrence of the original tumor from a growth backward from the nerve (see Fig. 18–11). In two of the 10 patients, the reappearance of tumor did not take place for 12 and 15 years; we do not know how many of the 237 may yet grow tumor. Reports in many cases do not include histologic study of the posterior cut end of the nerve.

Table 18–2 reveals that in the 15 patients in whom the glioma was confined to one optic nerve and was known to be incompletely excised, it recurred in at least seven of them. In three, the status of the patient is not known, and the four without recurrence at 1 to 15 years later were all given radiotherapy. Table 18–3 summarizes the poor results in six patients who refused any treatment and three who accepted radiation therapy only after major deficits developed. Table 18–4 summarizes the satisfactory results in 12 patients whose tumor proved to be confined to the optic canal and orbit. Table 18–5 reveals that a possibly incomplete intraorbital excision may also be followed for many

*References 5, 9, 19, 36, 42, 43, 48–50, 57, 60, 70, 76, 85, and 88–110.

years without recurrence. In Table 18–6 in 21 patients from 18 articles tumor spread, usually intracranial, occurred.

We also summarize from these tables all 35 patients with clear absence of tumor at the cut posterior end of the nerve. No recurrence occurred in any of them.[5, 19, 85, 93, 98] Marejeva and colleagues[98] reported their results in 47 patients with definite tumor in the prechiasmal cut nerve end: None of the 47 received radiation, and only 4 had recurrences. Three other patients, one each from Groswasser and colleagues,[42] Wright and colleagues,[19] and Wulc and colleagues,[85] had evidence of recurrence after not having radiation. Six others, in addition to the 40 from Marejeva and colleagues,[98] did not have recurrences, even though they did not have radiotherapy (WH Sweet: Unpublished data, 1993).[19, 85, 100] None of the 12 patients who had radiotherapy and had positive cut ends had recurrences,[99–101] that is, a perfect record for those with no histologic evidence of tumor at the level of neural transection or for those in whom tumor at that level was treated by radiation therapy and there was no recurrence.

The tiny streamer of tumor that can gradually spread backward within the nerve to the chiasm cannot be seen by the best MRI available. Fog and associates[121] reported on one case of an intraorbital glioma in which the optic foramen and the intracranial portion of the optic nerve appeared normal. The posterior ends of the nerve cut at the chiasm showed microscopic evidence of tumor, however.

A remarkable patient illustrating the value of prompt surgery was reported by Goodman and colleagues.[122] A 6-year-old boy with normal visual findings in all respects except for papilledema, an enlarged blind spot, and minimal proptosis proved to have a huge glioma throughout one optic nerve, which when resected just in front of the chiasm showed a terminal 1 mm of normal nerve.

Although there is almost unanimous agreement that juvenile pilocytic astrocytomas (also called *polar spongioblastomas*) that continue to grow cannot be distinguished by light microscopy from those that do not, Borit and Richardson,[49] in their detailed analysis of 30 patients, noted that some tumors with well-localized and apparently quiescent growth also had small areas of unusually dense cellularity. Few reports exist of electron microscopically evaluated ultrastructure in these cases, and we found none correlating subsequent growth patterns with any aspect of such structure.

The now-proven propensity of grade I optic nerve gliomas to grow and, in many instances, to be arrested in size by radiation therapy leads us to conclude that surgery, radiotherapy, or both should be reconsidered because the microscopic streamers growing from nerve back into chiasm and hypothalamus may be present when the gross mass of tumor is still asymptomatic and otherwise undetectable. Although grade I optic nerve glioma may grow slowly in the optic nerve, it is dangerously close to important parts of the brain. The safest way to rid the patient of this lesion is surgical excision. Although radiation can be valuable, we suggest reserving it for patients with microscopic or macroscopic tumor in the prechiasmal end of the nerve, especially in younger children.

Exceptions to this recommendation are early cases of neurofibromatosis. In such patients, independent tiny foci of tumor may be present elsewhere in the anterior visual

**TABLE 18–1 ■ GLIOMA CONFINED TO ONE OPTIC NERVE: MACROSCOPICALLY COMPLETE EXCISION FROM VARIABLE DISTANCES IN FRONT OF CHIASM TO GLOBE**

| Reference | No. of Cases | No. with Reference | Outcome* |
|---|---|---|---|
| Rand et al[88] | 1 | | 1 cystic tumor |
| Cuneo and Rand[89] | 1 | | OK 13 years later |
| Hanbery[90] | 1 | 1 | Chiasm looked normal; death 8 months later with huge glioma arising in chiasm spreading to hypothalamus |
| Jain[91] | 1 | 1 | Removal in front of chiasm in 2 stages in right eye (no microscopy; posterior cut end of nerve) followed by radiation treatment. Dose not stated. 17.5 months after right optic nerve out, new enlargement left optic foramen, left eye nearly blind from recurrence |
| Bane and Long[92] | 1 | | No recurrence at 22 mo |
| Richards and Lynn[93] | 4 | | No tumor in posterior cut end of nerve; no recurrence |
| Matson[5] | 7 | | 6 certainly and 1 possibly totally removed<br>No recurrence; 5 followed up 4–18 yr |
| Wong and Lubow[50] | 12 | | No recurrence in 3–14 yr; no radiation |
| Lloyd[95] | 8 | | No recurrence 1–14 yr |
| Myles and Murphy[9] | 4 | 1 | 1 postoperative death before 1932; 3 OK at 14 mo, 17 yr, and 19 yr |
| Chang and Wood[94] | 3 | 3 | Grossly total removal originally of 3 intraorbital gliomas. Recurred several years later in orbit or extended intracranially |
| Miller et al[48] | 11 | | 2 died postoperatively: 1 with seizure and cardiac arrest; 1 meningitis. All complete resections; no mention of microscopy at cut end of nerves |
| Heiskanen et al[60] | 5 | | Total excisions: 3 of 5 irradiated; other eye normal 4–18 yr later |
| DeSousa et al[96] | 3 | | Two alive; 1 dead of malignant trigeminal schwannoma years later |
| Karaguiosov[97] | 10 | | No recurrences 3–23 yr |
| Marejeva et al[98] | 57 | 4 | 57 optic nerves (cut just in front of chiasm posterior to area of grossly visible tumor); microscopic tumor in posterior cut end in 44 of 57. Recurrence in 4 of 44 at 1 to 12 yr |
| Visot et al[99] | 4 | | No recurrence, all > 10 yr; radiotherapy in all 4 for histologic invasions in posterior cut end of nerve |
| Charles et al[36] | 1 | | 1 cystic hemorrhagic tumor in orbit removed only from orbit, although approached transfrontally |
| Kalifa et al[100] | 3 | | 3 microscopic tumors in posterior end of optic nerve; 0 had no such tumor; 1 irradiated 5000–5300 rads; no recurrence at 10, 10, or 4 yr<br>5 microscopic tumors in posterior cut end of optic nerve, all irradiated; no recurrence in 5–20 yr follow-up |
| Tenny et al[102] | 29 | | 9 with irradiation also; all alive |
| Groswasser et al[42] | 1 | 1 | Visual evoked potentials in temporal field of fellow eye grossly prolonged latency for 4.5 yr, then return to work, i.e., spontaneous recovery |
| Helcl and Petraskova[57] | 4 | | Aged 6–13 yr; no recurrence |
| Flickinger et al[43] | 5 | 1 | After complete resection of tumor in 5 patients, tumor in 1 chiasm 2.7 yr later, then radiated with no progression 12 yr later |
| Gabibov et al[103] | 28 | 1 | 1 recurrence at 3 yr from stump of nerve near globe |
| Wulc et al[85] | 6 | 1 | 1 lateral orbital approach, posterior cut end of nerve in orbit—microscopic grade II astrocytoma 4 yr later |
| Wright et al[19] | 3 | 1 | 3 patients, all grade II tumors in posterior cut ends of optic nerves; subsequent tumor growth in 1, then no change for 5 years with vision 6/6 for 7 yr after craniectomy. This patient also had orbital recurrence from tumor left attached to globe |
| | 6 | | In 6, no tumor in posterior cut end of nerves; no recurrence at 2, 3, 5, 9, 10 yr. All grade 1 astrocytomas |
| Sweet, 1993 | 13 | 1 | Aged 5 mo–10 yr at first symptom, average, 5 yr; follow-up, 6–34 yr, average 24 yr; 1 recurrence at chiasm 15 yr postoperatively<br>Posterior cut end of nerve: for 8, inadequate data; follow-up, 18–36 yr; average, 24 yr; 1 tumor recurrence (already noted); 3 clearly free of tumor, follow-up, 6–13 yr, average, 9.5 yr; no recurrences, 2 clearly contained tumors, follow-up, 10–42 yr, average 26 yr; no recurrences these 2 groups (those with and without tumor) |

*Summary: 237 grossly total removals, 16 recurrences, 3 deaths after operation in earlier decades.

## TABLE 18–2 ■ GLIOMA CONFINED TO ONE OPTIC NERVE: MACROSCOPICALLY INCOMPLETE EXCISION IN FRONT OF CHIASM TO GLOBE

| Reference | No. of Cases | No. with Recurrence | Outcome* |
|---|---|---|---|
| Suarez et al[104] | 4 | 0 | 4 microscopic and macroscopic infiltrations of chiasm or even tract by tumor; all irradiated; all without recurrence 15, 14, 2, and 1 yr later |
| Spencer[76] | 1 | 1 | Removal of tumor in front of chiasm to just behind entrance of central retinal artery. Tumor still in oculobulbar part of nerve: 4 recurrences of intraorbital tumor in this patient 7, 2, 3, and 1 yr later—all benign astrocytomas |
| Gaini et al[101] | 1 | 1 | Tumor left in optic canal, regrew in both directions 11 yr later |
| Tenny et al[102] | 7 | 3 | Deaths from intracranial tumor at 3 mo, 3 yr, and 4 yr; no follow-up data on recurrence without death |
| Sweet, 1993 | 2 | 2 | One globe invaded by tumor recurrence at 15 mos; 1 chiasm invaded by tumor recurrence at 6 yr; average follow-up, 3.3 yr |

*Summary: Histologic examination posterior end of cut optic nerve is important. In 7 of 15 cases, there was known recurrence after incomplete removal. There was inadequate follow-up in most cases. Data do not permit evaluation of radiation for microscopic infiltration of posterior cut end of nerve.

## TABLE 18–3 ■ GLIOMA OF ONE OPTIC NERVE: NO EXCISION

| Reference | Outcome* |
|---|---|
| Jefferson[105] | First eye symptoms at 18 mos; blind OD age 5; always at top of class until age 12, then rapid downhill course to death. Autopsy: glioma of right optic nerve, chiasm, brain stem |
| Wong and Lubow[50] | 2 patients with several-year follow-ups; no progression |
| Smith[106] | 2-year-old boy with neurofibromatosis: OD 2-mm proptosis, 20/25 vision with central field depression. 10 months later, vision 20/30 or 20/40. CT scan showed optic glioma OD. At surgery, tumor into chiasm, radiation with little response |
| Wright et al[107] | 5-year-old girl. No neurofibromatosis. Blind OS with 3-mm proptosis; OD vision and VEP normal. 1 yr later, VEP-nasal fibers OD involved. Age 8, tumor at surgery in both optic nerves, chiasm, and hypothalamus. After radiation, no progression 4 yr later |
| Borit and Richardson[49] | Intraorbital tumor, operation refused; 5 years later operation accepted but chiasm involved |
| Wong et al[70] | 1 patient remained stable 9.5 years after diagnosis |
| Flickinger et al[43] | 1 patient had no treatment, moderate decrease in acuity in 1 eye at 10 years. 1 patient nearly blind in 1 eye after radiotherapy (Jehovah's Witness); no further visual loss 13 years later |

*Summary: Tumor spread in visual pathways in 5 cases, only slightly in a sixth case. No progression in 3 cases.

OD, right eye; CT, computed tomography; OS, left eye; VEP, visual evoked potential.

## TABLE 18–4 ■ GLIOMA OF ONE OPTIC NERVE: INTRAORBITAL EXCISION THOUGHT COMPLETE

| Reference | No. of Cases | Outcome* |
|---|---|---|
| Lloyd[95] | 1 | Normal optic foramen; normal nerve at each end of intraorbital glioma |
| Klug[108] | 3 | OK 14 mos, 17 yr, and 19 yr |
| Wright et al[107] | 1 | 20-year-old woman with glioma in orbit only, transfrontal operation; no tumor |
| Gaini et al[101] | 3 | Glioma in orbit only; no recurrence in follow-ups of < 5 to > 20 yr |
| Sweet, 1993 | 4 | Aged 1–14 yr at first symptom, average, 6.1 yr; intracranial optic nerve looked normal; removed behind optic canal; no recurrence at 7–37.5 yr, average, 25 yr |

*Summary: A few tumors are confined to orbit and canal.

pathway, as in Martuza's case reported earlier and the cases reported by Lewis and colleagues.[80] In such cases, frequent follow-up is required to determine when, where, and how to intervene. Our patient (see Case Report 5) with neurofibromatosis type 1 was given 15 years of life after the removal of an optic nerve glioma before four more gliomas killed him. In particular, the advisability of a course of immediate radiation therapy once minor microscopic tumor strands are seen in the posterior cut end of the nerve in a patient with neurofibromatosis type 1 is uncertain.

## SURGERY

Once surgery is determined to be necessary, the subfrontal transcranial approach to the intracranial, intracanalicular, and intraorbital portions of the optic nerve is the procedure of choice. Housepian's[123, 124] account of refinements of the original Dandy approach emphasizes diagonal division of the origin of the levator palpebrae superioris muscle just anterior to the annulus of Zinn and medial to the superior rectus, with resuture of the annulus and muscle after the removal. (See the excellent series of figures in his chapter

## TABLE 18–5 ■ GLIOMA OF ONE OPTIC NERVE: INCOMPLETE (?) INTRAORBITAL EXCISION, NO RECURRENCE

| Reference | No. of Cases | Outcome* |
|---|---|---|
| Knapp[109] | 3 | Large optic canals but only intraorbital operation well with good vision in other eye 15–18 yr later |
| Bane and Long[92] | 1 | 4-year-old girl followed up for 37 yr |
| Chutorian et al[110] | 16 | Followed up to 24 yr; normal vision in other eye |
| Spencer[76] | 1 | Proptosis 4–11 mm in 18 mos; no recurrence 5 yr after orbitotomy |
| Wong and Lubow[50] | 2 | Followed up for years |
| Wright et al[107] | 1 | Followed up 4 yr |
| Sweet, 1993 | 2 | Intraorbital excision known incomplete; 1 patient followed up 14 yr |

*Summary: 26 patients (7 articles), no recurrence.

## TABLE 18–6 ■ GLIOMA OF ONE OPTIC NERVE: INCOMPLETE (?) INTRAORBITAL EXCISION: RECURRENCE

| Reference | Recurrence | Outcome* |
|---|---|---|
| Szokalski[62] | 1 | 5 yr later, intraorbital recurrence size of small apple—removed; meningitis; death. Autopsy: walnut-sized tumor on chiasm |
| Goldzieher[63] | 1 | Orbital recurrence, 1 case |
| Byers[54] | 1 | Orbital recurrence at 1 yr; exenteration; death in 8 yr of huge intracranial glioma |
| Barraquer[64] | 1 | Intracranial extension 9 yr after operation |
| Pagenstecher[65] | 1 | Orbital recurrence 25 yr later; death from meningitis after second removal. Autopsy: tumor did not reach chiasm |
| Seefelder[111] | 1 | Intraorbital recurrence at 2 yr, again 1 yr later |
| Davis[112] | 1 | 1 case, distal half of right optic nerve removed; slow progression, enlargement of optic foramen, tumor into intracranial optic nerve, chiasm 4 yr later. Autopsy: Independent large tumor anterior and medial right temporal lobe |
| Levitt[113] | 1 | 1 case, 9-year-old girl, 4 yr later in semicoma, atrophy of other optic disk; extension of tumor to chiasm and hypothalamus |
| Christensen and Andersen[114] | 2 | 2 of 11 with glioma of nerve or nerve plus chiasm: reoperation 1 and 2 times. Intraorbital as well as intracranial recurrences |
| Zulch and Nover[115] | 1 | Intraorbital removal at age 3; chiasmal growth operated on at age 28 |
| Yanoff et al[116] | 1 | 5-year-old boy; enucleation; intraorbital removal 4 times in 1 yr; death at 6 yr from huge chiasmal glioma spreading to anterior and middle fossas. All orbital tumors juvenile pilocytic astrocytomas, 1 specimen this patient only rare mitoses and more cells than usual |
| Rougier et al[117] | 1 | 30-year-old woman 3 years after excision loss in contralateral eye of inferior temporal quadrant with arc central scotoma in other 3 quadrants; optic foramen much larger in ipsilateral eye |
| Mullaney et al[118] | 1 | 4-year-old boy, 48 yr later, gross proptosis for many years. Intraorbital reoperation only; histology: malignant features |
| Nicole et al[119] | 1 | 6 children: 4 good results 15, 14, 13, and 2 yr; 1 died 6 mo of unknown cause; 1 intracranial spread at 8 yr |
| Iraci et al[120] | 1 | 6-year-old girl, normal optic foramen, intraorbital removal, 3 yr later optic foramen enlarged, suprasellar mass, vision decreased other eye |
| Borit and Richardson[49] | 4 | 14 children: 4 orbital recurrences; 1 patient had 3 such recurrences with intracranial spread |
| Wulc et al[85] | 1 | 64-year-old woman with left eye signs progressive for 1 year. Lateral orbital approach to remove grade II astrocytoma: cut off tumor and nerve extending into conus and apex. 4 yr later, recurrence in orbit, tumor removed to chiasm with tumor at cut posterior end. Well but only 1-yr follow-up |

*Summary: 21 patients with recurrence (17 articles).

on intraorbital tumors in this text.) We recommend preliminary verification by histologic examination of a biopsy specimen. Luccarelli[125] described two patients in whom the gross appearance was of swelling confined to the anterior optic pathways. In one, a 39-year-old woman, only the full extent of one optic nerve was involved. In the other patient, a 32-year-old woman, the swelling involved both optic nerves and the chiasm. Histologic examinations revealed a highly radiosensitive ectopic pinealoma, more properly termed a *dysgerminoma*, only after the optic nerve had been resected in one of the patients. Excision of an optic glioma, usually in one stage, should occur from globe to chiasm. Care should be taken to leave attached to the chiasm the medial 2 mm of the nerve, which may contain a loop of fibers from the other eye. In view of reported recurrences when the intracanalicular portion of the nerve has been left behind, we disagree with Housepian's[124] statement that it is not essential to remove this part of the nerve in the treatment of these gliomas.

In 1947, Walsh[126] concluded, "The fact that a glioma, incompletely removed, may occasionally cease to grow does not seem sufficient reason for doing an incomplete operation." The results of long follow-ups in the ensuing 39 years support the wisdom of that advice. How to treat the patient when the eye is minimally involved remains a matter of uncertainty and partly depends on the accuracy with which the latest generations of CT and MRI scanners can detect growth of these tumors once they are discovered. Maisongrosse and coworkers'[127] solution was to give radiotherapy to a child whose acuity was 7/10 or less in the affected eye.

## Gliomas of the Chiasm, Optic Nerves, and Adjoining Brain

Most optic gliomas involve some combination of the chiasm, optic nerves, and adjoining brain. Whether or not they should be operated on is a question to be carefully weighed in each case. The decision about open operation and its extent should be guided by the following considerations.

Because of the hazards and little likelihood of a good result, many critics favor no surgery for these tumors. Opponents of surgery point out that Martin and Cushing[128] had three deaths within 48 hours of operation and no useful results in the four other patients treated in this way. In addition, Dandy's[53] four patients all died soon after surgery. Such results are irrelevant today because they occurred many years before the controllability of hypothalamopituitary deficits, infection, and cerebral edema as well as the use of the operating microscope. Housepian and colleagues at the New York Neurological Institute recommend attempting to reach a presumptive diagnosis of such tumors without surgery so that radiation therapy can begin immediately. Wright and associates[107] usually advise against surgery when the chiasm is involved, as did Throuvalas and associates[129] and Jefferson.[105] Robertson and Brewin[130] stated that in chiasmal gliomas "the effect of surgery (on vision) will almost inevitably be to make it immediately and permanently worse." They concluded that survival "is probably not affected by surgery or by radiotherapy."[130]

Many researchers think that the clinical and radiographic features of pituitary tumors, Hodgkin's disease, reticulum cell sarcomas, suprasellar ganglioneuromas, and ectopic pinealomas (dysgerminomas) cannot be distinguished with certainty from those of optic gliomas unless the patient has neurofibromatosis.[3, 48, 99] In fact, four reports exist of a misdiagnosis of craniopharyngioma.[43, 131–133] In one, a tongue projecting from a craniopharyngioma had enlarged an optic canal, simulating a glioma.[131] An inflammatory pseudotumor and a lymphoma are two other erroneous diagnoses reported from prominent institutions.[43, 48] The preoperative diagnosis of *chiasmatic hypophyseal glioma* in a case reported by Giuffré and coworkers[134] proved to be radionecrosis of this region caused by $^{60}$Co therapy to the pituitary gland many months before (R Giuffré: Personal communication, 1986).

For all of these reasons, many clinicians favor operative exposure. Pitfalls of surgery include one described by Miller and colleagues[48] of two cases in which the neurosurgeon's biopsy specimens of enlarged intracranial optic pathways were misdiagnosed as glioma by the surgeon and the first pathologist. More extensive tumor material revealed Hodgkin's sarcoma in one case and reticulum cell sarcoma in the other. The need for caution in the face of unexpectedly normal neural appearances was pointed out by Wright and associates.[107] In one patient with an enlarged optic foramen, the intracanalicular and intracranial portions of the optic nerve were excised but contained neither glial hyperplasia nor glioma. The need for caution, even in the face of the expected gliomatous appearance, has already been mentioned in a discussion of two cases in which the tumor proved to be a dysgerminoma.

When only a small biopsy specimen is taken, one must attempt to remove it from a portion of the visual pathway related to a blind area of the visual field to avoid the experience reported by Montgomery and colleagues,[135] in which 75% of their 15 patients undergoing biopsy suffered a surgically related increase in visual field deficit.

By using a Cavitron ultrasonic surgical aspirator while monitoring visual evoked potential responses, Albright and Sclabassi[136] removed 60% to 85% of two chiasmal gliomas without worsening of already severely impaired vision. This tactic deserves widespread emulation.

## Features Favorable for Partial or More Complete Resection

### Edema Without Neoplastic Invasion

Some optic gliomas clearly have surgically remediable aspects. The first of these was seen by Walsh.[126] At intra-

dural exposure, the left optic nerve was the size of the surgeon's middle finger, and the ipsilateral two thirds of the chiasm was greatly swollen. The affected nerve was excised from the chiasm forward into normal nerve. On histologic examination, the tumor proved to have been completely removed; the chiasmal swelling was not neoplastic. After 7 years, the vision in the other eye was still normal. Walsh wrote, "Resection of the nerve is indicated whether or not the chiasm is swollen and appears to be affected and whether or not the patient is a child."[126]

### Cystic or Hemorrhagic Component

Another favorable but infrequent finding is cystic fluid compressing the optic pathways. Kahn and coworkers[10] described a 9-year-old girl who in 1961 had advanced primary optic atrophy of the left eye, a visual acuity of only 20/400 in the left eye and 20/50 in the right, and a right homonymous hemianopia in each eye. A semilunar calcification was present 15 mm above and slightly behind the sella turcica. At surgery, the posterior part of the left optic nerve, the left half of the chiasm, and the left optic tract were grossly swollen with a *blue-domed* cyst bulging inferolateral to these structures. The surgeon aspirated 4 ml of yellow fluid, whereupon the swelling in the nerve, chiasm, and tract collapsed. The biopsy specimen from the tract revealed glioma. The findings after examination of the patient's eyes in March 1981 were the same except that visual acuity had improved (20/30 in the right eye). The patient's general health was excellent. CT scans showed a normal-sized optic chiasm, left optic tract, and medial left temporal lobe and no abnormality except multiple tiny calcifications. Myles and Murphy[9] evacuated a cyst involving the chiasm and one optic nerve with a good result that remained 10 years later. Pellet and associates[137] and Visot and associates[99] also recommended surgery for a major cyst.

Uihlein and Rucker[138] reported on the removal of a blood clot caused by a *telangiectatic* astrocytoma that had ballooned out much of the right chiasm and the right optic nerve. The visual acuity of the left eye and much of the temporal field in that eye, previously lost, recovered. The right eye remained blind. These are infrequent occurrences.

Karnaze and colleagues[139] described MRI scans of cystic degeneration in two of four chiasmal gliomas as hypointense on $T_1$-weighted images and as hypointense as cerebrospinal fluid on $T_2$-weighted images. Wulc and associates[85] described cystic degeneration in all six of optic nerve gliomas they reported. Fletcher and coworkers[7] reported that 3 of 22 patients who had tumors invading the chiasm developed cysts after substantial doses of radiation. Hoyt and coworkers[140] and Wilson and coworkers[61] described large cystic components of gliosis invading the brain, which as Kahn theorizes, may be of help to the aggressive surgeon. None of these authors mentions assistance the surgeon may receive from the larger cysts.

### Exophytic Growth of Tumor

Much more common but not widely enough recognized is the tendency of optic gliomas to break through their pial sheath and grow more readily in the subarachnoid space, as noted in 1940 by Wolff.[141] In the same symposium at the Royal Society of Medicine, this growth pattern was confirmed in a specimen from a 1-year-old child shown by Neame.[142] Cogan[143] stated, "The glioma itself may invade the subarachnoid space and extend a considerable distance forward or backward about a portion of the nerve which itself shows minimal neoplasia." Walter[144] and Stern and colleagues[145] made essentially the same statement. In the latter article, the contention was that the "tumor eruption and proliferation in the subarachnoid space correlated with the presence of neurofibromatosis."[145] Neurofibromatosis was not the diagnosis of our six cases with this growth pattern, however. Borit and Richardson[49] commented, "In the chiasmatic group the tumor always extended into the chiasmatic cistern and frequently involved the interpeduncular fossa and the lumen of the third ventricle. In most cases ... with minimal evidence of invasion of brain tissue."

Neurosurgeons should take advantage of these possibilities. Northfield[146] observed that the intracranial portion of an optic nerve glioma may compress and displace the chiasm without invading it. Bynke and associates[8] (Fig. 18–12) recorded a favorable example of this. In a patient with severe impairment of the fields and acuity in both eyes, an exophytic glioma arose by a mere 3-mm attachment to the medial caudal aspect of the right optic nerve. It pushed apart both nerves and the chiasm and was attached nowhere else, and its removal restored visual acuity and fields to normal on the left and nearly to normal on the right. Further improvement was seen 5 years later. Heiskanen and colleagues[66] described a similar case of a glioma arising from the front of the chiasm. Lèhlein and Tènnis[147] reported on a mushroom-like cap of tumor overlying the chiasm but arising from one optic nerve more than 5 mm in front of its junction with the chiasm. The tumor was successfully removed.

One of the authors (Sweet) has sought to use this compression phenomenon in seven patients in whom it was not

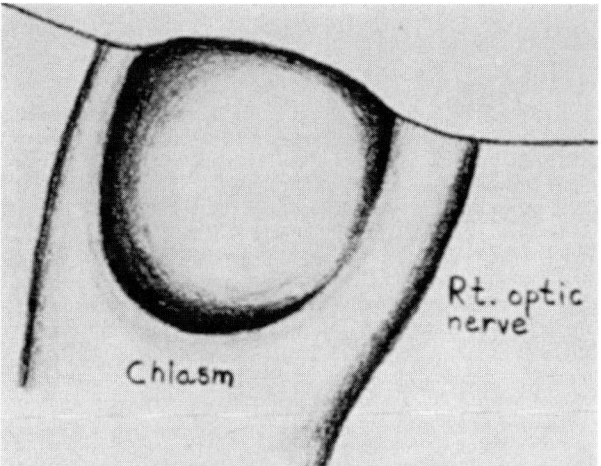

FIGURE 18–12 ■ Bynke's diagram of his patient with a completely exophytic glioma attached to the right optic nerve. (From Bynke H, Kagstrom E, Tjernstrom K: Aspects on the treatment of gliomas of the anterior visual pathways. Acta Ophthalmol 55:276, 1977.)

as severe. The most striking case was described in Case Report 1. The patient described in Case Report 6 illustrates another attractive feature of this growth pattern—that as the exophytic mass expands, it may compress the adjacent optic pathway, even to the point of slowly separating itself from the neural bundle rather than infiltrating it.

## Case Report 6

The patient, aged 4 years at the time of surgery on April 4, 1970, had a large intracranial glioma that showed the same growth behavior discussed in other cases. He had a proptotic blind right eye and a temporal defect in the left eye, and his right intracranial optic nerve expanded into a circular tangerine-sized mass 5 cm in largest diameter. This structure engulfed the chiasm but had severed its connection with the right optic tract, which was not visible. Figure 18–13A is a diagram of the two remarkably similar tumors, one in this patient and the other in the patient discussed in Case Report 7. Figure 18–13B shows the bed after tumor removal in this case. The extremely elongated left optic nerve had a rough gray area for a few millimeters on its medial aspect where the neoplastic chiasm had not separated itself totally from the nerve. After surgery, the lateral fibers of this optic nerve did not function, and an uncertain reduction in the field and acuity of the left eye preoperatively was converted to blindness. We waited for 7 months for some recovery of vision before removing the intraorbital and intracanalicular portions of the right optic nerve and tumor as well as the now infiltrated left optic nerve intracranially.

We saw the patient again 6 years later for retro-orbital headaches of increasing severity for 6 weeks. A broad, irregularly calcified suprasellar mass diagnosed as recurrent tumor was accompanied by massive enlargement of all four ventricles on the pneumoencephalogram but with no subarachnoid air passing above the prepontine cistern. A ventriculoatrial shunt restored the ventricles to normal size but did not help the headaches. Figure 18–13C shows how the rectangular fibrous mass with rough calcified inclusions looked at subfrontal operation on November 1, 1976. When this relatively circumscribed fibrocalcific mass had been removed, a smooth bed remained on the floor of the sellar and parasellar area. No neoplastic elements were identified histologically in the specimen. The headaches were greatly reduced. We cannot find any similar reports in the literature.

Ten years after this operation and 16 years after the tumor removals, the patient was leading a dramatically effective life. In a statewide competition, he had won one of a few scholarships for gifted students and did A-minus work in his first year of university. CT scans with and without contrast in October 1983 that had improved resolution and included direct coronal scans discriminated five small separate islands of suprasellar calcification and small soft tissue nodules (see Fig. 18–13D). These remained unchanged on CT scans and MRI scans obtained in August 1986.

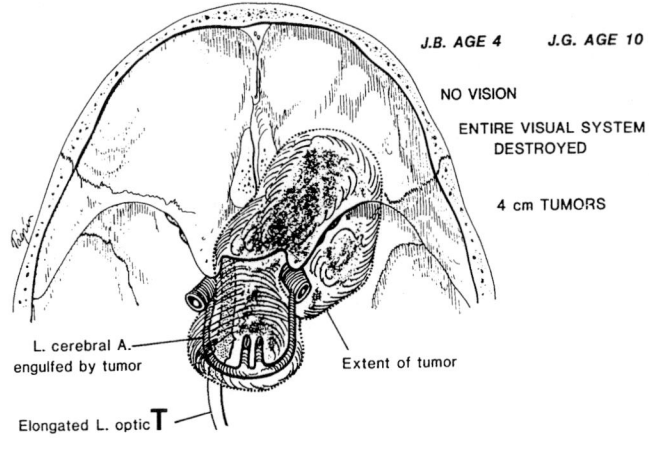

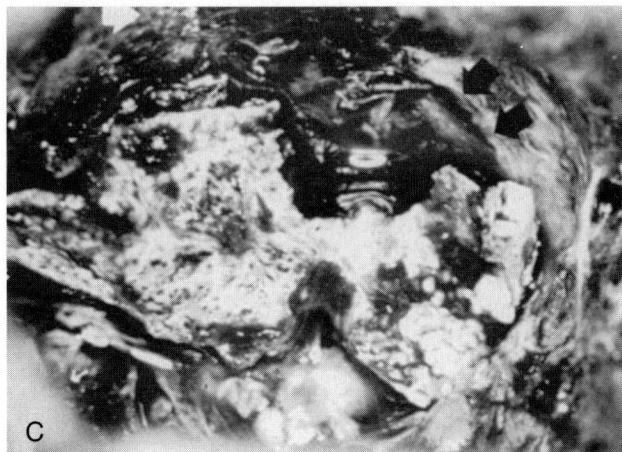

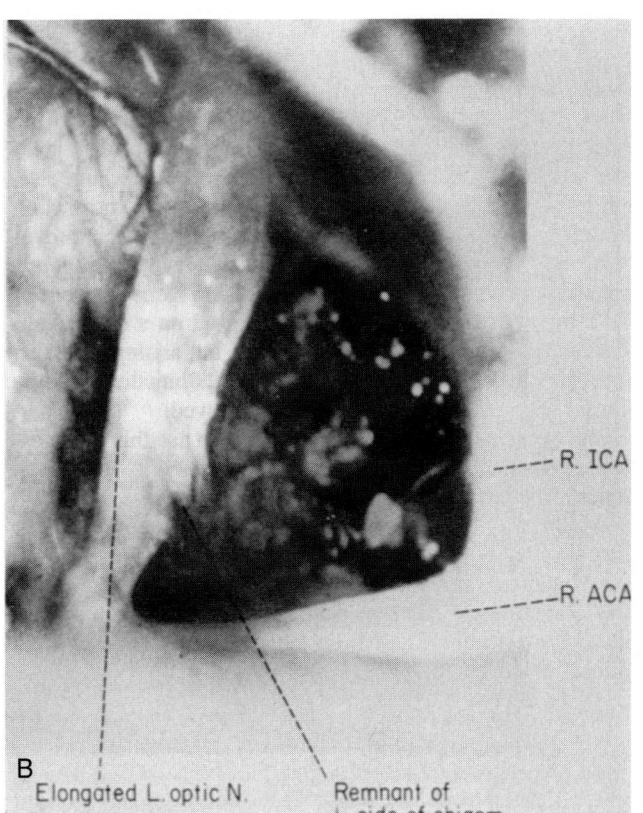

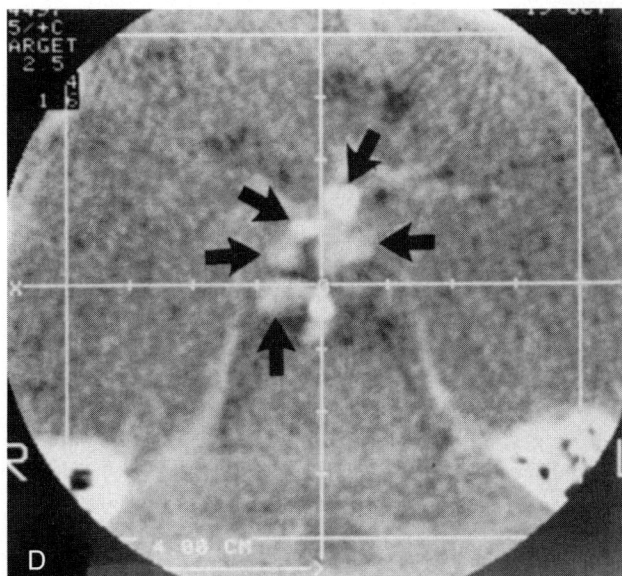

FIGURE 18–13 ■ *A*, Diagram of the remarkably similar tumors in Case Reports 6 and 7. *B*, Case Report 6. An intraoperative photograph obtained April 8, 1970, after the main tumor was removed. Note the ragged area on the medial aspect of the left optic nerve, which was the site of attachment of the grossly swollen chiasm to the somewhat swollen nerve, compared with the optic tract. *C*, Case Report 6. Intraoperative photograph obtained on November 1, 1976. The suprasellar region is exposed during this subfrontal operation; almost no normal structures are visible. The glistening irregular jagged features are calcific masses embedded in fibrous tissue. (*Black arrow*, posterior edge of the lesser wing of the right sphenoid bone; *white arrows*, planum sphenoidale.) *D*, Case Report 6. A contrast-enhanced computed tomography scan obtained on October 19, 1983. The *arrows* point to five separate islands of suprasellar calcification and soft tissue nodules (these were unchanged in the CT and magnetic resonance imaging scans obtained 3 years later).

## Case Report 7

The patient, aged 10 years at his first operation on January 3, 1970, had a clinical picture and treatment sequence (an initial two-stage operation) that was remarkably similar to that of the patient described in Case Report 6. His tumor, somewhat larger than the one in Case Report 6, had rendered him bilaterally blind before surgery, and he did not recover any vision in the left eye even though the left optic nerve looked fairly normal and had only tiny nubbins of obvious tumor at the left chiasmal remnant. He made a good adjustment to his blindness and is in excellent general health. The results of a CT scan obtained in July 1983 were normal. At age 25, he had completed a college degree and was training with the U.S. Internal Revenue Service.

## Case Report 8

The patient, a 9-year-old boy, had been completely blind in the right eye for at least 3 years. He was found to have low-normal intelligence after he had failed a year in school. A pneumoencephalogram outlined a large mass in the region of the right optic nerve, from which 3 ml of light yellow fluid were aspirated during surgery on July 29, 1960. The tumor, which covered all of the optic structures and extended above and beyond them in all directions, was removed piecemeal until it could be demonstrated that it was expanding only the right optic nerve, the right side of the chiasm, and the anterior end of the right tract. This nubbin seemed to separate cleanly from the normal-sized portions of the chiasm and the tract. Figure 18–14 illustrates the intracranial visual pathways that remained after the tumor was removed. The visual field of the left eye before surgery was reduced by a temporal hemianopia. Acuity and general performance remained satisfactory in the 23 years since, but we do not have detailed follow-up data.

## Case Report 9

A 17-year-old girl had steadily lost vision in both eyes for 10 years to an acuity of 20/100 in the right eye and 20/200 in the left eye, with only small seeing fields in the nasal quadrants of each eye. Numerous small suprasellar calcified areas had led to the diagnosis of craniopharyngioma. At surgery on July 5, 1966, the frontal lobes were eased readily off of a fluctuant, encapsulated tumor mass that bulged upward between the laterally displaced optic nerves. Aspiration yielded 1.8 ml of yellow fluid. After a reddish gray neoplasm was gently sucked out of the interior, continuous attachments to both optic nerves and to the chiasm were seen with the operating microscope. The normal-looking portions of the chiasm and both optic nerves were preserved (Fig. 18–15).

**PRESERVED NASAL FIELD    LEFT EYE**

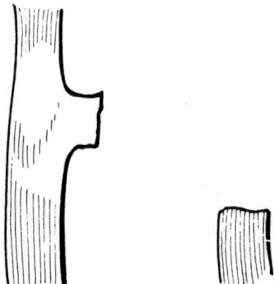

FIGURE 18–14 ■ Case Report 8. Diagram of the appearance of the left lateral chiasm and right optic tract after almost complete amputation of those portions invaded by the tumor.

Although postoperatively the patient had no vision in the right eye, the nasal field of the left eye remained larger, and its visual acuity was still 20/200 17 years later. Almost none of the suprasellar calcification was removed at surgery. The concern that this calcium might represent residual tumor seemed untenable to us in the light of the operative findings. The patient returned to work 2 months after surgery and 18 years later was working a 65-hour week. A CT scan obtained in June 1984 showed no tumor; she remained well and was functioning accordingly in December 1992, 26.5 years after tumor removal.

## Case Report 10

The patient, aged 18 years, who had a visual acuity of 20/60 in the right eye and a right nasal field defect, had a huge right optic foramen, and the intraorbital mass extended to the chiasmal region, according to findings on pneumoencephalogram. At surgery on January 15, 1973, a 2.2-cm dark red mass covered the visual structures and both internal carotid arteries (Fig. 18–16A). It could be separated easily from all of these normal structures, with the exception of where it expanded into the right optic nerve. Posteriorly, a large overhang superior to the right optic tract was

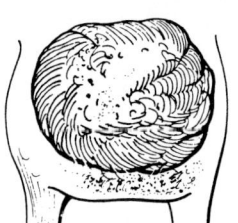

**PRESERVED NASAL FIELD**

**LEFT EYE**

FIGURE 18–15 ■ Case Report 9. Diagram of the appearance of the tumor at surgery.

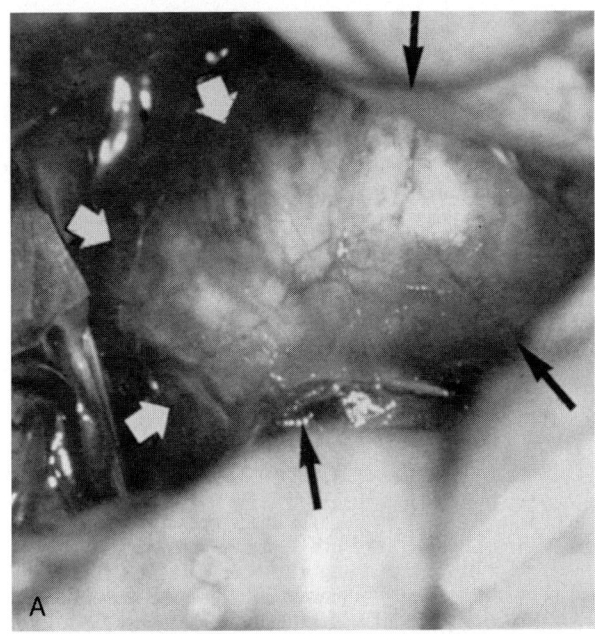
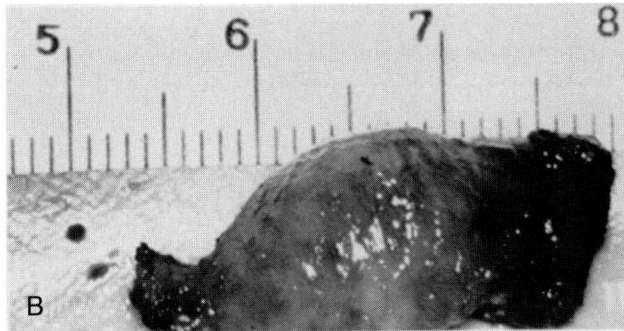
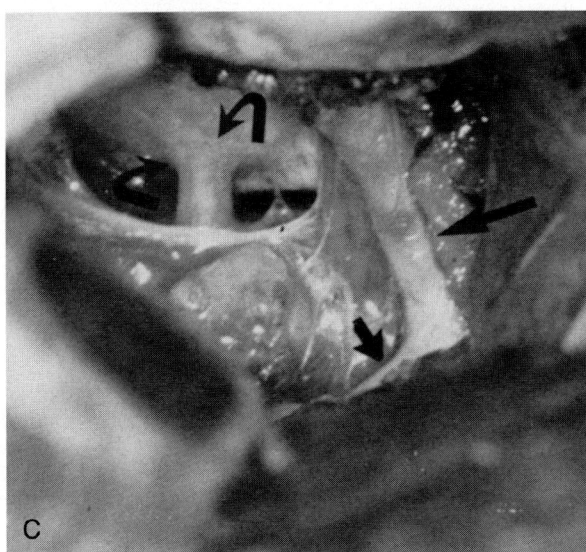

PRESERVED COMPLETE VISUAL FIELD        LEFT EYE

ACUITY 20/20

2.4 cm TUMOR

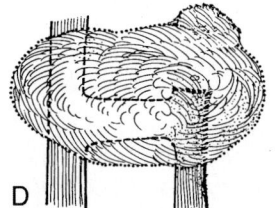

**FIGURE 18–16 ■** Case Report 10. *A,* Subfrontal exposure of the tumor (bounded by *white* and *black arrows*) covering the normal parasellar structures. *B,* The excised intracranial portion of the tumor expanding the right optic nerve; the huge optic foraminal end of tumor is to the right. *C,* After the tumor is removed, the normal structures can be seen in glistening intact arachnoid. (*Long straight arrow,* right internal carotid artery; *short straight arrow,* right anterior cerebral artery; *curved arrow,* pituitary stalk.) The left optic nerve, chiasm, and right optic tract are so grossly displaced by the tumor that they are covered by brain in this view. *D,* A diagram of the relationship of the intracranial portion of the tumor to the visual pathways.

present, but only a small attachment of tumor to the lateral aspect of the tract and chiasm existed. Most of these two structures looked normal. Removal was facilitated by transection of the intracranial mass just behind the optic foramen and at the junction of the optic nerve and chiasm. The main intracranial portion of the tumor (see Fig. 18–16) having been lifted out, the critical final dissection of tumor from the posterior visual pathways was more precise (see Fig. 18–16D). The roof of the optic canal and the orbit were then removed, and the anterior end of the tumor to behind the globe was dissected out as a separate specimen. The full visual field and acuity of the left eye were normal, and the patient has maintained an excellent work record since the operation. CT scans with and without contrast material obtained on January 11, 1984, showed no tissue suggestive of neoplasm in the suprasellar cistern. A single, low, suprasellar clip interferes with the resolution in its vicinity in CT and MRI scans. (We do not use metal clips for hemostasis in these patients now.) The patient was well and working full-time in September 1993, 20.6 years after operation.

## Hypothalamic Invasion

All of the foregoing patients had no intimation of a hypothalamic or other cerebral invasion by tumor. Only in the case of a Chinese man, aged 21 years when first diagnosed, have we had a fruitful result from a partial removal of a tumor invading the hypothalamus.

### Case Report 11

In contrast to the tumors whose primary origin in the visual pathways leads to initial symptoms of visual disturbance, this patient had had increasing polydipsia and polyuria for 2 years and visual impairment for only 6 months when we saw him. Although his irregular field defects were largely confined to the inferior temporal quadrants, his visual acuity was down to 20/200 in each eye. A pneumoencephalogram showed an anteriorly situated mass, about 2.5 cm in diameter, in the third ventricle. The patient's optic nerves and anterior chiasm looked normal on February 3, 1967, but the lamina terminalis and the posterior chiasm were covered with a gray mass, which, as seen from the right side, largely spared the optic tract (Fig. 18–17). The gray tissue within the anterior third ventricle was removed up to and including a 7-mm hole in the hypothalamic floor, through which the arachnoid covering the pons could be seen. The pathologic diagnosis was astrocytoma grade I.

Four weeks postoperatively, the patient was reading J2 slowly with the right eye and J4 with the left; the field defects were about the same. Kjellberg gave the patient 15 Gy of proton radiation at the Bragg peak at a single sitting—roughly equivalent to 30 Gy of gamma rays. The patient's visual acuity worsened slowly, down to 20/50 in each eye, and by August 1967 was 20/200 in the right eye and less than 20/400 in the left, with a nearly complete right homonymous

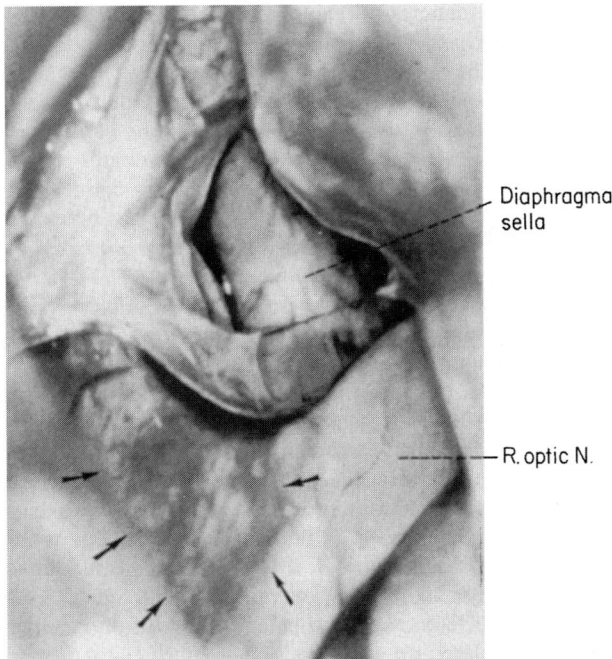

FIGURE 18–17 ■ Case Report 11. Subfrontal exposure. Before its removal, the gray tumor can be seen invading the lamina terminalis and much of the chiasm. The *small black arrows* mark the tumor boundaries. The chiasm is markedly postfixed.

hemianopia. No increase in tumor size was apparent on pneumoencephalogram. No more radiation was given. The visual acuity improved to J1 on the right and J3 on the left by February 1977. The patient's field defects still precluded his driving a car, however. In the ensuing 27 postoperative years, he became an energetic, effective businessman who traveled extensively.

Slowly growing gliomas invading the chiasm and one growing also into the hypothalamus in six children were radically removed. Each patient grew to be a productive adult who was followed from 15 to 27 years (average, 20 years) with no evidence of regrowth of tumor. Radiation, 15 Gy of protons at the Bragg peak, was given only to the patient with the hypothalamic invasion.

Other aggressive removals of the anterior portions of huge tumors invading nerves, chiasm, and hypothalamus in patients blind or virtually so have failed to achieve a useful result. One patient died postoperatively; another, although living 17 years later, had a poor quality of life. He is incontinent, unable to feed himself, and has limited speech. Two of our colleagues have had similar experiences, with one case each. Sweet's third case seemed at first similar to Case Reports 6 and 7. A 15-ml cyst in the right sylvian fissure continued into solid glioma of the right optic nerve and chiasm but then also invaded the left optic tract and hypothalamus, which were left behind. The boy had a disappointing course, which led to death 12 years later. In 18 other chiasmal or hypothalamic gliomas of our colleagues and in two more of Sweet's cases, we thought the situation called for no more intervention than a biopsy. The favorable outcomes of six more cases add to the evidence that operative exploration is the most certain means of determining operability of a tumor. These operations were all performed before 1974, usually without the benefit of an operating microscope.

## EXPERIENCES OF OTHER PARTIAL OR MAJOR REMOVALS

Many other accounts of one or more good results of major removals of gliomas invading the chiasm are in the literature. Ray[148] reported on a 13-year-old boy whose tumorous right half of the chiasm and adjacent segments of the right nerve and tract were resected by Cushing in 1929. Vision was preserved in the nasal field of the left eye until the patient died of another cause 32 years later. A postmortem examination revealed a tiny nodule of tumor at the chiasm.

Gaini and coworkers[101] did "a macroscopically complete removal," as demonstrated by CT, of a tumor invading one optic nerve and the chiasm on the same side. The child, blind in the left eye with a hemianopia in the other, had no evidence of recurrence 4 years later. CT was also used for documentation in one case from Helcl and Petraskova.[57]

Wulc and associates[85] described a 31-year-old woman with neurofibromatosis type 1 whose biopsy of a grade I astrocytoma invading the chiasm was followed by radiation therapy. The patient was free of symptoms for 7 years. Rapid proptosis on the left side led to exenteration of that orbit and another course of radiotherapy. A right temporal hemianopia with increased intracranial pressure 1 year later was followed by a left frontal lobectomy and subtotal resection of malignant cerebral glioma. The patient was well 2 years later, with good vision and no change in the visual field of the remaining eye, apparently another example of the astonishing variability in spontaneous and manipulated course of these tumors.

Myles and Murphy[9] (9 cases) and Helcl and Petraskova[57] (11 cases) performed partial or subtotal removal of tumors where considerable extension of tumor existed outside the visual pathways. Baram and colleagues[149] used acute or subacute visual deterioration as the basis for a partial surgical removal in three children; vision improved in one eye in two of them. Full details are not given in these three accounts.

Sufficient detail is given in other reports in which a worthwhile result ensued after near-total removal: Posner and Horrax[150] (three cases), Lèhlein and Tènnis[147] (three cases), and Matson[5] (two cases) as well as Boudet and colleagues,[151] Francois,[152] Karaguiosov,[97] MacCarty and colleagues,[153] and Helcl and Petraskova,[57] with one case each. If a portion of the tumor lies outside of visual and hypothalamic tissues or fails to enlarge some of the chiasm or opposite nerve, we see no good reason for leaving it in. It is usually avascular and readily removable. Chang and Wood[94] pointed out that small optic gliomas respond better to radiation than do large ones, which is an additional reason for partial extirpation rather than no removal.

Koos and colleagues[154] stated that, under the operating microscope, they can distinguish both tumor tissue and vessels from intact optic neural elements and normal vessels on longitudinal opening of the tight nerve sheath.

Under high magnification, "tumor was differentiated from compressed neural tissue and resected safely." By selective coagulation of tumor vessels, they provoked degeneration of unresectable tumor remnants. They reported that, in 10 children aged 3 to 5 years, such operations for spongioblastomas of the optic system yielded "unexpected and rapid improvement of vision as a persistent finding."[154] In two other children aged 3 to 5 years, extensive hypothalamic spongioblastomas were similarly resected "with rapid improvement in level of consciousness and endocrine disturbances."[154] The vision improvement in one eye remained constant in one of the two patients 3 years after surgery. They indicated that in one patient, an intrinsic rather than an exophytic tumor of right optic nerve and chiasm was attacked. Four years after partial removal of this *optic spongioblastoma*, the 6-year-old boy continues to have improved acuity in the right eye and normal vision in the left.

We agree with Matson's[5] 1969 dictum, to which many other authorities subscribe, that establishing the degree of operability by surgical exploration of the optic chiasm is of primary importance in every case. Up until 1996, we had seen no article by a neurosurgeon that gave details of major partial or complete removals of these tumors. Are we missing opportunities to help some of these patients?

## RADIATION THERAPY

It is now accepted that many of these tumors invading the chiasm and beyond are helped by radiation therapy. The effective dose, however, often exceeds 4500 cGy in approximately 1.8-Gy fractions. Data showing that these doses for whole-brain therapy are dangerous to cognitive and related functions in children deserve attention. An increased long-term survival from substantial dose increases has been accompanied by sustained declines in high-level cerebral functions, according to several retrospective studies.[155–158] Bamford and associates[159] noticed this effect, especially in children whose radiation treatment occurred before they reached 11 years of age. Hirsch and colleagues[155] reported that of 30 retrospectively studied children, intelligence was superior in 3, average in 10, and below average in 4; special educational methods were required in 11; and 2 were severely impaired. These concerns have led to efforts to find lower dose levels that are both safe and effective.[160] Extrapolation of data from children with acute lymphocytic leukemia treated by cranial radiation therapy in the lower doses of 1800 to 2400 cGy has been questioned because of the intrathecal methotrexate the patients had received. Declines in the full-scale intelligence quotient (FSIQ) of 18 patients were measured three times. Of the 18 children, 11 showed a decrement in FSIQ of more than 10 points between the first and third tests. The decrease was more marked in children aged 2 to 5 years when treated with the low standard dose of 2400 rads and was evident only 3 or more years after treatment.[161]

In the prospective and best-controlled study of the problem by Packer and coworkers,[156] 21 children aged 36 months to 18 years (median, 7.7 years) with malignant primary central nervous system tumors received radiotherapy. The lesions were mainly medulloblastomas and tumors in the pineal region and definitely did not involve the cerebral cortex, subcortical white matter, or deep gray masses. The patients were given 3600 cGy to the whole brain plus a boost of 1800 to 2000 cGy to the tumor site. A lower dose of 2400 cGy to the whole brain and 2400 to 2600 more to the tumor site was given to three children aged 18 to 36 months. They were matched by a group of 14 patients aged 18 months to 16.8 years (median, 7.7 years) whose cerebellar astrocytomas had been totally excised. A huge battery of neuropsychologic tests varying with the age of the patient was carried out before radiation or suboccipital craniectomy and was repeated thereafter. Fine motor, visuomotor integration, visuoperceptual function, memory, language, and arithmetic abilities were evaluated. All clinical details, especially those relevant to any complications of the illness and their treatments, were included in the assessments.

The declines in performance from the pretreatment baseline were dramatic, especially in the younger children. The three children younger than 36 months of age whose whole-brain radiation was only 2400 cGy had declines of 34, 36, and 37 points in FSIQ between baseline and testing 2 years later, to levels of 50, 68, and 87. Children aged 7 years or younger at diagnosis had a mean decline of 25 points in FSIQ 2 years later; the entire malignant tumor group dropped 14 points in FSIQ in the 2 years, whereas the excised astrocytoma control group gained 1 FSIQ point in that interval. The other tests showed varying degrees of impairment; memory was frequently impaired, and in 4 of 12 children, a further decline in memory function occurred over time; academic performance in school was also far worse in the radiated group. This excellent study has been described in detail because it presents the most convincing evidence that a well-fractionated dose of 3600 cGy to the whole brain of children younger than 10 years old is probably dangerous to cognitive functions. The firmness of this conclusion is impaired by the possibility in this series that the chemotherapy, too, may have had a deleterious role. Thirteen of the 18 children who had radiotherapy also received full courses of chemotherapy with cisplatin and vincristine.

In the 15 children younger than 11 years of age with slowly growing optic gliomas followed for more than 1 year, 8 received the adult dose of 5000 cGy, and 7 received from 3400 to 4600 cGy.[70] After doses of 49.5 to 52 Gy, three children aged 3.9 to 13 years developed panhypopituitarism or seizures. No studies of cognitive function were carried out. Kalifa and colleagues[100] radiated the tumors of 57 children aged 9 months to 15 years with 50 to 60 Gy. Surgical removal of an optic nerve–containing tumor, carried out in three cases, was followed by radiation of 50 to 53 Gy because the chiasm was invaded in all three. Follow-up occurred for 4, 10, and 10 years. Among 42 survivors, 26 had major mental retardation, especially in the very young group and in those with so large a tumor that the radiation field included some cerebral cortex.

## OTHER IMPORTANT STUDIES

Three other especially important studies have been conducted on low-grade gliomas of the optic chiasm, hypothal-

amus, or both, describing radical resection of such tumors. In Gillett and Symon's[162] seven patients (mean age, 20.3 years), the lesions were all mainly hypothalamic (i.e., retrochiasmatic), despite the fact that there were no major postoperative complications and no major worsening of symptoms in any of these patients. Radiotherapy was given to six of the seven patients. After follow-ups from 6 months to 6 years, five of the patients remain well. Wisoff and associates[163] have carried out similar aggressive surgery in 16 children. The three children younger than 1 year of age all died as a result of continuing growth of tumor. Of 13 children older than 1 year of age, however, 11 were well without clinical or radiographic progression 4 months to 4.5 years after surgery. No radiation therapy was given to six of them after a mean follow-up of 27 months in the hope that such therapy could be postponed until the child reached an age at which he or she would be less vulnerable to the effects of radiation. The study conducted by Albright and Sclabassi[136] is important in that the value of following visual evoked potentials during removal of 60% to 85% of two childhood chiasmal gliomas with a Cavitron ultrasonic surgical aspirator was shown.

## SUMMARY

1. A mass in the anterior visual pathways is nearly always a neoplasm. The concept that the slowly changing lesions are hamartomas has been disproved; the potential for unpredictable growth remains. The explanation for the extremely variable course in these lesions probably lies in an unusual tendency toward mutations in the growth-controlling genes—a hypothesis suggested by the spontaneous regression or disappearance of these tumors.

2. Calcification may develop not only within, but also outside the tumor. The latter locus should be identified to avoid the mistaken assumption of recurrence of tumor.

3. MRI at close spatial intervals provides essential critical diagnostic and postoperative follow-up information. CT scans give better information about calcification. Visual evoked potential responses, especially those with a checkerboard pattern stimulus, have proved their worth and should be used more widely.

4. A glioma confined to one optic nerve should be treated by neurectomy from the chiasm to the globe via a subfrontal approach as soon as it is diagnosed in most symptomatic patients. Exceptions to this rule are mainly patients with neurofibromatosis type 1.

5. More extensive probable gliomas should be explored transfrontally to confirm the diagnosis and to remove some or nearly all of the tumor in the few patients susceptible to such attack. Some large tumors partially amputate their connections with the normal visual pathways rather than infiltrate them. Metal clips for hemostasis at surgery should be avoided because they disturb interpretation of both CT scans and MRI.

6. Cautious radiation therapy of residual gross tumor is indicated, and careful clinical and neuroradiologic

follow-ups determine optimal dosage schedules. The radiation fields should be confined to the areas near the tumor. More data are needed on long-term effects of radiotherapy on cognitive functions.

## ACKNOWLEDGMENT

*Dr. Sweet expresses his gratitude to the Neuro-Research Foundation for its support during the preparation of this chapter.*

## REFERENCES

1. Dandy WE: Orbital Tumors. New York: Oskar Press, 1941, p 168.
2. Dandy WE: Results following the transcranial operative attack on operative tumors. Arch Ophthalmol 25:191–213, 1941.
3. Lloyd LA: Gliomas of the optic nerve and chiasm in childhood. In Smith JL (ed): Neuro-Ophthalmology Update. New York: Masson Publishing, 1977, pp 185–197.
4. Henschen F: Tumoren des Zentral nervensystems. In: Handbuch der Speiziellen Pathologishe Anatomica 1955, pp 817–816.
5. Matson DD: Neurosurgery of Infancy and Childhood. Springfield, IL: Charles C Thomas, 1969, pp 533–536.
6. Schuster G, Westberg G: Gliomas of the optic nerve and chiasm. Acta Radiol 6:221–232, 1967.
7. Fletcher WA, Imes RK, Hoyt WF: Chiasmal gliomas: Appearance and long-term changes demonstrated by computerized tomography. J Neurosurg 65:154–159, 1986.
8. Bynke H, Kagstrom E, Tjernstrom K: Aspects on the treatment of gliomas of the anterior visual pathways. Acta Ophthalmol 55:269–280, 1977.
9. Myles ST, Murphy SB: Gliomas of the optic nerve and chiasm. Can J Ophthalmol 8:508–514, 1973.
10. Kahn EA, Crosby EC, Schneider RC, et al: Correlative Neurosurgery. Springfield, IL: Charles C Thomas, 1969, pp 111–113.
11. Weiss L, Sagerman RH, King GA, et al: Controversy in the management of optic nerve glioma. Cancer 59:1000–1004, 1987.
12. Beyer RA, Paden P, Sobel DF, et al: Moyamoya pattern of vascular occlusion after radiotherapy for glioma of the optic chiasm. Neurology 36:1173–1178, 1986.
13. Cavazzuti V, Fischer EG, Welch K, et al: Neurological and psychophysiological sequelae following different treatments of craniopharyngioma in children. J Neurosurg 59:409–417, 1983.
14. Jakobiec FA, Depot MJ, Kennerdell JS, et al: Combined clinical and computed tomographic diagnosis of orbital glioma and meningioma. Ophthalmology 91:137–155, 1984.
15. Byrd SE, Harwood-Nash DC, Fitz CR, et al: Computed tomography of intraorbital optic nerve gliomas in children. Radiology 129:73–78, 1978.
16. Gorter CJ: Paramagnetic Relaxation. Amsterdam: Elsevier, 1947.
17. Del Regata JA: Frances Henry Williams. Int J Radiat Oncol Biol Phys 9:739–749, 1983.
18. Daniels DL, Herfkins R, Gager WE, et al: Magnetic resonance imaging of the optic nerves and chiasm. Radiology 152:79–83, 1984.
19. Wright JE, McNab AA, McDonald WI: Optic nerve glioma and the management of optic nerve tumours in the young. Br J Ophthalmol 73:967–974, 1989.
20. Hoyt WF, Meshel LG, Lessell S, et al: Malignant optic glioma of adulthood. Brain 96:121–132, 1973.
21. Barbaro NM, Rosenblum ML, Maitland CG, et al: Malignant optic glioma presenting radiologically as a "cystic" suprasellar mass: Case report and review of the literature. Neurosurgery 11:787–789, 1982.
22. Pomeranze SJ, Shelton JJ, Tobias J, et al: MR of visual pathways in patients with neurofibromatosis. AJNR Am J Neuroradiol 8:831–836, 1987.
23. Brown EW, Riccardi VM, Mawad M, et al: MR imaging of optic pathways in patients with neurofibromatosis. AJNR Am J Neuroradiol 8:1031–1036, 1987.
24. Packer RJ, Sutton LN, Bilaniuk LT, et al: Treatment of chiasmatic/hypothalamic gliomas of childhood with chemotherapy: An update. Ann Neurol 23:79–85, 1988.
25. Lin W, Tkach JA, Haacke EM, et al: Intracranial MR angiography: Application of magnetization transfer contrast and fat saturation to short gradient-echo, velocity-compensated sequences. Radiology 186:753–761, 1993.
26. Stern J, Jakobiec FA, Housepian EM: The architecture of optic nerve gliomas with and without neurofibromatosis. Arch Ophthalmol 98:505–511, 1980.
27. Azar-Kia B, Naheedy M, Elias DA, et al: Optic nerve tumors: Role of magnetic resonance imaging and computed tomography. Radiol Clin North Am 25:561–581, 1987.
28. Seiff SR, Brodsky MC, MacDonald G, et al: Orbital optic glioma in neurofibromatosis. Arch Ophthalmol 105:1689–1692, 1987.
29. Imes RK, Hoyt W: Magnetic resonance imaging signs of optic nerve gliomas in neurofibromatosis 1. Am J Ophthalmol 111:729–734, 1991.
30. Atlas S (ed): Magnetic Resonance Imaging of the Brain and Spine. New York: Raven Press, 1991, pp 744–745.
31. Strong JA, Hatten HP, Brown MT, et al: Pilocytic astrocytoma: Correlation between the initial imaging features and clinical aggressiveness. AJR Am J Roentgenol 1612:1369–1372, 1993.
32. Cohen BH, Bury E, Packer RJ, et al: Gadolinium-DTPA-enhanced magnetic resonance imaging in childhood brain tumors. Neurology 39:1178–1183, 1989.
33. Maitland CG, Abiko S, Hoyt WF, et al: Chiasmal apoplexy. J Neurosurg 56:118–122, 1982.
34. McLeod AR: Acute blindness in childhood optic glioma caused by hematoma. J Pediatr Ophthalmol Strabismus 20:31–33, 1983.
35. Applegate LJ, Pribam HFW: Hematoma of optic nerve glioma—cause for sudden proptosis. J Clin Neuroophthalmol 9:15–19, 1989.
36. Charles NC, Nelson L, Brookner AR, et al: Pilocytic astrocytoma of the optic nerve with hemorrhage and extreme cystic degeneration. Am J Ophthalmol 92:691–695, 1981.
37. Gomori JM, Grossman RI, Goldberg HI, et al: Intracranial hematomas: Imaging by high-field MR. Radiology 157:87–93, 1985.
38. Curatolo P, Cusmai R: Optic gliomas in children with neurofibromatosis. Lancet 1:1140, 1987.
39. Aron AM, Taff I, Wallace SA, et al: Neurofibromatosis and chiasmal glioma: Reappraisal for future management. Ann Neurol 20:399–400, 1986.
40. Cohen ME, Duffner PK, Kuhn JP, et al: Neuroimaging in neurofibromatosis. Ann Neurol 20:444, 1986.
41. Hurst RW, Newman SA, Cail WS: Multifocal intracranial MR abnormalities in neurofibromatosis. AJNR Am J Neuroradiol 9:293–296, 1988.
42. Groswasser Z, Friss A, Halliday AM, et al: Pattern and flash-evoked potentials in the assessment and management of optic nerve gliomas. J Neurol Neurosurg Psychiatry 48:1125–1134, 1985.
43. Flickinger JC, Torres C, Deutsch M: Management of low-grade gliomas of the optic nerve and chiasm. Cancer 61:635–642, 1988.
44. Williams M, Verity CM, Broadbent V, et al: Optic nerve gliomas in children with neurofibromatosis. Lancet 1:1318–1319, 1987.
45. Majorchik VE, Arkhipova NA, Bokeriia ZO: Visual evoked potentials in children with gliomas of the optic nerve and chiasm. Zh Vopr Neirokhir 1:20–24, 1988.
46. Hoyt WF, Baghdassarian SA: Optic glioma of childhood: Natural history and rationale for conservative management. Br J Ophthalmol 53:793–798, 1969.
47. Glaser JS, Hoyt WF, Corbett J: Visual morbidity with chiasmal glioma: Long-term studies of visual fields in untreated and irradiated cases. Arch Ophthalmol 85:3–12, 1971.
48. Miller NR, Iliff WJ, Green WR: Evaluation and management of gliomas of the anterior visual pathways. Brain 97:743–754, 1974.
49. Borit A, Richardson EP: The biological and clinical behaviour of pilocytic astrocytomas of the optic pathways. Brain 105:161–187, 1982.
50. Wong IG, Lubow M: Management of optic glioma of childhood: A review of 42 cases. In Smith JL (ed): Neuroophthalmology, Vol 6. St. Louis: CV Mosby, 1972, pp 51–60.
51. Donahue HC: An exceptional lesion of the orbit. Arch Ophthalmol 54:259–261, 1955.
52. Hudson AC: Primary tumors of the optic nerve. Royal London Ophthalmology Hospital Reports 18:317–349, 1912.
53. Dandy WE: Prechiasmal intracranial tumors of the optic nerves. Am J Ophthalmol 5:169–188, 1922.

54. Byers WGM: Primary intradural tumours of the optic nerve: Fibromatosis nervi optici. In: Studies from the Royal Victoria Hospital Montreal. Toronto: JA Carveth & Company, 1901, pp 3–82.

55. Reese AB: Tumors of the Eye, 3rd ed. Hagerstown, MD: Harper & Row, 1976, pp 134–145.

56. Brand WN, Hoover SV: Optic glioma in children: Review of 16 cases given megavoltage radiation therapy. Childs Nerv Syst 5:459–466, 1979.

57. Helcl F, Petraskova H: Gliomas of visual pathways and hypothalamus in children—a preliminary report. Acta Neurochir Suppl (Wien) 35:106–110, 1985.

58. Sugita K, Kageyama N: Treatment and follow up studies of the optic gliomas: Infant and child types. No Shinkei Ginka 2:97–103, 1977.

59. Kanamori M, Shibuya M, Yoshida J, et al: Long-term follow-up of patients with optic glioma. Childs Nerv Syst 1:272–278, 1985.

60. Heiskanen O, Raitta C, Torsti R: The management and prognosis of gliomas of the optic pathways in children. Acta Neurochir (Wien) 43:193–199, 1978.

61. Wilson WB, Feinsod M, Hoyt WF: Malignant evolution of childhood chiasmal pilocytic astrocytoma. Neurology 26:322–325, 1976.

62. Szokalski V: Tumeur squorho-cance reuse du nerf optique. Ann Ocul 46:43–50, 1861.

63. Goldzieher W: Die Geschwulste des Sehnerven. Graefes Arch Clin Exp Ophthalmol 19:119–144, 1873.

64. Barraquer J: Mixoma quistico del nervio optico de la papila y retina derechas y de la cavidad craneal y orbita izquierda. Arch Oftal Hispanoam 2:132–139, 1902.

65. Pagenstecher AH: Ueber Opticustumoren. Graefes Arch Clin Exp Ophthalmol 54:300–336, 1902.

66. Anderson DR, Spencer WH: Ultrastructural and histochemical observations of optic nerve gliomas. Arch Ophthalmol 83:324–335, 1970.

67. Alvord EC, Lofton S: Gliomas of the optic nerve or chiasm: Outcome by patient's age, tumor site, and treatment. J Neurosurg 68:85–98, 1988.

68. Armitage P: Statistical Methods in Medical Research. Oxford: Blackwell Scientific Publications, 1971, pp 408–414.

69. Berkson J, Gage RP: Calculation of survival rates for cancer. Mayo Clin Proc 25: 270–286, 1950.

70. Wong JYC, Uhl V, Wara W, et al: Optic gliomas: A reanalysis of the University of California, San Francisco experience. Cancer 60:1847–1855, 1987.

71. Derenzini M, Pession A, Trere D: Quantity of nucleolar silver-stained proteins is related to proliferating activity in cancer cells. Lab Invest 63:137–140, 1990.

72. Radhakrishnam VV: Nucleolar organizing regions in meningiomas. Br J Neurosurg 7:377–382, 1993.

73. Burnstine MA, Levin LA, Louis DN, et al: Nucleolar organizer regions in optic gliomas. Brain 116(Pt 6):1465–1476, 1993.

74. Louis DN, Meehan SM, Ferrante RJ, et al: Use of the silver nucleolar organizer region (AgNOR) technique in the differential diagnosis of central nervous system neoplasia. J Neuropathol Exp Neurol 51:150–157, 1992.

75. Spencer WH, Borit A: Diffuse hyperplasia of the optic nerve in von Recklinghausen's disease. Am J Ophthalmol 64:120–124, 1967.

76. Spencer WH: Primary neoplasms of the optic nerve and its sheaths: Clinical features and current concepts of pathogenetic mechanisms. Trans Am Ophthalmol Soc 70:490–528, 1972.

77. Pfeiffer RL: Personal communication to Taveras, Mount and Wood. Radiology 66:518–528, 1956.

78. Reese AB: Tumors of the Eye, 2nd ed. New York: Harper & Row, 1963, pp 171, 191, 192.

79. Horwich A, Bloom HJG: Optic gliomas: Radiation therapy and prognosis. Int J Radiat Oncol Biol Phys 11:1067–1079, 1985.

80. Lewis RA, Gerson LP, Axelson KA, et al: von Recklinghausen neurofibromatosis. II: Incidence of optic gliomata. Ophthalmology 91:929–935, 1984.

81. Tym R: Piloid gliomas of the anterior optic pathways. Br J Surg 49:322–331, 1961.

82. Venes JL, Latack J, Kandt RS: Postoperative regression of opticochiasmatic astrocytoma: A case for expectant therapy. Neurosurgery 15:421–423, 1984.

83. Berke RN: A modified Krönlein operation. Arch Ophthalmol 51:609–632, 1954.

84. Hird B: Discussion on tumours of the optic nerve. Proc R Soc Med 33:690–692, 1940.

85. Wulc AE, Bergin DJ, Barnes D: Orbital optic nerve glioma in adult life. Arch Ophthalmol 107:1013–1016, 1989.

86. Marx J: Learning how to suppress cancer. Science 261:1385–1387, 1993.

87. Jacoby LB: Clonal origin of nervous system tumors. In Schmidek HH, Levine AJ (eds): Molecular Genetics of Nervous System Tumors. New York: Wiley-Liss, 1993, p 211.

88. Rand CW, Inui R, Raines DL: Primary glioma of the optic nerve. Arch Ophthalmol 21:799–816, 1939.

89. Cuneo HM, Rand CW: Brain Tumors in Childhood. Springfield, IL: Charles C Thomas, 1952, pp 126–143.

90. Hanbery JW: Gliomas of the optic nerve. Stanford Med Bull 14:34–50, 1956.

91. Jain NS: Two-stage intracranial and orbital operation for glioma of the optic nerve. Br J Ophthalmol 45:54–58, 1961.

92. Bane WM, Long JC: Glioma of the optic nerve. Am J Ophthalmol 57:649–654, 1964.

93. Richards RD, Lynn JR: The surgical management of gliomas of the optic nerve. Am J Ophthalmol 62:60–65, 1966.

94. Chang CH, Wood EH: The value of radiation therapy for gliomas of the anterior visual pathway. In Brockhurst RJ, Boruchoff SA, Hutchinson BT, et al (eds): Controversy in Ophthalmology. Philadelphia: WB Saunders, 1977, pp 878–886.

95. Lloyd LA: Gliomas of the optic nerve and chiasm in childhood. Trans Am Ophthalmol Soc 71:488, 1973.

96. De Sousa AL, Kalsbeck JE, Mealey J Jr, et al: Optic chiasmatic glioma in children. Am J Ophthalmol 87:376–381, 1979.

97. Karaguiosov L: Surgical treatment of gliomas of the optic nerve and chiasma. Acta Neurochir Suppl (Wien) 28:411–412, 1979.

98. Marejeva TG, Rostotskaya VI, Sokolova ON, et al: Tumours of the optic nerve and chiasma in children: Diagnosis and surgical treatment. Acta Neurochir Suppl (Wien) 28:409–410, 1979.

99. Visot A, Rougerie J, Derome PJ, et al: Gliomes optochiasmatiques. Neurochirurgie 26:181–192, 1980.

100. Kalifa C, Ernest C, Rodary C, et al: Les gliomes du chiasma optique chéz l'enfant: Étude retrospective de 57 cas traites par irradiation. Memoires Originaux. Arch Fr Pediatr 38:309–313, 1981.

101. Gaini SM, Tomei G, Arienta C, et al: Optic nerve and chiasm gliomas in children. J Neurosurg Sci 26:33–39, 1982.

102. Tenny RT, Laws ER Jr, Younge BR, et al: The neurosurgical management of optic glioma: Results in 104 patients. J Neurosurg 57:452–458, 1982.

103. Gabibov GA, Blinkov SM, Tcherekayev VA: The management of optic nerve meningiomas and gliomas. J Neurosurg 68:889–893, 1988.

104. Suarez J, Garzon F, Schuster G, et al: Gliomas del nervio y quiasma optico en la infancia. Acta Neurol Latinoam 17:46–55, 1971.

105. Jefferson G: Discussion on tumours of the optic nerve. Proc R Soc Med 33:688, 692, 1940.

106. Smith JL (ed): Neuro-ophthalmology Update. New York: Masson Publishing, 1977.

107. Wright JE, McDonald WI, Call NB: Management of optic nerve gliomas. Br J Ophthalmol 64:545–552, 1980.

108. Klug GL: Gliomas of the optic nerve and chiasm in children. Aust N Z J Surg 47:596–600, 1977.

109. Knapp A: On the intracranial extension of optic nerve tumors. In: Contributions to Ophthalmic Science. Menasha, WI: George Banta Publishing Company, 1926, pp 69–73.

110. Chutorian AM, Schwartz JF, Evans RA, et al: Optic gliomas in children. Neurology 14:83–95, 1964.

111. Seefelder R: Beitrage zu den Gliomen des Sehnerven. Wien Klin Wochenschr 44:838–840, 1931.

112. Davis FA: Primary tumors of the optic nerve. Arch Ophthalmol 23:735–821, 1940.

113. Levitt JM: Discussion of Davis: Primary tumors of the optic nerve. Arch Ophthalmol 23:1019–1021, 1940.

114. Christensen E, Andersen SR: Primary tumors of the optic nerve and chiasm. Acta Psychiatr Scand 27:5–16, 1952.

115. Zulch KJ, Nover A: Die Spongioblastome des Sehnerven. Graefes Arch Clin Exp Ophthalmol 161:405–419, 1960.

116. Yanoff M, Davis RL, Zimmerman LE: Juvenile pilocytic astrocytoma ("glioma") of optic nerve: Clinicopathologic study of sixty-three cases. In Jakobiec FA (ed): Ocular and Adnexal Tumors. Birmingham, AL: Aesculapius, 1978, pp 685–707.

117. Rougier J, Rambaud G, Joyeux O: Spongioblastome du nerf optique:

A propagation chiasmatique. Oto-Neurol-Ophthalmol 45:53–58, 1973.

118. Mullaney J, Walsh J, Lee WR, et al: Recurrence of astrocytoma of optic nerve after 48 years. Br J Ophthalmol 60:539–543, 1976.

119. Nicole S, Palma L, Giuffre R, et al: 31 primary orbital lesions in infancy and childhood. Childs Nerv Syst 6:255–261, 1980.

120. Iraci G, Gerosa M, Tomazzoli L, et al: Gliomas of the optic nerve and chiasm: A clinical review. Childs Nerv Syst 8:326–349, 1981.

121. Fog J, Seedorff HH, Vaernet K: Optic glioma: Clinical features and treatment. Acta Ophthalmol 48:644, 1970.

122. Goodman SJ, Rosenbaum AL, Hasso A, et al: Large optic nerve glioma with normal vision. Arch Ophthalmol 93:991–995, 1975.

123. Housepian EM: Intraorbital tumors. In Schmidek HH, Sweet WH (eds): Operative Neurosurgical Techniques: Indications, Methods, and Results. New York: Grune & Stratton, 1982, pp 227–244.

124. Housepian EM: The surgical treatment of optic nerve sheath meningiomas. Mod Technol Surg Neurosurg 21:1–14, 1981.

125. Luccarelli G: Ectopic pinealomas of the optic nerves and chiasma: Report of two personal cases. Acta Neurochir (Wien) 27:205–221, 1972.

126. Walsh FB: Tumors ocular and intracranial and related conditions. In: Clinical Neuro-Ophthalmology. Baltimore: Williams & Wilkins, 1947, p 1140.

127. Maisongrosse G, Blanchard M, Antiphon R, et al: Gliomes du nerf optique et du chiasma: A propos de 10 cas. Bulletin of the French Society of Ophthalmology 82:207–210, 1982.

128. Martin P, Cushing H: Primary gliomas of the chiasm and optic nerves in their intracranial portion. Arch Ophthalmol 52:209–241, 1923.

129. Throuvalas N, Bataini P, Ennuyer A: Les gliomes du chiasma et du nerf optique. Bull Cancer (Paris) 56:231–264, 1969.

130. Robertson AG, Brewin TB: Optic nerve glioma. Clin Radiol 31:471–474, 1980.

131. Block MA, Goree JA, Jimenez JP: Craniopharyngioma with optic canal enlargement simulating glioma of the optic chiasm. J Neurosurg 39:523–527, 1973.

132. Desoretz DE, Blitzer PH, Wang CC, et al: Management of glioma in the optic nerve and/or chiasm: An analysis of 20 cases. Cancer 45:1467–1471, 1980.

133. Kovalic JJ, Grigsby PW, Shepard MJ, et al: Radiation therapy for gliomas of the optic nerve and chiasm. Int J Radiat Oncol Biol Phys 18:927–932, 1990.

134. Giuffré R, Bardelli AM, Taverniti L, et al: Anterior optic pathway gliomas. J Neurosurg Sci 26:61–72, 1982.

135. Montgomery AB, Griffin T, Parker RG, et al: Optic nerve glioma: The role of radiation therapy. Cancer 40:2079–2080, 1977.

136. Albright AL, Sclabassi RJ: Cavitron ultrasonic surgical aspirator and visual evoked potential monitoring for chiasmal gliomas in children. J Neurosurg 63:138–140, 1985.

137. Pellet W, Rakotobe A, Paillas JE: Evolution tardive des gliomes du chiasma traites par operation et irradiation. Rev Otoneuroophthalmol 43:241–249, 1971.

138. Uihlein A, Rucker CW: The neurosurgeon's role in acute visual failure. Arch Ophthalmol 60:223–229, 1958.

139. Karnaze MG, Sartor K, Winthrop JD, et al: Suprasellar lesions: Evaluation with MR imaging. Radiology 161:77–82, 1986.

140. Hoyt WF, Fletcher WA, Imes RK: Chiasmal gliomas: Appearance and long-term changes demonstrated by computerized tomography. Prog Exp Tumor Res 30:113–121, 1987.

141. Wolff E: Discussion on tumours of the optic nerve. Proc R Soc Med 33:687–688, 1940.

142. Neame H: Discussion on tumours of the optic nerve. Proc R Soc Med 33:692, 1940.

143. Cogan DG: Tumors of the optic nerve. Handbook Clin Neurol 17:350–374, 1974.

144. Walter GF: Kleinhirnastrocytome und Opticusgliome-eine vergleichende feinstrukturelle Untersuchung. Virchows Arch A Pathol Anat Histopathol 380:59–79, 1978.

145. Stern J, DiGiacinto GV, Housepian EM: Neurofibromatosis and optic glioma: Clinical and morphological correlations. Neurosurgery 4:524–528, 1979.

146. Northfield DWC: The Surgery of the Central Nervous System. Oxford: Blackwell Scientific, 1973, pp 183–185.

147. Léhlein W, Tonnis W: Die operative Behandlung der das Foramen opticum uberschreitenden Sehnervengeschwulste. Graefes Arch Ophthalmol 149:318–354, 1949.

148. Ray BS: Surgical lesions of optic nerves and chiasm in infants and children. In Smith JL (ed): Neuro-ophthalmology, Vol 3. St. Louis: CV Mosby, 1967, pp 77–99.

149. Baram TZ, Moser RP, van Eys J: Surgical management of progressive visual loss in optic gliomas of childhood. Ann Neurol 20:398, 1986.

150. Posner M, Horrax G: Tumors of the optic nerve: Long survival in three cases of intracranial tumor. Arch Ophthalmol 40:56–76, 1948.

151. Boudet A, Arnaud, Bullier, et al: Gliome du chiasma optique: A propos de quartre cas. Bull Soc Ophtalmol Fr 75:1045–1050, 1975.

152. Francois J: Gliome du chiasma. J Fr Ophtalmol 1:125–131, 1978.

153. MacCarty CS, Boyd AS, Childs DS: Tumors of the optic nerve and optic chiasm. J Neurosurg 33:439–444, 1970.

154. Koos WT, Bock FW, Salah S, et al: Microsurgery of gliomas of the optic nerves, the optic chiasm, and the hypothalamus. In Koos WT, Bock FW, Spetzler RF (eds): Clinical Microneurosurgery. Stuttgart: Georg Thieme, 1976, pp 58–63.

155. Hirsch JF, Reiner D, Czernichow P, et al: Medulloblastoma in childhood: Survival and functional results. Acta Neurochir (Wien) 48:1–15, 1979.

156. Packer RJ, Sutton LN, Atkins TE, et al: A prospective study of cognitive function in children receiving whole-brain radiotherapy and chemotherapy: 2-year results. J Neurosurg 70:707–713, 1989.

157. Raimondi AJ, Tomita T: Advantages of "total" resection of medulloblastoma and disadvantages of full head postoperative radiation therapy. Childs Nerv Syst 5:50–59, 1979.

158. Duffner PK, Cohen ME, Thomas PRM, et al: The long term effects of cranial irradiation in the central nervous system. Cancer 56:1841–1846, 1985.

159. Bamford FN, Jones PM, Pearson D, et al: Residual disabilities in children treated for intracranial space-occupying lesions. Cancer 37:1149–1151, 1976.

160. Tomita T, McLoue DG: Medulloblastoma in childhood with results of radical resection and low dose neuraxis radiation therapy. J Neurosurg 64:238–242, 1986.

161. Meadows AT, Massari DJ, Fergusson J, et al: Declines in IQ scores and cognitive dysfunctions in children with acute lymphocytic leukemia treated wtih cranial irradiation. Lancet 2:1015–1018, 1981.

162. Gillett GR, Symon L: Hypothalamic glioma. Surg Neurol 28:291–300, 1987.

163. Wisoff JH, Abbott R, Epstein F: Surgical management of exophytic chiasmatic-hypothalamic tumors of childhood. J Neurosurg 73:661–667, 1990.

# SECTION IV

# Anterior Skull Base

# CHAPTER 19

# Transbasal Approach to Tumors Invading the Skull Base

■ STÉPHANE GAILLARD, ANDRÉ VISOT, and PATRICK J. DEROME

For years, the complete removal of tumors invading the middle area of the skull base was considered impossible because they were located in a "no-man's land" for the different surgical specialties. When explored, these cases were approached successively through narrow exposures, and tumor removal was often incomplete.

In 1960, Tessier[22] asked Guiot for help in reducing his first case of hypertelorism. This new approach to the anterior skull base was first applied for the correction of craniofacial malformations like hypertelorism and craniofacial dysostosis. It was then adapted for the surgical removal of basal tumors. The first description of this approach, published in 1972, reported 16 cases of sphenoethmoidal lesions.[4]

## GOALS WITH THE TRANSBASAL APPROACH

The first goal with the transbasal approach is complete removal of the tumor. Some tumors are located at the midline, but most extend laterally toward the orbital walls, the lesser and greater sphenoid wings, and the middle fossa. The second goal is to free the cranial nerves and to open the optic foramens, the sphenoidal fissures, and even the foramen rotundum and foramen ovale, areas that cannot be reached through narrow anterior approaches. If the anterior and, possibly, the middle fossas need to be exposed, an anterior subdural and extradural approach is required. Anosmia, which often is present before the procedure, is the only side effect. Procedures that conserve structures of the cribriform area and the olfactory placode have been described, but their applicability depends on the tumor's location.[20] The combination of the transbasal approach with the other anterior transfacial approaches is discussed later.

## HAZARDS OF THE TRANSBASAL APPROACH

The most important complication of the transbasal approach is creation of a communication between the subarachnoid spaces and the upper air-filled cavities of the face (Fig. 19–1). Resection of an ethmoidosphenoidal mass widely opens the frontal sphenoid sinuses and the ethmoid air cells. The floor of the nasal fossas and the pharyngeal or cavum mucosa can be reached through the cranial approach. Meningeal tears and dural defects occur frequently, resulting in pneumatoceles, cerebrospinal fluid leaks, ascending infections, and meningitis.

The three structures between the intradural spaces and the air-filled cavities of the face are the dura, the bone involved by the tumor, and the rhinopharyngeal mucosal plane. After tumor removal, these structures must be repaired carefully to prevent complications. The dura must be closed tightly (which may require a pericranial graft) and the base of the skull must be reconstructed to eliminate a dead space that can lead to meningoceles, encephaloceles, postoperative extradural hematomas, or postoperative infections (Fig. 19–2). The mucosal plane must be preserved or reconstructed for the closure of the nasal fossas. Living tissue is necessary to feed the bone grafts used for the repair of the skull base.

When these dicta are strictly applied, the transbasal approach remains a benign and helpful procedure.

## SURGICAL TECHNIQUES

### Preparation

Prophylactic antibiotic therapy is strongly recommended, and is started with anesthesia induction and continued for 24 hours.

The patient is placed in the dorsal decubitus position with the head fixed in a three-point headrest. Some cases are operated on without fixation of the head so that all aspects of the positioning may be modified during surgery.

The operating microscope should be used near the neurovascular structures or around the cranial nerves, particularly for decompression of the optic nerves.

The frontal lobe must be retracted to expose the base of the skull. Assisted ventilation with negative pressure, mannitol, and continuous intraoperative lumbar drainage are all used routinely. Because the procedure may be a very

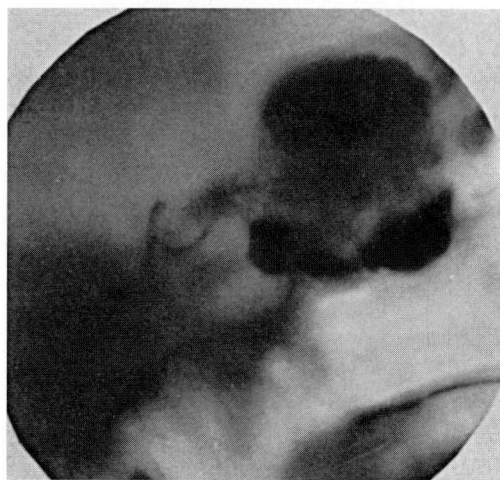
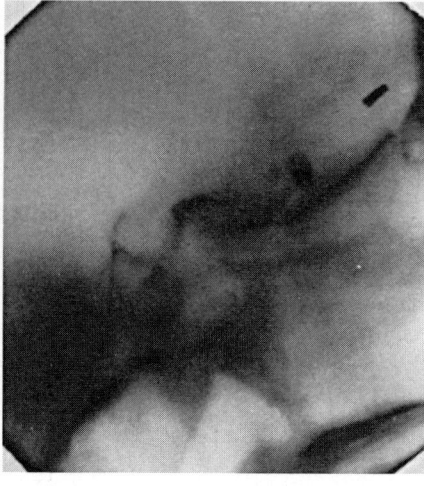

FIGURE 19-1 ■ Resection (*left* and *right*) of an ethmoidosphenoidal tumor (osteoma ?) opens the upper air cavities of the face widely.

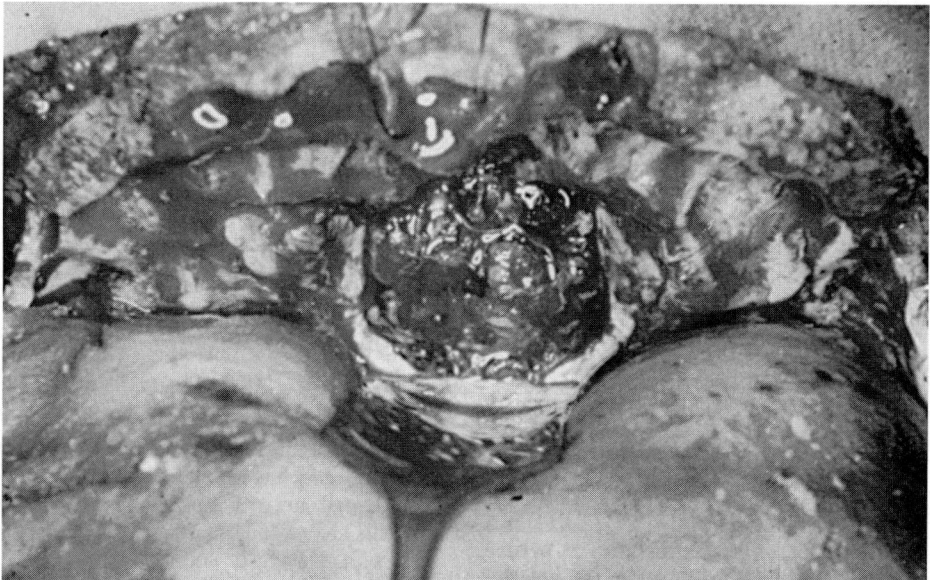

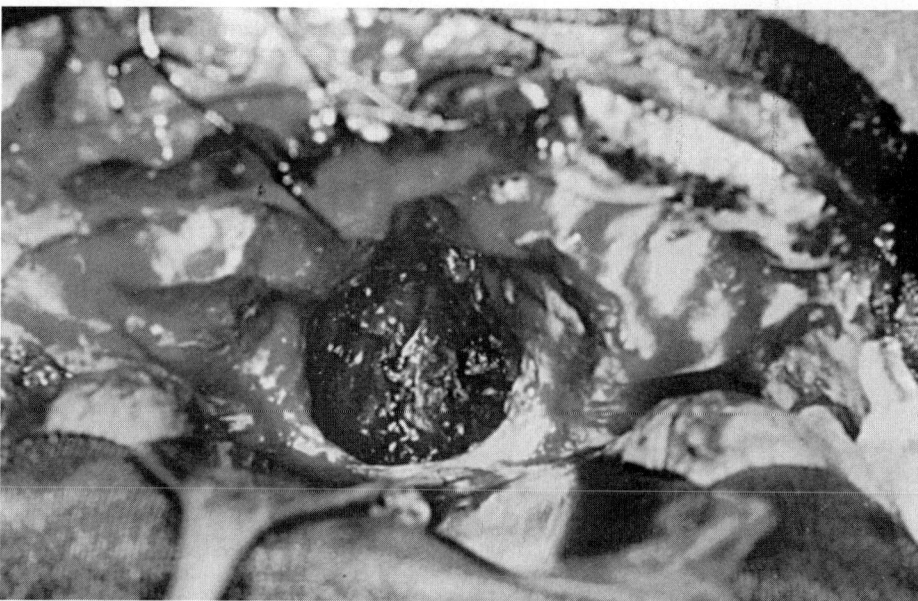

FIGURE 19-2 ■ Intraoperative view (*top*) of an ethmoidosphenoidal chordoma responsible for extradural compression of both optic nerves. The orbital roofs are partially removed. After the tumor has been removed (*bottom*), a large dead space extends to the nasal fossae and the deeper aspects of the pharyngeal mucosae. Note the free optic nerves.

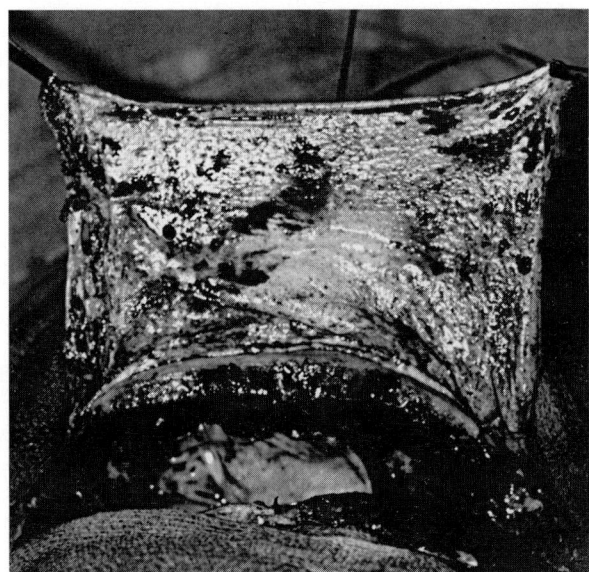

**FIGURE 19–3 ■** A large anterior pericranial flap is raised at the beginning of the operation; it will close the basal defect and may be considered as a "new mucosae plane."

long one, the anesthesiologist must maintain the patient as normothermic. Blood losses are carefully replaced and strict hemostasis applied at each step. If the tumor is vascular, preoperative embolization may be used.

## Mucosal Plane

Preserving the mucosal plane is always difficult. With a surgical approach from above, the sinus mucosa is dissected after tumor removal. Depending on the type of tumor, the mucosa may be involved by disease. In noninvasive tumors, the sinus mucosa is usually preserved, but this plane disappears in the ethmoidal area where the nasal fossas are widely opened and the turbinates visible. The best solution for closure of this area is a large anterior pericranial flap prepared at the beginning of the surgical procedure. This flap is cut along the temporal crests, as far as necessary, and turned anteriorly (Fig. 19–3); its supraorbital vascularization is preserved. At the end of the procedure, it is turned down to close the nasal fossas and the basal defect, and its posterior edge is sutured to the furthest limits of the subfrontal dura. Insertion of a bone graft in the basal defect is often sufficient to ensure a perfect closure without a posterior fixation of this new "mucosal plane."[5–7]

## Exposing the Skull Base

A temporotemporal incision is made just behind the hairline. The scalp is turned forward, taking care to not injure the frontotemporal branch of the facial nerve. The pericranial incision follows both temporal crests laterally to reach or overlap the coronal sutures, preserving a large anterior pericranial flap, which is curved upward. If more lateral exposure is necessary, the temporalis muscle is dissected

from the temporal fossa and retromalar area to the zygomatic process. A bifrontal free bone flap is fashioned with an inferior margin that is strictly supraorbital, without consideration for the size of frontal sinuses. If these sinuses are wide, their posterior walls and mucosas are removed, and their ostia are closed with bone grafts. After the subfrontal dura is dissected, the anterior fossa is exposed. This dissection is fairly easy, except for the area of both olfactory grooves. Sometimes it is possible to avoid meningeal tears by doing a primary resection of the crista galli and cutting the olfactory nerves one by one. The dissection must reach the posterior limits of the anterior fossa: the posterior edge of the lesser sphenoid wings, the tuberculum sellae, and the base of the anterior clinoid processes. A partially invaded dura or a tumor growing through the meninges into the intradural spaces may cause some problems. The subfrontal and intracerebral parts of the tumor are removed through a classic intradural approach before the subfrontal dura around the basal insertion of the tumor is dissected.

## Meningeal Repair

The dura is closed before the base is resected and the upper air-filled cavities are opened. There are three possibilities for repair:

1. The dura is preserved, but there are a few meningeal tears in the area of the olfactory grooves. The tears can be sutured with very fine sutures, but strengthening the dura at the midline with other material is advisable (Fig. 19–4).
2. There is a true dural defect, which must be closed with a dural substitute more than twice the size of the defect. This substitute is sutured to the dura at the furthest margins of the anterior fossa (Fig. 19–5).
3. The defect is exceptionally large, and the posterior dura has totally disappeared in front of the optochiasmatic cistern; in this case, it is impossible to

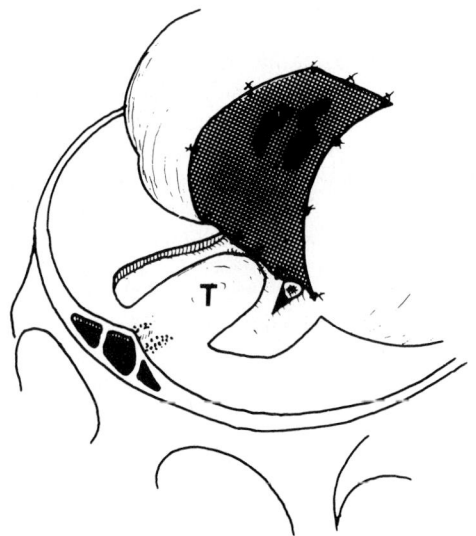

**FIGURE 19–4 ■** Strengthening of the subfrontal dura at the midline with a pericranial graft. (T, tumor.)

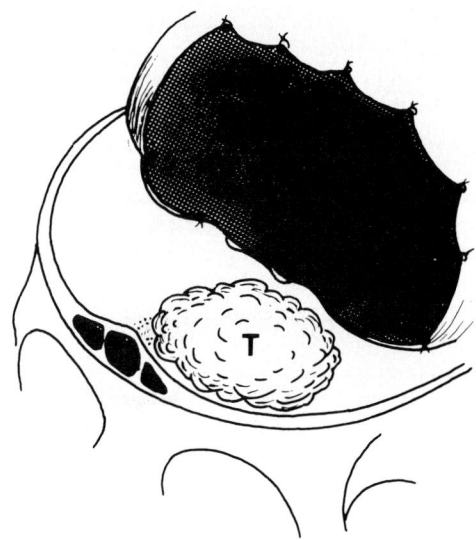

FIGURE 19–5 ■ A dural defect closed with a large graft. Note the suture at the remote edges of the anterior fossa. (T, basal insertion of the tumor.)

suture the dural substitute posteriorly (Fig. 19–6). This often occurs in tumors invading the posterior aspect of the anterior base up to the tuberculum sellae. In such cases, the graft is sutured only laterally and folded like a leaf of a book on the posterior third of the skull base (Fig. 19–7; see Fig. 19–9) a few weeks or months later, the subfrontal dura will be totally reconstituted and a new extradural transbasal approach will allow the removal of the invaded base and the tumor invading the nasal fossas without any intraoperative cerebrospinal fluid (CSF) leak.

The choice of a dural substitute depends on many factors. The material must be thick and tight enough to prevent leaks and ascending infection, it must be supple enough to permit brain re-expansion, and it must revascularize rapidly for quick adherence and to feed the bone grafts used to reconstruct the base of the skull. In our experience, a pericranial autograft is preferable to prosthetic materials or fascia lata.

A pericranial autograft has the same properties as periosteum. For a thicker graft and to preserve the anterior pericranium (covering the bifrontal free flap at the end of the procedure), the graft should be taken from the biparietal area through the same scalp incision (Fig. 19–8). If necessary, the sample can be as large as the entire subfrontal dura. We use this type of pericranial graft in almost all cases. Its periosteal face is placed toward the basal reconstruction.

The dural substitute used by Tessier in his first few cases of cranial malformation surgery was a dermic graft; this substitute was quickly forsaken for the pericranial autograft.

Subsequent steps in the removal of a tumor invading the anterior skull base and developed intracranially and extracranially depend on the quality of the dural repair. Two-step operations are strongly recommended when a watertight repair of the subfrontal dura is not obtained after intracranial tumor removal. Two or 3 months are necessary

to ensure the watertight closure of the dura. During this waiting period, a piece of inert material (Silastic) is inserted between the base and the pericranial graft (Fig. 19–9); it protects the grafts against hypothetical tumor invasion and makes the second extradural approach easier, at which time the tumor is removed.

Such a pericranial graft also may be used to close a clival dural defect (Fig. 19–10).

## Removal of the Basal Tumor

The difficulties encountered in removing a basal tumor vary according to the location, extension, and consistency of the tumor. All types of rongeurs and drills can be used to remove pathologically involved bone.

Tumors in the ethmoid area can be easily removed because there are no structures in the vicinity that can be injured. The nasal fossas are quickly reached, where the turbinates, septum, septal mucosas are identified and preserved if they are not invaded by tumor.

In the sphenoid area, the first step is to locate both optic nerves (Fig. 19–11A, B). Partial resection of the orbital roofs is the first step after the periorbita has been separated through an orbital approach. Therefore, the frontal bone is scraped to the upper margin of the orbits. When the supraorbital foramens are closed, resection of their lower rims helps to preserve the supraorbital vessels and nerves. The optic canals then are opened, and the extradural part of the optic nerves is identified. The tumor is attacked between the nerves (Fig. 19–12A). After intratumoral resection, the margins of bone are progressively removed. The medial walls of both orbits and the entire body of the sphenoid are then resected, if necessary, down to the pharyngeal and sinus mucosas (see Fig. 19–12B). The medial rim of the sphenoidal fissure can be opened from the midline (Fig. 19–13), and the foramen rotundum and the vidian canal in the root of the pterygoid can be reached.

Laterally, if the tumor involves the lesser and greater wings of the sphenoid, resection of the orbital roof is extended to the temporal dura so that the lesser wing and the upper margin of the sphenoidal fissure disappear. Working between the sphenoidal fissure and the optic foramen, the anterior clinoid process is progressively removed. This resection must be done very carefully because of the proximity of the internal carotid artery and the insertion of the small circumference of the tentorium just below the dura. Resection of the greater wing, between the periorbita and the temporal dura, is now easy and opens the inferior margin of the sphenoidal fissure, leading toward the floor of the middle fossa, the foramen rotundum, and the foramen ovale (see Fig. 19–13). At the end of this procedure, all upper cranial nerves are free. Posteriorly, it is now possible to reach the clivus after the tuberculum sellar area and the vertical part of the seller floor have been removed. Some bleeding may occur in this area because the dura of the sella is extremely vascular. Generally, this bleeding usually is not significant. Proceeding downward, the clivus is removed and the clival dura dissected to the anterior margin of the foramen magnum, which is opened. If dissection of the pharyngeal mucosa follows, the precervical space, the anterior arch of the atlas, and even the bodies of

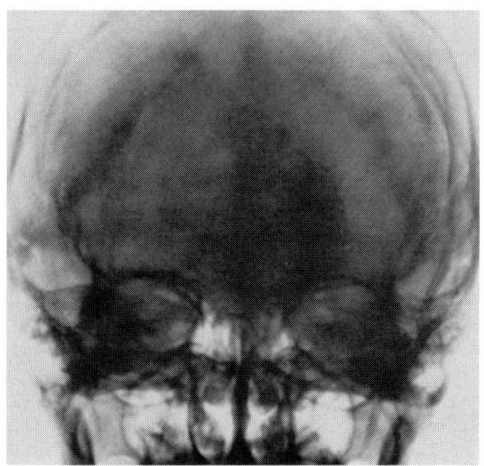
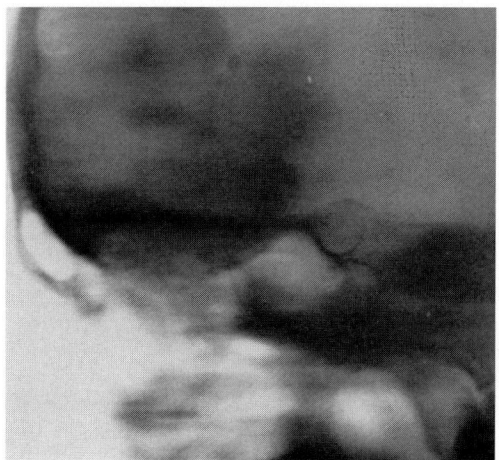

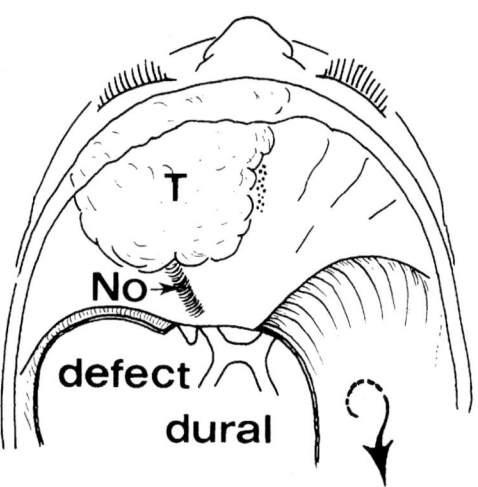

FIGURE 19–6 ■ An ossifying fibroma with a large intracranial extension. (T, basal insertion of the tumor; No, extradural portion of the left optic nerve.) After the intracranial portion of the tumor is removed, the optochiasmatic cistern is opened widely. An immediate watertight repair of the subfrontal dura is not possible.

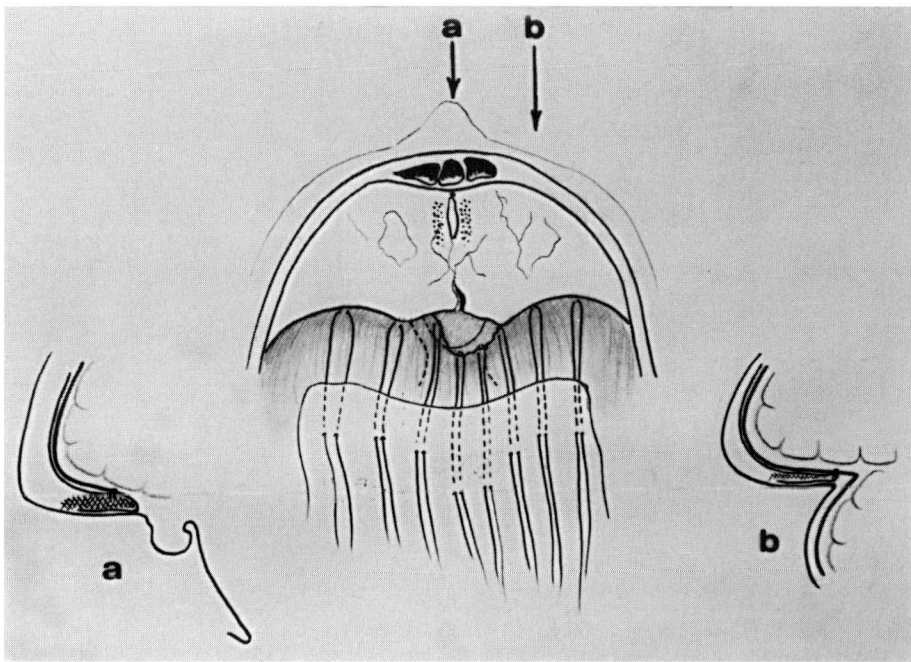

FIGURE 19–7 ■ The pericranial graft is folded posteriorly as a leaf of a book when the posterior sutures are not available. (a, medial cut; b, lateral cut [in a traumatic case].)

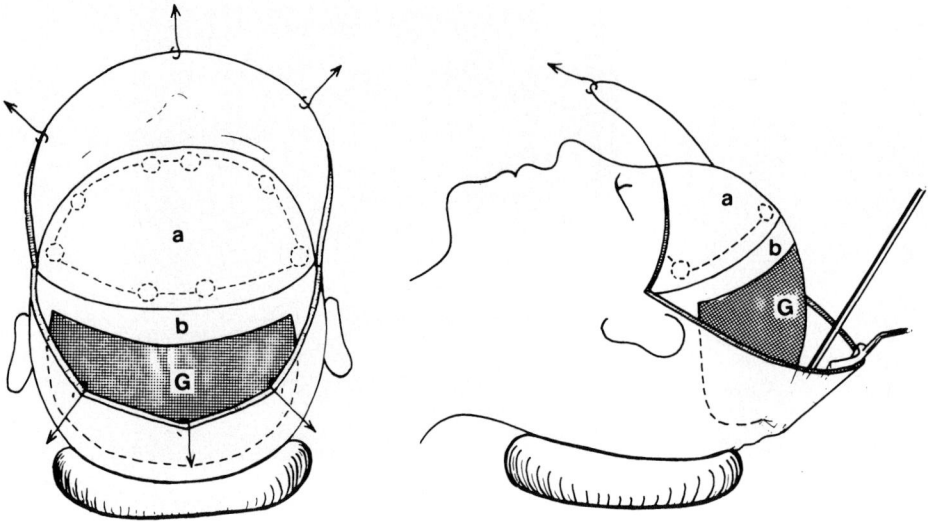

FIGURE 19–8 ■ Extraction of a pericranial graft. (a, anterior pericranium; G, graft; b, pericranial band preserved to allow sutures to be placed at the end of the procedure.)

C2 and C3 can be reached (Fig. 19–14). After this wide dissection, the base of the skull looks very different: the bony tissue has disappeared and the soft tissues of the orbits are attached only to the frontal and temporal dura by the optic nerves and sphenoidal fissures, and between them there is a large dead space bounded by the rhinopharyngeal mucosas. Of course, the extent of the basal resection depends on the kind of tumor with which we are dealing.

## Repair of the Skull Base

Repair of the skull base is not necessary if the basal defect is relatively limited. However, reconstruction of the bony

plane is one more guaranty against the risk of CSF leak; it protects the intracranial structures in transfacial or ear-nose-throat operations for recurrences of facial tumors. Repair of the skull base is strongly recommended in three circumstances: a large medial dead space; a large lateral orbital removal (thereby avoiding enophthalmos and pulsation of the eyeball); and an extension of the resection toward the orbitofrontal rim, the supraorbital margins, and the frontal area (for cosmetic reasons).

Autogenous bone is the best material for closure of the air-filled cavities of the face that have been widely opened, and are considered contaminated spaces. Grafts can be taken from the iliac bone, where it is possible to get a large specimen in one procedure. The iliac graft has the additional advantage that it provides cancellous rather than

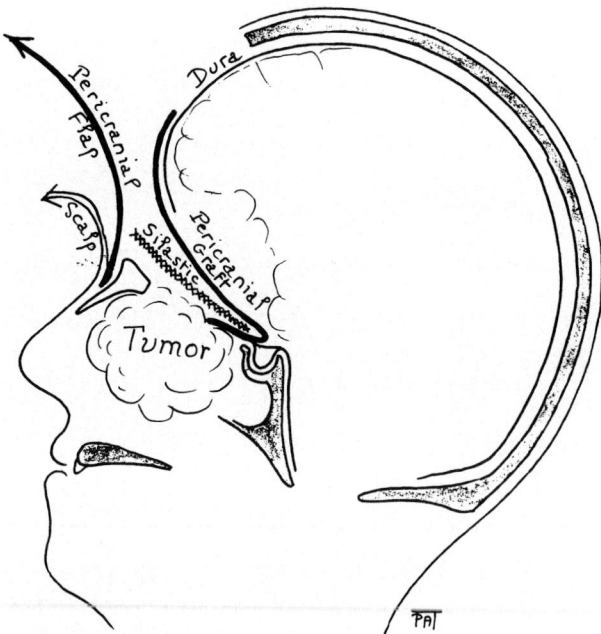

FIGURE 19–9 ■ Two-step operation. During the waiting time, a piece of an inert material is inserted between the pericranial graft repairing the subfrontal dura and the remaining basal tumor *(multiple crosses)*.

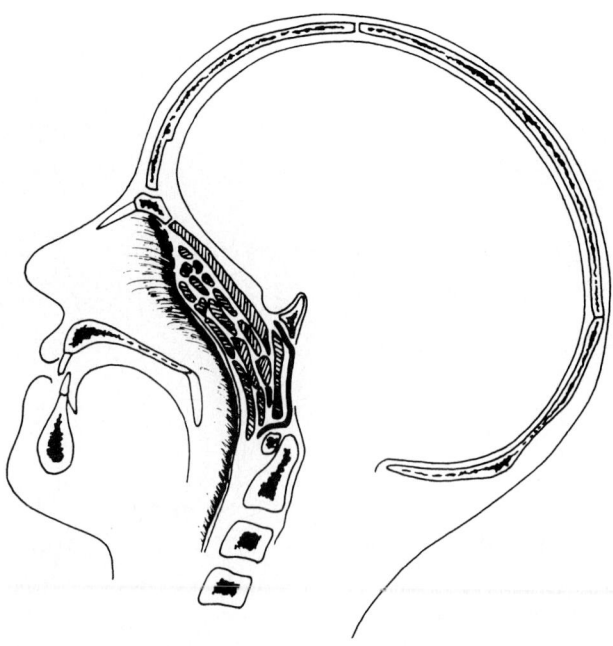

FIGURE 19–10 ■ Repair of a clival dural defect. The graft is applied to the bone reconstruction.

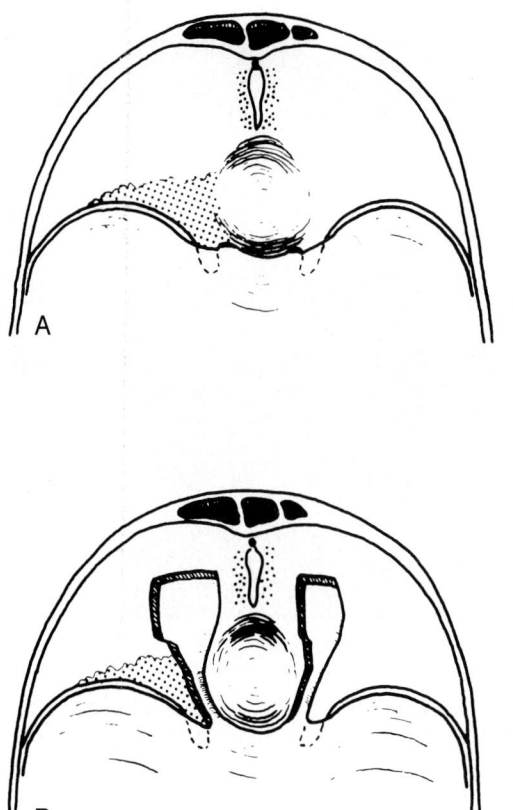

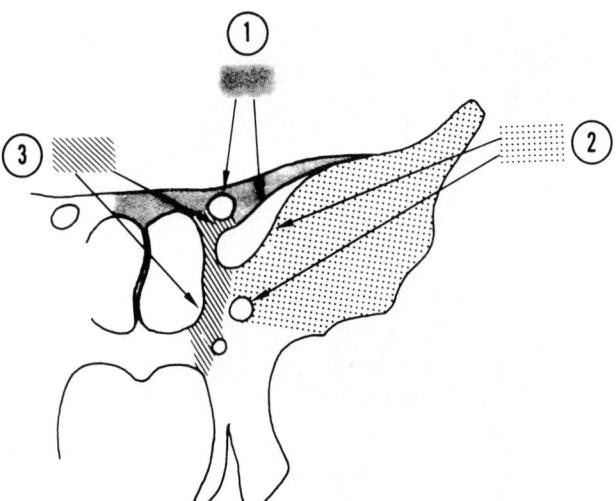

FIGURE 19-11 ■ *A,* Fibrous dysplasia involving the body and the left lesser wing of the sphenoid. *B,* Opening of the optic canals.

FIGURE 19-13 ■ (1) Vertical attack; (2) medial attack; (3) lateral attack.

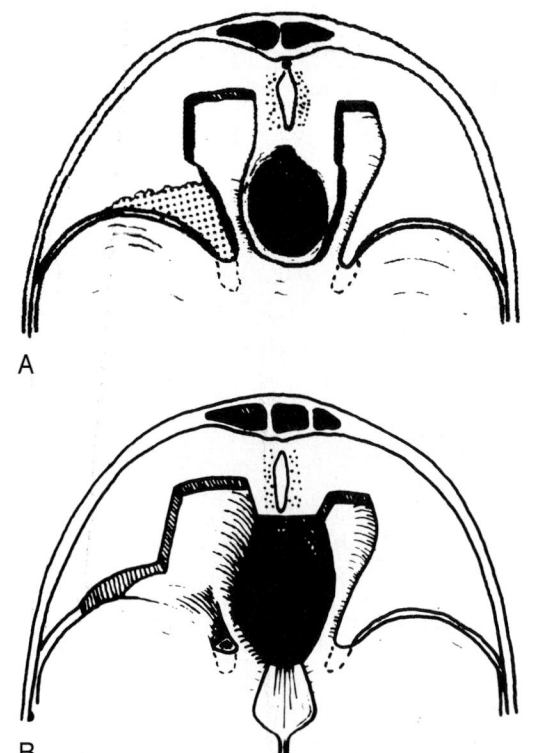

FIGURE 19-12 ■ *A,* Intratumoral resection between the optic nerves. *B,* Total removal of the sphenoid body leading to the pharyngeal mucosae. Opening of the left sphenoidal fissure and resection of the left anterior clinoid process.

cortical bone. Grafts taken from the vault, using the inner table of the bone flap (or extracted posteriorly if the bifrontal flap is involved by disease), are increasingly being used. Bone dust is also an excellent material that may be harvested with partial-thickness bur holes behind the posterior margin of the bifrontal free flap.

When the whole anterior fossa has been resected medially and laterally, after the medial walls and the roofs of the orbits have been repaired with two single grafts or one modeled graft, the dead space should be packed with cancellous bone. A final cortical graft can be used to close the ethmoidosphenoidal area. It should be implanted between the nasion and the clivus, beneath the horizontal portion of the sellar floor. If the clivus also has been removed, the graft should be applied as a near-vertical graft, fitted between the floor of the sella and the anterior margin of the foramen magnum or the anterior arch of the atlas. The optic nerves must remain completely free. Last, bone dust should be packed intracranially to provide a tight closure. (Figs. 19–15 to 19–18 illustrate the principles of this reconstruction.) Such reconstruction is required after resection of bone lesions, particularly in extensive fibrous dysplasia. Commonly, however, the basal repair is much easier; a bone graft is fitted in the basal defect, above the pericranial flap and closing the nasal fossas (Fig. 19–19*A, B*), after which bone dust is packed to suppress the dead space below the pericranial graft reconstructing the subfrontal dura.

## Closure

The bifrontal free flap is replaced using dural suspensions and cranioplasty of the bur holes.

If the tumor also invaded a part of the flap, the pathologically involved bone must be resected and a cranioplasty performed at the same stage. Again, a bone autograft is preferred to prosthetic material. (The possible need for such reconstruction must be anticipated when grafts are being obtained.)

If not used for closure of the nasal fossas and repair

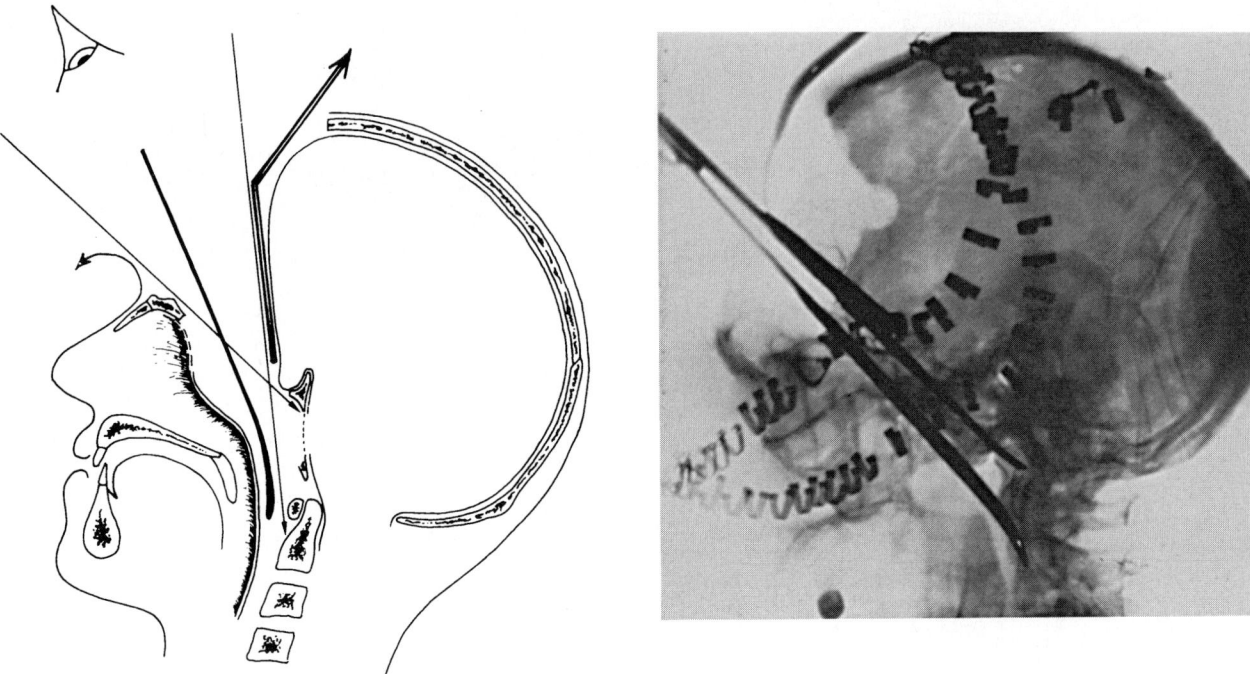

FIGURE 19–14 ■ Through the transbasal approach (*left*), it is possible to reach the clivus, the anterior arch of the atlas, and the bodies of C1 and C2. Notice the preservation of the pharyngeal mucosae. An intraoperative radiogram (*right*). The tips of the instruments are located at the anterior margin of the foramen magnum and the body of C2.

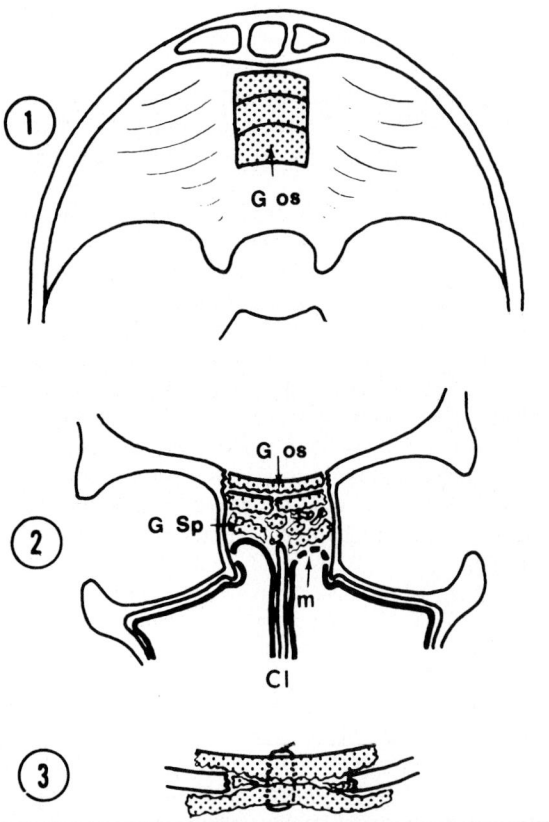

FIGURE 19–15 ■ Ethmoidal reconstruction. (1) Endocranial view of the anterior floor. (G os, split rib grafts.) (2) Frontal section. (G sp, cancellous bone grafts; m, mucosae; C1, nasal septum.) (3) Stud-like technique ensuring the closure of a defect when the bone is thin.

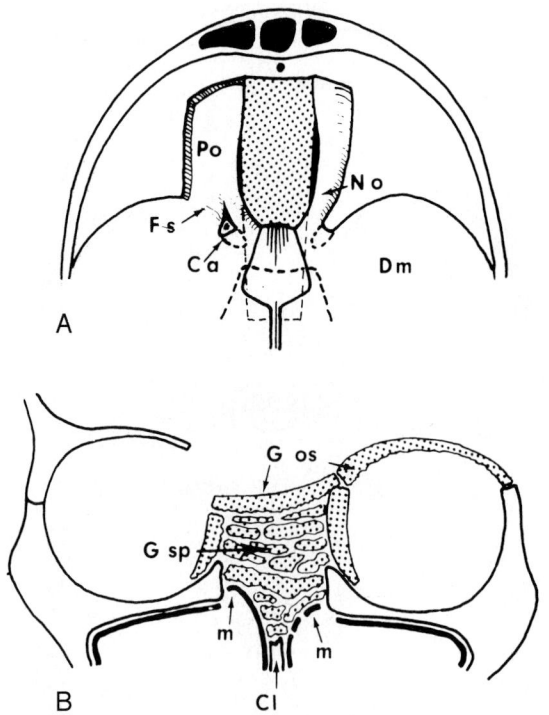

FIGURE 19–16 ■ Ethmoidosphenoidal reconstruction. *A,* Endocranial view. (Po, periorbita; No, optic nerve; Fs, sphenoidal fissure; Ca, anterior clinoid process; Dm, dura.) *B,* Frontal section. (G os, cortical bone grafts; G sp, cancellous bone grafts; m, mucosae; C1, nasal septum.) Note the simultaneous repair of an orbit roof.

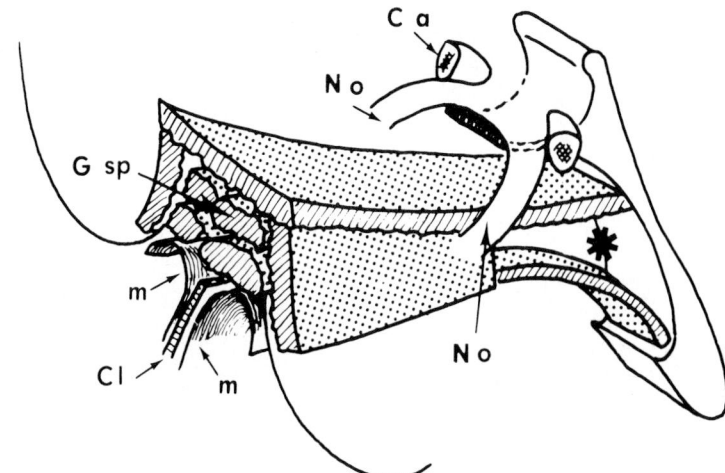

**FIGURE 19–17** ■ Sphenoethmoidal reconstruction at the midline. The dead space is packed with cancellous bone grafts between the new orbital walls and the large upper graft packed below the sellar floor. Notice that both optic nerves are free. (G sp, cancellous bone grafts; No, optic nerve; Ca, anterior clinoid process; m, mucosae; C1, nasal septum.)

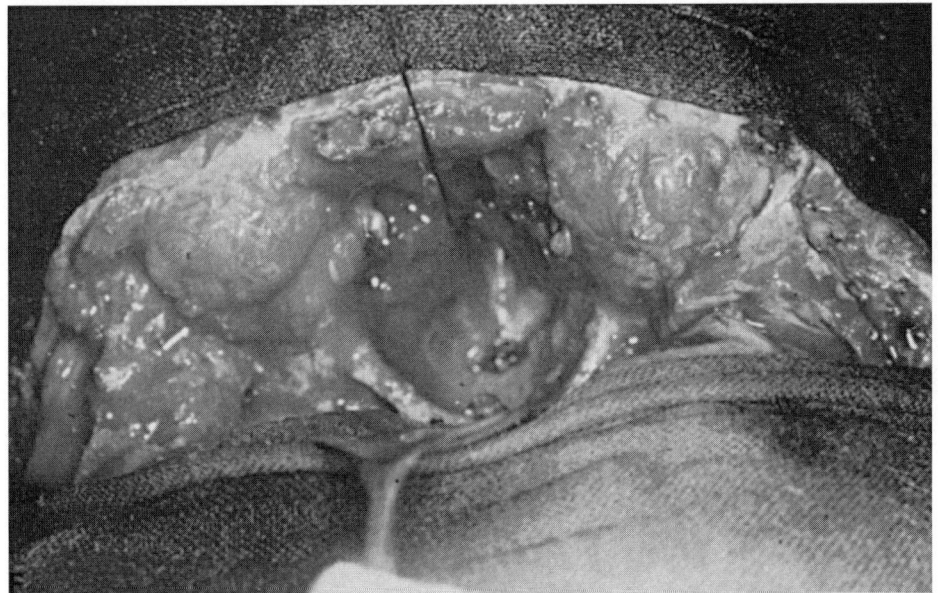

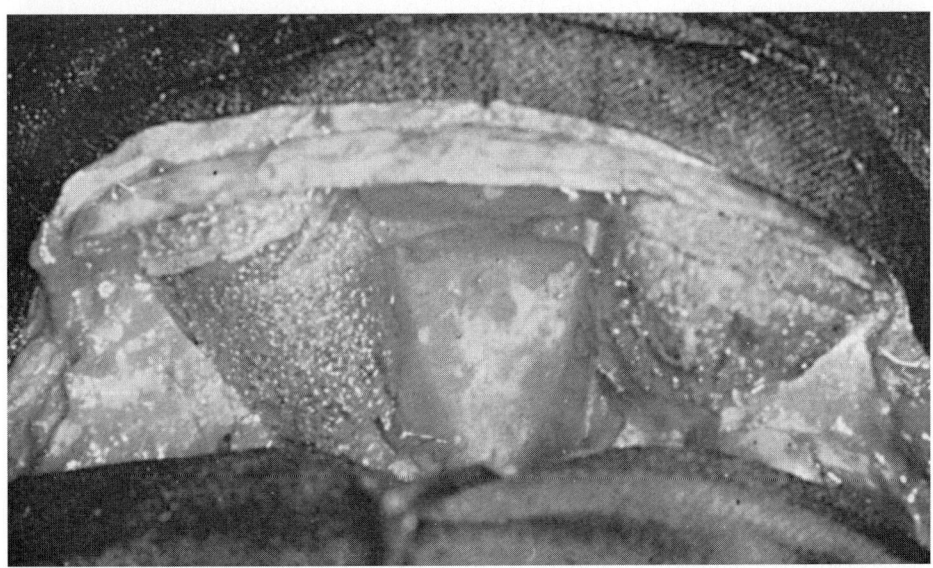

**FIGURE 19–18** ■ Extensive removal and basal reconstruction in a case of fibrous dysplasia (*top*). Intraoperative view of the removal of the entire anterior fossa. The upper orbital margins, roofs, and medial walls; the ethmoid; the body and lesser wings of the sphenoid; and the anterior clinoid processes have been resected. Medially, this resection leads to the nasal fossae and pharyngeal mucosae. Both optic nerves are totally free, and the sphenoidal fissures are opened. *Bottom,* An intraoperative view of the reconstruction. Both upper orbital margins have been repaired with a single-wired split rib graft. Note the large medial graft between the reconstruction of both orbits.

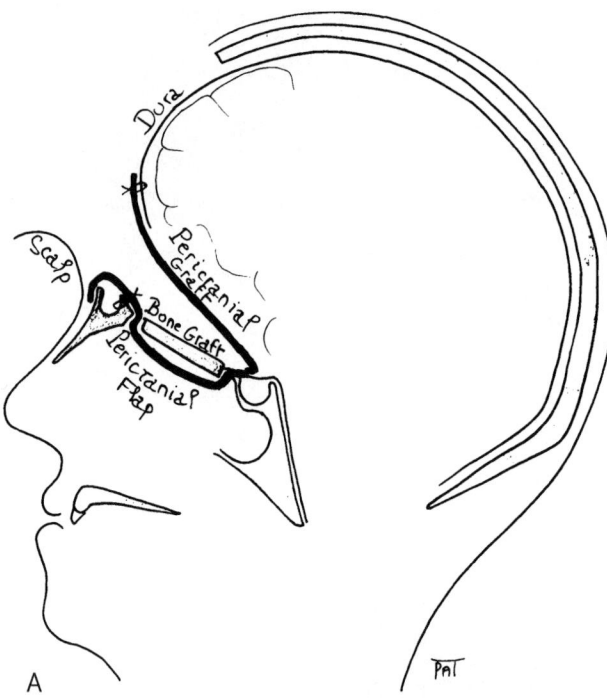

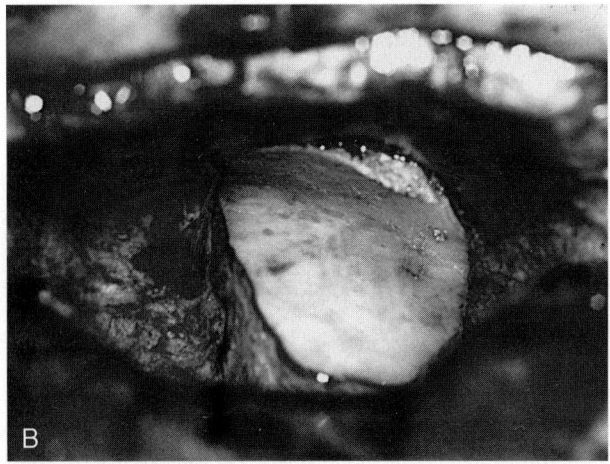

FIGURE 19–19 ■ *A* and *B*, Basal repair. *A*, A bone graft is fitted in the defect above the pericranial flap, which is also used for the closure of the frontal sinuses. *B*, An intraoperative view of the anterior fossa repair. (From Sekhar LN [ed]: Surgery of Cranial Base Tumors. New York: Raven Press, 813–815.)

of the mucosal plane (two-step operations), the anterior pericranial flap is turned down to cover the bifrontal free flap. Two drains are placed before the scalp is sutured, one extradurally in the subfrontal area and the other in the parietal area where the pericranial graft was extracted.

## LIMITS OF THE TRANSBASAL APPROACH AND THE COMBINATION OF SEVERAL APPROACHES

First described for basal osteotomies in craniofacial malformations, the subfrontal approach was successfully applied for the removal of bony lesions or extracranial/intracranial

tumors destroying or invading the skull base. Two aspects of this pathologic process must be considered: the possibilities for resection of bone and the tumoral limits that can be reached. Bone resection does not present problems. The entire anterior fossa and the largest part of the middle fossa can be resected. It is possible to free the vessels and nerves that pass through the optic canals, the sphenoidal fissures, the foramen rotundum, and the foramen ovale (Fig. 19–20). The posterior limit is the petrous bone, which can be reached through a posterolateral approach. Resection of a pathologic anterior and middle skull base involving the greater sphenoidal wing preserves all upper cranial nerves except for the olfactory tracts.

Problems arise when the adjacent soft tissues are involved. In the orbital area, the transbasal approach provides an excellent exposure. The anterior and inferomedial aspects of the cavernous sinus may be reached extradurally, but, except for few encapsulated lesions, its involvement constitutes one of the limits of the single transbasal approach. Inferiorly, the removal of a medial tumor is possible down to the turbinates and the palate, but this approach does not provide access if the tumor extends laterally to the maxillary sinuses. Posteriorly, the possibilities for removing the clivus through different anterior approaches are summarized in Fig. 19–21; the transcervical[21] and transoral approaches provide access only to its lower half; the rhinoseptal route is convenient for gaining access to the sella and the upper half of the clivus on the midline, but this approach remains narrow and lateral structures are not visible; and the transbasal approach allows an extended resection of the clivus except for the vision angle below the sella. Therefore, depending on the location and main extension of the tumor, the transbasal approach can be modified or combined with another surgical approach.

Many modifications have been proposed to enlarge the posterior visual field and potentially decrease the amount of frontal brain retraction; all these approaches enlarge the bony resection or osteotomies toward the middle face and orbits.[2, 10–19] Based on their extent, they are called the subfrontal, subfrontoextradural, frontonasal, fronto-orbito-

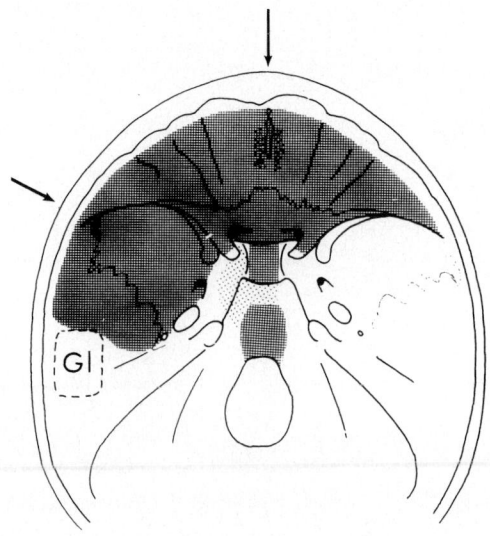

FIGURE 19–20 ■ Limits of basal resection through a bifrontal approach.

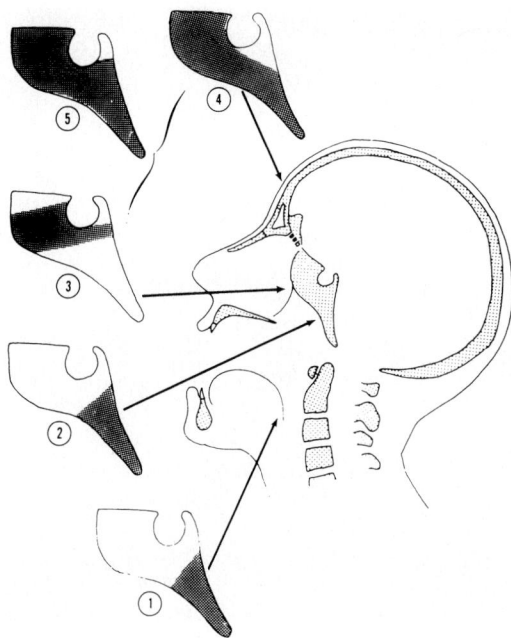

**FIGURE 19–21** ■ Limits of sphenoidal and clival resection through anterior approaches. (1) transcervical approach; (2) transoral approach; (3) rhinoseptal approach; (4) transbasal approach; (5) combination of transbasal and rhinoseptal approaches.

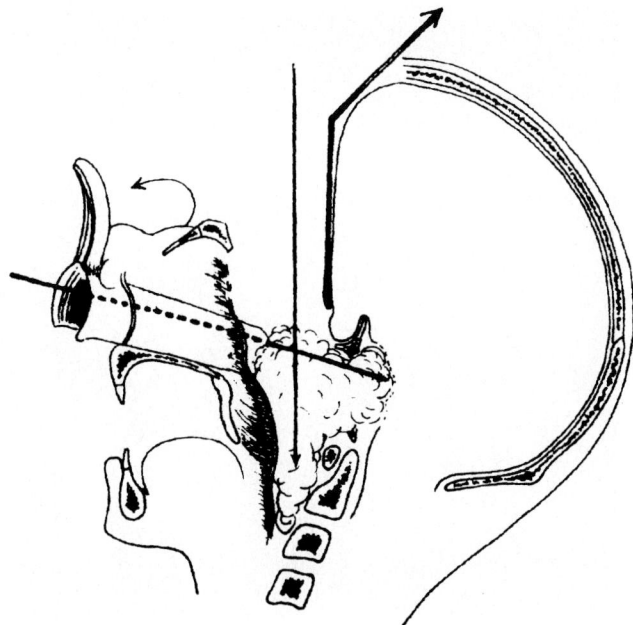

**FIGURE 19–23** ■ Combination of a rhinoseptal and transbasal approach in one-step procedure.

nasal, and the extended transbasal approch. Another possibility remains the combination in a one-step procedure of the transbasal and a transfacial approach, particularly for inferior and lateral facial extensions of the tumor[15–23] (Fig. 19–22). In our experience, combining a rhinoseptal route and a transbasal approach is very helpful in sphenoidal tumors that involve both the anterior cranial base and the posterior clival area (Fig. 19–23). This combination is particularly useful and successful in chordomas and chondromas (Fig. 19–24A, B).

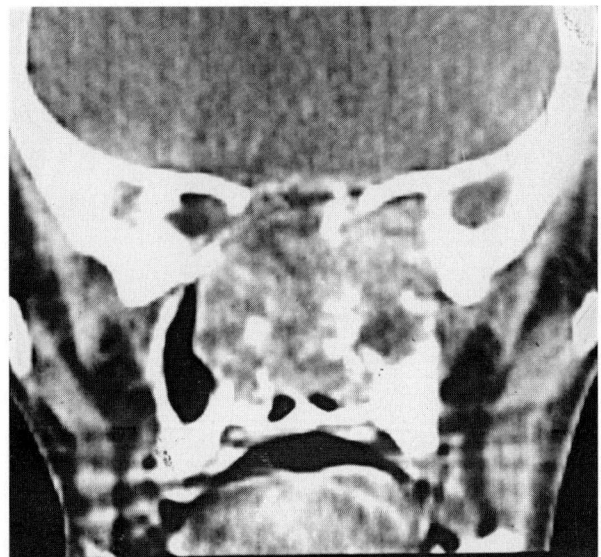

**FIGURE 19–22** ■ Case of an adenocarcinoma of the nasal fossae invading the anterior skull base and extending laterally in which an association of a transbasal and transfacial approach is recommended.

## INDICATIONS FOR THE TRANSBASAL APPROACH

A transbasal approach is not necessary to gain access to all tumors at the skull base. Its use depends on the exact anatomic location of the lesion. The transbasal approach should be used to increase the chances for total removal of a tumor. Table 19–1 summarizes cases in which this approach seemed absolutely necessary.

Diagnosis of a tumor invading the skull base does not routinely lead to a uniform treatment strategy. The choice between complete removal, decompression, or radiationtherapy without surgery must be based on the histologic characteristics and extent of the lesion. These factors must be assessed during the preoperative examination.

Computed tomography is more useful for the study of bone and magnetic resonance imaging for visualizing extension of the tumor in the cranial, nasal, or sinusal cavities. If a vascular lesion is suspected, angiographic study is necessary and may lead to preoperative embolization. The nature of the lesion may be very difficult to diagnose, in which case rhinoseptal biopsy is suggested. Biopsy prevents errors. Some invasive adenomas and sphenoidal mucoceles are often confused, clinically and radiologically, with destructive chordomas.

Lesions involving the skull base can be divided into three groups: (1) tumors of intracranial origin, such as meningiomas; (2) primary bone tumors; and (3) tumors or rhinopharyngeal origin, which are usually mailgnant.

### Meningiomas

Meningiomas invade the skull base in three different ways. First, the anterior fossa can be ruptured at its weakest point, the ethmoidal area and cribriform plates, as with

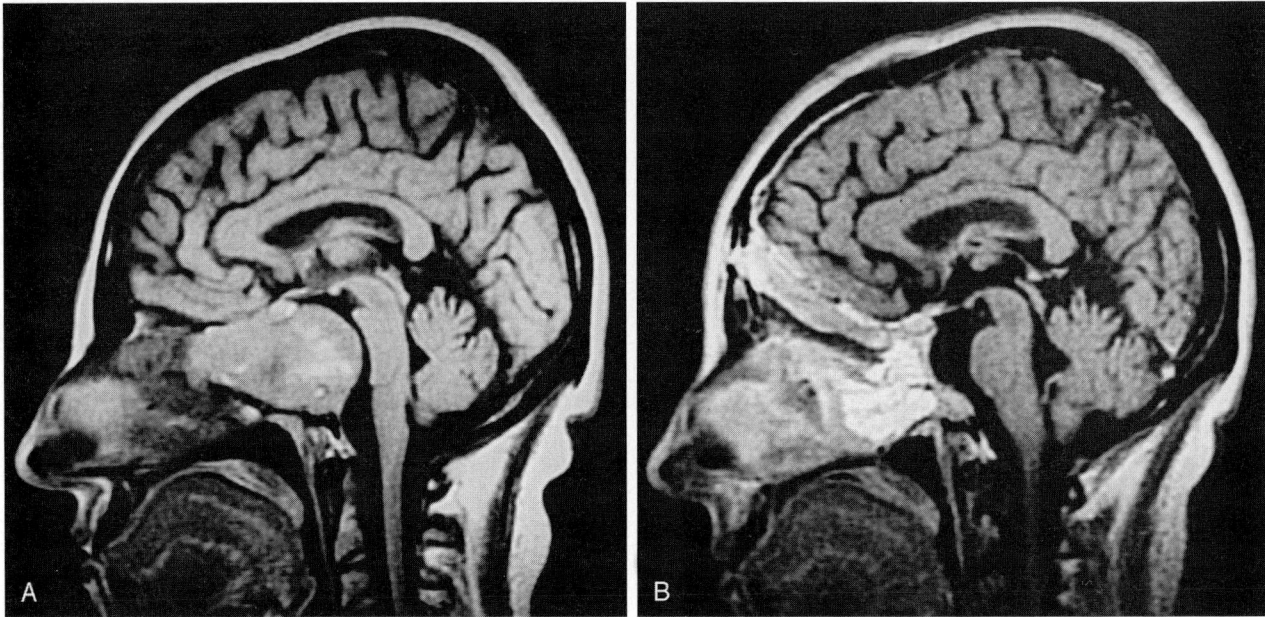

FIGURE 19–24 ■ Preoperative *(A)* and postoperative *(B)* magnetic resonance imaging (MRI scan) in a case of chordoma after a combined one-stage transbasal and transsphenoidal removal. (From Sekhar LN [ed]: Surgery of Cranial Base Tumors. New York: Raven Press, pp 813–815.)

intranasal extension of olfactory meningiomas,[4, 6, 7, 14] in which no true bone invasion occurs (Fig. 19–25). Second, with an en plaque meningioma,[1, 4, 9, 18] the dural tumor is less important than hyperostosis, which is not single reaction but a true tumoral infiltration of bone. Hyperostosis is responsible for the entire clinical syndrome and compression of the optic nerve into the optic canal. The dural plaque as well as the bone must be removed to avoid recurrence. A pterional location is not an indication for the transbasal approach. This approach is necessary and useful, however, when the lesion overlaps the optic canal and involves the sphenoidal area medially. Third, a bone reaction may be found close to the basal insertion of some en masse meningiomas.[6] The pathologic features of such a reaction are difficult to confirm, but it may be a true invasion that will result in the basal malignancy recurring several years after the intracranial part has been removed. Basal invasion by a meningioma must be removed along with the intradural mass in one or two stages, depending on the size of the dural defect and the duration of the intracranial procedure.[6]

## Primary Bone Tumors Involving the Skull Base

Bone tumors include many types of lesions[3]: some are malignant, such as sarcomas or metastases, whereas many are benign, such as osteomas, osteoblastomas, hemangiomas, ossifying fibromas,[4, 7, 12, 15, 18] or fibrous dysplasia.[5, 13, 16] Fibrous dysplasia, although not a tumor, can be consid-

TABLE 19–1 ■ **CASES IN WHICH A TRANSBASAL APPROACH WAS USED (TO DECEMBER 1997)**

| Tumor | No. of Patients |
|---|---|
| Fibrous dysplasia | 60 |
| Meningioma | 43 |
| Malignant ear-nose-throat tumor | 15 |
| Chordoma | 12 |
| Olfactory placode tumor | 8 |
| Chondroma | 6 |
| Ossifying fibroma | 6 |
| Osteoblastoma | 4 |
| Nasopharyngeal fibroma | 4 |
| Cylindroma | 4 |
| Osteoma | 3 |
| Sarcoma | 3 |
| Hemangiopericytoma | 1 |
| Craniopharyngioma | 1 |
| Osteopetrosis | 1 |
| **Total** | **171** |

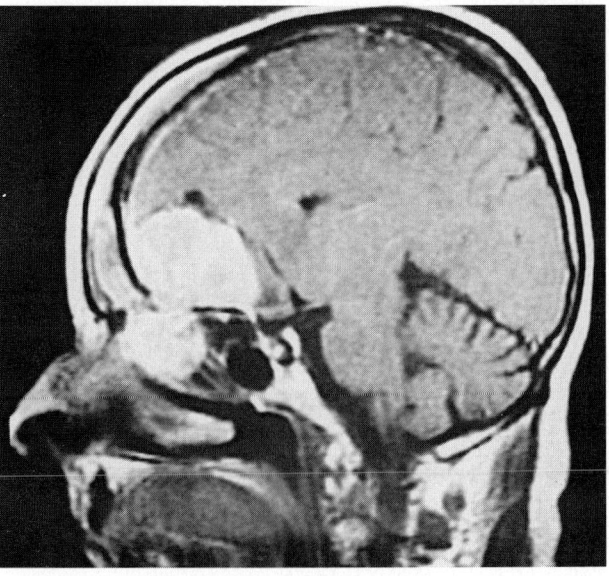

FIGURE 19–25 ■ Olfactory meningioma invading the nasal fossae.

ered one clinically, and is sometimes responsible for visual disturbances. It is very difficult to predict the evolution of this lesion, which is often found in young patients; however, progressive fibrous dysplasia with rapid visual loss is common. Our experience suggests that surgery is required if the fibrous dysplasia is progressive or the area of the optic foramen is involved.

Some bone tumors are difficult to classify because their pathologic potential is doubtful. Some of these tumors are malignant, but their malignancy is localized and it is impossible to remove them completely. Examples of these tumors include giant cell tumors,[8] chondromas,[7] and chordomas.[4, 11] Surgery is advised for chondromas because radiation therapy is ineffective. These tumors are more or less encapsulated, and they probably can be removed almost completely, even when they develop in the cavernous sinus. With chordomas, an aggressive surgical strategy is indicated; the transbasal approach (alone or in association with a transsphenoidal route) was useful in 15% of our cases in achieving the most complete removal of the tumor. Complementary irradiation with proton beam or gamma knife, rather than conventional radiation therapy, is recommended and gives the patient the best chance for long-term survival.

## Tumors of Rhinopharyngeal Origin

Among the rhinopharyngeal tumors that involve skull base, very few are benign (i.e., benign olfactory placode tumors[3] [esthesioneurocytomas] or nasopharyngeal fibromas). These tumors usually are malignant carcinomas or epitheliomas, and the approach to each varies. If the tumor extends toward the anterior fossa, the intracranial approach is suggested, but often in combination with a transfacial route.[17, 23] Extensive removal in these cases is more important than reconstruction. Unfortunately, when a patient with this type of tumor is seen by the neurosurgeon, it is often too late to accomplish a complete removal of all tumorous tissue. These patients must be seen very early in the course of tumor development, and to do so requires close cooperation between neurosurgical, ear, nose, and throat, and maxillofacial teams.

## REFERENCES

1. Castellano F, Guidetti B, Olivecrona H: Pterional meningiomas en plaques. Neurosurgery 9:188, 1952.
2. Cophignon J, George B, Marchac D, Roux FX: Voie transbasale élargie par mobilisation du bandeau fronto-orbitaire médian. Neurochirurgie 29:407, 1989.
3. Dahlin D: Bone Tumors. Springfield, IL: Charles C Thomas, 1964.
4. Derome P, Akerman M, Anquez L, et al: Les tumeurs sphenoethmoidales: Possibilités d'exerese et reparation chirugicales. Rapport de la Societe de Neurochirurgie de Langue Francaise. Neurochirurgie 15 (Suppl 1):1, 1972.
5. Derome PJ, Visot A, Akerman M, et al: Fibrous dysplasia of the skull. Neurochirurgie 29 (Suppl 1):1–114, 1983.
6. Derome PJ, Visot A: Bony reaction and invasion in meningiomas. In Al-Mefty O (ed): Meningiomas. New York: Raven Press, 1991, p 169.
7. Derome PJ, Visot A: Osseous lesions of anterior and middle base. In Seckhar LN, Janecka IP (eds): Surgery of Cranial Base Tumors. New York: Raven Press, 1993, p 809.
8. Geissinger JD, Siqueira ED, Rose ER: Giant cell tumors of the sphenoid bone. J Neurosurg 32:665, 1970.
9. Guiot G, Derome P: A propos des méningiomes en plaques du ptérion: Le traitement chirurgical des méningiomes hyperostosants. Ann Chir 20:CC 1109, 1966.
10. Jane JA, Park TS, Pobereskin LH, et al: The supra-orbital approach: Technical note. Neurosurgery 11:537, 1982.
11. Krayenbuhl H, Yasargil MG: Cranial chordomas. Prog Neurol 6:380, 1975.
12. Lehrer HZ: Ossifying fibroma of the orbital roof: Its distinction from blistering or intraosseus meningioma. Arch Neurol 20(5):536–541, 1969.
13. Liechtenstein L, Jaffe HL: Fibrous dysplasia of bone: A condition affecting one, several or many bones the graver of which may represent abnormal pigmentation of skin, premature sexual development, hyperthyroidism, or still other extraskeletal abnormalities. Arch Pathol 33:777, 1942.
14. Pertuiset B, Beciric T: La voie intracranienne dans l'exerese du prolongement nasal des meningiomes olfactifs. Presse Med 63:1863, 1958.
15. Plewes JL, Jacobson I: Familial frontonasal dermoid cysts: Report of four cases. J Neurosurg 34:683, 1971.
16. Reynaud J, Courson B: A propos des osteodysplasies et osteopathies fibreuses craniofaciales et de leur traitement. Ann Chir Plast Esthet 15:312, 1970.
17. Saunders WH, Miglets A: Surgical techniques for eradicating far advanced carcinoma of the orbital ethmoid and maxillary areas. Trans Am Acad Ophthalmol Otolaryngol 7:426, 1967.
18. Scott M, Peale AR, Croissant PD: Intracranial midline anterior fossae ossifying fibroma invading orbits, paranasal sinuses, and right maxillary antrum. J Neurosurg 34:827, 1971.
19. Seckhar LN, Nanda A, Synderman CN, Jacnecka IP: The extended frontal approach to tumors of the anterior middle and posterior skull base. J Neurosurg 76:198, 1992.
20. Spetzler RF, Herman JN, Beals S, et al: Preservation of olfaction in anterior craniofacial approaches. J Neurosurg 79:48, 1993.
21. Stevenson GC, Stoney RJ, Perkins RK, et al: A transcervical, transclival approach to the ventral surface of the brainstem for removal of a clivus chordoma. J Neurosurg 24:544, 1966.
22. Tessier P. Guiot G, Derome P: Orbital hypertelorism. II: Definite treatment of orbital hypertelorism by craniofacial or by extracranial osteotomies. Scand J Plast Reconstr Surg 7:39, 1973.
23. Van Buren JM, Ommaya AK, Ketcham AS: Ten years' experience with radical combined craniofacial resection of malignant tumors of the paranasal sinuses. J Neurosurg 28:341, 1968.

# Craniofacial Resection for Anterior Skull Base Tumors

■ GAVIN W. BRITZ and FRANCIS JOHNSTON

Skull base tumors are by definition tumors that arise from or are located in the bony structures at the base of the brain. They may originate from a variety of extracranial or intracranial tissues, or directly from the skull base. The usual extracranial sources include areas such as the paranasal sinuses, nasopharynx, and surrounding connective tissues whose tumors secondarily invade the skull base. The intracranial sources include basal meningiomas, pituitary tumors, and metastatic tumors that erode into the base of the skull. Osteosarcomas, chordomas, and chondrosarcomas are tumors that originate directly from the skull base

Despite this diversity in origin, they behave in a rather uniform way: they are frequently benign or only locally malignant, they rarely metastasize, and they prove refractory to radiation therapy or chemotherapy; thus, radical surgical resection is the treatment of choice in their management.[1] This procedure ideally involves an en bloc surgical resection of the tumor,[2-4] although this was often limited to partial removals because of the multitude of problems encountered in the treatment of skull base tumors.[5]

Several advances have occurred that have significantly altered the management of these tumors. Newer imaging techniques such as computed tomography and magnetic resonance imaging have led to improved delineation of the tumors, thus aiding in the preoperative evaluation and surgical planning (Figs. 20–1 and 20–2). Improvements in neuroanesthesia have allowed for greater control in the management of intraoperative cerebral swelling, thus improving the ultimate outcome.

In surgical treatment, the rate-limiting step in achieving the goal of radical surgical resection has been obtaining access to and exposure of these tumors. These tumors are difficult in that they lie ventral to the brain and posterior to the facial skeleton and aerodigestive system. Advances in surgical techniques, however, have resulted in the development of multiple different approaches that often involve a multidisciplinary team including neurosurgeons, plastic surgeons, maxillofacial surgeons, and otolaryngologists. The different approaches are used to obtain access to and exposure of skull base tumors in different locations, based on preoperative imaging studies and surgical planning. More recently, with the advent of surgical navigational

systems, surgical planning has further evolved to include preoperative computerized visualization of the procedure.

Surgical aids such as the microscope have allowed for improved surgical technique, and the ultrasonic aspirator permits a less traumatic and more complete removal of these tumors. Surgical navigational systems allowing for improved intraoperative visualization of both tumor and normal anatomy make the operation safer and permit a more complete removal of these tumors.[6]

The surgical management and choice of the surgical approach to skull base tumors depends largely on the location of the tumor. Each approach provides various angles and degrees of access along the skull base. This chapter concentrates on the management of anterior skull base tumors using the direct midline ventral approaches to

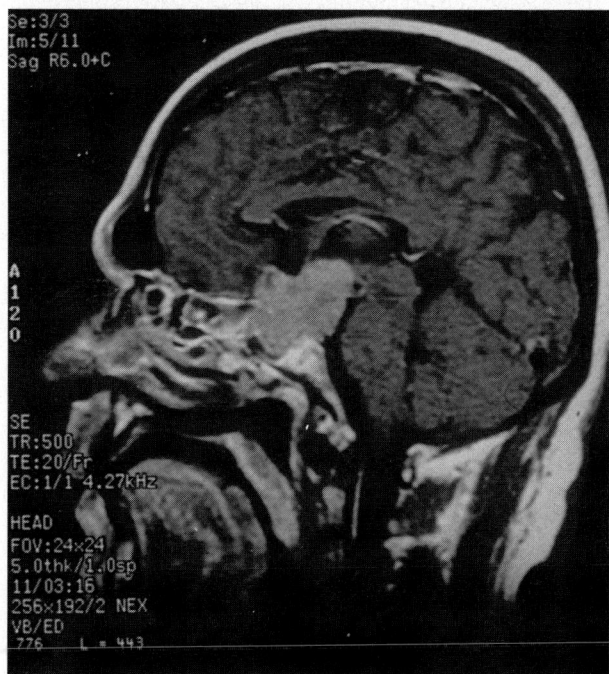

FIGURE 20–1 ■ A sagittal $T_1$-weighted gadolinium-enhanced magnetic resonance imaging scan demonstrating a chordoma that involves the superior clivus, the sphenoid sinus, and the sellar region with a suprasellar extension.

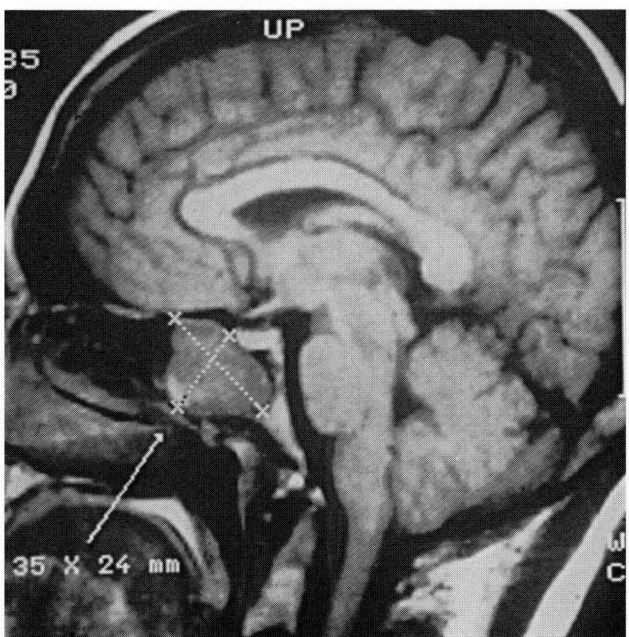

FIGURE 20–2 ■ A sagittal $T_1$-weighted gadolinium-enhanced magnetic resonance imaging scan demonstrating a chordoma that originates in the clivus and involves the sphenoid sinus.

these tumors in the region of the clivus. These approaches are particularly attractive because they are unencumbered by cranial nerves or major blood vessels.[7] Direct midline ventral approaches can be transnasal, transoral, or transfacial, and are modified according to the location of the tumor.

The transnasal or transsphenoidal route provides good access to the sellar region and rostral third of the clivus, but is limited in more extensive lesions in that region.[7, 8] The pure transoral route provides a direct approach to the anterior rim of the foramen magnum.[7, 9] This may then be modified by extending the approach with different maneuvers to improve the access to and exposure of tumors in the anterior skull base. Dividing the soft or hard palate in the transpalatal approach allows for access to the lower and middle third of the clivus.[10, 11] The Le Fort I osteotomy with mobilization of the hard palate and maxilla inferiorly allows for visualization of the whole clivus.[1, 12, 13] An extended maxillotomy combines a Le Fort I osteotomy with splitting of the hard and soft palate, and allows for exposure of the whole clivus and the craniocervical junction.[7, 14] In the transfacial approach, removal of the midface gives access to the paranasal sinuses and upper two thirds of the clivus.[15] These different approaches can also be combined with intracranial approaches, if necessary, to obtain a complete tumor resection.

## TRANSSPHENOIDAL APPROACH

Lesions involving the sellar region and the upper third of the clivus can be dealt with using the sublabial–rhinoseptal–transsphenoidal approach[8] (Fig. 20–3). This approach is simply an extension of pituitary surgery, which

is now widely performed. After oral intubation, the head is placed on a headrest slightly extended, with the surgeon next to the chest and positioned perpendicular to the plane of the imaging intensifier to allow for the correct intraoperative orientation. An antiseptic is then applied to the nose and mouth and the surrounding area is draped with sterile towels. The sphenoid sinus can be approached by either the sublabial or the rhinoseptal route; we prefer the latter approach, and describe it here.

After infiltration with local anesthetic containing 1:200,000 epinephrine and 0.5% lidocaine at the junction between the skin and the mucosa of the right naris, which is retracted with a Senn retractor, an incision is made into the mucosa to the nasal septum. A mucoperichondrial plane is then developed between the nasal mucosa and the septum and followed posteriorly to the posterior boundary of the cartilaginous septum, where the bony septum derived from the superior portion of the vomer and the inferior portion of the perpendicular plate of the ethmoid is identified. A speculum is then introduced and opened, fracturing the inferior portion of the perpendicular plate of the ethmoid and allowing for visualization of the midline and both sides of the anterior wall of the sphenoid sinus, with its keel-like appearance. Confirmation of location should be obtained with the imaging intensifier, which should confirm access and exposure to the sellar region through the sphenoid sinus, and the upper third of the clivus. The operating microscope is then introduced and used for the rest of the procedure.

The anterior wall of the sphenoid sinus is then opened with a 1-mm Kerrison punch, either starting at the ostia of the sinus located laterally, or after fracturing the wall with a small osteotome. The sinus is opened to the lateral, superior, and inferior aspect of the sella. The mucosa of the sinus is then stripped and removed and bleeding controlled with coagulation. The direction of approach can then be adjusted with angulation of the speculum and correlation of the image on the image intensifier. After deciding on the angle of approach, the speculum is advanced into the sinus directed toward the area of interest, and opened. Care should be taken not to use force to open the speculum because fractures of the sphenoid bone may occur. Occasionally tumors may have eroded through the anterior wall of the sphenoid sinus, and then the sinus is opened around the tumor.

The remainder of the operation depends largely on the surgical goals and the location of the tumor. Using the microscope, lesions in the midline involving the sphenoid sinus, sellar region, and rostral clivus can be removed. Lesions within the sella or that have involved the sella may require opening of the anterior wall of the sella. This is performed with a small osteotome placed on the wall to initiate the opening, which is then extended with a 1-mm Kerrison punch. The opening is extended laterally to the cavernous sinus, inferiorly to the sellar floor, and superiorly to the intercavernous sinus. This exposure of the sellar region allows for a good decompression of the optic chiasm, and patients presenting with chiasmal compression can be expected to have some improvement in vision.[8] In situations in which the dura has been violated, such as when the tumors have involved the dura or when the dura has been inadvertently opened, human-derived fibrin glue

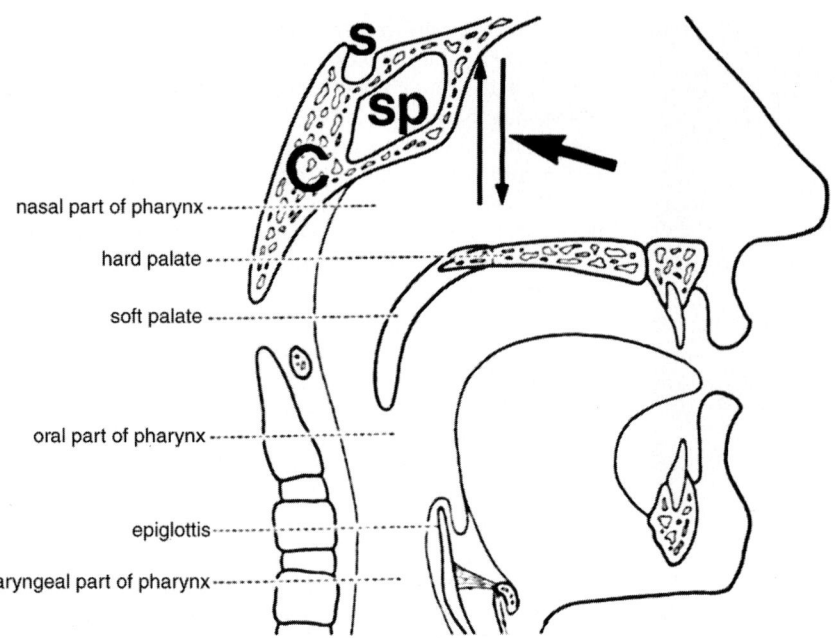

nasal part of pharynx

hard palate

soft palate

oral part of pharynx

epiglottis

laryngeal part of pharynx

**FIGURE 20–3** ■ A schematic representation of the extent of access and exposure (*vertical arrows*) to the sphenoid sinus (sp), sellar region (s) and superior clivus (C), which is possible with a transsphenoidal route.

(Tisseel; Immuno AG, Vienna, Austria) should be placed over the defect. Continuous lumbar cerebrospinal fluid (CSF) drainage should also be done for 5 days after surgery to facilitate repair and help prevent a CSF leak.

## TRANSORAL APPROACHES

The various transoral approaches allow the surgeon access to the whole clivus and craniocervical junction, and are ideally situated to expose midline extradural lesions. Depending on the type of transoral procedure, different regions along this plane can be accessed, and these different approaches are individually described. However, common to all the approaches is the need to perform the procedure through the mouth; the palatal-sparing transoral approach is described first, and serves as an example for the general approach to transoral procedures.

### Transoral (Palatal Sparing)

The palatal-sparing transoral approach provides access to the anterior rim of the foramen magnum and thus is ideally suited to midline lesions in and around the basion (Fig. 20–4). Because the procedure is done through the mouth, the first step is to ensure that this is possible. To place the required instruments in the mouth, an interdental distance greater than 25 mm is required.[16] In patients with diseases of the mouth or jaw (e.g., temporomandibular disease) in whom this gap cannot be obtained, median mandibular splitting with a midline glossotomy is required, allowing the tongue halves to be retracted laterally and inferiorly and thus making the operation feasible.[17, 18] It is also important preoperatively to assess the oral cavity and, if necessary, advise dental extractions before surgery; sepsis can arise from the teeth, leading to wound abscess and even death

from sepsis.[16] Gum guards can also be used to prevent damage to the teeth from the retractor systems.[16]

It is not necessary to perform a preoperative tracheotomy in all patients, and it should be reserved for patients with preoperative bulbar palsies and those who will require prolonged airway care.[19] A fiberoptic nasotracheal airway should be placed, with the patient awake if the cervicomedullary junction is compromised by the mass. A nasogastric tube or feeding tube is placed at this time to allow for aspiration of gastric contents during the early postoperative phase, and for nutritional support before the patient can initiate oral feeds. The patient is then placed on the Mayfield horseshoe in mild extension, and the mouth is pre-

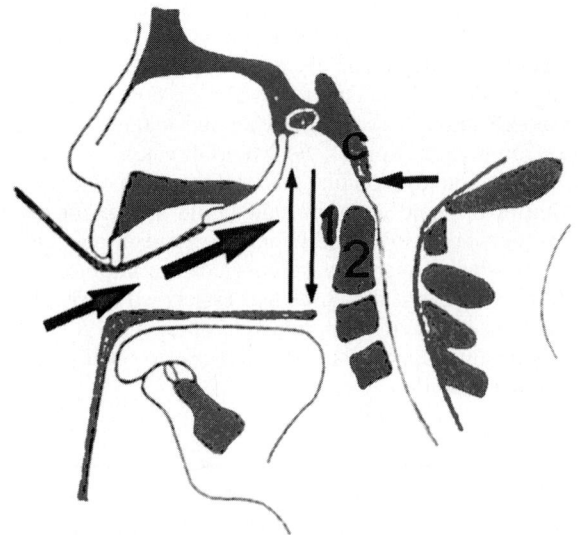

**FIGURE 20–4** ■ A schematic representation of the extent of access and exposure (*vertical arrows*) to the inferior clivus (C), the anterior foramen magnum (*small arrow*), the anterior arch of the atlas (1), and the body of the axis (2), which is possible with a palatal-sparing transoral approach (*large arrows*).

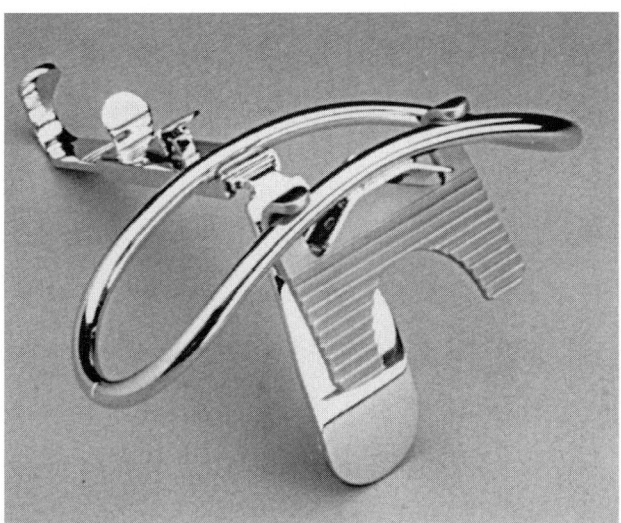

FIGURE 20–5 ■ A photograph of the Crockard self-retaining retractor system, which allows for retraction of the tissues without the need for stay sutures. (Codman & Shurtleff, Johnson & Johnson, Randolph, MA).

pared with povidone-iodine solution. In this approach, the soft palate need not be split, but instead is retracted into the nasopharynx with passage of a Jacques catheter intranasally and sutured in the region of the uvula.[20] A retractor system is then placed; we prefer the Crockard self-retaining retractor system (Codman & Shurtleff; Johnson & Johnson Co., Randolph, MA; Figs. 20–5 and 20–6), which allows for retraction of the tissues without the need for stay sutures.

The posterior pharyngeal wall is then palpated and the anterior tubercle of the atlas is identified as a landmark. After infiltration of local anesthetic containing 1:200,000 epinephrine and 0.5% lidocaine into the median raphe, the posterior pharyngeal wall is incised. The longus colli and longus capitus muscles are then reflected laterally to expose the anterior longitudinal ligament, the caudalmost clivus,

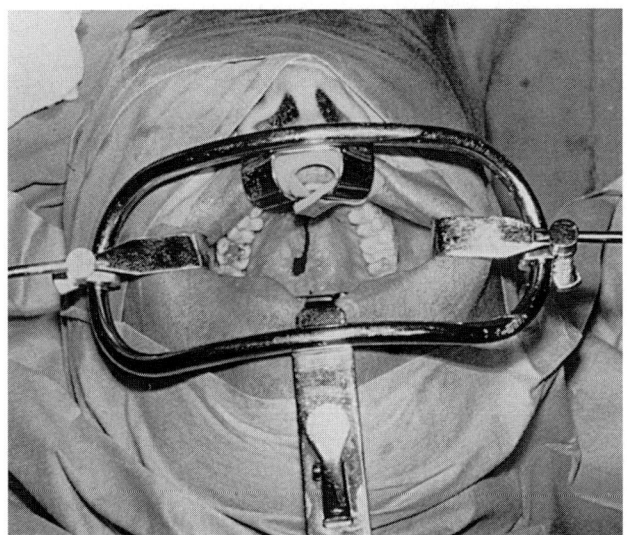

FIGURE 20–6 ■ An intraoperative photograph demonstrating the Crockard self-retaining retractor system in use allowing for retraction of the soft tissues during transoral surgery.

the anterior arch of C1, and the anterior surface of C2. To prevent injury to the hypoglossal nerves, the eustachian tubes, or the vertebral arteries, it is important to remain within 1.5 cm of the midline on each side. The caudalmost clivus, the anterior arch of C1, and the odontoid can then be removed with a high-speed drill, allowing for removal of the tumor and decompression of the neural system, depending on the tumor's location. A pulsatile tectorial membrane signifies completion of the extradural decompression. The longus colli and longus capitis muscles and the posterior pharyngeal wall are then closed with absorbable suture. At the end of all transoral procedures, the mandible should be moved to assess for temporomandibular joint dislocation, which can easily be corrected at the operation, but if missed necessitates another anesthetic.[16]

The subarachnoid space may be entered from this transoral approach to facilitate removal of intradural lesions in the region of the craniocervical junction.[21] Inadvertent entry may also occur in extradural lesions such as large clival chordomas because the dura may be invaded by the tumor, or it may be damaged as the tumor is removed.[16] Because postoperative CSF leakage, often complicated by infection, is the most serious sequela of transoral surgery, this is to be avoided at all costs, and methods have been designed to minimize this complication. First, in all intradural tumors and all situations in which the potential exists for violation of the dura, a large-bore lumbar catheter should be inserted to allow for postoperative CSF drainage. A CSF drainage rate of 10 to 20 ml/hr should be allowed for. This should be continued for at least 5 days to decrease hydrostatic pressure and allow wound healing.[20, 21] It has also been suggested that conversion to a lumbar-peritoneal shunt should be done after 5 days in patients with large dural defects,[21] although that is not our practice. The reason for this drainage is that dural closure in this region is difficult, often impossible, and drainage allows for healing to occur without continuous CSF pressure on the wound. In addition to lumbar drainage, repairing the defect with two layers of Lyodura, one layer inside and the other on the outside of the defect, held together with human-derived fibrin glue (Tisseel), aids in preventing postoperative CSF leak. The use of rotational flaps, either pharyngeal or sternocleidomastoid muscle, has also been described to prevent and treat CSF leaks after transoral surgery.[16, 22] The postoperative complication of tongue swelling can also be avoided by carefully ensuring the tongue is free from the retractors and is coated with 1% hydrocortisone before and after surgery.

After surgery, the patient should not be permitted oral intake for at least 3 to 5 days to allow for healing of the posterior pharyngeal wall; the oral intake can then be gradually increased from clear fluids to solids over a period of 2 to 3 days. Nutritional support should be provided with intravenous fluids and enteral feeds through the nasogastric tube/feeding tube that was placed after intubation. In those patients who underwent tracheotomy, the nasotracheal tube should be left in place for at least the first 24 hours to minimize the chance of upper airway obstruction from postoperative swelling.

## Transpalatal

The transpalatal approach is essentially an extension of the transoral procedure described previously. However, with the additional splitting of the hard and soft palates, access to a longer rostral-to-caudal field is provided that includes the lower half of the clivus, the anterior arch of C1, and the anterior surface of C2. This approach, however, remains limited in its lateral extent. Several variations in the transpalatal approach have been described; here we discuss the one with which we are most familiar.

The mucosa over the hard palate is incised from approximately 4 cm from the junction of the hard and soft palate, and then extended into the soft palate down toward the base of the uvula. At the base of the uvula the incision is then pushed off the midline to one side to preserve the base of the uvula. The hard palate is then removed, providing visualization of the vomer, which may then be removed. The Crockard self-retaining retractor system is then inserted and the operation continues as described in the palatal-sparing transoral approach, except that access is improved to include the lower half of the clivus, allowing for the removal of tumors that also involve this structure. A two-layer closure is then performed, with an absorbable suture to close the muscle and one to close the mucosa.

The potential complications of this procedure are similar to those of the palatal-sparing approach described earlier, although the additional splitting of the hard and soft palate produces some further potential problems. Oronasal fistulas may occur, particularly at the junction of the hard and soft palates.[16] These require secondary suturing and almost always heal over time.

Velopharyngeal dysfunction is more of a problem, and patients present with nasal regurgitation. Patients with purely extradural lesions and those without lower cranial nerve palsies have a much lower incidence of this problem, which may explain its pathogenesis. First, integrity of the posterior pharyngeal wall and the soft palate is necessary during phonation and swallowing to form a barrier between the nasopharynx and oropharynx.[21] With removal of a large amount of bone—and thus posterior pharyngeal wall support—such as in resection of the more extensive intradural tumors, patients have a higher incidence of this complication.[21] Posterior pharyngeal flaps, Teflon injections into this area,[21] and a "bone baffle"[23] have been described to provide more support in this area. Second, patients with neurogenic swallowing problems demonstrated on swallowing studies also have a higher incidence of this problem, reflecting the need for muscle coordination in the oropharynx and nasopharynx. Despite an improved understanding of its pathogenesis, patients with velopharyngeal dysfunction still present a serious problem that needs to be studied further.

## Le Fort I Osteotomy

The Le Fort I osteotomy was first described for the removal of a nasopharyngeal tumor in 1867, and now is a common operation in the realm of maxillofacial surgery.[24] Anatomically, a direct line of vision to the entire clivus without obstruction by intervening soft tissues is obtained by displacing the maxilla inferiorly (Fig. 20–7). This prompted the use of this approach for access to the clivus, and it was described in the transclival surgical treatment of aneurysms of the vertebrobasilar system with good results.[13] At the

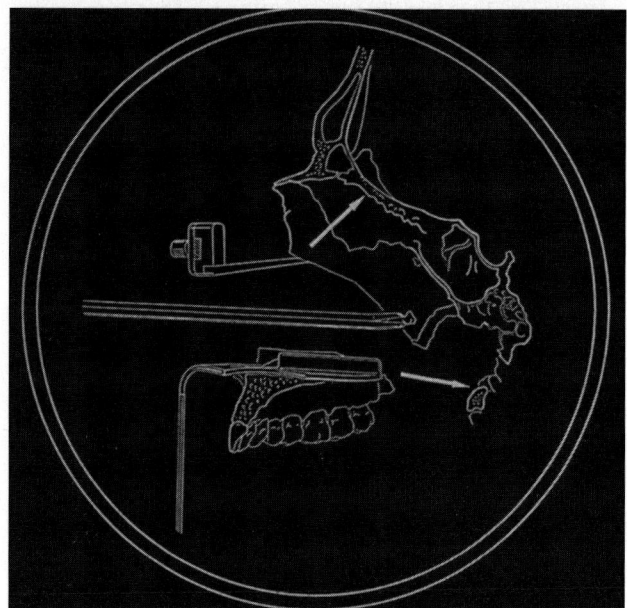

FIGURE 20–7 ■ A schematic representation of the extent of access and exposure (*arrows*) to the sphenoid sinus, sellar region, whole clivus, anterior foramen magnum, and upper cervical spine, which is possible with a Le Fort I maxillotomy surgical approach.

same institution, this procedure was used to treat midline skull base tumors.[1] This approach is ideally suited for both intradural and extradural midline lesions that can involve the whole clivus, because the whole clivus is exposed with this approach.

As with other transoral procedures, oral or nasotracheal intubation may be performed, with tracheotomies reserved for patients with compromised airways or severe bulbar palsies. All patients have a lumbar drain placed that is opened after surgery to allow for CSF drainage if dural violation occurs. The patient is then placed supine on a Mayfield headrest with the head elevated 15 degrees. After preparing the mouth with povidone-iodine solution, an incision is made above the mucogingival reflection extending from one upper molar to other, with the soft tissues reflected back subperiosteally to expose the maxilla. At this stage, the compression plates used to fixate the maxilla to the face at the end of the operation are marked off. This is important because precise relocation is necessary to prevent postoperative malocclusion. A standard Le Fort I osteotomy is then performed using a sagittal saw to cut through the malar buttresses to the maxillary tuberosities (Fig. 20–8). This exposes the nasal floor and pterygomaxillary fissure. The nasal septum is then divided from the maxilla in the midline, a curved chisel is used to separate the lateral pterygoid laminas from their maxillary attachments, and the maxilla is fractured downward[1] (Fig. 20–9). The blood supply to the maxilla is preserved with the greater palatine arteries and the mucosal supply of the faucial pillars.

The nasal mucosa is then stripped to expose the nasal septum and vomer. This is followed by removal of the inferior turbinates and the vomer. A modified Dingman gag is then inserted that retracts the cheeks laterally and the maxilla downward, exposing the posterior pharyngeal wall[1]

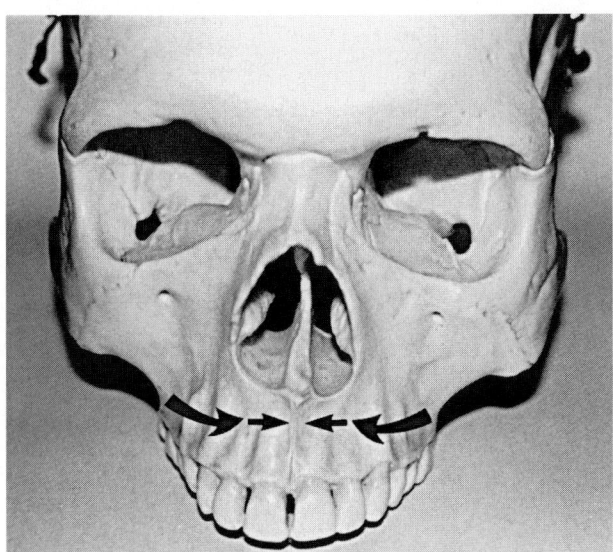

FIGURE 20–8 ■ A photograph demonstrating a standard Le Fort I osteotomy (*arrows*) that is performed with a sagittal saw cutting through the malar buttresses to the maxillary tuberosities, exposing the nasal floor and a pterygomaxillary fissure.

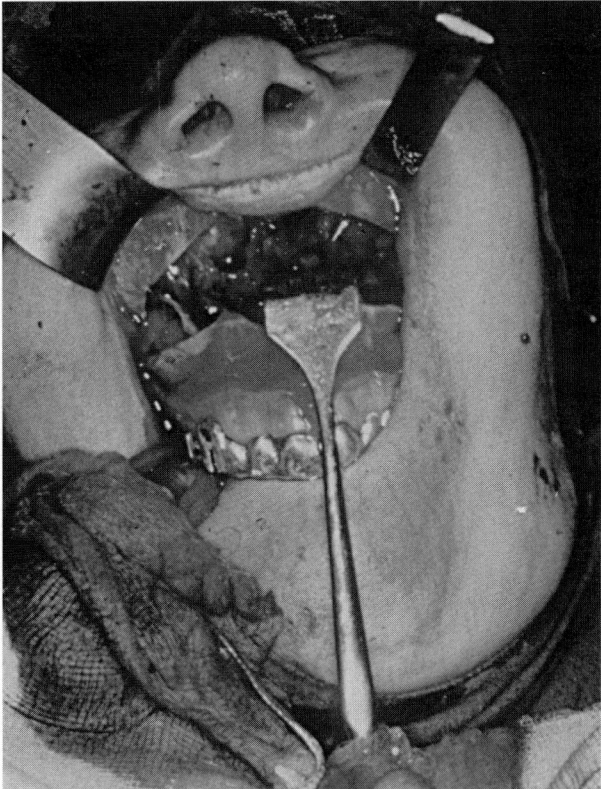

FIGURE 20–9 ■ An intraoperative photograph taken after the nasal septum has been divided from the maxilla in the midline. A chisel is used to separate the lateral pterygoid laminae from their maxillary attachments, which then allows the maxilla to be fractured downward.

(Figs. 20–10 and 20–11). This allows for exposure from the middle ethmoids to the anterior arch of the atlas, with the whole clivus between these structures (Fig. 20–12). After infiltration of local anesthetic containing 1:200,000 epinephrine and 0.5% lidocaine into the median raphe, the posterior pharyngeal wall is incised and reflected laterally to expose the whole clivus and the anterior arch of the atlas. Depending on the location of tumor, the high-speed drill can be used to remove the clivus to obtain access to the tumor, which can then be removed. In tumors that require an intradural exposure, the dura is opened with a small-bladed knife.

At completion of tumor removal, the dura is often difficult to close primarily and thus can be repaired with Lyodura as described previously, with lumbar drainage continued after surgery. The posterior pharyngeal wall is then repaired with absorbable suture. The maxilla is secured with minicompression plates and the mucosa repaired with absorbable suture. The postoperative course is as described previously.

## Extended "Open-Door" Maxillotomy

One disadvantage of the Le Fort I osteotomy is that the down-fractured maxilla may impede access to the craniocervical junction. This may be important if tumors involve the craniocervical junction in addition to the clivus, and thus require a larger area of access. Patients may also have an abnormal anatomic relationship between the clivus and craniocervical junction, impeding exposure. In these situations, the extended or "open-door" maxillotomy as described by Harkey and colleagues[25] and James and Crockard[26] is indicated. In this procedure, the Le Fort I osteotomy is combined with midline sagittal splitting of the maxilla and soft palate and their lateral displacement, thus allowing for exposure from the sphenoid to the third cervical vertebra.[27]

Orotracheal or nasotracheal intubation or tracheotomy is decided on as described previously, as is lumbar drainage. The patient is then placed supine on a Mayfield headrest with the head mildly extended to allow for access to the palate. After preparing the mouth with povidone-iodine

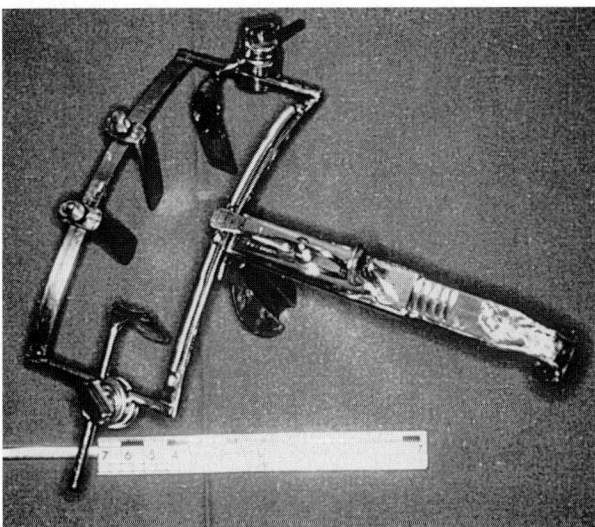

FIGURE 20–10 ■ A photograph of a modified Dingman gag that is used during the Le Fort I osteotomy, thus allowing for retraction of the cheeks laterally and the maxilla downward, exposing the posterior pharyngeal wall.

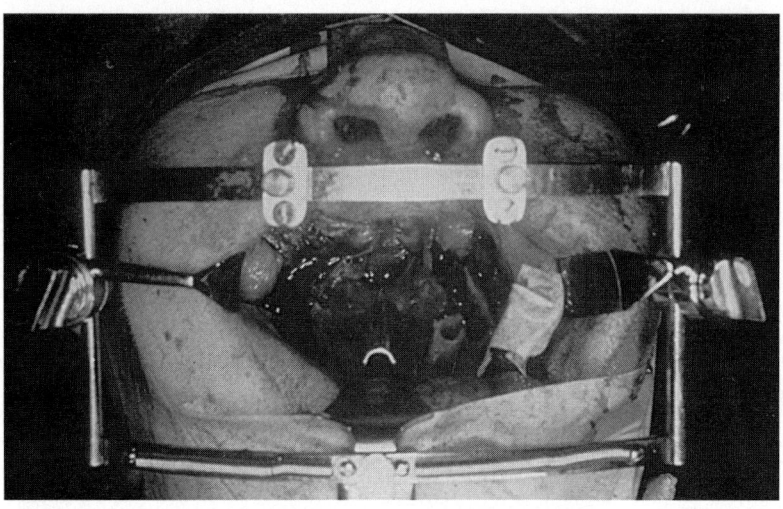

FIGURE 20–11 ■ An intraoperative photograph with the modified Dingman gag in use demonstrating the exposure of the posterior pharyngeal wall.

solution, an incision is made above the mucogingival reflection extending from one upper molar to other, with the soft tissues reflected back subperiosteally to expose the maxilla. As with the standard Le Fort I procedure, the compression plates used to fix the maxilla to the face at the end of the operation are marked off to ensure precise relocation. A midline sagittal incision is then made into the palatal mucoperiosteum and alveolar margin and is reflected off the underlying bone laterally. Care must be taken to ensure vascularity of the maxilla by not stripping the mucoperiosteum too far laterally. A standard Le Fort I osteotomy is then performed with a sagittal saw to cut through the malar buttresses to the maxillary tuberosities. This exposes the nasal floor and pterygomaxillary fissure. The nasal septum is then divided from the maxilla in the midline, and a curved chisel is used to separate the lateral pterygoid laminas from their maxillary attachments, after which the maxilla is fractured downward.[1] The nasal mucosa is then stripped to expose the nasal septum and vomer, and the inferior turbinates and vomer are removed. A Crockard retractor system is then inserted to permit exposure of the middle ethmoids, the entire clivus, and the craniocervical junction. After infiltration of local anesthetic containing 1:200,000 epinephrine and 0.5% lidocaine into the median raphe, the posterior pharyngeal wall is incised and reflected laterally. A high-speed drill is used to remove the clivus and associated bone necessary for access, and the tumor is resected. In intradural tumors, the dura is opened and then repaired with Lyodura as described previously, with lumbar drainage continued after surgery. The posterior pharyngeal wall is then repaired with absorbable suture. The two halves of the maxilla are secured with miniplates and the maxilla is secured with minicompression plates at the predetermined locations. The mucosa is repaired with absorbable suture. The postoperative course is as described previously for the other transoral procedures.

## TRANSFACIAL APPROACH

In tumors beneath the midface that include the anterior skull base, the transfacial route can be used to gain access with appropriate maxillectomy and ethmoidectomy. Exposure of the midface is the initial step in using the transfacial routes, and can be done either by a lateral rhinotomy (Weber-Fergusson incision) or by using the midface degloving technique made popular by Conley, Price, and colleagues,[15, 28, 29] but originally described by Casson and associates in 1974.[30] The advantage of using the midface degloving technique in the transfacial route for treating tumors in and around the sphenoid sinus and clivus is that the exposure and access are superior to those with the traditional procedures that require facial incisions that can

FIGURE 20–12 ■ An intraoperative photograph demonstrating the exposure obtained after the maxilla has been fractured downward in this patient, ranging from the middle ethmoids to the anterior arch of the atlas, with the whole clivus between these structures.

leave unsightly scars. Although the lateral exposure is less generous with the degloving technique than with the Weber-Fergusson incision, the bilateral exposure is an advantage in larger midline lesions such as in clival tumors.[15] Because of the advantages of the degloving approach in midline anterior skull base tumors, this approach is discussed as described by Price, Conley, and colleagues.[15, 28, 29]

Under general anesthesia, an oral endotracheal tube is placed and secured in the midline. A tarsorrhaphy is performed to prevent irritation of the eye, and topical cocaine is inserted on pledgets intranasally and 1:2000 epinephrine injected into the junction between the skin and the mucosa of the nose, gingival sulcus, and canine fossas. The nasal tip is separated from the nasal dorsum by intercartilaginous incisions, and the incision is continued around the pyriform margin to complete a circumvestibular release. A sublabial incision is then made that extends from the molars on each side. The soft tissues of the face and the nasal tip are then elevated subperiosteally to expose the inferior orbital rims to their lateralmost extent. The upper lip and nasal columella, nasal tip, and alar cartilages are then retracted over the nose to the infraorbital rim. Osteotomy of the infraorbital foramen is then performed, allowing for preservation of the infraorbital complex. The medial and inferior portions of the orbit are then freed and extended laterally to mobilize the face further.

The maxillary antrum is then entered and the anterior wall removed on both sides to provide access to the ethmoids. Osteotomies are then performed over the superior and inferior pyriform margins, allowing for completion of a medial maxillectomy. The nasal septum is exposed and released to the cribriform plate after ethmoidectomy and sphenoidotomy are performed. After removal of the posterior wall of the maxillary antrum and the ascending process of the palatine process, the nasopharynx, sphenoid sinus, and clivus are exposed. Tumor removal can then proceed, with the lateral limit of the dissection being the coronoid process of the mandible, and posteriorly the carotid arteries on the lateral aspect of the sphenoid sinus. The inferior resection is limited by the palate, although this can be extended by performing a palatectomy or maxillectomy if required.

On closure, the face is reapproximated anatomically, with the nasal tip repositioned with a transfixation suture and one placed at the base of the columella. The vestibular skin is then sutured to the pyriform margin, the frenulum carefully approximated, and the sublabial incision sutured. Packing is inserted into the cavity with antibiotic-saturated petroleum jelly and rhinoplastic taping is applied.

## CONCLUSION

Skull base tumors are rare tumors that originate from a variety of tissues, extracranially, intracranially, or directly from the skull base. Radical surgical resection is the treatment of choice in their management because they are frequently benign or only locally malignant, and are refractory to radiation therapy or chemotherapy.

These tumors are difficult to treat surgically, lying ventral to the brain and posterior to the facial skeleton and aerodigestive system; however, advances in surgical techniques involving the creation of multidisciplinary surgical teams have improved outcomes. Surgical management and choice of surgical approach to skull base tumors depends largely on the location of the tumor, with each approach providing various angles and degrees of access along the skull base. For anterior skull base tumors, the direct midline ventral approaches are particularly attractive because they are unencumbered by cranial nerves or major blood vessels.

The transnasal or transsphenoidal route provides good access to the sellar region and rostral third of the clivus. The transoral route provides a direct approach to the anterior rim of the foramen magnum, and may then be modified to improve access and exposure. Dividing the soft or hard palate in the transpalatal approach allows for access to the lower and middle third of the clivus. A Le Fort 1 osteotomy with mobilization of the hard palate and maxilla inferiorly allows for visualization of the whole clivus, and this can be further modified by splitting the hard and soft palates, allowing for exposure of the entire clivus and the craniocervical junction. In the transfacial approach, removal of the midface permits access to the paranasal sinuses and upper two thirds of the clivus. Another important aspect of these direct midline ventral approaches is that they can also be combined with different intracranial approaches to facilitate a more complete removal of tumor.

## REFERENCES

1. Uttley D, Moore A, Archer DJ: Surgical management of midline skull-base tumors: A new approach. J Neurosurg 71:705–710, 1989.
2. Cheesman AD, Lund VJ, Howard DJ: Craniofacial resection for tumors of the nasal cavity and paranasal sinuses. Head Neck Surg 8:429–435, 1986.
3. Westbury G, Wilson JSP, Richardson A: Combined craniofacial resection for malignant disease. Am J Surg 130:463, 1976.
4. Ketchum AS, Van Buren JM: Tumors of the paranasal sinuses: A therapeutic challenge. Am J Surg 150:406, 1985.
5. Shah JP, Galicich JH: Craniofacial resection for malignant tumors of the ethmoid and anterior skull base. Arch Otolaryngol 103:514–517, 1977.
6. Golfinos JG, Fitzpatrick BC, Smith LR, Spetzler RF: Clinical use of a frameless stereotactic arm: Results of 325 cases. J Neurosurg 83:197–202, 1995.
7. Crockard HA: Transclival surgery. Br J Neurosurg 5:237–240, 1991.
8. Laws ER: Transsphenoidal surgery for tumors of the clivus. Otolaryngol Head Neck Surg 92:100, 1984.
9. Mullan LI, Naunton R, Hekmat-Panah J, et al: The use of an anterior approach to ventrally placed tumors in the foramen magnum and vertebral column. J Neurosurg 24:536–543, 1966.
10. Pasztor E, Vajda J, Piffko P: Transoral surgery for craniocervical space occupying process. J Neurosurg 60:276–281, 1984.
11. Crockard HA: Anterior approaches to lesions of the upper cervical spine. Clin Neurosurg 34:389–416, 1988.
12. Brommer RB: The history of the Le Fort osteotomy. J Maxillofac Surg 14:119–122, 1986.
13. Archer DJ, Young S, Uttley D: Basilar aneurysms: A new transclival approach via maxillotomy. J Neurosurg 67:54–58, 1987.
14. Harkey HL, Crockard HA, Stevens JM, et al: The operative management of basilar impression in osteogenesis imperfecta. Neurosurgery 27:782–786, 1990.
15. Price JC, Holliday MJ, Johns ME, et al: The versatile midface degloving approach. Laryngoscope 98:291–295, 1988.
16. Crockard HA, Johnston F: Development of transoral approaches to lesions of the skull base and craniocervical junction. Neurosurg Q 3:61–82, 1993.

17. Arbit E, Patterson RH Jr: Combined transoral and median labioman-dibular glossotomy approach to the upper cervical spine. Neurosur-gery 8:672–674, 1981.
18. Delgado TE, Garrido E, Harwick RD: Labiomandibular transoral approach to chordomas in the clivus and upper cervical spine. Neuro-surgery 8:675–679, 1981.
19. Crockard HA: The transoral approach to the base of the brain and upper cervical cord. Ann R Coll Surg Engl 67:321–325, 1985.
20. Spetzler RF, Selman WR, Nash CL, et al: Transoral microsurgical odontoid resection and spinal cord monitoring. Spine 4:506–510, 1979.
21. Crockard HA, Sen CN: The transoral approach for the management of intradural lesions at the craniovertebral junction: A review of 7 cases. Neurosurgery 28:88–98, 1991.
22. Kenndy DW, Papel I, Holliday N: Transpalatal approach to the skull base. Ear Nose Throat J 65:48–58, 1986.
23. Bonkowski JA, Gibson RD, Snape L: Foramen magnum meningioma: Transoral resection with a bone baffle to prevent CSF leakage. J Neurosurg 72:493–496, 1990.
24. Moloney F, Worthington P: The origin of the Le Fort 1 maxillary osteotomy: Cheever's operation. Oral Surg 39:731–734, 1981.
25. Harkey HL, Crockard HA, Stevens JM, et al: The operative manage-ment of basilar impression in osteogenesis imperfecta. Neurosurgery 27:782–786, 1990.
26. James D, Crockard HA: Surgical access to the base of the skull and upper cervical spine by extended maxillotomy. Neurosurgery 29:411–416, 1991.
27. Anand VK, House JR 3d, al-Mefty O: Management of benign neo-plasms invading cavernous sinus. Laryngoscope 101:557–564, 1991.
28. Conley J, Price JC: Sublabial approach to the nasal and nasopharyn-geal cavities. Am J Surg 138:615–618, 1979.
29. Price JC: The midfacial degloving approach to the central skull base. Ear Nose Throat J 65:46–53, 1986.
30. Casson PR, Bonnano PC, Converse JM: The midface degloving procedure. Plast Reconstr Surg 53:102–113, 1974.

C H A P T E R   2 1

# Orbitozygomatic Infratemporal Approach for Parasellar Meningiomas

■ KENJI OHATA, BASSEM SHEIKH, TOSHIHIRO TAKAMI, and AKIRA HAKUBA

Lesions located high in the parasellar region and the interpeduncular fossa are challenging and often difficult to approach, owing both to the deep position and to the surrounding vital structures that obscure the view. In 1977, we developed a new surgical approach, the orbitozygomatic infratemporal approach,[1] consisting of an orbitozygomatic osteotomy, a frontotemporo-orbital craniotomy, and removal of the posterolateral wall of the orbital bone and major sphenoid wing lateral to the foramen spinosum. This approach provides a good exposure of the infratemporal fossa, permits access obliquely upward to the parasellar region and the interpeduncular fossa, and permits safe manipulation of parasellar and interpeduncular lesions via the shortest distance.

## OPERATIVE TECHNIQUE

The patient is placed in the "park bench" position. By using a three-pin headholder, the head is kept in an extended position at the craniovertebral junction about 40 degrees, and the neck is tilted toward the side opposite the lesion, keeping the vertex of the head about 35 degrees downward. Then the head of the operating table is elevated so that the temporal region is kept almost in the horizontal plane.

A bicoronal scalp incision is made to gain sufficient exposure of the zygomatic arch and superior and lateral orbital margins, starting at the inferior end of the base of the earlobe, running along the anterior margin of the ear cartilage, extending upward and forward, and running within the hairline to a level 2 cm above the upper margin of the contralateral zygomatic arch. Care is taken to avoid injury of the superficial temporal artery and vein, especially when the need for reconstruction of the base of the skull is expected. The skin flap is reflected anteriorly with the frontal pericranium, which is elevated about 2 cm above the superior orbital margin, and the superficial temporal fascia, which is divided obliquely from the lateral end of the frontal pericranial incision down to the anterior margin

of the external auditory canal and separated from the deep temporal fascia to prevent injury of the frontal branch of the facial nerve.[2, 3] To preserve the temporal and zygomatic branches of the facial nerve, the fascia covering the temporomandibular joint capsule is carefully pulled away, and the periosteum covering the outer surface of the zygomatic arch is incised vertically just in front of the tuberculum articulare. The entire outer surface of the zygomatic arch from its frontal process to its pedicle is then fully exposed subperiosteally. The superior and lateral orbital margins are then exposed, maintaining continuity of the pericranium and the periorbita. The superior and lateral periorbita are separated from the superior and lateral posterior walls of the orbit.

Six bur holes are made: the first in the lateral frontal bone just behind the frontal process of the zygomatic bone, *key bur hole*; the second at the pterion; the third in the temporal bone just above the pedicle of the zygomatic process; the fourth in the squamous suture about 3 cm above the zygomatic arch; the fifth in the coronal suture about 6 cm above the zygomatic arch; and the sixth in the frontal bone 3 cm above the orbital ridge (Fig. 21-1). The anterior and posterior ends of the zygomatic arch are then cut using a sagittal saw, and it is retracted downward hinged on the masseter muscle.

The supraorbital canal is opened by a chisel to protect the supraorbital nerve. The second, third, fourth, fifth, and sixth bur holes are then connected with a craniotome (see Fig. 21-1). Using a reciprocating saw, osteotomy of the lateral and superior walls of the orbit is performed from the inferior orbital fissure. The orbital content is protected by a spatula during this osteotomy. The frontotemporal bone flap and the orbitozygomatic flap are kept in saline solution containing an antibiotic. While protecting the periorbita and the dura mater with self-retaining retractors with tapering Sugita's spatulas, the remaining major sphenoid wing lateral to the foramen spinosum, forming the posterolateral orbital wall and the anterolateral part of the middle fossa, and the posterior portion of the orbital roof lateral to the superior orbital fissure are divided, using either a sagittal saw or small chisel (see Fig. 21-1). The remaining

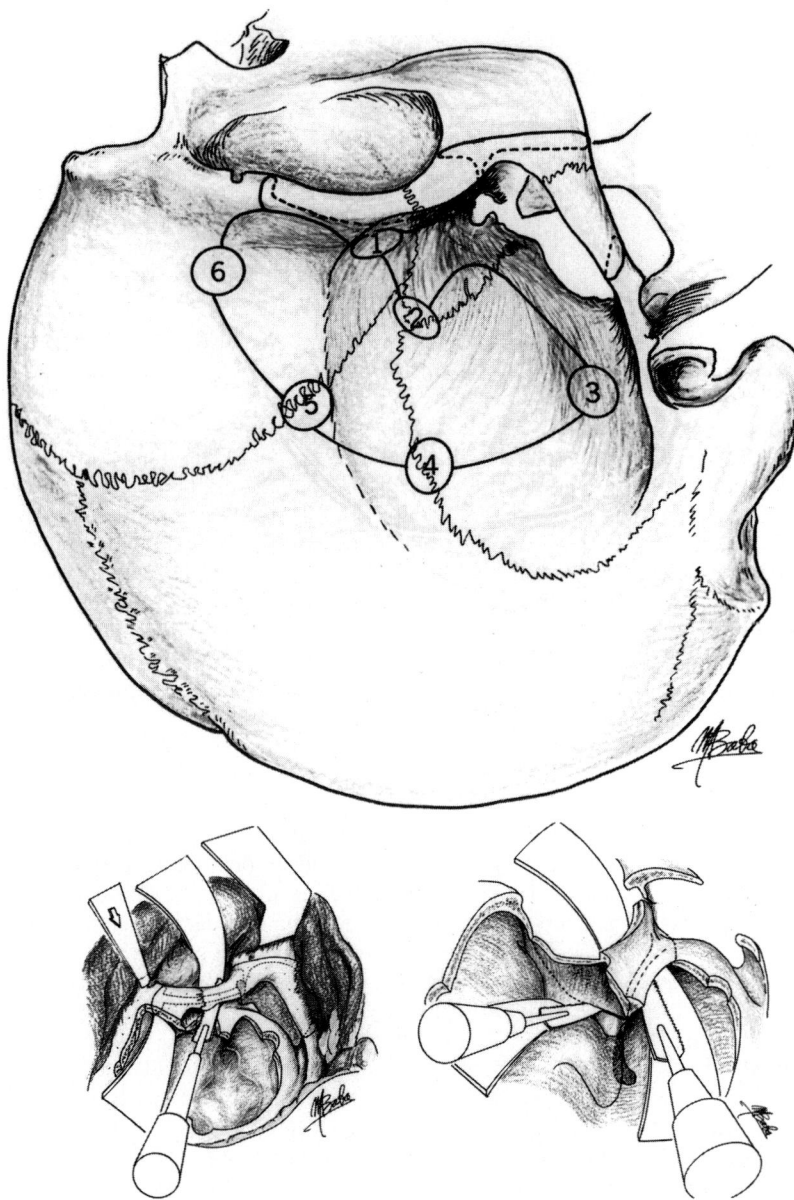

**FIGURE 21–1** ■ *Upper,* Location of the bur holes and the extent of cranitomy; the first bur hole is made at the frontal bone just behind its zygomatic process "key bur hole," the second at the pterion, the third on the temporal bone just above the pedicle of the zygomatic arch, the fourth in the squamous suture, the fifth in the coronal suture, and the sixth in the frontal bone 3 cm above the orbital ridge. *Lower left,* An orbitozygomatic osteotomy; the zygoma has been well exposed down to the zygomaticofacial canal. The supraorbital canal has been opened by a chisel to prevent its nerve from stretching. The osteotomy of the lateral and superior wall of the orbit is done from the inferior orbital fissure using a reciprocal saw. The orbital content is protected with a spatula during this procedure (the temporal muscle is not drawn). *Lower right,* Osteotomy of the greater sphenoid wing. The dura mater of the frontal base and temporal pole are retracted to expose the greater and lesser sphenoid wings. The line of osteotomy passes 5 to 10 mm lateral to the lateral margin of the superior orbital fissure. (From Oheta K, Baba M: Orbitozygomatic infratemporal approach. In Hakuba A [ed]: Surgical Anatomy of the Skull Base. Tokyo: Miawa Shoten, 1996, pp 1–35.)

medial part of the minor sphenoid wing is then partially removed with an air drill and a bone rongeur. The bone fragments are kept in the saline solution to be replaced at the end of the procedure.

The exposed frontotemporal dura mater is opened in semicircular fashion, from the medial superior orbital margin to the midportion of the inferior temporal region. The orbital contents are retracted medially downward by retracting the anterior dural fringe forward.

The operative microscope is now introduced, and either a trans-sylvian approach or a subtemporal approach can be taken with minimal retraction of the brain. In the trans-sylvian approach, the sylvian fissure is widely opened, with preservation of the bridging veins coming from the tip of the temporal lobe. The parasellar region as well as the interpeduncular fossa can be reached at a short distance through the space formed via this approach.

When the tumor is invading the cavernous sinus (CS),[2] the CS is explored by a combined orbitozygomatic infratemporal epidural and subdural approach, which has been described elsewhere.[4–6] The periosteal reflection, which is continuous with the periorbita, is divided at the superior and inferior margins of the superior orbital fissure by sharp dissection using either microscissors or a knife; then the temporal dura propria, forming the superficial layer of the CS, can be separated from the content of the superior orbital fissure (Fig. 21–2). The lateral part of the anterior clinoid process is shelled out leaving a thin layer of its cortical bone. The optic canal is then opened along its length (see Fig. 21–2). The cortical bone of the anterior clinoid process and the optic strut are removed by a bone-cutting forceps and a small diamond drill. After resection of the optic strut, the anteromedial triangle (Dolenc's triangle) is exposed in the epidural space (see Fig. 21–2). The dural incision passes along the sylvian fissure to the superior surface of the optic nerve sheath forward, then turns laterally at a right angle. It passes backward at a right angle and runs along the medial part of the distal carotid ring, then along the carotid artery 2 mm apart from the artery (see Fig. 21–2). Opening of the medial triangle (Hakuba's triangle, which is a triangle in the subdural space) starts from the distal ring along the medial side of the triangle to the posterior clinoid process and turns laterally at a right angle along the posterior side of this triangle to the dural entrance of the third cranial nerve. The lateral dural fringe of the medial triangle is elevated. Then the remaining outer layer of the CS is separated further backward from the inner layer of the lateral wall of the CS consisting of the nerve sheaths of the third through fifth cranial nerves, and the entire CS is unveiled. Bleeding from the CS is simply controlled by elevating the head side of the table, and the opened venous pathway in the CS is immediately sealed off by either insertion of Biobond-soaked oxidized cellulose (Oxycel) or insertion of fibrinogen-soaked Gelfoam sponge and thrombin-soaked Gelfoam sponge into the CS and a bipolar coagulation. Because the intracavernous internal carotid artery (ICA) has its own dural sheath,[7] the plane between the ICA and the tumor is usually found relatively easily, and the tumor is freed from the ICA if it is not invasive. When the artery is torn during dissection, 8–0 monofilament nylon interrupted sutures are applied while trapping this segment

of the artery between two temporary clips at both C3 and either C5 or the intrapetrous portions of the ICA with intravenous administration of barbiturates for brain protection[8] (pentobarbital 4 mg/kg as the initial dose, followed by 2 mg/kg/hr).

## CLOSURE OF THE OPENED PARANASAL SINUS AND DURAL DEFECT

If laceration of the paranasal sinus mucosa is large, it is better to open this sinus wall maximally, and the mucosa of the opened sinus should be removed entirely to prevent postoperative sinusitis and empyema. The opened sinus is closed with a piece of the abdominal fat fixed with fibrin glue. The large bony defect of the paranasal sinus is closed by using either a reflected basal dural flap with its broad base connecting with the remaining dura mater or the pericraniomusculofascial flap with the superficial temporal arteriovenous stalk. In the former case, the newly developed dural defect is closed by a free pericranial graft. If the laceration of the sinus mucosa is small, the defect is closed by application of the small piece of the temporal muscle. If the mucosa is intact, the bony defect is closed simply with insertion of either a sheet of the temporal fascia or the fascia lata in the epidural space. For watertight closure of the dura mater, fibrin glue is applied after approximation of the margins of the graft to the edges of the dura mater using interrupted 8–0 monofilament nylon sutures. Miniplates are used for adequate bone closure to fix the bone flaps to bone edges.

## SUMMARY OF CASES

Since 1977, 104 cases were treated using the orbitozygomatic approach either alone or combined with other approaches, such as the *oticocondylar approach*[9] or *transpetrosal approach*.[4] These cases included 24 parasellar meningiomas, 20 pituitary adenomas, 19 basilar tip aneurysms, 12 trigeminal neurinomas, 5 chordomas, 5 carotid cavernous aneurysms, 3 craniopharyngiomas, 3 CS cavernomas, and 13 other lesions. Of 24 parasellar meningiomas, 11 patients were men and 13 women. Age ranged from 35 to 67 years (mean of 50.2 years). Total removal of the tumor was accomplished in 19 cases, subtotal removal in 4, and partial removal in 1. Postoperative bacterial meningitis and either an epidural or a subdural hematoma were seen in three cases, wound infection in two, and pneumonia in one. In the cases of the tumors involving CS, impairment of extraocular movement was seen postoperatively in five cases, trigeminal nerve injury in four, and ipsilateral blindness in two. There was no mortality, but four patients developed disturbance of their conscious level (severely disabled in one case and moderately disabled in three). The operative results were classified as follows: excellent, when the patients have no neurologic deficit; good, when the patients have normal activity in daily life with minor neurologic dysfunction; fair, when the patients are moderately disabled but independent with major neuro-

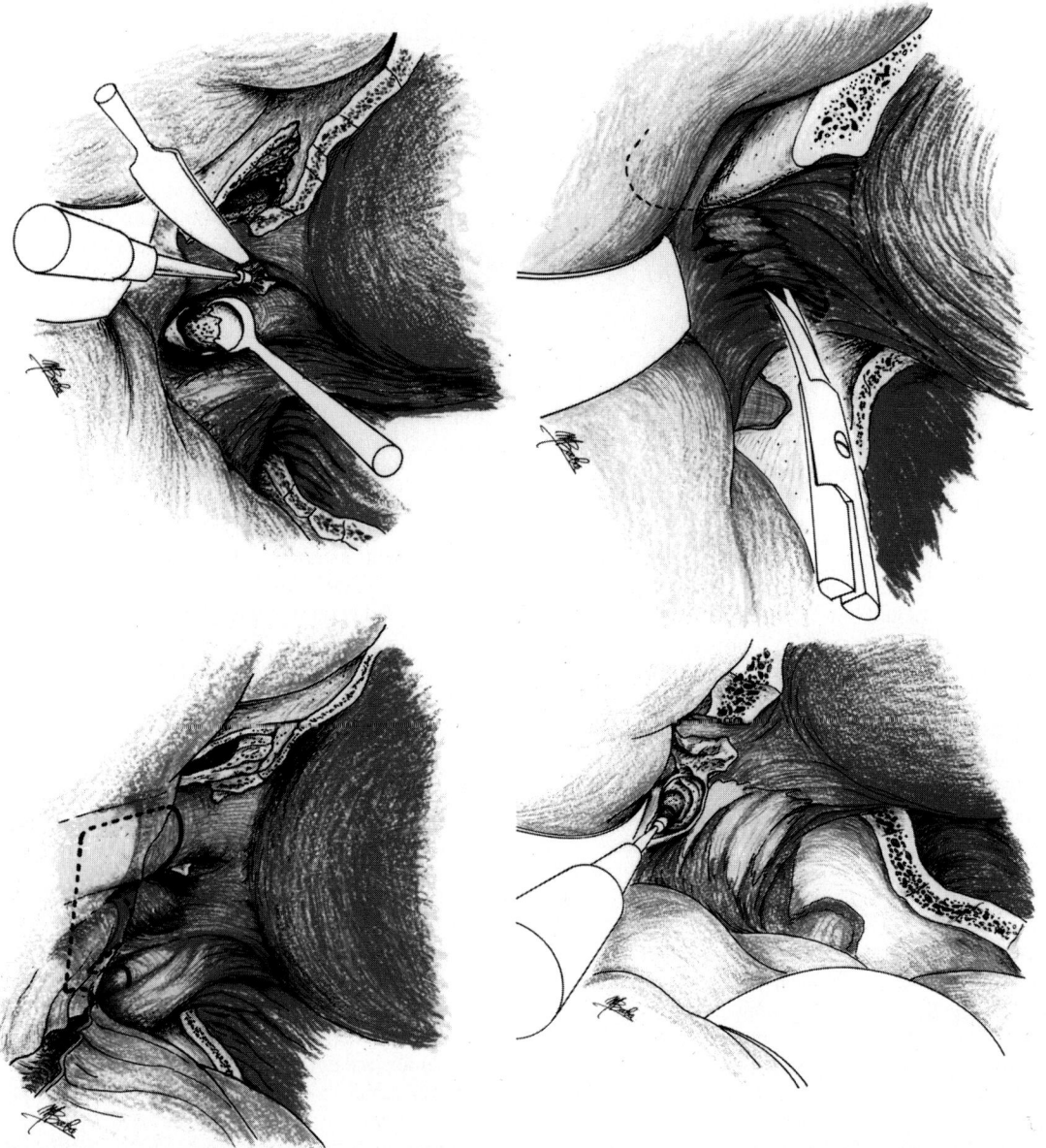

**FIGURE 21–2** ■ *Upper right,* The periosteal reflection, which is continuous with the periorbita, is divided at the superior and inferior margins of the superior orbital fissure by sharp dissection using either microscissors or a knife. Then the temporal dura propria, forming the superficial layer of the cavernous sinus, can be separated from the content of the superior orbital fissure. *Lower right,* Drilling of the anterior clinoid process. The lateral part of the anterior clinoid process has been shelled out leaving a thin layer of its cortical bone. The optic canal has been opened through its length. *Upper left,* Drilling of the optic strut. The cortical bone of the anterior clinoid process and the optic strut are being removed by a bone curet and a small diamond drill, respectively. *Lower left,* Dural opening around the paracavernous region. The *dotted line* shows the dural incision that passes along the sylvian fissure to the superior surface of the optic nerve sheath forwards and is then turned laterally at a right angle. It then passes backwards at a right angle and runs along the medial part of the distal carotid ring and then along the carotid artery (the optic strut has been resected and the anteromedial triangle [Dolenc's triangle] has been exposed). It then runs along the medial side to the posterior clinoid process and finally along the posterior side of the medial triangle (Hakuba's triangle) to the dural entrance of the oculomotor nerve. (From Oheta K, Baba M: Orbitozygomatic infratemporal approach. In Hakuba A [ed]: Surgical Anatomy of the Skull Base. Tokyo: Miawa Shoten; 1996, pp 1–35.)

logic deficit; and poor, when the patients are severely disabled and totally dependent. The operative results were excellent in 5 and good in 15 patients. Three of the remaining four patients were fair postoperatively as a result of bacterial meningitis in one; hypothalamic damage, which had been seen preoperatively, in one; and a combined epidural and subdural hematoma in one. The last one was poor because of a postoperative epidural hematoma. Two representative cases are described briefly.

# CASE REPORTS

## Case 1

The right orbitozygomatic infratemporal approach with a combined epidural and subdural (medial triangle) approach was used on a 57-year-old, right-handed man with a large right parasellar meningioma who had total ophthalmoplegia after partial removal of the tumor in the past (Fig. 21–3). A large tumor occupied the entire CS with encasement of the intracavernous segment of the right ICA. The tumor extended backward subdurally behind the upper clivus with marked compression of the pons and extended inferiorly into the right sphenoid sinus. All the cranial nerves were encased and invaded by the tumor in the CS and had to be sacrificed and removed with the tumor. The intracavernous ICA was carefully dissected out and preserved. The upper basilar artery and its tributaries, which were displaced backward

and partially encased, were also well preserved, with total removal of the tumor (Fig. 21–4). The patient had moderate left hemiparesis, which lasted 2 weeks postoperatively; he was neurologically intact except for permanent total ophthalmoplegia at 4 months.

## Case 2

A 57-year-old woman presented with progressive visual deterioration of the left eye. Radiologic study showed a large left parasellar meningioma (Fig. 21–5). A left orbitozygomatic approach was used for total removal of the tumor. The tumor was engulfing the ICA, but it could be easily separated from it because of the presence of arachnoid space between the artery and the tumor. The tumor extended into the left optic canal and compressed the optic nerve. The canal was opened for excision of that part of the tumor. The anterior part of the lateral wall of the CS was invaded by the tumor, but intracavernous structures were not involved by the tumor. The pituitary stalk was shifted and flattened by the tumor. All these structures were preserved, and total removal of the tumor was achieved (Figs. 21–6; see also Fig. 21–5). Postoperatively the patient showed mild left oculomotor palsy, which improved gradually.

# DISCUSSION

Radical removal of parasellar meningiomas usually involves difficult surgical procedures. Via the orbitozygo-

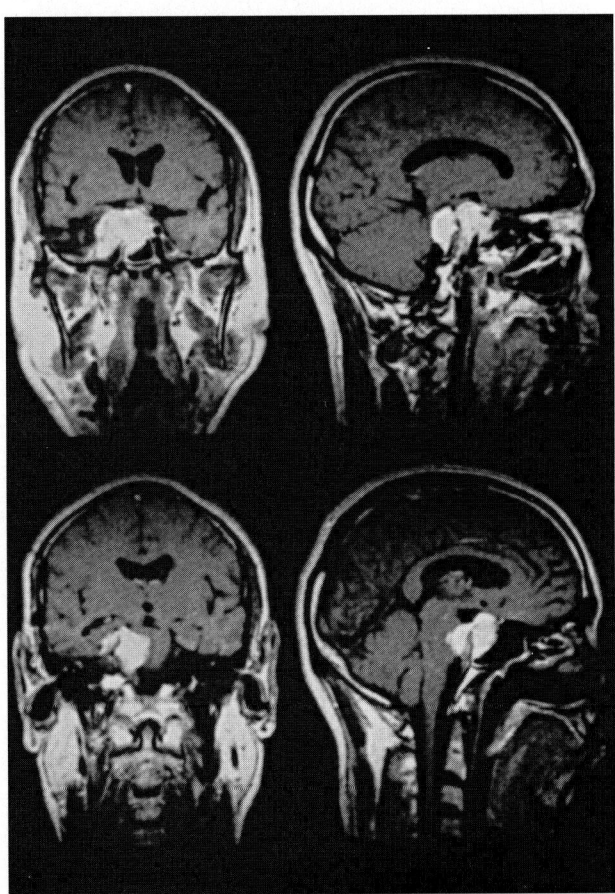

FIGURE 21–3 ■ Preoperative $T_1$-weighted magnetic resonance imaging scan with contrast of a case of right parasellar meningioma that was partially removed in the past. The tumor is encasing the right internal carotid artery and extending to the sphenoid sinus anteriorly: It also extends posteriorly, compressing the pons.

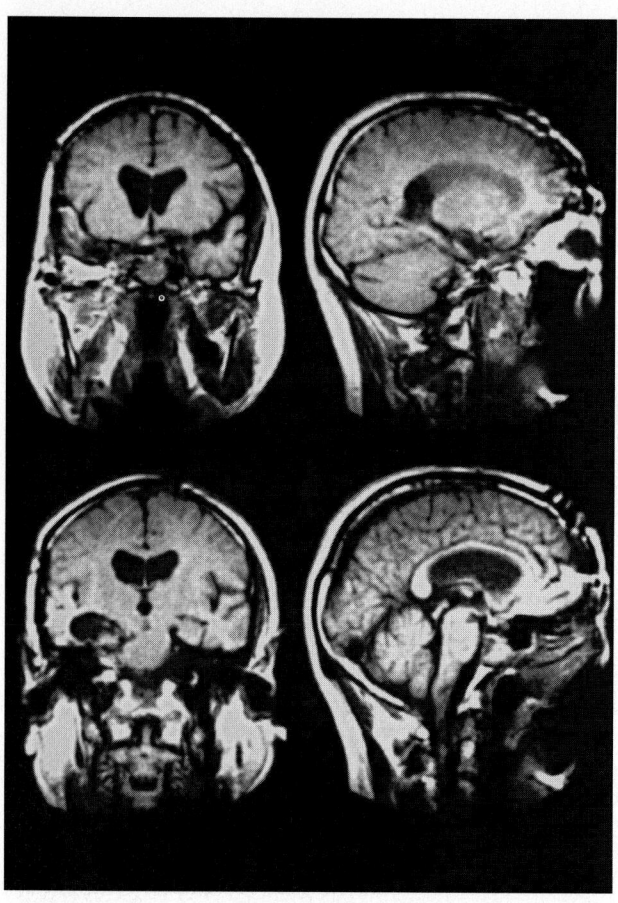

**FIGURE 21–4** ■ Postoperative study showing the complete removal of the tumor. The sphenoid sinus is repaired with a vascularized temporal musculofascial flap.

matic infratemporal approach, the working distance to the lesions in the parasellar region and the interpeduncular fossa is about 3 cm shorter and the angle to the lesions about 1 to 3 cm lower than via either the pterional or the subtemporal approach. Via the combined orbitozygomatic infratemporal epidural and medial triangle approach, the intracanal portion of the optic nerve is well exposed, so that much wider space between the optic nerve and the carotid artery can be obtained. Via this combined approach, the parasellar region, including the CS, and the interpeduncular fossa can be accessed in the shortest possible distance with minimal retraction of the temporal lobe. Manipulation of the vital structures is much easier and safer, even with large parasellar meningiomas, than via the conventional operative approaches.

The intracavernous portion of the ICA, 1 cm long, is epidurally exposed with removal of the petrosal apex at the posterior portion of the trigeminal impression medial to the great petrosal nerve groove by using an air drill. Therefore, when parasellar tumors extend into the CS, the intracavernous portion of the procedure is performed relatively safely while trapping the intracavernous portion of the ICA between its petrosal and C3 portions if necessary.[8] Because the petrosal bone is removed, both medial to the intrapetrosal portion of the ICA and anterior to the internal auditory meatus and cochlea, a transzygomatic preauricular transpetrosal approach[6] can be readily carried out. Therefore, parasellar tumors extending into the posterior fossa can be totally removed at one stage via this combined epidural and subdural approach.

If the sphenoparietal sinus is not involved by the parasellar meningiomas, sylvian vein should be preserved. This preservation can be done via the described combined orbitozygomatic infratemporal epidural and medial triangle approach delimited medially to the foramen rotundum because sylvian vein runs within the dura propria of the temporal lobe and drains usually into the sphenoparietal sinus, which is located lateral to the foramen ovale; that is, the dura propria of the temporal lobe forming the outer layer of the lateral wall of the CS medial to the foramen rotundum is separated from the inner layer consisting of the dural sheaths of the third and fourth cranial nerves and the first and second branches of the fifth cranial nerve. This dura propria is elevated and retracted backward together with the lateral leaf of the medial triangle opened along its medial and posterior sides. By this means, the infratemporal approach to the interpeduncular fossa can be taken via the temporopolar epidural space without cutting the temporopolar bridging veins.

To preserve the peripheral facial nerve in such low craniotomies, it is necessary to know its topographic anatomy.[10] After exiting from the stylomastoid foramen, the facial nerve crosses the posterior margin of the mandible about 2 cm below the inferior base of the earlobe and enters the parotid gland from behind, where it is situated between the superficial and deep portions of the gland. The branches leave the gland at its superior, anterior, and inferior borders, forming a pattern of rami located superficial to Bichat's fat and underneath the facial muscles, entering them from their deep surface. The temporal and zygomatic

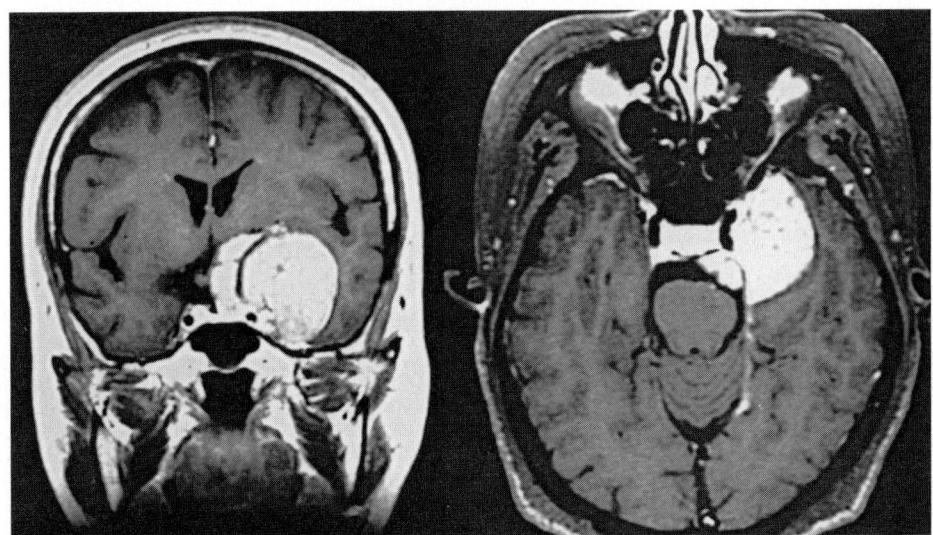

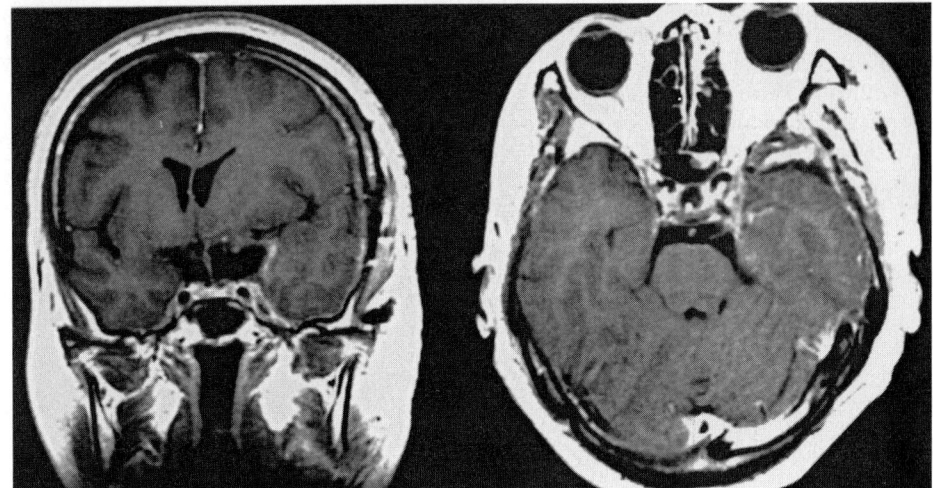

FIGURE 21-5 ■ *Upper,* Preoperative study of case 2; coronal and axial T$_1$-weighted magnetic resonance imaging scan with contrast injection showing the parasellar meningioma encasing the internal carotid artery and extending to the interpeduncular cistern. *Lower,* Postoperative study after total excision of the meningioma.

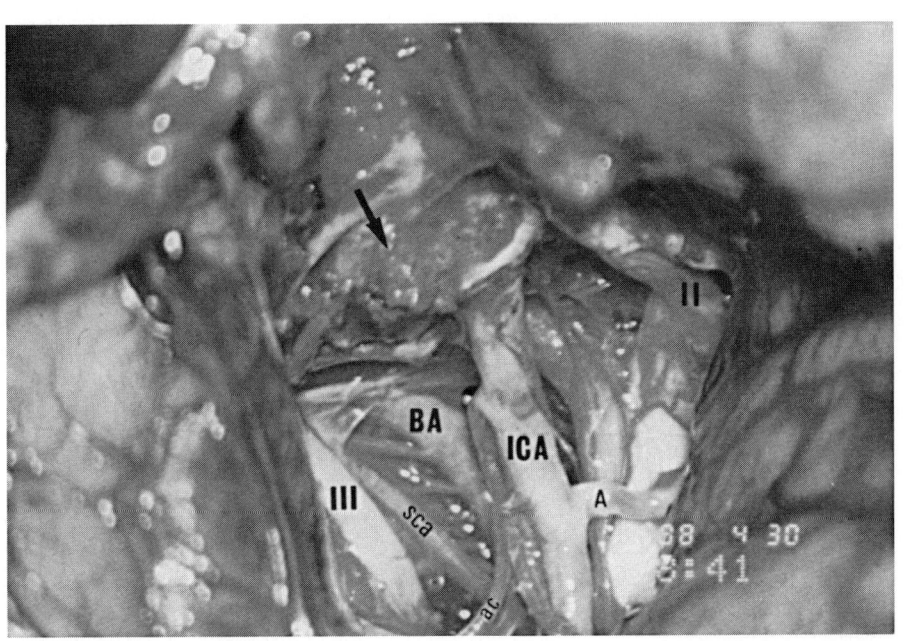

FIGURE 21-6 ■ Operative photograph after total excision of the tumor via the orbitozygomatic infratemporal approach with resection of the anterior clinoid process and opening the medial triangle to remove the tumor, involving the lateral wall of the cavernous sinus. (ICA, internal carotid artery; BA, basilar artery; II and III, second and third cranial nerves; sca, superior cerebellar artery; A, anterior cerebral artery.) Notice the presence of the accessory middle cerebral artery (ac) in this case. The lateral wall of the cavenous sinus is sealed with fibrin glue–soaked Helistat (*arrow*).

rami cross the zygomatic arch about 2 cm anterior to the anterior margin of the external auditory canal: Therefore, it is safe to make the skin incision along the anterior margin of the ear cartilage. The temporal and zygomatic rami of the ipsilateral facial nerve are usually well preserved by elevating the superficial temporal fascia together with the skin flap and subperiosteally dissecting the zygomatic arch and zygomatic bone.

## CONCLUSION

An orbitozygomatic infratemporal approach to the parasellar region, including the CS, and interpeduncular fossa has been presented and evaluated. We believe that an orbitozygomatic infratemporal approach may provide a better anatomic assessment of the lesions in the parasellar region and interpeduncular fossa and their surrounding structures than the conventional approach. This operation, however, is technically more demanding because familiarity with the use of chisels and sagittal saw, in addition to microsurgical techniques, is essential to its execution.

## REFERENCES

1. Hakuba A, Liu SS, Nishimura S: The orbitozygomatic infratemporal approach: A new surgical technique. Surg Neurol 26:271–276, 1986.
2. Ammirati M, Spallone A, Ma J, et al: An anatomical study of the temporal branch of the facial nerve. Neurosurgery 33:1038–1043, 1993.
3. Ohata K, Baba M: Orbitozygomatic infratemporal approach. In Hakuba A (ed): Surgical Anatomy of the Skull Base. Tokyo, Miwa Shoten, 1996, pp 1–35.
4. Hakuba A: Surgical approaches to the cavernous sinus via the medial triangle: Report of an aneurysm at the C4-C5 junction of the internal carotid artery [Japanese]. Geka Shinryo 26:1385–1390, 1965.
5. Hakuba A, Matsuoka Y, Suzuki T, et al: Direct approaches to vascular lesions in the cavernous sinus via the medial triangle. In Dolenc VV (ed): The Cavernous Sinus. New York: Springer-Verlag, 1987, pp 272–284.
6. Hakuba A, Tanaka K, Suzuki T, et al: A combined orbitozygomatic infratemporal epidural and subdural approach for lesions involving the entire cavernous sinus. J Neurosurg 71:699–704, 1989.
7. Ohata K, Hakuba A, Branco SJ: Development of the Meninges: Application to microneurosurgery [Japanese]. In: Surgical Anatomy for Microneurosurgery. Tokyo, SIMED Publications, 1997, pp 58–64.
8. Bruder N, Ravussin P, Young WL, et al: Anethesia for surgery of intracranial aneurysms. Ann Fr Anesth Reanim 13:209–220, 1994.
9. Ohata K, Baba M: Otico-condylar approach. In Hakuba A (ed): Surgical Anatomy of the Skull Base. Tokyo, Miwa Shoten, 1996, pp 37–75.
10. Millesi H: Extratemporal surgery of the facial nerve-palliative surgery. In Krayenbuehl H, et al (eds): Advances and Technical Standards in Neurosurgery, Vol 8. Vienna: Springer Verlag, 1980, pp 180–308.

## SUGGESTED READINGS

Hakuba A, Nishimura S, Jang BJ: A combined retroauricular and preauricular transpetrosal-transtentorial approach to clivus meningiomas. Surg Neurol 30:106–116, 1988.
Hakuba A, Nishimura S, Shirakata S, et al: Surgical approaches to the cavernous sinus: Report of 19 cases [Japanese]. Neurol Med Chir 22:295–306, 1982.

# Surgical Management of Olfactory Groove Meningiomas

■ ROBERT G. OJEMANN

In his classic monograph published in 1938, Harvey Cushing[1] described the origin, symptomatology, pathology, and surgical treatment of olfactory groove meningiomas based on careful observations in 29 patients. He clearly described the principles of surgical management, including internal decompression of the tumor before attempting to dissect the capsule, possible involvement of the anterior cerebral arteries, and repair of the defect in the floor of the frontal fossa with a fascial graft.

I have discussed the clinical presentation, radiographic features, and surgical management of olfactory groove meningiomas as part of several publications on meningiomas.[2–11] This chapter is based on those publications, a review of the literature, and personal experience with this tumor.

## SURGICAL ANATOMY

Olfactory groove meningiomas arise in the midline of the anterior fossa over the cribriform plate of the ethmoid bone and the area of the suture joining this structure and the sphenoid bone. The tumor may involve any of the area from the crista galli to the planum of the sphenoid bone and may be symmetric around the midline or extend predominantly to one side.

The primary blood supply comes from branches of the ethmoidal, meningeal, and ophthalmic arteries through the midline of the base of the skull. The A2 segments of the anterior cerebral arteries are usually separated from the tumor by a rim of cerebral tissue or arachnoid. In large tumors, these arteries may be involved with the tumor capsule. Frontopolar and small branches of the anterior cerebral arteries may be adherent into the posterior and superior tumor capsule and can be taken with the tumor.[5]

With small tumors, the olfactory nerves are displaced laterally on the surface of the tumor, and preserving at least one of these nerves may be possible. When the tumor is large, the olfactory nerve is so adherent and spread out on the capsule of the tumor that it cannot be saved, and the optic nerves and chiasm may be displaced downward and posteriorly.

## CLINICAL PRESENTATION

These tumors usually grow slowly, gradually compress the frontal lobe, and cause edema in the adjacent cerebral tissue. In Bakay's[12] series of 36 patients seen between 1950 and 1983, the complaints that led to evaluation in 19 patients were failing vision in 12, dementia in 3, headache in 3, and urinary incontinence in 1.

In my series of 19 patients seen from 1975 through 1992, 14 were women and 5 were men, ranging in age from 24 to 73 years, with 3 older than 70 years of age.[7] The complaints that led to evaluation in 17 patients were mental or personality change in 8, visual loss in 4, visual and mental symptoms in 1, headache and visual loss in 2, headache in 1, and seizure in 1. In two patients, the tumor was asymptomatic and was found on computed tomography (CT) scanning conducted for evaluation of a sinus problem. Many patients had a history of headache, but it was usually not this symptom that led to evaluation.

Because of the ability of the cerebral tissue to adapt to slow compression and the relative lack of focal functional cortical regions in the adjacent cerebral tissue, these meningiomas can often grow large before causing symptoms. In my series, 13 of the 19 tumors were large (more than 3 cm and usually over 4 cm). Even when symptoms begin, the patient, family, and colleagues tend to ignore mild and subtle symptoms. Such was the case with two physicians in my series.

Anosmia had not been an important symptom. Cushing[1] reported that loss of the sense of smell was possibly the primary symptom in only 3 of his 29 patients, and he questioned the reliability of the records in this regard. In my series, one patient reported on questioning that loss of sense of smell was the first symptom and, in retrospect, had been present for approximately a year before subtle changes in personality were noted. In Bakay's[12] series, all symptomatic patients had anosmia on examination, but in none was it a symptom that led to the diagnosis. He noted that patients are not usually concerned when they gradually lose their sense of smell over a long period of time.

## EVALUATION OF RADIOLOGIC STUDIES IN PLANNING THE OPERATION

For many years, the diagnosis of olfactory groove meningiomas was established by CT, and angiography was used to define the general relationship of the anterior cerebral arteries and the blood supply to the tumor. Several years ago, I stopped doing angiography in patients with smaller tumors (<3 cm) because I did not find that this study gave me additional information for planning the operation. I subsequently stopped using it even in larger tumors.

Magnetic resonance imaging (MRI) with gadolinium enhancement is the preferred radiologic study because it shows the extent of the tumor in all directions, the relationship of the tumor to the underlying ethmoid and sphenoid sinuses, the amount of edema in the surrounding brain, and, in many patients, the relationship of the optic nerves and anterior cerebral arteries to the tumor capsule (Figs.

22–1 and 22–2). MR angiography has been used but usually has not added essential information. Preoperative embolization has not been indicated in these patients.

## GENERAL ASPECTS OF SURGICAL MANAGEMENT

The objective of the operation is total removal of the olfactory groove meningioma, including the dural attachment and occasionally the involved bone, with preservation and improvement of neurologic function. In most patients with olfactory groove meningiomas, complete removal can

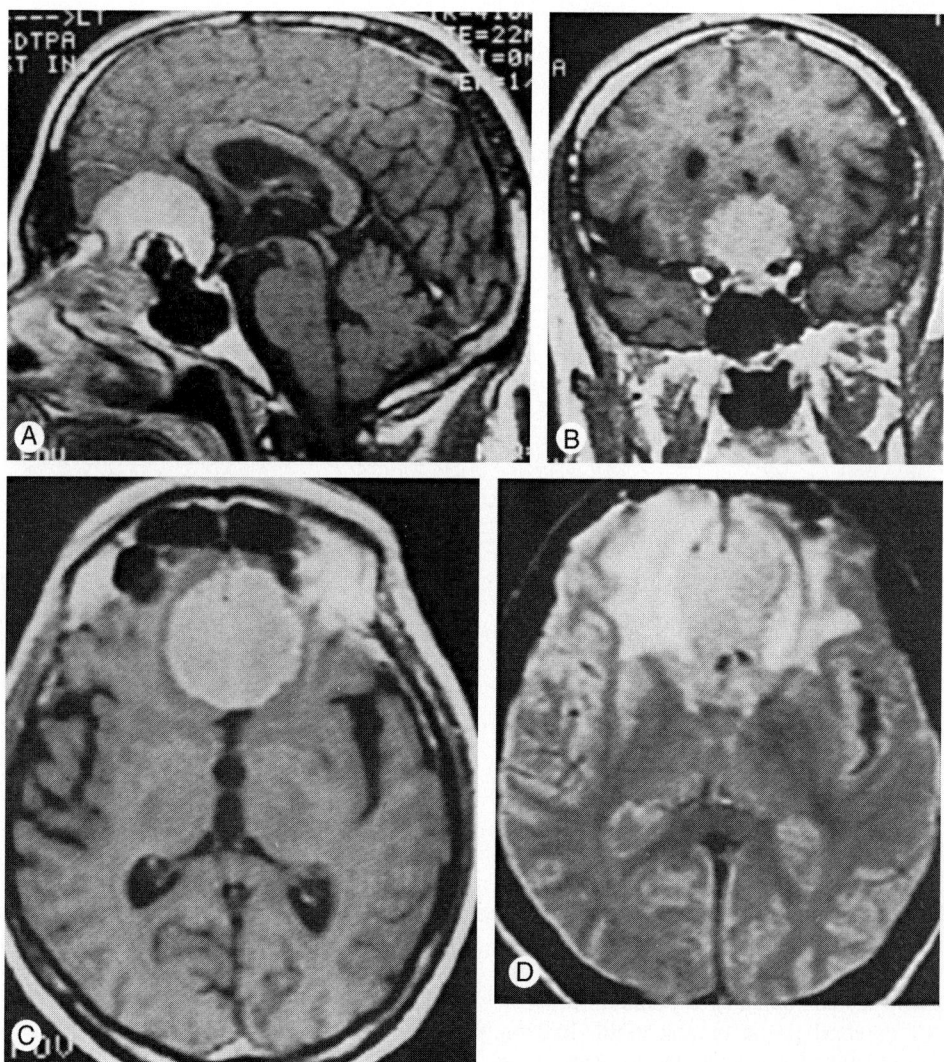

FIGURE 22–1 ■ An olfactory groove meningioma in a 59-year-old man who presented with a 3-year history of subtle changes in personality and mental function. Magnetic resonance images: *A,* Sagittal image (T1) after gadolinium enhancement. This midline view shows the anteroposterior and superior extent of the tumor. There is an unusual projection of bone containing an extension of the air sinus that leads into the base of the tumor. The posteroinferior edge of the tumor is lying on the tuberculum and projects down between the optic nerves. There appears to be a cerebrospinal fluid cistern on the posterior surface of the tumor. The anteroinferior tumor edge projects into the cribriform plate region. *B,* Coronal image (T1) after gadolinium enhancement. This image through the posterior edge of the tumor shows the tongue of tissue projecting down between the internal carotid arteries and over the optic nerves. Other coronal images show that the lateral extent of the tumor has not extended into the air sinuses. *C,* Axial image (T1) after gadolinium enhancement. The lateral extent of the tumor is defined. Edema or a gliotic reaction in the adjacent brain surrounds the tumor. *D,* Axial image (T2) without enhancement. The extent of the edema in tissue adjacent to the tumor is defined. The A2 segments of the anterior cerebral arteries are adjacent to the tumor capsule. At operation, the A2 segment of the anterior cerebral artery was separated from the superoposterior capsule by a thin layer of gliotic tissue, and in the midportion of the posterior capsule, the artery was in an arachnoid cistern and loosely adherent to the capsule with small arterial branches. Total removal of the tumor was accomplished, and the patient made a full recovery.

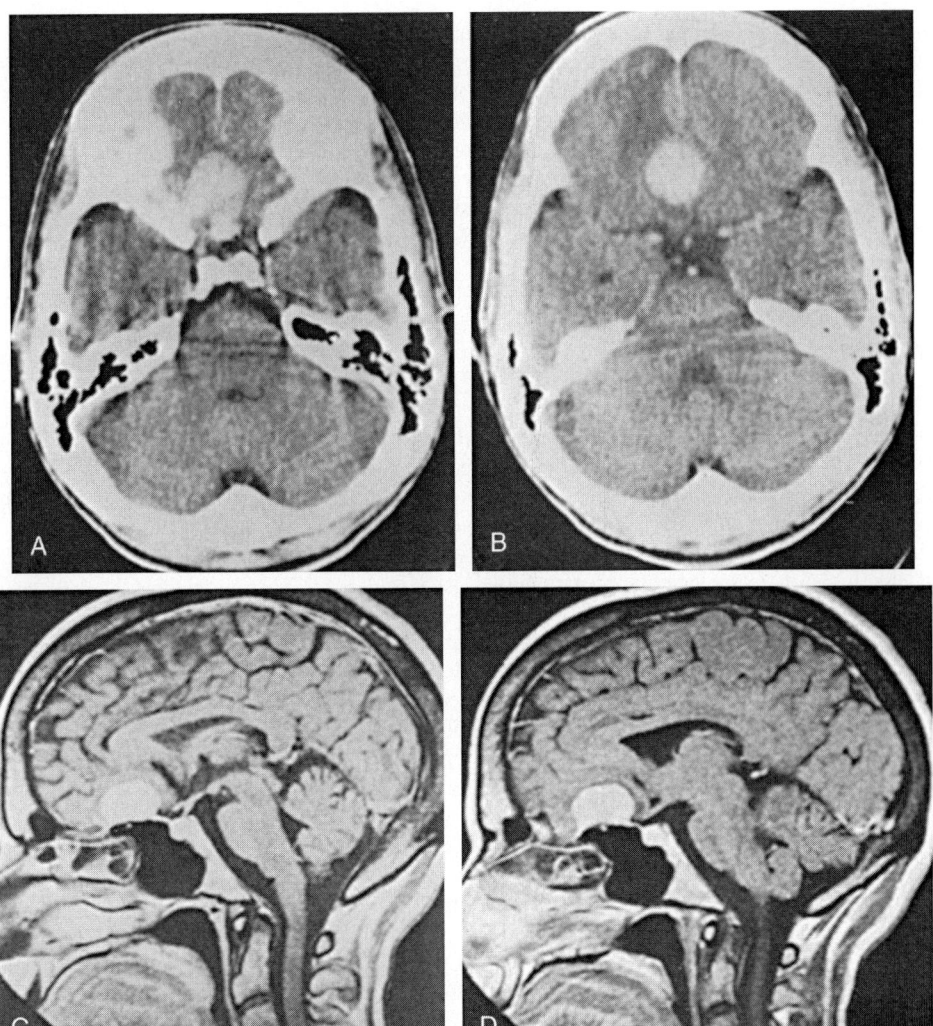

**FIGURE 22–2** ■ An olfactory groove meningioma in a 47-year-old woman who had a computed tomography (CT) scan to evaluate a sinus problem. There were no neurologic symptoms. *A* and *B,* CT images with contrast show the enhancing lesion in the posterior midline of the floor of the frontal fossa with extension to the right side. There is significant edema in the right frontal lobe. *C* and *D,* Magnetic resonance images (T1) with gadolinium enhancement. The midline image (*C*) shows the posterior placement of the tumor, the separation from the region of the anterior cerebral arteries, and the chiasm. The image to the right of midline (*D*) shows the proximity of the right optic nerve to the tumor.

be done with low morbidity and good recovery of function. However, in some patients in whom total removal carries a significant risk because of involvement of the major anterior cerebral artery branches, some tumor should be left, and the patient should be followed up with periodic scans. Radiation therapy may be used if the tumor starts to grow.

Age alone is not a factor in the decision for surgery. In my series of 19 patients, 9 were in their seventh decade and 3 in their eighth. In my overall series of meningiomas in patients older than 70 years of age, surgery was done if general health was reasonable and neurologic disability was worsening.[13] The incidence of operative morbidity has been low in this group of patients.

On examination, the sense of smell is usually absent but, if it is still present, as it may be in a small tumor, the patient should be warned about the loss of this function. This symptom is more troublesome after acute loss than it is after gradual loss associated with compression from the tumor.

In most patients, steroids have been started sometime before operation because of edema. When the patient arrives in the operating room, intravenous antibiotics are given and continued during the operation and for 24 hours

afterward. If the patient is not already on steroids and anticonvulsant medication, these are started.

After induction of anesthesia and insertion of a catheter into the bladder, 10 to 20 mg of furosemide (Lasix) is given, and during the operative exposure, 100 g of mannitol is administered intravenously. Cooperation of a skilled neuroanesthesiologist helps reduce operative morbidity and mortality.

## BIFRONTAL APPROACH

### General Considerations

For patients with large tumors (see Fig. 22–1), I prefer a bifrontal craniotomy. This approach is associated with the least amount of retraction on the frontal lobes, it gives direct access to all sides of the tumor, and it allows decompression of the tumor while the surgeon is working along the base of the skull to interrupt the blood supply. There is no problem from ligation of the anterior aspect of the superior sagittal sinus or coagulation of draining veins in this region. If the frontal sinus is appropriately handled, there should be no complication from entering the sinus.

Hassler and Zentner[14] reported that in 1938 Tönnis described a midline fronto-orbital approach with division of the anterior sagittal sinus and falx and preservation of frontal brain tissue. A bifrontal approach for large tumors is also used by Logue,[15] Long,[16] MacCarty and associates,[17] McDermott and Wilson,[18] Ransohoff and Nockels,[19] and Symon.[20]

## Operative Technique

The patient is carefully placed in the supine position with the knees slightly flexed and the head elevated, slightly extended, and held with the Mayfield-Kees three-point skeletal fixation headrest. A coronal incision is made through the galea, and care is taken to preserve the pericranial tissue (Fig. 22–3). The skin along the posterior aspect of the incision is elevated approximately 2 cm, and the pericranial tissue is then incised. This step gives extra pericranial tissue to cover the floor of the anterior fossa and to use to patch the convexity dura as needed. The skin flap and the pericranial tissue are then turned down together. The temporalis muscle is opened to expose the bone just below the anterior end of the superior temporal line. Bur holes are placed at this point and on each side of the sagittal sinus anterior to the skin incision. The dura is separated from the bone using a Penfield No. 3 dissector. The bone flap is usually cut in one piece. For the bone cut just above the supraorbital ridge, the craniotome is used to make a cut on each side as far medially as possible. Usually, this maneuver leaves 1 cm or less of bone in the midline. Because of the irregular bone projecting from the inner table of the skull in this area, cutting completely

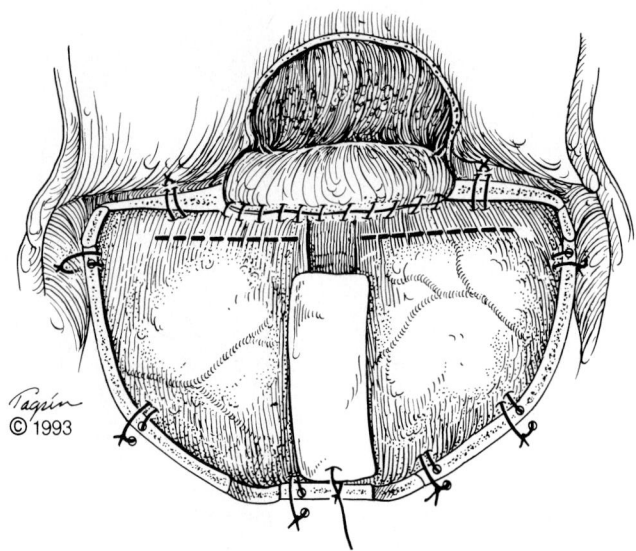

FIGURE 22–4 ■ The opening over the frontal sinus has been covered with a flap of pericranial tissue sutured to the adjacent dura. Before this step, the mucosa of the frontal sinus was removed, and the sinus was packed with Gelfoam soaked with an antibiotic solution. (Copyright © 1993, Edith Tagrin.)

across the area is usually not possible. The outer table is cut with a small bur on a high-speed air drill, and then the inner table is broken as the bone is elevated and the free bone flap is removed. An alternate method is to cut a right frontal bone flap first and then free the sagittal sinus and cut a second bone flap across the midline to the left side.

The frontal sinuses are almost always entered. The mucosa is removed, and the sinuses are packed with antibiotic-soaked absorbable gelatin sponge (Gelfoam). A flap of pericranial tissue from the back of the skin flap is turned down over the sinus and sewn to the adjacent dura (Fig. 22–4). Sutures are placed along the edge of the craniotomy to control epidural bleeding.

The dural incision is made over each medial inferior frontal lobe just above the anterior edge of the craniotomy opening. This incision need not extend more than 3 to 4 cm to each side and is carried medially near the edge of the sagittal sinus (see Fig. 22–4), thereby allowing good exposure yet protecting most of both frontal lobes during the operation. Bridging veins from the anterior frontal lobe to the midline area are coagulated and divided. The frontal lobes are carefully retracted, the sagittal sinus is divided between two silk sutures, and the falx is cut (Fig. 22–5). The frontal lobes are then carefully retracted laterally and slightly posteriorly with the Greenberg self-retaining retractor system. The tumor will come into view in the midline and at times grow into the region of the crista galli and falx. The cerebral cortex is carefully separated from the tumor capsule by division of arachnoid and small vascular attachments. The self-retaining retractors are repositioned.

The anterior capsule of the tumor is then opened, and a biopsy is performed. The anterior and midline portions of the tumor are then removed. The attachments of the tumor in the midline along the base of the frontal fossa are gradually divided, interrupting the blood supply that enters the tumor through numerous openings in the bone in this

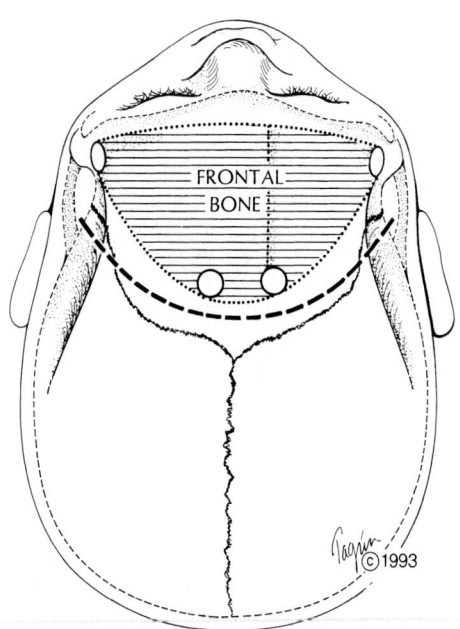

FRONTAL
BONE

FIGURE 22–3 ■ Bifrontal approach to an olfactory groove meningioma. The position of the skin incision (*dashed line*), bur holes, and free bone flap (*dotted line*) are outlined. (Copyright © 1993, Edith Tagrin.)

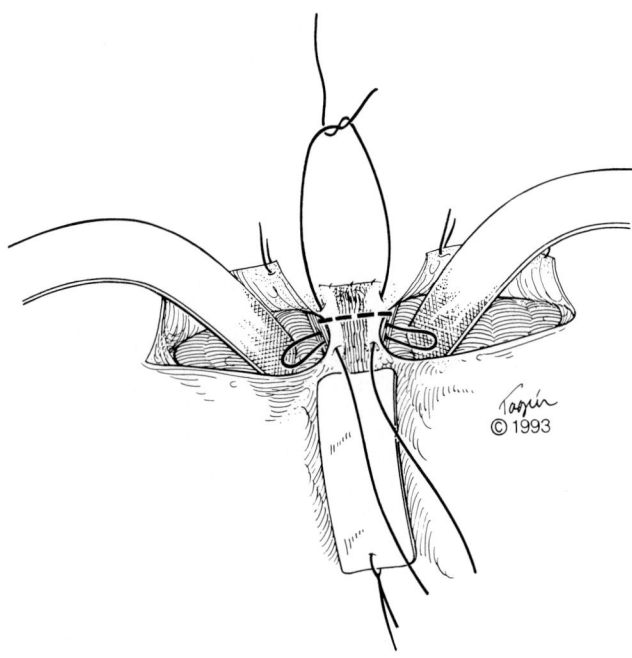

**FIGURE 22–5** ■ Ligation of the anterior sagittal sinus. (Copyright © 1993, Edith Tagrin.)

area (Fig. 22–6). These feeding arteries are occluded with coagulation and, occasionally, bone wax. Monopolar coagulation on a coated Penfield No. 4 can be a very effective method of occluding the arteries as they come out of the bone.

The dissection along the base is alternated with internal decompression of the tumor gradually to bring into view the base and to remove the bulk of the tumor. The Cavitron or cautery loops are very effective in performing decompression. The capsule now can be reflected into the area of the decompression with minimal pressure on the adjacent frontal lobes (Fig. 22–7). Self-retaining retractors keep the frontal lobes from falling into the decompression area. Great care is taken during the dissection of the posterior portion of the capsule, which is reflected anteriorly while

the surgeon looks for the pericallosal branch of the anterior cerebral artery complex. Usually, a rim of cerebral cortex or arachnoid separates the main trunk of the arteries from the tumor, although occasionally the artery may be embedded in the tumor. The frontopolar branch and other small branches are often adherent to the tumor or enter the capsule and may need to be divided (see Fig. 22–7). Symon[20] states, and I agree, that occluding these arteries does not cause a problem. Following the tumor capsule back to the sphenoid wing and then working medially usually enables the surgeon to identify the anterior clinoid processes and then the optic nerves. At times, seeing the optic nerves may be difficult because of the posterior and inferior compression and the thickened arachnoid. However, under magnification, the tumor can be reflected off the optic nerves (Fig. 22–8). A tongue of tumor may grow down over the dura on the tuberculum (see Fig. 22–1).

Once the bulk of the tumor is removed, the dural attachment is totally excised (Fig. 22–9). If the bone is not involved, removal of the dura is all that is necessary, and the area is covered with a sheet of gelatin sponge.

If hyperostosis is present, should it be removed? This area contains many of the feeding arteries, and Symon[20] stated that the recurrence rate of these tumors was so low that extensive removal of the hyperostosis and entering the ethmoid sinus are not usually indicated. I agree that an extensive resection of bone is not usually needed, but an area of hyperostosis should be drilled off to a point where a layer of bone is left. I recommend covering the area with gelatin sponge and a graft of pericranial tissue if the ethmoid sinus is thought to have been entered.

A special problem occurs if the tumor has grown through the bone into the ethmoid sinus. Derome and Guiot[21] reported that this problem occurred in approximately 15% of their patients, but it did not occur in my series. They recommended resection. Long[16] removes the involved bone and tumor with a high-speed drill, Cavitron, or laser. The defect is then covered by several compressed thicknesses of gelatin sponge and then fascia lata. The fascia is tacked into place if insertion of a watertight suture to the adjacent dura is not possible. Gelatin sponge is placed over the fascia.

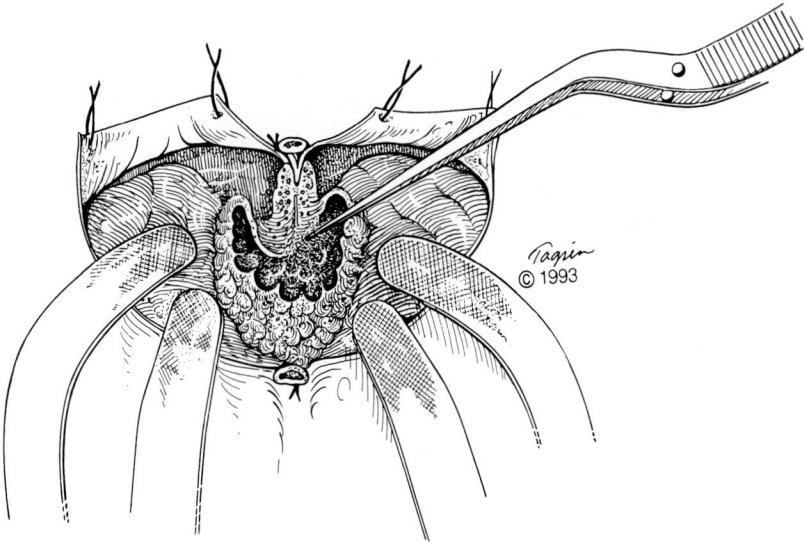

**FIGURE 22–6** ■ The anterior capsule of the tumor has been removed, and internal decompression has been started. The blood supply coming through the midline of the frontal fossa is being occluded. (Copyright © 1993, Edith Tagrin.)

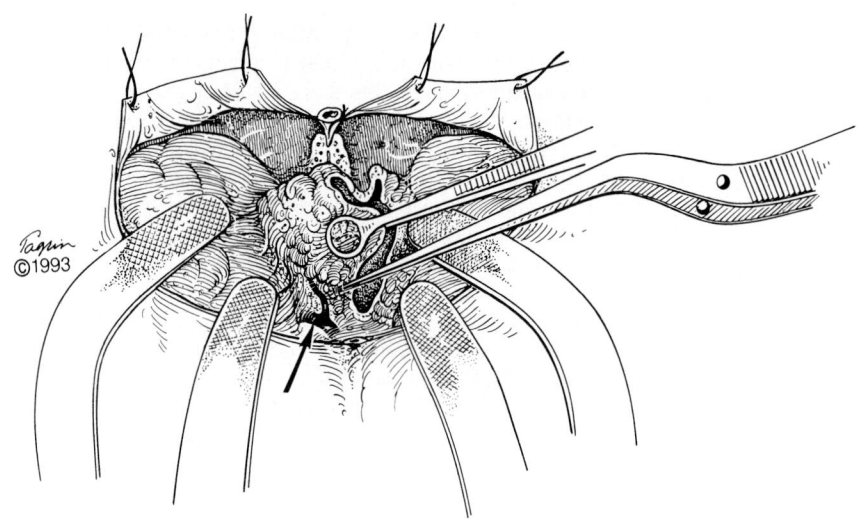

FIGURE 22–7 ■ The capsule of the meningioma is being displaced into the area of internal decompression, and attachments to the frontal lobe are being divided. Minimal retraction is required on the frontal lobe. The frontopolar artery is often adherent to the tumor and may need to be divided. (Copyright © 1993, Edith Tagrin.)

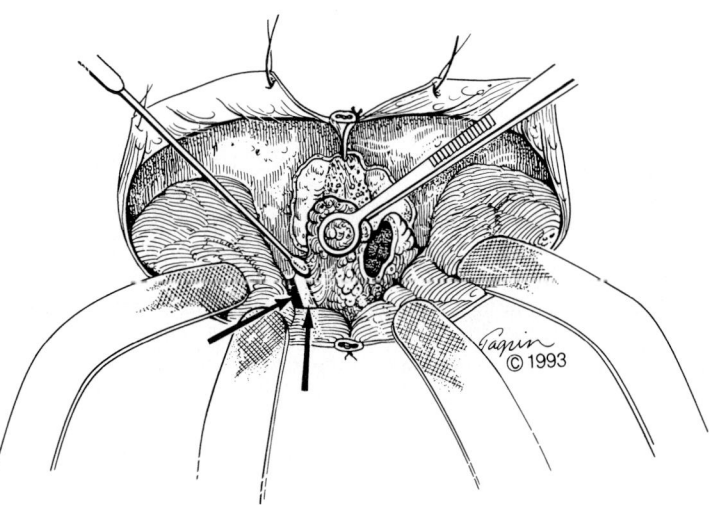

FIGURE 22–8 ■ The capsule of the meningioma has been followed along the floor of the anterior fossa to the region of the anterior clinoid after detachment of most of the base. The left optic nerve and internal carotid artery (arrows) have been exposed. The tumor is being separated from the arachnoid over the nerve. (Copyright © 1993, Edith Tagrin.)

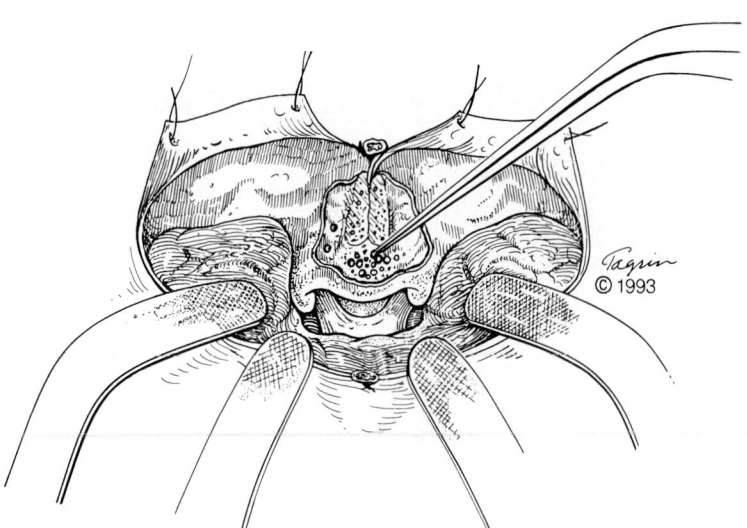

FIGURE 22–9 ■ The tumor has been removed. Multiple holes are seen in the bone where the arterial blood supply entered the tumor. (Copyright © 1993, Edith Tagrin.)

The convexity dura is closed with a free graft of pericranial tissue. The dura and graft are covered with gelatin sponge and the bone flap is wired into place. A wire is placed across each bur hole, and the holes are filled with acrylic cranioplasty material. The operative area is then thoroughly irrigated with antibiotic solution before closure.

## UNILATERAL SUBFRONTAL APPROACH

### General Considerations

For small tumors (see Fig. 22–2), a right subfrontal approach is usually used unless the tumor is located predominantly on the left side. The approach is from laterally over the orbital roof, with elevation of the frontal lobe. Kempe[22] described this approach, in which the patient's head was turned approximately 60 degrees to the side opposite the craniotomy. Symon[20] uses a unilateral approach for tumors of moderate size, with the head vertically positioned, and he may resect part of the frontal lobe, as does Logue.[15] McDermott and Wilson[18] also use a unilateral subfrontal approach for smaller tumors.

Some neurosurgeons use this approach for all olfactory groove meningiomas. Solero and colleagues[23] reported using a unilateral frontal craniotomy and resection of part of the frontal lobe. Seeger[24] combines a bifrontal craniotomy with a unilateral basal approach and partial division of the falx. Hassler and Zentner[14] described a pterional approach as a modification of Seeger's technique. DeMonte and Al-Mefty[25] use a unilateral or bifrontal exposure with resection of the orbital rim on one side. Babu and colleagues[26] prefer a unilateral frontal craniotomy with orbital osteotomy. Mayfrank and Gilsbach[27] use a unilateral frontal craniotomy with an interhemispheric approach.

### Operative Technique

The patient is carefully placed in the supine position with the right shoulder slightly elevated. The head is elevated and rotated approximately 60 degrees to the opposite side and held with the Mayfield-Kees skeletal fixation headrest.

The skin incision is made just above the zygomatic process behind the anterior hairline and extends medially to end near the midline at the hairline (Fig. 22–10). If the incision is too far forward or extends below the zygomatic process, the frontal branch of the facial nerve may be injured. The skin, underlying temporalis muscle, and pericranial tissue are turned down together, exposing the anterior and lateral inferior frontal and anterior temporal bone. The temporalis muscle may be cut to expose the zygomatic process. A bur hole is placed just below the anterior end of the superior temporal line (see Fig. 22–10), which allows exposure of the floor of the anterior fossa. Depending on the surgeon's preference, other bur holes are placed as needed. I usually use two others, as illustrated in Figure 22–10. A free bone flap is then cut. The lateral portion of the sphenoid wing is removed, as is the bone over the anterosuperior temporal region. After drill holes are made around the craniotomy opening, dural sutures are placed to

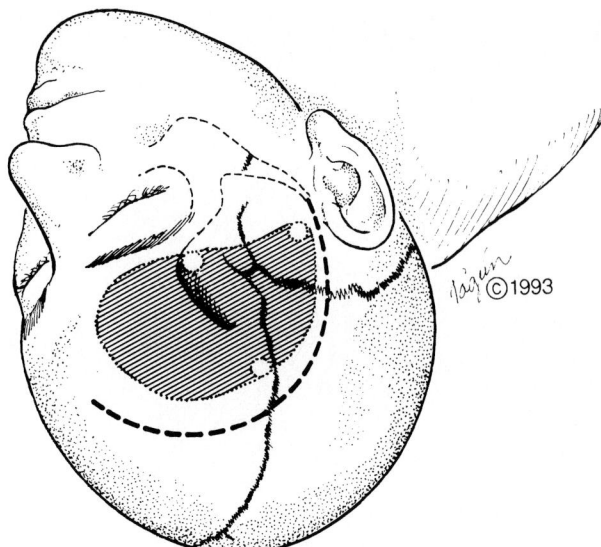

**FIGURE 22–10** ■ Right subfrontal approach to an olfactory groove meningioma. The position of the head, skin incision (*dashed line*), bur holes, and bone flap are seen. (Copyright © 1993, Edith Tagrin.)

control epidural bleeding. The dura is then opened over the inferior frontal and anterior temporal region (Fig. 22–11). Draining veins from the anterior temporal lobe along the sphenoid wing are divided, if necessary.

The frontal lobe is carefully elevated over the orbital roof, bringing the tumor into view (Fig. 22–12). The brain is protected, and self-retaining retractors are placed. The olfactory nerve may be displaced laterally and be densely involved with the surface of the tumor. The posterior cap-

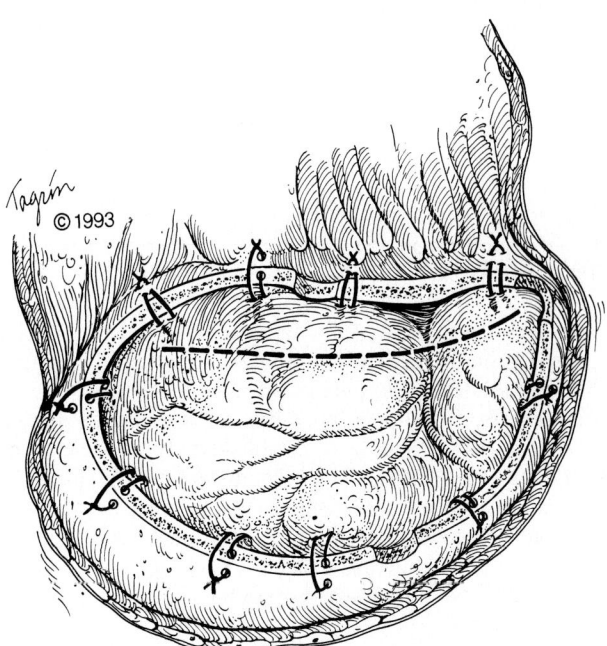

**FIGURE 22–11** ■ The skin and pericranial tissue have been turned down together. The bone flap has been elevated, and bone has been removed from the lateral sphenoid wing and over the anterior temporal region. The dural incision is shown (*dashed line*). (Copyright © 1993, Edith Tagrin.)

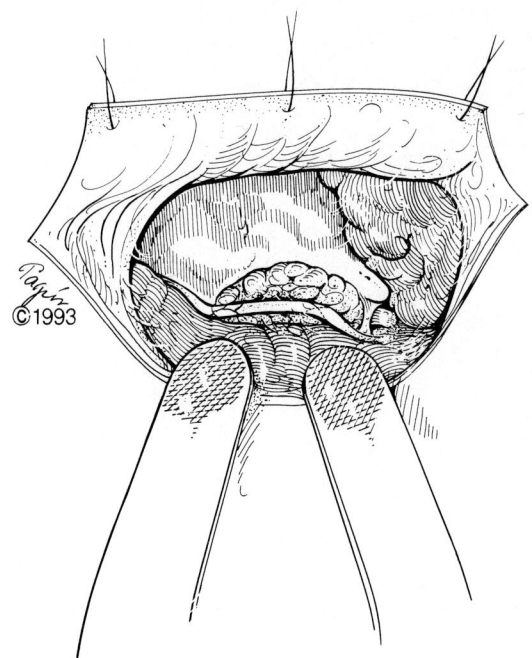

**FIGURE 22–12** ■ Exposure of the olfactory groove meningioma from the lateral subfrontal approach. The olfactory nerve is adherent to the tumor. The optic nerve is exposed posterior to the tumor. (Copyright © 1993, Edith Tagrin.)

sule is explored and the relationship of the optic nerve defined.

The principles of tumor removal are the same as described for the bifrontal approach. The tumor is internally decompressed, the blood supply is occluded along the base, and the tumor capsule is carefully withdrawn into the area of decompression, dividing attachments as they are encountered. Because these tumors are smaller, preserving the olfactory nerve on one side may be possible. Care is then taken to define the position of the optic nerves. The handling of the area of attachment of the tumor and the closure are the same as described for the bifrontal operation.

## IMMEDIATE POSTOPERATIVE MANAGEMENT

Steroid dosages are usually tapered over 5 to 10 days, depending on the patient's neurologic status and the extent of cerebral edema. Antibiotics are continued for 24 hours after surgery. How long anticonvulsant medication should be continued has not been established. If no history of seizures exists, I usually stop administering anticonvulsant medication within 2 to 3 months. If a seizure disorder has been present, anticonvulsants are continued for 6 months to 1 year, and sometimes longer. There is considerable difference of opinion about this point.

## COMPLICATIONS

The incidence of reported complications has been low since the advent of microneurosurgical techniques.[2–11, 14, 17, 19] The

major potential complications include worsening of mental function due to frontal lobe retraction or anterior cerebral artery injury, visual loss, cerebrospinal fluid leak, infection, and postoperative seizures. A cerebrospinal fluid leak through the ethmoid sinus can be closed through a transethmoidal repair.

In several series of patients treated since 1970, the operative mortality rate has also been low. Bakay[12] reported 1 death due to surgery in 11 patients, Symon[20] had no deaths in 18 patients, MacCarty and colleagues[17] reported 1 death in 27 patients, and Ransohoff and Nockels[19] had 2 deaths in 33 patients. In my series, 1 death occurred in 19 patients because of a pulmonary embolus.[7] Hassler and Zentner[14] had 1 death in 11 patients, also because of a pulmonary embolus.

## RESULTS

In most patients with olfactory groove meningioma, the tumor can be completely removed and the patient can resume a nearly normal life. Disturbance in mental function and personality changes that were present before surgery or transiently in the postoperative period usually disappear completely. In my series, all patients with preoperative mental symptoms or personality changes made a good recovery.

Patients with preoperative visual symptoms usually recover after surgery. In no patients in my series was the vision worse, and headache was usually relieved. Postoperative seizures have not been a problem.

MacCarty and colleagues[17] reported that the survival rate was higher for olfactory groove meningiomas than for any other meningioma sites. Data regarding recurrence were not given. Symon,[20] although not giving a specific figure, reported a very low recurrence rate. Chan and Thompson[28] reported no recurrence during a 9-year average follow-up. Ransoff and Nockels[19] had no recurrence in patients with benign meningiomas. We have not had a recurrence in our patients to date, and this result has been documented in most patients by follow-up MRI or CT.

## MANAGEMENT OF PATIENTS WITH ASYMPTOMATIC OLFACTORY GROOVE MENINGIOMAS

With the increasing use of CT and MRI for evaluation of sinus problems and other diseases, an asymptomatic lesion occasionally is found. When evaluating such a patient, the neurosurgeon needs to consider the size of the lesion, the presence or absence of edema in the adjacent brain, the lesion's proximity to the optic nerves, the age and general health of the patient, and the patient's psychological response to the presence of the tumor.

We have treated two patients with olfactory groove meningiomas in whom the lesion was found during evaluation for a sinus problem. One is illustrated in Figure 22–2. Surgery was recommended and performed because of edema in the adjacent brain structure and the proximity of the lesion to the optic nerves. Both patients made a full recovery.

# REFERENCES

1. Cushing H, Eisenhardt L: Meningiomas: Their Classification, Regional Behaviour, Life History, and Surgical End Results. Springfield, IL: Charles C Thomas, 1938.
2. Ojemann RG: Meningiomas of the basal parapituitary region: Technical considerations. Clin Neurosurg 27:233–262, 1980.
3. Ojemann RG: Surgical management of meningiomas of the tuberculum sellae, olfactory groove, medial sphenoid wing and floor of the anterior fossa. In Schmidek HH, Sweet WH (eds): Operative Neurosurgical Techniques. New York: Grune & Stratton, 1982, pp 869–889.
4. Ojemann RG: Meningiomas: Clinical features and surgical management. In Wilkins RH, Rengachary SS (eds): Neurosurgery. New York: McGraw-Hill, 1985, pp 635–654.
5. Ojemann RG: Olfactory groove meningiomas. In Al-Mefty O (ed): Meningiomas. New York: Raven Press, 1991, pp 383–394.
6. Ojemann RG: Surgical management of olfactory groove and medial sphenoid wing meningiomas. In Schmidek HH (ed): Meningiomas and Their Surgical Management. Philadelphia: WB Saunders, 1991, pp 242–259.
7. Ojemann RG: Management of cranial and spinal meningiomas. Clin Neurosurg 40:321–383, 1993.
8. Ojemann RG: Surgical management of anterior basal meningiomas. In Schmidek HH, Sweet WH (eds): Operative Neurosurgical Techniques, 3rd ed. Philadelphia: WB Saunders, 1995, pp 393–402.
9. Ojemann RG: Supratentorial meningiomas: Clinical features and surgical management. In Wilkins RH, Rengachary SS (eds): Neurosurgery. New York: McGraw-Hill, 1996, pp 873–890.
10. Ojemann RG, Swann KW: Meningiomas of the anterior cranial base. In Sekhar LN, Schramm VSS (eds): Tumors of the Cranial Base: Diagnosis and Treatment. Mount Kisco, NY: Futura, 1987, pp 279–294.
11. Ojemann RG, Swann KW: Surgical management of olfactory groove, suprasellar and medial sphenoid wing meningiomas. In Schmidek HH, Sweet WH (eds): Operative Neurosurgical Techniques, 2nd ed. Orlando, FL: Grune & Stratton, 1988, pp 531–545.
12. Bakay L: Olfactory meningiomas: The missed diagnosis. JAMA 251:53–55, 1984.
13. McGrail KM, Ojemann RG: The surgical management of benign intracranial meningiomas and acoustic neuromas in patients 70 years of age and older. Surg Neurol 42:2–7, 1994.
14. Hassler W, Zentner J: Pterional approach for the surgical treatment of olfactory groove meningiomas. Neurosurgery 25:942–947, 1989.
15. Logue V: Surgery of meningioma. In Symon L (ed): Operative Surgery: Neurosurgery. London: Butterworth, 1979, pp 138–173.
16. Long DM: Meningiomas of the olfactory groove and anterior fossa. In Long DM (ed): Atlas of Operative Neurosurgical Technique, Vol 1: Cranial Operations. Baltimore: Williams & Wilkins, 1989, pp 238–241.
17. MacCarty CS, Piepgras DG, Ebersold MJ: Meningeal tumors of the brain. In Youmans JR (ed): Neurological Surgery, 2nd ed. Philadelphia: WB Saunders, 1982, pp 2936–2966.
18. McDermott MW, Wilson CB: Meningiomas. In Youmans JR (ed): Neurological Surgery, 4th ed. Philadelphia: WB Saunders, 1996, pp 2782–2825.
19. Ransohoff J, Nockels RP: Olfactory groove and planum meningiomas. In Apuzzo MLJ (ed): Brain Surgery Complication Avoidance and Management. New York: Churchill Livingstone, 1993, pp 203–219.
20. Symon L: Olfactory groove and suprasellar meningiomas. In Krayenbuhl H (ed): Advances and Technical Standards in Neurosurgery, Vol 4. Vienna: Springer-Verlag, 1977, pp 67–91.
21. Derome PJ, Guiot G: Bone problems in meningiomas invading the base of the skull. Clin Neurosurg 25:435–451, 1978.
22. Kempe LG: Operative Neurosurgery, Vol 1. New York: Springer-Verlag, 1968, pp 104–108.
23. Solero CL, Giombini S, Morello G: Suprasellar and olfactory meningioma: Report of a series of 153 personal cases. Acta Neurochir (Wien) 67:181–194, 1983.
24. Seeger W: Microsurgery of the Cranial Base. New York: Springer-Verlag, 1983.
25. DeMonte F, Al-Mefty O: Management of meningiomas. In Tindall GT, Cooper PR, Barrow DL (eds): The Practice of Neurosurgery. Baltimore: Williams & Wilkins, 1996, pp 691–714.
26. Babu R, Barton A, Kasoff SS: Resection of olfactory groove meningiomas: Technical note revisited. Surg Neurol 44:567–572, 1955.
27. Mayfrank L, Gilsbach JM: Interhemispheric approach for microsurgical removal of olfactory groove meningiomas. Br J Neurosurg 10:541–545, 1996.
28. Chan RC, Thompson GB: Morbidity, mortality and quality of life following surgery for intracranial meningiomas: A retrospective study in 257 cases. J Neurosurg 60:52–60, 1984.

CHAPTER 23

# Surgical Management of Tuberculum Sellae and Sphenoid Ridge Meningiomas

■ VALLO BENJAMIN and BRUCE McCORMACK

Tuberculum sellae and medial sphenoid ridge menin-giomas present difficult technical challenges to the neurosurgeon because of their close proximity to the anterior visual pathways, arteries of the anterior circulation, and the hypothalamus.[1] Much has been written about these tumors, but little new information has been added to Cushing and Eisenhardt's classic work with regard to their study of anatomy, behavior, and classification.[2] Great strides, however, have been made in microneurosurgical techniques that enable resection of these tumors with a modest rate of morbidity and mortality when compared with the pioneer-ing efforts of Cushing and earlier surgeons. In this chapter, we discuss the surgical management of tuberculum sellae and medial sphenoid ridge meningiomas. These tumors are discussed separately because of differences in their ana-tomic relationship to the surrounding vital structures as well as surgical technical considerations.

## TUBERCULUM SELLAE MENINGIOMA

### Pathologic Anatomy and Classification

Cushing performed the first complete removal of a tubercu-lum sellae meningioma in 1916, but he did not report it until 1929.[3] Dandy[4] published the results of the first eight cases of surgical removal in 1922. In 1938, Cushing and Eisenhardt[2] reported 28 cases of tuberculum sellae menin-gioma and proposed a classification of four stages ac-cording to size. In their often-quoted text, Cushing and Eisenhardt used the term *suprasellar* in their description of tumors arising from dura over the tuberculum sellae. This term has led to much confusion in the literature because subsequent publications have included tumors arising from different locations, such as anterior clinoid, optic foramen, olfactory groove, and planum sphenoidale, under the rubric of suprasellar.[5–8] We believe that tuberculum sellae tumors should and can be distinguished in most cases from other so-called suprasellar tumors.

The tuberculum sellae is a slight bony elevation in front of the pituitary fossa that measures several millimeters in height and width. Tumors arising from this region are usually 2 to 4 cm in diameter at the time of clinical presentation. Because of the relatively small dimensions of the sellae, the dural attachment of these tumors often ex-tends anteriorly to the sphenoid limbus (anterior border of prechiasmatic sulcus) and posteriorly to involve the diaphragm sellae to the infundibulum. It is not useful to subclassify further tumors arising within these boundaries because with continued growth, all cause elevation of the optic nerves and chiasm and produce the same clinical picture. Although we recognize that the microscopic point of tumor origin may be at either the tuberculum or dia-phragma sellae, we refer to these tumors as *tuberculum sellae meningiomas.*[9]

Cushing and Eisenhardt[2] subclassified tuberculum sellae tumors into four groups: (1) initial stage, (2) presymptom-atic, (3) favorable for surgery, and (4) late or essentially inoperable. They not only recognized tuberculum sellae meningiomas as a distinct clinical entity, but also clarified the importance of tumor growth in relationship to the optic apparatus and the potential for surgical resection. The introduction of the operating microscope allowed neurosur-geons to understand better the relationship of tumor to surrounding structures. We discuss the relationship of tu-mor growth to the arachnoid membrane, pituitary stalk, optic apparatus, and arteries of the anterior circulation in the next section.

Although meningiomas may invade bone and cause hy-perostosis, they predominantly arise and grow in the sub-dural compartment but remain outside the arachnoid (epi-arachnoid). As the tuberculum sellae meningioma grows, the arachnoid of the floor of the chiasmatic cistern is pushed up and stretched over the tumor. With continued growth, the tumor encroaches on adjacent cisterns and becomes involved with various layers of arachnoid. The walls of the arachnoid cisterns provide a natural barrier between the meningioma and the arteries and nerves that course within the subarachnoid space.

The optic nerves are displaced and stretched superiorly and laterally by the tumor. Because the nerves are fixed at the optic foramen, they become angulated and compressed at this site. These tumors may grow eccentrically and involve one optic nerve to a greater degree than the other, and one or both of the nerves may be completely enveloped by tumor. The internal carotid arteries (ICA) are displaced laterally but usually less than the optic nerves, and tongues of tumor may insinuate themselves between these two structures. Large tumors may completely encase the carotid vessels. Generally the anterior cerebral arteries, which are located dorsal to the optic chiasm, are stretched, but on rare occasions, they may be encased by tumors larger than 4 cm. With further growth, tumor extends behind the sella turcica into the interpeduncular cistern. The pituitary stalk is usually displaced posteriorly. Extremely large tumors may compress the third ventricle and cause hydrocephalus. Less commonly, tumor can extend into the cavernous sinus. Tuberculum sellae tumors may spill over the planum sphenoidal. These tumors are distinguished from growths arising primarily from the planum because they elevate the anterior visual pathways, whereas the planum sphenoidal tumors depress the anterior visual pathways. Likewise, olfactory groove meningiomas also depress the anterior visual pathways. Anterior clinoid and medial sphenoid ridge meningiomas displace the optic apparatus medially and are discussed later.

## Clinical Presentation

Tuberculum sellae meningiomas constitute 4% to 10% of intracranial meningiomas.[2, 5, 10] The actual incidence is difficult to ascertain because in most series, the tumor has not been distinguished from other so-called suprasellar tumors. As with meningiomas in other locations, tuberculum sellae meningiomas occur much more frequently in women than men, with a predominance in the 30s and 40s.[8, 12]

In the series by Grisoli et al[14] of 28 patients with tuberculum sellae meningiomas and in other larger series of so-called suprasellar meningiomas, visual failure was the most common complaint in 93% to 100% of patients.[6–8] The incidence of headache, the second most common symptom, varied from 12% to 45%.[5–7, 15] In 1984, Symon and Rosenstein[7] reviewed their series of 101 patients with so-called suprasellar meningiomas and reported that the most common signs on admission were visual field defects (100%), loss of visual acuity (99%), and optic atrophy (85%). Papilledema, Foster Kennedy syndrome, and oculomotor nerve palsy were rare findings. Signs of hypothalamic-hypophyseal dysfunction are also reported to be rare.[5, 7] Mental changes, anosmia, neurologic deficits, and seizures are uncommon, and their incidence may, in part, reflect series with more heterogeneous tumor locations.[5, 7] In our own experience with nine patients who were operated on by the senior author from 1983 to the present, all patients presented with visual deterioration, whereas none demonstrated motor deficits, endocrinopathy, or cognitive dysfunction.

Cushing and Eisenhardt[3] called attention to the chiasmal syndrome produced by tuberculum sellae meningioma. They noted a tendency toward bitemporal field defects, but more commonly the fields were asymmetric, and one eye often was blind. This situation occurred in adult patients with optic atrophy and a normal sellae on plain skull x-ray study. Schlezinger and colleagues[16] focused on a prechiasmal syndrome in which incongruity and asymmetry of the field defects are a common finding when the chiasm is displaced upward and back, which is technically more correct. The most common pattern of vision loss is gradual or rapid progressive loss of vision in one eye, followed by gradual decrease in the acuity of the contralateral eye.[17] Diagnosis is delayed for an average of 2 years from the onset of symptoms to diagnosis.[6, 14] The visual disturbance is often misdiagnosed as retrobulbar neuritis.[18] Pregnancy may aggravate the symptoms.[6–8] The prompt diagnosis of these lesions requires a high index of suspicion by an ophthalmologist, particularly in elderly women with failing vision and optic atrophy.

## Preoperative Evaluation

Magnetic resonance imaging (MRI) with gadolinium enhancement is the diagnostic study of choice because the extent of dural involvement is best visualized with this method. Vascular relationships and, in particular, vascular encasement[19] are also best detected with MRI (Fig. 23–1A).

Gadolinium-enhanced MRI allows tumors arising from the tuberculum sellae to be distinguished from other so-called suprasellar tumors with a greater degree of accuracy than with computed tomography (CT). It may be difficult, however, to distinguish between a pituitary macroadenoma with suprasellar extension and a tuberculum sellae meningioma with intrasellar extension. The imaging characteristics that are consistently seen in MRI studies of tuberculum sellae meningiomas[20] but that are absent in those of pituitary macroadenomas are homogeneous enhancement with gadolinium, a suprasellar epicenter, and a tapered dural base (see Fig. 23–1B).

The typical CT scan shows a densely enhancing round mass in the midline above the sella extending laterally and anteriorly. CT scanning is reserved for patients with suspected hyperostosis of the skull base, which is best appreciated with a coronal CT scan with bone windows.

Cerebral angiography is helpful but has been largely replaced by MRI and magnetic resonance angiography. Elevation of both anterior cerebral arteries is the most common finding. The intracranial portion of the ICA may be displaced laterally, and a tumor blush may be seen. These angiographic findings are indistinguishable from the findings of a pituitary adenoma with suprasellar extension.

All patients should be examined preoperatively by an ophthalmologist to document central visual acuity and to perform visual field examination. If hypothalamic-hypophyseal dysfunction is present, a complete series of endocrinologic studies should be obtained, and the patient should have a consultation with an endocrinologist.

## Patient Selection and Decisions in Management

Optimal treatment of tuberculum sellae meningiomas is total surgical removal, including the dura and invaded bone, if possible. Conventional or stereotactic radiation therapy is not advocated for initial treatment.[21] Radiation

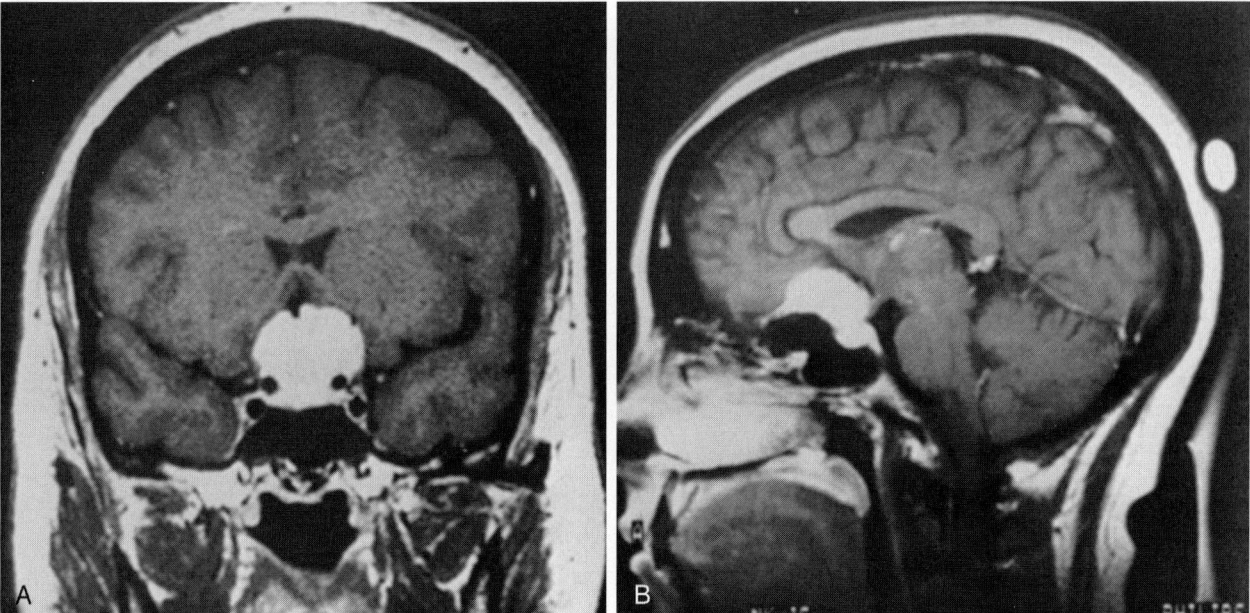

FIGURE 23–1 ■ *A*, Coronal contrast-enhanced magnetic resonance imaging scan of the sellar region in a patient with a tuberculum sellar meningioma. The carotid arteries are partially engulfed by tumor. *B*, Sagittal view of the same patient shows tumor extension on to the planum sphenoidale with a tapered dural base.

therapy may be an adjuvant treatment for a recurrent or residual tumor that is deemed surgically inaccessible or in an elderly or medically compromised patient. Preoperative embolization is not feasible because the tumor's arterial supply originates from the internal carotid circulation via branches of the ophthalmic artery.

These tumors may be approached through three cranial bone openings: the bifrontal, unilateral frontal, and pterional.[2, 3, 5, 6, 8, 10, 12, 17, 21–25] Advocates of the subfrontal approach believe it provides maximal exposure of the sellar region. Disadvantages include the risk of damage to the olfactory nerve and the potential for infection and cerebrospinal fluid (CSF) rhinorrhea as a result of opening of the frontal sinus. Others recommend removing the supraorbital arch with the subfrontal approach for optimal exposure of the sella.[21, 23] We resect tuberculum tumors via a pterional craniotomy. This approach does not jeopardize the olfactory nerves, and it does not subject the patient to the risks of CSF rhinorrhea or infection from transgression of the frontal sinus. Generous removal of the sphenoid ridge and a wide dissection of the sylvian fissure allow access to the suprasellar region with less brain retraction compared with the subfrontal approach. The only disadvantage is that the undersurface of the ipsilateral optic nerve and chiasm are not as well visualized as with the subfrontal approach. In our opinion, this minor disadvantage does not warrant exposing the patient to the risks and potential complications of a bifrontal craniotomy and anosmia. Generally the craniotomy flap is on the side of the nondominant hemisphere. If the tumor extends eccentrically between the optic nerve and carotid artery on one side, however, we approach the lesion from the ipsilateral side. This approach permits optimal surgical exposure for resection with no significant risk of injury to either the carotid artery or the optic nerve. If one eye is blind, the approach is from the amblyopic side because this method permits optimal exposure for decompression of the less involved optic nerve.

## Surgical Technique

At surgery, steroids, anticonvulsants, and a single dose of a broad-spectrum antibiotic are administered. Also, a spinal drain is inserted. The patient is placed supine, and the operating table is flexed to place the head above the level of the heart to facilitate venous drainage. The head is rotated 35 degrees, bringing the medial half of the sphenoid ridge to a vertical position. To minimize brain retraction and achieve maximal exposure of the skull base, the head is extended approximately 25 degrees. It is secured in position with a three-pin fixation device.

We use a standard pterional craniotomy, as described by Yasargil.[26] The incision is started at the zygomatic arch, less than 5 mm anterior to the tragus to avoid injury to the frontal branch of the facial nerve, which courses over the zygomatic arch more anteriorly. The incision curves upward and forward within the hairline and loops backward for 1 or 2 cm on the opposite side of the midline. This approach provides adequate cranial exposure and keeps the incision off the forehead. The plane of dissection during reflection of the scalp flap is between the two layers of the true temporalis muscle fascia at the fat pad to avoid injury to the frontal nerve branch, which courses in the superficial fascia. The temporalis muscle and its true fascia are incised by electrocautery and reflected inferiorly and posteriorly over the ear.

A bur hole is made at the frontozygomatic suture. The second hole is made in the squama of the temporal bone just behind the greater wing of the sphenoid. The greater sphenoid wing is then thinned with a high-speed drill and removed with a rongeur, and a free frontotemporal bone flap is cut with the craniotome. The remaining portion of the sphenoid wing is drilled out extradurally to allow an unobstructed exposure of the skull base. The dura is then opened parallel to the skull base and reflected posteriorly to expose the sylvian fissure.[1]

From this point on, the operating microscope is used. The arachnoid of the sylvian fissure must be opened widely to expose the tumor through the fissure, rather than from underneath the frontal and temporal lobes. The distal fissure is opened first, then dissected proximally. A single retractor is used to elevate the frontal lobe and expose the tumor. Temporal lobe retraction is not needed. CSF can be withdrawn through the spinal drain to facilitate exposure. Exposed brain is covered with rubber Penrose drains, which we have found to be helpful in preventing cortical injury.

Surgical resection of a tuberculum sellae tumor is depicted in sequential intraoperative photographs in Figure 23–2A to D. After the tumor is exposed, high-power magnification is used to identify the optic nerves, which are located on the anterolateral surface of the tumor. With large tumors, the optic nerves may be difficult to identify owing to thinning of these nerves from extreme compression.

The arterial feeders to the tumor attachment are coagulated before debulking the tumor. These vessels travel along the planum sphenoidal and the lesser wing of the sphenoid. Generally the safest point to start internal decompression is in the midline, at the anterior limit of the tumor. The optic nerves are least likely to be injured at this point. If, however, the patient has long-standing blindness in one eye, the nerve may be sectioned at its entrance into the optic canal to facilitate tumor removal and preservation of the intact contralateral optic nerve.

The overlying arachnoid is cut with microscissors, and conventional high-power suction and bipolar coagulation are adequate for debulking the interior of the tumor. The ultrasonic aspirator may be difficult to use because it requires an awkward angle. A laser is not used because of the close proximity and varied location of vessels that may be inadvertently injured. During the initial decompression, a 2- to 3-mm carpet of tumor should be cauterized and left at the dural attachment. This procedure avoids troublesome bleeding from the bone that may result when tumor and involved dura are stripped off the skull.

The interior of the tumor is gutted, leaving an outer rim of tumor tissue. The contralateral optic nerve and carotid artery are easier to decompress with the pterional approach. The operation should first begin with dissection of these structures. The surgeon then proceeds in a circumferential

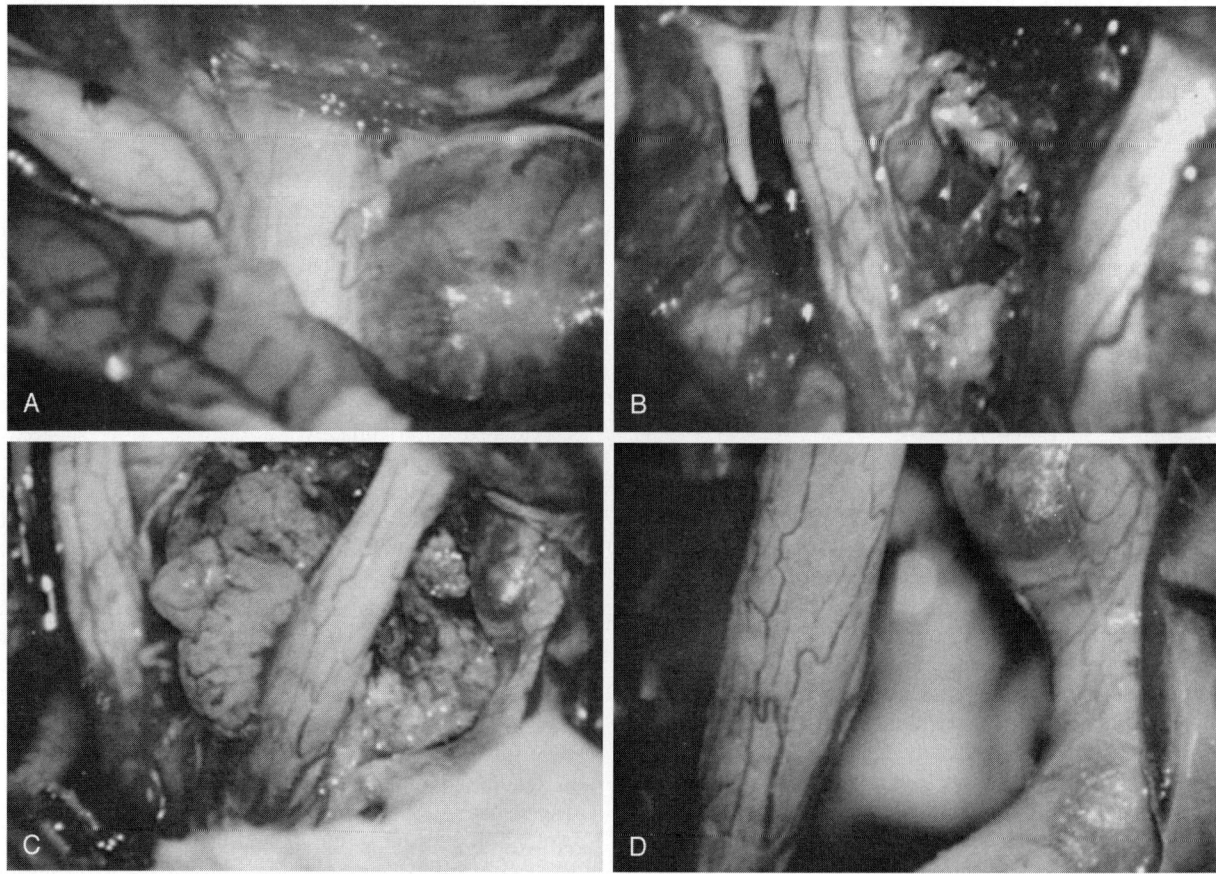

FIGURE 23–2 ■ Sequential microphotographs depicting steps in surgical resection. *A,* Photograph of right trans-sylvian exposure of a right tuberculum sellar meningioma showing the tumor covering the internal carotid artery. *B,* The tumor has been resected from the planum and the left optic nerve and internal carotid artery are freed of the tumor. The *short arrow* points to the origin of the posterior communicating artery. *C,* The tumor has been dissected and mobilized from the vertebral aspect of the ipsilateral optic nerve, and the internal carotid artery is visualized. The chiasm is also well seen. *D,* High-power magnification of the ipsilateral optic nerve and internal carotid artery following gross total removal of the tumor. The basilar artery can be seen out of focus in the interpeduncular cistern, as well as the middle cerebral artery to the right of the internal carotid artery.

fashion to remove tumor from underneath the optic chiasm. The tumor on the ipsilateral carotid artery and optic nerve is removed last because visualization of these structures is less optimal with the pterional approach. At this point, most of the tumor will have been removed, which relaxes the arachnoid-tumor interface and facilitates dissection. Dissection of the tumor from the carotid arteries and optic nerves is performed by grasping the tumor with microring forceps and gently pulling away from these structures while cauterizing (with low-power and continuous saline irrigation) and shrinking the tumor. The bits of cauterized tumor are removed piecemeal with microdissectors. The interface between tumor and arachnoid should be identified using high-power magnification. The surgeon should avoid violating the arachnoid membrane as much as possible and perform the dissection in the plane between the tumor and the arachnoid to preserve vessels and nerves that lie in the subarachnoid space. Angled microdissectors, angled bipolar forceps, and dental mirrors are helpful in removing tumor from the undersurface of the ipsilateral carotid artery and optic nerve. After decompression of the optic apparatus and carotid arteries, the pituitary stalk, which has a reddish orange color, is identified and preserved. Removal of the most posterior aspect of the tumor exposes the arachnoid of the interpeduncular cistern (Liliequist's membrane). Extension into the optic foramen may require drilling of the anterior clinoid and the roof for additional exposure.

After the tumor has been removed, the dural attachment and remnants of tumor at the base of the skull should be coagulated and, if possible, resected. Involved bone should be removed using a diamond drill. If the sphenoid sinus is entered, the defect is repaired with an appropriate piece of temporalis muscle, which is secured in position with autologous fibrin glue.

At the conclusion of the procedure, the dura is closed, and the remaining closure is handled in a routine manner. A subgaleal drain is left in place for 24 hours. The spinal drain is removed unless there is potential for CSF fistula, in which case a tunneled drain is left in place for several days.

After surgery, the patients should be closely monitored for diabetes insipidus. We closely follow urine volume and specific gravity as well as serum electrolytes and osmolarity. Steroids are slowly tapered, and the patients should be followed closely for pituitary dysfunction. A postoperative MRI scan is crucial for determining the completeness of surgical resection (Fig. 23–3A, B).

## Results

A review of various studies of so-called suprasellar meningioma demonstrates operative mortality rate ranging from 3% to 67%.[2, 5, 8, 10, 17, 18, 23, 24] Higher mortality rates were recorded before 1970, particularly in older series, when catastrophic vascular injury was frequent.[2, 5, 10] Most studies using microsurgical methods have reported 0% to 7% mortality rates.[6, 22, 24] A series in 1985, however, reported an 18% mortality rate from medical complications in advanced cases.[15] A considerable increase in the rates of mortality, morbidity, and failure of visual improvement occurs in cases in which the tumor size exceeds 3 cm.[5, 7, 8, 12, 13, 23] Postoperative morbidity is common in all series of so-called suprasellar meningioma and includes visual loss, diabetes insipidus, panhypopituitarism, anosmia, rhinorrhea, meningitis, cerebral infarction, and diencephalic dysfunction.

A review of operative series since 1979 indicates that the percentage of patients with suprasellar meningioma having complete excision has varied from 40% to 100%.[7] Recurrence rates, when reported, are generally less than 10%. Tumor recurrence is related to incomplete surgical resection. The most commonly cited reason for incomplete resection was to avoid major vascular injury.[10, 11, 22]

With regard to visual function, Grisoli et al[14] reported

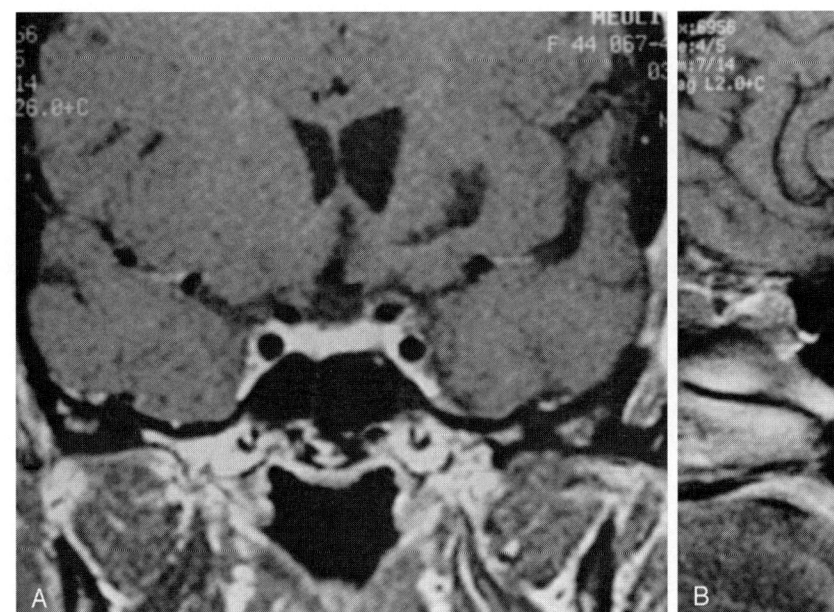
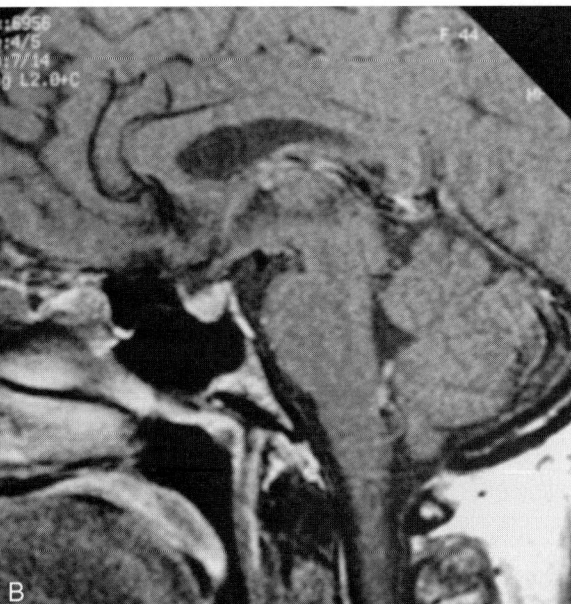

**FIGURE 23–3** ■ Coronal (A) and sagittal (B) magnetic resonance imaging scans with contrast enhancement of the sellar region following resection of a tuberculum sellar meningioma.

that except for patients with total blindness, improvement of visual acuity was the rule, even in cases of long-term duration. Best results were obtained in patients who had been operated on within 1 year of the onset of visual symptoms. Postoperative visual deterioration has been reported to vary from 5% to 38%[7, 12, 17] and may be due to a variety of problems, including inadequate tumor decompression, direct surgical trauma or compromise of vascular supply to the optic apparatus, and postoperative suprasellar hematoma.

Our series include nine patients with tuberculum sellae meningiomas varying from 2 to 4 cm in largest diameter who were operated on from 1983 to 2000. The first patient, aged 78, died in the immediate postoperative period from overwhelming pulmonary sepsis. Eight tumors were totally resected. Postoperative MRI detected a small residual tumor fragment within the cavernous sinus in one patient that was not visualized at surgery. Of the 16 patients with involved optic nerves, 8 had normal visual acuity, which was preserved after surgery. Moderate-to-severe acuity loss was present in the remainder, of which 50% improved, 25% remained the same, and 25% were made worse with surgery. With regard to visual fields, four improved, two remained the same, and two were made worse with surgery. Postoperative visual deterioration occurred in two eyes (one eye of two patients), which were severely compromised before surgery (visual acuity, 20/800). One patient who had full visual fields preoperatively maintained these fields after surgery. There were no other complications.

## MEDIAL SPHENOID RIDGE MENINGIOMA

### Pathologic Anatomy and Classification

Cushing and Eisenhardt[2] were the first to describe medial sphenoid ridge meningiomas accurately. They distinguished between global tumors, which are somewhat spherical in shape, and hyperostosing (en plaque) tumors, which are flat and cause bony reaction along the entire ridge. Global tumors may grow from any point along the ridge and were divided into three groups: (1) inner or clinoidal, (2) middle or alar, and (3) outer or pterional. Only the medial global variety is discussed here. These tumors present a much more complex and difficult surgical problem than do lateral sphenoid ridge meningiomas because they invariably involve arteries of the anterior circulation, the anterior visual pathways, and other cranial nerves. Although some medial sphenoid ridge meningiomas invade the cavernous sinus, other meningiomas originate within the cavernous sinus. These meningiomas, which present with extraocular motor nerve palsies, involve the visual pathways to a much smaller degree and require different management. They are excluded from this discussion. Small tumors of the optic foramen, which are often discovered early in their course and do not involve the carotid artery, are not considered within the medial sphenoid ridge group. Such lesions are classified as meningiomas of the optic canal or foramen.

Cushing and Eisenhardt's[1] original description of medial sphenoid ridge meningiomas was based on the relationship of the tumor to the bony ridge. We place more emphasis on the tumor's relationship to the various arachnoid cisterns, vascular structures, and optic apparatus to understand the gross pathologic anatomy and develop a strategy for their surgical resection. In large tumors that occupy the entire length of the ridge, it may be difficult to distinguish between lateral and medial growths for this reason. Tumors that involve the carotid artery and other vessels are considered to be true medial ridge meningiomas.

Medial sphenoid ridge meningiomas arise from the dura over the frontal and temporal aspects of the lesser sphenoid wing as well as the anterior clinoid. With large growths, the dural attachment extends to the petroclinal ligament and tentorium. Involvement of the dura of the tuberculum sellae and cavernous sinus is less frequent. As described previously with tuberculum sellae tumors, meningiomas arising from the medial sphenoid ridge grow in the subdural space but remain outside the arachnoid. Despite the fact that the cranial nerves and arteries are completely encircled by the growing neoplasm, the thick arachnoid and constant flow of CSF in the basal cisterns form a separable interface around these structures. Less commonly, tumor is directly adherent to these structures. This may occur with large and neglected tumors. The intracavernous cranial nerves and carotid artery lack an arachnoid investment, as does the initial 2- to 3-mm segment of the ICA as it arises from the cavernous sinus. Tumor may adhere at these sites. This arachnoid-CSF interface is also absent in previously operated patients because it is disrupted at the time of the first procedure.

The carotid artery and optic nerve are displaced medially by the tumor. With further growth, the tumor ultimately engulfs the ICA and middle cerebral artery (MCA), the anterior cerebral artery (ACA), and their central perforating branches. The tumor can be divided into an anterolateral and a posteromedial section in relation to the arterial tree. The small perforators are always in a cleft of arachnoid between the anterior and posterior portion of the tumor. With large growths, the ipsilateral optic apparatus may be paper thin, displaced medially, and often engulfed by the tumor.

Tumor may extend into the optic foramen and superior orbital fissure and invade the orbit. With extremely large growths, the tumor grows anteriorly into the frontal fossa, elevating the frontal lobe, and posteriorly over the tentorium and posterior clinoid region, and it may extend into the posterior fossa. The dura of the petroclinoid fold and lateral wall of the cavernous sinus is frequently involved and, less commonly, the cavernous sinus itself.[1]

### Clinical Presentation

Sphenoid ridge meningiomas account for approximately 20% of supratentorial meningiomas, of which less than half arise from the medial ridge.[27] There is a preponderance of middle-aged women in all series.[27–30, 33, 34] The onset of symptoms is insidious, usually developing over a 2-year period.[27, 32] In our series of 20 patients and in other series, visual loss is the most common presenting complaint.[2, 28, 32] Vision loss is usually unilateral and may often progress to blindness, but it is infrequent in the contralateral eye. Visual field abnormali-

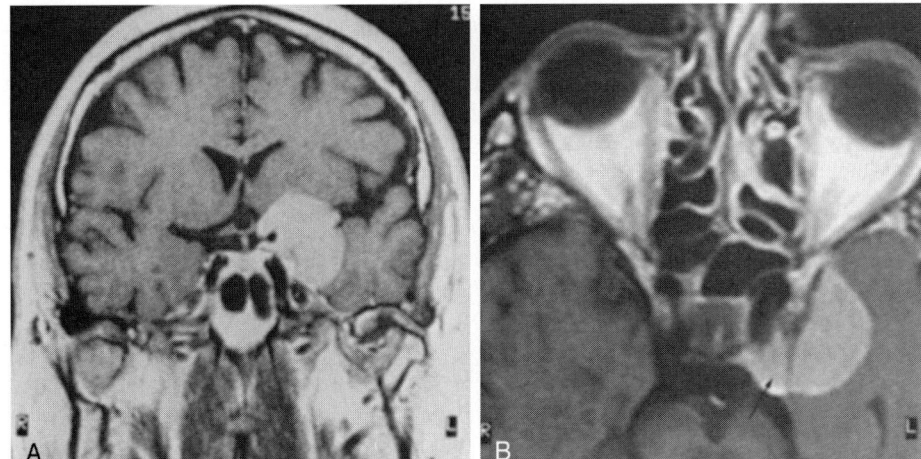

FIGURE 23–4 ■ *A,* Coronal magnetic resonance imaging scan with contrast enhancement of 3.5-cm meningioma of the left medial sphenoid ridge. The carotid artery is surrounded by the tumor. *B,* Axial view of the same patient, with an *arrow* pointing to tumor extension around the third cranial nerve in the region of posterior clinoid and petroclinal ligament.

ties are variable, depending on the involvement of the chiasm and the optic tract. Funduscopic examination commonly reveals optic atrophy and, less frequently, contralateral papilledema (Foster Kennedy syndrome).[2, 32] Oculomotor dysfunction and facial hypoesthesia occur when tumor involves the cavernous sinus and superior orbital fissure. Exophthalmos is due to tumor extension into the orbit and cavernous sinus. Headache and orbital pain may precede visual symptoms by many years. Intellectual deterioration and changes in cognition are frequently observed, particularly in elderly patients in whom the tumor is on the same side as the dominant cerebral hemisphere. Hemiparesis, aphasia, and seizures are seen less frequently.[28, 29, 32, 33]

## Diagnostic Studies

MRI with gadolinium contrast is the best preoperative examination to delineate accurately the tumor and its dural attachment as well as its extension into the orbit, cavernous sinus, and tentorial incisura (Fig. 23–4*A, B*). MRI also defines the relationship between tumor and major intracranial arteries[19] and is the procedure of choice in postoperative follow-up (Fig. 23–5*A, B*). The position of the optic nerve and chiasm can be seen on $T_1$-weighted images, particularly

in tumors less than 3 cm in size. $T_2$-weighted images best delineate the amount of cerebral edema. A CT scan with bone window is performed on patients in whom MRI demonstrates invasion of bone and hyperostosis of the skull base.

Cerebral angiography should be performed in tumors larger than 3 cm to determine the status of the intracranial arteries and define the blood supply to the tumor. With tumors smaller than 3 cm, in which MRI with gradient echo imaging has ruled out an aneurysm, preoperative angiography is not necessary. When indicated, cerebral angiography should include selective internal and external carotid catheterization to evaluate the anterior cerebral circulation and the dural blood supply of the tumor. Collateral circulation should be assessed so that in the event of an intraoperative vascular injury, the surgeon knows the optimal point at which to interrupt the vessel. Angiography shows elevation and stretching of the ICA, MCA, and ACA on the anteroposterior and lateral views. In large tumors, segmental narrowing or irregularity of the vessels may be seen, but complete vessel occlusion is rarely noted. The ICA often supplies blood to the neoplasm through the recurrent meningeal artery (a branch of the ophthalmic artery) and through the cavernous branches from the inferior lateral trunk (the ramus sinus cavernosi). The extracra-

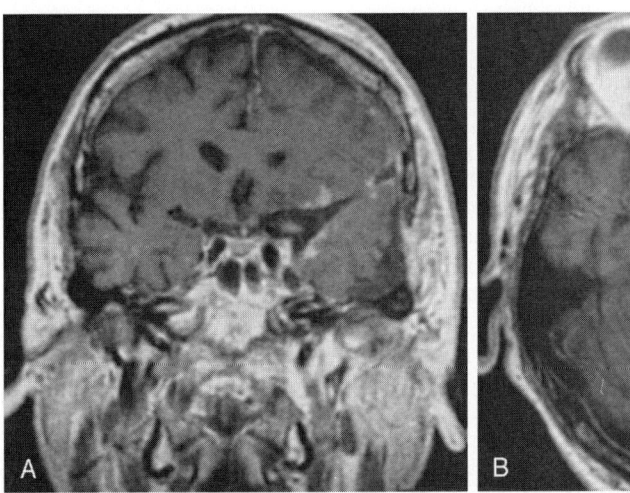
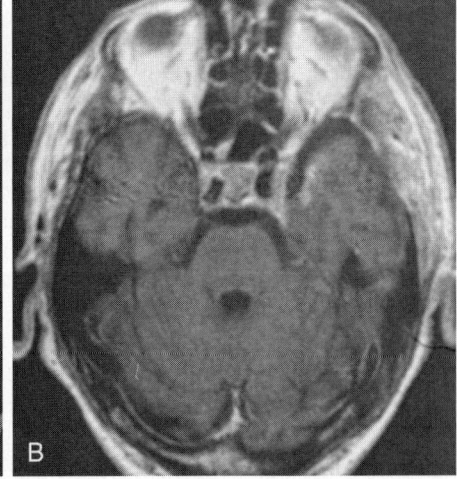

FIGURE 23–5 ■ Postoperative coronal (*A*) and axial contrast-enhanced (*B*) magnetic resonance imaging scan 1 week following surgery in the same tumor depicted in Figure 23–4.

nial dural blood supply includes the middle meningeal artery, the artery of the foramen rotundum, and the accessory meningeal and deep temporal arteries, and it is demonstrated by superselective catheterization of the external carotid artery. Embolization of the external carotid blood supply helps minimize blood loss in large and hypervascular tumors.

When dissection of the cavernous sinus is indicated, a preoperative temporary balloon occlusion test with neurologic monitoring and xenon/CT measurements of cerebral blood flow is mandatory to define the risk of ICA occlusion.[31, 37] Neurologic deficits produced by test occlusion are an indication that the patient is at high risk for cerebral infarction if the carotid artery were to be occluded. Those who clinically tolerate temporary occlusion but who have reductions in cerebral blood flow in the range of 15 to 35 ml/100 g/min are at moderate risk for cerebral infarction should permanent occlusion of the carotid be necessary.

As with tuberculum sellae meningiomas, documented visual field and acuity examinations are mandatory in the preoperative evaluation of these patients. A thorough general medical evaluation is important, especially in elderly patients, because these operations are lengthy and may require induced hypotension when hypervascular tumors are resected.

## Patient Selection and Decisions in Management

Many surgeons who have become cautious as a result of the high morbidity and mortality rates of radical resections of medial sphenoid ridge meningiomas have been content with partial removal.[2, 27, 28, 36] These tumors frequently recurred and were treated with repeated surgery and radiation therapy. Reoperation is associated with significantly higher rates of morbidity and mortality because the tumor adheres to vital structures.[34-36] Tumors may regrow despite radiation therapy,[38, 40, 41] and in our experience, radiation is less effective if a large amount of tumor is left behind. Al-Mefty[32] and others[31] have advocated aggressive surgical resection of these tumors with dissection of the cavernous sinus. It is not clear whether in the long-term the patient benefits most from more extensive surgery, with its increased risk of morbidity, or whether a radical removal of tumor, leaving the intracavernous portion behind, followed by radiation therapy, is the best treatment.[31]

We attempt a gross total resection. The initial procedure is the best opportunity for cure. We believe that dissection of tumor from the cavernous sinus is not warranted in patients with intact third nerve function for fear of permanent damage to this nerve. In this instance, patients should receive adjuvant stereotactic radiation therapy to the small portion of the neoplasm left behind. Patients with small benign irradiated tumors can survive for many years with no evidence of regrowth.[38, 39, 41] In elderly patients and in those with poor medical health, a less radical excision is acceptable.

## Surgical Technique

The cranial exposure is similar to that outlined in the section on tuberculum sellae meningiomas. More temporal fossa exposure is needed for resection of medial sphenoid ridge meningiomas, and more of the greater sphenoid wing is removed. Extensive cranial base exposures (orbitozygomatic infratemporal approach) have been described for these tumors,[42, 43] but in our experience, it has not been necessary to use these approaches.

The frontal and temporal lobes are often compressed by large tumors. The sylvian fissure must be opened widely to avoid brain retraction. After a wide microdissection of the sylvian fissure and exposure of the tumor, the vascularized dura surrounding the lateral tumor attachment on both sides of the sphenoid ridge is thoroughly coagulated with bipolar forceps. This procedure significantly reduces the blood supply to the neoplasm and helps reduce blood loss. Excision of the meningioma, however, should not be started at the base of the tumor because the ICA and its branches are difficult to visualize and are at risk of injury there. The surgical strategy is first to identify proximal branches of the MCA in the sylvian fissure and follow the branches into the tumor to the carotid bifurcation. While keeping constant surveillance of the arterial tree, the tumor is gutted and removed piecemeal. Surgical removal of a medial sphenoid ridge tumor is depicted with sequential intraoperative photographs in Figure 23–6A to D. The tumor located anterior and lateral to the arterial tree, which is usually larger, should be removed first, to expose and protect the MCA, ICA, and ACA. The arachnoid covering this portion of the tumor is incised with microscissors, and the surface is coagulated at a safe distance from major vessels. The tumor interior is then removed in a piecemeal fashion using suction and bipolar cautery. Microdissection, as described previously in the section on tuberculum sellae meningioma, is used to free the tumor from the arachnoid enveloping the sylvian vessels. With large tumors, the involved intracranial arteries may supply the tumor directly. In this case, the vessels are dissected within the tumor and coagulated and cut on the tumor side of the arachnoid, leaving a coagulated stump on the parent artery. This approach avoids thrombosis of the parent vessel and tearing the feeder from the parent vessel. If tumor directly involves the adventitia of the ICA, small coagulated bits of tumor may be left on the vessel without significant risk of recurrence. The MCA, ICA, and ACA are exposed. The origins of the posterior communicating artery and the anterior choroidal artery are then identified and followed distally.

After resection of tumor located anterior and lateral to the arterial tree, the remaining tumor, which is posterior and medial to the M1 segment of the MCA and A1 segment of the ACA and the ICA, is removed. Angle-tipped bipolar forceps are helpful in manipulating the anatomy around the perforating vessels, which are found in a cleft of arachnoid between the anterior and posterior portions of the tumor. The neoplasm can be freed from these vessels using minimal bipolar coagulation because the tumor is now devascularized as a result of its detachment from the sphenoid ridge. After exposure of the carotid artery and its major branches, the optic apparatus is freed of neoplasm. The optic nerve is best identified at its fixed point at the optic foramen. The optic apparatus is invariably elevated and displaced medially by tumor medial to the carotid artery. The tumor is carefully separated from the optic nerve, and traction is applied to pull it gently away from the arachnoid

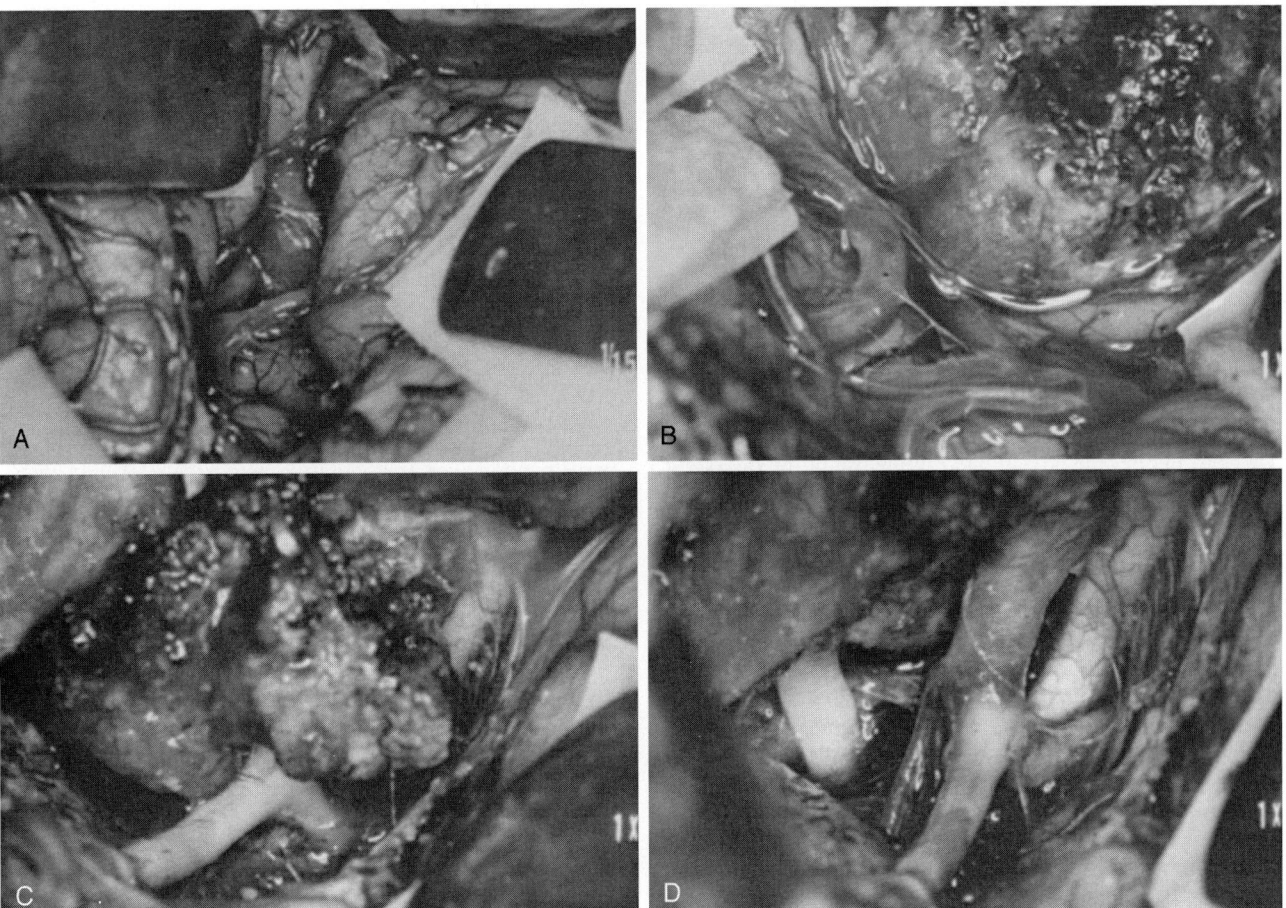

FIGURE 23–6 ■ Sequential photographs depicting steps in surgical resection of the medial sphenoid ridge meningioma shown in Figure 23–4. *A*, Intraoperative photograph of trans-sylvian exposure of a left medial sphenoid ridge meningioma. The sylvian fissure has been opened widely. Retractors are on the frontal and temporal lobes. The proximal branches of the middle cerebral artery (*long arrows*) are entangled with a tumor. *Arrowheads* point to the arachnoid and trabecular layer covering the tumor surface. *B*, The tumor anterior and lateral to the middle cerebral artery has been partially resected. *Open arrows* point to the groove on the tumor made by the middle cerebral artery. Note that the arachnoid layer covering this section of tumor is left intact. The *arrowhead* points to arachnoid strands attached to the adventitia of the middle cerebral artery. *C*, The tumor has been dissected and removed from the middle cerebral artery, anterior communicating artery, and carotid bifurcation. The optic and olfactory nerves are exposed. The remaining tumor is medial and posterior to the internal carotid artery. *D*, The normal anatomy of the medial sphenoid ridge region is shown after gross total resection of the tumor.

of the optic and chiasmatic cisterns, rather than retracting the optic apparatus. The superior hypophyseal arteries coursing medially from the carotid artery supply arterial blood to the optic nerves and should be preserved. When the tumor extends into the optic canal, the dura over the canal and the anterior clinoid process is excised widely and the roof and lateral wall of the orbit are removed with a high-speed drill. Diamond burs are safer and carry a low risk of tearing the underlying sleeve of the optic nerve. The dural sleeve of the optic nerve is opened with microscissors under high magnification, and the intraorbital tumor is removed.

Tumor extending along the tentorium is reached by lateral elevation of the medial temporal lobe. If the neoplasm extends beyond the tentorial edge into the posterior fossa, the tentorium is coagulated and sectioned behind the tumor. The fourth cranial nerve is exposed and preserved, if possible. The tumor is then removed from the upper clival region. If tumor extends into the cavernous sinus and the patient has a complete third nerve palsy, dissection of

tumor from the sinus is performed. This dissection is best performed as a staged procedure after recovery from initial surgery. Extracranial-intracranial bypass should be performed if the patient cannot tolerate carotid artery occlusion, as previously discussed.

Finally, the remaining fragments of neoplasm attached to the sphenoid ridge are removed. The involved dura is thoroughly coagulated or excised. If the sphenoid sinus is entered, it is repaired with a graft of temporalis fascia, which is secured over the defect with fibrin glue. At the conclusion of the procedure, the dura is closed in routine fashion. A subgaleal drain is left in place for 24 hours. The spinal drain is removed unless there is potential for CSF fistula, in which case a tunneled drain is left in place for several days. Postoperatively, patients should be closely monitored in an intensive care unit. In our experience, many of these patients have hydrocephalus and may require a shunting procedure at some point. Details of our surgical technique are described in *Neurosurgical Operative Atlas* by Rengachary and Wilkins.[1]

## Results

Surgical series of patients with medial sphenoid ridge meningiomas have reported high morbidity and mortality rates.[2, 27, 28, 30, 33, 34] In Cushing's original series of 13 patients, there were two perioperative deaths. Total removal was possible in only three cases. Most of the surviving patients had significant neurologic morbidity, and five eventually died of recurrence. Cushing and Eisenhardt[2] noted that "the crux of the removal lies in freeing the growth from its entanglement with the vessels at the carotid bifurcation" and they cautioned surgeons about the hazards of entering the carotid field. Injury to the major vessels of the anterior circulation has been the major cause of operative mortality and morbidity in all subsequent surgical series even after the advent and routine use of the operating microscope. In 1953, Uihlein and Weyand[33] reported their findings on a series of 52 patients with an operative mortality of 33%.[28] In 1970, Bonnal and associates[28] reported three operative mortalities in seven patients treated with only subtotal resection. In 1979, Konovalov and colleagues[30] reported an operative mortality of 19% in a series of 70 patients, all of whom were operated on with the use of the microscope. The surgical morbidity for medial sphenoid ridge meningioma includes hemiplegia, hypothalamic infarction, aphasia, neurovegetative disorders, visual loss, and diplopia. In one study, 23% of surviving patients were severely impaired.[27] More recent reports have shown improvement in the rates of operative mortality and morbidity and chances for cure.[29, 31, 32] The rate of recurrence for medial sphenoid ridge meningioma is one of the highest for intracranial meningiomas.[44] Recurrence is related to residual tumor that is left behind at the time of initial surgery. In the study conducted by Mirimanoff and colleagues[45] the rate of recurrence or progression was 34% at 5 years and 54% at 10 years for medial ridge tumors compared with 3% and 25% at 5 and 10 years for convexity meningiomas.

There are very few data concerning visual function after resection of these tumors. Most patients present with visual abnormalities. In one series, of 20 of the 24 patients who presented with visual disturbances, only 2 had visual improvement after tumor removal.[32] The author concluded that "recovery of vision in clinoidal meningiomas is poor."

In the senior author's personal series of 20 patients with medial global tumors ranging from 2 to 7 cm in size, 16 growths (80%) were completely removed. Of the four incomplete resections, surgery was terminated for medical problems in two patients and in the other two, intracavernous tumor was electively left to avoid oculomotor palsy. There was no surgical mortality. Also, there was no incidence of injury to arteries of the anterior circulation, although there were two silent infarcts of the anterior caudate nucleus. There was one permanent third nerve injury. After a mean follow-up of 4.5 years, 16 patients had improved, 2 were unchanged, and 2 were neurologically worse after surgery. Vision improved in 50% of patients who were not blind before surgery. Tumor has not recurred in patients who had undergone total removal. Two patients with residual intracavernous tumor were treated with adjuvant radiation therapy and have not shown further growth at 1 and 5 years after surgery.[2]

## Intraoperative Complications and Their Management

The major intraoperative complications of surgery for tuberculum sellae and medial sphenoid ridge meningioma are optic nerve and vascular injury. Blindness and worsening of vision can occur from excessive surgical manipulation or devascularization of the optic apparatus. High-power magnification should be used to identify and preserve enveloping arachnoid and blood vessels supplying the optic apparatus. Manipulation is minimized during tumor removal by applying countertraction to the surrounding chiasmatic arachnoid rather than to the nerves.

Injury to major vessels can occur from sharp dissection, a cautery loop, or excessive coagulation. Partially injured vessels may cause postoperative hemorrhage. Major bleeding is controlled with temporary vascular clips. A Sundt clip or 10–0 suture may be applied to the site of the injury, and, if necessary, the vessel is clipped and a vascular bypass graft is considered. For this reason, the superficial temporal artery should be identified and preserved during cranial exposure.

## ACKNOWLEDGMENT

*The authors thank Dr. Werner Doyle, for his editorial assistance and help in the preparation of this manuscript.*

## REFERENCES

1. Benjamin V, Nazzaro J: Medial sphenoid ridge meningiomas. In Rengachary SS, Wilkins RH (eds): Neurosurgical Operative Atlas. Baltimore: Williams & Wilkins, 1993, pp 285–297.
2. Cushing H, Eisenhardt L: Suprasellar meningiomas. In Meningiomas, Their Classification, Regional Behavior, Life History and Surgical End Results. Springfield, IL: Charles C Thomas, 1938, p 224.
3. Cushing H, Eisenhardt L: Meningiomas arising from the tuberculum sellae with the syndrome of primary optic atrophy and bitemporal field defects combined with a normal sellae turcica in a middle-aged person. Arch Ophthalmol 1:1–41, 1929.
4. Dandy WE: Prechiasmal intracranial tumors of the optic nerves. Am J Ophthalmol 5:169–188, 1922.
5. Solero CL, Giombini S, Morello G: Suprasellar and olfactory meningiomas: Report on a series of 153 personal cases. Acta Neurochir 67:181–194, 1983.
6. Andrews BT, Wilson CB: Suprasellar meningiomas: The effect of tumor location on postoperative visual outcome. J Neurosurg 69:523–528, 1988.
7. Symon L, Rosenstein J: Surgical management of suprasellar meningioma: Part 1. The influence of tumor size, duration of symptoms, and microsurgery on surgical outcome in 101 consecutive cases. J Neurosurg 61:633–641, 1984.
8. Finn JE, Mount LA: Meningiomas of the tuberculum sellae and planum sphenoidale: A review of 83 cases. Arch Ophthalmol 92:23–27, 1974.
9. Kinjo T, Al-Mefty O, Ciric I: Diaphragma sellae meningiomas. Neurosurgery 36:1082–1092, 1995.
10. Kadis GN, Mount LA, Ganti SR: The importance of early diagnosis and treatment of the meningiomas of the planum sphenoidale and tuberculum sellae: A retrospective study of 105 cases. Surg Neurol 12:367–371, 1979.
11. Sato M, Matsumoto M, Kodama N: Treatment of skull base meningiomas encasing the main cerebral artery. No Shinkei Geka 25:239–254, 1997.
12. Symon L, Jakubowski J: Clinical features, technical problems, and results of treatment of anterior parasellar meningiomas. Acta Neurochir Suppl (Wien) 28:367–370, 1979.
13. Jen SL, Lee LS: Suprasellar meningiomas: Analgesics of 32 cases. Chung Hua I Hsueh Tsa Chih (Taipei) 59:7–14, 1997.

14. Grisoli F, Diaz-Vasquez P, Riss M, et al: Microsurgical management of tuberculum sellae meningiomas: Results in 28 consecutive cases. Surg Neurol 26:37–44, 1986.
15. Al-Mefty O, Holoubi A, Rifai A, Fox JL: Microsurgical removal of suprasellar meningiomas. Neurosurgery 16:364–371, 1985.
16. Schlezinger NS, Alpers BJ, Weiss BP: Suprasellar meningiomas associated with scotomatous field defects. Arch Ophthalmol 35:624–642, 1946.
17. Gregorius KF, Hepler RS, Stern WE: Loss and recovery of vision with suprasellar meningiomas. J Neurosurg 42:69–75, 1975.
18. Grant FC, Hedges TR: Ocular findings in meningiomas of the tuberculum sellae. AMA Arch Ophthalmol 56:163–170, 1956.
19. Young SC, Grossman RI, Goldberg HI, et al: MR of vascular encasement in parasellar masses: Comparison with angiography and CT. AJR Am J Roentgenol 9:35–38, 1988.
20. Taylor SL, Barakos JA, Harsh GR, Wilson CB: Magnetic resonance imaging of tuberculum sellae meningiomas: Preventing preoperative misdiagnosis as pituitary macroadenoma. Neurosurgery 31:621–627, 1992.
21. Al-Mefty O, Smith RR: Tuberculum sellae meningiomas. In Al-Mefty O (ed): Meningiomas, New York: Raven Press, 1991, pp 395–411.
22. Jefferson A, Azzam N: The suprasellar meningiomas: A review of 19 years experience. Acta Neurochir Suppl (Wien) 28:381–384, 1979.
23. Jane JA, Park TS, Pobereskin LH, et al: The supraorbital approach: Technical note. Neurosurgery 11:537–542, 1982.
24. Ojemann RG: Meningiomas of the basal parapituitary region: Technical considerations. Clin Neurosurg 27:233–262, 1980.
25. Koos WT, Kletter G, Schuster H, Perneczky A: Microsurgery of suprasellar meningiomas. Adv Neurosurg 2:62–67, 1975.
26. Yasargil MG: General operative techniques. In Yasargil MG (ed): Microsurgery, Vol 1. New York: Thieme-Stratton, 1984, pp 208–271.
27. Fohanno D, Bitar A: Sphenoidal ridge meningioma. In Symon L (ed): Advances and Technical Standards in Neurosurgery, Vol 14. New York: Springer-Verlag, 1986, pp 137–174.
28. Bonnal JP, Thibaut A, Brotchi J, Born J: Invading meningiomas of the sphenoid ridge. J Neurosurg 53:587–599, 1970.
29. Ojemann RG: Meningiomas: Clinical features and surgical management. In Wilkins RH, Rengachary SS (eds): Neurosurgery. New York: McGraw-Hill, 1985, pp 635–654.
30. Konovalov AN, Fedorov SN, Faller TO, et al: Experience in the treatment of the parasellar meningiomas. Acta Neurochir Suppl (Wien) 28:371–372, 1979.
31. Sekhar LN, Sen CN, Jho HD, Janecka IP: Surgical treatment of intracavernous neoplasms: A four-year experience. Neurosurgery 24:18–30, 1989.
32. Al-Mefty O: Clinoidal meningiomas. J Neurosurg 73:840–849, 1990.
33. Uihlein A, Weyand RD: Meningiomas of anterior clinoid process as a cause of unilateral loss of vision: Surgical considerations. Arch Ophthalmol 49:261–270, 1953.
34. Olivecrona H: The surgical treatment of intracranial tumors. In Olivecrona H, Tonnis W (eds): Handbuch der Neurochirurgie. Berlin: Springer-Verlag, 1967, pp 1–301.
35. MacCarty CS, Taylor WF: Intracranial meningiomas: Experiences at the Mayo Clinic. Neurol Med Chir (Tokyo) 19:569–574, 1979.
36. Probst C: Possibilities and limitations of microsurgery in patients with meningiomas of the sellar region. Acta Neurochir (Wien) 84:99–102, 1987.
37. Spetzler RF, Carter LP: Revascularization and aneurysm surgery: Current status. Neurosurgery 16:111–116, 1985.
38. Barbaro NM, Gutin PH, Wilson CB, et al: Radiation therapy in the treatment of partially resected meningiomas. Neurosurgery 20:525–527, 1987.
39. Peele KA, et al: The role of postoperative irradiation in the management of sphenoid wing meningiomas: A preliminary report. Ophthalmology 103:1761–1766, 1996.
40. Wara WM, Sheline GE, Newman H, et al: Radiation therapy of meningiomas. AJR Am J Roentgenol 123:453–458, 1975.
41. Carella RJ, Ransohoff J, Newall J: Role of radiation therapy in the management of meningioma. Neurosurgery 10:332–339, 1982.
42. Al-Mefty O: Surgery of the Cranial Base. Boston, Kluwer Academic Publishers, 1989.
43. Al-Mefty O: Supraorbital-pterional approach to skull base lesions. Neurosurgery 21:474–477, 1987.
44. Mathiesen T, et al: Recurrence of skull base meningiomas. Neurosurgery 39:2–7, 1996.
45. Mirimanoff RO, Dosoretz DE, Linggood RM, et al: Meningioma: Analysis of recurrence and progression following neurosurgical resection. J Neurosurg 62:18–24, 1985.

# CHAPTER 24

# Sphenoid Ridge Meningiomas

■ ARMANDO BASSO, ANTONIO G. CARRIZO, and CHRISTOPHER DUMA

Meningiomas that grow from any point along the sphenoid ridge constitute approximately 14% to 20% of intracranial meningiomas.[1, 2] These tumors represent a complex and difficult surgical problem because they can involve arteries of the anterior circulation, anterior visual pathways, and oculomotor nerves.[1] For sphenoid ridge meningiomas, higher morbidity, mortality, and recurrence rates have been observed than for meningiomas in other locations.[1–4] Two main types can be recognized according to their presentation: nodular and en plaque.[3] The nodular meningioma is an encapsulated tumor of variable size that displaces or encircles intracranial arteries or cranial nerves. Generally, this tumor has a dural site of implantation through which it receives its blood supply. Meningioma en plaque has distinct characteristics that make it a different pathologic entity from the nodular type of sphenoidal meningioma. In the en plaque tumors, the pathologic cells fill the haversian canals and may spread into the pterion; orbital walls; malar bone; and zygomatic, temporal, and middle cranial fossae.[3–5] In this way, these tumors produce typically a hyperostotic reaction of these structures, which produces exophthalmos and temporal bowing. Less frequently, conversely, an osteolytic lesion can be found. In addition, an intracranial meningomatous plaque is always present.[3, 5]

According to Cushing and Eisenhardt,[3] the nodular or globoid meningiomas are classified depending on their site of implantation along the sphenoid wing as inner third, middle third, or outer third tumors. Tumors from the inner third are subdivided into sphenocavernous tumors (implanted in the external wall of the cavernous sinus [CS]) and clinoidal tumors (implanted on the corresponding clinoid process and projecting toward the anterior cranial fossa).[1, 6] Tumors from the middle third of the sphenoid ridge (alar meningiomas) occur less frequently and are difficult to diagnose early. Nodular meningiomas from the outer third of the sphenoid ridge, or sphenotemporal meningiomas, cause neurologic symptoms primarily because of compression of adjacent structures. In large tumors that occupy the entire length of the bony ridge, it is difficult to establish the exact site of origin of the tumor; this difficulty could explain the different classifications that have been proposed for sphenoid wing meningiomas.[3] Petit-Dutaillis divided them into lesser wing and greater wing meningiomas.[3] Bonnal and colleagues[4, 7] classified these tumors into five groups. Al-Mefty[6] distinguished three subgroups of

clinoidal meningiomas based on the presence or absence of an interfacing arachnoidal membrane between the cerebral vessels and the neoplasm. Sekhar and Altschuler[8] described five grades of intracavernous meningioma according to the extension of CS and internal carotid artery (ICA) involvement. The diversity of presentation of sphenoid ridge meningiomas and their complexity make surgical treatment a challenge that varies from case to case. If all the possibilities of presentation described were taken into consideration, almost a dozen types of sphenoid ridge meningiomas would have to be accepted, but such exhaustive classification is not practical for the analysis of a clinical series. For our presentation, we follow the classic Cushing division of these tumors, subdividing those of the deep or inner third into clinoidal and sphenocavernous varieties.[1]

## ANATOMIC CONSIDERATIONS

The sphenoidal wings belong to various regions and are anatomically complex: The posterior edge of the lesser wing represents the limit between the middle and the anterior skull base fossae and is related to the orbit, the sylvian fissure, and the tip of the temporal lobe. The external face of the greater wing is in the temporal and zygomatic fossae, next to the temporal muscle. The lesser wing is part of the roof of the orbit, and the greater wing belongs to the external wall. These compartments communicate through the optic canal, where the optic nerve and the ophthalmic artery pass, and through the superior orbital fissure. The oculomotor nerve, the first division of the trigeminal nerve, and the ophthalmic vein pass through this fissure connecting the orbit with the CS.[1] An understanding of the microsurgical anatomy of this structure is essential for the management of sphenocavernous meningiomas. In certain cases, the CS can be considered the limit of resection.

The lateral, superior, and posterior walls are constituted by two dural layers, whereas the medial wall is formed by a single layer. The ICA lies within the CS surrounded by a venous plexus; the main intracavernous branches of the ICA are the meningohypophyseal trunk and the inferolateral trunk. At the exit of the ICA from the CS, two fibrous rings that represent the dura enclosing the anterior clinoid process can be observed. These fibrous rings are important landmarks for the access of the intracavernous ICA, after resection of the clinoid process. The lateral wall of the CS has a thick outer layer, which continues the dura of the middle cranial fossa, and a thinner layer, which encloses cranial nerves III, IV, V-1, and V-2. The sixth cranial nerve and the sympathetic trunk cross the CS lateral to the ICA.[8]

The orbit and skull also communicate by the leptomeningeal sheath, which accompanies the optic nerve along its orbital course to the posterior pole of the ocular globe. This sheath is a direct prolongation of the inner layer of the dura and leptomeningeal layers of the skull. The outer layer of the dura is in continuity with the periorbita, which is similar in its histologic structure, throughout the optic canal and the superior orbital fissure. Meningiomas are the tumors most frequently located in this region. They have a tendency either to involve the meninges, bone, periorbit, and muscles or to displace and compress brain and orbital contents.[1]

## CLINICAL PRESENTATIONS

In early stages, sphenoid ridge meningiomas produce characteristic findings for each location from which they arise; however, detection of the site of origin of these lesions is difficult when the tumor has enlarged beyond a certain stage of development.[3, 9]

### Inner Third Sphenoid Wing Meningiomas

Clinoidal and sphenocavernous meningiomas are distinct varieties of tumor. Clinoidal meningiomas produce a progressive decrease in visual acuity and changes in the visual fields beginning with ipsilateral nasal hemianopsia. As the tumor grows, a superior temporal field defect occurs, and eventually the eye may become blind. Primary optic atrophy may be evident on the side of the tumor, and in tumors producing increased intracranial pressure, the contralateral optic disk may be swollen and edematous (Foster Kennedy syndrome).[1, 3, 6]

In patients with sphenocavernous meningiomas, oculomotor palsies occur frequently and usually start as abducens palsy. The symptoms slowly evolve and result in total ophthalmoplegia with hypesthesia in the distribution of the ophthalmic branch of the trigeminal nerve, which is secondary to the nerve's compression along the lateral wall of the CS. Exophthalmos may occur, owing to venous compression within the CS; this condition may be more evident with tumor progression toward the orbital apex.[1]

### Middle Third or Alar Meningiomas

Meningiomas of the middle third of the sphenoid ridge are characteristically larger than those in the inner third before detection. Middle third tumors initially produce increased intracranial pressure, headache, and papilledema, which is more evident on the side of the lesion. Dysfunction of the olfactory nerve, contralateral homonymous hemianopsia, personality changes, visual and olfactory hallucinations,

contralateral facial palsy, hemiparesis, and seizures are other symptoms that occur as the tumor increases in size.[2, 3]

### External Third or Pterional Meningiomas

Meningiomas en plaque are predominantly bony growths that must be differentiated from the globoid tumor, which has a far greater degree of intracranial involvement. The pterional meningioma produces a slowly evolving proptosis. This proptosis is caused by: (1) hyperostosis of the orbital walls, (2) the presence of an intraorbital tumor, (3) periorbital tumor infiltration, or (4) venous stasis secondary to ophthalmic vein compression when the tumor enters the CS. Another characteristic of these tumors, probably related to venous stasis and to obstruction of lymphatic drainage, is chronic palpebral edema. Skull deformities may be caused by temporal bone hyperostosis, and, in some cases, the temporal muscle is infiltrated by the tumor. As with inner third meningiomas, loss of visual acuity occurs gradually, and blindness may develop in advanced cases of pterional meningioma. Diplopia is not a constant symptom, but when present it is probably related to mechanical changes within the orbit and, less frequently, to involvement of the oculomotor nerves and muscles. Epiphora, photophobia, and focal or generalized seizures may also occur. Early and frequent symptoms of globoid pterional meningioma include hemicranial headaches, seizures, contralateral hemiparesis, and increased intracranial pressure. This tumor behaves as either a temporal or a frontal mass. Signs of orbital involvement are not constant but are similar to those found in the en plaque variety.[1, 3, 5, 9]

## RADIOGRAPHIC STUDIES

Approximately 90% of sphenoid ridge meningiomas are diagnosed by the use of conventional radiographic studies. Lateral, inclined posteroanterior, and axial views for the skull base and temporo-orbital projections of the optic canals are used. Radiologic features of sphenoid ridge meningiomas include focal hyperostosis, sclerosis, and erosion at the area of tumor attachment. These lesions are seen mainly in the internal table of the skull. Other features may include widening of the vascular grooves, sphenoparietal sinus, and superior orbital fissure; narrowing of the optic canal; and, rarely, enlargement of the foramen spinosum with hypertrophy of the middle meningeal artery. Although hyperostosis may not be present radiographically in a small percentage of inner and middle third meningiomas, it is an almost constant finding in the pterional en plaque meningioma (Fig. 24–1). This finding needs to be differentiated from fibrous dysplasia. In fibrous dysplasia, the hyperostotic alterations can be larger and tend to cross the midline more frequently than in the case of sphenoid ridge meningiomas. Bone becomes several times thicker, and alterations are more evident in the external table and diploë. Widening of the vascular grooves may also be seen.[1, 5, 18, 19]

Although hypocycloidal tomography has been almost completely replaced by computed tomography (CT) to de-

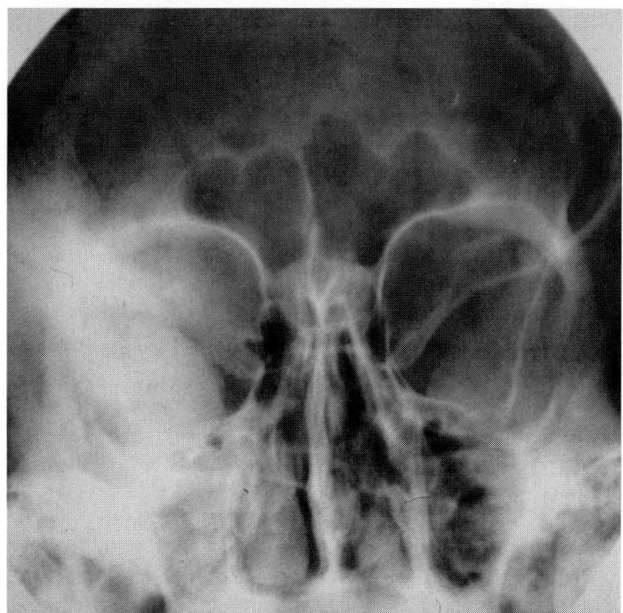

FIGURE 24–1 ■ A plain radiograph showing hyperostosis of the right sphenoid wing.

lineate these lesions, it was used to determine precisely the tumor's bony extension and the appearance of the superior orbital fissure and to examine the optic canal for evidence of encroachment. This information is used to determine the possible limits of the surgical procedure.

Cerebral gammagraphic studies with $^{99m}$Tc, $^{113}$In, or $^{197}$Hg yield positive results in 90% of meningiomas. In meningiomas of the sphenoid ridge, frontotemporal, retro-orbital, and supraorbital uptake is observed, overlapping skull base activity. Gammagraphic studies provide information about the intracranial tumors, peritumoral edema, and bony invasion by the tumors.[9] These data are scarcely useful compared with those furnished by current neuroimaging methods.

## Cerebral Arteriography

Selective catheterization of the ICA and external carotid artery was used in most meningiomas of the sphenoid ridge before surgery. These meningiomas act radiologically as temporal or frontotemporal masses. The anterior cerebral artery exhibits anteroposterior displacement toward the opposite side, which is usually mild in character and is related to the tumor's volume. The slow-growing mass may allow the brain to adapt to the volume changes. On the anteroposterior view of the carotid arteriogram, the middle cerebral artery (MCA) is not parallel to the sphenoid wing, but rather the M1 and M2 segments of the MCA curve to surround the meningioma, indicating its site of attachment. Clinoidal meningiomas show an elevation of the horizontal segment of the MCA, and alar meningiomas show inversion of the sylvian elbow. In pterional meningiomas, the second segment of the MCA is inwardly displaced. In subfrontal locations, the sylvian triangle is displaced backward on the lateral projections. In pretemporal tumor locations, the sylvian triangle is elevated. On frontotemporal

locations, the sylvian triangle is displaced upward and backward. When tumors are well vascularized, the tumor stain of the mass is seen (see Fig. 23–6), and by selective catheterization, contributions to the tumor's blood supply by the ICA and external carotid artery can be determined.

Selective study of the ophthalmic artery demonstrates the presence of an intraorbital mass by staining, blush, or vessel displacement. Partial feeding of intracranial tumor in inner varieties can be seen from an ophthalmic branch, which passes through the superior orbital fissure. In other cases, additional vascularization is found through the anterior meningeal artery, anterior ethmoidal branch, and ophthalmic branches. A preponderant supply from the intracavernous carotid artery is also found through the meningohypophyseal trunk and inferolateral trunk in sphenocavernous meningiomas. A well-developed superficial temporal artery in the external carotid system is observed in most cases, especially when the temporal muscle is invaded. Some cases show an enlarged middle meningeal artery feeding the lesion. Highly vascular tumors can be embolized preoperatively (a portion irrigated by the external carotid artery system), allowing tumor resection without excessive blood loss.[1, 9] Magnetic resonance angiography (MRA) and computed tomographic angiography are replacing digital subtraction angiography in the preoperative evaluation of this pathology except in cases in which embolization is desired.

## Computed Tomography

CT shows the different planes and compartments occupied by the tumor. CT scans must be performed in axial and coronal projections. Significant thickening of the roof and the lateral wall of the orbit is common in hyperostotic pterional meningiomas. This thickening can extend to the malar bone and anterior part of the middle cranial fossa. Osteolytic lesions are rare. Meningiomatous plaque is likely to appear as a thin hyperdense image overlapping the adjacent bone; in other cases, the intradural component develops a nodular configuration. The orbit can be examined to determine the factors producing exophthalmos: hyperostosis, periorbital infiltration by tumor, or intraorbital nodular tumor. Evidence of bone involvement by middle third sphenoid ridge meningiomas is usually less clear. The tumor can be seen as a well-defined mass demonstrating homogeneous enhancement with contrast agents. Edema of the temporal lobe and centrum semiovale can often be seen on the CT scan. This edema is attributed to middle cerebral vein and sphenoparietal sinus compression or occlusion, findings that can be verified by cerebral arteriography. With the use of CT scans, inner third sphenoid ridge meningiomas may be clearly categorized into clinoidal tumors and sphenocavernous tumors. Clinoidal tumors are almost always associated with hyperostosis of the anterior clinoid process or of the whole lesser wing of the sphenoid, with narrowing of the optic canal and, less frequently, of the superior orbital fissure. Characteristically the tumor mass grows predominantly upward, is subfrontal, has well-defined boundaries, and is rounded in shape. Sphenocavernous tumors are attached mainly to the external wall of CS, are anteroposteriorly oriented, and extend toward the posterior fossa through the free margin of the tentorium or anteriorly through the superior orbital fissure into the orbital apex, usually as a diffuse infiltration instead of as a well-defined mass. Hyperostosis is usually a less prominent feature of this tumor than in clinoidal tumors.[1, 2]

## Magnetic Resonance Imaging

Magnetic resonance imaging (MRI) cannot demonstrate bony architecture as well as CT. Intracranial calcifications noted on skull films or CT can be missed by MRI. MRI surpasses CT, however, in demonstrating normal and pathologic intracranial anatomy.

Meningiomas may have signal intensity similar to that of brain tissue on $T_1$-weighted and $T_2$-weighted sequences. The signal intensities of meningiomas vary widely, and some are hyperintense on $T_2$-weighted images because there are a number of histologic varieties of meningiomas. Usually, syncytial and angioblastic meningiomas present higher signal intensity on $T_2$-weighted images than transitional cell or fibroblastic meningiomas. Meningiomas tend to enhance uniformly after gadolinium injection. There may be some lack of homogeneity in the appearance of meningiomas related to calcifications and cyst formations, which can appear in some cases. Sphenoidal wing meningiomas are prone to causing hyperostosis of adjacent bone. The hyperostosis, most commonly involving the greater and lesser sphenoid wings and clinoid processes, is not as well seen as with CT, as mentioned previously.

MRI can identify the position of the ICA, MCA, and other vessels by flow void, and it can define the relationship of the ICA to the tumor better than digital subtraction angiography. A few meningiomas have visible vessels within them, seen as small curvilinear flow voids.

Gadolinium enhancement allows good anatomic definition of the CS. It is also useful in defining the extent of the meningiomatous plaque, which on CT scan can be difficult to distinguish from the adjacent hyperostosis and the thickening of adjacent dura (dura tail sign). In cases of parasellar or CS meningioma, the ICA may be encased and may become narrowed or occluded.

At present, MRA may be considered an important complement of MRI, which can be performed simultaneously. It can replace digital subtraction angiography in the preoperative assessment of sphenoidal meningiomas. It is generally not a satisfactory method of showing tumor vascularity; however, the circle of Willis and large intracranial vessels are well depicted.

## TREATMENT

Surgery is the primary treatment for meningiomas. Although it is difficult in most sphenoid ridge meningiomas, radical excision of the tumor is the aim of surgical intervention.[6, 8, 10] Meningiomas of the sphenocavernous or clinoidal type that involve the inner third of the sphenoid ridge present problems different from those of tumors of the outer third of the sphenoid ridge.[1, 6, 8] Sphenocavernous meningiomas arise from the external wall of the CS, in-

volve the oculomotor or trigeminal nerve, penetrate the CS, and constrict the ICA in a ring-like fashion. In these cases, total resection of the tumor is impossible. A resection of the nodular portion and coagulation of the wall of the CS (Simpson II grade) is advised in patients whose ocular motility is not definitely altered. Conversely, excision of the nodular part, microsurgical carotid dissection, and resection of the tumor's osteodural attachment (Simpson I grade) are possible in patients with a pure clinoidal tumor.[1, 11] Patients with pterional meningiomas en plaque have proptosis, frontotemporal bowing, and palpebral edema. The tumor, which originates in the pterion, spreads to proliferate in the dura, periorbital tissues, and zygomatic fossa. In these cases, complete resection can be performed except if the CS or the orbital apex is infiltrated by the lesion. Some classic papers propose that no surgical intervention be undertaken in patients with slow-growing, non–life-threatening tumors.[12] Guiot and coworkers[13, 14] recommended surgery to preserve vision, to effect orbital decompression, and to reduce proptosis except in cases of periorbital meningiomas, in which a complete resection is possible. More recently, some authors proposed a radical resection of these tumors, including the intracavernous component together with the encased ICA, with or without saphenous vein graft reconstruction.[15–17] There is no unanimous agreement with this attitude, and the matter is still open to debate.

## SURGICAL TECHNIQUE

### Pterional Meningiomas

In pterional meningiomas, surgery is performed with the head slightly elevated, to improve the venous return, and positioned 30 to 45 degrees away from the side of the lesion. A frontotemporal approach is used through a hemicoronal incision concealed behind the hairline. This approach permits a wide superior orbital edge exposure and allows one to obtain a pericranial graft, which may be used to close the dura later during the operation. The thickened pterion is resected starting with bur holes and rongeurs, then high-speed drills are employed to remove the hyperostosis progressively, excising the roof and lateral wall of the orbit and carrying the surgery into the floor of the middle cranial fossa. The superior orbital fissure is decompressed, as is the optic canal, if necessary. All of the bone in this area can be resected (Figs. 24–2 and 24–3). Once the involved bone is removed, a frontal craniotomy is performed enlarging the dural exposure as necessary, according to the extension of the tumor.[1, 5]

Next the orbital contents are explored. Three principal appearances are possible: (1) diffuse thickening of periorbital tissue, (2) nodular tumor formation, or (3) micronodular infiltration of the elements of the apex. Total excision is likely with the first two possibilities but not when the tumor has infiltrated the structures at the orbital apex.[1]

After opening of the dura of the anterior cranial fossa, the intracranial tumor mass is identified. If a small plaque of tumor is attached to thickened dura and covers the sphenoid ridge, dura and tumor are en bloc resected. Alter-

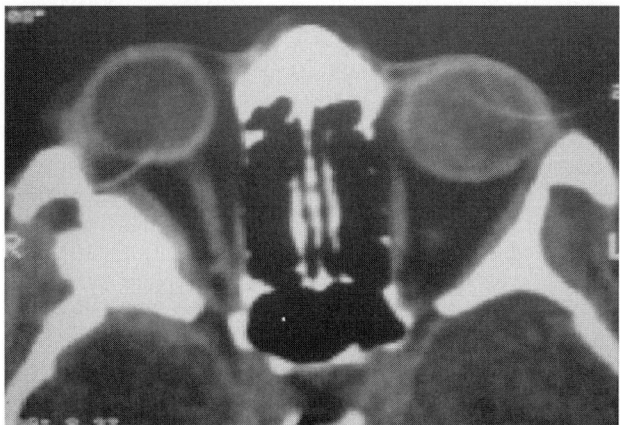

FIGURE 24–2 ■ A computed tomography scan with an axial view of a hyperostosing en plaque meningioma.

natively the tumor mass may be nodular and extend deeply into the sylvian fissure, displacing the temporal lobe and, to a lesser degree, the frontal lobe. Microsurgical techniques allow the careful dissection of tumor from the MCA and its branches. The ICA and optic nerve may be hidden by the lesion if the tumor has grown medially. Intradural tumor excision should be performed in a piecemeal fashion with the use of bipolar coagulation, microdissection, and ultrasonic aspiration. The infiltrated dura is resected to its medial limits. We have used dermal grafts from the buttocks to replace resected dura; however, this technique is bothersome and time-consuming. We have also used lyophilized dura for the same purpose. This material is relatively rigid, and its use presents more potential problems, such as the delayed development of Creutzfeldt-Jakob disease.[20, 21] We have used a periosteal flap fashioned from the tissues in the proximity of the craniotomy to close the dura. The periosteal graft is sutured to the dural defect and can then be further sealed, to obtain a watertight closure, with either fibrin glue or cyanoacrylate. No cerebrospinal leaks, collections of other fluids, or infections have occurred when we have used this technique to close the dura. At the beginning of our series, bony reconstruction was achieved with ribs that have been harvested, then split longitudinally through their cancellous portion. Each cortical fragment was fashioned to the bony defect and lateral wall of the orbit and was attached to the neighboring bone with stainless steel sutures. The use of methyl methacrylate has shortened the surgical procedure significantly by eliminating the need to harvest the rib grafts and to fashion several pieces of rib to the defect. If the pterional defect is small, it can be covered with the temporal muscle alone; however, if it is larger, it can also be repaired with either rib grafts, as initially in our series, or methyl methacrylate.[1, 5, 9] We have not employed iliac bone graft as it was proposed.[22, 23]

A different strategy is necessary for tumors that have spread to the zygomatic fossa and lower segments of the orbit or for tumors directly invading the malar bone. We have used an inferolateral access to the orbit instead of enlarged transcranial approaches at the beginning of our series.[22, 23] The transmalar approach is performed through a subciliary incision made in the lower lid that is extended

horizontally for approximately 3 cm. The subcutaneous plane is dissected from the orbicular muscle, exposing the lateral and inferior orbital rim, where the periosteum is divided. After the periosteal incision, the malar bone is widely exposed. A medial and anterior osteotomy is performed following the maxillozygomatic suture, using an oscillating saw; another osteotomy is made posteriorly and laterally in the zygomatic arcade; and another is made superiorly on the malar articulation with the frontal orbital process. The malar bone is removed in one piece, exposing the orbital inferolateral sectors and the zygomatic fossa. Tumoral tissue is extirpated up to the apex, reaching the site of the transcranial access. When the malar bone is normal, it is replaced using titanium low-profile bone plates and screws at the osteotomy sites to restore the form of the orbital cavity. When the malar bone is macroscopically infiltrated by tumor, the area can be reconstructed with rib grafts or with methyl methacrylate. After routine closure, temporary tarsorrhaphy is performed to protect the eye.[1, 5, 9] At present, thanks to earlier diagnosis, malar invasion is rarely found, and this technique is exceptionally employed.

## Inner and Middle Third Meningiomas

Inner third sphenoid ridge meningiomas are divided into clinoidal and sphenocavernous tumors.[1, 6, 8] The clinoidal tumors have a dural attachment on the upper part of the anterior clinoid process, whereas the sphenocavernous tumors are attached in the sphenocavernous angle. For operations on tumors of this location, the patient is placed in a supine position, and the head is slightly raised and turned 45 degrees to the side opposite the lesion. A pterional or frontopterional craniotomy is recommended. Depending on the tumor size, the lesser wing of the sphenoid is resected to the superior orbital fissure, allowing exposure of the lesion with a minimum of brain retraction. After the dura is opened, the tumor capsule is identified and coagulated with a bipolar unit. The capsule is opened, and the bulk of the tumor is removed with the use of curets, scissors, bipolar coagulation, ultrasonic aspirator, or the carbon dioxide laser. The site of dural implantation is identified, and the tumor's feeding vessels are coagulated. These vessels are almost always meningeal branches from the internal

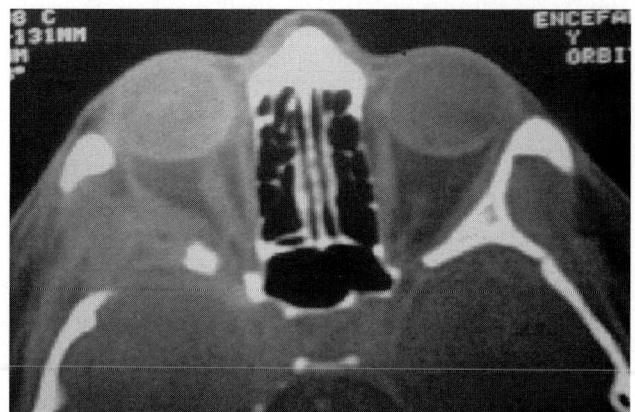

FIGURE 24–3 ■ A postoperative computed tomography scan of the same patient showing the extent of bone resection.

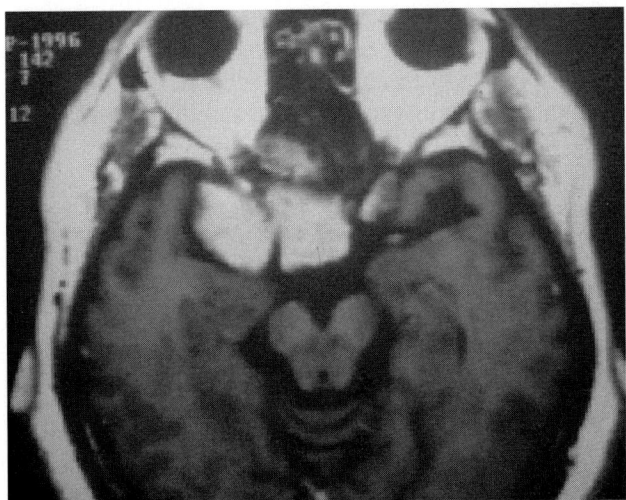

FIGURE 24–4 ■ A T₁-weighted magnetic resonance imaging scan of a clinoidal meningioma with encasement of the internal carotid artery.

maxillary artery and intracavernous branches of the ICA that supply the tumor. The supraclinoidal ICA and the MCA trunk and its branches must be handled carefully to avoid injury. The grade I Simpson technique of radical extirpation of a clinoidal meningioma is nearly always possible (Figs. 24–4 and 24–5). This technique involves complete macroscopic excision of the tumor and its osteodural implant. For sphenocavernous tumors with which a neurologic deficit has occurred because of abnormalities of ocular movements, extracavernous extirpation with coagulation of the dural attachment is advised (Simpson II technique).[11, 24] In sphenocavernous meningiomas with CS invasion, complete ophthalmoplegia, and involvement of trigeminal nerve, radical surgery is necessary to extirpate the lesion. In these cases, after the lesser wing of the sphenoid is resected, one must unroof the orbit, remove the anterior clinoid process, open the optic canal, and approach the CS through its superior wall to reach the intracavernous nodular portion of the meningioma.[25] The

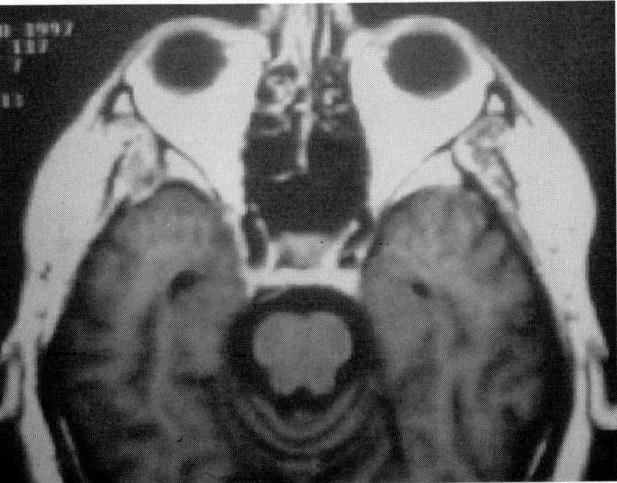

FIGURE 24–5 ■ A postoperative magnetic resonance imaging scan of the same case demonstrating complete resection sparing the internal carotid artery.

tumor is then removed with an ultrasonic aspirator or vaporized with the carbon dioxide laser. This technique does not guarantee that the tumor will not recur as a result of meningiomatous cells lying in the dural base.[26] Cerebrospinal fluid leakage and infection can be avoided by the use of a watertight closure of the dura, which may involve the use of pericranium and fibrin glue.[1, 9]

## RESULTS

In the past 25 years, 105 patients with sphenoid ridge meningiomas have been treated at the Hospital Santa Lucia, Buenos Aires, Argentina. This hospital is the regional ophthalmologic and neurosurgical institute that deals with tumors of the skull base and of the visual system. Of the 105 patients, 36 had meningiomas of the inner third of the sphenoid ridge, 21 had meningiomas of the middle third of the sphenoid ridge, and 48 had meningiomas at the pterion. Patients included 86 women and 19 men, most of whom were in their 40s.

Immediately after operation, the patients were classified into one of four categories according to their results: good (no sequelae), fair (minor sequelae), poor (severe sequelae), or death. Of the patients with inner third meningiomas, 29 patients (80.55%) had good results, 2 had fair results, 1 had poor results, and 4 died. In the middle third type, 14 patients (66%) had good results, 3 had fair results, 2 had poor results, and 2 died. In the pterional type, 43 patients (89.58%) had good results, 4 (8.33%) had fair results, 1 had poor results, and no one died. Of the entire patient group, 81.90% had good results, and an overall operative mortality rate of 5.71% was noted. These results are consistent with other reports that consider the surgical technique and stress the difficulties involved in the radical resection of sphenocavernous angle meningiomas, especially in relation to the supraclinoid ICA and its branches. Of the six deaths in our series, four resulted from a cerebral infarction as a consequence of a carotid or sylvian lesion, and the other two were from irreversible postoperative cerebral edema. This series spanned a long period of time, and most complications and deaths occurred at the beginning of the series. The use of microsurgical techniques has improved mortality and morbidity rates in our experience as well as in other series from the literature.[8, 15, 27, 28] The main causes of fair and poor results were extraocular muscle dysfunction, generally partial or transient; persistent exophthalmos; hemiparesis; and, less frequently, visual impairment.

Tumor recurrence is an important issue, mainly for the inner third location. From our experience and according to most authors, meningiomas from the skull base are associated with the highest rate of tumor recurrence.[29] This high recurrence rate is due to the particular anatomic characteristics of skull base meningiomas, especially those located at the sphenoid ridge, with their wide base of dural attachment, invasion of the CS, invasion of the underlying bone, and propagation of the tumor through the foramens and fissures of the skull base into the orbit and zygomatic fossa. Sixty-two of our patients (53 women and 9 men) were followed for 5 to 20 years postoperatively. Among these patients, 26 had inner third meningiomas, 8 had middle third meningiomas, and 28 had external third meningiomas. Seven recurrences were found in the first group (26.92%), two were found in the second group (25%), and five were found in the third group (17.85%). These findings represent a 22.58% recurrence rate at 10 years for the 62 patients who underwent surgery for meningiomas of the sphenoid ridge. Twelve of the patients with recurrences were reoperated on, and all of them received radiotherapy, which appears to halt the growth of the tumor.[30] The mean time of tumor recurrence was 6.2 years after surgery.

For recurrent meningiomas, reoperation is the most effective treatment. Alternative treatments, such as radiosurgery, high-energy radiotherapy, hormone therapy, and ultraselective catheterization for local injection of cytostatic drugs, can also be used as adjuvants.

## RADIOSURGERY

The microneurosurgeon is reaching the realistic limits of his or her surgical abilities for tumors within the CS. The difficulty of achieving complete resection compounded with the desire to maintain good clinical postoperative performance of the patient makes the task of complete tumor excision grand, if not impossible. Infiltration of tumor into the cranial nerves within the CS has been reported[20] requiring excision of the nerve or voluntary incompleteness of resection. The carotid artery has proved to be the ultimate deciding factor with regard to a surgeon's ability to resect these tumors completely. Kotapka and coworkers[31] reported 8 of 19 patients in their series had pathologic infiltration of the carotid artery, which led to the morbidity of their surgical resection as well as incompleteness of tumor removal. O'Sullivan and associates[32] in their series of 39 patients reported that the "degree of resectability is based on the degree of ICA involvement."

Tumor recurrence rates reported from series have ranged from 9% to 25% with 3.5-year median follow-ups.[33–36] The obvious shortcoming of these follow-up series is their limited follow-up. This shortcoming is substantiated by the long-term follow-up series of Mathiesen and colleagues.[37] In a 35-year follow-up series (from 1947 to 1982) for tumors of the skull base that were radically resected, 4% recurred within 5 years, and of grade III to IV tumors, 5-year recurrence was 25% to 45%. If followed for more than 5 years, the recurrence rate was 16% for grade I tumors, 20% for grade II, and "the majority" for grades IV/V; at 20 years, all tumors grade IV/V had recurred. If followed long enough, these tumors recur after incomplete surgical excision. For this reason, a biologic technique, such as radiosurgery, has an advantage over surgical resection if the tumor is appropriate for this technique.[38, 39]

Stereotactic radiosurgery is a potentially effective alternative to microsurgical removal of parasellar meningiomas. The goal of radiosurgery is preservation of neurologic function and prevention of further tumor growth.

Between May 1988 and January 1992, 34 patients (27 women and 7 men) with CS meningiomas underwent stereotactic radiosurgery using the 201-source $^{60}$Co Gamma knife at the University of Pittsburgh Medical Center, Pittsburgh, Pennsylvania. Patients were accepted for radiosurgery if the average tumor dimension was less than 35 mm in average diameter, if the tumor was sufficiently far from the optic nerves or tracts (usually >3 mm), and if primary or additional microsurgery was rejected (by physician, patient, or both) for fear of unacceptable risk.

## Clinical Response

Clinical evaluations after radiosurgery were performed by the treating or referring physician for all patients. The median clinical follow-up was 5.8 years (range, 0.5 to 10 years). Twenty-three patients (67%) were unchanged. Eight patients (24%, including one patient at 77 months) were improved after radiosurgery: Three had improved oculomotor nerve function, three had improvement of facial sensation, and two had both.

## Imaging Response

The median imaging follow-up interval for all 34 patients was 5.9 months (range, 2 to 10 years). No patient had evidence of tumor growth after radiosurgery (tumor control rate of 100%). Nineteen tumors (56%) regressed. Tumor regression became evident an average of 1.2 years after radiosurgery. Loss of central tumor contrast enhancement (presumed tumor necrosis) occurred in eight patients (24%); development of high T2 signal in the surrounding brain was observed in three patients (Figs. 24–6 and 24–7).

Under radiosurgical treatment, tumor control rates varied from 84% to 98%. The tumor control rate in the selected series of 34 patients followed for a median of 5.8 years was 100%. The 100% tumor control rate may be due to tumor selection, experience, and technique. The median tumor volume treated in this series was 4 cm³, smaller than in most series reported.

Mortality and morbidity rates of surgery are higher than

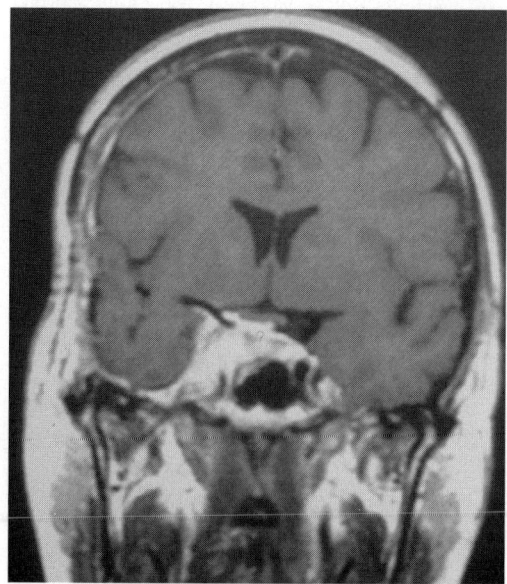

FIGURE 24–6 ■ A T₁-weighted magnetic resonance imaging scan with a coronal view of a right intracavernous meningioma.

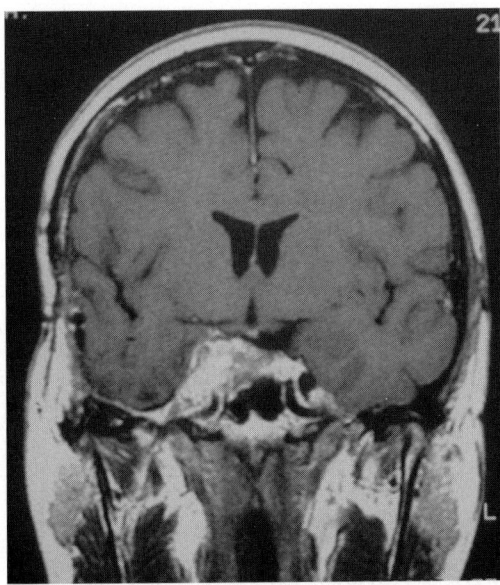

**FIGURE 24–7 ■** A magnetic resonance imaging scan of the same patient 8 months after radiosurgery showing a moderate reduction in the size of the tumor and a decrease in the central density of the mass.

those of radiosurgery. In our series, no patients died as a result of tumor progression or radiosurgery. This result contrasts sharply with the results of the surgical series. Taking into account that most surgical series that get published are those from the hands of experts in the field of skull base microsurgery, the morbidity and mortality rates are high, given the current standard of care from the radiosurgery series. In a study by Proust and colleagues[40] in a series of 39 skull base tumors treated microsurgically, 7.6% mortality and 10.3% morbidity rates were reported.

The general surgical morbidity resulting from microsurgical removal of these tumors varies. There are risks to the cranial nerves, risk to normal brain tissue during protracted retraction, and risk of stroke because of carotid manipulation (excision of tumor around the carotid or from bypass operations). The morbidity related to cranial nerves is also high in the surgical reports. This high morbidity is understandable and probably unavoidable given the anatomic relationship of these nerves to the tumors. O'Sullivan and associates[32] reported an 18% cranial nerve morbidity rate.

The resilience of the cranial nerves and intracranial carotid artery to high-dose, single-fraction radiosurgery has been reported in the past.[41–43] Leber and coworkers[44] in a series of 50 patients who had undergone Gamma knife radiosurgery for skull base meningiomas reported a zero optic neuropathy rate, at a median follow-up of 40 months, if the nerve and chiasm received less than 10 Gy.

There has been interest in using fractionated stereotactic radiation therapy to treat tumors in this region. Given the poor long-term historical results of fractionating radiation to meningiomas and the exceptionally high tumor control rates and low morbidity rates of Gamma knife radiosurgery, LINAC-based fractionated treatments need to prove their worth with similar long-term follow-up. These treatments are also more expensive than single-fraction radiosurgery using Gamma knife technique.

Chemotherapy has been used for meningiomas as well as progesterone-blocking hormonal therapies in recalcitrant cases of meningiomatosis. Promising results with the use of hydroxyurea for the treatment of recalcitrant meningiomas has been reported. Schrell and coworkers[45] in a small series of four patients over a 2-year follow-up, report a 100% tumor control rate with a zero complication rate.

Experienced skull base microneurosurgeons in centers where Gamma knife radiosurgery exists are increasingly becoming aware of the synergistic potential of expert microsurgery coupled with "mop-up" Gamma knife radiosurgery for residual or recurrent tumors. These same centers (20, which at one time devoted their use of radiosurgery to LINAC-based systems) have given up LINAC systems for Gamma knife technique because of increased ability to conform to the tumor with multiple isocenters, increased tumor control rates, and lower cranial neuropathy rates. Gamma knife technique appears by all reports to be the gold standard to which all other noninvasive techniques will be compared.

## REFERENCES

1. Basso A, Carrizo A: Sphenoid ridge meningiomas. In Schmidek H (ed): Meningiomas and Their Surgical Management. Philadelphia: WB Saunders, 1991, pp 233–241.
2. Benjamin V, McCormack B: Surgical management of tuberculum sellae and sphenoid ridge meningiomas. In Schmidek H, Sweet W (eds): Operative Neurosurgical Techniques. Philadelphia: WB Saunders, 1995, pp 403–413.
3. Cushing H, Eisenhardt L: Meningiomas: Their Classification, Regional Behavior, Life History, and Surgical End Results. Springfield, IL: Charles C Thomas, 1938, pp 298–319.
4. Bonnal J, Sedan R, Paillas J: Problemes cliniques, évolutifs et thérapeutiques souleves par les meningiomes envahissant de la base du crane. Neurochirurgie 7:l08–117, 1961.
5. Carrizo A, Basso A, Dickman G, et al: Combined approach to spheno-orbital tumors. (Abstract) 7th International Congress of Neurological Surgery, Munich, 1981, p 36.
6. Al-Mefty O: Clinoidal meningiomas. In Al-Mefty O (ed): Meningiomas. New York: Raven Press, 1991, pp 427–443.
7. Bonnal J, Thibaut A, Brotchi J, Born J: Invading meningiomas of the sphenoid ridge. J Neurosurg 53:587–599, 1980.
8. Sekhar L, Altschuler E: Meningiomas of the cavernous sinus. In Al-Mefty O (ed): Meningiomas. New York: Raven Press, 1991, pp 445–459.
9. Basso A, Carrizo A, Kreutel A, et al: La chirurgie des tumeurs spheno-orbitaires. Neurochirurgie 24:71–82, 1978.
10. Cook A: Total removal of large global meningiomas at the medial aspect of the sphenoid ridge. J Neurosurg 34:107–113, 1971.
11. Simpson D: The recurrence of intracranial meningiomas after surgical treatment. J Neurol Neurosurg Psychiatry 20:22–39, 1957.
12. Castellano F, Guidetti B, Olivecrona H: Pterional meningiomas en plaque. J Neurosurg 9:188–196, 1952.
13. Guiot G, Tessier P, Godon A: Faut-il operer les meningiomes en plaque de l'arete sphenoidale? Neurochirurgie 14:293–304, 1970.
14. Derome P, Guiot G: Bone problems in meningiomas invading the base of the skull. Clin Neurosurg 25:435–451, 1978.
15. Sekhar L, Moller A: Operative management of tumors involving the cavernous sinus. J Neurosurg 64:879–889, 1986.
16. Sekhar L, Sen C, Jho H: Saphenous vein graft bypass of the cavernous internal carotid artery. J Neurosurg 72:35–41, 1990.
17. Fukushima T, Díaz Day J: Surgical management of tumors involving the cavernous sinus. In Schmidek H, Sweet W (eds): Operative Neurosurgical Techniques. Philadelphia: WB Saunders, 1995, pp 493–510.
18. Brihaye J, Hofman G, Francois J: Les exophtalmies neurochirurgicales. Neurochirurgie 14:188–487, 1968.
19. Guyot J, Vouyouklakis D, Pertuiset B: Meningiomes de l'arete sphenoidale. Neurochirurgie (Paris) 13:571–584, 1967.
20. Lane K, Brown P, Howell D, et al: Creutzfeldt-Jakob disease in a

pregnant woman with an implanted dura mater graft. Neurosurgery 34:737–740, 1994.

21. Yamada S, Aiba T, Endo Y, et al: Creutzfeldt-Jakob disease transmitted by cadaveric dura mater graft. Neurosurgery 34:740–744, 1994.

22. Pellerin P, Lesoin F, Dhellemes R, et al: Usefulness of the orbito-fronto-malar approach associated with bone reconstruction for frontotemporosphenoid meningiomas. Neurosurgery 15:715–718, 1984.

23. Mickey B, Close L, Schaeffer S, et al: A combined frontotemporal and lateral infratemporal fossa approach to the skull base. J Neurosurg 68:678, 1988.

24. Cophignon J, Lucena J, Clay C, et al: Limits to radical treatment of spheno-orbital meningiomas. Acta Neurochir Suppl (Wien) 28:375–380, 1979.

25. Dolenc V: Microsurgical removal of large sphenoidal bone meningiomas. Acta Neurochir Suppl (Wien) 28:391–396, 1979.

26. Adegbite A, Khan M, Paine K, Tan L: The recurrence of intracranial meningiomas after surgical treatment. J Neurosurg 58:51–56, 1983.

27. Konovalov A, Fedorov S, Faller T, et al: Experience in the treatment of the parasellar meningiomas. Acta Neurochir (Suppl) 28:371–372, 1979.

28. Pompili A, Derome P, Visot A, Guiot G: Hyperostosing meningiomas of the sphenoid ridge. Surg Neurol 17:411–416, 1982.

29. Philippon J, Bataini J, Cornu P, et al: Les meningiomes recidivants. Neurochirurgie 32(Suppl 1):l–84, 1986.

30. Barbaro N, Gutin P, Wilson C, et al: Radiation therapy in the treatment of partially resected meningiomas. Neurosurgery 20:525–527, 1987.

31. Kotapka MJ, Kalia K, Martinez AJ, et al: Infiltration of the carotid artery by cavernous sinus meningioma. J Neurosurg 81:252–255, 1994.

32. O'Sullivan MG, van Loveren HR, Tew JM Jr: The surgical resectability of meningiomas of the cavernous sinus. Neurosurgery 40:238–244, 1997.

33. Adegbite AB, Khan MI, Paine KWE, et al: The recurrence of intracranial meningiomas after surgical treatment. J Neurosurg 58:51–56, 1983.

34. Melamed SH, Sahar A, Beller AJ: The recurrence of intracranial meningiomas. Neurochirurgie 22:47–51, 1979.

35. Miraminoff RO, Dosoretz DE, Linggood RM, et al: Meningioma: Analysis of recurrence and progression following neurosurgical resection. J Neurosurg 62:18–24, 1985.

36. Philippon J, Cornu P: The recurrence of meningiomas. In Al-Mefty O (ed): Meningiomas. New York: Raven Press, 1991, pp 87–105.

37. Mathiesen T, Lindquist C, Kihlstrom L, et al: Recurrence of cranial base meningiomas. Neurosurgery 39:2–7, 1996.

38. Ojemann RG: Skull base surgery: A perspective. J Neurosurg 76:569–570, 1992.

39. Suzuki M, Mizoi K, Yoshimoto T: Should meningiomas involving the cavernous sinus be totally resected? Surg Neurol 44:3–10, 1995.

40. Proust F, Verdure L, Toussaint P, et al: Intracranial meningioma in the elderly: Postoperative mortality, morbidity and quality of life in a series of 39 patients over 70 years of age. Neurochirurgie 43:15–20, 1997.

41. Duma CM, Lunsford LD, Kondziolka D, et al: Stereotactic radiosurgery of cavernous sinus meningiomas as an addition or alternative to microsurgery. Neurosurgery 32:699–705, 1993.

42. Nilsson A, Wennerstrand J, Leksell D, et al: Stereotactic gamma irradiation of basilar artery in cat: Preliminary experiences. Acta Radiol Oncol 17:150–160, 1978.

43. Tishler RB, Loeffler JS, Lunsford LD, et al: Tolerance of cranial nerves of the cavernous sinus to radiosurgery. Int J Radiat Oncol Biol Phys 27:215–221, 1993.

44. Leber KA, Bergloff J, Pendl G: Dose-response tolerance of the visual pathways and cranial nerves of the cavernous sinus to stereotactic radiosurgery. J Neurosurg 88:43–50, 1998.

45. Schrell UMH, Rittig MG, Anders M, et al: Hydroxyurea for treatment of unresectable and recurrent meningiomas. II: Decrease in the size of meningiomas in patients treated with hydroxyurea. J Neurosurg 86:840–844, 1997.

# Cavernous Sinus (Lateral Sellar Compartment)

# CHAPTER 25

# Anatomy of the Lateral Sellar Compartment (Cavernous Sinus)

■ DWIGHT PARKINSON

Within a shallow compartment, bounded by a double layer of dura laterally and superiorly and the periosteum of the sphenoid bone inferiorly and medially, lie the parasellar carotid and its branches; some veins; some autonomic nerves; portions of cranial nerves III, IV, V, and VI with accompanying meninges; and some adipose and connective tissue. Because the venous component is not singular, cavernous, or a true sinus, it is proposed that this area be called the *lateral sellar compartment* (LSC), Its coverings and contents are discussed in this chapter.

The biggest obstacle to understanding the anatomy and function of this anatomic area containing arteries, veins, myelinated and unmyelinated nerves, and adipose tissue is the persistence of the label *cavernous sinus*. The term is given two meanings at present. *Tumors* of the cavernous sinus can refer only to primary or secondary tumors within the compartment, whereas *thrombosis* of the cavernous sinus can refer only to the vessels within the compartment. The term *cavernous sinus* was given to this compartment by Winslow.[1] His descriptive term may have been based on Galen's[2] finding of the parasellar rete mirabile[3–5] in lower animals, which he then erroneously transposed to humans. Although Vesalius[6] corrected many of Galen's errors, he apparently did not examine this extradural compartment.

## COVERINGS AND SHAPE

The LSC is a slender extradural envelope that is a segmental enlargement of the extradural space along the neural axis from the sacrum to the orbit. The general contours of this compartment are determined by the medial aspect and lesser wing of the sphenoid bone, the superior orbital fissure, the anterior and posterior clinoids, and the tip of the petrous pyramid. Its average measurements are anteroposterior, 2 cm; transverse depth, 0.7 cm; and vertical depth, 1.3 cm. The double-layered dura of the clivus below the dorsum becomes part of the posterior wall of this space. Anteriorly, the compartment tapers and twists about 20 degrees on its vertical axis to continue through the superior orbital fissure into the orbit (Fig. 25–1). Posteriorly and superiorly, this compartment twists nearly 90 degrees to continue as a shallow space over the dorsum containing the basilar plexus of veins along with some adipose tissue to the foramen magnum, where it becomes continuous with the spinal epidural space containing adipose tissue and a plexus of veins known as *Batson's plexus* (see Figs. 25–1B and 25–5). Inferiorly and laterally the LSC funnels into a sleeve around the carotid through the foramen lacerum (see Figs. 25–1A–C and 25–3B–E), beneath whose sleeve there is also a plexus of veins with surrounding fat (see Fig. 25–5).

The two-layered dura along the floor of the middle fossa is slightly adherent to the bone except at the various foramina and fissures and at the clinoids, where it is firmly attached. At the upper border of the second division of cranial nerve V, the two layers of dura elevate from the surface of the middle fossa to form the lateral wall of the LSC. The outer layer of this lateral wall is much thicker than the inner layer (see Fig. 25–1E).[16, 17] The lateral wall continues upward, then forms the roof as it joins with the thickened tentorial extensions attaching to the posterior clinoid and then to the anterior clinoid. There is a small groove between these thickened tentorial attachments, into which the third and frequently the fourth nerves enter (see Fig. 25–1D). Medial to their entrance, lateral to the pituitary, and behind the carotid exit, which is firmly attached, the roof is thin, providing one of several surgical approaches. Further anteriorly the roof thickens into a tough, fibrous encirclement of the departing carotid artery. Medially the roof is continuous with the diaphragma sella (see Fig. 25–1D). The coverings of the pituitary, the lattermost of which form part of the medial wall of the LSC, may be of separate origin. All walls of this compartment contain appropriately sized nutrient vessels continuous with the adjacent meningeal systems from both the internal and the external carotid branches. The lower posterior limit usually includes the upper portion of the gasserian ganglion and extends along the upper margin of the second division of cranial nerve V. Anteriorly the lower limit runs along the first division of cranial nerve V (see Fig. 25–1A and E).

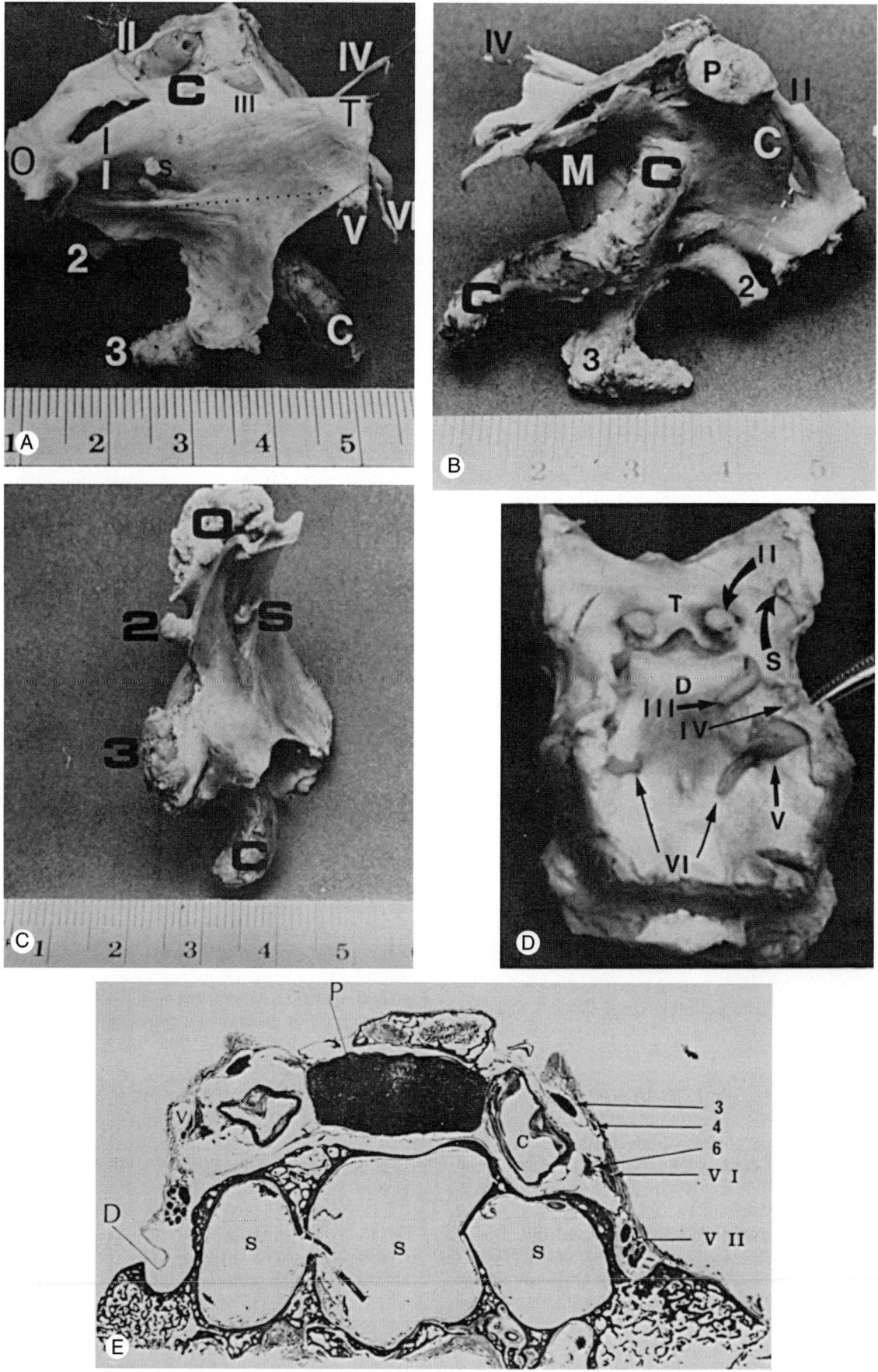

FIGURE 25–1 ■ *See legend on opposite page*

# NERVES

Anatomy texts vary enormously in that they show different spacings between cranial nerves III, IV, V, and VI. One author stated that the relationship is "actually of no clinical importance as the nerves are grouped so closely that a lesion is apt to affect all together,"[12] overlooking Jefferson's[13] findings. The third and fourth nerves always enter this compartment from above (see Fig. 25–1D), whereas the fifth and sixth nerves enter much lower down in the posterior fossa (see Fig. 25–1D and E). The entrance of the fifth cranial nerve from the posterior fossa looks as though a three-fingered hand had been pushed forward and downward, dragging with it the posterior fossa meninges, including the subarachnoid space, which form a pocket known as *Meckel's cave*. In some individuals, this meningeal pouch extends along the three divisions beyond the gasserian ganglion, and in others, it ends at the ganglion.[18] The medial wall of this pocket is much thinner than the outer wall, which becomes incorporated in the lateral wall of the LSC (see Fig. 25–1E). The entrances of the third, fourth, and sixth nerves are also accompanied by meningeal sleeves for varying distances. Thus, there are several extensions of arachnoid into the LSC. Beyond their arachnoid sleeves, the third, fourth, and fifth nerves are all firmly adherent in their dural tunnels, which are formed entirely from the thin inner layer of the two-layered lateral wall. (There are three layers of dural origin over these nerves.)

The sixth nerve is relatively loose in the LSC (see Fig. 25–1E). From their dural entrances, the parallel third and fourth nerves form the upper border of a triangle,[9] whereas the first division of the fifth nerve, within the dura, and the sixth, within the LSC, form the lower border as they all converge to exit at the superior orbital fissure. The base of this triangle is the dura of the clivus (see Fig. 25–1A and

D). This triangular space provides the most direct approach to the LSC.[14, 15]

The difficulty with the anatomy texts and some articles[11, 12] is that they were using specimens in which the nerves were dissected free of their surroundings, or skeletonized. In this situation, the nerves tend to hang down from whatever position the specimen was held. The correct relationship of cranial nerves III, IV, VI, and the first division of V is shown in Figures 25–1A, D and 25–2B. The space between cranial nerves III and IV above and V and VI below is evident. This distance is the base of the triangular space as the nerves converge forward to exit at the superior orbital fissure. The coronal section (see Fig. 25–1E) demonstrates the space between cranial nerves III and IV above and the first division of V and VI below at the midpituitary coronal level.

# ARTERIES

Before entering this compartment, the carotid artery is enclosed in a thick, tough fibrous sheath, which, in turn, is firmly adherent to the surrounding bone and fibrous tissue of the foramen lacerum. This sheath is continuous with the walls of the LSC (see Figs. 25–1A–C and 25–3B, C). Within the LSC, the carotid is slightly adherent to the medial wall proximally, then becomes relatively free along the anterior siphon. In most specimens, there are a few slender fibrous strands anchoring this segment of the carotid artery to the compartment walls. The veins go around these strands; none of the strands appears to go through any of the veins. At point of exit, the carotid is again enclosed in a fibrous encirclement formed in the roof of the LSC.

Despite complete trapping (the common method of treatment previously), some lateral sellar carotid venous (cav-

---

**FIGURE 25–1** ■ *A*, An adult male. The Left lateral sellar compartment (LSC) is removed from bone with sufficient soft tissue margin for orientation, lateral view. (Black 1, the position of the first division entering the superior orbital fissure. The *white 1* below completes the fissure extent. 2, second division emerging from the inferior boundary of the LSC; 3, third division entering the otic ganglion; II, IV, V, VI, the corresponding cranial nerves; III, third cranial nerve; S, sylvian vein entering the lateral wall.) *Black C* is placed just below the exit of the carotid above the dura. *White C* represents the carotid sheath where it would be going through foramen lacerum. *Black O* represents the posterior orbit being entered by optic nerve, which is above the space for the optic strut. The proximal cut end of the optic nerve is just below 11. Between and above III and IV is seen the sloping dorsum and basis, which continues with the same slope behind the tentorium, T. (*Dotted line,* average lower margin of the LSC along the upper edge of the second division anteriorly and across the gasserian ganglion posteriorly).

*B*, Medial aspect of the same specimen. (*White dotted line,* superior orbital fissure). *Black C* is the carotid artery sheathed in an extension of the LSC through the foramen lacerum. The uppermost black C marks the entrance of the carotid from the foramen into the LSC. *White C* marks the contour of the anterior carotid syphon within the LSC. (P, medial aspect of the pituitary sectioned in the mid-sagittal plane; M, Meckel's cave within the LSC. Immediately above M is the continuation of the LSC space into the basilar plexus space. 11, Optic nerve, going through the optic canal above the space for the orbital strut, then appearing again in the amputated posterior orbital cone.

*C*, An anterior view of the same specimen. (C, carotid artery within the sheath through the foramen lacerum; S, sylvian vein entrance; O, posterior surface of amputated orbit; 2, second division; 3, otic ganglion as the third division joins it.)

*D*, View from above the parasellar structures. (II to VI, arrows to the respective cranial nerves; T, tuberculum; D, dorsum; S, sylvian vein going down to enter the lateral wall of the LSC. Forcep holds out the cut margin of the tentorium laterally. (From Smith J [ed]: Neurophthalmology. St. Louis; Mosby-Year Book, 1972.)

*E*, Coronal section of LSC, in a 60-year-old man. (S, sphenoid sinuses; P, Pituitary gland; C carotid arteries, both of which have large atheromatous plaques. The numbers 3, 4, and 6 represent the cranial nerves. Note that 3 and 4 are within a dural sleeve formed from the thin inner layer of the lateral wall, which is best seen at the arrow tip for 3. The numbers V I and V II represent the first and second divisions of fifth cranial nerve. D represents the dura, which has separated from the bone on the left. It consists of two layers throughout the lateral wall. The floor of the LSC consists of the periosteum of the sphenoid bone. The coverings of the pituitary itself, part of which constitute part of the medial wall of the LSC, may have an entirely separate origin. Some thin veins are visible along the floor of the sella. (V, sylvian vein on the left on its way through the lateral wall to enter the plexus of veins in LSC.) In addition to the slender veins continuing along the floor of the sella, there are more beneath the right carotid artery, as well as larger veins above and lateral to both carotid arteries. The adipose tissue is minimal. The space between 4 and 6 represents the midportion of the triangular space.

ernous) fistulas may persist and increase. Such cases indicate that there are normally present collateral branches to and from the trapped segment of internal carotid. They must be normally present because the existence of a fistula does not cause new vessels to grow into or out of the lumen of a major artery such as the carotid. It was easy to demonstrate the existence of such collateral circulation by appropriate ligation and water injection studies on cadavers,[14, 19] but finding these anastomotic vessels was not so easy because they were thin walled, transparent, and adherent to the carotid artery for a considerable distance beyond their origin (Fig. 25–2A). Once physicians learned how and where to look, however, these collateral branches were found consistently.[20] Almost simultaneously, some were demonstrated at another center.[21] The parasellar carotid branches have been discussed elsewhere (see Fig. 25–2B), and their presence and many variations have been verified by several investigators, some with different terminology,[22–24, 29, 30, 45, 65] using cadaver dissection, operating room exposure, and angiographic definition.[22, 24] The significant feature is that collateral arteries exist between the two parasellar carotid arteries as well as between these segments and the external system. If they are cut, these vessels bleed equally from either end. Casts of the circulatory systems of stillborn infants in the Hunterian Museum in the Royal College Building in London (specimens K-391-1 and K-427-2) that are more than 200 years old show parasellar carotid branches, which have not been mentioned by Hunter or apparently by any subsequent curator.

Although some authors have attempted to classify these arteries embryologically,[25] their developmental origin remains unknown. My colleagues and I have corresponded extensively with Paget[30] and have sent her all our work. She finally concluded that she did not think they represented any of the standard developmental arteries of the region. The adherence of these thin-walled branches to or even within the adventitia of the carotid artery often misleads investigators into describing separate departures a few millimeters from the actual origins. In Basset's[31] stereoscopic atlas, some of these vessels can be seen, although they are not mentioned.

The dorsal meningeal artery and the inferior hypophysial artery, two constant branches of the meningohypophysial artery, form an anastomotic circle around the dorsum. When McConnell's (capsular) artery[32] is present across the floor of the sella, it completes a figure-eight configuration of anastomosis (see Fig. 25–2C). All of these arteries except McConnell's artery have direct external carotid connections as well as the obvious intercarotid artery anastomoses. It is immediately evident that there are two types of fistulas that could spill arterial blood into the parasellar veins: (1) an opening in the carotid itself and (2) a tear in one of these anastomotic branches. No amount of trapping or embolization of the internal carotid could control the distal flow in the second type of fistula, which is a dural wall type of fistula. Because some of these branches, particularly the dorsal meningeal artery, come into more intimate contact with bone than does the carotid artery itself, they may be more susceptible to tears when trauma occurs.

If a surgically or endovascularly trapped carotid artery segment includes a patent ophthalmic artery, a fistula is free to steal from the retinal perfusion pressure with the attendant risk of permanent blindness.[33–35] The small lateral sellar arteries usually are not large enough to offset this steal (see Fig. 25–2C). In such situations, the ophthalmic artery should be occluded first, even if for only a few minutes. The external carotid ophthalmic collateral artery is adequate for retinal circulation.[35]

Once it was examined with care, the anatomy of this space was self-evident and was confirmed by several investigators with general agreement on the findings. Two areas remain in dispute or unknown—the sympathetic anatomy and the venous anatomy.

## SYMPATHETIC PATHWAYS

The LSC sympathetic anatomy remains incompletely defined. There are even more variations here than in the vascular anatomy, variations that become more apparent with more numerous dissections (Fig. 25–3). The classic textbook depiction is of a loosely woven plexus on the adventitia of the carotid artery continuing along the ophthalmic artery. From this plexus, branches are shown to the various structures along the way. Finally, from this carotid plexus or its continuation along the ophthalmic artery, a branch is drawn going through the ciliary ganglion to the pupil (usually this branch is illustrated by dotted lines). The pathways controlling skin temperature and sweating to the head are assumed to follow the external carotid branches. Several factors can be viewed as evidence that this depiction is incorrect: (1) I have never observed, read, or heard of a report of Horner's syndrome resulting from clipping and even sectioning the ophthalmic artery, unless additional damage exists.[36, 37] (2) I as well as others[36, 37] have witnessed complete transection of the parasellar carotid, and Horner's syndrome did not result. (3) Elsewhere in the body, blood vessels receive their sympathetic supply at intervals via the peripheral nerves with which the autonomic fibers are traveling. (4) In the other extremities, if a peripheral nerve is sectioned, sympathetic changes within the distribution of that nerve result. If a peripheral blood vessel is sectioned, there are no corresponding sympathetic changes. I have found that the carotid sympathetic nerve from the superior sympathetic ganglion follows the carotid artery and is slightly adherent to the adventitia, giving off branches to the carotid artery and other structures intracranially. Then most of the dwindling residual of the nerve usually joins the sixth cranial nerve (see Fig. 25–3A–E).[39] A few fibers may continue beyond the carotid artery,[38, 39, 41] and some may join the third nerve. (Monro[40] drew this identical sixth nerve connection in 1732, and it was apparently soon overlooked and forgotten.) Next I have found that these sympathetic fibers merely adhere to the sixth nerve for a few millimeters, then usually leave it to join the first division of the fifth nerve at or just before the two nerves enter the superior orbital fissure.[39, 41] The sympathetics may leave the sixth nerve in one large bundle or in several small threads. These connections are visible but are not mentioned in the article by Conesa and associates[16] on the blood supply to the cranial nerves. I have been unable to follow the greatly dispersed sympathetics further within the first division, although in one specimen,

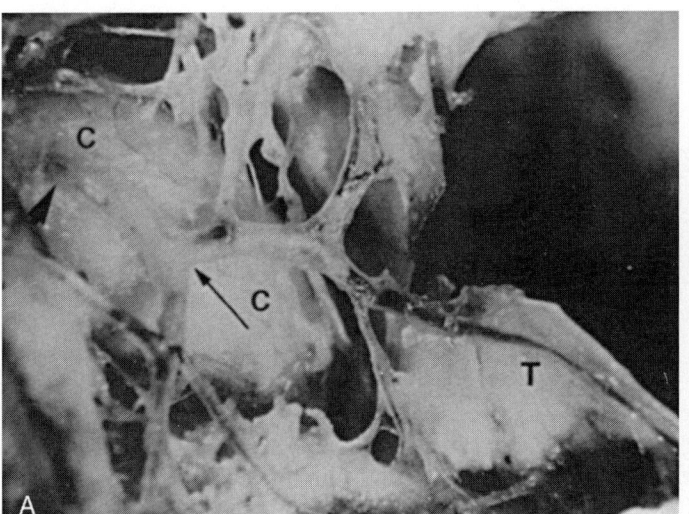

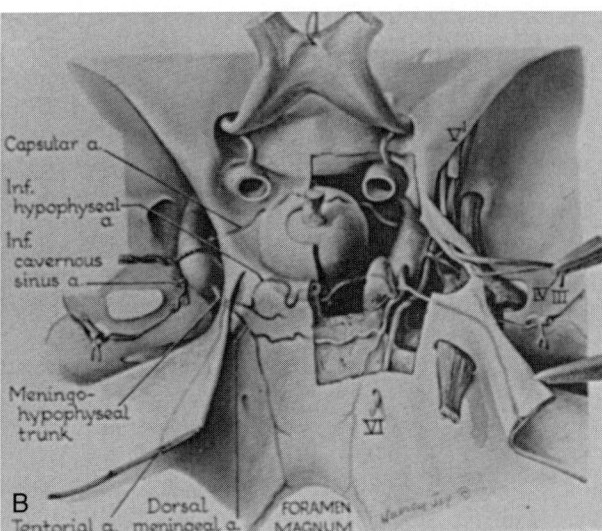

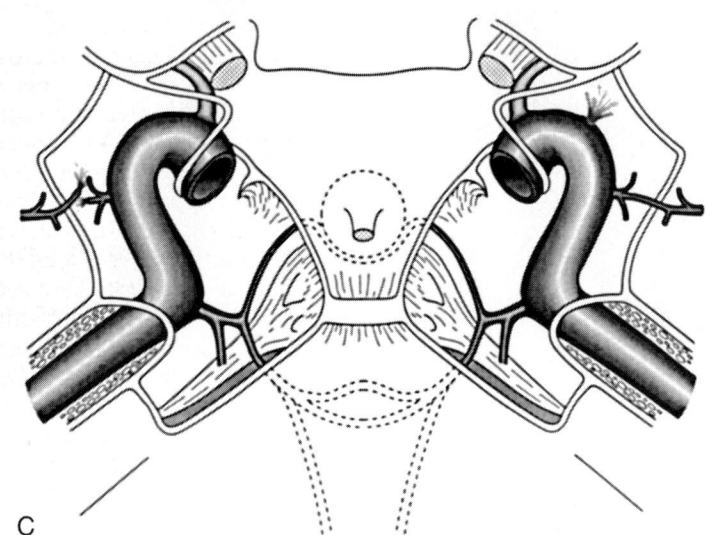

FIGURE 25–2 ■ Dissection of the right lateral sellar compartment (LSC) is pulled open and viewed from above, showing intermittently filled meningohypophysial trunk and branches. The *thick arrowhead* represents the departure of the meningohypophysial trunk from the carotid (C). The thin arrow lying on the carotid points to the first bifurcation. The left branch becomes the dorsal meningeal artery, which in this case gives rise to the inferior hypophysial artery going back up beneath the shaft of the *thick arrow*. The right branch becomes primarily the tentorial artery running above the T, which labels the tentorium. Note that the empty segments of these intermittently filled arteries resemble translucent connective tissue fibers, which are easily mistaken for trabeculae. Numerous venous channels and irregular bits of adipose tissue complete the picture.

*B,* The average position and connections of the branches of the parasellar carotid arteries, together with their relationship to the cranial nerves. The essential feature is the direct anastomosis between the two parasellar carotids and with the external system; the inferior lateral compartment artery to the middle meningeal artery seen on left is best example. The dorsal meningeal anastomoses directly with branches of the posterior fossa and cervical meningeal arteries. The cranial nerve arrangement is accurately shown on the right, with III and IV entering above and V and VI entering below. The triangular space is evident following these nerves forward. (From Parkinson D: Collateral circulation of cavernous carotid artery: Anatomy. Can J Surg 7:251–268, 1964.)

*C,* Diagram of the parasellar collaterals and the meningohypophyseal, which are capable of the perpetuating a fistula. The LSC is drawn as being devoid of veins. On the right, a tear in the carotid itself, which is a type 1 fistula, is shown. It is evident that if distal occlusion for trapping is above the ophthalmic, then retinal perfusion pressure is at risk. On the left, a tear in one of the anastomotic channels, a type 2 fistula, is shown. Usually, it appears within the dura.

Steal is insignificant from either hemisphere or eye, even if the carotid is occluded, but trapping will not cure this fistula.

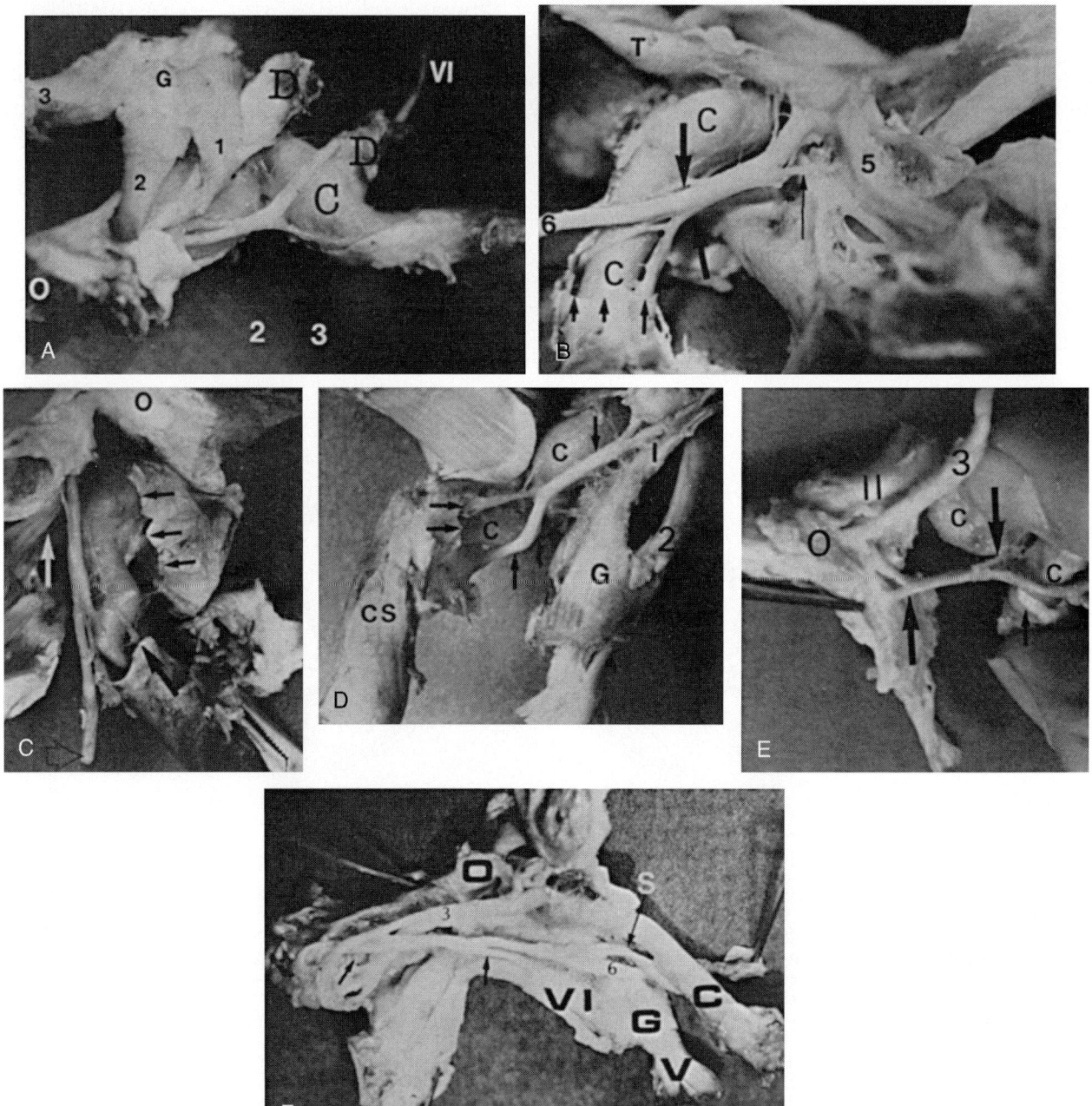

**FIGURE 25–3** ■ *See legend on opposite page*

multiple ganglion cells were found within the first division just after the sympathetic joined it, presumably an ectopic ciliary ganglion.[39]

This finding and the knowledge that the sympathetic pathways in the rest of the body follow the distribution of the peripheral nerves lead one to suspect that this pathway results in the eye abnormalities of Horner's syndrome when it is interrupted.[41] I also suspect that interruption of this pathway would result in decreased sweating within the distribution of the first division of the fifth cranial nerve because it is probable that the supply to the skin vessels and sweat glands follows the divisions of the fifth nerve. Both hypotheses are difficult to prove histologically and are impossible to prove on macroscopic examination. The closest example I have seen in 42 dissections is shown in Figure 25–3*F*. Proof will probably depend on two, as yet undiscovered, clinical syndromes as shown in Figure 25–4. Myles,[42] an ophthalmologist, has found one such patient, who has palsy of the sixth nerve, small pupils, a narrow fissure, normal sensation, and decreased sweating in the first division and who has some additional anhydrosis outside the distribution of the ipsilateral first division and is known to have a malignant tumor. Since publications by

my colleagues and I on this matter, there has been no further demonstration of these fibers or of their function beyond the putative syndromes.[41, 43, 44] Any autonomic supply to the cerebral vessels must accompany them from their dural entrance onward.[58, 59]

## VEINS

Because long-established fistulas result in thickened venous channels, it became apparent that a surgeon could be within this dural LSC, commonly called the *cavernous sinus*, and *outside* the venous channels.[14, 18] These surgical findings suggested that the normal anatomy is not a trabeculated venous cavern surrounding the carotid but rather a plexus of veins, as others have suspected.[47, 50] In cases of so-called carotid cavernous fistulas with slow trickles of contrast material and early films, angiography often demonstrates a discrete venous channel leaving the arterial opening. This channel might then go selectively in one or more of four main directions, which is unlikely if the artery were spilling

---

FIGURE 25–3 ■ Some common variations in the sympathetic pathways within the lateral sellar compartment (LSC) are shown. The sympathetic fibers are frequently flattened in one diameter, thus projecting larger or smaller than their true volume. The fat veins and most of the dural walls are removed.

*A,* Black 1, 2, and 3 represent the first division attached, second and third divisions sectioned of cranial nerve V with gasserian ganglion (G) hinged upward on the first division. White 2 and 3 represent positions that the respective division would occupy normally. If repositioned into the normal relationship, G would overly C. C represents the carotid with the sixth cranial nerve above being joined by the carotid sympathetic nerve from below, which has just emerged from the diagonally cut carotid dural sheath of the foramen lacerum. Proceeding forward *(lt),* the sympathetic nerve is then seen to leave the sixth cranial nerve as the uppermost branch and to enter the undersurface (medial) of the first division of the fifth cranial nerve. (Ds, tags of adherent dura, the lower of which (the sixth cranial nerve) is entering from the posterior fossa; O, amputated proximal orbit.)

*B,* The right LSC. In the lower left, *small arrows* that point upward represent the cut margin of the dural sleeve (sheath) surrounding the carotid artery in the foramen lacerum, beyond which the dural coverings of the LSC are removed. The largest of these three *arrows* points to the carotid sympathetic nerve emerging to join with the sixth cranial nerve (6) at the two opposing *large arrows.* The *Horizontal arrow* at the lower left shows the cut margin of the carotid sheath at the point where a secondary branch of the carotid sympathetic is emerging to cross the carotid artery (C) and join the primary sympathetic branch. The *thin vertical arrow* indicates the sympathetic component leaving the sixth cranial nerve to join the first division of the fifth cranial nerve (5), which is slightly out of focus. Beneath this area are some empty veins. (T, third cranial nerve.)

*C,* The right LSC is viewed from behind with part of the lateral wall removed. (*Solid horizontal arrows* indicate the cut edges.) This dural wall would be continuous with the dural sleeve, which sheaths the carotid in the foramen lacerum (above the forceps). The *large oblique black arrow* points to the cut margin of the carotid sheath. Emerging at the arrow tip is the carotid sympathetic nerve, most of which continues along the carotid artery, but just above this filament are two that fuse and then join the sixth cranial nerve, the proximal end of which is labeled with an *open arrow.* One of several small sympathetic fibers is then seen to leave the sixth cranial nerve and join the first division of the fifth cranial nerve *(white arrow),* which is held up. (O, optic nerve in the dural canal above the space for the optic strut.)

*D,* The right LSC. (CS, carotid sheath in the foramen lacerum; Cs, carotid arteries; G gasserian ganglion pulled down; 1 and 2, first and second divisions of the fifth cranial nerve. [The third division is removed.] The entire dural wall is removed down to its continuation as the carotid sheath *(horizontal arrows).* At the tip of the uppermost *horizontal arrow,* the carotid sympathetic nerve is seen emerging from the dural sheath to join with the sixth cranial nerve *(vertical arrows)* curving around the carotid from below. Continuing to the right, the sympathetic is seen to leave the sixth cranial nerve to join the first division, which is pulled down and out. The nerve joining the first division appears to be [but actually is not] larger than the sixth cranial nerve itself, which is turning upward.

*E,* The left LSC is viewed from the side. Fat, veins, and most of dura are removed. (O, posterior orbit; II, second cranial nerve just proximal to the orbit; 3, third cranial nerve; upper C, carotid syphon; lower C, carotid artery emerging from the cut margin of the carotid sheath within the foramen lacerum *(small vertical arrow).* Just beneath lower C is the sixth cranial nerve wrapping around the carotid. The left *vertical large arrow* pointing up lies on the first division of the fifth cranial nerve, indicating the departure of sympathetic fibers from the sixth cranial nerve to enter the first division. Distortion causes the continuing sixth cranial nerve to turn sharply upward to exit with the third cranial nerve. This distortion is caused by holding the first division down and out. The right *large vertical arrow* pointing downward points to a few of the sympathetic strands leaving the carotid artery to join the sixth cranial nerve. The sympathetic fibers look larger leaving than when they join the sixth cranial nerve, because all those fibers that are joining are not visible. They also appear to have twisted 180 degrees, because the first division of the fifth is turned down and out.

*F,* The right LSC and the posterior orbit. Of the 42 such dissections we have performed since our original article, this is the only one with a branch of the first division of the fifth cranial nerve joining the sixth cranial nerve instead of the sympathetic fibers leaving the sixth cranial nerve to join the first division. (Left, anterior; right, posterior.) Crossing a small branch of the third cranial nerve (3) going to the ciliary ganglion is an *oblique arrow* that ends on the ganglion. (6, sixth cranial nerve seen again at the far right entering the dura held with the forceps.) The number V I represent the first division of the fifth cranial nerve turned down and out, except for the solitary branch *(thick arrow),* which leaves to join the sixth cranial nerve (presumably therein picking up the sympathetic, which, in other specimens, leaves the sixth cranial nerve to join V I). This branch (nasociliary) continues through the orbital fissure and eventually gives a branch to the ciliary ganglion. (G, gasserian ganglion with the second and third divisions removed.) The second cranial nerve (O) is pulled and rotated laterally after entering the orbit. (C, carotid just before the sympathetic nerve departs to join the sixth cranial nerve.) A line connects the *thick vertical arrow* and represents the position of the superior orbital fissure.

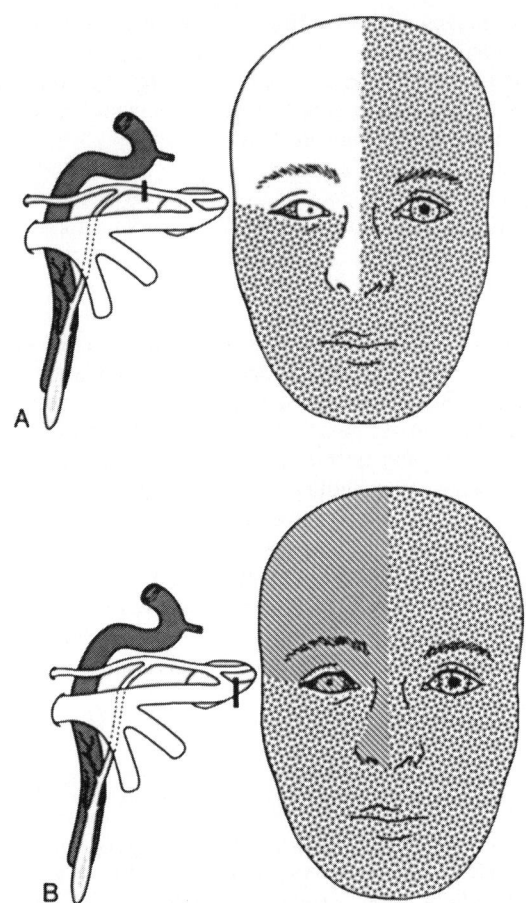

FIGURE 25–4 ■ *A,* The cross-hatching represents analgesia; the circles represent normal sweating. The syndrome is predicted from the discrete lesion *(black bar)* of the sixth cranial nerve in the segment joined by the sympathetic nerve. Sixth palsy and eye signs of Horner's syndrome include a small pupil, conjunctival injection, and narrow fissure. Anhydrosis within first division of fifth cranial nerve is seen. The patient has normal sensation. *B,* The syndrome is predicted from the discrete lesion *(black bar)* of the fifth cranial nerve just beyond the sympathetic junction from the sixth cranial nerve. Eye signs of Horner's syndrome include anhydrosis and analgesia in distribution of the first division of the fifth cranial nerve.

its contents into a surrounding venous cave with four equally accessible major outflow connections.

Embryologically the venous channels in this region begin as a plexus of slender veins surrounded by an abundance of adipose tissue,[52–54] which has been shown in a 20-cm fetus by Knosp and associates.[28] The venous channels are enlarged, and the adipose tissue is reduced in adults (see Figs. 25–1*E* and 25–7*A–E*). (The true dural sinuses develop and mature as sinuses without adipose tissue between the lumen and the dural wall.) Specimen K-429-1 in the Hunterian Museum of the Royal College of Surgeons Building in London shows a parasellar venous plexus with remarkable resemblance to casts made by my colleagues and me. Across the hall in the Welcome Museum, in specimen K-429, the venous pattern is also similar. (There is a persistent trigeminal artery that apparently had been not noticed by any of the curators through the centuries.)

My colleagues and I as well as other investigators, such as Taptas,[46, 47] have been unable to demonstrate trabeculae within the venous channels in the area. Occasionally, there

are connective tissue strands, which consist mainly of adipose tissue, between some of the venous channels, but they are never found going through or within a vein. Anatomy texts refer to this space as the cavernous sinus based on Winslow's[1] erroneous assumption that it is a trabeculated venous space resembling the corpora cavernosa of the penis (which is not a trabeculated venous space either). On further examination, however, there is no similarity in the structures (see Fig. 25–9). The descriptions of the corpora cavernosa contained in anatomy books are not accurate. They contain statements such as "from the internal surface of the fibrous envelope numerous trabeculae arise crossing in all directions dividing the space into a number of cavernous spaces giving an over all spongy appearance" or merely "comprised of erectile tissue," a case of an inaccurate description of one organ erroneously transposed to another.

Although some books accurately illustrate the venous anatomy of the LSC as a plexus, the text usually describes a trabeculated venous cavern surrounding the carotid artery.[55, 56] In 1902, Langer[56] described a plexus of veins, whereas an anatomy book published in 1901[57] illustrates a cross section attributed to Langer in which the carotid artery lies in a surrounding venous cavern. Ferner and colleagues[54] have drawn a plexus in this compartment that is continuous with the basilar plexus and the plexus about the carotid artery in the foramen. They also accurately draw the connecting superior sphenoidal sinus as a single uniform channel, yet they label the plexus of veins in the compartment as the *cavernous sinus.* In venous casts made by my colleagues and I (Fig. 25–5),[58] there were five consistent findings:

1. No two were alike, even from side to side in the same specimen.
2. Although there were some specimens with a predominantly larger vein lying superiorly, there were no specimens with a solitary lateral sellar venous channel. There were always multiple venous channels, no one of which resembled any of the smooth, uniform, regular intracranial dural sinuses.
3. In no specimen was the carotid completely surrounded by veins; there were always bare patches, which were occupied by nerves and fat.
4. There was no evidence of intravascular trabeculae.
5. Posteriorly the LSC veins continue on with the basilar plexus veins, which also have interspersed adipose tissue. (This plexus, in turn, is continuous with the extradural spinal plexus [Batson's], which is surrounded by considerable fat.)

Anteriorly the LSC plexus of veins coalesces and continues as the orbital veins, which are surrounded by considerable fat.[60] Posteroinferiorly the LSC plexus of veins with accompanying fat is continuous with a thin plexus along the carotid through the foramen lacerum (see Fig. 25–5). Laterally the superficial middle cerebral (sylvian) vein, which is devoid of fat, usually empties directly into the LSC venous plexus (see Fig. 25–1*A–E*). The LSC veins are continuous with the sphenoidal and petrosal sinuses, in cases in which there is no surrounding fat, as well as with the veins of the floor of the middle fossa dura, which have no fat. When the dura and fat are dissolved away, the

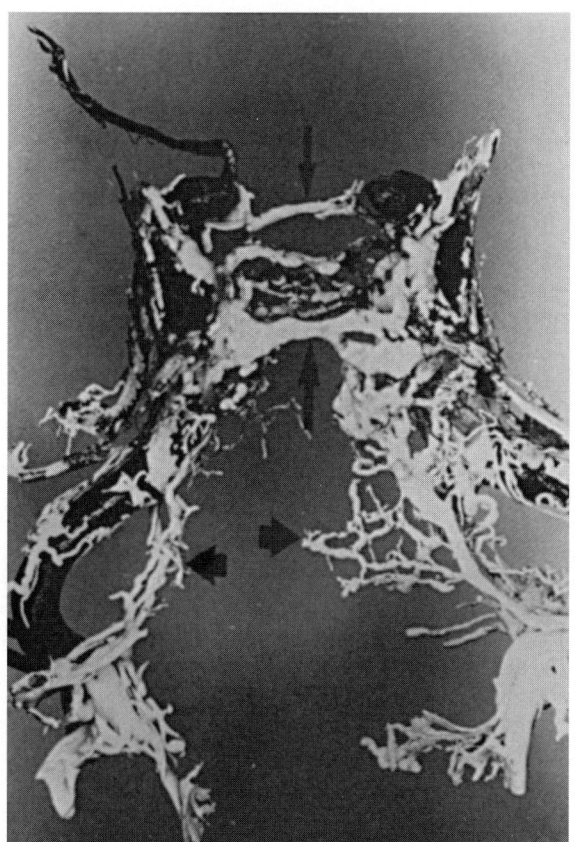

**FIGURE 25–5** ■ A corrosion specimen. A bilateral parasellar artery *(black)* and vein *(white)* injection are viewed from above. The right ophthalmic artery is broken off. The uppermost horizontal vein *(vertical arrow* pointing down) connects the plexi in the lateral sellar compartment anterior to the pituitary stalk. The next horizontal vein connects the two plexi posterior to the pituitary stalk. The inferior hypophyseal artery anastomosis is visible beneath this vein. Just beneath this area is the large vein *(vertical arrow* pointing up) running through the bony hole in the dorsum. Beneath this area on the left, branches of the dorsal meningeal artery are seen. The basilar plexus *(horizontal thick arrows)* is incompletely filled. The thin venous plexus about the internal carotid artery through the foramen lacerum is seen particularly well on the left.

tion of the carotid artery from the sphenoid by thin veins (see Fig. 25–1E). In addition to the venous connections around the pituitary stalk and beneath the pituitary gland, there is a canal through the dorsum sella connecting the LSC plexus in 70% of the specimens (see Fig. 25–5).[62] There is an accurate depiction of the true venous schema in a drawing accompanying an article by Spaziante and colleagues[63] on transsphenoidal pituitary surgery.

It is not possible to determine whether or not intravascular trabeculae exist just because they do not appear in casts and microscopic slides. Competent observers report finding trabeculae, thus there must be some basis for their findings.[61, 65] Connective tissue strands connect the carotid artery to the walls of this compartment; the veins go around these strands. If the entire compartment is assumed to be a venous cavity, the veins themselves could mislead an observer because they appear as thin, branching, translucent strands when empty and are easily mistaken for trabeculae (Fig. 25–6). Another possible explanation is that when any of these veins are stretched even minimally, the walls fenestrate, leaving septa or trabeculae. In two-dimensional preparations, the common wall of adjacent veins in cross section appears as a strand of connective tissue, or a trabecula, covered with endothelium (as such walls would have to be if they were intravascular) (Fig. 25–7C). A vein that is sectioned tangentially would also appear to be a strand of connective tissue. Enormous variations in the arterial anatomy are seen in our own specimens and in the many dissections of others,[3, 25–27, 65] especially in the second and third branchings within this compartment; when empty, these branches may appear to be strands of connective tissue (see Fig. 25–2A). Occasionally, some of them go through some of the larger veins and could be misinterpreted as intravenous trabeculae. The multiple autonomic branches traversing this space[38, 39, 43, 44] may explain some of the so-called trabeculae (see Fig. 25–3A–E). A study of photographs by Krivosic[64] leads to the belief that the structure labeled *interstitial connective tissue* is a tangential cut through the wall of a vessel. From the configuration shown, however, the structure is probably the meningohypophysial trunk (see Fig. 25–2C).

Two questions immediately arise if one is to accept the plexus type of anatomy as opposed to the classic single sinus cavity surrounding the carotid artery.[48, 49, 51] First, how can these thin-walled veins withstand the sudden burst of arterial flow of a traumatic carotid fistula? Second, how can one explain the apparent single spot of contrast material in most angiograms focusing on the lateral sellar region? In answer to the first question, these thin-walled veins are supported by noncompressible fluid (blood) and fat in all the adjacent structures contained in the relatively rigid dural compartment. There is no space within which a vein could suddenly distend and hence rupture. In answer to the second question, the superimposition of the multiple small veins viewed in any plane would appear as a single spot. If one carefully studies angiograms of good quality stereoscopically, more than one channel is visible in the area, and these channels are superimposed on each other (Fig. 25–8). An alternative explanation is that the contrast material may be filling only one of the larger, superiorly placed veins within the LSC. By venous cast, microscopic sections, gross inspection of the venous anatomy within the

patterns of the continuing venous channels are similar to a road map in which the state boundaries have been erased. There is no characteristic change that might indicate a sinus border. Moreover the veins of the floor of the middle fossa and the venous sinuses (see Fig. 25–8) are *within* the double-layered dura, whereas the venous plexus and accompanying fat within the LSC and its extensions along the carotid artery and down the dorsum are *extradural between* the double-layered dura and the periosteum of the sphenoid bone. Microscopically the LSC venous channels have extremely thin walls, little more than intima. When they are not immediately adjacent to each other, the venous channels are separated mostly by fat (see Fig. 25–7). Postmortem examination of thrombi in the LSC reveals the lumens of varying sized veins, never a single larger mass and never impaled with trabeculae.

Two authors[61, 66] describe only four venous channels; however, in several casts and cross-sections made by my colleagues and me, 10 fairly large veins may be identified. Our studies of cross sections often show complete separa-

*Text continued on page 339*

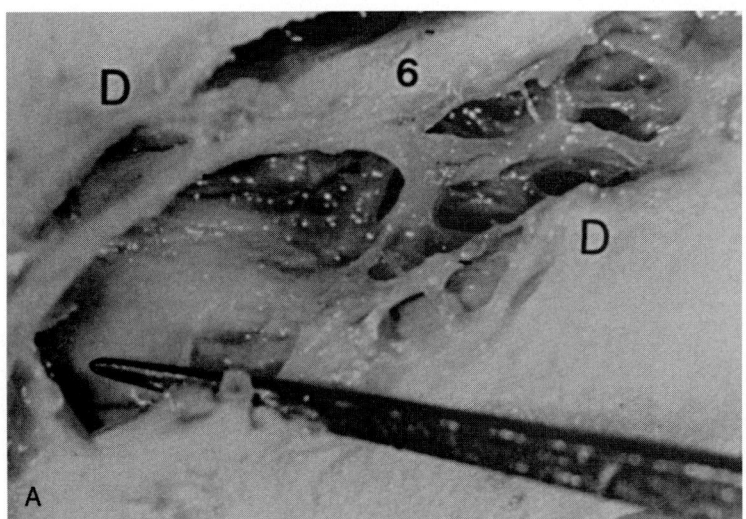

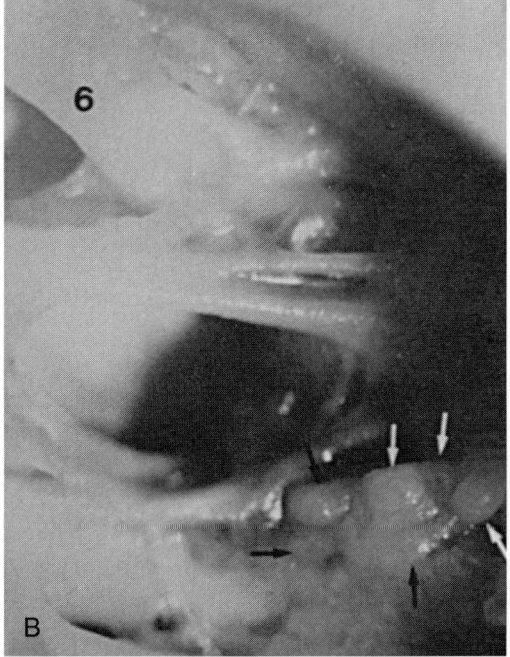

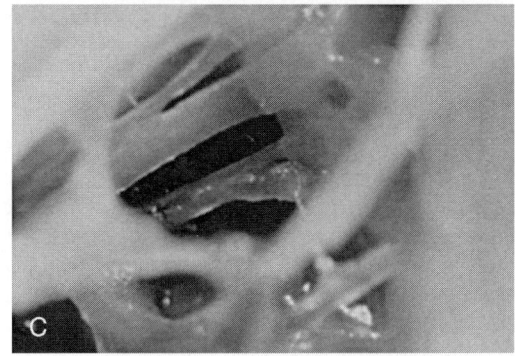

**FIGURE 25–6 ■** *A,* The right lateral sellar compartment (LSC). The dural wall *(D)* is opened and gently retracted. Some of the adipose tissue has been removed. Multiple venous channels are visible, one of which is held with the forceps so that an open cut end is visible. (6, sixth cranial nerve.) *B,* Veins of the right LSC in an adult. The dural wall is opened and gently retracted, exposing multiple venous channels. Some adipose tissue remains (surrounded by *black* and *white arrows*). In both *A* and *B,* if the area is retracted any further, the veins become thin translucent strands or tear and fenestrate and are easily mistaken for trabeculae. *C,* Multiple, empty translucent veins (in an adult) with adjacent fat removed.

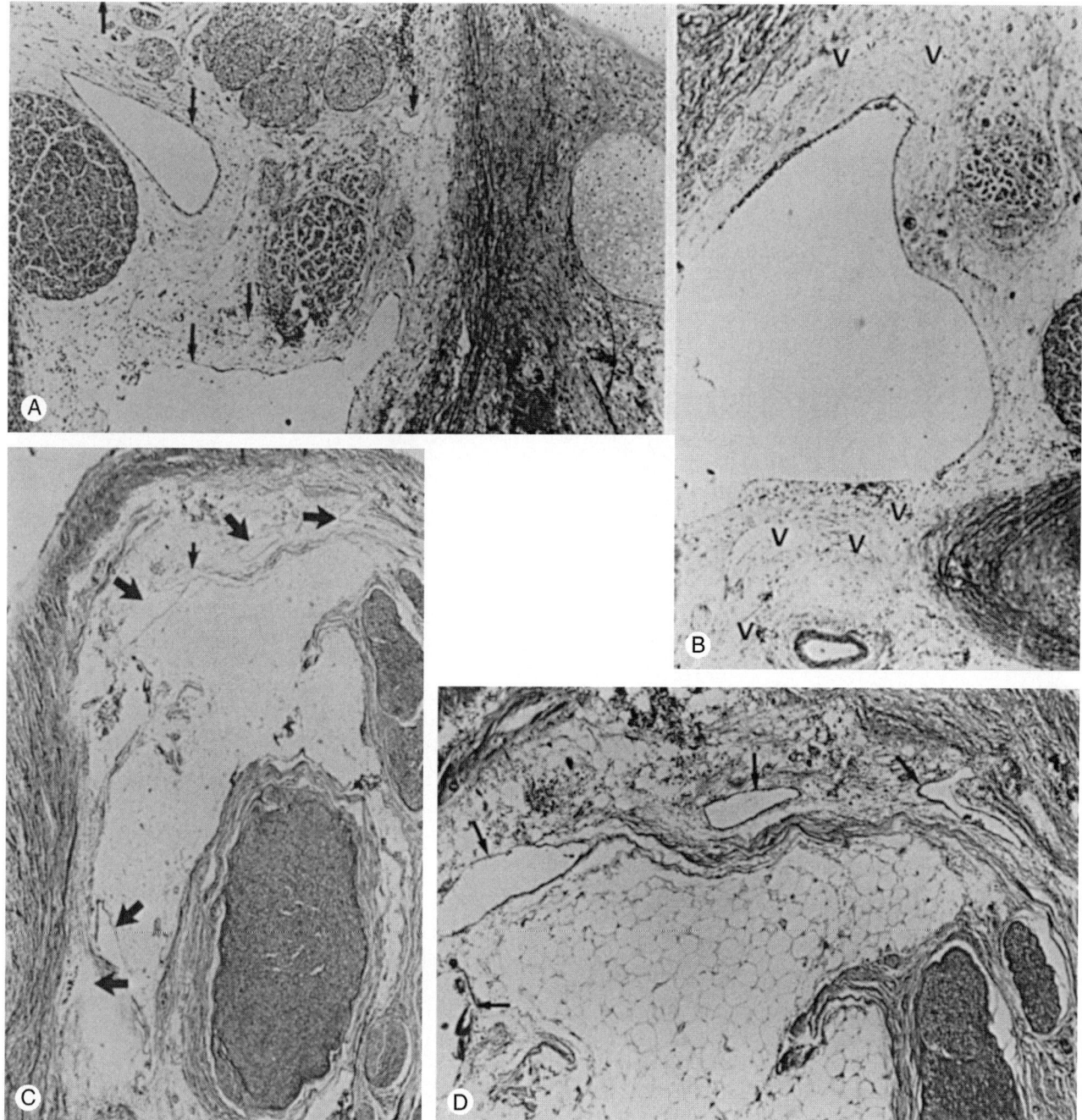

**FIGURE 25–7** ■ Multiple, random, coronal sections of the lateral sellar compartment demonstrating the abundant adipose tissue and multiple thin-walled veins in the developmental stages. Compare this with Figure 25–1E.

*A,* A 15-week-old fetus. (H & E, ×160 stain of coronal section of parasellar space) Body of cartilage is visible on the right. Note the multiple, variably sized, extremely thin-walled venous channels (six of which are marked with *arrows*) with large amounts of adjacent adipose tissue. Myelinated and unmyelinated nerve branches are also present.

*B,* Full-term male. (H & E, ×320.) Multiple small veins about one much larger vein. Abundant surrounding adipose tissue. A comparatively thin-walled artery lies at bottom. Compare this with the corpora cavernosa artery shown in Figure 25–9.

*C,* A 9-year-old male. (H & E, ×160.) Slightly thicker walled veins and comparatively less adipose tissue than that shown in B. The third vein from the top *(smaller arrow)* has an adjacent vein separated only by endothelium. Cranial nerve branches are encircled with more connective tissue.

*D,* Upper portion of Figure 25–7C. (H & E, ×420). Compare Figure 25–7A to D with Figure 25–9. The greatest similarity between the two structures is the absence of intravascular trabeculae in both.

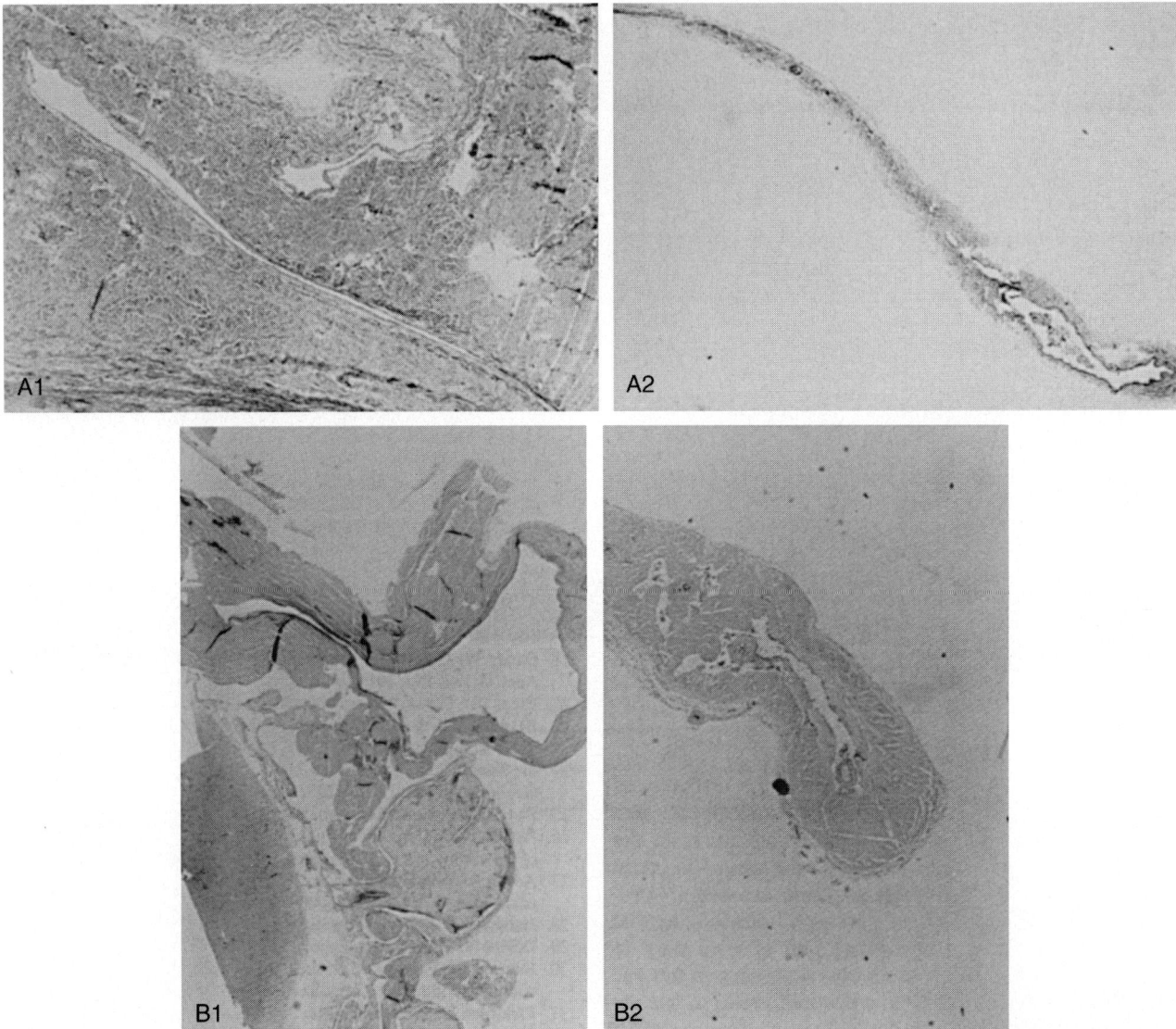

**FIGURE 25–8** ■ *A,* A 9-week-old infant. The superior (collapsed to a slit) and inferior sagittal sinus. There is no adipose tissue. *B,* A cross-section of the superior and inferior sagittal sinus in an adult. In both views, the vein lies within the dural wall with no surrounding adipose tissue. Note the arachnoid villa adjacent to the superior sinus and the unexplained artery within the inferior adult sinus. Accessory venous channels are present in each specimen.

space, angiographic studies, and configuration of thrombi at autopsy, the venous anatomy is that of a plexus of veins with varying amounts of surrounding adipose tissue lying not within but beneath the double layer of dura of the lateral wall of the LSC. Thus, it seems that the venous pathways within this compartment are not cavernous, trabeculated, singular, or a true sinus. They do not resemble the anatomy of the corpora cavernosa in any way (Fig. 25–9).

Changing the terminology used to refer to this compartment would immediately resolve some of the difficulty in understanding it. If Winslow had only examined the area more carefully, he would have seen no justification for the term *cavernous sinus*. Taptas[46, 47] suggests the use of the term *parasellar osteodural chamber*. Knosp and associates[28] propose the term *cavernous venous plexus*, acknowledging that the word *cavernous* is inappropriate and is used only to designate the position. Kehrli and associates[66] use LSC in their title yet conclude that the veins are true dural sinuses yet describe them as extradural and associated with adipose tissue. Weninger and coworkers[67] divide the compartment into three subdivisions but recognize that the structure is *extradural*. Because the plexus of veins is one

of several structures in this area, I use the inclusive term *LSC* for the compartment and *parasellar veins* for the venous channels therein. The LSC is a segmental enlargement of the lengthy continuous extradural strip of adipose tissue containing arteries, veins, and nerves, extending from the sacrum and including the orbit.

## REFERENCES

1. Winslow JB: Exposition anatomique de la structure du corps humain, Vol 2. London: Prevast, 1734, p 31.
2. Galen (150 AD), as quoted by Margotta R: In Lewis P (ed): An Illustrated History of Medicine. Middlesex: Hamlin Publishing Group, 1968, p 96.
3. Goshal N, Khamas WAH: Gross and histomorphological study on the rostral epidural rete mirabile of the pig. Ind J Anim Sci 55:304–310, 1985.
4. DeGutierrez-Mahoney GCG, Schechter MM: The myth of the rete mirabile in man. Neuroradiology 4:141–148, 1972.
5. Parkinson D: Rete mirabile, the marvelous network. Can J Neurol Sci 1:121–123, 1974.
6. Vesalius A: In Garrison FH (ed): History of Medicine. Philadelphia: WB Saunders, 1966, p 219.
7. Destrieux C, Kakou MK, Velut S, et al: Microanatomy of the hypophyseal fossa boundaries. J Neurosurg 88:743–752, 1998.
8. Xu Z, Wei X, Zhao C: Microsurgical anatomy of the wall of the cavernous sinus. Chung Hua I Hsueh Tsa Chih 76:855–858, 1996.
9. Reisch R, Vutskits L, Patonay L, Fries G: The meningohypophyseal trunk and its blood supply to different intracranial structures: An anatomical study. Minim Invasive Neurosurg 39:78–81, 1996.
10. Umansky F, Valarezo A, Elidan J: The superior wall of the cavernous sinus: A microanatomical study. J Neurosurg 81:914–920, 1994.
11. Kehrili P, Ali MM, Maillot C, et al: Comparative anatomy of the lateral wall of the 'cavernous sinus' in humans and the olive baboon. Neurol Res 19:571–576, 1997.
12. Hollinshead WH: Anatomy for Surgeons, Vol 1. New York: Hoeber Harper, 1954, p 560.
13. Jefferson G: The vascular aneurysms of the internal carotid artery in the cavernous sinus. Br J Surg 26:267–302, 1938.
14. Parkinson D: A surgical approach to the cavernous portion of the carotid artery: Anatomical studies and case report. J Neurosurg 23:474–483, 1965.
15. Dolenc VV: Direct neurological repair of intracavernous vascular lesions. J Neurosurg 58:524–584, 1983.
16. Conesa HA, Zadorecki EA, Lozano MC: Gross anatomy of the cavernous region. In Dolenc V (ed): The Cavernous Sinus. New York: Springer-Verlag, 1987, pp 43–55.
17. Umansky F, Nathan H: The cavernous sinus: An anatomical study of its lateral wall. In Dolenc V (ed): The Cavernous Sinus. New York: Springer-Verlag, 1987, pp 56–66.
18. Kehrli P, Maillot C, Wolff MJ: Anatomy and embryology of the trigeminal nerve and its branches in the parasellar area. Neurol Res 19:57–65, 1997.
19. Parkinson D: Collateral circulation of cavernous carotid. Presentation at the Royal College of Physicians and Surgeons of Canada, Edmonton, Alberta, 1962.
20. Parkinson D: Collateral circulation of the cavernous carotid artery: Anatomy. Can J Surg 7:251–257, 1962.
21. Schnurer LB, Statin S: Vascular supply of the intracranial dura from the internal carotid artery with special references to its angiographic significance. Acta Radiol 1:441–450, 1963.
22. Wallace S, Goldberg GI, Leeds ME, Mishlin MM: The cavernous branches of the internal carotid artery. Am J Roentgenol Radium Ther Nucl Med 1:34–36, 1967.
23. Willinsky R, Lasjaunias P, Berenstein A: Intracavernous branches of the internal carotid artery. Surg Radiol Anat 9:201–215, 1987.
24. Lasjaunias P, Doyon D, Vignaud J, et al: Progress in the arteriographic study of the cavernous sinus disease. In Salamon G (ed): Advances in Cerebral Angiography. New York: Springer-Verlag, 1975, pp 324–330.
25. Brassier G, Lasjaunias P, Guegan Y, Pecker J: Microsurgical anatomy of collateral branches of the intracavernous internal carotid artery. In Dolenc V (ed): The Cavernous Sinus. New York: Springer-Verlag, 1987, pp 81–103.

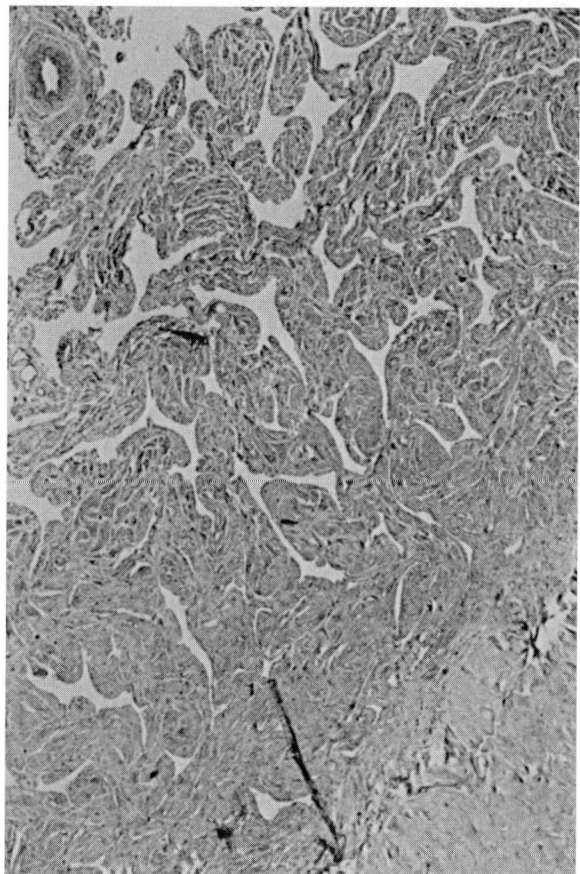

**FIGURE 25–9** ■ A stain of the corpora cavernosa of an adult penis (H & E, ×160). Note the thick muscular-walled, tightly coiled venous sinusoids of fairly uniform diameter, which is progressively narrower and more compact as the surrounding tunica is approached (lower right). Note the thick-walled artery in the upper left. There is no adipose tissue and no trabecula. Compare with the meningohypophyseal artery in Figure 25–7B. The anatomy of the two structures bears no similarity at all, except that there are no intravascular trabeculae in either case.

26. Krisht A, Barnett DW, Barrow DL, Bonner G: The blood supply of the cranial nerves: An anatomic study. Neurosurgery 34:275–279, 1994.
27. Jiminez-Castelllano J, Carmona A, Catalina-Herrera CJ: Anatomical study of the branches emerging along the intracavernous course of the internal carotid artery in humans. Acta Anat 148:157–161, 1993.
28. Knosp E, Muller G, Perneczky A: Anatomical remarks on the fetal cavernous sinus and on the veins of the middle cranial fossa. In Dolenc V (ed): The Cavernous Sinus. New York: Springer-Verlag, 1987, pp 104–116.
29. Dandy W, Goetsche E: The blood supply of the pituitary body. Am J Anat 11:137–150, 1911.
30. Paget DH: Personal communication, 1961.
31. Basset DL: A Stereoscopic Atlas of Human Anatomy. Baltimore: Williams & Wilkins, 1954 (stereoscopic slides).
32. McConnell EM: The arterial blood supply of the human hypophysis cerebri. Anat Rec 15:175–203, 1953.
33. Hoyt WF: Personal communication, 1968.
34. Parkinson D: Carotid cavernous fistula: Direct repair with preservation of the carotid artery. J Neurosurg 38:99–106, 1973.
35. Adson AW: Surgical treatment of vascular diseases altering the function of the eyes. J Am Acad Ophthalmol 46:95–111, 1942.
36. Hamby WB: Personal communication, 1976.
37. Dolenc V: Personal communication, 1990.
38. Johnson JH, Parkinson D: Intracranial sympathetic pathways associated with the sixth nerve. J Neurosurg 40:236–240, 1974.
39. Parkinson D, Johnson J, Chaudhuri A: Sympathetic connections of the fifth and sixth cranial nerves. Anat Rec 191:221–226, 1978.
40. Monro A: The Anatomy of the Humor, Bones and Nerves. Edinburgh: Hamilton & Balfour, 1746, p 363.
41. Parkinson D: Bernard, Horner syndrome and others. Surg Neurol 11:221–223, 1979.
42. Myles WM: Personal communication, 1993.
43. Lyon DB, Lemke BN, Wallow IH, Dortzbach RK: Sympathetic nerve anatomy in the cavernous sinus and retrobulbar orbit of the cynomolgus monkey. Ophthalmic Plast Reconstr Surg 8:1–12, 1992.
44. Mariniello G: Microsurgical anatomy of the sympathetic fibers running inside the cavernous sinus. J Neurosurg Sci 38:1–10, 1994.
45. Ruskell GL, Simons T: Trigeminal pathways to the cerebral arteries in monkeys. J Anat 155:23–37, 1987.
46. Taptas NJ: La loge du sinus caverneux rev. Acta Neurophthalmol 21:193–199, 1949.
47. Taptas NJ: La loge osteo-durale parasellaire et les elements vasculaires et nerveux qui la traversent. Une conception anatomique qui doit remplacer celle du sinus caverneus des classiques. Neurochirurgie 36:201–208, 1990.
48. Bonnet P: Physiologie pathologique de l'exophthalmos pulsatile. Arch Ophthalmol 13:233–251, 1953.
49. Bryhaye J: Pathogenesis and symptomatology of the carotid cavernous fistula. Third postgraduate course in neurosurgery. Pecs, July 1976.
50. Hamby WB, Dohn DF: Carotid cavernous fistula: Report of 36 cases and discussion of their management. Clin Neurosurg 11:150–170, 1964.
51. Narita Y, Watanabe Y, Hoshino T, et al: Myelopathy due to large veins draining recurrent spontaneous carotid cavernous fistula. Neuroradiology 34:433–435, 1992.
52. Solasol A, Zidunc C, Slimanc-Taleb S, et al: The veins of the cavernous sinus in the four month old human fetus. C R Assoc Anat 149:1009–1015, 1966.
53. Bol'Shakow OP: Macroscopical structure of the cavernous sinus. Fed Proc 23(trans suppl):308, 1960.
54. Ferner H, Monsen H, Pernkopf E (eds): Atlas of Topographic and Applied Human Anatomy, Vol 1. Philadelphia: WB Saunders, 1963.
55. Spalteholz W: Hand Atlas of Human Anatomy, Vol 2, 7th ed. Philadelphia: JB Lippincott, 1935.
56. Langer C (1902), quoted by Taptas, 1990.
57. Poirier P, Charpy A: Traite D'Anatomie Humaine. Paris: Masson, 1901, pp 968–981.
58. Parkinson D: Anatomy of the cavernous sinus. In Pia HW, Langmaid C, Zierski J (eds): Cerebral Aneurysms. New York: Springer-Verlag, 1979, pp 224–228.
59. Lang J, Kageyama I: Clinical anatomy of the blood spaces and blood vessels surrounding the siphon of the internal carotid artery. Acta Anat (Basel) 139:320–325, 1990.
60. Kubic S: Tumors of the sellar and parasellar area in adults. In Youmans JR (ed): Neurological Surgery, Vol 5. Toronto: WB Saunders, 1982, p 3112.
61. Bonneville JF, Catin F, Racie A, et al: Dynamic CT of the laterosellar extradural venous spaces. AJNR Am J Neuroradiol 10:535–542, 1989.
62. Schnitzlein HN, Murtagh FR, Arrington JA, Parkinson D: The sinus of the dorsum sellae. Anat Rec 213:587–589, 1985.
63. Spaziante R, De Divitiis E, Cappabianca P: Reconstruction of the pituitary fossa in transsphenoidal surgery: An experience of 140 cases. Neurosurgery 17:453, 1985.
64. Krivosic I: Histoarchitecture of the cavernous sinus. In Dolenc V (ed): The Cavernous Sinus. New York: Springer-Verlag, 1987, pp 117–129.
65. Tran Din H: Cavernous branches of the internal carotid artery: Anatomy and nomenclature. Neurosurgery 20:205–210, 1987.
66. Kehrli P, Maillot C, Wolff MJ: The venous system of the lateral sellar compartment (cavernous sinus): An histological and embryological study. Neurol Res 18:387–393, 1996.
67. Weninger WJ, Streicher J, Muller GB: Anatomical compartments of the parasellas region: Adipose tissue bodies represent intracranial continuations of extracranial spaces. J Anat 191:269–275, 1997.

# Surgical Management of Aneurysms and Fistulas Involving the Cavernous Sinus

■ ARTHUR L. DAY and C. MICHAEL CAWLEY

The intracavernous segment (CavSeg) of the internal carotid artery (ICA) has classically been defined as the segment that begins as the vessel emerges from the carotid canal at the foramen lacerum and ends as the artery penetrates the dura near the anterior clinoid (AC) process to enter the subarachnoid space. The CavSeg has been divided into five parts[1]: the posterior vertical portion,[2] the posterior bend,[3] the horizontal portion,[4] the anterior bend, and the anterior vertical portion.[1, 5]

Removal of the AC extradurally, however, exposes a segment of the carotid artery that is neither within the cavernous sinus nor the subarachnoid space (Fig. 26–1A, B).[1, 2] This vessel segment, herein called the clinoidal segment (ClinSeg), corresponds to the distal part of the anterior vertical portion of the CavSeg. Although some anatomists believe that this segment is invested by a collar of

the cavernous sinus dura, nonetheless, it exists as a clinically distinct and relevant portion of the ICA.[3] The ClinSeg is delineated distally (or superiorly) by dural reflections from the roof of the AC that extend medially toward the optic nerve and canal. The point where the ICA penetrates this dural plane to enter the subarachnoid space is known as the dural ring (DR), upper ring, or Perneczky's ring.

Proximally, the ClinSeg is delineated by a thin extension of the periosteum covering the undersurface of the AC. This membrane, extending from the ICA to the oculomotor nerve and called the carotico-oculomotor membrane (COM) or membranous ring, separates this segment from the cavernous sinus. An anatomic study by Rhoton and colleagues suggests that this membrane may actually form a collar through which the ICA penetrates the roof of the cavernous sinus.[3] Although this theory is still controversial,

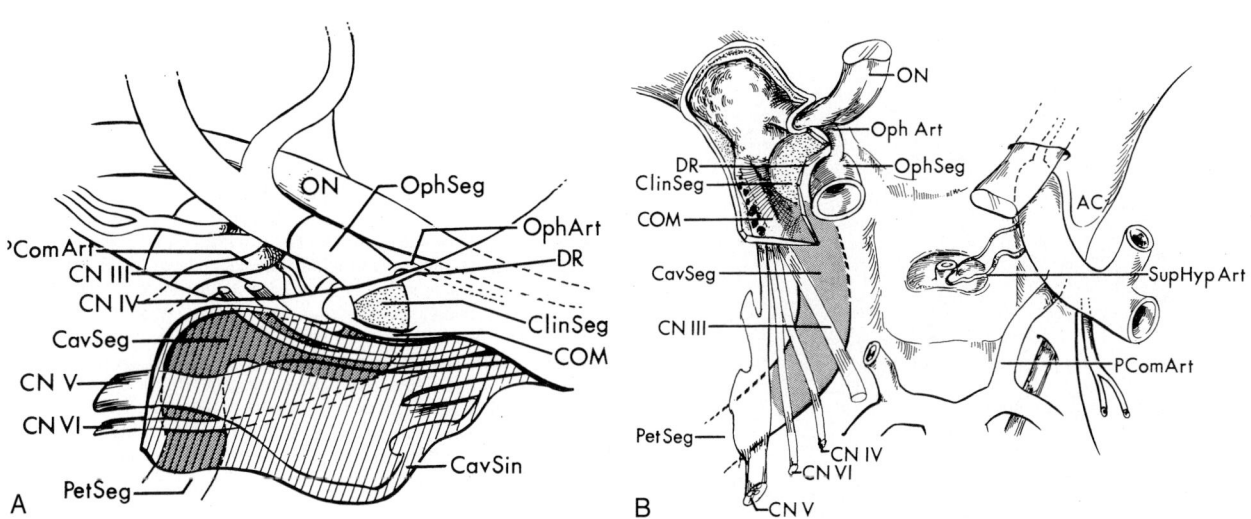

**FIGURE 26–1** ■ Cavernous sinus anatomy and terminology. Lateral *(A)* and dorsal *(B)* views. Note the two portions of the carotid artery considered to be within the cavernous sinus: (1) The cavernous segment (CavSeg) lies within the large venous channel of the cavernous sinus (CavSin), and (2) the clinoidal segment (ClinSeg), which corresponds to the anterior vertical segment of the cavernous carotid artery. Both segments lie below the dural ring and outside the subarachnoid space. (DR, dural ring; COM, carotid-oculomotor membrane; ON, optic nerve; OS, optic strut; AC, anterior clinoid process; OphSeg, ophthalmic segment; PetSeg, petrous segment; OphArt, ophthalmic artery; PComArt, posterior communicating artery; SupHypArt, superior hypophyseal artery; CN III, oculomotor nerve; CN IV, trochlear nerve; CN V, trigeminal nerve; CN VI, abducens nerve.)

Rhoton believes that venous tributaries in this collar indicate that the ClinSeg is technically intracavernous. In practice, however, the ClinSeg represents a distinct portion of the supracavernous ICA with both clinical and surgical implications.

Vascular lesions of the intracavernous carotid artery can be broadly divided into two groups: (1) nonfistulous arterial aneurysms and (2) carotid-cavernous fistulas.

# NONFISTULOUS ARTERIAL ANEURYSMS

Cavernous sinus region aneurysms account for approximately 3% to 5% of all angiographically identified intracranial aneurysms and about 15% of all aneurysms originating from the internal carotid artery.[4, 5] Intracavernous aneurysms may be divided into four types on the basis of their genesis and clinical course: (1) saccular (congenital), (2) arteriosclerotic (fusiform), (3) infectious, and (4) traumatic.

## Saccular and Arteriosclerotic Aneurysms

The numerous similarities between arteriosclerotic and saccular intracavernous aneurysms allow them to be discussed as a single clinical entity. Most intracavernous aneurysms are saccular and are believed to arise from congenital defects in the vessel wall at the site of actual or vestigial branches. The intracavernous branches most commonly thought to act as origin for such aneurysms are the meningohypophyseal trunk, the inferolateral trunk, and McConnell's capsular arteries. Intracavernous aneurysms are much more common in women, and symptoms generally begin in the fifth and sixth decades.[6, 7] Several clinical investiga-

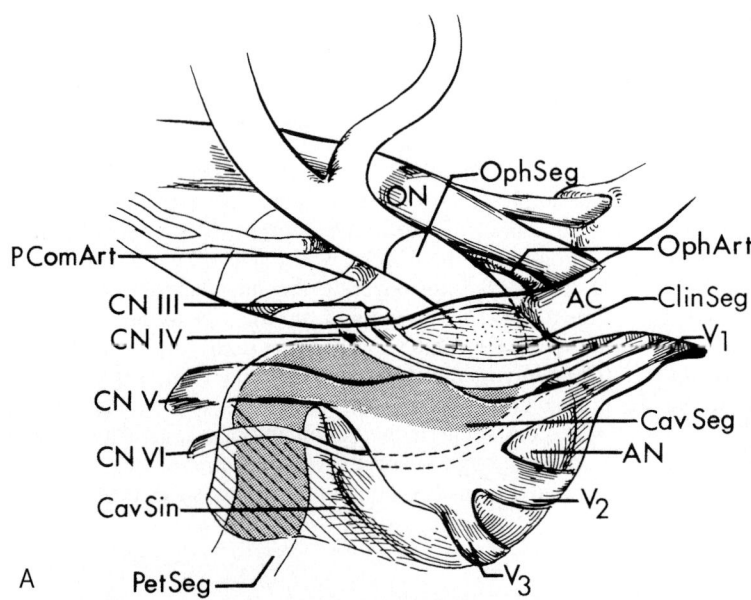

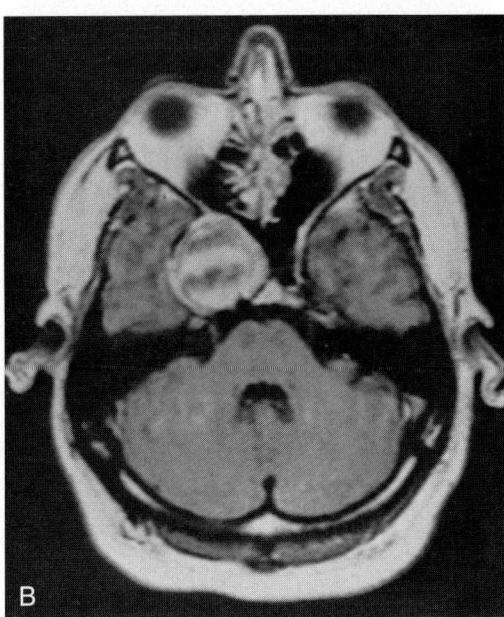

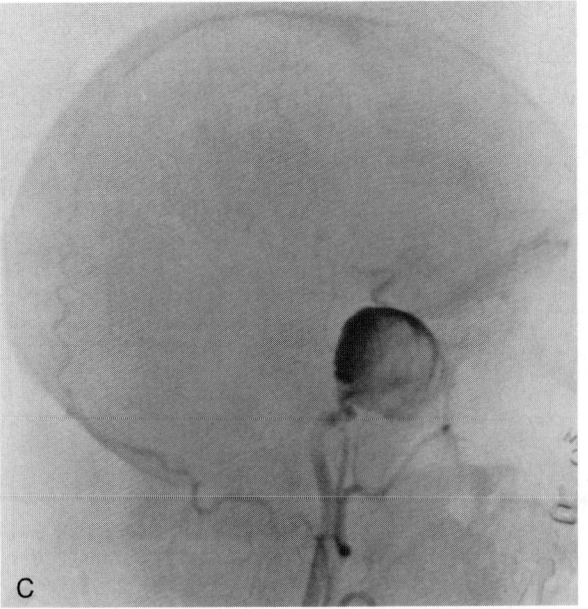

FIGURE 26–2 ■ True cavernous aneurysm. *A,* Lateral view (schematic): The cavernous segment (CavSeg) *(shaded area)* has an intimate association with the cranial nerves within the cavernous sinus (CavSin). Aneurysms (AN) of this segment invariably present with clinical deficits related to compression of these structures. (ON, optic nerve; AC, anterior clinoid process; OphSeg, ophthalmic segment; PetSeg, petrous segment; OphArt, ophthalmic artery; PComArt, posterior communicating artery; CN III, oculomotor nerve; CN IV, trochlear nerve; CN V, trigeminal nerve (three divisions: V1-3); CN VI, abducens nerve.) *B,* A computed tomography scan in 30-year-old man with facial pain and complete cavernous sinus syndrome. Note the giant aneurysm in the right parasellar area, burrowing beneath the sphenoid ridge toward the superior orbital fissure. *C,* This preoperative arteriogram (lateral view) demonstrates a giant intracavernous aneurysm with delayed filling of the intracranial carotid artery.

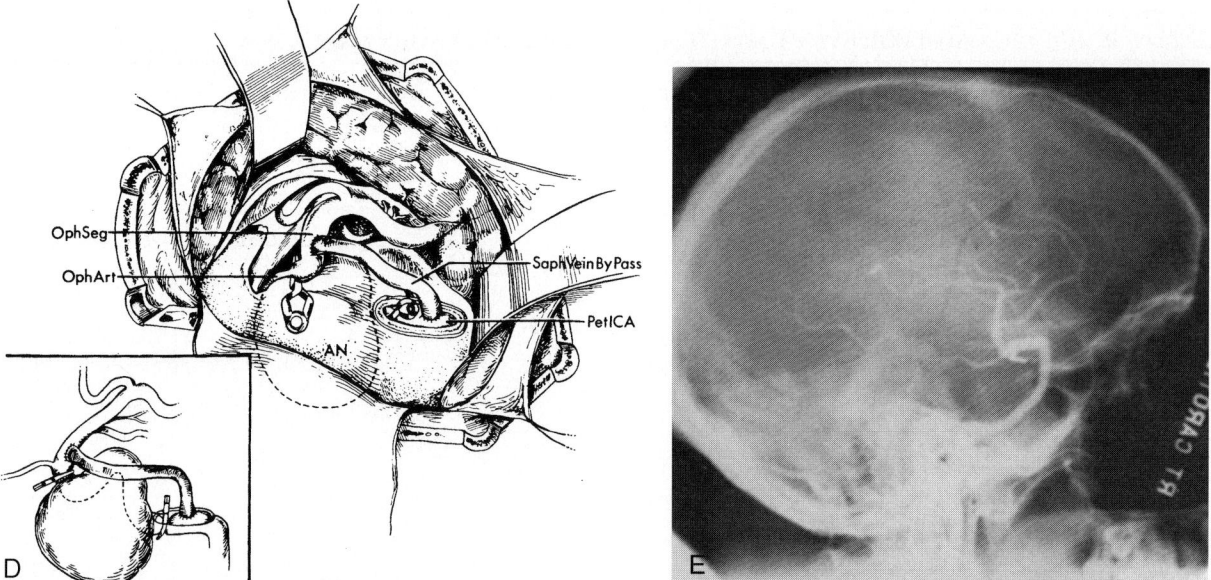

**FIGURE 26–2** ■ *Continued. D,* A petrosal to supraclinoidal carotid artery bypass (schematic): The petrous carotid artery has been exposed by drilling off the bone just posterior and slightly lateral to the foramen ovale. A saphenous vein graft spans over the bulging aneurysm, connecting the petrous and ophthalmic segments of the internal carotid artery. The aneurysm is thereafter trapped *(insert)* by clips on the distal petrous and clinoidal segments of the carotid artery. The contents of the cavernous sinus are not disturbed by the procedure. *E,* Postoperative arteriogram (lateral view). Note the excellent filling of the distal carotid artery from the short segment bypass. The patient subsequently had complete resolution of clinical symptoms other than mild abducens palsy apparent to extreme lateral gaze.

tions have demonstrated clearly different natural histories and treatment options between those aneurysms arising from the anterior vertical segment of the cavernous carotid artery (within the ClinSeg) and those arising from the more proximal ICA (within the CavSeg); thus, each will be considered separately.[6–9]

**True Intracavernous (CavSeg) Aneurysms.** Aneurysms arising from this ICA segment account for the majority of those identified as intracavernous. The hemodynamic forces exerted on this aneurysm type usually produce a lesion that burrows anteriorly and laterally beneath the sphenoid ridge, toward the superior orbital fissure. Most remain asymptomatic until reaching giant proportions (approximately 2.5 cm), at which point symptoms are caused by local mass effect against adjacent structures and may include isolated or combined deficits of the oculomotor, trochlear, abducens, trigeminal, and sympathetic nerves (Fig. 26–2A).[6, 7] Subarachnoid hemorrhage (SAH) or epistaxis is rare because, in addition to its own arterial wall, the aneurysm is covered by the venous structures within the sinus and by the overlying dura and surrounding bony structures.

In the symptomatic patient, computed tomography (CT) or magnetic resonance imaging (MRI) invariably demonstrates a round or oblong anterior extradural parasellar mass expanding anteriorly and laterally into the middle cranial fossa, beneath the sphenoid ridge and AC (see Fig. 26–2B).[6, 9] The definitive diagnosis is established by arteriography. When performed, this study should include careful assessment of the ipsilateral external carotid artery (ECA) for potential donor vessels, in the event that carotid ligation and extracranial-intracranial bypass are to be considered (see Fig. 26–2C).[11, 12] Intraluminal thrombosis often

occurs in large lesions and can cause an underestimation of the lesion's true size unless correlated with CT or MRI.

When symptoms are mild and confined to oculomotor or trigeminal dysfunction in the typical 65-year-old woman, aggressive intervention is sometimes not advised, because many patients will have a benign clinical course.[13] Visual loss (rare with this lesion type) or severe intractable facial pain are stronger indications for therapeutic intervention. SAH and epistaxis should be considered as neurologic emergencies and treated aggressively.

Treatment options, when indicated, include common carotid artery (CCA) ligation,[1, 2] ICA ligation (using either a detachable balloon or a gradually occluding clamp) often combined with a bypass procedure,[3] direct clipping, and endovascular coiling with ICA preservation[4] (Table 26–1).

***Common Carotid Artery Ligation.*** This treatment is generally performed with a gradual occluding device placed on the CCA several centimeters below the cervical bifurcation. After the clamp is installed and the artery partially narrowed during surgery, the patient is awakened and followed clinically as the clamp is progressively closed over the next several days. During the occlusion and for several days thereafter, the patient is kept well hydrated, and blood pressure is maintained at high-normal levels. The incidence of prolonged ischemic deficits following CCA ligation is significantly lower than that for selective ICA ligation.[14] Systemic anticoagulation probably reduces the risks of thromboembolic complications but may also restrict aneurysmal thrombosis.

Stabilization or improvement of symptoms occurs in most patients following CCA ligation.[15] Because the ICA remains patent with back flow from the ECA, however, this method is not always effective, and the degree of

TABLE 26–1    ■    ICA LIGATION FOR SYMPTOMATIC TRUE INTRACAVERNOUS ANEURYSM

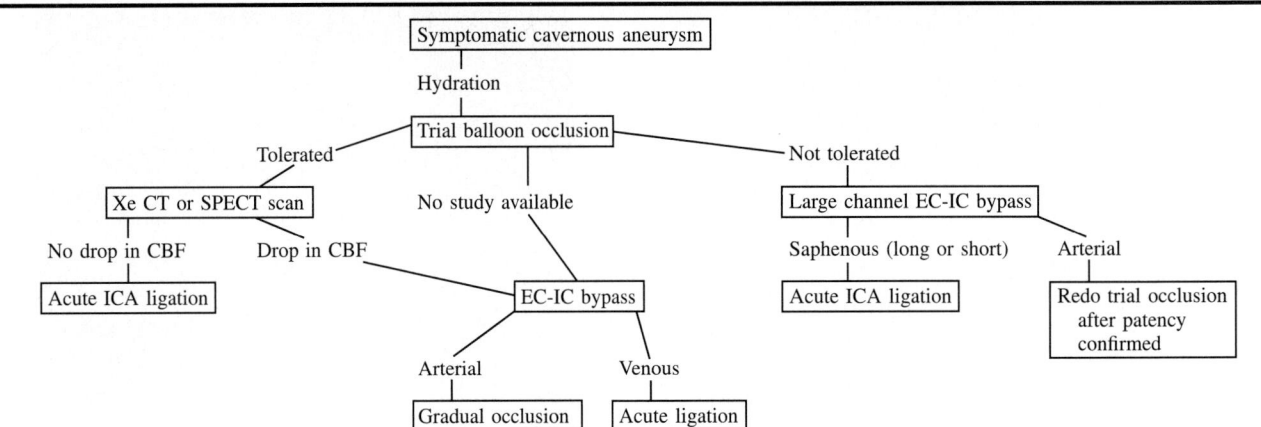

ICA, internal carotid artery; Xe CT, xenon computed tomography; CBF, cerebral blood flow; EC-IC, extracranial-intracranial.

oculomotor recovery may be less.[16–18] We generally reserve this treatment for actively symptomatic elderly (chronologic or physiologic) patients whose risks of ICA ligation appear excessive (see next section).

***Internal Carotid Artery Ligation.*** ICA ligation is the preferred option for most patients with true symptomatic intracavernous aneurysms, provided that the risks can be lowered to acceptable levels.[19] In most cases, proximal ICA ligation alone achieves aneurysmal thrombosis. Trapping should be performed in all cases with prior bleeding (SAH or epistaxis) to completely exclude the lesion from the circulation, or when the aneurysm and its compressive symptoms persist after proximal ligation.

When ICA ligation is contemplated, the surgeon should have a high degree of certainty that flow to the ipsilateral hemisphere will be well maintained via collateral channels. Ischemic symptoms may be delayed for hours or days afterward and may occur despite a well-tolerated Matas test or trial ICA balloon occlusion test under local anesthesia.[11, 17, 20] To more accurately assess ischemic risks, the patient is intravenously hydrated for 24 hours before a brief (15 to 30 minutes) trial involving ICA balloon occlusion.[21] A clinically successfully trial (no new hemispheric symptoms) may be further confirmed by a brief period of induced systemic hypotension.[22] A cerebral blood flow study (single photon emission computed tomography [SPECT]) or xenon computed tomography [Xe CT] is usually done thereafter to provide quantitative estimations of sufficient collateral channels (Fig. 26–3).[11, 20, 22]

If no significant clinical or hemispheric blood flow changes occur during the trial occlusion, a detachable balloon can usually be safely inflated near the aneurysm origin to ligate the ICA, without the need for surgical flow augmentation.[22, 24] Occlusion of the parent artery that includes the entire aneurysm neck prevents both anterograde and retrograde flow into the lesion. Many patients with symptomatic CavSeg aneurysms are elderly, and the option of the detachable balloon eliminates the need for general anesthesia or an intracranial procedure, while providing excellent relief of compressive symptoms. Patients with longer life expectancies or those with marginal blood flow values are treated with acute ICA ligation (trapping) combined with an extracranial-intracranial arterial bypass, ideally using the superficial temporal artery as the donor source.[23]

Some patients have poor collateral circulation (clinical intolerance to trial balloon occlusion or obvious focal decreases in flow on SPECT or Xe CT) and cannot undergo acute ICA ligation without a high risk of stroke. A long saphenous vein graft, connecting the ECA to a major middle cerebral artery trunk and combined with a trapping procedure, provides immediate flow replacement. In our experience, such procedures have higher risks and lesser long-term patency than do artery-to-artery anastomoses.[25] A preliminary extracranial-intracranial arterial bypass, followed days later by delayed subacute ICA ligation using clinical and blood flow monitoring, may reduce these risks but may also reduce anastomosis patency rates by not creating hemodynamic "demand" during the early postoperative period. Obviously, the decision to use either of these options should be weighed carefully against the patient's complaints and the natural history of the untreated lesion.

ICA ligation can also be combined with a short-segment saphenous vein bypass that immediately provides excellent distal ICA flow.[26–28] After extradural removal of much of the greater sphenoid wing, the entire lesser sphenoid wing, and the AC, a frontotemporal flap is turned and the sylvian fissure is widely split. The temporal lobe is mobilized and retracted to expose the dural floor of the middle cranial fossa. The dura is then opened from an intradural approach and stripped medially until the foramen spinosum and greater superficial petrosal nerve are encountered. After the middle meningeal artery is coagulated and cut, bone is drilled off posterior and lateral to the foramen ovale to expose the petrous ICA segment (PetSeg). A short-segment saphenous vein bypass connecting the petrous ICA with the ophthalmic segment of the vessel is then performed, combined with trapping of the vessel segment harboring the aneurysm (see Fig. 26–2D, E).

The advantages of the short-segment petrosal bypass are theoretically compelling and include the benefits of a short length graft, the replacement of the sacrificed vessel with

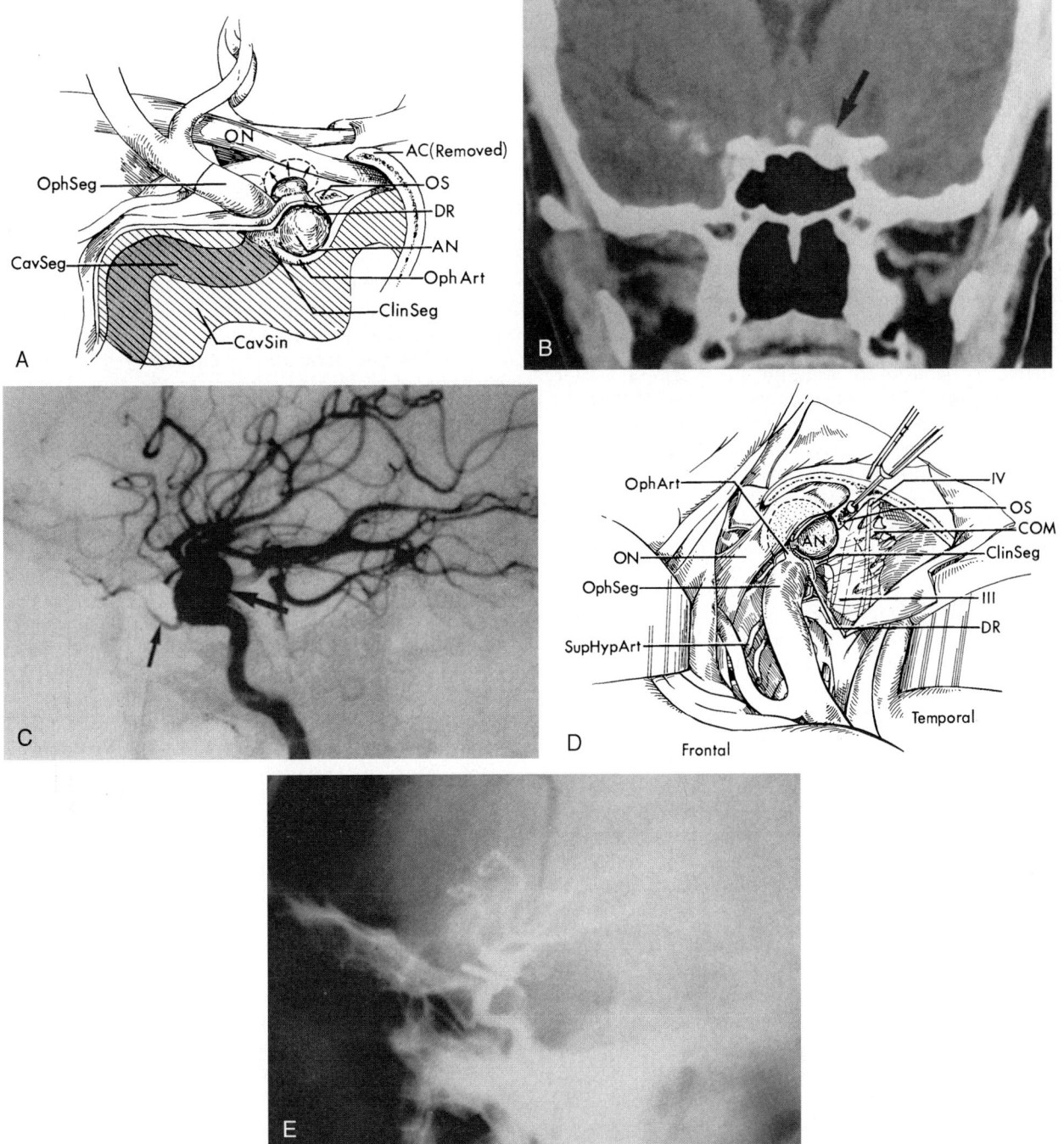

**FIGURE 26–3** ■ Clinoidal segment aneurysm. *A,* Operative view (schematic). Note the aneurysm (AN) arising in the clinoidal segment (ClinSeg) in conjunction with a similar origin of the ophthalmic artery (OphArt). ClinSeg aneurysms project above the plane of the cranial nerves within the cavernous sinus (CavSin) and present with either visual loss from optic nerve (ON) compression or subarachnoid hemorrhage following extension through the dura into the subarachnoid space *(arrows).* (AC, anterior clinoid process; DR, dural ring; OS, optic strut; OphSeg, ophthalmic segment.) *B,* A computed tomography scan of a clinoidal segment aneurysm *(arrow).* Note the aneurysm arising below and medial to the anterior clinoid process, indicating its origin within the clinoidal segment. *C,* A preoperative arteriogram (lateral view). Note the origin of the ophthalmic artery *(small arrow)* and the clinoidal segment (ClinSeg) aneurysm *(large arrow)* well below the plane of the anterior clinoid process, from the anterior vertical portion of the cavernous carotid artery (ClinSeg). Note the superior bulging of the aneurysm out of the ClinSeg into the subarachnoid space. This lesion should prompt strong considerations for simultaneous cervical internal carotid artery exposure, and intradural rather than extradural anterior clinoid process removal. *D,* Operative exposure (schematic) of the clinoidal segment (ClinSeg) aneurysm (AN). Note that the entire lesser wing of the sphenoid bone, including the anterior clinoid process, has been removed. The roof, side, and floor of the optic canal have been drilled away, as has the optic strut (OS), to completely define the dural ring (DR) and carotid-oculomotor membrane (COM). The dura adjacent to the ring is then sectioned circumferentially to allow mobilization of the internal carotid artery and to allow unimpeded clip placement on the aneurysm neck without compromise of the parent vessel lumen. (ON, optic nerve; III, oculomotor nerve; IV, trochlear nerve; OphArt, ophthalmic artery; OphScg, ophthalmic segment; SupHypArt, superior hypophyseal artery.) *E,* Postoperative arteriogram demonstrating excellent patency of the internal carotid artery, with complete obliteration of the aneurysm. Note the proximal origin of the ophthalmic artery.

another that maintains normal flow directions intracranially, and avoidance of direct manipulation of the nerves within the cavernous sinus. This procedure is, however, technically more difficult than convexity bypass procedures, and the exposure is often substantially limited by the bulging aneurysm. In addition, elderly patients often have arteriosclerotic intracranial vessels that do not respond well to temporary clipping or end-to-side anastomosis. In general, we reserve this procedure for younger patients in good medical health and without significant arteriosclerosis.

***Direct Clipping.*** Direct clipping of CavSeg aneurysms can be performed, but the procedure is limited by the lesion's size, shape, associated arteriosclerosis and thrombosis, and morbidity to cranial nerves, and the difficulty in reconstructing the ICA lumen while in the middle of a large venous channel.[29, 30] Recent advances in the use of profound hypothermia (and cardiac standstill, if necessary) have made this technique a highly useful adjuvant in the treatment of certain difficult aneurysms, but the hazards of the method when it is applied to a CavSeg lesion may not compare favorably to its natural history or the risks of less complex therapeutic modalities, especially in elderly patients.

***Interventional Techniques.*** By the time that they become symptomatic, CavSeg aneurysms often have very large necks that communicate widely with the parent vessel. Detachable balloons are not as effective in eliminating cavernous sinus (CavSin) aneurysms unless the parent vessel is simultaneously sacrificed, but endovascular (GDC) coils may be useful for some lesions.[31, 32] GDC coils work best when the aneurysm neck is small, and this modality, therefore, often has limited potential in the treatment of large intracavernous aneurysms.[33] Smaller CavSin aneurysms are more likely to have more narrow necks and be much more amenable to this technology. Because smaller intracavernous aneurysms are invariably asymptomatic and have no demonstrable risk of bleeding, however, treatment is probably not warranted.

**Clinoidal Segment Aneurysms.** ClinSeg aneurysms have been identified as a distinct entity with clinical and anatomical features that are very different from those arising on more proximal intracavernous portions.[8, 9] These lesions arise in the interval between the carotid-oculomotor membrane and the DR, from the anterior vertical segment of the intracavernous ICA, often in association with an ophthalmic or superior hypophyseal artery origin within this segment. With enlargement, hemodynamic forces project the aneurysm fundus superiorly, away from the cranial nerves in the cavernous sinus, and against the overlying dura, AC, and optic strut.

Because ClinSeg aneurysms originate below the ICA's penetrance into the subarachnoid space, small ClinSeg aneurysms are usually asymptomatic. Because of their superior projection, the cranial nerves within the cavernous sinus are usually not affected by the lesion's growth, although small lesions may project into the optic canal and cause optic nerve compression and visual loss. With enlargement (1 cm or greater), ClinSeg aneurysms may erode through the dura into the subarachnoid space, at which time they mimic ophthalmic segment (OphSeg) lesions

(Fig. 26–4A). SAH from an intracavernous aneurysm is almost always attributable to this variant.

Unlike OphSeg aneurysms, the neck of ClinSeg lesions is located below the DR, making preoperative recognition essential for safe treatment planning. Focal erosion of the optic strut or AC demonstrated on CT or MRI often marks the lesion's proximal origin (see Fig. 26–4B).[8] Arteriographically, ClinSeg aneurysms invariably originate below the plane of the ophthalmic artery (see Fig. 26–4C). Two clinical variations, based on site of aneurysm origin and direction of projection from the ClinSeg, have been clarified. One originates from the anterior lateral surface of the ClinSeg and may extend upward into, through, or medial to the AC. This type may cause optic nerve compression either within the optic canal extradurally or within the subarachnoid space after penetrating the dura. The other originates from the medial ClinSeg surface and may erode through the lateral sphenoid sinus wall to produce epistaxis or into the lateral sella beneath the diaphragma sella to mimic a pituitary tumor. Once exceeding 1 cm, either type may produce SAH, as the likelihood that the aneurysm has eroded through the dural roof of this segment and is projecting into the subarachnoid space is much higher.

***Direct Clipping.*** Asymptomatic lesions smaller than 1 cm should probably be observed unless the ClinSeg is to be exposed for other reasons. Larger or symptomatic lesions can be clipped in most cases, with preservation of ICA patency. Because proximal control of the ClinSeg lies within the cavernous sinus, the operative field should include sterile preparation of the cervical carotid bifurcation region. When the aneurysm has bled, we routinely open the neck incision, because the intracranial exposure necessary to clip the aneurysm carries significant risks of intraoperative rupture.

Adequate exposure of ClinSeg aneurysms begins with extensive extradural removal of the lateral sphenoid ridge and posterior orbital roof (see Fig. 26–4D). Because ClinSeg aneurysms are adherent and may actually erode through the AC, the most medial extent of the lesser wing of the sphenoid bone is not removed extradurally. The dura is opened, and the sylvian fissure is widely split, allowing the subarachnoid extension of the aneurysm to be directly visualized. The AC is then removed using an intradural approach. The optic canal roof and lateral wall are also carefully drilled away with a diamond drill, and the dural sheath overlying the optic nerve is opened to allow its mobilization. Finally, the optic strut is drilled down flush to the wall of the sphenoid sinus. Any bleeding from the sinus can be controlled easily with Gelfoam or Surgicel.

After the optic nerve has been freed and the branches of the OphSeg have been identified (ophthalmic and superior hypophyseal arteries), the dural attachments of the ICA at the DR are sectioned circumferentially, providing unimpeded clip access to the ClinSeg. The anterolateral type is usually best obliterated with a gently curved clip, whereas the medial type invariably requires a right-angled fenestrated clip that encircles the ICA. We routinely use intraoperative arteriography to document that the clip is in the proper position and that the ICA is patent before the wound is closed (see Fig. 26–4E).

Care should be taken to avoid injury to the oculomotor

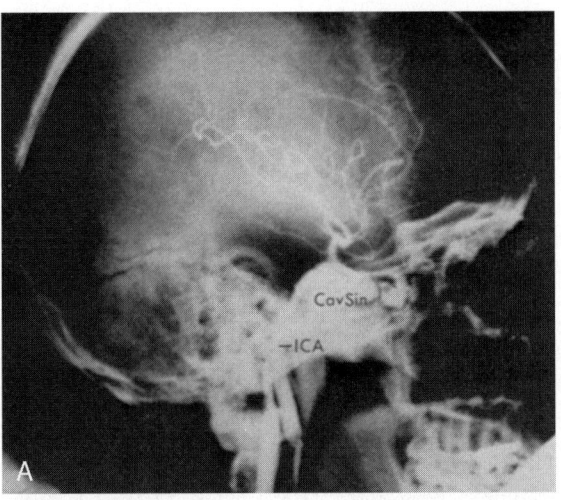
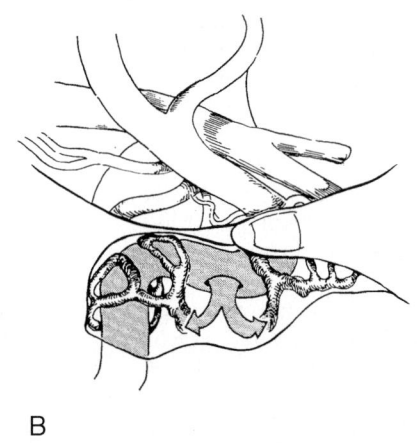
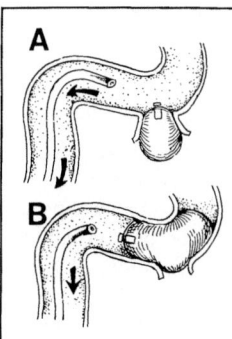

**FIGURE 26–4** ■ High-flow carotid cavernous fistula. *A,* A preoperative arteriogram (lateral view) in a young man who developed the subacute onset of a bruit and cavernous sinus syndrome following a closed head injury. Note the large arteriovenous fistula between the carotid artery (ICA) and the cavernous sinus (CavSin). *B,* Detachable balloon treatment of high-flow carotid-cavernous fistula (schematic). Note the tear in the carotid artery, with arterial flow proceeding directly into adjacent veins. A balloon-tipped flow-directed catheter is passed into the fistula and the balloon is detached, preserving the carotid lumen (insert A: upper right) or occluding the carotid lumen (insert B: lower right).

nerve (which sits at the lateral edge of the COM), either during the exposure or as the clip blades are being advanced to secure the proximal aneurysm neck. The oculosympathetic fibers exit from the ICA in the ClinSeg, and extensive dissection often results in a mild ptosis and miosis. Bone defects into the basal sinuses are often encountered while drilling the optic strut. To prevent postoperative cerebrospinal fluid rhinorrhea, these must be recognized and repaired, usually with a combination of muscle, Gelfoam, and tissue adhesive or methyl methacrylate.

***Interventional Techniques.*** ICA sacrifice should accomplish thrombosis of most ClinSeg aneurysms but carries the risk of hemispheric ischemia. GDC coils may have a role in the treatment of many of these lesions, because their necks are usually quite narrow. Surgical exposure to allow direct clipping of ClinSeg aneurysms can be safely performed in most patients, with only slightly higher operative risks than those associated with OphSeg lesions. In our opinion, most symptomatic or larger ClinSeg lesions should be directly viewed by a surgeon experienced in this area before an interventional technique is considered, unless medical risks contraindicate an open procedure.

## Infectious Aneurysms

Infectious aneurysms may affect the cavernous ICA either by septic embolization or by extension of an adjacent septic focus within the venous sinus or skull base.[34] Ultimately, the arteritis produced by the infection may lead to arterial thrombosis, aneurysm formation, or rupture. The primary treatment of such lesions should be appropriate antimicrobial drugs, with aggressive intervention reserved for persistent symptomatic lesions. When necessary, therapy should generally include ICA ligation, using the same precautions to prevent stroke as for the saccular variety.

## Traumatic Nonfistulous Aneurysms

Traumatic ICA aneurysm formation following closed head injury occurs predominantly in the intracavernous portion of that vessel. This type of aneurysm may also develop following penetrating injuries to the orbit or brain when the wall of the cavernous carotid artery is injured. The typical patient initially presents with a skull fracture of the anterior skull base, accompanied by unilateral blindness, anosmia, or other cranial neuropathies.[13] The aneurysm itself may not be symptomatic initially. Others may be heralded by unexplained arterial bleeding following parasphenoidal procedures that disrupt the ICA or one of its branches.[35–37] Massive epistaxis may develop immediately when nasal packing is removed or may occur later after the patient has been discharged seemingly free of problems. If epistaxis does occur, almost 50% of patients die before a diagnosis is established or adequate treatment is rendered.[37–39]

Aggressive therapy should be strongly considered following angiographic identification, because the mortality rate with lesions presenting with epistaxis is so high. Surgical trapping with simultaneous intracranial and cervical carotid ligation, or balloon occlusion at the site of the arterial injury, accelerates thrombosis and lessens the chances of collateral circulation development. Extracranial-intracranial bypass surgery, using an arterial donor to obviate need for systemic anticoagulation, should be considered when time and the patient's clinical state and anatomy permit.

## CAROTID-CAVERNOUS FISTULAS

Fistulous diversion of arterial flow in the region of the cavernous sinus can produce various clinical signs, including exophthalmos, orbital or cephalic bruit (or both), ocular pulsations, headache, chemosis, extraocular palsies, visual failure, or bleeding.[38, 40–42] Catastrophic complications such as SAH, epistaxis, or severe orbital bleeding are uncommon in untreated lesions.[43, 44] The pattern of venous drainage is a major determinant of the signs and symptoms produced by the fistula, regardless of the site or size of the arterial injury. The multiple venous outflow channels from the cavernous sinus allow the arterialized blood to be diverted anteriorly into the ipsilateral, contralateral, or bilateral orbital venous system or posteriorly into parenchymal veins within the brain.[45]

Carotid-cavernous fistulas (CCFs) can be categorized based on pathologic, hemodynamic, and arteriographic criteria, including (1) post-traumatic versus spontaneous (dependent on the presence or absence of head injury temporally related to onset), (2) high flow versus low flow (the size of the arteriovenous communication), (3) direct versus indirect or dural (arterial flow directly from the ICA, or from dural branches of the ICA or ECA), and (4) typical versus atypical (venous drainage into the dural sinuses or through parenchymal veins).[40, 41, 46, 47] The options and results of intervention are determined by a composite assessment of each of these criteria. Complete arteriography, including bilateral selective external and internal carotid injections and at least one vertebral injection, should be performed prior to treatment selection, because some fistulas have unusual arterial feeding patterns or venous drainage.

High-flow fistulas are usually post-traumatic in origin, although a few develop following intracavernous aneurysm rupture.[40, 41, 47] The typical patient is a young man with a pronounced and rapidly progressive cavernous sinus syndrome appearing shortly after sustaining a significant head injury.[13] The arterial supply to the fistula originates directly from the cavernous ICA, and distal carotid flow is often impaired. Venous drainage proceeds forward through the ipsilateral superior ophthalmic vein into the orbit. Sponta-

neous thrombosis of the fistula or of adjacent veins is rare, and most cases require aggressive intervention.

Low-flow fistulas typically arise in middle-aged or elderly women, are invariably spontaneous in origin, and usually coexist with a prior venous sinus thrombosis. Symptoms are usually mild and rarely evolve to a full-blown exophthalmos and panophthalmoplegia syndrome so characteristic of the high-flow variety.[40, 41, 47] Arterial supply to the fistula originates from dural branches of the ICA or ECA, and blood flow into the hemisphere is normal. Because arterial inflow is low, and there is already some impedance to venous outflow from prior sinus thrombosis, spontaneous regression is frequent, especially when compared with high-flow lesions.[40, 43, 46–48]

The goals of therapy for a CCF include preservation of vision, elimination of the bruit, and restoration of the orbit and its contents to normal while avoiding cerebral ischemic complications. The ideal treatment should obliterate the fistula while maintaining patency of the carotid artery. Interventional endovascular techniques have greatly facilitated the treatment of many of these lesions. Such methods include both arterial and venous-side occlusion and are generally considered first before any open surgical intervention is contemplated.

## High-Flow Fistulas

**Interventional Neuroradiologic Procedures.** Detachable balloon systems are the procedure of choice for most high-flow CCFs, because they offer the advantages of direct fistula occlusion without an open cervical or intracranial procedure.[40, 41, 49, 50] Angiography characteristically demonstrates early and dense opacification of the enlarged cavernous sinus and poorer-than-expected opacification of the cerebral arterial system (Fig. 26–5A). Although the high-flow, high-pressure shunt often makes the exact point of

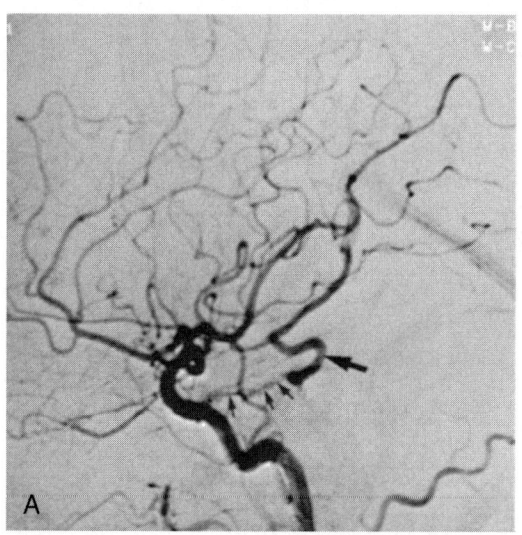

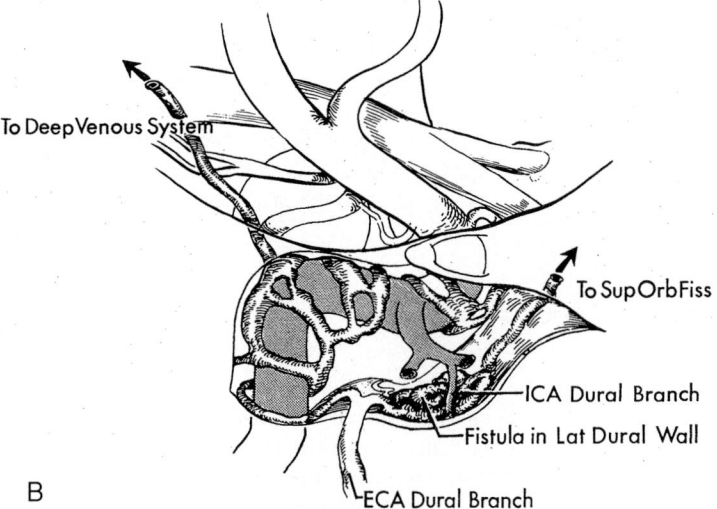

To Deep Venous System

To SupOrbFiss

ICA Dural Branch

Fistula in Lat Dural Wall

ECA Dural Branch

A                                                    B

**FIGURE 26–5 ■** Low-flow carotid cavernous fistula. *A,* A preoperative arteriogram (lateral view) in a 55-year-old man who had a recent severe headache suggestive of subarachnoid hemorrhage. Note the small dural fistula in the region of the cavernous sinus (multiple *small arrows*), with venous drainage *(large arrow)* bridging the tentorium and subarachnoid space to enter the deep venous system (atypical variant). *B,* A schematic representation of a dural fistula on the lateral cavernous sinus dural wall. Note the potential arterial filling from both the external and internal carotid dural branches. Venous drainage usually proceeds anteriorly into the ophthalmic veins (typical variant). In the actual case *(A),* the dura containing the fistula and the vein draining into the parenchyma were coagulated. Subsequent arteriography confirmed the complete obliteration of the fistula.

arteriovenous communication difficult to demonstrate, these factors greatly facilitate the ease and safety of passing a flow-directed detachable balloon directly into the fistula (see Fig. 26–5B).

In this fistula type, blood flow from the ipsilateral ICA is already largely diverted directly into the venous system without contributing substantially to brain perfusion. If simultaneous ICA sacrifice is required, it is generally well tolerated, as long as the fistula is simultaneously obliterated.[51, 52] If the balloon is detached below the fistula, or if ipsilateral proximal carotid thrombosis occurs from any other cause, several major problems are created, including: (1) persistence of the fistula (now filled retrograde from intracranial communications), (2) cortical steal (flow from collaterals that were supplying the distal hemisphere is now diverted toward the fistula), and (3) limited transarterial catheter access. In such circumstances, the fistula is still treatable by exposing the ClinSeg intracranially, temporarily clipping the ICA below the ophthalmic artery origin, and passing a detachable balloon-tipped catheter through the wall of the ClinSeg towards the fistula. When the temporary clip is released, retrograde flow will carry the balloon into the fistula. Trial inflation, monitored with transocular and transcranial Doppler and direct observation of the pulsating sinus, will confirm proper balloon placement and shunt obliteration. Once the fistula and its effects disappear, the balloon is detached, and a permanent clip is left in place on the ClinSeg.

**Direct Surgical Intervention.** Using adjunctive hypothermia and circulatory arrest, Parkinson exposed the intracavernous carotid artery through the lateral cavernous sinus wall.[52, 53] Dolenc and others also described a direct operative approach to high-flow CCF, using the same exposure described for petrous-to-supraclinoid ICA bypass for intracavernous aneurysms.[27–29] During such procedures, the ICA is very difficult to distinguish from the surrounding arterialized veins, and identification of the exact fistula site can be extremely tedious. Because of the technical difficulties of these approaches and their associated morbidity to the cranial nerves and brain, direct procedures should probably be restricted to those rare circumstances in which interventional techniques with detachable balloons or coils are not applicable.[54, 55]

## Low-Flow Fistulas

**Transarterial Procedures.** Most spontaneous fistulas are low-flow, low-pressure dural shunts that receive blood from several sources. The ECA frequently supplies this type of fistula, primarily through terminal meningeal branches of the internal maxillary artery and also from other contributing branches including the ascending pharyngeal and pterygopalatine arteries.[39, 40] The inferolateral and the meningohypophyseal trunks are the usual sources when the ICA supplies the fistula. Contralateral arterial dural contributions are also frequent.

The more benign symptoms, lesser likelihood of major visual complications, and greater tendency for spontaneous thrombosis justify conservative management of most spontaneous fistulas. Because the fistula originates from multiple, smaller dural branches of the ICA or ECA, detachable balloon techniques have little or no value. When intervention is indicated, particulate embolization with polyvinyl alcohol or other agents introduced into the ECA can produce excellent results with low risks.[40, 47] Occasionally, the hemodynamic changes caused by only partial ECA embolization are adequate to lead to spontaneous resolution of the entire fistula. ICA feeder embolization is more difficult and obviously more hazardous, and embolic procedures within this vessel should probably be delayed until all treatments through the ECA have been maximally exercised.

**Transvenous Approaches.** Thrombogenic materials, introduced into the cavernous sinus directly through Parkinson's triangle or indirectly through a draining vein (e.g., the superior ophthalmic vein) or sinus (e.g., the petrosal sinuses), can effectively thrombose these lesions with low morbidity and a high likelihood of ICA preservation.[56–58]

Although venous drainage of spontaneous CCF is usually through the ipsilateral lateral ophthalmic veins, variations are not uncommon. Arterialized outflow proceeding through parenchymal veins places these lesions at risk for hemorrhage, and more aggressive intervention is warranted (see Fig. 26–5A). Using a frontotemporal craniotomy, the lateral wall of the cavernous sinus may be exposed, along with the arterialized draining veins bridging the subarachnoid space. The fistula, usually readily apparent within the dura, is coagulated with low-power bipolar cautery (see Fig. 26–5B). The veins exiting the sinus into parenchyma are also coagulated and sectioned, thus restricting any residual sinus arterialization from reaching weaker parenchymal veins.

**Stereotactic Radiosurgery.** Several reports have indicated that dural arteriovenous fistulas may resolve following stereotactic-focused radiation (radiosurgery), including several small series of lesions in the cavernous sinus area.[59–61] Such treatments generally require months or years to effect obliteration but may be considered in select cases in which the fistula is well circumscribed and other options are inadvisable.

## REFERENCES

1. Inoue T, Rhoton AL Jr, Theel D, Barry ME: Surgical approaches to the cavernous sinus: A microsurgical study. Neurosurgery 26:903–932, 1990.
2. Day AL: Aneurysms of the ophthalmic segment: A clinical and anatomic analysis. J Neurosurg 72:677–691, 1990.
3. Seone E, Rhoton AL, de Oliveira E: Microsurgical anatomy of the dural collar (carotid collar) and rings around the clinoidal segment of the internal carotid artery. Neurosurgery 42:869–886, 1998.
4. Locksley HB: Natural history of subarachnoid hemorrhage, intracranial aneurysms, and arteriovenous malformation. J Neurosurg 25:219–239, 1966.
5. Sahs AL, Perret GE, Locksley HB, Nishioka H: Intracranial Aneurysms and Subarachnoid Hemorrhage: A Cooperative Study Philadelphia: JB Lippincott, 1969, p 296.
6. Linskey ME, Sekhar LN, Hirsch W, et al: Aneurysms of the intracavernous carotid artery: Clinical presentation, radiographic features, and pathogenesis. Neurosurgery 26:71–79, 1990.
7. Kupersmith MJ, Hurst R, Berenstein A, et al: The benign course of cavernous carotid artery aneurysms. J Neurosurg 77:690–693, 1992.
8. Day AL, Knego RS, Masson RL: Aneurysms of the Clinoidal Segment: A Clinicoanatomic Study. Presented at the American Associa-

tion of Neurological Surgeons Annual Meeting, Boston, Massachusetts, April 1993.

9. al-Rodhan NR, Piepgras DG, Sundt TM Jr: Transitional cavernous aneurysms of the internal carotid artery. Neurosurgery 33:993–996, 1993.

10. Hirsh WL, Hyrshko FG, Sekhar LN, Brunberg J: Comparison of MRI imaging, CT, and angiography in the evaluation of the enlarged cavernous sinus. Am J Radiol 151:1015–1023, 1988.

11. Linskey ME, Sekhar LN, Horton JA, et al: Aneurysms of the intracavernous carotid artery: A multidisciplinary approach to treatment. J Neurosurg 75:525–534, 1991.

12. Serbinenko FA, Filatov JM, Spallone A, et al: Management of giant intracranial ICA aneurysms with combined extracranial-intracranial anastomosis and endovascular occlusion. J Neurosurg 73:57–63, 1990.

13. Day AL, Rhoton AL Jr: Aneurysms and arteriovenous fistulae of the intracavernous carotid artery and its branches. In Youmans JR (ed): Neurological Surgery. Philadelphia: WB Saunders, 1990, pp 1807–1830.

14. Nishioka H: Report on the Cooperative Study of Intracranial Aneurysms and Subarachnoid Hemorrhage: Results of the treatment of intracranial aneurysms by occlusion of the carotid artery in the neck. J Neurosurg 25:660–682, 1966.

15. Swearingen B, Heros RC: Common carotid artery occlusion for unclippable carotid aneurysms: An old but still effective operation. Neurosurgery 21:288–295, 1987.

16. Lombardi G, Passerini A, Mighavacca F: Intracavernous aneurysms of the internal carotid artery. Am J Radiol 89:361–371, 1963.

17. Pozzati E, Fagioli L, Servadei F, Gaist G: Effect of common carotid ligation of giant aneurysms of the internal carotid artery. J Neurosurg 55:527–531, 1981.

18. Morley TP, Barr HWK: Giant intracranial aneurysms: Diagnosis, course, and management. Clin Neurosurg 16:73–94, 1968.

19. Drake CG, Peerless SJ, Ferguson GG: Hunterian proximal arterial occlusion for giant aneurysm of the carotid circulation. J Neurosurg 81:656–665, 1994.

20. Linskey ME, Jungreis CA, Yonas H, et al: Stroke risk after abrupt internal carotid artery sacrifice: Accuracy of preoperative assessment with balloon test occlusion and stable xenon-enhanced CT. Am J Neuroradiol 15:829–843, 1994.

21. Polin RS, Shaffrey ME, Jensen ME, et al: Medical management in the endovascular treatment of carotid-cavernous aneurysms. J Neurosurg 84:755–761, 1996.

22. Lewis AI, Tomsick TA, Tew JM Jr: Management of 100 consecutive direct carotid-cavernous fistulas: Results of treatment with detachable balloons. Neurosurgery 36:239–244, 1995.

23. Barnett DW, Barrow DL, Joseph GJ: Combined extracranial-intracranial bypass and intraoperative balloon occlusion for the treatment of intracavernous and proximal carotid artery aneurysms. Neurosurgery 35:92–97, 1994.

24. Fox AJ, Vinuela F, Pelz DM, et al: Use of detachable balloons for proximal artery occlusion in the treatment of unclippable cerebral aneurysms. J Neurosurg 66:40–46, 1987.

25. Diaz FG, Ausman A Pearce JE: Ischemic complications after combined internal carotid artery occlusion and extracranial–intracranial anastomosis. Neurosurgery 10:563–570, 1982.

26. Sekhar LN, Linskey ME, Sen CN, Altschuler EM: Surgical management of lesions within the cavernous sinus. Clin Neurosurg 37:440–489, 1991.

27. Sekhar LN, Sen CN, Jho HD: Saphenous vein graft bypass of the cavernous internal carotid artery. J Neurosurg 72:35–41, 1990.

28. Spetzler RF, Fukushima T, Martin N, Zabramski JM: Petrous carotid-to-intradural carotid saphenous vein graft for intracavernous giant aneurysm, tumor, and occlusive cerebrovascular disease. J Neurosurg 73:496–501, 1990.

29. Dolenc VV: Direct microsurgical repair of intracavernous vascular lesions. J Neurosurg 58:824–831, 1983.

30. Diaz FG, Ohaegbulam S, Dujovny M, Ausman JI: Surgical alternatives in the treatment of cavernous sinus aneurysms. J Neurosurg 71:846–853, 1989.

31. Higashida RT, Halbach VV, Dowd C, et al: Endovascular detachable balloon embolization therapy of cavernous carotid artery aneurysm: Results in 87 cases. J Neurosurg 72:857–863, 1990.

32. Guglielmi G, Vinuela F, Briganti F, Duckwiler G: Carotid-cavernous fistula caused by ruptured intracavernous aneurysm: Endovascular treatment by electrothrombosis with detachable coils. Neurosurgery 31:591–5996, 1992.

33. Guglielmi G, Vinuela F, Dion J, Duckwiler G: Electrothrombosis of saccular aneurysms via endovascular approach. Part 2: Preliminary clinical experiences. J Neurosurg 75:8–14, 1991.

34. Rout D, Sharma A, Mohan P, Rao VRK: Bacterial aneurysms of the intracavernous carotid artery. J Neurosurg 60:1236–1242, 1984.

35. Lister JR, Sypert GW: Traumatic false aneurysm and carotid-cavernous fistula: A complication of sphenoidotomy. Neurosurgery 5:473–475, 1979.

36. Robbins JB, Fitz-Hugh GS, Jane JA: Intracranial carotid catastrophies encountered by the otolaryngologist. Laryngoscope 86:893–902, 1976.

37. Baviszski G, Killer M, Knosp E, et al: False aneurysm of the intracavernous carotid artery: Report of 7 cases. Acta Neurochir (Wien) 139:37–43, 1997.

38. Handa J, Handa H: Severe epistaxis caused by traumatic aneurysm of cavernous carotid artery. Surg Neurol 5:241–243, 1976.

39. Liu MY, Shih CJ, Wang YC, Tsai SH: Traumatic intracavernous carotid aneurysm with massive epistaxis. Neurosurgery 17:569–573, 1985.

40. Barrow DL, Spector RH, Braun IF, et al: Classification and treatment of spontaneous carotid-cavernous sinus fistulas. J Neurosurg 62:248–256, 1985.

41. DeBrun GM, Vinuela F, Fox AJ, et al: Indications for treatment and classification of 132 carotid cavernous fistulas. Neurosurgery 22:285–289, 1988.

42. Martin JD Jr, Mabon RF: Pulsating exophthalmos: Review of all reported cases. JAMA 121:330–334, 1943.

43. Dohrmann PJ, Batjer HH, Samson D, Suss RA: Recurrent subarachnoid hemorrhage complicating a traumatic carotid cavernous fistula. Neurosurgery 17:480–483, 1985.

44. Lee SH, Burton CV, Chan GH: Posttraumatic ophthalmic vein arterialization. Surg Neurol 4:483–484, 1974.

45. Bickerstaff ER: Mechanisms of presentation of carotico-cavernous fistulae. Br J Ophthalmol 54:186–190, 1970.

46. Peeters FLM, Kroger R: Dural and direct cavernous sinus fistulas. Am J Radiol 132:599–606, 1979.

47. Vinuela F, Fox AJ, DeBrun GM, et al: Spontaneous carotid-cavernous fistulas: Clinical, radiological, and therapeutic considerations. J Neurosurg 60:976–984, 1984.

48. Newton TH, Hoyt WF: Dural arteriovenous shunts in the region of cavernous sinus. Neuroradiology 1:71–81, 1970.

49. Berenstein A, Krichoff 1, Ransohoff J: Carotid-cavernous fistula: Intraarterial treatment. AJNR Am J Neuroradiol 1:449–457, 1980.

50. DeBrun GN4, LaCour P, Vinuela F, et al: Treatment of 54 traumatic carotid-cavernous fistulas. J Neurosurg 55:678–692, 1981.

51. Tomsick TA, Tew JM, Lukin RR, Johnson JK: Balloon catheters for aneurysms and fistulae. Clin Neurosurg 31:135–164, 1983.

52. Parkinson D: Carotid cavernous fistula: Direct approach and repair of fistula and preservation of the artery. In Morley TP (ed): Current Controversies in Neurosurgery. Philadelphia: WB Saunders, 1976.

53. Parkinson D: Carotid cavernous fistula: Direct repair with preservation of carotid. J Neurosurg 38:99–106, 1973.

54. Tu YK, Liu HM, Hu SC: Direct surgery of carotid-cavernous fistulae and dural arteriovenous malformations of the cavernous sinus. Neurosurgery 41:798–805, 1997.

55. Day JD, Fukushima T: Direct microsurgery of dural arteriovenous malformation type carotid-cavernous sinus fistulas: Indications, technique, and results. Neurosurgery 41:1119–1124, 1997.

56. Mullan S: Experiences with surgical thrombosis of intracranial berry aneurysms and carotid cavernous fistulae. J Neurosurg 41:657–670, 1974.

57. Mullan S: Treatment of carotid-cavernous fistulae by cavernous sinus occlusion. J Neurosurg 50:131–144, 1979.

58. Miller NR, Monsein LH, Debrun GM, et al: Treatment of carotid-cavernous fistulas using a superior ophthalmic vein approach. J Neurosurg 83:838–842, 1995.

59. Chandler HC Jr, Friedman WA: Successful radiosurgical treatment of a dural arteriovenous malformation: Case report. Neurosurgery 33:139–142, 1993.

60. Barcia-Salorio JL, Soler F, Barcia JA, Hernandez G: Radiosurgery of carotid-cavernous fistulae. Acta Neurochir Suppl (Wien) 62:10–12, 1994.

61. Guo WY, Pan DH, Wu HM, et al: Radiosurgery as a treatment alternative for dural arteriovenous fistulas of the cavernous sinus. Am J Neuroradiol 19:1081–1087, 1998

CHAPTER 27

# Surgical Management of Tumors Involving the Cavernous Sinus

■ TAKANORI FUKUSHIMA and J. DIAZ DAY

Until 1965, when Parkinson's landmark article describing the direct surgical approach to carotid-cavernous fistulas was published, little reference was made in the neurosurgical literature to direct operative attack on lesions of the cavernous sinus.[1] This lack of information was largely a result of the inability in the premicrosurgical era to effectively deal with the extreme risks of significant hemorrhage and damage to the cranial nerves in the region. This anatomic locale has long been considered a true "no man's land" for direct surgical approaches. The modern era of microneurosurgery has realized expanded capabilities in microsurgical technique and has fostered the work of several neurosurgeons who have made great strides in effectively approaching this region with reduced morbidity.[2–14] In particular, the work of Dolenc should be recognized for the development of his combined epidural and subdural approach, which has become the standard method used to treat lesions in this region.[6]

## INDICATIONS

The indications for direct operative attack on neoplastic lesions arising in or involving the cavernous sinus have been a matter of recent debate. New forms of therapy, such as stereotactic radiosurgery, are providing alternatives in our armamentarium for treating these difficult tumors.[15–17] A firmer set of indications for operative intervention has been evolving. We briefly consider the presently acceptable indications for a direct operation on these lesions.

The presence of a mass in the cavernous sinus, of course, does not itself constitute an indication for a direct operation. Many factors must be taken into account, including the age and medical condition of the patient, imaging characteristics, adjacent structures involved, time course of the process, and functional severity of symptoms. Many patients, because of poor medical condition or refusal to undergo surgery, may not be candidates for intracavernous microsurgery. Recent reports have demonstrated that stereotactic radiosurgery presents a viable alternative in patients with small intracavernous meningiomas.[17] Most pa-

tients who are able to undergo general anesthesia and who harbor lesions that appear to be amenable to a total resection are offered an operation. Most of these patients have lesions that are consistent with benign tumors of the region (e.g., neurinomas, cavernous hemangiomas, pituitary adenomas, dermoids, chordomas, and chondrosarcomas). These tumors are well-encapsulated masses that are dissectible from the surrounding structures.

Patients with apparent meningiomas of the cavernous sinus, although their tumors are benign, are placed in a separate category for indications for operation. Patients who are able to undergo surgery who have debilitating symptoms, such as rapid visual loss or painful ophthalmoplegia, are offered an immediate operation. The goal of such an operation is decompression of the involved structures, with a total resection attempted only when circumstances are favorable. Patients with asymptomatic, small meningiomas are followed up with serial scans until they exhibit enlargement of the mass or neurologic symptoms. A few patients with minimal symptoms who have tumors that typically are treated conservatively are offered an operation. This decision is made because the resection is easier owing to the size of the tumor and lack of invasion into critical structures. These decisions rely on the judgment of the surgeon experienced with tumors in this area.

Difficult decisions are made in cases in which cavernous sinus involvement occurs by extensions of malignant processes from the paranasal sinuses and pharynx. Procedures treating such disorders are palliative because of the characteristically aggressive nature of these tumors, such as squamous cell carcinoma. En bloc resection of the cavernous sinus and adjacent areas may represent merely a heroic effort on the patient's behalf, with little realistic chance of long-term survival. Localized malignancies are an entirely different prospect in most cases. Local invasion by chordomas or chondrosarcomas may be effectively resected almost totally in many cases, with long-term recurrence-free survival, even though these tumors are incurable.[13]

Regardless of the process, surgery for these lesions is a formidable undertaking. As experience with these lesions grows, the indications will change according to technologic developments and growing surgical capabilities. This discussion outlines the methods for operative intervention when such an approach is deemed appropriate.

## SURGICAL ANATOMY

Recent work focusing on the microsurgical anatomy of the cavernous sinus and its adjacent structures has made a critical contribution to our understanding and capabilities in dealing with neoplasms involving the cavernous sinus.[7, 18–22] The individual surgeon's facility with the anatomic details of this complex region cannot be underemphasized as a basis for successful surgical therapy. The anatomy as presented in conventional texts, although an important initial basis, provides insufficient knowledge for the neurosurgeon operating in this region. An intimate comprehension of the multiple entry corridors and their specific anatomic substrates and boundaries is critical to the safe implementation of these procedures. Adequate preparation, including judicious use of the cadaver dissection laboratory, enhances the chances for a successful approach to these lesions.

The cavernous sinus is a tetrahedron-shaped space that is bounded on all sides by dura mater. It is located on either side of the sella turcica at the convergence of the anterior fossa, middle fossa, sphenoid ridge, and petroclival ridge. The contents of the sinus are contained within a membranous structure. Inferiorly and medially, this membrane consists of a periosteal layer of dura that covers the middle fossa and sella turcica. The superior and lateral portion of this outer cavernous membrane is contiguous with the connective tissue sheaths of cranial nerves III, IV, and V. This "true," or outer, cavernous membrane contains the structures within the cavernous sinus. A heavy venous plexus with connections to the ophthalmic veins, the pterygoid plexus, the superior and inferior petrosal sinuses, the basilar venous plexus, and the superficial middle cerebral veins via the sphenoparietal sinus is contained in the space. The internal carotid artery and its branches, accompanied by a sympathetic plexus of nerves, pass through the sinus. Also, cranial nerve VI travels through the cavernous sinus to enter the superior orbital fissure under the ophthalmic division of cranial nerve V.

The anatomy of the intracavernous carotid artery deserves special attention. The artery enters the cavernous sinus, piercing the true cavernous membrane, at the foramen lacerum. It is surrounded here by a thickening of this connective tissue, which forms a fibrous ring around the artery. The artery then bends anterosuperiorly toward the superior orbital fissure. Just distal to this bend, the meningohypophyseal trunk typically arises on the superomedial side. This trunk has three branches: (1) the tentorial (Bernasconi-Cassinari), (2) the dorsal meningeal, and (3) the inferior hypophyseal arteries, all of which display some variability. The carotid artery usually gives rise to the artery of the inferior cavernous sinus on its lateral side as it courses anteriorly. This vessel traverses the sinus, usually crossing over cranial nerve VI, and anastomoses with several branches of the internal maxillary artery. These anastomoses include: (1) the recurrent meningeal artery at the superior orbital fissure, (2) the artery of the foramen ro-

tundum, (3) the accessory meningeal artery at the foramen ovale, and (4) the middle meningeal artery at the foramen spinosum. The tentorial artery is absent from the meningohypophyseal trunk in some cases, and in these situations, a marginal tentorial artery is typically found arising from the artery of the inferior cavernous sinus.[19] In a few patients (approximately 10%), branches off the medial side of this segment (known as McConnell's capsular arteries) supply the capsule of the pituitary gland.[19]

The artery makes another bend in the anterior portion of the cavernous sinus superomedially. This segment of the artery exits the cavernous sinus and pierces the enveloping membrane. The membrane in this region is called the carotico-oculomotor membrane, because it spans the gap between the oculomotor nerve in the medial wall of the cavernous sinus and the carotid artery.[19, 23] This loop is then completed in the extracavernous, extradural space under the anterior clinoid process. This loop has been designated the *siphon segment*, or clinoidal segment, and continues posteriorly a short distance before piercing the dura. Here, it is surrounded by a fibrous ring of dura, and the ophthalmic artery typically originates just inside this fibrous dural ring.[23–25]

The internal carotid artery has been assigned nomenclature that divides it into several segments by different authors. We have been using the system described by Fisher in 1938, which numbers the segments beginning from the carotid bifurcation.[26] We make a small modification to the original system with regard to numbering the petrous carotid segment (Fig. 27–1). The C1 segment begins at the carotid bifurcation and extends to the origin of the posterior communicating artery. C2 is the ophthalmic segment described by Day, stretching from the posterior communicating artery to the fibrous dural ring.[23] The extradural, extracavernous clinoid segment is given the designation of C3. C4 is the true intracavernous segment of the artery and is delimited by the carotico-oculomotor membrane anteriorly and the origin of the meningohypophyseal trunk posteriorly. From the meningohypophyseal trunk, the artery is designated as C5 until it has passed under the trigeminal nerve. The intrapetrous portion begins at the point at which V3 crosses over the artery and extends to its entrance into the carotid canal in the infratemporal fossa. This segment is designated as C6.

Crucial to the surgeon's understanding of the relevant surgical anatomy of the cavernous sinus is a thorough working knowledge of the multiple triangular-shaped entry corridors into the region. The various entry points have been described by various authors and were brought together into a unified geometric construct of the region in 1986 by Fukushima.[7] This scheme is illustrated in Figure 27–2.

**Anterior Triangle.** The anterior triangle describes an epidural space that contains the C3 portion of the internal carotid artery. It is exposed by removal of the anterior clinoid process, either intradurally or extradurally. The boundaries of the triangle are the extradural optic nerve, the fibrous dural ring, and the medial wall of the superior orbital fissure.[4–6, 27] The C3 carotid segment enters this space by piercing the carotico-oculomotor membrane. It is important to bear in mind the proximity of the oculomotor

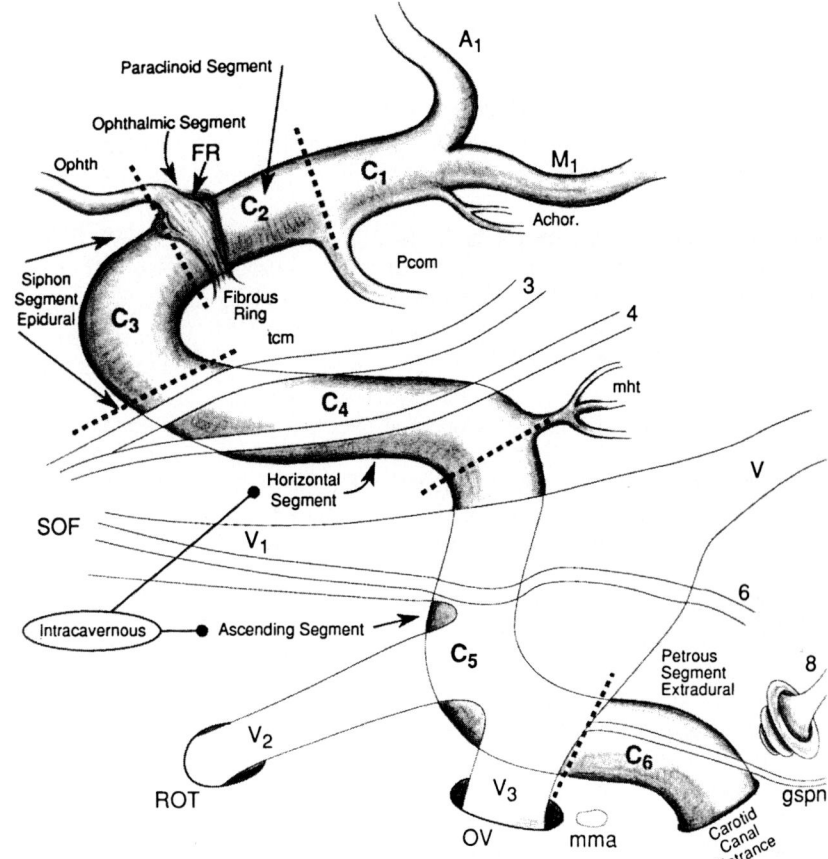

**FIGURE 27–1** ■ Illustration of the segmental nomenclature of the intracranial internal carotid artery. The divisions are indicated by the *dashed lines*. C1 begins at the bifurcation and extends to the origin of the posterior communicating artery. C2 extends to the fibrous dural ring, making C1 and C2 the two intradural segments of the vessel. C3 corresponds to the extradural, extracavernous carotid siphon segment, which is delimited by the fibrous dural ring and the carotico-oculomotor membrane. C4 is truly intracavernous and extends to the take-off of the meningohypophyseal trunk. The C5 segment is mainly inferior to the trigeminal complex and extends from the meningohypophyseal trunk to the posterolateral fibrous ring, at which point the carotid artery becomes extracavernous. The C6 segment is the horizontal intrapetrous carotid artery. (Modified from Fischer E: Die Lagabweichrugan der vorderen Hirnarterie in Gefassbild. Zentralb Neurochir 3:300–312, 1938.)

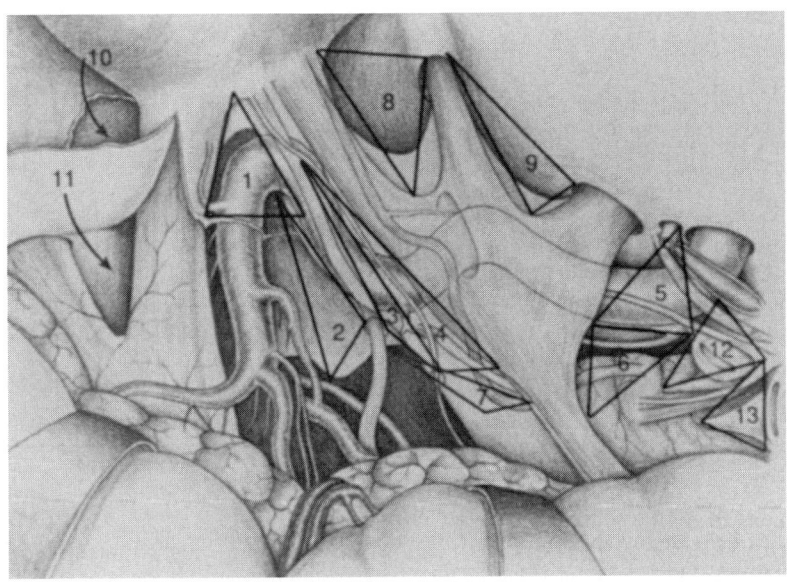

**FIGURE 27–2** ■ A geometric construct of the entry corridors to the cavernous sinus region. (1, anterior triangle; 2, medial triangle; 3, superior triangle; 4, lateral triangle; 5, posterolateral triangle; 6, posteromedial triangle; 7, posteroinferior triangle; 8, anterolateral triangle; 9, far lateral triangle; 10, anterior tip of the cavernous sinus route; 11, extended transsphenoidal route; 12, premeatal triangle; 13, postmeatal triangle.)

nerve, which runs in the medial wall of the superior orbital fissure, thus in apposition to the lateral boundary of this space.

**Medial Triangle.** The medial triangle is delimited by the intradural carotid artery, the posterior clinoid process, the porus oculomotorius, and the siphon angle of the carotid artery.[9] This space is the primary corridor of access to the C4 portion of the carotid and thus is used for the direct approach to most intracavernous aneurysms. This space is also critical in terms of exposure for most intracavernous tumors.

**Superior Triangle.** The medial and lateral boundaries of the superior triangle are cranial nerves III and IV, respectively.[7] The posterior margin is the edge of the dura along the petrous ridge. This triangle is the entry corridor used to locate the meningohypophyseal trunk.

**Lateral Triangle.** Described by Parkinson in 1965, the lateral triangle is a very narrow space that is delimited by the trochlear nerve medially and by the ophthalmic division of the trigeminal nerve laterally.[1] Again, the dura of the petrous ridge forms the posterior margin. This triangle may be opened to expose cranial nerve VI as it crosses the C5 segment of the carotid artery.

**Posterolateral Triangle.** The posterolateral triangle, first described by Glasscock in 1968, describes the location of the horizontal intrapetrous carotid artery.[28] Exposure of the artery in this space is a critical maneuver in gaining proximal control of the carotid artery. The foramen ovale, foramen spinosum, posterior border of the mandibular division of the trigeminal nerve, and cochlear apex define this space. Removal of the bone of this triangle exposes approximately 10 mm of the C6 segment of the carotid artery.[29]

**Posteromedial Triangle.** The posteromedial triangle describes the anterior petrous projection of a volume of bone that may be removed to make a window in the petrous apex to the posterior fossa. First described by Kawase and colleagues, this space is delimited by the cochlea, the porus trigeminus, and the posterior border of V3 at the posterior apex of the posterolateral triangle.[30, 31] If this triangle is used to make a window in the petrous bone, the anterior brain stem and root of the trigeminal nerve may be accessed without encountering neural or vascular structures in the bone.

**Posteroinferior Triangle.** The porus trigeminus, posterior clinoid, and entrance to Dorello's canal define this triangle. An incision in this area exposes the petrosphenoidal ligament (Gruber's ligament), which forms the roof of Dorello's canal. Cranial nerve VI can be observed in this space making the first of its two bends, the second occurring as it crosses the intracavernous carotid artery.

**Anterolateral Triangle.** The anterolateral triangle is defined by the area between the first and second divisions of the trigeminal nerve as they exit the middle cranial fossa. The anterior border of the triangle is an imaginary line drawn from the lateral edge of the superior orbital fissure to the medial lip of the foramen rotundum. This space is the entry point for exposure of the superior orbital vein and cranial nerve VI and is used to access carotid-cavernous fistulas.[32]

**Lateralmost Triangle (Lateral Loop).** Analogous to the anterolateral triangle, this space is bounded by V2, V3, and an imaginary line from the foramen rotundum to the foramen ovale. Lateral extensions of cavernous sinus tumors are also accessed through this route. In some patients, the sphenoidal emissary foramen and vein are found here, communicating the cavernous sinus with the pterygoid venous plexus.[19]

**Anterior Tip of the Cavernous Sinus.** This entry corridor is affected through an anterior transbasal approach to the cavernous sinus, which exposes the apical portion of the region. Bilateral exposure of the carotid siphon and the C4 segment is obtained through this strategy.

**Back of the Cavernous Sinus.** Through an extended transsphenoidal approach, the posteroinferior aspect of the cavernous sinus is appreciated from the underside. The bilateral C4 segments are seen after wide removal of the sellar floor toward the carotid eminence. This exposure is useful in cases of large pituitary adenomas that extend into the cavernous sinus.

**Premeatal Triangle.** The premeatal triangle is used to help define the location of the cochlea from the middle fossa angle of view. The boundaries are the medial lip of the internal acoustic meatus, the intrapetrous carotid genu, and the geniculate ganglion. The cochlea is located in the basal portion of this triangle. This triangle is important in cases in which the petrous apex is removed through the extradural middle fossa approach.[29]

**Postmeatal Triangle.** The postmeatal triangle delimits the volume of bone located between the internal auditory canal and the superior semicircular canal and is used to maximize bone removal of the petrous apex through an extradural middle fossa approach.[29] The boundaries are the geniculate ganglion, the lateral lip of the internal acoustic meatus, and the posterior end of the arcuate eminence.

A thorough working knowledge of these triangular-shaped entry corridors is a reasonable prerequisite to operating in the region. Because of the complicated anatomy and the potential for difficult hemostasis, this construct organizes the region in such a way that provides an anatomic foundation for the operative principles outlined herein.

Table 27–1 presents a morphometric analysis from our laboratory of the critical relationships between the major landmarks of the cavernous sinus (unpublished data). These measurements provide a gauge of the areas to be encountered through each of the triangular entry corridors to the region.

## ANESTHETIC AND MONITORING TECHNIQUES

The ability of modern neuroanesthesia to facilitate operative procedures by providing increased relaxation of neural tissue and pharmacologic protection against ischemia has realized great improvements. Several maneuvers are used in our cases to help maximize exposure while minimizing retraction of the brain. Administration of osmotic diuretic

## TABLE 27-1 ■ MORPHOMETRIC ANALYSIS OF THE ANATOMICAL TRIANGLES OF THE CAVERNOUS SINUS (NO. = 30 SIDES)

| Triangle | Border Length (mm) | ± SD | Range (mm) |
|---|---|---|---|
| **Anterior** | | | |
| Posterior (fibrous ring length) | 6.30 | 1.01 | 5.0–8.0 |
| Medial | 6.88 | 1.52 | 4.5–9.0 |
| Lateral | 8.72 | 1.00 | 6.5–9.8 |
| **Medial** | | | |
| Posterior | 5.41 | 1.24 | 3.6–7.2 |
| Medial | 10.63 | 1.28 | 8.2–12.5 |
| Lateral | 8.04 | 0.93 | 6.0–10.0 |
| **Superior** | | | |
| Posterior | 7.61 | 1.94 | 5.8–9.5 |
| Medial | 8.73 | 1.65 | 5.9–10.2 |
| Lateral | 10.48 | 2.34 | 6.9–12.8 |
| **Lateral** | | | |
| Posterior | 6.94 | 2.78 | 3.5–8.0 |
| Medial | 10.48 | 2.34 | 6.9–12.8 |
| Lateral | 11.79 | 2.52 | 7.0–13.3 |
| **Anterolateral** | | | |
| Anterior | 5.83 | 1.22 | 4.2–7.4 |
| Medial | 10.63 | 2.29 | 7.2–15.1 |
| Lateral | 10.36 | 2.51 | 5.9–15.0 |
| **Lateralmost** | | | |
| Anterior | 10.53 | 2.58 | 7.0–15.9 |
| Medial | 10.03 | 2.43 | 6.7–13.8 |
| Lateral | 7.54 | 3.13 | 4.0–11.0 |
| **Posterolateral** | | | |
| Medial | 20.06 | 3.15 | 15.0–25.8 |
| Lateral | 14.42 | 2.52 | 9.5–19.0 |
| Posterior | 13.90 | 2.14 | 10.8–17.5 |
| **Posteromedial** | | | |
| Anterior | 13.90 | 2.14 | 10.8–17.5 |
| Posterior | 8.66 | 2.02 | 7.5–12.5 |
| Lateral | 9.48 | 2.22 | 7.8–13.2 |
| **Premeatal** | | | |
| Anterior | 8.09 | 1.57 | 5.0–9.2 |
| Medial | 10.72 | 1.89 | 8.0–14.0 |
| Lateral | 13.11 | 2.02 | 9.5–16.5 |
| **Postmeatal** | | | |
| Medial | 13.11 | 2.02 | 9.5–16.5 |
| Lateral | 14.39 | 1.84 | 10.0–16.0 |
| Posterior | 12.99 | 3.73 | 9.2–18.5 |

SD, standard deviation.

agents is routine at the beginning of each surgery. We infuse 20% mannitol solution (0.5 mg/kg) along with furosemide (20 to 40 mg) at the time of skin incision. Further relaxation is attained by maintenance of end-tidal carbon dioxide in the range of 25 to 30 mm Hg. In some cases, these maneuvers alone may not be adequate to provide adequate relaxation, necessitating the use of cerebrospinal fluid (CSF) drainage. This procedure is performed either through a ventricular catheter or a lumbar drain. We rarely use lumbar drainage of CSF in our cases, mainly because of personal preference. Patients with significant elevation of intracranial pressure are not well served by insertion of a lumbar drain at the beginning of the operation. The safest and least complicated method is insertion of a catheter into the frontal horn of the lateral ventricle, which provides ample and accurate drainage of CSF throughout the operation.

Neurophysiologic monitoring is routinely used in all cases. The specific configuration is tailored to each case, with the operative approach and the neural and vascular structures likely to be compromised taken into consideration. Somatosensory evoked potentials and electroencephalographic data are always recorded when the potential for temporary occlusion of the carotid artery exists. When the operative approach involves exposure of any part of the facial nerve, facial nerve monitoring is employed.[33] We are also interested in using the technique of extraocular muscle electrodes implanted to monitor the oculomotor, trochlear, and abducens nerves.[34] It shows promise in the preservation of those structures. Visual and brain stem auditory evoked potentials have not found much application in our cases of tumors involving primarily the cavernous sinus.

Before planned occlusion of the carotid artery, a suppressive agent (e.g., propofol) is administered to the point of electroencephalographic burst suppression. Burst suppression is then maintained for the entire period of occlusion. Even with burst suppression, the best results are obtained when occlusion time is minimal. Any attenuation of response is an indicator that tolerance to occlusion may be limited, and preservation of the evoked potentials predicts tolerance to ischemia induced by occlusion. However, this is not always the case.

One addition to our armamentarium is a cerebral blood flow monitor, which is used intraoperatively.[35] The flow probe is applied directly to the pial surface and is capable of measuring flow through those vessels. We place the flow probe in an area known to be supplied by the occluded vessel and follow cerebral blood flow before and during the occlusion. Blood flow that drops below 30 ml/100 g/min is unlikely to be tolerated and also gives information regarding the availability of collateral flow to the area being monitored.

## SURGICAL APPROACHES

The cavernous sinus region may be approached through several different corridors. The appropriate choice of surgical approach is dictated mainly by the extent and character of involvement of adjacent structures. Some lesions are fairly well confined within the bounds of the cavernous sinus and require only a straightforward dissection of the region. Other lesions require the combination of two or more standard approaches to adequately access the lesion. Others are best handled by some variation of one of the standard approaches, and this is a point that we wish to emphasize. Because of the high potential for morbidity associated with these operations, we approach each lesion individually, tailoring our approach according to the exposure expected to be necessary. Maneuvers that put particular structures at unnecessary risk and lengthen operating time are not used.

Surgical strategy is dictated mainly by the specific entry corridors to the cavernous sinus expected to be used to resect the lesion. The cavernous sinus can be divided into four separate quadrants. Lesions involving the anteromedial region are approached via the anteromedial and anterolat-

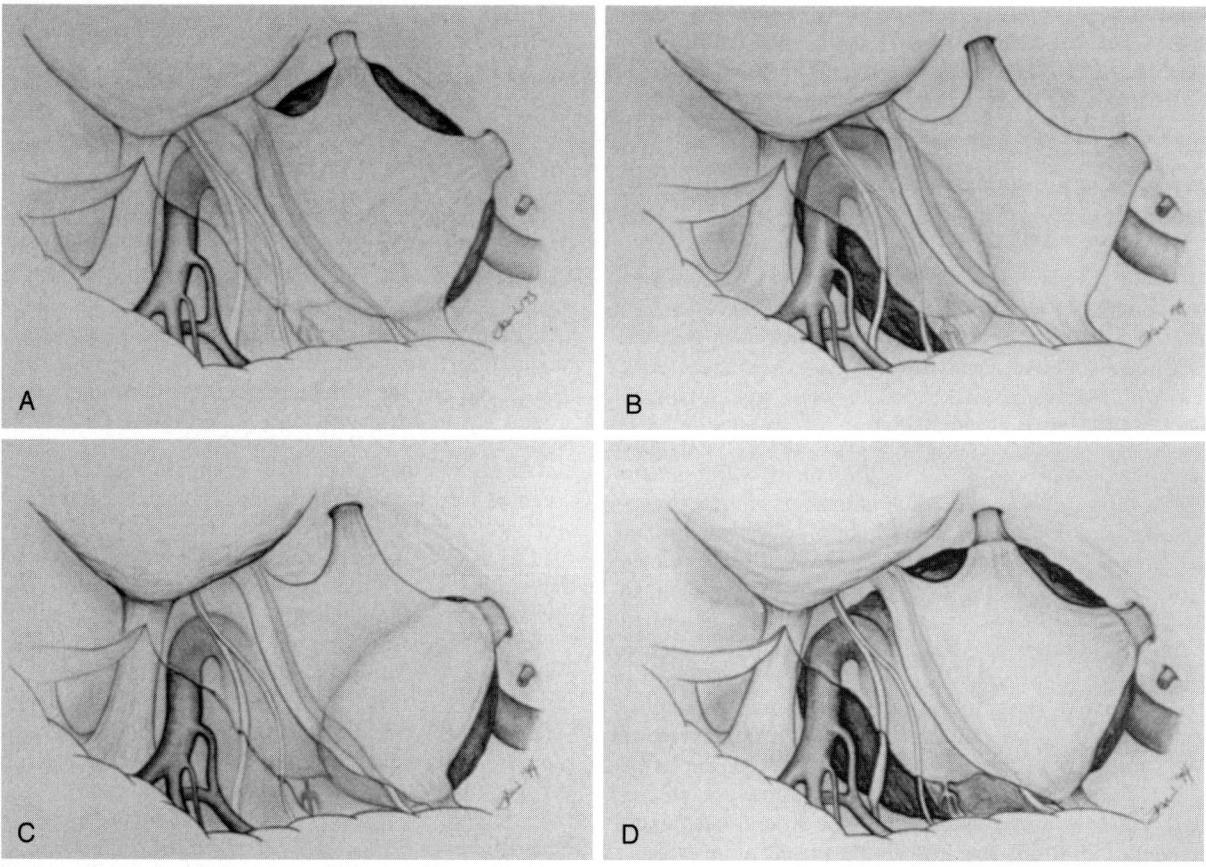

FIGURE 27–3 ■ A, Tumors with their primary component located in the anterolateral quadrant of the cavernous sinus may often be approached exclusively through an extradural route to open the anterolateral and far lateral triangles. The mass illustrated may also require exposure via the posterolateral or posteromedial triangles but still remain extradural. B, This tumor is located in the posteromedial and anteromedial quadrants, which would require intradural exposure and dissection via the medial, superior, and lateral cavernous triangles. The anteromedial component could be resected via an extradural exposure of the anterior triangle. C, Masses with their greatest bulk in the posterolateral quadrant of the cavernous sinus are best handled via a lateral approach, again entirely extradural. D, Extensive lesions that involve all quadrants of the cavernous sinus and extend to the posterior fossa or the para/suprasellar regions require a combined approach for adequate exposure.

eral triangles. Because these two triangles are exposed extradurally, in selected cases (e.g., neurinoma of V2), opening the dura might not be necessary in resecting such a lesion. This concept similarly applies to lesions located in the anterolateral quadrant, approached via the lateral loop and posterolateral triangles (Fig. 27–3A). More posterior lesions, involving the posteromedial and posterolateral regions of the cavernous sinus, usually require exposure through the medial, superior, and lateral triangles (see Fig. 27–3B). These triangles, although possible to open through an extradural route, are typically entered intradurally. Masses confined mainly to the posterolateral quadrant of the region are best approached laterally through the middle fossa (see Fig. 27–3C). Lesions involving more than one of these four areas, for example, a mass with extensive posterior cavernous involvement with extension into the posterior fossa, may require a combined approach for adequate exposure (see Fig. 27–3D). This type of lesion requires a combined strategy via an anterolateral and middle fossa transpetrosal approach. Many lesions require more than one of the standard approaches for satisfactory exposure, and the experience and judgment of the surgeon are necessary to adequately plan the procedure. We outline the standard approaches to intracavernous neoplasms used in

our practice and discuss the general indications for their use.

## Frontotemporal Epidural and Subdural Approach to the Cavernous Sinus

Dolenc is credited with the initial development and use of the combined epidural and subdural frontotemporal approach (anteromedial transcavernous approach), originally used to directly approach intracavernous aneurysms.[4, 6] This technique has become the standard by which lesions within the cavernous sinus are approached. This strategy effectively exposes lesions confined to the cavernous sinus and those with extension to the supratentorial compartment. Lesions with extension into the petroclival area and the posterior fossa are not well exposed by this approach. The method is, however, easily combined with a more lateral approach (e.g., middle fossa transpetrosal) to access such posterior extensions of tumor. Dolenc's combined epidural and subdural strategy has been modified in several ways.[27, 36–38] These modifications largely center around the bone flap used and the extent of extradural bone removal at the skull base. The following discussion presents these modifications as alternatives to the basic approach; the modifications are selected on the basis of the exposure expected to be necessary.

## Positioning

After induction of general endotracheal anesthesia, the patient is placed in the supine position on the operating table. The table is flexed approximately 30 degrees, and the patient's legs are propped up on one or two pillows. The Mayfield pin headrest is applied with the two-pin arm on the dependent side. We place the posteriormost pin at the inion and rotate the arm such that the anterior pin comes to rest on the body of the mastoid. The single pin is placed inside the hairline, near the contralateral pupillary line. The head position is fixed and is rotated approximately 30 degrees, with the vertex oriented slightly downward (Fig. 27–4). When in the proper orientation with respect to rotation, the malar eminence is the highest point of the head. We call this position the "head-hanging" position. The back of the table is then tilted such that the head is at, or slightly above, the level of the heart. The patient is now ready for the final skin preparation and draping.

## Incision and Flap Elevation

We use three different methods of initial scalp incision and elevation, the choice of which depends mainly on the

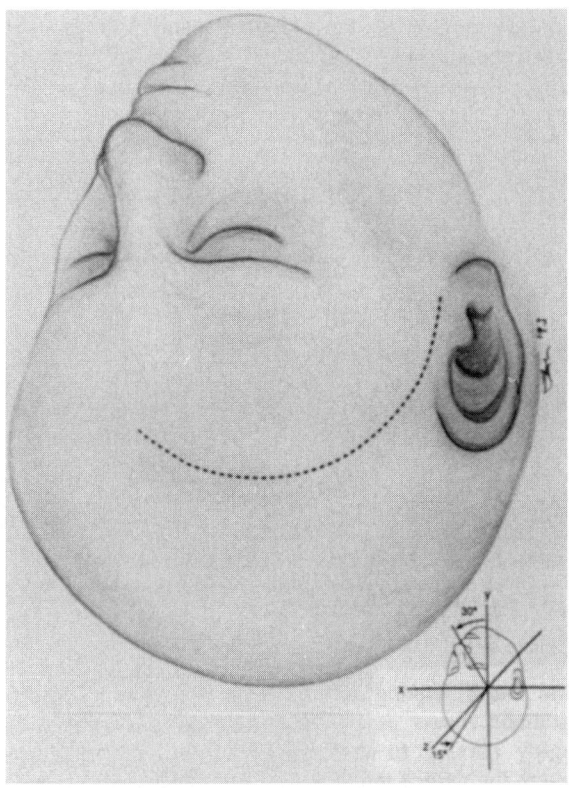

**FIGURE 27–4** ■ Head position for the standard frontotemporal approach to the cavernous sinus. The head-hanging position is demonstrated with the head turned 30 degrees and tilted downward approximately 15 degrees. This position is also used for the temporopolar approach.

amount of inferior-to-superior exposure desired. Also, three different methods of craniotomy are used, again depending on the degree of inferior-to-superior exposure necessary.

### SINGLE-LAYER TECHNIQUE

The standard one-layer technique is used when the requirement for extradural bone removal is minimal, and a limited inferior-to-superior viewing angle will be necessary. Also, this technique does not include the creation of a vascularized pericranial flap for use at closure. We begin the incision just anterior to the tragus at the level of the zygoma root and proceed superiorly, inside the hairline. The incision curves gently forward, ending in the midline. The temporalis muscle and fascia are incised. Particular attention is paid to the area around the zygoma root. The temporalis muscle is freed from its attachment to the zygoma root, which yields increased elevation of the muscle anteriorly. Use of monopolar cautery in this area should be restrained because of the proximity of the frontalis branch of the facial nerve. The pericranium medial to the superior temporal line is elevated with the temporalis muscle and fascia. This myocutaneous flap is elevated anteriorly to expose the frontozygomatic recess and is held in place with large hooks.

### HALF-AND-HALF TECHNIQUE

The half-and-half method is used when vascularized pericranial flap is desired and obtaining a high degree of inferior-to-superior exposure is not necessary. After the skin incision is made, the flap is elevated medial to the superior temporal line in two layers by sharp dissection of the areolar connective tissue layer between the pericranium and the galea. Care must be exercised to avoid damaging the supraorbital nerve, which lies adherent to the inner surface of the galea and can be mistakenly included in the pericranial layer. At the superior temporal line, the pericranium is incised. The temporalis muscle and fascia are then elevated with the scalp and reflected anteriorly, just as in the single-layer technique. The pericranium is then elevated from the bone to the supraorbital rim and reflected anteriorly. We protect this flap by wrapping it in wet gauze, and we keep it moist during the operation.

### TWO-LAYER TECHNIQUE

The two-layer technique is used when increased inferior-to-superior trajectory is necessary, because this technique results in reflection of the temporalis muscle inferiorly and laterally. This method rotates the muscle away from the orbital rim and frontozygomatic recess, thus preventing the muscle mass from creating an obstruction when the microscope is radically rotated to obtain a more rostral view. The skin incision is typically started slightly more inferiorly, exposing the entire zygomatic root. Beginning medially, the galeal layer is elevated from the pericranium, and the areolar bands, which span the two layers, are sharply divided. Again, the supraorbital and supratrochlear nerves must be preserved with the galeal layer. As the superior temporal line is reached, the areolar connective tissue that is continuous with the pericranial layer is ele-

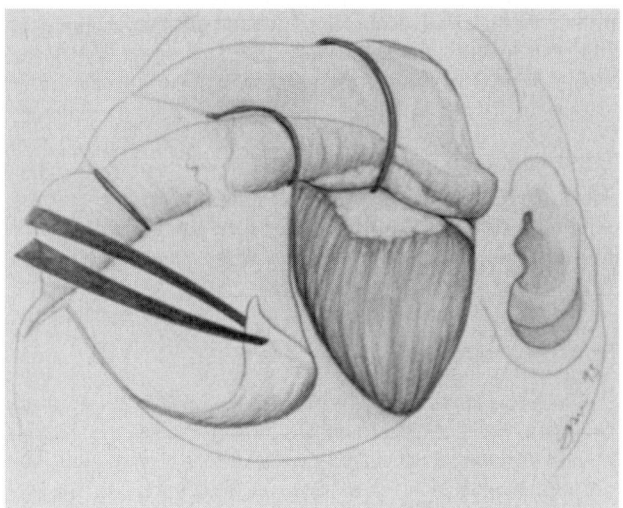

FIGURE 27–5 ■ The two-layer scalp flap technique is illustrated, preserving the frontalis branches of the facial nerve by splitting the superficial and deep temporal fat pads. This technique preserves a vascularized periosteal flap, which is used in closure of the skull base. Note the preservation of the supraorbital nerve.

vated with the galea, which exposes bare temporalis fascia. The critical step in this maneuver is handling the temporal fat pad. This fat pad consists of superficial and deep components. The superficial fat pad is surrounded by the loose areolar connective tissue overlying the temporalis fascia and contains the frontalis branches of the facial nerve. The fat pad is elevated with the areolar tissue and the galeal layer. The galeal layer is elevated to expose the supraorbital rim, lateral orbital rim, and entire zygomatic process, which is covered by fascia. The deep fat pad is situated over the inferior portion of the temporalis muscle as it passes under the zygomatic arch and is covered by fascia. This pad of fat is left in place and retracted with the muscle (Fig. 27–5).

The temporalis muscle is now elevated, and monopolar cautery is used as necessary. This elevation is begun anteriorly at the lateral orbital rim, and the periosteum is incised so as to leave a cuff for reattachment of the fascia. The muscle is elevated without any incision being made in this structure and is reflected inferiorly and posteriorly. The vascularized pericranial flap is next elevated and reflected anteriorly as described earlier for the half-and-half technique.

## Craniotomy and Extradural Bone Removal

As with the elevation of the skin flap, the degree of inferior-to-superior exposure and the posterior limits of the expected dissection determine the type of bone flap to be used. A routine pterional bone flap is sufficient for masses limited to the anterior and anterolateral cavernous sinus. Tumors with much more extensive involvement posteriorly and those that escape the confines of the region require a more generous cranial opening for adequate exposure.

### FRONTOTEMPORAL CRANIOTOMY

This is the most frequently used bone flap and provides satisfactory exposure in most cases. Two or three bur holes

are made, preferably with the pediatric-sized bur hole drill bit. The first hole is placed in the keyhole area in an attempt to straddle the sphenoid ridge. The second hole is placed directly posterior, just below the superior temporal line, at the posterior limit of the exposed bone. The third hole is optional and is placed inferiorly, in the temporal squama, just above the floor of the middle fossa. Typically, the flap is made with a more generous frontal exposure than that typically used for an anterior circulation aneurysm. The dimensions are usually approximately 7 to 8 cm by 5 cm, centered one third above and two thirds below the superior temporal line. The temporal squama remaining inferiorly is removed, resulting in a flat angle of view along the middle fossa floor. The dura is then tacked to the posterosuperior bone margin with fine suture through obliquely drilled wire-pass holes.

With a generous frontal extension toward the midline, the frontal sinus is frequently encountered. An open frontal sinus must be handled properly to avoid an annoying complication from a CSF leak or postoperative infection. We recommend use of a high-speed drill and a diamond bur to exenterate the mucosa of the sinus. This procedure must be meticulously performed to avoid formation of a mucocele. Next, the ostia are carefully occluded, usually with a piece of temporalis muscle, and the sinus is then packed with fat. The packed sinus will be covered with pericranium, or other fascia, at the conclusion of the case.

### TRANSZYGOMATIC CRANIOTOMY

After the galeal layer is reflected by use of the two-layer technique, the periosteum of the zygomatic process and the lateral orbital rim is incised and elevated. We make this incision in such a way that leaves a cuff of tissue for later reapproximation. The temporalis muscle is freed from the temporal squama and of its attachment to the inner surface of the zygoma. The zygoma is now cut with a sagittal or reciprocating saw (Fig. 27–6). The anterior cut is made parallel to the lateral orbital rim, beginning at the frontozy-

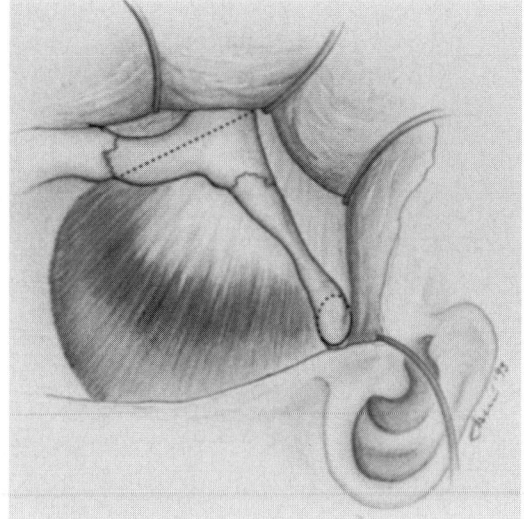

FIGURE 27–6 ■ The osteotomies used for the transzygomatic craniotomy are demonstrated. This method results in what is called a T-bone cut, maximizing inferior temporalis retraction.

gomatic suture, leaving as little bone overhanging the frontozygomatic recess as possible. The posterior cut is made roughly parallel to the surface of the temporal squama through the root of the temporal zygomatic process, and care is taken to avoid invasion of the temporomandibular joint. This technique results in what we call a "T-bone" cut and maximizes inferior temporalis muscle retraction, resulting in an increased ability to gain an inferior-to-superior view. A frontotemporal craniotomy is now made as described earlier. The remaining temporal squama is removed to obtain a flat viewing angle along the middle cranial fossa floor.

## ORBITOZYGOMATIC CRANIOTOMY

This craniotomy technique results in maximal inferior-to-superior trajectory and allows the widest access to the cavernous sinus up toward the brain base. The scalp flap needs to be made in two layers, and elevation of the pericranium is extended to include the periorbital fascia. The periorbital fascia is elevated from the midline superiorly to the inferolateral aspect of the orbit. This tissue must be freed to a depth of approximately 1.5 cm inside the orbit. If the supraorbital nerve travels through a supraorbital foramen, freeing the nerve is necessary. By use of a small osteotome, the bone of the foramen is removed in a wedge to free the nerve and allow forward reflection with the pericranium.

Two bur holes are then made, one in the keyhole area and the second about 5 cm posteriorly, inferior to the superior temporal line. Next, the thick bore that connects the anterior temporal base to the orbital wall is drilled away. Then, a cut is made with the craniotome beginning at the posterior bur hole, proceeding inferiorly toward the middle fossa floor, then curving upward over the temporal line to meet the pterional bur hole (Fig. 27–7). A sagittal or reciprocating saw is now used to cut the zygoma root parallel to the squamosal surface, as described earlier (Fig. 27–8). The next cut is made roughly parallel to, and several millimeters above, the zygomaticomaxillary suture, cutting

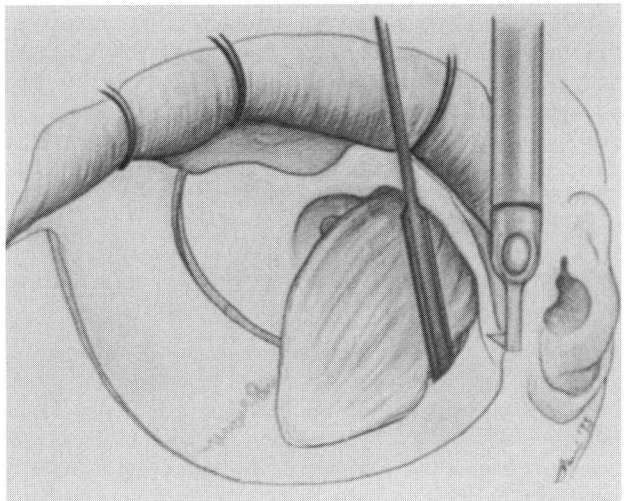

**FIGURE 27–8** ■ The root of the zygomatic process is cut parallel to the surface of the temporal squama to prevent any obstructing process to maximal inferior temporalis retraction.

into the lateral wall of the orbit. The medial supraorbital rim is cut and continued posteriorly several millimeters into the orbital roof. The orbital wall is next incised, either with the sagittal saw or a small osteotome, from medial to lateral, thus freeing the supraorbital and lateral orbital rims (Fig. 27–9). The final cut made is through the articulation of the zygomatic and sphenoid bones from posterior. These bone incisions free the flap as a single unit (Fig. 27–10). Sometimes, the flap needs to be freed from some remaining attachment of the sphenoid wing, which is easily accomplished via fracturing of that remaining attachment.

## Extradural Bone Removal

Extradural removal of bone at the cranial base provides several advantages. Primarily, reduction of cranial base bone volume reduces the degree of necessary retraction of

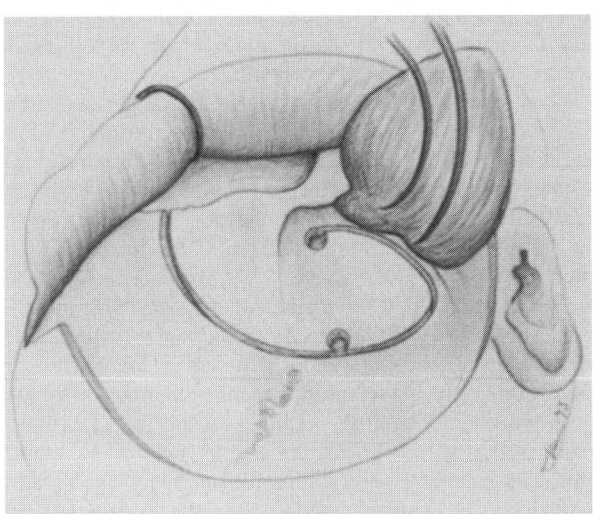

**FIGURE 27–7** ■ The initial craniotome osteotomy is illustrated, extending through the medial orbital rim.

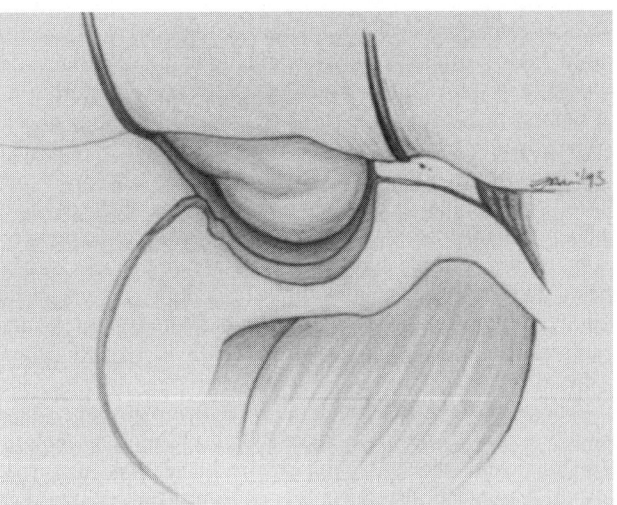

**FIGURE 27–9** ■ Intraorbitally, the osteotomy is made at a depth of approximately 10 to 15 mm. The zygoma is incised just superior to the zygomaticofrontal foramen (shown) and the zygomaticomaxillary suture.

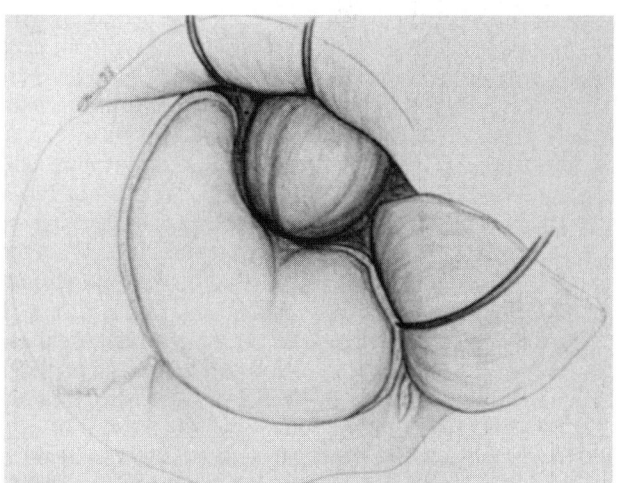

**FIGURE 27–10** ■ The bone flap is removed in a single piece after first fracturing any remaining attachment at the sphenoid ridge.

neural structures. Second, removal of bone surrounding neural structures as they pass through bone canals results in mobility of these structures without impingement against bone surfaces, which may result in pressure-induced ischemia. Third, transposition of neural and vascular structures from their bone canals results in wider corridors of access. In this chapter, we describe the technique for maximal removal of the anterolateral base; however, the extent of removal of the cranial base is individualized for each case. Risk is associated with every degree of bone removal at the skull base, and for this reason, determination of the exposure for each particular case is an important step in surgical planning.

The initial step in this procedure is reduction of the sphenoid wing. The dura is elevated and retracted with 4-mm, tapered retractors. Under constant irrigation, the sphenoid wing is reduced with a high-speed drill. Initially, the wing is flattened down to the level of the meningo-orbital artery as it joins the dura at the superior orbital fissure apex. Bone irregularities of the frontal floor are reduced with a diamond bur, resulting in a smooth contour of the orbital roof. The superior orbital fissure is skeletonized to expose approximately 10 mm of periorbital fascia, and the foramen rotundum is unroofed to the infratemporal peripheral branches to expose 5 to 8 mm of V2. When lateral cavernous exposure is desired, the foramen ovale is similarly unroofed to mobilize V3. The orbit may now be skeletonized, leaving only a thin shell of bone adherent to the periorbital fascia. The meningo-orbital artery, typically at the superior orbital fissure apex, is coagulated and divided. The adhesion of the dura at the superior orbital fissure apex is divided approximately 4 to 5 mm. This goal can be achieved without risk to cranial nerves III and IV.

The next stage of extradural bone removal, optic canal unroofing, is the most technically demanding. It is helpful to first locate the exit point of the nerve from the optic canal. A very short segment (about 1 mm) can be identified as it spans the gap between bone and dura. On the medial side, care must be taken to avoid entering the sphenoid sinus, which lies just medial to the optic canal. If the sinus

is opened, it must be carefully exenterated of its mucosa and packed with either muscle or fat. The sinus may likewise be entered on the lateral side when the surgeon drills between the optic canal and anterior clinoid, while reducing the optic strut.

The anterior clinoid process is next removed on the lateral side of the optic canal. Optimal technique is critical because the anterior clinoid process is surrounded by the optic nerve, internal carotid artery, and contents of the superior orbital fissure.

Under constant cooling from irrigation, the anterior clinoid process is hollowed out with the diamond drill. This structure must never be removed in a single piece. The sides are thinned to the point at which the sides can be lightly fractured and dissected free from the dura. The very tip of the anterior clinoid is usually removed with the aid of small alligator forceps, and the small (1 to 2 mm) tip is gently twisted free after careful dural dissection. When the anterior clinoid is hollowed out, the surgeon must be ever cognizant of the relative positions of the optic nerve, the carotid artery, and the superior orbital fissure contents. The optic nerve is medial; the carotid artery, anterior and inferior; and cranial nerve III, lateral in the medial superior orbital fissure wall. At times, this removal is complicated by the presence of a bridge between the anterior and posterior clinoid processes, forming a caroticoclinoidal foramen. Under such circumstances, completing the resection of this structure intradurally may be necessary. Occasionally, with final removal of the anterior clinoid, bleeding from the cavernous sinus occurs, typically from disruption from the carotico-oculomotor membrane. This bleeding is controlled by packing one or two small pieces of Surgicel in the defect. Bipolar cautery should not be used because it is ineffective, and current may spread to the oculomotor nerve.

Next, the full anterolateral cranial base is skeletonized, and the neural structures are able to be mobilized, after being freed from the constraints of their respective bone foramina (Fig. 27–11). Hemostasis is attained with the use of bone wax and monopolar cautery. Monopolar cautery should be used only in areas that do not have underlying sensitive structures. A typical example is in the middle fossa in the region of the tegmen tympani. Heat transfer through bone here can damage cranial nerve VII or the hearing apparatus.

When extradural exposure of the intrapetrous carotid artery is desired, it is appropriately exposed in the posterolateral triangle (Fig. 27–12). The dura must be elevated from the middle cranial fossa to expose the greater superficial petrosal nerve running in the major petrosal groove. The middle meningeal artery must be coagulated and divided as it exits the foramen spinosum. This vessel is usually surrounded by a plexus of veins, which must be effectively coagulated. With the greater superficial petrosal nerve exposed, the landmarks delineating the position of the carotid artery are apparent because the artery lies under the nerve and is running parallel, toward V3. Drilling is begun posterior to V3, just medial to the foramen spinosum. The greater superficial petrosal nerve is typically divided near V3 and reflected posteriorly for greater exposure of the internal carotid artery. Bone over the artery is removed from the tensor tympani muscle lateral to bone

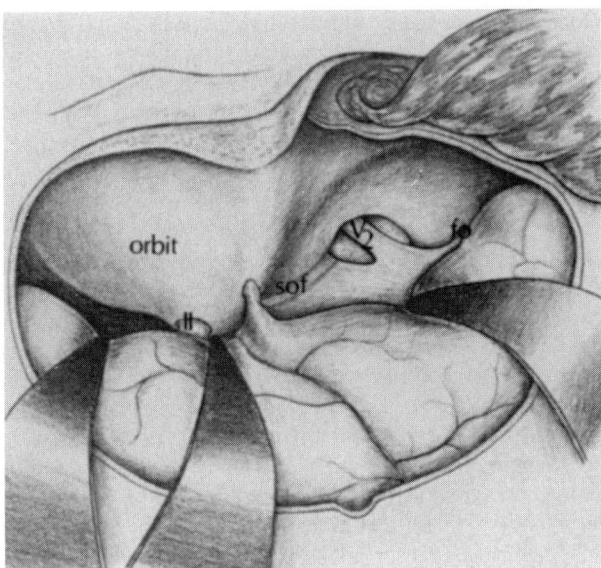

**FIGURE 27–11** ■ This figure illustrates the view of the anterior and middle cranial base at the completion of the extradural bone dissection to unroof the maxillary division of the trigeminal (V2), the superior orbital fissure (sof), and the optic nerve (II). (fo, foramen ovale.)

that lies under V3. The greatest danger in this procedure is violation of the cochlea, which lies 1 to 2 mm from the carotid genu. Excessive bone removal posterior to the carotid genu carries significant risk for cochlear violation.

### INTRADURAL TRANSCAVERNOUS DISSECTION

Neoplastic lesions that escape the bounds of the cavernous sinus typically require intradural exposure of adjacent regions. In these cases, the cavernous sinus may be opened through the medial, superior, and lateral triangles via an intradural dissection. This intradural approach to the cavernous sinus begins with opening of the dura using a T-shaped incision. The incision starts at the anterior frontal corner of the exposure and curves downward, close to the posterior bone margin, toward the anterior temporal corner. A cut is then made along the dura that covers the sylvian

fissure and proceeds toward the optic nerve dura, completing the T. The dural flaps are retracted forward and tacked down with fine suture.

Arachnoid dissection usually begins with splitting of the sylvian fissure. Dividing the anterior 3 to 4 cm is sufficient in most cases and provides adequate retraction of the frontal and temporal lobes while minimizing retractor pressure. It is often necessary to coagulate and divide the bridging veins of the temporal tip to satisfactorily mobilize the temporal lobe. The arachnoid surrounding the optic nerve and intradural carotid artery is then sharply divided, and damage to small perforating arteries is carefully avoided. Arachnoid division continues posteriorly to the tentorial edge, dividing the membrane of Liliequist to expose the oculomotor nerve as it enters the porus oculomotorius. The lateral dural wall of the cavernous sinus is now visible at this point of the dissection from the anterior margin of the middle fossa to the tentorial edge posteriorly.

The medial triangle of the cavernous sinus is readily opened at its apex after the carotid artery is sharply liberated of its attachment at the fibrous dural ring. The dura over the triangle can then be incised toward the posterior clinoid, a procedure that produces a tremendous amount of bleeding, except when the region is filled with tumor. Bleeding is controlled by judicious packing with Surgicel. Medial and posterior packing can be fairly generous to close off the connections to the basilar venous plexus and inferior petrosal sinus. Lateral packing must be more modest to avoid compression of cranial nerve III.

Dissection of the superior triangle is best performed after opening of the medial triangle and liberation of cranial nerve III by opening the porus oculomotorius, reflecting the dura from the outer cavernous membrane over cranial nerve III, and incising the outer cavernous membrane to free the nerve. The triangle can then be entered medial to cranial nerve IV. This triangle contains the meningohypophyseal trunk, which is subject to compression by overzealous packing of the space to control hemorrhage. Vigorous packing posteriorly and laterally can also result in compression of cranial nerve VI. Analogous to the maneuver made to open this triangle, the lateral triangle is similarly opened by reflecting the middle fossa dura from

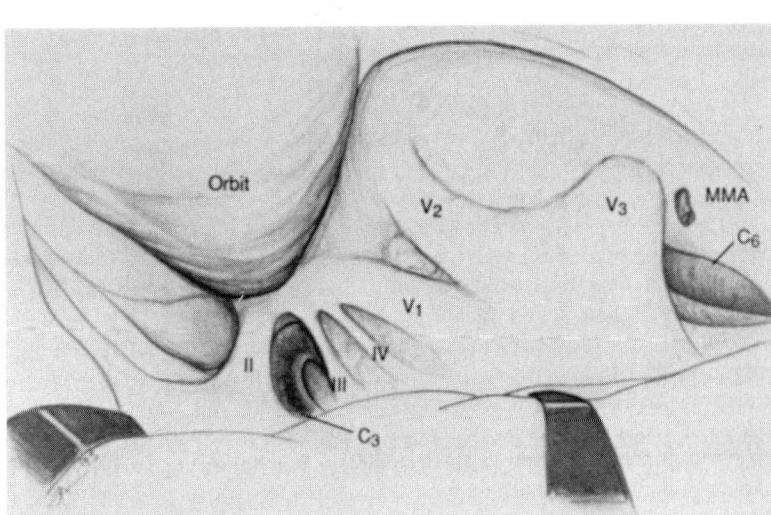

**FIGURE 27–12** ■ The dura propria is reflected from the outer cavernous membrane to expose the trigeminal complex, the trochlear, and the oculomotor nerves. With extradural resection of the anterior clinoid process, the carotid siphon is well exposed (C3). The extradural exposure of the intrapetrous carotid artery (C6) exposes approximately 10 mm of the vessel in the middle fossa.

the true cavernous membrane over cranial nerve IV and continuing to the trigeminal first branch and semilunar ganglion. The lateral triangle can then be entered and cranial nerve VI exposed as it crosses over the intracavernous carotid artery. Packing for hemostasis in this triangle must avoid compression of the carotid artery and cranial nerve VI.

At the completion of the dissection, the anteromedial, anterolateral, and posteromedial quadrants of the cavernous sinus are exposed. The posterolateral portion is usually incompletely exposed via this dissection because of obstruction by the trigeminal complex. Intradurally, cranial nerve III is visible from the interpeduncular fossa to its entrance into the superior orbital fissure. Cranial nerve IV is seen from near its entrance into the incisural edge, crossing the cavernous sinus to enter the superior orbital fissure on top of cranial nerve III. Lateral to the trochlear nerve, in the lateral triangle, deflection of the ophthalmic division of the trigeminal nerve exposes cranial nerve VI crossing the intracavernous carotid artery. Incision of the incisural edge between the porus trochlearis and the porus trigeminus widely opens the posteroinferior triangle and Dorello's canal. Tumor is resected by use of the techniques outlined in the subsequent section on specific intracavernous methods.

## CLOSURE

Closure in these procedures is at times complicated. The goal of closure at the skull base is complete separation of the intradural compartment from extradural structures. A watertight dural closure is critical to the successful avoidance of postoperative complications secondary to CSF leakage and contamination, and fascial patch grafts are used as necessary to meet this goal. Even the most meticulous closure has the potential for small leaks. Therefore, all potential routes of communication should be closed off with autologous fat grafts and fascial barriers. As discussed earlier, opened paranasal sinuses must be exenterated of mucosa to avoid mucocele formation. Then, any ostia are obliterated and the sinus is occluded with muscle or fat. The fat or muscle graft is then best sealed from the dural closure by covering with an additional vascularized pericranial flap and strategically placing tacking sutures prevents migration. We use titanium plates for securing the bone flap because of the superior cosmetic results obtained.

## Anterolateral Temporopolar Transcavernous Approach

This approach provides access to the cavernous sinus from a more lateral trajectory than the standard frontotemporal method.[36] The technique makes use of extradural retraction of the frontal and temporal lobes, both to protect the cortical surface and to preserve the venous drainage of the temporal tip. The extensive extradural dissection provides a very wide corridor of access to the cavernous sinus region, as well as wide access to the infrachiasmatic and upper clival areas. In contrast to the standard frontotemporal approach, the cavernous sinus triangles are opened from an extradural route, using minimal intradural dissection.

Integral to the basis of this technique is an understanding of the anatomy of the lateral wall and roof of the cavernous sinus. The dura covering the cavernous sinus, on the undersurface of the temporal lobe, is adherent to the outer cavernous membrane. The outer (or "true") cavernous membrane is formed by the connective tissue sheaths of cranial nerves III, IV and V and is continuous with periosteum at the bone margins. This membrane envelopes the structures in the cavernous sinus. Thus, the dura can be elevated from the outer cavernous membrane with minimal hemorrhage if no large tears are created in this membrane. The ability to expose the cavernous sinus in this way is the key element of this approach.

Employment of a vascularized pericranial flap is typically required for closure; therefore, the two-layer scalp flap technique is necessary. The incision is a generous frontotemporal incision, beginning at, or just below, the root of the zygomatic process. Either of the three bone flaps described earlier may be used for this approach. Again, the degree of inferior-to-superior trajectory that will be required dictates the use of the transzygomatic or orbitozygomatic flaps. Extradural bone removal proceeds as outlined earlier. The novel aspects of the approach begin when extradural bone removal is complete and the dura is ready to be opened.

Beginning at the superior orbital fissure apex, the meningo-orbital fibrous band is coagulated and divided. The temporal dura is retracted posteriorly. Elevation of the dural margin begins at the superior orbital fissure and extends laterally to the foramen ovale. At the junction of the periorbital fascia and dura, the cleavage plane is sharply developed, and the connective tissue fibrils bridging the dura and the outer cavernous membrane are divided, as the dura is retracted posteriorly. In this way, the dura is reflected from the outer cavernous membrane toward the petrous ridge (see Fig. 27–12). If performed properly, little bleeding occurs from the cavernous sinus. Cavernous sinus bleeding from small tears in the outer cavernous membrane is stopped by packing small pieces of Surgicel into the openings. The anteromedial limit in dural elevation is the tentorial edge, which is handled after the dura is opened.

The dura is now ready to be opened. An L-shaped incision is made beginning along the dura covering the sylvian fissure, approximately 5 cm from its attachment to the carotid artery. The incision is extended through optic nerve sheath dura and is then carried medial across the tuberculum sellae for 2 to 3 cm (Fig. 27–13). The retractors are replaced to provide posterior retraction on both the frontal and temporal lobes, and the fibrous dural ring surrounding the carotid artery is sharply freed from the vessel. The lateral portion of this fibrous ring is met by the tentorial edge, formed by a fold in the dura. The two layers composing this fold are then split. This maneuver elevates the temporal dura from the outer cavernous membrane over the medial triangle and effectively frees the medial margin of temporal dura, resulting in full lateral and posterior retraction. Some arachnoidal dissection around the porus oculomotorius is typically a prerequisite to this move. At this juncture, the structures of the lateral wall of the cavernous sinus should be plainly visible through the thin veil of the outer cavernous membrane, from the sella to the trigem-

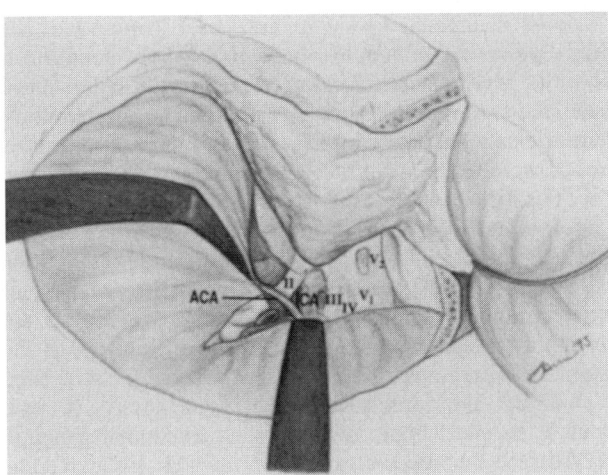

FIGURE 27–13 ■ The dura is opened in an L-shaped incision to expose the sylvian fissure and intradural internal carotid artery. The sylvian fissure is split approximately 2 cm for additional retraction. (ACA, anterior cerbral artery; CA, carotid artery.)

inal third division. The medial, superior, and lateral triangles are well delineated (Fig. 27–14).

Splitting of the sylvian fissure is usually performed to decrease the required retractor pressure, even though the degree of frontal and temporal lobe retraction is somewhat lessened with this approach. No more than the anterior 1 to 2 cm of the fissure need be split in most cases. During the dissection, it will be clear that the temporal tip bridging veins need not be sacrificed with this approach because the temporal dura is retracted with the temporal lobe, obviating sacrifice of these vessels. The arachnoid is opened over the optic nerve and chiasm, as well as the carotid artery to expose the A1 and M1 segments (Fig. 27–15). The medial and anterolateral portions of the cavernous sinus are exposed at this point of the dissection, and tumor resection may proceed.

At the conclusion of the case, dural closure must be performed in as complete a manner as possible. Closure requires the use of a pericranial or fascial graft, and if any bone sinuses were opened during the extradural bone removal, these must be exenterated and packed with a fat or muscle graft. A problem area of closure is that around the optic nerve. The incision in the optic nerve sheath dura

is not closed with suture because of the risk of damage to the nerve from compression or direct trauma. Fascial patch grafts are used to close the incision around the nerve, and then fat is placed around the nerve area. The fascial graft is tacked such that it will prevent migration of the fat graft, and the area is finally sealed with fibrin glue. For superior cosmetic results the bone flaps are secured with one of the titanium plating systems.

## Lateral Approach to the Posterior Cavernous Sinus Region (Rhomboid Approach)

Although the posterior cavernous sinus region may be accessed strictly through an anterior trajectory, the exposure is narrow, and cranial nerve V is an obstacle to adequate vision. This narrow corridor provides limited access to the posteroinferior triangle and region surrounding the porus trigeminus. For this reason, a more lateral and posterior approach is indicated, either subtemporal or transpetrosal, that provides a wider operative corridor and access inferolateral to the trigeminal complex. The extradural middle fossa transpetrosal approach provides such exposure through a subtemporal route and is easily combined with the frontotemporal approach.[29–31, 39, 40] At our institution, we call this method the rhomboid approach, named for the complex of middle fossa floor landmarks that delineate the anterior transpetrosal window of bone through which the posterior cavernous sinus and petroclival areas are exposed. When bone removal through this approach is maximized, near-total resection of the petrous apex results.[29]

Avoidance of complication from this technique depends mainly on an intimate knowledge of the internal anatomy of the petrous bone and the relationships between internal structures and surface landmarks. The major potential complications of the procedure are hearing loss resulting from cochlear or bone labyrinth violation and compromise of facial nerve integrity and function. In an attempt to simplify the technique, we have devised a geometric construct of key middle fossa landmarks that delineates the volume of bone to be resected. This construct helps to locate, and thus avoid, internal structures of the petrous pyramid.[29]

The approach is performed with the head in the 90-degree lateral position, through a 4 × 4 cm temporal craniotomy centered two thirds anterior and one third posterior over the external auditory meatus. When performed

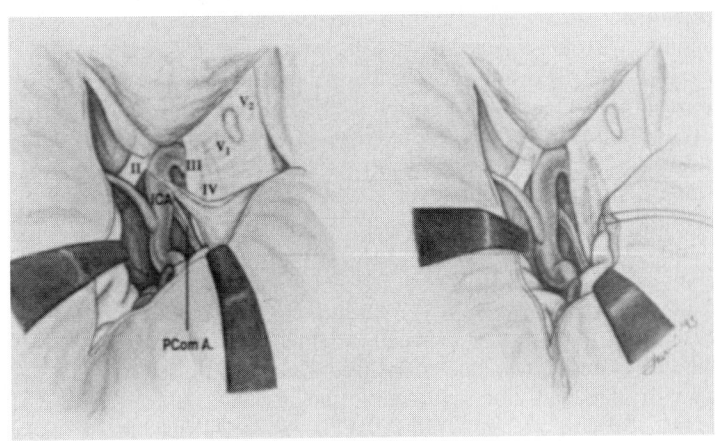

FIGURE 27–14 ■ The opening of the fibrous dural ring and the porus oculomotorius with splitting of dural leaves composing the tentorial edge are shown. This maneuver allows lateral retraction of this dural edge and opening of the medial triangle. This also leads into the opening of the superior triangle in similar fashion. (PCom A, posterior communicating artery; ICA, internal carotid artery.)

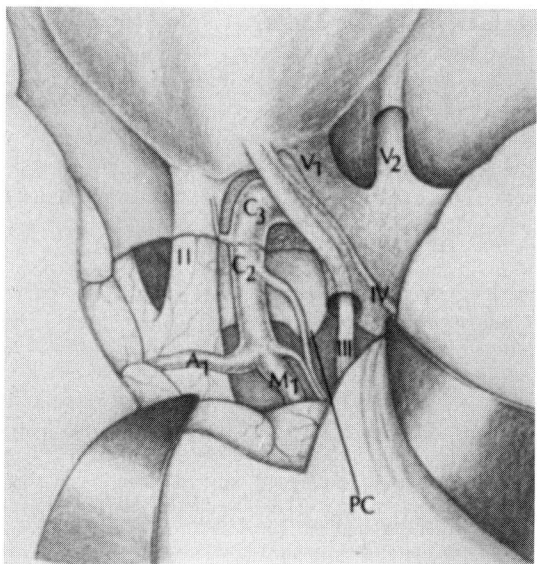

FIGURE 27-15 ■ The final exposure of the anteromedial and posteromedial cavernous sinus via the temporopolar approach.

in combination with a frontotemporal approach, a more generous temporal extension of the craniotomy must be made that reaches posterior to the root of the zygomatic process. The head is rotated about 60 degrees toward the contralateral side, either initially or by later rotation of the table. Middle fossa dural elevation begins posteriorly and laterally, over the petrous ridge, and continues anteromedially to the foramen ovale. Dura is elevated in this manner to avoid traction on the greater superficial petrosal nerve (GSPN), which may result in facial nerve compromise. The GSPN lies in the major petrosal groove of the middle fossa floor and is covered by a thin layer of periosteum. The middle meningeal artery and surrounding venous plexus are coagulated and divided near the artery's exit from the foramen spinosum. The dura is then separated from the trigeminal complex at the foramen ovale, continuing posteriorly toward the porus trigeminus. Tapered retractors are used to retract the dura medially and posteriorly to expose the entire middle fossa floor (Fig. 27-16).

At this juncture, the landmarks necessary to begin the bone dissection are identifiable. The volume of bone that will be resected corresponds to a rhomboid-shaped complex of landmarks of the middle fossa floor. This geometric construct is defined by: (1) the intersection of the GSPN and V3, (2) the intersection of lines projected along the axes of the GSPN and the arcuate eminence (AE), (3) the arcuate eminence intersection with the petrous ridge, and (4) the porus trigeminus. Obliquely projecting this construct through the petrous bone to the inferior petrosal sinus delimits the volume of petrous bone that has no neural or vascular structures.

Bony resection begins with the exposure of the internal auditory canal (IAC). By use of a high-speed diamond drill, the IAC is found 3 to 4 mm deep to the middle fossa floor along the bisection axis between lines projected along the GSPN and the arcuate eminence. We call this bisection axis Brackmann's line, and drilling begins along its midpoint. The entire length of the IAC is exposed. Next, the

GSPN is uncovered lateral to the facial hiatus, until the geniculate ganglion is exposed. A thin shell of bone is left over the ganglion for protection. The GSPN is sectioned near V3 and reflected laterally to increase intrapetrous carotid exposure. The carotid is exposed in the posterolateral triangle from V3 to the tensor tympani muscle. Then, the bone between the IAC and carotid can be safely removed to expose posterior fossa dura (Fig. 27-17). Great care must be taken to avoid the cochlea during this portion of bone dissection. The cochlea is located in the base of the premeatal triangle, which is defined by the carotid genu, the geniculate ganglion, and the medial lip of the internal auditory meatus.[29] Resection of apical petrous bone is continued inferiorly to the level of the inferior petrosal sinus. The apical bone inferior to the trigeminal ganglion can be removed by coring out of the petrous apex. The wedge of bone remaining that lies lateral to the IAC can be removed, to result in an almost 270-degree exposure of the IAC. This lateral wedge of bone is defined by the postmeatal triangle, which is bounded by the geniculate ganglion, the arcuate eminence, and the lateral lip of the internal auditory meatus. It is often helpful to blue-line the superior semicircular canal during removal of this bone to avoid entering the vestibule.

With the bone dissection complete, the posterior and inferolateral cavernous sinus can be widely accessed. The limits of this exposure are the foramen of Dorello medially and the inferior petrosal sinus below. The trigeminal complex may be completely freed of dura and then elevated or retracted medially. This exposure provides visualization of the C5 and C6 portions of the carotid artery. A prerequisite to this maneuver for increasing the exposure of the posterior cavernous sinus is extradural liberation of the V2 and V3 divisions in their respective bone canals. Elevation of the trigeminal complex in this way allows full exposure of the posterior cavernous sinus and complete petrous apex

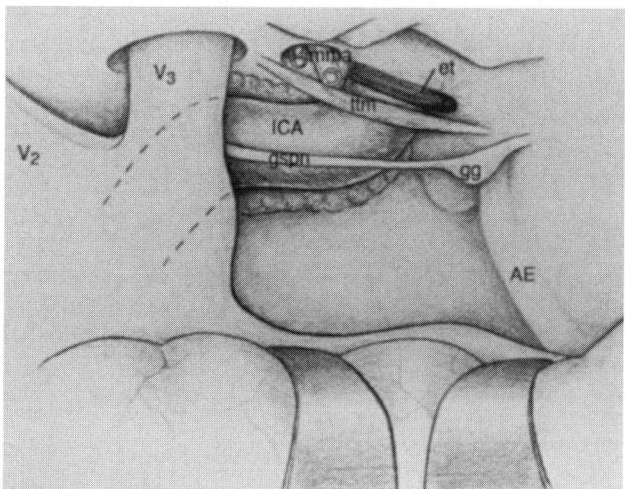

FIGURE 27-16 ■ This middle fossa floor is exposed via the extended middle fossa approach. The landmarks to begin the extradural bone removal are visible at this point in the procedure. (AE, arcuate eminence; et, eustachian tube; gg, geniculate ganglion; gspn, greater superficial petrosal nerve; ICA, internal carotid artery; mma, middle meningeal artery; ttm, tensor tympani muscle; V2 and V3, mandibular and maxillary divisions of the trigeminal.)

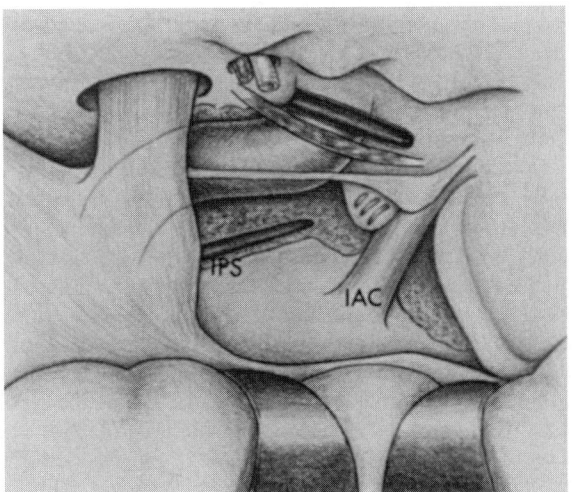

**FIGURE 27–17 ■** After the extradural bone resection is completed, the posterior fossa dura to the level of the inferior petrosal sinus (IPS) is exposed. The internal auditory canal (IAC) is skeletonized approximately 270 degrees. The posterior cavernous sinus is exposed via this route by elevating and medially translocating the trigeminal complex, opening the outer cavernous membrane inferior to the trigeminal ganglion.

resection extradurally under direct vision (unpublished data).

The dura is opened at the porus trigeminus above the superior petrosal sinus. This incision is carried laterally as far as the arcuate eminence and exposes the superior surface of the tentorium. A parallel incision is then made inferior to the superior petrosal sinus. The superior petrosal sinus is ligated with small vascular clips and divided at its medial aspect. The retractors can then be placed on the undersurface of the tentorium, and the temporal lobe is retracted more superiorly under its protection. The trigeminal root is also liberated from its dural attachment at the porus trigeminus. Mobilizing the trigeminal complex medially and superiorly provides a corridor to the posterior cavernous sinus and the entrance of cranial nerve VI into Dorello's canal. To expose the intracavernous carotid artery, it is necessary to open the outer cavernous membrane between the trigeminal ganglion and the posterolateral fibrous ring surrounding the carotid's entrance to the cavernous sinus at the foramen lacerum. In this way, the intracavernous carotid may be exposed to the crossing point of cranial nerve VI. This strategy provides full access to the posterolateral quadrant of the cavernous sinus, and tumor resection may proceed. The main venous connections of the posterolateral cavernous sinus are to the pterygoid venous plexus via the sphenoidal emissary, the inferior petrosal sinus, and the basilar venous plexus. Effective hemostasis is obtained via packing oxidized cellulose in the direction of these venous connections.

Closure requires the use of a vascularized musculofascial flap fashioned from the temporalis muscle and fascia. This flap is laid across the middle fossa floor and the petrous bone defect. Attaining a watertight dural closure in the posterior fossa dura is very difficult; therefore, it is often helpful to place a fascial graft in the defect in the petrous apex supported by a fat graft.

## SPECIAL TECHNIQUES OF INTRACAVERNOUS SURGERY

### Intracavernous Tumor Resection

Proper instrumentation is one of the major assets to successful resection of cavernous sinus neoplasms. A full array of dissectors, including microring curets, is useful. A wide selection of cottonoids is also necessary for protection of neural and vascular structures and dissection of tumor. An extremely useful tool is a pressure-attenuable suction tip that is invaluable for working around delicate structures to prevent damage induced by traction. The pressure-adjustable sucker is used for retraction and dissection as well as suction of blood and CSF. Proper instrumentation is key to application of the technical principles of tumor resection in this region.

The techniques used for resection of these tumors vary, depending on the degree of invasiveness and adherence to neural and vascular structures. Tumors such as trigeminal neurinomas that are well encapsulated and nonadherent can be relatively uncomplicated to remove. After exposure of tumor capsule through one of the triangular entry corridors, tumor debulking is performed with suction, ring curets, and alligator biopsy forceps. Developing a plane between tumor capsule and the neural and vascular structures is usually possible within the confines of the cavernous sinus. This dissection is typically performed by use of a combination of fine dissectors and long, thin cottonoids. The capsule is dissected free, continually collapsing solid tumor at the periphery into the center. Adjacent entry corridors may need to be accessed to completely free the tumor capsule. Usually, tumor is primarily resected from one or two triangular spaces, and adjacent portals are entered to dissect tumor and to push or sweep the mass toward the primary route of resection. When the capsule is freed, it is removed from the cavernous sinus, and hemostasis is attained with judicious use of Surgicel packing. This same general technique is used for any well-encapsulated, nonadherent tumor.

Invasive and adherent tumors present an entirely different surgical challenge. In these cases, the outcome with regard to morbidity depends mainly on the judgment and experience of the surgeon. Attempts at dissection of tumor from cranial nerves often result in damage either directly or from interruption of the nerves' blood supply. In some cases, when the cranial nerves have already been rendered nonfunctional by tumor invasion, the nerves may be resected with tumor to gain a more complete resection. This possibility is always considered and discussed with the patient before surgery.

Tumors such as meningiomas are approached initially with the primary intent of interrupting the blood supply to the tumor. These tumors can be quite tenacious and invasive, qualities that can prevent total resection without significant morbidity. Invasion of the intracavernous carotid artery may require a bypass procedure for total tumor resection. The dural origin and surrounding margin are resected in cases in which a complete resection is performed.

Invasive, malignant processes, such as squamous cell

cancer, involve a very extensive procedure for removal. In these cases, the affected cavernous sinus and adjacent structures are removed en bloc. This procedure requires wide exposure of the cavernous sinus and adjacent regions as well as a bypass procedure to permit resection of the affected carotid artery.

## Techniques of Hemostasis

Complete hemostasis throughout the surgical procedure is one of the primary determinants of the success or failure of any direct approach to the cavernous sinus. The potential for tremendous bleeding from the cavernous sinus requires familiarity and practice with certain techniques before such a surgical undertaking. A complete understanding of the anatomy and the elements of the triangular-shaped entry corridors is requisite to maintaining a dry operative field. Compulsive hemostasis begins with the skin incision and is maintained until final skin closure.

Preparation for the maintenance of hemostasis begins with the selection of instruments and the arrangement of materials by the scrub nurse. Bipolar cautery forceps should be available in a wide range of lengths and tip sizes. We prefer to use high settings during the initial phases of the operation to more effectively treat bleeding from scalp and muscle. As structures vulnerable to damage from the spread of heat or current are neared, the settings are reduced. Monopolar cautery is used frequently during the initial phases of these operations and is very useful to stop bleeding from bone at the skull base. When the bone of the middle fossa floor and sphenoid ridge is drilled, hemostasis is attained by several methods. Bone wax is judiciously used to seal off bleeding from porus bone. In addition to monopolar cautery, a high-speed drill, fitted with a diamond bur, cauterizes bone when used without irrigation. Bone bleeding at the skull base can often be persistent; therefore, patience and effective use of these techniques are necessary.

As the foramina of the cranial nerves are approached, the technical strategy changes. Heat and current from the monopolar cautery can spread for several millimeters through bone and can damage the nerves. Bone bleeding around neural foramina is controlled more with bone wax than with cautery or the diamond drill. Bleeding from the cavernous sinus also occurs via tiny rents in the cavernous membrane when the dura is separated from the margins of the foramina. This bleeding can be controlled by packing tiny pieces of Surgicel into the open cavernous membrane and covering for 1 or 2 minutes with a small cottonoid. Coagulating the Surgicel for 1 to 2 seconds with the bipolar after it is packed in the hole is sometimes helpful. Bleeding can occur from a tear in the cavernous membrane during the final stages of removal of the anterior clinoid process. Although possible to remove without bleeding, more frequently, the carotico-oculomotor membrane develops a small tear that can bleed profusely. A small piece of Surgicel suffices when packed into the opening and covered with a cottonoid for 1 to 2 minutes. An important principle in hemostatic technique in the cavernous sinus is patience. Much is gained by packing an area, moving to another area

to work, then coming back later to the original bleeding site.

The geometric construct describing the entry corridors to the cavernous sinus region serves as a foundation for effective hemostasis. Knowledge of the nature and communications of the venous plexus residing within each triangle, as well as the proximity of anatomic structures, is critical. In cases of tumor resection, the tumor mass often tamponades the cavernous venous plexus. Surgicel packing for hemostasis then begins after the tumor mass is removed from the area. In the anterior triangle, packing lateral and medial must be conservative because of the position of cranial nerve III and the optic nerve. Anteroinferior packing is less constrained; however, constriction of the carotid siphon must obviously be avoided. The anterolateral triangle typically contains the anastomosis of the superior orbital vein with the cavernous venous plexus and, therefore, can produce brisk bleeding when opened. The main concern in this triangle is avoidance of overpacking in the direction of cranial nerve VI, because the abducens nerve is entering the superior orbital fissure on its underside. The lateralmost triangle can also produce significant bleeding if a sphenoid emissary vein is present beside the mandibular branch that exits the foramen ovale. This sphenoid emissary is seen only in a few patients; however, when present, it can be quite large.

The medial cavernous triangle can bleed tremendously when opened. Packing must be conservative laterally, in the direction of cranial nerve III; however, inferomedial packing can be quite generous. Here, the cavernous sinus communicates with the basilar venous plexus along the clivus and the inferior petrosal sinus. Therefore, a large amount of Surgicel may be packed in their direction without compromise of any vital structures. The superior triangle does not have such an area that may be so generously packed. The meningohypophyseal trunk is found in this triangle and is vulnerable to overzealous packing. The lateral triangle is the space entered to expose cranial nerve VI as it crosses over the C4 segment of the carotid artery. Surgicel placement must be modest, except in the inferomedial direction toward the clivus.

Exposure of the intrapetrous carotid artery in the posterolateral triangle does not usually produce significant bleeding. This segment of the carotid is, however, often covered by a venous plexus that is an extension of the cavernous venous plexus. This plexus must be coagulated with bipolar cautery before work with this segment begins. The posteromedial triangle similarly is not a major concern for significant hemorrhage. When bone deep in this space is removed, the inferior petrosal sinus is encountered and must be occluded. Also, deep drilling to the clivus usually results in encountering the basilar venous plexus, which must be packed and coagulated. The posteroinferior triangle can also produce a fair amount of hemorrhage from connections with the basilar venous plexus and inferior petrosal sinus. In the floor of this space runs Dorello's canal and cranial nerve VI. Hemostasis in this space must be performed carefully to avoid compression of this structure.

## Closure Techniques

Avoidance of complications in these procedures includes meticulous attention to dural closure to prevent CSF leakage and subsequent contamination. Judicious use of fascial grafts is important in meeting this goal. Typically, abdominal fat and rectus fascia are harvested in these cases for dural closure and sealing of opened paranasal sinuses. In areas of difficult dural closure, such as around the optic nerve, fat grafts are placed and secured with fine sutures tamponading them against the open area. This arrangement is then covered with a layer of fibrin glue to hasten the fibrotic process. Muscle or fat is also tacked to areas where dural edges are unable to be tightly apposed. Also, at the corner areas of complex dural incisions, fat or muscle is used to completely plug any small holes. Fibrin glue is applied to the entire dural surface at the completion of dural closure.

As discussed, open paranasal sinuses commonly result from extensive removal of bone at the skull base. Any open sinus must be meticulously exenterated of any mucosa. We prefer to use a high-speed drill fitted with a diamond bur for this purpose. The heat generated by the drill provides extra assurance of destroying any mucous-producing epithelial cells. Ostia are then occluded with muscle or bone wax to prevent communication with bacteria-laden adjacent sinus cavities. The sinus is then packed with autologous fat. We then cover the opening to the packed sinus with a vascularized pericranial flap and carefully tack the edges to adjacent surfaces to prevent migration.

The ultimate cosmetic result of these procedures is partially dependent on the proper reattachment of the bone flap, especially in cases in which a transzygomatic or orbitozygomatic flap has been used. One of the titanium plating systems now available provides superior cosmetic results over those obtained with wire or suture. We prefer to use one of the low-profile systems, especially at points where only skin is covering the bone surface to be approximated.

Another cosmetic consideration relates to the reattachment of the temporalis muscle. If the muscle is not supported in some manner along the superior temporal line, it tends to sink into the temporal fossa, resulting in a poor appearance. To combat this, oblique wire-pass holes are made along the superior temporal line before the bone flap is replaced. The superior edge of the muscle can then be sutured to the superior temporal line, maintaining its position during the healing process.

## Skull Base Carotid Bypass Procedures

Invasive tumors often require sacrifice of the internal carotid artery if they are to be completely removed. Balloon test occlusion is performed before surgery to determine tolerance to occlusion of the involved internal carotid artery.[41] Patients who tolerate occlusion without incident may be treated without bypass, thus avoiding the potential major complications of thromboembolic sequelae and anticoagulation associated with these procedures. In cases in which occlusion is not tolerated, the carotid flow can be preserved by performing a bypass procedure.[8, 18, 20, 42, 43] This procedure was first performed in 1986 by Fukushima to treat a giant intracavernous aneurysm.[7, 8, 44] Over time, the procedure has evolved to include three variations. The most common form is a bypass between the C3 and C6 segments

of the carotid. The second important variation is an anastomosis from the high cervical portion of the internal carotid artery to the C3 segment.[8, 45]

The C3-to-C6 bypass procedure requires exposure of those two segments in sufficient length to perform the anastomosis procedure. The C3 portion is exposed in the anterior triangle through removal of the anterior clinoid process and detachment of the fibrous dural ring. The C6 segment is exposed in the posterolateral triangle.[46] It is usually helpful to free the dura from the posterior trigeminal complex, as discussed earlier, to gain several additional millimeters of exposure. Clips can then be placed to trap the intracavernous carotid segments. A saphenous vein graft is harvested from the upper thigh and prepared for anastomosis. Any loose adventitia is stripped from the vein, and tributaries are ligated with fine suture. The graft is flushed with heparinized saline solution, and proper orientation is maintained by marking either end of the graft. The distal anastomosis is then performed, either end to end or end to side, with 8–0, 9–0, or 10–0 suture. Suture selection depends on the wall thickness of both the graft and the carotid artery. Control of carotid flow is maintained either by a temporary clip near the genu or by exposure in the neck. The proximal anastomosis is performed between the origins of the ophthalmic artery and the posterior communicating artery. In some cases, the anastomosis may be performed in an end-to-end fashion if the tumor resection leaves a carotid stump including the ophthalmic origin or the ophthalmic artery is taken with tumor resection in the orbit. The anastomosis is performed under electroencephalographic burst suppression induced by barbiturates. Patients are given low-dose heparin therapy for several days postoperatively, and they are then given aspirin or warfarin (Coumadin) for approximately 3 months.

In cases of en bloc cavernous sinus resection, resecting carotid artery well into the infratemporal fossa and petrous bone may be necessary. In this case, the carotid is bypassed from the high cervical segment, near the origin at the carotid bifurcation. Saphenous vein is again harvested from the upper thigh in an appropriate length. The graft is anastomosed in end-to-end fashion and tunneled through the infratemporal fossa to enter the cranial vault subtemporally. The proximal end is then anastomosed to the C3 segment as outlined earlier.

## SUMMARY

Direct operative treatment of intracavernous neoplasms has realized great strides in the past decade. Several experienced centers have had success with treating these patients more aggressively, while limiting morbidity. Advances in microsurgical technique, neuroanesthesia, imaging techniques, neurovascular reconstruction, and microanatomic knowledge have all provided significant contributions to the successful surgery of these lesions. However, the therapeutic approach to these difficult tumors is still debated. The appropriate role of surgery in the overall management of these patients is still evolving as we continue to refine our management strategies.

The techniques and strategies outlined in this chapter

have evolved over an experience with these lesions, beginning in 1983. This series encompasses 146 cases of cavernous sinus neoplasms. Forty-eight cases in the series, patients who had benign encapsulated tumors, such as neurinomas, had the most satisfying results. Total resection in this group of patients is almost always a realistic expectation, with a minimum of morbidity. The commonest lesion treated was meningioma, accounting for 72 cases. As experience has accumulated, a less aggressive approach has been taken with meningiomas of the cavernous sinus because of our inability to remove these tumors completely without the risk of cranial nerve morbidity. Treating patients with invasive tumors has also contributed the most to our understanding of the important factors involved in revascularization of the internal carotid artery. Balloon test occlusion with measurement of cerebral blood flow is currently the best tool for determining the need for revascularization.

We anticipate that direct surgery will continue to play a prominent role in the treatment of these tumors, although it is increasingly combined with adjuvant therapies that present less risk to the cranial nerves while increasing the effectiveness of treatment. The indications for these procedures are still evolving as different centers gain wider experience with direct surgery, stereotactic radiosurgery, and endovascular techniques. Clearly, much room for improvement remains in the overall results of treating these difficult lesions.

## REFERENCES

1. Parkinson D: A surgical approach to the cavernous portion of the carotid artery: Anatomical studies and case report. J Neurosurg 23:474–483, 1965.
2. Al-Mefty O, Smith RR: Surgery of tumors invading the cavernous sinus. Surg Neurol 30:370–381, 1988.
3. Cioffi FA, Bernine FP, Punzo A, et al: Cavernous sinus meningiomas. Neurochirurgia (Stuttg) 30:40–47, 1987.
4. Dolenc V: A combined epi- and subdural direct approach to carotid-ophthalmic artery aneurysms. J Neurosurg 62:667–672, 1985.
5. Dolenc VV, Kregar R, Ferluga M, et al: Treatment of tumors invading the cavernous sinus. In Dolenc VV (ed): The Cavernous Sinus: Multidisciplinary Approach to Vascular and Tumorous Lesions. Wien: Springer-Verlag, 1987, pp 377–391.
6. Dolenc VV: Cavernous sinus masses. In Apuzzo MLJ (ed): Brain Surgery: Complication Avoidance and Management. New York: Churchill Livingstone, 1993, pp 601–614.
7. Fukushima T: Direct operative approach to the vascular lesions in the cavernous sinus: Summary of 27 cases. Mt Fuji Workshop Cerebrovasc Dis 6:169–189, 1988.
8. Fukushima T, Day JD, Tung H: Intracavernous carotid artery aneurysms. In Apuzzo MLJ (ed): Brain Surgery: Complication Avoidance and Management. New York: Churchill Livingstone, 1993, pp 925–944.
9. Hakuba A, Matsuoka Y, Suzuki T, et al: Direct approaches to vascular lesions in the cavernous sinus via the medial triangle. In Dolenc VV (ed): The Cavernous Sinus. Wien: Springer-Verlag, 1987, pp 272–284.
10. Hakuba A, Suzuki T, Jin TB, Komiyama M: Surgical approaches to the cavernous sinus: Report of 52 cases. In Dolenc VV (ed): The Cavernous Sinus. Wien: Springer-Verlag, 1987, pp 302–327.
11. Lesoin F, Jomin M, Boucez B, et al: Management of cavernous sinus meningiomas: Report of twelve cases and review of the literature. Neurochirurgia (Stuttg) 28:195–198, 1985.
12. Lesoin F, Jomin M: Direct microsurgical approach to intracavernous tumors. Surg Neurol 28:17–22, 1987.
13. Sekhar LN, Ross DA, Sen C: Cavernous sinus and sphenocavernous neoplasms. In Sekhar LN, Janecka IP (eds): Surgery of Cranial Base Tumors. New York: Raven Press, 1993, pp 521–604.
14. Sephernia A, Samii M, Tatgiba M: Management of intracavernous tumours: An 11-year experience. Acta Neurochir Suppl (Wien) 53:122–126, 1991.
15. Barbaro NM, Gutin PH, Wilson CB, et al: Radiation therapy in the treatment of partially resected meningiomas. Neurosurgery 20:525–528, 1987.
16. Carella RJ, Ransohoff J, Newall J: Role of radiation therapy in the management of meningioma. Neurosurgery 10:332–339, 1982.
17. Duma CM, Lunsford LD, Kondziolka D, et al: Stereotactic radiosurgery of cavernous sinus meningiomas as an addition or alternative to microsurgery. Neurosurgery 32:699–705, 1993.
18. Al-Mefty O, Khalil N, Elwany MN, Smith RR: Shunt for bypass graft of the cavernous carotid artery: An anatomical and technical study. Neurosurgery 27:721–728, 1990.
19. Harris FS, Rhoton AL: Anatomy of the cavernous sinus: A microsurgical study. J Neurosurg 44:169–180, 1976.
20. Sekhar LN, Burgess J, Akin O: Anatomical study of the cavernous sinus emphasizing operative approaches and related vascular and neural reconstruction. Neurosurgery 21:806–816, 1987.
21. Umansky F, Elidan J, Valarezo A: Dorello's canal: A microanatomical study. J Neurosurg 75:294–298, 1991.
22. Umansky F, Nathan H: The lateral wall of the cavernous sinus with special reference to the nerves related to it. J Neurosurg 56:228–234, 1982.
23. Day AL: Aneurysms of the ophthalmic segment. J Neurosurg 72:677–691, 1990.
24. Perneczky A, Knosp E, Borkapic P, Czech T: Direct surgical approach to infraclinoidal aneurysms. Acta Neurochir (Wien) 76:36–44, 1983.
25. Perneczky A, Knosp E, Czech T: Para- and infraclinoidal aneurysms. Anatomy, surgical technique and report on 22 cases. In Dolenc VV (ed): The Cavernous Sinus. Wien: Springer-Verlag, 1987, pp 252–271.
26. Fischer E: Die Lagabweichrugan der vorderen Hirnarterie in Gefassbild. Zentralb Neurochir 3:300–312, 1938.
27. Dolenc V, Skrap M, Sustersic J, et al: A transcavernous-transsellar approach to the basilar tip aneurysms. Br J Neurosurg 1:251–259, 1987.
28. Glasscock ME: Exposure of the intra-petrous portion of the carotid artery. In Hamberger CA, Wersall J (eds): Disorders of the Skull Base Region: Proceedings of the Tenth Nobel Symposium, Stockholm, 1968. Stockholm: Almqvist & Wicksell, 1969, pp 135–143.
29. Day JD, Fukushima T, Giannotta SL: Microanatomical study of the extradural middle fossa approach to the petroclival and posterior cavernous sinus region: Description of the rhomboid construct. Neurosurgery 34:1009–1016, 1994.
30. Kawase T, Shiobara R, Toya S: Anterior transpetrosal-transtentorial approach for sphenopetroclival meningiomas: Surgical method and results in 10 patients. Neurosurgery 28:869–876, 1991.
31. Kawase T, Toya S, Shiobara R, Mine T: Transpetrosal approach for aneurysms of the lower basilar artery. J Neurosurg 63:857–861, 1985.
32. Mullan S: Treatment of carotid-cavernous fistulas by cavernous sinus occlusion. J Neurosurg 50:131–144, 1979.
33. Traynelis VC, Gantz BJ: Intraoperative facial nerve monitoring. In Loftus CM, Traynelis VC (eds): Intraoperative Monitoring Techniques in Neurosurgery. New York: McGraw-Hill, 1994, pp 157–163.
34. Moller AR: Monitoring techniques in cavernous sinus surgery. In Loftus CM, Traynelis VC (eds): Intraoperative Monitoring Techniques in Neurosurgery. New York: McGraw-Hill, 1994, pp 141–157.
35. Carter LP: Continuous monitoring of cortical blood flow. In Loftus CM, Traynelis VC (eds): Intraoperative Monitoring Techniques in Neurosurgery. New York: McGraw-Hill, 1994, pp 53–61.
36. Day JD, Giannotta SL, Fukushima T: Extradural temporopolar approach to lesions of the upper basilar artery and infrachiasmatic region. J Neurosurg (in press).
37. Fujitsu K, Kuwabara T: Zygomatic approach for lesions in the interpeduncular cistern. J Neurosurg 62:340–343, 1985.
38. Hakuba A, Tanaka K, Suzuki T, Nishimura S: A combined orbitozygomatic infratemporal epidural and subdural approach for lesions involving the entire cavernous sinus. J Neurosurg 71:699–704, 1989.
39. Hitselberger WE, Horn KL, Hankinson H, et al: The middle fossa transpetrous approach for petroclival meningiomas. Skull Base Surg 3:130–135, 1993.
40. House WF, Hitselberger WE, Horn KL: The middle fossa transpetrous approach to the anterior-superior cerebellopontine angle. Am J Otol 7:1–4, 1986.

41. Horton JA, Jungreis CA, Pistoia F: Balloon test occlusion. In Sekhar LN, Janecka IP (eds): Surgery of Cranial Base Tumors. New York: Raven Press, 1993, pp 33–36.

42. Linskey ME, Sekhar LN, Sen C: Cerebral revascularization in cranial base surgery. In Sekhar LN, Janecka IP (eds): Surgery of Cranial Base Tumors. New York: Raven Press, 1993, pp 45–68.

43. Sekhar LN, Sen CN, Jho HD: Saphenous vein bypass of the cavernous internal carotid artery. J Neurosurg 72:35–41, 1990.

44. Spetzler RF, Fukushima T, Martin N, Zabramski JM: Petrous carotid-to-intradural carotid saphenous vein graft for intracavernous giant aneurysm, tumor, and occlusive cerebrovascular disease. J Neurosurg 73:496–501, 1990.

45. Miyazaki S, Fukushima T, Fujimaki T: Resection of high-cervical paraganglioma with cervical-to-petrous internal carotid artery saphenous vein bypass: Report of two cases. J Neurosurg 73:141–146, 1990.

46. Glasscock ME III, Smith PG, Whitaker SR, et al: Management of aneurysms of the petrous portion of the internal carotid artery by resection and primary anastomosis. Laryngoscope 93:1445–1453, 1983.

47. Hakuba A, Nishimura S, Jang BJ: A combined retroauricular and preauricular transpetrosal-transtentorial approach to clivus meningiomas. Surg Neurol 30:108–116, 1988.

48. Harsh GR, Sekhar LN: The subtemporal, transcavernous, anterior transpetrosal approach to the upper brain stem and clivus. J Neurosurg 77:709–717, 1992.

49. Parkinson D: Transcavernous repair of carotid-cavernous fistula: Case report. J Neurosurg 26:420–424, 1967.

# Pituitary Tumors

# Transsphenoidal Approaches to Lesions of the Sella

■ W. JEFFREY ELIAS and EDWARD R. LAWS, JR.

A variety of approaches to the sella turcica have been developed since the first pituitary operation, a temporal craniotomy, by Paul, a Liverpool surgeon in 1882.[1] Several extracranial procedures were used to access the sella via facial incisions, until Cushing[2] embraced and modified the transnasal approach in 1909. Further contributions to this approach included the endonasal technique used by Hirsch,[3] the x-ray image intensifier used by Guiot,[4] and microsurgical selective tumor removal introduced by Hardy.[5] Contemporary transsphenoidal surgery represents the compilation of techniques pioneered by these and other surgeons and is used in the surgical treatment of more than 90% of pituitary adenomas and for other sellar lesions, such as craniopharyngiomas, cysts, metastatic carcinomas, and other less common entities (Tables 28–1 to 28–3). Our current transsphenoidal approach has evolved from experience with more than 3000 sellar lesions since 1972. We employ three transsphenoidal surgical approaches in the treatment of sellar pathology.

Most sellar lesions at our institution are operated on through a unilateral endonasal approach. The cosmetic endonasal incision is not associated with dental anesthesia, involves minimal surgical dissection, and has a short recovery time. For larger tumors with suprasellar or parasellar extension, a sublabial conversion is made to maximize exposure. Finally, reoperations and operations in children are performed predominantly with an endonasal septal pushover technique. The advent of minimally invasive neurosurgery has resulted in our use of adjunctive procedures, including endoscopy and frameless stereotaxis, in a continued effort to increase accuracy and reduce morbidity.

## CLINICAL PRESENTATION

The most common problems affecting the pituitary gland that require surgical intervention involve pituitary adenomas, which present in three ways. Most common is the tumor that presents with mass effect. These slow-growing, benign tumors enlarge within the sella turcica and, as they extend superiorly into the intracranial compartment, produce compression of the optic chiasm with visual loss that is usually bitemporal in nature. Headache is not always a component of the symptom complex in these patients, and often the enlarging tumor mass compresses the normal pituitary gland and presents with slowly progressive hypopituitarism. Another subset of pituitary adenomas consists of the lesions that overproduce normal pituitary hormones. These include acromegaly with excessive production of growth hormone, prolactinomas, adrenocorticotropic hormone (ACTH) adenomas that result in either Cushing's disease or Nelson's syndrome, and the more infrequent active thyroid-stimulating hormone secreting pituitary adenoma that presents with secondary hyperthyroidism. Finally, many pituitary tumors are discovered as incidental lesions in patients when imaging is obtained for the evaluation of headaches, nasal sinus difficulty, or head injury or in patients who present with clinical manifestations of hypopituitarism or disturbances of electrolyte balance, usually hyponatremia and syndrome of inappropriate antidiuretic hormone.

In childhood, patients with pituitary disorders usually present either with failure of growth and sexual maturation or with evidence of excessive hormone production resulting in gigantism or Cushing's disease. Some pituitary lesions present with diabetes insipidus as a major symptom. These patients can have a variety of pituitary disorders other than a simple adenoma, including craniopharyngiomas, germinomas, Langerhans' cell granulomas, and metastatic tumors. With the exception of patients who have hyperfunctioning pituitary tumors, the differential diagnosis of a

TABLE 28–1 ■ CLINICAL ENTITIES TREATED BY TRANSSPHENOIDAL MICROSURGERY, 1972–1997

| Clinical Entity | No. of Patients |
|---|---|
| Pituitary adenoma | 2665 |
| Craniopharyngioma | 98 |
| Empty sella/arachnoid cyst | 75 |
| CSF rhinorrhea | 72 |
| Clivus chordoma | 27 |
| Miscellaneous lesions | 124 |
| *Total* | 3061 |

CSF, cerebrospinal fluid.

**TABLE 28–2 ■ PITUITARY ADENOMAS TREATED BY TRANSSPHENOIDAL MICROSURGERY, 1972–1997**

| Clinical Entity | No. of Patients |
| --- | --- |
| Functioning adenomas | |
|   Acromegaly | 468 |
|   Prolactin-secreting adenomas | 871 |
|   Cushing's disease | 381 |
|   Nelson-Salassa syndrome (postadrenalectomy ACTH) | 62 |
| Nonfunctioning adenomas (includes FSH/LH, null cell) | 855 |
| Miscellaneous pituitary adenomas | 24 |
| Total pituitary adenomas | 2665 |

ACTH, adrenocorticotropic hormone; FSH, follicle-stimulating hormone; LH, luteinizing hormone.

sellar lesion is broad, and careful preoperative laboratory evaluation and imaging studies are necessary before surgical treatment.

## INDICATIONS FOR SURGICAL MANAGEMENT

Pituitary apoplexy is a dramatic and often urgent indication for surgical intervention. These patients present with either hemorrhage into an existing pituitary tumor or acute necrosis of the tumor with subsequent edema. Such patients can have precipitous visual loss, usually associated with headache, and frequently collapse from acute adrenal insufficiency. These patients need steroid supplementation on an urgent basis and are frequently misdiagnosed as having subarachnoid hemorrhage, myocardial infarction, or stroke. If visual loss is severe and progressive, emergent surgical intervention, usually by the transsphenoidal approach, is indicated.[6, 7] If the patient has a relatively mild form of apoplexy and is clinically stable, it is prudent to measure the serum prolactin because some patients with prolactinomas present in this fashion and can occasionally be successfully treated with medical therapy.

A much more common indication for surgery of pituitary adenomas is a macroadenoma that is producing mass effect

**TABLE 28–3 ■ MISCELLANEOUS LESIONS TREATED BY TRANSSPHENOIDAL MICROSURGERY**

| | |
| --- | --- |
| Nasal glioma | Colloid cyst |
| Meningioma | Basilar impression |
| Sphenoid sinus carcinoma/sarcoma | Pilocystic astrocytoma (sellar) |
| Sphenoid sinus cyst | Lymphoma |
| Ganglioglioma | Cholesteatoma |
| Cavernous angioma (parasellar) | Hemangiopericytoma |
| Myeloma/plasmacytoma | Hemangiosarcoma |
| Fibrous dysplasia (parasellar) | Chondroma |
| Carotid-cavernous fistula | Chondrosarcoma |
| Tolosa-Hunt syndrome (granuloma) | Neuroendocrine carcinoma |
| Germinoma/teratoma | Esthesioneuroblastoma |
| Hypothalamic hamartoma | Aspergilloma |
| Schwannoma | Mucormycosis |
| Hemangioblastoma | Langerhans' cell histiocytosis |
| Metastatic carcinoma | Wegener's granulomatosis |
| Inflammatory disease/hypophysitis | Fibrosarcoma |
| Melanoma | |

in the form of progressive visual loss. These patients should always have a serum prolactin determination because dramatic shrinking of prolactinomas can occur with appropriate medical management in a relatively short period of time.[8] More often the prolactin is only modestly elevated, and the patient has a clinically nonfunctioning pituitary tumor that has enlarged to the point of compressing the optic apparatus. Large tumors can affect the brain itself producing hypothalamic symptoms, epilepsy, and motor or sensory loss. Parasellar extensions of pituitary adenomas can affect the cranial nerves within the cavernous sinus, resulting in craniofacial pain or numbness, diplopia, pupillary irregularity, or ptosis. The transsphenoidal approach is usually successful in reversing mass effect in the suprasellar compartment and in the cavernous sinuses. Some patients with large tumors extending toward the frontal or temporal lobes cannot be successfully treated by a transsphenoidal approach, and these patients are candidates for craniotomy.

In some cases, surgical management may be necessary to establish an accurate diagnosis. A large number of lesions can mimic pituitary adenomas, producing elevation in prolactin by interfering with the transport of dopamine from the hypothalamus through the pituitary stalk to the anterior pituitary lactotrophs.[9] When the pathology is uncertain, it may be essential to obtain an accurate histologic diagnosis. Craniopharyngiomas and Rathke's cleft cysts can mimic pituitary adenomas. Aneurysms of the carotid artery may likewise produce symptoms similar to those of a pituitary tumor. A variety of other tumors, such as meningiomas, germinomas, and dermoid tumors, can occur in this region, as does the occasional metastatic carcinoma or primary malignant tumor (see Table 28–3).

Among the hyperfunctioning pituitary adenomas, those producing Cushing's disease, especially in adults, are currently best managed by transsphenoidal exploration and removal of a pituitary microadenoma when detected. At present, medical management for Cushing's disease is not optimal, and the surgical approach provides the best means for obtaining a prompt, lasting remission of the disease. A selective transsphenoidal approach provides results in children that are currently similar to those of radiation therapy and may give a child the chance of avoiding long-term hypopituitarism, which usually follows conventional radiation therapy. For reasons that are not clear, the recurrence rate for ACTH adenomas in children is significantly higher than that seen in adults.[10]

Active acromegaly is currently considered an indication for surgical management, primarily because of the promptness with which growth hormone decreases.[11] Selective microsurgical removal of a pituitary tumor has been particularly effective in acromegalics, providing excellent rates of long-term control and a low recurrence rate.[11]

The failure of prior therapy often represents an indication for surgical intervention. Some patients treated with radiation therapy have a favorable initial response, then develop recurrence, either in the form of mass effect or as recurrent hormonal hypersecretion (prolactin, growth hormone, or ACTH). Some patients with presumed prolactinomas have normalization of prolactin after medical therapy but progressive growth of tumor. These patients at surgery usually have lesions other than prolactinoma. Some patients with prolactinomas and high prolactin levels have a suboptimal response to medical therapy, with persistent abnormal prolactin levels. Surgery as an adjunct may further reduce prolactin levels and may improve the response to adjunctive therapy by decreasing tumor burden. Occasionally a patient with a prolactinoma truly intolerant of medical therapy requires surgery.

## PREOPERATIVE EVALUATION AND MANAGEMENT

At our institution, the preoperative evaluation represents a combination of neurosurgical and endocrinologic assessment of pituitary function. A complete discussion of the endocrinologic evaluation is beyond the scope of this chapter.[12] Briefly, serum laboratory studies routinely include baseline pituitary hormone levels, and women receive pregnancy testing when appropriate. Serum calcium and glucose levels are measured to detect occult cases of type I multiple endocrine neoplasia. Provocative testing of the pituitary includes an oral glucose tolerance test for acromegalics and dexamethasone suppression testing for patients with Cushing's disease. In the latter group, we rely heavily on 24-hour urine levels of cortisol for diagnosis and occasionally obtain inferior petrosal sinus sampling in equivocal situations.

Visual field testing is necessary before and after surgery in patients with optic nerve involvement. Surgical planning depends on magnetic resonance imaging (MRI) to determine the location of the carotid arteries and the extent of tumor expansion. The relationship of the pituitary lesion with respect to the normal gland and optic nerves is also crucial in selecting the surgical approach. When we use frameless stereotaxy, a preoperative computed tomography (CT) scan with fiducial markers in place is necessary and provides information regarding nasal sinus anatomy, which is particularly useful in reoperative situations in which normal bony landmarks are disrupted or absent.

Patients are hospitalized the night before surgery to administer antibiotics and stress dose steroids (i.e., 100 mg hydrocortisone intravenously every 6 hours) because the pituitary-adrenal reserve may be impaired even in mild cases of hypopituitarism. This regimen applies in all cases except Cushing's disease patients, who do not receive steroids preoperatively or postoperatively because of their excessive endogenous steroids. Their serum cortisol levels are measured the night before surgery and every 6 hours subsequently, so that the trend can be recorded after tumor resection; postoperative assessment of tumor removal and cure depends on proven hypocortisolemia.

## POSITIONING AND NASAL PREPARATION

Patient positioning and nasal preparation are identical for each of the three approaches. After anesthetic induction and oral intubation, the oropharynx is packed with moist gauze to prevent swallowing of blood and secretions. The patient is placed in a comfortable semirecumbent position, which not only diminishes venous pressure, but also pre-

vents blood from occluding the surgeon's field of view. A horseshoe headrest is used rather than skull fixation to maintain flexibility and allow subtle intraoperative head movements. The left ear is cocked toward the left shoulder, and the head is slightly flexed such that the nasal bridge is parallel to the floor. An oblique angle between the head and the body now exists, and the operating table is positioned such that the head is perpendicular to the walls of the room to enhance the surgeon's orientation with regard to the midline and to make positioning of the x-ray image intensifier more straightforward (Fig. 28–1).

The nasal preparation begins immediately after intubation with the intranasal administration of a decongestant spray. The nasal mucosal surfaces are treated with cotton pledgets soaked in 0.05% oxymetazoline. The face is prepared with an aqueous antiseptic solution, and the nasal pledgets are removed so that the mucosal surfaces can be injected with 0.5% lidocaine with 1:200,000 epinephrine. The initial submucosal injections are performed with a 25-gauge needle and include both sides of the septum as well as the sublabial mucosa. Much of the initial nasal dissection occurs with the proper injection of the mucosa, which blanches as it is lifted from the septum. Deeper injections can be done with a spinal needle. The entire nasal preparation and dissection to the face of the sphenoid sinus is performed with the nasal speculum, loupe magnification, and a headlight.

Before the incision, the right lower quadrant of the abdomen is prepared in case a fat graft is needed to seal a cerebrospinal fluid leak. The details of the anesthetic management have been previously described[13]; we do not routinely use an arterial line, Foley catheter, or compression stockings. A lumbar drain is placed in cases of large tumors with suprasellar extension.

## ENDONASAL APPROACH

Most transsphenoidal procedures at our institution are performed through one nostril via the endonasal approach. Selection of this approach depends on the tumor size and exposure requirements, and tumors extending above the sella often can be effectively removed (Fig. 28–2). Rarely, this approach is limited by the size of the adult nares, but it does require the use of a low-profile endonasal speculum (Fig. 28–3). This exposure involves a few simple steps with relatively few instruments and can be routinely performed by the neurosurgical service (see Fig. 28–3).

The columella is retracted laterally exposing the glistening tip of the cartilaginous septum. The hemitransfixion incision can be made in either nare, but we prefer the right nostril because it is usually easier for a right-handed surgeon to elevate a right anterior mucosal tunnel (Fig. 28–4). The incision should be extended inferiorly and laterally within the ala to reduce the tension on the mucosal flap when the retractor is placed. An alar incision can be made but requires a meticulous closure with fine sutures. We rarely perform an alotomy because we convert to a sublabial approach when additional exposure is necessary.

Initially the Cottle knife is used to dissect the mucosa from the cartilage, thus creating an anterior tunnel. Adher-

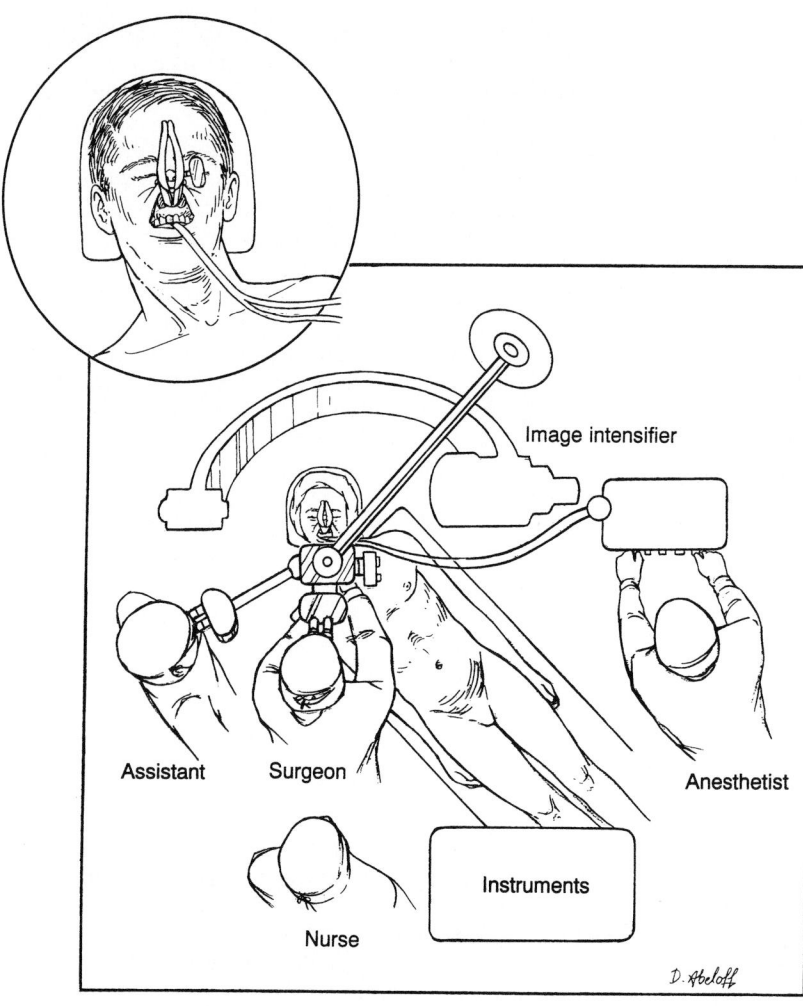

D. Abeloff

**FIGURE 28–1** ■ Patient positioning and the operating room set-up for transsphenoidal surgery.

ent attachments of the mucosa to the nasal spine exist and require sharp separation with the Cottle dissector or fine scissors (see Fig. 28–6). This maneuver should sweep mucosa from the vertical septum onto the floor to release a mucosal flap adequate for later retraction. Along the junction of the bony and cartilaginous septum, blunt dissection

with the Cottle elevator easily establishes an ipsilateral posterior tunnel (Fig. 28–5).

The cartilaginous septum is incised vertically at its junction with the perpendicular plate of the ethmoid and is disarticulated bluntly from the bony septum and swept to the contralateral side as it separates from the nasal spine

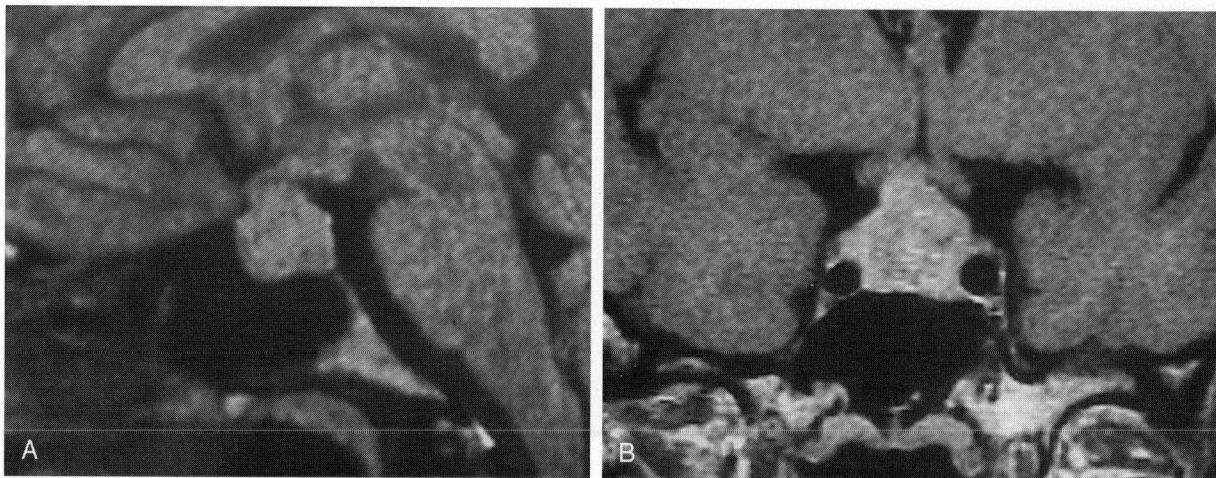

**FIGURE 28–2** ■ Sagittal (*A*) and coronal T$_1$-weighted magnetic resonance images (*B*) of a pituitary macroadenoma removed using the endonasal approach.

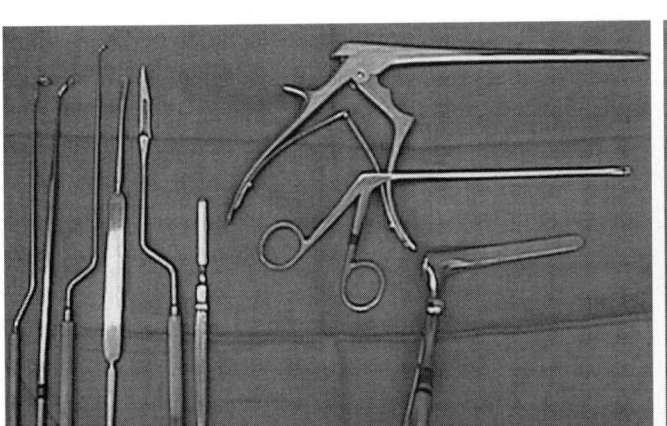
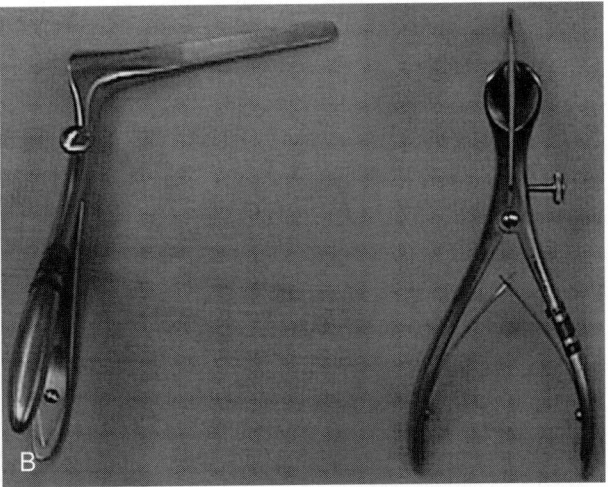

FIGURE 28–3 ■ Instruments (A) and a low-profile speculum (B) are required for the endonasal approach.

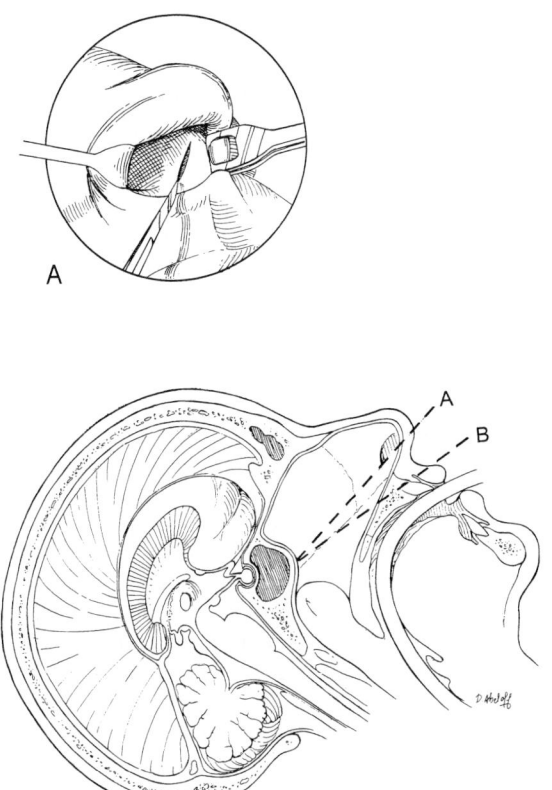

FIGURE 28–4 ■ Hemitransfixion incision (A) and trajectories (B) to the sella with the endonasal and sublabial approaches.

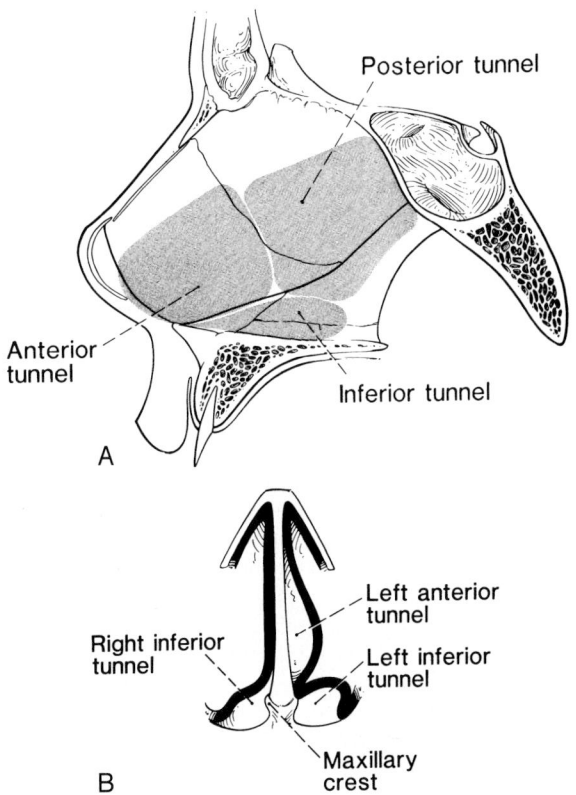

Posterior tunnel

Anterior tunnel

Inferior tunnel

A

Left anterior tunnel

Right inferior tunnel

Left inferior tunnel

Maxillary crest

B

FIGURE 28–5 ■ A and B, Diagram of the tunnels created by elevating the nasal mucosa. The anterior tunnel can be created either on the right or the left of the cartilaginous septum.

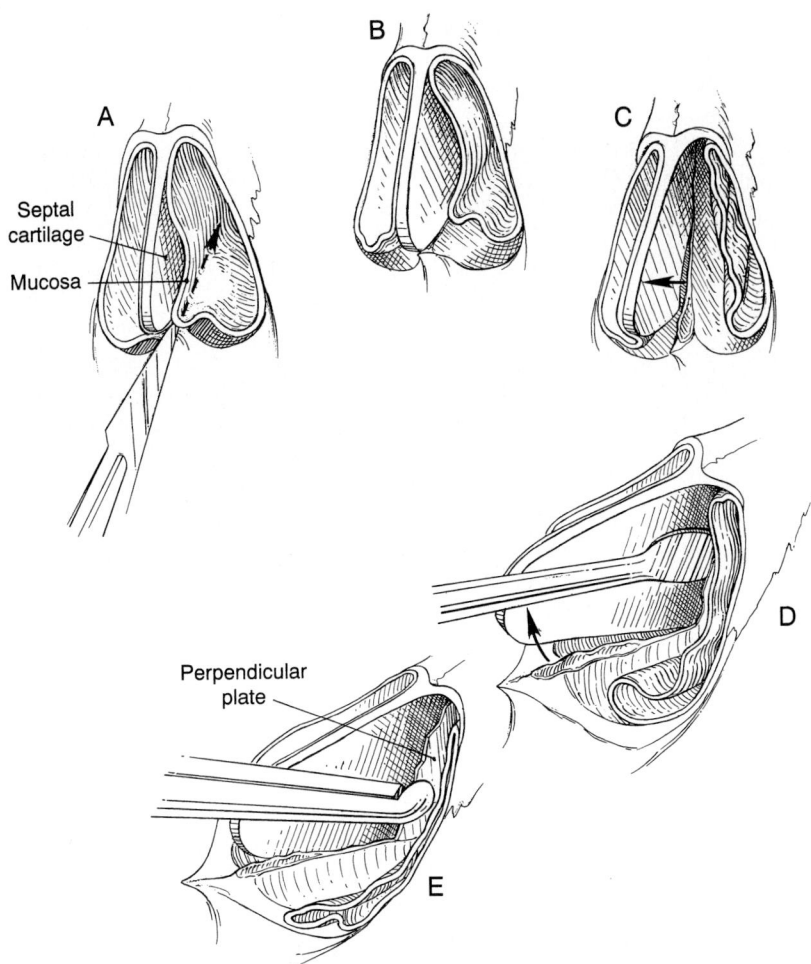

FIGURE 28–6 ■ The nasal tunnels connected (*A*) and elevated (*B*). Displacement of the nasal septum to the right (*C*) and disarticulation from the maxillary ridge (*D*). Removal of the perpendicular plate of the ethmoid (*E*).

Septal cartilage
Mucosa
Perpendicular plate

(Fig. 28–6). The mucosa on the contralateral side of the bony septum is elevated, establishing bilateral posterior submucosal tunnels. The endonasal speculum can now be inserted medial to the displaced cartilaginous septum and straddling the bony septum. Further posterior submucosal dissection can be done by gently opening the speculum as it is advanced.

The bony septum is removed with Knight scissors or is deliberately fractured with a Takahashi forcep, and this bone is saved for reconstruction of the sellar floor. Care should be taken not to fracture the septum too far superiorly because the anterior cranial fossa may be entered. Similarly the approach should follow the floor of the nasopharynx to avoid a misdirected entry into the cranium. Lateral exposure is improved by outfracturing the turbinates. As the face of the sphenoid sinus and its lateral ostia come into view, the keel of the vomer and the rostrum of the sphenoid provide midline orientation (Fig. 28–7). Position and trajectory are confirmed with videofluoroscopy before introducing the operating microscope.

The sphenoid sinus is entered with a chisel or by grasping the area above the vomer between the sphenoid ostia with a Ferris Smith forcep, and the entrance is enlarged with a Kerrison rongeur. The sphenoid ostia reside high on the anterior wall of the sinus, so that additional bone removal initially extends from them in an inferomedial direction. The sphenoid mucosa is stripped to reduce infec-

tion and bleeding and to prevent the formation of a postoperative mucocele.

The sellar floor now comes into view, and its sagittal dimensions are confirmed with fluoroscopy before proceeding. We use a 350-mm focal length on the microscope with at least 12.5 times magnification, so that the sella fills the entire field of view. Frequently, pituitary tumors erode the floor of the sella, or it may be thinned similar to an eggshell. We attempt to enter the sella without creating a durotomy by gently grasping the floor with a forcep or by working a blunt hook through the bone. When the sellar floor is of normal thickness, a chisel or high-speed air drill may be necessary. The remainder of the floor is removed widely to the margin of each cavernous sinus with a Kerrison rongeur so that the sellar dura is fully visualized. It is best to avoid extensive superior removal of bone because there is usually dense attachment of the sellar dura at the junction with the anterior fossa, and violation here can produce a spinal fluid leak.

The dural surface is cauterized with a monopolar suction device before a rectangular durotomy is excised with a bayoneted knife (Fig. 28–8). The dura can also be opened in a cruciate, X-shaped, or elliptical fashion. It is prudent to review the imaging studies before dural opening to note the position of the carotid arteries. With microadenomas or in situations in which large venous channels exist, such as a prominent intercavernous sinus in a patient with Cushing's

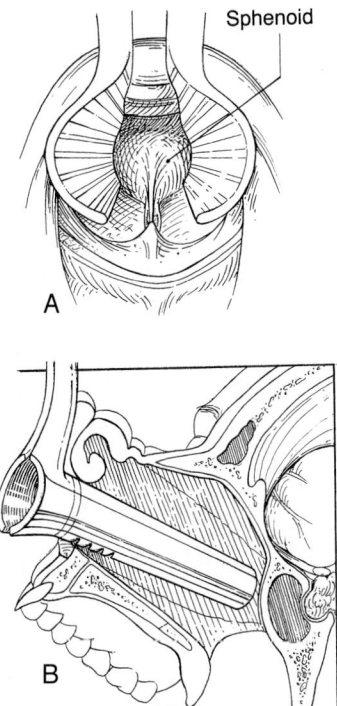

FIGURE 28–7 ■ Anterior wall of the sphenoid sinus with the midline vomer keel as visualized through sublabial retractor placement.

disease, the dura is carefully coagulated and incised horizontally. Venous bleeding between the dural sleeves is controlled with an angled bipolar cautery. Often tumor extrudes through the dura immediately, but it is helpful first to develop a subdural plane with a blunt nerve hook.

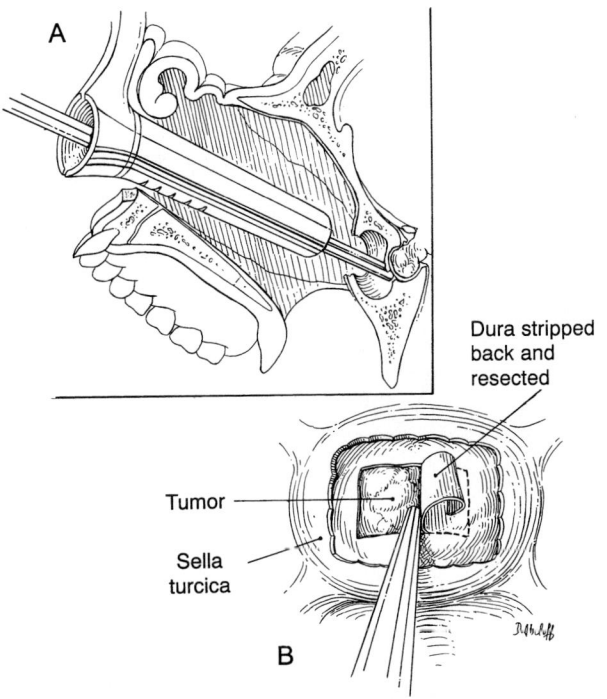

FIGURE 28–8 ■ Removal of the floor of the sella (A) and rectangular durotomy (B).

The excised dural specimen is studied pathologically for evidence of tumoral invasion.[14, 15]

The tumor removal of a pituitary adenoma is initiated by entering the capsule with a ring curet (Fig. 28–9), and, once loosened, the fragments are removed with small cupped forceps from the central inferior aspect of the open sella. Next, lateral tumor is removed by using a blunt ring curet to dissect along the medial cavernous sinus walls and the carotids. Tumor should never be grasped laterally and pulled away for fear of producing serious hemorrhage. Finally, the superior portions of the tumor are resected, and suprasellar fragments often collapse into the sella as the expanded diaphragm descends into the sella.

Suprasellar extensions are removed by carefully advancing a large, right-angled, ring curet above the sella and gently pushing it in a posterior fashion from the dorsum sellae until the tumor falls into intrasellar space. The diaphragma sellae can be easily torn with this step, resulting in a cerebrospinal fluid leak. Further suprasellar decompression can be obtained by prolapsing the tumor's superior capsule and diaphragm by injecting 10 to 25 ml of air into a lumbar drain placed preoperatively. This prolapse can be reversed by aspirating cerebrospinal fluid from the drain. Alternatively a Valsalva maneuver by the anesthesiologist or bilateral jugular vein compressions accomplish the same increase in intracranial pressure. We use the endoscope as an adjunctive technique to inspect the suprasellar resection.

Optic nerve decompression from a transsphenoidal approach has proved to be highly effective in preserving vision (Table 28–4).[7, 16] The insertion of a 30-degree angled endoscope into the suprasellar space provides visualization of the subchiasmatic region for assessing the adequacy of decompression and the extent of tumor resection.

Normal anterior pituitary gland may appear as a thin ribbon of tissue in the sella as it is displaced by a large macroadenoma. Its appearance should be distinct on gross inspection from the more friable, grayish adenoma. Aggressive intrasellar resection is possible because only about 15% of the anterior lobe is required to maintain pituitary function.[17] The posterior lobe of the pituitary is not normally present in cases with macroadenomas. In microadenomas, its appearance is characteristic, and minimal manipulation of the posterior lobe and the pituitary stalk is mandatory if one is to avoid diabetes insipidus.

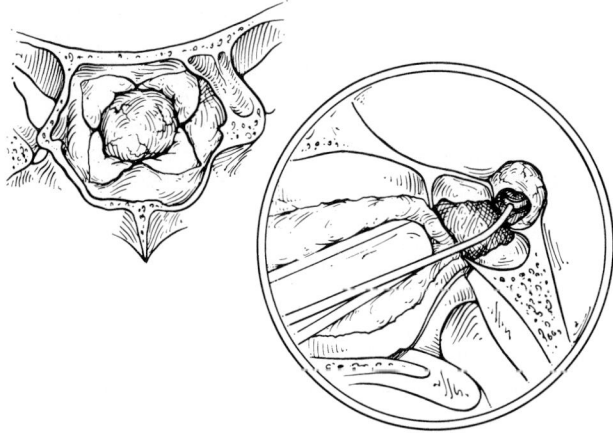

FIGURE 28–9 ■ Internal resection of a pituitary adenoma with the ring curet.

## TABLE 28–4 ■ RESULTS OF TRANSSPHENOIDAL SURGERY IN PATIENTS WITH PREOPERATIVE VISUAL FIELD DEFECTS

| Postoperative Vision | Patients (%) |
| --- | --- |
| Improved | 81 |
| Unchanged | 13 |
| Worse | 6 |

Data from Laws ER Jr, Kern EB: Complications of transsphenoidal surgery. Clin Neurosurg 23:401, 1976; Laws ER Jr, Kern EB: Complications of transsphenoidal surgery. In Tindall GT, Colins WF (eds): Clinical Management of Pituitary Disorders. New York: Raven Press, 1979, pp 435–445.

In patients with Cushing's disease, a pituitary adenoma may not be apparent when the dura is opened, and so a transverse incision is made into the pituitary gland proper. Once this incision is made, subdural dissection of the lateral wings of the pituitary gland is started, first on one side, then on the other, with Hardy dissectors. If the incision into the gland has been made deeply enough, lateral pressure with a Hardy dissector usually causes the microadenoma to herniate into the operative field. Its location can be delineated, its cavity entered, and its removal completed by use of a small ring curet and cup forceps. All tissue that appears suspicious is removed, and a biopsy specimen is occasionally obtained from the residual, presumed normal, pituitary gland.

The technique of hypophysectomy for metastatic carcinoma or diabetic retinopathy is mainly of historical interest but is similar to that described for microadenomas.[16] The pituitary gland is dissected subdurally; first, the lateral wings are dissected, then the inferior aspect of the gland. The subdural plane of dissection is maintained, and considerable pressure is used to strip the lateral aspects of the gland, from anterior to posterior, away from the walls of the cavernous sinus. This procedure is performed cautiously and gradually, working first on one side, then the other, then on the inferior aspect of the gland, repeating this sequence many times. The gland shrinks, and once some mobility has been achieved, the superior aspect of the gland can be dissected, then depressed, permitting the pituitary stalk to come into view. The stalk is cauterized with a bipolar, then transected with an alligator scissor or a No. 11 blade knife. Once this has been accomplished, a Hardy dissector is placed along the floor of the sella, then used to dissect behind and over the superior surface of the gland to free it completely. In some cases, the dissection does not go smoothly, and the gland may have to be removed piecemeal, in which case, the sella must be searched thoroughly for retained fragments of the gland. Total hypophysectomy must be achieved for optimal results.

This technique can also be used in the surgical management of Cushing's disease, if an anticipated microadenoma is not readily discovered. Sequential excisional biopsy specimens of the pituitary are obtained, first the central wedge, then the lateral lobes. A stub of gland is left attached to the pituitary stalk, then the posterior lobe is carefully explored.

Cerebrospinal fluid leaks can occur early in the procedure when sharply opening the dura in the setting of an anterior cerebrospinal fluid diverticulum, which occurs in 17% of normal individuals.[18] Weeping cerebrospinal fluid leaks may be apparent by a blackened hue in the blood as the two fluids mix. After tumor removal, the dead space of the tumor cavity is ordinarily obliterated with the gelatin sponge material (Gelfoam). With cerebrospinal fluid leaks, however, the closure requires occlusive packing with abdominal fat taken from the right lower quadrant. This tissue is soaked in 1 g chloramphenicol/100 ml saline and briefly dried with cotton fibers before being rolled in fibrillar collagen (Avitene). An appropriate size is selected for the sella (Fig. 28–10A), and the remainder is packed into the sphenoid sinus. A rectangular strut or plate of nasal bone placed in the epidural or subdural space is used to secure the intrasellar graft while reconstructing the floor of the sella (see Fig. 28–10B). We do not routinely close cerebrospinal fluid defects with fibrin glue, unless the leak is recurrent or recalcitrant, and we do not use routine postoperative lumbar drainage.

The significant morbidity associated with intrasellar hemorrhage can be diminished if managed appropriately. Attempts to avoid separating the dural leaves when entering the sella can prevent the cavernous sinus from being opened. If opened, the cavernous sinus can be occluded with small cottonoids held in place by the suction cannula until the procedure and resection are complete. More difficult bleeding requires packing the sinus with Gelfoam, but overaggressive packing can be associated with transient or permanent cranial nerve palsies. The head may be further elevated to decrease venous pressure, but attention must be paid to the possibility of venous air embolism. The sella can be packed with the abdominal fat graft technique described earlier, and in cases of persistent bleeding, muscle packing provides superior hemostasis.

Arterial bleeding from a carotid injury represents an immediate life-threatening situation. Hemostasis without compromising the artery's distal flow is quite difficult. We have experienced three such situations and were able to gain hemostasis in two with muscle autografts; the third patient expired from cerebral ischemia after the bleeding was controlled with a balloon catheter. Carotid artery injuries should be immediately evaluated postoperatively with

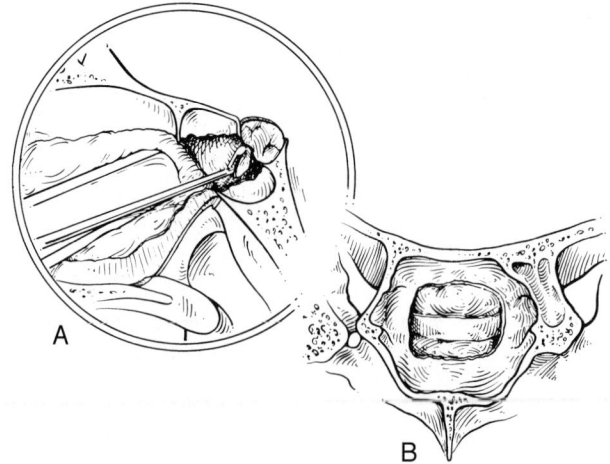

FIGURE 28–10 ■ A, Intrasellar packing with an abdominal fat graft. B, Sellar floor reconstruction with a nasal bone strut.

angiography to determine if a pseudoaneurysm or carotid-cavernous fistula exists.

On completion of the tumor removal, the sphenoid sinus is left patent in the absence of cerebrospinal fluid leakage, and the retractor is withdrawn while examining the mucosal flaps for evidence of tears. Unilateral tears should heal, but septal perforations result from bilateral tears. The mucosal flaps are reapproximated at the midline, and the cartilaginous septum is repositioned over the nasal spine before closing the mucosal incision with several interrupted absorbable sutures. We pack the nasopharynx bilaterally with tagged cotton nasal packing in the fingers of a rubber glove lubricated with antibiotic ointment so that the mucosal flaps are in intimate contact with the septum and the nasal floor.

Complications from transsphenoidal surgery of the sella are uncommon (Table 28–5).[19, 20] The current mortality rate is less than 1%, and serious morbidity, such as carotid injuries, intracranial hemorrhages, stroke, and visual loss, occurs in fewer than 2% of patients.[21]

## SUBLABIAL CONVERSION

The sublabial conversion approach is so named because in our practice it is preceded by endonasal dissection. It is used in situations in which wider exposure is desired preoperatively or if the endonasal exposure is unsatisfactory. Although the entire procedure can be performed through the sublabial incision, we perform the initial exposure endonasally because of the ease of direct dissection of the septum and the diminished likelihood of mucosal tears. Once the anterior and posterior submucosal tunnels are created, the cartilaginous septum is disarticulated, and a contralateral posterior tunnel is developed. The sublabial incision is made at this stage in the buccogingival junction between the canines (Fig. 28–11A). The mucosa is elevated superiorly from the maxillary crest to the anterior nasal spine medially and laterally along the margins of the piriform aperture. Bilateral inferior floor tunnels are created along the downward-sloping maxilla. Sharp dissection separates the adhesions between anterior and inferior mucosal flaps along the nasal spine. The cartilaginous septum must be swept laterally from the nasal spine to create an adequate submucosal space for insertion of a Hardy, Landolt, or Hubbard speculum. As with the endonasal speculum, the retractors should be slowly advanced past any mucosal tears. Intraoperative videofluoroscopy or computerized image-guided techniques confirm the positioning of the retractor before proceeding into the sphenoid sinus.

## ENDONASAL SEPTAL PUSHOVER

The endonasal septal pushover approach is used in reoperative situations in which the usual landmarks are disrupted and in an effort to preserve remaining septal and mucosal tissue.[22] This technique is especially helpful in recurrent cases of Cushing's disease because the tissue is extremely friable and prone to bleeding and in children, in whom the anatomic structures are small. This basic approach can be used for any midline sellar lesion and can be modified for endoscopic pituitary surgery.[23–26]

A speculum is inserted into the nostril deep to the cartilaginous septum in an attempt to identify a segment of bony septum covered by mucous membrane. If such a remnant exists, it is usually apparent as part of the superior perpendicular ethmoid plate, and a vertical mucosal incision is begun here and carried downward, then anteriorly along the base of the nasal septum toward the nasal spine of the maxilla. The inferior border of the nasal septum is disarticulated from the maxillary ridge starting posteriorly until adequate relaxation and visualization of the face of the sphenoid is obtained. Some elevation of a contralateral inferior mucosal tunnel may be helpful (Fig. 28–12). Attempts are made to recreate posterior tunnels by separating the mucosa from the perpendicular plate of the ethmoid. This attempt can be quite difficult, and, more commonly, the posterior aspect of the septum, which is absent of bone, can be displaced with the cartilaginous portion.

The surgical position is confirmed frequently with videofluoroscopy, and we have relied on frameless stereotaxy for continuous feedback regarding three-dimensional location and trajectory (Fig. 28–13). The retractors are advanced cautiously into the sphenoid sinus as scar tissue is removed with cupped forceps to expose the face of the sella.

TABLE 28–5 ■ **COMPLICATIONS OF TRANSSPHENOIDAL SURGERY (2562 CASES)**

| Complication | No. of Patients |
|---|---|
| Operative mortality (30-day) | |
|   Hypothalamic injury/hemorrhage | 5 |
|   Meningitis | 2 |
|   Vascular injury/occlusion | 4 |
|   CSF leak, pneumocephalus, SAH/spasm, MI | 1 |
|   Postoperative MI—postoperative seizure | 1 |
| Total | 14 (1.05%) |
| Major morbidity | |
|   Vascular occlusion/spasm/SAH (stroke) | 5 |
|   Visual loss (new) | 11 |
|   Vascular injury (repaired) | 8 |
|   Meningitis (nonfatal) | 8 |
|   Sellar abscess | 1 |
|   Sellar pneumatocele | 1 |
|   Sixth nerve paralysis | 2 |
|   Third nerve paralysis | 1 |
|   CSF rhinorrhea | 49 |
| Total | 86 (3.4%) |
| Lesser morbidity | |
|   Hemorrhage, intraoperative or postoperative | 9 |
|   Postoperative psychosis | 5 |
|   Nasal septal perforation, webbing | 16 |
|   Sinusitis, lip infection, postoperative | 5 |
|   Transient third or sixth nerve palsy | 5 |
|   Diabetes insipidus (usually transient) | 35 |
|   Cribriform plate fracture | 2 |
|   Maxillary fracture | 2 |
|   Hepatitis | 1 |
|   Symptomatic SIADH | 37 |
| Total | 117 (4.6%) |

CSF, cerebrospinal fluid; SAH, subarachnoid hemorrhage; MI, myocardial infarction; SIADH, syndrome of inappropriate antidiuretic hormone.

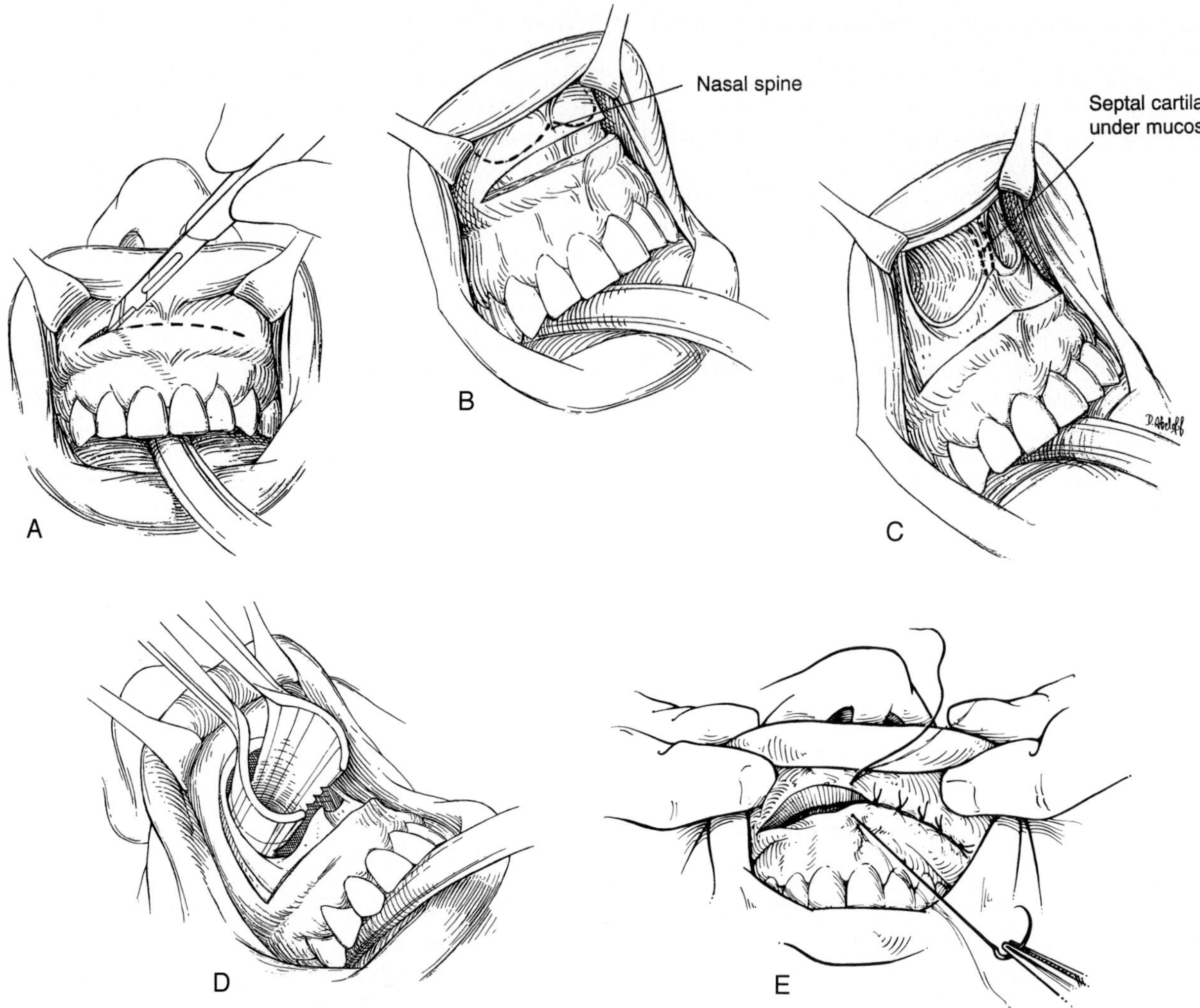

FIGURE 28-11 ■ The sublabial approach: incision (*A*), mucosal elevation (*B, C*); placement of the speculum (*D*); and closure (*E*).

## POSTOPERATIVE CARE

Postoperatively, patients ordinarily return to the neurosurgical ward and not to the intensive care unit. Fluid balance, urine specific gravity, and daily serum sodium values are meticulously recorded. A Foley catheter is rarely necessary.

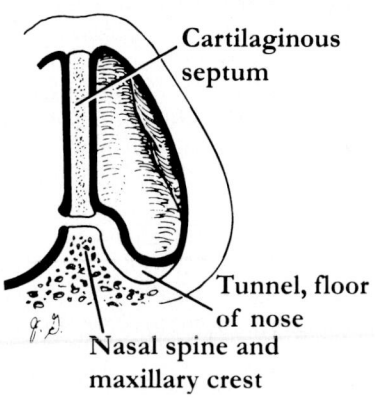

FIGURE 28-12 ■ Endonasal septal pushover technique utilized in reoperative and pediatric patients.

Eighteen percent of patients may experience transient diabetes insipidus,[21] indicated by a nadir of urinary specific gravity to 1.000 and urinary outputs greater than 300 ml/hr. We allow patients to compensate for fluid loss with oral intake, but in symptomatic cases of polyuria and when progressive hypernatremia occurs, we administer vasopressin by a subcutaneous, intranasal, or oral route. Delayed hyponatremia may occur, probably as part of a triphasic response to pituitary injury, and is treated with fluid restriction.[28] In unusual cases of recalcitrant hyponatremia, we use intravenous urea to promote diuresis with frequent measurements of serum chemistries.[29]

Antibiotics are administered until the nasal packing is removed at 24 to 48 hours. Intravenous nafcillin is started preoperatively and converted to oral clindamycin when oral intake resumes postoperatively. Over the next few days, minor sanguineous rhinorrhea is controlled with intranasal vasoconstrictors, and the nasopharynx is cleaned with saline spray. We are occasionally faced with the question as to whether this rhinorrhea represents a cerebrospinal fluid leak. If this is the case, plain skull radiographs or CT may demonstrate intracranial air, and dynamic spinal fluid testing using a lumbar puncture does not show a compensatory rise in intracranial pressure with Valsalva or Quecken-

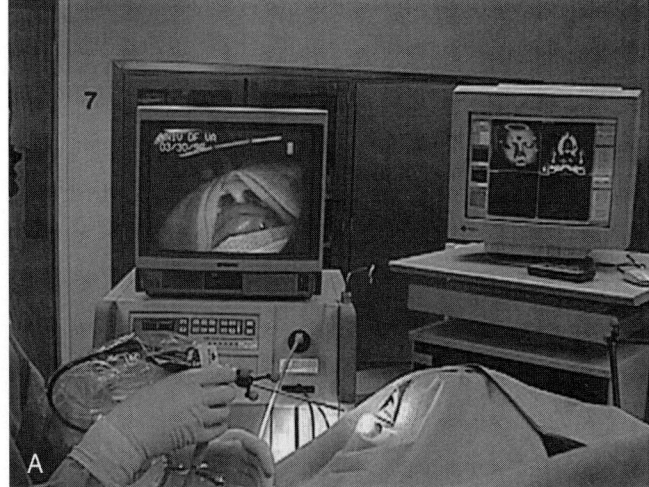

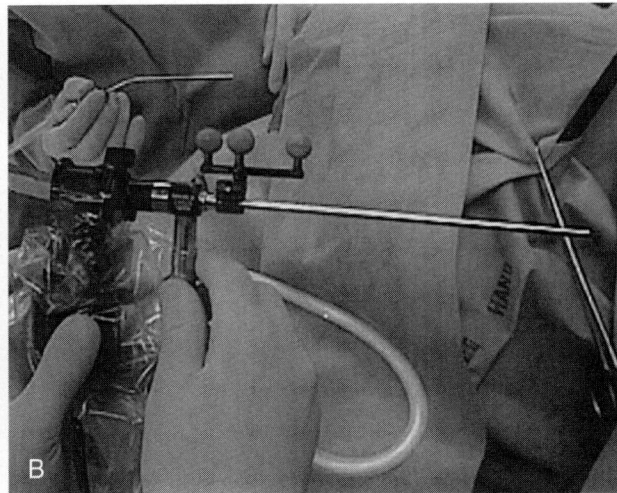

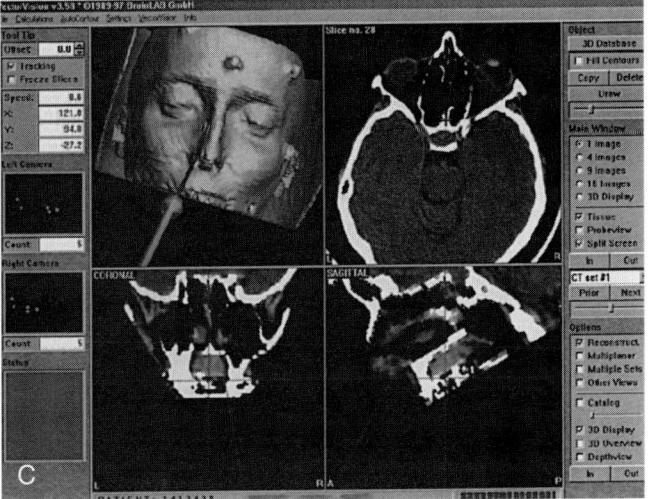

FIGURE 28–13 ■ *A–C,* The neuroendoscope is adapted with a frameless stereotaxy.

stedt maneuvers because a cerebrospinal fluid fistula decompresses the subarachnoid space. Currently, we test the rhinorrhea for the presence of tau-transferrin, a marker unique to the cerebrospinal fluid.[30, 31] Postoperative spinal fluid leaks are treated initially with a short trial of bed rest and lumbar drainage, but our current policy is one of early definitive reoperation to close the leak.

By postoperative day 1 or 2, the appropriate baseline pituitary hormones are again studied, and replacement therapy, including testosterone in men and estrogen in women, is initiated when necessary. Morning cortisol levels are obtained 24 hours after the cessation of perioperative corticosteroids to determine the need for replacement corticosteroids. The incidence of iatrogenic hypopituitarism in patients harboring microadenomas is now less than 3% in our experience. Cushing's disease patients are monitored closely for signs of adrenal insufficiency with frequent vital signs, orthostatic measurements, and serum cortisol levels every 6 hours. Data suggest that postoperative adrenal insufficiency in these patients indicates complete tumor removal and a lasting surgical remission.

Most patients are discharged from the hospital by the third postoperative day, and by this time, the need for replacement hormonal therapy has been determined. Patients are reassessed 6 weeks later, and definitive postoperative imaging studies (MRI) are obtained 3 months after surgery. Pregnancy after transsphenoidal surgery for microadenomas has been achieved in 84% of women.[32]

## CONCLUSION

Contemporary transsphenoidal surgery represents the primary method of treatment for pituitary adenomas and many other lesions affecting the sella. It is now being performed with a low risk of serious complications by experienced neurosurgeons. The endonasal approach affords excellent access to the sella with minimal invasiveness to the patient. Newer techniques, such as endoscopy and stereotaxis, are being developed and used to reduce further the morbidity of the procedure.[33]

## ACKNOWLEDGMENTS

*The authors are grateful to Diane Abeloff and William Westwood, who prepared the illustrations, and to Dr. Tord Alden, who assisted with the photographs.*

# REFERENCES

1. Caton R, Paul FT: Notes of a case of acromegaly treated by operation. BMJ 2:1421, 1893.
2. Cushing H: Partial hypophysectomy for acromegaly: With remarks on the function of the hypophysis. Ann Surg 50:1002–1017, 1909.
3. Hirsch O: Symptoms and treatment of pituitary tumors. Arch Otolaryngol 55:268–306, 1952.
4. Guiot G: Transsphenoidal approach in surgical treatment of pituitary adenomas: General principles and indications in non-functioning adenomas. Excerpta Medica International Congress Series 303:159–178, 1973.
5. Hardy J: Transsphenoidal microsurgery of the normal and pathological pituitary. Clin Neurosurg 16:185–214, 1969.
6. Bills DC, Meyer FB, Laws ER Jr, et al: A retrospective analysis of pituitary apoplexy. Neurosurgery 33:602–609, 1993.
7. Laws ER Jr, Trautmann JC, Hollenhorst RW Jr: Transsphenoidal decompression of the optic nerve and chiasm: Visual results in 62 patients. J Neurosurg 46:717–722, 1977.
8. Thorner MO, Martin WH, Rogol AD, et al: Rapid regression of pituitary prolactinomas during bromocriptine treatment. J Clin Endocrinol Metab 51:438–445, 1980.
9. Smith MV, Laws ER Jr: Magnetic resonance imaging measurements of pituitary stalk compression and deviation in patients with nonprolactin-secreting intrasellar and parasellar tumors: Lack of correlation with serum prolactin levels. Neurosurgery 34:834–839, 1994.
10. Leinung MC, Kane LA, Scheithauer BW, et al: Long term follow-up of transsphenoidal surgery for the treatment of Cushing's disease in childhood. J Clin Endocrinol Metab 80:2475–2479, 1995.
11. Davis DH, Laws ER Jr, Ilstrup DM, et al: Results of surgical treatment for growth hormone-secreting pituitary adenomas. J Neurosurg 79:70–75, 1993.
12. Landolt AM, Vance ML, Reilly PL: Pituitary Adenomas. New York: Churchill Livingstone, 1996.
13. Messick JM, Laws ER Jr, Abboud CF: Anesthesia for transsphenoidal surgery of the hypophyseal region. Anesth Analg 57:206–214, 1978.
14. Scheithauer BW, Kovacs KT, Laws ER Jr, et al: Pathology of invasive pituitary tumors with special reference to functional classification. J Neurosurg 65:733–744, 1986.
15. Thapar K, Kovacs K, Scheithauer BW, et al: Proliferative activity and invasiveness among pituitary adenomas and carcinomas: An analysis using the MIB-1 antibody. Neurosurgery 38:99–107, 1996.
16. Laws ER Jr, Randall RV, Kern EB, et al (eds): Management of Pituitary Adenomas and Related Lesions with Emphasis on Transsphenoidal Microsurgery. New York: Appleton-Century-Crofts, 1982.
17. Page RB: The anatomy of the hypothalamo-hypophysial complex. In Knobil E, Neill JD (eds): The Physiology of Reproduction, 2nd ed. New York: Raven Press, 1994, pp 1527–1619.
18. Renn WH, Rhoton AL Jr: Microsurgical anatomy of the sellar region. J Neurosurg 43:288–298, 1975.
19. Laws ER Jr, Kern EB: Complications of transsphenoidal surgery. Clin Neurosurg 23:401, 1976.
20. Laws ER Jr, Kern EB: Complications of transsphenoidal surgery. In Tindall GT, Collins WF (eds): Clinical Management of Pituitary Disorders. New York: Raven Press, 1979, pp 435–445.
21. Ciric I, Ragin A, Baumgartner C, et al: Complications of transsphenoidal surgery: Results of a national survey, review of the literature, and personal experience. Neurosurgery 40:225–237, 1997.
22. Wilson WR, Laws ER Jr: Transnasal septal displacement approach for secondary transsphenoidal pituitary surgery. Laryngoscope 102:951–953, 1992.
23. Cappabianca P, Alfieri A, de Divitiis E: Endoscopic endonasal transsphenoidal approach to the sella: Towards functional endoscopic pituitary surgery. Minim Invasive Neurosurg 41:66–73, 1998.
24. Heilman CB, Shucart WA, Rebeiz EE: Endoscopic sphenoidotomy approach to the sella. Neurosurgery 41:602–607, 1997.
25. Jho HD, Carrau RL: Endoscopic endonasal transsphenoidal surgery: Experience with 50 patients. J Neurosurg 87:44–51, 1997.
26. Yaniv E, Rappaport ZH: Endoscopic transseptal transsphenoidal surgery for pituitary tumors. Neurosurgery 40:944–946, 1997.
27. Sethi DS, Pillay PK: Endoscopic management of lesions of the sella turcica. J Laryngol Otol 109:956–962, 1995.
28. Kelly DF, Laws ER Jr, Fossett D: Delayed hyponatremia after transsphenoidal surgery for pituitary adenoma. J Neurosurg 83:363–367, 1995.
29. Reeder RF, Harbaugh RE: Administration of intravenous urea and normal saline for the treatment of hyponatremia in neurosurgical patients. J Neurosurg 70:201–206, 1989.
30. Nandapalan V, Watson ID, Swift AC: Beta-2-transferrin and cerebrospinal fluid rhinorrhoea. Clin Otolaryngol 21:259–264, 1996.
31. Reisinger PW, Hochstrasser K: The diagnosis on the basis of detection of beta 2-transferrin by polyacrylamide gel electrophoresis and immunoblotting. J Clin Chem Clin Biochem 27:169–172, 1989.
32. Laws ER Jr, Fode NC, Randall RV, et al: Pregnancy following transsphenoidal resection of prolactin-secreting pituitary tumors. J Neurosurg 58:685–688, 1983.
33. Elias WJ, Chadduck JB, Alden TD, et al: Frameless stereotaxy for transsphenoidal surgery. Neurosurgery 45:271–277, 1999.

# Endoscopic Transsphenoidal Surgery

■ HAE-DONG JHO

Since neuroendoscopy was first implemented in choroid plexus surgery in a patient with hydrocephalus almost a century ago, its progress has been slow with only sporadic anecdotal reports until recent years. With the advent of ventricular shunt systems, the enthusiasm for ventricular endoscopy fizzled. Ventricular endoscopy was revived for third ventriculostomies in selected patients with obstructive hydrocephalus. A few leading endoscopic neurosurgeons have expanded the use of endoscopy in neurosurgery to include ventricular tumor surgery, intra-axial brain surgery with stereotactic guidance, extra-axial intracranial surgery, endoscope-assisted microsurgery, endonasal transsphenoidal surgery, and spinal surgery. Concurrently, endoscopic optics, better video imaging systems, proper endoscopic accessory attachments for neurosurgical application, adoption of frameless stereotaxis and computer image–guided systems, and new appropriate surgical instruments have all been continuously developing. Although neuroendoscopy is still in its fledgling stage, its future potential, when compared with microscopic neurosurgery, seems to be enormous.

Sinonasal endoscopy was initiated 2 decades ago in Europe and imported to the United States 1 decade ago. Sinonasal endoscopy has brought radical changes in the concepts of pathophysiology and treatment of sinonasal ailments as well as surgical techniques.[1] Rather than to strip the infected sinus mucosa as conventional sinus surgery did in the past, endoscopic sinus surgery aims to restore physiologic mucous drainage by eliminating obstructive pathoanatomy and is called *functional endoscopic sinonasal surgery*. Endoscopic sinus surgery has rapidly replaced conventional sinus surgery. Interest in the use of endoscopy in transsphenoidal surgery spontaneously arose because of how easily the sphenoidal sinus could be entered with sinonasal endoscopy. Sinonasal endoscopy has been used for insertion of transsphenoidal retractors, through a transseptal route or endonasal route, in preparation for the microscopic removal of a pituitary adenoma, for a simple biopsy of a sellar lesion, and for endoscopic pituitary tumor surgery. This chapter describes endoscopic transsphenoidal surgery, which is not just endoscope-assisted microscopic surgery but is rather an operation done completely with an endoscope that also does not require a transsphenoidal retractor or nasal speculum and postoperative nasal packing.[2–8] Endoscopic transsphenoidal surgery uses an endonasal route to the rostrum of the sphenoidal sinus and an anterior sphenoidotomy about 1.5 to 2 cm in size. This endonasal endoscopic pituitary surgery has advanced to the point of application in the surgical treatment of midline pathologies at the anterior fossa, clivus, and posterior fossa as well as pathologies in the optic nerve and cavernous sinus. The approximate 2-cm width of the midline skull base can be approached with endoscopic endonasal techniques from the crista galli to the foramen magnum.

## HISTORY

Guiot and colleagues[9] in 1963 were the first in the literature to report the use of an endoscope during sublabial transsphenoidal surgery. With the advent of functional sinonasal endoscopy, cerebrospinal fluid (CSF) leaks were repaired endoscopically either at the anterior fossa or at the sphenoidal sinus. The first endoscopic pituitary surgery was reported by Jankowski and associates in 1992.[10] Three patients with pituitary adenomas were treated endoscopically through a middle turbinectomy approach. This endoscopic endonasal middle turbinectomy technique was later replaced by a conventional transseptal technique. Shikani and Kelly[11] in 1993 reported endoscopic biopsy of the sellar lesion. They later performed tumor resection as a second stage by a conventional microscopic technique. Wurster and Smith[12] in 1994 mentioned in a letter that they performed endoscopic pituitary surgery in two patients. Gamea and coworkers[13] in 1994 described the adjunctive use of an endoscope during microscopic sublabial transsphenoidal surgery. Sethi and Pillay[14] in 1995 reported endoscopic pituitary surgery with a transsphenoidal retractor placed through a transseptal approach. Helal[15] in 1995 reported the adjunctive use of endoscopy during transseptal microscopic pituitary surgery. Jho and Carrau and their coworkers[4, 8] in 1996 reported endoscopic pituitary surgery through an endonasal route. My technique differs from the others in that the sinonasal anatomy is not disrupted except for a small anterior sphenoidotomy. It also differs in that a transsphenoidal retractor or nasal speculum is not used, and the pituitary tumor resection is performed completely with endoscopy. When the operation is finished, nasal packing is not necessary. Many pituitary surgeons use angled-lens endoscopes to inspect anatomic corners that are hidden from microscopic view during conventional microscopic pituitary surgery.

The use of an endonasal route is not new in pituitary surgery. When Hirsch in Vienna in 1909 performed his first pituitary surgery, he approached the sella though an endonasal route with multiple-stage sinonasal operations.[16] After his first and successful transsphenoidal surgery, Hirsch changed his endonasal approach to a transseptal submucosal approach, probably in fear of the chance of surgical infection through such a wide communication made between the nasal and the cranial cavity. This endonasal route was revisited by Griffith and Veerapen in 1987.[17] They inserted a transsphenoidal retractor through the patient's natural nasal airway to the sphenoidal rostrum for microscopic pituitary surgery. Cooke and Jones[18] in 1994 reported a lack of sinonasal and dental complications when an endonasal route was adopted for microscopic pituitary surgery. My endoscopic pituitary surgery technique uses exactly the same surgical route between the middle turbinate and the nasal septum. My technique, however, does not require a straight tubular corridor as microscopic pituitary surgery does, eliminating the use of a transsphenoidal retractor.

## PREOPERATIVE MANAGEMENT AND SURGICAL INDICATIONS

As with microscopic pituitary surgery, all patients with pituitary adenomas undergo formal endocrine evaluations and visual examinations preoperatively and postoperatively. A magnetic resonance imaging (MRI) scan of the brain with and without contrast enhancement is also obtained for every patient. Occasionally a computed tomography (CT) scan of the brain is obtained. Bone windowed CT scans, axial and coronal views, disclose the bony anatomy of the paranasal sinuses in detail. Although the detailed anatomic information of the paranasal sinuses was helpful, it proved not to be necessary in most patients. When an MRI scan cannot be obtained for patients with claustrophobia or extreme obesity, a CT scan is obtained that includes thinly sliced coronal views at the pituitary fossa. Hypopituitarism is treated preoperatively. Although stress doses of a steroid were used intraoperatively and perioperatively in the earliest patients, an intraoperative or perioperative steroid is no longer used when the patient's pituitary-adrenal function is normal preoperatively. Instead, a morning cortisol level is measured the day after surgery to confirm that it is higher than 18 $\mu$g/dl. If the morning cortisol level is less than 18 $\mu$g/dl, perioperative treatment is instituted with oral hydrocortisol, 20 mg every morning and 10 mg every night, until the pituitary-adrenal axis is proven to be normal. For patients with Cushing's disease, dexamethasone is administered postoperatively 1 mg orally twice a day. Serum cortisol and urinary free cortisol levels can be measured to judge the postoperative outcome of Cushing's disease when

dexamethasone is used instead of hydrocortisol. Postoperatively, oral antibiotics (clarithromycin, 500 mg twice a day) are given arbitrarily for 5 days because the endonasal approach trespasses the semicontaminated sinonasal cavity.

Surgical indications for patients with pituitary adenomas to undergo endoscopic transsphenoidal surgery are similar to those for conventional microscopic transsphenoidal surgery. Patients with hormonally inactive pituitary adenomas are operated on when the tumors cause symptomatic compression of the optic nerve system, hypopituitarism, pituitary apoplexy, or severe frontotemporal headaches. Patients with hormonally active pituitary adenomas causing acromegaly, hyperthyroidism, and Cushing's disease are operated on as the first choice of treatment. Patients with prolactinomas are operated on only when they do not respond to dopaminergic medications, they develop intolerable side effects to the medications, or they choose against dopaminergic medications. Other mass lesions at the pituitary fossa are operated on for a simple biopsy or for resection. Contrary to conventional microscopic surgery, a large suprasellar tumor can be directly visualized, enhancing the chance for total resection. If further exploration at the planum sphenoidale is required for the suprasellar portion of the tumor, it can be done easily by extending bony exposure rostrally. This endoscopic transsphenoidal approach can eliminate the need of a transcranial approach for pituitary adenomas.

I have not yet encountered a patient whose nostril or nasal airway was too small or narrow to undergo endoscopic transsphenoidal surgery. Patients with Cushing's disease often have a narrow nasal airway because of swollen hypertrophic mucosa, which also easily bleeds. Among 130 patients who have undergone endoscopic transsphenoidal surgery, 2 patients with Cushing's disease required a two-nostril technique. An endoscope was inserted through one nostril and the surgical instruments were inserted through the other. Reoperation by endoscopic techniques for patients who have undergone previous transsphenoidal surgery is relatively easy because an anterior sphenoidotomy has already been done as part of the previous surgery, and submucosal dissection is not required. Reoperation can be done as many times as needed.

## PERTINENT SINONASAL ANATOMY

To perform endoscopic pituitary surgery, functional physiology and anatomy of the sinonasal cavity have to be understood. In the paranasal sinus, mucociliary movement is orchestrated by the delivery of mucus flow to the sinus ostia. From the sinus ostia, nasal mucosal ciliary movement is also directed to establish the physiologic flow of mucus to the nasopharynx and nostrils. When the tract of physiologic mucus flow is interrupted mechanically or functionally, the paranasal sinuses retain stagnant mucus, which can be easily infected causing sinusitis. The confluence of the drained mucus from the frontal sinus, anterior ethmoidal sinus, and maxillary sinus is located anteriorly at the middle meatus. Mucosal drainage of the posterior ethmoidal sinus and sphenoidal sinus occurs at the spheno-ethmoidal recess, which is located between the posterolateral aspect of the middle turbinate and the rostrum of the sphenoidal sinus. Any pathology interrupting this mucus flow is detrimental to the sinuses. The endoscopic pituitary surgery described here approaches the area between the middle turbinate and the nasal septum. The surgical anatomy involved during this surgical approach is not complex because the sphenoidal sinus is located between the middle turbinate and septum. The sinonasal anatomy located anteriorly and laterally to the middle turbinate is important for sinonasal function. Those structures should not be traumatized or disrupted. Anterior to the middle turbinate is the uncinate process, behind which is a groove called the *hiatus semilunaris*. Along the posterorostral bank of the hiatus semilunaris is the ethmoidal bullae. As mentioned earlier, the mucus from the frontal sinus and anterior ethmoidal air cells drains to the hiatus semilunaris. The maxillary sinus ostium is located at the caudal end of the hiatus semilunaris just lateral to the middle turbinate. When endoscopic endonasal pituitary surgery is finished, normal anatomy has to be restored. To minimize disruption of the sphenoidal sinus mucosa, the mucosal removal is made only at the anterior sphenoidotomy hole and anterior wall of the sella. When a pituitary tumor is removed, reconstruction is made at the anterior wall of the sella. The sphenoidal sinus is left as an air-filled cavity as normal. No foreign surgical material is left in the sphenoidal sinus cavity. The middle turbinate is placed back medially so as not to block the mucosal drainage through the maxillary sinus ostium.

The posterior septal artery arises from the sphenopalatine branch of the internal maxillary artery and passes to the posterior nasal septum at the inferior medial aspect of the posterior middle turbinate. When surgical access is obtained between the middle turbinate and nasal septum for an anterior sphenoidotomy, the posterior septal artery has to be coagulated and divided to prevent unwanted intraoperative or postoperative nasal bleeding. Delayed copious nasal bleeding after transsphenoidal surgery is often caused by rebleeding from this artery. When the sphenoidal sinus is entered with an endoscope, the complex anatomy is visualized in panoramic fashion. The clival indentation is seen at the bottom midline, the bony protuberances covering the internal carotid arteries are lateral to the clival indentation, the sella is at the center, the cavernous sinuses are seen lateral to the sella, the tuberculum sella is at the top, and the bony protuberances of the optic nerves are seen laterally.

## SURGICAL PROCEDURE

### Surgical Instruments

Appropriate surgical equipment is necessary to perform adequate endoscopic pituitary surgery. Attempting an endoscopic operation of this nature with a borrowed otolaryngologic endoscope results only in frustration. An endoscopic surgical technique is different from that of microscopic surgery. Being well trained in microscopic surgery does not preclude the need for practice in endoscopy. The required surgical instruments are endoscopes with 0-, 30-, and 70-degree lenses (Fig. 29–1A) and their appendages, including a video-imaging system and light source connections, an endoscope lens cleansing device, a rigid endoscope holder, and various surgical instruments specifically designed for endoscopic surgery. The diameter

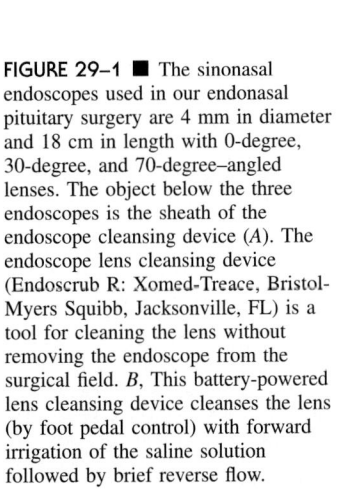
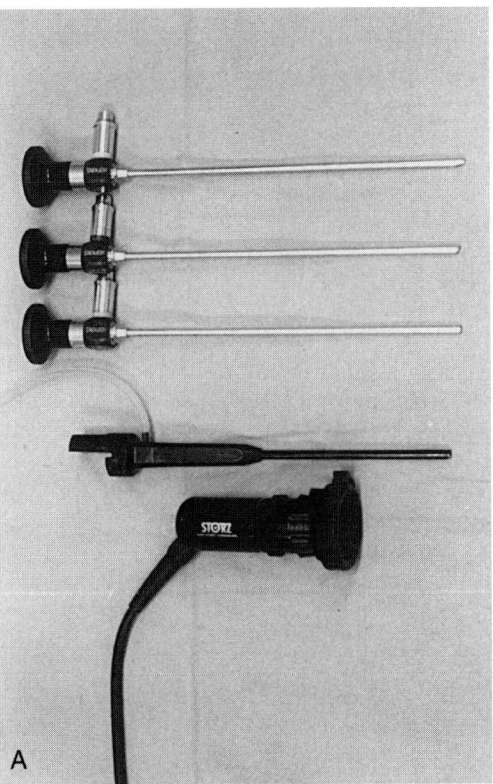
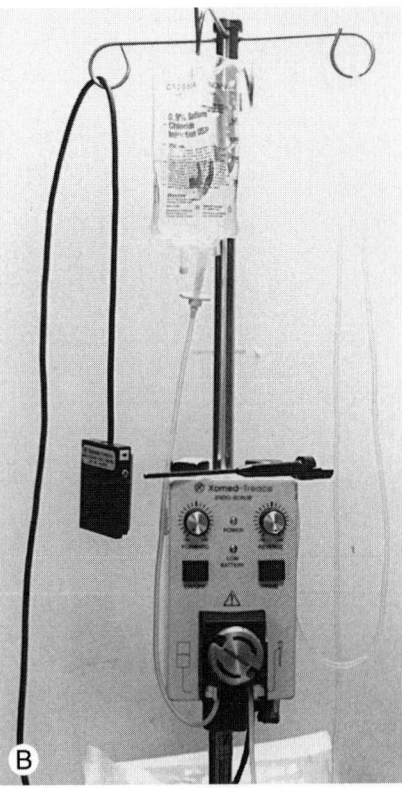

**FIGURE 29–1** ■ The sinonasal endoscopes used in our endonasal pituitary surgery are 4 mm in diameter and 18 cm in length with 0-degree, 30-degree, and 70-degree–angled lenses. The object below the three endoscopes is the sheath of the endoscope cleansing device (*A*). The endoscope lens cleansing device (Endoscrub R: Xomed-Treace, Bristol-Myers Squibb, Jacksonville, FL) is a tool for cleaning the lens without removing the endoscope from the surgical field. *B*, This battery-powered lens cleansing device cleanses the lens (by foot pedal control) with forward irrigation of the saline solution followed by brief reverse flow.

A

B

of an endoscope must be 4 to 5 mm because the quality of the video image drops when its diameter is reduced to 3 mm or less. A fiberoptic endoscope is of no use for the same reason. The length of an endoscope has to be 18 cm or longer. When an 18 cm-long endoscope was used for removal of a posterior fossa tumor through an endonasal transclival approach, it proved to be marginally short and restricted the surgeon's operating space between the endoscopic appendages and the patient's face.

An endoscopic lens cleansing device is required to cleanse the lens so that the surgeon can operate without interruption (see Fig. 29–1B). I use a device with a battery-powered motor and disposable irrigation tubing and endoscope cleansing sheath. The irrigation tubing is inserted into a saline bag, which is hung on a pole. The irrigation tube is passed through a battery-powered motor that has two knobs controlling the intensity of irrigation, one for forward and one for reverse. This motor-powered irrigation device, controlled by a foot pedal, pushes saline forward. When the foot pedal is released, the motor reverses its rotary direction and draws the saline back for 1 or 2 seconds. The forward flow of irrigation saline cleans the lens, and the reverse flow clears water bubbles at the end of the endoscope. Although this device is not completely satisfactory yet, it helps the surgeon significantly in the task of keeping the endoscope lens clean. The main problems with this device that have been noted so far are the short reverse flow interval and the easily damaged seal at the proximal end of the endoscope sheath. Inserting the endoscope through the cleansing sheath produces friction, even with lubrication, and no matter how delicately handled often damages the small rubber ring seal, which leads to water bubbles obscuring the video image. A more dependable endoscope lens cleansing device needs to be developed.

An appropriate holder for the endoscope is another piece of essential equipment required to perform this operation successfully (Fig. 29–2A, B). An endoscope holder needs to hold the endoscope extremely rigidly. Its holding terminal must be compact and slender enough so as not to detract from the adequate operating space around the endoscope shaft needed for the surgeon to maneuver surgical instruments. The endoscopic holder currently available commercially is not adequate. Two different types are currently in the process of development. One is a simple manual holder with multiple joints that can be tightened by hand. The other is a holder with joints that are tightened or released by one button powered by nitrogen gas. The latter, although more expensive, will be a promising and convenient device once fully developed. An endoscope holder must be mounted to the operating table as well as to various neurosurgical head-holding devices. Endoscope holders not only provide fixed video imaging on a video monitor, but also allow a surgeon to use both hands freely. Fluoroscopic guidance, which was used in earlier patients, is no longer used in routine pituitary surgery. It is still used in anterior fossa and posterior fossa surgery as well as occasional pituitary tumor patients in which complexity of the sinonasal anatomy is anticipated.

Among various surgical instruments, a monopolar Bovie suction No. 8 French or No. 9 French cannula, a bipolar suction No. 8 French or No. 9 French cannula, and a single-blade bipolar coagulator are useful. They are all disposable. A monopolar bovie-suction cannula is malleable and insulated. It is useful in preparing the nasal cavity as bloodless during an anterior sphenoidotomy. A bipolar suction cannula and a single-blade bipolar coagulator that has two cables producing bipolar functioning with one at the core and the other at the shell are also used. These bipolar instruments are used for dural or intradural hemostasis. Suction No. 5 French and No. 7 French cannulas vary in curvature for sellar operations. As a dural suturing

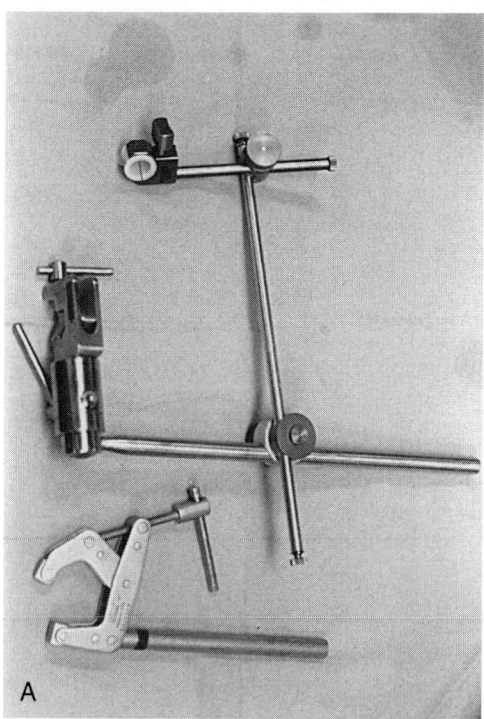

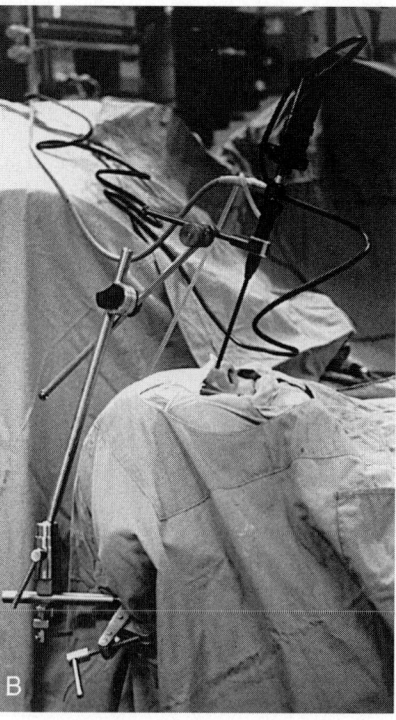

A        B

FIGURE 29–2 ■ *A* and *B,* Our manual endoscope holder consists of a combination of a Greenberg retractor mounting system and our own custom-made distal joint. It provides rigid fixation of the endoscope so that the surgeon can have continuous stable video images as well as having both hands free to use surgical instruments.

device, microclips have been used, but further development is required for adequate dural suturing. Other instruments used are a micropituitary rongeur, pituitary rongeur, ethmoid rongeurs, high-speed drill, micro-Kerrison rongeurs, pituitary ring curets, Jannetta 45-degree microdissector, single-blade Kurze scissors, and a specially designed septal breaker. A high-speed drill is useful when the sphenoidal sinus is small and not well pneumatized. For drilling, the endoscope has to be mounted to the endoscope holder. A high-speed drill and a suction cannula can be inserted next to the endoscope shaft without difficulty. A suction cannula has to be placed next to the drill bit to prevent dusting of the endoscope lens.

## Myths in Sinonasal Surgery

In earlier patients, topical application of a vasoconstrictor and local infiltration of lidocaine with epinephrine were used in the belief that their use would reduce intraoperative as well as postoperative bleeding. Sometimes a piece of polytetrafluoroethylene (Teflon) or Gelfoam sponge was left at the middle meatus in the hope that it would minimize postoperative bleeding and postoperative mucosal adhesions. It turned out to provide only a false sense of security. Gradually, all those techniques were eliminated. When the topical use of a vasoconstrictor and local injection of lidocaine with epinephrine were completely eliminated in my surgical practice, postoperative nasal bleeding was noted much less than when they were used. Meticulous hemostasis using monopolar coagulation at the rostrum of the sphenoidal sinus has minimized the incidence of postoperative nasal bleeding. The use of vasoconstrictors may lessen bleeding intraoperatively; however, postoperative nasal bleeding was more notable probably because of intraoperative vasoconstriction of the nasal mucosa leading to inadequate intraoperative hemostasis and postoperative vasodilatation when vasoconstrictor effects wore off.

When meticulous hemostasis was obtained with electrocoagulation at the rostrum mucosa and anterior sphenoidotomy site, the placement of Gelfoam sponge or Teflon was completely unnecessary. When an anterior sphenoidotomy was performed, care was taken not to strip off the mucosa at the sphenoidal sinus. When the sphenoidal mucosa is stripped off from the sinus cavity, not only can excessive bleeding occur interfering with the operation, but also the healing of the sinus is nonphysiologic. When the bony opening of an anterior sphenoidotomy is made, only the corresponding mucosa at the anterior sphenoidotomy hole is opened to enter the sphenoidal sinus. The mucosa at the anterior wall of the sella is removed with electrocoagulation. The remaining mucosa of the sphenoidal sinus is kept intact as much as possible. When a pituitary tumor operation is finished, the anterior wall of the sella is reconstructed. The sphenoidal sinus is left intact without any packing. Once healed, the sphenoidal sinus is open with widened anterior sphenoidotomy and lined with normal mucosa.

## Positioning

The patient is positioned supine. The torso is elevated about 20 degrees, and the head is positioned with the forehead-chin line set horizontally. The level of the head is placed a little higher than that of the heart in the hope that the cavernous sinus venous pressure stays low to minimize venous bleeding. This horizontally leveled head positioning allows the surgeon to access the middle turbinate easily and naturally when the endoscope is inserted at 25 degrees cephalad. When the anterior fossa is explored, the head is extended approximately 15 degrees. Conversely, 15-degree flexion is applied when the clival or posterior fossa region is explored. The head is rotated toward the surgeon at 10 to 20 degrees. A head pin fixation device can be used but is not necessary. The hip and knee joints are gently flexed for patient comfort. A soft pillow is placed underneath the knee joints. A Foley catheter is inserted occasionally in selective patients who are expected to undergo longer operating hours or for the possible occurrence of diabetes insipidus. Fluoroscopic C-arm imaging is now used only selectively in patients with anterior fossa or posterior fossa tumors or with patients with complex sinonasal anatomy. Ophthalmic eye ointment is placed on the cornea and conjunctiva. The eyelids are closed and sealed with soft vinyl adhesives. The oropharynx is packed with a 2-inch gauze roll to prevent aspiration from accumulated stagnant blood at the time of extubation.

The video monitor is placed a few feet away from the patient's head to face the surgeon directly. The lens cleansing motor is placed next to the video monitor. When a fluoroscopic C-arm is used, the video monitor is placed at the right side of the C-arm and the lens cleansing motor at the left side. A scrub nurse is positioned behind the surgeon. The nasal cavity, entire face, and abdominal wall are prepared and draped in an aseptic manner. When fat graft material is required to fill the tumor resection cavity, an appropriate amount of the abdominal fat tissue is obtained through a 1- to 2-cm infraumbilical transverse skin incision. Clindamycin is mixed with the endoscope's irrigation fluid. As a regimen of intraoperative antibiotics, 1 g of cephazolin is given intravenously in the operating suite before the start of the operation.

## Surgical Approaches

An endoscopic endonasal approach to the sella can be made by a *paraseptal, middle meatal,* or *middle turbinectomy approach.* The paraseptal approach is made between the nasal septum and the middle turbinate. The middle turbinate is squeezed laterally, and the nasal septum is fractured away contralaterally at the sphenoidal rostrum. The fractured nasal septum is pushed away by submucosal dissection at the contralateral side of the sphenoidal rostrum. The paraseptal approach to the anterior fossa skull base accesses the anterior skull base directly under fluoroscopic C-arm guidance between the nasal septum and the middle turbinate. The middle meatal approach is made lateral to the middle turbinate. It provides direct access to the anterior aspect of the cavernous sinus and the optic nerve by a posterior ethmoidectomy. It also allows access to the unilateral anterior fossa by an anterior ethmoidectomy. When a larger operating space is required, the middle turbinectomy approach can be used by resection of the middle turbinate. Although it provides a wider corridor to the sella, the lack of middle turbinate structures can be problematic when a supportive structure is required for skull base reconstruction.

## Surgical Technique of Endoscopic Transsphenoidal Pituitary Surgery

Once the patient is positioned, the nasal cavity, entire face, and abdominal wall are prepared and draped in an aseptic manner. When the nasal cavity is prepared with Q-tips, the size of the nasal airway is probed to determine which nostril is to be used. Because the nasal septum is usually somewhat deviated to either side, the nostril with the wider nasal airway is used for the surgical approach. The size of the nasal airway can be measured in advance by reviewing an axial MRI scan of the nasal cavity. When both nasal cavities are comparable in size, the contralateral nostril is used in patients with microadenomas that are located laterally. This endonasal approach is a few degrees off from the midline, and it is relatively easy to visualize the contralateral side of the sella and the cavernous sinus. When the patient's head is positioned horizontally with the forehead-chin line parallel to the floor, the middle turbinate is spontaneously visualized by the tip of the endoscope when it is inserted into the nasal cavity.

When an endoscope is inserted, the inclined angle of the endoscope shaft is about 25 degrees, which has proven to be a comfortable and easy position for the surgeon who stands at the side of the patient looking cephalad. The endoscope is held in the surgeon's nondominant hand for the intranasal procedure of the operation. When the anterior sphenoidotomy is completed, the endoscope is mounted to the endoscope holder. When the endoscope is held in the hand, the palm and last three digits are used to grab the endoscope, and the index finger and thumb are used to steer the video camera to maintain anatomic orientation of the video images. During the operation, the video camera has to be continuously steered to maintain correct orientation of the video images. When the middle turbinate is identified, two to four ½ × 3 inch cotton patties are inserted between the middle turbinate and the nasal septum to widen the space in between (Figs. 29–3A, B and 29–4A, B). The cotton patties have to be pushed down to the rostrum of the sphenoidal sinus. The anterior sphenoidotomy to be made ranges from the inferior margin of the middle turbinate to the sphenoidal sinus ostia, which is about 1 to 1.5 cm rostral from the inferior margin of the middle turbinate. The consistent anatomic landmark for an anterior sphenoidotomy is the inferior margin of the middle turbinate. Although the sphenoidal sinus ostia can be visualized directly (see Fig. 29–4C), that visualization is not necessary for performing an anterior sphenoidotomy. When the sphenoidal sinus is entered near the level of the inferior margin of the middle turbinate, any further rostral exposure can be easily made relative to the exposed sellar floor. When an anterior sphenoidotomy is prepared for and attempted rostrally first, the surgeon may erroneously enter the anterior cranial fossa. The inferior margin of the middle turbinate leads to the clival indentation at about 1 cm below the level of the sellar floor.

Care must be taken not to traumatize the mucosa in the nasal cavity while surgical instruments are inserted and removed. The degree of surgical trauma to the nasal mucosa is a determining factor for postoperative nasal bleeding. When a sharp-edged surgical instrument is inserted, the instrument tip has to be guided by direct endoscopic visualization.

The cotton patties are then removed. Often, mucosal bleeding follows when the cotton patties are removed. Mucosal bleeding from the rostrum of the sphenoidal sinus between the middle turbinate and nasal septum is controlled with electrocoagulation using monopolar suction. The mucosa at the rostrum of the sphenoidal sinus is completely coagulated to be divided vertically approximately 1.5 cm in length rostrally from the level of the inferior margin of the middle turbinate. The posterior lateral septal artery arises from the sphenopalatine artery and passes at the inferolateral corner of the sphenoethmoidal recess, which is approximately the medial posterior corner of the inferior margin of the middle turbinate. The posterior lateral septal artery has to be coagulated and divided to prevent intraoperative and postoperative nasal bleeding. The nasal septum and vomer are fractured from the rostrum of the sphenoidal sinuses using the septal breaker, which is an instrument I designed specifically for this endoscopic operation. The rostral nasal septum is relatively easy to break; however, the caudally located vomer is often too thick to break without using the specially made septal breaker. The fractured nasal septum is pushed contralaterally, and the contralateral rostrum of the sphenoidal sinus is dissected submucosally. The anterior aspect of the sphenoidal rostrum is exposed bilaterally.

By penetration with a suction cannula, the sphenoidal sinus is entered on either side. Attention is paid not to strip the sphenoidal sinus mucosa because inadvertent stripping causes unwanted oozing of blood from the bony sinus wall. The anterior wall of the sphenoidal sinus is removed performing an anterior sphenoidotomy at about 1.5 to 2 cm in size. For an anterior sphenoidotomy, ethmoid rongeurs and Kerrison punches or a high-speed drill can be used.

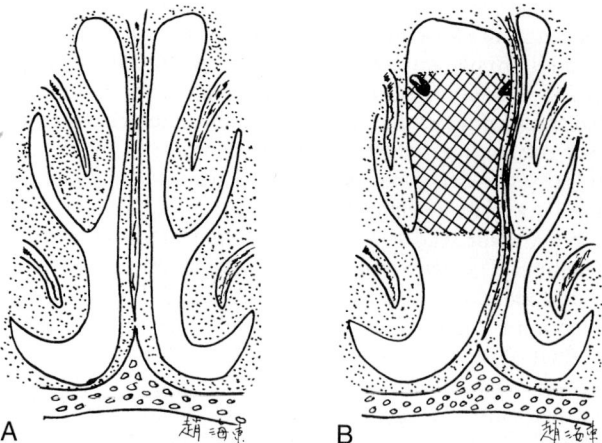

**FIGURE 29–3 ■** This schematic drawings demonstrate the area where an anterior sphenoidotomy is going to be made (A, B). The consistent landmark leading to the floor of the sella is the inferior margin of the middle turbinate. The inferior margin of the middle turbinate leads to the area that is approximately 1 cm below the floor of the sella in the sphenoidal sinus.

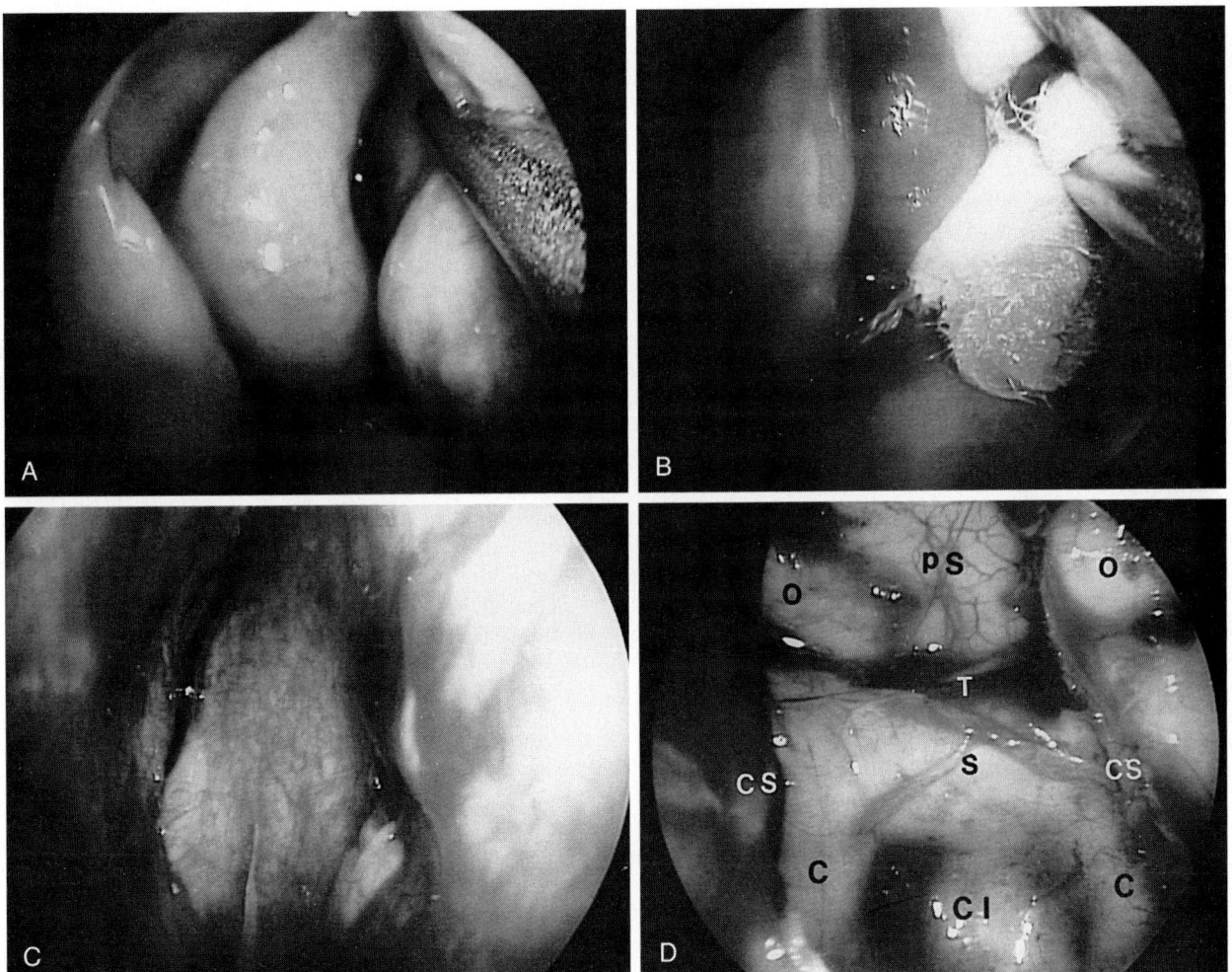

**FIGURE 29–4** ■ Under the 0-degree endoscope, the right-sided middle turbinate is exposed at the center of the surgical field *(A)*. A few cotton patties, 1/2 × 3 inches, are inserted between the middle turbinate and the nasal septum in front of the rostrum of the sphenoidal sinus *(B)*. The rostrum of the sphenoidal sinus is exposed. Bilateral sphenoidal ostia are visible on either side *(C)*. An anterior sphenoidotomy is made about 1.5 to 2 cm in size with ethmoidal rongeurs and Kerrison rongeurs or a high-speed drill. When the endoscope is advanced into the sphenoidal sinus, a panoramic view of the sphenoidal sinus *(D)* demonstrates the clival indentation (CI), internal carotid arteries (C), sella (S), cavernous sinuses (CS), tuberculum sella (T), planum sphenoidale (PS), and optic protuberances (O).

When a high-speed drill is used, the endoscope has to be mounted to the endoscopic holder. Once an anterior sphenoidotomy is performed, the sphenoidal mucosa is opened in appropriate size along the margin of the anterior sphenoidotomy. The sphenoidal sinus septum is trimmed, and further rostral extension of the anterior sphenoidotomy is performed accordingly, relative to the sella. Often the sella is exposed from the tuberculum sella to the clival indentation in the vertical dimension and from cavernous sinus to cavernous sinus in the transverse dimension. At this point, endoscopic view demonstrates the tuberculum sella rostrally, optic protuberances at 11 and 1 o'clock locations, the bony wall covering the cavernous sinus and carotid artery laterally, clival indentation caudally, and the internal carotid arteries at 7 and 5 o'clock locations (see Fig. 29–4D). The endoscope is mounted to the endoscope holder, and the endoscope tip is advanced for a close-up view of the sella.

Using a bipolar suction coagulator, the sphenoidal mucosa at the anterior wall of the sella is coagulated and removed. A small hole is made at the inferolateral corner

of the anterior bony wall of the sella. The anterior bony wall of the sella is removed with a 1-mm Kerrison punch circumferentially, from cavernous sinus to cavernous sinus and from the sellar floor to the tuberculum sella. The dura mater is coagulated along the periphery circumferentially with a single-blade bipolar coagulator. The dural opening is made along the inferior margin at the floor of the sella using a Jannetta 45-degree microdissector. The anterior dural wall is incised and removed circumferentially for biopsy. An alternative is a cross incision of the dura mater. In case of a microadenoma covered by normal pituitary tissue, the pituitary tissue is sliced or split with a Jannetta 45-degree microdissector to find the tumor tissue.

When the tumor is identified, it is curetted out first. At the tumor resection cavity, a thin layer of the normal pituitary tissue is shaved off to accomplish complete resection of the tumor because microadenomas that require surgical resection are usually hormonally hyperactive tumors. In case of a macroadenoma, the adenoma tissue often spills out when the dura mater is opened. Care has to be taken not to lose any of the tumor specimen by suctioning.

The tumor tissue is sampled for pathologic examination. Once enough of the tumor specimen is collected, the tumor is removed with a suction cannula at the central portion of the sella for debulking. Two No. 5 French or No. 7 French suction cannulas can be used for tumor removal. When the tumor is fibrotic, either from previous medical or surgical treatments or by its intrinsic nature, the tumor tissue is gently curetted with a pituitary ring curet held in one hand, in addition to being suctioned with a suction cannula held in the other hand. When the tumor resection cavity is created at the central portion of the pituitary fossa, a 45-degree angled curet is used first followed by a 90-degree angled curet to remove the lower portion of the tumor from the floor of the sella. A downwardly angled pituitary ring curet is used in one hand and a downwardly curved suction canula in the other hand for removal of the lower portion of the tumor.

The dura mater of the floor of the sella is exposed directly when the lower portion of the tumor is removed. Next the lateral portion of the tumor is removed with a suction cannula angled upwardly and upwardly angled pituitary ring curets, 45 degrees as well as 90 degrees. The medial wall of the cavernous sinus is exposed when the lateral portion of the tumor is removed. The rostral portion of the tumor is removed circumferentially with variously upwardly curved and angled suction cannulas and pituitary ring curets. When normal pituitary gland tissue is identified, the pituitary gland tissue is preserved as much as possible. The tumor is removed either with suction cannulas in each hand or with a suction cannula in one hand and a pituitary ring curet in the other. When the diaphragm sella is identified along the peripheral edge of the rostral portion of the tumor, the tumor is continuously removed circumferentially toward the center. When the tumor is removed along the edge of the diaphragma sella, the suprasellar portion of the tumor progressively descends through the central opening of the diaphragma sella. The suprasellar portion of the tumor that is progressively descending is continuously removed with either two upwardly curved suction cannulas or a suction cannula and a pituitary ring curet, both angled upwardly.

Thinned pituitary tissue is often identifiable rostrally when the suprasellar portion of the tumor has been removed. When the pituitary tissue is severely stretched out, the rostrally located pituitary tissue appears to be a transparent membrane similar to the arachnoid membrane. When this rostral tissue is penetrated, the arachnoid membrane may rupture resulting in a CSF leak. Sometimes the arachnoid membrane bulges down along the anterior edge of the diaphragma sella in front of the thinned pituitary tissue. The last piece of the pituitary tumor is often located at the insertion point of the pituitary stalk. When this last piece of the tumor is removed at the reversed dimple of the pituitary stalk, the transparent and thinned pituitary tissue descends down looking like a lily with a dimple at the center. It continuously bulges downward with pulsation toward the floor of the sella. The tumor resection cavity in the sella has to be filled and supported with an abdominal fat graft to prevent postoperative CSF leak by delayed rupture of the membrane, which can happen when the patient exhales a held breath or repeatedly coughs during extubation or anytime postoperatively.

When the tumor is so solid and fibrotic that the suprasellar portion of the tumor does not descend spontaneously, the suprasellar portion can be exposed directly by a 30-degree lens endoscope or by further removal of the bone at the tuberculum sella or planum sphenoidale. When the arachnoid membrane is ruptured, the optic nerves and chiasm, anterior cerebral artery system, and inferior aspect of the hypothalamus are under direct view with a 30-degree lens endoscope (Fig. 29–5A, B). When CSF leakage does not occur intraoperatively and the tumor is a microadenoma, an abdominal fat graft is not necessary. After removal of a macroadenoma, the tumor resection cavity is supported with an abdominal fat graft. Occasionally a piece of Gelfoam sponge is used instead of an abdominal fat graft when a sufficient amount of the pituitary tissue still remains rostrally. An abdominal fat graft is harvested via a 1- to 2-cm transverse skin incision just inferior to the umbilicus. The anterior wall of the sella is reconstructed using autogenous bone saved at the time of the anterior sphenoidotomy (Fig. 29–6A). When autogenous bone is not available, a piece of thin titanium mesh is placed (see Fig. 29–6B). No foreign material is laid in the sphenoidal

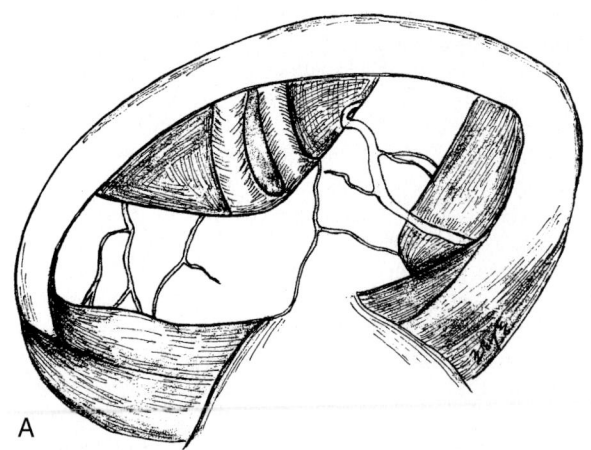
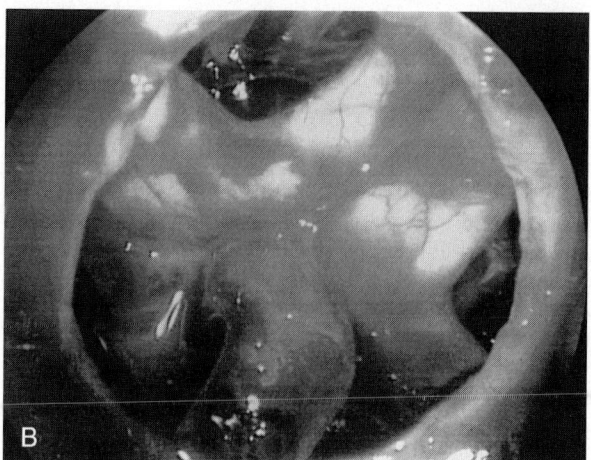

FIGURE 29–5 ■ When the suprasellar portion of the tumor is removed, the optic nerves, chiasm, and anterior cerebral arterial system are under direct 30-degree lens endoscopic view. (A, a schematic drawing; B, a 30-degree endoscopic view after removal of a suprasellar craniopharyngioma.)

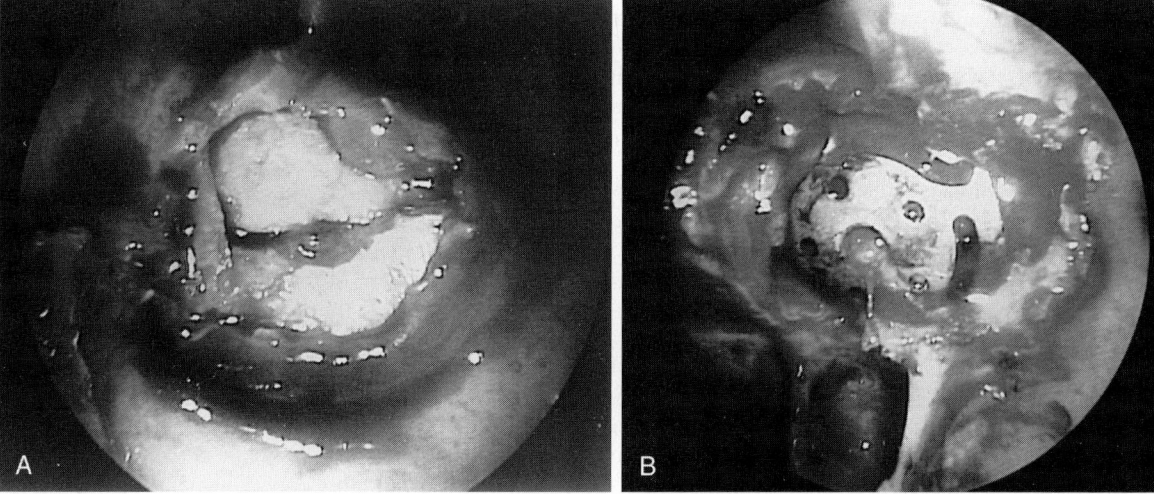

FIGURE 29–6 ■ A small piece of abdominal fat graft is placed at the tumor resection cavity when the tumor resection cavity is too large or cerebrospinal fluid leakage is encountered intraoperatively. The anterior wall of the sella is reconstructed with autogenous bone *(A)* or titanium mesh *(B)*.

sinus or nasal cavity. The endoscope is hand-held again, the nasopharynx and nasal cavity are inspected, and any stagnant blood is removed with a suction cannula. The middle turbinate is placed back to its normal position. The abdominal incision is closed in subcuticular fashion and covered with a small bandage. The operation is finished.

## Surgical Approach to the Anterior Fossa Skull Base

For meningiomas located in the olfactory groove, planum sphenoidale, or tuberculum sella or for repair of CSF leakage at the anterior fossa, the endoscopic endonasal approach to the anterior fossa skull base has been employed (Fig. 29–7A). This approach is also useful for suprasellar

craniopharyngiomas or large suprasellar pituitary tumors with fibrotic solid natures. For CSF leak repair, either a paraseptal or a middle meatal approach can be used. For tumor removal, a paraseptal approach is used. As with the approach to the anterior fossa skull base, a fluoroscopic C-arm image is used for intraoperative guidance.

The head is positioned in 15-degree extension of the forehead-chin line to maintain the endoscope insertion angle at about 25 degrees, which is, as mentioned before, comfortable and easier for the surgeon. Otherwise the patient is prepared in the same manner as described earlier with pituitary surgery. For the middle meatal approach, the middle turbinate is pushed medially and anterior, or a posterior ethmoidectomy is performed to reach the anterior skull base. A CSF leak is often directly visible. The mucosa is dissected around the skull base defect, and an abdominal

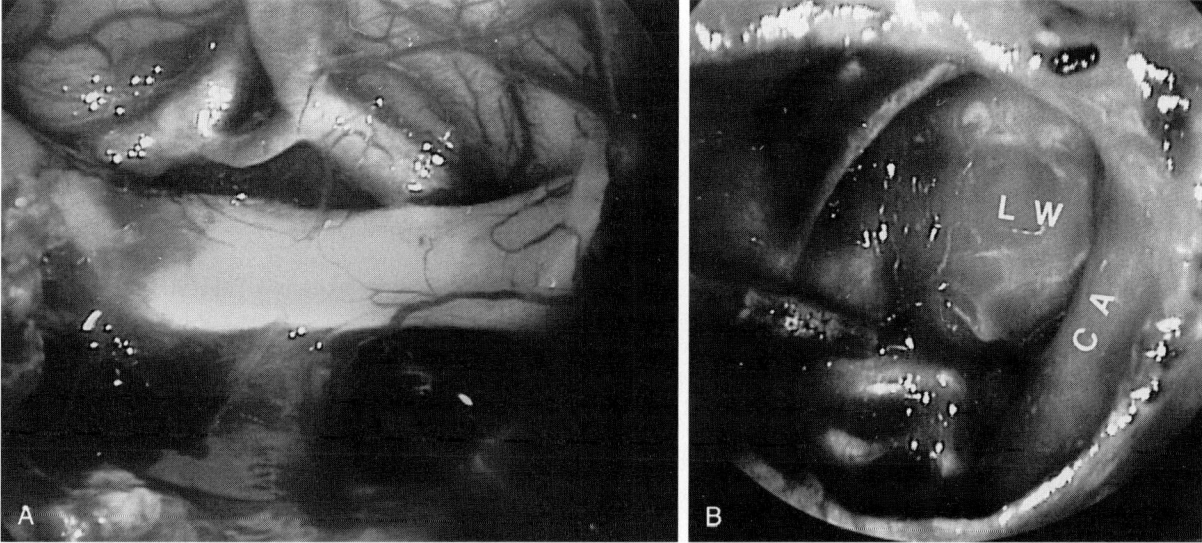

FIGURE 29–7 ■ When a meningioma at the planum sphenoidale was removed by an endoscopic endonasal anterior skull base approach, the pituitary stalk, optic system, and anterior cerebral artery system were directly visualized in a 0-degree lens endoscope *(A)*. When a pituitary tumor encasing the carotid artery in the cavernous sinus was removed *(B)*, the carotid artery (CA) and lateral wall of the cavernous sinus (LW) are visualized directly under the 30-degree lens endoscope.

fat graft is inserted into the cranial cavity. When a whole piece of fat graft is inserted into the cranial cavity, a portion of the fat is grabbed and pulled gently to wedge it into the skull defect. A piece of thin titanium mesh is laid at the skull defect. The middle turbinate is placed back to its normal position.

For anterior fossa tumor surgery, a paraseptal approach is used. For tumors located at the tuberculum sella or planum sphenoidale, the surgical approach is similar to the aforementioned pituitary operation except that further rostral exposure is required. The middle turbinate is laterally displaced, and the nasal septum is fractured contralaterally. A rostral anterior sphenoidotomy is performed to enter the sphenoidal sinuses first, then the sella and tuberculum sella are identified. Under fluoroscopic guidance, further rostral exposure is made at the anterior skull base removing the posterior ethmoid sinuses. This approach itself interrupts anterior or posterior ethmoidal arteries during exposure resulting in complete devascularization of the meningioma. Approximately a 2-cm wide portion of the midline anterior skull base can be exposed with this technique. The skull base bone is removed with a high-speed drill or Kerrison punch. The dura mater is opened, the tumor is removed, then central debulking is followed by peripheral dissection. The skull base defect is reconstructed with dural graft placement and autogenous bone graft or titanium mesh placement. Abdominal fat grafts have also been used. Fat graft material laid at the tumor resection cavity can be a concern, however, of possibly becoming a compressive mass to the optic nerve system. The dural reconstruction has been performed with microclips, but the currently available clips require instrumental and functional improvement. The main potential problem in this technique is CSF leak and subsequent meningitis. The middle turbinate is placed back to its normal position, and the operation is finished.

## Surgical Approach to the Cavernous Sinus or Optic Nerve

Although surgical indication for the decompression of the optic nerve is a controversial issue, the optic nerve at the optic canal can be easily exposed using this endoscopic endonasal approach. The surgical approach to the cavernous sinus is similar to that to the optic nerve. This endoscopic approach to the cavernous sinus is best suited for pituitary adenomas invading the cavernous sinus. Tough fibrotic tumors, such as meningiomas, are difficult to remove by an endoscopic technique. Biopsy for the histologic diagnosis of cavernous sinus lesions can be performed with this technique. The endonasal endoscopic approach to the cavernous sinus is an anteromedial approach to the cavernous sinus. The fact that cavernous cranial nerves are located at the lateral wall of the cavernous sinus makes this approach advantageous. Pituitary adenomas can involve the cavernous sinus by mechanical compression, by lateral tumor bulging, by intrusion into the cavernous sinus through a defect of the medial wall of the cavernous sinus, or by direct extension from dural invasion. A laterally bulged tumor can be removed by the pituitary approach described earlier and does not need any further particular maneuvering. The 30-degree lens endoscope discloses the

medial wall of the cavernous sinus well when the lateral portion of the tumor is completely removed. Tumors that have intruded into the cavernous sinus by a defect of the medial wall can be removed completely under direct endoscopic visualization. The cavernous carotid artery is exposed during this procedure. Invasive pituitary adenomas of an infiltrating nature may not be completely resectable; however, they can be debulked to reduce the size of the tumor so that Gamma knife surgery can be performed for the residual portion of the tumor postoperatively.

The cavernous sinus or the optic nerve can be approached via a paraseptal, middle meatal, or middle turbinectomy approach. When a paraseptal approach is used, it visualizes the contralateral cavernous sinus better than it does the ipsilateral. It exposes the anteromedial aspect of the cavernous sinus. The optic nerve also can be better approached when the contralateral nostril is used. The middle meatal approach with a posterior ethmoidectomy provides a straight anterior approach to the cavernous sinus. The middle turbinectomy approach renders a larger corridor that can reach the cavernous sinus or the optic nerve. The paraseptal approach has been sufficient for approaching the cavernous sinus or the optic nerve. As mentioned earlier, a contralateral approach is preferred to make an anteromedial approach to the cavernous sinus or to the optic nerve. The surgical approach is similar to that of the pituitary adenoma surgery described earlier. When an anterior sphenoidotomy is made, submucosal dissection at the contralateral side of the sphenoidal rostrum is extended further laterally, and the anterior sphenoidotomy is performed generously at the contralateral side of the sphenoid sinus. It exposes the contralateral cavernous sinus laterally up to the medial anterior temporal fossa. The bone is removed from the anterior aspect of the sella as well as from the cavernous sinus, and unroofing the medial internal carotid artery is completed if necessary. The sellar portion of the pituitary tumor is removed first before attacking the tumor portion in the cavernous sinus. For an isolated cavernous sinus tumor, the tumor is approached directly by opening the dura mater medial to the carotid siphon. The tumor is removed with various pituitary ring curets and suction cannulas. Attention has to be paid not to traumatize the lateral wall of the cavernous sinus to prevent ocular cranial nerve dysfunction. The carotid artery is directly visible with its pulsation. Tumor resection is performed medially and posteriorly to the carotid siphon, which is arced in a C shape with the convexity anterior toward the surgeon. When the tumor is completely removed, the lateral wall of the cavernous sinus can be completely visualized (see Fig. 29–7B). An abdominal fat graft is necessary to protect the cavernous carotid artery. The carotid artery is wrapped with a fat graft. If necessary, the sphenoid sinus is filled with an abdominal fat graft to protect the carotid artery. In that case, the sphenoidal sinus mucosa is removed completely before the fat graft is placed.

## Surgical Approach to the Clivus and Posterior Fossa

The advantage of the endoscopic technique in the surgical approach to the clivus and posterior fossa over a microscopic technique in transsphenoidal surgery is the flexibility

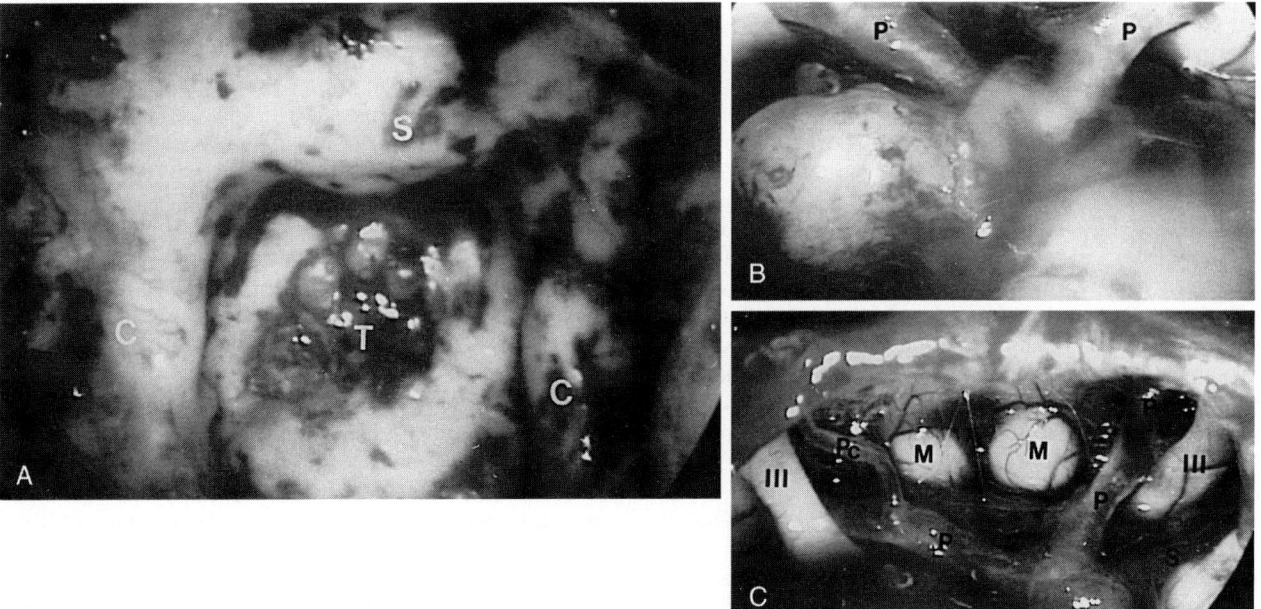

FIGURE 29–8 ■ The clivus is exposed by an endonasal endoscopic approach for removal of the clival and posterior fossa chordoma. The sella (S), internal carotid arteries (C), and the tumor at the center of the clivus (T) are demonstrated by a 0-degree lens endoscope *(A)*. When a tumor in the posterior fossa encasing the basilar artery *(B)* was removed, the basilar bifurcation, posterior cerebral arteries (P), posterior communicating arteries (Pc), superior cerebellar arteries (S), mammillary bodies (M), and bilateral oculomotor nerves (III) were demonstrated through a 70-degree lens endoscope *(C)*.

of endoscopic visualization, which ranges from the crista galli at the anterior fossa to the foramen magnum. This endoscopic approach exposes the entire clivus from the floor of the sella to the foramen magnum in a width of approximately 2 cm (Fig. 29–8A). The internal carotid artery is the lateral limit of this exposure. This technique has been used for radical resection of clival chordomas and midline clival meningiomas. A paraseptal approach is used, but the middle turbinectomy approach can be used when a larger surgical corridor is required. A fluoroscopic C-arm image is used for guidance to the vertical dimension. The clival bone is removed with a high-speed drill between the internal carotid arteries in the transverse dimension and from the floor of the sella to the foramen magnum or to the lower clival level as needed. The chordoma is then removed with suction cannulas and pituitary rongeurs. Bone is shaved at the tumor resection margin until normal bone is clearly documented. Often the limitation of this technique is the inability for further extension of the tumor margin laterally or cephalad toward the posterior clinoid or dorsum sella. Intradural tumor is then resected. When intradural tumor is resected, the pons and medulla can be visualized. A 30- or 70-degree lens endoscope visualizes the further rostral aspect of the brain stem or cranial nerves laterally (see Fig. 29–8B, C). Dural defects are repaired with an abdominal fat graft; however, direct dural repair by a dural graft is the ideal method to reconstruct the dura once relative surgical instruments have improved. The dural microclips currently available include applicators that are too short in the shaft to be used for this purpose.

## POSTOPERATIVE MANAGEMENT

Patients are kept in a regular hospital room overnight. If they do well, they are discharged home the next day.

Postoperative discomfort is minimal and often does not require strong analgesics. Postoperative nasal bleeding has also been minimal since the techniques of meticulous hemostasis and elimination of intraoperative use of vasoconstrictors were adopted. In earlier patients, postoperative diuresis was an annoying problem that often prolonged patients' hospital stays to more than 1 night. Because the use of intraoperative intravenous fluid has been judicious in the volume given, postoperative diuresis induced by excessive intravenous fluid use has not occurred. Vasopressin (Pitressin) is used immediately when diabetes insipidus is confirmed by exhibition of the classic symptoms of polyuria and polydipsia, clear diluted urine with low urinary specific gravity, and increased serum osmolarity and sodium concentration. Postoperative CSF leakage is a potential complication in transsphenoidal surgery. When a CSF leak has been confirmed, the leak is repaired immediately with endoscopic re-exploration and the placement of an abdominal fat graft. Immediate repair of a CSF leak enhances rapid recovery, lessens the chance of meningitis, and shortens the patient's hospital stay compared with a less aggressive treatment, such as lumbar spinal drainage. Formal endocrine evaluation, visual examination, nasal examination, and postoperative MRI scans are all performed a few weeks postoperatively.

## SURGICAL RESULTS

Endoscopic endonasal operations have been performed in more than 130 patients at this institution. Among 100 patients who had undergone operations from September 1993 through October 1997, 58 were women and 42 were men, with an age range of 14 to 88 years (median, 38 years). Eighty-five patients had pituitary adenomas, and 15 had other skull base lesions. Among 85 patients with pituitary adenomas, 25 patients had microadenomas, 22 had intrasellar macroadenomas, 24 had macroadenomas with suprasellar extension, and 14 had invasive macroadenomas involving the cavernous sinus in addition to suprasellar extension. Forty-three adenomas were hormonally hyperactive (12 caused Cushing's disease, 26 were prolactinomas, and 5 caused acromegaly). Two patients were operated on as outpatients, and 66 patients stayed in the hospital overnight postoperatively. Postoperative discomfort was minimal. Ten patients with Cushing's disease improved clinically with normal urinary cortisol levels. Two patients with incompletely treated Cushing's disease were treated by Gamma knife. Among 26 patients with prolactinomas, 16 improved clinically with normal postoperative prolactin levels, 4 improved clinically with mildly elevated postoperative prolactin levels, and 6 had residual tumors in the cavernous sinuses. Among 42 patients with hormone-inactive adenomas, 34 underwent total resection, and 8 had subtotal removal with residual tumors in the cavernous sinuses. Three patients developed postoperative CSF leaks, which were immediately repaired with endoscopic abdominal fat graft placement.

## POTENTIAL COMPLICATIONS AND THEIR AVOIDANCE

Postoperative CSF leakage has been a major potential complication in transsphenoidal surgery. In the first patient at this institution who underwent an endonasal endoscopic procedure, and who had metastatic adenocarcinoma to the sella, CSF leakage occurred postoperatively. To make a histologic diagnosis, the patient underwent an endonasal endoscopic biopsy. A small piece of tumor tissue was procured with a pituitary rongeur in the sella. No fat graft was placed. A CSF leak was not noted intraoperatively; however, the patient developed postoperative CSF leakage a day after the operation. The CSF leak was immediately repaired with endonasal endoscopic placement of an abdominal fat graft. Another patient with a recurrent pituitary adenoma after a previous transsphenoidal operation developed a postoperative CSF leak. Despite the intraoperative concern of a possible postoperative CSF leak because of a wide defect of the bone and dura mater at the anterior wall and the floor of the sella from the previous operation, the placement of the fat graft at the tumor resection cavity had to be tailored so as not to cause compression of the optic system. Surrounding supportive structures to hold an abdominal fat graft were lacking. Pieces of bone were not available for bone reconstruction because of the previous transseptal approach. Use of titanium mesh could have prevented CSF leak in this patient, however. Packing too large of a portion of fat graft into the sella might have caused optic compression. Despite the placement of a generously sized fat graft into the sella, the patient developed a postoperative CSF leak. The CSF leak was repaired with placement of a larger fat graft into the sella and sphenoid sinus on the second postoperative day. Every effort has been made to reconstruct the anterior bony wall of the sella in all patients with the patient's own bone or titanium mesh. In a third patient who underwent resection of a

macroadenoma who did not show CSF leak intraoperatively, an abdominal fat graft was not performed at the tumor resection cavity despite the arachnoid membrane descending and bulging down into the tumor resection cavity in the sella. The patient developed a CSF leak postoperatively, and it was repaired with endoscopic re-exploration and abdominal fat graft placement. During surgery for microadenomas, a fat graft was not placed. Although fibrin glue has not been used in cases here, the usage of fibrin glue made out of the patient's own blood may facilitate a watertight seal of the dural opening. Postoperative CSF leakage was one of the reasons for prolonged patient hospitalization.

Most patients were able to be discharged the day following the operation mostly because they did not require obstructive nasal packing. Two patients with microadenomas were discharged from the hospital a few hours after operation per their wishes. As mentioned previously, the most common cause of delay in the patients' discharge in this series was postoperative diuresis requiring a differential diagnosis from diabetes insipidus. Judicious intraoperative fluid management has reduced the incidence of postoperative diuresis. Delayed electrolyte imbalances can occur for so many days postoperatively that routine patient hospitalization for a certain number of days is not warranted. The length of the patient's hospitalization should be individualized depending on the patient's endocrine and electrolyte conditions. Other complications encountered in our group of patients at this institution included temporary diabetes insipidus in two patients, expected permanent diabetes insipidus in a patient with a craniopharyngioma, worsening of anterior pituitary function in six patients, asymptomatic synechia of the nasal mucosa in one patient, and chronic sphenoid sinusitis in one patient. The chronic sphenoid sinusitis was noted in a routine postoperative visit at 6 weeks and successfully treated with a 5-day course of antibiotics.

## ADVANTAGES AND DISADVANTAGES OF THE ENDONASAL ENDOSCOPIC TECHNIQUE

Avoidance of postoperative nasal packing seems to be a significant advantage for patient comfort, quick recovery, and early release from the hospital. This endoscopic approach through a natural nasal airway not requiring use of a transsphenoidal retractor eliminates the need of any sort of postoperative nasal packing. Postoperative pain and discomfort are also minimal. Quick postoperative recovery and short hospitalizations in the patients at this institution were made possible by the selection of this natural endonasal route without use of a transsphenoidal retractor. I have not yet encountered a patient who has had too narrow a nasal pathway to undergo the endonasal endoscopic technique. This endonasal technique does not require sublabial incisions or nasal transfixion incisions and subsequently minimizes the chance of dental, gingival, and sinonasal complications. Because the endoscopic technique does not use ethmoidectomy or resection of the middle turbinate and stripping of the sphenoidal sinus mucosa, normal sinonasal physiologic anatomy is well maintained postoperatively.

The main advantage of the endoscopic technique is that the 30-degree angled lens can visualize hidden anatomic corners as well as the diaphragma sella and the suprasellar region directly. The optic system, hypothalamus, and intracranial vessels can be directly demonstrated with the angled endoscope after removal of the suprasellar portion of the tumor. By rotating the angled lens endoscope, the corners of the sella and sphenoidal sinus can also be visualized directly. The endoscope can provide a panoramic view of the sphenoid sinus demonstrating the bony protuberance of the optic nerves and carotid arteries. This panoramic view of the sphenoidal sinuses eliminates the need of using an intraoperative fluoroscopic C-arm image. Although risk of injury to the carotid artery, the optic system, and the hypothalamus is low with conventional microscopic transsphenoidal surgery, the capability of the endoscope to visualize those structures directly may further reduce incidence of such a rare catastrophe. A close-up endoscopic view at the juncture of tumor and pituitary gland tissue has appeared to be much clearer than the remote view provided by an operating microscope. This close-up view at the tumor-pituitary juncture enhances the chance of complete resection of the tumor. The capability of an angled view by an endoscope enables surgical resection of the tumor from the cavernous sinus, anterior fossa, and posterior fossa under the direct visualization.

The disadvantages of endoscopic pituitary surgery when compared with conventional microscopic surgery are the two-dimensional monitor-generated flat images and the reduced clarity and sharpness of the monitored images. Endoscopic video images are still inferior to those of direct microscopic visualization. A digitally enhanced camera has improved the picture quality to some degree. High-definition cameras and monitors would further improve the quality of endoscopic views. Another disadvantage is the learning curve for neurosurgeons who are already well trained in conventional microscopic surgery. Despite a neurosurgeon's painstaking training in microsurgery, most are not used to endoscopic surgical maneuvers and need to spend extra time getting used to new endoscopic surgical skills. The endoscope shaft occupying the surgical corridor often interferes with the surgeon's maneuvering surgical tools until he or she masters these surgical skills. Maneuvering surgical instruments during endoscopic endonasal transsphenoidal surgery is somewhat similar to the way one picks up food with one chopstick held parallel in each hand. One of the major concerns often imparted by microscopic pituitary surgeons has been the possibility of uncontrollable bleeding within a limited exposure. As with microscopic pituitary surgery, significant bleeding has been encountered from the tumors with high vascularity. The endoscopic endonasal technique has not been a handicap in particular when dealing with this type of tumor. Venous sinus bleeding occasionally became cumbersome, but there has not been a single case that has needed to be aborted. Because of the intrinsic learning curve, the operation time for endoscopic surgery was initially longer than that for microscopic surgery. Once the surgeon becomes accustomed to this endoscopic technique, the operation time will become comparable or even shorter.

## CONCLUSIONS

The endoscopic endonasal transsphenoidal approach has been described for the surgical treatment of pituitary adenomas as well as for other skull base lesions located at the midline anterior fossa, cavernous sinus, optic nerve and midline clivus, and posterior fossa.

## ACKNOWLEDGMENTS

*The author thanks Arthur P. Nestler, B.S.N., and Robin A. Coret, B.A., for their assistance in preparation of this manuscript.*

## REFERENCES

1. Stammberger H: Endoscopic endonasal surgery—concepts in treatment of recurring rhinosinusitis. II: Surgical technique. Otolaryngol Head Neck Surg 94:147–156, 1986.
2. Jho HD: Endoscopic endonasal pituitary surgery: Technical aspects. Contemp Neurosurg 6:1–7, 1997.
3. Jho HD, Carrau RL, Ko Y: Endoscopic pituitary surgery. In Wilkins RH, Rengachary SS (eds): Neurosurgical Operative Atlas, Vol 5. Baltimore: Williams & Wilkins, 1996, pp 1–12,
4. Jho HD, Carrau RL: Endoscopy assisted transsphenoidal surgery for pituitary adenoma: Technical note. Acta Neurochir (Wien) 138:1416–1425, 1996.
5. Jho HD, Carrau RL: Endoscopic endonasal transsphenoidal surgery: Experience with 50 patients. J Neurosurg 87:44–51, 1997.
6. Jho HD, Carrau RL, Mclaughlin ML, Somaza SC: Endoscopic transsphenoidal resection of a large chordoma in the posterior fossa. Acta Neurochir (Wien) 139:343–348, 1997.
7. Jho HD, Carrau RL, Ko Y, Daly M: Endoscopic pituitary surgery: An early experience. Surg Neurol 47:213–223, 1997.
8. Carrau RL, Jho HD, Ko Y: Transnasal-transsphenoidal endoscopic surgery of the pituitary gland. Laryngoscope 106:914–918, 1996.
9. Guiot G, Rougerie J, Fourestler A, et al: Une nouvelle technique endoscopique: Exploration endoscopiques intracraniennes. Presse Med 71:1225–1228, 1963.
10. Jankowski R, Auque J, Simon C, et al: Endoscopic pituitary tumor surgery. Laryngoscope 102:198–202, 1992.
11. Shikani AH, Kelly JH: Endoscopic debulking of a pituitary tumor. Am J Otolaryngol 14:254–256, 1993.
12. Wurster CF, Smith DE: The endoscopic approach to the pituitary gland (Letter). Arch Otolaryngol Head Neck Surg 120:674, 1994.
13. Gamea A, Fathi M, El-Guindy A: The use of the rigid endoscope in trans-sphenoidal pituitary surgery. J Laryngol Otol 108:19–22, 1994.
14. Sethi DS, Pillay PK: Endoscopic management of lesions of the sella turcica. J Laryngol Otol 109:956–962, 1995.
15. Helal MZ: Combined micro-endo trans-sphenoid excisions of pituitary macroadenomas. Eur Arch Otorhinolaryngol 252:186–189, 1995.
16. Landolt AM: History of transsphenoidal pituitary surgery. In Landolt AM, Vance ML, Reilly PL (eds): Pituitary Adenomas. New York: Churchill Livingstone, 1996, pp 307–314.
17. Griffith HB, Veerapen R: A direct transnasal approach to the sphenoid sinus: Technical note. J Neurosurg 66:140–142, 1987.
18. Cooke RS, Jones RAC: Experience with the direct transnasal transsphenoidal approach to the pituitary fossa. Br J Neurosurg 8:193–196, 1994.

C H A P T E R    3 0

# Repair of the Sella Turcica After Transsphenoidal Surgery

■ RENATO SPAZIANTE, ENRICO DE DIVITIIS, and PAOLO CAPPABIANCA

The transsphenoidal approach to the sella turcica is influenced at each step of its execution by the regional anatomy. Specifically, to rebuild the pituitary fossa and nasal and paranasal structures, traditional neurosurgical methods—obtaining hemostasis by coagulation of the operative site under direct visual control, suspending and suturing the dura mater, and fusing the bone flap—cannot be used. Alternative methods have been devised to deal with the transsphenoidal approach, and they are discussed in this chapter.

## GENERAL PRINCIPLES

The fundamental goals of reconstruction of the region of the sella follow.

1. Hemostasis
2. Reduction of intrasellar dead space
3. Support for suprasellar structures (the diaphragma sellae, chiasmal cistern, optic structures, and third ventricle)
4. Prevention or arrest of cerebrospinal fluid (CSF) leakage
5. Reconstitution of the integrity of the sellar floor.

To satisfy these aims, the sellar cavity must be adequately packed and the breech in the bone and dura in its floor sealed.

## PACKING OF THE PITUITARY FOSSA

An intrasellar tumor often causes an increase in the size of the sella turcica, ranging from being barely perceptible in the case of a microadenoma up to being huge in the case of giant adenomas. During its development, an intrasellar lesion first stretches and then causes atrophy or even the disappearance of the diaphragma sellae that normally covers the pituitary fossa, dividing it from the cranial fossa, the chiasmal cistern, and the optic structures.

Removal of a sellar tumor (or the normal pituitary in cases of hypophysectomy) leaves a free space within the pituitary fossa (Fig. 30–1). The walls of this space are potentially hemorrhagic; unless it is obliterated, the space will tend to fill with blood. Therefore, there is the danger of intrasellar hematoma formation with a mass effect. Meningitis or an intrasellar abscess may also occur because of the communication of the sellar space with the sphenoidal sinus. When the pituitary fossa is not properly separated from the intracranial contents either because of congenital incompetence of the diaphragma sella or, more commonly, because of its secondary atrophy, the pulsatile action of the brain can force the arachnoid of the chiasmal cistern down toward the sellar floor; it can then involve the optic nerves and cause their downward displacement. In the most serious cases, the third ventricle may herniate into the sellar cavity. The onset or worsening of a CSF fistula is greatly favored.[1]

To avoid these problems, the free intrasellar space is obliterated by packing it with substances that will ensure hemostasis, provide both immediate and future support for the suprasellar structures, and create a barrier between the inside and the outside of the pituitary fossa (Fig. 30–2). The substances that best fulfill these requirements are subcutaneous fat, fascia, or muscle, which are usually harvested from the thigh or the abdomen[2, 3]; fragments of cartilage and bone from the nasal septum or the sphenoid[2]; reabsorbable materials such as fibrin sponge, oxidized cellulose hemostat, Gelfoam, collagen, and fibrin glue[4–6]; and lyophilized dura mater.[3, 7] These various substances can be used alone or in combination. The prepared (commercially available) reabsorbable substances and lyophilized dura mater are the easiest to use and are used most frequently, with bone-cartilage fragments being added when necessary. When the surgical situation requires the packing to be particularly effective, the best materials are muscle or subcutaneous fat, even though to harvest them is a time-consuming procedure that may even be a source of contamination.[8] Fat is preferable to muscle, because it undergoes less necrosis and less scar retraction that would result in a reduction in the volume of the packing. This could be a problem when the packing is insufficient or if an excessive amount of material needs to be inserted to compensate for later loss in volume.[9, 10]

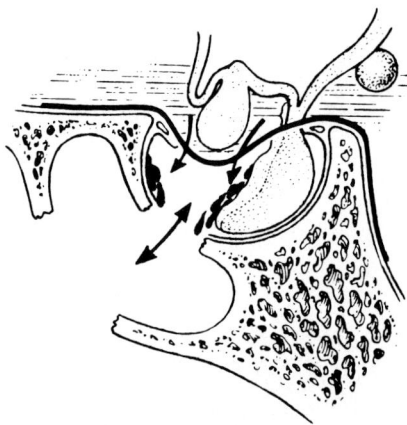

FIGURE 30–1 ■ The conditions that frequently need to be corrected after removal of pituitary fossa lesions. The surgical site is bloody because of many small hemorrhages that arise from the cut surface of the hypophysis and the dura mater covering the sellar floor and the cavernous sinuses. The suprasellar structures tend to be pushed toward the sellar floor because of the ineffectiveness of the sellar diaphragma. Preoperative adhesions, surgical damage, or downward distention of the chiasmal cistern favor the development of cerebrospinal fluid leaks *(upper arrows)*. Communication with the septic sphenoidal sinus may lead to contamination of the sellar cavity *(double-faced arrow)*.

## CLOSURE OF THE SELLAR FLOOR

Classically,[2] the pituitary fossa is reached by removing a 1-cm² segment of the floor of the sella, opening the dura in a cruciate fashion, and coagulating its edges for hemostasis and to provide wider access to the sella. The resultant bone defect must be repaired in order to support the materials that will eventually be used to fill the pituitary fossa and to create an effective barrier between the intrasellar and extrasellar spaces. Only rarely should the sellar floor be left open.

Closure of the dura mater is customarily deemed need-

less and is almost impossible to accomplish. Nevertheless, it has been suggested that a watertight closure of the dura with special suture-tying instruments and a needle and a suitable practical technique may be obtained even through a small hole into a narrow, deep surgical field such as the transsphenoidal area. Direct closure, when dural edges have not been retracted because of coagulations or torn margins and they can be approximated, or, more often, patch-graft closure can be used.[11] If opening of the dura of the sellar floor is made in a reversed U shape (as we at present do), a small flap that is hinged downward is obtained that gives a wide, regular, and perfectly sized access to the pituitary fossa. It can be successively replaced, providing a first, highly efficacious component for rebuilding the sellar floor.

The simplest and most effective method of restoring the sellar floor is to use a disk of cartilage or bone harvested from the nasal septum or paranasal structures during the initial stages of the surgical exposure.[2] This material is cut to the correct shape and size and is inserted below the edges of the opening in the bone, in the epidural space, so that pressure from the dura mater will help maintain its position until healing provides a true union (Fig. 30–3). Analogous results can be obtained with disks of lyophilized dura mater or fascia lata.[12] Using the unilateral septal technique, a substitute of the nasal cartilage is often required to obliterate the bone window. Prostheses of synthetic histoacrylic resin, ceramic, and lyophilized bone have been used.[13–15] A silicone plate, which possesses a hardness very similar to that of cartilage, may be a very suitable substitute.[16] Furthermore, for fusion of the plug (whatever its nature), histoacrylic biologic glues or natural derivatives have been used.[3, 6, 17, 18]

In cases in which the floor of the sella is paper thin, it can be opened by cutting two small lateral bone flaps, which can be turned to the side (Fig. 30–4); when the floor is reconstructed, the bone flaps are returned to their original position and secured either by fixing them to each other and to the edges of the breech in the bone or by threading a strip of cartilage beneath the upper and lower margins of the hole in the bone, bridging the medial edge of the two juxtaposed bone flaps (Fig. 30–5). Because the bone edges fit together perfectly and the periosteum has been preserved, the chances for physiologic union of the sella floor are improved.[19]

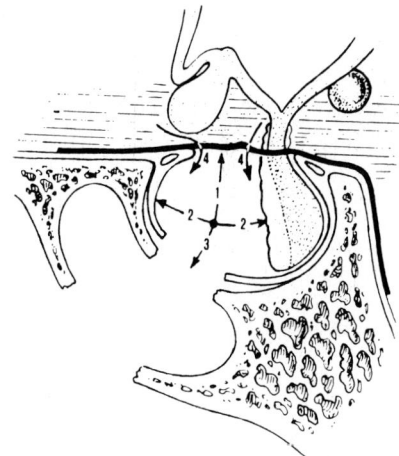

FIGURE 30–2 ■ The basic problems at which packing of the pituitary fossa is aimed (in addition to reducing the amount of intrasellar dead space): (1) to support the diaphragma sellae, the chiasmal cistern, and the suprasellar structures; (2) to ensure hemostasis of the surgical bed by contact and light compression; (3) to seal the intrasellar space against external (sphenoidal) agents; and (4) to prevent or arrest cerebrospinal fluid leaks.

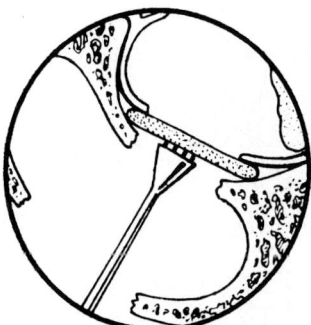

FIGURE 30–3 ■ The sellar floor is usually easily closed by slipping a disk of cartilage or bone (or lyophilized dura mater or synthetic materials) into the extradural space. This disk generously overlaps the breech in the bone and in the dura on all sides.

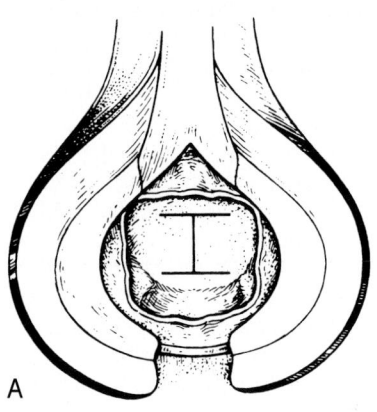
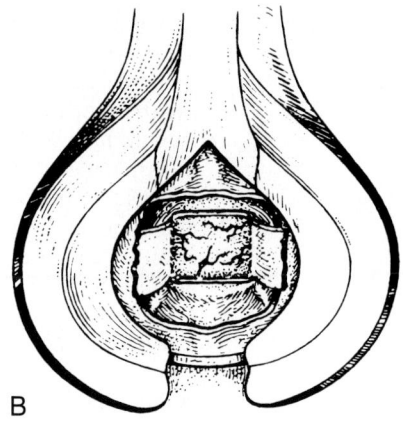

**FIGURE 30–4** ■ *A,* Lines along which the sellar floor can be cut if it has a paper-like consistency. *B,* Two small flaps are reflected to the sides, parallel to the carotid artery grooves.

## PACKING AND CLOSURE OF THE SPHENOIDAL SINUS

Packing of the sphenoidal sinus is not universally accepted to be mechanically useful,[20, 21] but we use this technique to support the sellar floor when it is particularly stretched and inconsistent ("ghost" sella) and to create a less septic postoperative environment by using reabsorbable substances soaked in an antibacterial solution.

The same materials are used as for packing the pituitary fossa. The simplest method is to use a fibrin or gelatin sponge soaked in antibiotic solution, together with residual bone-cartilage fragments. The largest fragment can be used to approximately reconstruct the anterior wall of the sphenoidal sinus and separate it from the nasal fossa. Hermetic closure of the sphenoidal sinus by synthetic materials, bone cements, or resins does not prevent the aforementioned mechanical complications or CSF leakage and adds the risks of foreign body reaction and chemical osteitis.[20, 22] Moreover, it prohibits or greatly impedes reoperation by the transsphenoidal route, which may be necessary either if, despite careful rebuilding of the sellar region, mechanical complications arise or, later, because of the progression of the pituitary disease.

There are some conditions in which it may be useful to avoid any filling of the sphenoidal sinus, as well as any closure of the sellar floor. This is the case when hemostasis at the operative site is inadequate; a permeable sphenoidal sinus is an excellent way of draining blood that may collect in the pituitary fossa during the first hours after surgery. Likewise, not packing the pituitary fossa facilitates the spontaneous delivery of residual intrasellar and suprasellar tumor, such as an hour-glass adenoma or cystic craniopharyngioma in which only an intracapsular removal has been performed. In these cases, a free sphenoidal sinus is absolutely necessary to allow further emptying of the sellar tumor.[12, 23]

## RECONSTRUCTION OF NASAL STRUCTURES

Reconstruction of nasal structures is usually limited to either (nonobligatory) reapposition of the cartilage of the nasal septum, in cases in which this has been removed, or returning the nasal septum to the midline, in the case of a unilateral transseptal approach.[24] The two nostrils are filled with medicated, nonadhesive gauze. In the transnasal approach, the columella is held by three or four sutures, of which one transfixes deeply. If a transnasal unilateral approach is performed, no suture is required, the nasal mucosa being simply replaced on the septum. When the transoral route is used, the gingival mucosa can be reapposed with a few stitches or can even be left open.

### Methods for Reconstructing the Pituitary Fossa

The underlying lesion and conditions encountered during surgery determine the manner in which the sellar region is

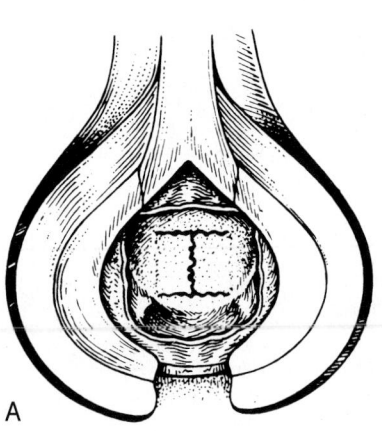
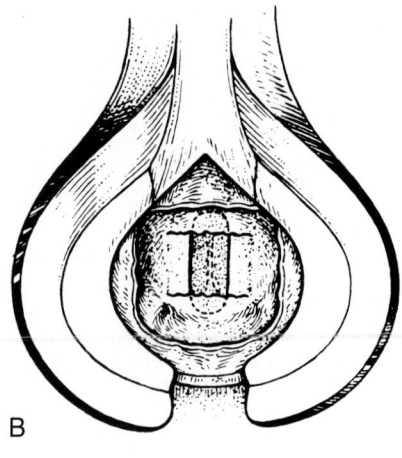

**FIGURE 30–5** ■ To reconstruct the sellar floor after it is opened as noted in Figure 30–4, the bone flaps are returned to their natural position. They can be secured by fitting them into each other and to the edges of the sellar opening *(A).* When this approach proves unreliable, a strip of cartilage can be threaded beneath the edges of the hole in the bone bridging the medial edge of the two juxtaposed bone flaps *(B).*

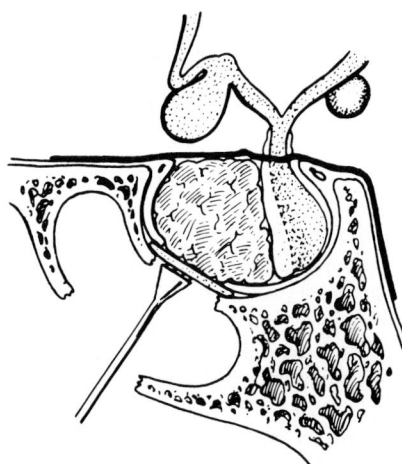

**FIGURE 30–6** ■ Simple intradural packing. The packing materials are inserted intradurally, completely filling the intrasellar space. A disk of cartilage or similar material is fitted extradurally to close the sellar floor. (From Spaziante R, de Divitiis E, Cappabianca P: Reconstruction of the pituitary fossa in transsphenoidal surgery: An experience of 140 cases. Neurosurgery 17:453, 1985.)

reconstructed. Although the needs of each case during surgery are the main guide, general criteria can be formulated for the principal methods.

## Simple Intradural Packing

Simple intradural packing is the fundamental method suggested in most classic descriptions of transsphenoidal surgery.[2] Materials for packing the sellar cavity are introduced into the intradural space, and the plug that closes the floor is fixed into the epidural space (Fig. 30–6). This is easily and rapidly performed and is the ideal solution when the empty space left at the end of the operation is no larger than the sella turcica.

This approach has two main limitations: (1) The packing cannot be very tight, even when this is needed, because the pressure developing within the sella is transmitted to suprasellar and parasellar structures; and (2) the packing material is not solidly adherent to the walls of the fossa and can move about.

## Anchored Intradural Packing

To avoid the limitations of simple intradural packing, the packing material can be fixed to the floor of the sella so that it is more stable and offers more complete closure.

There are two slightly different methods by which this can be accomplished; both are based on the same principles. The first consists of interposing the disk of cartilage used to close the sella between two muscle fragments that are larger than the hole in the sella.[25] One is placed intradurally, and the other is placed in the sphenoidal sinus (Fig. 30–7A). A suture, which previously has been passed through the entire packet, is then tied, consolidating the mass and fixing it to the sellar floor so that it cannot move either into the sella nor outward. A later variant consists of interposing a large muscle fragment between two cartilage disks, one intradural and the other intrasphenoidal (see Fig. 30–7B).[26] A suture that previously has been passed through all the components is tightened and tied. As well as securely anchoring the packing to the sellar floor, the ligature pushes the muscle centrifugally, thus filling the lateral recesses of the pituitary fossa and providing better hemostasis of the wall of the cavernous sinus.

## Extradural Packing

The dura covering the sellar floor can be detached easily from the floor and elevated as far as the insertion to the cavernous sinus, of which it forms the medial wall, preventing further elevation. The wide space thus obtained can then be packed with the same materials as mentioned earlier (Fig. 30–8), which are interposed between two large

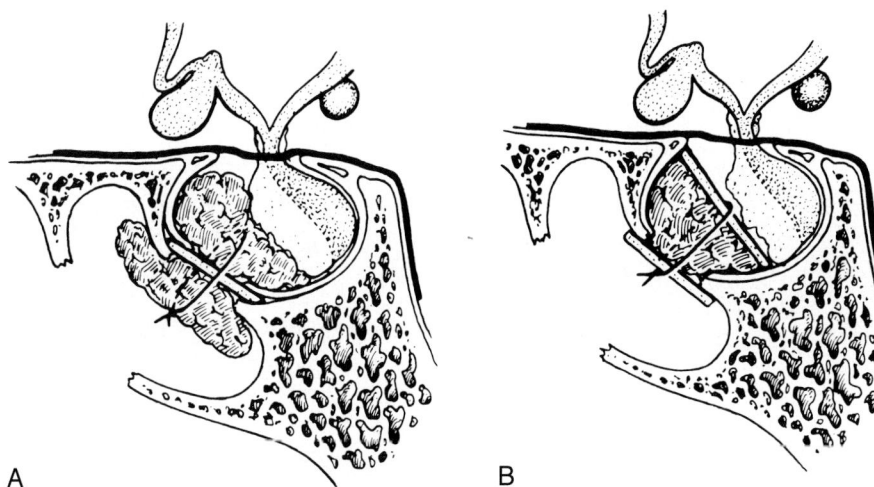

A                                        B

**FIGURE 30–7** ■ Anchored intradural packing. *A,* The disk of cartilage closing the sellar floor is interposed between two large muscle fragments, one inside and the other outside the sella. By tying a suture previously passed through them, the mass is consolidated and firmly fastened to the sella. *B,* Two cartilage disks, one intradural and the other intrasphenoidal, sandwich a large muscle fragment and close the breach in the sella. The packet is solidly anchored by tightening a suture previously passed through the disks and muscles; in addition, the muscle splits laterally, filling the lateral recesses of the sellar cavity. (From Spaziante R, de Divitiis E, Cappabianca P: Reconstruction of the pituitary fossa in transsphenoidal surgery: An experience of 140 cases. Neurosurgery 17:453, 1985.)

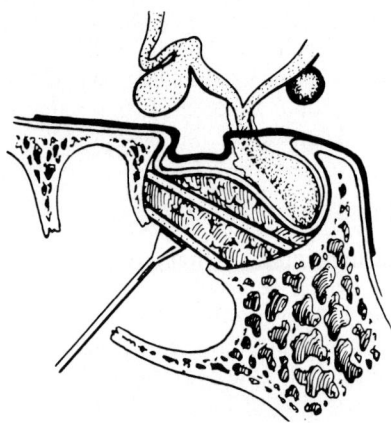

**FIGURE 30–8** ■ Extradural packing. Intradural free space is greatly reduced by detaching the dura mater from the sellar floor. The extradural space is filled with the usual materials interposed between the two cartilage disks, the larger one in contact with the dura mater, the other closing the hole in the sella. (From Spaziante R, de Divitiis E, Cappabianca P: Reconstruction of the pituitary fossa in transsphenoidal surgery: An experience of 140 cases. Neurosurgery 17:453, 1985.)

bone-cartilage disks—one corresponding with the dural hole, the other to the breech in the bone.[27–29]

This type of packing can be particularly tight and hermetic because the elastic forces produced by distending the dura mater make it more compact and stable. Furthermore, there is no risk of introducing an excessive amount of packing material because the dura cannot be interrupted or elevated beyond the limits imposed by its own elasticity (unless exceptionally violent maneuvers are used). Thus, there is no risk of excessive pressure being transmitted to perisellar structures (Fig. 30–9).

### Combined Extradural-Intradural Packing

Extradural packing is advantageous from many points of view; it does not allow a particularly large residual cavity to be packed completely, however, because there is a limit to the degree of dural movement at the sellar floor. In this situation, the ideal solution is to make part of the packing

intradural (producing volume) and part extradural (providing stability, solidity, and watertight closure) (Fig. 30–10).

### Packing in the Case of Cerebrospinal Fluid Leakage

The method of sellar reconstruction for repair of a CSF leak must be meticulous, because such a leak can create serious postoperative problems.[30–32] A strip of fascia lata or lyophilized dura is placed to protect the arachnoid and the diaphragma sellae; the sellar cavity is then partially filled with muscle or subcutaneous fat inserted into the intradural space. A second strip of fascia or lyophilized dura is used on the inner surface of the dura mater to close it.[2, 3, 5, 22, 28, 33] A particularly precise extradural packing is then performed (Figs. 30–11 and 30–12). Continuous CSF lumbar drainage is highly recommended for at least 72 hours to allow the plugging material to consolidate, thus diverting the CSF flow from the fistula and decreasing the CSF pressure. Its working rates must be carefully checked, however, to avoid risk of pneumocephalus, which may even turn into a tension pneumocephalus.[34]

## INDICATIONS IN RELATION TO THE MOST FREQUENT SELLAR DISEASES

Several factors determine the technique used to reconstruct the pituitary fossa. The possibilities range from situations in which no packing or reconstruction of the sellar walls is necessary to those in which they must be performed with obsessive precision.

### Pituitary Microadenoma

The size and topographic relationships of pituitary microadenomas mean that there is hardly ever any need to pack the residual cavity after their removal. Hemostasis usually occurs a few minutes after the lesion is removed.

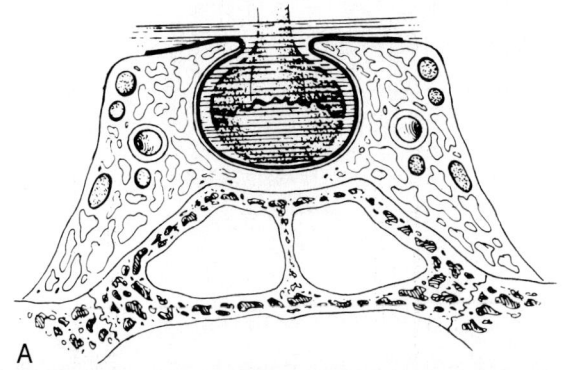
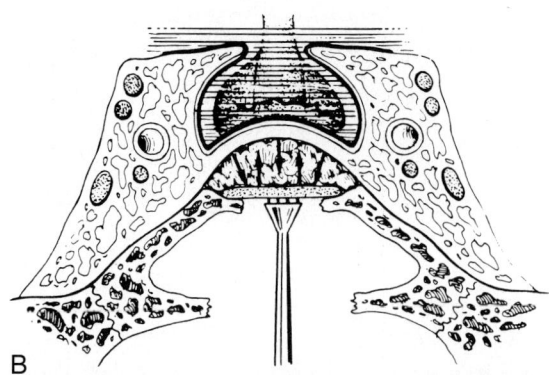

**FIGURE 30–9** ■ Cross-section of the pituitary fossa along a coronal plane before *(A)* and after *(B)* extradural packing. The dura mater of the sellar floor is joined to the walls of the cavernous sinuses. When it is detached from the floor and pushed upward, its distention creates elastic forces that compress the packing materials. The risk of overpacking is avoided because the dura cannot be elevated to an unlimited degree; increased pressure inside the packed space is not transmitted to suprasellar and perisellar structures. (From Spaziante R, de Divitiis E, Cappabianca P: Reconstruction of the pituitary fossa in transsphenoidal surgery: An experience of 140 cases. Neurosurgery 17:453, 1985.)

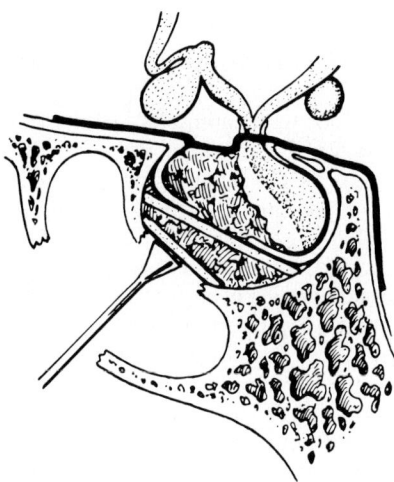

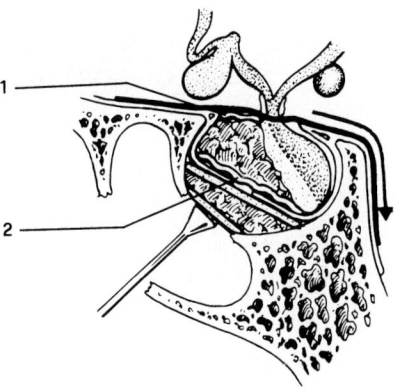

**FIGURE 30–10** ■ Combined extradural-intradural packing. The free space within the pituitary fossa is partly filled intradurally; extradural packing, as mentioned earlier, is performed afterward. (From Spaziante R, de Divitiis E, Cappabianca P: Reconstruction of the pituitary fossa in transsphenoidal surgery: An experience of 140 cases. Neurosurgery 17:453, 1985.)

**FIGURE 30–11** ■ General rules for packing to treat cerebrospinal fluid leakage. The first strip of fascia lata or lyophilized dura mater reinforces the diaphragma sellae and arachnoid of the chiasmal cistern (1). Partial intradural packing is performed, and the dura mater of the sellar floor is closed and reinforced with a second strip of fascia or lyophilized dura (2). Reconstruction of the sella is completed by extradural packing. The *arrow* running along the dorsum sellae demonstrates the usefulness of continuous spinal lumbar drainage during the operation and for the first few postoperative days.

**FIGURE 30–12** ■ An intraoperative fluoroscopic image. *A,* Intraoperative cerebrospinal fluid leakage after complete removal of a pituitary tumor with intrasellar and suprasellar extensions is clearly demonstrated by spontaneous entrance of air into the suprasellar cistern. *B,* Combined extradural-intradural packing of the sellar cavity. The first strip of lyophilized dura (not visible and indicated by the asterisk) reinforces the arachnoid. A second strip of lyophilized dura marked with iodinated contrast medium reinforces the dura mater of the sellar floor *(open arrow).* The packing is completed extradurally *(arrows).*

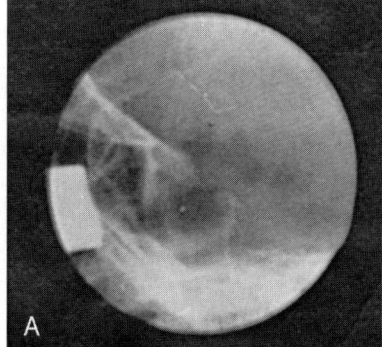

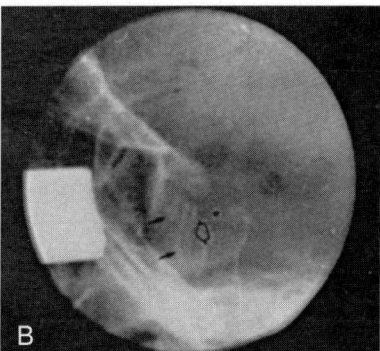

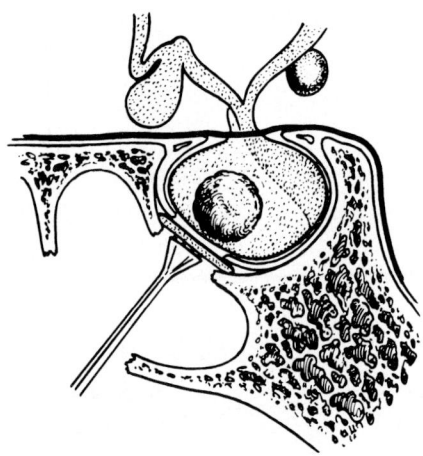

**FIGURE 30–13** ■ After removal of a microadenoma, there is usually no need to fill the sellar cavity because of the relationships between the residual cavity and the surrounding anatomic structures. However, plugging the sellar floor with a cartilage disk fitted extradurally may be advisable to restore the sellar wall.

Suprasellar structures are not involved by the adenoma and are supported naturally (Fig. 30–13). Reconstruction of the sellar floor with a cartilaginous plug fixed in the epidural space is useful for separating the pituitary fossa from the sphenoidal sinus (Fig. 30–14). Two situations, however, may require effective packing: (1) extension of the microadenoma toward the cavernous sinus with persistent hemorrhage after its removal,[35] and (2) a coexisting spontaneous or intraoperatively formed intrasellar arachnoidocele, which rarely occurs. In the event of CSF leakage (which frequently occurs when *radical* removal is pursued), the provisions already outlined would have to be implemented.[36]

## Intrasellar Adenomas

In cases of intrasellar adenomas (adenomas confined to the sella or slightly indenting the chiasmal cistern), the sellar cavity is wider than normal and can be very large (e.g., in the case of giant adenomas developing downward). The diaphragma sellae is usually atrophied as a result of pressure from the adenoma; nonetheless, suprasellar structures (the cisterns and optic pathways) are virtually unaffected by the growth of the adenoma. Packing the cavity is useful both in ensuring hemostasis of the large cavity and in

supporting the suprasellar structures, which could otherwise herniate downward and cause immediate or delayed onset of the empty sella syndrome. Because there is much downward distention of the dura of the sella (Fig. 30–15), extradural packing can be very easy and efficacious and does not carry the risk of overpacking (Fig. 30–16). If intradural packing is used, its upward extent must be checked fluoroscopically (Fig. 30–17) to ensure that the packing does not extend above the interclinoid plane.[3, 5]

## Adenoma with Large Suprasellar Extension

After a large tumor with suprasellar extension is removed, the residual cavity is very large and most of it is out of direct visual control. The diaphragma sellae is incompetent, and there is compression, stretching, and adherence of the dome of the adenoma to suprasellar and cerebral structures; in some places, adenomatous tissue may reach beyond the capsule. The sella turcica is larger than normal, although its volume is not always proportionate to the overall volume of the adenoma. These are the most suitable conditions for the development of mechanical complications. CSF leakage can develop because of an interruption in the continuity of the chiasmatic cistern by the adenoma, its accidental rupture during surgery, or as a result of excessive stretching postoperatively.

Adequately packing this space can be a difficult problem. To fill the cavity completely (Fig. 30–18) would create the same consequences as those caused by the adenoma.[12, 17, 37] To prevent overpacking, filling must be strictly limited to the intrasellar space, its upper limit remaining well beneath the interclinoid plane. Such packing, which is disproportionate to the volume of the residual cavity, risks being mobile and thus ineffective. These difficulties can be greatly reduced after the adenoma has been removed by returning the chiasmal cistern to its natural position. This can occur spontaneously (21%;[38] 58% of cases, according to Nakane and associates[39]), or it can be achieved (61% of our cases;[38] 20% of cases of Nakane and associates[39]) by introducing either a small amount of air or Ringer's solution into the subarachnoid space via a lumbar catheter (perioperative pneumoencephalography) or by compressing the jugular vein in the neck for a few seconds (Fig. 30–19). Greater amounts of air may be injected in more resistant cases (forced cistern air dissection or "pumping" technique[38]). When the capsule of the adenoma returns to the sellar cavity, the situation becomes analogous to that of an

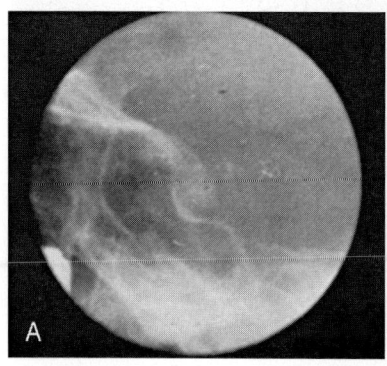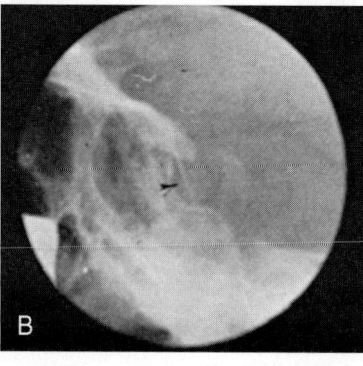

**FIGURE 30–14** ■ An intraoperative fluoroscopic image. *A,* The residual cavity is filled with a sponge soaked in iodinated medium after removal of a microadenoma. *B,* An extradural cartilage disk *(arrowhead)* closes the sellar floor and reduces the intradural free space.

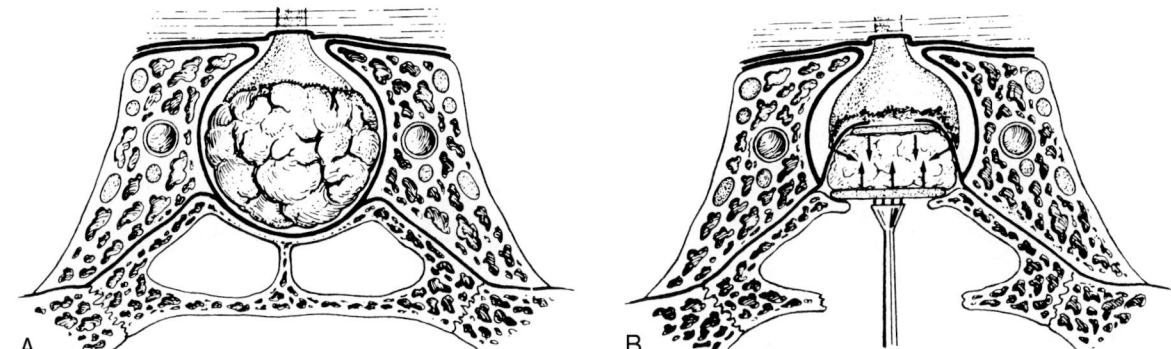

**FIGURE 30–15** ■ A cross-section of the pituitary fossa along a coronal plane before *(A)* and after *(B)* removal of a large intrasellar adenoma, followed by extradural packing of the residual cavity. Because the dura mater of the sellar floor has been greatly distended, it can be detached very easily and extensively raised before the walls of the cavernous sinus are tightened. Almost the entire intrasellar residual cavity can be filled in this way.

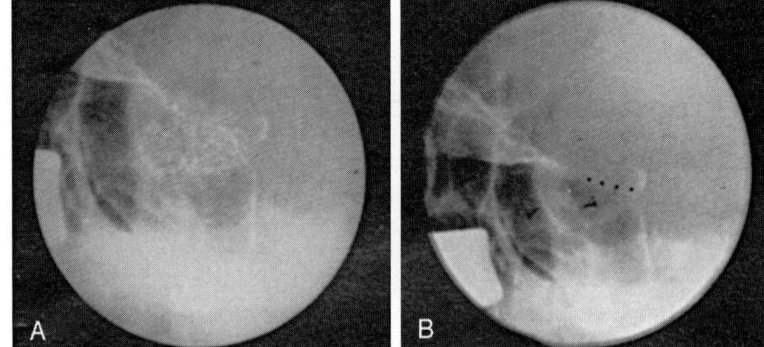

**FIGURE 30–16** ■ An intraoperative fluoroscopic image. *A,* The residual cavity after removal of a large intrasellar adenoma is visualized by a radiopaque cottonoid. *B,* The outside and inside limits of extradural packing *(open arrowheads)*. The correct position of the diaphragma sellae is outlined by the air bubble remaining within the pituitary fossa *(dotted line)*.

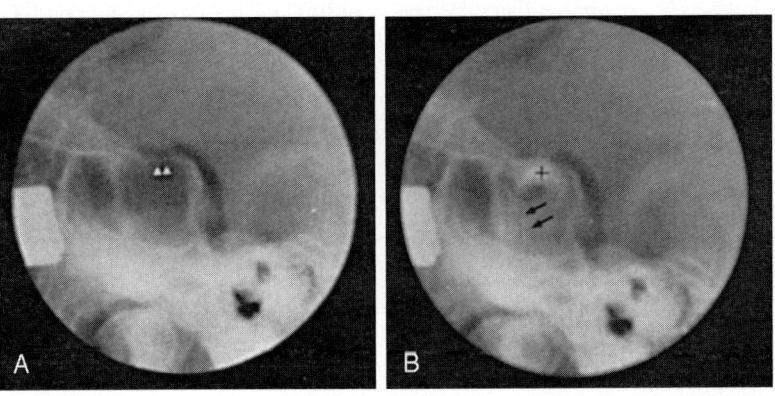

**FIGURE 30–17** ■ An intraoperative fluoroscopic image of the removal of a large intrasellar adenoma. *A,* The diaphragma sellae *(white arrowheads)* is outlined by an air bubble within the pituitary fossa, while the chiasmal cistern is visualized by means of perioperative pneumoencephalography (PEG). *B,* Intradural filling of the defect with reabsorbable materials, the upper limit of which is marked with a sponge soaked in iodinated contrast medium *(cross)*. The sellar floor is closed with numerous bone and cartilage fragments that have been inserted extradurally *(arrows)*.

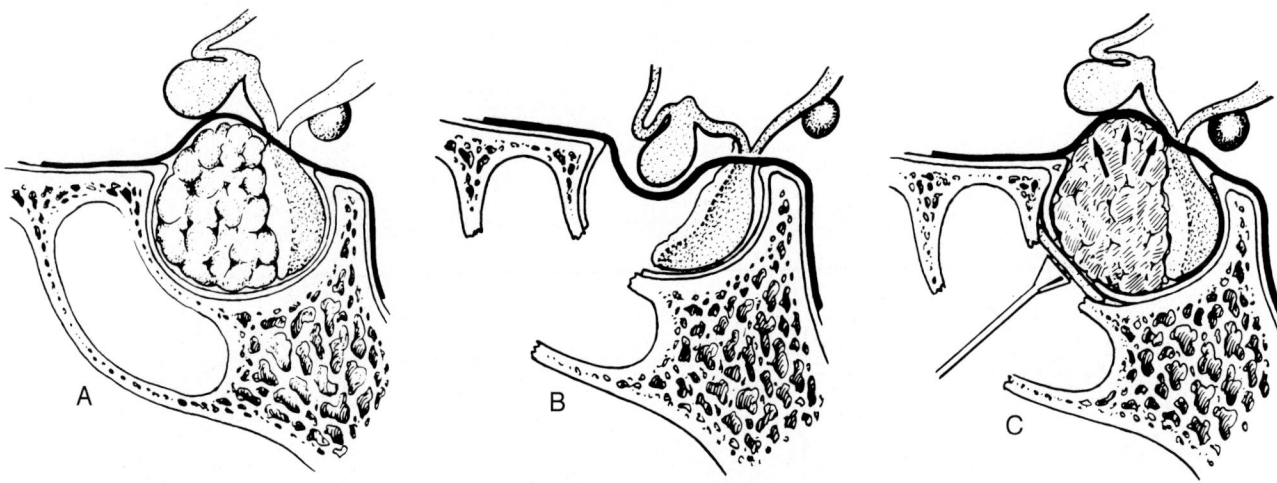

FIGURE 30–18 ■ After removal of an adenoma with suprasellar extension *(A),* there are many features that predispose the patient to postoperative mechanical complications, such as empty sella syndrome, cerebrospinal fluid rhinorrhea, and hemorrhage *(B).* An effective intradural tamponade carries the risk of being too tight, causing compression of the suprasellar structures similar to that produced by the growth of the adenoma *(C).* (From Spaziante R, de Divitiis E, Cappabianca P: Reconstruction of the pituitary fossa in transsphenoidal surgery: An experience of 140 cases. Neurosurgery 17:453, 1985.)

intrasellar adenoma, although it must be remembered that the diaphragma sellae is completely incompetent. If the capsule remains raised, however (Fig. 30–20), packing will be necessary, also to eliminate the possibility that, at some point in time, the dome of the adenoma will invert its curve and descend into the sellar cavity.[17, 27, 40] It is then best to perform anchored intradural packing or mixed intradural-extradural packing (Fig. 30–21).[41] In the same way, one must check during the operation to determine whether or not the capsule spontaneously descends into the sellar cavity (Figs. 30–22 and 30–23). Special consideration must be given to cases of hourglass adenoma, in which removal of the suprasellar portion is inevitably incomplete. To encourage descent into the sellar cavity of the residual suprasellar portion with a view to further surgery or radiotherapy or to obtain better optic decompression, it may be useful not to do any packing or to close the floor but simply to sterilize the sphenoidal sinus.[12, 23] Although there are risks, this approach may prove to be the most advantageous.

## Empty Sella

A pituitary adenoma may often be accompanied by an intrasellar arachnoidocele as a consequence of spontaneous necrosis or previous treatment.[1] During removal of the adenomatous tissue the arachnoid must be protected and elevated and put back in its natural position[2, 5] to avoid risk of CSF leakage and to prevent the serious complications that an empty sella can provoke with time.[28, 42] Packing must be of sufficient volume, consistency, and stability to avoid recurrence of the empty sella. Extradural mixed packing is probably the best type of repair in this situation, because the arachnoid is protected with a strip of lyophilized dura before being very carefully elevated.[41]

Correction of a pure empty sella presents different problems. The aims of such an operation are to elevate the chiasmatic cistern and optic structures; to prevent progressive stretching and erosion of the sellar floor (involving dura and bone) as a result of transmission by the CSF of the pulsatile action of the brain; to prevent compression and distortion of the pituitary and its stalk, repositioning them in an anatomic position; to prevent (or arrest) CSF leakage; and to prevent late recurrence.[1, 32, 43] The packing in this situation must be well proportioned, carried out with minimal trauma, and very stable. The ideal is an extradural repair (Fig. 30–24).[29, 43] Elevation of the dura mater will greatly reduce the space within the sella-intrasellar structure, and suprasellar structures are lifted without being damaged by the surgical maneuvers, because the arachnoid

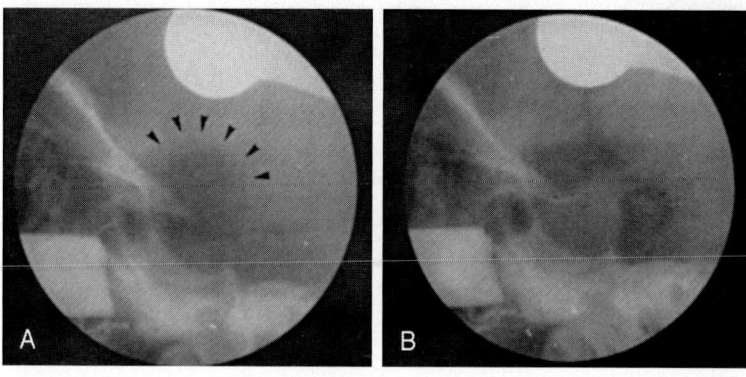

FIGURE 30–19 ■ An intraoperative fluoroscopic image. *A,* Following removal of an adenoma with an extensive suprasellar extension, the dome of the tumor remains raised *(arrowheads). B,* Injection of fractionated amounts of air through a lumbar spinal catheter pushed it downward, refilling the chiasmal cistern and dissecting the loose adhesions from surrounding structures.

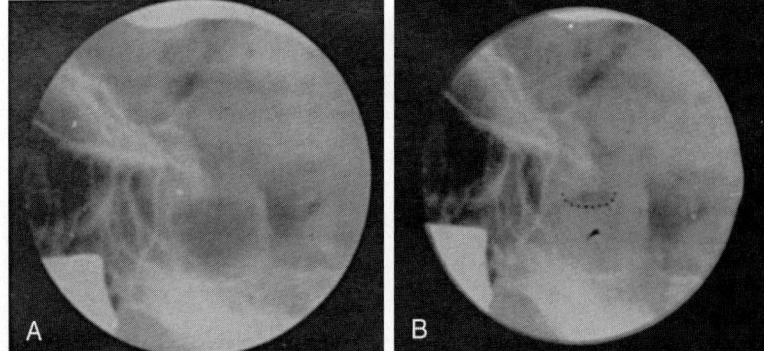

FIGURE 30–20 ■ An intraoperative fluoroscopic image. *A,* After complete removal of an adenoma with suprasellar extension, its dome collapsed, as demonstrated by perioperative pneumoencephalography (PEG). *B,* Combined intradural-extradural packing. The upper limit beneath the interclinoid plane is outlined by an air bubble remaining inside the pituitary fossa *(dotted line).* The *arrowhead* points out the bone disk that constitutes the inner surface of the extradural packing.

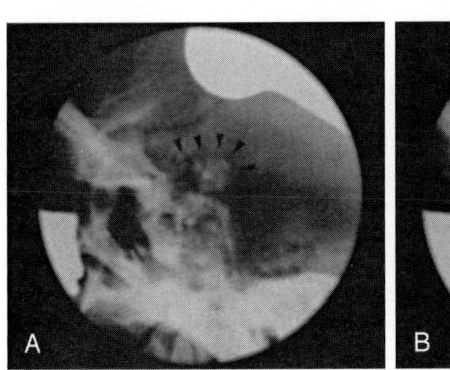 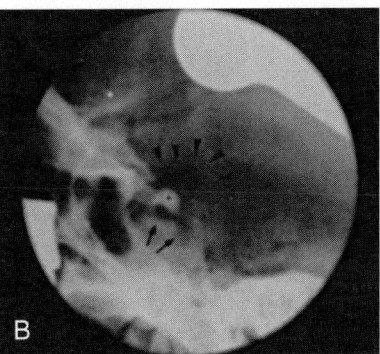

FIGURE 30–21 ■ An intraoperative fluoroscopic image. *A,* Adenoma with suprasellar extension *(arrowheads)* visualized by diluted water-soluble nonionic contrast medium that was injected into it before the dura mater was opened. *B,* The dome of the tumor *(arrowheads)* failed to descend despite repeated maneuvers to collapse it. A proper tamponade was achieved by combined intradural (the upper limit is marked with a sponge soaked in iodinated contrast medium) and, for the most part, extradural packing *(arrows).*

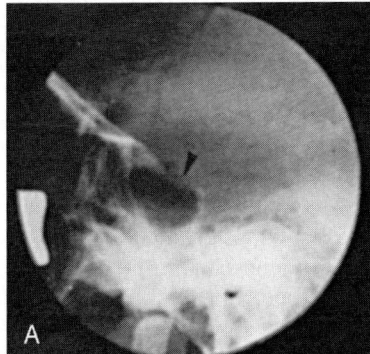 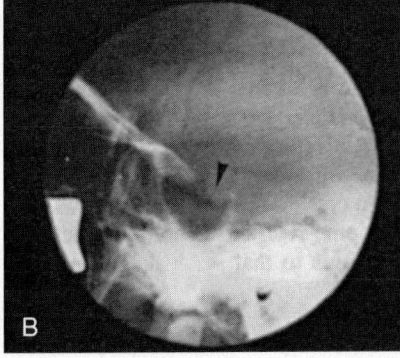 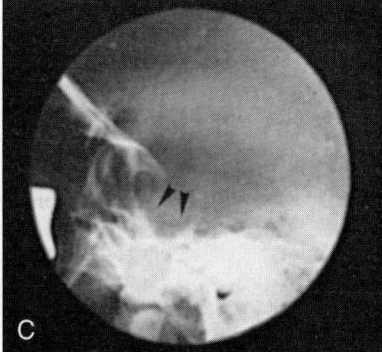

FIGURE 30–22 ■ An intraoperative fluoroscopic image. After complete removal of a pituitary cystic tumor with extensive suprasellar extension, the dome of the tumor *(arrowhead)* spontaneously returned to the interclinoid plane *(A).* Afterward, it appeared in the sellar cavity *(B);* soon afterward, it descended deep toward the sellar floor *(C).*

FIGURE 30–23 ■ An intraoperative fluoroscopic image. *A,* A pituitary adenoma with a suprasellar extension visualized by diluted water-soluble nonionic contrast medium that was injected into it before the dura mater was opened. *B,* After removal of the adenoma, the diaphragma sellae spontaneously descended deep into the sellar cavity *(arrowheads).* (From Spaziante R, de Divitiis E, Cappabianca P: Reconstruction of the pituitary fossa in transsphenoidal surgery: An experience of 140 cases. Neurosurgery 17:453, 1985.)

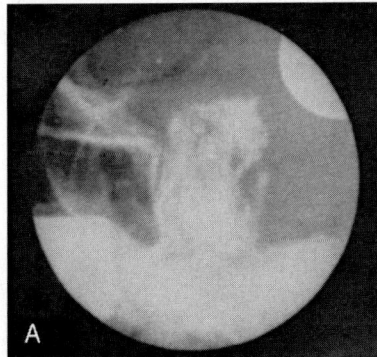 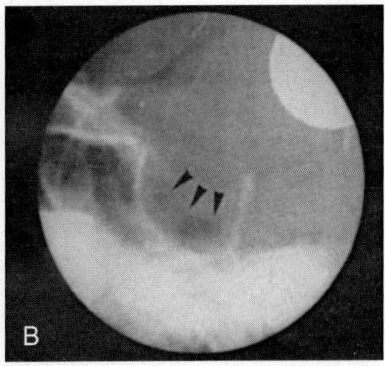

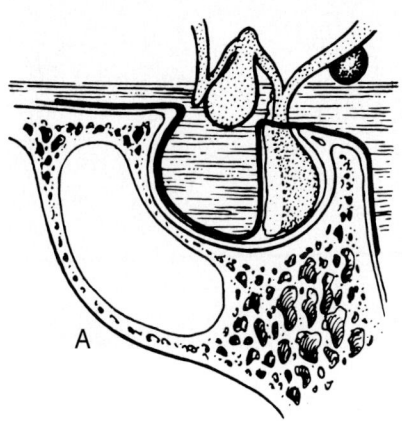
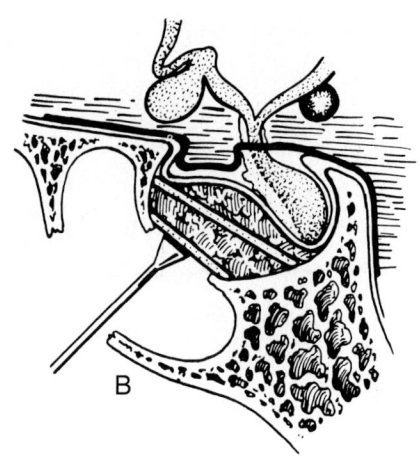

FIGURE 30-24 ■ *A*, The most suitable method for achieving the primary goals of the surgical treatment of a pure empty sella (reduction of arachnoidocele, chiasmapexy, protection of the pituitary gland and sellar floor against pulsatile action of cerebrospinal fluid [CSF], and prevention of CSF leakage) is extradural packing *(B)*. Besides being very stable and well proportioned, it does not carry the risk of intrasellar and suprasellar structures being damaged by the surgical maneuvers.

pocket protects them; the sellar floor is protected against cerebral pulsation. The best packing material to use for this purpose is either subcutaneous fat or bone-cartilage fragments, which will not undergo much necrosis or retraction with time so that the initial volume will not excessively decrease later. In consideration of the peculiar features involved with this approach, which are aimed at obtaining a definitive filling of the pituitary fossa, methods using prosthetic material have also been devised, such as an inflatable detachable balloon for intravascular embolization[44, 45] or a Silastic tube for draining devices arranged in an ovoidal or circular form, which we performed in one case (Fig. 30-25). Percutaneous endoscopic gastrostomy (PEG) fluoroscopic visualization of the chiasmal cistern and of the intrasellar diverticulum during the entire procedure (Fig. 30-26) is almost indispensable.[9]

## Ghost Sella

Ghost sella is a special problem because the large size of the sella and the flimsiness of the floor may prevent efficient performance of any of the methods of repair described.[41] This problem occurs very rarely, but when it is encountered, it may be necessary to resort to intradural packing (Fig. 30-27), combined with packing of the sphenoidal sinus with muscle, fat, and bone-cartilage fragments.[28, 33]

## Other Sellar Lesions

Other lesions more rarely approached by the transsphenoidal route (e.g., arachnoid cysts, dermoid cysts, meningiomas, chondromas, metastases) involve intraoperative factors similar to those of the more common conditions and can be treated in an analogous manner.

Arachnoidal cysts have both intrasellar and suprasellar growth and features similar to those of pituitary adenomas with suprasellar extension (Fig. 30-28); however, their walls do not readily heal solidly postoperatively and they can communicate with the subarachnoid space through a unidirectional valve mechanism, favoring the entry and accumulation of CSF under pressure and the subsequent development of CSF rhinorrhea.[46] Postoperative mechanical complications are, therefore, more frequent.[47]

Special problems arise in cases of cystic craniopharyngiomas with relevant suprasellar extension. Removal through the transsphenoidal route must often be restricted to emptying the tumor cyst without completely removing the capsule, because it has adhered too firmly to the boundaries. The main goal of treatment in such cases is to obtain total and definitive collapse of the tumor capsule, creating a way for permanent draining of the cyst contents, waiting for the effects of radiotherapy when this is planned. Provided there is no communication with the cerebral space or passage of CSF across the tumor wall, a hermetic closure of the sellar floor must be avoided. Instead, to allow the cyst cavity to

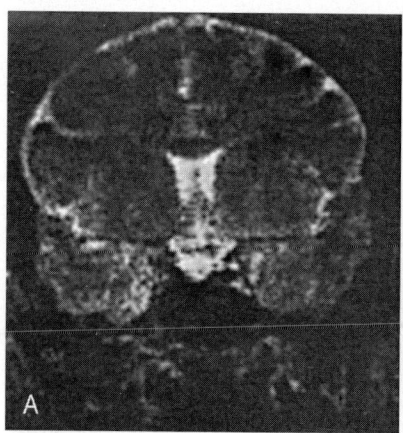
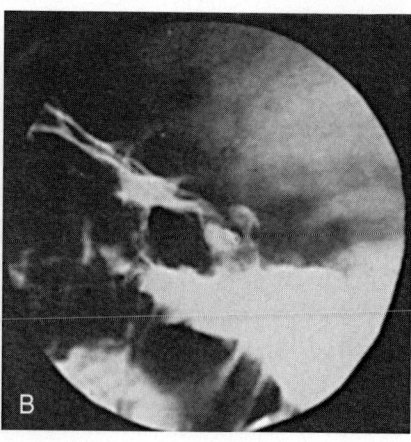

FIGURE 30-25 ■ *A*, A magnetic resonance image showing a post-traumatic empty sella (with slight enlargement of the sella turcica) in a patient suffering from progressive, serious narrowing of the visual field. *B*, A roentgenogram of the sella turcica (lateral view) 1 month after a transsphenoidal operation. Extradural packing of the pituitary fossa has been achieved by means of a Silastic tube (commonly used for cerebrospinal fluid drainage systems) arranged in a spiral configuration. Its resultant elastic action was very useful in raising, smoothly and perpetually, the dura to compel arachnoidpexy and chiasmapexy.

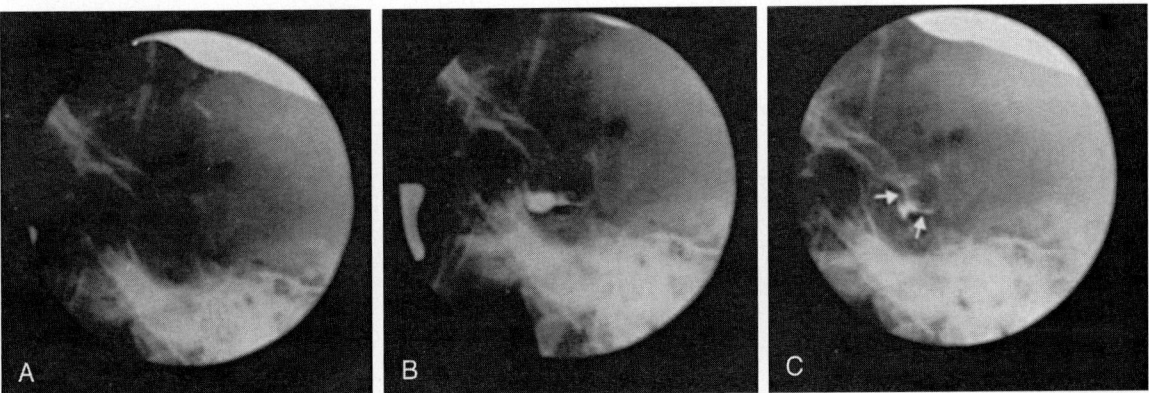

**FIGURE 30–26** ■ An intraoperative fluoroscopic image. *A,* An empty sella visualized by perioperative pneumoencephalography (PEG). *B,* A small amount of nonionic water-soluble contrast medium was injected through a thin needle into the dura mater within the arachnoid pouch to mark its bottom. *C,* The sellar cavity was packed extradurally, raising the arachnoid diverticulum and delineating the pituitary gland *(white arrows).*

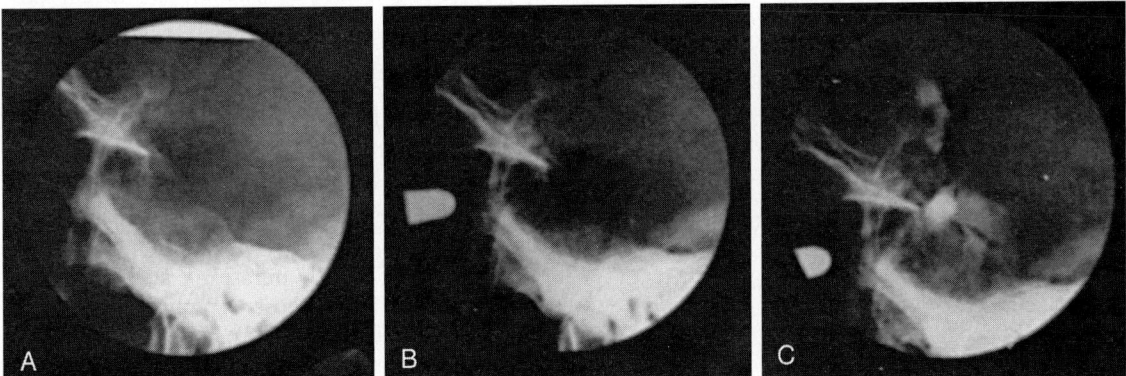

**FIGURE 30–27** ■ An intraoperative fluoroscopic image. *A,* A giant pituitary adenoma with extensive suprasellar extension. The sella turcica has completely disappeared. *B,* The residual cavity after removal of the tumor spontaneously filled with air. *C,* Widespread intradural packing with fat lightly soaked in water-soluble nonionic iodinated contrast medium to avoid the risk of overpacking. Some contrast has escaped into the cisternal spaces through an apparently spontaneous disruption of the subarachnoid layer. (Preoperatively, the patient complained of a spontaneous intratumoral hemorrhage.)

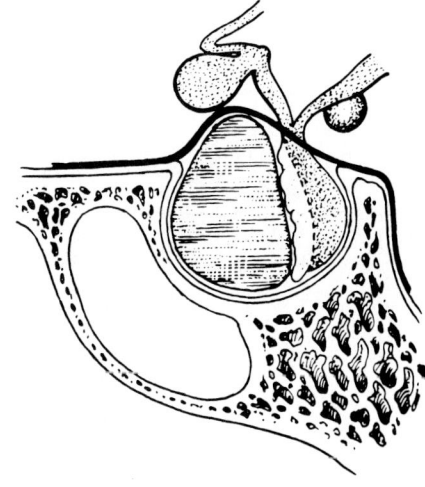

**FIGURE 30–28** ■ An intrasellar and suprasellar arachnoid cyst. The anatomic conditions are similar to those of an adenoma with suprasellar extension (see also Fig. 30–18). Even if emptying is surgically more favorable, the structural characteristics of the cyst wall and its relationship with cerebrospinal fluid pathways may favor the development of postoperative mechanical complications.

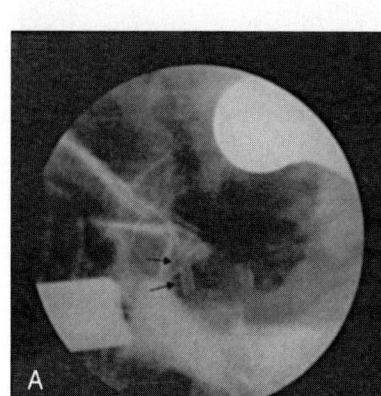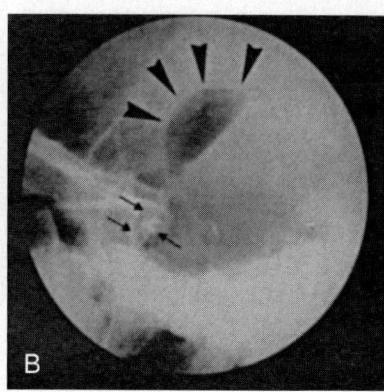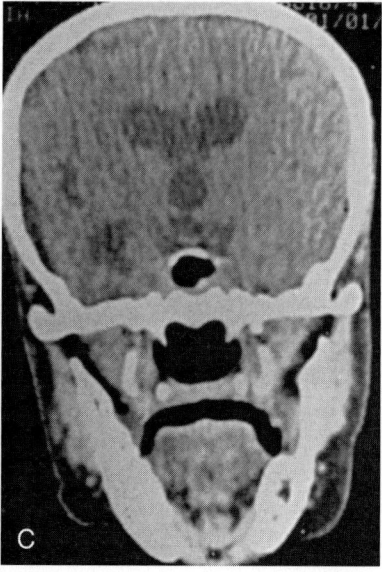

FIGURE 30–29 ■ *A,* The dome of this cystic craniopharyngioma with suprasellar extension collapsed when it was completely emptied, as demonstrated by perioperative pneumoencephalography (PEG). A short Silastic tube was used to establish a permanent communication between the cyst and the sphenoid sinus *(arrows). B,* Two days later, the cyst cavity was empty, but its dome retained its suprasellar extension *(arrowheads). C,* One month after surgery, the tumor cavity was empty, as is evident on this computed tomography scan, and occupied only the intrasellar region.

communicate with the sphenoidal sinus to improve drainage of the contents of the cyst and avoid its recurrence, a Silastic tube may be inserted through the surgical defect in the sellar floor, creating a permanent fistula (Fig. 30–29).[48]

## FUNCTIONAL HYPOPHYSECTOMY

The residual cavity is small after functional hypophysectomy, and its reconstruction may be unnecessary. There are two exceptions to this rule: (1) when there is diffuse hemorrhage caused by the wide dissection surface of the gland, and (2) when there is CSF leakage caused by a section of the pituitary stalk in total hypophysectomy (Fig. 30–30). This problem arises in about 11% of cases.[49] In view of the satisfactory condition of the diaphragma sellae,

intradural packing and closure of the sellar floor constitute an adequate repair.[2, 28]

## CEREBROSPINAL FLUID RHINORRHEA

Frequently, but not exclusively, a nontraumatic CSF rhinorrhea occurs as the consequence of the development of an empty sella or a pituitary adenoma. This is perhaps the most difficult condition to be treated by the transsphenoidal approach.[30, 31] It can occur as an intraoperative complication in 6% to 20% of cases, depending on the characteristics of the sellar lesion.[50, 51] Furthermore, it can occur as an immediate or delayed postoperative complication in 3% to 6.4% of cases,[33, 52, 53] requiring reoperation in 1.5% to 2% of cases,[28, 32, 36, 47] although the frequency is decreasing in

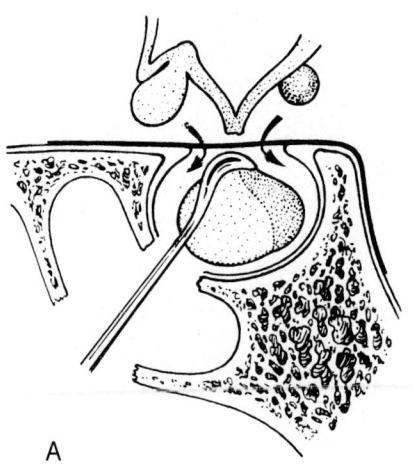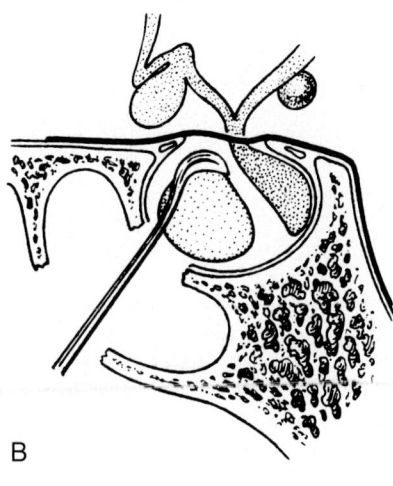

A                                    B

FIGURE 30–30 ■ Total *(A)* and anterior *(B)* selective functional hypophysectomy. In *A,* a section of the pituitary stalk is a factor predisposing the patient to cerebrospinal fluid leakage *(arrows)* and requires proper treatment.

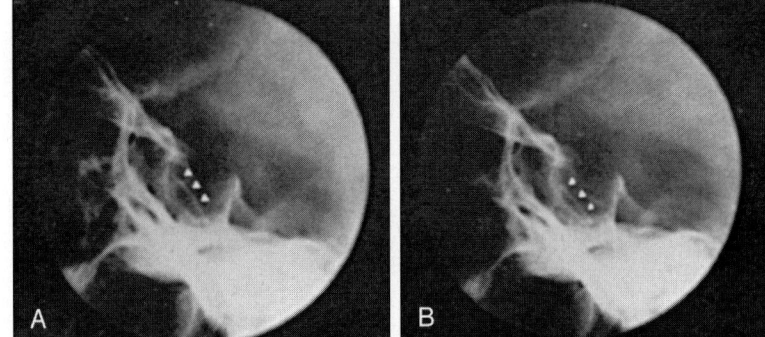

**FIGURE 30–31** ■ A roentgenogram of the sella turcica (lateral view). *A,* Five days and 3 months *(B)* after a transsphenoidal operation. The bone fragment limiting the extradural packing *(arrowheads)* is lowered because of scarring and retraction of the packing material.

recent clinical series. The success of an operation or reoperation for CSF rhinorrhea remains disappointing, with cure rates of approximately 80%, even in patients who have undergone multiple operations.[21, 31]

## ERRORS AND COMMON COMPLICATIONS

Reconstruction of the pituitary fossa may be ineffective, because either a nonsuitable method was chosen or the volume of packing material inserted was inadequate, either from the outset or because of its subsequent retraction or necrosis (Fig. 30–31) or because it was excessive.[9, 14] The consequences can be: (1) an intrasellar hematoma, (2) contamination of the cavity, (3) postoperative empty sella, or (4) CSF leakage. Care must be taken not to interpret a hyperdense lesion seen on an early postoperative computed tomography (CT) scan as a true postoperative hematoma (the actual frequency of which is less than 1% of cases[51]) (Fig. 30–32), because materials such as oxidized cellulose, Avitene, and fibrin sponge absorb blood and have an appearance on CT scans similar to that of a true blood clot.[14, 51, 54, 55] Also, a certain degree of intrasellar arachnoidocele

is a common finding on postoperative radiographic studies and is not a complication unless there are symptoms of an empty sella syndrome,[14] but this is a rare occurrence.[37]

CSF rhinorrhea can be transitory or prolonged. Prolonged CSF rhinorrhea persists for days after surgery, and when it does not improve despite suitable provisions, it requires surgical intervention (using the transsphenoidal, transethmoidal, or transcranial routes or even a CSF shunting procedure).[31, 32] Transitory CSF leakage is frequently seen in the early postoperative period but usually stops within a few hours or days, either spontaneously or after continuous CSF drainage.[36] We believe that this measure should be used whenever a CSF leak occurs, whether it is before, during, or immediately after surgery.[56, 57] We routinely insert a lumbar spinal subarachnoid catheter at the outset of the operation in all patients operated on by a transsphenoidal route, except those with a true microadenoma unless problems related to CSF leakage are anticipated.

Excessive packing of the sella is a less frequent event; its most serious and perhaps most common consequence is extension into the suprasellar cistern (Fig. 30–33), which recreates de novo chiasmal compression and alteration in the visual fields.[35, 37, 55] Besides the case of unperceived

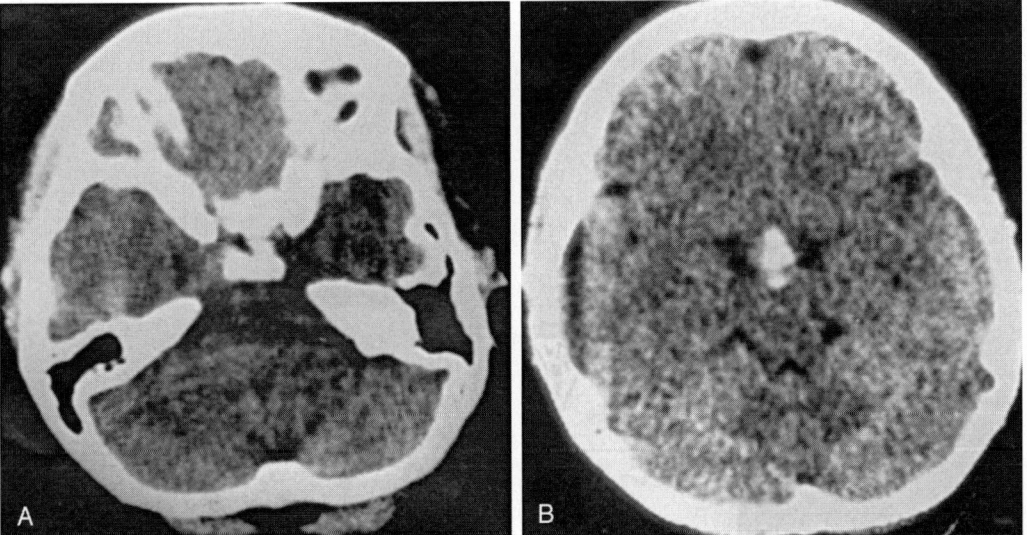

**FIGURE 30–32** ■ A computed tomography scan obtained 24 hours after a transsphenoidal operation for an adrenocorticotrophic hormone–secreting intrasellar and suprasellar adenoma demonstrating a bloody hyperdensity simulating a hematoma within the tumor bed that appears to be both intrasellar *(A)* and suprasellar *(B)*. Because the patient was complaining of worsening vision, she was operated on again. A hemostatic sponge was found.

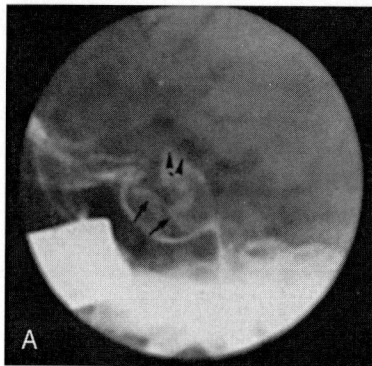
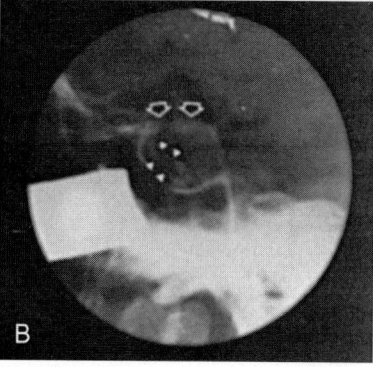

**FIGURE 30–33** ■ An intraoperative fluoroscopic image. *A,* An intrasellar adenoma bulging into the chiasmal cistern. Combined extradural *(arrows)* and intradural packing. There is so much intradural packing material (lightly soaked in iodinated contrast medium) that its upper limit *(arrowheads)* indents the suprasellar cistern demonstrated by means of perioperative pneumoencephalography (PEG). *B,* The amount of packing was reduced, freeing the chiasmal cistern. Its upper limit *(open white arrows)* is at the interclinoid plane. The *white arrowheads* outline the extradural packing.

introduction of overabundant filling materials, overpacking is usually a consequence of an attempt to cure intraoperative CSF leakage, a diffuse hemorrhage from a cut surface, or a severe hemorrhage originating from a cavernous sinus. If moderate in amount, the consequences of overpacking may regress because of the expected reduction in the volume of packing materials; otherwise, it is best to reoperate and remove this material rather than risk a useless and probably damaging wait. Excessive intrasellar compression, excessive traction, or distortion of the dura mater of the sellar floor and of the wall of the cavernous sinus may cause paresis of the oculomotor nerves,[51, 58] postoperative trigeminal syndrome,[5] or intense and persistent postoperative headaches. More exceptional complications caused by overpacking of the sella include compression or spasm of the carotid artery in its intracavernous segment.[53, 58]

## SUMMARY

Although the transsphenoidal approach to the pituitary fossa and removal of the lesion are carried out by all surgeons in a virtually identical fashion, there is little agreement concerning reconstruction of the surgical site. Conflicting ideas remain about the usefulness of careful reconstruction and hermetic closure of the sella, which, for some authors, is advisable only in cases with elements of high risk.[12, 23, 59]

The relative rarity of mechanical complications with this type of surgery has led to little consideration being given to this aspect. It should not be underestimated, because although such complications are rare, they are very difficult to treat and may be more incapacitating and more severe than the original lesion. Preventing them with such sophisticated surgery is, therefore, imperative.[28, 43]

Our experience is based on the 352 transsphenoidal operations summarized in Table 30–1. Tables 30–2, 30–3, and 30–4 show the procedure used, the risk factors that influenced surgery, and the postoperative complications observed, respectively. These findings have convinced us that the sellar region must routinely be reconstructed in the most careful and opportune way unless there are very specific reasons for a different approach.[60] Among the first 15 patients, we encountered one case of secondary empty sella and the reappearance of visual problems in another patient (Fig. 30–34), probably because of overpacking,[46]

certainly as a result of an unsuitable method of packing. In follow-up of 150 cases,[61] there were no serious mechanical complications, even though the conditions in many of the cases were particularly unfavorable (e.g., invasive giant adenoma, associated empty sella, spontaneous preoperative CSF rhinorrhea). Only one patient had to undergo repeat surgery; following a slight subjective deterioration of vision, a postoperative CT scan suggested the presence of an intrasellar hematoma that on reoperation turned out to be a blood-soaked hemostatic sponge (see also Fig. 30–32). In a previous report,[61] we maintained that this reoperation was unnecessary and the patient's visual function recovered spontaneously. However, subsequent experience in two identical cases has proved to us that in such occurrences

**TABLE 30–1** ■ **SYNOPSIS OF 352 TRANSSPHENOIDAL SURGICAL PROCEDURES PERFORMED FROM 1978 THROUGH 1992**

| Cause | No. of Cases |
|---|---|
| **Pituitary Tumors** | |
| Microadenoma | 70 |
| Intrasellar adenoma | 49 |
| Intrasellar adenoma indenting the chiasmal cistern | 28 |
| Suprasellar adenoma | 116 |
| Giant invasive adenoma | 20 |
| Total | 283 |
| **Other Sellar Tumors** | |
| Craniopharyngioma | 15 |
| Meningioma of the diaphragma sellae | 5 |
| Metastasis | 2 |
| Epidermoid tumor | 1 |
| Neurohypophyseal tumor | 1 |
| Chondrosarcoma | 1 |
| Total | 25 |
| **Empty Sella** | 10 |
| **Benign (Arachnoidal) Cyst Reoperation for Recurrence** | 4 |
| Pituitary adenoma (suprasellar) | 21 |
| Epidermoid tumor | 1 |
| Total | 22 |
| **Reoperation for Postoperative Complications** | |
| CSF rhinorrhea | 3 |
| Empty sella syndrome | 1 |
| Hematoma | 3 |
| Hemorrhagic infiltration | 1 |
| Total | 8 |

## TABLE 30–2 ■ FACTORS INFLUENCING THE SURGICAL PROCEDURE

| Factor | No. of Cases |
|---|---|
| Intrasellar Arachnoidocele Associated with Pituitary Tumor | 24 |
| Preoperative or Intraoperative CSF Leakage | 36 |
| **Previous Treatment** | |
| Transsphenoidal surgery | 11 |
| Transcranial surgery | 5 |
| External radiotherapy | 3 |
| External radiotherapy plus transsphenoidal surgery | 4 |
| External radiotherapy plus transcranial surgery | 3 |
| Total | 26 |

## TABLE 30–4 ■ SUMMARY OF THE TECHNIQUES OF SELLAR PACKING PERFORMED IN 352 TRANSSPHENOIDAL PROCEDURES

| Technique | No. of Cases |
|---|---|
| No packing | 93 |
| Intradural packing | 116 |
| Intradural-extradural packing | 62 |
| Extradural packing | 53 |
| Intradural with sphenoidal sinus packing | 28 |

there is not a strict correlation between surgical findings and outcomes. In all three cases, in fact, at reoperation, a few blood-soaked hemostats and blood clots were found, without any pressure effect. These findings were not those of a true hematoma exerting pressure effects on the surrounding structures, so that reoperation seemed useless; in all cases, on the contrary, visual disturbances disappeared completely in the immediate postoperative course. On the other hand, early postoperative CT scans very often show bloody collections reproducing the preoperative shape and size of the adenoma, even after the complete removal of a tumor and the patient being completely free of symptoms. The appearance of these features is caused by blood, fluid, packing, or hemostatic substances that may collect within the residual cavity, mainly when the tumor capsule fails to collapse. Early postoperative CT scans are, in other words, so difficult to evaluate[54] that they are not conclusive for a true diagnosis of postoperative *hematoma*: Indications for

## TABLE 30–3 ■ POSTOPERATIVE MECHANICAL COMPLICATIONS

| Complication | No. of Cases |
|---|---|
| **Requiring Reoperation** | |
| CSF rhinorrhea | 3 |
| Empty sella syndrome | 1 |
| Hematoma | 3 |
| Hemorrhagic infarction | 1 |
| Total | 8 |
| **Not Surgical** | |
| Hemorrhagic infarction | 1 |
| CSF rhinorrhea | 9 |
| Visual field defect | 2 |
| Diplopia | 3 |
| Diabetes insipidus | 5 |
| Total | 20 |
| **Mortality** | |
| Mechanical complications | |
| Hemorrhagic infarction | 2 |
| Other | |
| Pulmonary embolism | 1 |
| Extrapituitary disease | 1 |
| Respiratory failure | 1 |
| Total | 5 |

reoperation are based mainly on clinical findings. CT and magnetic resonance imaging (MRI) have a decisive role, on the contrary, in recognizing cases in which hemorrhage occurred not within the tumor cavity but as a hemorrhagic infiltration of a residual suprasellar tumor impinging the surrounding cerebral formations, caused by surgical manipulation. Such a serious and likely fatal complication (which occurred in two cases in our series) did not benefit from a transsphenoidal reoperation. In our more recent experience, based on 187 cases, the incidence of complications did not decrease, despite increasing confidence in the surgical technique. This is not surprising considering that a more aggressive approach was used that was aimed at more complete tumor removal and cases with very adverse features were admitted to transsphenoidal surgery (e.g., aging patients, huge recurring tumors), in which almost all complications occurred.

Of the most feared complications of transsphenoidal surgery, intrasellar abscess and related infectious complications are rare.[62–64] The possibility of a CSF leak with related dangers of septic meningitis, on the other hand, should be considered more frequently as well.

Multiple risk factors favor postoperative complications; therefore, reconstruction of the region should be performed meticulously. The most important risk factors follow.

1. Preoperative or intraoperative CSF leakage
2. A large residual cavity[37, 43]
3. Marked suprasellar extension of the lesion[27, 43, 52, 59]
4. Anomalous positioning of the dome of the adenoma after the removal of neoplastic tissue[22, 43]
5. A coexisting preoperative or intraoperative empty sella
6. Persistent bleeding after removal of an adenoma, even after prolonged compression and irrigation
7. Precarious preoperative visual function because of involvement of the chiasm
8. Previous surgery or radiotherapy[5, 8, 32, 65]
9. Ghost sella[28, 33, 41, 59]
10. Age

Natural biologic substances obtained during surgery or common reabsorbable materials used in neurosurgery fulfill the packing requirements in almost every situation.[28] Extradural packing, used on its own or together with intradural packing, constitutes the best method for producing a solid, stable closure of the sella, both immediately and with the passage of time. The consolidation is so effective that patients are often seen in which all the extradural packing undergoes pronounced ossification (Figs. 30–35 and 30–36).

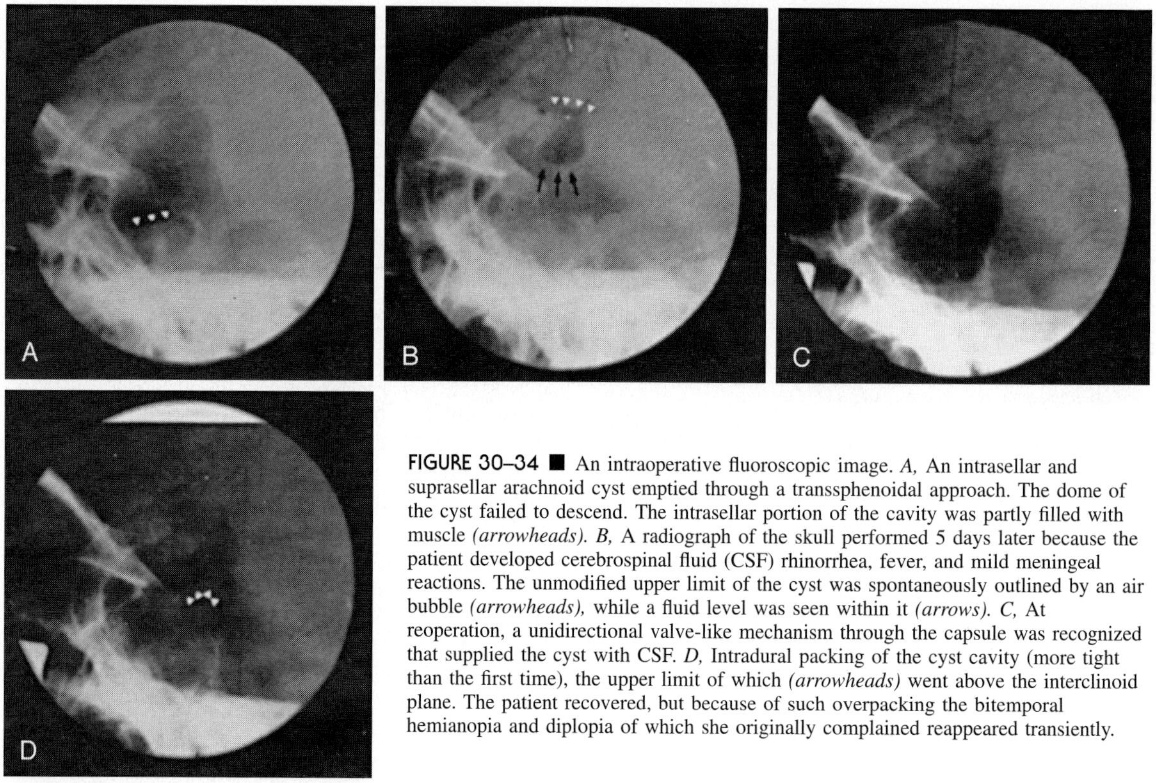

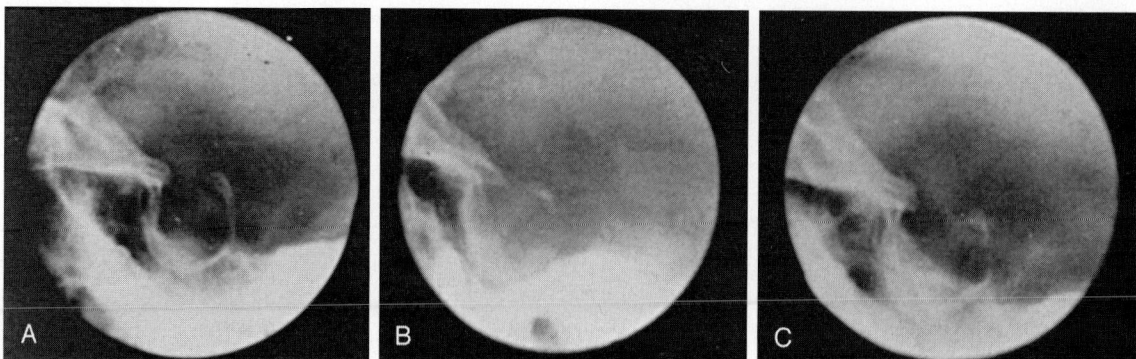

**FIGURE 30–34** ■ An intraoperative fluoroscopic image. *A,* An intrasellar and suprasellar arachnoid cyst emptied through a transsphenoidal approach. The dome of the cyst failed to descend. The intrasellar portion of the cavity was partly filled with muscle *(arrowheads)*. *B,* A radiograph of the skull performed 5 days later because the patient developed cerebrospinal fluid (CSF) rhinorrhea, fever, and mild meningeal reactions. The unmodified upper limit of the cyst was spontaneously outlined by an air bubble *(arrowheads)*, while a fluid level was seen within it *(arrows)*. *C,* At reoperation, a unidirectional valve-like mechanism through the capsule was recognized that supplied the cyst with CSF. *D,* Intradural packing of the cyst cavity (more tight than the first time), the upper limit of which *(arrowheads)* went above the interclinoid plane. The patient recovered, but because of such overpacking the bitemporal hemianopia and diplopia of which she originally complained reappeared transiently.

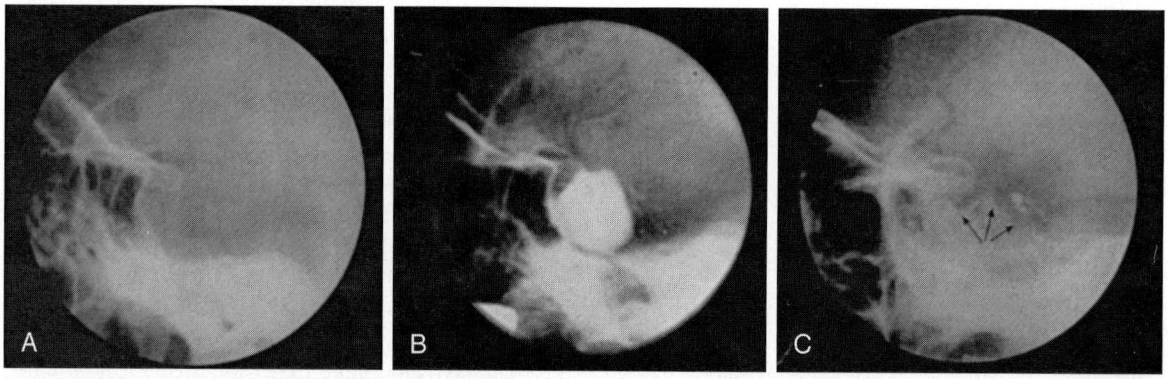

**FIGURE 30–35** ■ *A,* A preoperative radiograph of the skull showing an enlarged and eroded sella turcica with disappearance of the dorsum in a case of a growth hormone–secreting intrasellar adenoma. *B,* An intraoperative fluoroscopic image. The dimensions of the adenoma are shown by a sponge soaked in iodinated contrast medium introduced into the residual cavity. *C,* A radiograph of the skull was obtained 3 years later. The sellar boundaries and the dorsum sellae are recalcified. The materials used for intradural and extradural packing *(arrows)* are thinly calcified and ossified, as are the bone fragments lying in the sphenoidal sinus.

**FIGURE 30–36** ■ A roentgenogram of the skull before *(A)*, 1 year after *(B)*, and 3 years after *(C)* a transsphenoidal operation for empty sella with cerebrospinal fluid rhinorrhea that was cured with extradural packing. Progressive ossification of the packing material is clearly visible.

It would be extremely difficult to conceive a better result than this.

## ACKNOWLEDGMENTS

*The authors wish to thank Mr. Antonio D'Agostino, who lovingly and patiently prepared the drawings; Mr. Ciro Varchetta, who carefully prepared the photographs; and Mrs. Juliet Houlden, who checked the English translation with gracefulness and efficiency.*

## REFERENCES

1. de Divitiis E, Spaziante R, Stella L: Empty sella and benign intrasellar cysts. In Krayenbuhl H (ed): Advances and Technical Standards in Neurosurgery, Vol 8. Berlin: Springer-Verlag, 1981, pp 3–74.
2. Hardy J: Transsphenoidal microsurgery of the normal and pathological pituitary. Clin Neurosurg 16:185, 1969.
3. Laws ER Jr: Transsphenoidal approach to lesions in and about the sella turcica. In Schmidek HH, Sweet WH (eds): Current Techniques in Operative Neurosurgery. New York: Grune & Stratton, 1977, pp 161–172.
4. Ciric IS, Tarkington J: Transsphenoidal microsurgery. Surg Neurol 2:207, 1974.
5. Wilson CB, Dempsey LC: Transsphenoidal microsurgical removal of 250 pituitary adenomas. J Neurosurg 48:13, 1978.
6. Armenise B, Montinaro A: The prevention of nasal liquorrhea caused by transsphenoidal surgery for pituitary adenomas. J Neurosurg Sci 29:57, 1985.
7. Ludecke D, Kautzky R, Saeger W, et al: Selective removal of hypersecreting pituitary adenomas? Acta Neurochir 35:27, 1976.
8. Faria MA Jr, Tindall GT: Transsphenoidal microsurgery for prolactinomas. In Givens JR (ed): Hormone-Secreting Pituitary Tumors. Chicago: Year Book Medical Publishers, 1982, pp 275–297.
9. Hudgins WR, Raney LA, Young SW, et al: Failure of intrasellar muscle implants to prevent recurrent downward migration of the optic chiasm. Neurosurgery 8:231, 1981.
10. Peer LA: The neglected "free fat graft": Its behavior and clinical use. Am J Surg 92:40, 1956.
11. Guity A, Young PH: A new technique for closure of the dura following transsphenoidal and transclival operations. J Neurosurg 72:824, 1990.
12. Griffith HB: Transsphenoidal pituitary surgery. In Symon L (ed): Operative Surgery. London: Butterworths, 1979, pp 187–194.
13. Afshar F, Thomas A: Bromocriptine-induced cerebrospinal fluid rhinorrhea. Surg Neurol 18:61, 1982.
14. Kaplan HC, Baker HL Jr, Houser OW, et al: CT of the sella turcica after transsphenoidal resection of pituitary adenomas. AJNR Am J Neuroradiol 6:723, 1985.
15. Kobayashi S, Sugita K, Matsuo K, et al: Reconstruction of the sellar floor during transsphenoidal operations using alumina ceramic. Surg Neurol 15:196, 1980.
16. Kubota T, Hayashi M, Kabuto M, et al: Reconstruction of the skull base using a silicone plate during transsphenoidal surgery. Surg Neurol 36:360, 1991.
17. Nicola G: Transsphenoidal surgery for pituitary adenomas with extrasellar extension. In Krayenbuhl H, Maspes PE, Sweet WH (eds): Progress in Neurological Surgery. Basel: S. Karger, 1975, pp 142–199.
18. Young WC, Gates GA: The use of cyanoacrylate in transsphenoidal hypophysectomy. Laryngoscope 88:1784, 1978.
19. de Divitiis E, Spaziante R: Osteoplastic opening of the sellar floor in transsphenoidal surgery: Technical note. Neurosurgery 20:445, 1987.
20. Mickey BE, Samson D: Neurosurgical applications of the cyanoacrylate adhesives. Clin Neurosurg 28:429, 1981.
21. Ommaya AK: Spinal fluid fistulae. Clin Neurosurg 23:363, 1976.
22. Landolt AM, Strebel P: Technique of transsphenoidal operation for pituitary adenomas. In Krayenbuhl H (ed): Advances and Technical Standards in Neurosurgery, Vol 7. Berlin: Springer-Verlag, 1980, pp 119–177.
23. Rand RW: Fifteen years experience with transnasal transsphenoidal operation for pituitary tumours. In Brock M (ed): Modern Neurosurgery 1. Berlin: Springer-Verlag, 1982, pp 173–180.
24. Tindall GT, Collins WF Jr, Kirchner JA: Unilateral septal technique for transsphenoidal microsurgical approach to the sella turcica. J Neurosurg 49:138, 1978.
25. Weiss MH, Kaufman B, Richards DE: Cerebrospinal fluid rhinorrhea from an empty sella: Transsphenoidal obliteration of the fistula. J Neurosurg 39:674, 1973.
26. Landolt AM: Therapeutic aspects of the empty sella syndrome. In Glaser JS (ed): Neuro-ophthalmology, Vol 9. St. Louis: CV Mosby, 1977, pp 229–235.
27. Guiot G, Derome P, Demailly P, et al: Complications inattendue de l'exerese complete de volumineux adenomes hypophysaires. Rev Neurol 118:164, 1968.
28. Derome PJ, Visot AM, Delalande O, et al: Mechanical complications after the transsphenoidal removal of pituitary adenomas. In Derome PJ, Jedinak CP, Peillon F (eds): Pituitary Adenomas. Paris: Asclepios, 1980, pp 233–235.
29. Olson DR, Guiot G, Derome P: The symptomatic empty sella. Prevention and correction via the transsphenoidal approach. J Neurosurg 37:533, 1972.
30. Garcia-Uria J, Carrillo R, Serrano P, et al: Empty sella and rhinorrhea: A report of eight treated cases. J Neurosurg 50:466, 1979.
31. Hubbard JL, Mc Donald TJ, Pearson BW, et al: Spontaneous cerebrospinal fluid rhinorrhea: Evolving concepts in diagnosis and surgical management based on the Mayo Clinic experience from 1970 through 1981. Neurosurgery 16:314, 1985.
32. Laws ER Jr, Fode NC, Redmond MJ: Transsphenoidal surgery following unsuccessful prior therapy: An assessment of benefits and risks in 158 patients. J Neurosurg 63:823, 1985.
33. Landolt AM: Cerebrospinal fluid rhinorrhea: A complication of therapy for invasive prolactinomas. Neurosurgery 11:395, 1982.
34. Altinörs N, Arda N, Kars K, et al: Tension pneumocephalus after transsphenoidal surgery: Case report. Neurosurgery 23:516, 1988.
35. Hardy J, Beauregard H, Robert F: Prolactin-secreting pituitary adenomas: Transsphenoidal microsurgical treatment. Clin Neurosurg 27:38, 1980.
36. Black PMcL, Zervas NT, Candia GL: Incidence and management of complications of transsphenoidal operation for pituitary adenomas. Neurosurgery 20:920, 1987.
37. Laws ER Jr, Kern EB: Complications of transsphenoidal surgery. In Tindall GT, Collins WF (eds): Clinical Management of Pituitary Disorders. New York: Raven Press, 1979, pp 435–445.
38. Spaziante R, de Divitiis E: Forced subarachnoid air in transsphenoidal excision of pituitary tumors. J Neurosurg 71:864, 1989.
39. Nakane T, Kuwayama A, Watanabe M, et al: Transsphenoidal approach to pituitary adenomas with suprasellar extension. Surg Neurol 16:225, 1981.
40. Goldman JA, Hedges TR III, Shucart W, et al: Delayed chiasmal decompression after transsphenoidal operation for a pituitary adenoma. Neurosurgery 17:962, 1985.
41. Wilson CB: Neurosurgical management of large and invasive pituitary tumors. In Tindall GT, Collins WF (eds): Clinical Management of Pituitary Disorders. New York: Raven Press, 1979, pp 335–342.
42. Spaziante R, de Divitiis E, Stella L, et al: The empty sella. Surg Neurol 16:418, 1981.
43. Guiot G, Derome P: Surgical problems of pituitary adenomas. In Krayenbuhl H (ed): Advances and Technical Standards in Neurosurgery, Vol 3. Berlin: Springer-Verlag, 1976, pp 3–33.
44. Nagao S, Kinusaga K, Nishimoto A: Obliteration of the primary empty sella by transsphenoidal extradural balloon inflation: Technical note. Surg Neurol 27:455, 1987.
45. Cybulski GR, Stone JL, Geremia G, Anson J: Intrasellar balloon inflation for treatment of symptomatic empty sella syndrome. Neurosurgery 24:105, 1989.
46. Spaziante R, de Divitiis E, Stella L, et al: Benign intrasellar cysts. Surg Neurol 15:274, 1981.
47. Baskin DS, Wilson CB: Transsphenoidal treatment of non-neoplastic intrasellar cysts: A report of 38 cases. J Neurosurg 60:8, 1984.
48. Laws ER Jr: Transsphenoidal microsurgery in the management of craniopharyngioma. J Neurosurg 52:661, 1980.
49. Tindall GT, Payne NS, Nixon DW: Transsphenoidal hypophysectomy for disseminated carcinoma of the prostate gland: Results in 53 patients. J Neurosurg 50:275, 1979.
50. Balagura S, Derome P, Guiot G: Acromegaly: Analysis of 132 cases treated surgically. Neurosurgery 8:413, 1981.
51. Hardy J, Mohr G: Le prolactinomes. Aspects chirurgicaux. Neurochirurgie 27(Suppl 1):41, 1981.

52. Ciric I, Mikhael M, Stafford T, et al: Transsphenoidal microsurgery of pituitary macroadenomas with long-term follow-up results. J Neurosurg 59:395, 1983.
53. Horwitz NH, Rizzoli HV: Postoperative Complications of Intracranial Neurological Surgery. Baltimore: Williams & Wilkins, 1982, p 472.
54. Nelson PB, Robinson AG, Hirsch W: Postoperative computed tomography evaluation of patients with large pituitary tumors treated with operative decompression and radiation therapy. Neurosurgery 28:238, 1991.
55. Dolinskas CA, Simeone FA: Transsphenoidal hypophysectomy: Postsurgical CT findings. AJNR Am J Neuroradiol 6:45, 1985.
56. Findler G, Sahar A, Beller AJ: Continuous lumbar drainage of cerebrospinal fluid in neurosurgical patients. Surg Neurol 8:455, 1977.
57. Loew F, Pertuiset B, Chaumier EE, et al: Traumatic, spontaneous and post-operative CSF rhinorrhea. In Symon L (ed): Advances and Technical Standards in Neurosurgery, Vol 11. Berlin: Springer-Verlag, 1984, pp 171–207.
58. Laws ER Jr: Complications of transsphenoidal microsurgery for pituitary adenoma. In Brock M (ed): Modern Neurosurgery 1. Berlin: Springer-Verlag, 1982, pp 181–186.
59. Nicola GC, Tonnarelli GP, Griner AC: Complications of transsphenoidal surgery in pituitary adenomas. In Derome PJ, Jedinak CP, Peillon F (eds): Pituitary Adenomas. Paris: Asclepios, 1980, pp 237–240.
60. Spaziante R, de Divitiis E, Cappabianca P: Reconstruction of the pituitary fossa in transsphenoidal surgery: An experience of 140 cases. Neurosurgery 17:453, 1985.
61. Spaziante R, de Divitiis E, Cappabianca P: Techniques of reconstruction of the sella and related structures. In Schmidek HH, Sweet WH (eds): Operative Neurosurgical Techniques. New York: Grune & Stratton, 1988, pp 321–337.
62. Robinson B: Intrasellar abscess after transsphenoidal pituitary adenomectomy. Neurosurgery 12:684, 1983.
63. Nelson PB, Hirsch BE, De Vries EJ: Abscess of the sphenoid sinus after transsphenoidal surgery. Neurosurgery 28:152, 1991.
64. Onishi H, Haruhide I, Kuroda E, et al: Intracranial mycotic aneurysm associated with transsphenoidal surgery to the pituitary adenoma. Surg Neurol 31:149, 1989.
65. Baskin DS, Boggan JE, Wilson CB: Transsphenoidal microsurgical removal of growth hormone-secreting pituitary adenomas: A review of 137 cases. J Neurosurg 56:634, 1982.

# Transcranial Surgery for Pituitary Macroadenomas

■ CHRIS B. T. ADAMS

## INDICATIONS FOR TRANSCRANIAL SURGERY FOR PITUITARY TUMORS

Pituitary tumors are usually treated by the transsphenoidal approach for several reasons: It is a less intrusive operation; the surgeon comes straight down onto the tumor and can preserve the normal pituitary tissue; there is negligible risk of epilepsy; and recovery of vision and the visual fields is quicker because the optic nerves and chiasm are not manipulated. In some circumstances, transsphenoidal surgery is contraindicated or insufficient. The procedure is insufficient when the surgery fails to remove adequate amounts of tumor, particularly to decompress the optic chiasm. The alternative is the transcranial approach.

The transcranial approach is indicated when transsphenoidal surgery is contraindicated. The usual reason is doubt about diagnosis. If the lesion may *not* be a pituitary adenoma but perhaps a meningioma or craniopharyngioma, a craniotomy is advisable. Occasionally an entirely intrasellar meningioma or craniopharyngioma can be removed by the transsphenoidal route, but in general these lesions are more safely removed transcranially. A clue to a meningioma is seeing a *tongue* of pathologic tissue extending particularly along the floor of the anterior cranial fossa. A clue to a craniopharyngioma is a presentation with diabetes insipidus. Diabetes insipidus is indicative of a hypothalamic disorder, and pituitary adenomas do not cause diabetes insipidus initially.

Another indication for the transcranial approach is failed transsphenoidal surgery. There are several reasons for this failure. One is that the pituitary adenoma is too tough. Transsphenoidal surgery relies on the surgeon removing the intrasellar component, then the suprasellar component falling into the cavity created. A few adenomas are tough. In those circumstances, I advise taking no more than a biopsy specimen and obliterating the sphenoid sinus. The latter action may seem unnecessary with a large tough tumor between the nasal cavity and the cerebrospinal fluid, but I have regretted not obliterating the sphenoid sinus in these (unusual) circumstances when subsequently performing transcranial surgery. It is the consistency of the tumor, not the size, that limits the effectiveness of transsphenoidal surgery.

Failure of the suprasellar extension to descend is another reason for failed transsphenoidal surgery. The usual cause is that a component of the tumor is extending superiorly, laterally, or anteriorly (Fig. 31–1). If the suprasellar extension has pushed vertically, it usually falls into the tumor cavity created by the transsphenoidal surgeon. If an extension of tumor hooks around the optic nerve or carotid artery, this extension prevents descent of the tumor, and the tumor extension above the carotid artery or chiasm is inaccessible. The anterior extension is particularly troublesome for the transsphenoidal surgeon, being just at the wrong angle to the line of approach (Fig. 31–2). Finally, recurrent pituitary adenomas may not fall down satisfactorily because of adhesions between the tumor and the sur-

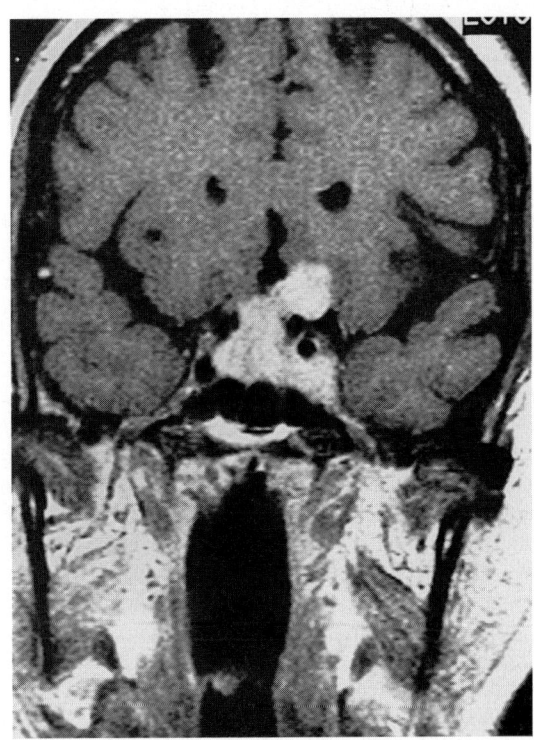

FIGURE 31–1 ■ A magnetic resonance imaging scan showing the suprasellar extension hooking laterally and preventing the descent of the tumor during transsphenoidal surgery.

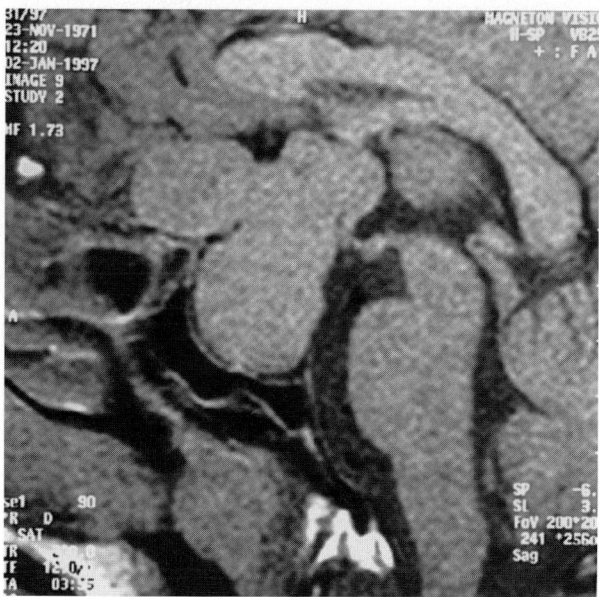

FIGURE 31–2 ■ A magnetic resonance imaging scan to show the suprasellar extension of a growth hormone–secreting tumor that extends anteriorly. A radical removal was achieved by a transcranial approach. Note the position of the anterior communicating artery.

rounding brain. In these circumstances, the combined transcranial/transsphenoidal approach may be the best way of total eradication of the tumor, which may be justified if the tumor has recurred despite previous irradiation. Radical surgery is also indicated for a hormone-secreting adenoma, such as acromegaly (or Cushing's syndrome), in which hormonal cure depends on total removal of the tumor.

## PREOPERATIVE CONSIDERATIONS

All patients should have a magnetic resonance imaging (MRI) scan. This scan shows the vessels well so that formal angiography is not usually indicated. The visual fields should be formally recorded, and pituitary function tests should be performed. The transcranial route almost inevitably causes hypopituitarism because the normal pituitary tissue is pushed superiorly under the diaphragma sella, and it is this tissue that is coagulated and cut by the surgeon en route to the tumor (Fig. 31–3). Two pints of blood should be crossmatched. Epilepsy is possible after transcranial surgery, and anticonvulsants such as a hydantoin should be started preoperatively. The patient should be warned of this possibility and the effect this might have on driving, working with machinery, or ascending heights. The patient should be warned of the risks of surgery, both general and specific. General risks are those of any operation, such as deep vein thrombosis, bleeding into the operative cavity, infection, the anesthetic, and epilepsy when a craniotomy is carried out. The specific risks are those of damage to the optic nerve or nerves (impaired vision or visual fields), damage to the blood vessels (internal carotid artery or anterior cerebral arteries), and damage to the pituitary stalk (hypopituitarism and diabetes insipidus). Ce-

rebrospinal fluid rhinorrhea occasionally occurs and anosmia, especially if excessive retraction of the frontal lobe is needed.

## PREFIXED CHIASM

The length of the intracranial optic nerves varies from patient to patient. The tumor extension influences the distance of the optic nerves to the tuberculum sella. If the suprasellar extension thrusts between the optic nerves, it pushes the chiasm upward and backward, allowing good access for the surgeon. Sometimes the suprasellar extension pushes the chiasm upward and forward, however, severely limiting the surgeon's access. This is called *prefixed chiasm*. The position of a chiasm can be predicted on the sagittal MRI scan by finding the anterior communicating artery (shown in the sagittal MRI section as a black dot—see Fig. 31–3), which denotes the position of the chiasm.

## AIMS OF SURGERY

The aims of pituitary surgery are ultimately to cure the patient of the tumor, without damage to the pituitary; to relieve the symptoms and the signs that have been caused by the tumor; and to achieve this relief without damage to the patient. When the tumor is hormone secreting, total extirpation of the tumor is necessary to achieve a cure. A nonfunctioning tumor does not necessarily require total removal, especially if the risks of such an attempt are significant. In these circumstances, the aims should be an adequate debulking of the tumor to produce chiasmal and optic nerve decompression before radiotherapy or radiosurgery.

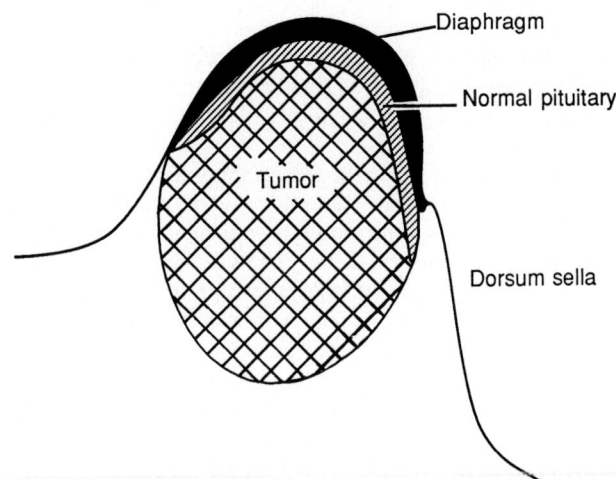

FIGURE 31–3 ■ Diagram to show how the adenoma pushes the normal pituitary superiorly as a thin rind. This makes the normal pituitary tissue particularly vulnerable during transcranial surgery, whereas it is relatively protected with transsphenoidal surgery.

## TECHNIQUE OF TRANSCRANIAL PITUITARY SURGERY

I advise a pterional craniotomy[2]; it is unnecessary in general to use a bifrontal approach. In determining which side to operate on, there are two main factors. If one eye is already blind, I would operate on the side of the blind eye because the ipsilateral optic nerve (to the craniotomy) is most vulnerable to operative manipulation. The other factor is the lateral extension of the tumor. It makes more sense to operate on the side of maximal tumor extension.

The patient is positioned supine with the head turned about 40 degrees to the opposite side and slightly extended. An incision is marked out just behind the hairline from the zygomatic arch to the midline.[2] I turn a pterional free bone flap; I still prefer making drill holes and using a Gigli saw because I believe it is safer. I nibble the sphenoid wing away, then open the dura. If the tumor is large, I ask the anesthetist to administer mannitol or a diuretic to shrink the brain. If the tumor is blocking the third ventricle or foramina of Monro, causing hydrocephalus, a ventricular drain can be inserted.

The dura is opened in a gentle curve just above the eyebrow and hitched up. I then introduce the operating microscope and split the sylvian fissure. This is a key maneuver and allows the main middle cerebral artery, the anterior cerebral artery, and the internal carotid artery to be identified and safeguarded. I cover the exposed frontal lobe with absorbable fabric (Surgicel). This covering protects the brain and allows cotton strips or patties to be placed on and peeled off without damaging the brain surface. A retractor should never be placed on bare brain but always on a pattie. While the sylvian fissure is split, cerebrospinal fluid is gently sucked away relieving intracranial pressure. Having traced back to the internal carotid artery, the optic nerve is then identified.

The next step is to debulk the tumor. If there is sufficient space, this debulking is done by working between the optic nerves. If a chiasm is prefixed, it may be easier to work between the optic nerve and the chiasm (Fig. 31–4). Early in the operation, the surgeon should avoid working near the ipsilateral optic nerve and concentrate on debulking the tumor. I do this using bipolar coagulation and cutting out the contents with scissors. If soft, the tumor center can be sucked out, which is easier for the surgeon. I find the ultrasonic aspirator too bulky and potentially dangerous. Angled curets, Bronson Ray type, are helpful. As the debulking proceeds, the opposite optic nerve and internal carotid artery are identified. I avoid coagulating and cutting vessels running to the chiasm if possible; I also avoid taking vessels when working between the optic nerves and carotid artery, often these being perforating vessels.

As debulking proceeds, the tumor capsule (the compressed tumor and thinned diaphragma sella) can be gradually drawn down and excised. I find the sucker (held in the left hand) is a useful instrument to bring the capsule down, especially if one makes a hole in the capsule and inserts the sucker in the hole. I start the capsule removal near the left (if operating on the right) optic nerve and internal carotid artery so that these vital structures become defined. Having done this, I work my way superiorly toward the chiasm. If the anterior cerebral artery is surrounded or severely distorted, this needs defining at an early stage. At this point, I trace the right (ipsilateral) anterior cerebral artery from the carotid bifurcation. By working from one side (laterally), then from the other side (medial side), I define the anterior communicating artery and the chiasm at the summit of the tumor.

Having delivered the summit of the tumor, the surgeon is in a better position to remove the most difficult part of the tumor: the ipsilateral component compressing the optic nerve and internal carotid artery on the side of the exposure. The only time I invariably use angled bipolar forceps is for this stage of the operation. These forceps are invaluable for coagulating the capsule *hidden* by the ipsilateral optic nerve.

Once the suprasellar component is delivered, I coagulate the capsule at the level of the dorsum sellae, amputating the suprasellar component from the intrasellar component. The pituitary stalk is almost invariably seen in the angle between the optic nerve and the carotid artery. It is easily recognized by the striated appearance of the long axis of pituitary stalk resulting from the portal venous system.[3]

Using angled curets, the intrasellar component is removed. Much of this removal is done blindly, the bleeding

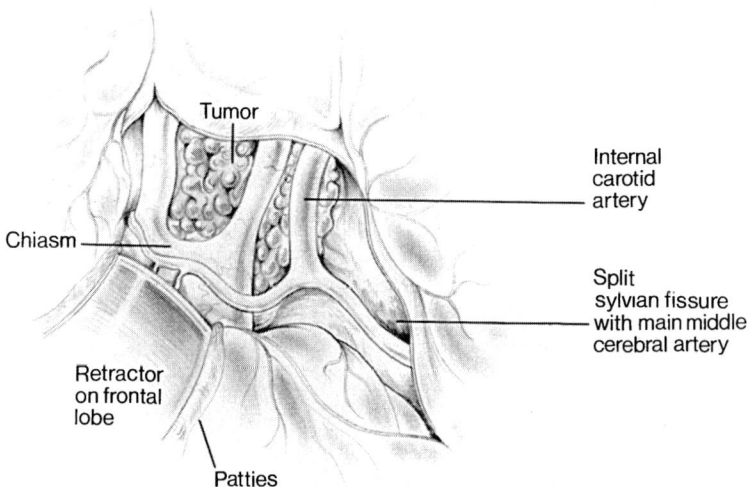

FIGURE 31–4 ■ A diagrammatic view of the usual anatomy. Note the approach between the optic nerve and the internal carotid artery to the pituitary adenoma.

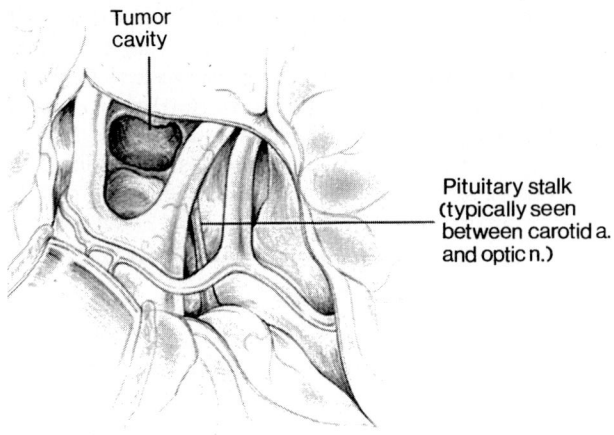

FIGURE 31–5 ■ The anatomy after the removal of the tumor. The pituitary stalk is usually seen between the optic nerve and the internal carotid artery.

controlled by pressure, patience, and Surgicel. If previous transsphenoidal surgery has been carried out and the sphenoid sinus has *not* been obliterated, pericranium and temporalis muscle are taken to produce a watertight cerebrospinal fluid closure of the pituitary fossa (Fig. 31–5).

I then close the wound in a routine fashion, checking hemostasis, replacing the cerebrospinal fluid that was sucked away with Ringer's solution, closing the dura, and replacing the bone flap. Particular care should be taken to inspect the frontal lobe; excessive retraction can occur too easily without the surgeon realizing it, while concentrating on the pituitary tumor down the microscope and not appreciating the degree of fixed retraction on the frontal lobe.

## RADICAL COMBINED TRANSCRANIAL AND TRANSSPHENOIDAL APPROACH

Occasionally, it is necessary to aim for a complete radical removal of the tumor, for instance, when a tumor has recurred despite radiotherapy. In these circumstances, I have completed removal of the suprasellar component, then drilled off the tuberculum sella between the optic nerves and the optic foramina (Fig. 31–6). The sphenoid sinus is entered, allowing the mucosa to be displaced and the anterior wall of the pituitary fossa to be removed. Removal of the sellar component can be achieved under direct vision except for the ipsilateral intrasellar tumor being less visible. Alternatively a separate transsphenoidal approach can be carried out, and that has the advantage of better bilateral tumor exposure but the disadvantage of possibly failing to see remaining tumor superiorly. Whichever method the surgeon uses, particular care must be taken to achieve a cerebrospinal fluid tight closure with obliteration of the sphenoid sinus.

## POSTOPERATIVE COMPLICATIONS

### General Complications

General complications include infection, bleeding into the operative cavity, epilepsy, and leakage of cerebrospinal fluid. These complications are common to any supratentorial craniotomy and are not considered further except cerebrospinal fluid leakage. This complication occurs in two circumstances. The first is if a previous transsphenoidal operation has been performed and an inadequate obliteration of the sphenoid sinus has been achieved. I have already alluded to the necessity to obliterate the sphenoid sinus during a transsphenoidal approach when a transcranial procedure is clearly going to be necessary in the future. This necessity is so even when no cerebrospinal fluid is seen. Failure to do so means cerebrospinal fluid rhinorrhea is extremely likely after the transcranial approach because the dural lining of the pituitary fossa has been penetrated during the transsphenoidal approach. In these circumstances, fascia and fat may be introduced into the pituitary fossa transcranially, but it is not easy to obtain a watertight closure this way. The second circumstance when cerebrospinal fluid rhinorrhea may be seen is when bone is drilled away from the skull base, thus entering an extension of the sphenoid sinus. If recognized, a fat and fascia repair is necessary. Rhinorrhea usually ensures when such an occurrence has not been recognized.

### Frontal Lobe Damage

Frontal lobe damage is perhaps the commonest complication, although often unappreciated because its manifestations may be subtle. It is particularly likely to occur in the elderly and is due to excessive frontal lobe retraction. The elderly especially take longer to recover from this surgery than after transsphenoidal surgery. There may be subtle changes of memory, judgment (on a social or professional level), concentration, and personality. These changes can be minimized by gentle technique and especially minimal brain retraction. A pattie or cotton strip should always be placed between the brain and the retractor. The retractor should be moved frequently and removed when it is not needed. Splitting the sylvian fissure to separate the frontal and temporal lobes also minimizes the amount of retraction. If there is evidence of an area of soft blue brain at

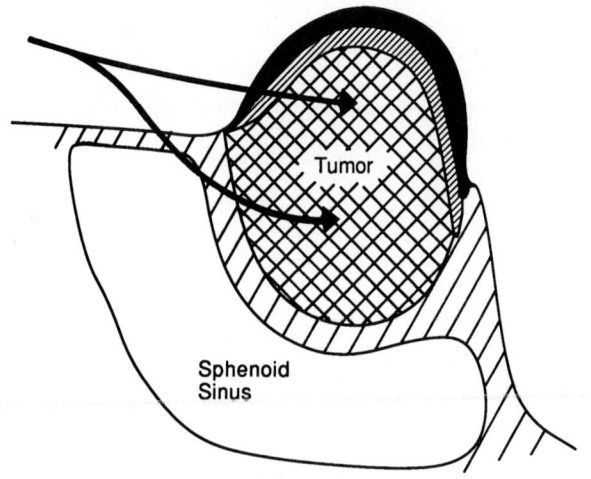

FIGURE 31–6 ■ The combined transcranial, transsphenoidal approach for the radical removal of a pituitary adenoma.

the end of the operation, the surgeon should beware. This area may represent hemorrhagic infarction and often causes postoperative bleeding and deterioration. Such areas should be removed surgically before closing the dura.

## Frontal Lobe Cyst Formation

Cystic enlargement of an area of frontal lobe damage sufficient to act as a space-occupying lesion may occur. I have described one such case and speculated on the causal mechanism.[2]

## Anosmia

Unilateral or bilateral anosmia often reflects the vigor of frontal lobe retraction. If there is a significant subfrontal extension of the pituitary tumor, anosmia is inevitable.

## Perioperative Optic Nerve Damage

If an eye is blind preoperatively, it will not recover postoperatively. If vision is severely impaired preoperatively, it is also unlikely to recover, and if such a nerve is manipulated at all, vision is likely to be lost altogether postoperatively. The patient should be thus warned.

The most vulnerable nerve is the ipsilateral optic nerve. The only rule is not to touch or manipulate it, but this is rarely possible to achieve. Before teasing tumor away, the tumor should be debulked as much as possible and only at the last stage when space has been created should the remaining tumor be rolled away from the optic nerve. Meningiomas creep down the optic foramen, but in my experience, pituitary tumors do not behave in that fashion.

The blood supply of the optic nerve, nerves, and chiasm varies. The chiasm is supplied by small vessels from the anterior communicating artery, and these must be preserved. The rule is not to coagulate or cut any significant-looking vessel running to the chiasm or optic nerves. In general, however, I suspect that it is manipulation of these structures that usually causes the damage rather than ischemia.

## Damage to the Internal Carotid, Anterior Cerebral, or Anterior Communicating Arteries

One of the most unpleasant occasions of my neurosurgical career was cutting the internal carotid artery. The patient was elderly, had undergone two previous craniotomies and radiotherapy for the pituitary tumor, and the artery was embedded in scar tissue. I did not see the artery; this, however, is not an excuse because I should have picked up the middle cerebral artery and traced it proximally. This tracing can be extremely difficult. On another occasion, I damaged both anterior cerebral arteries. The tumor was firmly adherent to these vessels, and I should have stopped the operation leaving tumor behind around the vessels; this was an error of judgment.

Although the literature describes such vascular damage repaired by fine sutures, I have been unable to achieve such repairs in these circumstances. I try to place aneurysm clips so as to occlude the hole in the vessel without occluding the vessel; this has occasionally worked. Usually, however, I end up having to occlude the vessel to stop the bleeding.

Occasionally one pulls a small vessel out of the side of a larger vessel. It can be difficult to stop the bleeding, but I find that placing the finest bipolar forceps on either side of the hole and using low bipolar coagulation seals the hole without occluding the main vessel.

## Hypothalamic Damage

Hypothalamic damage is rare after removal of a pituitary adenoma. It is easily caused by overenthusiastic removal of a craniophyaryngioma. With hypothalamic damage, the patient loses sense of thirst and hunger. Fluid control can be achieved only by weighing the patient, and excessive weight gain is usual. Hypothalamic wasting or a precocious puberty occurs in the presence of tumors, usually hypothalamic gliomas, and not after surgical trauma. To remove or not to remove a craniopharyngioma intimately involved in the hypothalamus demands the finest surgical judgment, with the desire to achieve a total removal yet the need to avoid devastating hypothalamic damage. Any publication addressing the results of craniopharyngioma surgery that does not include dispassionate assessment of endocrine and psychological tests (especially for memory) is not worth reading.

## Pituitary Damage, Including Diabetes Insipidus

Damage to anterior pituitary function is common after transfrontal surgery because the normal pituitary gland is usually pushed superiorly against the diaphragma sella rather like a rind around the tumor (see Fig. 31–3). The diaphragma is the first thing to be coagulated and cut when removing such tumor transcranially, hence destroying normal function. Pituitary replacement hormone therapy maintains reasonable health, but the patient never returns to normal. The patient seems sluggish both physically and mentally and gains weight. The standard hormone replacement therapy does not include growth hormone or other hormones given in the physiologically pulsatile fashion. Perhaps there are other hormones yet to be discovered.

Fluids should be restricted to 2 L/day for 48 hours postoperatively. A postoperative diuresis is normal, especially in patients cured of acromegaly. If the urinary output is more than 200 ml/h for 3 hours, plasma and urinary osmolality are measured. If the former is more (and the latter less) than 295 mOsm/kg, desmopressin should be administered. The osmalality measurements should be repeated in 24 hours.

## Salt-Losing Syndrome

Salt-losing syndrome is rare. It is alarming and usually occurs 1 to 2 weeks after the operation.[4–7] My patient developed a headache, then lapsed rapidly into a coma and on admission had a low sodium value. The mechanism is unknown, but salt-losing syndrome is assumed to be due to inappropriate antidiuretic hormone secretion. It is difficult to measure antidiuretic hormone and so not enough is known about this rare condition. I advise placing a central venous line to determine if it is primarily a low sodium (low venous pressure) or water overload (high venous pressure). I treated (successfully) my patient empirically with rapid infusions of fluids and salt, then restricted fluids to increase the serum sodium. Until more is known about this mysterious condition, it can be treated only empirically. Kelly et al[6] recommend using urea for salt-losing syndrome, pointing out that urea enhances sodium reabsorption at the kidney. I have no experience using urea but would try it if again faced with this problem.

## Postoperative Visual Deterioration (Table 31–1)

Acute visual deterioration within hours of surgery is usually due to a postoperative hematoma in the tumor cavity. The best way to avoid this situation is to be sure to remove the tumor in its entirety. If, however, the tumor invades the clivus, bleeding from the cancellous bone can be difficult to stop, although bone wax, Surgicel, and patience are usually sufficient. Reoperation is necessary.

Olsen and coworkers[15] have described acute deterioration after transsphenoidal surgery resulting from herniation of a chiasm into the pituitary fossa. This condition is amazingly rare, considering how, after transsphenoidal surgery, the diaphragma rapidly descends to the floor of the pituitary fossa on many occasions without visual impairment. The question can be asked if herniation per se (apart from Guiot's unique case) can cause visual deterioration.

Occasionally, and in my experience this has been just after transsphenoidal surgery (but I do not see why it should *not* happen after transcranial surgery), a unilateral loss of vision occurs about 8 days after surgery. Morello and Frera[12] describe a similar patient. I agree with their conclusion that ischemic damage is the most likely explanation.

Insidious visual deterioration is almost always due to recurrent tumor, which usually reproduces the original visual field deficit (ie, a bitemporal hemianopia). Another possibility is radiation damage to the optic nerves or chiasm after radiotherapy. This visual deterioration usually occurs 9 to 18 months after radiotherapy and is often

### TABLE 31–1 ■ CAUSES OF POSTOPERATIVE VISUAL FAILURE

| Immediately postoperatively | Hematoma |
| | Operative damage |
| | Acute empty sella syndrome |
| Subacute (usually 8 days postoperatively) | Unilateral; probably ischemic |
| Months after operation/irradiation | Recurrent tumor |
| | Irradiation damage |
| | ?Empty sella syndrome—doubtful |
| | ?Scarring of chiasm without displacement—doubtful |

### TABLE 31–2 ■ CLASSIFICATION OF RESULTS

| Type | Size (mm) | % Cure Rate After Transsphenoidal Approach |
| --- | --- | --- |
| Microadenoma | <10 | 80 |
| Mesoadenoma | 10–20 | 80 |
| Macroadenoma | >20 | 40 |

sudden and unilateral. The mechanism is vascular damage and hence similar to stoke. Some improvement may occur. Guy et al[8] suggest gadolinium-enhanced MRI scanning to confirm the diagnosis of radiation damage.

A third possibility has been suggested: herniation of the chiasm into the pituitary fossa as described previously, acutely. I believe most of these cases have been due to radiation damage. There is also confusion in much of the literature regarding damage resulting from scarring around the optic nerve and chiasm (without necessarily any significant herniation into the fossa) and actual displacement of the optic nerves and chiasm. I am not convinced of visual deterioration by the so-called empty sella syndrome. At the time of writing, there are no studies with controls (i.e., MRI studies of chiasmal or optic nerve positions on postoperative patients without visual deterioration). Those interested should consult references.[9–26]

## RESULTS

There are no modern meaningful results for transcranial surgery because such an approach is usually carried out only when the standard transsphenoidal approach fails. The older literature provides the sort of results obtained by transcranial surgery.[27–38] In general, my results from transsphenoidal surgery mirror the size of the tumor. I use a simple classification (Table 31–2). I recommend the introduction of a group, *mesoadenoma*, signifying tumors 1 to 2 cm maximum diameter as measured on MRI. Often, these are classified by other authors as *macroadenomas*, but the surgical results are similar to microadenomas, and they should be delineated from macroadenomas. Invasive adenomas are usually macroadenomas, and the few exceptions to this rule do not justify more complicated classifications.[1] Dolenc[39] has advocated the direct exploration of a cavernous sinus. I suspect, however, that gamma knife radiosurgery will be the treatment of choice for extensions within the cavernous sinus, although further evaluation of both of these techniques is required.

## REFERENCES

1. Adams CBT: The management of pituitary tumours and postoperative visual deterioration. Acta Neurochir (Wien) 94:103–116, 1988.
2. Adams CBT: A Neurosurgeon's Notebook. Oxford: Blackwell Scientific, 1998.
3. Harris GW: Neural control of the pituitary gland: II. The adenohypothesis. BMJ 2:627–634, 1951.
4. Andrews BT, Fitzgerald PA, Tyrell JB, Wilson CB: Cerebral salt wasting after pituitary exploration and biopsy: Case report. Neurosurgery 18:469–471, 1986.

5. Siva Kumar V, Raj Shekhar V, Chandy MJ: Management of neurosurgical patients with hyponatremia and natriuresis. Neurosurgery 34:269–274, 1994.
6. Kelly DF, Laws ER Jr, Fossett D: Delayed hyponatremia after transsphenoidal surgery for pituitary adenoma: Report of nine cases. J Neurosurg 83:363–367, 1995.
7. Olson BR, Gumowski J, Rubino D, Oldfield EH: Pathophysiology of hyponatremia after transsphenoidal pituitary surgery. J Neurosurg 87:499–507, 1997.
8. Guy J, Mancuso A, Beck R, et al: Radiation-induced optic neuropathy: A magnetic resonance imaging study. J Neurosurg 74:426–432, 1991.
9. Buys SN, Kerns TC: Irradiation damage to the chiasm. Am J Ophthalmol 44:483–486, 1957.
10. Crompton MR, Layton DD: Delayed radionecrosis of the brain following therapeutic x-radiation of the pituitary. Brain 83:85–101, 1961.
11. Colby MY Jr, Kearns TP: Radiation therapy of pituitary adenomas with associated visual impairment. P Mayo Clin Proc 37:15–24, 1962.
12. Morello G, Frera C: Visual damage after removal of hypophyseal adenomas: Possible importance of vascular disturbances of the optic nerve and chiasm. Acta Neurochir (Wien) 15:1–10, 1966.
13. Lee WM, Adams JE: The empty sella syndrome. J Neurosurg 28:351–356, 1968.
14. Mortara R, Norrell H: Consequences of a deficient sellar diaphragma. J Neurosurg 32:565–573, 1970.
15. Olson DR, Guiot G, Derome P: The symptomatic empty sella: Prevention and correction via the transsphenoidal approach. J Neurosurg 37:533–537, 1972.
16. Hodgson SF, Randall RV, Holman CB, Maccarthy CS: Empty sella syndrome: Report of 10 cases. Med Clin North Am 56:897–907, 1972.
17. Harris JR, Levene MB: Visual complications following irradiation for pituitary adenomas and craniopharyngiomas. Radiology 120:167–171, 1976.
18. Lee FK, Richter HA, Tsai FY: Secondary empty sella syndrome. Acta Radiol Suppl (Stockh) 347:313–326, 1976.
19. Aristizabal S, Caldwell WL, Avila J: The relationship of time-dose fractionation factors to complications in the treatment of pituitary tumours by irradiation. Int J Radiat Oncol Biol Phys 2:567–573, 1977.
20. Basauri L, Castro M, Garcia JA: The empty sella syndrome: Analysis of 10 cases. Acta Neurochir (Wien) 38:111–120, 1977.
21. Atkinson AB, Allen IV, Gordon DS, et al: Progressive visual failure in acromegaly following external pituitary irradiation. Clin Endocrinol 10:469–479, 1979.
22. Hodgson SF, Randall RV, Laws ER: Empty sella syndrome. In Youmans J (ed): Neurological Surgery, 2nd ed. Philadelphia: WB Saunders, 1982, p 3176.
23. Sheline GE: Radiation therapy of pituitary tumours. In Givens JR (ed): Hormone Secreting Tumours. Chicago: Year Book Medical Publishers, 1982, p 139.
24. McFadzean RM: The empty sella syndrome: A review of 14 cases. Trans Ophthal Soc UK 103:537–541, 1983.
25. Grossman A, Cohen BL, Charlesworth M, et al: Treatment of prolactinomas with megavoltage radiotherapy. BMJ 288:1105–1109, 1984.
26. Jones A: Radiation oncogenesis in relation to the treatment of pituitary tumours. Clin Endocrinol 35:379–397, 1991.
27. Halstead AE: Remarks on the operative treatment of tumours of the hypophysis. Surg Gynecol Obstet 10:494–502, 1910.
28. Cushing H: The Pituitary Body and Its Disorders. Philadelphia: JB Lippincott, 1912.
29. Cairns H: The prognosis of pituitary tumours I. Lancet 2:1310–1311, 1935.
30. Cairns H: The prognosis of pituitary tumours II. Lancet 2:1363–1364, 1935.
31. Henderson WR: The pituitary adenomata: A follow up study of the surgical results in 338 cases (Dr. Harvey Cushing's series). Br J Surg 26:811, 1939.
32. Bakay L: The results of 300 pituitary adenoma operations (professor Herbert Olivecrona's series). J Neurosurg 7:240, 1950.
33. Obrador AS: Adenomas of the pituitary based on a neurosurgical experience of 65 operated patients. Rev Clin Esp 81:396–401, 1961.
34. Jefferson AA: Chromophobe pituitary adenomata: The size of the suprasellar portion in relation to the safety of operation. J Neurol Neurosurg Psychiatry 32:633, 1969.
35. Stern WE, Batzdorf U: Intracranial removal of pituitary adenomas: An evaluation of varying degrees of excision from partial to total. J Neurosurg 33:564, 1970.
36. Ray BS, Patterson RH Jr: Surgical experience with chromophobe adenomas of the pituitary gland. J Neurosurg 34:726, 1971.
37. Symon L, Jakubowski J: Transcranial management of pituitary tumours with suprasellar extension. J Neurol Neurosurg Psychiatry 42:123, 1979.
38. Rand RW: Transfrontal transsphenoidal craniotomy in pituitary and related tumours. In Rand RW (ed) Microneurosurgery, 3rd ed. St. Louis: CV Mosby, 1984.
39. Dolenc VV: Transcranial epidural approach to pituitary tumours extending beyond the sella. Neurosurgery 41:542–552, 1977.

# Surgical Management of Endocrinologically Silent Pituitary Tumors

■ ANDRÉ VISOT, STÉPHANE GAILLARD, and PATRICK J. DEROME

Improvements in the survey of hypophyseal hormones have considerably modified our knowledge of so-called nonfunctional pituitary adenomas, also called nonfunctioning silent, endocrine-inactive or nonsecretory adenomas. It is now known that, after immunocytochemical staining, most of these nonfunctioning adenomas are true gonadotrope adenomas secreting one or many hormonal products.[1, 2] However, true gonadotrope adenomas and silent tumors have similar clinical and therapeutic features. The secreting character of the tumor is most often established in surgically removed specimens.

In the past, pituitary tumors producing one or more of the glycoproteins, thyroid-stimulating hormone (TSH), Luteinizing hormone (LH), follicle-stimulating hormone (FSH), and the α-glycoprotein subunit were thought to be rare. However, using modern immunocytochemical and molecular biologic techniques, increasing numbers of these tumors are being detected.[1, 3–5] Many of them produce α- and β-glycoprotein subunits in addition to intact glycoprotein. Their hormone production is often low compared with the size of the tumor, and serum hormone levels may not be elevated.

Tumors that produce the gonadropins LH or FSH, or the α-subunit, account for most clinically nonfunctioning adenomas. They do not cause a specific clinical syndrome and usually exhibit symptoms of a large mass lesion or hypopituitarism. In surgical series, gonadotrope adenomas account for 12% to 17% of operated pituitary adenomas.[1, 3] Tables 32–1 and 32–2 demonstrate the current prevalence of gonadotrope adenomas in a series of secreting and endocrinologically silent pituitary adenomas operated at the Hôpital Foch.

## ANATOMOCLINICAL CONSIDERATIONS

### Clinical Features

The most common presenting complaint is usually loss of vision or a peripheral field abnormality (77% in our series).

These complaints are found in all the reported series: in 84% of cases in Taiwan,[3] 74% in Montreal,[6] 72% in the American series reported by Laws and colleagues,[7] 44% in Arafah's series,[8] 60% in a Spanish series,[9] and more than 60% in the report by Black and associates.[1] The visual impairment sometimes is severe, especially in the oldest patients, and may consist of unilateral blindness and visual field cut in the opposite eye. This is due to the insidious growth of the tumor and concomitant progressive visual deterioration. Occasionally, a distinct ophthalmologic problem, such as glaucoma or cataract, has delayed the correct diagnosis, and some of our patients have been operated on for a potential ophthalmologic problem. Bitemporal hemianopsia remains the main criterion for differentiating between an ophthalmologic disease and chiasmal compression. Sometimes, the initial visual symptoms are acute and usually reach the oculomotor nerves. In these cases, the clinical presentation is similar to that of a subarachnoid hemorrhage, with headache, meningism, and unilateral ophthalmoplegia, with or without visual impairment (9% in our series). These cases result from a sudden necrotic or hemorrhagic transformation of the tumor, which is always identified in surgery.

Endocrinologic symptoms are the second characteristics exhibited by patients with such pituitary adenomas. In our experience, these symptoms are present in 75% of cases, but only 35% exhibit clinical symptoms considered to be due to hypopituitarism, subsequently confirmed by laboratory tests. These symptoms include amenorrhea, loss of libido, hypothyroidism, and symptoms of inadequate pro-

TABLE 32–1 ■ SURGICAL SERIES OF PITUITARY ADENOMAS: 1960–1997:4277 CASES (HÔPITAL FOCH, NEUROSURGICAL DEPARTMENT)

| | |
|---|---|
| Prolactin adenomas | 1503 cases (37%) |
| Growth hormone adenomas | 1050 cases (24%) |
| Nonfunctioning adenomas | 997 cases (23.6%) |
| Cushing and Nelson adenomas | 707 cases (15%) |
| Thyroid-stimulating hormone adenomas | 20 cases (0.4%) |

TABLE 32–2 ■ SURGICAL SERIES OF PITUITARY
ADENOMAS: IN 1 YEAR (1994): 189 CASES
(HÔPITAL FOCH, NEUROSURGICAL DEPARTMENT)

| | | |
|---|---|---|
| Prolactinomas | 86 | 45% |
| Growth hormone adenoms | 41 | 22% |
| Corticotropic adenomas | 34 | 18% |
| Gonadotropic adenomas | 22 | 12% |
| Thyrotropic adenomas | 2 | <1% |
| Null cell adenomas | 4 | 2% |
| **Total** | **189** | **100%** |

duction of adrenal steroids sometimes leading to lethargy, fever, and abdominal pain with hyponatremia due to adrenal insufficiency. None of our patients had preoperative diabetes insipidus, which, if present, requires careful review of the diagnosis of pituitary adenoma.[10] In the rare cases of proven pediatric nonfunctioning pituitary adenomas,[11, 12] primary amenorrhea and the arrest of growth and sexual development are the initial clinical symptoms.

The third presenting feature is the incidental discovery of pituitary adenomas on brain imaging, computed tomography (CT), or magnetic resonance imaging (MRI). This is increasing with the improvement in neuroimaging procedures. However, screening for hormone overproduction by these tumors must be done. These cases may constitute a difficult therapeutic challenge.[4, 13]

## Radiologic Considerations

Magnetic resonance imaging has proven to be the most useful brain imaging technique for the study of a nonfunctioning pituitary adenoma. $T_1$-weighted MRI should be performed in the sagittal and coronal planes, without and then with gadolinium. Dynamic sequences are useful, especially in microadenomas, which are rarely nonfunctioning. If MRI is contraindicated because of a pacemaker or intraocular foreign body, CT scanning, without and then with contrast material, must be obtained, especially in the coronal section. Most of the pertinent data concerning the characteristics of a pituitary adenoma may be obtained by careful study of MRIs.

## Size and Extension of the Adenoma

At diagnosis, most nonfunctioning pituitary adenomas are already macroadenomas.[6, 8, 13–15] All symptomatic "silent" macroadenomas have extended beyond the confines of an enlarged sella, and the most common form of expansion can be represented as a medial suprasellar expansion filling the suprasellar space. We usually distinguish three types of medial suprasellar expansion:

- Type 1 (14% in our series) is a suprasellar expansion presenting as a bulge in the diaphragma sellae that extends into the suprasellar space and reaches the lower part of the optic tract.
- Type 2 expansion fills all the suprasellar space and chiasmal compression is obvious.

- Type 3 expansion reaches the foramen of Monro. Visual symptoms are present; hydrocephalus is possible.

Types 2 and 3 constitute 86% of our cases.

Sphenoidal extension is often combined with suprasellar extension but may be isolated, and usually takes the form of a bulging of a thin sellar floor into the sphenoid sinus. However, if the sellar floor has been destroyed, the dura may be invaded and the invasive adenoma can then reach and extend into the sphenoid sinus and posteriorly into the spongy sphenoid bone.

It is important to recognize the other types of intracranial tumor expansion because they may modify the therapeutic strategy, particularly the operative approach. Subfrontal expansion can occur medially between the optic nerves and extend above the sphenoidal planum, lifting up the frontal lobes. This kind of expansion cannot reasonably be reached by a transsphenoidal approach, except in cases of visual decompression and incomplete removal in an elderly patient who cannot be operated by a cranial approach. Retrochiasmatic expansion is a type of expansion that occurs in cases of optic nerve shortening. Such expansion extends the tumor into the interpeduncular cistern and upward as far as the foramen of Monro. Occasionally, an adenoma is found behind the dorsum sellae and the clivus, stretching the brain stem.

Cavernous involvement by a pituitary adenoma is often questionable. A true invasion is identified as a perforation of the dura of the cavernous sinus with involvement extending into the sinus, around the carotid artery. In these cases, unilateral progressive oculomotor palsies are common. More frequently, the macroadenoma displaces the intact dural wall of the cavernous sinus laterally over a great distance without invading the dura. Last, the most specific signs of cavernous sinus invasion are internal carotid artery encasement and lateral bulging of the external wall of the cavernous sinus.[16]

Middle fossa expansion of a macroadenoma consists of a lateral cranial extension of the tumor between the optic nerve and supraclinoid carotid artery, or between the carotid artery and third nerve or ipsilateral optic bundle. Such tumor expansion can be reached only by a pterional cranial approach.

### Enclosed or Invasive Macroadenomas

Most nonfunctioning macroadenomas remain enclosed adenomas. In these cases, MRI shows a well-shaped, round tumor that stretches the adjacent structures without disrupting the dura or the sellar walls. Total removal is then considered possible. In one third of the cases,[6] invasion clearly extends into the cavernous sinus, sphenoid body, or cranial space by perforation of the diaphragma sellae. The tumor is surgically unresectable unless the invasion is local and the surgeon is prepared for a cerebrospinal fluid (CSF) leak (Fig. 32–1).

Brain imaging by CT or MRI is also useful for preoperative evaluation of possible intraoperative surgical problems, including vascular injury if the carotid arteries are bulging into the sella, CSF leakage in cases of extreme distorsion of the diaphragma sellae, or an irregularly shaped upper part of the tumor, indicating possible rupture of the arach-

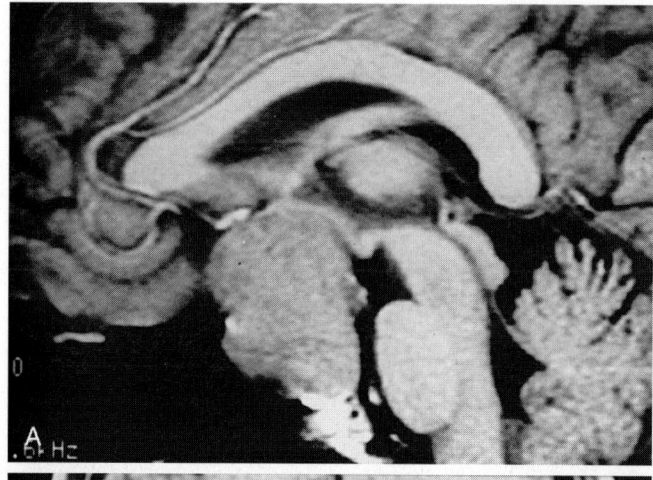

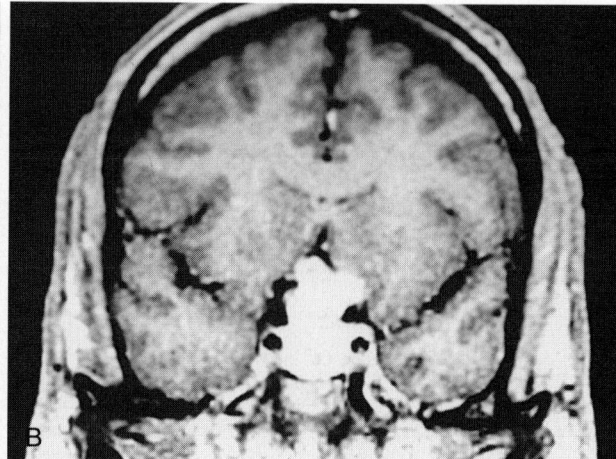

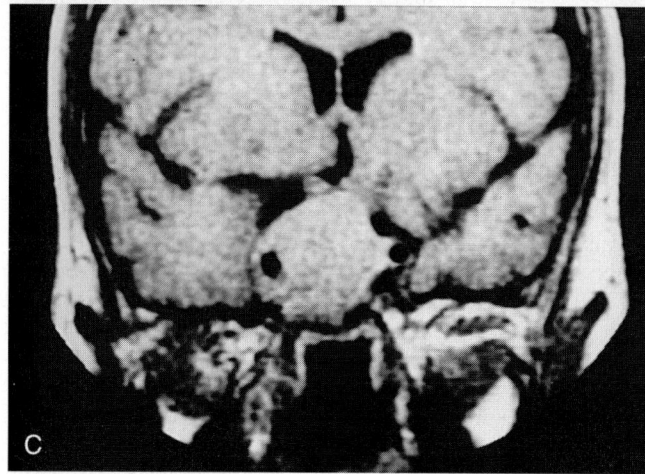

**FIGURE 32–1** ■ Invasive endocrinologically silent pituitary adenomas. *A,* Invasive suprasellar sphenoidal tumor. *B,* Suprasellar multilobulated expansion. *C,* Invasive cavernous sinus tumor.

noid membrane. Hemorrhage from a fibrous adenoma can be suspected before surgery in patients exhibiting marked contrast enhancement on radiography or vascular blush supply on angiography. Routine cerebral angiography is not performed in our institution unless the diagnosis is doubtful. MR angiography is now considered of little value for preoperative evaluation of the consistency of the adenoma. In our series of nonfunctioning pituitary adenomas, 72% were considered by the surgeon to be soft tumors, sometimes fluid or necrotic, and the other 28%, had a fibrous, hemorrhagic, or semifibrous appearance.

## ENDOCRINE EVALUATION

For patients with nonfunctioning adenomas, endocrine evaluation should include measurement of the levels of serum prolactin, growth hormone, cortisol, triiodothyronine, thyroxine, FSH, and LH. In approximately 71% of these adenomas, preoperative partial hypophyseal insufficiency has been demonstrated.[6, 9, 15] Moderate hyperprolactinemia (<200 ng/ml) is usual (50% to 65%). Negative immunocytochemical staining in these cases argues strongly for hypothalamohypophyseal disconnection.[6, 8, 9, 17] α-Subunit and TSH levels should also be tested; even if they are often normal, they might be useful markers for follow-up if their levels are elevated.

Although most nonfunctioning pituitary adenomas are

shown by immunocytochemical staining to be gonadotropic adenomas, they are commonly considered silent. The levels of plasma gonadotropins or their subunits are usually low. Increased basal FSH seems to be more common, especially in men.[18–22] Increased basal LH is rare and is often combined with an excess of α-subunit.[17, 19, 21, 23, 24] Overproduction of α-subunit is frequent, but overproduction of basal LH β-subunit is rare.[19–22]

## SURGICAL MANAGEMENT

### Goals of Surgery

#### Visual Prognosis

Because most nonfunctioning pituitary adenomas are macroadenomas, usually accompanied by visual symptoms, the first goal of surgery is resolution of the visual state. Postoperative results are usually good or excellent, especially after transsphenoidal surgery.[6, 7, 13, 25] In our institution, visual results after trans-sphenoidal surgery for nonfunctioning adenomas are as follows:

Improvement: 80%
No change: 13.8%
Worsening: 6.2%
- 2.8% after first surgery
- 18% after second surgery for recurrence

Improvements in visual symptoms concern visual field and visual acuity, and depend on preoperative visual status, operative approach, and duration of symptoms. Postoperative worsening of visual symptoms is much more predictable in older patients with poor preoperative vision. In macroadenoma extending into the suprasellar space but involving no evident visual deficit, the indication for transsphenoidal surgery to prevent visual symptoms is questionable.

## Endocrinologic Prognosis

Preoperative antehypophyseal insufficiency is often present in patients with nonfunctioning pituitary adenomas. After transsphenoidal surgery, the endocrinologic status is often unchanged and requires substitution therapy, but it may also be either worsened or improved.[6, 9, 13, 15]

Pituitary insufficiency can be improved if surgery is not delayed too long and if the insufficiency is due to compression of normal tissue.[8] The goal of surgery is to preserve pituitary function and sometimes to achieve partial restoration.

## Total Removal: Goal and Challenge

In patients with nonfunctioning pituitary adenomas, we advocate complete tumor removal[4] because there is no proven effective medical therapy and radiation therapy is known to be harmful, especially in elderly patients. Total removal must therefore be the goal of surgery, because the tumor is soft, noninvasive, and well delimited by normal tissue (Fig. 32–2). Even in large adenomas, a clean surgical plane can be found at the beginning of the procedure and progressively followed and separated from the adjacent compressed normal structures. This procedure is valid for the transsphenoidal approach. On the other hand, pituitary adenomas operated through a cranial approach are always invasive tumors and are totally unresectable without major postoperative complications. The goal of surgery using a cranial approach is subtotal removal and decompression of the optic nerves and chiasm.

## Cranial Approaches

Indications for a cranial approach in patients presenting with a nonfunctioning pituitary adenoma are infrequent (2.3% in our series). In fact, craniotomy is indicated only in patients with visual symptoms not improved by medical therapy and an adenoma that is unresectable by the transsphenoidal route. Such cases are mostly encountered when the intracranial part of an extension is separated from the intrasellar part by a narrow neck, or when the intracranial extension is huge and multidirectional (Fig. 32–3). Extensions that are subfrontal, lateral middle fossa, retroclival, or suprasellar with a narrow neck can be indications for a primary cranial approach, but the latter may also be indicated as the second stage of a two-step procedure after trans-sphenoidal surgery. The choice and side of the cranial approach depend on the location and size of the adenoma as seen on MRI.

*Bifrontal medial craniotomy,* such as that used in olfactory groove meningiomas, is recommended for the removal of huge subfrontal tumors.

*The pterional approach* is commonly used when the tumor fills the suprasellar medial and lateral cisterns.

*The subtemporal approach* is advocated for subtemporal retroclival and infratentorial extensions.

*The transbasal subfrontal approach* is not indicated for pituitary tumors, even when extensive, because this approach is entirely extradural, and the larger part of the adenoma threatening the visual pathways is intradural.

*Approaches to the cavernous sinus,* as described by some authors,[26, 27] do not, apart from exceptional cases, seem to be of any value for the surgical management of nonfunctioning pituitary adenomas. The main reason is that a pituitary adenoma extending into the cavernous sinus as a space-occupying lesion is an invasive, unresectable tumor.

## Complications of the Cranial Approach

Complications of this approach are well known.[28] They are closely related to elevation of the frontal or temporal lobes, dissection of major arteries and perforating vessels, and

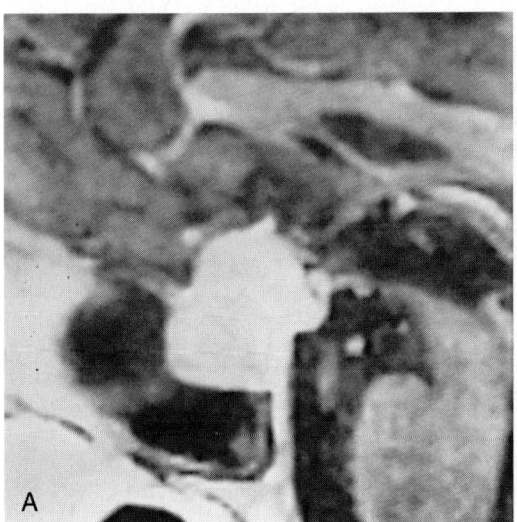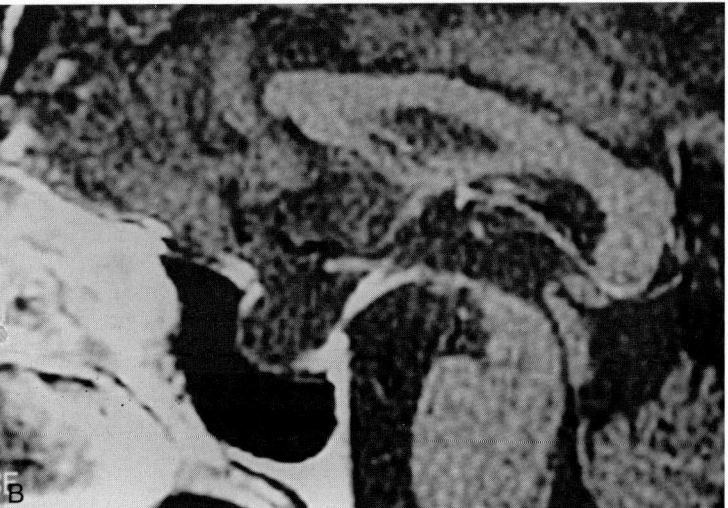

**FIGURE 32–2** ■ The goal of surgery is complete removal. *A,* Preoperative magnetic resonance imaging scan of a nonsecreting pituitary adenoma. *B,* Complete removal after transsphenoidal surgery.

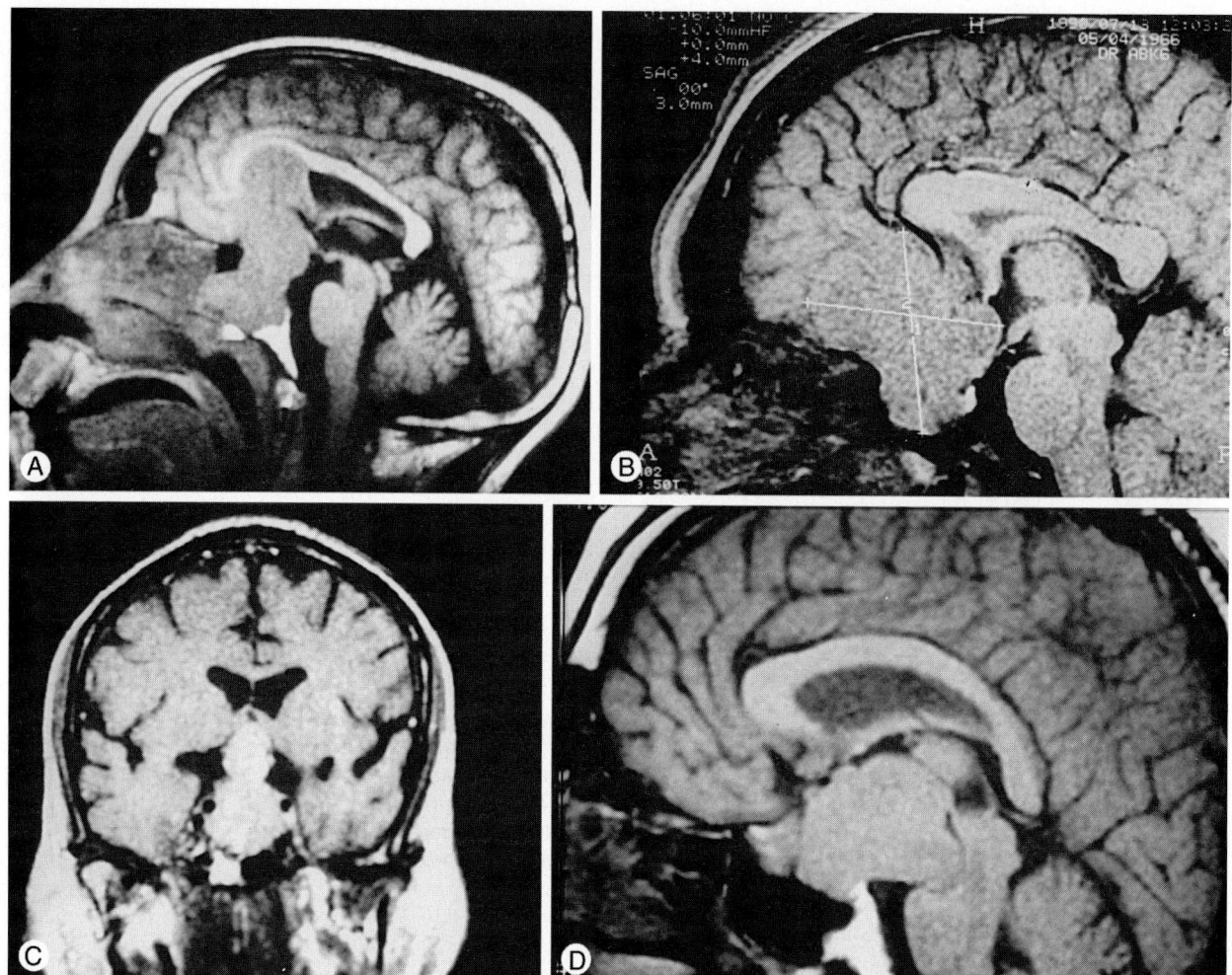

**FIGURE 32–3 ■** Indications for a cranial approach in endocrinologically silent pituitary tumors. *A,* Huge suprasellar expansion. *B,* Subfrontal expansion. *C,* Suprasellar expansion with a narrow neck linking with the intrasellar expansion. *D,* Retrochiasmatic expansion.

manipulations of the optic tract and oculomotor nerves. One particular feature of cranial surgery for nonfunctioning pituitary adenomas should be stressed: when such adenomas are operated through a cranial approach, they are usually huge, heterogeneous, fibrous, or hemorrhagic. Therefore, as with meningiomas in the same area, close adhesions to vascular and adjacent brain structures are encountered. Not infrequently, rupture of the arachnoidal plane is noted, so that dissection behind the optic chiasm involving the posterior wall of the carotid artery and optic bundle becomes hazardous and often leads to incomplete tumor removal. After a cranial approach, manipulation of the optic tract or partial devascularization of the optic nerves or chiasm leads to more frequent postoperative worsening of visual status than after trans-sphenoidal surgery.

Every attempt should be made to preserve the pituitary stalk, which often adheres closely to the tumor. As in craniopharyngiomas, the choice is then between cutting the stalk and leaving the residual tumor in place.

## TRANSSPHENOIDAL APPROACH

The surgical technique for the removal of pituitary adenomas by the transsphenoidal approach has remained almost identical to the one Cushing[29] used initially, with the addition of improvements by Kanavel[30] and Hirsch,[31] and as modified by Halstead,[32] who first used the sublabial incision. As he developed the techniques of intracranial surgery, Cushing abandoned the transsphenoidal route, and it was forgotten by most of his students, with the notable exception of Dott.[33] With the technical advances introduced by Guiot[34] and Hardy,[35] the transsphenoidal approach has been commonly used for the surgical treatment of pituitary adenomas and other tumors of the sellar area.[36] The different steps in the procedure are described in detail in Chapter 28, as well as in many well documented reports.[34–37] However, we wish to stress certain aspects of transsphenoidal surgery we have observed in our institution, where it was initially practiced under the direction of Guiot.

Preoperative hormonal substitution therapy is routinely used for nonfunctioning pituitary adenomas; it consists of administering 50 mg of succinate hydrocortisone intramuscularly, 1 hour before surgery, and 25 mg every 6 hours thereafter. Twenty milligrams of oral hydrocortisone is given 18 hours after the first injection.

Perioperative antibiotic medication consists of lincomycin, 10 mg/kg every 8 hours, and gentamicin, 1 mg/kg over 24 hours.

Preoperative review of CT and MRI scans is essential to demonstrate the configuration of the sphenoid bone and the position of the carotid arteries, particularly in cases of reoperation.

Even in macroadenomas, a lumbar drain is not inserted, because surgery is performed under a C-arm fluoroscope so that the progression of instruments can be followed at each step in the procedure. When tumor removal is almost complete, the operative cavity fills up with air, and the position and prolapse of the diaphragma sellae are controlled on a television screen. Bilateral jugular vein compression is usually enough to help debulk a soft suprasellar tumor and make the diaphragma sellae prolapse into the sella. It is thought that raising the intracranial pressure is not safe for the optic nerves or chiasm, which are already compressed, especially in fibrous adenomas.[38, 39]

Except for reoperation, when the endonasal approach may be an effective alternative method to avoid the scar made by previous surgery, the conventional sublabial approach is favored at our instutition. For many years, the sublabial incision has not been sutured at the end of the procedure, without any adverse consequence. The sublabial incision has two main advantages:

1. Enlargement of the piriform sinus to avoid fracture of the turbinates as the retractor is opened
2. A wide exposure of the sellar floor, an essential condition for exposing the dura as far as possible laterally in relation to the cavernous sinus

The mucosa inside the sphenoid sinus is usually removed because it may be extensive, and its removal probably reduces the risk of postoperative infection or mucocele.

The dura is not coagulated before opening, because this can induce its shrinkage, and extradural bleeding.

The lateral and suprasellar parts of the tumor are usually removed without direct visual inspection, thanks to two anatomic landmarks, the transverse sinus, running upward, and the cavernous sinus on each side of the sphenoid bone. These parts of the tumor are removed with "home-made" instruments, i.e., malleable and variously angled curets and suckers. These instruments permit constant but gentle contact with the walls of the sella and the operative cavity.

After tumor removal, normal pituitary tissue can be identified, even with macroadenomas. This tissue is compressed against the wall of the sella as a pink, adhesive tissue. Sometimes, however, the normal pituitary is not visible, and this is always noted in the surgical report as an important item of information for further endocrinologic follow-up. The absence of any residual tumor is confirmed by microscopic examination, flexible fiberoptic endoscopy, and aspiration toward the walls with variously angled instruments.

Hemostasis is ensured with Gelfoam, although even then bleeding from the intradural venous sinus is significant. Hemostasis must be obtained carefully, especially in cases of subtotal removal. We have had rare but memorable experiences of postoperative rebleeding into the operative cavity from a residual tumor. For a trained pituitary surgeon, this rebleeding is most predictable in cases of huge suprasellar fibrous adenomas without collapse of the diaphragma sellae during surgery (semifibrous or fibrous adenomas constitued 28% of the nonfunctioning pituitary adenomas in our series).

After the adenoma is removed and hemostasis obtained, a piece of Gelfoam is usually left in the operative cavity.

A piece of bone, extracted from the nasal septum, is inserted below the edges of the opening of the anterior wall of the sella.

In our institution, surgery is performed by the neurosurgeon alone. The mean duration of the procedure is 1 hour.

## Postoperative Management

Immediately after surgery, the patient's water balance and urinary output and density should be measured every hour and, for 2 days thereafter, every 3 hours. Serum electrolyte levels should be monitored daily. Diabetes insipidus most be detected quickly to institute medical therapy. In cases of nonfunctioning pituitary adenomas, the patient is always discharged with steroid hormonal substitution therapy until the postoperative endocrinologic evaluation on day 8 after surgery. The patient also must be tested at home for delayed hyponatremia by systematic staining.

## Complications

The Complications of Transsphenoidal Surgery observed in our institution are listed in Tables 32–3 and 32–4. Many well documented papers have been published on the subject.[36, 37, 40–42] Here, we stress only some important possible complications.

A CSF fistula may occur in cases of nonfunctioning pituitary adenoma if the diaphragma sellae is injured or invaded by an invasive tumor, which can be suspected by an irregularly shaped suprasellar extension. This situation also may be predictable in patients who have undergone previous transcranial or transsphenoidal surgery, and radiation therapy.[41–43] In such cases, two distinct situations are possible.

First, a distorted diaphragma sellae can sustain a minor tear, which can be routinely repaired by clipping the two edges of the tear together with a bayonnet clip holder and inserting a piece of fascia lata under the diaphragma. Watertight closure of the sella is completed by introduction of muscle to support the fascia lata, and by a bone graft that closes the sella.

The second possibility, complete laceration of the dia-

---

TABLE 32–3 ■ **COMPLICATIONS OF THE TRANS-SPHENOIDAL APPROACH IN A SERIES OF 4000 CASES (HÔPITAL FOCH, NEUROSURGICAL DEPARTMENT)**

Surgical mortality
  Before 1985: 1%
  Last decade (1986–1996): 0.2%
Mechanical complications: <2%
  Cerebrospinal fluid leak: 2% (1% reoperated)
  Secondary empty sella: 0.2% (0% last decade, 1986–1996)
Transient oculomotor palsy: 1.5%
Visual worsening
  In microadenoma: 0%
  In macroadenoma
   • First surgery: 2.8%
   • Reoperation: 18%
Endocrinologic complications
  Rare but difficult to summarize because of usual partial preoperative pituitary insufficiency

TABLE 32–4 ■ NONFUNCTIONING PITUITARY ADENOMAS: MORTALITY AMONG 395 CASES WITH LONG-TERM FOLLOW-UP* (HÔPITAL FOCH, NEUROSURGICAL DEPARTMENT)

| Mortality | No. of Cases | % | Causes |
|---|---|---|---|
| Early | 3 | 0.7 | Two cases with lung embolism<br>One unknown (1 month after transsphenoidal surgery) |
| Secondary | 4 | 1 | Traffic accident: one case<br>Two cases with brain radionecrosis (2 and 4 years after radiation therapy)<br>One case with cerebral ischemia (after 4 years of follow-up) |
| Late | 3 | 0.7 | Two cases 20 years after the onset of symptoms<br>One case 28 years after the onset of symptoms, multiple surgery, radiation therapy, and shunt procedure |

*Overall mortality rate: 2.5% (10 cases).

phragma sellae, requires a more aggressive procedure to close the fistula and avoid resurgery. A piece of fascia lata is sutured to the anterior dura just under the transverse sinus with a long needle holder used in heart surgery, and then pushed upward to "reconstruct" the diaphragma sellae. This fragment is maintained in position by meticulous packing of the sella with muscle and fat. Closure of the sella is easy if the firm, bony part of the anterior wall remains intact, in which case a piece of bone grafted extradurally ensures permanent closure. On the other hand, if the anterior wall and floor of the sella have already been destroyed by the adenoma because of sphenoidal extension or an invasive sphenoidal adenoma, no osseous structure is available to keep the bone graft in place, in which case packing of the sphenoidal sinus is mandatory using the same materials as mentioned previously (e.g., muscle, fat, and glue). Spongy bone extracted from the iliac crest can be useful for constructing a watertight closure of the sphenoid sinus. The insertion of any foreign material into the sphenoid sinus is prohibited in our department because of the risk of infection. In such cases, postoperative lumbar drainage is used for 6 or 7 days. Despite this meticulous procedure, cases of recurrent CSF rhinorrhea have been described,[42] and in our experience 1% of patients (of a series of 4000 cases) had to be reoperated for CSF leakage. We stress that:

1. A perioperative CSF fistula in patients with macroadenoma must be treated and closed in a single operation.
2. Postoperative CSF rhinorrhea after transsphenoidal surgery must be detected and closed as soon as possible using the same approach.
3. Insertion of a permanent CSF shunt is a rescue procedure.

The secondary empty sella syndrome may occur under three conditions: (1) an enlarged sella, (2) a large suprasellar extension, and (3) adherences between the distended diaphragma sellae and optic tract. This rare syndrome, described in the early period of transsphenoidal surgery,[39, 40, 44] has not been observed for many years because it has been prevented by extradural packing of the sellar floor.[41, 44]

Suspected postoperative hematoma after transsphenoidal surgery is difficult to manage, particularly in elderly patients with marked impairment of preoperative vision. Early brain CT or MRI scans are difficult to evaluate because they often reproduce the preoperative size of the tumor. We have come to the conclusion that postoperative worsening of visual status without improvement after 3 hours of high-dose corticosteroid therapy is an absolute indication for reoperation, which, however, often gives disappointing findings. It involves the gentle removal of noncompressive clots until the pulsations of the upper part of the hematoma are obvious. Nevertheless, it must be stated that this reoperation is often quickly successful as regards vision. Such reoperations can be prevented by meticulous hemostasis, particularly in cases of fibrous adenoma or proven residual tumor, or in elderly patients with marked impairment of preoperative vision.

## RADIATION THERAPY

Although the indications for postoperative radiation therapy are not open to question in cases of proven residual tumor, controversy persists between the supporters and opponents of systematic postoperative irradiation, even if there is no obvious residual adenoma.[45] In patients with nonfunctioning pituitary adenomas, systematic postoperative radiation therapy led to a mean rate of recurrence of 11% (Table 32–5), whereas in patients who underwent surgery alone, this rate was 27%. These data argue in favor of the value of postoperative irradiation for the prevention of recurrence. On the other hand, all pituitary adenomas do not display the same behavior. The growth of pituitary adenomas, particularly the endocrine inactive type, is usually slow, but may be faster with more recurrences, especially in young patients.

The final decision regarding radiation therapy would be easier if markers of aggressivity and invasiveness were available. Routinely, these markers cannot yet be used, but the first results of studies based on the use of genetic molecular markers seem promising.[46] Because the goal of radiation therapy is to deliver the maximal dose to the target and the minimal dose to adjacent structures, different methods of irradiation can be proposed, including heavy particles, Gamma knife surgery, or x-ray irradiation, either conventional or delivered by linear accelerator. The control rates for nonfunctioning pituitary adenomas after adjuvant radiation therapy seem to be high, at nearly 85%[47] and 90.3% for 10-year progression-free survival.[48] However, with adjuvant radiation therapy, the mean rate of recurrence is 11% (see Table 32–5). In our institution, 15 of 104 patients with nonfunctioning pituitary adenomas (14%) who had postoperative radiation therapy with a mean 10-year follow-up had a recurrence. Irradiation does not prevent recurrence, but merely delays it.

Radiation therapy may have pernicious effects, and the

## TABLE 32–5 ■ PERCENTAGE OF RECURRENCE OF ENDOCRINOLOGICALLY SILENT PITUITARY ADENOMAS REPORTED IN THE LITERATURE

| Authors (References) | Surgery Alone | | | Surgery + Radiation Therapy | | |
| --- | --- | --- | --- | --- | --- | --- |
| | Total No. of Cases | No. of Recurrences | % | Total No. of Cases | No. of Recurrences | % |
| Ebersold et al.[7] | 42 | 5 | 12 | 50 | 9 | 18 |
| Jaffrain-Réa et al.[64] | 33 | 9 | 27 | 24 | 2 | 8.8 |
| Hayes et al.[68] | 29 | 13 | 45 | 42 | 9 | 21 |
| Sheline[67] | 29 | 20 | 69 | 80 | 9 | 11 |
| Ciric et al.[57] | 32 | 9 | 28 | 67 | 4 | 6 |
| Chun et al.[65] | 60 | 9 | 15 | 54 | 4 | 7 |
| Vlahovitch et al.[66] | 89 | 14 | 16 | 46 | 4 | 8 |
| **Total** | **285** | **79** | **27** | **363** | **41** | **11** |

progressive onset of hypopituitarism in a few months or years is a well-known complication.[49, 50]

The rate of pituitary insufficiency is higher if the radiation dose is 50 Gy or more. Other complications of radiation therapy have been reported and were observed in our series. They included:

1. Subacute incompletely regressive encephalitis[51, 52]
2. Delayed brain radionecrosis[53]
3. Radiation-induced brain tumors, including glioma,[54] astrocytoma,[55] and meningioma[55]

We observed one radiation-induced glioblastoma and one skull base sarcoma several years after conventional radiation therapy for nonfunctioning pituitary adenomas. Symptomatic bilateral supraclinoid carotid artery stenosis was also observed in one patient 15 years after conventional radiation therapy for pituitary adenoma.

The pernicious neuropsychological effects of radiation therapy are well known in children, but not in adults.

Because the complications of postoperative radiation therapy are known, its advantages and risks must be carefully weighed, especially in older patients, if pituitary function is normal and if there is no obvious residual tumor. In the past, radiation therapy was always proposed in our department after surgery for nonsecreting pituitary adenomas, even if total removal was visually achieved by the neurosurgeon. However, because of the increasingly frequent complications reported after radiation therapy, and above all thanks to the development of brain imaging, we have gradually changed our policy. Our attitude now is to weigh up the pros and cons according to the age of the patient and size of the residual tumor, as follows:

1. If there is no obvious residual tumor on delayed, controlled MRI, radiation therapy is not performed.
2. If there is a documented residual tumor:
   • If the tumor is less than 10 mm in diameter and separated from the optic tract, Gamma knife surgery or linear accelerator radiation is proposed.
   • If the tumor is more than 10 mm in diameter, conventional radiation therapy is proposed, with a lower dose for older patients.

## RECURRENCES

The mean rate of recurrence for nonfunctioning pituitary adenomas after surgery alone is approximately 30% (range,

10% to 69%). Table 32–5 summarizes the results for reported surgical series. These cases were reoperated or had adjuvant irradiation. Because nonfunctioning pituitary adenomas cannot be followed up on the basis of hormonal criteria, CT or MRI criteria must be used. The schedule for postoperative brain imaging usually includes:

1. A first postoperative check-up 2 or 3 months after surgery. This waiting period avoids the usual early postoperative changes seen on CT or MRI[56] (Fig. 32–4).
2. The second follow-up study is performed 6 months later, and if there is no obvious residual tumor, the study is repeated every year.
3. The interval after which further morphologic studies are performed has not been clearly defined, but because the largest number of recurrences occurred between 4 and 8 years after surgery,[6, 57–59] the follow-up period must be extended for many years.

The absence of late recurrences in some follow-up series is surprising, and is probably due to the limitation of the observation period. In our department, 55 recurrent nonfunctioning pituitary adenomas were observed of 395 cases (14%) with a long-term follow-up of more than 10 years. Summarized data for this series are listed in Table 32–6. From the results, it can be concluded that, as stated previously, radiation therapy does not prevent recurrence but delays it. Ninety percent of our patients experienced new visual symptoms at the time of recurrence, probably because the morphologic follow-up had not been suffi-

## TABLE 32–6 ■ FIFTY-FIVE (14%) RECURRENT NONFUNCTIONING PITUITARY ADENOMAS OF 395 CASES WITH LONG-TERM FOLLOW-UP (HÔPITAL FOCH, NEUROSURGICAL DEPARTMENT)

| | |
| --- | --- |
| Mean age at time of recurrence | 60 yr |
| Sex | 38 M |
| | 19 F |
| Mean time to recurrence after surgery | |
| Less than 5 yr | 21 cases |
| 5–10 yr | 17 cases |
| More than 10 yr | 17 cases |
| Mean time to recurrence | |
| With previous radiation therapy | 15 yr |
| Without radiation therapy | 6 yr |

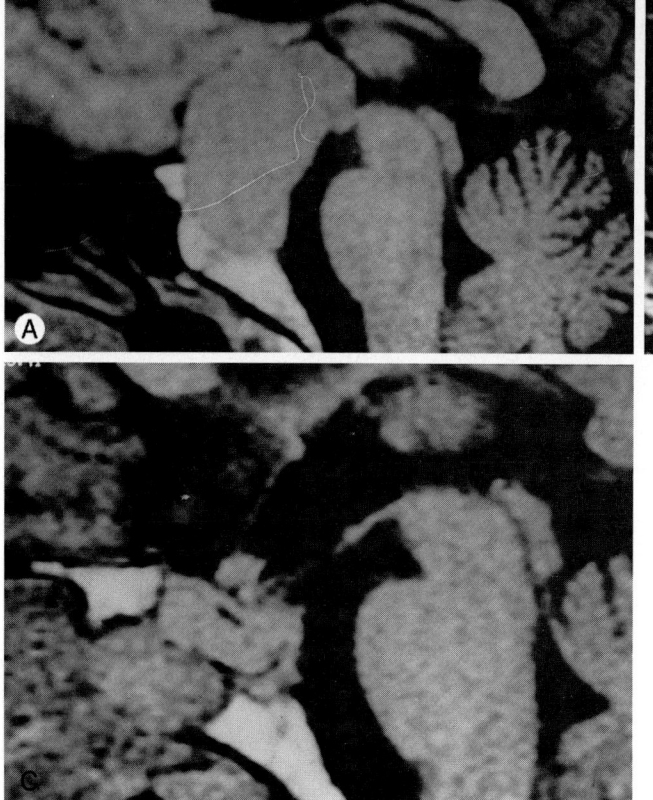

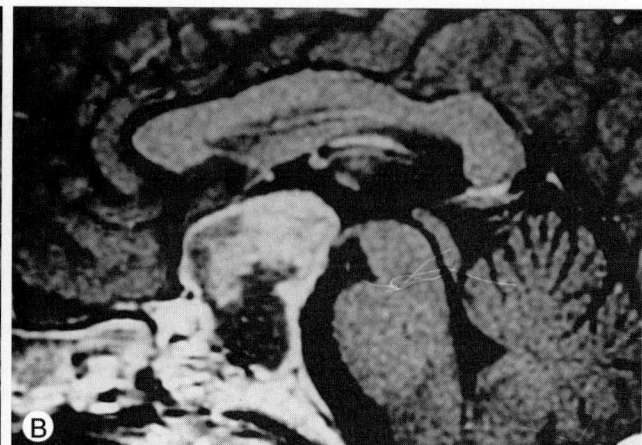

FIGURE 32–4 ■ Postoperative imaging. *A,* A preoperative magnetic resonance imaging seen of a huge adenoma. *B,* The same adenoma 4 days after transsphenoidal surgery. *C,* Same cases 2 months after surgery.

ciently meticulous, or patients had been lost to follow-up because of an uneventful clinical course. Forty-seven of these 55 cases of recurrence concerned macroadenomas, and 8 known residual tumors that had increased in size.

Table 32–7 summarizes the therapeutic management of these recurrent cases. Our experience leads to the following conclusions:

1. *Reoperation* is highly recommended if visual symptoms are present.
2. *The choice of surgical approach* is subject to the same rules as the first surgery.
3. *Prior radiation therapy and surgery* increase the fibrous component of the tumor.
4. *Reoperation* led to incomplete removal in 40% of our cases.
5. *Reoperation by the transsphenoidal approach* in cases of recurrent nonfunctioning pituitary adenomas leads to more frequent complications:
   - Twenty percent postoperative visual worsening (instead of 3.1% after initial surgery in our department)
   - Nine percent CSF fistula (instead of 3.6% at the first surgery)

Table 32–8 gives the results of follow-up after treatment for recurrences.

## SURGICAL STRATEGY

As stated in this and other documented reports by pituitary surgeons throughout the world, radiation therapy should be

considered an adjuvant treatment for endocrinologically silent pituitary adenomas, and medical therapy is not yet routinely effective. The main challenge in treating these adenomas is the surgical strategy. Because, in experienced hands, the transsphenoidal approach is relatively benign, is of short duration, and gives good results, it has for many years been the first choice in the surgical treatment of nonfunctioning pituitary adenomas. It was performed in 95% of our cases regardless of the size of the adenoma. Inferior sphenoidal extension of the tumor is an absolute indication for the transsphenoidal approach. However, for removal by this approach, a suprasellar medial extension has to have widespread connections with the intrasellar part, thus enabling the instruments to reach the uppermost portion of the tumor without risk, because the adenoma is encapsulated, allowing the suprasellar portion to descend to the sellar floor after the sella has been evacuated. In general, when there is a narrow neck between an intrasellar

TABLE 32–7 ■ THERAPEUTIC MANAGEMENT OF 55 RECURRENT NONFUNCTIONING PITUITARY ADENOMAS (HÔPITAL FOCH, NEUROSURGICAL DEPARTMENT)

| | | |
|---|---|---|
| Reoperation: 50 cases | Transsphenoidal approach: | 50% |
| | Cranial approach: | 50% |
| Twenty cases incomplete removal → 16 of radiation therapy | | |
| Thirty cases of subtotal or total removal | | |
| Radiation therapy: 4 cases | | |
| Medical treatment: 1 case | | |

TABLE 32–8 ■ **FOLLOW-UP OF 55 RECURRENT NONFUNCTIONING PITUITARY ADENOMAS AFTER TREATMENT OF THE RECURRENCE (HÔPITAL FOCH, NEUROSURGICAL DEPARTMENT)**

Five patients died (two of brain radionecrosis)
Fifty patients are still alive after several surgical procedures and radiation therapy

and a suprasellar medial or lateral extension, transsphenoidal surgery allows only the removal of the intrasellar part of the tumor.

Therefore, the transsphenoidal approach may constitute the first step in a two-stage procedure comprising the transsphenoidal and cranial approaches. This strategy must be carefully considered when a cranial extension is unresectable by the transsphenoidal route (i.e., in cases of a subfrontal, subtemporal, or suprasellar extension of the tumor with a narrow connection with its intrasellar part). The transsphenoidal approach should usually be proposed as the first step because:

1. It allows the removal of the intrasellar part of the tumor and the subsequent acquisition of important

information on tumor consistency, and confirms the silent, nonfunctioning character of the adenoma by immunocytochemical studies. This information is very important to ensure that no postoperative medical treatment is indicated.
2. Above all, this approach allows meticulous closure of the sella, thus ensuring the absence of CSF leakage after cranial surgery.

The transsphenoidal approach may also be proposed after craniotomy to preserve normal hypophyseal tissue (Fig. 32–5).

Evidence of residual tumor in the cavernous sinus after transsphenoidal surgery is not an indication for secondary cranial surgery because tumor removal might in any case be incomplete. Usually, 1 or 2 months separate the two steps of the combined procedure. This period allows the immunocytochemical results to be obtained, as well as postoperative visual evaluation and watertight closure of the sella.

In some large, nonfunctioning pituitary adenomas, transsphenoidal surgery can be intentionally repeated.[60] This strategy may not be considered often, but has proved effective in some of our cases. It consists of the following: during the first transsphenoidal surgery, the upper part of

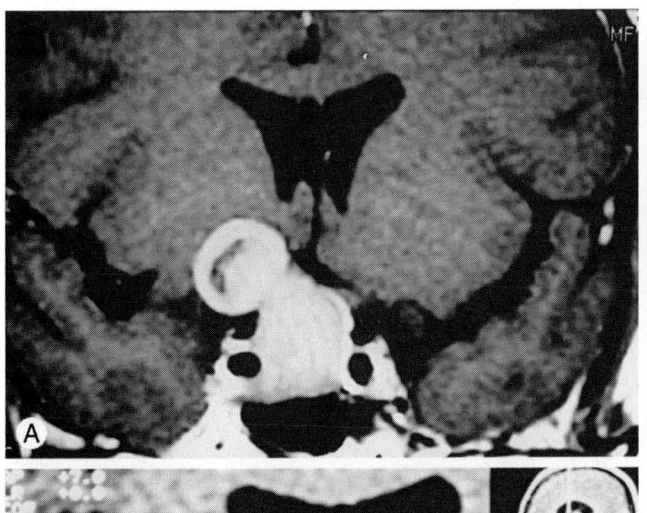
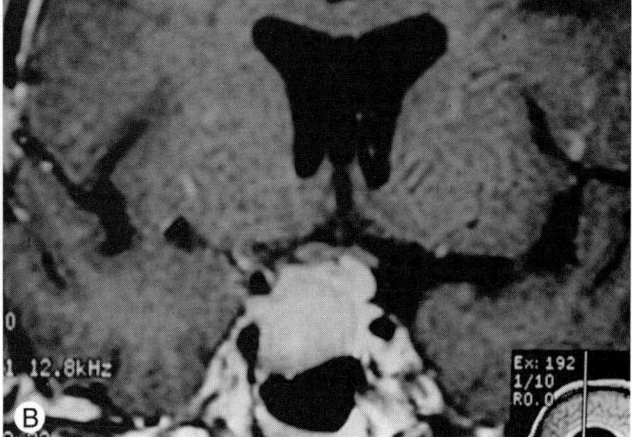
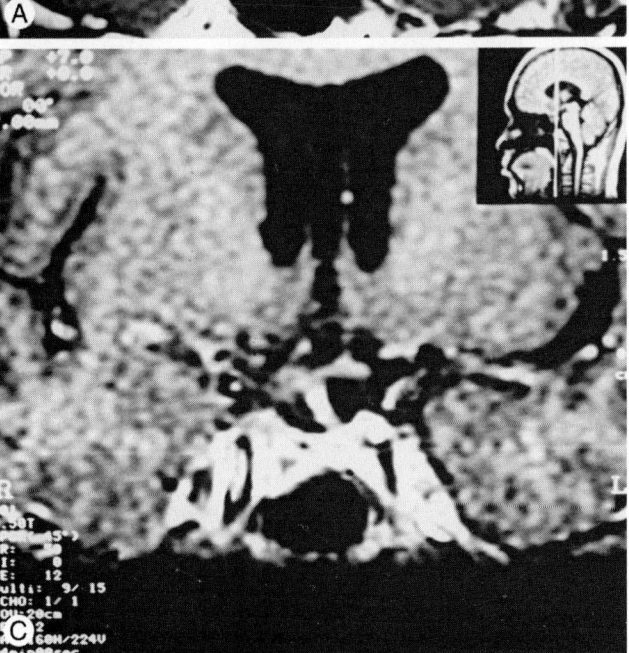

FIGURE 32–5 ■ Nonfunctioning pituitary tumors: cranial and transsphenoidal surgery in two steps. *A,* Lateral expansion with a narrow neck, which is an indication for a cranial approach. *B,* A magnetic resonance imaging (MRI) scan 3 months after the craniotomy. *C,* The same case with an MRI scan 6 months after secondary surgery using a transsphenoidal approach.

the tumor does not prolapse into the sella, either spontaneously or by the artificial means of jugular compression. If its removal is thought to be hazardous, the tumor is left in place after meticulous hemostasis. After this decompressive surgery, visual recovery usually is observed. Two or 3 months after surgery, MRI may show evidence of the descent of the residual upper part of the tumor into the sella, thus making a second transsphenoidal operation a reasonable indication (Figs. 32–6 and 32–7). The goal of this strategy is to achieve complete removal in two stages while preserving, if possible, the normal hypophyseal tissue and avoiding radiation therapy. The mandatory anatomic condition for the upper part of the tumor to prolapse secondarily into the sella is a wide link between its intrasellar and suprasellar extensions. This technique must not be used for lateral suprasellar extensions, which must be removed by a cranial approach.

## PITUITARY INCIDENTALOMA

The finding of pituitary incidentaloma has become more frequent (by 13%)[14] since brain CT scanning or MRI has been more routinely performed for unrelated reasons.

In such cases, endocrinologic evaluation is recommended. It should indicate hormonal overproduction in cases of secreting but "silent" adenomas such as prolactinoma, growth hormone adenoma, or corticotropic adenoma. The therapy indicated for each specific tumor type may therefore be necessary. If there is no evidence of hormone overproduction, pituitary function should be evaluated by screening for hypopituitarism. Water deprivation and urinary excretion should be measured to detect diabetes insipidus, because if this is present, the pituitary tumor is probably not an adenoma. A microadenoma usually exhibits normal pituitary function. Therefore, when a nonsecreting incidental microadenoma is discovered, first-intention surgery does not seem to be indicated because the risk of significant tumor growth is small.[61, 62] However, brain imaging has to be repeated every year and surgery proposed if there is clearly documented enlargement of the adenoma. In cases of nonfunctioning incidental macroadenoma, surgery is highly advisable if there are marked visual symptoms or hypopituitarism. In the absence of these symptoms, it is possible to wait 6 months and then re-evaluate the situation, but the patient and his or her family must be aware that surgery may be necessary. Of course, in such cases, the clinical verdict determines the final decision, especially for older patients with a concomitant ophthalmologic disease.

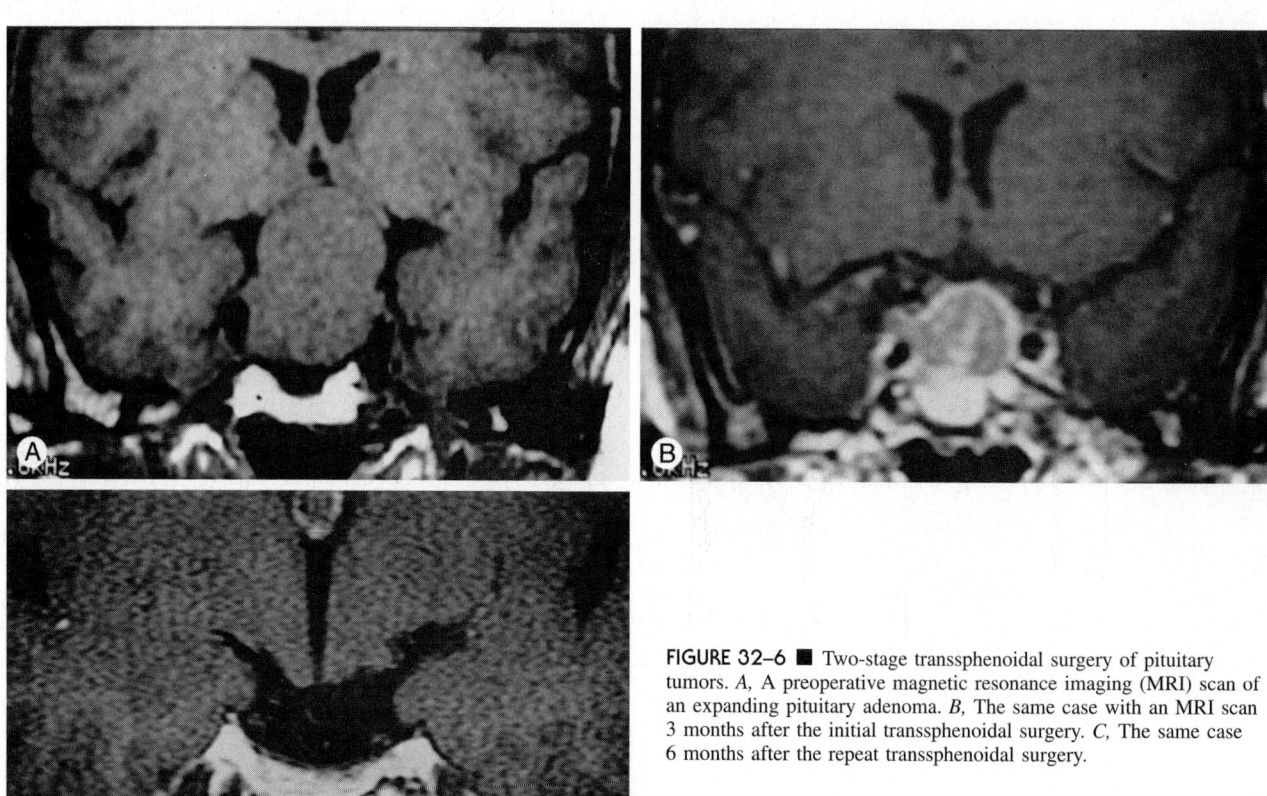

FIGURE 32–6 ■ Two-stage transsphenoidal surgery of pituitary tumors. *A*, A preoperative magnetic resonance imaging (MRI) scan of an expanding pituitary adenoma. *B*, The same case with an MRI scan 3 months after the initial transsphenoidal surgery. *C*, The same case 6 months after the repeat transsphenoidal surgery.

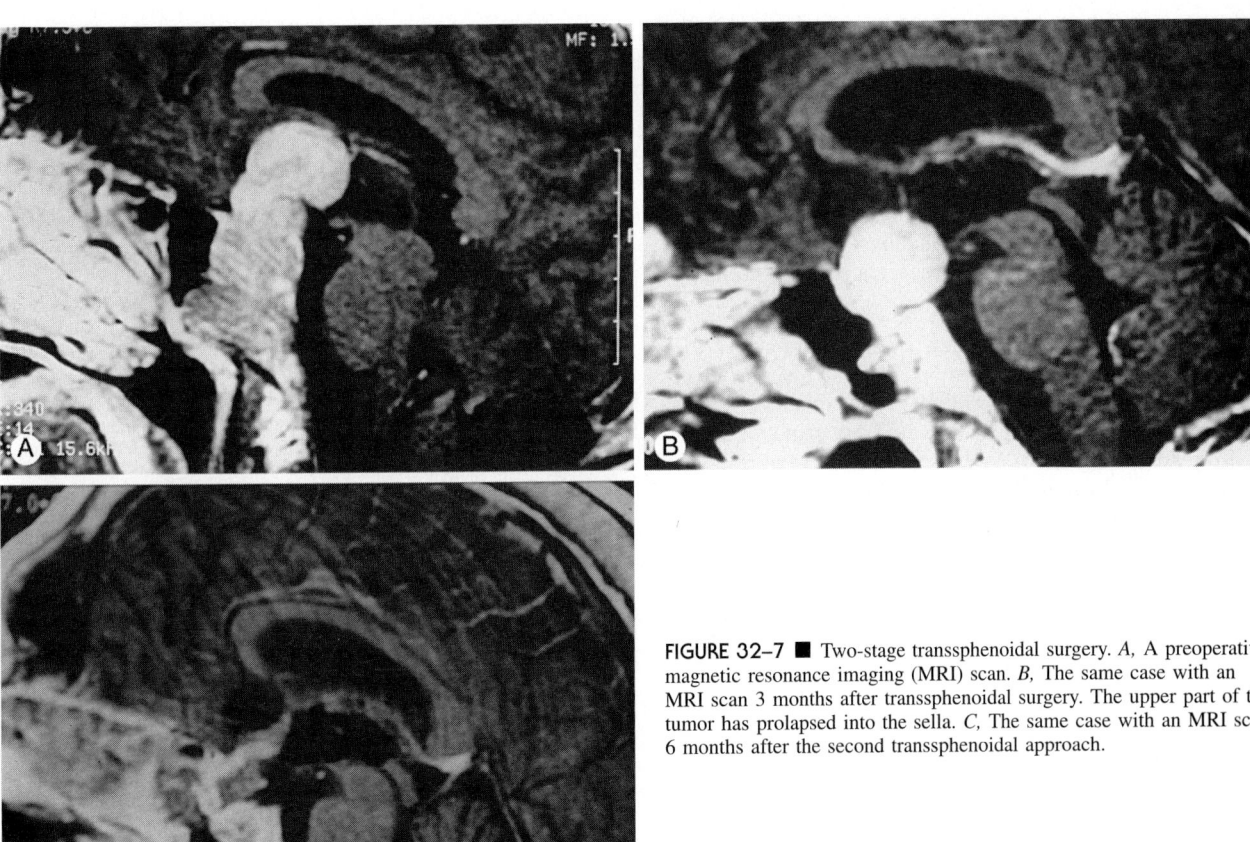

FIGURE 32–7 ■ Two-stage transsphenoidal surgery. *A,* A preoperative magnetic resonance imaging (MRI) scan. *B,* The same case with an MRI scan 3 months after transsphenoidal surgery. The upper part of the tumor has prolapsed into the sella. *C,* The same case with an MRI scan 6 months after the second transsphenoidal approach.

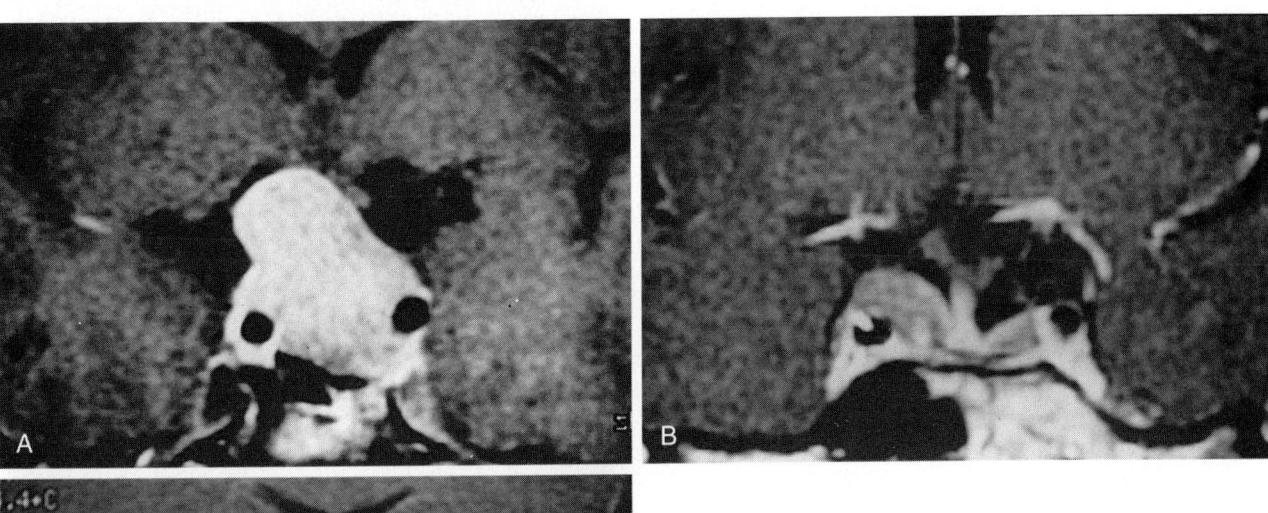

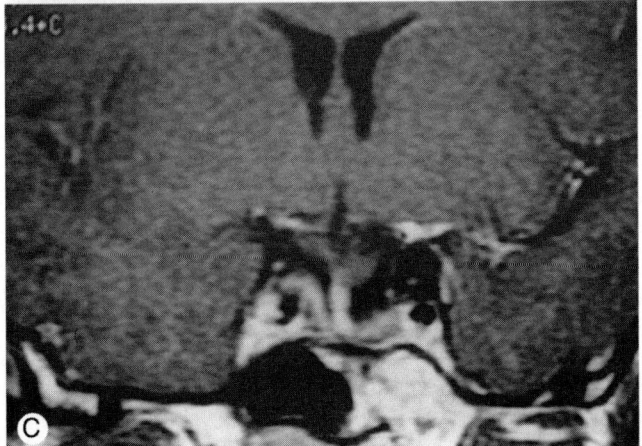

FIGURE 32–8 ■ A nonfunctioning pituitary adenoma: combined transsphenoidal and radiosurgery. *A,* A pituitary adenoma before surgery. *B,* The same case with a magnetic resonance imaging (MRI) scan 4 months after incomplete removal of the paracavernous part of the tumor. *C,* The same case with an MRI scan 1 year after radiosurgery by Gamma knife.

## THE FUTURE

Because of the occurrence of giant tumors, invasiveness, unusual tumor consistency, a tendency toward recurrence, the risk of radiation therapy, and the absence of effective medical treatment, some of nonsecreting pituitary adenomas still constitute a difficult challenge for the neurosurgeon. What are the reasonable prospects for the future?

- *Extensive surgery* is thought to be of little use, even in the most experienced hands, and even if there are further developments in neuronavigation. Extensive surgery cannot claim to achieve total removal of an invasive macroadenoma without damage to the adjacent structures, vessels, nerves, brain stem, and hypothalamus, and does not avoid the need for subsequent radiation therapy.
- *New trends in the field of medical therapy* will probably constitute the most significant advances. At present, neither dopaminergic agonists nor somatostatin analogues should be proposed as first therapy if visual symptoms are present, unless surgery is strongly contrainidicated. However, drugs can be useful as adjuvant therapy in patients not cured by surgery. More extensive use of new scintigraphic studies of dopaminergic receptors might be promising.[63]
- *Radiosurgery* is probably underused, especially in Europe, and should replace conventional radiation therapy, on condition that the neurosurgeon leaves residual tumor suitable for radiosurgery (Fig. 32–8).

## REFERENCES

1. Black PM, Hsu DW, Klibanski A, et al: Hormone production in clinically nonfunctioning pituitary adenomas. J Neurosurg 66:244–250, 1987.
2. Jameson JL, Klibanski A, Black PM, et al: Glycoprotein hormone genes are expressed in clinically nonfunctioning pituitary adenomas. J Clin Invest 80:1472–1478, 1987.
3. Ming-Tak D, Hsu E, Ting LT, et al: The clinicopathological characteristics of gonadotroph cell adenoma: A study of 118 cases. Hum Pathol 28:905–911, 1997.
4. Wilson CB: Surgical management of pituitary tumors: Extensive personal experience. J Clin Endocrinol Metab 82:2381–2385, 1997.
5. Thapar K, Kowacs K, Laws ER, et al: Pituitary adenomas: Current concepts in classification, histopathology and molecular biology. Endocrinologist 3:39–56, 1993.
6. Comtois R, Beauregard M, Somma M, et al: The clinical and endocrine outcome to transsphenoidal microsurgery of non secreting pituitary adenomas. Cancer 68:860–866, 1991.
7. Ebersold MJ, Quast LM, Laws ER Jr, et al: Long term results in transsphenoidal removal of nonfunctioning pituitary adenomas. J Neurosurg 64:713–719, 1986.
8. Arafah BM: Reversible hypopituitarism in patients with large nonfunctioning pituitary adenomas. J Clin Endocrinol Metab 62:1173–1179, 1986.
9. Marazuela M, Astigarraga B, Vicente A, et al: Recovery of visual and endocrine function following transsphenoidal surgery of large nonfunctioning pituitary adenomas. J Endocrinol Invest 17:703–707, 1994.
10. Chanson P, Petrossians P: Les Adénomes Hypophysaires Non fonctionnels. Paris: John Libbey. Eurotext (Eds), 1998, pp 5–127.
11. Dyer H, Civit T, Visot A, et al: Transsphenoidal surgery for pituitary adenomas in children. Neurosurgery 34:207–212, 1994.
12. Mindermann T, Wilson CB: Pediatric pituitary adenomas. Neurosurgery 36:259–269, 1995.
13. Harris PE, Afshar F, Coates P, et al: The effects of transsphenoidal surgery on endocrine function and visual fields in patients with functionless pituitary tumors. QJM 71:417–427, 1989.
14. Molitch ME: Evaluation and treatment of the patient with a pituitary incidentaloma. J Clin Endocrinol Metab 80:3–6, 1995.
15. Greenman Y, Tordjman K, Kisch E, et al: Relative sparing of anterior pituitary function in patients with growth hormone secreting macroadenomas: Comparison with nonfunctioning macroadenomas. J Clin Endocrinol Metab 80:1577–1583, 1995.
16. Scotti G, Yu C-Y, Dillon WP, et al: MR imaging of cavernous sinus involvement by pituitary adenomas. AJR Am J Roentgenol 151:799–806, 1988.
17. Boute D, Dewailly D, Fossati P: Adénomes gonadotropes. Ann Med Interne (Paris) 69:42–52, 1990.
18. Kwekkeboom DJ, Dejong FH, Lamberts SWJ: Gonadotrophin release by clinically nonfunctioning and gonadotroph pituitary adenomas in vivo and vitro: Relation to sex and effects of thyrotropin releasing hormone, gonadotropin releasing hormone and bromocriptine. J Clin Endocrinol Metab 68:1128–1135, 1989.
19. Danesdoost L, Gennarelli TA, Bashey HM, et al: Identification of gonadotroph adenomas in men with clinically nonfunctioning adenomas by the luteinizing hormone beta subunit response to thyrotropin releasing hormone. J Clin Endocrinol Metab 77:1352–1355, 1993.
20. Snyder PJ: Gonadotroph cell adenomas of the pituitary. Endocr Rev 6:552–563, 1985.
21. Oppenheim DS, Kana AR, Sanghar JS, et al: Prevalence of alpha subunit hypersecretion in patients with pituitary tumors: clinically nonfunctioning and somatotroph adenomas. J Clin Endocrinol Metab 70:859–664, 1990.
22. Chanson P, Pantel J, Young J, et al: Free luteinizing hormone beta subunit in normal subjects and patients with pituitary adenomas. J Clin Endocrinol Metab 82:1397–1402, 1997.
23. Klibanski A, Deutsch PJ, Jameson JL, et al: Luteinizing hormone secreting pituitary tumor: Biosynthetic characterization and clinical studies. J Clin Endocrinol Metab 64:536–542, 1987.
24. Trouillas J, Girod C, Sassolas G, et al: The human gonadotropic adenoma: Pathologic and hormonal correlations in 26 tumors. Semin Diagn Pathol 3:42–57, 1986.
25. Sassolas G, Trouillas J, Treluyer C, et al: Management of nonfunctioning pituitary adenomas. Acta Endocrinol 129 (Suppl 1):21–26, 1993.
26. Sekhar LN, Chen CN, Jho HD, et al: Surgical treatment of intracavernous neoplasm. Neurosurgery 24:18–30, 1989.
27. Almefty O, Smith RR: Surgery of tumors invading the cavernous sinus. Surg Neurol 30:370–381, 1988.
28. Guiot G, Derome PJ: Surgical problems of pituitary adenomas. Tech Stand Neurosurg 3:3–33, 1976.
29. Cushing H: Surgical experience with pituitary disorders. JAMA 63:1515–1525, 1914.
30. Kanavel AB: Removal of tumors of the pituitary body by an infranasal route. JAMA 53:1704, 1909.
31. Hirsch O: Endonasal method of removal of hypophyseal tumors with a report of two cases. JAMA 55:772, 1910.
32. Halstead AE: Remarks on the operative treatment of tumors of hypophysis: Two cases operated on by an oronasal route. Trans Am Surg Assoc 27:75, 1910.
33. Dott N, Bailey P: A consideration of the hypophyseal adenomata. Br J Surg 13:314–366, 1925.
34. Guiot G: Transsphenoidal approach in surgical treatment of pituitary adenoma: General principles and indications in nonfunctioning adenomas. International Congress Series Vol 303. Amsterdam: Excerpta Medica, 1973, pp 159–178.
35. Hardy J: Transsphenoidal surgery of the normal and pathological pituitary. Clin Neurosurg 16:185–217, 1969.
36. Laws ER Jr: Transsphenoidal approach to pituitary tumors. In Schmidek HH, Sweet WH (eds): Operative Neurosurgical Techniques, 3rd ed. Philadelphia: WB Saunders, 1995, pp 283–292.
37. Landolt AM: Surgical management of recurrent pituitary tumors. In Schmidek HH, Sweet WH (eds): Operative Neurosurgical Techniques, 3rd ed. Philadelphia: WB Saunders, 1995, pp 315–326.
38. Barrow DL, Tindall GT: Loss of vision after transsphenoidal surgery. Neurosurgery 27:60–68, 1990.
39. Decker RE, Chalif DJ: Progressive coma after the transsphenoidal decompression of a pituitary adenoma with marked suprasellar extension: Report of two cases. Neurosurgery 28:154–158, 1991.
40. Derome PJ, Visot A, Delalande O, et al: Mechanical complications after transsphenoidal removal of pituitary adenomas. In Derome PJ, Jedynak CP, Peillon F (eds): Pituitary Adenomas. Paris: Asclepios, 1980, pp 233–235.

41. Spaziante R, de Devitiis E, Cappabianca P: Repair of the sella following transsphenoidal surgery. In Smidek HH, Sweet WH (eds): Operative Neurosurgical Techniques, 3rd ed. Philadelphia: WB Saunders, 1995, pp 327–345.
42. Laws ER, Fode NC, Redmond MJ: Transsphenoidal surgery following unsuccessful prior therapy. J Neurosurg 63:823–829, 1985.
43. Nicola GC, Tonnarelli G, Griner AC, et al: Surgery for recurrence of pituitary adenomas. In Faglia G, Beck-Peccoz P, Ambroso B, et al (eds): Pituitary Adenomas: New Trends in Basic and Clinical Research. International Congress Series Vol 961. Amsterdam: Excerpta Medica, 1991, pp 329–336.
44. Olson DR, Guiot G, Derome P: The symptomatic empty sella: Prevention and correction via the transsphenoidal approach. J Neurosurg 37:533–537, 1972.
45. Bradley KM, Adams CBT, Potter CPS, et al: An audit of selected patients with nonfunctioning pituitary adenomas treated by transsphenoidal surgery without irradiation. Clin Endocrinol 41:655–659, 1994.
46. Bates AS, Farrel WE, Bicknell EJ, et al: Allelic deletion in pituitary adenomas reflects aggressive biological activity and has a potential value as a prognostic marker. J Cllin Endocrinol Metab 82:818–824, 1997.
47. Tran LM, Blount L, Horton D: Radiation therapy in pituitary tumors: Results in 95 cases. Am J Clin Oncol 14:25–29, 1991.
48. Zangg M, Adaman O, Pescia R, et al: External irradiation of macroinvasive pituitary adenomas with telecobalt: A retrospective study with long term follow up in patients irradiated with doses mostly of between 40–45 Gy. Int J Radiat Oncol Biol Phys 32:671–680, 1995.
49. Snyder PJ, Fowble BF, Schatz NJ, et al: Hypopituitarism following radiation therapy of pituitary adenomas. Am J Med 81:457–462, 1986.
50. Shalet SM: Radiation therapy and pituitary dysfunction (Editorial). N Engl J Med 328:131–132, 1993.
51. Delattre JY, Poisson M: Complications neurologiques de la radiothérapie cérébrale: Apport des études expérimentales. Bull Cancer 77:715–724, 1990.
52. Créange A, Felten D, Kiesel I, et al: Lecoencephalopathie subaiguë du rhombocéphale après radiothérapie hypophysaire. Rev Neurol 150:704–708, 1994.
53. Al-Mefty O, Kersh JE, Routh A, et al: The long term side effects of radiation therapy for benign tumors in adults. J Neurosurg 73:502–512, 1990.
54. Tsang RW, Laperriére NJ, Simpson WJ, et al: Glioma arising after radiation therapy for pituitary adenoma: A report of four patients and estimation of risk. Cancer 72:2227–2233, 1993.
55. Brada M, Ford D, Ashley S, et al: Risk of second brain tumor after conservative surgery and radiotherapy for pituitary adenoma. BMJ 304:1343–1346, 1992.
56. Rodriguez O, Mateos B, De La Predaja R: Postoperative follow up of pituitary adenomas after transsphenoidal resection: MRI and clinical correlation. Neuroradiology 38:747–754, 1996.
57. Ciric I, Mikhael M, Stadfort T, et al: Transsphenoidal microsurgery of pituitary macroadenomas with long term follow up results. J Neurosurg 59:395–401, 1983.
58. McCullough WM, Marcus RB Jr, Rhoton AI, et al: Long term follow up of radiotherapy for pituitary adenoma: The absence of late recurrence after 45 Gy. Int J Radiat Oncol Biol Phys 21:607–614, 1991.
59. Derome PJ, Visot A, Delalande O, et al: Pituitary adenomas: Our experience of tumoral recurrence after surgery. In Faglia G, Beck-Peccoz P, Ambrosi B, et al (eds): Pituitary Adenomas: New Trends in Basic and Clinical Research. International Congress Series Vol 961. Amsterdam: Excepta Medica, 1991, 321–327.
60. Saito K, Kuwayama A, Yamamoto N, et al: The transsphenoidal removal of nonfunctioning pituitary adenomas with suprasellar extensions: The open sella method and intentionally staged operation. Neurosurgery 36:668–676, 1995.
61. Reincke M, Allolio B, Saeger W, et al: The "incidentaloma" of the pituitary gland: Is neurosurgery required? JAMA 263:2772–2776, 1990.
62. Donovan LE, Corenblum B: The natural history of the pituitary incidentaloma. Arch Intern Med 155:181–183, 1995.
63. De Herder WW, Reijs AE, Kwekkeboom DJ, et al: In vivo imaging of pituitary tumors using a radiolabelled dopamine $D_2$ receptor radiologand. Clin Endocrinol 45:755–767, 1996.
64. Jaffrain-Réa ML, Derome P, Bataini JP, et al: Influence of radiotherapy on long term relapse in clinically non secreting pituitary adenomas: A retrospective study (1970–1988). Eur J Med 2:398–403, 1993.
65. Chun M, Masko GB, Hetelekidis S: Radiotherapy in the treatment of pituitary adenomas. Int J Radiat Oncol Biol Phys 15:305–309, 1988.
66. Vlahovitch B, Reybaud C, Rhiati J, et al: Treatment and recurrences in 135 pituitary adenomas. Acta Neurochir (Wien) 42 (Suppl):120–123, 1988.
67. Sheline GE: Proceedings: Treatment of nonfunctioning chromophobe adenomas of the pituitary. Am J Roentgenol Radiat Ther Neurol Med 120:553–561, 1974.
68. Hayes TP, Davis RA, Raventos A: The treatment of pituitary chromophobe adenomas. Radiology 98:149–153, 1971.

CHAPTER 33

# Surgical Management of Growth Hormone–Secreting and Prolactin-Secreting Pituitary Adenomas

■ MARK D. KRIEGER, ARUN P. AMAR, WILLIAM T. COULDWELL, and MARTIN H. WEISS

## MANAGEMENT OF GROWTH HORMONE–SECRETING PITUITARY ADENOMAS

Somatotropes, or growth hormone (GH)-producing cells of the pituitary gland, comprise approximately 50% of the normal adenohypophysial cell population and are located in the lateral wings of the anterior lobe. GH is a 191–amino-acid polypeptide hormone that opposes the effect of insulin, stimulates the uptake of amino acids, and causes a release of free fatty acids from tissue storage sites. In the liver and other tissues, GH also mediates the synthesis of somatomedins (also called insulin-like growth factors), which induce protein synthesis in the skeleton and in muscle, and glucose oxidation in adipose tissue; they also stimulate cell replication at these sites. The secretion of GH is stimulated by GH-releasing hormone (GHRH) and inhibited by somatostatin. GH and somatomedin-C (also known as insulin-like growth factor-1 [IGF-1]) stimulate the release of somatostatin, thereby downregulating the secretion of GH. GH is secreted in episodic surges occurring every 3 to 4 hours; in young people, the greatest peaks occur after the onset of deep sleep. Stimuli of GH secretion include insulin-induced hypoglycemia, arginine, exercise, L-dopa, clonidine, propranolol, and GHRH.

Acromegaly and gigantism are the result of oversecretion of GH into the somatic circulation. Collectively, they are second in frequency to hyperprolactinemia as pituitary hypersecretory syndromes. They are almost always caused by a somatotroph (i.e., GH-secreting) adenoma of the pituitary (>99% of cases) as opposed to somatotroph hyperplasia from excess secretion of ectopic GHRH.[1] Although most of these pituitary tumors exhibit a moderate growth rate, they often present relatively early in their growth because of the detection of a hypersecretory syndrome. In our personal series, more than 70% were microadenomas on presentation.[2] However, they can present as macroadeno-

mas with extrasellar extension and focal destruction.[3, 4] (In other series, as many as 85% to 90% of patients present with macroadenomas and 10% to 15% with microadenomas.[1]) Younger patients with acromegaly often harbor larger and more rapidly growing tumors.[5] Acromegalic tumors may contain and also secrete prolactin (PRL) or the α-subunit (common to all the glycoprotein adenohypophysial hormones) and, rarely, thyroid-stimulating hormone (TSH) in addition to GH.[3] Most patients with large tumors have mixed GH and PRL hypersecretion,[6] which results in concomitant hyperprolactinemia in 20% to 40% of patients.[3, 5] PRL is most often secreted from a tumor containing a mixed population of somatotroph and lactotroph cells (an acidophilic stem cell tumor), but occasionally from a bipotential mammosomatotroph adenoma.[4] In patients harboring mammosomatotroph adenomas, the two hormones, by definition, are present within the same cell, the same secretory granule, or both, and are usually secreted in a similar dynamic pattern.[5]

The total amount of GH secreted in a 24-hour period is variable among patients harboring GH-secreting tumors and depends on cell activity, but it roughly correlates with the size of the tumor.[7] GH oversecretion results in elevated plasma IGF-1 levels[3] that are fairly stable and reflect the integrated pulsatile 24-hour secretion of GH. As GH levels increase, IGF-1 rises linearly until GH reaches approximately 20 ng/ml, after which the IGF-1 level plateaus. As a corollary, to achieve any measure of successful treatment, GH must decrease to a level below 20 ng/ml for IGF-1 levels to drop or clinical improvement to occur.[1] However, there is a poor correlation between plasma GH levels and clinical manifestations of acromegaly, presumably because of variable responsiveness of peripheral tissues to GH excess.[3]

### Clinical Manifestations and Diagnosis

The clinical manifestations of excess secretion of GH depend on the age of the patient. If the excess secretion

438

occurs in childhood or adolescence, before the epiphyses of long bones have fused, the result is gigantism; people with such a condition may attain great height if the disease progresses unchecked (often >7 ft). After fusion of the epiphyses, excess GH produces the syndrome of acromegaly in adults, with soft tissue and bony enlargement in characteristic locations. Clinical manifestations of these soft tissue changes include coarsening of facial features, laryngeal enlargement, goiter, thick heel pads, acanthosis nigricans, cardiomegaly, and hepatomegaly. Bony changes are extensive, producing prognathism (enlargement of the mandible with increased spacing between the teeth) and bony enlargements of hands and feet. Soft tissue and bony changes may produce compressive neuropathies and arthropathies. Metabolic manifestations include associated hypertension, diabetes mellitus and goiter, and commonly hyperhidrosis. Deficiencies in corticotropin-releasing hormone and TSH are found in less than 10% to 20% of patients. Hypogonadism occurs in 30% to 40% of patients, but it may be attributable to associated hyperprolactinemia[3] and may result in osteoporosis. Acromegaly affects men and women with approximately equal frequency.

The diagnosis is made by assessing GH secretion. A basal fasting GH level greater than 10 ng/ml is present in 90% of acromegalic patients. However, because GH is secreted in several peaks throughout the day, a single fasting level may fail to demonstrate an elevated level in some patients. Therefore, the suspected diagnosis is confirmed by the glucose suppression test. In the acromegalic person, an oral administration of 100 g of glucose fails to suppress the serum GH level to less than 5 ng/ml at 60 minutes. The measurement of serum IGF-1 levels are elevated in acromegalic patients and proves to be a more reliable measure of the disease and its response to treatment. Radiographic imaging (magnetic resonance imaging [MRI], computed tomography [CT], or both) demonstrates the presence of a pituitary adenoma in greater than 90% of patients with endocrinologically documented acromegaly. High-field, thin-section MRI scans are the most sensitive imaging method for preoperative localization of pituitary adenomas. On unenhanced images, focal glandular hypodensity identified on coronal images is the most sensitive predictor of adenoma location. Radiographic evaluation should consist of coronal, sagittal, and axial MRI, with large tumors usually having similar signal intensity to that of brain on $T_1$-weighted images. The normal pituitary gland, infundibulum, and cavernous sinuses enhance immediately after administration of gadolinium-diethylenetriamine-penta-acetic acid (DTPA), allowing contrast between the enhancing normal glandular tissue and the low-intensity adenomas. A $T_1$-weighted image after the infusion of gadolinium-DTPA is the method of choice for the delineation of intrasellar disease. Shortly after administration, the normal vascular pituitary increases in signal intensity, and a pituitary tumor is visible but remains less intense, being slower to perfuse with the contrast agent.

## Indications for Therapy and Goals of Treatment

Excess secretion of GH should be considered a malignant endocrinopathy, which may result in life-threatening medical complications, and thus should be treated aggressively once diagnosed. Left untreated, the mortality rate is double that of healthy age-matched control subjects, from complications including hypertension, cardiac disease, diabetes, pulmonary infections, and associated malignancies.[8–11] The goals of therapy in management of a GH-secreting pituitary adenoma include: (1) resolution of tumor mass effect, (2) restoration of normal GH physiology (absolute normalization of GH and somatomedin C [IGF-1] levels), and (3) replacement of any associated hormone deficiencies.

To date, there are no generally accepted criteria for assessment of cure of acromegaly.[9, 12–14] Various biochemical tests have been proposed in the postoperative period, including basal GH level, mean GH levels, GH response to the oral glucose tolerance test, GH response to thyrotropin-releasing hormone, and IGF-1 (somatomedin C) levels. Each of these tests has been found limited in determining cure. Many authors now believe that criteria for successful therapy (chemical cure) include 24-hour integrated GH concentration of no more than 2.5 ng/ml, together with normalization of the circulating IGF-1 level.[4, 15]

In our institution, we use normalization of the IGF-1 level as the ultimate determinant of successful therapy (chemical cure). We have found that, in 99% of cases, an early postoperative growth hormone level of 2 ng/ml or less correlates with long-term normalization of the IGF-1 level and thus long-term disease remission. However, higher levels of GH rarely indicate long-term chemical cure.[2]

## Microadenomas

In the patient harboring a GH-secreting microadenoma, if he or she is medically stable enough to undergo a surgical procedure, surgical resection should be considered the optimal first choice of management. Trans-sphenoidal microsurgical adenomectomy is currently the most accepted and efficient first-line therapy for the GH-secreting tumors of acromegaly.[9, 16–27] Some authors indicate that the transnasal dissection in the acromegalic patient with associated soft tissue and bony changes may present an added challenge for the surgeon. However, in our experience, this has never been a limiting factor in the use of the trans-sphenoidal approach. Such tumors may be cured by chemical criteria in most cases. A large, combined analysis of 1360 acromegalic patients by Ross and Wilson[24] documented an overall postoperative cure rate of 60.4%. Microadenomas have an even higher rate of cure, exceeding 76% to 84% in large surgical series.[9, 16, 19–21, 26–28] In our personal series, 78% of patients with microadenomas undergoing trans-sphenoidal resection achieved normal long-term IGF-1 levels, and were considered cured. This rate was determined using very stringent criteria for cure: a postoperative growth hormone level not greater than 2 ng/ml, a normal 5-year IGF-1, and clinical evidence of disease remission at 5 years.[2] Postoperative persistent elevation of GH or IGF-1 levels would be an indication for pharmacotherapy or radiation therapy (see later).

## Macroadenomas

The patient harboring a GH-secreting macroadenoma poses a more difficult management dilemma. Certainly, the likelihood of cure is low in cases of large tumors with frank cavernous sinus invasion; in our series, only 31% of all patients with a macroadenoma achieved chemical cure by surgery alone.[2] Pharmacotherapy or radiation therapy should thus be considered as integral components in the overall management plan. In these cases, initial pharmacotherapy may be indicated; however, surgical resection may be helpful in decreasing the tumor load to effect an absolute normalization of IGF-1 levels by pharmacotherapy.

## Pharmacotherapy

Pharmacotherapy should be considered in (1) patients in whom surgery is contraindicated; (2) patients whose GH and IGF-1 levels are still elevated after surgery, as an alternative to radiation therapy at this stage; and (3) patients with elevated GH and IGF-1 levels after surgery and radiation therapy.[1] Medical therapy may be administered in conjunction with radiation therapy to provide interim GH suppression while awaiting the beneficial effects of the radiation.

## Somatostatin Analogues

### PHYSIOLOGY

Native somatostatin is believed to control GH secretion by suppression of GH release from the pituitary gland and GHRH from the hypothalamus.[29] At present, there is only one Food and Drug Administration (FDA)-approved analogue appropriate for clinical use, octreotide (Sandostatin; Sandoz, East Hanover, NJ; previously designated as SMS 201-995).[30] Octreotide contains the active sequence of somatostatin, and it appears to control GH secretion similarly by suppression of GH release from the pituitary gland and by suppression of GHRH from the hypothalamus.[29] Compared with the native hormone, it has enhanced binding affinity to the somatostatin receptor and a prolonged half-life of 110 minutes after subcutaneous injection of a 50- to 100-μg dose, providing an overall duration of effect of 6 to 8 hours.[31] A single injection of octreotide produces a decrease in GH levels within 30 to 60 minutes, with maximum suppression of GH levels occurring in 2 to 4 hours.[32] Analogues are under investigation that have greater biologic potency than octreotide and are more specific for the pituitary gland.[4]

### TUMOR SOMATOSTATIN RECEPTOR STATUS

Large numbers of specific somatostatin-binding sites in human GH-secreting pituitary adenomas have been demonstrated.[33–35] There appears to be heterogeneity with regard to the number of somatostatin receptors between tumors and in their distribution within a particular tumor. Most tumors contain somatostatin receptors in densities that are comparable with those in normal somatotrophs[35] and respond normally to somatostatin.[36] However, 10% to 30% of GH-secreting tumors have reduced numbers of somatostatin receptors; patients with such tumors exhibit diminished in vivo responses to octreotide.[35]

### DOSE AND MODE OF ADMINISTRATION

The usual initial dose is 100 μg subcutaneously every 8 hours, and this dose should be increased until adequate suppression is achieved. In acromegalic patients treated with octreotide, a close correlation has been found between the mean 24-hour GH and IGF-1 levels before and during therapy.[37–40] Therefore, regular IGF-1 measurements on an outpatient basis enable optimization of the daily dose and number of octreotide injections needed for each individual patient.[38, 40] Most patients achieve control with 300 to 600 μg/day.[32] In a national survey, doses of 750 μg/day resulted in increased frequency of tumor shrinkage without adding any biochemical or clinical benefit.[41] Over a 6-month period, the size of the pituitary tumor was reduced in 34% of patients receiving this latter dose versus 17% of patients receiving 300 μg/day. The maximum recommended dose is 1500 μg/day.[4] As much as 50% of patients can be maintained on a twice-daily regimen,[42] but some patients may achieve better control by receiving the same daily dose every 6 hours instead.[4] In this regard, continuous subcutaneous pump infusion of 100 to 600 μg/day has been shown to provide superior and more stable suppression of mean 24-hour GH levels.[43]

### EFFICACY

Seventy-five to 90% of acromegalic patients experience some biochemical, clinical, and metabolic improvement with octreotide therapy. Clinical improvement may be heralded by the disappearance or the amelioration of excessive sweating, headaches, paresthesia, soft tissue swelling, and joint pain improvement of nerve entrapment symptoms, together with a general sense of well-being.[4, 41] Immediate and prolonged relief of headaches is experienced in some patients with acromegaly, usually in those with evidence of suprasellar tumor extension.[44] Visual field improvement has been noted, in many cases without demonstrable change in tumor size (see later).[4] In some patients, dose- and time-related symptoms indicative of drug dependency occur,[45] which may be mediated by the binding of octreotide to opioid receptors.[4]

Effective decreases of GH and IGF-1 levels occur in 30% to 53% and in 40% to 68% of patients, respectively, according to various studies.[4, 31, 32, 41, 46, 47] In most patients, IGF-1 levels fall within 1 week of the start of treatment and tend to normalize in 37% to 81% of patients with continued therapy.[41, 42, 48–50] GH and IGF-1 levels have been shown to continue to decrease with long-term treatment of 1.5 to 2 years compared with levels at 6 to 12 months.[51] Long-term responsiveness can be predicted by the acute GH suppression effect of a single test injection of 50 μg of octreotide. The mean hourly GH level from 2 to 6 hours after drug injection exhibits a high degree of correlation with the 24-hour integrated GH level after long-term (1- to 2-year) therapy.[52] The plasma IGF-1 and GH level responses 2 hours after drug injection or any time during subcutaneous infusion are also useful predictors of efficacy.[4] Plasma PRL levels in patients with mixed GH/PRL-containing tumors have been shown to be suppressed by octreotide in approximately one half of cases.[51] Elevated concentrations of the α-subunit, which can be found in approximately 35% of acromegalic patients,[53] respond to octreotide in a similar fashion to GH level.[32]

Preoperative treatment with octreotide causes the tumor to become soft and to exhibit a grayish-red color at surgery.[54] Several neurosurgical groups have concluded that pretreatment with octreotide to soften the adenoma has facilitated surgical resection.[54, 55] Long-term octreotide therapy produces a slight decrease in pituitary tumor size in approximately 20% to 50% of acromegalic patients.[38, 39, 41, 56] Complete tumor shrinkage has been reported in isolated cases.[57] Tumor size may increase soon after the drug is stopped,[58] but in occasional patients, a period off the drug may subsequently permit comparable control to be achieved at a lower dose. This phenomenon is possibly explained by a reversal of somatostatin receptor downregulation.[4]

### HISTOLOGIC CHANGES

Shrinkage of adenomas during octreotide therapy might reflect a decrease in the size of individual tumor cells.[32] Electron microscopy of adenomas pretreated with octreotide revealed small necrotic cells and a greater number of macrophages, whereas normal pituitary cells showed an accumulation of lipoprotein and secretory granules.[59] These morphologic findings were primarily consistent with chronic suppression of GH release.

### SIDE EFFECTS

Although octreotide is usually well tolerated, several side effects have been reported. Within the first few days of administration, a transient decrease in gastrointestinal motility and slowed absorption occur in most patients. The patient may experience transient abdominal pains and bloating. Steatorrhea, presumably due to a reduction in pancreatic exocrine secretion,[21] occurs less frequently but may persist with long-term therapy. Treatment with pancreatic enzymes, if necessary, is usually effective.[1]

Nutritional deficiency has not been reported. Toxic hepatitis has occurred very infrequently. Inhibition of insulin secretion can lead to hyperglycemia, although the concomitant improvement in glucose tolerance as a consequence of a decrease in GH secretion is usually sufficient to prevent this. Although somatostatin inhibits TSH secretion, hypothyroidism has not been reported during long-term octreotide therapy.[38, 39, 48] The side effect of greatest concern is cholelithiasis due to suppression of cholecystokinin secretion and a resulting decrease in bile flow. The incidence of gallstone formation in patients on long-term octreotide therapy is 40% to 50%[15, 60]; thus, all patients should be screened regularly for the development of gallstones during treatment.[42] No allergic problems related to octreotide have been reported, although antibodies to octreotide have been detected in one patient.[6] Tachyphylaxis and desensitization have not been observed during long-term treatment.[32] Although the injections are often painful, the pain may be minimized by slow injection of the drug.[1]

## Dopaminergic Analogues

### PHYSIOLOGY

Dopamine agonists stimulate GH secretion from normal subjects through a central nervous system–mediated mechanism that increases GHRH secretion,[61] and possibly through the regulation of somatostatin secretion.[4] In contrast, in acromegalic patients, dopamine agonists suppress GH secretion in at least one half of patients[62] through a PRL-dependent $D_2$ receptor mechanism.[63] Dopamine agonists are primarily effective in GH-secreting tumors that also secrete PRL.[4] Unfortunately, many acromegalic tumors contain few or no $D_2$ receptors, which is reflected by a poor clinical response to these drugs.

### DOSE AND MODE OF ADMINISTRATION

All available agents are members of the ergoline family of compounds. Both bromocriptine (Parlodel; Sandoz) and pergolide (Permax; Lilly, Indianapolis, IN) are available for use in the United States. Newer dopamine agonists do not seem to offer any major advantage over bromocriptine in these patients.[4] Bromocriptine is administered orally every 8 to 12 hours.[4] Up to 20 to 30 mg bromocriptine per day has been used to obtain maximum benefit, a dose that has been frequently associated with side effects.[1, 4] To avoid the occurrence of side effects when initiating therapy, a low dose of 1.25 mg should be administered at bedtime. Gradual increases in increments of 1.25 mg should be made every 3 to 4 days until the desired effect is reached.[1] The medication should be taken with meals.[64]

### EFFICACY

Amelioration of signs and symptoms of GH excess occurs in 70% of treated acromegalic patients, although GH levels are reduced to 10 ng/ml or less in only 50% and to 5 ng/ml or less in only 20% of these patients.[4] Only 8% of patients achieve normal IGF-1 levels, which is the only reliable parameter for assessing overall normality of pulsatile GH secretion.[1] Less favorable results are seen with larger tumors and if initial GH levels are above 50 ng/ml.[63] Tumor shrinkage is uncommon, occurring in only 10% to 15% of patients.[4, 65]

The only known factor predicting responsiveness to dopaminergic agonists is coexistence of PRL hypersecretion. Even in such patients, it is not unusual to achieve total suppression of PRL secretion with only partial or no suppression of GH.[4] A single test dose of bromocriptine (2.5 mg orally) followed by hourly plasma GH levels for 4 to 6 hours may be used to assess therapeutic efficacy. Caution should be observed during this test because side effects may occur after the administration of this dose.

### HISTOLOGIC CHANGES

At a morphologic level, bromocriptine produces almost no change in human GH-secreting adenomas, except for an increase in the stromal tissue volume with occasional occurrence of vacuolation and single-cell necrosis.[66]

### SIDE EFFECTS

Significant side effects of bromocriptine include malaise, nausea, vomiting, and postural hypotension. Less commonly, headache, abdominal cramps, constipation, nasal congestion, and depression have been described. Hallucinations have been reported in 1.3% of patients[67] and, rarely, cold-induced vasospasm, most pronounced in the digits, may occur.[1]

## Combined Use of Bromocriptine and Octreotide

Few patients who do not respond to either octreotide or bromocriptine alone respond to the combination of octreotide and bromocriptine.[32, 51, 68, 69]

## Radiation Therapy

With the advent of a pharmacotherapeutic agent effective in a large percentage of these tumors, it is hoped that the need for radiation therapy in these patients will diminish. At our institution, radiation therapy is considered only for those patients in whom chemical cure through surgery has not been achieved and in whom medical therapy is contraindicated, not tolerated, or demonstrated to be ineffective.

Radiation therapy has been advocated for the management of pituitary tumors since 1907.[70] Radiation therapy per se, however, should not be considered a completely benign therapy or an equivalent alternative to microsurgical resection.[71] Adverse effects from radiation in this region may range from mild to severe. It carries a significant risk of worsening of pre-existing hypopituitarism, with an overt 10% to 15% frequency of panhypopituitarism[72]; may increase the rate of atherogenesis in the major vessels in the field; and it may cause visual impairment.[71] These complications increase as a function of total treatment dose.[73] The visual impairment may result from one of several mechanisms, including empty sella syndrome, treatment failure, and direct radiation damage to optic pathways. The latter complication is seen with significant frequency with daily fractionation of greater than 220 cGy.[73] Other minor complications from radiation therapy include epilation, scalp swelling, and otitis.[74]

Should radiation therapy be indicated in an acromegalic patient, a dose of 4000 cGy by external beam is considered optimal by most radiation therapists.[73, 75] In a reported series of 12 patients treated with radiation therapy alone, Chun and colleagues[71] described a 50% recurrence rate, with a 75% incidence of local control after salvage treatment. Other authors report a local control rate of 50% to 79%, with an adequate salvage in cases of recurrence.[76, 77] The rationale for the use of postoperative radiation therapy is to reduce the incidence of recurrence, with several studies suggesting improved tumor control with the combination of surgery plus radiation therapy[71, 72, 78, 79] This is especially true in large and invasive lesions, which exhibit an increased rate of recurrence. This treatment, however, by no means ensures recurrence-free survival, but the time to recurrence may be prolonged. Valtonen and Myllymaki[80] have reported a surprisingly high 36% recurrence rate in patients with so-called "total removal" after transfrontal craniotomy and postoperative radiation therapy, with recurrences occurring up to 18 years after therapy. Thus, published recurrence rates may be misleading in series with short follow-up times.

The development of focal radiation therapy techniques (i.e., stereotactic radiosurgery) offers a potentially improved method in delivering accurate lethal dosages of radiation to the tumor while limiting toxicity to the surrounding visual and neural structures. Clinical trials are under way.

## Follow-Up

As noted earlier, most patients with microadenomas experience postoperative amelioration of their endocrinopathy. Overall, 78% of patients with microadenomas and 64% of all patients (microadenomas and macroadenomas) in our personal series attained normal postoperative IGF-1 levels.[2]

Although the surgical experience with microadenomas has been satisfying, cure with restoration of intact pituitary function is rarely achieved with large macroadenomas.[63] In our series, only 31% of patients with macroadenomas achieved a chemical cure from surgery alone.[2] Even when normal postoperative GH levels are achieved, normal pulsatile secretion of GH and glucose suppression often are not restored.[4] Clinically, the physical manifestations of acromegaly are rarely reversed; however, there appears to be little progression of the clinical manifestations of disease when GH levels are below 5 ng/ml.

All acromegalic patients, regardless of initial tumor size, must be followed assiduously for recurrence of their endocrinopathy after surgery. This vigilance is mandated by the increased morbidity and mortality associated with persistent disease. Physical examination for progression of acromegaly and for the development of hypopituitarism is indicated. Whereas GH levels less than 5 ng/ml are not usually associated with persistent clinical disease, levels greater than 2 ng/ml indicate a risk for recrudescent disease and must be monitored closely. After an initial postoperative IGF-1 level obtained at 6 weeks, follow-up measurements of GH or IGF-1 should be performed every 6 months.[3] If octreotide is administered after irradiation, it is withdrawn for 2 weeks every 1 to 2 years, and GH and IGF-1 levels are measured. If they are normal, the drug should be discontinued.[1]

## MANAGEMENT OF PROLACTIN-SECRETING PITUITARY ADENOMAS

The mammotropes, also called lactotropes, secrete PRL in the normal pituitary and represent 15% to 25% of the adenohypophysial cells. They are located in the lateral gland, and they accumulate during pregnancy and lactation and after estrogen therapy. PRL is a 198–amino-acid polypeptide known to facilitate the development of breast tissue to ensure the production of milk. PRL secretion is stimulated by thyrotropin-releasing hormone, estrogens, stress, and exercise. Dopamine is acknowledged to be the principal PRL-inhibitory factor.

Prolactin-secreting adenomas are the most common type of secretory pituitary tumor and are second in frequency only to null-cell adenomas in overall incidence.[64] In the pediatric population, however, they represent the most frequent type of adenoma overall.[81]

## Clinical Manifestations and Diagnosis

Although these tumors are found pathologically at autopsy with equal frequency in men and women, they are clinically significantly more common in women. They are also more common in girls than boys.[81] Hyperprolactinemia causes galactorrhea in women and hypogonadism, which are exhibited as anovulatory infertility in the woman and impotence in the man.[82, 83] Presumed abnormalities in pulsatile secretion of GHRH and gonadotropins precipitate a relative estrogen deficiency.[84, 85] This hypogonadal state is associated with osteoporosis in women[86] and both cortical and trabecular osteopenia in men.[87]

In a series of some 392 PRL-secreting pituitary tumors operated on by one of us (MHW), 321 (82%) were in female patients.[88] The most common presenting symptom in this group was the development of secondary amenorrhea (72%); only approximately 50% of those with amenorrhea had associated galactorrhea.[88] Epidemiologically, approximately 5% of women with primary amenorrhea and 25% of women with secondary amenorrhea (other than those who are pregnant) harbor a PRL-secreting pituitary tumor as the cause of their clinical symptoms. Because of this readily identifiable symptom, these patients usually present relatively early in the course of evolution of the tumors; this is unfortunately not true in the male population. Because the primary symptom of a PRL-secreting tumor in the male patient is usually a decrease in libido well before true impotence is observed, this problem is frequently ascribed to the aging process or functional causes. Approximately two thirds of men with hyperprolactinemia due to a PRL-secreting tumor have a low serum testosterone level[89]; this condition may be secondary to hyperprolactinemia per se or to mechanical compression of adjacent normal pituitary gland. Thus, men often present at a more advanced age and later in the course of their disease with chiasmal compression and visual compromise. In our series, visual loss ranging in duration from 2 to 24 months was the initial complaint in 60% of men but only 10% of women.[88] For the same reasons, large tumors associated with hypothyroidism and adrenal insufficiency are more common in men.[89] In the pediatric population, boys tend to have much larger tumors and higher preoperative PRL levels than girls, and they frequently present with focal neurologic deficit or other signs of significant mass effect.[81]

The diagnosis is secured by radiographic evidence of a pituitary lesion with an elevation of serum PRL. As with GH-secreting tumors, high-field, thin-section MRI is the most sensitive imaging method for preoperative localization of pituitary adenomas. There exists a rough correlation between the size of the lesion radiographically and pathologically and the serum level of PRL. In addition, local invasion of the tumor into the adjacent venous cavernous sinuses is associated with a marked increase in serum PRL. The diagnosis of pathologic PRL excess should be based on serial blood measurements[63]; PRL levels greater than five times the upper limit of normal are usually associated with a PRL-secreting pituitary tumor.[90] In the endocrinologic evaluation of the patient suspected of harboring a PRL-secreting tumor, it must be appreciated that larger tumors of any endocrine basis may cause a mild to moder-

ate hyperprolactinemia resulting from the so-called "stalk section effect" (disconnection hyperprolactinemia stalk compression causing loss of dopaminergic inhibition to tonic PRL release),[91] which must be distinguished from a true prolactinoma. Under such circumstances, it is rare to see PRL levels in excess of 100 ng/ml. However, we encountered a patient with a preoperative prolactin level above 600 ng/ml, confirmed by serial laboratory testing, that was attributed to stalk section effect on the basis of immunohistochemical analysis of the tumor, which failed to stain for prolactin.[92] In general, large tumors (>2 cm in diameter) associated with PRL levels less than 150 ng/ml (certainly those <100 ng/ml) should be suspected of being nonsecretors when planning management strategies. Such nonsecretors would not be expected to respond to chemical reductions of serum PRL.

A number of reports suggest that neither tumor size nor PRL levels change over a number of years in most women with microprolactinomas.[93, 94] In fact, it has been observed that few microprolactinomas progress to macroadenomas.[90] In one of our earlier series, for example, only 3 of 27 women harboring microadenomas demonstrated significant tumor growth over a 6-year interval of observation.[95] In contrast, macroadenomas, which for reasons described earlier frequently occur in men, may behave in an aggressive manner.[63] They may be associated with invasion of the cavernous sinuses and diffuse invasion of the base of the skull, and they commonly extend to the suprasellar region.[96] Hemorrhage or cyst formation within the tumor may also occur.

The levels of elevated PRL in a diagnosed pituitary adenoma are of great help in determining subsequent management because the ability successfully to extirpate the tumor is reduced with large or invasive lesions (see later).

## Indications for Therapy and Goals of Treatment

Bromocriptine is the first-choice drug for therapy of PRL-secreting tumors. The efficacy of bromocriptine (a dopaminergic agonist) in reducing serum PRL, in addition to reducing tumor size and inhibiting further tumor growth, is well established (see later). The central considerations related to treating such patients are the ability of the patient to tolerate the medication, the realization that the treatment must continue for the duration of the patient's life, and the implications for fertility.

With PRL-secreting microadenomas, therapeutic options include medical or surgical management. In our series, 225 of 262 patients (86%) undergoing surgery for tumors less than 1 cm in size had normal (<20 ng/ml) postoperative PRL levels (i.e., chemical cure).[88] The operative mortality rate was zero, and associated morbidity was low. The experience of other centers corroborates this high rate of surgical success.[97–103] Strong consideration should thus be given to surgical intervention in patients harboring smaller tumors without significant hyperprolactinemia.

In cases of larger tumors, however, surgical chemical cures (i.e., postoperative serum PRL <20 ng/ml) are much less frequent. Those tumors associated with PRL levels greater than 200 ng/ml recur in over 50% of cases after surgery alone[82]; the rate of recurrence of hyperprolactinemia after surgery for macroadenomas (with PRL levels >250 ng/ml) exceeds 70%.[82, 104] In our series, only 63 of 130 (49%) of those patients with tumors greater than 1 cm had chemical cure. Although no medical therapy results in cure of a PRL-secreting macroadenoma, only a minority of these patients remain free of their disease after surgery alone. Therefore, bromocriptine should be considered as initial therapy for those patients in whom surgical resection resulting in chemical cure is deemed unlikely.[105] On the other hand, some surgeons recommend operative removal in most macroadenomas.[102]

It is our practice to place all patients with large or invasive pituitary tumors with endocrinologically documented PRL secretion on a therapeutic trial of bromocriptine initially, and to monitor clinical status and the lesion's radiographic appearance accordingly. All solid primary PRL-secreting tumors should respond to the medication, both by a reduction in tumor size and by a reduction in PRL level. One exception to this management is larger primary cystic tumors, which are much less likely to respond to pharmacotherapy.

The goals of treatment include: (1) reduction of the tumor mass, (2) correction of the hyperprolactinemic state, and (3) preservation of anterior pituitary function.[82] The tenet of therapy should be absolute normalization of PRL levels because a prolonged hyperprolactinemic state may be associated with significant osteoporosis and infertility. Surgical resection of these lesions is indicated in patients who are intolerant of the side effects of the medication, unable to afford the cost of the medication for a prolonged period, or in whom sustained tumor reduction is not effected. Furthermore, the FDA recommends discontinuing the medication as soon as pregnancy has been established because of concerns about its safety to the mother and fetus.[106] As discussed later, expansion of the tumor and compression of the optic structures has been reported in patients while off bromocriptine during gestation.[106] Thus, the desire for fertility constitues another indication for surgical resection, and in our experience, 72 of 96 women (75%) who wanted to achieve pregnancy did so after transsphenoidal surgery.[88] Collectively, these reasons necessitate surgery in approximately 20% to 25% of patients with microadenomas, whereas the remaining patients can be successfully treated with bromocriptine alone.[97, 103, 107] Among patients with macroadenomas, however, Wilson[102] and others recommend operative removal in most cases.

Subsequent to surgery, if hyperprolactinemia is persistent to some extent, the patient may be able to tolerate greatly reduced doses of bromocriptine to effect long-term control, or the use of postoperative radiation therapy should be considered to bring the residual tumor under control. In our series, all patients who had endocrinologic recurrence (relapse of hyperprolactinemia after initial hormonal normalization) or immediate endocrinologic failure (serum prolactin levels > 20 ng/ml on the morning after surgery) were able to resume bromocriptine at much lower doses than they had taken before surgery. All of them tolerated this reduced dose, and although the serum prolactin level was not always restored to normal, no patient has required postoperative radiation therapy.[88]

After radiation therapy for prolactinomas, PRL levels fall slowly over many years, but they rarely reach the normal level[82]; thus, these patients may benefit from adjuvant medical therapy with bromocriptine.

## Pharmacotherapy with Dopaminergic Analogues

### Physiology

Bromocriptine is a dopamine agonist that suppresses PRL production and release by the stimulation of dopamine receptors. This orally active dopamine agonist is a semisynthetic ergot alkaloid that was specifically developed as an inhibitor of PRL secretion. It directly stimulates neuronal and pituitary cell membrane dopamine receptors.[108] A single dose of 2.5 mg results in suppression of serum PRL for up to 14 hours.[109] The biologic effect, however, may persist for more than 24 hours in some patients.[64]

The FDA has approved the use of cabergoline (Dostinex), a synthetic ergoline derivative with high specificity and affinity for the $D_2$ dopaminergic receptor.[110–114] With effects persisting up to 120 days after administration,[115] this long-lasting and potent agonist is typically dosed once or twice a week, thus leading to improved compliance compared with bromocriptine, which often must be taken up to three times a day. Furthermore, in other comparative studies, cabergoline has been shown to be more effective than bromocriptine in both normalizing serum prolactin and restoring gonadal function.[112, 113] Cabergoline is also better tolerated than other ergot derivatives[112] and may demonstrate efficacy in patients who are refractory to bromocriptine.[113] However, the teratogenic potential of cabergoline has not been extensively investigated.[112] Consequently, the drug is generally not considered first-line therapy for the treatment of infertility associated with hyperprolactinemia, and its current application may be limited to patients who have failed treatment with, or are intolerant of, bromocriptine.[112]

Several other dopamine agonists, including two ergot derivatives (pergolide mesylate and lisuride) and one quinolone (quinagolide), have been shown to suppress serum prolactin and reduce tumor size, but have not been approved by the FDA for the treatment of prolactinomas.[110]

### Dose and Mode of Bromocriptine Administration

Bromocriptine has proved safe and effective in 20 years of widespread use in the treatment of prolactinomas since its approval in 1978.[64] Initiation of bromocriptine therapy is as described in the previous section for use in GH/PRL-secreting adenomas. Bromocriptine is usually given in a dose of 2.5 mg three times daily. In some patients with large tumors in whom the tumor size does not decrease or the PRL level is not suppressed by more than 80% of pretreatment levels with the aforementioned dose, much larger doses are required, up to 15 to 20 mg/day.[64, 82] However, in certain cases, the dose may be decreased after achievement of adequate suppression.[64] Other authors have reported that if reduction in tumor size has not occurred within a 3-month period after starting bromocriptine, it is unlikely that it will occur and medical therapy should be abandoned.[82] It has been our observation that patients who do not respond by 6 weeks are unlikely to respond by 3 months, so our current practice is to obtain an MRI scan 6 weeks after initiating medical therapy to document tumor reduction.

In the bromocriptine-treated patient who responds to medication but fails to normalize his or her serum PRL levels and does not achieve restoration of gonadal function, a combined surgical and medical approach should be considered. After the surgical procedure, hyperprolactinemia is often more responsive to medical therapy, requiring lower doses for control of PRL.[82] As mentioned earlier, reduced doses of bromocriptine have been effective in controlling our patients who were not surgically cured, and adjuvant radiation has not been necessary.[88]

Dopamine agonist therapy must be given chronically. In most patients, withdrawal of the drug results in a return of hyperprolactinemia and re-expansion of the tumor.[116, 117] Occasionally, patients with a microadenoma or an unidentifiable tumor do not experience a recurrence after discontinuation of therapy.[64] In a patient with a microadenoma, bromocriptine can be discontinued every 2 years on a trial basis to determine the need for continued therapy.[69]

## Efficacy

After adequate bromocriptine therapy, the PRL levels are usually lowered by over 80% or are normalized.[82] The PRL-reducing response to therapy in patients with microadenomas and with macroadenomas is similar, with the exception that in the latter group, the time required for effective lowering of PRL is usually longer.[64] In addition, in over 80% of patients, bromocriptine and other dopamine agonists are effective in reversing visual abnormalities and restoring gonadal and anterior pituitary functions.[82, 90] Most female patients begin menstruation within 6 months of initiating therapy. The restoration of fertility in women with bromocriptine has been well documented.[118] However, as stated previously, the continuation of bromocriptine during pregnancy is contraindicated, and patients who wish to become pregnant should undergo surgery.[106]

In addition to reducing PRL secretion, bromocriptine is effective at decreasing tumor size.[119–121] The reduction of the tumor may occur very rapidly, within days of initiation of therapy, and result in dramatic decompression of the optic chiasm and resolution of headaches and other signs and symptoms of raised intracranial pressure.[82] Some tumors are very responsive to bromocriptine and shrink by more than 80% within 6 weeks of initiation of therapy.[82] Although most patients have a satisfactory biochemical and clinical response to medical therapy, there have been isolated case reports of lack of response or progression of disease during bromocriptine therapy.[122–124] Therefore, close monitoring of serum prolactin levels and serial MRI is mandatory. In women, once hyperprolactinemia has been corrected and the menstrual cycle normalized, fertility is usually re-established and the pregnancy rates are the same as those of normal women in the same age group.[125, 126] Although it is tempting intuitively to suggest that pretreatment with bromocriptine may shrink the tumor and facilitate surgical resection, no study has yet reported higher surgical cure rates after such preoperative treatment with bromocriptine.[127, 128] Conversely, as discussed later, some surgeons believe that bromocriptine produces adverse effects on the consistency of the adenoma that impede tumor resection,[119] although this has not been our experience.[120]

## Histologic Changes

Bromocriptine therapy of human prolactinomas for a period of 2 weeks has been shown to induce cell shrinkage and degenerative, necrotic, and fibrotic changes in the tumor; the secretory granules within a cell increase in number but not in volume.[66] Others have demonstrated that the cytoplasmic and nuclear volumes are reduced. In the cytoplasm, the amount of rough endoplasmic reticulum and size of the Golgi apparatus are greatly reduced, and the cell changes from appearing highly active to quiescent. These changes are reversed after bromocriptine withdrawal.[82]

## Medical Management and Pregnancy

Pregnant women with microprolactinomas rarely experience complications related to tumor expansion, the reported risk being less than 0.5% to 1%.[64, 82] However, in pregnant women with macroprolactinomas, the situation is different; the risk for development of symptoms related to tumor enlargement, such as headache, visual field disturbances, and ophthalmoplegia, is approximately 15%, and that for development of asymptomatic tumor enlargement is 9%.[129] These complications appear to occur with equal frequency during all trimesters.[125] Therefore, measures to reduce tumor size such as surgery and radiation are recommended before conception in female patients with macroadenomas who desire to become pregnant. In the event that the tumor enlarges during pregnancy, bromocriptine has been shown to be safe and effective.[130–132] Its administration during pregnancy has not increased the risk of congenital anomalies, spontaneous abortion, or multiple births.[133, 134] Motor and psychological development of children born to women treated with bromocriptine during pregnancy were normal.[134]

If a patient plans to become pregnant while on bromocriptine therapy, a coordinated schedule of follow-up must be observed by the patient, endocrinologist, and neurosurgeon. It is recommended that a woman with a prolactinoma, regardless of tumor size, who wishes to become pregnant while on bromocriptine therapy use mechanical contraceptive precautions for 3 months. During this period, she should undergo complete endocrine, neuroradiologic, and neuro-ophthalmologic evaluations. After achieving three regular menstrual cycles, she should discontinue the contraceptive precautions. Pregnancy should be suspected when the menses are 2 days overdue, and at that time, the serum β-human chorionic gonadotropin level should be measured; once pregnancy is confirmed, bromocriptine should be discontinued immediately. The woman should then be followed closely for signs and symptoms of tumor expansion. Should visual field abnormalities develop, bromocriptine therapy would be indicated as the clinical situation warrants.[64] After termination of pregnancy, headaches and visual field defects acquired because of tumor expansion resolve as the tumor becomes smaller in all cases.

## Side Effects and Complications

Commonly occurring side effects of bromocriptine therapy have been discussed earlier in the section on the GH-secreting pituitary tumor. A rare complication in patients with large prolactinomas is the development of a cerebrospinal fluid leak during treatment caused by shrinkage of the tumor.[69] In women, galactorrhea may persist even though the PRL level is lowered to the normal range.[135] It has been reported that if bromocriptine is given for more than 3 months, the tumor may become fibrous in consistency, which may cause difficulty with surgical resection,[119] although this has not been our personal experience.[120]

Occasionally, patients who initially respond to bromocriptine with a reduction in tumor size and normalization of serum PRL may subsequently experience recrudescence of the tumor as medical therapy is continued.[136–138] In some cases, patient compliance may be responsible, whereas in others, the tumor may undergo a process of dedifferentiation whereby it becomes refractory to dopamine agonist action, as evidenced by the in vitro resistance of cultured lactotrophs to high concentrations of bromocriptine.[137]

Similarly, a discrepancy in the clinical response as judged by tumor size and circulating PRL levels may develop during the course of treatment. Despite marked reduction in serum PRL throughout the duration of bromocriptine therapy, for instance, some patients may experience continued tumor expansion and progressive symptoms from mass effect.[139, 140] Conversely, others may simulate the development of bromocriptine resistance, with steady elevations in serum PRL levels after an initial suppression, despite serial imaging studies that show continual regression in tumor size.[141] Reports of acquired bromocriptine resistance or dissociation between tumor growth and serum PRL measurements are rare, however, and the true incidence of these phenomena is not known.

## Radiation Therapy

The reader is referred to the sections on management of GH-secreting pituitary tumors—analogous comments regarding the use of radiation therapy in these pituitary tumors can be made.

## Follow-Up

After surgery in a patient harboring a microprolactinoma in whom total resection was thought to be achieved, postoperative measurement of PRL levels are the most sensitive measure of completeness of resection and any recurrence. Because of the short half-life of endogenous PRL, postoperative levels may be checked as early as the morning after surgery. This measurement is repeated at 6 weeks, and it should be performed at routine intervals (every 3 months) in the early postoperative period. Depending on the clinical course, the intervals may be increased accordingly.

We have reported the prognostic value of serum PRL levels obtained immediately after trans-sphenoidal surgery.[88] Our practice is to assess fasting morning PRL levels on postoperative day (POD) 1 and random serum levels sampled at 6 weeks, 12 weeks, and then every 6 months for a minimum of 5 years. Levels less than 10 ng/ml on POD 1 predict long-term endocrinologic cure, in patients with microadenomas (100%) as well as those with macroadenomas (93%). In contrast, patients with "normal" levels of 10 to 20 ng/ml on POD 1 remain at risk for endocrinologic recurrence, especially if preoperative tumor size exceeds 10 mm (100% in our series). However, none of our patients with a microadenoma has had relapse.[88]

In other series, recurrence of hyperprolactinemia after initial hormonal normalization has been reported in 10% to 50% of patients after trans-sphenoidal resection, depending on the preoperative size of the tumor and the length of follow-up.[97–99, 101, 103, 142] Differences in surgical technique may also underlie this variation. For example, based on the hypothesis that delayed recurrences result in situ from residual tumoral cells at the periphery of an adenoma, Grisoli and colleagues[107] have proposed performing an "enlarged" rather than selective adenomectomy by removing a layer of normal pituitary gland at the outer edge of the tumor as well as the pituitary capsule in contact with the sellar meninges. Using this technique in 26 patients with tumors less than 20 mm in diameter, they obtained normal serum PRL levels in all cases after an average of 16 months. This length of follow-up is short, however, and it remains to be proven whether this technique results in a lower incidence of delayed recurrence.

Relapses usually occur within the first few years after surgery, although they have been reported after more than 10 years of follow-up.[88, 97, 99] Often, such recurrences are asymptomatic, but even in patients without overt clinical manifestations, treatment may be indicated to prevent osteoporosis.[97, 142] As stated earlier, reduced levels of bromocriptine are usually well tolerated and often effective in preventing significant enlargement of recurrent tumors.[88, 97]

In most cases, however, imaging of the sella turcica fails to reveal residual or recurrent adenoma, and surgical re-exploration is unlikely to achieve chemical cure.[88, 97, 98, 142] This observation may reflect the fact that, with vigilant protocols for sampling postoperative PRL levels, most tumor recurrences are detected early. In our series, for instance, no recurrence was greater than 55 ng/ml.[88] Alternatively, this observation may imply that there are other reasons for recurrent hyperprolactinemia besides regrowth of residual tumor remnants, such as a secondary empty sella or a disordered hypothalamic-pituitary axis.[97, 98, 143]

The clinical response in impotent men with hyperprolactinemia treated with testosterone is often unsatisfactory until the PRL levels are lowered.[83] It is presumed that elevated PRL levels interfere with the peripheral effect of testosterone.

## REFERENCES

1. Ho PJ, Barkan AL: Acromegaly. In Bardin CW (ed): Current Therapy in Endocrinology and Metabolism, 4th ed. Philadelphia: BC Decker, 1991, pp 38–43.
2. Krieger MD, Couldwell WTC, Weiss MH: Assessment of surgical cure of acromegaly. J Neurosurg 86:351A, 1997.
3. Baumann G: Acromegaly. Endocrinol Metab Clin North Am 16:685–702, 1987.
4. Frohman LA: Therapeutic options in acromegaly. J Clin Endocrinol Metab 72:1175–1181, 1991.

5. Serri O, Robert F, Comtois R, et al: Distinctive features of prolactin secretion in acromegalic patients with hyperprolactinaemia. Clin Endocrinol 27:429–436, 1987.
6. Wass JAH: Octreotide treatment of acromegaly. Horm Res 33 (Suppl 1): 1–6, 1990.
7. Randall RV: Acromegaly and gigantism. In DeGroot LJ (ed): Endocrinology, 2nd ed. Philadelphia: WB Saunders, 1991, pp 330–350.
8. Bengtsson BA, Eden S, Ernest I, et al: Epidemiology and long term survival in acromegaly. Acta Med Scand 223:327–335, 1988.
9. Melmed S: Acromegaly. N Engl J Med 322:966–977, 1990.
10. Nabarro JDN: Acromegaly. Clin Endocrinol 26:481–512, 1987.
11. Wright AD, Hill DM, Lowry C, Fraser TR: Mortality in acromegaly. QJM 39:1–16, 1970.
12. Arafah BM, Rosenzweig JL, Fenstermaker R, et al: Value of growth hormone dynamics and somatomedin C (insulin-like growth factor I) levels in predicting the long-term benefit after transsphenoidal surgery for acromegaly. J Lab Clin Med 109:346–354, 1987.
13. Barkan AL: Acromegaly. Trends Endocrinol Metab 3:205–210, 1992.
14. Giannella-Neto D, Wajchenberg BL, Mendonca BB, et al: Criteria for the cure of acromegaly: Comparison between basal growth hormone and somatomedin C plasma concentrations in active and non-active acromegalic patients. J Endocrinol Invest 11:57–60, 1988.
15. Ho KY, Weissberger AJ, Marbach P, Lazarus L: Therapeutic efficacy of the somatostatin analog SMS 201–995 (octreotide) in acromegaly. Ann Intern Med 112:173–181, 1990.
16. Arafah BH, Brodkey JS, Kaufman B, et al: Transsphenoidal microsurgery in the treatment of acromegaly and gigantism. J Clin Endocrinol Metab 50:578–585, 1980.
17. Aron DC, Tyrrell JB, Wilson CB: Pituitary tumors: Current concepts in diagnosis and management. West J Med 162:340–352, 1995.
18. Baskin DS, Boggan JE, Wilson CB: Transsphenoidal microsurgical removal of growth hormone-secreting pituitary adenomas: A review of 137 cases. J Neurosurg 56:634–641, 1982.
19. Buchfelder M, Brockmeier S, Fahlbusch R, et al: Recurrence following transsphenoidal surgery for acromegaly. Horm Res 35:113–118, 1991.
20. Davis DH, Laws ER, Ilstrup DM, et al: Results of surgical treatment for growth hormone-secreting pituitary adenomas. J Neurosurg 79:70–75, 1993.
21. Fahlbusch R, Honegger J, Buchfelder M: Surgical management of acromegaly. Endocrinol Metab Clin North Am 21:669–692, 1992.
22. Hardy J, Somma M: Acromegaly: Surgical treatment by transsphenoidal microsurgical removal of the pituitary adenoma. In Tindall GT, Collins WF (eds): Clinical Management of Pituitary Disorders. New York: Raven Press, 1979, pp 209–217.
23. Laws ER, Fode NC, Redmond MJ: Transsphenoidal surgery following unsuccessful prior therapy. J Neurosurg 63:823–829, 1985.
24. Ross DA, Wilson CB: Results of transsphenoidal microsurgery for growth hormone-secreting pituitary adenoma in a series of 214 patients. J Neurosurg 68:854–867, 1988.
25. Serri O, Somma M, Comtoid R, et al: Acromegaly: Biochemical assessment of cure after long term follow-up of transsphenoidal selective adenomectomy. J Clin Endocrinol Metab 61:1185–1189, 1985.
26. Tindall GT, Oyesiku NM, Watts NB, et al: Transsphenoidal adenomectomy for growth hormone-secreting pituitary adenomas in acromegaly: Outcome analysis and determinants of failure. J Neurosurg 78:205–215, 1993.
27. Tucker HS, Grubb SR, Wigand JP, et al: The treatment of acromegaly by transsphenoidal surgery. Arch Intern Med 140:795–802, 1980.
28. Leavens ME, Samaan NA, Jesse RH, Byers RM: Clinical and endocrinological evaluation of 16 acromegalic patients treated by transsphenoidal surgery. J Neurosurg 47:853–860, 1977.
29. Masuda A, Shibasaki T, Kim YS, et al: The somatostatin analog octreotide inhibits the secretion of growth hormone (GH)-release hormone, thyrotropin and GH in man. J Clin Endocrinol Metab 69:906–1000, 1989.
30. Bauer W, Briner U, Doepfner W, et al: SMS 201-995: A very potent selective octapeptide analogue of somatostatin with prolonged action. Life Sci 31:1133–1140, 1982.
31. Barnard LB, Grantham WG, Lamberton P, et al: Treatment of resistant acromegaly with a long-acting somatostatin analogue (SMS 201-995). Ann Intern Med 105:856–861, 1986.
32. Lamberts SWJ: The role of somatostatin in the regulation of anterior pituitary hormone secretion and the use of its analogs in the treatment of human pituitary tumors. Endocr Rev 9:417–436, 1988.
33. Moyse E, Le Dafniet M, Epelbaum J, et al: Somatostatin receptors in human growth hormone and prolactin-secreting pituitary adenomas. J Clin Endocrinol Metab 61:98–103, 1985.
34. Ikuyama S, Nawata H, Kato K, et al: Specific somatostatin receptors on human pituitary adenoma cell membranes. J Clin Endocrinol Metab 6:666–671, 1985.
35. Reubi JC, Landolt AM: The growth hormone responses to octreotide in acromegaly correlate with adenoma somatostatin receptor status. J Clin Endocrinol Metab 68:844–850, 1989.
36. Kelijman M, Williams TC, Downs TR, Frohman LA: Comparison of the sensitivity of growth hormone secretion to somatostatin in vivo and in vitro in acromegaly. J Clin Endocrinol Metab 67:958–963, 1988.
37. Oppizzi G, Petroncini MM, Dallabonzana D, et al: Relationship between somatomedin-C and growth hormone levels in acromegaly: Basal and dynamic evaluation. J Clin Endocrinol Metab 63:1348–1353, 1986.
38. Lamberts SWJ, Uitterlinden P, del Pozo E: SMS 201-995 induces a continuous decline in circulating growth hormone and somatomedin-C levels during therapy of acromegalic patients for over two years. J Clin Endocrinol Metab 65:703–710, 1987.
39. Barkan AL, Kelch RP, Hopwood NJ, Beitins IZ: Treatment of acromegaly with the long-acting somatostatin analog SMS 201-995. J Clin Endocrinol Metab 66:16–23, 1988.
40. Lamberts SWJ, Uitterlinden P, Verleun T: Relationship between growth hormone and somatomedin-C levels in untreated acromegaly, after surgery and radiotherapy and during medical therapy with Sandostatin (SMS 201-995). Eur J Clin Invest 17:354–359, 1987.
41. Ezzat S, Snyder PJ, Young WF, et al: Octreotide treatment of acromegaly: A randomized, multicenter study. Ann Intern Med 117:711–718, 1992.
42. Page MD, Millward ME, Hourihan M, et al: Long-term treatment of acromegaly with octreotide (Sandostatin). Horm Res 33 (Suppl 1):20–31, 1990.
43. Christensen SE, Weeke J, Orskov H, et al: Continuous subcutaneous pump infusion of somatostatin analogue SMS 201-995 versus subcutaneous injection schedule in acromegalic patients. Clin Endocrinol 27:297–306, 1987.
44. Williams G, Ball J, Lawson R, et al: Analgesic effect of somatostatin analogue (octreotide) in headache associated with pituitary tumors. BMJ 295:247–248, 1987.
45. Popovic V, Paunovic VR, Micic D, et al: The analgesic effects and development of dependency to somatostatin analogue (octreotide) in headache associated with acromegaly. Horm Metab Res 20:250–251, 1987.
46. Sandler LM, Burrin JM, Williams G, et al: Effective long-term treatment of acromegaly with a long-acting somatostatin analog (SMS 201-995). Clin Endocrinol (Oxf) 26:85–95, 1987.
47. Mcknight JA, McCance DR, Sheridan B, et al: Long-term dose-response study of somatostatin analogue (SMS 201-995, octreotide) in resistant acromegaly. Clin Endocrinol 34:119–125, 1991.
48. Lamberts SWJ, Uitterlinden P, Verschoor L, et al: Long-term treatment of acromegaly with the somatostatin analogue SMS 201-995. N Engl J Med 313:1576–1580, 1985.
49. Barkan A, Lloyd RV, Chandler WF, et al: Treatment of acromegaly with SMS 201-995 (sandostatin): Clinical, biochemical and morphologic study. In Lamberts SWJ (ed): Sandostatin in the Treatment of Acromegaly. New York: Springer-Verlag, 1988, pp 103–108.
50. Harris AG, Prestele H, Herold K, et al: Long-term efficacy of sandostatin (SMS 201-995, octreotide) in 178 acromegalic patients: Results from the International Multicenter Acromegaly Study Group. In Lamberts SWJ (ed): Sandostatin in the Treatment of Acromegaly. New York: Springer-Verlag, 1988, pp 117–125.
51. Lamberts SWJ, del Pozo E: Somatostatin analog treatment of acromegaly: New aspects. Horm Res 29:115–117, 1988.
52. Lamberts SWJ, Van Koetsveld P, Hofland L: A close correlation between the inhibitory effects of insulin-like growth factor-1 and SMS 201-995 on growth hormone release by acromegalic pituitary tumours in vitro and in vivo. Clin Endocrinol (Oxf) 31:401–410, 1989.
53. White MC, Newland P, Daniels M, et al: Growth hormone secreting pituitary adenomas are heterogeneous in cell culture and commomly secrete glycoprotein hormone alpha-subunit. Clin Endocrinol (Oxf) 25:173–179, 1986.

54. Spinas GA, Zaph J, Landolt AM, et al: Pre-operative treatment of 5 acromegalics with a somatostatin analogue: Endocrine and clinical observations. Acta Endocrinol (Copenh) 114:249–256, 1987.

55. Landolt AM, Osterwalder V, Jantzer R, Stuckmann G: Pre-operative treatment of acromegaly with SMS 201-995: Surgical and pathological observations. Neuro Endocrinol Lett 7:94, 1985.

56. Jackson I, Barnard LB, Lamberton P: Role of long-acting somatostatin analogue (SMS 201-995) in the treatment of acromegaly. Am J Med 81 (Suppl 6):94–100, 1986.

57. Sadoul J-L, Thyss A, Freychet P: Invasive mixed growth hormone/prolactin secreting pituitary tumour: Complete shrinking by octreotide and bromocriptine and lack of tumour growth relapse 20 months after octreotide withdrawal. Acta Endocrinol (Copenh) 126:179–183, 1992.

58. Charest L, Comtois R, Beauregard H, Serri O: Growth hormone rebound after cessation of SMS 201-995 treatment in acromegaly. Can J Neurol Sci 16:442–445, 1989.

59. George SR, Kovacs K, Asa SL, et al: Effect of SMS 201-995, a long-acting somatostatin analogue, on the secretion and morphology of a pituitary growth hormone cell adenoma. Clin Endocrinol (Oxf) 26:395–405, 1987.

60. Wass JAH, Anderson JV, Besser GM, Dowling RH: Gall stones and treatment with octreotide for acromegaly. BMJ 299:1162–1163, 1989.

61. Vance ML, Kaiser DL, Frohman LA, et al: Role of dopamine in the regulation of growth hormone secretion: Dopamine and bromocriptine augment GHRH-stimulated growth hormone secretion in normal man. J Clin Endocrinol Metab 64:1136–1141, 1987.

62. Wass JAM, Thorner MO, Morris DV, et al: Long-term treatment of acromegaly with bromocriptine. BMJ 1:875–878, 1977.

63. Alford FP, Arnott R: Medical management of pituitary tumors. Med J Austr 157:57–60, 1992.

64. Vance ML, Thorner MO: Prolactinomas. Endocrinol Metab Clin 16:731–753, 1987.

65. Oppizzi G, Liuzzo A, Chiodini P, et al: Dopaminergic treatment of acromegaly: Different effects on hormone secretion and tumor size. J Clin Endocrinol Metab 58:988–992, 1984.

66. Mori H, Maeda T: Changes in prolactinomas and somatotropinomas in humans treated with bromocriptine. Pathol Res Pract 183:580–583, 1988.

67. Turner TH, Cookson JC, Wass JAH, et al: Psychotic reactions during treatment of pituitary tumors with dopamine agonists. BMJ 289:1101–1103, 1984.

68. Chiodini PG, Cozzi R, Dallabonzana D, et al: Medical treatment of acromegaly with SMS 201-995, a somatostatin analog: A comparison with bromocriptine. J Clin Endocrinol Metab 64:447–453, 1987.

69. Klibanski A, Zervas NT: Diagnosis and management of hormone-secreting pituitary adenomas. N Engl J Med 324:822–831, 1991.

70. Gramegna A: Un cas d'acromegalie traité par la radiothérapie. Rev Neurol 17:15, 1909.

71. Chun M, Masko GB, Heterlekidis S: Radiotherapy in the treatment of pituitary adenomas. Int J Radiat Oncol Biol Phys 15:305–309, 1988.

72. Noell KT: Prolactin and other hormone producing pituitary tumors: Radiation therapy. Clin Obstet Gynecol 23:441–452, 1980.

73. Aristzabal S, Caldwell WL, Avila J: The relationship of time-dose fractionation factors to complications in the treatment of pituitary tumors by irradiation. Int J Radiat Oncol Biol Phys 2:667–673, 1977.

74. Baglan R, Marks J: Soft-tissue reactions following irradiation of primary brain and pituitary tumors. Int J Radiat Oncol Biol Phys 7:455–459, 1981.

75. Sheline GF: Treatment of non-functioning chromophobe adenomas of the pituitary. AJR Am J Roentgenol 120:553–561, 1974.

76. Kramer S: The value of radiation therapy for pituitary and parapituitary tumors. CMAJ 99:1120–1127, 1968.

77. Urdaneta N, Chessin H, Fisher JJ: Pituitary adenomas and craniopharyngiomas: Analysis of 99 cases treated with radiation therapy. Int J Radiat Oncol Biol Phys 1:895–902, 1975.

78. Bloom HTG: Radiotherapy of pituitary tumors. In Jenkins JS (ed): Pituitary Tumors. London: Butterworth, 1973, pp 165–197.

79. Ciric I, Mikhael M, Stafford T, et al: Transsphenoidal microsurgery of pituitary macroadenomas with long-term follow-up results. J Neurosurg 59:395–401, 1984.

80. Valtonen S, Myllymaki K: Outcome of patients after transcranial operation for pituitary adenoma. Ann Clin Res 18 (Suppl 47):43–45, 1986.

81. Mindermann T, Wilson CB: Pediatric pituitary adenomas. Neurosurgery 36:259–268, 1995.

82. Thorner MO: Prolactinoma. In Bardin CW (ed): Current Therapy in Endocrinology and Metabolism, 4th ed. Philadelphia: BC Decker, 1991, pp 35–38.

83. Evans WS, Thorner MO: Mechanisms for hypogonadism in hyperprolactinemia. Semin Reprod Endocrinol 2:9–22, 1984.

84. Leyeendecker G, Struve T, Plotz EJ: Induction of ovulation in chronic intermittent (pulsatile) administration of LH-RH in women with hypothalamic and hyperprolactinemic amenorrhea. Arch Gynecol 229:177–190, 1980.

85. Jacobs HS, Franks S, Murray MAF, et al: Clinical and endocrine features of hyperprolactinemic amenorrhea. Clin Endocrinol (Oxf) 5:439–454, 1976.

86. Klibanski A, Greenspan SL: Increase in bone mass after treatment of hyperprolactinemic amenorrhea. N Engl J Med 315:542–546, 1986.

87. Greenspan SL, Oppenheim DO, Klibaski A: Importance of gonadal steroids to bone mass in men with hyperprolactinemic hypogonadism. Ann Intern Med 110:526–531, 1989.

88. Amar AP, Chen JCT, Couldwell WT, Weiss MH: Predictive value of immediate serum prolactin levels following transsphenoidal surgery (Abstract). J Neurosurg 88:392A–393A.

89. Hulting AL, Muhr C, Lundberg PO, Werner S: Prolactinoma in men: Clinical characteristics and the effect of bromocriptine treatment. Acta Med Scand 217:101–109, 1985.

90. Cunnah D, Besser M: Management of prolactinomas. Clin Endocrinol (Oxf) 34:231–235, 1991.

91. Lees PD, Pickard JD: Hyperprolactinemia, intrasellar pituitary tissue pressure, and the pituitary stalk compression syndrome. J Neurosurg 767:192–196, 1987.

92. Albuquerque FC, Hinton DR, Weiss MH: Excessively high prolactin level in a patient with a non-prolactin secreting adenoma. J Neurosurg (in press).

93. Schlechte J, Dolan K, Sherman B, et al: The natural history of untreated hyperprolactinemia: A prospective analysis. J Clin Endocrinol Metab 68:412–418, 1989.

94. Sisam DA, Sheehan JP, Sheeler LR: The natural history of untreated microprolactinomas. Fertil Steril 48:67–71, 1987.

95. Weiss MH, Teal J, Gott P, et al: Natural history of microprolactinomas: Six year follow-up. Neurosurgery 12:180–182, 1983.

96. Lundin P, Nyman R, Burman P, et al: MRI of pituitary macroadenomas with reference to hormonal activity. Neuroradiology 34:43–51, 1992.

97. Massoud F, Serri O, Hardy J, et al: Transsphenoidal adenomectomy for microprolactinomas: 10 to 20 years of follow-up. Surg Neurol 45:341–346, 1996.

98. Laws ER: Comment on paper by Massoud et al. Surg Neurol 45:344–345, 1996.

99. Thomson JA, Davies DL, McLaren EH, Teasdale GM: Ten-year follow up of microprolactinoma treated by transsphenoidal surgery. BMJ 309:1409–1410, 1994.

100. Giovanelli M, Losa M, Mortini P, et al: Surgical results in microadenomas. Acta Neurochir Suppl (Wien) 65:11–12, 1996.

101. Webster J, Page MD, Bevan JS, et al: Low recurrence rate after partial hypophysectomy for prolactinoma: The predictive value of dynamic prolactin function tests. Clin Endocrinol (Oxf) 36:35–44, 1992.

102. Wilson CB: A decade of pituitary microsurgery. J Neurosurg 61:814–833, 1984.

103. Molitch ME: Pathologic hyperprolactinemia. Endocrinol Metab Clin North Am 21:877–901, 1992.

104. Adams CBT: The management of pituitary tumours and post-operative visual deterioration. Acta Neurochir (Wien) 94:103–116, 1988.

105. Serri O, Rasio E, Beauregard H, et al: Recurrence of hyperprolactinemia after selective transsphenoidal adenomectomy in women with prolactinoma. N Engl J Med 309:280–283, 1983.

106. Physicians' Desk Reference, 51st ed. Montvale, NJ: Medical Economics Company, 1997, pp 2411–2413.

107. Grisoli F, Brue T, Graziani N, et al: Enlarged adenomectomy for enclosed prolactinomas: A preliminary study of 26 cases. Acta Neurochir (Wien) 103:92–98, 1990.

108. Corrodi H, Fuxe K, Hokfelt T, et al: Effect of ergot drugs on central cathecolamine neurons: Evidence for stimulation of central dopamine neurons. Pharm Pharmacol 25:409–412, 1973.

109. Thorner MO, Schran HF, Evans WS, et al: A broad spectrum of

prolactin suppression by bromocriptine in hyperprolactinemic women: A study of serum prolactin and bromocriptine levels after acute and chronic administration of bromocriptine. J Clin Endocrinol Metab 50:1026–1033, 1980.

110. Shimon I, Melmed S: Management of pituitary tumors. Ann Intern Med 129:472–483, 1998.

111. Bevan JS, Davis JR: Cabergoline: An advance in dopaminergic therapy. Clin Endocrinol 41:709–712, 1994.

112. Rains CP, Bryson HM, Fitton A: Cabergoline: A review of its pharmacological properties and therapeutic potential in the treatment of hyperprolactinemia and inhibition of lactation. Drugs 49:255–279, 1995.

113. Webster J, Piscitelli G, Polli A, et al: A comparison of cabergoline and bromocriptine in the treatment of hyperprolactinemic amenorrhea. N Engl J Med 331:904–909, 1994.

114. Muratori M, Arosio M, Gambino G, et al: Use of cabergoline in the long-term treatment of hyperprolactinemic and acromegalic patients. J Endocrinol Invest 20:537–546, 1997.

115. Ciccarelli E, Grottoli S, Razzore P, et al: Long-term treatment with cabergoline, a new long-lasting ergoline derivate, in idiopathic or tumorous hyperprolactinemia and outcome of drug-induced pregnancy. J Endocrinol Invest 20:547–551, 1997.

116. Thorner MO, Perryman RL, Rogol AD, et al: Rapid changes of prolactinoma volume after withdrawal and reinstitution of bromocriptine. J Clin Endocrinol Metab 53:480–483, 1981.

117. Zarate A, Canales ES, Cano C, Pilonieta CJ: Follow-up of patients with prolactinomas after discontinuation of long-term therapy with bromocriptine. Acta Endocrinol (Copenh) 104:139–142, 1983.

118. Vance ML, Evans WS, Thorner MO: Drugs five years later: Bromocriptine. Ann Intern Med 100:78–91, 1984.

119. Landolt AM: Surgical treatment of pituitary prolactinomas: Postoperative prolactin and fertility in seventy patients. Fertil Steril 35:620–625, 1981.

120. Weiss MH, Wycoff RR, Yadley R, et al: Bromocriptine treatment of prolactin-secreting tumors: Surgical implications. Neurosurgery 12:640–642, 1983.

121. Zervas NT: Surgical results for pituitary adenomas: Results of an international survey. In Black PMcL, Zervas NT, Ridgeway EC (eds): Secretory Tumors of the Pituitary Gland. New York: Raven Press, 1984, pp 377–385.

122. Breidahl HD, Topliss DJ, Pike JW: Failure of bromocriptine to maintain reduction in size of a macroprolactinoma. BMJ 287:451–452, 1983.

123. Crosignani PG, Mattei A, Ferrari C, et al: Enlargement of a prolactin-secreting pituitary macroadenoma during bromocriptine. Br J Obstet Gynaecol 89:169–170, 1982.

124. Martin NA, Hales M, Wilson CB: Cerebellar metastasis from a prolactinoma during treatment with bromocriptine. J Neurosurg 55:615–619, 1981.

125. Gemzell C, Wang CF: Outcome of pregnancy in women with pituitary adenoma. Fertil Steril 31:363–372, 1979.

126. Skrabanek P, McDonald D, Meager D, et al: Clinical course and outcome of thirty-five pregnancies in infertile hyperprolactinemic women. Fertil Steril 33:391–395, 1980.

127. Fahlbusch R, Buchfelder M, Schrell U: Short-term preoperative treatment of macroprolactinomas by dopamine agonists. J Neurosurg 67:807–815, 1987.

128. Hubbard JL, Scheithauer BW, Abboud CF, Laws ER Jr: Prolactin-secreting adenomas: The preoperative response to bromocriptine treatment and surgical outcome. J Neurosurg 67:816–821, 1987.

129. Molitch ME: Pregnancy and hyperprolactinemic woman. N Engl J Med 312:1364–1370, 1985.

130. Canales ES, Garcia IC, Ruiz JE, et al: Bromocriptine as prophylactic therapy in prolactinoma during pregnancy. Fertil Steril 36:524–526, 1981.

131. Konopka P, Raymond JP, Merceron RE, et al: Continuous administration of bromocriptine in the prevention of neurological complications in pregnant women with prolactinomas. Am J Obstet Gynecol 146:935–938, 1983.

132. Van Roon E, Van der Vijver JCM, Gerretsen G, et al: Rapid regression of a suprasellar extending prolactinoma after bromocriptine treatment during pregnancy. Fertil Steril 36:173–177, 1981.

133. Turkalj I, Braun P, Krupp P: Surveillance of bromocriptine in pregnancy. JAMA 247:1589–1591, 1982.

134. Raymond JP, Goldstein E, Konopka P, et al: Follow-up of children born of bromocriptine-treated mothers. Horm Res 22:239–246, 1985.

135. Thorner MO, McNeilly AS, Hagen C, et al: Long-term treatment of galactorrhea and hypogonadism with bromocriptine. BMJ 2:419–422, 1974.

136. Bevan JS, Webster J, Burke C, Scanlon MF: Dopamine agonists and pituitary tumor shrinkage. Endocr Rev 13:220–240, 1992.

137. Breidahl HD, Topliss DJ, Pike JW: Failure of bromocriptine to maintain reduction in size of a macroprolactinoma. BMJ 287:451–452, 1983.

138. Bannister P, Sheridan P: Continued growth of a large pituitary prolactinoma despite high dose bromocriptine. Br J Clin Pract 41:712–713, 1987.

139. Crosignani PG, Mattei A: Enlargement of a prolactin-secreting pituitary microadenoma during bromocriptine treatment. Br J Obstet Gynaecol 89:169–170, 1982.

140. Kupersmith MJ, Kleinberg D, Warren FA, et al: Growth of prolactinoma despite lowering of serum prolactin by bromocriptine. Neurosurgery 24:417–423, 1989.

141. Ahmed SR, Shalet SM: Discordant responses of prolactinoma to two different dopamine agonists. Clin Endocrinol 24:421–426, 1986.

142. Buchfelder M, Fahlbusch R, Schott W, Honegger J: Long-term follow-up results in hormonally active pituitary adenomas after primary successful transsphenoidal surgery. Acta Neurochir Suppl (Wien) 53:72–76, 1991.

143. Maira G, Anile C, DeMarinis L, Barbarino A: Prolactin-secreting adenomas: Surgical results and long-term follow-up. Neurosurgery 24:736–743, 1989.

C H A P T E R     3 4

# Surgical Management of Cushing's Disease

■ BROOKE SWEARINGEN and NICHOLAS T. ZERVAS

C ushing originally focused attention on pituitary basophilism as the cause of the "polyglandular disorder" in his 1932 monograph.[1] This led to Naffziger's attempt at surgical therapy via a transcranial hypophysectomy in 1933. Naffziger's patient initially improved, but her disease recurred despite radiation therapy, and she died 7 years later.[2] Although pituitary irradiation was sometimes performed, therapy was usually directed to the adrenal glands, and subtotal bilateral adrenalectomy was the recommended treatment until the 1960s. This focus may have been partly due to the difficulty in distinguishing pituitary from adrenal causes of hypercortisolism and to the complicating incidence of basophilic adenomas in patients without clinical disease.[3] Advances in the management of Cushing's disease have included the development of endocrinologic diagnostic techniques capable of localizing the clinical syndrome to a pituitary source and improvements in surgical results through the transsphenoidal approach.

## ENDOCRINE DIAGNOSIS

Endocrine evaluation of Cushing's syndrome requires: (1) biochemical confirmation of hypercortisolism and (2) localization of hormone overproduction (pituitary, adrenal, or ectopic). Confirmation of hypercortisolism can be obtained by measurements of elevated basal levels of 24-hour urine-free hydrocortisone or hydrocortisone metabolites (17-hydroxysteroids). Urine-free cortisol levels above 100 g/24 hr or 17-hydroxysteroid levels above 12 mg/24 hr are suggestive of Cushing's syndrome. Because hydrocortisone levels vary diurnally (highest at 8:00 AM, lowest between 6:00 PM and midnight), randomly obtained hydrocortisone levels are rarely useful. Loss of diurnal variation is seen in Cushing's syndrome, and midnight hydrocortisone levels higher than 8 g/dl are also suggestive of the disease.

Suppression testing is useful to confirm the diagnosis of Cushing's syndrome and to assist with the localization of hormone overproduction. The best screening test for Cushing's syndrome is the 1-mg overnight dexamethasone suppression test, in which the patient is given 1 mg of dexamethasone orally at 11:00 PM and is tested at 8:00 AM for serum hydrocortisone level. Levels less than 5 g/dl rule out the diagnosis of Cushing's syndrome. Elevated levels of more than 5 g/dl neither confirm the diagnosis nor assist in localizing the abnormality because failure to suppress may result from neoplastic sources of corticotropin-releasing hormone (CRH) or hydrocortisone as well as other causes of elevated hydrocortisone levels: drug-related causes (e.g., phenytoin and estrogens), stress, alcohol, depression, and, possibly, hypothalamic causes. Further suppression testing is required for serum hydrocortisone levels in this range. Presumably, in Cushing's disease, the pituitary set point for feedback inhibition of glucocorticoids on CRH production is raised but not eliminated; this is the rationale for the responses seen with low- and high-dose dexamethasone testing.[4] For low-dose testing, the patient is given 0.5 mg four times daily for 2 days; in normal individuals, the urine-free hydrocortisone and 17-hydroxysteroid values fall to less than 50% baseline. If no suppression occurs, the patient is given the high-dose test: 2 mg dexamethasone orally four times daily for 2 days. Failure to suppress with high doses is most consistent with an ectopic source of CRH or an adrenal tumor. In 1992, new criteria for suppression were proposed[5]: with low-dose testing, urine-free hydrocortisone and 17-hydroxysteroid levels should fall to less than 20 Fento (Fg) and less than 4 mg, respectively, whereas with high-dose testing, the urine-free hydrocortisone level should fall to 90% of baseline. A modified version of the high-dose test has been proposed, in which a single dose of 8 mg is given at midnight, and plasma hydrocortisone is measured at 8:00 AM[6]; urine-free hydrocortisone levels in 92% of patients with pituitary Cushing's syndrome suppress to 50% of baseline.

Thus, suppression with high-dose dexamethasone but not with low-dose is considered the hallmark of Cushing's disease and indicates a CRH-producing pituitary adenoma that is partially responsive to feedback inhibition. Because the tumor in these cases is overproducing CRH, one might expect to see marked elevations in plasma CRH levels; however, this is usually not the case, and CRH levels are often only slightly increased or even normal (in these cases, presumably the syndrome results from the loss of diurnal variation or from intermittent hypersecretion). Marked elevation of CRH levels is more commonly seen with ectopic CRH-producing tumors, usually oat cell carcinoma or carcinoid. With adrenal hydrocortisone-producing tumors, CRH production is completely suppressed by feedback inhibition, and plasma CRH levels are very low. However, the actual diagnosis is at times at variance with the responses predicted from the classic suppression tests. Some patients with Cushing's disease fail to show suppression with the standard high-dose dexamethasone test,[7] and some ectopic tumors are suppressible.[8] In uncertain cases, computed tomography (CT) of the lung or adrenal glands is useful for visualization of an ectopic source. The sensitivity of the standard suppression testing can also be enhanced by combining it with CRH stimulation. Because CRH-producing adenomas are stimulated by CRH, and because normal corticotropic cells are suppressed by hypercortisolemia, patients with Cushing's disease exhibit increased CRH and hydrocortisone secretion in response to administered CRH. Although some ectopic tumors respond to CRH and some pituitary adenomas do not, enhanced diagnostic sensitivity (100%) and specificity (98%) have been achieved when this test is combined with suppression testing.[9]

Because some patients with ectopic CRH-producing tumors have suppression test results identical to those seen in pituitary adenomas, incorrect diagnoses are sometimes made. The ability to confirm a pituitary source has been improved significantly by the introduction of simultaneous, bilateral inferior petrosal venous sinus catheterization.[10] This technique permits the measurement of CRH levels directly from the pituitary in comparison with peripheral CRH (mixed venous) levels by catheterizing and simultaneously sampling blood from both inferior petrosal sinuses and the vena cava. If the ratio of petrosal to peripheral adrenocorticotropic hormone (ACTH) was greater than 2:1, a pituitary source was confirmed in 95% of patients with Cushing's disease.[10] When it was combined with CRH stimulation, the diagnostic accuracy was increased further; all patients in a National Institutes of Health series who had a petrosal-to-peripheral ratio greater than 3:1 had Cushing's disease, whereas the ratio was less than 3:1 in all patients with ectopic CRH-producing tumors or adrenal disease.[11] This test may also help lateralize the tumor within the sella because a right-to-left CRH concentration ratio of 1.4:1 or greater predicted tumor laterality with 70% accuracy; if tumor is not found on the side predicted, however, an intensive effort must be made to explore the entire gland.

## RADIOLOGIC EVALUATION

Magnetic resonance imaging has largely replaced CT scanning in the radiologic evaluation of pituitary tumors. At best, the sensitivity of CT scanning for corticotropin-secreting tumors was 63%.[12] With high field strength magnetic resonance imaging (MRI), using high-resolution technique (3-mm slice thickness), numerous series have reported sensitivities of 75% to 100% for microadenomas in general.[13, 14] For Cushing's disease specifically, MRI has an overall sensitivity of 71% and a specificity of 87%.[15] The most reliable indicator is a focal hypointensity on coronal

images; convexity of the gland and stalk deviation are less sensitive predictors.

## THERAPEUTIC OPTIONS

### Surgery

The therapy of choice for Cushing's disease remains transsphenoidal microsurgery. Numerous surgical series since 1982 reported remission rates of 70% to 90% after such surgery.[16–23] In general, remission rates are highest in cases in which an intrasellar microadenoma is found at exploration and is selectively removed. Cases in which tumor is found but remission does not occur may result from cavernous sinus or dural invasion by the tumor, pituitary hyperplasia, misdiagnosis of an ectopic or adrenal tumor, or tumor rests missed by the exploration. In cases in which no tumor is found at surgery, remission occurs less frequently (69%)[20]; small microadenomas not actually visualized at operation may nonetheless be successfully removed by hemihypophysectomy or total hypophysectomy. Remission is less likely to be achieved in cases of macroadenomas (54%).[20] On the basis of these results, we currently recommend selective adenomectomy as the initial surgical procedure. If remission is not achieved, we recommend a second procedure for complete hypophysectomy. If no tumor is seen at the initial operation, we perform a hemihypophysectomy based on lateralization data from the petrosal sinus catheterization. Because these data are only 70% accurate, we explore the entire gland before removing the presumably involved half, and we recommend reoperation for hypophysectomy if no remission occurs.

Postoperatively, prolonged hypocortisolism is seen after successful adenomectomy; this state may last 6 to 12 months[24, 25] and requires steroid replacement until recovery of the pituitary-adrenal axis occurs. Hydrocortisone levels that normalize quickly (within the first few weeks) may be associated with an early recurrence. Remission is assessed by measuring fasting hydrocortisone and urine-free hydrocortisone levels 5 days after surgery; the patient's condition is maintained on small doses of dexamethasone, which do not interfere in the hydrocortisone assay, to prevent hypocortisolism. Serum hydrocortisone and urine-free hydrocortisone levels should be low; if remission has not been achieved, we recommend early re-exploration. If the data are equivocal, hydrocortisone levels can be reassessed in a few weeks because rare cases of delayed fall in postoperative hydrocortisone levels are seen.[26]

Recurrence rates of 3% to 10% after initially successful adenomectomy have been reported.[15–22] Reoperation after recurrence or a failed initial procedure was successful in achieving an overall remission in 73%.[27] If recurrent adenoma was again found and selectively removed, the remission rate was 95%; if no tumor was found, and semihypophysectomy or complete hypophysectomy was performed, the remission rate was 42%, with surgically induced hypopituitarism in 50%.

The overall complication rate of transsphenoidal surgery is reported to be approximately 3%.[28] In the operative series of Cushing's disease, complication rates vary between 1%

and 9%.[15–22] The most common complications include diabetes insipidus, cerebrospinal fluid leaks with meningitis, and postoperative visual deficits. The mortality rate ranges from 0% to 1% and is usually related to perioperative cardiac complications.

## Medical Therapy

Although limited control of hypercortisolism can be achieved by pharmacologic means, such treatment is considered primarily adjunctive therapy in patients not cured by surgery or awaiting radiation effects. Drug therapy can be directed at blocking the adrenal production of hydrocortisone or the adenoma's production of corticotropin. Adrenal blockade can be achieved with mitotane, ketoconazole, metyrapone, or aminoglutethimide. Ketoconazole blocks steroidogenesis at multiple sites and is generally well tolerated.[29] Its use may lead to abnormal liver function and, rarely, to hepatic failure. Mitotane and metyrapone block the 11-hydroxylase enzyme, thereby inhibiting steroidogenesis.[30, 31] Use of mitotane is associated with gastrointestinal side effects and, possibly, teratogenicity, and complete blockade may lead to hypocortisolism that requires steroid replacement.[32] Its effects may persist for weeks to months after discontinuation of the drug, presumably by direct adrenal cytotoxicity. Metyrapone is effective in blocking 11-hydroxylase, and its use is associated with gastrointestinal symptoms, hypertension, and hirsutism.[29, 33] It currently is no longer available in the United States. Aminoglutethimide blocks several steps in steroidogenesis but has been associated with central nervous system effects as well as skin rashes.[34, 35] Combination therapy with these agents may minimize side effects and enhance effectiveness; ketoconazole is usually the initial agent of choice.

Direct inhibition of CRH production has been attempted through the use of cyproheptadine, a serotonin antagonist, and bromocriptine, a dopamine agonist. Cyproheptadine has been reported to be effective in some patients, but therapy for 3 to 6 months is required before this improvement is evident, and its use is associated with multiple side effects.[36] Bromocriptine is only occasionally effective.[37]

## Radiation Therapy

Radiation therapy has been used as both primary and adjunctive therapy since Cushing's original description. Conventional fractionated therapy at doses of 4000 to 5000 cGy is effective in about 50% of cases,[38] and a remission rate of 85% has been reported in children with juvenile Cushing's disease.[39] The major disadvantages of this treatment are its delayed effectiveness (6 to 24 months may elapse before a response is seen) and the risk of panhypopituitarism.

To provide interim control, radiation should be combined with steroid blockade.[40] Stereotactic radiosurgery with a proton beam has been more effective, with remission rates of 85% at 12 years, although the rate is only 55% at 2 years.[41] Similar results have been obtained with alpha particles[42] and the focused cobalt units.[43] A significant incidence of hypopituitarism is associated with radiation

therapy, seen in up to 55% of patients receiving focused cobalt treatment. There is also some risk of visual field disturbance with radiosurgery, especially if fractionated radiation has been previously given.

## Adrenalectomy

Until the early 1970s, bilateral adrenalectomy with pituitary irradiation was the mainstay of treatment for Cushing's disease. Its role is now limited to patients for whom transsphenoidal surgery has failed and whose condition cannot be controlled pharmacologically while they await radiation effect. It carries a mortality rate of 4% and may lead to the development of Nelson's syndrome because the original pituitary adenoma may continue to enlarge. Adrenalectomy patients require lifelong glucocorticoid and mineralocorticoid replacement and must be followed up for both the development of Nelson's syndrome and the recurrence of hypercortisolism because, rarely, adrenal remnants may respond to ongoing corticotropin stimulation.

## SUMMARY

Transsphenoidal neurosurgery remains the treatment of choice for Cushing's disease, with selective adenomectomy whenever possible. If the patient is not in remission after the initial procedure, we usually recommend re-exploration for hypophysectomy. In cases of persistent disease, we suggest adrenalectomy or radiation therapy with pharmacologic blockade, and we recommend adrenalectomy in cases in which blockade is ineffective, a delay in control of the hypercortisolism is intolerable, or the risk of radiation-induced hypopituitarism and possible loss of fertility is unacceptable. Stereotactic radiosurgery may well offer significant benefit to patients who fail to respond to transsphenoidal surgery or are not surgical candidates and can tolerate pharmacologic blockade while awaiting radiation benefits.

## REFERENCES

1. Cushing HW: The basophilic adenomas of the pituitary body and their clinical manifestations (pituitary basophilism). Bull Johns Hopkins Hosp 50:137–195, 1932.
2. Lisser H: Hypophysectomy in Cushing's disease. J Nerv Ment Dis 99:727–733, 1944.
3. Boggan JE, Wilson CB: Cushing's disease and Nelson's syndrome. In Wilkins RH, Rengachary SS (eds): Neurosurgery, Vol 1. New York: McGraw-Hill, 1985, pp 859–863.
4. Liddle GW: Tests of pituitary-adrenal suppressibility in the diagnosis of Cushing's syndrome. J Clin Endocrinol 20:1539, 1960.
5. Flack MR, Oldfield EH, Cutler GB, et al: Urine free cortisol in the high-dose dexamethasone suppression test for the differential diagnosis of the Cushing syndrome. Ann Intern Med 116:211, 1992.
6. Tyrrell JB, Findling JW, Aron DC, et al: An overnight high-dose dexamethasone suppression test for rapid differential diagnosis of Cushing's syndrome. Ann Intern Med 104:180–186, 1986.
7. Grossman AB, Howlett TA, Perry L, et al: CRF in diagnosis of Cushing's syndrome: A comparison with the dexamethasone suppression test. Clin Endocrinol (Oxf) 29:167–178, 1988.
8. Mason AMS, Ratcliffe JG, Buckle RM, Mason AS: ACTH secretion by bronchial carcinoid tumors. Clin Endocrinol (Oxf) 1:3–25, 1972.

9. Nieman LK, Chrousos GP, Oldfield EH, et al: The corticotropin releasing hormone stimulation test and the dexamethasone suppression test in the differential diagnosis of Cushing's syndrome. Ann Intern Med 105:862–887, 1986.
10. Oldfield EH, Chrousos G: The preoperative lateralization of ACTH secreting pituitary microadenomas by bilateral and simultaneous inferior petrosal venous sinus sampling. N Engl J Med 213:100–103, 1985.
11. Oldfield EH, Doppman JL: Petrosal sinus sampling with and without corticotropin releasing hormone for the differential diagnosis of Cushing's syndrome. N Engl J Med 325:897–905, 1991.
12. Marcovitz S, Wee R, Chan J, Hardy J: The diagnostic accuracy of preoperative CT scanning in the evaluation of pituitary ACTH-secreting adenomas. AJR Am J Roentgenol 149:803–806, 1987.
13. Kucharczyk W, David SO, Kelly WM, et al: Pituitary adenomas: High resolution MR imaging at 1.5 T. Radiology 161:761–765, 1987.
14. Kulkarni MV, Lee KF, McArdle CB, et al: 1.5 T MR imaging of pituitary microadenomas: Technical considerations and CT correlation. AJNR Am J Neuroradiol 9:511, 1988.
15. Peck WW, Dillon WP, Norman D, et al: High resolution MR imaging of pituitary microadenomas at 1.5%: Experience with Cushing's disease. AJR Am J Roentgenol 152:145–151, 1989.
16. Hardy J: Cushing's disease: 50 years later. Can J Neurol Sci 9:375–380, 1982.
17. Fahlbusch R, Buchfelder M, Muller OA: Transsphenoidal surgery for Cushing's disease. J R Soc Med 79:262–269, 1986.
18. Carpenter PC: Cushing's syndrome: Update of diagnosis and management. Mayo Clin Proc 61:495–498, 1986.
19. Chandler WF, Schteingart DE, Lloyd R, et al: Surgical treatment of Cushing's disease. J Neurosurg 66:204–212, 1987.
20. Nakane T, Kuwayama A, Watanabe M, et al: Long term results of transsphenoidal adenomectomy in patients with Cushing's disease. Neurosurgery 21:218–222, 1987.
21. Mampalam TJ, Tyrrell JB, Wilson CB: Transsphenoidal microsurgery for Cushing's disease: A report of 216 cases. Ann Intern Med 109:487–493, 1988.
22. Tindall GT, Hering CJ, Clark RV, et al: Cushing's disease: Results of transsphenoidal microsurgery with emphasis on surgical failures. J Neurosurg 72:363–369, 1990.
23. Post KD, Habas J: Cushing's disease: Results of operative treatment. In Cooper PR (ed): Contemporary Diagnosis and Management of Pituitary Adenomas. Park Ridge, IL: American Association of Neurological Surgeons, 1991, pp 139–150.
24. Fitzgerald PA, Aron DC, Findling JW, et al: Cushing's disease: Transient secondary adrenal insufficiency after selective removal of pituitary microadenomas: Evidence for a pituitary origin. J Clin Endocrinol Metab 54:413–422, 1982.
25. Chrousos GP, Schulte HM, Oldfield EH, et al: The corticotropin releasing factor stimulation test: An aid in the evaluation of patients with Cushing's disease. N Engl J Med 310:622–626, 1984.
26. McDonald SD, Von Hofe SE, Dorfman SG, et al: Delayed cure of Cushing's disease after transsphenoidal surgery of pituitary microadenomas: Report of two cases. J Neurosurg 49:593–596, 1978.
27. Friedman RB, Oldfield EH, Nieman LK, et al: Repeat transsphenoidal surgery for Cushing's disease. J Neurosurg 71:520–527, 1989.
28. Black PM, Zervas NT, Candia GL: Incidence and management of complications of transsphenoidal operation for pituitary adenomas. Neurosurgery 20:920–924, 1987.
29. Sonino N, Boscaro M, Merola G, Mantero F: Prolonged treatment of Cushing's disease by ketoconazole. J Clin Endocrinol Metab 61:718–722, 1985.
30. Brown RD, Nicholson WE, Chick WT, et al: Effect of o,p'DDD on human adrenal steroid 11 beta-hydroxylation activity. J Clin Endocrinol Metab 36:730–733, 1973.
31. Dickstein G, Lahav M, Shen-Orr Z, et al: Primary therapy for Cushing's disease with metyrapone. JAMA 255:1167–1169, 1986.
32. Luton JP, Mahoudeau JA, Bouchard P, et al: Treatment of Cushing's disease by o,p'DDD: Surgery of 62 cases. N Engl J Med 300:459–464, 1979.
33. Jeffcoate WJ, Rees LH, Tomlin S, et al: Metyrapone in long term management of Cushing's disease. BMJ 2:215–217, 1977.
34. Fishman LN, Liddle GW, Island DP, et al: Effects of aminoglutethimide on adrenal function in man. J Clin Endocrinol Metab 27:481–490, 1967.
35. Misbin RI, Canary J, Willard D: Aminoglutethimide in the treatment of Cushing's syndrome. J Clin Pharmacol 16:645–651, 1976.
36. Couch RM, Smail PJ, Dean HJ, et al: Prolonged remission of Cushing's disease after treatment with cyproheptadine. J Pediatr 104:906–908, 1984.
37. Boscaro M, Benato M, Mantero F: Effect of bromocriptine in pituitary dependent Cushing's syndrome. Clin Endocrinol (Oxf) 19:485–491, 1983.
38. Orth DN, Liddle GW: Results of treatment of 108 patients with Cushing's syndrome. N Engl J Med 285:243–247, 1971.
39. Jennings AS, Liddle GW, Orth DN: Results of treating childhood Cushing's disease with pituitary irradiation. N Engl J Med 297:957–962, 1977.
40. Schteingart DE, Tsao HS, Taylor CI, et al: Sustained remission of Cushing's disease with mitotane and pituitary irradiation. Ann Intern Med 92:613–619, 1980.
41. Kjellberg RN, Kliman B, Swisher B, Butler W: Proton beam therapy of Cushing's disease and Nelson's syndrome. In Black PM, Zervas NT, Ridgway EC, et al (eds): Secretory Tumors of the Pituitary Gland. New York: Raven Press, 1984, pp 295–307.
42. Fabrikant JI, Levy RP: Radiation therapy of pituitary tumors. In Barrow DL, Selman W (eds): Neuroendocrinology. Baltimore: Williams & Wilkins, 1992, pp 367–393.
43. Degerblad M, Rahn T, Bergstrand G, Thoren M: Long-term results of stereotactic radiosurgery to the pituitary gland in Cushing's disease. Acta Endocrinol (Copenh) 112:310–314, 1986.

# Surgical Management of Recurrent Pituitary Tumors

■ ALEX M. LANDOLT

The results of pituitary adenoma reoperation do not match those of primary operations. The physician and the surgeon caring for patients who require these procedures must therefore carefully weigh the advantages and disadvantages of repeat surgery against radiation therapy and medical treatment, which share the advantage that their effectiveness does not depend on the previous surgical intervention. Often, however, a combination of different treatment modalities must be used. This renders the treatment of recurrent pituitary adenomas a truly interdisciplinary problem, involving neurosurgeons, endocrinologists, and radiation therapists.

## INCIDENCE OF ADENOMA RECURRENCE

Pituitary adenomas are usually benign tumors and can be cured by surgery and radiation therapy. Henderson[52] found that 87% of the patients who were operated on by Harvey Cushing and who had undergone postoperative radiation therapy remained asymptomatic after 5 years. Thirteen percent of adenomas in Cushing's patients recurred. Symptoms of recurrence appeared within 3 years in 70% and within 5 years in approximately 95% of this group. No recurrence developed later than 8 years after the operation. In several series, the greatest number of recurrences occurred from 4 to 8 years after surgery.[24, 26, 80, 82] This suggests the existence of a time limit after which the patient may be reasonably safe from recurrences. On the other hand, an analysis of the Mayo Clinic data presented by MacCarty and colleagues[78] suggests that the incidence of recurrences even after a follow-up of 19 years does not show a trend toward an upper limit, but rather seems to represent a linear function of time (Fig. 35–1), a view supported also by Wirth and associates.[125] The author suspects that the absence of late recurrences (later than 5 to 10 years) in a number of follow-up studies is primarily due to a limitation in the observation time.

Table 35–1 summarizes the results of surgical follow-up studies reported in the literature. The variation of the individual results is evident. Radiation therapy, however, reduces the incidence of recurrences in all but two series.[32, 118]

The difference between the number of recurrences after surgery and surgery followed by radiation therapy is highly significant ($P < .005$ by the Kruskal-Wallis test). Transcranial surgery has been associated with a higher recurrence rate (30%) than transsphenoidal surgery (5%); however, this is probably because larger adenomas are more often operated on transcranially.[79] It is surprising that no substantial progress seems to have been made in the treatment results since the 1950s; however, such comparisons of series are hazardous because of the development of improved techniques to detect recurrent adenomas, selection of patients submitted to radiation therapy, and changes in statistical techniques. Only few authors use life tables to present their data.[43, 82]

## BIOLOGIC ASPECTS OF ADENOMA RECURRENCE

The histologic tumor examination, at least in the case of the surgeon, is primarily performed to obtain information about the tumor's *prognosis*. In pituitary adenomas, histo-

FIGURE 35–1 ■ Results of long-term follow-up of transcranially operated pituitary adenomas treated at the Mayo Clinic. (Data from MacCarty CS, Hanson EJ, Randall RV, Scanlon PW: Indications for and results of surgical treatment of pituitary tumors by the transfrontal approach. In Kohler PO, Ross GT [eds]: Diagnosis and Treatment of Pituitary Tumors. Amsterdam: Excerpta Medica, 1973, pp 139–145.)

## TABLE 35-1 ■ INCIDENCE OF RECURRENCES AFTER PITUITARY ADENOMA SURGERY

| Author (Surgeon, if Different from First Author) | Reference | Year | Surgical Technique | No. of Patients | Without Radiation Therapy (%) | With Radiation Therapy (%) | Follow-Up (yr) |
|---|---|---|---|---|---|---|---|
| Cairns | 20 | 1935 | C | 50 | 18 | — | — |
| Henderson (Cushing) | 52 | 1939 | C, S | 205 | 56 | 13 | 5 |
| Davidoff and Feiring | 28 | 1948 | C | 19 | 50† | 17.6 | 0.5–17 |
| Bakay (Olivecrona) | 7 | 1950 | C | 232 | — | 10.2 | 5 |
| Tönnis et al. | 117 | 1952 | C | 137 | 10.2‡ | — | — |
| Mogensen | 83 | 1957 | C | 52* | 14.3 | 20 | 3 |
| Guillaume and Caron | 45 | 1958 | C | 141 | 10.6 | — | 1–16 |
| Heimbach (Krayenbühl) | 51 | 1959 | C | 75 | — | 12 | 1–17 |
| Marguth and Nover | 79 | 1964 | C | 476 | 8.6‡ | — | — |
| Martins et al. (Kempe) | 81 | 1965 | C | 54 | — | 6 | — |
| Elkington and McKissock (McKissock) | 33 | 1967 | C | 226 | — | 7.5 | 2–25 |
| Svien and Colby | 111 | 1967 | C, S | 213* | 8 | 4.8 | 1–11 |
| Burian et al. | 19 | 1970 | C, S | 118 | 29.7‡ | — | 1–9 |
| Stern and Batzdorf | 110 | 1970 | | 64 | 9.4 | — | 5.5 |
| Ray and Patterson | 93 | 1971 | C | 164 | 22 | 8 | 1–20 |
| MacCarty et al. | 78 | 1973 | C | 96 | 31.8 | 3 | 5–19 |
| Sheline (Boldrey) | 107 | 1973 | C | 84* | 86 | 11.3 | 4–38 |
| Wirth et al. (Schwartz) | 125 | 1974 | C | 157 | 25.8 | 11.7 | 5.3 |
| Pistenma et al. | 90 | 1975 | C, S | 24 | — | 25 | 0–16 |
| Muhr et al. (Hugosson) | 85 | 1980 | C | 19 | — | 21 | 5–10 |
| Salmi et al. (Valtonen) | 97 | 1982 | C, S | 56 | — | 19.6 | 5 |
| Symon et al. | 112 | 1982 | C | 270 | 22 | 3 | 5–30 |
| Ciric et al. | 24 | 1983 | S | 99 | 28 | 6 | — |
| Ebersold et al. (Laws) | 32 | 1986 | S | 100* | 12 | 18 | 6 |
| Valtonen and Myllymäki | 118 | 1986 | C | 111 | 41 | 39 | 14–33 |
| Guidetti et al. | 44 | 1987 | C, S | 237 | 8.3 | 4.6 | 6 |
| Vlahovitch et al. | 121 | 1988 | C, S | 135 | 16 | 8.3 | 20 |
| Grigsby et al. (Schwartz) | 43 | 1989 | C, S | 121 | — | 15.7 | 10–30 |
| Comtois et al. (Hardy) | 26 | 1991 | S | 71* | 21 | — | 6.4 |
| McCoullough et al. (Rhoton) | 82 | 1991 | C, S | 76 | — | 9.2 | 5–20 |
| Van Lindert et al. | 119 | 1991 | C | 50* | 36 | 0 | 5.4 |

*Endocrine inactive adenomas only.
†Recurrences excluded.
‡Number of irradiated and nonirradiated patients not included.
C, transcranial; S, transsphenoidal.

logic examination provides little information about prognosis because aggressive and rapidly growing adenomas may show a benign histologic pattern, whereas benign adenomas may show an aggressive pattern.[31, 57]

A number of factors are known to promote recurrence. Large adenomas are often more difficult to remove radically than are small ones. Forty-four to 94% of adenomas grow into the dura surrounding the sella, the cavernous sinus, the suprasellar structures, and the sphenoid sinus.[71, 103, 105] Large adenomas invade the basal sella dura more often than do small ones; however, even microadenomas may invade the dura[103] (Fig. 35-2). Invasive growth is also related to the *tumor growth rate* (see later),[71, 86] another factor possibly leading to increased tumor recurrence rate. A relation between invasive growth and adenoma recurrence has been found in adenomas with macroinvasion seen by computed tomography (CT), magnetic resonance imaging (MRI), and during surgery (Hardy's grades III and IV[49]).[26]

## TUMOR GROWTH

Tumor growth is the net result of the difference between cell multiplication and cell death. Both are not necessarily constant during the lifetime of a tumor. A number of factors can influence them, such as tumor size, tumor vascularization, tumor differentiation or dedifferentiation, and the endocrine environment. Further changes may be caused by treatment. Bromocriptine may reduce the growth fraction (i.e., the percentage of tumor cells engaged in the cell division cycle) of prolactinomas as long as the drug is present.[21, 66] Octreotide (a synthetic, long-acting somatostatin analogue) has the same effect.[72] Radiation therapy does not appear to affect the growth rate but rather the rate of cell death,[72] as reported by morphometric studies, which demonstrate increased numbers of necrotic cells in irradiated pituitary adenomas.[4, 96]

## MALIGNANT PITUITARY TUMORS AND PITUITARY CARCINOMAS

Pituitary carcinomas grow rapidly and invade the structures surrounding the sella (cavernous sinus, sphenoid sinus, ethmoid sinuses, maxillary sinus, epipharynx, clivus, cranial nerves, and the brain). Their microscopic appearance is not a reliable diagnostic criterion, nor can invasive

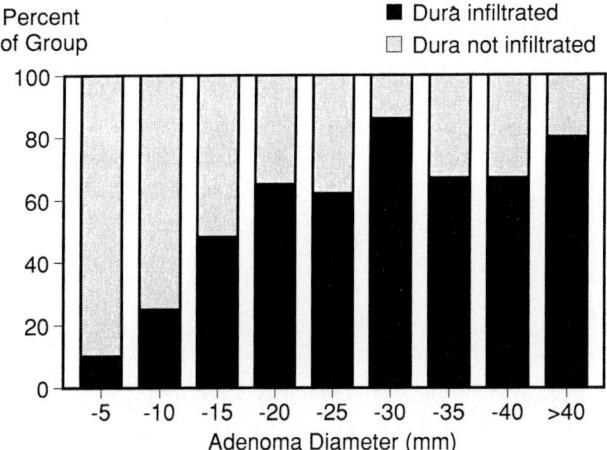

Percent of Group

■ Dura infiltrated
☐ Dura not infiltrated

FIGURE 35–2 ■ Incidence of basal sella dura invasion by pituitary adenomas, as found by routine light microscopic examination of biopsy specimens of a personal, previously published series of 182 pituitary adenomas. The difference in the diameters of invasive and noninvasive adenomas is highly significant ($P < .00001$). (Data from Landolt AM, Shibata T: Growth, cell proliferation, and prognosis of pituitary adenomas. In Faglia G, Beck-Peccoz P, Ambrosi B, et al [eds]: Pituitary Adenomas: New Trends in Basic and Clinical Research. International Congress Series, Vol 961. Amsterdam, Excerpta Medica, 1991, pp 169–178.)

growth alone be used as a criterion for malignancy—otherwise, most pituitary adenomas would have to be re-classified. The malignant nature of pituitary carcinomas is exhibited by metastatic spread to the cerebrospinal fluid (CSF), the brain parenchyma, and extraneural sites, including the regional lymph nodes, lung, liver, bone, kidney, bladder, uterus, and heart.[57, 58, 64, 98] Spread by CSF occurs only after transcranial tumor extirpation.

## FOLLOW-UP OF PITUITARY ADENOMAS

*Endocrinologically active adenomas* are followed by regular determination of a few marker hormones. No imaging examinations are needed as long as the endocrine data remain within normal limits.

In acromegaly, the easiest parameter to follow is the insulin-like growth factor 1 (IGF-1) level (also termed *somatomedin C*). Simple growth hormone (GH) determinations are not reliable because of their diurnal variation and reaction to stress. They must be supplemented by functional tests because single values can be above the upper limit of normal in healthy people because GH is normally secreted in bursts.[91] Measurement of IGF-1 is less labile and is related to the overall daily GH secretion. Postoperative GH dynamics during an oral glucose tolerance test or thyroid hormone-releasing hormone test, as well as measurement of IGF-1 activity, are prognostic factors.[17, 95, 102] No recurrences were detected in 43 acromegalic patients in whom a GH suppression to less than 2 μg/L was achieved during the oral glucose tolerance test, whereas four recurrences were noted 1 to 3 years after surgery in 18 patients with GH levels below the normal upper limit of 5 μg/L that could not be suppressed to 2 μg/L.[17]

Higher growth and recurrence rates are found in patients with *Cushing's disease* than in those with the other types of pituitary adenoma.[72] Recurrence rates of 8% to 21% (follow-up of 10 to 72 months) have been reported. The best parameter to follow in Cushing's disease is the free urinary cortisol in a 24-hour sample. Single corticotropin-releasing hormone values are not reliable.[59] A cooperative follow-up study showed that patients experiencing a postoperative phase of adrenal insufficiency needing glucocorticoid replacement have a significantly lower risk of later relapse (4.3% versus 26.3% in a follow-up period of up to 10 years).[14]

*Prolactinomas*, particularly *pseudoprolactinomas*, are more difficult to follow because prolactin (PRL) values may be misleading and no good functional test exists for differentiating hyperprolactinemia caused by an adenoma and functional disturbances of the normal gland. The follow-up must be based on serum PRL levels and on radiographic studies. Prolactinomas causing only slight hyperprolactinemia and endocrinologically inactive adenomas causing hyperprolactinemia by interfering with hypothalamic PRL inhibition (pituitary stalk compression) may reach considerable sizes without showing elevated PRL values. Some patients with early postoperative recurrence of modest hyperprolactinemia (<100 μg/L) may remain stable during years of follow-up and show no trace of a recurrent adenoma on MRI scans performed years after surgery. Prolactinomas with preoperative PRL values above 100 to 200 μg/L are easier to follow, behaving like other endocrine active adenomas.

Reports concerning the recurrence of prolactinomas present highly divergent data (Table 35–2). The data suggest a higher recurrence rate of macroprolactinomas, but this cannot be proved because of the wide variation in results. In addition, recurrence of hyperprolactinemia is not equivalent to recurrence of the adenoma, and even prolonged radiographic follow-up of patients with recurrent hyperprolactinemia often fails to demonstrate tumor regrowth.[5, 99] Re-establishment of normal dynamic reactions to domperidone and thyroid-releasing hormone is a good prognostic sign for a low recurrence rate.[23] No recurrences were found in a personal series followed for 7 to 10 years after an interval of 4 years.[68]

The follow-up of *endocrinologically inactive adenomas* depends on CT and MRI scans because the reappearance of visual disorders (affecting the visual field and visual acuity) is usually a late sign appearing only after the tumor has reached a considerable size. In addition, these signs are nonspecific and also may be due to scar formation combined with postoperative empty sella syndrome[89] or radiation damage.[47, 48, 65, 113]

We use the following schedule for postoperative MRI or CT scans in endocrinologically inactive adenomas:

- A *baseline examination* is performed approximately 2 to 3 months after surgery. This postoperative interval has been chosen to allow reabsorption of a hematoma in the tumor cavity (see later).[108, 114]
- The *second follow-up study* is performed 1 year later.
- The *third study* is performed after an additional interval of 2 years if the 1-year control study was identical to the baseline study. An interval of only 1 year is chosen if the 1-year control study results are suspect for recurrence.

TABLE 35–2 ■ **RECURRENCES AFTER SURGERY OF PROLACTINOMAS**

| First Author | Reference | Year | Adenoma Diameter (mm) | No. of Patients | Recurrences (%) | Follow-Up (yr) Range, Average |
|---|---|---|---|---|---|---|
| Bertrand | 10 | 1983 | | 30 | 10 | >1 |
| Serri | 104 | 1983 | ≤10 | 24 | 50 | 2–6 |
| | | | >10 | 5 | 80 | 2–3 |
| Rodman | 94 | 1984 | ≤10 | 29 | 17 | 0.5–1.4 |
| | | | >10 | 5 | 20 | 6.5 |
| Buchfelder | 18 | 1985 | ≤10 | 50 | 16 | >5 |
| | | | >10 | 18 | 22.5 | >5 |
| Charpentier | 22 | 1985 | ≤10 | 100 | 10 | 0.5–4.7 |
| | | | >10 | 22 | 9 | 0.5–4.7 |
| Arafah | 5 | 1986 | ≤10 | 67 | 7 | 1.3–8 |
| | | | >10 | 29 | 34.5 | 1.3–8 |
| Schlechte | 99 | 1986 | | 37 | 39 | 5 |
| Ciccarelli | 23 | 1990 | ≤10 | 18 | 33 | 4–15 |
| | | | >10 | 4 | 50 | 4–7 |
| Webster | 124 | 1992 | | 21 | 14 | 4.25 |
| Landolt | 68 | 1996 | | 40 | 17 | 7–10 |

- *Further studies* are delayed for 4 or more years if the previous studies are negative.

## SYMPTOMS OF PITUITARY ADENOMA RECURRENCE

The patient usually experiences a reappearance of the symptoms (i.e., visual problems, endocrine disorders, headaches) that affected him or her previously. Headaches are an unreliable manifestation of an adenoma recurrence but must not be neglected. The author performs a neuroradiologic re-examination if headaches appear unexpectedly in a patient who has already undergone surgery. This may also relieve the patient of any concerns about possible tumor recurrence.

The reasons for reoperation in a group of 131 patients treated by Laws and colleagues[75] were pituitary hyperfunction in 63, visual loss in 50, other mass effects in 5, and CSF rhinorrhea in 13 (or combinations of these). Nicola and coworkers[88] operated a second time on 26 patients because of visual symptoms, in 7 because of endocrine symptoms, and in 23 because of both.

## PREOPERATIVE EVALUATION

### Endocrinologic Examination

The preoperative endocrinologic examination includes assay for hypersecreted hormones and to establish the function of the remaining normal hypophysis. The assay is useless in patients with pre-existing insufficiency. The author uses a combined intravenous stimulation with four hypothalamic releasing hormones.[106] It may seem trivial to mention that the endocrine type of an adenoma remains unchanged; however, exceptions to this rule have been noted.[35, 64, 123]

Recurrent adenomas, particularly in Cushing's disease, may be minute. The value of recurrent Cushing's adenoma localization with inferior petrosal sinus sampling, including a corticotropin-releasing factor stimulation test,[74] is not yet established.[101]

### Radiographic Examination

Radiographic evaluation of suspected pituitary adenoma recurrence is difficult unless the tumor is large. The examination must show the size, localization, and possible invasiveness of the recurrence, and the topography of the sella, which has been changed by the previous tumor and surgical intervention.

Magnetic resonance imaging of recurrent adenomas must include images with and without gadolinium enhancement. The images must be compared with those obtained before the first intervention because recurrent adenomas often maintain the imaging characteristics of the original tumor. Small recurrences localized in the cavernous sinus can be detected only by careful comparison of the gadolinium-enhanced venous channels of the cavernous sinuses (Fig. 35–3).

Particular attention must be paid to the *transplanted material* (gelatin foam, muscle, fascia, fat) in the interior of the former tumor cavity, which undergoes characteristic changes with time.[108] Gelatin foam appears as an intrasellar, hypodense mass with an enhancing rim that shrinks or disappears after 4 to 15 months. Muscle forms enhancing masses that may have an appearance similar to an adenoma; however, its texture is often inhomogeneous. Comparison with muscle tissue transplanted into the sphenoid sinus and adenoma extensions into the cavernous sinus or the parasellar area, if present, may be helpful for diagnosis. A correct diagnosis often can be reached only with follow-up examinations showing progressive enlargement, shrinkage, or a stable but questionable mass. This explains the importance of early postoperative baseline studies. Tissue transplanted into the sphenoid sinus shows as inhomogeneous masses on MRI examination with a tendency to

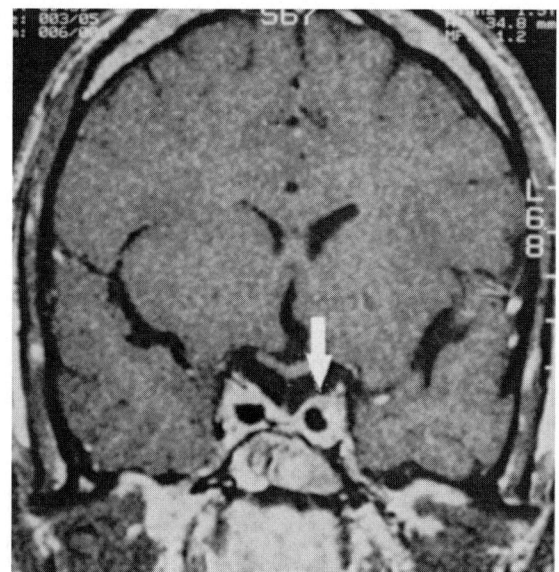

FIGURE 35–3 ■ A magnetic resonance imaging (MRI) scan of a recurrent microadenoma causing acromegaly (*white arrow*). Note the small tumor fragment in the interior of the cavernous sinus (no demonstration of venous channels after contrast enhancement).

shrink on follow-up studies. After contrast enhancement, remaining or regenerating mucosa appears as a bright line surrounding the sinus cavity.[108]

Computed tomography is less helpful than MRI for localizing recurrent pituitary adenomas, with the exception of macroadenomas.[30, 114] CT is needed primarily to demonstrate the bony configuration of the sphenoid, particularly if the primary operation was performed at another institution. This helps the surgeon to identify the landmarks for correct identification of the approach, particularly if the sphenoid sinus was filled with fat during the previous intervention.

## TREATMENT OF RECURRENT ADENOMAS

### Therapeutic Options

#### Surgery

It is often impossible to obtain a better result with reoperation than with the primary intervention because reoperation is performed under more difficult circumstances; therefore, other forms of therapy must be considered that may offer better results.

Bilateral adrenalectomy cures persistent or recurrent Cushing's disease in most instances. However, Nelson's syndrome[87] can be expected to develop in 10% to 38% of patients because of loss of cortisol-dependent feedback inhibition of the corticotropic adenoma.[25, 54]

#### Medical Therapy

*Antisecretory drugs* (dopamine agonists, somatostatin analogues) primarily influence the secretory activity of the adenoma, but may also affect tumor size.

The *dopamine agonists* bromocriptine, lisuride, cabergoline, and quinagolide can normalize hyperprolactinemia regardless of whether the prolactinoma being treated is primary or recurrent. *Bromocriptine* normalizes hyperprolactinemia in 54% of patients with macroprolactinomas and 82% of patients with microprolactinomas.[38] Tumor shrinkage amounting to more than 50% of the pretreatment volume has been observed in up to 80% of patients[13, 61]; however, adenoma shrinkage and correction of the hyperprolactinemia are reversible after discontinuation of the drug. The drug does not cure patients, with a few exceptions.[34] Unpleasant side effects (e.g., nausea, stomach pain, loss of appetite, nasal congestion, headache, sedation, dizziness, emotional problems) occur, at least temporarily, in up to one third of patients and, if they persist, may lead to drug discontinuation, followed by a rapid reincrease of PRL levels and re-expansion of the tumor.[13, 115] *Quinagolide* (CV 205-502; Norprolac), a recently introduced, long-acting, non–ergot-derived dopamine agonist, may be used in patients with bromocriptine intolerance because of its better efficacy and improved tolerance.[53]

*Octreotide* (SMS 201-995; Sandostatin), a synthetic octapeptide somatostatin analogue with a half-life of 80 to 90 minutes, offers a new treatment of acromegaly.[11] The drug is injected in doses of 50 to 100 μg every 8 hours (rarely every 12 hours) to maintain a GH serum level suppression and normal IGF-1 values.[92] Pretreatment GH levels are reached within a few days to weeks if the treatment is interrupted.[62] Octreotide lowered the GH levels in 94% and normalized them in 45% of 189 acromegalic patients who took part in a cooperative study.[120] In some patients, continuous subcutaneous infusion has been used for improving GH suppression.[84] This, however, became obsolete with the introduction of a long-acting octreotide incorporated into microspheres (Sandostatin LAR) that provides controlled, slow release of the drug, thus eliminating the rather inconvenient twice- or thrice-daily injections of the previously available drug preparation. The drug is injected once every 4 weeks and causes a more stable lowering of the otherwise fluctuating GH values.[63] The extent of adenoma shrinkage caused by octreotide varies. Lamberts and del Pozo[60] found a slight reduction of adenoma size in three of four patients, whereas Barkan and colleagues[8] described a tumor volume reduction of 20% to 54% in all treated patients. The positive effect of octreotide may be increased by simultaneous bromocriptine treatment, particularly in acromegalic patients with concomitant hyperprolactinemia or adenomas containing PRL.[9, 60]

Medical treatment of primary or recurrent Cushing's disease can be tried with drugs that interfere with steroid production, such as aminoglutethimide, metyrapone, o,p′-mitotane DDD, or ketoconazole (for review, see Boscaro and Sonino[15]).

Medical treatment of endocrinologically inactive adenomas is rarely successful. Luteinizing hormone-releasing hormone superagonists have been used. However, changes in tumor size were reported only rarely (for review, see Liuzzi and associates[76]). Warnet and colleagues,[122] however, reported a favorable effect of octreotide, with improvement of visual disturbances within 4 days in 10 of 23 patients. This rapid effect may help in the selection of patients who may eventually benefit from conservative treatment if surgery cannot be performed or must be delayed.

It has been suggested that rapidly growing pituitary tumors be treated with *cytostatic agents*; however, there is only one report describing a woman with a rapidly recurring pituitary adenoma with acromegaly who benefited from combined treatment with doxorubicin (Adriamycin) and lomustine (CCNU).[55]

## Radiation Therapy

Radiation therapy is an efficient method for treating primary or recurrent pituitary adenomas (see Table 35–1). It often represents the first therapeutic choice. A dose of 4000 cGy high-voltage radiation is applied in fractions of no more than 200 cGy in patients who have not undergone previous radiation. A higher dose (some authors use 5000 cGy or more) carries the risk of postactinic necrosis of the optic chiasm, hypothalamus, and temporal lobes.[3, 6, 37, 65] Optic neuropathy starts 6 months to 2 years after radiation therapy and cannot be influenced. MRI is indispensable for early diagnosis of this complication because the changes are not seen on CT.[47, 113]

*Reirradiation* of previously irradiated adenomas is possible.[36, 100] However, there is a significant risk of radiation damage to the optic nerves and temporal lobes that must be taken into account. The permitted dose for reirradiation has to be calculated carefully taking into account the repair the patient's body has undergone since the first radiation treatment. Retreatment causes the almost certain complete loss of remaining pituitary function.

Direct implantation of radioactive [125]I seeds during reoperation is another option that may be used to destroy the remaining tumor. However, no patient studies have been published summarizing any experience. The danger of carotid wall necrosis has to be considered.[56]

## Stereotactic Radiosurgery

Stereotactic radiosurgery (Gamma knife surgery) is an adjunctive therapeutic option in patients with recurrent pituitary adenomas; because of its precision, it may be used in previously irradiated patients if the dose is reduced according to projected radiation dose tolerance estimates.[36, 100, 109]

The single-dose radiosurgery treatment can deliver a higher dose than fractionated radiation therapy because of its higher precision (steep fall-off of the dose at the margin of the isocenter), which means that the dose applied to the optic nerves is lower, and because it delivers a dose with higher biologic effectiveness.[40]

Normal GH secretion was documented 12 months after treatment in three of four acromegalic patients and normal corticotropin-releasing hormone in 1 of 6 patients with Cushing's disease.[109] The author's follow-up study of 16 patients with uncured or recurring acromegaly showed, compared with a similar group of 50 patients treated with fractionated radiation therapy, a significantly faster lowering of the GH and IGF-1 levels after Gamma knife treatment[69] (Fig. 35–4). Half of the Gamma knife–treated patients had normal hormone parameters after 1.3 years, whereas the same percentage was reached only 7.1 years after fractionated radiation therapy.

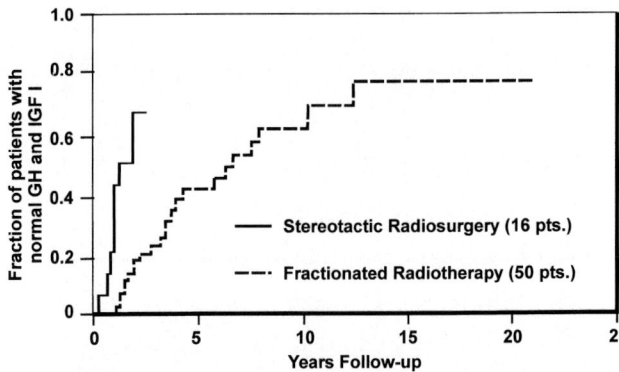

FIGURE 35–4 ■ This graph shows the cumulative distribution function (Kaplan-Meier estimate) of 50 acromegalic patients (pts.) treated with fractionated radiotherapy (40 Gy in fractions of 2 Gy) and 16 acromegalic patients treated with stereotactic (Gamma knife) radiosurgery (50 Gy to the center, 25 Gy to the tumor margin). (From Landolt AM, Haller D, Lomax N, et al: Stereotactic radiosurgery for recurrent surgically treated acromegaly: Comparison with fractionated radiotherapy. J Neurosurg 88:1002–1008, 1998.)

The Pittsburgh group reported normal GH levels in 72% 29 months after treatment, whereas normal IGF-1 values were seen in only 27% after 15 months.[126] PRL levels were lowered to only 18% to 69% of the initial value after 7 to 37 months. None was normal without additional dopamine agonist treatment. Normalization of the pituitary-adrenal axis was reached in 52% over 4 to 39 months in 21 patients with Cushing's disease. Tumor growth control was achieved in 94% and a volume decrease in 46% of the patients. Proximity of the adenoma to the optic nerve may render a pretreatment debulking of the tumor mass necessary to keep the doses applied to the optic nerves below 9 Gy.

## SURGICAL TECHNIQUE

Surgery of recurrent pituitary adenomas is influenced by the technique used in the preceding operation. Every neurosurgeon performing the first adenoma operation is aware that pituitary adenomas may recur and that he or she may have to reoperate for tumor recurrence. This means that the surgeon must preserve or restore as many anatomic landmarks as possible. The sella floor must be reconstructed with septum bone or cartilage whenever possible. The rostrum and the floor of the sphenoid sinus must be opened wide enough to allow a full view of the sella floor, but no more. Previous filling of the sphenoid sinus renders reoperation difficult, and therefore is performed only when the diaphragma sellae has been injured and CSF escapes.

The author uses the direct endonasal approach described by Griffith and Veerapen[42] as a transsphenoidal approach in all patients. The nose is prepared for 24 hours with neomycin drops in patients with signs of infection or extensive crust formation. The operation is done with the patient in a semisitting position.[73]

Both nasal cavities are filled with cotton swabs soaked in a solution of 10 ml of 1% lidocaine containing 10 drops of 0.1% epinephrine at the start of the operation. This

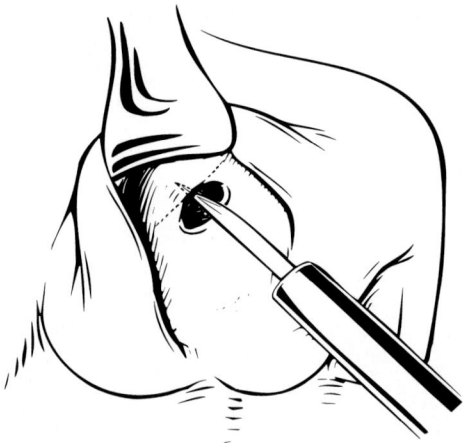

**FIGURE 35–5** ■ Incision of the nasal septum in a patient with a septum perforation caused by a previous intervention.

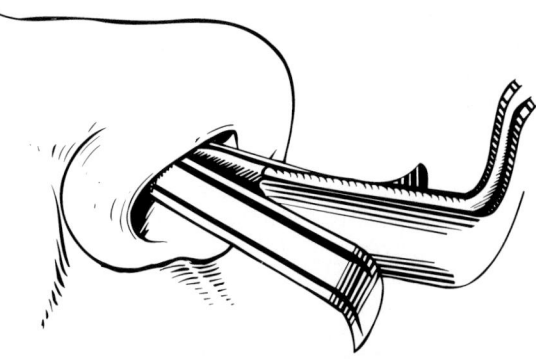

**FIGURE 35–7** ■ Insertion of the nasal speculum between the two brain retractors (see Fig. 35–6). The tip of the speculum is pushed down until its anterior edge reaches the anterior surface of the sphenoid bone.

procedure reduces capillary bleeding and improves visualization of the nasal cavity by decongesting the mucosa.

The right nostril is held open with a lid retractor or Killian nasal speculum. The septum is incised along the posterior edge of an existing perforation, which is enlarged (Fig. 35–5), or, in case of an intact septum, at a distance of approximately 1 cm in front of the sphenoid floor. The two mucosa sheaths are separated with the aid of a fine (3-mm) dissecting suction tube or a fine dissector. The direction of the approach is repeatedly checked with lateral fluoroscopy. The interest of the surgeon is focused during the separation of the two mucosal layers on the inferior edge of the previous opening in the sinus, particularly the inferior remnant of the previous rostrum, which is a key landmark for the entire operation because it confirms the exact midline direction of the approach. The dissection is advanced to a level corresponding to the previous rostrum. This method is easier to use in patients in whom the sinus was not previously filled with fat.

Two flat 12-mm blades are inserted between the two mucosal flaps (Fig. 35–6). This procedure facilitates the introduction of the pituitary speculum (Fig. 35–7). Fluoroscopic control is used to avoid insertion of the speculum tips deep into the interior of the sphenoid sinus (Fig. 35–8).

The sella floor, if it was reconstructed with septal bone or cartilage during the previous operation, may appear to be intact in patients with a recurrent microadenoma. A fine chisel or a drill and fine punches are used to gain access to the sellar contents, although the bony sella floor is usually missing in recurrent macroadenomas and the basal sella dura is replaced by scar tissue.

The consistency of the adenoma is usually similar to that at the first operation unless the adenoma has been irradiated or if a prolactinoma was previously treated with dopamine agonists; both measures lead to tumor fibrosis.[4, 12, 70] The normal pituitary gland is easily identified because it is orange-yellow, which differs markedly from the grayish-red, finely granular adenoma. The dissection is performed more aggressively than in the primary operation. A generous resection of marginal tissue between the recurrent adenoma and the normal gland is performed if the volume of the remaining normal tissue permits.

Hemostasis is easy in most instances. The tumor cavity is filled with fat or fascia. Fascia is used in patients in whom the diaphragma sellae was injured and CSF escapes.

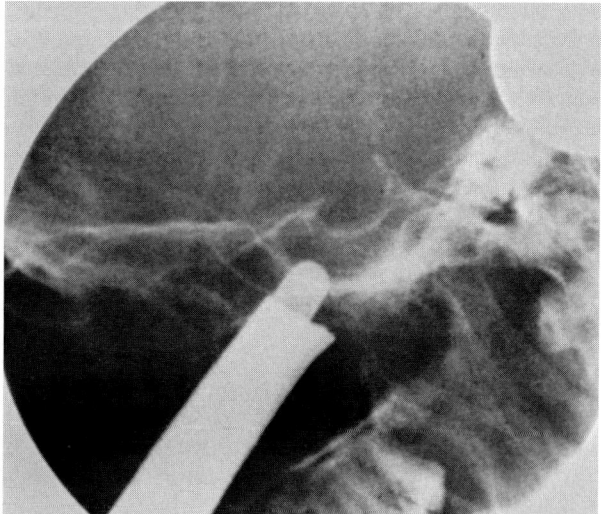

**FIGURE 35–8** ■ Radiofluoroscopy control during insertion of the pituitary speculum. Note that the brain retractors are too far advanced; their tips are located within the sphenoid sinus. (Image distortion is caused by the photographic process.)

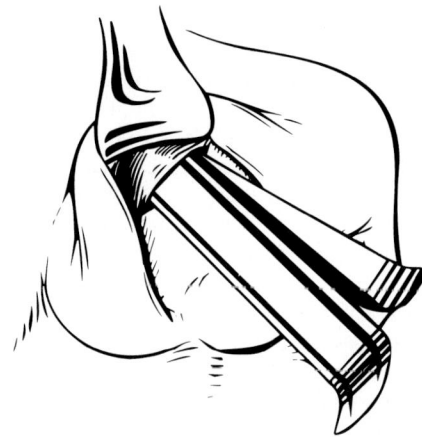

**FIGURE 35–6** ■ Insertion of two brain retractors between the mucosal flaps in the posterior sentum.

The tumor cavity may be drained with a plastic drain (No. 8 French gauge, with continuous suction generated by a water column of approximately 1 m) in patients with difficult hemostasis and continuing diffuse, light oozing (Fig. 35–9). The sella floor is reconstructed with septum, if available. The leaflets of the mucous membrane are attached to each other with fibrin glue. The incision is not sutured. Tamponade of the nasal cavities is needed rarely. Antibiotic prophylaxis is obtained with a daily infusion of 2.2 g of amoxicillin beginning before surgery and discontinued on the first or second postoperative day.

## Special Situations

Patients who have undergone transcranial adenoma extirpation previously are more difficult to treat by a subsequent transsphenoidal procedure because the diaphragma sellae is totally or partially missing. The adenoma and its surrounding scar tissue can adhere to the optic system and the hypothalamus, which renders an endocrine cure impossible. The procedure is therefore used primarily for decompressing the nervous structures and debulking the tumor before radiation therapy. Special care is taken in the dissection of the suprasellar portion of the tumor. It may be helpful to outline the contour of this portion with an intraoperative lumbar subarachnoid injection of 10 to 20 ml of air with fluoroscopy. Debulking may lead to empty sella syndrome with downward herniation of the chiasm because of adhesions.[89] To prevent this, the author uses bone obtained from the sphenoid floor partially to fill the empty sella.

Craniotomy in patients who have had previous transsphenoidal surgery does not usually present major problems; on the contrary, this is a safe procedure in large adenomas because the sphenoid sinus has been safely obliterated, preventing postoperative CSF rhinorrhea. It is usually easier to operate transcranially after a previous transsphenoidal operation than vice versa. The situation is similar to that with tumors that must be removed with a two-step combined procedure. In this situation, the transsphenoidal operation is performed first.[46]

To avoid exploration through a region of adhesions between the brain, the optic nerves, and the dura covering the skull base, the surgeon performing a craniotomy for a

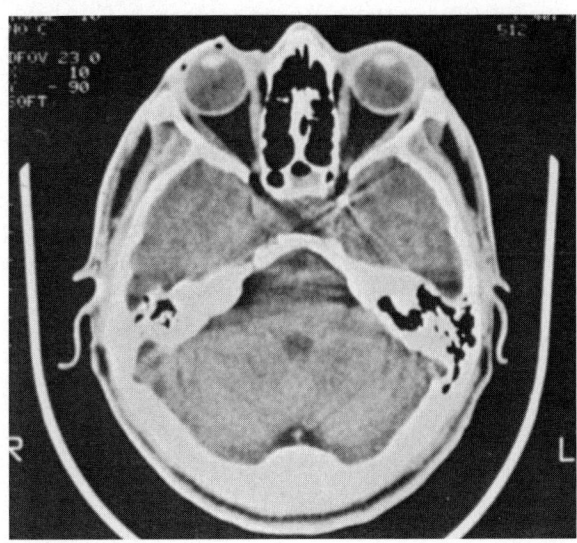

FIGURE 35–10 ■ An intraoperative control computed tomography scan (without contrast) performed because of deviation from the midsagittal approach. The orientation clip is localized within the left cavernous sinus, lateral to the carotid.

second time may consider another approach, such as a transfrontal approach, instead of a pterional approach.

## Pitfalls and Complications of Surgery

The most dangerous problem occurring during transsphenoidal pituitary reoperation is deviation from the midline. Large openings in the floor of the sphenoid sinus and a presellar sphenoid sinus that offer little opportunity to identify the sella are dangerous, particularly if the sinus has previously been filled with fat. Complete loss of orientation can occur. Careful dissection may uncover a carotid artery. However, it may remain unclear whether the lateral or the medial aspect of the sinus knee is exposed. The only way to become oriented in this situation is to place a metal clip in the surgical field, remove the pituitary speculum, perform a provisional wound closure, and obtain an intraoperative CT scan (Fig. 35–10). Reinsertion of the pituitary speculum with correction of the approach toward the recurrent adenoma is then possible.

Deviation from the midline may lead to an injury of the internal carotid artery, the optic nerve crossing the superolateral aspect of the sphenoid sinus in the optic canal, and the cranial nerves in the lateral wall of the cavernous sinus (see Fig. 35–10). Injury of the *internal carotid artery* is an immediate, life-threatening situation. The massive arterial bleeding is controlled by lowering the arterial pressure with nitroprusside or a similar drug, compressing the carotid artery in the neck, and plugging the injury with muscle. Care must be taken that the muscle is not inserted completely into the vessel because this may lead to embolization into a smaller cerebral vessel. The muscle is fixed with fibrin glue; the sella floor is reconstructed, if possible; and the sphenoid sinus is tightly filled with muscle, fascia, and fat. Removal of the tumor usually must be abandoned in this situation.[67] Intraoperative balloon occlusion of the vessel has been described as an

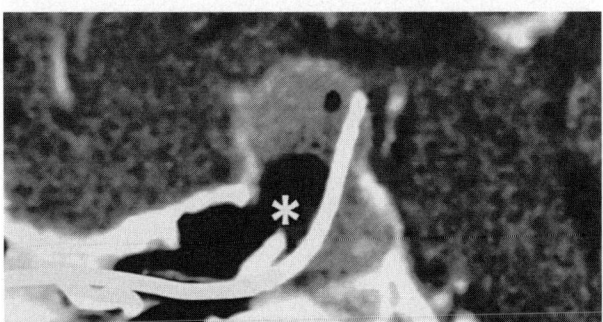

FIGURE 35–9 ■ Suction drainage of the surgical cavity obtained on the first postoperative day after a partial pituitary adenoma extirpation. The *asterisk* marks the fat used for the inferior closure of the surgical cavity.

alternative.[16] A possible late consequence of a carotid injury is the formation of a false arterial aneurysm or a carotid-cavernous fistula.[2]

The *optic nerve* may be injured in the region of the optic canal because of deviation from the midline, or particularly after a previous transcranial operation because of a perforation of the diaphragma sellae with local adhesions between the adenoma and the chiasm. Intraoperative recording of visual evoked responses has been suggested to prevent optic nerve damage in this situation.[27]

A *CSF fistula* may occur if the diaphragma sellae is injured, particularly in patients who had undergone previous transcranial surgery and radiation therapy. Routine closure of intraoperative CSF leaks is performed with fascia, a fat transplant, fibrin tissue glue, and use of postoperative lumbar CSF drainage for approximately 1 week.[46, 50, 67, 116] The prognosis for closure of the CSF fistula is not necessarily good. Laws and colleagues[75] operated on 21 patients with CSF rhinorrhea a second time after previous adenomectomy. Fistula closure was successful in 16 (76%). Three patients needed tertiary interventions (third transsphenoidal operation, craniotomy, transethmoidal repair, and CSF shunts), and the fistula persisted in two (10%) of these patients even after these measures were instituted.

The author has modified his technique of CSF fistula repair after unsuccessful attempts with the usual technique in an endocrinologically inactive macroadenoma; histologic examination demonstrated necrosis of the transplanted tissue 3 weeks after intrasphenoid transplantation. The fat and fascia do not contain a particularly high density of transplantable fibroblasts. Successful closure was obtained after covering the diaphragma sellae opening with periosteum obtained from the iliac crest and filling the sella and part of the sphenoid sinus with red cancellous bone from the pelvis. The transplants were fixed with fibrin glue, and the remaining sinus cavity was filled with fat.

The complication rate of pituitary adenoma reoperations is higher than that reported for primary procedures. Laws and colleagues[75] reported on a group of 158 transsphenoidal reoperations (127 adenomas, 31 other lesions) with a mortality rate of 2.5%. Two patients had stroke, 2 excessive hemorrhage, 2 meningitis, 9 CSF rhinorrhea, 1 a palsy of cranial nerve VI, 11 permanent diabetes insipidus, 13 new hypopituitarism, and 2 had new septal perforations. Among 56 reoperated patients, Nicola and coworkers[88] noted 2 with palsies of cranial nerve VI and 2 with CSF rhinorrhea requiring a third operation.

## RESULTS

The results of surgery of recurrent pituitary adenomas show fundamental differences between endocrinologically active and inactive tumors because improvement of neurologic defects by debulking of intrasellar and suprasellar masses is much easier to achieve than normalization of endocrine hyperfunction, which depends on complete or almost complete elimination of the abnormally secreting tissue. Minute remnants may cause failure of the operation.

Improvement of visual symptoms was achieved by Laws and colleagues[75] in 61% of 54 reoperated patients. Deterioration of vision occurred in 2% of patients. Derome and associates[29] described improvement of vision in 68%, unchanged vision in 18%, and deterioration in 14% of 30 patients. Nicola and coworkers[88] reported improvement in 51%, equality in 33%, and deterioration in 16% of 49 patients who underwent a second operation.

In a series of 126 patients (follow-up of 1 to 16 years) with endocrinologically inactive adenomas, Comtois and associates[26] found that *second recurrences* appeared in 7 of 15 patients up to 10 years after the reoperation, despite radiation in 7 and more aggressive surgery in all. They found a higher second recurrence rate in patients receiving radiation therapy (five of seven) than in patients who were not irradiated (two of eight). The difference, however, is not significant. In a series of 158 reoperations, of which 31 were done for other tumors of the sellar region, Laws and colleagues[75] found that 26 patients (17%) required a third surgical intervention after a mean follow-up of 37 months.

The endocrine results in most of the series reported are inferior to the neurologic results (Table 35–3). Neurologic improvement, however, can be achieved by partial tumor extirpation, whereas endocrine normalization requires far more radical tumor removal. Giovanelli and coworkers[41] consider, with the exception of a few special cases, reoperation for acromegaly not to be curative. Abe and Lüdecke,[1] on the other hand, consider reoperation a good option if MRI reveals a well circumscribed (enclosed) adenoma remnant. In 16 of 18 enclosed adenoma recurrences (89%), they describe normal postoperative GH and IGF-1 levels, whereas none of 10 adenomas with invasive growth had normal GH and IGF-1 serum levels after reoperation. Table 35–3 presents the endocrine results reported in different published series. The results do not match those obtained

## TABLE 35–3 ■ ENDOCRINE RESULTS OF SURGERY OF SECRETING, RECURRENT PITUITARY ADENOMAS

| First Author | Reference | Year | Acromegaly* | Prolactinomas* | Cushing's Disease* | Nelson's Syndrome* |
|---|---|---|---|---|---|---|
| Laws | 75 | 1985 | 5 (12) | 12 (41) | 1 (4) | 5 (24) |
| Friedman | 39 | 1989 | | | 24 (33) | |
| Derome | 29 | 1991 | 3 (8) | 2 (6) | 2 (8) | 1 (5) |
| Lüdecke | 77 | 1991 | | | 7 (11) | |
| Nicola | 88 | 1991 | 5 (10) | 5 (8) | 1 (2) | |
| Abe | 1 | 1998 | 16 (28) | | | |
| Total | | | 29 (58) 50% | 19 (55) 34% | 35 (58) 60% | 6 (29) 20% |

*Normalized patients (total patients).

by primary operations (see Chapters 24 to 26). This is not surprising. The data also show that patients with Nelson's syndrome do significantly less well than those with adenomas of Cushing's disease.

A major problem, however, is represented by the group of patients who have been operated on, have undergone a full course of radiation therapy, do not or no longer respond to drugs, and have recurring neurologic symptoms. In this situation, the surgeon must be satisfied with debulking the tumor as a palliative measure.

## REFERENCES

1. Abe T, Lüdecke DK: Recent results of secondary transnasal surgery for residual or recurrent acromegaly. Neurosurgery 42:1013–1022, 1998.
2. Ahuja A, Guterman LR, Hopkins LN: Carotid cavernous fistula and false aneurysm of the carotid artery: Complications of transsphenoidal surgery. Neurosurgery 31:774–779, 1992.
3. Al-Mefty O, Kersch JE, Routh A, et al: The long-term side effects of radiation therapy for benign brain tumors in adults. J Neurosurg 73:502–512, 1990.
4. Anniko M, Wersäll J: Morphological effects in pituitary tumours following radiotherapy. Virchows Arch 395:45–58, 1982.
5. Arafah BM, Brodkey JS, Pearson OH: Gradual recovery of lactotroph responsiveness to dynamic stimulation following surgical removal of prolactinomas: Long-term follow-up studies. Metabolism 35:905–912, 1986.
6. Aristizabal S, Caldwell WL, Avila J: The relationship of time-dose fractionation factors to complications in the treatment of pituitary tumors by irradiation. Int J Radiat Oncol Biol Phys 2:667–673, 1977.
7. Bakay L: The results of 300 pituitary adenoma operations (Professor Herbert Olivecrona's series). J Neurosurg 7:240–255, 1950.
8. Barkan AL, Lloyd RV, Chandler WF, et al: Preoperative treatment of acromegaly with long-acting somatostatin analog SMS 201-995: Shrinkage of invasive pituitary macroadenomas and improved surgical remission rate. J Clin Endocrinol Metab 67:1040–1048, 1988.
9. Barkan AL, Kelch RP, Hopwood NJ, et al: Treatment of acromegaly with the long-acting somatostatin analog SMS 201-99. J Clin Endocrinol Metab 66:16–23, 1988.
10. Bertrand G, Tolis G, Montes J: Immediate and long-term results of transsphenoidal microsurgical resection of prolactinomas in 92 patients. In Tolis G, Stefanis C, Mountokalakis T, Labrie F (eds): Prolactin and Prolactinomas. New York: Raven Press, 1983, pp 441–452.
11. Besser GM, Wass JAH: Somatostatin octapeptide analogue (octreotide) in the medical management of acromegaly. In Landolt AM, Heitz PU, Zapf J, et al (eds): Advances in Pituitary Adenoma Research. Oxford: Pergamon Press, 1988, pp 221–225.
12. Betzold M, Saeger W, Riedel M, Lüdecke DK: Microscopical effects of radiotherapy on pituitary adenomas in acromegaly. Acta Endocrinol 117 (Suppl):287, 1988.
13. Bevan JS, Webster J, Burke CW, Scanlon MF: Dopamine agonists and pituitary tumor shrinkage. Endocr Rev 13:220–240, 1992.
14. Bochiccio D, Losa M, Buchfelder M: Factors influencing the immediate and late outcome of Cushing's disease treated by transsphenoidal surgery: A retrospective study by the European Cushing's Disease Survey Group. J Clin Endocrinol Metab 80:3114–3120, 1995.
15. Boscaro M, Sonino N: Cushing's disease: Medical treatment. In Landolt AM, Vance ML, Reilly PL (eds): Pituitary Adenomas. New York: Chrchill Livingstone, 1996, pp 417–430.
16. Britt RH, Silverberg GD, Prolo DJ, et al: Balloon catheter occlusion for cavernous carotid artery injury during transsphenoidal hypophysectomy: Case report. J Neurosurg 55:450–452, 1981.
17. Buchfelder M, Brockmeier S, Fahlbusch R, et al: Recurrence following transsphenoidal surgery for acromegaly. Horm Res 35:113–118, 1991.
18. Buchfelder M, Lierheimer A, Schrell U, et al: Recurrence of hyperprolactinemia detected in long-term follow-up of surgically normalized microprolactinomas. In Auer LM, Leb G, Tscherne G, et al (eds): Prolactinomas: An Interdisciplinary Approach. Berlin: Walter de Gruyter, 1985, pp 183–187.
19. Burian K, Pendl G, Salah S: Über die Rezidivhäufigkeit von Hypo-

20. physen-Adenomen nach transfrontaler, transsphenoidaler oder zweizeitig kombinierter Operation. Wien Med Wochenschr 120:833–836, 1970.
20. Cairns H: Prognosis of pituitary tumours. Lancet 2:1310–1311, 1935.
21. Carboni P, Detta A, Hitchcock ER, Postans R: Pituitary adenoma proliferative indices and risk of recurrence. Br J Neurosurg 6:33–40, 1992.
22. Charpentier G, de Plunkett T, Jedynak P, et al: Surgical treatment of prolactinomas. Horm Res 22:222–227, 1985.
23. Ciccarelli E, Ghigo E, Miola C, et al: Long-term follow-up of "cured" prolactinoma patients after successful adenomectomy. Clin Endocrinol 32:583–592, 1990.
24. Ciric I, Mikhael M, Stafford T, et al: Transsphenoidal microsurgery of pituitary macroadenomas with long-term follow-up results. J Neurosurg 59:395–401, 1983.
25. Cohen KL, Noth RH, Pechinski T: Incidence of pituitary tumors following adrenalectomy: A long-term follow-up study of patients treated for Cushing's disease. Arch Intern Med 138:575–579, 1978.
26. Comtois R, Beauregard H, Somma M, et al: The clinical and endocrine outcome to transsphenoidal microsurgery of nonsecreting pituitary adenomas. Cancer 68:860–866, 1991.
27. Costa e Silva I, Wang AD, Symon L: The application of flash visual evoked potentials during operations on the anterior visual pathways. Neurol Res 7:11–16, 1985.
28. Davidoff LM, Feiring EH: Surgical treatment of tumors of the pituitary body. Am J Surg 75:99–136, 1948.
29. Derome PJ, Visot A, Delalande O, et al: Pituitary adenomas: Our experience with tumoral recurrence after surgery. In Faglia G, Beck-Peccoz P, Ambrosi B, et al (eds): Pituitary Adenomas: New Trends in Basic and Clinical Research. International Congress Series Vol 961. Amsterdam: Excerpta Medica, 1991, pp 321–327.
30. Dolinskas CA, Simeone FA: Transsphenoidal hypophysectomy: Postsurgical CT findings. AJNR Am J Neuroradiol 6:45–50, 1985.
31. Earle KM, Dillard SH: Pathology of adenomas of the pituitary gland. In Kohler PO, Ross GT (eds): Diagnosis and Treatment of Pituitary Tumors. Amsterdam: Excerpta Medica, 1973, pp 3–16.
32. Ebersold MJ, Quast LM, Laws ER, et al: Long-term results in transsphenoidal removal of nonfunctioning pituitary adenomas. J Neurosurg 64:713–719, 1986.
33. Elkington SG, McKissock W: Pituitary adenoma: Results of combined surgical and radiotherapeutic treatment in 260 patients. BMJ 1:263–266, 1967.
34. Eversmann T, Fahlbusch R, Rjosk HK, von Werder K: Persisting suppression of prolactin secretion after long-term treatment with bromocriptine in patients with prolactinomas. Acta Endocrinol 92:413–427, 1979.
35. Felix I, Asa SL, Kovacs K, Horvath E: Changes in hormone production of a recurrent silent corticotroph adenoma of the pituitary: A histologic, immunocytochemical, ultrastructural, and tissue culture study. Hum Pathol 22:719–721, 1991.
36. Flickinger JC, Deutsch M, Lunsford LD: Repeat megavoltage irradiation of pituitary and suprasellar tumors. Int J Radiat Oncol Biol Phys 17:171–175, 1989.
37. Flickinger JC, Rush SC: Linear accelerator therapy of pituitary adenomas. In Landolt AM, Vance ML, Reilly PL (eds): Pituitary Adenomas. New York: Chrchill Livingstone, 1996, pp 475–483.
38. Flückiger E, del Pozo E, von Werder K: Prolactin: Physiology, Pharmacology and Clinical Findings. Monographs on Endocrinology, Vol 2. Berlin: Springer-Verlag, 1982.
39. Friedman RB, Oldfield EH, Nieman LK, et al: Repeat transsphenoidal surgery for Cushing's disease. J Neurosurg 71:520–527, 1989.
40. Ganz JC: Gamma knife treatment of pituitary adenomas. In Landolt AM, Vance ML, Reilly PL (eds): Pituitary Adenomas. New York: Chrchill Livingstone, 1996, pp 461–474.
41. Giovanelli M, Losa M, Mortini P: Acromegaly: Surgical results and prognosis. In Landolt AM, Vance ML, Reilly PL (eds): Pituitary Adenomas. New York: Chrchill Livingstone, 1996, pp 333–351.
42. Griffith H, Veerapen R: A direct transnasal approach to the sphenoid sinus: Technical note. J Neurosurg 66:140–142, 1987.
43. Grigsby PW, Simpson JR, Fineberg B: Late regrowth of pituitary adenomas after irradiation and/or surgery: Hazard function analysis. Cancer 63:1308–1312, 1989.
44. Guidetti B, Fraioli B, Cantore GP: Results of surgical management of 319 pituitary adenomas. Acta Neurochir (Wien) 85:117–124, 1987.

45. Guillaume J, Caron JP: Remarques cliniques et chirurgicales relatives aux adénomes hypophysaires. Neurochirurgie 4:338–343, 1958.
46. Guiot G: Transsphenoidal approach in surgical treatment of pituitary adenomas: General principles and indications in non-functioning adenomas. In Kohler PO, Ross GT (eds): Diagnosis and Treatment of Pituitary Tumors. Amsterdam: Excerpta Medica, 1973, pp 159–178.
47. Guy J, Manusco A, Beck R, et al: Radiation-induced optic neuropathy: A magnetic resonance imaging study. J Neurosurg 74:426–432, 1991.
48. Hammer HM: Optic chiasmal radionecrosis. Trans Ophthalmol Soc U K 103:208–211, 1983.
49. Hardy J: Transsphenoidal surgery of hypersecreting pituitary tumors. In Kohler PO, Ross GT (eds): Diagnosis and Treatment of Pituitary Tumors. Amsterdam: Excerpta Medica, 1973, pp 179–194.
50. Hardy J: Atlas of Transsphenoidal Microsurgery in Pituitary Tumors. New York: Igaku-Shoin, 1991.
51. Heimbach SB: Follow-up studies on 105 cases of verified chromophobe and acidophilic pituitary adenomata after treatment by transfrontal operation and x-ray irradiation. Acta Neurochir (Wien) 7:101–155, 1959.
52. Henderson WR: The pituitary adenomata: A follow-up study of the surgical results in 338 cases (Dr. Harvey Cushing's series). Br J Surg 25:811–921, 1939.
53. Homburg R, West C, Brownell J, Jacobs HS: A double-blind study comparing a new non-ergot, long-acting dopamine agonist, CV 205-502, with bromocriptine in women with hyperprolactinemia. Clin Endocrinol 32:565–571, 1990.
54. Hopwood NJ, Kenny FM: Incidence of Nelson's syndrome after adrenalectomy for Cushing's disease in children: Results of a nationwide survey. Am J Dis Child 131:1353–1356, 1977.
55. Kasperlik-Zaluska AA, Wiskawski J, Kaniewska J, et al: Cystostatics for acromegaly: Marked improvement in a patient with an invasive pituitary tumor. Acta Endocrinol 116:347–349, 1987.
56. Kaufman B, Lapham LW, Shealy CN, Pearson OH: Transsphenoidal yttrium 90 pituitary ablation: Radiation damage to the internal carotid. Acta Radiol Ther Phys Biol 3:17–25, 1966.
57. Kernohan JW, Sayre GP: Tumors of the pituitary gland and infundibulum. In Atlas of Tumor Pathology, Section X, Fascicle 3. Washington, DC: Armed Forces Institute of Pathology, 1956, pp 37–42.
58. Kovacs K, Horvath E: Tumors of the pituitary gland. In Hartmann WH, Sobin LH (eds): Atlas of Tumor Pathology, 2nd Series, Fascicle 2. Washington, DC: Armed Forces Institute of Pathology, 1986, pp 217–224.
59. Krieger DT: Cushing's Syndrome. Monographs on Endocrinology, Vol 2. Berlin: Springer-Verlag, 1982, pp 124–126.
60. Lamberts SWJ, del Pozo E: Somatostatin analog treatment of acromegaly: New aspects. Horm Res 29:115–117, 1988.
61. Lamberts SWJ, MacLeod RM: Prolactinomas: Medical treatment. In Landolt AM, Vance ML, Reilly PL (eds): Pituitary Adenomas. New York: Churchill Livingstone, 1996, pp 431–441.
62. Lamberts SWJ, Uitterlinden P, del Pozo E: SMS 201-995 induces a continuous decline in circulating growth hormone and somatomedin-C levels during therapy of acromegalic patients for over two years. J Clin Endocrinol Metab 65:703–710, 1987.
63. Lancranjan I, Bruns C, Grass PO, et al: Sandostatin LAR: A promising therapeutic tool in the management of acromegalic patients. Metabolism 45 (Suppl 1):67–71, 1996.
64. Landolt AM: Ultrastructure of human sella tumors. Acta Neurochir (Wien) 22 (Suppl):1–167, 1975.
65. Landolt AM: Hazards of radiotherapy in patients with pituitary adenomas. In Derome P, Jedynak CP, Peillon F (eds): Pituitary Adenomas: Biology, Physiopathology and Treatment. Paris: Rueil-Malmaison, Asclepios Publishers, 1980, pp 235–232.
66. Landolt AM: Clinical problems in prolactinomas from the neurosurgical standpoint. In Hoshino K (ed): Prolactin Gene Family and its Receptors: Molecular Biology to Clinical Problems. International Congress Series Vol 819. Amsterdam: Excerpta Medica, 1988, pp 433–440.
67. Landolt AM: Transsphenoidal surgery of pituitary tumors: Its pitfalls and complications. Prog Neurol Surg 1:1–30, 1990.
68. Landolt AM: The role of surgery in prolactinoma treatment. In von Werder K, Fahlbusch R (eds): Pituitary Adenomas: From Basic Research to Diagnosis and Therapy. Amsterdam: Elsevier, 1996, pp 331–340.
69. Landolt AM, Haller D, Lomax N, et al: Stereotactic radiosurgery for recurrent surgically treated acromegaly: Comparison with fractionated radiotherapy. J Neurosurg 88:1002–1008, 1998.
70. Landolt AM, Osterwalder V: Perivascular fibrosis in prolactinomas: Is it increased by bromocriptine? J Clin Endocrinol Metab 58:1179–1183, 1984.
71. Landolt AM, Shibata T, Kleihues P: Growth rate of human pituitary adenomas. J Neurosurg 67:803–806, 1987.
72. Landolt AM, Shibata T: Growth, cell proliferation, and prognosis of pituitary adenomas. In Faglia G, Beck-Peccoz P, Ambrosi B, et al (eds): Pituitary Adenomas: New Trends in Basic and Clinical Research. International Congress Series Vol 961. Amsterdam: Excerpta Medica, 1991, pp 169–178.
73. Landolt AM, Strebel P: Technique of transsphenoidal operation for pituitary adenomas. Adv Tech Stand Neurosurg 7:119–171, 1980.
74. Landolt AM, Valavanis A, Girard J, Eberle AN: Corticotropin-releasing factor test used with bilateral, simultaneous inferior petrosal sinus blood-sampling for the diagnosis of pituitary-dependent Cushing's disease. Clin Endocrinol 25:687–696, 1986.
75. Laws ER Jr, Fode NC, Redmond MJ: Transsphenoidal surgery following unsuccessful prior therapy. J Neurosurg 63:823–829, 1985.
76. Liuzzi A, Zingrillo M, Ghigi MR, et al: Endocrine inactive adenomas: Medical treatment. In Landolt AM, Vance ML, Reilly PL (eds): Pituitary Adenomas. New York: Chrchill Livingstone, 1996, pp 443–452.
77. Lüdecke DK, Heinrichs M, Saeger W: Recurrences after transnasal adenomectomy in Cushing's disease. In Faglia G, Beck-Peccoz P, Ambrosi B, et al (eds): Pituitary Adenomas: New Trends in Basic and Clinical Research. International Congress Series Vol 96. Amsterdam: Excerpta Medica, 1991, pp 337–348.
78. MacCarty CS, Hanson EJ, Randall RV, Scanlon PW: Indications for and results of surgical treatment of pituitary tumors by the transfrontal approach. In Kohler PO, Ross GT (eds): Diagnosis and Treatment of Pituitary Tumors. Amsterdam: Excerpta Medica, 1973, pp 139–145.
79. Marguth F, Nover A: Morphologie und Klinik der Hypophysenadenom-Rezidive. Acta Neurochir (Wien) 11:716–730, 1964.
80. Marguth F, Oeckler R. Recurrent pituitary adenomas. Neurosurg Rev 8:221–224, 1985.
81. Martins AN, Kempe LG, Hayes GJ: Pituitary adenomas: Current concepts based on twenty years' experience at Walter Reed General Hospital. Acta Neurochir (Wien) 13:469–494, 1965.
82. McCollough WM, Marcus RB Jr, Rhoton AL Jr, et al: Long-term follow-up of radiotherapy for pituitary adenoma: The absence of late recurrence after > 4500 cGy. Int J Radiat Oncol Biol Phys 21:607–614, 1991.
83. Mogensen EF: Chromophobe adenoma of the pituitary gland: A follow-up study on 60 surgical patients with special reference to endocrine disturbances. Acta Endocrinol 24:135–152, 1957.
84. Møller N, White MC, Chatterjee S, et al: High dose, long-term, continuous subcutaneous infusion of SMS 201–995 (Sandostatin) in acromegaly. In Landolt AM, Heitz PU, Zapf J, et al (eds): Advances in Pituitary Adenoma Research. Oxford: Pergamon Press, 1988, pp 233–234.
85. Muhr C, Bergström K, Enoksson P, et al: Follow-up study with computerized tomography and clinical evaluation 5 and 10 years after surgery for pituitary adenoma. J Neurosurg 53:144–148, 1980.
86. Nagashima T, Murovic JA, Hoshino T, et al: The proliferative potential of human pituitary tumors in situ. J Neurosurg 64:588–593, 1986.
87. Nelson DH, Meakin JW, Dealy JB Jr, et al: ACTH-producing tumor of the pituitary gland. N Engl J Med 259:161–164, 1958.
88. Nicola GC, Tonnarelli G, Griner AC, et al: Surgery for recurrence of pituitary adenomas. In Faglia G, Beck-Peccoz P, Ambrosi B, et al (eds): Pituitary Adenomas: New Trends in Basic and Clinical Research. International Congress Series Vol 961. Amsterdam: Excerpta Medica, 1991, pp 329–336.
89. Olson DR, Guiot G, Derome P. The symptomatic empty sella: Prevention and correction via the transsphenoidal approach. J Neurosurg 37:533–537, 1972.
90. Pistenma DA, Goffinet DR, Bagshaw MA, et al: Treatment of chromophobe adenomas with megavoltage irradiation. Cancer 35:1574–1582, 1975.
91. Quabbe HJ, Buch K, Solbach HG, et al: Treatment of acromegaly by transsphenoidal operation, 90-yttrium implantation and bromocriptine: Results in 230 patients. Clin Endocrinol 16:107–119, 1982.

92. Quabbe HJ, Plöckinger U: Dose-response study and long-term effect of the somatostatin analog octreotide in patients with therapy-resistant acromegaly. J Clin Endocrinol Metab 68:873–881, 1989.

93. Ray BS, Patterson RH: Surgical experience with chromophobe adenomas of the pituitary gland. J Neurosurg 34:726–729, 1971.

94. Rodman EF, Molitch ME, Post KD, et al: Long-term follow-up of transsphenoidal selective adenomectomy for prolactinoma. JAMA 252:921–924, 1984.

95. Roelfsema F, van Dulken H, Frölich M: Long-term results of transsphenoidal pituitary microsurgery in 60 acromegalic patients. Clin Endocrinol 23:555–565, 1985.

96. Saeger W, Betzold M, Lüdecke DK: Äderung der Differenzierung von Hypophysenadenomen durch Strahlentherapie? Ultrastrukturell-morphologische Untersuchungen. Verh Dtsch Ges Pathol 72:453, 1988.

97. Salmi J, Grahne B, Valtonen S, Pelkonen R: Recurrence of chromophobe pituitary adenomas after operation and postoperative radiotherapy. Acta Neurol Scand 60:681–689, 1982.

98. Scheithauer BW, Kovacs KT, Laws ER, Randall RV: Pathology of invasive pituitary tumors with special reference to functional classification. J Neurosurg 65:733–744, 1986.

99. Schlechte JA, Sherman BM, Chapler FK, et al: Long-term follow-up of women with surgically treated prolactin-secreting pituitary tumors. J Clin Endocrinol Metab 62:1296–1301, 1986.

100. Schoenthaler R, Albright NW, Wara WM, et al: Reirradiation of pituitary adenoma. Int J Radiat Oncol Biol Phys 24:307–314, 1992.

101. Schulte HM, Allolio B, Doppman JL, Oldfield EH: Value of hormone measurement in blood from inferior petrosal sinuses. In Faglia G, Beck-Peccoz P, Ambrosi B, et al (eds): Pituitary Adenomas: New Trends in Basic and Clinical Research. International Congress Series Vol 961. Amsterdam: Excerpta Medica, 1991, pp 193–198.

102. Schuster LD, Bantle JP, Oppenheimer JH, et al: Acromegaly: Reassessment of the long-term therapeutic effectiveness of transsphenoidal pituitary surgery. Ann Intern Med 95:172–174, 1981.

103. Selman WR, Laws ER, Scheithauer BW, et al: The occurrence of dural invasion in pituitary adenomas. J Neurosurg 64:402–407, 1986.

104. Serri O, Rasio E, Beauregard H, et al: Recurrence of hyperprolactinemia after selective transsphenoidal adenomectomy in women with prolactinoma. N Engl J Med 309:280–283, 1983.

105. Shaffi OM, Wrightson P: Dural invasion by pituitary tumours. N Z Med J 81:386–390, 1975.

106. Sheldon WR, DeBold CR, Evans WS, et al: Rapid sequential intravenous administration of four hypothalamic hormones as a combined anterior pituitary function test in normal subjects. J Clin Endocrinol Metab 60:623–630, 1985.

107. Sheline GE: Treatment of chromophobe adenomas of the pituitary gland and acromegaly. In Kohler PO, Ross GT (eds): Diagnosis and Treatment of Pituitary Tumors. Amsterdam: Excerpta Medica, 1973, pp 201–216.

108. Steiner E, Knosp E, Herold CJ, et al: Pituitary adenomas: Findings of postoperative MR imaging. Radiology 185:521–527, 1992.

109. Stephanian E, Lunsford LD, Coffey RJ, et al: Gamma knife surgery for sellar and suprasellar tumors. Neurosurg Clin North Am 3:207–218, 1992.

110. Stern WE, Batzdorf U: Intracranial removal of pituitary adenomas: An evaluation of varying degrees of excision from partial to total. J Neurosurg 33:564–573, 1970.

111. Svien HJ, Colby MY: Treatment for Chromophobe Adenoma. Springfield, IL: Charles C Thomas, 1967, pp 33–40.

112. Symon L, Logue V, Mohanty S: Recurrence of pituitary adenomas after transcranial operation. J Neurol Neurosurg Psychiatry 45:780–785, 1982.

113. Tachibana O, Yamaguchi N, Yamashima T, et al: Radiation necrosis of the optic chiasm, optic tract, hypothalamus, and upper pons after radiotherapy for pituitary adenoma, detected by gadolinium-enhanced, T1-weighted magnetic resonance imaging: Case report. Neurosurgery 27:640–643, 1990.

114. Teng MMH, Huang CI, Chang T: The pituitary mass after transsphenoidal hypophysectomy. AJNR Am J Neuroradiol 9:23–26, 1988.

115. Thorner MO, Perryman RL, Rogol AD, et al: Rapid changes of prolactinoma volume after withdrawal and reinstitution of bromocriptine. J Clin Endocrinol Metab 53:480–483, 1981.

116. Tindall GT, Barrow DL: Disorders of the pituitary. St. Louis: CV Mosby, 1986, pp 389–394.

117. Tönnis W, Oberdisse K, Weber E: Bericht über 264 operierte Hypophysenadenome. Acta Neurochir (Wien) 3:113–130, 1952.

118. Valtonen A, Myllymäki K: Outcome of patients after transcranial operation for pituitary adenoma. Ann Clin Res 18 (Suppl):4743–4745, 1986.

119. Van Lindert EJ, Grotenhuis JA, Meijer E: Results of followup after removal of non-functioning pituitary adenomas by transcranial surgery. Br J Neurosurg 5:129–133, 1991.

120. Vance ML, Harris AG: Long-term treatment of 189 acromegalic patients with the somatostatin analog octreotide: Results of the international multicenter acromegaly study group. Arch Intern Med 151:1573–1578, 1991.

121. Vlahovitch B, Reynaud C, Rhiati J, et al: Treatment and recurrences in 135 pituitary adenomas. Acta Neurochir (Wien) 42 (Suppl):120–123, 1988.

122. Warnet A, Harris AG, Renard E, et al: A prospective multicenter trial of octreotide in 24 patients with visual defects caused by nonfunctioning and gonadotropin-secreting pituitary adenomas. Neurosurgery 41:786–797, 1997.

123. Watanobe H, Kudo K, Okushima T, et al: A null cell adenoma of the pituitary detected seven years after removal of a prolactinoma: Recurrence or de novo tumourigenesis? Acta Endocrinol 125:700–704, 1991.

124. Webster J, Page MD, Bevan JS, et al: Low recurrence rate after partial hypophysectomy for prolactinoma: The predictive value of dynamic prolactin function tests. Clin Endocrinol 36:35–44, 1992.

125. Wirth FP, Schwartz HG, Schwetschenau PR: Pituitary adenomas: Factors in treatment. Clin Neurosurg 21:8–25, 1974.

126. Witt TC, Kondziolka D, Flickinger JC, et al: Gamma knife radiosurgery for pituitary tumors. Prog Neurol Surg 14:114–127, 1998.

# Stereotactic Radiosurgery for Pituitary Adenomas and Craniopharyngiomas

■ ERIK-OLOF BACKLUND

Radiosurgical techniques are increasingly used for tumors in the sellar region, either alone or as additional treatment after subtotal surgery.[1–8] Apart from the classic radiosurgical tool, the Gamma knife, various systems based on linear accelerator techniques are now used routinely.[9] The number of pituitary adenomas and craniopharyngiomas that have been treated by Gamma knife only is estimated to be approximately 7000 cases worldwide. Radiosurgery as part of the neurosurgeon's armamentarium is no longer a controversial issue.

## PITUITARY ADENOMAS: THE GAMMA KNIFE

The moderate size and usually well-defined anatomic boundaries of a pituitary adenoma make such a tumor an ideal object for stereotactic radiosurgery. This was the rationale for attempts during the 1950s and 1960s to treat intrasellar tumors with various radioactive implants. A significant rate of serious complications, however, made this technique less attractive, particularly when transsphenoidal microsurgery was introduced as a safe and effective mode of treatment.

With the advent of the Gamma knife,[11] a noninvasive, precise obliteration of minute intracranial tissue volumes became possible, using radiation but without the risks inherent in the implantation techniques. This stimulated the pioneering group in Stockholm to include pituitary patients in the first group to be treated with the Gamma knife. The first two tumors ever treated this way were a craniopharyngioma[12] and a pituitary adenoma. The patient with an adenoma had had a so-called "chromophobe tumor" removed by the author in 1967 by a standard intracapsular enucleation through the transfrontal route. When prophylactic postoperative irradiation was planned, which was the routine management at that time, single-dose Gamma knife irradiation was considered a new and potentially superior alternative. The case was thoroughly discussed with the oncologists, and in January 1968, 28 Gy was given to the center of the sella. The dose was chosen based on the assumed radiation tolerance of the optic nerves, 5 to 6 Gy.

After this pilot case, 19 patients with adenomas were treated during a 4-year period, representing a very heterogeneous mixture of indications and pathologic processes. Many of these patients had had less radical surgery. *A multitarget concept was adopted early* as a method to overcome one of the inherent limitations of the first Gamma knife, the very small, disc-shaped radiation fields, too small for the volumes of many of the tumors. In fact, the multitarget alternative was used in most of these cases. This early case material was never systematically analyzed and thus never published as a series. Nonetheless, eight were selected for a report in 1979[13] because each of these cases illustrated biologic or clinical phenomena of interest for the continuation of the project. For example, a reduction of tumor volume was achieved even when the radiation field was nonhomogeneous. Regression of clinical disturbances was also recorded in many cases (for example, amelioration of visual field loss) concomitant with the decrease in tumor volume. Some patients with hypersecreting tumors showed improvement of their endocrine state (Fig. 36–1).

In one case, an early radiation effect was studied postmortem. The patient died from an intercurrent emergency 10 days after Gamma knife treatment, when 70 Gy had been given to each of two targets in his large suprasellar tumor. The border of a necrotic area, obviously radiation induced, corresponded surprisingly well with the 10% isodose level, indicating that as low a dose as 7 Gy could be lethal for adenoma cells. In the patient with the longest follow-up, the tumor size remained unchanged during an observation time of almost 10 years. This course is surprising because a very low radiation dose was used, a maximum of 15 Gy to four isocenters, corresponding to an edge dose of only 7 Gy.

### Corticotropin-Releasing Hormone–Producing Adenomas

Based on these first experiences, a prospective study on corticotropin-releasing hormone (CRH)–producing tumors

## PROLACTINOMAS - STEREOTACTIC RADIOSURGERY

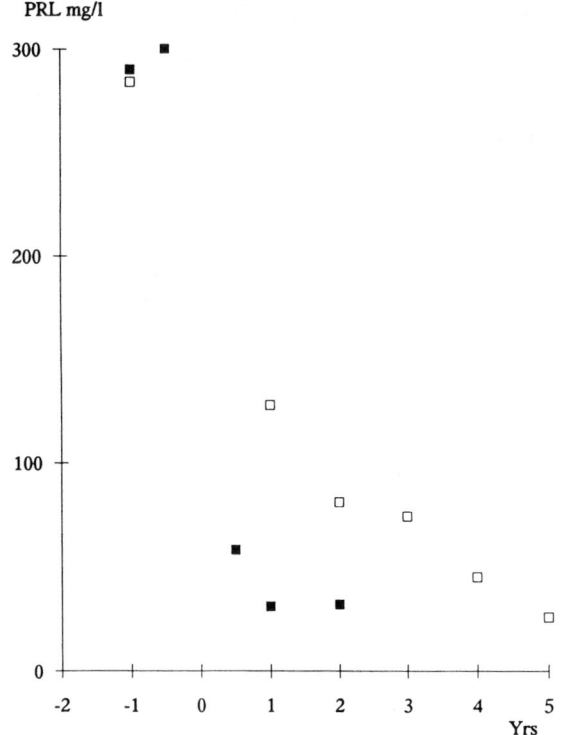

**FIGURE 36–1** ■ The diagram shows the serum prolactin values for two female patients with prolactinomas who were treated during the early 1970s. Using the 14-mm collimator of Gamma knife II, a maximum dose of 70 Gy was given to one patient (*solid squares*) and 50 Gy to the other (*open squares*). The follow-up periods are short (2 and 5 years, respectively), but the prolactin values show an increasing tendency to stay close to normal (25 mg/L). Zero time on the abscissa is the date of irradiation.

was initiated by the Stockholm group,[14] and over the years, some unique experience has been gained.

A thorough long-term study of 29 consecutive patients with Cushing's disease was published in 1986.[15] In this series, which encompassed only intrasellar tumors, a special policy was followed. Initially, the medioposterior part of the anterior lobe, at that time assumed to be the site of predilection for CRH-producing adenomas, was irradiated. If there was no response to this first irradiation, the protocol included a stepwise second, third, or even fourth irradiation, first to the medioanterior, and subsequently to either the right or the left lateral part of the anterior lobe. The effect of each irradiation was thoroughly evaluated before the patient received further radiosurgery to the tumor.

The net result of this study was that 22 patients (76%) were cured by no more dramatic means than Gamma knife treatment, albeit in 8 only after more than one irradiation. During the course of the study, five of the nonresponders needed a bilateral adrenalectomy, whereas two were in better condition and warranted expectant management. No recurrences took place. On the other hand, hormonal insufficiencies appeared gradually over the postoperative years in approximately 50% of those who were cured exclusively by Gamma knife treatment.

The Stockholm group also published a second series of

77 patients with Cushing's disease in whom Gamma knife treatment was the first choice.[16] Fifty-nine patients from this series were followed for 2 to 15 years. In 51 patients, the stereotactic localization of the tumor was made by cisternography, computed tomography (CT), or both, and in the most recent eight patients, localization was made by stereotactic magnetic resonance (MR). The total cure rate in this series of 59 was 82%, although in 6 patients cure was achieved only after adrenalectomy. The eight patients in whom the adenoma was localized with stereotactic MR are all cured. This technical alternative is today the method of choice.[17]

## Acromegaly: an Early Long-Term Study

Between 1969 and 1989, 38 patients with acromegaly were treated with the Gamma knife in Stockholm. Seventeen of these patients were from foreign countries, but the remaining 21 (14 women, 7 men) were accessible for a thorough follow-up.[18]

In seven patients, radiosurgery was the only treatment, whereas Gamma knife treatment was preceded by surgical tumor removal in six patients and surgery followed by radiation therapy in seven others. In one patient, radiation therapy was the only treatment given before radiosurgery. These pretreatment therapies had been given 1 to 10 years (mean, 4.3 years) before Gamma knife treatment. The indication for the latter was active acromegaly in all 21 patients. The dose given to the center of the tumor varied between 30 and 70 Gy, the lower dosage being used in four patients previously treated with radiation therapy.

The observation time after radiosurgery was 1 to 21 years. Virtual cure was obtained in two patients only; both were young. In eight, the acromegalic symptoms and growth hormone levels were reduced, but not to normal levels. The remaining 11 patients were essentially unchanged at follow-up. In 2 of the 13 patients without previous radiation therapy, pituitary insufficiency had developed at follow-up.

The poor results might be partly explained by the fact that the series included tumor residues after surgery and invasive adenomas in which radiologic delineation is notoriously difficult. The authors suggest that in spite of the less rewarding results presented, the availability of dramatically improved localization techniques justifies a resumption of the project in acromegalic patients in whom surgery has failed. The results from a more recent report support this treatment alternative.[19]

## More Recent Experiences: Mixed Series

A publication from Pittsburgh describes 18 patients with adenoma who had various pathologic lesions.[20] The results are summarized in Table 36–1. Sixteen patients had recurrent tumor after surgery, and in five, radiation therapy had been given before Gamma knife treatment. The control of tumor growth was quite satisfactory. In this study, the multitarget alternative was used. The one tumor with volume increase had a unilateral expansion into the cavernous sinus, the region where delineation of tumor border for

TABLE 36–1 ■ **THE PITTSBURGH EXPERIENCE***

| | No. of Patients |
|---|---|
| **Changes in Tumor Size After Treatment** | |
| Shrinkage | 8 |
| Unchanged | 9 |
| Increase | 1 |
| | |
| **Changes in Endocrine Pathology** | |
| GH—producing tumors | 4 |
| Normalized | 3 |
| Unchanged | 1 |
| CRH—producing tumors | 6 |
| Improvement | 3 |
| Unchanged | 3 |

*$N = 18$. Previous treatment, surgery ($n = 16$) and radiation therapy ($n = 5$). CRH, corticotropin-releasing hormone; GH, growth hormone.

dose planning is notoriously difficult. The series is too small to allow firm conclusions concerning the chances for endocrinologic cure after Gamma knife treatment. A pleasing feature of this series, however, is the absence of deterioration of pituitary function.

Visual impairment occurred in two patients. The Pittsburgh group accepted a somewhat higher tolerance level for the optic nerves than that practiced by other groups. Allowance was made for previous radiation therapy, but the authors give no account of how this element relates to the complications reported in the paper.

One study from the University of Bergen, Norway, includes 14 patients, all with hypersecreting adenomas.[21] The follow-up period ranged from 2.5 to 4.5 years (Table 36–2). In all cases, there was evidence of control of neoplastic growth after Gamma knife treatment, with signs of necrosis or regression of tumor on CT. Moreover, there was striking improvement of the endocrine dysfunction in nine patients, but only three were cured exclusively by Gamma knife treatment. In two, radiosurgery had no effect on the endocrinopathy. The volumes irradiated were fairly small and, in many cases, only one isocenter was used (Fig. 36–2). Stereotactic MR localization was not used in this series.

In the acromegalic patients, an interesting correlation was found between dosage and effect. The one cured patient received 25 Gy to the tumor edge; the two improved patients, 20 Gy; and the unchanged one, 13 Gy only.

TABLE 36–2 ■ **THE BERGEN EXPERIENCE: ACTIVE ADENOMAS***

| | Endocrinopathy After Treatment | | | |
|---|---|---|---|---|
| | n | − | (+) | + |
| Acromegaly | 4 | 1 | 2 | 1 |
| Cushing's disease | 4 | 2 | 2† | — |
| Nelson's syndrome | 3 | — | 2 | 1 |
| Prolactinoma | 3 | — | 3 | — |
| Total | 14 | 3 | 9 | 2 |

*$N = 14$. Follow-up ≥ 18 months. Tumor growth was controlled in all 14 patients.
†Cured after subsequent transsphenoidal operation.
−, cured; (+), improved; +, unchanged.

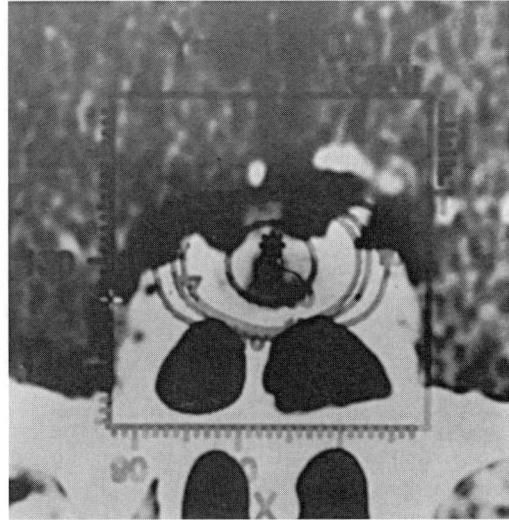

FIGURE 36–2 ■ In this patient with Nelson's syndrome, it was decided to treat the whole tissue volume corresponding to the anterior part of the sella with the Gamma knife. The picture shows the dose diagram calculated for this; the concentric dark circles with numbers corresponding to the 10, 50, 70, and 90 isodose levels. There is an optimal agreement between the 90% isodose level and the borders of the volume selected for irradiation. The superimposed scale is measured in millimeters.

In the Cushing disease group, all patients received 25 Gy to the tumor edge. Two were cured, and the other two improved, with complete cure after subsequent microsurgical adenoma removal. In spite of persistent endocrinopathy after Gamma knife treatment and before surgery, these two patients showed clear-cut radiologic evidence of reduction in tumor size, with loss of central contrast enhancement on CT.

In patients with Nelson's syndrome, the dosage given to the edge of tumor was somewhat more aggressive, from 25 to 35 Gy. In two patients, the tumor decreased in size, and the plasma CRH level normalized, but not to fully normal levels. One patient was unchanged.

The patients with prolactinoma were treated primarily to arrest aggressive parasellar tumor growth after failed surgery in two cases and as a primary treatment in one. In the two postoperative cases, the tumor shrank and showed signs of central necrosis on CT. In all three patients, the hyperprolactinemia, which was refractory to treatment before Gamma knife treatment, was cured with tolerable doses of bromocriptine.

## Summary: Pituitary Adenomas

Control of neoplastic growth of pituitary adenomas with the Gamma knife is obtained provided that the minimum dose to any part of the tumor is in excess of 12 to 15 Gy. When endocrine cure is evaluated after treatment with a similar protocol, the prospects are promising, provided that optimal localization technique is used. So far, Gamma knife treatment seems to apply best to small, CRH-producing tumors.

A great deal of work has yet to be conducted. The radiosensitivity of the visual pathways needs to be determined, and possible differential sensitivity of the different tumor types needs to be explored. Further analysis of the relationship between the irradiation parameters used and the results is also needed. Nonetheless, certain trends may already be emerging. The use of the Gamma knife in the treatment of residual tumor after surgery is increasing (Fig. 36–3). This development may make conventional, fractionated radiation therapy, which is less precise, obsolete as supplementary treatment after subtotal removal. Above all, the rapid improvement in imaging techniques strongly indicates that localization difficulties, which still may hamper the technique, will soon be overcome.

# CRANIOPHARYNGIOMAS

## Therapeutic Problem Defined

If the literature on this topic is examined in detail, even the most experienced craniopharyngioma surgeons report widely varying rates of achievement of total or nearly total removal. More recent papers reveal a diverging spectrum of views regarding the possibility of a real cure of a craniopharyngioma.[22–24] With "average" surgery, the frequency of virtually total removal seems to be approximately one in two cases (see Backlund and colleagues[25] for review).

Difficulties during craniopharyngioma surgery often relate to the size of the tumor, which occasionally can be grotesque. Cystic parts of a large tumor may be teased away from the brain by delicate microsurgical technique. However, radical removal of a large tumor with a more polymorphic architecture can be a far more formidable

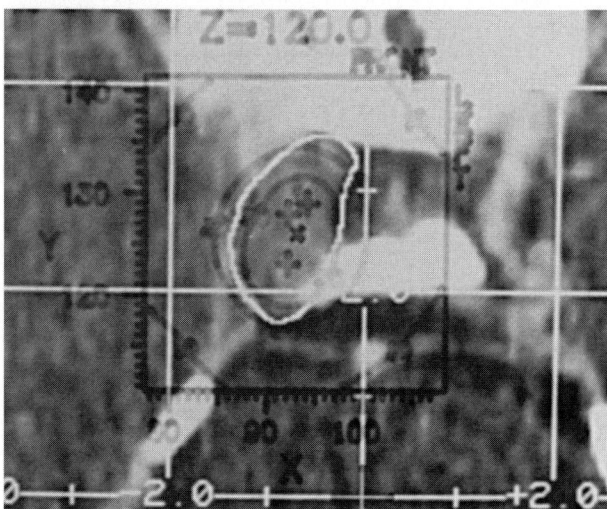

FIGURE 36–3 ■ A soft tissue mass, remaining after transsphenoidal surgery in this patient with acromegaly, is outlined by the white contour. The posterior part of the mass was assumed by the surgeon to be adenoma tissue left at the operation. The concentric lines correspond with the 10%, 30%, and 50% dose levels used when three lesions are produced in a cluster arrangement by the Gamma knife. The edge of the assumed hypersecreting tissue volume is well covered by 50% of the maximum dose. Both treatments were performed by the same surgeon. The case discussed here illustrates the crucial importance of using the Gamma knife as a surgeon's tool.

surgical undertaking. In a short series, the results after such extensive surgery may seem acceptable, but all published series in which the number of patients and the length of the observation time allow firm conclusions to be drawn include between 10% and 20% of cases that are "fundamentally hopeless," that is, impossible to cure in the long term regardless of the type of therapy used. This factor must be taken into account when various management policies are discussed.

Most craniopharyngiomas are cystic, often with one large, solitary cyst, occasionally with a volume exceeding 100 ml. Of the total tumor bulk, also in a tumor with more than one cyst, 80% to 90% of the mass may be cystic, with the solid part constituting a relatively insignificant part of the tumor's total volume. The threat that a craniopharyngioma poses for the patient is probably related to the total volume of the tumor. Thus, permanent obliteration of the cyst or cysts would be a valuable contribution to the therapy.

Stereotactic injection of radioactive colloidal solutions into a craniopharyngioma cyst has induced permanent obliteration.[26] Moreover, the possibility of obliterating solid tumor parts with the Gamma knife was shown early.[12, 27] This latter technique is far superior to, essentially not comparable with, and obviously less risky than more conventional types of external irradiation, which still are occasionally recommended after subtotal microsurgical removal. The value of a combination of conservative microsurgery and Gamma knife radiosurgery has been emphasized.[28] The currently used computerized dose planning allows the normal structures adjacent to the tumor to be protected.[29, 30]

The intrinsic safety of stereotactic methods must never be disregarded. In 1932, considering the formidable problems in craniopharyngioma surgery, Cushing hoped for a future method "whereby the usually multilocular epithelial lesion can be destroyed or inactivated in situ."[31] The stereotactic methods offer therapeutic alternatives of precisely that kind (Fig. 36–4). Moreover, in both human and economic terms, a stereotactic procedure, routinely performed under local anesthesia only, involves a much shorter hospital stay and time off work than does an open operation.

## Multimodality Therapeutic Approach

The treatment in any craniopharyngioma case may be tailored to the requirements of the individual patient (i.e., with regard to the anatomy of the tumor). In practice, this means that a multimodality treatment protocol is a logical approach.[32] Four therapeutic options may then be included, either alone or in combination:

1. Microsurgical removal
2. Stereotactic puncture of a cyst or cysts, with injection of an obliterating substance, such as radioactive $^{90}Y$ in a colloidal solution
3. Radiosurgery with stereotactically directed single-dose irradiation, using the Gamma knife, for example
4. In a few selected cases, radiation therapy using a linear accelerator

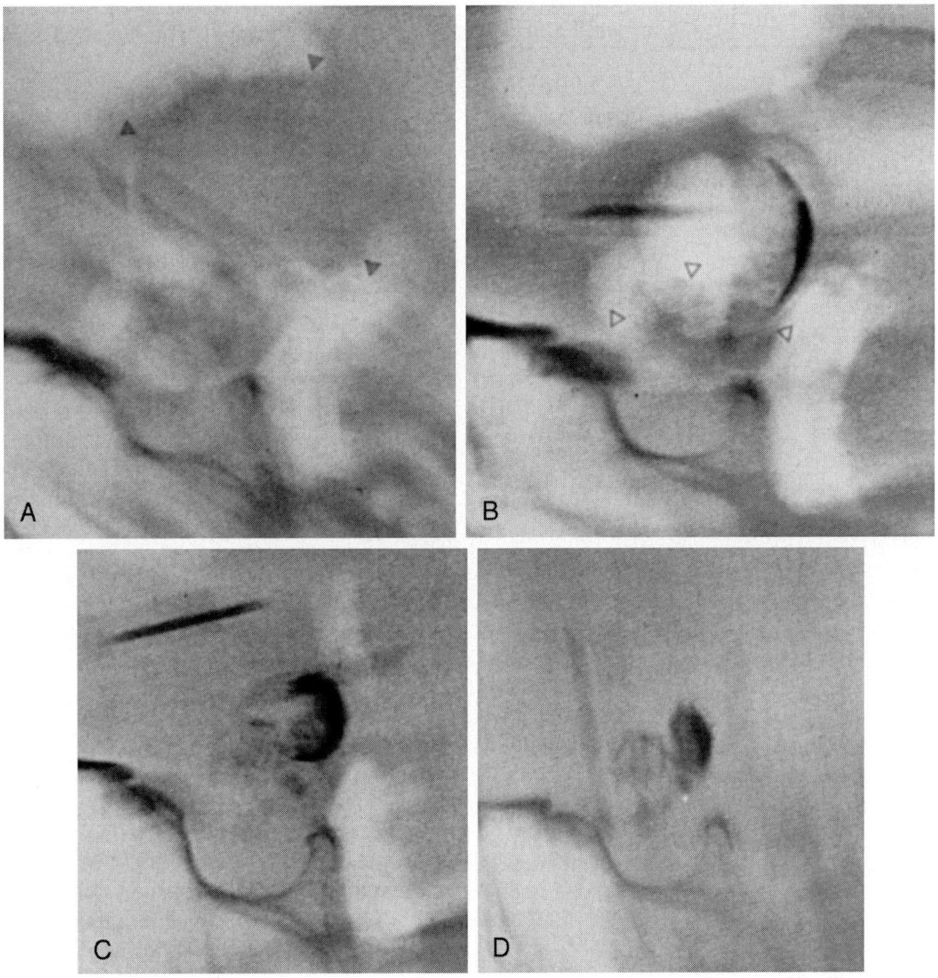

**FIGURE 36–4** ■ In this patient with a craniopharyngioma, which was a recurrent tumor after previous microsurgical removal, encephalography (*A*) shows a larger, superior tumor part (*solid arrowheads*) suspected to be cystic. A smaller part, immediately above the sella, is more irregular and calcified, indicating a solid tumor. This morphology was confirmed by stereotactic puncture and biopsy. In connection with this study, $^{90}$Y was injected into the cystic part, which harbored two cysts. One month later (*B*), when the cysts were reduced in size, some air and contrast medium were injected to outline the solid part (*open arrowheads*), which was treated with the Gamma knife. Follow-up x-ray studies 1 (*C*) and 4 (*D*) years after the treatment show a progressive shrinkage of the whole tumor mass. The state shown in *D* was found completely unchanged at a 15-year follow-up computed tomography scan. The patient is leading a normal life more than 20 years after the first stereotactic operation.

Crucial therapeutic decisions should be made by matching these therapeutic options with four types of tumor appearance, such as the following categorization long used by the author:

A. A predominantly cystic tumor with one large, even huge, solitary cyst and with a solid tumor component of limited or even insignificant size, located basally
B. The whole tumor of limited size (<2 cm), which is a reasonable object for radical removal with minimum risk
C. A larger, usually pleomorphic tumor, with more than one cyst
D. A very large tumor with an appreciable solid component, often with many (smaller) cysts

The four therapeutic options mentioned have been used, alone or in combination, by the author since the early 1960s. The first 43 patients have been described in detail (follow-up, 10 to 23 years) in two papers from 1989.[25, 33] Table 36–3 shows the therapeutic choices in these 43 cases, based completely on the anatomy of each individual tumor. All patients had no previous therapy and represent a consecutive, unselected series from 1964 to 1976.

With regard to the title of this chapter, note that the Gamma knife alternative seldom was used exclusively (see Table 36–3). On the other hand, careful study of each tumor's anatomy led the surgeon to choose surgery alone, a combination of modalities, or, a choice that was obvious in cases with a large monocyst, intracystic treatment.

The overall results in this long-term study were gratifying and are summarized in Table 36–4. The results obtained with this multimodality protocol indicate that an optimal

---

TABLE 36–3 ■ **THE MULTIMODALITY PROTOCOL IN PRACTICE: TREATMENTS USED IN 43 CONSECUTIVE CASES**

| Morphologic Type | No. of Patients | Treatment Modality | |
|---|---|---|---|
| A | 18 | Intracavitary isotope ($^{90}$Y) | 18 |
| B | 13 | Total removal | 9 |
| | | Radiosurgery (Gamma knife) | 4 |
| C | 9 | Subtotal removal after bulk reduction by intracavitary isotope | 4 |
| | | Radiosurgery and intracavitary isotope combined | 4 |
| | | Intracavitary isotope and LINAC | 1 |
| D | 3 | Partial removal and postoperative linac | 2 |
| | | LINAC only | 1 |

LINAC, linear accelerator radiation therapy.

## TABLE 36–4 ■ FOLLOW-UP FOR CRANIOPHARYNGIOMAS, 1964–1976*

| Group | Death Due to Recurrence (n) | Death with No Recurrence (n) | Alive and Well (n) |
|---|---|---|---|
| A (n = 18) | 0 | 3 | 15 |
| B (n = 13) | 1 | 1 | 11 |
| C (n = 9) | 3 | 0 | 6 |
| D (n = 2) | 2 | 0 | 0 |
| Total (n = 42) | 6 | 4 | 32 |

*N = 43. Follow-up, 10 to 23 years. One patient lost to follow-up.

management in *any* case of craniopharyngioma should include two elements.

First, a detailed study of the tumor anatomy should be performed with CT and MR, with the primary aim of disclosing cysts that are suitable for intracavitary irradiation. The proportions between solid and calcified tumor components, soft tissue parts, and cystic compartments should be assessed and quantified. The aim should be to appreciate the relative bulk effect of each of these components as a basis for treatment design. A particular aspect in this context is the fact that neither CT nor MR may give fully reliable information concerning the tumor's inner anatomy. Craniopharyngioma cysts may have attenuation on CT, and may be mistaken for solid tumor. Thus, any large, rounded tumor compartment may be a cyst, which can be proven by an exploratory stereotactic puncture. If this procedure is performed with preparations for radioisotope injection, the entire therapy can be given during one session.

Second, stereotactic treatment should be the first choice if more than approximately 50% of the total bulk of the tumor is cystic and the number of cysts is reasonable, that is, not more than three. Open craniotomy with microsurgical removal of monocystic tumors, especially if they are huge, may be difficult to justify today, even if this procedure can be performed with very little risk. The completely nondramatic, intracavitary isotope treatment, which induces a safe and permanent obliteration of such tumors, must never be forgotten as a superior therapeutic alternative. Moreover, this treatment excludes *any* argument for shunting or drainage procedures, such as the insertion of reservoir devices for bleomycin installation, which is far from unrisky.

## Summary: Craniopharyngiomas

With the stereotactic techniques now established as a neurosurgical treatment paradigm, we must now more than ever carefully compare various treatment options and tailor a management program for each patient, which may include more than one modality. It is a matter of common sense that a low-risk, simple, cost-effective but nevertheless curative procedure should also define the optimal treatment for a patient with craniopharyngioma. However, a relative indifference toward stereotactic approaches rules among many colleagues today, probably explained by the regrettable fact that many influential neurosurgeons still have limited personal experience with stereotactic operations. This has led to a situation in which stereotactic techniques are considered "competing" alternatives to major surgery, used by special groups or departments only. This is a serious misconception. The idea that all problems related to radical tumor or vascular surgery in the brain can always be solved by the exclusive use of the operating microscope represents an obsolete therapeutic attitude. The technical sophistication of various therapeutic systems and, not least, of imaging techniques, has set the stage for a future in which *multimodality therapeutic programs* represent *methodologic optima* for many problematic diseases in the central nervous system. A good example is the current policy in arteriovenous malformation management, in which microsurgery, embolization, and radiosurgery are often used in combination.

The complete spectrum of surgical alternatives, microsurgery as well as stereotaxy, should be available in any department, making it possible for the surgeon to make the choice of treatment freely, and in relation to the specific problems each patient presents. When the surgeon is personally familiar with more than one therapeutic technique, he or she is able to design treatment protocols with a minimum of bias. This is a most important prerequisite for the progress of craniopharyngioma surgery.

## REFERENCES

1. Ganz JC: Gamma knife treatment of pituitary adenomas. Stereotact Funct Neurosurg 64 (Suppl 1):3–10, 1995.
2. Motti ED, Losa M, Pieralli S, et al: Stereotactic radiosurgery of pituitary adenomas. Metabolism 45 (8 Suppl 1):111–114, 1996.
3. Park YG, Kim EY, Chang JW, et al: Volume changes following gamma knife radiosurgery of intracranial tumors. Surg Neurol 48:488–493, 1997.
4. Ikeda H, Jomura H, Yoshimoto T: Gamma knife radiosurgery for pituitary adenomas: Usefulness of combined transsphenoidal and gamma knife radiosurgery for adenomas invading the cavernous sinus. Radiat Oncol Investig 6:26–34, 1998.
5. Lim YL, Leem W, Kim TS, et al: Four years' experiences in the treatment of pituitary adenomas with gamma knife radiosurgery. Stereotact Funct Neurosurg 70 (Suppl S1):95–109, 1998.
6. Martinez R, Bravo G, Burzaco J, et al: Pituitary tumors and gamma knife surgery: Clinical experience with more than two years of follow-up. Stereotact Funct Neurosurg 70 (Suppl S1):110–118, 1998.
7. Morange-Ramos I, Régis J, Dufour H, et al: Gamma knife surgery for secreting pituitary adenomas. Acta Neurochir (Wien) 140:437–443, 1998.
8. Pan L, Zhang N, Wang E, et al: Pituitary adenomas: The effect of gamma knife radiosurgery on tumor growth and endocrinopathies. Stereotact Funct Neurosurg 70 (Suppl S1):119–126, 1998.
9. Yoon SC, Suh TS, Jang HS, et al: Clinical results of 24 pituitary macroadenomas with linac-based stereotactic radiosurgery. Int J Radiat Oncol Biol Phys 41:849–853, 1998.
10. Ho RTK: Report from the Leksell Gamma Knife Society. 1997.
11. Leksell L: Stereotaxis and Radiosurgery: An Operative System. Springfield, IL: Charles C Thomas, 1971.
12. Backlund EO: Stereotaxic treatment of craniopharyngiomas. In Hamberger CA, Wersäll J (eds): Nobel Symposium 10: Disorders of the Skull Base Region. Stockholm: Almqvist & Wiksell, 1969, pp 237–244.
13. Backlund EO, Bergstrand G, Hierton-Laurell U, et al: Tumor changes after single dose irradiation by stereotactic radiosurgery in "nonactive" pituitary adenomas and prolactinomas. In Szikla G (ed): Stereotactic Cerebral Irradiation. Amsterdam: Elsevier-North Holland, 1979, pp 109–206.
14. Thorén M, Rähn T, Hall K, et al: Treatment of pituitary dependent Cushing's syndrome with closed stereotactic radiosurgery by means of Co-60 gamma radiation. Acta Endocrinol (Copenh) 88:7–17, 1978.

15. Degerblad M, Rähn T, Bergstrand G, et al: Long-term results of stereotactic radiosurgery to the pituitary gland in Cushing's disease. Acta Endocrinol (Copenh) 112:310–314, 1986.

16. Rähn T, Thorén M, Werner S: Stereotactic radiosurgery in pituitary adenomas. In Faglia G, Peck-Peccoz P, Abriosi B, et al (eds): Pituitary Adenomas: New Trends in Basic and Clinical Research. Amsterdam: Excerpta Medica, 1991, pp 303–312.

17. Seo Y, Fukuoka S, Takanashi M, et al: Gamma knife surgery for Cushing's disease. Surg Neurol 43:170–176, 1995.

18. Thorén M, Rähn T, Guo WY, et al: Stereotactic radiosurgery with the cobalt-60 gamma unit in the treatment of growth hormone-producing pituitary tumors. Neurosurgery 29:663–668, 1991.

19. Landolt AM, Haller D, Lomax N, et al: Stereotactic radiosurgery for recurrent surgically treated acromegaly: Comparison with fractionated radiotherapy. J Neurosurg 88:1002–1008, 1998.

20. Stephanian E, Lunsford LD, Coffey RJ, et al: Gamma knife surgery for sellar and suprasellar tumors. Neurosurg Clin N Am 3:207–218, 1992.

21. Ganz JC, Backlund EO, Thorsen F: The effects of gamma knife surgery of pituitary adenomas on tumor growth and endocrinopathies. Stereotact Funct Neurosurg 61 (Suppl 1):30–37, 1993.

22. Sanford RA: Craniopharyngioma: Results of survey of the American Society of Pediatric Neurosurgery. Pediatr Neurosurg 21 (Suppl 1):39–43, 1994.

23. Laws ER: Transsphenoidal removal of craniopharyngioma. Pediatr Neurosurg 21 (Suppl 1):57–63, 1994.

24. Broggi G (ed): Craniopharyngioma: Surgical Treatment. Berlin: Springer-Verlag, 1995.

25. Backlund EO, Axelsson B, Bergstrand CG, et al: Treatment of craniopharyngiomas: The stereotactic approach in a ten to twenty-three years' perspective. I: Surgical, radiological and ophthalmological aspects. Acta Neurochir (Wien) 99:11–19, 1989.

26. Backlund EO: Studies on craniopharyngiomas. III: Stereotaxic treatment with intracystic yttrium-90. Acta Chir Scand 139:237–247, 1973.

27. Backlund EO: Studies on craniopharyngiomas. IV: Stereotaxic treatment with radiosurgery. Acta Chir Scand 139:344–351, 1973.

28. Inoue HK, Fujimaki H, Kohga H, et al: Basal interhemispheric supra- and/or infrachiasmal approaches via superomedial orbitotomy for hypothalamic lesions: Preservation of hypothalamo-pituitary functions in combination treatment with radiosurgery. Childs Nerv Syst 13:250–256, 1997.

29. Chung WY, Pan HC, Guo WY, et al: Protection of visual pathway in gamma knife radiosurgery for craniopharyngiomas. Stereotact Funct Neurosurg 70 (Suppl S1):139–151, 1998.

30. Leber KA, Berglöff J, Pendl G: Dose-response tolerance of the visual pathways and cranial nerves of the cavernous sinus to stereotactic radiosurgery. J Neurosurg 88:43–50, 1998.

31. Cushing H: Intracranial Tumors. Notes upon a Series of Two Thousand Verified Cases with Surgical Mortality Percentages Pertaining Thereto. Springfield, IL: Charles C Thomas, 1932.

32. Backlund EO: Treatment of craniopharyngiomas: The multimodality approach. Pediatr Neurosurg 21 (Suppl 1):82–89, 1994.

33. Sääf M, Thorén M, Bergstrand CG, et al: Treatment of craniopharyngiomas: The stereotactic approach in a ten to twenty-three years' perspective. II: Psychosocial situation and pituitary function. Acta Neurochir (Wien) 99:97–103, 1989.

# Craniopharyngiomas and Other Intracranial Cystic Lesions

C H A P T E R    3 7

# Craniopharyngiomas: A Summary of Data

■ WILLIAM H. SWEET

By far the most comprehensive published account of craniopharyngioma is the major monograph by Choux and colleagues.[1] Although most of the monograph is in French, it includes extensive summaries in English, including the legends to all figures. It is based primarily on data from 474 patients younger than 16 years of age. These data were collected from members of the Société de Neurochirurgie de Langue Française and the International Society for Pediatric Neurosurgery and are described as the ISPC-91 series. Many of the tables include data from all age groups and many nations, as attested by the 579 references cited by the authors. The symposium organized by Epstein and colleagues at New York University and held on December 17 through 19, 1993, in which 24 authors from all over the world presented their findings will become the most broadly based source of expert information on the subject. Most of the presentations concentrated on the authors' personal data. Its organizers have kindly supplied me with most of the manuscripts so that a supplemental account to Samii's valuable chapter (see Chapter 39) can be included in these volumes.

and coworkers,[4] who in 1973 reported that an oropharyngeal type of squamous epithelial cell without calcification found in 11 of 12 adults and only 1 of 28 children was associated with a much better prognosis than the faster growing type. This cell is said to have distinctive histologic features: groups of radially arranged columnar cells around aggregates of round or polygonal cells. These central masses may become transparent or die. This appearance of dead cells, the authors say, "has reminded some observers of the earliest fetal tooth buds. . . . The discrete areas of dead cells often underwent slow calcification."[4] Although Adamson and associates[5] have confirmed these findings, other thorough studies, such as those of Miller[6] and Petito and colleagues,[7] have failed to do so. Light microscopic and electron microscopic appraisals conducted by Lisczak and coworkers,[8] even those showing "aggressive growth patterns," failed to agree with what actually occurred.[9] Although Giangaspero and associates[10] described six adults who had tumors and the appearance of a favorable prognosis, three of them actually had a short downhill course to death, and the other three had been followed up for only 8 months or less.[10]

## PATHOLOGY

Agreement has long existed that almost none of the cells in craniopharyngiomas displays malignant features. Peet reported on a case of a child whose tumor, which was mainly "adamantinomatous," had some carcinomatous features.[2] Nelson and colleagues[3] reported on a patient who, 35 years after the first operation, also showed malignant zones in the tumor.[3] The widely ranging types of parenchymal cells need concern us no further because their blood supply of all types is so meager as never to interfere with removal. Differentiation of various types of cells that at times predominate in these tumors led to the terms *adamantinoma* and *ameloblastoma*, which are applied to embryonic cells of the dental enamel organs. Epithelial cells are common; even cholesteatomatous and teratomatous areas occur. Trying to correlate specific histologic features with any other behavioral aspect of interest has proved to be fruitless. The most successful attempt is that of Kahn

## CAPSULE

The detailed structure and extent of the cells often surrounding the actual tumor do not represent the usual kind of capsule. This feature is the surgeon's most commonly unsolved problem. Critchley and Ironside,[11] in one of the earlier comprehensive accounts, describe "the glial tumor reaction in the surrounding structures" as a consistent third element of the lesion along with the epithelial elements and connective tissue stroma. They say that "the glial proliferation forms a sort of capsule," invading extensively in a few cases, even into the central portion of the tumor. They also say that "transection through the capsule reveals a definitely laminated system of connective tissue elements composed externally of neuroglia and internally of fibrous tissue. Within these coverings, there is usually a fine epithelial stratum made up of two or more layers of stratified epithelium." Thus, they say that in one of their cases,

477

"The tumor was surrounded by a fibrous capsule except where it was united to the anterior surface of the infundibulum from the upper part of which it seemed to arise." This external glial layer was reported also by Bailey and coworkers[12] to be invaded by epithelial neoplastic streamers, often with the glial layer so substantial and perhaps so tenacious that the plane of cleavage would be more likely to lie in the normal hypothalamus. Ingraham and Scott,[13] however, although describing large cysts as often having a tough fibrous capsule, also say that "the solid masses of the craniopharyngiomas are usually separated from neighboring brain or hypophyseal tissue by only a thin layer of gliosis and possess no well defined capsule." These three descriptions present the problem "in capsule form," so to speak, namely, do these patients have a sufficiently complete glial investment where it is needed against normal brain to permit a delicate and complete removal of tumor plus a normally functioning brain?

Some pathologists,[5] including Miller,[6] described the finger-like epithelial streamers invading the glial layer as invasions of brain. This is not brain any more than solid glioma is brain.

I saw the autopsy of a patient in the 1940s who during life had been subjected to repeated cyst aspirations; the firm-walled entire tumor could be gently lifted away from the brain after some tiny avascular strands of tissue were cut. Bartlett[14] states that "a slow growing tumor usually fell out of its bed at autopsy," whereas "fast growing tumors excited a gliotic or collagenous reaction." By 1948, I had decided that one should explore every resectable-sized craniopharyngioma so as not to leave in situ any readily removable mass. My first such patient was a 14-year-old boy; the cystic portion of his tumor lay lateral to the left optic nerve, compressing it and its blood vessels so that it was white. Aspiration of the cyst permitted the nerve to resume its normal shape and its blood vessels to fill. The solid parts of the tumor were removed from between the left internal carotid artery and the nerve, including a left inferoposterolateral extension into the cerebellopontine angle. The tumor capsule, which had no tenacious adherence to neighboring structures, was sturdy enough to permit a probable total removal. We did not know enough about supplemental corticosteroid to administer any. Probably, no pressure was exerted on the hypothalamus, and the patient recovered smoothly and fully. Forty-five years later, he continued to work full time as a certified nurse's aid.

This lucky result led me to reinvestigate accounts of the pathologic characteristics of the capsule. There was and remains general agreement that a reactive gliosis commonly occurs whenever the tumor is in contact with or invading hypothalamus, and the publications on this issue continue to emanate from several distinguished neuropathologists.[15–18] Those whom I consulted in 1951 gave me no encouragement, however, that this layer might permit innocuous dissection by the neurosurgeon. They emphasized its density and the general toughness of glial scars.

In early 1952, a neurology colleague, Quadfasel, referred to me a close and favorite relative only on the condition that I remove her tumor completely, even if during the operation I estimated the risk of death to be over 90% if I continued the removal. He had arrived at this decision because the relentless downhill course of these patients treated by discouraging successive cyst aspirations, shunts, and partial removals would have been intolerable to this highly intelligent lady. Our endocrinologists were informed about the merits of cortisone, but I also described to him the capsule problem. He nevertheless urged taking the unknown degree of risk involved. Her tumor, which filled most of the third ventricle, had pushed the chiasm forward to be flush with the tuberculum sellae. Removal via the lamina terminalis between the optic tracts required easing some right-sided tumor medially under the right tract, resulting in a partial hemianopia. The tumor in the upper posterior part of the third ventricle crept downward and forward with minimal surgical urging. In my experience, this type of tumor has only minor adhesions to the posterior part of the third ventricle, a view of Matson's with which I agree. Because the main adhesions are to brain and vessels anteroinferiorly, the likeliest site of the cells of origin, it is safer to deal with these through the lamina terminalis than by a superior transventricular route. The patient had a delightful first postoperative week, so encouraging that our endocrinologist abruptly stopped the cortisone late one day and left the hospital. This action was followed by a precipitous fall in blood pressure. We did not spot the trouble until hours of cerebral ischemia had ruined her higher mental functions. Fortunately, she died 4 months later, having rendered a vitally important service, namely, showing that the capsule can be of surgically useful character, even when it lies against much of the third ventricular wall.

My initial experience, which is encouraging regarding tumor removal without mortal injury to the brain, is presumably related to a safety factor of the glial layer. The tendency of glial proliferation to occur with these tumors can be so pronounced that the lesion may seem to be a glioma of the visual pathways. I have had two such patients and was saved from leaving the tumor in situ only by the assiduity of the neuropathologist Richardson, who looked through many sections of operative biopsy samples until he found a cluster of epithelial cells. Removal of such a tumor in one patient resulted in complete recovery of her visual fields and acuity from a grossly impaired preoperative level. In another patient, the glial investment appeared grossly to be soft white matter, yet happily turned out microscopically to contain no neurons or nerve fibers.

In one patient, a very thin layer of pseudocapsule was still intact in one area of the surgical specimen, yet he recovered and had no recurrence and no disability in 18 years of follow-up.[19]

Conversely, we treated a patient whose tissue from the posterior edge of his chiasm looked normal. Both with macroscopic techniques and even with the operating microscope, this area was indistinguishable from the rest of the chiasm. Hematoxylin and eosin staining showed mostly astrocytes but with small epithelial rests. The remainder of the largely third ventricular tumor had been removed, but I feared major visual impairment if I removed more chiasm. The patient worked effectively in the family butcher shop for 10 years, when after 2 months of recurrent symptoms we found almost all of his third ventricle to be reoccupied by tumor. At our reoperation, Crowell and I clearly left a small amount of tumor. His further course was described again in 1980 by Sweet[9]; it was at first satisfactory as a result of careful regulation of his hormonal supplement (as is discussed later) but by 1988 had steadily deteriorated to level "poor."[19]

Confirmation that the glial reactive layer facilitates the surgeon's dissection has been noted by Hoffman and colleagues,[20] Kahn and colleagues,[4] Katz,[19] and Symon.[21] Kobayashi and associates[22] conducted the most extensive pathologic study of the surface of this tumor vis-à-vis the brain in seven patients who went to autopsy without previous surgery. Their serial sections revealed that significant cystic portions of the tumors had a connective tissue membrane between the tumor inside and its smooth attachment to the adjacent glial barrier outside. A distinct layer of gliosis lay between the cyst wall and viable ganglion cells in the hypothalamus and thalamus that ranged in thickness from several hundred micrometers to a few millimeters. Degenerated neurons and demyelinated fibers in this layer were largely replaced by Rosenthal fibers and fibrillary astrocytes (Fig. 37–1). However, the solid portions of the tumors had no connective tissue membrane; protrusions of

tumor invaded the gliotic zone. In some areas, tumor cells were only a few micrometers away from viable neurons of hypothalamus or thalamus, and no glial reaction occurred. Prevention of significant hypothalamic injury remains the surgeon's principal problem.

## RADIOLOGIC EVALUATION

The ability to determine the precise location and volume of cystic and solid components of the tumor has greatly improved treatment by all modalities, especially those involving stereotaxis.

Magnetic resonance imaging (MRI) and MR angiography are responsible for the discovery of a new syndrome, fusiform dilatation of the carotid artery. Sutton[23] has described an unusual complication resulting from neurosurgeons' attempts to dissect the last bit of tenacious adherences to the supraclinoid internal carotid artery of craniopharyngioma (nine patients) or chiasmatic-hypotha-

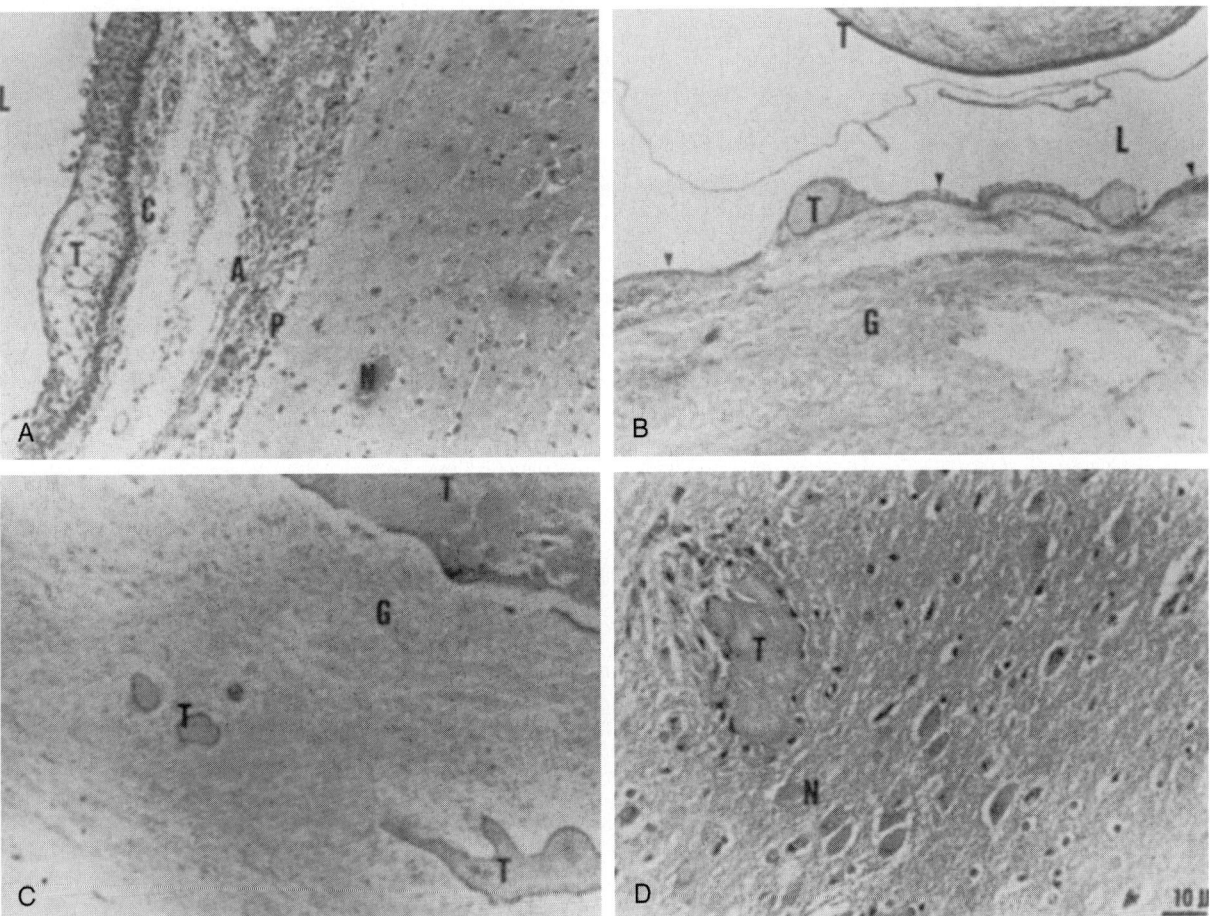

**FIGURE 37–1** ■ *A,* The wall of a cystic portion of the tumor's surface showing a connective tissue membrane between the inside of the tumor and its smooth attachment to the adjacent arachnoid and pia. No gliosis appears in the adjoining brain. *B,* Cystic portion of tumor (L); this layer of scattered tumor cells is next to extensive glial reaction between tumor and brain. *C,* The solid portions of tumor have no outer connective tissue membrane. Papillary protrusions of tumor invaded the gliotic zone. With and without the connective tissue layer, the layer of gliosis varied in thickness from several hundred microns to a few millimeters. *D,* The exceptional situation of a cluster of epithelial cells within viable neurons of hypothalamus with no glial reaction is seen. (With thanks to Kobayashi T, Kageyama N, Yoshida J, et al: Pathological and clinical basis of the indications for treatment of craniopharyngiomas. Neurol Med Chir [Tokyo] 21:39–47, 1981, who did serial sections on the interface between tumor and brain in seven patients who came to autopsy having had no previous surgery in the tumor area.) (L, lumen; T, tumor; C, connective tissue; A, arachnoid; P, pia; N, normal brain; G, glia; F, normal nerve fibers.)

lamic glioma (two patients). The complication consists of the delayed appearance of aneurysmal dilatation of the entire circumference of the vessel. Figure 37–2A is a normal digital subtraction angiogram obtained preoperatively in a patient with a hypothalamic astrocytoma. Figure 37–2B is the right carotid arteriogram of the same patient that was obtained 10 years after right pterional craniectomy and radiation therapy. It shows striking dilatation of the entire supraclinoid internal carotid. None of the nine patients with craniopharyngioma had a hemorrhage or any other symptom referable to the lesion, and no treatment has been given. MRI proton-density weighted spin-echo sequences demonstrate a flow void that depicts the dilated artery (see Fig. 37–2C). MR angiography also shows the lesion well and confirms flowing blood within it. The lesion was found 6 to 12 months after operation in the patients with craniopharyngiomas and several years after operation and radiation in those with gliomas. However, of the two patients with fusiform dilatation of the carotid artery that was discovered 8 and 11 years after operation for glioma, one experienced headaches and possibly a hemorrhage. Opera-

tion for the lesion yielded a poor result, and no further operations have been performed in the asymptomatic patients.

## ENDOCRINE ABNORMALITIES

Sklar[24] describes endocrine abnormalities seen at the first presentation, at which only a few children with craniopharyngiomas complain of symptoms of hormonal deficiency. However, 80% to 90% of them prove to have such inadequacies, along with their common symptoms of headache, vomiting, and visual problems.[24] A summary of laboratory measurements[25–28] is shown in Table 37–1. Almost half of the patients are short in stature, and growth rate is subnormal in most of these patients. Sorva[26] found that the growth records showed impairment in 19 of 22 children with craniopharyngioma and preceded the diagnosis by an average of 4 years. An alert pediatrician spotted this feature in a 17-year-old young man as the only sign or symptom of

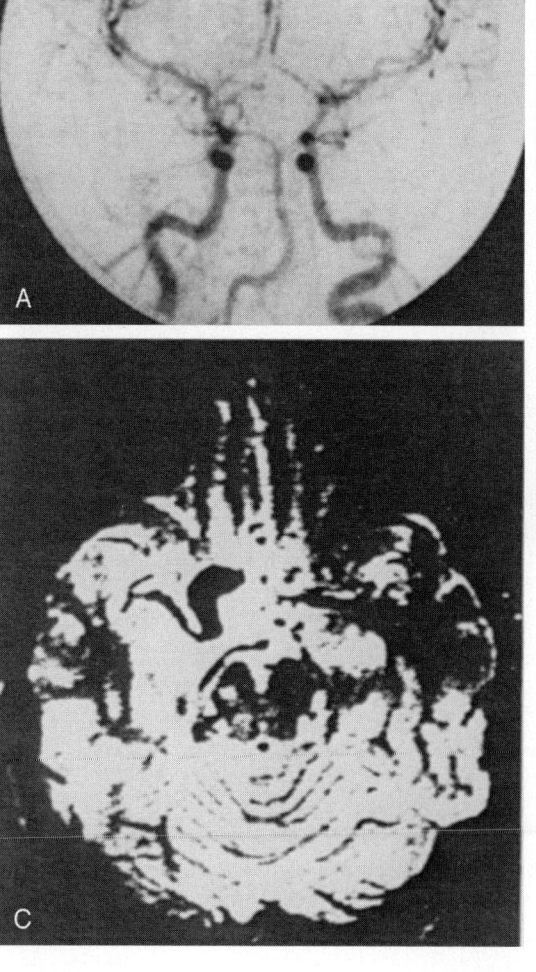

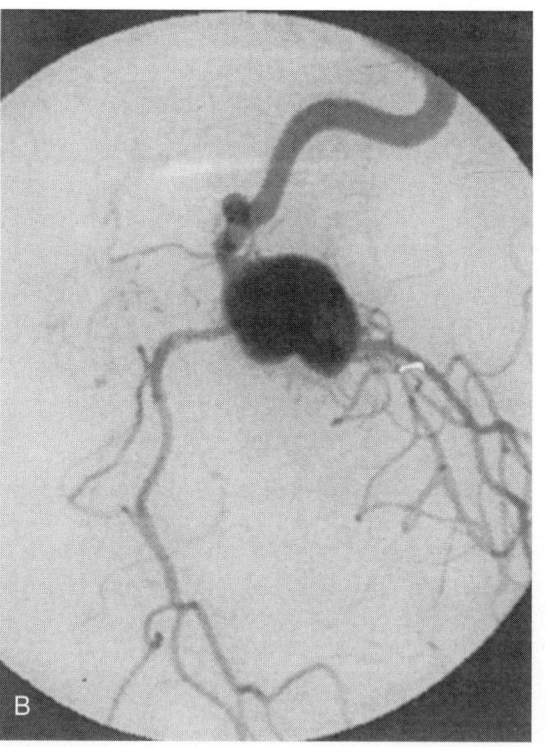

FIGURE 37–2 ■ A, Digital subtraction angiogram performed as part of the original preoperative evaluation of a patient with a hypothalamic astrocytoma. No carotid artery abnormality is seen. B, Right carotid arteriogram performed on the same patient 10 years after right pterional craniotomy and radiation therapy shows marked aneurysmal dilatation of the entire supraclinoid carotid artery segment. C, Proton density–weighted magnetic resonance image, demonstrating a flow void within a dilated supraclinoid carotid artery on the right side.

TABLE 37–1 ■ **CRANIOPHARYNGIOMA: HYPOTHALAMIC-PITUITARY FUNCTION BEFORE TREATMENT**

| Abnormality | Incidence (%) |
| --- | --- |
| Growth hormone deficient | 75 |
| Luteinizing hormone, follicle-stimulating hormone deficient | 40 |
| Adrenocorticotropin deficient | 25 |
| Thyroxine-stimulating hormone deficient | 25 |
| Increased prolactin | 20 |
| Antidiuretic hormone deficient | 9–17 |

Data from Thomsett MJ, Conte FA, Kaplan SL, Grumbach MM: Endocrine and neurologic outcome in childhood craniopharyngioma. J Pediatr 97:728–735, 1980; Sorva R: Children with craniopharyngioma. Acta Pediatr Scand 77:587–592, 1988; Stahnke N, Grubel G, Lagenstein I, Willig RP: Long-term follow-up of chidren with craniopharyngioma. Eur J Pediatr 142:179–185; Blethen SL: Growth in children with a craniopharyngioma. Pediatrician 14:242–245, 1987.

his modest-sized third ventricular tumor. This tumor was readily removed by Sweet, and the patient achieved a good record at university and thereafter.

A raised prolactin level suggests damage to hypothalamic areas, which normally inhibit release of prolactin. Although diabetes insipidus is common after a major or radical removal of the tumor, it is found in only a few before operation. As became apparent in the early 1950s, preoperative testing for corticotropin-adrenal insufficiency and assessment of sodium and water balance are vitally important. Even if these results are normal, any operative trauma to the hypothalamus requires prophylactic administration of large doses of glucocorticosteroids. The necessity of continuing administration of cortisone and regular studies on the entire hormone picture of these patients led our endocrinologists to emphasize to patients and parents the imperative need for frequent monitoring of the endocrine status and immediate supplemental medication, even with such minor stress as a common cold. This approach has resulted in a great reduction in the late postoperative endocrine-related deaths described by Matson and Crigler.[29] The burgeoning understanding of the importance of administering hormonal supplements in the management of surgical and any other form of stress has yielded gratifying results.

One of the many metabolic effects of cortisone is that it decreases polyuria and increases urine osmolality in patients with diabetes insipidus of central origin, thus tending to obscure that diagnosis. Moreover, high-dose glucocorticoids can decrease the secretion of growth hormone, corticotropin, thyroid-stimulating hormone, thyroxine, and prolactin. Also, the commonly used prophylactic anticonvulsants phenytoin and carbamazepine may cause reduced levels of thyroid-stimulating hormone and thyroxine, both total and free.[30, 31] Carbamazepine also rarely causes diabetes insipidus. The complexity of these hormonal interactions is evidenced also by the variable changes in growth rate occurring in the first postoperative year. The rate may be increased, normal, or decreased, with about equal numbers in each of the groups. Those with excessive growth in height also gain weight; they had hyperinsulinism, normal immunoreactive insulin-like growth factor-1 level, elevated prolactin level, and delayed thyroid-stimulating hormone response to thyroid-stimulating hormone-

releasing hormone, which indicate a hypothalamic lesion. The one third of patients growing at a normal rate had low insulin levels, with values of the other hormones the same as those in the fast growers. Those growing too slowly had low levels of insulin, insulin-like growth factor-1, prolactin, and thyrotropin.[32] The value of the endocrinologist is illustrated by the case of the patient discussed earlier, who had become less active and heavier on our postoperative discharge regimen of thyroxine, 0.2 mg/day, and hydrocortisone, 25 mg/day. He continued to have visual acuity of J1 and J4 and small inferior temporal field defects. The endocrinologist rightly suspected that we were giving him too much glucocorticosteroid, gradually reduced his prednisone to 3 mg in the morning and 1 mg in the evening, changed his pitressin tannate in oil to desmopressin acetate, increased the dosage of thyroxine from 0.2 mg to 0.3 mg/day, and added 5 mg/day of amphetamine (Dexedrine). The symptoms I was attributing to recurrence vanished. The patient lost 16 kg, dropping to 66 kg; his visual fields and acuity improved to nearly normal; and he was again earning his living as a meat cutter. I trust that the neurosurgeon will require no further evidence that the collaboration of an exceedingly well-informed endocrinologist is necessary to follow up and treat these patients for a very long time.

## VISUAL PROBLEMS

That visual problems deserve special attention is indicated by a 1990 statement of Yasargil and colleagues: "The destructive effects of these tumors on the optic pathways were disastrous in two thirds of the patients in this series and were especially pronounced in the children."[33] Pierre-Kahn and coworkers[34] addressed this problem in 16 children who had severe loss of vision, severe papilledema with hemorrhage, or episodes of transient amaurosis. With the objective of prompt amelioration of pressure against the anterior visual pathways achieved with a minimum of general stress he sought to puncture a sizable cyst and slowly drain it into a reservoir, which he left in situ for an average of 50 days in 12 children before performing his principal operation. In the other 4 children, he was unable to enter a cyst. In 18 children with less visual loss or cysts too small to identify, he proceeded to immediate tumor removal. Tumor removal was total in 25 of the 30 cases. In the children who had repeated puncture of the cyst through the reservoir, the visual acuity improved in 7 of 17 eyes and worsened or stayed the same in 12 of 20. The authors also point out that the surgeon must take care that the interopticocarotid space is adequately widened by tumor before this area is dissected lest he or she injure tiny arteries from the internal carotid passing superomedially to optic nerve and chiasm.

## TREATMENT

### Observation

In the ISPC-91 series, 11 children with only endocrine symptoms were at first merely observed. Of these, the symptoms of two progressed, and the patients had operations 2 years later.[1] Follow-up data are provided for only two other patients, who showed no further growth 4 and 10 years later, respectively.

## Surgery

Since 1970, a gradual, and more recently, a rapid swing has occurred toward the objective of achieving a total or near-total removal of these tumors at the first operation. The route chosen depends on the principal site of the tumor; the great variability on this score is illustrated and the corresponding variations in approach are discussed by Samii and coworkers in this volume and by Yasargil and coworkers,[33] Symon and coworkers,[35, 36] and Lapras and coworkers.[37]

### Transsphenoidal Approach

We owe our most authoritative information on this tactic to Laws.[38] A summary of his presentation at the Epstein symposium follows: Craniopharyngiomas arising below the sella diaphragm produce progressive enlargement of the sella, giving a radiographic picture seen in 30% to 60% of previously reported series. The diaphragm usually remains as an effective barrier that prevents intimate tumor attachment to any of the important overlying intracranial structures. However, the tumor usually fuses with the diaphragm, which must usually be removed. The floor of the sella is also removed as widely as possible to create the greatest possible working area. The necessary careful reconstruction of the sella after the tumor has been removed is described by Laws as "a major challenge of this operative approach." Likewise, similar tumor attachments to the medial dural wall of both cavernous sinuses need to be stripped away "with bleeding from the sinus, damage of the intracavernous carotid artery or trauma to the cranial nerves in the cavernous sinuses." Laws routinely dissects the tumor from the pituitary stalk "with minimal trauma" and finds that he can remove via the sphenoid route most tumors associated with enlarged sellas. In 65% of these patients, major suprasellar and parasellar extensions were present. He has also approached transsphenoidally some predominantly suprasellar craniopharyngiomas, usually with only a palliative goal.

From 1973 to 1993, Laws performed transsphenoidal removals on 76 such tumors. Of the 29 patients treated primarily by this route and followed up over 5 years, total removal was achieved in 27, with one operative death, one living disabled patient, 25 well patients, and two who had recurrences, one of whom is well and the other disabled. Of the 17 patients in whom only subtotal removal was achieved, 11 were well, five disabled, and one dead from other causes. Of the 18 such patients treated secondarily by the transsphenoidal route, the results were almost as good as those in the primary subtotal removals. In Laws' 89 operations, only two deaths occurred. Anyone wishing to emulate or improve on the record of this skillful, thoughtful man would do well to begin with some personal tutorial sessions with him.

## Stereotactic Methods of Focal Radiation

By far the most successful proponent of stereotactic methods of focal radiation is Backlund,[39, 40] who has brought to fruition Leksell's two pioneering concepts. First, the larger cysts are treated by the instillation of pure electron, beta-emitting isotope $^{90}$Y or $^{32}$P. The former, which has a 62-hour half-life and 2.3 MeV electrons, is slightly less convenient and penetrates deeper compared with the 14.3-day half-life and 1.74 MeV electrons of $^{32}$P. The electrons at these energies are unlikely to damage visual or hypothalamic structures beyond the fibrous connective tissue and gliotic layers forming the cyst wall. Second, the solid components are treated by photons from $^{60}$Co admitted to the target area via air-containing channels in a lead helmet that are directed to a focal target area. This tactic does not have the effective cutoff of radiation beyond the target provided by particle radiation with electrons, protons, or helium atoms.

However, Backlund has included in his standard therapeutic protocol an open microsurgical total removal if "the size and shape of the tumor" indicate that safe surgery with a problem-free postoperative course could be expected. In 1993, he reported the results from his first 43 consecutive patients who had no previous therapy and who were treated between 1964 and 1976.[40] Of the 13 patients selected for tumor removal, the nine who underwent open operations described earlier and the four who underwent focused photon treatment (Gamma knife) had a smooth post-treatment course and tumor elimination. Colloidal $^{90}$Y was the primary treatment in 18 patients with a large, usually monocystic, tumor. In the remaining 12 patients, different combinations of treatment were used. In four, initial intracystic radiation to reduce bulk was followed by open subtotal removal; in four others, focused photons to the solid tumor followed intracystic $^{90}$Y administration; in one patient, the cystic radiation was followed by linear accelerator radiation. In the nine patients with very large tumors, linear accelerator radiation was paired with partial surgical removal in only two.

Follow-up revealed that six patients (15%) died of their tumors, and 4 died of autopsy-proven other causes. However, in one of these four, the autopsy revealed a subarachnoid hemorrhage from an erosion of the posterior communicating artery—likely to be related to the treatment of the tumor. Only one patient was lost to follow-up, leaving 32 who were all "alive and well." The thoroughness of the staff of the Karolinska Institute and Sweden's social security system have resulted in an unusually complete appraisal of the status of the survivors. Of 29 patients younger than 65 years of age, 23 (79%) work regularly, and 21 work full time. Of the 4 with disability pensions, two had cognitive and neurologic deficits related to radiation in childhood, and one had poor endocrine follow-up findings. Of those treated in childhood, only two were married, and they had no children. Comparison of days off work per year and days of hospitalization per year between the craniopharyngioma survivors and the general Swedish population revealed a slight advantage in terms of lesser disability for the group of 23 tumors.

From these results, we may conclude that when one considers the near-certain improvement from heavy-particle focused radiation and microsurgical removal by the most skilled neurosurgeons, one can hope for improvement in the results.

Although the number of patients in whom the advantages of microsurgical removal is likely higher than the 9 of 43 (21%) recorded here, the place for stereotactically controlled radiation is also firmly established by these carefully assembled data.

## Stereotactic Control of Radiation Treatments

Procedures involving *stereotactic radiosurgery* are defined as methods for delivering a single dose to distinct volumes that are determined by precise imaging. *Stereotactic radiotherapy* refers to the same general tactic for the distinction, usually of larger volumes by fractionation. Tarbell and associates[41] gave a full account of methodology for achieving these two closely related objectives. Patients are treated on a prototype linear accelerator that delivers radiation in multiple coplanar arcs through small circular collimators measuring 0.5 to 50 mm. Reproducibility of the precise position of the frame attached to the head is a requirement for treatment in repeated fractions. In over 3300 sets of multiple scalp readings, individual measurements between fittings varied only 0.31 mm. The facility opened June 1, 1992, and had treated 10 craniopharyngiomas by late 1993.

## Chemotherapy for Cysts

Umezawa and coworkers[42] found that the antibiotic bleomycin is toxic to squamous cell cancer cells. Because benign squamous epithelial cells often occur in craniopharyngiomas, Kubo and colleagues[43] checked the toxicity of bleomycin in cultures of these cells. The results encouraged Takahashi and colleagues[44] to carry out multiple such injections into the cysts of seven patients; they had three excellent and one poor result in predominantly cystic tumors, and three deaths occurred in solid or mixed tumors. Broggi and coworkers[45] described the disappearance of 13 cysts and the decrease in size of five cysts in 18 patients followed up from 3 to 31 months. Fischer and associates,[46] however, having used the agent both in a cyst and systemically, evoked progressive blindness and hemiparesis gradually over 2 years without radiographic evidence of recurrence. Several conferees at the Epstein symposium derived cautious encouragement from their experiences.

## Comparison of the Two Customary Methods of Treatment

Intensive efforts to reach well-founded conclusions on this subject are not helped by the mental agility of many of us in presenting the data on our own favored tactic in the most alluring fashion. In the words of Brada and Thomas, "The results are . . . often retrospective, not standardized and frequently colored in favor of the treatment modality reported."[47] For example, Table 37–2, Degree of Disability After Treatment, contains the footnote "Does not include patients dead from disease or complications."[54] No other part of the original article gives this information. Numerous authors emphasize the necessity of long follow-ups with full information on the extent of deficits in all of the visual, endocrine, metabolic, and neuropsychological areas so likely to be affected. The well-known major problems in the treatment of these tumors lead to referrals at long distances, making intensive follow-up on these aspects the more difficult and proper vigilance in endocrine support less likely. The sketchy definitions of classes of recovery also obscure comparisons between reports. For example, total blindness can usually be compensated for by an otherwise normal person but may lead to total disability in the presence of moderate mental or psychosocial retardation.

## Subtotal Surgical Resection Only

Subtotal surgical resection can be dismissed now on the basis of many publications, of which only six are cited here.[48–53] Many early, rapidly growing recurrences are the almost universal experience.

## POLL OF NEUROSURGEONS

As a component of the monograph of Choux and colleagues,[1] the philosophy of craniopharyngioma management in children was solicited from 17 prominent neurosurgeons. Microscopic complete removal, when possible, is the first choice of 13 (Basso, Fukushima, Hoffman, Kobayashi, Konovalov, Lapras, Laws, Mori, Samii, Symon, Takahashi, Takakura, Yasargil). Backlund, Lunsford, and Steiner, all pupils of Leksell, follow his pioneering technique of using $^{90}$Y or $^{32}$P radiation on the cystic component and focused gamma radiation on the solid component.

TABLE 37–2 ■ **DEGREE OF DISABILITY AFTER TREATMENT***

| | Surgery (No. = 15) | | Surgery and Radiotherapy (No. = 31) | |
| --- | --- | --- | --- | --- |
| | *No Recurrence* No. (%) | *Recurrence* No. (%) | *No Recurrence* No. (%) | *Recurrence* No. (%) |
| 1—No disability | 3(20) | 3(20) | 18(58) | 0(0) |
| 2—Mild handicap | 1(7) | 3(20) | 7(23) | 0(0) |
| 3—Major disability | 2(15) | 3(20) | 2(6) | 4(13) |
| 4—Incapable of self-care | 0(0) | 0(0) | 0(0) | 0(0) |

*Does not include patients dead from disease or complications.
From Scott RM, Hetelekidis S, Barnes P, et al: Surgery, Radiation, and Combination Therapy in the Treatment of Childhood Craniopharyngioma—a 20-year experience. Presented at the Symposium on Craniopharyngioma: The Answer. New York, New York Medical Center, December 17–19, 1993. Reprinted with permission from S. Karger, AG, Basel.

Derome is the most conservative, favoring initial observation in children[1] "especially if the tumor is calcified." This is a startling statement because most children show calcium in tumor on CT scanning. Derome thinks that radiation should be postponed until after the first decade of life. Although most publications by neurosurgeons agree with the huge majority of 76% recorded in the poll, a few neurosurgeons, including, interestingly, the successors of Matson at the Boston Children's Hospital and the group at the University of California, San Francisco (UCSF), as well as radiation oncologists, are giving radiation therapy a steadily increasing role. After the death of Matson in 1969, the next publication on the subject from the Boston Children's Hospital by Fischer and colleagues[53] reported on 37 children treated between 1972 and 1984. Total removal was thought to be accomplished in 8 of 14 initial attempts to excise the tumor; 23 other patients were initially irradiated. At the Epstein symposium, Scott and colleagues[54] from the Boston Children's Hospital continued the same emphasis on irradiation as the usual initial therapy and reported on 15 patients who had initial extensive surgery and 37 who had lesser surgery plus radiation. The surgeon thought that total removal was achieved in 10, but recurrence took place in nine of them. Scott and coworkers,[54] in Table 37–2, show the degree of disability in the two groups.

The University of California, San Francisco, group, represented by Wara and associates[55] at the Epstein symposium, summarized their view of the literature as appears in Table 37–3. These figures may be compared with the more detailed data from the ISPC-91 series of 454 patients, in which an operative mortality rate of 3.7% was reported, and with the data from Choux and coworkers' article, which includes individual figures for 17 services from 1975 through 1991.[1] In five services that performed 167 operations, the mortality rate was 0%; it varied from 12% to 15% in the five services that performed 155 operations and that had the highest mortality rate. Mortality rate averaged 6.7% in the seven intermediate services. In general, as the surgeon's experience increased, the mortality rate declined: for example, my rate of 7.5% for my whole series of radical removals fell from 10% for the first 28% to zero for the last 12.

Again, in the ISPC-91 series, in which follow-ups lasted longer than 3 years, in 53 children who underwent operation plus radiation, six (11.3%) died, whereas in the 239 children who had operation only, 14 (5.8%) died. French investigators have emphasized the danger of brain injury from radiation in childhood. Comprehensive appraisals of performance under the general heading of psychosocial adjustment were classified by Pierre-Kahn as indicating normal performance in 81% of patients not irradiated, but in only 22% of patients who had irradiation early or as a complement to surgery.[56] The intelligence quotient averaged 88 after surgical treatment only and was only 75 in the irradiated patients reported by Pierre-Kahn and associates. This discrepancy in the results of the irradiations and the extirpations points to the need for more critically assembled data.

Although the short range of the beta-emitting $^{90}Y$ and $^{32}P$ makes radiation of the cysts attractive, focused gamma radiation for the solid tumor is more dangerous because of the vulnerability of the hypothalamic and visual systems, which are usually in direct contact with tumor. However, see the article by Backlund and colleagues[39] for contrary evidence.

The actual completeness of the initial removal varies greatly. In Russia, in Konovalov's far-flung catchment area, which spread through nine time zones, approximately one third of his more than 500 craniopharyngiomas were of "giant" size (>5 cm in diameter).[57] There is general agreement that the morbidity and mortality rates are significantly higher in this "giant" group; Yasargil's operative mortality rate was seven of eight in tumors larger than 6 cm in diameter. The degree of determination to get the tumor out balanced against eagerness to prevent brain damage is bound to be variably assessed by different surgeons. The risk of external radiation, especially in children in this particular situation, is poorly known. The modes of handling the recurrences involve differing decisions as to: (1) the minimally or asymptomatic lesions demonstrated by surgery, (2) the age of the patient, (3) the variably crucial invaded brain, and (4) the neurologic and general medical status of the patient.

Although drawing conclusions from the entire world literature is difficult, I venture to try to appraise my own experience of 40 patients who underwent a radical removal. Regarding the three immediate postoperative deaths, I would not repeat the mistake I made of trying to dissect tumor away from an artery in two of them. During operation, I would also send for histologic examination any specimen with an appearance suggestive of neural tissue to be guided on the wisdom of further removal. As the length of observation has increased, the number of deaths relatively unrelated to tumor has increased more than the number of those resulting from recurrence. Thus, all deaths in the six who died of recurrence occurred 112 to 1412 years after their initial operation. Of the 10 whose deaths were of causes unrelated to tumor, five died in the zero to 15-year survival group, and the remaining five lived from 16 to 26.9 years (mean, 22.3 years). The patients in whom recurrences have taken place were in four of six cases in the good or excellent category at first. However, 6 of the patients who had recurrences have died, and 4 of the 5 still living have deteriorated to the fair-to-poor category. Fifteen of the 19 still living are in the good or excellent category. In the same categories were 8 of the 10 who died of

TABLE 37–3 ■ **RADIATION ONCOLOGISTS' VIEWPOINT ON CRANIOPHARYNGIOMA OUTCOME**

| | Incidence (%) | |
|---|---|---|
| *Outcome Measure* | *Total Resection* | *Subtotal Resection and Radiotherapy* |
| Death | 10 | 1–2 |
| Recurrence | 40–50 | 20–30 |
| Total removal | 60–70 | — |
| Morbidity | 30 | 10 |
| New tumor or vascular complication | — | 1–2 |

Modified from Brada M, Thomas DG: Craniopharyngioma revisited. Int J Radiat Oncol Biol Phys 27:471–475, 1993. With kind permission from Elsevier Science Ltd, The Boulevard, Langford Lane, Kidlington OX5 1GB, UK.

unrelated causes and 4 of 6 before their fatal recurrence. The main good feature of the series is that the status of 23 of the 40 patients was good to excellent in reference to their craniopharyngiomas; the patients died of other causes. The main weak feature of the series is the progression to the failed III and IV groups, or death in 10 of the 11 recurrences. I would now recommend that the primary objective of total removal be maintained but that clinical imaging studies be performed every 6 months for the first several years. Focal proton radiation should be given as soon as clear-cut recurrence develops, unless there is good reason to expect that the tumor can be removed totally at reoperation.

## ACKNOWLEDGMENTS

*The author wishes to express his appreciation to the Neuro-Research Foundation for its support in the preparation of this manuscript and Deborah Wallace for her intelligent assistance.*

## REFERENCES

1. Choux M, Lena G, Genitori L: Le craniopharyngiome de l'enfant. Neurochirurgie 37(Suppl 1):1–174, 1991.
2. Peet MM: Pituitary adamantinomas: Report of three cases. Arch Surg 15:829–854, 1927.
3. Nelson GA, Bastian FO, Schlitt M, White RL: Malignant transformation in craniopharyngioma. Neurosurgery 22:427–429, 1988.
4. Kahn EA, Gosch HH, Seeger JF, Hicks SP: Forty-five years' experience with the craniopharyngiomas. Surg Neurol 1:5–12, 1973.
5. Adamson TE, Wiestler OD, Kleihues P, Yasargil MG: Correlation of clinical and pathological features in craniopharyngiomas. J Neurosurg 73:12–17, 1990.
6. Miller DC: Pathology of craniopharyngiomas: Clinical import of pathological findings. Presented at the Symposium on Craniopharyngioma: The Answer. New York, New York Medical Center, December 17–19, 1993.
7. Petito CK, DeGirolami E, Earle K: Craniopharyngiomas: A clinical and pathological review. Cancer 37:1944–1952, 1976.
8. Lisczak T, Richardson EP, Phillips JP, et al: Morphological, biochemical, ultrastructural, tissue culture and clinical observations of typical and aggressive craniopharyngiomas. Acta Neuropathol (Berl) 43:191–203, 1978.
9. Sweet WH: Recurrent craniopharyngiomas: Therapeutic alternatives. Clin Neurosurg 27:214–224, 1980.
10. Giangaspero F, Osburne DR, Burger PC, Stein RB: Suprasellar papillary squamous epithelioma ("papillary craniopharyngioma"). Am J Surg Pathol 8:57–64, 1984.
11. Critchley M, Ironside RN: The pituitary adamantinomata. Brain 49:437–481, 1926.
12. Bailey P, Buchanan DN, Bucy PC: Intracranial Tumors of Infancy and Childhood. Chicago: University of Chicago Press, 1939, pp 349–375.
13. Ingraham FD, Scott HW: Craniopharyngiomas in children. J Pediatr 29:95–116, 1946.
14. Bartlett JR: Craniopharyngiomas—a summary of 85 cases. J Neurol Neurosurg Psychiatry 34:37–41, 1971.
15. Van den Bergh R, Brucher JM: L'abord transventriculaire dans les cranio-pharyngiomes du troisième ventricule: Aspects neurochirurgicaux et neuro-pathologiques. Neurochirurgie 16:51–65, 1970.
16. Ghatak NR, Hirano A, Zimmerman HM: Ultrastructure of a craniopharyngioma. Cancer 27:1465–1475, 1971.
17. Grcevic N, Yates PO: Rosenthal fibers in tumors of the central nervous system. J Pathol 73:467–472, 1957.
18. Zülch KJ: Brain Tumors: Their Biology and Pathology, 2nd ed. New York: Springer, 1965
19. Katz EL: Late results of radical excision of craniopharyngiomas in children. J Neurosurg 42:86–90, 1975.
20. Hoffman HJ, Hendrick EB, Humphreys RP, et al: Management of craniopharyngioma in children. J Neurosurg 47:218–227, 1977.
21. Symon L: Radical excision of craniopharyngioma: Results in 20 patients. J Neurosurg 62:174–181, 1985.
22. Kobayashi T, Kageyama N, Yoshida J, et al: Pathological and clinical basis of the indications for treatment of craniopharyngiomas. Neurol Med Chir (Tokyo) 21:39–47, 1981.
23. Sutton LN: Vascular Complications of Surgery for Craniopharyngioma and Hypothalamic Glioma. Presented at the Symposium on Craniopharyngioma: The Answer. New York, New York Medical Center, December 17–19, 1993.
24. Sklar CA: Craniopharyngioma: Endocrine abnormalities at presentation. Presented at the Symposium on Craniopharyngioma: The Answer. New York, New York Medical Center, December 17–19, 1993.
25. Thomsett MJ, Conte FA, Kaplan SL, Grumbach MM: Endocrine and neurologic outcome in childhood craniopharyngioma. J Pediatr 97:728–735, 1980.
26. Sorva R: Children with craniopharyngioma. Acta Pediatr Scand 77:587–592, 1988.
27. Stahnke N, Grubel G, Lagenstein I, Willig RP: Long-term follow-up of children with craniopharyngioma. Eur J Pediatr 142:179–185, 1984.
28. Blethen SL: Growth in children with a craniopharyngioma. Pediatrician 14:242–245, 1987.
29. Matson DD, Crigler JF Jr: Management of craniopharyngiomas in childhood. J Neurosurg 30:377–390, 1969.
30. Smith PJ, Surks MI: Multiple effects of 5,5(-diphenylhydantoin on the thyroid hormone system. Endocr Rev 5:514–524, 1984.
31. Isojarvi JIT, Pakarinen AJ, Myllyla VV: Thyroid function in epileptic patients treated with carbamazepine. Arch Neurol 46:1175–1178, 1989.
32. Bucher H, Zapf J, Torresani T, et al: Insulin-like growth factors I and II, prolactin and insulin in 19 growth hormone-deficient children with excessive, normal or decreased longitudinal growth after operation for craniopharyngioma. N Engl J Med 309:1142–1146, 1983.
33. Yasargil MG, Curcic M, Kis M, et al: Total removal of craniopharyngiomas. J Neurosurg 73:3–11, 1990.
34. Pierre-Kahn A, Sainte-Rose C, Renier D: Surgical Approach to Children with Craniopharyngiomas and Severely Impaired Vision. Presented at the Symposium on Craniopharyngioma: The Answer. New York, New York Medical Center, December 17–19, 1993.
35. Symon L, Pell MF, Habib AHA: Radical excision of craniopharyngioma by the temporal route: A review of 50 patients. Br J Neurosurg 5:539–549, 1991.
36. Symon L: Adult Craniopharyngioma: A Different Problem? Presented at the Symposium on Craniopharyngioma: The Answer. New York, New York Medical Center, December 17–19, 1993.
37. Lapras C, Patet JD, Mottolese C, et al: Craniopharyngiomas in childhood: Analysis of 42 cases. Prog Exp Tumor Res 30:350–358, 1987.
38. Laws E: Transsphenoidal Approach to Craniopharyngiomas. Presented at the Symposium on Craniopharyngioma: The Answer. New York: New York Medical Center, December 17–19, 1993.
39. Backlund E, Axelsson B, Bergstrand CG, et al: Treatment of craniopharyngiomas—the stereotactic approach in a ten to twenty-three years' perspective. Acta Neurochir (Wien) 99:11–19, 1989.
40. Backlund E: Treatment of Craniopharyngiomas: The multi-modality approach. Presented at the Symposium on Craniopharyngioma: The Answer. New York, New York Medical Center, December 17–19, 1993.
41. Tarbell NJ, Barnes P, Scott M, et al: Advances in Radiation Therapy for Craniopharyngiomas. Presented at the Symposium on Craniopharyngioma: The Answer. New York, New York Medical Center, December 17–19, 1993.
42. Umezawa H, Maeda K, Takeuchi T, et al: New antibiotics bleomycin A and B. J Antibiot (Tokyo) 19:200–209, 1966.
43. Kubo O, Takakura K, Miki Y, et al: Intracystic therapy of bleomycin for craniopharyngioma—Effect of bleomycin on cultured craniopharyngioma cells and intracystic concentration of bleomycin. No Shinkei Geka 2:683–688, 1974.
44. Takahashi H, Nakazawa S, Shimura T: Evaluation of postoperative intratumoral injection of bleomycin for craniopharyngioma in children. J Neurosurg 62:120–127, 1985.
45. Broggi G, Giorgi C, Franzini A, et al: Preliminary results of intracavitary treatment of craniopharyngioma with bleomycin. J Neurosurg Sci 33:145–148, 1989.

46. Fischer EG, Welch K, Shillito J, et al: Craniopharyngiomas in children: Long-terms effects of conservative surgical procedures combined with radiation therapy. J Neurosurg 73:534–540, 1990.
47. Brada M, Thomas DG: Craniopharyngioma revisited. Int J Radiat Oncol Biol Phys 27:471–475, 1993.
48. Hoogenhoot J, Otten B, Kazem I, et al: Surgery and radiation therapy in the management of craniopharyngiomas. Int J Radiat Oncol Biol Phys 10:2293–2297, 1984.
49. Manaka S, Teramoto A, Takakura K: The efficacy of radiotherapy for craniopharyngioma. Br J Radiol 58:480–482, 1985.
50. Sung DI, Chang CC, Harisiadis L, Carmel PW: Treatment results of craniopharyngiomas. Cancer 47:847–852, 1981.
51. Weiss M, Sutton L, Marcia V, et al: The role of radiation therapy in the management of childhood craniopharyngioma. Int J Radiat Oncol Biol Phys 17:1313–1321, 1989.
52. Wen BC, Hussey DH, Staples J, et al: A comparison of the roles of surgery and radiation therapy in the management of craniopharyngiomas. Int J Radiat Oncol Biol Phys 16:17–24, 1989.
53. Fischer EG, Welch K, Belli JA, et al: Treatment of craniopharyngiomas in children: 1972–1981. J Neurosurg 62:496–501, 1985.
54. Scott RM, Hetelekidis S, Barnes P, et al: Surgery, radiation, and combination therapy in the treatment of childhood craniopharyngioma—a 20-year experience. Presented at the Symposium on Craniopharyngioma: The Answer. New York, New York Medical Center, December 17–19, 1993.
55. Wara WM, Sneed PK, Larson DA: The role of radiation therapy in the treatment of craniopharyngioma. Presented at the Symposium on Craniopharyngioma: The Answer. New York, New York Medical Center, December 17–19, 1993.
56. Pierre-Kahn A, Brauner R, Renier D, et al: Traitement des craniopharyngiomes de l'enfant: Analyse retrospective de 50 observations. Arch Fr Pediatr 45:163–167, 1988.
57. Konovalov AN: Techniques and strategies of direct surgical management of craniopharyngiomas. In Apuzzo M (ed): Surgery of the Third Ventricle. Baltimore: Williams & Wilkins, 1987, pp 542–552.

CHAPTER 38

# Management of Craniopharyngiomas: Additional Comment

■ CHRIS B.T. ADAMS

The management of craniopharyngiomas is a matter of dispute. Two camps exist—one advocating radical excisional surgery, the other conservative surgery followed by external radiotherapy. The controversy is not helped by the publishing of optimistic surgical results in neurosurgical journals and similar results for radiotherapy and conservative surgery in radiotherapy journals. One problem is the variable and often prolonged natural history of these lesions.[1] This makes assessment of results difficult. These results are probably best expressed as "progression-free survival" rates for 5, 10, 15, and 20 years. The results of aggressive surgery aiming at complete excision are characterized by Yasargil's series.[2] In the primary surgical group (i.e., the first operation rather than surgery for a recurrence), 98% total removal rate was achieved. The operative mortality was 10% and the morbidity was 13%; these figures were related to the size of the lesion as indeed was the quality of the outcome. Eighty percent required hormone replacement therapy. Patients with small (<2 cm) lesions had a mortality of 6% and a good outcome in 94%, whereas those patients at the other end of the scale (>6 cm) had an 88% mortality and a 13% good outcome. These are the results of an expert microneurosurgeon. The overall recurrence rate was 7% in this series, but other series (after "complete excision") report a higher recurrence rate, such as Hoffman's series[3] in which there was a 39% recurrence; 16 of 28 surviving patients had cognitive impairment, but there was only a 2% mortality. The results of limited surgery followed by radiotherapy are well summarized by Brada's group.[4-8] Incomplete surgery alone has a higher recurrence rate. Conservative surgery and external beam radiotherapy using conventional doses produced 5, 10, and 15 years progression-free survival rates with 79%, 72%, and 72%, respectively.[4] The role of surgery is to obtain a biopsy, evacuate cysts, relieve hydrocephalus by a shunt, or debulk the main mass. During radiotherapy treatment, surgery may be urgently required to relieve hydrocephalus or to evacuate a cyst that may enlarge during radiotherapy. The mortality is zero (other than that of conservative treatment), and the morbidity is low. Impaired pituitary function is the commonest, but this is lower than that for surgery.

There is a 2% chance of other tumors at 20 years owing to radiotherapy.[8]

Although it is easy to compare the results of excisional surgery and conservative surgery with radiotherapy, direct comparison is, as yet, impossible because each treatment group contains selected patients. No prospective randomized trial has been done, or is likely to be done in the future, owing to the strongly held views. However, I think the following conclusions and guidelines may be formulated.

1. Excision surgery may be attempted in patients with small (<2 cm) craniopharyngiomas, particularly in those whose pituitary function has already been destroyed, and especially those craniopharyngiomas confined to the pituitary fossa. It is less easy when pituitary function is preserved and the patient is a child. In my experience, conservative treatment (i.e., cyst aspiration) does not improve pituitary function and sooner, rather than later, the pituitary function deteriorates. There are good reasons to avoid irradiation in the prepubertal child. Irradiation, especially in children younger than 7 years of age, damages intellectual development. Furthermore, at any age, irradiation causes delayed pituitary damage. In this group, I perform conservative surgery in the hope of preserving pituitary function until puberty; then, if a recurrence arises, I perform definitive surgery. I do not feel confident omitting radiotherapy at the initial stage, but I do so.

2. I believe that conservative surgery, in order to obtain a biopsy, evacuate cysts, debulk solid craniopharyngioma tissue, or introduce a shunt for hydrocephalus followed by radiotherapy, is the best definitive treatment for most craniopharyngiomas, especially those larger than 2 cm. Certainly, attempts at removing a large craniopharyngioma are associated with unacceptable mortality and morbidity. As a young surgeon, I was extremely proud of having totally removed a large craniopharyngioma in a 12-year-old boy. The result was disastrous owing to hypothalamic damage. The

487

boy developed an uncontrolled appetite and lost his ability to feel thirst. His fluid intake could be controlled only by weighing him. I did that boy and his parents no favors.

## REFERENCES

1. Bartlett JR: Craniopharyngiomas—a summary of 85 cases. J Neurol Neurosurg Psychiatry 34:37–41, 1971.
2. Yasargil M, Curic M, Kis M, et al: Total Removal of Craniopharyngiomas: Approaches and long term results in 144 patients. J Neurosurg 73:3–11, 1990.
3. Hoffman HJ, Silva de M, Humphreys RP, et al: Aggressive surgical management of craniopharyngiomas in children. J Neurosurg 76:47–52, 1992.
4. Jose CC, Rajan B, Ashley S, et al: Radiotherapy for the treatment of recurrent craniopharyngioma. Clin Oncol 4:287–289, 1992.
5. Brada M, Thomas DGT: Craniopharyngioma revisited. Int J Radiat Oncol Biol Phys 27:471–475, 1993.
6. Rajan B, Ashley S, Gorman C, et al: Craniopharyngioma—long term results following limited surgery and radiotherapy. Radiother Oncol 26:1–10, 1993.
7. Rajan B, Brada M: Craniopharyngioma controversy. Crit Rev Neurosurg 6:92–96, 1996.
8. Rajan B, Ashley S, Thomas DGT, et al: Craniopharyngioma: Improving outcome by early recognition and treatment of acute complications. Int J Radiat Oncol Biol Phys 3:517–521, 1997.
9. Jones A: Radiation oncogenesis in relation to the treatment of pituitary tumours. Clin Endocrinol 10:494–502, 1991.

# Surgical Management of Craniopharyngiomas

■ MADJID SAMII and AMIR SAMII

Craniopharyngiomas are benign, slow-growing, well encapsulated tumors of variable consistency (solid or cystic, with or without calcification) that involve primarily the sellar region. These tumors grow by expansion, although glial reaction and small papillary tumor projections into the glial undersurface may falsely lead to the impression of tumor invasion. In general, there are two histologically distinct types of craniopharyngioma: the adamantinous and the squamous-papillary type.

Radical microsurgical removal is the treatment of choice to effect a cure. However, the sellar region is a crossroad for major cerebral blood vessels and several cranial nerves that govern vision and eye movement, and contains structures central to the endocrinologic and autonomic systems and the emotional sphere of our being. These structures can be affected by the tumor, making the surgical procedure a challenge requiring a skilled and experienced team familiar with this extremely vulnerable region.

Alternative treatment options, such as nonradical surgery followed by radiation therapy, stereotactic cyst puncture with or without intracavitary radioisotope instillation, and stereotactic radiosurgery, are available. In general, these alternatives fail to solve the patient's problems over the long term. However, in combination with conservative surgery, radiation therapy, for example, appears significantly to prolong the progression/recurrence-free interval compared with conservative surgery only, but not compared with radical removal, where tumor-free survival rates of 100% have been reported.[1-3]

## CLASSIFICATION

It is of fundamental importance to the surgeon to possess a clear anatomic definition of the tumor and its relationship to the third ventricle.

In 1962, Rougerie[4, 5] was the first to propose a surgical classification for craniopharyngiomas. He defined five anatomic forms: prechiasmatic craniopharyngiomas, intrasellar craniopharyngiomas, retrochiasmatic craniopharyngiomas, "les formes géantes," and atypical craniopharyngiomas. In 1975, Pertuiset[6] recommended the following classification:

intrasellar craniopharyngiomas, suprasellar (prechiasmatic, subchiasmatic, and retrochiasmatic) craniopharyngiomas, intrasellar and suprasellar craniopharyngiomas, and intraventricular craniopharyngiomas. Konovalov[7] has classified craniopharyngiomas as follows: endosuprasellar craniopharyngiomas, suprasellar-extraventricular craniopharyngiomas, intraventricular craniopharyngiomas, and giant craniopharyngiomas.

Kobayashi[8] singled out four types: type I, anterior; type II, intrasellar; type III, ventricular; and type IV, posterior. Steno[9] offered the following classification: intrasellar and suprasellar, and suprasellar: extraventricular, intraventricular, and mixed. Hoffman[10] described three types of craniopharyngiomas: intrasellar, prechiasmatic, and retrochiasmatic.

However, independent of the numerous historical and current classifications, many authors suggest that the axis of tumor growth in craniopharyngiomas, which in the first instance is in a vertical projection, is the essential selection criterion for the various surgical approaches.[11-14] Based on this and taking into consideration the different classification proposals and possible tumor extension to the anterior, middle, and posterior fossas, as well as into the ventricular system and the sphenoid sinus, we propose the following classification. Vertical tumor extension can be classified into five grades of severity, from grade I to grade V (Fig. 39-1):

- In grade I, the tumor is located purely in the intrasellar or infradiaphragmatic region.
- In grade II, the tumor is localized in the cistern with or without an intrasellar component.
- In grade III, the tumor extends into the lower half of the third ventricle.
- In grade IV, the tumor expands to the upper half of the third ventricle.
- In grade V, the tumor dome reaches the septum pellucidum or extends into the lateral ventricle(s).

With regard to tumor growth in the horizontal plane, lateral and sagittal extensions can be described, respectively. Infrasellar extension into the sphenoid sinus with destructive sellar expansion (S) may be present. Lateral extension (L) includes temporal skull base invasion, and

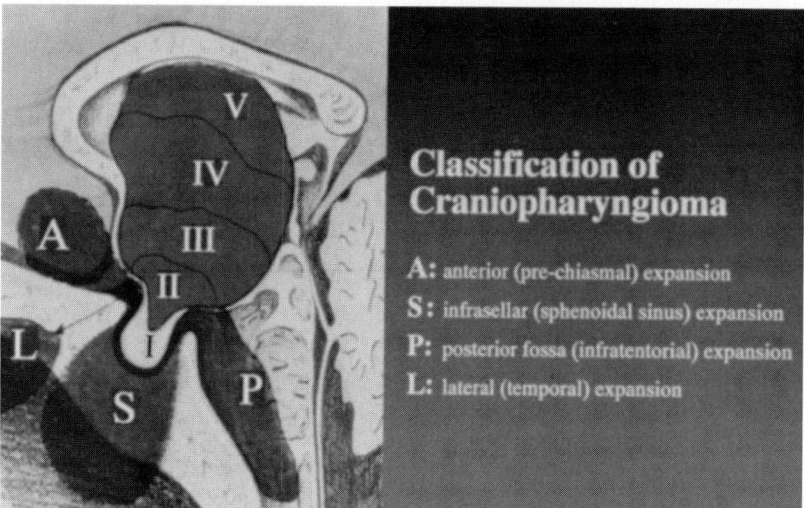

FIGURE 39–1 ■ This drawing is representative of the grading of craniopharyngiomas. The main focus is on the vertical tumor extension. (Grade I, intrasellar tumor; Grade II, intracisternal tumor, with or without intrasellar component; Grade III, intracisternal tumor extending into the lower half of the third ventricle; Grade IV, intracisternal tumor extending into the upper half of the third ventricle; Grade V, intracisternal tumor extending to the septum pellucidum or into the lateral ventricles.)

involvement of the corpus striatum or the temporal lobe itself in paraventricular expansion. Finally, sagittal extension manifests as midbrain compression in the posterior protrusion or even as growth into the posterior fossa (P), and interhemispheric fissure or frontal lobe invasion characterizes an anterior expansion (A).

Atypical craniopharyngiomas may be located in the pharynx or limited entirely to the sphenoid sinus, or may even be found in the pineal region.[15]

## CLINICAL FEATURES AND PREOPERATIVE EVALUATION

Craniopharyngiomas, by virtue of their location, can produce a combination of neurologic and endocrine symptoms. The main presenting symptoms are visual disturbances. In 70% of patients, visual field defects are present, whereas in 89.9% decreased visual acuity is found.[16, 17] In approximately 50%, increased intracranial pressure is clinically evident, and papilledema occurs in 18.5% of patients.[18] Selective hormonal disturbances can precede neuro-ophthalmologic symptoms. The frequency of endocrine manifestations ranges from 24% to 53% in patients from 2 to 15 years of age, and in patients older than 15 years, it increases to approximately 75%. At the time of diagnosis, the signs of hypophysial-hypothalamic involvement are usually those of growth retardation (33%), obesity (25%), diabetes insipidus (20%), and delayed puberty (50%).[18]

Magnetic resonance imaging (MRI), computed tomography (CT), endocrine studies, and neuro-ophthalmologic and neuropsychological evaluation are the standard tools for diagnosis and planning of surgical treatment of craniopharyngiomas. MRI with and without paramagnetic contrast (gadolinium) administration is the prime imaging tool for diagnostic screening, whereas CT is mandatory for evaluating changes in the bony structures of the skull base and determining the presence of tumor calcifications. Large craniopharyngiomas almost always stretch and sometimes engulf the surrounding arteries; therefore, preoperative angiography can be helpful to establish the surgical strategy.

MR angiography is a reliable noninvasive procedure that has increasingly replaced conventional angiographic studies.

Typically, 50% of patients with craniopharyngiomas demonstrate intracranial calcifications and 30% have hydrocephalus.[18] The tumor never seems to deform the planum sphenoidale without enlarging the sella turcica. Furthermore, the optic canals usually are not enlarged.[15] In our experience, when we suspected infiltration of the cavernous sinus on the basis of the preoperative neuroradiologic studies, it was not confirmed intraoperatively. Endocrine deficits are reported as follows: growth hormone (GH; 60%), luteinizing hormone/follicle-stimulating hormone (LH/FSH; 60%), adrenocorticotropic hormone (ACTH; 30%), and thyroid-stimulating hormone (TSH; 30%).[18]

## PATIENT SELECTION AND MANAGEMENT DECISIONS

There is abundant controversy among physicians regarding the treatment of choice for craniopharyngioma. Depending on personal specialty and experience, different treatment modalities have been proposed. Most neurosurgeons consider total surgical tumor excision as the treatment of choice. Other neurosurgeons experienced with stereotactic methodology advocate stereotactic aspiration and drainage of cystic craniopharyngiomas and, as an additional option, implantation of β-emitting isotopes. Another stereotactic treatment modality is the intracavitary instillation of bleomycin. Others suggest that external fractionated radiation or radiosurgery or subtotal tumor removal combined with radiation therapy should be performed. However, in combination with conservative surgery, radiation therapy appears significantly to prolong the progression/recurrence-free interval compared with conservative surgery only, but not compared with radical removal, for which tumor-free survival rates of 100% have been reported.[1–3] Because radical tumor excision carries a very low rate of morbidity,[9, 18, 19] we advocate the radical removal of craniopharyngiomas as the method of choice, with early surgery after the diagnosis.

This approach may reduce the incidence of irreversible defects at the level of the optic pathway, mesodiencephalon, and frontal lobes.

## REGIONAL SURGICAL ANATOMY

Purely intrasellar craniopharyngiomas are uncommon; they expand in the sella and compress the pituitary, producing endocrinopathies before compressing the optic nerve. More frequently, the tumor grows by pushing the diaphragm upward, breaking through it, and extending in any direction. In relation to the optic chiasm, the tumor may extend anteriorly in the direction of the subfrontal space (prechiasmatic craniopharyngioma). These are frequently cystic tumors and achieve large sizes before being diagnosed. When the tumor grows posterior to the chiasm (retrochiasmatic craniopharyngioma), it displaces the pituitary stalk forward and the chiasm forward and upward, making the optic nerve appear falsely prefixed (pseudoprefixity of the optic chiasm). Cystic retrochiasmatic craniopharyngiomas may reach an enormous size by expanding into the posterior fossa and the prepontine cistern.

Tumor extension down to the cervical spine has been described.[20] The tumor may also displace the chiasm upward (subchiasmatic craniopharyngioma) and the pituitary stalk backward. Both retrochiasmatic and subchiasmatic craniopharyngiomas are frequently solid tumors, and they usually press against the third ventricle as they grow, causing compression of the hypothalamus and obstruction of the foramen of Monro. When it is pushed upward by the tumor, the floor of the third ventricle becomes paper thin and tears so that the tumor protrudes directly into it. Craniopharyngiomas may also grow laterally into the subtemporal space, producing compression of the temporal lobe.

Craniopharyngiomas may arise directly from the floor of the third ventricle. This is essentially a retrochiasmatic tumor, but it may extend anteriorly to the prechiasmatic space, superiorly into the lumen of the third ventricle, posteriorly to the interpeduncular and prepontine cisterns, and laterally to the basal ganglia and temporal lobe.

Although large craniopharyngiomas frequently grow into the third ventricle, purely intraventricular craniopharyngiomas are exceptional.[21] A review of the literature revealed only 24 cases.[22] Intraventricular craniopharyngiomas have been hypothesized to arise from a pars tuberalis containing squamous epithelial rests or remnants of Rathke's pouch and then to grow along the pituitary stalk, extending to the infundibulum or tuber cinerum in the floor of the third ventricle.[23, 24]

Craniopharyngiomas usually adhere to the major arteries at the skull base and to the small perforating arteries arising from the anterior communicating artery, posterior communicating artery, and branches from the anterior choroidal artery and thalamoperforating vessels.[19, 24] Vascular adhesions are one of the most important reasons for incomplete tumor removal. Attempts at radical dissection of the tumor capsule from the arterial wall have been associated with weakening of the adventitia by injuring the vasa vasorum, causing fusiform dilatations of the carotid artery.[25]

The anterior part of the tumor is supplied by perforators from the anterior communicating artery and proximal anterior cerebral artery. The lateral part of the tumor receives branches from the posterior communicating artery, and the intrasellar portion is usually supplied from intracavernous meningohypophysial vessels. Craniopharyngiomas do not usually receive a blood supply from the posterior cerebral arteries or from the basilar artery unless the anterior blood supply for the lower hypothalamus and floor of the third ventricle is absent (anatomic variant).

## CHOICE OF SURGICAL APPROACH

Many different surgical approaches have been used in the treatment of craniopharyngiomas (Fig. 39–2). According to the localization and expansion of the tumor, different approaches have characteristic advantages and disadvantages. Therefore, the best surgical approach can be selected only after careful evaluation of the topography of the tumor, based on detailed neuroradiologic studies.

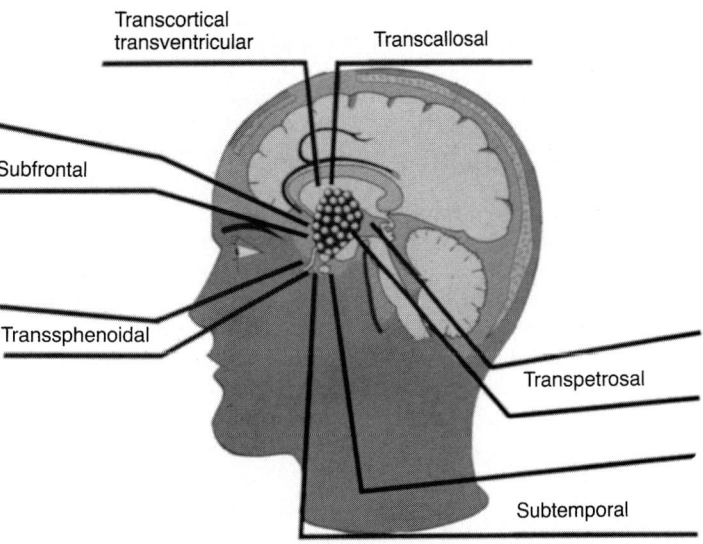

FIGURE 39–2 ■ Different approach options are given for the removal of craniopharyngiomas.

Some approaches may be superior in specific situations, such as the transsphenoidal approach route for grade I, purely intrasellar tumors, whereas purely intraventricular tumors can be excised by a transventricular approach, small retrochiasmatic tumors by the subtemporal route, and large retrochiasmatic tumors with extension along the clivus by a transpetrosal-transtentorial approach.

Based on our experience, we prefer the subfrontal unilateral or bilateral route to treat grade III, IV, and V tumors because these tumors originate from remnants of Rathke's pouch, which is a midline structure. Thus, the surrounding elements are displaced from the midline in any direction, and therefore a midline approach to the suprasellar area is the best primary approach to the tumor center for sufficient tumor enucleation to permit a good overview of all surrounding structures for further total removal.

In cases of a prefixed chiasm and a retrosellar tumor expanding into the interpeduncular-pontine cistern and the third ventricle, the lamina terminalis represents a window through which these extensions can be removed.

The choice of whether to perform a unilateral or bilateral approach depends on the size and the lateral expansion of the tumor. Because of variations in the anatomic relationships of the suprasellar structures, the surgeon should be prepared to extend a unilateral approach into a bilateral one for more complete tumor removal. In removing grade I and II tumors, the transsphenoidal approach usually is taken.

## SURGICAL TECHNIQUES

### Subfrontal Approach

For this approach, the patient is positioned supine, with slight flexion of the trunk and knees. The patient's head is placed in a fixation device with the head elevated above the heart for venous drainage. The vertex is tilted down with slight extension of the neck to allow the frontal lobes to fall away without excessive retraction. This position provides a comfortable working setting for the surgeon and offers exposure of the entire frontal fossa floor to the basilar apex.

The subfrontal unilateral approach begins with a bitemporal coronal incision. For cosmetic reasons, we prefer this to a circumscribed flap incision on the forehead. Three bur holes usually are sufficient for the craniotomy (Fig. 39–3). First, the lateral bur hole is placed at the root of the zygomatic process of the frontal bone, which forms a palpable ridge at its junction with the infratemporal fossa. The hole should be placed approximately 1 to 1.5 cm above the frontozygomatic suture. A small slit can be made in the aponeurosis of the temporal muscle to expose the bony ridge at the temporal fossa. The bur hole is placed directly on that ridge. As the hole is drilled, care is taken not to enter the bony orbit, which would injure Tenon's capsule, and to keep the hole as close as possible to the floor of the anterior cranial fossa. This approach also allows troublesome bony overlapping to be avoided later on. The second, medial bur hole is situated approximately 4 cm from the lateral hole. We try to place this hole as low as

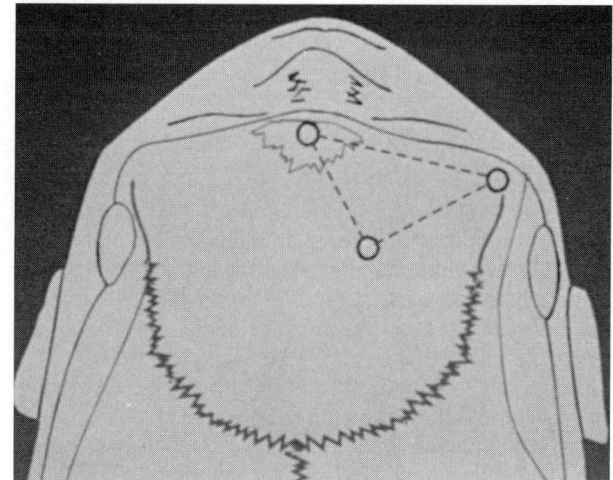

FIGURE 39–3 ■ Placement of the three bur holes for a unilateral frontal craniotomy.

possible (at the level of the glabella) and close to the midline. This procedure can be carried out even with a large frontal sinus that extends far superiorly. When the frontal sinus is opened, its mucosal lining is stripped downward so that the drill can be advanced through the posterior sinus wall without damaging the mucosa. We mention this detail because it is of importance in preventing the spread of pathogenic organisms from the paranasal sinuses into the cranial cavity and obviates the need for tube drainage of the frontal sinus into the nasal cavity in case the frontal sinus has been widely opened and a portion of mucosa has been removed. After the frontal sinuses have been exposed, the mucosa is cleaned out and the sinuses are packed with antibiotic gauze until the end of the operation. The third, superior bur hole is placed approximately 3 cm above and midway between the lateral and medial perforations. For the bilateral approach (Fig. 39–4), two lateral bur holes are

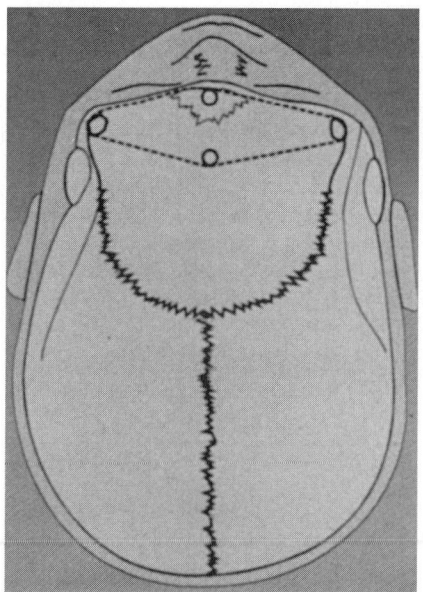

FIGURE 39–4 ■ Placement of the four bur holes for a bifrontal craniotomy.

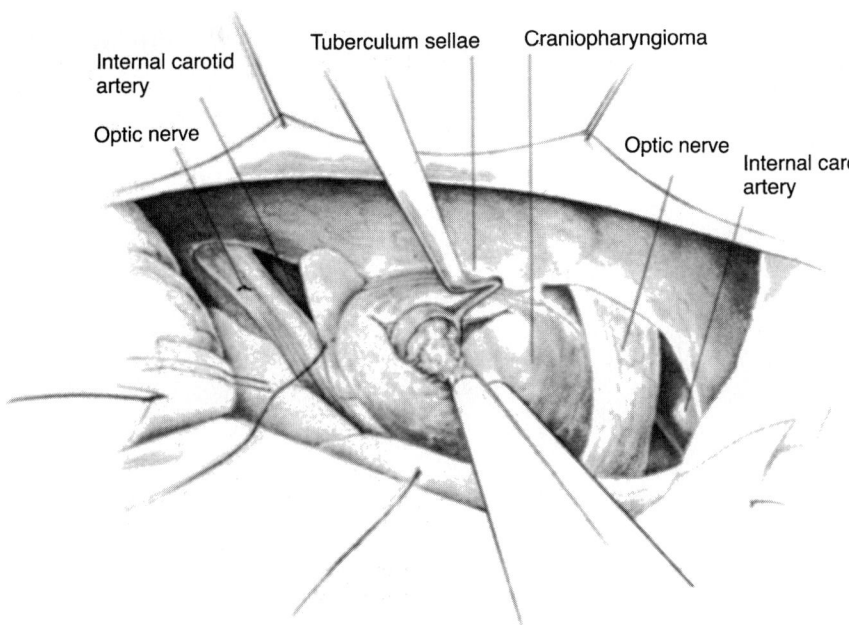

FIGURE 39–5 ■ Intraoperative findings in the case of a postfixed optic chiasm. After retraction of the right frontal lobe, the suprasellar tumor capsule is identified in the anterior angle of the optic chiasm and is opened. A piecemeal enucleation of the tumor is performed with a curet and suction tip. (From Samii M: Surgery of the Skull Base. Berlin: Springer-Verlag, 1989, p 277.)

placed as described, a third hole is placed above the glabella, and the fourth one is positioned 3 cm higher.

In the unilateral approach, the dura is then opened with a frontobasal incision lateral to the superior sagittal sinus. Intradural exposure is carried out in standard fashion, facilitating frontal lobe retraction by progressively opening the arachnoid and draining cerebrospinal fluid (CSF). It has proved useful and advantageous to expose the anterior skull base from the lateral side, using the lesser sphenoid wing as a landmark. The olfactory nerves are identified, exposed, and preserved in continuity without exerting traction. Microdissection begins until both optic nerves have been exposed. The basal cisterns are then opened to remove more CSF. For an optimal overview of the suprasellar structures and the tumor, the arachnoidal sheet of both optic nerves and the optic chiasm is dissected (Fig. 39–5).

The condition of the chiasm, which cannot be completely evaluated neuroradiologically, determines whether we proceed subchiasmatically or through the lamina terminalis, or by both routes. In cases of a postfixed chiasm (Fig. 39–6), tumor removal is first performed between the optic nerves; removal of this part of the tumor decompresses the optic pathway, which allows the surgeon to visualize the pituitary stalk. If the pituitary stalk has not been infiltrated, it should be preserved (see Fig. 39–6). If it is cystic, the contents should be drained by puncture. Feeding vessels to the capsule should be coagulated. When the chiasm is prefixed (Fig. 39–7), which occurs in large, predominantly retrochiasmatic tumors, removal is performed through the lamina terminalis (Figs. 39–8 and 39–9), which offers easy access to the inferior part of the third ventricle. This bifrontal approach permits a panoramic, multidirectional dissection of the most adherent parts of the tumors, which can be manipulated anterior to the chiasm, through the lamina terminalis, and also through the opticocarotid space of both sides (Fig. 39–10). A further option is to drill the tuberculum sellae to improve the view into the sella (Fig. 39–11). Here, opened ethmoid cells do not present a problem because they can be covered with free muscle grafts or with the same galea-periosteal flap used to close the frontal sinuses. Fibrin glue is used as sealant.

## Transsphenoidal Approach

See Chapter 31 for a discussion of the trans-sphenoidal approach.

## Pterional Approach

The frontotemporal or pterional approach may be used alone or in combination with a transsphenoidal or transcallosal approach to remove large craniopharyngiomas.

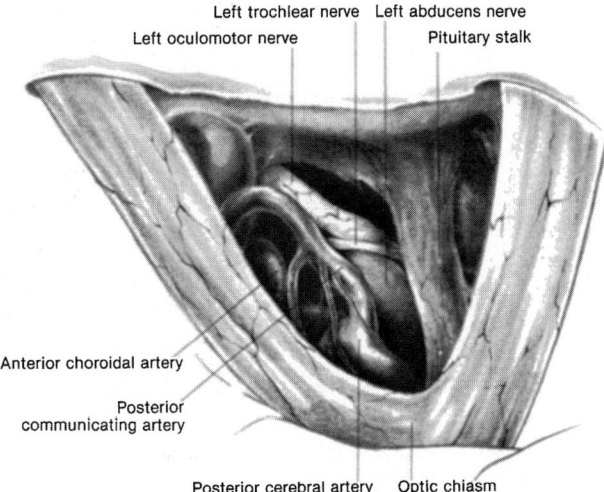

FIGURE 39–6 ■ Surgical cavity after the tumor has been removed. Microanatomy as viewed through the anterior angle of the optic chiasm. The pituitary stalk is intact. (From Samii M: Surgery of the Skull Base. Berlin: Springer-Verlag, 1989, p 277.)

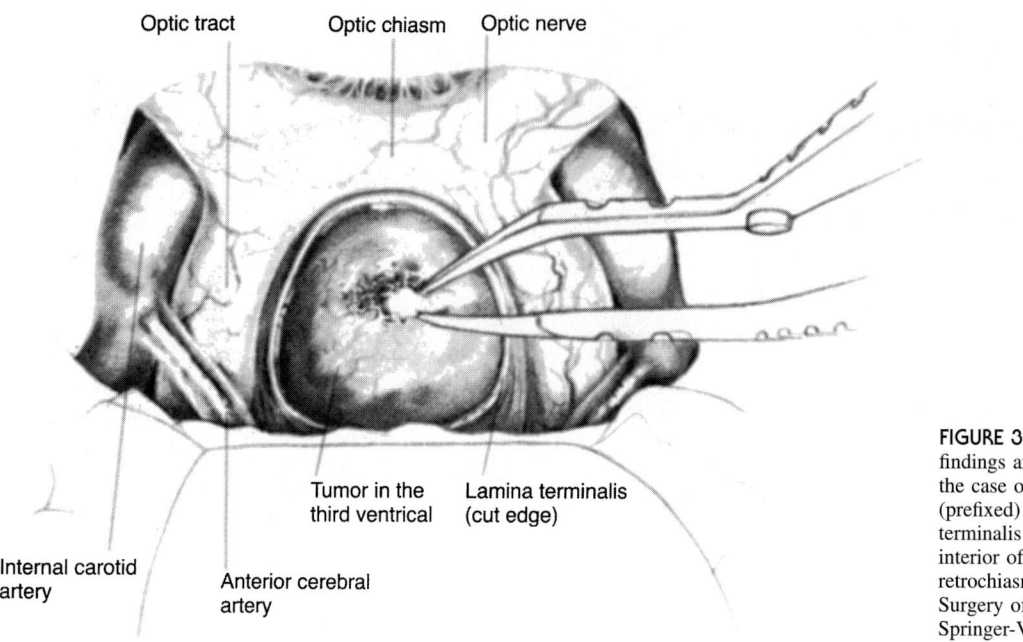

Optic tract    Optic chiasm    Optic nerve

Tumor in the          Lamina terminalis
third ventrical       (cut edge)

Internal carotid
artery

Anterior cerebral
artery

**FIGURE 39–7** ■ Intraoperative findings after a bifrontal craniotomy in the case of an anteriorly displaced (prefixed) optic chiasm. The lamina terminalis is opened for removal of the interior of the tumor through the retrochiasmal angle. (From Samii M: Surgery of the Skull Base. Berlin: Springer-Verlag, 1989, p 279.)

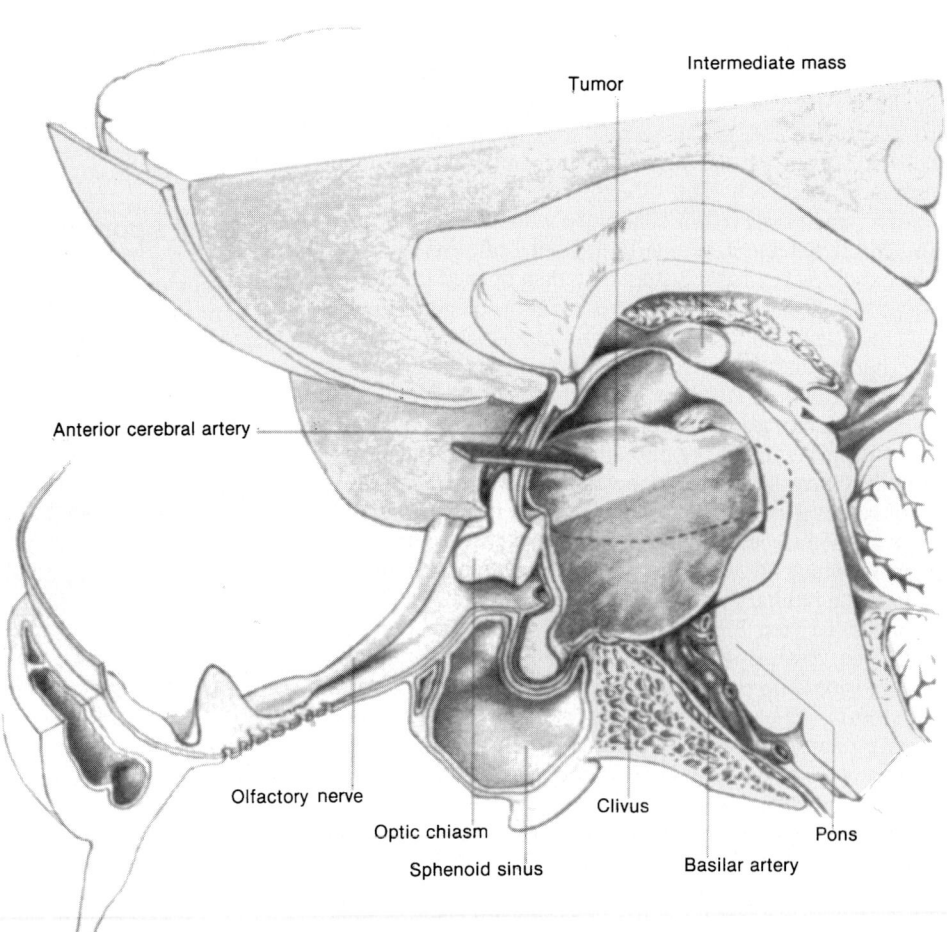

Tumor          Intermediate mass

Anterior cerebral artery

Olfactory nerve          Clivus

Optic chiasm          Pons

Sphenoid sinus          Basilar artery

**FIGURE 39–8** ■ Three-dimensional representation of the extent of the tumor in the transverse and sagittal planes, including the route of surgical access. (From Samii M: Surgery of the Skull Base. Berlin: Springer-Verlag, 1989, p 280.)

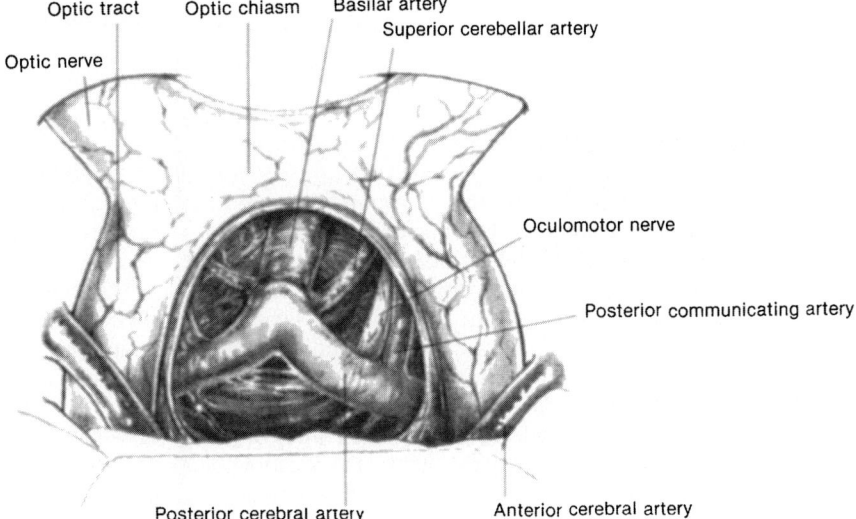

**FIGURE 39–9** ■ View into the prepontine space showing the microsurgical anatomy after the tumor has been removed through the lamina terminalis. (From Samii M: Surgery of the Skull Base. Berlin: Springer-Verlag, 1989, p 280.)

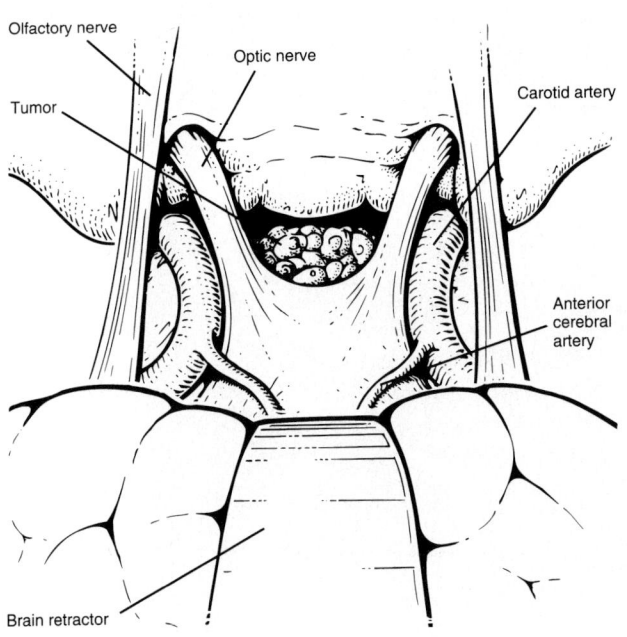

**FIGURE 39–10** ■ Intraoperative picture after a bifrontal craniotomy, and exposure of the sellar region in a patient with a craniopharyngioma.

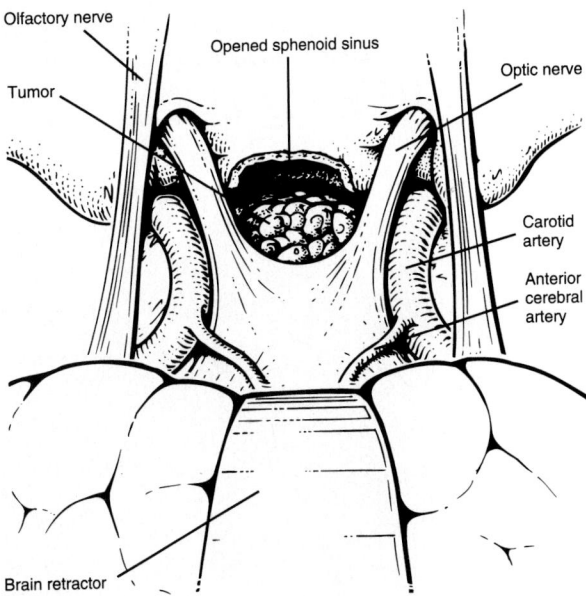

**FIGURE 39–11** ■ Intraoperative finding in the case of a prefixed optic chiasm in which the tuberculum sellae is removed and the sphenoid sinus is seen.

A frontotemporal craniotomy is performed. The lower margin of the opening has to be positioned well in relation to the floor of the middle cranial fossa. The tumor is dissected in the parachiasmal spaces such as the prechiasmatic, opticocarotid, and carotidotentorial spaces, the triangle superior to the carotid bifurcation, and through the opening of the lamina terminalis.[14] The technique of tumor removal is the same as that used with the subfrontal approach.

## Transcallosal Approach

Transcallosal exposure is possible through a small paramedian frontal craniotomy. The posterior margin of the craniotomy is just behind the coronal suture line. The dural flap is turned over the superior sagittal sinus, and the approach is made along the falx with minimal lateral retraction of the frontal lobe away from the falx. The corpus callosum is exposed; it is usually very thin as a result of obstructive hydrocephalus. A transcallosal incision of approximately 2 cm is made between or just immediately lateral to the pericallosal arteries above the location of the foramen of Monro, 1 cm anterior to the interauricular line. This approach provides access into the lateral ventricles through the dilated foramen of Monro. The tumor capsule is easily visualized. Internal decompression of the tumor by aspiration of cystic contents and piecemeal removal of calcified parts is carried out. The fornix, the anterior commissure, the choroid plexus, the choroidal ar-

teries, and the veins of the wall and floor of the third ventricle are key structures to preserve to minimize iatrogenic morbidity.

# C A S E   R E P O R T S

## Case Report 1

A 12-year-old boy was referred to our department after having been operated on 3 years previously. Originally, he presented with deteriorating visual acuity and ataxia. A CT scan of the head revealed a suprasellar cystic tumor that was partly removed through a right frontal approach. This resulted in improvement of his visual acuity. The boy was able to return to bike riding.

Three years later, a physical examination at school detected a renewed deterioration of his visual acuity bilaterally. One month later, hyperphagia, hyperdipsia, drowsiness, headache, nausea, and discrete ataxia were evident. At our department, an endocrine screening confirmed an almost complete breakdown of the adrenotropic and gonadotropic function of the anterior lobe of the pituitary gland. The hormonal dysregulation was treated with compensatory endocrine substitution therapy. A CT scan revealed a large suprasellar cystic tumor occupying the entire third ventricle, with obstructive hydrocephalus (Fig. 39–12A). A shunt was placed, ameliorating the patient's nausea and headaches. One week later, a bifrontal

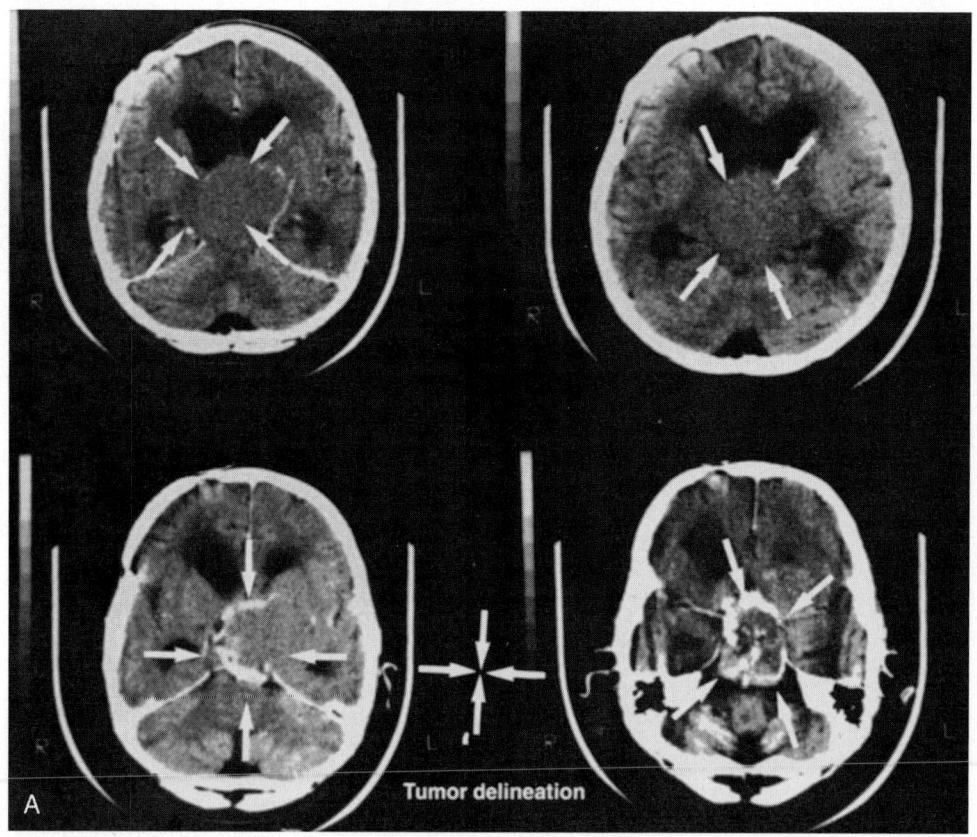

**FIGURE 39–12** ■ A 12-year-old boy (Case Report 1). *A*, A preoperative computed tomography scan (axial plane) demonstrating a large solid, cystic, and calcified craniopharyngioma with occlusion—hydrocephalus and periventricular edema. Condition after right frontal craniotomy.

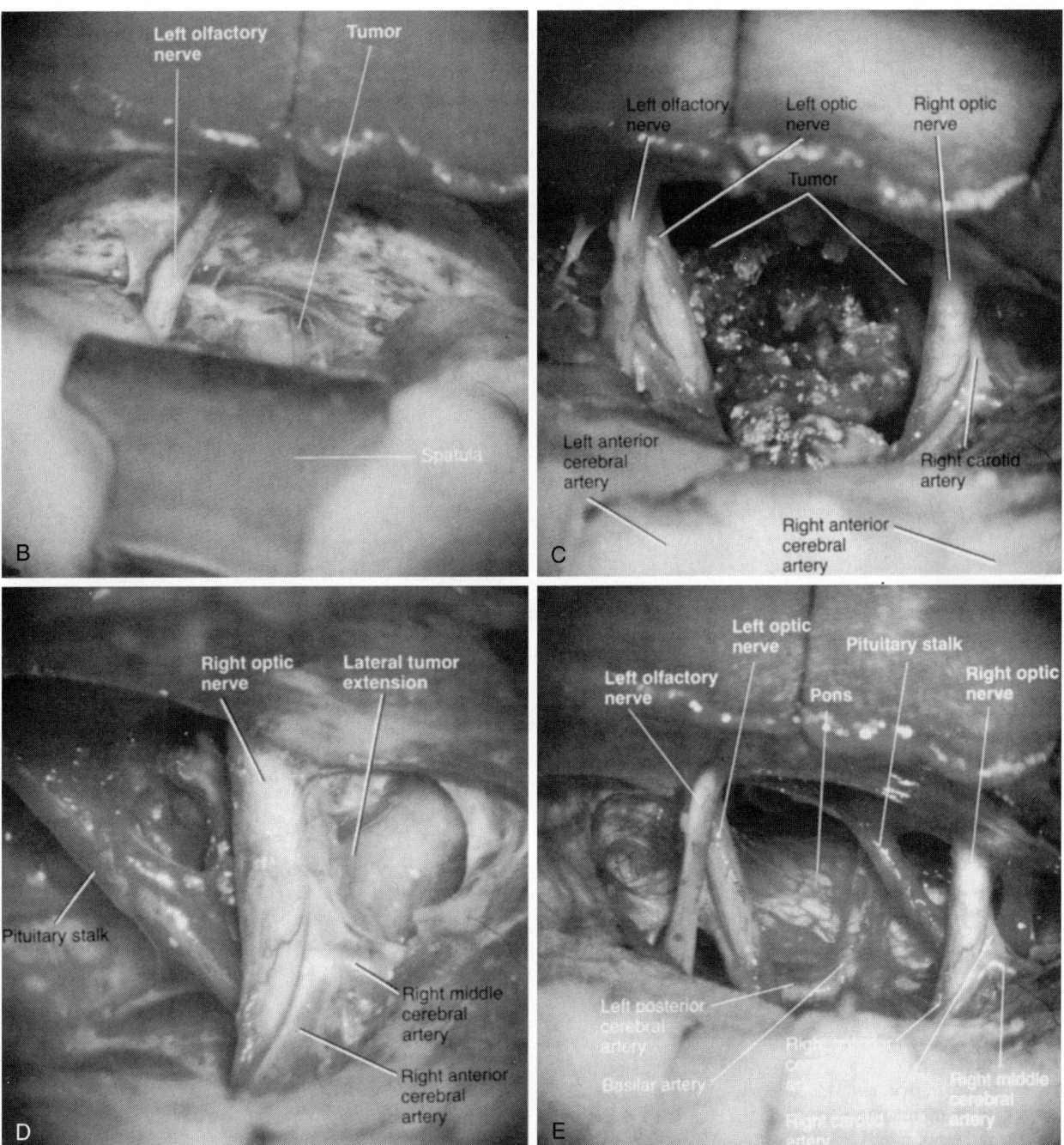

**FIGURE 39–12 ■** *Continued. B,* Intraoperative findings after a bifrontal craniotomy opening of the dura, and ligation and transection of the superior sagittal sinus. The right olfactory nerve was sacrificed during the first operation; the left olfactory nerve is preserved and exposed. The brain spatula is retracting the frontal lobe; the anterior part of the tumor is visible. *C,* The intraoperative picture after partial removal of the tumor. Both optic nerves are freed from the tumor's tissue. The right carotid, middle cerebral, and anterior cerebral arteries are demonstrated. *D,* The parasellar extension of the tumor into the middle fossa as well as the preserved infundibulum are shown. *E,* The surgical site after total removal of the tumor. All surrounding structures are preserved (i.e., optic nerves, carotid artery, basilar artery and its branches, pituitary stalk, left olfactory nerve).

osteoplastic craniotomy was performed with preservation of the left olfactory nerve (the right olfactory nerve having been sacrificed at the first operation; see Fig. 39–12B, C). A large cystic tumor was completely removed, preserving the pituitary stalk (see Fig. 39–12D, E). After surgery, the patient's hormonal status did not recover and he was maintained on endocrine substitution therapy. The boy was discharged in good general condition and was able to resume his education.

### Case Report 2

A 50-year-old locksmith had complained of severe bifrontal headache for 2 years. He was often tired and lacking in motivation. For 1 year, he was hoarse and ataxic, and his visual acuity deteriorated predominantly in his left eye to the point where he could detect only outlines. Polydipsia, polyuria, and nocturia then developed. A CT scan revealed a suprasellar tumor, which was operated on through a subtemporal route. Abnormalities in the patient's vital signs during surgery prevented the surgeon from removing the tumor. The patient was referred to our department as an emergency case, and he was found to be somnolent and obese with panhypopituitarism. The patient was immediately treated with hormonal substitution and subsequently was operated on (Fig. 39–13A, B). Using a bifrontal approach with preservation of both olfactory nerves, the cystic parts of the tumor were aspirated and the tumor was removed radically, leaving the surrounding structures intact (see Fig. 39–13C). The patient's visual acuity did not improve after the operation. His postoperative diabetes insipidus was treated with desmopressin. Hormonal substitution therapy was continued, and the patient was discharged in a good general condition.

## MAJOR INTRAOPERATIVE COMPLICATIONS AND THEIR MANAGEMENT

Since the early 1980s, the subfrontal approach has been our approach of choice for removing craniopharyngiomas. The following remarks focus on this approach.

Starting with the skin incision, the surgeon must be careful to avoid damaging the frontal branch of the facial nerve. The scalp incision should be positioned no more than 1 cm anterior to the tragus. In detaching the scalp from the orbital rim, the supraorbital nerve has to be identified, the supraorbital foramen should be opened, and the supraorbital nerve should be moved slightly downward, to prevent damaging the nerve(s) during the craniotomy.

The frontal sinus, if opened, should be exenterated to prevent formation of a mucocele. If there is a bleeding tendency or oozing into the frontal sinus, the opening to the nasal cavity should be enlarged to provide optimal drainage and reduce the risk of a postoperative hematoma in the frontal sinus area.

After the dura is opened, very careful handling is abso-

lutely requisite for the preservation of the olfactory nerves during microsurgery. The surgeon must refrain from manipulating the nerves directly. He or she should dissect only the arachnoid around the nerve and not coagulate feeding vessels. Extreme caution with the aspiration and suction instrument is advisable because this cranial nerve is particularly vulnerable to injury.

The following aspects minimize the risk of iatrogenic cerebral contusion:

- The patient should be shunted before surgery if hydrocephalus is present.
- The patient should receive adequate hormonal substitution therapy.
- Neuroanesthesiologic "brain relaxation" techniques are used during the intervention.
- The frontal craniotomy must provide an optimal view to the skull base without shifting and compressing the forebrain unnecessarily.
- The exposure of the anterior fossa should be performed stepwise with increasing CSF drainage so that the frontal lobe can fall back gently with minimum compression.

In the microsurgical era, iatrogenic lesions of the optic nerve and optic pathway are preventable. First, the surgeon enucleates the tumor through removal of solid parts or puncture of the cyst before dissection of the tumor capsule is started along the optic pathway. The same principle is also applicable to handling of vessels around the tumor, especially small-caliber vessels. An optimal postoperative outcome depends on preservation of the perforating vessels, particularly the perforators of the thalamus and hypothalamus.

In some cases, the pituitary stalk can be identified and preserved. Hypothalamic disturbances may occur if very large craniopharyngiomas engulf or infiltrate the pituitary stalk so that it cannot be identified early during surgery. Any pulling or pressure on the pituitary stalk can result in traction to the hypothalamus, which can produce lesions with severe postoperative complications, either through direct damage of the parenchyma or through microvascular rupture. Therefore, it is important that after the basic enucleation, a systematic exposure and resection of the tumor capsule are performed with utmost attention to identification of the pituitary stalk.

## POSTOPERATIVE MANAGEMENT

The most common postoperative complications in the management of craniopharyngioma are of endocrine origin. The following deficits are often observed: GH (95%), TSH (90%), ACTH (75%), and LH/FSH (95%). Diabetes insipidus occurs in 70% of patients.[18] All hormonal deficiencies are treated with replacement medication.

The incidence of postoperative hypothalamic syndromes such as hypersomnia, temperature dysregulation, profound amnesia, and disturbances of water, electrolyte, and caloric balance has been tremendously improved by the incorporation of microsurgical techniques. These syndromes do not result primarily from a direct iatrogenic trauma to this region, but rather from rupture or coagulation of the small

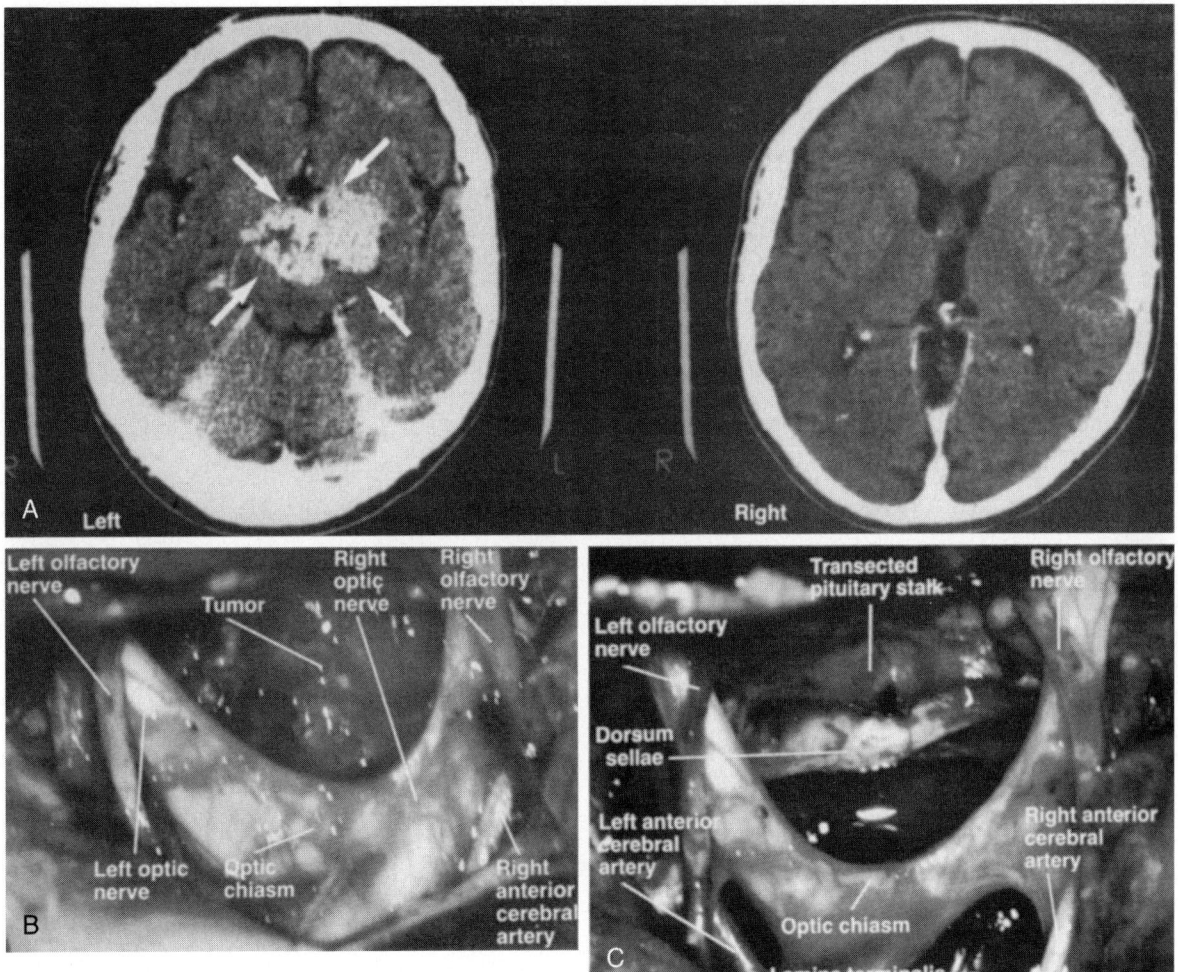

**FIGURE 39–13** ■ A 50-year-old man (Case Report 2). *A,* Preoperative (*left*) and postoperative (*right*) computed tomography scans (axial plane) of a large suprasellar, intraventricular craniopharyngioma. The arrows indicate tumor extension. *B,* Surgical exposure demonstrating both olfactory and optic nerves, the optic chiasm, and the anterior portion of the tumor. *C,* Intraoperative findings after total removal of the tumor. One can see the retrochiasmal opening of the lamina terminalis, both anterior cerebral arteries, diaphragma sellae with transected pituitary stalk, dorsum sellae, and both preserved olfactory nerves.

but important peritumoral vessels feeding the thalamus and hypothalamus.

## RECURRENT CRANIOPHARYNGIOMAS

Patients with recurrent craniopharyngiomas represent a substantial group who have initially undergone subtotal operations, and finally have to be operated on again because the tumor has progressed. These patients invariably return with worsening, recurrent, or new symptoms.

Subtotally resected tumors show a recurrence rate of 57%, whereas those that have been resected totally have a recurrence rate of 19%. A combined therapy of subtotal surgery and postoperative irradiation results in a recurrence rate of 29%. Most of the recurrences appear during the first 3 years after initial treatment.[18]

Radical reoperation in craniopharyngiomas has a higher morbidity rate because the tumor may be more adherent to the surrounding structures.[26] However, recurrent cases should be operated on radically, if possible, by an experienced surgeon to give the patient the best chance for a cure if his or her general condition is suitable for surgery. If not, cystic puncture with radionuclide implantation or radiation therapy should be considered in those patients in whom medical or surgical steps (e.g., shunting and hormone replacement) cannot achieve a stable and suitable condition for open microsurgical removal.

## RESULTS

The overall 10-year post-treatment survival rate for craniopharyngiomas is 92.5% after total removal and 85.6% after subtotal removal (if radiation therapy is combined with subtotal removal, the survival rate improves to 90%).[18]

Yasargil and colleagues[14] achieved total removal in 90% of 144 patients. In tumors smaller than 2 cm, the outcome was good (improved, totally independent) in 93% of patients. In intermediate-sized tumors (2 to 4 cm), 82.1% of patients were given a good postoperative rank. Of patients harboring large tumors (4 to 6 cm), 65% had a good outcome. Giant (>6 cm) craniopharyngiomas had a "good" result in only 12.5% of patients.

The following data from Yasargil and colleagues' series[14] suggest that primary surgery has a significantly better outcome than secondary surgery. In children, the clinical outcome was good in 72.5% after primary surgery, whereas after secondary surgery, only 31.6% of the children were in good condition. In adults, the clinical outcome was good in 80.3% after primary surgery, whereas the results after secondary surgery were good in only 38.5% of the patients.[14]

Regarding ophthalmologic outcome, Cabezudo and associates[27] showed that the prognosis for improvement of preoperative visual deficits is related to the preoperative symptoms. In patients in whom symptoms existed for less than 1 year, 87% had improved vision, whereas in patients in whom symptoms existed for more than 1 year, only 33% experienced visual improvement after surgery.

After surgical treatment, the endocrine status of these patients is often worse. Thirty-three percent of patients become obese, 70% have diabetes insipidus, and 33% of the pediatric patients undergo paradoxical spontaneous growth during some months. Hormonal deficits are usually observed as follows: GH (95%), TSH (90%), ACTH (75%), and LH/FSH (95%).[18]

Postoperative neuropsychological disorders occur in 30% to 60% of children.[18] Pierre-Kahn and colleagues[28] noted that social integration of children after therapy without radiation is normal in 88% of patients, whereas after radiation therapy (either alone or combined with surgery), it is normal in only 22% of patients.

"Giant" craniopharyngiomas are especially difficult to remove surgically and are associated with rates of postoperative morbidity and mortality of up to 87.5%.[14]

Between 1984 and 1991, 10 giant craniopharyngiomas (with a maximum diameter of over 5 cm) were surgically removed at our institution (Table 39–1). The age of these patients ranged from 1 to 48 years (mean age of 15.4 years). All patients showed massive vertical extension of a retrochiasmal tumor occupying the third ventricle. Six were grade V (vertical growth up to the septum pellucidum or into the lateral ventricle), and four were grade IV (vertical growth up to the upper half of the third ventricle). As for the additional subgroups, there was one patient with lateral expansion to the middle fossa; one with posterior fossa expansion; two with lateral expansion to the middle fossa and posterior fossa expansion; one with anterior prechiasmal expansion, lateral expansion to the middle fossa, and posterior fossa expansion; one with infrasellar sphenoid expansion and lateral expansion to the middle fossa; and two with anterior prechiasmal expansion and lateral expansion to the middle fossa.

The lamina terminalis route was used in eight patients through a bilateral subfrontal approach. In one patient, an extended pterional approach combined with a presigmoid exposure was chosen for massive posterior fossa expansion. In another patient, a transsphenoidal exposure was used for an infrasellar extension. The tumors were totally removed in seven patients who underwent primary radical surgery; total resection could not be achieved in two of three recurrent giant tumors, resulting in subtotal resections. There was no postoperative mortality among these patients, and

## TABLE 39–1 ■ PRINCIPAL CLINICAL SIGNS AND SYMPTOMS OF 10 GIANT CRANIOPHARYNGIOMAS

| Age (yr) Sex | Preoperative Signs/Symptoms (Time of Onset of First Sign Before Diagnosis) | Visual Field | | Preoperative Endocrine Status | Postoperative Endocrine Substitution |
| | | Pre-operative | Post-operative | | |
| --- | --- | --- | --- | --- | --- |
| 11 f | Tiredness, apathy, nausea, vertigo, vomiting (3 wk) | Left:  B Right: B | Left:  B Right: B | Normal | Corticoids, thyroxines, DDAVP |
| 17 f | Headache, tiredness, vomiting, forgetfulness, amenorrhea (remission with glycerol therapy), double vision (5 mo) | Left:  A Right: B | Left:  A Right: A | Estradiol ↓ | Corticoids, thyroxines, DDAVP |
| 8 f | Tiredness, sleep disturbance, headache, vomiting, inappetence, oculomotor palsy (1 yr) | Left:  B Right: B | Left:  B Right: B | Substitutions*: DDAVP, corticoids, thyroxine | Corticoids, thyroxines, DDAVP |
| 11 m | Headache (5 mo) | Left:  A Right: B | Left:  A Right: B | Normal | Corticoids, thyroxines, DDAVP |
| 4 f | Inappetence, drop attacks, excitation, loss of weight, hemiparesis on entire right side (2 yr) | Left:  D Right: C | Left:  D Right: B | Substitutions*: thyroxines, DDAVP | Corticoids, thyroxines, DDAVP |
| 2 m | Ataxia, reduced general status, hydrocephalus (4 mo) | Left:  D Right: D | Left:  D Right: D | Corticoids ↑ | Corticoids, DDAVP |
| 10 m | Severe headache, vertigo, vomiting, cushingoid appearance (1 yr) | Left:  A Right: A | Left:  A Right: A | Growth hormone ↓, corticoids ↓ | Corticoids, thyroxines, DDAVP |
| 48 f | Severe temporal visual field defect on the right eye (3 mo) | Left:  A Right: D | Left:  A Right: D | Substitutions*: thyroxines, corticoids | Corticoids, thyroxines, estradiol |
| 38 f | Headache, drowsiness, vomiting, amnesia (since 1 wk before operation) (2 mo) | Left:  A Right: A | Left:  A Right: A | Luteinizing hormone ↓, follicle-stimulating hormone ↓, estradiol ↓ | Corticoids, thyroxines |
| 8 f | Headache, vomiting, vertigo, tiredness (6 mo) | Left:  B Right: C | Left:  B Right: C | Normal | Corticoids, thyroxines, DDAVP |

*Patient previously had a subtotal operation elsewhere.

A, Normal; B, slight deficit (+); C, moderate–accentuated deficit (+ +); D, blind; DDAVP, 1-deamino (8-D-arginine) vasopressin.

all survived in the mean follow-up period of 6.5 years (2 to 9.5 years) without recurrence.

## SUMMARY

At the turn of the century, radical excision of craniopharyngiomas is considered the method of choice, delivering the best outcome for the patient without sacrificing functional outcome.[11–13, 29–33]

What hurdles may make total excision impossible? The effectiveness of an attempt at total removal can be evaluated by three factors: morbidity, recurrence, and mortality. These three points are conditioned by three objective and one very individual aspect. The three objective conditioners are size (e.g., which structures are involved?), the consistency of the tumor, and the adhesions between the tumor and the surrounding structures (e.g., calcified adhesion to the carotid artery or optic pathway). Nevertheless, the fundamental variable is the skill and experience of the surgeon. The optimal surgical approach for the removal of craniopharyngiomas is clearly influenced by the surgeon's experience.[19, 34–42] A good approach for tumor removal through real or potential spaces must allow a good overview and control of nearby vital neurovascular structures throughout the procedure.[40, 42, 43] The subfrontal approach and primarily the bifrontal exposure with sparing of the olfactory nerves allow an unobstructed access to subfrontal extensions, controlling both optic nerves and both internal carotid arteries. Furthermore, the retrochiasmatic component may be removed by opening the lamina terminalis or by working in the opticocarotid space, or both. The advantage of opening the lamina terminalis is that the surgeon may carefully excise that part of the tumor in its retrochiasmatic location at the level of the third ventricle. Based on our experience, even large tumors can be approached through a subfrontal route without an increased rate of morbidity or postoperative complications. The surgical anatomy encountered allows good visualization of the area. Through the different spaces or portals, complete removal of the tumor is possible.

The other main surgical approaches are the transsphenoidal route, the subtemporal or extended pterional approach, the transventricular route, and the transpetrosal-transtentorial exposure.

The transsphenoidal route is the approach of choice for grade I and II craniopharyngiomas. Low surgical morbidity and improvement of preoperative visual field deficits and hyperprolactinemia have been reported.[44] If suprasellar calcifications are found, complete tumor removal is unlikely, and a subfrontal approach is necessary to accomplish as complete an excision as possible. Special attention must be given to avoid trauma to the optic nerves and the chiasm. Tumors with significant suprasellar extension and attachments to the optic chiasm, hypothalamus, and vascular structures should not be approached by the transsphenoidal route.

The pterional, or frontotemporal approach, allows better exposure of the interopticocarotid space, and if it is extended posteriorly and combined with a superior retraction of the temporal lobe, it may expose somewhat better the

lateral tumor portion in the space between the third cranial nerve and the posterior communicating artery inferiorly and the optic tract superiorly. However, with regard to morbidity, third nerve palsies are not rare; fluctuating hemiparesis resulting from involvement of the intrinsic vascular hemispheric supply and homonymous visual field defects may occur. The transventricular route, which is an approach that descends from above, determines that the surgeon either must incise some cortical tissue or split a part of the corpus callosum and work at a considerable depth, passing the foramen of Monro.[45] This may constitute a handicap. Therefore, there is greater risk that the neurovascular structures (e.g., the optic nerve, the internal carotid artery, and the anterior cerebral artery) eventually may be engulfed and iatrogenic lesions may occur, especially during dissection of the tumor capsule.

By means of proper preoperative evaluation, microsurgical technique, prevention of hormone insufficiency, and maintenance of the fluid-electrolyte balance, cure can be achieved in this challenging and "baffling problem to neurosurgeons," as Cushing[46] described craniopharyngioma surgery in 1932.

Total removal of craniopharyngiomas as the method of choice should not be interpreted as "radicality by all means." Unnecessary risks should not be taken if unfavorable situations become evident during surgery. Neurosurgeons should refrain from planning a primary subtotal removal of the tumor with adjuvant radiation therapy. The overall recurrence rate for this type of combined therapy is approximately 29%, whereas the recurrence rate in totally resected craniopharyngiomas is 19%. Evidence indicates that reoperation of these recurrent tumors has the worst outcome in terms of morbidity and mortality (20.5%).[18]

A combined therapy of surgery and irradiation should be considered as a method of "second choice," reserved for extremely difficult cases in which total removal was attempted but could not be achieved.

## REFERENCES

1. Crotty TB, Scheithauer BW, Young WF, et al: Papillary craniopharyngioma: A clinicopathological study of 48 cases. J Neurosurg 83:206–214, 1995.
2. Zuccaro G, Jaimovich R, Mantese B, Monges J: Complications in paediatric craniopharyngioma treatment. Childs Nerv Syst 12:385–390, 1996.
3. Rajan B, Ashley S, Thomas DG, et al: Carniopharyngioma: Improving outcome by early recognition and treatment of acute complications. Int J Radiat Oncol Biol Phys 37:517–521, 1997.
4. Rougerie J: What can be expected from the surgical treatment of craniopharyngiomas in children? Report of 92 cases. Childs Brain 5:433–449, 1979.
5. Rougerie J, Raimondi AJ: Craniopharyngiomas. In Amador LV (ed): Brain Tumors in Young. Springfield, IL: Charles C Thomas, 1983, pp 599–618.
6. Pertuiset B: Craniopharyngiomas. In Vinken PJ, Bruyn GW (eds): Handbook of Clinical Neurology, Vol 18. Amsterdam: North Holland Publishing, 1975, pp 531–572.
7. Konovalov AN: Microsurgery of tumours of diencephalic region. Neurosurg Rev 6:37–41, 1983.
8. Kobayashi T: Recent progress in the treatment of craniopharyngioma. Neurosurgery 3:101–112, 1984.
9. Steno J: Microsurgical topography of craniopharyngiomas. Acta Neurochir (Wien) 35 (Suppl):94–100, 1985.
10. Hoffman HJ: Pediatric tumors—craniopharyngioma. In Long DM (ed): Current Therapy in Neurological Surgery. Philadelphia: BC Decker, 1989, pp 82–84.

11. Ammirati M, Samii M, Sephernia A: Surgery of large retrochiasmatic craniopharyngiomas in children. Childs Nerv Syst 6:13–17, 1990.
12. Bhagwati SN, Deopujari CE, Parulekar GD: Lamina terminalis approach for retrochiasmal craniopharyngiomas. Childs Nerv Syst 6:425–429, 1990.
13. Klein HJ, Rath SA: Removal of tumors in the third ventricle using the lamina terminalis approach: Three cases of isolated growth of craniopharyngiomas in the third ventricle. Childs Nerv Syst 5:144–147, 1979.
14. Yasargil MG, Curcic M, Kis M, et al: Total removal of craniopharyngiomas: Approaches and long-term results in 144 patients. J Neurosurg 73:3–11, 1990.
15. Raimondi AJ: Pediatric Neurosurgery. Berlin: Springer-Verlag, 1987, pp 277–291.
16. Symon L: Experiences with radical excision of craniopharyngioma. In Samii M (ed): Surgery of the Sellar Region and Paranasal Sinuses. Berlin: Springer-Verlag, 1991, pp 373–380.
17. Fu X, Wang H: Ocular symptoms of tumors at sella turcica region. Yen Ko Hsueh Pao 12:166–168, 1996.
18. Choux M, Lena G, Genitori L: Le craniopharyngiome de l'enfant. Neurochirurgie 37 (Suppl):1–174, 1991.
19. Samii M, Bini W: Surgical treatment of craniopharyngiomas. Zentralbl Neurochir 52:17–23, 1991.
20. Baba M, Iwayama S, Jimbo M, et al: Cystic craniopharyngioma extending down into the upper cervical spinal canal. No Shinkei Geka 6:687–693, 1978.
21. Fukushima T, Hirakawa K, Kimura M, et al: Intraventricular craniopharyngioma: Its characteristics in magnetic resonance imaging and successful total removal. Surg Neurol 33:22–27, 1990.
22. Iwasaki K, Kondo A, Takahashi JB: Intraventricular craniopharyngioma: Report of two cases and review of the literature. Surg Neurol 38:294–301, 1992.
23. Arwell WJ: The development of the hypophysis cerebri in man, with special reference to the pars tuberalis. Am J Anat 37:159–193, 1926.
24. Symon L, Sprich W: Radical excision of craniopharyngioma: Results in 20 patients. J Neurosurg 62:174–181, 1985.
25. Sutton LN, Gusnard D, Bruce DA, et al: Fusiform dilatations of the carotid artery following radical surgery of childhood craniopharyngiomas. J Neurosurg 74:695–700, 1991.
26. Konovalov AN: Microsurgery of craniopharyngiomas. In Rand RW (ed): Microneurosurgery, 3rd ed. St. Louis: CV Mosby, 1985, pp 196–213.
27. Cabezudo Artero JM, Vaquero Crespo J, Bravo G, et al: Status of vision following surgical treatment of craniopharyngiomas. Acta Neurochir (Wien) 73:165–177, 1984.
28. Pierre-Khan A, Brauner R, Renier D, et al: Traitement des craniopharyngiomes de l'enfant: Analyse retrospective de 50 observation. Arch Fr Pediatr 45:163–167, 1988.
29. Hoffman HJ, Hendrick ZB, Humphreyes RP, et al: Management of craniopharyngioma in children. J Neurosurg 47:218–227, 1977.
30. Sweet WH: Radical surgical treatment of craniopharyngioma. Clin Neurosurg 23:52–70, 1976.
31. Weiner HL, Wishoff JH, Rosenberg ME, et al: Craniopharyngiomas: A clinicopathological analysis of factors predictive of recurrence and functional outcome. Neurosurgery 35:1001–1010, 1994.
32. Anderson CA, Wilkening GN, Filley CM, et al: Neurobehavioral outcome in pediatric craniopharyngioma. Pediatr Neurosurg 26:255–260, 1997.
33. Honegger J, Barocka A, Sadri B, Fahlbusch R: Neuropsychological results of craniopharyngioma surgery in adults: A prospective study. Surg Neurol 50:19–28, 1998.
34. Fujitsu K, Kuwabara T: Zygomatic approach for lesions in the interpeduncular cistern. J Neurosurg 62:340–343, 1985.
35. Hakuba A, Nishimura S, Inove Y: Transpetrosal-transtentorial approach and its application in the therapy of retrochiasmatic craniopharyngiomas. Surg Neurol 24:405–415, 1985.
36. Kobayashi T, Nakane T, Kageyama N: Combined trans-sphenoidal and intracranial surgery for craniopharyngioma. Prog Exp Tumor Res 30:341–349, 1987.
37. Konig A, Lüdecke DK, Hermann HD: Transnasal surgery in the treatment of craniopharyngiomas. Acta Neurochir (Wien) 83:1–7, 1986.
38. Laws ER: Transsphenoidal microsurgery in the management of craniopharyngioma. J Neurosurg 52:661–666, 1980.
39. Long DM, Leibrock L: The transcallosal approach to the anterior ventricular system and its application in the therapy of craniopharyngiomas. Clin Neurosurg 27:160–168, 1980.
40. Mori T, Kodoma N, Takaku A, et al: Bifrontal approach for craniopharyngioma, and postoperative follow-up study. Acta Neurochir (Wien) 51:138–144, 1979.
41. Bini W, Sepehrnia A, Samii M: Some technical considerations regarding craniopharyngioma surgery: The bifrontal approach. In Samii M (ed): Surgery of the Sellar Region and Paranasal Sinuses. Berlin: Springer-Verlag, 1991, pp 373–380.
42. Shillito J: Craniopharyngiomas: The subfrontal approach, or none at all? Clin Neurosurg 27:188–205, 1980.
43. Suzuki J, Katakura R, Mori T: Interhemispheric approach through the lamina terminalis to tumors of the anterior part of the third ventricle. Surg Neurol 22:157–163, 1984.
44. Honegger J, Buchfelder M, Fahlbusch R, et al: Transsphenoidal microsurgery for craniopharyngioma. Surg Neurol 37:189–196, 1992.
45. King TT: Removal of intraventricular craniopharyngiomas through the lamina terminalis. Acta Neurochir (Wien) 45:277–284, 1979.
46. Cushing H: Intracranial Tumors: Notes upon a Series of Two Thousand Verified Cases with Surgical-Mortality Percentages Pertaining Thereto. Springfield, IL: Charles C Thomas, 1932, pp 93–98.

# Transsphenoidal Microsurgery for Craniopharyngioma

■ RUDOLF FAHLBUSCH, JÜRGEN HONEGGER, and MICHAEL BUCHFELDER

The history of transsphenoidal surgery for craniopharyngioma is almost as old as the history of the transsphenoidal approach itself. Two years after the first transnasal removal of a pituitary adenoma by Schloffer in 1907, Halstead[1] performed a successful transsphenoidal operation for a craniopharyngioma. In 1932, however, Cushing[2] critically reviewed his own series of 14 craniopharyngiomas treated by transsphenoidal surgery. In view of the unsatisfying outcome, he considered this approach for craniopharyngiomas a therapeutic mistake. After Cushing had abandoned the transsphenoidal operation, the tradition of transsphenoidal surgery was continued by Norman Dott and by Oscar Hirsch. Hirsch,[3] working originally in Vienna and later in Boston, reported on 12 transsphenoidal operations for craniopharyngiomas. Surgical results had improved with the advent of antibiotic therapy and steroid replacement. In 1967, Hamlin[4] from Stockholm advocated transsphenoidal surgery for craniopharyngiomas and reported on long-term cures in his series covering 1946 to 1966. With the advances in microsurgical operating technique and the x-ray image intensifier introduced by Guiot and Hardy in Paris in the 1960s, transsphenoidal surgery revived and spread throughout the world. Now, selective tumor removal was feasible.

The use of the transsphenoidal approach for diseases other than pituitary adenomas was still being questioned, however. Hardy and colleagues[5, 6] showed that transsphenoidal surgery of craniopharyngioma is possible even in giant craniopharyngioma without major morbidity. In 1980, Laws[7] reviewed the large Mayo Clinic experience, delineated the indications and limitations of the approach, and detailed his surgical technique. He demonstrated that complete excision is possible in a high percentage of cases during a transsphenoidal procedure with low morbidity and mortality.[7, 8] Today, 30% to 40% of patients with craniopharyngiomas undergo transsphenoidal operations.[9, 10]

## PREOPERATIVE EVALUATION

In addition to the clinical examination, the preoperative evaluation is based on endocrinologic, ophthalmologic, and neuroradiologic investigations.

## Endocrinologic Evaluation

Most of our patients who underwent transsphenoidal surgery for craniopharyngioma presented with endocrine symptoms, although panhypopituitarism was a relatively rare finding. Sophisticated endocrinologic evaluation is important for adequate perioperative management. Perioperative hydrocortisone replacement is imperative in cases of an insufficient hypothalamic-pituitary-adrenal axis. If hypothyroidism is diagnosed, patients undergoing elective surgery should first be started on replacement therapy and should be in euthyroid state at the time of surgery to reduce the risk of surgery. Delayed puberty and growth retardation are characteristic endocrinologic symptoms in children with craniopharyngiomas. The finding of diabetes insipidus suggests a craniopharyngioma. The presence of diabetes insipidus is therefore helpful in the differential diagnosis, but preoperative diabetes insipidus was found in 23% of all our cases, and in only 2.9% of our transsphenoidal cases.[10]

## Ophthalmologic Evaluation

Ophthalmologic assessment includes visual acuity and visual field examination (Goldmann perimetry or computerized perimetry). Funduscopy may show optic atrophy. Oculomotor nerve function is assessed by clinical examination. Careful ophthalmologic examination is necessary to distinguish chiasmal syndrome from frequently found independent eye disease.

## Neuroradiologic Evaluation

Magnetic resonance imaging (MRI), the imaging technique of choice, depicts tumor size and configuration. It is the only imaging technique that precisely shows the relationship of the craniopharyngioma to the surrounding structures. Plain skull radiographs are still very helpful for showing the size of the pituitary fossa, bony erosions, and calcifications. Computed tomography (CT) is used to assess further the extent of calcifications of a craniopharyngioma. The localization of vessels is shown by MRI in a two-dimensional plane. MRI angiography provides information about the course and the relationship of vessels. For differential diagnosis, its demonstration of large aneurysms is particularly important. Aneurysms may be calcified and, therefore, may be mistaken for craniopharyngiomas; however, small aneurysms cannot be reliably demonstrated by MRI angiography. Arterial digital subtraction angiography is performed in patients who had prior surgery for the craniopharyngioma. This technique provides a more precise angiogram and may show small iatrogenic aneurysms that can result from prior surgery.

## INDICATIONS FOR A TRANSSPHENOIDAL APPROACH

For intrasellar craniopharyngiomas, the only practicable approach is the transsphenoidal route. The transsphenoidal approach is also appropriate for craniopharyngiomas with intrasellar and suprasellar extension if the neuroradiologic and ophthalmologic evaluations suggest an infradiaphragmatic location. A smooth, well-circumscribed, symmetric suprasellar extension suggests an infradiaphragmatic location of a tumor arising from the pituitary fossa. A subdiaphragmatic location is suspected if a chiasmal pattern of visual fields defects with bitemporal hemianopia is detected, whereas atypical visual field defects suggest a supradiaphragmatic extension of the craniopharyngioma.

Sellar enlargement indicates that the tumor originates within the pituitary fossa. Enlargement of the pituitary fossa by the tumor has been considered a critical feature allowing for transsphenoidal management.[7] In our experience, however, the pituitary fossa is only slightly enlarged in most subdiaphragmatic craniopharyngiomas. The sella turcica may even be normal in craniopharyngiomas that

arise from the pituitary fossa.[10, 12] In our opinion, the transsphenoidal approach for subdiaphragmatic craniopharyngioma is not precluded by the presence of a normal sella, unless there is an obvious discrepancy between a small intrasellar portion and a large suprasellar portion of tumor. The criteria for using a transsphenoidal approach are often the same as in pituitary adenomas, particularly because the precise pathologic classification of the lesion is commonly unclear before surgery. Pituitary adenoma and Rathke's cyst are common differential diagnoses. In our series of 35 patients with craniopharyngiomas undergoing primary transsphenoidal surgery, features highly suggestive of a craniopharyngioma, such as diabetes insipidus (8 patients) and neuroradiologic evidence of calcifications (6 patients), were found in only a minority of cases.

Since 1983, we have operated on 50 craniopharyngiomas by the transsphenoidal route among 168 patients undergoing surgery for craniopharyngiomas (including stereotactic cyst drainage). The total series of the first author consists of 60 transsphenoidal operations for craniopharyngiomas. Since the mid-1970s, large infradiaphragmatic and supradiaphragmatic craniopharyngiomas have been operated on using a two-stage transcranial and transsphenoidal procedure for complete resection.

Secondary transsphenoidal surgery is indicated for a recurrent or residual tumor after a prior transcranial or transsphenoidal operation. A secondary transsphenoidal approach may also be used for palliation in advanced disease for tumor debulking or for cyst drainage.

## SURGICAL TECHNIQUE

The routine transsphenoidal technique used in our department is described here in detail. We point out the general

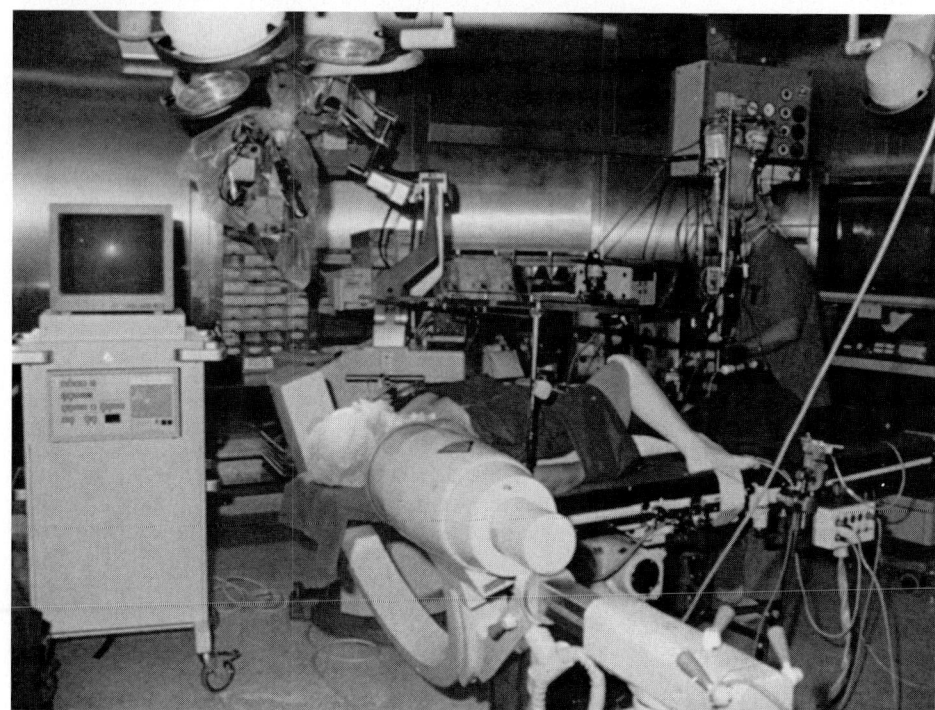

FIGURE 40–1 ■ Arrangement of the equipment in the operating room and positioning of the patient.

principles of the approach that are similar in different centers despite slight technical variations.

Approach and tumor removal are illustrated by intraoperative photographs from a patient who had an intrasellar and suprasellar craniopharyngioma. Explanatory drawings are added.

## Approach

In general, we use a sublabial, unilateral rhinoseptal approach although pernasal paraseptal and direct pernasal approaches to the wall of the sphenoid sinus also are performed increasingly. Following Cushing's original method, the patient is positioned supine (Fig. 40–1). The head is positioned straight along the body axis and then slightly tilted downward (10 to 15 degrees). Before final draping, the vestibulum oris and the nasal mucosa are infiltrated with ornipressin solution diluted in saline. The surgeon stands behind the patient's head and the assistant to the left side. First, the upper lip is retracted with a small Langenbeck retractor (Fig. 40–2A). A horizontal 3- to 4-mm mucosal incision is made approximately 5 mm from the mucosal reflection at the vestibulum oris on the inside of the upper lip. Next, the soft tissue is gently stripped off just above the anterior surface of the cartilaginous nasal septum and the anterior nasal spine, and a perpendicular incision of the perichondrium of the cartilaginous septum is made. Careful dissection with a sharp rasp is necessary

to find a cleavage plane between cartilage and perichondrium (see Fig. 40–2B). A mucosal tunnel can be created easily with the dissector with low risk of tearing the mucosa only in this layer. Next, the ligaments between the cartilaginous septum, the anterior spine of the maxilla, and the mucosa are carefully incised to extend the mucosal tunnel down to the medial inferior border of the piriform aperture. The anterior maxillary spine is resected with a rongeur. A diamond drill is useful to occlude bleeding from bone arteries. Once the basal cartilaginous septum is mobilized, it is gently pushed to the opposite side. At this stage, a small conical retractor (Cushing type) is inserted, and the operating microscope is used.

A mucosal corridor is created by enlarging the mucosal tunnel down to the sphenoid sinus, the direction of the exposure being guided by x-ray image intensifier. The cartilage is bluntly separated from the bony nasal septum, and the mucosa is detached from the bony septum on both sides with a microdissector. Within this corridor, the bony nasal septum is removed with a straight forceps. The floor of the sphenoid sinus is exposed (Fig. 40–3A, B). The sphenoid sinus is opened with the diamond drill. The opening can be enlarged with a rongeur or with the drill just beyond the blades of the self-retaining retractor. At this stage, a larger retractor (Hardy-type speculum) is inserted to allow a wider opening of the blades. The blades of the retractor must be placed just outside the sphenoid sinus to prevent fractures and should be opened gently. Opening of the retractor is facilitated with increasing opening of the

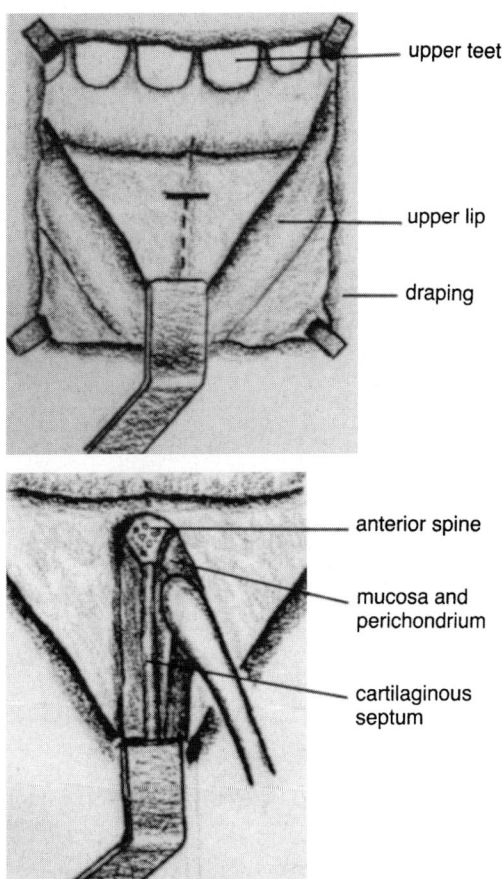

FIGURE 40–2 ■ *A,* Retraction of the upper lip. The *straight horizontal line* indicates a skin incision; the *broken line* signifies the direction of blunt dissection. *B,* Unilateral dissection of the mucosal tunnel.

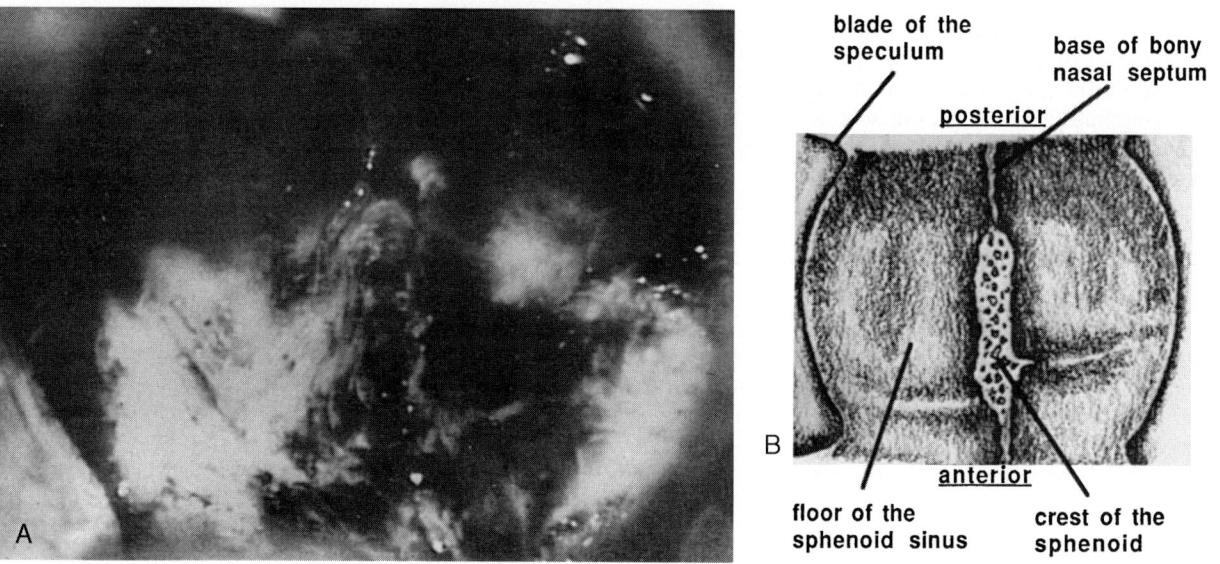

FIGURE 40–3 ■ *A* and *B*, Exposure of the floor of the sphenoid sinus.

sinus. A wide opening of the sphenoid sinus (Fig. 40–4) is crucial for sufficient illumination of the surgical field. Ideally, an overview from the planum sphenoidale to the middle clivus is provided (Fig. 40–5*A*, *B*). The mucosa of the sphenoid sinus is removed (see Fig. 40–4). If the sphenoid sinus is poorly pneumatized, the outline of the sella must be exposed by drilling away the sphenoid bone. Poor pneumatization of the sphenoid bone is mainly a problem in the dorsal portion of the sphenoid, requiring bone removal until the sella is fully exposed. Reduced or missing pneumatization of the sphenoid, as found in children, is not a contraindication to the transsphenoidal approach. The sellar floor is opened with an air drill in the midline, and resection is completed with rongeurs to the medial wall of the cavernous sinus, to the reflection at the clivus, and close to the anterior fossa (see Fig. 40–4 and Fig. 40–6*A*, *B*). Again, a large opening is imperative.

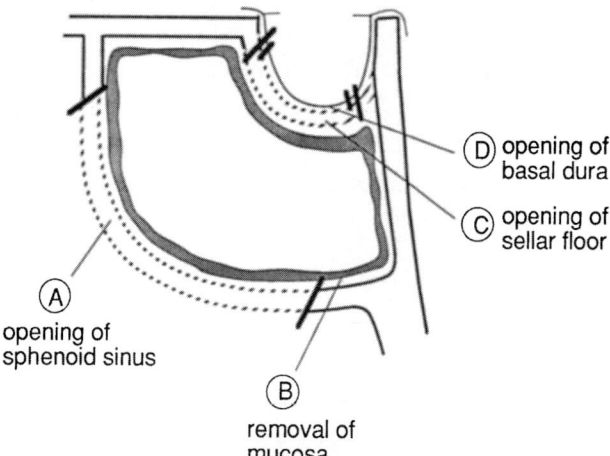

FIGURE 40–4 ■ The midline section demonstrates the successive steps of the approach and the extent of resection of the anatomic structures. *A*, Opening of the sphenoid sinus. *B*, Removal of the mucosa from the sphenoid sinus. *C*, Opening of the sellar floor. *D*, Opening of the basal dura.

The dura is opened with microscissors in a cruciate manner, and the dura retracts by coagulation (see Fig. 40–4).

## Tumor Removal

Once the basal dura is widely opened, the sellar content is exposed. Different locations of the pituitary gland are encountered: the pituitary gland may be compressed anterior to the craniopharyngioma (Figs. 40–7 and 40–8*A*). This feature is typical of craniopharyngiomas. The preoperative MRI scan shown in Figure 40–7 is from the patient illustrated in the operative photographs. The pituitary is then split in the vertical midline plane with microscissors, and bleeding is carefully coagulated. As soon as the pituitary layer is divided, the tumor capsule is visualized (Fig. 40–9*A*, *B*). Alternatively, the pituitary gland may be displaced posteriorly (see Fig. 40–8*B*), and the craniopharyngioma is visible after removal of the basal dura.

In cystic craniopharyngiomas, the cyst may be punctured with a sharp needle and cyst fluid aspirated at this stage of surgery. Care must be taken to prevent puncturing of the diaphragm and subsequent cerebrospinal fluid (CSF) leakage. As the cyst collapses, the tumor pressure is reduced. Further dissection is not always facilitated, however, particularly if the diaphragm enters the sella prematurely. The capsule is opened with microscissors. Intracapsular necrotic or solid tumor is debulked with curettes (Fig. 40–10*A*, *B*).

Usually, the capsule can be gradually mobilized with blunt dissection. The capsule is pulled to the midline with a microforceps while it is detached externally from the surrounding structures (i.e., pituitary gland, cavernous sinus) with a microdissector. Mobilized capsule is excised in a stepwise fashion. This excision may be facilitated by prior bipolar coagulation. Often, the capsule is firmly adherent to the diaphragm. Sharp excision of this portion of the tumor from the diaphragm is required to accomplish complete resection. Not infrequently, rupture of the dia-

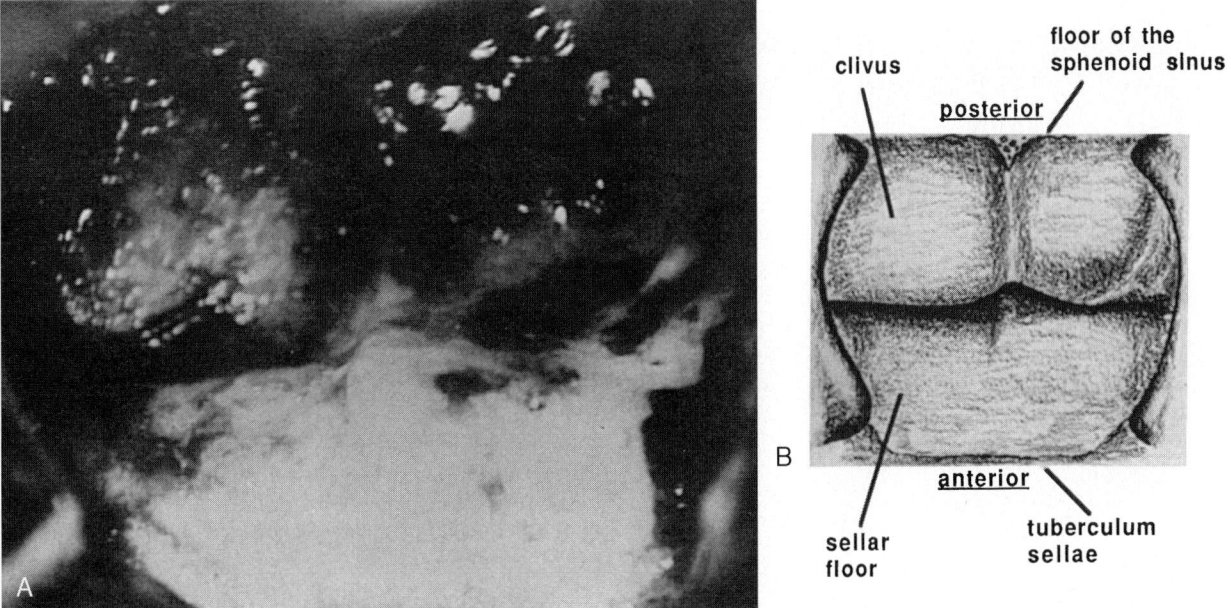

FIGURE 40–5 ■ *A* and *B*, Exposure of the sellar floor and the clivus.

phragm occurs at this stage of surgery, and CSF may escape into the operative field. If the upper surface of the capsule cannot be separated from the diaphragm, excision of these adherences is required. The diaphragm is incised with microscissors lateral to the tumor adherence. The diaphragm can then be depressed with a pituitary hook, and the excision of the craniopharyngioma capsule together with the diaphragm is completed.

Another crucial structure is the pituitary stalk, from which the tumor often originates. Tight connection of the capsule to the pituitary stalk is commonly encountered. In such cases, sharp excision of the capsule from the stalk is also necessary for radical tumor excision. The stalk had to be entirely sacrificed in only one of our cases. Dissection of the capsule is the crucial step of the operation and

renders the procedure more difficult than in pituitary adenomas. During tumor removal, the diaphragm usually descends into the pituitary fossa (Fig. 40–11*A*, *B*). If the suprasellar tumor portion does not enter the pituitary fossa spontaneously, it usually can be made to descend by an increase in intracranial pressure with bilateral jugular vein compression and by positive end-expiratory pressure ventilation. We believe that intraoperative lumbar instillation of saline solution or air is not helpful when the patient is in a supine position.

A calcified shell of the craniopharyngioma is sometimes not completely resectable, whereas crumbling calcifications can be removed.

Craniopharyngiomas that arise from the caudal end of the stalk may grow underneath the diaphragma sellae and

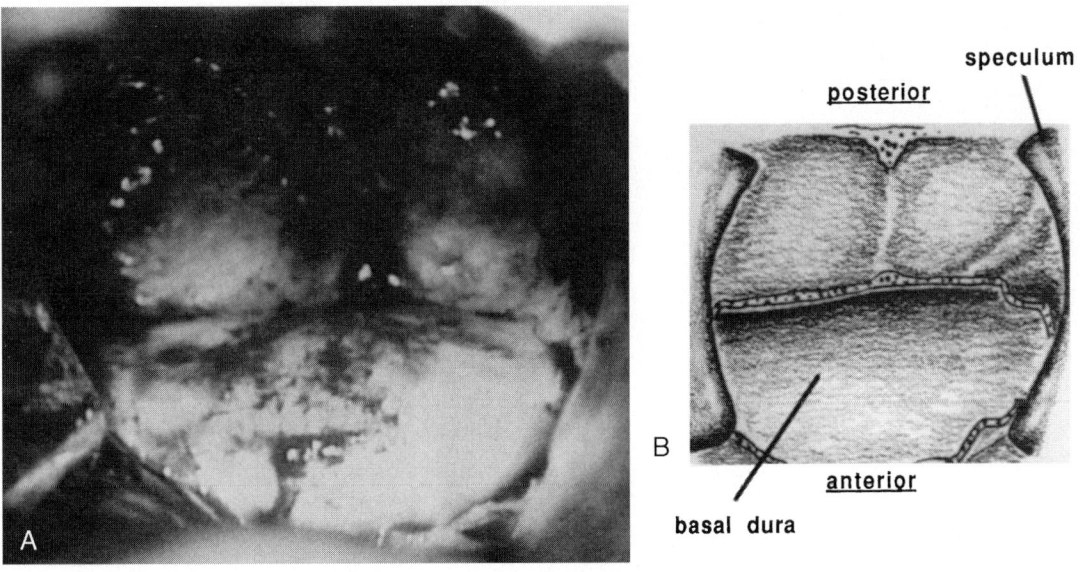

FIGURE 40–6 ■ *A* and *B*, The sellar floor has been removed.

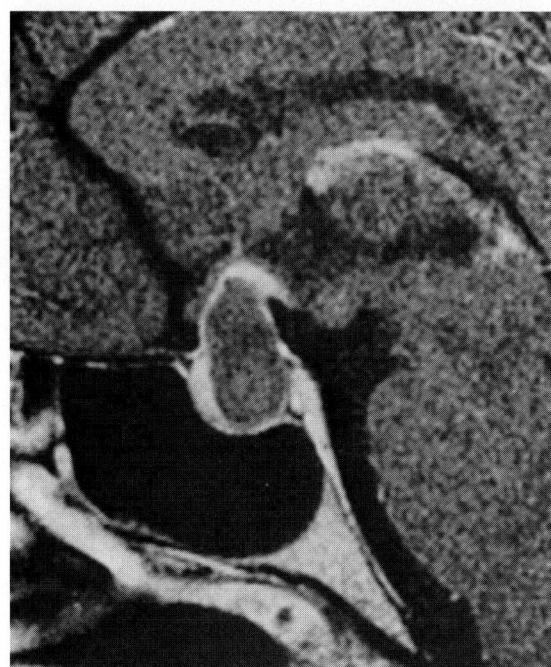

FIGURE 40–7 ■ A magnetic resonance imaging scan of a craniopharyngioma that displaces the pituitary gland anteriorly.

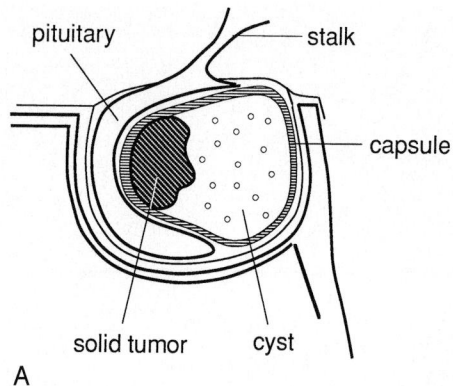

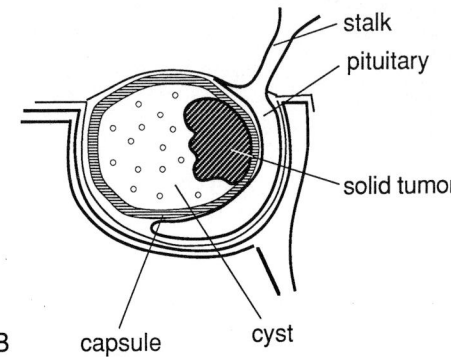

FIGURE 40–8 ■ *A*, Anterior compression of the pituitary by the craniopharyngioma. *B*, Posterior displacement of the pituitary by the craniopharyngioma.

are classified with the subdiaphragmatic craniopharyngiomas that we deal with in this chapter. Craniopharyngiomas may arise at the site where the pituitary stalk penetrates the diaphragm. Growth in both the supradiaphragmatic space and infradiaphragmatic space is then possible. This tumor origin accounts for a large gap of the diaphragm at the site of the tumor and explains why, in rare instances, a small supradiaphragmatic portion can be mobilized through a diaphragmatic opening and removed transsphenoidally. In general, however, only infradiaphragmatic tumor should be removed by the transsphenoidal approach.

Laws[7] proposed placement of a Silastic tube into cystic lesions during transsphenoidal surgery for permanent cyst drainage into the nasopharynx. He used the method in secondary surgery if it was necessary to leave the capsule behind.

Use of a rigid endoscope offers a better panoramic overview of the sphenoid sinus, especially in reoperations,

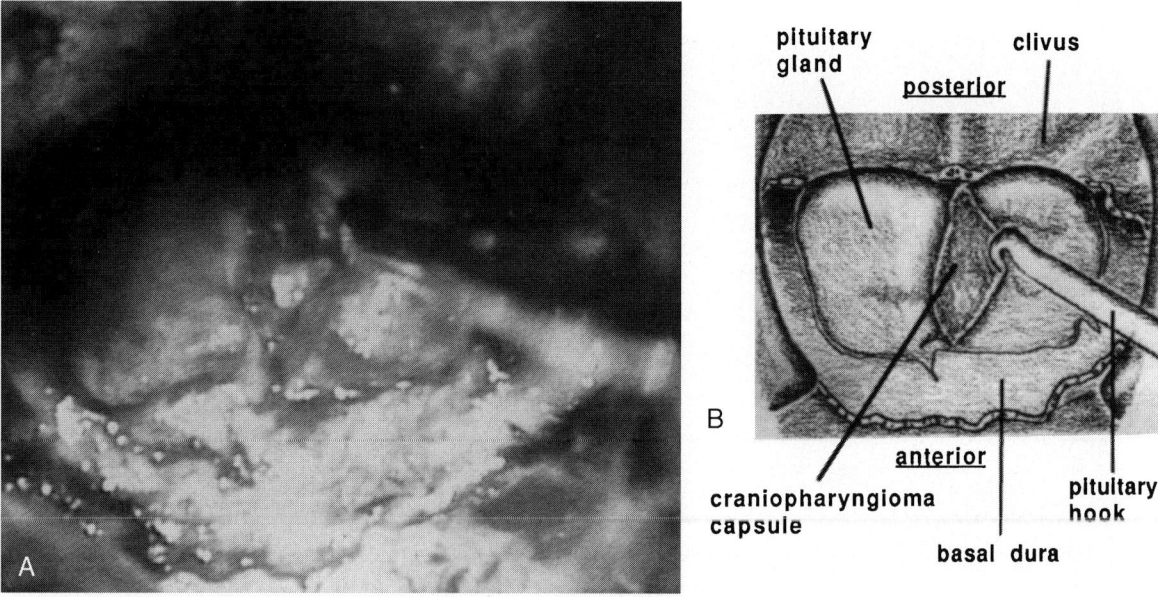

FIGURE 40–9 ■ *A* and *B*, The pituitary gland has been split in the midline. The craniopharyngioma capsule is visualized.

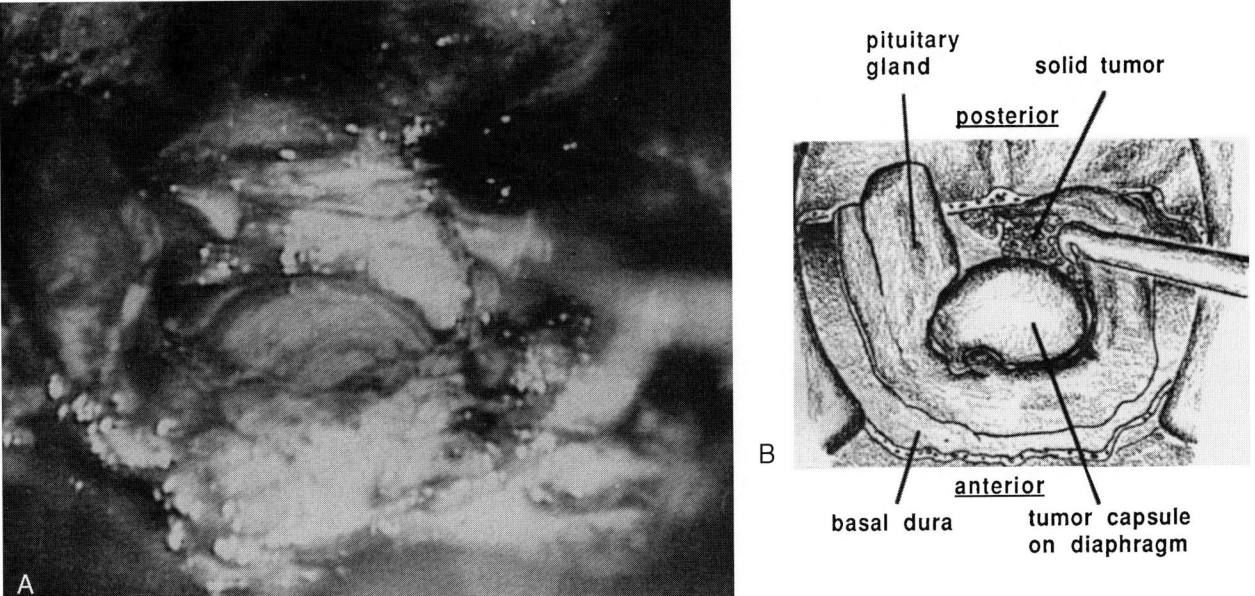

FIGURE 40-10 ■ *A* and *B*, The capsule has been opened. The suprasellar capsule enters the pituitary fossa.

an improved view of parasellar extension versus the displaced cavernous sinus, and good identification of the tumor location/origin at the pituitary stalk and the elevated diaphragm. Even tiny CSF leaks can be easily identified.

## Closure

The surgical opening and any CSF leak (Fig. 40-12*A*) are sealed with fascia lata, and fibrin glue is applied as adhesive. One piece of fascia is placed at the level of the diaphragm. A second, larger strip of fascia covers the exposed surgical field (i.e., the clivus, the sella, and the planum sphenoidale) (see Fig. 40-12*B*). If excision of the diaphragm is required for complete tumor resection, a

significant intraoperative CSF leak is produced. In these cases, we also plug the sphenoid sinus with muscle or fat from the thigh to hold the fascia in place.

We have had experience with 150 cases of sellar lesions in which we performed endoscopic-assisted microsurgery, 7 of which were craniopharyngiomas.

## COMPLICATIONS

The operative morbidity rate among the 35 patients who underwent primary surgery in our series was 5.7% (one case of meningitis, one nasal CSF fistula). The risk of secondary surgery is higher because of a distorted anatomy

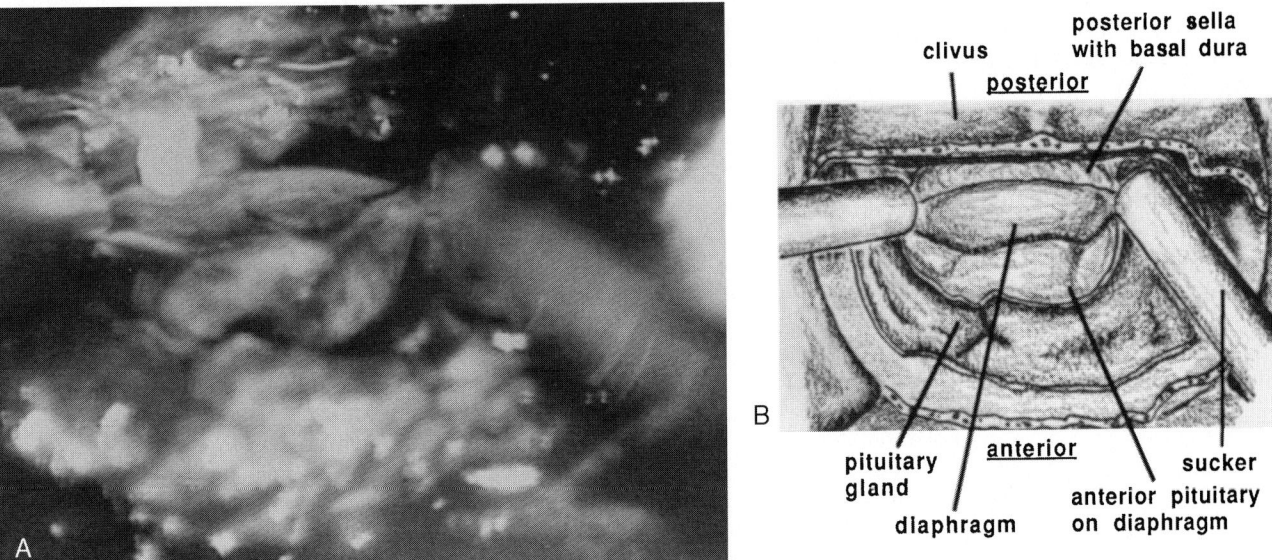

FIGURE 40-11 ■ *A* and *B*, The craniopharyngioma has been removed, and the diaphragm has descended to the sellar floor.

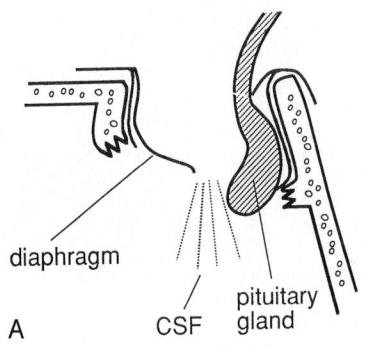

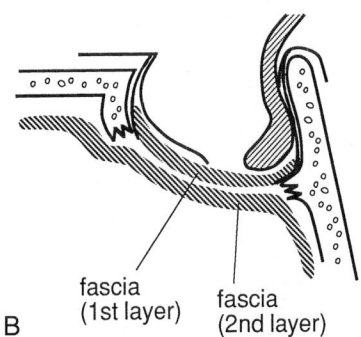

FIGURE 40–12 ■ *A*, Leakage of cerebrospinal fluid (CSF) after tumor removal. *B*, Closure of the CSF leak and the surgical opening with fascia.

and scar formation with adherence to vital structures. In this group the same two complications raised the morbidity rate to 13.2%. After primary transcranial surgery, another patient experienced visual deterioration. In one patient, the procedure was abandoned because of subarachnoid hemorrhage. No operative mortality was encountered in our series. Our findings confirm the low complication rate reported in other large series.[8, 13] A postoperative CSF leak is the most common complication reported in the literature. If the data from the Rochester, Hamburg, Zürich, and our own series are compiled, a mortality rate of 3% results.[7, 10, 13, 14]

## POSTOPERATIVE MANAGEMENT

In the event of an intraoperative CSF leak, a lumbar CSF drainage is inserted immediately after surgery while the patient is still under anesthesia. Over a period of 3 to 5 days, 20 ml of CSF is drained three times daily to prevent postoperative leakage.

In the immediate postoperative period, patients are routinely observed in the recovery room for 2 to 4 hours before being returned to the surgical ward.

Hydrocortisone, 100 mg/24 hours intravenously (i.e., 50 mg during surgery and 50 mg until the next morning), is administered to patients with adrenal insufficiency and to patients in whom the preservation of pituitary function

is uncertain. The dosage of hydrocortisone is then gradually tapered to a final oral dose of 25 mg daily. Endocrine reassessment 1 week after surgery reveals whether replacement therapy can be discontinued. Replacement of the other anterior pituitary functions can be adjusted according to endocrine reassessment 1 week and 3 months after surgery. Fluid balance (fluid intake and urine output) and urine specific gravity are carefully monitored to detect diabetes insipidus. Diabetes insipidus is treated by desmopressin (DDAVP) intramuscularly for the first 5 to 6 days, until the nasal mucosa has recovered sufficiently for nasal administration.

Neuroradiologic reassessment with MRI (plus CT) is performed 3 months after surgery. Ophthalmologic reassessment is carried out 1 week and 3 months after surgery. The patients are then followed at annual or biennial intervals.

## RESULTS

With primary surgery, complete removal was accomplished in 85.7% of our 35 patients. Resection was incomplete in three patients mostly because of a nondescending diaphragm and in one patient because of an unexpected supradiaphragmatic tumor portion. The tumor residue was removed by an additional transcranial operation in these four cases. Similar results were attained by Laws,[7] with complete excision in 9 of 14 patients. Others have favored subtotal tumor removal without excision of the capsule from the stalk to prevent damage to the pituitary stalk.[13] In our opinion, complete tumor removal should be given priority. Pituitary deficiency can be easily replaced, and even reproductive function can be medically restored.

In half of our patients undergoing a transsphenoidal approach after previous surgery, total tumor removal was feasible.

Calcifications may hinder tumor removal or even render it impossible,[15] even if the sellar mass is drilled using the microdrill. A calcified suprasellar, subdiaphragmatic tumor portion is less likely to collapse into the pituitary fossa during surgery. In our group undergoing primary surgery, two craniopharyngiomas with preoperative evidence of calcifications were incompletely removed because of a nondescending suprasellar portion.

### Ophthalmologic Results

The ophthalmologic outcome of transsphenoidal surgery is more favorable than that of transcranial surgery.[10, 13] Recovery of vision is attained in most patients (86.7% showed improvement after primary surgery), and postoperative deterioration of vision is a rare exception. Craniopharyngiomas suitable for transsphenoidal surgery are not expected to encroach directly on the optic chiasm. In contrast to the transcranial approach, direct manipulation of the optic pathways is avoided in the transsphenoidal approach. This fact is another reason for the excellent visual outcome of transsphenoidal surgery.

## Endocrinologic Results

Few publications give a detailed account of endocrinologic outcome. A high rate of new postoperative diabetes insipidus, sixfold more than before surgery,[11] in our series agrees with the literature.[6, 14] However, there are discordant results with respect to anterior pituitary function. In our experience, anterior pituitary function is usually preserved after transsphenoidal surgery, but a pre-existing deficiency rarely recovers.

Landolt and Zachmann's[14] review of the literature and our own experience[10] confirm a low relapse rate after transsphenoidal removal of craniopharyngiomas.

## SUMMARY

The recurrence rate after partial removal of craniopharyngioma is high. Patients benefit from adjunctive radiation therapy, but this does not guarantee long-term control of residual tumor. Therefore, tumor removal should be as radical as possible. The low morbidity and mortality and the favorable endocrinologic outcome of the transsphenoidal approach justify attempting complete resection in intrasellar and suprasellar subdiaphragmatic tumors. Removal of adherent capsule from the diaphragm and pituitary stalk is the technically demanding step of the operation.

The indications for a transsphenoidal operation after prior surgery and the extent of resection in these cases should be considered carefully because of a higher operative risk.

## REFERENCES

1. Halstead AE: Remarks on the operative treatment of tumors of the hypophysis. Surg Gynecol Obstet 10:494–502, 1910.
2. Cushing H: Intracranial Tumors: Notes upon a Series of Two Thousand Verified Cases with Surgical-Mortality Percentages Pertaining Thereto. Springfield, IL: Charles C Thomas, 1932.
3. Hirsch O: Hypophysentumoren—ein Grenzgebiet. Acta Neurochir (Wien) 5:1–10, 1957.
4. Hamlin H: Discussion of Leksell L, Backlund EO: The treatment of craniopharyngiomas. Acta Neurol Scand 43:240, 1967.
5. Hardy J, Lalonde JL: Exérèse par voie trans-sphénoïdale d'un craniopharyngiome géant. Union Med Can 92:1124–1129, 1963.
6. Hardy J, Vezina JL: Transsphenoidal neurosurgery of intracranial neoplasm. Adv Neurol 15:261–274, 1976.
7. Laws ER: Transsphenoidal microsurgery in the management of craniopharyngioma. J Neurosurg 52:661–666, 1980.
8. Laws E: Transsphenoidal removal of craniopharyngioma. Pediatr Neurosurg 21 (Suppl 1):57–63, 1994.
9. Baskin DS, Wilson CB: Surgical management of craniopharyngiomas: A review of 74 cases. J Neurosurg 65:22–27, 1986.
10. Fahlbusch R, Honegger J, Paulus W, et al: Surgical treatment of craniopharyngiomas: Experience with 168 patients. J Neurosurg 90:237–250, 1999.
11. Honegger J, Buchfelder M, Fahlbusch R: Surgical treatment of craniopharyngiomas: Endocrine results. J Neurosurg 90:251–257, 1999.
12. Grisoli F, Vincentelli F, Farnarier P, et al: Trans-sphenoidal microsurgery in the management of nonpituitary tumors of the sella turcica. In Brock M (ed): Modern Neurosurgery 1. Berlin-Heidelberg: Springer-Verlag, 1982, pp. 193–201.
13. König A, Lüdecke DK, Herrmann HD: Transnasal surgery in the treatment of craniopharyngiomas. Acta Neurochir (Wien) 83:1–7, 1986.
14. Landolt AM, Zachmann M: Results of transsphenoidal extirpation of craniopharyngiomas and Rathke's cysts. Neurosurgery 28:410–415, 1991.
15. Nagpal RD: Trans-sphenoidal excision of craniopharyngiomas. J Postgrad Med 37:97–101, 1991.

# Surgical Management of Arachnoid, Suprasellar, and Rathke's Cleft Cysts

■ DIETER HELLWIG, BERNHARD L. BAUER, THOMAS RIEGEL, HENRY H. SCHMIDEK, and WILLIAM H. SWEET

Most of the intracranial cystic lesions that occur in adults are related to neoplasms, bacterial or parasitic infections, or loss of tissue owing to malformation, infarction, or injury, including that resulting from surgical resection of brain tissue. These topics are discussed in other chapters of this book; however, an additional group of cystic intracranial lesions are encountered in neurosurgical practice and three of these lesions are discussed in this chapter: the arachnoid, suprasellar, and Rathke's cleft cyst. Of particular interest is that the management of these lesions continues to evolve with the development of endoscopic neurosurgical techniques.[1-7]

## INTRACRANIAL ARACHNOID CYSTS

Arachnoid cysts are intra-arachnoid benign cystic lesions filled with cerebrospinal fluid (CSF).[8] According to Cohen,[2] in 1831 Bright was the first to describe the intra-arachnoid location of intracranial arachnoid cysts. These lesions are probably developmental in origin and become symptomatic either because of their progressive enlargement or because of hemorrhage into the cyst. The enlargement of arachnoid cysts had been discussed controversially and is up to now a point of discussion. There are different hypotheses to explain the growth of arachnoid cysts: (1) active fluid secretion from the cyst wall,[9, 10] (2) fluid accumulation caused by an osmotic pressure gradient,[11] (3) pumping of CSF through a persistent communication between the cyst and the arachnoid space due to vascular pulsation,[12] and (4) the so-called slit-valve mechanism, which is described later.[1, 13, 14] Arachnoid cysts occur throughout the neuraxis, and generally, no communication is demonstrable between the cyst and the subarachnoid space, although occasionally during surgery, an arachnoid cyst is observed being filled through an apparent one-way valve.[15] Arachnoid cysts may be asymptomatic throughout life, and rarely, they may spontaneously regress[16]; however, if they do become symptomatic, the progression results from compression on the underlying brain, overlying bone, or both. There is an ongoing discussion whether space-occupying asymptomatic cysts should be operated on to prevent a hindrance to normal brain development and function.[8, 17] If the indication for surgery is questionable, intracranial pressure (ICP) monitoring should be performed to prove ICP elevation or pathologic pressure waves.[3]

### Case Report 1

A 14-year-old boy was admitted with aggressive attitudes, loss of motivation, headache, and nausea. The neurologic examination was normal. An electroencephalogram showed a left-sided reduction of activity in the parieto-occipitoretrotemporal region. Computed tomography (CT) demonstrated a large left parieto-occipital arachnoid cyst with a slight mass effect (Fig. 41–1). Epidural ICP measurement during a period of 24 hours revealed normal values (Fig. 41–2). We concluded that the cyst was not related to the patient's symptoms, and no further intervention was performed. Ten years of follow-up examinations show that the patient is in good neurologic condition with normal age-related capacity.

The clinical symptoms resulting from these arachnoid cysts depend greatly on their location—whether over the sylvian fissure; over the cerebral convexity; in the interhemispheric region; in the sella and suprasellar region; around the optic nerve, the quadrigeminal plate, or the cerebellopontine angle; in the region of the clivus; over the cerebellar vermis or cerebellar hemisphere; or within the lateral or fourth ventricle.[18-20] Arachnoid cysts have also been described extending across the region of the foramen magnum from the posterior cranial fossa into the upper cervical spine posterolateral to the spinal cord.[21] The midline lesions often lead to an obstruction of the CSF and result in focal symptoms and raised ICP.[22-25]

The arachnoid cyst wall is histologically indistinguishable from normal arachnoidal membrane. Moderate thickening of the arachnoid and an increase in connective tissue

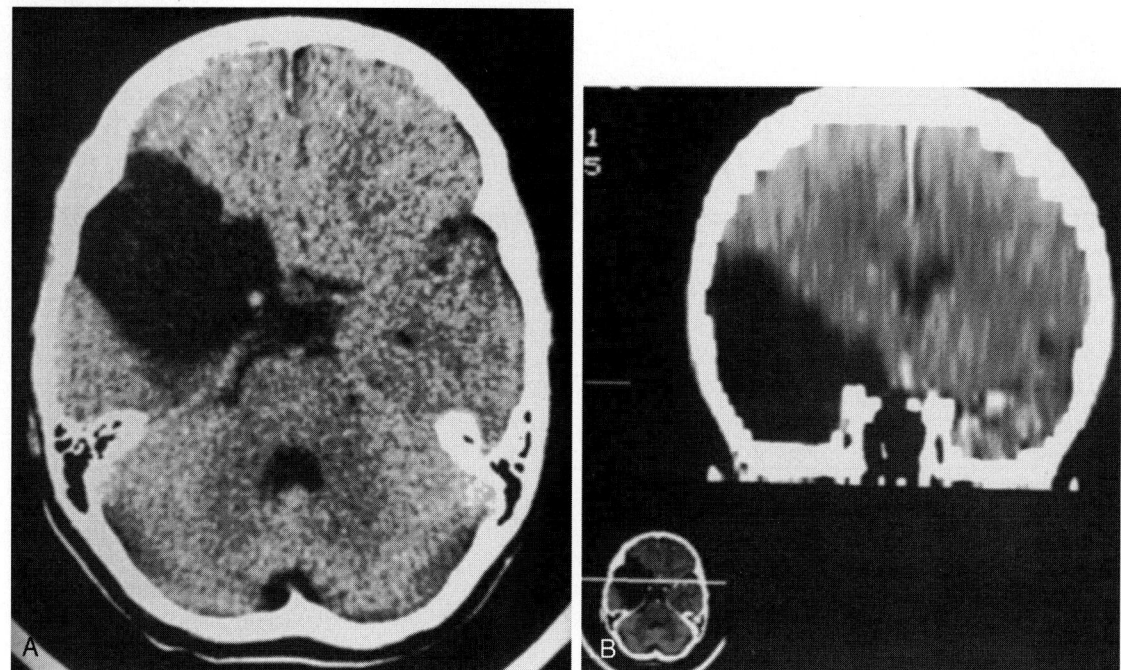

FIGURE 41–1*A* and *B* ■

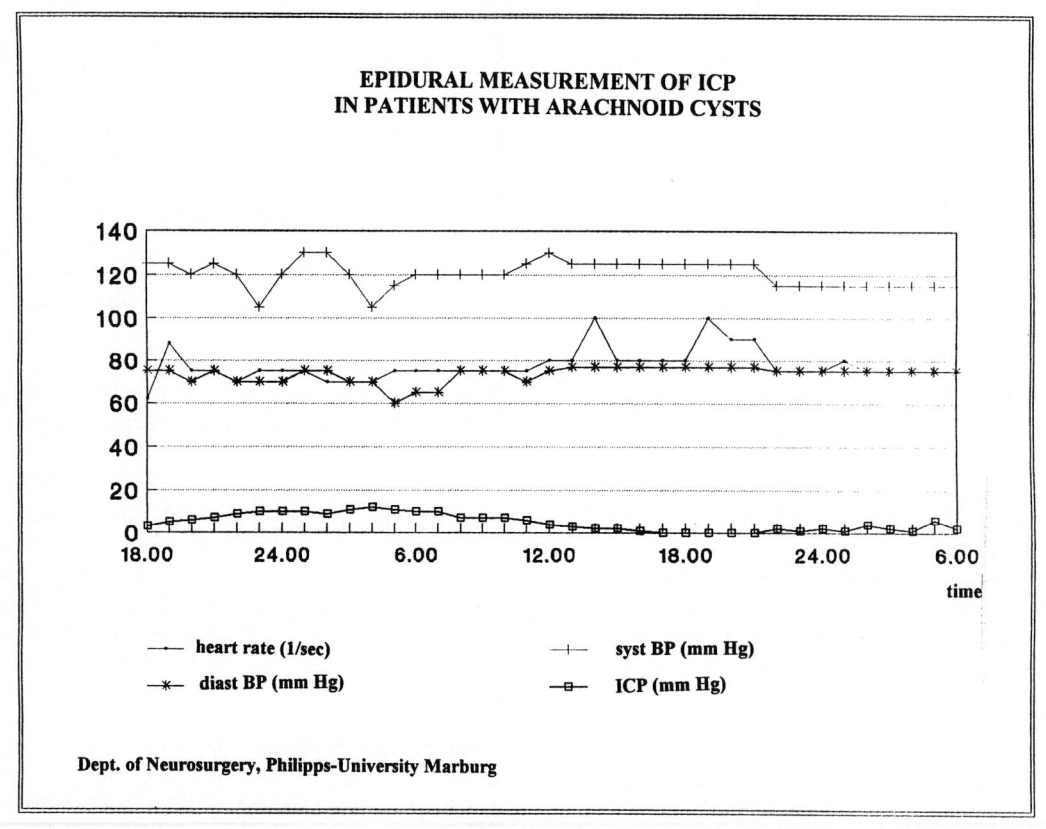

FIGURE 41–2 ■

are common (Fig. 41–3).[26] Ultrastructural studies confirm the similarity of the cyst membrane with the normal meningeal counterpart, including the cell-cell connections and the occurrence of basal laminal structures. Quantitative differences in the contribution of the single components have been found both between different cysts and between cysts and normal arachnoid.

A special kind of arachnoid cyst formation consists of a luminal epithelial layer connected with a glial sheet, followed peripherally by a thin connective tissue covering (Fig. 41–4). The glial nature of parts of the cyst lining can be shown by glial fibrillary acidic protein (GFAP) staining. Some authors have called these cysts "glioependymal."[27]

## Case Report 2

This 72-year-old woman suffered from headache, stupor, and right hemiparesis. A large left hemispheric cystic process with a midline shift was diagnosed by CT and magnetic resonance imaging (MRI) examination (Fig. 41–5A, B). Using three-dimensional stereotactic trajectory and target-point calculation, the cyst membrane was approached endoscopically through a right frontal bur hole. The gray membrane was opened by radiofrequency coagulation, and biopsies were taken (see Fig. 41–5C). The cyst contained CSF-like fluid. There was no evidence of tumor or other pathology. The histopathologic diagnosis was that of an epithelial cyst. The cyst was opened endoscopically to the left lateral ventricle. After surgery, the CT scan showed that the midline shift was greatly reduced. The left frontal horn was enlarged again (see Fig. 41–5D). A few days after the intervention, the patient was alert and she was discharged with only a slight hemiparesis.

In many cases, arachnoidal cysts are incidental findings noted on CT scanning or MRI of the head performed for a reason unrelated to the cyst. Such patients are informed about the radiographic finding; provided with a copy of the study so they can present it to a physician at a later date, if necessary; and followed up annually. In approximately 15% of middle fossa arachnoid cysts, an asymptomatic

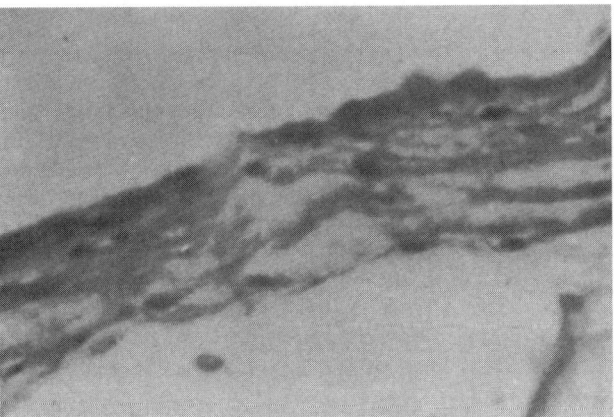

**FIGURE 41–3 ■** Lining of subarachnoid cysts consisting of a single layer of arachnoid and adjacent loose subarachnoid network and psammoma body. H & E stain. (From Youmans JR: Neurological Surgery, 2nd ed, Vol 3. Philadelphia: WB Saunders, 1982, p 1437.)

lesion may become symptomatic as a result of bleeding in association with the cyst and raised ICP. This event may occur after minor head trauma.[28–30]

## Case Report 3

A 12-year-old boy had been hit on the head by a hockey stick. He suffered from headaches, and 2 weeks later, his consciousness was impaired. MRI examination showed a left chronic subdural hematoma (Fig. 41–6A) related to a temporal arachnoid cyst (see Fig. 41–6B). The subdural hematoma was drained through a silicone catheter. On CT examination, the subdural hematoma was greatly reduced with no signs of raised ICP or mass effect (see Fig. 41–6C). We decided to leave the arachnoid cyst without further operative intervention. The patient did not develop complications during the postoperative course. Over a follow-up period of 9 years, the arachnoid cyst has remained unchanged.

In a report of six cases of subdural hematoma occurring in 18 patients with previously asymptomatic middle cranial fossa arachnoid cysts, Rogers and colleagues[31] recommend a cystoperitoneal shunt to treat the cyst after evacuation of the hematoma. Auer and coworkers[32] also recommend evacuation of the hematoma and the cyst's wall in one procedure. Handa and associates[33] reported on the two-stage removal of bilateral cysts and hematomas. They recommend that the hematomas be drained initially through bur holes and that 3 months later, the cyst wall be resected and a cystoperitoneal shunt inserted. Markakis and colleagues[34] also recommend a two-stage approach to the management of large arachnoidal cysts, beginning with a shunt procedure, which is followed several weeks later by the resection of the cyst wall and a ventriculostomy. Another treatment option is to evacuate the hematoma through an endoscopic bur hole approach and perform a cystostomy to the CSF space in one procedure.[35]

Cerebral convexity cysts occurring in adults present as seizures, headache, raised ICP, and sometimes, marked reactive thickening of the overlying skull with erosion of the inner table. These cases can be managed by the wide excision of the membranes and the establishment of communication between the cyst interior and the CSF of the subarachnoid space. The same approach has been used in the treatment of symptomatic interhemispheric arachnoid cysts and cysts in the region of the quadrigeminal plate that produce aqueductal obstruction that leads to hydrocephalus. Before the advent of MRI, arachnoid cysts of the cerebellopontine angle often presented a diagnostic dilemma that required differentiation from other mass lesions located in the cerebellopontine angle.[18] Cysts of the cerebellopontine angle may mimic other lesions in this location and may cause hearing loss and cerebellar signs. These cysts may present as intermittent downbeat nystagmus with an associated hydrocephalus or as vague symptoms, including hearing loss and dysequilibrium, contralateral trigeminal neuralgia, or hemifacial spasm.[36–39]

Surgical options for the management of symptomatic arachnoid cysts include the endoscopic resection of the cyst wall with opening of the membranes, which establishes communication with the hemispheric or ventricular CSF

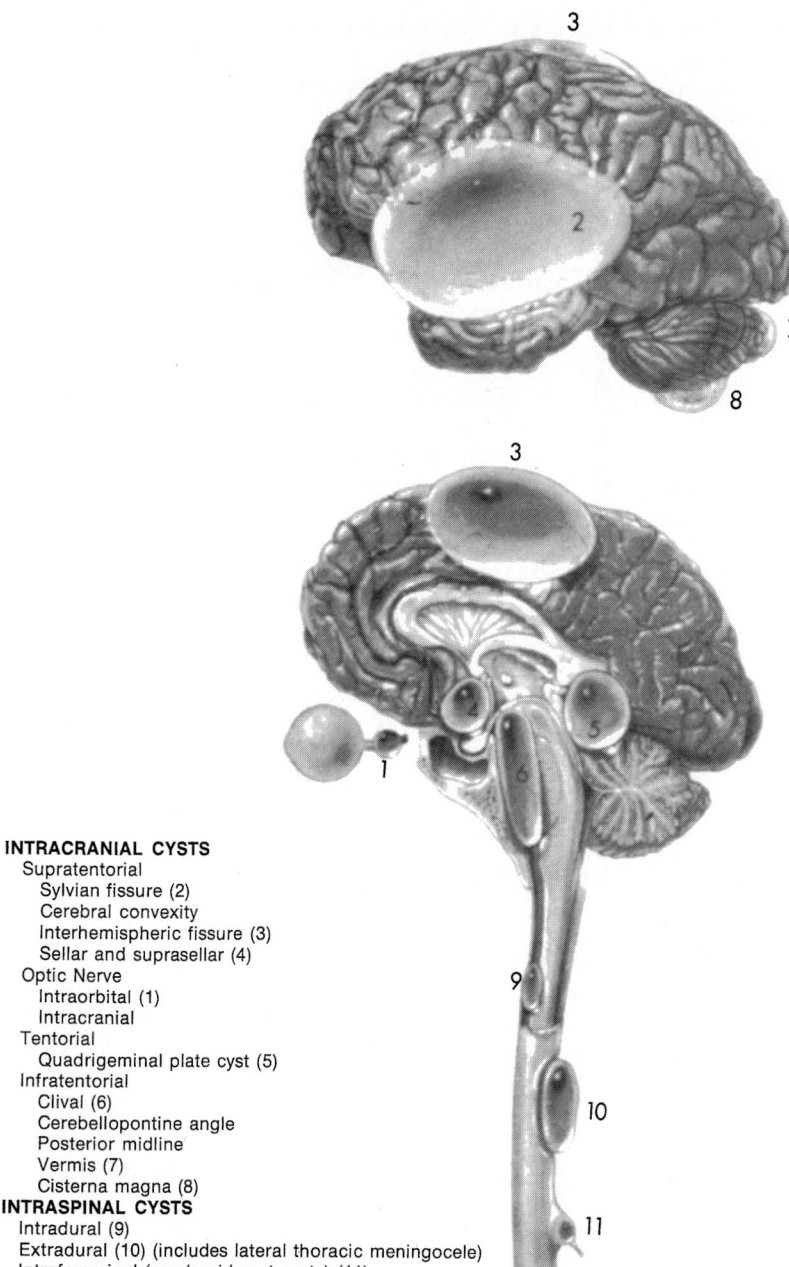

**INTRACRANIAL CYSTS**
  Supratentorial
    Sylvian fissure (2)
    Cerebral convexity
    Interhemispheric fissure (3)
    Sellar and suprasellar (4)
  Optic Nerve
    Intraorbital (1)
    Intracranial
  Tentorial
    Quadrigeminal plate cyst (5)
  Infratentorial
    Clival (6)
    Cerebellopontine angle
    Posterior midline
    Vermis (7)
    Cisterna magna (8)
**INTRASPINAL CYSTS**
  Intradural (9)
  Extradural (10) (includes lateral thoracic meningocele)
  Intraforaminal (arachnoid root cysts) (11)

**FIGURE 41–4** ■ So-called glioependymal cyst with arachnoid, connective tissues, and glial sheet lining forming the cyst wall. Cresyl violet stain, ×125. (From Youmans JR: Neurological Surgery, 2nd ed, Vol 3. Philadelphia: WB Saunders, 1982, p 1439.)

pathways.[3, 6] Subsequent shunting can be performed in cases where a concomitant hydrocephalus exists and the endoscopic procedure is insufficient. Other options are stereotactic cyst aspiration,[40, 41] shunt drainage or drainage of the lesion through a bur hole, craniectomy with resection of the cyst walls, and craniectomy and ventriculostomy of the cyst.[8, 17, 42] In a cooperative European study of the management of arachnoid cysts in children, total excision or marsupialization emerged as the first choice surgical procedure, and shunting procedures were often applied to cysts located in deeper locations. Among the 285 patients, from birth to 15 years of age, there was a resultant reduction of the size of the cyst in approximately two thirds of the cases, and in 205, the cyst had disappeared completely on follow-up CT scanning.[43] Another study of the relative merits of different approaches to the management of arachnoid cysts in children is based on an analysis of 40 children treated between 1978 and 1989 at the University of California, San Francisco. Of 15 patients with cysts that were treated initially by fenestration alone, 67% showed no clinical or radiographic improvement and subsequently required cyst-peritoneal or ventriculoperitoneal shunting. All of these patients improved postoperatively, although shunt revision was required in approximately one third of cases as a result of the recurrence of a cyst. These authors concluded that irrespective of the location of the lesion, cyst-peritoneal or cyst-ventriculoperitoneal shunting is the treatment of choice.[17] Two groups reported about their results in neuroendoscopic treatment of arachnoid cysts. In a prospective study, Schroeder and coworkers[7] treated

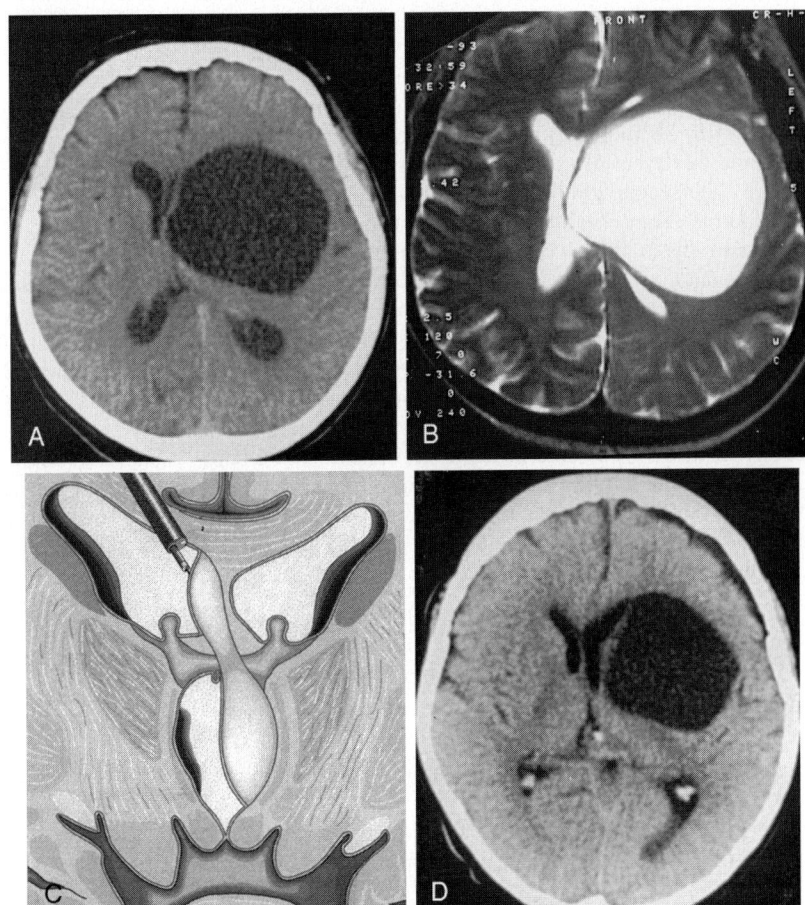

**FIGURE 41–5***A–D* ■ Electrosurgical technique for cystoventriculostomy. The rigid endoscope is placed into the right frontal horn, 5 mm distant from the cyst's surface. The electrosurgical coagulation and cutting probe is forwarded through the endoscope's working channel. With the tip of the probe, the cystoventriculostomy is performed in a contact mode.

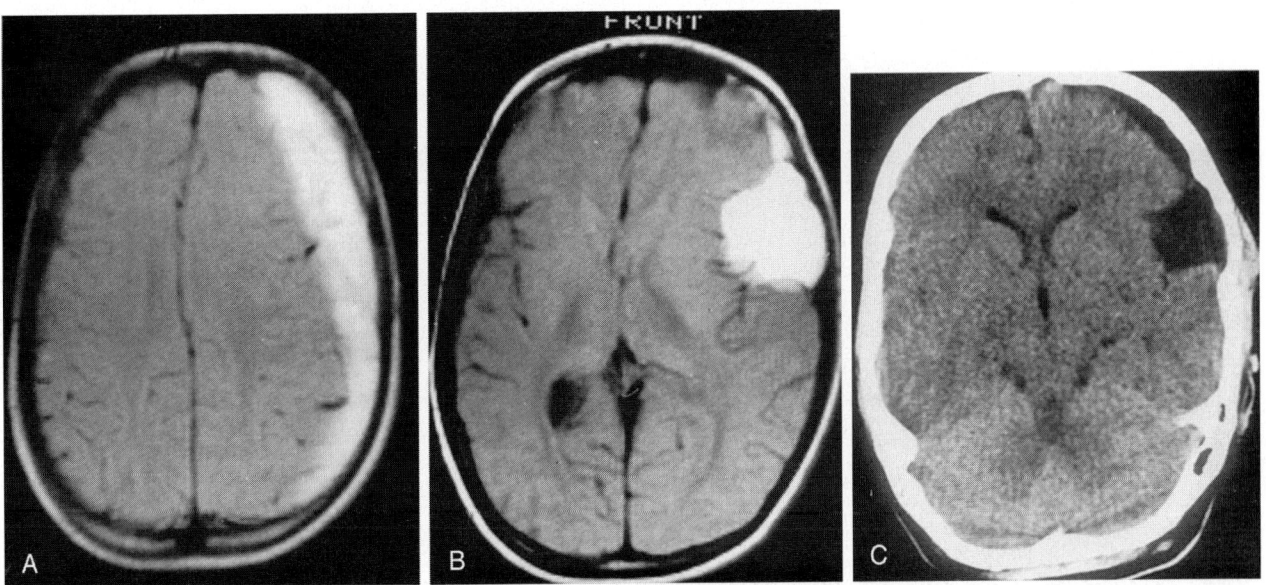

**FIGURE 41–6***A–C* ■

seven consecutive patients with symptomatic arachnoid cysts in different locations endoscopically. The authors performed cystocisternostomies and ventriculocystostomies via bur holes with the aid of a universal neuroendoscopic system. Symptoms were relieved in five patients and improved in one patient, whereas the size of the cyst decreased in six patients. Although the follow-up period was short (15 to 30 months), the authors recommend neuroendoscopic treatment of arachnoid cyst as the first therapy of choice. The second study has been conducted by Hopf and coworkers.[6] They evaluated 24 patients with intracranial arachnoid cysts that were treated endoscopically. Their surgical strategy was to create broad communication between the cyst and the subarachnoid space. Different techniques were used; that is, endoscopic fenestration (10 cases), endoscopic controlled microsurgery (five patients), and endoscopy assisted microsurgery (nine cases). In all patients sufficient fenestration of the cysts could be achieved with a favorable outcome in 17 patients. Operative complications included infection (three patients), bleeding into the cyst (one patient), and subdural fluid collections (four patients). The authors conclude that different endoscopic techniques do provide sufficient treatment of selected arachnoid cysts.

## Neuroendoscopic Instrumentation and Operative Technique in Treatment of Arachnoid Cysts

### Endoscopes

Different rigid and flexible endoscopes are available to perform cystostomy, cystoventriculostomy, or cystocister-noventriculostomy. The advantages of rigid lens scopes are the brilliant and bright pictorial quality and the guidance via a predetermined direct trajectory. Angled rigid scopes are used together with microscopes and neuronavigational devices in endoscopy assisted microsurgery.

They offer the possibility to look around corners. Flexible neuroscopes have the advantage of steerability and maneuverability, which make inspection and interventions on multifocal and multiseptated cystic lesions easier.

### Guidance

There are different methods to perform endoscopic interventions on arachnoid cysts. The easiest and most time-sparing technique is the "free-hand method." The approach is a single bur hole, and during the intervention the surgeon orients on anatomic landmarks. The advantage is to be free from holding and guiding devices; however, the operative approach and the targeting could be inaccurate.

Frame-based stereotactic guidance provides high accuracy and ensures orientation but could be time-consuming and restricts endoscope movements.

Newly developed neuronavigation systems provide image guidance, which is interactive and precise. These systems can be applied in a "free-hand" mode or in combination with holding and guiding devices (Fig. 41–7A–C).

### Instruments

Moving neuroendoscopic working instruments within preformed or pathologic central nervous system (CNS) cavities, as arachnoid cysts are, is not easy and requires training for several reasons: distances might be estimated incor-

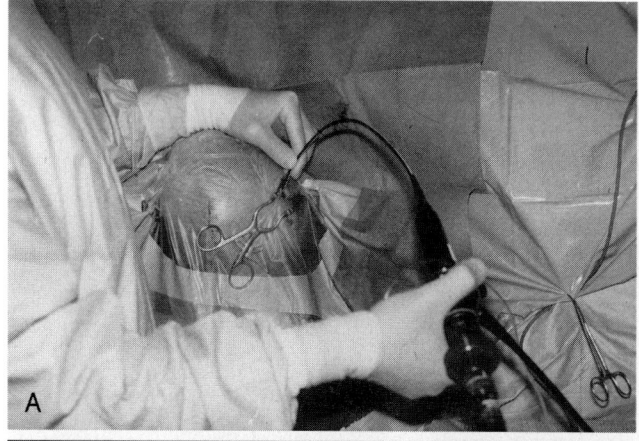

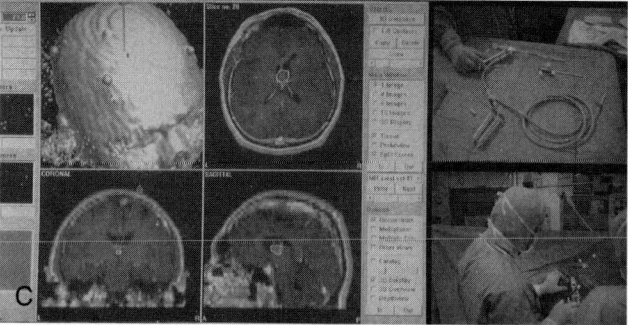

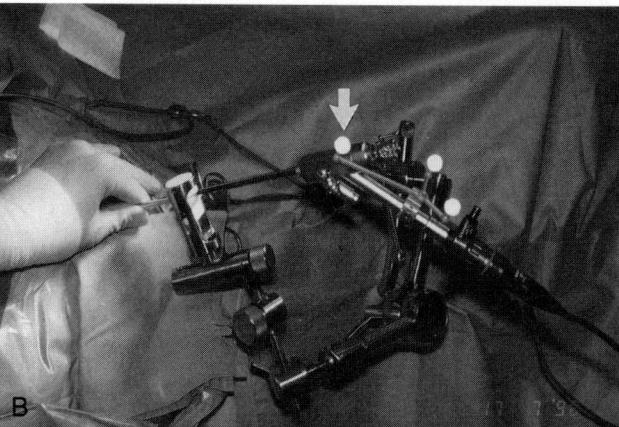

FIGURE 41–7 ■ Different neuroendoscopy guiding techniques. *A,* Free-hand technique with the flexible steerable endoscope. *B,* Fixed technique with the rigid endoscope (Zeppelin Co.) adjusted to a stereotaxy holding and guiding device in combination with neuronavigational guidance (see the white star–shaped instrument adapters [*arrow*]). *C,* Neuronavigation assembly for three-dimensional calculation and real-time visualization of the endoscopic approach to a ventricular cystic lesion.

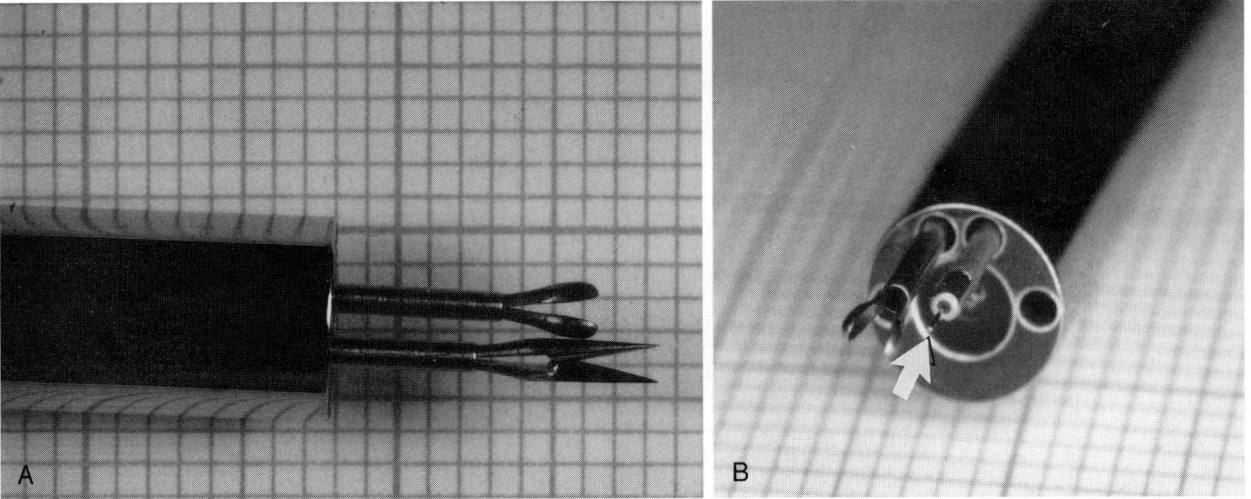

FIGURE 41–8 ■ Supplementary endoscopy working instruments. *A*, Microscissors and grasping forceps guided through the rigid endoscope's working channel. *B*, Biopsy forceps and the tip of the bipolar coagulation and cutting microelectrode, which has a diameter of 0.9 mm (Erbe Co.) *(arrow)*.

rectly; the instrument may enter the viewing field from the side or is out of view; the surgeon controls the procedure at a video screen, and not directly as in microsurgery.

Different instruments are available for endoscopic interventions on arachnoid cysts. Microforceps and scissors are helpful to open and resect cyst membranes (Fig. 41–8A). In many cases, it is advisable to open the arachnoid cysts using electrosurgical devices. In cooperation with Erbe Company, we have developed a bipolar cutting and coagulation microprobe, which is controlled automatically by an electrosurgical unit. The regulated energy release avoids thermal damage to vulnerable structures. Safe hemostasis is ensured by pinpoint accuracy and effective coagulation of small vessels. The cutting depth is freely adjustable up to 3 mm. The cutting needle can be retracted into the endoscope's working channel. The probes are available for both rigid and flexible endoscopes with diameters of between 0.9 and 1.5 mm (see Fig. 41–8B). Balloon catheters (Fogarty, double-balloon) are very useful to enlarge the stomas in an atraumatic fashion.

## Imaging

Intraoperative digital dynamic subtraction cystography (cystoventriculography) is performed routinely to show the communication of the arachnoid cyst to the adjoining CSF compartments and the restoration of normal CSF flow (Fig. 41–9A, B). After the endoscopic intervention postoperative electrocardiogram (ECG)-gated dynamic MRI examination demonstrates the normalized CSF flow under real-time conditions (Fig. 41–10A, B).

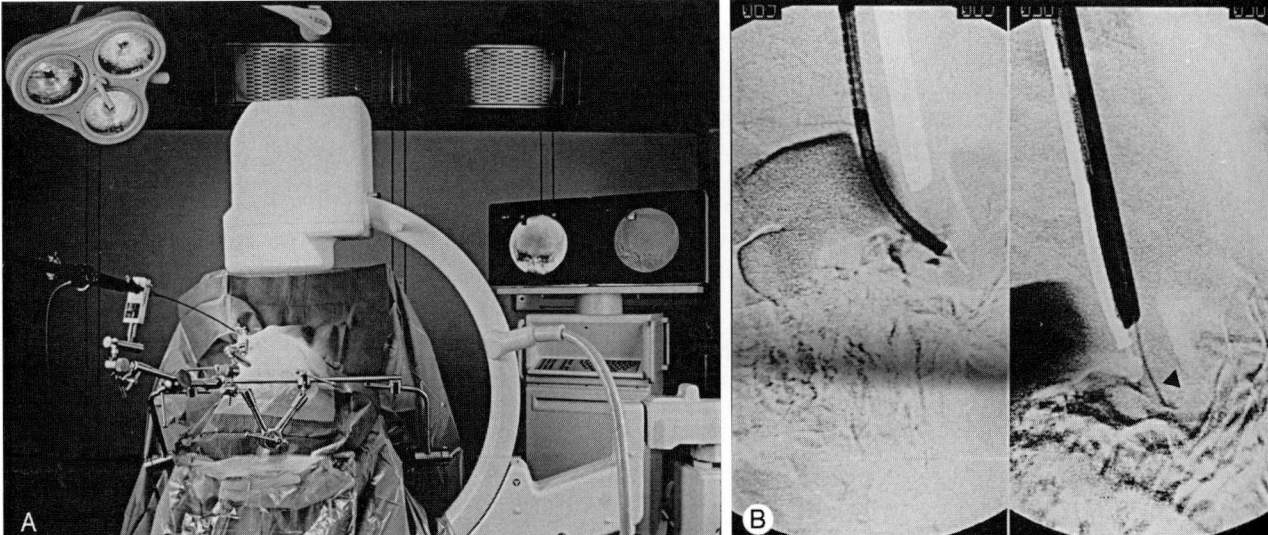

FIGURE 41–9 ■ Intraoperative fluoroscopy. *A*, An intraoperative setup with a fluoroscopy unit. The flexible, steerable endoscope is fixed to the Marburg neuroendoscopy holding and guiding system. *B*, Intraoperative digital dynamic subtraction ventriculography offers a real-time movement control of the endoscope and the working instruments. The flexible, steerable endoscope is guided to the sellar region using a road mapping technique. At the tip of the endoscope, the bipolar electrode is forwarded *(black arrow)*.

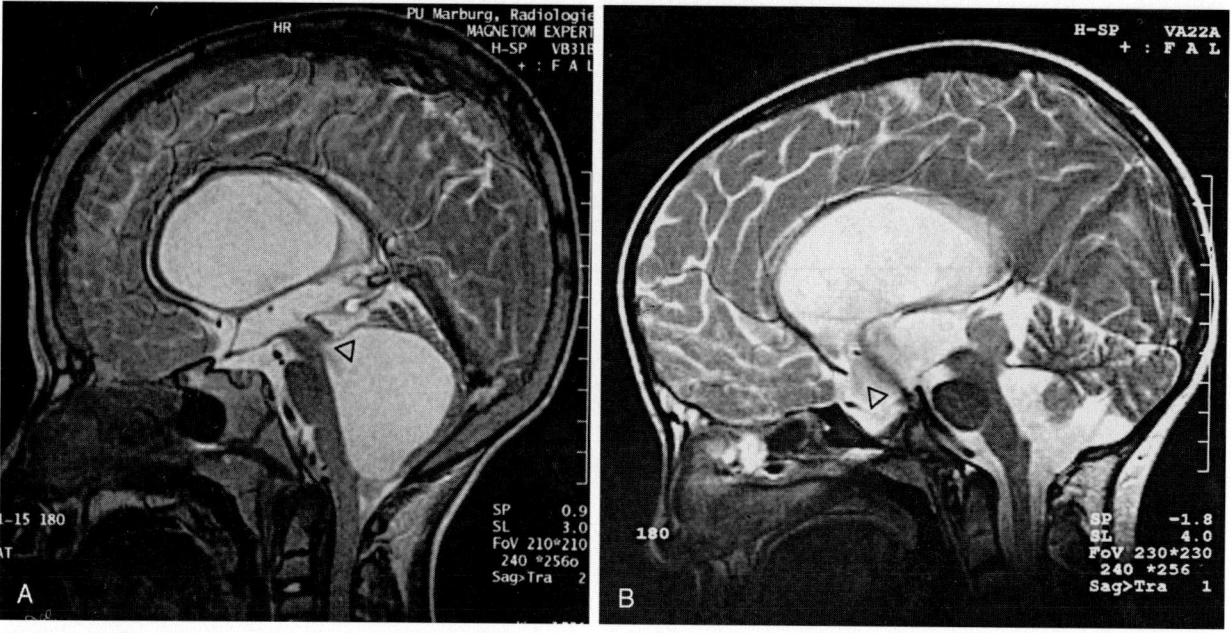

FIGURE 41–10 ■ An electrocardiogram-gated dynamic magnetic resonance imaging (MRI) examination. *A*, Typical cerebrospinal fluid flow signal of the aqueduct of Sylvius *(arrow)* from the third ventricle to the cystic enlarged fourth ventricle. The cyst is caused by adhesive occlusions of the foramina of Luschka and Magendi after the resection of a cerebellar pilocytic astrocytoma. *B*, After third ventriculostomy (see the flow signal from the third ventricle to the interpeduncular cistern *[arrow]*), the size of the fourth ventricle has been greatly decreased.

## SUPRASELLAR CYSTS

Suprasellar cysts are arachnoid cysts that occur in the sella region and become symptomatic as locally expanding lesions. Arachnoid cysts in relation to the sella turcica represent 10% of all cases.[46] The term *suprasellar cyst,* formerly a synonym for craniopharyngioma, designates a small group of lesions, usually congenital, with a thin, even transparent wall that is filled with clear, colorless, or light yellow fluid. The congenital effect from these cysts, which constitute fewer than 1% of all intracranial mass lesions, was severe enough to cause symptoms in the first two decades in 46 of the 54 reports collated by Hoffman and coworkers.[47] The lesion evolves as a consequence of prevention of CSF circulation into the chiasmatic cistern or laterally from the interpeduncular cistern beneath the hypothalamus and behind the pituitary stalk and optic chiasm. The presence of CSF from below the pontine cistern then pushes the hypothalamic floor upward and thins it greatly so that above the arachnoid dome are only at most a few glial and ependymal cells, as described by Harrison[48] in three of four cases. In many of the cases, thin, even transparent, connective tissue is the only lining to the cyst. As arachnoid cysts in other locations, suprasellar arachnoid cysts may enlarge over time. This change could be effected by active secretion of the membrane[49] or from ectopic choroid-like structures[9] or osmotic pressure gradients.[11] Another theory for the enlargement of suprasellar arachnoid cysts is based on the endoscopic and cine-mode evidence of a slit valve,[1, 13, 14] formed by an arachnoid membrane around the basilar artery. This valve is supposed to open and close with arterial pulsations and lead to an inflow of CSF into the cyst forced by a pressure gradient.

By the time that the diagnosis is made, much or all of the third ventricle is usually filled by the cyst, causing an obstruction of one or both foramina of Monro, lateral ventricular dilatation, and a huge head. Indeed, the dome of the cyst is usually much higher than that shown in Figure 41–11, lying just beneath the corpus callosum. One possible mechanism for this block is excessive development of an arachnoidal curtain that extends from the posterior hypothalamus to the dorsum sellae below, originally described by Key and Retzius.[50] Its presence, confirmed by Lillequist[51] and by Fox and Al-Mefty,[52] becomes a menace when it and the arachnoid lateral to it become imperforate. Another mechanism of pathogenesis, proposed by Starkman and coworkers,[53] is that intra-arachnoidal spaces in the embryo persist and expand exclusively within the arachnoid. This event was demonstrated incidentally at autopsy in a careful dissection of an intact suprasellar cyst by Krawchenko and Collins.[8] Most suprasellar arachnoid cysts occur in children with a male prevalence.[2] The clinical picture often includes, in addition to hydrocephalus with a big head and ataxia, disturbed visual acuity and fields, because of forward and upward displacement of the chiasm, and hypopituitarism, because of pressure in the hypothalamus and pituitary stalk. These symptoms caused by a suprasellar cystic lesion had been first described by Pieter Pauw, a Dutch anatomist, in the 16th century.[54]

A constant forward and backward nodding of the head and neck, the bobble-head doll syndrome, is an inconstant sign.[55–57] An unusual symptom is precocious puberty.[46, 58] Headache may occur in older patients. On CT scans, the cyst has the density of CSF; its wall shows neither enhancement nor calcification and is often mistaken for a dilated third ventricle. According to Cohen,[2] suprasellar arachnoid cysts appear as midline round or oval hypodense lesions adjacent to the dilated frontal horns. They have a typical "Mickey Mouse" configuration on axial CT scans or MRI.

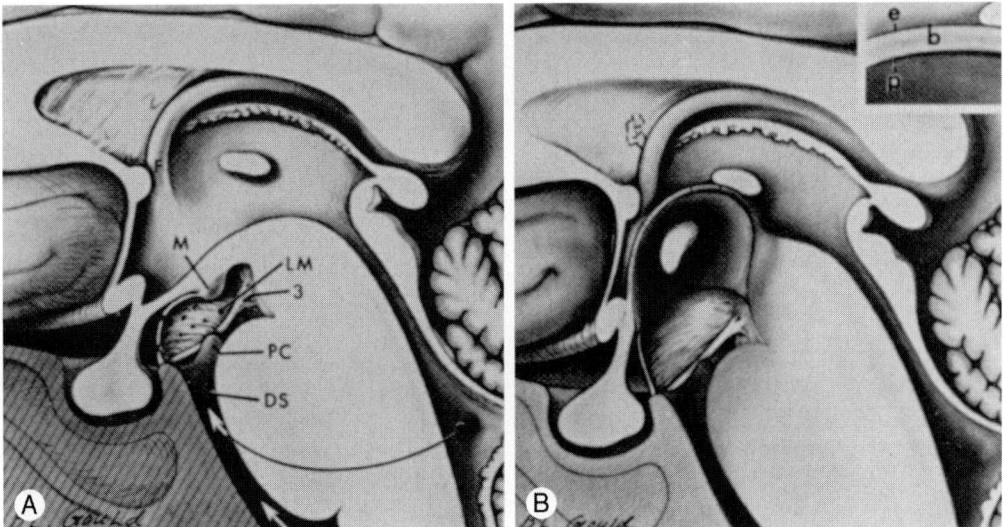

FIGURE 41-11 ■ Anatomy of a suprasellar cyst. *A*, Artist's conception of the sagittal section of a normal brain and the sellar region, looking to the right. (F, fornix; M, mammillary body; LM, Lillequist's membrane; 3, right oculomotor nerve; PC, right posterior clinoid process; DS, dorsum sellae; arrows, normal flow of cerebrospinal fluid through the prepontine and interpeduncular cisterns.) *B*, The membrane of Lillequist has ballooned forward and backward, compressing the floor of the third ventricle to the level of the massa intermedia. The left base of the almost-three-dimensional cyst has been cut away to show the right oculomotor nerve. *Inset*, Enlargement of the compressed cyst-ventricular floor junction. (e, Ependymal lining of the floor of the third ventricle; b, brain parenchyma of the compressed hypothalamus; p, pia.) (From Fox JL, Al-Mefty O: Suprasellar arachnoid cysts: An extension of the membrane of Lillequist. Neurosurgery 7:617, 1980.)

Effective surgical treatment, which would seem to require simply making a big opening between the cyst and a normal CSF compartment, proves to be surprisingly difficult. Various combinations have been tried, including the transfrontal removal of the lower anterior wall of the cyst beneath the chiasm, a transcorticoventricular or transcallosal approach to remove much of the dome, the insertion of catheters between the cyst and ventricle or chiasmatic cistern, and the insertion of shunts from the lateral ventricles. Any one of these operations alone has a poor chance of sustained success. Agreement seems to be converging on the insertion of a combination of shunts from the lateral ventricles to the peritoneal cavity, with either a transcallosal route to remove the cystic dome, which was used with sustained success by Hoffman in five cases, or subfrontal removal of the anterior cyst wall. This latter tactic was successful in two cases from Gonzalez and colleagues,[59] three cases from Raimondi and colleagues,[60] and two cases from Murali and Epstein.[61] However, the lower opening closed, and symptoms recurred in one case of each of the last two groups and in one of Hoffman's cases. The fact that shunts from the ventricles alone may not suffice was demonstrated in a case from Murali and Epstein, in a child in whom a neonatal shunt kept the ventricles small but who also required opening of a suprasellar cyst to control bilateral visual loss 9 years later. Ventriculoperitoneal shunting alone was satisfactory in Raimondi's fourth case. Each of the traditional approaches has been associated with a high rate of recurrence of cysts.[2]

Upcoming neuroendoscopic techniques seem to solve some of the major surgical problems in treatment of suprasellar arachnoid cysts. Pierre-Khan and associates[57] were the first to publish their results after performing endoscopic ventriculocystostomy of suprasellar arachnoid cysts. They used a monopolar electroprobe to create the wide stoma between the cyst and the ventricular cistern (ventriculocys-

tostomy [VC]). In contrast to them, Caemaert and associates[1] prefer to use the neodymium:yttrium aluminum garnet (Nd:YAG) laser to open the cyst to the ventricular system and the basal cisterns (ventriculocystcisternostomy [VCC]). None of the patients had postoperative complications or need for a secondary shunting procedure. Additional authors have published similar successful results.[2, 6, 14, 62, 63]

## Neuroendoscopic Technique in Treatment of Suprasellar Arachnoid Cysts

Preoperatively, it is advisable to plan the operative approach whether stereotactically or by neuronavigation. Through a frontal precoronar bur hole approach, the surgeon enters the frontal horn of the lateral ventricle with the endoscope.[64] Usually, the cyst dome is bulging through the foramen of Monro. Ventriculocystostomy is performed using microscissors and microforceps as well as the bipolar coagulation and cutting device. It is advisable to create a large stoma (10 to 15 mm in diameter). After inspection of the parasellar region, it is absolutely necessary to open the membrane of Lillequist (cystocisternostomy), which forms the inferior wall of the cyst toward the prepontine cistern, using the basilar artery as a landmark. Our bipolar coagulation and cutting electrode proves to be the best instrument to make bloodless openings and avoids thermal effects to the surrounding nerval tissue.[65]

Because many patients are severely impaired by the time of initial diagnosis, prompt aggressive effort and close follow-ups are required.

### ▌ Case Report 4

An 8-year-old girl presented with signs of raised ICP, ataxia, and a cognitive disorder. MRI showed a hydrocephalus caused by a large suprasellar cyst with brain stem compression (Fig. 41–12A). The girl was operated on with the neuroendoscopic technique using the frontal transventricular bur hole approach. Six days after the intervention, the girl's clinical condition was good, and she was discharged. A control MRI, taken 1 year after the intervention, shows that the cystic lesion has reduced greatly in volume, and free CSF communication exists between the ventricular system and the basal cisterns, which is documented by a postoperative ECG-gated dynamic MRI (see Fig. 41–12B). The girl still has no neurologic signs.

## RATHKE'S CLEFT CYSTS

Rathke's pouch, the superiorly directed evagination from the stomodeum of the 4-week-old human embryo, becomes obliterated at all but its cranial portion by the seventh week of gestation. The anterior wall of the remaining small cavity, "the pituitary pouch," develops into the anterior lobe of the pituitary gland, and its posterior wall proliferates much less to become the pars intermedia of the gland. At autopsy, Shanklin[66] found that a residual lumen between a portion of these two structures persisted in 22 of 100 normal pituitary glands. Small, asymptomatic, fluid-containing cysts were found in 13 of these 22 specimens. Such cysts of Rathke's cleft were recorded in 26% of routine autopsy series in five publications.[67–70] Infrequently, these cysts enlarge enough to produce symptoms. These residual clefts of Rathke's pouch are usually lined with cuboidal or columnar epithelial cells, which are often ciliated and include mucin-secreting goblet cells that stain positively by the periodic acid–Schiff method. Stratified or pseudostra-

tified squamous epithelium may also be present and may rest on a collagenous connective tissue stroma.

By November 1989, Voelker and coworkers[71] had collected a total of 155 histologically confirmed symptomatic cases from the world literature, including their own eight cases. The increased recognition of the disorder is evident from the total of only 35 cases found in the literature in 1977 by Yoshida and associates.[72] The Rathke cleft cyst was both intrasellar and suprasellar in 90 patients, intrasellar in 22, suprasellar in 15, and intrasphenoidal in one. The cyst capsule varies in thickness and may be any color. Common colors of the more watery fluids are yellow, blue, or green, at times with cholesterol crystals. The content of the cyst may vary from watery or serous (in 15 cases) to mucoid, gelatinous, and caseous, like motor oil, to white and creamy. This last appearance may be suggestive of pus. The content of one of the cysts was so tough as to require a rongeur for removal.[73] Although in these series reported with only a few patients a limited range of abnormal appearances may be described in CT scans and MRI, the extreme differences in the cystic content of protein and other chemicals are matched by similar variation in the scans, as pointed out by many authors.[74–79] However, the size and location of the lesion were delineated in approximately 100% of the MRI studies and 90% of the CT scans. Image features such as a sellar epicenter, smooth contour, absence of calcification, absence of internal enhancement, and homogeneous attenuation or signal intensity within the lesion suggest the diagnosis of a Rathke cleft cyst.[80]

Kleinschmidt and associates[81] proposed a new pathognomonic MR feature—the posterior ledge sign—of Rathke's cleft cysts. Ross and colleagues[73] stated that the diagnosis can be made at operation after the cystic cavity is irrigated. The lining of Rathke's cleft cyst is smooth and transparent; that of a craniopharyngiomatous or a pituitary adenomatous cyst is lined at least at some point by tumor.

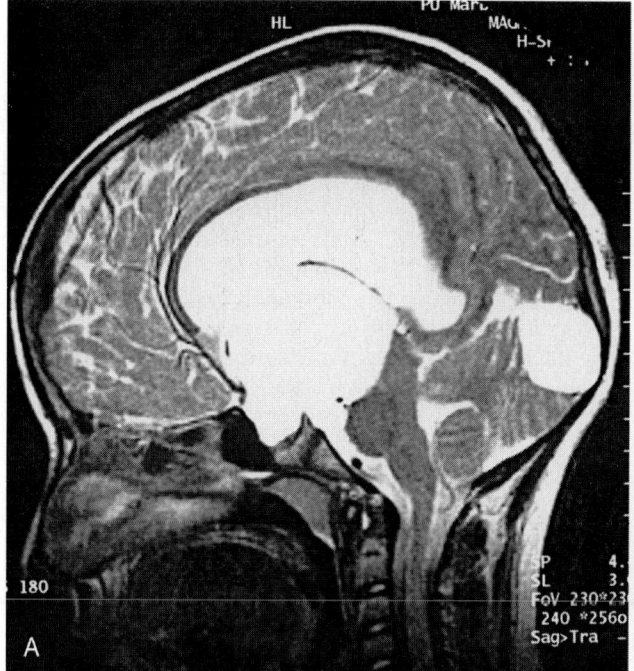
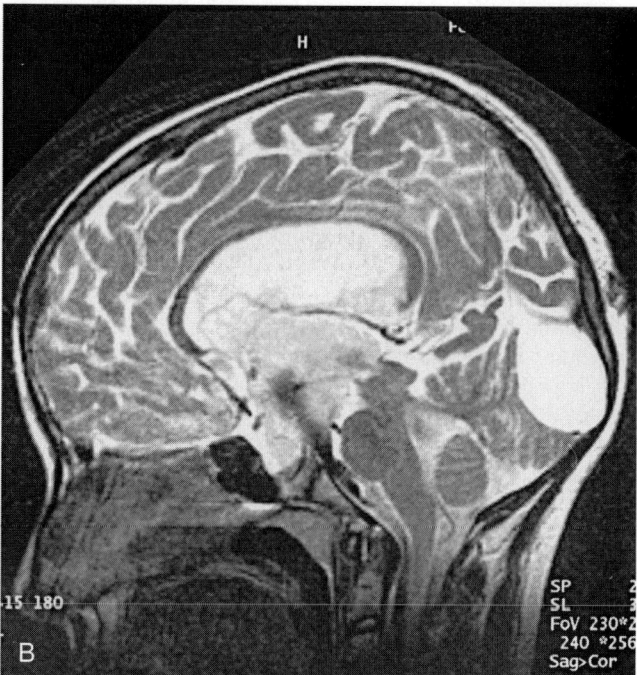

FIGURE 41–12A and B ■

## Case Report 5

This 62-year-old woman was admitted with a progressive bitemporal hemianopia and agitated psychosis (Karnofsky score of 30%). On MRI, a large cystic suprasellar space-occupying lesion with a blockage of foramen of Monro (Fig. 41–13A, B) was noted. Endoscopic stereotactic cyst evacuation was performed as an emergency procedure. The cystic lesion was reached through a right frontal bur hole. The gray membrane that bulged into the foramen of Monro was coagulated and was opened by microscissors. The sticky yellow contents of the cyst were aspirated. The remaining cyst membrane was vaporized using a laser. The histopathologic diagnosis was of a low-grade astrocytoma. Visual loss and the psychological disturbances of the patient normalized immediately after the procedure. A postoperative MRI showed that the cystic process was totally evacuated (see Fig. 41–13C, D). The patient was discharged 12 days after the procedure (Karnofsky score of 90%).

## CLINICAL DATA

Fager and Carter,[82] who had the earliest reported series of five living patients, found no solid abnormal tissue other than the thin wall in any of them. Visual fields and acuity, grossly abnormal in four of the patients preoperatively, improved greatly after the operation. The authors did not remove the cyst wall completely, but no symptoms recurred in any of the patients, who were followed up for as long as 9 years. They, therefore, regard total excision of the wall as unnecessary, concluding that a less radical approach suffices for these purely cystic intrapituitary or parapituitary lesions containing milky or mucoid fluid.

The following data are taken mainly from the reviews by Voelker and associates.[71] The female:male ratio was greater than 2:1, and the patients ranged in age from 4 to 78 years, with a mean age of 38 years and the highest frequency in the sixth decade. The preoperative duration of symptoms was from 3 days to 18 years, with an average of 34.9 months. Clinical presentation of patients is charac-

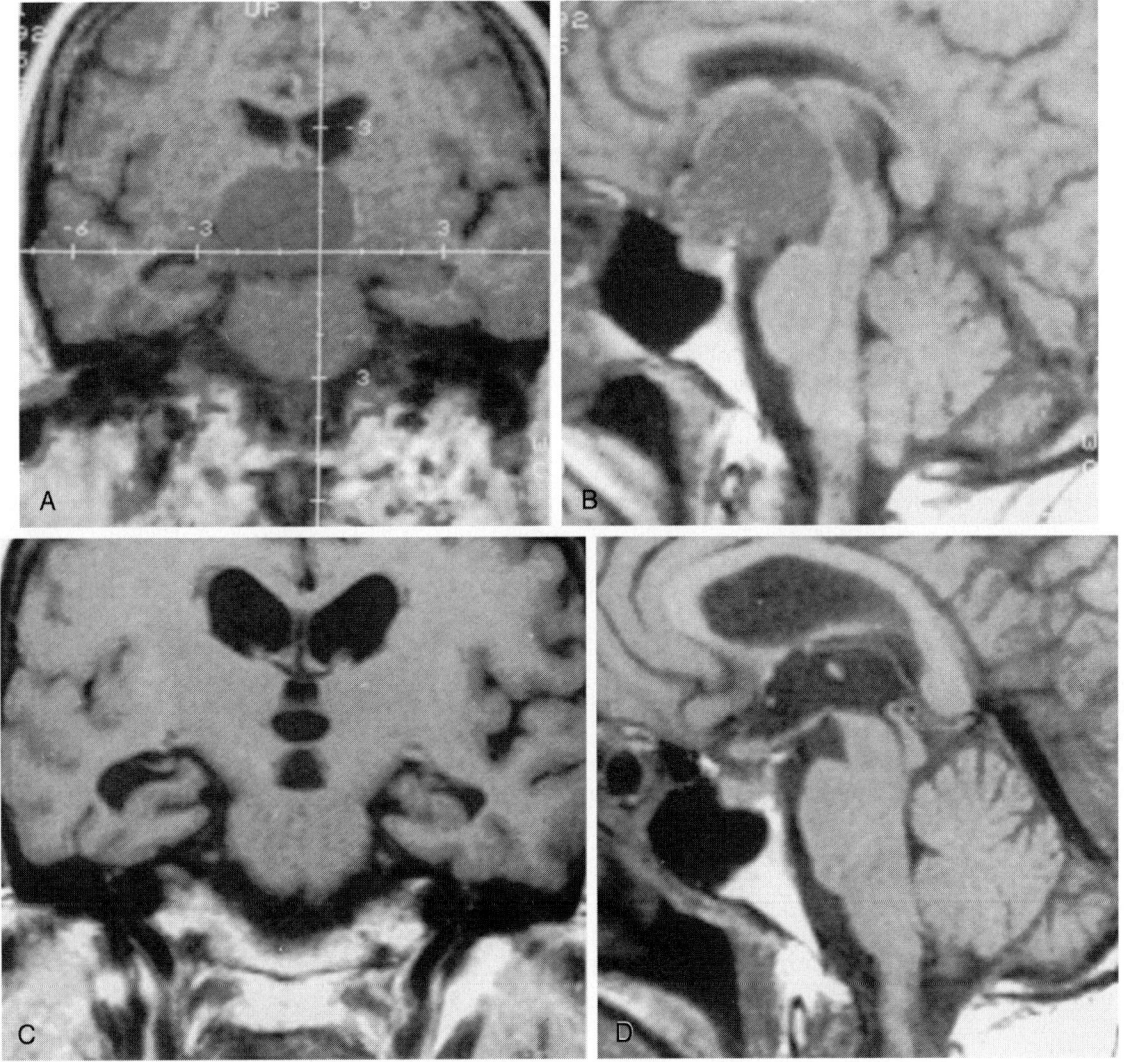

**FIGURE 41–13A–D** ■

terized by the triad: pituitary dysfunction, visual impairment, and headache.[78] The commonest symptoms were those caused by pituitary hypofunction. Dwarfism occurred in more than 70% of those younger than 18 years of age. Of the 37 patients with amenorrhea-galactorrhea, 14 had also a pituitary adenoma. Hyperprolactinemia might have occurred whether or not the amenorrhea-galactorrhea syndrome was present. Half of the patients had visual field defects, and about one fourth had decreased visual acuity. Almost half of the patients had headaches, which were often frontal headaches. Nausea and vomiting were noted in only 18 patients. Bouts of aseptic meningitis, although infrequent, should be recognized and are discussed later. A few patients described vertigo, diplopia, lethargy, or syncope. Intermittent episodes of fever in only six cases were, at least in the patient of Van Hilten and colleagues,[83] an unusual symptom of hypothalamic involvement. Attacks of fever at approximately 2-week intervals sometimes woke her at night or occurred randomly. They lasted for 6 hours, during which she had a rectal temperature of 39°C, followed by 3 hours of excessive sweating and a gradual return of temperature to normal. This picture proved to result from a $20 \times 20 \times 20$ mm suprasellar cyst extending up to the foramina of Monro and causing dilatation of both lateral ventricles and increased ICP. After lasting drainage of the cyst (three operations), all symptoms virtually disappeared.

Surgical excision of the cyst (usually partial) was carried out in 137 of the 155 patients, the remaining 18 cysts having been found at necropsy. The approach was by craniotomy in 60 cysts and via the sphenoid sinus in 59 cysts. Ross and coworkers[73] used the transsphenoidal route in 40 of 43 patients. The three patients with suprasellar lesions involving the pituitary stalk had transcranial approaches. The 10 patients of Midha and coworkers[84] were all operated on transsphenoidally as well as the 28 patients of El Mahdy and Powell.[78] This route was selected in only three of Voelker and coworkers' eight patients, all of whom had suprasellar extensions from the main intrasellar mass.[71] Operative mortality was zero in each of these four series. The recurrence rate after a craniotomy is approximately twice as high as that following the transsphenoidal route. Furthermore, if the cyst wall is removed only partially at craniotomy, the material secreted by the remnant may provoke an aseptic meningeal reaction. However, headache is not satisfactorily controlled by the partial removal of cyst wall advocated by the neurosurgeon Wilson and colleagues.[73] Of their 32 patients whose preoperative symptoms included headaches, 21 obtained relief. Of 14 patients in whom headache was the only preoperative symptom, the headache persisted after operation in seven patients. No correlation existed between the size of the lesion and the incidence of headache or the likelihood of disappearance of the headache after operation. The two patients with the largest lesions (23 and 25 mm) did not have a headache. However, of the 17 patients who had preoperative hyperprolactinemia, only three have continued to have prolactin levels above normal after operation. No data have been collated on the results on these scores after craniotomies.

Ross and coworkers[73] advocate the extremely conservative simple drainage of the cyst transsphenoidally "accompanied by biopsy of the cyst wall, when this is possible without entering the subarachnoid space or damaging normal structures." In fact, they took no operative pathologic specimen to confirm the diagnosis in 17 of their 40 patients. El Mahdy and Powell[78] performed a partial excision of the cyst wall and drainage of the contents into the sphenoid sinus. In seven patients with an intraoperative CSF leakage, they used fascia lata or fat grafts.

Midha and associates[84] obtained biopsies of the cyst wall in eight patients and removed all of it in two. The preoperative symptoms and signs in all 10 had disappeared, except those related to pituitary dysfunction and in three patients with visual problems. Although Ross and colleagues[73] followed up their patients for a mean of 68 months, with the longest follow-up at 126 months, they have seen only one symptomatic recurrence.

Totally benign behavior is far from invariable, however. One Japanese patient presented with acute adrenal insufficiency, which capped the hypopituitarism secondary to the intrasellar Rathke cleft cyst.[85] There is one report of an acute hemorrhage into a Rathke cleft cyst.[86] Another report is of hemosiderin deposits in the calcified epithelium of Rathke's cleft cyst,[87] which emerged with an abrupt onset of severe headache and gave rise to an enhancing intrasellar and suprasellar mass. The mass was successfully removed transsphenoidally. One of Yoshida and associates' patients had a small nodule on her cyst wall that was scraped out with a curet.[72] Only part of the cyst wall was removed, and a serious recurrence took place within 1 year. Raskind and coworkers' patient, whose cyst contained a clear, colorless fluid, experienced a recurrence requiring reoperation 26 years later.[88] The patient reported by Berry and Schlezinger[89] had only a fragment of the cyst wall removed at the first craniotomy. At a major recurrence 37 months later, the cyst was three times the original size but contained the same clear, colorless mucoid fluid. The recurrences described by Yoshida and colleagues,[72] Iraci and colleagues,[90] and Matsushima and colleagues[91] were in patients with solid components to their lesions that contained stratified epithelium. In Matsushima's case, although the cyst was filled with the typical mucinous, pus-like material and some of its lining was ciliated, mucin-containing columnar cells, most of it consisted of stratified squamous epithelium. This last component determined the outcome, namely death from recurrent tumor 20 months after its subtotal removal. Clearly, the solid portion of the tumor more than the appearance of the cystic fluid determines the prognosis. Two patients of Marcincin and Gennarelli[92] and one of Rout and colleagues[93] experienced recurrences in 4 months to 2 years after transsphenoidal evacuation of the cysts, even though the cyst fluid and wall were typical of pure Rathke's cleft lesions. A permanent visual loss ensued in one of the patients. The lesion was approached intracranially at recurrence in the second patient, and the entire cyst wall was removed. Two more recurrences after craniotomy have been reported by Yamamoto and coworkers[94] and by Leech and Olafson,[95] and four more have been reported after transsphenoidal approaches by Roux and coworkers,[96] Midha and coworkers,[84] Ross and coworkers,[73] and El Mahdy and Powell.[78] Surprisingly, Mukherjee and associates[97] describe a re-expansion rate of 33% in 12 patients with Rathke's cleft cysts during a follow-up time from 1 to 168 months (median of 30 months). They propose to evaluate the role of radiotherapy for recurrent symptomatic tumors.

As the reports have accumulated, it has become clear that many patients have transitional lesions or even highly unusual accompanying lesions. Russell and Rubenstein[98] were among the first to point this out, describing in two patients dumbbell cysts, the intrasellar portion of which was lined by a single layer of ciliated epithelium that changed abruptly at the diaphragma sellae to the squamous epithelium characteristic of a craniopharyngioma for the suprasellar portion. In a case reported by Yoshida and associates,[72] there was a tumor nodule with an inner lining of columnar cells that covered many layers of stratified squamous epithelium. Tajika and coworkers[99] found some areas of stratified epithelium in two of their three patients with Rathke's cleft cysts; in one of the two patients, cholesterol crystals, calcification, and brown fluid were present. Conversely, some ciliated, combined with columnar, cell areas were found in two other patients with histologic findings otherwise typical of a craniopharyngioma. This underlines the assumption that Rathke's cleft cysts may originate from squamous cell rests along the craniopharyngeal canal, resulting in a spectrum of cystic lesions in this area ranging from simple Rathke's cleft cysts to complex craniopharyngiomas.[78]

## Case Report 6

A 28-year-old patient suffering from a secondary amenorrhea was admitted to our department. An MRI scan showed a cystic lesion growing up from the sellar region and bulging into the third ventricle (Fig. 41–14A). We decided to perform primarily an endoscopic cyst evacuation using the frontal transventricular bur hole approach. The cyst was totally evacuated, and the cyst membrane was partly resected (see Fig. 41–14B). The histopathologic diagnosis of the cyst membrane and its contents was ambiguous; some

cells showed characteristics of craniopharyngioma cells, whereas others seemed to be of epithelial origin. Crystalloid and amorphic material was found in the contents of the cyst. The established histopathologic diagnosis was that of Rathke's cleft cyst; the differential diagnosis was a craniopharyngioma.

Goodrich and coworkers[100] described a suprasellar soft necrotic tumor rather than a fluid-containing tumor that contained many ciliated cuboidal or columnar cells typical of the lesion under discussion; however, other parts of the tumor included masses of squamous epithelium. Another Rathke's cleft cyst was reported that had characteristics of an epidermoid cyst.[101] Harrison and associates[102] suggested that Rathke's cleft cysts, epithelial cysts, epidermoid cysts, dermoid cysts, and craniopharyngiomas represent a continuum of ectodermally derived epithelial cystic epithelial lesions. In another group, the solid tumor of a chromophobe adenoma was associated with the typical histologic form of Rathke's cleft cyst.[103-108] The more solid tissue there is associated with the cyst, the more likely it is to include a chronic inflammatory process or the stratified epithelium of a craniopharyngioma or of the glandular tissue of a pituitary adenoma. These tissues are likely to show enhancement in a scan.

These lesions are also more likely to have a major or completely suprasellar portion. Yuge and coworkers[109] have added two more exclusively suprasellar Rathke's cleft cysts to the 15 cysts collected by Voelker and coworkers.[71] In the patients from Miyagi and coworkers,[105] the lesions extended into the third ventricle. The patients in each of two publications[109, 110] actually presented with hypothalamic tumors, one as a noncystic hypothalamic mass. This patient had an x, x, y karyotype in all cells (Klinefelter's syndrome). These larger tumors were not totally removed. In the case from Itoh and Usui,[111] the subepithelial tissue consisted of normal pituitary gland. The Rathke cleft cyst reported by Onda and associates[112] was associated with an arachnoid cyst; the cyst reported by Ikeda and colleagues[113]

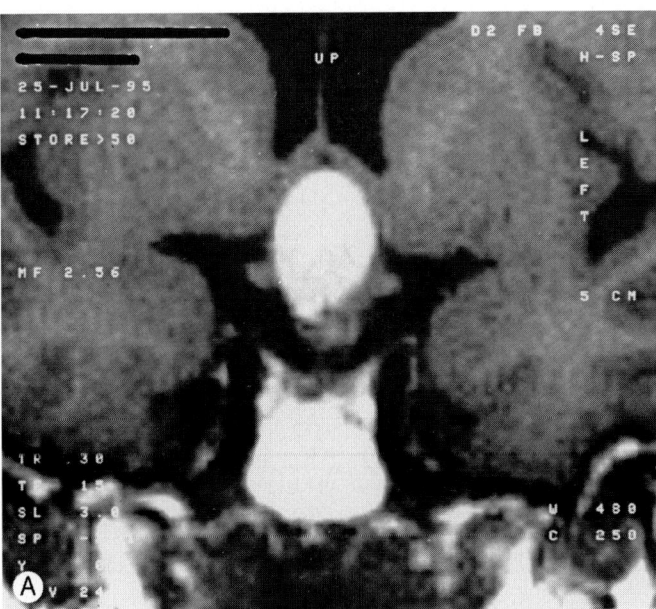
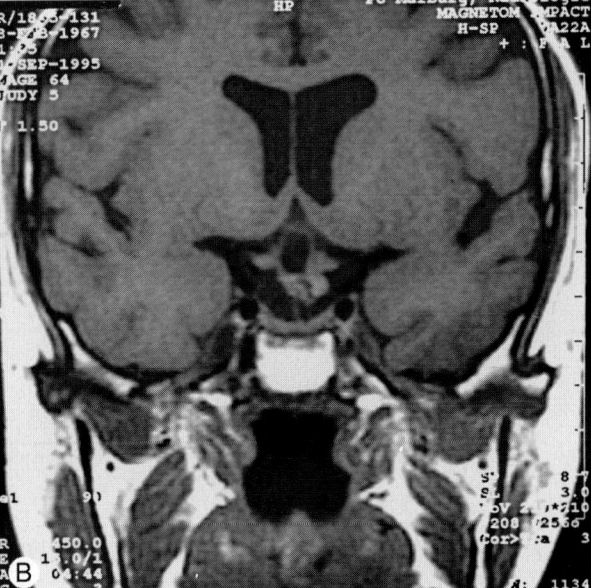

**FIGURE 41–14A** and *B* ■

was associated with an eosinophil (acromegalic) adenoma. Arita and coworkers[114] described a case of Cushing's disease accompanied by Rathke's cleft cyst, and Ersahin and associates[115] presented a case of Rathke's cleft cyst with diabetes insipidus. Two papers have reported chronic (granulomatous) hypophysitis related to Rathke's cleft cyst.[116, 117]

Cannova and associates[118] found a granulomatous sarcoidotic lesion of the hypothalamic-pituitary region associated with a Rathke cleft cyst. More distant accompanying lesions have been described by Koshiyama and colleagues,[119] in the form of Hashimoto's thyroiditis with diabetes insipidus and by Kim and colleagues,[120] as a maldevelopmental mass with absence of pituitary gland, a rudimentary prosencephalon; two other cysts, one a pigmented epithelial cyst (possibly a rudimentary eye) and the other a dorsal ependymal cyst, plus several other congenital abnormalities.

A single case report was published of a large suprasellar tumor extending downward to attach to the anterior wall of the pituitary gland. The cyst wall of the tumor was consistent with Rathke's cleft cyst in many places, but both its immunohistochemical and ultrastructural features were indistinguishable from colloid cysts of the third ventricle.[121] The cyst wall was totally removed via a subfrontal approach, and the authors achieved an excellent clinical result. Shuangshoti and colleagues[122] have also presented evidence that the intrasellar epithelial cysts are histologically and histochemically indistinguishable from the higher neuroepithelial or colloid cysts. Graziani and associates[123] assumed a common embryologic origin of suprasellar neurenteric cysts, the Rathke cleft cyst and the colloid cyst.

## Case Report 7

A 50-year-old man had a sudden frontal headache and a loss of consciousness. In the emergency unit, he was stuporous with weak motor activity. CCT and MRI revealed a cystic lesion in the third ventricle with obstructive hydrocephalus (Fig. 41–15A, B). Through a right frontal bur hole, an endoscopic stereotactic cyst perforation and evacuation of the colloidal mate-

rial was performed. The histopathologic diagnosis was a colloid cyst. The cyst wall was shrunk using the bipolar microelectrode. Membranous material adherent to the ventricular ependyma was left in situ. This was confirmed by a postoperative CCT examination (see Fig. 41–15C). One day after the intervention, the patient was alert without neurologic deficit. Ten days after the intervention, the patient was discharged without any deficit. Four years after the operation, the patient shows no clinical or radiologic signs of cyst recurrence.

The reports of recurrences after mere evacuation of cysts have provided support for those who, from the first, included readily removable cyst wall as part of the surgical objective. In a 1984 publication (when high-resolution CT scanning was available), Shimoji and coworkers[124] noted enhanced capsules around low-density cysts in all three of their patients. They, therefore, elected to remove "as much as possible of the capsule" in all three and achieved good clinical results. Specimens from all three patients showed a histologic pattern typical of Rathke's cleft cyst, with the addition of squamous epithelium in the third case. Swanson and coworkers[107] also used the presence of capsular enhancement at CT scanning of an intrasellar mass to guide them to a transfrontal excision of the cyst wall. Nonfunctional pituitary adenomatous cells constituted a part of that wall; therefore, they gave the patient a course of radiation therapy. This patient represented the sole reported case thus treated. The transsphenoidal route has been favored for most cases, especially when the suprasellar portion shows minimal enhancement.

In our experience with nontumorous cystic midline lesions, involving more than 50 patients, it is not necessary to resect the whole cyst membrane to prevent a recurrence. As an example, we have operated on 20 colloid cysts of the third ventricle in neuroendoscopic technique using the frontal bur hole approach. The cysts were evacuated and the membranes were resected subtotally. During a follow-up period from 6 months to 5 years, there was not one recurrence.

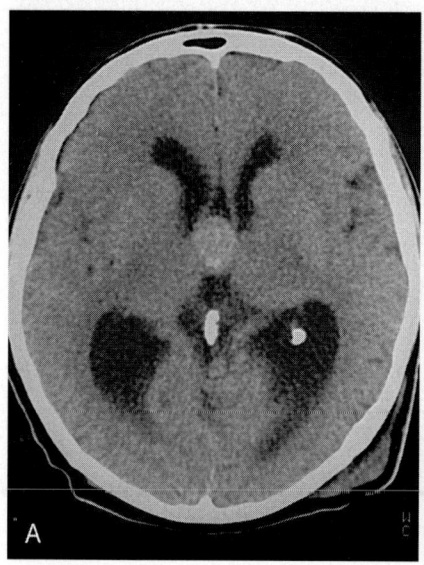 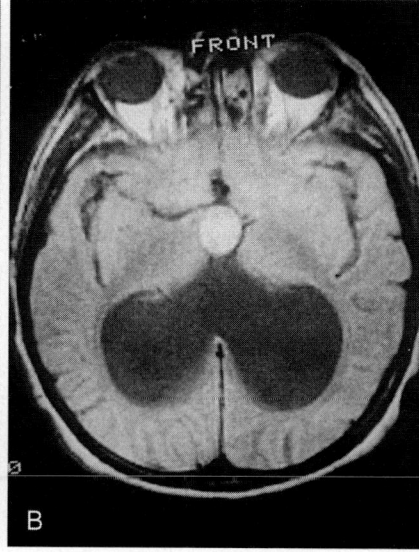 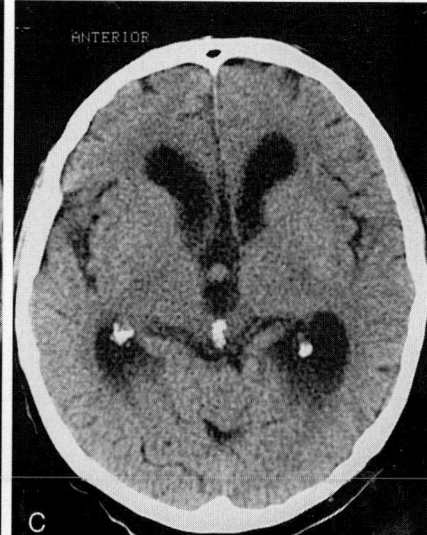

**FIGURE 41–15A–C** ■

## INTRASELLAR OR SUPRASELLAR ABSCESS

Gomez Perun and associates[125] stated in 1981 that 50 intrasellar abscesses had been reported; usually, the infection was propagated from a neighboring air or vascular sinus. The uninfected content of Rathke's cleft cyst may be a thick, white, or yellowish pus-like fluid that was mistaken for pus by the authors. Typically, the cellular reaction in the CSF is predominantly lymphocytic, and culture results of the "pus" and CSF are repeatedly negative. The patient is reacting to a "foreign body" that he himself has secreted, as described in the following section.

### Case Report 8

The 63-year-old woman suffered from a progressive left-sided loss of vision and a feeling of a swollen cheek. CT showed a space-occupying process in the left maxillary sinus, sphenoid sinus, and pterygopalatine fossa with destruction of the bottom of the sella turcica and a small suprasellar expansion (Fig. 41–16). During surgery, a transsphenoidal endoscopic-assisted approach was used. This approach proved to be helpful not only in transsphenoidal pituitary surgery but also in treatment of brain abscesses as pathologic cavity in different localization.[126] Intraoperatively, we found a pyomucocele of the maxillary and sphenoid sinuses that had affected an intrasellar partly suprasellar abscess. The maxillary and sphenoid sinuses were fenestrated, and sticky purulent contents were aspirated. The cavities were rinsed, and a tamponade was applied. Microbial investigation revealed infection with Staphylococcus aureus, and the patient was treated with antibiotics. Two days after the intervention, the patient's vision improved greatly. The patient was discharged to home 2 weeks

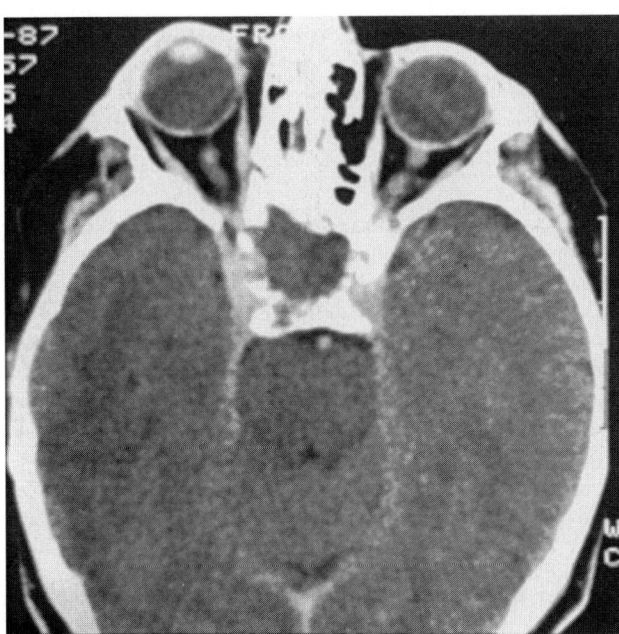

**FIGURE 41–16 ■**

later without a visual field defect or other neurologic deficits.

## BOUTS OF CHEMICAL MENINGITIS: THE SYNDROME OF THE TOXIN-LEAKING CNS CYST

An important point emerges from collation of the data from scattered individual case reports of patients with curious repeated febrile episodes, often with CSF pleocytosis. A culture was obtained from an organism in only one case. Attacks of a recurrent chemical febrile meningitis in a craniopharyngioma, presumably from a leakage of keratin or cholesterol, are a rare but well-authenticated occurrence.[127]

### Case Report 9

The 44-year-old patient had two febrile episodes with headache and opisthotonos 2 years before admission. Repeated CSF punctures revealed a slight pleocytosis. The first MRI scan showed no evidence of an intracranial space-occupying lesion. Later, it was suggested that these symptoms were the result of an aseptic meningitis after spontaneous perforation of a cystic craniopharyngioma. An MRI scan that was performed 3 months after the second febrile attack showed a cystic process in the anterior part of the third ventricle growing up from the suprasellar region (Fig. 41–17A, C). The cyst was approached by three-dimensional stereotactic calculation under direct endoscopic control. The cyst wall was coagulated using bipolar radiofrequency (RF), and the cyst was opened using microscissors. The cyst consisted of a thick yellow fluid. The cyst was emptied, and the capsule was coagulated. The postoperative follow-up was uneventful. On MRI, the residual tumor membrane is visible (see Fig. 41–17B, D). The patient was discharged 12 days after the intervention without neurologic symptoms or psychological disorder (Karnofsky score of 100%). The patient decided to undergo Gamma knife treatment for the remaining tumor capsule.

In the first such case of Rathke's cleft cyst, reported as an abscess by Obenchain and Becker,[128] the patient had five episodes in 3 years of severe headaches, nausea, vomiting, general malaise, and fever, all leading to hospital admissions but resolving spontaneously a few days later. Finally, blurring of vision in her inferior temporal quadrants led to the diagnosis of her intrasellar and minimally suprasellar mass, from which, via a subfrontal route, 2 ml of "purulent" fluid was aspirated. S. epidermidis was cultured from this fluid, and the patient was given penicillin, isoniazid, and ethambutol for 1 month. Then, via the transsphenoidal route, 3 ml of "pus" was aspirated, and the capsule was removed. Histologically, the wall was fibrous and lined by columnar epithelium with chronic inflammatory cells. The patient's recovery was excellent and sustained. The absence of acute inflammatory cells and the spontaneously subsiding brief attacks that had occurred for 3 years cast doubt on the role of the staphylococci.

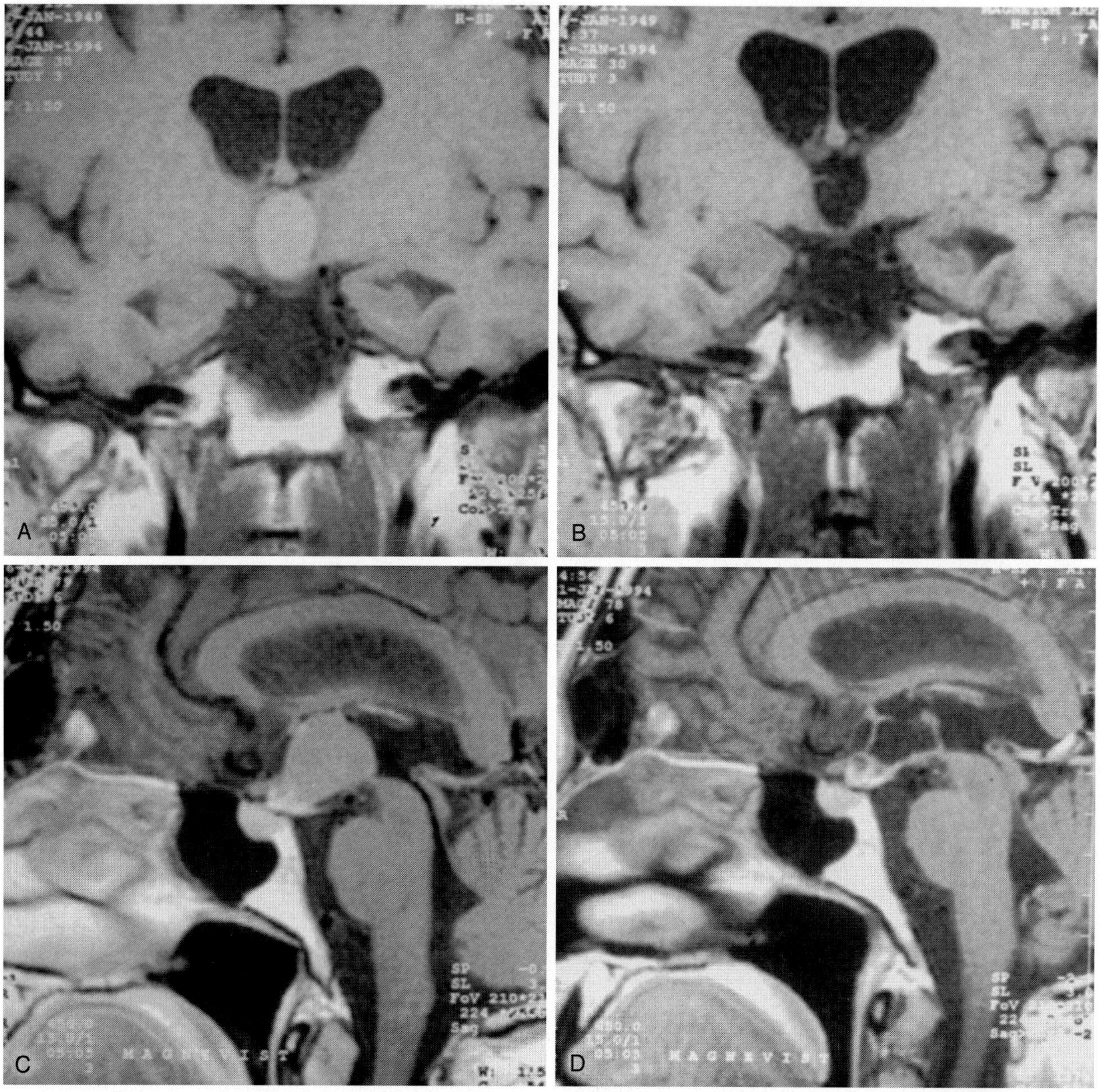

**FIGURE 41–17A–D ■**

In the next reported case,[129] similar recurrent brief episodes occurred. These episodes each lasted only 2 or 3 days and were characterized by intense supraorbital pain, fever to 39°C or 40°C, and about 50 clear-cut temporal lobe seizures a day. These seizures each lasted for several seconds and occurred mainly during the bouts of fever. These mysterious episodes continued for 10 years, during which time the patient's weight increased from 50 to 72 kg. Although the patient did not develop nuchal rigidity in the attacks, a lumbar puncture finally performed in 1977 revealed a largely lymphocytic pleocytosis and a normal protein level. Demonstration of an infratemporal quadrantanopia was followed by pneumography, which revealed a suprasellar mass. At a subfrontal exposure, thick, pus-like fluid was removed from a subchiasmatic cyst, the capsule of which was largely removed. The cyst wall was

heavily vascularized and infiltrated with inflammatory cells but lined with the typical ciliated columnar and cuboidal epithelium. The patient had also developed the symptoms and laboratory findings of deficient thyroid-stimulating hormone, adrenocorticotropic hormone, and luteinizing hormone-releasing hormone. The febrile episodes involving a headache stopped at once after operation, and the patient gradually made a full recovery. The seizures continued to require phenobarbital and valproic acid for control.

The following year, Verkijk and Bots[101] described a patient in whom meningeal reactions developed after surgery on a cyst; these reactions resolved spontaneously in 9 months. In the case reported by Steinberg and coworkers,[130] the initial symptoms pointed to a pituitary origin because of defects in visual acuity and fields, but then over the next 2 years, the patient was in the hospital numerous times with bouts of severe headache, nausea, vomiting, confusion, stiff neck, decreased visual acuity, and ataxic gait. On different occasions, the CSF showed pleocytosis, an increased protein level, and elevated pressure. All culture results were always negative. The episodes either resolved spontaneously or disappeared promptly after increases in the dosage of dexamethasone. Decreases in this dosage were followed by a recurrence of the symptoms. The sella was found to be enlarged and to contain a mass without suprasellar extension; the sella was, however, partially empty, with its anterior portion filling with air. These findings were apparently considered to be incidental. The lateral and third ventricles became increasingly dilated, and egress of contrast was delayed through the aqueduct and out of the fourth ventricle. The hydrocephalus was treated by ventriculoatrial shunt in 1972. Intracranial obstruction of the shunt required two revisions; each time, the symptoms promptly resolved. The patient died 1 year later of pneumonia. At autopsy, the Rathke cleft cyst occupying the entire sella was filled with thick, yellow-green fluid. The cyst epithelium was largely ciliated and columnar, squamous in one area and keratinized in others. The leptomeninges adjacent to the chiasm and third ventricle were "moderately fibrotic with mild chronic inflammation."

Episodes of severe meningeal symptoms and signs, also with completely negative culture results, characterized a patient reported on by Gomez Perun and coworkers.[125] One episode in May 1977 was especially severe. When a suprasellar lesion was demonstrated and explored 6 months later, the cyst contained a thick, white fluid, which had an intense inflammatory reaction, and numerous vessels in the cyst wall, along with a lining of ciliated columnar epithelium. Also, an extensive frontal basal arachnoiditis was present that was not noted in the other cases. The "pus" was sterile, and the patient made a prompt recovery but soon regressed, with similar episodes of aseptic meningitis. Despite three more operations, he too died; no organism was ever grown.

The patient reported on by Sonntag and coworkers[131] had only two episodes of a lymphocytic aseptic meningeal reaction before his intrasellar-suprasellar mass was subfrontally exposed. Seven milliliters of "pus" was aspirated, and the cyst wall was subtotally removed. The aspirate was sterile, but rare gram-negative rods were seen, and chloramphenicol was administered for 1 week. The symptoms recurred in 1 month, leading to transsphenoidal drainage of 5 ml of "pus" and "extensive removal of its wall." Culture results from this fluid were also negative. Therapy with chloramphenicol was continued for 1 month, and the patient has remained well for almost 2 years.

Shimoji and associates[124] described three clear-cut cases of chemical meningitis. In the first, brief episodes of headache, nausea, vomiting, and fever were accompanied by enough eye signs to point to the sellar region and its cyst. At craniotomy, the "abscess like viscous fluid" was sterile. As much cyst wall as possible was removed, and an excellent result persisted 2 years later. In the second case, a 52-year-old woman, four episodes of aseptic meningitis were required before a transsphenoidal evacuation of "milky, abscess-like viscous fluid" occurred and "as much as possible" of the cyst wall was removed. She, too, made an excellent recovery, which continued at 2 years. Both pa-

tients were also given 3000 cGy of $^{60}$Co radiation. In the third case, an intermittent fever to 38°C on hospitalization rose to 39°C after pneumoencephalography; the patient, a 42-year-old woman, had meningeal signs and a CSF pleocytosis of 456 neutrophils and 74 lymphocytes. No growth occurred on culture. A week of antibiotic therapy brought no change, but 30 mg/day of prednisolone given in addition to the antibiotics dropped the temperature to normal the next day. The yellowish-white gelatinous cyst fluid and, "as far as possible," its capsule, were removed via craniotomy. The periodic acid–Schiff-positive stratified squamous epithelium was heavily infiltrated with inflammatory cells. Good recovery persisted at 28 months.

Thick, yellow, pus-like material and a cyst wall accompanied by squamous epithelium and thick connective tissue infiltrated with inflammatory cells was described in two other reports.[93, 132]

One more clear-cut case of a foreign body reaction to the content of Rathke's cleft cyst has been reported by Albini and associates.[133] The 19-year-old woman developed headache, galactorrhea, and a few months later, amenorrhea. Bitemporal hemianopia and deficiencies in thyroid-stimulating hormone, adrenocorticotropic hormone, luteinizing hormone, and releasing hormone were identified. There had never been any episodes of fever or other suggestion of an aseptic meningeal reaction. The sella was enlarged, and while in the hospital, the patient developed a partial right third nerve paresis along with polydipsia and polyuria. At right pterional craniotomy, a large cyst seen on CT scan arising from the sella turcica was emptied of its thick, white fluid, and the cyst wall was insofar as possible removed. An excellent clinical result was obtained. The cyst wall was lined by the ciliated columnar and squamous epithelium of a Rathke cleft cyst. The rest of the specimen was infiltrated with lymphocytes, plasmacytes, and multinucleated giant cells among islands of preserved pituitary tissue. No organisms were ever demonstrated. Apparently, the cystic fluid never seeped into the subarachnoid space. At 3-year follow-up, the patient had had no more headache and no mass observed by CT.

From the service of Bognàr and coworkers[134] comes the report of two more patients with symptomatic histologically typical Rathke's cleft cysts and no preoperative episodes, which suggested aseptic meningitis. In both of them, the cyst contents were removed via the sphenoid sinus. Inflammatory cells and bacteria were recognized in the operative specimen, but technical problems were said to have prevented identification of organisms. Antibiotics were used, and one patient recovered uneventfully. In the other patient, transsphenoidal partial removal was followed by worsening in 2 weeks, leading to a frontolateral craniotomy, which likewise did not eliminate all of the abnormal tissue. *S. aureus* and *Streptococcus pyogenes* grown from the specimen at the second operation were treated by antibiotics, but they failed to avert death on the ninth postoperative day. This sequence suggests that the cyst content facilitated the bacterial growth seen only after the second operation. Because of the diagnosis of infection, neither of these patients was given large doses of corticosteroids. Both patients may have been reacting primarily to the chemicals in the cyst fluid.

At least four reports have been published of spontaneous

rupture of cystic craniopharyngiomas into the subarachnoid space that gave rise to a major but sterile meningeal reaction. This reaction was not different from those associated with Rathke's cleft cyst in that a predominantly neutrophilic, rather than lymphocytic, reaction occurred in the severe cases.[124, 135–137] Intracranial epidermoid tumors also rarely show this behavior (two cases[137]; one case[138]). There is also at least one dermoid cyst in this category.[139]

In conclusion, Rathke's cleft cysts tend to occur mainly within the sella; their precise extent can now be determined by modern CT and MRI scanning. Most of these cysts are best approached transsphenoidally; however, approximately 10% that are wholly suprasellar should be removed via craniotomy. Whether transsphenoidal aspiration of the cyst and biopsy suffice, as urged by Ross and colleagues,[73] or whether removal of as much cyst wall as seems safe is preferable is currently unclear. The neurosurgeons who favor a more aggressive stance will need to show that they achieve better relief of symptoms such as significant headache as well as fewer recurrences. The suprasellar component may need to be removed to the full extent dictated by safety because a repeat craniotomy is probably more hazardous than a second transsphenoidal approach.

At least 11 patients in less than 250 have Rathke's cleft cysts and demonstrate recurrent episodes of systemic or usually meningeal febrile illness. This finding suggests that some of these typically thin-walled cysts may contain a peculiar chemical irritant that can leak out enough to contaminate the CSF and possibly the bloodstream at intervals and produce these dangerous responses. In our experience, after endoscopic cyst evacuation (Rathke's cleft cyst, craniopharyngioma, colloid cyst), the contents that contact the CSF compartments lead to a temporary increase in body temperature owing to aseptic meningitis, which lasts for almost 24 hours and recurs spontaneously.

## REFERENCES

1. Caemaert J, Abdulah J, Calliauw L, et al: Endoscopic treatment of suprasellar arachnoid cysts. Acta Neurochir (Wien) 119:68–73, 1992.
2. Cohen A, Perneczky A: Endoscopy and the management of third ventricular lesions. In Apuzzo MLJ (ed): Surgery of the Third Ventricle, 2nd ed. Baltimore: Williams & Wilkins, 1998, pp 922–927.
3. Gaab MR, Schroeder HWS: Arachnoid cysts. In King W, Frazee J, DeSalles A (eds): Endoscopy of the Central and Peripheral Nervous System. New York: Thieme, 1998, pp 136–147.
4. Grotenhuis JA: The use of endoscopes during surgery of the suprasellar region. In Hellwig D, Bauer BL (eds): Minimally Invasive Techniques for Neurosurgery. Heidelberg: Springer-Verlag, 1998, pp 107–110.
5. Hellwig D, Bauer BL, List-Hellwig E: Stereotactic endoscopic interventions in cystic brain lesions. Acta Neurochir Suppl (Wien) 64:59–63, 1995.
6. Hopf NJ, Resch KDM, Ringel K, Perneczky A: Endoscopic management of intracranial arachnoid cysts. In Hellwig D, Bauer BL (eds): Minimally Invasive Techniques for Neurosurgery. Heidelberg: Springer-Verlag, 1998, pp 111–119.
7. Schroeder HW, Gaab MR, Niendorf WR: Neuroendoscopic approach to arachnoid cysts. J Neurosurg 85:293–298, 1996.
8. Krawchenko J, Collins GH: Pathology of an arachnoid cyst: Case report. J Neurosurg 50:224–228, 1979.
9. Go KG, Houthoff HJ, Blaauw EH, et al: Arachnoid cysts of the sylvian fissure: Evidence of fluid secretion. J Neurosurg 60:803–813, 1984.
10. Little J, Gomez M, MacCarty C: Infratentorial arachnoid cysts. J Neurosurg 39:380–386, 1973.
11. Hanieh, A, Simpson DA, North JB: Arachnoid cysts: A critical review of 41 cases. Childs Nerv System 4:92–96, 1988.
12. Williams D, Gutkelch AN: Why do central arachnoid pouches expand? J Neurol Neurosurg Psychiatry 37:1085–1092, 1974.
13. Santamarta D, Aguas J, Ferrer E: The natural history of arachnoid cysts: Endoscopic and cine-mode MRI evidence of a slit-valve mechanism. Minim Invasive Neurosurg 38:133–137, 1995.
14. Schroeder HW, Gaab MR: Endoscopic observation of a slit-valve mechanism in a suprasellar prepontine arachnoid cyst: Case report. Neurosurgery 40:198–200, 1997.
15. Hornig GW, Zervas NT: Slit defect of the diaphragma sellae with valve effect: Observation of a "slit valve." Neurosurgery 30:265–267, 1992.
16. Weber R, Voit T, Lumenta C, Lenard HG: Spontaneous regression of a temporal arachnoid cyst. Childs Nerv Syst 7:414–415, 1991.
17. Ciricillo SF, Cogen PH, Harsh GR, et al: Intracranial arachnoid cysts in children: A comparison of the effects of fenestration and shunting. J Neurosurg 74:230–235, 1991.
18. Brooks ML, Mayer DP, Staloff RT, et al: Intracanalicular arachnoid cyst mimicking acoustic neuroma: CT and MRI. Comput Med Imaging Graph 16:283–285, 1992.
19. Floris R, Pastore FS, Silvestrini M, et al: Supracerebellar arachnoid cyst and reversible tonsillar herniation: Magnetic resonance imaging and pathophysiological considerations. Neuroradiology 34:404–406, 1992.
20. Turgut M, Ozcan OE, Onol B: Case report and review of the literature: Arachnoid cyst of the fourth ventricle presenting as a syndrome of normal pressure hydrocephalus. J Neurosurg Sci 36:55–57, 1992.
21. Bhatia S, Thakur RC, Devi BI, et al: Craniospinal intradural arachnoid cyst. Postgrad Med J 68:829–830, 1992.
22. Punzo A, Conforti R, Martiniello D, et al: Surgical indications for intracranial arachnoid cysts. Neurochirurgia 35:35–42, 1992.
23. Pagni CA, Canavero S, Vinci V: Left trochlear nerve palsy, unique symptom of an arachnoid cyst of the quadrigeminal plate: Case report. Acta Neurochir (Wien) 105:147–149, 1990.
24. Kurokawa Y, Sohma T, Tsuchita H, et al: A case of intraventricular arachnoid cyst: How should it be treated? Childs Nerv Syst 6:365–367, 1990.
25. Arai H, Sato K: Posterior fossa cysts: Clinical, neuroradiological and surgical features. Childs Nerv Syst 7:156–164, 1991.
26. Miyagami M, Tsunokawa T: Histological and ultrastructural findings of benign intracranial cysts. Noshuyo Byori 10:151–160, 1993.
27. Friede RL, Yasargil MG: Supratentorial intracerebral epithelial (ependymal) cysts: Review, case reports and fine structure. J Neurol Neurosurg Psychiatry 40:127–137, 1977.
28. Olsen NK, Madsen HH: Arachnoid cyst with complicating intracystic and subdural haemorrhage. Röntgen Blätter 43:166–168, 1990.
29. Servadei F, Vergoni G, Frattarelli M, et al: Arachnoid cyst of middle cranial fossa and ipsilateral subdural haematoma: Diagnostic and therapeutic implications in three cases. Br J Neurosurg 7:249–253, 1993.
30. Passero S, Filosomi G, Cioni R, et al: Arachnoid cysts of the middle cranial fossa: A clinical, radiological and follow-up study. Acta Neurol Scand 82:94–100, 1990.
31. Rogers MA, Klug GL, Siu KH: Middle fossa arachnoid cysts in association with subdural haematomas: A review and recommendations for management. Br J Neurosurg 4:497–502, 1981.
32. Auer L, Gallhofer B, Ladurner G, et al: Diagnosis and treatment of middle cranial fossa arachnoid cysts and subdural hematoma. J Neurosurg 54:366–369, 1981.
33. Handa J, Okamato K, Sato M: Arachnoid cysts of the middle cranial fossa: Report of bilateral cysts in siblings. Surg Neurol 10:127–130, 1981.
34. Markakis E, Heyer R, Stoeppler L, et al: Die Aplexie der perfsylvi- achen Region. Neurochirurgia 22:211–220, 1979.
35. Hellwig D, Riegel T: Endoscopic evacuation of intracerebral and septated chronic subdural hematomas. In Jimenez D (ed): Endoscopic Intracranial Neurosurgery. Park Ridge, IL: AANS Publications Committee, 1998, pp 185–197.
36. Chan T, Logan P, Eustace P: Intermittent downbeat nystagmus secondary to vermian arachnoid cyst with associated obstructive hydrocephalus. J Clin Neuroophthalmol 11:293–296, 1991.
37. Haberkamp TJ, Monsell EM, House WF, et al: Diagnosis and treatment of arachnoid cysts of the posterior fossa. Otolaryngol Head Neck Surg 103:610–614, 1990.

38. Babu R, Murali R: Arachnoid cyst of the cerebellopontine angle manifesting as contralateral trigeminal neuralgia: Case report. Neurosurgery 28:886–887, 1991.

39. Higashi S, Yamashita J, Yamamoto Y, et al: Hemifacial spasm associated with a cerebellopontine angle arachnoid cyst. Surg Neurol 37:289–292, 1992.

40. Iacono RP, Labadie EL, Johnstone SJ, et al: Symptomatic arachnoid cyst at the clivus drained stereotactically through the vertex. Neurosurgery 27:130–133, 1990.

41. Pell MF, Thomas DG: The management of intratentorial arachnoid cysts by CT-directed stereotactic aspiration. Br J Neurosurg 5:399–403, 1991.

42. Lange M, Oeckler R, Beck OJ: Surgical treatment of patients with midline arachnoid cysts. Neurosurg Rev 3:35–39, 1990.

43. Oberbauer RW, Haase J, Pucher R: Arachnoid cysts in children: A European co-operative study. Childs Nerv Syst 8:281–286, 1992.

44. Bauer BL, Hellwig D: Minimally invasive endoscopic neurosurgery: A survey. Acta Neurochir Suppl 61:1–12, 1994.

45. Hellwig D, Benes L, Bertalanffy H, Bauer BL: Endoscopic stereotaxy: An eight year's experience. Stereotact Funct Neurosurg 68:90–97, 1997.

46. Rengachary SS, Watanabe I: Ultrastructure and pathogenesis of intracranial arachnoid cysts. J Neuropathol Exp Neurol 40:61–83, 1981.

47. Hoffman HJ, Hendrick EB, Humphreys RP, et al: Investigation and management of suprasellar arachnoid cysts. J Neurosurg 57:597–602, 1982.

48. Harrison MJG: Cerebral arachnoid cysts in children. J Neurol Neurosurg Psychiatry 34:316–323, 1971.

49. Dei-Anang K, Voth D: Cerebral arachnoid cysts: A lesion of the child's brain. Neurosurg Rev 12:59–62, 1989.

50. Key A, Retzius G: Studien in der Anatomie des Nervensystems und des Bindegewebes, Vol 1, plate III. Stockholm: P.A. Norsted and Soner, 1875.

51. Lillequist B: The anatomy of the subarachnoid cisterns. Acta Radiol 48:61, 1956.

52. Fox JL, Al-Mefty O: Suprasellar arachnoid cysts: An extension of the membrane of Lillequist. Neurosurgery 7:615–618, 1980.

53. Starkman SP, Brown TC, Linell EA: Cerebral arachnoid cysts. J Neuropathol Exp Neurol 17:484–500, 1958.

54. Kivela T, Pelkonen R, Oja M, Heiskanen O: Diabetes insipidus and blindness caused by a suprasellar tumor: Pieter Pauw's observations from the 16th century. JAMA 279:48–50, 1998.

55. Benton, J, Nellhaus G, Huttenlocher P, et al: The bobble head doll syndrome: Report of a unique truncal tremor associated with third ventricular cyst and hydrocephalus in children. Neurology 16:725–729, 1966.

56. Albright L: Treatment of bobble-head doll syndrome by transcallosal cystectomy. Neurosurg 8:593–595, 1981.

57. Pierre-Khan A, Capelle L, Brauner R, et al: Presentation and management of suprasellar arachnoid cysts. J Neurosurg 73:355–359, 1990.

58. Sugawara A, Ebina K, Sawataishi J, et al: Suprasellar arachnoid cyst associated with precocious puberty: Report of an operated case and review of the literature. No Shinkei Geka 20:1107–1112, 1992.

59. Gonzalez CA, Villarejo FJ, Blazquez MG, et al: Suprasellar arachnoid cysts in children: Report of three cases. Acta Neurochir (Wien) 60:281–296, 1982.

60. Raimondi AJ, Shimoji T, Gutierrez FA: Suprasellar cysts: Surgical treatment and results. Childs Nerv Syst 7:57–72, 1980.

61. Murali R, Epstein F: Diagnosis and treatment of suprasellar arachnoid cyst. J Neurosurg 50:515–518, 1979.

62. Dhooge C, Govaert P, Martens F, et al: Transventricular endoscopic investigation and treatment of suprasellar arachnoid cysts. Neuropediatrics 23:245–247, 1992.

63. Decq P, Brugieres P, Le Guerinel C, et al: Percutaneous endoscopic treatment of suprasellar arachnoid cysts: Ventriculocystostomy or ventriculocisternostomy? Technical note. J Neurosurg 84(4):696–701, 1996.

64. Hellwig D, Riegel T, Bertalanffy A: Neuroendoscopic techniques in treatment of intracranial lesions. Minim Invas Ther Allied Technol 7:123–135, 1998.

65. Hellwig D, Haag R, Bartel V, et al: Application of new electrosurgical devices and probes in endoscopic neurosurgery. Neurol Res 21:67–72, 1999.

66. Shanklin WM: The incidence and distribution of cilia in the human pituitary with a description of microfollicular cysts derived from Rathke's cleft. Acta Anat (Basel) 11:361–382, 1951.

67. Bayoumi ML: Rathke's cleft and its cysts. Edinb Med J 55:745–749, 1948.

68. Gillman T: The incidence of ciliated epithelium and mucous cells in the normal Bantu pituitary. S Afr Med Sci 5:30–40, 1940.

69. McGrath P: Cysts of sella and pharyngeal hypophyses. Pathology 3:123–131, 1971.

70. Rasmussen AT: Ciliated epithelium and mucous-secreting cells in the human hypophysis. Anat Rec 41:273–283, 1929.

71. Voelker JL, Campbell RL, Muller J: Clinical, radiographic and pathological features of symptomatic Rathke's cleft cysts. J Neurosurg 74:535–544, 1991.

72. Yoshida J, Kobayashi T, Kageyama N, et al: Symptomatic Rathke's cleft cyst: Morphological study with light and electron microscopy and tissue culture. J Neurosurg 47:451–458, 1977.

73. Ross DA, Norman D, Wilson CB: Radiologic characteristics and results of surgical management of Rathke's cysts in 43 patients. Neurosurgery 30:173–179, 1993.

74. Asari S, Ito T, Tsuchida S, et al: MR appearance and cyst content of Rathke cleft cysts. J Comput Assist Tomogr 14:532–535, 1990.

75. Christophe C, Flamant-Durand J, Hanquinet S, et al: MRI in seven cases of Rathke's cleft cyst in infants and children. Pediatr Radiol 23:79–82, 1993.

76. Ito H, Nishizaka T, Kajiwara K, et al: Pituitary nonadenomatous tumor (Rathke's cleft cyst). Nippon Rinsho 51:2711–2715, 1993.

77. Nakasu Y, Isozumi T, Nakasu S, et al: Rathke's cleft cyst: Computed tomographic scan and magnetic resonance imaging. Acta Neurochir (Wien) 103:99–104, 1990.

78. El Mahdy WE, Powell M: Transsphenoidal management of 28 symptomatic Rathke's cleft cysts, with special reference to visual and hormonal recovery. Neurosurgery 42 (1):7–16, 1998.

79. Oka H, Kawano N, Suwa T, et al: Radiological study of symptomatic Rathke's cleft cysts. Neurosurgery 35:632–636, 1994.

80. Naylor MF, Scheithauer BW, Forbes GS, et al: Rathke cleft cyst: CT, MR, and pathology of 23 cases. J Comput Assist Tomogr 19:853–859, 1995.

81. Kleinschmidt Demasters BK, Lillehei KO, Steaaars JC: The pathologic, surgical, and MR spectrum of Rathke cleft cysts. Surg Neurol 44:19–26, 1995.

82. Fager CA, Carter H: Intrasellar epithelial cysts. J Neurosurg 24:77–81, 1966.

83. Van Hilten BJ, Roos RAC, de Bakker HM, et al: Periodic fever: An unusual manifestation of a recurrent Rathke's cleft. J Neurol Neurosurg Psychiatry 43:533, 1990.

84. Midha R, Jay V, Smyth HS: Transsphenoidal management of Rathke's cleft cysts. Surg Neurol 35:441–454, 1991.

85. Tanigawa K, Yamashita S, Namba H, et al: Acute adrenal insufficiency due to symptomatic Rathke's cleft cyst. Intern Med 31:467–469, 1992.

86. Onesti ST, Wisniewski T, Post KD: Pituitary hemorrhage into a Rathke's cleft cyst. Neurosurgery 27:644–646, 1990.

87. Wagle VG: Hemorrhage into Rathke's cleft cyst. Neurosurgery 28:335, 1991.

88. Raskind R, Brown HA, Mathis J: Recurrent cyst of the pituitary: 26-year follow-up from first decompression. J Neurosurg 28:595–599, 1968.

89. Berry RG, Schlezinger NS: Rathke cleft cysts. Arch Neurol 1:48–58, 1959.

90. Iraci G, Girodano R, Gerosa M, et al: Ocular involvement in recurrent cyst of Rathke's cleft: Case report. Ann Ophthalmol 11:94–98, 1979.

91. Matsushima T, Fukui M, Ohta M, et al: Ciliated and goblet cells in craniopharyngioma: Light and electron microscopic studies at surgery and autopsy. Acta Neuropathol (Berl) 50:199–205, 1980.

92. Marcincin RP, Gennarelli TA: Recurrence of symptomatic pituitary cysts following transsphenoidal drainage. Surg Neurol 18:448–451, 1982.

93. Rout DL, Das L, Rao VRK, et al: Symptomatic Rathke's cleft cysts. Surg Neurol 19:42–45, 1983.

94. Yamamoto M, Takara E, Imanaga H, et al: Rathke's cleft cyst: Report of two cases. Neurol Surg 12:609–616, 1984.

95. Leech RW, Olafson RA: Epithelial cysts of the neuraxis. Presentation of three cases and a review of the origins and classification. Arch Pathol Lab Med 101:196–202, 1977.

96. Roux FX, Constans JP, Monsaingeon V, et al: Symptomatic Rathke's cleft cysts: Clinical and therapeutic data. Neurochirurgia (Stuttg) 31:18–20, 1988.

97. Mukherjee JJ, Islam N, Kaltsas G, et al: Clinical, radiological and pathological features of patients with Rathke's cleft cysts: Tumors that may recur. J Clin Endocrinol Metab 82(7):2357–2362, 1997.

98. Russell DS, Rubinstein LJ: Pathology of Tumors of the Nervous System, 3rd ed. Baltimore: Williams & Wilkins, 1971.

99. Tajika Y, Kubo O, Kamiya M, et al: Clinicopathological features of 5 cases of pituitary cyst including Rathke's cleft cyst. Neurol Surg 10:1055–1064, 1982.

100. Goodrich JT, Post KD, Duffy P: Ciliated craniopharyngioma. Surg Neurol 24:105–111, 1985.

101. Verkijk A, Bots GT: An intrasellar cyst with both Rathke's cleft and epidermoid characteristics. Acta Neurochir (Wien) 51:203–207, 1980.

102. Harrison MJ, Morgello S, Post KD: Epithelial cystic lesions of the sellar and parasellar region: A continuum of ectodermal derivates? J Neurosurg 80:1018–1025, 1994.

103. Hiyama H, Kubo O, Yato S, et al: A case of pituitary adenoma combined with Rathke's cleft cysts. Neurol Surg 14:435–440, 1986.

104. Matsumori K, Okuda T, Nakayama K, et al: A case of calcified prolactinoma combined with Rathke's cleft cysts. Neurol Surg 12:833–838, 1984.

105. Miyagi A, Iwasaki M, Shibuya T, et al: Pituitary adenoma combined with Rathke's cleft cyst—case report. Neurol Med Chir (Tokyo) 33:643–650, 1993.

106. Nishio S, Mizuno J, Barrow DL, et al: Pituitary tumors composed of adenohypophysial adenoma and Rathke's cleft cyst elements: A clinicopathological study. Neurosurgery 21:371–377, 1987.

107. Swanson SE, Chandler WF, Latack J, et al: Symptomatic Rathke's cleft with pituitary adenoma: Case report. Neurosurgery 17:657–659, 1985.

108. Troukedes KM, Walfish PG, Holgate RC, et al: Sellar enlargement with hyperprolactinemia and a Rathke's pouch cyst. JAMA 240:471–473, 1978.

109. Yuge T, Shigemori M, Tokutomi T, et al: Entirely suprasellar symptomatic Rathke's cleft cyst. No Shinkei Geka 19:273–278, 1991.

110. Wenzel M, Salcman M, Kristt DA, et al: Pituitary hyposecretion and hypersecretion produced by a Rathke's cleft cyst presenting as a noncystic hypothalamic mass. Neurosurgery 24:424–428, 1989.

111. Itoh J, Usui K: An entirely suprasellar symptomatic Rathke's cleft cyst: Case report. Neurosurgery 30:581–585, 1992.

112. Onda K, Tanaka R, Takeda N, et al: Symptomatic Rathke cleft cyst simulating arachnoid cyst: Case report. Neurol Med Chir (Tokyo) 29:1039–1043, 1989.

113. Ikeda H, Yoshimoto T, Katakura R: A case of Rathke's cleft cyst within a pituitary adenoma presenting with acromegaly: Do "transitional cell tumors of the pituitary gland" really exist? Acta Neuropathol (Berl) 83:211–215, 1992.

114. Arita K, Uozumi T, Takechi A, et al: A case of Cushing's disease accompanied by Rathke's cleft cyst: The usefulness of cavernous sinus sampling in the localization of microadenoma. Surg Neurol 42:112–116, 1994.

115. Ersahin Y, Ozdamar N, Demirtas E, Mutluer S: A case of Rathke's cleft cyst presenting with diabetis insipidus. Clin Neurol Neurosurg 97:317–320, 1995.

116. Wearne MJ, Barber PC, Johnson AP: Symptomatic Rathke's cleft cyst with hypophysitis. Br J Neurosurg 9:799–803, 1995.

117. Roncaroli F, Bacci A, Frank G, Calbucci F: Granulomatous hypophysitis caused by a ruptured intrasellar Rathke's cleft cyst: Report of a case and review of the literature. Neurosurgery 43:141–149, 1998.

118. Cannova S, Romano C, Buffa R, Faglia G: Granulomatous sarcoidotic lesion of hypothalamic-pituitary region associated with Rathke's cleft cyst. J Endocrinol Invest 20:77–81, 1997.

119. Koshiyama H, Kato Y, Masutani H, et al: A case of Rathke's cleft cyst associated with diabetes insipidus and Hashimoto's thyroiditis. Jpn J Med Sci Biol 28:406–409, 1989.

120. Kim TS, Cho S, Dickson DW: Aprosencephaly: Review of the literature and a report of a case with cerebellar hypoplasia, pigmented epithelial cyst and Rathke's cleft cyst. Acta Neuropathol (Berl) 79:424–431, 1990.

121. Wolfsohn AL, Lach B, Benoit BG: Suprasellar xanthomatous Rathke's cleft cyst. Surg Neurol 38:106–109, 1992.

122. Shuangshoti S, Netsky M, Nashold BS Jr: Epithelial cysts related to the sella turcica: Proposed origin from neuroepithelium. Arch Pathol 90:444–450, 1970.

123. Graziani N, Dufour H, Figarella Branger D, et al: Do the suprasellar neurenteric cyst, the Rathke's cleft cyst and the colloid cyst constitute a same entity? Acta Neurochir (Wien) 13:174–180, 1995.

124. Shimoji T, Shinohara A, Shimizu A, et al: Rathke cleft cysts. Surg Neurol 21:295–310, 1984.

125. Gomez Perun J, Eiras J, Carcavilla LI: Abcès intrasellaire au sein d'un kyste de la poche de Rathke. Neurochirurgie 27:201–205, 1981.

126. Hellwig D, Riegel T: Stereotactic endoscopic treatment of brain abscess. In Jimenez DF (ed): Intracranial Endoscopic Neurosurgery. Park Ridge, IL: AANS Publications Committee, 1998, pp 199–207.

127. Martin JB: Case records of the Massachusetts General Hospital: Case 17—1980. N Engl J Med 302:1015–1023, 1980.

128. Obenchain TG, Becker DP: Head bobbing associated with a cyst of the third ventricle. J Neurosurg 37:457, 1972.

129. Menault F, Sabouraud O, Javalet A, et al: Kyste de la fente de Rathke. Rev Otoneuroophtamol 51:383–390, 1979.

130. Steinberg GK, Koenig GH, Golden JB: Symptomatic Rathke's cleft cysts. J Neurosurg 56:290–295, 1982.

131. Sonntag VKH, Lenge KL, Balis MS, et al: Surgical treatment of an abscess in a Rathke's cleft cyst. Surg Neurol 20:152–156, 1983.

132. Okamoto S, Handa H, Yamashita J, et al: Computed tomography in intra and suprasellar epithelial cysts (symptomatic Rathke cleft cysts). AJNR Am J Neuroradiol 6:515–519, 1985.

133. Albini CH, MacGillivray MH, Fisher JE, et al: Triad of hypopituitarism, granulomatous hypophysitis and ruptured Rathke's cleft cyst. Neurosurgery 22:133–136, 1988.

134. Bognàr L, Szeifert GT, Fedoresàk I, et al: Abscess formation in Rathke's cleft cyst. Acta Neurochir (Wien) 117:70–72, 1992.

135. Russell RWR, Pennybacker JB: Craniopharyngioma in the elderly. J Neurol Neurosurg Psychiatry 24:13, 1978.

136. Patrick BS, Smith RR, Bailey TO: Aseptic meningitis due to spontaneous rupture of craniopharyngioma cyst: Case report. J Neurosurg 41:387–390, 1974.

137. Lloyd MH, Belchetz PE: The clinical features and management of pituitary apoplexy. Postgrad Med 53:82–85, 1977.

138. De Klerk DJJ, Spence J: Chemical meningitis with intracranial tumours. S Afr Med J 48:131–135, 1974.

139. Schwartz JF, Balentine JD: Recurrent meningitis due to an intracranial epidermoid. Neurology 28:124–129, 1978.

140. Cantu RN, Kjellberg RN, Moses JM, et al: Aseptic meningitis due to dermoid tumor: Case report and confirming test. Neurochirurgia (Stuttg) 11:94–98, 1968.

# Endoscopic Neurosurgery

# Endoscopic Neurosurgery

■ JACQUES CAEMAERT

In the last decade, endoscopic neurosurgery has undergone a rapid growth in indications and applications. The ideas and the techniques of endoscopic neurosurgery are not new, but today they had not gained wide acceptance owing to a lack of suitable instruments and to the limitations of neuroradiology. With the tremendous progress in computed tomography (CT) and magnetic resonance (MR), lesions have been revealed that are appropriate for an endoscopic approach. Particularly important are the lesions confined to or adjacent to the ventricle. The last 10 years have been very fruitful in defining both the indications and developing instruments so that the endoscope is now a valuable neurosurgical tool. It is important to realize that endoscopic neurosurgery is a technique, not a "solution," and is also not a "subspecialty" but is rather an instrument analogous to the operating microscope, the ultrasonic aspirator, and neuronavigation devices.

This chapter is orientated at a practical level and is based on 14 years of experience in endoscopic neurosurgery. There are two different concepts regarding the use of a neuroendoscope: (1) endoscopic neurosurgery, and (2) endoscopy-assisted microsurgery. In the first technique, the surgery is performed in a cavity through the channels of the endoscope inserted in the ventricular system or in other cystic structures. The second technique, endoscopy-assisted microsurgery, uses the endoscope as an optic device to guide microsurgical instruments that are used alongside this optic element. This can be done in various subarachnoid spaces, such as the cerebellopontine angle or the basal cisterns.

## HISTORY

Endoscopic neurosurgery[37, 103, 226] dates to 1910 when Lespinasse,[52, 142] a urologist, who treated two children with hydrocephalus by endoscopic coagulation of the choroid plexus. The same procedure was adopted by Dandy who, in 1922, reported avulsion of the choroid plexus in hydrocephalic children under cystoscopic control.[50, 51] One year later, Mixter,[159] using a small urethroscope introduced through the anterior fontanel, relieved an obstructive hydrocephalus by performing an endoscopic third ventriculostomy. This was followed in the same year by Fay and Grant's[61] first endoscopic photographs of the cerebral ventricles. In 1936, Putnam[192, 193] and Scarff[208, 209] described their results with the endoscopic coagulation of choroid plexus for the treatment of hydrocephalus. With the development in 1949 by Nulsen, Spitz, and Holter of the valve system for shunting, the further attempts at endoscopic control of hydrocephalus were abandoned in favor of lower morbidity procedures. In Utrecht, Holland, Bosma was an early pioneer in modern endoscopy. Since 1962, Bosma has applied 8-mm film registration in interventions for hydrocephalus and tumors. The construction of solid rod lens systems by Hopkins was a milestone in the development of neuroendoscopy. This technique was applied by Griffith for endoscopic third ventriculostomy and choroid plexus coagulation.[78–81] In 1963, Guiot[87] introduced the use of solid quartz rod lenses, whose internal reflective properties are fitted with an external light source that provides a very bright light. Olinger and Ohlhaber[171] designed a 17-gauge needle endoscope for spinal endoscopy. In the 1970s, Fukushima[69–72] described and used flexible endoscopy with fiberglass optics applied to different situations.

## Indications

Paralleling the development of these techniques, insight is growing into the real indications for their usage (Table 42–1). The choice of endoscopic approach is determined by the potential benefit to the patient. Endoscopic neurosurgery is not easy; it is time-consuming and is associated with definite risks. The advantage should be in the enhanced safety for the patient and the diminished invasiveness of the method. The application of an endoscope requires the presence of a cavity—either the ventricular system or a cystic structure. The performance of endoscopic surgery in the parenchyma of the brain is absolutely contraindicated.

## GENERAL TECHNIQUE

When we started our work in 1986 no suitable dedicated endoscopic instrument was available for neurosurgery, whereas in recent years numerous neuroendoscopes have

## TABLE 42-1 ■ ENDOSCOPIC NEUROSURGICAL INDICATIONS

*Hydrocephalus:* third ventriculostomy, septostomy, desobstruction, choroid plexus coagulation
  Obstructive: Aqueduct
              Foramina of Magendie and Luschka
              Foramina of Monro
  Asymmetric hydrocephalus
  Multilocular hydrocephalus
  Malresorptive hydrocephalus
*Cystic lesions:* fenestration, biopsy, partial or total removal
  Arachnoid cysts
    Suprasellar
    Convexity
    Sylvian fissure
    Cerebellopontine angle
    Quadrigeminal cistern
  Ependymal cysts
    Paraventricular
    Cavum septi pellucidi
    Cavum veli interpositi
  Epidermoid cysts
    New
    Recurrent
  Colloid cysts
  Cystic tumors
  Pineal cysts
  Degenerative cysts
    Post radiosurgery
    Post brachytherapy
    Post meningoencephalitis
  Parasitic cysts

*Tumors:* biopsy, partial or total removal
  Bulging into the ventricles
  Confined to the ventricles
  Cystic parts
  Craniopharyngioma
*Catheter*
  Insertion, denudation, repositioning, and removal
*Hemorrhage*
  Intracerebral hematoma
  Acute subdural hematoma
  Septated chronic subdural hematoma
  Intraventricular hemorrhage
*Spinal*
  Syringomyelia
  Lumbar disk herniation
  Thoracic disk herniation
  Traumatic spinal hematoma
*Endoscopy-assisted microsurgery*
  Aneurysm
  Sellar and suprasellar region
  Acoustic neuroma
  Transsphenoidal pituitary surgery
  Cerebellopontine angle surgery
*Miscellaneous*
  Carpal tunnel release
  Transventricular hippocampectomy
  Craniosynostosis

been developed worldwide.* Along with the Richard Wolf Company, Drongen, Belgium, in association with Richard Wolf Knittlingen, Germany,[30] we developed a multipurpose endoscope that was safe and simple and had a rigid round shaft long enough to be compatible with all existing stereotactic systems. The endoscope had a maximum outer diameter of 6 mm, a smoothly rounded tip, and four channels of which two irrigation channels (in and out) reached the tip of the instrument. The instrument was to have a wide working channel and an optimal image quality. The side channels were to join the main shaft at an angle that would allow instruments to be introduced through them. During the next 6 years, changes were made to five successive prototypes and these were then tested in a series of endoscopic procedures. The final instrument was tried for 1

*See references 6, 14, 15, 19–21, 30, 41, 43, 48, 53, 56, 68, 73, 78, 82, 85, 86, 96, 102, 104, 169, 189, 229, and 234.

year before being presented at the Second Congress of Minimally Invasive Neurosurgery in Marburg, Germany, in 1993. This instrument (Fig. 42–1) consists of a 30.5-cm rigid shaft with an outer diameter of 6 mm and contains four channels (Fig. 42–2). The largest channel (internal diameter [ID], 3 mm) is dedicated to the optic element (the "telescope"), which consists of a solid rod lens system. At the proximal end, an eyepiece permits attachment of an objective to the video camera (Fig. 42–3*A, B*). At the distal tip, a "lens angle" of 5 degrees brings the viewing field coaxial with the working field so that the action always takes place in the center of the image. When working at an appropriate distance (mainly 1 to 1.5 cm), the working instruments are seen in the middle of the circle. The field that is seen through the telescope measures 120 degrees. The second channel, the working channel (outer diameter [OD], 2.5 mm), permits introduction of instruments (see Fig. 42–14) and is situated above the viewing element.

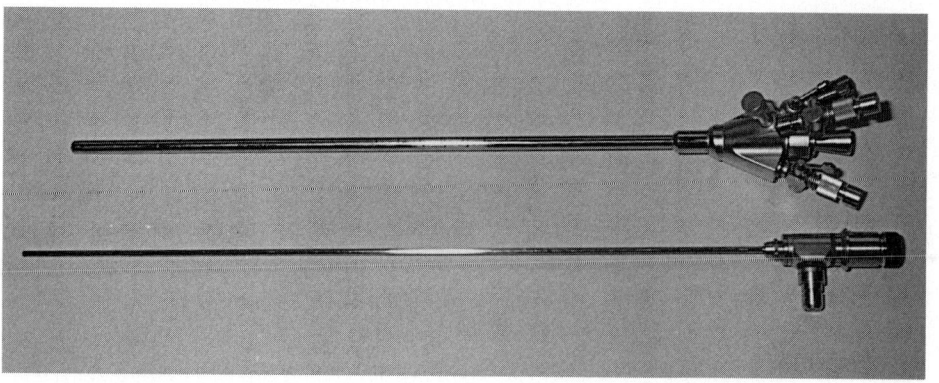

FIGURE 42–1 ■ The multipurpose Caemaert rigid endoscope (Richard Wolf, Drongen, Belgium, Knittlingen, Germany).

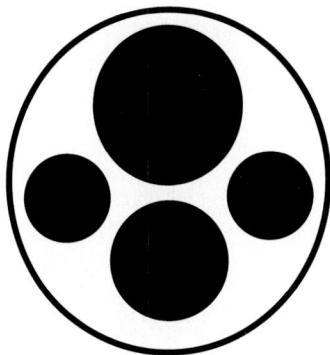

FIGURE 42–2 ■ A cross-section of the shaft with four channels.

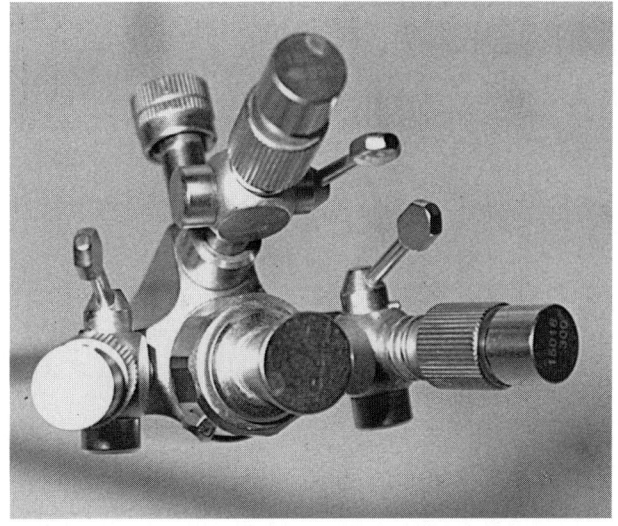

FIGURE 42–4 ■ Four inlet adapters at the proximal end of the endoscope.

Two irrigation channels (ID, 1.67 mm) permit irrigation and aspiration (Fig. 42–4). The inlet tubing is usually attached to the left adapter, although it can be changed if required. The outlet tubing can be disconnected, and this channel can be used to introduce small instruments, such as a laser fiber, ultrathin grasping forceps, and scissors. This feature allows an operator to work with two instruments simultaneously.

The rinsing solution (Ringer's solution) is kept at 36°C by warming it in a special oven. We have tried several warming devices (e.g., blood warming instruments) and abandoned them because none were able to follow the changes rapidly enough from slowly dripping to freely streaming. The changing of the 1-L bags must be done carefully to avoid infection. The outlet tubing is led to a recipient that is installed at the zero calibration level of the intracranial pressure (see Fig. 42–7) to prevent a siphoning effect resulting in ventricle collapse, which obliterates the view and potentially tears cortical veins resulting in a subdural hematoma. If siphoning does occur, the outlet

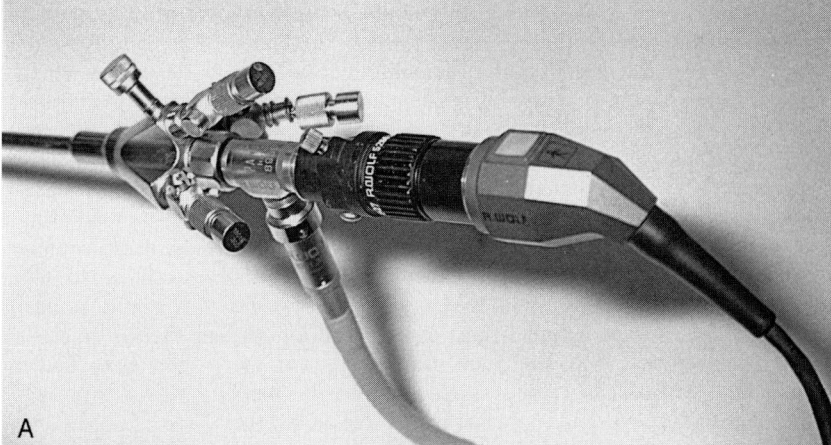

A

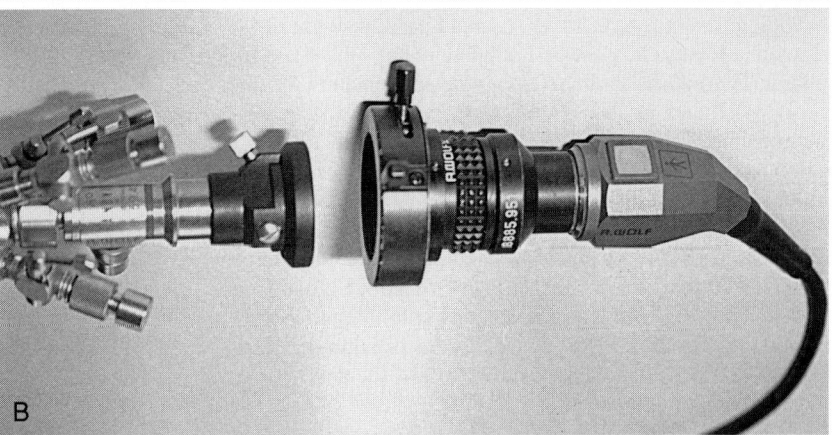

B

FIGURE 42–3 ■ The attachment of the camera to the ocular of the endoscope with a small objective (A) and with a big objective and eyepiece adapter (B).

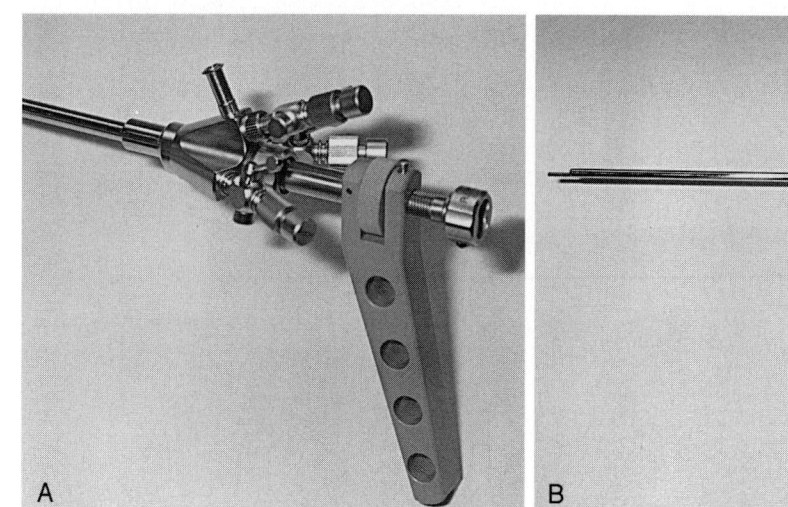

FIGURE 42–5 ■ *A,* Shorter version of the ventriculoscope with a depth screw to advance the optic element with a 70-degree angulated lens. *B,* A shorter version with a 70-degree optic element in place.

stopcock is closed immediately and irrigation is started to refill the ventricles. Both inlet and outlet tubing should be taped to the camera with Steri-Strips to prevent them from kinking. Constant irrigation is absolutely necessary, because small amounts of bleeding occur. This is not dangerous as such but can obliterate the image. At the beginning of the procedure, one can often see blood running down from the roof of the ventricles where the shaft penetrates the ependyma. This bleeding stops after sufficient irrigation but can restart if the intraventricular pressure is too low. Acceleration of the rinsing usually stops the bleeding quickly. Irrigation should not be started through the endoscope before the instrument reaches the ventricle, because severe cerebral edema of the white matter and tearing of brain tissue can result.

The instrument with the 30.5-cm shaft is compatible for use with every existing stereotactic system. A 19-cm version has been produced (Fig. 42–5) for free-hand use. This instrument is provided with a depth screw that permits stepwise advancement of the optic element. The optic element can be angulated 30 to 70 degrees, which allows the operator to look around a corner (e.g., to the posterior part of the third ventricle with the main shaft fixed near the foramen of Monro). The camera is mounted on the head of the instrument and could otherwise be blocked by the stop and guide carrier. The usual stop and guide from the stereotactic system have to be replaced by one single guide with an eccentrically burred channel (Fig. 42–6). This permits alternately to bring the working channel or the viewing channel in the central stereotactic axis. The fact that the inner channel of the guide is eccentric does not permit one to use a separate stop and guide, because the slightest rotation from one to the other would obstruct or at least hinder the introduction of the instrument. The single guide should be made of metal, because the metal-to-metal friction allows the surgeon to feel slight differences in resistance indicating, for example, that the ependyma is perforated. Plastic guides do not provide the same feeling. Another advantage of the length of the shaft is that even in free-hand conditions, the movements at the top will be minimized by a longer shaft. Movement of the

upper part of the endoscope over 1 cm affects much more the position of the tip in a shorter shaft than in a longer shaft.

Early in our work, intraventricular or epidural pressure monitoring was performed during the procedure. This was abandoned because the intracranial pressure does not reach an unacceptable level with an appropriate use of the endoscope. The outlet must be inspected regularly to ensure that it remains patent. Cerebrospinal fluid (CSF) can also come out of the ventricle alongside the working instruments through the working channel. Only working through a narrow foramen of Monro or in the depth of a cystic lesion, in which only a small hole has been made, requires extra attention to avoid building up pressure.

Endoscopic procedures can take place in a standard well-equipped neurosurgical operating room (Fig. 42–7).[167] The patient is positioned with the bur hole at the highest part of the operating field to prevent CSF from leaking out and air from entering the head. A catastrophic pneumocephalus could ensue from lower placement of the bur hole. The surgeon stands at the head end of the operating table slightly to the right. The assistant stands at the surgeon's left side. The instrument nurse and the instrument tables

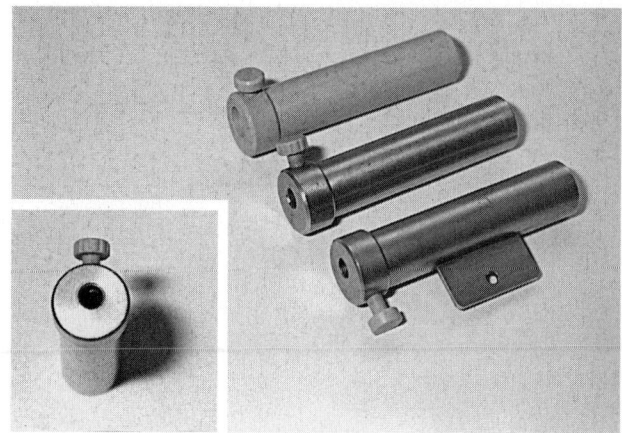

FIGURE 42–6 ■ A stereotactic guide (single).

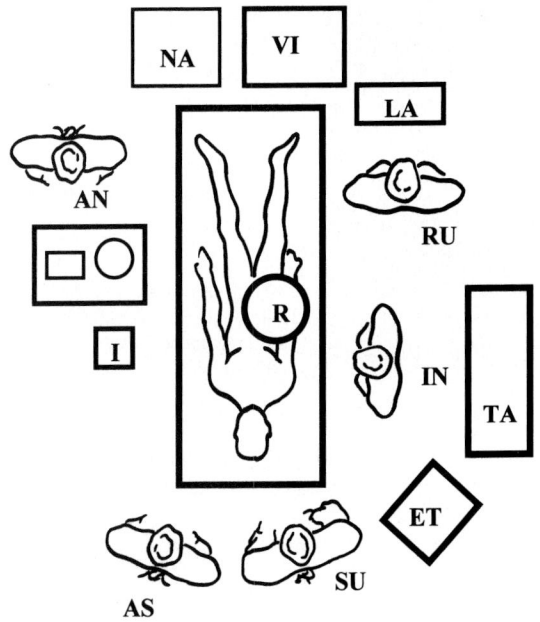

FIGURE 42-7 ■ An operating theater setting.

are at the right side of the operating table. The laser source is at the right foot end. The video tower (Fig. 42–8) with the monitor on top is in the middle at the foot of the operating table. The anesthesiologist and the respirator are on the left side of the operating table. If the microscope is used, it fits best in the corner at the left top end of the operating table. The irrigation fluid bags can be hung onto the respirator and should be accessible for the circulating nurse. There should always be two rinsing bags, which are connected to Y-tubing, so that the bag can be changed immediately when it is empty. The dripping chamber of the tubing should be empty to gain good visual control over the irrigation flow. The neuronavigation computer and monitor tower are positioned to the left of the video tower.

## Rigid or Flexible Neuroendoscopes?

The experience of most authors is that rigid endoscopes are far superior to flexible endoscopes. The image quality of the flexible glass fibers is far below that of the solid rod lens systems of the rigid endoscope, and the small outer diameter in flexible endoscopes is overshadowed by the lack of enough irrigation channels of sufficient inner diameter. It is absolutely necessary to have a separate inlet and outlet irrigation channel that both reach the top of the instrument.[64, 68, 75, 108, 112, 126, 167, 189] The irrigation fluid should be able to flow in freely. In some flexible endoscopes, the irrigating fluid must sometimes be injected and aspirated through the same channel. In addition, a flexible endoscope requires much more attention to orientation, and this instrument should be tested outside the brain before it is introduced. Afterwards, some reference indicator should be used to be sure about the orientation in the brain. Moreover, after repeated use, many flexible endoscopes cannot be straightened. In addition, with flexible endoscopes, it is difficult to be certain what happens behind the lens, be-

cause after repeated use the tip remains curved to a certain degree. These instruments should be introduced through an introductory sheath,[150] because white matter can be damaged if the endoscope is not completely straightened when it is retracted.

"Steerability" does not actually exist with flexible endoscopes—it is not possible to navigate with these instruments through several holes that are not aligned along one trajectory. The term steerability of flexible endoscopes is very misleading. The flaccid shaft is a problem rather than an advantage. With the rigid endoscope, one can always be sure that the shaft of the instrument is straight behind the lens, whereas with flexible endoscopes, in the best of cases you see what you see but you don't see what you do. One can never see the movements of the shaft proximal to the lens. Moreover, looking around the corner may seem attractive, but in itself does not yet permit working around a corner (Fig. 42–9). The working channels of flexible endoscopes are too small in many cases to introduce instruments that are large enough to perform real work. We have designed a very small flexible endoscope (Fig. 42–10) for use through the working channel of the rigid endoscope. The idea was to introduce it under direct visual control of the camera on the rigid instrument and at the same time to have the opportunity to look around the corner. The image quality of this small flexible endoscope is so inferior to

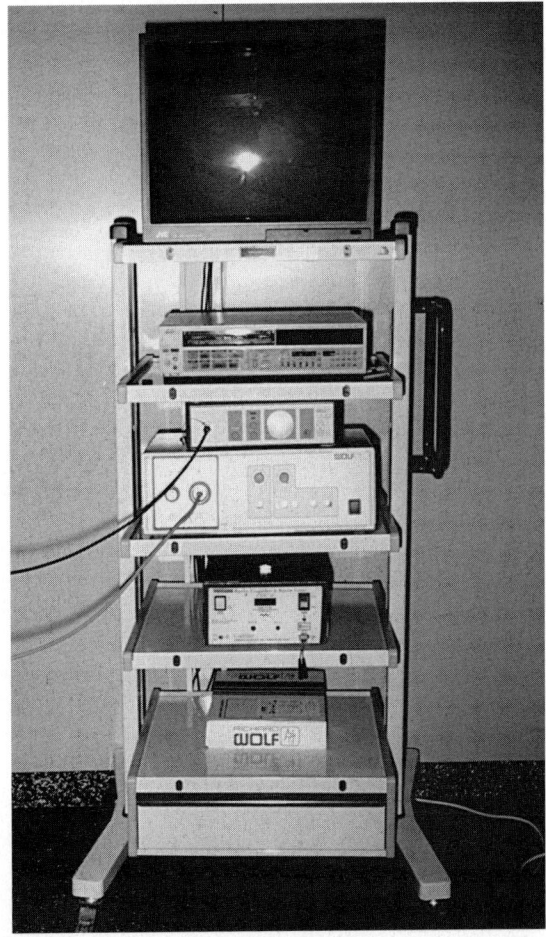

FIGURE 42-8 ■ The video tower with (from top to bottom) television monitor, videorecorder, camera unit, light source, bipolar coagulator.

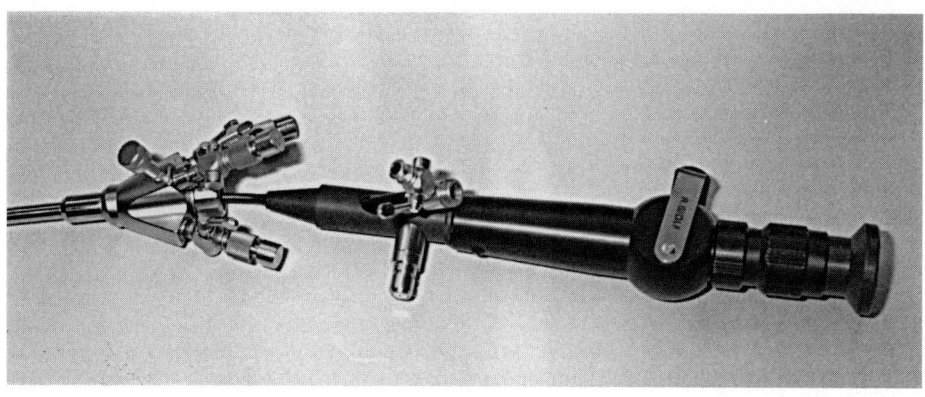

FIGURE 42-9 ■ A small flexible endoscope for use through the working channel of the rigid endoscope.

that of the rigid lens system that it is dangerous if not impossible to work with.

## Pediatric Neuroendoscope System

A dedicated pediatric endoscope system was designed by Hopf[107, 108] and produced by the Richard Wolf Company (Fig. 42–11 *A, B*). It has an extraordinarily small outer diameter (oval cross-section: 4.4 × 3.3 mm or 6.1 × 4.8 mm), which makes it valuable for intraventricular endoscopic procedures in newborn babies and children. It has telescopes with a lens angle of 5 degrees, 25 degrees, and 70 degrees and a 2.7-mm diameter. There are different sheets and working elements with working channels, two irrigation channels, and an insert for steering instruments at the tip.

## Check Before Starting

It is very important to check every part of the equipment before inserting the endoscope into the brain. The camera should be connected to the camera unit and activated; the video recorder and video monitoring should be tuned on. A trial registration should be done, and the automatic white

balance should be performed. The surgeon can focus the image in his or her closed left hand, because this mimics the size of the cavities in which the surgeon will have to work. The shaft is wetted before it is inserted into the cortex.

## Introduction of the Instrument

An 8-mm bur hole should be made somewhat conically to permit movement of the shaft. When the intracranial pressure is high, it is advisable to make only a linear dural incision, otherwise a cruciform incision has to be made. A 6-mm linear cortical coagulation and incision is performed, and a 6-mm wet cotton pledget is inserted to keep the entrance open while the endoscope is being assembled.

The instrument can be introduced free-hand or stereotactically. We are using the free-hand technique more frequently in case the size of the ventricles permits safe introduction, based on an estimation of the appropriate angles on preoperative MR. When the ventricular system is small and where the angles of approach are important, we highly recommend stereotactic guidance or neuronavigation (Fig. 42–12*A*). This is the case in most of the colloid cysts and in lesions in the posterior part of the third ventricle, such as pineal tumors. However, in these cases,

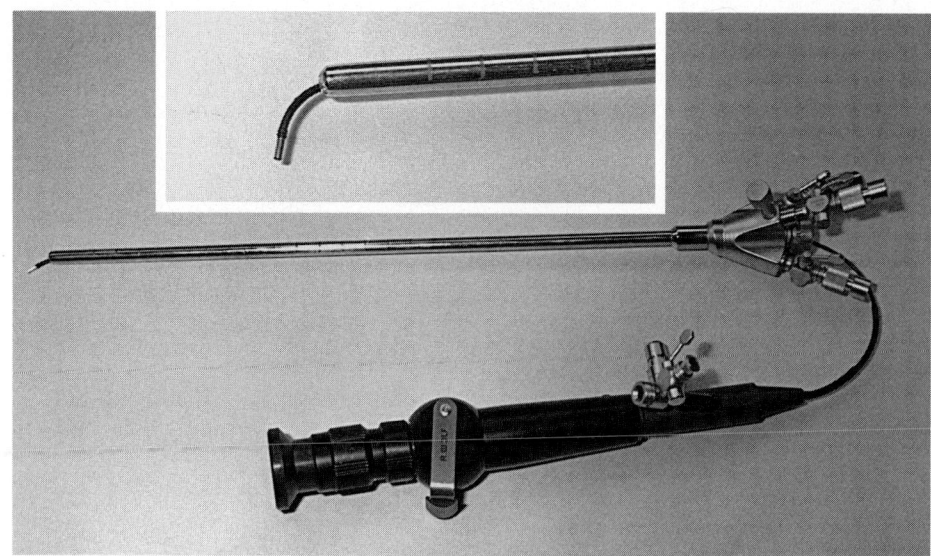

FIGURE 42-10 ■ A flexible endoscope 2.2 mm O.D. inserted in the working channel.

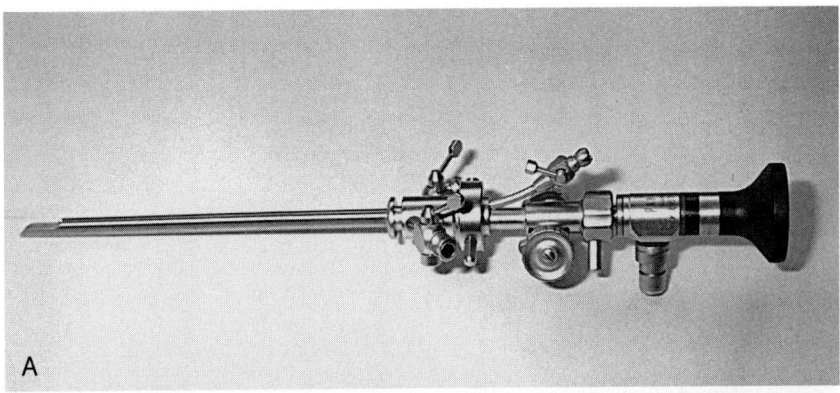

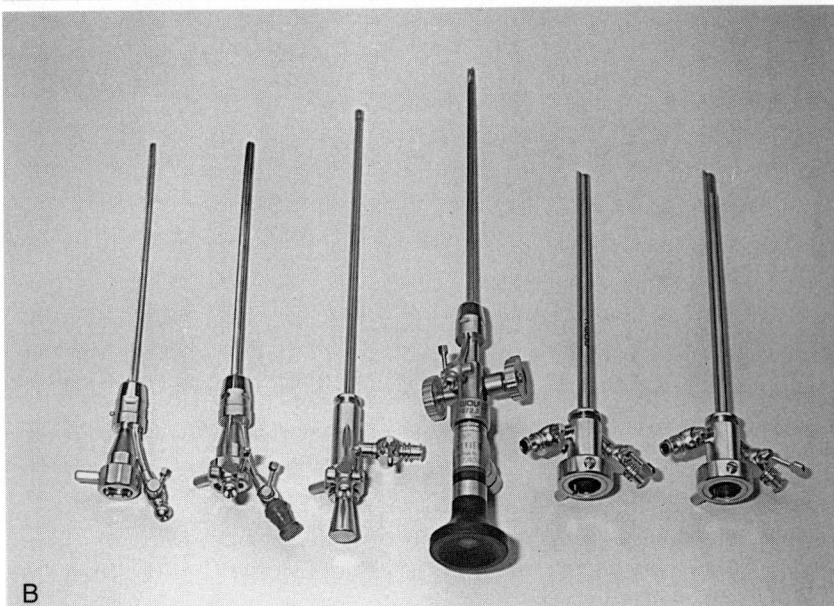

FIGURE 42–11 ■ *A,* Pediatric Hopf ventriculoscope (Richard Wolf, Knittlingen). *B,* Instrument set for the Hopf pediatric ventriculoscope.

the use of stereotactic guidance is limited to the introduction of the instrument. Once the ventricle has been reached, the instrument is detached from the stereotactic instrument carrier and the operation is continued free-hand from then onward (see Fig. 42–12*B*). The stereotactic arc can sometimes be used as a support for the hands, but we do not leave the shaft connected to the stereotactic arc because one should be able to make tiny movements to allow frequent correction of the position and the direction of the endoscope. For rigid intraventricular endoscopy, we are absolutely opposed to using a holding device. Its use involves a loss of time to lock and unlock the device each time when one has to change direction. There is no substitute for a well-trained assistant holding the endoscope. The assistant keeps his or her left hand resting on the patient's skull, holds the shaft between the thumb and the index fingers, and presses the shaft against the bony edge of the bur hole. This provides good stability. The camera and the head of the endoscope are held in the assistant's right hand. With the surgeon's guidance, the assistant should follow the delicate movements that are necessary for working. The assistant should feel the surgeon's intention to move in the sagittal and frontal plane and to change angles. The surgeon will steer the endoscope at the level of the camera and the inlet adapters with his left hand, while his right hand remains free to handle the working instruments. Of-

ten, left index finger and thumb will guide a second instrument simultaneously.

A self-retaining holding device can be very useful in endoscopy-assisted microsurgery. A special mechanical arm has been designed by the Marburg group.[15] A pneumatic holding arm has been devised by the Mainz group and produced by Aesculap, and an adaptation of the Leylla retractor with a double arm has been designed by Hopf (Fig. 42–13). Neuronavigation and robotic systems can be attached to the endoscopic shaft for the same purpose as the stereotactic guidance used during introduction.[10, 19, 58, 109, 143, 156, 199, 204, 238]

The guide through which the instrument is introduced stereotactically can be advanced upward over the shaft and fixed with a small screw so that it remains attached to the upper part of the shaft. To change the depth of introduction, the surgeon gives a verbal message to the assistant to go deeper or to retract. Under no circumstances should the assistant take the initiative to move, introduce, or retract the instrument.

The tip of the instrument is smoothly rounded when the channels are filled with their mandrins during introduction into the white matter. The optic element is put in place instead of the mandrin of the optic channel so that one is able to immediately detect the penetration of the ependyma and the entrance into the ventricle. One can most often see

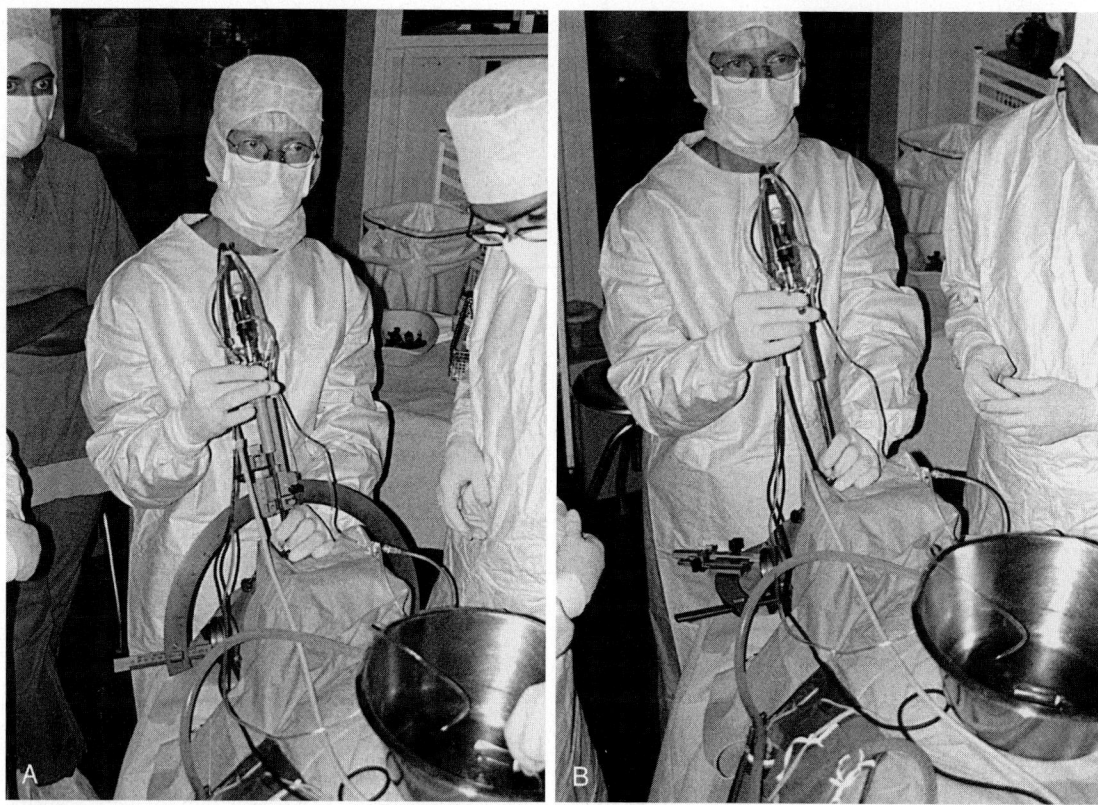

**FIGURE 42–12** ■ *A,* Introduction of the endoscope under stereotactic guidance. *B,* Free-hand continuation of the operation after detaching from the stereotactic arc.

the color of the white matter change from ivory white to a slightly bluish color as the ventricle is nearly approached. It then opens suddenly like a curtain.

## Working Instruments

A number of suitable neuroendoscopes are commercially available. The challenge is to construct new instruments to work through the different channels.[21, 30, 100, 181, 195–221] These various instruments are discussed in some detail (Fig. 42–14*A–R*).

### Aspiration Catheters

Aspiration catheters have to be thin-walled with a wide lumen and have a Luer-lock connector at their proximal end. There can be side holes, and the tip can be cut off obliquely (see Fig. 42–14*J*) to gain some sharpness for penetration of tough membranes or cyst capsules. If penetration is not easy, it should be preceded by bipolar or laser coagulation. Smaller very flexible catheters (see Fig. 42–14*H*), also with Luer-lock connectors, can be introduced through one of the side channels for aspiration of air bubbles, selective aspiration of small blood clots, or aspiration of the blood directly from the site of a damaged vessel, so that this blood does not contaminate the ventricle during attempts at coagulation of the bleeding vessel. Highly suitable catheters can be found among the catheters that are used in cardiac catheterization. When it is useful to work somewhat out of the straight direction of the

working channel, one can use a catheter with a prebent tip that curves as soon as it leaves the shaft.

## Grasping Forceps

Several types of grasping forceps can be introduced through the main working channel. Some of them have dentations (see Fig. 42–14*O*) to have a firm grip on membranes. This enables one to stretch the membranes while cutting them with a laser fiber that is introduced through one of the side channels. Other grasping forceps have a cup shape (see Fig. 42–14*N, M*) that permits sampling biopsy specimens. Very tiny grasping forceps (see Fig. 42–14*I*) can be introduced through one of the side channels and permit simultaneous working with two instruments. After 14 years of experience, we prefer the cup-shaped grasping forceps for biopsies. One should not open the jaws of these forceps before retraction out of the endoscope, otherwise one might lose a piece of tissue and cause an aqueduct obstruction.

## Scissors

Two types of scissors are available. The big one (see Fig. 42–14*R*) fits into the working channel and has one straight leg that is fixed forward and one moving leg that cuts. The straight leg can be introduced into a small hole, and the direction of the cut can be determined by turning the moving leg in this direction before closing. The very tiny scissors (see Fig. 42–14*Q*) fit into one of the side irrigation channels.

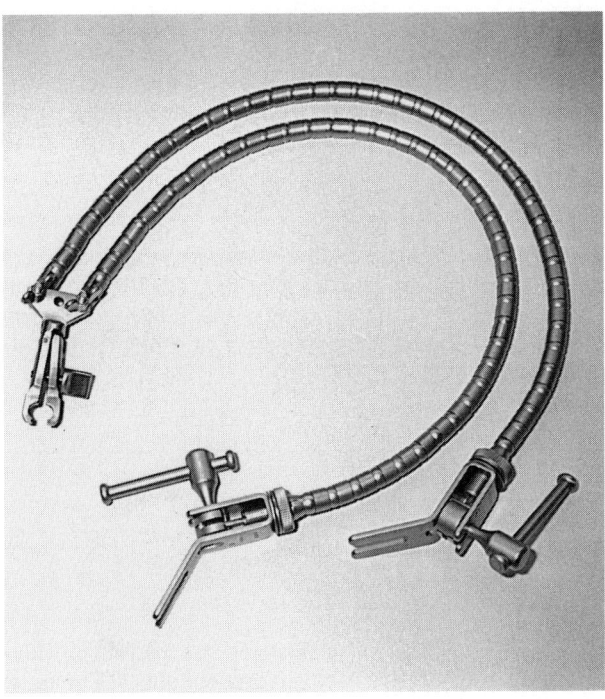

FIGURE 42–13 ■ A holding device according to Hopf.

## Laser

In ventricular endoscopy, one always works under water and therefore we prefer the neodymium:yttrium aluminum

garnet (Nd:YAG) laser for coagulation and cutting. For coagulation, blunt fibers (hemispheric fibers) (see Fig. 42–14A) can be used in a nontouch mode, and the energy is delivered from 1.5 to 2 mm from the tissue surface. Fibers of 400, 600, and 800 μm can be used. They fit into the working channel as well as in the irrigation channels. The energy applied depends on the color of the tissue that is coagulated. Darker tissues such as blood vessels or a bluish cyst dome require less energy than whiter surfaces such as the ventricular wall. The laser light is reflected by these ivory white surfaces, and a higher power has to be used.

Laser cutting can be obtained by small blunt fibers (400 μm) or conically shaped fibers (see Fig. 42–14B) (600 μm). Here the energy is concentrated in the sharp tip, which must be used in the contact mode. Each time that one switches from coagulating to cutting, it is necessary to switch the fibers. Once the tissue has been touched by the coagulating fibers, they lose their coagulation capacity but they can still be used as cutting or vaporizing fibers. Laser energy can penetrate the surface for 6 to 7 mm and should never be used when the underlying tissue is functional neural tissue. For the coagulation of blood vessels in a membrane or for the coagulation of a tumor surface, it is an ideal instrument. The cutting laser gives less dissipation of energy and produces fine superficial cuts.

## Bipolar Coagulation

Three types of bipolar coagulation probes are available. The most frequently used is one with two parallel cups separated by a thin septum (see Fig. 42–14E). To coagulate

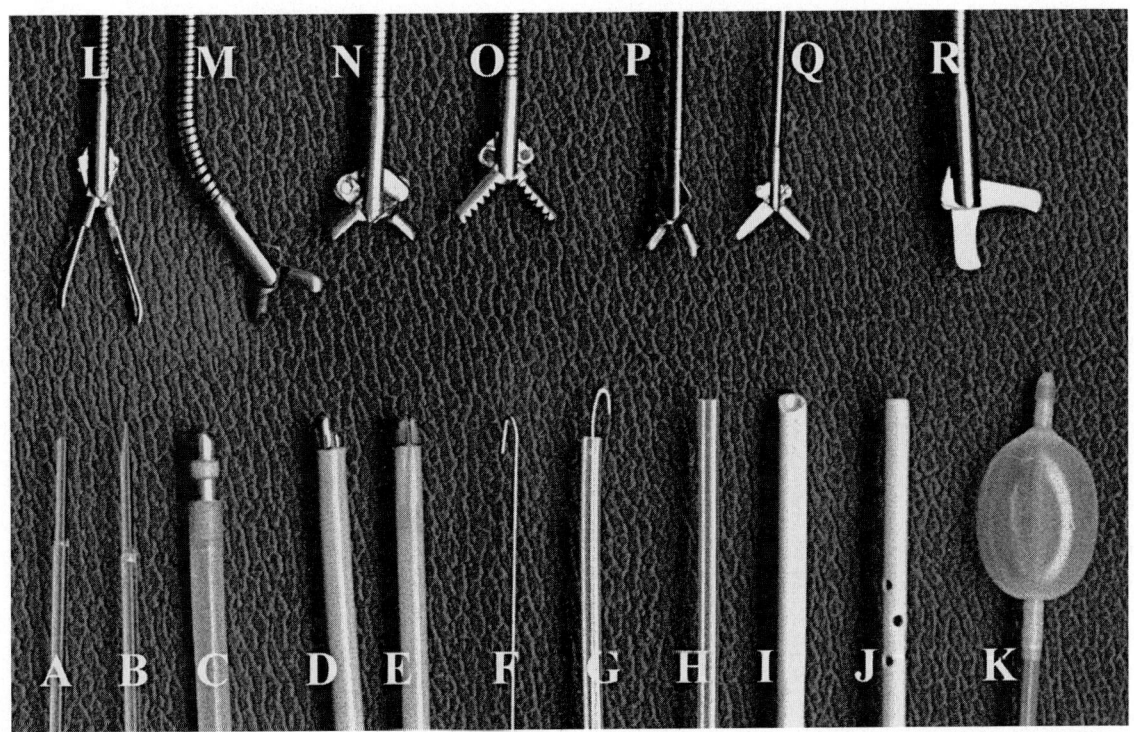

FIGURE 42–14 ■ Working instruments for use through the working channel. A, Coagulating laser fiber. B, Cutting laser fiber. C, Bipolar probe with two rings. D, Bipolar probe with unequal legs. E, Bipolar probe with equal caps. F, Hooklet. G, Insulated hooklet. H, Small aspiration catheter. I, Aspiration catheter with an oblique tip. J, Aspiration catheter with side holes. K, Inflatable balloon catheter. L, Wire loop grasping device. M, Pre-bend grasping forceps. N, Cup-shaped grasping and biopsy forceps. O, Indented grasping forceps. P, Micro grasping forceps for use through the side channel. Q, Micro scissors. R, Scissors.

a vessel, one should bring both poles into contact with the vessel before firing. During coagulation, the irrigation should be minimized because otherwise it dissipates the energy and the coagulation process is impaired. Immediately after coagulation, abundant irrigation can be continued. It is advisable to continue the coagulation while retracting the probe from the tissue. This action reduces the risk of the instrument sticking to the tissue. For the coagulation of structures that can only be reached tangentially (e.g., choroid plexus from an occipital bur hole), a bipolar probe exists where the poles are two metal rings so that the coagulation occurs at the side surface of the probe (see Fig. 42–14C). A third type of bipolar coagulator has one short leg and one long leg (see Fig. 42–14D). This type is very useful to pick up a bleeding blood vessel or a bleeding edge of a tissue and apply some stretching before coagulating.[204]

### Balloon Catheter

An inflatable balloon catheter is an atraumatic and useful instrument (see Fig. 42–14K) that permits one to enlarge a perforation into a bigger hole. It is the instrument of choice for third ventriculostomy. It may also be used to create holes in membranes, which can be interconnected by scissors. For a fenestration, the hole obtained by a balloon catheter is usually too small. We prefer the Fogarty type of balloon catheters that have one single inflatable belly. We have tested the eight-shaped balloon catheters that have two bellies and a narrowing in the middle. The drawback of these catheters is that the two halves are not always equally inflated, and the distal half becomes invisible by inflation of the proximal half. Moreover, the central narrowing is not distensible enough to create a significant hole. In one operation, the balloons exploded after a few inflations.

### Manwaring Saline Torch

This instrument is comparable to the laser in its use and effects,[93, 151] and the same precautions should be taken as with the laser. This saline radiofrequency irrigator, or saline torch, uses saline as an electrically conductive medium between the recessed electrode and the face of the ceramic tube. When a membrane is touched by the ceramic tube, a hole is vaporized in the wall of the membrane that is the exact dimension of the catheter tip. Alternatively, the sharp tungsten tip can be advanced for cutting tissue.

### Ultrasound Probe

This probe offers real-time control during endoscopic procedures. Systems for endoneurosonography are described by Auer[8]; Resch and Reisch,[197] Bauer and Hellwig,[15] Yamakawa and associates,[230] Yamasaki and coworkers.[231]

### Computerized Ultrasonic Aspiration (CUSA)

Removal of endoscopic tumor can be facilitated with the use of a micro-CUSA probe, as reported by Oka (personal communication). The advantages over the grasping forceps is that one does not have to retract the instrument continu-

ously after each bit. The problem, however, is that ultrasonic aspiration in itself does not control the bleeding but can actually cause bleeding. A combination with an electrical coagulation device at the tip of the same probe would probably be ideal.

### Hooklet

If the tip of a Fogarty mandrin is bent, the result is a handsome homemade hooklet (see Fig. 42–14F) that can be insulated (by means of a long thin infusion catheter) (see Fig. 42–14G) for the application of a monopolar cutting current.

## SPECIFIC INDICATIONS

### Obstructive Hydrocephalus

#### Third Ventriculostomy

Indications for third ventriculostomy are present in noncommunicating (obstructive) hydrocephalus.* The most frequent cause is aqueductal stenosis due to congenital, hereditary, or idiopathic causes. Acquired aqueductal stenosis is found in tumors of the posterior fossa, post intraventricular hemorrhage, and postinfectious ventriculitis. MR (Fig. 42–15) shows supratentorial hydrocephalus and a

---

*See references 13, 40, 49, 63, 72, 87, 120–122, 124, 125, 130, 134, 139, 140, 147, 149, 151, 162, 175, 178, 182, 183, 205–208, 210, 216, 220, 225.

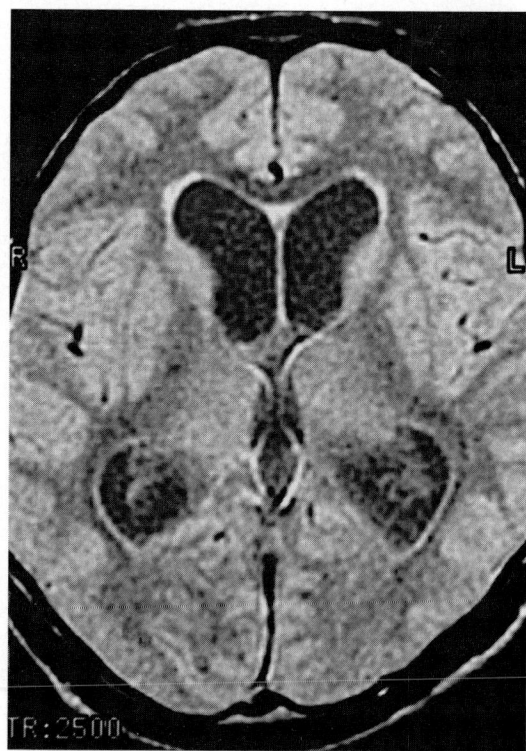

**FIGURE 42–15** ■ Preoperative magnetic resonance imaging in obstructive hydrocephalus.

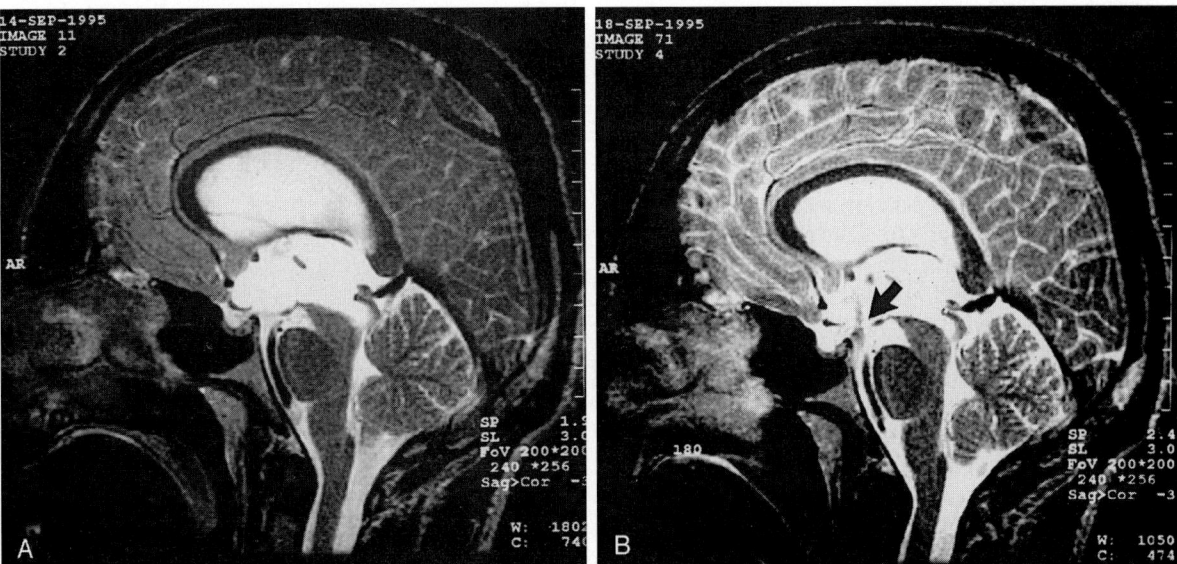

FIGURE 42–16 ■ *A,* T$_2$-weighted magnetic resonance image (MRI) of preoperative bulging of the floor of the third ventricle and prestenotic dilatation of the aqueduct. *B,* A postoperative T$_2$-weighted MRI with flow void through third ventriculostomy. Disappearance of the bulging of the floor and reduction of the prestenotic dilatation in obstructive hydrocephalus.

prestenotic dilatation of the proximal part of the aqueduct (Fig. 42–16). The obstruction can be membranous, and this is the only indication for aqueductoplasty. The stenosis or occlusion can be short or long, depending on the etiology. Postoperatively, one can see a flow void through the stoma in the floor of the third ventricle and a reduction of the ventricular dilatation[168] (Fig. 42–17), which is usually less than after shunting operations. Slit ventricles are not seen, but exceptionally subdural collections can occur postoperatively.[161] Another indication for third ventriculostomy is the obstruction of the foramina of Magendi and Luschka. Here MR reveals a wide open aqueduct with a flow void and a large fourth ventricle. Another group of indications is in

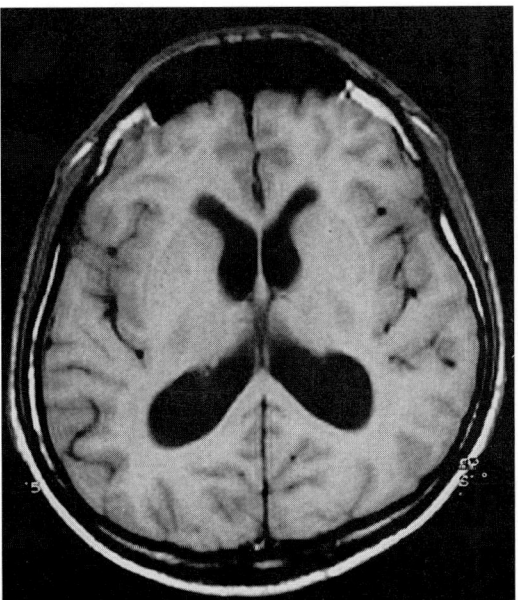

FIGURE 42–17 ■ Postoperative magnetic resonance image after third ventriculostomy in obstructive hydrocephalus.

shunt failure in patients with a prior cardiac or peritoneal shunt. In these cases, an endoscopic internal shunt can make the patient shunt free. Approximately 65% of the patients can remain shunt free in this way.

A prerequisite to performing a third ventriculostomy is that there should be a bulging in the floor of the third ventricle (see Fig. 42–16). In a real obstructive hydrocephalus, one can see a downward protrusion of the floor sometimes into the sella turcica and mainly also behind the dorsum sellae in the interpeduncular and prepontine cisterns. The exact site for the perforation (Fig. 42–18, see color section) lies between the infundibular recess anteriorly and the mamillary bodies posteriorly. The former is easy to recognize by the reddish vascular rete staining the anterior floor of the third ventricle. The latter are recognizable because they remain as white dots posterior to the more bluish translucent thinned floor of the ventricle. The underlying arterial blood vessels often shine through and protrude upward into the ventricle. These are the posterior cerebral arteries. The cardiac pulsations are recognized. The trajectory should be studied meticulously on preoperative MR or CT. The entry point should be close enough to the midline so that, going through the foramen of Monro, the floor of the third ventricle is reached on the midline. If the operator approaches too laterally, the result would be an approach that is too lateral to the floor, which may cause an injury to the underlying oculomotor nerve. In the sagittal plane, the entry point lies most often in the precoronary region. Except when there is an extremely wide ventricular system, it is unwise to try to perforate the floor of the third ventricle and to perform an aqueductoplasty from the same bur hole. One should make the choice between these two techniques beforehand. In cases where a third ventriculostomy is combined with a biopsy of a tumor in the posterior part of the third ventricle (e.g., pineal tumor), it is necessary in most cases to make two bur holes—one in the precoronary region and one much more anteriorly. It is one of the only cases in which two trajectories are needed. Theoretically, a flexible endoscope would offer some advantage in this indication, but practically it is quite hazardous and difficult to work around the corner through a flexible endoscope introduced in the third ventricle through the foramen of Monro. In many cases, the floor of the ventricle is so thin and stretched that it can be perforated without any preparation with a blunt balloon catheter. Sometimes, however, the membrane is quite tough and difficult to perforate. In these cases, a small short bipolar coagulation dot helps to create a rough surface and to make the beginning of the perforation that can be fulfilled by the Fogarty catheter. The use of laser is absolutely contraindicated at this site, because of the danger of perforating the underlying arterial vessels. After the initial perforation, repeated inflation of the balloon catheter progressively enlarges the hole (Fig. 42–19, see color section). As soon as the perforation is obtained, the floor becomes flaccid and moves up and down with cardiac and respiratory movements. The edges of the opening can sometimes be smoothed by using the grasping forceps. When the stoma is big enough (Fig. 42–20, see color section), it is important to inspect the underlying arachnoid space. In some cases, the arachnoid membrane must be perforated, and adhesions have to be destroyed by the balloon catheter. If one were to neglect this, it would certainly enhance the failure rate in control of the hydrocephalus. Only when a clear image (Fig. 42–21, see color section) is obtained of the basilar artery and the clivus is the third ventriculostomy considered as technically satisfactory. It then depends on the resorptive capacities as to whether the operation is sufficient. Between 65% and 75% of the cases can remain shunt-free after third ventriculostomy. In all series, the percentage of success is lower in the first year of life and in meningomyelocele patients with Arnold-Chiari malformation. Subarachnoid and intraventricular hemorrhages and infections are unfavorable prognostic factors, although none of them is an absolute contraindication. In both groups, we have seen successful cases. Complications are mainly caused by incorrect positioning of the stoma. If the perforation is done too far anteriorly, the result can often be transient diabetes insipidus. However, if the perforation is done too posteriorly, the coagulation and perforation can damage the mamillary bodies and result in a memory deficit. If the perforation is done too laterally, damage may be done to the oculomotor nerve. Furthermore, if the surgeon goes too deep along the clivus to open the arachnoid space, this action can be dangerous for the abducens nerve. Overdrainage of the CSF with slit ventricles and subdural collections or hematomas is seldom seen.

## Asymmetric Hydrocephalus

When there is no communication between the left and right lateral ventricles, a fenestration in the septum pellucidum (septostomy) can be made.[129, 224] A relatively avascular area is selected; the septal vessels are coagulated by laser or bipolar probe in a circular array; and special attention is paid to vessels on the opposite side of the septum, which if not coagulated can bleed while fenestrating the septum.

The roundel is then cut out by a laser or scissors (Fig. 42–22). It remains attached by a fine stalk to prevent it

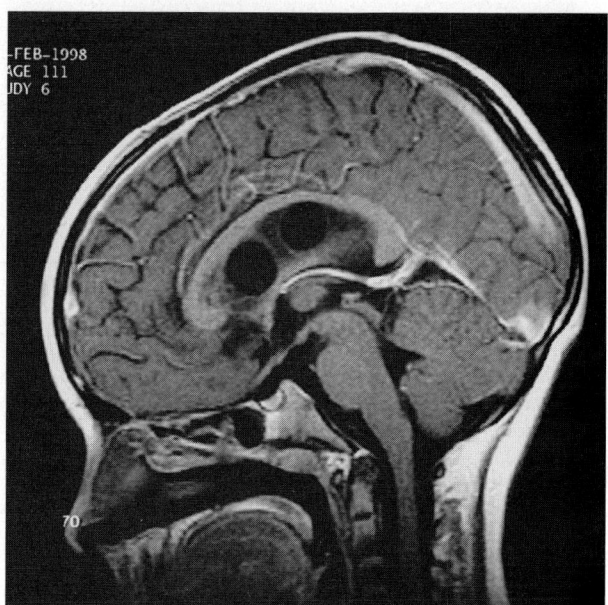

FIGURE 42–22 ■ Sagittal magnetic resonance image after a septostomy: two holes of about 2 cm.

from falling into the ventricle and is finally avulsed by the grasping forceps and extracted.

## MALRESORPTIVE HYDROCEPHALUS

### Coagulation of the Choroid Plexus

In malresorptive hydrocephalus it may be advantageous to lower the production of CSF. The real indication for this technique is in those patients in which a delicate disequilibrium exists between production and resorption of CSF.[26, 80, 81, 184, 193, 205, 206, 209, 211] There are two limiting factors: (1) the CSF is not only produced by the choroid plexus but also reaches the ventricles transependymally, and (2) one can only reach the plexus of the lateral ventricles, whereas the remaining plexus in the roof of the third ventricle and in the fourth ventricle can continue to produce CSF. Technically, it is possible to coagulate the entire choroid plexus of the lateral ventricles. The entry points are bilateral bur holes in the high occipital region. The patient lies face down so that the bur holes are in the uppermost part of the operating field as required. The distance to the midline can be determined on preoperative CT or MR. A short trajectory through the cortex and the white matter leads to the corpus of the lateral ventricle from where both the frontal and temporal horns can be reached.

Where the frontal and temporal parts of the choroid plexus merge with each other, they can be coagulated by the most frequently used bipolar probe. For the more anterior situated parts, it should be done with a double-ring probe that permits tangential coagulation of the plexus. Care should be taken not to coagulate the underlying tissue, which may be fornix, thalamus, hippocampus. It is advisable to move the plexus away from these structures and allow it to coagulate while sliding it against the coagulating probe. After the coagulation is complete, abundant irrigation is necessary to wash out cellular debris that originates from the coagulations. We do not leave an external ventricular catheter at the end of the operation. Closure of the bur hole is extremely important in these cases, because failure to control hydrocephalus would entail leakage of CSF. A patch of dura substitute is inserted in between the patient's dura and the bone, about 5 mm beyond the bony edges. In this way, raised intracranial pressure will press this dura roundel against the bone if hydrocephalus is not controlled by the endoscopic intervention. The bur hole is then filled with a mixture of bone filings and organic glue (Tissucol, Baxter). On top, we place a piece of Surgicel (Johnson & Johnson). Finally, the scalp is sutured meticulously.

# PARAVENTRICULAR AND INTRAVENTRICULAR CYSTIC LESIONS

Many different cystic lesions are confined to the ventricular spaces or bulge into the ventricles (see Table 42–1). The relationship between the brain tissue, the cysts, and the ventricular system is clearly demonstrated by CT and MRI. The symptomatology can be due to the secondary hydrocephalus or may be related to their location and local pressure. Periventricular cysts often affect the limbic system with neuropsychological impairment.

## Paraventricular and Intraventricular Arachnoid Cysts

Although arachnoid cysts always originate from the surface of the brain, they can be very deep seated or acquire such a volume that they come into close contact with the ventricular system. Examples of superficially located arachnoid cysts are those of the sylvian fissure, the cerebellopontine angle, the brain convexity, and the interhemispheric fissure. Other cysts originate from deeper arachnoid spaces, such as the quadrigeminal cistern or the optochiasmatic and prepontine cisterns. It is important to realize that many arachnoid cysts remain asymptomatic throughout life and do not require treatment.[174] However, when they become symptomatic by local or general elevated intracranial pressure or by neurologic deficit or epilepsy, they should be treated.[16, 29, 31, 74, 98, 105, 106, 173, 190] Microsurgical operations are often large interventions that are fraught with complications, such as the collapse of the brain, subsequent development of a subdural hematoma, and secondary closure and recurrence of the cyst. In many cases, internal shunting (cystoatrial or cystoperitoneal) is a good alternative.

Endoscopic approaches have proved to be very efficient during the last 10 years. They require close contact of the arachnoid cyst membrane with either a wide subarachnoid space or the ventricular system. This makes some arachnoid cysts very suitable candidates for endoscopic treatment, whereas others tend to recur because the fenestrations could not be made large enough. The latter is often the case in arachnoid cysts in the sylvian fissure. The openings that can be made in the cyst walls toward the basal cisterns around the circle of Willis are often too small

and tend to heal. Other cases offer the opportunity to make a large fenestration of up to 2 cm; here the results are very good and stable in the long term.

## General Technique

The choice of the approach to the cyst is very important. Because the endoscope is a rigid instrument, all fenestrations should be planned in one straight line. According to necessity, one may come first through the ventricular cavity and open the cyst wall (or vice versa) to come through the arachnoid cyst and penetrate toward the ventricle. Depending on the size of the ventricles, they can be approached stereotactically, by neuronavigation, or by freehand. Often it is not difficult at all to enter an arachnoid cyst; however, once inside the cyst, there are no more anatomic landmarks and it becomes difficult to decide where the fenestration should be. This is particularly the case when the ventricular spaces are small. However, it remains possible to detach the endoscope from the stereotactic arc to permit the delicate movements necessary for fenestration. When several membranes must be perforated, reinsertion of the endoscope into the stereotactic instrument carrier can be done. The cyst wall often presents as a bluish dome with small to moderately sized vessels at its surface (Fig. 42–23, see color section). These vessels can be coagulated first either by laser in the noncontact mode (40 to 60 W of power) or by bipolar coagulation. We mainly prefer the laser, because we do not have to fear the penetration of laser energy in the depth. At the opposite side of the membrane, there is only CSF. By coagulation, one can see some shrinkage of the membranes before penetration. After a circular roundel (Fig. 42–24, see color section) has been defined by coagulation spots, this can be cut out by the conically shaped cutting laser fiber or by using scissors that interconnect several holes made by the bipolar probe (Fig. 42–25, see color section). At the end, the roundel remains attached by a fine stalk to prevent it from falling into the ventricle. It is then extracted with the large grasping forceps. (Fig. 42–26, see color section). The membrane is often too big to fit into the working channel, and it is then advisable to pull it against the lens and back up the whole endoscope through the chimney in the white matter. This trajectory remains open for a time that is usually sufficient to reintroduce the shaft under visual control through the same route.

## Results and Complications

When properly performed, the endoscopic fenestration usually provides a cure for arachnoid cysts. Early in our experience we had to make some re-interventions, because the hole was too small (it had been performed by bipolar coagulation and enlarged by a Fogarty inflatable balloon catheter). Those holes measured about 6 mm. On re-exploration at a later date, the first hole was not always completely closed. Although a residual opening of about 2.5 mm remained, the cysts were again bulging and distended. We soon realized that openings should be at least 10 mm and preferably 20 mm in diameter. In many cases, it is also

TABLE 42–2 ■ **SYMPTOMS IN SUPRASELLAR ARACHNOID CYSTS**

| General Symptoms | Neurologic Findings | Ophthalmologic Examination |
|---|---|---|
| Head circumference >P97 | Seizures | Altered vision |
| Headache | Mental retardation | Paralysis of upward gaze |
| Vomiting | Headbobbing | Optic atrophy |
| Muscular weakness | Intention tremor | |
| Inattention | Dysmetry | |

advisable to make a second hole at the other end of the cyst to permit constant flow of CSF through the cyst. Blood vessels can sometimes be located at the opposite side of the cyst wall; These vessels are not always visible through the membrane. While cutting, these vessels can be opened and bleed profusely. For these cases, a special bipolar probe with one long leg and one short leg is designed to pick up the edge of the tissue and coagulate the bleeding vessel. Constant abundant irrigation is mandatory. Small bleeds can often be controlled by simple rinsing until clear vision is restored. Bipolar and laser coagulation in the noncontact mode can be used. During coagulation, the irrigation should be diminished for a while, because it produces an inhibitory effect on the coagulation. Immediately after coagulation, the rinsing should be restored to maximum to control the bleeding site and to restore the surgeon's vision. When there is any doubt about the completeness of hemostasis, an external drain can be left in place for a few days. In the worst case, one should be prepared to switch to an open craniotomy and, therefore, the patient should be positioned and draped so that this remains a possibility. In cases where arachnoid cysts cause obstructive hydrocephalus, this can be relieved by the fenestration of the cyst provided that the resorptive capacities over the convexity are normal. When there is also a malresorptive hydrocephalus, the fenestration is very useful to create a single cavity, which is then shunted.

## SUPRASELLAR ARACHNOID CYSTS

Large suprasellar arachnoid cysts can cause hydrocephalus in children. Typical symptoms are summarized in Table 42–2. The symptoms are due to hydrocephalus or to a local compression, mainly of the thalamic region and the quadrigeminal plate region. They often have a typical Mickey-Mouse appearance (Fig. 42–27). Hydrocephalus can be mild or pronounced and asymmetric. The cyst itself presents as a large round or oval formation in the suprasellar region. The third ventricle is displaced upward and posteriorly. It remains visible only as a small cleft on an MRI (Fig. 42–28A, B).

Various treatment modalities have been proposed.[105, 194] Open surgical interventions can be complicated by severe neuropsychological impairment or by collapse of the brain with subsequent bilateral chronic subdural hematomas. Shunting of the cyst often requires bilateral shunting, because there is no left-to-right communication. After the hydrocephalus has been treated successfully, the cyst can continue to grow; therefore, shunting of the cyst itself is proposed. The cyst walls are often tough and difficult to penetrate. The catheter slides tangentially over the surface of the cyst.

The clinical and paraclinical investigations have been described in detail by Pierre-Kahn[182] and others, who have proposed treatment under endoscopic control or an endoscopic approach.[16, 29, 53] Initially, we made a bipolar penetration and enlarged the hole by repeatedly inflating a Fogarty catheter; however, these openings were too small (about 6 mm) and tended to heal. Two children had to be operated on again when their cysts were re-expanding and the symptoms relapsed, although the initial hole had not entirely closed. Therefore, we now use the laser to obtain 10-to-20 mm fenestrations. The angle of approach is very important (Fig. 42–29A–C). In the frontal plane, one should choose

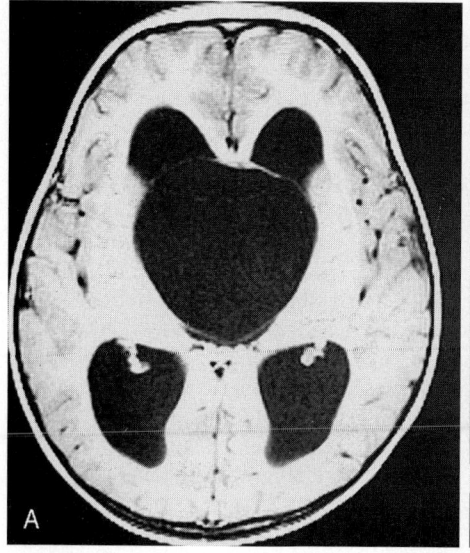
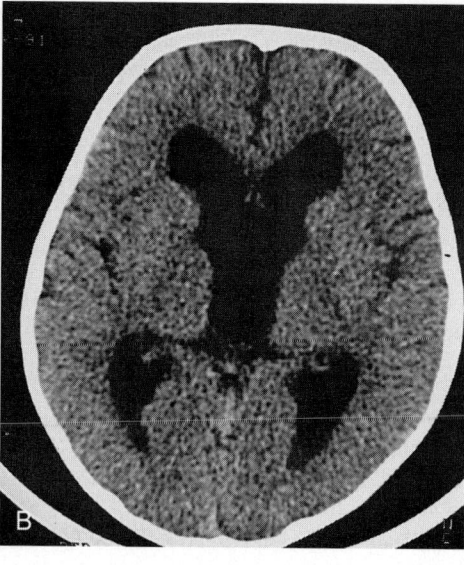

**FIGURE 42–27** ■ *A*, A preoperative magnetic resonance image (MRI) in a suprasellar arachnoid cyst in case 1. *B*, Postoperative MRI in a suprasellar arachnoid cyst in case 1.

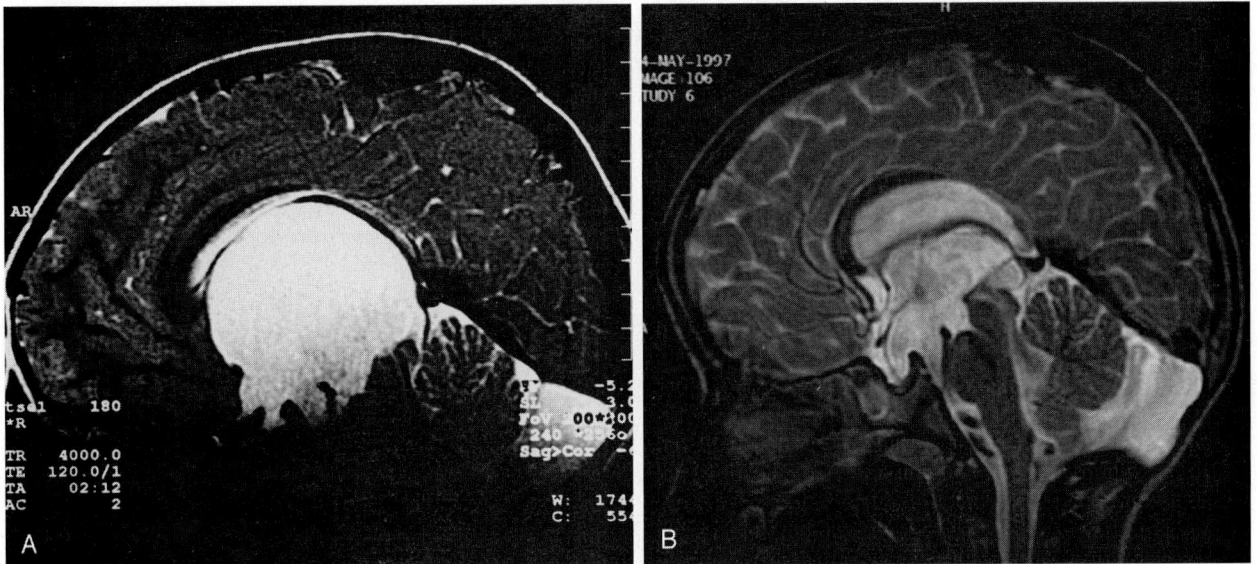

FIGURE 42–28 ■ *A,* Preoperative sagittal magnetic resonance image (MRI) in a suprasellar arachnoid cyst. *B,* Postoperative sagittal MRI in a suprasellar arachnoid cyst showing the opening (with flow void) of the sylvian aqueduct and the collapse of the cyst dome.

a trajectory that starts close to the midline, so that the lowest point of the trajectory comes onto the midline. In the sagittal plane, the trajectory should end in the prepontine area and start in the precoronal region. In cases where the ventricles are only slightly dilated, stereotactic guidance is advisable. The target point should then be the basilar artery in the depth of the cyst. Through a right coronal bur hole, the dome of the cyst is reached. Most often this is a bluish membrane that is crossed by tiny vessels (see Fig. 42–28). In some cases, blood vessels connect the cyst wall to the ependyma across the ventricle. When the ventricles are rather small, one enters the frontal horn quite close to the cyst dome. One starts by pushing away the membrane from the tip of the endoscope with a blunt instrument, such as the bipolar coagulation probe or the closed grasping forceps. A coagulating laser fiber can then be introduced through the right irrigation channel to coagulate the vessels in the nontouch mode. By doing this, one can observe a considerable shrinkage of the membrane, so that it detaches itself from the fornix and a longer distance is obtained from the tip of the endoscope to the membrane. This makes it much easier to work. One can also use two trajectories, but this is certainly not the first choice.

The coagulating laser probe is used in the nontouch mode to coagulate the vessels in a circular pattern. It is not advisable to coagulate the whole circle (see Fig. 42–24). It is sufficient to coagulate only the vessels. Coagulation is also applied at sites where a blood vessel is translucent through the membrane at its opposite side. By means of the cutting laser in the contact mode, the roundel is then cut out (see Fig. 42–25) but remains attached by a fine stalk to prevent it from falling into the cyst or into the ventricle (see Fig. 42–26). The roundel is then grasped and avulsed. To bring it out it is often necessary to pull out the whole endoscope, holding the membrane firmly against the lens. Re-insertion of the endoscope through the same trajectory offers no problems.

After the first fenestration, we prefer to enter the cyst. Here, an astonishing view is seen of the suprasellar region

structures (Fig. 42–30, see color section): The termination of the basilar artery into the posterior cerebral arteries, numerous branches in the interpeduncular fossa going toward the brain stem, both oculomotor nerves, and the posterior communicating arteries are visible. More anteriorly, the internal carotid artery, sometimes the A1 segment and the recurrent artery of Heubner, can be seen. In the middle, the pituitary gland is seen as a pink plate from which the pituitary stalk climbs upward to the roof of the cyst that pushes the floor of the third ventricle upward. In the depth of the cyst around the basilar artery, a constant finding is a slit valve (Fig. 42–31, see color section), which might be part of the pathogenetic mechanism by which the cyst enlarges.[228] At every beat of the heart, one can see this slit opening and closing again. We try to destroy this slit valve mechanism. A first attempt can be made to avulse parts of the membrane with the grasping forceps. When this is difficult to accomplish, additional enlargement of the opening can be obtained by the inflatable Fogarty catheter. In most cases the opening is still not large enough, and by climbing up along the clivus, we find the membrane stretched over the dorsum sellae in a totally avascular area. It is easy to grasp the membrane over the dorsum sellae and tear an opening in it. This opening can be enlarged by the Fogarty balloon catheter. By means of scissors and grasping forceps, it can be extended toward the hole that was already created at the original slit valve. The membrane can also be hooked up to a small hooklet that is used to stretch it, after which a blunt cutting fiber can be introduced through the side channel to cut the membranes in the concavity of the hooklet (Fig. 42–32, see color section). By doing so the risk of damage to the basilar artery is minimized. One can enlarge the fenestration toward the frontal horn of the lateral ventricle by making additional cuts or cut out more of the membrane. This may be more difficult when the membranes are already waving and floppy. To overcome this problem, one can use the bipolar or laser coagulation probes to make several holes that can be connected by scissors.

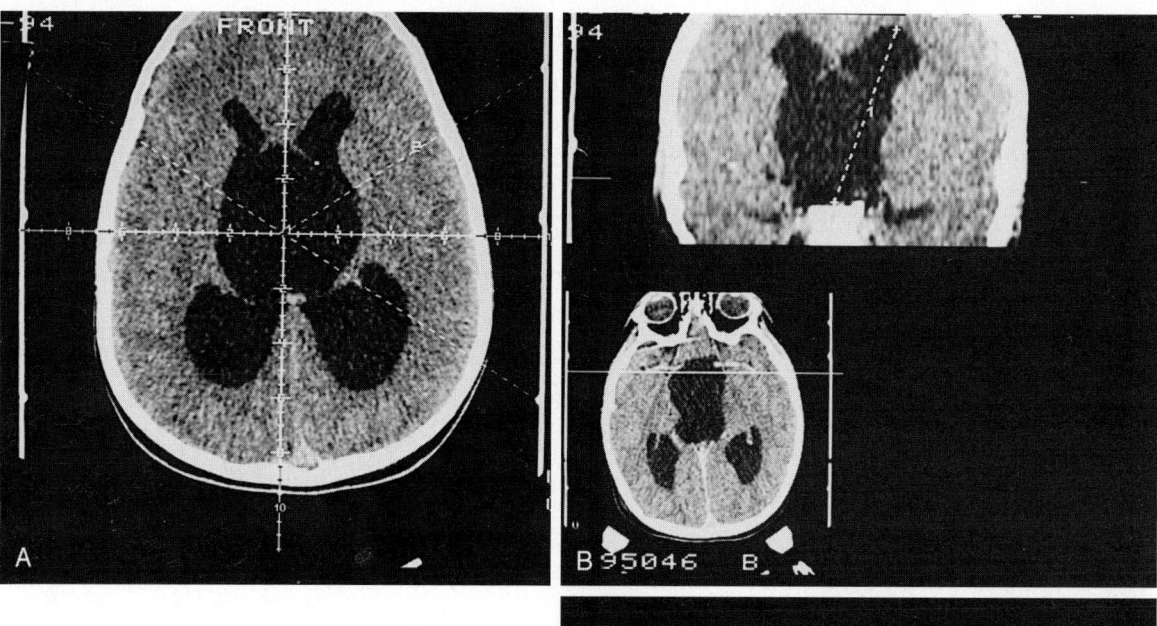

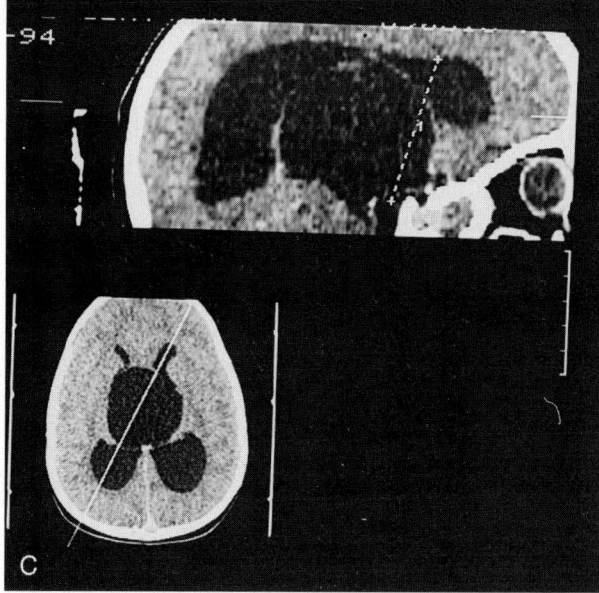

FIGURE 42–29 ■ *A,* Stereotactic targeting on the dome of the cyst bulging in the left frontal horn in a suprasellar arachnoid cyst. *B,* Planning of the trajectory on frontal stereotactic computed tomography (CT) in a suprasellar arachnoid cyst. *C,* Planning of the trajectory on stereotactic sagittal reconstruction. CT in a suprasellar arachnoid cyst for fenestration and opening of the floor of the cyst around the basilar artery.

We have treated eight children with suprasellar cysts in this way. The symptoms of intracranial hypertension improved dramatically in all of these patients as did the headbobbing, tremor, and dysmetria caused by local compression. In one girl, long-standing mental retardation and hormonal disturbances were not affected, although the hydrocephalus and the cyst were cured. Postoperative MRI shows a decompression of the thalamic region bilaterally (Fig. 42–33). Instead of a distended balloon, one can observe a more flaccid cavity. The cyst never disappears entirely, but it is reduced significantly in size. The tissue defect always remains visible, but the tension is relieved. An advantage over shunting operations is the absence of the shunt material, slit ventricle syndrome, and subdural collections. There was no mortality, and the morbidity was limited to seizure 6 hours after the operation following which the patient made a full recovery.

## Arachnoid Cysts of the Brain Convexity

This localization is rather rare, but some arachnoid cysts of the convexity are big enough to come into close contact with the ventricular ependyma so that they can be treated by fenestration toward the ventricle. In these cases, one enters the cyst first and perforates the cyst wall toward the ventricle. The opening should be as large as possible.

## Arachnoid Cysts of the Sylvian Fissure

Many temporal arachnoid cysts that extend into the sylvian fissure are asymptomatic and do not require treatment.[174] In cases with pronounced headache and treatment-resistant epilepsy, some form of treatment is mandatory. Often this has involved the microsurgical fenestration of the cyst

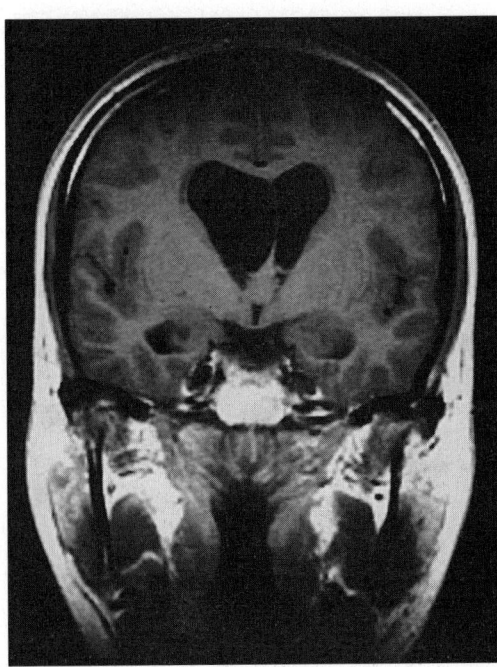

FIGURE 42–33 ■ Asymmetric hydrocephalus and bulging of the septum pellucidum in a colloid cyst obstructing the foramina of Monro.

toward the basal cisterns and resection of part of the wall; however, closure of these openings may lead to a recurrence. A valuable alternative is shunting of the cyst over a low-pressure valve. The drawback of this method is the presence of foreign material and the shunt-related complications. In cases in which MRI reveals a rather big area in which the cyst wall is in contact with the suprasellar and parasellar subarachnoid spaces, an endoscopic operation can be considered. Through a temporal bur hole the dura is opened; the lateral cyst wall is perforated; and the endoscope is advanced toward the midline. Often the big arterial vessels of the circle of Willis, the branches of the middle cerebral artery, and the oculomotor nerve are already discernible through the cyst membrane. The fenestration is started at a point free of arterial vessels. Bipolar coagulation, grasping forceps, scissors, and the hooklet are the instruments of choice. A cutting laser can be used to cut membranes that are stretched by one of these instruments. A coagulating laser is contraindicated because of the vessels on the opposite side of the membrane.

## Arachnoid Cysts of the Cerebellopontine Angle

These cysts can be reached by a retrosigmoid bur hole as for the approach of an acoustic neuroma. The specific problems in this kind of cyst arise from the presence of the cranial nerves IX, X, and XI and more anteriorly cranial nerves VII, VIII, and V.[191] A trajectory should be planned inferolaterally to superomedially, and an opening should be made as large as possible toward the parapontine basal cisterns. Care should be taken for the small vasa nervorum, such as the labyrinthine artery. They can be confused on preoperative imaging with epidermoid cysts.

## Arachnoid Cysts of the Quadrigeminal Cistern

These cysts tend to produce obstructive hydrocephalus by compressing the sylvian aqueduct. They have an anterior extension in the third and sometimes in one or both of the lateral ventricles. Their inferior extension compresses the cerebellum downward so that it has an excavated aspect on MRI. Depending on their posterior extension, these cysts can be approached anteriorly or posteriorly. When the cyst is less than 2 cm from the dura under the confluens sinuum, it can be approached posteriorly. Under the microscope, the cerebellum is pushed downward slightly to permit the introduction of the endoscope through a paramedially placed bur hole. The posterior wall can be opened by classical microsurgical instrumentation. Through this opening, the endoscope is introduced and advanced forward toward a place where a large fenestration can be made to the third or the lateral ventricle. Postoperatively, one can observe a reopening of the aqueduct and the expansion of the cerebellum, which regains its typical appearance.

## Cysts of the Cavum Septi Pellucidi and Cavum Veli Interpositi

These midline cysts can be asymptomatic when they are small. These findings are not rare on CT or MRI; however, some of these cysts tend to grow and expand. The lateral walls of the cysts are then ballooned with compression of the surrounding structures and thinning of the corpus callosum. They can be approached from the lateral ventricle. Stereotactic guidance is preferable in most cases, because of the narrow spaces. The cysts of the cavum septi pellucidi should be fenestrated starting from the frontal horn. The cysts of the cavum veli interpositi should be fenestrated, starting from the trigonum or corpus of the lateral ventricle. One can try to plan a laterolateral trajectory so that it is possible to fenestrate both walls of the cyst.

## Paraventricular Ependymal Cysts

These cysts can be seen along the lateral ventricles and sometimes in the thalamic region beside the third ventricle.[17, 222] Such a paraventricular ependymal cyst can cause intermittent headache and diplopia. In a typical case, a fenestration was performed starting from the right frontal horn through a normal foramen of Monro. A small rim of brain tissue covering the top of the cyst had to be removed. The patient recovered fully without side effects and without recurrence on MR in the follow-up period of 5 years.

## Epidermoid Cysts

Total resection of the epidermoid membrane of these cysts is ideal; however, in many cases this is not possible, and in recurrences of epidermoid cysts it is unwise to try to remove the entire membrane.

The cysts can be approached according to their position, either directly or through the ventricle. The typical snow-white contents may be aspirated using a stiff polyurethane catheter connected to the vacuum. The tubing should be arranged so that the aspiration can be stopped abruptly to avoid damage to vulnerable structures (e.g., cranial nerves). A grasping forceps can sometimes be used to mobilize the contents. When possible, parts of the epidermoid membrane can also be removed, but no attempt should be made to remove them completely. Epidermoid cysts of the cerebellopontine angle can be confused with arachnoid cysts.

## Colloid Cysts

A colloid cyst is often revealed by hydrocephalus owing to an obstruction of the foramen of Monro. These cysts can remain asymptomatic for a long time and then give only intermittent symptomatology. They can cause sudden death owing to an acute obstructive hydrocephalus.[203] The ventricular dilatation is often asymmetric, and one can see a bulging of the septum pellucidum toward the less affected side. This may be the signature of a colloid cyst in cases of isodense cysts on a CT scan.[188] More recently, they are very easily recognized on MR (Fig. 42–34A, B) as hyperintense structures on $T_1$-weighted images and by contrast enhancement after the administration of gadolinium. On $T_2$-weighted images, they present as round black dots. Different treatment modalities have been described, including ventricular shunting, stereotactic puncture and aspiration,[24, 160, 201] and microsurgical removal. We believe that this lesion can easily be controlled by an endoscopic approach. We have tried stereotactic puncture of the cysts in the past. The cysts are often small, and the danger exists of damaging the fornix, choroid plexus, thalamostriate vein, septal veins, and small vessels at the surface of the cyst capsule. They often contain viscous or semisolid contents that are difficult to aspirate through thin stereotactic needles.[137] Thicker needles do not penetrate the capsule with-

out prior coagulation. As a result, the stereotactic method usually ends in only partial removal. Although these patients are often helped in the immediate postoperative period, the cysts tend to recur.*

Since 1986, there has been an evolution in our technique for removal of colloid cysts.[32] Our approach involves one bur hole and one trajectory, but often two instruments are used simultaneously through the working channel and through one of the irrigation side channels. In most cases we use stereotactic guidance or neuronavigation for the initial introduction, because the angle of approach is very important (Fig. 42–35A–C). One should be able to approach the wall of the cyst by laterally sliding tangentially over the head of the caudate nucleus and frontally in order to penetrate the third ventricle beneath the fornix. The foramen of Monro is more parasagittal than axial, and the endoscope has to pass through a cleft-like opening. One should also be able to move upward to reach the septum pellucidum in case a septostomy is needed. In some cases with wide ventricles, it is sufficient to plan the trajectory on frontal and sagittal MR images. In cases of pronounced asymmetric hydrocephalus, the choice between a left- or right-sided approach is determined by the widest ventricle. In symmetric cases, the nondominant side is preferred. The place of the bur hole has to be far anterior, even on the front, and 2.5 to 3 cm from the midline. The bur hole should be at the highest point of the operating field to prevent air from entering the ventricles and CSF from leaking outward. As soon as the ventricle is reached, the cyst dome becomes visible as a green protrusion through the foramen of Monro (Fig. 42–36A, see color section). After removal of the mandrins, irrigation is started and the endoscope is detached from the stereotactic arc. The first step is to look around for precise orientation and to inspect the relationship between the cyst, choroid plexus, septal

---

*See references 4, 28, 32, 36, 38, 47, 54–56, 77, 89, 91, 95, 138, 145, 146, 153, 154, 166.

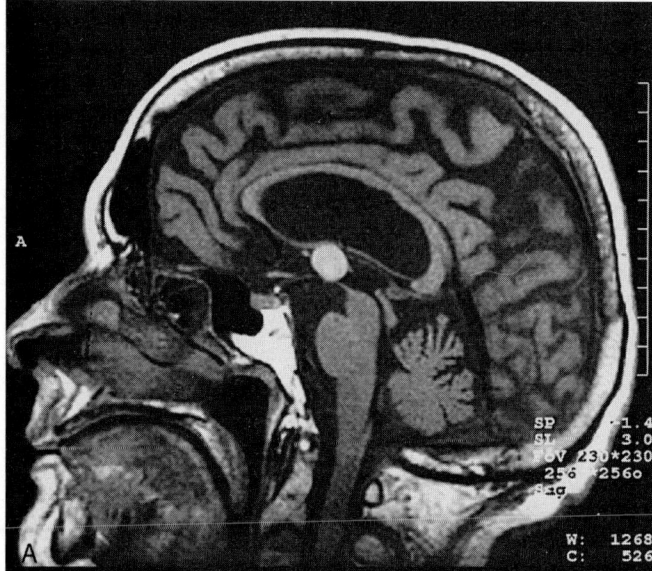
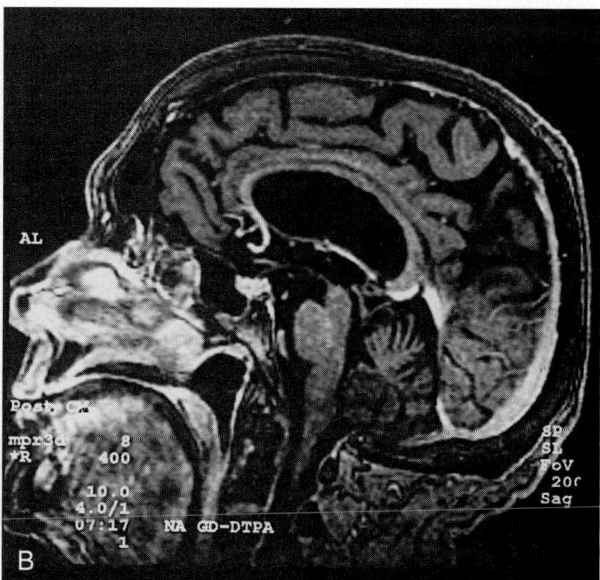

FIGURE 42–34 ■ A, A preoperative mediosagittal magnetic resonance image (MRI) in a colloid cyst. B, Postoperative mediosagittal MRI after the removal of a colloid cyst.

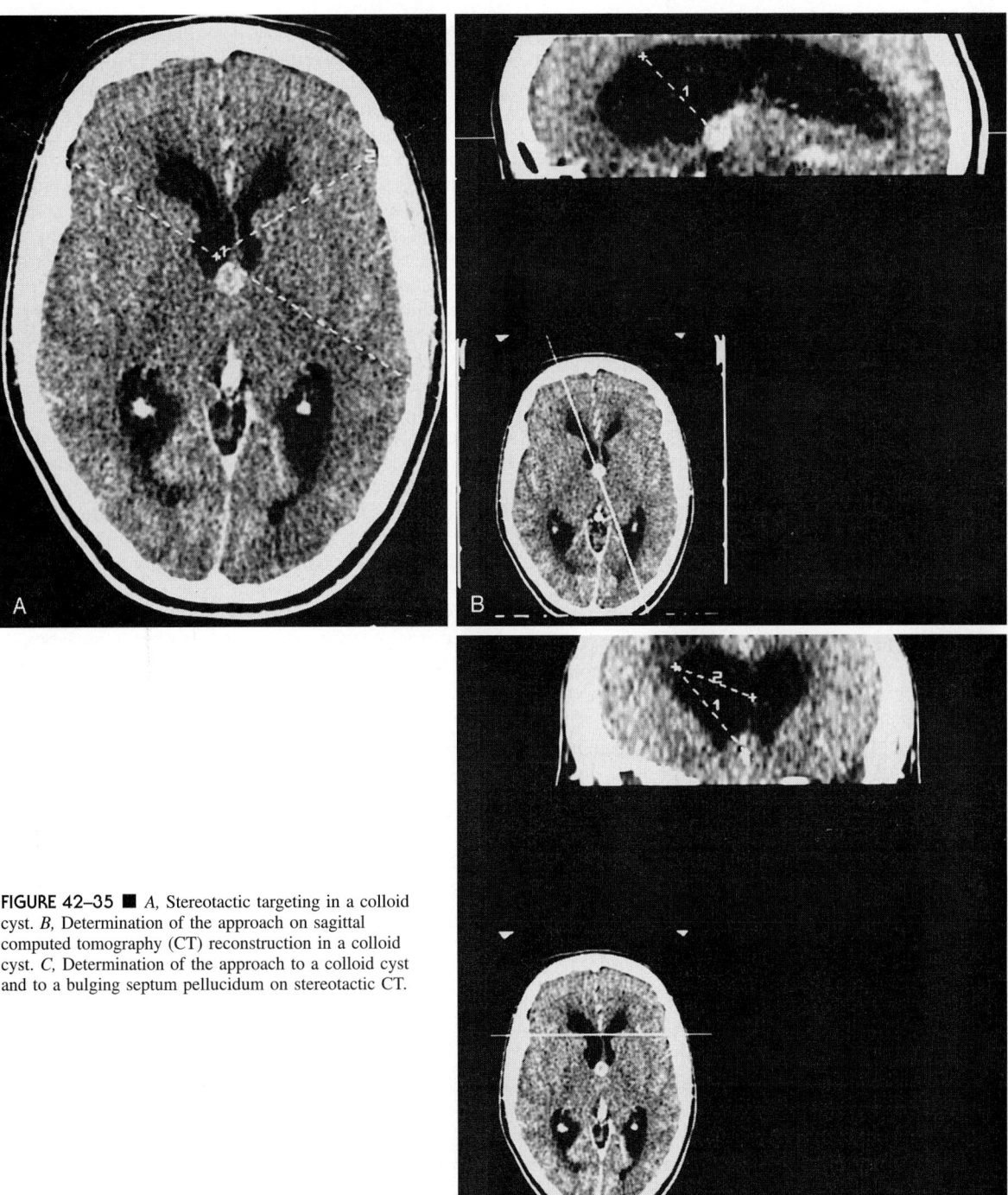

**FIGURE 42–35** ■ *A,* Stereotactic targeting in a colloid cyst. *B,* Determination of the approach on sagittal computed tomography (CT) reconstruction in a colloid cyst. *C,* Determination of the approach to a colloid cyst and to a bulging septum pellucidum on stereotactic CT.

vein, and thalamostriate veins. In many cases, a small cleft remains visible between the cyst wall and the fornix, which explains why the symptomatology of colloid cysts is often intermittent over a long period. From the very beginning, continuous irrigation is mandatory to keep the ventricles in their original size. If the pressure is lowered, the result is oozing from the veins in the roof of the ventricle where the ependyma covers the surface of the corpus callosum. The next step is determined by the individual presentation of the lesion. Small vessels over the surface must be coagulated using a laser in the nontouch mode (see Fig.

42–36*B,* in color section). If the choroid plexus overlies the cyst, it should be coagulated too; care should be taken to avoid the thalamostriate vein, which can be hidden by the plexus. The maximum area of cyst capsule is exposed. With the cutting laser a hole is made in the capsule, and the stiff aspiration catheter with a 45-degree oblique tip is inserted into the working channel to remove the contents (see Fig. 42–36*C,* in color section). The aspiration is supplied by using a 10-mm syringe. The contents are usually very viscous and it is necessary to remove and re-introduce the tip of the catheter several times (see Fig. 42–36*D,* in color section). A grasping forceps (see Fig. 42–36E, in color section) is used to mobilize the semisolid contents. At this stage of the operation, one can see a flaccid translucent cyst wall (see Fig. 42–36F, in color section) and a large decompression of the foramen of Monro. The capsule should be coagulated, and further shrinkage of the capsule can be obtained. From time to time the edge of the partially emptied capsule is grasped. By applying gentle traction, one can pull out more and more of the capsule through the foramen of Monro (see Fig. 42–36G, in color section). In this way, surprising amounts of residual capsule and contents can become visible and reachable. The tearing of the capsule should always be done very carefully because excessive traction can result in bleeding around the corner and out of reach. Once a vessel is bleeding, it is easier to coagulate the vessel by the bipolar probe than by the coagulating laser. The effect of the bipolar coagulation is also less penetrating in the depth, which is particularly important in the coagulation of the choroid plexus. Often it is advisable to use two instruments simultaneously—one through the large working channel and one through an irrigation channel (see Fig. 42–36H, in color section). According to necessity, the left or right irrigation channel can be used to introduce a tiny instrument while the other is used for the inlet tubing. In these circumstances, the irrigation fluid is running through the working channel alongside the instrument. The conically shaped cutting fibers should not be used through the side channels, because the delicate tips may break and fall into the ventricle. To overcome this problem, either the cutting fiber is used through the wide working channel and the very thin grasping forceps is used through the irrigating channel or grasping forceps are used through the working channel and a thin blunt fiber is used through one of the side channels as a cutting device in the contact mode. The other irrigation channel should be used for continuous rinsing while working through the other two.

The foramen of Monro is opened widely (see Fig. 42–36I, in color section). Only a small rim of coagulated capsule remains at its posterior edge where it merges with the surrounding tissue. The most difficult part of the surgery is freeing the capsule from the posterior inferior side of the column of the fornices to which it may adhere. In large colloid cysts and when an asymmetric hydrocephalus is seen, we prefer to make a septostomy (see Fig. 42–36J, in color section) to ensure a good left-to-right communication. We believe that this may postpone or avoid a reoperation in case of a recurrence. In the septum pellucidum, an area is selected that is relatively free of blood vessels. A circular pattern of small coagulations is created by the coagulating laser fiber, after which this roundel is cut out by the laser in contact mode. It is not necessary to coagulate the whole circle, because coagulation causes blanching of the tissue, and thus more energy is needed for the laser cutting. The laser light is reflected by white tissues, thus a higher cutting power is needed. As usual in fenestrations, the roundel remains attached by a fine stalk that is finally grasped with a forceps and pulled out, if necessary by extracting the whole endoscope. The trajectory remains open and permits easy reintroduction of the shaft through the white matter. The reintroduction is necessary to accomplish a final irrigation and inspection. No external ventricular catheter is used after the procedure.

Based on 10 years of experience, we find that the endoscopic resection can be as complete as with a microsurgical transventricular approach. A transcallosal interhemispheric approach may enhance the certainty of total removal but, in our opinion, is too invasive a procedure compared with the endoscopic method using one bur hole. In an early case in our series in which only partial removal was obtained, we made an interesting observation: The first postoperative MRI showed partial removal, whereas an MRI 14 months later showed further shrinkage of the cyst remnants. Instead of a recurrence, the CSF may have washed out the contents progressively through the fenestration in the wall. The patient is still doing well 7½ years after the intervention.

Using an appropriate technique, the endoscopic resection of colloid cysts involves only a few complications. Complications that are described in the literature include damage to the fornix, ventriculitis, epilepsy, bleeding, and failure to cut the capsule. Particular attention should be paid to the assessment of the patient's memory functions before and after the operation. Clinically, we have seen no worsening of memory functions in our patients. The only morbidity we noted was some slowness when one patient awakened from general anesthesia. This might have been caused by the use of normal saline for irrigation. The normal saline might have disturbed the $Ca^{2+}$ and $K^+$ ions that are important for neural transmission. This patient recovered fully after 24 hours.

## Cystic Tumors

This section deals with tumors that contain large cystic parts. Sometimes it may be difficult to obtain conclusive biopsy specimens from these tumors, because the wall is too thin. It is possible to enter the tumor cyst endoscopically and biopsy the wall from inside, which enhances the certainty that a conclusive specimen is taken for pathologic examination and also allows irrigation of the contents of the cyst and eventually aspiration of them to reduce the size of the space-occupying lesion.

## Pineal Cysts

Pineal cysts may remain asymptomatic or they may enlarge and obstruct the sylvian aqueduct. They can present with diplopia or vertical gaze paralysis due to compression of the quadrigeminal plate. These cysts can be tumorous, degenerative, or posthemorrhagic (Fig. 42–37). They can be approached from the nondominant frontal horn of the lateral ventricle. Because these lesions become symptomatic owing to hydrocephalus, the foramen of Monro is widened. The bur holes should be placed anteriorly enough to reach the posterior part of the third ventricle. According to its position, one can work under or above the interthalamic commissure. By means of the bipolar coagulation or laser coagulation, the anterior part of the wall may be coagulated and removed. The contents can be aspirated to prevent them from escaping into the ventricle. When the compression was not too long-standing, the aqueduct re-

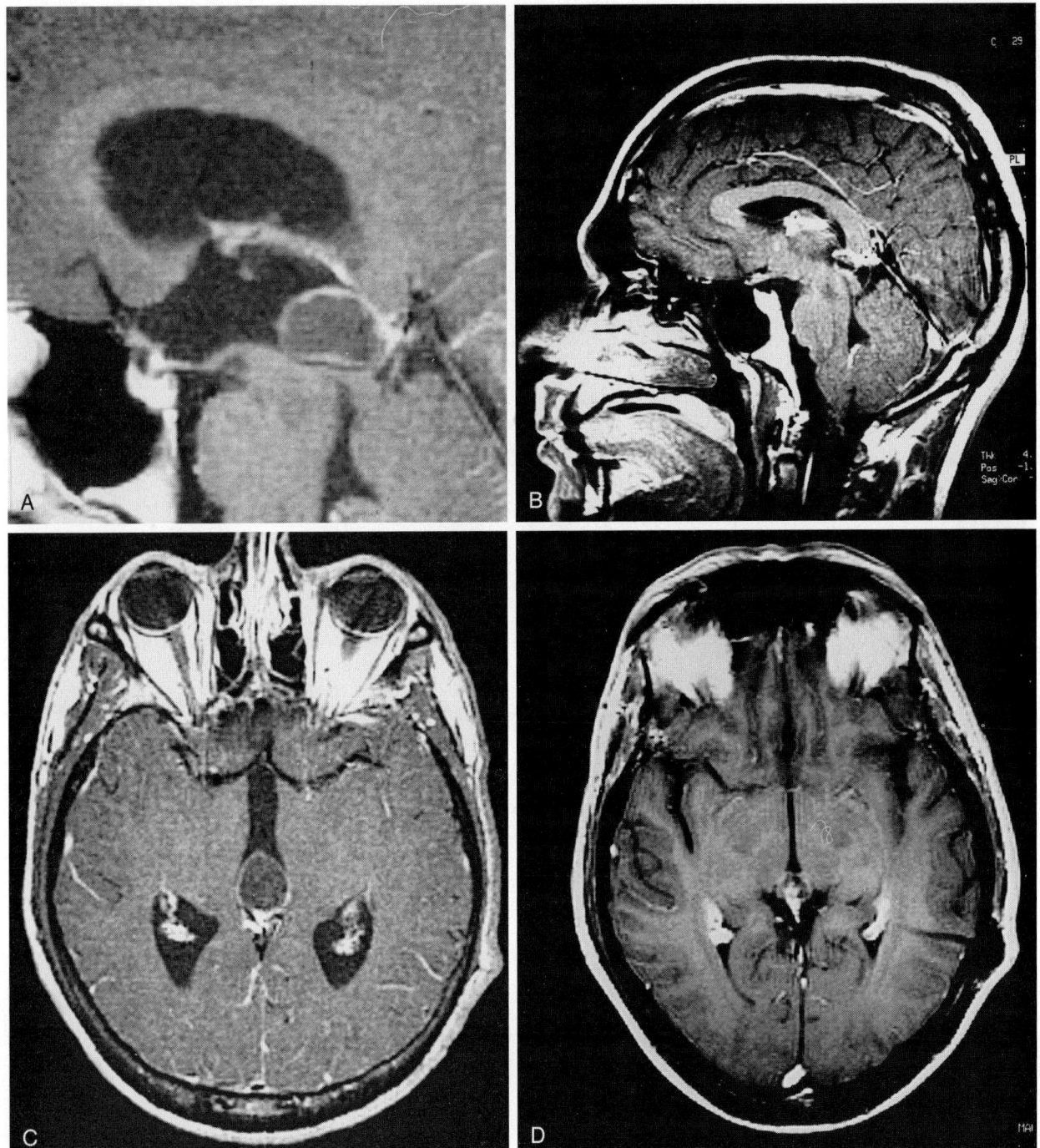

**FIGURE 42–37** ■ *A,* Preoperative sagittal magnetic resonance image (MRI) of a pineal cyst. *B,* Postoperative sagittal MRI of a pineal cyst. *C,* Preoperative axial MRI of a pineal cyst. *D,* Postoperative sagittal MRI of a pineal cyst.

opens and no third ventriculostomy or shunting operation is necessary.

## Degenerative Cysts

**Postradiosurgery Cysts.** These cysts have been described years after the radiosurgical treatment of arteriovenous malformations (AVMs).[90] Although the original lesion is cured, benign glial cysts may develop. A young woman was treated for a deep-seated temporal AVM. Twelve years

later, she developed temporal lobe epilepsy and a severe memory disorder. MR revealed a huge cyst elevating the hippocampus and compressing the small temporal horn of the lateral ventricle. A stereotactic approach was used posteriorly. The ventricle was entered, and the target was the part of the cyst wall that was bulging into the ventricle. A blunt instrument was used through the working channel to push the membrane away from the tip of the endoscope to be able to see and to work in this narrow space. A fenestration was performed, and the contents of the cyst were aspirated and irrigated. In the anterior part of the

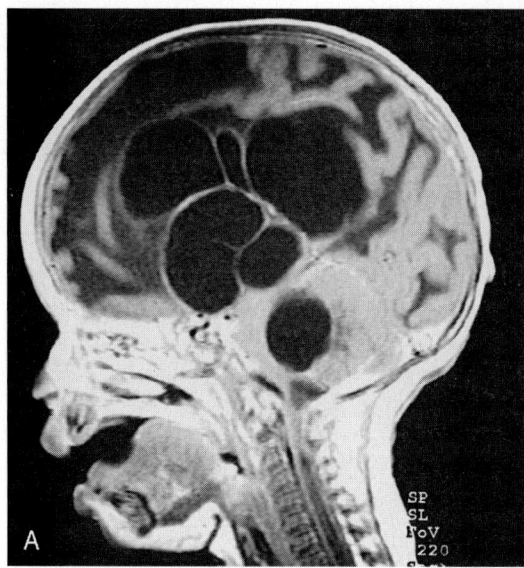
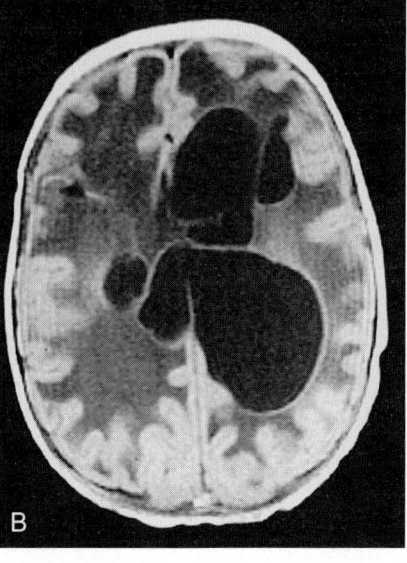

FIGURE 42–38 ■ *A*, and *B*, Sagittal and axial magnetic resonance images of a multiloculated post-meningoencephalitis cyst.

cyst, at its medial side, a biopsy was taken from the wall and it showed only gliotic tissue. Postoperatively, there was a marked reduction in the size of the defect. The patient's clinical symptoms subsided quickly.

**Postbrachytherapy Cysts.** These cysts can originate after treatment of tumors with ¹²⁵I. In most successful cases the tumor shrinks or even disappears, whereas in others, the necrotic tumor becomes cystic. These cysts tend to enlarge gradually.

A young girl was treated for an inoperable oligodendroglioma in the central region with ¹²⁵I. After 1 year, her original symptoms had subsided but she developed some headache. A new MR scan showed the presence of a huge cystic degeneration of the irradiated area. Serial biopsies were taken at seven different places in the wall of this cystic formation, and all showed radionecrosis and no viable tumor tissue. After the biopsy, the cyst contents that proved to be entirely liquid were aspirated in the hope that this would be sufficient. However, after an initial period of stabilization, the cyst distended again. When the patient developed progressive hemiparesis and memory and character disturbance, we decided to make a fenestration toward the lateral ventricle. In one place the wall of the necrotic cyst was bulging into the lateral ventricle. This place was selected as the target. Stereotactic guidance was necessary, because we approached the membrane from within the cyst, which reached the upper surface of the brain in the parietal region. By entering such a tumor cyst, one completely loses every orientation because there is no more recognizable anatomy.

Knowing where to go by the stereotactic guidance, we saw a small area where the wall was thin. First we made a small hole by bipolar coagulation. Close inspection showed that this led into the lateral ventricle. The opening was enlarged with a Fogarty balloon catheter, laser coagulation, and cutting device. A large fenestration connected the cyst with the ventricle; it produced a spectacular reduction of the cyst distention and total remission of the symptoms. This girl is attending normal school and Girl Scouts now 4 years after the endoscopy.

**Postmeningoencephalitis Cysts.** Infections can cause huge multiloculated cysts (Fig. 42–38*A*, *B*) that originate in the ventricles and extend in all directions. Thin membranes separate the different cavities, and their expansivity often causes hydrocephalus.[147, 148, 151, 165] In the past, it was necessary to insert several ventricular catheters and eventually several valves to treat the condition (Fig. 42–39). Endoscopically, one can intercommunicate all the cysts by large fenestrations of the walls. A trajectory is used on which the membranes are lined up and eventually we use more trajectories that originate from the same bur hole. Some of these cysts have a very high protein content, and it is advisable to aspirate and irrigate the contents of the cyst through a separate aspiration catheter before the fenestration. In some cases, it is sufficient to connect all the cysts

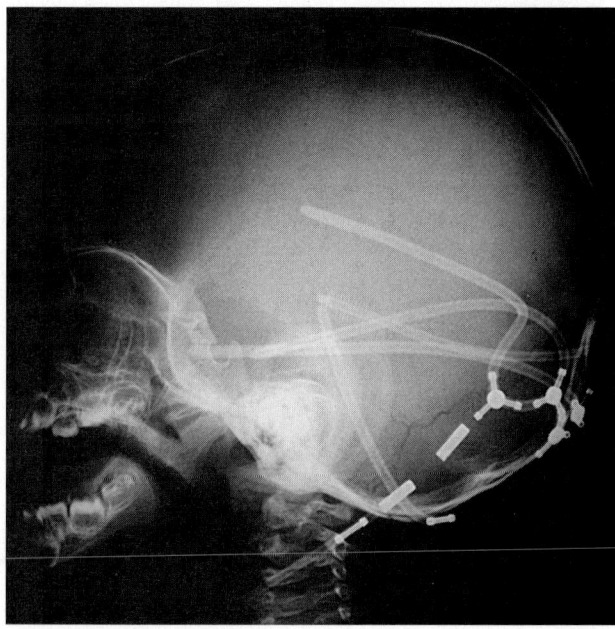

FIGURE 42–39 ■ Pre-endoscopy edge. Treatment for multilocular hydrocephalus.

to each other and to the ventricular system; in this way an obstructive hydrocephalus can be solved. In other cases the resorptive capacity over the convexity for CSF has been impaired, and it is necessary to insert a shunt. Nevertheless, the endoscopic procedure remains useful for creating one communicating cavity so that hydrocephalus can be treated with a single ventricular catheter. The clinical picture remained excellent.

## Parasitic Cysts

In cysticercosis multiple cysts can obstruct the ventricles. Endoscopic evacuation is possible.[5, 18, 45, 163]

## TUMORS

The role of endoscopic techniques in tumors is quite restricted. Many tumors bulge into the ventricles or are confined to the ventricular system. If their operability is questionable or absent, they can be approached endoscopically. The main goals are to perform a biopsy,[59] sometimes with partial removal but seldom with total removal.[9, 33, 62, 76, 88, 110] The endoscope can be introduced free-hand when the ventricles are wide enough. Stereotactic guidance is used when the depth of penetration and the direction are critical. Some tumors bulge into the ventricles but have an unclear delineation toward the parenchyma. In these cases (often benign astrocytomas), one can never be certain that one can obtain a complete resection by microsurgical methods. In these cases, we prefer an endoscopic biopsy followed by [125]I brachytherapy. A blind transventricular stereotactic biopsy can be dangerous to attempt, because there is no surrounding tissue to give tamponade and prevent venous oozing after the biopsy has been taken. Small vessels at the surface of the tumor can be coagulated with the bipolar coagulation probe. After this, a biopsy can be performed either by use of an aspiration catheter or with the help of grasping forceps. The biopsy should not be taken from the coagulated area. The instrument can be introduced under the surface of the tumor to obtain viable conclusive tissue samples. Often one can see a total or almost total obstruction of the foramen of Monro. In cases of acute or severe intracranial overpressure, deblocking the foramen of Monro can be the goal. Where there is a homogeneous avascular-looking surface, no coagulation is needed before entering the tumor to take the biopsy. In many cases one can observe infiltration into the surrounding tissue, which is very compromising for total resection as well in open microsurgery as in endoscopic surgery. As in stereotactic biopsy, it is advisable to take serial samples to prevent undergrading. Small venous bleedings can be easily controlled by simple rinsing. Tumors in the posterior part of the third ventricle (e.g., pineal tumors) can be easily reached with the rigid endoscope (Fig. 42–40). The trajectory should be planned on sagittal MR or on sagittal CT reconstructions (Fig. 42–41). The bur hole will have to be quite frontal. If one enters through the frontal horn of the lateral ventricle, one can observe the foramen of Monro, fornix, choroid plexus, septal veins, and thalamostriate veins (Fig. 42–42, see color section). On approaching the foramen, one can see the interthalamic commissure appearing in the depth. Advancing slowly permits visualization of the tumor, and the choice should be made whether to go above or under the interthalamic commissure. Small vessels at the surface of the tumor will have to be coagulated. Figures 42–43, 42–44, and 42–45 show two cases that are quite similar on MR but have a totally different pathologic diagnosis: Figure 42–40 is a pinealoblastoma, and Figures 42–43 to 42–45 are a germinoma. Their preoperative endoscopic appearance is very different (Figs. 42–46 and 42–47, see color section). With the endoscope, more malignant areas are sometimes discernible mainly in benign tumors. This heterogeneous na-

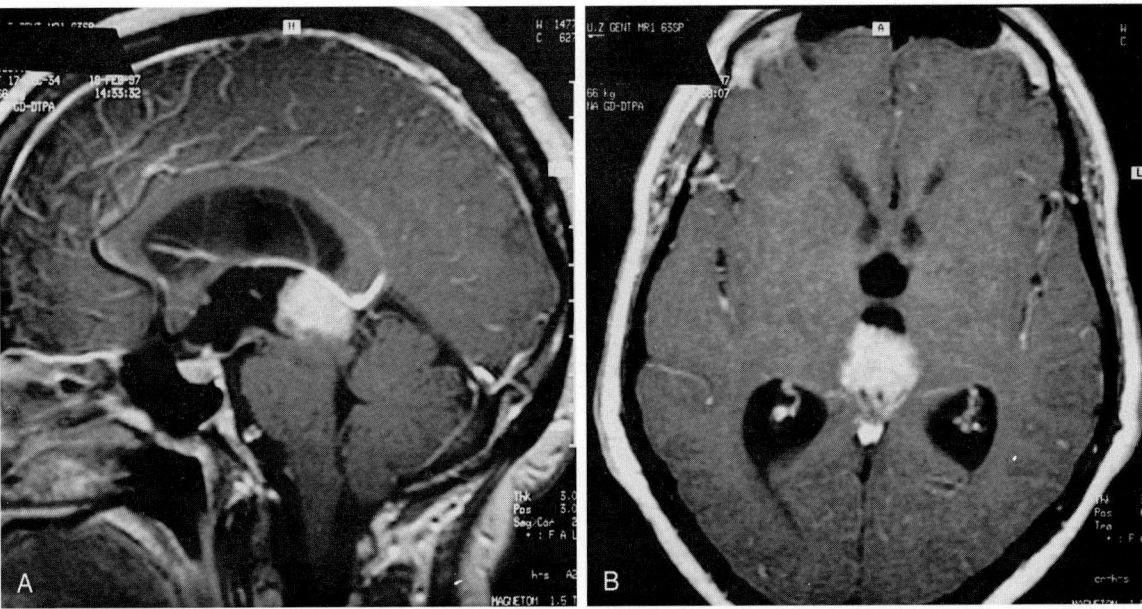

**FIGURE 42–40** ■ *A,* and *B,* Sagittal and axial magnetic resonance images of a pineal gland tumor (pinealoblastoma).

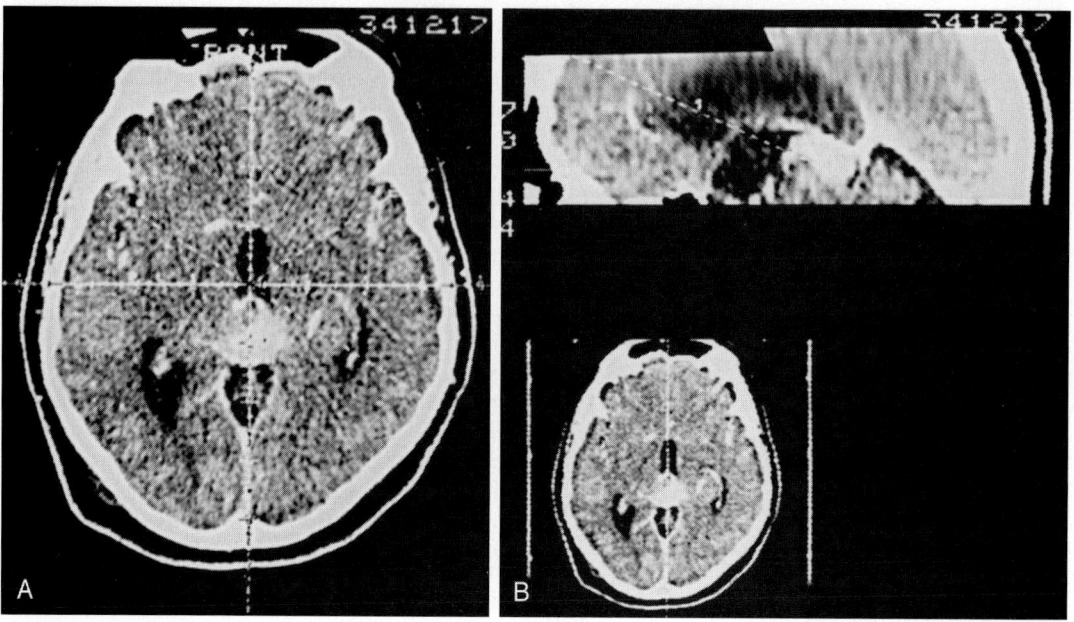

FIGURE 42–41 ■ *A,* Axial stereotactic computed tomography scan of a pineal tumor (pinealoblastoma). *B,* Sagittal stereotactic reconstruction for biopsy of a pineal gland tumor.

ture can be recognized by differences in color and vascular patterns. Biopsies of these different areas often result in more profuse venous oozing that requires hemostasis by bipolar or laser.

## CRANIOPHARYNGIOMA

Although microsurgery is often the treatment of first choice in craniopharyngiomas, some patients are suitable candidates for an endoscopic approach.[1] Among the indications are small craniopharyngiomas that obstruct the foramen of Monro. In patients in poor general condition and also in some recurrent craniopharyngiomas, it is often possible to do partial resections of cystic and solid components to alleviate the symptoms. In large cystic recurrences, we prefer to first treat the patient with intracavitary $^{30}$Y irradiation.[11, 12]

Two cases are presented to illustrate the possibilities. Figure 42–48 (*A–F*) shows a 70-year-old lady in a bad fragile condition with a solid craniopharyngioma, which also contains semisolid necrotic and calcified parts. She was admitted with a history of gait disturbance, memory loss, diabetes insipidus, and increasing obesity for 2 months. Clinical examination showed a well, conscious but

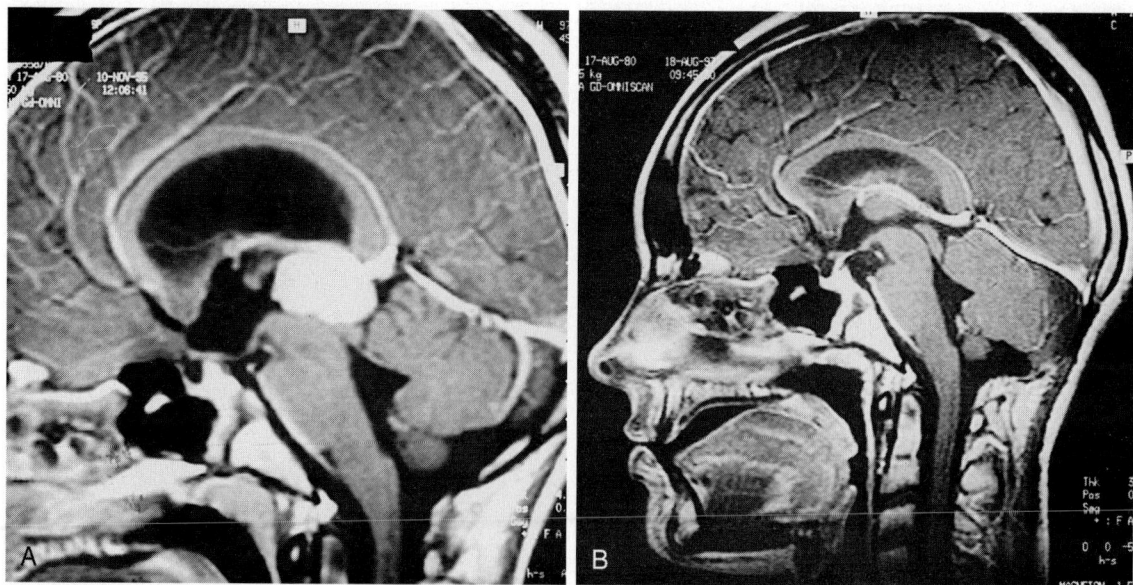

FIGURE 42–43 ■ *A,* Sagittal magnetic resonance image (MRI) of a pineal germinoma. *B,* Sagittal MRI of a pineal germinoma after an endoscopic biopsy and external radiotherapy.

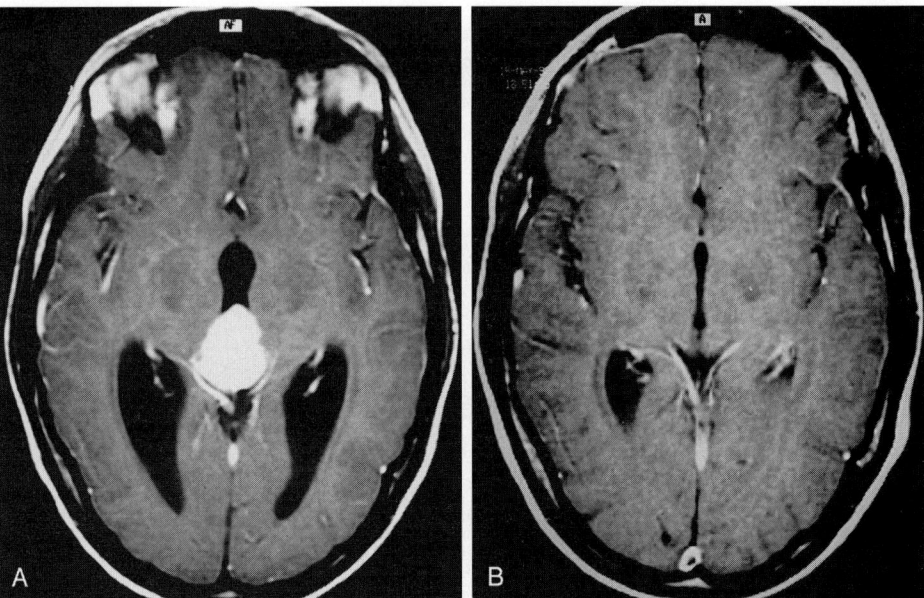

**FIGURE 42–44 ■** *A,* An axial magnetic resonance image (MRI) of a pineal germinoma preoperatively. *B,* An axial MRI of a pineal germinoma postoperatively.

confused patient. There was no motor or sensory neurologic deficit. She had tetrapyramidal symptoms. Blood examination showed electrolyte disturbances. MR showed a well-delineated oval craniopharyngioma in the suprasellar region. The first endoscopic intervention was limited to a biopsy and evacuation of the fluid motor-oil like component. After initial improvement of gait and memory disturbance, the symptomatology relapsed and the MR showed an increasing lesion in the suprasellar area that extended up to the third ventricle and caused hydrocephalus. A new endoscopic operation was performed with total macroscopical removal (Fig. 42–49 *A–F,* see color section). The immediate postoperative period was complicated by a severe electrolyte disturbance that subsided in 2 weeks. After this, the patient became confused; this was attributed to an aresorptive hydrocephalus. A ventriculoatrial shunt was

inserted after a CSF perfusion test showed decreased resorptive capacities. During the whole procedure continuous irrigation is necessary to wash out the motor oil–like substance that was intermingled with the semisolid contents, although the lesion was not really cystic. Part of the lesion could be aspirated after an initial coagulation of the capsula. She recovered and left the hospital with hormonal substitution. Control MR showed total macroscopic removal until she died 2 years later of bacterial pneumonia, which was not related to the initial pathology.

A second case was a 28-year-old man who had already been treated for his craniopharyngioma in the past 9 years after a stereotactic diagnostic and evacuative puncture of a cystic craniopharyngioma. He was treated by stereotactic $^{90}$Y instillation. About 1 year later, a partial resection of the solid tumor was performed. Four years later, a new

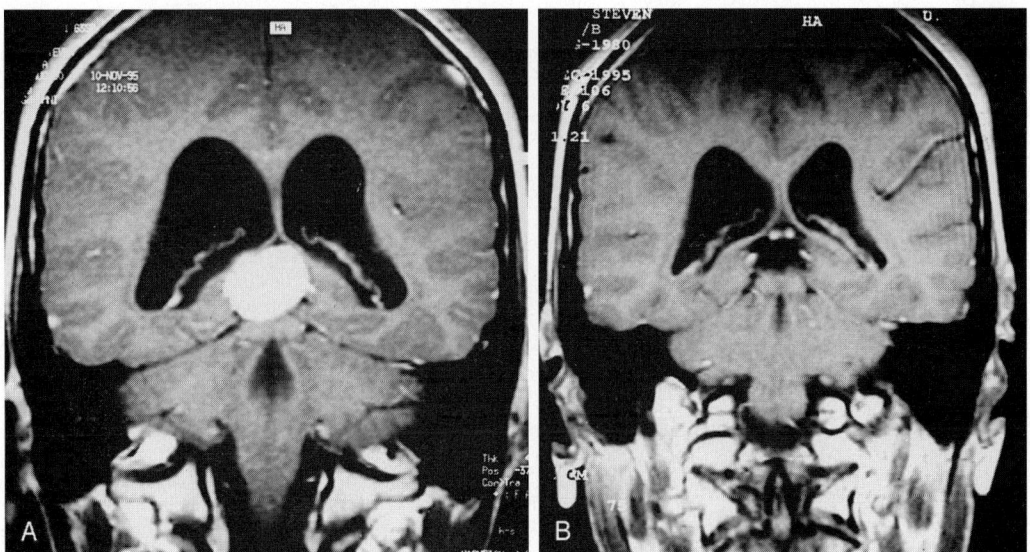

**FIGURE 42–45 ■** *A,* A frontal magnetic resonance image (MRI) of a pineal germinoma. *B,* A frontal MRI of a pineal germinoma after an endoscopic biopsy and external radiotherapy.

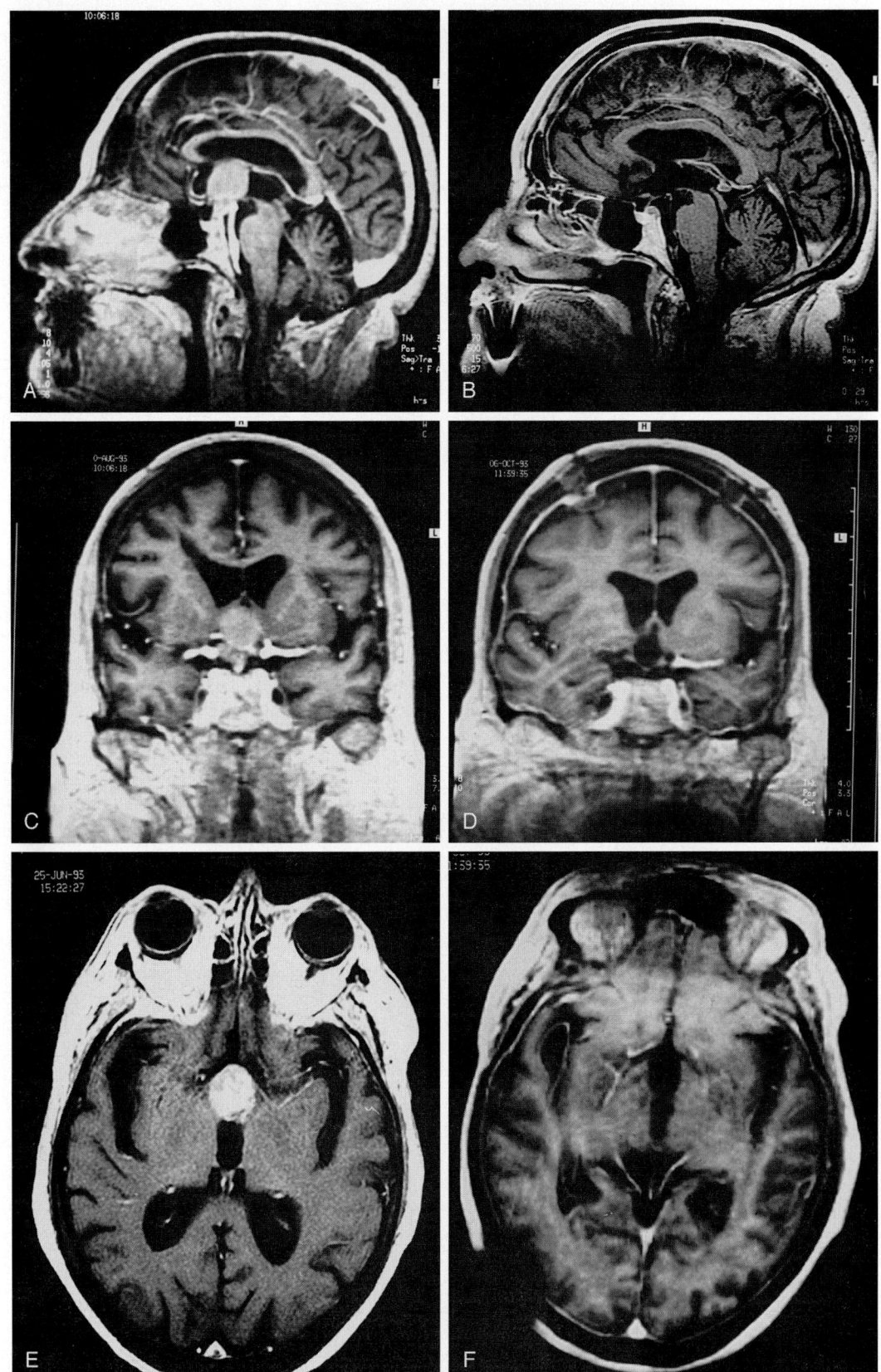

**FIGURE 42–48** ■ *A–F,* Pre- and postoperative sagittal frontal and axial magnetic resonance images of a craniopharyngioma that was removed endoscopically.

cyst was again treated by instillation of yttrium followed by evacuative puncture. Another 4 years later, worsening of the visual field, memory disturbance, and hormonal disturbance led to a control MR that showed a huge solid and cystic recurrence (Fig. 42–50A). Because former attempts at total removal did not succeed, we decided to remove the tumor endoscopically as far as possible. We opened the upper large cyst and removed the posterior half of the wall. The posterior half of the solid part was then removed. Finally, the lower cyst was dissected free from the basilar artery and largely opened, evacuated, and partially removed (see Fig. 42–50B). There was clear improvement postoperatively in the visual field and symptoms of raised intracranial pressure.

## ENDOSCOPIC PLACEMENT OF VENTRICULAR CATHETER

### Insertion

In the management of hydrocephalus with ventricular catheters, endoscopic techniques are sometimes useful.[113, 134, 150, 217] In most cases, one should be able to insert a ventricular catheter properly free-hand, guided by classical anatomic landmarks. In difficult cases, stereotactic guidance can be helpful. However, even the most experienced neurosurgeon is sometimes faced with malposition of a ventricular catheter. The most common cause of a shunt malfunction is obstruction of the proximal catheter by ingrowth of the choroid plexus. This can be avoided by using the so-called "mandrin endoscope" (Caemaert-Richard Wolf, Fig. 42–51). The instrument is 10 cm long and has a 1.1-mm outer diameter. This thin rigid endoscope is used as the mandrin of a ventricular catheter that is put in place during introduction. In the tip of the catheter, a small incision is made through which the mandrin endoscope protrudes

slightly. This permits visualization of the intraventricular structures and allows placement of the catheter at a distance from the choroid plexus. The mandrin is then retracted to connect the ventricular catheter to the shunt system.

Obstructed ventricular catheters are sometimes difficult to remove without tearing the ingrown choroid plexus. In these cases, denudation of the catheter can be performed through the endoscope under direct visual control using laser and scissors, until the catheter is completely free and can be removed.[227] One option would be to leave the catheter in place, but this is excluded in the case of shunt infections. A new catheter can be inserted immediately following removal of the first catheter under the same endoscopic control.

Catheters that are not obstructed, but are malpositioned, can be repositioned by grasping them with the grasping forceps. They can be pulled back and re-entered in the frontal horn of the lateral ventricles anterior to the foramen of Monro.

## ENDOSCOPIC MANAGEMENT OF INTRACRANIAL HEMORRHAGES

### Intracerebral Hematoma

Deep-seated intracerebral hematomas do not always require evacuation; however, if local compression or progressive symptomatology requires intervention and no underlying vascular malformation is demonstrated, one can consider the use of an endoscope for this purpose.[7] The shaft is introduced inside the hematoma. Starting from the center, the coagulated blood is evacuated by means of wide aspiration catheters, grasping forceps, and abundant irrigation. The blood clots may be very tough and adherent, but progressively they can be washed out. It is not necessary to evacuate the entire hematoma. It is sufficient to remove

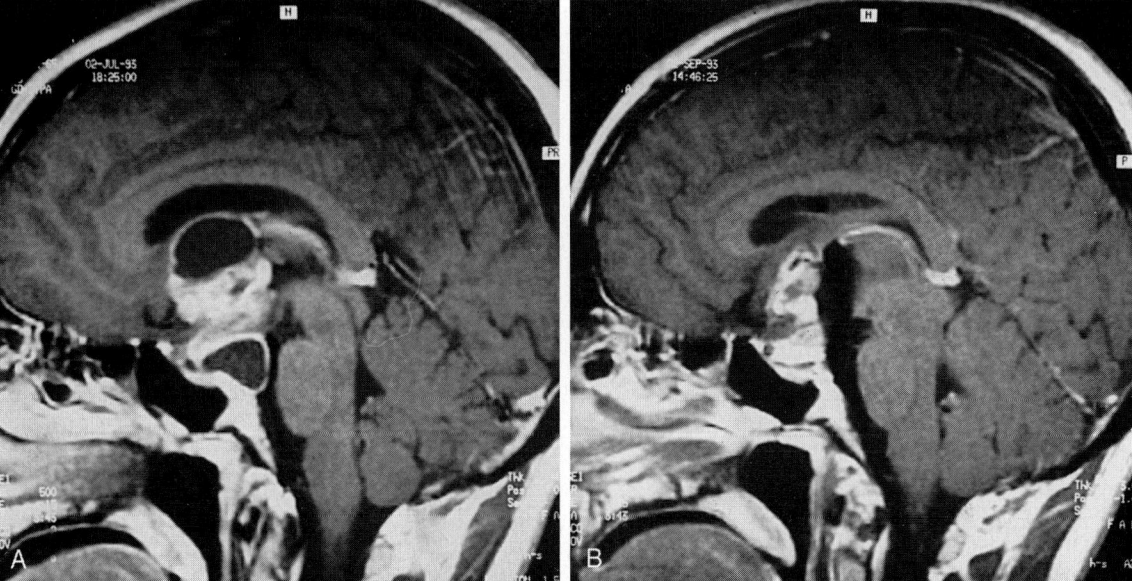

FIGURE 42–50 ■ A, Recurrent craniopharyngioma with two cysts and a solid part. B, Restoration of cerebrospinal fluid flow after partial endoscopic removal of a recurrent craniopharyngioma.

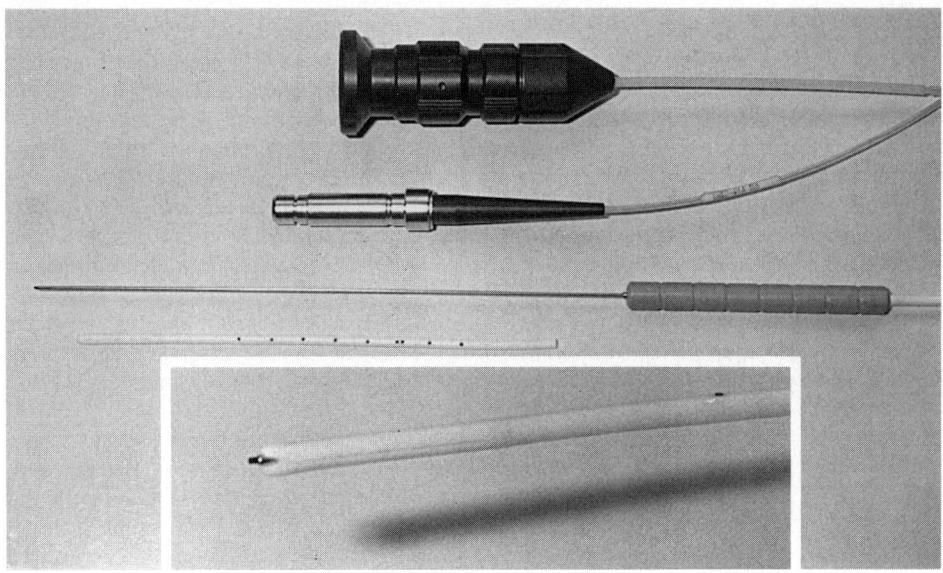

FIGURE 42–51 ■ A mandrin endoscope.

a critical volume for internal decompression rather than take the risk of preoperative rebleeding. With the current endoscopic instruments for hemostasis, intraoperative arterial bleeding can potentially produce some very serious problems.

## Traumatic Intracranial Hematoma

Acute subdural hematoma often requires a large decompressive craniotomy. The underlying contusion and edema are often the problem rather than the hematoma itself. An interhemispheric acute subdural hematoma is difficult to reach by classical trepanation. It can be removed through one single precoronal bur hole close to the midline. Insertion of the endoscope in the interhemispheric fissure permits the complete evacuation of such a hematoma (Fig. 42–52A–D). Some extradural hematomas can be evacuated endoscopically.[128]

## Septated Chronic Subdural Hematoma

Some chronic subdural hematomas are septated and consist of separate cavities so that irrigation and drainage cannot evacuate the whole hematoma. Insertion of a rigid or flexible endoscope permits one to wash out the liquified hematoma and to fenestrate the membranes that constitute the septa, thus creating a single chamber into which an external drain can be left in place to permit re-expansion of the brain.[100]

## Intraventricular Hematoma

In some acute and subacute intraventricular hemorrhages, it may be helpful to remove the blood through the ventriculoscope. Large organized clots can sometimes be extracted through the endoscopic trajectory by pulling out the whole endoscope that holds the blood clot against the lens with the grasping forceps. Reintroduction through the same trajectory offers no problems.

## SPINAL ENDOSCOPY[23, 27, 127, 131, 135, 186, 187, 210]

### Syringomyelia

Syringomyelia can present as a multiloculated form seen on MR as an intramedullary cyst interrupted by several septations (Fig. 42–53A, B). A small laminectomy is performed over the lowest extension of the syrinx. After opening of the dura, a small medullary incision is made at the thinnest part of the cyst; a flexible (2.5 mm) endoscope (Fig. 42–54) is introduced and slowly advanced upward. While rinsing, through the small irrigating channel, one can distinguish the septations that can be opened by blunt perforation with the tip of the endoscope. After all the cavities have been interconnected, the endoscope is retracted slowly and a small Silastic drain is inserted into the syrinx and sutured to the arachnoid membrane.[111, 112] The interconnected cysts collapse (see Fig. 42–53B).

### Epiduroscopy

Inspection of the epidural space by means of a thin flexible endoscope has been proposed as an adjunct to the adhesiolysis in cases of failed back surgery or for diagnostic purposes.

### Endoscopy in the Thoracic Spine

Endoscopic thoracic disk removal is possible with a collapsed lung at the side of the approach.[57, 114, 202, 211]

### Endoscopic Lumbar Diskectomy[92, 135, 143, 155, 233, 239]

Dedicated instruments have been designed by Yeung for endoscopic percutaneous lumbar diskectomy. The tech-

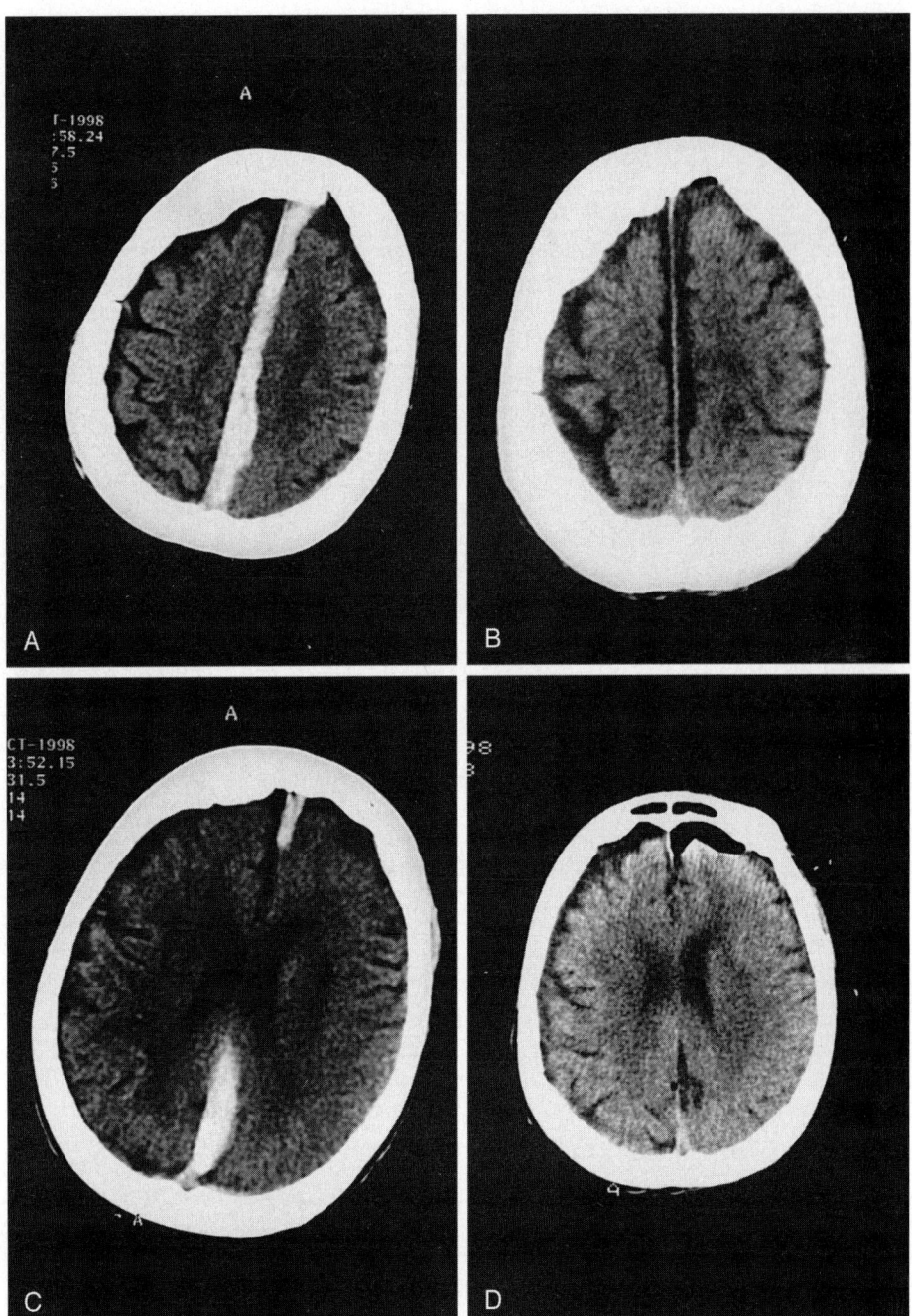

**FIGURE 42–52** ■ Traumatic interhemispheric acute subdural hematoma in a 72-year-old lady. *A*, Preoperative axial computed tomography (CT) high slice. *B*, Postoperative axial CT high slice. *C*, Preoperative axial CT low slice. *D*, Postoperative axial CT low slice.

nique has similarities with the percutaneous nucleotomy techniques and is used if the herniation is contiguous with the disk space without free fragments. Radiologic consideration in each individual patient will determine whether the disk space and the spinal canal are accessible. A multichannel 20-degree oval spinescope with a 2.7-mm working channel and integrated continuous irrigation allows maximum visual clarity and minimum bleeding. Inflow and outflow ports are connected to the scope tip and working channel. The 1-mm channel can also accommodate a laser fiber as an adjunct to the working channel. A lateral uniportal or biportal approach leads to the compressed nerve root, which is dissected free under direct visual control. Intradiskal fragmentectomy is possible. A 70-degree angu-

lated optic element permits working around the corner. Instruments for facetectomy and foraminotomy are available. The patient is mildly sedated, and an anesthesiologist is present during the procedure. Local medication is used generously so that only a minimal amount of sedation is required. Fluoroscopy is used during the entire procedure on an intermittent basis to ensure proper positioning of the instrument.

Another set of instruments has been designed by Knight for widening the lumbar exit route foramina using an endoscope-assisted laser technique. A uniportal posterolateral approach and a side-firing holmium laser probe are used. Under direct visual control, epidural scarring, extruded and sequestered disks, and osteophytes are removed

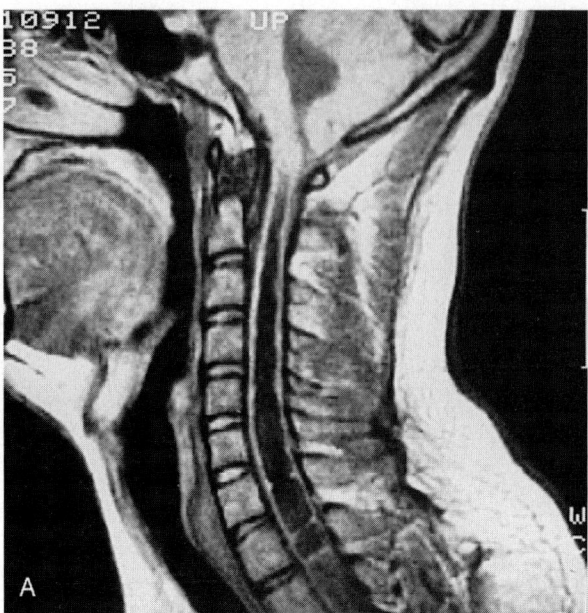

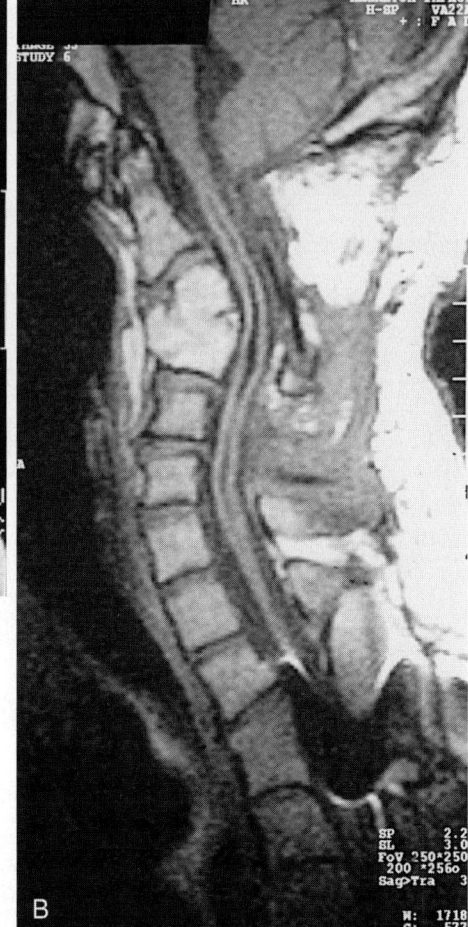

FIGURE 42–53 ■ A preoperative magnetic resonance image in septated syringomyelia.

by holmium laser ablation. The integrity of the nerve root can be monitored constantly. Satisfactory results are obtained in 72% of the primary treated group, 58% of a revision group after keyhole surgery, and 33% in revision after more extended surgery.

## MISCELLANEOUS

### Endoscopic Decompression of Carpal Tunnel

The endoscopic release of the median nerve entrapment in the carpal tunnel may be performed either as a single portal technique or as a two portal technique.[25, 35, 117, 119, 157, 198] The carpal tunnel is canalized by a slotted cannula that guides a hook knife that cuts the ligament under endoscopic control. The technique requires a tourniquet and a bloodless field. In the large series mentioned earlier, the degree of success is higher than 90%. (Note that the complication rate to date of endoscopic carpal tunnel release (ECTR) is at least as great as with the open procedure, and when it occurs there is greater functional severity.)

## ENDOSCOPY-ASSISTED MICROSURGERY

The use of an endoscope to enhance visual control during microsurgery differs from the use of an endoscope in a

ventriculoscopy. With the endoscope the light is brought down in the depth of small clefts where the illumination of the microscope is insufficient; the magnification factor is much higher because one can get much closer to the region of interest.[3, 42, 66, 132, 133, 136, 176, 177, 179, 180] It is possible to work around the corner by means of angulated lenses of 30 and 70 degrees in combination with the angle of view of 120 degrees. This permits the surgeon to inspect structures that cannot be seen through the microscope. Here the

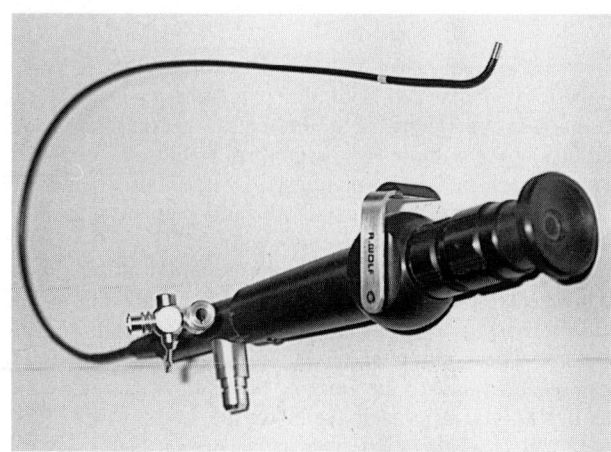

FIGURE 42–54 ■ A 2.5-mm flexible myeloscope.

endoscope functions as an optic element and not as a working instrument. The main pioneer of this technique is Perneczky.[180] His "keyhole" concept[179] and his use of angulated endoscopes add a new dimension to microsurgery. Small craniotomies give access to "windows" through which deep-seated structures can be reached.[66, 67, 179, 180] The anatomic knowledge for these approaches is magnificently illustrated in Perneczky's atlas.[178] Perneczky designed a thin bayonet-shaped endoscope with a curved end, which can be inserted into very small clefts and offers very good optical quality. It is amazing to see how the endoscopic images can enhance what is seen through the microscope. Contrary to the microscope, it is possible to introduce an endoscope from a different direction through a separate trajectory that can even be perpendicular to the viewing axis of the microscope. Alternating and simultaneous use of a microscope and an endoscope are also possible.[84] In the video monitor, a picture-in-picture setting is very useful, and projection of this double information in a head-mounted viewing system facilitates eye-hand coordination.[156, 218] For the introduction of the angulated lens scopes, microscope control is mandatory because they are progressing in a different direction than the viewing axis. This could be very dangerous for damage of structures lying anterior to the tip of the endoscope. Specific indications for endoscopy-assisted microsurgery follow.

## Aneurysm Surgery

Endoscopes with angulated lenses permit safer dissection of arterial aneurysms and inspection of the neck before clipping. This avoids entrapment of small branches or arterial loops.

## Endoscope-Assisted Microsurgery of the Sellar and Suprasellar Region

Small supraorbital craniotomies give access to the suprasellar region by one of the approaches proposed by Perneczky.[177, 178, 219] For some pathologies, it may be advisable to start the approach from the opposite side and cross the midline. Pituitary tumors, craniopharyngiomas, tuberculum sellae meningiomas, and optic gliomas are among the most common pathologies here. Correct positioning of the patient's head with some overextension causes spontaneous retraction of the frontal lobes to permit working in the subarachnoid spaces.

## Endoscope-Assisted Transsphenoidal Pituitary Surgery

The pioneers of this technique are Yaniv and Rappaport,[232] Jho,[115, 116] and Heilman and associates.[94] They described an approach through one nostril crossing the sphenoid sinus, opening the sellar floor, and working inside the sella turcica. This results in an atraumatic operation comparable with microsurgical transsphenoidal pituitary surgery.[34] The main advantage is the possibility of looking around the

corner with angulated lenses to inspect the lateral walls of the sella turcica and the medial walls of the cavernous sinuses. In this way, a residual tumor can be detected and removed with angulated instruments under visual control.

## ENDOSCOPY-ASSISTED MICROSURGERY OF THE CEREBELLOPONTINE ANGLE

Endoscopes may reduce the extent of the surgical approach for acoustic neuromas, microvascular decompression of cranial nerves V and VII and CPA epidermoid cysts.[132, 185, 191, 218] The main advantage of this technique in the cerebellopontine angle is the inspection of the internal auditory canal for remnants of tumor tissue in the depth of the canal during excision of a vestibular schwannoma.

## ACKNOWLEDGMENTS

*I wish to thank the following people: Mrs. Beatrijs Janssens, Mrs. Linda Van Langenhove, Mrs. Lea Van Gheluwe, Mrs. Antonine Colle, Mrs. Myriam François, and Mr. Peter Dierickx for their excellent help in the preparation of the text and the figures. Special thanks to Mr. Eric Vandevelde, who produced the black and white pictures, and to Mr. Roger Vanden Broecke, who provided invaluable help with the video documentation.*

## REFERENCES

1. Abdullah J, Caemaert J: Endoscopic management of craniopharyngiomas: A review of 3 cases. Minim Invas Neurosurg 38:79–84, 1995.
2. Ahn SS, Ro KM: Endoscopy of the sympathetic nervous system. In King WA, Frazee JG, De Salles AAF (eds): Endoscopy of the Central and Peripheral Nervous System. New York: Thieme 15:164–171, 1998.
3. Apuzzo MLJ, Heifetz MD, Weiss MH, Kurze T: Neurosurgical endoscopy using a side viewing telescope (Technical note). J Neurosurg 46:398–400, 1977.
4. Apuzzo MLJ, Chandrasoma PT, Zelman V, et al: Computed tomographic guidance stereotaxis in the management of lesions of the third ventricular region. Neurosurgery 15:502–508, 1984.
5. Apuzzo MLJ, Dobkin WR, Zee CS, et al: Surgical considerations in treatment of intraventricular cysticercosis: An analysis of 45 cases. J Neurosurg 60:400–407, 1984.
6. Auer LM, Holzer P, Ascher PW, Heppner F: Endoscopic neurosurgery. Acta Neurochir (Wien) 90:1–14, 1988.
7. Auer LM, Deinsberger W, Niederkorn K, et al: Endoscopic surgery versus medical treatment for spontaneous intracerebral hematoma: A randomized study. J Neurosurg 70:530–535, 1989.
8. Auer LM: Ultrasound stereotaxic endoscopy in neurosurgery. Acta Neurochir 54(Suppl):34–41, 1992.
9. Auer LM: Endoscopy of intraaxial lesions. In King WA, Frazee JG, De Salles AAF (eds): Endoscopy of the Central and Peripheral Nervous System. New York: Thieme, 1998, pp 91–119.
10. Auer LM, Auer DP: Virtual endoscopy for planning and simulation of minimally invasive neurosurgery. Neurosurgery 43:529–548, 1998.
11. Backlund EO: Studies on craniopharyngiomas: Stereotactic treatment with intracystic yttrium 90. Doctor thesis, Stockholm, Bröderna Lagerström Publishers and Acta Chir Scand 139:237–247, 1973.
12. Backlund EO, Axelsson B, Bergstrand CG, et al: Treatment of craniopharyngiomas: The stereotactic approach in a ten to twenty-three year perspective. Acta Neurochir 99:11–19, 1989.
13. Barlow P, Ching HS: An economic argument in favour of endoscopic

third ventriculostomy as a treatment for obstructive hydrocephalus. Minim Invas Neurosurg 40:37–39, 1997.

14. Bauer B, Hellwig D: Minimally invasive endoscopic neurosurgery—a survey. Acta Neurochir 61(Suppl):1–12, 1994.

15. Bauer BL, Hellwig D: Intracranial and intraspinal endoscopy. In Schmidek HH, Sweet WH: Operative Neurosurgical Techniques. Philadelphia: WB Saunders, 1995, pp 695–713.

16. Bauer BL, Hellwig F, Sweet WH, et al: The management of intracranial arachnoid, suprasellar and Rathke's cleft cysts. In Schmidek HH, Sweet WH: Operative Neurosurgical Techniques. Philadelphia: WB Saunders (in press).

17. Baysefer A, Erdogan E, Gezen F, et al: Cyst of the mesencephalon (neuroepithelial cyst?): Review and case report. Minim Invas Neurosurg 40: 148–150, 1997.

18. Baysefer A, Erdogan E, Gönül E, et al: Primary multiple cerebral hydatid cysts: Case report with CT and MRI study. Minim Invas Neurosurg 41:35–37, 1998.

19. Benabid AL, Lavallee S, Hoffman D, et al: Potential use of robots in endoscopic neurosurgery. Acta Neurochir 54(Suppl):93–97, 1992.

20. Bergsneider M, Frazee JG: Ventricular endoscopy. In De Salles AAF, Lufkin RB: Minimally Invasive Therapy of the Brain, Vol 20. New York: Thieme, 1997, pp 254–267.

21. Bergsneider M: Transendoscopic instrumentation and techniques. In King WA, Frazee JG, De Salles AAF: Endoscopy of the Central and Peripheral Nervous System, Vol 3. New York: Thieme, 1998, pp 16–22.

22. Birkett DH: Three-dimensional endoscopy. In King WA, Frazee JG, De Salles AAF: Endoscopy of the Central and Peripheral Nervous System, Vol 19. New York: Thieme, 1998, pp 232–236.

23. Blomberg RG: Epiduroscopy and spinaloscopy: Endoscopic studies of lumbar spinal spaces. Acta Neurochir 61(Suppl):106–107, 1994.

24. Bosch DA, Rähn T, Backlund EO: Treatment of the contents of the third ventricle by stereotactic aspiration. Surg Neurol 9:15–18, 1978.

25. Brown RA, Gelberman RH, Seiler JG III, et al: Carpal tunnel release: A prospective, randomized assessment of open and endoscopic methods. J Bone Joint Surg 75A:1265–1275, 1993.

26. Buchholz RD, Pittman MD: Endoscopic coagulation of the choroid plexus using the Nd:Yag laser: Initial experience and proposal for management. Neurosurgery 28:421–427, 1991.

27. Burman MD: Myeloscopy or the direct visualization of the spinal canal and its contents. J Bone Joint Surg 13:695, 1931.

28. Caemaert J, Calliauw L: Surgical techniques in the management of colloid cysts of the third ventricle: A note on the use of a modern endoscope. Adv Tech Stand Neurosurg 17:149–153, 1990.

29. Caemaert J, Abdullah J, Calliauw L, et al: Endoscopic treatment of suprasellar arachnoid cysts. Acta Neurochir (Wien) 119:68–73, 1992.

30. Caemaert J, Abdullah J, Calliauw L: A multipurpose cerebral endoscope and reflections on techniques and instrumentation in endoscopic neurosurgery. Acta Neurochir (Wien) 61(Suppl):49–53, 1994.

31. Caemaert J, Abdullah J, Calliauw L: Endoscopic diagnosis and treatment of para- and intra-ventricular cystic lesions. Acta Neurochir 61(Suppl):69–75, 1994.

32. Caemaert J, Abdullah J: Endoscopic management of colloid cysts. Tech Neurosurg 1:185–200, 1995.

33. Camacho A, Kelly PJ: Volumetric stereotactic resection of superficial and deep-seated intra-axial brain lesions. Acta Neurochir 54(Suppl):83–88, 1992.

34. Cappabianca P, Alfieri A, de Divitis E: Endoscopic endonasal transsphenoidal approach to the sella: Toward functional endoscopic pituitary surgery (FEPS). Minim Invas Neurosurg 41:66–73, 1998.

35. Chow JCY: Endoscopic release of the carpal ligament: A new technique for carpal tunnel syndrome. Arthroscopy 5:19–24, 1989.

36. Clark WC, Woodall W, Nicoll JA, Coakham HB: Intracerebral epithelial cyst: Immunohistological diagnosis and endoneurosurgical treatment. Br J Neurosurg 3:507–512, 1989.

37. Cohen AR: The history of neuroendoscopy. In Manwaring KH, Crone KR (eds): Neuroendoscopy, Vol 1. New York: Mary Ann Liebert, 1992, pp 3–8.

38. Cohen AR: Ventriculoscopic management of colloid cysts of the third ventricle. In Manwaring KH, Crone KR (eds): Neuroendoscopy, Vol 1. New York: Mary Ann Liebert, 1992, pp 109–118.

39. Cohen AR: Endoscopic ventricular surgery. Pediatr Neurosurg 19:127–134, 1993.

40. Cohen AR: Endoscopic laser third ventriculostomy. N Engl J Med 328:552, 1993.

41. Cohen AR: Ventriculoscopic surgery. In Loftus CM (ed): Clinical Neurosurgery. Baltimore: Williams & Wilkins, 41, 1993, pp 546–562.

42. Cohen AR, Perneczky A, Rodziewics GS, Gingold SI: Endoscope-assisted craniotomy: Approach to the rostral brain stem. Neurosurgery 36:1128–1130, 1995.

43. Cohen AR: Endoscopic ventricular anatomy. In Cohen AR, Haines SJ (eds): Minimally Invasive Techniques in Neurosurgery: Concepts in Neurosurgery. Baltimore: Williams & Wilkins 7:14–24, 1995.

44. Cohen AR: Endoscopic neurosurgery. In Wilkins R, Rengachary SS (eds): Neurosurgery, Vol 51, 2nd ed. New York: McGraw-Hill, 1996, pp 539–546.

45. Couldwell WT, Apuzzo MLJ: Management of cysticercosis cerebri. Contemp Neurosurg 19:1–6, 1989.

46. Crone KR: Endoscopic technique for removal of adherent ventricular catheters. In Manwaring KH, Crone KR (eds): Neuroendoscopy, Vol 1. New York: Mary Ann Liebert, 1992, pp 41–46.

47. Crone KR, Miller MN: Colloid cysts: Endoscopy vs. microneurosurgical treatment. In King WA, Frazee JG, De Salles AAF: Endoscopy of the Central and Peripheral Nervous System, Vol 8. New York: Thieme, 1998, pp 78–83.

48. Crue BL: Needle scope attached to stereotactic frame for inspection of cisterna magna during radiofrequency trigeminal tractotomy. Appl Neurophysiol 39:58–64, 1977.

49. Dalrymple SJ, Kelly PJ: Computer-assisted stereotactic third ventriculostomy in the management of noncommunicating hydrocephalus. Stereotact Funct Neurosurg 59:105–110, 1992.

50. Dandy WE: Cerebral ventriculoscopy. Johns Hopkins Hosp Bull 33:189–190, 1922.

51. Dandy WE: The Brain. New York: Harper & Row, 1969, p 241.

52. Davis L: Neurological Surgery. Philadelphia: Lea & Febiger, 1939, p 405.

53. Decq P, Brugières P, Le Guerinel C, et al: Percutaneous endoscopic treatment of suprasellar arachnoid cysts: Ventriculocystostomy or ventriculocystocisternostomy (Technical note). J Neurosurg 84:696–701, 1996.

54. Decq P, Le Guerinel C, Brugières P, et al: Endoscopic management of colloid cysts. Neurosurgery 42:1288–1296, 1998.

55. Deinsberger W, Böker DK, Bothe HW, et al: Stereotactic endoscopic treatment of colloid cysts of the third ventricle. Acta Neurochir 131:260–264, 1994.

56. Deinsberger W, Böker DK, Samii M: Flexible endoscopes in treatment of colloid cysts of the third ventricle. Minim Invas Neurosurg 37:12–16, 1994.

57. Dickman CA: Endoscopy for thoracic spine disease. In King WA, Frazee JG, De Salles AAF: Endoscopy of the Central and Peripheral Nervous System, Vol 16. New York: Thieme, 1998, pp 172–197.

58. Dorward NL, Alberti O, Zhao J, et al: Interactive image-guided neuroendoscopy: Development and early clinical experience. Minim Invas Neurosurg 41:31–34, 1998.

59. Drake JM: Neuroendoscopy tumor biopsy. In Manwaring KH, Crone KR (eds): Neuroendoscopy, Vol 1. New York: Mary Ann Liebert, 1992, pp 103–108.

60. Farouk A, Abdullah J: Endoscopic neurosurgery: Report of the first five cases done in Malaysia using the Caemaert-Abdullah method. Minim Invas Neurosurg 41:74–78, 1998.

61. Fay T, Grant FC: Ventriculoscopy and intraventricular photography in internal hydrocephalus. JAMA 80:461–463, 1923.

62. Ferrer E, et al: Neuroendoscope management of pineal region tumours. Acta Neurochir (Wien) 139:12–21, 1997.

63. Forjaz S, Martelli N, Latuf N: Hypothalamic ventriculostomy with catheter (Technical note). J Neurosurg 29:655–659, 1968.

64. Frank EH, Ragel BR: A malleable endoscopic instrument (Technical note). Minim Invas Neurosurg 41:79–80, 1998.

65. Frazee JG, Shah AS: Interactive surgery and telepresence. In King WA, Frazee JG, De Salles AAF: Endoscopy of the Central and Peripheral Nervous System, Vol 21. New York: Thieme, 1998, pp 243–251.

66. Fries G, Reisch R: Biportal neuroendoscopic microsurgical approaches to the subarachnoid cisterns: A cadaver study. Minim Invas Neurosurg 39:99–104, 1996.

67. Fries G, Perneczky A: Endoscope-assisted brain surgery. II: Analysis of 380 procedures. Neurosurgery 42:226–232, 1998.

68. Fukushima T, Ishijima B, Hirakawa K, et al: Ventriculofiberscope: A new technique for endoscopic diagnosis and operation. J Neurosurg 38:251–256, 1973.

69. Fukushima T, Schramm J: Klinischer Versuch der Endoskopie des Spinalkanals: Kurzmitteilung. Neurochirurgia 18:199–203, 1975.

70. Fukushima T: Endoscopic biopsy of intraventricular tumors with the use of a ventriculofiberscope. Neurosurgery 2:110–113, 1978.

71. Fukushima T: Endoscopy of Meckel's cave, cisterna magna, and cerebellopontine angle. J Neurosurg 48:302–306, 1978.

72. Fukushima T: Flexible endoneurosurgical therapy for aqueductal stenosis (Letter). Neurosurgery 34:379, 1994.

73. Gaab MR: A universal neuroendoscope: Development, clinical experience, and perspectives (Abstract). Childs Nerv Syst 10:481, 1994.

74. Gaab MR, Schroeder HWS: Arachnoid cysts. In King WA, Frazee JG, De Salles AAF: Endoscopy of the Central and Peripheral Nervous System, Vol 12. New York: Thieme, 1998, pp 137–147.

75. Gaab MR, Schroeder HWS: Endoscopy for intraventricular lesion. In King WA, Frazee JG, De Salles AAF: Endoscopy of the Central and Peripheral Nervous System, Vol 7. New York: Thieme, 1998, pp 68–77.

76. Gaab MR, Schroeder HWS: Neuroendoscopic approach to intraventricular lesions. J Neurosurg 88:496–505, 1998.

77. Ghatak NR, Kasoff I, Alexander E: Further observation on the fine structure of a colloid cyst of the third ventricle. Acta Neuropathol 39:101–107, 1977.

78. Griffith HB: Technique of fontanelle and persutural ventriculoscopy and endoscopic ventricular surgery in infants. Child's Brain 1:359–363, 1975.

79. Griffith HB: Endoneurosurgery: Endoscopic intracranial surgery. Adv Tech Stand Neurosurg 14:2–24, 1986.

80. Griffith HB, Jamjoom AB: The treatment of childhood hydrocephalus by choroid plexus coagulation and artificial cerebrospinal fluid perfusion. Br J Neurosurg 4:95–100, 1990.

81. Griffith HB: Endoscopic choroid plexus coagulation and cerebrospinal fluid perfusion in the treatment of infantile hydrocephalus. In Manwaring KH, Crone KR (eds): Neuroendoscopy, Vol 1. New York: Mary Ann Liebert, 1992, pp 91–96.

82. Grotenhuis JA, Tacl S: The use of flexible micro-endoscopes for visualization of blind corners during microneurosurgical procedures. Abstractbook 1st International Congress on Minimal Invasive Techniques in Neurosurgery, Wiesbanden, 16, 1993.

83. Grotenhuis JA, de Vries J, Tacl S: Angioscopy-guided placement of balloon-expandable stents in the treatment of experimental carotid aneurysms. Minim Invas Neurosurg 37:56–60, 1994.

84. Grotenhuis JA: Endoscope-assisted craniotomy. Tech Neurosurg 3:201–212, 1995.

85. Grotenhuis JA: Manual of Endoscopic Procedures in Neurosurgery. Nijmegen, The Netherlands: Machaon, 1995.

86. Grunert P, Perneczky A, Resch K: Endoscopic procedures through the foramen intraventriculare of Monro under stereotactical conditions. Minim Invas Neurosurg 37:2–8, 1994.

87. Guiot G: Ventriculocisternostomy for stenosis of the aqueduct of Sylvius. Acta Neurochir (Wien) 28:275–289, 1973.

88. Gutierrez-Lara F, Patino R, Hakim S: Treatment of tumors of the third ventricle: A new and simple technique. Surg Neurol 3:323–325, 1975.

89. Hall WA, Lunsford LD: Changing concepts in the treatment of colloid cysts: An 11-year experience in the CT era. J Neurosurg 66:186–191, 1987.

90. Hara M, Nakamura M, Shiokawa Y, et al: Delayed cyst formation after radiosurgery for cerebral arteriovenous malformation: Two case reports. Minim Invas Neurosurg 41:40–45, 1998.

91. Heikkinen ER: Stereotactic neurosurgery: New aspects of an old method. Ann Clin Res Suppl 47:73–83, 1986.

92. Heikkinen ER: "Whole body" stereotaxy: Application of stereotactic endoscopy to operations of herniated lumbar discs. Acta Neurochir Suppl 54:89–92, 1992.

93. Heilman CB, Cohen AR: Endoscopic ventricular fenestration using a "saline torch." J Neurosurg 74:224–229, 1991.

94. Heilman CB, Shucart WA, Rebeiz EE: Endoscopic sphenoidotomy approach to the sella. Neurosurgery 41:602–607, 1997.

95. Hellwig D, Bauer BL, List-Hellwig E, et al: Stereotactic endoscopic procedures on processes of the cranial midline. Acta Neurochir Suppl 53:23–32, 1991.

96. Hellwig D, Bauer BL: Minimally invasive neurosurgery by means of ultrathin endoscopes. Acta Neurochir 54(Suppl):63–68, 1992.

97. Hellwig D, Bauer BL, Dauch WA: Endoscopic stereotactic treatment of brain abscesses. Acta Neurochir 61(Suppl):102–105, 1994.

98. Hellwig D, Bauer BL, List-Hellwig E: Stereotactic endoscopic interventions in cystic brain lesions. Acta Neurochir 64(Suppl):59–63, 1995.

99. Hellwig D, Riegel T, Bauer BL, et al: Endoneurosurgery of skull base processes: The frontal transventricular approach. In Samii M (ed): Skull base surgery. Basel: Karger, (in press).

100. Hellwig D, Thomas JK, Bauer BL, List-Hellwig E: Endoscopic treatment of septated chronic subdural hematoma. Surg Neurol 45:272–275, 1996.

101. Hellwig D, et al: Application of new electrosurgical devices and probes in endoscopic Neurosurgery. Neurol Res 21:67–72, 1999.

102. Hellwig D, Riegel T, Sure U, et al: First application of a flexible, steerable 3D-endoscope for surgical interventions. 49th Annual meeting of the German Society of Neurosurgery (Johann Ambrosius Barth) 144, 1998.

103. Hellwig D: Neuroendoscopy of the spinal canal historical review, indications and results. Zentralbl Neurochir 49. Jahrestagung der Deutschen Gesellschaft für Neurochirurgie—49th Annual meeting of the German Society of Neurosurgery (Johann Ambrosius Barth): 74, 1998.

104. Hirsch JF: Percutaneous ventriculocisternostomies in noncommunicating hydrocephalus. Monogr Neural Sci 8:170–178, 1982.

105. Hoffmann HJ, Hendrick EB, Humphreys RP, et al: Investigation and management of suprasellar arachnoid cysts. J Neurosurg 57:597–602, 1982.

106. Hopf NJ, Resch KDM, Ringel K, Perneczky A: Endoscopic management of intracranial arachnoid cysts. In Hellwig D, Bauer BL (eds): Minimally Invasive Techniques for Neurosurgery. Berlin: Springer-Verlag, 1998, pp 111–119.

107. Hopf NJ, Perneczky A: Endoscopic neurosurgery and endoscope-assisted microneurosurgery for the treatment of intracranial cysts. Neurosurgery 43:1330–1336, 1998.

108. Hopf NJ: Endoscopic neurosurgery around the corner with a rigid endoscope (Technical note). Minim Invas Neurosurg 42:27–37, 1999.

109. Hopf NJ, Busert C, Darabi K, et al: Neuronavigation and stereotaxy applied to endoscopic neurosurgery. Zentralblatt für Neurochirurgie, 49. Jahrestagung der Deutschen Gesellschaft für Neurochirurgie—49th Annual meeting of the German Society of Neurosurgery (Johann Ambrosius Barth): 144, 1998.

110. Hor F, Desgeorges M, Rosseau GL: Tumour resection by stereotactic laser endoscopy. Acta Neurochir 54(Suppl):77–82, 1992.

111. Hüwel N, Perneczky A, Urban V, Fries G: Neuroendoscopic technique for the operative treatment of septated syringomyelia. Acta Neurochir 54(Suppl):59–62, 1992.

112. Hüwel N, Perneczky A, Urban V: Neuro-endoscopic techniques in operative treatment of syringomyelia. Acta Neurochir 123:216, 1993.

113. Jamal MT, Kerry RC: Endoscopically guided shunt placement. Tech Neurosurg 3:159–167, 1995.

114. Jho HD: Endoscopic microscopic transpedicular thoracic discectomy (Technical note). J Neurosurg 87:125–129, 1997.

115. Jho HD, Carrau RL: Endoscopic endonasal transsphenoidal surgery: Experience with 50 patients. J Neurosurg 87:44–51, 1997.

116. Jho HD, Carrau RL, Ko Y, Daly MA: Endoscopic pituitary surgery: An early experience. Surg Neurol 47:213–223, 1997.

117. Jimenez DF: Endoscopy for carpal tunnel decompression. In King WA, Frazee JG, De Salles AAF: Endoscopy of the Central and Peripheral Nervous System, Vol 18. New York: Thieme, 1998, pp 215–231.

118. Jimenez DF, Barone CM: Endoscopic craniectomy for early surgical correction of sagittal craniosynostosis. J Neurosurg 88:77–81, 1998.

119. Jimenez DF, Gibbs S, Clapper AT: Endoscopic treatment of carpal tunnel syndrome: A critical review. J Neurosurg 88:817–826, 1998.

120. Jones RFC, Stening WA, Brydon M: Endoscopic third ventriculostomy. Neurosurgery 26:86–92, 1990.

121. Jones RFC, Teo C, Stening WA, Kwok BCT: Neuroendoscopic third ventriculostomy. In Manwaring KH, Crone KR (eds): Neuroendoscopy 1. New York: Mary Ann Liebert, 1992, pp 63–77.

122. Jones RFC, Stening WAS, Kwok BCT, Sands TM: Third ventriculostomy for shunt infections in children. Neurosurgery 32:855–860, 1993.

123. Jones RFC, Tep C, Currie B, et al: The antisiphon device—its value in preventing excessive drainage. In Matsumoto S, Tamaki N (eds): Hydrocephalus: Pathogenesis and Management. Berlin: Springer-Verlag, 1991, pp 383–390.

124. Jones RFC, Kwok BCT, Stening WA, Vonau M: The current status of endoscopic third ventriculostomy in the management of non-communicating hydrocephalus. Minim Invas Neurosurg 37:28–36, 1994.

125. Jones RFC, Kwok BCT, Stening WA, Vonau M: Neuroendoscopic third ventriculostomy: A practical alternative to extracranial shunts in non-communicating hydrocephalus. Acta Neurochir 61 (Suppl):79–83, 1994.

126. Karakhan VB: Endofiberscopic intracranial stereotopography and endofiberscopic neurosurgery. Acta Neurochir 54(Suppl):11–25, 1992.

127. Karakhan VB, Filimonov BA, Grigoryan YA, Mitropolsky VB: Operative spinal endoscopy: Stereotopography and surgical possibilities. Acta Neurochir Suppl 61:108–114, 1994.

128. Karakhan VB, Khodnevich AA: Endoscopic surgery of traumatic intracranial haemorrhages. Acta Neurochir 61(Suppl):84–91, 1994.

129. Kehler U, Gliemroth J, Arnold H: Asymmetric hydrocephalus: Safe endoscopic perforation of septum pellucidum (Technical note). Minim Invas Neurosurg 40:101–102, 1997.

130. Kelly PJ: Stereotactic third ventriculostomy in patients with non-tumoral adolescent/adult onset aqueductal stenosis and symptomatic hydrocephalus. J Neurosurg 75:873–875, 1991.

131. Kessel G, Böcher-Schwarz HG, Ringel K, Perneczky A: The role of endoscopy in the treatment of acute traumatic anterior epidural hematoma of the cervical spine: Case report. Neurosurgery 41:688–690, 1997.

132. Khodnevich AA, Karakhan VB: New kinds of microneuroprotectors for microsurgery and endoscopy of cerebellopontine angle neurovascular decompression. Acta Neurochir 61(Suppl):40–42, 1994.

133. King WA: Endoscopy of the cranial base. In De Salles AAF, Lufkin RB: Minimally Invasive Therapy of the Brain, Vol 21. New York: Thieme, 1997, pp 268–273.

134. Kleinhaus S, Germann R, Sheran M, et al: A role for endoscopy in the placement of ventriculoperitoneal shunts. Surg Neurol 18:179–180, 1982.

135. Knight MTN, Vajda A, Jakab GV, Awan S: Endoscopic laser foraminoplasty on the lumbar spine—early experience. Minim Invas Neurosurg 41:5–9, 1998.

136. Knosp E, Perneczky A, Koos WT, et al: Meningiomas of the space of the cavernous sinus. Neurosurgery 38:434–444, 1996.

137. Kondziolka D, Lunsford LD: Stereotactic management of colloid cysts: Factors predicting success. J Neurosurg 75:45–51, 1991.

138. Kondziolka D, Lunsford LD: Stereotactic techniques for colloid cysts: Roles of aspiration, endoscopy and microsurgery. Acta Neurochir 61(Suppl):76–78, 1994.

139. Kunz U, Goldman A, Bader CL, et al: Endoscopic fenestration of the 3rd ventricular floor in aqueductal stenosis. Minim Invas Neurosurg 37:42–47, 1994.

140. Lapras C, Bret P, Patet JD, et al: Hydrocephalus and aqueductal stenosis: Direct surgical treatment by interventriculostomy (aqueductal cannulation). J Neurosurg Sci 8:321–325, 1981.

141. Lawton MT, Heiserman JE, Coons SW, et al: Juvenile active ossifying fibroma: Report of four cases. J Neurosurg 86:279–285, 1997.

142. L'Espinasse VL: In Davis L (ed): Neurological Surgery, 2nd ed. Philadelphia: Lea & Febiger, 1943, p 442.

143. Levy ML, Day JD, Albuquerque F, et al: Heads-up intraoperative endoscopic imaging: A prospective evaluation of techniques and limitations. Neurosurgery 40:526–531, 1997.

144. Levy ML, Lavine SD, Mendel E, et al: The endoscopic stylet: Technical notes. Neurosurgery 35:335–336, 1994.

145. Lewis AI, Crone KR, Taha J, et al: Surgical resection of third ventricle colloid cysts: Preliminary results comparing transcallosal microsurgery with endoscopy. J Neurosurg 81:174–178, 1994.

146. Lewis AI, Crone KR: Advances in neuroendoscopy. Contemp Neurosurg 16:1–6, 1994.

147. Lewis AI, Keiper GL, Crone KR: Endoscopic treatment of loculated hydrocephalus. J Neurosurg 82:780–785, 1995.

148. Lewis AI, Larson JJ, Crone KR: Endoscopic treatment of complex hydrocephalus. Tech Neurosurg 1:168–175, 1995.

149. Manwaring KH, Rekate H, Klaplan A: Hydrocephalus management by endoscopy. Ann Neurol 26:488, 1989.

150. Manwaring KH: Endoscope-guided placement of the ventriculoperitoneal shunt. In Manwaring K, Crone KR (eds): Neuroendoscopy 1. New York: Mary Ann Liebert, 1992, pp 29–40.

151. Manwaring KH: Endoscopic ventricular fenestration. In Manwaring K, Crone KR (eds): Neuroendoscopy 1. New York, Mary Ann Liebert, 1992, pp 79–89.

152. Manwaring KH, Manwaring ML, Moss SD: Magnetic field guided endoscopic dissection through a burr hole may avoid more invasive craniotomies. Acta Neurochir 61(Suppl):34–39, 1994.

153. Mathiesen T, Grane P, Lindquist C, et al: High recurrence rate following aspiration of colloid cysts in the third ventricle. J Neurosurg 78:748–752, 1993.

154. Mathiesen T, Grane P, Lindgren L, Lindquist C: Third ventricle colloid cysts: A consecutive 12-year series. J Neurosurg 86:5–12, 1997.

155. Mayer HM, Brock M, Berlien H-P, Weber B: Percutaneous endoscopic laser diskectomie (PELD): A new surgical technique for non-sequestrated lumbar discs. Acta Neurochir Suppl 54:53–58, 1992.

156. McGregor JM: Enhancing neurosurgical endoscopy with the use of "virtual reality" headgear. Minim Invas Neurosurg 40:47–49, 1997.

157. Menon J: Endoscopic carpal tunnel release: Preliminary report. J Arthrosc Related Surg 10:31–38, 1994.

158. Miller MN: Organization of the neuroendoscopy suite. In Manwaring KH, Crone KR (eds): Neuroendoscopy, Vol 1. New York: Mary Ann Liebert, 1992, pp 9–16.

159. Mixter WJ: Ventriculoscopy and puncture of the floor of the third ventricle. Boston Med Surg J 188:277–278, 1923.

160. Mohadjer M, Teshmar E, Mundinger F: CT stereotaxic drainage of colloid cysts in the foramen of Monro and the third ventricle. J Neurosurg 67:220–223, 1987.

161. Mohanty A, Anandh B, Reddy MS, Sastry KVR: Contralateral massive acute subdural collection after endoscopic third ventriculostomy: A case report. Minim Invas Neurosurg 40:59–61, 1997.

162. Natelson SE: Early third ventriculostomy in meningomyelocele infants—shunt independence? Childs Brain 8:321–325, 1981.

163. Neal JH: An endoscopic approach to cysticercosis cysts of the posterior third ventricle. Neurosurgery 36:1040–1043, 1995.

164. Neugebauer E, Ure BM, Lefering R, et al: Technology assessment of endoscopic surgery. Acta Neurochir 61(Suppl):13–19, 1994.

165. Nida TY, Haines SJ: Multiloculated hydrocephalus: Craniotomy and fenestration of intraventricular septations. J Neurosurg 78:70–76, 1993.

166. Nitta M, Symon L: Colloid cysts of the third ventricle: A review of 36 cases. Acta Neurochir 76:99–104, 1985.

167. Oka K, Tomonaga M: Instruments for flexible endoneurosurgery. In Manwaring KH, Crone KR (eds): Neuroendoscopy, Vol 1. New York: Mary Ann Liebert, 1992, pp 17–28.

168. Oka K, Go Y, Kin Y, et al: The radiographic restoration of the ventricular system after third ventriculostomy. Minim Invas Neurosurg 38:158–162, 1995.

169. Oka K, Tomonaga M: Instrumentation: Tech Neurosurg 1:151–158, 1995.

170. Okutsu I, Ninomiya S, Takatori Y, et al: Results of endoscopic management of carpal tunnel syndrome. Orthop Rev 22:81–87, 1993.

171. Olinger CP, Ohlhaber RL: Eighteen-gauge microscopic-telescopic needle endoscope with electrode channel: Potential clinical and research application. Surg Neurol 2:151–160, 1974.

172. Otsuki T, Jokura H, Nakasoto N, Yoshimoto T: Stereotactic endoscopic resection of angiographically occult vascular malformations. Acta Neurochir Suppl 61:98–101, 1994.

173. Paladino J, Rotim K, Heinrich Z: Neuroendoscopic fenestration of arachnoid cysts. Minim Invas Neurosurg 41:137–140, 1998.

174. Parsch CS, Kraub J, Hofman E, et al: Arachnoid cysts associated with subdural hematomas and hygromas: Analysis of 16 cases, long-term follow-up, and review of the literature. Neurosurgery 40:483–490, 1997.

175. Patterson RHJ, Bergland RM: The selection of patients for third ventriculostomy based on experience with 33 operations. J Neurosurg 29:252–254, 1968.

176. Perneczky A, Knosp E, Matula C: Cavernous sinus surgery: Approach through the lateral wall. Acta Neurochir 92:76–82, 1988.

177. Perneczky A: Planning strategies for the suprasellar region: Philosophy of approaches. Proc Jpn Congress Neurol Surgeons 11:343–348, 1992.

178. Perneczky A, Tschabitscher M, Resch KDM: Endoscopic Anatomy for Neurosurgery. Stuttgart: Thieme, 1993.

179. Perneczky A, Müller-Forell W, van Lindert E: Keyhole Concept in Neurosurgery with Endoscope-Assisted Microsurgery: 25 Case Studies. Stuttgart: Thieme, 1998.

180. Perneczky A, Fries G: Endoscope-assisted brain surgery. I: Evolution, basic concept, and current technique. Neurosurgery 42:219–225, 1998.

181. Piek J, Wille C, Warzok R, Gaab MR: Waterjet dissection of the brain: Experimental and first clinical results (Technical note). J Neurosurg 89:861–864, 1998.

182. Pierre-Kahn A, Capelle L, Brauner R, et al: Presentation and management of suprasellar arachnoid cyst: Review of 20 cases. J Neurosurg 73:355–359, 1990.

183. Pierre-Kahn A, Renier D, Bombois B, et al: Place de la ventriculocisternostomie dans le traitement des hydrocephalies non communicantes. Neurochirurgie 12:557–569, 1975.

184. Pittmann T, Bucholz RD: Endoscopic choroid plexectomy. In Manwaring KH, Crone KR (eds): Neuroendoscopy, Vol 1. New York: Mary Ann Liebert, 1992.

185. Poe DS, Heilman CB, Youssef TF: Neurootologic endoscopy. In King WA, Frazee JG, De Salles AAF: Endoscopy of the Central and Peripheral Nervous System, Vol 14. Stuttgart: Thieme 1998, pp 156–163.

186. Pool JL: Direct visualization of dorsal nerve roots of the cauda equina by means of a myeloscope. Arch Neurol Psychiatr 39:1308–1312, 1938.

187. Pool JL: Myeloscopy: Intraspinal endoscopy. Surg Clin North Am 37:1401–1402, 1957.

188. Powell MP, Torrens MJ, Thompson JLG, Horgan G: Isodense colloid cysts of the third ventricle: A diagnostic and therapeutic problem resolved by ventriculoscopy. Neurosurgery 13:234–237, 1983.

189. Powers SK: Fenestration of intraventricular cysts using a flexible steerable endoscope and the argon laser. Neurosurgery 18:637–641, 1986.

190. Powers SK: Fenestration of intraventricular cysts using a flexible, steerable endoscope. Acta Neurochir (Wien) 54(Suppl):42–46, 1992.

191. Prott W: Cisternoscopy-endoscopy of the cerebellopontine angle. Acta Neurochir (Wien) 31:105–113, 1974.

192. Putnam TJ: The surgical treatment of infantile hydrocephalus. Surg Gynecol Obstet 76:171–182, 1943.

193. Putnam TJ: Treatment of hydrocephalus by endoscopic coagulation of the choroid plexus. N Engl J Med 210:1373–1376, 1934.

194. Raimondi AJ, Shimoji T, Gutierrez FA: Suprasellar cysts: Surgical treatment and results. Childs Brain 7:57–72, 1980.

195. Reidenbach HD: Technical fundamentals of endoscopic hemostasis. Acta Neurochir Suppl (Wien) 54:26–33, 1992.

196. Resch KDM, Perneczky A, Tschabitscher M, Kindel ST: Endoscopic anatomy of the ventricles. Acta Neurochir 61(Suppl):57–61, 1994.

197. Resch KDM, Reisch R: Endo-neuro-sonography: Anatomic aspects of the ventricles. Minim Invas Neurosurg 40:2–7, 1997.

198. Resnick CT, Miller BW: Endoscopic carpal tunnel release using subligamentous two portal technique. Contemp Orthop 22:269–277, 1991.

199. Rhoten RLP, Luciano MG, Barnett GH: Computer-assisted endoscopy for neurosurgical procedures (Technical note). Neurosurgery 40:632–638, 1997.

200. Riegel T, Hellwig D, Bauer BL, Mennel HD: Endoscopic anatomy of the third ventricle. Acta Neurochir 61(Suppl):54–56, 1994.

201. Rivas JJ, Lobato RD: CT-assisted stereotaxic aspiration of colloid cysts of the third ventricle. J Neurosurg 62:238–242, 1985.

202. Rosenthal D, Rosenthal R, de Simone A: Removal of a protruded thoracic disc using microneurosurgical endoscopy: A new technique. Spine 19:1087–1091, 1994.

203. Ryder JW, Kleinschmidt-De Masters BK, Keller TS: Sudden deterioration and death in patients with benign tumours of the third ventricle area. J Neurosurg 64:216–223, 1986.

204. Saenz A, Zamorano L, Matter A, et al: Interactive image guided surgery of the pineal region. Minim Invas Neurosurg 41:27–30, 1998.

205. Sainte-Rose C: Third ventriculostomy. In Manwaring KH, Crone KR (eds): Neuroendoscopy, Vol 1. New York: Mary Ann Liebert, 1992, pp 47–62.

206. Sainte-Rose C, Chumas P: Endoscopic third ventriculostomy. Tech Neurosurg 1:176–184, 1995.

207. Sayers MP, Kosnik EJ: Percutaneous third ventriculostomy: Experience and technique. Childs Brain 2:24–30, 1976.

208. Scarff JE: Third ventriculostomy as the rational treatment of obstructive hydrocephalus. J Pediatr 6:870–871, 1935.

209. Scarff JE: Endoscopic treatment of hydrocephalus: Description of a ventriculoscope and preliminary report of cases. Arch Neurol Psychiatr 35:853–860, 1936.

210. Scarff JE: Evaluation of treatment of hydrocephalus: Reports of third ventriculostomy and endoscopic cauterization of choroid plexuses compared with mechanical shunts. Arch Neurol 14:382–391, 1966.

211. Scarff JE: The treatment of nonobstructive (communicating) hydrocephalus by endoscopic cauterization of the choroid plexus. J Neurosurg 33:1–8, 1970.

212. Segal S: Endoscopic anatomy of the ventricular system. In King WA, Frazee JG, De Salles AAF: Endoscopy of the Central and Peripheral Nervous System, Vol 5. Stuttgart: Thieme, 1998, pp 38–58.

213. Shelden CH, Jacques S, Lutes HR: Neurologic endoscopy. In Schmidek HH, Sweet WH (eds): Operative Neurosurgical Techniques. Philadelphia: WB Saunders, 1988, pp 423–430.

214. Silbergeld DL, Vollmer DG, Tantuwaya VS, et al: Endoscopic transventricular hippocampectomy. J Epilepsy 8:68–73, 1995.

215. Stern EL: The spinascope: A new instrument for visualizing the spinal canal and its contents. Med Record 143:31–32, 1936.

216. Stookey B, Scarff J: Occlusion of the aqueduct of Sylvius by neoplastic and non-neoplastic processes with a rational surgical treatment for relief of the resultant obstructive hydrocephalus. Bull Neurol Inst N Y 5:348–377, 1936.

217. Taha JM, Crone KR: Endoscopically guided shunt placement. Tech Neurosurg 1:159–167, 1995.

218. Taneda M, Kato A, Yoshini T, Hayakawa T: Endoscopic-image display system mounted on the surgical microscope. Minim Invas Neurosurg 38:85–86, 1995.

219. Taniguchi M, Perneczky A: Subtemporal keyhole approach to the suprasellar and petroclival region: Microanatomic considerations and clinical application. Neurosurgery 41:592–601, 1997.

220. Teo C: Endoscopy for the treatment of hydrocephalus. In King WA, Frazee JG, De Salles AAF: Endoscopy of the Central and Peripheral Nervous System. Stuttgart: Thieme, 1998, pp 59–67.

221. Vandertop WP, Verdaasdonk RM, Van Swol CFP: Laser-assisted neuroendoscopy using a neodymium-yttrium aluminium garnet or diode contact laser with pretreated fiber tips. J Neurosurg 88:82–92, 1998.

222. Van Lindert E, Hopf N, Perneczky A: Endoscopic treatment of mesencephalic ependymal cysts: Technical case report. Neurosurgery 43:1234–1241, 1998.

223. Veto F, Horvath Z, Doczi T: Biportal endoscopic management of third ventricle tumors in patients with occlusive hydrocephalus (Technical note). Neurosurgery 40:871–877, 1997.

224. Vinas FC, Castillo C, Diaz FG: Microanatomical considerations for the fenestration of the septum pellucidum. Minim Invas Neurosurg 41:20–26, 1998.

225. Vries J: An endoscopic technique for third ventriculostomy. Surg Neurol 9:165–168, 1978.

226. Walker ML: History of neuroendoscopy. Tech Neurosurg 1:148–150, 1995.

227. Whitfield PC, Guazzo EP, Pickard JD: Safe removal of retained ventricular catheters using intraluminal choroid plexus coagulation. J Neurosurg 83:1101–1102, 1995.

228. Williams B, Guthkelch AN: Why do central arachnoid pouches expand? J Neurol Neurosurg Psychiatry 37:1085–1092, 1974.

229. Yamakawa K, Kondo T, Yoshioka M, Takakura K: Application of superfine fiberscope for endovasculoscopy, ventriculoscopy and myeloscopy. Acta Neurochir 54(Suppl):47–52, 1992.

230. Yamakawa K, Kondo T, Yoshioka M, Takakura K: Ultrasound guided endoscopic neurosurgery: New surgical instrument and technique. Acta Neurochir 61(Suppl):46–48, 1994.

231. Yamasaki T, Moritake K, Takaya M, et al: Intraoperative use of Doppler ultrasound and endoscopic monitoring in the stereotactic biopsy of malignant brain tumors (Technical note). J Neurosurg 80:570–574, 1994.

232. Yaniv E, Rappaport H: Endoscopic transseptal transsphenoidal surgery for pituitary tumors. Neurosurgery 40:944–946, 1977.

233. Yeung AT: Arthroscopic microdiscectomy for discogenic pain: On the cutting edge of surgical option. Arthroscopy (submitted).
234. Zamorano L, Chavantes C, Dujovny M, et al: Stereotactic endoscopic interventions in cystic and intraventricular brain lesions. Acta Neurochir Suppl 54:69–76, 1992.
235. Zamorano L, Chavantes C, Moure F: Endoscopic stereotactic interventions in the treatment of brain lesion. Acta Neurochir 61(Suppl):92–97, 1994.
236. Zamorano L, Chavantes C, Jiang Z, et al: Stereotactic neuroendoscopy. In Cohen AR, Haines SJ (eds): Minimally Invasive Techniques in Neurosurgery: Concepts in Neurosurgery, Vol 7. Baltimore: Williams & Wilkins, 1995, pp 49–65.
237. Zamorano L, Jiang Z, Grosky W, et al: Telepresence and virtual reality in computer assisted neurological surgery: Basic theory and a prototype. J Vir Real Med 1:54–59, 1997.
238. Zamorano L, Jiang C, Chavantes C, Diaz FG: Stereotactic and interactive image-guided neuroendoscopy. In De Salles AAF, Lufkin RB: Minimally Invasive Therapy of the Brain, Vol 19. Stuttgart: Thieme, 1997, pp 241–253.
239. Zucherman JF, Implicito DA, Hsu K: Endoscopy for lumbar spine disease. In King WA, Frazee JG, De Salles AAF: Endoscopy of the Central and Peripheral Nervous System, Vol 17. Stuttgart: Thieme, 1998, pp 199–214.

SECTION IX

# Hydrocephalus

# CHAPTER 43

# Current Systems for Cerebrospinal Fluid Shunting and Management of Pediatric Hydrocephalus: Endoscopic and Image-Guided Surgery in Hydrocephalus

■ JAMES M. DRAKE and MARK R. IANTOSCA

## CLINICAL PRESENTATION OF HYDROCEPHALUS

Hydrocephalus is one of the most common complications of virtually any insult to the neonatal, infant, or child's nervous system. It occurs in approximately 1 in 2000 births and is associated with approximately one third of all congenital malformations of the nervous system.[1, 2] It is also a common complication of intraventricular hemorrhage, brain tumors, infections, and head injury.[3] The causes of hydrocephalus in 345 children undergoing a first shunt insertion in the randomized shunt design trial[26] are listed in Table 43–1. The median corrected age of the patients was 55 days, indicating that this is a problem seen most commonly in infancy. An estimated 33,000 shunts are placed in patients of all ages annually in the United States, with an estimated shunt prevalence of more than 56,000 in children younger than 18 years old.[1]

The diagnosis of hydrocephalus is based on clinical and radiologic features. As seen in Table 43–1, children most commonly present with symptoms of irritability, delayed development, vomiting, and headache and on examination have increasing head circumference and a bulging fontanelle. Magnetic resonance imaging (MRI) has the best diagnostic utility in terms of establishing the cause and defining the site of obstruction but may be combined with computed tomography (CT), particularly if looking for evidence of intracranial calcification. Ultrasound is quite practical in critically ill premature infants with intraventricular hemorrhage or in patients with myelomeningocele in whom the cause is not in doubt. In patients with mild ventricular enlargement, evidence of transependymal flow of cerebrospinal fluid (CSF) usually suggests that the process is more acute. Other signs of progressive hydrocephalus—enlargement of the temporal horns, dilation of the third ventricle, and effacement of the sulci—are not absolutely specific. In cases in which there is doubt, careful observation with serial images, rather than subjecting the patient to the known risks of shunt failure, is prudent.

## TREATMENT WITH CEREBROSPINAL FLUID SHUNTS

### History of Shunts

The history of hydrocephalus is a fascinating one and dates back to the dawn of civilization. Early attempts at management failed because of ignorance about the pathogenesis, primitive surgical techniques, and lack of appropriate equipment and biocompatible materials. Early 20th century attempts at achieving closed ventricular drainage included gold, glass, silver, and rubber tubes; catgut; and linen threads passed from the ventricle to the subdural space.[4–7] Similar techniques were used to connect the lumbar thecal sac to the peritoneum or renal pelvis.[8–10] After attempts at third ventriculostomy[11, 12] and choroid plexectomy,[13] shunts from the lateral ventricle to cisterna magna, Torkildsen shunts,[14] and shunts from the lumbar to ureter came into more widespread use.

The treatment of hydrocephalus was revolutionized when Nulsen and Spitz[15] reported in 1952 the successful use of a ventriculojugular shunt using a spring and stainless steel ball valve. The two valves were housed in rubber intravenous tubing, which acted as a flushing device, and connected to polyethylene tubing at either end. Occlusion of the venous catheter by blood clot was a frequent problem.

Holter's shunt was the first to employ silicone, and he designed a multiple slit valve out of silicone for use in his son who developed hydrocephalus.[16] Almost at the same time, Pudenz[17] also concluded that silicone was the best

## TABLE 43–1 ■ CAUSE AND CLINICAL PRESENTATION IN 344 PEDIATRIC PATIENTS

| | |
|---|---|
| Corrected age (median) | 55 days |
| Hydrocephalus causes | |
| Intraventricular hemorrhage | 24.1% |
| Myelomeningocele | 21.2% |
| Tumor | 9.0% |
| Aqueduct stenosis | 7.0% |
| CSF infection | 5.2% |
| Head injury | 1.5% |
| Other | 11.3% |
| Unknown | 11.0% |
| Two or more causes | 8.7% |
| Presenting symptoms | |
| Irritability | 26.6% |
| Delayed developmental milestones | 19.8% |
| Nausea or vomiting | 19.0% |
| Headache | 17.5% |
| Lethargy | 17.5% |
| New seizures or change in seizure pattern | 6.6% |
| Diplopia | 5.8% |
| Worsening school performance | 4.2% |
| Fever | 2.6% |
| Presenting signs | |
| Increase head circumference | 81.3% |
| Bulging fontanelle | 70.6% |
| Delayed developmental milestones | 20.9% |
| Loss of upward gaze | 15.8% |
| Decreased level of consciousness | 12.6% |
| Other focal neurologic deficit | 12.4% |
| Papilledema | 12.0% |
| 6th nerve palsy | 4.6% |
| Hemiparesis | 3.8% |
| Nuchal rigidity | 1.8% |

CSF, cerebrospinal fluid.

material and designed two valves to use as ventriculoauricular shunts.

## Mechanical Principles and Available Shunt Components

CSF shunts regulate flow by means of one-way valves. The standard valves that have been in use for decades simply open or close depending on the pressure across them (Fig. 43–1A).[17–21] They can be grouped into four general design categories: silicone rubber slit valves, silicone rubber diaphragm valves, silicone rubber miter valves, and metallic spring ball valves.[20] The pressure at which they open is termed the *opening pressure*, and typically there are low, medium, and high designations, which generally correspond to 5, 10, and 15 mm $H_2O$ pressure, but there are no universal standards. Once open, the valves have little resistance to flow and let large quantities of CSF through the shunt. When patients stand up, this situation can lead to *siphoning* as CSF drains out of the head under the effect of gravity into the abdomen. Large negative intracranial pressures and low-pressure headache and subdural hematomas can result.[18, 19, 22]

Other valve designs have tried to limit this siphoning effect and include siphon-reducing devices. These have a mobile membrane that moves to narrow an orifice in response to a negative pressure inside the shunt system (see Fig. 43–1B).[23, 24] Examples are the antisiphon device and

the Delta valve (Medtronic PS Medical, Goletta, CA). A flow-limiting valve has a flexible diaphragm that moves along a piston of increasing diameter (see Fig. 43–1C). This flexible diaphragm reduces the flow orifice, dramatically increasing the resistance to flow. This increase in resistance results in little increase in flow rate despite progressive rise in pressure—essentially a flow limit. The Orbis Sigma NMT (Boston, MA) is an example of this valve.[25]

Other valves try to reduce the effects of gravity by changing their configuration according to how they are positioned (see Fig. 43–1D). In some designs, metallic balls rest on top of a standard spring ball valve to increase the opening pressure when the valve (and patient) are vertical. In another, a single metallic ball rests in an asymmetric valve seat in upright position, increasing the resistance.

There are also several externally adjustable valves. The simplest involves moving metallic balls along Silastic sleeves, to open or occlude two parallel valve systems (see Fig. 43–1E). This leads to four settings: low, medium, high, and off. Other designs uses a magnetized rotor to adjust the tension on a spring ball valve. The rotor may have 3 to 18 pressure settings and be controlled by an external bar magnet, or electromagnet. The magnetized systems are susceptible to external magnetic fields, including those of MRI. Verification of the pressure setting by means of an x-ray study is usually required.

Although several different ventricular and peritoneal catheters exist, there is little to choose among them. There are a number of ways of connecting the ventricular catheter to the distal system, including bur hole reservoirs, right angle connectors, right-angled guides, and preshaped catheters, and some systems come in a completely unitized fashion. In closed-ended peritoneal catheters, the adjacent slits act as a valve.

## Shunt Selection

Currently, no data recommend one particular shunt over another. In fact, a randomized trial on CSF shunt design that compared a standard valve to the Delta valve and the Orbis-Sigma valve failed to show any difference in terms of overall shunt failure.[26] There are important considerations to be taken into account, however, when considering the individual patient, including age, weight, skin thickness, head size, size of the ventricles, pathogenesis of hydrocephalus, acuteness of the illness, presence of internal lines or gastrostomy, tracheotomy openings, status of the distal drainage site, and plans for further surgery.

For example, a premature infant with thin skin stretched further by a rapidly expanded head cannot handle adult-size equipment without the risk of skin erosion. If the same infant has blood in the ventricles, immediate implantation of a valve with a narrow flow-limiting orifice might increase the risk of early obstruction. If one ventricle is significantly larger than the other, placing the ventricular catheter on that side is easier. In patients with large ventricles and large skulls with fused sutures, placing a flow-limiting or siphon-reducing device might decrease the risk of subdural hemorrhage.

If there are loculations within the ventricular system, fenestrating them endoscopically at the time of shunt insertion would at least attempt to keep the number of shunts to one. If a patient is expected to have a number of subsequent and important MRI studies, metallic shunt components or magnetic programmable valves might interfere with the interpretation of these images. Finally, if a patient is scheduled to have further intra-abdominal surgery—for example, to close a colostomy or to reconstruct the bladder, this might influence the choice of site of distal drainage.

For most routine cases, it is probably better to use a shunt system with which one is quite familiar. In this setting, the authors prefer a two-piece system, with a non-flanged ventricular catheter, connected to flat-bottomed valve with a reservoir, with open-ended distal tubing.

## Surgical Technique—Initial Shunt Insertion

Although shunt surgery is often regarded with some disdain by staff and trainee neurosurgeons alike—"plumbing"—it has the highest failure rate of any neurosurgical procedure, and nothing is less forgiving of any technical errors than a shunt operation. Shunts often fail from tissue occluding the upper or lower end. Parenchymal ventricular catheters, extraperitoneal distal catheters, and spontaneously disconnected or migrated shunts have happened in virtually every neurosurgery service. These complications are avoidable. The authors believe that shunt surgery should command great respect, require meticulous attention to detail, and be carried out in a skilled and expeditious fashion.

Body wash and shampoo the night before and again before surgery with an antiseptic solution (i.e., chlorhexidine) is recommended. In the operating room, the patient is positioned under general endotracheal anesthesia, with the head rotated to the side opposite the shunt and the neck extended so that there is almost a straight line between the scalp and abdominal incisions. A number of meta-analyses have shown that prophylactic antibiotics are effective,[27] and they are strongly recommended. Cloxicillin, 50 mg/kg administered 0.5 hour before surgery, is often used. For patients in whom an abdominal trochar is being used, the bladder should be emptied either by a Credé maneuver or by urinary catheter. Hair is clipped (not shaved) in the operating room if desired to assist with skin closure and bandage application. Hair removal has never been shown to decrease the risk of infection, however.[28]

The patient should be positioned so that there is a flat plane between the upper and lower incision sites, so that the shunt can be passed easily. For an occipital bur hole, this means rotating the head to the opposite side and extending the neck, usually with a rolled towel (Fig. 43–2A). The site of the bur hole and abdominal incisions should be selected and marked before draping, before the surface landmarks are obscured. Occipital bur holes are usually on the flat part of the occiput 3 to 4 cm from the midline along the course of the lambdoid suture. In patients with Dandy-Walker malformation or huge arachnoid cysts of the posterior fossa, the transverse sinus can be placed much higher than in normal subjects. In these patients, the position of the transverse sinus should be identified preoperatively by MRI, and the placement of the bur hole

should be modified according to the results of this examination. Frontal bur holes are along the coronal suture 2 to 3 cm from the midline. The issue of frontal versus occipital bur hole has never been resolved.[29]

The skin is meticulously prepared with a slow-release iodine solution. Disposable, adhesive drapes are used to cover the patient and the operating table entirely except for a small band of skin from the bur hole site to the abdomen (see Fig. 43–2B). The drapes may need to be stapled to the hair-bearing areas of the scalp. Small skin incisions are adequate (see Fig. 43–2C). It is better to position the incision so that the hardware is not afterward directly underneath. The bur hole need not be a standard size, and a twist drill is adequate unless using a bur hole reservoir or intraoperative ultrasound. In infants, particularly if premature, an opening between the splayed sutures at either frontal or occipital sites is all that is required. The dura does not need to be opened widely, and in patients with thinned cortical mantles, a wide dural opening may allow CSF to escape around the ventricular catheter into the subcutaneous tissues, promoting a CSF leak. The brain pia is cauterized and nicked.

The abdominal incision is simultaneously opened by an assistant. The method and site are unimportant. Paraumbilical and upper midline sites are common. One needs to be sure that the peritoneum has truly been opened and not just the preperitoneal space. Passing a blunt dissector easily well into the abdominal cavity verifies this (see Fig. 43–2D). A pursestring suture around the peritoneum tends to prevent omentum from herniating but is not absolutely necessary. The authors prefer to use abdominal trochars in *virgin* abdomens from a paraumbilical location. Opening the rectus sheath through a tiny incision and visualizing the posterior wall of the sheath facilitates placement. The posterior sheath is then picked up by the tip of the trochar, then the tip is angled inferiorly and off the midline to avoid hitting the great vessels (see Fig. 43–2E). A gentle pop is felt as the peritoneum is penetrated. A blunt instrument can also be passed along the trochar sheath to verify peritoneal entry.

Care must be taken when tunneling. If the metal tube is too deep, either the chest or the posterior fossa can be entered. One has to be particularly careful in patients who have had an occipital craniectomy because it is possible to pass the device into the bone opening by mistake. If the tunneling device is too superficial, a skin laceration, which may be initially unrecognized, can occur. A gentle curve to the tunneling instrument allows one to direct the tip posteriorly when coming over the anterior chest into the neck, then by rotating 180 degrees, the tip anteriorly toward the occiput (see Fig. 43–2F). Significant resistance is usually felt at the posterior nuchal line. Firm pressure, making sure that the pointed central stylet has not backed out, and guarding against plunging usually allow this fascia to be penetrated. If one is using excessive force, a separate incision should be made in the neck.

If passing to a frontal bur hole, an intervening incision is needed over the occiput. There appears to be no logical reason to tunnel down the back of the patient. Not only is it awkward, but also with time a fibrous cord similar to a bow string forms, which is unsightly and can even affect neck mobility. The cord also remains if the shunt hardware

# Standard Differential Pressure Valve

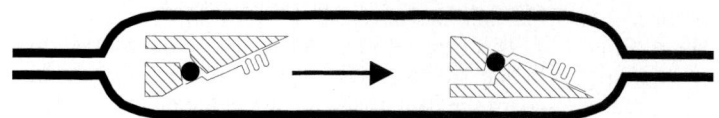

## Mechanism

Spring-ball valve

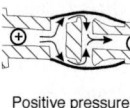

Valve closed

Valve open

A

## Pressure Flow Characteristics

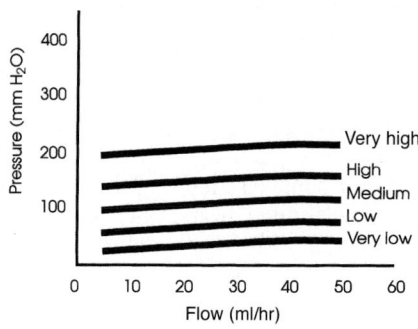

# PS Medical Delta Valve

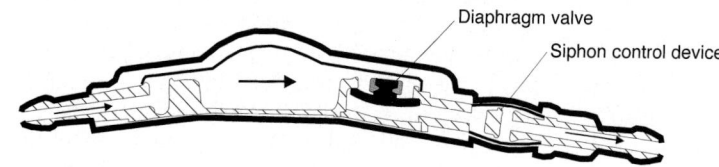

## Mechanism

Diaphragm Valve

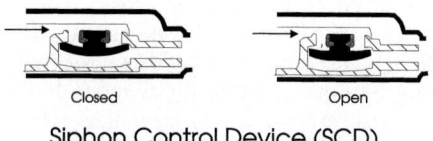

Closed          Open

### Siphon Control Device (SCD)

Positive pressure
Diaphragm open
Low resistance

Negative pressure
Diaphragm closed
High resistance

B

## Pressure Flow Characteristics

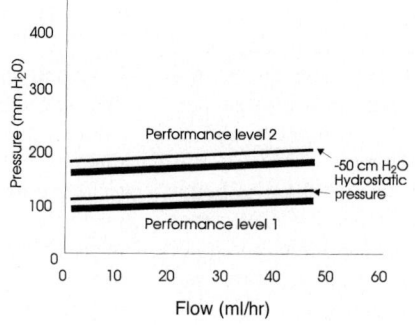

**FIGURE 43–1 ■** Shunt valve designs. *A*, Standard differential pressure shunt, spring valve. Flow increases rapidly once opening pressure is exceeded. *B*, Siphon-reducing device distal to a standard differential pressure valve, diaphragm type. The effects of gravity are reduced in the upright position.

is removed. The tunneling device is rigid enough when in place to compress the chest of small children so that the anesthetist typically notes an increase in airway pressure. It should not be left in place too long. The device can also tear the scalp, particularly in small infants, in whom one is trying to bring the straight tunneling tube around the curved skull.

The peritoneal tubing, with or without the attached valve, is then passed along the tube, attaching suction to the distal end and irrigating. The valve should then be attached and irrigated to fill it with fluid, usually the antibiotic solution soaking the shunt equipment. It is not necessary to test the opening pressure of the shunt in the operating room. Merely handling the valve changes its performance charac-

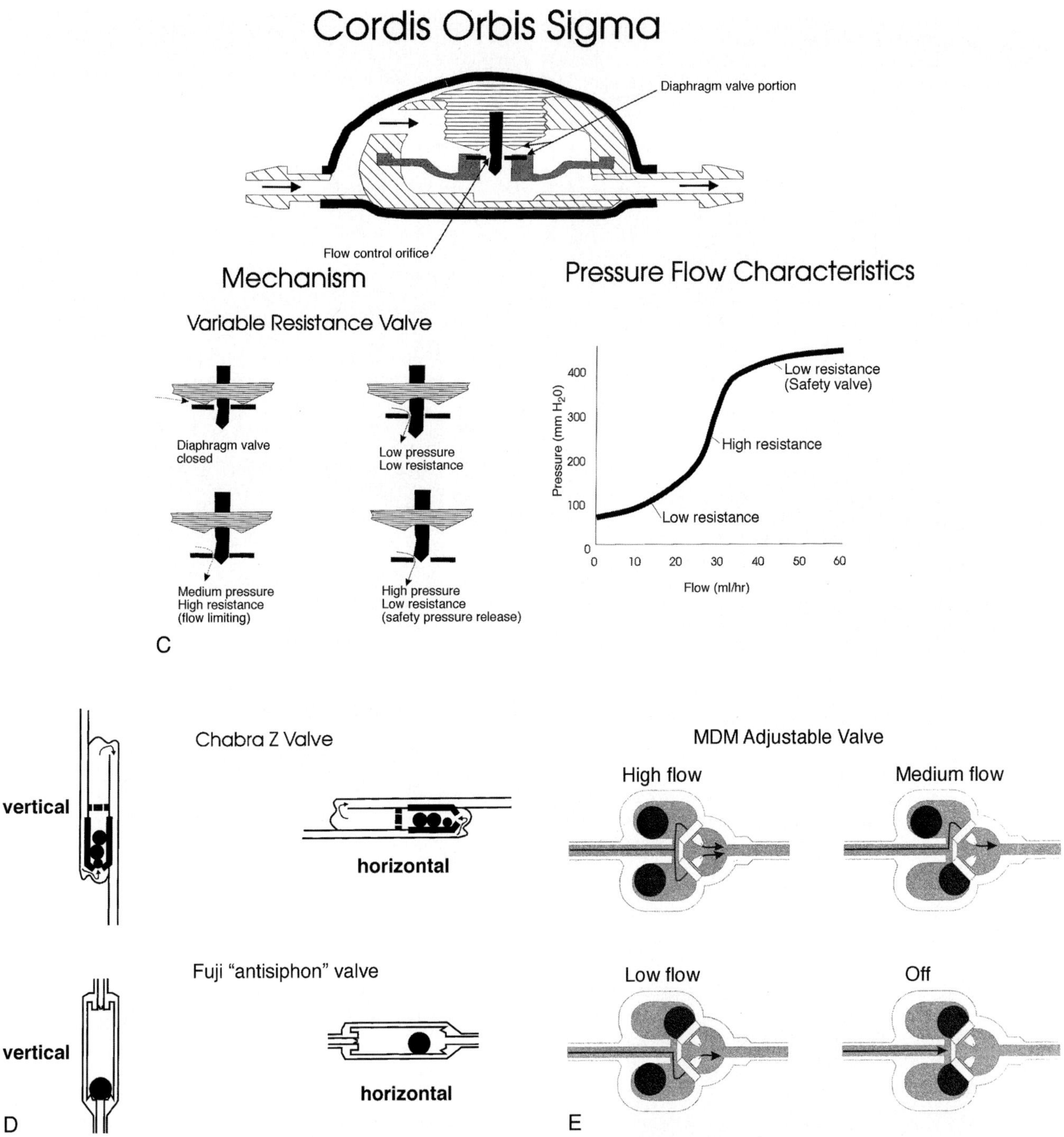

# Cordis Orbis Sigma

## Mechanism

### Variable Resistance Valve

## Pressure Flow Characteristics

C

D

E

**FIGURE 43–1** *Continued* ■ *C*, A flow-limiting valve with a variable resistance orifice leading to flow limit as seen in flow pressure curve. *D*, Two gravity actuated devices that increase the opening pressure *(above)*, or the resistance *(below)* in the vertical position. *E*, A percutaneous adjustable valve that can be completely occluded. (*A–C*, From Drake JM, Kestle J: Determining the best cerebrospinal fluid shunt valve design: The pediatric valve design trial. Neurosurgery 38:604–607, 1996. *D* and *E*, From Drake JM, Sainte-Rose C: The Shunt Book. New York: Blackwell Scientific, 1995, p 1.)

teristics for days, and air bubbles can also affect these measurements. It is important to connect the valve in the right direction.

The ventricular catheter trajectory is then determined according to external landmarks (see Fig. 43-2G). From a frontal bur hole, traditional landmarks for the foramen of Munro or the intersection of the planes through the pupil and the external auditory meatus (or simply being perpendicular to the skull) are used. From the occipital location,

a target at the midpoint of the forehead just at the normal hair line ensures that the catheter proceeds into the frontal horn instead of the temporal horn. There is no proven ideal location for the ventricular catheter. Evidence from the pediatric shunt design trial suggests that frontal or occipital locations are better than in the body of the ventricle or in the third ventricle.[30] Hitting small ventricles is easier from a frontal location. In these patients, ultrasound or even stereotaxis may assist with successful ventricular cannula-

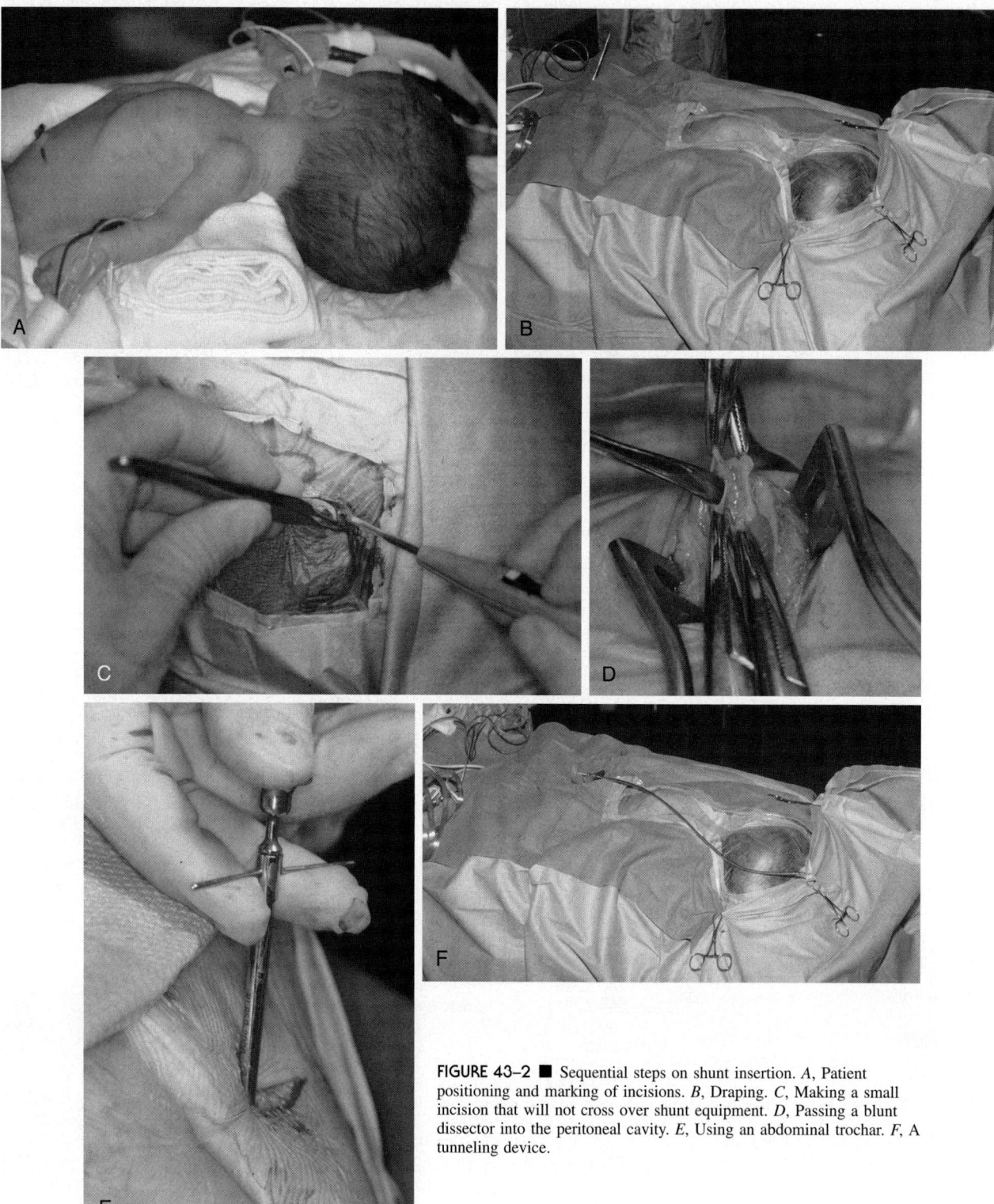

**FIGURE 43–2** ■ Sequential steps on shunt insertion. *A*, Patient positioning and marking of incisions. *B*, Draping. *C*, Making a small incision that will not cross over shunt equipment. *D*, Passing a blunt dissector into the peritoneal cavity. *E*, Using an abdominal trochar. *F*, A tunneling device.

tion. The authors routinely use ultrasound either through the shunt bur hole or, in infants, through the open fontanelle (see Fig. 43–2*H*). An endoscopic stylet can also be used to place the shunt (see Fig. 43–2*I*). Whether assisted placement results in improved outcome is the subject of an ongoing clinical trial. With these techniques, the surgeon is as certain as possible that the catheter is in good position

at the end of the case and not in one of the *unusual* sites, such as the sylvian fissure or quadrigeminal cistern.

The ventricular catheter can usually be felt to pop once the ependyma is breached with concomitant gush of CSF. Gently irrigating the catheter may show pulsatile CSF flow into and out of the catheter. Withdrawing vigorously simply draws brain tissue into the catheter and plugs the shunt if

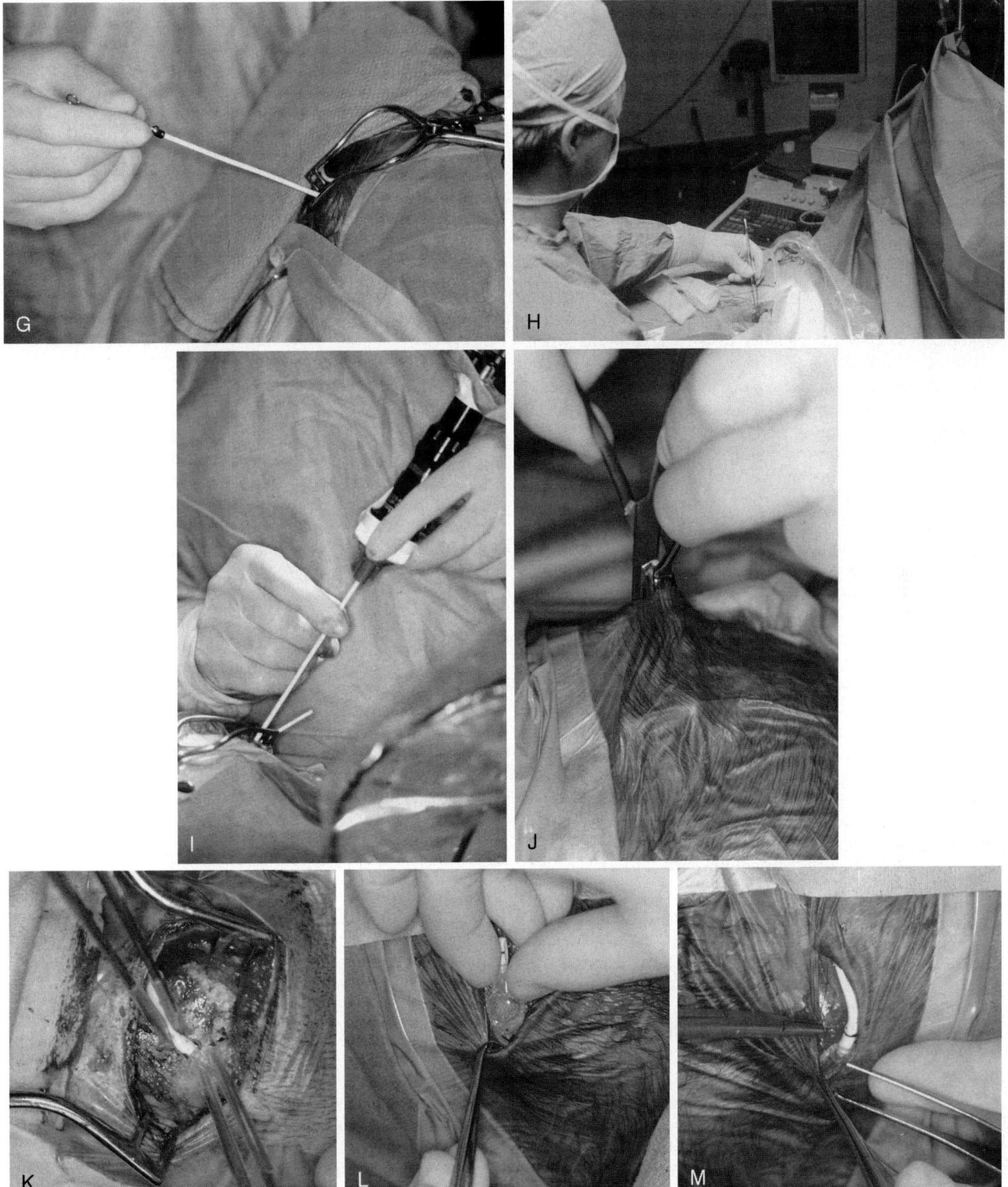

**FIGURE 43–2** *Continued* ■ *G*, Cannulating the ventricle according to landmarks. *H*, Using ultrasound guidance to place the ventricular catheter. *I*, Using a shunt scope to place the ventricular catheter. *J*, Making the subcutaneous pocket for the valve. *K*, Silastic sleeved forceps coaxing the tubing onto the connector. *L*, Placing the valve into its pocket. *M*, Suturing the valve to the pericranium.

one is in the parenchyma. Although there is no official limit on the number of passes, after two, the authors use ultrasound. A little fresh blood that clears is not unusual and one reason to recommend a separate ventricular catheter, so that blood and debris can be cleared before attaching to the valve. Extensive hemorrhage should prompt extensive irrigation until it clears. Installing a narrow-orifice, high-resistance valve is this setting is likely to result in rapid occlusion.

There are a number of ways of getting the ventricular

catheter around the bur hole corner; all are somewhat awkward. Simply bending the catheter, using the forces of the brain, bur hole, and dura, is fine, but the inherent stiffness of the catheter tends to move the tip in the opposite direction. In patients with large ventricles and thin cortical mantles, the catheter can take an almost vertical trajectory. Right-angled guides avoid this. When attaching bur hole reservoirs (usually with contained valves), the ventricular catheter must be withdrawn, then readvanced. The attachment site is usually below the cortical surface, where it becomes adherent, and losing the catheter at a subsequent revision is possible.

When using a flat-bottomed valve, a pocket must be created along the distal path. This pocket must be exactly along the course of the catheter or the valve binds when attempting to slide it along (see Fig. 43–2J). This binding can be an enormous nuisance, particularly if the ventricular catheter is already connected. When attaching the ventricular catheter to the valve, one should avoid using metal instruments directly on the tubing forcefully because they can lacerate it, and the tubing can subsequently leak or break. We put Silastic sleeves over forceps and snaps (see Fig. 43–2K) or use a clean gauze sponge. Similarly, when tying the catheter over the connector, having the tie directly over the neck of the connector, tight enough not to allow spontaneous disconnection or, alternatively, not too tight to lacerate the tubing, is vital. The valve system is then placed into its pocket by gently tugging on the peritoneal catheter from below (see Fig. 43–2L). The shunt system should then be secured to the pericranium (see Fig. 43–2M). It is incredible how unsecured systems can migrate. Post fossa catheters are particularly difficult to secure and have a high tendency to move. A three-way connector in this site also seems to come under excessive stress with neck motion and be prone to fracture.

Once in place, the system should be checked that it is flowing, either spontaneously or with gentle pumping of the reservoir. If there is any doubt, the system should be disconnected to verify that both ends are patent. This verification avoids the patient returning from the recovery room directly back to the operating room. The distal catheter is then inserted, making sure that is goes easily. If the catheter keeps backing out of the abdomen, it may be coiling up in the preperitoneal space. The surgeon needs to ensure that he is truly intraperitoneal. The pursestring suture is then tied snugly, and the abdominal layers are reapproximated.

Skin closure is critical. Any CSF leak predisposes to wound breakdown or infection. Normally the skin is closed in two layers, with careful apposition of the skin edges. The fragile skin of premature infants may fray and leak CSF through large needle holes. An occlusive dressing, which also resists attempts by small children to remove it; is also recommended for 48 hours. Positioning in the postoperative period is important. In patients with large ventricles, early mobilization may risk a subdural hemorrhage. In patients with high-resistance valves, placing them in an upright posture may promote CSF drainage and prevent accumulation under the skin.

The postoperative hospital stay is typically 2 to 3 days. Prophylactic antibiotics are normally given intravenously preoperatively and sometimes for a few doses postopera-

tively only. Prolonged antibiotic treatment in the postoperative period in an uncomplicated shunt patient is unwarranted. Shunted patients typically have immediate resolution of acute symptoms. In infants, a sunken fontanelle with standard valves is typical. Low-pressure headache can occur in older patients, particularly if the hydrocephalus is long-standing. An initial postoperative CT or MRI study, unless there was some particular problem intraoperatively, is unlikely to be helpful. Normally, patients are seen in follow-up at approximately 3 months postoperatively with a CT or MRI scan at this time and at 1 year with repeat imaging because the ventricles do not reach their final size on average until 1 year, at least in children.[30]

## Ventriculopleural Shunts

Pleural shunts are a second choice to peritoneal shunts. Contraindications include previous chest surgery and adhesions, active pulmonary disease including infection, or borderline pulmonary function in patients in whom a significant pleural effusion might push them into respiratory failure. Infants are more likely to develop a significant effusion temporarily. The pleural space can be entered at a variety of sites. Along the anterior axillary line, in the fourth to sixth interspace is often convenient. A muscle-splitting approach along the upper border of the rib (to avoid the neurovascular bundle) reveals the translucent pleura and the lung moving with ventillation.

The pleura is opened sharply, as with the peritoneum. There is no need to ask the anesthetist to collapse the lung because it moves away slightly as atmospheric pressure enters the chest cavity. The distal catheter is then introduced gently, being careful to guide it along the chest wall, not into the lung parenchyma. The catheter may need to be cut to length to avoid putting excess tubing, even allowing for growth, into the chest. There is no need to place a pursestring suture, and a Valsalva maneuver by the anesthetist inflates the lung adequately. Rapidly closing the muscles with a few sutures avoids further air entry into the chest.

A small pneumothorax is seen on the mandatory postoperative film. It resolves over the next few days, whereas the CSF usually accumulates as a small pleural effusion, especially in infants. These patients need to be monitored for any evidence of respiratory distress and with serial chest films.[31, 32] Usually the intrapleural fluid disappears over the next several weeks. In patients in whom the pleural fluid progressively accumulates, leading to respiratory distress with significant shift of the mediastinum, percutaneous drainage of the fluid and moving the distal tubing to another site are required.

## Ventriculocardiac Shunts

Cardiac shunts are third choice among the distal sites because of the serious complications of cor pulmonale and shunt nephritis.[33, 34] Catheter embolization is also a possibility. With growth, the shunts tend to block as they pull out of the right atrium, so that a small child might need several revisions for growth-related failure. The shunt

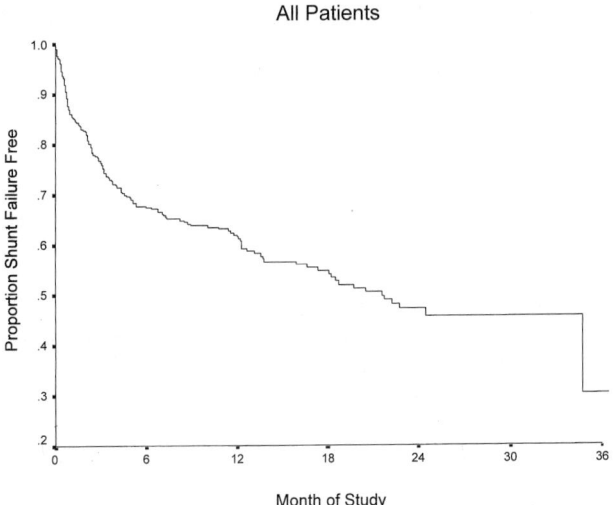

All Patients

FIGURE 43–3 ■ Shunt failure from the time of the first shunt insertion. Most failures occur within 6 months. The 2-year failure rate is 50%. (From Drake JM, Kestle J, Milner R, et al: Randomized trial of cerebrospinal fluid shunt valve design in pediatric hydrocephalus. Neurosurgery 43:294–305, 1998.)

tip should lie in the superior vena cava just above the triscuspid valve. There are a number of ways of achieving this position. Entrance to the jugular vein is usually achieved via the common facial vein, which is tied proximally and held with a stay suture distal to the venotomy site. The catheter is then advanced down the jugular vein into the superior vena cava, which is much easier to do on the right side. Percutaneous methods into the jugular and subclavian vein have also been described.[35] Positioning the tip can be done under fluoroscopy or even ultrasound.[36, 37] Fluoroscopy is useful because occasionally the catheter can be seen traveling out the subclavian vein. Alternatively, one can use the tip of the catheter as an electrocardiogram lead and look for a change in P wave polarity.

## MANAGEMENT OF SHUNT FAILURE

In most centers, the frequency ratio of shunt revision to initial shunt insertion surgery is 2:1. Having a sound grasp of the nuances of managing patients with failing CSF shunts is extremely important, and shunt revision surgery can be at times quite challenging.

### Clinical Presentation and Diagnosis

#### Mechanical Failure

Shunt mechanical complications may occur at any time, from in the recovery room immediately after the shunt operation to years later; at this time, the patient and the family may have all but forgotten about the shunt or falsely believed that the shunt is no longer necessary. The most common time for a shunt to fail is in the first 6 months after insertion (Fig. 43–3).[38] In the shunt design trial, the overall 1-year failure rate was 39%, including an 8% infection rate.[26]

Common to most mechanical complications is the obstruction of CSF shunt flow and the accompanying rise in intracranial pressure. This rise leads most commonly to headache, nausea and vomiting, and lethargy. The clinical signs and symptoms of 150 patients presenting with shunt failure are listed in Table 43–2. The onset of symptoms may be quite variable, ranging from sudden and severe to slow and insidious. A rapid and severe rise in intracranial pressure leads ultimately to unconsciousness. Less obvious signs of shunt mechanical malfunction include irritability, deterioration in school performance, or delay in achievement of developmental milestones. Occasionally, new or increased seizure frequency may be a symptom of mechanical shunt dysfunction.

Patients may also complain of double vision, or families may notice loss of conjugate gaze with sixth nerve palsies. Loss of vision from chronic papilledema may be insidious, particularly in small children. The only sign may be the child moving closer and closer to the television and subsequently "bumping into things."

Signs of mechanical dysfunction relate to the clinical

## TABLE 43–2 ■ SHUNT FAILURE PRESENTATION

|  | Mechanical (No. = 122) (%) | Infection (No. = 28) (%) |
|---|---|---|
| Symptoms |  |  |
| Headache | 16.2 | 11.5 |
| Nausea or vomiting | 39.3 | 30.8 |
| Irritability | 35.9 | 34.6 |
| New seizure or change in seizure pattern | 1.7 | 3.8 |
| Loss of developmental milestones | 8.5 | 3.8 |
| Worsening school performance | 1.7 | 0.0 |
| Abdominal pain |  | 19.2 |
| Signs |  |  |
| Papilledema | 2.6 | 3.8 |
| Bulging fontanelle | 42.7 | 23.1 |
| Increased head circumference | 38.5 | 19.2 |
| Decreased level of consciousness | 18.8 | 7.7 |
| Nuchal rigidity | 0.0 | 3.8 |
| 6th nerve palsy | 2.6 | 3.8 |
| Loss of upward gaze | 6.0 | 0.0 |
| Fluid tracking along shunt | 23.1 | 15.4 |
| CSF leak that necessitates shunt revision | 3.4 | 15.4 |
| Shunt reservoir cannot be depressed | 5.1 | 3.8 |
| Shunt reservoir does not refill | 12.0 | 0.0 |
| Fever | 2.6 | 69.2 |
| Meningismus |  | 8.0 |
| Wound erythema |  | 26.9 |
| Skin erosion |  | 23.1 |
| Purulent wound discharge |  | 7.7 |
| Abdominal mass (pseudocyst) |  | 3.8 |
| Peritonitis |  | 15.4 |
| Test results |  |  |
| Enlarging ventricles | 70.9 | 30.8 |
| Disruption/migration on x-ray study | 13.7 | 0.0 |
| Shunt flow study showing obstruction | 2.6 | 0.0 |
| Positive bacterial culture CSF and/or shunt material |  | 92.3 |

CSF, cerebrospinal fluid.

manifestations of raised intracranial pressure as well as abnormalities of the performance of the shunt hardware. Examination of the mental status of the patient may show variation from subtle intellectual deterioration to coma. On physical examination infants often present with a bulging fontanelle, split sutures, and abnormally increased head circumference. Despite the absence of infection, nuchal rigidity may be present from herniation of the tonsils through the foramen magnum. Papilledema appears in patients with closed sutures. Sixth nerve palsy, which may be bilateral, often accompanies papilledema. Loss of vertical gaze is also common. With impending brain herniation, decerebrate posturing, apnea, bradycardia, and pupillary dilatation ensue.

Examination of the site of the shunt equipment implantation may provide confirmatory evidence of shunt dysfunction. Although pumping of the shunt reservoir is a time-honored technique, in fact, this is often misleading.[39] A patient in whom a reservoir fills slowly may simply have small ventricles. Shunts whose reservoirs remain umbilicated for prolonged periods of time or even permanently, however, are often blocked proximally. A reservoir that is difficult to depress or refills apparently instantaneously frequently indicates a distal obstruction. Some shunt reservoirs contain proximal and distal occluders (or, less satisfactory, two valveless reservoirs). By occluding the distal reservoir and depressing and allowing the reservoir to refill, one can imply that the proximal catheter is patent. Similarly, by occluding the proximal reservoir and flushing distally, one can imply patency of the distal catheter. In this situation, the reservoir should remain umbilicated if the occluder is working properly.

Fluid collecting around the shunt, particularly if it firmly distends the skin, is progressive, and tracks along the distal catheter is often a sign of shunt occlusion. When shunts fracture, CSF often continues to track along the fibrous sheath. In this scenario, one can often feel a small amount of fluid and a space where the shunt has come apart. It may be difficult, however, to distinguish an empty sheath from a sheath containing shunt tubing, particularly if the shunt has been implanted for some years or the tract is calcified. A fluid thrill can sometimes be felt at the site of a distal catheter disruption, with pumping of the proximal reservoir.

Patients with shunt overdrainage may complain of postural headache—headache that begins with the assumption of the upright posture and disappears with recumbency. Patients with subdural hematoma may present with signs of raised intracranial pressure, but there may some true localizing signs, such as hemiparesis. Patients with loculated CSF compartments also tend to present with signs of increased pressure. Patients with loculated fourth ventricles may present specifically with bulbar paralysis and apnea. Sometimes, symptoms and signs of syringomyelia, particularly in shunted myelomeningocele patients, may be a manifestation of shunt obstruction. The clinical features of shunt mechanical dysfunction may also be intermittent. This occurs not only in the slit ventricle syndrome, but also with partially occluded proximal or distal catheters.

### Diagnostic Tests

Imaging studies are normally the first investigation undertaken. CT, MRI, or ultrasound scanning can determine the size and shape of the ventricles as well as any other collections or loculated compartments. The position and course of the ventricular catheter can also be seen best on CT. Dilatation of the ventricles compared with a previous image when the shunted patient was well is the simplest and clearest evidence of shunt dysfunction. Some patients, however, may have small ventricles or demonstrate minimal enlargement in the presence of shunt obstruction, and the ventricular size alone, in the absence of previous images, may be quite misleading in terms of shunt function (Fig. 43–4A, B). This situation is true particularly in children, in whom growth and development of the brain and congenital malformations alter one's notions of what normal ventricular size is.

Plain anteroposterior and lateral films of the skull, chest, and abdomen demonstrate whether the shunt is in continuity or has come apart of fractured (see Fig. 43–4C). For this reason, all shunt apparatus should be easily seen on x-ray studies. These x-ray studies may also demonstrate a peritoneal catheter that has migrated out of the abdomen with growth or obvious misplacement of the ventricular or peritoneal catheter. The films must often be scrutinized quite closely to detect small separations at connectors or along tubing. Calcification along the tubing is common in old shunts, which are prone to fracture. Common sites of shunt fracture are at connectors between the valve and the peritoneal catheter, where the hard connector repeatedly stresses the soft tubing, and in the neck, where fracture is presumably related to movement.

Uncertainty about the status of the shunt in a patient with symptoms compatible with shunt obstruction often leads to other diagnostic tests. The simplest test is the shunt tap. Under sterile conditions, the reservoir can be punctured with a 25-gauge butterfly needle catheter. Free flow of fluid indicates patency of the proximal catheter. The tubing can be used as a manometer to measure the pressure in the ventricle system. If the reservoirs is distal to the proximal valve, flow of CSF back into the shunt gives an indication of the patency of the distal catheter. A shunt tap can also be therapeutic and life-saving in critically ill shunted patients. Aspiration of 5 to 10 ml of fluid frequently dramatically improves a deteriorating shunted patient while preparations for surgery are made. In life-threatening situations, when the proximal catheter is blocked and no CSF can be aspirated, passing a lumbar puncture needle through the shunt, bur hole, and brain into the ventricle may be life-saving. This needle often destroys the proximal portion of the shunt but is of little consequence given the gravity of the situation and the forthcoming shunt revision. Other measurements of shunt patency include the use of radionuclide injections[40] or contrast agents.

## Surgical Technique—Shunt Revision

The surgery for shunt revision is not that different from an initial shunt insertion, but there are a few important points. Unless one is planning on removing the shunt for an infection, the patient should be prepped and draped as for a shunt insertion, including upper and lower incisions. This prep is necessary even if one strongly suspects one or the

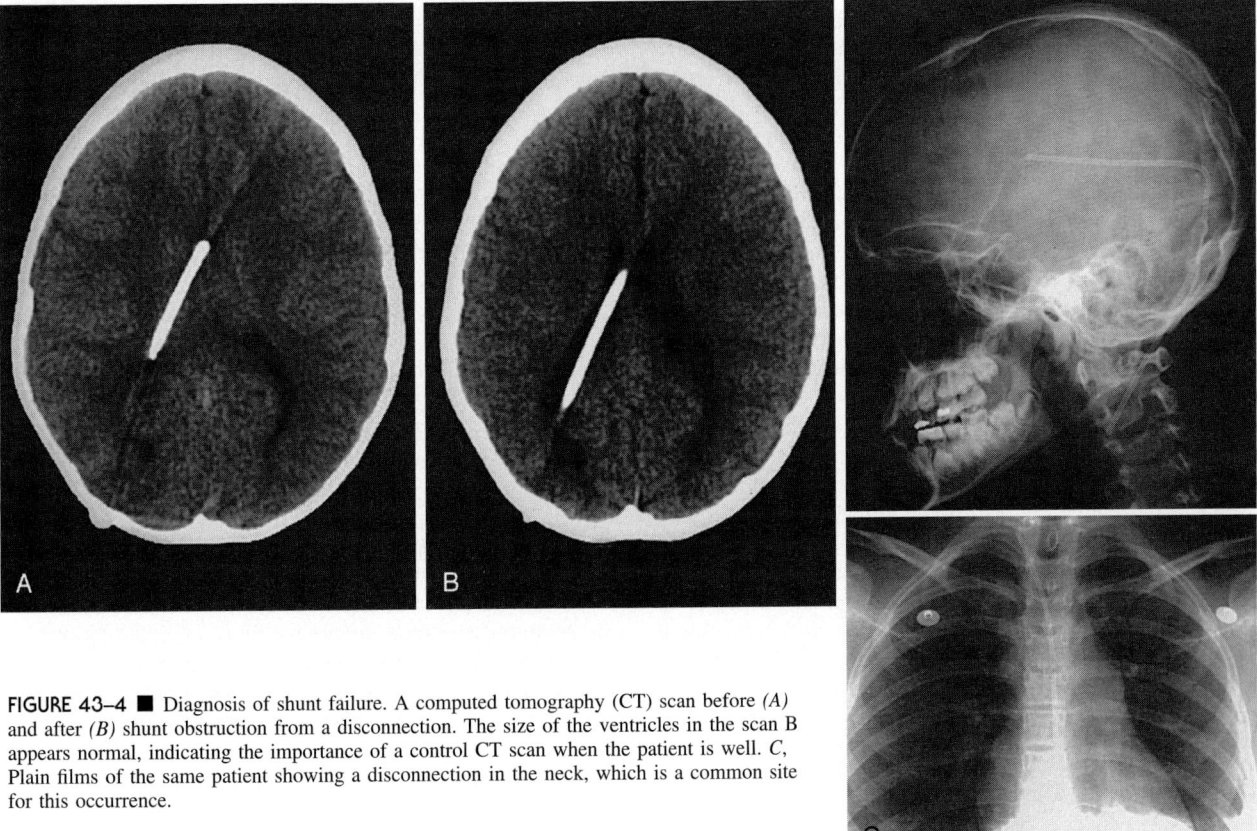

FIGURE 43–4 ■ Diagnosis of shunt failure. A computed tomography (CT) scan before *(A)* and after *(B)* shunt obstruction from a disconnection. The size of the ventricles in the scan B appears normal, indicating the importance of a control CT scan when the patient is well. *C,* Plain films of the same patient showing a disconnection in the neck, which is a common site for this occurrence.

other end of the shunt because these suspicions can turn out to be wrong.

The authors normally explore the upper end of the shunt first because one can test both ends from the same location, and piecemeal replacement of the lower end from an abdominal site using connectors is to be discouraged. Once the skin is incised, cutting cautery can be used to expose the shunt hardware easily with minimal bleeding (Fig. 43–5A). Care must be taken with bur hole reservoir systems, particularly when there is a tie on the ventricular catheter that resides below the pial surface. This tie becomes stuck, and it is easy to lose the catheter when it

separates. These lost catheters are extremely difficult to find, and one should probably introduce a ventriculoscope into the ventricle, rather than searching blindly in the parenchyma. For this reason, the authors rarely recommend bur hole systems. The equipment should then be inspected carefully for signs of damage, CSF egress, or infection.

Disconnecting the ventricular catheter from the valve allows patency of the upper end to be determined as well as the opportunity to take a CSF sample. Slow drops from the upper end often indicate an incomplete but clinically significant ventricular catheter obstruction, as evidenced by the gush of high-pressure CSF when the catheter is re-

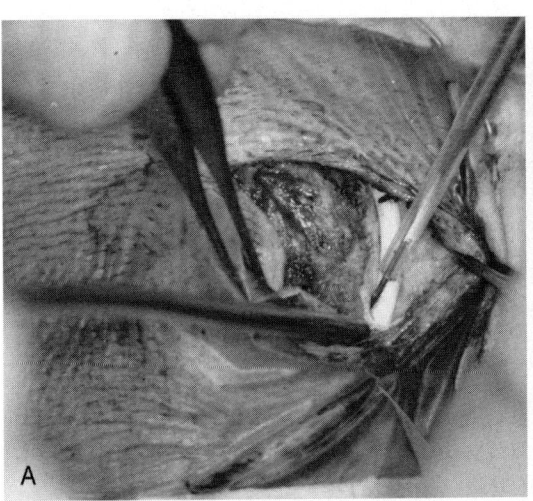

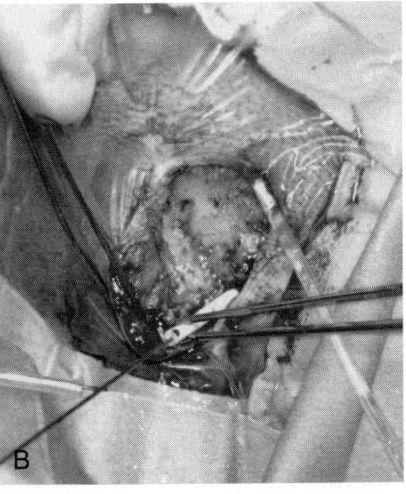

FIGURE 43–5 ■ *A,* Dissecting the shunt apparatus during a shunt revision with a cutting cautery, which will not harm the Silastic material. *B,* Applying cautery to the ventricular catheter stylet in order to free a stuck ventricular catheter.

placed. If there is doubt, the catheter can be gently manipulated, or a manometer using clear Silastic tubing and a straight connector can be attached to demonstrate free to-and-fro flow.

The lower end is then tested by connecting the clear Silastic tubing manometer to the valve and watching for spontaneous drainage. The distal system may need to be irrigated, but if flow is poor, the lower end should probably be explored. It is possible to reopen the same lower end incision and, using the cutting cautery, expose the tubing as well as its fibrous tract. Stay sutures on the tract allow the tubing to be removed from the abdomen, then the same or a new catheter can be passed down the same tract, avoiding a separate laparotomy.

If the upper end of the shunt is the culprit, the ventricular catheter should be gently removed and a new catheter introduced in rapid sequence, being careful not to lose too much CSF because the ventricles collapse. The standard landmarks are again employed, but as with an initial shunt insertion, ultrasound, endoscopy, or stereotaxis can be employed as aids. Preferably, one uses the metal stylet to direct the catheter, although with small ventricles, sliding the limp catheter down the old tract may suffice. One has no control over the trajectory of the catheter without the stylet, and astonishing catheter positions can result.

If the ventricular catheter is stuck, gently rotating the catheter may free it. Otherwise the metal stylet can be advanced down the lumen to the tip and cautery applied to the metal stylet while rotating the ventricular catheter (see Fig. 43–5B).[41] Badly stuck catheters should probably be left in place rather than produce a serious intraventricular hemorrhage. If hemorrhage does occur, manifested as frankly bloody CSF, the ventricle should be copiously irrigated with warm irrigation fluid. Failure of the CSF to clear should prompt placement of an external ventricular drain and abandoning the shunt revision.

Lower end obstruction is less common, and its cause should be always be sought. Distal slit valves may accumulate debris, which forms a column inside the shunt eventually blocking the slits. Unclogging the tip or just cutting it off may suffice. If the peritoneal catheter has fractured or is too short, the authors recommend replacing the entire aging system rather than piecing it together. The latter may result in further disruption in short order. Connectors should not be placed anywhere along the path of the peritoneal catheter below the skull in growing children. They become adherent to the surrounding tissues, and the catheter breaks with growth. If there appears to be an outflow problem into the peritoneum, the catheter should be removed to another site, rather than placing it down the same tract. If the problem is the valve or if one is changing a valve onto the same peritoneal catheter, care should be taken when pulling the peritoneal catheter up into the wound, then repassing it back down from above. It is possible for the catheter to kink or coil out of site, impeding shunt flow. It is preferable to expose the valve rather than extract and reinsert blindly.

## Shunt Infection

Shunt infection remains an important, distressing cause of shunt failure.[42, 43] Shunt infection puts the patient at in-

creased risk of intellectual impairment, the development of loculated CSF compartments, and even death. Despite intensive efforts to prevent shunt infection for decades, most centers report infection rates on the order of 5% to 10%. Although the mechanism of shunt contamination seems relatively straightforward, the exact intervention that has led to lower rates in some centers remains elusive.[43–45]

Shunt infection remains in some cases remarkably difficult to establish, even in retrospect. A simple working definition is unequivocal evidence of infection of the shunt equipment, the overlying wound, the CSF, or distal drainage site related to the shunt. *Unequivocal evidence* requires demonstration of the organism on Gram stain or culture from material in, on, or around the shunt or from fluid withdrawn from the shunt.

Shunt infection is probably best classified in terms of site:

1. Wound infection—an incision or shunt track with signs of inflammation, purulent discharge, and organisms seen on Gram stain or culture.
2. Meningitis—fever, meningismus, CSF leukocytosis, and organisms seen on Gram stain or culture.
3. Peritonitis—fever, abdominal tenderness (abdominal pseudocyst and abdominal abscess may present with mass with or without fever), and organisms seen on Gram stain or culture. For vascular shunts, findings are fever, leukocytosis, positive blood culture, with or without evidence of shunt nephritis or cor pulmonale.
4. Infected shunt apparatus—minimal signs of CSF contamination with bacteria recovered from purulent exudate in or on shunt material, Gram stain of CSF withdrawn from the shunt, or positive culture on fluid aspirated from the shunt under sterile conditions.[46] Organisms that grow only from the shunt equipment or CSF on broth culture are probably contaminants.

Most shunt infections appear within 2 months of surgery. Delayed infections with skin commensal organisms are possible.[47] Contamination of the shunt can occur from other surgical procedures that expose it, such as bladder augmentation with peritoneal shunts; however, it is unusual for remote sepsis to contaminate the shunt.

The most common organisms infecting CSF shunts are staphylococci—approximately 40% of shunt infections are caused by *Staphylococcus epidermidis* infections and 20% by *Staphylococcus aureus*.[42, 48, 49] Other species isolated from infected shunts include the coryneforms, streptococci, enterococci, aerobic gram-negative rods, and yeasts. Because these organisms are commonly part of the normal skin flora, and shunt infection usually occurs within 2 months of surgery, endogenous spread from the patient or surgical staff is the logical route of infection.

Bacteria colonize the shunt in the form of a continuous biofilm. This biofilm is composed of bacterial cells, either singly or in microcolonies, all embedded in an anionic matrix of bacterial exopolymers and trapped macromolecules.[50] The biofilm offers protection against many common antibacterial agents, including antibodies, white blood cells, surfactants, and antibiotics. For this reason, treatment of shunt infections by the exclusive use of systemic or intraventricular antibiotics[42, 51] has been ineffective.

## Clinical Presentation

Most shunt infections present within 2 months of shunt insertion.[26] The clinical features depend on the site of infection. Wound infections are usually manifested as fever reddening of the incision site or shunt tract; and, with progression, discharge of pus from the incision. In chronic wound infections, the shunt may become exposed as the wound breaks down. Table 43–2 indicates the clinical presentation of shunt infection in 28 patients from the shunt design trial.[26] Erosion of the thin skin in infants, particularly premature infants, from pressure also results in a wound infection. Any leak of CSF from the incision because of a high-resistance valve or poor distal flow also often results in contamination of the shunt and subsequent infection.

Patients with meningitis or ventriculitis usually present with fever, headache, or irritability and often with some neck stiffness if not nuchal rigidity. Peritonitis is less common. Patients typically present with fever, anorexia or vomiting, and abdominal tenderness. The severity of the symptoms depends to some extent on the infecting organism. Patients infected with S. epidermidis may look remarkably well and may have intermittent fever and irritability only. They may also present with signs of a typical shunt obstruction without fever or leukocytosis. Patients with abdominal pseudocysts (which are invariably infected) may present with a mass only. Small pseudocysts may be difficult to detect on abdominal examination. Historically, patients with ventriculoatrial shunts, in addition to presenting with signs of a septicemia, could manifest shunt nephritis or cor pulmonale.

The infection often involves more than one compartment or progresses to multiple compartments, as in a patient who develops a wound infection that progresses to meningitis. Shunts have been demonstrated to be impervious to bacterial migration across the shunt wall, so that spread occurs along the inside or outside the shunt. Although the possibility of retrograde bacterial movement up the lumen of the shunt has been disputed, clear evidence of spread of infection from the peritoneal cavity to the brain has been reported.

In terms of differential diagnosis, all patients with suspected shunt infection should have a thorough history and physical examination to rule out other possible infections or identify possible sources of infection. This differential diagnosis is particularly important in children, in whom any of the common childhood febrile illnesses can resemble a shunt infection, such as otitis media and, particularly in myelomeningocele patients, urinary tract infection. Patients with an uninfected shunt obstruction can have nuchal rigidity resulting from tonsillar herniation and occasionally a low-grade fever.

## Diagnostic Tests

Routine blood tests frequently reveal a polymorphonuclear leukocytosis. Blood culture is perhaps less important in patients with ventriculoperitoneal shunts but should be performed in febrile patients. Culture of the urine or other obvious sites of infections, for example, the wound, should also be taken. Plain film examination of the shunt system reveals whether the shunt system is still intact, whether an abdominal viscus may have been perforated, and whether or not there are any extraneous pieces of shunt equipment from previous revisions that may also be contaminated. A CT or MRI scan of the head is also important to display the size of the ventricles not only as part of determining whether or not the shunt is obstructed, but also how the size and configuration of the ventricles may influence decisions to remove the shunt and insert an external ventricular drain (EVD). Placing an EVD in a patient with a functioning but infected shunt with slit ventricles may be quite difficult. Rarely, evidence of ventriculitis or even more uncommonly brain abscess may be revealed on cerebral images.[52, 53] Abdominal ultrasound should be performed in any patient with abdominal pain or tenderness or a mass or in patients suspected of having a distal obstruction.

All patients without obvious wound infection or cutaneously extruded hardware should have the shunt system aspirated through an existing reservoir. Examination of the CSF for cell count, Gram stain, and culture confirms the diagnosis of shunt infection and quickly gives an index of the probable infecting organism. Shunt aspiration should be done with meticulous aseptic technique so as not to contaminate a shunt system that is, in fact, sterile or to introduce a second organism in shunts that are already infected. Shunt aspiration provides a high diagnostic yield of shunt infection of approximately 95% and is quite safe. Lumbar puncture or ventricular puncture gives a much lower yield (7% to 26%). Although CSF leukocytosis of 50 to 200 cells per ml, is common, a normal CSF count may not rule out a colonized shunt, and CSF protein and glucose are often normal. In patients with a wound infection, care should be taken not to contaminate the interior of the shunt when aspirating the collection surrounding the shunt system.

Because about 30% of patients who prove to be infected also have a shunt obstruction, at the time of surgery, ventricular CSF should be resampled. Sending all the hardware to the microbiology laboratory results in overdiagnosis of shunt infections because skin commensals contaminating the shunt during removal show up on broth culture. It is recommended that any purulent material on the shunt be swabbed for microscopy and culture. Subsequently a local area of the shunt should be swabbed with alcohol and fluid aspirated from the lumen of the shunt with a sterile syringe and needle. If no aspirate is obtained, the shunt component should be irrigated with sterile saline.

## Treatment

Shunt removal with interval antibiotic treatment (usually with external ventricular drainage) carries the highest shunt infection cure rate and the lowest mortality rate.[51] CSF shunt removal with immediate replacement carries an almost equal shunt infection cure rate with a higher morbidity and mortality rate. Antibiotic treatment alone has the lowest cure rate and the highest mortality rate. These findings seem sensible given what is now known about bacterial biofilms. Every attempt should be made to remove all existing hardware, even lost ventricular and peritoneal catheters. These can act as a nidus for a repeat infection after treatment.

Normally the EVD is left in place for approximately 1 week. This time provides an opportunity to examine the CSF daily, to verify that the CSF has become sterile, and to verify that the antibiotics in use are appropriate given the organism's antibiotic sensitivity. Intraventricular antibiotic injection and antibiotic level measurement can also be performed with an EVD. At the time of shunt reinsertion after an interval EVD, the EVD is usually clamped for 8 to 12 hours (provided that the patient can tolerate it) to allow the ventricles to expand and facilitate ventricular cannulation with the new shunt.

Organisms that cause meningitis in the general population and that infect patients with shunts or cause hydrocephalus and are discovered at time of shunt insertion can usually be treated with antibiotics alone. This includes *Haemophilus influenzae* and *Streptococcus pneumoniae*.[54, 55] Incumbent in this form of treatment is that the CSF be resampled to verify sterilization. Failure to clear the CSF within 48 to 72 hours should prompt removal of the shunt equipment.

Given the considerable morbidity, let alone financial cost, of shunt infections, prevention is the leading consideration for the future. Several studies have instituted procedures aimed at risk reduction (such as restricting operating room personnel, operating early in the day, soaking the shunt in antibiotics, and using prophylactic antibiotics) and reported a reduction in shunt infection from 7.75% to 0.17%[44] in one series and from 12.9% to 3.8%[56] in another, using historical controls from the same institution. These studies leave doubt as to which of the deliberately altered factors is important.

## Management of the Difficult Shunt Patient

Difficult shunt patients seem to fall into two general categories. One category is patients with intractable symptoms, usually headache, in whom doubt about the functional status of the shunt exists.[57–59] The other is patients who present repeatedly with shunt malfunction for no apparent reason. Both sets of patients can be difficult to manage. The patients often otherwise lead normal lives and are completely disabled or continuously in the hospital with their shunt problem.

A detailed history, including all the previous shunt surgeries, is mandatory. Previous operating room notes from the hospital where the surgery was done should be sought. The relevant imaging, which should be related to the patient's clinical status at the time the images were obtained, should also be carefully studied. This whole process often requires creating a spreadsheet or log to keep track of the multiple interventions. All culture reports should also be sought, looking for an unrecognized or partially treated infection. A thorough physical examination, including the shunt equipment, follows. Current imaging should be complete, including plain X-ray films of the shunt equipment.

In patients with chronic headache, an idea of whether the headache is postural can often be obtained by the history. Other exacerbating and relieving symptoms as well as concomitant features should be sought. Determining the functional status of the shunt by pumping the reservoir is notoriously unreliable.[39] If the shunt's functional status by

standard imaging is still uncertain, a flow study using a radioisotope or other contrast agent should be done. If the reservoir is above the valve, reflux into the ventricles confirms that the upper end is patent. Otherwise, it may be more difficult to decide which end is blocked. Sitting the patient up or pumping the reservoir helps to determine what effect these manipulations have on the shunt system. Collection of contrast material in a localized cyst in the abdomen can also be seen with this technique and confirmed with ultrasound. These flow studies are not infallible, and both false-positive and false-negative results are possible.

If all information suggests the shunt is working, intracranial pressure monitoring is usually the next step. Using a separate intraparenchymal probe is warranted because it provides the most accurate information. The patient should be monitored for 48 to 72 hours to ensure that prolonged periods of sleep and wakefulness, in various postural positions, are recorded. The patient or family should also keep a timed log to record any headaches, so that they can be related to the pressure recordings. Slightly negative intracranial pressure when upright is normal. In patients with symptomatic postural hypotension, large negative pressures associated with the headache are sought. Patients with slit ventricle syndrome usually have plateau waves of 20 or 30 minutes with pressures frequently greater than 20 mm Hg and usually when asleep at night.

Patients with postural hypotension usually respond to placement of either a siphon-reducing device or a flow-limiting valve. Verification that both ends of the shunt are functioning properly at surgery is mandatory before replacing the valve. Leaving the pressure monitor in place for a few days ensures that the new valve is functioning as expected. If the patient continues to experience headache, the relationship to the new pressure profile can help to sort this out.

Patients with slit ventricle syndrome are more difficult to deal with.[60–64] The authors replace any standard differential valve with a flow-limiting valve, provided that the system is shown to be completely patent at surgery. This action often dilates the ventricles slightly and, more importantly, demonstrates progressive decline in plateau waves during sleep.[25] If that fails, one is usually faced with expanding the intracranial compartment. Subtemporal decompression has not stood the test of time for this condition, and although much more extensive, a cranial vault expansion is usually required. One can temporize before embarking on this extensive surgical procedure with antimigrainous drugs (which can be tried before any of these interventions) while the patient and surgeon reconsider the wisdom of this operation.

In patients in whom the pressure monitoring is normal or bears no relationship to headache, surgical restraint is wise. These patients are unlikely to be helped by further shunt surgery, and each attempt increases the risk that they will suffer a surgical complication that will only exacerbate the situation. Assessment by a chronic pain or headache specialist team consisting of physicians and psychiatrists or psychologists is important, particularly if the patient is dependent on narcotic analgesics. Various forms of psychotherapy may dramatically improve the patient's condition. As a last resort, particularly if the opinion of the team is that the headache is organic, the shunt can be explored or changed, but patients have to realize that likely nothing will be found.

In patients with repetitive obstruction for no apparent reason, every search for a possible indolent infection should be made, including anaerobic cultures. Encysted fluid collections in the abdominal cavity, even in the absence of positive cultures, strongly point to an infection. If there is any doubt, the whole shunt system, including any retained hardware (the exception being fragments in the chest wall not in communication with the abdomen) should be removed and an external drain placed. A new system should be placed at new sites in the head and abdomen.

If there are repetitive proximal obstructions, the ventricular catheter may be traveling down a sheath of gliotic tissue to the same site, only to be replugged. Placing the ventricular catheter under ultrasound or endoscopic guidance into a completely different site (even the opposite ventricle) obviates this problem. If the patients have slit ventricles when the shunt is functioning, changing the valve to a flow-limiting one may slightly expand the ventricles and possibly lead to a reduced rate of obstruction. Another possibility is to place a programmable shunt, so that the opening pressure can be changed once implanted.[65] Finally, particularly if the patient has a history of aqueduct stenosis, an endoscopic third ventriculostomy (ETV) may render the patient shunt-free entirely, as discussed in the next section.[66] Dissatisfaction with the long-term outcome and significant failure rates of conventional CSF shunting systems has resulted in a resurgence of interest in the earliest form of treatment for hydrocephalus, ventriculostomy.[67, 68]

## ENDOSCOPIC THIRD VENTRICULOSTOMY

### History

The earliest endoscopic treatment for hydrocephalus was choroid plexus fulguration performed by Lespinasse in 1910.[69] Dandy[70] subsequently described an open technique for third ventriculostomy for the treatment of noncommunicating hydrocephalus. A percutaneous ventriculostomy technique employing an endoscope was first described by Mixter in 1923.[71] Fay and Grant[71a] published the first intraventricular photographs that same year, providing the first visual record of endoscopic anatomy. Because of the limited illumination and large size of early endoscopes, open ventriculostomy procedures as well as percutaneous fluoroscopic and later CT-guided techniques remained popular for many years. Hopkins provided the technical advances necessary for the revival of neuroendoscopy.[71b] Hopkins' innovative solid rod lens and coherent quartz fiber lens systems underlie the basic design of all modern rigid and flexible endoscopic systems. The improved optics and illumination and reduced size of modern endoscopes have greatly increased their utility and reduced associated morbidity and mortality.

### Patient Selection

Third ventriculostomy is intended to treat noncommunicating hydrocephalus with patent subarachnoid spaces and adequate CSF absorption. Results of endoscopic third ventriculostomy (ETV) are related to the cause of hydrocephalus encountered as well as clinical and radiographic features of the individual patient. Table 43–3 lists causes of obstructive hydrocephalus divided according to reported success rates of ETV (see outcomes later). Patients with acquired aqueductal stenosis or tumors obstructing third or fourth ventricular outflow have demonstrated the highest success rates, exceeding 75% in carefully selected series of patients.[72–75] Previously shunted patients with or without myelomeningocele and patients with congenital aqueductal stenosis or cystic abnormalities leading to obstruction (i.e., arachnoid cyst, Dandy-Walker malformations) have shown intermediate response.[73, 74, 76–78] Further study of this intermediate group is likely to identify subgroups with higher success rates. Infants presenting with hydrocephalus associated with myelomeningocele, hemorrhage, or infection have demonstrated poor response to ventriculostomy,[72, 79, 80] and despite limited reports of success in such patients,[74, 76, 77, 81–84] they are more controversial candidates for this procedure. The procedure is not advisable in patients who have undergone prior radiation therapy because of the extremely poor response rates, altered anatomy (i.e., thickened third ventricular floor), and increased risk of bleeding.[74, 76, 80]

Several clinical features may influence the outcome of third ventriculostomy (Table 43–4). There appears to be a significant association between increasing patient age and a more favorable outcome.[73, 74, 76, 85] Evidence suggests that this association applies to the age at which hydrocephalus initially developed as well as age at the time of ventriculostomy.[74, 85] Several studies show success rates of approximately 50% in patients younger that 2 years old, regardless of cause.[73, 74, 77] Results are even poorer in patients younger than 6 months old.[85]

Many studies have demonstrated a trend toward more successful ventriculostomy outcome in patients with existing shunt systems.[73, 77, 85] In fact, third ventriculostomy

---

TABLE 43–3 ■ **VENTRICULOSTOMY SUCCESS RATES BY HYDROCEPHALUS CAUSE**

High success rates (≥75%)
   Acquired aqueductal stenosis
   Tumor obstructing ventricular outflow
      Tectal
      Pineal
      Thalamic
      Intraventricular
Intermediate success rates (50%–70%)
   Myelomeningocele (previously shunted, older patients)
   Congenital aqueductal stenosis
   Cystic abnormalities obstructing CSF flow
      Arachnoid cysts
      Dandy-Walker malformation
   Previously shunted patients with difficulties
      Slit ventricle syndrome
      Recurrent or intractable shunt infections
      Recurrent or intractable shunt malfunctions
Low success rates (<50%)
   Myelomeningocele (previously unshunted, neonatal patients)
   Posthemorrhagic hydrocephalus
   Postinfectious hydrocephalus (excluding aqueductal stenosis of infectious origin)

TABLE 43–4 ■ **FAVORABLE CLINICAL AND RADIOGRAPHIC FEATURES FOR ENDOSCOPIC THIRD VENTRICULOSTOMY**

**Clinical**
Cause of hydrocephalus in high or intermediate success group (see Table 43–3)
Age >6 months at time of hydrocephalus diagnosis
Age >6 months at time of procedure
No prior radiation therapy
No history of hemorrhage or meningitis
Patient previously shunted

**Radiographic**
Clear evidence of ventricular noncommunication
  Obstructive pattern of HCP
  Aqueductal anatomic obstruction
  Lack of aqueductal flow void on T$_2$ MRI
Favorable third ventricular anatomy
  Width and foramen of Monro sufficient to accommodate endoscope
    Rigid > 7 mm
    Flexible > 4 mm
  Thinned floor of third ventricle
  Downward bulging floor, draped over clivus
  Basilar posterior to mammillary bodies
Absence of structural anomalies impeding procedure
  AVM or tumor obscuring third ventricular floor
  Enlarged massa intermedia
  Insufficient space between mammillary bodies and basilar and the clivus
  Basilar artery ectasia

AVM, arteriovenous malformation; HCP, hydrocephalus; MRI, magnetic resonance imaging.

has been found to be useful in the treatment of intractable shunt infections and malfunctions and even slit ventricle syndrome refractory to other treatments.[66, 72, 76, 86–89] Other series of ventriculostomy in previously shunted patients have been less promising.[78, 90] These contradictory results may reflect the mix of patients in small series. The improved outcome in previously shunted patients is commonly attributed to increased CSF absorptive capacity; however, the effect of the shunt itself on CSF absorption is difficult to distinguish from the effect of increased age in these patients.

Preoperative assessment of CSF absorptive capacity has been advocated by some authors,[91, 92] but these techniques have not been widely accepted.[74, 85] Because the patency of CSF pathways is one of the assumptions on which the procedure is based, a preoperative CSF absorption study would be invaluable in identifying patients who would likely benefit from ventriculostomy. The observed delay between operation and decrease in ventricular size (see outcomes), however, suggests that CSF absorption may increase slowly postventriculostomy. Therefore, preoperative assessment of CSF absorptive capacity may fail to identify all appropriate patients.[74] Until an accurate functional predictor of this capacity is practical, radiographic assessment of the obstructive pattern of hydrocephalus by MRI will likely remain the preoperative diagnostic procedure of choice.

Table 43–4 depicts preoperative radiographic criteria frequently cited for improving outcome and limiting morbid-

ity of ETV. Preoperative MRI optimally demonstrates all relevant anatomic features and should be obtained for all proposed third ventriculostomy patients. Initially, confirmation of noncommunicating hydrocephalus of favorable cause should be established by the pattern of ventricular dilatation. Anatomic obstruction of CSF pathways between the aqueduct and the fourth ventricular outflow foramina may be visible on T$_2$ or T$_1$ contrast images. Additionally, T$_2$ images should reveal absence of the aqueductal CSF flow void frequently present in normal individuals.

Once the patient's suitability for the procedure has been established, the neurosurgeon must clarify the details of third ventricular anatomy that are likely to affect morbidity. First, the width of the third ventricle and diameter of the foramen of Monro must be sufficient to accommodate the endoscope of choice (see technique). Additionally the thickness of the third ventricular floor and the anatomy of the proposed puncture site in relationship to vital structures, particularly the basilar artery and its branches, must be assessed. A downward bulging third ventricular floor draped over the clivus has been cited as a prerequisite for this procedure in the past, but others have not found this to be necessary.[74, 80] Ultimately the surgeon must be satisfied that there is no structural lesion (i.e., tumor of arteriovenous malformation) or anatomic variation that would render the procedure unduly difficult or hazardous. In cases of doubt, it is reasonable to visualize the floor of the third ventricle and abandon the procedure if the floor is unsuitable.

## Technique

An ever-increasing variety of endoscopic equipment is currently available for neuroendoscopic procedures. For uncomplicated third ventriculostomy, a 0- or 30-degree rigid scope offers superior optics and anatomic orientation. The Gaab endoscope (Johnson & Johnson, Randolph, MA), inserted through a 7-mm rigid cannula, provides the advantage of two working ports with a third for continuous irrigation. A 4-mm flexible steerable endoscope (Johnson & Johnson, Randolph, MA) introduced through a No.12 French peel-away sheath allows for improved maneuverability within the ventricular system, at the expense of some image quality. Flexible scopes are useful for accessing more remote portions of the ventricular system (i.e., pineal recess, aqueduct). Several miniature fiberoptic endoscopes are also now available. These scopes can be inserted through a standard ventricular catheter; however, their inferior optics and lack of an irrigating or working channel limit their potential applications (i.e., ventricular catheter placement).

A miniature video camera is attached to the endoscope, and orientation is adjusted before insertion. The monitor should be placed at a comfortable distance and height for viewing throughout the case. Use of the camera allows the senior surgeon, trainee, and operating room staff to view the entire case, greatly enhancing the opportunities for learning without added morbidity.

Adequate continuous irrigation is imperative for proper visualization, particularly if bleeding is encountered. This irrigation is provided by running Ringer's lactate through blood-warming apparatus, with a shut-off valve on the scope. An uninterrupted release pathway for irrigation fluid is equally essential to avoid dangerous elevations of intracranial pressure. A separate channel for fluid release can be intermittently or partially blocked to provide transient pressure tamponade for control of bleeding. Direct pressure using the scope cannula itself can also be useful for homeostasis.

ETV can be performed with either a flexible or a rigid endoscope. The patient is positioned supine in a horseshoe headrest with the neck flexed 15 to 20 degrees. A bur hole is made over the right coronal suture, 2 to 2.5 cm lateral to the midline. Optimal positioning of the bur hole varies slightly depending on the proposed trajectory as determined from preoperative MRI. The bur hole is placed more anteriorly to provide access to the posterior third ventricle if desired. The dura is opened in cruciate fashion, and the pial surface is coagulated and incised. A 3-mm diameter, blunt-tipped brain needle is inserted into the right frontal horn, directed toward the foramen of Monro. After CSF sampling and intracranial pressure assessment, the needle is withdrawn, and the same tract is used for insertion of the endoscope sheath or cannula. This technique allows for blunt separation of the ependymal layer and progressive enlargement of this opening, minimizing ependymal bleeding, a common cause of poor intraventricular visualization.

Once insertion of the endoscope into the lateral ventricle has been achieved, the foramen of Monro is located by identification of the choroid plexus and septal and thalamostriate veins (Figs. 43–6A, B and 43–7A). After passage of the endoscope through the foramen of Monro, the optic chiasm, infundibulum, mamillary bodies, massa intermedia, and aqueduct can all be observed along the floor of the third ventricle from anterior to posterior, depending on trajectory (see Figs. 43–6C, D and 43–7B, G). A flexible scope is generally necessary to view the lamina terminalis, suprapineal recess, or third ventricular roof. In cases of obstructive hydrocephalus, a diamond-shaped transparent membrane is commonly seen between the mamillary bodies and infundibulum. The dorsum sellae, clivus, and basilar artery are often visible through this membrane (see Fig. 43–7B). This area of the third ventricular floor between the clivus and the basilar artery is the ideal site for third ventriculostomy.

Numerous methods of perforating the third ventricular floor have been described that employ the scope itself, a cautery unit, laser, or endoscopic instrument.[73, 76, 80, 93–95] The authors use a closed blunt biopsy forceps for initial fenestration and a 4-French Fogarty balloon catheter for enlargement of the ventriculostomy (see Fig. 43–7C, D, E). Care is taken to inflate the balloon only under direct vision within the opening because blindly withdrawing an inflated balloon from the basal cisterns carries a significant risk of injury to perforating vessels. After adequate enlargement of the ventriculostomy, the scope can be advanced to inspect the prepontine and interpeduncular cisterns (see Fig. 43–7F).

Postoperative management of patients after ETV must be individualized to address the unique preoperative and intraoperative details of each case. Patients with subacute

hydrocephalus presentations and uneventful procedures may require only short-term postoperative observation, whereas patients with acute presentations or significant intraoperative bleeding often require an external ventricular drain with continuous intracranial pressure monitoring in an intensive care unit setting. Patients undergoing a simultaneous endoscopic tumor biopsy or removal of a prior existing shunt system require particularly close observation and monitoring.

In the past, postoperative CSF shunting has been recommended to promote expansion of pericerebral CSF spaces and to improve absorption.[81, 83, 90] Compelling evidence suggests, however, that CSF flow through the ventriculostomy maintains its patency, and shunts can lead to closure of the opening.[72, 90] The authors do not recommend a coexisting CSF shunt and ETV.

## Outcome

The goal of ETV and, to date, the best objectively quantifiable measure of a successful outcome, is shunt independence. ETV has yielded a higher success rate with lower morbidity and mortality than earlier methods of third ventriculostomy. Mortality rates for open ventriculostomy procedures varied between 5% and 27% with success rates of 37% to 75%.[11, 72, 80, 82, 90, 96] Percutaneous X-ray and later CT-guided techniques reduced this mortality rate to 2% to 7% with a 44% to 75% rate of shunt independence.[72, 79, 80, 83, 90, 97] Studies using modern endoscopic techniques and equipment, with or without stereotactic CT or MRI guidance, have reported low morbidity (3% to 12%) and essentially no mortality, with success rates greater than 75% for carefully selected patient groups. Table 43–5 depicts the results of ETV studies with success rates by cause where this information is available. The current challenge is to define appropriate indications and devise objective measures for preoperative and postoperative assessment of these patients.

One of the most confusing aspects of outcome evaluation in ETV patients is the failure of the ventricles to return to normal size. Most studies report a gradual decrease in the ventricular size over months to years postoperatively, with resolution of periventricular edema and increased extracerebral spaces, coinciding with clinical improvement.[72–75, 90, 94] One series of patients treated with either CSF shunts or ETV showed no difference in intellectual outcome despite enlarged ventricles in the ETV group.[94] Multiple authors have reported *late failures*, in which the ventriculostomy closes sometimes years postoperatively.[74, 86] Radiographic evaluation of suspected closure is confounded by the presence of persistently enlarged ventricles, and closure must often be suspected based on clinical evidence alone.

Studies detailing the serial measurements of multiple radiographic indices of ventricular size postoperatively show that the third ventricular size responds more quickly (usually within 3 months) than the lateral ventricular size (2 years).[98, 99] Additionally, third ventricular size appears to correlate most closely with outcome in these patients.[75, 98, 99]

Several newer modalities appear promising as potential objective measures of ventriculostomy function. MRI de-

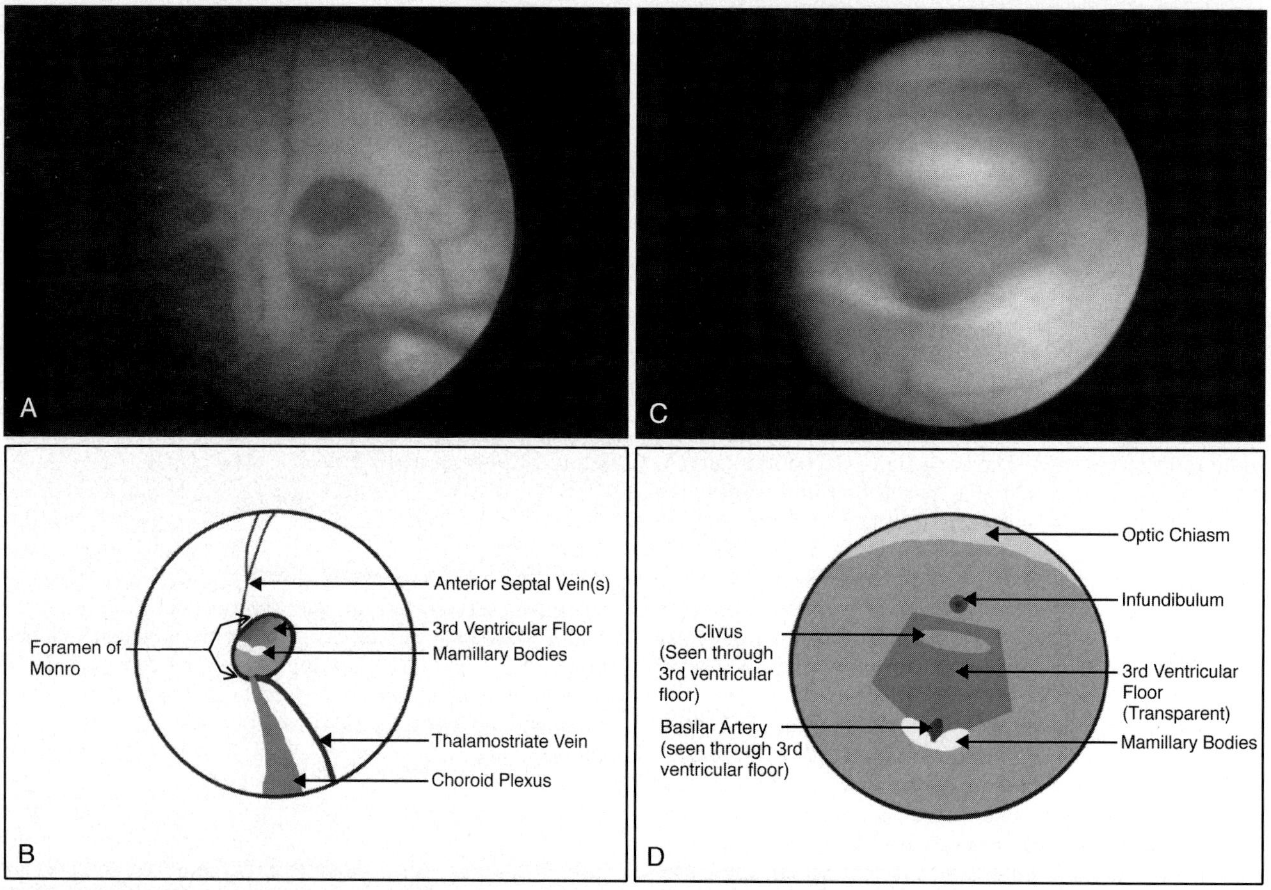

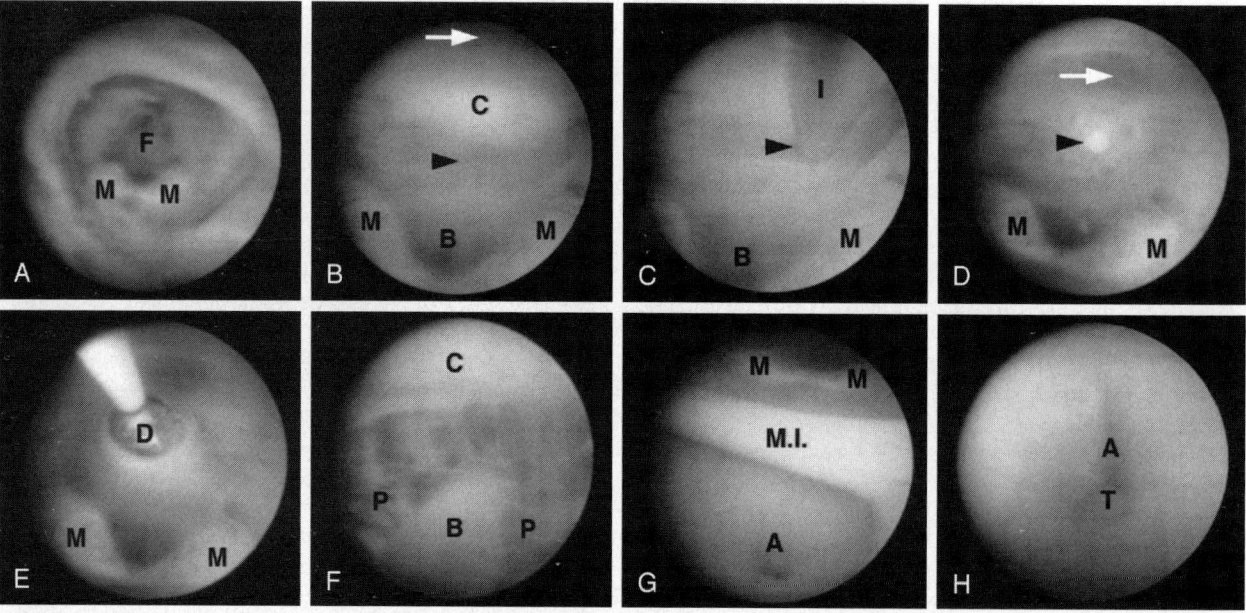

**FIGURE 43–6** ■ Anatomy of the foramen of Monro as viewed from the lateral ventricle, operative photograph *(A)*, and the diagram *(B)*. A close-up view of anatomy of the third ventricular floor, an operative photograph *(C)*, and a schematic diagram *(D)*.

**FIGURE 43–7** ■ A series of operative photographs demonstrating the endoscopic third ventriculostomy procedure. *A,* Entrance is through the foramen of Monro from the right lateral ventricle. *B,* A close-up of the third ventricular floor; an *arrowhead* depicts the proposed ventriculostomy site. *C,* Blunt forceps piercing the third ventricular floor. *D,* View of the initial ventriculostomy opening. *E,* Dilatation of the ventriculostomy using a Fogarty balloon catheter. *F,* View of basal cisterns through the ventriculostomy opening. *G,* View of the mid-third ventricular floor. *H,* View of the aqueduct demonstrating an obstruction by a tectal tumor. Mamillary bodies (M); floor of third ventricle (F); clivus (C); basilar artery (B); ventriculostomy site *(black arrowhead)*; blunt forceps (I); infundibular recess *(white arrow)*; Fogarty balloon (D); basilar perforators (P); massa intermedia (M.I.); aqueduct (A); tectal tumor (T).

## TABLE 43–5 ■ SUMMARY OF ENDOSCOPIC THIRD VENTRICULOSTOMY TRIALS

| Author/Year | Procedure | Patients (n) | Overall Success | Morbidity | Procedure Abort Rate | Follow-Up (mean) | Success (Shunt Independence) by Cause (n) | | | | | | |
|---|---|---|---|---|---|---|---|---|---|---|---|---|---|
| | | | | | | | AS | MMC | Tumor | SVS | Shunt | PHH | Other |
| Hirsch et al/1986[106] | ETV | 114 | 70% | — | — | — | 70% (114) | — | — | — | — | — | — |
| Jones et al/1990[76] | ETV | 24 | 50% | 8% | 16% | NS | 57% (14) | 40% (5) | 67% (3) | — | — | — | 0% (2) |
| Kelly/1991[72] | SETV | 16 | 94% | 0% | 0% | 1–5 yr (3.5 yr) | 94% (16) | — | — | — | — | — | — |
| Dalrymple and Kelly/1992[107] | SETV | 85 | 87% | — | — | 1–66 mo | — | — | — | — | — | — | — |
| Jones et al/1992[73] | ETV | 54 | 60% | 7% | 9% | 3 mo–7 yr (27 mo) | 65% (31) | 40% (10) | 86% (7) | — | 75% (4) | 0% (2) | — |
| Goodman/1993[108] | MRETV | 3 | 100% | 0% | 0% | 6–14 mo (10 mo) | 100% (3) | — | — | — | — | — | — |
| Jones et al/1994[74] | ETV | 101 | 61% | 5% | 6% | NS | 78% (9) | 52% (21) | 81% (16) | — | — | — | — |
| Sainte-Rose and Chumas/1996[75] | ETV | 82 | 81% | NS | NS | (1.8 yr) | 67% (111) | — | > 80% (53) | — | — | — | — |
| | RTV and STV | 104 | 68% | — | — | (5.7 yr) | — | — | — | — | — | — | — |
| Teo and Jones/1996[77] | ETV | 69 | 72% | 3% | 9% | 1–17 yr (32 mo) | — | 72% (69) | — | — | — | — | — |
| Goumnerova and Frim/1997[101] | ETV | 23 | 73% | 9% | — | 7–44 mo (17 mo) | 69% (13) | — | 71% (7) | — | — | 0% (1) | 100% (2) |
| Baskin et al/1998[66] | ETV | 16 | 63% | 12% | — | (18.8 mo) | — | — | — | 63% (16) | — | — | — |
| Brockmeyer et al/1998[78] | ETV | 97 | 49% | 6% | 26% | 15–69 mo (24.2 mo) | 56% (16) | 50% (16) | 61% (18) | 50% (4) | — | 0% (4) | 38% (13) |

ETV, endoscopic third ventriculostomy; SETV, stereotactic (CT-guided) endoscopic third ventriculostomy; MRETV, stereotactic (MR-guided) endoscopic third ventriculostomy; RTV, x-ray-guided third ventriculostomy; STV, stereotactic (CT-guided) third ventriculostomy; AS, aqueductal stenosis; MMC, myelomeningocele; SVS, slit-ventricle syndrome; shunt, intractable shunt infection or malfunction; PHH, posthemorrhagic hydrocephalus; NS, not significant.

tection of T2 flow void around the ventriculostomy has been correlated with clinical outcome in ETV.[100–102] This observation has proven most helpful in confirming ventriculostomy patency postoperatively, particularly in patients with persistent ventriculomegaly.[101, 102] Actual quantification of flow velocity through ventriculostomies has also been demonstrated by phase-contrast MRI and Doppler ultrasonography.[103, 104] Intraventricular pressure has been observed to return to normal over 3 months in a patient after third ventriculostomy who underwent concurrent implantation of a telemetric intracranial pressure monitor.[105] It is hoped that methods of quantifying ventriculostomy function will allow neurosurgeons to refine further the techniques necessary to improve outcome. Radiographic confirmation may also help define indications with more subjective outcomes, for example, the observation of less fulminant shunt malfunctions in patients after ventriculostomy.[76]

## Complications

Several series of ETV report no mortality and low morbidity (see Table 43–5).[66, 72–78, 101, 106–108] The most common serious complications are related to structures in and around the floor of the third ventricle. In patients with aqueductal obstruction, the third ventricular floor is usually thinned out and transparent, with the hypothalamic nuclei displaced laterally. When the floor is not thinned or the ventriculostomy is not performed at the preferred midline site, injury to the hypothalamus or bleeding can result.

These complications have been attributed to direct pressure from the perforating instrument, elevated CSF temperature from cautery or the light source, or distention of the third ventricle from continuous irrigation without adequate drainage.[75] Reported complications from injury to this area include the syndrome of inappropriate secretion of antidiuretic hormone, diabetes insipidus, loss of thirst, amenorrhea, and trance-like states.[106, 109] These complications are usually transient. Bradycardia is also observed on occasion when perforating a thickened third ventricular floor, and a near-fatal cardiac arrest has been reported.[110] Transient postoperative fevers, which frequently occur in these patients, are commonly attributed to irritation of the ependyma from blood or manipulation of the hypothalamus.[94]

Other structures at risk in this area include the third and sixth cranial nerves, fornix, and caudate. Injuries to all of these structures, usually transient or clinically silent, have been reported.[106, 109] The major life-threatening risk during the procedure is injury to the basilar artery and its branches. The basilar bifurcation is usually visible through the thinned third ventricular floor. Extreme caution should be taken to avoid injuring these vessels, particularly when preoperative imaging suggests a thickened ventricular floor or aberrant location (i.e., anterior to the mamillary bodies) of these vessels. The authors perform the initial fenestration with a blunt instrument rather than the cautery or laser to minimize the risk of arterial damage. Injury to these vessels can result in catastrophic hemorrhage, stroke, or pseudoaneurysm formation.[111]

Other routine complications, associated with most neurosurgical procedures, have also been observed. Superficial wound infections as well as meningitis and ventriculitis, subdural hematomas, and CSF leaks have all been described.[75, 106, 109]

## OTHER ENDOSCOPIC APPLICATIONS

Endoscopic techniques, with and without the addition of stereotactic assistance, are increasingly used for treating a variety of conditions and complications related to hydrocephalus. In stereotactic-guided techniques, the scope target can be selected and intervening structures (i.e., the foramen of Monro) chosen as part of the trajectory.[72, 112] CT-based or MRI-based frame systems or the newer frameless stereotactic systems can be easily adapted for use with a rigid endoscope. These systems are particularly useful when planning the trajectory in patients with small ventricles, distorted anatomy as a result of prior shunting procedures or infection, or approaching intraventricular lesions. They are also helpful when operating in large ventricles where the light is diffused, in loculated ventricles where there is essentially no recognizable anatomy, and in CSF turbid from debris or blood when scope image is poor. Collapse of the ventricular system or cystic cavities can rapidly render the preoperative imaging data useless.

Intracranial cysts and loculated regions of the ventricular system have been successfully treated with these techniques.[93, 113, 114] Endoscopic procedures for colloid cysts and suprasellar arachnoid cysts have been particularly successful.[115–117] Several studies have examined the role of ventriculoscopic shunt catheter placement[118, 119]; however, prospective, randomized study of the usefulness of this procedure is under way. Likewise, treatment of intraventricular tumors and their associated hydrocephalus with endoscopic techniques requires further study, particularly in midline posterior fossa tumors.[75] Ventriculoscopic procedures for pineal, suprasellar, and tectal lesions have proven most useful to date.[120–123] Further study and technical refinements will lead to many more potential uses for these procedures in the treatment of hydrocephalus and its associated causes. The challenge for neurosurgeons is to define the indications and outcomes and refine the techniques for safely performing these useful procedures.

## REFERENCES

1. Bondurant CP, Jimenez DF: Epidemiology of cerebrospinal fluid shunting. Pediatr Neurosurg 23:254–259, 1995.
2. Bondurant CP, Jimenez DF: Epidemiology of cerebrospinal fluid shunting. Pediatr Neurosurg 23:254–258, 1997.
3. Aronyk KE: The history and classification of hydrocephalus. Neurosurg Clin North Am 4:599–609, 1993.
4. McCullough DC: A history of the treatment of hydrocephalus. Concepts Neurosurg 3:1–10, 1990.
5. Fisher RG: Surgery of the Congenital Anomalies. Baltimore: Williams & Wilkins, 1951.
6. Davidoff LE: Treatment of hydrocephalus. Arch Surg 18:1737–1762, 1929.
7. Sharpe W: The operative treatment of hydrocephalus: A preliminary report of forty-one patients. Am J Med Sci 153:563–571, 1917.
8. Cushing H: The special field of neurological surgery. Cleveland Med J 4:1–25, 1905.
9. Ferguson AH: Intraperitoneal diversion of the cerebrospinal fluid in cases of hydrocephalus. N Y Med 67:902, 1898.
10. Nicholl JH: Case of hydrocephalus in which peritoneo-meningeal drainage has been carried out. Glasgow Med J 63:187–191, 1905.
11. Dandy WE: Diagnosis and treatment of strictures of the aqueduct of Sylvius (causing hydrocephalus). Arch Surg 51:1–14, 1945.
12. Mixter WJ: Ventriculoscopy and puncture of the floor of the third ventricle. Boston Medical and Surgical Journal 188:277–278, 1923.
13. Dandy WE: Extirpation of the choroid plexus of the lateral ventricles in communicating hydrocephalus. Ann Surg 68:569–579, 1918.
14. Torkildsen A: A new palliative operation in cases of inoperable occlusion of the sylvian aqueduct. Acta Chir Scand 82:117–124, 1939.
15. Nulsen FE, Spitz EB: Treatment of hydrocephalus by direct shunt from ventricle to jugular vein. Surg Forum 399–403, 1952.
16. Wallman LJ: Shunting for hydrocephalus: An oral history. Neurosurgery 11:308–313, 1982.
17. Pudenz RH: The surgical treatment of hydrocephalus—an historical review. Surg Neurol 15:15–26, 1981.
18. Fox JL, McCullough DC, Green RC: Effect of cerebrospinal fluid shunts on intracranial pressure and on cerebrospinal fluid dynamics. 2: A new technique of pressure measurements: Results and concepts. 3: A concept of hydrocephalus. J Neurol Neurosurg Psychiatry 36:302–312, 1973.
19. Fox JL, Portnoy HD, Shulte RR: Cerebrospinal fluid shunts: An experimental evaluation of flow rates and pressure values in the anti-siphon valve. Surg Neurol 1:299–302, 1973.
20. Drake JM, Sainte-Rose C: The Shunt Book. New York: Blackwell Scientific, 1995.
21. Watts C, Keith HD: Testing the hydrocephalus shunt valve. Childs Brain 10:217–228, 1983.
22. Chapman PH, Cosman ER, Arnold MA: The relationship between ventricular fluid pressure and body position in normal subjects and subjects with shunts: A telemetric study. Neurosurgery 26:181–189, 1990.
23. Horton D, Pollay M: Fluid flow performance of a new siphon-control device for ventricular shunts. J Neurosurg 72:926–932, 1990.
24. Portnoy HD, Schulte RR, Fox JL, et al: Anti-siphon and reversible occlusion valves for shunting in hydrocephalus and preventing post-shunt subdural hematomas. J Neurosurg 38:729–738, 1973.
25. Sainte-Rose C, Hooven MD, Hirsch JF: A new approach to the treatment of hydrocephalus. J Neurosurg 66:213–226, 1987.
26. Drake JM, Kestle J, Milner R, et al: Randomized trial of cerebrospinal fluid shunt valve design in pediatric hydrocephalus. Neurosurgery 43:294–305, 1998.
27. Langley JM, LeBlanc JC, Drake J, Milner R: Efficacy of antimicrobial prophylaxis in placement of cerebrospinal fluid shunts: Meta-analysis. Clin Infect Dis 17:98–103, 1993.
28. Horgan MA, Piatt JH Jr: Shaving of the scalp may increase the rate of infection in CSF shunt surgery. Pediatr Neurosurg 26:180–184, 1997.
29. Bierbauer KS, Storrs BB, McLone DG, et al: A prospective, randomized study of shunt function and infections as a function of shunt placement. Pediatr Neurosurg 16:287–291, 1990.
30. Tuli S, O'Hayon B, Drake JM, Kestle JRW: Change in ventricular size and effect of ventricular catheter placement in pediatric shunted hydrocephalus. Neurosurgery 1998 (in press).
31. Sanders DY, Summers R, DeRouen L: Symptomatic pleural collection of cerebrospinal fluid caused by a ventriculopleural shunt. South Med 90:345–346, 1997.
32. Beach C, Manthey DE: Tension hydrothorax due to ventriculopleural shunting. J Emerg Med 16:33–36, 1998.
33. Lam CH, Villemure JG: Comparison between ventriculoatrial and ventriculoperitoneal shunting in the adult population. Br J Neurosurg 11:43–48, 1997.
34. Lundar T, Langmoen IA, Hovind KH: Fatal cardiopulmonary complications in children treated with ventriculoatrial shunts. Childs Nerv Syst 7:215–217, 1991.
35. Decq P, Blanquet A, Yepes C: Percutaneous jugular placement of ventriculo-atrial shunts using a split sheath: Technical note. Acta Neurochir 136:92–94, 1995.
36. McGrail KM, Muzzi DA, Losasso TJ, Meyer FB: Ventriculoatrial shunt distal catheter placement using transesophageal echocardiography: Technical note [see comments]. Neurosurgery 30:747–749, 1992.
37. Szczerbicki MR, Michalak M: Echocardiographic placement of cardiac tube in ventriculoatrial shunt: Technical note. J Neurosurg 85:723–724, 1996.

38. Drake JM, Kestle J: Determining the best cerebrospinal fluid shunt valve design: The pediatric valve design trial. Neurosurgery 38:604–607, 1996.
39. Piatt JH Jr: Pumping the shunt revisited: A longitudinal study. Pediatr Neurosurg 25:73–76, 1996.
40. Vernet O, Farmer JP, Lambert R, Montes JL: Radionuclide shuntogram: Adjunct to manage hydrocephalic patients. J Nucl Med 37:406–410, 1996.
41. Steinbok P, Cochrane DD: Shunt removal by choroid plexus coagulation (Letter; comment). J Neurosurg 85:981, 1996.
42. Drake JM, Kulkarni AV: Cerebrospinal fluid shunt infections. Neurosurg Q 3:283–294, 1993.
43. Borgbjerg BM, Gjerris F, Albeck MJ, Borgesen SE: Risk of infection after cerebrospinal fluid shunt: An analysis of 884 first-time shunts. Acta Neurochir 136:1–7, 1995.
44. Choux M, Genitori L, Lang D, Lena G: Shunt implantation: Reducing the incidence of shunt infection. J Neurosurg 77:875–880, 1992.
45. Renier D, Lacombe J, Pierre-Kahn A, et al: Factors causing acute shunt infection: Computer analysis of 1174 operations. J Neurosurg 61:1072–1078, 1984.
46. Bayston R, Hart CA, Barnicoat M: Intraventricular vancomycin in the treatment of ventriculitis associated with cerebrospinal fluid shunting and drainage. J Neurol Neurosurg Psychiatry 50:1419–1423, 1987.
47. Schiff SJ, Oakes WJ: Delayed cerebrospinal-fluid shunt infection in children. Pediatr Neurosci 15:131–135, 1989.
48. Langley JM: Design for a study of the risk factors for cerebrospinal fluid shunt infection. Master's Thesis, McMaster University, Hamilton, Ontario, 1989.
49. Meirovitch J, Kitai-Cohen Y, Keren G, et al: Cerebrospinal fluid shunt infections in children. Pediatr Infect Dis J 1987; 6:921–924, 1987.
50. Brydon HL, Bayston R, Hayward R, Harkness W: Reduced bacterial adhesion to hydrocephalus shunt catheters mediated by cerebrospinal fluid proteins. J Neurol Neurosurg Psychiatry 60:671–675, 1996.
51. James HE, Walsh JW, Wilson HD, et al: Prospective randomized study of therapy in cerebrospinal fluid shunt infection. Neurosurgery 7:459–463, 1980.
52. Fischer G, Goebel H, Latta E: Penetration of the colon by a ventriculoperitoneal drain resulting in an intra-cerebral abscess. Zentralbl Neurochir 44:155–160, 1983.
53. Nadvi SS, Parboosing R, van Dellen JR: Cerebellar abscess: The significance of cerebrospinal fluid diversion. Neurosurgery 41:61–66, 1997.
54. Petrak RM, Pottage JC Jr, Harris AA, Levin S: Haemophilus influenzae meningitis in the presence of a cerebrospinal fluid shunt. Neurosurgery 18:79–81, 1986.
55. Klein DM: Shunt infections. In Scott RM (ed): Hydrocephalus. Baltimore: Williams & Wilkins, 1990, p 88.
56. Kestle JRW, Hoffman HJ, Soloniuk D, et al: A concerted effort to prevent shunt infection. Childs Nerv Syst 9:163–165, 1993.
57. James HE, Nowak TP: Clinical course and diagnosis of migraine headaches in hydrocephalic children. Pediatr Neurosurg 17:310–316, 1991.
58. Dahlerup B, Gjerris F, Harmsen A, Sorensen PS: Severe headache as the only symptom of long-standing shunt dysfunction in hydrocephalic children with normal or slit ventricles revealed by computed tomography. Childs Nerv Syst 1:49–52, 1985.
59. Stellman-Ward GR, Bannister CM, Lewis MA, Shaw J: The incidence of chronic headache in children with shunted hydrocephalus. Eur J Pediatr Surg 7:12–14, 1997.
60. Di Rocco C: Is the slit ventricle syndrome always a slit ventricle syndrome? Childs Nerv Syst 10:49–58, 1994.
61. Coker SB: Cyclic vomiting and the slit ventricle syndrome. Pediatr Neurol 3:297–299, 1987.
62. Epstein F, Lapras C, Wisoff JH: 'Slit-ventricle syndrome': Etiology and treatment. Pediatr Neurosci 14:5–10, 1988.
63. Sgouros S, Malluci C, Walsh AR, Hockley AD: Long-term complications of hydrocephalus. Pediatr Neurosurg 23:127–132, 1995.
64. Walker ML, Fried A, Petronio J: Diagnosis and treatment of the slit ventricle syndrome. Neurosurg Clin North Am 4:707–714, 1993.
65. Reinprecht A, Dietrich W, Bertalanffy A, Czech T: The Medos Hakim programmable valve in the treatment of pediatric hydrocephalus. Childs Nerv Syst 13:588–593, 1997.
66. Baskin JJ, Manwaring KH, Rekate HL: Ventricular shunt removal:
The ultimate treatment of the slit ventricle syndrome. J Neurosurg 88:478–484, 1998.
67. Sainte-Rose C, Hoffman HJ, Hirsch JF: Shunt failure. Concepts Pediatr Neurosurg 9:7–20, 1989.
68. Hoppe-Hirsch E, Laroussinie F, Brunet L, et al: Late outcome of the surgical treatment of hydrocephalus. Childs Nerv Syst 14:97–99, 1998.
69. Grant JA: Victor Darwin Lespinasse: A biographical sketch. Neurosurgery 39:1232–1237, 1996.
70. Dandy WE: An operative procedure for hydrocephalus. Bull Johns Hopkins Hosp 33:189–190, 1922.
71. Mixter W: Ventriculoscopy and puncture of the floor of the third ventricle. Boston Med Surg J 188:277–278, 1923.
71a. Fay T, Grant FC: Ventriculoscopy and intraventricular photography in internal hydrocephalus. JAMA 80:461–463, 1966.
71b. Griffith HB: Technique of fontanel and persutural ventriculoscopy in infants. Childs Brain 1:359–363, 1975.
72. Kelly PJ: Stereotactic third ventriculostomy in patients with nontumoral adolescent/adult onset aqueductal stenosis and symptomatic hydrocephalus (see comments). J Neurosurg 75:865–873, 1991.
73. Jones RF, Teo C, Stening WA, Kwok CT: Neuroendoscopic third ventriculostomy. In Manwaring KH, Crone KR (eds): Neuroendoscopy. New York: Mary Ann Liebert, 1992, pp 63–77.
74. Jones RF, Kwok BC, Stening WA, Vonau M: The current status of endoscopic third ventriculostomy in the management of noncommunicating hydrocephalus. Minim Invasive Neurosurg 37:28–36, 1994.
75. Sainte-Rose C, Chumas P: Endoscopic third ventriculostomy. Tech Neurosurg 1:176–184, 1996.
76. Jones RF, Stening WA, Brydon M: Endoscopic third ventriculostomy. Neurosurgery 26:86–91, 1990.
77. Teo C, Jones R: Management of hydrocephalus by endoscopic third ventriculostomy in patients with myelomeningocele. Pediatr Neurosurg 25:57–63, 1996.
78. Brockmeyer D, Abtin K, Carey L, Walker ML: Endoscopic third ventriculostomy: An outcome analysis. Pediatr Neurosurg 28:236–240, 1998.
79. Jaksche H, Loew F: Burr hole third ventriculo-cisternostomy: An unpopular but effective procedure for treatment of certain forms of occlusive hydrocephalus. Acta Neurochir (Wien) 79:48–51, 1986.
80. Drake JM: Ventriculostomy for treatment of hydrocephalus. Neurosurg Clin North Am 4:657–666, 1993.
81. Natelson SE: Early third ventriculostomy in meningomyelocele infants—shunt independence? Childs Brain 8:321–325, 1981.
82. Patterson RH Jr, Bergland RM: The selection of patients for third ventriculostomy based on experience with 33 operations. J Neurosurg 29:252–254, 1968.
83. Sayers MP, Kosnik EJ: Percutaneous third ventriculostomy: Experience and technique. Childs Brain 2:24–30, 1976.
84. Vries JK, Friedman WA: Postoperative evaluation of third ventriculostomy patients using 111in-DTPA. Childs Brain 6:200–205, 1980.
85. Jones RF, Kwok BC, Stening WA, Vonau M: Neuroendoscopic third ventriculostomy: A practical alternative to extracranial shunts in noncommunicating hydrocephalus. Acta Neurochir Suppl 61:79–83, 1994.
86. Jones RF, Stening WA, Kwok BC, Sands TM: Third ventriculostomy for shunt infections in children. Neurosurgery 32:855–859, 1993.
87. Yamamoto M, Oka K, Ikeda K, Tomonaga M: Percutaneous flexible neuroendoscopic ventriculostomy in patients with shunt malfunction as an alternative procedure to shunt revision. Surg Neurol 42:218–223, 1994.
88. Perlman BB: Percutaneous third ventriculostomy in the treatment of a hydrocephalic infant with aqueduct stenosis. Int Surg 49:443–448, 1968.
89. Reddy K, Fewer HD, West M, Hill NC: Slit ventricle syndrome with aqueduct stenosis: Third ventriculostomy as definitive treatment (see comments). Neurosurgery 23:756–759, 1988.
90. Hoffman HJ, Harwood-Nash D, Gilday DL: Percutaneous third ventriculostomy in the management of noncommunicating hydrocephalus. Neurosurgery 7:313–321, 1980.
91. Foltz EL: Treatment of hydrocephalus by ventricular shunts (letter). Childs Nerv Syst 12:289–290, 1996.
92. Pudenz R, Foltz E: Hydrocephalus: Overdrainage by ventricular shunts—a review and recommendations. Surg Neurol 35:200–212, 1991.

93. Heilman CB, Cohen AR: Endoscopic ventricular fenestration using a "saline torch." J Neurosurg 74:224–229, 1991.
94. Sainte-Rose C: Third ventriculostomy. In Manwaring KH, Crone KR (ed.): Neuroendoscopy. New York: Mary Ann Liebert, 1992, pp 47–62.
95. Crone KR: Endoscopic technique for removal of adherent ventricular catheters. In Manwaring KH, Crone KR (eds): Neuroendoscopy. New York: Mary Ann Liebert, 1992, pp 41–46.
96. Scarff JE: Evaluation of treatment of hydrocephalus: Results of third ventriculostomy and endoscopic cauterization of choroid plexuses compared with mechanical shunts. Arch Neurol 14:382–391, 1966.
97. Forjaz S, Martelli N, Latuf N: Hypothalamic ventriculostomy with catheter: Technical note. J Neurosurg 29:655–659, 1968.
98. Oka K, Go Y, Kin Y, et al: The radiographic restoration of the ventricular system after third ventriculostomy. Minim Invasive Neurosurg 38:158–162, 1995.
99. Schwartz TH, Yoon SS, Cutruzzola FW, Goodman RR: Third ventriculostomy: Post-operative ventricular size and outcome. Minim Invasive Neurosurg 39:122–129, 1996.
100. Jack CR Jr, Kelly PJ: Stereotactic third ventriculostomy: Assessment of patency with MR imaging. AJNR Am J Neuroradiol 10:515–522, 1989.
101. Goumnerova LC, Frim DM: Treatment of hydrocephalus with third ventriculocisternostomy: Outcome and CSF flow patterns. Pediatr Neurosurg 27:149–152, 1997.
102. Wilcock DJ, Jaspan T, Worthington BS, Punt J: Neuro-endoscopic third ventriculostomy: Evaluation with magnetic resonance imaging. Clin Radiol 52:50–54, 1997.
103. Lev S, Bhadelia RA, Estin D, et al: Functional analysis of third ventriculostomy patency with phase-contrast MRI velocity measurements. Neuroradiology 39:175–179, 1997.
104. Wilcock DJ, Jaspan T, Punt J: CSF flow through third ventriculostomy demonstrated with colour Doppler ultrasonography. Clin Radiol 51:127–129, 1996.
105. Frim DM, Goumnerova LC: Telemetric intraventricular pressure measurements after third ventriculocisternostomy in a patient with noncommunicating hydrocephalus. Neurosurgery 41:1425–1428, 1997.
106. Hirsch JF, Hirsch E, Sainte-Rose C, et al: Stenosis of the aqueduct of Sylvius: Etiology and treatment. J Neurosurg Sci 30:29–39, 1986.
107. Dalrymple SJ, Kelly PJ: Computer-assisted stereotactic third ventriculostomy in the management of noncommunicating hydrocephalus. Stereotact Funct Neurosurg 59:105–110, 1992.
108. Goodman RR: Magnetic resonance imaging-directed stereotactic endoscopic third ventriculostomy. Neurosurgery 32:1043–1047, 1993.
109. Teo C, Rahman S, Boop FA, Cherny B: Complications of endoscopic neurosurgery. Childs Nerv Syst 12:248–253, 1996.
110. Handler MH, Abbott R, Lee M: A near-fatal complication of endoscopic third ventriculostomy: Case report. Neurosurgery 35:525–527, 1994.
111. McLaughlin MR, Wahlig JB, Kaufmann AM, Albright AL: Traumatic basilar aneurysm after endoscopic third ventriculostomy: Case report. Neurosurgery 41:1400–1403, 1997.
112. Zamorano L, Chavantes C, Moure F: Endoscopic stereotactic interventions in the treatment of brain lesions. Acta Neurochir Suppl 61:92–97, 1994.
113. Lewis AI, Keiper GL Jr, Crone KR: Endoscopic treatment of loculated hydrocephalus. J Neurosurg 82:780–785, 1995.
114. Cohen AR: Endoscopic ventricular surgery. Pediatr Neurosurg 19:127–134, 1993.
115. Rappaport ZH: Suprasellar arachnoid cysts: Options in operative management. Acta Neurochir 122:71–75, 1993.
116. Decq P, Brugieres P, Le Guerinel C, et al: Percutaneous endoscopic treatment of suprasellar arachnoid cysts: Ventriculocystostomy or ventriculocystocisternostomy? Technical note. J Neurosurg 84:696–701, 1996.
117. Lewis AI, Crone KR, Taha J, et al: Surgical resection of third ventricle colloid cysts: Preliminary results comparing transcallosal microsurgery with endoscopy (see comments). J Neurosurg 81:174–178, 1994.
118. Ure BM, Holschneider AM: Ventriculoscopic implantation of ventricular shunts in children with hydrocephalus. Eur J Pediatr Surg 7:299–300, 1997.
119. Kellnar S, Boehm R, Ring E: Ventriculoscopy-aided implantation of ventricular shunts in patients with hydrocephalus. J Pediatr Surg 30:1450–1451, 1995.
120. Ellenbogen RG, Moores LE: Endoscopic management of a pineal and suprasellar germinoma with associated hydrocephalus: Technical case report. Minim Invasive Neurosurg 40:13–15, 1997.
121. Drake J: Neuroendoscopy Tumour Biopsy. New York: Mary Ann Leibert, 1992.
122. Ferrer E, Santamarta D, Garcia-Fructuoso G, et al: Neuroendoscopic management of pineal region tumours. Acta Neurochir 139:12–20, 1997.
123. Oka K, Yamamoto M, Nagasaka S, Tomonaga M: Endoneurosurgical treatment for hydrocephalus caused by intraventricular tumors. Childs Nerv Syst 10:162–166, 1994.

CHAPTER 44

# Surgical Management of Hydrocephalus in Adults

■ MEL H. EPSTEIN and JOHN A. DUNCAN III

The use of cerebrospinal fluid (CSF) shunts to treat hydrocephalus in both children and adults has made hydrocephalus one of the most treatable neurologic conditions. Before the use of ventricular shunts, neurosurgical procedures used to attempt to control ventricular size included choroid plexectomy, which could be performed endoscopically or an open procedure, such as that described by Dandy.[1] In the 1940s, White and Michelsen,[2] Dandy and Stookey and Scarff performed open third ventriculostomy, which yielded somewhat better results until ventricular shunts became much more successful.[3, 4] Percutaneous endoscopic third ventriculostomy was first described by Mixter[5] with poor results. Recently, however, third ventriculostomy has re-emerged as another option in the treatment of hydrocephalus, especially when stereotactic or endoscopic techniques are used to facilitate this procedure.[6–9]

The introduction and use of ventricular shunts without question changed the prognosis for individuals with hydrocephalus, and most attain fairly normal intelligence. Improvement in survival and outcome has come, however, at a price. Many new problems related to shunting, including the creation of shunt dependency, have occurred. The natural history of untreated hydrocephalus reported by Lawrence and Coates showed a 46% 10-year survival and intellectual impairment in 62%.[9] After shunting, however, Foltz and Shurtleff demonstrated a 10-year survival of almost 95% and with intellectual impairment in only 30% of shunted children.[10] Furthermore, the syndrome of occult or normal-pressure hydrocephalus (NPH) in adults is now a well-recognized, although rare, cause of gait disturbance and dementia,[11–13] whose symptoms can often be improved after shunting. However, differentiating NPH from ventricular enlargement that results from atrophy and aging is still quite difficult. The ability to predict the response to shunting adult hydrocephalus depends on clinical, radiologic, and CSF biomechanical studies. These studies can help to determine which adults will improve after a shunt is placed.

This chapter reviews the pathophysiology of hydrocephalus in adults. The indications and technical aspects of shunting and shunt revisions are detailed, as well as problems that have been created by shunt dependency, such as the slit ventricle syndrome. Adult hydrocephalus, including the treatment of NPH, is discussed. Nonshunting alternatives, specifically endoscopic third ventriculostomy, are also reviewed.

## ETIOLOGY AND PATHOPHYSIOLOGY

Hydrocephalus is excessive accumulation of CSF within the ventricles. Often, this ventricular enlargement is accompanied by elevation in intracranial pressure (ICP). However, in adult clinical practice, enlarged ventricles are not always associated with elevated ICP; therefore, these states must be differentiated as indications for shunting vary. Some conditions associated with normal- or low-pressure ventricular enlargement include low-pressure ventricular dilatation, cerebral atrophy, porencephalic cysts, and adult NPH. NPH is characterized by progressive gait disturbance, dementia, and incontinence, often presenting in this order. NPH is treated by shunt placement but must be differentiated from other causes of dementia if symptoms are to improve after surgery.

Congenital malformations account for a large percentage of childhood hydrocephalus. Aqueductal stenosis is the most common type of congenital hydrocephalus. The lateral and third ventricles are enlarged, and the fourth ventricle is normal in size and configuration. Most cases of aqueductal stenosis causing hydrocephalus are diagnosed in the first few years of life, because they present with typical signs of elevated ICP such as macrocephaly. Because of the frequent use of in utero ultrasound during pregnancy, aqueductal stenosis can also be diagnosed before a child is born, and a planned shunt can be inserted after birth. However, the first appearance of hydrocephalus due to aqueductal stenosis can be in late adolescence or in the adult, who presents with chronic headaches and visual disturbance and usually has a head that is relatively large. There may also be a history of school problems and learning disabilities throughout childhood. Sometimes, aqueductal stenosis is first diagnosed after a mild-to-moderate head injury that seems to precipitate new signs of elevated ICP.

The Chiari malformations can cause both childhood and

adult hydrocephalus. Type I Chiari malformation with cerebellar tonsillar ectopia is seen without associated myelomeningocele. Symptoms are usually referable to compression of the lower medulla and upper cervical spine, but hydrocephalus can occasionally be responsible for the initial presenting symptoms and hindbrain radiographic findings. If hydrocephalus is not recognized before posterior fossa decompression for a Chiari I malformation, serious complications, including pseudomeningocele, wound CSF leak, and meningitis, can occur. Similarly, in patients with a symptomatic syrinx, Chiari I malformation, and hydrocephalus, the hydrocephalus should be treated first by insertion of a ventriculoperitoneal shunt.

The Chiari II malformation is usually a cause of hydrocephalus in children with myelomeningocele. In children with myelomeningocele, all have an associated Chiari II malformation and early hydrocephalus. Approximately 80% of these children will develop progressive hydrocephalus that will require shunt placement.

Hydrocephalus can also be caused by cysts, such as porencephalic cysts within the brain adjacent to the ventricle or arachnoid cysts in the subarachnoid space or ventricle. In particular, arachnoid cysts of the suprasellar region obstruct the third ventricle, and quadrigeminal cysts of the dorsal midbrain compress the posterior third ventricle and cerebral aqueduct, causing hydrocephalus. The use of intraoperative ultrasound or improved stereotactic techniques can direct shunt catheters into both the arachnoid cysts or the ventricles, thus enabling shunting of necessary compartments. Stereotactic fiberoptic ventriculoscopy has been used to visualize the tough capsule of these arachnoid cysts and to puncture them, leading to accurate catheter placement and cyst decompression. This procedure can also communicate the arachnoid cysts with the ventricle, forming a single common compartment that can be shunted.

The Dandy-Walker cyst is a posterior fossa cyst in communication with an enlarged fourth ventricle that is associated with hypoplasia of the cerebellar vermis. When this cyst is symptomatic and exists with ventricular enlargement, a shunt must be placed. Our practice in adults is to shunt the lateral ventricle first and then the posterior fossa cyst, if necessary, connecting both catheters to form a single distal shunt system. The results of direct shunting are superior to those of craniotomy and fenestration of the cyst. In infants, however, placement of a single fourth ventricular shunt is often successful in decompressing all ventricles and should be considered before placement of a standard ventriculoperitoneal shunt. This approach often avoids development of the isolated or trapped fourth ventricle, which can occur after conventional lateral ventriculoperitoneal shunts in these young children.

Acquired hydrocephalus in adults has many causes. Tumor-related hydrocephalus is most commonly associated with posterior fossa tumors, suprasellar tumors, and tumors of the third ventricle and pineal region. Although controversial, our practice is to not perform a preoperative shunt, to temporize with preoperative high-dose dexamethasone (Decadron), and in rare cases, to use a temporary ventriculostomy. The major goal of the tumor surgery is to re-establish normal CSF pathways, frequently avoiding a shunt. With this strategy, a shunt is needed in only 20% to 30% of cases postoperatively.

Vascular causes of hydrocephalus include vascular malformations such as vein of Galen malformations, giant midline aneurysms, and subarachnoid hemorrhages. Hydrocephalus follows subarachnoid hemorrhage in approximately 25% of cases. Other vascular causes of hydrocephalus include thrombosis of the dural sinuses, bilateral jugular vein disruption, such as in radical neck surgery or in superior vena cava obstruction owing to tumors or long-standing indwelling catheters.[14] These occlusive disorders, however, often produce a pseudotumor-like picture of a swollen brain and small ventricles. Occasionally, progressive ventricular enlargement is seen.

## CEREBROSPINAL FLUID DYNAMIC TESTING

The measurement of a patient's CSF hydrodynamic profile is often useful in the evaluation of several syndromes. This form of testing can measure ICP and intraventricular pressure acutely or over an extended period, indirectly measure CSF absorption through measurement of resistance to CSF absorption (R), and measure neural axis volume buffering capacity as an indication of brain compliance. The sum of these techniques has several purposes. First, in some cases of ventricular enlargement such as atrophy, a shunt is not clearly required. However, symptoms may not be classic, and clear-cut progressive ventricular enlargement may not be present. Measurement of ICP, CSF absorption as R, and pressure-volume index (PVI) as an indication of compliance allows for comparison of the measured results from normal values and differences from known biomechanical profiles in active hydrocephalic syndromes (Table 44–1).[15–18] This approach is beneficial for adults with NPH, in whom an abnormal biomechanical profile can predict a good response to shunting, as opposed to those with hydrocephalus ex vacuo, in whom shunting would not improve symptoms.[19–20] These techniques involve the placement of a catheter into the CSF, usually intraventricular. The lumbar subarachnoid space can sometimes be used, if communicating hydrocephalus is present. Once a pressure tracing is obtained, the measurement of ICP is the first and most straightforward parameter. Normal ICP in children should not exceed 10 mm Hg in infants, 15 mm Hg in older children, and 20 mm Hg after 15 years of age (see Table 44–1). Once an initial ICP is measured, a multiple-day continuous measurement of ICP is useful because it frequently discerns abnormal pressure phenomena, including Lundburg A waves, which can rise to 80 to 100 mm Hg, and Lundburg B waves, which can rise up to 40 to 50 mm Hg and can occur at a rate of one per minute. Several investigators have correlated better responses to shunting adults who have NPH with an increased frequency of observing B waves.[21, 22] In addition, in children who are shunt dependent and may have intermittent signs of elevated ICP with headaches, ICP monitoring techniques can be useful in the identification of those with true pressure abnormalities versus chronic headaches, which may be either psychological in origin or unrelated to abnormal CSF pressures.

**TABLE 44-1 ■ BIOMECHANICAL PROFILE OF THE VARIOUS CLINICAL GROUPS OF HYDROCEPHALUS**

| | Intracranial Pressure (mm Hg) | Pressure-Volume Index (ml) | Resistance to CSF Absorption (mm Hg/ml/min) |
|---|---|---|---|
| Normal child | 3–12 | 8–22* | <3 |
| Normal adult | 10–15 | 25 | <3 |
| Childhood hydrocephalus | 10–20 | 28.1 | 7.2 |
| Shunted hydrocephalus | 0–10 | 18.4 | Range, 2–30† |
| Normal-pressure hydrocephalus | 10–15 | 16 | 17 |

*Dependent on the size of the intracranial and intraspinal compartments (see normograms in references 18 and 19).
†Resistance to cerebrospinal fluid (CSF) absorption range becomes dependent on intracranial pressure and is not constant in shunted hydrocephalus.[17]

## NORMAL-PRESSURE HYDROCEPHALUS

NPH was described in 1965 by Adams and coworkers[11] as occult hydrocephalus associated with normal CSF pressure (180 mm $H_2O$ or less). The clinical syndrome included gait disturbance, dementia, and urinary incontinence. Furthermore, CSF shunting reversed these symptoms to a variable extent. The obvious importance of recognizing NPH is in distinguishing this form of dementia and gait abnormalities from other forms of senile dementia as a treatable entity. Many studies have subsequently tried to predict the type of patient most likely to respond to shunting based on various parameters.[23–25] The gait disturbance is characterized by a "magnetic" gait, with small steps and minimal movement of the feet, sometimes called a gait apraxia. In patients who responded best to shunting, gait disturbance was the initial and most disabling of the three symptoms. A variable amount of dementia is present with NPH. In contrast to the findings with gait apraxia, when dementia was the predominant feature, the response to shunting was minimal. Urinary incontinence is the third feature of NPH and is usually a frontal release sign often associated with a general loss of accepted social behavior. This incontinence can respond to shunting, but the improvement in urinary function is less than the improvement in gait. The methods used to investigate NPH for possible shunting involve ICP and CSF dynamic measurements, imaging studies, radioisotope cisternography, and a trial of CSF drainage.

ICP measurements are often normal in NPH. However, long-term monitoring can show the presence of A waves or B waves. One early and still useful test for evaluating NPH is the Katzman infusion test, in which a CSF catheter is placed in the lumbar space, and a constant infusion of fluid is performed to determine the rate of rise of CSF pressure and the time required to reach a new steady-state pressure.[19, 20] This test, therefore, depends on both pressure-volume characteristics and on CSF absorption factors to determine the rate at which ICP rises and reaches a new steady-state pressure, if at all. Coupling the ICP monitoring with determination of R resistance to CSF absorption by bolus or infusion techniques[3, 19, 20, 26] is an excellent way to obtain this information all in one monitoring period.

DiChiro and colleagues[27] introduced radioisotope cisternography to describe a characteristic pattern in NPH. Radioactive iodinated serum albumin is introduced into the lumbar subarachnoid space, and cerebral radioisotope scanning is performed at 6, 24, and 48 hours later. Nor-

mally, CSF should flow from the lumbar space up over the convexities of the hemispheres and subsequently be absorbed into the sagittal sinus. The supposed characteristic pattern for NPH demonstrates failure of the isotope to ascend over the cerebral convexities as well as prolonged reflux of the isotope into the ventricles. When this pattern is seen, it is interpreted as a pattern typical for NPH, and shunting is often recommended. Multiple studies, however, have failed to demonstrate this as the best test, and patients with the typical syndrome who respond well to shunting can have negative results on radioisotope cisternography. It is, however, useful information about CSF dynamics and helps guide clinical decision making.

Occasionally, a determination of response to shunting is made by withdrawal of a large volume of CSF and observation of the clinical response of the patients. This procedure can be performed with a lumbar puncture in which CSF is removed until the opening pressure is reduced to half its original value, or it can be accomplished with continuous lumbar drainage. Collectively, these techniques are only fair predictors of the response to shunting and must be interpreted cautiously. Good clinical judgment and consistent support test patterns are often the key to correct diagnosis.

The results of ventricular shunting of NPH, however, can be quite dramatic. Often, despite all of these predictive tests, one cannot accurately determine which patient will respond well to shunting. In addition, an initial excellent response with improvement of symptoms often gives way to a re-emergence of symptoms several months later. Stein and Langfitt[28] reported improvement in 64% of patients, which then decreased to 24% sustained improvements. Laws and Morki[29] found 50% improvement, with 64% improvement in patients with the classic triad of NPH. Black[30] reported a 47% overall improvement, with a 60% improvement in those with the triad. Patients with a predominance of gait apraxia generally respond best, and those with dementia respond least, to shunting. In our hands, a shunt is performed if the classic clinical triad is present with a gait disturbance as the predominant finding, supported by one or more predictive tests.

## INDICATIONS FOR SURGERY

Adults can present with either NPH or hydrocephalus caused by similar conditions as those seen in children, such as aqueductal stenosis or intracranial mass lesion. Adults usually have obvious signs of elevated ICP, with severe headaches, papilledema, and vomiting. In this situation, the decision to proceed with a shunt is clear-cut. Shunting is considered to treat NPH in older adults with the triad of dementia, gait disturbance, and incontinence. The previous discussion outlines the decision of who receives a shunt with NPH.

## Ventricular Shunting for Hydrocephalus

The vast array of shunting devices has many similar features. Current shunt systems have a valve incorporated within the shunt with an opening and closing pressure, so that all currently used valves are pressure regulated. Given the fact that shunts all drain CSF relatively quickly when the patient is in the upright position as a result of siphoning, most of the flow characteristics of currently available shunts are relatively unimportant, as recently demonstrated in a pediatric multicenter trial. However, other technical aspects of the initial shunting procedure and choice of hardware affect the success of the shunt and decrease the incidence of shunt malfunction. Shunt valves can be located proximally and distally. Distal slit valves are now to be avoided because of the high frequency of distal shunt malfunction and unpredictable flow characteristics. The currently used valve mechanisms today include spring-ball valves, and diaphragm valves.[31] Siphoning occurs when the patient is in the upright position, in which a negative pressure is exerted that is related to the vertical distance between the inlet and the outlet of the shunt.[32, 33] Although siphoning is often not a detrimental factor in young childhood and may even be necessary for adequate neonatal shunt function, adults can have significant problems related to siphoning because of the longer length of the shunt in the vertical position and the presence of a rigid skull at the time that the shunt is initially placed. For this reason, siphoning may cause low-pressure symptoms and subdural

hematoma formation more frequently in the adult-shunted hydrocephalus population.[34] As a result, antisiphon devices are commonly used. These devices hypothetically disrupt siphoning in situ by allowing positive atmospheric pressure to occlude negative shunt pressure when present, thus stopping CSF flow. Whether or not antisiphon devices actually work remains to be proved because overdrainage and subdural hematoma can and do occasionally occur in patients with these shunt systems.

Although the individual flow characteristics of any shunt may not be particularly important, a partially unitized shunt system (valve and distal catheter) is advantageous because it is easier to insert, decreases operative time, and avoids the possibility of shunt disconnection or disintegration associated with a connector. A separate ventricular catheter facilitates placement. Brisk return of CSF is quickly recognized; CSF is easily sampled; and ventriculoscopy can be performed as needed using this system. Only one connection is needed and should employ a side connector or inlet. This feature enables the surgeon to have easy access to the shunt catheter and avoids the surgeon's having to work underneath a reservoir with a catheter that has become embedded in the brain. A premeasured right angle ventricular catheter is advantageous when the cortical mantle is thin, preventing unwanted catheter migration with a severely dilated ventricle. The valve system should have incorporated into it some sort of flushing or tapping chamber to enable access to CSF, as well as the ability to pump and test a shunt to assess its function.

The patient's position is important to the correct implantation of the shunt. The head is turned sharply to the left, and the shunt is placed initially in the right occipital area (Fig. 44–1). By use of a Hudson brace or power craniotome, a bur hole is placed approximately 4 cm up from the inion and 3 to 4 cm off the midline (Fig. 44–2). This occipital placement allows a relatively straight pass into the body of the ventricle, so that the shunt catheter is mainly within the ventricle. This trajectory avoids the risk

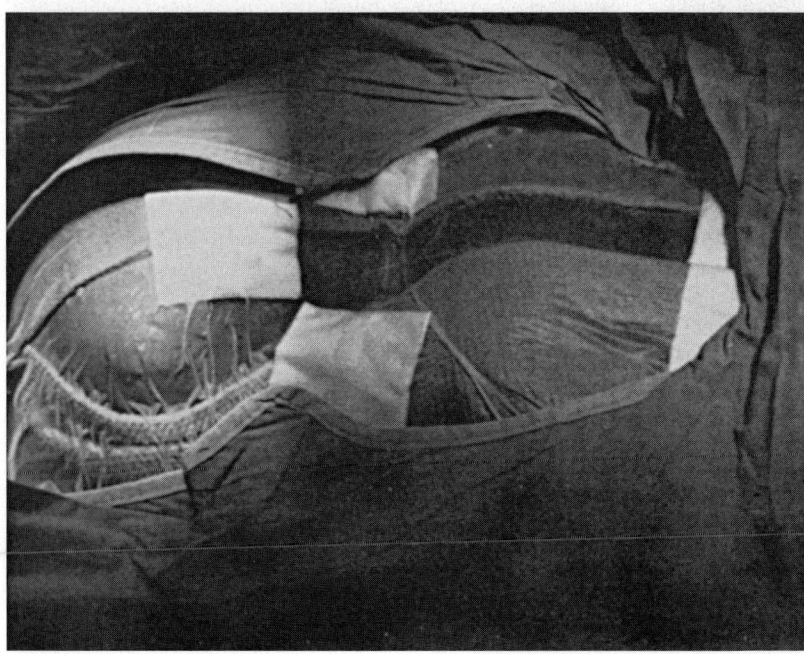

**FIGURE 44–1 ■** A plastic drape not only decreases skin contact but also helps to maintain the body temperature of small children.

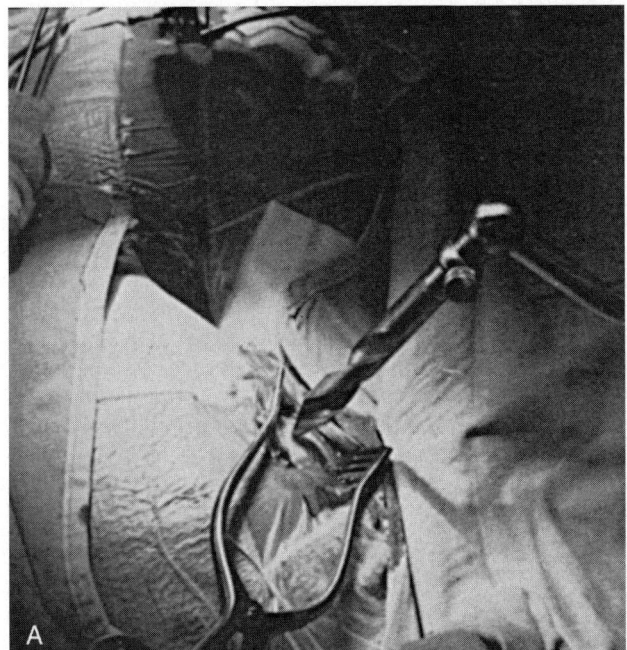

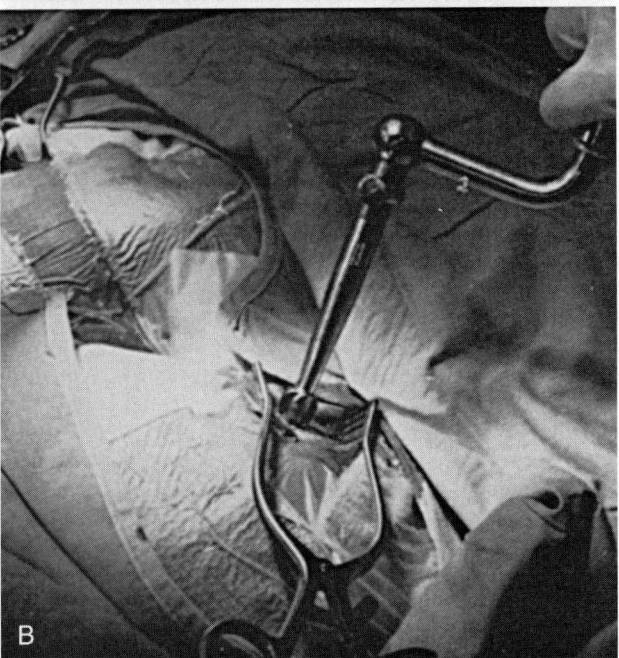

**FIGURE 44–2** ■ *A*, The bur hole for the flushing device must be made carefully, because the bit does not lock in the normal fashion within the skull of young children. *B*, It is important that the bur hole is large enough to accommodate the flushing device if it is the type that is seated in the bur hole. This lowers the profile and decreases the risk of a decubitus ulcer.

of too low an entry through the internal capsule, which can happen with shunt placement sites that are more lateral and inferior, such as at Kean's point. An adequate length of ventricular catheter must be selected, so that the tip is anterior to the foramen of Monro, away from the choroid plexus. Generally, a 6-cm catheter is used in a small newborn, an 8-cm catheter in an older infant and young child, and a 10-cm catheter is used in children older than 18 months and in adults. Because of risk of injury to the

internal capsule, a frontal ventricular approach is often recommended in adults, especially when dilatation of the frontal horns predominate. In this case, a frontal bur hole is placed over the coronal suture, 2 to 3 cm off midline. The catheter trajectory is perpendicular to all adjacent skull surfaces and a 5- to 6-cm catheter is needed to reach the foramen of Monro. We also routinely soak the shunt in bacitracin solution, avoid handling the hardware, and use perioperative antibiotics, believing that this plays an important role in reducing shunt infections, although this is a controversial point in literature.[35–38]

A rolled towel is placed across the shoulder blades to elevate the chest and neck and to allow for a straight passage of the shunt passer, with no secondary incisions between the head and the abdomen. The abdominal incision is a horizontal incision, below the rib cage and lateral to the midline or umbilicus. Once the shunt is laid in position, the dura is opened with cautery to cause an opening just big enough to allow the passing of the shunt catheter. A large dural opening should be avoided because it allows CSF to flow around the shunt and cause a subcutaneous fluid collection. The ventricular catheter is then passed directly into the occipital horn of the lateral ventricle using a stylet. A shunt ventriculoscope can be used instead of a stylet or inserted after the ventricle is cannulated to confirm the location of the catheter tip and to avoid the choroid plexus. Fluid should then be sampled from the ventricular catheter, all connections made, and CSF should be visualized from the lower end of the shunt to ensure that the valve system is opened and functioning spontaneously. It is placed into the peritoneal cavity. The full length of the peritoneal catheter can be placed to allow for subsequent growth. In our practice, use of abdominal trocars are avoided for distal peritoneal placement.

A ventriculoperitoneal shunt is often the initial shunt of choice for adults with hydrocephalus. However, because of siphoning, subdural hematoma or low-pressure headaches may be a more common finding in adults with very large ventricles and a rigid calvarium. In these cases, a ventriculoatrial shunt may be a useful first option in adult hydrocephalus, because the shorter shunt between the head and the heart provides less siphoning effect. A medium-pressure valve is usually chosen for shunting in adults.

To perform a ventriculoatrial shunt, the surgeon makes an incision across the anterior border of the sternomastoid muscle, and the common facial vein is identified. Our practice is to isolate the vein both proximally and distally with ligatures and to tie the vein off distally. A small opening is made into the facial vein and the shunt is passed down the jugular vein into the right atrium of the heart. On the right side, this step is easily performed with electrocardiographic control: An alligator clip is attached to the stylet of the distal tubing, and it is connected to lead II of the anesthesia electrocardiographic machine.[39] The atrium is indicated by the P wave configuration becoming more and more upright, and when it becomes a biphasic P wave, the tip has entered the right atrium. The catheter must be pulled back if cardiac arrhythmia is encountered. A chest radiograph taken in the recovery room should confirm that the catheter is at the T6 level. On the left side, where there are more turns of the venous anatomy, fluoroscopic control with a flexible wire is useful for proper placement of the distal shunt in the right atrium. With ventriculoatrial shunts, lengthening should be considered when the shunt tip rises above the T4 level, because above that level, distal malfunction is significantly more common.

A pleural shunt is a very good option if the peritoneum cannot be used. This shunt is especially useful in patients older than 8 years of age who cannot have a ventriculoperitoneal or ventriculoatrial shunt.

We have had recent success with a ventriculocholecystatic shunt when all serosal surfaces were impaired secondary to adhesion, infection, or sclerosis. In these cases, the right atrium is not accessible secondary to thrombosis, abnormal venous anatomy, or scarring.

## COMPLICATIONS

### Proximal Shunt Malfunction and Revision

Because ventricular shunting usually produces shunt dependency, the diagnosis of a shunt malfunction is obvious because of overt signs of elevated ICP, including headaches, vomiting, and lethargy. This mode of presentation occurs in approximately 70% of those who receive shunts.[16] In the other 30% of cases, however, signs of deterioration may be subtle and may include neuropsychological changes and other cognitive or behavioral symptoms.[15] In adults with NPH, a shunt malfunction may cause a re-emergence of the triad of symptoms.

When a shunt malfunction is suspected, evaluation begins with a CT scan to compare ventricular size and look for interval enlargement of the ventricles. A shunt series can be performed to determine continuity of the shunt and shunt placement. In adults with NPH, the ventricles often do not change very much in size, so that a radionucleotide shunt flow study is often useful to establish the fact that the shunt is draining fluid from the ventricle into the peritoneum. With a suspected distal shunt malfunction, the surgeon should look carefully for signs of infection and formation of a pseudocyst, which is a common cause of distal shunt malfunction. A shunt tap is useful to measure ICP, to test both proximal and distal portions of the shunt, and to exclude a shunt infection. Table 44–2 gives the frequency of some common shunt complications.

The most common shunt malfunction is proximal occlusion of the shunt, occurring approximately 80% of the time. In an attempt to prevent proximal shunt problems,

the surgeon should place the shunt catheter anterior to the foramen of Monro in the lateral ventricle. This placement can be accomplished with an adequate length of ventricular catheter through an occipital placement or with a 5- to 6-cm ventricular catheter in a frontal catheter placement with the bur hole at the coronal suture. The frontal route is especially useful when the occipital horns are not significantly dilated. The replaced ventricular catheter is connected to the distal shunt assembly after distal shunt function is tested. During a proximal revision, the ventricular catheter may be difficult to remove. When the ventricular catheter is stuck, several attempts can be made to relieve the adherence. First, the ventricular catheter can be grasped with a hemostat and rotated, which may free the catheter with a sudden give in the resistance. If twisting the catheter does not free it, the next step is to place the stylet down the shunt catheter and touch the Bovie cautery to the stylet. This procedure can sometimes coagulate the choroid plexus at the tip of the catheter, thus releasing it. If resistance is still a problem, the catheter should be left in place; a new bur hole should be placed next to the existing one; and a new ventricular catheter should be used. Ventricular endoscopy can free the catheter tip from the adherent choroid plexus and remove the retained catheter under direct vision (Fig. 44–3).

When more than one recent proximal shunt occlusion has occurred, different steps must be taken to prevent further malfunction. Low-grade shunt infection by organisms such as *Staphylococcus epidermidis, Corynebacterium parvum,* or *Propionibacterium acnes* must be excluded and if present treated appropriately with shunt removal, external drainage, and appropriate antibiotic therapy. In other cases of recurrent shunt failure, endoscopy has shown that often a new catheter is placed into a sheath of scar tissue that is likely to occlude within the next several days to weeks. We therefore use a different site for placement, which is often the frontal route, with recurrent proximal occlusions.

When a proximal revision must be performed in the setting of relatively small ventricles, certain steps are taken. It is frequently wise to place a new catheter at a frontal site, leaving a blocked occipital catheter in place. A second

TABLE 44–2 ■ **COMPLICATIONS OF SHUNTS AND THEIR FREQUENCY IN 380 CHILDREN WITH SHUNTS**

| Complication | Number/% |
| --- | --- |
| Infection | 41/11* |
| Seizures | 55/14.5 |
| Subdural hematoma | 12/3.0 |
| Loculated ventricles | 26/7.0 |
| No complications | 220/58.0 |
| Slit ventricle syndrome | 43/11.5 |

*Infection rate per shunt operation is 5%.

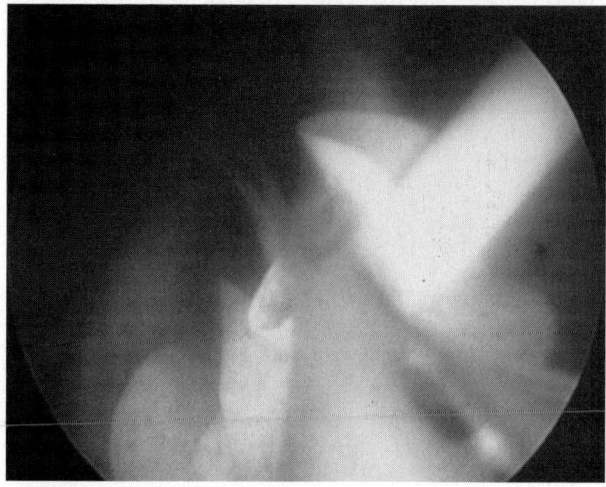

FIGURE 44–3 ■ The retained flanged ventricular catheter adheres to the choroid plexus and the scar.

alternative is to attempt to slide a new ventricular catheter down the same tract after the old ventricular catheter is removed. No attempt should be made to place the catheter by use of a stylet or brain needle, because it may veer off the existing tract and miss the ventricle. If the catheter does not find its way into the ventricle, then a single attempt with a brain needle can be made to try to cannulate the small ventricle. If this attempt is unsuccessful, repeated attempts should not be made, and the operation should be aborted. The patient should be watched closely for signs of elevated ICP, and serial CT scans and the proximal shunt revision should be subsequently performed when the ventricle has dilated. Alternatively, a small ventricle can often be cannulated with the aid of a ventriculoscope; however, multiple blind approaches are again to be avoided.

During proximal revision, when the surgeon encounters moderately blood-tinged CSF after the new ventricular catheter is placed, an effort should be made to clear the ventricular system of new hemorrhage. The new catheter is irrigated with saline until it begins to clear. This process often requires patience because up to 20 minutes of gentle irrigation of saline may be needed. Once the CSF clears, a new ventricular catheter should replace the catheter through which irrigation was being performed. If the blood does not clear, it may be wise to place a temporary ventriculostomy for several days until the CSF is clear.

## Distal Shunt Malfunction and Revisions

Distal shunt malfunctions can be related to a short distal catheter usually secondary to continued somatic growth, shunt fracture, and distal shunt occlusion. Distal shunt occlusions are most often seen in shunt infections, which can lead to impaired CSF absorption from the peritoneum and the formation of an abdominal pseudocyst. CSF should be sampled in patients with distal shunt problems to exclude infection and to allow the fluid to be analyzed in the laboratory for a long time, because diphtheroids may not grow in culture media in the first 2 to 5 days, necessitating culture for 7 to 10 days. Distal shunts have also been known to erode into various abdominal viscera,[40] and some shunts have eroded into the intestine, bladder, and vagina, and have even protruded from the anus. Most of these complications were seen with the spring-loaded distal shunt tubing, which is now avoided.

## Shunt Infections

Despite efforts to avoid infection with preoperative antibiotics and special routines for preparing and draping a patient for a shunt operation, each shunt operation is associated with a 2% to 8% rate of postoperative shunt infection.[35, 37, 38] Overall, between 5% and 15% of shunts can be expected to become infected over the life of the shunt. Approximately 66% of shunt infections are diagnosed within 1 month after surgery, and close to 80% manifest by 6 months.[35] Shunt infections can cause signs of meningitis, as well as other external signs, such as redness or fluctuance along the path of the shunt. The most common agents

are staphylococci, but gram-positive bacilli and enterobacilli can also infect shunts. The methods of treating shunt infections include:

1. Antibiotics alone, both intravenous and, in rare cases, intrathecal
2. Shunt removal with delayed reinsertion
3. Antibiotics, shunt removal, and immediate shunt replacement
4. Shunt removal, antibiotics, and external ventricular drainage followed by delayed shunt reinsertion

Because most individuals with shunts are shunt dependent, shunt removal alone often does not allow adequate treatment of the hydrocephalus. The most successful and predictable treatment of a shunt infection is administration of intravenous antibiotics, removal of all shunt hardware, and placement of a temporary ventriculostomy for approximately 1 week. Once the infection is cleared, a new ventriculoperitoneal shunt is placed, either on the same side or at a different site. Antibiotics are continued for an additional several days and then discontinued. If signs of peritonitis or distal shunt failure are present, the shunt may need to be removed emergently. However, an individual with sepsis may be too great an anesthetic risk and is best treated with antibiotics until vital signs have stabilized.

In cases in which a nonfulminating shunt infection is present without signs of sepsis, or shunt failure, an attempt can be made to treat the shunt in situ and using intravenous or intrathecal antibiotics alone.[41, 42] Both *Haemophilus influenzae* and *Streptococcus pneumoniae* infections have been reported to be treated successfully in this fashion. However, the families must understand that this treatment may fail in approximately 40% of cases.

In patients with ventriculoatrial shunts, shunt nephritis is a unique complication.[43] This condition presents with proteinuria, hematuria, and progressive decline in kidney function. Shunt nephritis should be considered diagnostic of shunt infection. Often, the only positive culture results are obtained with culture of the shunt hardware.

## Shunt Alternatives—Endoscopic Third Ventriculostomy

Endoscopic third ventriculostomy has been used successfully in the treatment of **noncommunicating** hydrocephalus. Kelly reported[7] a series of adults and adolescents with late-onset aqueductal stenosis in which only 1 of 16 patients required placement of a shunt after third ventriculostomy. This observation has now been confirmed in a large series of patients worldwide, and it is estimated that 85% to 90% of patients with late-onset aqueductal stenosis can be treated safely and effectively with this technique. In addition to the low morbidity and decreased risk of overdrainage and subdural hematoma formation, third ventriculostomy has also been used successfully to treat shunt infections and even slit ventricles in patients with aqueductal stenosis. Unfortunately, this technique has been shown to be much less effective for patients with noncommunicating hydrocephalus secondary to myelodysplasia, congenital aqueductal stenosis, or prior infection. The success rate for infants with congenital aqueductal stenosis is less than 50%. On the other hand, tumors of the tectum,

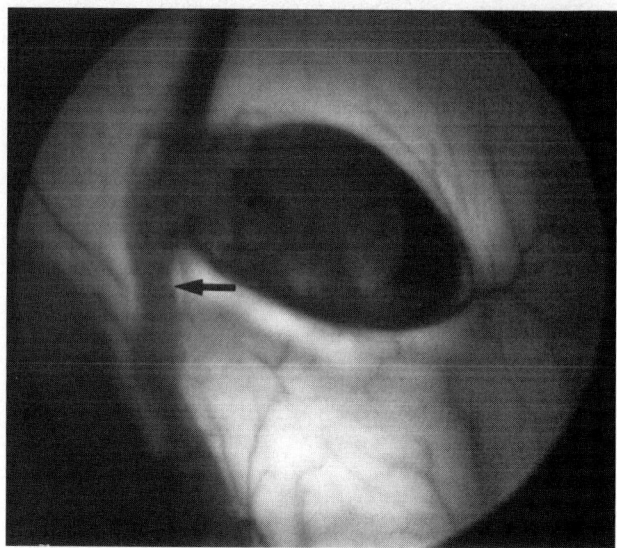

FIGURE 44–4 ■ The foramen of Monro, choroid plexus *(arrow)*.

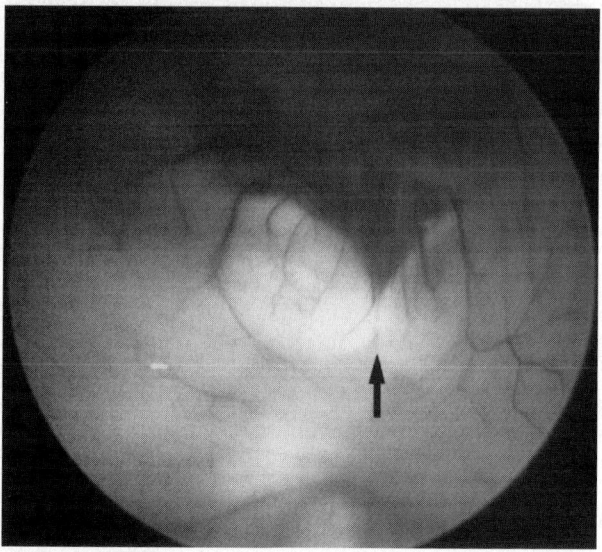

FIGURE 44–6 ■ The posterior floor of the third ventricle, mamillary bodies *(arrow)*, basilar and posterior cerebral arteries.

pineal region, or within the ventricle can be biopsied, and the hydrocephalus can be managed in a significant number of patients using this technique. Therefore, patient selection is the key to its success.[44]

Before surgery, all patients considered for third ventriculostomy should undergo magnetic resonance imaging of the brain in both axial and sagittal planes. Good candidates are those with clear aqueductal stenosis and, most important, severe thinning of the floor of the third ventricle in which the third ventricle is expanded and the floor nearly invisible radiographically.

The patient is brought to the operating room and placed supine on the table. We prefer to use a rigid endoscope that has an external diameter of less than 4 mm. A self-retaining mechanical clamp is fixed to the operating room table that allows hands to be free after the scope has been inserted. An open working channel and a second irrigation channel are needed. The eyepiece is attached to a video camera and monitor, which is located within easy view of the surgeon.

A bur hole is placed over the right coronal suture, 2 cm off midline. A No. 12 French peel-away catheter with a stylet or other trephine is gently passed into the right lateral ventricle to the foramen of Monro. This portion of the procedure may be stereotactically assisted if need be, although we have found this to be unnecessary secondary to the marked degree of ventricular dilatation. Once the introducer is inserted, the ventriculoscope is passed into the lateral ventricle under direct vision. The choroid plexus, thalamostriate vein, septal vein, and foramen of Monro are identified. The scope is then passed into the third ventricle, and the thinned interthalamic adhesion, mamillary bodies, optic chiasm, and tuber cinereum can be visualized. The

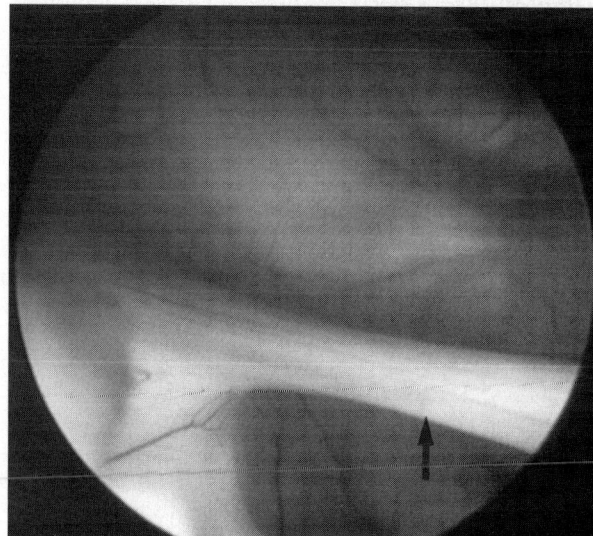

FIGURE 44–5 ■ The third ventricle, interthalamic adhesion *(arrow)*.

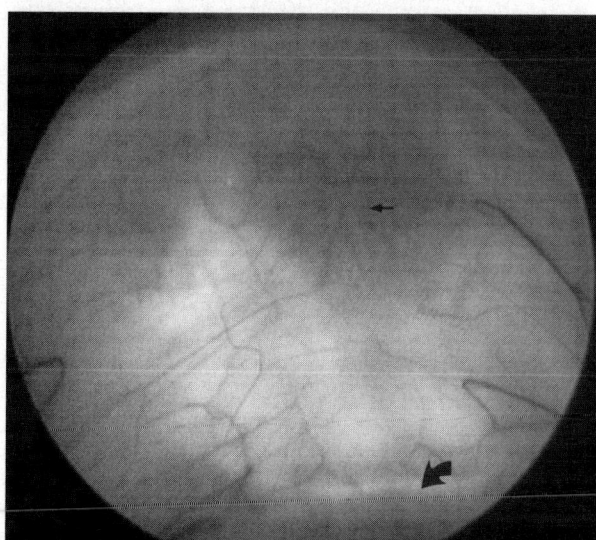

FIGURE 44–7 ■ The anterior floor of the third ventricle, the basilar artery *(arrow)*, and the infundibulum *(small arrow)*. Place the ventriculostomy between the infundibulum and the basilar artery.

clivus and basilar artery can be seen beneath the translucent floor (Figs. 44–4 to 44–7).

The floor of the third ventricle will pulsate with the heartbeat and respiration. If it is not mobile or transparent, the procedure should be terminated secondary to increased risk of hypothalamic and vascular injury. If the basilar artery can be visualized, the floor of the third ventricle is fenestrated between the clivus and the basilar artery in blunt fashion using either the scope itself or preferably blunt biopsy forceps. Cautery (laser or electric) should be avoided. The fenestration can then be enlarged by passing the scope or No. 2 to 4 French Fogarty balloon catheter through the opening. All minor bleeding will cease with gentle saline irrigation. The scope and introducer are removed, and the wound is closed. A temporary external ventricular catheter can be used if necessary.

Complications include injury to the basilar artery, hypothalamus, and optic apparatus. Care must be taken to avoid injury and serious complications. Ventricular decompression is often not seen even after symptoms improve. Ventriculostomy patency can often be visualized with magnetic resonance imaging CSF flow sequences.

# REFERENCES

1. Dandy WE: The diagnosis and treatment of hydrocephalus resulting from strictures of the aqueduct of Sylvius. Surg Gynecol Obstet 31:340–358, 1920.
2. White JC, Michelsen JJ: Treatment of obstructive hydrocephalus in adults. Surg Gynecol Obstet 74:44–109, 1942.
3. Becker DP, Nulsen FE: Control of hydrocephalus by valve-regulated venous shunt: Avoidance of complications in prolonged shunt maintenance. Neurosurgery 28:215–226, 1968.
4. Stookey B, Scarff J: Occlusion of the aqueduct of Sylvius by neoplastic and non-neoplastic processes with a rational surgical treatment for relief of the resultant obstructive hydrocephalus. Bull Neurol Inst N Y 5:348–377, 1936.
5. Mixter WJ: Ventriculoscopy and puncture of the floor of the third ventricle. Boston Med Surg J 188:277–278, 1923.
6. Hoffman HJ, Harwood-Nash D, Gilday DL: Percutaneous third ventriculostomy in the management of noncommunicating hydrocephalus. Neurosurgery 7:313–321, 1980.
7. Kelly PJ: Stereotactic third ventriculostomy in patients with nontumoral adolescent/adult onset aqueductal stenosis and symptomatic hydrocephalus. J Neurosurg 75:865–873, 1991.
8. Jones RFC, Teo C, Stening WA, et al: Neuroendoscopic third ventriculostomy. In Manwaring KH, Crone KR (eds): Neuroendoscopy, Vol 1. New York: Mary Ann Liebert, 1992, pp 63–77.
9. Lawrence KM, Coates S: The natural history of hydrocephalus: Detailed analysis of 182 unoperated cases. Arch Dis Child 37:345–362, 1962.
10. Foltz EL, Shurtleff DB: Five year comparative study of hydrocephalus in children with and without operation. Neurosurgery 20:1064–1079, 1963.
11. Adams RD, Fisher CM, Hakim S, et al: Symptomatic occult hydrocephalus with normal cerebrospinal fluid pressure. N Engl J Med 273:117–126, 1965.
12. Hammock MK, Milhorat TH, Baron IS: Normal pressure hydrocephalus in patients with myelomeningocele. Dev Med Child Neurol 18(Suppl 37):55–68, 1976.
13. Ojemann RG, Fisher CM, Adams MD, et al: Further experience with the syndrome of normal pressure hydrocephalus. J Neurosurg 31:279–294, 1969.
14. Symonds CP: Thrombophlebitis of the dural sinuses and cerebral veins. Brain 60:531–533, 1937.
15. Fried A, Shapiro K: Subtle deterioration in shunted childhood hydrocephalus: A biomechanical and clinical profile. J Neurosurg 65:211–216, 1986.
16. Shapiro K, Fried A: Pressure-volume relationships in shunt-dependent childhood hydrocephalus: The zone of pressure instability in children with acute deterioration. J Neurosurg 64:390–396, 1986.
17. Shapiro K, Fried A, Marmarou A: Biomechanical and hydrodynamic characterization of the hydrocephalic infant. J Neurosurg 63:69–75, 1985.
18. Shapiro K, Marmarou A, Shulman K: Characterization of clinical CSF dynamics and neural axis compliance using the pressure-volume index: The normal PVI. Am Neurol 7:508–514, 1980.
19. Hussey F, Shanzer B, Katzman R: A simple constant infusion manometric test for measurement of CSF absorption. II: Clinical studies. Neurology 20:665–680, 1970.
20. Katzman R, Hussey F: A simple constant-infusion manometric test for measurement of CSF absorption: Rationale and method. Neurology 20:534–544, 1970.
21. Martin G: Lundberg's B waves as a feature of normal pressure hydrocephalus. Surg Neurol 8:247–249, 1978.
22. Symon L, Dorsch NWC: Use of long-term intracranial pressure measurements to assess hydrocephalic patients prior to shunt surgery. J Neurosurg 42:258–273, 1975.
23. DiRocco C, DiTrapani G, Maira G, et al: Anatomical-clinical correlations in normotensive hydrocephalus. J Neurol Sci 33:437–452, 1977.
24. Huckman MS: Normal pressure hydrocephalus: Evaluation of diagnostic and prognostic tests. Am J Neuroradiol 2:385–395, 1981.
25. Salmon JH: Adult hydrocephalus: Evaluation of shunt therapy in 80 patients. J Neurosurg 37:423–428, 1972.
26. Marmarou A, Shulman K, Roende RM: A nonlinear analysis of the cerebrospinal fluid system and intracranial pressure dynamics. J Neurosurg 48:332–344, 1978.
27. DiChiro G, Reames PM, Matthews WB: RISA ventriculography and RISA-cisternography. Neurology 14:185–191, 1964.
28. Stein SC, Langfitt TW: Normal pressure hydrocephalus. J Neurosurg 41:463–470, 1974.
29. Laws ER, Morki B: Occult hydrocephalus: Results of shunting correlated with diagnostic tests. Clin Neurosurg 24:316–333, 1977.
30. Black P: Idiopathic normal pressure hydrocephalus. J Neurosurg 52:371–377, 1980
31. Portnoy HD, Tripp L, Croissant PD: Hydrodynamics of shunt values. Childs Nerv Syst 2:242–256, 1976.
32. McCullough DC: Symptomatic progressive ventriculomegaly in hydrocephalics with patent shunt and antisiphon devices. Neurosurgery 19:617–621, 1986.
33. Portnoy HD, Schutte RR, Fox JL, et al: Antisiphon and reversible occlusion values for shunting in hydrocephalus and preventing post shunt subdural hematomas. J Neurosurg 38:729–737, 1973.
34. Samuelson S, Long DM, Chou SN: Subdural hematomas as a complication of shunting procedures for normal pressure hydrocephalus. J Neurosurg 37:548–551, 1972.
35. Choux M, Genitori L, Lang D, Lena G: Shunt implantation: Reducing the incidence of shunt infection. J Neurosurg 77:875–880, 1992.
36. George R, Leibrock L, Epstein MH: Long-term analysis of cerebrospinal fluid shunt infections. J Neurosurg 51:804, 1979.
37. Haines S, Taylor F: Prophylactic methicillin for shunt operations: Effect on incidence of shunt malfunction and infection. Childs Nerv Syst 9:10–22, 1982.
38. Walters BC, Hoffman HJ, Hendrick EB, et al: Cerebrospinal fluid shunt infection: Influences on initial management and subsequent outcome. J Neurosurg 60:1014–1021, 1984.
39. McLaurin RL, Glass IH, Kaplan S: Ventriculoatrial shunt for hydrocephalus: Electrocardiographic control for accurate placement. Am J Dis Child 105:216–218, 1963.
40. Grosfeld JL, Cooney DR, Smith J, Campbell RL: Intraabdominal complications following ventriculoperitoneal shunt procedures. Pediatrics 54:791–796, 1974.
41. Mates S, Glaser J, Shapiro K: Treatment of CSF shunt infections with medical therapy alone. Neurosurgery 11:781–783, 1982.
42. McLaurin RL, Frame PT: The role of shunt externalization in the management of shunt infections. Concepts Pediatr Neurosurg 6:133–146, 1985.
43. Wald SL, McLaurin RL: Shunt associated glomerulonephritis. Neurosurgery 3:146–150, 1978.
44. Drake J: Ventriculostomy for treatment of hydrocephalus. Neurosurg Clin North Am 4:657–666, 1993.

# CHAPTER 45

# Lumboperitoneal Shunting

■ ROBERT DUTHEL, CHRISTOPHE NUTI, M. J. FOTSO, P. BEAUCHESNE, and JACQUES BRUNON

The treatment of hydrocephalus using lumboperitoneal shunts was first mentioned by Ferguson 100 years ago and performed in a patient who did not survive.[2] Cushing published 12 cases in which he connected the subarachnoid space to the peritoneal cavity with mediocre results.[2] In 1971, Kushner and associates[11] reported a series of 80 shunts and showed an increased incidence of kyphoscoliosis linked to the laminectomy and of serious inflammatory reactions associated with the use of polyethylene shunts. In 1975, Spetzler and associates[17] reported a simplified percutaneous method for shunt replacement that rendered the laminectomy unnecessary. During the 1980s, we noted a relatively high rate of complications with ventricular shunts, such as subdural hematoma and intracerebral hematoma mainly in elderly patients in precarious health with idiopathic hydrocephalus.

The lumboperitoneal shunt appears to have a lower complication rate than other shunts and is useful in the treatment of communicating hydrocephalus.

## TECHNIQUE

### Valve Systems

Although the first lumboperitoneal shunts used a simple connection between the tubes above and below the insertion point,[2] at present a valve is interposed in the system. This valve reduces the flow when the patient is erect. The H.V. Cordis lumbar valve is self-adjusting to postural changes in the upright or prone position. The valve consists of a ball and spring entry valve to control pressure in the horizontal position. The exit valve is made up of a system of superimposed balls, which adds to the action of the entry valve and allows for the regulation of even greater pressure. The systems are color-coded to identify the pressure combinations.

|        | Horizontal | Vertical          |
| ------ | ---------- | ----------------- |
| Blue   | 85–125     | 205–285 mm $H_2O$ |
| Yellow | 85–125     | 265–365 mm $H_2O$ |
| Red    | 50–80      | 170–240 mm $H_2O$ |
| White  | 50–80      | 230–320 mm $H_2O$ |

The horizontal pressure range is chosen as a function of the degree of ventricular dilatation. Although there are six color codes in practice, we almost always use either the "red" or the "white" valve systems.

The ASSE valve is a variable resistance valve ensuring automatic regulation of the flow from the prone to the upright position. The resistance varies form 50 mm $H_2O$ when the patient is prone to 250 mm $H_2O$ when the patient is upright. The valve is implanted vertically. There are two types of valve—one for the right side (R. valve) and one for the left side (L. valve). Because the valves above and below the insertion point are horizontal, one must take care that the tubes follow a curved path and that there are no kinks or bends in them.

Both the tubes are made of Silastic, and the one above the insertion point measures 60 cm with a 1.6-mm external and 0.76-mm internal diameter. The tube's distal extremity is multiperforated. This catheter is passed through a 14-gauge Tuohy needle. The peritoneal catheter measures 122 cm and can be shortened when required.

## Surgical Technique

The operation is usually carried out on the left side with the patient in the lateral decubitus position,[4, 17] under general anesthesia. Both of the patient's knees are brought up to the chest, and a small cushion is placed under the abdomen to ensure that the umbilicus remains in the median position.

The lumbar, iliac, and periumbilical regions of the patient are prepared and draped. A 2- to 3-mm incision is made in the intervertebral space (at either L3-L4 or L4-L5), and a 14-gauge Tuohy needle is positioned in the subarachnoid lumbar space with its bevel facing upward (Fig. 45–1). The proximal catheter is then passed through the needle. If the cerebrospinal fluid (CSF) is flowing freely from the catheter, the Touhy needle can be removed. The length of tube originally put in place must be long enough so that when the needle is removed, the perforated portion of the catheter remains in the subarachnoid space without leaking. An incision is then made in the axillary line at the same level as the lumbar puncture. The subcutaneous tract site is prepared; using a Salmon tube, the subarachnoidal catheter is introduced into the area and connected to a valve. The valve is then fixed carefully in position (Fig. 45–2). The valve has different rates of flow in the horizontal and vertical positions. A short paraumbilical incision

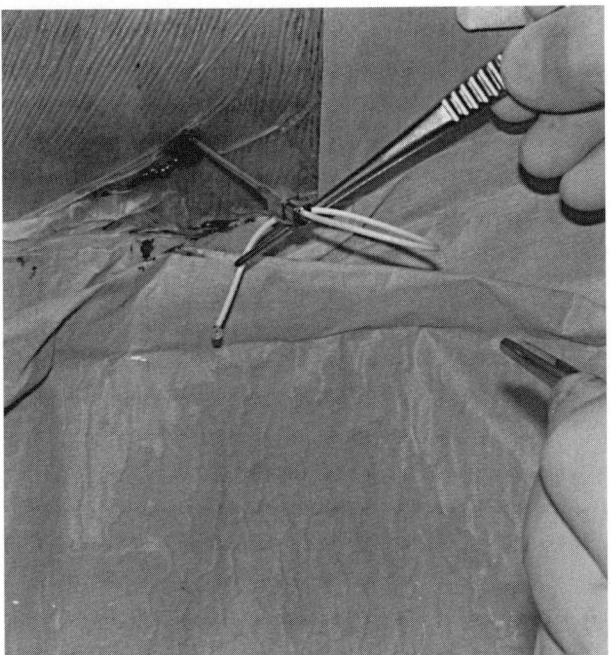

FIGURE 45–1 ■ The Tuohy needle is in position for catheterization of the tube above the insertion site. The cerebrospinal fluid can flow freely from the end of the tube.

health with respect to walking independently, disappearance of sphincter problems, and an improvement in intellectual capacities.

The change in the results seen over the long term is not a function of this technique but arises from the complexity of chronic hydrocephalus.[8] In our series of 115 patients (apart from those patients with chronic idiopathic hydrocephalus), our series includes patients with hydrocephalus secondary to a subarachnoid hemorrhage (37 patients), cranial trauma (9 patients), meningitis (4 patients), and tumor (8 patients). Other indications included control of papilledema in benign intracranial hypertension and one patient with intracranial hypertension after a depressed fracture over the torcular. The clinical symptoms of intracranial hypertension and papilledema improved rapidly, and this improvement has been maintained for over 10 years. Three patients benefitted from a lumboperitoneal shunt used to treat a benign intracranial hypertension. The ophthalmologic signs disappeared after the shunt procedure. In these latter cases, the lumboperitoneal shunt is preferred because the small cerebral ventricles make insertion of a ventricular catheter more technically difficult.

Other uses of lumboperitoneal shunting involve slit ventricle syndrome and for post-traumatic rhinorrhea after the failure of surgical repair[10] or if the site of the leak is not accessible.

on the right side allows the distal catheter to be placed in the peritoneal cavity using either a blunt trocar or a short surgical incision.[17, 18] This catheter is tunneled subcutaneously and connected to the spinal catheter (Fig. 45–3).

## INDICATIONS

The lumboperitoneal shunt can be considered as a "continuous" lumbar puncture, and contraindications to a lumbar puncture are also contraindications to a lumboperitoneal shunt (hydrocephalus related to a brain tumor, obstructive hydrocephalus).

As with any shunt, the lumboperitoneal shunt can only drain a CSF that is sterile and reasonably clear. When the CSF is hemorrhagic or has a high-protein content, the valve may be obstructed. Idiopathic hydrocephalus is the problem most frequently treated with a lumboperitoneal shunt in our department, and its innocuousness has led us to propose this treatment as our first choice with this type of pathology.

In our series of 46 patients with idiopathic hydrocephalus (normal pressure hydrocephalus), 67.5% had good early results but these results diminished over time to approximatly 35%, whereas the 65.5% of initially good results seen in patients with "secondary" chronic hydrocephalus remain at this level. In the report by Bret and Chazal,[3] good results were obtained for 52.6% of patients with a wide range of etiologies and independent of the technique used to treat the hydrocephalus. The percentage of good results in the literature varies enormously and ranges from 24% (Stein) to 90% (Varsilouthis), with a "good" result involving a patient who has returned to his former state of

## Complications of Lumboperitoneal Shunts[13]

In our series of 195 patients, there was a 20.5% complication rate (40 cases). Neither the underlying pathology nor

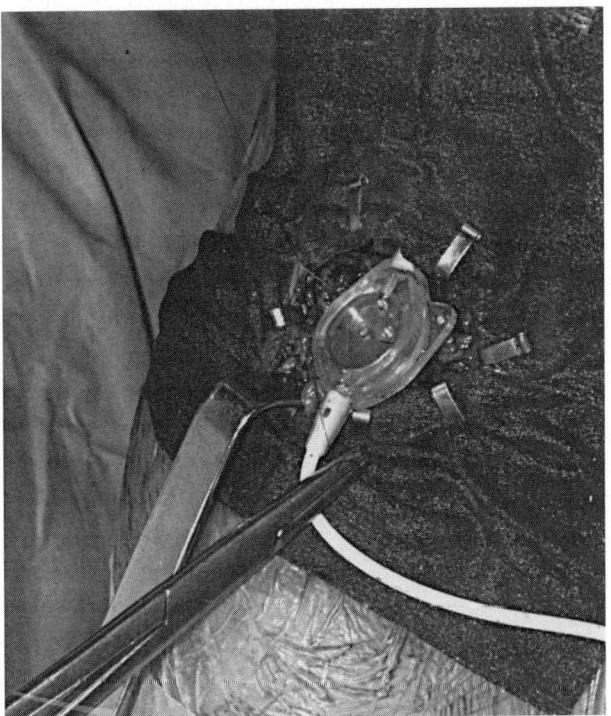

FIGURE 45–2 ■ An ASSE type of valve is ready to be placed in the correct position. The tube leaving downward from the insertion site will then pass subcutaneously.

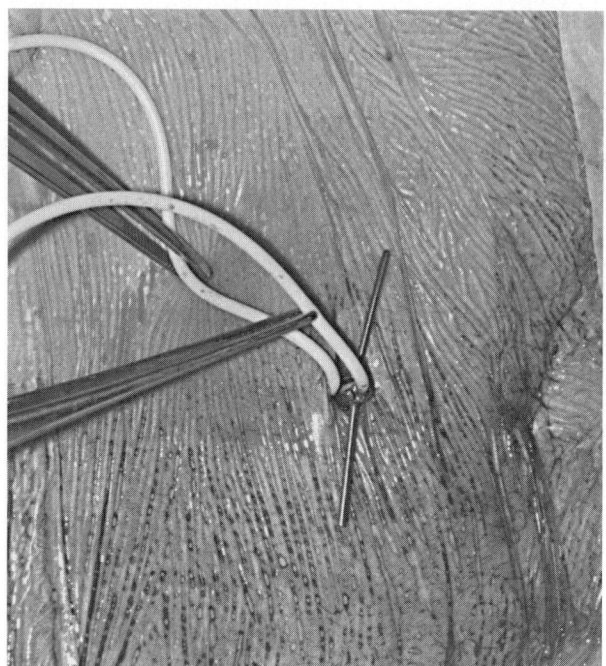

**FIGURE 45–3** ■ ■ The tube passing downward from the insertion point is placed in position in the peritoneal cavity after its subcutaneous passage.

the type of valve had bearing on these complications. The nonspecific complications include death from septic meningitis (0.5%); obstruction or obturation or displacement of the catheters (14.3%); infection (5.1%), which included one death; and subdural hematoma.

Philippon and associates[15] reported on a series of 46 adult patients with a 22% rate of mechanical complications, 2% meningitis, 2% subdural hematoma and seven cases (15%) of postural cephalalgia.

In a series of 207 patients, Aoki[1] reported 52 complications (25%): 25% were mechanical; 3% involved subdural hematoma; 1% were due to infection; 5% involved radiculopathy; 2% were attributed to Arnold-Chiari syndrome; and 1% involved pneumocephalus. Aoki[1] compared this series of 207 lumboperitoneal shunt cases with a series of 120 cases of ventriculoperitoneal shunts. The complication rate in the latter series was 52% comprising intracerebral and intraventricular hemorrhages and slit ventricles. In Bret and Chazal's study[3] of 225 shunts for idiopathic hydrocephalus (including 197 ventriculoperitoneal shunts and 28 lumboperitoneal shunts), there was a 35.5% complication rate of cases and 5.3% mortality rate. Their review of the literature showed a complication rate ranging from 10% to 40% and a mortality rate of up to 12.5%.

In our experience, mechanical complications are the most frequent but are less frequent than with ventriculoperitoneal shunts. Complications caused by infection also appear to be less frequent than those reported with ventricular shunts. In the absence of any antibioprophylaxis, we observed a 5.1% incidence of meningitis.[2]

Subdural collections may be "spontaneous" or arise as the result of trauma. It is, therefore, difficult to know what role the shunt plays. In the literature, the rate varies from 2.5% to 20%.[1, 5, 9, 15] The rate of subdural extravasation is lower after lumboperitoneal shunt than after a ventriculoperitoneal shunt. We have not seen slit ventricles, intracerebral hematoma, or intraventricular hemorrhage as a complication of lumboperitoneal shunting.

## Specific Complications

In our series, two patients experienced sciatica, and we removed the catheter in one patient because of the intensity of the pain. When the hydrocephalic symptoms reappeared, a new lumboperitoneal shunt was inserted. There was a dramatic improvement with no further radiculopathy.

Scoliosis or kyphoscoliosis following a lumboperitoneal shunt has been documented in children and may be associated with an idiopathic syringomyelia.[11] Arachnoiditis, which was reported with polyethylene tubing, has disappeared with the advent of Silastic catheters.

Tonsillar herniation is seen particularly in children[6, 7] after shunting and may be the result of a chronic pressure gradient between the cerebral and spinal fluid. The resultant tonsillar herniation may be symptomatic and accompanied by syringomyelia. In adults, tonsillar herniation seems to be rarer, and a very long interval may elapse after insertion of the lumboperitoneal shunt before it occurs. Payner and colleagues[14] reported 23 cases, of which 18 occurred in patients younger than 15 years of age. Chazal commenting on his series reported two such cases.[9] Because most cases of tonsillar herniations and scoliotic deformities are seen in patients younger than 15 years of age, we recommend a lumboperitoneal shunt as an initial intervention only in adults.

## CONCLUSIONS

The lumboperitoneal shunt is a simple technique that has a lower complication rate than occurs with ventricular-type shunts. Specific flow-regulated valves must be used. This is the procedure of choice for patients with idiopathic hydrocephalus, particularly those who are elderly or in poor health, with hydrocephalus after subarachnoid hemorrhage, meningitis, or surgery. It is also the preferred treatment for benign intracranial hypertension and with the CSF fistula recurring after treatment.

In children, the lumboperitoneal shunt is used when the ventricular shunt is not possible and particularly when there is a slit ventricle syndrome.

## REFERENCES

1. Aoki N: Lumboperitoneal shunt: Clinical applications, complications and comparison with a ventriculoperitoneal shunt. Neurosurgery 26:998–1004, 1990.
2. Bret P, Lapras C, Twose G, et al: La dérivation lombopéritonéale: Indications et résultats à propos de 80 observations. Neurochirurgie 28:13–20, 1982.
3. Bret P, Chazal J: Hydrocéphalie chronique de l'adulte. Neurochirurgie, 36 (Suppl 1):159, 1990.
4. Brunon J, Motuo-Fotso MJ, Duthel R, Huppert J: Traitement de l'hydrocéphalie chronique de l'adulte par dérivation lombo-péritonéale. Neurochirurgie 37:173–178, 1991.

5. Choux M, Genitori L, Lang D, Lena G: Shunt implantation: Reducing the incidence of shunt infection. J Neurosurg 77:875–880, 1992.
6. Chumas P, Kulkarni AV, Drake JM, et al: Lumboperitoneal shunting: A retrospective study in the pediatric population. Neurosurgery 32:376–383, 1993.
7. Chumas P, Armonstrong DC, Drake JM, et al: Tonsillar herniation: The rule rather than the exception after lumboperitoneal shunting in the pediatric population. J Neurosurg 78:568–573, 1993.
8. Clarfeld AM, Danis MB: Normal pressure hydrocephalus: Saga or swamp? JAMA 262:2592–2593, 1989.
9. Duthel R, Nuti C, Motuo-Fotso MJ, et al: Complications des dérivations lombo-péritonéales. Neurochirurgie 42:83–90, 1996.
10. Huppert J, Bret P, Lapras C, Fischer G: Utilisation de la dérivation lombo-péritonéale dans les fistules de LCR de la base du crâne persistantes ou récidivantes. Neurochirurgie 33:220–223, 1987.
11. Kushner J, Alexander E, Courtland H, Kelly D: Kyphoscoliosis following lumbar subarachnoid shunts. J Neurosurg 34:783–791, 1971.
12. Lorenzetti Cl, Ramadan A, Mamie C, et al: Prévention des infections des drainages ventriculaires pour hydrocéphalie. Neurochirurgie 40:233–241, 1994.
13. Lund-Johansen M, Svendsen F, Wester K: Shunt failure and complications in adults as related to shunt type, diagnosis and the experience of the surgeon. Neurosurgery 35:839–844, 1994.
14. Payner TD, Prenger E, Berger TS, Crone KR: Acquired Chiari malformations: Incidence, diagnosis and management. Neurosurgery, 34:429–434, 1979.
15. Philippon J, Duplessis E, Dorwling-Carter D, et al: Dérivation lombo-péritonéale et hydrocéphalie à pression normale des sujets âgés. Rev Neurol 145:776–780, 1989.
16. Selman WR, Spetzler RF, Wilson CB, Grollmus JW: Percutaneous lumboperitoneal shunt: Review of 130 cases. Neurosurgery 6:255–257, 1980.
17. Spetzler RF, Wilson CB, Grollmus JM: Percutaneous lumboperitoneal shunt. J Neurosurg 43:770–773, 1975.
18. Spetzler R, Wilson CB, Schulte R: Simplified percutaneous lumboperitoneal shunting. Surg Neurol 7:25–29, 1977.

# Advanced Technologic Systems for Intracranial Surgery

CHAPTER 46

# Image-Guided Neurosurgery

■ RONALD E. WARNICK and JAMES S. BATH

Medicine has experienced significant technologic advances in conjunction with the rapid evolution of computers and medical imaging. The power and graphics capabilities of today's computer workstations, coupled with high-resolution imaging modalities, provide unprecedented visualization of patient anatomy for diagnosis and therapeutic interventions. Image-guided surgery (IGS) draws from these advances and takes it a step further, creating three-dimensional (3-D) interactive image representations for surgical navigation. "Virtual" is now reality.

Since its beginnings in the early 1970s, computed tomography (CT) has opened up the inner world of the patient. The development of magnetic resonance imaging (MRI) further enhanced anatomic definition. Newer modalities, such as positron emission tomography and single photon emission CT, give life to planar images by recording real-time changes in quantifiable metabolic tissue activity or targeted radiotracer uptake fused with anatomic data.

Most planar scan images, although providing excellent information on anatomic definition and activity, are limited by their two-dimensionality in the 3-D surgical world. In the past, the surgeon was required to create and maintain mental reconstructions of complex structures and surgical trajectories in three dimensions, while accounting for dynamic anatomic changes created by surgical intervention.

The computer, like digital imaging, has quickly become a necessary device in a physician's arsenal for improving the standard of patient care. Innovative software programs enable medical professionals to quantify, qualify, and manipulate data sets derived from a wide range of diagnostic and therapeutic processes. New developments in computer networking allow data and images to be conveniently transmitted throughout the hospital, the local area, and, in an increasing number of instances, the world through advances in telemedicine.

Image-guided interactive surgical navigation combines these powerful technologies in one system. The result is a truly interactive surgical planning and navigation tool. IGS systems automatically create and display the third dimension from planar images, allowing visualization of patient anatomy in multiple planes, localization of critical structures, and planning of optimal surgical paths before initiating surgical treatment. During surgery, the systems become an interactive guide, showing the precise location of surgical instrumentation en route to the target structure, as displayed on the reconstructed computer images.

Specifically, the systems incorporate powerful computer workstations to process and display patient scan images, which can then be viewed from multiple image planes. Preoperative image processing allows further structural delineation through sophisticated tissue segmentation and graphic volume rendering algorithms for targeting and treatment planning. The systems become interactive when the patient image data are correlated, or "registered," to patient anatomy in the operating room by using a precision positional digitizer to select predefined points on the anatomy. Digitizers identify the exact location and orientation of specialized surgical instruments in the surgical field and the patient using one of a number of innovative digital technologies, such as optical camera arrays, magnetic field positioners, or passive robotic arms. The predefined or "fiducial" points are adhesive markers, bony landmarks, or any immobile point on the anatomy that appears on the scan and can be selected with a tracked probe in the operating room.

Once the patient and data set are registered, the system is then able to track surgical probes and, consequently, patient anatomy throughout the preoperative and intraoperative processes with millimetric accuracy. The combined result of interactive surgical planning, visualization, and tracking with these systems is enhanced confidence and expedience of treatment delivery for the physician. Ultimately, patients benefit from reduced trauma due to smaller incisions, more accurate tissue removal, and reduced dissection of surrounding tissue, as well as reduced operative times and the potential for improved surgical outcomes and shorter hospital stays.

This chapter describes the use of image guidance in daily neurosurgical practice. It also highlights the areas of advancement that may help reveal the future of image guidance. The initial sections provide a system overview and describe the flow of the image-guided procedure. Subsequent sections incorporate case studies describing image-guided craniotomy and tumor resection, skull base operations, and trajectory-based procedures. The approaches described in this chapter reflect the authors' experience and should not be interpreted as the only applications for frameless stereotactic techniques in neurosurgery.

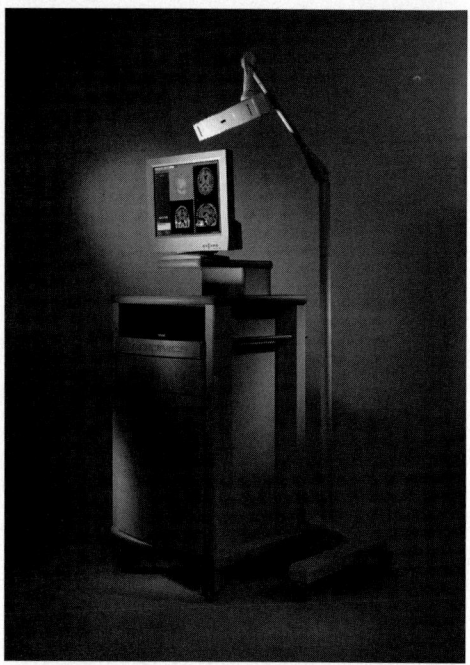

FIGURE 46–1 ■ The Optical Tracking System from Radionics (Burlington, MA).

## SYSTEM OVERVIEW

Most current IGS systems consist of an infrared camera array, a computer workstation, and numerous tracking instruments. Other technologies, such as passive robotic arms and magnetic and sonic localization, have been developed and provide similar tracking capabilities.[1–6] This chapter describes the use of the Optical Tracking System, or OTS (Radionics, Burlington, MA; Fig. 46–1), but the components and procedures described are representative of most IGS systems.

## Camera Array

The camera array is a highly accurate, linear array composed of three one-dimensional CCD (charge-coupled device) sensors in a compact housing (Fig. 46–2). The camera

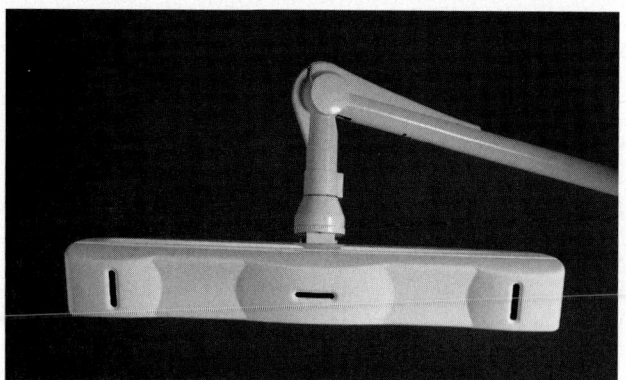

FIGURE 46–2 ■ Compact camera array with three infrared sensors.

array was specifically developed for medical measurement in an operating room environment. The camera, which is mounted on a mobile stand, detects highly focused pinpoints of infrared light pulsed from light-emitting diodes (LEDs) on the tracked instruments in the surgical field.

An alternative camera array that may be used by the system consists of two, two-dimensional (2-D) CCD cameras functioning in a configuration that can detect actively emitted or passively reflected infrared light. In passive reflective mode, infrared emitters located in the camera array flood the surgical field with infrared light. The light reflects off spheres coated with reflective tape and affixed to the tracked instrument. The reflected light is detected and digitized by the array. The system is able to determine the precise location of the spheres using an algorithm to calculate the centroid of the reflected spheres.

The location of the LEDs or spheres is then sent to the camera digitizer, housed in the system console, which processes the information and transfers the positional data of the instruments to the system computer (Fig. 46–3).

## Computer Workstation

A powerful computer, such as the OTS Hewlett-Packard workstation, is housed in a mobile console that provides storage for system peripherals and components, making it easy to position in the operating room. The system can interface with the hospital network through an Ethernet connection using DICOM software to transfer patient scans from the hospital scanner to the operating room. The computer system also has numerous peripheral drives, such as an optical disk, digital audio tape (DAT), and ¼-inch tape to ensure compatibility with most scanners.

The IGS program software is located on the system computer. The software is written in C++ for a UNIX platform and has been designed for ease of use and versatility; its Windows-like environment minimizes keyboard use and allows the user to point and click with the mouse to navigate easily through the program's functions. The software interface uses visual icons to display graphically all necessary functions (i.e., image transfer, application programs, system diagnostics) for users who are unfamiliar with computer interfaces (Fig. 46–4).

The software is designed so the user can move through the program in a linear fashion. Each screen has a small message window that instructs the user to perform a function and then move to the next screen. The patient's images are automatically reconstructed from the original axial image set into a 3-D view and the three orthogonal views (i.e., axial, sagittal, and coronal planes). The system offers trajectory-based views, called Plane-of-Probe and Probe's Eye views, for more intuitive assessment of direction during surgery. On the same screen, the user can select the case type (i.e., cranial, spinal, ear-nose-throat, or image-based stereotactic) and adjust image magnification and gray-scale levels. The user can move through all levels of the image volume to identify the lesion and critical structures and define optimal surgical trajectories before the case begins. Multiple trajectories can be defined depending on the complexity of the case.

Spine implant planning and trajectory simulation are best

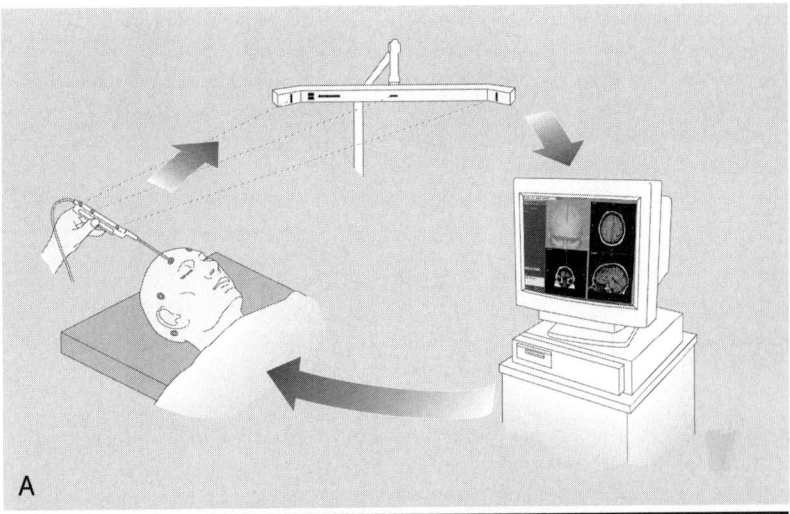

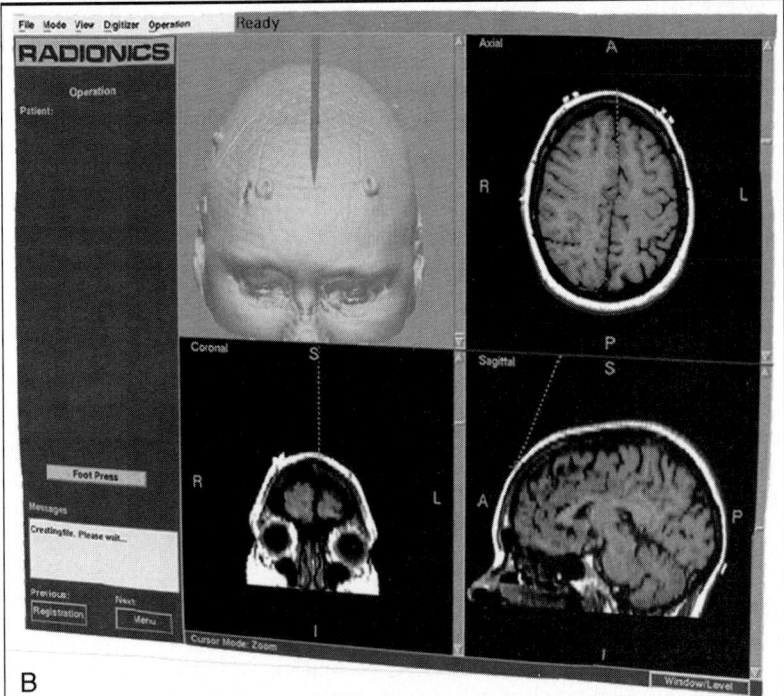

**FIGURE 46–3** ■ *A* and *B*, Relationship between the camera, computer, and patient.

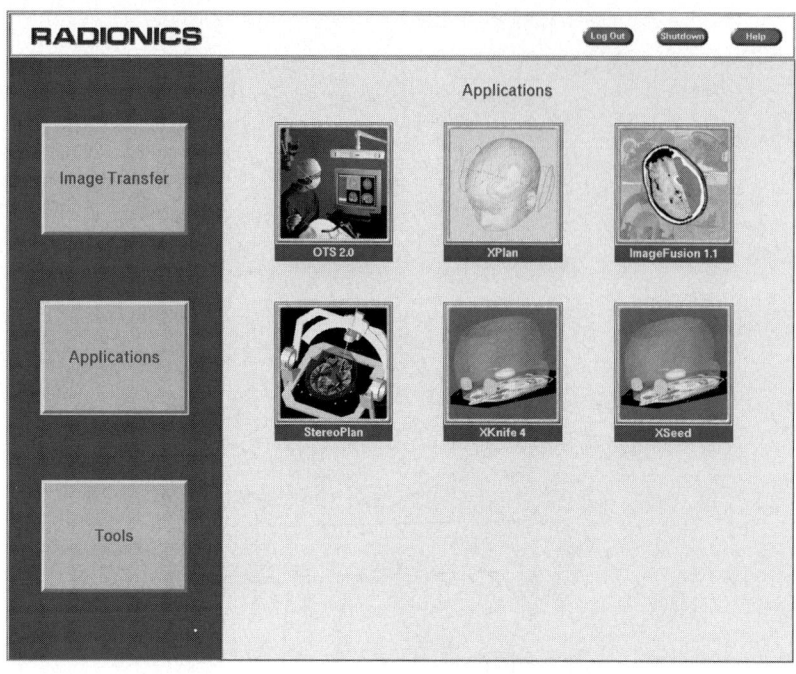

FIGURE 46–4 ■ QuickScreen software interface.

performed before surgery, using the trajectory planning features of the software. For pedicle screws, an optimal trajectory can be visualized using orthogonal images and drawn graphically by selecting entry and end points that best follow the longitudinal axis of the pedicle. The software allows the user to define the width and length of the virtual trajectory to determine the appropriate implant size for the selected trajectory. The graphics can be displayed through the course of the procedure as a 3-D guide while the surgeon navigates the implant into place. In cranial applications, the ability preoperatively to assess the intended surgical path has also proved useful for trajectory-based procedures such as ventricular catheter placement, epilepsy electrode placement, and frameless biopsy.

Pointer-as-a-Mouse is a unique feature of the OTS that allows the user to access and change software options during surgery without breaking sterility or requiring an assistant at the computer (Fig. 46–5). The user moves the tracked probe a short distance from the surgical exposure to open the software menu. Because the coordinate space and the probe origination are known, the system can easily correlate the orientation of the probe to a linear arrangement of menu options. By moving the probe like the hands of a clock, the surgeon selects the desired option, such as changing viewing layouts, performing intraoperative registrations, and displaying trajectory plans. The menu automatically closes when the probe is moved into the surgical exposure, at which point interactive navigation resumes.

Other available features on the market or in development also seek to facilitate surgeon control of the software from the surgical field. These include touch-screen monitors, sterilizable remote controls, touch pads, and voice-activated software. Like Pointer-as-a-Mouse, each attempts to provide the surgeon with a direct, easy-to-use interface.

## Tracking Instruments

As mentioned previously, the instruments incorporate active LEDs or reflective spheres that emit or reflect infrared light to the camera array. The system determines orientation and direction of the instrument by timed emittance sequence or geometric configuration of the LEDs/reflectors in space.

The LEDs/reflectors are positioned on the system probes in a predetermined, rigid geometric pattern. A pattern file is created in the camera processor so the pattern can be recognized in any 3-D orientation, provided the LEDs/spheres are in view of the camera array. Size of the geometric pattern is limited by the camera's ability to recognize each LED/sphere as a distinct point at a defined distance from the others around it.

Instruments with active LEDs are available in two configurations: tethered by a thin coaxial cable, or remotely powered by an on-board battery. In the wired configuration, the power and strobe signals are generated by the system controller, whereas all functions in the wireless battery configuration are controlled by an on-board circuit board.

Advances in the area of infrared-tracked instrumentation may reduce and ultimately eliminate bulky light arrays from the instruments, which can disrupt instrument balance and ergonomics. Reflective tape and adhesive LEDs are two methods that are being investigated. Other research focuses on pattern recognition of instrument surface markings by real-time video acquisition. Such advances may allow seamless integration of tracking technology to almost any instrument. Work with magnetic systems may allow for a single miniature sensor to be placed at the tip of the instrument as an unobtrusive means of localizing the instrument tip. At the time of writing, the accuracy of magnetic technology is still adversely affected by proximity to ferrous metals in the surgical field, although efforts are being made to correct magnetic field disruption through software.

The standard OTS instrument set consists of two straight probes for registration and navigation and two Depth Probes. The Depth Probe is a device that allows the user to simulate, from the surgical field, trajectories through the

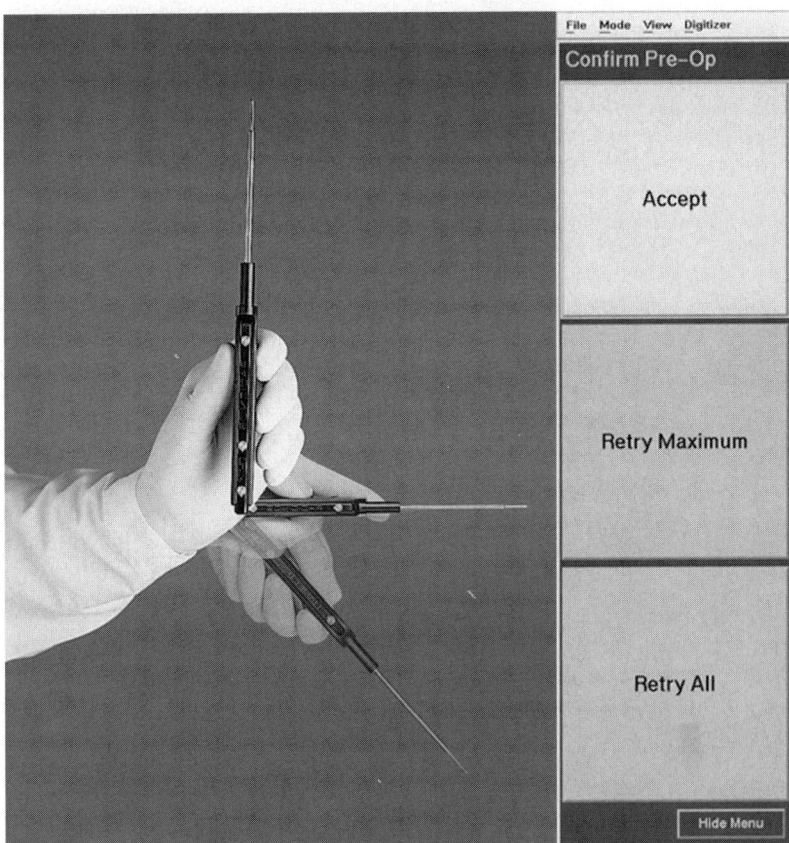

FIGURE 46-5 ■ Pointer-as-a-Mouse, enabling the surgeon to access and change software options from the surgical field.

anatomy displayed on the images. The stylet of the Depth Probe slides through the body of the probe (Fig. 46–6) as it is pressed against the actual patient anatomy, telling the computer to proceed through the anatomy as if following the surgical path. With this unique device, the user can identify preoperatively the tumor location, tumor margins, critical anatomy, incision location, and craniotomy size. Because the Depth Probe automatically advances the image slices, it gives the surgeon control from the surgical field without requiring an assistant to manipulate the software at the computer.

The Dynamic Reference Frame* (DRF), essential to any optical IGS system, tracks patient movement after patient registration (Figs. 46–7 and 46–8). When matching

*Dynamic Reference Frame is a registered trademark of Image Guided Technologies, Inc., Boulder, Colorado.

the patient to preoperative scans, the OTS creates stereotactic space around the patient anatomy in a way similar to that with a stereotactic space created by a standard stereotactic frame. The user can select any point in that space and accurately match that point to the same point on the scan image, or vice versa. To correct for movement, the DRF is a small, rigid, light arrangement fixed to the patient

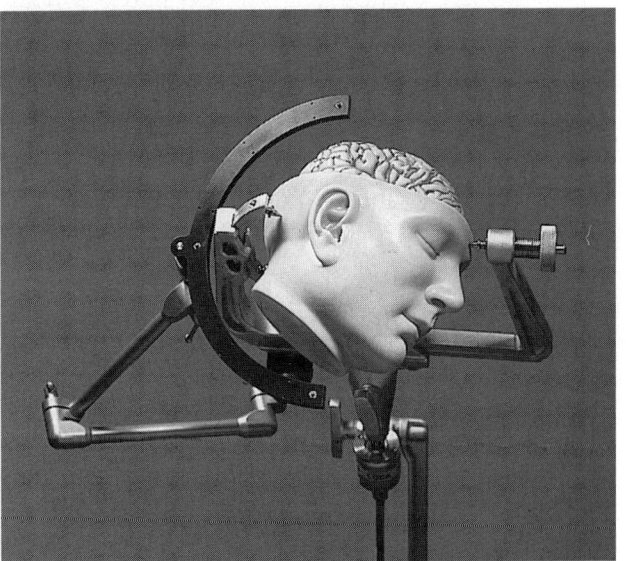

FIGURE 46-7 ■ Cranial Dynamic Reference Frame, which is utilized to track any movement by the patient, operating table, or camera during the procedure.

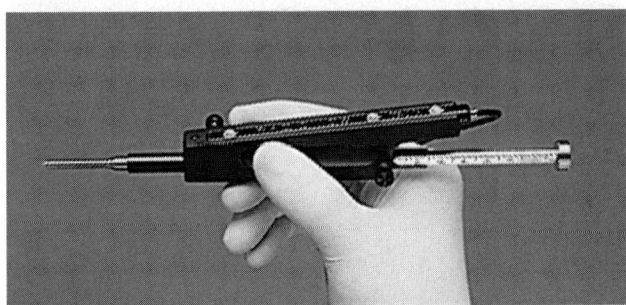

FIGURE 46-6 ■ Depth Probe with the stylet retracted through the probe body to simulate passage through the anatomy.

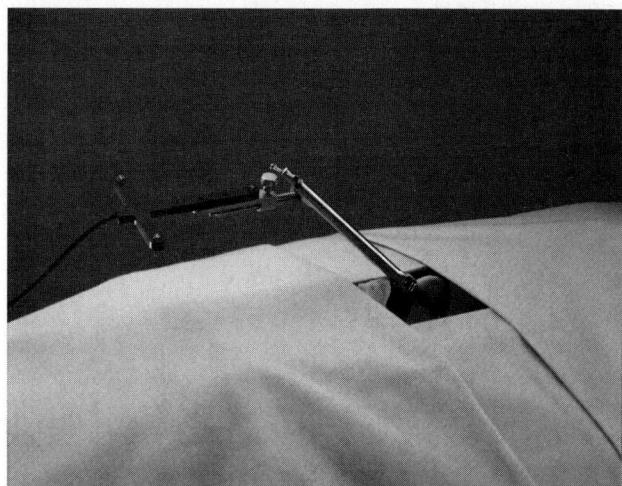

**FIGURE 46–8 ■** Spinal Dynamic Reference Frame.

by the headholder or, in spine cases, clamped to the vertebra; it emits infrared light throughout the procedure. If either the patient or the camera moves, the system detects a change in the position of the DRF and updates the system accordingly.

Once the probe and DRF are connected to the system, the user can quickly register the patient by selecting the points, either fiducial markers or anatomic landmarks, on the patient anatomy. The system automatically displays the points as selected on the images during image registration. The computer then correlates the image set to the patient set by performing rigid-body transformation, which seeks to minimize the average distances by rotating and translating the point set until a best fit is achieved. The software then displays the registration accuracy. When the registration accuracy is satisfactory, the user accepts the value and proceeds to navigation.

Because many other instruments are used during the course of surgery, modules have been developed for "universal instrument" registration. This utility allows the user to affix a compact array of lights to virtually any rigid hand-held instrument and register the instrument to the system for tracking during surgery. The registration sequence defines both the tip and trajectory of the instrument for optimal tracking through the anatomy. Instruments that have been tracked include endoscopes, ultrasonic aspirators (Fig. 46–9), spine instruments, suction tips, and drills. This module allows the user to track a wide range of instruments as needed throughout the procedure.

To register a surgical instrument, the user simply affixes one of several light arrays in a position least disruptive to instrument ergonomics. Each light array has a different clamp configuration and the set covers a wide range of surgical instrument geometries. The standard OTS probe is used to calibrate a registration tool in the surgical field. This is accomplished by transferring the known OTS probe tip location and trajectory to the calibration tool by placing the probe into the tool and registering the location in the software. This effectively localizes a divot (tip) location in the center of the tool and a mechanical vertical axis defined by an adjustable shaft aligned perpendicularly to the central divot. Then, by placing an instrument with a light array

into the calibration tool, as performed with the OTS probe, the computer correlates the tip location and trajectory of the tool to the light array on the instrument. Because the registration tool remains in the surgical field for the duration of the procedure, any instrument/light array combination can be registered during the case.

## CASE FLOW OF AN IMAGE-GUIDED SURGERY PROCEDURE

An image-guided procedure consists of several steps, including image acquisition, data transfer, operating room setup, system calibration, graphic display, and operative use. The success of the procedure relies on the coordinated efforts of the IGS team, which usually consists of radiologic technologists, operating room staff, and the neurosurgeon.

### Image Acquisition

The basis of IGS lies in the ability to correlate patient anatomy to preoperative scans. To achieve this, there must be an identical set of reference or fiducial markers that appear on both the scan and the patient. The points can be adhesive or bone-fixed radiopaque markers, bony landmarks, or other rigid, immobile anatomic points. Several studies demonstrate the relative accuracy of various fiducial points.[7–9]

For cranial work, these points are often special radiopaque markers developed for IGS that provide a distinct point of reference and, therefore, are considered more accurate than anatomic landmarks. For procedures in which markers are not available or desired, precise selection of anatomic landmarks such as the tragus, inner and outer canthes, and nasion can result in acceptable registration accuracy.

Experience has shown that skin markers provide little correlation to the spinal column because of skin shift relative to the target vertebrae occurring between the scanner

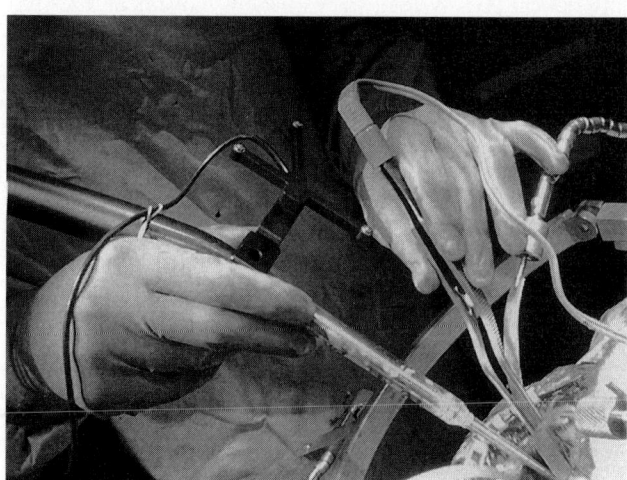

**FIGURE 46–9 ■** Universal Instrument Registration light array affixed to the ultrasonic aspirator.

and operating table. Distinct bony protrusions such as the spinous process, facets, and transverse processes are commonly used for their prominence and accessibility in the exposure.

The markers are noted on the scan before the start of the procedure. The markers on the patient are then localized using the tracked probe in the surgical field. With the two sets of data points, the system can correlate all points on the anatomy to their corresponding points on the scan images. The first step is to acquire the patient images and transfer the data set to the workstation.

When scanning for a cranial procedure with fiducial markers, the procedure begins with placement of several such markers on the patient's scalp before scanning. At least four fiducial markers are required for system calibration; however, six or more markers are used for most OTS procedures. The placement of fiducial markers is important in determining the accuracy of the system. For optimal accuracy, the fiducial markers should be applied in a noncolinear configuration to form a plane passing through the target of interest. In practice, however, standard fiducial placement that does not require any hair removal can be performed easily by radiologic technologists, and provides sufficient accuracy for most neurosurgical procedures. Four doughnut-shaped fiducials are placed over the forehead, temporal region, and mastoid (Fig. 46–10). The underlying skin is marked through the center hole of the fiducial marker so that the fiducial can be accurately reapplied if dislodged.

Computed tomography or MRI can be used for IGS; most cranial procedures rely on MRI, whereas spine scans typically use CT. CT is preferred when visualization of bony anatomy is essential. Image acquisition is performed with a constant field of view and consistent slice spacing. The scan includes the entire anatomic volume and all potential markers, using 1- to 3-mm contiguous slices that allow the IGS computer to provide an accurate 3-D reconstruction. The patient is instructed not to move during the scan to avoid interference with the stereotactic image acquisition. An image-guided procedure should not be attempted with an agitated or otherwise uncooperative patient. Newer scanners incorporating volumetric and helical scanning acquisition are reducing scan time and increasing postscan processing to optimize image resolution.

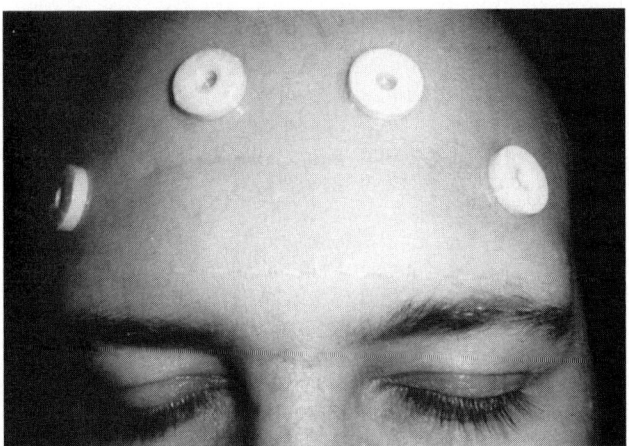

FIGURE 46–10 ■ Position of fiducial markers on the patient.

The ability to fuse multiple image sets allows the system to coregister CT and MRI, and alternate between the sets during planning and navigation. This is very useful during cranial and spinal applications where critical transitions occur from bone to soft tissue.[10] Several studies describe the utility of fusing functional images to standard scans to localize critical areas of the brain. Although useful, such scanners are not yet commonly available, and the imaging protocols are nonstandard relative to normal stereotactic imaging.

## Data Transfer

The imaging data can be transferred to the operating room computer workstation by magnetic tape, disk, or network connection. The radiologic technologist commonly downloads the OTS MRI or CT data onto a 4-mm DAT tape that accompanies the patient to the operating room. The tape is then loaded into the DAT tape reader and transferred to the OTS computer for reconstruction of the scan into 2-D and 3-D views. The imaging data can also be transferred directly over an Ethernet system and uploaded into the OTS computer through a network connection in the operating room. It is expected that network transfer will be the common interface in the coming years, using a DICOM format, as hospital networks are modernized and scanner-dependent file parameters are standardized.

## Operating Room Setup

The patient is placed in the operative position with the head fixed in the Mayfield head clamp for cranial procedures. Special care is taken during pin placement to avoid displacement of the scalp fiducials, which could introduce significant calibration error. Patients undergoing spinal procedures are positioned in a conventional manner, with care taken to minimize differential spine flexion on the table versus the position in which the patient was scanned.

In the case of cranial applications, the DRF is attached to the Mayfield headholder in such a way that it also has a direct line of sight with the camera but does not obstruct the operative field. For standard spine navigation, the DRF is placed directly on the vertebra after the incision and surgical exposure has been performed.

The position of the IGS console and camera stand relative to the patient is unique to each operation and must be carefully planned by the surgeon. In general, the system console should be positioned so the surgeon can easily view the graphic display during the operation with minimal movement (Fig. 46–11A). Most important, the system requires a direct line of sight between the LED probe and the camera array. Therefore, possible obstructions, such as a microscope, overhead instrument table, and other team members should be positioned so that the tracked instruments can be seen by the camera array (see Figure 46–11B).

## System Calibration

The system is calibrated by registering the patient to the scan images. First, the fiducial markers or anatomic land-

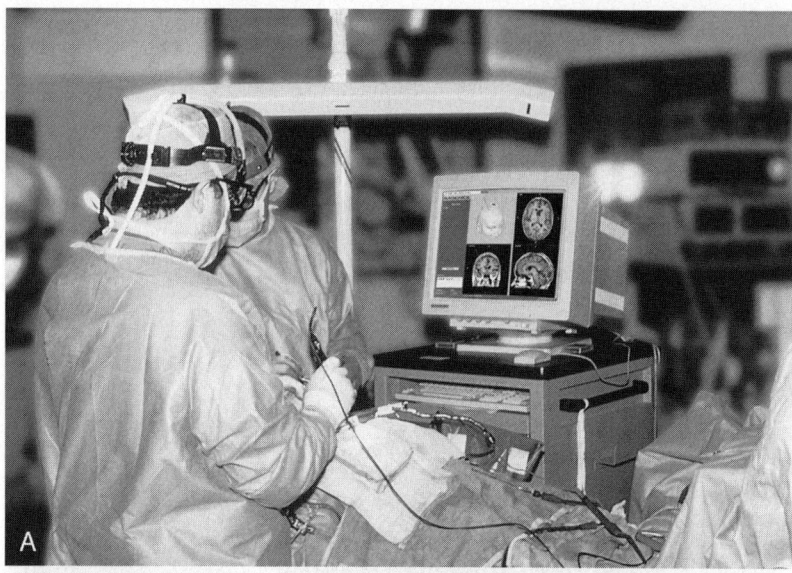

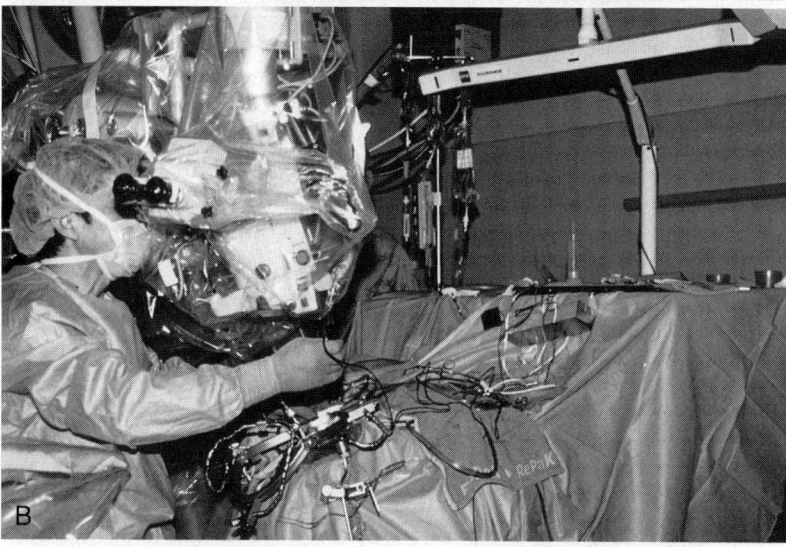

FIGURE 46–11 ■ *A*, Surgeon with an unobstructed view of the system monitor. *B*, Proper positioning of the camera with a microscope in use.

marks are identified on the 2-D and 3-D images generated by the IGS software. A distinct part of each fiducial or landmark is selected by using the mouse to deposit a cursor at that point. The system is then calibrated by using the system probe to register each of the markers or landmarks in a sequence defined by the system (Fig. 46–12). This step establishes a direct link between the patient's anatomy and the imaging information.

Advances are underway to automate the registration process. Automatic software recognition of specialized markers on the scan images and on the patient may obviate the need for preoperative image registration and probe marker selection. The net result is a faster, more intuitive, potentially more accurate process that saves valuable operating room time.

The computer calculates, displays, and records the estimated calibration error by computing the difference between the spatial coordinates of the fiducials from the configured image set and the actual registration of the fiducials with the LED probe. The error reflects the accuracy of fiducial transformation and usually ranges from 1 to 3 mm. If the error exceeds this range, the surgeon has

the option of either recalibrating or eliminating one or more markers from the registration set. The accuracy of calibration can be confirmed visually by touching the LED probe to the fiducial markers and anatomic landmarks and by noting the proximity of the cursor on the screen to the landmarks displayed on the imaging studies.

In cases where fiducials are not used for reasons of convenience, cost, or efficiency, and a higher degree of registration is required than typically obtained with anatomic markers, the user can select the surface matching feature. Surface matching algorithms were incorporated to facilitate patient registration while obviating the need for scanning with fiducial markers. Surface matching uses several anatomic landmarks to orient the patient anatomy to the overall scan data set. The user then selects random points over the anatomic surface (70 to 90 for cranial and 30 to 50 for spinal) with the OTS probe. The software transforms the surface points to the stereotactic space of the roughly registered data set. The software then rotates and translates the set of points until they best correlate to the surface of the 3-D reconstruction. The software seeks to minimize the distance between corresponding anatomic

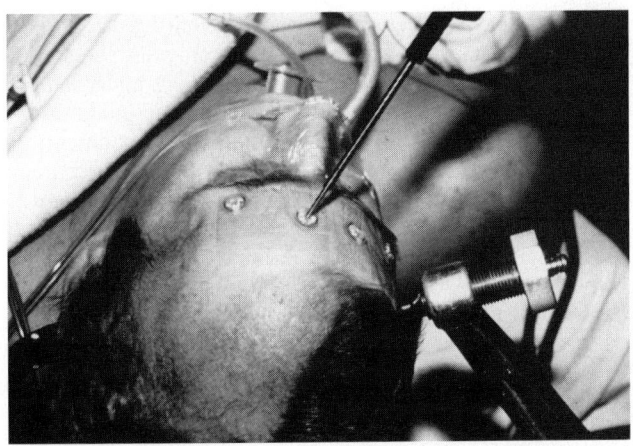

**FIGURE 46–12** ■ Marker selection using a probe for patient registration.

and image set points. The current algorithms, however, require further refinement to better handle large, quasi-spherical objects, such as the cranium, and to accommodate for skin shift. In cranial cases where accuracy is paramount, fiducial markers provide better accuracy.[9] Surface matching tends to be more effective when registering a vertebra because of the intricate geometry of the bone. The benefit here lies in eliminating the difficulty in accurately locating distinct, vertebral landmarks in exposures obscured by blood and soft tissue.

One deviation from point-to-point correlation is video registration using a laser striping system.[11] This method acquires 3-D data points created and captured by inter-secting laser light and optical rays on the anatomic surface. If perfected, this method has the potential for providing automatic, noncontact cranial registration. Like surface matching, the points created by the intersecting beams are localized in space and transformed to a surface map that is matched to the 3-D reconstruction on the patient image set. Current limitations include the inability of the video sensor to realize points from the quadrants of the head and the presence of hair, corrupting acquisition of the surface points.

## Graphic Display

Once the system is calibrated, the camera array continuously tracks the position of the instrument tip and trajectory and graphically displays the location on reconstructed 2-D and 3-D images. The software allows the surgeon to select a variety of imaging displays, including continuous mode (axial, sagittal, coronal), static orthogonal views, and probe views (Fig. 46–13).

Presurgical planning for cranial applications is usually performed with the Depth Probe, which allows the surgeon to navigate the intracranial contents in three imaging planes as the probe is advanced against the head, simulating intracranial penetration (Fig. 46–14). This provides the ability to simulate passage through patient anatomy and to visualize critical structures to plan the optimal skin incision, craniotomy flap, and surgical trajectory before surgery. In probe views, the coronal and sagittal planes are replaced with Plane-of-Probe view and Probe's Eye view. The Plane-of-Probe view reconstructs the patient's images to show the

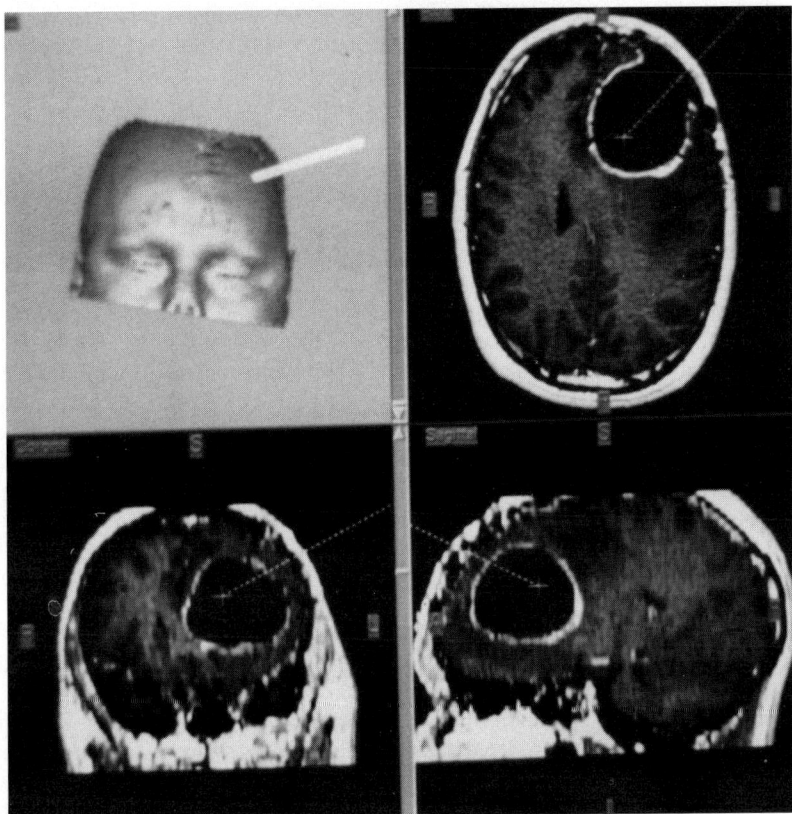

**FIGURE 46–13** ■ Views offered by an image-guided surgery system.

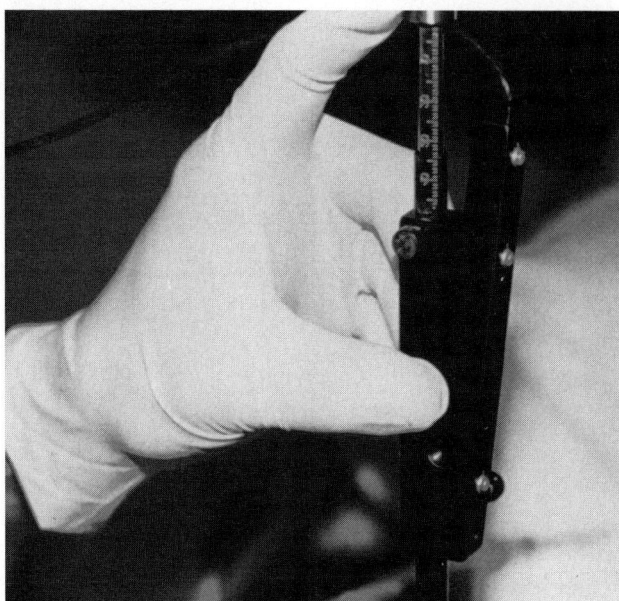

FIGURE 46–14 ■ Presurgical planning using the Depth Probe to simulate intracranial navigation.

actual plane the probe creates as it passes through various image slices. This view displays the intracranial contents that are traversed if the probe is advanced along that trajectory. The Probe's Eye view allows the surgeon to "look" directly through the center of the probe. These views are particularly helpful for trajectory-based procedures.

## OPERATIVE USE OVERVIEW

### Cranial Applications

Once the patient is registered to the system, the cranial DRF is covered with a translucent drape, with special care taken to avoid folds that would obscure the LEDs. A sterile Depth Probe is then connected to the system and used during surgery to check the position and extent of the bone flap and dural opening, and to confirm the approach to the lesion. The patient's head position can be changed at any time because the DRF maintains a fixed position to the head and allows the computer to account for changes without the need for recalibration. Intraoperative calibration may also be performed as a backup in the event that the DRF is accidentally moved relative to the head. After the craniotomy is performed, the surgeon recalibrates the system using internal landmarks such as the dural retention holes in the surrounding skull. This calibration is saved in the system memory and can be recalled and used for recalibration in case of DRF failure, DRF movement, or computer lockup.

The OTS has proven useful in a wide variety of cranial cases. Intrinsic tumors, brain metastases, and vascular malformations are easily localized through small skin, bone, and cortical incisions and are approached along optimal trajectories. Skull lesions are rapidly identified and easily

removed. For extremely small lesions requiring direct visualization for resection, the IGS system can guide the neurosurgeon to the lesion. In general, any patient undergoing a craniotomy can benefit from the use of image guidance.

During actual tumor resection, the OTS provides information about the extent of resection. Anatomic accuracy consists of maintaining the preoperative target position as much as possible during surgery. Measures that could lead to excessive change in brain volume, such as mannitol, furosemide, hyperventilation, and lumbar drainage, should be minimized or titrated to need. Tumor cysts or the ventricular system should not be entered early in the procedure to avoid excessive loss of fluid (i.e., remove solid components first). Because cerebrospinal fluid loss and lesion debulking cause shifts in brain structure, the surgeon must anticipate the decreasing accuracy of the OTS as surgery proceeds. Dissection/resection should begin closest to the most critical or eloquent brain tissue, with lesions in non-eloquent regions approached last. Maneuvering the probe around the resection bed while observing the monitor provides feedback about possible residual tumor through a range of approaches. In a similar manner, the probe can aid in determining when a gross total volumetric resection is complete. Closure time is minimized because bone and skin incisions are small.

In performing conventional stereotactic brain biopsies, a stereotactic frame is applied to the patient before the scan. However, these frames are uncomfortable for the patient and can be cumbersome for the neurosurgeon. In addition, trajectory planning with these systems is often complicated and nonintuitive. Frameless image guidance can be used in a variety of trajectory-based procedures, obviating the need for frame-based stereotaxy. Compared with frame-based stereotactic systems, the advantages of image guidance are patient acceptance (no ring placement), less cumbersome hardware, and easier trajectory planning.

An IGS system can also replace frame-based stereotactic techniques to drain a hematoma or abscess cavity, place a catheter into a cyst or slit ventricle, or guide a rigid endoscope to an intraventricular target. Procedures aimed at lesions smaller than 1 cm in diameter or those requiring a high degree of accuracy (e.g., functional procedures) should be performed using a frame-based stereotactic system because the current 3-D positioners do not provide sufficient stability for these applications.

For image-guided biopsies, the patient's head must be fixed in the Mayfield headholder during surgery, which usually necessitates the use of general anesthesia, with its attendant risks. In addition, the accuracy of biopsy using OTS is limited by the ability of the 3-D positioner to precisely and rigidly fix the LED probe. Further refinement is needed before the OTS can be used in functional procedures or to access small lesions in critical locations (e.g., brain stem biopsy).

### Spinal Applications

Image-guided spine surgery has natural application in the directed navigation of implants such as pedicle screws, cervical transarticular screws, odontoid or lateral plating screws, or interbody fusion hardware.[12–14] Although a posterior approach facilitates DRF fixation and registration, anterior and transthoracic approaches are being investigated using modified DRF fixation hardware and surface matching registration. Many believe that image guidance is not useful in first-time fusion cases, where anatomic landmarks and conventional reference angles are readily apparent, because of a small cost-benefit ratio. Instead, image guidance proves most useful in cases where landmarks have been shifted, deformed, or removed, as with scoliotic spines, spondylolisthesis, trauma, and corrective fusion surgery.

Advances in spinal navigation will increase the application of minimally invasive methods for a wide variety of open spine procedures. Integration of fluoroscopic images for visualization and instrument tracking in place of CT data can provide real-time intuitive image sets. Technology exists to perform ultrasonographic registration by correlating a 3-D image set derived with standard ultrasound with the 3-D image reconstruction. Others are investigating percutaneous placement of fiducial markers that will allow point-to-point registration without creating an exposure. Such methods of percutaneous registration may allow minimally invasive placement of screws, cages, or stimulators with continuous, nonfluoroscopic guidance.

Because initial registration takes place after the surgical incision to expose the spinal column, much of spine IGS is performed under sterile conditions. As such, the sterile spine dynamic reference frame is securely affixed to the target vertebra because this will be the anatomy tracked during the procedure. Some have suggested that positioning the DRF on adjacent vertebral bodies adds convenience by moving the DRF away from the working space, with minimal affect on the overall accuracy. Vertebrae, however, unless previously fused, move independent of one another during the procedure and are in a different relative position from scan to operating room because of overall flexion of the spinal column. Both factors can lead to significant errors if the DRF is not placed on the vertebra registered to the system.

In the future, software might be used to transform the orientation of adjacent segments to correlate with that of the preoperative image set, thus obviating the need to treat vertebrae as independent bodies. Because it is recommended that the DRF be affixed to the spinous process for optimal mechanical purchase, the laminectomy is performed after image-guided placement of an implant. If the patient has had a previous laminectomy, the DRF may be placed laterally on the transverse process. Once affixed to the vertebra, the registration process proceeds using marker registration and surface matching, as described earlier.

The standard OTS probe is used to localize the spinal cord tumor or desired entry point through the pedicle, lamina, or vertebral body, depending on the surgical approach and treatment method. If the system is being used for tumor localization, the standard probe can be used throughout to localize the margin and assist with optimal resection. For implant placement, the surgeon can then switch to universal instrument registration to track probes, drills or drill guides, taps, and screwdrivers. The tracked instrument is then aligned with the preoperative trajectory plan using either the orthogonal or trajectory views offered by the system software. The path can be continually re-viewed by observing the updated image on the system monitor as the instrument passes through the cancellous bone to its final position.

After placing the first implant set of a multilevel fusion, the DRF is moved to the next vertebra and the level is registered to the system. The software permits the surgeon to preregister the images of all levels before the case and simply use the Pointer-as-a-Mouse to switch to the next registration set when ready to select the corresponding points with the probe.

## LIMITATIONS

As with all surgical instruments, there are limitations to IGS during the surgical procedure. Because the IGS system relies on optical signals from the probe to the tracking cameras, a direct visual path must exist between these two components. Objects disrupting this direct line of sight can constrain the use of image guidance. The surgeon must also keep in mind that the accuracy of image-guided technology (which relies on presurgical images) decreases as the case progresses because of fluid and tissue shifts. This is particularly true for extensive resection of a large tumor.

The advance and integration of intraoperative imaging methods have already begun, providing real-time solutions for tissue shift. A growing number of sites use intraoperative CT or MRI to assess better the extent of resection and accommodate for tissue shift occurring over the course of the procedure.[15-18] Coupling the intraoperative scanner to the image-guided system allows the surgeon to use updated image sets during navigation after the intraoperative scan has been performed. A DICOM link transfers the image set to the IGS workstation. The image set is then uploaded to the program software and reconstructed in three dimensions. In some cases, the scanner is already in stereotactic image space, providing a registered image set on acquisition. In other cases, the surgeon places radiopaque markers around the craniotomy opening that can be identified on the scans and then on the patient, using a tracked instrument. In either case, the new image set is registered and navigation can resume in and around the resected area, with an image set no longer degraded by brain shift or anatomic changes due to surgical intervention.

In the future, lower-cost, compact scanners will greatly facilitate inclusion of intraoperative imaging in a broader array of neurosurgical procedures. Many advances have already been made to minimize the field strength adjacent to an intraoperative MRI device, requiring fewer changes to instrumentation and ancillary equipment. Lower emission, mobile CT scanners add the benefit of portability, which can also be cost-justified over numerous departments.[18] This also provides the ability to bring the scanner to the patient, further minimizing disruption of the case flow to acquire a new image set. While overall image quality continues to improve, scanner manufacturers continue to reduce the tradeoffs inherent to acquisition speed and lower field strength/emissions versus high-resolution images. Image-guided systems will need to streamline the standard transfer process by loading, processing, and registering image sets automatically. This will eliminate software manipulation by the user and save valuable operating time.

It is often inconvenient to alternate between a surgical instrument and the standard tracked pointing probe when working under the microscope. Universal instrument registration solves this problem by allowing the attachment of LEDs to virtually any surgical instrument; this instrument then, in effect, becomes the OTS probe after appropriate calibration. For example, an ultrasonic aspirator with the LED attachment can be used to remove the tumor *and* assess the extent of resection (see Fig. 46–9).

An optional module enables the user to calibrate the microscope focal point, transforming the microscope into the tracking instrument. This can reduce the need to draw attention away from the exposure to a remote monitor. Ongoing collaboration between leading microscope and IGS system manufacturers will provide the market with numerous microscope tracking options; the collaborations have greatly improved the quality of integration as well as the breadth of systems the surgeon has to choose from when evaluating image guidance systems. Most systems are now able to track the microscope focal point, automatically update for changes in focus and zoom, and display critical image information in the microscope ocular over a range of microscope models. As improvements in the surgical microscopes emerge, such as refined robotic stands and advanced electronic controls, image-guided systems will use these capabilities to microadjust the microscope position in a hands-free manner and display a wider array of information in the ocular.

To look beyond the realm of the surgical microscope as the primary means of bringing anatomic information closer to the surgeon, clinical investigation of heads-up displays seeks to expand visualization capabilities through digital processing integration of image-related and monitoring data sets.[19] Advances in product design may also result in added comfort and freedom of movement over the course of the procedure. Holographic displays will then add a third dimension to the planar information overlays in microscopes and head-mounted displays.

## APPLICATIONS AND CASE STUDIES

### Craniotomy

#### CASE STUDY

A 45-year-old, right-handed man presented with a generalized seizure followed by a several-day period of postictal dysphasia. He was neurologically normal after institution of corticosteroids. MRI showed a 1.5-cm enhancing lesion in the left posterior temporal lobe with surrounding edema (Fig. 46–15A). Systemic evaluation revealed a primary lung carcinoma. The patient underwent image-guided craniotomy. After system calibration, the Depth Probe was used to map the location of the tumor and the adjacent transverse sinus (see Fig. 46–15B). A small, lazy-S skin incision and trephine craniotomy were performed to expose

the tumor. The tumor was then localized on the cortical surface and a sulcal trajectory was selected using the orthogonal images as displayed (see Fig. 46–15C, D). A complete tumor resection was performed and the patient was neurologically intact after surgery. He was discharged the following day.

### Skull Base Surgery

Image guidance is well suited for skull base lesions because they are relatively fixed and brain shift is minimal compared with cortical or subcortical lesions. Specific uses in skull base surgery include the identification of underlying surface structures (e.g., venous sinuses) and bony structures (e.g., occipital condyle), as well as assessment of extent of resection. The choice of imaging studies is based on the individual case.

#### CASE STUDY

A 39-year-old man presented with a 2-week course of severe hoarseness and difficulty swallowing. Initial neurologic examination revealed bilateral 10th and 12th cranial nerve dysfunction. MRI demonstrated a 4 × 4 × 3 cm clival extra-axial mass compressing the brain stem (Fig. 46–16A). A CT scan showed destruction of the lower clivus, foramen magnum, and left occipital condyle. The lesion was consistent with either a chordoma or chondrosarcoma. After treatment options were discussed with the patient, a transoral approach was performed using the OTS to guide the surgical trajectory, bony exposure, and extent of resection. The OTS was helpful in maintaining the appropriate trajectory at the posterior oropharynx (see Fig. 46–16B) and demonstrated that the most rostral portion of the tumor was inaccessible by this exposure (see Fig. 46–16C). Therefore, a bilateral maxillotomy and palatal split were performed to reach the superior border of the tumor and the clivus. This procedure was accomplished using OTS guidance, which provided a margin of safety in determining a midline orientation, as well as delineating the ventral and dorsal aspects of the tumor (see Fig. 46–16D). Frozen-section evaluation confirmed a low-grade chordoma. The tumor infiltrated the bone, soft tissue, and posterior longitudinal ligament but did not penetrate the dura. The OTS was used extensively to judge the extent of tumor resection in the rostral-caudal directions and dorsally along the brain stem. The patient had an uncomplicated postoperative course and the postoperative MRI scan demonstrated excellent tumor resection with decompression of the brain stem (see Fig. 46–16E).

### Trajectory-Based Procedures

For trajectory-based procedures, the Depth Probe is used to locate the planned entry point on the patient's head, and the underlying skin is marked. A small area of hair is shaved and the patient is prepared and draped in the usual

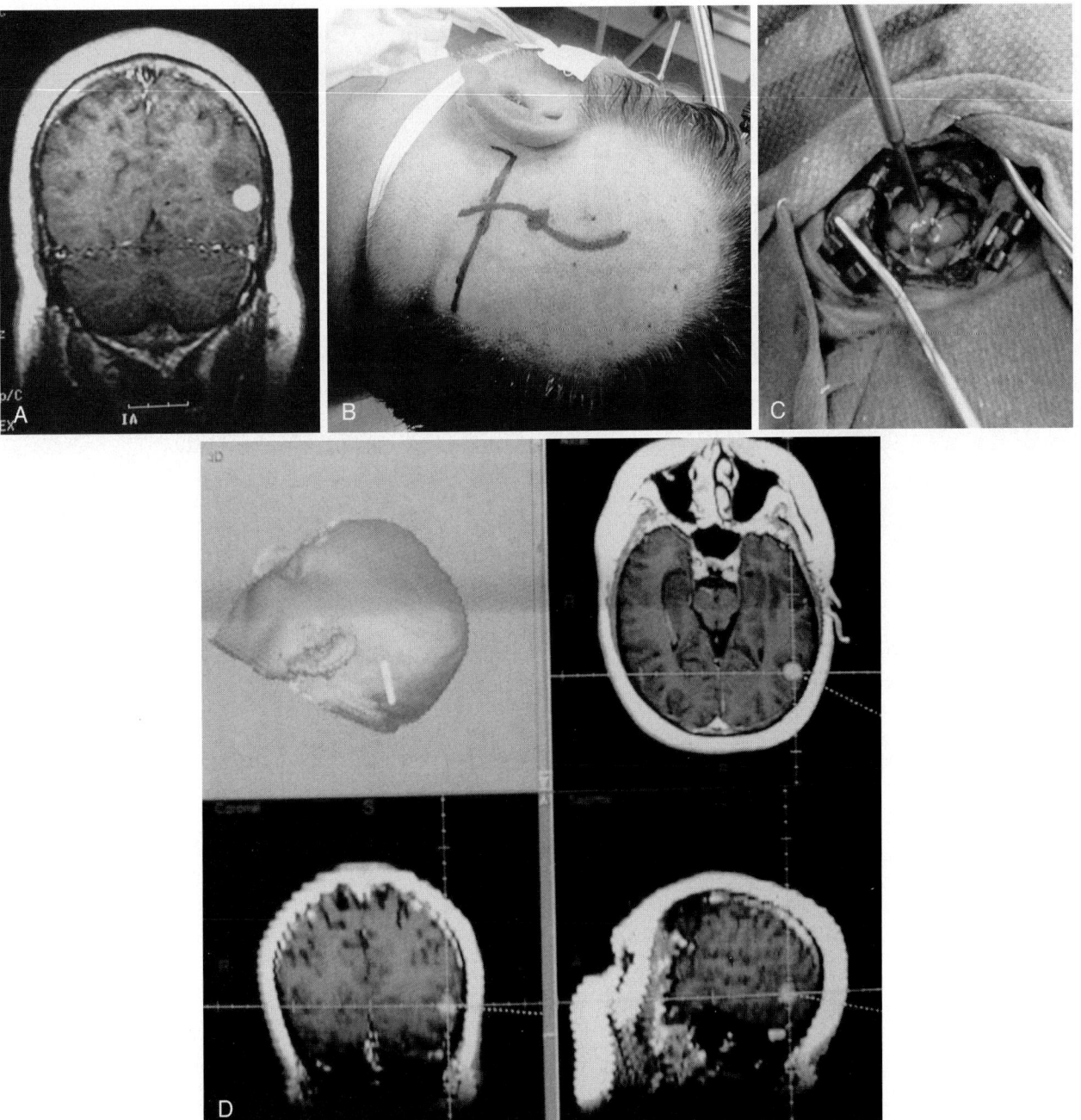

FIGURE 46–15 ■ *A*, A magnetic resonance imaging scan shows a 1.5-cm enhancing lesion in the left posterior temporal lobe with surrounding edema. *B*, Depth Probe is used to map the location of the tumor and the adjacent transverse sinus. *C* and *D*, The tumor is localized on the cortical surface; a sulcal trajectory was selected using the orthogonal images.

fashion for an IGS procedure. A skin incision and bur hole are made using standard techniques. At this point, the 3-D positioner snake arm is attached to the side rail of the operating table and the OTS Depth Probe is secured to the distal end. The IGS probe is positioned over the bur hole such that the real-time trajectory superimposes on the pre-planned trajectory as visualized on the system console. The 3-D positioner is then locked and the screen double-checked to ensure that the final trajectory is acceptable on the three orthogonal views. If the surgeon wants to access different views (e.g., probe views) while the tracked probe is fixed in the 3-D positioner, the LED cartridge can be

temporarily removed from the probe handle and used as the mouse to select menu items. The Depth Probe pointer is then replaced with the appropriate Radionics stereotactic guide tube.

For tumor biopsy, the Nashold needle is set to a depth of 23 cm, as measured from the bottom of the plastic depth stop to the center of the side-cutting window. In the case of catheter placement, the depth of 23 cm is measured to the tip of the catheter. The needle or catheter is then passed through the guide tube to the intracranial target. Biopsy sampling or cyst aspiration proceeds in the standard fashion. The system monitor is checked frequently to ensure

FIGURE 46–16 ■ *A*, Magnetic resonance imaging demonstrated a 4 × 4 × 3 cm clival extra-axial mass compressing the brain stem. *B*, The Optical Tracking System (OTS) was helpful in maintaining the appropriate trajectory at the posterior oropharynx. *C*, The OTS demonstrated that the most rostral portion of the tumor was inaccessible by this exposure.

that the tracked probe has not deviated from the desired trajectory.

## C A S E   S T U D Y

A 72-year-old, right-handed man presented with a 1-month history of progressive, right-sided weakness. He was noted to have a 4/5 right hemiparesis on neurologic examination. MRI revealed a ring-enhancing lesion in the left posterior frontal lobe that appeared to involve the motor cortex (Fig. 46–17*A*). An OTS stereotactic biopsy was recommended before the initiation of adjuvant therapy. At the time of surgery, the patient underwent general anesthesia and the head was fixed in the Mayfield three-pin head-holder. The OTS was calibrated and used to determine the target, entry point, and trajectory for the tumor biopsy (see Fig. 46–17*B, C*). Quadrant samples were taken (see Fig. 46–17*D*) and frozen section confirmed glioblastoma. The patient had an uncomplicated postoperative course and was discharged the following morning.

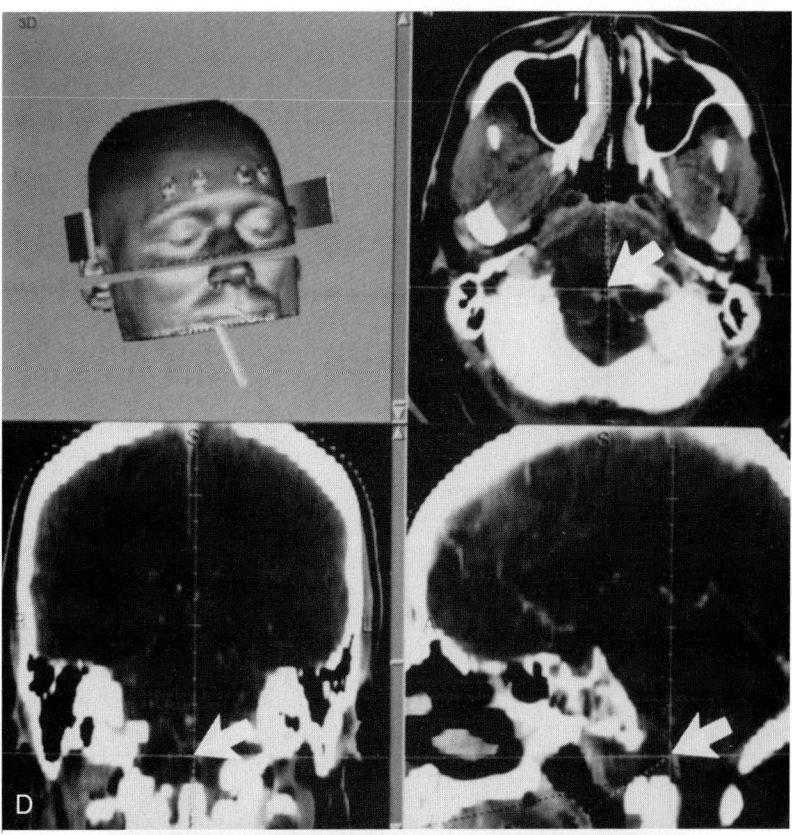

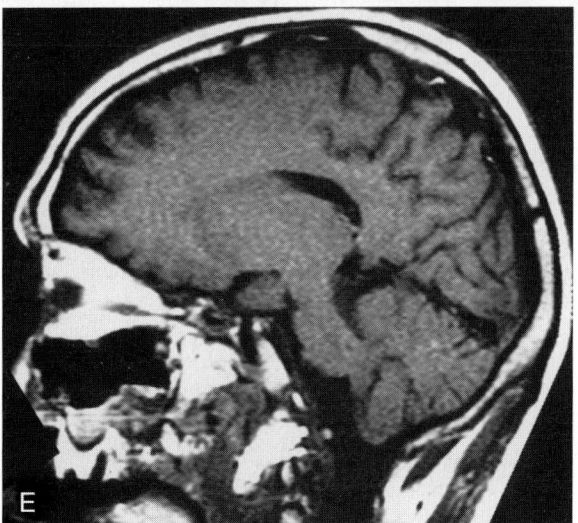

FIGURE 46–16 ■ *Continued. D*, A bilateral maxillotomy and palatal split were performed to reach the superior border of the tumor and the clivus. This procedure was accomplished using OTS guidance, which provided a margin of safety in determining a midline orientation as well as delineating the ventral and dorsal aspects of the tumor. *E*, A postoperative magnetic resonance imaging scan demonstrated an excellent tumor resection with decompression of the brain stem.

## CONCLUSION

Although IGS systems remain a capital expense, improvements are expected to enhance system versatility to aid in cost justification over a breadth of specialties. Most systems currently support neurosurgical, orthopedic,[20–22] otolaryngologic,[23–26] and craniomaxillofacial[27] applications, and may soon offer viable products for interventional radiology. Still other treatment modalities share computer platforms for frame-based functional neurosurgical planning and radiation therapy.

Systems are being developed by a number of surgical device companies with the promise of future developments

that will further advance the field of IGS. Programs are underway to develop software and hardware solutions to alleviate current technologic limitations in digital, preoperative image-based guidance systems such as brain shift during the surgery. Development of intraoperative CT and MRI scanners could provide the next level of interactive, minimally invasive surgical navigation by coupling real-time imaging with dynamic instrument tracking. In effect, multiple visual and digital image-based guidance technologies will be combined to offer unprecedented visualization inside the human body.

It has been said that image guidance allows the physician to see the unseen—a statement indicative of the technology. Advances in image guidance appear to be limited only by

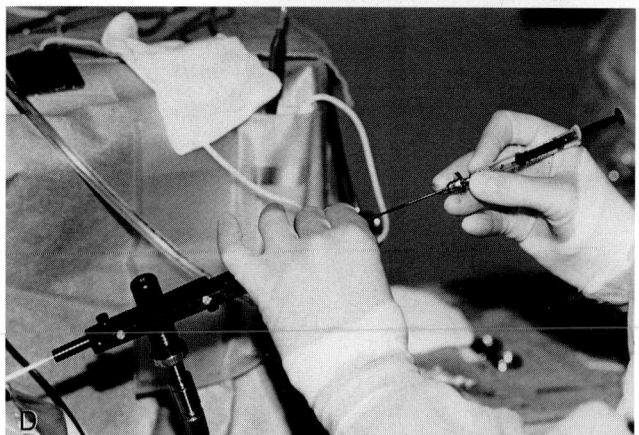

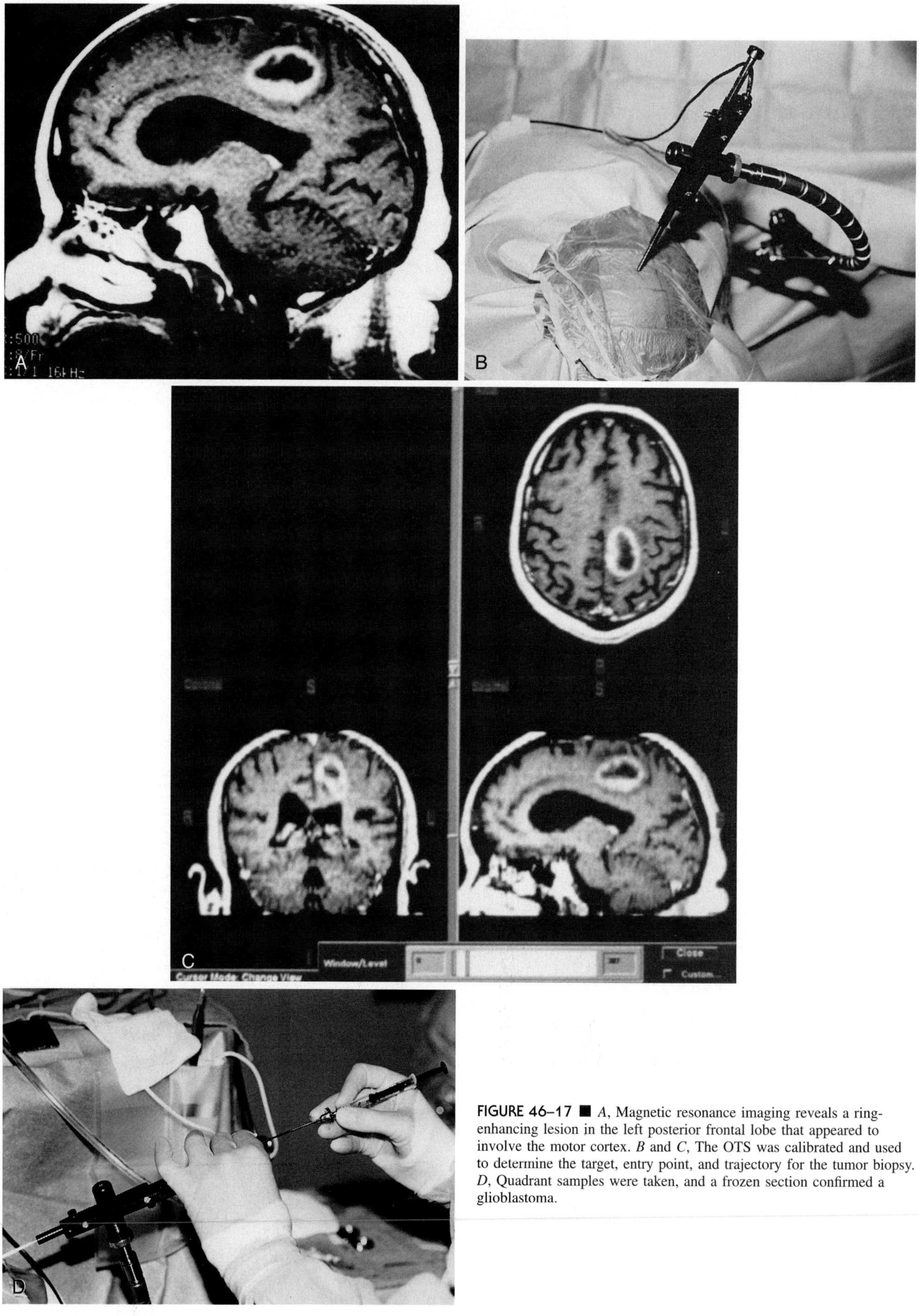

**FIGURE 46–17** ■ *A,* Magnetic resonance imaging reveals a ring-enhancing lesion in the left posterior frontal lobe that appeared to involve the motor cortex. *B* and *C,* The OTS was calibrated and used to determine the target, entry point, and trajectory for the tumor biopsy. *D,* Quadrant samples were taken, and a frozen section confirmed a glioblastoma.

the innovation and imagination of medical professionals and medical device manufacturers.

## ACKNOWLEDGMENTS

*The authors thank the following for their contributions to this project: John R. Adler, MD, Steven D. Chang, MD, and David Martin, MD, Stanford Medical Center, Stanford, California; and Andrew J. Kokkino, MD, and John M. Tew, Jr., MD, University of Cincinnati Medical Center, Cincinnati, Ohio.*

## REFERENCES

1. Sandeman DR, Gill SS: The impact of interactive image guided surgery: The Bristol experience with the ISG/Elekta Viewing Wand. Acta Neurochr Suppl (Wien) 64:54–58, 1995.
2. Marmulla R, Hilbert M, Niederdellmann H: Intraoperative precision of mechanical, electromagnetic, infrared and laser-guided navigation systems in computer-assisted surgery. Mund Kiefer Gesichtschr 1:S145–S148, 1998.
3. Guthrie BL, Adler JR Jr: Frameless stereotaxy: Computer-interactive neurosurgery. In Barrow DL (ed): Perspectives in Neurological Surgery. St. Louis: Quality Medical Publishing, 1991, Chapter 2, pp 1–19.
4. Guthrie BL: Graphic-interactive cranial surgery: The operating arm system. In Pell MF, Thomas DGT (eds): Handbook of Stereotaxy: Using the CRW Apparatus. Baltimore: Williams & Wilkins, 1994, pp 193–211.
5. Barnett GH, Kormos DW, Steiner CP, et al: Intraoperative localization using an armless, frameless stereotactic wand. J Neurosurg 78:510–514, 1993.
6. Pell MF, Brennan JW: Computer-assisted and frameless stereotaxy: The initial Australian experience. J Clin Neurosci 5:40–45, 1998.
7. Maciunas RJ, Fitzpatrick JM, Galloway RL, et al: Beyond stereotaxy: Extreme levels of application accuracy are provided by implantable fiducial markers for interactive image-guided neurosurgery. In Maciunas RJ (ed): Interactive Image-Guided Neurosurgery. Park Ridge, IL: American Association of Neurological Surgeons, 1993, pp 17–44.
8. Alp MS, Dujovny M, Misra M, et al: Head registration techniques for image-guided surgery. Neurol Res 20:31–37, 1998.
9. Sipos EP, Tebo SA, Zinreich J, et al: In vivo accuracy testing and clinical experience with the ISG Viewing Wand. Neurosurgery 39:194–202, 1996.
10. Ganslandt O, Steinmeier R, Kober H, et al: Magnetic source imaging combined with image-guided frameless stereotaxy: A new method in surgery around the motor strip. Neurosurgery 41:621–627, 1997.
11. Gleason PL, Kikinis R, Altobelli D, et al: Video registration virtual reality for nonlinkage stereotactic surgery. Stereotact Funct Neurosurg 63:139–143, 1994.
12. Lavallee S, Sautot P, Troccaz J, et al: Computer-assisted spine sur-
gery: A technique for transpedicular screw fixation using CT data and a 3-D optical localizer. J Image Guided Surg 1:65–73, 1995.
13. Welch WC, Subach BR, Pollack IF, et al: Frameless stereotactic guidance for surgery of the upper cervical spine. Neurosurgery 40:958–963, 1997.
14. Kim KD, Masciopinto JE, Johnson JP: Frameless stereotaxy for thoracic pedicle screw placement. Presented at the meeting of the American Association of Neurological Surgeons/Congress of Neurological Surgeons, Section on Disorders of the Spine and Peripheral Nerves, Rancho Mirage, California, February 11–14, 1998.
15. Wirtz CR, Tronnier VM, Staubert A, et al: Successful reregistration of image guided neurosurgery with intraoperative MRI. Presented at the Fifth Scientific Meeting of the International Society for Magnetic Resonance in Medicine, Vancouver, British Columbia, Canada, April 12–18, 1997.
16. Wirtz CR, Bonsanto MM, Knauth M, et al: Intraoperative magnetic resonance imaging to update interactive navigation in neurosurgery: Method and preliminary experience. Comput Aided Surg 2:172–179, 1997.
17. Black P: The intraoperative MRI: A radical new tool for neurosurgery. Presented at the 49th Annual Meeting of the German Society of Neurosurgery, Hanover, Germany, June 12–16, 1998.
18. Koos W, Roessler K, Matula C, et al: Combinations of intraoperative computed tomography (CCT) and image-guided neurosurgery. In Proceedings of the 11th International Congress of Neurological Surgery. Moduzzi Editore (in press).
19. Barnett GH, Steiner CP, Weisenberger J: Adaptation of personal projection television to a head-mounted display for intra-operative viewing of neuroimaging. J Image Guided Surg 1:109–112, 1995.
20. Sati M, de Guise JA, Drouin G: Computer assisted knee surgery: Diagnostics and planning of knee surgery. Comput Aided Surg 2:108–123, 1997.
21. Tockus L, Joskowicz L, Simkin A, et al: Computer-aided image-guided bone fracture surgery: Modeling, visualization, and preoperative planning. In Wells WM, Colchester A, Delp S (eds): Lecture Notes in Computer Science, Medical Image Computing and Computer-Assisted Intervention First International, MICCAI '98. Conference, Cambridge, Massachusetts, October, 1998. Berlin: Springer, 1998, pp 29–38.
22. Tso CY, Ellis RE, Rudan J, et al: A surgical planning and guidance system for high tibial osteotomies. In Wells WM, Colchester A, Delp S (eds): Lecture Notes in Computer Science, Medical Image Computing and Computer-Assisted Intervention, MICCAI '98. First International Conference, Cambridge, Massachusetts, October, 1998. Berlin: Springer, 1998, pp 39–50.
23. Ecke U, Klimek L, Muller W, et al: Virtual reality: Preparation and execution of sinus surgery. Comput Aided Surg 3:45–50, 1998.
24. Anon JB: Computer-aided endoscopic sinus surgery. Laryngoscope 108:949–961, 1998.
25. Klimek L, Mosges R: Computer-assisted surgery in the ENT specialty: Developments and experiences from the first decade. Laryngorhinootologie 77:272–282, 1998.
26. Metson R, Gliklich RE, Cosenza M: A comparison of image guidance systems for sinus surgery. Laryngoscope 108:1164–1170, 1998.
27. Bohner P, Holler C, Hassfeld S: Operation planning in craniomaxillofacial surgery. Comput Aided Surg 2:152–161, 1997.

# CT/MRI-Based Computer-Assisted Volumetric Stereotactic Resection of Intracranial Lesions

■ HOWARD L. WEINER and PATRICK J. KELLY

Before the era of modern neuroimaging, neurosurgical approaches for resection or biopsy of intra-axial brain tumors typically employed large craniotomy flaps, which would be of sufficient size so as to ensure adequate exposure of the lesion in question. Such openings were often imprecise and frequently led to the exposure and potential damage of normal structures. Tumor stereotaxis developed partially as a result of modern neuroradiologic techniques, which provided very precise anatomic localization of the location and volumetric extent of such neoplasms. Furthermore, the explosion of modern computer technology over the past 20 years facilitated the transfer of this information into a database that could be utilized not only for surgical planning but also for the execution of the actual surgical procedure. As a result, operative procedures could be more precise, minimizing potential morbidity, duration of hospital stay, and, ultimately, cost. Minimally invasive computer-assisted stereotactic tumor surgery, therefore, developed as a method of precise image-guided intracranial navigation for the safe removal of intra-axial brain tumors. It became a technique for gathering, storing, and reformatting image-derived three-dimensional volumetric information that defined a lesion with respect to the surgical field. It enabled the neurosurgeon to plan and simulate the operative procedure ahead of time (the "virtual" craniotomy) such that the safest and least invasive approach could be employed. Moreover, this technology allowed the surgeon to visualize exactly the border between the tumor and the surrounding brain. The necessity for stereotactic volumetric approaches became even more critical with the advent of truly minimally invasive "keyhole" approaches, in which surgeons could no longer rely on visualized intracranial landmarks. The advantages of this technology to the surgeon, the patient, and third-party payers became apparent.

With the original advent of computed tomography (CT) scanning, many neurosurgeons began to rethink classical approaches to common intracranial tumors.[2, 3, 11, 22] Compared with projection radiography and ventriculography, which were used in functional stereotactic procedures, CT was a natural data source for tumor stereotaxis. It provided a precise three-dimensional database that could easily be incorporated into a stereotactic coordinate system. In addition, for the first time surgeons could actually see the intracranial tumor target volume directly. Magnetic resonance imaging (MRI) also became a most valuable addition to the stereotactic preoperative database.

CT-based, and later MRI-based, point-in-space stereotactic biopsy procedures for the diagnosis of intracranial tumors became commonplace.[2, 6, 25, 26] In addition, point stereotaxis could also be used to drain a tumor cyst, to place multiple radionuclide catheters within a CT/MRI-defined tumor, and to center a craniotomy precisely over a superficial lesion or to locate a deep one. However, point-in-space stereotactic techniques could not be used to identify tumor margins, which were clearly visible on the imaging studies. The volumetric stereotactic method, in which a tumor volume is represented in stereotactic space by computer reconstruction of planar tumor boundaries defined by stereotactic CT and MRI, was developed in order to facilitate the intraoperative identification of CT- and MRI-defined tumor borders and to maintain a surgeon's three-dimensional orientation during the resection of an irregularly shaped neoplasm.[19, 23, 24, 28, 29]

We began performing CT/MRI-based stereotactic volumetric resections of deep-seated intracranial lesions in January 1980.[22] This procedure has been very useful in the resection of superficial as well as deep-seated intra-axial lesions. As clinical experience was developed, technical innovations increased the facility and accuracy with which these operations were performed. In particular, the operating room computer system and appropriate software replaced cumbersome manual methods used in the early procedures. The computer was used for the transposition of volumetric information derived from axial stereotactic CT scans and MR images into three-dimensional space and to monitor and display the position of stereotactically directed instruments in relation to computer-generated reconstructions of the tumor volume. In this chapter we discuss the state-of-the-art aspects of this approach as well as newer developments made possible by the recent revolution in imaging and computer technology.

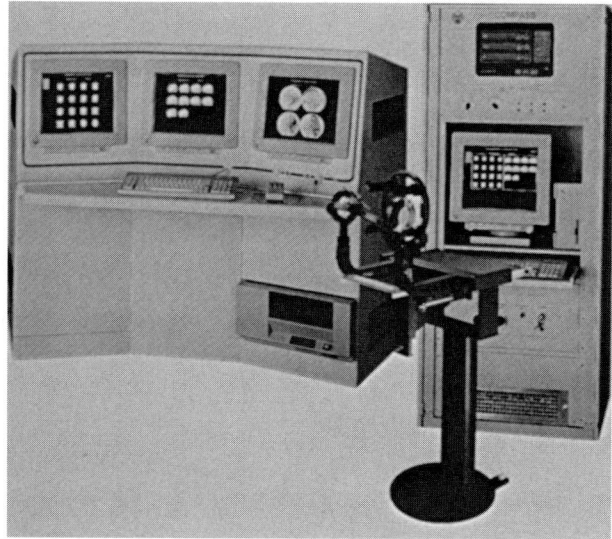

FIGURE 47–1 ■ Modern COMPASS stereotactic system includes a three-screen workstation console (*left*), electronic control panel with digital readout for stereotactic coordinates (*right*), and an arc-quadrant stereotactic frame with cartesian robotic slide mechanism and optical encoder position sensors.

## INSTRUMENTATION

### Stereotactic Frame

Although other stereotactic frames could be modified for volumetric stereotactic procedures, the COMPASS stereotactic system (COMPASS International, Rochester, MN) was designed specifically for volumetric tumor stereotaxis. It evolved from modifications made to a standard Todd-Wells stereotactic frame. These modifications were then incorporated into an intermediate system (the so-called Kelly-Goerss frame) which, following some clinical experience, was further modified into the COMPASS system.[27] In addition, basic software for data acquisition, surgical planning, and interactive surgery evolved over an 8-year period and was rewritten for functionality on evolutionary computer and image-processing platforms. The sole purpose of the computer hardware and software was to render volumetric stereotactic procedures more convenient and time efficient.

The contemporary version of the COMPASS stereotactic frame consists of a fixed arc-quadrant three-dimensional slide and removable headholder (Fig. 47–1). It can be fixed onto a semipermanent base unit or mounted onto the lateral support rails of a standard operating table. In addition, data acquisition hardware (localization systems for CT, MRI, and digital subtraction angiography [DSA]) and computer support hardware and software are also considered to be part of the system.

### Headholder

The headholder (Fig. 47–2) consists of a round base ring, four vertical supports, and a skull fixation system. The headholder attaches to the patient's skull by means of flanged carbon fiber pins that are inserted into four holes drilled in the outer table of the patient's skull into the diploë.

Detachable micrometers are used to measure the distance between the end of the carbon fiber pins and the outer face of the vertical supports. These measurements and the fact that the pins are replaced in previously drilled holes in the skull provide a method for accurate replacement of the stereotactic headholder. Thus, data acquisition and surgery do not need to be performed on the same day, and additional procedures can be performed later on using the same database.

### Arc-Quadrant

The 160-mm radius arc-quadrant attaches to horizontal arms that extend from the base plate of the three-dimensional slide. Probes and retractors are directed by an attachment on the upper face of the arc. The arc-quadrant provides two angular degrees of freedom for approach trajectories: a collar angle (from the horizontal plane) and an arc angle (from the vertical plane).

### Three-Dimensional Positioning Slide

The headholder fits into a support yoke of a three-dimensional slide that moves the patient's head within the fixed

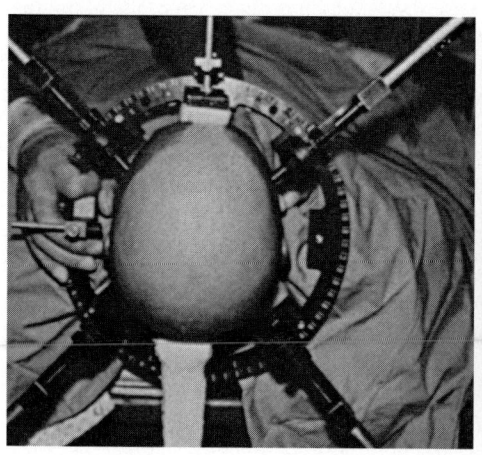
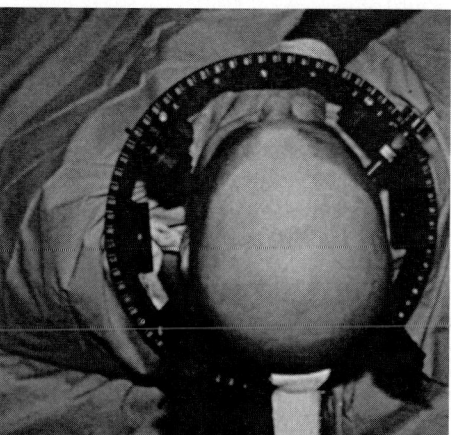

FIGURE 47–2 ■ The COMPASS stereotactic headframe with (*left*) and without (*right*) attached micrometers. Note the indexing marks on the base ring of the headholder. The headholder fixes to the patient's skull by means of four fixed-length flanged carbon fiber pins that insert into twist drill holes made in the outer table of the skull. Micrometers measure the extension of the carbon fiber pin beyond the plane of the vertical support and provide a mechanism for precise frame reapplication.

arc-quadrant (Fig. 47–3). Each axis of the three-dimensional slide is moved by worm gear and a computer-controlled stepper motor that is activated at a remote control console located outside the surgical field. Hand cranks are provided on each of the three axes for manual backup.

Stereotactic coordinates on the slide are detected by optical encoders on the X, Y, and Z axes that transmit the coordinates to digital readout scales and to the computer. In addition, vernier scales on each axis for direct reading of stereotactic coordinates are provided as a backup to the optical encoders.

## Computer System

The computer, although not absolutely necessary, saves a great deal of time when calculating target points, interpolating imaging-defined tumor volumes, cross-registering points and volumes between CT, MR images, and digital angiography (DA) and in real-time interactive image displays during the surgical procedure. The computer makes volumetric stereotactic procedures practical and time efficient.

## Hardware

The COMPASS stereotactic frame is supported by a SUN SPARC 10 (SUN Microsystems, Mountainview, CA) with three X terminal display monitors mounted in a custom-

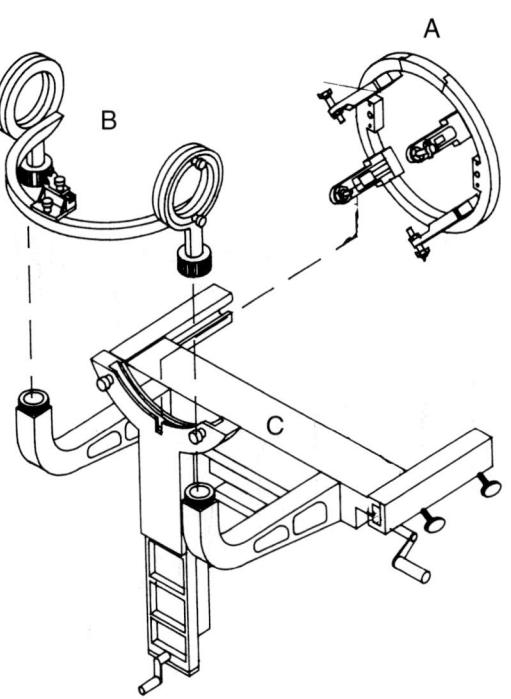

**FIGURE 47–3** ■ This schematic of a simplified COMPASS stereotactic frame demonstrates the circular headholder (A), the 160-mm radius arc-quadrant (B), and slide mechanism containing three axes (C), which attaches to a semipermanent floor stand or to a standard operating room table. Hand cranks, which provide mechanical back-ups to three-axis computer-controlled stepper motors, are shown.

designed ergonometrically efficient workstation style console (COMPASS International, Rochester, MN).

## Software

Data acquisition, surgical planning, and interactive display software run by mouse/cursor and menu interactive devices and voice recognition systems allows user-friendly interaction with the operating room computer system before and during surgery. Stereotactic tumor resections are possible using manual methods for calculation of stereotactic coordinates and cross-correlation of target points between the different imaging modalities.

## Laser

The carbon dioxide ($CO_2$) laser has been found to have very limited application in the resection of superficial lesions but has several advantages in the stereotactic resection of deep tumors. First, the laser is convenient for removing tissue from a deep cavity and is relatively hemostatic. Second, the laser removes tissue by means of a narrow beam of light; thus, there is one less instrument that must be inserted into a narrow surgical field. At present, a Sharplan 1100 $CO_2$ Laser System (Medical Industries, Tel Aviv, Israel) is used in stereotactic resections.

## Stereotactic Retractors

An arc-mounted stereotactic retractor system comprises cylindrical retractors, dilators, and an arc-quadrant adapter. The retractor is a thin-walled hollow cylinder that is 140 mm in length and 2 cm in diameter. The retractor cylinder is directed toward the focal point of the stereotactic arc-quadrant. Dilators that fit inside the retractor cylinder are 1 cm longer than the retractor. The distal end of the dilator is wedge-shaped and spreads an incision to the diameter of the retractor so that the retractor cylinder can be advanced. The retractor is used not only to maintain exposure but also to provide a fixed stereotactic reference structure within the stereotactic surgical field.

## Accessory Instruments

Extra-long bipolar forceps with a shaft length of 150 mm are required to control bleeding in the surgical field when working through the stereotactic retractors. In addition, 150- to 160-mm-long suction tips, dissectors, and alligator scissors are also used.

## Heads-up Display for the Operating Microscope

In a specially designed heads-up display unit (similar to that used in jet fighter aircraft), the image output of a small video monitor mounted on the operating microscope is optically superimposed on the surgical field viewed through the microscope. The computer-generated image displayed on the video monitor is scaled by a system of lenses to the desired size. Thus, the surgeon sees the actual surgical field with the computer-generated rendition of that field based on CT and MRI, which are superimposed.

## MATERIALS AND METHODS

Computer-assisted volumetric stereotactic resections are performed in three phases: (1) database acquisition, (2) treatment planning, and (3) interactive procedure.

### Data Acquisition

A CT-MRI–compatible stereotactic head frame is placed on the patient's head and secured by carbon fiber pins inserted into ⅛-inch twist drill holes through the outer table of the skull into the diploë. For frame replacement, detachable micrometers are used to measure the carbon fiber fixation pins with respect to the fixed vertical support elements of the headholder. This provides a mechanism for accurately replacing the frame for subsequent data acquisition or surgical procedures.

After frame application, the stereotactic CT scan, MRI scan, and angiographic examinations as shown in Figure 47–4 follow.

A CT table adaptation plate receives the stereotactic headholder CT-localization system, which consists of nine carbon fiber localization rods that are arranged in the shape of the letter "N" on either side of the head and anteriorly to create nine reference marks on each CT slice. Stereotactic CT scanning is done on a General Electric 9800 CT scanning unit, which gathers 5-mm slices through the lesion and uses a medium body format. In some patients, a stereotactic MRI examination is also done.

The MRI localization system consists of capillary tubes filled with copper sulfate solution, which also create nine reference marks on each MR image.

DSA is used for the localization of important blood volumes that must be preserved in the surgical approach and tumor resection. A DF table adaptation plate receives the stereotactic headholder on the General Electric DF 5000 DA unit. The localization system consists of four lucite plates, which each contain nine radiopaque reference marks located on either side of the head anteriorly and posteriorly. This creates 18 reference marks on each antero-posterior and lateral DA image. The mathematical relationships between the fiducial marks and their locations on the DA images are the basis from which stereotactic coordinates for intracranial vessels can be calculated and stereotactic target points derived from CT and MRI can be displayed on angiographic images. DA is performed using a femoral catheterization technique. Angiography is carried out under the direction of New York University, Division of Interventional Neuroradiology.

### Surgical Planning

After data acquisition, the archived computer data tapes from the CT, MRI, and DA examinations are read into the operating room computer system. The nine reference marks on each CT slice and MRI scan are detected automatically by an intensity detection algorithm. This suspends the position of each slice in a three-dimensional computer image storage matrix.

### Volume Reconstruction

Volumes defined by CT contrast enhancement, CT low attenuation, and $T_1$ and $T_2$ signal abnormalities on MRI scans are each established in the computer matrix as follows. First, the surgeon, who is seated at the computer console, digitizes the tumor by tracing around the outline of the lesion defined by CT contrast enhancement; sometimes, the surgeon traces around that defined by CT hypodensity, by the $T_1$- and $T_2$-weighted signal abnormalities of the MRI scan. Then each of these digitized contours is suspended in a separate computer image matrix. Finally, a computer program interpolates intermediate slices at 1-mm intervals between the digitized contours and creates separate volumes in space by filling in each of these slices with 1-mm cubic voxels.[26]

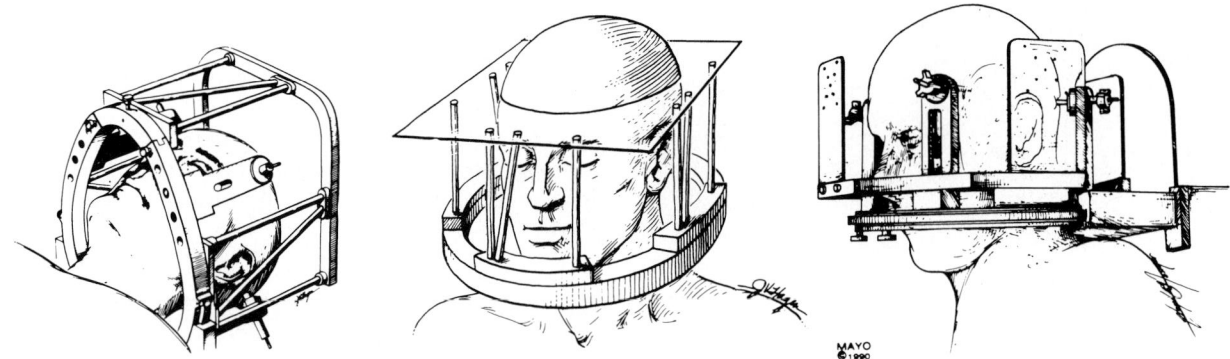

FIGURE 47–4 ■ Stereotactic localization device for computed tomography (CT) and magnetic resonance imaging (MRI) (*left*) contains nine rods arranged in the shape of the letter "N." These produce nine reference marks on each CT slice from which stereotactic coordinates are calculated (*middle*). Stereotactic digital angiography fiducial reference plates fix the base ring of the COMPASS stereotactic frame bilaterally, anteriorly, and posteriorly (*right*). These create a set of 18 reference marks for the calculation of stereotactic coordinates from angiograms and the cross-registration of CT and MRI data onto the angiographic images. (Reprinted with permission of the Mayo Clinic, © 1990.)

## Surgical Trajectory

The actual surgical approach (or view line) is expressed in stereotactic frame adjustments (collar: angle from the horizontal plane; arc: angle from the vertical plane) that access a selected point with the interpolated tumor volumes from an entry point on the surface of the brain. In general, the surgical approach selected takes into account the three-dimensional shape of the lesion, important overlying cortical regions, subcortical white matter pathways, and vascular structures that must be preserved. In most cases, the stereotactic surgical approach to the lesion is selected on anteroposterior and lateral DSA images on which the digitized tumor volume has been displayed.

## Patient Rotation

The COMPASS stereotactic headholder has indexing marks inscribed around its circumference that align to an indexing mark in the headholder receiving yoke of the three-dimensional slide system. Thus, the patient's head can be rotated to any position that will provide a comfortable working position for the surgeon. In addition, in order to avoid possible spatial shifts of the intracranial contents, the surgeon must rotate the patient's head in the stereotactic headholder so that the trephine opening will be at the least dependent position in the surgical field (i.e., on top). This places the proposed trephine in the most superior position within the surgical field, and the spatial integrity of the brain is maintained by the intact skull that encases it. This is similar to opening a jar of liquid. The top is directed in the least dependent position, and the liquid within the jar doesn't move.

In order to illustrate this point, the following example is provided. An approach is planned to a posterior dorsal thalamic tumor through the superior parietal lobule (Fig. 47–5). Here, a patient rotation of 180 degrees is selected

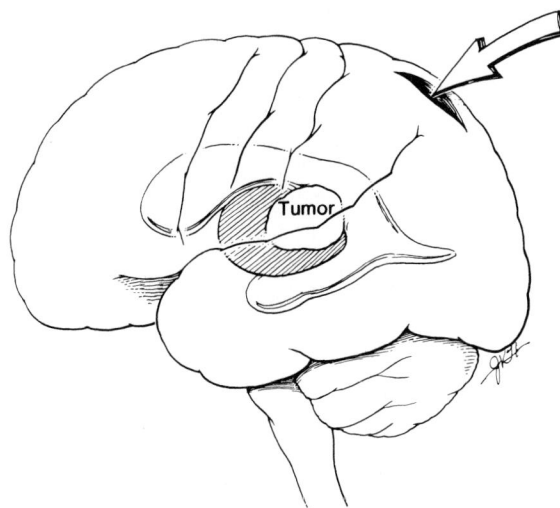

## POSTERIOR-SUPERIOR APPROACH

FIGURE 47–5 ■ Dorsal thalamic tumor is approached through the superior parietal lobule and the atrial region of the lateral ventricle.

with appropriate collar and arc angles (approximately 35 degrees on the collar and 0 degrees on the arc) (Fig. 47–6). The patient's body is placed in the park bench position. The head in the COMPASS stereotactic headholder is turned to 180 degrees, and the operating room table is elevated to approximately 35 degrees in a reverse Trendelenburg position.

## Surgical Procedures

The technical aspects of the surgical procedure depend on whether the lesion is superficial or deep. In the approach to superficial lesions, the stereotactic instrument is used to center a circular trephine of known diameter over the tumor. The relationship between the computer display of the circular trephine superimposed by the heads-up display onto the actual trephine in the surgical field and slices from the CT or MRI-defined tumor volumes will orient the surgeon during dissection around and removal of the neoplasm with the $CO_2$ laser. Deep tumors are removed through a cylindrically shaped stereotactically directed retractor using a $CO_2$ laser.

## Superficial Lesions

**Procedural Aspects.** The patient is anesthetized with general endotracheal anesthesia. The stereotactic head frame is replaced employing the same pin holes in the skull, pin placements, and frame micrometer settings used during the data acquisition phase. The patient is then positioned in the stereotactic frame. In the COMPASS system, the patient's head in the stereotactic headholder may be rotated to any position that will provide not only a comfortable working situation for the surgeon but will also minimize brain shifts as described in the previous section. The headholder rotation angle has usually been determined during the surgical planning phase, but if this has been modified for some reason (e.g., when encountering a previously made surgical incision), the new rotation is entered into the computer program, and the computer calculates new stereotactic frame adjustments that place the center of the tumor into the focal point of the stereotactic arc-quadrant and accounts for the modified patient rotation. The head of the operating room table is raised to place the position of the intended trephine in the least dependent portion of the surgical field (usually equivalent to the collar angle).

After preparing and draping the head, the stereotactic arc-quadrant is positioned. The selected arc and collar approach angles are set on the instrument. Through an incision in the scalp, a pilot hole is drilled in the outer table of the skull by a stereotactically directed 1/8-inch drill. The scalp is then opened with a linear incision. A craniotomy is performed using a power trephine centered on the pilot hole. The size of the trephine selected is equal to or slightly larger than the largest cross-sectional area of the tumor as viewed from the selected surgical approach angles that were determined during the planning phase.

The computer displays the configuration of the trephine in relationship to the reformatted tumor outlines into the heads-up display unit of the operating microscope (Fig.

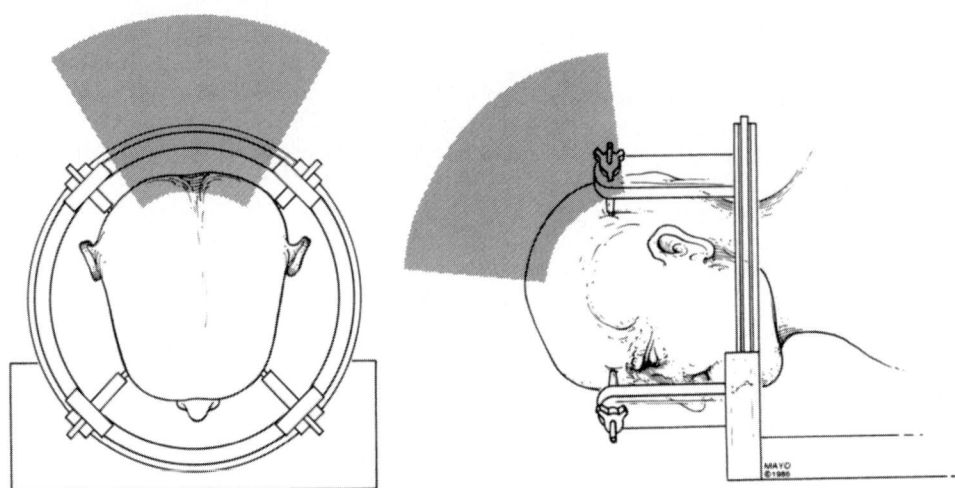

**FIGURE 47–6** ■ Patient rotation of 180 degrees is used for parasagittal approaches in which collar angles of 0 to 80 degrees and arc angles from +15 to −15 can be used (*shaded area*). A three-quarter prone body position is employed. (By permission of the Mayo Foundation.)

47–7). The surgeon then superimposes the graphic image of the trephine over the actual trephine in the surgical field using the most superficial computer-generated tumor slice as a template. A section of cortex that has the same size and configuration as a superficial computer-generated slice image is removed with bipolar forceps and scissors. We have found that cortex is nonviable when tumors extend to within 1 cm of the surface. A plane is then developed around the tumor using suction and bipolar forceps.

During tumor resection, the computer displays 1-mm-thick slice configurations of the lesion at successively deeper levels in the correct spatial relationship to a circle, which represents in size and position the location of the stereotactically placed trephine within the surgical field. It is best to first isolate the lesion from surrounding brain tissue and keep the specimen intact. Computer displays of deep tumor slices along the view line provide information on the expected configuration of the tumor as it is encoun-

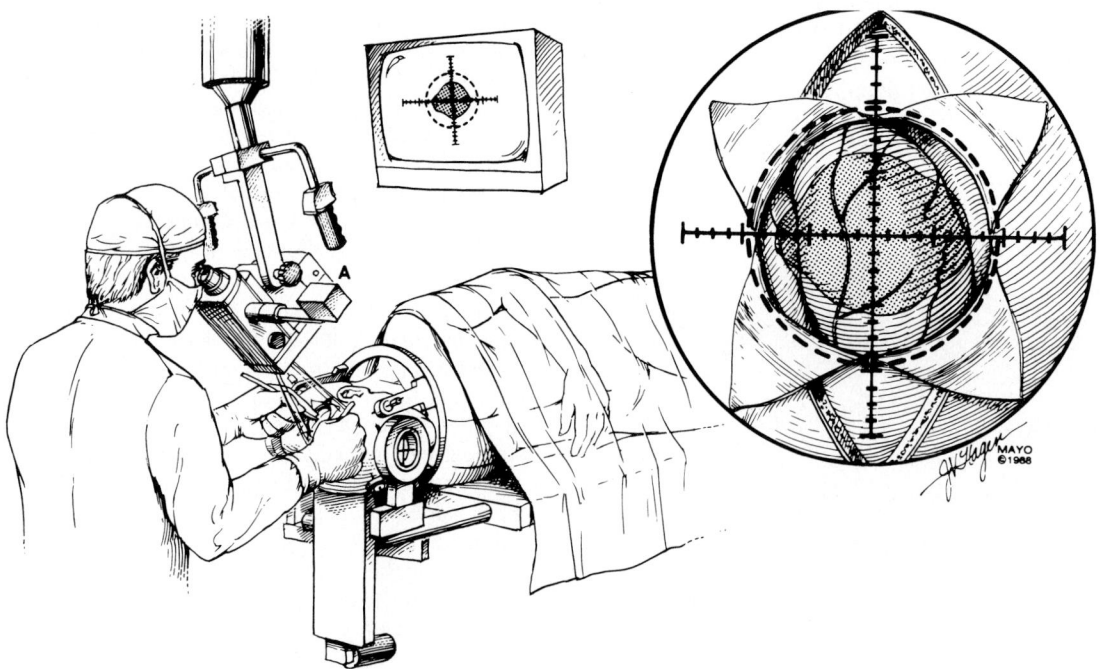

**FIGURE 47–7** ■ Illustration of the method used for the stereotactic resection of a superficial tumor. A trephine opening of the skull is performed centered on a pilot hole drilled by means of the stereotactic frame. The computer displays the position of a tumor slice in proper position with respect to the location of the trephine at a specified distance along the viewline on the display monitor and into the heads-up display unit of the operating microscope (A). The image is scaled in the heads-up display, and the microscope is moved until the configuration of the trephine in the image display is exactly the same size as the actual trephine in the surgical field and aligns to the trephine. The surgeon then uses the tumor slice image as a template that will aid in identification of the surgical plane between the computed tomography and magnetic resonance imaging defined tumor and surrounding brain tissue. This facilitates isolation of the tumor from the surrounding brain tissue. (From Kelly PJ: Volumetric stereotactic surgical resection of intra-axial brain mass lesions. Mayo Clin Proc 63:1186–1198, 1988.)

tered during the procedure. Measurements may be taken from the edges of the trephine opening and compared with the tumor-generated slice images. Slice depth can be determined by measuring from the level of the cranium at the edge of the trephine to the depth in the brain at which the surgeon is working. This is simply measured on the bipolar forceps with a millimeter ruler. This measurement, added to the distance from the outer surface of the probe carrier assembly on the stereotactic arc-quadrant, is subtracted from 135 mm (the distance from the outer surface of the probe carrier assembly to the focus of the arc-quadrant) and will provide the distance in millimeters from the plane of the surgical field to the focal point plane of the stereotactic arc-quadrant. The computer-generated tumor slice image corresponding to this plane may then be displayed. If the surgeon notes that hyperventilation, mannitol, or loss of subarachnoid fluid has resulted in the brain collapsing away from the dura and inner table of the skull, this amount of collapse can be measured and the depth of the slice images can be updated accordingly.

Compared with classical neurosurgical internal tumor decompressions, volumetric resection mandates that the interior of the lesion should not be entered until late in the procedure, because the walls of the lesion may collapse and render subsequent computer-generated slice images no longer accurate. Employing this method, we have found that intermediate- and high-grade gliomas can be totally removed as intact specimens with negligible bleeding. In addition, infiltrated areas of brain parenchyma in low-grade gliomas located in nonessential brain tissue can also be resected in this way. In fact, we have found that the intraoperative heads-up display of the reconstructed tumor volume has enhanced the surgeon's technical ability to develop a surgical plane around a specified lesion.

## Deep Tumors

Volumetric stereotactic resection of periventricular, basal ganglia, or thalamic tumors requires stereotactic retractors, extra-long bipolar forceps, and dissecting instruments.

The stereotactic retractors are mounted on the stereotactic arc-quadrant. The position of these retractors is also indicated on the computer display terminal in the operating room and in the heads-up display unit of the operating microscope (Fig. 47–8). The position of the cylindrical retractor is shown as a circle in the computer display in relationship to the tumor slice. During surgery, the computer-generated image of the retractor is superimposed on the actual view of the retractor in the operating microscope.

Various surgical approaches have been developed for various deep tumor locations. These approaches include transcortical, trans-sulcal, trans-sylvian, and interhemispheric exposure. The actual approach selected depends on the proximity of the tumor to deep sulci that can be split microsurgically and spread wide enough to provide adequate exposure. The approach to thalamic tumors depends on whether they are located anteriorly (and thus approached from the anterosuperior position), posterodorsally (and exposed through the lateral ventricle by way of the superior parietal lobule), or posteroventrally (and approached from posterior laterally). The issue is the preservation of normal

thalamic tissue. Multiplanar MRI is invaluable in defining the anatomic relationships between a tumor and normal structures to select the best surgical approach trajectory for stereotactic craniotomy.

The stereotactic resection of deep tumors is performed under general anesthesia. The patient is placed in the stereotactic headholder and positioned in the stereotactic frame. The selected target point within the tumor volume is positioned into the focal point of the stereotactic arc-quadrant.

In cystic tumors, intraventricular tumors, or tumors near the ventricular system, the monitoring of possible movements of the tumor during the procedure may be necessary. This is accomplished by means of a series of 0.5-mm stainless steel reference balls that are deposited at 5-mm intervals along the surgical view line in the tumor by a stereotactically directed biopsy cannula inserted through a 1/8-inch drill hole in the skull. Anteroposterior and lateral radiographs are obtained. The position of these steel balls on subsequent radiographs after exposure of the lesion may indicate shifts in the position of the tumor that can be adjusted in the computer software for updated accurate tumor slice images.

The scalp is opened with a linear or slightly curved incision. A 1.5-inch trephine craniotomy is performed, and a cruciate opening of the dura is accomplished. A linear incision is made in the cortex, and then the subcortical white matter incision is progressively deepened with the stereotactically directed $CO_2$ laser. Alternatively, a convenient sulcus can be split microsurgically, and the cortical incision can be made in the depths of this sulcus.

The direction of the subcortical incision should be through nonessential brain tissue and in a direction parallel to major white matter fibers. As the incision is deepened, the stereotactic retractor is advanced to maintain the developing exposure.

The computer has calculated the range of the tumor along the surgical view line. At the outer border of the tumor, the laser beam is deflected laterally; a dilator is placed through the retractor; and the retractor is advanced. This creates a shaft from the surface to the outer border of the tumor. Using the computer display, which demonstrates the relationship of the computer-generated tumor slice images to the edges of the retractor as a guide, the surgeon creates a plane of dissection around the lesion with the laser or with suction and bipolar forceps. The length of the suction and bipolar forceps is 10 to 15 mm longer than the stereotactic retractor; thus, the plane between tumor and brain tissue can be developed for 10 to 15 mm beyond the end of the retractor using the computer-generated slice images as a guide, which helps the surgeon to identify and develop that plane. Once the plane has been developed entirely around the tumor to a uniform depth, tumor tissue within the retractor is then removed with 65 to 85 W of defocused laser power. In general, a tumor is removed slice by slice, extending from the most superficial slices to the deepest ones. Hemostasis is secured using the extra-long bipolar forceps.

When stainless steel reference balls have been placed (because of concern over spatial shifting of the tumor), anteroposterior and lateral teleradiographs are obtained and compared with the initial pictures to record possible move-

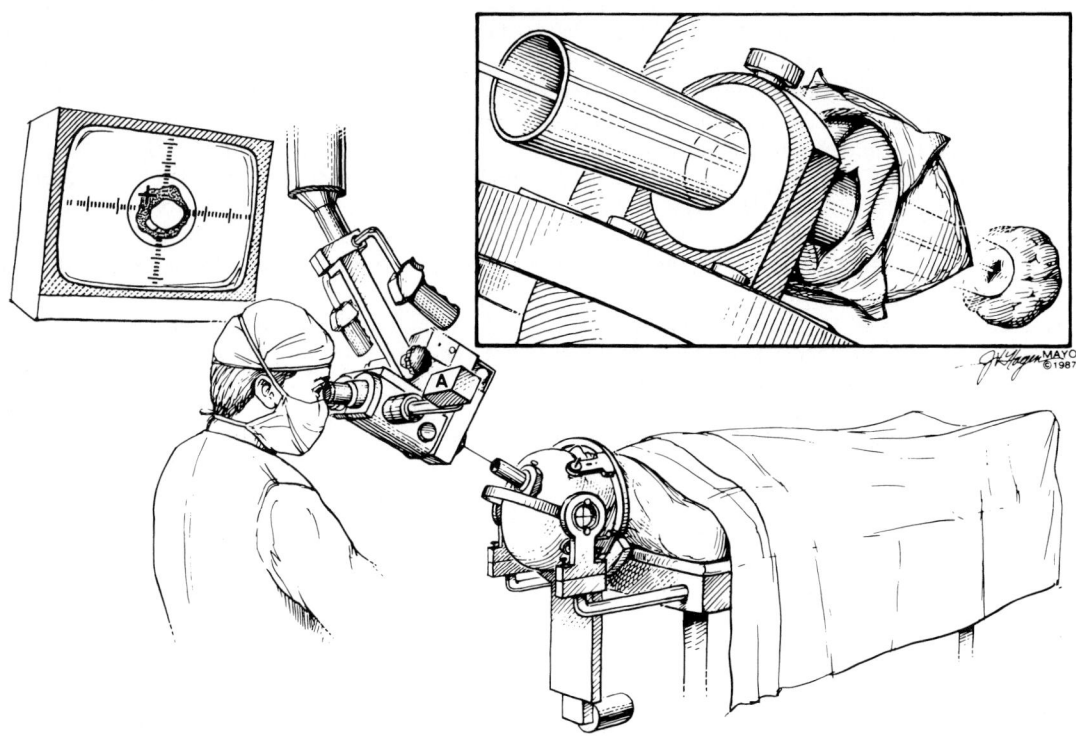

**FIGURE 47–8** ■ The stereotactic cylindrical retractor is employed during the resection of deep-seated lesions. The computer displays the configuration of a cross-section of the retractor (*circle*) with respect to a selected slice through the tumor volume cut perpendicular to the surgical viewline. This information is displayed on a computer monitor in the operating room as well as in the heads-up display unit of the operating microscope (A). (From Kelly PJ: Volumetric stereotactic surgical resection of intra-axial brain mass lesions. Mayo Clin Proc 63:1186–1198, 1988.)

ments of the reference balls. In our experience, shifting of a deep tumor occurs rarely unless it is associated with a tumor cyst that is entered early in the procedure or adherent to the walls of the lateral or third ventricle, which are opened with the loss of ventricular fluid.

Tumors that are larger than the retractor opening can be removed as follows. First, one side of the tumor is positioned under the retractor and the surgeon creates a plane between this side of the tumor and brain tissue with the laser. The display image is then translated on the computer display terminal to position the other side of the lesion under the retractor (Fig. 47–9). The computer calculates new stereotactic frame adjustments, which are duplicated on the servomotor-driven slide mechanism of the frame by remote control. This side of the tumor is then separated from brain tissue with the laser. After isolating the lesion from surrounding brain tissue, it may then be vaporized by a laser or removed by biopsy forceps and suction as previously described.

## Tumors of the Posterior Parahippocampal Gyrus

We have described a novel, computer-assisted volumetric stereotactic approach for resecting tumors of the posterior parahippocampal gyrus.[39] This approach illustrates the novel ways in which volumetric stereotaxis can be exploited for removal of lesions in difficult locations. Earlier attempts to resect lesions in this location were limited by a significant risk of injury to lateral temporal lobe cortical (language, visual) and vascular (vein of Labbé) structures.

To avoid these problems, we designed a lateral occipital-subtemporal trajectory, which is essentially under this region of the brain. Originally described in seven patients, this technique has now been utilized in more than 25 such operations for various intra-axial neoplasms of the brain. We found that it was advantageous to avoid unnecessary brain resection or retraction, thus reducing the risk of injury to lateral temporal lobe structures and helping to maintain precise spatial and anatomic orientation for the surgeon. Furthermore, like all computer-assisted volumetric approaches, we delineated the margin between the tumor and the surrounding neural tissue.[39]

## Patient Selection for Stereotactic Resection

In general, the techniques outlined can be used to resect any intracranial tumor. However, in some regions, there is little need to employ the volumetric method; for example, in the resection of skull base lesions where one can easily find the tumor and discern its boundaries. In addition, the volumetric stereotactic technique is not appropriate for lesions located in frontal, temporal, or occipital poles because these can be managed with a standard lobectomy. For most other locations, however, the volumetric stereotactic method can be useful. However, because glial neoplasms represent the most common tumor type for which these procedures are indicated, the selection of appropriate surgical coordinates is imperative. Metastatic tumors, intraventricular lesions, vascular malformations, and many others can be performed by employing this minimally invasive surgical approach.

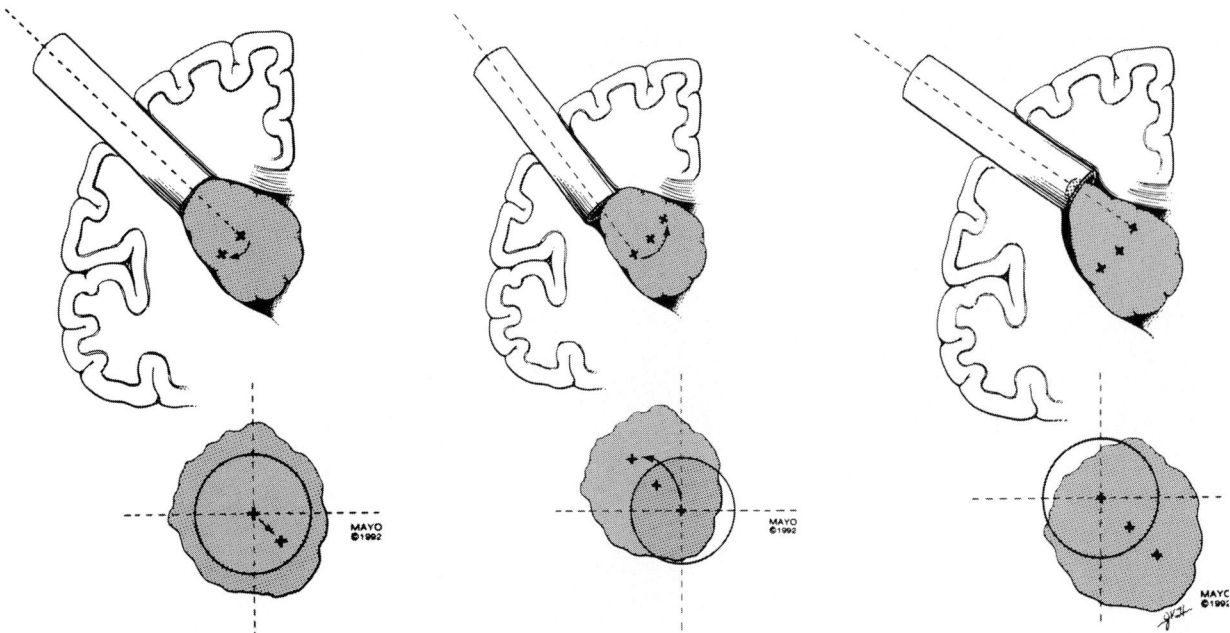

**FIGURE 47–9** ■ Tumors that are larger than the cross-sectional diameter of the retractor are removed by first translating to a new target point within the tumor volume in order to place a new target point beneath the retractor opening (*left*). In principle, the surgeon first isolates the tumor from surrounding brain tissue before removing it. The computer indicates the computed tomography/magnetic resonance imaging defined edge of the tumor with respect to the edge of the cylindrically shaped retractor (*middle*). A plane between the tumor and the surrounding brain tissue is established using the computer-generated slice images as a guide. Then, another part of the tumor is translated under the retractor, and the computer image is correspondingly updated (*right*). (By permission of the Mayo Foundation.)

## Spatial Types of Glial Tumors

Glial neoplasms can be classified into three types based on the growth patterns and presence or absence of tumor tissue, with or without surrounding tumor cell–infiltrated parenchyma.

**Type I.** Tumor tissue only with no surrounding parenchymal isolated tumor cell infiltration (Fig. 47–10). In general, type I tumors include gangliogliomas, most juvenile pilocytic astrocytomas, many xanthoastrocytomas, rare proto-

plasmic astrocytomas, and some oligodendrogliomas in young patients. Complete surgical resection can, in theory, cure these patients (Fig. 47–11).

**Type II.** Tumor tissue parenchyma is surrounded by isolated infiltrating tumor cells (Fig. 47–12). These cells are frequently high-grade gliomas. Low-grade tumors can also have a mass of tumor tissue that is hypodense within a field of infiltrated parenchyma. Surgical resection of the tumor tissue mass will benefit the patient in direct relationship to the proportion of the lesional volume that the tumor tissue proper comprises (Fig. 47–13). Resection of a small mass of tumor tissue within a large field of infiltrated parenchyma is of questionable benefit.

**Type III.** Parenchyma is infiltrated with isolated tumor cells only and no tumor tissue (Fig. 47–14). Type III tumors are more frequently low-grade gliomas. However, rare grade IV astrocytomas can present as type III tumors. However, these are usually hypodense or isodense on CT scanning. Resection of these lesions essentially involves resection of viable, albeit infiltrated, brain tissue.

## Surgical Patient Selection in Glial Neoplasms

Precision removal by means of computer-assisted volumetric stereotaxis of the imaging-defined intracranial tumor is dependent on the ability to recognize tumor boundaries on imaging studies. The technique is not appropriate for all glial neoplasms. Patient selection for computer-assisted volumetric resection in glial neoplasms, as in all surgeries, is based on a risk:benefit ratio and the following guidelines.

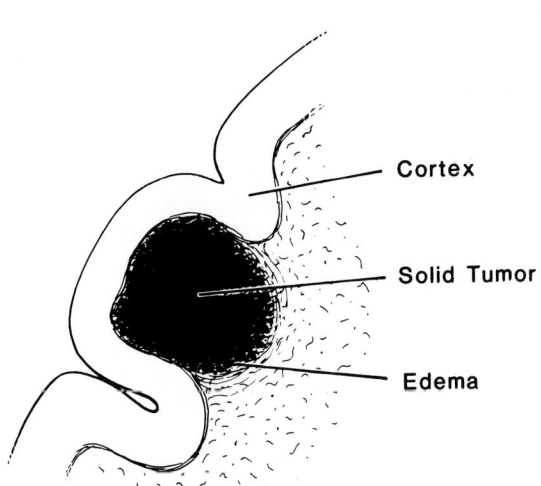

Cortex

Solid Tumor

Edema

**FIGURE 47–10** ■ Type I glial neoplasm comprises solid tumor tissue only, usually presents as a contrast-enhancing mass, and can be completely resected.

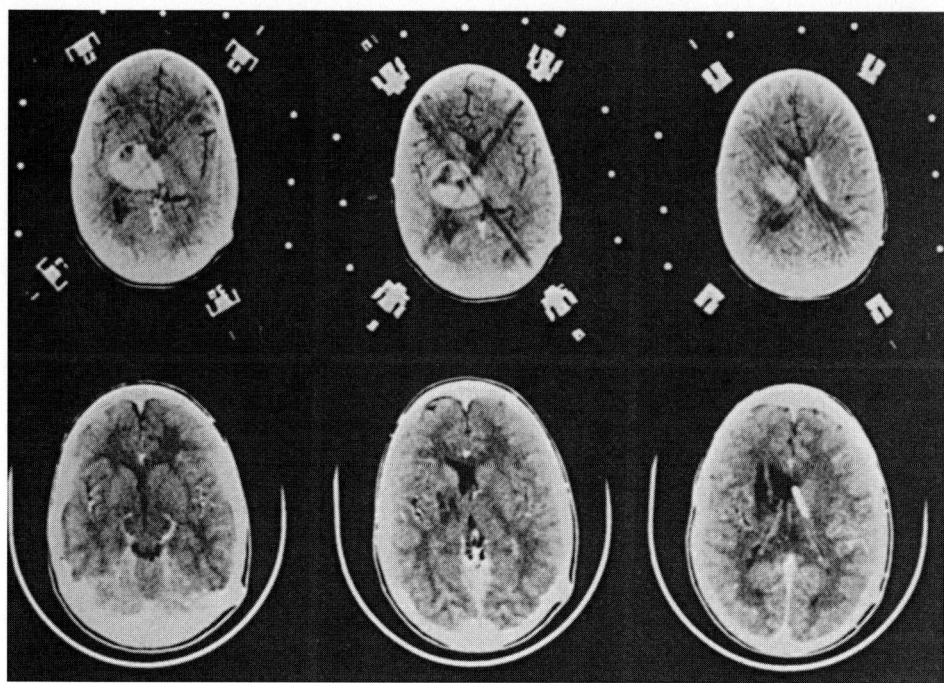

FIGURE 47–11 ■ Preoperative (*top*) and postoperative (*bottom*) computed tomography scans of a 7-year-old girl with a pilocytic astrocytoma involving the right thalamus, internal capsule, and basal ganglia. The patient had a mild hemiparesis preoperatively that was essentially unchanged postoperatively.

## Contrast-Enhanced Lesions

If the tumor volume defined by contrast enhancement on CT scanning (or gadolinium enhancement on MRI) is approximately equal to the volume defined by the $T_2$-weighted image of the MRI (or the volume of perilesional hypodensity on a CT scan), the lesion is frequently a type I tumor. This, in most cases, can (and should) be resected. The postoperative results will be good, and the morbidity will be low.

However, in a type II lesion, the volume defined by gadolinium enhancement on MRI or CT contrast enhancement is less than the volume defined by $T_2$ prolongation on MRI. An important exception can be noted in type I lesions in patients with seizures: The perilesional hypodensity or surrounding regions of $T_2$ prolongation in these cases may represent edema and not infiltrated parenchyma.

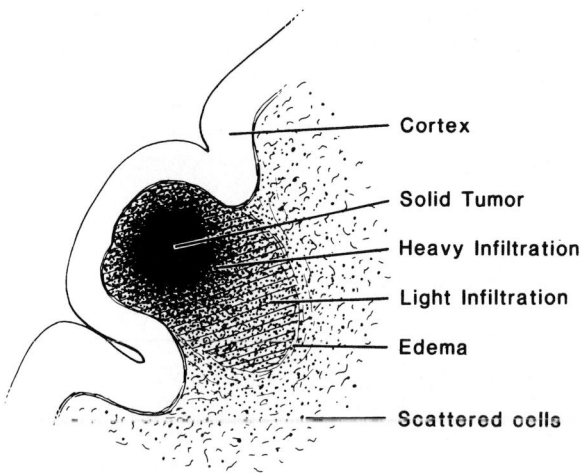

FIGURE 47–12 ■ Type II glial tumor featuring a solid tumor tissue mass surrounded by parenchyma infiltrated by isolated tumor cells.

A stereotactic serial biopsy can be performed to exclude the presence of infiltrating tumor cells prior to consideration for definitive surgery. One study indicates that patients harboring grade 4 gliomas undergoing computer-assisted volumetric resection followed by radiation therapy have a better chance of survival than do those who have radiation therapy following a biopsy alone.[9] Resection provides not only internal decompression but also significant tumor cell reduction and sets the stage for more effective radiation therapy and chemotherapy.

In nonessential brain regions, volumetric stereotactic resection of the entire volume of tumor tissue as well as infiltrated brain tissue can provide very significant cytoreduction and should theoretically prolong survival in high- and low-grade glial tumors.[18]

## Nonenhancing Tumors

No imaging method can prospectively differentiate solid tumor tissue from parenchyma infiltrated by isolated tumor cells in tumors that do not exhibit contrast enhancement. In most cases, the absence of contrast enhancement usually indicates that the lesion comprises isolated tumor cells within parenchyma only. Resection of the imaging-defined lesional volume is, in fact, resection of intact and usually functional brain parenchyma, and a neurologic deficit is usually the result. Therefore, in many of these cases, stereotactic biopsy and (when appropriate) radiation therapy may represent the only surgical and therapeutic options.

In some low-grade glial tumors, tumor tissue is present and hypodense. A serial stereotactic biopsy procedure can establish whether the lesion comprises tumor tissue, infiltrated parenchyma, or both. Some CT hypodense nonenhancing tumor tissue lesions can be resected from essential brain regions with low morbidity (Fig. 47–15).

In particular, low-grade oligodendrogliomas, dysembryoplastic neuroepithelial tumors (DNETs), and some gangli-

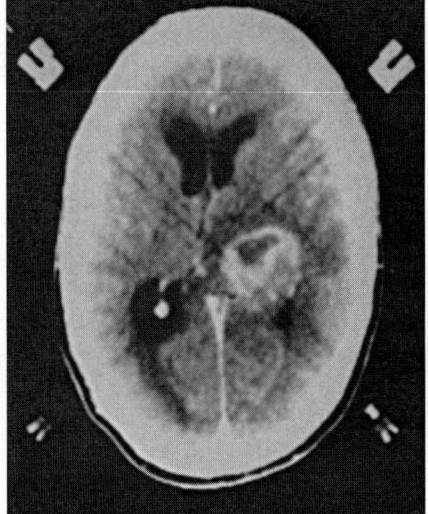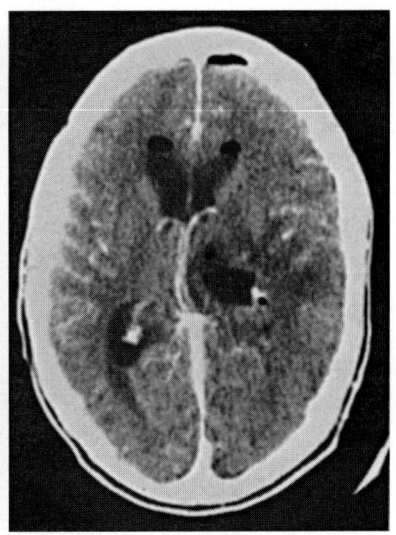

FIGURE 47–13 ■ In essential brain regions, resection of the only tumor tissue mass in a type II glioma is possible as in this 43-year-old man with a left posteriordorsal thalamic grade 4 astrocytoma. Preoperative (*left*) and postoperative (*right*) contrast-enhanced computed tomography scans are shown.

ogliomas in young patients (usually presenting with seizures) will manifest a solid tumor tissue mass that is hypodense and nonenhancing on CT scanning. Serial biopsies in these lesions will show only tumor tissue with minimal or no surrounding infiltrated parenchyma (type I tumor).

Tumors located in eloquent brain, which on biopsy are found to comprise isolated tumor cells within parenchyma with or without tumor tissue (type II or type III, respectively), should not be resected unless careful cortical mapping techniques establish that the involved parenchyma is "silent" (Fig. 47–16).

Hypodense type II or type III tumors, which are located in nonessential brain tissue, can be completely resected. Low-grade oligodendrogliomas, mixed gliomas, and astrocytomas located in frontal or anterior or medial temporal lobes or superior parietal lobules can be selectively resected

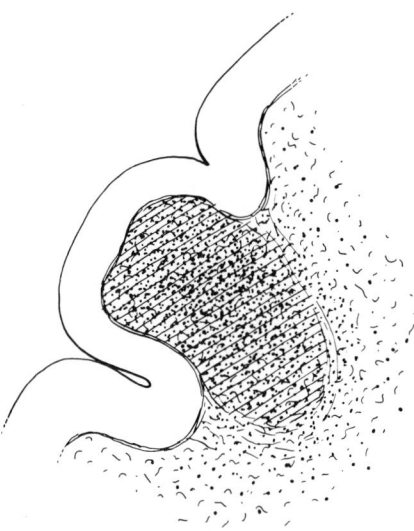

FIGURE 47–14 ■ Type III gliomas consist of isolated tumor cells, which reside in and infiltrate a volume of intact brain tissue. Resection of these lesions is, in fact, resection of functioning (albeit diseased) brain parenchyma.

by imaging-based volumetric stereotactic methods with rewarding postoperative results.

## RESULTS

One thousand, one hundred, and sixty-five (1165) patients underwent computer-assisted, volumetric stereotactic resection procedures at the Mayo Clinic (from August 1984 to September 1993) and at New York University Medical Center (from September 1993 to December 1994) over a 10-year period between August 1984 and December 1994. Overall surgical morbidity was 6.5%, and mortality was less than 1%. Postoperative imaging studies confirmed complete resection of the radiographically defined target volume in more than 90% of cases. Postoperative and follow-up results have been published previously in a series of publications.[1, 7, 8, 17, 19–31, 34, 36, 39] Moreover, the average global charges (physician-related plus hospital-related) for tumor resection by volumetric, minimally invasive stereotaxis was 67% of the charges for patients undergoing classical craniotomy for similar lesions.

### Morbidity and Mortality

Forty-three patients were neurologically worse after the operation: 14 patients were neurologically normal before and had deficits afterward, and 29 additional patients experienced worsening of a deficit noted on the preoperative neurologic examination. Postoperative deficits resulted from the surgical approach or from local perilesional trauma. In 18 of 43 patients, postoperative neurologic deficits were consistent with neuronal injury along the surgical approach. For instance, 14 patients with mediotemporal or posteroventral thalamic lesions sustained a permanent contralateral superior quadrantopsia, and two others had a homonymous hemianopsia following the temporo-occipital approach that was necessary to resect their lesions. The trans-sylvian exposure of a left subinsular metastatic tumor produced a contralateral arm dyspraxia in another patient.

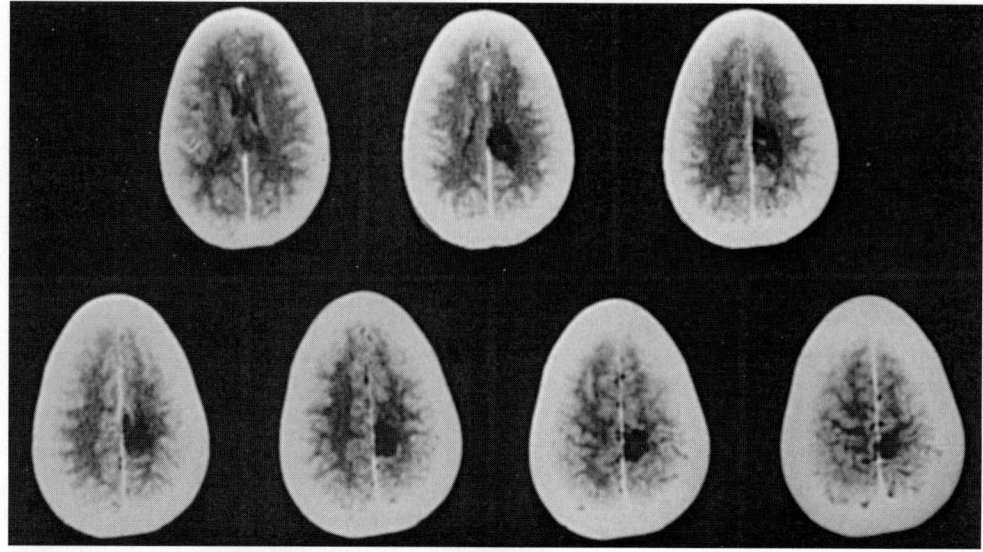

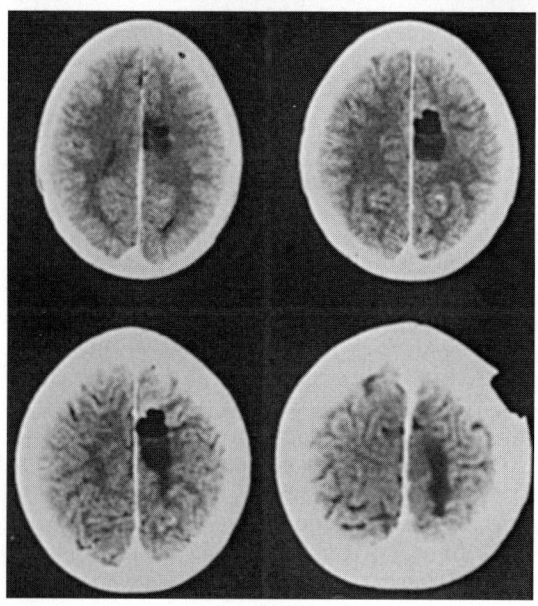

FIGURE 47–15 ■ Preoperative computed tomography scan (*top*) in a 3-year-old boy with a subcortical oligodendroglioma located beneath the postcentral convolution. The tumor comprises solid tumor tissue only and was completely resected (*bottom*) with no postoperative neurologic deficit.

Finally, a transvermian exposure of a midline cerebellar thrombosed arteriovenous malformation resulted in increased gait apraxia.

The remaining 25 patients who were worse after surgery sustained deficits consistent with local trauma inflicted in resecting the neoplasm or disruption of the parenchymal blood supply. Most often, this occurred in high-grade glial neoplasms with peritumoral tumor cell infiltration. However, deficit followed resection in some low-grade, apparently circumscribed lesions. For example, a 27-year-old woman noted worsening of a postoperative hemiparesis following resection of a 3-cm thrombosed arteriovenous malformation that was located in the left lateral basal ganglia. Six patients with thalamic pilocytic astrocytomas noted worsened preoperative hemiparesis postoperatively, which was slight in four patients and moderate in two patients.

In a series of 657 patients, operated on between August 1984 and December 1991 (Table 47–1), six deaths occurred within 1 month of surgery. One death was the result of massive brain stem edema after removal of a ventral thalamic mixed pilocytic/fibrillary astrocytoma with brain stem infiltration apparent on the MRI and two from massive pulmonary embolization (one 2 weeks after resection of a large left lateral ventricle meningioma and the other 6 days after resection of a thalamic glioblastoma). Another patient underwent a herniation syndrome and died owing to a subdural hygroma, which had developed 2½ weeks after resection of a larger intraventricular neurocytoma. Two additional patients with grade 4 astrocytomas continued to deteriorate neurologically owing to tumor progression despite tumor resection; these patients died within 30 days of the surgical procedure.

## High-Grade Glial Tumors

Computer-assisted stereotactic resection can remove all CT-defined contrast-enhancing portions of high-grade glial neoplasms from neurologically important subcortical areas

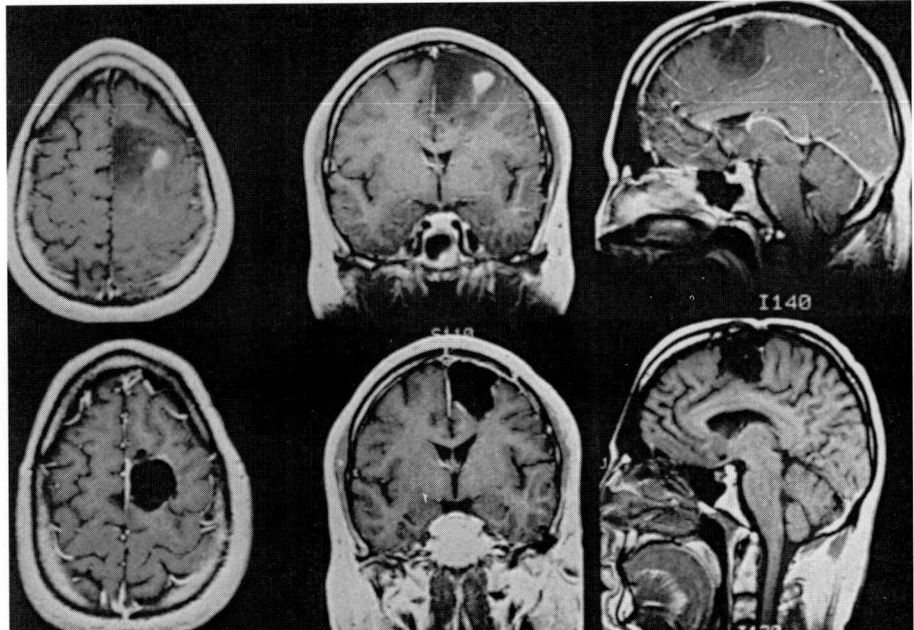

**FIGURE 47–16** ■ Preoperative (*top*) and postoperative (*bottom*) results in a 39-year-old man presenting with intractable seizures and an infiltrating grade 2 oligodendroglioma in the posterior third of the left superior frontal convolution, which was resected using a stereotactically placed trephine and the volumetric resection technique. The patient's neurologic examination was normal before and after surgery.

with acceptable levels of mortality and morbidity.[8, 19, 24, 29] Postoperative CT studies usually demonstrate an absence of contrast enhancement around the surgical defect. Nevertheless, the mean postoperative survival time for our patients harboring grade 4 astrocytomas treated with postoperative external beam radiation therapy (50 to 65 Gy) was 50.6 weeks. This survival rate compares favorably with a consecutive series of patients harboring grade 4 gliomas who underwent radiation therapy following a biopsy alone (mean survival of 33 weeks).[31] However, following resection, new areas of contrast enhancement on CT scanning

developed within low-density areas surrounding the surgical defect within 6 to 9 months of the procedure.

Computer-assisted volumetric stereotactic resection allows safe and complete resection of the contrast-enhancing mass lesion in high-grade gliomas. However, preoperative stereotactic MRI (especially the $T_2$-weighted image) in high-grade glial tumors always demonstrates much larger areas of abnormality than those indicated by contrast enhancement on CT scanning.[25, 26] An examination of stereotactic serial biopsy specimens obtained in patients with high-grade gliomas from these MRI-defined abnormalities outside the contrast-enhancing tumor mass reveals a larger area of intact edematous brain parenchyma infiltrated by aggressive isolated tumor cells.[4, 6, 7, 25, 26] In fact, this edematous infiltrated parenchyma usually extends as far as (and in some cases beyond) the area of signal prolongation abnormality on the $T_2$-weighted MRI.[25, 26] It would be technically possible using volumetric stereotaxis to resect the volume defined by the MRI abnormality and this, in theory, would substantially prolong postoperative survival.[15, 16] However, unacceptable neurologic deficits would result from removal of the intact albeit infiltrated parenchyma.

A similar problem exists for patients with grade 3 astrocytomas, mixed gliomas, and oligodendrogliomas. Although the cellular elements within these tumors are not as mitotically active as in the grade 4 tumor, isolated tumor cells also infiltrate intact and surrounding edematous parenchyma[25, 26] and defy surgical attempts to cure them. In addition, grade 3 gliomas, particularly astrocytomas, tend to have larger infiltrative components with respect to tumor tissue components than do grade 4 lesions. Thus, the benefit of resecting a relatively small tumor tissue mass in the face of a large volume of infiltrated parenchyma is questionable.

## Low-Grade Astrocytomas

The resectability of these tumors depends on the degree of histologic circumscription. In adults, low-grade astrocyto-

### TABLE 47–1 ■ LOCATION OF TUMORS IN 657 PATIENTS UNDERGOING STEREOTACTIC RESECTION (AUGUST 1984–DECEMBER 1991)

| Location | Total | Right | Left |
|---|---|---|---|
| **Supratentorial** | | | |
| Central | 63 | 32 | 31 |
| Basal ganglia | 31 | 19 | 12 |
| Thalamus | 55 | 19 | 36 |
| Third ventricle | 37 | — | — |
| Posterior/deep frontal | 142 | 66 | 76 |
| Parietal | 108 | 51 | 57 |
| Occipital | 26 | 10 | 16 |
| Temporal | 67 | 33 | 34 |
| Temporo-occipital | 15 | 6 | 9 |
| Temporoparietal | 20 | 7 | 13 |
| Parieto-occipital | 11 | 7 | 4 |
| Corpus callosum | 3 | — | — |
| Lateral ventricle | 25 | 17 | 8 |
| Total | 603 | | |
| **Infratentorial** | | | |
| Deep cerebellar hemisphere | 23 | | |
| Vermis | 7 | | |
| Mesencephalon | 8 | | |
| Pons | 11 | | |
| Medulla | 5 | | |
| Total | 54 | | |

mas are usually manifest by an area of low density on CT scanning and prolongation of signal on MRI.[25] Stereotactic serial biopsy studies of these so-called fibrillary astrocytomas reveal that the tumor consists almost entirely of infiltrated intact parenchyma with little tumor tissue proper.[25, 26] Therefore, resection of the tumor by stereotactic craniotomy involves resection of intact but infiltrated parenchyma defined by the low-density areas on CT scanning and signal prolongation on MRI. However, in important brain areas, this results in a postoperative neurologic deficit, and stereotactic resection is therefore rejected as an option.[19, 29] In some cases, the lesion is confined to expendable brain tissue, such as the posterior portion of the superior frontal convolution.

Juvenile pilocytic astrocytomas, conversely, which tend to occur in children and young adults, are histologically circumscribed. Despite the fact that many are located in the thalamus and other important subcortical locations, they can be completely resected by computer-assisted stereotactic technique with excellent postoperative results.[19, 29, 33] These lesions exhibit prominent contrast enhancement on CT or on MRI with gadolinium, and the histologic borders are defined accurately by the contrast enhancement.

## Metastatic Tumors

Many surgeons have had the unsettling experience of trying unsuccessfully to locate deep subcortical metastatic lesions during a conventional craniotomy. In fact, reported surgical series of metastatic tumors removed at nonstereotactic craniotomies report a certain percentage of patients with incomplete resections.[12, 32, 35, 40] Metastatic tumors are usually located at the gray-white junction subcortically. They can be located superficially near the crown of a gyrus. They can also be located at the gray-white junction in the depths of a deep sulcus, and they can be difficult to find at conventional craniotomy. Other tumors may be deep to the insular cortex, deep to the mesial occipital cortex, or under the cortex of the interhemispheric fissure.

Stereotactic techniques can be advantageous in the resection of the superficial metastases as well as the deeply

situated lesions.[30] First, stereotactic point localization helps to center small cranial trephines directly over superficial lesions (the trephine need be no larger than the cross-sectional area of the neoplasm). The approach is, therefore, selective and direct, and no more brain need be exposed than is absolutely necessary. With volumetric stereotaxis and intraoperative image displays, identification of the plane between the tumor and the brain is straightforward and, in fact, simple. These lesions can be completely resected by the computer-assisted stereotactic craniotomy.

Our postoperative morbidity for stereotactic resection of centrally located and deep-seated metastatic tumors (mortality rate of 0; morbidity rate of 4.3%), compares favorably with that associated with conventional craniotomy for these lesions in the past (mortality rate of 11%).[12, 32, 35, 38, 40]

## Vascular Malformations

Angiographically, occult arteriovenous malformations and cavernous hemangioma are well-circumscribed lesions that can be completely removed stereotactically with relatively low risk. A byproduct of establishing the histology is that cessation or significant reduction of seizures, when present, usually results.

Small deep-seated active arteriovenous malformations may also be resected using similar techniques (Fig. 47–17). The position of the feeding vessels is established in the three-dimensional surgical planning matrix and is approached and clipped or coagulated before the remainder of the lesion is dissected away from the surrounding parenchyma.

## Intraventricular Lesions

A more limited but direct approach to intraventricular lesions can be made stereotactically. Brain and ventricular incisions need to be only large enough to remove the lesion. Thus, intraventricular lesions are removed through a 1.5-inch trephine and 2-cm cylindrical retractor (Fig. 47–18).

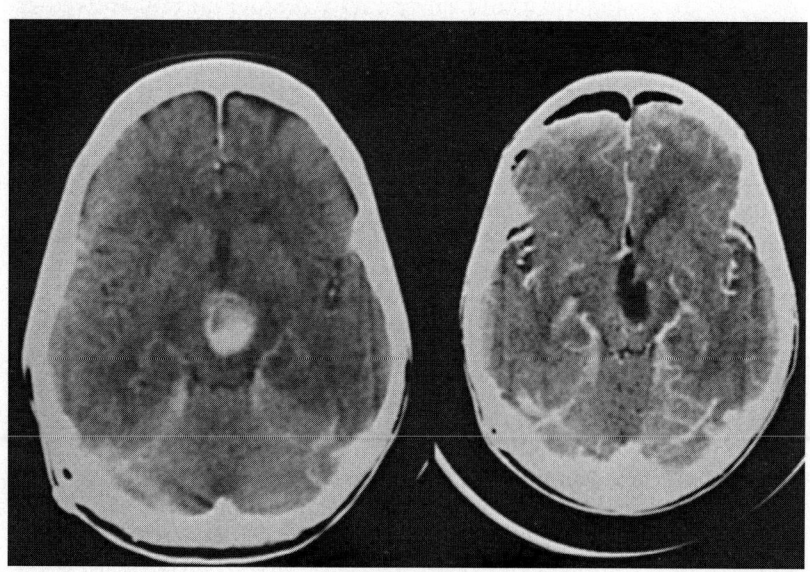

FIGURE 47–17 ■ Preoperative (left) and postoperative (right) computed tomography scans in a 29-year-old woman with a mesencephalic arteriovenous malformation (AVM) with a hemorrhage. The hematoma and AVM were resected using the 2-cm-diameter stereotactic retractor. The patient was lethargic and had Weber's syndrome preoperatively. She made an excellent neurologic recovery following evacuation of the hematoma and resection of the AVM.

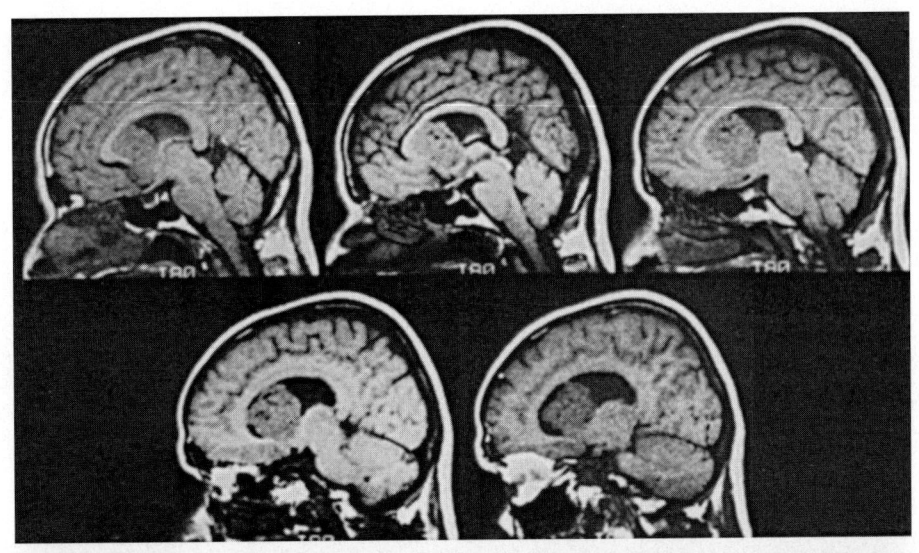

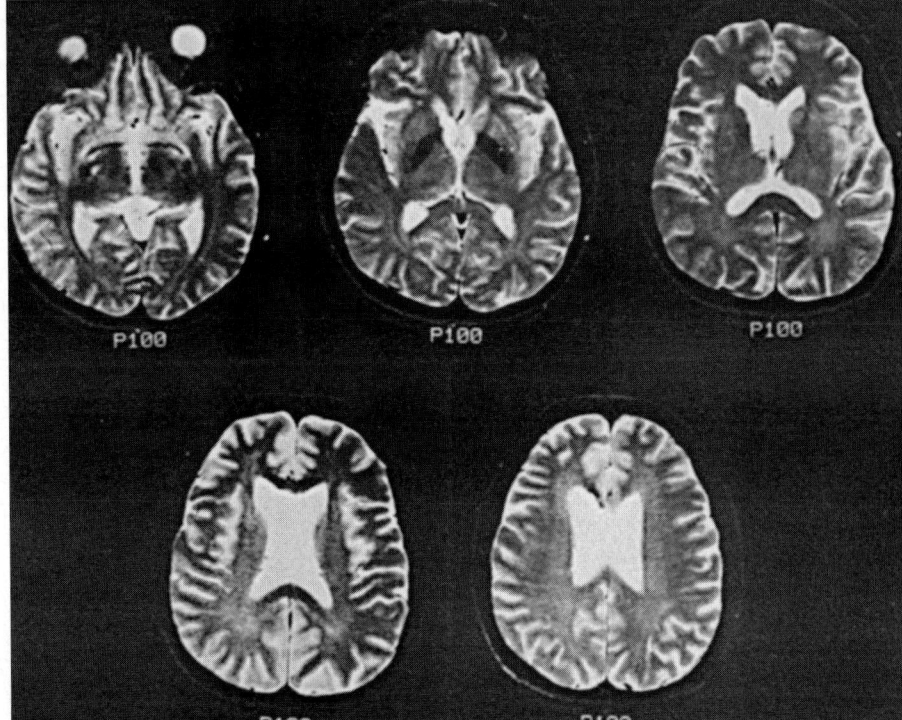

FIGURE 47–18 ■ Preoperative (*top*) and postoperative (*bottom*) magnetic resonance imaging studies in a 58-year-old woman with a large intraventricular subependymal astrocytoma and associated hydrocephalus. The lesion was totally resected using a 2-cm stereotactic retractor and multiple translations. A gross total excision of the lesion was accomplished. The patient did not require a shunt.

Colloid cysts are approached through the lateral ventricle and foramen of Monro into which the cyst extends. The approach features an anterior trephine craniotomy (about at the frontal hairline), splitting of the superior frontal sulcus, and exposure of the cyst in the foramen of Monro by means of the 2-cm-diameter stereotactic retractor (Fig. 47–19). This approach does not violate epileptogenic brain tissue and provides an anterior vantage point for dealing with the attachment of the cyst. We have resected 28 colloid cysts in this manner without permanent complications.[1]

Large third ventricular lesions are usually approached through the right lateral ventricle, unless the lesion has significantly enlarged the left foramen of Monro. In the latter instance, the lesion would be approached from the left side (Fig. 47–20). One fornix can be incised to extend the stereotactic retractor into the third ventricular lesion, where an internal decompression of the lesion is performed with a $CO_2$ laser until only a thin rim of the capsule remains. The computer display of the cross-sections of the digitized CT/MRI-defined tumor volume is extremely useful in this step, because the surgeon, knowing where tumor stops and third ventricular wall begins, can be aggressive within the tumor with no risk of extending through the capsule and damaging the walls of the third ventricle. After this internal decompression, the retractor is withdrawn to the level of the roof of the third ventricle, and the capsule is carefully dissected from the walls of the third ventricle. The tumor capsule can be contracted using the defocused laser, which facilitates the dissection of the capsule from the wall of the third ventricle.[34]

## NEW DIRECTIONS IN MINIMALLY INVASIVE COMPUTER-ASSISTED STEREOTACTIC NEUROSURGERY

The advantages of computer-assisted stereotactic neurosurgery have become evident over the past several years, as have the ease and applicability of computer technology. These developments have enabled us to embark on several new projects that have rapidly become incorporated into our neurosurgical armamentarium. It has become clear that computers can be used to monitor and display to the surgeon the position of surgical instruments within a stereotactically defined work environment. This makes possible a trend toward even more minimally invasive as well as endoscopic surgery, not only in subarachnoid and intraventricular spaces but also for intra-axial target volumes.

### Frameless Stereotaxis

Computers make possible instrumentation for on-line registration of surgical instrument position within the surgical work envelope by transmitting the position of a surgical tool to an operating room computer system. Several frameless systems are currently available and in use at our institution. These include multiple-jointed, articulated arm digitizers. These may be cumbersome and require frequent repositioning during the operative procedure. In addition, image-guided, stereotactic navigational microscopes, based on optical digitizing methods utilizing a system of light-emitting diodes (LEDs), have also been introduced. These, however, are limited by "line-of-sight" considerations, which often only become apparent during real-time operations, when the patient is positioned on the operating table and the entire team of surgeons, anesthesiologists, and

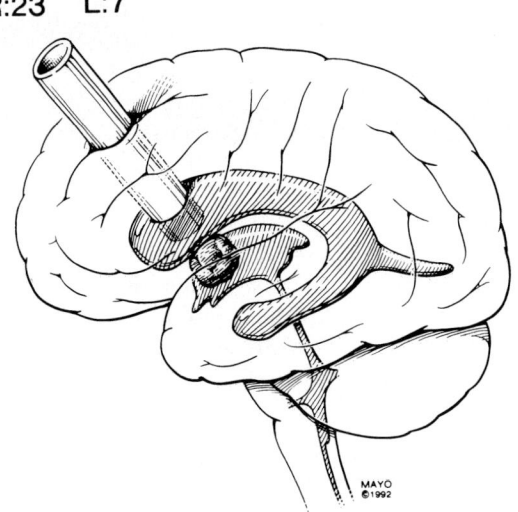

R:23   L:7

FIGURE 47–19 ■ Exposure of the anterior third ventricular lesion. A stereotactic retractor is placed through a microsurgically opened superior frontal sulcus and subcortical incision into the lateral ventricle. The ipsilateral fornix can be sacrificed if the foramen of Monro must be enlarged in order to extend the retractor into the third ventricle itself. (By permission of the Mayo Foundation.)

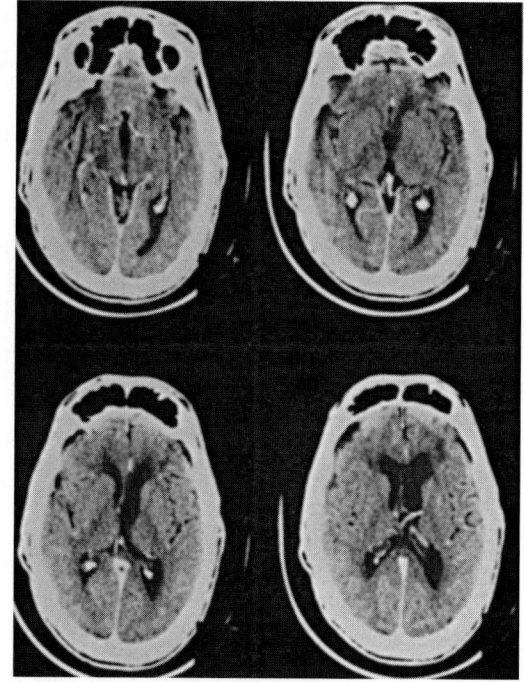

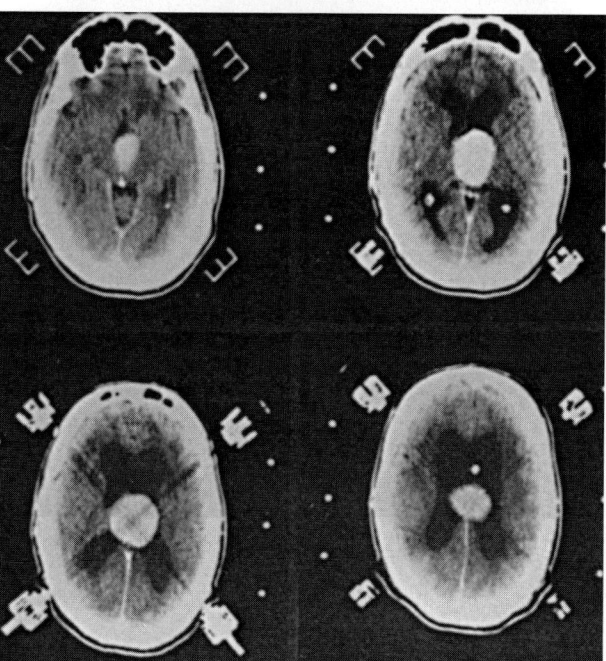

FIGURE 47–20 ■ Preoperative (*top*) and postoperative (*bottom*) contrast-enhanced computed tomography scans in a 56-year-old man who presented with a recent memory deficit and hydrocephalus due to a giant, partially calcified colloid cyst of the third ventricle. He was neurologically intact postoperatively; his recent memory had improved to better than preoperative levels by 3 months after surgery.

nurses are at work. Alternatively, we have developed magnetic field digitizers to cross-register points from the imaging database to the actual surgical field. Sensors on this device are connected to a wire similar to that attached to bipolar forceps. With tuning of the magnetic field and computer-generated distortion corrections, we have reliable and reasonable accuracy with this instrument as a pointing device. We have also incorporated a suction device and a heads-up display to this unit in order to increase its utility in the operating room. The REGULUS and, more recently, the CYGNUS systems (COMPASS International, Rochester, MN) have been developed to give surgeons more freehand efficiency. The latter system is the first portable image-guided surgery system, which is operated from a laptop computer, with a network image-acquisition interface, thus reducing the costs of this technology significantly. In our institution, this system is actually shared between affiliated hospitals. We are currently objectively and mathematically comparing all three prototypical image-guided navigational systems that are in use at our institution for actual precision and accuracy.

## Integration of Stereotaxis and Endoscopy

We have incorporated computer-assisted, frameless stereotaxis into our free-hand endoscopic procedures over the last several years. In the first author's experience in pediatric neurosurgery, intraventricular anatomy may frequently be distorted and devoid of normal anatomic landmarks, rendering such surgical procedures unacceptably risky. With the integration of the visual information obtained endoscopically and the navigational information provided by stereotaxis, we have been able to successfully place ventricular catheters in complex hydrocephalus, fenestrate irregular cysts and loculated ventricles, retrieve retained catheters, and perform endoscopic septostomy and third ventriculostomy. We can biopsy and resect intraventricular lesions, such as tumors and colloid cysts, with improved accuracy, confidence, and safety.

## Integration of Functional Brain Mapping in Image-Guided Neurosurgery

Magnetoencephalography (MEG) is a noninvasive, accurate, and reproducible method for the preoperative assessment of patients with lesions associated with eloquent sensory and motor cortex.[17, 36] We have incorporated the interactive use of MEG functional mapping in our stereotactic, volumetric resections, allowing for safer approaches for resection of eloquent cortex lesions. We have, therefore, developed MEG-mapping-derived functional risk profiles that were used as powerful tools for both presurgical planning and intraoperative guidance. We developed a process for transforming the MEG-derived sensorimotor localization coordinates into the COMPASS stereotactic coordinate system. This, in turn, is incorporated into the stereotactic database, enabling the simultaneous visualization of functional and anatomic data. The results of this technique have appeared in several publications.[17, 36]

## Stereotaxis and Molecular Neurosurgery

With new molecular biologic advances in the field of neuro-oncology, stereotactic methods combined with modern computing power and imaging databases provide powerful options for molecular neurosurgery. Point-in-space and volumetric computer-assisted imaging-based tumor stereotactic procedures can be easily modified for the preplanned and precise delivery of genetic and chemotherapeutic agents to an imaging-defined anatomic target volume. These techniques could provide more uniform coverage and dose levels of the therapeutic material within the defined target structure.[21]

## CONCLUSION

With the computer-assisted volumetric stereotactic method described, it is theoretically possible to resect all tumors detected by CT or MRI. The procedure has been found to be most effective for the resection of well-circumscribed lesions in deep-seated intra-axial locations. For instance, juvenile pilocytic astrocytomas can be totally removed with minimal morbidity from any subcortical location, such as the thalamus, by this method. Furthermore, patients with other circumscribed glial tumors, metastatic tumors, and thrombosed vascular malformations can derive significant benefit from this procedure.

Without volumetric stereotaxis the surgeon may become lost, resulting in unnecessary tissue damage. This may lead to neurologic deficits and a prolonged and expensive recovery period. Furthermore, the border between tumor and surrounding normal brain may not be obvious, possibly leading to the resection of normal tissue in eloquent brain regions. The neurosurgeon benefits from this technology by being able to localize the lesion, visualize the border between the lesion and surrounding tissue, conceptualize the three-dimensional character of the neoplasm, and plan the safest approach preoperatively, based on the neural and vascular anatomy. The patient benefits from a smaller skin incision, craniotomy flap, and brain exposure, resulting in reduced operative morbidity, shorter hospitalization, and reduced cost.

In conclusion, computer-assisted volumetric stereotactic craniotomy provides several advantages over conventional freehand neurosurgical techniques in the management of intra-axial mass lesions. First, the stereotactic method maintains surgical orientation as the procedure extends below the cortical surface, and the approach is preplanned to disrupt as little important brain tissue as possible. Beyond the gross appearance of a tumor at surgery and its apparent margins on visual inspection, the computer display images provide additional information to the surgeon regarding where tumor boundaries lie in relationship to surrounding brain tissue. The method allows us to resect as much of a lesion as we choose to remove. However, limitations in malignant glial neoplasms lie in the biology of the disease process itself—unresectable intact parenchyma that is infiltrated by isolated tumor cells. The best candidates for computer-assisted stereotactic volumetric resection, therefore, are patients with histologically circumscribed glial and nonglial tumors and non-neoplastic lesions.

## REFERENCES

1. Abernathey CD, Davis DH, Kelly PJ: Treatment of colloid cysts of the third ventricle by stereotaxic microsurgical laser craniotomy. J Neurosurg 70:525–529, 1989.

2. Apuzzo MLJ, Sabshin JK: Computed tomographic guidance stereo-taxis in the management of intracranial mass lesions. Neurosurgery 12:277–285, 1983.
3. Brown RA: A computerized tomography–computer graphics approach to stereotaxic localization. Neurosurgery 50:715–720, 1979.
4. Burger PC, Dubois PJ, Schold SC Jr, et al: Computerized tomographic and pathologic studies of the untreated, quiescent, and recurrent glioblastoma multiforme. Neurosurgery 59:159–168, 1983.
5. Clarke RH, Horsley V: On a method of investigating the deep ganglia and tracts of the central nervous system (cerebellum). BJJ 2:1799–1800, 1906.
6. Daumas-Duport C, Monsaingeon V, Szenthe L, et al: Serial stereotac-tic biopsies: A double histological code of gliomas according to malignancy and 3-D configuration, as an aid to therapeutic decision and assessment of results. Appl Neurophysiol 45:431–437, 1982.
7. Daumas-Duport C, Scheithauer BW, Kelly PJ: A histologic and cyto-logic method for the spatial definition of gliomas. Mayo Clin Proc 62:435–449, 1987.
8. Devaux BC, O'Fallon JR, Kelly PJ: Resection, biopsy and survival in malignant glial neoplasms: A retrospective study of clinical param-eters, therapy and outcome. J Neurosurg 78:767–775, 1993.
9. Frankel SA, German WJ: Glioblastoma multiforme: Review of 219 cases with regard to natural history, diagnostic methods, and treat-ment. Neurosurgery 15:489–503, 1958.
10. Gehan EA, Walker MD: Prognostic factors for patients with brain tumors. NCR Monogr 46:189–195, 1977.
11. Goerss S, Kelly PJ, Kall B, et al: A computed tomographic stereotac-tic adaptation system. Neurosurgery 10:375–379, 1982.
12. Haar F, Patterson RH Jr: Surgery for metastatic intracranial neoplasm. Cancer 30:1241–1245, 1972.
13. Hitchock E, Sato F: Treatment of malignant gliomata. J Neurosurg 21:497–505, 1964.
14. Horsley V, Clarke RH: The structure and function of the cerebellum examined by a new method. Brain 31:45–124, 1908.
15. Hoshino T: A commentary on the biology and growth kinetics of low grade and high grade gliomas. J Neurosurg 27:388–400, 1984.
16. Hoshino T, Barker M, Wilson CB, et al: Cell kinetics of human gliomas. Neurosurgery 37:15–26, 1972.
17. Hund M, Rezai AR, Kronberg E, et al: Magnetoencephalographic mapping: Basic of a new functional risk profile in the selection of patients with cortical brain lesions. Neurosurgery 40:936–942, 1997.
18. Jelsma R, Bucy PC: The treatment of glioblastoma multiforme of the brain. Neurosurgery 27:385–400, 1967.
19. Kelly PJ: Volumetric stereotactic surgical resection of intra-axial brain mass lesions. Mayo Clin Proc 63:1186–1198, 1988.
20. Kelly PJ: Tumor Stereotaxis. Philadelphia: WB Saunders, 1991.
21. Kelly PJ: Stereotactic procedures for molecular neurosurgery. Exp Neurol 144:157–159, 1997.
22. Kelly PJ, Alker GJ Jr: A stereotactic approach to deep seated CNS neoplasms using the carbon dioxide laser. Surg Neurol 15:331–334, 1981.
23. Kelly PJ, Alker GJ Jr, Goerss S: Computer-assisted stereotactic laser microsurgery for the treatment of intracranial neoplasms. Neurosur-gery 10:324–331, 1982.
24. Kelly PJ, Alker GJ Jr, Kall B, et al: Precision resection of intra-axial CNS lesions by CT-based stereotactic craniotomy and computer monitored $CO_2$ laser. Acta Neurochir 68:1–9, 1983.
25. Kelly PJ, Daumas-Duport C, Kispert DB, et al: Imaging-based stereo-tactic serial biopsies in untreated intracranial glial neoplasms. J Neu-rosurg 66:865–874, 1987.
26. Kelly PJ, Daumas-Duport C, Scheithauer BW, et al: Stereotactic histologic correlations of computed tomography and magnetic reso-nance imaging defined abnormalities in patients with glial neoplasms. Mayo Clin Proc 62:450–459, 1987.
27. Kelly PJ, Goerss SJ, Kall BA: Evolution of contemporary instrumen-tation for computer-assisted stereotactic surgery. Surg Neurol 30:204–215, 1988.
28. Kelly PJ, Kall BA, Goerss SJ: Transposition of volumetric informa-tion derived from computed tomography scanning into stereotactic space. Surg Neurol 21:465–471, 1984.
29. Kelly PJ, Kall B, Goerss S, et al: Computer-assisted stereotaxic resection of intra-axial brain neoplasms. J Neurosurg 64:427–439, 1986.
30. Kelly PJ, Kall BA, Goerss SJ: The results of CT based computer-assisted stereotactic resection of metastatic intracranial tumors. Neu-rosurgery 22:7–17, 1988.
31. Kelly PJ, Hunt C: The limited value of cytoreductive surgery in elderly patients with malignant gliomas. Neurosurgery 34:62–66, 1994.
32. MacGee EE: Surgical treatment of cerebral metastases from lung cancer: The effect on quality and duration of survival. J Neurosurg 35:416–420, 1971.
33. McGirr SJ, Kelly PJ, Scheithauer BW: Stereotactic resection of juve-nile pilocytic astrocytomas of the thalamus and basal ganglia. Neuro-surgery 20:447–452, 1987.
34. Morita A, Kelly PJ: Resection of intraventricular tumors via com-puter-assisted volumetric stereotactic approach. Neurosurgery 32:920–927, 1993.
35. Raskind R, Weiss SE, Manning JJ, et al: Survival after surgical excision of single metastatic brain tumors. AJR Am J Roentgenol 111:323–328, 1971.
36. Rezai AR, Hund M, Kronberg E, et al: The interactive use of magnet-oencephalography in stereotactic image-guided neurosurgery. Neuro-surgery 39:92–102, 1996.
37. Spiegel EA, Wycis HT, Marks M, et al: Stereotaxic apparatus for operation on the human brain. Science 106:349–350, 1947.
38. Van Eck JHM, Go KG, Ebels EJ: Metastatic tumors of the brain. Psychiatr Neurol Neurochir 68:443–462, 1965.
39. Weiner HL, Kelly PJ: A novel computer-assisted volumetric stereo-tactic approach for resecting tumors of the posterior parahippocampal gyrus. J Neurosurg 85:272–277, 1996.
40. Yardeni D, Reichenthal E, Zucker G, et al: Neurosurgical manage-ment of single brain metastasis. Surg Neurol 21:377–384, 1984.

# Open Magnetic Resonance Imaging–Guided Neurosurgery Focusing on Intracranial Gliomas

■ VOLKER SEIFERT, MICHAEL ZIMMERMANN, CHRISTOS TRANTAKIS, JENS-PETER SCHNEIDER, and JÜRGEN DIETRICH

Preservation of brain function while maximizing resection is the main goal of glioma surgery. The period of survival and the quality of life have been found to correlate with the degree of glioma removal.[1, 5] Monitoring of eloquent brain areas can be facilitated at the time of surgery using cortical stimulation to identify motor or language cortex.[5, 14] Somatosensory evoked potentials help to localize the sensory cortex or a phase reversal across the central sulcus to identify the motor cortex.[39]

In the 1990s, navigational devices have provided an unprecedented degree of surgical guidance during neurosurgical procedures. The development of image-guided neurosurgery represents a substantial improvement in the microsurgical treatment of tumors, vascular malformations, and other intracerebral lesions. It allows a greater accuracy in the localization of the lesion, a more accurate determination of its margins, and a safer surgical removal, avoiding injury of the surrounding brain tissue. Available systems of image-guided surgery include both frame-based and frameless technologies. They transfer preoperative diagnostic image data to the surgical field with the aid of a digitized articulating arm or detectors that track devices emitting ultrasound or infrared light. All these systems use images acquired before surgery to create a three-dimensional space on which navigation during the whole neurosurgical procedure is based.[2, 3, 7, 12, 13, 15, 21, 28, 34, 37, 38, 40] However, none of the current devices can provide the neurosurgeon with information about the dynamic changes (brain shift) that occur during the progress of the surgical procedure owing to tumor removal, brain edema, and loss of cerebrospinal fluid. In addition, these systems are unable to detect intraoperative adverse events and complications (e.g., intracranial hemorrhage). Black and colleagues[6] were instrumental in the development and implementation of the 0.5-tesla, vertical open magnetic resonance imaging (MRI) system for intraoperative guidance during different neurosurgical procedures, including surgery of brain tumors, drainage of intracranial cysts, spinal surgery, and interstitial hyperthermia. Using 0.5-T MRI guidance, Martin and associates[22] described their experience with the removal of low-

grade gliomas. Complete resection of the tumor mass using intraoperative guidance was achieved in 72% of their patients and a subtotal removal was achieved in 28%. Intraoperative imaging in these patients revealed residual tumor involving deep brain structures, speech center, or motor cortex. By merging MRI with frameless stereotactic procedures, navigational tools, and multimodality image fusion, it has become possible to combine all available three-dimensional information with real-time image updating. Definition of correct tumor margins, comprehension of the full extent of the tumor, and accurate definition of anatomic landmarks may improve surgical efficiency and diminish invasiveness. Complete resection of tumors, decreased vulnerability of surrounding tissues, and avoidance of critical structures should improve clinical outcome and reduce complication rates.[22] In this context, we present current experiences with MRI-guided neurosurgical procedures focusing on intracranial gliomas.

## TECHNICAL CONDITIONS FOR MAGNETIC RESONANCE IMAGING–GUIDED NEUROSURGERY

Since late 1996, a number of surgical procedures, including biopsies, craniotomies, transsphenoidal surgery, and interstitial minimally invasive laser procedures have been performed using a 0.5-T superconducting MR system, the Signa SP (General Electric Medical Systems, Milwaukee, WI; Fig. 48–1). Its open-configuration magnet provides the space for surgery. Images are viewed on monitors located in the gap, allowing for accurate intraoperative guidance and correlation between instrument position and anatomic brain structures.[24, 29, 33, 36]

For radiofrequency transmission and reception, a flexible head coil is used (Fig. 48–2A). The dimensions of the two coil loops connected at one side are 23 × 19 cm. Because access to the lesion might be through a small bur hole, craniotomy, or transsphenoidal approach, it is possible to attach the coil in a variety of configurations to the patient's

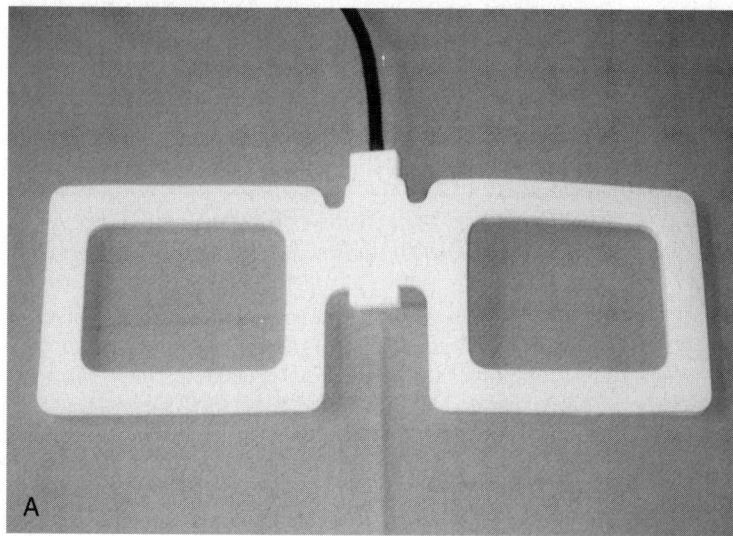

FIGURE 48-1 ■ A vertical opened 0.5T magnetic resonance tomograph "SIGNA SP" (General Electric Medical Systems, USA) with two in bore displays.

head (see Fig. 48-2B). Coil flexibility is necessary for such a procedure, but flexibility can also result in unstable coil fixation to the patient's head. However, with increasing experience, a method of fixation was developed using drapes, pads, and plasters, so that the head coil could be fixed in a relatively rigid position to the patient's head. Sterile coil drapes specially manufactured for this purpose are also available.

Liquid crystal display monitors mounted above the image region allow the neurosurgeon to view intraoperative images without leaving the MRI device. To permit interactive selection of the image plane, a special light-emitting diode (LED) tracking system, the Flashpoint Position Encoder (Image Guided Technologies, Boulder, CO) is inte-

grated into the system. It is therefore possible to determine a scan plane and to control the position of an instrument rigidly connected to the tracking system, such as a biopsy needle (Fig. 48-3A) or a blunt pointer (see Fig. 48-3B). Using a common single-slice gradient-echo sequence with an acquisition time of 3 seconds per image, the delay due to reconstruction time between a change in the tracking system position and display of the corresponding image is approximately 7 seconds. This interactive mode could be used to provide nearly real-time control for biopsies, and for intraoperative guidance for all other microneurosurgical procedures.

The patient is positioned in the MRI scanner in such a way that the suspected lesion is situated near the isocenter between the magnets, and good access is provided for the surgeon to the target area. For localization of the lesion, fast $T_2$-weighted spin-echo sequences and $T_1$-weighted spin-echo sequences before and after injection of gadolinium-diethylaminetriamine-penta-acetic acid (DTPA) are used. Thereafter, the continuous interactive imaging mode with a gradient-echo sequence is applied, for which a $T_1$-weighted, fast multiplanar spoiled gradient echo (TR = 24 to 30 msec, TE = 8 to 9 msec, flip angle 45 degrees, reversible band width 16.6 kHz) with a single, 10-mm-thick slice is used. Using this configuration, a new image could be obtained every 3 to 4 seconds. Alternatively, a more $T_2$*-weighted gradient-echo sequence (TR = 35 msec, TE = 12.7 msec, flip angle 90 degrees, slice thickness 10 mm, 7 sec/image) can be used for better visualization of the ventricle system and intracerebral vessels. As a result of these preoperative scans, the planned bur hole or craniotomy can be directly centered over the lesion.

In the first patients, craniotomy was carried out outside the magnet because some instruments were not yet avail-

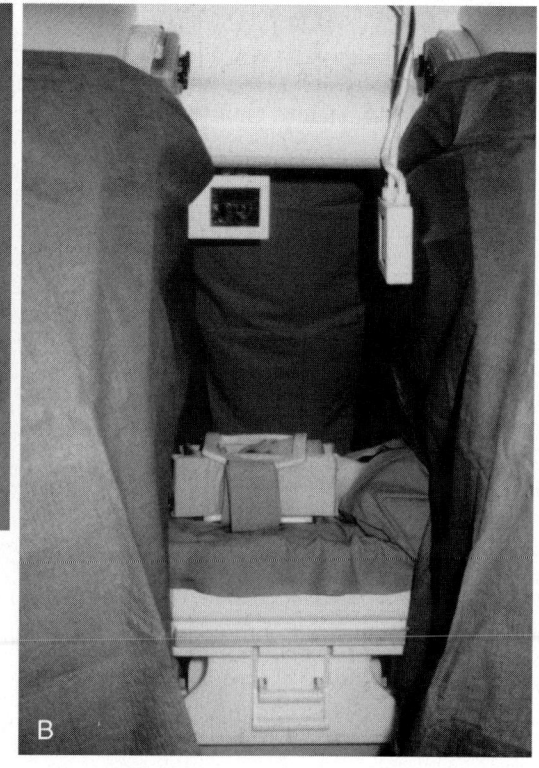

FIGURE 48-2 ■ Flexible transmit/receive coil. A, Two loops opened. B, Fixed to the patient's head before sterile draping of the operation field.

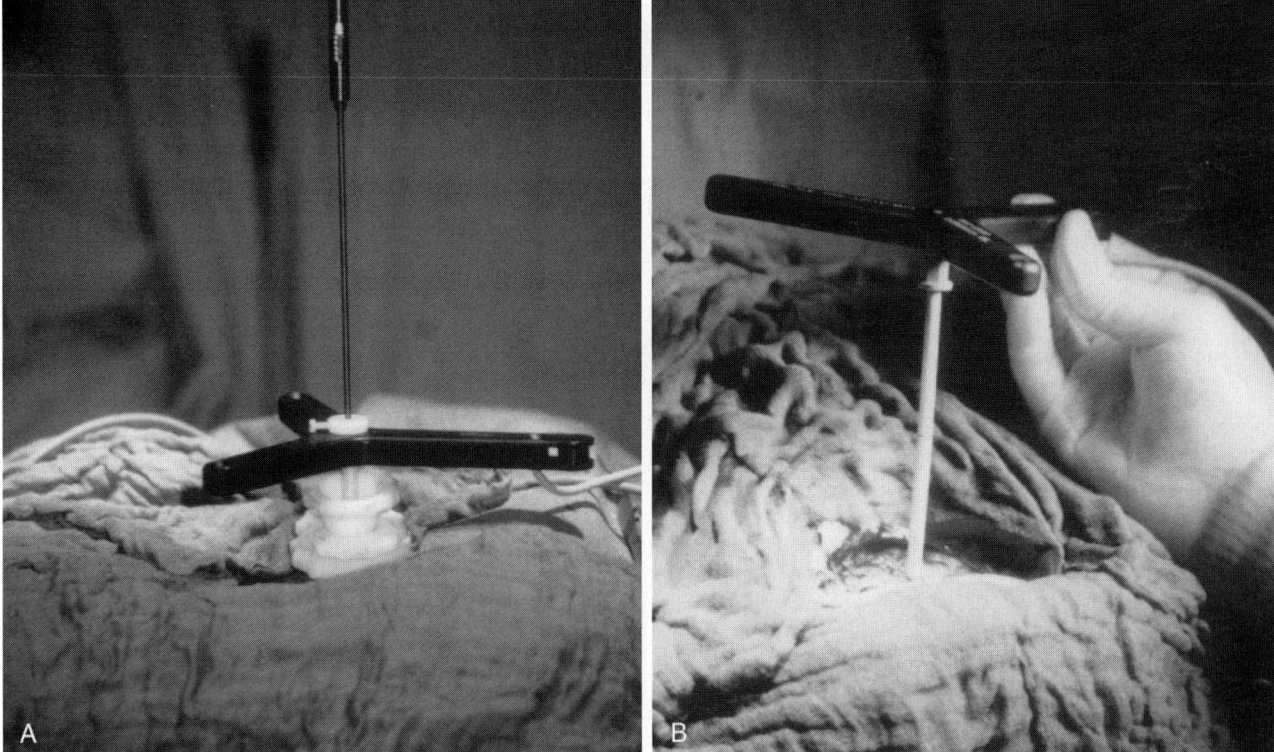

**FIGURE 48–3** ■ *A,* The use of LED-based optical tracking in combination with the bur hole snapper (Fa. Magnetic Vision, Switzerland) for the intraoperative guidance of the biopsy cannula (Sedan side-cutting needle, Fa. Elekta, Sweden). *B,* LED-flashpoint and the blunt pointer in situ. The magnetic resonance imaging (MRI) compatible blunt pointer can be filled with water or gadolinium, depending on the MRI sequence.

able in MR-compatible materials. Once a full range of MR-compatible equipment became available (e.g., the Midas Rex pneumatic drill system [Midas Rex Pneumatic Tools, Quierschied, Germany], the ICC-350 MRI electrocautery unit [Fa. Erbe, Tübingen, Germany], an ultrasonic aspirator [Fa. Elekta, Sweden], and several neurosurgical instruments [Aesculap, Germany; Codman]), the whole procedure could be carried out within the MRI unit. Tumor removal was carried out under microneurosurgical conditions using an MR-compatible microscope (Fa. Studer, Rheinfal, Switzerland; Fig. 48–4). Anesthesia is started outside the MR room. An MR-compatible patient monitoring system and respirator were necessary conditions for general anesthesia in the scanning room. The Multigas Monitor (MR-Equipment Corporation, Munich, Germany) and the Servo Ventilator 900 C (Siemens, Erlangen, Germany) are used to continue anesthesia inside the MRI unit.

## MAGNETIC RESONANCE IMAGING–GUIDED MICROSURGERY OF INTRACRANIAL TUMORS

The first craniotomy for resection of an intracranial tumor was performed in August 1997. Subsequently, 44 craniotomies have been performed using intraoperative MRI guidance. Craniotomy and tumor removal were performed completely within the interventional MRI scanner using nonmagnetic surgical instruments. In 33 patients, histologic evaluation revealed low- or high-grade gliomas. In 26 pa-

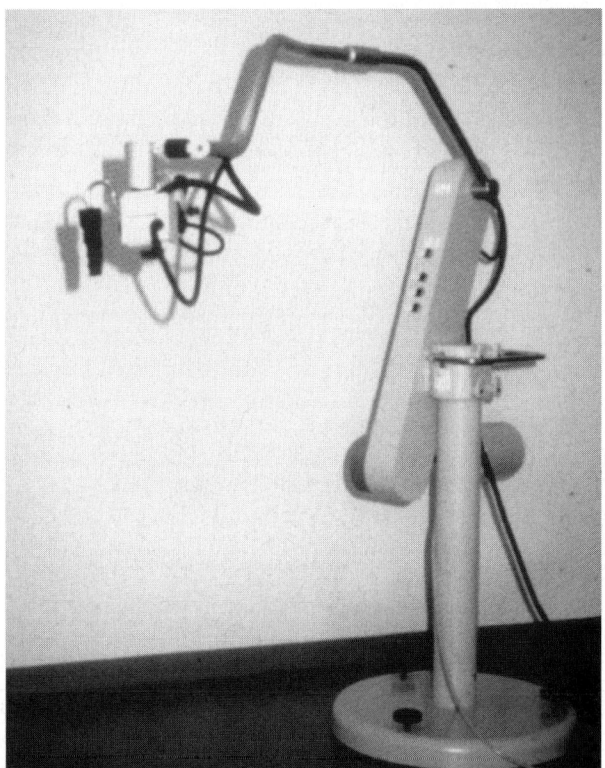

**FIGURE 48–4** ■ A magnetic resonance imaging–compatible microscope with various fixed-focus lenses (250, 300, and 350 mm). The magnification can be changed gradually. It can be moved in all directions.

**TABLE 48–1 ■ HISTOLOGIC RESULTS, MORBIDITY, MORTALITY, AND EXTENT OF TUMOR REMOVAL IN 33 PATIENTS WITH INTRACRANIAL GLIOMAS OPERATED USING INTERVENTIONAL MAGNETIC RESONANCE IMAGING**

| Histology | Grade* | No. | Complete | Incomplete | Morbidity | Mortality |
|---|---|---|---|---|---|---|
| | | | Removal | | | |
| Astrocytoma | II | 11 | 9 | 2 | 3 | 0 |
| Astrocytoma | III | 2 | 2 | 0 | 1 | 0 |
| Oligodendroglioma | II | 4 | 3 | 1 | 0 | 0 |
| Oligodendroglioma | III | 2 | 1 | 1 | 0 | 0 |
| Subependymoma | I | 1 | 1 | 0 | 0 | 0 |
| Dysembryoblastoma | I | 1 | 1 | 0 | 0 | 0 |
| Glioblastoma | IV | 12 | 9 | 3 | 2 | 0 |
| | | Σ = 33 | Σ = 26 | Σ = 7 | Σ = 6 | Σ = 0 |

*World Health Organization classification.

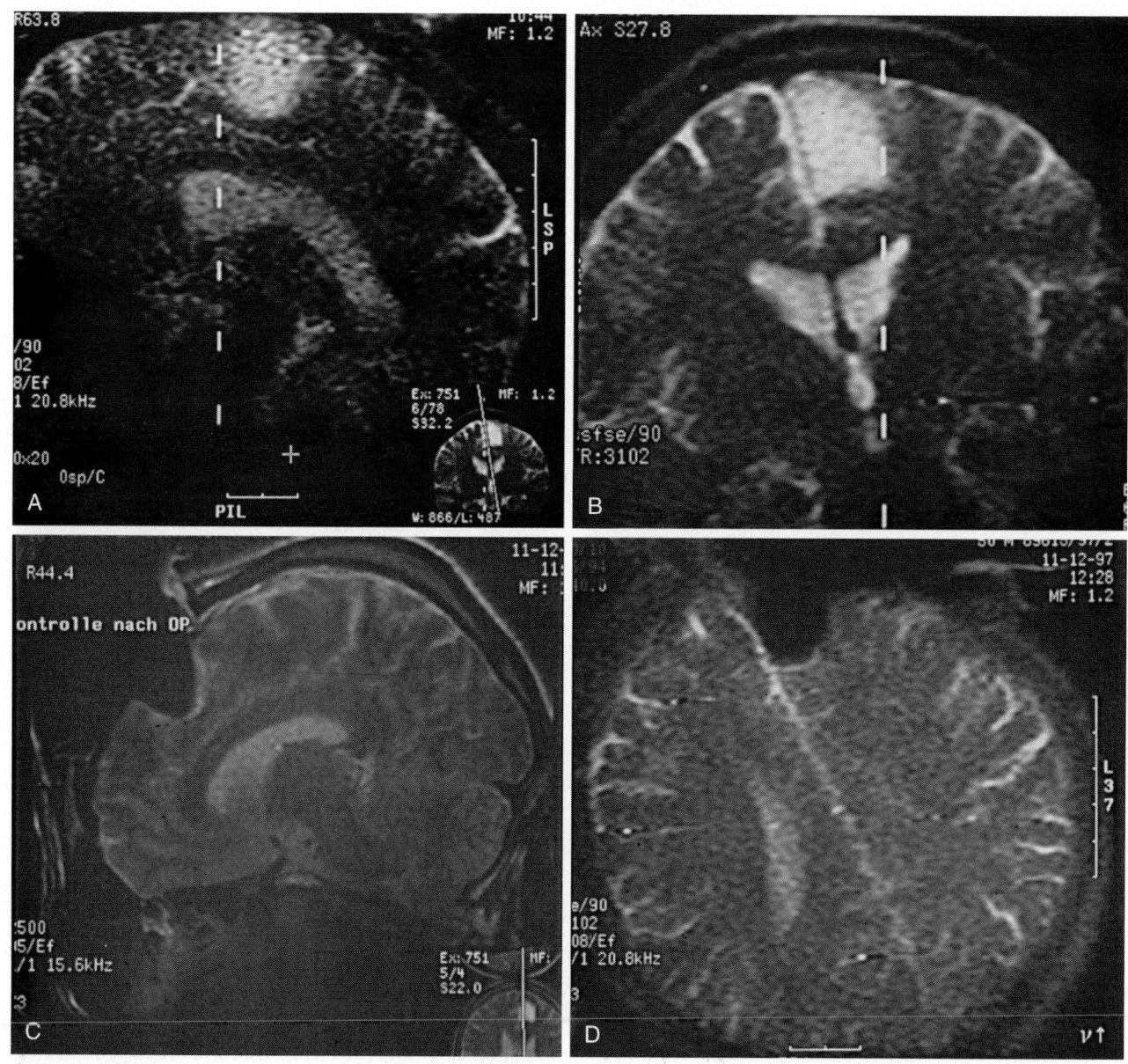

FIGURE 48–5 ■ Interactive image guidance with the optical LED-tracking system in a patient with a low-grade astrocytoma. Marking of the lateral (coronal T$_2$-weighted magnetic resonance [MR] image) (A) and anterior tumor border (sagittal T$_2$-weighted MR image) (B). C and D, Intraoperative MRI was obtained to demonstrate complete tumor removal.

tients (79%), complete tumor removal was achieved with the aid of MRI guidance. In seven cases (21%), only subtotal tumor removal was achieved (Table 48–1). Intraoperative images in these patients revealed residual tissue abnormalities involving or encroaching on deep brain structures or motor/language cortex. The initial MRI allows precise localization of the intracranial lesion in relation to the patient's head and the surrounding brain tissue using the LED tracking system (Fig. 48–5). It is also useful for planning the craniotomy and trajectory of access to the lesion in relation to the surrounding normal brain. During removal of the lesion, serial images are used to guide the tumor resection as well as control the radicality of tumor removal (Figs. 48–6 and 48–7). The use of gadolinium-DTPA may be helpful to determine the extent of resection in cases of high-grade gliomas, meningiomas, and metastasis (Fig. 48–8). During tumor removal, a slight enhancement may occur at the border of the surrounding brain, which can be clearly differentiated from evidence of a

solid tumor remnant. Intraoperative MRI is also a helpful tool for detection of intraoperative complications (e.g., hemorrhage). In this regard, in one patient an epidural hematoma was detected by intraoperative MRI at the end of the surgical procedure. The hematoma was immediately removed and the patient transferred to the intensive care unit without neurologic deterioration from this intraoperative complication. After surgery, 6 (18%) of 33 patients had neurologic deficits, which were transient in 5 cases (paresis, dysphasia). In these patients, the tumors were located in or near eloquent brain areas (sensorimotor cortex/speech center). In one patient, the bone flap had to be removed because of an infection.

## DISCUSSION

Interactive MRI-guided brain biopsy was introduced in the course of 1 year as a routine clinical method after experi-

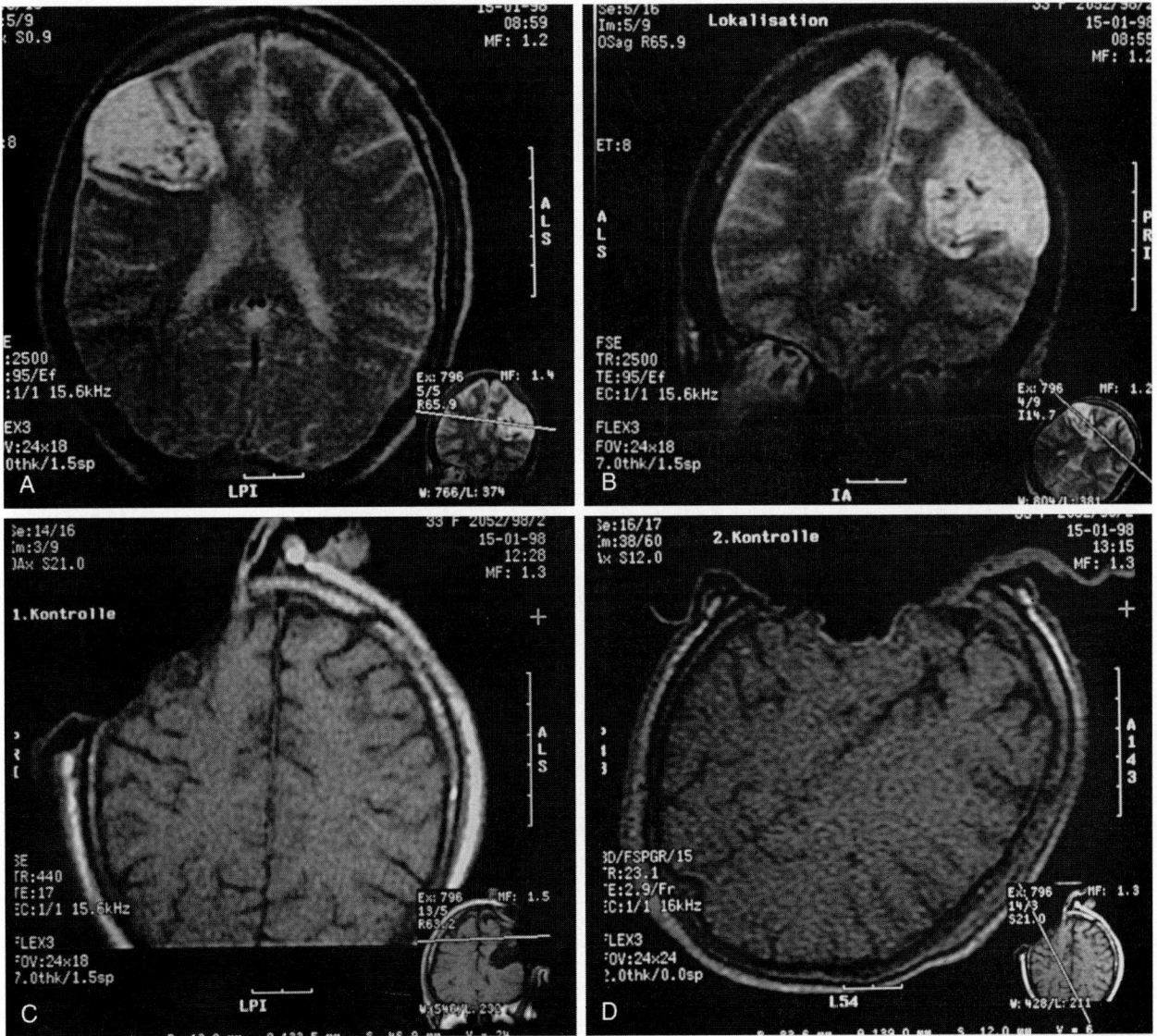

FIGURE 48–6 ■ Magnetic resonance images show a craniotomy performed to remove a ganglioblastoma (WHO I) in a 34-year-old woman suffering from seizures. *A* and *B,* These images (axial and coronal T$_2$-weighted, without gadolinium) were obtained after positioning the patient and after coil fixation. *D,* This image shows a small residual tumor, which was histologically verified and removed immediately.

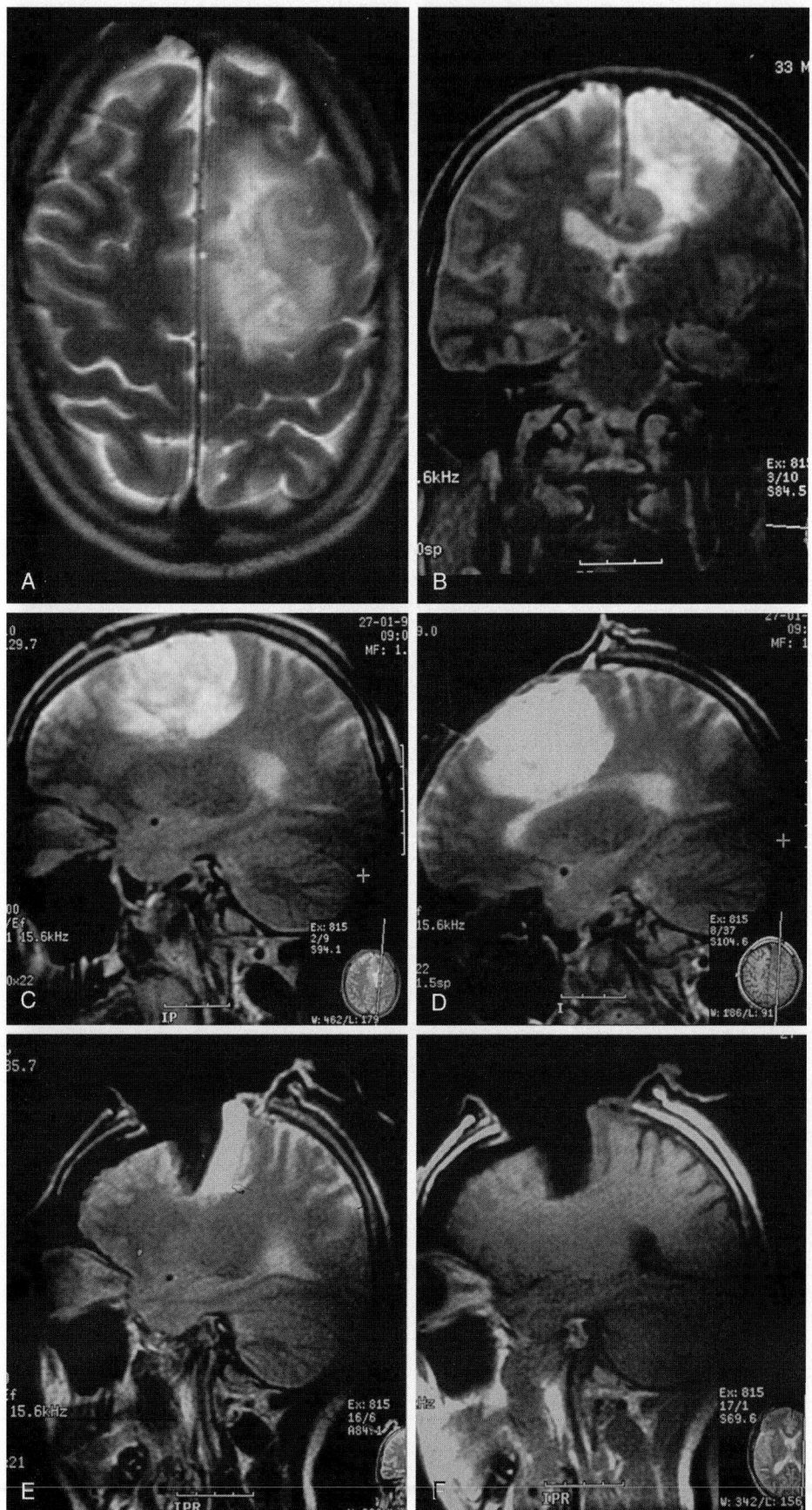

FIGURE 48–7 ■ Magnetic resonance (MR) images demonstrating a low-grade astrocytoma (WHO II) in a 34-year-old male patient. *A–C,* These images (T$_2$-weighted intraoperative MR images) demonstrate a large frontal tumor adjacent to the motor cortex. *D,* This image was obtained after a craniotomy and opening of the dura. T$_2$-weighted MR images (*E*) and T$_1$-weighted MR images (*F*) were obtained during tumor removal, showing some residual tumor adjacent motor cortex. These images also demonstrate the brain shift that occurs during progressive tumor removal.

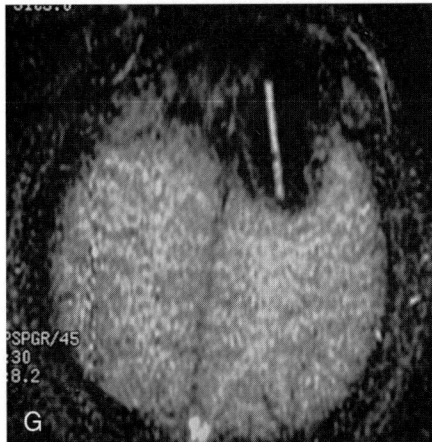

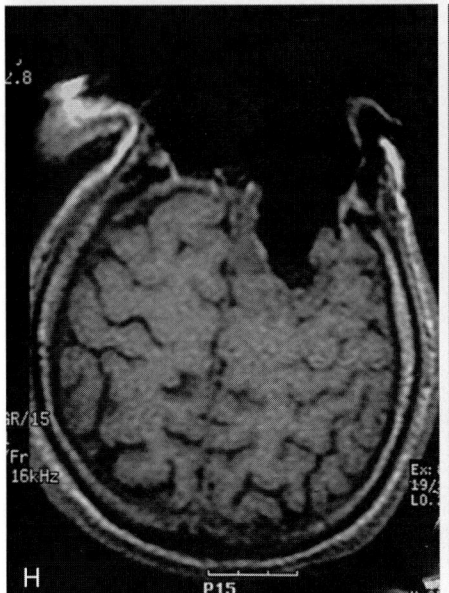

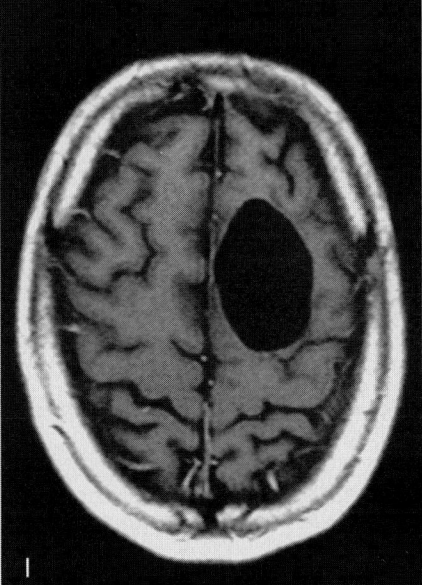

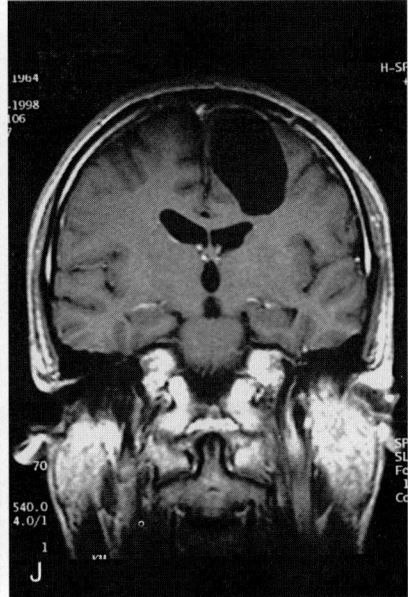

**FIGURE 48–7** *Continued* ■ In the course of tumor removal near real-time images (T1w fast multiplanar spoiled gradient echo, TR = 24-30 ms, TE = 8-9 ms, flip angle of 45 degrees, rbw 16.6 kHz) were obtained using a blunt pointer, which was filled with gadolinium. In this interactive mode, almost a real-time control of tumor removal was achieved (*G*). *H,* No residual tumor is seen. *I* and *J,* These images demonstrate the postoperative result 3 months after complete removal of the tumor.

ence was gained in using the scanning and tracking systems and after some auxiliary equipment was developed (e.g., holding device, microscope, surgical instruments). In a second step, microneurosurgical procedures, such as microsurgery of brain tumors or transsphenoidal procedures, could be completely performed in the interventional MRI device once MR-compatible equipment became available. The whole procedure can be carried out in the vertical open MR system. Intraoperative MRI provides near—real-time images that enable the surgeon to modify the pre-planned approach during the actual surgery. The use of LED-based optical tracking of surgical instruments (e.g., needles, pointers, microsurgical instruments) combined with changes in the MRI planes provides continuous interactive feedback between the surgical maneuvers and the corresponding images.[29, 33] The indications for surgery of suspected intracerebral lesions result from the development of optimized treatment strategies for some tumors and from the pressure to find such therapeutic concepts for other diseases. In the 1990s, an increasing number of minimally invasive techniques for diagnostic brain biopsy and microneurosurgery of brain tumors and vascular lesions have been developed.[8, 10, 23, 25, 31]

The treatment of low-grade gliomas remains controver-

sial. Treatment options have included observation alone, biopsy sampling for confirmation of diagnosis followed by observation, and surgical resection at the time of diagnosis, at the time of increased growth, or when symptoms worsen. Radiation has been both recommended and discouraged, and chemotherapy is recommended for some classes of gliomas. Variations in the biologic activity of low-grade gliomas have contributed to the difficulty in making treatment decisions.[9, 17, 20, 26, 27, 32, 35] Studies have shown that surgical resection of low-grade gliomas can result in an improved survival time for patients, and that the degree of resection correlates with a better outcome.[1, 4, 5, 28]

Because of its superior imaging modalities and optimal contrast differentiation for the detection of intracerebral lesions, MRI is the ideal imaging system for intraoperative guidance in neurosurgery. However, because of the configuration of MRI systems and the lack of MR-compatible auxiliary equipment and surgical instruments, it was very difficult until recently to perform microneurosurgical procedures inside the MRI device. Since the development of so-called "open" MRI-systems since the mid-1990s, new perspectives for MRI-guided and controlled procedures, some of which have become reality in specialized centers, have evolved.[11, 16, 18, 19, 33, 36] The configuration of the Signa

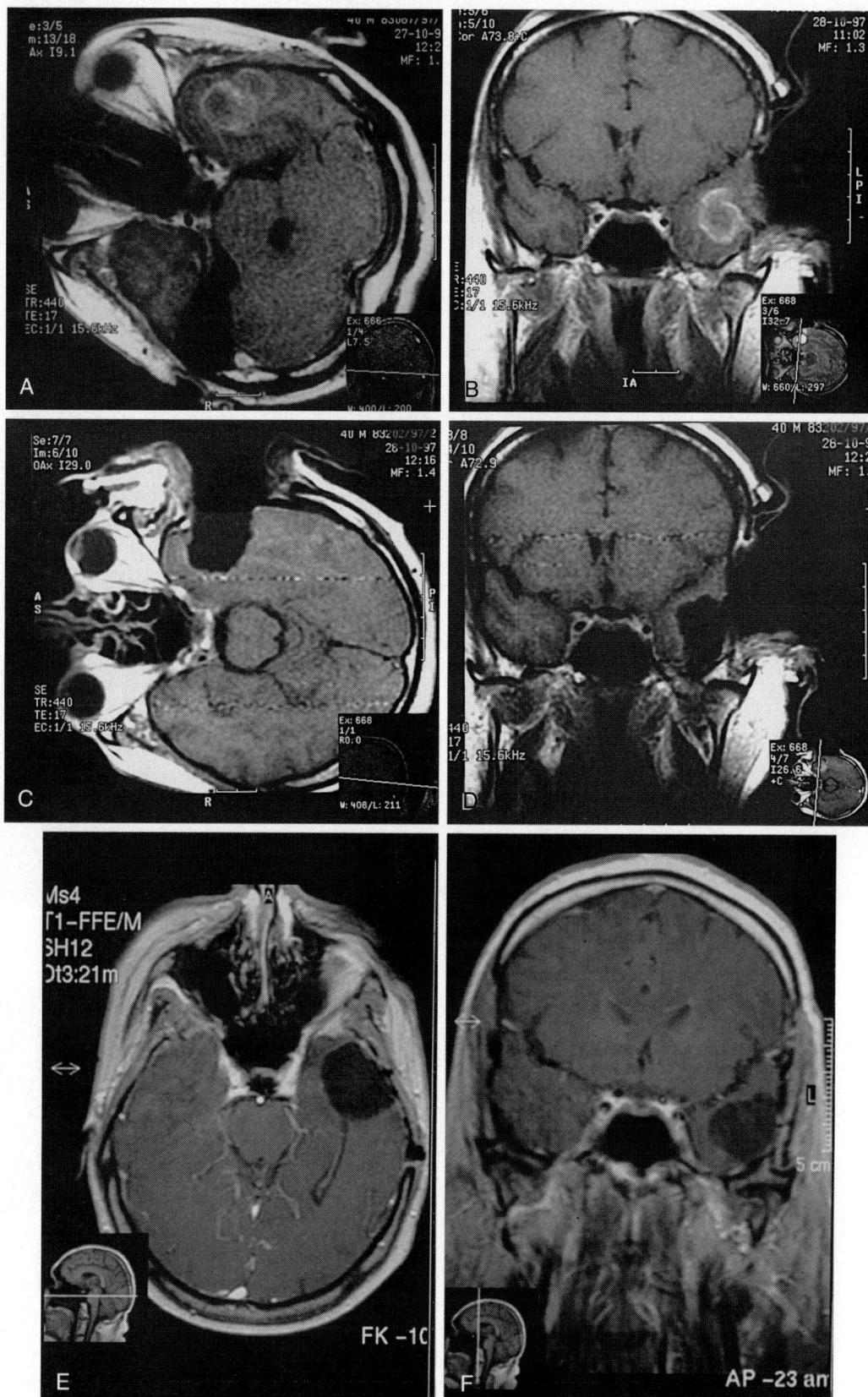

**FIGURE 48-8** ■ Gadolinium-enhanced T$_1$-weighted MR-images of a 56-year-old patient with a left temporal glioblastoma (WHO IV), before (*A* and *B*) and after complete removal of the tumor (*C* and *D*). *E* and *F,* These images were obtained 6 months after surgery and radiation therapy. No tumor recurrence is indicated.

SP system allows accurate, interactive MRI-guided targeting in several regions of the body.[6, 16, 24, 30, 33, 36] Because of good contrast between a lesion and the surrounding tissue in the brain and the lack of motion artifacts, this method is also practicable for neurosurgical procedures.[6, 16]

With regard to intraoperative accuracy, no problem occurred in the detection of lesions with a diameter of 0.8 cm or larger detected by a standard computed tomography or MRI examination. Despite the lower resolution and contrast compared with those obtained with a conventional 1.5-T scanner, all suspected lesions were visible on $T_1$- or $T_2$-weighted images using the open system and the flexible transmission/reception coil.

Essential for good image quality was the position of the patient and coil in relation to the homogeneous part of the magnetic field. It was necessary to achieve this while still providing a good access for the neurosurgeon. In every case, we tried to position the patient's head in a such way that the lesion came near to the isocenter and near to the center of the volume framed by the two coil loops. Freehand use of the three-LED tracking handpiece in combination with a single-slice gradient-echo sequence ($T_1$ or $T_2$* weighted) in continuous, near–real-time imaging mode was used for planning the best location of the craniotomy. A helpful instrument for guiding the instrument exactly to the target area was a computer-simulated virtual needle.

Nevertheless, during the first procedures some problems arose resulting from components of the MRI system or the auxiliary equipment. They rendered the operation more difficult or prolonged the procedure. Another problem was the limited mobility of the holding device in a first prototype version. We also had difficulties with targeting in cases of suspected lesions without any contrast enhancement, and a blurred demarcation on native $T_1$-weighted images in low-grade astrocytomas. These tumors were visible with fast $T_2$-weighted spin-echo sequences. But neither faster $T_2$-weighted spin-echo sequences nor a $T_2$*-weighted gradient-echo sequence was able to differentiate between the tumor and surrounding edema. Using prescribed gradient-echo sequences in the continuous imaging mode, detection of lesions was very difficult, and we therefore performed tumor removal without interactive scanning in such cases. In our opinion, a clear differentiation between tumor and surrounding structures near–real-time images is of great importance for the result and accuracy of the surgery. Intraventricular targets have been reached safely and cystic structures in various locations have been drained under continuous image control. The potential advantages of precise localization and optimization of the access route have also been demonstrated by combining an operative microscope with MRI-guided resection of deep-seated, small tumors. During the resection of large, deep-seated tumors, brain structures may move and become deformed, negating the value of preoperative images. Using intraoperative optical tracking and updating of volumetric images, surgeons are able not only to locate the tumor margins but to resect the tumor completely while preserving the integrity of surrounding normal brain. A multimodality representation of morphology can be created by integrating information from preoperative CT or MRI with functional physiologic data (transcranial magnetic stimulation, MR angiography,

and functional MRI) and metabolic information (single photon emission CT or positron emission tomography). These combined data can then be registered simultaneously with intraoperative real-time MRI data. Navigational tools can be used for localization, targeting, and correlation of anatomic models and surgical procedures. Real-time updating of the image database is necessary to follow the progress of the procedures and to find exact tumor margins within deformable tissue structures.

Immediate intraoperative monitoring is also helpful in the case of complications due to surgery (e.g., hemorrhage). If such an event is recognized immediately on intraoperative imaging, the neurosurgeon can deal with the problem– for example, by reopening the craniotomy and evacuating the hematoma, with the operative field still within the MRI magnet. In one patient with a brain metastasis, an epidural hematoma was recognized at postoperative MRI after wound closure while the patient was still in the magnet. The hematoma was immediately evacuated and the result demonstrated by intraoperative MRI. The risk of clinical sequelae secondary to such a bleeding episode is thereby minimized.[6]

## CONCLUSION

Image-guided therapy using open MRI technology offers the possibility of improving the safety, efficacy, and cost effectiveness of existing procedures and may result in the development of new procedures that currently cannot be performed outside this new surgical environment. Intraoperative MRI is helpful for navigation as well as determining tumor margins to achieve a complete and safe resection of intracranial lesions. Complications related to the surgical procedure are reduced and the risk of neurologic deterioration due to tumor removal and postoperative complications is diminished. The intraoperative application of interventional MRI technology may represent a major step forward in the field of neurosurgery.

## REFERENCES

1. Ammirati M, Vick N, Liao YL, et al: Effect of the extent of surgical resection on survival and quality of life in patients with supratentorial glioblastomas and anaplastic astrocytomas. Neurosurgery 21:201–206, 1987.
2. Apuzzo MLJ, Sabshin JK: Computed tomographic guidance stereotaxis in the management of intracranial mass lesions. Neurosurgery 12:277–285, 1983.
3. Barnett GH, Kormos DW, Sator K, Weisenberger J: Use of a frameless, armless stereotactic wand for brain tumor localization with two-dimensional and three-dimensional neuroimaging. Neurosurgery 32:674–678, 1993.
4. Berger MS, Deliganis AV, Dobbins J, Keles GE: The effect of extent of resection on recurrence in patients with low grade cerebral hemisphere gliomas. Cancer 74:1784–1791, 1994.
5. Berger MS, Kincaid J, Ojemann GA, Lettich E: Brain mapping techniques to maximize resection, safety, and seizure control in children with brain tumors. Neurosurgery 25:786–792, 1989.
6. Black PM, Moriaty T, Alexander EA, et al: Development and implementation of intraoperative magnetic resonance imaging and its neurosurgical applications. Neurosurgery 41:831–845, 1997.
7. Bucholz RD, Smith KR, Henderson J: Intraoperative localization using a three dimensional optical digitizer. Proc SPIE 1894:312–322, 1993.

8. Carter BS, Harsh GR: Diagnosis of suspected intracranial metastases: Role of direct tissue examination. Neurosurg Clin North Am 7:425–433, 1996.

9. Cohadon F, Auoad N, Rougier A, et al: Histologic and non-histologic factors correlated with survival time in supratentorial astrocytic tumors. J Neurooncol 3:105–111, 1985.

10. Ebel H, Rust DS, Scheuerle A: Value of stereotaxy in neurosurgery: Indications and analysis of results of 71 cases. Nervenarzt 67:650–658, 1996.

11. Friebe M, Grönemeyer D: Der Kernspintomograf als Therapiegerät. Krankenhaus Technik 4:56–62, 1995.

12. Galloway RL, Marcinuas RJ, Latimer JW: The accuracies of four stereotactic frame systems: An independent assessment. Biomed Instrum Technol 25:457–460, 1991.

13. Guthrie BL, Adler JR: Computer-assisted preoperative planning, interactive surgery, and frameless stereotaxy. Clin Neurosurg 38:112–131, 1995.

14. Haglund MM, Berger MS, Shamseldin M, et al: Cortical localization of temporal lobe language sites in patients with gliomas. Neurosurgery 34:567–576, 1994.

15. Heilbrun MP, Roberts TS, Apuzzo MLJ, et al: Preliminary experience with Brown-Roberts-Wells (BRW) computerized tomography stereotaxic guidance system. J Neurosurg 59:217–222, 1983.

16. Kettenbach J, Silverman SG, Schwartz RB, et al: Aufbau, klinische Eignung und Zukunftsaspekte eines 0,5-T-MR-Spezialsystems für den interventionellen Einsatz. Radiologe 37:825–834, 1997.

17. Laws ER, Taylor WF, Clifton MB, Okazaki H: Neurosurgical management of low-grade astrocytoma of the cerebral hemispheres. J Neurosurg 61:665–673, 1984.

18. Lenz GW, Dewey C: Interventional MRI. Electromedica 63:41–45, 1995.

19. Lufkin RB: Interventional MR imaging. Radiology 197:16–18, 1996.

20. Lunsford LD, Somaza S, Kondziolka D, Flickinger JC: Survival after stereotactic biopsy and irradiation of cerebral nonanaplastic, nonpilocytic astrocytoma. J Neurosurg 82:523–529, 1995.

21. Marcinuas RJ, Galloway RL, Fitzpatrick JM: A universal system for interactive image-directed neurosurgery. Stereotact Funct Neurosurg 58:108–113, 1992.

22. Martin C, Alexander EA, Wong T, et al: Surgical treatment of low-grade gliomas in the intraoperative magnetic resonance imager. Neurosurg Focus 4:8, 1998.

23. Matsumoto K, Tomita S, Higashi H, et al: Image guided stereotactic biopsy for brain tumors: experience of 71 cases. No Shinkei Geka 23:897–903, 1995.

24. Moriaty TM, Kikins R, Jolesz FA, et al: Magnetic resonance imaging therapy. Neurosurg Clin North Am 7:323–331, 1996.

25. Moringlane JR, Voges M: Real-time ultrasound imaging of cerebral lesions during "target point" stereotactic procedures through a burr hole. Acta Neurochir (Wien) 132:134–137, 1995.

26. Philippon JH, Clemenceau SH, Fauchon FH, Foncin JF: Supratentorial low grade astrocytomas in adults. Neurosurgery 32:554–559, 1993.

27. Piepmeier J, Christopher S, Spencer D, et al: Variations in the natural history and survival of patients with supratentorial low-grade astrocytomas. Neurosurgery 38:872–879, 1996.

28. Roberts DW, Strohbehn JW, Hatch JF, et al: A frameless stereotaxic integration of computerized tomographic imaging and the operating microscope. J Neurosurg 65:545–549, 1986.

29. Schenk JF, Jolesz FA, Roemer PB, et al: Superconducting open configuration MRI system for image-guided therapy. Radiology 195:805–814, 1995.

30. Schmidt F, Schneider JP, Thiele J, et al: Holding device for MR-guided biopsies. Fortschr Rontgenstr 166:177, 1997.

31. Scholz M, Schwechheimer K, Hardenack M, et al: MIN-biopsy of brain tumors: Operative technique and histomorphological results. Minim Invasive Neurosurg 39:12–16, 1996.

32. Shaw EG, Daumas-Duport C, Scheithauer BW, et al: Radiation therapy in the management of low-grade supratentorial astrocytomas. J Neurosurg 70:853–861, 1989.

33. Silverman SG, Collick BD, Figueira MR, et al: Interactive MR-guided biopsy in an open-configuration MR imaging system. Radiology 197:175–181, 1995.

34. Smith KR, Frank KJ, Bucholz RD: The NeuroStation: A highly accurate, minimally invasive solution to frameless stereotactic neurosurgery. Comput Med Imaging Graph 18:247–256, 1994.

35. Soffietti RCA, Giordana MT: Prognostic factors in well-differentiated cerebral astrocytomas in the adult. Neurosurgery 24:686–692, 1989.

36. Steiner P, Schoenberger AW, Penner EA, et al: Interactive stereotaxic interventions in superconducting, open 0.5-Tesla MRI tomography. Fortschr Rontgenstr 165:276–280, 1996.

37. Watanabe E, Mayangi Y, Kosugi Y, et al: Open surgery assisted by the neuronavigator: A stereotactic, articulated, sensitive arm. Neurosurgery 28:792–800, 1991.

38. Watanabe E, Watanabe T, Manaka S: Three-dimensional digitizer (neuronavigator): New equipment of computed tomography-guided stereotactic surgery. Surg Neurol 27:543–547, 1987.

39. Wood CC, Spencer DD, Allison T, et al: Localization of human sensorimotor cortex during surgery by cortical surface recording of somatosensory evoked potentials. J Neurosurg 68:99–111, 1988.

40. Zinreich JS, Tebo SA, Long DM, et al: Frameless stereotactic integration of CT imaging data: Accuracy and initial applications. Radiology 188:735–743, 1993.

# CHAPTER 49

# Technique of Gamma Surgery

■ DHEERENDRA PRASAD and LADISLAU STEINER

History is replete with examples of the individual mind changing the direction of thinking in a manner so radical that it takes generations to assess the implications of the change. When Leksell[1] proposed that neurosurgeons give up opening the skull in selected cases and use a different physical agent to achieve their ends through the patient's intact skull, he triggered a murmur of dissent that has not yet died down. And yet, despite the slow acceptance of his ideas, radiosurgery has increasingly been used for different neurosurgical conditions with accruing data on its efficacy and safety. The Gamma knife has sparked development of other, similar technologies that are now collected under the rubric of radiosurgery. In reemphasizing the initial choice and motivation of Leksell to design an alternative tool for the neurosurgeon, we paraphrase our activity as *Gamma surgery*: neurosurgery performed with the Gamma knife. We use *Gamma surgery* in place of *radiosurgery* to restrict Leksell's original definition to the only tool strictly adhering to his principles. No less controversial than the technology itself has been the name that Leksell chose to give it—the *Gamma knife*. Although technically a misnomer, it carries with it Leksell's statement of intent. Hence, out of respect for him, we continue to use it.

## PHYSICAL BASIS OF GAMMA SURGERY

### Agent: Ionizing Radiation

Radiation capable of producing ions by ejecting electrons from molecules in target tissue is referred to as *ionizing radiation*. Typical binding energies for electrons in biologic tissues are of the order of 10 eV, and therefore photons exceeding 10 eV in energy are considered ionizing. Visible light is in the 2-eV range and ultraviolet light occupies the 2- to 10-eV range; beyond 10 eV are, successively, x-rays and gamma rays.

Electromagnetic radiation may be viewed as either a waveform or a particle. In the energy range applicable to gamma rays, it is more convenient to view them as particles, called *photons*. A photon has no mass and no charge; it is simply an energy packet. The energy in one photon (E) is equal to the product of the frequency ($\nu$) of the radiation and Planck's constant (h):

$$E = h\nu \qquad (1)$$

It is this energy that produces effects on biologic tissues.

## Basis of Biologic Effects: Interactions of Radiation with Matter

Akin to a collision in the macroscopic world, the interaction of a photon with matter results in energy transfer from photon to matter. Depending on the energy of the photon, one of three phenomena occurs: (1) the photoelectric effect, (2) Compton scattering, or (3) pair production.

The photoelectric effect predominates when low-energy photons (100 KeV or less) such as those of ultraviolet rays interact with tissue. Pair production is typical of radiation with photon energies greater than 2 MeV. At intermediate beam energies (150 KeV to 2 MeV), Compton scattering results in ejected electrons carrying off part of the energy, with generation of a secondary photon of lesser energy. This process results in a cascade of electrons, photons, and ionized molecules that results in biologic effects. Gamma ray photons from a $^{60}$Co source have energies of 1.17 and 1.33 MeV. Compton scattering is therefore the primary mode of energy transfer to tissues from gamma rays.

## Taming the Photon: Beam Collimation

After extensive research at the Gustav Werner Institute at Uppsala, Sweden, using a 120-MeV proton beam, the characteristics and biologic effects of a single high dose of radiation were defined. Leksell used this information to design a tool that replaced the single beam of the cumbersome particle accelerator by an array of $^{60}$Co sources.

The geometry of the sources as well as their minimum number were governed by the need to achieve a high enough dose rate at the focal point (isocenter) and to minimize scatter. By itself, any single gamma beam from any of the sources, despite collimation by a series of collimators, remains a divergent albeit narrow beam as a result of Compton scattering. Although the overall dimensions of this beam are defined by the collimator used, it is incapable of focusing in the conventional sense (as with light and a lens in optics). What Leksell realized, however, was that if several of these beams converge at the same

657

point (isocenter), then a zone of high dose concentration and rate is achieved around that point. This convergence phenomenon is what *focused* connotes in the definition of radiosurgery. The isocenter thus becomes the radiosurgical focal point. Later, we discuss in more detail the accuracy and precision with which the isocenter can be defined using the Gamma knife.

## Creating Sharp Boundaries: Conformal Dose Distribution

When multiple beams of photons are used to treat a spherical target, the only variable that needs to be adjusted is the size of the collimator. Aligning the geometric center of the target with the isocenter of the treatment source ensures precise coverage of the target with predictable fall-off of dose in surrounding tissues. Nature, however, rarely presents spherical targets, and irregular targets require that the irradiation geometry "conform" to the target. This can be achieved in several ways.

One method is to choose a combination of isocenters (with differently sized collimators as needed) and adjust their geometric positions and relative weights to achieve a high-dose field that conforms to the target. This was the method used in the Gamma knife from the beginning, and is only now becoming possible to a lesser extent in some photon-based radiosurgical systems.

Another method is to shape the beams themselves to conform to the two-dimensional target profile in a plane perpendicular to the incident beams. This is the principle used in the design of the multileaf collimators and micromultileaf collimators that are now available for use with linear accelerators modified for radiosurgery.

Finally, compensators can be used to shape the beams. Photon beams in general are minimally affected by compensators, and when multiple beams are used simultaneously as in the Gamma knife, compensation is impractical as well. Compensation is most useful in particle accelerator–based radiosurgery.

The choice of methods to ensure conformity is therefore a function of the technology used to perform radiosurgery. The relative advantages of the different approaches have not been rigorously studied.

## INSTRUMENTATION FOR GAMMA SURGERY

### Gamma Knife

The Gamma knife system (Fig. 49–1) comprises three different parts:

1. The Gamma knife
   a. The radiation unit, which houses the $^{60}$Co sources
   b. A treatment couch with the collimator helmets attached to it
   c. The control panel and the couch driving mechanism (hydraulic or electric)
2. Stereotactic frame for target localization and for supporting the patient's head during treatment
3. Computerized dose planning system

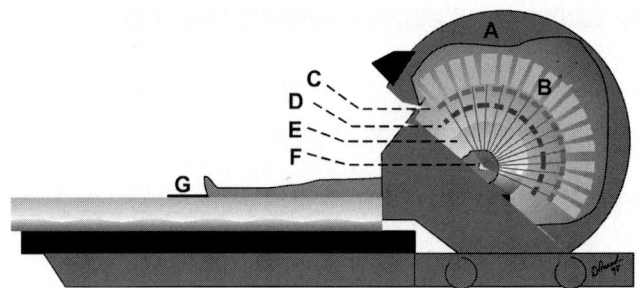

**FIGURE 49–1** ■ Schematic cross-section of the Model U Gamma Unit. The central body (A) houses the sources (B) and the fixed inner collimators (C and D). The outermost innermost collimator (E) is interchangeable and attached to the retractable couch (G). To effect the treatment, the target (F) is positioned at the unit center point.

### Radiation Source

The radioactive isotope $^{60}$Co is produced by bombarding the stable isotope $^{59}$Co in a nuclear reactor. When the radioactive isotope decays, it emits an electron and two quanta of gamma radiation. In the Gamma knife, the electrons are absorbed before they can reach the patient. The half-life of the isotope is 5.26 years and the end product is $^{60}$Ni. Thus, every 5.26 years the dose rate of the Gamma knife is halved and the radiation time doubled for a given dose. There is no evidence to suggest that changes in dose rate occurring within two half-lives of the isotope have any clinical significance, but because of the long radiation times for certain treatments, replacement of the sources is suggested 7 to 10 years after original loading.

Pellets of $^{60}$Co (1 mm in diameter and 1 mm long) are stacked axially in a cylindrical stainless steel capsule that is welded shut. This capsule is contained in another sealed stainless steel capsule, and an aluminum container provides the outer covering. The whole assembly is referred to as the *source*. The specific activity of each pellet varies and the capsules are filled with 12 to 20 pellets to ensure an equal contribution to the total activity from each source. The total activity of the Gamma knife is approximately 6000 Ci at the initial loading of sources. As mentioned earlier, as a result of Compton scattering, there is a penumbra around the collimated edge of the beam that cannot be made any narrower than 1.5 mm.

### Spatial Source Distribution: Implementation of Collimation

The radiation sources are housed in a hemisphere called the *central body* inside the radiation unit, and are symmetrically distributed around the perimeter of the central body. The central body has conical channels for each of the sources and the gamma ray beams diverge through these to channels that lead toward the unit center point. The *unit center point* is defined as the point of intersection of the axes of each of the individual source beams. It corresponds to the isocenter of a radiation therapy device with a rotating gantry, such as a linear accelerator. Inside the central body, the part of the channel closest to the radiation source is made of tungsten and the second part of lead. Focusing or collimation of the beams occurs in the channels. The helmet on the treatment couch makes up the third part of the

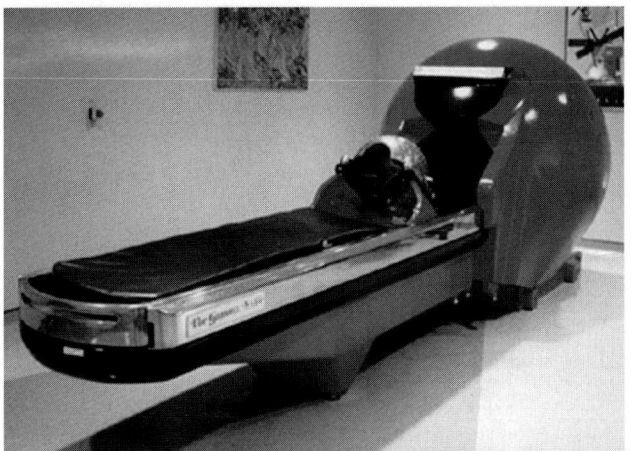

FIGURE 49–2 ■ Gamma knife model U.

beam channel when the couch is in the treatment position and the collimators of the helmet are aligned with their counterparts in the central body. This outermost helmet determines the ultimate size of the focal spot generated at the unit center point or in the target. It is made of 96% tungsten alloy. The individual collimators on the helmets are removable and interchangeable because they have conical channels of equal size for a given size of collimator. There are four different collimator helmets distinguished by differences in the diameter of their circular aperture projected on a surface perpendicular to the beam axis at the unit center point. These diameters or collimator sizes are 4, 8, 14, and 18 mm. Any intermediate collimator can be simulated by firing two different collimators at the same isocenter (e.g., a 4- and an 8-mm collimators can be combined to form a 6-mm collimator). When necessary, one or more of these collimators can be replaced with solid *plugs* with no aperture that are 60 mm thick, thus blocking the radiation from that particular source.

There are three models of the Gamma knife available, model U (Fig. 49–2), model B (Fig. 49–3), and model C. All have 201 radiation sources. They differ in the spatial distribution of the radiation sources in the central body, and therefore the resulting radiation dose profiles differ somewhat in the transaxial, coronal, and sagittal planes. These differences are of no consequence for clinical utility

or results. The B model, which is a later development, has the advantage of easier source replacement.

The C prototype represents the latest in technological development of the Gamma unit. This model is characterized by a central control system that allows the planning computer to communicate directly with the treatment unit. This transfers the coordinates and exposure timings for each isocenter directly from the workstation to the console. Modifications of the couch make it ergonomically superior. The collimators are color coded and designed with a new fitting to make plugging easier. The console commands an automated positioning system that changes over from one isocenter to another automatically, thereby shortening the setup time for each "shot." The basic principle and the final effectiveness in terms of clinical outcome, however, remain the same.

## Patient Positioning and Movement

At the time of treatment, the patient is positioned on the treatment couch and the stereotactic frame, which is fixed to the patient's head and attached inside the helmet so that the intended target point in the brain coincides with the unit center point. Shielding doors of the radiation unit then open and the treatment couch slides into the treatment position; alignment is achieved when the couch collimator docks with the intermediate collimator of the unit. The precision of this docking is regulated with microswitches. On the least resistance to docking, the treatment is automatically aborted and the couch withdraws from the radiation unit.

## Console Functions

The console provides the operator with an audiovisual telemonitoring system to observe the patient during the treatment. It has two timers that are set to the treatment exposure time as prescribed by the treatment protocol. The timers also are interlocked, with one counting up and the other down. Treatment does not commence unless the two timers are set to identical treatment times. An array of indicators report the status of the equipment to the operator.

## Technical Specifications of the Gamma Knife

The Gamma knife satisfies a number of accuracy and safety requirements expected of a stereotactic procedure[2]:

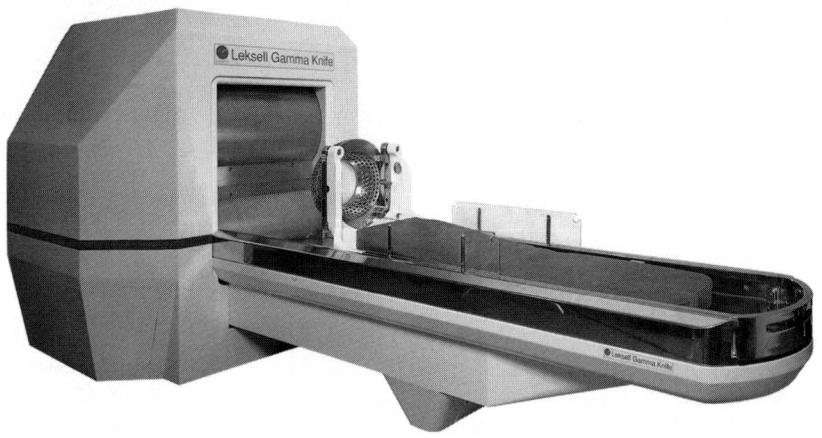

FIGURE 49–3 ■ Gamma knife model B.

1. It should be possible to align the target point with the unit center point to within 0.5 mm.
2. The axes of all beams should intersect at the unit center point within 0.3 mm.
3. The dose rate anywhere in the target should not be significantly lower than 0.5 Gy/min.
4. Stray radiation from the unit should not be hazardous to the patient or the staff.

*Precision* relates to the smallest sphere within which all beams of the Gamma knife intersect. *Accuracy* relates to the distance between the unit center point and the point of the maximum absorbed dose from the radiation field of the Gamma knife. In clinical practice, the accuracy of Gamma knife surgery also depends on the resolution of the imaging modalities used for target localization. Magnetic resonance imaging (MRI) allows a resolution of 1 mm and computed tomography (CT), 0.5 mm.

## Stereotactic Frame

### Modified Model "G" Frame

The Leksell stereotactic frame (Fig. 49–4) is a specially constructed unit with a rectangular base ring that carries engraved coordinates.[1, 3] The stereotactic frame is applied to the skull in the operating room under full aseptic precautions. In the basic frame kit, the user is provided with earplugs that attach to the base through an adapter to hold the frame level during the fixation process. For a patient who is not anesthetized, however, this can be very unpleasant and painful. We are using a locally devised disposable drape with Velcro fasteners that holds the frame in position on the head without the use of the ear plugs. This simple device reduces patient discomfort significantly. It is fixed to the patient's skull through four rigid corner uprights to

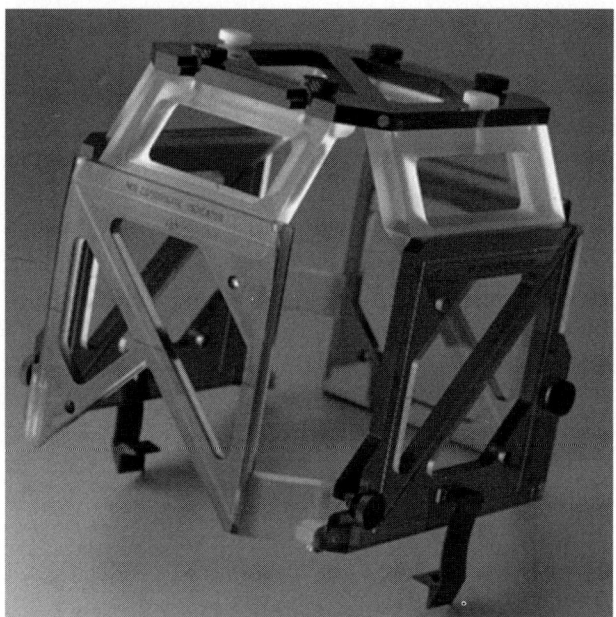

FIGURE 49–5 ■ A magnetic resonance imaging (MRI) indicator box, which when attached to the frame will generate markers (fiducials) on the image that permit registration of the images into the Leksell space.

maintain its position throughout the entire surgical procedure. A variety of coordinate boxes (Fig. 49–5) made of Perspex can then be fixed onto the base ring and carry fiducial markers that are used for localization in MRI, CT, and angiography equipment.

Gamma surgery is performed by attaching graduated gauges to the frame base ring that allow setting of the Z and Y coordinates. These gauges attach to the trunions of the Gamma unit to support the patient as well as localize the isocenter at the unit center point. The same base ring also accepts other stereotactic devices like the arc used for biopsies and other open stereotactic procedures, should one of these need to be performed in conjunction with gamma surgery.

### Defining the Location of the Skull in the Frame

The patient's skull and its position in the stereotactic space needs to be defined for calculating the radiation dose distributions. This definition is made using the so-called "Gamma knife skull scaling instrument," which is a sphere with 24 drilled holes through which the distance form the surface of the sphere to the skull surface can be measured. The measurements are obtained using a calibrated dipstick with the scaling instrument attached to the stereotactic frame.

### Dose Planning Hardware and Software

#### Computer

To calculate the equations necessary to form dose distributions, manipulate images from multiple modalities, and store all relevant data in a retrievable form requires considerable computing power. The current platform for this

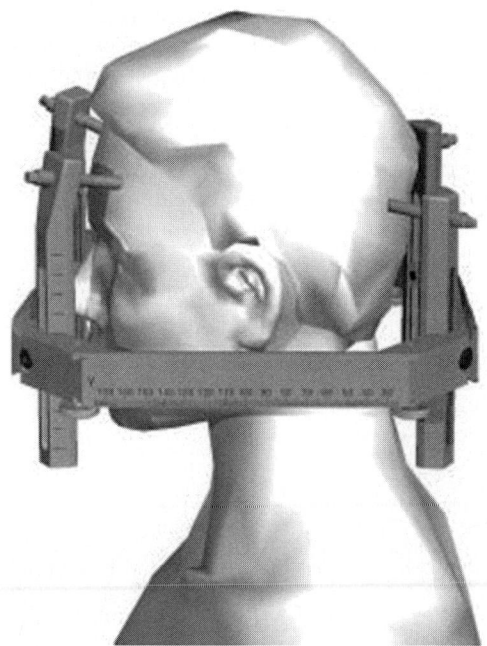

FIGURE 49–4 ■ The Leksell stereotactic frame model G, demonstrating the mode of fixation on the head.

process is a Hewlett-Packard UNIX workstation. Efficient use of the planning software requires a local area network (LAN), connecting this machine to the CT scanner and MRI. Conventional cut-film angiographic images must be scanned into the system using a flatbed scanner. If digital subtraction angiographic (DSA) is used, DSA images may be transferred over the LAN. Suitable storage, such as DAT tape or magneto-optical disk, should be available for archiving cases.

## Dose Calculation Algorithms

The computer uses mathematical models to compute the dose distribution and generate the isodose curves that represent the radiation field in the brain. Although a detailed treatment of these algorithms is beyond the scope of this text, the general concepts are discussed.

In absolute terms, for any fixed radiation source it is possible to determine the dose at one specific point; this dose is referred to as the *reference dose* ($D_R$). All other points in space receive an actual dose ($D_A$) that can be related to this reference dose, if all the factors that can modify $D_R$ are known.

$$D_A = D_R \times \text{factors} \quad (2)$$

Because $D_R$ is arrived at by measurement at a fixed distance from the source in a phantom (typically the center of the phantom) of ideal and fixed geometry, one of the first factors that relate $D_R$ to $D_A$ is the distance of the reference point to the actual point (d) where the dose is being measured. Because radiation attenuates following the inverse square law, this term in the equation is referred to as the *inverse square term* $(1/d)^2$:

$$D_A = D_R \times (1/d)^2 \times \text{factors} \quad (3)$$

The next element is the influence that tissue (or the tissue phantom) exerts on the beam by absorbing part of its energy. For gamma rays, this loss is approximately 4% per centimeter. The influence of this component on the dose is therefore called the *tissue phantom ratio* (T):

$$D_A = D_R \times (1/d)^2 \times T \times \text{factors} \quad (4)$$

As the radiation beam passes through the collimator system, it experiences scatter. The effect of this scatter is that only the energy vectors along the long axis of the beam channel are able to continue along the path; the rest are lost. The size of the collimator therefore changes the percentage of radiation energy able to pass (less for smaller collimators), and this is referred to as the *output factor* (O):

$$D_A = D_R \times (1/d)^2 \times T \times O \times \text{factors} \quad (5)$$

Finally, so far we have assumed that the target point and the reference point are both located along the beam axis (central ray). If the point of interest is displaced along the transverse axis of the beam, an off-axis compensation has to be made (X):

$$D_A = D_R \times (1/d)^2 \times T \times O \times X \quad (6)$$

In a simplified fashion, the solution in Equation 6 typifies point dose calculations in radiosurgery in general and gamma surgery in particular.

The computer has stored in its memory the spherical dose distribution from a single source of any given collimator size. This distribution is arrived at by measuring the dose at a depth of 400 mm from the source using a water phantom and measuring doses in a sphere of 80 mm radius at a depth of 10 mm from the surface of the phantom. Because all 201 sources are identical, the computer can use this distribution for the entire source array to calculate the resultant dose distribution in the brain. Using these data and incorporating the parameters specific to the patient, the dose distribution is calculated.

In the practice of gamma surgery, we need to know the dose distribution in the entire target, not just at a point. This is achieved by calculating the dose at each point in a matrix of $31 \times 31 \times 31$ points, which means Equation 6 is solved 29,791 times for each isocenter. Next, the individual dose matrices for each shot (isocenter) are superposed and normalized to the matrix center chosen by the operator. The distance between the adjacent points of the matrix is kept as small as possible (chosen by the operator), but should be large enough to cover the lesion and any neighboring structures of interest. Graphic subroutines can then display the normalized dose contours for the plan to be evaluated by the operator. These contours are generated by connecting voxels calculated to receive the same dose.

## User Interface: Gamma Plan Software

The most important aspect of gamma surgery is that most of the functions described previously should be possible to perform through a user-friendly, intuitive interface. With the growing use of the personal computer, it is reasonable to expect the neurosurgeon to have a basic familiarity with computers, but it should not be essential for him or her to be trained in UNIX to make a dose plan. This objective is well served by the software Gamma Plan (Elekta Instruments, Atlanta, GA). The following key functions are available:

A. Database functions
   1. Patient registration
   2. Archiving of data
   3. Restoring archived data
B. Image handling
   1. Importing image data from network, scanner, or tape
   2. Registration of stereotactic images
   3. Adjusting viewing level and window settings
   4. Fusing image sets
   5. Reconstructing multiple planes of images from one set
   6. Viewing multiple studies at a time
C. Dose planning
   1. Visual on-image planning using multiple modalities at the same time
   2. Selection of dose matrix
   3. Real-time display of isodose contours in any plane
   4. Region of interest delineation
   5. Accurate dose measurements at any point or in any volume
   6. Shielding of critical structures, with generation of required plug patterns
   7. Optimization of the user-generated dose plan
   8. Automated filling of target volume with shots

D. Three-dimensional (3-D) capabilities
   1. Generation of a 3-D model of target and other defined objects
   2. 3-D representation of the dose plan
   3. Manipulation of the 3-D image to inspect the dose plan from any vantage point
E. Documentation
   1. Generation of a printed treatment plan
   2. Graphic printout of the on-screen view of the dose plan

## IMAGING FOR GAMMA SURGERY

The success of radiosurgery depends intrinsically on the accuracy of the radiologic definition of the target. In purely physical terms, the key parameters that define the quality of a stereotactic image are resolution and distortion. Whereas resolution is essential for distinguishing pathologic and normal tissue, elimination of distortion is the key to accurate localization. For example, MRI provides the best soft tissue resolution in the brain but is more prone to distortion than CT. The combination of imaging modalities therefore not only gives additional valuable information for planning but enhances the overall accuracy of the treatment plan.

### Stereotactic Magnetic Resonance Imaging

Magnetic resonance imaging is the imaging modality used most commonly for localizing most lesions. Most current MRI machines are equipped with an adapter that receives the Leksell stereotactic frame. The manufacturers of the Gamma knife make fiducial boxes to fit the various head coils in use. Because space is at a premium, the fiducial box is designed to fit very closely to the skull, a point of special importance when the frame is displaced to one side at time of placement for the treatment of laterally located lesions. The neurosurgeon performing radiosurgery should be aware of these limitations. Stereotactic adapters need periodic checks and alignment to ensure accurate scans.

The fiducial box generates dot-like fiducials on the image. These are used to register the image into the radiosurgical planning system. Direct transfer of the images from the MRI computer to the planning system computer is highly recommended. This is not only faster but allows better resolution than scanned images, and also avoids any distortion that might occur while scanning the images.

Greatest spatial accuracy is achieved with spin-echo sequences. Images obtained before and after administration of gadolinium contrast using $T_1$-weighted spin-echo sequences are therefore the mainstay of imaging for gamma surgery. As a rule, these are performed with thin slices (2 to 3 mm) with no interslice gap or overlap. Additional sequences that are used occasionally are continuous interference steady state (CISS) and magnetization-prepared rapid gradient echo (MPRAGE). We have found CISS particularly useful in defining the trigeminal nerve in cases of trigeminal neuralgia and in identifying neurovascular structures at the porus acusticus in small vestibular schwannomas.

Magnetic resonance imaging also plays a role in planning treatment of vascular lesions by providing the third dimension to the visualization of the malformation. There are, however, many unanswered issues such as reliable demonstration of flow, distinction of nidus from surrounding draining veins, and the failure of MR angiography to be time-selective like conventional angiography. MRI permits the precise delineation of the relationship of the malformation to the adjacent soft tissue structures and allows the use of the dosimetry software to determine the exact dose delivered. It is recommended that an independent assessment of the extent of the malformation on the MRI scan be made and then compared with the angiographic nidus. Gamma Plan has a built-in feature that allows this cross-comparison to be made. Although its true value is yet to be established, this feature nevertheless is a valuable learning tool. In our experience with large arteriovenous malformations (AVMs), for which we perform both angiography and MRI, we have seen that MRI tends to overestimate the nidus because the draining veins cannot be distinguished from the nidus.

### Stereotactic Computed Tomography

Despite its higher spatial accuracy, the use of CT for radiosurgery suffers from two problems. The currently used metallic quick-fix screws that are used to affix the frame to the skull are MR compatible but do produce an artifact with CT. Second, the soft tissue definition obtained with CT is poorer than with MRI. We use CT only if MRI is not feasible because of metallic implants, pacemakers, or physical constraints in a given patient, such as kyphosis or excessive weight.

Some reduction in artifact can be obtained by using multislice spiral interpolation techniques.

### Stereotactic Angiography

The recommended method is a combination of rapid, serial cut-film angiography with manual subtraction angiography and DSA. The rate of filming for cut-film angiography is typically of the order of three frames per second. Even so, some of the very-high-flow malformations and fistulas require faster filming speeds or the use of DSA equipment in the continuous mode fully to understand the nidus. To obtain accurate stereotactic angiograms, a head holder with receptacles for the frame is used to position the patient. The x-ray tubes and the film are positioned strictly orthogonal (Fig. 49–6), and collimation is used to keep the field of view limited to the cranium and stereotactic frame. The orientation of the patient to the radiographic apparatus is standardized and maintained, as are the magnification factors in the frontal and lateral projections. This serves to minimize any distortion of the markers on the film. Because filming is possible only in the two orthogonal planes using this arrangement, if it is anticipated that the delineation of a particular target requires a special view, such as Towne's, then the patient's neck will need to be flexed at the time of frame placement. The neurosurgeon must understand the requirements of the angiographic team to anticipate such

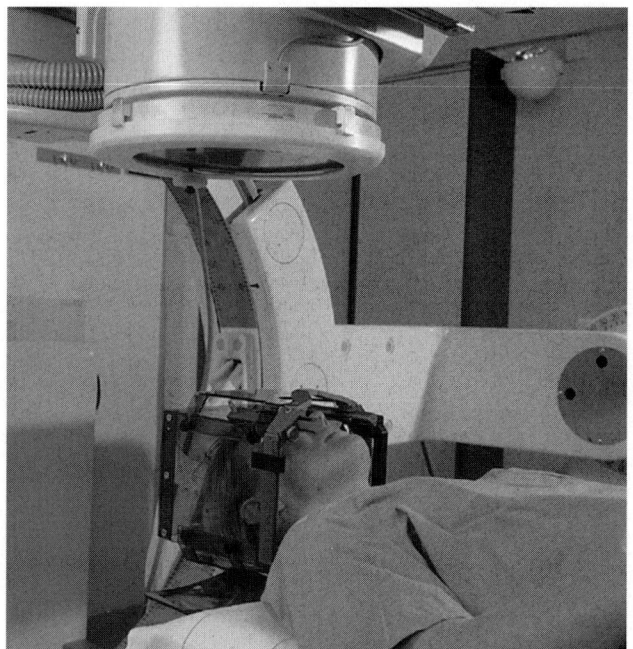

**FIGURE 49–6** ■ Patient position in the angiography suite, with a biplane unit. Observe that an adapter receives the stereotactic head frame and fixates it in strict orthogonal alignment to the x-ray tube.

situations. Care has to be exercised when subtracting the images so as not to subtract the markings on the frame and the fiducials completely.

Digital subtraction angiography in its present form cannot be used primarily for radiosurgical planning because of the inherent spatial distortion of the image intensifier. The distortion can be quantified by using a water phantom and a mathematical matrix developed for correction. Nevertheless, this is a potential error factor that should best be avoided. DSA is valuable, however, for identifying the dynamics of very fast shunts and complex malformations, and therefore should be performed whenever possible along with conventional stereotactic angiography.

The cut-film angiograms thus generated are scanned (Fig. 49–7) into the radiosurgical planning system using a digital scanner, which needs periodic calibration to avoid inaccuracies. Commercially available angiographic equipment has optional attachments available for digital output that can permit direct access to angiographic films through a computer-based network, and could eliminate the need for scanning. A number of available picture archiving systems provide a centralized high-resolution scanning utility that can be used to input the angiographic images into the network.

The principal objective of the entire procedure is to localize the nidus of the malformation as accurately as possible. Marking the nidus on stereotactic films for radiosurgery is an acquired art that requires experience, and all neurosurgeons and neuroradiologists in training must seek the opportunity to learn this technique. The ideal angiographic phase for the delineation of the target is one in which the nidus is well opacified and the draining veins are just beginning to fill. Every effort should be made to identify the fistulas that comprise a malformation. Indeed, if all such fistulas in a given malformation could be identi-

fied, it would theoretically be possible to cure the malformation by treating the fistulas alone.

The stereotactic angiogram film has external landmarks in the form of proximal and distal scale markings that maintain their position relative to the AVM on the frontal and lateral projections. A conscious effort must be made to correlate the coordinates on the two projections. The Z or vertical coordinate can be visualized on both frontal and lateral films. If the limits for the target on the Z axis, as delineated on the two projections, do not match, the validity of the target delineation should be questioned. The other factor important to keep in mind is that the actual magnification of objects within the frame varies in a nonlinear fashion between the proximal and distal scales for a given projection, although this can be ignored in approximate determination of the coordinates for the purpose of target delineation, provided that the focus-film distance is 1000 mm or more.

## PLANNING FOR GAMMA SURGERY

### Fundamentals

An optimal radiosurgical dose plan prescribes the steepest possible isodose gradient to the periphery of the target volume. This means that the margin of the target volume receives a high dose and the normal tissue next to it as low a dose as possible. There are situations in which it is more desirable to chose a less steep gradient and a lower isodose line at the periphery. The distribution of the dose in the target volume can also be varied to some extent. In radiation therapy, the principle is to achieve a homogeneous dose distribution in the target volume. Whether this should also be an important principle for the smaller radiosurgical target volumes is under debate; it probably depends on the pathologic process in the target volume. For example, there is no reason to believe that an inhomogeneous dose distribution is in any way beneficial for the treatment of an AVM of the brain, whereas a malignant tumor with a poorly oxygenated tumor center may actually benefit from a dose distribution with a high central dose. A higher average dose to the target volume results from a dose plan with a higher maximal dose compared with a dose plan with the same peripheral dose but with a smaller maximal dose. It has therefore been contended that the risk of complications is higher with an inhomogeneous dose distribution to the target volume. However, the experience from Gamma knife surgery is that the average dose delivered to the normal brain determines the risk, and this dose is not directly related to the average dose to the target volume when the peripheral dose gradient is steep.

The nature of the lesion determines the minimal effective dose. This dose should be delivered to the outer boundary of the target volume. The goal of treatment planning is to prescribe this dose to all parts of the surface of the target volume with a surface dose gradient steep enough to minimize the dose and thus the risk to adjacent normal structures. In some situations, such as in planning the treatment for tumors pushing on the optic chiasm, it may be necessary to compromise and plan the dose distribution so that

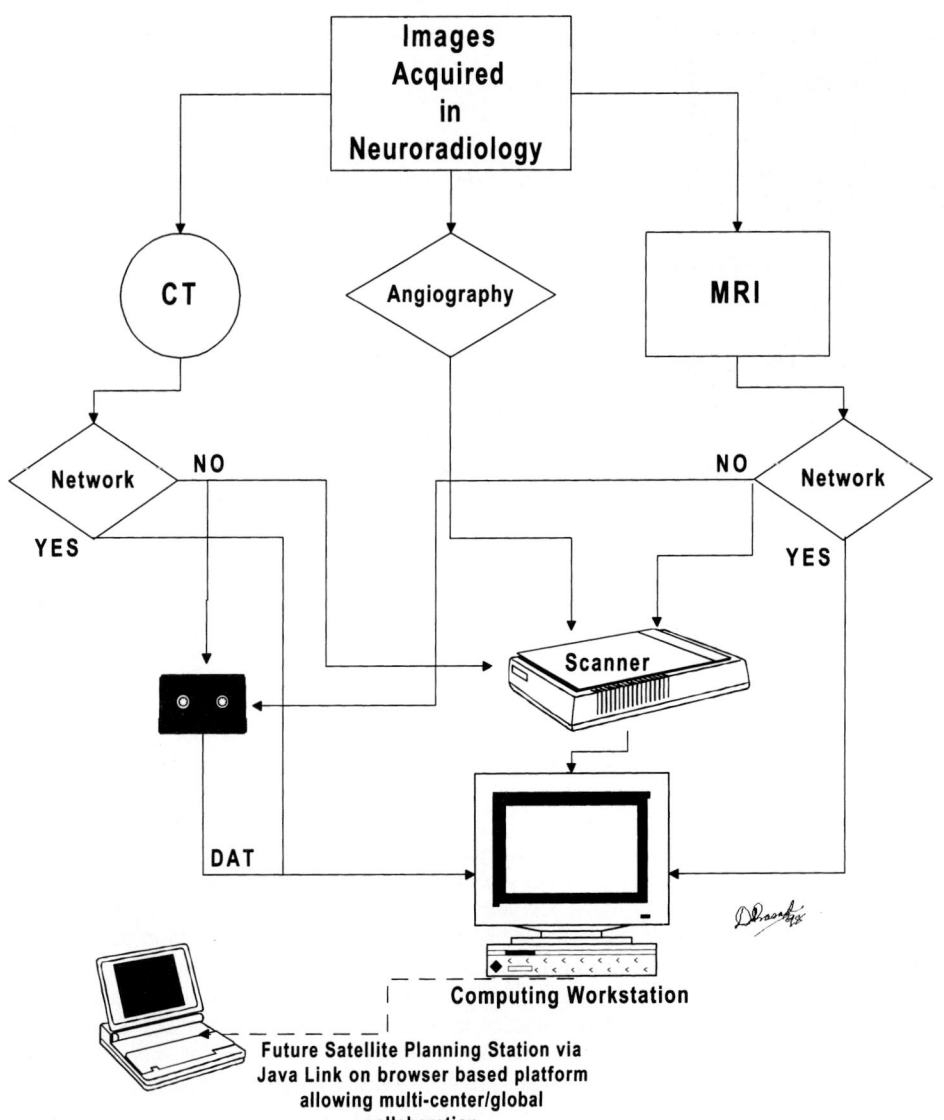

FIGURE 49–7 ■ Flowchart depicting image transfer from radiology to the Gamma surgery planning suite.

the surface of the target volume locally receives less than the optimal dose.

The dose delivered to a certain volume in the skull is determined by the radiation exposure time. The exposure time for a given dose is determined by the distance of the volume from the radiation sources and the amount of tissue the radiation beams must traverse before reaching the target. The distribution of the dose can be varied in four ways:

1. By choice of collimator helmet
2. By using multiple isocenters with similar or different collimators
3. By adjusting the relative weight assigned to the isocenters
4. By plugging selected beam channels in a collimator helmet

## The Planning Process

A dose planning session (Fig. 49–8) always begins by importing the relevant radiographic data (images) into the computer (see Fig. 49–7). Each set of images then has to be processed to identify the stereotactic fiducials for the computer (registration). Once this step is completed, the computer is able to locate any point on the images in cartesian space and display Leksell frame coordinates for it.

## Image Manipulation

Stereotactic CT images are imported as transaxial images and MRIs as transaxial, coronal, and sagittal images. The window and level settings of the gray-scale mapping of the images can be varied to optimize the visibility of regions of interest. Reformatting in planes other than those of the data acquisition can also be performed. Thus, transaxial CT and MRI can be used to reconstruct coronal and sagittal images. Positioning a centering cross-hair on one image in any projection automatically updates all images and projections on view and displays the coordinates of the center of the cross-hair. Reconstruction of coronal and sagittal planes is important for CT images, where the imaging technique permits only transaxial images to be ob-

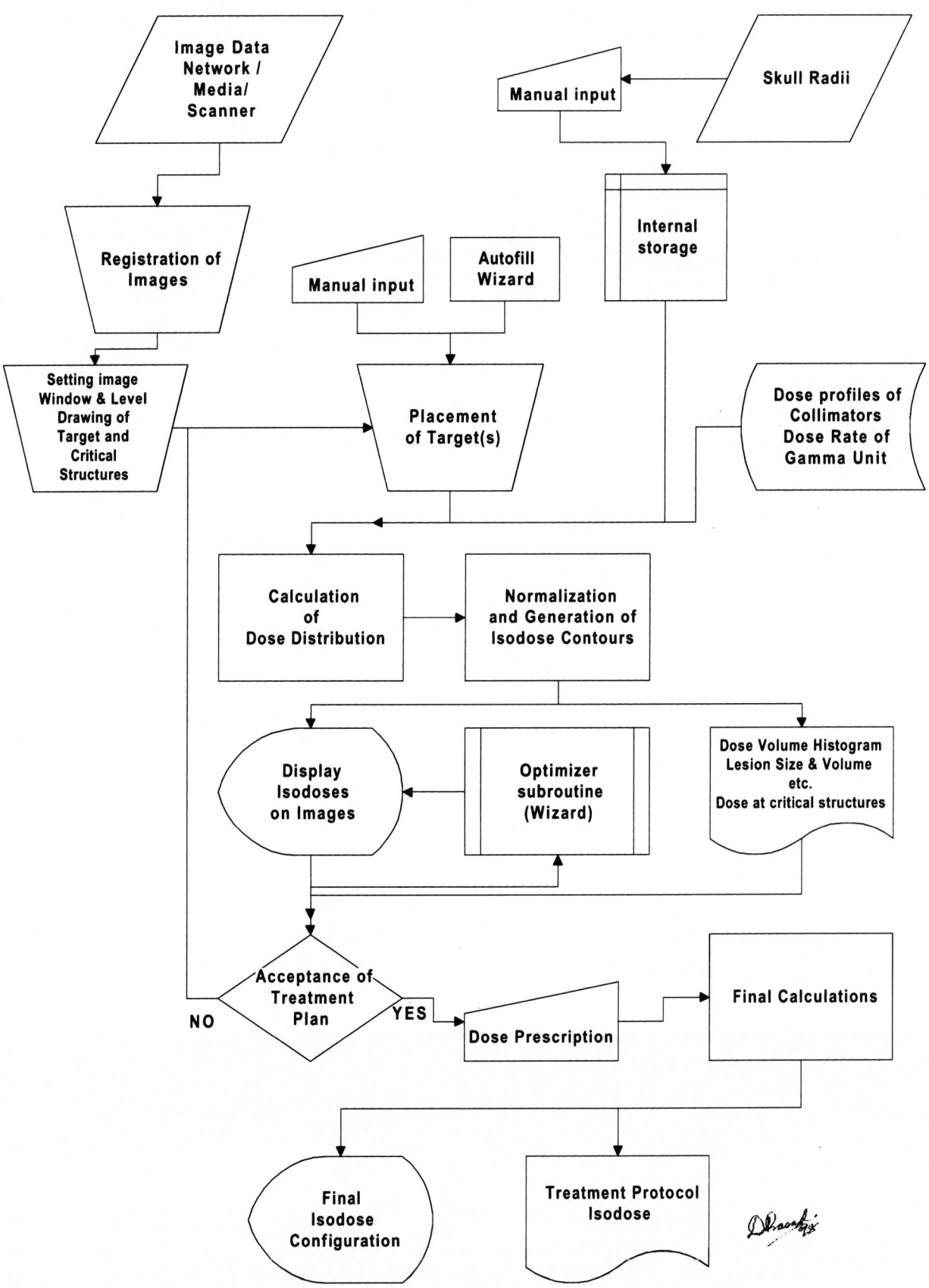

FIGURE 49–8 ■ Flowchart of the planning process.

tained. Reconstruction is also important for MRI because Z-coordinate determinations from stereotactic coronal MRIs are unreliable owing to distortion, which is not present in the transaxial images.

## Image Fusion

Images obtained stereotactically by different imaging modalities can be exactly fused. This technique may be of value to enhance delineation of a tumor and its neighboring structures. Thus, the advantages of the better soft tissue delineation of MRI can be combined with the bone window information from CT. MR angiography raw data can be fused with $T_1$-weighted spin-echo images to superpose flow data on structural detail.

## Defining the Target Volume and Three-Dimensional Reconstruction

The drawing tool of the software is used to define the borders of the target volume as well as any eloquent structures in the proximity of the intended radiation volume. 3-D reconstructions (Fig. 49–9) of these structures can then be displayed and manipulated to inspect their interrelationships. The surgeon must bear in mind that this is merely a 3-D representation of two-dimensional data; in the future, it is hoped that true 3-D data will be used by planning software. The defined structure and target boundaries are projected to all other image sets as well, even across platforms, such as from angiography to MRI and vice versa. This feature should be used to supplement one imaging modality with information from another.

## Placement of Isocenters

The dose plan is created directly on the target volume. The operator uses the mouse interactively to place one isocenter (shot) after another to generate (virtually instantaneously) the isodose contours that will result from the selected shots. The number, location, size, and assigned weight for each shot are set and modified as needed until a contour that conforms to the target volume is obtained. As a rule, more isocenters result in better conformity (and longer treatment time). Two smaller-sized shots are on the whole superior in terms of dose containment within abnormal tissue to one

larger one. Except for very small or perfectly spherical targets, therefore, two or more isocenters are the rule.

### AUTOMATED PLACEMENT AND OPTIMIZATION OF ISOCENTERS

A recent addition to Gamma Plan is software (Wizard; Elekta, Inc., Atlanta, GA) that allows the user to define the target volume and choose a collimator size. The program then performs an autofill routine that populates the target with isocenters. This interesting new facet of the software has yet to be evaluated for its practicability and clinical usefulness.

An additional feature of the Wizard is the ability mathematically to optimize the relative positions and assigned weights of the shots to satisfy criteria that define conformity and dose homogeneity for the computer. Once again, clinical application of this added feature has not been extensively evaluated.

## Shielding Critical Structures

In some situations, beam channels can be plugged to modify the dose distribution and avoid radiation exposure to sensitive structures. Plugging particularly affects the periphery of the radiated volume (i.e., the distributions of the 10% to 30% isodoses). Using the shielding tool in the software, the computer can automatically generate the pattern of beam channels to block to protect the structure covered by the shield that has been placed by the operator. This does not, however, mean that it is possible to shield structures that are in contact with the target. Such an attempt results in undertreatment of a part of the tumor. As shielding is invoked in the course of planning, the isodose contours on the target will also change, requiring readjustment of the isocenters. Based on current experience, we are able to reduce exposure of the optic pathways in cases of suprasellar and parasellar tumors from the order of 15% of the maximum dose to approximately 2% of the maximum dose.

## Dose Prescription

Several parameters of the dose plan generated as described previously are then analyzed before a dose prescription can be made.

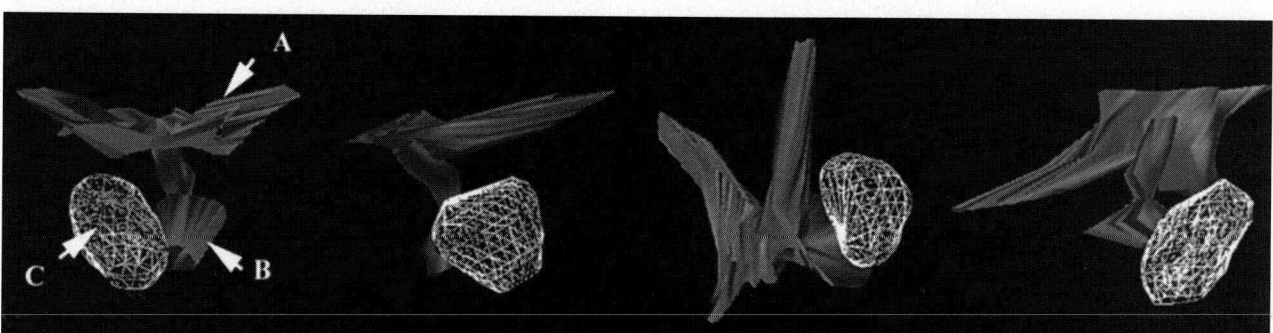

**FIGURE 49–9** ■ Three-dimensional reconstruction (of two-dimensional data) allows visual inspection of the anatomy from several angles. Here the relationships of the optic chiasm (A), pituitary gland (B), and pituitary adenoma (C) are evaluated from four different vantage points. The mesh around the tumor volume depicts the radiation field.

1. The total target volume is one factor. In simplified terms, the higher the volume the less the maximum dose that can be used with the same likelihood of untoward effects. This is so because as the volume of the target increases, more isocenters or larger collimators need to be used. Despite the focusing effect of multiple convergent sources, the larger target volume corresponds to a larger volume in isodoses outside the target (including normal tissues).

2. Distribution of dose within the target is assessed using the dose volume histogram (DVH; Fig. 49–10). The DVH is a plot of the radiation dose delivered versus the tissue volume included in a given dose. The maximum dose delivered to any target is in fact delivered to a point in the target (usually its epicenter), but the tissue volume included in the maximum dose is theoretically zero. From there, the included volumes increases to the periphery of the target. Thus, the minimum dose that would be responsible for biologic effects is the dose at the margin of the target (Fig. 49–11). Finally, the DVH shows the volume of tissue outside the target included in the lower isodose lines.

3. Dose received by critical structures (measurable literally with the click of a mouse; Fig. 49–12) affects the maximum dose that can be prescribed to the target. In addition to the absolute dose tolerance of such structures, it is important to consider their functional state (as evidenced by neurologic examinations) as a potential factor that could lower their ability to withstand radiation. Although empirical, this is a judgment call that surgeons are used to making in the operating field, and there is no substitute for personal and published experience in making these decisions.

4. The nature of the lesion. Variations in prescribed dose for different lesions are described in Chapter 50.
    v. The anatomic location of the target.
    vi. History of prior radiation. In conjunction with fractionated external beam radiation, radiosurgery is used to provide a localized boost to the pathologic area. In such situations, the dose that was delivered by the conventional method has to be considered when prescribing the radiosurgical dose. Although the exact conversion equivalence between single-dose and fractionated radiation is not known, the presumption that a single dose is approximately 2.5 to 3 times as effective as the same total dose delivered with fractionated techniques is probably close to the truth.

## PERFORMING GAMMA SURGERY

### Verification of the Protocol

The operator planning the procedure generates a printed document detailing the selected isocenters, along with the appropriate timings for exposure. This document also details the maximum dose, the minimum dose, and the isodose to which the prescription was made. In cases where plugging is used, the protocol also includes the pattern of channels to be plugged. This protocol should be verified to ensure correctness of all parameters.

### Verification of Patient Position, Plug Pattern, and Timing

Two independent observers should control the position of the isocenter, one setting the carriers on the frame and the other reading the coordinate, writing it down, and cross-checking it with the protocol. The same applies for the pattern of channels plugged, the size of collimator chosen, and, finally, the treatment time set on the timers.

### Protection of the Ocular Lens

The lens of the eye is radiosensitive, and passage of primary beams from the source could result in cataracts. Therefore, any sources incident on the eye lens are blocked. In the U model Gamma knife, it is possible to identify the sources that need to be plugged by shining a flashlight through the aperture in the collimator and confirming the point of incidence on the skull. In the B model, however, there are sources around the occiput whose beams would reach the lens after intersecting at the isocenter. To calculate the location of these sources, the planning software has a built-in subroutine. If the manual approach is used, the exposure time for the relevant shot has to be readjusted to compensate for the loss of the blocked source. This can be done either by applying the plug to the pattern in the computer, or by a simple hand calculation, provided the number of additional plugs does not exceed 10:

$$Tc = T \times So/(So - n) \qquad (7)$$

where $Tc$ = corrected shot time, $T$ = original shot time, $So$ = sources open before applying lens plugs, and $n$ = number of lens plugs.

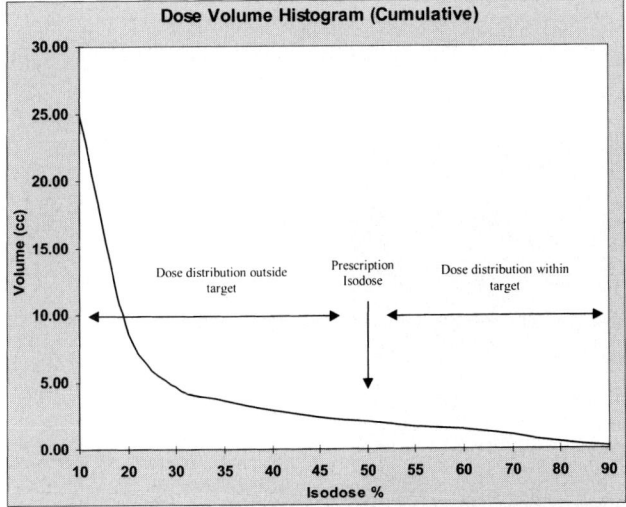

FIGURE 49–10 ■ The dose volume histogram (DVH) for the entire dose matrix serves as a good indicator of the dose distribution within and outside the target. Depending on the pathology the requirements for the slope of the curve differ for the portion inside the target. For the part outside the target the sharpest fall off possible is desirable.

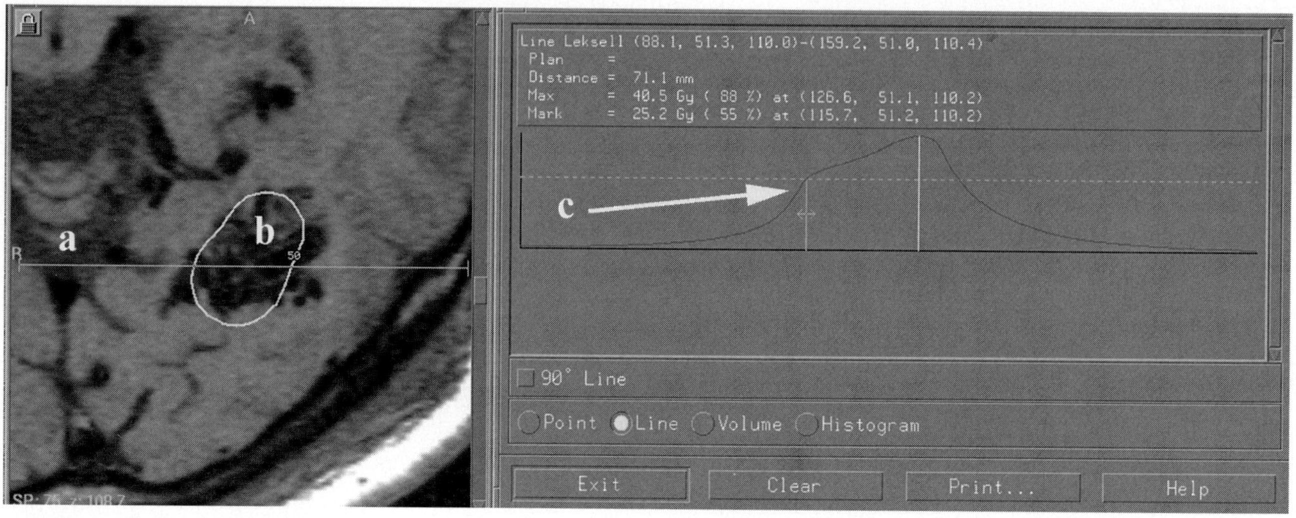

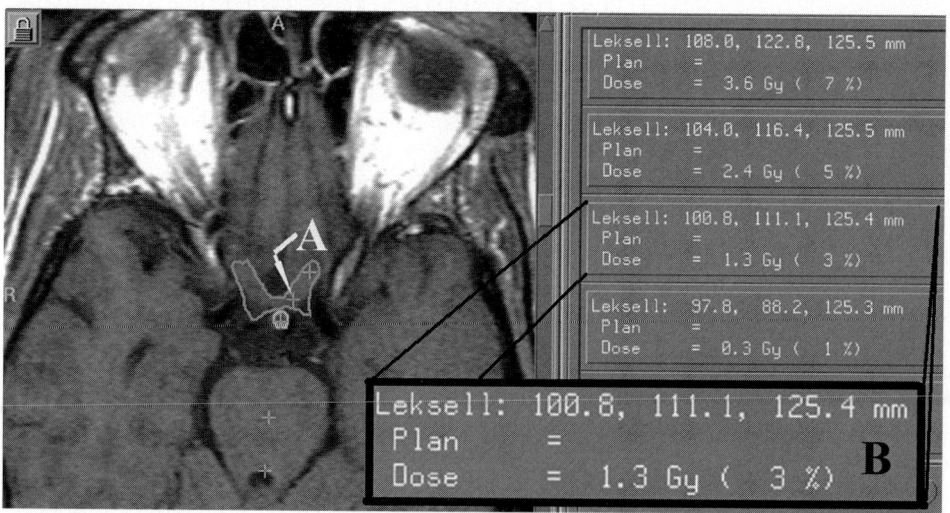

**FIGURE 49–11** ■ Dose profile through a cross-sectional line (a) drawn through an arteriovenous malformation (b) demonstrates the sharp fall off of the radiation dose at each edge of the lesion (c).

## Patient Position and Comfort

Within limits, it is possible to flex or extend the patient's neck by changing the selected gamma angle, thus allowing the patient's comfort level to be optimized. Because this means revision of the plan protocol, it requires repetition of some of the aforementioned steps. Most patients appreciate some padding under the neck for comfort and background music for distraction, particularly when the exposures are long.

In the U model of the Gamma knife, it is sometimes necessary to position patients prone when treating lesions that are posteriorly located, to avoid collision of the frame and the collimator helmet. In other instances, the treatment of a far lateral lesion requires removal of the front vertical post on the opposite side to avoid a collision. When removal of a post is necessary, the other three post screws should be checked to ensure that they are secure because loss of more than one point of fixation will result in displacement of the frame and consequently render the treatment plan and imaging studies useless.

## Removal of the Frame

After completion of the treatment, the stereotactic frame is removed under standard aseptic precautions in the gamma suite. We have observed that most patients complain of some discomfort from the decompression that they experience as the screws are removed. This can be associated with pain if the frame moves during removal as it comes loose off the skull. It has been our strategy to have the patient hold the frame steady while we remove the screws, which tends to minimize the pain because the patient's sensations serve as a feedback loop for him or her to hold it in the least uncomfortable position. Also, when loosening the screws, a few turns at a time for each screw is better tolerated than removing them one at a time completely.

## CONCLUSION

The increasing speed of available computers and the ability rapidly to transfer and store large volumes of data will

**FIGURE 49–12** ■ Point dose measurements are made by clicking at the point of interest (A) with a mouse. The *inset* (B) shows that the readout includes the Leksell coordinates of the point of measurement, the absolute dose received, and the percentage of the maximum dose received at that this point.

doubtless continue to refine the planning process. The next logical step is toward a platform-independent interface that will be usable over a web browser and allow interactive planning between centers with large experience and newer, less experienced ones. Even though the machine itself will be modified, it seems unlikely that Leksell's creative genius will be surpassed in its simple yet elegant implementation of radiosurgery.

## REFERENCES

1. Leksell L: The stereotaxic method and radiosurgery of the brain. Acta Chir Scand 102:316–319, 1951.
2. Arndt J, Backlund E-O, Larsson B, et al: Stereotactic irradiation of intracranial structures: Physical and biological considerations. Inserm Symp 12:81–92, 1979.
3. Leksell L: A stereotaxic apparatus for intracerebral surgery. Acta Chir Scand 99:229–233, 1949.

# Gamma Surgery in Cerebral Vascular Lesions, Malformations, Tumors, and Functional Disorders

■ LADISLAU STEINER, BRYAN RANKIN PAYNE, DHEERENDRA PRASAD, CHRISTER LINDQUIST, and MELITA STEINER

The Gamma knife is a neurosurgical tool used either as a primary or adjuvant procedure for treatment of intracranial pathologic processes. It was developed in the late 1960s as an alternative to open stereotactic lesioning for functional disorders. Variations in anatomy and the need for physiologic confirmation of the target limited its early usefulness for these indications. However, the technology proved effective in the management of structural disorders as well. The limited scope of the pathologic process treated with the Gamma knife (intracranial) and its unique technology make the Gamma knife an extension of the neurosurgeon's therapeutic arsenal, and not a separate specialty. It should not be mistaken for a form of radiation therapy because it differs conceptually from the radiation oncologist's idea of tumor treatment, which is based on variable tissue response to fractionated radiation. It is a single-session, stereotactically guided procedure for various neurosurgical pathologic processes that restricts radiation exposure as much as possible to the lesion only.

It has been shown that the Gamma knife can palliate some ocular tumors. In a more limited application of the concept, the treatment of extracranial tumors, such as liver and pancreas, may evolve. Obviously, these lesions will not be treated by a neurosurgeon. However, when it is used for neurosurgical lesions, no one is more qualified to apply it. It is the operator and the pathologic process that define the use of a technology. When Walter Dandy placed a cystoscope in a ventricle for the first time, he was not performing a urologic procedure.[1] The microscope, when used by the neurosurgeon, ophthalmologist, or otolaryngologist, is a neurosurgical, ophthalmologic, or otolaryngologic instrument, respectively.

It is remarkable how difficult it was, and still is, for some neurosurgeons to accept for use as a neurosurgical tool a physical agent to which they are not accustomed. Some of the causes of this reticence can be identified:

1. Lack of historical perspective. Some neurosurgeons do not realize that Leksell's concept was rooted in the philosophy of the founders of neurosurgery, which included recognition of technologic advances and their application to neurosurgical practice. The early adoption by Cushing of the x-ray machine, his use of the "radium bomb" in glioma treatment,[2] and his introduction of the use of radiofrequency lesions are just a few examples of "technology transfer."

2. The difficulty of accepting a neurosurgical procedure without opening the skull, despite the fact that every neurosurgeon knows that trephination is itself a minor part of the neurosurgical act. The laser beam, the bipolar coagulator, and the ultrasound probe are accepted without resistance because they are used after skull trephination. The recently introduced "photon radiosurgery," with its limited scope compared with gamma surgery, is accepted widely as "neurosurgery" because it reaches the target through a small bur hole.

3. The loss of the thrill and glamor provided by the open surgical act.

4. The deeply rooted acceptance of the dogma that where ionizing beams are involved, a radiation therapist is needed. Developments since the late 1970s have demonstrated that a neurosurgeon can acquire the necessary grounding in radiation physics and radiobiology to handle ionizing beams. This is much easier than for a radiation oncologist to master neuroanatomy and management of neurosurgical lesions, and thus to exclude bias when deciding whether to use the microscope or the Gamma knife in each particular case.

The trend in surgery has been toward less traumatic and more physiologic surgery. These may be achieved by new technology and with increased skill on the part of operators. If in the course of this evolution aspects of the procedure are modified or even eliminated, the procedure is still neurosurgical. To relegate less invasive procedures to non-surgeons is to argue that the only aspect of a patient's care that is unique to a surgeon is purely technical. This is patently untrue; it is the surgeon's responsibility to maintain the standard of surgical care by adapting to new technologies.

670

There is no substitute at this time for the physical extirpation of a mass lesion in terms of cure or control of either vascular or oncotic pathologic processes. The attractiveness of radiosurgery is not that it supplants open neurosurgical procedures, but that it allows treatment of lesions treated earlier only with unacceptable morbidity or mortality. There is, and likely always will be, a gray area where the benefits of various modalities are debated. Only through the evaluation of long-term results of these various therapies, as well as their availability and cost, the experience of the operators, and individual patient preferences, will the "best" therapy in any given case be decided.

In this chapter, we describe the results of our experience with the Gamma knife as well as the published results of other centers, where required.

Table 50–1 lists all the cases treated with the Gamma knife worldwide through 1997. Many of the indications listed are not universally accepted as appropriate for Gamma surgery. In this chapter, we give our version of the facts for each indication.

# HISTORY

Clarke and Horsley[3] developed the first stereotactic system, and the method was first applied clinically by Spiegel and

colleagues.[4] It allowed for the localization of intracranial structures by their spatial relationship to cartesian coordinates relative to a ring rigidly affixed to the skull. This was a prerequisite to the development of radiosurgery by Lars Leksell. His ambition was to develop a method of destroying localized structures deep in the brain without the degree of coincident brain trauma associated with open procedures. The convergence of multiple beams of ionizing radiation at one stereotactically defined point was the result. A nominal dose is delivered to the paths of each incident beam. However, at the point of intersection of the beams, a dose proportional to the number of individual beams is delivered. The physical specifications of the device would be designed to ensure sharp drop-off of delivered radiation at the edge of the intersection point. This would allow precise selection of the targeted lesion and minimization of trauma to surrounding tissue. Leksell termed this concept *radiosurgery* in 1951.

Various sources of ionizing radiation were tried. Leksell first used an orthovoltage x-ray tube coupled to a stereotactic frame in the treatment of trigeminal neuralgia and for cingulotomy in obsessive-compulsive disorders.[5] A cyclotron was used as an accelerated proton source to treat various pathologic processes[6, 7] but was too cumbersome and expensive for widespread application. A linear accelerator was evaluated but was deemed not to have the inherent precision necessary for this work. Fixed gamma sources of $^{60}$Co and a fixed stereotactic target fulfilled the requirements of precision and compactness. The first Gamma knife was built between 1965 and 1968.

The use of a single high dose of ionizing beams to treat neurosurgical problems was a novel and creative concept in the late 1960s and changed the direction of development in many fields of neurosurgery. However, a creative innovation is never perfect in its inception, and the Gamma knife was no exception. Contributions of excellence by numerous neurosurgeons and physicists, using advances in computer technology to improve the software used in planning, have over the years defined the current use of the tool. For instance, improvements in the planning system now allow for systematic exclusion of the optic apparatus from exposure during treatment of parasellar masses. In lesions only 2 to 5 mm away, the dose to sensitive structures can be limited to less than 2% to 7% of the maximum dose. However, despite all the changes in application of gamma surgery, the underlying concepts behind it have not changed since its inception. This speaks for the sagacity of Lars Leksell and his invention.

Doses delivered and indications for the various lesions treated were all initially empiric. In the subsequent discussions, this should be taken into consideration when doses, both minimal and maximal, are discussed, as well as results.

## TABLE 50–1 ■ NUMBER OF CASES TREATED WITH THE GAMMA KNIFE WORLDWIDE FROM 1968 TO 1997

| Diagnosis | No. | Percentage |
|---|---|---|
| **Vascular** | 18,188 | 23.0 |
| Arteriovenous malformation | 17,442 | 22.0 |
| Aneurysm | 94 | 0.1 |
| Other vascular | 652 | 0.8 |
| | | |
| **Tumor** | 57,889 | 73.1 |
| *Benign* | | |
| Acoustic neuroma | 8307 | 10.5 |
| Meningioma | 9969 | 12.6 |
| Pituitary | 7806 | 9.8 |
| Pineal | 1152 | 1.5 |
| Craniopharyngioma | 1058 | 1.3 |
| Hemangioblastoma | 451 | 0.6 |
| Chordoma | 465 | 0.6 |
| Trigeminal neuroma | 469 | 0.6 |
| Other benign tumors | 608 | 0.8 |
| | | |
| *Malignant* | | |
| Metastasis | 17,221 | 21.6 |
| Glioma | 7958 | 10.1 |
| Chondrosarcoma | 91 | 0.1 |
| Glomus tumor | 233 | 0.3 |
| Ocular melanoma | 355 | 0.4 |
| NPH carcinoma | 420 | 0.5 |
| Hemangiopericytoma | 288 | 0.4 |
| Other malignant tumors | 625 | 0.8 |
| | | |
| **Functional** | 3073 | 3.9 |
| Intractable pain | 204 | 0.3 |
| Trigeminal neuralgia | 1521 | 1.9 |
| Parkinson's disease | 607 | 0.8 |
| Psychoneurosis | 68 | <0.1 |
| Epilepsy | 539 | 0.7 |
| Other | 134 | 0.2 |
| | | |
| Total | 79,150 | 100 |

From Elekta Radiosurgery, Inc., Atlanta, 1998.

# PATHOPHYSIOLOGY

The effects of single high-dose gamma radiation on pathologic and normal tissue have been studied on clinical human and experimental animal tissue. These studies are incomplete because the human material tends to come from treatment failures and the experimental material from normal animals. However, some conclusions as to the method of effectiveness and of tissue tolerances can be drawn.

## Normal Tissue

The relative radioresistance of normal brain relates to its low mitotic activity. Also, the rate at which a total dose of radiation is applied affects the damage caused by the dose. This is due to the ability of the cell to effect repairs during the actual time of irradiation. A higher dose rate (same total dose applied over a shorter period of time) consequently increases the lethality of the dose. The normal tissue surrounding the stereotactically targeted pathologic tissue receives a markedly lower dose but over the same time. Therefore, not only is the total dose lower but the dose rate is lower. This effect is seen most clearly at doses above and below 1 Gy/min.[8] This radiobiologic phenomenon explains part of the relative safety of single-dose radiation with steep gradients at the edge of targeted tissue on the surrounding structures. There are likely additional mechanisms at play in such sparing.

The steep gradient of dose and consequently dose rate does not exist in conventional radiation therapy. When treating tumors, the radiation oncologist uses "fractionation" or division of the total dose into smaller portions, which allows for repair of normal tissue as well as transition of dormant cells in the target to a mitotic phase (at which time they are more sensitive to radiation). Creating a dose gradient at the lesion's margin not only eliminates the need for fractionation but improves the effectiveness of the delivered dose within the target (high-dose-rate zone) by 2.5 to 3 times that of the same dose delivered in a fractionated manner. The Gamma knife stereotactically excludes normal tissue from the high-dose-rate zone area as much as possible. It may also take advantage of the natural difference in susceptibility of pathologic versus normal tissue.

To understand the radiobiology of a single high dose of radiation on normal brain, the parietal lobes of rats treated by a Gamma knife were studied at our center. We found that a dose of 50 Gy caused astrocytic swelling without changes in neuronal morphology or breakdown of the blood-brain barrier at 12 months. There was fibrin deposition in the walls of capillaries. At 75 Gy, necrosis and breakdown of the blood-brain barrier were seen at 4 months. More vigorous morphologic changes were seen in astrocytes, and hemispheric swelling coincident with the necrosis occurred at 4 months. With the dose increased to 120 Gy, necrosis was seen at 4 weeks, but it was not associated with hemispheric swelling. Astrocytic swelling occurred at only 1 week postirradiation.[9] These findings are consistent with earlier reports on the effective dose for producing well-defined lesions in the thalamus in patients treated with the Gamma knife.[10, 11]

## Tumor Response

Little is known about the pathophysiologic changes induced by gamma surgery at the cellular level in tumors.

Division of tumor cells is presumably inhibited by radiation-induced damage to DNA. Also, it has been shown that the microvascular supply to tumors is inhibited by changes resulting from gamma surgery. Meningiomas treated by gamma surgery showed reduction of blood flow over time, and tumors responding early showed the greatest reduction in blood flow.[12] Other investigators have proposed that the induction of apoptosis by gamma radiation in proliferating cells may be responsible for at least a portion of the effect of gamma surgery on tumors.[13] Although such contentions may be premature, they suggest directions for future research.

The objective of gamma surgery is therefore not necessarily tumor necrosis. For this, higher doses than typically used would be needed, and pathologic changes in adjoining normal tissue may occur with such an approach. Some authors believe these changes, seen months after high-dose gamma surgery and most clearly in the white matter, represent vasogenic edema. This has not been conclusively demonstrated, however. Ideally, after gamma surgery, tumors begin to shrink without changes in the normal tissue. The rate of shrinkage in general is slower in more benign tumors.

The effectiveness of the therapy depends most on the ability to define and treat the entire lesion. Malignant gliomas respond poorly to any surgical technique, including gamma surgery, because of the inability to include all of the microscopic disease within the treated area. Individual metastatic deposits and small benign tumors are well handled with both open resection and the Gamma knife because the tumor margin can be defined. The similarity to open surgical techniques is striking.

To cover the target conformally, more than one isocenter is nearly always used (see Chapter 49). When multiple radiation fields are made to overlap in this manner, the radiation dose distribution becomes inhomogeneous. The resulting areas of local maxima are called *hot spots*. Controversy exists as to whether the presence of hot spots in gamma surgery is beneficial or detrimental. Although an even dose distribution is an essential and basic concept in radiation therapy, there is some evidence that these local maxima may be of benefit in gamma surgery. The factors behind this line of reasoning are as follows: because of radiation geometry, hot spots are usually located in the deep portions of the target. In tumors, this is usually the area that receives the poorest blood supply and is therefore relatively hypoxic. Furthermore, the ability of a cell to respond to otherwise sublethal dosages of radiation can be affected by its own condition as well as by the state of the cells near it. Cells that are sublethally injured and are in the vicinity of similar cells recover more often than cells that are in the vicinity of lethally injured cells. The hot spots therefore create islands of lethally injured cells that enhance the cell kill in the sublethal injury zone.[14] Oxygen is a radiosensitizer, and the relatively high dose rate of the hot spots acts to offset any loss of efficacy in the hypoxic core of the target. This position is supported by the work of other researchers.[15]

## Cranial Nerves

The susceptibility of cranial nerves to injury from gamma surgery is of great interest. Tolerance depends on the particular nerve and the individual nerve's involvement by the pathologic process requiring treatment. Because of these factors, it is difficult to extrapolate exact numbers in many cases, but some statements can be made with some certainty.

The optic and acoustic nerves are the most sensitive of the cranial nerves to radiation. They are thought to be more vulnerable because they are central nervous system tracts, contain oligodendrocytes, and carry complex information. These tracts are unable to regenerate after injury. Optic neuropathy has been reported as a complication after single doses greater than 8 Gy.[16]

On the other hand, the trigeminal and facial nerves are significantly more resilient. In the treatment of trigeminal neuralgia with radiosurgery in which 50 to 100 mm$^3$ of the trigeminal roots at the entry zone were treated with 60 to 80 Gy, only one mild facial hypoesthesia was reported.[17] In a larger group of small-sized acoustic neuromas not distorting the trigeminal nerve treated with radiosurgery with peripheral doses of 10 to 25 Gy, the incidence of facial hypoesthesia was 19%. This seems to indicate that it is the length of nerve exposed that is the critical determinant in injury. In the same 254 patients, the incidence of facial paresis was 17%, although this was in all cases transitory.

The cranial nerves in the cavernous sinus are relatively robust. Neuropathies have not been seen with doses up to 40 Gy.[16]

## Normal Cerebral Vasculature

There is both clinical and experimental data on the effect of single high-dose gamma irradiation of normal cerebral vasculature. In treating 1917 arteriovenous malformations (AVM), we have seen only two incidences of clinical syndromes possibly associated with the stenosis of normal vessels. This low incidence was seen even though normal vessels occasionally were included in the treatment field. One case of a middle cerebral artery occlusion was reported after treatment of a glioma with 90-Gy gamma surgery followed by 40 Gy of fractionated whole-brain irradiation.[18] Steiner and colleagues[19] described two cases in which disproportionate white matter changes could be ascribed to venous stenosis and occlusion. In a case of diencephalic AVM, marked edema was associated with venous outflow occlusion. This patient had visual and cognitive deficits, but over the course of months his neurologic status returned to baseline. Because veins in this region can obliterate spontaneously, it is difficult to assess the contribution of the gamma surgery to this process (Fig. 50–1).

In the treatment of pituitary adenomas with cavernous sinus extension, or of meningiomas near the medial sphenoid wing, we are aware of no published or unpublished cases of occlusion of normal vasculature. This absence of stenosis is noted even though the internal carotid artery or portions of the circle of Willis, or its proximal branches, are often included in the treatment field. Our single instance of treatment of an intracranial aneurysm with the Gamma knife did lead to narrowing and eventual occlusion of the adjacent small posterior communicating artery segment; whether this was associated with the obliteration of the

aneurysm neck or primary changes in the artery is unknown. It is possible that the incidence of occlusion of smaller vessels is more common than recognized because the occlusion would occur slowly and compensatory changes could take place, preventing clinical syndromes from occurring. Regardless of the process, the clinical impact is minimal.

Experimental studies done on normal vasculature in the brains of rats[20] and cats[21] showed similar findings. The primary injury was endothelial necrosis and desquamation, muscular coat hypertrophy, and fibrosis at lower doses (25 to 100 Gy). At doses up to 300 Gy, necrosis of the muscular layer was seen in cats. In only one instance, a rat anterior cerebral artery treated with 100 Gy, was occlusion of a vessel seen. Follow-up of 2 to 20 months was allowed. Similar studies on hypercholesterolemic rabbits treated with 10 to 100 Gy showed no histologic changes in the basilar arteries and no instances of occlusion after 2 to 24 months.[22]

## Arteriovenous Malformations

The moderate changes in the normal cerebral vasculature after high doses of gamma radiation, and their minimal clinical effects, are in sharp contrast to the response of AVM vessels. Complete radiographic obliteration of an AVM can be achieved after appropriate gamma surgery. The effects of ionizing radiation and a role for it in the management of AVMs was first reported in 1928 by Cushing.[23] During craniotomy for an AVM, he had to interrupt surgery because of major hemorrhage from the lesion. He then treated the patient with fractionated radiation. At reoperation 5 years later, only an obliterated avascular mass was discovered. This early success was overshadowed by numerous series of failures.[24–30] Only Johnson[31] reported reasonable results with a 45% angiographic obliteration rate. The introduction of the Gamma knife rekindled interest in the treatment of AVMs with radiation.[32] The pathologic changes in AVMs treated with the Gamma knife have been described by several authors.[33–35] The earliest change is damage to the endothelium with swelling of the endothelial cells and subsequent denudation or separation of the endothelium from the underlying vessel wall. The most important changes are seen later in the intima, with the appearance of loosely organized spindle cells (myofibroblasts) and an extracellular matrix containing type IV collagen, which is not seen in the intima of untreated vessels. Expansion of the extracellular matrix and cellular degeneration define the final stage before luminal obliteration. The occlusion of the vessels is not a thrombotic process but rather the culmination of a concentric narrowing of the vessel by an expanding vessel wall. Subsequent recanalization of an angiographically proven obliterated AVM has not occurred in our experience.

## VASCULAR MALFORMATIONS

### Arteriovenous Malformations

In AVMs, the indications for gamma surgery versus other treatment options are often unclear at best. Small, asymp-

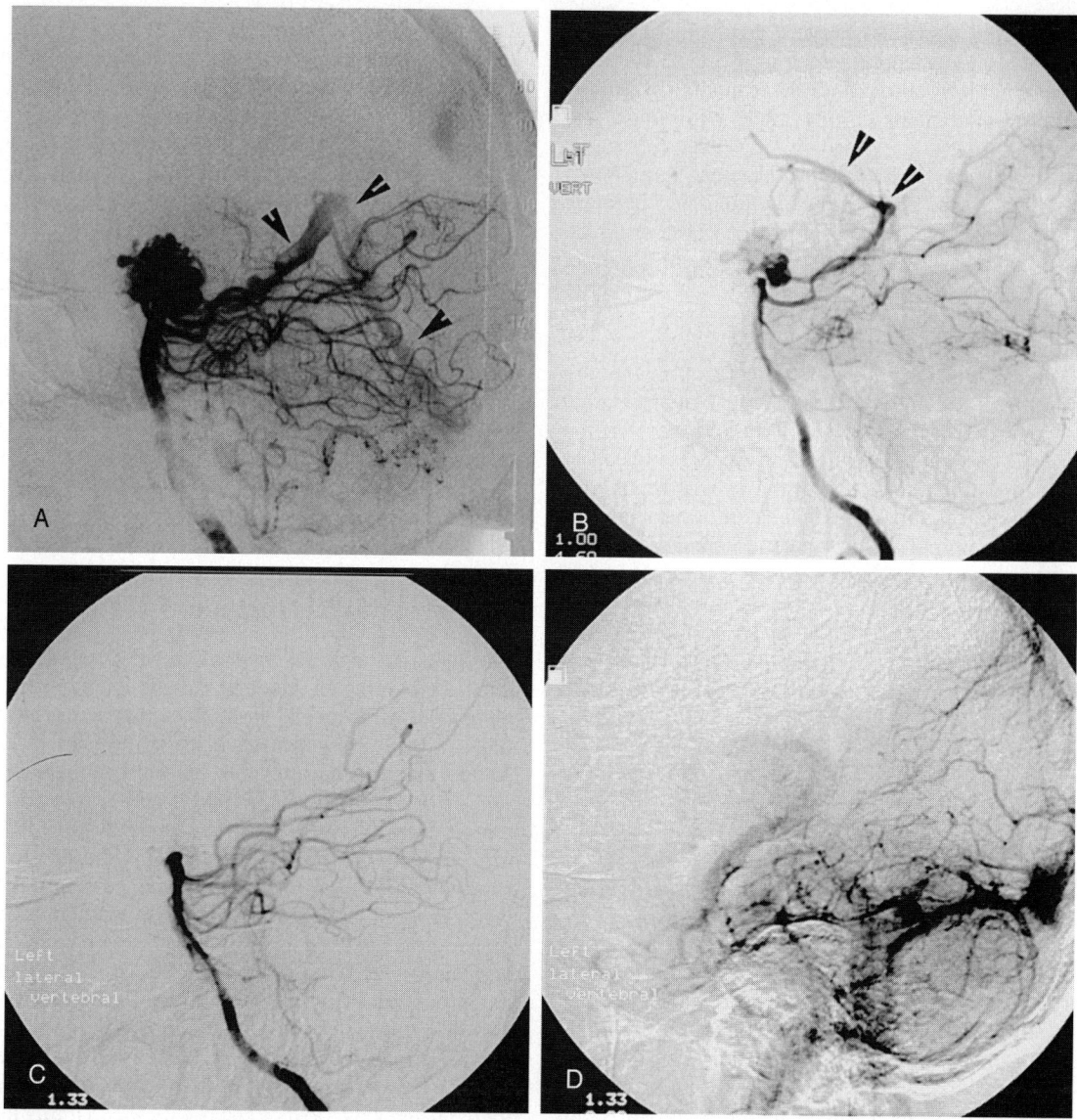

**FIGURE 50–1** ■ A thalamic arteriovenous malformation (AVM) is shown with lateral vertebral arteriography *(A)*. A similar view was obtained 17 months after. Gamma surgery shows partial obliteration of the nidus *(B)*. The basal vein of Rosenthal, the vein of Galen, and the straight sinus were not visualized. Venous drainage of the residual AVM appears to be through the ascending choroidal veins and the internal cerebral veins. Early *(C)* and late *(D)* filling vertebral arteriograms were obtained 37 months after. Gamma surgery shows obliteration of the AVM and the complete absence of the deep venous system.

tomatic, inoperable AVMs are clearly best treated with the Gamma knife, whereas AVMs with a large, symptomatic hemorrhage in noneloquent, superficial portions of the brain are best treated with open surgery. The risk-benefit ratio is clear in both of these situations; in other situations, it is not as clear. A knowledge of the capabilities of various treatments to effect cure, the associated morbidity and mortality associated with the treatment, and the natural history of the disease after various treatments is necessary to prescribe the most efficacious treatment plan. Unfortunately, these are unknown in most instances. The natural history of AVMs is not fully understood. Some authors believe that size matters, with smaller AVMs bleeding at a higher rate than larger ones,[36–39] or at a lower rate.[40, 41] There is also evidence that size is independent of the hemorrhage rate.[42–46] Similarly, the rate of hemorrhage of an AVM after a previous hemorrhage is thought to be

higher than the rate in unruptured AVMs by some authors,[37, 43, 45, 47] but not by others.[38, 48, 49] The effects of age, sex, pregnancy, and AVM location also confound the question of rupture risk.[36–38, 42–45, 48, 50, 51]

The published results of microsurgery tend to come from centers of surgical excellence, and the patients they treat with open surgery are, by definition, more amenable to this treatment. The effectiveness of microsurgical treatment and its comorbid results are known shortly after surgery. The short-term morbidity of treatment with the Gamma knife is nil, but because the benefits and potential complications require time to become apparent, follow-up of these patients is problematic. The quality of the AVMs treated with the Gamma knife also varies in large series compared with those treated by microsurgery. All of these factors make comparison of the modalities difficult. When the additional risks and benefits of preoperative embolization are taken into account, the matter is even less clear. It is paramount for the physician treating a patient with an AVM to be aware, as much as possible, of the options that are available and the magnitude of the risks and benefits associated with each.

## Methods

### PERIOPERATIVE MANAGEMENT

Patients are routinely admitted the day before radiosurgery. Preoperative consultations are obtained as necessary, including evaluation by the neuroradiology service. The patients are loaded with antiseizure medications and levels drawn before therapy. Patients already on medication for seizures also have their levels evaluated. Although we have never had a patient have a seizure during therapy, the small but serious risk of a generalized seizure while the patient is secured in the gamma unit makes every precaution reasonable. Patients are also started on systemic dexamethasone the evening before therapy, and this is continued until the following evening. The use of high-dose perioperative dexamethasone is empirical. Although we have used steroids throughout our experience with the Gamma knife, their original indication, to minimize vasogenic edema at the time of therapy, has never been documented as a problem. Hence, their prophylactic use is debatable.

### FRAME PLACEMENT

Placement of the head frame is done in the operating room. Patients are given intravenous sedation, usually short-acting narcotics and propofol, until they are no longer responsive to verbal or moderate physical stimuli. The anesthesia service monitors the patient throughout the procedure. We have found this far superior to the previous practice of applying the frame using only local anesthesia. Patients treated both before and since we have applied the frame in this way have clearly stated their preference for frame placement under anesthesia.

We have fashioned a simple strap with Velcro ends that is placed across the patient's head and then fastened above the frame after it has been lowered into position. This holds the frame in position while the pins are secured and eliminates the need for the earplugs in the auditory canal, which can be painful.

The space available within the Gamma knife unit is limited, as is the three-dimensional coordinate system within the frame itself. Therefore, care must be taken to skew the placement of the frame in the direction of the lesion if it is far off the center of the brain. This includes having the frame base at the level of the zygomatic arch for skull base and posterior fossa lesions and to the side of the head for lesions that are more than a short distance off the midline. Care must be taken not to compress the ear against the frame. For posterior fossa lesions, the frame should be as posterior as possible to prevent having to perform the treatment in the prone position.

### IMAGING AND DOSE PLANNING

In planning the treatment of an AVM, both stereotactic arteriography and stereotactic magnetic resonance imaging (MRI) are used. This requires cooperation between the treating neurosurgeon and the radiologist performing the examination. With angiography, the only views applicable to the planning of treatment are standardized, anteroposterior and lateral views exactly orthogonal to the frame. The frame is placed in a fixed holder and a Perspex box carrying fiducial markers is applied to it. The relevant films are then manually scanned into the planning station or, if available, they can be electronically downloaded. The relative position of the fiducials and AVM allows localization of the AVM relative to the frame. If evaluation of previous films indicates that any other view is necessary to visualize the AVM, then the frame's position must be adjusted.

Digital subtraction angiography may be helpful in understanding the anatomy of an AVM, but it cannot be used in the planning of treatment. Distortion of the radiograph by the image intensifier is too great to allow for the precision necessary for radiosurgery.

The stereotactic MRI allows better visualization of the dimensions of nonspherical targets in the axial plane. It helps to define the shape of the AVM and confirms angiographically obtained information. It is difficult to differentiate the nidus from the draining veins on MRI, so MRI tends to overestimate the size of the AVM. The capability to incorporate MR angiographic data into the planning process is expected to be available in future releases of Gamma Plan software.

For details of planning, see Chapter 49.

### THE GAMMA KNIFE

The Gamma knife consists of a body that contains the radiation sources and a treatment couch that delivers the patient into the unit. Within the body are 201 $^{60}$Co source capsules aligned with two internal collimators that direct the gamma radiation toward the center of the unit. A third, external collimator helmet is attached to the treatment couch. Four external collimator helmets are provided; they have fixed-diameter apertures that create isocenters of 4, 8, 14, or 18 mm in diameter. By changing external collimator helmets, the diameter of the roughly spherical isocenter can be varied. The 201 individual collimators within the helmet are machined to exact standards to direct the 201 beams of gamma radiation to a common point of intersection, creating the isocenter. The frame attached to the patient's head is adjusted in the collimator helmet so that the area to be treated is at that point of intersection. For a more detailed description, see Chapter 49.

### TREATMENT

After the treatment plan has been made, the patient is moved on to the Gamma knife couch and the Y and Z coordinates for the first exposure are set on the frame attached to the patient's head. The patient's head is then placed in the collimator helmet and secured on either side by trunions, and the X coordinate is set. Visual confirmation of correct settings must be made by the operator *in addition to the person who sets the coordinates*. The head at this point is suspended by the frame within the helmet, and for comfort, the neck should be supported with towels or an equivalent material. The exposure time of the corresponding isocenter is entered at the control panel twice for confirmation and the session then commences with the entire couch being mechanically pulled into the body of the unit. The external collimator helmet locks into place with the internal collimators. After each exposure, the patient is withdrawn from the collimator helmet and the process is repeated. Necessary changes to the collimator helmet are made as needed according to the plan. Newer versions of the Gamma knife make direct entry of data from the planning station to the control panel possible, as well as mechanical adjustments of coordinates without removing the patient from the collimator helmet. Improved ergonomics and an integrated collimator helmet changer are also planned. Obviously, these changes will not affect the efficacy of the treatment, but will make the process simpler for the operator.

At the end of treatment, the frame is removed from the head in the suite. There is usually a sensation of tightening and discomfort reported by the patient during removal. At least two pairs of hands should be available to steady the frame and prevent injury by a pin as they are removed. Venous bleeding, if it occurs, can be controlled by manual pressure for several minutes. The occasional arterial bleeder usually requires a hemostatic suture, which should be readily available. The suture is removed the following morning. After frame removal, the pin sites are dressed in a sterile fashion and a modest head wrap applied.

## Results

We have treated 2155 vascular malformations, 1917 of which were AVMs, with the Gamma knife since 1970. As experience with this tool grows, the capabilities and limitations of the Gamma knife are being defined. Serendipitously, the first AVMs were treated by prescribing a 25-Gy periphery dose, which means that the edge of the AVM received this dose and this was the minimum dose received by the entire AVM. Subsequent changes in protocol showed a significant decrease in success with doses less than 25 Gy, and small improvements in obliteration rates but significantly more radiation-associated complications with higher doses. Optimally, we therefore treat most AVMs with 25 Gy at the margin.

As in microsurgery, when performing gamma surgery feeding arteries or draining veins should be left alone and only the nidus should be treated. In very large AVMs that were only partially treated because of the excessive dose necessary for optimal treatment, occasional cures have been achieved. This is thought to be due to fortuitous inclusion of all the pathologic shunts within the higher-dose treatment field. Targeting only the feeding vessels to the AVM has had very limited success because of recruitment of small, angiographically occult feeding arteries. However, the first patient ever treated had only the feeding vessels targeted, and a cure was obtained. The early success with this strategy has not been reproduced.

The results of gamma surgery on AVMs are affected by the minimum dose applied to the AVM and the size of the AVM. These two factors are interdependent. It has been shown that the limitation to the allowed marginal dose imposed by the size of the malformation decreases the rate of obliteration. Some reports contend that low-dose gamma

surgery with large malformations results in obliteration rates comparable with those in smaller lesions treated with a larger marginal dose. It is doubtful that these results will hold up in larger series. To date, in our experience larger AVMs have a lower obliteration rate.

Between 1970 and 1990, 880 patients were optimally treated. *Optimally* is defined as at least 25 Gy at the margin of the entire nidus of the AVM. The age range of these patients was 3 to 76 years; approximately 15% were pediatric patients (<17 years of age).

The presenting symptoms were hemorrhage (70%), seizures (16%), headache (5%), neurologic deficits not associated with acute hemorrhage (4%), and other (2%).

Most of the referrals were for AVMs deemed operable only with unacceptable morbidity, explaining the fact that 73% of the AVMs were located in deep areas of the brain (20% in the basal ganglia or thalamus, 16% around or within the ventricular system, 11% within the brain stem) or within eloquent cortex. Eighty-five percent were supratentorial, and of these, 62% were located on the right side, 37% on the left side, and 1% were centrally located.

In this series, the patients treated earlier were subjected to a vigorous protocol of repeated angiograms. Later, with the introduction of computed tomography (CT) and then MRI, angiography was not performed until the nidus was no longer evident on these screening examinations.

### IMAGING OUTCOME

Of the 880 patients treated, 461 had adequate angiographic follow-up (Table 50–2). Of these 461 patients, 80% were cured within 2 years. In patients with MRI examinations that showed no residual nidus, roughly one third were found on subsequent follow-up angiography to be cured, one third to be subtotally obliterated (no residual nidus but early filling vein present on angiography), and one third to be partially obliterated (nidus smaller but still present).

Angiographic changes precede obliteration. The diameter of the nidus as well as the feeding arteries and occasionally draining veins become smaller. The nidus decreases in size and the shunt is reduced. We have classified angiographic changes as either no change, partial obliteration (decrease in the size of the nidus) (Fig. 50–2), subtotal obliteration (no evidence of nidus but with a persistent early draining vein) (Fig. 50–3), and total obliteration (Figs. 50–4 to 50–6).

At the time of the last evaluation of our results, only 5% of patients who had had follow-up angiograms had no

### TABLE 50–2 ■ OUTCOME OF RADIOSURGERY FOR ARTERIOVENOUS MALFORMATIONS

| Series | No. of Cases | % Obliterated at 24 mo* |
|---|---|---|
| Bunge et al.† | 374 | 82 |
| Forster et al.[138] | 160 | 76 |
| Kawamoto et al.[139] | 144 | 70 |
| Kondziolka et al.[84, 133] | 402 | 71 |
| Steiner et al.[140] | 461 | 80 |

*Angiographically proven obliteration.
†H. Bunge, personal communication, 1993.

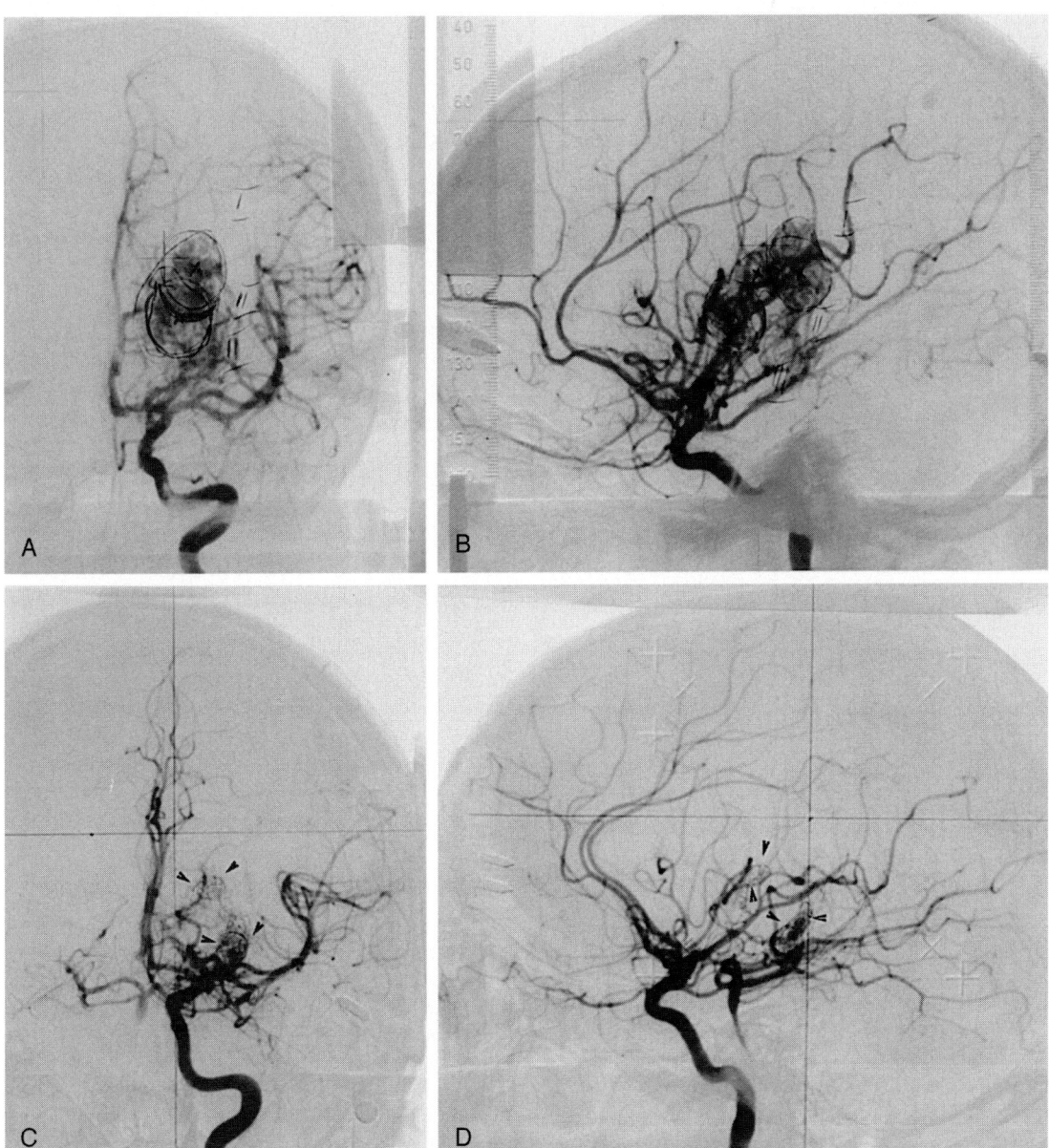

**FIGURE 50–2** ■ Partial obliteration of an arteriovenous malformation (AVM). Left sylvian AVM shown in the anteroposterior *(A)* and lateral *(B)* views of a left carotid angiogram. The same views 4 years later *(C and D)* show a decrease in the size of the nidus but persistent shunting of blood through the partially obliterated malformation *(arrowheads)*. The residual AVM was recently re-treated.

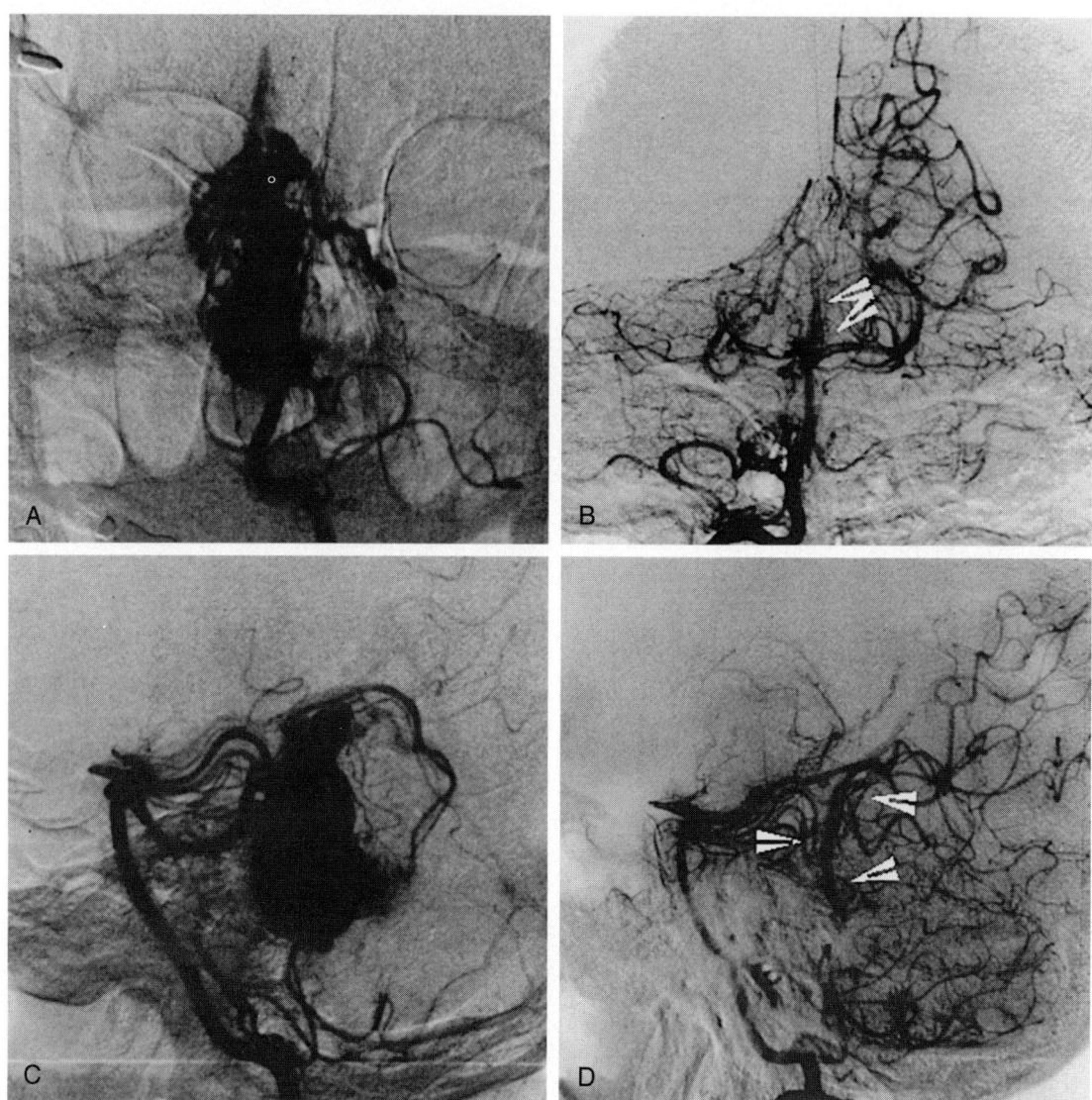

FIGURE 50–3 ■ Subtotal obliteration of an arteriovenous malformation (AVM) after gamma surgery. The anteroposterior *(A)* and lateral *(C)* vertebral angiograms demonstrate an AVM located within the vermis of the cerebellum. Control angiography with the same views *(B and D)* obtained 3 years after gamma surgery shows no demonstrable nidus but the presence of an early filling vein *(arrowheads).*

change in the status of their AVMs. Eighty percent were cured, 10% had subtotal obliteration, and 5% had partial obliteration. The angiogram should be complete and of high quality, and should be reviewed by an experienced and interested neuroradiologist or neurosurgeon. No patient with an angiographically proven obliterated AVM has ever hemorrhaged in our experience, nor has a patient with a subtotally obliterated AVM. Regardless of this, we do not consider a patient cured until he or she has total obliteration of the AVM. The early draining vein represents persistence of the shunt.

In this group of patients, obliteration rates were affected by the size of the nidus. The rate for AVMs less than 1 cm³ in volume was 88%. For 1 to 3 cm³, it was 78%, and for greater than 3 cm³, 50%.

Evaluation of patients treated suboptimally (periphery dose <23 to 25 Gy) shows a sharp decline in obliteration rates (Fig. 50–7). Doses greater than 25 Gy were associated with little improvement in obliteration rate.

Of the 1917 patients we have treated, 277 underwent embolization of the AVM before gamma surgery. Only 53 had follow-up angiograms. Of these, 43 (81%) were cured. The low rate of follow-up angiography in this subset is due disproportionately to evidence of flow voids on follow-up MRI scans. We are now undertaking a study of this subgroup, including patients treated up to 2 years previously. It is clear, however, that the ability of the embolization procedure to improve obliteration rates with gamma surgery depends on shrinking the size of the nidus. If embolization only decreases flow or splits the AVM into multiple portions, it is unlikely to alter the outcome of gamma surgery.

Gamma surgery was performed on 218 patients to treat residual nidus after microsurgery. Of these patients, 182 had an angiogram at 2 years after gamma surgery and 153 (85%) were cured.

The criticism has been leveled against radiosurgery series for AVMs reported in the literature that the results are

*Text continued on page 682*

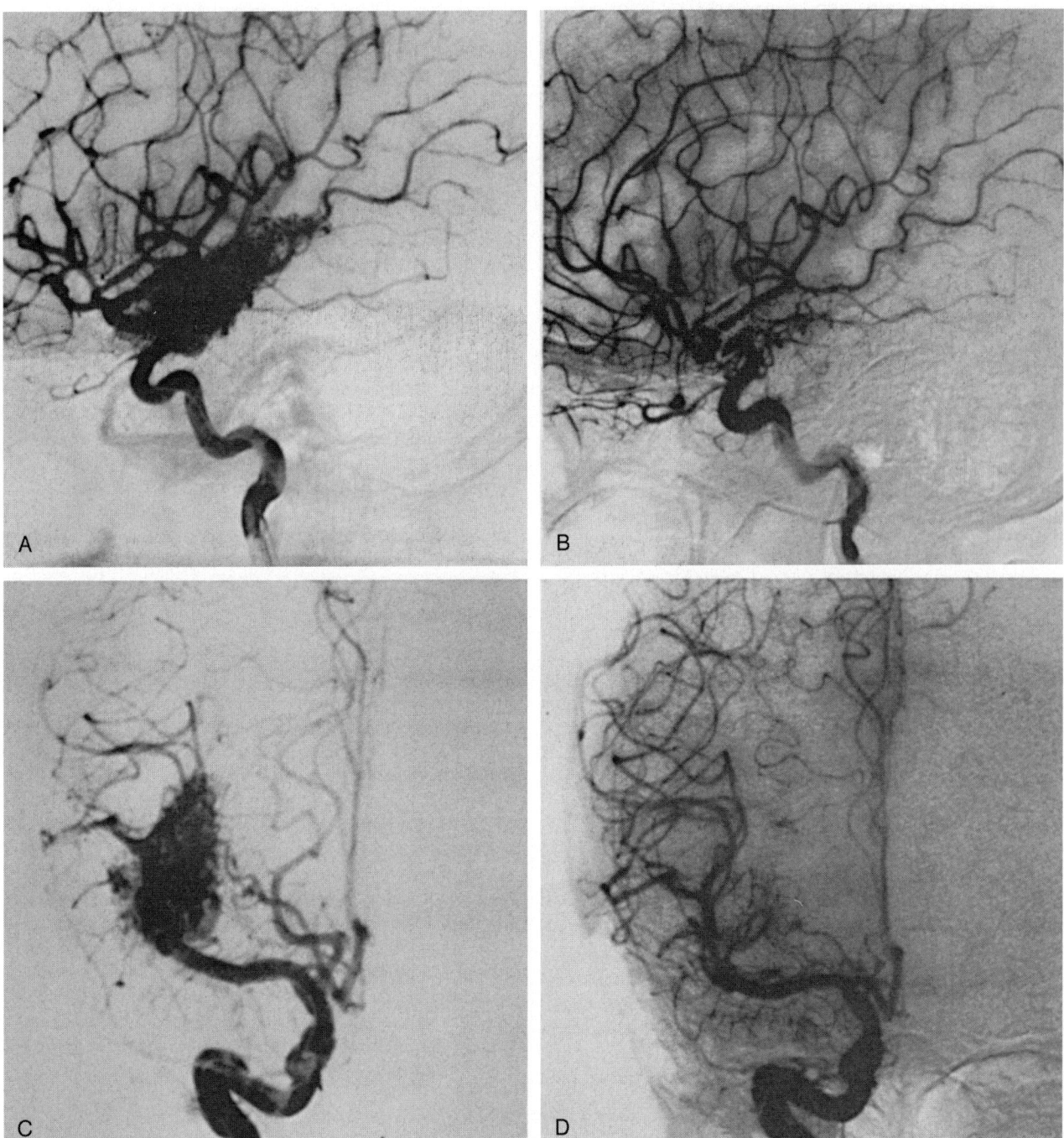

**FIGURE 50–4** ■ Total obliteration of an arteriovenous malformation (AVM) following gamma surgery. The AVM in the right sylvian region is shown after partial embolization in the *(A)* lateral and *(B)* frontal projections before and 2 years after gamma surgery, showing complete obliteration of the malformation in the *(C)* lateral and *(D)* frontal projections.

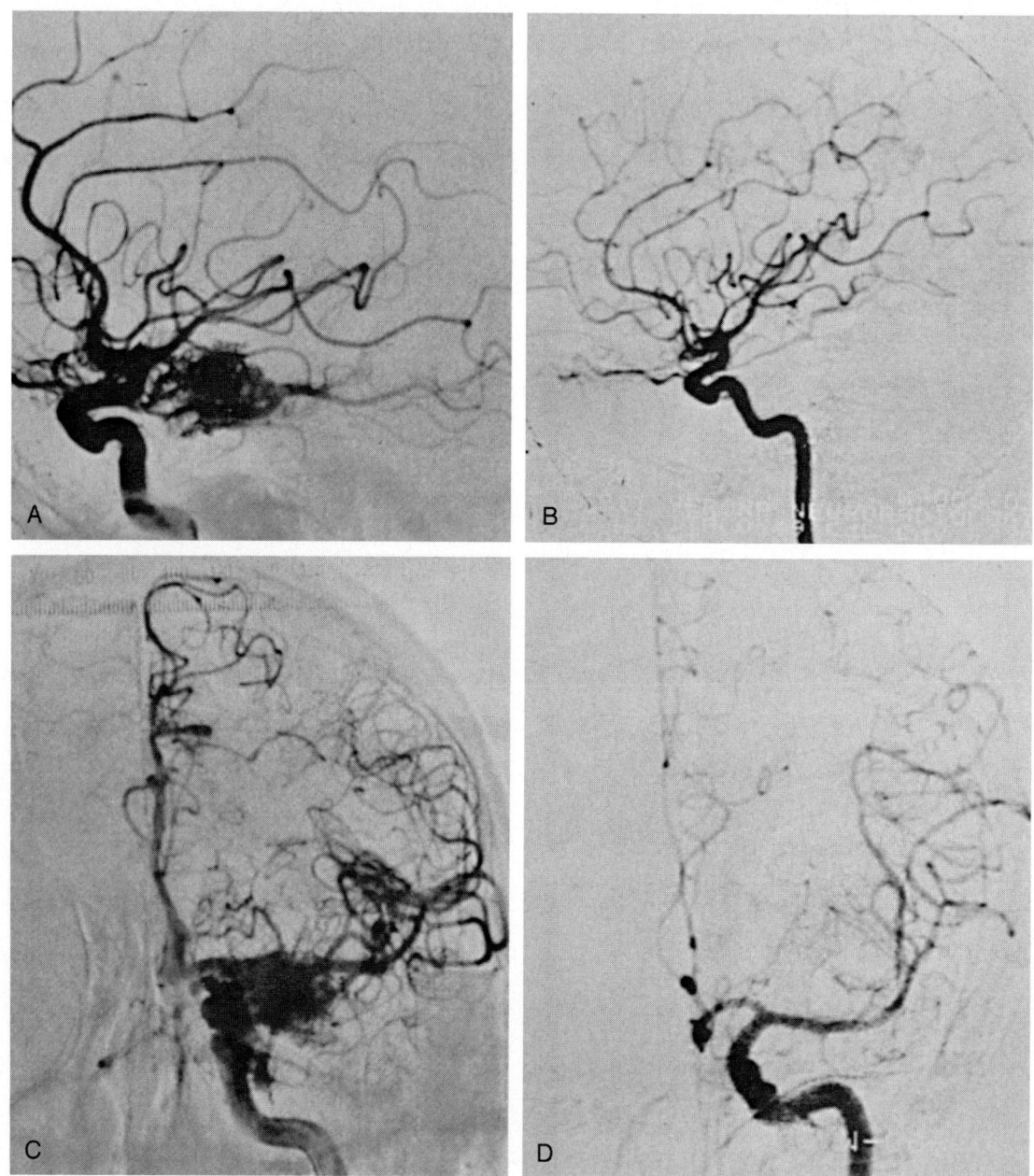

FIGURE 50–5 ■ Early obliteration of an arteriovenous malformation (AVM) following gamma surgery. This left internal carotid angiogram shows the lateral *(A)* and frontal *(B)* views of the malformation before and 6 months after *(C and D)* gamma surgery. In this case, early angiography was prompted by a magnetic resonance imaging scan, which showed no flow voids in the region of the treated AVM.

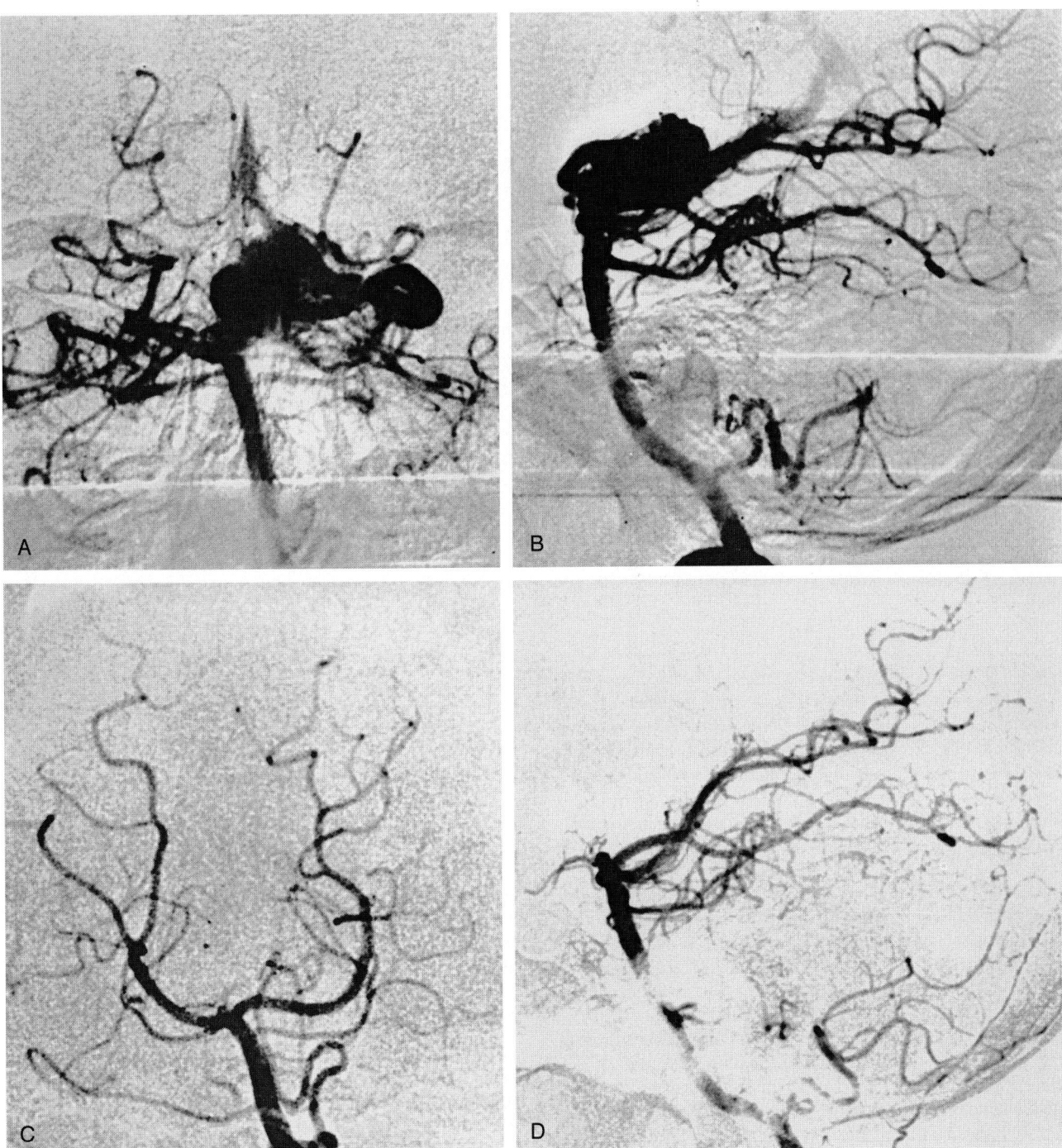

**FIGURE 50–6** ■ Obliteration of a midbrain arteriovenous malformation (AVM). Vertebral arteriogram showing frontal *(A)* and lateral *(B)* views before and 2 years after *(C and D)* gamma surgery. No neurologic deficit was present.

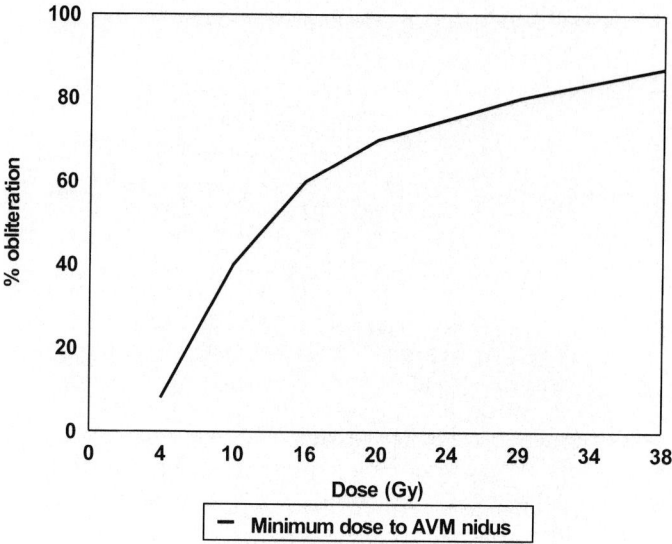

FIGURE 50–7 ■ The dose-response curve of arteriovenous malformations.

biased because angiography is performed only after there is no evidence of residual nidus on MRI. In addition, because the reported obliteration rate is for patients who had follow-up angiograms, the reported numbers are biased toward a favorable group. To a limited extent, this is true. Evaluation of the group of 880 patients showed that by assuming the worst-case scenario in which every patient with an MRI but not an angiogram was considered not cured, the final percentages of obliteration dropped by less than 1%.

## CLINICAL OUTCOME

A review of the long-term clinical outcome after gamma surgery was carried out on 247 patients we treated between 1970 and 1983.[52] The presenting symptoms varied widely, and 94% of the patients had hemorrhaged before therapy. Ninety-eight of these patients had chronic headaches, and 66% had complete relief after gamma surgery. An additional 9% improved. Twenty-six percent had seizures before therapy; 19% of these became seizure free and 51% improved. Eleven patients (5% of patients without a prior seizure) had at least one seizure after therapy. Resolution or significant improvement was also seen in 53 of 74 patients with motor deficits (72%), 19 of 46 with a sensory deficit (41%), 23 of 44 with memory disturbance (52%), and 26 of 35 with language dysfunction (74%).

We have analyzed in detail the outcome of seizures in our patients by questionnaire. Of 1200 respondents, there were 178 patients with seizures as a preoperative symptom. At the time of analysis, 62% were seizure free, with almost half of these off medication. An additional 24% were improved.

The cause for clinical improvement after gamma surgery in such a large number of patients is unknown. The natural tendency of neurologic deficits to improve over time must be presumed to play a major role. The improvement in regional blood flow after AVM obliteration may also be responsible for a portion of the gains made by the patients. Whatever the reason, significant improvement is seen in many patients.

## HEMORRHAGE RISK IN THE TREATMENT-RESPONSE INTERVAL

The annual incidence of hemorrhage in untreated AVMs is reported by various authors as between 2% and 5%. From research based on our own material, we reached several other conclusions: the risk of hemorrhage increases with age and is also higher in women during the fertile years.[46]

Whether gamma surgery without obliteration of the nidus provides partial protection from hemorrhage is still controversial. Some authors have demonstrated that there may be some degree of protective effect.[52–54] Because the incidence of hemorrhage in a matched group of untreated patients will likely never be known, and the timing of obliteration is not known except as occurring between diagnostic scans, it is a difficult position to support.

The incidence of hemorrhage during the first 2 years after gamma surgery was studied in 1604 of our patients and reported by Karlsson and colleagues.[55] There were 49 hemorrhages, for an annual incidence of 1.4%. This is significantly lower than the generally accepted rate of 3% to 4% per year, but includes all 1604 patients, including those known and not known to have obliterated AVMs. Of these hemorrhages, 14 were fatal (annual rate of 0.4%) and 9 resulted in permanent neurologic deficits (annual rate of 0.3%).

In 113 patients with subtotal obliteration of the AVM,

## TABLE 50–3 ■ PERMANENT NEUROLOGIC DEFICITS AFTER RADIOSURGERY FOR ARTERIOVENOUS MALFORMATIONS

| Series | Radiation-Induced Complications | Rebleeding |
| --- | --- | --- |
| Bunge et al.* | 4 | 5 |
| Sutcliffe et al.[132] | 3.8 | 3.8 |
| Kawamoto et al.† | 3.7 | 4.2 |
| Kondziolka et al.[133] | 3.1 | 5.2 |
| Steiner et al.[52] | 3.1 | 2.3 |

*H. Bunge, personal communication, 1993.
†S. Kawamoto, personal communication, 1994.

we observed no hemorrhages. No hemorrhage occurred during 948 risk years (average, 8.5 years). Assuming a natural risk of hemorrhage of 4%, there should have been 34 hemorrhages in this interval. These observations should be tested on larger patient populations before final conclusions are made.

## COMPLICATIONS

Acute post-treatment nausea and vomiting occur occasionally and are not associated with any lasting effects. These may be treated symptomatically.

Rare seizures have occurred in our experience, all in the post-treatment period and in patients with a previous seizure disorder. None of our patients experienced a seizure while the head was secured in the gamma unit. However, this possibility should not be discounted because of the risk of cervical spine injury associated with the head being fixed in the unit.

The results of a series of 816 patients treated for AVMs with gamma surgery with follow-up CT (630 patients) or MRI (239 patients) showed white matter changes in a significant number of cases.[56] CT showed hypointensity changes in 11% of cases, and MRI showed increased signal on the $T_2$-weighted images in 37%. The higher percentage of changes in MRI scans reflects the higher sensitivity of this imaging modality. The earliest onset of these changes was 3 months, and 92% occurred within 15 months. Resolution of these changes was the usual course, on average within 5 months (range, 1 to 17 months; Fig. 50–8). Clinical symptoms were associated with these changes in 6% of the entire group and resolved completely in half. Therefore, 3% of patients had a fixed neurologic deficit after gamma surgery for AVM (Table 50–3).

A rare occurrence after gamma surgery for AVM is the development of an expansive cyst at or adjacent to an obliterated AVM, first reported in 1992[33] in 2 patients of a series of 40. We have seen this event twice in our material.

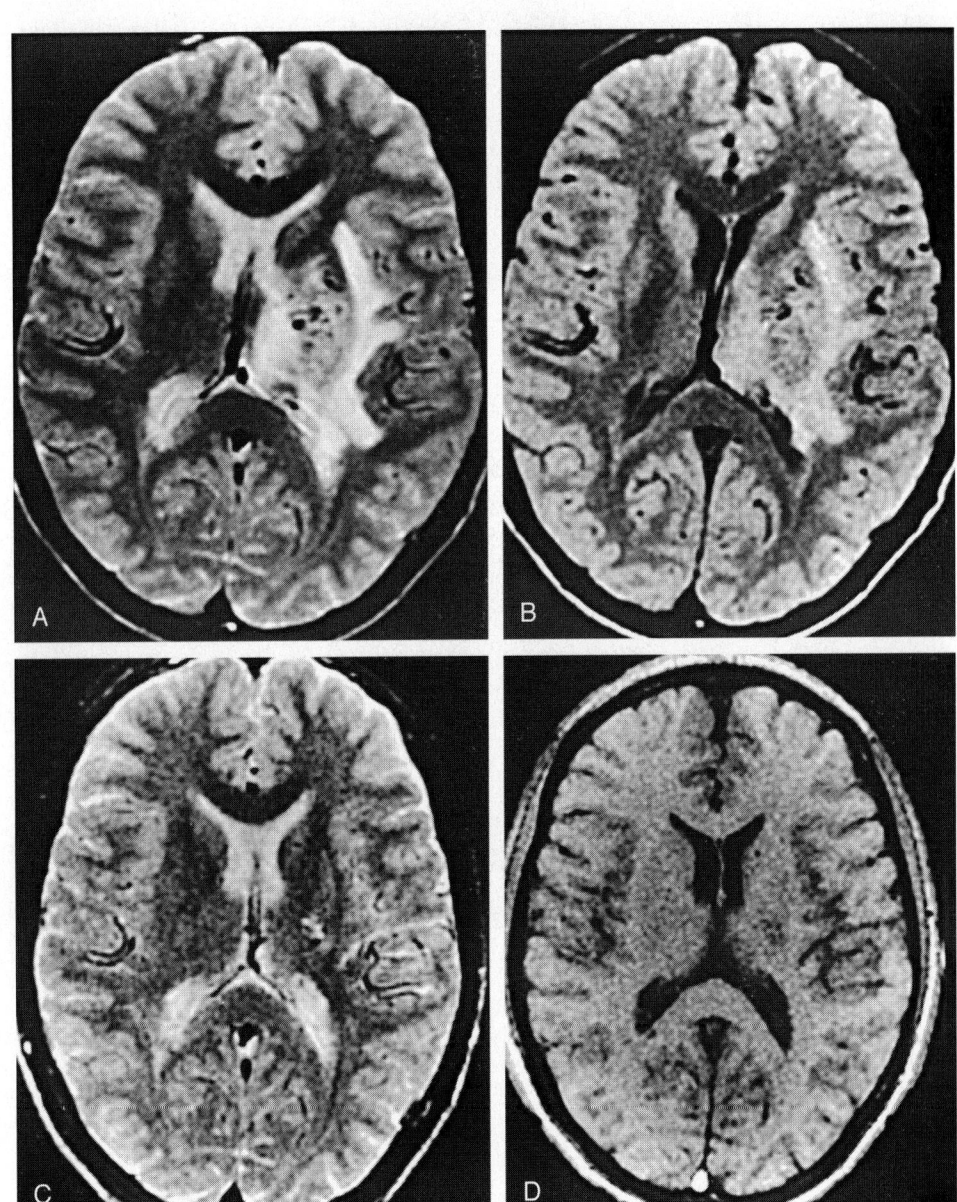

FIGURE 50–8 ■ The onset and resolution of radiation-induced changes of normal brain tissue. Radiation-induced changes 6 months after radiosurgical treatment of a left basal ganglia arteriovenous malformation (AVM) with a margin dose of 20 Gy. The appearance on $T_2$-weighted (A) and a $T_1$-weighted (B) MRI. These changes showed progressive regression of the AVM and its complete disappearance at 2 years after the onset (C and D). Angiography documented total obliteration of the AVM.

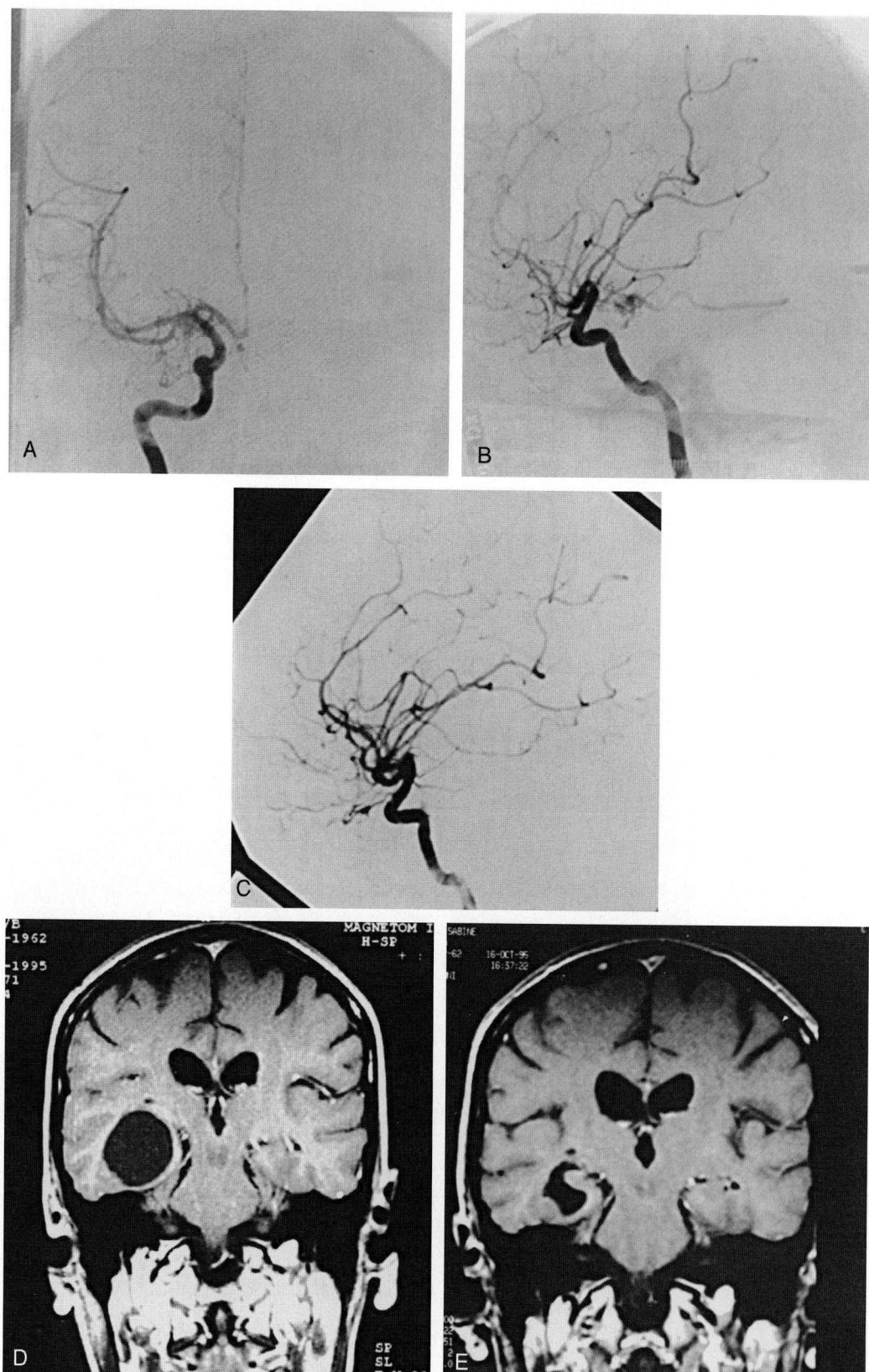

**FIGURE 50–9  ■**  The delayed occurrence of cyst formation following gamma surgery for an arteriovenous malformation (AVM). This small right-sided AVM visualized on anteroposterior (A) and lateral carotid arteriography (B) was cured as shown on this control angiogram, which was obtained 2 years after gamma surgery (C). The development of headaches and personality changes prompted a magnetic resonance imaging (MRI) examination 7 years after gamma surgery (D and E). This cyst was surgically decompressed. The biopsy of the cyst wall did not reveal any evidence of a tumor. (Follow-up MRI courtesy of Professor J. Camaert, Chairman, Department of Neurosurgery, Gent, Belgium.)

These occur 5 to 10 years after treatment and occasionally are symptomatic due to mass effect, requiring extirpation. The etiology of these cysts is unclear. We are aware of seven cases worldwide, five of which were operated on, usually because of mass effect. There was no evidence of malignancy in any of these cases. All those reported were in patients imaged solely by angiography at the time of treatment, and the condition of the surrounding brain at the time of gamma surgery was not documented by CT or MRI (Fig. 50–9).

## Dural Malformations

Dural malformations with or without associated AVMs are uncommon lesions. Optimal treatment is unknown, although reasonable cure rates can be achieved with smaller lesions using gamma surgery. Larger lesions, unless wholly inoperable, should be managed with at least partial open surgical or endovascular treatment before radiosurgery.

We have treated 58 dural malformations with gamma surgery. The incidence of cure decreased with increasing length of the fistula. Of the 19 fistulas under 15 mm in length, 10 had angiographic follow-up and 7 (70%) were cured (Fig. 50–10). Of those between 15 and 25 mm in length, six had adequate follow up and three were obliterated. There were 14 patients with lesions greater than 25 mm in length and 7 had angiograms, which showed 5 cures.

Three patients hemorrhaged after treatment (none with

neurologic deficit). In two of these patients, fistulas are still patent.

## Spontaneous Carotid-Cavernous Sinus Fistulas

Large, symptomatic fistulas require prompt intervention; endovascular treatment is often used. Ideally, treatment obliterates the fistula while maintaining patency of the carotid artery, but this often is not possible with endovascular techniques and certainly not with open surgical therapy.

We have treated nine patients with carotid cavernous sinus fistulas using gamma surgery. The age range was 20 to 62 years. There was no acute reversible symptomatology in these cases. Six of these patients have had follow-up angiography and five were found to be cured while maintaining carotid artery patency. Gamma surgery should be considered in the treatment of this entity when acute ablation of the fistula is not mandated by the clinical syndrome, and the eye is not threatened with excessive intraocular pressures.

## Vein of Galen Malformations

We have treated eight patients with vein of Galen malformations. The patients ranged in age from 4 to 72 years of age. Three are cured and two have shown partial obliteration by angiography (Fig. 50–11). One patient has no

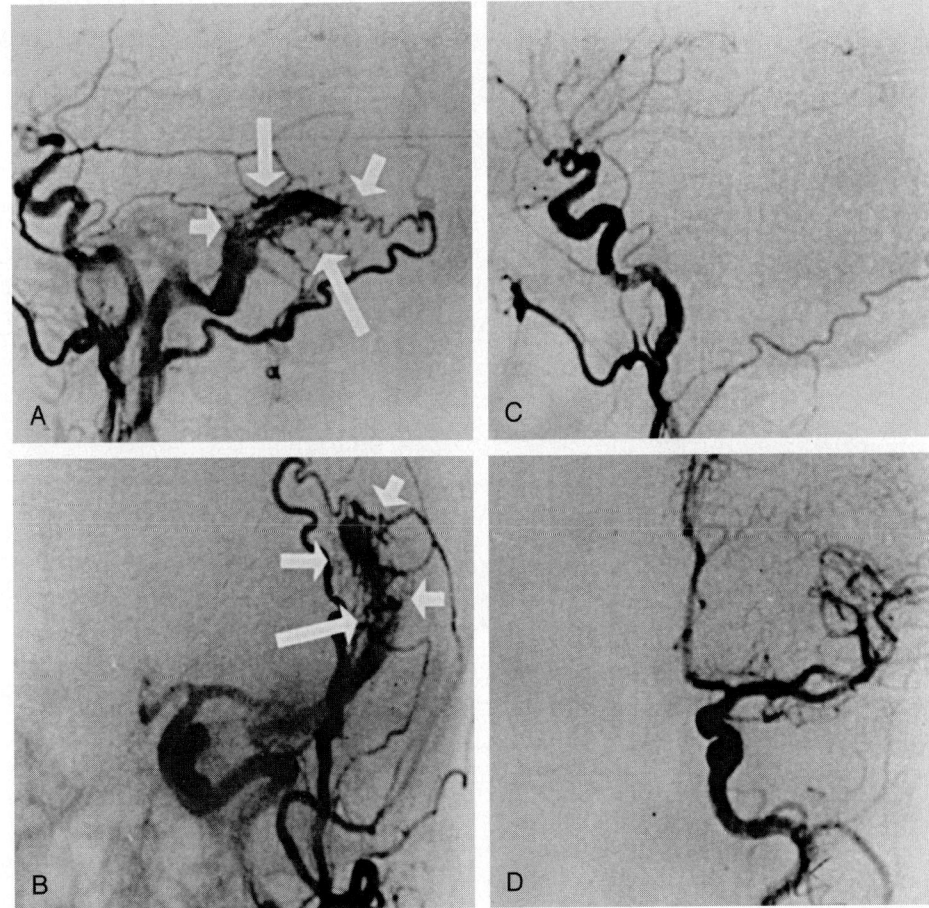

FIGURE 50–10 ■ Total obliteration of a dural arteriovenous malformation (AVM) following gamma surgery. Left common carotid angiogram lateral *(A)* and frontal *(B)* projections of a dural AVM in the region of the left transverse sinus. Complete obliteration is demonstrated at 2 years after gamma surgery in the lateral *(C)* and frontal *(D)* projections.

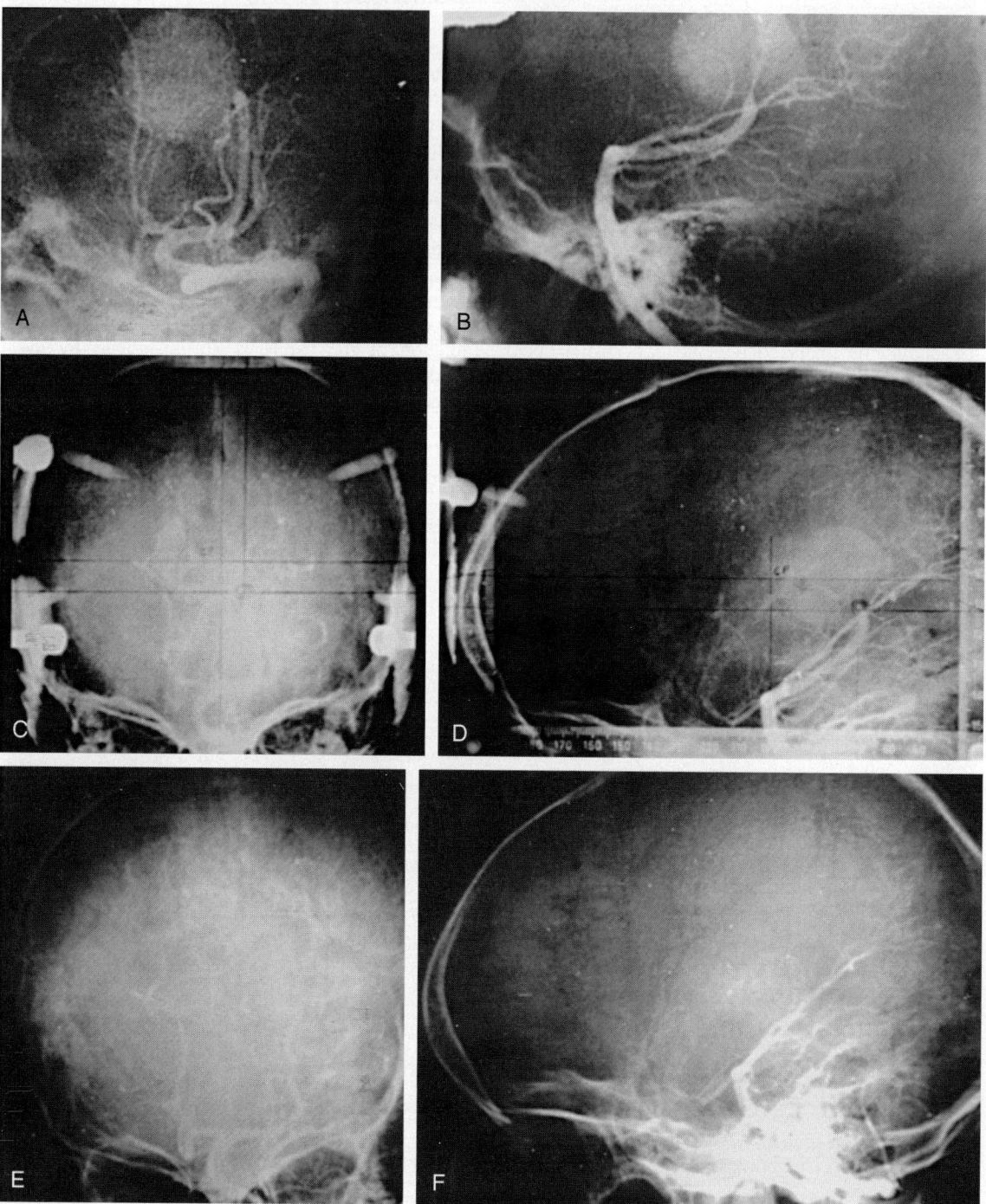

**FIGURE 50–11** ■ Gamma surgery for a vein of Galen malformation. Anteroposterior *(A)* and *(B)* lateral vertebral angiograms show direct shunting of blood into the primitive precursor (promesencephalic vein) of the vein of Galen. A stereotactic angiogram *(C* and *D)* obtained at the time of treatment is shown. Control angiography obtained 1 year later *(E* and *F)* demonstrate cure of the malformation. (Courtesy of Hernan Bunge MD, Clinica del Sol, Buenos Aires, Argentina.)

residual malformation on MRI and awaits confirmatory angiography, and another has had no recent follow-up imaging. One patient showed no response by MRI at 20 months.

## Cavernous Hemangiomas

The success in treating AVMs prompted the treatment of cavernous hemangiomas (angiographically occult vascular malformations [AOVMs]) with the Gamma knife. Their tendency to be small, with a lack of intervening normal brain tissue and relatively low rate of clinically significant hemorrhage, made cavernomas a natural target for the Gamma knife. The rate of hemorrhage for cavernomas is widely disparate in the neurosurgical literature, reported as between 0.1% and 32%.[57–61] This is largely due to semantic differences in defining a hemorrhage, with some authors counting the presence of a hemosiderin ring on MRI as evidence of a hemorrhage, and others recognizing only hemorrhages brought to attention by neurologic changes.

Gamma surgery of cavernous malformations appears to have a histologic effect on them that is not evident on imaging studies. In one patient,[62] a gamma surgery–treated cavernous hemangioma followed for 5 years showed no change on MRI studies. Histologic examination after surgical removal of the lesion showed it to be effectively obliterated (Fig. 50–12).

A total of 23 patients have been treated by us for cavernous hemangiomas, all between 1985 and 1996, 22 of whom are available for follow-up evaluation.[63] The patients presented either with epilepsy (6) or hemorrhage (16). The maximum treatment dose varied from 11 to 60 Gy (mean, 33 Gy). The minimum, or periphery dose, varied from 9 to 35 Gy (mean, 18 Gy).

Nine symptomatic hemorrhages occurred in this group after therapy, for an annual incidence of 8%. Four of these patients subsequently underwent surgery. There was a statistical trend ($P = .17$) for higher peripheral doses to be associated with greater likelihood of post-treatment

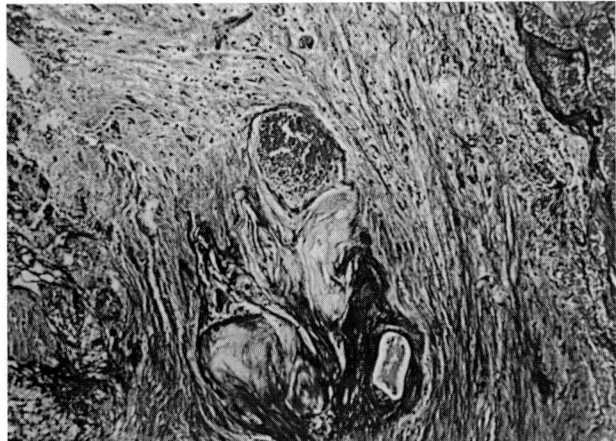

**FIGURE 50–12** ■ Hematoxylin and eosin–stained histologic section of a cavernous malformation that was treated with gamma surgery. Because no change was observed on serial magnetic resonance imaging examinations over 5 years, the lesion was excised. Except for a single persistent capillary channel (*arrow*), the malformation was obliterated.

hemorrhage. There was no relationship between lesion location and occurrence of hemorrhage.

Six patients experienced neurologic decline secondary to radiation-induced changes, which was permanent in five. Two also had a post-treatment hemorrhage. Radiation-induced changes were defined as radionecrosis or edema seen on CT or MRI associated with clinical decline. Two patients subsequently underwent surgery. Thus, the radiation-induced complication rate is 22%, nearly 8 times higher than expected for a similarly treated group of patients with AVM. As expected, there was a significant ($P = .005$) relationship between peripheral radiation dose and the occurrence of radiation-associated complications.

The high incidence of post-treatment hemorrhage and radiation-induced complications is greater than the expected morbidity rate from an untreated group. For this reason, the routine use of the Gamma knife in the treatment of cavernous hemangiomas cannot be supported at this time.

Published observations demonstrate a protective effect of gamma surgery on the rate of hemorrhage in these lesions. Based on 38 cases with AOVMs, Kondziolka and associates[64] maintain that radiosurgery offers benefit to these patients. They report that six patients (15%) had significant reduction in size, with a 13% hemorrhage rate; 10 of the patients (26%) had neurologic deficit, and two of these underwent surgery and succumbed to the illness. The rate of complications, combined with the fact that only 15% of the patients in this series had any reduction in the size of the lesion, does not, in our opinion, constitute grounds for justifying radiosurgery for an AOVM. Furthermore, their contention that the complications reported by us[65] may in part be due to the high doses used in treatment is not supported by their statistics with a lower dose.

These 38 patients were a part of a later report on 47 patients from the same authors detailing the outcome. They found a postradiosurgery annual hemorrhage rate of 8.8%, which, compared with the risk reported by the same authors at 0.6% to 4.5%, is high, even if the difference is not statistically significant. They chose, however, to compare their postradiosurgery hemorrhage rates with the preradiosurgery rate in the same subjects, making the assumption that the rate could be based on an epoch starting from first observation or first hemorrhage. This is fallacious, because the malformation was present before the presenting hemorrhage and most likely from birth. Recomputed on this basis, the preradiosurgery annual bleed rate comes to 5.9%, which is more congruent with the expected natural history. Once again, the incidence of hemorrhages postradiosurgery seems spuriously higher. It is certainly unlikely that radiosurgery could increase the propensity to or frequency of hemorrhage, but it seems to offer no protection, or some protection at a high cost of side effects.

## Developmental Venous Anomalies

The natural history of developmental venous anomalies (previously called *venous angiomas*) is benign,[66] and clearly they are not surgical lesions. Before clear elucidation of this prognosis, we treated 19 patients for this entity. One patient was cured and three had partial obliterations.

Three patients had radionecrosis and one had symptomatic edema. One patient with radionecrosis underwent subsequent débridement. A 5% cure rate with a 30% complication rate for a benign entity is unacceptable.

## TUMORS

Treatment of tumors with gamma surgery introduces a new approach to the evaluation of the end point of treatment. Unlike microsurgery, no actual debulking of tissue occurs, and in the short term there are no visible changes. Success is, therefore, established by a pattern of reduced tumor size or a lack of growth over serial follow-up studies.

In an attempt to eliminate some of the subjectivity of naked-eye observations and the obvious fallacy resulting from the estimation of a three-dimensional object on the basis of three linear measurements in orthogonal planes, we have developed software at the University of Virginia Neurosurgical Visualization Laboratory that allows estimation of lesion volume based on MRI or CT images. The procedure involves scanning the study into a computer program and outlining the pathologic area in each slice. The computer then measures the area within the contour and calculates a volume based on slice thickness; the process is repeated for each slice and the total volume calculated by integrating the individual slice volumes. The error of this method was estimated by scanning balloons filled with a known volume of fluid, and it was found to be ±0.5% to 2% for tumors greater than 1 cm$^3$ and up to ±7% for tumors less than 1 cm$^3$, provided the study slice thickness remains below 7.5 mm. We now require all follow-up studies to be performed with a slice thickness of 3 mm with zero overlap or gap between adjacent slices. Even though the technique of volume estimation has a high level of accuracy, we prefer to ignore changes of less than 15% as insignificant.

### Pituitary Adenomas

The efficacy of radiation in the treatment of pituitary adenomas was well documented before gamma surgery was used for this disease.[67, 68] Reduced fractionation techniques had been shown to have effectiveness in the treatment of Cushing's disease and were the impetus for the use of

radiosurgery. MRI has replaced less exact, invasive localization procedures (cisternography) and CT in the planning of gamma surgery in patients with pituitary adenomas. There still remain difficulties with the use of gamma surgery. The periphery dose that can be delivered for macroadenomas is limited if optic nerve structures are in contact with the tumor. Localization of microadenomas can be difficult with even the best MRI examinations, and amelioration of hypersecretory syndromes is delayed.

One of the best indications for gamma surgery for secreting or nonsecreting pituitary adenomas is residual tumor that is not removable with microsurgical techniques (i.e., within the cavernous sinus). If it is known before microsurgery that the cavernous sinus is involved and a debulking procedure is considered, then every effort to clear the tumor away from the optic nerves and chiasm should be made to make postoperative gamma surgery more effective. A suprasellar approach should be considered if there is doubt that this can be accomplished through a transsphenoidal approach. There is some difficulty in differentiating residual tumor from postoperative changes on MRI, but this cannot be helped. A thorough operative note concerning any foreign material or grafts left behind is important, as well as a high-quality preoperative scan for comparison.

Another indication for gamma surgery is persistence or recurrence of elevated hormone levels after microsurgery. In either instance, the tumor that cannot be removed, either because of its location or inability to localize the tumor within the sella, may be treated by gamma surgery. Tumor in the cavernous sinus can be treated as with other macroadenomas. Difficulty in localizing the tumor usually requires targeting all the contents within the sella. If the patient has already undergone aggressive microsurgical treatment, he or she is often already experiencing panhypopituitarism. If not, this is a possible complication of gamma surgery. If the patient has a secreting microadenoma but the symptomatology is not urgent, and microsurgery is for some reason not considered, then gamma surgery can be used as the primary therapy.

### Results

We have treated 202 pituitary tumors, all macroadenomas and locally invasive (Table 50–4). There were five malignant tumors. All had been previously treated one or more times by some other modality. Microsurgery alone was used in 90.3%, radiation therapy and microsurgery in 8.2%,

TABLE 50–4 ■ OUTCOME FOR GAMMA SURGERY FOR PITUITARY ADENOMAS

| Tumor Type | No. | Size Decreased | Unchanged | Increased | Endocrine Remission |
|---|---|---|---|---|---|
| Nonsecreting | 30 | 19 | 10 | 1 | — |
| Secreting | 77 | 50 | 19 | 8 | — |
| Growth hormone | 21 | 18 | 3 | 0 | 43% |
| Prolactin | 16 | 11 | 3 | 2 | 44% |
| Corticotropin-releasing hormone | 36 | 19 | 11 | 6 | 57% |
| Pleurihormonal | 4 | 2 | 2 | 0 | — |
| Total | 107 | 69 | 29 | 9 | — |

and radiation therapy alone in 1.5%. Tumor volume ranged from 0.9 to 32 cm³, with an average volume of 11 cm³.

Tumors were treated with a maximum dose of 6 to 60 Gy (average, 37.5 Gy). This discrepancy is due to variations in patient profile. Patients who had received previous radiation therapy or had a tumor close to the optic apparatus received in general lower doses. Newer software (Gamma Plan) allows for very specific shielding of the optic nerves and chiasm, and this has allowed for higher doses to be given when these structures are nearby. Periphery doses ranged from 3 to 28 Gy (average, 15 Gy).

### NONSECRETING TUMORS

We have treated 53 nonsecreting pituitary tumors, 30 of which have had radiographic follow-up after a minimum of 6 months and an average of more than 2 years. Of these, 19 (63%) showed a decrease in tumor volume. Ten had no change in the size (34%), and one increased in size (3%). The only indication we have to date for treating these tumors is for postoperative residual tumors to lower the incidence of tumor progression or progression in spite of previous radiation therapy. Only one tumor that we have treated has increased in size, demonstrating the efficacy of gamma surgery for these indications.

### CORTICOTROPIN-RELEASING HORMONE–SECRETING TUMORS

Fifty-nine patients with corticotropin-releasing hormone (CRH)-secreting tumors have been treated by us. These tumors had all been treated with microsurgery before consultation. Radiographic follow-up is available for 36 of these patients and shows a decrease in the size of the tumor in 19 cases (53%), no change in 11 (30%), and an increase in 6 (17%). Because most CRH-secreting tumors are symptomatic and potentially very dangerous because of hypercortisolism, the control of endocrine abnormalities is a more important measure in tumor control than size. In 52 cases, endocrine follow-up evaluation is available. In 57%, cortisol levels decreased, in 37% they were unchanged, and 6% had increased levels.

The results from 35 patients treated at the Karolinska Institute have been reported.[69] Of the 29 patients who were followed for up to 9 years, 22 had normalization of their endocrine abnormalities, 10 within 1 year and the remainder within 3 years.

### GROWTH HORMONE–SECRETING TUMORS

We have treated 59 patients with growth hormone–secreting tumors. Endocrine follow-up is available for 38 of these patients. There was normalization in 43% of cases and no change in 57%. No patient had an elevation in growth hormone level.

### PROLACTIN-SECRETING TUMORS

Of the 22 prolactin-secreting tumors treated by us at Virginia, 16 have had radiographic follow-up of 6 months or more. Eleven (69%) had a decrease in the size of their tumor, three were unchanged (19%), and two showed an increase in size (12%). Endocrine follow-up was available for all 22 patients. There was remission in 44% of cases and no change in the remaining 56%.

## Craniopharyngiomas

Craniopharyngiomas are very difficult tumors to treat. Their histologically benign behavior is misleading. The near impossibility of resecting them completely and their usual location in and around the hypothalamus make them difficult to cure. Various medical therapies have been used in the treatment of craniopharyngiomas. Microsurgery, intracystic instillation of radioisotopes, radiation therapy, and now radiosurgery have all been used. Long-term evaluation of patients with craniopharyngiomas is available after various treatment protocols.[70, 71] The general consensus is that as complete a surgical resection as possible, without creating significant morbidity, should be performed; this is followed by radiation therapy and gives reasonable long-term survival. The ill effects on children after receiving fractionated brain irradiation are well known.[72–76] Good results with resection alone have been achieved, but only in the hands of a few neurosurgeons. Even so, long-term results in children with subtotal resection followed by radiation therapy have been shown to be superior to complete resection alone,[70] and the deficits incurred with aggressive surgery can be considerable.

Gamma surgery as an adjunct to microsurgical resection has been used in lieu of or in addition to radiation therapy at several centers. The instillation of radioisotopes into large, nonloculated cystic components of the tumor and gamma surgery for the solid portion is the treatment policy for craniopharyngiomas at our center (Fig. 50–13).

We have treated 31 craniopharyngiomas in Virginia with gamma surgery, some of whom were reported on earlier.[77] Maximum dose was 25 to 50 Gy (average 34.2) with a periphery dose of 9 to 16.7 Gy (average of 13 Gy). Since the introduction of more advanced software for planning treatment, shielding has been incorporated for the treatment of all lesions in this region to protect the optic apparatus and uninvolved hypothalamus. This has become more refined with the introduction of more sophisticated planning systems (Gamma Plan software), but the maximum dose in all cases was kept below 8 Gy.

Of the 31 patients, two patients died at 6 and 15 months after gamma surgery. Three of the tumors increased in size, and one has unchanged. Five (16%) disappeared radiographically, and 19 (61%) decreased in size. One patient was lost to follow-up (Figs. 50–14 and 50–15).

Several other series using gamma surgery in the treatment of craniopharyngiomas have been reported,[78, 79] with results similar to ours. As larger series with longer follow-up times become available, it is likely that gamma surgery will either take the place of less discriminate radiation therapy or be a useful adjunct to it.

## Meningiomas

Meningiomas are usually benign, circumscribed tumors that arise from the coverings of the central nervous system

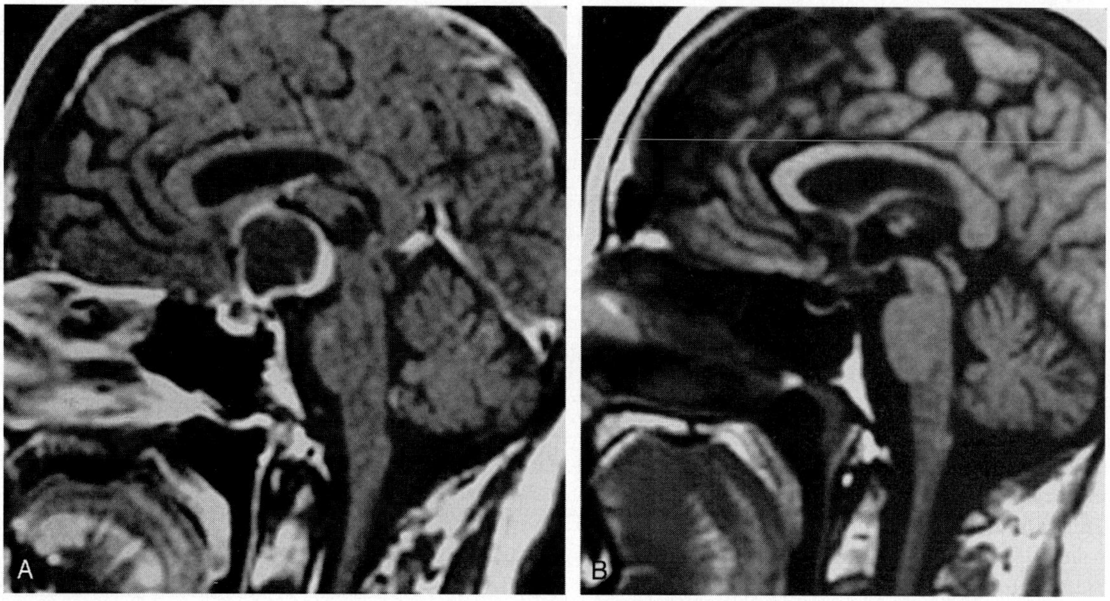

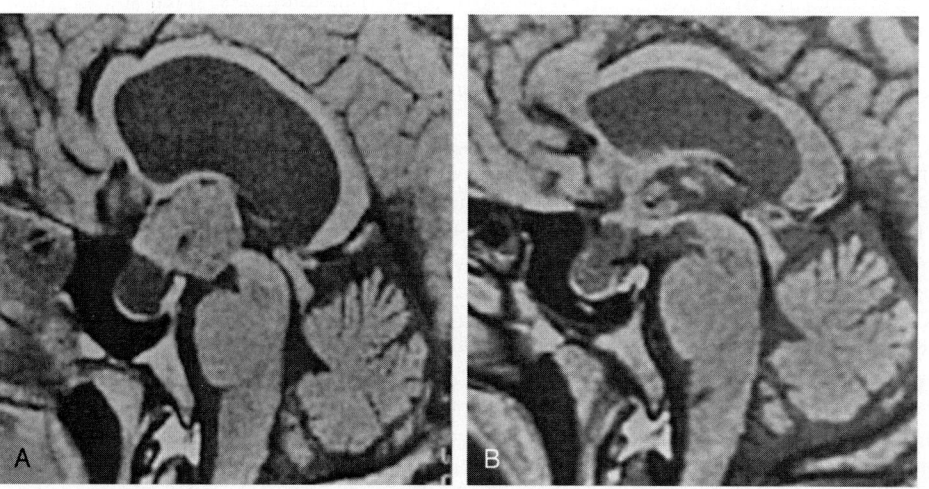

**FIGURE 50–13** ■ Craniopharyngioma shown in a post-contrast $T_1$-weighted saggital magnetic resonance imaging (MRI) scan *(A)* 12 months after gamma surgery and stereotactic instillation of $^{32}P$ *(B)*. The most recent follow-up MRI is taken after 5 years and the tumor decreased 73% in size.

**FIGURE 50–14** ■ Craniopharyngioma treated with gamma surgery following three microsurgical resections. A sagittal $T_1$-weighted magnetic resonance imaging (MRI) scan of a suprasellar craniopharyngioma in a 34-year-old man *(A)* demonstrating a marked reduction at 30 months after radiosurgery *(B)*. The patient recovered his visual acuity; his visual field defect resolved; and he returned to his job as a policeman.

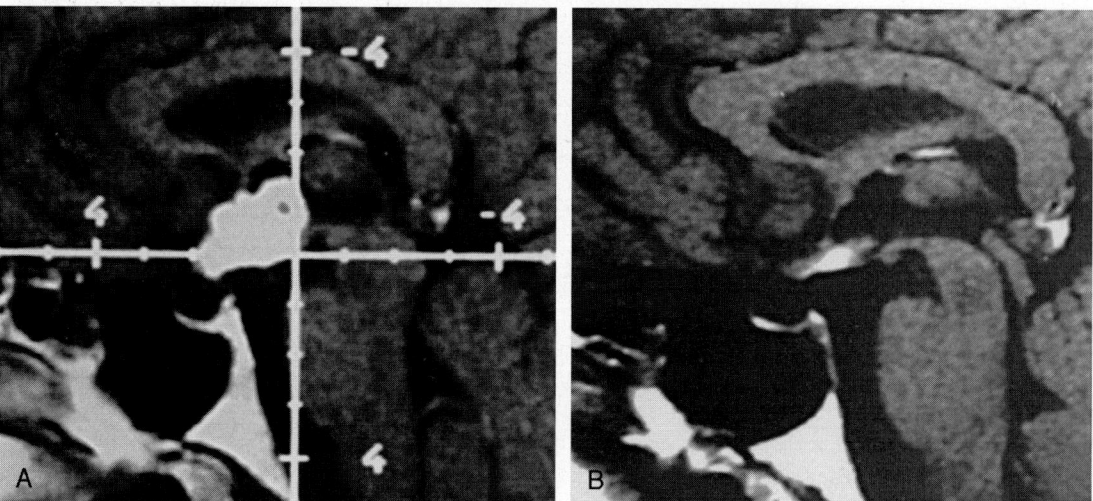

**FIGURE 50–15** ■ Reduction in size of a craniopharyngioma treated with gamma surgery. Residual craniopharyngioma following microsurgery was treated with the gamma knife. Contrast-enhanced $T_1$-weighted images before *(A)* and 4 months after *(B)* treatment. The size of the tumor was greatly reduced. The patient has a normal neurologic examination and endocrine profile.

and therefore tend to be superficial. Because of these attributes, microsurgical extirpation of the entire tumor as well as any involved meninges is the treatment of choice. Unfortunately, many meningiomas do not have one or more of the aforementioned attributes. Aggressive, locally invasive tumors, especially those invading or involving critical or difficult-to-control neural or vascular structures, and those at the skull base, can be problematic to remove completely. The use of radiation to lower recurrence rate after microsurgical removal of meningiomas was shown to be beneficial.[80–82] Recurrence rates were found to be dramatically decreased, and for patients with residual tumor after surgery, the progression of tumor growth was significantly decreased (Table 50–5).

We have treated 329 meningiomas at the University of Virginia since 1989. The most recent evaluation of our material was for 206 patients with a follow-up of 1 to 6 years. Tumor volume ranged from 1 to 32 cm$^2$. These patients received an average maximum dose of 38 Gy (range, 20 to 60 Gy) and an average periphery dose of 14 Gy (range, 10 to 20 Gy). There were 142 patients treated for residual tumor and 64 treated with gamma surgery primarily. Radiographic follow-up was available for 151 patients. Of the evaluated patients, 94 (63%) showed a decrease in the volume of their tumor of greater than 15%. No change in size was seen in 40 (26%), and an increase in size was seen in 17 (11%). The results of other centers reported in the literature are similar[83–85] (see Table 50–3).

Tumors in the cavernous sinus can be difficult to remove microsurgically without significant morbidity. Residual tumor attached to still patent vascular or neural structures can be targeted with gamma surgery, permitting less radical microsurgical resection and a lower morbidity rate.

In our group of meningiomas treated by gamma surgery, 112 were within the cavernous sinus. In 68%, the tumor either disappeared (Fig. 50–16) or shrank, in 30% it remained the same size, and in 2% it grew larger. Petroclinoid meningiomas involving the cavernous sinus were not included in this series and will be evaluated in the future.

We now have long-term follow-up of 10 to 21 years in 31 meningiomas treated with the Gamma knife. Two thirds of these tumors have either shrunk significantly or remained stable (Fig. 50–17).

We have begun to obtain a stereotactic angiogram before gamma surgery for large tumors. This allows treatment to include the vascular supply for large tumors when ideal treatment is not possible because of radiation dose constraints imposed by the treatment volume. This has resulted in significant tumor shrinkage and a lasting effect even in the long term.

We had no clinical complications treating meningiomas. However, a tumor without a histologic diagnosis and with equivocal imaging characteristics in the pineal region was treated as a presumed meningioma, and bilateral edema of the basal ganglia occurred. This resulted in cognitive disturbances with incomplete recovery.

The primary therapy for meningiomas is microsurgery. The advantages of histologic diagnosis, debulking, and a reasonable chance of cure secure surgical extirpation as the procedure of choice for this tumor. The tumors most amenable to gamma surgery treatment are less than 10 to 15 cm$^3$ in volume. The ability of gamma surgery effectively to treat small tumors with low morbidity argues strongly, however, for minimizing morbidity during open procedures. The option to treat residual tumor in critical or hard-to-reach locations should temper the enthusiasm for total surgical removal. This is especially true in locations where complete meningeal resection is impossible and thus the chance of recurrence is high.

## Vestibular Schwannomas

Although this lesion has historically and incorrectly been referred to as an *acoustic neuroma*, we prefer the designation of *vestibular schwannoma*, which recognizes the anatomic and histologic origins of these tumors.[86] There may be no other disease about which the proper treatment arouses as much angst as the vestibular schwannoma. Neurosurgeons cite the series of surgeons with enormous experience removing these tumors to justify suboccipital removal, whereas otolaryngologists sacrifice the inner ear during the translabyrinthine approach in an attempt better to expose the facial nerve. Radiosurgery's proponents cite excellent tumor control and low morbidity, but must acknowledge that although the tumor often shrinks, it is still there and the long-term history remains unknown. Therefore, it is in the best interest of our patients that long-term outcome in patients treated with various modalities be evaluated openly, and that small series, anecdotal evidence, and personal beliefs not weigh too heavily in our minds.

## TABLE 50–5 ■ OUTCOME OF RADIOSURGERY FOR MENINGIOMAS

| Series | No. of Patients | Size | | | | Follow-Up (mo) | Complications | Improved |
| | | Slight Decrease | Significant Decrease | Increase | Unchanged | | | |
|---|---|---|---|---|---|---|---|---|
| Bunge et al.* | 16 | 3 | 0 | 1 | 7 | 6–36 | — | — |
| Forster et al.† | 3 | 2 | 0 | 1 | 0 | ≤24 | — | — |
| Kondziolka et al.[84] | 81 | 19 | — | 5 | 27 | 6–48 | 3 | 9 |
| Rähn et al.‡ | 82 | 11 | 1 | 3 | 8 | 3–120 | — | 12 |
| Steiner et al.§ | 151 | — | 94 | 17 | 40 | 6–252 | 0 | 12 |

*H. Bunge, personal communication, 1993.
†D. M. C. Forster, personal communication, 1993.
‡T. Rähn, personal communication, 1993.
§L. Steiner, refers to information in this chapter and reflects current data.

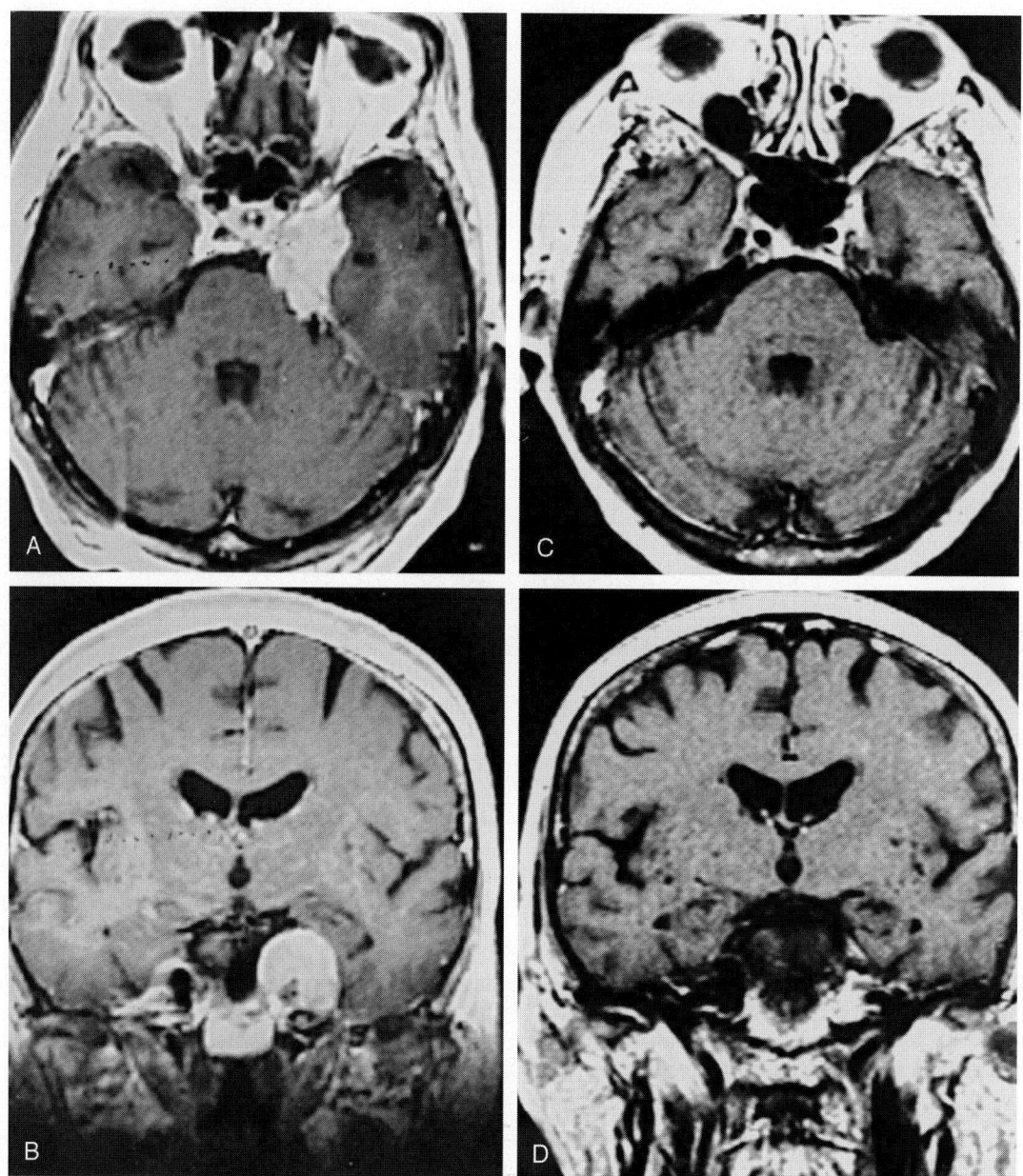

**FIGURE 50–16** ■ A large left parasellar meningioma residual after microsurgery is visualized on post-contrast $T_1$-weighted *(A)* axial and coronal *(B)* magnetic resonance imaging (MRI) scans. An MRI obtained 6 months following gamma surgery shows that the tumor has disappeared *(C and D)*. Repeated control MRI examinations for 5 years show no recurrence of the tumor.

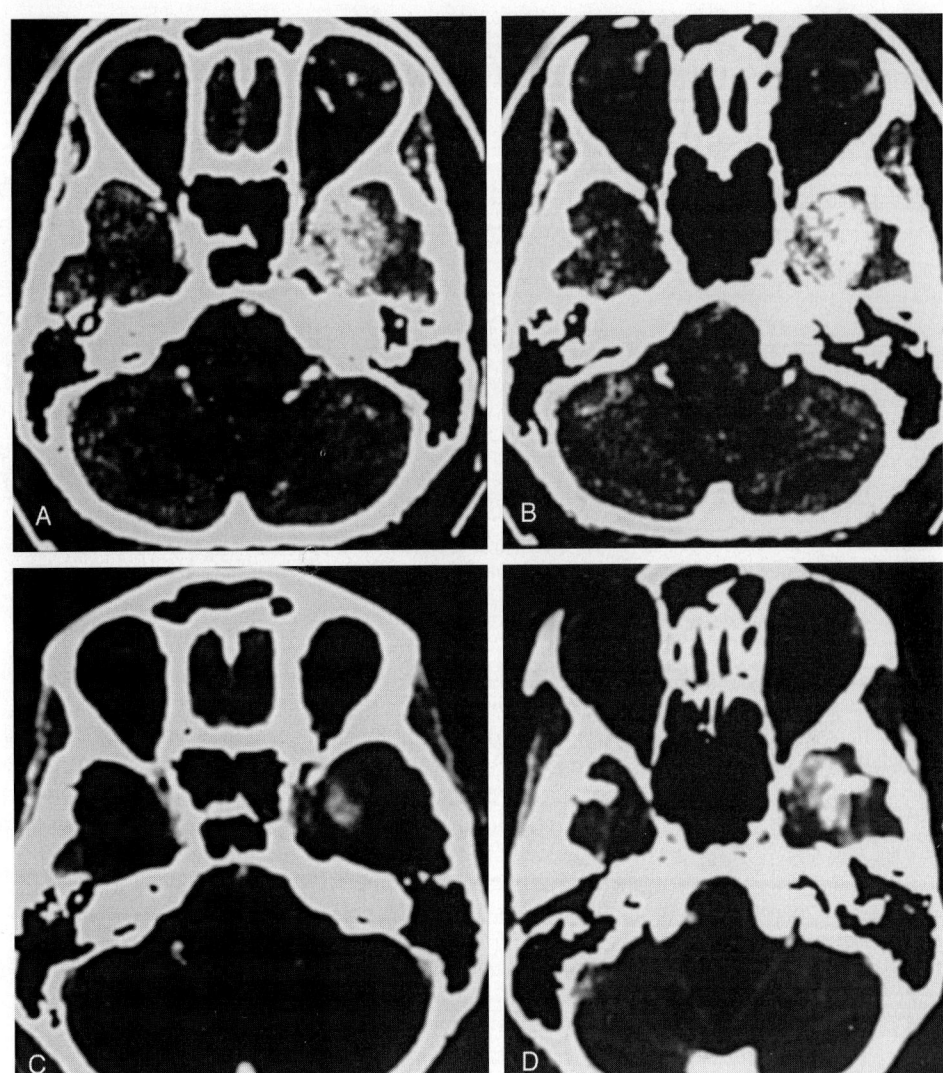

**FIGURE 50–17** ■ Long-term result of gamma surgery for meningioma. Computed tomography (CT) scans of a right parasellar meningioma treated with a tumor margin dose of 8.75 Gy *(A and B)*. The tumor regressed greatly in size, and the last follow-up 12 years after gamma surgery is shown *(C and D)*. The patient had complete relief from her pretreatment partial-complex (déja vù) seizures.

The first vestibular schwannoma treated with the Gamma knife was by Leksell and Steiner in 1969.[87] Since then, 8307 have been treated around the world through 1997. The clearest indications for gamma surgery for this tumor are in medically high-risk patients, for postoperative residual tumor, and when the patient refuses microsurgery. The usefulness of irradiation in the postoperative period was shown by Wallner and colleagues[88] in 1987; in their series, external-beam irradiation lowered the recurrence rate from 46% to 6%. By then, gamma surgery was already being widely applied to this disease under many circumstances.

The advent of MRI has made planning for this procedure much more exact. With a high-quality MRI scan and a relatively small tumor, the seventh cranial nerve can occasionally be visualized and carefully excluded from the treatment field. The trigeminal nerve can nearly always be identified except with the largest tumors, which in most cases should not be treated primarily with gamma surgery.

Small collimators are used to match better the isodose configuration to the size and shape of the tumor. We have had no brain stem–related complications. Previously, we used minimum periphery doses up to 20 Gy and maximum doses up to 70 Gy, but now use a margin dose of 11 to 15

Gy at the 30% to 50% isodose curve. The incidence of cranial nerve palsies rose considerably at the higher doses without significant improvement in tumor control.

We have treated 171 patients with vestibular schwannomas from 1989 to 1998. Ninety-four of these patients with greater than 6 months' follow-up have been reported.[89] Radiosurgery was the primary treatment in 62 of these patients and adjuvant (after microsurgery) in 45. The volume of the treated tumors ranged from 0.5 to 13.2 cm³.

Of the patients treated primarily with gamma surgery, a decrease in tumor size was seen in 76%, no change in 19%, and an increase in size in 5%. Among the 41 patients with a decrease in the size of their tumors, the decrease was greater than 75% in 6, 50% to 75% in 10, 25% to 50% in 10, and 15% to 25% in 15. It is our policy not to consider decreases in size of less than 15% significant. This is true of all tumors and vascular malformations that we treat. Duration of radiologic follow-up for these patients ranged from 1 to 7 years.

Of the patients treated with gamma surgery after microsurgery, a decrease in tumor size was seen in 68%, no change in 22%, and an increase in size in 10%. Among the 27 patients with a decreased tumor size, the decrease

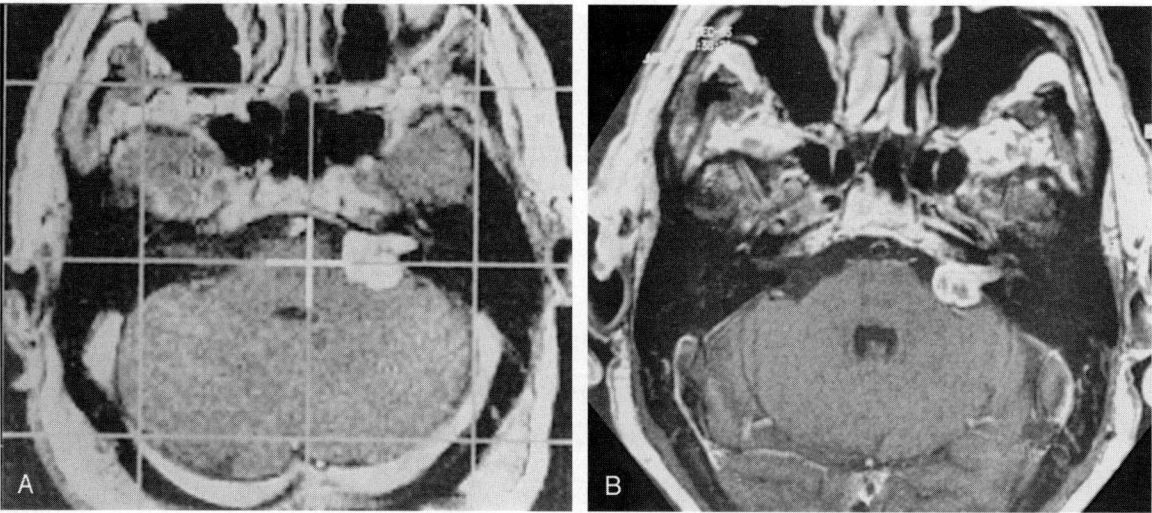

**FIGURE 50–18** ■ Reduction in the size of a vestibular schwannoma after gamma surgery. A contrast-enhanced T₁-weighted magnetic resonance imaging scan *(A)* of a left vestibular schwannoma, showing reduction in size 12 months after radiosurgery with a margin dose of 15 Gy *(B).*

was greater than 75% in 6, 50% to 75% in 5, 25% to 50% in 9, and 15% to 25% in 7 (Fig. 50–18).

Of the 171 patients we treated, there were 5 with transient changes in trigeminal sensation and 3 with facial paresis. One of the patients with facial weakness was operated on shortly after gamma surgery and was lost to follow-up. Another patient recovered completely in 6 weeks, and the third has nearly completely recovered at 10 months. The incidence of worsened hearing in our patients with useful hearing before gamma surgery was 9% at 2 years. Later evaluation of this complication with longer follow-up (manuscript in preparation) showed that approximately 60% of patients with useful hearing before gamma surgery lose it within 5 years, whereas 5% will actually experience an improvement. The reminder retain useful hearing.

Other centers report similar rates of tumor control, with no change or a decrease in tumor size in 89% to 94% of patients[17, 90] (Table 50–6).

Evaluation of the material from the Karolinska group included evaluation of radiographic changes in addition to size.[17] The most common change was loss of central enhancement in the tumor on contrast-enhanced MRI or CT images. This occurred in 70% of patients within 6 to 12 months after the treatment, although these changes were reversible. Another change that we have often seen is a transient increase in the size of the tumor during the first 6 months after gamma surgery. Such tumors then commonly regress to their original size or smaller (Fig. 50–19).

The previously published incidence of cranial neuropathies at other centers was 17% at Karolinska and 29% at Pittsburgh for facial paresis, which in most cases was transient or mild. The trigeminal nerve was affected in various ways in 33% at Pittsburgh, most commonly with a mild hypoesthesia. Complication rates at these centers are comparable with those in our series.

We have not seen one case of cerebellar edema or hydrocephalus requiring spinal fluid diversion after gamma surgery for vestibular schwannomas, but both of these have been reported elsewhere.[17, 90]

## Astrocytomas

The treatment of astrocytomas, whether low or high grade, is largely defined by the ability effectively to reduce the tumor burden and to lower the rate of recurrence. Except in the case of pilocytic astrocytoma, cure is rare. Classically, the goal of reducing tumor burden is obtained by gross total resection with a margin of "normal" brain when possible and postoperative radiation in cases with more malignant tumors. The indications for radiation therapy for intermediate-grade tumors, chemotherapy, repeat surgical debulking, and other therapies depend on several factors, many of which are not clearly defined. Into this cornucopia of choices, gamma surgery has been introduced. Intellectually, we have difficulty accepting the application of a focused technique for an infiltrative process. Nevertheless,

TABLE 50–6 ■ **OUTCOME OF RADIOSURGERY FOR ACOUSTIC NEUROMAS**

| Series | No. of Patients | Size | | | Follow-Up (mo) |
| | | *Decreased* | *Static* | *Increased* | |
| --- | --- | --- | --- | --- | --- |
| Kawamoto et al.* | 69 | 22 | 43 | 4 | 3–24 |
| Linskey et al.[134] | 89 | 20 | 65 | 4 | 4–36 |
| Norén et al.[17] | 209 | 121 | 56 | 34 | 2–206 |
| Prasad et al.[89] | 94 | 76 | 19 | 5 | 6–60 |

*S. Kawamoto, personal communication, 1994.

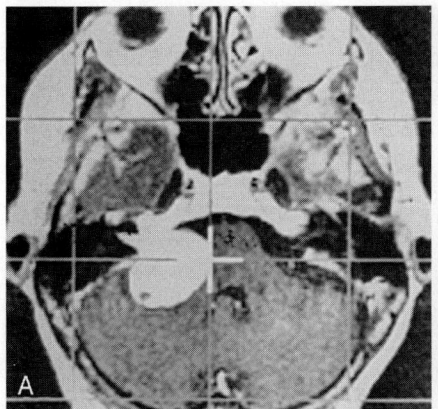 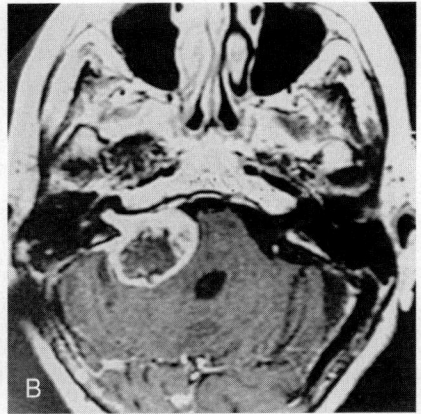 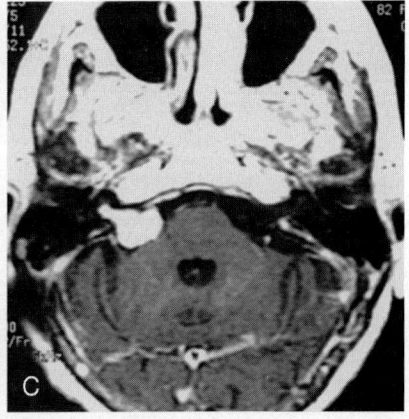

**FIGURE 50–19** ■ A right vestibular schwannoma with a volume of 9.3 cm³ shown on a post-contrast $T_1$-weighted axial magnetic resonance imaging (MRI) scan prior to gamma surgery *(A)*. The same lesion 6 months after treatment shows central nonenhancement and no change in the size of the lesion *(B)*. Thirty-six months after treatment, the lesion is again homogeneously enhancing and is significantly smaller (69%) *(C)*. Control MRI examinations for 6 years show that the lesion has remained stable.

recent results showing improved survival rates indicate that this negative attitude may be inappropriate.

In the case of low-grade tumors, gamma surgery can be used in place of surgical resection when the tumor is in an inaccessible location (e.g., brain stem) or when the patient chooses this alternative. The small size and relative circumscription of these tumors makes planning straightforward, and fairly good results have been obtained.

For high-grade tumors, gamma surgery may be used in several ways. If the tumor is small and in an inaccessible location (e.g., thalamus), gamma surgery is used to treat the tumor primarily. Focal or whole-brain irradiation is also used as an adjunct therapy. The incidence of radionecrosis is relatively high when aggressive protocols are used, and differentiating recurrence from this phenomenon can be problematic. Gamma surgery can also be used as an adjunct to surgical resection. The incidence of residual postoperative tumor is unfortunately not uncommon after "total" surgical resections, and care is often taken when the tumor abuts eloquent brain not to create neurologic deficit even at the expense of incomplete gross tumor resection. In

these cases, gamma surgery can be used to treat the residual tumor. Whole or focal radiation therapy has been used to lower the recurrence rate after these surgical therapies have been undertaken.

## Results

### LOW-GRADE ASTROCYTOMAS

We have treated 56 benign astrocytomas. The general indication was a deep-seated tumor not amenable to surgical resection or for which the patient insisted on gamma surgery.

We have treated 15 patients with grade I astrocytomas with greater than 1 year's follow-up available. Tumor size proved important, with best results in patients with a tumor volume of less than 3 cm². Of these patients, the tumor disappeared in one case (7%), shrank in eight (53%), and increased in six (40%; Fig. 50–20). Two patients subsequently underwent surgery, one for an increase in tumor size and one for a hemorrhage and radiation-induced

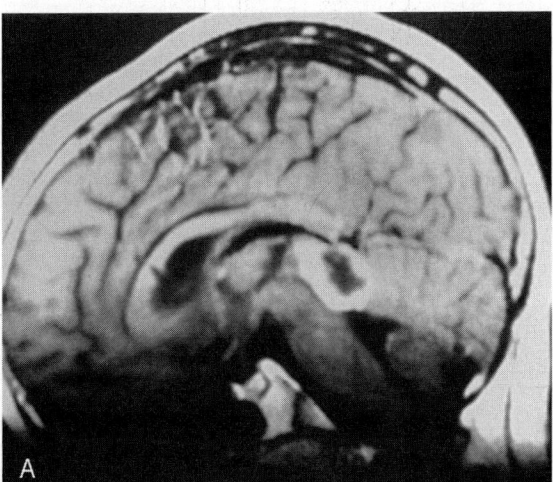 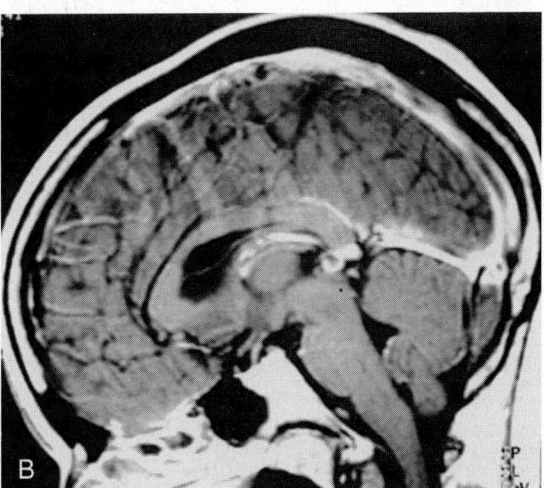

**FIGURE 50–20** ■ A pilocytic astrocytoma is shown on a post-contrast $T_1$-weighted sagittal magnetic resonance imaging (MRI) scan *(A)*. Annual control MRI examinations were obtained, and the latest made 9 years after gamma surgery is shown *(B)*.

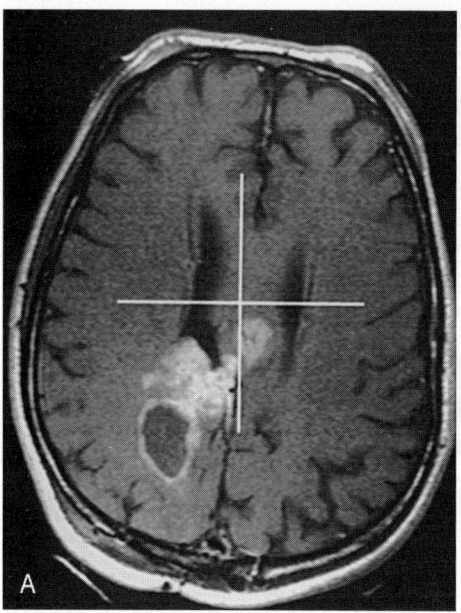
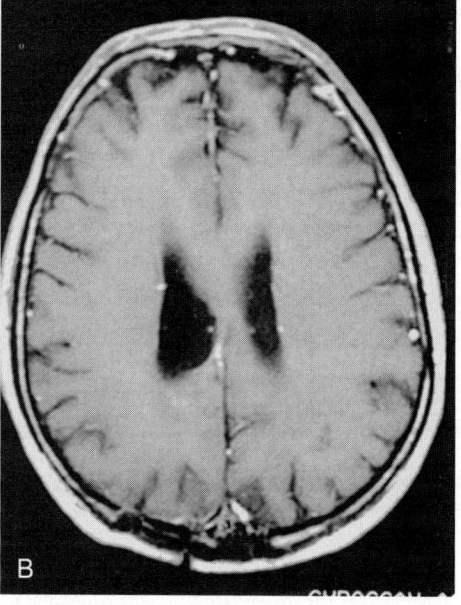

**FIGURE 50–21** ■ A post-contrast T$_1$-weighted axial magnetic resonance imaging (MRI) scan demonstrating a right parietal glioblastoma multiforme and associated cyst on post-contrast T$_1$-weighted axial MRI *(A)*. The same patient 11 months after gamma surgery shows complete radiographic disappearance of the lesion *(B)*.

changes. In two patients, a cyst associated with the tumor enlarged while the solid portion became smaller. One of these patients is the only patient to have had a decline in neurologic function after gamma surgery.[91]

We have follow-up of over 1 year for 17 patients operated on for grade II astrocytomas. Three (18%) disappeared, seven (41%) shrank, two (12%) remained unchanged, and five (31%) increased in size. One patient died from progression of his disease at 46 months after treatment. No relationship was found between pretreatment tumor size and outcome. These results are similar to those of other reported series.[92]

### HIGH-GRADE ASTROCYTOMAS

We have treated 56 malignant astrocytomas. Our experience has been similar to that of other reported series,[93, 94]

with most patients showing an initial decrease in size or remaining stable for a period (Fig. 50–21); however, recurrence and progression are the rule with these tumors, and no therapy is curative. Because of the differences in histologic type and the wide variety of therapies and protocols available for these tumors, it is difficult to judge the benefit of gamma surgery. Although we have observed a statistically significant prolongation of life expectancy in the group of patients undergoing radical tumor debulking, radiation therapy, chemotherapy, and gamma surgery (24 months versus 6 months for biopsy and radiation therapy), we doubt these results will be borne out in a larger series. The limit of the benefit that radiation can contribute to the treatment of these lesions seems to have been reached; hence, it is assumed that dose escalation with the Gamma knife in the treatment protocol of this disease will only marginally change the clinical outcome.

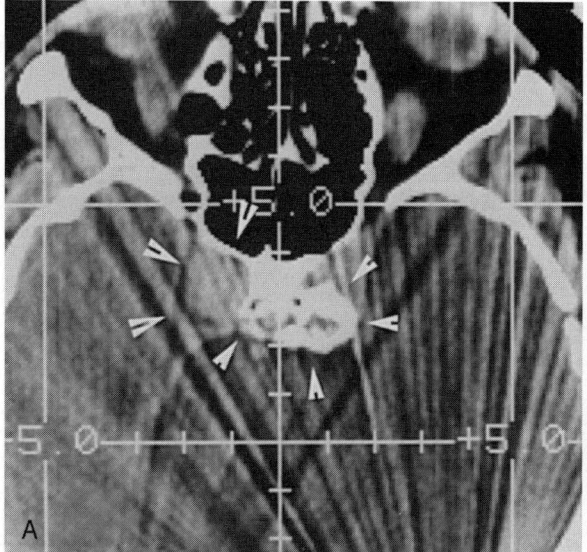
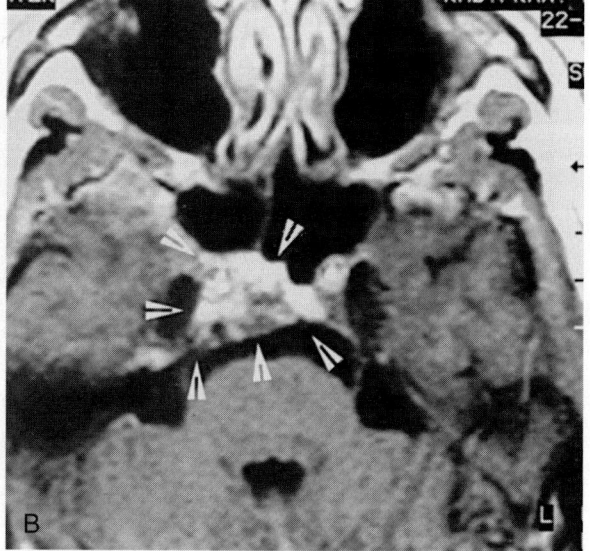

**FIGURE 50–22** ■ Gamma surgery for a residual chordoma. A post-contrast axial computed tomography image at the time of treatment *(A)*. A post-contrast T$_1$-weighted axial magnetic resonance imaging (MRI) scan obtained 7 years after gamma surgery demonstrates a 35% reduction in tumor volume *(B)*.

## Chordomas

Chordomas at the level of the clivus or elsewhere in the skull base are difficult to remove surgically and have a high recurrence rate. The use of postoperative radiation with heavy particles was shown to be associated with a significant increase in long-term survival but with only a modest reduction in tumor size.[95, 96]

We treated 10 patients with chordomas, with follow-up greater than 2 years available in 6. Two tumors shrank (Fig. 50–22), two increased in size, and the remaining two are unchanged.

Linear accelerator–based radiosurgery results for chordomas have been published. Thirteen patients followed for an average of 32 months (range, 4 to 80 months) were evaluated. All but one patient, who died of tumor progression at 4 months, were alive. The rate of local tumor control was 69% (tumor unchanged or smaller) and there was one significant complication (pituitary dysfunction requiring replacement therapy).[97]

## Chondromas and Chondrosarcomas

These are rare tumors in the skull base. We have treated four chondromas and seven chondrosarcomas with gamma surgery. Response in some cases was very good (>50% reduction in size), and none has progressed over a follow-up of 1 to 5 years (Fig. 50–23).

Muthukumar and colleagues[98] treated 15 patients (9 with chordomas and 6 with chondrosarcomas) with gamma surgery and reported their results with an average follow-up of 4 years. Four of their patients had died; only two deaths were related to progression of disease, and both of these had progression outside of the treated area. Only one of the surviving 11 had tumor progression, and five had shrunk. Gamma surgery seems to be a reasonable treatment alternative for these tumors, but longer follow-up times and larger series are required before definitive statements can be made.

## Metastatic Tumors

Except for solitary lesions, the treatment of metastatic brain tumors is primarily palliative. In cases of solitary metastasis long-term survival is not unknown, although in general the guiding philosophy is palliation, aiming at reversal of neurologic deficits and maintenance of quality of life. There has been some disagreement regarding the total number and volume of tumors that can be treated with gamma surgery in cases of multiple metastases. Our general guideline is not to treat more than three if that is known to be the case. We have treated more, but usually when additional lesions were discovered on the treatment MRI. The integral dose that the remainder of the brain receives is difficult to determine when making more than one treatment plan. Studies indicate that treating more than three lesions at the same time increases the integral dose to the brain to levels requiring lowering of the prescription dose to the individual lesions, thus reducing the efficacy of the treatment.[99] However, given the limited survival expectation in these patients, the pertinence of a rigid consideration of the integral dose is debatable.

If metastatic deposits are spatially located very far from one another, treating them all with the same frame placement may be difficult because of the space limitations within the treatment helmet. This needs to be taken into account when considering placement of the frame.

Surgical extirpation of a solitary brain metastasis has been shown significantly to prolong survival if the primary disease is controlled. Likewise, whole-brain irradiation has been show to be of benefit for some tumor types. These conclusions and the well-defined limits, both physical and radiographic, of most metastatic lesions make them very amenable to gamma surgery. For these reasons, as well as the high incidence of these lesions, the treatment of metastatic tumors is a frequent indication for gamma surgery worldwide.

Most reports of gamma surgery for metastatic tumors report a 7- to 10-month survival after treatment[100–103] (Table 50–7). The authors do not divide the patients whose tumors had shrunk from those that were unchanged. The histologic types, radiation dosages, and previous treatments vary considerably in the literature. Most centers use a maximum dose of at least 50 Gy and a periphery dose of 28 to 30 Gy. These doses are adjusted down if whole-brain irradiation has already been given, although dose reduction for tumors that appear after whole-brain irradiation may not be necessary or desirable. The use of adjuvant whole-brain

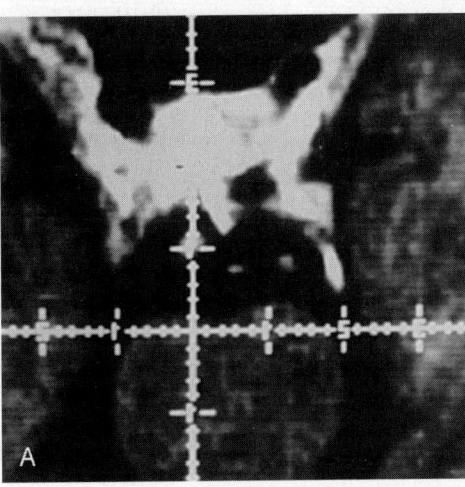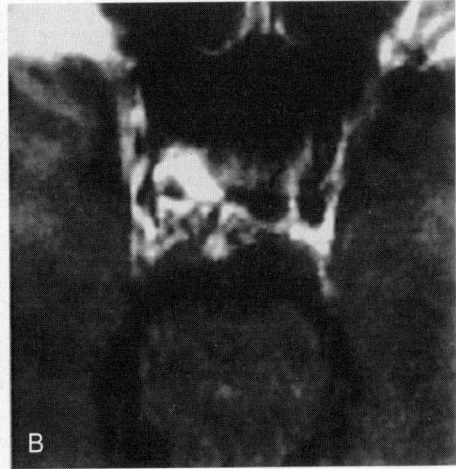

FIGURE 50–23 ■ Gamma surgery for a residual chondrosarcoma. Computed tomography scans of a 32-year-old man with a postoperative residual chondrosarcoma in the sellar region before (A) and 18 months after (B) gamma surgery. Note the regression in the size of the residual. The patient has no neurologic deficits.

TABLE 50–7 ■ **OUTCOME OF GAMMA SURGERY FOR METASTATIC TUMORS**

| Series | No. Metastatic Lesions | % Decreased/Unchanged | % Increased | Median Survival (mo) |
|---|---|---|---|---|
| Shiau et al.[106] | 219 | 82* | 16 | 10 |
| Baardsen et al.[135] | 45 | 90 | 10 | 17 |
| Young[136] | 669 | 91 | 9 | 7 |
| Gerosa et al.[137] | 343 | 88† | 12 | 9.5 |
| Kihlstrom et al.[103] | 105 | 94 | 6 | 7‡ |

*At 6 months (93% for lesions treated with >18 Gy).
†At 12 months.
‡Mean survival.

irradiation is empiric in some instances. There has been no benefit shown for melanoma, and if these lesions are treated, they should either be extirpated or treated with gamma surgery. For tumors with a propensity toward multiple brain metastases (e.g., most lung carcinomas), whole-brain irradiation may be appropriate. The relative benefit for each histologic tumor type and the role of gamma surgery for single or multiple metastases await detailed analyses of large series of patients.

We have treated 226 patients for metastatic tumors to the brain. Individual histologic types were analyzed only in a few instances. Evaluation of our series demonstrated an 83% control rate for treated lesions (disappeared, shrunk, or unchanged without recurrence) and a median survival of 7 months. Eleven percent disappeared, 63% shrank, and 10% were unchanged (Figs. 50–24 and 50–25). Sixteen percent increased in size. The usual cause of death was systemic disease.

The various primary tumor types in some instances have been evaluated separately. A series of 17 patients with 30 renal cell carcinoma metastases to the brain was evaluated (manuscript in preparation) and treated by us at the University of Virginia. The average survival was 15 months. An unmatched control group of 10 patients who received external-brain radiation therapy had an average survival of 5.5 months. Factors associated with longer survival in the group treated with gamma surgery included a higher Karnofsky performance status, absence of extracranial metastases, adjuvant whole-brain radiation therapy, and prior surgical resection. Surprisingly, size and number of metastases did not have a significant effect on survival, although in cases of a single metastasis with controlled local disease, long-term survival could be achieved (Fig. 50–26).

Of 32 metastatic melanomas treated by Somaza and coworkers,[104] 97% disappeared, shrank, or remained unchanged. Average survival in their series was 9 months, with systemic disease the cause of death in almost all cases. Three patients remained alive at 13 to 38 months after gamma surgery. Seung and colleagues[105] treated 55 patients with 140 metastatic melanomas and reported an average survival just short of 8 months. Freedom from progression was seen in 89% of tumors at 6 months and 77% at 1 year. Survival was related inversely to total tumor burden and less to the number of metastases.

A large series of patients with metastatic disease to the brain was reported by Shiau and associates.[106] They showed that melanomas had shorter freedom-from-progression intervals than other histologic types (e.g., adenocarcinoma, renal cell carcinoma), and that certain imaging characteristics were associated with survival. Multivariate analysis showed that longer control of treated lesions was significantly associated with higher prescribed dose, a homoge-

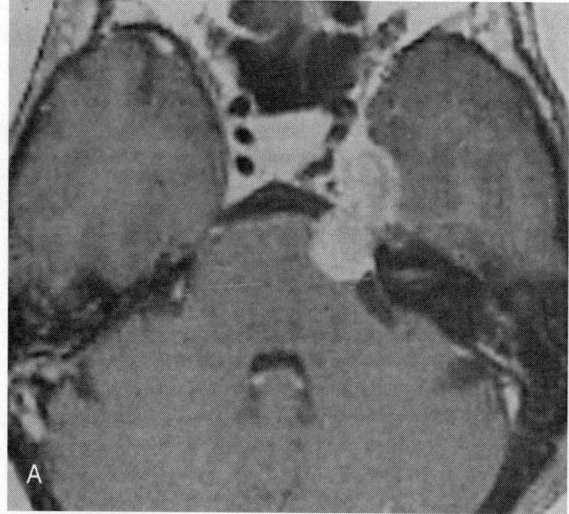
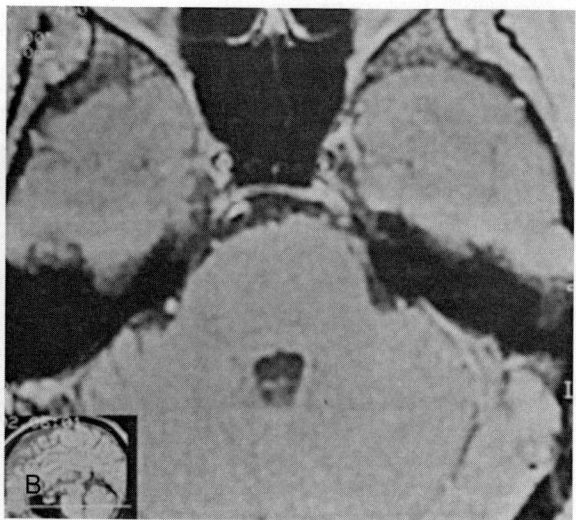

FIGURE 50–24 ■ A patient with a metastasis from breast carcinoma to the region of Meckel's cave and the gasserian ganglion. A contrast-enhanced T₁-weighted magnetic resonance imaging (MRI) scan before *(A)* and 6 months after *(B)* gamma surgery. Total regression of the tumor occurred, and 4 years after the treatment the latest MRI reveals no tumor.

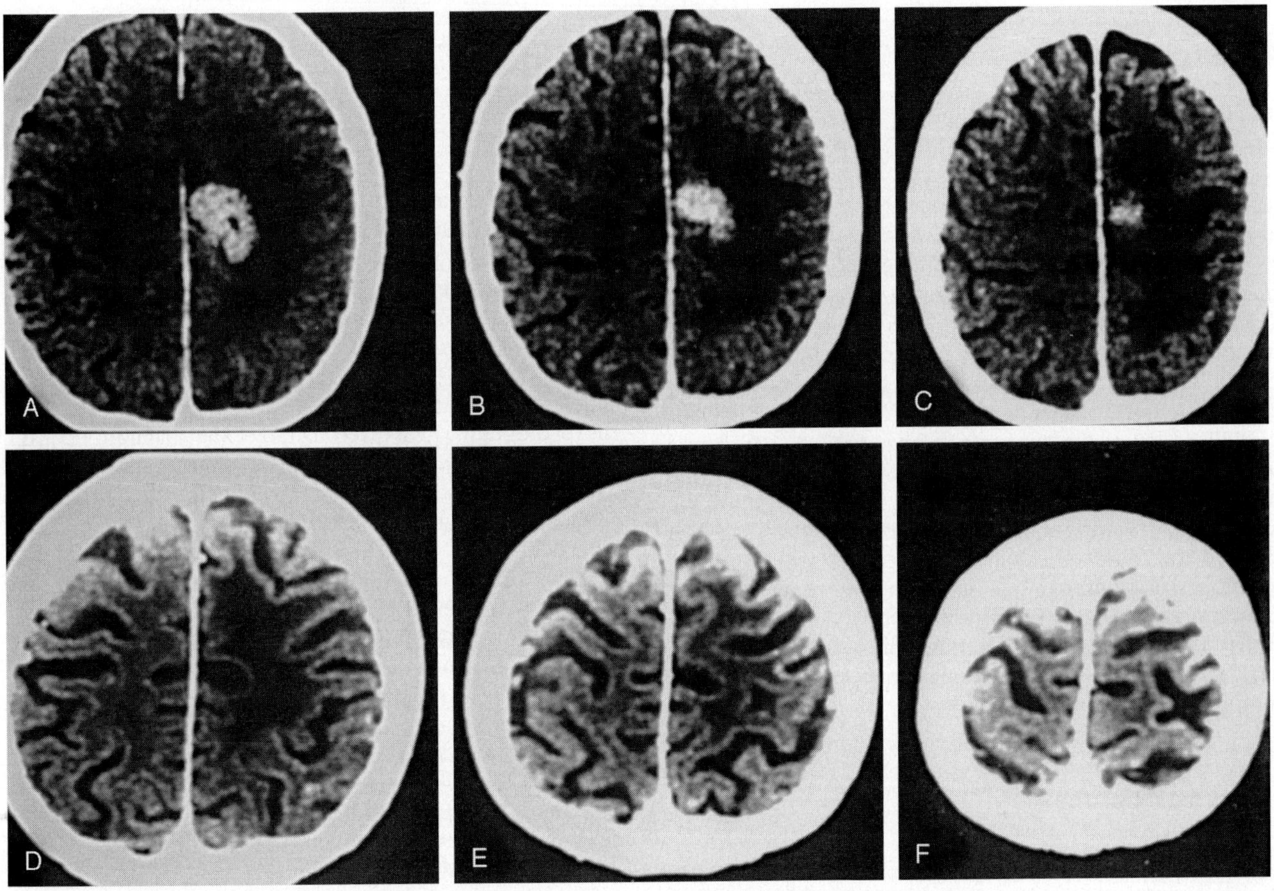

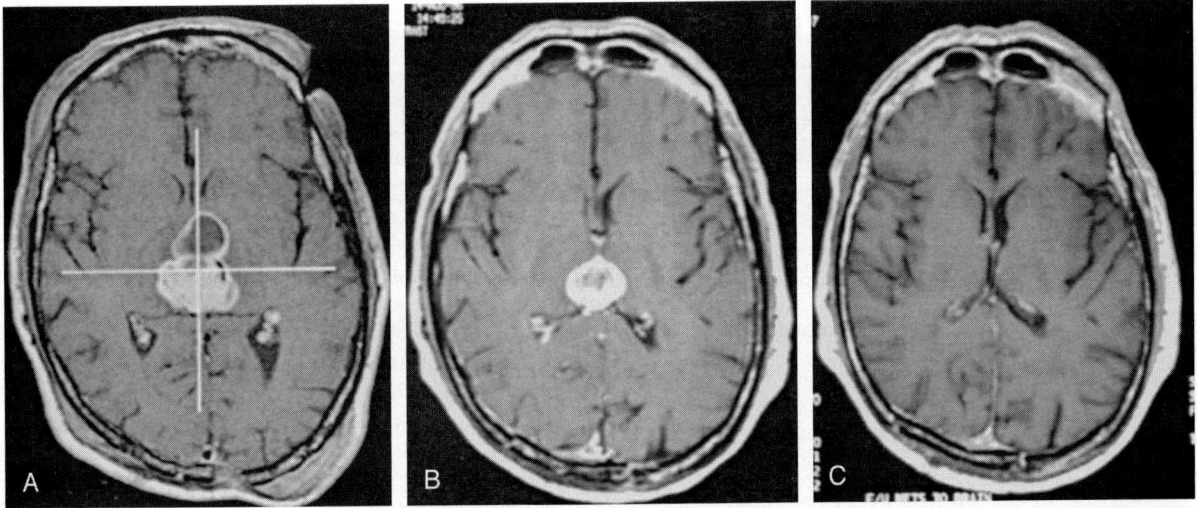

**FIGURE 50–25** ■ Gamma surgery for cerebral metastasis from systemic lymphoma. A 66-year-old man with cerebral lymphoma metastasis is shown before *(A–C)* and 2½ months after gamma surgery *(D–F)*. The tumor disappeared completely.

**FIGURE 50–26** ■ Gamma surgery for renal cell carcinoma. A post-contrast axial $T_1$-weighted magnetic resonance imaging scan at the time of treatment *(A)*, at 3 months *(B)*, and at 1 year *(C)* after gamma surgery. This patient developed two additional metastases that were subsequently treated successfully with gamma surgery. The patient survived 17 months before succumbing to metastatic deposits outside the brain.

neous pattern of contrast enhancement, and a longer interval between primary diagnosis and gamma surgery.

## Hemangioblastomas

The gold standard for treatment of hemangioblastomas is surgical resection of the solid component of the tumor. If it is present, it is not necessary to resect the cystic portion of the tumor. Similarly, we have treated only the solid portion of these tumors with gamma surgery. The results of 11 of our patients with hemangioblastomas have been reported.[107] Four of these patients had von Hippel-Lindau disease. These patients were followed for an average of 27 months and were treated with a maximum dose of 28 to 60 Gy and a peripheral dose of 11 to 20 Gy. The usual course was either a decrease in the size of the solid component (7 of 10) of the tumor or no change (3 of 10). It was not uncommon, however, for the cystic portion of the tumor to grow larger regardless of the behavior of the solid portion. During follow-up, four patients required open surgery for relief of expanding cysts and two for unresponding solid tumors.

Although several patients responded well, the high incidence of second, open procedures indicates that the microsurgical removal of hemangioblastomas is in most cases the initial procedure of choice.

## Uveal Melanomas

The most common surgical treatment for uveal melanomas is enucleation, but several centers report relatively large series of patients with these tumors treated with gamma surgery.[108, 109] Other therapeutic options include radium plaque therapy and proton beam therapy. The first uveal melanoma treated with gamma surgery was in Buenos Aires,[110] and gamma surgery has become a more frequently used procedure for this unusual lesion. The use of gamma surgery and its stereotactic technique requires that the eyeball be fixated relative to the stereotactic frame. This is accomplished with retrobulbar blocks and external fixative sutures that are attached to the frame. At the University of Vienna, a specially designed suction device that is attached to the frame is used.[111]

The Sheffield group reported a series of 29 patients treated and followed for an average of 14 months. The average periphery dose was 73 Gy corresponding to the 50% isodose line. The dose was delivered in two sessions not more than 8 days apart. All but two patients had good local control. The two failures required later enucleation. Three patients died of metastatic disease.[109]

Of the three patients treated by us, there has either been no change or a slight decrease in the size of the tumor with at least 2 years of follow-up. When necessary, we placed a spacer to elevate the eyelid to prevent radiation injury to the lid. One of our three patients was treated with two sessions to protect the eyeball from acute increased intraocular pressure, which can be a problem after radiation exposure. The experience in treating uveal melanomas with gamma surgery has shown that it is effective for short-term

local control. Longer follow-up is required to determine if this procedure is superior to other therapies.

## FUNCTIONAL SURGERY

### Pain

The lack of anatomic and pathophysiologic background knowledge of the mechanisms of pain makes the management of pain by open or closed stereotactic techniques largely unsatisfactory.

Early results using gamma surgery to produce thalamotomies for pain control were published by Steiner and colleagues.[11] All of the 52 patients treated had terminal cancer and were treated before the advent of CT or MRI. Pneumoencephalography was used to target the thalamic centrum medianum-parafasciculus complex. Good pain relief was obtained in 8 patients and moderate pain relief in 18. The patients had in general only temporary relief of pain. Of those with good pain relief, five died without recurrence of pain between 1 and 13 months after the procedure and three had recurrence of pain at 3, 6, and 9 months, respectively. Doses between 100 and 250 Gy were tested. Observation of an actual lesion was possible only in 21 of 36 patients who had a postmortem examination. Not surprisingly, the presence of a lesion was associated with relief. Lesions were reliably created only with doses greater than 160 Gy. The collimators used were 3 × 5 and 3 × 7 mm. The most effective lesions were more medially located near the wall of the third ventricle, and the greatest relief was for pain in the face or arm.

These results were not very encouraging. However, with improvements in neuroimaging and alternate target selection, it is possible that more effective lesions can be produced. More recent reports seem to support this expectation.[112]

### Trigeminal Neuralgia

Radiosurgery was first used to treat trigeminal neuralgia when Leksell treated three patients with an orthovoltage stereotactic technique, obtaining long-term relief of symptoms. With the introduction of the Gamma knife, a series of 46 patients was treated at Stockholm with less encouraging results (S. Hakansson, personal communication, 1993). The target in these cases was the gasserian ganglion, and targeting was by bony landmarks or cisternography. With advances in neuroimaging, most notably MRI, gamma surgery for trigeminal neuralgia was revisited. However, the focus of treatment shifted from the ganglion to the nerve root entry zone. A number of centers have since shown the safety and at least short-term pain relief afforded with this approach.

A multicenter trial with 50 patients showed "good" to "excellent" relief of pain in 88% of patients (54% pain free and 34% with significant relief) at 2 years. Complete relief was obtained in 72% of patients treated with 70 Gy or greater. We failed to reproduce the reported long-term results.[113]

Most patients in the series of 60 treated with gamma surgery by Regis and colleagues were pain free by 1 to 3 months (J. Regis, personal communication, 1998).

Six cases of refractory cluster headache (five chronic and one episodic) were treated by gamma surgery directed at the trigeminal nerve root entry zone. "Excellent" results were reported in four cases (off medication), "good" in one, and "fair" in the other with an 8- to 14-month follow up.[114]

## Movement Disorders

Thalamotomy for tremor in Parkinson's disease remains one of the most gratifying procedures in functional neurosurgery and has a firm place in the therapeutic armory for those common cases in which drugs fail to stop the tremor. However, to avoid the potential risks of open thalamotomies, the prototype Gamma knife was used by Leksell for the production of thalamic lesions in five cases of tremor between 1968 and 1970. At that time, the intended target could not be visualized but was indirectly determined using derived coordinates relative to the anterior and posterior commisures visualized by pneumoencephalography. Verification that a lesion had been produced could not be obtained because neither CT nor MRI was available. Fixation of the patient's head for the radiosurgical procedure was also unsatisfactory because the stereotactic frame used for target localization was too large to fit into the collimator helmet. Instead, fixation devices were applied onto a plaster-of-Paris helmet previously molded on the patient's head. It is therefore not surprising that beneficial results were not obtained. In 1986, MRI was introduced at Karolinska Hospital, and better anatomic visualization of the target volume became possible. A new stereotactic frame compatible with MRI that also served as the fixation device in the Gamma knife was introduced.[115]

These improvements paved the way for new attempts to relieve parkinsonian tremor by gamma thalamotomy, and the first two cases was treated using this improved methodology.[116] The procedure was performed using an 8-mm collimator, and the volume of the resulting lesion was much larger than intended (1.5 cm³). The tremor began to dwindle after 2 months, but a transient hemiparesis and mild speech disturbance ensued secondary to edema. The eventual outcome was, however, satisfactory, and 4 years after treatment the patient returned free of tremor contralateral to the side of the thalamic lesion, asking for a second procedure to stop the tremor that had developed on the other side.

The second patient was treated using a 4-mm collimator, which produced a thalamic lesion of smaller volume. In this case, the clinical result was not satisfactory. She was treated a second time, still without relief of tremor. It is not clear whether the lack of effect was due to the atypical clinical picture in this patient or to the lack of physiologic corroboration of the target. In spite of experience from centers active in this field indicating that modern imaging techniques, especially MRI, may obviate the need for physiologic target definition, this remains controversial. Lim and associates[117] showed a high incidence of delayed internal capsule stroke in patients treated with stereotactic radio-frequency lesioning who had a previous history of vascular disease. If these results are reproduced, then gamma surgery may become the treatment of choice at least for that subgroup most at risk for stroke.

Rand has treated 18 cases of movement disorder with radiosurgery (R. Rand, personal communication, 1994). Of the seven patients with resting tremor, four responded to a nucleus ventralis lateralis lesion with marked improvement in the tremor, and in two patients rigidity improved as well. Eight other patients underwent radiosurgical pallidotomy for rigidity, and four had significant improvement. Two of three patients treated with a nucleus ventralis lateralis lesion for intention tremor showed dramatic improvement. Results termed "good," "excellent," or "complete" relief of tremor by the authors were obtained in 63% of 34 patients treated with thalamic lesioning by Duma and colleagues,[118] and similar results have been reported by Young and associates,[119] Ohye and colleagues,[120] and Hirai and coworkers (T. Hirai, personal communication, 1999).

A pertinent change in the surgical management of movement disorders, particularly parkinsonian tremor, was the introduction of deep brain stimulation, which allows the amelioration of symptoms without a destructive lesion. Good results have been obtained with this technique and it may supplant destructive lesions as the surgical procedure of choice in most patients.[121, 122]

## Obsessive-Compulsive Neurosis

Despite therapeutic progress, conventional treatment of anxiety disorders fails or has only a temporary effect in 20% of patients. These disorders are often severely disabling and are associated with rates of suicide comparable with those of depression. First described by Leksell,[123] psychosurgery targeting the frontolimbic connections in both anterior internal capsules (capsulotomy) is a valuable therapeutic method for selected severe cases. The first procedures using the Gamma knife to create the lesions were also performed by Leksell.

Mindus and colleagues[124] at the Karolinska Institute reported the effects of such procedures on anxiety symptoms and personality characteristics, in conjunction with results of imaging studies using MRI and positron emission tomography (PET). The patient material comprised two series of patients with a 15-year mean duration of psychiatric illness, all of whom had undergone various extensive treatment trials. One series consisted of 24 patients subjected to capsulotomy by a conventional thermocoagulation technique and followed for 1 year. The other series comprised seven patients treated by gamma surgery and followed for 7 years. The clinical effects of these treatments were evaluated subjectively by two independent observers and also rated on the Comprehensive Psychopathological Rating Scale. Ratings were performed 10 days before and 2, 6, and 12 months after surgery. The effects on personality were evaluated by the Karolinska Scales of Personality, which were developed to measure traits related to frontal lobe dysfunction and to reflect different dimensions of anxiety proneness.

At the 12-month follow-up, statistically and clinically significant improvement was noted in all assessments of symptomatic and psychosocial function. Freedom from symptoms or considerable improvement was noted in 79% of patients, and none was worse after the operation. Negative effects on the personality were not noted. Behind these numbers are numerous examples of dramatic improvements in individual lifestyles. A number of patients had been unable to work or function socially owing to such problems as preoccupation with personal cleanliness and the inability to use public transportation, with resulting domestic confinement, aggravated psychological problems, deterioration of family relationships, and devastation of personal economy. After surgery, these patients were able to return to their previous occupation and a normal social function. The results of gamma capsulotomy were comparable with those obtained with capsulotomy performed by the thermocoagulation technique. Only in five of the seven patients could a lesion be demonstrated by MRI, and those were the patients who benefited from the procedure. The lowest effective target dose was 160 Gy, whereas 100, 120, and 152 Gy failed to produce lesions.

Treatment of a new series of 10 patients was started in 1988, using stereotactic MRI for more accurate anatomic target localization and the new Gamma knife model B to produce the lesions. In this series, the lesions were produced using a 4-mm collimator and three isocenters on each side for overlapping fields, creating a cylindrical lesion. The maximum dose within the target volume was 200 Gy. Although it is too early to evaluate the long-term psychological effects in this series of patients, important radiologic information, which will serve to plan future treatments, is already available. The development of the lesions has been followed by MRI and CT scans every 3 months. Not unexpectedly, MRI has been found to be particularly valuable for these follow-up studies. On $T_2$-weighted images, a high-intensity signal appears in the target area after approximately 3 months. This signal is most likely produced by local edema. The edema extends to a maximal volume at approximately 9 months and then slowly subsides. The edema is directly related to the dose and to the volume irradiated. The preliminary impression is that the results equal those obtained in the earlier series.

A comparison of the radiobiologic effects between these two series unfortunately is not possible because neither MRI nor CT was available when the lesions developed in the first series of patients. In the second series, the edema was extensive in a few patients, and it may therefore be wise to adjust the dose or decrease the volume exposed to necrotizing doses in the future. It may be sufficient to use only one isocenter and the 4-mm collimator. With these treatment parameters and a maximal dose of 180 Gy, a lesion measuring approximately 50 $mm^3$ can be expected within several weeks with only minimal transient edema.

Gamma capsulotomy offers several important clinical as well as scientific advantages over capsulotomy using an open technique. The most important is patient tolerance. It is our experience that this psychologically vulnerable group of patients is much more willing to undergo a closed stereotactic procedure, which, in contrast to open surgery, leaves no external marks. Theoretically, the gradual development of the radiolesion may also allow the patient to make a better psychological adjustment to his or her new situation. The psychological rehabilitation phase is an important part of any psychosurgical procedure.

If it proved ethically acceptable, a control group of patients could be subjected to spending time in the collimator helmet without radiation. At a later stage, if this sham procedure was shown to provide no result compared with the real procedure, the control group would receive the appropriate treatment. Such a controlled study is probably necessary before the capsulotomy procedure is generally accepted. Further efforts should also be made to study the biology of the developing lesions. Important questions include, When does the functional effect of the radiation start, and what are the characteristics of the MRI and CT images at this time? Even the issue of dose-volume relationships needs to be addressed further. The PET scanner may help to answer some of these questions, and pretreatment and post-treatment evaluation is planned for further series of patients.

## Epilepsy

Seizure was the presenting symptom in 59 of the 247 patients with AVM of the brain treated by Steiner and colleagues[52] with gamma surgery between 1970 and 1984. The treatment resulted in the relief of some or all seizures in 52 of these patients. Eleven were successfully taken off anticonvulsant medication. Interestingly, in three patients the seizure disorder stopped although the AVM itself was unaffected by the radiation.[52] These observations and those made by others[125–127] prompted the idea of testing focal irradiation as a treatment modality for focal epilepsy.

At the Neurosurgery Department at the University of Virginia, basic science research was done on changes in neuroexcitability after irradiation. The brains of rats treated with the Gamma knife were found to have a higher seizure threshold than those of control rats when placed in solutions of varying concentrations of penicillin. This effect was lost at high concentrations (S. Henson, personal communication, 1998). Subsequent ongoing in vivo animal research using a hippocampal rat epilepsy model seems to be providing results similar to those obtained in the in vitro studies (Z. Chen, personal communication, 1999).

Biochemical analysis of changes in rat brains after gamma surgery done by Regis and colleagues[128] showed changes in the concentrations of excitatory and inhibitory amino acids, particularly γ-aminobutyric acid (GABA). Warnke and coworkers[129] showed that patients with low-grade astrocytomas and associated epilepsy had significant relief from seizures after interstitial radiosurgery. Single photon emission CT scanning showed a reduced number of GABA receptors before treatment in both the tumors and surrounding brain. Levels of these receptors increased after therapy.[129] These early studies show that functional changes may occur at the cellular level without gross structural damage. The implications of this for functional neurosurgery are intriguing.

Epilepsy has been treated with the Gamma knife at many centers, but there have been few published results. We have treated six patients, three of whom had structural lesions. The early results for the first three patients was encouraging, with significant reduction in seizure activity, but these results were not durable in the long term.

Barcia-Salorio and associates[130] treated 11 patients with idiopathic epilepsy. Preoperative invasive electrodiagnostic confirmation of the epileptogenic focus was performed and treatment was with low-dose (10 to 20 Gy) radiosurgery. Complete relief from seizures was obtained in four patients and significant reduction in seizure activity in five. The effect of the treatment was not seen for several months in most instances. Regis and colleagues[131] reported a case of mesial temporal lobe epilepsy treated with gamma surgery using 25 Gy given to the 50% isodose line. The patient was seizure free after the treatment. At 10 months, a lesion was evident on both CT and MRI that conformed to the 50% isodose line (amygdala and hippocampus). Whether actual gross structural lesioning with this method is associated with better results or more complications is unknown. Further results of 23 patients treated by Regis and colleagues (J. Regis, personal communication, 1998) show that the 3 patients with greater than 2 years of follow-up are seizure free and that most with 6 to 9 months of follow-up are improved. One patient was cured of his seizures before any changes were evident on MRI examination.

The potential for a less invasive, nondestructive therapy to treat epilepsy should obviously be investigated. However, its feasibility and effectiveness in the long term need to be proved. Furthermore, the need for physiologic monitoring to determine conclusively the epileptogenic focus cannot be entirely discarded. Future developments of noninvasive physiologic monitoring will influence the development of gamma surgery for epilepsy.

## CONCLUSIONS

The indications and usefulness of gamma surgery are being defined more carefully with the passage of time. The advances of the past several decades have paralleled improvements in neuroimaging. The identification of discrete thalamic, hypothalamic, and basal ganglia nuclei with acceptable confidence may allow the use of gamma surgery in a wider variety of functional disorders. This will require a better understanding of the relationship of anatomy and function, as well as improved spatial definition of these nuclei. With existing technology, the treatment of some functional disorders such as Parkinson's disease, obsessive-compulsive disorder, and chronic pain is being evaluated.

Technical advances and improvements of the gamma unit will increase the ease of use of the machine, and better defined protocols should improve the clinical results obtained. Other advances in fields such as pharmacology may allow the selective sensitization of tumors or provide protective effect to normal tissue, increasing the efficacy and safety of tumor treatment. In the first stage of development of gamma surgery, it is mandatory to define its usefulness in various pathologic processes. The elimination of its use when it is not clinically indicated and the expansion of its use into new areas when it has been shown to have efficacy are important goals. The rapidly accumulating material from patients who have been treated will define the place of the Gamma knife in the armory of neurosurgery.

## REFERENCES

1. Dandy WE: Cerebral ventriculoscopy. Bull Johns Hopkins Hosp 33:189, 1922.
2. Schulder M, Loeffler JS, Howes AE, et al: Historical vignette: The radium bomb: Harvey Cushing and the interstitial irradiation of gliomas. J Neurosurg 84:530–532, 1996.
3. Clarke R, Horsley V: One method of investigating the deep ganglia and tracts of the central nervous system (cerebellum). BMJ 2:1799–1800, 1906.
4. Spiegel E, Wycis H, Marks M, et al: Stereotaxic apparatus for operations on the human brain. Science 106:349–350, 1947.
5. Leksell L: The stereotaxic method and radiosurgery of the brain. Acta Chir Scand 102:316, 1951.
6. Larsson B, Leksell L, Rexed B: The use of high-energy protons for cerebral surgery in man. Acta Chir Scand 125:1, 1963.
7. Leksell L, Larsson B, Andersson B: Lesions in the depth of the brain produced by a beam of high energy protons. Acta Radiol 54:251–264, 1960.
8. Hall EJ, Marchese M, Hei TK, et al: Radiation response characteristics of human cells in vitro. Radiat Res 114:415–424, 1988.
9. Kamiryo T, Kassell NF, Thai QA, et al: Histological changes in the normal rat brain after gamma irradiation. Acta Neurochir (Wien) 138:451–459, 1996.
10. Flickinger JC, Lunsford LD, Kondziolka D: Dose-volume considerations in radiosurgery. Stereotact Funct Neurosurg 57:99–105, 1991.
11. Steiner L, Forster D, Leksell L, et al: Gammathalamotomy in intractable pain. Acta Neurochir (Wien) 52:173–184, 1980.
12. Hawighorst H, Engenhart R, Knopp MV, et al: Intracranial meningiomas: Time- and dose-dependent effects of irradiation on tumor microcirculation monitored by dynamic MR imaging. Magn Reson Imaging 15:423–432, 1997.
13. Tsuzuki T, Tsunoda S, Sakaki T, et al: Tumor cell proliferation and apoptosis associated with the Gamma knife effect. Stereotact Funct Neurosurg 66:39–48, 1996.
14. Hopewell JW, Wright EA: The nature of latent cerebral irradiation damage and its modification by hypertension. Br J Radiol 43:161–167, 1970.
15. Verhey LJ, Smith V, Serago CF: Comparison of radiosurgery treatment modalities based on physical dose distributions. Int J Radiat Oncol Biol Phys 40:497–505, 1998.
16. Tishler RB, Loeffler JS, Lunsford LD, et al: Tolerance of cranial nerves of the cavernous sinus to radiosurgery [see comments]. Int J Radiat Oncol Biol Phys 27:215–221, 1993.
17. Noren G, Greitz D, Hirsch A, et al: Gamma knife surgery in acoustic tumours. Acta Neurochir Suppl (Wien) 58:104–107, 1993.
18. Szikla G, Betti O, Blond S: Data of late reactions following stereotactic irradiation of gliomas. INSERM Symp 12:167–174, 1979.
19. Steiner L, Greitz T, Backlund E, et al: Radiosurgery in arteriovenous malformations of the brain: Undue effects. INSERM Symp 12:257–270, 1979.
20. Kamiryo T, Lopes MBS, Berr SS, et al: Occlusion of the anterior cerebral artery after gamma knife irradiation in a rat. Acta Neurochir (Wien) 138:983–990, 1996.
21. Nilsson A, Wennerstrand J, Leksell D, et al: Stereotactic gamma irradiation of basilar artery in cat: Preliminary experiences. Acta Radiol Oncol Radiat Phys Biol 17:150–60, 1978.
22. Kihlström L, Lindquist C, Adler J, et al: Histological studies of gamma knife lesions in normal and hypercholesterolemic rabbits. In Steiner L (ed): Radiosurgery: Baseline and Trends. New York: Raven Press, 1992, pp 111–119.
23. Cushing H, Bailey P: Tumors Arising from the Blood Vessels of the Brain. Springfield, IL: Charles C Thomas, 1928, p 46.
24. Wegemann H-J: Das Schicksal operierter Patienten mit arteriovenösem Aneurysma des Gehrins. Zurich: Juris Druck and Verlag, 1969.
25. Krayenbühl H. Discussion des Rapports sur "Les Angiomes Supratentoriels." Bruxelles: Congrès International de Neurochirurgie, 1957.
26. Olivecrona H, Ladenheim J: Congenital Arteriovenous Aneurysms of the Carotid and Vertebral Systems. Berlin: Springer-Verlag, 1957, p 91.

27. McKissock W, Hankinson J: The Surgical Treatment of Supratentorial Angiomas. Bruxelles: Congrès International de Neurochirurgie, 1957.
28. Pool J: Aneurysms and Arteriovenous Anomalies of the Brain: Diagnosis and Treatment. New York: Harper and Row, 1965.
29. Jefferson G: Les hemorrhagies sous-arachnoidiennes par angiomes et aneurysms chez le jeune. Rev Neurol (Paris) 80:413–432, 1948.
30. Ray B: Cerebral arteriovenous aneurysms. Surg Gynecol Obstet 73:614–648, 1941.
31. Johnson J: Cerebral Angiomas: Advances in Diagnosis and Therapy. Berlin: Springer-Verlag, 1975, pp 256–258.
32. Steiner L, Leksell L, Greitz T, et al: Stereotaxic radiosurgery for cerebral arteriovenous malformations: Report of a case. Acta Chir Scand 138:459–464, 1972.
33. Yamamoto M, Jimbo M, Kobayashi M, et al: Long-term results of radiosurgery for arteriovenous malformation: Neurodiagnostic imaging and histological studies of angiographically confirmed nidus obliteration. Surg Neurol 37:219–230, 1992.
34. Schneider BF, Eberhard DA, Steiner L: Histopathology of arteriovenous malformations after gamma knife radiosurgery. J Neurosurg 87:352–357, 1997.
35. Szeifert GT, Kemeny AA, Timperley WR, et al: The potential role of myofibroblasts in the obliteration of arteriovenous malformations after radiosurgery. Neurosurgery 40:61–65, 1997; discussion 65–66.
36. Albert P, Salgado H, Polaina M, et al: A study on the venous drainage of 150 cerebral arteriovenous malformations as related to haemorrhagic risks and the size of the lesion. Acta Neurochir (Wien) 103:30–34, 1990.
37. Graf CJ, Perret GE, Torner JC: Bleeding from cerebral arteriovenous malformations as part of their natural history. J Neurosurg 58:331–337, 1983.
38. Itoyama Y, Uemura S, Ushio Y, et al: Natural course of unoperated intracranial arteriovenous malformations: Study of 50 cases. J Neurosurg 71:805–809, 1989.
39. Spetzler RF, Hargraves RW, McCormick PW, et al: Relationship of perfusion pressure and size to risk of hemorrhage from arteriovenous malformations [see comments]. J Neurosurg 76:918–923, 1992.
40. Jomin M, Lesoin F, Lozes G: Prognosis for arteriovenous malformations of the brain in adults based on 150 cases. Surg Neurol 23:362–366, 1985.
41. Pasqualin A: Natural Risk of Hemorrhage from Cerebral Arteriovenous Malformations: A Long Term Evaluation in 168 Patients. Presented at CNS Meeting, San Francisco: 1995.
42. Brown RD Jr, Wiebers DO, Forbes G, et al: The natural history of unruptured intracranial arteriovenous malformations. J Neurosurg 68:352–357, 1988.
43. Crawford PM, West CR, Shaw MD, et al: Cerebral arteriovenous malformations and epilepsy: Factors in the development of epilepsy. Epilepsia 27:270–275, 1986.
44. Forster DM, Kunkler IH, Hartland P: Risk of cerebral bleeding from arteriovenous malformations in pregnancy: The Sheffield experience. Stereotact Funct Neurosurg 61:20–22, 1993.
45. Fults D, Kelly DL Jr: Natural history of arteriovenous malformations of the brain: A clinical study. Neurosurgery 15:658–662, 1984.
46. Karlsson B: Gamma knife surgery of arteriovenous malformations. Ph.D. Thesis. Stockholm: Karolinska Institute, 1996.
47. Forster DM, Steiner L, Hakanson S: Arteriovenous malformations of the brain: A long-term clinical study. J Neurosurg 37:562–570, 1972.
48. Ondra SL, Troupp H, George ED, et al: The natural history of symptomatic arteriovenous malformations of the brain: A 24-year follow-up assessment [see comments]. J Neurosurg 73:387–391, 1990.
49. Sadasivan B, Malik GM, Lee C, et al: Vascular malformations and pregnancy. Surg Neurol 33:305–313, 1990.
50. Harbaugh KS, Harbaugh RE: Arteriovenous malformations in elderly patients. Neurosurgery 35:579–584, 1994.
51. Robinson JL, Hall CS, Sedzimir CB: Arteriovenous malformations, aneurysms, and pregnancy. J Neurosurg 41:63–70, 1974.
52. Steiner L, Lindquist C, Adler JR, et al: Clinical outcome of radiosurgery for cerebral arteriovenous malformations [see comments]. J Neurosurg 77:1–8, 1992.
53. Kjellberg RN, Davis KR, Lyons S, et al: Bragg peak proton beam therapy for arteriovenous malformation of the brain. Clin Neurosurg 31:248–290, 1983.
54. Steiner L, Lindquist C, Adler JR, et al: Outcome of radiosurgery for cerebral AVM (Letter). J Neurosurg 77:823, 1992.
55. Karlsson B, Lindquist C, Steiner L: The effect of gamma knife surgery on the risk of rupture prior to AVM obliteration. In Gamma Knife Surgery in Cerebral Arteriovenous Malformations. PhD Thesis. Stockholm: Karolinska Institute, 1996, pp 34–52.
56. Guo WY: Radiological aspects of gamma knife radiosurgery for arteriovenous malformations and other non-tumoural disorders of the brain. Acta Radiol Suppl 388:1–34, 1993.
57. Aiba T, Tanaka R, Koike T, et al: Natural history of intracranial cavernous malformations. J Neurosurg 83:56–59, 1995.
58. Curling OD, Kelly DL, Elster AD, et al: An analysis of the natural history of cavernous angiomas. J Neurosurg 75:702–708, 1991.
59. Garner TB, Del Curling O Jr, Kelly DL Jr, et al: The natural history of intracranial venous angiomas. J Neurosurg 75:715–722, 1991.
60. Kondziolka D, Lunsford L, Kestle J: The natural history of cavernous malformations. J Neurosurg 83:820–824, 1995.
61. Robinson JR, Awad IA, Little JR: Natural history of the cavernous angioma. J Neurosurg 75:709–714, 1991.
62. Steiner L, Prasad D, Lindquist C, et al: Clinical aspects of gamma knife stereotactic radiosurgery. In Gildenberg P, Tasker R, Franklin P (eds): Textbook of Stereotactic and Functional Neurosurgery. New York: McGraw-Hill, 1998, pp 763–803.
63. Karlsson B, Kihlstrom L, Lindquist C, et al: Radiosurgery for cavernous malformations. J Neurosurg 88:293–297, 1998.
64. Kondziolka D, Lunsford LD, Flickinger JC, et al: Reduction of hemorrhage risk after stereotactic radiosurgery for cavernous malformations. J Neurosurg 83:825–831, 1995.
65. Weil S Jr, Tew JM Jr, Steiner L: Comparison of radiosurgery and microsurgery for treatment of cavernous malformations of brain stem (Abstract). J Neurosurg 72:336A, 1990.
66. Garner TB, Curling JOD, Kelly DL, et al: The natural history of intracranial venous angiomas. J Neurosurg 75:715–722, 1991.
67. Kjellberg RN, Shintani A, Frantz AG, et al: Proton beam therapy in acromegaly. N Engl J Med 278:689–695, 1968.
68. Levy RP, Fabrikant JI, Frankel KA, et al: Charged-particle radiosurgery of the brain. Neurosurg Clin N Am 1:955–990, 1990.
69. Rahn T, Thorén M, Hall K. Stereotactic radiosurgery in the treatment of MB Cushing. INSERM Symp 12:207–212, 1979.
70. Hetelekidis S, Barnes PD, Tao ML, et al: 20-year experience in childhood craniopharyngioma [see comments]. Int J Radiat Oncol Biol Phys 27:189–195, 1993.
71. Rajan B, Ashley S, Gorman C, et al: Craniopharyngioma: Long-term results following limited surgery and radiotherapy. Radiother Oncol 26:1–10, 1993.
72. Mulhern RK, Kepner JL, Thomas PR, et al: Neuropsychologic functioning of survivors of childhood medulloblastoma randomized to receive conventional or reduced-dose craniospinal irradiation: A Pediatric Oncology Group study. J Clin Oncol 16:1723–1728, 1998.
73. Chadderton RD, West CG, Schuller S, et al: Radiotherapy in the treatment of low-grade astrocytomas. II: The physical and cognitive sequelae [published erratum appears in Childs Nerv Syst 11:715, 1995]. Childs Nerv Syst 11:443–448, 1995.
74. Yang TF, Wong TT, Cheng LY, et al: Neuropsychological sequelae after treatment for medulloblastoma in childhood: The Taiwan experience. Childs Nerv Syst 13:77–80, 1997; discussion 81.
75. Ilveskoski I, Pihko H, Wiklund T, et al: Neuropsychologic late effects in children with malignant brain tumors treated with surgery, radiotherapy and "8 in 1" chemotherapy. Neuropediatrics 27:124–129, 1996.
76. Chapman CA, Waber DP, Bernstein JH, et al: Neurobehavioral and neurologic outcome in long-term survivors of posterior fossa brain tumors: Role of age and perioperative factors. J Child Neurol 10:209–212, 1995.
77. Prasad D, Steiner M, Steiner L: Gamma knife surgery for craniopharyngioma. Acta Neurochir (Wien) 134:167–176, 1995.
78. Coffey RJ, Lunsford LD: The role of stereotactic techniques in the management of craniopharyngiomas (Review) [published erratum appears in Neurosurg Clin N Am 1:7, 1990]. Neurosurg Clin N Am 1:161–172, 1990.
79. Backlund E-O: Solid craniopharyngiomas treated by stereotactic radiosurgery. INSERM Symp 12:271–282, 1979.
80. Barbaro NM, Gutin PH, Wilson CB, et al: Radiation therapy in the treatment of partially resected meningiomas. J Neurosurg 20:525–528, 1987.

81. Taylor BW, Marcus RBJ, Friedman WA, et al: The meningioma controversy: Postoperative radiation therapy. Int J Radiat Oncol Biol Phys 15:299–234, 1988.
82. Goldsmith BJ, Wara WM, Wilson CB, et al: Postoperative irradiation for subtotally resected meningiomas: A retrospective analysis of 140 patients treated from 1967 to 1990 (Review) [published erratum appears in J Neurosurg 80:777, 1994]. J Neurosurg 80:195–201, 1994.
83. Steiner L, Lindquist C, Steiner M: Meningiomas and gamma knife radiosurgery. In Al-Mefty O (ed): Meningiomas. New York: Raven Press, 1991, pp 263–272.
84. Kondziolka D, Lundsford L, Linskey M, et al: Skull base radiosurgery. In Alexander E III, Lundsford LD (eds): Stereotactic Radiosurgery. New York: McGraw-Hill, 1993, pp 175–188.
85. Kondziolka D, Lunsford LD, Coffey RJ, et al: Stereotactic radiosurgery of meningiomas. J Neurosurg 74:552–559, 1991.
86. Henshen F: Über Geschwülste der hinteren Schädelgrube insbesondere des Kleinhirnbrückenwinkels. In Pathologisch-anatomischen. Stockholm: Karolinska Institute, 1910, p 283.
87. Leksell L: A note on the treatment of acoustic tumours. Acta Chir Scand 136:763–765, 1971.
88. Wallner K, Sheline GE, Pitts LH, et al: Efficacy of irradiation for incompletely excised acoustic neurilemomas. J Neurosurg 67:858–863, 1987.
89. Prasad D, Phillips CD, Steiner M: Gamma surgery for acoustic neurinomas (Abstract). J Neurosurg 84:372A, 1996.
90. Flickinger JC, Lunsford LD, Linskey ME, et al: Gamma knife radiosurgery for acoustic tumors: Multivariate analysis of four year results. Radiother Oncol 27:91–98, 1993.
91. Szeifert GT, Prasad D, Kamiryo T, et al: The role of the gamma knife in the therapy of intracranial astrocytomas. In Shibata S (ed): Surgery of Gliomas. Osaka: Medica Publishers, 1998, pp 254–278.
92. Pozza F, Colombo F, Chierego G, et al: Low-grade astrocytomas: Treatment with unconventionally fractionated external beam stereotactic radiation therapy. Radiology 171:565–569, 1989.
93. Gutin PH, Wilson CB: Radiosurgery for malignant brain tumors (Editorial; Comment). J Clin Oncol 8:571–573, 1990.
94. Loeffler JS, Alexander Ed, Shea WM, et al: Radiosurgery as part of the initial management of patients with malignant gliomas [see comments]. J Clin Oncol 10:1379–1385, 1992.
95. Suit HD, Goitein M, Munzenrider J, et al: Increased efficacy of radiation therapy by use of proton beam. Strahlenther Onkol 166:40–44, 1990.
96. Austin-Seymour M, Munzenrider J, Goitein M, et al: Fractionated proton radiation therapy of chordoma and low-grade chondrosarcoma of the base of the skull. J Neurosurg 70:13–17, 1989.
97. Latz D, Gademann G, Hawighorst H, et al: The initial results in the fractionated 3-dimensional stereotactic irradiation of clivus chordomas [German]. Strahlenther Onkol 171:348–355, 1995.
98. Muthukumar N, Kondziolka D, Lunsford LD, et al: Stereotactic radiosurgery for chordoma and chondrosarcoma: Further experiences. Int J Radiat Oncol Biol Phys 41:387–392, 1998.
99. Davey P, O'Brien P: Disposition of cerebral metastases from malignant melanoma: Implications for radiosurgery [see comments]. Neurosurgery 28:8–14, 1991; discussion 14–15.
100. Coffey RJ, Lunsford LD: Stereotactic radiosurgery using the 201 cobalt-60 source gamma knife. Neurosurg Clin N Am 1:933–954, 1990.
101. Coffey RJ, Flickinger JC, Bissonette DJ, et al: Radiosurgery for solitary brain metastases using the cobalt-60 gamma unit: Methods and results in 24 patients. Int J Radiat Oncol Biol Phys 20:1287–1295, 1991.
102. Flickinger JC, Kondziolka D, Lunsford LD, et al: A multi-institutional experience with stereotactic radiosurgery for solitary brain metastasis [see comments]. Int J Radiat Oncol Biol Phys 28:797–802, 1994.
103. Kihlstrom L, Karlsson B, Lindquist C: Gamma knife surgery for cerebral metastases: Implications for survival based on 16 years experience. Stereotact Funct Neurosurg 61:45–50, 1993.
104. Somaza S, Kondziolka D, Lunsford LD, et al: Stereotactic radiosurgery for cerebral metastatic melanoma. J Neurosurg 79:661–666, 1993.
105. Seung SK, Sneed PK, McDermott MW, et al: Gamma knife radiosurgery for malignant melanoma brain metastases [see comments]. Cancer J Sci Am 4:103–109, 1998.
106. Shiau CY, Sneed PK, Shu HK, et al: Radiosurgery for brain metastases: Relationship of dose and pattern of enhancement to local control. Int J Radiat Oncol Biol Phys 37:375–383, 1997.
107. Niemela M, Young J, Jääskeläinen J, et al: Gamma knife radiosurgery in 11 haemangioblastomas. J Neurosurg 85:591–596, 1996.
108. Marchini G, Gerosa M, Piovan E, et al: Gamma knife stereotactic radiosurgery for uveal melanoma: Clinical results after 2 years. Stereotact Funct Neurosurg 66:208–213, 1996.
109. Rennie I, Forster D, Kemeny A, et al: The use of single fraction Leksell stereotactic radiosurgery in the treatment of uveal melanoma. Acta Ophthalmol Scand 74:558–562, 1996.
110. Chinela A, Zambrano A, Bunge H, et al: Gamma knife surgery in uveal melanomas. In Steiner L (ed): Radiosurgery: Baselines and Trends. New York: Raven Press, 1992, pp 161–169.
111. Zehetmayer M, Menapace R, Kitz K, et al: Suction attachment for stereotactic radiosurgery of intraocular malignancies. Ophthalmologica 208:119–121, 1994.
112. Young RF: Functional neurosurgery with the Leksell gamma knife. Stereotact Funct Neurosurg 66:19–23, 1996.
113. Kondziolka D, Lunsford LD, Flickinger JC, et al: Stereotactic radiosurgery for trigeminal neuralgia: A multiinstitutional study using the gamma unit. J Neurosurg 84:940–945, 1996.
114. Ford RG, Ford KT, Swaid S, et al: Gamma knife treatment of refractory cluster headache. Headache 38:3–9, 1998.
115. Leksell L, Lindquist C, Adler JR, et al: A new fixation device for the Leksell stereotaxic system: Technical note. J Neurosurg 66:626–629, 1987.
116. Lindquist C, Kihlstrom L, Hellstrand E: Functional neurosurgery: A future for the gamma knife? Stereotact Funct Neurosurg 57:72–81, 1991.
117. Lim JY, De Salles AA, Bronstein J, et al: Delayed internal capsule infarctions following radiofrequency pallidotomy: Report of three cases. J Neurosurg 87:955–960, 1997.
118. Duma CM, Jacques DB, Kopyov OV, et al: Gamma knife radiosurgery for thalamotomy in parkinsonian tremor: A five-year experience [see comments]. J Neurosurg 88:1044–1049, 1998.
119. Young RF, Vermeulen SS, Grimm P, et al: Electrophysiological target localization is not required for the treatment of functional disorders. Stereotact Funct Neurosurg 66:309–319, 1996.
120. Ohye C, Shibazaki T, Hirato M, et al: Gamma thalamotomy for parkinsonian and other kinds of tremor. Stereotact Funct Neurosurg 66:333–342, 1996.
121. Tasker RR: Deep brain stimulation is preferable to thalamotomy for tremor suppression. Surg Neurol 49:145–153, 1998; discussion 153–154.
122. Duff J, Sime E: Surgical interventions in the treatment of Parkinson's disease (PD) and essential tremor (ET): Medial pallidotomy in PD and chronic deep brain stimulation (DBS) in PD and ET. Axone 18:85–89, 1997.
123. Bingley T, Leksell L, Meyerson BA, et al: Long-term results of stereotactic anterior capsulotomy in chronic obsessive-compulsive neurosis. In Sweet WH, Obrador S, Martin-Rodriguez JG (eds): Neurosurgical Treatment in Psychiatry, Pain, and Epilepsy. Proceedings of the Fourth World Congress of Psychiatric Surgery, Sept 7–10, 1975, Madrid, Spain. Baltimore: University Park Press, 1977, pp 287–299.
124. Mindus P: Capsulotomy in Anxiety Disorders: A Multidisciplinary Study. Stockholm: Karolinska Institute, 1991.
125. Elomaa E: Focal irradiation of the brain: An alternative to temporal lobe resection in intractable focal epilepsy? Med Hypotheses 6:501–503, 1980.
126. Barcia Salorio JL, Roldan P, Hernandez G, et al: Radiosurgical treatment of epilepsy. Appl Neurophysiol 48:400–403, 1985.
127. Rossi GF, Scerrati M, Roselli R: Epileptogenic cerebral low-grade tumors: Effect of interstitial stereotactic irradiation on seizures. Appl Neurophysiol 48:127–132, 1985.
128. Regis J, Kerkerian-Legoff L, Rey M, et al: First biochemical evidence of differential functional effects following gamma knife surgery. Stereotact Funct Neurosurg 66:29–38, 1996.
129. Warnke PC, Berlis A, Weyerbrock A, et al: Significant reduction of seizure incidence and increase of benzodiazepine receptor density after interstitial radiosurgery in low-grade gliomas. Acta Neurochir Suppl (Wien) 68:90–92, 1997.
130. Barcia-Salorio JL, Barcia JA, Hernandez G, et al: Radiosurgery of

epilepsy: Long-term results. Acta Neurochir Suppl (Wien) 62:111–113, 1994.

131. Regis J, Peragui JC, Rey M, et al: First selective amygdalohippo-campal radiosurgery for "mesial temporal lobe epilepsy." Stereotact Funct Neurosurg 64:193–201, 1995.

132. Sutcliffe JC, Forster DM, Walton L, et al: Untoward clinical effects after stereotactic radiosurgery for intracranial arteriovenous malformations. Br J Neurosurg 6:177–185, 1992.

133. Kondziolka D, Lundsford L, Flickinger J: Gamma knife stereotactic radiosurgery for cerebral vascular malformations. In Alexander E III, Lundsford LD (eds): Stereotactic Radiosurgery. New York: McGraw-Hill, 1993, pp 136–146.

134. Linskey ME, Lunsford LD, Flickinger JC, et al: Stereotactic radiosurgery for acoustic tumors. Neurosurg Clin N Am 3:191–205, 1992.

135. Baardsen R, Larsen JL, Wester K, et al: Cerebral metastases treated with stereotaxic gamma radiation. 6-year experience with the "gamma knife" at the Haukeland hospital [Norwegian]. Tidsskr Nor Laegeforen 117:1591–1595, 1997.

136. Young RF: Radiosurgery for the treatment of brain metastases. Semin Surg Oncol 14:70–78, 1998.

137. Gerosa M, Nicolato A, Severi F, et al: Gamma knife radiosurgery for intracranial metastases: From local tumor control to increased survival. Stereotact Funct Neurosurg 66:184–192, 1996.

138. Forster DM, Kunkler IH, Hartland P: Risk of cerebral bleeding from arteriovenous malformations in pregnancy: The Sheffield experience. Stereotact Funct Neurosurg Suppl 1:20–22, 1993.

139. Kawamoto S: Radiosurgery of cerebral AVMs: An update. No To Shinke: 48:129–141, 1996.

140. Steiner L, Lindquist C, Adler JR, et al: Outcome of radiosurgery for cerebral AVM. J Neurosurg 77:823, 1992.

CHAPTER 51

# Stereotactic Interstitial Radiosurgery in the Management of Brain Tumors

■ G. REES COSGROVE, JAY S. LOEFFLER, and NICHOLAS T. ZERVAS

Shortly after its discovery in 1898, Curie suggested that radium could be inserted directly into a tumor with beneficial effect.[6] Interstitial irradiation has since been used in many different organ systems for the treatment of neoplasia.[13] With the introduction of stereotactic techniques in neurosurgery, it became possible accurately to place radioactive sources into brain tumors, and the term *interstitial brachytherapy* was introduced to differentiate this from standard external radiation treatment, or *teletherapy.*

More recently, radiosurgical techniques using focused external beams have been developed that deliver a single, high dose of ionizing radiation to a target volume noninvasively.[20, 25] Whereas external radiosurgery delivers its energy over minutes to hours, interstitial brachytherapy provides focal intratumoral irradiation over a period of hours or days.[27, 34] In both therapeutic modalities, the objective is to deliver a high dose of radiation to a well defined target volume with minimal exposure to surrounding normal brain structures.

Interstitial radiosurgery implies the delivery of ionizing radiation interstitially to the tumor (as in brachytherapy) in a high-dose single fraction (as in radiosurgery), and hence the name. In this chapter, we present our experience using a miniature x-ray generator that can be placed stereotactically into intracranial tumors to deliver a single fraction of high-dose interstitial irradiation in less than an hour. The physical characteristics of the Photon Radiosurgical System (PRS; Photoelectron Corporation, Waltham, MA) are described, and the early clinical experience as well as possible future applications discussed.

## RADIOBIOLOGIC CONSIDERATIONS

Conventional irradiation uses dose fractionation over time to take advantage of the differences in radiosensitivity between neoplastic and normal tissues. Dose fractionation allows repair of sublethal damage in normal tissues, which therefore receive a lesser radiobiologic effect and are rela-

tively spared. Neoplastic tissues receive a relatively greater radiobiologic effect with fractionation because of reoxygenation, cell cycle redistribution, and repopulation of tumor cells.[20, 25, 33] Dose fractionation also allows for larger volumes of tissue to be irradiated.

The major radiobiologic advantage of any form of interstitial brachytherapy is due to intratumoral placement of the radioactive isotope. With standard-energy isotopes, the radiation dose is attenuated in tissue and a dose decline rate proportional to $1/r^2$ yields a sharp dose fall-off. This allows for a high dose to be delivered to the tumor while minimizing exposure to the surrounding normal brain.[7] Because the photons produced by the PRS are low in energy, their absorption characteristics are different from those of standard brachytherapy sources. The "soft x-rays" of the device are attenuated rapidly in tissue and a dose decline rate of $1/r^3$ is obtained rather than $1/r^2$ as seen for standard, higher-energy interstitial radioactive sources. The steep dose fall-off permits treatment of larger target volumes than would be possible with conventional external radiosurgical systems.

The total radiation dose required to produce a given biologic effect in tissue depends on the time over which the tissue is irradiated.[26, 27] This dose rate is a major determinant of the biologic effect of a given dose of ionizing radiation. In general, lowering the dose rate (and increasing the exposure time) reduces the biologic effect of a given dose of radiation.[7, 30] High dose rates of approximately 1 to 2 Gy/min are possible with the PRS, and rates can reach up to 500 Gy/min at the tumor center.[15] In addition, the irradiation dose rate varies across the target volume according to the radiation technique used. The dose rate of conventional radiation therapy varies by approximately 5% to 10%, whereas that of external-beam radiosurgery or the PRS may vary by 50% across the target volume.

Stereotactic radiosurgery uses accurate target localization and steep dose gradients to deliver a single, high-dose fraction of irradiation. The radiobiology of interstitial radiosurgery is probably similar to that of external radiosurgery in that both deliver a high dose of radiation in a single fraction over a period of perhaps 15 minutes to 1 hour.[19]

Standard interstitial brachytherapy using conventional implanted radionuclides usually requires days to weeks for completion of the treatment.[21, 27] The PRS combines the short treatment times of radiosurgery with the dose delivery advantages of an interstitial source.

## DEVICE DESCRIPTION

The PRS is a new, miniature x-ray generator capable of delivering a prescribed therapeutic radiation dose directly to small brain lesions.[15] The device weighs 3.8 lb and is designed to be compatible with current stereotactic frames (Fig. 51–1). It contains a small electron gun that creates a 40-μA electron beam (approximately 0.5 mm wide). The beam is accelerated through a high-voltage field (range, 15 to 40 kV in 5-kV increments) and then passes through a deflection chamber that controls beam position and ensures beam straightness. After traveling down the evacuated, magnetically shielded, rigid probe (3 mm in diameter and 100 mm in length), the electron beam strikes a thin gold foil target (0.5 μm) at the probe tip, producing x-ray photons whose effective energies are in the 10- to 20-keV range. The gold foil is thick enough to stop the electrons but thin enough to allow the x-rays thus generated to pass through. The last 20 mm of the probe tip is constructed from beryllium, which is transparent to these low-energy x-ray photons. The x-rays are emitted from the tip in a spherical symmetric pattern, resulting in a dose rate in tissue of up to 120 Gy/hr at a 10-mm radius. Two scintillation counters monitor radiation; one is within the device housing and one is positioned on the stereotactic frame to detect the small number of photons that pass through the skull. Although 99.9% of the energy created by the electron collision with the gold foil is in the form of heat and only 0.1% is generated as x-rays, hyperthermia has been excluded as a possible tumoricidal factor by limiting the power of the electron beam to maintain the temperature at the tumor margin to less than 45°C. The system is operated from an electronic control box powered through a standard wall socket. A cable from the control box provides the low-voltage electrical power to the unit. Packing of all high-voltage components in a grounded housing result in a compact device with total electrical isolation for the patient's safety.[5, 10, 15, 16, 36]

## Dosimetry

The PRS produces a radiation field similar to that of a conventional high-dose-rate interstitial brachytherapy source[28] but has the advantage of electronic control. In addition, no special handling or storage techniques are required. The probe tip delivers point-source emission of low-energy photons only when activated, with adjustable intensity and peak energies.[15] The x-ray beam behaves essentially as a point isotropic source. Ionization chamber measurements determined that the dose rate in water for the PRS x-ray beam with a current of 40 μA and voltage of 40 kV is 15 Gy/min at a distance of 10 mm. The absolute dose is estimated to be ±10%.[4, 5, 16] Because the PRS produces low-energy photons with a dose decline rate of $1/r^3$, a 30% dose reduction per millimeter of unit tissue is created, which results in an extremely steep dose fall-off (Fig. 51–2). Because of the extremely sharp dose fall-off, it is possible to deliver radionecrotic doses to larger treatment volumes than with conventional external radiosurgical systems.

To evaluate the dosimetry provided by the PRS against other available technologies, dose-volume histograms generated for the PRS, linear accelerator (LINAC) radiosurgery, and proton beam radiation therapy were compared.[16] All three treatment plans prescribed a dose to a 2-cm diameter spherical lesion using a three-dimensional treatment planing system. The PRS plan used a single probe at the center of the lesion. The linac radiosurgery plan used a 6-MV linear accelerator with four arcs. The proton treatment plan used three circular beam portals. The linac and proton treatment plans were prescribed so that the 80% and 90% isodose lines, respectively, covered the treatment volume. The PRS plan prescribed 100% of the dose to the tumor volume, plus a 2-mm margin of presumed normal tissue beyond the defined tumor border.[16] Comparison of dose-volume histograms from the proton beam, linac, and PRS treatment plans (Fig. 51–3) demonstrated relative normal tissue sparing with the PRS plan beyond that provided with the proton or linac radiosurgery plans for treatment

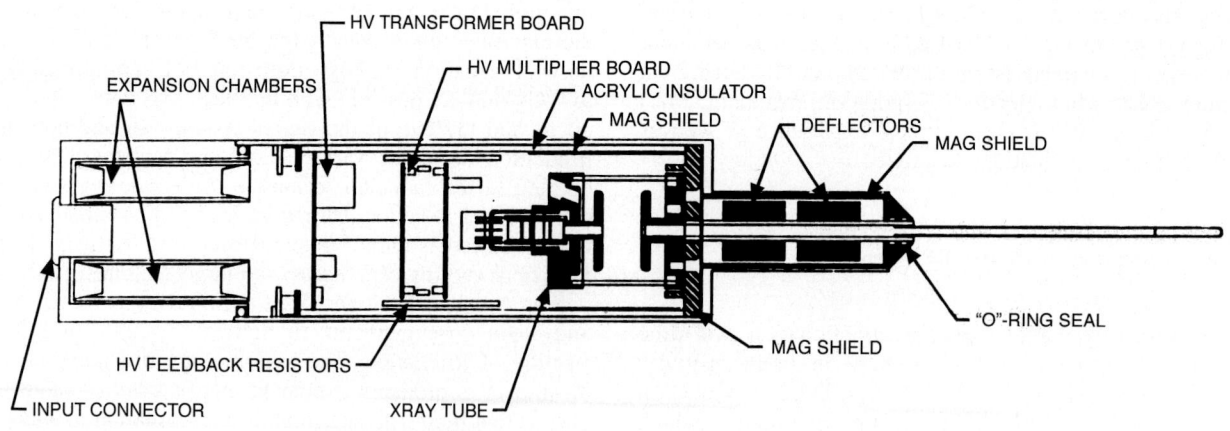

FIGURE 51–1  ■  Internal diagram of the Photon Radiosurgical System.

volumes of less than 50 ml. The high-dose region in the PRS dose curve is due to the point-source nature of the PRS treatment with its dependence on treatment radius. In conclusion, the dosimetry provided with the PRS treatment plan appears similar to, and perhaps better than that achieved with proton beam or linac three-dimensional treatment planning for small, spherical intracranial lesions.

## SURGICAL TECHNIQUE

The PRS is designed for use with stereotactic frames and initial experience has been acquired using the CRW system

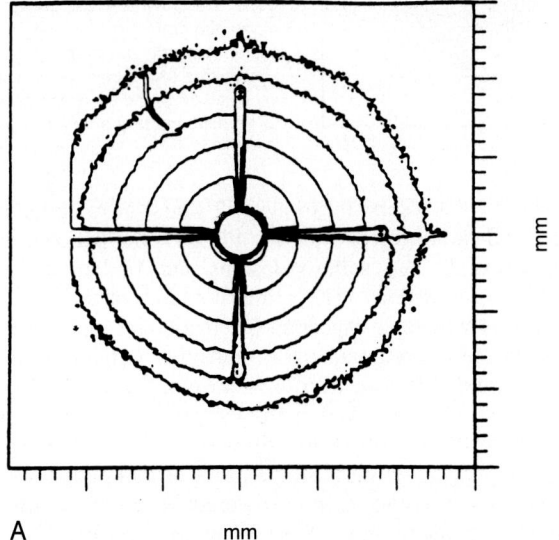

A                    mm

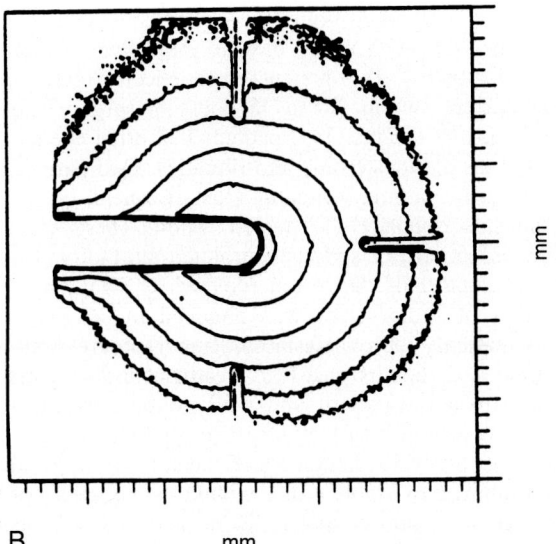

B                    mm

FIGURE 51–2 ■ Spherical isodose contours of the Photon Radiosurgical System along the probe axis *(A)* and in the plane of the probe axis *(B)*. (From Beatty J, Biggs PJ, Gall KP, et al: A new miniature x-ray device for interstitial radiosurgery: Dosimetry. Med Phys 23:53–62, 1996.)

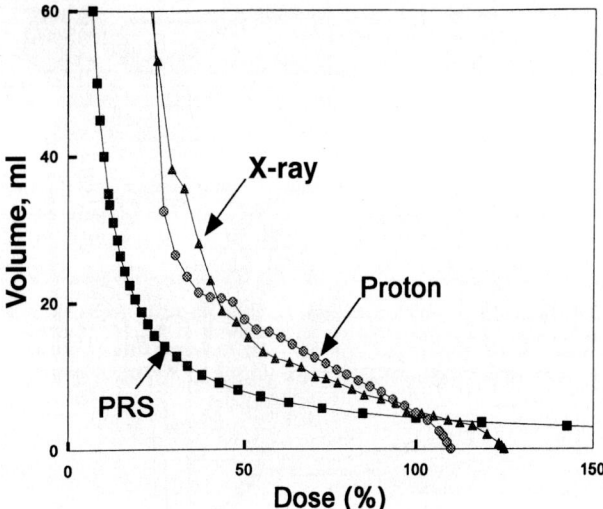

FIGURE 51–3 ■ Dose-volume curves from the LINAC (x-ray), proton beam, and Photon Radiosurgical System (PRS) demonstrate that with the PRS treatment, high doses are delivered to small volumes with some normal tissue sparing for volumes less than 50 ml compared with the linac or proton beam therapy plans. (From Douglas RM, Beatty J, Gall K, et al: Dosimetric results from a feasibility study of a novel radiosurgical source for irradiation of intracranial metasases. Int Radiat Oncol Biol Phys 36:443–450, 1996.)

(Radionics, Burlington, MA). After fixation of the frame to the patient, a stereotactic computed tomography (CT) scan with contrast is obtained using 1.5-mm contiguous slices through the tumor. The anteroposterior, lateral, and vertical dimensions of the tumor are determined and target coordinates are calculated for the center of the lesion. If appropriate, a standard stereotactic biopsy is then performed through a bur hole and specimens from the target are submitted for pathologic analysis.

If intraoperative frozen section analysis confirms the diagnosis of tumor, then the irradiation treatment can be instituted at the same sitting. First, the biopsy needle tract is dilated slightly to accommodate the probe tip (3-mm diameter) using a graduated series of dilators. The PRS device is then mounted on the arc of the CRW stereotactic apparatus and advanced along the biopsy tract to the target coordinates (Fig. 51–4). In general, lesions less than 2.0 cm in diameter are prescribed 18 Gy and lesions greater than 3.0 cm are prescribed 15 Gy. The exact lesion dimensions obtained from the contrast-enhanced CT are combined with dose/depth and isodose curves of the PRS to determine the optimal radiation treatment plan. The probe tip position, beam voltage, and current are used to calculate the duration of treatment required to administer the prescribed dose to the periphery of the tumor with a 2-mm margin. With all components connected to the control box, the prescribed voltage and current parameters are selected, and the timer is set to the calculated treatment time. The device is activated by starting the timer and automatically terminates after completion of the selected treatment time. The PRS probe is then removed, and the incision is closed in standard fashion. The procedure is carried out under local anesthesia with intravenous sedation to minimize patient discomfort.[10, 11, 16, 27]

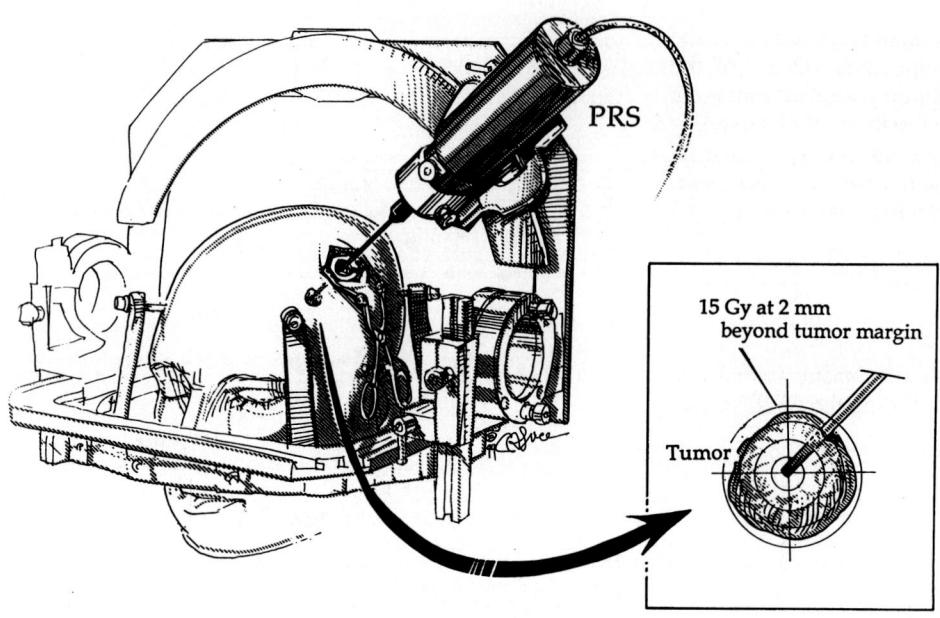

**FIGURE 51–4** ■ The Photon Radiosurgical System (PRS) is mounted on the arc carrier of the CRW frame that stereotactically places the probe tip at the target center. After the device has been activated, a low-energy x-ray beam emanates from the tip of the probe to irradiate the lesion target *(inset)*.

## CLINICAL EXPERIENCE

We have been performing interstitial radiosurgery with the PRS at the Massachusetts General Hospital since December 1992. Case selection has been limited to those patients with either primary or secondary malignant brain tumors who were not considered suitable for conventional surgical treatment. Initially, lesions had to be 3 cm or less in greatest dimension and supratentorial in location, but since 1997, we have expanded our criteria to include lesions up to 4 cm in size and cerebellar in location.

All patients have undergone detailed clinical evaluation, Karnofsky Performance Scale (KPS) rating, and contrast-enhanced CT scan or magnetic resonance imaging (MRI) prior to treatment. All patients return at regular intervals for follow-up clinical evaluation and imaging studies to document any changes in lesion size. Tumor response was graded independently by a neuroradiologist with direct measurement of the maximal tumor dimensions as seen on the last post-treatment MRI study and compared with pretreatment studies. Reduction or stabilization of tumor size was accepted as local control, whereas enlargement of the tumor indicated local failure. Clinical and radiologic outcomes were measured at the last follow-up visit or at the time of death. If the tumor showed signs of progression at any time after treatment, alternative methods of treatment were used as clinically necessary. Patients with metastases who had not received whole-brain radiation therapy (WBRT) before interstitial radiosurgery were given 30 Gy in 10 fractions after treatment. Patients with primary malignant gliomas were given WBRT up to 5700 cGy in conventional fashion after interstitial radiosurgery.

## RESULTS

To date, 40 patients with cerebral metastases and 5 patients with malignant primary tumors (26 men, 19 women; age range, 37 to 80 years; mean age, 62 years) have undergone interstitial radiosurgery with the PRS. Of the patients with metastases, 22 had solitary lesions and 18 had multiple (from 2 to 7) lesions. The primary source of the cerebral metastases was lung cancer in 25, malignant melanoma in 10, renal cell carcinoma in 3, and other carcinoma in 2. Lesions ranged in size from 4 to 40 mm (mean, 16.8 mm) in greatest diameter and were located in various lobes. Treatment diameter (lesion diameter + 2-mm margin) ranged from 8 to 44 mm. Single doses of radiation between 10 and 20 Gy (mean, 15.8 Gy) were administered, with an average treatment time of 19.5 minutes (range, 4 to 75 minutes). Fourteen patients with cerebral metastases had received prior WBRT, and the remainder received 30 Gy in 10 fractions within 2 weeks of PRS treatment.

All patients tolerated the procedure well and most patients were discharged home the day after treatment. Follow-up has ranged from 10 days to more than 30 months (mean, 7 months). Two patients experienced isolated focal motor seizures within 24 to 48 hours of surgery and required anticonvulsants. Two patients had brain edema that resolved on corticosteroids and diuretics. One patient had a subdural hematoma 3 months after treatment, but it was on the side opposite the treated lesion. There were no deaths, infections, or serious neurologic morbidity.

Local control of the lesion (defined as stabilization or reduction of tumor size) was obtained in 36 (90%) of the 40 patients with metastases. Tumor progression was observed at 3 months post-PRS treatment in two patients, at 6 months in one patient, and at 10 months in one patient. Surgical resection was performed in all four patients and pathologic analysis demonstrated central necrosis along with a thin rim of viable tumor around the periphery of the lesion in two patients, and radiation necrosis only in the other two. Two patients had postmortem examination. One patient with malignant melanoma who died 12 months after treatment had no tumor cells in the treated lesion. The second patient with adenocarcinoma of the lung died 20 months after treatment and demonstrated no tumor cells in the treated frontal lesion, but rare viable tumor cells were detected in the treated temporal lesion.

At last follow-up, 34 patients with cerebral metastases have died: 26 from systemic disease (between 12 days and 31 months after treatment), 7 from distant central nervous system (CNS) metastases (between 5 and 14 months after treatment), and 1 patient 10 days after percutaneous gastrostomy for recurrent aspiration pneumonia. Six patients with cerebral metastases are alive and well. Median survival was 13 months.

Of the five patients who were thought to have unresectable primary brain tumors, three had malignant gliomas. In each case, although there was satisfactory control of the lesion within the treatment volume, infiltrative tumor grew into the surrounding cortex, resulting in progressive and unremitting disease. One patient was diagnosed with a primary CNS lymphoma and has had complete and long-term control of the lesion at the treatment area, but recurrent lymphoma in other lobes successfully treated with methotrexate. The final patient was believed to have a malignant glioma based on clinical presentation, radiologic findings, and intraoperative pathologic analysis. Subsequent pathologic evaluation suggested that the abnormal glial cells and necrosis were not due to tumor but were probably reactive astrocytes adjacent to an area of ischemic necrosis. Only necrotic tissue was irradiated and the patient has had no adverse effects from treatment.

## DISCUSSION

Intracerebral metastases are common and occur in up to 15% of patients with cancer.[14] The relatively well circumscribed, noninvasive nature of brain metastases, compared with the diffuse, infiltrating primary brain tumors, makes them appropriate candidates for focal therapy.[12, 29] Focal irradiation has been used successfully for both newly diagnosed and recurrent brain metastases, and can administer a lethal tumor dose while minimizing exposure to normal brain.[2, 6, 17, 20, 22, 31, 37]

The goal of any radiosurgical procedure is to deliver accurately a large single fraction of radiation to a small target volume while minimizing exposure to surrounding tissue.[23] With external radiosurgical systems, the desired dose-volume distribution is obtained when the focused beams intersect and summate at the target point after traversing cranial tissue from varied angles.[11] Conventional interstitial brachytherapy obtains its desired dose-volume distribution by placing a radiation source directly in the tumor. Dose rates for conventional implanted radionuclides are in the range of 0.5 to 2.0 cGy/min and the treatment takes many hours to several days.[28] The dose rate during radiosurgery, with either linac or Gamma knife, is typically several hundred centigrays per minute, with treatment times averaging 15 to 60 minutes.[27]

The PRS has operational characteristics that combine the short treatment times of external-beam radiosurgery with the radiobiologic advantages of interstitial brachytherapy.[10] The major radiobiologic advantage of interstitial brachytherapy is related to intratumoral placement of the radioactive isotope. The emitted dose is attenuated in tissue with increasing distance ($1/r^2$) from the source, which results in maximal delivery of radiation to the tumor with relative sparing of the surrounding normal brain.[7] Of two commonly used isotopes, $^{125}I$ generates low-energy photons (28 to 35 keV) but has a very low dose rate, typically requiring treatment times of several days. Radioisotopes with very low dose rates may require permanent implantation.[10, 11] $^{192}Ir$ emits high-energy photons (300 to 610 keV) and higher dose rates that can shorten treatment times, but has less sharply defined dosimetry.[34] These conventional radioactive isotopes have been effective in the treatment of certain brain tumors but do decay in activity during storage and require special facilities and procedures for their safe handling and disposal. Protective shielding of health personnel must also be considered. Compared with interstitial brachytherapy using standard implanted radionuclides, the PRS treatment has significant advantages because of the adjustable dose rate and steeper dose gradient—and hence less dose to normal tissue outside the target—it provides. Also, PRS treatment eliminates the need to handle radioactive sources.[5]

Unlike external radiosurgical systems, which require very large and expensive facilities, the portable PRS provides a unique, cost-effective opportunity for providing interstitial radiation therapy immediately after histologic confirmation of malignancy in patients undergoing biopsy of intracranial lesions.[16] Moreover, the dosimetry provided by the PRS is similar to, and perhaps better than that achieved with proton beam or linac three-dimensional treatment planning for small, spherical intracranial lesions.[16]

An obvious difference between interstitial approaches (brachytherapy and PRS) and other noninvasive radiosurgical techniques (Gamma knife, linac, or proton beam therapy) is that with the former, a catheter or probe tip must be placed into the tumor. This imparts a small but definite risk of hemorrhage, injury to the surrounding brain, or infection. Given the need for tissue diagnosis before many forms of radiation treatment, however, the added risk of the treatment procedure can be minimized by inserting the probe at the time of the stereotactic biopsy. The PRS should not impart any more risk than conventional interstitial procedures, and because the procedure is performed over a very short time, the risk of infection is less.[11, 27]

Potential inaccuracies involving target selection and volume determination exist with any radiosurgical system, but the extremely sharp dose distribution curves of this device require targeting accuracy. Opening of the cranial vault with shift of intracranial structures may induce additional targeting error. Placement of the probe itself could displace the tumor volume from its imaged position and may increase the inaccuracy related to dose distribution. The same problem of mechanical perturbation of tissues exists with interstitial brachytherapy using temporary $^{125}I$ implants. The ability, however, to check the actual position of the implanted sources with postoperative radiographs and to modify the source positions by placing or adjusting the catheters positions, may be a potential advantage of the $^{125}I$ catheter implant system.[10, 27, 31]

The spherical and noninfiltrative nature of cerebral metastases makes them ideal candidates for interstitial brachytherapy and radiosurgical treatment.[20, 27, 37] WBRT in patients with cerebral metastases extends median survival time to between 3 and 6 months depending on the type of primary cancer, extent of systemic disease, and a variety of other factors, but overall prognosis is poor.[8] Patients with solitary cerebral metastases who undergo surgical excision plus WBRT experience improved overall survival (10 to 12 months) and better local control rates compared with WBRT alone.[32, 35, 38] Resection of multiple metastases may also lead to improved survival in those patients with controlled systemic disease, but resective surgery necessitates hospitalization and operative risk, which could be minimized by less invasive techniques. Palliation of symptoms and improvement in long-term survival have already been demonstrated in patients with both new and recurrent solitary brain metastases using $^{125}$I implants.[31] If the PRS device is similarly effective, it could represent an attractive alternative to conventional surgery in this population of patients.[10, 11]

Treatment that provides local control of single, multiple, or recurrent brain metastases imparts clinical benefit in terms of quality of life and survival.[3, 24, 32] Patchell and colleagues[32] demonstrated that the combination of surgery and radiation therapy for solitary brain metastases improved local control from 48% to 80% and increased median survival from 15 to 40 weeks. Alexander and coworkers[3] demonstrated local control rates of 89% and median survival of 9.4 months in 248 radiosurgically treated patients with brain metastases. The results of radiosurgery are encouraging and suggest that radiosurgery can be an effective alternative to surgery in patients with single, multiple, or recurrent cerebral metastases.[1, 3, 9, 16–18]

Interstitial radiosurgery using the photoelectron device offers a safe alternative for the treatment of brain metastases. Results of treatment using the PRS technique demonstrate a 90% local control rate and median survival of 13 months, which are within the ranges reported by others and appear to be comparable with results of other radiosurgical modalities.

When tissue diagnosis is required, the ability to perform stereotactic biopsy and interstitial radiosurgery at the same procedure could be advantageous and cost effective. However, the PRS is unlikely to replace conventional radiosurgery devices such as Gamma knife, linac, or proton beam, especially in the treatment of patients with arteriovenous malformations or acoustic neurinomas.[11]

Interstitial radiosurgery imparts less dose to nontarget normal tissue than other forms of radiosurgery. This reduction in dose at larger volumes may represent a clinical advantage for selected cases and may allow for treatment of metastases too large to be treated with external radiosurgery. It is not yet clear what role the photoelectron device will have in the treatment of primary brain tumors. Malignant and even low-grade gliomas are usually larger than 3 to 4 cm at the time of diagnosis and tend to infiltrate locally along white matter tracts. However, the device may be of use in small, deep gliomas or recurrences, and treatment plans incorporating multiple isocenters are feasible.[10, 11]

Perhaps its most useful role will be for intraoperative irradiation during open neurosurgical procedures in a fashion similar to that used by other surgical specialties. The probe tip can be easily shielded to allow for unidirectional irradiation of resection cavities, tumor margins, dural attachments, or skull base lesions. Conversely, sensitive neural structures could be shielded by thin, radiopaque metals to prevent radiation injury during treatment. It may have even broader application in other surgical subspecialties, including breast cancer surgery, urology, gynecology, orthopedics, and otolaryngology.[10, 11]

## CONCLUSIONS

The PRS is a novel device for the interstitial radiosurgical treatment of cerebral metastases and possibly other brain tumors. It offers a convenient and cost-efficient method for providing interstitial radiation therapy in patients undergoing diagnostic biopsy of intracranial lesions. When treating small, circumscribed, nearly spherical intracranial lesions, the PRS treatment appears to offer superior dosimetric advantages over linac, Gamma knife, or proton beam therapy in sparing the surrounding normal brain tissue. Given its operational characteristics and dosimetry profile, it compares favorably with current external radiosurgical devices and has certain logistical advantages over standard interstitial brachytherapy.

## REFERENCES

1. Alder JR, Cox RS, Kaplan I, et al: Stereotactic radiosurgical treatment of brain metastases. J Neurosurg 76:444–449, 1992.
2. Alesch F, Hawliczek R, Koos WT: Interstitial irradiation of brain metastases. Acta Neurochir (Wien) 63:29–34, 1995.
3. Alexander E, Moriarty TM, Davis RB, et al: Stereotactic radiosurgery for definitive, noninvasive treatment of brain metastases. J Natl Cancer Inst 87:34–40, 1995.
4. Hakim A, Zervas NT, Hakim F, et al: Initial characterization of the dosimetry and radiobiology of a device for administering interstitial stereotactic radiosurgery. Neurosurgery 40:510–517, 1997.
5. Beatty J, Biggs PJ, Gall KP, et al: A new miniature x-ray device for interstitial radiosurgery: Dosimetry. Med Phys 23:53–62, 1996.
6. Bernstein M, Cabanotg A, LaPerriere N, et al: Brachytherapy for recurrent single brain metastases. Can J Neurol Sci 22:13–16, 1995.
7. Bernstein M, Gutin PH: Interstitial irradiation of brain tumors: A review. Neurosurgery 9:741–750, 1981.
8. Cairncross JG, Kim JH, Posner JB: Radiation therapy for brain metastases. Ann Neurol 7:529–541, 1980.
9. Coffey RJ, Flickinger JC, Bissonette DJ, et al: Radiosurgery for solitary brain metastases using the cobalt-60 gamma unit: Methods and results in 24 patients. Int J Radiat Oncol Biol Phys 20:1287–1295, 1991.
10. Cosgrove GR, Hochberg FH, Zervas NT, et al: Interstitial irradiation of brain tumors using a miniature radiosurgery device: Initial experience. Neurosurgery 40:5518–525, 1997.
11. Cosgrove GR, Zervas NT: Interstitial radiosurgery. In Gildenburg PH, Tasker RR (eds): Textbook of Stereotactic and Functional Radiosurgery. New York: McGraw-Hill, 1998, pp 619–624.
12. Cull A, Gregor A, Hopwood P, et al: Neurological and cognitive impairment in long-term survivors of small cell lung cancer. Eur J Cancer 30a:1067–1074, 1994.
13. Danlos H: Quelques considerationes sur le traitement des dermatoses par le radium. J Physiother 3:98–106, 1905.
14. DeAngelis LM: Management of brain metastases. Cancer Invest 12:156–165, 1994.
15. Dinsmore M, Hart KJ, Sliski AP, et al: A new miniature x-ray source for interstitial radiosurgery: Device description. Med Phys 23:45–52, 1996.
16. Douglas RM, Beatty J, Gall K, et al: Dosimetric results from a feasibility study of a novel radiosurgical source for irradiation of intracranial metastases. Int J Radiat Oncol Biol Phys 36:443–450, 1996.

17. Engenhart R, Bernhard NK, Hover KH, et al: Long-term follow-up for brain metastases treated by percutaneous stereotactic single high-dose irradiation. Cancer 71:1353–1361, 1993.
18. Flickinger JC, Kondziolka D, Lunsford LD, et al: A multi-institutional experience with stereotactic radiosurgery for solitary brain metastases. Int J Radiat Oncol Biol Phys 28:797–802, 1994.
19. Flickinger JC, Lunsford LD, Kondziolka D: Dose prescription and dose volume effects in radiosurgery. Stereotact Radiosurg 3:51–59, 1992.
20. Flickinger JC, Loeffler Js, Larson DA: Stereotactic radiosurgery for intracranial malignancies. Oncology 8:81–98, 1994.
21. Gutin PH, Philips TL, Wara WM, et al: Brachytherapy of recurrent malignant brain tumors with removable high-activity iodine-125 sources. J Neurosurg 60:61–68, 1984.
22. Heros DO, Kasdon DL, Chun M: Brachytherapy in the treatment of recurrent solitary brain metastases. Neurosurgery 23:733–737, 1988.
23. Hudgins WR: What is radiosurgery? Neurosurgery 23:272–273, 1988.
24. Kanady K, Choi N, Efird J, et al: Efficacy of postoperative fractionated external beam radiation in the treatment of solitary NSCLC brain metastases. Int J Radiat Oncol Biol Phys 30:294, 1994.
25. Luxton G, Petrovich Z, Jozsef G, et al: Stereotactic radiosurgery: Principles and comparison of treatment methods. Neurosurgery 32:241–258, 1993.
26. Marks LB, Spencer DP: The influence of volume on the tolerance of the brain to radiosurgery. J Neurosurg 75:177–180, 1991.
27. McDermott MW, Cosgrove GR, Larson DA, et al: Interstitial brachytherapy for intracranial metastases. Neurosurg Clin N Am 7:485–495, 1996.
28. Meigooni A, Meli J, Nath R: A comparison of solid phantoms with water for dosimetry of $^{125}$I brachytherapy sources. Med Phys 15:695–701, 1988.
29. Nieder C, Berberich W, Nestle U, et al: Relation between local result and total dose of radiotherapy for brain metastases. Int J Radiat Oncol Biol Phys 33:349–355, 1995.
30. Noell KT, Herskovic AM: Principles of radiotherapy of CNS tumors. In Wilkins RH, Rengachary SS (eds): Neurosurgery. New York: McGraw-Hill, 1985, pp 1084–1095.
31. Prados M, Leibel S, Barnett CM, et al: Interstitial brachytherapy for metastatic brain tumors. Cancer 63:657–660, 1989.
32. Patchell RA, Tibbs PA, Walsh JW, et al: A randomized trial of surgery in the treatment of single metastases to the brain. N Engl J Med 322:494–500, 1990.
33. Philips MH (ed): Physical Aspects of Stereotactic Radiosurgery. New York: Plenum, 1993.
34. Scharfen CO, Sneed PK, Wara WM, et al: High activity iodine-125 interstitial implant for gliomas. Int J Radiat Oncol Biol Phys 24:583–591, 1992.
35. Smalley SR, Laws ER, O'Fallon JR, et al: Resection for solitary brain metastases: Role of adjuvant radiation therapy and prognostic variables in 229 patients. J Neurosurg 75:531–540, 1992.
36. Smith D, Silski A, Beatty J, et al: A new miniature x-ray device for stereotactic radiotherapy: Treatment methodology. Med Phys 20:1291, 1993.
37. Thornton AF, Harsh GR: Recommendations for treatment of brain metastases. Neurosurg Clin N Am 7:559–564, 1996.
38. Vecht CJ, Haaxma-Reiche H, Noordijk EM, et al: Treatment of single brain metastasis: Radiotherapy alone or combined with neurosurgery. Ann Neurol 33:583–590, 1993.

# Tumors on the Cerebral Convexities

# CHAPTER 52

# Surgical and Radiotherapeutic Management of Brain Metastasis

■ PERRY BLACK

Brain metastases have become the commonest intracranial tumors, slightly outnumbering primary intracranial neoplasms.[1] An estimated 20% to 40% of cancer patients develop intracranial metastases at some stage of their disease.[2-5] The apparently high incidence of brain metastasis reflects the longer survival of patients with cancer in response to improved methods of treatment; it may also be a function of improved detection with high-resolution neuroimaging techniques.

## PATHOLOGIC ASPECTS

### Origin of Metastases

Common sources of metastases to the brain are tumors of the lung, breast, and kidney and malignant melanomas.[6] Metastases from other sources, including the gastrointestinal tract, thyroid, uterus, ovary, pancreas, and prostate as well as sarcomas, are relatively uncommon.[7-13] Although melanoma is not the commonest tumor metastasizing to the brain, it ranks highest in its proclivity to spread to the brain[14] and has a greater tendency for metastasis to the brain in males than in females.[15]

In some series of brain metastasis, about 50% of the patients present with neurologic symptoms or signs as the first manifestation of malignant disease.[11, 13, 16, 17] The primary origin in these cases is usually discovered later (see Figs. 52–1 and 52–2), but occasionally the primary tumor cannot be identified, even at autopsy. In patients in whom the primary tumor is unknown initially, more than half are subsequently found to have bronchogenic carcinoma.[16]

### Distribution in Brain

#### Solid Metastases

About two thirds of intracranial metastases are located within the brain parenchyma (intracerebral) (Figs. 52–1 to 52–3). The remaining one third are situated in the subdural or extradural space and may compress, but not necessarily invade, the brain (Fig. 52–4). Metastases in brain parenchyma, in more than 60% of cases, are located at the gray-white junction in the vascular border zone regions; this supports the concept that metastatic emboli tend to lodge in vessels at the site of sudden reduction of vascular caliber (gray-white junction) and in the distal vascular bed (border zone).[18]

In some series, a predominance of parenchymal metastases has been observed in the distribution of the middle cerebral artery,[9, 13] a finding that has been explained on the basis of laminar arterial flow.[19] The cerebellum has also been reported as a site of predilection[7, 21]; this appearance may be related to the fact that mass lesions in the cerebellum tend to manifest themselves clinically earlier than those in relatively silent areas, such as the frontal lobes. Wide variability exists in the location of brain metastases. Tumor emboli may settle in any part of the brain, and the distribution probably reflects the relative mass of the different areas of the brain.[22, 23]

### Leptomeningeal Metastases

Leukemia and lymphoma constitute another major category of central nervous system metastases. They generally invade the leptomeninges in a diffuse or multifocal manner,[24] usually with widespread seeding of tumor cells in the cerebrospinal fluid rather than as solid tumor deposits (Fig. 52–5). Although hematologic malignancies contribute the largest proportion of cases of leptomeningeal metastases, an increasing number of solid tumors—especially carcinoma of the breast—is being found as a source of this form of central nervous system metastasis.

### Single Versus Multiple Brain Metastases

A brain metastasis is regarded as being single when only one metastasis is present in the brain, regardless of the presence of extracranial cancer (Figs. 52–6 and 52–7; see also Figs. 52–1 and 52–4). A solitary brain metastasis is a single brain metastasis in which no known cancer exists elsewhere in the body (see Figs. 52–1 and 52–2).[25] Single or solitary metastases occur in 50% to 65% of cases when the diagnosis is made while the patient is alive.[14, 22] Metastases from the colon, breast, and kidney are generally

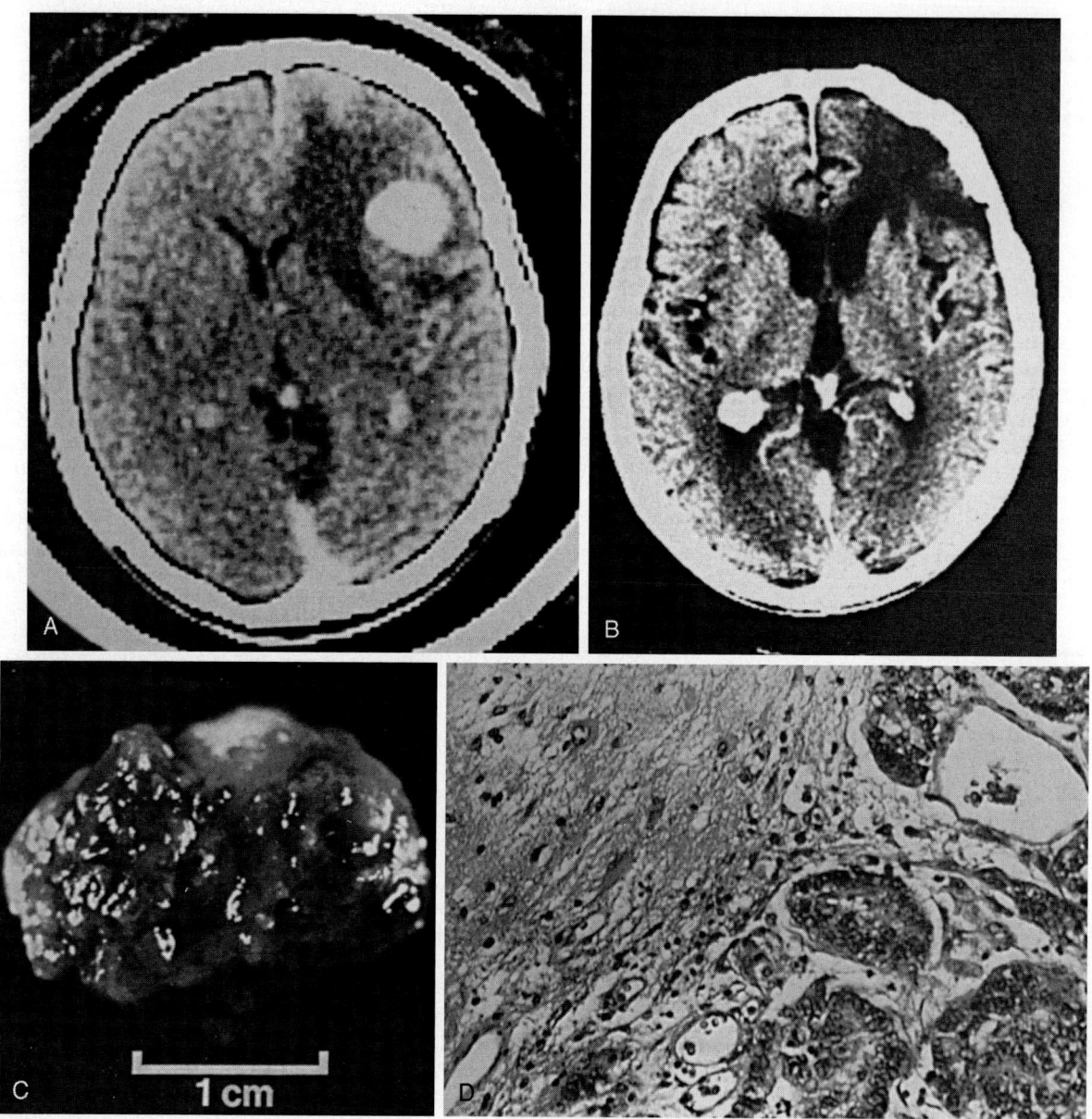

**FIGURE 52–1** ■ Solitary brain metastasis in a patient whose initial presentation was related only to cerebral symptoms. Despite a search for a possible primary source, the bronchogenic site of origin did not become apparent until 8 months after surgical excision of the brain metastasis, when the patient began to have chest pain. *A,* A computed tomography (CT) scan with contrast showing a frontal mass that was surgically excised and proved to be metastatic, but the primary tumor was unknown. After surgery, the patient received a course of whole-brain radiotherapy. *B,* A CT scan of the same patient 1 year later; there is no evidence of recurrence of brain metastasis, but the patient's general condition declined secondary to the bronchogenic carcinoma. *C,* Gross photograph of the mass removed from the frontal region. *D,* Histopathologic section of lesion showing well to moderately differentiated adenocarcinoma infiltrating the brain tissue, narrow bands of which are visible between the epithelial elements. (Original magnification × 420.) (Pathologic interpretation courtesy of Dr. Jeffrey Stead, Hahnemann University Hospital, Philadelphia.)

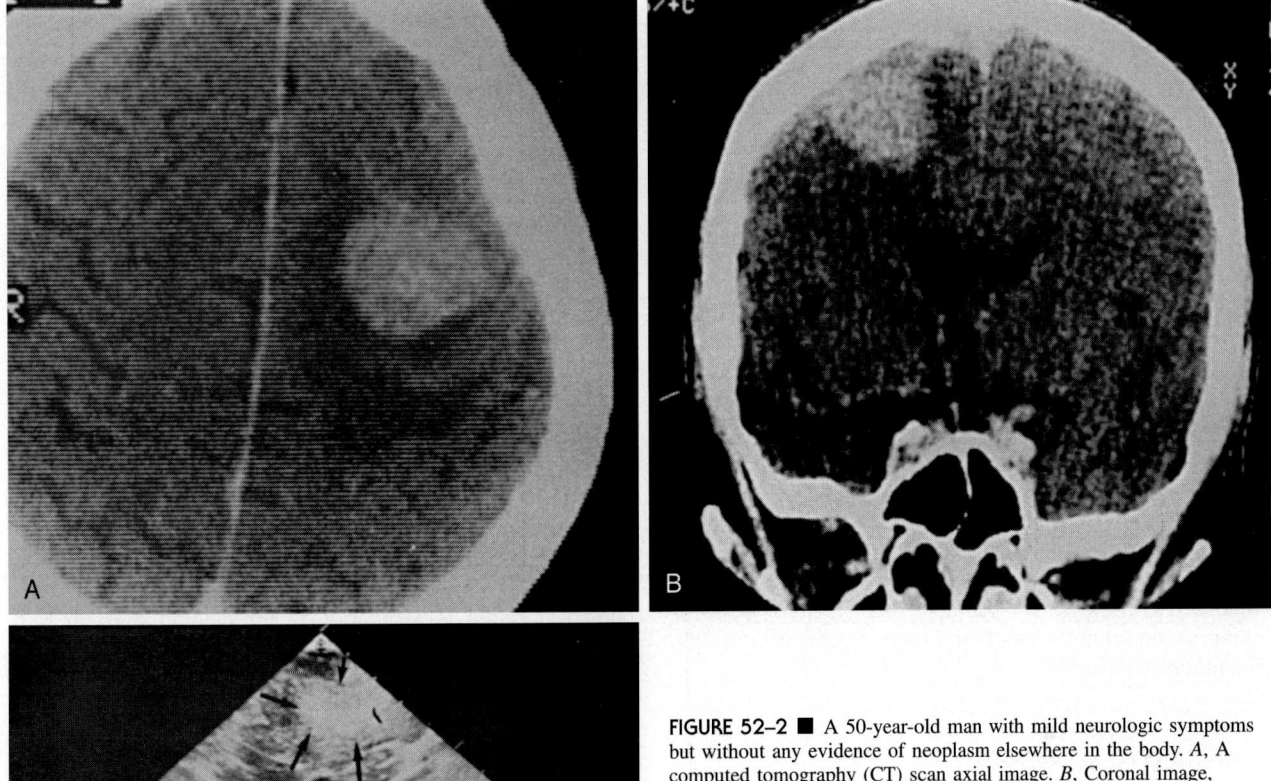

**FIGURE 52–2 ■** A 50-year-old man with mild neurologic symptoms but without any evidence of neoplasm elsewhere in the body. *A,* A computed tomography (CT) scan axial image. *B,* Coronal image, showing a lesion in the left frontotemporal area, which is suspicious for metastasis; note that the lesion is relatively circumscribed and surrounded by moderate edema. *C,* An excisional biopsy, rather than a stereotactic biopsy, was undertaken because the lesion was close to the surface; it was readily accessible, and there was no suspicion of brain abscess. The cortex appeared normal, and intraoperative ultrasound was used to precisely localize the lesion (*arrows*) and thus aid in placement of the cortical incision. An alternative to the use of ultrasound at the time of the craniotomy would have been stereotactic localization of the tumor site.

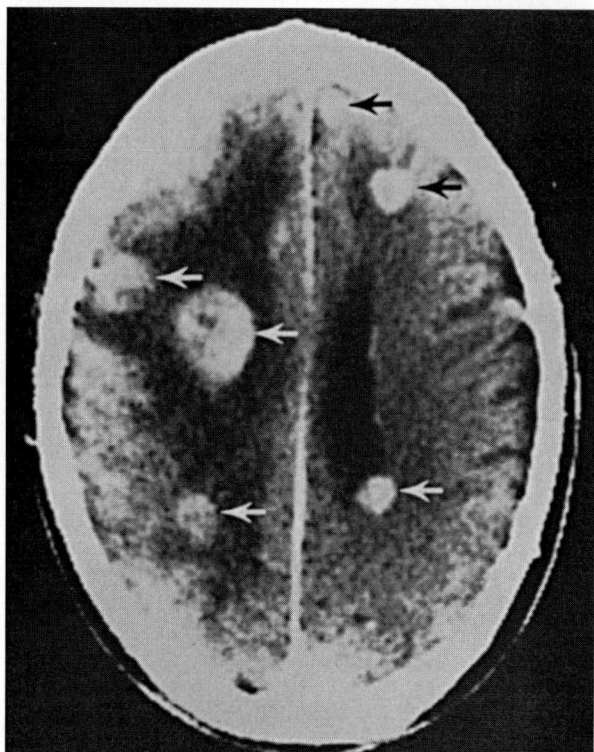

FIGURE 52–3 ■ A computed tomography (CT) scan showing multiple intracranial metastases (*black* and *white arrows*). The patient had bronchogenic carcinoma.

associated with single (or solitary) brain lesions, whereas melanoma and lung cancer are more prone to multiple intracranial metastases.[4]

## Characteristics of Lesions

Intracerebral metastases generally are soft, nodular, circumscribed masses, often with central necrosis (see Fig. 52–1). They vary in size from minute (requiring microscopic identification) to centimeters in diameter (see Fig. 52–4). Even small metastases are characteristically associated with enormous surrounding reactive edema, which further compresses the brain tissue and increases neurologic symptoms and signs (see Fig. 52–1).

## LATENT INTERVAL

Wide variability exists in the interval between the clinical appearance of the primary cancer and that of the cerebral metastasis. As mentioned previously, a cerebral metastasis commonly presents as the first manifestation of a malignant neoplasm in the body. The appearance of the primary and the metastatic lesion at widely separated intervals is referred to as *metachronous* metastasis (see Figs. 52–1, 52–2, 52–5, and 52–6), in contrast with *synchronous* metastasis, in which the primary and metastatic lesions become manifest roughly simultaneously (see Figs. 52–4 and 52–7). For example, in different series, an intracranial lesion was the

first manifestation of malignancy in 14% to 40% of patients with brain metastasis from lung cancer, and the primary lung lesion was detected months to years later.[17, 25, 26] The reverse may also be true, with the symptoms of cerebral metastasis appearing months to 15 years after the diagnosis of the primary tumor.[16, 22]

The interval between the appearance of the primary tumor and the metastasis tends to be a function of the tissue of origin; the average interval between the diagnosis of lung carcinoma and the development of brain metastasis is 4 to 10 months,[17] whereas the average interval between the diagnosis of breast cancer and the development of brain metastasis is 3 years.[16] Although metastases are generally regarded as rapidly growing lesions, they can rarely grow so slowly that calcification may occur.[27]

## DIAGNOSIS

Contrast-enhanced computed tomography (CT) and enhanced magnetic resonance imaging (MRI) are equally sensitive in detecting brain metastases that are 1.5 cm or greater in size.[28] In a series of brain metastasis from small cell lung carcinoma, however, MRI was clearly superior to CT for smaller lesions (particularly those <5 mm diameter) and for lesions of all sizes in the posterior fossa.[29] In 60% of patients with brain metastasis, double-dose contrast administration is more effective than single-dose contrast administration in detecting multiple metastases; with double doses of contrast medium, no difference in lesion detection was noted as a function of the magnet strength standard (0.5, 1.0, or 1.5 Tesla), and double-dose contrast administration was not associated with adverse effects.[30] Scanning with thallium single photon emission computed tomography (SPECT) is of relatively little value in the detection and differential diagnosis of brain metastasis.[31]

The combination of history, physical and neurologic examination, and neuroimaging generally enables differentiation of metastatic tumor from other lesions, including primary brain tumors, abscess, infarction, and hemorrhage. In a study of brain metastasis, needle biopsy of brain lesions in patients with known extracranial cancer revealed nonmetastatic lesions in 11% of the cases, even after contrast-enhanced CT or MRI.[29] This finding underscores the need to establish a histologic diagnosis without assuming that a brain lesion is metastatic, despite the presence of a known malignancy elsewhere (Figs. 52–8 and 52–9).

For patients in whom brain metastasis is suspected but who do not have a history of systemic malignancy, diagnostic work-up should include chest radiograph study (see Fig. 52–7). This study reveals a mass lesion in the lung in more than 60% of patients with brain metastasis, reflecting either primary bronchogenic carcinoma or a metastasis to the lung from a primary tumor elsewhere.[32] If the chest radiograph study is unrevealing, CT of the chest may show a lung lesion. In a study comparing a chest radiograph study with a chest CT scan in search of a lung primary, the chest radiograph study was nonspecific or negative in almost 40% of the cases, but the chest CT scan proved positive; the mean size of the lung lesion in these cases was 2.5 cm, by comparison with 4.2 cm in cases with positive chest

*Text continued on page 724*

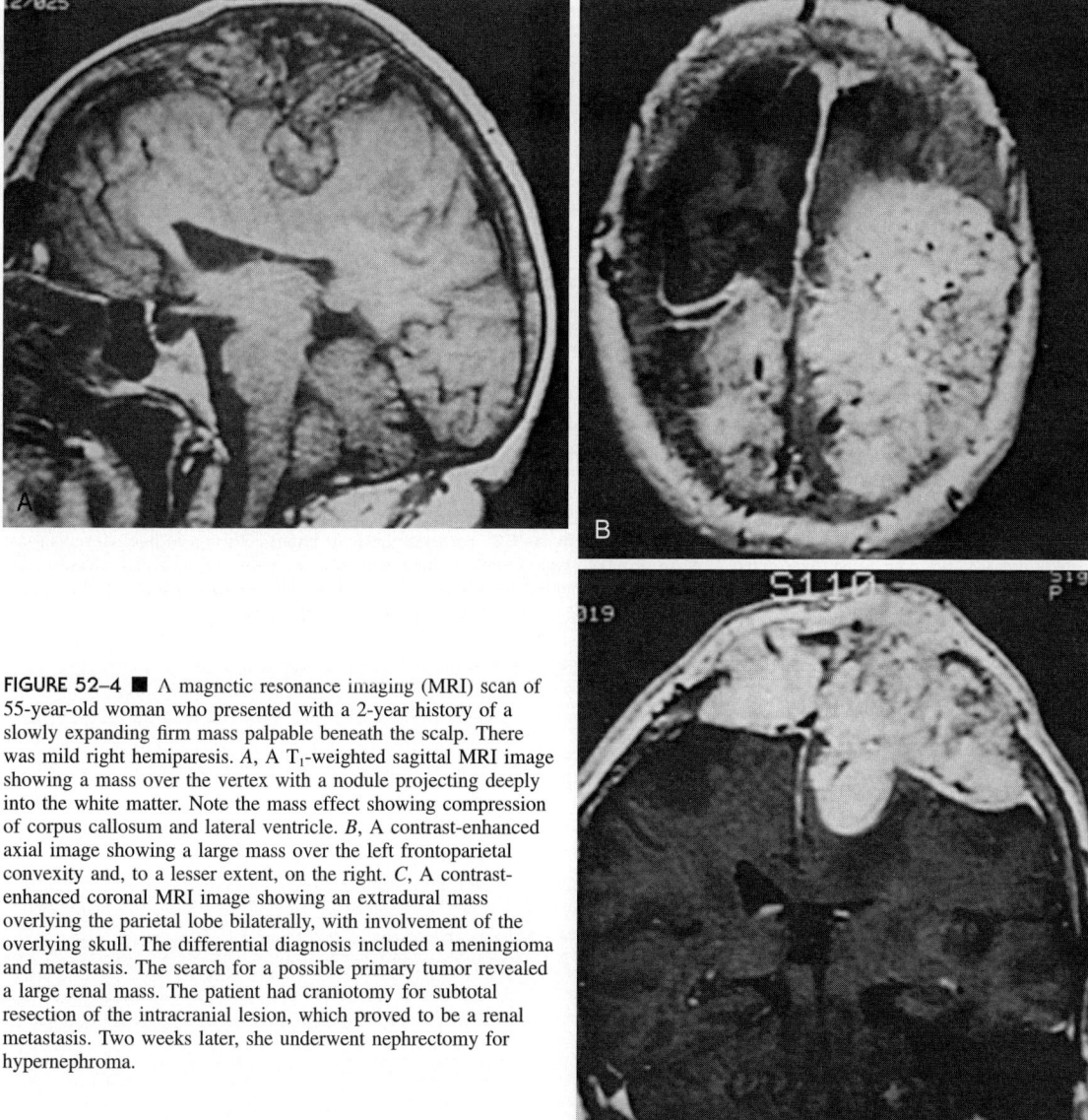

FIGURE 52–4 ■ A magnetic resonance imaging (MRI) scan of
55-year-old woman who presented with a 2-year history of a
slowly expanding firm mass palpable beneath the scalp. There
was mild right hemiparesis. *A,* A T₁-weighted sagittal MRI image
showing a mass over the vertex with a nodule projecting deeply
into the white matter. Note the mass effect showing compression
of corpus callosum and lateral ventricle. *B,* A contrast-enhanced
axial image showing a large mass over the left frontoparietal
convexity and, to a lesser extent, on the right. *C,* A contrast-
enhanced coronal MRI image showing an extradural mass
overlying the parietal lobe bilaterally, with involvement of the
overlying skull. The differential diagnosis included a meningioma
and metastasis. The search for a possible primary tumor revealed
a large renal mass. The patient had craniotomy for subtotal
resection of the intracranial lesion, which proved to be a renal
metastasis. Two weeks later, she underwent nephrectomy for
hypernephroma.

**FIGURE 52–5 ■** *A*, A computed tomography (CT) scan of a 47-year-old woman with a history of breast carcinoma, which was treated 2 years earlier with a mastectomy and chemotherapy. She then presented with a 3-month history of headaches, confusion, and lethargy. Other than papilledema, the neurologic examination was normal. The CT scan showed symmetric hydrocephalus with no evidence of a mass lesion. Meningeal carcinomatosis (carcinomatous meningitis) was suspected, thus a lumbar puncture was performed. Precautions were taken to have a twist-drill set available at the bedside to permit a ventricular puncture in the event of cerebral herniation. Although the patient's cerebrospinal fluid (CSF) pressure was elevated, she tolerated the spinal tap without incident. *B*, Cytopathologic examination of the CSF revealed sheets of tumor cells compatible with metastasis from the patient's primary breast tumor. The patient was given a course of whole-brain radiation therapy, as well as intraventricular methotrexate via an implanted ventricular (Ommaya) reservoir. She did not respond to this therapy and continued to decline until she died 6 weeks later. Although this patient did not respond to this mode of therapy, some others with meningeal carcinomatosis do show improvement.

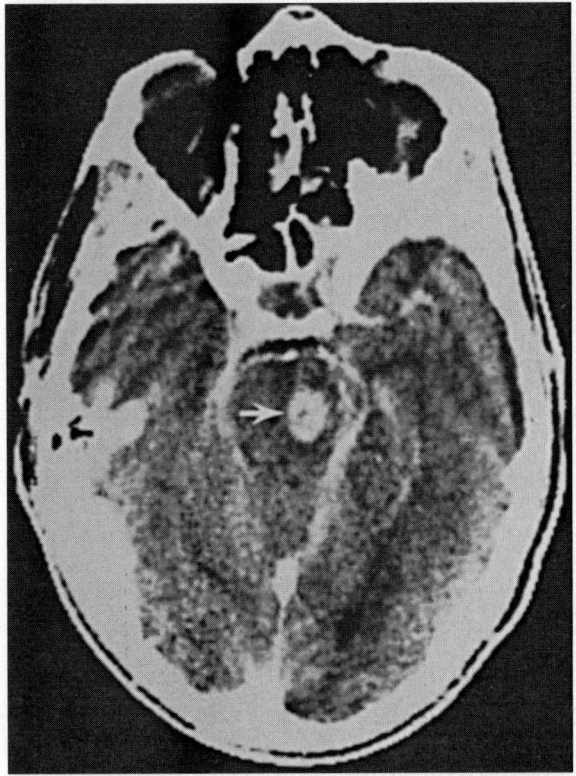

**FIGURE 52–6 ■** A computed tomography (CT) scan of a 51-year-old man with mild hemiparesis who had a history of bronchogenic carcinoma that was diagnosed 3 months earlier. The scan revealed an inoperable enhancing lesion, presumably metastasis, in the midbrain (*arrow*). In this situation, further diagnostic or therapeutic measures appear to be futile.

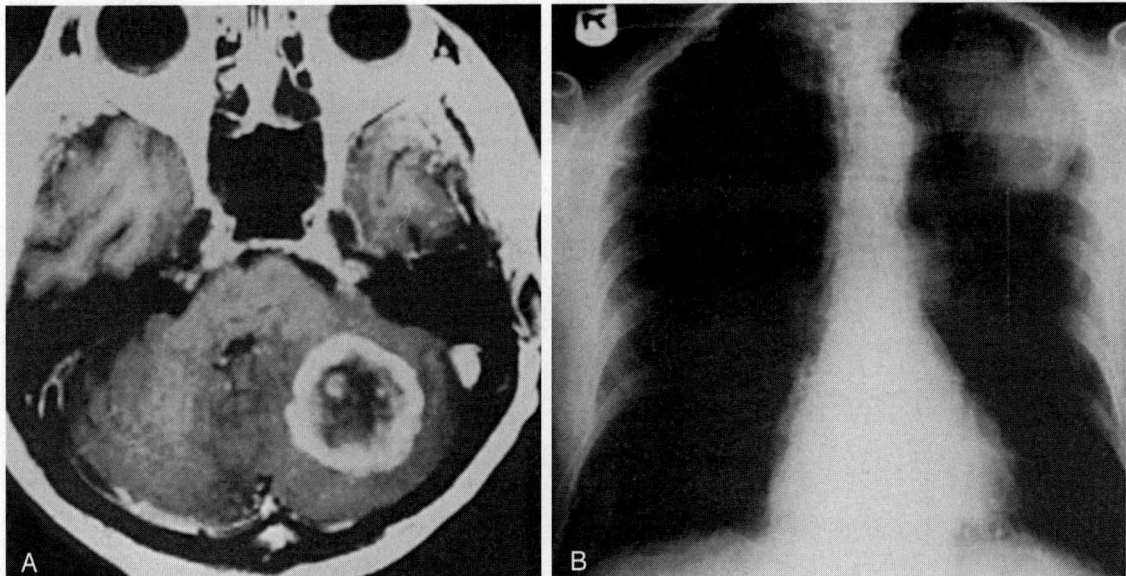

**FIGURE 52–7** ■ A 70-year-old man presented with 6-week history of headaches and 1-week history of nausea and vomiting. On examination, he had a gait disturbance with a tendency to stagger to the left. *A,* A contrast-enhanced axial $T_1$-weighted magnetic resonance imaging (MRI) scan showed a large ring-enhancing left cerebellar mass with compression and shift of the fourth ventricle. The supratentorial images showed mild hydrocephalus. *B,* A chest x-ray study showed a large mass in the left upper lobe. In view of the life-threatening nature of the cerebellar mass, surgical excision was carried out, and the lesion proved to be metastatic. The patient subsequently underwent a thoracotomy for resection of the left upper lobe; histologic examination revealed non–small cell bronchogenic carcinoma.

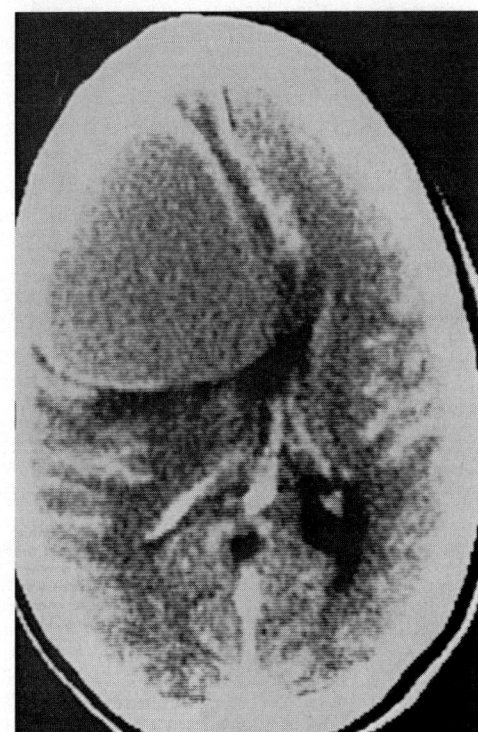

**FIGURE 52–8** ■ A computed tomography (CT) scan of a woman, age 55, with a history of squamous cell carcinoma of the lung, for which she had had a left lower lobectomy 1 month earlier. She now presented with a history of progressive lethargy lasting several days, frontal headache, and mild left hemiparesis, as well as nausea and vomiting. A CT scan of the head with contrast enhancement showed a homogeneous, relatively isodense right frontal mass with rim enhancement. To rule out the possibility that the mass could be a hematoma, a right frontal twist-drill trephine was made, with needle evacuation of 100 ml of dark blood. To reduce the chance of further bleeding, which was presumed to be from an adjacent tumor metastasis, thrombin (5000 U) was instilled into the hematoma cavity. A catheter was left in the hematoma cavity for drainage overnight. Her neurologic condition improved considerably. This case illustrates the desirability of establishing a definitive diagnosis of the brain lesion, even in cases of known malignancy elsewhere.

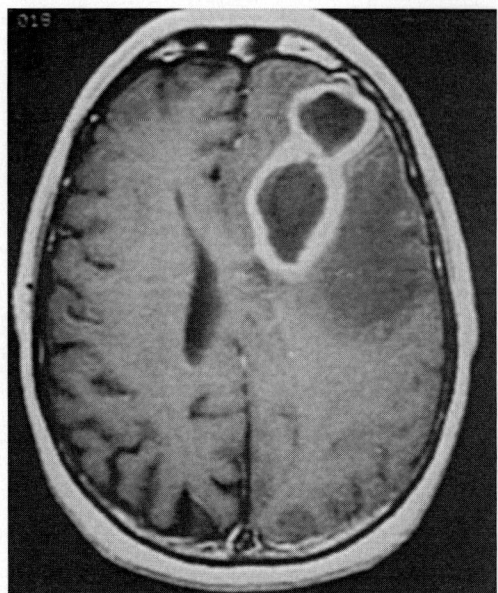

FIGURE 52–9 ■ A contrast-enhanced axial $T_1$-weighted magnetic resonance imaging (MRI) scan in a 55-year-old man with history of prior resection of a non–small cell lung carcinoma 3 years earlier. The multilocular nature of the ring-enhancing lesion in the left frontoparietal area suggests possibility of brain abscess, which was proved by stereotactic biopsy and aspiration. A stereotactic biopsy is preferable to excisional biopsy when there is suspicion of a brain abscess; this applies even for superficial lesions, because both the diagnosis and treatment can be achieved without the need for craniotomy.

x-ray study.[33] If the CT scan of the chest is negative, an examination of the breast (mammography) or prostate (to determine serum level of prostatic-specific antigen) is performed. CT scanning of the abdomen and pelvis is the next diagnostic step in search of the primary tumor (Fig. 52–10), and upper and lower gastrointestinal series may be needed. Beyond these diagnostic measures, further search for a primary site is not likely to be fruitful, and a biopsy (excisional or stereotactic) of the brain lesion may be required to establish a histologic diagnosis.

## MANAGEMENT

### Evaluation of Treatment Modalities

Management of metastasis to the brain is almost always palliative, with cure the rare exception. Because the results of therapy (in terms of survival and restoration or maintenance of neurologic function) are usually limited, considerable controversy exists regarding the appropriate mode of therapy and whether any therapy is warranted at all. Evaluation of various therapeutic modalities—radiation, surgery, or chemotherapy—was confounded by a lack of controlled, randomized studies whereby the relative merits of the respective modalities could be assessed objectively.

### Randomized Clinical Trials

Four randomized, controlled studies have been reported. Two of these studies compared surgery plus whole-brain radiotherapy versus radiotherapy alone for single metastasis in patients in good condition. The combination of surgical excision followed by radiation therapy was found to be superior to radiation therapy alone, in terms of duration and quality of survival (Table 52–1).[29, 34] The third study showed no difference in survival between the two groups.[35] The fourth randomized study in patients with single brain metastasis compared complete surgical resection plus whole-brain radiotherapy versus surgery alone.[36] Recurrence of tumor at the site of the original metastasis or elsewhere in the brain was less frequent in the surgery plus radiotherapy group than in the group with surgical resection alone. Although patients who received radiotherapy were less likely to die of neurologic causes, there was no difference between the two groups in duration of functional independence or length of survival.

Except for the randomized clinical trials cited here, reports on the management of cerebral metastasis have generally been limited by a failure to control for critical variables, such as the stage of the systemic disease, the degree of neurologic deficit, the number or location of metastatic lesions, the cell type, and the radiosensitivity of the primary lesion. Reported studies have also tended to be confounded by the use of a combination of treatment modalities.

Despite these limitations, progress is being made in the identification of patients for whom therapy is likely to benefit quality (remission of symptoms) and duration of survival. For purposes of rough comparison, the respective therapeutic modalities are shown in Table 52–1 in relation to a baseline of *no treatment*, in which case the median survival is approximately 1 month.

### Steroid Therapy

Administration of corticosteroids reduces neurologic symptoms and signs in about two thirds of patients with intracranial metastasis.[37] The benefits are often evident within 24 hours. Steroids are believed to exert a beneficial effect primarily by reducing cerebral edema surrounding the tumor; to a lesser extent, a direct oncolytic effect may be exerted on the tumor itself.[37] Corticosteroids decrease permeability of tumor capillaries caused by radiation.[38] The type of glucocorticoid does not have a significant influence on the effect.

Steroid therapy is generally started at least 24 hours before the initiation of radiation therapy or surgery. When dexamethasone is used, the recommended dose has been 16 mg daily in divided doses, but higher doses may be used if no clinical response occurs.[39] A more recent randomized clinical trial in patients with brain metastasis, using varying doses of dexamethasone, has shown that 4 mg/day is as effective as 16 mg/day.[40] Steroid doses may be safely tapered after radiotherapy. The use of steroids alone in the management of brain metastasis can prolong median survival from 1 month (without treatment) to 2 months; the palliative benefit of steroids is short lived (see Table 52–1).[20]

### Radiation Therapy

#### Conventional Whole-Brain Radiotherapy

Aside from the use of steroids to control cerebral edema, radiotherapy is the most commonly used therapeutic mod-

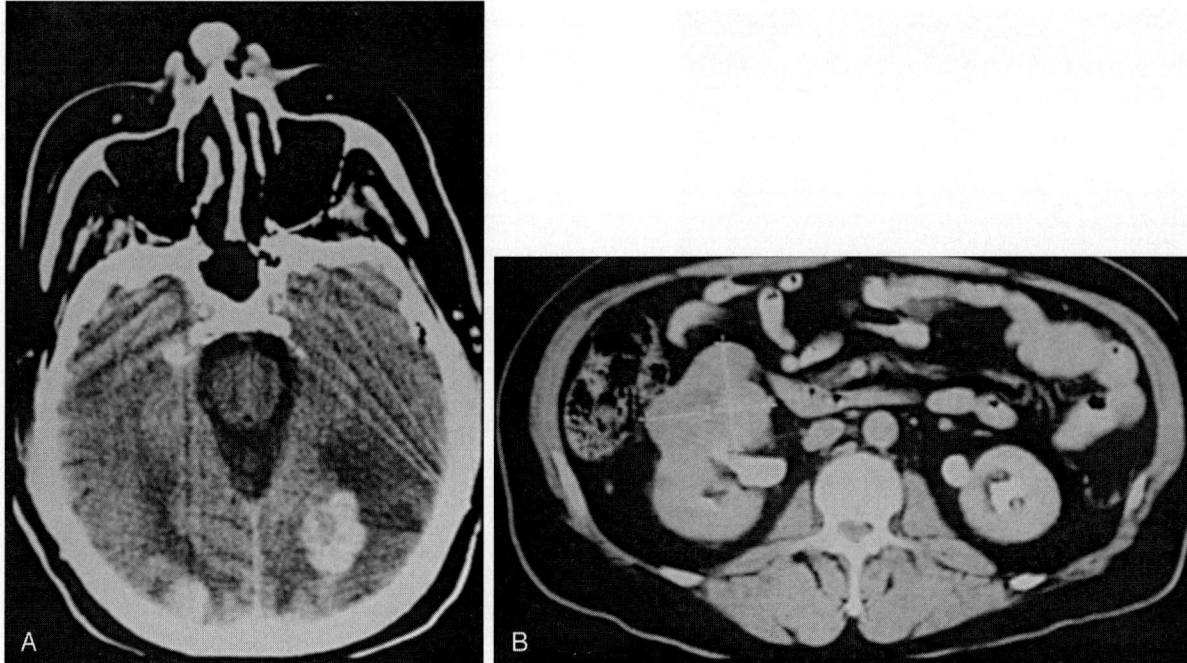

**FIGURE 52–10 ■** *A*, A contrast-enhanced computed tomography (CT) scan of 61-year-old man with a history of headaches lasting several months, showing a circumscribed enhancing mass in each occipital lobe. *B*, A contrast-enhanced abdominal CT scan showing large right renal mass. Despite the presence of two separate brain lesions, which were thought to be metastases from hypernephroma, the cerebral lesions appeared accessible and were both removed by separate craniotomies performed 2 weeks apart; ultrasound was used intraoperatively to aid localization. Histologically, both lesions were metastases, whose origin was compatible with hypernephroma. The craniotomies were performed at separate times in order to determine whether visual impairment would occur after the first craniotomy, in which case the remaining lesion would have been treated with radiotherapy only. Vision remained bilaterally intact after both procedures.

ality for cerebral metastases (Fig. 52–11), particularly in the management of multiple intracranial metastatic lesions. Radiotherapy also plays an important role in the postoperative treatment of patients with intracranial metastasis who have had surgical excision. Whole-brain therapy (rather than regional or stereotaxic therapy limited to the tumor area) is generally recommended for such patients. The rationale for whole-brain radiation is based on the assumption that, in addition to the single or multiple metastases evident on CT or MRI scans, approximately half of the patients have additional scattered metastases in the brain that are too small to be visualized by neuroimaging techniques.

With respect to the dose of radiation, a study in patients with unresected single brain metastasis was conducted in which a whole-brain dose of 32 Gy was administered in 1.6-Gy fractions twice daily, with an interfraction interval of 4 to 8 hours.[41] A boost dose (sparing the cervical spinal cord and cerebellum) was then escalated to total doses of 48, 54.4, 64, or 70.4 Gy. In this randomized study, the investigators found that a total dose of at least 54.4 Gy (using accelerated hyperfractionated radiation therapy) pro-

## TABLE 52–1 ■ BRAIN METASTASIS: COMPARISON OF SURVIVAL BY TREATMENT MODALITIES

| Study | Therapeutic Modality | Median (mo) | 1 Year (%) | >2 Years (%) |
|---|---|---|---|---|
| Posner[20] | No treatment | 1 | — | — |
| Posner[20] | Steroids alone | 2 | — | — |
| Posner[20, 64]; Shapiro and Posner[37] | WBRT alone | 3–6 | 2–3 | 4–8 |
| Haar and Patterson[7]; Raskind et al[9]; Posner[20, 64] | Surgery alone* | 5–6 | 22–31 | 3–7 |
| Ransohoff[8]; Sundaresan et al[17]; Shapiro and Posner[37] | Surgery and WBRT and/or chemotherapy | — | — | — |
| Ransohoff[8]; Sundaresan et al[17]; Shapiro and Posner[37]; Galicich et al[75] | Retrospective studies | 6–12 | 38–53 | 25 |
| Patchell et al[29]; Vecht et al[34]; Mintz et al[35]; Patchell et al[36] | Prospective randomized studies (surgery and WBRT) | 10–12 | — | — |
| Mehta et al[49]; Coffey et al[50] | Surgery, WBRT, and radiosurgery | 6.5–10 | 33 | — |
| Posner[20] | Chemotherapy | Benefit not established | | |
| Posner[20] | Immunotherapy | Benefit not established | | |

*Single metastasis.
WBRT, whole-brain radiation therapy.

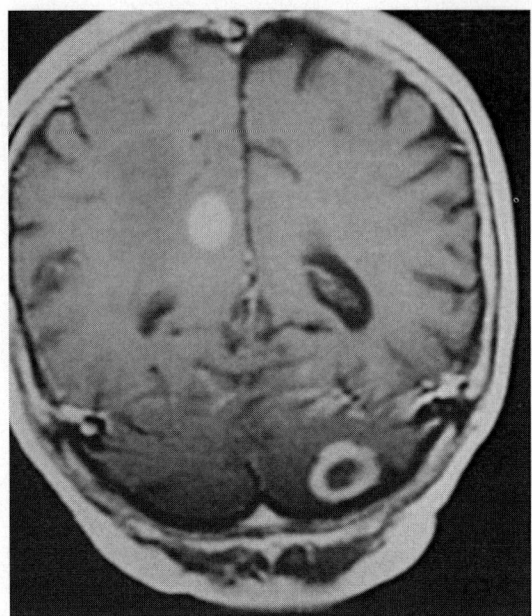

FIGURE 52–11 ■ A contrast-enhanced coronal $T_1$-weighted magnetic resonance imaging (MRI) scan of a 45-year-old woman with clinically stable bronchogenic carcinoma. Note the small circumscribed lesion in the parasagittal right parietal lobe and another lesion in the left cerebellum. A computed tomography (CT)–guided stereotactic biopsy of the right parietal lesion confirmed metastatic disease. The patient then received whole-brain radiotherapy followed by a stereotactic radiosurgery boost localized to each of the metastases.

vided the best outcome: With a dose of 54.4 Gy, the median survival was 5.4 months, and the 1-year survival rate was 33%. At 64 Gy, the median survival was 7.2 months, and the survival rate was 28%. When the total dose was increased to 70.4 Gy, survival was increased to 8.2 months, with a 1-year survival rate of 37%. Improvement in neurologic function also increased with dose escalation. As reported in the latter study, radiation administered in 1.6-Gy fractions may reduce the neurotoxicity previously reported with higher doses per fraction. For example, with a fractionation schedule of 3 Gy/day, 11% of patients who survived for 1 year developed dementia.[42]

In a wide variety of radiotherapy fractionation schedules for patients with brain metastases,[43] among them was a study of accelerated hyperfractionation (1.6 Gy twice a day) to a total dose of 54.5 Gy compared with an unconventional regimen of 30 Gy in 10 fractions. The accelerated hyperfractionation regimen showed no benefit over the conventional dosage schedule.

Surgical resection plus intraoperative radiotherapy has been reported to result in the same survival as patients who have surgery followed by conventional postoperative radiotherapy.[44] The intent of intraoperative radiotherapy is to minimize the risk of neurotoxicity associated with conventional transcranial radiation.

Prophylactic low-dose cranial irradiation has been suggested as a method of preventing brain metastasis. In two series of patients with small cell lung cancer in remission, low total dose (approximately 25 Gy) provided prophylaxis against brain metastasis with minimal neurotoxicity.[45, 46]

The role of reirradiation for progressive or recurrent brain metastases has been controversial. In one retrospec-

tive study, the median dose of the first course of treatment was 30 Gy. The median dose of the second course was 20 Gy.[47] The median survival after re-irradiation was 4 months with no significant radiation toxicity in most patients. With respect to prognostic indicators, there is a broad consensus from various trials of radiotherapy for brain metastasis that improved survival can best be expected in patients with good pretreatment performance (Karnofsky) status and absent or inactive extracranial tumor.[48]

## Stereotactic Radiosurgery

Brain metastases are regarded as ideal lesions for stereotactic radiosurgery because of their usual spherical shape. Lesions that are smaller than 3 cm in diameter are most amenable to this technique, which entails the use of the stereotactically guided linear accelerator (see Fig. 52–11)[49] or the 201-source[60] Co Gamma unit (Gamma knife) (see Table 52–1).[50] Either of these two techniques entails delivery of a single, high dose of radiation, although multiple doses may be given.

An immunohistochemical study was carried out to determine the proliferative potential of tumor present at the site of a metastasis previously treated with radiosurgery.[51] Persistent or residual tumor was found to be less viable than tumors not exposed to radiosurgery.

Median survival in a group of patients with one or more brain metastases treated with linear-accelerator stereotactic radiosurgery was 6.5 months, and this survival was associated with improved quality of life and neurologic function (see Table 52–1).[49] In a series of patients with single brain metastasis treated with the Gamma knife, median survival was 10 months, and the 1-year survival rate was 33%.[50] Because the dose of focused radiation is relatively high with either of the two types of stereotactic radiosurgery, this form of radiation therapy can be expected to effectively control tumors otherwise considered to be resistant to conventional radiotherapy, while sparing surrounding normal brain.

A course of conventional whole-brain radiotherapy is generally given first and is followed by "boost radiosurgery" limited to the tumor site. Either form of stereotactic radiosurgery (Gamma knife or linear accelerator) can be given at the time of recurrence after surgical excision or after relapse in a previously irradiated field.[51, 53] When used as a supplement to whole-brain radiation, radiosurgery has been reported to be superior to radiosurgery alone.[55] A retrospective study of stereotactic radiosurgery in conjunction with whole-brain radiotherapy for a single brain metastasis was reported to result in median survival of 56 weeks.[53] The authors state that these results are comparable to randomized trials of surgical resection and whole-brain radiotherapy.[29, 34] For melanoma metastases to brain, the combination of stereotactic radiosurgery and whole-brain radiotherapy resulted in a median survival after diagnosis of 9 months (range, 3 to 38 months).[54] Radiosurgery can be directed to multiple metastatic lesions during the same radiosurgical session.[55] Temporary clinical worsening after stereotactic radiosurgery, presumably resulting from transient edema, has been reported in 10% of patients, and delayed radionecrosis has been reported in 3%.[52, 56]

Despite the reduced potential for radiation toxicity when

lower doses per fraction are used,[41] the possibility of dementia after whole-brain radiotherapy remains a concern. Clinical trials may be worthwhile to test the efficacy of stereotactic radiosurgery alone, without whole-brain radiotherapy. Results from a randomized clinical trial in patients with a single brain metastasis[36] have shown that surgery without postoperative radiotherapy results in a higher incidence of recurrence than surgery combined with postoperative whole-brain radiotherapy; there was no difference in survival or duration of quality of life in the two groups. It appears reasonable to defer postoperative radiotherapy until there is evidence of tumor recurrence. Although this approach poses the risk that previously unsuspected metastases may appear, they can likely be detected while still quite small on serial CT or MRI (perhaps every 2 to 3 months postoperatively). Such lesions might then be amenable to further doses of stereotactic radiosurgery (or surgical excision), obviating the potential toxicity of whole-brain radiotherapy.

Stereotactic radiosurgery for single brain metastasis has been reported as having results similar to those of surgical resection.[57] A cost analysis suggested that stereotaxic radiosurgery was also more cost-effective than surgery.

## Surgery

### Indications

The consensus among neurosurgeons concerning cerebral metastatic disease has been that surgical excision should generally be restricted to patients with a single intracerebral metastasis and whose general medical status is satisfactory. With the evolution of neurosurgical experience with brain metastasis over the years, this traditional restriction to a single metastasis has been changing. Excision may be considered for a life-threatening metastasis, even in the presence of one or more additional metastatic deposits in the brain.[58, 59] Surgery for more than one metastatic lesion may be carried out, even if this may require two separate craniotomies, particularly for radioresistant lesions (see Fig. 52–10).[60, 61] A report from the University of Texas M.D. Anderson Cancer Center described an aggressive approach to surgical removal of multiple metastases in selected patients.[61] Reported survival was similar to that of patients with excision of a single metastasis.

Surgical removal is applicable particularly for tumors that are radioresistant, such as melanoma, renal cell carcinoma, thyroid carcinoma, and metastases from the gastrointestinal tract. Radiosensitive tumors, such as lymphomas and small cell lung cancer, are generally treated with radiotherapy alone. Tumors of intermediate radiosensitivity, such as breast carcinoma and non–small cell lung cancer, are borderline situations. For such tumors, surgical excision may be considered if the tumors are surgically accessible, particularly if they are life-threatening. Surgery may be favored in patients with slow-growing tumors, as suggested by the natural history of the disease or by a long latency period after diagnosis of the primary malignancy.[62] A long latency period may signify good host defense mechanisms against the primary tumor, and survival after surgical excision of the cerebral metastasis may be increased.[8]

Surgical intervention is recommended for patients who are presumed to have metastatic disease but the nature of the primary extracranial tumor is unknown (Fig. 52–12; see also Figs. 52–1, 52–8, and 52–9). The need to establish a tissue diagnosis is imperative if the intracranial lesion is single, so that the possibility of a benign, curable lesion, such as meningioma, hematoma (see Fig. 52–8), or abscess (see Fig. 52–9), can be ruled out.[29] In the case of a patient with a confirmed primary malignancy elsewhere in the body, a single intracranial lesion is probably metastatic, but stereotactic or excision biopsy (when surgically feasible) is desirable.

Metastatic lesions deep in the dominant hemisphere generally are not amenable to safe surgical excision.[8] This restriction also applies to thalamic lesions in either hemisphere,[8] although the transcallosal approach is being used increasingly for biopsy or excision of various types of thalamic tumors.[63] An inoperable metastasis in the brain stem is shown in Figure 52–6.

### Surgical Excision Alone

The median survival after excision of a single metastasis (in most reported cases, without radiotherapy) is 5 to 6 months (see Table 52–1).[7, 9, 64] The median and 1-year survival statistics from surgery alone appear to be approximately the same as for radiation alone. Strictly speaking, it is not appropriate to make a direct comparison between these two therapeutic modalities because patients selected for surgery are more likely to be in better general condition than patients offered radiotherapy alone.

### Combined Therapy: Surgery Plus Radiotherapy

The combination of surgery followed by radiotherapy for brain metastasis evolved from the concept that radiation therapy is most effective in the presence of a relatively small number of actively growing, well-oxygenated tumor cells.[63] The center of the tumor contains a large number of hypoxic cells, which tend to be more resistant to destruction by radiation than actively growing, well-oxygenated cells located closer to the periphery of the tumor. Surgery has the advantage of removing the relatively resistant hypoxic core of the tumor. Residual actively growing tumor cells on the periphery have been reported in about one third of surgical cases, however, even in those in whom complete gross resection is performed.[21, 22, 62, 66] The combination of surgery and radiation thus compensates for the deficiencies of either modality alone.

In keeping with the theoretical advantage of combined therapy, many retrospective studies on single brain metastasis in the past decade have suggested that the combination of surgery and radiotherapy is superior to radiotherapy alone, with respect to survival and recurrence of the brain metastasis.[17, 67–69] In one of these retrospective studies, which involved patients with brain metastases from non–oat cell lung cancer, favorable prognostic variables included absence of local and systemic disease at time of craniotomy, aggressive treatment of the primary lung cancer, and metachronous onset of the brain metastasis.[17] Another of the studies, also limited to single metastasis from non–small cell lung cancer, included a comparison of pa-

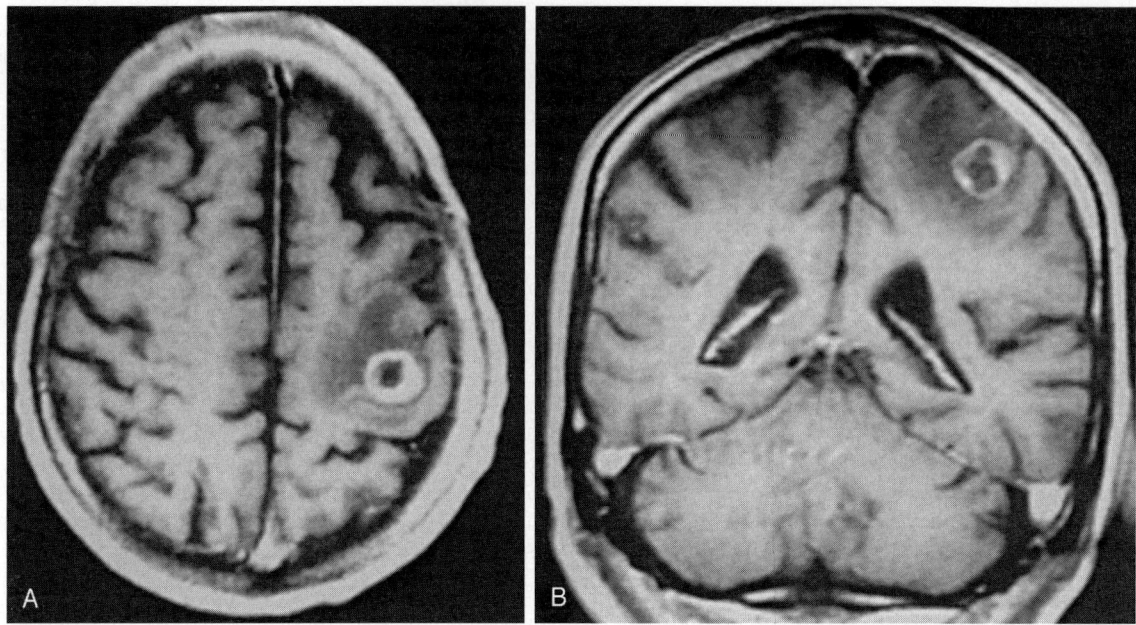

**FIGURE 52–12** ■ An axial (*A*) and coronal (*B*) contrast-enhanced T$_1$-weighted magnetic resonance imaging (MRI) scan of a 75-year-old man presenting with 1-month history of mild headaches and right hemiparesis. The small ring-enhancing mass in the left parietal area at the gray-white junction was suspicious for a solitary metastasis. Metastatic work-up revealed no evidence of an extracranial malignancy. An excisional biopsy was carried out; placement of the craniotomy bone flap was facilitated by stereotactic guidance to pinpoint the location of the scalp incision. After exposure of the cortex, the stereotactic probe was again used to target the entry point on the cortex to approach the subcortically placed lesion. Histologic examination revealed metastatic carcinoma, which was compatible with a primary bronchogenic lesion.

tients treated with surgery followed by radiation versus a small group of patients first treated with radiation followed by surgery; the group consisting of surgery followed by radiotherapy had a longer median survival.[69]

## Surgical Technique

### OPEN RESECTION BY CRANIOTOMY

Metastatic tumors are commonly circumscribed, although not encapsulated, and can often be totally separated from surrounding brain tissue (see Figs. 52–1, 52–2, 52–7, 52–10, and 52–12).[8, 22] For intracerebral metastases, intraoperative ultrasound is invaluable in localizing the lesion, which is usually subcortical (see Fig. 52–2C). After the location of the lesion is identified, the cortical incision is preferably made in the depths of the sulcus overlying the tumor, to minimize damage to the adjacent gyrus. When the tumor pseudocapsule is reached, dissection is similar to that for excision of a meningioma. As the dissection progresses, cottonoids are inserted in the plane between the tumor capsule and the surrounding normal brain. The tumor is gradually enucleated from its bed. Placement of one or more self-retaining brain spatulas may be helpful, but the retraction tension on brain is kept to a minimum. If the tumor is large, resection in one piece may not be feasible, and the central core of the tumor is debulked before completing circumferential dissection of the tumor capsule. Meticulous hemostasis of the tumor bed is carried out. The tumor bed is lined with pledgets of a topical hemostatic agent, such as oxidized regenerated cellulose (Surgicel; Johnson & Johnson Patient Care, New Brunswick, NJ). Systemic steroids are maintained for several days postoperatively, then tapered, if feasible.

There are instances, mainly with large metastatic tumors, in which the tumor is only partially circumscribed, and a plane of cleavage between some portions of the tumor and brain cannot be found. In this situation, tumor debulking is carried out comparable to the technique used in resecting malignant glioma.

### AWAKE CRANIOTOMY FOR BRAIN MAPPING

When the lesion lies close to the frontal or temporal speech area, local anesthesia is preferred, to enable speech localization by means of cortical electrical stimulation while the patient is awake. When localizing motor cortex (if identification of the speech area is not necessary) (see Fig. 52–12), however, mapping of the motor area can be achieved with the patient under general anesthesia, with modification in the selection of anesthetic agents. Inhalational anesthetics, such as nitrous oxide and the halogenated agents, are avoided because they depress cortical activity. Instead, intravenous agents are used during motor mapping. Muscle relaxants are avoided so that the motor responses may be observed.

### Residual or Recurrent Tumor

At autopsy, the completeness of tumor resection has been confirmed in about 75% of the cases, and the remainder show tumor infiltration in the surrounding brain parenchyma.[22] In another autopsy study, no residual tumor was found at the site of the previous surgical excision in 58% of cases, although many of these patients were found to have metastases elsewhere in the brain.[21] Postoperative radiation was not used in either of the latter two series.[21, 22] The approximately 60% to 75% chance of eliminating the local metastasis by surgical excision is encouraging, and the addition of postoperative radiation may be expected to improve these results further (see Fig. 52–1).

## Stereotactic Biopsy

CT-guided or MRI-guided stereotactic biopsy is carried out for deep lesions or when surgical excision of a relatively superficial lesion is not feasible. Stereotactic biopsy is also advisable when abscess is a diagnostic consideration. If an abscess is found, diagnosis and definitive treatment (aspiration) are achieved without craniotomy.

When stereotactic guidance is used, it is best to identify an entry point on the scalp directly over the lesion at right angles to the skull. This method increases the accuracy of the stereotactic trajectory and permits access to the lesion via the shortest distance through brain tissue. For superficially located lesions, use of the conventional stereotactic entry points (coronal suture for more anterior lesions or posterior parietal entry point for the more posterior lesions) might result in a tangential trajectory for the biopsy probe, which makes stereotactic targeting more difficult. Approach to temporal lesions via a coronal suture entry point near the vertex of the skull carries the risk of severing branches of the middle cerebral artery. This risk is significantly diminished by a lateral temporal approach perpendicular to the temporal bone.

Tumor seeding in the brain along the biopsy probe after stereotactic biopsy has been reported.[70] The risk of such iatrogenic seeding becoming clinically manifest nodules may be minimized by postbiopsy regional or whole-brain radiotherapy.

## Surgical Mortality and Morbidity

In the past 2 decades, mortality within 30 days after surgery for single metastases in most studies has ranged from 2% to 9%.[17, 29, 34, 68, 71] A study from multiple institutions reported a mortality of 9%[34]; in this study, two of the three deaths that occurred were in patients with posterior fossa metastases. Postoperative morbidity (complications) in various studies ranges from 8% to 28%.[17, 29, 61, 68, 69] Complications included neurologic worsening, meningitis, pulmonary embolism, intracranial hematoma, and cerebral infarction.

## Chemotherapy and Immunotherapy

The use of CDDP (cis-diamminedichloroplatinum) as an adjuvant has been reported to prolong survival significantly after surgical excision of a brain lesion metastatic from lung.[72] There are few other reports of benefit of chemotherapy or immunotherapy in the management of cerebral metastasis. The failure of antitumor drugs has been partly attributed to the inability of most of these drugs to cross the blood-brain barrier.[73] The lipid-soluble nitrosoureas that cross this barrier are of some value in the management of primary brain tumors (gliomas), but these agents have not been found useful for the management of brain metastases.[20] An exception is choriocarcinoma, which responds well to a combination of radiation therapy and chemotherapy.[37]

## MENINGEAL CARCINOMATOSIS

Metastatic involvement of the leptomeninges implies that the entire neuraxis is exposed to the malignancy, as illustrated by the presence of tumor cells in the cerebrospinal fluid (see Fig. 52–5). Without treatment, survival is usually limited to about 6 weeks. The survival can be improved by treatment that combines radiotherapy and chemotherapy. Young and associates[74] recommended delivering radiotherapy to the major site of the neurologic symptoms (the brain or spine) and treating the remainder of the neuraxis with intrathecal drugs (methotrexate, arabinosylcytosine, or both). The drugs are given in repeated doses by lumbar puncture or via an indwelling ventricular catheter with a subcutaneous reservoir under the scalp (Ommaya device; Heyer-Schulte Corporation, Goleta, CA). The ventricular route is preferable because it entails simply puncturing the scalp with a needle for penetration of the subcutaneous reservoir, which is better tolerated than repeated lumbar punctures. The ventricular route also has the advantage of better cerebrospinal fluid dispersion of the antitumor agent. In the series treated by Young and associates, patients with lymphoma and, to a lesser degree, those with breast carcinoma responded well to this combined therapy: The median survival extended to about 5 months.[74] The response of bronchogenic carcinoma, melanoma, and other malignancies is less predictable.

## GUIDELINES FOR PATIENT SELECTION FOR SURGICAL INTERVENTION

With increasing exceptions, surgical excision of brain metastases is generally limited to patients with a single metastasis. Although single metastases occur in about 50% of patients, it has been estimated that only half of the patients with single metastases have lesions that are surgically accessible; only approximately 25% of all patients with brain metastases are candidates for surgical resection.[69] Those with surgically inaccessible lesions are considered for radiotherapy alone or no treatment at all. Apart from surgical resection of a metastatic lesion, stereotactic biopsy may need to be considered for the purpose of establishing a histologic diagnosis. Guidelines for selection of patients for surgical intervention follow.

## Surgically Accessible Metastasis

Implicit in the decision regarding surgical accessibility of a presumed metastasis is the expectation that its excision would not leave the patient with a severe neurologic deficit. Surgery is recommended for patients with relatively superficial single lesions, preferably those that are thought to be relatively radioresistant (e.g., melanoma or metastasis from kidney, gastrointestinal tract, or thyroid) because radiosensitive tumors (e.g., lymphoma) may be treated with radiotherapy alone. Excision of a metastatic lesion that is immediately life-threatening or incapacitating may be considered, even in the presence of more than one metastatic brain lesion; this concept may be extended to the removal of multiple metastatic brain tumors if they are surgically accessible. Based on the improved results of combined therapy, surgical excision of one or more metastatic lesions is followed by a course of radiotherapy (see Figs. 52–1, 52–4, 52–7, 52–10, and 52–12).

## Status of the Primary Tumor

Surgical excision is favored when the primary tumor can or has been treated or is symptomatically quiescent, and the immediate threat to life is the intracranial metastasis. Under the latter circumstances, management of the brain metastasis takes precedence over treatment of the primary tumor.

## Extracranial Metastases

The patient is a better candidate for surgical intervention if no metastases are present elsewhere in the body. The presence of extracranial metastases that are under satisfactory control represents a borderline situation; surgical excision may be considered, especially if the intracranial lesion is life-threatening, such as a cerebellar metastasis causing brain stem or fourth ventricular compression (see Fig. 52–7).

## General Condition and Life Expectancy

Excision of a suspected brain metastasis may be performed if the patient's general condition, in terms of surgical risk, is satisfactory. Craniotomy performed with the patient under local anesthesia may be considered to avoid the risks of general anesthesia (see Fig. 52–12). Various authors have used a minimum life expectancy of 2[29] to 6 months[21, 34] as a factor in determining a patient's suitability for excision of a metastasis. In one surgical series, excision of a single brain metastasis was considered beneficial if the patient's condition was not likely to be made worse and if the patient was expected to survive for at least 6 months.[21] In another series, craniotomy was thought to be worthwhile if the patient could lead a functional home life, did not require continuous nursing care, and could have a normal daily life.[62]

## Uncertain Diagnosis

Excisional or stereotactic biopsy may be necessary to establish a tissue diagnosis, which is important in management planning. For example, the patient may have a history of a malignancy that had presumably been cured; the presence of a single intracerebral mass lesion does not necessarily indicate a metastasis (see Figs. 52–8 and 52–9). An intracranial lesion in a patient with a known malignancy may prove to be an unrelated benign or treatable process, as illustrated by the intracerebral hematoma in Figure 52–8. When brain abscess is a serious diagnostic consideration, stereotactic biopsy (for possible aspiration of the abscess) is preferable to excisional biopsy, even when the lesion is superficial (see Fig. 52–9). In cases in which the MRI or CT scan is suggestive of either brain metastasis or brain abscess, it is desirable at the time of surgical excision or stereotactic biopsy to obtain a culture of the necrotic core of the lesion.

## Shunt for Hydrocephalus

Patients with hydrocephalus secondary to obstruction of the cerebrospinal fluid pathway by tumor or edema can be offered a shunt procedure that can provide significant temporary relief of symptoms. The shunt can be inserted in conjunction with excision of a metastatic tumor, or the shunt can be used as an adjunct to radiation therapy. Although the theoretical risk of dissemination of the malignancy via the shunt exists, this concern is generally not clinically significant.

# QUALITY OF SURVIVAL: HOSPICE CARE

In some circumstances, withholding active therapy of any kind is reasonable, as in cases in which the patient is terminally ill, with expected survival limited to a matter of days or weeks. The decision is readily made to withhold treatment in a terminally ill patient with widespread metastases outside the nervous system. At times, the primary goal is management of pain rather than tumor control. Regardless of life expectancy, surgical intervention does not seem warranted in the presence of profound neurologic deficit except for the purpose of biopsy when the diagnosis is in doubt. The chance of reversing profound neurologic deficit with either surgery or radiotherapy is remote. Although borderline situations exist in which a course of radiotherapy and steroids might be considered, such patients are probably best treated symptomatically with hospice care. This treatment includes administering medication for the relief of specific symptoms, such as pain and nausea, rather than attempting to prolong life but with little hope of quality survival.

# SUMMARY

For most patients with cerebral metastasis, radiotherapy is the primary modality of treatment. This modality applies to patients with multiple intracranial metastases as well as those with single metastases that are surgically inaccessible. Approximately 25% of all patients with brain metastasis are candidates for surgical excision of a suspected metastatic lesion. In some instances, excision of more than one surgically accessible lesion or excision of a life-threatening mass may be considered, even in the presence of one or more other metastases elsewhere in the brain. Surgical excision is considered in cases of relatively radioresistant metastatic tumors, whereas radiosensitive lesions are better managed with radiotherapy alone. Patients may be considered as suitable candidates for surgical excision if their life expectancy is at least 2 to 6 months. Surgical excision is followed by a course of whole-brain radiation or possibly limited to local or regional radiotherapy. For lesions smaller than 3 cm, conventional radiotherapy may be followed by a boost of stereotactic radiosurgery (linear accelerator or Gamma knife) directed to the tumor site. Apart from surgical intervention for excision of a brain metastasis, stereotactic biopsy is often indicated to establish a tissue diagnosis, even in cases in which the patient has a known systemic malignancy.

Advances in the past decade have shown that the combination of surgical excision followed by radiotherapy is superior to either modality alone. Refinements in radiotherapy, with respect to dose per fraction and total dose, as well as stereotactic radiosurgery have added to the slightly improved outlook for selected patients with brain metastasis. Furthermore, the full potential of stereotactic radiosurgery remains to be defined.

## ACKNOWLEDGMENTS

*The author gratefully acknowledges the assistance of Mary F. McCabe, M.A., and Emily Morton.*

## REFERENCES

1. Walker AE, Robins M, Weinfeld FD: Epidemiology of brain tumors: The national survey of intracranial neoplasms. Neurology 35:219, 1985.
2. Aronson SM, Garcia JH, Aronson BE: Metastatic neoplasms of the brain: Their frequency in relation to age. Cancer 17:558, 1964.
3. Deviri E, Schachner A, Halery A, et al: Carcinoma of the lung with a solitary cerebral metastasis: Surgical management and review of the literature. Cancer 52:1507, 1983.
4. Delattre JY, Krol G, Thaler HT, et al: Distribution of brain metastases. Arch Neurol 45:741, 1988.
5. Cairncross JG, Posner JB: The management of brain metastases. In Walker MD (ed): Oncology of the Nervous System. Boston: Martinus Nijhoff, 1983, pp 341–377.
6. Black P: Metastatic tumors of the central nervous system: Cerebral metastasis. In Abeloff MD (ed): Complications of Cancer: Diagnosis and Management. Baltimore: Johns Hopkins University Press, 1979, pp 283–312.
7. Haar F, Patterson RH Jr: Surgery for metastatic intracranial neoplasm. Cancer 30:1241, 1972.
8. Ransohoff J: Surgical management of metastatic tumors. Semin Oncol 2:21, 1975.
9. Raskind R, Weiss ST, Manning JJ, et al: Survival after surgical excision of single metastatic brain tumors. AJR Am J Roentgenol 111:323, 1971.
10. Richards P, McKissock W: Intracranial metastases. BMJ 1:15, 1963.
11. Simionescu MD: Metastatic tumors of the brain: A follow-up study of 195 patients with neurosurgical considerations. J Neurosurg 17:361, 1960.
12. Taylor HG, Lefkowitz M, Skokog SJ, et al: Intracranial metastases in prostate cancer. Cancer 53:2728, 1984.
13. Veith RG, Odom GL: Intracranial metastases and their neurosurgical treatment. J Neurosurg 23:375, 1965.
14. Walker MD: Brain and peripheral nervous system tumors. In Holland JF, Frei E (eds): Cancer Medicine, Vol 3. Philadelphia: Lea & Febiger, 1973, pp 1385–1407.
15. Madajewicz S, Karakousis C, West CR, et al: Malignant melanoma brain metastases: Review of Roswell Park Memorial Institute experience. Cancer 53:2550, 1984.
16. Van Eck JHM, Ebels EJ, Go KG: Metastatic tumours of the brain. Psychiatr Neurol Neurochir 68:443, 1965.
17. Sundaresan N, Galicich JH, Beattie EJ: Surgical treatment of brain metastasis from lung cancer. J Neurosurg 58:666, 1983.
18. Hwang TL, Close TP, Grego JM, et al: Predilection of brain metastases in gray and white matter junction and vascular border zones. Cancer 77:1551–1555, 1996.
19. Kindt GW: The pattern of location of cerebral metastatic tumors. J Neurosurg 21:54, 1964.
20. Posner JB: Management of central nervous system metastases. Semin Oncol 4:81, 1977.
21. Lang EF, Slater J: Metastatic brain tumors: Results of surgical and nonsurgical treatment. Surg Clin North Am 44:865, 1964.
22. Stortebecker TP: Metastatic tumors of the brain from a neurosurgical point of view: A follow-up study of 158 cases. J Neurosurg 11:84, 1954.
23. Olson ME, Chernik NL, Posner JB: Infiltration of the leptomeninges by systemic cancer: A clinical and pathologic study. Arch Neurol 30:122, 1974.
24. Patchell RA: Brain metastases: Neurologic complications of systemic cancer. Neurol Clin 9:817, 1991.
25. Macchiarini P, Bounaguid IR, Hardin M, et al: Results and prognosis factors of surgery in the management of non-small cell lung cancer with solitary brain metastasis. Cancer 68:300–304, 1991.
26. Salvati M, Cervoni L, Tarantino R, et al: Solitary cerebral metastasis as first symptom of lung cancer. Neurochirurgie 40:256–258, 1994.
27. Murray JJ, Houston MC: Calcified intracranial metastases from breast carcinoma with a therapeutic response to tamoxifen therapy. South Med J 79:253, 1986.
28. Nomoto Y, Miyamoto T, Yamaguchi Y: Brain metastasis of small cell lung carcinoma: Comparison of Gd-DTPA enhanced magnetic resonance imaging and enhanced computerized tomography. Jpn J Clin Oncol 24:258–262, 1994.
29. Patchell RA, Tibbs PA, Walsh JW, et al: A randomized trial of surgery in the treatment of single metastases to the brain. N Engl J Med 322:494, 1990.
30. Tatsuno S, Hata Y, Tada S: Double-dose Gd-DTPA: Detectability of intraparenchymal brain metastasis. Nippon Igaku Hoshasen Gakkai Zasshi 56:855–859, 1996.
31. Dierckx RA, Martin JJ, Dobbeleir A, et al: Sensitivity and specificity of thallium-201 single-photon emission tomography in the functional detection and differential diagnosis of brain tumors. Eur J Nucl Med 21:621–633, 1994.
32. Bentson JR, Steckel RJ, Kagan AR: Diagnostic imaging in clinical cancer management: Brain metastases. Invest Radiol 23:335–341, 1988.
33. Latief KH, White CS, Protopapas Z, et al: Search for a primary lung neoplasm in patients with brain metastasis: Is the chest radiograph sufficient? AJR Am J Roentgenol 168:1339–1344, 1997.
34. Vecht CJ, Haaxma-Reiche H, Noordijk EM, et al: Treatment of single brain metastasis: Radiotherapy alone or combined with neurosurgery? Ann Neurol 33:583, 1993.
35. Mintz AH, Kestle J, Rathbone MP, et al: A randomized trial to assess the efficacy of surgery in addition to radiotherapy in patients with a single cerebral metastasis. Cancer 78:1470–1476, 1996.
36. Patchell RA, Tibbs PA, Regine WF, et al: Postoperative radiotherapy in the treatment of single metastases to the brain: A randomized trial. JAMA 280:1485–1489, 1998.
37. Shapiro WR, Posner JB: Corticosteroid hormones: Effects in an experimental brain tumor. Arch Neurol 30:217, 1974.
38. Jarden JO, Dhawan V, Poltorak A, et al: Positron emission tomographic measurement of blood-to-brain and blood-to-tumor transport of $^{82}$Rb: The effect of dexamethasone and whole-brain radiation therapy. Ann Neurol 18:636, 1985.
39. Renaudin J, Fewla D, Wilson CD: Dose dependency of Decadron in patients harboring brain tumors. J Neurosurg 39:302, 1973.
40. Vecht CJ, Hovestadt A, Verbiest HB, et al: Dose-effect relationship of dexamethasone on Karnofsky performance in metastatic brain tumors: A randomized study of doses of 4, 8, and 16 mg per day. Neurology 44:675–680, 1994.
41. Epstein BE, Scott CB, Sause WT, et al: Improved survival duration in patients with unresected solitary brain metastasis using accelerated hyperfractionated radiation therapy at total doses of 54.4 gray and greater. Cancer 71:1362–1367, 1993.
42. DeAngelis LM, Delattre JY, Posner JD: Radiation-induced dementia in patients cured of brain metastases. Neurology 39:789, 1989.

43. Murray KJ, Scott C, Greenberg HM, et al: A randomized phase III study of accelerated hyperfractionation versus standard in patients with unresected brain metastases: A report of the Radiation Therapy Oncology Group (RTOG) 9104. Int J Radiat Oncol Biol Phys 39:571–574, 1997.

44. Nakamura O, Matsutani M, Shitara N, et al: New treatment protocol by intra-operative radiation therapy for metastatic brain tumors. Acta Neurochir 131:91–96, 1994.

45. Arriagada R, Le Chevalier T, Borie F, et al: Prophylactic cranial irradiation for patients with small-cell lung cancer in complete remission. J Natl Cancer Inst 87:183–190, 1995.

46. Rubenstein JH, Dosoretz DE, Katin MJ, et al: Low doses of prophylactic cranial irradiation effective in limited stage small cell carcinoma of the lung. Int J Radiat Oncol Biol Phys 33:329–337, 1995.

47. Wong WW, Schild SE, Sawyer TE, et al: Analysis of outcome in patients reirradiated for brain metastases. Int J Radiat Oncol Biol Phys 34:585–590, 1996.

48. Berk L: An overview of radiotherapy trials for the treatment of brain metastases. Oncology 9:1205–1212, 1995.

49. Mehta MP, Rozental JM, Levin AB, et al: Defining the role of radiosurgery in the management of brain metastases. Int J Radiat Oncol Biol Phys 24:619, 1992.

50. Coffey RJ, Flickinger JC, Bissonette DJ, et al: Radiosurgery for solitary brain metastases using the Cobalt-60 Gamma unit: Methods and results in 24 patients. Int J Radiat Oncol Biol Phys 20:1287, 1991.

51. Harris OA, Adler JR: Analysis of the proliferative potential of residual tumor after radiosurgery for intraparenchymal brain metastases. J Neurosurg 85:667–671, 1996.

52. Engenhert R, Kimmig BN, Hover K-H, et al: Long-term follow-up for brain metastases treated by percutaneous stereotactic single high-dose irradiation. Cancer 71:1353, 1993.

53. Auchter RM, Lamond JP, Alexander E: A multiinstitutional outcome and prognostic factor analysis of radiosurgery for resectable single brain metastasis. Int J Radiat Oncol Biol Phys 35:27–35, 1996.

54. Somaza S, Kondziolka D, Lunsford LD, et al: Stereotactic radiosurgery for cerebral metastatic melanoma. J Neurosurg 79:661–666, 1993.

55. Fuller BG, Kaplan ID, Adler J, et al: Stereotaxic radiosurgery for brain metastases: The importance of adjuvant whole-brain irradiation. Int J Radiat Oncol Biol Phys 23:413, 1992.

56. Loeffler JS, Alexander E III, Kooy HM, et al: Radiosurgery for brain metastases. In DeVita VT, Hallman S, Rosenberg SA (eds): Cancer: Principles and Practice of Oncology. Philadelphia: JB Lippincott, 1993, pp 1–13.

57. Rutigliano MJ, Lunsford LD, Kondziolka D, et al: The cost effectiveness of stereotactic radiosurgery versus surgical resection in the treatment of solitary metastatic brain tumors. Neurosurgery 37:445–453, 1995.

58. French LA, Ausman JI: Metastatic neoplasms to the brain. Clin Neurosurg 24:41, 1977.

59. Posner JB: Surgery for metastases to the brain. N Engl J Med 322:544, 1990.

60. Hazuka MB, Burleson WD, Stroud DN, et al: Multiple brain metastases are associated with poor survival in patients treated with surgery and radiotherapy. J Clin Oncol 11:369, 1993.

61. Bindal RK, Sawaya R, Leavens ME, et al: Surgical treatment of multiple brain metastases. J Neurosurg 79:210–216, 1993.

62. MacGee EE: Surgical treatment of cerebral metastases from lung cancer: The effect on quality and duration of survival. J Neurosurg 3:416, 1971.

63. Shucart WA, Stein BM: Transcallosal approach to the anterior ventricular system. Neurosurgery 3:339, 1978.

64. Posner JB: Diagnosis and treatment of metastases to the brain. Clin Bull 4:47, 1974.

65. Bergonie J, Tribondeaut L: Interpretation of some results of radiotherapy and an attempt at determining a logical technique of treatment. Radiat Res 11:587, 1959.

66. Kelly PJ, Kall BA, Goerss SJ: Results of computed tomography-based computer-assisted stereotactic resection of metastatic intracranial tumors. Neurosurgery 22:7, 1988.

67. Sause WT, Crowley JJ, Morantz R, et al: Solitary brain metastasis: Results of an RTOG/SWOG protocol evaluation: Surgery + RT versus RT alone. Am J Clin Oncol 13:427, 1990.

68. Mandell L, Hilaris B, Sullivan M, et al: The treatment of single brain metastasis from non-oat cell lung carcinoma: Surgery and radiation versus radiation therapy alone. Cancer 58:641, 1986.

69. Patchell RA, Cirrincione C, Thaler HT, et al: Single brain metastases: Surgery plus radiation or radiation alone. Neurology 36:447, 1986.

70. Karlsson B, Ericson K, Kihlstrom L, et al: Tumor seeding following stereotactic biopsy of brain metastases: Report of two cases. J Neurosurg 87:327–330, 1997.

71. Salvati M, Cervoni L, Raco A: Single brain metastases from unknown primary malignancies in CT-era. J Neurooncol 23:75–80, 1995.

72. Nakagawa H, Fujita T, Izumimoto S, et al: cis-diamminedichloroplatinum (CDDP) therapy for brain metastasis of lung cancer. II: Clinical effects. J Neurooncol 16:69–76, 1993.

73. Wilson WL, de la Garza JG: Systemic chemotherapy for CNS metastases of solid tumors. Arch Intern Med 115:710, 1965.

74. Young DF, Shapiro WR, Posner JB: Treatment of leptomeningeal cancer. Neurology 25:370, 1975.

75. Galicich JH, Sundaresan N, Arbit E, et al: Surgical treatment of single brain metastasis: Factors associated with survival. Cancer 45:381, 1980.

C H A P T E R    5 3

# Parasagittal and Falcine Meningioma Surgery*

■ DARREN S. LOVICK and ROBERT E. MAXWELL

The designation *parasagittal* for meningiomas along the superior sagittal sinus was first suggested by Cushing in 1922.[1] The anatomic and surgical distinction between parasagittal and falx meningiomas is more critical than the clinical distinction based on symptoms. The term *parasagittal* implies that a tumor arising from the dura mater high on the convexity of the hemisphere involves the wall and possibly the lumen of the sagittal sinus. The falx meningioma arises from the falx cerebri and gains a secondary attachment to the walls of the sagittal sinus only if it is large or widely spread en plaque.[2] Although it is difficult to determine with certainty in all cases whether a large tumor is parasagittal or falcial, parasagittal meningiomas predominate, as is consistent with the predilection of meningiomas to arise where arachnoidal granulation tissue is most abundant. The practical operative criterion proposed by Cushing for distinguishing a primary tumor of the falx cerebri rests on its complete concealment by overlying cerebral cortex. The parasagittal meningiomas were approximately seven times more frequent than the falcial tumors in Cushing's series. Cushing found hyperostosis of the skull associated with one fourth of parasagittal meningiomas but not with meningiomas limited to the falx.[3] No appreciable difference has been found in the clinical presentation or symptoms of these two classes of meningiomas. They do, however, present different technical considerations for the surgeon.

Olivecrona[4] was the first to distinguish parasagittal meningiomas according to their site of origin along the sagittal sinus. He reported that 52% of parasagittal meningiomas involved the middle third of the sinus, 37% were attached to the anterior third of the sinus, and 11% were attached to the posterior third of the sinus. Thirteen of Olivecrona's 27 cases of parasagittal meningiomas showed evidence of bilateral growth.

Cushing found at the time of surgery that the frontal and occipital tumors were all sizable, but many tumors along the middle third of the sinus were small. He ascribed this finding to the tendency of tumors adjacent to the paracentral lobule to produce earlier and more obvious symptoms than those of occipital tumors and tumors in more frontal

locations. Olivecrona and Cushing emphasized that the symptomatic differences between parasagittal meningiomas depended on whether they were located along the anterior, middle, or posterior third of the sinus. The division of the sinus into thirds also proves useful in clarifying technical considerations that concern the operative management of the sagittal sinus itself when it is involved by tumor.

The sagittal sinus extends from the crista galli to the torcular Herophili. The anterior third of the sinus extends from the crista galli to the coronal suture, the middle third runs between the coronal and lambdoid sutures, and the posterior third encompasses the length of sinus from the lambdoid suture to the torcular Herophili. The middle third of the sagittal sinus lies adjacent to the paracentral lobule and the motor and sensory cortex for the foot and lower leg, which borders the rolandic fissure. This area is drained by a cortical vein, or group of veins, that is important to preserve if it is still patent at the time of surgery.

## SYMPTOMS

One of the more publicized brain tumors was that of General Leonard Wood, who came to Cushing in 1910 with focal jacksonian seizures of the left foot and progressive numbness and spasticity of the left lower leg. Subsequent surgery revealed a parasagittal meningioma involving the middle third of the sagittal sinus in the region of the paracentral lobule. The seizures may initially be motor or sensory, but they usually spread to include both motor and sensory involvement. Sometimes, loss of consciousness ensues, and the patient has residual Todd's paralysis. Signs and symptoms of increased intracranial pressure are not common because the patient usually is evaluated and the tumor is diagnosed before it attains great bulk. If the seizures are controlled with anticonvulsant medication and the spastic weakness of the contralateral lower extremity is ignored, the tumor may grow and extend laterally to compromise fibers from the arm area of the pararolandic cortex.

Meningiomas adjacent to the anterior third of the sagittal sinus tend to attain greater size before diagnosis and surgery because of the more insidious onset and progression of symptoms (Fig. 53–1). These tumors produce a frontal

*This chapter has been adapted from Schmidek H: Meningiomas and Their Surgical Management. Philadelphia: WB Saunders, 1991.

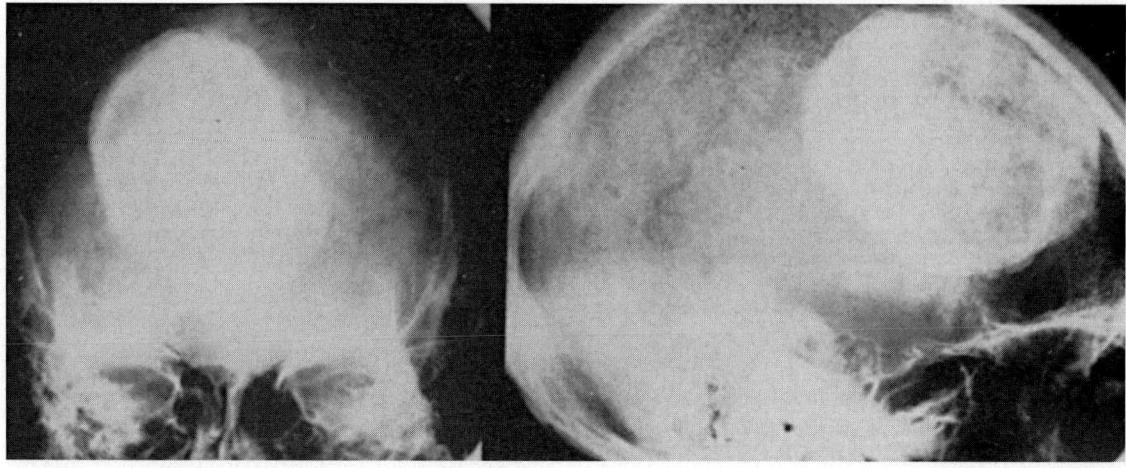

FIGURE 53–1 ■ Parasagittal and falx meningiomas adjacent to the anterior third of the sagittal sinus often grow large before they are diagnosed, because of the insidious onset and progression of symptoms. This meningioma is unusual because of the dense calcification on plain skull radiographs.

lobe syndrome with progressive dementia characterized by apathy and alterations of personality. Of patients with anterior third parasagittal meningiomas, 25% have seizures, but they are less frequent and nonfocal.[5] Symptoms and signs of increased intracranial pressure, including headache and papilledema or optic atrophy, accompany the dementia. Failing vision may prompt the patient to seek a medical opinion.

Patients with meningiomas involving the posterior third of the sagittal sinus usually have a chief complaint of headache. The characteristic localizing sign is a hemianopsia, the pattern of which depends on the size and precise location of the tumor. The visual field deficit is often so slowly progressive that it goes unnoticed by the patient, particularly if only the peripheral visual field is involved. Sometimes the patient is aware of visual hallucinations.

Patients with a long history of headaches are more likely to have complete homonymous hemianopsia because the tumor is large. Smaller tumors located above the calcarine fissure may cause anopsia of the inferior quadrant, and tumors adjacent to the tentorium cerebelli may spare the upper banks of the calcarine fissure and produce anopsia of the superior quadrant. Epilepsy, if visual hallucinations are not considered such, is uncommon with meningiomas involving the posterior third of the sagittal sinus.

## RADIOGRAPHIC INVESTIGATION

Radiographic evaluation includes plain skull radiographs, computed tomography (CT), magnetic resonance imaging (MRI), and angiography. The purpose of radiologic studies is to make a putative diagnosis and obtain anatomic information for surgical planning.

### Skull Radiographs

Plain skull x-ray films may demonstrate hyperostosis, enostosis, striations, and other evidence of tumor involving

the skull. Vascular markings give information about skull vascularity in the vicinity of the tumor and site of the craniotomy (see Fig. 53–1).

## Computed Tomography

CT imaging characteristics denoting a meningioma include a hypodense, dural-based mass that with contrast administration demonstrates intense, rapid, and homogeneous enhancement (Figs. 53–2 and 53–3). Calcification is present

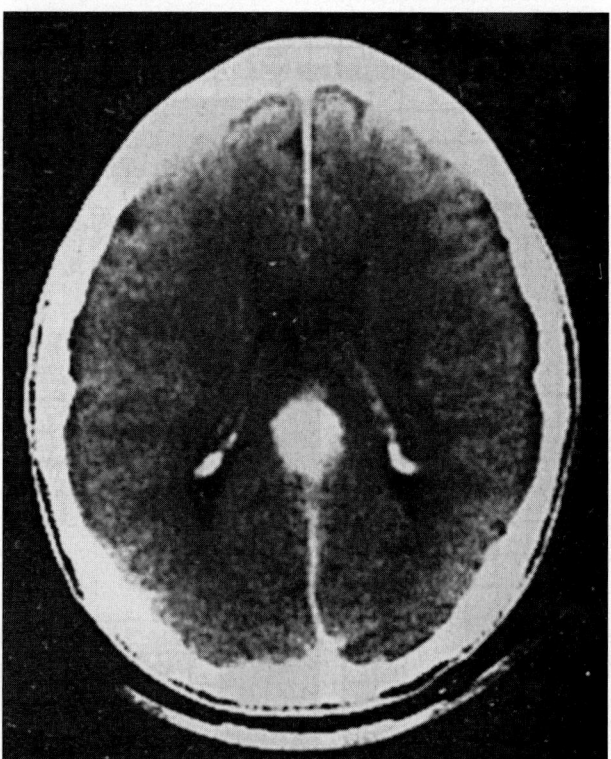

FIGURE 53–2 ■ A contrast-enhanced computed tomography scan demonstrating the bilateral configuration of a falcine meningioma.

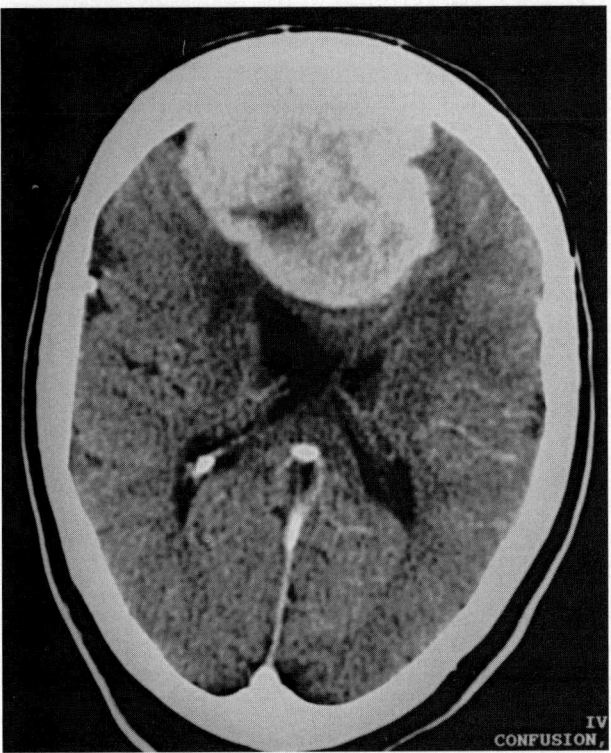

**FIGURE 53–3** ■ A computed tomography scan of the head with contrast demonstrating an enhancing bilateral parasagittal meningioma with effacement of the lateral ventricles and edema of the white matter. The following angiograms are of this tumor.

in almost 25% of meningiomas and ranges from a diffuse sand-like appearance to a dense sclerosis.[6] A spectrum of bony changes can occur at bone-tumor interface. Hyperostosis is not uncommon and pathologically represents bone infiltrated with nests of neoplastic cells.[7, 8] CT detects 85% of meningiomas without contrast enhancement and 95% of meningiomas with contrast enhancement.[9] Patients presenting with seizures or headaches resulting from meningiomas are frequently identified with CT and referred to the neurosurgeon for further evaluation. Although MRI provides superior soft tissue detail, CT with thin sections and coronal reconstructions demonstrates the extent of bony invasion.

## Magnetic Resonance Imaging

Multiplanar MRI with gadolinium enhancement provides imaging features to suggest the diagnosis of meningioma and to delineate the cortical and vascular anatomy for operative planning. Parasagittal and falcine meningiomas appear isointense to hypointense to gray matter on $T_1$-weighted images and may display a concentric sunburst pattern from a central arteriole feeder.[6] If the meningioma has not become too large, a rim of subarachnoid space may be preserved between the tumor margin and the underlying cortex (Fig. 53–4). Almost all meningiomas demonstrate rapid, homogeneous enhancement with gadolinium (Figs. 53–5 to 53–7).[10] Peritumoral edema is common surrounding meningiomas, especially those anterior to the coronal suture that attain a large size before diagnosis.[11, 12]

Hemorrhage is uncommon into a meningioma (Fig. 53–8).[13]

During the MRI scan, other detailed vascular and cortical anatomy may be elucidated via magnetic resonance angiography, magnetic resonance venography, and functional magnetic resonance. For preoperative planning, the cortical venous drainage, sinus patency, displacement of major arteries, and location of the central sulcus or speech regions relative to the tumor can be attained by a rapid, noninvasive means. In addition to preoperative information, the application of scalp markings and software allows MRI-guided frameless stereotaxy for use in the operating room. Barnett[14] reported frameless stereotaxy helpful in the resection of parasagittal and falcine meningiomas.

## Angiography

Digital subtraction angiography aids in diagnosis; provides dynamic vascular information critical for surgical planning; and offers therapeutic adjuncts, such as embolization. Meningiomas initially derive their blood supply from dural-based arterioles. External carotid injections are necessary to delineate the extracortical blood supply to the tumor. As the tumor grows, pial parasitization occurs,[15] and the neoplasm attains a dual blood supply, the tumor capsule from pial vessels and the core from meningial arteries.[16] The general angiographic features suggestive of a meningioma include a dural-based vascular pedicle often with angiographic pial parasitization. Meningiomas demonstrate the "mother-in-law sign," a blush of contrast enhancement that appears early but stays late into the venous phase (Figs. 53–9 to 53–13).[6]

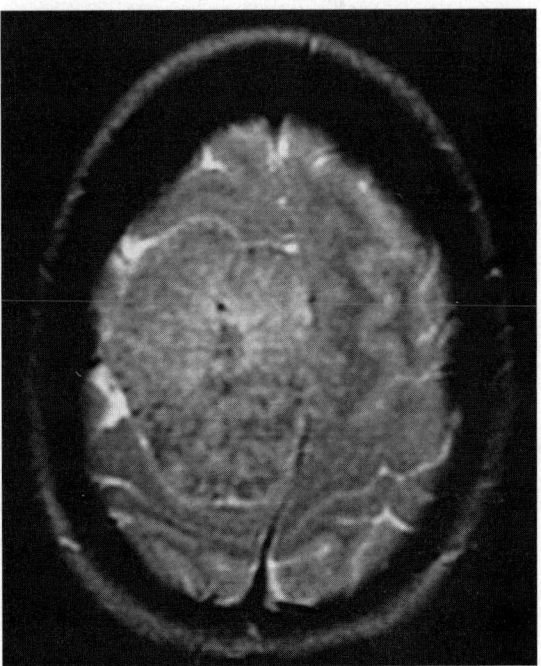

**FIGURE 53–4** ■ A $T_2$-weighted axial magnetic resonance imaging (MRI) scan demonstrating a meningioma with isointense signal to gray matter, a sunburst pattern from a central vessel, and rim of cerebrospinal fluid between the tumor and the pial interface.

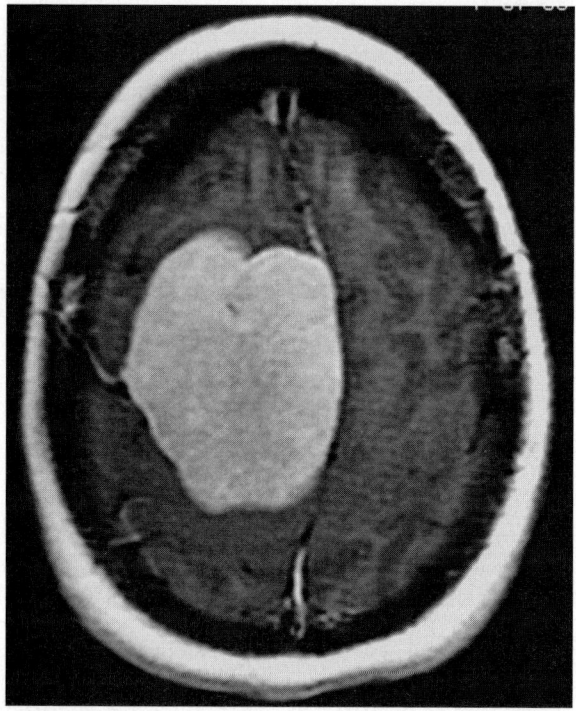

**FIGURE 53–5** ■ A T₁-weighted axial magnetic resonance imaging scan demonstrating a homogeneous gadolinium-enhancing parasagittal meningioma with mass effect displacing the falx to the left and a cortical vein entering laterally.

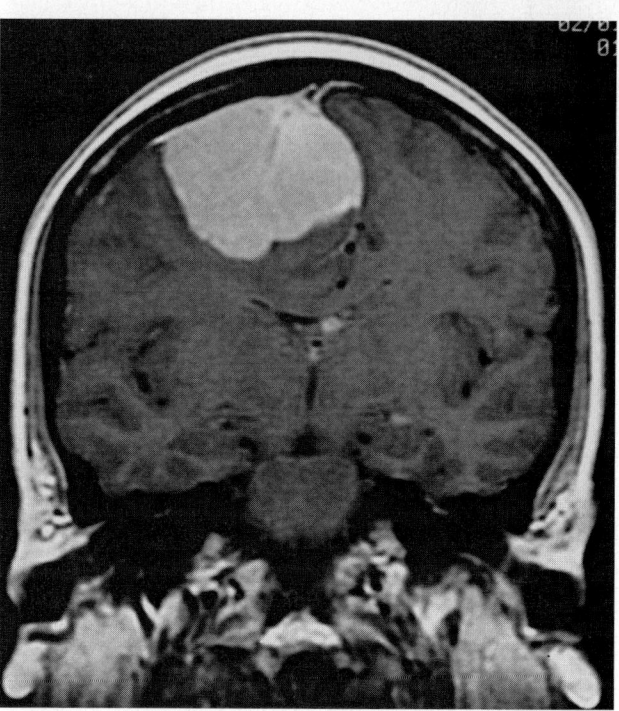

**FIGURE 53–6** ■ A T₁-weighted coronal magnetic resonance imaging scan demonstrating a homogeneous gadolinium-enhancing parasagittal meningioma. Note the enhancement of the ipsilateral wall of the sinus, the position of the anterior cerebral arteries, and the flow void within the superior sagittal sinus.

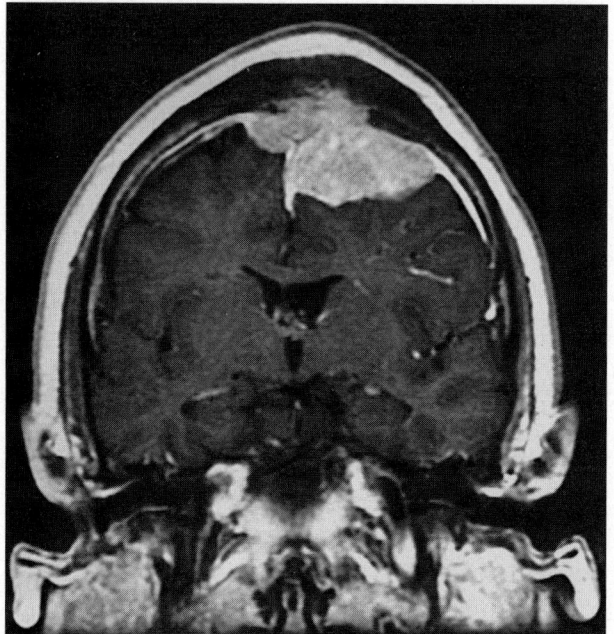

**FIGURE 53–7** ■ A T₁-weighted coronal magnetic resonance imaging scan demonstrating a bilateral parasagittal meningioma with invasion through the bone and loss of flow within the sagittal sinus.

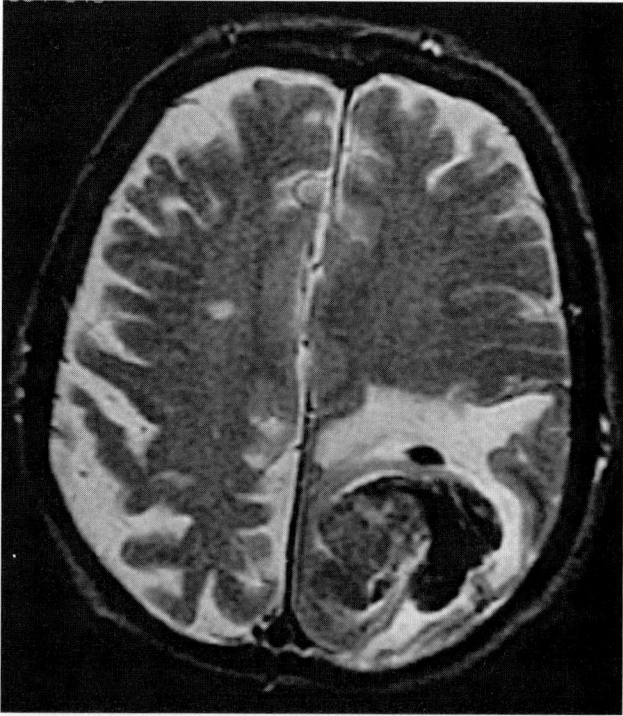

**FIGURE 53–8** ■ A T₂-weighted axial magnetic resonance imaging scan with a hypointense signal within the meningioma was found at operation to be a hemorrhage.

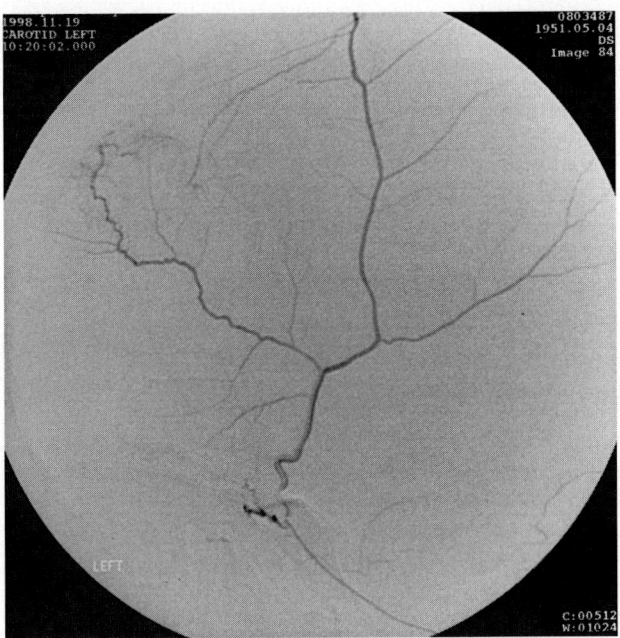

**FIGURE 53–9** ■ Digital subtraction angiography of the middle meningeal artery. The meningioma displays an early capillary blush.

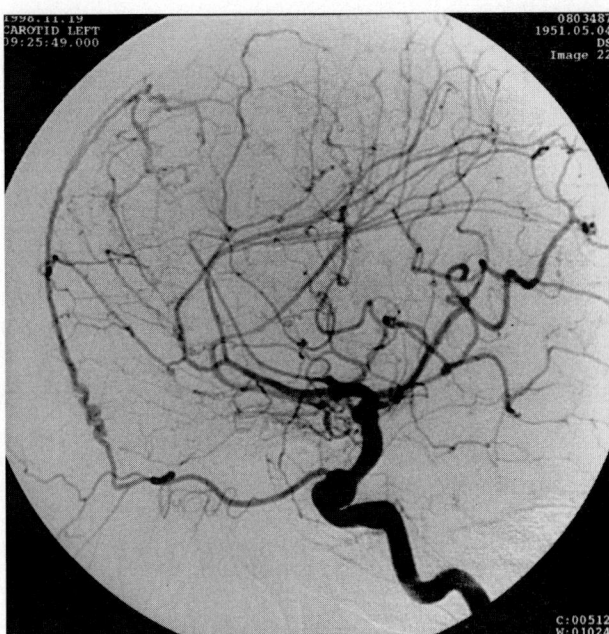

**FIGURE 53–11** ■ A lateral left internal carotid artery injection. The ophthalmic artery is large, and two large anterior falcine branches provide an additional dural supply to this meningioma. The anterior cerebral arteries distally are pushed caudal by the meningioma.

Information one must attain from the angiogram before resection includes the following:

1. What is the primary arterial supply to the meningioma, and where are these vessels located relative to the planned craniotomy exposure? What is the relationship of the branches from the anterior cerebral artery to the tumor?
2. How vascular is the tumor? Extremely vascular

angioblastic meningiomas are often difficult to excise without significant blood loss, unless en bloc dissection of a small tumor is feasible. One may consider preoperative embolization because it is shown to reduce intraoperative complications secondary to bleeding and the necessity for blood transfusion.[17]
3. Is the sagittal venous sinus widely patent, partially occluded, or completely occluded by tumor?
4. What is the relationship of major cortical draining

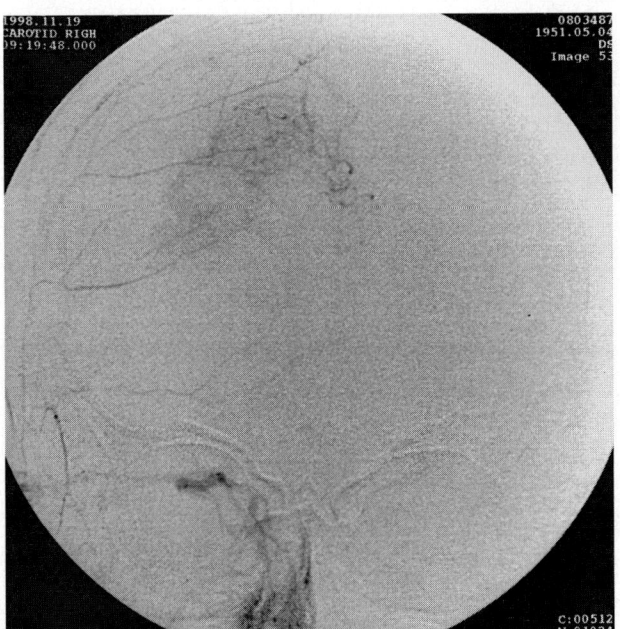

**FIGURE 53–10** ■ Venous phase of the angiogram in Figure 53–9. Notice that the prolonged "hang-up" of contrast within the meningioma, called the mother-in-law sign, comes early and stays late.

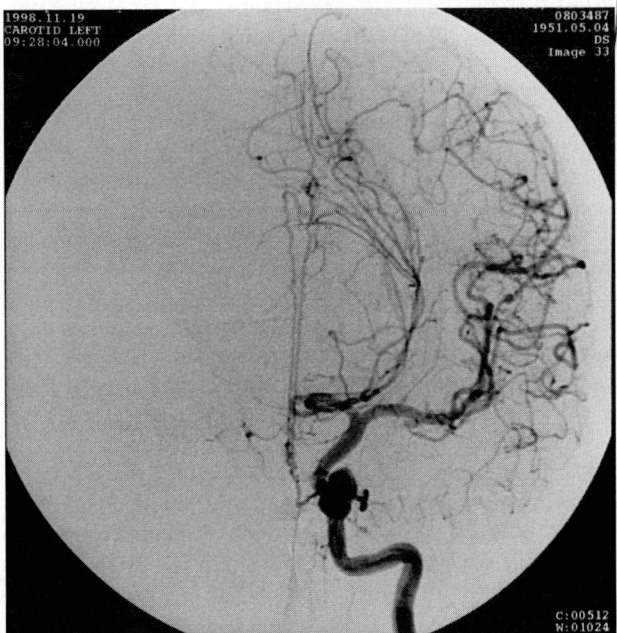

**FIGURE 53–12** ■ An anteroposterior left internal carotid artery injection. The falcine branches off the ophthalmic artery are noted in the midline, whereas the anterior cerebral artery is pushed laterally.

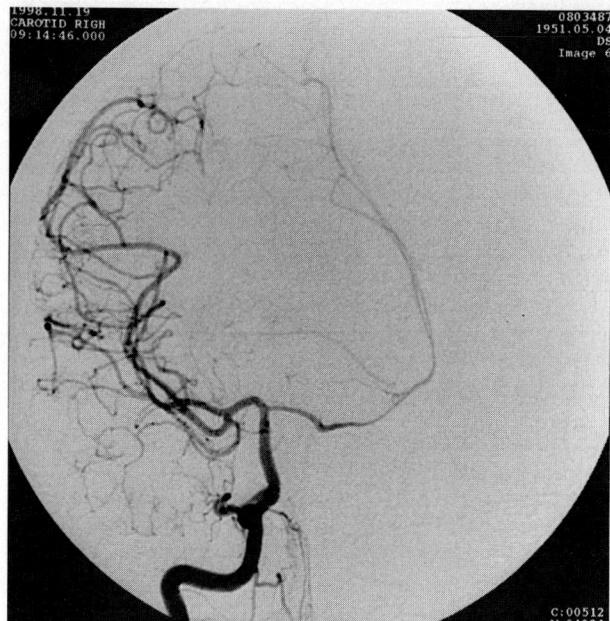

FIGURE 53–13 ■ An anteroposterior right internal carotid injection. The ophthalmic artery does not supply the falcine branches; however, the anterior cerebral arteries are again greatly displaced.

veins, such as the anastomotic vein of Trolard, to the tumor?

A critical principle is that large draining cortical veins entering the sagittal sinus and the sinus itself, if still patent, must be spared during exposure and excision of parasagittal or falcine meningiomas along the middle third or posterior third of the sinus. Attention should be given to the location of these large draining veins, and the surgery must be planned so that these vessels are spared. Acute surgical occlusion of the middle third of the sagittal sinus may result in spastic diplegia. Occlusion of the posterior third of a widely patent sinus may be fatal. The technical decision to effect a "cure" by total extirpation of a parasagittal meningioma by excision or reconstruction of the sinus by duraplasty or vein grafting may depend on the preoperative angiographic assessment of the patency of the superior sagittal sinus and on the presence of collateral anastomotic channels to the sylvian or meningeal veins.[18]

Numerous technical methods were devised to assess the patency of the superior sagittal sinus. Morris[19] recommended an oblique half-axial view to show the entire sinus. This view may be misleading if a segment of the sinus is not visualized. To overcome this problem, Yasargil and Damur[20] recommended half-axial oblique phlebography obtained by simultaneous bilateral injection of the internal carotid artery. Waga and Handa[21] recommend an alternative technique of using contralateral carotid compression during the injection of 10 to 12 ml of contrast medium for half-axial oblique phlebography. Subtraction angiography also is advised because the inner table of the skull can mimic an opacified superior sagittal sinus (Fig. 53–14).

Marc and Schechter[22] believe that occlusion of the superior sagittal sinus by a slowly growing tumor can be predicted with reasonable accuracy from the lateral projection of the venous phase of a carotid angiogram, provided that the findings include the following:

1. Nonvisualization of a segment of the superior sagittal sinus
2. Failure of cortical veins to reach the superior sagittal sinus
3. Delay of venous drainage in the area of obstruction
4. Reversal of the normal venous flow, with large collaterals connecting the anterior-superior sagittal sinus with the superior sagittal sinus at a site distal to the obstruction, the transverse sinus, or the middle cerebral vein

Nonvisualization of a segment of the superior sagittal sinus without the other signs on the lateral view could occur because the sinus is receiving a large volume of unopacified blood from the opposite cerebral hemisphere through a large cortical vein at that location.

Phlebography also may show collateral venous drainage through enlarged scalp veins.[21] These dilated scalp veins also are seen when the scalp is shaved and should be considered in planning the scalp incision and flap.

Walkenhorst[23] reviewed 79 parasagittal meningiomas involving the dural sinus angle and 35 falx meningiomas to determine whether angiography provided signs conclusive for differentiating the two tumor types preoperatively. He reported that a falx meningioma is excluded angiographically when the blood supply is from branches of the middle cerebral artery or when the external carotid artery contributes to the tumor circulation. Marked basal convex meandering of the pericallosal artery on the lateral angiogram is evidence for a falx rather than a parasagittal meningioma.

Selective injection of the external carotid artery may be

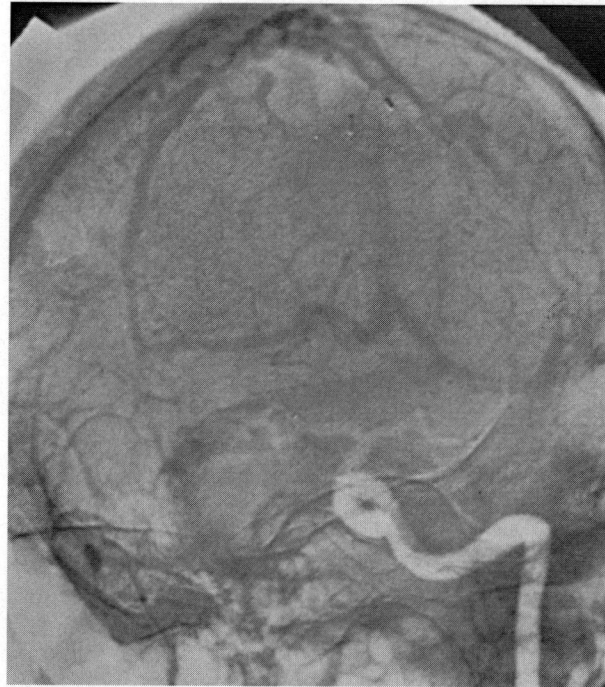

FIGURE 53–14 ■ Subtraction carotid angiography with contralateral carotid compression in which the half-axial oblique view, which is used during the venous phase, demonstrates occlusion of the superior sagittal sinus by a parasagittal meningioma.

helpful in determining the site of tumor attachment at the convexity or along the falx cerebri. The tentorial branches from the internal carotid artery may delineate the site of dural attachment of posterior falx meningiomas. Subtraction studies, angiotomography, and magnification also may improve definition of tumor vascularity. Internal carotid artery injection of contrast agents with digital subtraction angiography is an effective method for demonstrating venous anatomy and patency of the sagittal sinus.

## Sagittal Sinography

Sagittal sinography is mentioned for completeness and historically was considered when angiography did not provide a satisfactory venous phase for determining sinus patency with middle and posterior third parasagittal tumors. The procedure involved placing a bur hole in the exact midline 8 cm above the nasion. A No. 11 scalpel blade was used to fenestrate the sinus wall, and a fine catheter was inserted 3 cm into the sinus. Aspiration of venous blood confirmed the catheter position before the contrast medium was injected.

The disadvantages of direct sagittal sinography are that incomplete information regarding collateral venous flow is obtained and the cerebral pattern of venous drainage is not seen. The procedure may be technically troublesome, is time-consuming, and carries the risk of sinus thrombosis[24] and air embolism.[25]

## PREOPERATIVE MANAGEMENT

The typical preoperative medical evaluation includes a 12-lead electrocardiogram and chest radiographs. In addition, serum electrolytes, complete blood count, coagulation indices, and type and crossmatch for 2 units of packed red cells are obtained. Patients are loaded with phosphenytoin, and serum levels are confirmed before surgery. Patients are started on a regimen of corticosteroid therapy 1 to 3 days before surgery depending on the extent of vasogenic edema. Antibiotics are given on induction of general anesthesia.

## INDICATIONS FOR SURGERY

Patients with meningiomas present with a spectrum of indications for surgery. For tumors with mass effect and symptoms attributable to increased intracranial pressure, there seems little controversy for surgery. Elderly patients with small tumors or patients in poor systemic health may be observed with serial scans because some meningiomas demonstrate no to minimal growth.[26] Seizures appear to decrease for most patients after surgery, and anticonvulsants can eventually be tapered or discontinued.[27] Elderly patients with a good functional status preoperatively also appear to live longer and more independently after surgery.[28]

## OPERATIVE APPROACH AND TECHNIQUES

### Position

The head is positioned so that the sagittal plane of the head is parallel to the walls and perpendicular to the ceiling. For tumors along the anterior third of the sagittal sinus, the patient is supine, with the head of the table flat or slightly elevated. The head is supported in a donut head holder or by three-point skeletal fixation. Tumors involving the middle third of the sinus are more easily approached if the head is elevated a few degrees and the neck is slightly flexed so that the surgeon looks directly down on the vertex. Tumors between the lambdoidal suture and torcular Herophili can be approached with the patient in a three-quarter sitting position with the neck flexed and the head secured by three-point skeletal fixation (Fig. 53–15) or with the patient in the prone position in three-point skeletal fixation. The head must be able to be raised or lowered quickly to control sagittal sinus venous pressure in the event of bleeding from the sinus or the occurrence of air emboli.

### Scalp Incision

The incision is outlined on the shaved and prepared scalp with a sterile marking before draping but after positioning, so that no confusion arises regarding the relationship of the incision to key landmarks. The midline is identified with a crosshatch mark that can be seen easily.

The curvilinear or sinusoidal transverse scalp incision offers several advantages over the more traditional scalp flap. The incision is quickly opened and closed. It is readily extended on either side of the midline if more exposure is needed. The blood supply to the scalp is not compromised. The incision is less restrictive and can easily be adapted to additional surgery at a later date, if necessary. The transverse incision is in the plane bisecting the anteroposterior diameter of the tumor, and its extension is equidistant on either side of the tumor (Fig. 53–16).

### Bone Flap

A free bone flap is preferred to an osteoplastic or periosteal hinged flap high on the convexity or across the midline at the vertex. The skull is thick in this region and not easily fractured. No muscle or fascia needs to be removed from the bone, and the bone flap does not need to be secured. Troublesome bleeding from the bone is easier to control, and the flap can be manipulated more safely in the region of the sagittal sinus.

The bone flap is extended to or just across the midline for unilateral tumors. The bone flap is carried well across the midline to the extent dictated by the size and shape of the tumor when the CT scan shows a bilateral meningioma (see Fig. 53–16). The bone flap is centered over the tumor. Care is taken to make the bone flap particularly generous when the meningioma is adjacent to the paracentral lobule, so that functionally important sensory and motor cortex

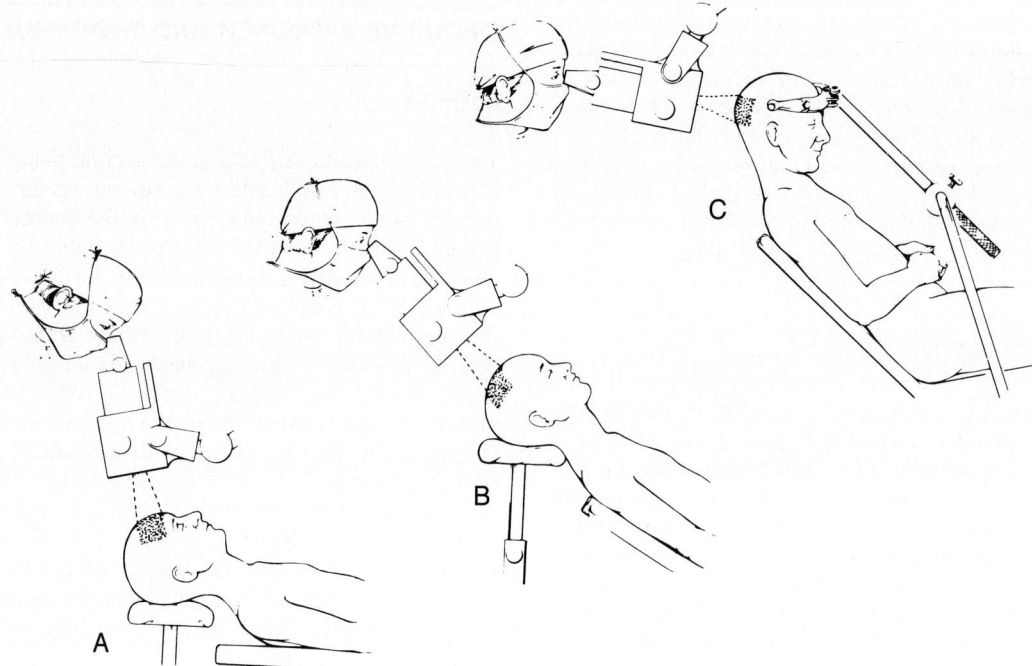

**FIGURE 53–15** ■ Head position of the patient for approaching meningiomas involving the anterior third (*A*), the middle third (*B*), and the posterior third (*C*) of the sagittal sinus.

does not have to be removed or manipulated for exposure of the tumor.

Bur holes are placed immediately on both sides of the sagittal sinus at the anterior margins of the bone flap but not directly over the sinus or the tumor (see Fig. 53–15). The dura mater and sinus are carefully separated from the

inner table of the skull with a dural separator. A Gigli saw or a high-speed air osteotome is used to connect the bur holes. The bone cuts across the sinus are performed last, and the anterior cut is made before the posterior cut.

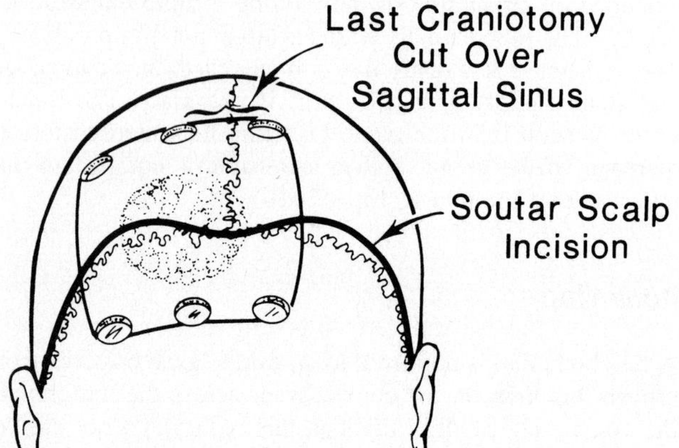

If the bone flap is attached to the dura mater or involved by tumor over or near the sagittal sinus, using a rongeur to cut the bone away is preferable to risking tearing of the sagittal sinus by avulsing the tumor with the bone. If, in advance, the tumor is known or strongly suspected to involve the skull over the sinus, the bone flap is not freed on all sides with the saw because the rocking action of the rongeur on the free bone flap that is tethered by tumor may tear the sagittal sinus or injure adjacent brain. Performing sequential outer table craniotomies for large parasagittal hyperostosing tumors is less attractive than in convexity meningiomas, unless the location of the sagittal sinus is known precisely in advance.[29]

Brisk venous bleeding from the sagittal sinus may occur and should be anticipated. Strips of oxidized cellulose or thrombin-soaked absorbable gelatin sponge that have been prepared in advance are placed over the bleeding sinus, and gentle pressure is applied with cotton strips. Dural and epidural bleeding is otherwise handled with bipolar coagulation and dural tacking stitches.

## Dural Opening and Tumor Excision

The sagittal sinus is readily identified, but bridging cortical veins just beneath the dura mater can be torn if they are not anticipated and carefully dissected off the dural flap as it is turned. The flap is hinged on the sagittal sinus to avoid damaging these important draining veins, which can cause serious neurologic deficit if interrupted at a site posterior to the coronal suture (Fig. 53–17).

**FIGURE 53–16** ■ The scalp incision bisects the anteroposterior plane of a parasagittal or falx meningioma. The free bone flap crosses the midline to the extent determined by the size and configuration of the tumor. Bur holes are placed on either side rather than directly over the sagittal sinus.

Last Craniotomy
Cut Over
Sagittal Sinus

Soutar Scalp
Incision

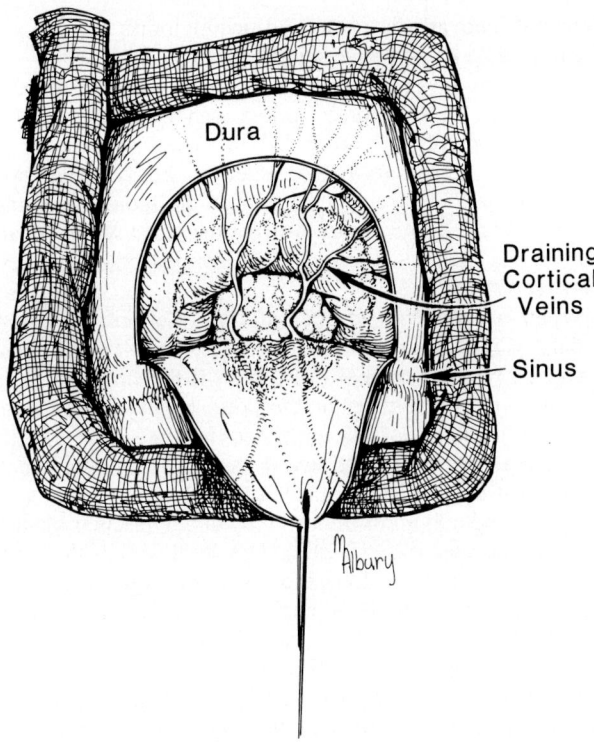

FIGURE 53–17 ■ The dura mater is carefully peeled away from a parasagittal meningioma. Bridging veins that drain the cerebral cortex and enter the sagittal sinus are spared.

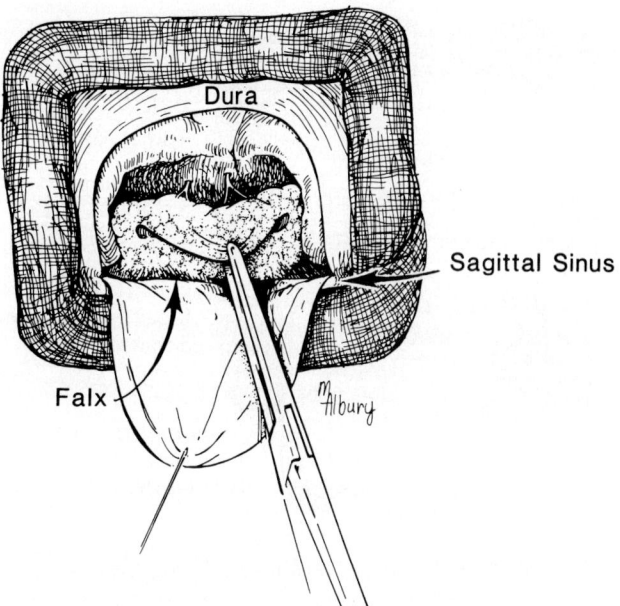

FIGURE 53–18 ■ A parasagittal meningioma is first debulked by intracapsular enucleation. The thin capsular wall is then delivered into the tumor cavity as arachnoidal adhesive bands and feeding vessels are divided. The capsule is removed piecemeal until only the attachment to the falx and the sagittal sinus remains.

Parasagittal meningiomas often can be palpated through the dura mater, and the dura is opened, so that unnecessary brain exposure is avoided. Abnormally thickened dura is resected to remove tissue infiltrated with meningioma cells.[30] Recurrence is associated with the extent of resection,[31] and multiple meningiomas appear to be from tumor spread of a single clone.[32, 33] The dura mater is peeled away from the tumor immediately and is not used to retract the tumor, as is suggested for convexity meningiomas because of the risk of initiating bleeding from the sinus or bridging cortical veins (see Fig. 53–17).

The capsule is partially exposed through the use of bipolar cautery to coagulate small vessels that are parasitized from the pia arachnoid over adjacent cortex. A cleavable pial-tumor plane is not always present. Sindou and Alaywan[34] studied 150 patients with preoperative angiography. Only 34.8% of meningiomas with evidence of pial parasitization had a cleavable pial-tumor interface. Conversely, in meningiomas with primarily a dural supply, 83.6% had a cleavable plane. This procedure is performed without excision of any cortex and with little retraction of surrounding brain. An intracapsular enucleation is performed, and the capsule is delivered into the tumor cavity. In general, if the tumor is not excessively vascular and if it aspirates well, the best way of proceeding is to deliver the tumor by invaginating the capsule (Fig. 53–18). After the tumor mass is removed, the attachment to the falx and sagittal sinus is excised and coagulated.

If a large meningioma invaginates the medial surface of the hemisphere along the middle third of the falx in the vicinity of the paracentral lobule, it may on rare occasion be preferable to expose the tumor by performing a wedge cortical resection that is well anterior to the motor cortex, rather than to attempt to expose the tumor through forceful retraction of the brain and interruption of cortical draining veins passing to the sagittal sinus (Fig. 53–19). Gentle retraction on the cortex is always attempted initially, however, to see if the tumor can be exposed and excised without brain section.

Bilateral tumors infiltrating the falx and presenting on the medial side of both cerebral hemispheres require resection of the falx along the anterior and posterior margins of

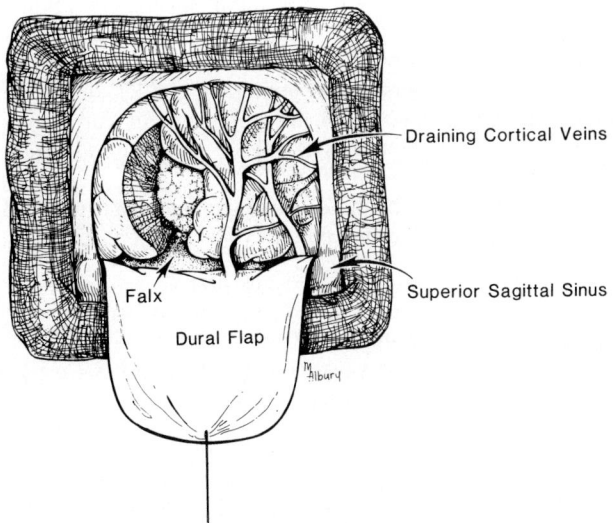

FIGURE 53–19 ■ A large meningioma of the falx invaginates the paracentral lobule beneath large draining cortical veins. An anterior wedge resection of premotor cortex adjacent to the falx provides access to the tumor without forceful retraction on the motor cortex or injury to the important bridging veins.

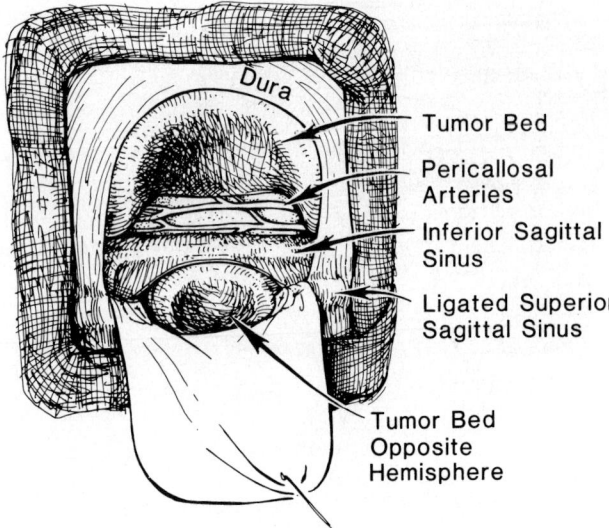

**FIGURE 53-20** ■ A bilateral parasagittal meningioma has been excised along with a segment of the involved falx and occluded sagittal sinus, which was first ligated and then divided. A collateral vein from the sagittal sinus proximal to the occlusion is spared along with the patent inferior sagittal sinus. The pericallosal arteries that supplied feeding branches to the tumor appear on the dorsal surface of the corpus callosum.

the tumor. The inferior sagittal sinus and pericallosal arteries are preserved because feeding vessels coming off the pericallosal branches are coagulated and divided (Fig. 53–20).

## SUPERIOR SAGITTAL SINUS INTERVENTIONS

Simpson[31] found that complete excision of a meningioma with its dural attachment is followed by fewer clinical recurrences (5% to 9%) than is complete removal of the tumor with coagulation of the dural attachment (17%), complete removal without treatment of the dural attachment (29%), or partial removal of the tumor (39%). The goal of surgery is gross total resection; sudden occlusion of the middle and posterior third of the sinus carries the potential dire consequences of spastic diplegia and death, however.

The management of the superior sagittal sinus involved with meningioma depends on three anatomic criteria:

1. From the angiogram, is the sinus patent?
2. Does the meningioma involve the anterior, middle, or posterior third of the sinus?
3. What portion of the sinus is involved: the lateral wall, roof, or combinations thereof?

There is agreement that the anterior third of the superior sagittal sinus, the segment in front of the coronal suture, can be ligated and divided for meningioma resection regardless of patency. In addition, there is little controversy regarding resection of an occluded sinus, provided that collateral venous channels, such as those passing through the falx to the inferior sagittal sinus or meningeal veins, are preserved. Conversely, several authors have put forth

technical innovations to manage meningiomas involving a patent middle or posterior sagittal sinus.

If a tumor involves the middle or posterior third of a patent sinus, one of three options can be exercised: (1) Resect the involved portion of the sinus and repair it primarily or with a graft; (2) resect the sinus and provide a bypass; or (3) leave this portion of the tumor, allowing tumor growth eventually to obstruct the sinus while collateral venous channels develop. Definitive resection is undertaken at a later time.

When a tumor is attached to one wall of the sinus without significant infiltration of the dura mater or lumen, it may be possible to peel the tumor off the sinus wall and coagulate the dura mater at the point of attachment (Fig. 53–21A). If the tumor has infiltrated the sinus lumen in the lateral angle but not obliterated the sinus, a feasible method is to grasp the superior and lateral wall of the sinus with the contained nubbin of tumor with curved vascular clamps or hemostats (see Fig. 53–21B). The dural wall of the sinus is excised by cutting along the inner curve of the clamps. The clamps are rotated one half turn, and a running vascular suture is used to perform the sinorrhaphy as the clamps are removed one at a time (Fig. 53–22).

A parasinus meningioma classification was first devised by Bonnal and Brotchi[35] and later modified by Hakuba[36] into eight subtypes depending on the number of sinus walls involved and sinus patency. These subtypes are well illustrated by Hakuba.[36] Briefly, in types I and II, the

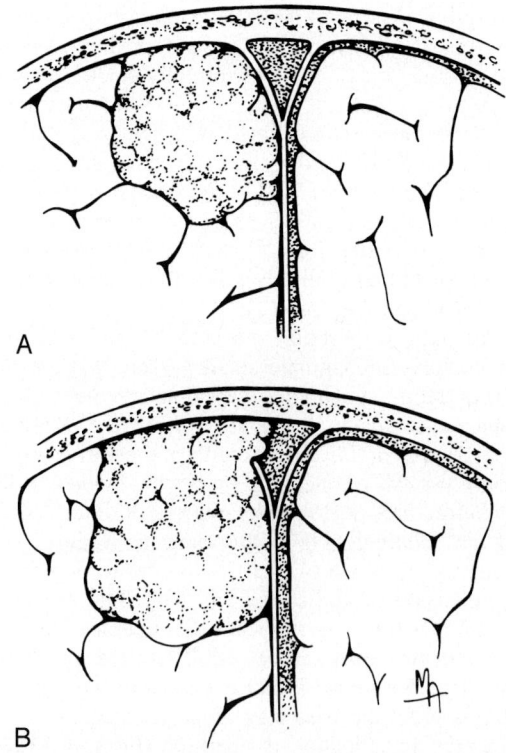

**FIGURE 53-21** ■ *A,* This coronal view of the superior sagittal sinus illustrates a meningioma involving one wall. A parasagittal meningioma usually infiltrates both layers of dura mater, whereas a falx meningioma may be attached to the outer layer only. *B,* This coronal view of the superior sagittal sinus illustrates a meningioma infiltrating the lateral wall and angle of the sinus and protruding into the lateral recess of the lumen.

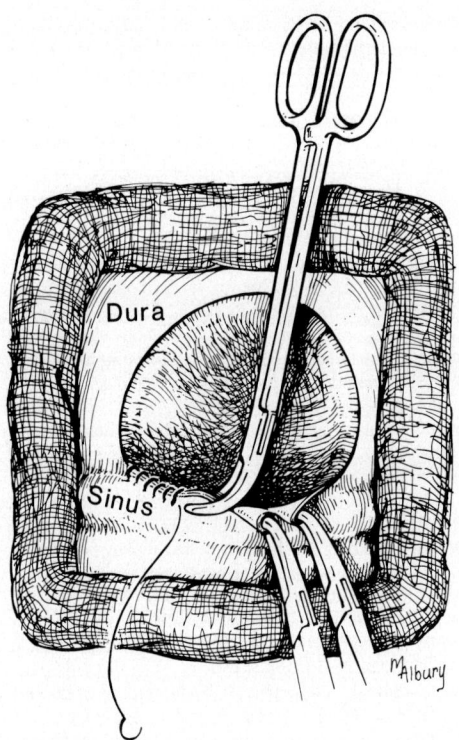

**FIGURE 53–22** ■ The patent sagittal sinus with a meningioma involving the lateral recess is opened longitudinally along the inside curve of vascular clamps. The clamps are applied sequentially as the dural walls forming the lateral angle are partially excised along with the contained tumor. The clamps are then removed in reverse order as sinorrhaphy is performed with a running vascular stitch.

meningioma can be resected and the patency of the sinus maintained without a graft. In types III through VIII, multiple walls of the sinus are involved, and a graft must be fashioned or tumor tissue left in situ.

Several authors have published case reports[37–39] and series[36] demonstrating techniques for measuring stump pressures[40] and fashioning vein bypass grafts. A delayed thrombosis reaches almost 50% with vein interposition[36, 41, 42] and perhaps higher with synthetic materials.[37] Ransohoff[43] describes using a laser to remove meningioma cells from the sinus wall until bleeding is encountered, then primarily repairing the wall.

If multiple sinus walls are involved with tumor, precluding total resection and primary repair, we prefer leaving residual tumor to occlude the sinus slowly and allow collateral venous channnels to develop. The patient is then followed with serial MRI scans to assess tumor growth and sinus patency. If resection is again warranted, the sinus is then taken and careful attention is paid to preserving cortical and meningeal venous channels.

Hartman and Klug[44] reported enclosing a patent sagittal sinus infiltrated by tumor in a sleeve fashioned from the falx and convexity dura. This sleeve of dura contains and directs any possible future recurrent growth of tumor in such a way that it eventually obliterates the sinus. Collateral circulation gradually develops, then the segment of sagittal sinus occluded by tumor can be excised with less risk.

## CLOSURE

The dura is closed primarily, or a patch graft is fashioned with pericranium, fascia lata, or a synthetic substitute according to the surgeon's preference. The epidural space is washed with saline and the bone flap secured with miniplates and screws. The galea is closed with an interrupted, inverted nonabsorbable suture and the skin with staples. Sterile dressings and a standard head wrap are applied.

## POSTOPERATIVE CARE

The primary concern in the postoperative period is that a venous thrombosis, hematoma, or brain edema could produce a focal or generalized increase in intracranial pressure, progressive neurologic dysfunction, and transtentorial herniation. The patient is observed closely in the recovery room and the intensive care unit for deterioration in the level of consciousness, focal neurologic deficit, or seizure activity. Vital signs, pulmonary function, blood gases, and fluid and electrolyte balance are monitored. The head is elevated 20 to 30 degrees. Corticosteroid therapy should be continued at full dose for 72 hours or through the expected period of maximal brain swelling, before a steroid taper is started. Seizure prophylaxis with parenteral diphenylhydantoin is continued. A CT scan without contrast enhancement is advisable to distinguish brain swelling and postoperative hematoma in a patient with persistent or progressive lethargy or obtundation or progressive focal neurologic deficit. MRI and magnetic resonance venography or angiography is indicated if an evolving venous thrombosis is suspected.

## ACKNOWLEDGMENTS

*The authors thank Edward Michel, M.D., and Charles Truwit, M.D., for providing and interpreting the radiographs illustrated throughout the chapter.*

## REFERENCES

1. Cushing H: The meningiomas (dural endotheliomas): Their source and favored seats of origin (Cavendish Lecture). Brain 45:282, 1922.
2. Northfield DWC: The Surgery of the Central Nervous System. Oxford: Blackwell, 1973, p 884.
3. Cushing H, Eisenhardt L: Meningiomas: Their Classification, Regional Behavior, Life History and Surgical End Results. Springfield, IL: Charles C Thomas, 1938, p 785.
4. Olivecrona H: Die Parasagittalen Meningiome. Leipzig: Georg Thieme, 1934.
5. Lund M: Epilepsy in association with intracranial tumours. Acta Psychiatr Scand 81(Suppl):149, 1952.
6. Osborne A: Meningiomas and other nonglial neoplasms. In Diagnostic Neuroradiology, St. Louis: CV Mosby, 1996, pp 579–625.
7. Pompili A, Derome PJ, Visot A, Guiot G: Hyperostosing meningiomas of the sphenoid ridge: Clinical features, surgical therapy and long-term observations: Review of 49 cases. Surg Neurol 17:411–416, 1982.
8. Bonnal J, Thibaut A, Brothci J, Boren J: Invading meningiomas of the sphenoid ridge. J Neurosurg 53:587–599, 1980.
9. New P, Aronow S, Hesselink J: National Cancer Institutes study: Evaluation of computed tomography: The diagnosis of intracranial neoplasms IV meningiomas. Radiology 136:665–675, 1980.

10. Fujii K, Fujita N, Hirabuki N, et al: Neuromas and meningiomas: Evaluation of early enhancement with dynamic MR imaging. AJNR Am J Neuroradiol 13:1215–1220, 1992.

11. Inamura T, Nishio S, Takeshita I, et al: Peritumoral brain edema in meningiomas: Influence of vascular supply upon its development. Neurosurgery 31:179–185, 1992.

12. Bitzer M, Helge T, Morgalla M, et al: Tumor-related venous obstruction and development of peritumoral brain edema in meningiomas. Neurosurgery 42:730–373, 1998.

13. Onesti S, Zahos P, Ashkenazi E: Spontaneous hemorrhage into a convexity meningioma. Acta Neurochir (Wien) 138:1250–1251, 1996.

14. Barnett G: Surgical management of convexity and falcine meningiomas using interactive image guided surgery systems. Neurosurg Clin North Am 7:279–284, 1996.

15. Tenner MS: The role of conventional neuroradiologic techniques in relation to computed tomography. In Sher JH, Ford DH (eds): Primary Intracranial Neoplasms. New York: SP Med and Sci, 1971, pp 71–85.

16. Osborne AG: The external carotid artery. In Introduction to Cerebral Angiography. Hagerstown: Harper & Row, 1980, pp 49–86.

17. Macpherson P: The value of preoperative embolization of meningiomas estimated objectively and subjectively. Neuroradiology 33:334–337, 1991.

18. Oka K, Go Y, Kimura H, Tomonaga M: Obstruction of the superior sagittal sinus caused by parasagittal meningiomas: The role of collateral venous pathways. J Neurosurg 81:520–524, 1994.

19. Morris L: Angiography of the superior sagittal and transverse sinuses. Br J Radiol 33:606, 1960.

20. Yasargil MG, Damur M: Thrombosis of the cerebral veins and dural sinuses. In Newton TH, Potts DG (eds): Radiology of the Skull and Brain, Vol 2. St. Louis: CV Mosby, 1974, p 2375.

21. Waga S, Handa H: Scalp veins as collateral pathway with parasagittal meningiomas occluding superior sagittal sinus. Neuroradiology 11:119, 1976.

22. Marc JA, Schechter MM: Cortical venous rerouting in parasagittal meningiomas. Radiology 112.85, 1974.

23. Walkenhorst A: Angiographic aspects of parasagittal meningiomas. Acta Neurochir (Wien) 31:288, 1974.

24. Krayenbühl H: Cerebral venous and sinus thrombosis. Clin Neurosurg 14:1, 1967.

25. Askenasy HM, Kosary IZ, Braham J: Thrombosis of the longitudinal sinus diagnosis by carotid angiography. Neurology 12:288, 1962.

26. Olivero W, Lister R, Elwood P: The natural history and growth rate of asymptomatic meningiomas: A review of 60 patients. J Neurosurg 83:222–224, 1995.

27. Chozick B, Reinert S, Greenblatt S: Incidence of seizures after surgery for supratentorial meningiomas: A modern analysis. J Neurosurg 84:382–386, 1996.

28. Pompili A, Callovini G, Delfini R, et al: Is surgery useful for very old patients with intracranial meningioma? Lancet 351:117–120, 1998.

29. Colon G, Ross D, Hoff J: Sequential outer table craniotomy in a hyperossified meningioma. J Neurosurg 88:346–348, 1998.

30. Nakau H, Miyazawa T, Tamai S, et al: Pathological significance of meningeal enhancement (Flare sign) on meningiomas in MRI. Surg Neurol 48:584–591, 1997.

31. Simpson D: The recurrence of intracranial meningiomas after surgical treatment. J Neurol Neurosurg Psychiatry 20:22, 1957.

32. Stangl A, Wellenreuther R, Lenartz D, et al: Clonality of multiple meningiomas. J Neurosurg 86:853–858, 1997.

33. Larson J, Tew J, Simon M, Menon A: Evidence for clonal spread in the development of multiple meningiomas. J Neurosurg 83:705–709, 1995.

34. Sindou M, Alaywan M: Most intracranial meningiomas are not cleavable tumors: Anatomic-surgical evidence and angiographic predictability. Neurosurgery 42:476–480, 1998.

35. Bonnal J, Brotchi J: Surgery of the superior sagittal sinus in parasagittal meningiomas. J Neurosurg 48:935, 1978.

36. Hakuba A: Reconstruction of dural sinus involved in meningiomas. In Al-Mefty O (ed): Meningiomas. New York: Raven Press, 1991, pp 371–382.

37. Bederson J, Eisenberg M: Resection and replacement of the superior sagittal sinus for treatment of a parasagittal meningioma: Technical case report. Neurosurgery 37:1015–1019, 1995.

38. Murata J, Sawamura Y, Saito H, Abe H: Resection of a recurrent parasagittal meningioma with a cortical vein anastomosis: A technical note. Surg Neurol 48:592–597, 1997.

39. Hakuba A, Huh C, Tsujikawa S, Nishimura S: Total removal of a parasagittal meningioma of the posterior third of the sagittal sinus and its repair by autologous vein graft: Case report. J Neurosurg 51:397–382, 1979.

40. Schmid-Elsaesser R, Steiger H, Yousssy T, et al: Radical resection of meningiomas and AVF involving critical dural sinus segments: Experience with intraoperative sinus pressure monitoring and elective sinus reconstruction in 10 patients. Neurosurgery 41:1005–1018, 1997.

41. Al-Mefty O, Yamamoto Y: Neurovascular reconstruction during and after skull base surgery. Contemp Neurosurg 15:1–9, 1993.

42. Sindou M: Reconstructive procedures of the intracranial venous system. Presented at the First International Workshop on Surgery of the Intracranial Venous System, Osaka, Japan, September 12–14, 1994.

43. Ransohoff J: Removal of convexity, parasagittal, and falcine meningiomas. Neurosurg Clin North Am 5:293–297, 1994.

44. Hartman K, Klug W: Recurrence and possible surgical procedures in meningiomas of the middle and posterior parts of the superior sagittal sinus. Acta Neurochir (Wien) 31:283, 1975.

# CHAPTER 54

# Convexity Meningioma Surgery*

■ DARREN S. LOVICK and ROBERT E. MAXWELL

*"To other than beginners much of what follows may seem trifling, but it is on a multiplicity of trifles, carefully observed, that the success of one of these operations depends."*

Harvey Cushing[1]

Cushing[1] coined the term *meningioma* to define and distinguish a class of neoplasms arising from the meninges of the brain and spinal cord. Meningiomas account for approximately 15% of central nervous system tumors. Most of these tumors have a benign histopathologic appearance and follow a similar clinical course.[2, 3] Atypical and malignant meningiomas constitute 7% and 2% of meningiomas.[4] Benign meningiomas occur more commonly in women,[5] and malignant meningiomas are perhaps slightly more frequent in men.[6] The peak incidence is between the ages of 50 and 70 years.[2] Among intracranial meningiomas, nearly 90% are supratentorial, 10% are in the posterior fossa, and fewer than 2% are intraventricular. Approximately one third of supratentorial meningiomas arise along the superior sagittal sinus or falx; one third over the convexity of the hemispheres; and one third from the basal regions, such as the sphenoid ridge, the perisellar region, and the olfactory grooves.[2, 7–10] This chapter discusses the classification, clinical presentation, radiologic appearance, preoperative medical management, and surgical techniques for treating patients with convexity meningiomas.

## CLASSIFICATION OF CONVEXITY MENINGIOMAS

Cushing and Eisenhardt[2] separated the convexity meningiomas into seven groups based on surgical considerations relevant to their radiographic localization, neurologic presentation, and prognosis. Cushing[10] first classified the convexity meningiomas according to location in 1922 as frontal, paracentral, parietal, occipital, and temporal. This classification proved inadequate for precise localization of these tumors because the frontal lobe includes the large region anterior to the rolandic fissure. Thirty-eight (70%) of 54 convexity meningiomas reported in 1938 by Cushing and Eisenhardt[2] were anterior to the rolandic fissure. Cushing[1] later reclassified the convexity meningiomas into seven categories by subdividing the frontal meningiomas into

precoronal, coronal, and postcoronal groups. This classification proved more relevant for surgical considerations based on the clinical and radiographic presentation.

## SYMPTOMS OF CONVEXITY MENINGIOMAS

### Precoronal Convexity Meningiomas

The mental symptoms that are seen in patients with anterior parasagittal or olfactory groove meningiomas are notably absent in patients with frontal convexity meningiomas. Dementia, personality change, and incontinence are much less common with frontal convexity meningiomas away from the midline. These tumors may grow to a large size before headache, seizure, or visual disturbances associated with papilledema bring the patient to a physician's attention.

### Coronal Convexity Meningiomas

Cushing[1] found in this series that one third of all convexity meningiomas were primarily attached along the coronal suture. Of these tumors, 29 were located at the pterion, and 17 were located between the pterion and bregma. Compared with frontal convexity meningiomas located further posteriorly, the coronal tumor remains symptomatically silent for long periods. These tumors become quite large and cause pressure symptoms. Visual blurring, diplopia, and choked disks or secondary atrophy may occur. A contralateral paresis of the arm and face eventually occurs, but the leg remains relatively spared. Focal motor seizures start in the hand or face. Paraphasia may occur with tumors compressing the dominant hemisphere. Cushing observed a tendency for meningiomas of the bregma and pterion at either end of the coronal suture to cause hyperostosis, but hyperostosis is unusual with convexity tumors arising along the central portion of the suture. En plaque meningiomas midway along the coronal suture may produce hyperostosis.

---

*This chapter has been adapted from Schmidek H: Meningiomas and Their Surgical Management. Philadelphia: WB Saunders, 1991.

## Postcoronal Convexity Meningiomas

Convexity meningiomas overlying Brodmann's areas 6 and 8 of the cerebral cortex often produce simple partial motor seizures, which are characterized by conjugate movement of the head and eyes with twitching of the contralateral face and arm. Some patients describe a sensory aura characterized by a sense of tingling or warmth in the contralateral face or arm. A contralateral, central facial and arm paresis eventually occurs.

## Pararolandic Meningiomas

The pararolandic region includes the sensory postcentral gyrus (Brodmann's areas 1, 2, and 3) and the motor precentral gyrus (Brodmann's area 4). Jacksonian seizures involving the contralateral arm and face combined with dysarthria when the dominant hemisphere is compressed characterize meningiomas over the convexity in this region. Cushing and Eisenhardt[2] noted that the seizures produced by pararolandic tumors usually have a motor rather than sensory aura initially. The nine cases they described were all on the dominant side and were prone to recurrence.

## Parietal Meningiomas

Most parietal meningiomas produce sensory seizures and compress or irritate the postcentral gyrus. Meningiomas located near the lambdoid suture (posterior portions of Brodmann's areas 5 and 7) are less epileptogenic.[1] The sensory auras experienced with convexity meningiomas over the parietal lobe are restricted to the contralateral face and arm, with sparing of the leg and foot initially. Receptive dysphasia is sometimes found with meningiomas over the dominant parietal cortex.

## Temporal Meningiomas

Convexity meningiomas compressing the outer surface of the temporal lobe, excluding pterional meningiomas arising along the outer third of the sphenoid wing, are relatively uncommon. Patients with these meningiomas have contralateral seizures and weakness involving the face and upper extremity. Later, when signs and symptoms of increased intracranial pressure are apparent, an ipsilateral spastic weakness of the leg may occur in association with a contralateral shift of the brain stem and compression of the opposite cerebral peduncle against the edge of the tentorium cerebelli. Visual disturbance usually is associated with choked disks or secondary optic atrophy. An incongruous, homonymous visual field deficit may be detected if the patient can cooperate and concentrate sufficiently for testing.

## Occipital Meningiomas

Occipital convexity meningiomas are rare. Cushing[1] found no tumors in this location among 54 convexity meningiomas. Signs and symptoms of increased intracranial pressure are associated with a congruous, homonymous hemianopsia and with visual hallucinations in patients with tumors in this location.

## PREOPERATIVE EVALUATION OF MENINGIOMAS

The preoperative management involves radiologic evaluation, systemic assessment pertinent for general anesthesia, and institution of medical therapy. One should determine whether the imaging characteristics are consistent with the diagnosis of meningioma. If not, what are the alternative pathologies, and how does this influence the surgical strategy? In addition to diagnosis, imaging studies provide anatomic information regarding the tumor's location relative to eloquent cortex, vascular structures, and bony landmarks for operative planning. The medical management includes a review of the patient's medical history, preoperative tests to determine eligibility for general anesthesia, and administration of an anticonvulsant and corticosteroids.

Head computed tomography (CT) with and without contrast administration is typically obtained before referral to the neurosurgeon or obtained as a screening imaging study. Noncontrast CT scans detect 85% of meningiomas, and contrast-enhanced CT scans detect 95% of meningiomas.[11] Without contrast enhancement, meningiomas appear as a hyperdense mass adjacent to the dura. Calcification is present in nearly 25% of meningiomas and ranges from a diffuse sand-like appearance to a dense sclerosis.[12] A spectrum of bone changes can occur at bone-tumor interface. Hyperostosis is not uncommon and pathologically represents bone infiltrated with nests of neoplastic cells.[13, 14] Conversely, other meningiomas invade the bone and may spread outside the calvaria (Fig. 54–1). Greater than 90% of meningiomas demonstrate dense, uniform enhancement.[12] Atypical, malignant, and benign meningiomas cannot be distinguished on CT.[15, 16] In addition to supporting the diagnosis, noncontrast CT is helpful in delineating the extent of bony involvement in preoperative planning.

Multiplanar magnetic resonance imaging (MRI) with gadolinium enhancement provides imaging features to confirm the diagnosis of meningioma and defines the cortical and vascular anatomy for operative planning. Images suggestive of meningiomas include a dural-based mass isointensive to hypointense to brain on T1-weighted images (Fig. 54–2),[12] an enhancing dural tail,[17, 18] a rim of subarachnoid space between the tumor margin and the underlying cortex (Fig. 54–3), and rapid homogeneous enhancement with gadolinium (Figs. 54–4 and 54–5). Two thirds of meningiomas are associated with peritumoral edema, and this is not strictly dependent on tumor size.[20, 21] Spontaneous hemorrhage within a meningioma is uncommon but does occur (Fig. 54–6).[22]

During the magnetic resonance study, other detailed vascular and cortical anatomy may be elucidated via magnetic resonance angiography, magnetic resonance venography, and functional magnetic resonance. For preoperative planning, cortical venous drainage, sinus patency, displacement of major arteries, and location of the central sulcus or speech regions relative to the tumor can be attained by

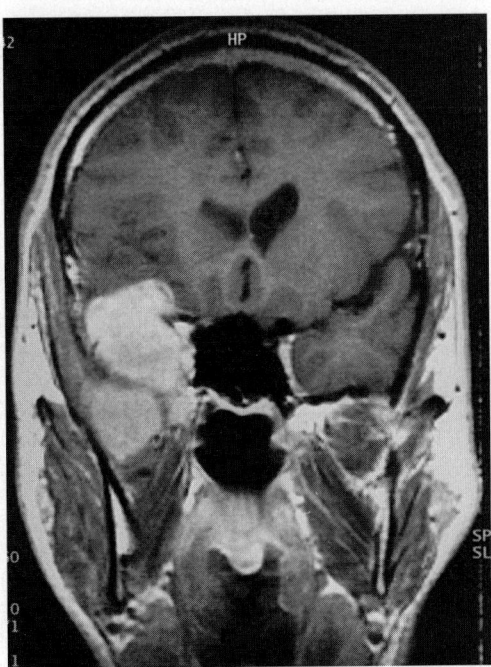

FIGURE 54–1 ■ A magnetic resonrance imaging scan of a sphenoid wing meningioma demonstrating bone invasion and spread into the infratemporal fossa.

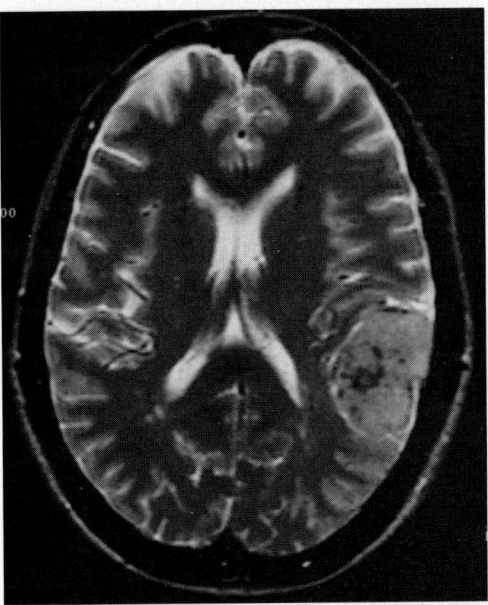

FIGURE 54–3 ■ An axial $T_2$-weighted magnetic resonance imaging scan demonstrating a convexity meningioma with an arachnoid plane separating the tumor and the pia.

a rapid, noninvasive means (Fig. 54–7). In addition to preoperative information, the application of scalp markings and specific software allows MRI-guided frameless stereotaxy for use in the operating room.

Angiography is useful if the tumor abuts or involves critical vascular structures or structures that may need to be sacrificed for total resection or spared better to preserve

function. Initially, convexity meningiomas derive their primary blood supply from dural arteries, usually the middle meningeal artery. After growing to about 2 cm in diameter, meningiomas begin to parasitize blood supply from adjacent pial vessels and possess a dual blood supply.[23] The meningioma's capsule is supplied from pial arterioles and the inner core from dural vasculature.[24] The tumor may show a sunburst pattern on angiograms resulting from a central perforating vessel. On late capillary and venous phase films, meningiomas demonstrate a prominent, homogeneous, prolonged vascular blush termed the "mother-in-

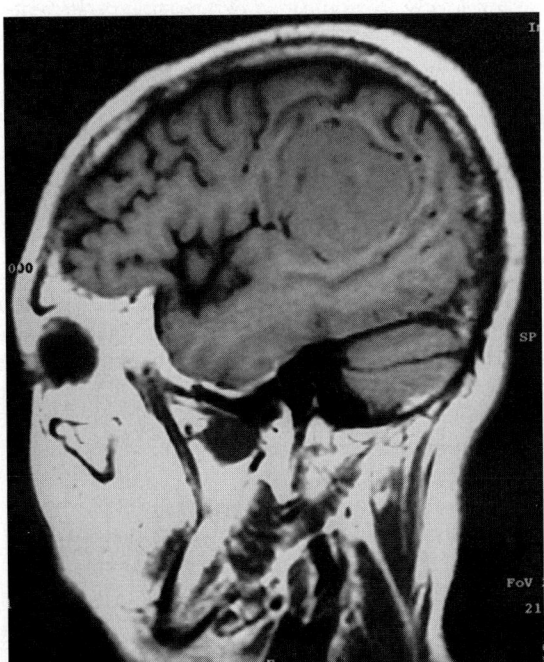

FIGURE 54–2 ■ A sagittal $T_1$-weighted magnetic resonance imaging scan demonstrating a convexity meningioma pushing into the posterior sylvian fissure that is isointense to gray matter.

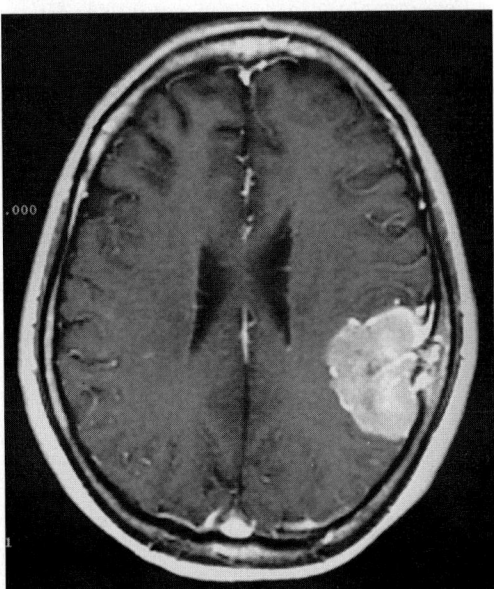

FIGURE 54–4 ■ Axial $T_1$-weighted magnetic resonance imaging scan with gadolinium demonstrating intense, homogeneous enhancement of the convexity meningioma.

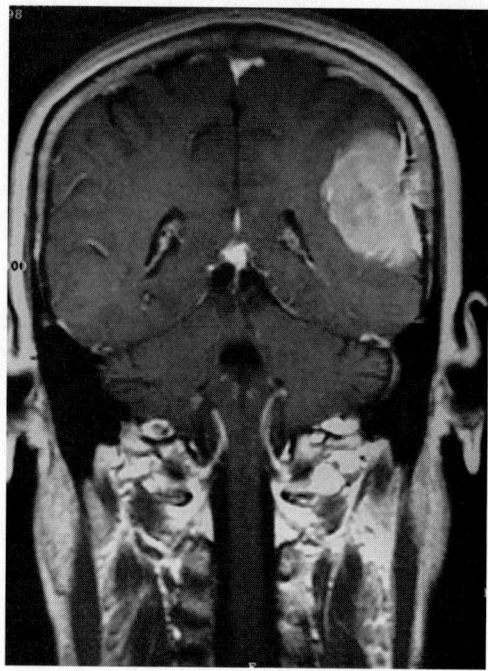

FIGURE 54–5 ■ Coronal T₁-weighted magnetic resonance imaging scan showing intense, homogeneous enhancement of the convexity meningioma.

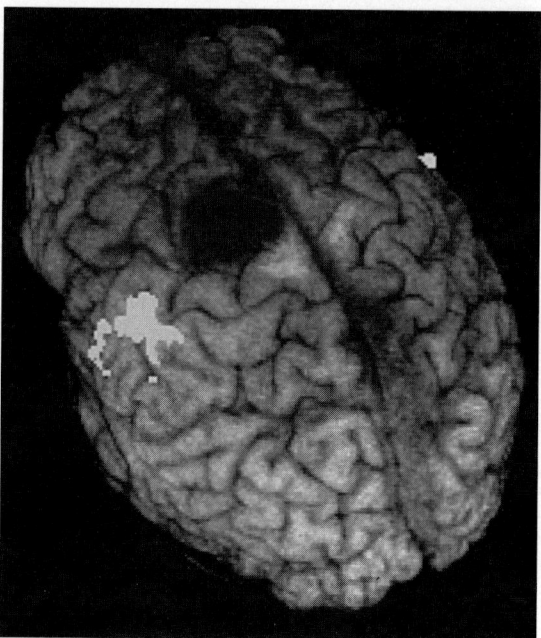

FIGURE 54–7 ■ A functional magnetic resonance imaging scan demonstrating the motor strip (*white*) in relation to the meningioma (*black*).

law sign,'' because it comes early and stays late (Fig. 54–8).[12]

The radiologic findings can mimic a high-grade glioma with extension to the cortical surface; a schwannoma of cranial nerve origin; or, in case reports, neurosarcoidosis.[12, 25] If radiologic findings inconsistent with meningioma are found, other pathologic diagnoses must be considered and their impact on the surgical procedure explored. Problems are best handled by anticipation rather than reaction after

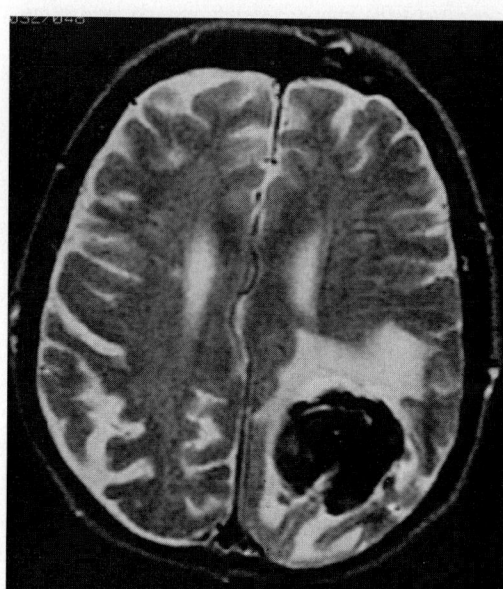

FIGURE 54–6 ■ T₁-weighted axial magnetic resonance imaging scan with a significant hypodense region that was found to be hemorrhage at the time of surgery.

the fact. Most importantly, it is the neurosurgeon's responsibility to determine whether the radiographic abnormality is commensurate with the clinical presentation. If not, more history and tests are necessary to reach a diagnosis and avoid operating on an incidental finding.

The typical preoperative medical evaluation includes a 12-lead electrocardiogram and chest radiographs, serum electrolytes, complete blood count, coagulation indices, and type and screen. Patients are loaded with phosphenytoin, and serum levels are confirmed before surgery. Patients are started on a regimen of corticosteroid therapy 1 to 3 three days before surgery depending on the extent of vasogenic edema. Antibiotics are given on induction of general anesthesia.

## PRINCIPLES OF MENINGIOMA SURGERY

The goal of surgery is total resection with preservation of function. The general principles of meningioma surgery are determined by tumor location, size, configuration, and vascularity. The preferred operative approach is one that provides options for dealing with technical contingencies that arise throughout the case.

### Localization

Accurate localization can be achieved via many methods and is imperative if one plans a small skin incision and bone flap. For experienced surgeons, the combination of an imaging study with bony landmarks suffices. Another simple technique involves placing several radiopaque markers parallel to one another in the sagittal plane on the

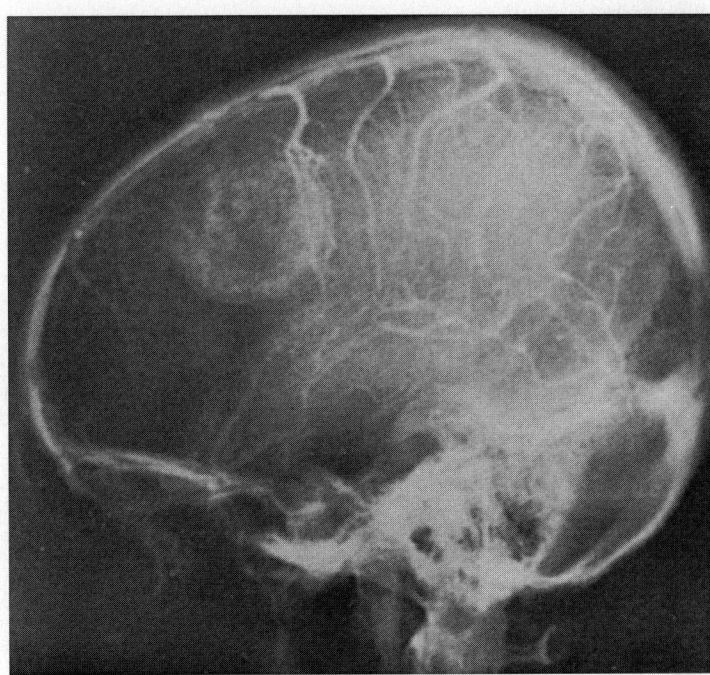

**FIGURE 54–8** ■ An angiogram showing a meningioma tumor stain that is characteristically diffuse and persistent into the venous phase. (From Maxwell RE, Chou SN: Preoperative evaluation and management of meningiomas. In Schmidek HH, Sweet WH [eds]: Operative Neurosurgical Techniques: Indications, Methods, and Results, Vol 1, 2nd ed. Philadelphia: WB Saunders, 1988, p 550.)

patient's scalp over the meningioma. Consequently the CT axial image is perpendicular to the markers. The tumor margins can be marked on the patient's scalp in the axial plane based on the CT slice and in the coronal plane in reference to the markers. Frameless stereotaxy may be helpful for localization and design of the skin incision and bone flap. Once intradural, however, frameless stereotaxy has been of marginal benefit for resection of convexity meningiomas.

## Position

Meningioma surgery may require several hours, and proper positioning is important for unimpeded venous return and the surgeon's ergonomic posture. The head should be higher than the heart, and excessive angulation or twisting of the neck should be avoided. The head should be secured in three-point pinion fixation and attached to the table to prevent motion during the procedure and allow movement of the patient's body and head as a single unit. Inadequate cranial fixation during the procedure can distort the operative exposure deterring microsurgical techniques, result in contamination of the field, or disturb the patient's airway. Pressure points on vulnerable areas, such as the eyes, brachial plexus, and peripheral nerves, should be prevented by careful positioning and padding. Care should be exercised so that scrub solutions do not run into the eyes or pool about the cautery plate, which could increase the risk of burns. The relationship of the tumor to the brain and other contiguous structures should be considered in advance so that gravity can be used to minimize the need for brain retraction. The head position and operati field are planned with consideration of the handedness of the surgeon and the optimal location for instruments such as self-retaining retractors and the operating microscope. Often, a surface on which to rest and steady the forearms is helpful

to the surgeon, particularly for working under the operating microscope in the sitting position.

## Scalp Incision

Factors one should consider in designing a skin incision are as follows: (1) the vascular supply to the scalp, (2) adequate exposure provided by the skin incision, (3) modification of the incision in the event that preoperative localization was inaccurate or access to critical structures during the surgery outside the flap is necessary (venous sinus), (4) modification of the incision if the meningioma recurs adjacent to the resection site for adequate exposure without compromising the vascular supply to the scalp, and (5) provision of pericranial or temporalis fascia flaps if a vascularized dural reconstruction is anticipated. A satisfactory cosmetic result is always an important consideration.

A scalp flap needs to be only slightly larger than the proposed bone flap, provided that the tumor location, size, and site of dural attachment are known in advance. If any doubt exists, one should err on the side of a scalp and bone flap that is too generous when exposing a meningioma.

The scalp is extremely vascular and rarely devascularized when good surgical principles are followed. Some meningiomas recur, and scalp incisions are reopened, extended, or revised. Linear and S-shaped incisions provide adequate exposure when centered on the lesion and offer the advantages of less total incisional length, reduced skin tension, and easy modification at second operation. The blood supply to the scalp is always considered, and flaps are based on their vascular pedicle. The length of a scalp flap should not exceed the width by more than a 3:2 ratio, and a flap should be designed to be widest at its base. Flaps prove more troublesome to modify than linear or S-shaped incisions.

The cosmetic result of an incisional scar should be

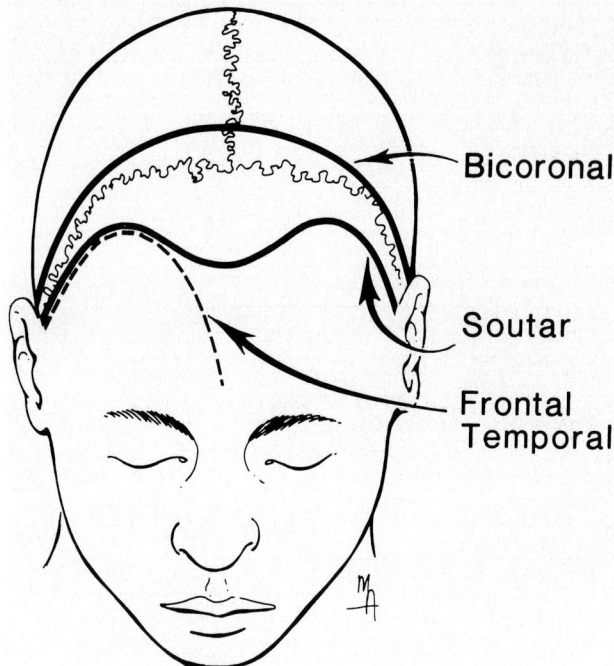

**FIGURE 54–9** ■ A bicoronal or Soutar scalp incision positioned behind the hairline provides wider exposure and less cosmetic deformity than a frontotemporal incision, in which the anterior limb of the incision crosses the forehead. (From Maxwell RE, Chou SN: Convexity meningiomas and general principles of meningioma surgery. In Schmidek HH, Sweet WH [eds]: Operative Neurosurgical Techniques: Indications, Methods, and Results, vol 1, 2nd ed. Philadelphia: WB Saunders, 1988, p 556.)

considered. A bicoronal or Soutar incision is preferable to a frontal or frontotemporal scalp flap in which the anterior limb of the incision crosses the forehead and leaves a cosmetic deformity (Fig. 54–9). The temporal branch of the facial nerve can be spared if the scalp incision extends no lower than the top of the zygomatic arch and is barely in front of the ear. This branch is also vulnerable in the temporalis fascia at the temporal fat pad and can be spared with reflection of the temporalis muscle with the skin at this location.[25] At other locations, a flap or linear incision provides similar cosmetic results, and use is at the dicretion of the surgeon.

The skin is incised sharply, and large arterioles and veins are controlled with bipolar cautery. Raney clips are placed to tamponade remaining bleeding, provided that the galea aponeurotica is included in the clip. The scalp is reflected leaving the pericranium intact and retracted with fishhooks attached to the drapes or a retracting bar.

The pericranium is used for duraplasty after the tumor is resected. The pericranium is incised with a monopolar cautery along the edges of the skin incision. It can be incised circumferentially, elevated, and soaked in saline or incised on three sides, reflected as a flap, placed under tension with dural stitches, and covered with a moist gauze sponge.

## Elevation of Bone Flap

Use of the true osteoplastic bone flap, in which the scalp, muscle, and skull bone are turned as a unit, is disadvanta-

geous in meningioma surgery for two reasons. First, it preserves the excessive blood supply from the branches of the external carotid artery. Second, the flap tends to be bulky and difficult to handle, and it limits exposure if the tumor and dura mater are attached to the bone flap. The choice between a free bone flap and a flap hinged on periosteum and muscle is governed by the location and other peculiarities of the specific tumor and by the preference of the surgeon. Free bone flaps more often are turned high on the convexity, near the vertex, and in the midfrontal region.

Bur holes are placed circumferentially outside the margin of the tumor (Fig. 54–10). The bone edges are waxed and the dura stripped from the inner surface of the calvaria only in the direction of the next bur hole. Stripping of the dura into the flap may produce bleeding from the tumor, making the flap difficult to elevate under direct vision. Stripping outside the proposed flap creates a tissue plane that is unused, bleeds, and slows the dissection. Bur holes are joined at their outer margins to ensure maximal exposure of the dura. The final bone cut is made on the side of the flap closest to a large dural venous sinus. If the dura and a venous channel are torn, the bone flap can be quickly turned, and the bleeding can be more rapidly controlled.

The bur holes can be connected via a variety of techniques. The Gigli saw removes less bone, has a guard to prevent dural tears, and cuts the bone with a bevel. The beveled cut reduces postoperative depression of the bone flap and improves the cosmetic result (Fig. 54–11). The air osteotome occludes diploic vascular channels with fine

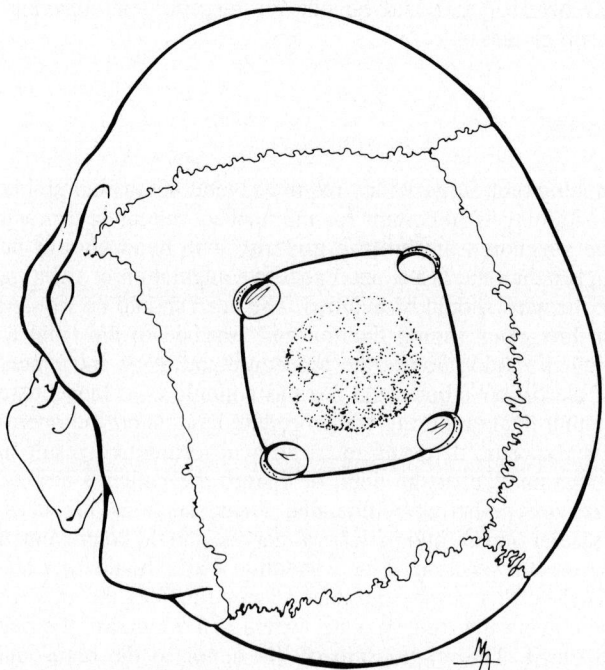

**FIGURE 54–10** ■ The bone flap over a convexity meningioma is wider than the tumor and is centered over the tumor. A free bone flap is turned high on the convexity or at the vertex. The saw cut adjacent to the sinus is made last so that the bone flap can be elevated quickly if bleeding occurs. (From Maxwell RE, Chou SN: Convexity meningiomas and general principles of meningioma surgery. In Schmidek HH, Sweet WH [eds]: Operative Neurosurgical Techniques: Indications, Methods, and Results, Vol 1, 2nd ed. Philadelphia: WB Saunders, 1988, p 557.)

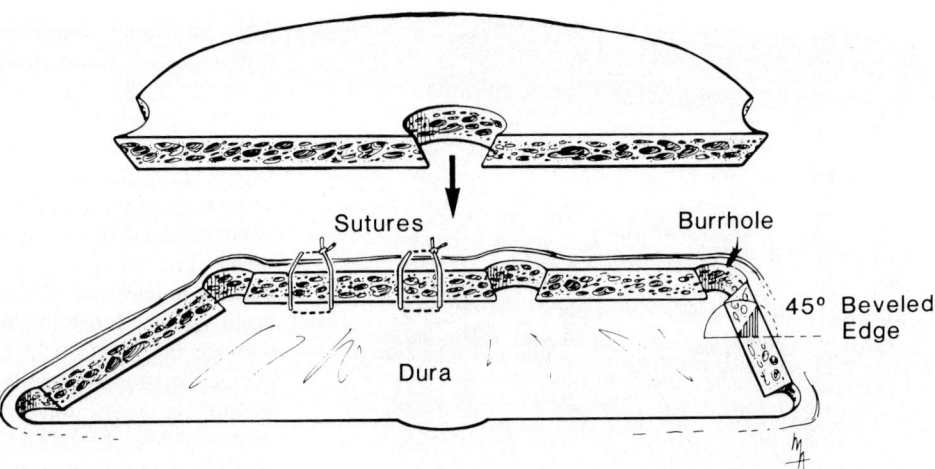

FIGURE 54–11 ■ The bone edge is beveled when cut to prevent the bone flap from sinking when it is sutured in place. The craniotomy cuts join the outer tangent of the bur hole to increase dural exposure. The dura is tacked up to reduce epidural bleeding. (From Maxwell RE, Chou SN: Convexity meningiomas and general principles of meningioma surgery. In Schmidek HH, Sweet WH [eds]: Operative Neurosurgical Techniques: Indications, Methods, and Results, Vol 1, 2nd ed. Philadelphia: WB Saunders, 1988, p 557.)

bone dust as it cuts and reduces bone bleeding. The cut is perpendicular to the skull and removes more bone, however. This disadvantage has been eliminated with the advent of miniplates and screws that allow the bone flap to be firmly fixed in the correct plane, achieving a good cosmetic outcome. Sequential outer table craniotomies can be undertaken to remove the bone in hyperossified meningiomas that have thickened the overlying bone, reducing the need for cranioplasty.[27]

The flap is elevated slowly under direct vision, and the dura is stripped from the inner table. By stripping the dura between the bur holes before elevating the bone flap, one ensures a dural edge to sew the duraplasty, even if the dura is tightly adherent to the inner table and is torn medially. Bleeding diploic channels are packed with wax. Troublesome oozing from arachnoid granulation tissue over dural sinuses or dura infiltrated by vascular tumor can be controlled by placing oxidized cellulose or absorbable gelatin sponge on the bleeding surface and applying gentle pressure with cotton strips. Bleeding from the epidural space, beneath the margins of the skull, can be controlled by placing pledgets of absorbable gelatin sponge between the dura and skull, then tacking the dura to the inner table of the skull to obliterate the epidural space (see Fig. 54–11). After hemostasis is achieved, the wound is irrigated; cotton pledgets are placed at the bone margins; and clean, dry skin towels are applied to the margins of the scalp wound before the dura is opened.

## Dural Opening

The dura mater is inspected and gently palpated to assess the location of the venous sinuses, meningeal vessels, and tumor and to assess the relative tightness of the underlying brain. Ultrasound is helpful in locating the tumor margin and venous sinuses. The dura should not opened until the brain is relaxed. Opening the dura with elevated intracranial pressure may result in normal cortex herniating through the dural defect, leading to cortical ischemia before the tumor can be excised. If all measures, such as steroids, mannitol, head elevation, and hyperventilation, are ineffective and the patient is well anesthetized and paralyzed, lateral ventriculostomy and cerebrospinal fluid diversion is

another option for reducing intracranial pressure. If the craniotomy is in an unusual location for ventriculostomy passage, ultrasound visualization of the ventricle may be helpful.

The dura mater is elevated at the margin rather than over the center of the tumor with a sharp hook and incised with a knife preserving the arachnoid. The dural incision is extended circumferentially about the margin of the tumor using blunt-tipped scissors (Fig. 54–12). Whenever possible, the dura and bone should be excised when involved by the tumor to reduce the possibility of recurrence. Nakau and associates[28] demonstrated in four of nine patients meningioma cells 4.5 mm from the tumor edge. Others have shown that multiple meningiomas likely represent a single clone that spread via the subarachnoid space.[29, 30] A margin of normal dura should be excised with meningioma. Cauterization of bone and dura is less effective, and the recurrence rate is higher. Dura mater involved by the tumor is

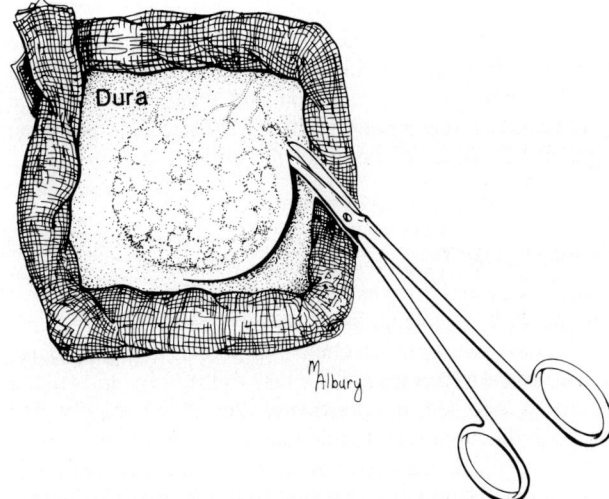

FIGURE 54–12 ■ The dural incision is extended circumferentially about the margin of the tumor with blunt-tipped scissors. Little cortex needs to be exposed during excision of convexity meningiomas. (From Maxwell RE, Chou SN: Convexity meningiomas and general principles of meningioma surgery. In Schmidek HH, Sweet WH [eds]: Operative Neurosurgical Techniques: Indications, Methods, and Results, Vol 1, 2nd ed. Philadelphia: WB Saunders, 1988, p 558.)

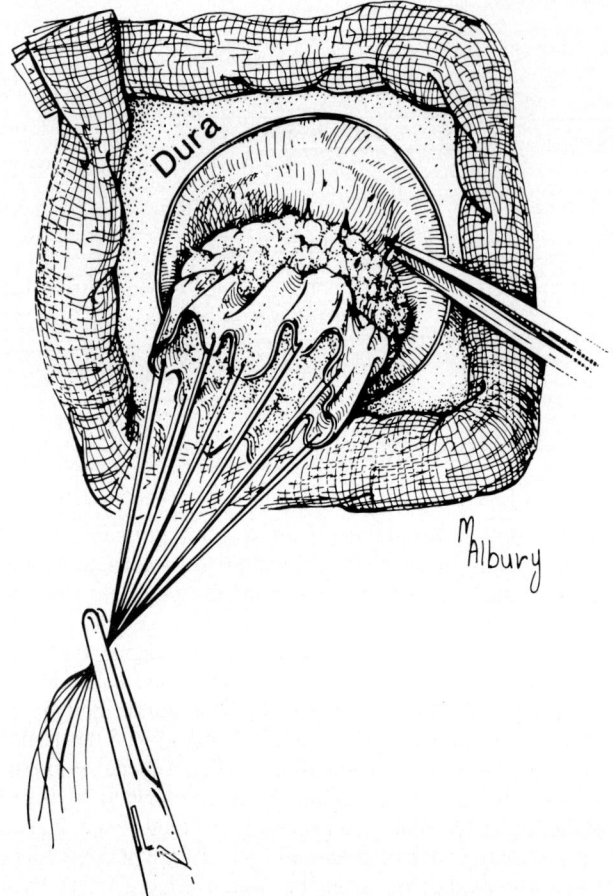

**FIGURE 54–13** ■ Dura mater left attached to a convexity meningioma provides a useful handle for retracting and manipulating the tumor. (From Maxwell RE, Chou SN: Convexity meningiomas and general principles of meningioma surgery. In Schmidek HH, Sweet WH [eds]: Operative Neurosurgical Techniques: Indications, Methods, and Results, Vol 1, 2nd ed. Philadelphia: WB Saunders, 1988, p 559.)

isolated from surrounding dura and left attached to the neoplasm. Sutures can be passed through the dura and used for indirect gentle traction and manipulation of the meningioma, reducing or eliminating the need for retraction applied directly to the tumor or the brain (Fig. 54–13).

## Tumor Excision

The priority in meningioma surgery is to preserve and restore function, and all technical principles and procedures are dedicated to this purpose. Injury to the brain and cranial nerves is avoided by preserving the blood supply and excising the tumor with minimal or no brain retraction. Every technical alternative to forceful brain retraction is explored as the situation dictates. Traction is applied to the tumor capsule or the dura attached to the tumor, as previously described, rather than to the adjacent brain. Position of the head should be adjusted so that gravity works to the surgeon's advantage. The most useful technique for removing all but the smallest meningiomas involves exenteration of the core of the tumor early in the resection.

This procedure creates a space into which the thinned tumor capsule can be retracted (Fig. 54–14).

At this stage, the magnification and cold light provided by the operating microscope are helpful adjuncts in the dissection and development of the arachnoidal plane between tumor and brain. The bipolar coagulator and microscissors can be used to take down fine arachnoidal adhesive bands and small tumor vessels parasitized from the pia mater (Fig. 54–15). If brain retraction is necessary, moist cotton sponges are placed between the retractors and the brain tissue. Self-retaining retractors produce less tissue damage than hand-held retractors, provided that they are not applied too forcefully for too long. The surgeon may, on rare occasions, judiciously elect to resect a small amount of brain tissue to expose the tumor, thereby obviating the need for forceful brain retraction.

Sindou and Alaywan[31] demonstrated in 150 patients that only one half to two thirds of meningiomas possess a cleavable tumor-pial plane for resection. Only 35% of meningiomas with and 83.6% of meningiomas without angiographic evidence of pial vessel parasitization had a cleavable plane. The spinal meninges possess an additional intermediate layer not present in human cerebral meninges that may improve the odds for a cleavable plane.[32]

Few technical difficulties are encountered during tumor excision if the tissue is accessible, soft, and relatively avascular or necrotic so that suction and curettage can be

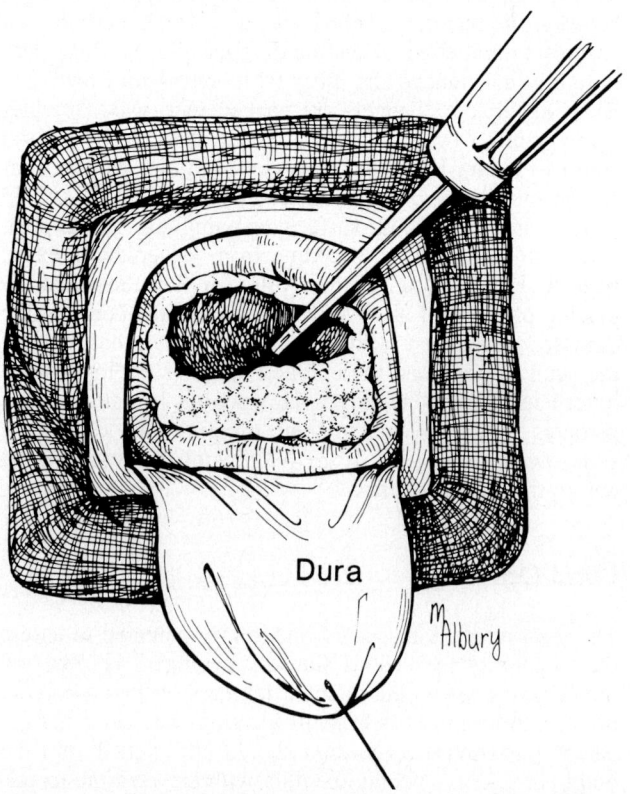

**FIGURE 54–14** ■ Intracapsular enucleation of tumor tissue permits invagination of the tumor capsule and development of the plane between the meningioma and the brain without forceful retraction. (From Maxwell RE, Chou SN: Convexity meningiomas and general principles of meningioma surgery. In Schmidek HH, Sweet WH [eds]: Operative Neurosurgical Techniques: Indications, Methods, and Results, Vol 1, 2nd ed. Philadelphia: WB Saunders, 1988, p 559.)

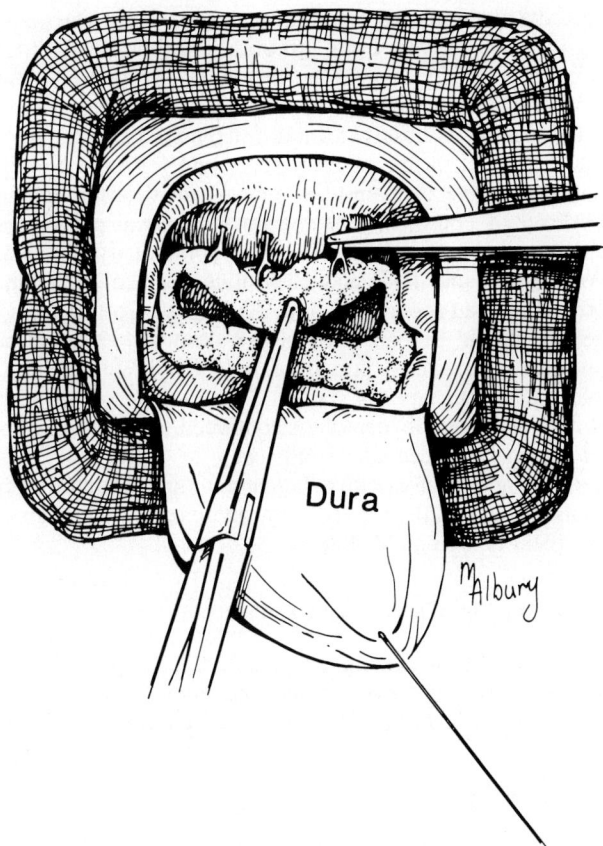

**FIGURE 54–15** ■ The bipolar coagulator and microscissors are used to take down arachnoidal adhesive bands and tumor-feeding vessels as a plane is developed between the cortex and the thinned tumor capsule. (From Maxwell RE, Chou SN: Convexity meningiomas and general principles of meningioma surgery. In Schmidek HH, Sweet WH [eds]: Operative Neurosurgical Techniques: Indications, Methods, and Results, Vol 1, 2nd ed. Philadelphia: WB Saunders, 1988, p 560.)

used to reduce the tumor bulk before the tumor capsule is delivered. A large tumor with tough, tenacious tissue that cannot be aspirated can be excised piecemeal with a cutting loop cautery. This technique carries the risk of damage to important nerves or vessels encompassed by or adjacent to the tumor. The ultrasonic aspirator and carbon dioxide laser sometimes facilitate the excision of firm, gritty, or vascular tumors.[33, 34]

The ultrasonic aspirator selectively fragments and aspirates tissue exposed at the tip of the instrument, which vibrates longitudinally at a frequency of 23,000 times per second. Fragmentation of tissue depends on the water content of the tissue; less power and exposure are required to fragment tissue with high water content, such as areolar tissue, than tissue with considerable collagen or elastic tissue, such as blood vessels.[33] This selective tissue removal permits the identification and elective preservation or coagulation of blood vessels. Visibility is improved because the tissue is shaved from the surface rather than cut from beneath the surface with cautery loops, spoon curets, or biopsy forceps. The simultaneous aspiration immediately removes blood from the tumor bed. Flamm and Ransohoff[35] reported the advantage of ultrasonic aspiration in the surgical removal of 30 meningiomas.

The carbon dioxide laser is also sometimes useful in brain tumor surgery.[34] Laser energy is converted to heat when it is absorbed by tumor tissue, and thermal coagulation occurs. If sufficient energy is absorbed, the tissue vaporizes. The advantages of surgical lasers include: (1) the ability to operate with smaller exposures, (2) reduced brain retraction, (3) a reduced amount of mechanical manipulation through vaporization of the tumor mass, (4) vaporization of the dural attachment after removal of the tumor, (5) improved operative precision, and (6) enhanced ability to remove meningiomas that might otherwise prove difficult to extirpate by conventional means.[36]

Beck[37] has suggested that combining the use of the carbon dioxide laser for cutting with that of the neodymium:yttrium-aluminum-garnet (Nd:YAG) laser for coagulation is advantageous. He prefers the Nd:YAG laser for use on tumors with a rich vascular supply, and he reported a decreased need for blood transfusions in patients undergoing operation with this laser. The Nd:YAG laser produces a homogeneous coagulation with an energy-dependent depth effect.[38] The penetration of the laser beam in tissues is controlled by the output wattage; the grade of coagulation is controlled by duration of radiation time and by the output wattage.[38] Tumor shrinkage and demarcation based on different absorption properties facilitate dissection and allow the preservation of healthy tissue.[40]

Hemostasis is a major problem when large, firm, extremely vascular meningiomas are encountered. Dandy[41] stated, "Because of the great dural vascularity, dura endotheliomas offer the most difficult battles in cranial surgery." Preoperative irradiation and embolization of feeding vessels from branches of the external carotid artery can reduce intraoperative bleeding of the tumor. Intraoperative arterial hypotension also can be induced with sodium nitroprusside to help control bleeding from the tumor and reduce turgor of the brain. When large feeding vessels to the tumor are accessible, they are coagulated before the tumor capsule is entered. If the site of attachment of the meningioma to the dura mater can be identified and exposed early in the resection, the major arterial feeders are coagulated and divided at this point.

Not only do meningiomas tend to be more vascular, but also they have reduced hemostatic properties in relation to other common brain tumors, such as gliomas. In gliomas, the local tissue factors favor the deposition of fibrin and the persistence of these deposits; in meningiomas, the amount of fibrin deposited is smaller, and the fibrin products are broken down more rapidly because of comparatively low thromboplastic activity and high fibrinolytic activity.[42] The fibrinolytic activity of intracranial tumors can be depressed by antiplasmin drugs to lessen bleeding from the tumor.[43]

The brisk intracapsular bleeding encountered during the resection of angioblastic meningiomas may not be controlled by simple pressure with cotton balls or pledgets. Thrombin-soaked absorbable gelatin sponge, oxidized cellulose, or microfibrillar collagen hemostat (Avitene) can be applied with gentle pressure to control tumor bleeding. Based on the size and location of the tumor, the condition of the patient, and the rate of bleeding, the surgeon must judge whether the most expedient course is to tolerate moderate bleeding to enucleate the tumor rapidly and thereby shorten the operating time and perhaps reduce the overall blood loss and chance of morbidity.

The operating microscope and microinstrumentation are helpful during the extracapsular tumor dissection but may be a hindrance during the intracapsular removal of the bulk of large tumors. The surgeon should not be distracted by insignificant oozing and anatomic trivia within the tumor stroma that is magnified out of proportion by the operating microscope. The microscope is essential, however, if important arteries, veins, or nerves are passing through crevices in the capsule of a multilobulated tumor. Although the operating microscope, bipolar coagulation, and microinstrumentation now make possible the precise dissection around important vessels and nerves, the primary objectives of preserving and improving function are not sacrificed in a heroic attempt for a cure.

## Wound Closure

The necessity of formally closing a dural defect by fashioning an autologous dural graft or inserting a dural substitute is open to question.[44] Experimental and clinical evidence shows that a neodural membrane forms in the absence of a graft. Many neurosurgeons prefer to close the dura and reconstitute the subdural space even when the surgery requires excision of dura because of involvement by the tumor. Abbott and Dupree[45] recommend dural closure to prevent cerebrospinal fluid leakage, brain herniation, wound infection, and cortical scarring and adhesions. The use of pericranium, temporalis fascia, and fascia lata is widespread for closing dural defects. These autologous materials have the advantages of being readily available and pliable. Also the use of lyophilized dura mater has been shown to be free of complications, and it precludes the need for additional incisions at the time of surgery.[44]

There appears to be little advantage other than ready accessibility in repairing the dura mater with inorganic or synthetic dural substitutes. Banerjee and associates[46] reported delayed postoperative subdural hematomas associated with bleeding from neovascularized membranes provoked by Silastic dural substitutes. Implanted synthetic foreign materials may also increase the risk of infection.

After closure of the dura, the bone flap is plated into position. An acrylic or wire mesh cranioplasty can be performed to repair a defect necessitated by the excision of bone involved by the meningioma. The cranioplasty occasionally is delayed and is performed as a second procedure. This approach may be indicated in cases of severe swelling of the brain or suspected contamination or if a patient in poor general health has had to endure a long period of anesthesia. Care should be taken to approximate the galea aponeurotica with an inverted, absorbable suture before closing the scalp incision.

## POSTOPERATIVE CARE

The primary concern in the postoperative period is that a hematoma or brain edema could produce a focal or generalized increase in intracranial pressure, progressive neuro-

logic dysfunction, and transtentorial herniation. The anesthesiologist strives for a smooth extubation without straining to avoid unnecessary elevation of blood pressure and intracranial pressure.

The patient is observed immediately for baseline function on arrival to the recovery room and followed closely in the intensive care unit for subsequent deterioration in the level of consciousness, the onset of focal neurologic deficit, or seizure activity. Vital signs, pulmonary function, blood gases, and fluid and electrolyte balance are monitored. The head is elevated 20 to 30 degrees. Corticosteroid therapy should be continued at full dose for 72 hours or through the expected period of maximal brain swelling, before a steroid taper is started. Seizure prophylaxis with parenteral diphenylhydantoin is continued. A CT scan without contrast enhancement is advisable to distinguish brain swelling and postoperative hematoma in a patient with persistent or progressive lethargy, obtundation, or progressive focal neurologic deficit.

## ACKNOWLEDGMENTS

*The authors thank Edward Michel, M. D., and Charles Truwit, M. D., for providing and interpreting the radiographs illustrated throughout the chapter.*

## REFERENCES

1. Cushing H: Meningiomas. Macewen Memorial Lecture, 1927. Glasgow: Jackson Wylie & Company, 1927.
2. Cushing H, Eisenhardt L: Meningiomas: Their Classification, Regional Behavior, Life History, and Surgical End Results. Springfield, IL: Charles C Thomas, 1938, p 785.
3. Zulch, KJ: Brain Tumors: Their Biology and Pathology. New York: Springer, 1965.
4. Maier, H, Ofner D, Hittamir A, et al: Classic, atypical, and anaplastic meningioma: Three histopathological subtypes clinical revelence. J Neurosurg 77:616, 1992.
5. McDermott MW, Wilson CB: Meningiomas. In Youmans J (ed): Neurologic Surgery, 4th ed. Philadelphia: WB Saunders, 1996, pp 2782–2825.
6. Salcman M: Malignant meningiomas. In Al-Mefty O (ed): Meningiomas. New York: Raven Press, 1991, pp 75–85.
7. Chan RC, Thompson GB: Morbidity, mortality, and quality of life following surgery for intracranial meningiomas; A retrospective study in 257 cases. J Neurosurg 60:52, 1984.
8. Jaaskelainen J: Seemingly complete removal of histologically benign intracranial meningioma: Late recurrence rate and factors predicting recurrence in 657 patients: A multivariate analysis. Surg Neurol 26:461, 1986.
9. Kallio M, Sankila R, Hakulinen T, et al: Factors affecting operative and excess long-term mortality in 935 patients with intracranial meningioma. Neurosurgery 31:2, 1992.
10. Cushing H: The meningiomas (dural endotheliomas): Their source and favored seats of origin (Cavendish lecture). Brain 45:282, 1922.
11. New P, Aronow S, Hesselink J: National Cancer Institute study: Evaluation of computed tomography: The diagnosis of intracranial neoplasms IV meningiomas Radiology 136:665–675, 1980.
12. Osborne A: Meningiomas and other nonglial neoplasms. In Diagnostic Neuroradiology. St. Louis: Mosby, 1996, pp 579–625.
13. Pompili A, Derome PJ, Visot A, Guiot G: Hyperostosing meningiomas of the sphenoid ridge: Clinical features, surgical therapy and long-term observations: Review of 49 cases. Surg Neurol 17:411–416, 1982.
14. Bonnal J, Thibaut A, Brothci J, Boren J: Invading meningiomas of the sphenoid ridge. J Neurosurg 53:587–599, 1980.
15. Servo A, Porras M, Jaaskelainen J, et al: Computed tomography and angiography do not reliably discriminate malignant meningiomas from benign ones. Neuroradiology 32:94–97, 1990.

16. Salcman M: Malignant meningiomas. In Al-Mefty O (ed): Meningiomas. New York: Raven Press, 1991; pp 75–85.

17. Goldsher D, Litt AW, Pinto RS, et al: Dural "tail" associated with meningiomas on Gd-DTPA-enhanced MR images: Characteristics, differential diagnostic value, and possible implications of treatment. Radiology 176:447–450, 1990.

18. Tien RD, Yang PJ, Chu PK, "Dural tail sign" a specific MR sign for meningioma? Case report. J Comput Assist Tomogr 15:64–66, 1991.

19. Fujii K, Fujita N, Hirabuki N, et al: Neuromas and meningiomas: Evaluation of early enhancement with dynamic MR imaging AJNR Am J Neuroradiol 13:1215–1220, 1992.

20. Inamura T, Nishio S, Takeshita I, et al: Peritumoral brain edema in meningiomas: Influence of vascular supply upon its development Neurosurgery 31:179–185, 1992.

21. Bitzer M, Helge T, Morgalla M, et al: Tumor-related venous obstruction and development of peritumoral brain edema in meningiomas. Neurosurgery 42:730–737, 1998.

22. Onesti S, Zahos P, Ashkenazi E: Spontaneous hemorrhage into a convexity meningioma. Acta Neurochir (Wien) 138:1250–1251, 1996.

23. Tenner MS: The role of conventional neuroradiologic techniques in relation to computed tomography. In Sher JH, Ford DH (eds): Primary Intracranial Neoplasms. New York: SP Med and Sci, 1971, pp 71–85.

24. Osborne AG: The external carotid artery. In Introduction to Cerebral Angiography. Hagerstown, MD: Harper & Row, 1980, pp 49–86.

25. Jackson R, Goodman J, Huston D, Harper R: Parafalcine and bilateral convexity neurosarcoidosis mimicking meningioma: Case report and review of the literature. Neurosurgery 42:635–638, 1998.

26. Fox J: Atlas of Neurosurgical Anatomy: The Pterional Perspective. New York: Springer-Verlag, 1989.

27. Colon G, Ross D, Hoff J: Sequential outer table craniotomy in a hyperossified meningioma. J Neurosurg 88:346–348, 1998.

28. Nakau H, Miyazawa T, Tamai S, et al: Pathological significance of meningeal enhancement (Flare sign) on meningiomas in MRI. Surg Neurol 48:584–591, 1997.

29. Stangl A, Wellenreuther R, Lenartz D, et al: Clonality of multiple meningiomas. J Neurosurg 86:853–858, 1997.

30. Larson J, Tew J, Simon M, Menon A: Evidence for clonal spread in the development of multiple meningiomas. J Neurosurg 83:705–709, 1995.

31. Sindou M, Alaywan M: Most intracranial meningiomas are not cleavable tumors: Anatomic-surgical evidence and angiographic predictability. Neurosurgery 42:476–480, 1998.

32. Salpietro F, Alafaci C, Lucerna S, et al: Do spinal meningiomas penetrate the pial layer? Correlation between MRI and microsurgical findings and intracranial tumor interfaces. Neurosurgery 41:254–258, 1997.

33. Hodgson W, Poddar P, Mencer E, et al: Evaluation of ultrasonically powered instruments in the laboratory and in the clinical setting. Am J Gastroenterol 72:133, 1979.

34. Saunders M, Young H, Becker D, et al: The use of the laser in neurological surgery. Surg Neurol 14:1, 1980.

35. Flamm F, Ransohoff J: Ultrasonic aspiration of intracranial tumors. Presented at the 47th Annual Meeting of the American Association of Neurological Surgeons, Los Angeles, CA, April 22–26, 1979.

36. Strait T, Robertson J, Clark W: Use of the carbon dioxide laser in the operative management of intracranial meningiomas: A report of twenty cases. Neurosurgery 10:464, 1982.

37. Beck O: The use of Nd-YAG and the $CO_2$ laser in neurosurgery. Neurosurgy Rev 3:261, 1980.

38. Beck O: The use of Nd-YAG laser in neurosurgery. Neurosurg Rev 7:151, 1984.

39. Handa H, Takeuchi J, Yamagami T: Nd-YAG laser as a surgical tool. Neurosurg Rev 7:159–164, 1984.

40. Beck O, Frank F: The use of the Nd-YAG laser in neurosurgery. Lasers Surg Med 5:345, 1985.

41. Dandy WE: The Brain. New York: Hoeber, 1965, p 514.

42. Tovi D, Pandolfi M, Astedt B: Local haemostasis in brain tumours. Experientia 31:977, 1975.

43. Koos W, Valencak E, Krause H, et al: L'active fibrinolytique relev'ee dans les tumeurs intra-craniennes. Neurochirurgie 17:549, 1971.

44. MacFarlane MR, Symon L: Lyophilized dura mater: Experimental implantation and extended clinical neurosurgical use. J Neurol Neurosurg Psychiatry 42:854, 1979.

45. Abbott WM, Dupree EL: The procurement, storage and transplantation of lyophilized human cadaver dura mater. Surg Gynecol Obstet 130:112, 1970.

46. Banerjee T, Meagher JN, and Hunt WE: Unusual complications with use of Silastic dural substitute. Am Surg 40:434, 1974.

# CHAPTER 55

# Surgical Management of Supratentorial Hemispheric Gliomas in Adults

■ HENRY H. SCHMIDEK

Surgery of gliomas is performed in order to accomplish several objectives. Central to the various considerations is an attempt to improve the quality as well as duration of the patient's life. From a technical perspective, the objective(s) include establishing a tissue diagnosis, cytoreduction, drainage of neoplastic cysts, removal of necrotic tissue producing a mass effect, and the introduction of radiotherapeutic or chemotherapeutic agents. This chapter addresses the techniques of radical and subtotal tumor resection by open operation.

In spite of the advances in surgical and in radiation therapy techniques over the last decade, the best therapeutic result in the management of high-grade gliomas has been accomplished by the removal of maximal amounts of tumor tissue followed by radiation therapy. The smaller the residual tumor, the longer the survival time and the lower the complication rate associated with the operation.

## ANAPLASTIC ASTROCYTOMA AND GLIOBLASTOMA MULTIFORME

Approximately 50% of intracranial neoplasms are gliomas. Of any 100 tumors in this group, 55 are glioblastomas, 20 to 30 are grade I and II astrocytomas, and 5 are oligodendrogliomas.[1-4] Glioblastomas are most common in men aged 50 to 60 years.[5] The recent studies in the molecular genetics of glial tumors indicate that the glioblastoma multiforme may arise either from the progression of anaplasia in a pre-existing astrocytoma or de novo. This tumor grows rapidly, and if it is left untreated, it is associated with a life expectancy of 2 months from the time of diagnosis.[6, 7] The frontal lobe is involved in 36.7% of patients, the temporal lobe in 33.9%, the parietal lobe in 25%, and the occipital lobe in 2.2%.[5] These tumors characteristically extend along the commissures and fiber tracts within the white matter; conversely, the cortex appears to constitute a barrier to the spread of the tumor. Glioblastomas are multiple in 2.5% to 4.9% of patients,[2, 3] and are bilateral in 11% to 47%.[6] Tumors originating above the level of the corpus

callosum tend to spread to the opposite hemisphere, resulting in the so-called butterfly glioma, whereas those originating below the level of the corpus callosum spread to involve the basal ganglia.[8] Tumors in the temporal lobe are least likely to spread and theoretically are the most suitable for resection. These tumors may invade the cerebral ventricles, but distant metastases are rare without previous surgical intervention.[9-12]

Although these tumors appear to be encapsulated, their margins are ill-defined and infiltrate adjacent brain tissue.[13, 14] These tumors are usually gray or pinkish with firm outer margins and a softer necrotic center. Cysts may be present, and occasionally, there are several. Foci of recent and old hemorrhage also may be seen. A subclass of encapsulated glioblastomas, which are usually 3 to 5 cm in diameter, grossly circumscribed with a gray-red surface, and frequently adherent to the dura, along with a propensity to occur in the temporal lobe, have been described.[15, 16]

## SUPRATENTORIAL LOW-GRADE ASTROCYTOMAS

Supratentorially located low-grade astrocytomas comprise approximately 30% of intracranial tumors. The onset of symptoms is at age 30 to 40 years in adults[4] with a male preponderance.[5] They are present in the frontal lobe (40% to 50%), temporal lobe (31% to 35%), parietal lobe (14% to 16%), and the occipital lobe (0% to 1.2%).[5] Their appearance is that of ill-defined, firm, white to pinkish gray lesions that merge imperceptibly into surrounding brain tissue and obliterate the distinction between the cortex and the white matter.

## CYSTIC CEREBRAL ASTROCYTOMA

Cystic pilocystic astrocytomas constitute about 3% of hemispheric gliomas and usually appear as a large cyst contiguous with the lateral ventricle and containing a small mural nodule, which enhances on computed tomography (CT) or magnetic resonance imaging (MRI) scans. The mean age of these patients is 18 years, and the average duration of the clinical history is 14 months. These patients present with seizures (68%), headache (63%), and vomiting (51%). The temporal lobe is involved in 49% of the cases, the parieto-occipital lobe in 35%, and the frontal lobe in 16%. The most important favorable prognostic variable is the total excision of the tumor nodule.[17]

## OLIGODENDROGLIOMAS

Oligodendrogliomas represent about 5% of intracerebral gliomas,[3, 4] particularly in men 30 to 50 years of age.[20, 21] Oligodendrogliomas occur most frequently in the frontal lobes (50%), most often extending to the opposite side, followed by parietal lobes (30.6%); and the temporal lobes (19.4% of cases)[5] and are frequently in close proximity to the ventricular wall. Occasionally, these tumors seed the cerebrospinal fluid (CSF) to spread to other parts of the nervous system.[20, 22, 23] Spontaneous intratumoral hemorrhage occurs in approximately 40% of patients. Gross calcification is present in 50% of patients, and histologic calcification is present in 75%.

At surgery, the tumor appears as a well-defined, globular, occasionally gelatinous mass that often is cystic and hemorrhagic.

Approximately 50% of oligodendrogliomas are mixed gliomas containing both astrocytic and oligodendrocytic elements.

## PREOPERATIVE ASSESSMENT

Often cerebral gliomas may present either with mental deterioration, personality change, grand mal seizures, headache, raised intracranial pressure, or a seizure or focal neurologic deficit. The initial complaint among patients with low-grade astrocytomas is headache in 32% to 35% of the cases, mental changes in 13% to 15%, visual failure in 3% to 15%, and vomiting in 6% to 8%.[5] Forty percent of the patients with glioblastomas had headache, 21% had mental changes, 12% had dysphasia, 12% had hemiparesis, 10% experienced vomiting, and 5% had miscellaneous

symptoms. Headache and mental changes were the initial symptoms in 17% of patients with oligodendrogliomas, and hemiparesis was an initial finding in 14%. The Brain Tumor Study Group found that in patients with glioblastomas, 31% had headaches as an initial symptom, 18% had seizures, 16% had personality changes, 13% motor symptoms, and 7% sensory symptoms. Among patients with all grades of gliomas, 38% of the National Hospital series had seizures, 35% had headache, 16% had mental changes, 10% had hemiparesis, and 8% experienced vomiting.

### Radiographic Assessment

MRI scanning with and without enhancement provides exquisite anatomic delineation of the lesions, and the appearance often is very suggestive of the diagnosis. However, at present the diagnosis of a malignant tumor cannot be made definitively without tissue confirmation. With current technology the enhanced MRI study is the most accurate technique for outlining the extent of the tumor and the peritumoral edema and detecting small lesions. In studies correlating the CT and MRI appearances with biopsy specimens, it has also been demonstrated that tumor may be detected up to 15 mm beyond the enhanced CT margin and beyond the abnormalities seen on the $T_2$-weighted MRI. This finding is important because it has also been found that in the vast majority of patients treated for malignant gliomas, recurrence occurs within 2 cm of the original disease site as documented by CT scanning.

Certain CT characteristics provide clues to the nature of the tumor. Calcification and homogeneous enhancement are more common in cases of oligodendrogliomas, and cerebral edema is less likely to occur than in other gliomas, whereas calcification and hydrocephalus are seen more frequently in low-grade gliomas, and irregular CT enhancement was more frequent in high-grade astrocytomas (Table 55–1).

It can be very difficult to distinguish between a cerebral infarct and a brain tumor on a CT scan. Up to 60% of recent cerebral infarcts (1 to 4 weeks) will show contrast enhancement.[22] However, this enhancement will decrease or disappear in an area of infarction, whereas it will either persist or increase in a neoplasm.

In the immediate postoperative period, CT and MRI scanning are a routine part of patient assessment. In Soloman's study comparing the results of 70 postoperative CT scans with the patient's clinical status, 46 scans showed

---

TABLE 55–1 ■ GLIOMAS: INCIDENCE OF MANIFESTATIONS IN EACH TYPE AND GRADE OF TUMOR

| | Astrocytoma (%) | | Oligodendroglioma (%) | | Total (%) |
|---|---|---|---|---|---|
| | Grades 1–2 | Grades 3–4 | Grades 1–2 | Grades 3–4 | |
| Calcification | 11 (31) | 9 (8) | 7 (70) | 5 (45) | 32 (18) |
| Edema | 30 (83) | 106 (90) | 5 (50) | 10 (91) | 151 (84) |
| Midline shift | 31 (86) | 95 (81) | 8 (80) | 9 (82) | 143 (80) |
| Obliteration of ventricle | 34 (94) | 109 (92) | 8 (80) | 11 (100) | 163 (91) |
| Hydrocephalus | 22 (61) | 37 (31) | 6 (60) | 3 (27) | 68 (38) |
| High attenuation | 7 (19) | 18 (15) | 2 (20) | 1 (9) | 28 (17) |
| Total | 135 | 374 | 36 | 39 | 585 |

From Claveria LE, Kendall BE, DuBoulay GH: Computerized axial tomography in supratentorial gliomas and metastases. In First European Seminar on Computerized Axial Tomography in Clinical Practice. Berlin: Springer-Verlag, 1977. With permission of the authors and publisher.

the patient's status was improved or unchanged from preoperative findings and these findings paralleled the patient's clinical course. Of 24 scans which had shown a worsened patient status, 62% of the patients deteriorated clinically.[12] These studies allow one to detect both the positive effect of surgical treatment in stable postoperative patients as well as alerting the surgeon to CT-demonstrated abnormalities mandating reoperation or therapy. Twenty percent of studies showed asymptomatic ventricular enlargement.

In the later postoperative period, tumor recurrence is diagnosed by the presence of new areas of contrast enhancement or an increase in peritumoral edema, or both. Biopsy of the enhancing ring in seven patients with glioblastoma who underwent surgery and radiation revealed that the enhancing ring represented viable tumor, whereas a tumor's hypodense center is often the result of cellular necrosis or radiation change.[26]

Distinguishing radiation necrosis from recurrent tumor can be difficult. One series, for example, included three cases of partial enhancement of a mass lesion that were indistinguishable from the enhancement that appeared in previously treated gliomas. A nonspecific avascular mass was seen on the angiograms, and this study was not helpful in arriving at a specific diagnosis.[27, 29] The appearance on CT of viral encephalitis, atrioventricular malformation, metastatic brain tumor, cerebral abscess, resolving intracerebral hematoma, and demyelinating disease[30] can all present as a mass lesion that is difficult to distinguish from gliomas.

The Wada intra-arterial sodium amytal test is occasionally used preoperatively when planning surgery in patients in whom resection could interfere with the patient's language ability.[29] From 150 to 200 mg of sodium amytal is injected over 1 to 2 seconds into the internal carotid artery while the patient's speech and motor power are examined repeatedly. If speech arrest occurs at the same time as a transient contralateral hemiplegia, speech is localized on the side of the injection. If speech becomes garbled after the onset of the contralateral hemiplegia and the patient is able to resume counting and naming objects within 15 to 20 seconds while the contralateral hemiplegia is still present, speech probably is localized on the opposite side. The same procedure then is performed on the opposite side for verification.

Patronas and colleagues reported on an experience with 45 patients with histologically proven, high-grade astrocytomas studied using positron-emission tomography (PET) with fluorine ($^{18}$F-)2-deoxyglucose (FDG).[30] This study showed that the mean survival time of patients with tumors exhibiting high glucose utilization was 5 months, whereas patients with lower glucose utilization had a mean survival time of 19 months. Enhanced CT scans performed on these patients revealed no consistent features that could be used to distinguish the very aggressive tumors from the less aggressive ones. Lilja and associates reported improved delineation of gliomas from surrounding edema using PET with L-methyl-C-methionine (C-L-methionine) compared with CT, angiography, and in some instances, PET with $^{68}$Ga-EPTA.[31, 49]

## Ophthalmologic Assessment

Formal neurophthalmologic examination, including a detailed visual field examination, should be performed on any cooperative patient in whom the tumor or the surgical approach might endanger the optic pathways. Temporal lobe tumor, except for those located at the temporal tip, frequently produce a complete or partial homonymous superior quadrantanopia. Occipital tumors usually produce a partial or complete homonymous hemianopia; however, a superiorly placed tumor can be associated with an inferior quadrantanopia just as inferiorly placed tumors can produce a superior quadrantanopia. Parietal tumors are less likely to produce a discrete field deficit, although large parietal lobe tumors may produce an inferior homonymous quadrantanopia.

## Neuropsychological Assessment

Patients undergoing resection of intracranial gliomas should be evaluated by neuropsychological testing before and after surgery. This is of help in counseling the patient and the family, and can alert the surgeon to subtle deficits that are difficult to delineate fully on routine neurologic examination.

The complexity of human abilities subserved by the cerebral hemispheres requires a battery of tests that can measure: (1) sensory perceptual functions (vision, hearing, touch); (2) speed and strength of motor function; (3) complex tests of psychomotor functions (i.e., patient's ability to organize and integrate sensory information with the motor output necessary to solve relatively complex problems); (4) language and communications skills; (5) visual-spatial abilities of various kinds; (6) areas of abstraction, analytical reasoning, and concept formation; and (7) memory. Because cerebral organization in humans more closely resembles a complex of integrations rather than a set of specific and independent locations of a function, a well-localized disease process can have far-reaching effects on total brain function. When treatments such as radiation and chemotherapy are used, the need for qualitative as well as quantitative assessment of higher brain function is clear. Specifically, one needs to know whether there is impairment of cognitive function, to what degree it exists, and how this impairment will alter the patient's ability to function in his or her environment. IQ testing alone does not adequately answer these questions. The full-scale IQ tends to return to premorbid or near premorbid levels shortly after insult to the brain; this may occur even when damage is severe and obvious impairment remains.

A neuropsychological evaluation consists of administration of either the Wechsler Adult Intelligence Scale (WAIS) or the Wechsler Intelligence Scale for Children (WISC-R), the Halstead-Reitan neuropsychological test battery, and the Minnesota Multiphasic Personality Inventory (MMPI).

To evaluate the emotional status of a patient, the MMPI provides quantitative scores for individual subjects on the basis of answers to a large number of questions. The test can be scored with respect to normative data on a series of scales that include hypochondriasis, depression, hysteria, psychopathic deviance, paranoia, psychoasthenia, schizophrenia, and hypomania. In addition to these scores, the test includes validational scales that provide assistance in judging whether the answers are consistent and reasonable and, therefore, open to valid interpretation.

## PREOPERATIVE MANAGEMENT

### Corticosteroids

An adult patient with a supratentorial glioma manifested by mass effect and edema is begun on dexamethasone, 8 mg IV or PO every 6 hours. Dexamethasone has the advantage of not retaining sodium and a 2- to 4-day biologic half-life. Neurologic improvement may occur within 4 hours of administration.[47-49] The side effects of short-term steroid administration (less than 4 weeks' duration) include psychic effects, increased appetite, leukopenia, and hyperglycemia. Long-term administration can lead to hypothalamus-pituitary-adrenal axis suppression, cushingoid appearance, hypertension, psychological disturbances, growth retardation, osteoporosis and aseptic hip necrosis, myopathy, infection, poor wound healing, glaucoma, and cataracts. The most immediate effect of steroid therapy is the reduction of cerebral edema, and there is evidence that the steroids may also inhibit the growth of tumor cells.

### Anticonvulsant Therapy

Patients with a supratentorial glioma often present with a seizure disorder or experience seizures at some time during their disease. The patient who is newly diagnosed and is in no neurologic distress is given a loading dose of diphenylhydantoin (Dilantin), which consists of 600 to 1000 mg in divided doses over 8 to 12 hours. This dosage provides effective plasma concentrations within 24 hours in most patients. Maintenance therapy is, in most adults, 300 to 400 mg/day. Blood levels are determined periodically and plasma concentrations adjusted to 10 to 20 mg/ml.[51] Chloramphenicol, dicumarol, disulfiram, isoniazid, and sulthiame can inhibit the inactivation of diphenylhydantoin and thus lead to an increase in plasma levels. Conversely, carbamazepine (Tegretol) may lower diphenylhydantoin levels. If the seizures persist despite adequate blood levels of either, carbamazepine frequently is used.

## INTRAOPERATIVE MANAGEMENT

Craniotomies for intracranial glioma are usually performed under general endotracheal anesthesia. All patients are monitored using an arterial line, electrocardiogram (ECG), central venous line, and Foley catheter. At the beginning of the operation the patient receives intravenous dexamethasone and prophylactic antibiotic. If the dura is tense when it is exposed, mannitol supplemented by furosemide (Lasix) is given concurrently. The dura is not incised until it is seen to pulsate well, which indicates that the intracranial pressure has been lowered.

## SURGICAL ALTERNATIVES

### Stereotactic Biopsy

Stereotactic biopsy of intracerebral mass lesions allows one to establish the nature of the tumor, drain its cystic

components, and instill therapeutic agents into a tumor cavity; however, a major issue in the management of malignant gliomas is the optimal extent of surgical resection that should be performed. The preponderance of the present evidence is that patients with a malignant glioma clearly benefit from cytoreductive surgery compared with stereotactic biopsy regarding life expectancy and quality of life. Although there is a selection bias, generally those patients treated by biopsy and radiation do less well than those subjected to subtotal resection and radiation. In addition, brain biopsy fails in about 10% of patients to obtain sufficient or representative material to allow the correct diagnosis to be established. Tissue sampling requires that one take specimens from the area of putative edema, the area of contrast-enhancement on the CT or MRI, and the center of the lesion. With the use of CT, MRI-based, frameless stereotaxis a trajectory can easily be planned that allows for obtaining several samples through the lesion and thereby achieving a higher yield.

### Internal Decompression

The extent of internal decompression has been compared with survival rates in the management of patients with anaplastic gliomas and glioblastomas in several series. These studies indicate that the more extensive the removal of tissue, the longer the survival, the better the quality of life, and the lower the rate of postoperative complications. Internal decompression with reduction of tumor mass is chosen when the specifics of the case, such as the location of the tumor, preclude radical tumor removal. In these cases, the approach is essentially the same as that described later but it is elected to remove smaller amounts of neoplasm.

## LOBECTOMY IN THE MANAGEMENT OF SUPRATENTORIAL CEREBRAL GLIOMAS

### Frontal Lobectomy

A frontal lobectomy represents the most complete form of surgical removal of cerebral glioma. Conceptually, this operation involves removal of the tumor and a margin of normal tissue beyond the boundaries of the tumor demonstrated by CT or MRI scan. This approach takes into consideration that tumor recurrence most commonly is seen within 2 cm of the mass demonstrated on the imaging studies. In the following discussion, the surgical management of a dominant hemisphere glioma is considered.

#### Surgical Positioning and Exposure

The patient is positioned on the back with the left shoulder elevated by a sponge wedge, allowing the head to be turned toward the right 20 to 40 degrees (Fig. 55-1). A transcoronal skin incision is made behind the hairline, extending the left limb of the incision to the zygoma and the right limb to the inferior temporal line (see Fig. 55-1). The facial nerve courses below the zygoma and is to be

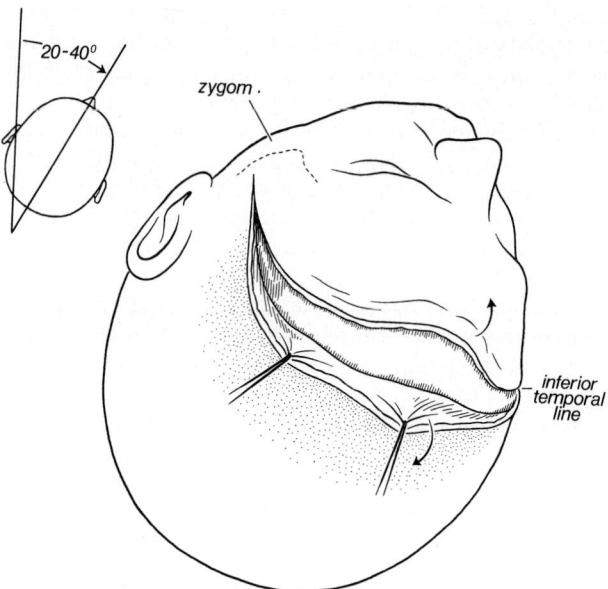

**FIGURE 55–1** ■ Transcoronal skin incision extending from just above the zygoma on the left to the inferior temporal line on the right. *Inset,* The patient's position with respect to the surgeon.

avoided (see Fig. 55–6). The area of anticipated incision is infiltrated with 0.5% lidocaine (Xylocaine) with epinephrine for hemostasis. The skin flap is reflected anteriorly over a roll of sponges and is held in place by fishhooks on elastic bands (Fig. 55–2). Disposable Raney clips are applied to the skin edge from a multiclip applicator. The temporalis muscle is incised with the cautery, leaving its insertion into the frontoparietal bone intact (see Fig. 55–2). It is reflected laterally and covered with a moist sponge. The bone flap is fashioned to allow exposure of the frontal

pole and the anterior portion of the sylvian fissure. Bur holes are placed and the bone is cut with the high-speed Midas Rex air drill (see Fig. 55–2). Medially, the bone flap extends to 1 to 1.5 cm lateral to the midline to avoid the superior sagittal sinus and its large draining veins. The posterior medial bur hole is placed immediately behind the coronal suture; the posterior lateral bur hole is 1 to 2 cm behind the suture. The inferior bur hole is placed immediately posterior to the pterion, and the anterior lateral bur hole is placed medial to the insertion of temporalis muscle, with care being taken to avoid entering the orbit. The anterior medial bur hole is placed 1 to 1.5 cm lateral to the superior sagittal sinus and as low on the frontal bone as possible without entering the frontal sinus. At the pterion, the Midas Rex drill is used to remove the lateral part of the sphenoid wing (Fig. 55–3). The bone flap is removed. If the dura is tense despite preoperative steroids and intraoperative hyperventilation, mannitol and furosemide (Lasix) are administered rapidly. If the tumor has a cystic component, the dura overlying the cyst is cauterized and the cyst tapped with a ventricular needle. The dura is now opened and the sagittal sinus and any draining veins are protected (see Fig. 55–3). The temporal tip, the sphenoid wing, the inferior frontal gyrus, and Brodmann's area localized in the posterior half of the inferior frontal gyrus are identified.

Intraoperative brain mapping is an extremely useful adjunct to radical tumor surgery. These techniques allow localization of the language cortex, the somatosensory cortex, and seizure foci, which then allows for maximal tumor resection adjacent to eloquent areas of brain.[48, 53]

In performing a frontal lobectomy, the cortical incision usually starts 7 to 8 cm from the frontal pole and extends laterally to the level of the lesser wing of the sphenoid. The pia-arachnoid is coagulated with the bipolar forceps and is cut with fine scissors. Large cortical vessels are isolated and coagulated (Fig. 55–4). The gray and white matter then are sectioned with a metal suction tip. It is important to keep the plane of dissection at the same depth

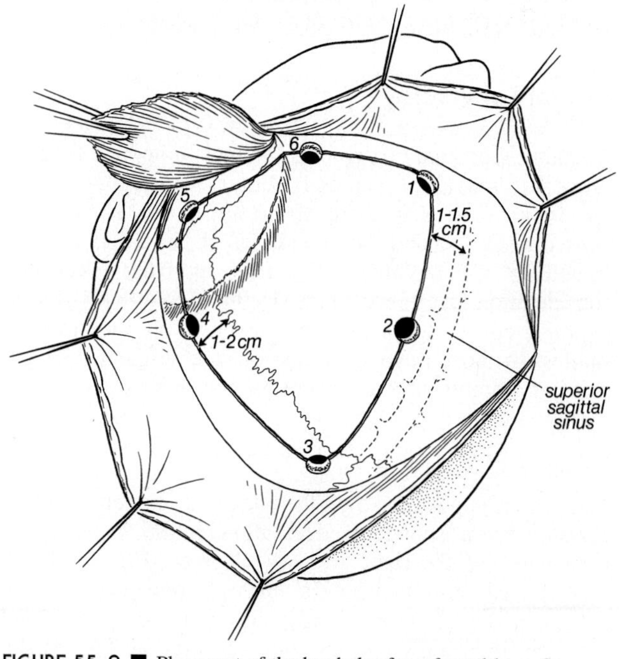

**FIGURE 55–2** ■ Placement of the bur holes for a frontal bone flap after the temporalis muscle has been reflected laterally. The medial extent is 1 to 1.5 cm lateral to the superior sagittal sinus.

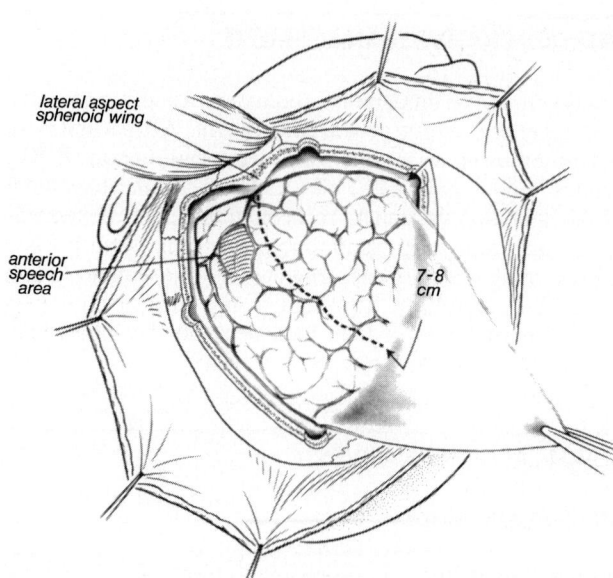

**FIGURE 55–3** ■ The line of incision showing the relationship of the anterior speech area to the lateral aspect of the sphenoid wing.

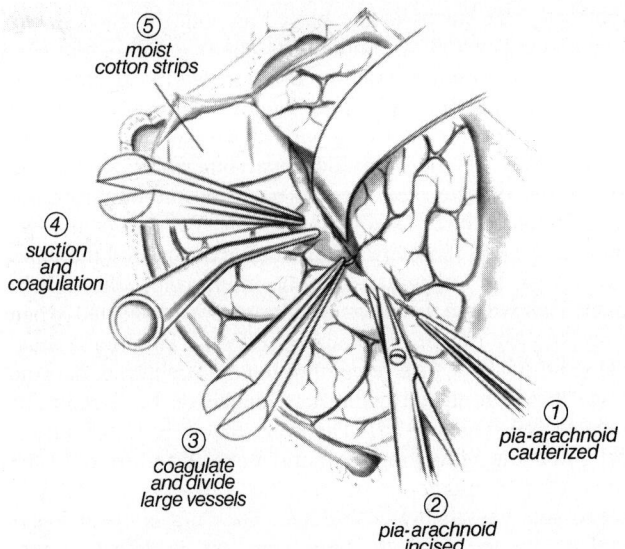

**FIGURE 55–4 ■** Steps in performing a cortical resection (see the text for details). Note the moist cotton strips protecting the area of the brain to the left.

throughout the length of the incision. Lining the posterior wall of the resection plane with moist cotton strips, the portion of the frontal lobe to be removed is retracted with a broad brain retractor. When the medial veins draining into the superior sagittal sinus are coagulated and sectioned, care should be taken to divide them close to the brain. As the incision is carried toward the base of the frontal lobe, the lateral ventricle is entered. To prevent bleeding into the ventricle a cotton ball should be placed gently over the ventricle. Should it not be desirable to open the ventricle, the medial aspect of the cortical incision is made at the level where the two hemispheres are clearly separate. This approach is anterior to the corpus callosum, the ventricle, and the anterior cerebral artery.

To perform a more complete lobectomy for tumors whose margins can be circumvented by such a resection, the anterior cerebral arteries from both sides must be identified. The ipsilateral frontopolar artery on the medial surface of the frontal lobe is then divided near the cortical surface. The contralateral frontopolar artery must be avoided. This artery is near the midline and can easily be mistaken for its opposite counterpart (Fig. 55–5). As the floor of the frontal fossa is approached, the olfactory tract lying in the olfactory groove is encountered. To avoid bleeding and the possibility of opening the cribriform plate and producing a CSF leak, this structure should be left in place. The frontal tip is now held only by the draining veins over the medial orbital surface and the tip of the frontal lobe. These vessels are coagulated and divided. If the tumor extends caudal to the line of resection, additional tumor is removed by suction, leaving the more infiltrating margins alone to prevent further injury to functioning brain.

Following removal of the resected tissue, the entire cavity is filled with wet cotton balls, to which suction is applied. These are left in place several minutes. Just before removal, they are irrigated with saline to prevent small vessels from adhering to the cotton. After removal, obvious remaining bleeding points are coagulated.

The dura is closed in a watertight fashion, which may require the interposition of a pericranial graft. Before the last several stitches are placed, the cavity is filled with saline to displace intracranial air. An epidural Jackson-Pratt drain is left in place in the epidural space, and the bone flap is replaced using microplating techniques and self-tapping screws. The reflected temporalis muscle is sutured to the muscle left on the bone flap.

## Potential Postoperative Deficits

The frontal lobectomy described earlier is designed to avoid the motor strip and Broca's speech area. Patients undergoing frontal lobectomy usually have no gross post-

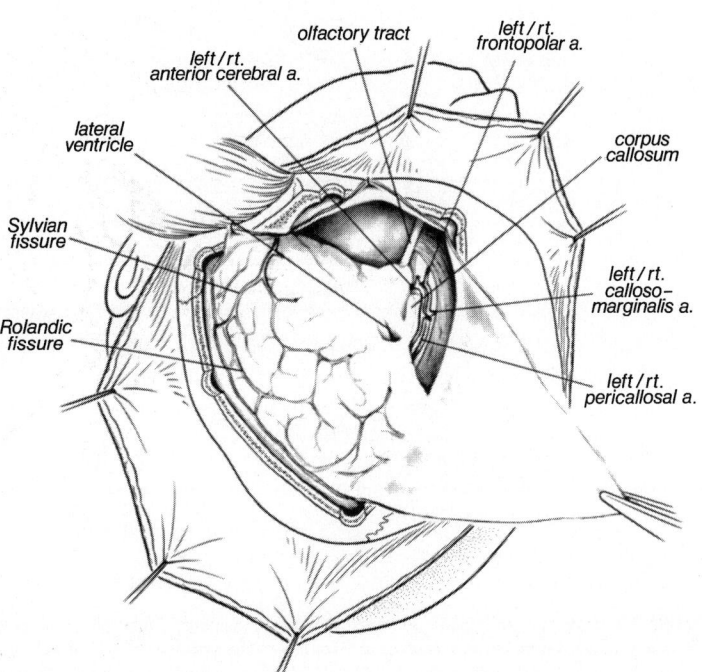

**FIGURE 55–5 ■** Structural relationships at the base and medial aspect of the frontal fossa after removal of the frontal tip.

operative sensorimotor deficits. It is possible, however, for such a patient to be apathetic and demonstrate a general slowing of the intellect, especially if the lobectomy has been on the dominant hemisphere. Occasionally, impairment of recent memory and of voluntary and serial memorization can occur.[35] Although lesions limited to the frontal pole region do not result in motor deficits, voluntary and more complex control can be impaired. The high motor deficit is usually associated with difficulty with serial, alternate, or novel tasks.[35]

## Temporal Lobectomy

A temporal lobectomy is usually performed with the patient's body in either a lateral or three-quarters lateral position, with the head to be in a full lateral position (Fig. 55–6). A question mark–shaped skin incision is commonly used. This incision starts above the zygoma, passes along the anterior margin of the pinna, and curves posteriorly so the incision is 3.5 cm behind the external auditory meatus (see Fig. 55–6). This incision spares the branch of the facial nerve to the frontalis muscle and the superficial temporal artery. The scalp flap is reflected anteroinferiorly. The temporalis muscle may be dealt with either as a separate flap or as part of an osteoplastic flap. If the osteoplastic flap is chosen, electrocautery is used to incise the muscle approximately 0.5 cm from its line of insertion. Then it is reflected laterally and placed under the same fishhooks as the skin. The bur holes are placed as with the osteoplastic flap and connected by craniotome. The free flap is removed and set aside until the end of the craniotomy. If an osteoplastic flap is chosen, three incisions are made in the temporalis muscle, allowing bur holes to be placed beneath it (see Fig. 55–6). Two additional bur holes are placed above the muscle (see Fig. 55–6). The anteroinferior bur hole is placed just posterior to the outer canthus of the eye and anterior to the pterion, allowing exposure of the anterior tip of the temporal lobe. The inferiormost bur hole is placed above the zygoma. Bur holes are connected when necessary by rongeuring bone beneath the temporalis muscle (Fig. 55–7A). The remaining bone is fractured, and the bone flap is reflected while it is hinged on the temporalis muscle (see Fig. 55–7B). The bone flap is reflected inferiorly, and the remaining temporal bone is removed to the floor of the middle fossa (see Fig. 55–7B). The middle meningeal vessels are coagulated. The dura is opened several millimeters from the bony edge and is reflected anteroinferiorly (Fig. 55–8A).

The cortical resection can involve removal of the anterior 5 to 6 cm of the temporal lobe; or alternatively, if intraoperative cortical mapping is not being employed, the vein of Labbé may be used as a landmark for the posterior extent of the resection. Both, however, can be misleading because of the variability of the position of the vein of Labbé and the size of the temporal lobe. More consistent landmarks, therefore, are recommended. The junction of the rolandic and sylvian fissures is the most reliable landmark. The

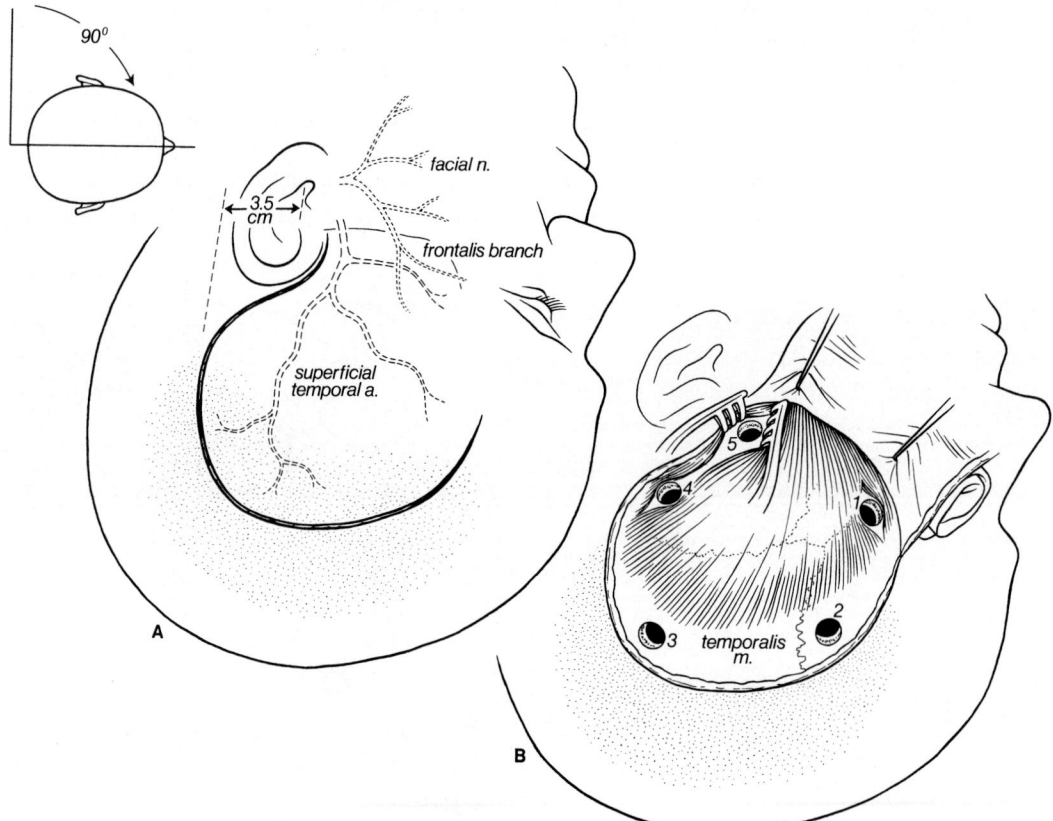

**FIGURE 55–6** ■ *A*, Skin incision for a left temporal lobectomy. Note the position of the zygoma, superficial temporal artery, and facial nerve. *B*, Placement of bur holes for an osteoplastic flap. *Inset*, The position of the patient relative to the surgeon.

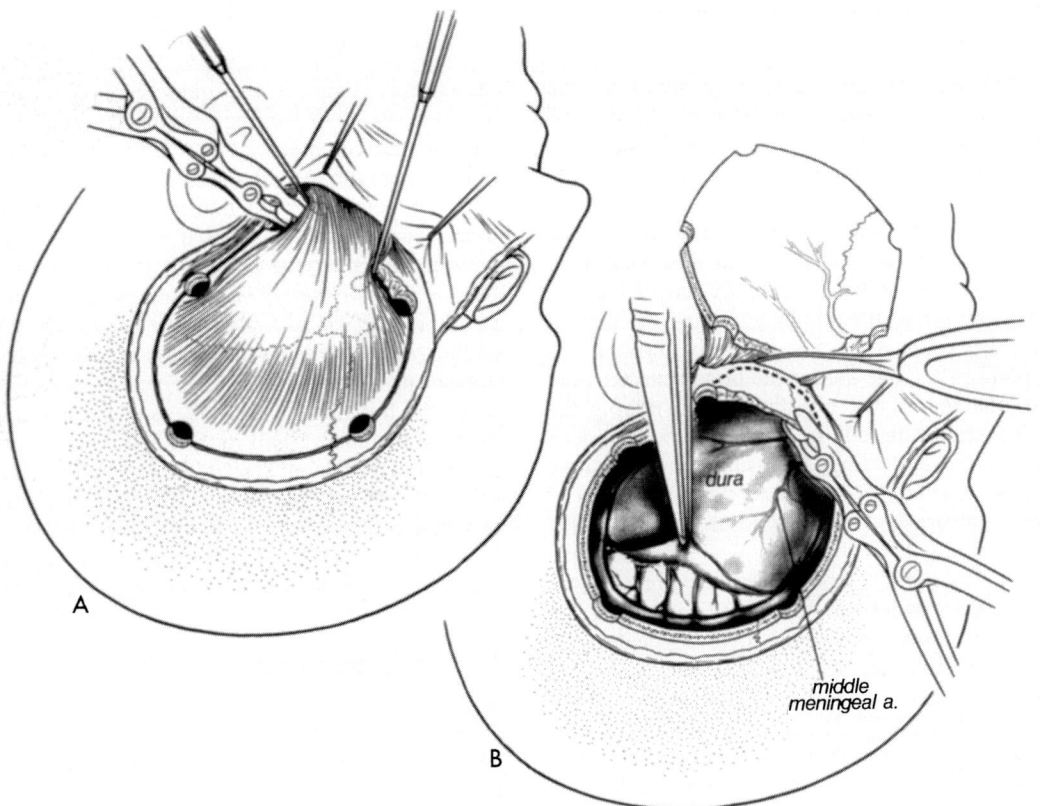

**FIGURE 55–7** ■ *A*, Connecting bur holes No. 1 and No. 5 beneath the temporalis muscles to allow the muscle to remain intact. *B*, Removal of the remaining temporal bone to expose the inferior to lateral aspect of the temporal bone. Dura reflected laterally after coagulation of the middle meningeal artery.

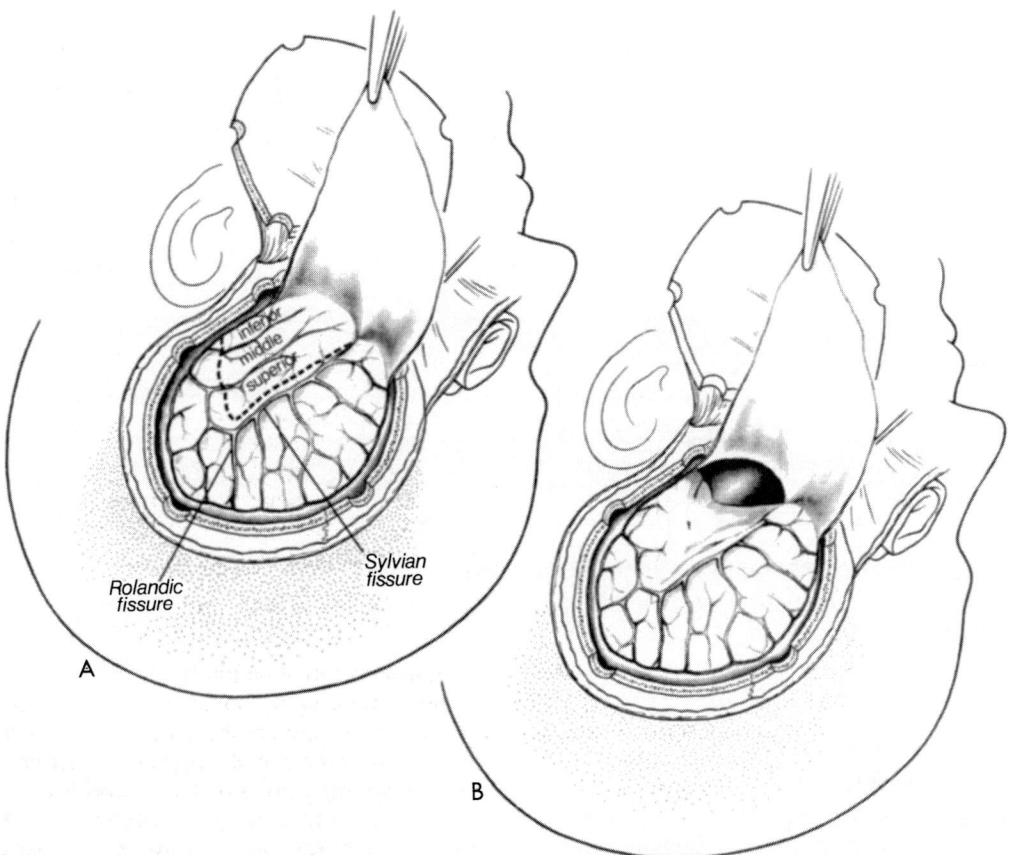

**FIGURE 55–8** ■ The left temporal lobectomy. *A*, A cortical incision, sparing the posterior speech area and the middle cerebral vessels (see the text). *B*, Operative site after removal of tissue.

first and second temporal convolutions posterior to that intersection are to be avoided. When starting the cortical dissection along the superior temporal gyrus, it is best to leave a thin layer of the superior temporal gyrus cortex to protect the middle cerebral vessels (see Fig. 55–8A).

The dissection is started at the anterior edge of the first temporal gyrus and carried posteriorly to the junction of the rolandic and sylvian fissures, where the line of incision turns inferiorly and across the middle and inferior temporal gyri. As the dissection is carried medially through the superior temporal gyrus, one incises the pia-arachnoid, gray matter, white matter, and the pia-arachnoid overlying the insula. The dissection proceeds so as not to cross the deep pia-arachnoid barrier protecting the insula and the middle cerebral vessels (Fig. 55–9). Failure to do so can lead to postoperative hemiparesis. After the insula has been exposed, the dissection is carried into the white matter of the temporal stem. Once the temporal stem is entered, the incision is directed downward through the uncus to the floor of the middle fossa. Attention is then directed to the posterior portion of the incision, which is extended from the superior temporal gyrus on the inferior aspect of the temporal lobe (see Fig. 55–9). The temporal horn is entered and covered with a cottonoid. Because these two incisions meet on the inferior surface of the temporal lobe, the

resection is complete; the draining veins, however, are still in place. At this time, the bridging veins over the anterior part of the temporal lobe are coagulated and cut near the brain, as are the medial and inferior veins, which drain into the cavernous sinus on the undersurface of the temporal lobe. Once the lobe is excised, the resultant cavity is dealt with as previously described. If the tumor extends toward the uncus, it is possible to remove the parahippocampal gyrus and the lateral aspect of the uncus. The medial aspect of the uncus is left in place to protect the optic tract. If the dissection is carried medially, care must be taken to preserve the third nerve, the posterior cerebral artery, and the cerebral peduncle (see Fig. 55–9). The transverse temporal gyrus of Heschl on the superior surface of the temporal lobe also is left intact. On nondominant temporal lobe resections, the posterior extent of the cortical incision can be carried out to the supramarginal and angular gyri. Closure of the wound is carried out as previously described.

## Occipital Lobectomy

### Surgical Positioning and Exposure

The three-quarters prone or a semisitting position may be used for easy access to the midline (Fig. 55–10). The skin

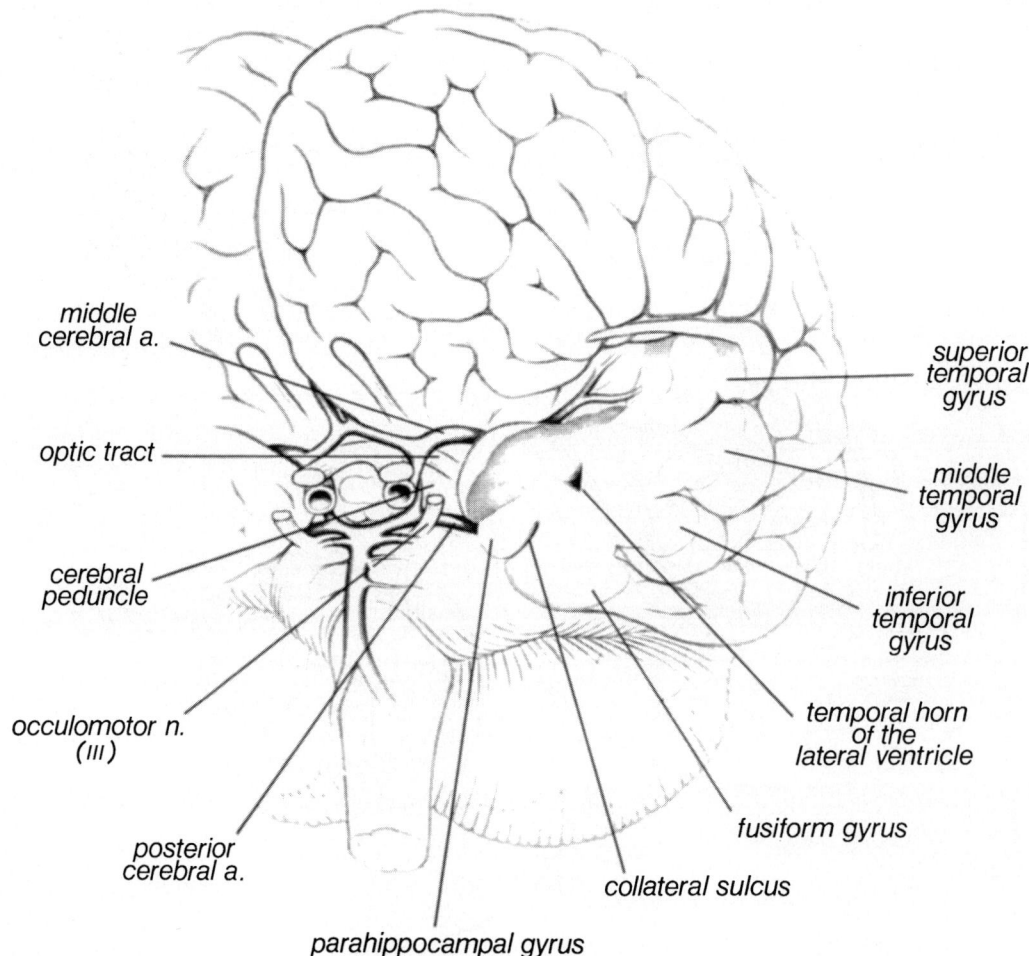

FIGURE 55–9 ■ A basal to lateral view of the left side of the brain with a partial temporal lobectomy. Note the proximity of the middle cerebral artery, optic tract, oculomotor nerve, posterior cerebral artery, and cerebral peduncle to the medial extent of the incision.

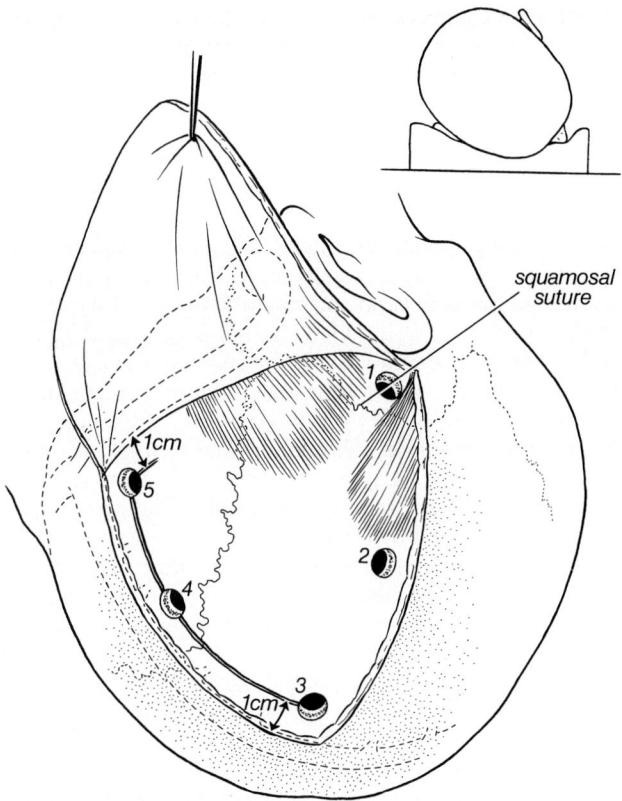

**FIGURE 55–10** ■ An occipital lobectomy skin incision and bur hole placement. *Inset*, The patient's position with respect to the surgeon.

sphere, damage to the cerebral hemisphere in the area of the junction of the parietal, occipital, and temporal lobes can produce dyslexia, dysgraphia, and acalculia. Van Buren has mapped the cortical areas in which electrical stimulation causes interference with speech and has shown that these extend into the angular and supramarginal gyri.[36] The position of the angular gyrus then was measured in 10 cadavers. The distance from the angular gyrus to the occipital pole is 3.5 cm and from the angular gyrus to the parietal-occipital midline is 2.4 cm (see Fig. 55–11).[36] In the dominant hemisphere, damage to the angular gyrus, Wernicke's area, and the surrounding parietal temporal cortex (Fig. 55–13) leads to deficits in recognition of complex visual and auditory symbols, including those of written and spoken language, defects in the visual-spatial-body image, and severe communication abnormalities. The general deficit is profound asymbolia.

## Decompression Without Lobectomy

Although not amenable to lobectomy, a glioma that occurs in areas of important neurologic function should be considered for radical removal because, first, the tumor mass may displace vital areas without actually infiltrating them so that dysphasia and hemiparesis caused by local compression and edema can be relieved or reduced. Second, if the tumor has infiltrated vital areas and rendered them

incision starts in the midline at the superior nuchal line, is carried forward on the midline, and swings laterally to end just below the squamosal suture (see Fig. 55–10). The skin flap is reflected inferiorly to preserve the occipital artery and the greater and lesser occipital nerves. Bur holes for the bone flap are made 1 cm lateral to the midline, 1 cm above the transverse sinus inferiorly, and in the posterior superior portion of the temporal bone (see Fig. 55–10). A free bone flap is removed. The dura is opened in a T fashion to allow reflection toward both the superior sagittal sinus and the transverse sinus (Fig. 55–11). In the dominant hemisphere, the cortical incision is started 3.5 cm from the occipital tip on the superior cortical margin to avoid damage to the angular gyrus. On the nondominant side, it is started 7 cm from the occipital tip (see Fig. 55–11). The cortical incision and subpial dissection is performed as previously described (section on frontal lobectomy). The occipital horn of the lateral ventricle may or may not be entered. It is covered with cotton fluffs. As the calcarine fissure is approached, the posterior cerebral artery can be seen in its depths (Fig. 55–12); this artery is coagulated and divided. Before removing the occipital lobe, the draining veins that enter the torcular are coagulated and cut near the cortex. Following removal of the occipital lobe, the cavity is filled with saline and the dura is closed. The remainder of the operation follows general neurosurgical practices.

## Potential Postoperative Deficits

Following occipital lobectomy, the patient will have contralateral homonymous hemianopia. In the dominant hemi-

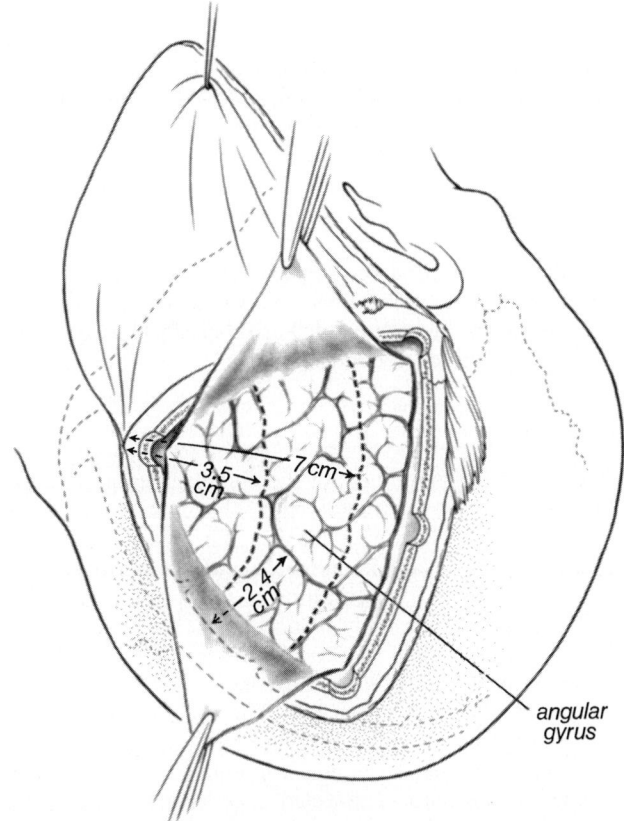

**FIGURE 55–11** ■ Reflection of the dura in a T shape to protect both the superior sagittal and transverse sinus. Cortical incisions for both dominant (3.5 cm) and nondominant (7 cm) hemispheres are shown. Note the proximity to the midline of the angular gyrus (see text).

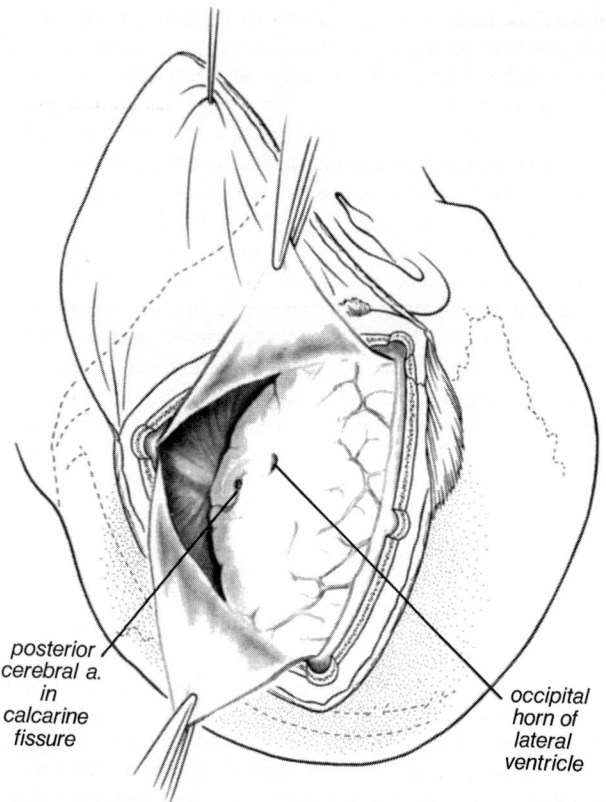

FIGURE 55–12 ■ The posterior cerebral artery as seen in the depths of the calcarine fissure after removal of the occipital pole.

nonfunctional, their surgical removal, if one stays within the limits of grossly evident tumor, should not increase the patient's neurologic deficit. However, there is evidence that functioning motor, sensory, or language tissue can be located within a tumor of the surrounding infiltrated brain. Intraoperative stimulation mapping techniques have identified patients who have shown functional tissue within the boundaries of infiltrative gliomas. Therefore, to maximize glioma resection in functional areas intraoperative mapping may be used to identify cortical or subcortical tissue within as well as adjacent to tumor.

## Exposure

When operating on tumors of the dominant temporal lobe, Broca's area, or the motor strip, the exact location of the tumor will determine the specific placement of the craniotomy. For example, in the case of a posterior temporal parietal tumor, a modification of the approach used for either temporal lobectomy or occipital lobectomy may be used. Tumors located in Broca's area can be approached either through a modification of the craniotomy used for frontal or temporal lobectomy. For tumors beneath the motor strip, a rectangular skin and free bone flap craniotomy centered over the tumor is preferred. After the skull is opened, the dura is reflected superiorly to protect the superior sagittal sinus. On opening the dura, the cortex is inspected. Rarely, a tumor nodule appears on the surface, or a subcortical tumor will widen the overlying gyri. Equally frequent, however, are broadened gyri secondary to edema

in the cortex adjacent to the tumor. Using the information gleaned from the preoperative CT and MRI (and, increasingly, proton magnetic resonance spectroscopy) in conjunction with image-guided stereotaxis, the tumor usually can be accurately delineated intraoperatively.

## Procedure

A small cortical incision is made, the tumor is located, and the cortical excision is expanded. Biopsies then are taken from both the peripheral and central portions of the tumor. If the tumor is necrotic, the resection may extend directly into motor and speech areas if the surgeon remains within the tumor mass. The necrotic and softened portions of the tumor are best removed by routine suction, or the ultrasonic aspirator. If the tumor is infiltrative and firm and the anatomy of the brain is preserved, resection should not be undertaken. In this instance an adequate decompression can usually be obtained by removal of the tumor up to, but not within, the vital area. If the infiltrative nature of the tumor precludes removing most of it, removal of adjacent frontal, temporal, or occipital tissue may provide necessary internal decompression.

If the tumor is cystic on initial insertion of the cannula, enough fluid is drained through the cannula to decompress the brain. Once the cyst is opened through the cortical incision, retractors are gently inserted into the interior of the cyst, which is inspected for tumor nodules. If they are present, the tumor nodules and the surrounding cyst walls are excised.

## POSTOPERATIVE CARE

Following craniotomy, patients are admitted to the intensive care unit. On the first postoperative day, epidural

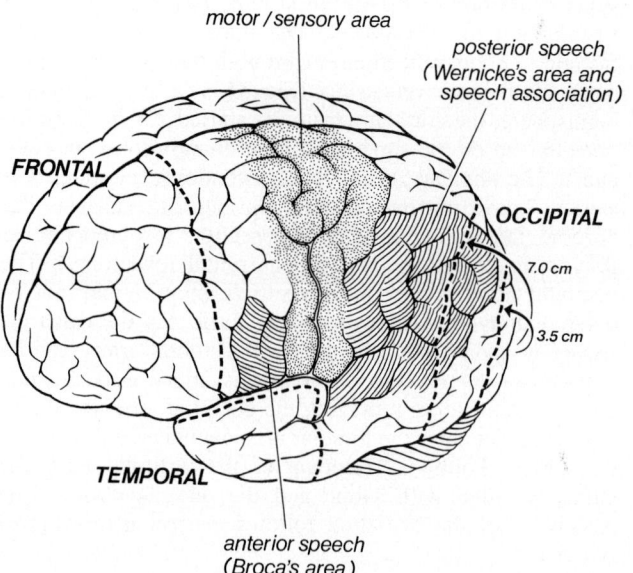

FIGURE 55–13 ■ Cortical incisions for dominant hemisphere lobectomies (occipital lobe nondominant hemisphere lobectomy also shown) and their relationships to precentral and postcentral gyri and speech areas.

drains are removed and a baseline postoperative CT scan is performed. Sutures are removed at 1 week, and radiation therapy is started any time thereafter. Steroids and anticonvulsants are routinely maintained for the first several weeks after surgery and throughout radiation therapy. Neuropsychological testing is repeated after completion of radiation therapy, and the patient's Karnofsky Performance Scale is established and plans made regarding further activities.

## REOPERATION FOR CEREBRAL GLIOMAS

The concept of reoperation for cerebral gliomas originated with Cushing.[37, 38] He described patients who had a tumor removed and then subsequently underwent a second operation for removal of a recurrence. One such patient had six operations.

Several series have addressed the issue of reoperation in management of patients with malignant gliomas. The majority of malignant gliomas recur within 2 cm of their original margins. Young reported on 24 reoperated patients with astrocytoma grades III or IV whose median survival time after reoperation was 14 weeks. The most important prognostic factor was the Karnofsky rating (KR) at the time of the second operation. Patients with a score of 60 or greater had a median survival time after the second surgery of 22 weeks. Patients with a KR of less than 60 had a median survival time of 9 weeks. Age, sex, and location of tumor were not significantly correlated with the duration of survival. This is in contrast to Soloman, who reported on 40 reoperated patients with glioblastoma.[39] Median survival after the second operation was 37 weeks; the patient's KR, tumor grade, interoperative interval, or age did not significantly affect the outcome. The influence of age on total survival was also reflected in the patient's undergoing reoperation. Median survival after the second operation was 36 weeks for the 23 patients older than 40 years and approximately 55 to 60 weeks for the 17 patients younger than 40; however, survival after the second operation was not significantly different in young and old patients. Harsh reported a series including 39 patients with glioblastoma and 31 patients with anaplastic astrocytomas. Median survival for patients with glioblastoma was 35 weeks (11 of the patients had a KR of 70 or greater) and was 84 weeks for patients with anaplastic astrocytomas. For patients with glioblastomas, both age and preoperative KR had a statistically significant effect on the duration of postoperative high-quality survival but not on postoperative survival independent of quality; for anaplastic astrocytomas only age was significant.

Reoperation can improve severe neurologic deficits if the recurrent tumor is compressing and not infiltrating vital structures. Radiation necrosis of the brain can be a diagnostic problem. CT, MRI, and PET studies may not allow one to distinguish between tumor recurrence and the effects of postoperative irradiation. In these situations multiple biopsies through the lesion along a trajectory through the mass is needed. Proton magnetic resonance spectroscopic imaging (MRSI), which allows in vivo measurements of the concentration of brain metabolites such as choline-containing phospholipids, has been used to differentiate recurrence from radiation effect. In two patients, in whom conventional neuroimaging was equivocal for such a distinction, metabolic images from MRSI showed a high choline signal in histologically proven tumor recurrence, and a low choline signal was present where radiation changes predominated.

In a second surgical approach the same skin flap as that used for the initial surgery should be used. If it is not, it must be extended so as not to compromise a major blood supply to the scalp, which already has been damaged by radiation.

The dura and the fibrous tissue growing from the dura frequently adheres to the bone flap at its margins and at the bur hole sites, and it needs to be separated gently. If there is any question of adequate exposure, extension of the bone flap is to be encouraged. The dura usually adheres to the cortex at the line of previous dural incision, and the two must be carefully separated. Sometimes this separation is best accomplished by creating a second dural opening in the same shape but slightly larger than the initial one, allowing the surgeon to develop a plane of dissection between unscarred cortex and the dura. This is particularly important if the line of incision is close to the motor or speech area. If the surgery is in the vicinity of the rolandic fissure, interoperative electric stimulation for identification of the motor strip may be useful because normal anatomic landmarks are frequently distorted or absent. Pool points out that recurrent tumor close to the motor strip may make it relatively insensitive to electrical stimulation. Identification of the recurrent tumor is not a problem with current neuroimaging techniques. As in the first operation, recurrent tumor should be removed as radically as possible. In patients in whom a large cystic cavity is found with a mural nodule, the nodule and the surrounding cyst wall are removed, the cystic fluid drained, and the cyst irrigated. Following these maneuvers we then line the site of tumor resection with seven to eight carmustine (Gliadel) wafers. The current evidence is that the median survival of patients with recurrent glioblastomas increased from 24 weeks with placebo to 32 weeks with the implanted wafers. The 6-month survival time in these cases increased from 38% with placebo to 58% with Gliadel treatment. The downside of this treatment modality is that the single package of Gliadel wafers costs the hospital pharmacy in excess of $10,000: thus, this issue deserves careful scrutiny by the neurosurgical community.

In general, reoperation should be reserved for patients harboring low-grade gliomas and mixed tumors in a surgically accessible area, whereas the reoperation of patients with glioblastoma should be carefully tailored to the patient's neurologic state and the likelihood of a functionally useful result being achieved that is likely to provide the patient with a better quality of survival than would have been accomplished without further operation. It is of considerable interest that, in a recent analysis, it was found that reoperation for supratentorial gliomas carries no greater operative morbidity or mortality rate than primary surgery.

## SUMMARY

The best reported surgical results in the management for supratentorial gliomas involve radical surgical excision followed by radiation and, recently, the use of Gliadel wafers to provide chemotherapy. Surgical resection accomplishes the most when it leaves the least amount of residual tumor. Current neuroimaging techniques allow a very good delineation of the tumor volume and provide an exquisite view of the regional anatomy; however, identifying the exact boundaries of an infiltrative glioma is a problem that has not yet been solved. In the majority of cases tumor recurrence occurs within 2 cm of the previous lesion. Recurrent glioma needs to be distinguished from a mass effect produced by radiation necrosis, and this may require biopsy of the lesion as well as decompression. The rates of morbidity and mortality of the reoperative cases are no higher than that with the primary operation; however, justification for this undertaking depends on the age of the patient, the interval since primary surgery, the performance status of the patient, and the specific symptoms. The best 5-year survival data among patients with supratentorial gliomas treated by surgery and radiation therapy according to current guidelines occur with pilocytic astrocytoma (100%), oligodendrogliomas (64%), and low-grade astrocytomas (36%), as compared with a 1-year survival rate following radical excision of malignant gliomas and 24% survival rate following partial resection and radiation therapy as the treatment of these lesions.

## REFERENCES

1. Preul MC, Leblanc R, Caramanos Z, et al: Magnetic resonance spectroscopy guided brain tumor resection: Differentiation between recurrent glioma and radiation change in two diagnostically difficult cases. Can J Neurol Sci 25:13–22, 1998.
2. Herholz K, Reulen HJ, von Stockhausen HM, et al: Preoperative activation and intraoperative stimulation of language-related areas in patients with gliomas. Neurosurgery 41:12253–12260, 1997.
3. Berger MS, Rostomily RC: Low grade gliomas: Functional mapping resection strategies, extent of resection, outcome. J Neurooncol 34:85–101, 1997.
4. Woodward DE, Cook J, Tracqui P, et al: A mathematical model of glioma growth: The effect of extent of surgical resection. Cell Prolif 29:269–288, 1996.
5. Skirboll SS, Ojemann GA, Berger MS, et al: Functional cortex and subcortical white matter located within gliomas. Neurosurgery 38:678–684, 1996.
6. Kiwit JC, Floeth FW, Bock WJ: Survival in malignant glioma: Analysis of prognostic factors with special regard to cytoreductive surgery. Zentralb Neurochir 57:76–88, 1996.
7. Hockberg FHI, Pruitt A: Assumptions in the radiotherapy of glioblastoma. Neurology 30:907, 1980.
8. Martins AN, Johnson JS, Henry JM, et al: Delayed radiation necrosis of the brain. J Neurosurg 47:336, 1977.
9. Wada J, Rasmussen T: Intracranial injection of sodium amytal for the lateralization of cerebral speech dominance. J Neurosurg 17:266, 1960.
10. Patronas NJ, DiChina G, Kufta C, et al: Prediction of survival in glioma patients by means of positron emission tomography. J Neurosurg 62:816, 1985.
11. Lilja A, Bergstron K, Hartvig P, et al: Dynamic study of supratentorial gliomas with L-methyl-11C-methionine and positron emission tomography. Am J Neuroradiol 6:505, 1985.
12. Soloman MJ, Kaplan RS, Duchen TB, et al: Effect of age and reoperation on survival in the combined modality treatment of malignant astrocytomas. Neurosurgery 10:454, 1982.
13. Taphoorn MJ, Heimans JJ, Snoek FJ, Lindeboom J: Assessment of quality of life in patients treated for low-grade glioma: A preliminary report. J Neurol Neurosurg Psychiatry 55:372–376, 1992.
14. Salcman M: Malignant glioma management. Neurosurg Clin North Am 1:49–63, 1990.
15. Florell RC, Macdonald DR, Irish WD, Bernstein M: Selection bias, survival, and brachytherapy for glioma. J Neurosurg 76:179–183, 1992.
16. Vecht CJ, Avezaat CJ, van Putten WL, Eijkenboom WM: The influence of the extent of surgery on the neurological function and survival in malignant glioma. A retrospective analysis of 243 patients. J Neurol Neurosurg Psychiatry 53:466–471, 1990.
17. Winger MJ, Macdonald DR, Cairncross JG: Supratentorial anaplastic gliomas in adults. The prognostic importance of extent of resection and prior low-grade glioma. J Neurosurg 71:487–493, 1989.
18. Lilja A, Lundqvist H, Olsson Y, et al: Positron emission tomography and computed tomography in differential diagnosis between recurrent and residual glioma and treatment-induced brain lesions. Acta Radiol 30:121–128, 1989.
19. Whittle IR, Denholm SW, Gregor A: Management of patients over 60 years with supratentorial glioma: Lessons from an audit. Surg Neurol 36:106–111, 1991.
20. Bricolo A, Turazzi S, Cristofori L, Gerosa M: Experience in "radical" surgery of supratentorial gliomas in adults. J Neurosurg Sci 34:297–298, 1990.
21. Walsh AR, Schmidt RH, Marsh HT: Cortical mapping and resection under local anesthetic as an aid to surgery of low and intermediate grade gliomas. Br J Neurosurg 4:485–491, 1990.
22. Tovi M, Lilja A, Bergstrom M, Ericsson A: Delineation of gliomas with magnetic resonance imaging using Gd-DTPA in comparison with computed tomography and positron emission tomography. Acta Radiol 31:417–429, 1990.
23. Sandeman DR, Sandeman AP, Buxton P, Hughes HH: The management of patients with an intrinsic supratentorial brain tumor. Br J Neurosurg 4:299–312, 1990.
24. Mosskin M, Ericson K, Hindmarsh T, von Holst H: Positron emission tomography compared with magnetic resonance imaging and computed tomography in supratentorial gliomas using multiple stereotactic biopsies as reference. Acta Radiol 30:225–232, 1989.
25. Whitton AC, Bloom HJ: Low-grade glioma of the cerebral hemispheres in adults: A retrospective analysis of 88 cases. Int J Radiat Oncol Biol Phys 18:783–786, 1990.
26. Berger MS, Kincaid J, Ojemann GA, Lettich E: Brain mapping techniques to maximize resection, safety, and seizure control in children with brain tumors. Neurosurgery 25:786–792, 1989.
27. Choksey MS, Valentine A, Shawdon H, Freer CE: Computed tomography in the diagnosis of malignant brain tumors: Do all patients require biopsy? J Neurol Neurosurg Psychiatry 52:821–825, 1989.
28. Fadul C, Wood J, Thaler H, et al: Morbidity and mortality of craniotomy for excision of supratentorial gliomas. Neurology 38:1374–1379, 1988.
29. Moser RP: Surgery for glioma relapse. Factors that influence a favorable outcome. Cancer 62:381–390, 1988.

# Surgical Management of Low-Grade Gliomas

■ RENATO GIUFFRÈ and FRANCESCO S. PASTORE

## CLASSIFICATION—PATHOLOGY

Astrocytomas, oligodendrogliomas, and mixed (oligoastrocytic) gliomas are low-grade, that is, grade I gliomas according to the classification of the World Health Organization (WHO). "The Yale Neuro-Oncology Tumor Data Bank reported an incidence of these oncotypes respectively of 60%, 23.3%, and 16.7% among all low-grade gliomas."[1]

Fibrillary, gemistocytic, protoplasmic, or mixed astrocytomas present different surgical problems according to whether they are solid or cystic. A solid astrocytoma has a hard or rubbery consistency, is sometimes cartilaginous, and is whitish in the fibrillary form; it is softer, gelatinous, and translucent in the gemistocytic and protoplasmic varieties. On the surface, the growth is either diffuse or apparently circumscribed. Under the surface, it usually has less consistency and tends to form either several small cysts or a single large one; a single large cyst is most often found in the fibrillary and gemistocytic varieties.[2] The pilocytic variety is rare among astrocytomas of the cerebral hemispheres and is found more often in the posterior fossa (cerebellum and brain stem), diencephalon, and anterior optic pathways. In most cases, cerebral pilocytic astrocytoma consists of a large unilocular cyst with a mural nodule; it differs from other forms of astrocytoma in biologic behavior and in a marked responsiveness to therapy.[3–5]

Oligodendroglioma is often very hard and gritty on section, because it contains palpable calcifications: It is grayish pink and has clear-cut limits on the surface (where it infiltrates the gyri, giving them a hypertrophied, "scalloped or garlanded" appearance) to become indistinct in depth, where small mucinous cysts may be found. Small nodules as hard as warts are found in the cortex and are detected by the surgeon on inspection or on palpation. When the tumor spreads through the leptomeninges, it forms large lumps that project beyond the surface like bluish-red fungi. In such cases, the tumor may adhere to the dura mater and may be mistaken at first sight for a meningioma.[2]

Mixed oligoastrocytomas do not differ in gross appearance from true oligodendrogliomas and constitute a purely histologic variety. Tumors such as pleomorphic xantho-astrocytomas and gangliogliomas are low-grade, usually resectable tumors with a very low incidence and will not be considered here.

Both oncotypes (astrocytoma and oligodendroglioma) occur preferentially in the frontal lobes, after which come the temporal, parietal, and occipital lobes, in this order. These diffusely infiltrative tumors do not respect boundaries, however, and most low-grade gliomas straddle the fissures to involve contiguous lobes.

There are no typical sites by oncotype, except perhaps the frontolateral region for oligodendroglioma. Both of these gliomas may be parasagittal, affecting the frontal and parietal lobes. Hard gliomas "of the edge," bordering on the sagittal fissure, develop along the medial gyri and may infiltrate the corpus callosum or spread contralaterally through the corpus callosum ("butterfly gliomas").

Whether these tumors emerge on the surface or are subcortical, they infiltrate the white substance diffusely and may spread in depth toward the ventricular system or basal nuclei. Gliomas arising from the diencephalon, which are distinguished by certain histologic and clinical features (occurrence of pilocytic astrocytomas, preference for youth) and which present peculiar biologic behavior and peculiar problems of treatment, are discussed in Chapter 61.

Any centrencephalic spread of a hemispheric glioma limits surgical resection, a point that is addressed under surgical technique. Such spread occurs along the projection fibers (Fig. 56–1). Seeger[6] recognized two other possible routes of tumor spread: (1) along the associative fibers (intrahemispheric spread), and (2) along the commissural fibers (interhemispheric spread). An example of the latter is the contralateral spread via the corpus callosum, as already mentioned. An example of intrahemispheric spread is the subcortical migration of neoplastic cells via the short associative U-shaped fibers between two adjacent gyri.

However, tumor progression is a process of dislocation or infiltration of the surrounding neural tissue, and these two patterns of growth may explain the neurophysiologic data showing "in toto" displacement of eloquent areas but also the occasional presence of neural activity in the tumor core.[7]

The WHO classification criteria are purely histopatho-

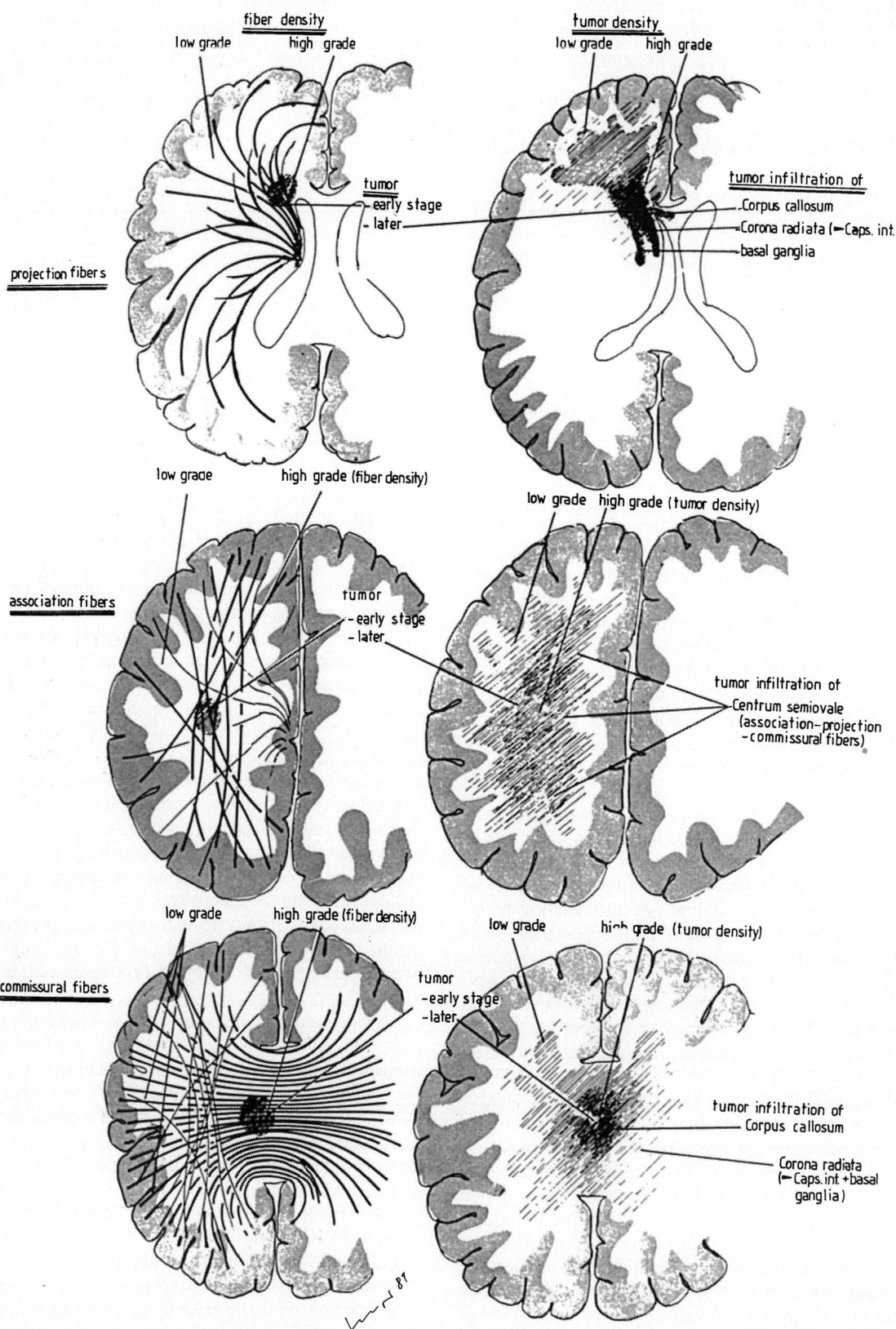

**FIGURE 56–1** ■ Patterns of tumor spread along the projection, association, and commissural fibers. (From Seeger W: Strategies of Microsurgery in Problematic Brain Areas. Vienna: Springer-Verlag, 1990, p 25.)

logic, and their limitations were highlighted in the 1980s and 1990s by the advances of immunohistochemistry, molecular biology, and neuroimaging. When classifying gliomas today, one must take account of specific markers of different cell types, parameters of cellular kinetics, and metabolic data relating to neoplastic tissue in vivo. Thus, tumor grading based solely on morphology is supplemented by neurodiagnostic grading (the presence or absence of contrast enhancement on computed tomograpy [CT] and magnetic resonance imaging [MRI]),[8] metabolic grading (increased glucose consumption on positron-emission tomography [PET]), and grading based on parameters of cellular molecular biology and kinetics.

On the last point, histologically similar tumors may exhibit differing proliferative potential. Subgroups of low-grade astrocytomas exist that have different proportions of cells in the S phase of DNA synthesis, expressed by different values of the labeling index (LI). One subgroup with a low LI (<1%) is characterized by slow growth, and another with the same or higher LI is biologically more aggressive, which partially explains the very different clinical behavior often seen in histologically similar tumors.[9] The proliferative potential of a given tumor (expressed in the LI) correlates with necrosis and tissue hypervascularization rather than with the number of mitoses and cellular anomalies (or monstrosities).[10, 11] This fact confirms the undue importance that was formerly attached to the mitotic count in gliomas as an index of growth rate. It is now known that mitoses may be lacking in a glioblastoma multiforme and may be present in a slow-growing oligodendroglioma.[12]

The PET tumor grading based on glucose consumption by area is also a better predictor of the long-term prognosis of gliomas than is histologic grading.[13]

The data on the biology of gliomas have been, in the last decade, increasing exponentially. These data will eventually form the basis of a new classification of the far from homogeneous group of low-grade gliomas.

Because low-grade gliomas do not constitute a homogeneous group, treatment clearly cannot be uniform in all cases, and the results are not easily comparable.

## CLINICAL AND BIOLOGIC FEATURES OF LOW-GRADE GLIOMAS

Low-grade gliomas of the cerebral hemispheres occur less frequently than malignant gliomas (glioblastomas, primitive neuroectodermal tumors [PNET]), affect a younger population, and have a better prognosis. Perhaps because of the lower frequency of these tumors and the fact that patients may remain well for a long time, few formal clinical trials have been mounted; therefore, the natural history of low-grade gliomas is less well known than is that of the high-grade varieties. In addition, the preoperative clinical history has changed substantially in recent years as a result of neuroimaging techniques, which have ensured much earlier diagnosis. In the pre-CT era, patients with low-grade hemispheric glioma often presented with headache, papilledema, and focal deficits, whereas today they undergo surgery after only a few episodes of convulsions and are absolutely normal neurologically. For exam-

ple, in the series of Laws and coworkers,[14] consisting of patients treated between 1915 and 1975, 40% had papilledema at the time of presentation; almost half complained of headache; and 51% exhibited motor deficits. In the series of Gol,[15] comprised of patients treated before 1960, 72% had a headache at the time of diagnosis; 59%, papilledema; 56%, hemiparesis; and 56%, seizures. By contrast, in Piepmeier's series,[16] in which all the patients were diagnosed by CT, 5% initially had a headache; 15%, motor weakness; and more than 90%, seizure activity (the frequency of papilledema was not stated). In addition, in the series of Vertosick and associates,[17] 16% had headache; 8% papilledema; 16% motor deficits; and 92%, seizures.

Epileptic activity in patients with low-grade cerebral gliomas is important not only clinically, because it is the earliest symptom, but also surgically. Electrocorticographic recordings in patients with a slow-growing glioma have revealed epileptogenic foci separate from the tumor.[18] This nontumoral cortex, although not marked by neuronal loss, nonetheless shows a change in neuronal subpopulations, that is, a reduction of neurons immunoreactive to γ-aminobutyric acid and to somatostatin,[19] which is an expression of local hyperexcitability. Hence, the seizures in these patients, which are often refractory to drugs, can be controlled only if the epileptogenic foci are removed along with the tumor. A patient with chronic epilepsy may thus have a glioma. Among 51 patients with epilepsy of 1 to 27 years' duration (mean duration of 11 years), Goldring and colleagues[20] found 40 gliomas, including 25 low-grade astrocytomas and 1 oligodendroglioma. In one patient with a 22-year history of epilepsy, they found a glioblastoma, evidently the outcome of secondary degeneration, as is discussed later. CT and, even better, MRI define the lesion, but these modalities have limitations: the lack of increase in lesion volume on serial CT scans does not exclude a tumor. The clinical features, warn Goldring and coworkers, may be very deceptive; a history typical of essential epilepsy does not exclude a tumor as the cause. For instance, generalized febrile convulsions in infancy followed by complex partial seizures—a history typical of temporal mesial sclerosis—was the history of some subjects with temporal glioma.

The biology (cellular kinetics and metabolism) of these nonsymptomatic tumors that have a long natural history (remaining silent or nonsymptomatic for years and then exploding dramatically) cannot be considered benign and certainly arouse scientific interest. Low-grade gliomas (astrocytomas, mixed gliomas, and ependymomas) have a lower percentage of cells in the S phase (LI = 2% to 6.7%) than do malignant gliomas (LI = 9.1% to 46.5%).[21] The growth fraction (GF) (i.e., the total number of cells involved in cellular proliferation as a proportion of the entire cell population of the tumor) is correspondingly low: GF = 0 to 4.5% in low-grade astrocytomas, and GF = 1.7% to 32.2% in glioblastomas.[22] Flow cytometry of nuclear DNA in well-differentiated gliomas shows that most of the cells have the same ploidy (as a rule, they are diploid), with little variation from one area of the tumor to another. Malignant gliomas, by contrast, display hyperploidy (up to octaploid cells) or aneuploidy, and the ploidy varies from one area of the tumor to another.[12] The disordered distribution of nuclear DNA evidently betrays the disordered reproduction of cells in malignant gliomas. As PET shows, low-grade gliomas are quantitatively comparable in blood flow, oxygen utilization, and glucose consumption to the adjacent normal brain tissue. Although no difference exists in blood flow between low-grade and high-grade gliomas,[23] glucose consumption is much higher in the latter.[24] PET also shows, through the uptake of [11]C-l-methionine, a much higher rate of protein synthesis in high- than in low-grade gliomas.[25]

A mature glioma takes much longer to grow than does a glioblastoma. Noninvasive estimates have been made on serial CT scans, but few data exist on mature gliomas. Tsuboi and associates[26] evaluated the doubling time in four grade II astrocytomas and mixed gliomas at 937.3 ± 66.5 days and compared this with 48.1 ± 20.9 days on 11 glioblastomas. In mature gliomas, the production of daughter cells must be almost exactly equal to cell loss and inactivation. Hoshino[27] supplied a theoretical basis for this clinical intuition. Determining the LI at necropsy in patients in whom it had been determined before operation, he found that, unlike immature gliomas, the well-differentiated varieties conserved the labeled cells for a long time. He, therefore, called this mode of cell proliferation of low-grade gliomas "conservative." In malignant gliomas, all the daughter cells proliferate, whereas in low-grade gliomas, one of two appears to retain the capacity for mitosis, whereas the other loses it. As a result, the proliferating pool grows moderately while sterile nonproliferating cells are continually being added to the cell population; therefore, the GF progressively slackens (Fig. 56–2).

However, the most worrying aspect of the biology of low-grade gliomas is the possibility alluded to earlier of malignant degeneration over time. In a study of 137 recurrent low-grade gliomas, Müller and coworkers[28] found that only 14% of grade I astrocytomas had not changed grade by the time of the recurrence, whereas 55.5% had become grade II, and 30.5% had become glioblastomas. Similarly, of 23 grade I oligodendrogliomas, 15 (65.1%) had recurred as grade II oligodendrogliomas, and two (8.6%) as glioblastomas.[29] Laws and associates[14] found that at least half of the 79 low-grade astrocytomas in their series that recurred after treatment had turned into grade III or grade IV. Zülch,[2] in a series of 104 supratentorial astrocytomas, found malignant degeneration in 23%. Rubinstein,[30] who studied 129 glioblastomas at necropsy, estimated that about 20% may have derived from the malignant degeneration of low-grade astrocytomas. Piepmeier found that over a median follow-up of 8 years, 50% of the astrocytomas and 10% of the oligodendrogliomas recurred as higher grade.[1]

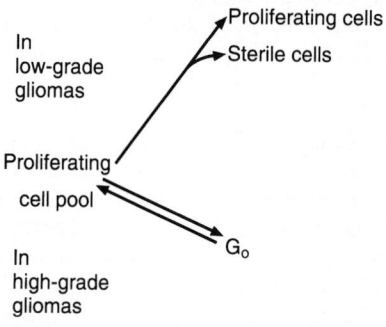

FIGURE 56–2 ■ Cytodynamic of low-grade gliomas.

In the series of Wallner and coworkers[31] 10 of the 29 patients with oligodendroglioma had a recurrence: at reoperation or at necropsy, only four had undergone no change, two had become glioblastomas, three had become grade III mixed gliomas, and one had become a grade II astrocytoma.

During the last 10 years, it has become evident that classification systems that are morphologically based are inadequate to describe either the biologic identity of these lesions or their biologic potential (malignant transformation).[32] The relevance of these features in the choice of therapeutic options and for determining a reliable prognosis has produced an overwhelming amount of studies on gliomas genetics and molecular biology, almost 75% of all the literature articles on the subject in recent years. A slow-growing tumor as the low-grade astrocytoma is expected to have a low proliferative activity. Many studies have identified as a measure of this activity the percentage of astrocytoma cells expressing the proliferation antigen Ki 67 MIB-1 (expressed during the entire cell cycle) and the proliferating nuclear antigen (PCNA) (only expressed during S1 phase). For a low-grade glioma the MIB-1 index should not exceed 4%.[33] MIB-1 expression reflects differences in biologic behavior, such as the rapid progression of a residual tumor or stable remaining tumor. MIB-1 LI is reported to be lower in "quiescent" tumors.[34]

However, it is a common experience that a variable percentage (50% to 85%) of low-grade gliomas undergo malignant transformation. The molecular neuropathologic basis of this process is the summation of significant genetic alterations.

These mutations concern two categories of genes: (1) oncosuppressors, and (2) oncogenes. As a consequence, the former will lose function in two stages. At the beginning, a copy of the gene is lost through an inactivating mutation, often a deletion. This situation may establish a predisposition to tumor formation. A second genetic event, however, is necessary for the complete inactivation of a suppressor gene. For oncogenes, mutations have an activating effect, and only one could be enough to induce a neoplastic phenotype.[35]

Cytogenetic analysis identified several alterations in pylocytic astrocytomas, but none is specific. In only few cases, a modification of oncosuppressor gene p53 has been described. Through a comparative genoma hybridization technique, detecting losses and gains of DNA copy number across the entire genoma, a constantly increased copy number of 8q emerged as the most frequent change in low-grade gliomas.[36]

Conversely, in diffuse astrocytomas, the p53 mutation is more frequent and may represent an indicator of malignant transformation. In fact, astrocytomas with a significant gemistocytic fraction, typically carrying a p53 mutation, seem to progress more rapidly.[37] Protoplasmic astrocytomas have low MIB-1 indices, and p53 reactivity is observed in a few of these tumors.[38]

p53 genes regulate the G1 phase of the cell cycle that activates p21, and its inactivation seems to play a relevant role in neoplastic progression, determining further genomic instability.[39] However, the function of p53 appears to prevent also DNA rupture, duplication errors, and anomalous regional genomic amplification, therefore deserving the appellative of DNA caretaker. In fact, the cell cycle is normally stopped by p53 to allow repair; if the latter is not possible, the cell undergoes apoptosis. Moreover p53 is claimed to function as genomic gatekeeper (i.e., regulate the expression of many genes).[40] There is evidence that the loss of only one allele for p53 increases the risk of tumorigenesis, suggesting that a decreased genic dosage is sufficient to compromise the surveillance function.[41] The implications for therapy of these data are evident. For instance, adenoviral vectors may carry a normal p53 gene in mutated tumoral cell nuclei.[42]

The cell kinetic of a low-grade glioma should differ only slightly from normal adult astrocytes, and the inactivation of p53 is a consequence not only of mutation or allelic loss but also of the so-called "transcriptional silencing".[43] The overexpression of MDM2, establishing a linkage to mutant or wild type p53 inhibits transcription.[44]

The overexpression of PDGFR (encoding for a growth factor) and the mutations of TP53, inactivating the p53, have often been indicated as responsible for the proliferative stimulus, with the contemporary inhibition of apoptosis. Bcl-2 is a proto-oncogene that also blocks apoptosis.[45] Apoptosis is a sequence of morphologic and biochemical changes that lead to cell death. Tumorigenesis is the consequence not only of cell proliferation but also of the loss of the ability to undergo apoptosis. These events provide the necessary genomic instability for further phenotype changes, cell cycle deregulation, and the selection of malignant cell clones. Although in slow-growing gliomas the cell cycle is not deregulated, grade II astrocytomas must have an unbalance between proliferative activity and apoptosis. Grade II astrocytomas have been divided in two groups with significantly different survival (1062 versus 1686 days), related to the value over or under 8% of the MIB LI. The presence of well-differentiated astrocytes with a high MIB LI suggests that cell cycle deregulation precedes further alterations with phenotypic transformation and that MIB LI might be used as a prognostic factor.[33]

There is still debate on the clonality of the resultant malignant tumors. The tumor is originated from confluent clones of multiple transformed cells or from a single cell clone. Polymerase chain reaction assay studies through amplification of a high polymorphic microsatellite marker locus suggested that low-grade and malignant gliomas are usually monoclonal and that tumor cell migration represents the basis for extensively infiltrating tumors.[46] Different populations of cells with diverse genetic alterations may coexist in the same tumor, but this appears to be a transitional state, because the cell clone with the more efficient features of growth will rapidly prevail.

Loss of heterozygosity (LOH) on chromosomes 19q and 1p are the commonest reported alterations in oligodendrogliomas. The loss of a chromosome region carrying the residual copy of an oncosuppressor gene is revealed by a contiguous marker absence, using DNA amplification.[47]

Many factors that are intrinsic or extrinsic to the cell microenvironment keep under control the replication and differentiation of the neuroepithelial cell. Growth and trophic factors are little proteic molecules identified in molecular biology studies that may represent potential pharmacologic agents to regulate neuroepithelial pathologic proliferation and differentiation. A peculiarity of this regulatory system is that the same factor may exert different and also opposite effects on neuroepithelial cells in different stages of differentiation or to neuroepithelial cells that belong to different parts of the nervous system.[48] This is probably the consequence of differences in number and type of growth factors receptors or of a fine modulatory intracellular process regarding transcription pathways of the signal generated after receptor-growth factor linkage. Therefore, tumors that are morphologically alike may differ substantially as far as their biologic behavior, only due to different receptor expression, thus disclosing further identification methods.

The transcriptional factors induce specific gene transcription, possibly modifying the cell phenotype. There are suggestions that activation of protein STAT 1 and STAT 2 by transcriptional factors allows differentiation toward an astrocytic phenotype of the neoplastic cells of the low-grade gliomas. Conversely, a differentiation to a high grade implies an inhibition of the pathway, determining lower levels of STAT proteins.[49] In view of future therapeutic application, this is evidence in favor of preservation of differentiation mechanisms also during oncogenesis.

Growth factors have been proved to determine the angiogenic potential of glioma cells, and angiogenesis has been used as a biologic marker for low-grade gliomas at risk of malignant transformation. Patients with more than seven microvessels counted on a 400 microscopic field of tumor tissue are reported to have a shorter survival time and a greater chance of tumor progression. Higher staining for vascular endothelial growth factor (VEGF) seems related to a worse prognosis.[50] Fibrillary astrocytomas, studied with determination of microvessel density and VEGF levels, appear not as a single pathologic entity but as a wide spectrum of tumors with a different attitude to malignant transformation. VEGF secretion may also represent the common pathway of microvascularization and progression to glioblastomas.[51] The p53 gene is thought to regulate VEGF and, consequently, tumor neovascularization.[52]

The recent progress in molecular neuropathology helped to discover anomalies of oncogenes and tumor suppressor genes, new sites for putative tumor suppressor genes (through microsatellite analysis), and peculiar molecular pathways for each tumor type. The presence of alterations in cell cycle regulatory genes of anaplastic gliomas may explain their amazing growth potential. Autocrine and paracrine growth factors and their respective protein receptors appear to contribute to glial and endothelial cell proliferation. The pattern of genetic alterations will help to further differentiate histopathologic entities into genetic distinct groups and to better define the mechanisms of angiogenesis. The common target is to establish a correlation between histopathologic, molecular, and clinical data.

## NEURODIAGNOSTIC IMAGING

The "typical" imaging features for the diagnosis of a low-grade glioma in an adult patient were considered: CT scan hypodensity, without contrast enhancement; lack of contrast enhancement on a CT scan; hypointensity on short TR $T_1$-weighted and hyperintensity on long TR $T_2$-

weighted MRI scans; no contrast enhancement on MRI.[53] Nevertheless, further experience has demonstrated the unreliability of these parameters also in high standard radiodiagnostics. Forty-eight biopsies performed by Bernstein contradicted the radiologic diagnosis in 31.3% of cases, and a refutation of neuroimaging-based hypotheses followed the 20 bioptic procedures of Kondziolka in 50% of cases. Unrecognized pathologies included higher grade gliomas, oligodendrogliomas, mixed astrocytomas, and inflammatory lesions. However, the opinions of these authors are not convergent when the treatment of these patients has to be considered: histologic diagnostic confirmation with biopsy is imperative for Kondziolka, whereas Bernstein reserves biopsy for lesions that are very likely to be treated surgically. Bernstein recommends observation for others.[53, 54]

Berger analyzed different MRI aspects of low-grade tumors while looking for a correlation with the histologic type. He concluded that neither the presence of a cyst, nor the degree of mass effect, nor the cortical or subcortical location, nor the ratio of tumor volume $T_1$-weighted/$T_2$-weighted, nor the diameter of the tumor, nor the presence of hemorrhage, nor vascular flow voids have any predictive value for histology. Only $T_1$ hypointensity seems to correlate well with the softness of a tumor at surgery. This could be explained by the loose structure of astrocytoma presenting with a microcystic mesh with some degree of mucinous degeneration. Less hypointense lesions express a firmer architecture as typically seen in oligodendrogliomas and mixed astrocytomas.[55]

Further steps in characterization of low-grade gliomas with a propensity to malignant transformation and in tumor boundary definition are represented by PET and high-resolution magic angle spinning proton (HRMS 1H) magnetic resonance.

11c Methionine PET has been reported to be useful to detect changes in the endothelium and blood-brain barrier related to malignant low-grade glioma transformation.[56] It proved to be better than fluorodeoxyglucose in delineating the borders of low-grade gliomas, but methionine uptake cannot differentiate anaplastic gliomas.[57]

A [201]TI SPECT scan has been claimed to enable differential diagnosis between low-grade and high-grade gliomas. Although less expensive than PET, it may give false-positive results in low-grade gliomas. It demonstrates high sensitivity for tumors with a bromodeoxyuridine LI equal or inferior to 5%.[58]

HRMAS 1H magnetic resonance spectroscopy produces well-resolved spectra of metabolites from an intact tissue specimen. The metabolic ratio presented the highest sensitivity in differentiating normal tissue from a tumor as well as in distinguishing between tumor groups. For instance, the resonance ratio of inositol to creatine may help to differentiate the tumor type.[59]

HRMAS 1H for choline showed that all progressive astrocytomas had elevated choline levels of more than 45%, whereas stable cases showed an elevation of less than 35%, no change, or even a decreased signal.[60]

1H NMR spectra of human brain tumor homogenates revealed a broad resonance at 5.3 to 5.4 ppm in glioblastomas and is not detectable in low-grade gliomas. This resonance has been identified as ceramide, a sphingosine–fatty acid combination portion of ganglioside (with an immunosuppressive activity), indicating an abundance of monounsaturated fatty acids. It is suggested that a role of aberrant ganglioside and ceramide precursors on the grade of malignancy and invasiveness.[61]

There is evidence that no major difference exists between the PET investigation of glucose metabolism and the less expensive SPECT measurement of amino acid uptake ([123]I α-methyl thyrosine, [123]IMT).[62]

## MANAGEMENT DECISIONS

With the advances in neurodiagnostics, the pathology that confronts the clinician today is different from what it was two decades ago, and this development requires new and more demanding decisions. In the days of angiography, encephalography, and radionuclide scanning, low-grade cerebral gliomas reached the surgeon after years of history, when they had grown large, with mass effect and signs of hypertension. These gliomas sometimes already contained foci of dedifferentiation inside. Today, at the first convulsive seizures, CT and MRI reveal small, less malignant tumors in patients who are neurologically intact. When it is considered that this pathology arises in young individuals on the convexity of a cerebral hemisphere, frequently beside "eloquent" cortical and subcortical areas, the magnitude of the dilemma facing the surgeon becomes clear.[63]

Although oncologic surgery should generally be performed as early and as radically as possible, some contend that an operation should be postponed when serial scanning shows no change in the volume or structure of the lesion. Others argue that biopsy plus radiotherapy is just as effective as surgical resection. Yet others[17] question the use of radiotherapy, because of its long-term detrimental effects, and assert that because these patients never die as a result of a progression of the low-grade tumor but instead of its malignant degeneration, a management strategy designed to prevent dedifferentiation would be just as effective as eradication of the original tumor. The point is highly controversial and must be examined from several perspectives (Table 56–1).

### TABLE 56–1 ■ SURGERY IN LOW-GRADE GLIOMAS

| Indications | Reasons Why Surgery is Questionable |
|---|---|
| Diagnosis and classification | Risk of postoperative deficits in a young, neurologically sound patient with a long life expectancy |
| Debulking the mass and alleviating symptoms | |
| Reducing the proliferating cell pool | Early surgery has not been proved to lengthen survival |
| Decreasing the number of cells inherently resistant to radiation therapy | There is no significant correlation between the extent of surgical resection and the length of survival |
| Preventing or reducing the risk of increase in malignancy | |
| Cytoreduction makes subsequent radiotherapy more effective | |
| Chemotherapy has proved ineffective in all cases | |

Surgery is questioned first because of the risk of postoperative deficits in a young, neurologically sound patient with a long life expectancy. This situation requires the utmost precision in the diagnosis of the anatomic limits of the tumor and the functional status of the most important adjacent nervous structures.

Second, early surgery has yet to be proved to improve survival. As is discussed later in the section on results, one of the factors in long-term survival is a long preoperative history. The follow-up study of Laws and coworkers,[64] which is one of the most important studies in terms of numbers and time span, makes this point.

Third, no proof exists that more generous resection correlates significantly with longer survival. A correlation of this kind, generally valid for any tumor, is argued by Salcman,[65] who cites Laws and associates.[14] However, although Laws and associates found a significantly higher 5-year survival rate among patients who had undergone total removal than among those who had undergone biopsy and subtotal removal or radical subtotal removal, statistical significance was not maintained at 15 years, total removal excluded. Furthermore, as these authors state, the most favorable lesions tend to be treated more radically, and the least favorable (deep-seated, infiltrative, noncystic), more sparingly. Weir and Grace,[66] Piepmeier,[16] and Vertosick and colleagues[17] deny any significant correlation between the extent of surgical resection and the length of survival.

All these points, which tend to undermine the importance of surgery in low-grade cerebral gliomas, are counterbalanced by the following considerations, according to which surgery is indicated: (1) for diagnosis and classification, (2) for debulking the mass and relieving symptoms, (3) for reducing the proliferating cell pool, (4) for preventing or reducing the risk of degeneration, (5) for decreasing the number of cells inherently refractory to radiotherapy, (6) because cell reduction makes subsequent radiotherapy more effective, and (7) because chemotherapy has proved ineffective.

Each of these assertions calls for comment. First, surgery is valuable as a diagnostic check on a patch of low density on a CT scan and on one of low intensity in the $T_1$ sequences and of increased intensity in the $T_2$ sequences of MRI. A tumor must be differentiated from an infective or vascular lesion, and the borders of the tumor must be demarcated from the surrounding edema. The tumor must be typed not only histologically but also, if possible, for proliferative potential by immunochemistry (antibromodeoxyuridine monoclonal antibodies for the LI and anti-Ki-67 antigen for the GF). For these purposes, stereotactic surgery may be preferred to open surgery, a point that is discussed in Chapter 52. Surgical resection is needed for debulking the mass and palliating symptoms when a glioma is discovered at a late stage and has already grown large. In any case, surgical resection reduces the proliferating pool and delays the growth of the tumor. As Hoshino[27] pointed out, low-grade gliomas differ from more malignant gliomas in the lack of cellular traffic between the nonproliferating pool and the proliferating pool (see Fig. 56–2). In low-grade gliomas, the conservative mode of proliferation ensures the continual addition to the cell population of sterile, permanently nonproliferating cells (for which there is no return to the reproductive cycle). In glioblastoma, by

contrast, frequent reciprocal traffic exists between nonproliferating and proliferating cells: its growth may be depressed by cell bunching; partial surgical resection may stimulate the cells in $G_0$ to return to the proliferating pool and thus end, paradoxically, by accelerating tumor growth. Nonetheless, surgical resection, however satisfactory, is always limited. As Sano[67] reminded us, 99% removal of a tumor corresponds with only a 2-log reduction of the number of cells that constitute a neoplastic population ($10^7$ to $10^8$).

As we have seen, at the time of a recurrence, low-grade gliomas exhibit increased malignancy and resistance to treatment. Because it is not known which cells will be subject to dedifferentiation or what factors contribute to the process, the risk is presumably proportional to the number of neoplastic cells. Therefore, the most extensive cytoreduction possible should be advantageous. In addition, no one has ever suggested that surgical resection may favor dedifferentiation. On the evidence of Vertosick and associates,[17] two points emerge: (1) patients who present dedifferentiation tended to be diagnosed at a younger age than did those who did not (mean of 33 versus 43 years), and (2) those who received radiotherapy underwent dedifferentiation an average of 5.4 years later than did those who did not (3.7 years later). However, these data are preliminary data and have not been statistically validated.

When does a low-grade glioma degenerate—that is, at what stage in its natural history? How can the change be detected in time? Clinical experience shows that dedifferentiation occurs several years after the initial symptoms of the tumor—on average 5 years after, in the 12 cases of Francavilla and coworkers,[68] with a range of 1.5 to 10 years. PET with $^{18}$Fluorodeoxyglucose is currently the most sensitive tool for detecting incipient malignant transformation, which manifests increased metabolism (increased glucose consumption), is focal (in agreement with the histologic data) and is similar to the hypermetabolic state observed in de novo malignant gliomas. One PET scan at one point in the natural history may not have predictive value, any more than does a histologic examination performed at that time. Serial PET scans are needed to identify variations in the biologic behavior of a tumor.

Apart from all the foregoing reasons, surgical resection is indicated in low-grade gliomas because no concrete alternative exists, given their biologic resistance to chemotherapy and scant sensitivity to radiotherapy. The cellular kinetics and metabolism of these oncotypes, which differ little from those of healthy nervous tissue, and the integrity of the blood-brain barrier prevent cytostatic agents from entering the tumor with a higher concentration gradient than that of the surrounding healthy tissue.[65] Radiotherapy is recommended in only a few cases, as is discussed later.

In conclusion, we can share in part the statements of Bernstein[69] regarding the presumed absence of negative prognostic factors in a patient younger than 40 years of age, with epilepsy but without neurologic deficits, harboring a low-density intrinsic lesion, without enhancement and without mass effect. As mentioned, molecular markers may enhance the predictive accuracy. For a patient older than 40 years, with or without neurologic deficits, mass effect, or enhancement, we think that more aggressive treatment should be considered. For lobar lesions, we recommend the most radical surgery followed by radiotherapy; for deeper or "diffuse" lesions (particularly if located in "eloquent" areas), stereotactic biopsy and radiotherapy should be the treatment of choice.

## PATIENT SELECTION AND CHOICE OF SURGICAL APPROACH

The factors in favor of surgical treatment for slow-growing gliomas outweigh those in favor of waiting or abstaining both in number and in importance.

The surgical choice is between open resection and stereotactic surgery followed by other treatment (irradiation or interstitial radiotherapy). The criteria for the stereotactic option depend, according to Salcman,[70] on the characteristics of: (1) the tumor (centrally sited, poorly demarcated, extremely small, containing a large cyst or changing character); (2) the patient (either too ill for a craniotomy or neurologically intact); and (3) subsequent treatment (catheter-based, requires repeated sampling). "In essence, the same criteria employed in the selection of open versus closed techniques can be applied to low-grade tumors, but with more stringent emphasis on neurologic condition and radiographic definition."[65] In summary, in the case of low-grade cerebral glioma, as for almost all other central nervous system diseases, surgical treatment must be tailored to the neurologic status and social needs of the patient, to the site and size of the lesion, to the ability of the surgeon, and to the facilities available to him or her. General directives can come only from randomized prospective studies conducted over a sufficiently long time by several institutions on series matched for pathology, patient selection, and management.

## PREOPERATIVE EVALUATION

The brain is a singular organ in that many of its main functions are represented on its surface. Areas of the cortex both near and distant are connected subcortically by short and long associative fibers. A surgeon preparing to approach a subcortical hemispheric glioma traditionally has the problem of tumor projection to the surface in relation to the functionally most important cortex and its principal projections. Neuroimaging now solves this problem noninvasively. The rolandic fissure, which delineates the sensorimotor cortex, has always been the pole star of the topography of the cerebral cortex, something that Giacomini intuited in Turin in 1878.[71] That the rolandic fissure is the pole star does not, of course, apply to polar so much as to "central" sites: it is no accident that in the English-speaking world, the rolandic fissure is the central sulcus and the rolandic convolutions, the pre- and postcentral gyri. On the basis of careful studies on cadavers, Giacomini found a way of projecting the central sulcus onto the skull surface by means of an ingenious pair of cardboard compasses. The transverse line from ear to ear, intercepted at the vertex by the sagittal midline, is divided into segments, one on either side. When the vertical leg of the compasses is centered on the central point of one segment, the other leg, inclined at 30 degrees, identifies the sulcus (Fig. 56–3). Constant in site, unlikely to be displaced, especially in its medial portion, the pararolandic cortex is now detectable

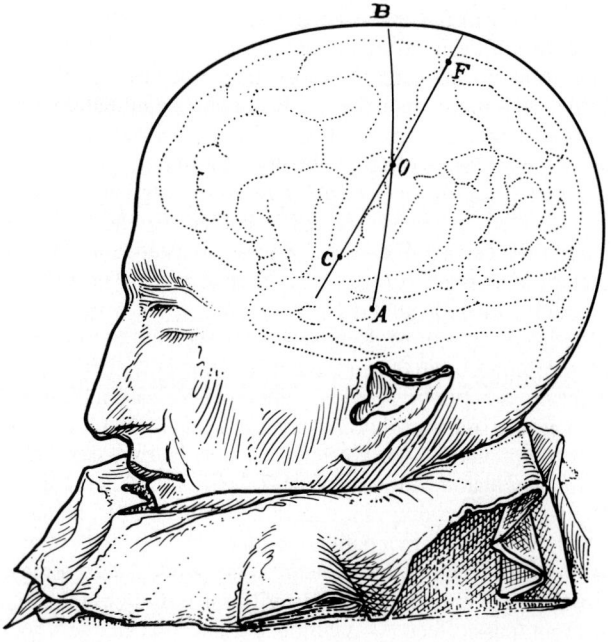
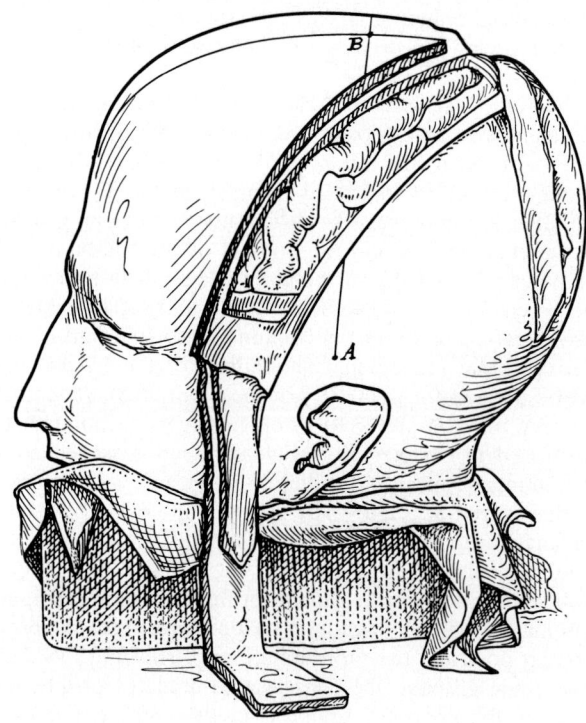

FIGURE 56–3 ■ Goniometric identification of the central sulcus. (From Giacomini C: Guida allo studio delle circonvoluzioni cerebrali dell'uomo, 2nd ed. Torino: E Loescher, 1884.)

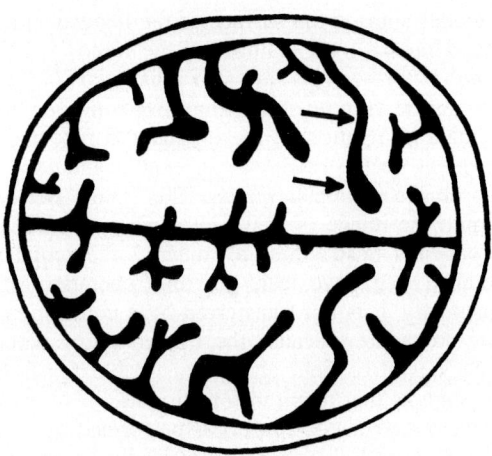

FIGURE 56–4 ■ Tomographic aspect of the central sulcus.

in the highest axial CT cuts (Fig. 56–4). Parasagittal MRI sections locate the central sulcus through the cingulate and marginal sulci. Less accurately, the lower half of the rolandic cortex is shown adjacent to the lateral sulcus: lateral sagittal MRI sections identify it with the perpendicular to the posterior roof of the insula (Fig. 56–5).[72] To identify the whole length of the central sulcus, three-dimensional MRI is needed.[73] Imaged on the lateral surface of the hemisphere are also the inferior frontal gyrus and the superior temporal gyrus, which in the left hemisphere comprise Broca's area and the auditory area, respectively. Thus, a large part of the cortex, which is known traditionally as being "eloquent," is located via the rolandic area.

This precise anatomic definition supplied by neuroimaging may not be sufficient for planning and performing the operation for several reasons. First, the anatomic structures may be displaced or distorted, especially by slow-growing space-occupying lesions, such as the ones that we are considering; therefore, the anatomic landmarks may be unreliable. The surgical damage feared by surgeons on the basis of the standard anatomic landmarks is, surprisingly and fortunately, not usually found in the postoperative course. Second, major centers and nervous pathways may

or may not be infiltrated, damaged, or interrupted by the neoplastic process; the surgeon should know their functional status. Third, although the sensorimotor cortex is more constant in its anatomy, the cortex related to language and cognitive functions has a much more variable and complex organization, hence the need to see the functional data for the various cortical areas alongside or superimposed on the anatomic images. PET and single photon emission computed tomography, which supply quantitative maps of physiologic, biochemical, and biophysical parameters but have poor spatial anatomic resolution, are superimposed on CT and MRI in the "computerized brain atlas."[74-77] The performance of various motor, verbal, and cognitive tasks or sensory stimulation is known to show a constant focal increase on PET, both in the glucose metabolism and in regional cerebral blood flow in certain areas of the cerebral cortex. For practical reasons, the regional blood flow has been investigated by use of $H_2^{15}O$. Once again, the rolandic cortex has proved to be the easiest to study, both on the motor side and on the sensory side: images are altered during either the performance of simple motor tasks involving a single limb or during sensory stimulation of it. Language, being a more complex function, still defies precise localization: numerous areas of the cortex and circuits are involved in the act of repeating words heard or of generating new ones; the nervous pathways activated in the production of new words and in getting used to them (repeating a list of names) are numerous. PET performed volunteers and the speech map obtained by Ojemann and coworkers[78] by intraoperative stimulation (arrest or error in naming known objects presented) agree on the following: (1) extreme individual variation, (2) language cannot be located reliably on purely anatomic criteria, and (3) the traditional area of Broca needs to be revised.

Nariai and colleagues[79] pointed out that a glioma may be located within a single gyrus without altering its external morphology. Alternatively, a tumor may cause swelling or distortion of the cortical surface of the gyrus. In the latter situation, three-dimensional MRI may not warrant the identification of "eloquent" areas, and the functional mapping

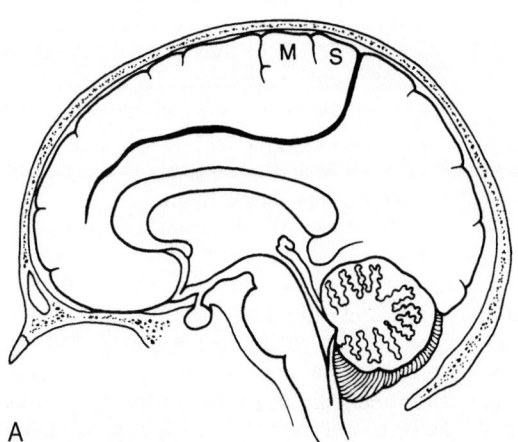

A

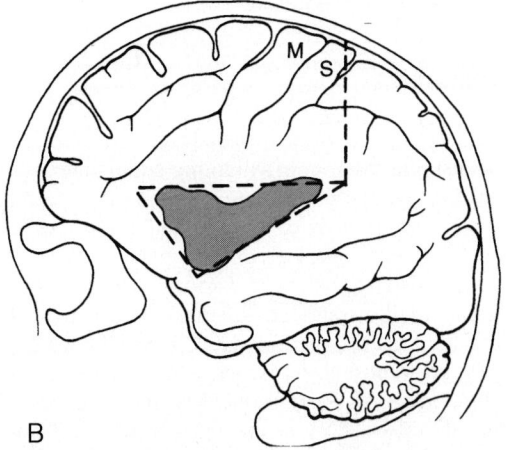

B

FIGURE 56–5 ■ Geometric identification of central sulcus on magnetic resonance imaging. *A*, The parasagittal plane: the cingulate sulcus ends superiorly as the marginal sulcus; *B*, The far lateral sagittal plane.

with PET 11C-methionine seems to offer the necessary accuracy.

## ANESTHETIC CONSIDERATIONS AND AIDS TO SURGERY

Craniotomy for cerebral glioma is almost always performed with the patient under general anesthesia and with monitoring of various parameters (e.g., electrocardiographic reading, arterial pressure, central venous pressure, and blood gas analysis) and checking of the fluid balance. Black and Ronner[80] and Walsh and associates[81] have mapped the sensorimotor and language cortex in a few cooperative patients by use of electrical stimulation while the patients were under local anesthesia. Systemic anesthetic agents were used occasionally on completion of the mapping studies. Ebeling and colleagues[82] localized the motor cortex intraoperatively with patients under general anesthesia and with temporary decurarization. However, these are all isolated experiments. Somatosensory evoked potentials are more widely used for illustrating the rolandic cortex when tumors are adjacent to it. They require appropriate screening of the operating room to reduce artifacts. For cortical mapping, Berger and colleagues,[83] operate on patients who are awake with mild fentanyl sedation, using a local anesthetic for the scalp. Alternatively, during bone flap removal, propofol provides a deep sedative effect that can be reversed in 10 minutes.

Obviously, the operating microscope and microsurgical instruments, bipolar cautery, ultrasonic aspirators, and laser equipment are now part of routine neurosurgical practice. B-mode ultrasound with surface ultrasound probes is also useful in cases of subcortical glioma, as is explained later.

Last, the spatial incompatibility between cumbersome neurodiagnostic machines (CT, MRI, and digital angiography) and operating room demands, and also between stereotactic frames and free-hand surgery, has been overcome at a few leading centers by means of sophisticated and complex equipment. The precision of stereotactic methods is often needed in the surgery for gliomas.

## SURGICAL TECHNIQUE

### Craniotomy

The importance of neuroimaging, especially with three-dimensional MRI, in highlighting simultaneously the tumor and the layout of the cortex of the entire cerebral hemisphere concerned with its main sulci and gyri has already been discussed. The cerebral hemisphere can, furthermore, be sectioned according to various planes on the computer display to illustrate the relations between the tumor and the deep-seated structures (e.g., internal capsule, basal nuclei, and ventricular cavities). MR angiography relies on "angiographic" pulse sequences that potentiate the signal from the blood flow at the expense of that from the static tissues. Thus, the relations between the tumor and the cerebral vascular network are studied on the three-dimen-

sional model both on the surface of the hemisphere and in sections. The structural features of the tumor (e.g., cysts, calcifications, or necrosis) are also illustrated.

Knowing the volume and spatial disposition of the neoplastic mass in relation to the eloquent cortex and to no less eloquent deep structures can enable simulation of a test flap on the computer screen. This image is then projected onto the image of the skull surface and transferred to the patient's head either by means of external points of reference (e.g., eye, ear, previous operation scar) or stereotactically. It is not transferred by a conventional stereotactic procedure, because the frame or ring would obstruct the operative field and is unsuitable for free-hand surgery, such as that required for gliomas.

Frameless stereotactic surgery is performed by means of a localizing arm.[84] The five-part jointed arm operated by the surgeon is connected to a graphic-oriented computer (Fig. 56–6). Its tip, which runs along the surface of the skull, records the coordinates of each point on it in relation to reference points consisting of three metal pins, which are lodged noncolinearly in sterile conditions (under local anesthesia) in the patient's scalp. These skull markers, which appear on the two CT scout scans (anteroposterior and lateral), likewise constitute the points of reference of the CT coordinates. Because the arm coordinates and CT coordinates are correlated in the same computer, after appropriate calibration, the tip of the localizing arm that runs along the skull surface is shown on the CT scan by a cursor. The optimal approach to the underlying tumor, even if it is small, can easily be centered. The craniotomy is thus targeted and personalized. It may consist of a trephine hole 4 to 5 cm in diameter. The chosen approach need not be the most direct, but it must be the safest for the neurologic integrity of the patient.

### Cortical Approach

In surgeries for subcortical lesions that do not emerge on the surface, the following procedure is used. After the dura mater is opened, the surgeon has to recognize the tumor, size up its spatial relations with the adjacent structures, and decide where to incise the cortex. B-mode ultrasound[85, 86] now replaces manual palpation: it localizes the tumor in relation to the cortex, to the underlying ventricle, to the falx, to the tentorium, or to the bony base; it also characterizes the tumor structure (calcifications or secluded cysts), specifies its volume,[87] and demarcates its margins. Although CT shows low-grade gliomas as hypodense, ultrasonography shows them as hyperechogenic.[86] The surrounding edema appears as hypoechogenic or very faintly echogenic against the healthy parenchyma.[87]

Even when the dura mater has been opened, recognition of the eloquent cortex and its relations with paracentral tumors is not necessarily straightforward. The smallness of the craniotomy opening, the extreme variability of the morphology of the cortical sulci even in normal individuals, and the asymmetry of a given sulcus in the two hemispheres may make recognition of the areas of reference difficult,[88] the more so because of the adjacent pathology. Once again, neurophysiologic methods are helpful, mainly in the topography of the rolandic cortex. Easiest to obtain

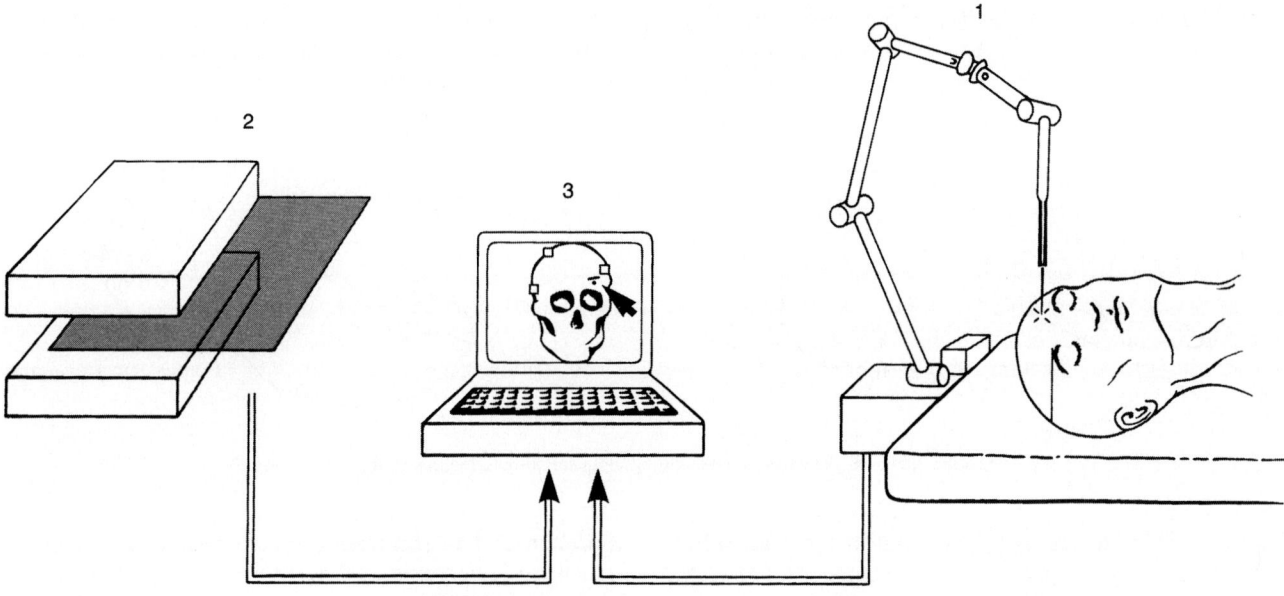

**FIGURE 56–6** ■ Frameless stereotactic surgery system.

and most constant (reproducible) is the cortical representation of the hand by somatosensory evoked potentials on stimulation of the contralateral median nerve. With the patient under general anesthesia, the topography of the hand is clear on both gyri separated by the central sulcus. The potentials are approximately mirrored in form on the two sides, the $P_{20}$–$N_{30}$ waves being of greater amplitude in the precentral area and the $N_{20}$–$P_{30}$ waves, in the postcentral area (Fig. 56–7).[89] Focal somatosensory evoked potentials of great amplitude have also been obtained from the posterosuperior bank of the sylvian fissure. Could this be a secondary somatosensory area?[90] Unfortunately, evoked potentials are not as helpful in identifying the visual and auditory cortex intraoperatively.

The cortex involved in the expression of language can only be demarcated by stimulation with the patient under local anesthesia. Electrostimulation of the cortex, pioneered by Bartholow[91] and Horsley[92] and later systematized by Penfield and Boldrey,[93] still has applications for delineation of speech areas,[78] as already discussed. Whatever the means used, the neurophysiologic identification of the eloquent cortex is not only an aid in the planning of an operation but also in its execution. Because of possible displacement by the tumor, the surgeon is freer to be more aggressive than if he or she is working only from anatomic landmarks.

However, is there really a "silent" cortex? Brodmann's areas 1 through 7, 17 through 19, 27 through 28, and (in the dominant hemisphere) 40 through 45, are considered to be eloquent (Fig. 56–8). The problem with the remainder of the cortex is that it gives no elementary responses to stimulation; rather it is involved in complex mechanisms of neurophysiologic and neuropsychological integration, and it does not give signals in laboratory animals that are easily applied to humans. Furthermore, although projection fibers (motor, special, or general sensory) underlie the eloquent cortex, short and long intrahemispheric associative fibers underlie the rest.

Desire to spare the lobar cortex and underlying fibers as

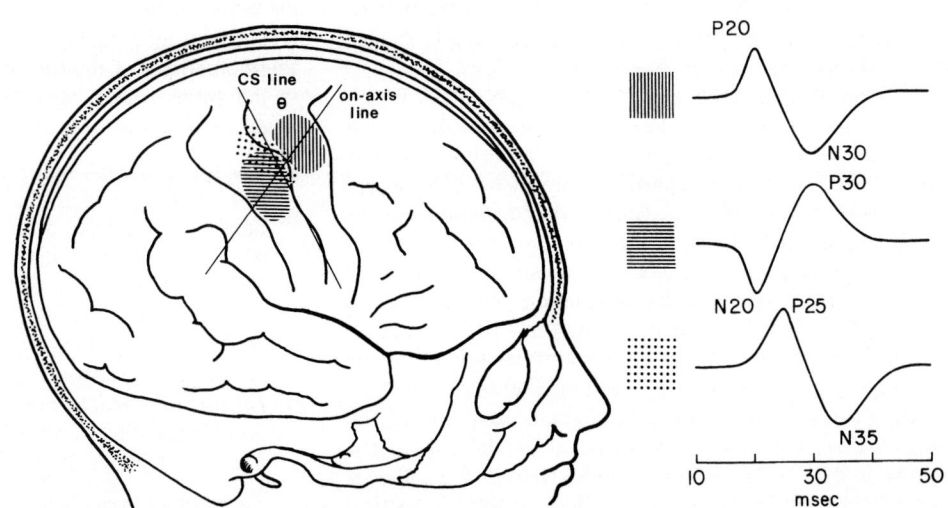

**FIGURE 56–7** ■ Somatosensory evoked potential–guided mapping of the cortical sensory motor area. (From Wood CC, Spencer DD, Allison T, et al: Localization of human sensory motor cortex during surgery by cortical surface recording of somatosensory evoked potentials. J Neurosurg 68:99–111, 1988.)

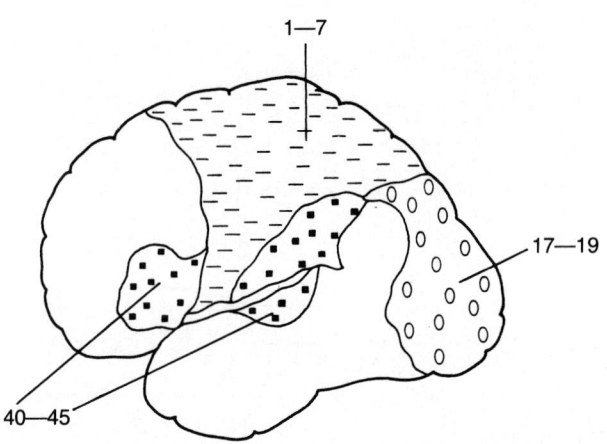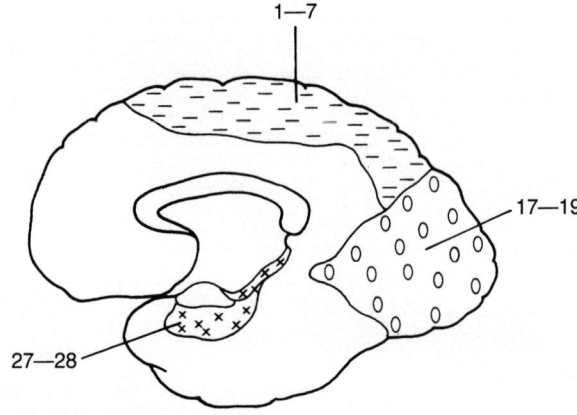

**FIGURE 56–8** ■ Schematic topography of eloquent cortical regions of the brain.

far as possible has led to the proposal of the trans-sulcal surgical approach[94, 95]: by using these natural corridors, the surgeon can go down 2 to 3 cm in pseudodepth without incising tissue, thus remaining outside the brain. Furthermore, because the sulci, especially the major ones, are full of fluid, their opening ensures decompressive depletion, hence the renewed interest in the anatomy of the cerebral sulci.[88, 96] Several varieties of sulci are recognized: limiting, axial, opercular, and complete (Fig. 56–9). Their extreme variation from one individual to another and between hemispheres in a single individual is confirmed, and efforts are being made to define the numerous ways in which one sulcus continues with another (full, partial, or simulated communication). The depth of some sulci has been measured on several specimens: the superior frontal sulcus is 17 to 24 mm deep; the superior temporal, 15 to 25 mm; and the junction of the interparietal with the postcentral sulcus, 20 to 27 mm.[97] The course of the blood vessels in the sulci is not uniform: some descend to the bottom of the sulcus before penetrating the brain substance, whereas others only cross the sulcus to rise to the top of the adjacent gyrus.[61] In either case, they are easily dissected between the arachnoid trabeculations of the sulcus or retracted toward one or the other gyrus with a spatula. An advantage of a transsulcal over a transgyral incision is that the cortex is less thick at the bottom of a sulcus than at the summit of a gyrus. A disadvantage is that an incision at the bottom of a sulcus interrupts the subcortical associative U-shaped fibers that connect two neighboring gyri.

On superficial inspection, deciding which sulcus to approach is not always easy. The arachnoid must be incised at several points to distinguish first the deep from the shallow sulci and from a sulcus-like impression of an artery on the cortex (Fig. 56–10).[6] Rarely, minute blood vessels obstruct access to a sulcus; if they do, they must be cauterized and cut (Fig. 56–11). Not only must the depth of the sulcus be noted but also its orientation with respect to the cortical plane. In normal brains, the sulci are almost perpendicular to the surface. A subcortical tumor diverts their course (Fig. 56–12). The tumor, therefore, must be sought via the compressed and oblique deep sulci. The incision does not have to be made at the bottom of the sulcus; it can be made in a lateral wall if the latter is closer to the tumor (Fig. 56–13).[6] Both in the trans-sulcal

approach and in the transgyral approach, the primary branches of the superficial arteries can still be dissected fairly comfortably because they remain outside the parenchyma in the Virchow-Robin space.

Because the operating microscope is an optical instrument, it is Yasargil's impression that the divergence of the light beams enables the surgeon to work at a depth of 10 to 12 cm through an opening 1.5 cm long and 0.5 cm wide (Fig. 56–14).[95] However small the cortical incision is, it nonetheless interrupts an enormous number of neurons and their connections and fibers. A wedge of cortex with a section that is 1 mm$^2$ and 2.5 mm deep contains up to 60,000 neurons. Neuronal density varies, of course, from one area of the cortex to another, being greatest in the striate area and lowest, perhaps, in the precentral gyrus.

## Tumor Resection

Microsurgical debulking of the tumor proceeds piecemeal from its center to its periphery. The resultant cavity is cleared with a spatula only when it allows gentle, nontraumatic retraction of the adjacent tissue. Last comes resection of the peripheral zone of tumor infiltration, which is biologically the most active because it is consists of the largest number of neoplastic cells proliferating and migrating into the adjacent tissue.

The operative plane is established according to the objective conditions of the tumor and subjective factors relating to the surgeon and the patient.[70] The following situations cover most cases (Fig. 56–15)[6]:

1. *Superficial tumor infiltrating only one gyrus*: tumor resection must spare the long fibers projecting to neighboring gyri and converging deep to the tumor margins. Preservation of vessels is the main problem.
2. *Tumor infiltrating more than one gyrus on the surface*: a larger number of long projection fibers is sacrificed, but other long fibers converging from the healthy cortex must be spared in depth.
3. *Diffuse subcortical tumor*: resection deafferents the underlying intact cortex and intercepts a certain number of intact fibers.

For solid gliomas diffusely infiltrating the centrum ovale,

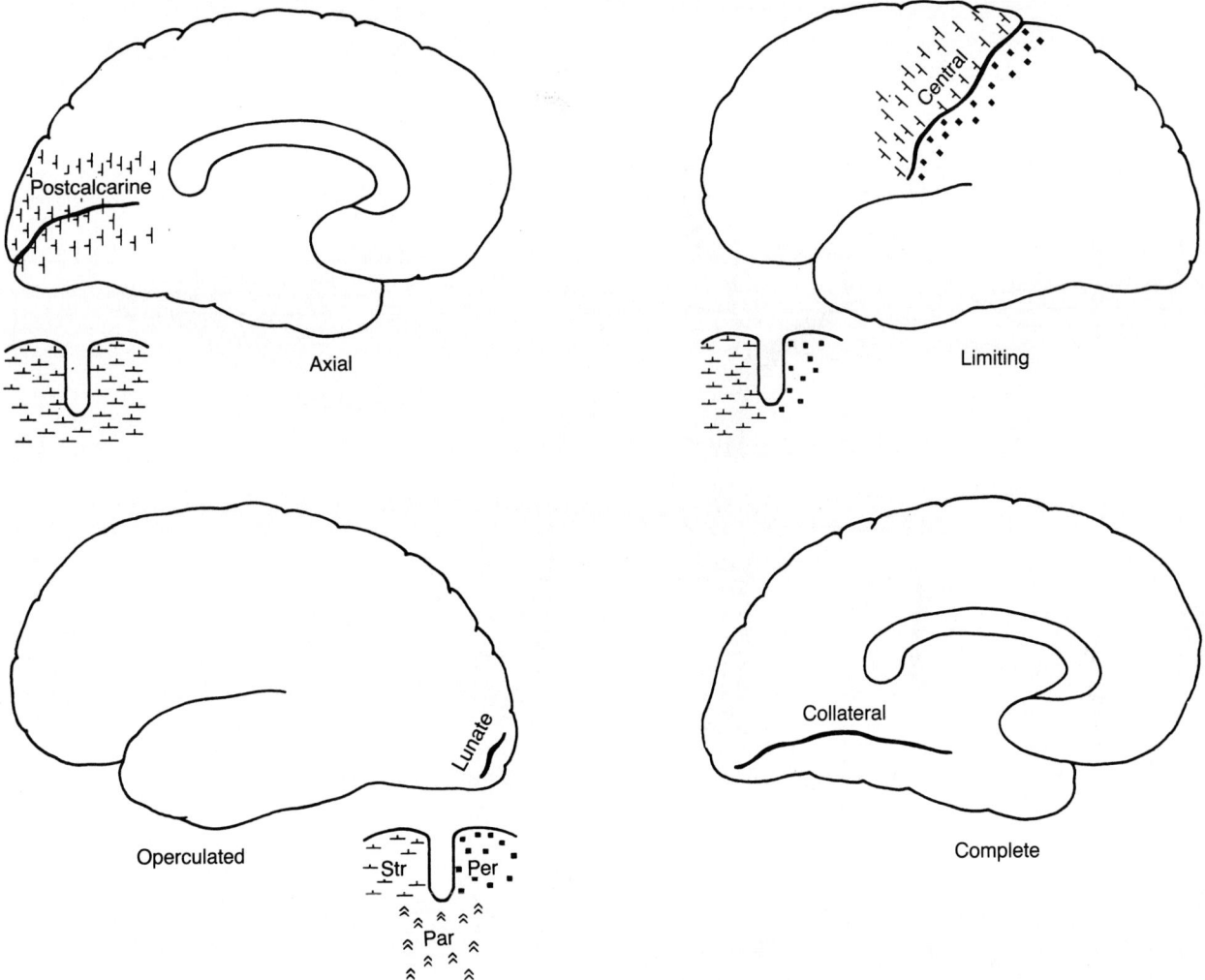

**FIGURE 56–9** ■ The four types of cortical sulci: *Axial*: an infolding in homogeneous areas. *Limiting*: separates the cortex into two areas different both for morphology and function. *Operculated*: separates distinct functional areas at its entrance, and often a third area of function is present in its floor (e.g., the lunate sulcus separating with its walls the striate, peristriate, and parastriate areas). *Complete*: that which is so deep that it produces an elevation in the ventricular walls.

a lobectomy is not indicated, because it does not prolong life and results in psychological deficits. This type of tumor develops deeper than the cortex. Under the cortex, the limits to resection are the allocortical areas, the basal nuclei, and the internal capsule. A selective tumorectomy, whether centrotumoral or including as much as possible of the marginal zone, affords the same survival and better health. The rare cystic astrocytomas of the cerebral hemispheres are much less of a surgical problem. The pilocytic variety is particularly favorable because simple resection of the mural nodule yields a good short-and long-term result, regardless of whether the cyst wall is completely removed. There are suggestions that contrast enhancement of the cyst wall at CT or MR requires its complete removal to ensure radicality.[98] Brachytherapy has been used for small tumors and restricted to selected areas of the brain. Sealed radioactive isotopes, such as [192]Ir or [125]I, are stereotactically positioned usually in cases of a recurrence of a postsurgical glioma.[99]

Ultrasonic aspiration[100] has several advantages over the former combined use of aspirating cannula and electric

loop in the debulking of a solid tumor. A single instrument leaves the operating field freer, minimizes mechanical damage to nervous tissue (traction), and eliminates damage resulting from heating. Observed in slow motion, the ultrasonic aspirator works in three stages: (1) fragmentation of the tissue adjacent to the vibrating tip within a radius of not more than 2 mm, (2) suspension of the fragmented tissue in irrigating fluid supplied by the instrument, and (3) aspiration of the aqueous emulsion. The power of the vibrating tip and of aspiration is adjustable. The speed of action depends on the consistency of the tissue to be removed. However, the lower the power of fragmentation, the less the damage will occur to the vascular framework. Fragmentation is selective for a tissue with a large aqueous component and spares the vessel walls, which have collagenous and elastic components. The tiny vessels are freed from the surrounding parenchyma and are easily cauterized without being torn. Hard or moderately calcified, poorly vascularized, low-grade gliomas are an elective indication for the ultrasonic aspirator. Because the instrument does not provide for hemostasis, this is handled by bipolar

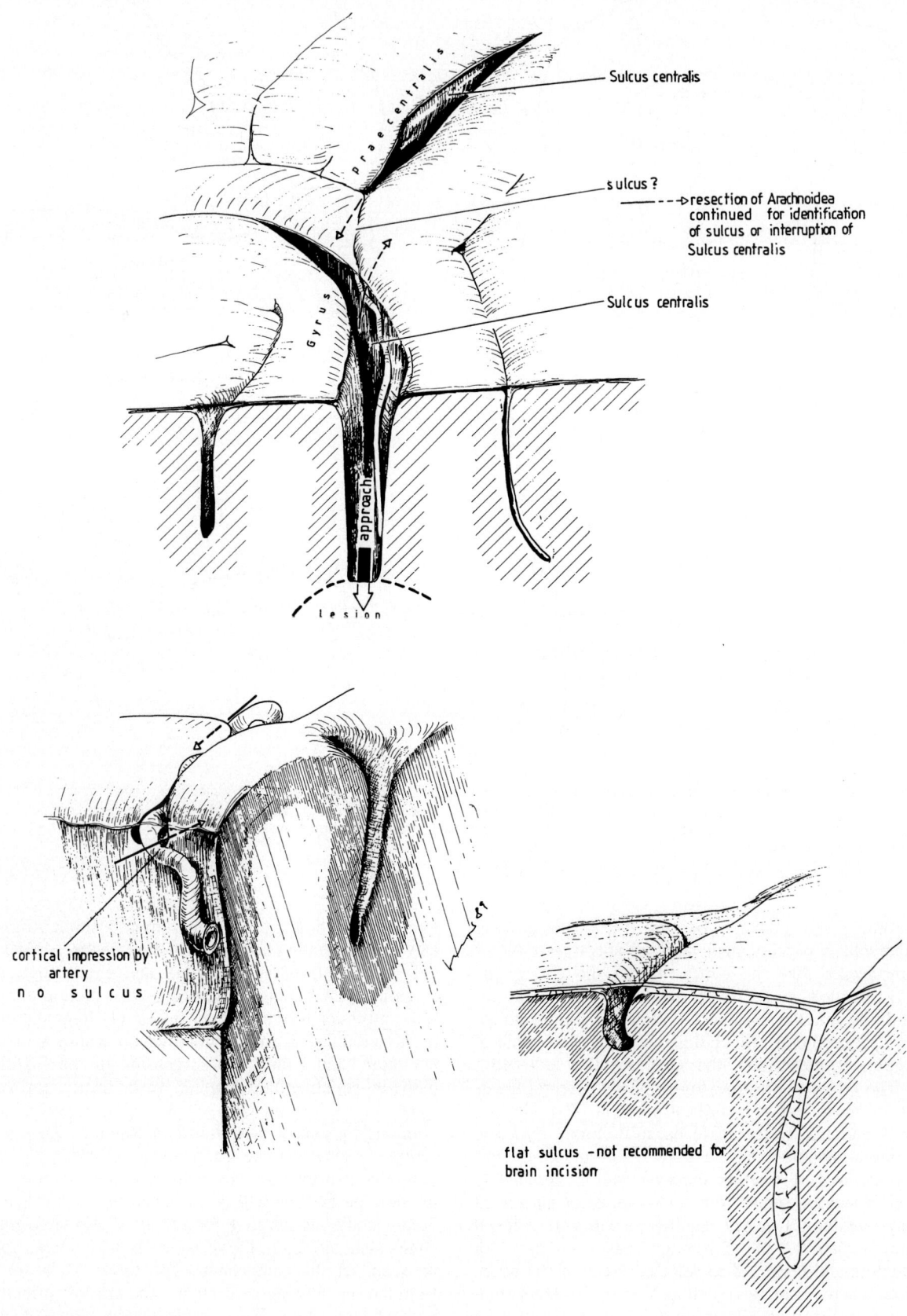

**FIGURE 56–10** ■ The arachnoid has to be incised at several points in order to distinguish the deep sulci from a sulcus-like impression of an artery on the cortex. (From Seeger W: Strategies of Microsurgery in Problematic Brain Areas. Vienna: Springer-Verlag, 1990, p 13.)

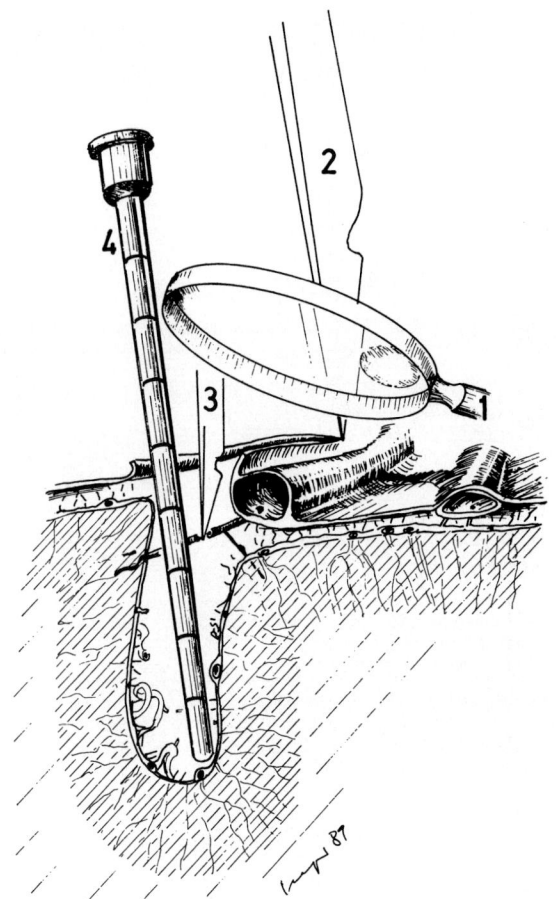

FIGURE 56–11 ■ Sulcal approach strategies. (From Seeger W: Strategies of Microsurgery in Problematic Brain Areas. Vienna: Springer-Verlag, 1990, p 11.)

coagulation. An aspirator with an ultrasonic vibrating tip is useful not only in the debulking of the central mass of a glioma but also in the dissection of its peripheral margins, which are very indistinct. The instrument gives the operator some tactile feedback on the tissue encountered and thus warns him or her of variations in resistance in the transition from the tumor to the surrounding edema or healthy tissue.

The 1970s brought another very useful aid to tumor resection—the laser beam. The carbon dioxide laser is preferred both for incising the cortex and for debulking the tumor.[101–103] Introduced by Patel in 1965, it operates at a wavelength of 10.6 m. It emits an invisible beam in the far infrared zone, which is absorbed by water and thus may be applied to all tissues. It vaporizes the water content of tissues; when appropriate, the penetration depth is only 0.2 mm into soft tissue. The advantages of this immaterial knife include: (1) precise dissection of the tumor mass; (2) speed; (3) vaporization of deep tumor processes with a nontouch technique; and (4) less risk of surgical infection because the laser knife has sterilizing effects as well as because it does not touch the tissues. In addition, because it has no electromagnetic field, it does not stimulate the nervous structures or interfere with the electrophysiologic monitoring equipment (e.g., electrocardiogram, electroencephalogram, and pulse rate). The disadvantages are the cumbersomeness of the equipment, the risk of explosion of anesthetic gases because of the high temperatures that the laser beam may reach (1700°C to 1800°C), and the restriction of hemostasis to vessels with a diameter of less than 0.5 mm. Because of the last feature, the carbon dioxide laser beam is indicated for low-grade gliomas. In more vascularized tumors (glioblastomas or angioblastic meningiomas), which require greater capacity for hemostasis, the neodymium:yttrium-aluminum-garnet laser is more suitable.

When a tumor is massive and superficial, it is best to use a focusing laser beam to shorten the vaporization time; in deep regions of the brain, the tumor should be vaporized with a defocused beam with continuous movement to avoid injury to the normal deep structures.

Last, laser technology has rekindled the recurrent interest in the possibility of inducing fluorescence by tissue photosensitizers to discover the tumor margins in the course of surgery. New generations of photosensitizing agents (phthalocyanine) have been proposed.[104]

Haglund and coworkers[105] developed a technique of optical image enhancement with intravenous injection of indocyanine green. This method enables the surgeon to differentiate normal brain, low-grade gliomas and high grade gliomas as an effect of different dynamics of optical signals. The technique also provides a clear image of the resection margins in malignant tumors during surgical removal. An analogous method developed by Allen and Maciunias at Vanderbilt University[55] involves the use of implanted fiducial markers combined with an infrared tracking system relating fiducial-based images to the position of the tip of an infrared probe, with an estimated error of less than 1 mm. Both the techniques are based on the different light penetration coefficient of tissues, owing to optical characteristics of the tissue and to the wave length of the light.

It has always been the surgeon's dream to have visual control of his or her work during the surgery. Some information is supplied by intraoperative ultrasound: Tumor residues are shown to be hyperechogenic. A close correspondence was demonstrated between low-grade glioma volumes evaluated with neuroimaging techniques and the volumes found intraoperatively using ultrasound-based methods.[87] However, previous radiation therapy may generate hyperecheogenic false-positive images due to gliosis.

Intraoperative neurophysiologic methods are likely to make a contribution that is of theoretical rather than practical interest. King and Schell[90] noted that somatosensory evoked potentials increase in amplitude as tumor debulking proceeds. Whether the phenomenon depends on improved cerebral perfusion (general effect) or on decompression of fibers of the internal capsule that project to the cortex lying against the tumor mass (local effect) is unknown.

Since 1985, the problem has been moving to a more brilliant solution, based on sophisticated imaging techniques.[106] The principle is similar to that of the Guthrie-Adler localizing arm. A jointed sensor arm tells a computer the position of its tip in the cranial cavity (Fig. 56–16). The preoperative CT (or MRI or angiographic) findings are projected on the computer display. The fiducial points are three metal markers (for CT) or three fat-filled capsules (for MRI) fixed to the nasion and the two tragi with adhesive tape (Fig. 56–17). After calibration, the machine

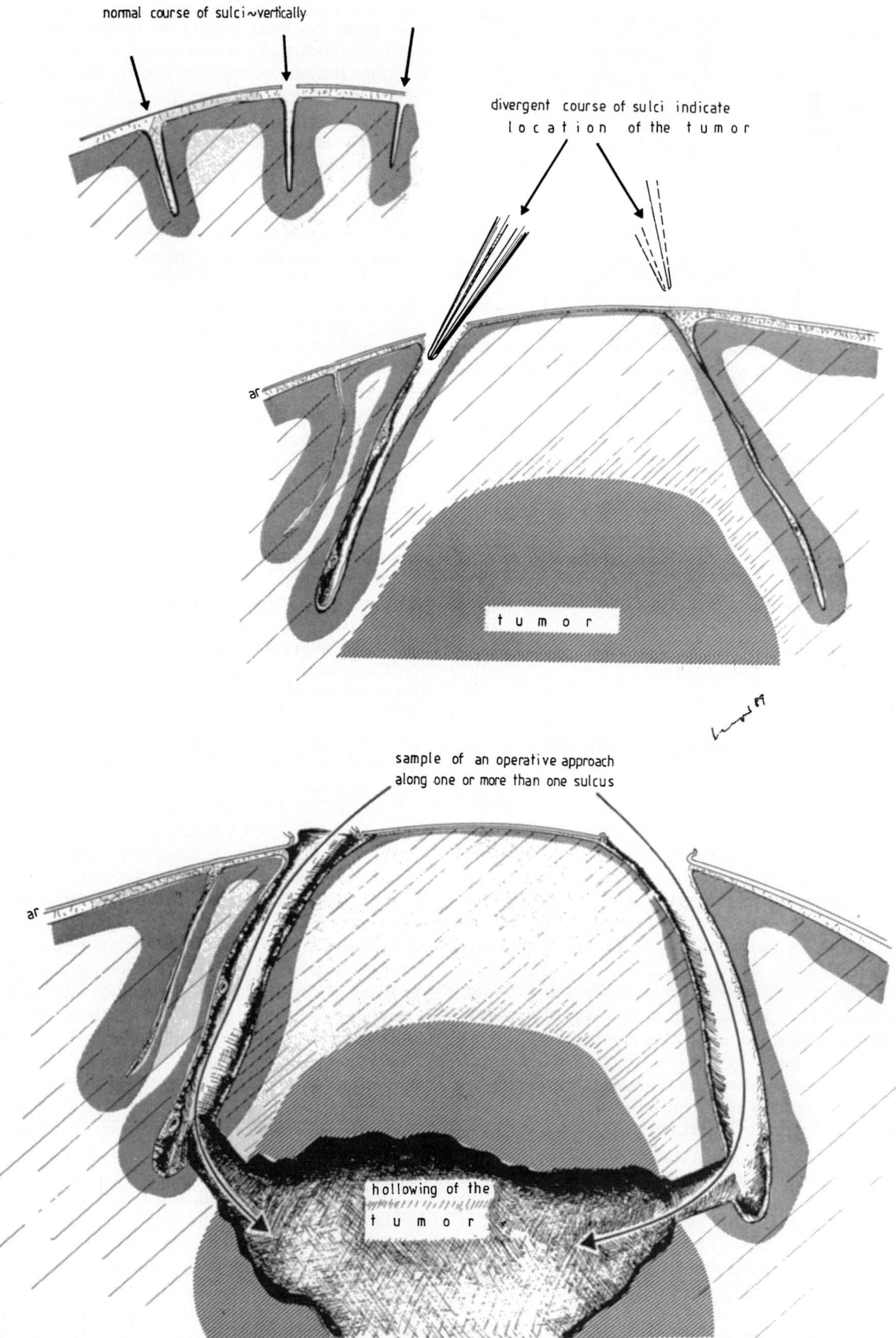

**FIGURE 56–12** ■ Tumoral distortion of the sulcal pattern of orientation. (From Seeger W: Strategies of Microsurgery in Problematic Brain Areas. Vienna: Springer-Verlag, 1990, p 15.)

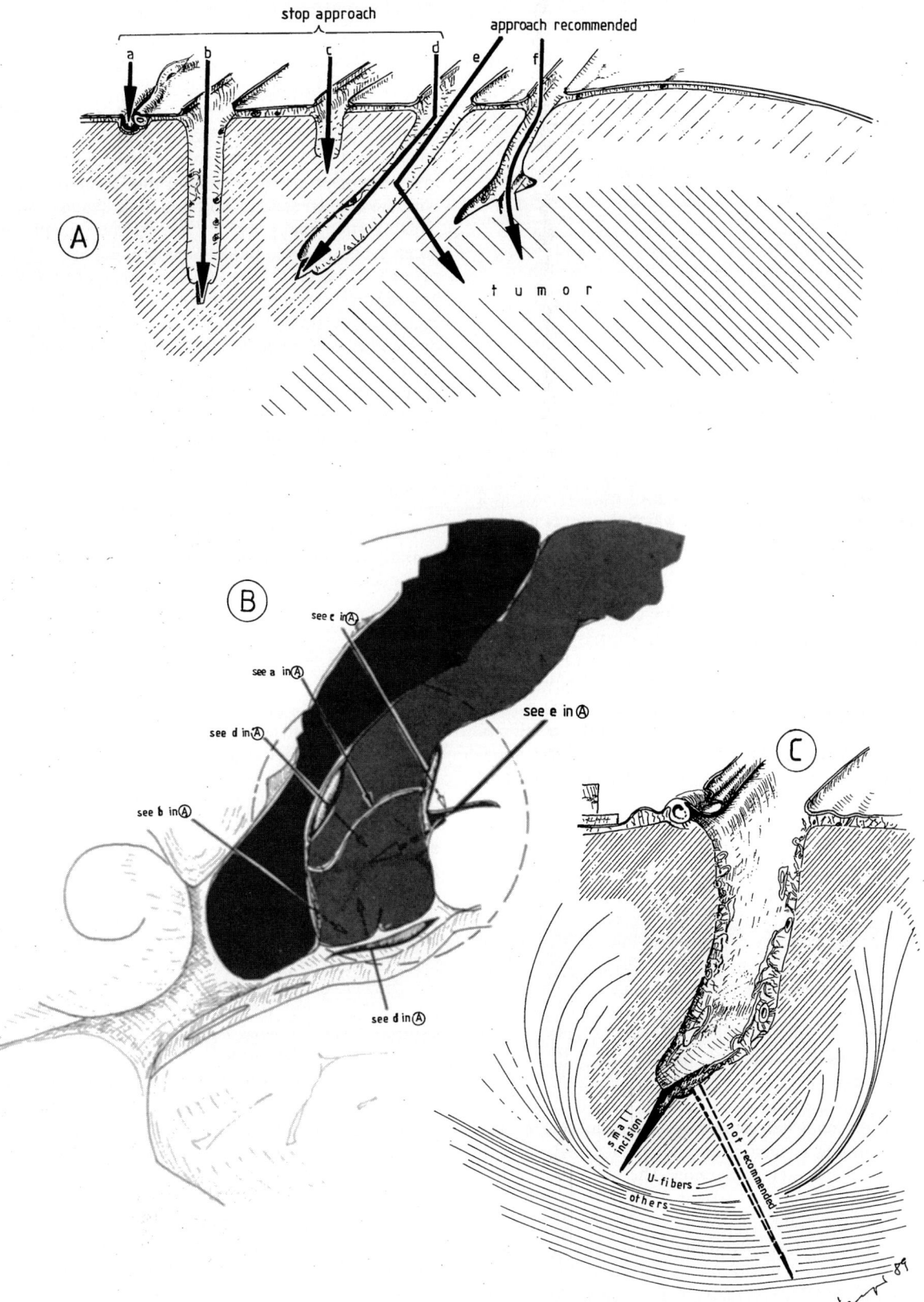

**FIGURE 56–13** ■ Sulcal approach strategies. (From Seeger W: Strategies of Microsurgery in Problematic Brain Areas. Vienna: Springer-Verlag, 1990, p 17.)

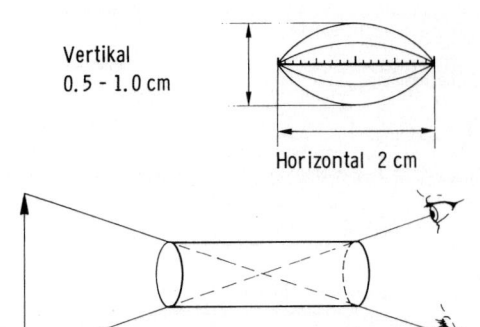

FIGURE 56–14    ■    Optic effect in the operating microscope. (From Yasargil MG, Cravens GF, Roth P: Surgical approaches to "inaccessible" brain tumors. Clin Neurosurg 34:42–110 1988. © Williams & Wilkins.)

gives the surgeon the spatial position of the tip of the sensor arm as it is moved over the neuroimages. The arm, fixed to the Mayfield headrest, is introduced into the operative field only when the surgeon wants to know the exact position of the tip. The margin of error is around 2 mm, negligible in open surgery, in which the target inevitably moves during the procedure (respiratory movements or vascular pulsations). Watanabe and associates[106, 107] called the instrument a "neuronavigator."

In recent years, although the routine use of this apparatus spread diffusely and many different models have been released by the industry; nevertheless, few reports appeared in the literature specifically regarding the surgical treatment of low-grade gliomas.

The spatial incompatibility between neurodiagnostic apparatus (CT, MRI, digital angiography) and the requirements of the operating room has been overcome by Kelly[108] by a complex organization centering on a heads-up display system, similar to that used on fighter aircraft, which projects the tumor sections obtained by the computer from CT or MRI data into the operating microscope. Kelly provides a detailed account in Chapter 49.

Another method is that proposed by Hassenbusch and colleagues.[109] Craniotomy is performed under a stereotactic frame; when the dura mater has been opened, two or three stereomarkers are introduced at the tumor margins (the ones most difficult to distinguish or situated in the most critical areas) according to the coordinates supplied by CT or MRI (Fig. 56–18). They are "micropatties" (0.6 × 0.6 cm), each with a string tail or silicone sheeting microtubes, either of which are introduced through a microbiopsy forceps with the ends left emerging from the cortex. The stereotactic frame is then removed, and the surgeon proceeds to free-hand tumor resection. The advantage of this method is that the markers remain lodged at the edges of the tumor (in the brain adjacent to it) despite shifts in the tumor or in the cerebral hemispheres resulting from cyst drainage or tumor debulking.

Berger[55] also reports the use of ultrasonic guidance to introduce catheters at the tumor boundaries as a "fence" to mark the limit of surgical resection. The proposed method of ultrasonic neuronavigation includes a program to calculate the shift of intracranial content occurring with tumor progressive debulking and cerebrospinal fluid re-

moval, performing a continuous correction of the initial spatial parameters.

## Associated Intractable Epilepsy

Often epileptic foci are associated to low-grade gliomas. Berger and coworkers[83] have registered intraoperatively this pathologic activity, establishing relevant correlations with the clinical status. Only in 6 of 45 patients studied did electrocorticography fail to demonstrate epileptic activity. Twenty-one patients harbored one epileptic focus, and 18 patients harbored at least two foci. Some of these foci were adjacent; others were far from the tumor. The latter were mainly associated with temporal lobe gliomas. Epileptiform discharges rose from temporal mesial structures even in tumors of the lateral cortex. The neural tissue of 90% of the identified foci were histologically free of tumor infiltration, which was usually normal and resulted only in a few cases with mild gliosis. Multiple epileptogenic foci were associated with a longer history of seizures. The authors stress the importance of tumor and epileptic focus resection under the guide of electrocorticography, particularly in children and for long-lasting epilepsy, with the goal to optimize seizure control and allow possible interruption or reduction of drug therapy.

## Hemostasis and Closure

Hemostasis is ensured in the usual way under the operating microscope by means of bipolar cautery, discontinuous irrigation with lukewarm isotonic saline solution, and dabbing of the walls with cottonoids. Even the smallest nontumoral vessels are spared. As little use as possible is made of foreign materials (e.g., fibrin sponge, oxidized cellulose net) for lining the cavity, which is then filled with physiologic saline.

An extended internal decompressive operation impinging on sound nervous tissue is now viewed with great circumspection, because any sacrifice of nervous tissue always involves neurologic or behavioral deficits, even if they are not detectable with the tests currently available. No such rule applies to the resection of epileptogenic cortical foci separate from the neoplastic mass, which is recommended by Ghatan and associates.[18]

Once the dural margins have been secured to the periosteum by interrupted sutures along the perimeter of the craniotomy, the dural flap is made watertight. The bone is replaced; because the craniotomy is small and its site is at the convexity, there is no point in removing the bone flap for decompression (the classic decompressive operation is to be performed at the base). If the surgeon desires, an epidural probe for prolonged intracranial pressure (ICP) recording is positioned by tunneling the cable beneath the scalp for a few centimeters and bringing it to the surface through a tiny incision in the scalp at a distance from the main wound.

In conclusion, although neurosurgery is not rejecting its origins (the foundations of surgical technique laid down by Cushing and Dandy), this specialty is preparing to take

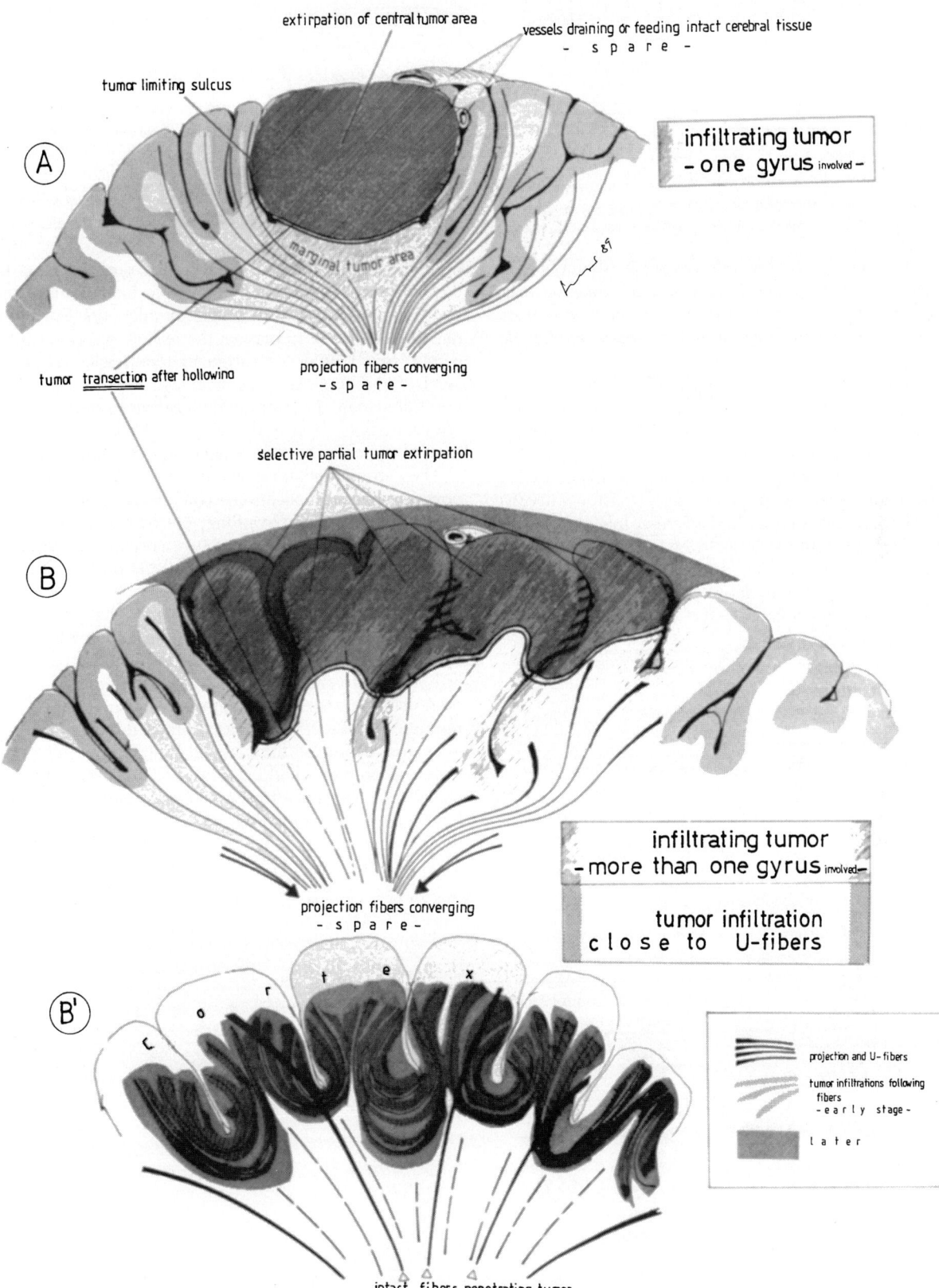

**FIGURE 56–15** ■ Different patterns of glioma infiltration. (From Seeger W: Strategies of Microsurgery in Problematic Brain Areas. Vienna: Springer-Verlag, 1990, p 21.)

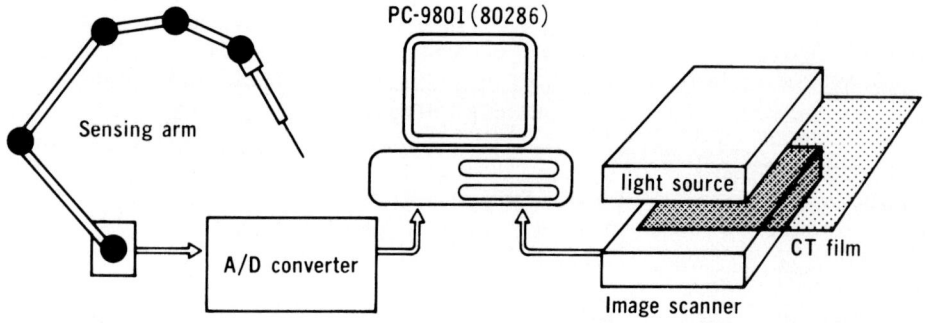

FIGURE 56–16 ■ Neuronavigator. (From Watanabe E, Mayanagy Y, Kasugi Y, et al: Open surgery assisted by the neuronavigator: A stereotactic, articulated, sensitive arm. Neurosurgery 28:792–800, 1991.)

a qualitative leap with the aid of image digitalization techniques. The firm establishment of neuroimaging technologies (which now form part of the operating room setup), the first clinical applications of robotics, and the computerized management of neurophysiologic monitoring systems (e.g., evoked potentials, PET, SPECT) have set the stage for a revision of technique. The main advantages are: (1) personalized instead of standardized craniotomy, (2) prior simulation and not just planning of the operation, and (3) intraoperative verification of the extent of resection so that no surprises occur postoperatively. Genuine tumorectomy replaces the former lobectomy, lobulectomy, and polectomy. In addition, tumorectomy does not have to be total. The surgeon's aim is to remove the tumor, but he or she will later decide between grossly total resection and subtotal resection according to the requirements of the case.

Stereotactic and open biopsies are addressed in other chapters.

## MAJOR INTRAOPERATIVE COMPLICATIONS AND THEIR MANAGEMENT

Improved anesthetic technique, the prophylactic use of corticosteroids, and the intraoperative use of a mannitol bolus before the dural incision if the dura mater is tense are the means whereby the operative field is made fit for surgical manipulation. The surgeon takes great care not to damage veins and to prevent the leakage of blood into the cerebrospinal fluid compartment (ventricles, cisterns, and sulci of the convexity). A spatula is used only if it does not traumatize the surrounding nervous tissue; scooping with retractors fixed to the Mayfield headrest is preferable to manual scooping, which is always discontinuous.

These conditions minimize the risk of intraoperative and postoperative complications. The intraoperative risks are lobar or hemispheric swelling, episodic or subcontinuous bleeding, and incarceration of cerebrospinal fluid in the operative cavity or in a ventricular pole or, less likely, in a cistern. Swelling of the operative field may be the result of hyperemia (increased cerebral blood volume) or edema; either may be local or diffuse. Hydrostatic edema may be caused by congestion of a vessel that results from a rise in capillary and venous pressure after distention of the walls of resistance vessels. Hyperemia may be associated with normal, decreased, or increased blood flow.

Determination of the cerebral blood flow still presents technical problems and furnishes only an overall picture of the blood perfusion of each cerebral hemisphere. Particularly useful are regional blood flow data, which PET and SPECT can supply, but not in the course of an operation. Thus, we still do not know how the blood flow and cerebral

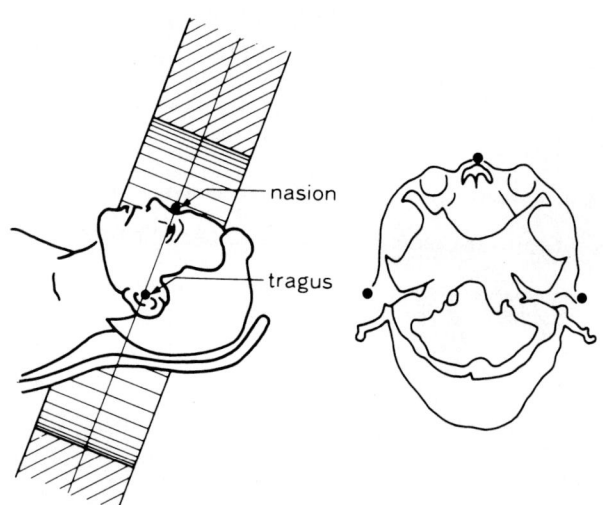

FIGURE 56–17 ■ Artificial coordinates method(s): fiducial points. (From Watanabe E, Mayanagy Y, Kasugi Y, et al: Open surgery assisted by the neuronavigator: A stereotactic, articulated, sensitive arm. Neurosurgery 28:792–800, 1991.)

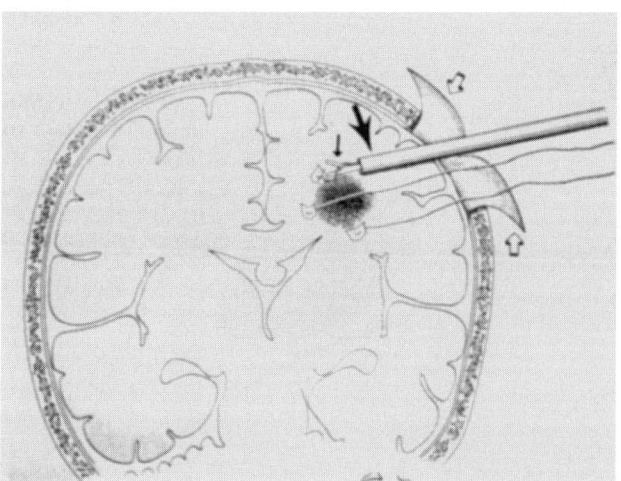

FIGURE 56–18 ■ Artificial coordinates method(s)—stereomarkers. (From Hassenbusch SJ, Anderson JS, Pillay PK: Brain tumor resection aided with markers placed using stereotaxis guided by magnetic resonance imaging and computed tomography. Neurosurgery 28:801–806, 1991.)

metabolism are regulated in single areas of the brain adjacent to space-occupying lesions or after they have been evacuated surgically, nor do we know what the regional response will be to drugs or to variations in pressure of the respiratory gases. An intravenous mannitol bolus (which increases the blood flow irrespective of the ICP), hyperventilation, and, on occasion, cautious withdrawal of cerebrospinal fluid are options if intraoperative congestion of the brain occurs. Initially, the surgeon must ensure that the swelling is not a result of anesthesia or a large tumor residue, of a clot deep in the operative cavity, or of incarcerated cerebrospinal fluid.

## POSTOPERATIVE MANAGEMENT

An operation on a cerebral glioma is not high-risk surgery; therefore, the immediate postoperative management is the same as that required for any other neurosurgical operation of average complexity. It has now been standardized after decades of experience.

The patient is kept in intensive care for the first 48 to 72 hours under close neurologic supervision and monitoring of autonomic parameters. Drainage, if applied, is removed after 24 hours. The ICP recording probe is removed on postoperative day 3. Antiedema osmotic treatment is discontinued on day 4, and corticosteroid therapy is titrated down a few days later. Prophylactic antibiotics are discontinued between days 4 and 6. CT scanning is performed on day 7 of an uneventful course, and a neurophysiologic (evoked potentials) and neuropsychological assessment is performed on day 10. Antiepileptic therapy or prophylaxis is given for years.

The immediate postoperative period may be marked by the same complications as those that may arise during the operation (e.g., brain swelling, bleeding, engorgement of cerebrospinal fluid) as well as infarction adjacent to the operative field or distant from it, resulting from the interruption of arteries or veins. Neuroimaging and continuous ICP recording are diagnostic. To differentiate swelling resulting from congestion from that resulting from edema, CT scanning is essential after contrast injection. The hypodensity found in the standard images increases by a few Hounsfield units if the blood volume is increased, an increase that is too small, however, to be appreciable on the CT scan. Even minimal bleeding in the operative cavity, either subdural or extradural, shows up clearly on CT and MRI. Regarding ICP, whether a given cerebral perfusion pressure is sufficient in a particular individual to ensure perfusion to all parts of the brain is unknown. Particularly vulnerable are those areas adjacent to the operative focus, whose vascular autoregulation is presumably altered. It has been decided arbitrarily that an ICP of over 20 mm Hg must be corrected by hyperventilation and antiedema osmotic agents. These measures are adopted only in severe neurologic conditions, which are rarely found in patients with low-grade cerebral glioma. If infiltration of deep structures occurs, the surgeon will choose a biopsy rather than extensive resection. Indeed, if surgical series since the introduction of CT are evaluated, the following situation is illustrative. Of the 25 patients that Vertosick and associ-

ates[17] operated on between 1978 and 1988, five underwent debulking; four had an open biopsy; and 16 had stereotactic biopsy, with zero operative mortality and zero morbidity. Of Piepmeier's[16] 50 patients operated on between 1975 and 1985, 19 underwent total resection; 17, subtotal resection; and 14, biopsy, with only one postoperative death. In the series of McCormack and coworkers,[110] of 53 patients (10 gross total resections, 34 subtotal resections, and nine biopsies) operated on between 1977 and 1988, only one died of myocardial infarction, in the postoperative period, and five died after the 30-day period but while the patients were still in hospital. Three patients who had been neurologically intact before surgery had mild deficits thereafter. In the series of McCormack and colleagues, 15 reoperations were necessary: three for shunts, three for cyst aspiration, two for infection, and seven for further tumor resection.

The role of radiotherapy in the management of low-grade gliomas is discussed in several excellent review articles.[111–113] Unfortunately, no uniform or systematic studies have been performed that would allow a firm judgment, but the number of patients receiving radiotherapy in the past few years has increased.[114] Retrospective analysis of past series, with all their limitations, seems to show that as far as astrocytomas are concerned: (1) patients who undergo surgery for pilocytic astrocytoma (even if incompletely) should not be irradiated; (2) patients with fibrillary or protoplasmic astrocytoma who have undergone gross total resection should not be irradiated but should be followed up closely with neuroimaging; (3) patients with these tumors who have undergone incomplete resection should receive conventional fractionated radiotherapy at doses of 4500 to 5500 cGy in a limited volume (dose to be reduced and commencement of radiotherapy deferred for patients younger than 2 to 3 years of age); and (4) patients with gemistocytic astrocytoma should receive postoperative radiotherapy regardless of the extent of resection.[115] With regard to oligodendrogliomas[116] and the rarer mixed gliomas, the published data are still more fragmentary and discordant. It does seem, however, that radiotherapy slows tumor regrowth.[114]

## GROWTH RESUMPTION

It is more appropriate to speak of growth resumption long after treatment than of recurrence, because an infiltrating tumor is never completely eradicated. The literature supplies data on the rates of recurrence, on the length of the interval since operation, and on the histologic differences on the second appraisal (at surgery or at necropsy) compared with the first. Very few opinions on the treatment of a recurrence have been published. Among the series explicitly discussing this topic, one refers to a long period and the other to the CT era: Laws and colleagues[64] reported on 151 recurrences of grade I and grade II astrocytomas that were treated surgically between 1915 and 1976. Of the recurrences, 105 were treated surgically (alone or associated with other therapy), 36 nonsurgically, and 10 were not treated. The 12-month survival rates were 45.7%, 46.1%, and 47.6%, which is virtually the same for the three groups. McCormack and associates[110] reported on 24 recurrences among 41 patients who survived total or subtotal removal: seven had a second operation, and 12 received chemotherapy. The mean survival of those who had a second operation was 12 months from the recurrence. The authors stated that neither reoperation nor chemotherapy prolonged postrecurrence survival. Such data increase the importance of the first management decision; at the time of recurrence, the tumors exhibit increased malignancy and resistance to treatment.

## RESULTS

The largest series (461 cases) and the one covering the longest time span (1915 to 1975) is that of the Mayo Clinic.[14, 64] Although the long-term results are obviously better in patients treated since 1950 as a result of improved surgical and anesthetic techniques and antiedema agents, the factors that correlate with longer survival are age under 20 years, good neurologic status before and after operation, epileptic seizures as the onset symptom, preoperative history of symptoms for not less than 6 months, grossly total surgical resection, and parietal or occipital tumor site. Sex, astrocytoma histologic grade I or II, the presence of an intratumoral cyst, the side affected, and surgical lobectomy (which in malignant astrocytoma improves the prognosis) had little or no impact on survival. Laws and coworkers combined patient age with six of the most important prognostic factors to score the probability of survival (Table 56–2). Operative mortality excluded, survival varies widely (Fig. 56–19): the 5-year survival rate ranges from 69% to 35%. At 15 years, the rate is over 50% in low-risk patients, versus 16% for the mean. The effectiveness of postoperative radiotherapy could not be assessed per se but only in relation to other parameters. Its value is proved only in patients older than 40 years of age with high scores (i.e., with several risk factors). Patient age proved to be by far the most important factor in prognosis, more important than all the other clinical factors and forms of treatment combined, and this aspect is confirmed by the experience of many authors.[69, 117, 118] The reason for this result is unclear, but what is clear is a difference in biologic behav-

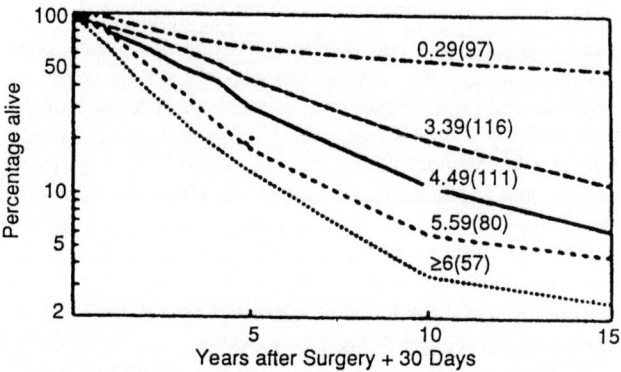

FIGURE 56–19 ■ Score-based survival curves of patients with low-grade hemispheric glioma. See Table 56–2 for basis of scoring system. (From Laws ER, Taylor WF, Clifton MB, Okazaki H: Neurosurgical management of low-grade astrocytoma of the cerebral hemispheres. J Neurosurg 61:665–673, 1984.)

ior of these oncotypes between the young and the adult host.

We dealt with the subject of different low-grade astrocytomas of the cerebral hemispheres as a whole, but we also mentioned that this pathologic entity includes three oncotypes: (1) the astrocytomas representing about 60%, (2) oligodendrogliomas approximately 23%, and (3) mixed oligo astrocytomas about 17%. Actually, the biologic and clinical features of these oncotypes are comparable if we consider the age at presentation, symptomatology, possibility of tumor progression to a higher grade, and absence of spinal diffusion or metastases. But with respect to long-term survival, pure oligodendrogliomas emerge more favorably, pure astrocytoma appear a worse, and mixed oligoastrocytomas display intermediate behavior. The series of Shaw and colleagues[119] of the Mayo Clinic, which was drawn from a 20-year period, compares the survival of pure and mixed oligodendrogliomas using univariate and multivariate analysis and examining 14 prognostic factors. The tumor grade emerged as the factor that was most significantly related to survival. Less significant was the extent of surgical resection. Younger age was also significantly related with a more favorable prognosis for both oncotypes so that, after gross total surgical resection, radiotherapy may not be required. Conversely, radiotherapy with doses of 5000 cGy is advocated in older patients and for partially resected tumors.

Reports confirm the importance of the length of clinical history among the clinical factors considered relevant for long-term prognosis. Tumors with a longer duration of symptoms and chronic epilepsy seem much less likely to progress toward malignancy over time.

The routine use of CT since the time of the series by Laws and colleagues has added a new factor to be evaluated in the long-term prognosis of low-grade cerebral gliomas: the absence of contrast enhancement (i.e., the integrity of the blood-brain barrier) is associated with a better prognosis.

The 1975 to 1985 experience of Yale University[16] shows that the only factors relevant to a better prognosis are age under 40 years and no contrast enhancement on the CT scan. The results of the 1977 to 1988 series at New York University[110] agree: Multivariate regression analysis dem-

## TABLE 56–2 ■ SCORING SYSTEM FOR LOW-GRADE HEMISPHERIC GLIOMAS

| Score = Age at Diagnosis 0.072 | |
| --- | --- |
| **+ 0** | **+ 1** |
| Surgery after 1949 | Surgery before 1949 |
| No personality change | Personality change |
| Normal consciousness | Altered consciousness |
| Total resection | Partial resection |
| Site other than the frontal or temporal lobe | Frontal or temporal lobe |
| Mild postoperative neurologic deficit | Moderate-to-severe postoperative neurologic deficit |

Scoring system based on the data by Laws ER, Taylor WF, Clifton MB, Okazaki H: Neurosurgical management of low-grade astrocytoma of the cerebral hemispheres. J Neurosurg 61:665–673, 1984.

onstrates that the most important prognosticators for improved survival are young age, absence of contrast enhancement of the original tumor on CT, and the performance status of the patient. The CT contrast enhancement of the original tumor is associated with a 6.8-fold increase in risk for a late recurrence. However the prognostic significance of contrast enhancement is questioned by some authors,[1] whose further experience contradicts the results obtained in the 75 to 85 decade series. Bernstein[69] still ascribes some value to the presence of contrast enhancement as related to malignant progression, but Philippon and coworkers[120] deny these findings.

The value of aggressive surgical behavior has also been questioned. The likelihood of malignant transformation has been demonstrated proportional to the preoperative tumor volume or to residual volume and the latter result inversely related to the time of recurrence.[121] On the other hand, Bernstein[69] emphasizes the unreliability of retrospective studies regarding tumors with different locations being treated differently: these limitations explain the dichotomy existing in the literature between supporters of aggressive surgery and supporters of "wait and see" behavior.

## SUMMARY

There has been a revival of scientific and clinical interest in low-grade gliomas, which were neglected for many years in the literature. Within this group of tumors, extraganglionic gliomas have attracted even less attention, and many surgical series group them together with those of the cerebellum, hypothalamus, brain stem, and anterior optic pathways. This grouping is inadvisable, because both histologically and biologically as well as from the diagnostic and therapeutic viewpoints, the latter gliomas are altogether different from those of the cerebral hemispheres.

One reason for this revival of interest is that in the neuroimaging age, the clinician is confronted with pathology that is different from what used to be seen two decades ago. The clinician now sees a small lesion in a young, neurologically intact subject whose only complaint is a short history of epileptic seizures. The lesion is of the cerebral convexity, is diffusely infiltrative, and may have connections with the higher functions of the hemisphere: eloquent cortex, its projections, and associative fibers.

For tumors that are indolent for years, one may legitimately wonder whether aggressive treatment—surgery or radiotherapy—is appropriate in all cases and whether the potential benefits of treatment may not be counterbalanced by its risks and adverse effects.[63, 122, 123] Retrospective studies are of little help in shaping judgment, for the reasons given already (unselected series of tumors much larger than those that are treated now), to which must be added: nonuniformity of pathologic classification criteria, the question of sampling errors, nonuniformity in classifying preoperative neurologic status (Karnofsky's performance scale), nonuniformity of the extent of surgical resection or of a dose of radiotherapy, and the lack of a contemporary group of matched control subjects who did not receive treatment. Lastly and fundamentally is the nonuniformity of biologic behavior of the tumor through time; it is subject

to dedifferentiation in a high percentage of cases in the course of its natural history. We have no sure data on which to form a judgment regarding the optimal treatment for low-grade cerebral gliomas. These data can come only from prospective, randomized studies of large series. Meanwhile, surgery has both a diagnostic and a therapeutic role. Its diagnostic role may well diminish with advances in neuroimaging procedures, like PET and SPECT, and the chemical quantification in vivo of metabolites in selected regions of the brain, such as can be obtained with proton MR spectroscopy.[124] On the therapeutic front, surgery may well maintain its hold, unless valid alternatives are developed. Although surgery has so far been limited by the risks of damage that it induces, the progress of technology will reduce the risk of undesired side effects and allow surgery to be more aggressive and safer.

## REFERENCES

1. Piepmeier JH: Criteria for patient selection: Low-grade gliomas. Clin Neurosurg 44:51–62, 1997.
2. Zülch KJ: Brain Tumors, 3rd ed. Berlin: Springer-Verlag, 1986.
3. Schisano G, Tovi D, Nordenstam H: Spongioblastoma polare of the cerebral hemisphere. J Neurosurg 20:241–251, 1963.
4. Palma L, Guidetti B: Cystic pilocytic astrocytomas of the cerebral hemispheres: Surgical experience with 51 cases and long-term results. J Neurosurg 62:811–815, 1985.
5. Afra D, Mu;auller W, Slowik F, Firsching R: Supratentorial lobar pilocytic astrocytomas: Report of 45 operated cases, including 9 recurrences. Acta Neurochir (Wien) 81:90–93, 1986.
6. Seeger W: Strategies of Microsurgery in Problematic Brain Areas, with Special Reference to NMR. New York: Springer-Verlag, 1990.
7. Skirboll SL, Ojemann GA, Berger MS, et al: Functional cortex and subcortical white matter located within gliomas. Neurosurgery 38:678–685, 1996.
8. Silverman C, Marks JE: Prognostic significance of contrast enhancement in low-grade astrocytomas of the adult cerebrum. Radiology 139:211–213, 1981.
9. Hoshino T, Rodriguez LA, Cho KG, et al: Prognostic implications of the proliferative potential of low-grade astrocytomas. J Neurosurg 69:839–842, 1988.
10. Germano IM, Ito M, Cho KG, et al: Correlation of histopathological features and proliferative potential of gliomas. J Neurosurg 70:701–706, 1989.
11. Labrousse F, Daumas-Duport C, Batorski L, Hoshino T: Histological grading and bromodeoxyuridine labeling index of astrocytomas: Comparative study in a series of 60 cases. J Neurosurg 75:202–205, 1991.
12. Hoshino T: Cell kinetics of brain tumors. In Salcman M (ed): Neurobiology of Brain Tumors. Vol 4: Concepts in Neurosurgery. Baltimore: Williams & Wilkins, 1991, pp 145–159.
13. Patronas NJ, Di Chiro G, Kufta C, et al: Prediction of survival in glioma patients by means of positron emission tomography. J Neurosurg 62:816–822, 1985.
14. Laws ER, Taylor WF, Clifton MB, Okazaki H: Neurosurgical management of low-grade astrocytoma of the cerebral hemispheres. J Neurosurg 61:665–673, 1984.
15. Gol A: The relatively benign astrocytomas of the cerebrum: A clinical study of 194 verified cases. J Neurosurg 18:501–506, 1961.
16. Piepmeier JM: Observations on the current treatment of low-grade astrocytic tumors of the cerebral hemispheres. J Neurosurg 67:177–181, 1987.
17. Vertosick FT, Selker RG, Arena VC: Survival of patients with well-differentiated astrocytomas diagnosed in the era of computed tomography. Neurosurgery 28:496–501, 1991.
18. Ghatan S, Berger MS, Ojemann GA, Dobbins J: Seizure control in patients with low-grade gliomas: Resection of the tumor and separate seizure foci. J Neurosurg 74:355A, 1991.
19. Haglund MM, Berger MS, Kunkel DD, et al: Changes in gamma-aminobutyric acid and somatostatin in epileptic cortex associated with low-grade gliomas. J Neurosurg 77:209–216, 1992.

20. Goldring S, Rich KM, Picker S: Experience with gliomas in patients presenting with a chronic seizure disorder. Clin Neurosurg 33:15–42, 1986.
21. Yoshii Y, Maki Y, Tsuboi K, et al: Estimation of growth fraction with bromodeoxyuridine in human central nervous system tumors. J Neurosurg 65:659–663, 1986.
22. Zuber P, Hamou MF, De Tribolet N: Identification of proliferating cells in human gliomas using the monoclonal antibody Ki-67. Neurosurgery 22:364–368, 1988.
23. Tachibana H, Meyer JS, Rose JE, Kandula P: Local cerebral blood flow and partition coefficients measured in cerebral astrocytomas of different grades of malignancy. Surg Neurol 21:125–131, 1984.
24. Di Chiro G, De La Paz RL, Brooks RA, et al: Glucose utilization of cerebral gliomas measured by [$^{18}$F] fluorodeoxyglucose and positron emission tomography. Neurology 32:1323–1329, 1982.
25. Bustany P, Chatel M, Derlon JM, et al: Brain tumor protein synthesis and histological grades: A study by positron emission tomography (PET) with $^{11}$C-l-methionine. J Neurooncol 3:397–404, 1986.
26. Tsuboi K, Yoshii Y, Nakagawa K, Maki Y: Regrowth patterns of supratentorial gliomas: Estimation from computed tomographic scans. Neurosurgery 19:946–951, 1986.
27. Hoshino T: A commentary on the biology and growth kinetics of low-grade and high-grade gliomas. J Neurosurg 61:895–900, 1984.
28. Müller W, Afra D, Schröder R: Supratentorial recurrences of gliomas: Morphological studies in relation to time intervals with astrocytomas. Acta Neurochir (Wien) 37:75–91, 1977.
29. Müller W, Afra D, Schröder R: Supratentorial recurrence of gliomas: Morphological studies in relation to time intervals with oligodendrogliomas. Acta Neurochir (Wien) 39:15–25, 1977.
30. Rubinstein LJ: The correlation of neoplastic vulnerability with central neuroepithelial cytogeny and glioma differentiation. J Neurooncol 5:11–27, 1987.
31. Wallner KE, Gonzales M, Sheline GE: Treatment of oligodendrogliomas with or without postoperative irradiation. J Neurosurg 68:684–688, 1988.
32. Piepmeier JM, Christopher S: Low-grade gliomas: Introduction and overview. J Neurooncol 34:1–3, 1997.
33. Schiffer D, Cavalla P, Chio A, et al: Proliferative activity and prognosis of low-grade astrocytomas. J Neurooncol 34:31–35, 1997.
34. Dirven CM, Koudstall J, Mooij JJ, Molenaar WM: The proliferative potential of the pilocytic astrocytoma: The relation between MIB-1 labeling and clinical and neuro-radiological follow-up. J Neurooncol 37:9–16, 1998.
35. Knudson AG Jr: Mutations and cancer: Statistical study of retinoblastoma. Proc Natl Acad Sci U S A 68:820–823, 1971.
36. Nishizaki T, Ozaki S, Harada K, et al: Investigation of genetic alterations associated with the grade of astrocytic tumor by comparative genomic hybridization. Genes Chromosomes Cancer 21:340–346, 1998.
37. Watanabe K, Tachibana O, Yonekawa Y, et al: Role of gemistocytes in astrocytoma progression. Lab Invest 76:277–284, 1997.
38. Prayson RA, Estes ML: MIB1 and p53 immunoreactivity in protoplasmic astrocytomas. Pathol Int 46:862–866, 1996.
39. Bogler O, Huang HJ, Cavenee WK: Loss of wild-type p53 bestows a growth advantage on primary cortical astrocytes and facilitates their in vitro transformation. Cancer Res 55:2746–2751, 1995.
40. Chernova OB, Chernov MV, Agarwal ML, et al: The role of p53 in regulating genomic stability when DNA and RNA synthesis are inhibited. Trends Biochem Sci 20:431–434, 1995.
41. Venkatachalam S, Shi YP, Jones SN, et al: Retention of wild-type p53 in tumors from heterozygous mice: Reduction of p53 dosage can promote cancer transformation. EMBO J 17:4657–4667, 1998.
42. Gomez Manzano C, Fueyo J, Kyritsis AP, et al: Adenovirus-mediated transfer of the p53 gene produces rapid and generalized death of human glioma cells via apoptosis. Cancer Res 56:694–699, 1996.
43. Fueyo J, Gomez-Manzano C, Bruner JM, et al: Hypermethylation of the CpG island of p16/CDKN2 correlates with gene inactivation in gliomas. Oncogene 13:1615–1619, 1996.
44. Ehrmann J Jr, Kolar Z, Vojtesek B, et al: Prognostic factors in astrocytomas: Relationship of p53, MDM-2, BCL-2 and PCNA immunohistochemical expression to tumor grade and overall patient survival. Neoplasma 44:299–304, 1997.
45. Carroll RS, Zhang J, Chauncey BW, et al: Apoptosis in astrocytic neoplasms. Acta Neurochir 139:845–850, 1997.
46. Kattar MM, Kupsky WJ, Shimoyama RK, et al: Clonal analysis of gliomas. Hum Pathol 28:1166–1179, 1997.
47. Reifenberger J, Ring GU, Gies U, et al: Analysis of p53 mutation and epidermal growth factor amplification in recurrent gliomas with malignant progression. J Neuropathol Exp Neurol 55:822–831, 1996.
48. Noble M, Mayer-Prochel M: Molecular growth factors, glia and gliomas. J Neurooncol 35:193–209, 1997.
49. Bonnie A, Sun Y, Nadal-Vicens M, et al: Regulation of gliogenesis in the central nervous system by the JAK-STAT signaling pathway. Science 278:477–483, 1997.
50. Abdulrauf SI, Edvardsen K, Ho KL, et al: Vascular endothelial growth factor expression and vascular density as prognostic markers of survival in patients with low-grade astrocytoma. J Neurosurg 88:513–520, 1998.
51. Jensen RL: Growth factor-mediated angiogenesis in the malignant progression of glial tumors: A review. Surg Neurol 49:189–195, 1998.
52. Takekawa Y, Sawada T: Vascular endothelial growth factor and neovascularization in astrocytic tumors. Pathol Int 48:109–114, 1998.
53. Kondziolka D, Lunsford LD, Martinez AJ: Unreliability of contemporary neurodiagnostic imaging in evaluating suspected adult supratentorial (low-grade) astrocytoma. J Neurosurg 79:533–536, 1993.
54. Bernstein M, Guha A: Biopsy of low-grade astrocytomas. J Neurosurg 80:776–777, 1994.
55. Berger MS: Surgery of low-grade gliomas:Technical aspects. Clin Neurosurg 44:161–180, 1997.
56. Herholz K, Holzer T, Bauer B, et al: 11C-methionine PET for differential diagnosis of low-grade gliomas. Neurology 50:1316–1322, 1998.
57. Kaschten B, Stevenaert A, Sadzot B, et al: Preoperative evaluation of 54 gliomas by PET with fluorine-18-fluorodeoxyglucose and/or carbon-11-methionine. J Nucl Med 39:778–785, 1998.
58. Tamura M, Shibasaki T, Zama A, et al: Assessment of malignancy of glioma by positron emission tomography with 18F-fluorodeoxyglucose and single photon emission computed tomography with thallium-201 chloride. Neuroradiology 40:210–215, 1998.
59. Cheng LL, Chang IW, Louis DN, Gonzalez RG: Correlation of high resolution magic angle spinning proton magnetic resonance spectroscopy with histopathology of intact brain tumor specimens. Cancer Res 58:1825–1832, 1998.
60. Tedeschi G, Lundbom N, Raman R, et al: Increased choline signal coinciding with malignant degeneration of cerebral gliomas: A serial proton magnetic resonance spectroscopy imaging study. J Neurosurg 87:516–524, 1997.
61. Lombardi V, Valko L, Valko M, et al: 1H NMR ganglioside ceramide resonance region on the differential diagnosis of low and high malignancy of brain gliomas. Cell Mol Biol 17:521–535, 1997.
62. Woesler B, Kuwert T, Morgenroth C, et al: Non-invasive grading of primary brain tumors: Results of a comparative study between SPET with 123I-alpha-methyl tyrosine and PET with 18F-deoxyglucose. Eur J Nucl Med 24:428–434, 1997.
63. Morantz RA: Controversial issues in the management of low-grade astrocytomas. In Wilkins RH, Rengachary SS (eds): Neurosurgery Update I. New York: McGraw-Hill, 1990, pp 245–251.
64. Laws ER, Taylor WF, Bergstralh EJ, et al: The neurosurgical management of low-grade astrocytoma. Clin Neurosurg 33:575–588, 1986.
65. Salcman M: Radical surgery for low-grade glioma. Clin Neurosurg 36:353–366, 1990.
66. Weir B, Grace M: The relative significance of factors affecting postoperative survival in astrocytomas, grades one and two. Can J Neurol Sci 3:47–50, 1976.
67. Sano K: Integrative treatment of gliomas. Clin Neurosurg 30:93–124, 1983.
68. Francavilla TL, Miletich RS, Di Chiro G, et al: Positron emission tomography in the detection of malignant degeneration of low-grade gliomas. Neurosurgery 24:1–5, 1989.
69. Bernstein M: Low-grade gliomas: In search of evidence-based treatment. Clin Neurosurg 44:315–330, 1997.
70. Salcman M: Surgical decision-making for malignant brain tumors. Clin Neurosurg 35:285–311, 1989.
71. Giacomini C: Topografia della scissura di Rolando. Torino: Vercellino Tip, 1878.
72. Berger MS, Cohen WA, Ojemann GA: Correlation of motor cortex brain mapping data with magnetic resonance imaging. J Neurosurg 72:383–387, 1990.

73. Hu X, Tan KK, Levin DN, et al: Three-dimensional magnetic resonance images of the brain: Application to neurosurgical planning. J Neurosurg 72:433–440, 1990.
74. Fox PT, Burton H, Raichle ME: Mapping human somatosensory cortex with positron emission tomography. J Neurosurg 67:34–43, 1987.
75. Levin DN, Hu X, Tann KK, et al: The brain: Integrated three-dimensional display of MR and PET images. Radiology 172:783–789, 1989.
76. Evans AC, Marrett S, Torrescorzo J, et al: MRI-PET correlation in three dimensions using a volume-of-interest (VOI) atlas. J Cereb Blood Flow Metab 11:A69–A78, 1991.
77. Martin N, Grafton S, Vinuela F, et al: Imaging techniques for cortical functional localization. Clin Neurosurg 38:132–165, 1992.
78. Ojemann G, Ojemann J, Lettich E, Berger M: Cortical language localization in left dominant hemisphere: An electrical stimulation mapping investigation in 117 patients. J Neurosurg 71:316–326, 1989.
79. Nariai T, Senda M, Ishii K, Maehara T, et al: Thre-dimensional imaging of cortical structure, function and glioma for tumor resection. J Nucl Med 38:1563–1568, 1997.
80. Black PMCL, Ronner SF: Cortical mapping for defining the limits of tumor resection. Neurosurgery 20:914–919, 1987.
81. Walsh AR, Schmidt RH, Marsh HT: Cortical mapping and resection under local anaesthetic as an aid to surgery of low and intermediate grade gliomas. Br J Neurosurg 4:485–491, 1990.
82. Ebeling U, Schmid UD, Reulen HJ: Tumour-surgery within the central motor strip: Surgical results with the aid of electrical motor cortex stimulation. Acta Neurochir (Wien) 101:100–107, 1989.
83. Berger MS, Saadi Ghatan BS, Haglund MM, et al: Low-grade gliomas associated with intractable epilepsy: Seizure outcome utilizing electrocorticography during tumor resection. J Neurosurg 79:62–69, 1993.
84. Guthrie BL, Adler JR: Computer-assisted preoperative planning, interactive surgery, and frameless stereotaxy. Clin Neurosurg 38:112–131, 1992.
85. Auer LM, Van Velthonen V: Intraoperative ultrasound imaging: Comparison of pathomorphological findings in US and CT. Acta Neurochir (Wien) 104:84–95, 1990.
86. Rubin JM, Chandler WF: Ultrasound in Neurosurgery. New York: Raven Press, 1990.
87. Leroux PD, Berger MS, Ojemann GA, et al: Correlation of intraoperative ultrasound tumor volumes and margins with preoperative computerized tomography scans: An intraoperative method to enhance tumor resection. J Neurosurg 71:691–698, 1989.
88. Ono M, Kubik S, Abernathey CD: Atlas of the Cerebral Sulci. New York: G Thieme Verlag, 1990.
89. Wood CC, Spencer DD, Allison T, et al: Localization of human sensorimotor cortex during surgery by cortical surface recording of somatosensory evoked potentials. J Neurosurg 68:99–111, 1988.
90. King RB, Schell GR: Cortical localization and monitoring during cerebral operations. J Neurosurg 67:210–219, 1987.
91. Bartholow R: Experimental investigations into the functions of the human brain. Am J Med Sci 67:305–313, 1874.
92. Northfield DWC: Sir Victor Horsley: His contributions to neurological surgery. Surg Neurol 1:131–134, 1973.
93. Penfield WG, Boldrey E: Somatic motor and sensory representation in the cerebral cortex of man as studied by electrical stimulation. Brain 60:389–443, 1937.
94. Pia HW: Microsurgery of gliomas. Acta Neurochir (Wien) 80:1–11, 1986.
95. Yasargil MG, Cravens GF, Roth P: Surgical approaches to "inaccessible" brain tumors. Clin Neurosurg 34:42–110, 1988.
96. Harkey HL, Al-Mefty O, Haines DE, Smith RR: The surgical anatomy of the cerebral sulci. Neurosurgery 24:651–654, 1989.
97. Szikla G, Bouvier G, Hori T, Petrov V: Angiography of the human brain cortex: Atlas of vascular patterns and stereotactic cortical localization. Berlin: Springer-Verlag, 1977.
98. Berger MS, Ojemann GA, Lettich E: Cerebral hemispheric tumors of childhood. Neurosurg Clin N Am 34:839–852, 1992.

99. Hellwig D, Bauer BL, List-Hellwig E, et al: Stereotactic-endoscopic procedures on processes of the cranial midline. Acta Neurochir Suppl 53:23–32, 1991.
100. Epstein F: The Cavitron ultrasonic aspirator in tissue surgery. Clin Neurosurg 31:497–505, 1984.
101. Gonghai C, Qiwu X: Carbon dioxide laser vaporization of brain tumors. Neurosurgery 12:123–126, 1983.
102. Ascher PW, Heppner F: CO₂ laser in neurosurgery. Neurosurg Rev 7:123–133, 1984.
103. Koivukangas J, Koivukangas P: Treatment of low-grade cerebral astrocytoma: New methods and evaluation of results. Am Clin Res 47 (Suppl):115–124, 1986.
104. Poon WS, Schomaker KT, Deutsch TF, Martuza RL: Laser-induced fluorescence: Experimental intraoperative delineation of tumor resection margins. J Neurosurg 76:679–686, 1992.
105. Haglund MM, Berger MS, Hockman DW: Enhanced optical imaging of human gliomas and tumor margins. Neurosurgery 38:308–317, 1996.
106. Watanabe E, Mayanagy Y, Kosugi Y, et al: Open surgery assisted by the neuronavigator, a stereotactic, articulated, sensitive arm. Neurosurgery 28:792–800, 1991.
107. Watanabe E, Watanabe T, Manaka S, et al: Three-dimensional digitizer (neuronavigator): New equipment for computed tomography-guided stereotaxic surgery. Surg Neurol 27:543–547, 1987.
108. Kelly PJ: Stereotactic imaging, surgical planning and computer-assisted resection of intracranial lesions: Methods and results. In Symon L (ed): Advances and Technical Standards in Neurosurgery. New York: Springer-Verlag, 1990, pp 77–118.
109. Hassenbusch SJ, Anderson JS, Pillay PK: Brain tumor resection aided with markers placed using stereotaxis guided by magnetic resonance imaging and computed tomography. Neurosurgery 28:801–806, 1991.
110. McCormack BM, Miller DC, Budzilovich GN, et al: Treatment and survival of low-grade astrocytoma in adults 1977–1988. Neurosurgery 31:636–642, 1992.
111. Garcia D, Fulling K, Marks JE: The value of radiation therapy in addition to surgery for astrocytomas of the adult cerebrum. Cancer 55:917–919, 1985.
112. Sheline GE: The role of radiation therapy in treatment of low-grade gliomas. Clin Neurosurg 33:563–574, 1986.
113. Morantz RA: Radiation therapy in the treatment of cerebral astrocytoma. Neurosurgery 20:975–982, 1987.
114. Marks JE: Ionizing radiation. In Salcman M (ed): Neurobiology of Brain Tumors. Vol. 4: Concepts in Neurosurgery. Baltimore: Williams & Wilkins, 1991, pp 299–320.
115. Weingart J, Olivi A, Brem H: Supratentorial low-grade astrocytomas in adults. Neurosurg Q 1:141–159, 1991.
116. Bullard D, Rawlings CE, Phillips B, et al: Oligodendroglioma: An analysis of the value of radiation therapy. Cancer 60:2179–2188, 1987.
117. Piepmeier J, Christopher S, Spencer D, et al: Variations in the natural history and survival of patients with supratentorial low-grade astrocytomas. Neurosurgery 38:872–879, 1996.
118. Vecht CJ: Effect of age on treatment decisions in low-grade glioma. J Neurol Neurosurg Psychiatry 56:1259–1264, 1993.
119. Shaw EG, Scheithauer BW, O'Fallon JR, Davis DH: Mixed oligoastrocytomas: A survival and prognostic factors analysis. Neurosurgery 34:577–582, 1994.
120. Philippon JH, Clemenceau SH, Fauchon FH, Foncin JF: Supratentorial low-grade astrocytomas in adults. Neurosurgery 32:554–559, 1993.
121. Berger MS, Deliganis AV, Dobbins J, Evren Keles G: The effect of the extent of resection on recurrence in patients with low-grade cerebral hemisphere gliomas. Cancer 74:1784–1791, 1994.
122. Cairncross JG, Laperriere NJ: Low-grade glioma: To treat or not to treat? Arch Neurol 46:1238–1239, 1989.
123. Laws ER: The conservative management of primary gliomas of the brain. Clin Neurosurg 36:367–374, 1990.
124. Sutton LN, Wang Z, Gusnard D, et al: Proton magnetic resonance spectroscopy of pediatric brain tumors. Neurosurgery 31:195–202, 1992.

# Surgical Management of Recurrent Gliomas

■ GRIFFITH R. HARSH

Renewed growth of a mass at the site of a previously treated brain glioma raises issues pertaining to the indications for and choices of treatment. Important considerations include the following: (1) Is the mass a recurrence of the original tumor, (2) why did the tumor regrow, (3) does this regrowth pose a threat to the patient's neurologic function and survival, and (4) what additional therapy is appropriate?

## CONFIRMATION OF RECURRENCE

When recurrent growth of a glioma is suspected either clinically or radiographically, the full set of imaging studies should be reviewed with careful attention directed toward detecting any change of imaging signals and documenting the size of the lesion. The original pathologic specimen should be reviewed.

### Differential Diagnosis

An enlarging lesion at the site of a previously treated glioma likely represents renewed growth of an incompletely eradicated initial tumor rather than the development of a new pathologic entity. Exceptions are infrequent, but they do occur, as is noted in the following list:

- A tumor of related histology may supplant the original tumor; for example, the astrocytic component may replace the oligodendrocytic component as the predominant subtype of a mixed glioma, or a gliosarcoma may arise from a previously treated glioblastoma.
- A distinctly new tumor may arise near the site of an eradicated tumor. This is more likely to occur if there is a genetic predisposition to tumor development shared by cells in the area; for example, multiple gliomas may occur in a patient with tuberous sclerosis or neurofibromatosis.
- Non-neoplastic lesions induced by treatment of the original tumor may mimic tumor growth; for example, an abscess may be found at the site of tumor resection, or radiation necrosis may follow focal high-dose irradiation.

These differential diagnoses must be excluded before prognosis is addressed and therapy chosen. Neurodiagnostic imaging usually permits accurate prediction of the diagnosis. Usually, recurrent gliomas have imaging features similar to those of the original lesion. A recurrent malignant glioma will likely have central low-density rim enhancement, and hypodense surrounding components on computed tomographic (CT) scans. On magnetic resonance imaging (MRI) scans, the center and surrounding area will be $T_1$-hypointense and $T_2$-hyperintense, and the rim will enhance.[9, 10] In some cases, however, attention to subtle differences may be required: a more spherical, sharply demarcated, highly enhanced rim may suggest an abscess rather than recurrent malignant glioma, and a more diffuse, irregularly marginated pattern of surrounding edema may indicate radionecrosis rather than recurrent tumor. Two scenarios, malignant progression and radiation effects, often pose particular diagnostic difficulty. In each case, alternative diagnoses often cannot be distinguished by imaging criteria alone.

### Malignant Progression

The first scenario is the renewed growth of a low-grade tumor. When low-grade gliomas regrow after therapy, approximately half remain nonanaplastic, but the other 50% progress to a more malignant form.[34, 43, 54, 55, 86] Molecular analyses have delineated genetic correlates of this progression.[82] Enlarging low-grade tumors usually resemble the original tumor on imaging studies. When a progression in grade has occurred, the new tumor may also resemble the old one, especially if the original tumor enhanced with contrast. Enhancement is highly predictive of recurrence; low-grade enhancing tumors are six to eight times as likely to recur as nonenhancing tumors.[53] Most commonly, new malignant growth enhances in a previously nonenhancing glioma and, thus, is readily identified. In one study, only 30% (16 of 42) of low-grade tumors enhanced initially, but 92% (22 of 24) enhanced at recurrence.[53] Occasionally, however, an enlarging malignant focus may not enhance. However, it might be apparent as a region of hypermetabolism on a 2-deoxyglucose positron-emission tomography (PET) study, increased activity on a thallium or iodine single photon emission CT (SPECT) scan, or an area of increased cerebral blood volume on a functional MRI scan.[1, 21, 44] The sensitivity of these modalities for detecting tumor recurrence is approximately 80%.[41, 76] Usually, however, histologic analysis after biopsy or resection is warranted to verify malignant transformation.

## Radiation Effects

The second scenario that causes diagnostic difficulty is renewed enlargement of a tumor mass following radiation. Usually only large, very malignant tumors grow sufficiently fast to show significant enlargement during, or within 3 months of completing, a course of radiation. When this does occur, the prognosis is particularly poor.[5] Radiation can cause tumor enlargement in three ways: (1) through an early reaction, which is likely to be edema occurring during or shortly after irradiation; (2) through an early delayed reaction that involves edema and demyelination arising a few weeks to a few months after radiation; and (3) through a late delayed reaction that occurs 6 to 24 months after radiation and reflects radiation-induced necrosis.[45]

Regional teletherapy at a dose of 60 Gy is the current standard radiation treatment for most gliomas.[83] Although this dose has a low risk of inducing radiation necrosis,[81] regional early and early delayed effects are relatively common. In most cases tissue swelling represents edema and is transient. Acute symptoms from early or early delayed effects of radiation usually respond quickly to a short course of corticosteroids. The low-density, $T_1$-hypointense, $T_2$-hyperintense regions of edema correspond to the area irradiated. Chronically, these volumes of brain will demonstrate parenchymal atrophy, enlargement of subarachnoid spaces, and ex vacuo ventricular dilatation. Dementia with apathy, inanition, and memory loss and decline in fine motor control are the clinical correlates. In the absence of new tumor growth, enhancement on CT and MRI beyond the initial tumor resection margin is infrequent; when it does occur, it is patchy, irregularly marginated, and easily distinguished from the more focal appearance of recurrent tumor.

In contrast, the late delayed effect of radiation-induced necrosis appears at about the time malignant tumors might be expected to recur.[69] The risk of radiation necrosis increases with the volume of tissue treated, the dose delivered, and the fraction size.[52] Radiation necrosis following fractionated treatment to doses of less than 70 Gy is rare, but it is much more common following brachytherapy and radiosurgery. These methods deliver high doses of radiation to relatively small volumes over a short time period.[2, 51, 69] A common protocol for brachytherapy is a 50- to 60-Gy boost (to 60 Gy of regional external beam radiotherapy) to a 0- to 5-cm tumor delivered over approximately 1 week. The radiosurgical equivalent is a 10- to 20-Gy boost to a 0- to 3-cm tumor delivered in less than 1 hour.[49] Necrosis is radiographically and pathologically evident in almost all cases and symptomatic in about half.

Whether arising from higher doses of fractionated radiotherapy, brachytherapy, or radiosurgery, radiation necrosis is often difficult to distinguish radiographically from recurrent tumor. It forms a ringlike contrast-enhancing mass that resembles a malignant tumor. It has a CT hypodense, $T_1$-hypointense, $T_2$-hyperintense center; an enhancing annular region; and a hypodense, $T_1$-hypointense, $T_2$-hyperintense surrounding area. The surrounding area corresponds to edema that strikingly conforms to the patterns of white matter tract radiations. The similarity of this appearance to that of recurrent tumors and the time course of its occurrence frequently necessitate additional measures to differentiate radiation-induced necrosis from recurrent tumor. A variety of functional neurodiagnostic imaging techniques are currently being studied for their ability to distinguish between these two possibilities. These techniques include PET scans, SPECT scans, and MRI cerebral blood volume mapping. Regions of high activity are thought to distinguish recurrent tumor from relatively metabolically inactive and hypovascular radiation necrosis.[1, 21, 44, 78] Although specificity for differentiation of tumor recurrence from radiation necrosis of up to 100% has been claimed, in many cases, the data from these studies are inconclusive and the diagnosis is revealed either by the clinical course or by analysis of a pathologic specimen.[11, 76]

When an enlarging mass that is recurrent tumor, radiation necrosis, or both becomes symptomatic, corticosteroid therapy is required.[22] About half of the patients receiving high-dose–rate brachytherapy and radiosurgery develop symptoms that either prove refractory to corticosteroids or require debilitating long-term steroid use.[49–51, 69] Surgery for resection of an enlarging, symptomatic mass is needed in 20% to 40% of patients following such brachytherapy or radiosurgery of a malignant glioma.[49–51, 69] At reoperation for presumed radiation necrosis following focal radiation treatment of a malignant glioma, necrosis was found in 5% of cases, tumor alone in 29%, and a mixture of radiation necrosis and tumor in 66%.[69] In almost all cases, the tumor that is seen is of reduced viability.[17, 65]

## CAUSES OF RECURRENCE

Renewed growth of a brain glioma following surgery and possibly radiation and chemotherapy indicates failure of these therapies to reduce the tumor mass to a size (approximately $10^5$ cells) that would permit its eradication by the patient's immune system (Fig. 57–1).[67, 70] Failure arises from a number of factors that limit the efficacy of each modality.

### Recurrence After Surgery

Surgery may fail because of anatomic considerations, pathologic features, or errors in judgment or technique. The involvement of critical structures may limit the initial resection. Tumor investment of the anterior or middle cerebral arteries; involvement of the optic pathway, the diencephalon, the internal capsule, or brain stem; or proximity to eloquent cortex warrants incomplete removal. Tumor recurrence, despite removal of all macroscopically evident tumor, can occur if there is microscopic infiltration of adjacent structures. Even low-grade cerebral gliomas are usually infiltrative, and microscopic foci of neoplastic cells are frequently found several centimeters from the densely

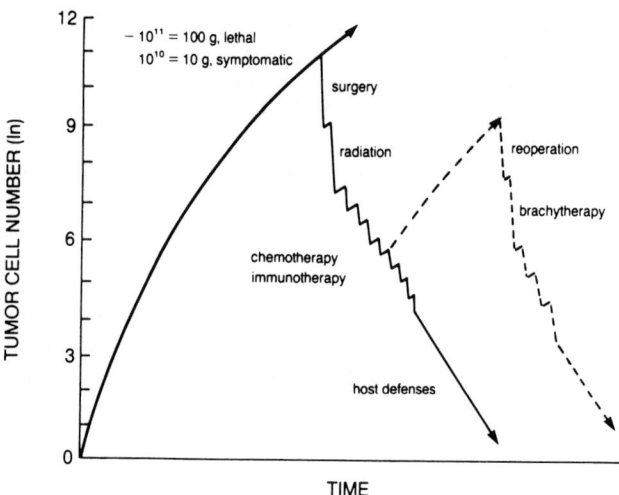

**FIGURE 57–1** ■ Multimodality therapy of malignant gliomas. Various therapeutic methods, including reoperation, are used in an attempt to reduce the number of tumor cells.

cellular tumor. Anaplastic astrocytomas and glioblastomas characteristically are widely invasive. Finally, errors in judgment, such as preoperatively underestimating the amount of tumor that can be safely removed or intraoperatively failing to remove tumor that was targeted, result in leaving potentially resectable tumor as a nidus of regrowth.

## Recurrence After Radiation

Radiation therapy may fail because of inadequate targeting, underutilization of tolerable dose, or radiation resistance of the tumor cells. The correlations between imaging abnormality and tumor extent are incomplete. Pathologic studies have shown that individual tumor cells can be found throughout and even beyond CT hypodense and MRI $T_2$-hyperintense areas of malignant glioma.[10, 35] The choice of field size for irradiation of such a lesion is difficult and relies as much on the trade-off between target volume and tolerable dose as on the accurate delineation of tumor boundaries. Failure to include an adequate annulus of tissue about the tumor to accommodate imaging uncertainty and technical error may leave tumor cells incompletely irradiated. Even if the maximal dose tolerated by infiltrative surrounding brain is delivered, tumor cells may remain viable. Hypoxic, nonproliferating cells are particularly radioresistant; with time or change in the physiologic conditions following therapy, re-entry of cells into the cell cycle permits the proliferation that results in clinically apparent tumor recurrence.[30] A recent study of high-dose fractionated proton irradiation following radical resection of glioblastomas showed the following: (1) a dose between 80 and 90 Gy is sufficient to prevent tumor regrowth; (2) outside this high-dose volume, tumor regrows, usually in areas receiving between 60 and 70 Gy; and (3) enlargement of the high-dose volume to include more peripheral areas is likely to be accompanied by unacceptably high levels of symptomatic radiation-induced necrosis.

## Recurrence After Chemotherapy

Chemotherapy fails as a result of inadequate drug delivery, toxicity, or cell resistance. The blood-brain barrier is deficient in the contrast-enhancing region of the tumor, but it is usually intact in surrounding brain; thus, lipid-insoluble drugs have limited access to tumor cells infiltrating peripheral regions. The margin between drug efficacy and neurotoxicity, bone marrow suppression, pulmonary injury, and intestinal side effects is often narrow. Noncycling cells are resistant to cell cycle–specific drugs, and potentially vulnerable cells often rapidly develop biochemical means of resistance to chemotherapeutic agents.[30, 39]

Even if these therapies significantly reduce the tumor burden, the patient's immune response may be rendered ineffective by chemotherapy and by the tumor's secretion of factors that are antagonistic to immune cytokines.[38] Each of these limitations of each component of multimodality therapy may contribute to failure to prevent tumor regrowth. At the time of tumor recurrence, consideration of these reasons for failure is essential to assessment of prognosis and to the choice of subsequent therapy.

# PROGNOSTIC IMPLICATIONS OF RESIDUAL AND RECURRENT TUMOR

In the management of a recurrent glioma, consideration of the prognostic implications of regrowth is essential. The presence of residual tumor and the occurrence of tumor regrowth likely have different prognostic implications.

## Residual Tumor

Radiologic demonstration of residual tumor after initial treatment may be consistent with preoperative goals and expectations; the prognosis would be that which was originally formulated. If, however, residual tumor is identified unexpectedly, the prognosis may need to be altered. The prognostic import of residual tumor is best seen in the relationship between the extent of resection and the likelihood of tumor recurrence.

Cytoreductive surgery is a fundamental part of the treatment of most systemic malignancies.[19] In most cases, there is a strong relationship between the extent of resection and outcome. For gliomas, the relationship between the extent of resection or, more significantly, the size of residual tumor, and outcome measures, such as interval to tumor progression and survival, is less clear.

Correlation of survival with the extent of resection for low-grade gliomas has been suggested by retrospective uncontrolled reviews and comparisons with historical reports.[43, 53, 80] One study of 461 adult patients with low-grade cerebral gliomas found that gross total surgical removal correlated with length of survival.[43] Another study reported a median survival of 7.4 years following maximal surgical resection. The median survival of a subgroup of hemispheric tumors compared favorably (10 years versus 8 years) with that of a comparable series treated with biopsy and radiation alone.[53, 80]

For high-grade gliomas, the correlations between the extent of resection at the initial operation and both the time to tumor recurrence and the duration of patient survival are disputed.[16] Historical reports and reviews of large series have noted the association of survival and the extent of resection for both astrocytomas and oligodendrogliomas.[12, 32, 57, 72, 83] Extensive reviews of the literature, however, have failed to locate randomized, controlled clinical trials comparing survival after biopsy with that after radical resection of malignant gliomas.[56, 63] Nevertheless, the benefit of surgical cytoreduction has been strongly suggested, as indicated by the following findings:

1. Reviews of multicentered trials have shown that the more complete the resection, the longer the patient lived.[70, 88]
2. In another study of 243 patients, multivariate regression analysis identified the extent of resection as an important prognostic factor ($P < .0001$) for survival.[79]
3. Single-center studies have confirmed this relationship: In one study containing 21 patients with glioblastomas and 10 patients with anaplastic astrocytomas, median survival time after gross total resection was 90 weeks versus only 43 weeks following subtotal resection, and the 2-year survival rates were 19% and 0%, respectively, even though the two groups were well matched for other prognostically significant variables.[3, 15] In another study, patients with a gross total resection of their malignant glioma lived longer (76 weeks versus 19 weeks) than those who underwent only a biopsy, even after correction for tumor accessibility and all other prognostically significant variables.[87]
4. In two larger series, patients with resected cortical and subcortical grade IV gliomas lived longer (50.6 weeks versus 33 weeks[20] and 39.5 weeks versus 32 weeks[40]) after surgery and radiation than those who underwent biopsy and radiation.
5. Small postoperative tumor volume has been shown to correlate with time to tumor progression after surgery[47] and longer patient survival.[5]

The data that exist for gliomas and experience with tumors outside the central nervous system suggest that cytoreduction, although less than ideal, does have a benefit when a near-total removal (1 to 2 log reduction of tumor cell number) of a glial tumor can be achieved. Thus, failure to identify and remove a readily accessible tumor mass at an initial operation might warrant reoperation before regrowth occurs.

## Recurrent Tumor

Regrowth of tumors after an initial response (diminution or stability) to surgery and radiation therapy is ominous. This is particularly true if the growth is more rapid or more infiltrative than that of the original tumor. Such growth often exhibits changes in the basic biology of the tumor that make it less responsive to subsequent therapy. A short interval between initial treatment and the recurrence of symptoms often indicates rapid regrowth and a poor prognosis. Factors to be considered in estimating prognosis include the biology of the tumor (its pathology, growth rate, and invasiveness), its resectability, its prior response to radiation and chemotherapy, and the age and performance status of the patient. Estimates of the recurrent tumor's size, growth rate, invasiveness, and location must be made in assessing its potential for causing both neurologic deficit and death. Reappearance of a slowly growing, well-demarcated frontal oligodendroglioma in a young patient in good neurologic condition after a 10-year interval of postsurgical quiescence clearly carries a much different prognosis than diffuse diencephalic spread of a glioblastoma multiforme in an elderly patient with a poor performance status 3 months after treatment with surgery, radiation, and chemotherapy.

## THERAPY OF RECURRENT TUMORS

The choice of therapy of a recurrent glioma is based on a comparison of the natural history of the regrowing tumor with the risk/benefit ratio of potential therapies. Gliomas that recur warrant aggressive multimodality therapy if the patient is in good neurologic and general medical condition and therapeutic options offer a realistic chance for significant increase in neurologic status or extension of survival.[68]

### Patterns of Recurrence

When gliomas recur, most do so locally. More than 80% of cases of recurrent glioblastoma multiforme arise within 2 cm of the original margin of contrast-enhancing tumor (Fig. 57–2).[29, 84] This tendency to recur locally is a function of tumor cell distribution. There is a gradient of tumor cell density in which tumor cell number decreases rapidly at increasing distances from the contrast-enhancing rim of solid tumor. Thus, although individual tumor cells are spread throughout the brain at great distances from the primary site, there are so many more cells locally that odds favor local reaccumulation of tumor mass.[9, 10, 35] Factors contributing to the likelihood of local recurrence include the following: (1) the relative predominance of tumor cell mass in the region, (2) the statistical likelihood that a local cell will be the cell that first develops a competitive proliferative advantage, and (3) the possibility that the physiologic milieu (hypervascularity, disrupted tissue architecture, and paracrine growth factor stimuli) at the site is particularly conducive to regrowth.

As tumor cell proliferation resumes at the initial tumor site, cells again spread rapidly and diffusely. Tumor cell proliferation resumes at distant sites as a result of the influx of these new, mitotically active cells or the renewed growth of cells that spread before the initial treatment.[14] Consequently, treatments targeting local recurrence alone are, at best, briefly palliative. Treatment of tumor recurrence thus usually involves a combination of modalities aimed at both local and distant disease.

### Multimodality Therapy

An enlarging lesion that was originally a low-grade glioma should undergo biopsy (stereotactically or, if resection is

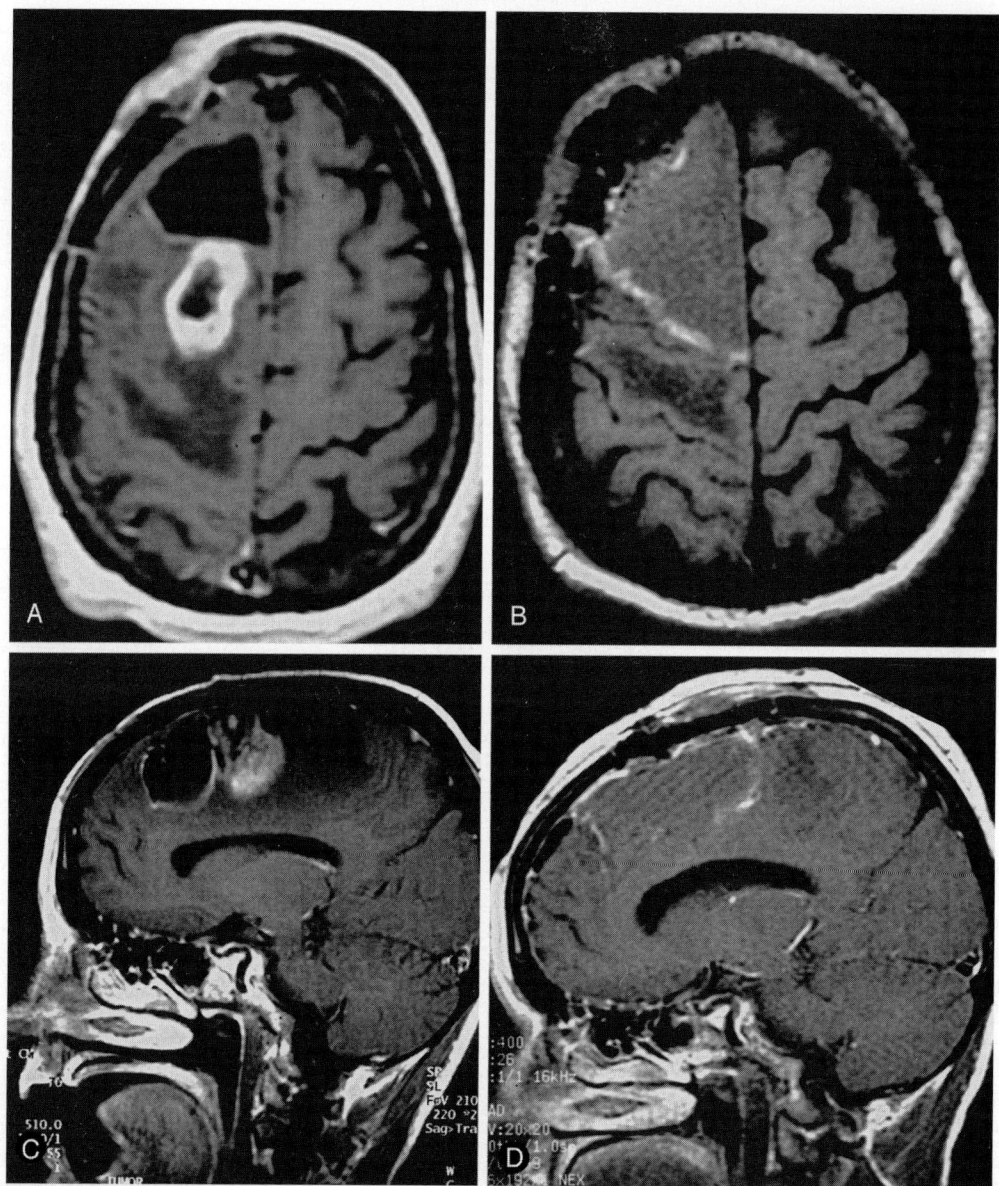

**FIGURE 57–2** ■ Recurrent malignant glioma. A 43-year-old woman developed right arm and leg weakness 11 months after complete resection and irradiation (60 Gy) of a right frontal glioblastoma. Preoperative axial *(A)* and sagittal *(C)* magnetic resonance imaging scans show ring contrast enhancement just posterior to the resection cavity. Reoperation, guided by intraoperative electrocorticographic mapping of the left primary motor area, accomplished gross total removal of the tumor and surrounding frontal lobe back to the prefrontal sulcus, as seen on postoperative axial *(B)* and sagittal *(D)* images. After the perioperative edema resolved, full strength returned to the patient's extremities.

anatomically feasible, by open craniotomy) to confirm its histology (Fig. 57–3). If the tumor remains low grade and a large part of the lesion can be resected without inflicting significant neurologic deficit, it should be removed; if the tumor was not irradiated initially the tumor bed and surrounding area should receive fractionated teletherapy. An interval of at least five years following an initial conservative dose may permit re-irradiation. If the tumor is inaccessible to surgery, radiation alone should be prescribed. If a previously irradiated low-grade tumor recurs as a low-grade glioma, it should be resected, if possible. If the tumor is inaccessible, stereotactically delivered focal radiation should be given.[59]

If the low-grade tumor recurs as a high-grade tumor, or if a high-grade tumor recurs, reoperation should be at-

tempted if the patient has a Karnofsky score of at least 70 and removal of all or almost all of the contrast-enhancing tumor is potentially attainable or if the tumor mass is causing neurologic symptoms that might be palliated by its reduction.[37] If the tumor was not irradiated previously, the tumor bed and its annular margin should receive regional teletherapy. Even when radiotherapy has been used initially, it is an option at recurrence.[31] Hypofractionated stereotactic radiotherapy (SRT, 5 Gy per fraction to doses ranging from 20 to 50 Gy) given to 29 patients with recurrent high-grade astrocytomas resulted in a median survival time after retreatment of 11 months.[73] Steroid-dependent toxicity occurred in 36% of patients, reoperation was required in 6%, and a total dose in excess of 40 Gy predicted radiation damage ($P < .005$).

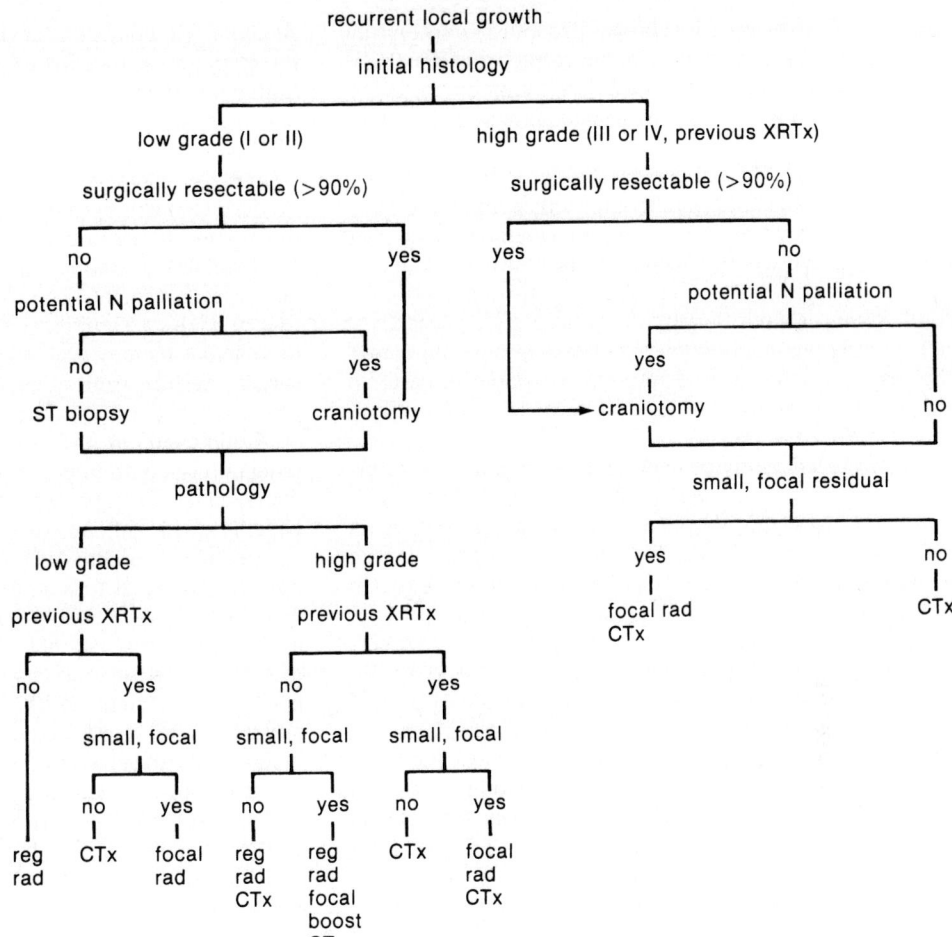

**FIGURE 57–3** ■ Management of recurrent gliomas. Decisions regarding the management of a recurrent tumor should consider grade, resectability, and prior therapy. (N, neurologic; reg rad, regional fractionated radiation therapy; focal rad/boost: stereotactic radiosurgery, brachytherapy, or radiotherapy; small, focal: less than 10 cm³, radiographically demarcated; CTx, chemotherapy.)

Others advocate that a stereotactically delivered focal boost of interstitial brachytherapy or radiosurgery should be given to any contrast-enhancing residual, particularly if the recurrent tumor is a glioblastoma.[2, 50, 69] Brachytherapy has proved valuable in treating glioblastomas, both initially and at the time of recurrence.[54, 60] The median survival following brachytherapy using temporary implantation of high-activity ¹²⁵I sources was 49 weeks for recurrent glioblastomas but only 52 weeks for anaplastic astrocytomas.[69] Patients receiving brachytherapy were highly selected; only about 20% of recurrent tumors met the criteria of appropriate size and focality. Almost 10% of patients suffered severe acute toxicity, and approximately 40% required reoperation for medically refractory neurologic deterioration and intracranial mass effect. Although tumor was identified in 95% of the specimens harvested at reoperation, reoperation was associated with longer survival time after brachytherapy (90 weeks versus 37 weeks for those not undergoing reoperation). The authors suggested that this rate of morbidity was justified by the prolongation of survival achieved in patients with glioblastomas but not by that for those with anaplastic astrocytomas.[69] Subsequent studies using low-activity ¹²⁵I sources implanted permanently at open operation have shown similar survival outcomes but lower rates of necrosis and reoperation after brachytherapy.[54]

Stereotactic radiosurgery is a less invasive way of induc-

ing tumor necrosis. Reported median survival following radiosurgery of recurrent glioblastomas is 40 weeks, and for recurrent anaplastic astrocytomas, it is at least 16 months. Here, too, patients were selectively treated, and significant radiation injury occurred frequently (21% of cases).[2] In a retrospective comparison of interstitial brachtherapy and radiosurgery, the median durations of survival times of the two groups were similar (11.5 months and 10.2 months, respectively). The actuarial risks of reoperation for necrosis at 12 and 24 months were 33% and 48%, respectively, after radiosurgery and 54% and 65%, respectively, after brachytherapy, with the caveat that the brachytherapy group had larger tumors and longer follow-up.[74] Other forms of focal radiation therapy such as photodynamic therapy (PDT), boron neutron capture therapy (BNCT), and intraoperative radiation (IORT) have been used sparingly for recurrent glioma.[25, 55]

Chemotherapy of recurrent astrocytomas is often valuable. Low-grade tumors will generally not have been treated by chemotherapy at the time of initial presentation unless a predominant oligodendrocytic component warranted procarbazine, CCNU, and vincristine (PCV) chemotherapy.[24] Adjuvant chemotherapy of malignant gliomas, in combination with radiation and surgery, increases the percentage of patients surviving at 1 year by 10% (a relative increase of 23.4%) and at 2 years by 8.6% (a 52.4% relative increase).[18, 23, 71] For grade IV tumors, bischloroethylnitrosourea bischloronitrosourea carmustine (BCNU) and PCV provide similar results, but the PCV combination is superior for grade III tumors.[23, 48] At the time of renewed growth of a high-grade tumor, if the tumor has not been exposed previously to a nitrosourea, then BCNU or the PCV combination should be tried.[61] A systematic review of 32 chemotherapy studies involving 1031 patients with recurrent malignant gliomas treated with chemotherapy identified nitrosoureas as the sole class of agents capable of significantly extending time to tumor progression.[31] If nitrosourea therapy is unsuccessful, alternatives such as carboplatin, cisplatin, or tamoxifen might be tried.[90] The response rates (partial response or stable disease) to such chemotherapy at the time of recurrence range from 20% to 50%.[62]

A more recent study of multimodality therapy for recurrent gliomas used multivariate statistical analysis to identify factors affecting response.[31] Fifty-one patients with recurrent malignant gliomas were treated in a phase II trial of multidrug chemotherapy. Of the 51 patients, 31 (61%) patients underwent reoperation consisting of radical tumor debulking before chemotherapy was begun. Disease stabilization or partial response occurred in 29 of the 51 (57%) patients. Median time to tumor progression (MTP) was 19 weeks for all pathologies, ranging from 32 weeks for patients with anaplastic astrocytomas to 13 weeks for those with glioblastoma multiforme. Median survival time (MST) was 40 weeks for all pathologies, 79 weeks for patients with anaplastic astrocytoma, and 33 weeks for those with glioblastoma multiforme. Thirty-five percent of patients had a serious chemotoxicity, but none had permanent morbidity or mortality. Factors associated with a longer MTP included a higher Karnofsky score, lower initial histologic grade, lack of prior chemotherapy, greater degree of myelotoxicity, smaller postoperative tumor volume, greater extent of resection, and a local rather than diffuse pattern of recurrence. Factors associated with a longer MST were a higher Karnofsky score, anaplastic astrocytoma rather than glioblastoma at recurrence, greater degree of myelotoxicity, and lobar rather than central location of the tumor.[31]

Alternative approaches have employed intracavitary or interstitial immunotherapy, chemotherapy, or gene therapy following reoperation for recurrent malignant gliomas.[8, 28, 64] One immunotherapy study employing lymphokine-activated killer cells and interleukin-2 described a median survial time of 53 weeks after reoperation and immunotherapy compared with 26 weeks following reoperation and chemotherapy.[28] The initial randomized, double-blind clinical trial with intracavitary BCNU wafers showed improved survival rates in the BCNU arm relative to the placebo arm at 6 months after treatment, but the survival curves converged at longer follow-up.[8] Preliminary gene therapy studies using ganciclovir activated by a thymidine kinase gene delivered by a retrovirus produced by a modified mouse fibroblast packaging cell line have proved feasible and safe but have not yet demonstrated either efficacy or proof of mechanism.[64]

## Rationale for Reoperation

Early reoperation, within months of the initial procedure, might be indicated for complications such as intracerebral,

subdural, or epidural hematoma; wound dehiscence and infection; or hydrocephalus and CSF leakage. Occasionally, failure to identify and remove an accessible tumor at a first operation might warrant reoperation. In the Royal Melbourne Hospital experience, 5 of 200 patients underwent early reoperation.[34]

More frequently, true tumor recurrence after an interval of response to the initial therapy is the reason for considering reoperation. Reoperation is justified if it produces sustained improvement of neurologic condition and quality of life, as well as significant enhancement of response rates to adjuvant therapy. Palliation of neurologic symptoms by surgery results from reduction of the local mass effect produced by the tumor and tumor-induced edema.

Multiple studies have shown that primary surgical cytoreduction can both improve neurologic deficits and promote maintenance of high-performance status. One review of 82 patients examined five categories of neurologic function in each patient. One hundred and ninety-one neurologic deficits were noted before surgery. After surgery, 151 deficits were improved or stable, and 40 were worse.[71] Another study showed that patients undergoing gross total resection of their malignant gliomas were likely to have improved neurologic outcome (97% of 36 patients had either improved or stable neurologic conditions), improved functional status (mean Karnofsky score improvement of 6.8%), and extended maintenance of good functional status (mean of 185 weeks).[3, 15] A third study confirmed that the extent of surgery correlated with better immediate postoperative performance, lower 1-month mortality rate, and longer survival: 43% of patients with malignant gliomas improved, 50% remained unchanged, and 7% suffered deterioration in their neurologic condition following resection of at least 75% of their tumor, as opposed to the outcomes of a more limited resection (28% improved, 51% were unchanged, and 21% were worse).[79]

Similar results can be achieved by reoperation. Forty-five percent of the patients had an improved Karnofsky score following reoperation in one series.[3, 64] In another series focusing on reoperation, when gross tumor resection was achieved, 82% (32 of 39) of patients had shown improvement or stability in their Karnofsky score.[85] In a third, patients with Karnofsky scores of 50 or less also underwent reoperation. Two thirds improved from a dependent to an independent state, and the median survival was similar to that for all patients undergoing reoperation.[75]

The doubling rate of malignant gliomas is so high, however, that the benefits gained by reoperation will be very brief unless adjuvant therapies are used to induce remission of tumor growth. Surgical resection is especially beneficial when reduction of tumor burden improves the response rate to such therapies. Studies from the University of California at San Francisco (UCSF), Memorial Sloan-Kettering, and the University of Washington at Seattle have shown that reoperation followed by chemotherapy leads to stabilization of the performance score for significant intervals (Fig. 57–4).[4, 7, 26] At UCSF, 44% of patients with glioblastomas maintained a performance level of at least 70 (a level consistent with self-care and judged to be survival of high quality[33] [Table 57–1]) for at least 6 months after reoperation; 18% maintained this level for at least a year; and three patients did so for longer than 3 years. Most patients

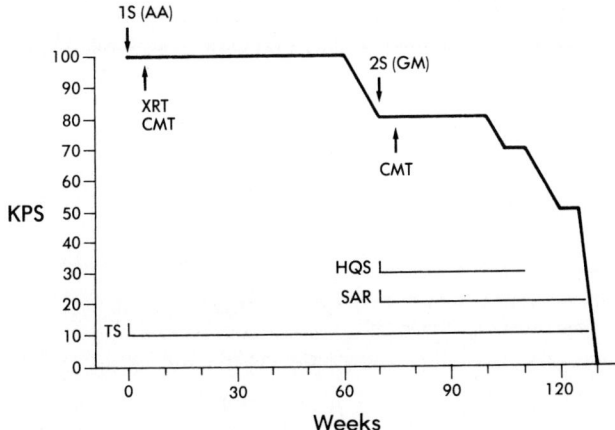

**FIGURE 57–4** ■ Quality of life considerations in the management of patients with malignant gliomas. Maintenance of high-performance status is a critical feature of outcome. The Karnofsky score (KPS) as a function of time indicates the quality of the survival time that follows each intervention. (1S, initial surgery; XRT, radiation theraphy; CMT, chemotheraphy; 2S, reoperation; TS, total survival; HQS, high-quality survival (K ≥70); SAR, survival after reoperation; AA, anaplastic astrocytoma; GM, glioblastoma multiforme.)

(52% of 31) with anaplastic astrocytomas maintained this performance level for at least 12 months after reoperation; 13% had more than 4 years of high-quality survival. Approximately 90% of the survival after reoperation for anaplastic astrocytoma was of high quality.[26] In the Memorial Sloan-Kettering group, the median duration of maintenance

## TABLE 57–1 ■ KARNOFSKY PERFORMANCE STATUS

| Definition | % | Criteria |
|---|---|---|
| Able to carry on normal activity and to work; no special care is needed | 100 | Normal; no complaints; no evidence of disease |
| | 90 | Able to carry on normal activity; minor signs or symptoms of disease |
| | 80 | Normal activity with effort; some signs or symptoms of disease |
| Unable to work; able to live at home, care for most personal needs; a varying amount of assistance is needed | 70 | Cares for self; unable to carry on normal activity or to do active work |
| | 60 | Requires occasional assistance, but is able to care for most needs |
| | 50 | Requires considerable assistance and frequent medical care |
| Unable to care for self; requires equivalent of institutional or hospital care; disease may be progressing rapidly | 40 | Disabled; requires special care and assistance |
| | 30 | Severely disabled, hospitalization is indicated although death is not imminent |
| | 20 | Very sick; hospitalization necessary; active supportive treatment necessary |
| | 10 | Moribund; fatal processess progressing rapidly |
| | 0 | Dead |

From Karnofsky D, Burchenal JH, Armistead GC Jr, et al: Triethylene melamine in the treatment of neoplastic disease. Arch Intern Med 87:477–516, 1951.

of independent status (a Karnofsky score of at least 80) was 34 weeks.[4] In the University of Washington series, patients with a Karnofsky score of at least 70 maintained this high level of function for an average of 37 weeks after reoperation for glioblastoma and for 70 weeks after reoperation for anaplastic astrocytoma.[7]

Aggressive surgical cytoreduction at the time of recurrence may increase the duration as well as the quality of patient survival. Support for reoperation is found in comparisons of the outcomes in cases in which different degrees of tumor removal were accomplished and in comparisons of the survival of patients following reoperation with that of historical control patients not undergoing reoperation. Patients in whom gross total resection of a glioblastoma is achieved survive longer (45.6 weeks versus 25.6 weeks) than do those receiving near-total or subtotal resections; for anaplastic astrocytomas, the effect of the extent of resection is similar (87.5 weeks versus 55.7 weeks).[7] In the Sloan-Kettering series that grouped glioblastomas and anaplastic astrocytomas together, a similar difference was found (51.2 weeks versus 23.3 weeks).[4] In the UCSF series, survival of patients undergoing reoperation and chemotherapy for either anaplastic astrocytoma or glioblastoma was longer than that of patients receiving chemotherapy alone at the time of tumor recurrence.[26]

The benefit of reoperative surgery is also suggested by experience with brachytherapy. Patients undergoing reoperation for tumor recurrence, radiation necrosis, or both following brachytherapy for glioblastomas either initially or at first recurrence survived longer than those not receiving reoperation: median total survival of 120 weeks versus 62 weeks for patients with primarily treated tumors, and 90 weeks versus 37 weeks for patients treated with brachytherapy at the time of first recurrence.[69]

Reoperation as a part of the multimodality treatment of recurrent gliomas is further supported by study of long-term survivors of glioblastoma multiforme. A review of the UCSF experience identified 22 of 449 (5%) patients with glioblastomas who survived at least 5 years after diagnosis. Sixteen of 22 patients had tumor recurrence that was treated; 9 underwent between one and three reoperations. For 8 of the 16 patients with treated recurrence, survival time after treatment of recurrence (median of 4.5 years) was longer than the remission produced by the initial treatment.[13]

The benefit to survival from reoperation is not above dispute. As noted, multivariate analyses of chemotherapy studies have found that extent of resection and smaller postopertive volume are associated with prolongation of time to tumor progression but not of survival.[66] A similar study of survival after progression of malignant gliomas identified high Karnofsky score and age less than 50 years as independent prognostic factors.[77] Those who underwent reoperation (58 of 143 patients) lived longer (median of 35 weeks versus 16 weeks, $P < .005$ in univariate analysis) after tumor recurrence than those treated without reoperation, but multivariate analysis identified only a trend toward reduction of risk of death (relative risk = 0.74; 95% confidence interval = 0.50–1.11; $P = .014$) following reoperation. Randomized controlled trials using MRC brain tumor prognostic indices for analysis of outcomes are needed to evaluate definitively the benefits of reoperation.[42]

## TABLE 57–2 ■ REOPERATION FOR RECURRENT GLIOMAS

| Author | No. of Patients | Pathology | SAR | HQS | Morb | Mort | ⁻K | Px Relations | Weeks |
|---|---|---|---|---|---|---|---|---|---|
| Young et al[89] | 24 | GM | 14 | | 52% | 17% | 25% | K-³ 60 → SAR | 22 v 9 |
| | | | | | | | | II > 12 m → SAR | 16.5 v 8.5 |
| Salcman et al[67] | 40 | MG | 37 | | | 0% | | Age < 40 → SAR | 57 v 36 |
| Ammirati et al[4] | 55 | 64% GM | 36 | 34 | 16% | 64% | 45% | K > 70 → SAR | 48.5 v 19 |
| | | | | | | | | Grade → SAR | 61 v 29 |
| | | | | | | | | Ext. resect. → SAR | 51.2 v 23.3 |
| Harsh et al[26] | 49 | GM | 36 | 10 | 8% | 5% | 5% | Age → SAR | |
| | | | | | | | | K-³ 70 → HQS | |
| Harsh et al[26] | 21 | AA | 88 | 83 | 3% | 3% | 10% | Age → HQS | |
| | | | | | | | | Grade → SAR | |
| Berger et al[7] | 56 | GM | | | | | | K-³ 70 → SAR | 70.7 v 36.5 |
| | | | | | | | | K-³ 70 → SQE | 36.6 v 8.4 |
| | | | | | | | | Age² 60 → SQE | 35.1 v 9.4 |
| | | | | | | | | II > 12m → SAR | 150 v 48 |
| Berger et al[7] | 14 | AA | | | | | | II > 12m → SOE | 99.5 v 22.4 |
| Kaye[34] | 50 | GM | | | 16% | 0% | | Age → SAR | |
| | | | | | | | | Grade → SAR | |
| | | | | | | | | II → SAR | |
| | | | | | | | | Age → HQS | |
| | | | | | | | | Grade → HQS | |
| | | | | | | | | II → HQS | |
| Barker et al[5] | 46 | GM | 36 | 18 | 23% | 0% | 28% | K → SAR | |

GM, glioblastoma multiforme; AA, anaplastic astrocytoma; SAR, survival after reoperation; SQE, same quality existence; HQS, high-quality survival (K = /³ 70); Morb, morbidity; Mort, mortality; ⁻K, increased performance score; Cx, complications; II, interoperative interval; Ext resect, extent of resection; Px, prognostic relations.

*Note*: For a description of Karnofsky performance ratings, see Table 57–1.

## Selection of Patients for Reoperation

Case selection is critical to outcome. The patient's profile of prognostic factors, his or her predicted tolerance of the procedure, and the feasibility of extensive tumor resection without undue risk of new neurologic morbidity must all be considered. Multiple characteristics have been identified as predictive of a good response to reoperation (Table 57–2). Foremost among these are tumor histologic type, patient age, performance status, interoperative interval, and extent of resection.[37]

The prognostic significance of tumor grade is evident in most series. Median survival after reoperation was 88 weeks for patients with anaplastic astrocytomas but only 36 weeks for those with glioblastomas at UCSF and was 61 weeks and 29 weeks, respectively, at Sloan-Kettering.[4, 27]

Age may be more significant than tumor grade. In one series, survival after reoperation was 57 weeks for those younger than 40 years but only 36 weeks for older patients.[68] Other authors found an association between youth and total survival after diagnosis and between youth and quality of survival after reoperation, but not between youth and duration of survival after reoperation.[4, 27]

The patient's preoperative performance score significantly affects the outcome of reoperation. At Kentucky, survival after reoperation was 22 weeks for patients with performance scores of at least 70 but only 9 weeks for more disabled patients.[89] In the University of Washington series, for glioblastomas, survival after reoperation was almost twice as long (71 weeks versus 36 weeks) for patients with Karnofsky scores of at least 70.[7]

The prognostic importance of the interval between initial treatment and recurrence is disputed.[86] The Kentucky series found survival time to be twice as long if the interval between operations exceeded 6 months. At the University of Washington, a three-fold difference (150 weeks versus 48 weeks for glioblastoma and 164 weeks versus 52 weeks for anaplastic astrocytomas) was noted when the time to progression exceeded 3 years.[7] Others, however, have found either no relation or an inverse relation between the interoperative interval and the survival time after reoperation.[4, 27, 68]

A more complete resection of recurrent tumor portends longer survival. At Sloan-Kettering, gross total resection afforded a median survival of 51.2 weeks versus 23.3 weeks for a more limited resection.[4, 85] Others have noted a strong trend in the correlation between a more complete removal of tumor and survival duration.[7] The ability to remove sufficient tumor mass to be of oncologic benefit depends on the location of the tumor and its physical characteristics. Removal is facilitated by a more superficial location in noneloquent areas; a discrete pseudoencapsulated mass is more easily removed than a less well margined, diffuse one; drainage of a cystic component often provides immediate reduction of mass, as well as an avenue for further resection of tumor.

During the interval between initial surgery and tumor recurrence, the patient usually undergoes therapy that might affect his or her tolerance of further surgery. The decision to reoperate must consider the patient's overall physical condition, tissue viability, blood coagulability, hematologic reserve, and immune function following surgery, radiation, corticosteroids, and chemotherapy. A high risk of multisystem failure, failure to thrive, intracranial hemorrhage, anemia, wound infection, pneumonia, or neurologic damage may exist. This risk should be assessed for each patient by obtaining preopertive chemical, hematologic, and radiographic studies.

In choosing patients for reoperation, consideration of the individual patient's profile of these prognostically significant factors permits a reasonable estimate of the likelihood that he or she will benefit from the procedure.

## Preparation for Reoperation

Before surgery, the patient usually receives corticosteroids; they should be continued. At the time of induction of anesthesia, the patient is fitted with elastic stockings and thigh-high intermittent compression air boots. He or she is given additional steroids, prophylactic antibiotics, an anticonvulsant, and osmotic and loop diuretics and is hyperventilated. In positioning the patient, the likelihood of elevated intracranial pressure makes elevation of the head above the level of the heart particularly important.

## Reoperative Exposure

In planning the needed exposure, the location of the tumor can be specified by its relationship to the margins of the craniotomy plate on a CT scan or to the cortical pattern of gyri and sulci on an MRI scan, or by intraoperative stereotactic localization techniques. The procedure should be planned in advance to ensure adequate skin opening, craniotomy, and durotomy to expose the recurrent mass. All may need to be shifted or enlarged relative to the original procedure because of the increased extent of the tumor or a desire to perform corticography for mapping of motor or speech function, or both.

The skin incision from the previous operation is usually used. The skin opening can be increased by introducing additional incisions. They should be external to the previous flap, avoid its base and other vascular pedicles, and intersect the previous incision at right angles. The margins of the prior craniotomy flap should be defined. Generally, this is best accomplished with a curet beginning at a prior trephination. Only rarely does the prior kurf need to be recut. Dissection in the epidural plane can be begun with a curet followed by a No. 3 and then a No. 2 Penfield dissector. The craniotomy plate is further elevated as the dura is stripped from its inner surface with a periosteal elevator. Epidural adhesions fixing dura to the craniotomy margin should be preserved as prophylaxis against postoperative extension of an epidural fluid collection unless the craniotomy needs to be enlarged. In this case, these adhesions are dissected with a curet and trimmed. After the dura has been stripped from the undersurface of the cranial plate, an additional segment of bone can be removed with a craniotome.

The durotomy may need to be enlarged, but often, it can be limited to part of the dural exposure. It should be planned to minimize traverse of cortical adhesions. For instance, in re-exposing a temporal lesion, the durotomy can be placed over the cyst remaining from the prior resection. Flapping the dura superiorly then allows adhesions to be put on traction such that they may be dissected from cortex, coagulated, and sharply divided. Extending a durotomy along an old incision line should be avoided. The prior incision line should be traversed perpendicularly and as infrequently as possible because it is often the site of the densest adhesions. Microdissection of larger vessels from dural attachments may be necessary.

Once the dura is opened and retracted, the exposed cortex is inspected for the surface presentation of the tumor; its abnormal color, consistency, and vascularity should be apparent.

Localization of the subcortical extent of the tumor is then undertaken. Again, the preoperative imaging studies and intraoperative computer-assisted stereotactic localization techniques are of value (Fig. 57–5).[36] Transcortical

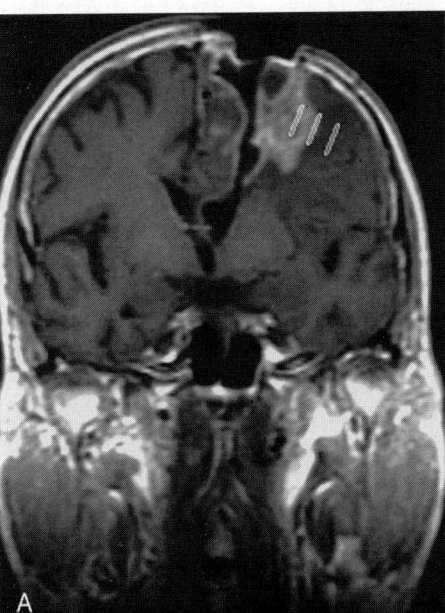
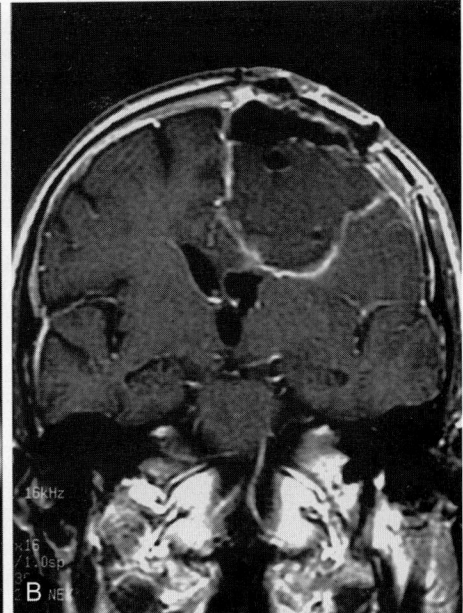

FIGURE 57–5 ■ Surgical technique. A 39-year-old man developed marginal recurrence about the cystic resection cavity left after removal and irradiation of an anaplastic astrocytoma 3 years earlier. As part of a gene therapy trial, three columns of vector-producing cells were infused within the tumor, at the tumor margin, and in surrounding infiltrated brain (A, coronal MRI). Five days later, the tumor and the infused tissue were removed to be analyzed. Care was taken to extend the resection to the margin of eloquent areas and to achieve watertight closure (B, coronal, immediately postoperative magnetic resonance imaging scan).

ultrasonography is often helpful, although this technique tends to overestimate the volume of recurrent tumor.[46] Tumor may also be found by locating a cystic resection cavity or encephalomalacic brain left after the previous operation. In that almost all tumors recur within 2 cm of the original tumor's margin, exposure of the initial tumor's surgical bed usually reveals at least part of the recurrent mass.

Electrocorticographic mapping of motor, sensory, and speech areas may reduce the chance of inflicting a neurologic deficit and may encourage a more extensive resection by revealing the relationship of the site of cortical traverse and of the subsequent subcortical dissection to eloquent brain (see Figs. 57–2 and 57–5).[6] This technique is often more difficult at the time of reoperation because of cortical disruption by the tumor and prior surgery. An intraoperative photograph from cortical mapping at the time of the initial craniotomy may suffice.

Generally, the appearance of the tumor itself is the best guide to its extent. Tumor-infiltrated cortex is likely to have increased vascular markings, a pink to gray color, and a firm consistency. Its central core may vary from yellow cystic fluid of low viscosity to high-viscosity, soupy, white necrosis that resembles pus to a yellow-gray, granular, honeycomb-like material. Generally, the center is relatively avascular, although it may be traversed by thrombosed blood vessels.

Some authors advocate incision into the tumor mass and internal debulking with an ultrasonic aspirator or laser as an initial step. However, this often induces significant hemorrhage. Enucleation by circumferential dissection in the pseudoplane about the rim of solid tumor is usually more satisfactory. Arteries supplying the tumor and veins draining it can be coagulated and divided as they enter the tumor mass much as the vascular supply of an arteriovenous malformation (AVM) is handled. Particularly in areas of noneloquent brain, the softened, necrotic, highly edematous white matter around the tumor provides an excellent plane of dissection. The use of bipolar cautery forceps and suction together accomplishes this dissection while reducing local mass. Beyond the encephalomalacic brain lies more normal brain that, although edematous and possibly injured by prior retraction and radiation therapy, is often functional and should be preserved.

Often, the tumor can be removed as a single specimen without the need for significant retraction of surrounding brain. In general, gentle, temporary displacement of a cottonoid patty lying on the margin of resection provides sufficient exposure of the dissection plane so that fixed, self-retaining retractors are unnecessary. Retraction of the tumor mass is preferable to retraction of surrounding brain. Often, identification of the appropriate plane for the circumferential dissection is facilitated by this retraction on the tumor; coherence of the tumor mass helps delineate the plane between solid tumor and tumor-infiltrated brain.

Once the tumor mass has been removed, the margins of resection should be inspected to verify that the excision is complete. The margins should be free of tumor that is more firm, glassy, opaque, and hypervascular. Biopsies of the surrounding edematous brain should be sent for frozen section analysis to verify absence of tumor. If solid tumor or tumor infiltrating into noneloquent areas remains, it

should be removed. In some cases, extension of tumor into eloquent areas or diencephalic structures precludes resection of the entire mass. In such cases, the tumor should be divided. This process often entails coagulation of numerous strands of small, thin-walled blood vessels, particularly if the extension is in the direction of the vascular supply, such as medial extension of a temporal lobe tumor toward the posterior aspect of the sylvian fissure. Care should be taken to coagulate and sharply divide these vessels. Tearing them without prior coagulation will leave a loose end that will retract and continue to bleed. Such loose ends should be directly coagulated rather than tamponaded with hemostatic packing, which may encourage deeper dissection of a hematoma.

After the resection has been completed, hemostasis should be confirmed by filling the tumor cavity with saline and, during a Valsalva maneuver, observing for wisps of continuing hemorrhage. This check should be performed with the patient's blood pressure at least as high as his or her normal level. The cavity is then aspirated, lined with a single layer of Surgicel, and filled again with irrigation fluid. Hyperventilation is then reversed to permit expansion of the brain during closure.

Watertight dural closure is essential (see Fig. 57–5B). Often, this can be attained by primary suturing, given the decompression by tumor removal. If the dura is incompetent, it may be supplemented by a pericranial graft. Peripheral and central dural tacking sutures are placed. The bone fragments are wired together, and then the craniotomy plate is fixed with nonabsorbable monofilament suture, stainless steel wire, or titanium miniplates. The wound is irrigated several times with antibiotic solution and then closed in layers with 2–0 absorbable suture in muscle, fascia, and galea. The galeal sutures should be inverted and the knots should be cut short to avoid superficial erosion. They should be placed in sufficient proximity so that tension-free closure of the skin is possible. Simple running 4–0 nylon skin sutures or staples provide adequate skin closure except at sites of attenuation, where horizontal mattress sutures may be less likely to compromise blood supply.

Postoperatively, the patient should be monitored closely for at least 72 hours for signs of increased intracranial pressure from hematoma or edema. Fluid restriction, dehydration, and corticosteroids should be continued throughout this period. The patient should be mobilized as soon as possible, and a gadolinium-enhanced MRI scan should be obtained as soon as he or she is able to tolerate it.

## ACKNOWLEDGMENT

*While Harsh quotes Karnofsky[33] as ranking level 70 on his scale for at least 6 months as a high-quality survival, on reference to that scale (see Table 57–1), one notes that the grade 70 patient is unable to carry on normal activity or do active work. However, this patient can care for himself or herself. Many of us would prefer not to survive at all if 6 months at that level were the best outcome that was likely. Wilson[11] has reported that 22 of 449 patients with glioblastomas treated at UCSF survived at least 5 years; 16 of those 22 experienced a recurrence. He believes that some entirely new agents or tactics must be developed. Harsh gives us excellent advice on what to do about the problem today pending such future development.*

*WILLIAM H. SWEET*

# REFERENCES

1. Alavi JB, Alavi A, Chawluk J, et al: Positron emission tomography in patients with gliomas. A predictor of prognosis. Cancer 62:1074–1078, 1988.
2. Alexander EA, Loeffler JS: Radiosurgery using a modified linear accelerator. Neurosurg Clin North Am 3:174–176, 1992.
3. Ammirati M, Vick N, Liao Y, et al: Effect of the extent of surgical resection on survival and quality of life in patients with supratentorial glioblastomas and anaplastic astrocytomas. Neurosurgery 21:201–206, 1987.
4. Ammirati M, Galicich JH, Arbit B: Reoperation in the treatment of recurrent intracranial malignant gliomas. Neurosurgery 21:607–614, 1987.
5. Barker FG, Chang SM, Gutin PH, et al: Survival and functional status after resection after resection of recurrent glioblastoma multiforme. Neurosurgery 42:709–723, 1998.
6. Berger MS, Ojemann GA, Lettich E: Neurophysiological monitoring during astrocytoma surgery. Neurosurg Clin North Am 1:65–80, 1990.
7. Berger MS, Tucker A, Spence A, Winn HR: Reoperation for glioma. Clin Neurosurg 39:172–186, 1992.
8. Brem H, Piantadosi S, Berger PC, et al: Placebo controlled trial of safety and efficacy of intraoperative controlled delivery by biodegradable polymers of chemotherapy for recurrent gliomas. Lancet 345:1008–1012, 1995.
9. Burger PC, Dubois PJ, Schold SC Jr, et al: Computerized tomography and pathologic studies of the untreated, quiescent, and recurrent glioblastoma multiforme. J Neurosurg 58:159–169, 1983.
10. Burger PC, Heinz ER, Shibata T, et al: Topographic anatomy and CT correlations in the untreated glioblastoma multiforme. J Neurosurg 68:698–704, 1988.
11. Carvalho PA, Schwartz RB, Alexander E III, et al: Detection of recurrent gliomas with quantitative thallium-201/technetium-99m HMPAO single-photon emission computerized tomography. J Neurosurg 77:565–70, 1992.
12. Chang CH, Horton J, Schoenfeld O, et al: Comparison of postoperative radiotherapy and combined postoperative radiotherapy and chemotherapy in the multidisciplinary management of malignant gliomas. Cancer 52:997–1007, 1983.
13. Chandler KL, Prados MD, Malec M, Wilson CB: Long-term survival in patients with glioblastoma multiforme. Neurosurgery 32:716–720, 1993.
14. Choucair AK, Levin VA, Gutin PH, et al: Development of multiple lesions during radiation therapy and chemotherapy in patients with gliomas. J Neurosurg 65:654–658, 1986.
15. Ciric I, Ammirati M, Vick N, et al: Supratentorial gliomas: Surgical considerations and immediate postoperative results. Gross total resection versus partial resection. Neurosurgery 21:21–26, 1989.
16. Coffey RJ, Lunsford LD, Taylor FH: Survival after stereotactic biopsy of malignant gliomas. Neurosurgery 22:465–473, 1988.
17. Daumas-Duport C, Blond S, Vedrenee C, Szikla G: Radiolesion versus recurrence: Bioptic data in 30 gliomas after interstitial implant or combined interstitial and external radiation treatment. Acta Neurochir 33 (Suppl):291–299, 1984.
18. Deutsch M, Green SB, Strike TA, et al: Results of a randomized trial comparing BCNU plus radiotherapy, streptozotocin, plus radiotherapy, BCNU plus hyperfractionated radiotherapy and BCNU following misonidazole plus radiotherapy in the postoperative treatment of malignant glioma. Int J Radiat Oncol Biol Phys 16:1389–1396, 1989.
19. Devita VT: The relationship between tumor mass and resistance to chemotherapy. Cancer 51:1209–1220, 1983.
20. Devaux BC, O'Fallon JR, Kelly PJ: Resection, biopsy, and survival in malignant gliomas: A retrospective study of clinical parameters, therapy, and outcome. J Neurosurg 78:767–775, 1993.
21. DiChiro G, Brooks R, Bairamian D, et al: Diagnostic and prognostic value of positron emission tomography using [18F] fluorodeoxyglucose in brain tumors. In Reivich M, Alavi A (eds): Positron Emission Tomography. New York: Alan R Liss, 1985, pp 291–309.

22. Edwards MS, Wilson CB: Treatment of radiation necrosis. In Gilbert HA, Kagan AR (eds): Radiation Damage to the Nervous System. A Delayed Therapeutic Hazard. New York: Raven Press, pp 120–143.
23. Fine HA, Dear KBG, Loeffler JS, et al: Meta-analysis of radiation therapy with and without adjuvant chemotherapy for malignant gliomas in adults. Cancer 71:2585–2597, 1993.
24. Glass J, Hochberg FH, Gruber ML, et al: The treatment of oligodendrogliomas and mixed oligodendroglioma-astrocytomas with PCV chemotherapy. J Neurosurg 76:741–745, 1992.
25. Hara A, Nishimura Y, Sakai N, et al: Effectiveness of intraoperative radiation therapy for recurrent supratentorial low grade glioma. J Neuro oncol 25:239–243, 1995.
26. Harsh GR, Levin VA, Gutin PH, et al: Reoperation for recurrent glioblastoma and anaplastic astrocytoma. Neurosurgery 21:615–621, 1987.
27. Harsh GR, Wilson CB: Neuroepithelial tumors in adults. In Youmans JR (ed): Neurological Surgery, 3rd ed. Philadelphia: WB Saunders, 1990, pp 3040–3136.
28. Hayes RL, Koslow M, Hiesiger EM, et al: Improved long term survival after intracavitary interleukin-2 and lymphokine-activated killer cells for adults with recurrent malignant glioma. Cancer 76:840–852, 1995.
29. Hochberg FH, Pruitt A: Assumptions in the radiotherapy of glioblastoma. Neurology 30:407–911, 1980.
30. Hoshino TA: A commentary on the biology and growth kinetics of low-grade and high-grade gliomas. J Neurosurg 61:895–900, 1984.
31. Huncharek M, Muscat J: Treatment of recurrent high grade astrocytoma: Results of a systematic review of 1,415 patients. Anticancer Res 18:1303–1311, 1998.
32. Jelsma R, Bucy PC: Glioblastoma multiforme: Its treatment and some factors affecting survival. Arch Neurol 20:161–171, 1969.
33. Karnofsky D, Burchenal JH, Armistead GC Jr, et al: Triethylene melamine in the treatment of neoplastic disease. Arch Intern Med 87:477–516, 1951.
34. Kaye AH: Malignant brain tumors. In Rothenberg RE (ed): Reoperative Surgery. New York: McGraw-Hill, 1992, pp 51–76.
35. Kelly PJ, Daumas-Duport C, Scheithauer B, et al: Stereotactic histologic correlation of computed tomography and magnetic resonance imaging defined abnormalities in patients with glial neoplasma. Mayo Clin Proc 62:450–459, 1987.
36. Kelly PJ: Stereotactic biopsy and resection in thalamic astrocytomas. Neurosurgery 25:185–195, 1989.
37. Kelly PJ, Rappaport ZH, Bhagwati SN, et al: Reoperation for recurrent malignant gliomas: What are your indications? Surg Neurol 47:39–42, 1997.
38. Kikuchi K, Neuwelt EA: Presence of immunosuppressive factors in brain tumor cyst fluid. J Neurosurg 59:790–799, 1983.
39. Kornblith PL, Walker M: Chemotherapy of gliomas. J Neurosurg 68:1–17, 1988.
40. Kreth FW, Warnke PC, Scheremet R, Ostertag CB: Surgical resection and radiation therapy in the treatment of glioblastoma multiforme. J Neurosurg 78:762–766, 1993.
41. Kuwert T, Woesler B, Morgenroth C: Diagnosis of recurrent glioma with SPECT and iodine-123-alpha-methyl tyrosine. J Nucl Med 39:23–27, 1998.
42. Latif AZ, Signorini D, Gregor A, et al: Application of the MRC brain tumour prognostic index to patients with malignant glioma not managed in randomised control trial. J Neurol Neurosurg Psychiatry 64:747–750, 1998.
43. Laws ER, Taylor WF, Clifton MB, Okazaki H: Neurosurgical management of low-grade astrocytoma of the cerebral hemispheres. J Neurosurg 61:665–673, 1984.
44. Le Bihan D, Douek M, Argyropoulou M, et al: Diffusion and perfusion magnetic resonance imaging in brain tumors. Top Magn Reson Imaging 5:25–31, 1993.
45. Leibel SA, Sheline GE: Radiation therapy for neoplasms of the brain. J Neurosurg 66:1–22, 1987.
46. LeRoux PD, Berger MS, Ojemann GA, et al: Correlation of intraoperative ultrasound tumor volumes and margins with preoperative computerized tomography scans. J Neurosurg 71:691–698, 1989.
47. Levin VA, Hoffman WF, Heilbron DC, et al: Prognostic significance of the pretreatment CT scan on time to progression for patients with malignant gliomas. J Neurosurg 52:642–647, 1980.
48. Levin VA, Silver P, Hannigan J, et al: Superiority of post radiotherapy adjuvant chemotherapy with CCNU, procarbazine, and vincristine

(PCV) over BCNU for anaplastic gliomas: NCOG 6G61 final report. Int J Radiat Oncol Biol Phys 18:321–324, 1990.

49. Loeffler JS, Alexander E III, Shea WM, Wen PY, et al: Radiosurgery as part of the initial management of patients with malignant glioma. J Clin Oncol 10:1379–1385, 1992.

50. Loeffler JS, Alexander E III, Hochberg FH, et al: Clinical patterns of failure following stereotactic interstitial irradiation for malignant gliomas. Int J Radiat Oncol Biol Phys 19:1455–1462, 1990.

51. Loeffler JS, Alexander E III, Wen PY, et al: Results of stereotactic brachytherapy used in the initial management of patients with glioblastoma. J Natl Cancer Inst 82:1918–1921, 1990.

52. Marks JE, Boylan RJ, Prossal SC, et al: Cerebral radionecrosis; incidence and risk in relation to dose, time, fractionation, and volume. Int J Radiat Oncol Biol Phys 7:243–252, 1981.

53. McCormich BM, Miller DC, Budzilovich GN, et al: Treatment and survival of low grade astrocytoma in adults, 1977–1988. Neurosurgery 31:636–642, 1992.

54. McDermott MW, Sneed PK, Gutin PH: Interstitial brachytherapy for malignant brain tumors. Semin Surg Oncol 14:79–87, 1998.

55. Muller PJ, Wilson BC: Photodynamic therapy for recurrent supratentorial gliomas. Semin Surg Oncol 11:346–354, 1995.

56. Nazzaro J, Neuwelt E: The role of surgery in the management of supratentorial intermediate and high-grade astrocytomas in adults. J Neurosurg 73:331–344, 1990.

57. Nelson DF, Nelson JS, Davis DR, et al: Survival and prognosis of patients with astrocytoma with atypical or anaplastic features. J Neurooncol 3:99–103, 1985.

58. Olmsted WW, McGee TP: Prognosis in meningiomas through evaluation of skull bone patterns. Radiology 123:375–377, 1977.

59. Ostertag CB: Biopsy and interstitial radiation therapy of cerebral gliomas. Ital J Neurol Sci 2(Suppl):121–128, 1983.

60. Prados MB, Gutin PH, Phillips TL, et al: Interstitial brachytherapy for newly diagnosed patients with malignant gliomas: The UCSF experience. Int J Radiat Oncol Biol Phys 24:593–597, 1992.

61. Prados MB, Gutin PH, Phillips TL, et al: Highly anaplastic astrocytoma: A review of 357 patients treated between 1977 and 1989. Int J Radiat Oncol Biol Phys 23:3–8, 1992.

62. Prados MD, Russo C: Chemotherapy of brain tumors. Semin Surg Oncol 14:88–95, 1998.

63. Quigley MR, Maroon JC: The relationship between survival and the extent of the resection in patients with supratentorial malignant gliomas. Neurosurgery 29:385–389, 1991.

64. Ram Z, Culver K, Oshiro E, et al: Summary of results and conclusions of the gene therapy of malignant brain tumors: A clinical study. J Neurosurg 82:343A, 1995.

65. Rosenblum ML, Chiu-Liu H, Davis RL, Gutin PH: Radiation necrosis versus tumor recurrence following interstitial brachytherapy: Utility of tissue culture studies. Proc Am Assoc Neurol Surgeons 53:264, 1985.

66. Rostomily RC, Spence AM, Duong D: Multimodality management of recurrent adult malignant gliomas: Results of a phase II multiagent chemotherapy study and analysis of cytoreductive surgery. Neurosurgery 35:378–388; discussion 388, 1994.

67. Salcman M, Kaplan RS, Samaras GM, et al: Aggressive multimodality therapy based on a multicompartmental model of glioblastoma. Surgery 92:250–259, 1982.

68. Salcman M, Kaplan RS, Durken TB, et al: Effect of age and reoperation on survival in the combined modality treatment of malignant astrocytomas. Neurosurgery 10:454–463, 1982.

69. Scharfen CD, Sneed PK, Wara WM, et al: High activity iodine-125 interstitial implant for gliomas. Int J Radiat Oncol Biol Phys 24:583–591, 1992.

70. Shapiro WR: Treatment of neuroectodermal brain tumors. Ann Neurol 12:231–237, 1982.

71. Shapiro WR, Green SB, Burger PL, et al: Randomized trial of three chemotherapeutic regimens in postoperative treatment of malignant glioma. J Neurosurg 71:1–9, 1989.

72. Shaw EG, Scheithauer BW, O'Fallon JR, et al: Oligodendrogliomas: The Mayo Experience. J Neurosurg 76:428–434, 1992.

73. Shepherd SF, Laing RW, Cosgrove VP: Hypofractionated stereotactic radiotherapy in the management of recurrent glioma. Int J Radiat Oncol Biol Phys 37:393–398, 1997.

74. Shrieve DC, Alexander E, Wen PC, et al: Comparison of stereotactic radiosurgery and brachytherapy in the treatment of recurrent glioblastoma multiforme. Neurosurgery 36:275–284, 1995.

75. Sipos L, Afra D: Reoperations of supratentorial anaplastic astrocytomas. Acta Neurochir 39:99–104, 1997.

76. Sonoda Y, Kumabe T, Takahashi T: Clinical usefulness of 11C-MET PET and 201T1 SPECT for differentiation of recurrent glioma from radiation necrosis. Neurol Med-Chir 38:342–347; discussion 347–348, 1988.

77. Stromblad LG, Anderson H, Malmstrom P: Reoperation for malignant astrocytomas: Personal experience and a review of the literature. Br J Neurosurg 7:623–633, 1993.

78. Valk PE, Budinger TF, Levin VA, et al: PET of malignant cerebral tumors after interstitial brachytherapy. Demonstration of metabolic activity and correlation with clinical outcome. J Neurosurg 69:830–838, 1988.

79. Vecht CJ, Avezaat CJ, van Patten WL, et al: The influence of the extent of surgery on the neurological function and survival in malignant glioma. A retro-operation analysis in 243 patients. J Neurol Neurosurg Physchiatry 53:466–471, 1990.

80. Vertosick FT, Selker RG, Arena VC: Survival of patients with well differentiated astrocytomas diagnosed in the era of computed tomography. Neurosurgery 28:496–501, 1991.

81. Vick NA, Coric IS, Eller TW, et al: Reoperation for malignant astrocytoma. Neurology 39:430–432, 1989.

82. Von Diemling A, Louis DM, Von Ammon K, et al: Subsets of glioblastoma multiforme defined by molecular genetic analysis. Brain Pathol 3:19–26, 1993.

83. Walker MD, Alexander E, Hunt WE, et al: Evaluation of BCNU and/or radiotherapy in the treatment of anaplasic gliomas. J Neurosurg 49:333–343, 1978.

84. Wallner KE, Galicich JH, Krol G, et al: Patterns of failure following treatment for glioblastoma multiforme and anaplastic astrocytoma. Int J Radiat Oncol Biol Phys 16:1405–1409, 1989.

85. Wallner KE, Galicich JH, Malkin MG: Inability of computed tomography appearance of recurrent malignant astrocytoma to predict survival following reoperation. J Clin Oncol 7:1492–1496, 1989.

86. Wilson CB: Reoperation for primary tumors. Semin Oncol 2:19–20, 1975.

87. Winger MJ, Macdonald DR, Cairncross JG: Supratentorial anaplastic gliomas in adults. The prognostic importance of extent of resection and prior low grade glioma. J Neurosurg 71:487–493, 1989.

88. Wood JR, Green SB, Shapiro WR: The prognostic importance of tumor size in malignant gliomas: A computed tomographic scan study by the Brain Tumor Cooperative Group. J Clin Oncol 6:338–343, 1988.

89. Young B, Oldfield EH, Markesberry WR, et al: Reoperation for glioblastoma. J Neurosurg 55:917–921, 1981.

90. Yung WKA, Mechtler L, Gleason MJ: Intravenous carboplatin for recurrent malignant glioma: A phase II study. J Clin Oncol 9:860–864, 1991.

# Tumors of the Brain Stem, Third Ventricle, and Lateral Ventricle

# C H A P T E R   5 8

# Surgical Management of Diencephalic and Brain Stem Tumors

■ ALEXANDER N. KONOVALOV, SERGEY K. GORELYSHEV, and ELENA A. KHUHLAEVA

S urgery of primary axial tumors of the brain—tumors of the brain stem, thalamic, and hypothalamic regions—presents serious problems. Until recently, most of these tumors have been considered unremovable and even untreatable. Lesions of the midline are more common in children than in adults. They represent approximately 57% of pediatric brain tumors.[1] Despite localization in deep-seated, vitally important structures of the brain, some of these tumors are reachable and, because of their benign nature and well-defined borders, can be removed. Modern diagnostic methods, such as computed tomography (CT) and magnetic resonance imaging (MRI), make possible the visualization of these tumors, and microsurgical technique permits their successful ablation.

The Moscow Burdenko Neurosurgical Institute is a major referral center where patients with severe brain lesions often come "as a court of last resort" after they have been treated elsewhere unsuccessfully. We operate on them, even if very strong contraindications to radical surgery on these patients exist.

The diencephalic region includes the hypothalamus (lamina terminalis, chiasma, tuber cinereum, and corpora mamillaris, as well as the hypophyseal stalk)[2]; the thalamus; and the roof of the third ventricle. We discuss three groups of midline primary brain tumors: tumors of the hypothalamus, the thalamus, and the brain stem.

We include in this analysis only those cases that were operated on by one neurosurgeon, because this permits a better understanding of the possibilities and limitations of surgery (Table 58–1).

## HYPOTHALAMIC GLIOMAS

Hypothalamic gliomas include tumors involving the chiasm and walls of the third ventricle. We differentiate these tumors using the system shown in Figure 58–1.

1. Tumors of the optic chiasm (group I) with predominant anterior expansion (Figs. 58–2 and 58–3).

Some of these tumors reach giant size and form masses that displace the frontal lobes. They may grow into the middle fossa as well. These tumors are often solid or partially cystic. In addition to real tumor cysts, large arachnoid cysts are seen in some cases, which develop as a result of disturbances in cerebrospinal fluid (CSF) circulation in the sylvian fissure and basal cisterns. Usually, these cysts, despite their huge size, are well delineated.

2. The second group (group II) consists of tumors that destroy the chiasm and grow anteriorly as well as penetrate into the third ventricle (Fig. 58–4). The anterior cerebral ($A_1$) and anterior communicating artery are a natural border between these two nodes.

3. The third group (group III) consists of tumors whose predominant growth is into the third ventricle. Some of these tumors have their origin in chiasma (group IIIa) (Figs. 58–5 and 58–6); others originate in the floor of the third ventricle (group IIIb) (Figs. 58–7 and 58–8), or infiltrate all the walls of the third ventricle including its roof (group IIIc). In the last two subgroups the chiasm, which shows no signs of infiltration, is stretched on the anterior pole of the tumor.

4. The last, relatively small, group consists of tumors that predominantly destroy half of the chiasm and grow along one or both optic tracts (Figs. 58–9 and 58–10).

This classification has practical importance because the surgical approach depends on the precise localization of

TABLE 58–1 ■ **DIENCEPHALIC AND BRAIN STEM TUMORS (No. = 473)**

| Localization | No. of Operations |
|---|---|
| Hypothalamic gliomas | 161 |
| Gliomas of the thalamus | 71 |
| Brain stem tumors | 241 |
| Total | 473 |

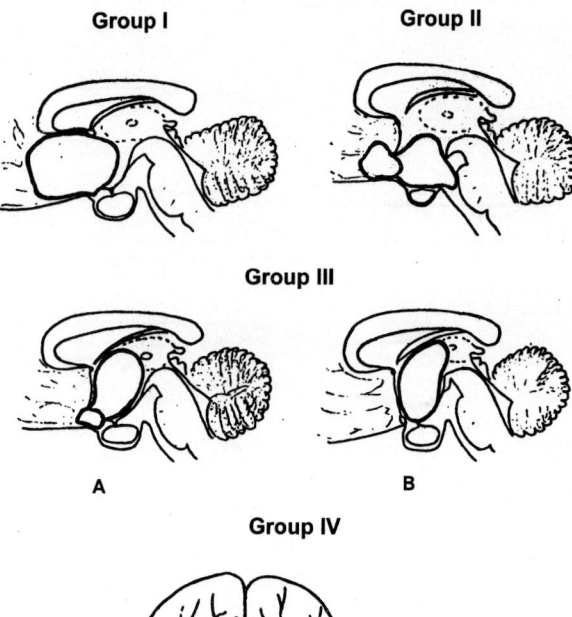

**Group I**  **Group II**

**Group III**

A                        B

**Group IV**

FIGURE 58–1 ■ Topography of hypothalamic tumors. Tumors of the optic chiasm with predominant anterior expansion (group I). Tumors with anterior growth and penetration into the third ventricle (group II). Predominant growth into the cavity of the third ventricle (group III) with infiltration of chiasm (A) or with gliomas (B) of the floor of the third ventricle (tumors of this group originate in the floor of the third ventricle; chiasm without signs of infiltration is stretched on the anterior pole of the tumor). Tumors that grow along the optic tract and predominantly destroy one half of chiasm (group IV).

the tumor. However, many other classifications have been developed by pathologists and neurosurgeons. The classification that to some extent resembles ours was described by Bregeat in 1978.[3]

## Clinical Picture

The clinical picture varies with the type of tumor (Table 58–2). The first symptoms in groups I, II, and IIIa are visual disturbances. At the time of the patient's admission, the disturbances are always grave, often asymmetric, and associated with primary atrophy of the optic nerves.

The manifestation of the disease in patients with gliomas

in groups IIIb and IIIc begins with intracranial hypertension and signs of hypothalamic insufficiency. The clinical picture is characterized by mild, symmetric visual disturbances with papilledema and hydrocephalus.

## Histology

In accordance with recent World Health Organization (WHO) classification of brain tumors, hypothalamic tumors in most cases are pilocytic astrocytomas. Previously, we included some of these tumors into the group of fibrillary astrocytomas. In some cases the patterns of malignancy were revealed in pilocytic astrocytomas: frequent mitosis, prominant endothelial proliferation, and necrotic foci. These tumors often infiltrate adjacent arachnoid and grow around the carotid artery and its branches, which become embedded into the tumor tissue.

## Computed Tomography and Magnetic Resonance Imaging Diagnostic Methods

CT and MRI are very effective diagnostic methods for detecting hypothalamic tumors. In most cases, CT allows discrimination between gliomas and other suprasellar tumors. Gliomas are usually homogeneous, hyperdense (see Fig. 58–8), and, occasionally, isodense (see Fig. 58–3B) or hypodense tumors. Nevertheless, some gliomas show the signs characteristic for craniopharyngiomas: large cysts (see Fig. 58–2B) and calcifications.

MRI allows the surgeon to clarify the relation of the tumor to the skull base and vital brain structures; for example, the brain stem, the third ventricle, and its roof.

---

TABLE 58–2 ■ **CLINICAL DIFFERENTIATION OF GLIOMAS INVOLVING THE CHIASM AND GLIOMAS OF THE VENTRICLE FLOOR**

|  | Location | |
|---|---|---|
|  | *Chiasm* | *Third Ventricle Floor* |
| Manifestation of disease | | |
| Visual disturbances | 70% | 20% |
| Hypertension | 8% | 50% |
| Pituitary insufficiency | 2% | 28% |
| Clinical picture | | |
| Visual disturbances | Grave (35% practically blind), asymmetric | Mild, symmetric |
| Eye fundus | | |
| Primary atrophy | 81% | 47% |
| Papilledema | 13% | 53% |
| Hydrocephalus (computed tomographic data) | 48% | 100% |

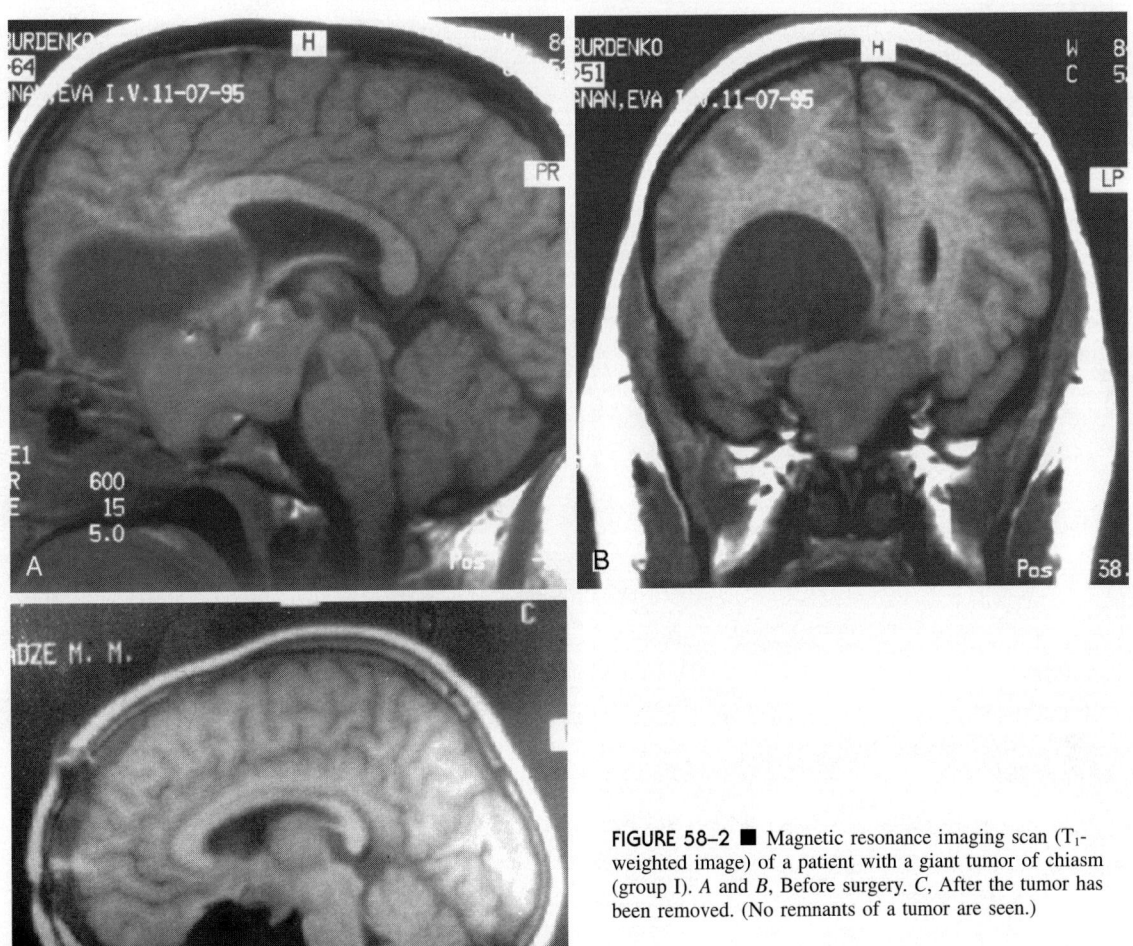

**FIGURE 58–2 ■** Magnetic resonance imaging scan ($T_1$-weighted image) of a patient with a giant tumor of chiasm (group I). *A* and *B,* Before surgery. *C,* After the tumor has been removed. (No remnants of a tumor are seen.)

MRI, used in combination with CT, makes defining the topographic type of tumor possible and thus enables the surgeon to choose the appropriate surgical approach. Hypothalamic gliomas usually look like high intense masses on $T_2$-weighted MRI scans (see Fig. 58–5*B*), whereas $T_1$ images show hypointense lesions (see Figs. 58–2*A*, 58–4*A*, and 58–5*A*). $T_1$-weighted MR image after gadolinium injection usually shows marked enhancement of the tumor (see Figs. 59–4*B* and 59–8*A*). A tumor cyst is characterized by low signals on $T_1$-weighted scans (see Fig. 58–2*B*).

## Surgery

Indications for direct surgery in cases of hypothalamic glioma are still uncertain, and many authors can echo the words of Gertrude Stein "There is no answer, There never was an answer, There never will be an answer. That's the answer."[38]

Experience of surgical removal of these tumors is rather limited. Several neurosurgeons advocate the radical (subto-

tal) removal as a first attempt of treatment of these tumors.[4, 27–48]

Hoffman and associates "advocate an aggressive surgical approach to these tumors for diagnostic and therapeutic purposes." They believe that patients with progressive visual and neurologic deterioration and a rapidly expanding suprasellar mass lesion should be treated surgically.[41–43]

According to Medlock and Scott, the indications for surgery are to debulk symptomatic tumors (>50 mm) that are exophytic or cystic and to relieve obstruction at the foramen of Monro.[38]

Radical (70% to 95%) resection without operative mortality was also achieved by Wisoff (11 of 16 patients)[44] and by Valdueza and associates (12 of 20 patients).[45]

Lapras[49] analyzed this problem at the European Congress in Moscow in 1991 and concluded that radical surgery is preferable to palliative methods and irradiation.

Some of the authors believe that radiotherapy is an effective adjuvant treatment modality[5–14, 27, 45–48]; others strongly advocate the role of chemotherapy.[16–26] Chemotherapy is used: (1) as initial treatment; (2) as a palliative

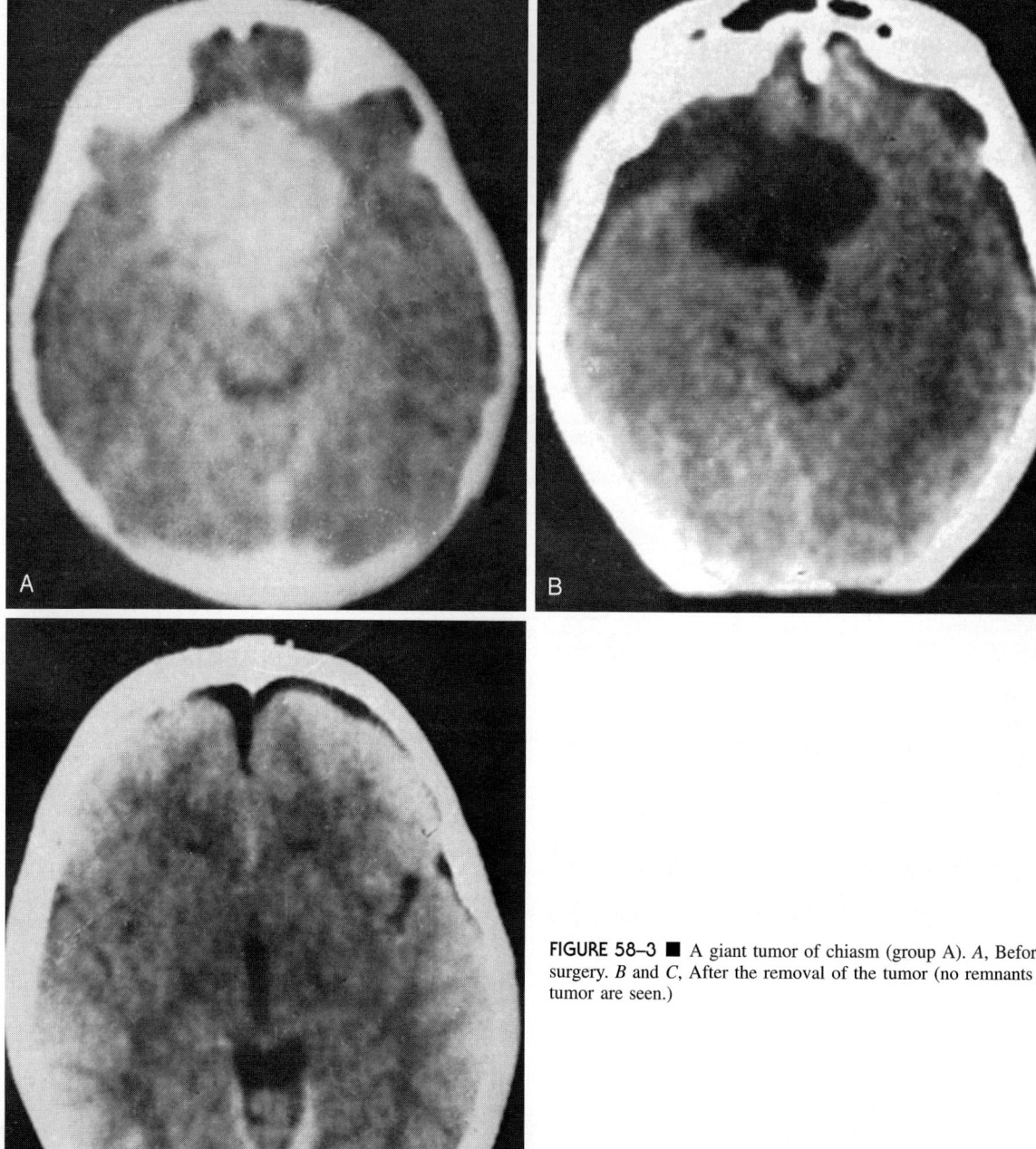

**FIGURE 58–3** ■ A giant tumor of chiasm (group A). *A,* Before surgery. *B* and *C,* After the removal of the tumor (no remnants of a tumor are seen.)

method, which can postpone the need for radiotherapy; and (3) in patients with recurrent chiasmatic-hypothalamic gliomas.

A preliminary report devoted to the Gamma knife treatment of diencephalic gliomas has been published.[15]

From 1982 to 1998, 161 patients with hypothalamic gliomas were operated on in the Burdenko Neurosurgical Institute (Moscow).

## Chiasmal Gliomas with Anterior Growth (Group I) (see Figs. 58–2 and 58–3)

A subfrontal unilateral approach is usually adequate for radical removal of chiasmal gliomas. After debulking the main part of the tumor with the ultrasonic aspirator, additional space appears, and almost all parts of the tumor are accessible.

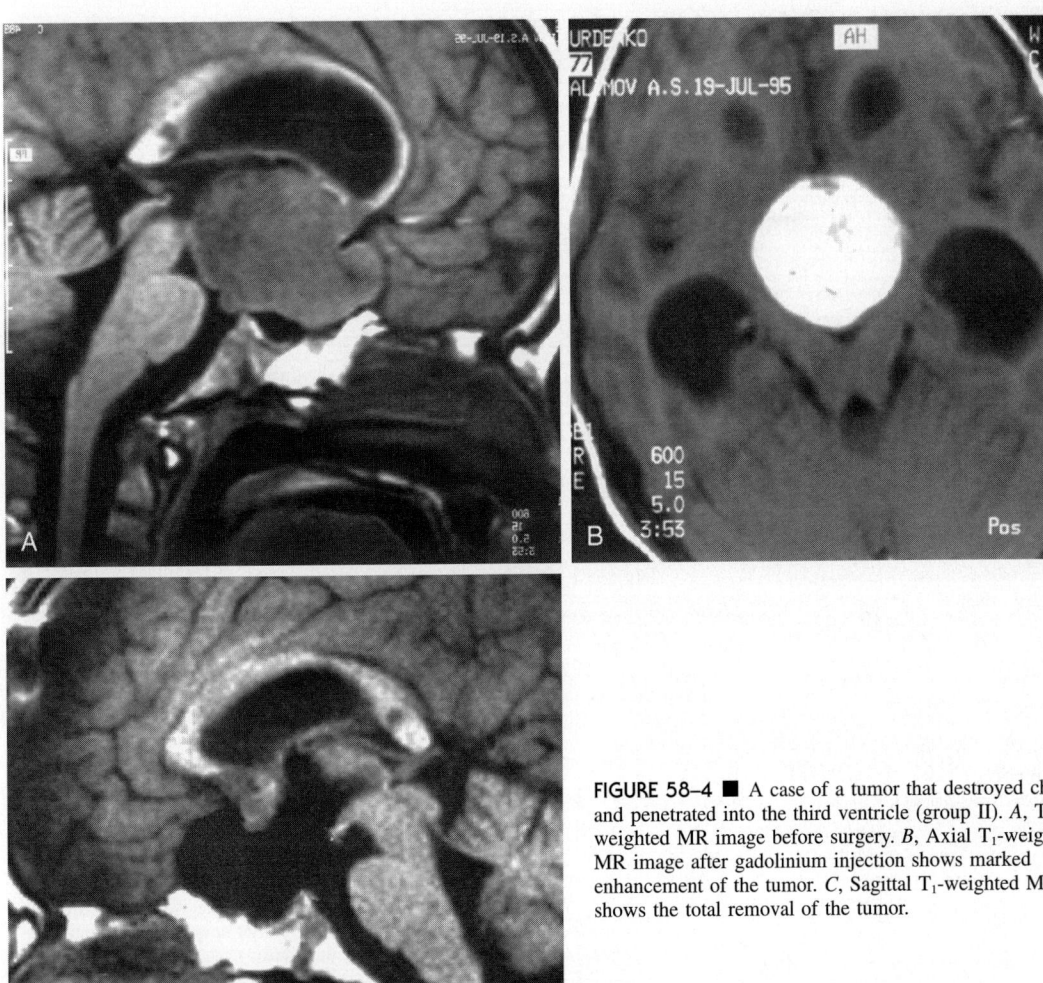

FIGURE 58–4 ■ A case of a tumor that destroyed chiasm and penetrated into the third ventricle (group II). *A*, T$_1$-weighted MR image before surgery. *B*, Axial T$_1$-weighted MR image after gadolinium injection shows marked enhancement of the tumor. *C*, Sagittal T$_1$-weighted MR image shows the total removal of the tumor.

Often, the tumor grows asymmetrically: one optic nerve and half of the chiasm are predominantly infiltrated by the tumor, whereas the other optic nerve is simply displaced. If the vision on the side of the predominant tumor growth is absent or very low, this optic nerve may be cut at the level of its entrance into the optic channel, which facilitates further tumor removal and helps to expose the ophthalmic artery, from which the main tumor feeders arise. Coagulation of these arteries diminishes blood loss during tumor ablation.

It is usually possible to differentiate, under the microscope, the normal tissue of the optic pathways and to separate it from the tumor. Care is necessary to reveal and preserve the pituitary stalk, which is usually displaced downward and backward by the tumor.

The most difficult stage of the surgery is usually the removal of a part of the tumor that is hidden behind the carotid bifurcation and the anterior cerebral arteries. It is necessary to manipulate in the narrow space between perforating arteries. The posterior part of the tumor, which penetrates in the cavity of the third ventricle, is softer and can usually be easily removed by aspiration. If the tumor

infiltrates the adjacent membranes and surrounding main arteries are embedded into the tumor tissue, surgery becomes more difficult and takes hours of meticulous dissection.

## Tumors with Predominant Growth into the Third Ventricle (Group III) (see Figs. 58–5 to 58–8)

Our experience shows that the transcallosal approach is the best approach to reach tumors with predominant growth into the third ventricle. This access is well described by several published reports.[32, 50, 51] We have used this approach in 75 cases. The corpus callosum is divided between the anterior cerebral arteries with an incision 1 to 1.5 cm long. The tumor can then be reached and removed through one or both foramina of Monro (in the last case, the septum pellucidum must be opened). The upper surface of a tumor can also be exposed by division of the columna fornicis.

Ultrasonic aspiration is helpful when removing the main bulk of a tumor. Tumors usually infiltrate the anterior wall and the floor of the third ventricle; in some cases, they

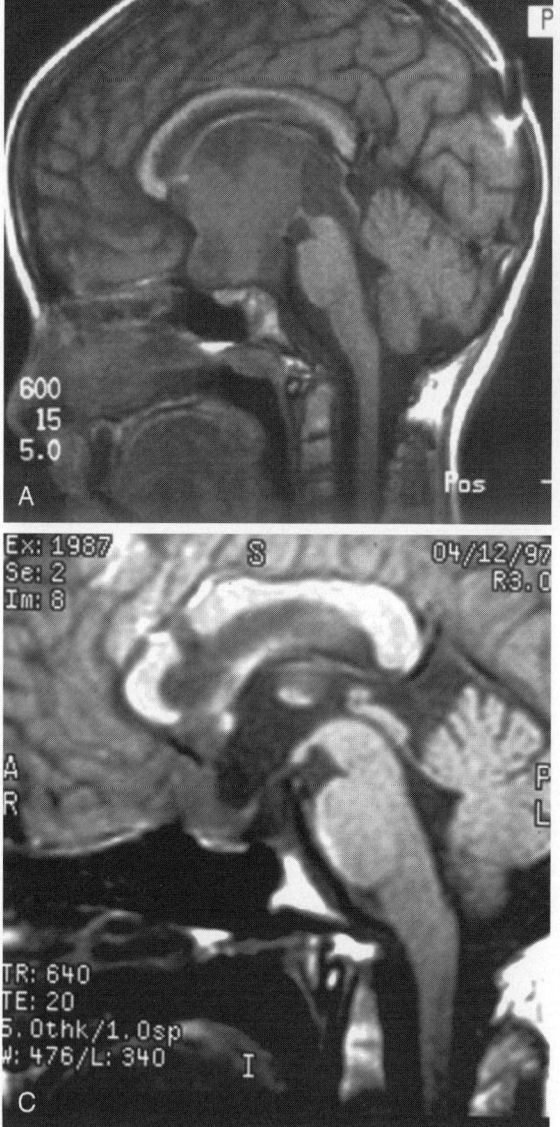

**FIGURE 58–5** ■ Magnetic resonance image of a tumor with predominant growth into the third ventricle cavity (group III). The tumor partly infiltrated the chiasm, and the main part is located in the cavity of the third ventricle. *A,* Before surgery (T$_1$). *B,* Before surgery (T$_2$). *C,* After surgery (small remnants of a tumor are seen near the chiasm).

also infiltrate the lateral walls and occlude the foramen of Monro. Even in these cases, subtotal tumor removal is usually possible, leaving only a thin layer of tumor that infiltrates the adjacent brain tissue. After the tumor has been removed through the hole in the floor of the third ventricle, the basilar artery and its branches (which lie behind the arachnoid membrane) can usually be seen.

Some of these tumors are richly supplied by vessels coming from the anterior wall and the ventricle floor. These vessels are coagulated during removal of the tumor.

### Tumors that Grow Anteriorly and Penetrate into the Third Ventricle (Group II) (see Fig. 58–4)

Tumors that infiltrate both chiasmata and invade into the third ventricle (group II) usually need a combined approach (either a transcallosal and subfrontal approach or a transcallosal and pterional approach) to remove them.

### Gliomas of the Optic Tract (Group IV)
(see Figs. 58–9 and 58–10)

Tumors of the optic tract have an asymmetric localization, and the main part of the tumor is hidden behind the carotid artery and its bifurcation. A pterional transsylvian approach is preferable for their removal. Although the operating field is narrow and the posterior communicating and anterior choroidal arteries hinder a wide exposure of the lateral surface of the tumor, it can be radically removed up to the border of normal-looking brain structures. The presence of cysts simplifies the removal of the tumor.

Some of these tumors cannot be removed by any means because they have spread (e.g., bilaterally along visual pathways) (Fig. 58–11).

Selection of the appropriate approach depends on the size and the precise location of a tumor. In one of our cases, a very unusual approach was chosen: The tumor was removed via the posterior fossa above the cerebellum and

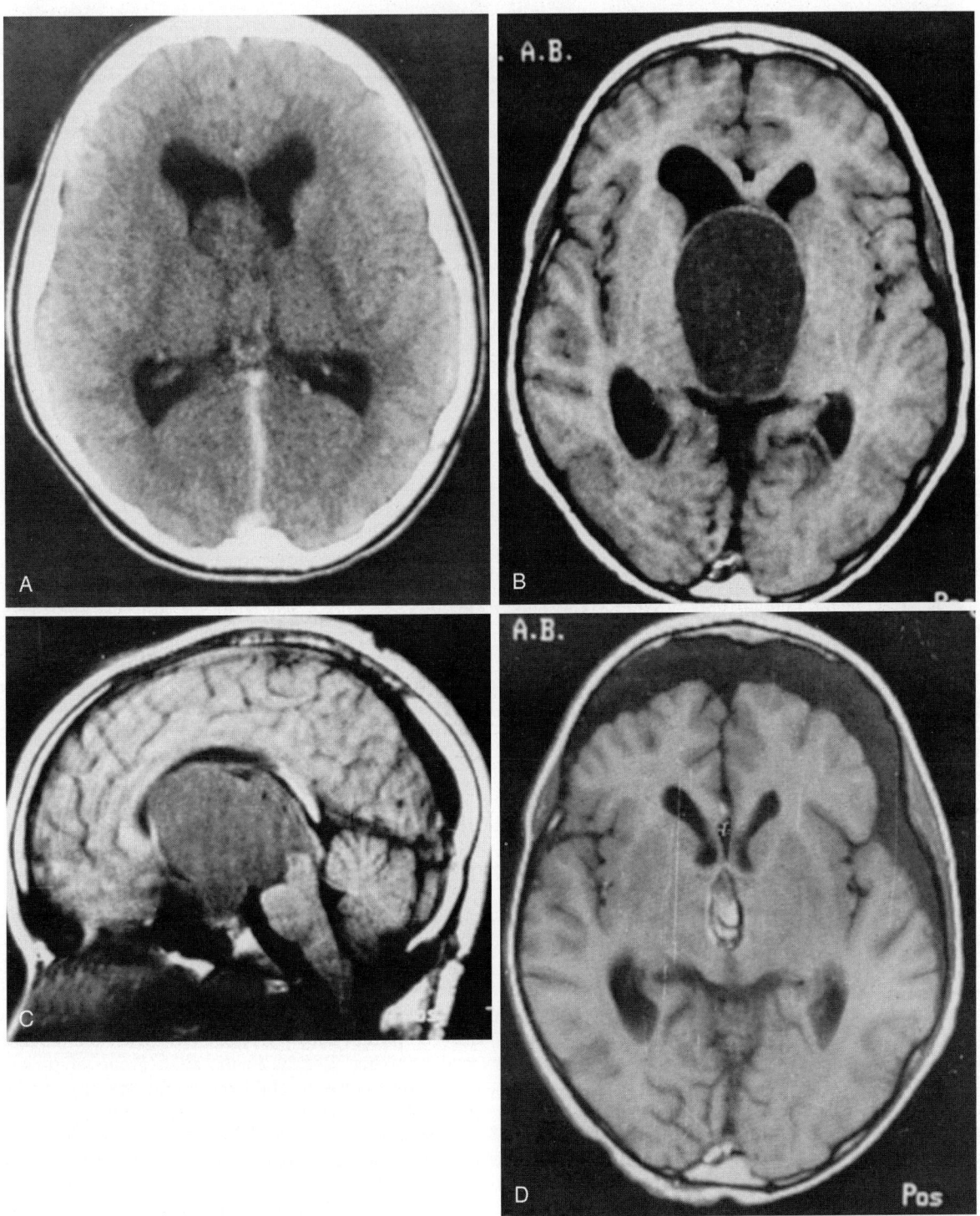

FIGURE 58–6 ■ *A*, A computed tomography (CT) scan of a tumor of the chaism. *B* and *C*, A magnetic resonance (MR) image taken 6 months after a shunting procedure shows rapid growth of the tumor (group IIIa). The tumor infiltrates the chiasm; the main part is in the cavity of the third ventricle. *D*, An MR image taken 2 weeks after surgery shows a small blood clot in the third ventricle and bilateral subdural fluid collections. (See the case study in the text.)

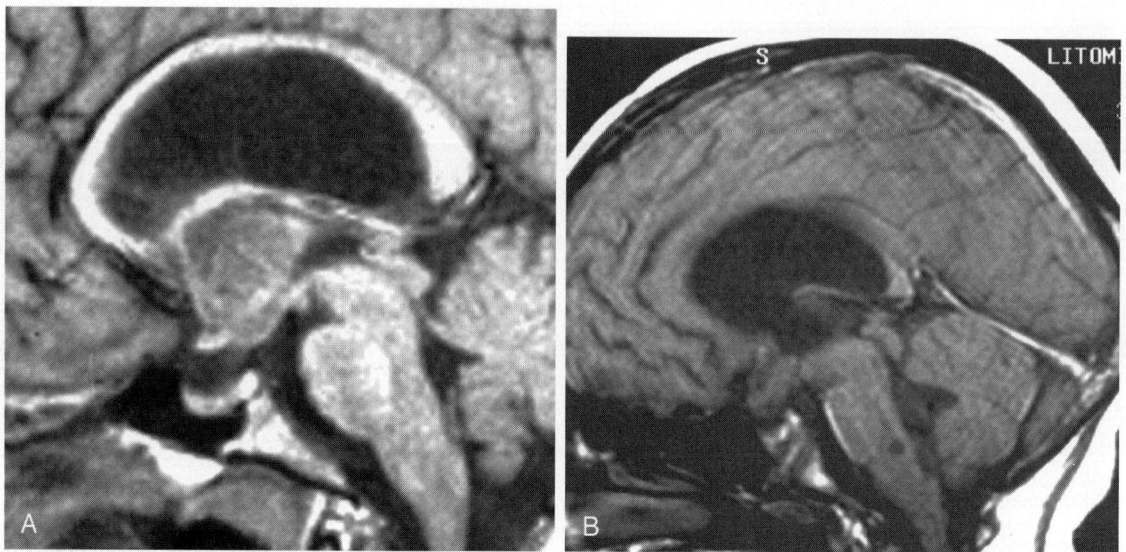

FIGURE 58–7 ■ Magnetic resonance image (T₁) of a glioma of the floor of the third ventricle (group IIIb). The tumor is entirely situated in the cavity of the third ventricle. During surgery, the chiasm without signs of infiltration was seen stretched on the anterior pole of the tumor. *A*, Before surgery. *B*, After the removal of the tumor (tiny remnants of a tumor are seen).

through the tentorial notch to reach the basal medial surface of the temporal lobe.

## Results

Surgery on diencephalic gliomas may provide astonishing results. We have operated on some patients who were in a desperate state: They were cachectic and had a severe hypothalamic insufficiency. Nevertheless, some of these patients (mainly children) not only survived the surgery but also showed a quick and marked improvement.

One of the cases that illustrates the difficulty of such surgery follows.

## Case Report 1

An 11-year-old boy was admitted to the pediatric department on September 17, 1992, with headaches and vomiting. CT revealed a large tumor of the third ventricle and hydrocephalus (see Fig. 58–6A). After shunting (Torkildsen's bilateral ventriculocisternostomy), the patient improved. Because of the stable clinical state of the patient and the absence of neurologic deficits, removal of the tumor of the third ventricle was postponed; however, a 6-month follow-up MRI showed marked progression of the tumor (see Fig. 58–6B, C). At this time, the patient's visual acuity was 0.3 in the right eye and 1.0 in the left eye, with a bitemporal hemianopsia. No other serious neurologic or endocrinologic signs were present. Intracranial pressure was normal. On MRI, the tumor was interpreted as a group III glioma with infiltration of the chiasm and predominant growth into the third ventricle (see Fig. 58–6B).

Surgery was performed on October 10, 1992, and the tumor was removed via a transcallosal transfornical approach. The tumor had infiltrated the walls of the third ventricle and chiasm. It was removed radically, except for the zone of peritumoral gliosis.

The postoperative period was dramatic. MRI revealed a small blood clot in the third ventricle and bilateral subdural fluid collections (see Fig. 58–6D). The patient needed intensive care for 2 months and was unconscious for about 2 weeks. Midbrain symptoms, memory disturbances, and diabetes insipidus occurred. Gradually, the patient became alert, but for long periods of time he was somnolent. Severe memory disturbances then became evident. During subsequent months, the boy made a dramatic improvement, and his behavior, memory, and other functions became practically normal.

For 6 years almost all the symptoms were absent, the boy was active, and he had no complaints. Visual acuity in the right eye was 0.2 and in the left eye was 1.0. Then the tumor recurred, and the boy was operated on again.

The results of surgery on hypothalamic gliomas are summarized in Table 58–3. Better results are achieved in the group of tumors with predominant localization in the chiasm, despite the fact that in this group, 37% of tumors are very large (>5 cm in diameter). Surgery on third ventricle gliomas produces more complications, and the mortality rate is higher. Results in the adult group of patients are worse than those in children. During the past 5 years the mortality rate for both children and adults for all types of tumors was absent (0%) (Fig. 58–12).

Causes of death from hypothalamic tumors are presented in Table 58–4. The main cause of death was hemorrhage into the remaining tumor. Disturbance of blood circulation with ischemic lesions in different vascular territories (which occurred in 5% of operated patients) was another important cause of serious complications.

Removal of hypothalamic tumors often results in changes in water-electrolyte regulation. Diabetes insipidus developed in 17% of cases. In contrast to patients with craniopharyngiomas (in whom diabetes insipidus is one of the commonest surgical complications), in those with

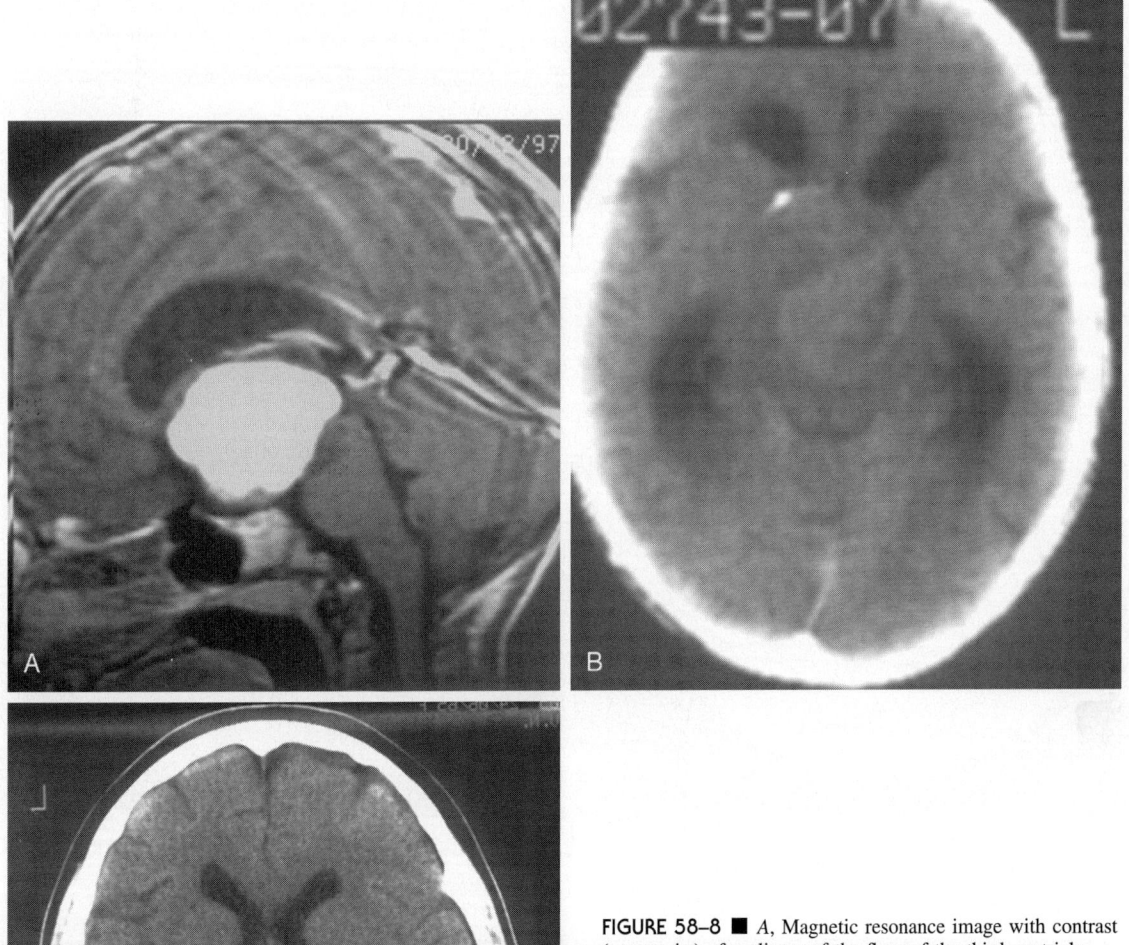

**FIGURE 58–8** ■ *A*, Magnetic resonance image with contrast (magnevist) of a glioma of the floor of the third ventricle (group IIIb) before surgery. The tumor is situated in the cavity of the third ventricle. *B*, Computed tomography scan of the same patient (isodense tumor). *C*, After the tumor has been removed.

hypothalamic gliomas we have observed the syndrome of water retention with brain edema and coma in some cases. Normalization of water-electrolyte disturbances results in a marked improvement in the patient's state.

Removal of hypothalamic gliomas often results in brain collapse, subdural CSF, and blood collections, which required additional surgical intervention in 7% of cases (external drainage or shunting procedures) (see Fig. 58–6D). Their appearance does not depend on surgical approach, and the risk factors likely to contribute to this complication were preoperative ventriculomegaly (frontal horn index >0.40) and tumor size (>5 cm in diameter).

Because these tumors can destroy the chiasm, we were afraid that surgery would produce additional serious impairment to visual acuity. However, analysis of our results shows that these concerns were overestimated: Worsening

of vision occurred in 22% of cases, whereas in 40% there were no changes; in 38% the vision improved.

Follow-up evaluation (mean of 7 years; range of 1 to 16 years) showed that the tumor recurred in only 14% of cases. A second surgery was performed in 13 cases.

Gamma-radiotherapy with rotation was performed in 17 patients with astrocytomas grades II and III. They received 48 to 54 Gy to the tumor volume; all of these patients are free of recurrence, and no neurologic sequelae related to the irradiation have occurred.

The results of our surgery can be improved with stricter indications for surgery. We have operated on several patients with enormous and widespread tumors that caused irreversible damage to vital brain structures. In such cases, a good result could not be expected.

With proper case selection, surgery of primary hypotha-

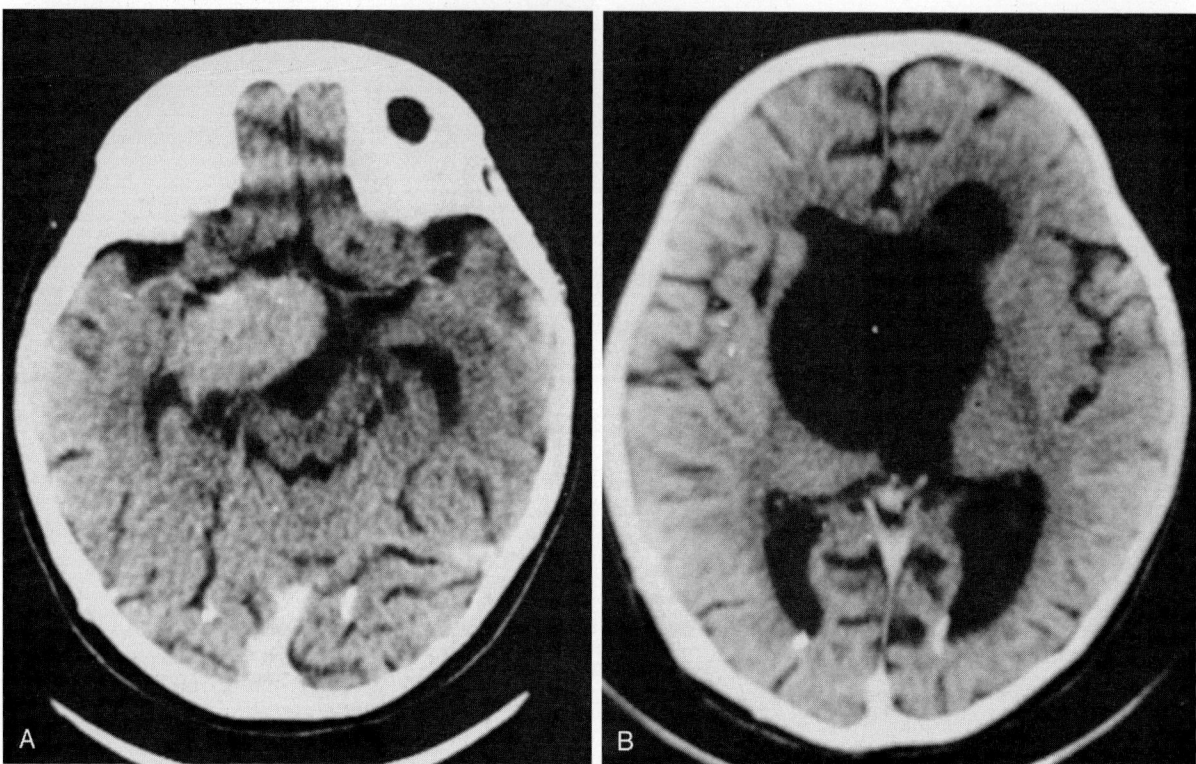

**FIGURE 58–9** ■ *A* and *B*, Glioma of the optic tract and chiasm (group IV). The tumor destroyed half of the chiasm, grew along the right visual tract, and formed a giant cyst that compressed the third ventricle.

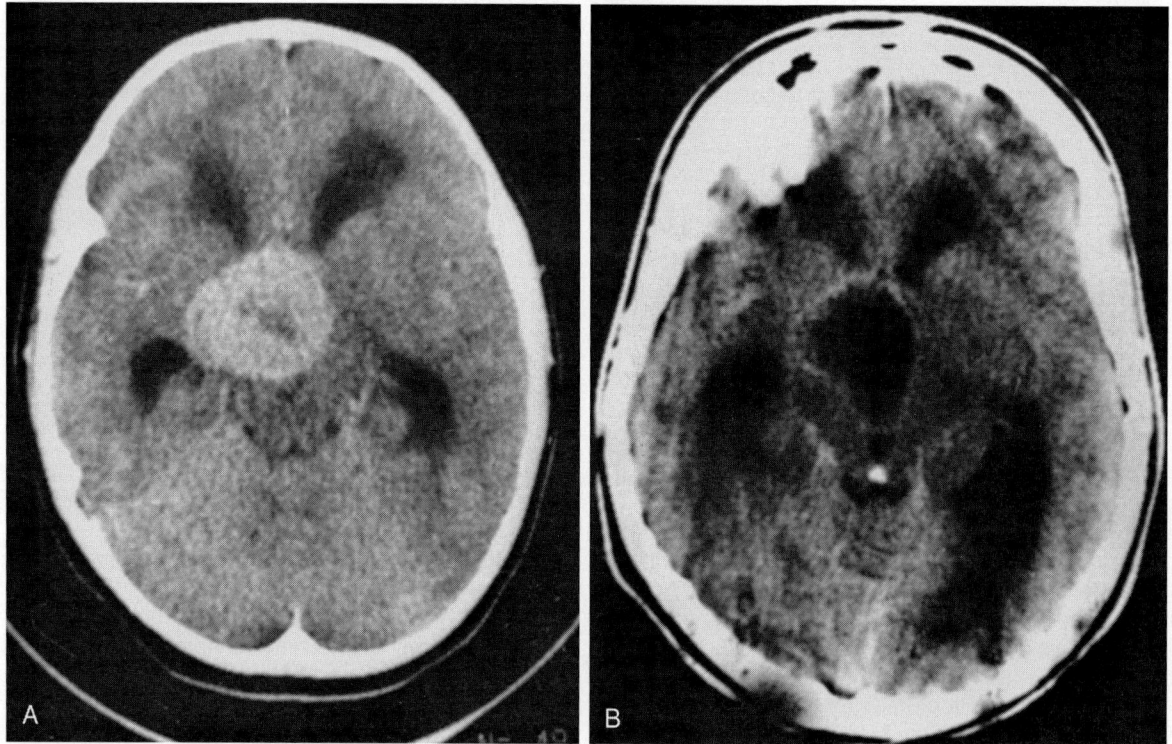

**FIGURE 58–10** ■ Glioma of the optic tract and chiasm (group IV). *A*, Before surgery. *B*, After the tumor has been removed.

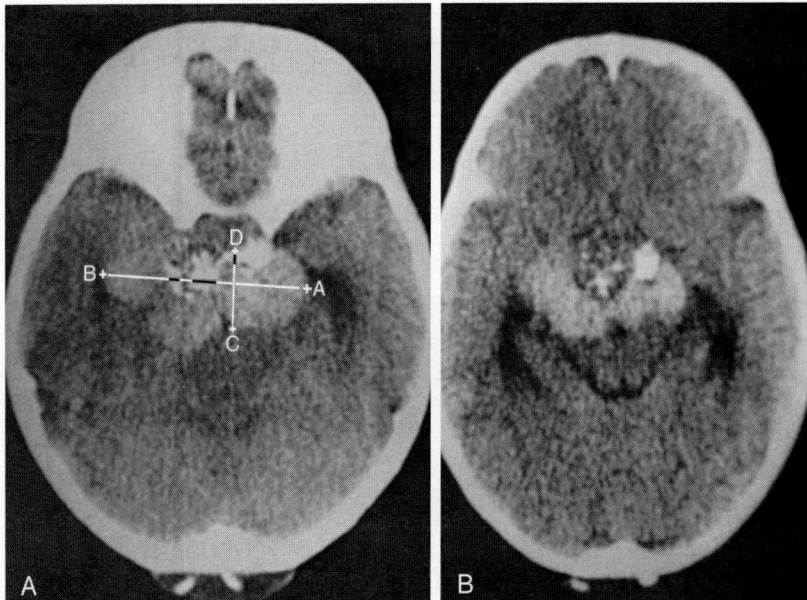

**FIGURE 58–11** ■ *A* and *B*, An example (computed tomography scan) of an unresectable tumor, which grew bilaterally along visual pathways.

lamic gliomas may result in the improvement or stabilization of visual functions, a long-term period free of recurrence, and a relatively favorable postoperative period.

## THALAMIC TUMORS

Indications for surgery on thalamic tumors are controversial. In adults these tumors are mostly malignant diffuse-growing, therefore possibilities of radical tumor removal are limited. On the other hand, among children, focal benign tumors are revealed quite often. This permits an attempt of their resection. Some authors show favorable

results after thalamic tumor surgery.[52–55] Kelly, using a stereotactic resection, achieved good results in 32 cases of circumscribed thalamic tumors.[56]

We consider that surgery is indicated in a focal thalamic lesion if the tumor is distinguished by infiltrative type of growth without clear tumor-brain interface. Indications of surgery are limited because only partial tumor ablation is possible.

In our practice, we differentiate several topographic variants of thalamic tumors: (1) anterior, when the tumor is localized on the level of the foramen of Monro; (2) posterior, when the tumor occupies the posterior part of the thalamus and the pulvinar; (3) lateral; and (4) total, when a voluminous tumor occupies the whole thalamus and spreads into adjacent structures. It is also reasonable to distinguish a group of tumors, which occupy both the thalamus and the midbrain. Tumor distribution according to these variants and histology are summarized in the Tables 58–5 and 58–6.

TABLE 58–3 ■ **LOCALIZATION, NUMBER OF OPERATIONS, AND MORTALITY RATE IN HYPOTHALAMIC GLIOMAS**

| Localization | Children Operation/ Mortality (%) | | Adults Operation/ Mortality (%) | |
|---|---|---|---|---|
| Tumors of the optic chiasm with predominant anterior expansion | 25/1 | 4% | 8/1 | |
| Tumors with anterior growth and penetration into the third ventricle | 26/0 | 0% | 6/1 | |
| Predominant growth into the third ventricle | 61/6 | 10% | 14/2 | |
| Tumors of chiasma and the third ventricle | | | | |
| Gliomas of the floor of the third ventricle | | | | |
| Tumors infiltrating the walls and roof of the third ventricle | | | | |
| Growth along the visual tract | 19/0 | 0% | 4/0 | |
| Total | 131/7 | 5.6% | 32/4 | 12.5% |

During the past 5 years, the mortality was zero (0%).

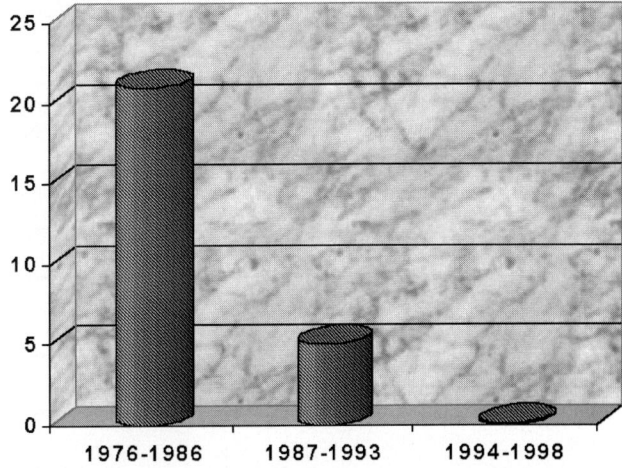

**FIGURE 58–12** ■ The diagram illustrates the dynamics of mortality since 1976 until the present time. During the last 5 years, mortality was absent.

## TABLE 58–4 ■ CAUSES OF DEATH ASSOCIATED WITH THE REMOVAL OF HYPOTHALAMIC TUMORS

| | |
|---|---|
| Hemorrhage into the remaining part of the tumor | 8 |
| Ischemic disturbances of blood circulation in the hemispheres and diencephanlon (occlusion of internal carotid artery) | 1 |
| Purulent leptomeningitis and periventrical encephalitis | 1 |
| Thomboembolism of the pulmonary artery | 1 |

## TABLE 58–6 ■ HISTOLOGY OF THALAMIC TUMORS (71 CASES)

| Histology | No. | % |
|---|---|---|
| Pilocytic astrocytoma | 8 | 12 |
| Fibrillary astrocytoma | 32 | 45 |
| Anaplastic astrocytoma | 19 | 28 |
| Glioblastoma | 5 | 6 |
| Ganglioastrocytoma | 2 | 3 |
| Others | 5 | 6 |

Clinical manifestation in some dimensions corresponds with tumor location. Tumors of the anterior part of the thalamus at an early stage occlude the foramen of Monro on the side of the lesion (or rarely on both sides), producing asymmetric lateral ventricles megaly. Posterior thalamic lesions primarily compress the aqueduct, which results in the development of symmetric dilatation of the lateral ventricles.

Clinical symptoms other than signs of intracranial hypertension mainly depends not on damage to the thalamus itself but on compression or invasion of the surrounding structures (e.g., internal capsule, quadrigeminal plate, peduncles). A definition of the aforementioned topographic groups in our point of view is important for selection of the most appropriate surgical approach.

## Surgery

As was mentioned earlier, we consider that an attempt at radical tumor resection should be made in all focal, slowly progressive tumors (mainly benign tumors). We also operate on malignant lesions that have no diffuse spreading into adjacent structures. In most cases the results of CT and MRI investigations permit us to distinguish between benign focal and diffuse malignant tumors. If clinical and neuroimaging data are not distinct, stereotactic biopsy is indicated.

Thalamic tumors may by accessed in many ways—transcallosally, transcortically, via a transsylvian fissure, or by using a posterior interhemispheric and combined approach.

In the case of anterior thalamic tumors, we prefer to explore using the transcallosal approach. It is necessary to maintain the microscope direction in the foramen of Monro projection. Orientation in the lateral ventricle may be difficult: The main landmarks—the foramen of Monro and the choroidal plexus—may by hidden by the bulging tumor. In that case, the position of the thalamostriate, septal, and nucleus caudatus veins helps to determine the position of the foramen of Monro.

A small incision in the thalamic superior surface (usually in front of the thalamostriate vein) is necessary to explore the tumor. We use retractors with 5-mm blades to support brain wound margins. Tumor ablation is performed mainly with ultrasound aspiration or bipolar coagulation and simultaneous aspiration of tumor tissue.

The radicality of tumor resection depends on the existence of a distinct brain-tumor interface. Even in the case of a left-sided tumor, we prefer right-sided transcallosal access. The opposite side approach, in some cases, is more convenient because the trajectory of the surgical approach is straighter and less brain retraction is necessary.

In the case of posterior thalamic and pulvinar tumors, we prefer the posterior occipital approach. The tentorium section is necessary when the tumor penetrates into the peduncle.

Large tumors that occupy the whole thalamus need for their resection transcortical exploration (frontotemporal or parietal). Ventriculomegaly has made such an approach feasible.

Pterional basal access provides limited exposure to the tumor through small spaces between branches of the carotid artery and optic tract. That is why it is necessary to combine this approach as with the upper transcallosal approach. Some of the tumors may be also reached by splitting the sylvian fissure. Some examples of thalamic tumor removal via different routes are illustrated in Figures 58–13 and 58–14.

## Ventricular Shunting

When tumors interfere with CSF circulation and produce ventricular dilatation, a shunt may be necessary. When dealing with focal resectable tumors, we prefer to start with direct tumor removal. In the case of a malignant tumor or a patient's critical condition owing to intracranial hypertension, it is necessary to start with a shunting procedure. Surgical results are summarized in Table 58–7.

Three patients died after surgery. One patient died as result of exacerbation of intracranial inflammation (the patient was previously shunted in another hospital and the surgery had been complicated by meningitis). In two other cases, death was caused by hemorrhage into the tumor remnants.

Clinical conditions improved in 50% of observations immediately after surgery, and further improvement was observed in another 20% of operated patients. In the pediat-

## TABLE 58–5 ■ TOPOGRAPHICAL VARIANTS OF THALAMIC TUMORS (71 CASES)

| Variant | No. | % |
|---|---|---|
| Anterior | 13 | 19 |
| Total | 18 | 25 |
| Lateral | 20 | 28 |
| Posterior | 10 | 14 |
| Thalamus and midbrain | 10 | 14 |

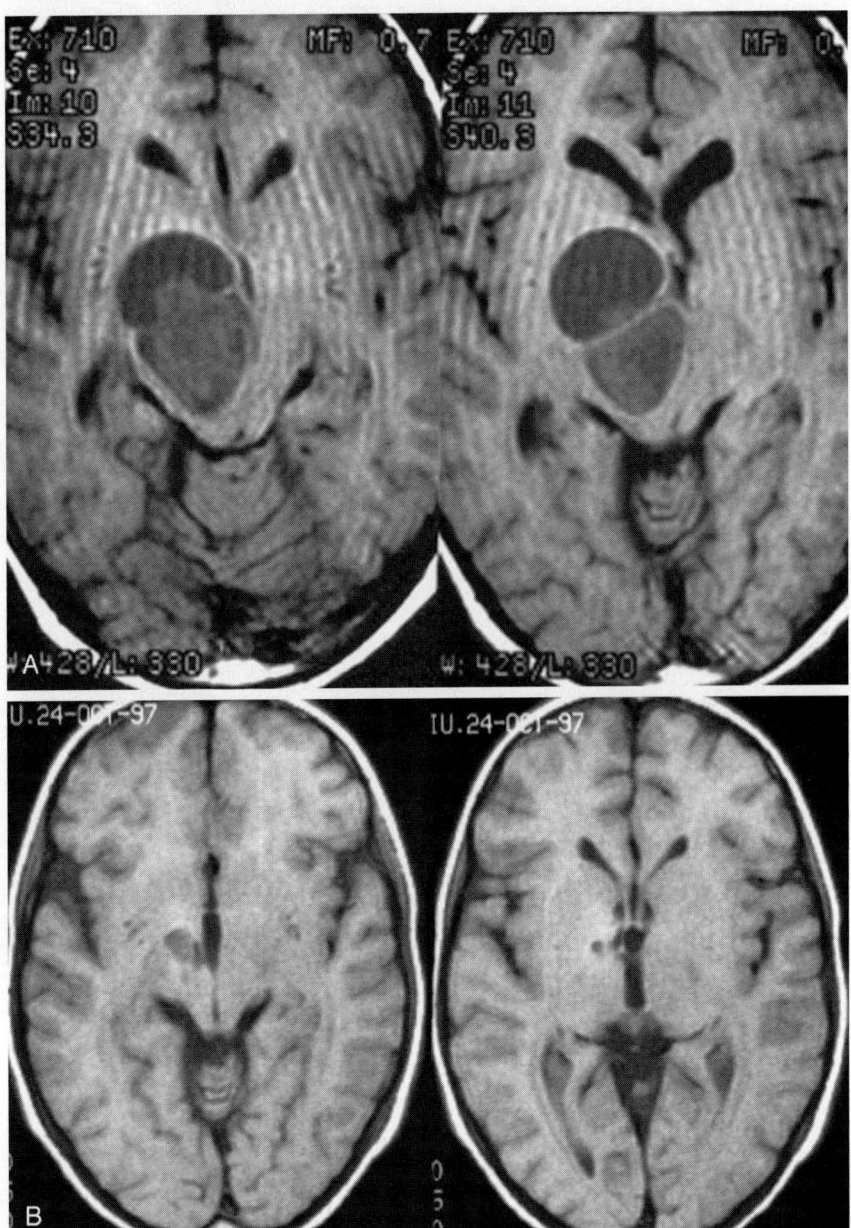

**FIGURE 58–13** ■ Magnetic resonance (MR) images revealing a cystic thalamic-midbrain tumor *(A)*. Postoperative MR images after subtotal removal of a pilocytic astrocytoma via the transcallosal approach *(B)*.

TABLE 58–7 ■ **RESULTS OF THALAMIC TUMOR SURGERY**

|  | No. of Cases (71 Cases = 100%) | Benign Tumors (47 Cases = 100%) | Malignant Tumors (24 Cases = 100%) |
|---|---|---|---|
| Total resection | 35 (49%) | 33 (70%) | 2 (8%) |
| Subtotal resection | 22 (31%) | 11 (23%) | 11 (46%) |
| Partial resection or open biopsy | 14 (20%) | 3 (7%) | 11 (46%) |
| Postoperative |  |  |  |
| Improvement | 33 (48%) | 24 (51%) | 9 (37%) |
| No change | 12 (16%) | 8 (17%) | 4 (17%) |
| Impairment | 23 (32%) | 13 (28%) | 10 (42%) |
| Death | 3 (4%) | 2 (4%) | 1 (4%) |
| Follow-up |  |  |  |
| Dead | 39 | 20 | 19 |
| Alive | 32 | 27 | 5 |
| Median survival (yrs) | 5.1 | 5.8 | 2.3 |

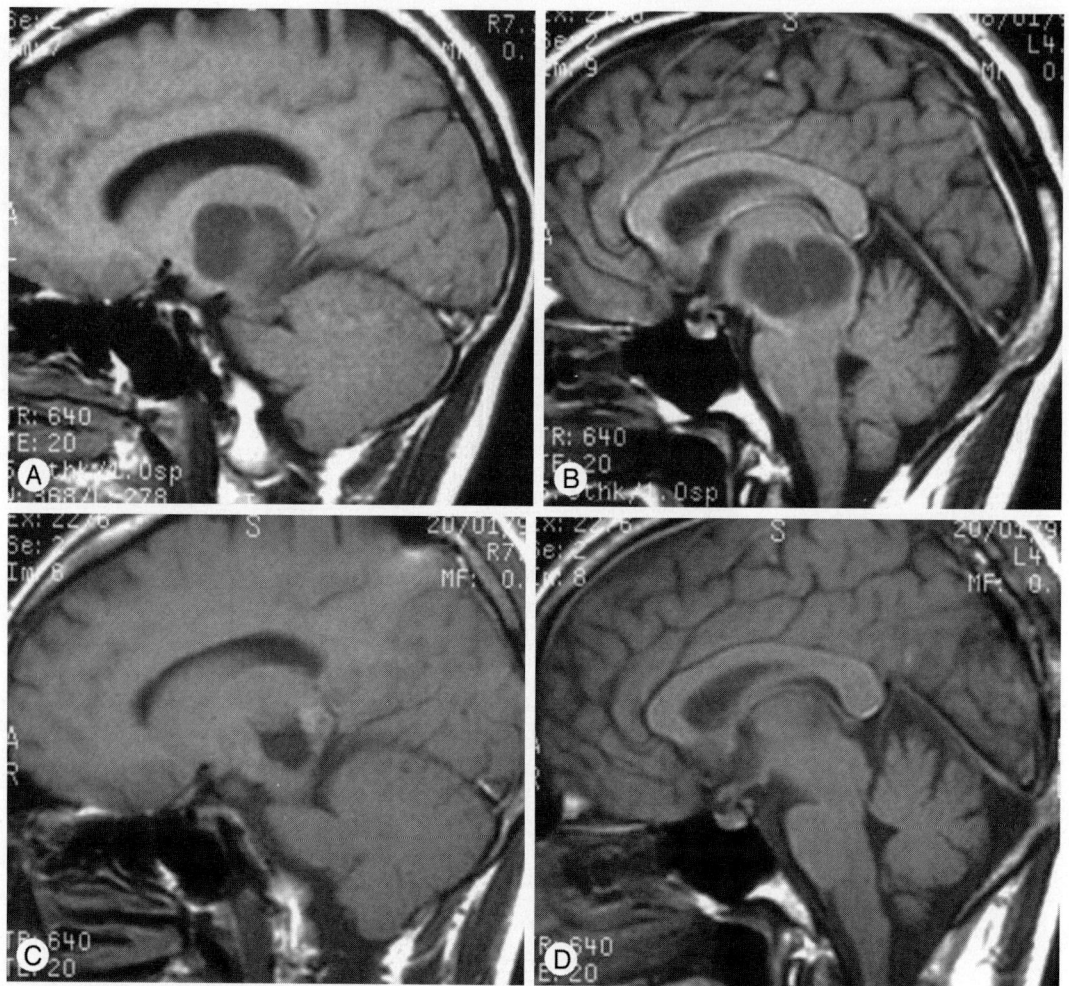

**FIGURE 58–14** ■ *A* and *B*, A preoperative magnetic resonance imaging (MRI) scan shows a posterior tumor of the thalamus. *C* and *D*, A postoperative MRI scan after radical resection through the interhemispheric occipital approach.

ric group, results were much better, mainly because focal thalamic tumors are common to pediatric pathology.

## BRAIN STEM TUMORS

Until recently, tumors of the brain stem were considered to be unremovable, and surgery was attempted either to biopsy the tumor or evacuate the cystic lesion. One of the first descriptions of brain stem tumor removal was that of Pool, who resected the tumor of the aqueduct in 1968.[57]

In 1986, Stroink and coworkers[58] presented the results of surgical treatment of brain stem tumors (BSTs) in 35 patients who underwent a suboccipital craniectomy for histologic evaluation, decompression, subtotal resection of the tumor, and/or cyst aspiration. They differentiated several groups of these tumors on the basis of the location of the tumor, whether it was intrinsic or extrinsic to the brain stem and its contrast-enhancing CT features. Surgery was considered in cases of contrast-enhancing tumors growing exophytically into the fourth ventricle, as well as in cases of focally intrinsic tumors with bright contrast enhancement.

In 1986, Epstein and McCleary[59] summarized their experience of radical excision of intrinsic nonexophytic brain stem gliomas in 34 children. They classified these tumors into focal, diffuse, and cervicomedullary subgroups and recommended primary radical excision only for cervicomedullary neoplasms, which were often benign. Such treatment could result in improvement in a patient's condition; radiation therapy, chemotherapy, or both were considered appropriate treatment for tumors located above the medulla. Later, a series of patients with successfully removed brain stem tumors was presented.[60–68] One of the most detailed descriptions of surgical technique for BST removal (especially for cervicomedullary tumors) was given by Constantini and Epstein.[69] However, despite intensive investigations and numerous publications devoted to indications for surgery of BSTs, this subject remains controversial.

In 1984, we started to operate on patients with primary BSTs in order to establish the indications and contraindications for surgery. Since then about 1000 patients with BSTs have been examined in the outpatient department of the Moscow Burdenko Neurosurgical Institute. In all of these cases, the diagnosis was verified with the help of CT, MRI, or both. In 241 patients, we attempted radical tumor removal. Only these cases are discussed in this chapter.

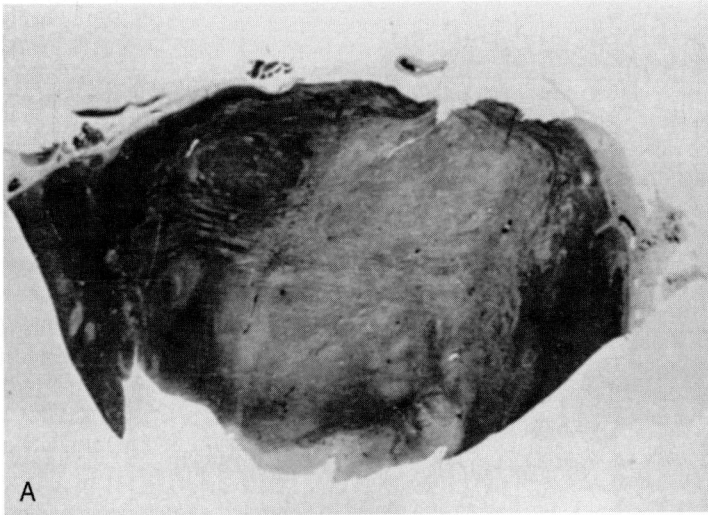
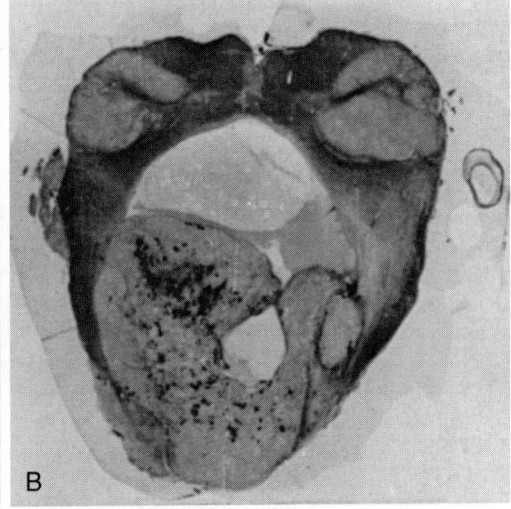

FIGURE 58–15 ■ Types of tumor growth. *A*, A diffuse-growing tumor in the pons. *B*, An expansive-growing tumor in the medulla oblongata.

One of the main goals of our investigators was to discover types of tumor growth. Pathologic examination was performed in 93 cases by Korshunov. These included patients that died (predominantly before 1984) without surgery, after exploration of the posterior fossa or after an attempt at partial removal of the BST. According to pathologic data, we identify three main types of tumor growth.

1. Diffuse-growing tumors (67%), which are not demarcated from surrounding brain stem structures. Neurons and axons of the brain stem tissue persist between tumor cells in different parts of the tumor (Fig. 58–15*A*). These tumors are astrocytic gliomas with different degrees of malignancy (I-IV).
2. Expansive-growing tumors (22%), in which the border of the tumor is well defined (see Fig. 58–15*B*) and brain stem structures are demarcated from the tumor by a compact layer of tumor astrocytes axons ("tumor capsula"). Pathologic examination reveals pilocytic astrocytomas (grade I). Of these tumors, 40% contain vascular hamartomas and are called *angioastrocytomas*.
3. Infiltrative-growing tumors (11%) look macroscopically like well-circumscribed tumors; however, in reality, the tumor cells infiltrate brain stem structures. Neural tissue in this zone is totally destroyed by the tumor (so-called *pseudofocal tumors*). Pathologically, these tumors were primitive neuroepithelial tumors (PNETs).

From the surgical point of view, it is important to outline cystic tumors that can be observed in the first and second groups. It is also important to differentiate tumors with the exophytic component (extrinsic tumors) and tumors that are located completely inside the brain stem (intrinsic tumors) and do not penetrate its surface (Fig. 58–16). Some diffuse tumors have an exophytic component that protrudes in the fourth ventricle or one of subarachnoid cisterns. It was noted that the exophytic component does not contain brain stem tissue (i.e., representing the focal component).

## Diagnosis

CT and MRI permit us to detect the delineation of the tumor's edges, the type of tumor growth, which is eventu-

ally verified only during surgery. According to these criteria, we define the following groups of BSTs.

1. *Diffuse tumors.* A CT scan shows the enlargement and deformation of the brain stem and different variants of precontrast density (isodensity, hypodensity, mixed density) without delineation of the tumor edges. Areas of increased density are considered to be the evidence of malignant degeneration in that part of the tumor or the sign of bleeding.[70, 71] Different types of contrast enhancement can be observed, but these tumors are usually nonenhancing lesions (Fig. 58–17). Diffuse tumors have a low signal on MR $T_1$-weighted images and an increased signal on MR $T_2$-weighted images (Fig. 58–18). Seventy percent of them show an absence or a low degree of gadolinium enhancement. Most diffuse tumors involve the large area of the brain stem: the pons as well as the midbrain or medulla oblongata. However, in rare occasions, diffuse tumors

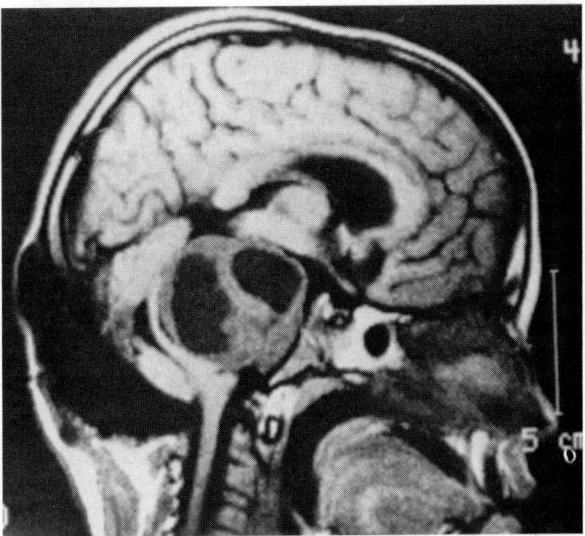

FIGURE 58–16 ■ A magnetic resonance imaging (MRI) scan ($T_1$) demonstrates an intrinsic brain stem tumor. The brain stem surface is not penetrated by the tumor.

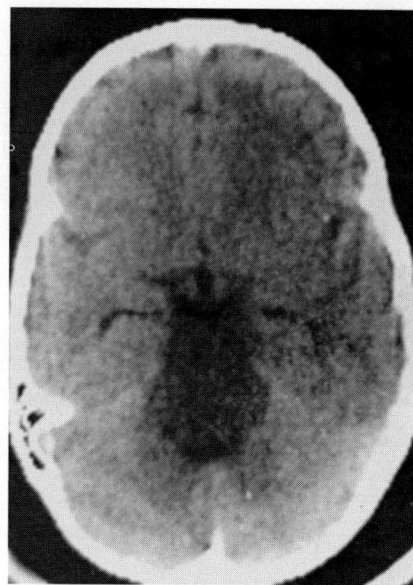

**FIGURE 58–17 ■** Diffuse tumor. A computed tomography (CT) scan shows a hypodense, nonenhancing intrinsic brain stem lesion.

can be small and can imitate the focal tumor (Fig. 58–19). Perhaps these cases represent the initial stage of benign diffuse tumor growth.

2. *Focal-diffuse tumors* (diffuse tumors with "focal" component). These tumors consist of a focal well-delineated intrinsic part or the exophytic component and the part where the tumor has a diffuse type of growth (see Fig. 58–25). If the tumor is poorly defined on a CT scan, MRI may be helpful.

3. *Focal tumors.* An enhanced CT scan shows a well-delineated hyperdense lesion in the brain stem with a cyst (in some cases) (Fig. 58–20). As was mentioned earlier, focal tumors are benign astrocytomas, and it is necessary to differentiate them from "pseudofocal" malignant infiltrating growing tumors (Fig. 58–21). Most focal benign tumors show evident contrast enhancement after gadolinium injection (see Fig. 58–24).

Other lesions of the brain stem that should be differentiated from brain stem gliomas are brain stem hematomas, hemangioblastomas, metastatic tumors, cholesteatomas, and granulomas. In cases in which the nature of the brain stem lesion is in doubt, direct surgery or stereotactic surgery is performed to establish the type of lesion.

## Clinical Manifestation

The clinical manifestation of these gliomas depends on factors such as the tumor location, type of growth, and degree of malignancy. Diffuse malignant tumors are characterized by a short duration of the disease, rapid deterioration of the patient's clinical state, and severe signs of brain stem damage, which include cranial nerve palsy and signs of long-term damage. Signs of intracranial hypertension are not common and appear usually in the late stage of the disease.

For focal tumors, slow progression of neurologic signs, corresponding to tumor location, is more typical. In some cases of benign tumors, local signs of brain stem damage are very mild. We found that different variants of hyperkinesis are typical for midbrain tumors. The main neurologic signs revealed at the time of admission have been analyzed in 120 patients and presented in Table 58–8.

## Indications for Surgery

We consider that surgery is indicated in all cases of focal tumors, focal-diffuse tumors with evident focal component, and cystic tumors. Other than that, we had to operate on some patients who had malignant predominantly diffuse tumors.

## Surgery

In the 14-year period from 1984 to July 1998, 241 patients were selected for surgery with the aim of radical tumor removal. These patients consisted of 81 adults and 160 children, who presented with a history of illness between 1 month and 25 years. The longest duration of the disease occurred in cases of benign focal tumors, such as angioastrocytomas. At the time of admission, most patients were severely disabled (see Table 58–8).

### Tumor Location Along the Brain Stem

For selection of the most adequate approach to the tumor, we identify several groups of BSTs according to their predominant location.

TABLE 58–8 ■ **BRAIN STEM TUMORS: NEUROLOGIC SIGNS IN 120 PATIENTS AT THE TIME OF ADMISSION**

| Caudal Brain Stem | | Rostral Brain Stem | |
|---|---|---|---|
| *Neurologic Signs* | *No. of Patients* | *Neurologic Signs* | *No. of Patients* |
| Hemiparesis | 26 | Hemiparesis | 32 |
| Monoparesis | 2 | Ataxia | 18 |
| Ataxia | 40 | Unilateral hyperkinesis | 16 |
| Ninth and tenth nerve deficit | 45 | Oculomotor disorders | 46 |
| Eighth nerve deficit | 17 | Parinaud's syndrome | 35 |
| Sixth nerve deficit | 28 | Behavioral problems | 22 |
| Lateral gaze palsy | 16 | High intracranial pressure* | 32 |
| High intracranial pressure* | 30 | | |

*In six patients, shunting was performed before admission.

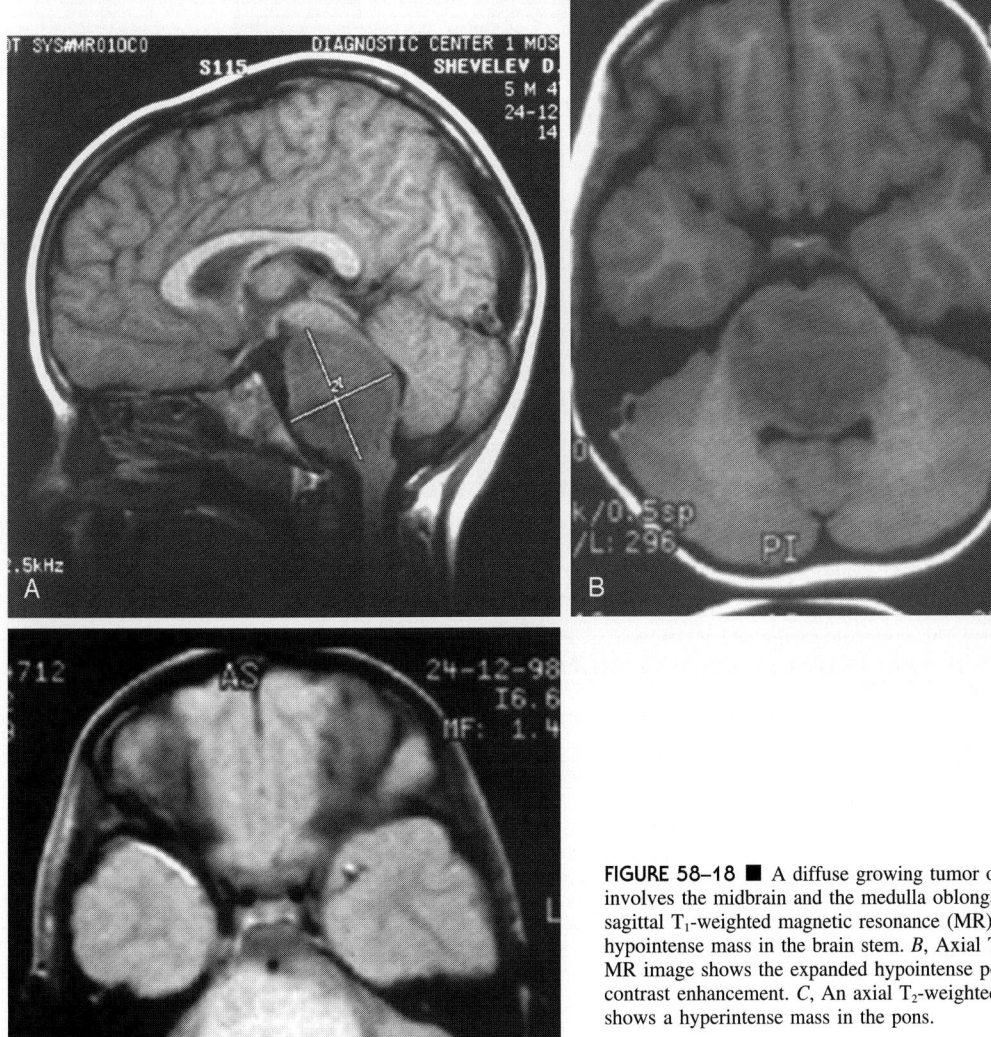

FIGURE 58–18 ■ A diffuse growing tumor of the pons that involves the midbrain and the medulla oblongata. *A*, A sagittal $T_1$-weighted magnetic resonance (MR) image shows a hypointense mass in the brain stem. *B*, Axial $T_1$-weighted MR image shows the expanded hypointense pons and no contrast enhancement. *C*, An axial $T_2$-weighted MR image shows a hyperintense mass in the pons.

1. Caudal BSTs: cervicomedullary, medullary, medullary-pontine, and pontine
2. Rostral BSTs: pontine-midbrain, midbrain tegmentum or peduncle, tectal plate, and aqueductal tumors. (In 17 cases, midbrain tumors spread into the posterior thalamus.)

In each of these groups we identified subgroups according to the intrinsic or extrinsic type of tumor growth. The number of patients in each of these groups is summarized in Table 58–9.

The exophytic part of the tumor is localized in the fourth ventricle (in 76 patients), cerebellopontine angle (in 24 patients), and cisterna ambiens (in 27 patients). The exact extension of the tumor was determined predominantly by MRI and to a lesser extent by enhanced CT and was being verified during surgery. It is necessary to mention that MRI is very valuable in cases of cervicomedullary tumors and intrinsic tectal plate tumors that are poorly diagnosed by CT.

## Surgical Technique

### Patient's Position

In most cases, we prefer to operate on patients with BSTs in the sitting position with all necessary precautions against air embolism. This position is most convenient when the tumor is located in the upper pons and midbrain. The prone position is preferable for small children and patients with extensive hydrocephalus.

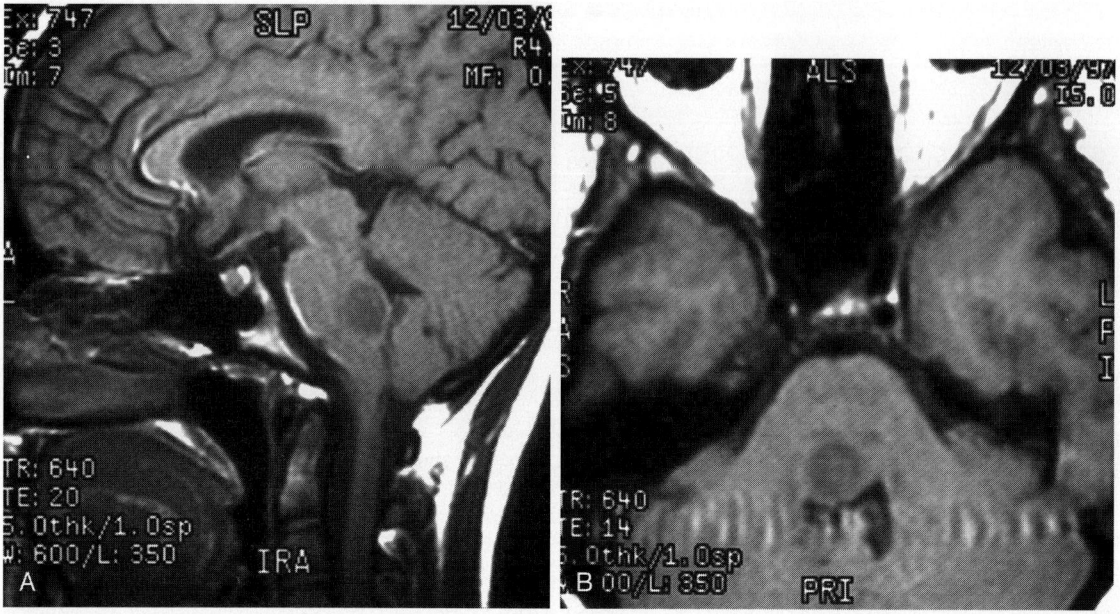

**FIGURE 58–19** ■ Small diffuse tumor of the pons. Pathologic examination of tumor tissue revealed the persistence of brain stem tissue among tumor cells (fibrillary astrocytoma) and confirmed the diffuse type of tumor growth. Sagittal *(A)* and axial *(B)* T₁-weighted magnetic resonance images show a small hypointense lesion in the pons tegmentum, imitating the focal tumor.

**TABLE 58–9** ■ **CAUDAL BRAIN STEM TUMORS: NEUROLOGIC STATUS 1.5 MONTHS\* AFTER SURGERY RELATED TO TUMOR LOCATION**

|  | Sp. Med | Med | Med P | Pons |
|---|---|---|---|---|
| Improved | 7 (41%) | 12 (48%) | 15 (38%) | 28 (53%) |
| Unchanged | 3 (18%) | 5 (20%) | 10 (25%) | 11 (21%) |
| Deterioration + improvement† | 3 (18%) | 1 (4%) | 4 (10%) | 6 (12%) |
| Deteriorated | 0 (0%) | 3 (12%) | 2 (5%) | 5 (10%) |
| Death | 4 (23%) | 4 (16%) | 9 (22%) | 2 (4%) |
| TOTAL   134 | 17 (100%) | 25 (100%) | 40 (100%) | 52 (100%) |

\*Mean time of discharge after surgery.
†Some neurologic symptoms increased, some decreased.
Sp. Med, spinomedullary BSTs; Med, medullary BSTs.

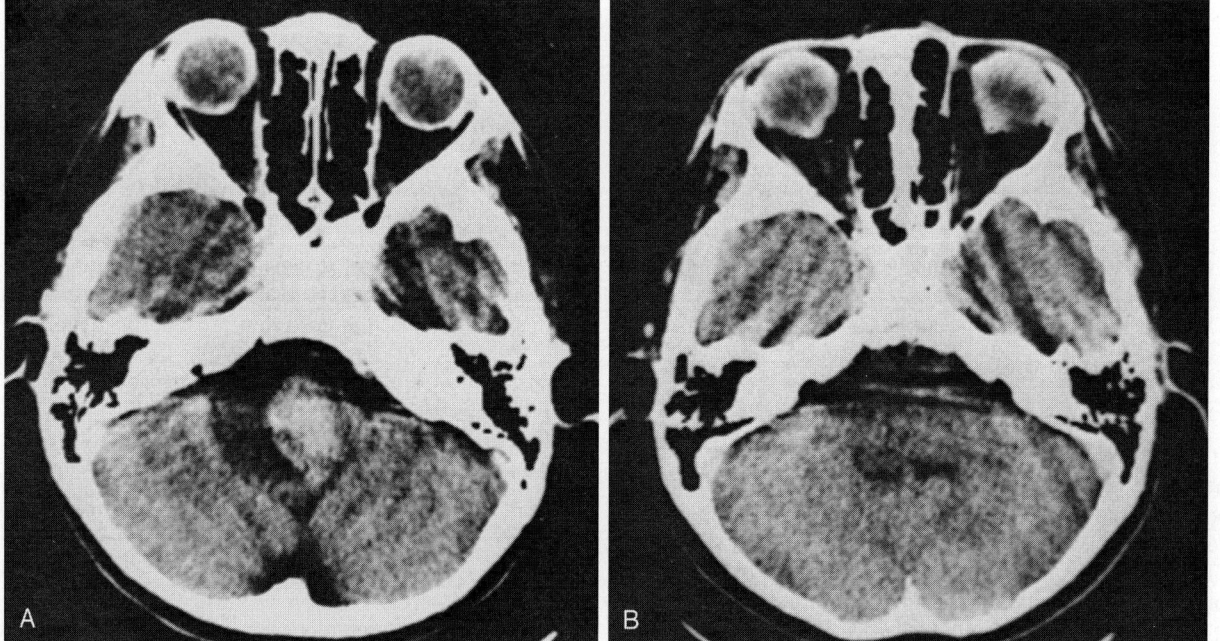

**FIGURE 58–20** ■ A focal tumor of the pons before *(A)* and after *(B)* surgery. *A,* The computed tomography (CT) scan shows a focal enhancing solid tumor and a cyst in the pons; *B,* CT scan taken 12 months after total removal of the tumor.

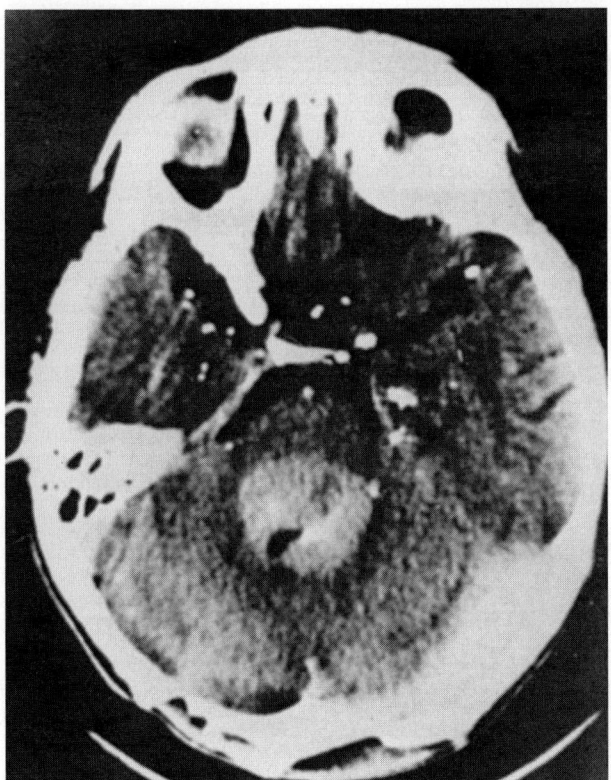

**FIGURE 58–21** ■ Pseudofocal tumor. This enhanced computed tomography (CT) scan demonstrates a well-delineated lesion of the pons. The pathologic examination revealed PNET.

## Brain Stem Function Monitoring

In order to control brain stem functions during surgery,[72, 73] we monitor the somatosensory evoked potential (SSEP) and the auditory evoked potential (AEP) and use direct stimulation of the motor nuclei of cranial nerves III, VI, VII, IX, X and XII.

According to our experience, registration of SSEP and AEP is not very reliable. More information comes from mapping from the floor of the fourth ventricle with the help of direct stimulation of the motor nuclei of the cranial nerves.

Tumor removal often causes hemodynamic reactions, such as bradycardia and an increase or decrease of blood pressure. Our experience shows that hemodynamic reactions usually happen during manipulation in the vicinity to the nuclei of cranial nerves V and IX and disappear when manipulation in that region ceases.

## Approaches

Surgical approaches depend strictly on the location and size of the tumor. Thorough investigation of the BST topography with the help of MRI is essential to select the best access.

Tumors located in the tectal plate were reached both with the supracerebellar subtentorial or occipital supratentorial route, with section of the tentorium lateral and along the rectus sinus.

Gliomas that predominantly occupy midbrain tegmentum, brain peduncle, or both can be approached by different ways—perhaps by the occipital transtentorial, lateral subtentorial, or subtemporal approach (Fig. 58–22).

If the tumor grows into the fourth ventricle or is identified as an aqueductal tumor, the medial posterior fossa access is preferable. Some tumors that grow in the region of the aqueduct were easily reached through the fourth ventricle. Figure 58–23 illustrates the tumor in this location before and after surgery.

In some cases, the combination of different approaches permits the surgeon to accomplish radical tumor ablation. For example, the supracerebellar route can be combined with the approach through the fourth ventricle; the occipital transtentorial approach can be combined with the supracerebellar; and so forth. In cases in which the tumor penetrates into the thalamus, the transcallosal way may be applied.

The most difficult task is to approach tumors that are located predominantly in the anterior part of the pons and the peduncle. In such cases, the pterional route, using a subtemporal approach with tentorial section, or the presigmoid route may be selected.

Caudal BSTs (involving the pons, medulla oblongata, and upper segments of the spinal cord) can be explored and removed using the osteoplastic posterior fossa approach.

In cases of spinomedullary tumors that occupy the cervical part of the spinal cord, we prefer a laminotomy with repositioning of the vertebral arches after tumor removal.

When we approach dorsally exophytic tumors that occupy the fourth ventricle, we do not cut the vermis. For adequate exploration of the fourth ventricle it is necessary only to coagulate and divide the plexus in the region of the foramen of Magendie.

## Technique of Tumor Removal

Ultrasound aspiration is the most efficient method for glial BST removal, especially if the tumor is solid. Softer tumors may be evacuated with bipolar coagulation and simultaneous aspiration of coagulated tissue. It is necessary to mention that coagulation changes the color and density of the tumor (it becomes more solid and pale), and for determination of the border between the tumor and brain stem structures, thorough aspiration of coagulated tissue is necessary. When dealing with brain stem lesions, we prefer not to use the retractor to open the brain stem wound.

If the tumor has the exophytic component, the surgery starts with its removal. Radicality of tumor ablation in such cases depends on the possibility of distinguishing the interface between the tumor and the surrounding brain (Fig. 58–24).

A special group of tumors is presented by so-called dorsally exophytic tumors growing into the fourth ventricle that can be successfully removed.[74]

Pollack and colleagues achieved favorable results in 18 patients with dorsally exophytic tumors.[75] These are fourth ventricle tumors with a broad attachment to the fourth ventricle floor. The exophytic part of the tumor is easily removed with Cavitron. However, if the definite tumor–brain stem interface is absent, complete resection of the tumor is not feasible (Fig. 58–25).

Our experience also shows positive results and a long-lasting effect after the ablation of this type of tumor. We observed a 25-year-old patient who was initially operated

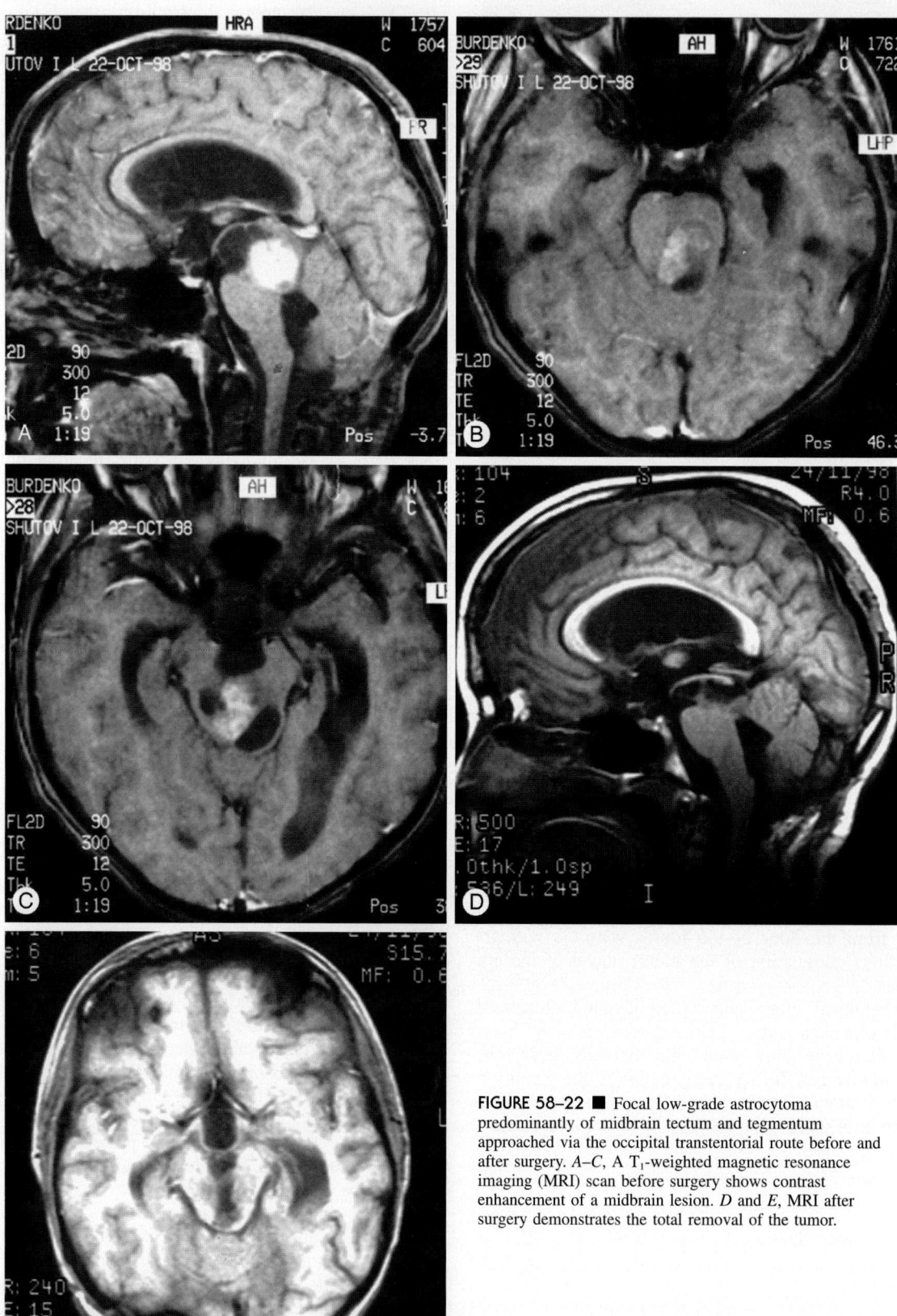

**FIGURE 58–22** ■ Focal low-grade astrocytoma predominantly of midbrain tectum and tegmentum approached via the occipital transtentorial route before and after surgery. *A–C,* A T$_1$-weighted magnetic resonance imaging (MRI) scan before surgery shows contrast enhancement of a midbrain lesion. *D* and *E,* MRI after surgery demonstrates the total removal of the tumor.

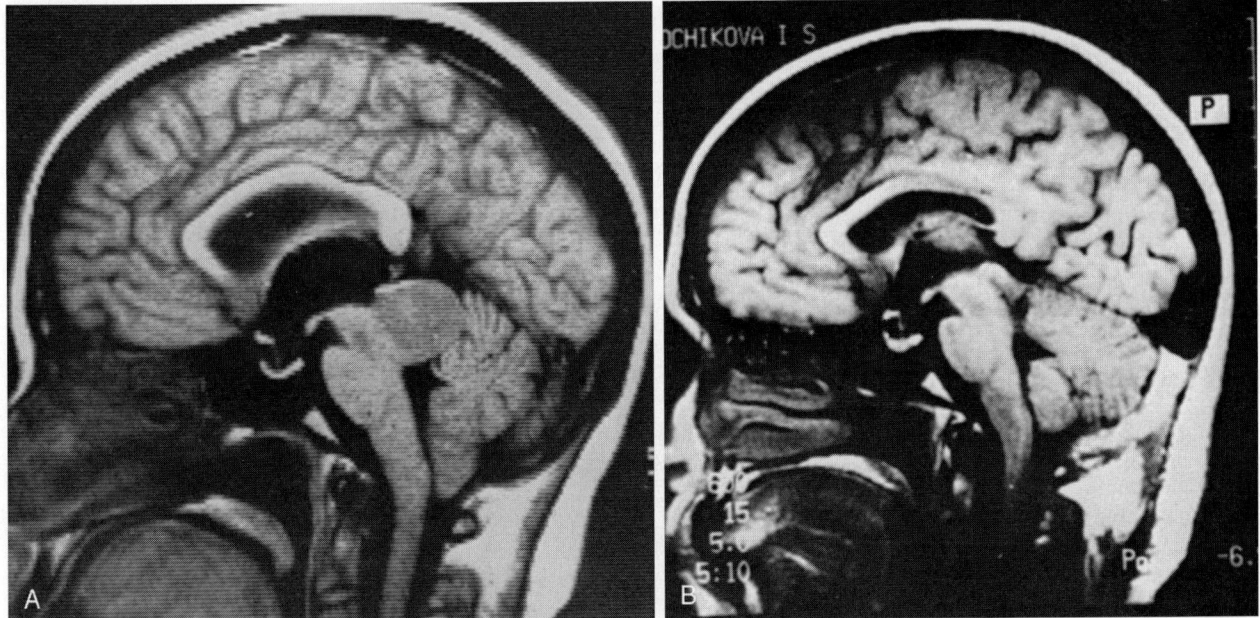

FIGURE 58–23 ■ The focal tumor of midbrain tegmentum removed through the fourth ventricle. *A,* A magnetic resonance imaging (MRI) scan (T₁) taken before surgery. *B,* MRI taken 3 weeks after the total removal of the tumor.

on 20 years earlier. A second surgery was performed because of the recurrence of the disease. In the patient's childhood, only partial removal of the fourth ventricle exophytic glial tumor was undertaken.

If the tumor contains a cyst or cysts, evacuation of cystic fluid greatly facilitates removal of the tumor because the surgeon gains additional space for manipulation. When the cavity after evacuation of a cyst or removal of a tumor is large, we utilize a spatula with narrow blades (3 to 5 mm width) just to support the cavity walls. Routinely we use as a retractor blades of bipolar coagulating forceps.

In approximately half of our cases, the tumor was intrinsic to the brain stem, and it was necessary to make an incision in the surface of the brain stem. The length of this incision may vary, but it is usually relatively small (≈1 cm). That is enough to reach and remove even large tumors.

In our practice, we try to put these incisions in the place nearest to the surface of the tumor. It is important to approach the tumor at a distance from the nuclei of cranial nerves VII, IX, and X. This location can be determined with the help of fourth ventricle floor mapping.

When the tumor penetrates into the subarachnoid space, it may come into contact with important arteries. In some cases, these vessels are included in the tumor tissue. The surgeon must be cautious when removing a tumor that penetrates into the ventral part of the brain stem and contacts vertebral or basilar arteries and their branches.

Some tumors are well supplied with blood, and these vessels must be coagulated while the tumor is being removed. In some cases, such coagulation may result in ischemic damage of the surrounding brain tissue.

Critical in the removal of brain stem gliomas is differentiation between tumor and brain tissue. If tumor infiltrates the brain stem, its removal may result in increased neurologic morbidity, with disturbances of vital neurologic functions. In such cases, radical tumor removal is impossible.

We do not want to describe in detail the risks of surgery in all groups of patients with BSTs. We only want to comment on our experience with cervicomedullary tumor surgery (in 17 patients).

Constantini and Epstein[69] described these tumors and they have emphasized that almost invariably they are low-grade tumors that are amenable to radical surgery. The rostral extension of the tumor is restricted by long tracts and the obex without infiltration of the medulla and the pons (Fig. 58–26). As in previous articles, they emphasized that surgery was especially effective and safe in this group of BSTs.

We also have favorable results in some patients in this group (Fig. 58–27). However, our experience is in some contradiction to the aforementioned data. In the majority of our observations of spinomedullary tumors there were neurologic or MRI signs of medulla oblongata involvement (Fig. 58–28) that made the radical surgery risky, and postoperative mortality in this group was dangerously high (23%). These authors also described a case of diffuse infiltrating astrocytoma of the cervicomedullary region.[76] It seems that careful analysis of clinical presentation and MRI data is of special importance for better operative planning and optimal management of this group of BSTs.

### Results

The results of BST removal are presented in Tables 58–9, 58–10, and 58–11. Some comments are in order.

1. The more unfavorable results are observed in the group of patients with spinomedullary tumors and gliomas of medulla oblongata and lower pons (see Table 58–9). The postoperative mortality is the highest in this group. Preoperative and postoperative disturbances of vital functions such as breathing and

*Text continued on page 834*

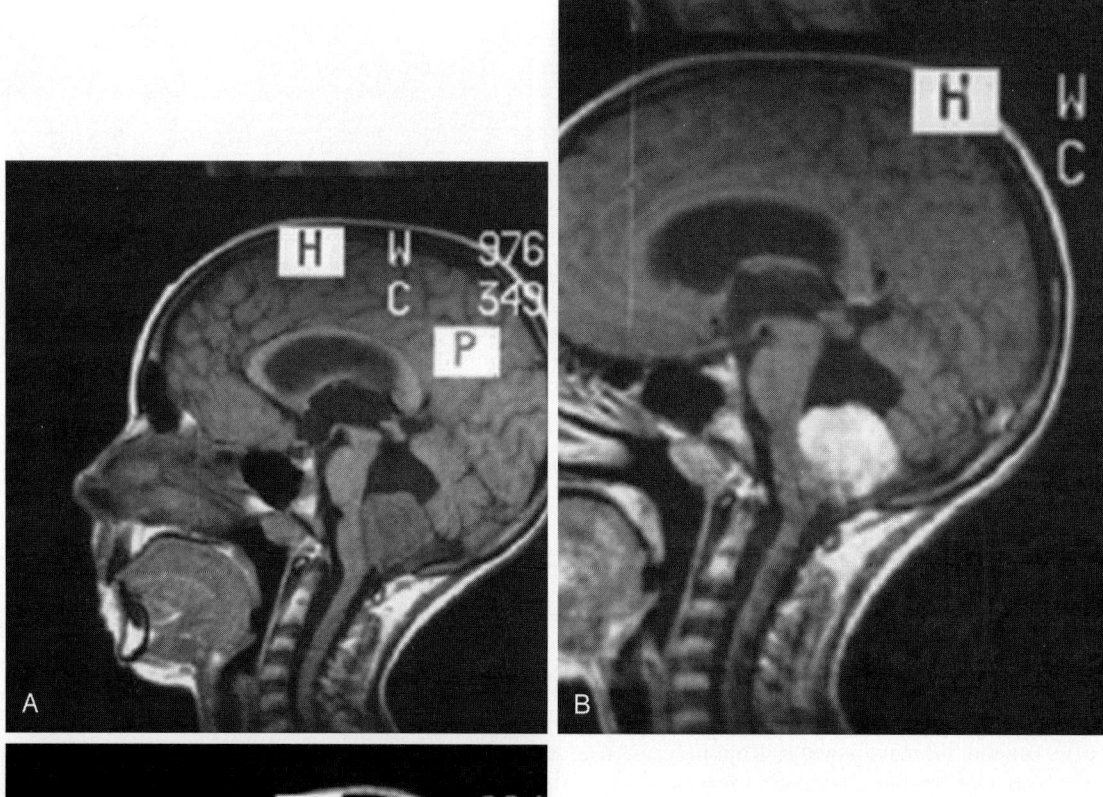

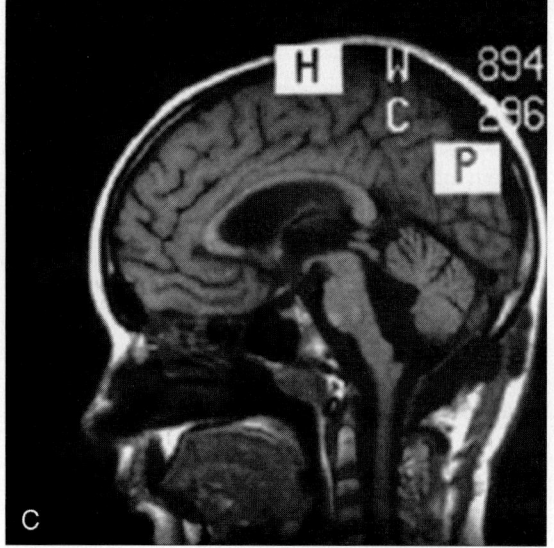

**FIGURE 58–24 ■** Dorsally exophytic pilocytic astrocytoma of the medulla oblongata in a 12-year-old girl suffering vomiting, nausea, and weight loss. The duration of the disease is not less than 10 years. A magnetic resonance imaging (MRI) scan before *(A)* and after *(B)* surgery. *A,* Sagittal $T_1$-weighted MRI shows a hypointense mass growing from the dorsal surface of the medulla oblongata. *B,* Sagittal $T_1$-weighted MRI scan after gadolinium injection shows marked enhancement of the tumor. *C,* Sagittal $T_1$-weighted MRI scan shows the total removal of the tumor.

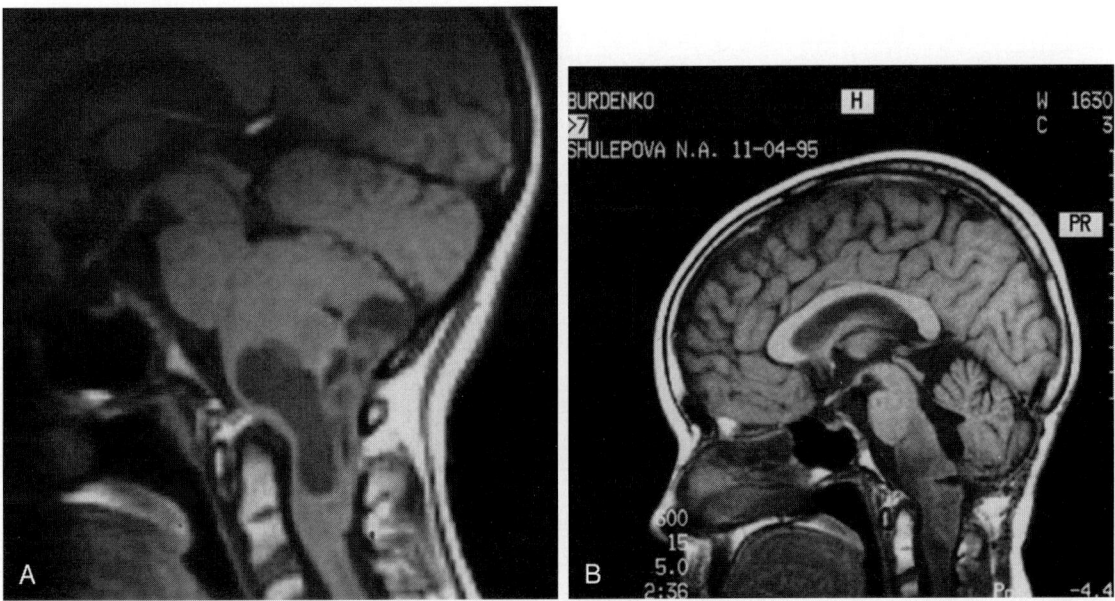

**FIGURE 58–25** ■ Dorsally exophytic focal-diffuse tumor arising from the medulla oblongata and upper segments of the spinal cord, occupying the fourth ventricle. *A,* A magnetic resonance imaging (MRI) scan before surgery. *B,* An MRI scan 10 months after surgery shows the removal of the exophytic part of the tumor and enlargement of the medulla oblongata infiltrated by the tumor (low-grade astrocytoma).

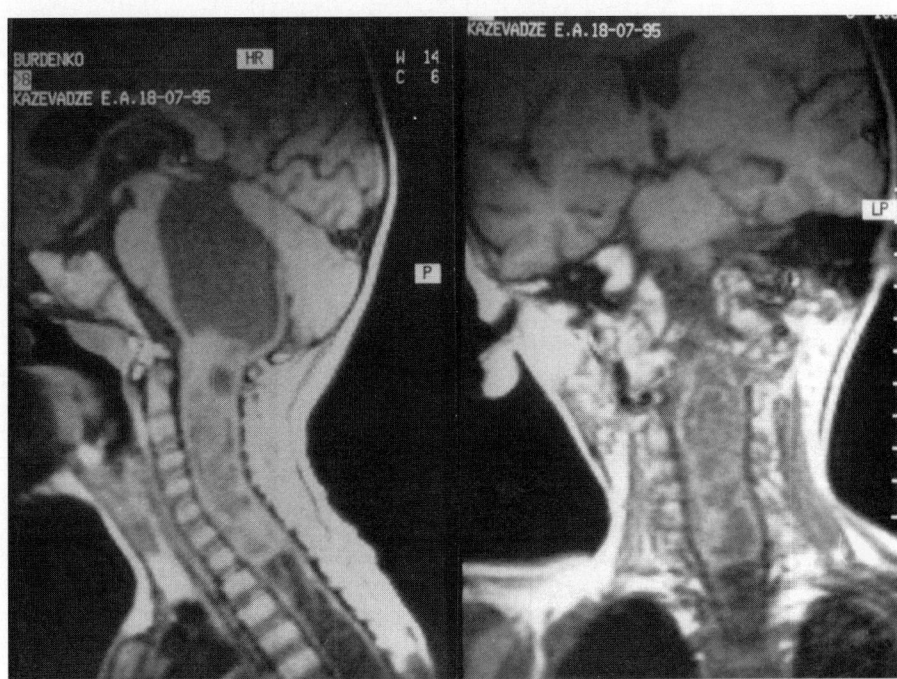

**FIGURE 58–26** ■ A spinomedullary tumor. The magnetic resonance imaging scan shows an upper cervical tumor with a rostral fourth ventricle cyst. Severe deficit of cranial nerves IX and X.

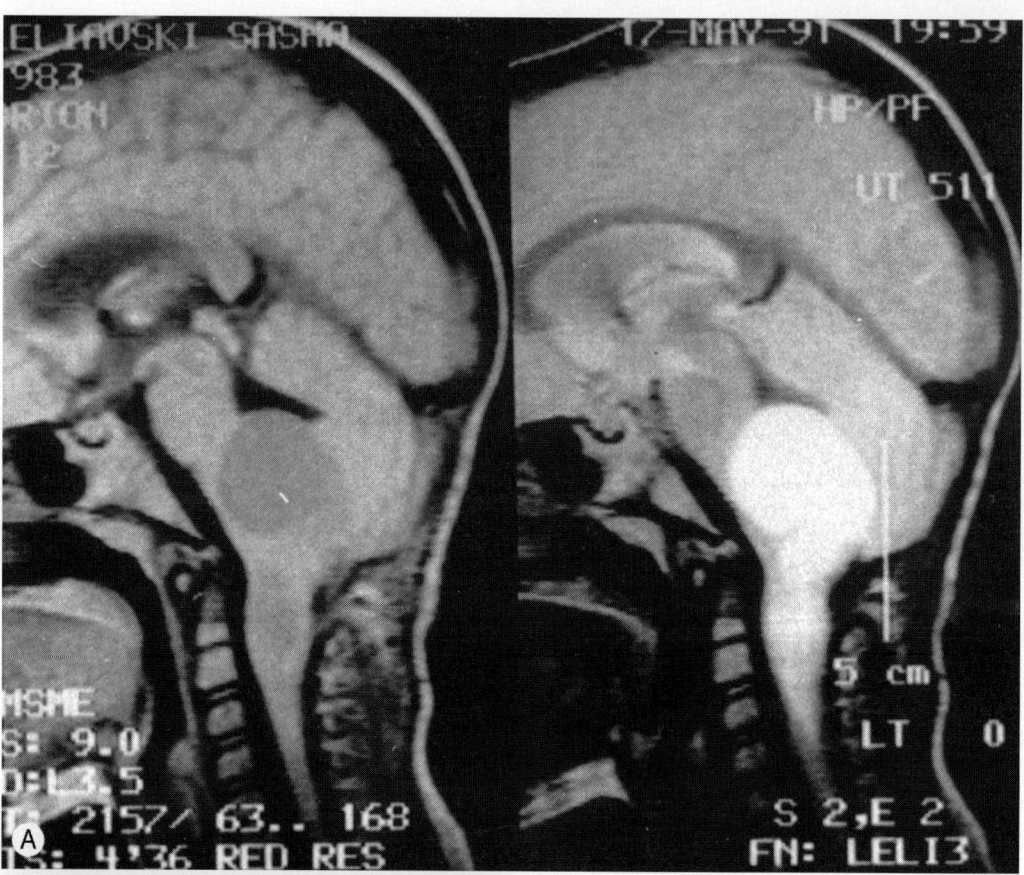

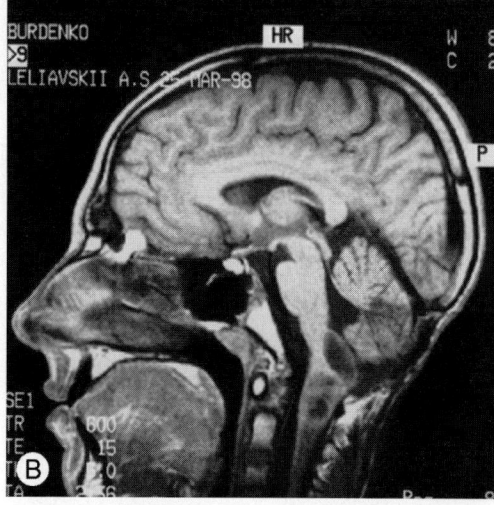

**FIGURE 58–27** ■ Spinomedullary tumor without signs of medulla oblongata infiltration. *A,* A magnetic resonance imaging (MRI) scan before surgery shows a predominantly solid upper cervical tumor with a cyst in the fourth ventricle. *B,* An MRI after surgery shows the removal of a cyst from the fourth ventricle. The follow-up period is 7.5 years without signs of recurrence.

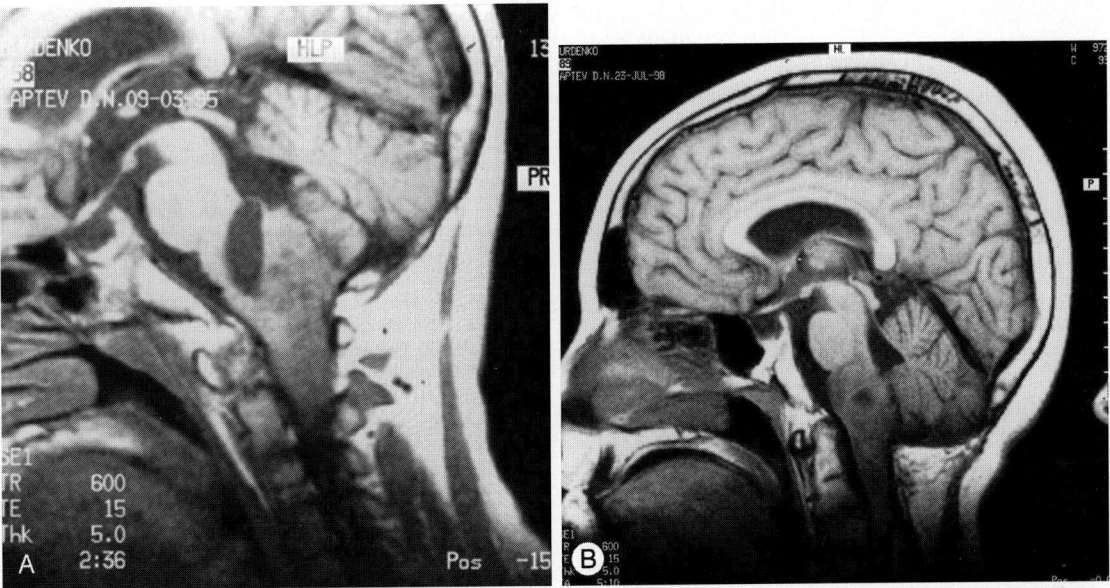

**FIGURE 58–28** ■ A predominantly solid spinomedullary focal-diffuse tumor, arising from the medulla oblongata and cervical part of the spinal cord. *A*, A magnetic resonance imaging (MRI) scan before surgery demonstrates the enlargement of the medulla oblongata and upper segments of the spinal cord. *B*, After partial removal of a fibrillary astrocytoma.

### TABLE 58–10 ■ ROSTRAL BRAIN STEM TUMORS: NEUROLOGIC STATUS 1.5 MONTHS* AFTER SURGERY RELATED TO TUMOR LOCATION

|  | P Mid | Mid | Tect |
|---|---|---|---|
| Improved | 26 (54%) | 18 (67%) | 17 (53%) |
| Changed | 9 (19%) | 1 (4%) | 8 (25%) |
| Deterioration + improvement† | 4 (8%) | 4 (15%) | 4 (13%) |
| Deteriorated | 6 (13%) | 2 (7%) | 2 (6%) |
| Death | 3 (6%) | 2 (7%) | 1 (3%) |
| TOTAL   107 | 48 (100%) | 27 (100%) | 32 (100%) |

*Mean time of discharge after surgery.
†Some neurologic symptoms increased, some decreased.
P Mid, pontine midbrain BSTs; Mid, tegmentum, crus cerebri BSTs; Tect, aqueductal, and tectal BSTs.

### TABLE 58–11 ■ BRAIN STEM TUMORS: NEUROLOGIC STATUS 1.5 MONTHS* AFTER SURGERY RELATED TO AGE AND TUMOR LOCATION

|  | Caudal BSTs | | Rostral BSTs | |
|---|---|---|---|---|
|  | *Children* | *Adults* | *Children* | *Adults* |
| Improved | 47 (52%) | 15 (35%) | 45 (65%) | 16 (42%) |
| Unchanged | 15 (16%) | 14 (33%) | 10 (15%) | 8 (21%) |
| Deterioration + improvement† | 10 (11%) | 4 (9%) | 5 (7%) | 7 (18%) |
| Deteriorated | 9 (10%) | 1 (2%) | 7 (10%) | 3 (8%) |
| Death | 10 (11%) | 9 (21%) | 2 (3%) | 4 (11%) |
| TOTAL   241 | 91 (100%) | 43 (100%) | 69 (100%) | 38 (100%) |

*Mean time of discharge after surgery.
†Some neurologic symptoms increased, some decreased.

### TABLE 58–12 ■ BRAIN STEM TUMORS: LONG-TERM RESULTS AFTER BRAIN STEM TUMOR REMOVAL IN 105 PATIENTS

| Location | Neurologic Signs* | | | Signs of Recurrence | No Information† |
|---|---|---|---|---|---|
|  | *Mild* | *Moderate* | *Severe* |  |  |
| Caudal brain stem (No. = 56) | 17 (30%) | 17 (30%) | 2 (4%) | 12 (21%) | 8 (15%) |
| Rostral brain stem (No. = 49) | 21 (43%) | 5 (10%) | 3 (6%) | 3 (6%) | 17 (35%) |

*No signs of recurrence.
†In 25 cases, we could get no information because of social and political changes in Russia.

swallowing often necessitate long-term artificial ventilation, which cannot be effective enough to save a patient's life. Much better results may be achieved in patients with rostral brain stem tumors (see Table 58–10).

2. Removal of malignant tumors produces worse results in comparison with removal of benign tumors. The survival of patients with gliomas (grade IV) and PNET did not exceed 6 months.
3. Results are best after the removal of focal tumors.
4. Surgery in adults is more dangerous than that in children (see Table 58–11).
5. The long-term results are much better in patients with rostral BSTs (Table 58–12), possibly because of the predominance of benign tumors in the midbrain. Follow-up (ranging from 6 months to 9 years) showed that caudal BSTs recurred in 21% of cases, whereas rostral BSTs recurred only in 6%.

We may conclude that surgical removal of primary BSTs is indicated in cases of focal and some focal-diffuse benign (cystic and solid) tumors. Surgery may result in marked long-lasting improvement.

# REFERENCES

1. Koos WT, Horaczek A: Statistics of intracranial midline tumors in children. Acta Neurochir Suppl (Wien) 35:1–5, 1985.
2. Lang J: Surgical anatomy of the hypothalamus. Acta Neurochir (Wien) 75:5–22, 1985.
3. Bregeat P: Quelques reflexions sur les gliomes hypothalamique. Adv Ophtal 36:130–137, 1978.
4. Raimondi AJ: Pediatric Neurosurgery. New York: Springer-Verlag, 1987.
5. Mohadjer M, Etou A, Milios E, et al: Chiasmatic optic glioma. Neurochirurgia (Stuttg) 34:90–93, 1991.
6. Bataini JP, Delanian S, Ponvert D: Chiasmal gliomas: Results of irradiation management in 57 patients and review of literature. Int J Radiat Oncol Biol Phys 21:615–623, 1991.
7. Capo H, Kupersmith MJ: Efficacy and complications of radiotherapy of anterior visual pathway tumors. Neurol Clin 9:179–203, 1991.
8. Gould RJ, Hilal SK, Chutorian AM: Efficacy of radiotherapy in optic gliomas. Pediatr Neurol 3:29–32, 1987.
9. Cohen ME, Duffner PK: Optic pathway tumors. Neurol Clin 9:467–477, 1991.
10. McLaurin RL, Breneman J, Aron B: Hypothalamic gliomas: Review of 18 cases. Concepts Pediatr Neurosurg 7:19–29, 1987.
11. Wechsler-Jentzsch K, Witt JH, Fitz CR, et al: Unresectable gliomas in children: Tumor-volume response to radiation therapy. Radiology 169:237–242, 1988.
12. Friedman HS, Oakes WJ: Recurrent brain tumors in children. Pediatr Neurosci 13:233–241, 1987.
13. Scott E, Mickle JP: Pediatric diencephalic gliomas—A review of 18 cases. Pediatr Neurosci 13:225–232, 1987.
14. Turpin G, Heshmati HM, Scherrer H, et al: Tumeurs hypothalamiques primitives (en dehors des cranio-pharyngiomes): Étude endocrinienne et evolutive post-radiotherapidue. A propos de 17 obserrvations. Ann Med Interne (Paris) 137:395–400, 1986.
15. Ganz JC, Smievoll Al, Thorsen F.: Radiosurgical treatment of gliomas of the diencephalon. Acta Neurochir Suppl (Wien) 62:62–66, 1994.
16. Bernstein M, Laperriere NJ: A critical appraisal of the role of brachytherapy for pediatric brain tumors. Pediatr Neurosurg 16:213–218, 1991.
17. Mohadjer M, Etou A, Milios E, et al: Chiasmatic optic glioma. Neurochirurgia (Stuttg) 34:90–93, 1991.
18. Kretschmar CS, Linggood RM: Chemotherapeutic treatment of extensive optic pathway tumors in infants. J Neurooncol 10:263–270, 1991.
19. Petronio J, Edwards MS, Prados M, et al: Management of chiasmal and hypothalamic gliomas of infancy and childhood with chemotherapy. J Neurosurg 74:701–708, 1991.
20. Packer RJ, Sutton LN, Bilaniuk LT, et al: Treatment of chiasmatic/hypothalamic gliomas of childhood with chemotherapy. Ann Neurol 23:79–85, 1988.
21. Shuper A, Horev G, Kornreich L: Visual pathway glioma: An erratic tumour with therapeutic dilemmas. Arch Dis Child 76:259–263, 1997.
22. Garvey M, Packer R: An integrated approach to the treatment of chiasmatic-hypothalamic gliomas. J Neurooncol 28:167–183, 1996.
23. Sutton LN, Molloy PT, Sernyak H: Long-term outcome of hypothalamic/chiasmatic astrocytomas in children treated with conservative surgery. J Neurosurg 83:583–589, 1995.
24. Chamberlain MC: Recurrent chiasmatic-hypothalamic glioma treated with oral etoposide. Arch Neurol 52:509–513, 1995.
25. Janss AJ, Grundy R, Cnaan A, et al: Optic pathway and hupothalamic/chiasmatic gliomas in children younger than age 5 years with 6 years follow-up. Cancer 75:1051–1059, 1995.
26. Nishio S, Morioka T, Takeshita I, et al: Chemotherapy for progresive pilocytic astrocytomas in the chiasmo-hypothalamic regions. Clin Neurol Neurosurg 97:300–306, 1995.
27. Symon L, Pell MF, Habib AH: Radical excision of craniopharyngioma by the temporal route: A review of 50 patients. Br J Neurosurg 5:539–549, 1991.
28. Gillett GR, Symon L: Hypothalamic glioma. Surg Neurol 28:291–300, 1987.
29. Apuzzo ML, Levy ML, Tung H: Surgical strategies and technical methodologies in optimal management of craniopharyngioma and masses affecting the third ventricular chamber. Acta Neurochir Suppl (Wien) 53:77–88, 1991.
30. Koos WT, Perraczky A, Horaczek A: Problems of surgical technique for the treatment of supratentorial midline tumors in children. Acta Neurochir Suppl (Wien) 35:31–41, 1985.
31. Gower DJ, Pollay M, Shuman RM, Brumback RA: Cystic optic glioma. Neurosurgery 26:133–136, 1990.
32. Carmel PW: Tumors of the III ventricle. Acta Neurochir (Wien) 75:136–146, 1985.
33. Stein BM: Third ventricle tumors. Clin Neurosurg 17:315–331, 1985.
34. Albright AL, Sclabassi RJ: Cavitron ultrasonic surgical aspiration and visual evoked potential monitoring for chiasmal gliomas in children. J Neurosurg 63:138–140, 1985.
35. Schuster H, Koos WT, Zaunbauer F: Results of microsurgical treatment of gliomas of the optic system and hypothalamus in children. Mod Probl Pediatr 18:211–215, 1977.
36. Maspes P, Geuna E: Resultats du traitement chirurgical de 182 cas de tumeurs du III ventricule. Neurochirurgie 12:633–636, 1966.
37. Pecker J, Faivre J, Guy G: Indications chirurgicales dans les tumeur du plancher du III ventricule. Neurochirurgie 12:653–660, 1966.
38. Medlock MD, Scott RM: Optic chiasm astrocytomas of childhood. Pediatr Neurosurg 27:129–136, 1997.
39. Konovalov AN, Gorelyshev SK, Serova NK: Surgery of guant gliomas of chiasm and III ventricle. Acta Neurochir (Wien) 130:71–79, 1994.
40. Konovalov AN, Gorelyshev SK: Surgical treatment of anterior third ventricle tumours. Acta Neurochir (Wien) 118:33–39, 1992.
41. Alshail E, Rutka GT, Becker LE, Hoffman HJ: Optic chiasmatic-hypothalamic glioma. Brain Pathol 7:799–806, 1997.
42. Rutka JT, Hoffman HJ, Drrake JM, Humphreys RP: Suprasellar and sellar tumors in children and adolescence. Neurosurg Clin N Am 3:803–820, 1992.
43. Hoffman HJ, Humphreys RP, Drake JM, et al: Optic pathway/hypothalamic gliomas: A dilemma in management. Pediatr Neurosurg 19:186–195, 1993.
44. Wisoff JH: Management of optic pathway tumors of childhood. Neurosurg Clin N Am 3:791–802, 1992.
45. Valdueza JM, Lohmann F, Dammann O, et al: Analysis of 20 primarily surgically treated chiasmatic/hypothalamic pilocytic astrocytomas. Acta Neurochirr (Wien) 126:44–50, 1994.
46. Erkal HS, Serin M, Cakmak A: Management of optic pathway and chiasmatic-hypothalamic gliomas in children with radiation therapy. Radiother Oncol 45:11–15, 1997.
47. Nishio S, Takeshita I, Fujiwara S, et al: Optico-hypothalamic glioma: An analysis of 16 cases. Child's Nervous System 9:334–338, 1993.
48. Rodriguez LA, Edwards MS, Levin VA: Management of hypothalamic gliomas in children: An analysis of 33 cases. Neurosurgery 26:242–246, 1990.
49. Lapras C: Presented at the 9th European Congress of Neurosurgery, Moscow, 1991.

50. Long DM, Chou SN, Shelley N: Transcallosal removal of the craniopharingiomas within the III ventricle. J Neurosurg 39:563–567, 1973.
51. Stein BM: Transcallosal approach to third ventricle tumors. In Schmidek HH, Sweet WH: Operative Neurosurgical Techniques. New York: Grune & Stratton, 1982.
52. Albright AL, Sclabassi RJ: Use of the Cavitron ultrasonic surgical aspirator and evoked potentials for the treatment of thalamic and brain stem tumors in children. Neurosurgery 17:564–568, 1985.
53. Drake JM, Joy M, Goldenberg A, Kreindler D: Computer- and robot-assisted resection of thalamic astrocytomas in children. Neurosurgery 29:27–33, 1991.
54. Hoffman HJ, Soloniuk DS, Humphreys RP, et al: Management and outcome of low-grade astrocytomas of the midline in children: A retrospective review. Neurosurgery 33:964–971, 1993.
55. Villarejo-F, Amaya-C, Perez-Diaz-C: Radical surgery of thalamic tumors in children. Child's Nerv Syst 10:111–114, 1994.
56. Kelly PJ: Stereotactic biopsy and resection of thalamic astrocytomas. Neurosurgery 25:185–195, 1989.
57. Pool JL: Gliomas in the region of the brain stem. J Neurosurg 29:164–167, 1968.
58. Stroink AR, Hoffman HJ, Hendric EB, et al: Diagnosis and management of pediatric brain stem gliomas. J Neurosurg 65:745–750, 1986.
59. Epstein F, McCleary EL: Intrinsic brain stem tumors in childhood: Surgical indications. J Neurosurg 64:11–15, 1986.
60. Konovalov AN, Atieh J: The surgical treatment of primary brain stem tumors. In Schmidek HH, Sweet WH (eds): Operative Neurosurgical Techniques, 2nd ed. New York: Grune & Stratton, 1988, pp 709–737.
61. Heffez DS, Zinreich SJ, Long DM: Surgical resection of intrinsic brain stem lesions: An overview. Neurosurgery 27:789–798, 1990.
62. Pendl G, Vorcapic P: Microsurgery of intrinsic midbrain lesions. Acta Neurochirurg Suppl (Wien) 53:137–143, 1991.
63. Bricollo A, Turrazzi S, Cristofori I, et al: Direct surgery for brain stem tumours. Acta Neurochirurg Suppl (Wien) 53:148–158, 1991.
64. Vandertop WP, Hoffman HJ, Drake JM, et al: Focal midbrain tumors in children. Neurosurgery 31:186–194, 1992.
65. Behnke J, Christen HJ, Bruck W, et al: Intra-axial endophytic tumors in the pons and/or medulla oblongata. II: Intraoperative findings, postoperative results, and 2-year follow-up in 25 children. Child's Nerv Syst 13:122–134, 1997.
66. Abbott R, Shiminski-Maher T, Epstein FJ: Intrinsic tumors of the medulla: Predicting outcome after surgery. Pediatr Neurosurg 25:41–44, 1996.
67. Xu QW, Bao WM, Mao RI, et al: Surgical treatment of solid brain stem tumors in adults: A report of 22 cases. Surg Neurol 48:30–36, 1997.
68. Freeman CR, Farmer JP: Pediatric brain stem gliomas: A review. Int J Radiat Oncol Biol Phys 40:265–271, 1998.
69. Constantini S, Epstein F: Surgical indication and technical considerations in the management of benign brain stem gliomas. Neuro oncol 28:193–205, 1996.
70. Zimmerman RA: Neuroimaging of primary brain stem gliomas: Diagnosis and course. Pediatr Neurosurg 25:45–53, 1996.
71. Fischbein NJ, Prados MD, Wara W: Radiologic classification of brain stem tumors: Correlation of magnetic resonance imaging appearance with clinical outcome. Pediatr Neurosurg 24:9–23, 1996.
72. Morota N, Deletis V, Epstein F, et al: Brain stem mapping: Neurophysiological localization of motor nuclei on the floor of the fourth ventricle. Neurosurgery 37:922–930, 1995.
73. Strauss C, Romstock J, Nimsky C: Intraoperative identification of motor areas of the rhomboid fossa using direct stimulation. J Neurosurg 79:393–399, 1993.
74. Hoffman HJ: Dorsally exophytic brain stem tumors and midbrain tumors. Pediatr Neurosurg 24:256–262, 1996.
75. Pollack IF, Hoffman HJ, Hemphreys RP, et al: The long-term outcome after surgical treatment of dorsally exophytic brain stem gliomas. J Neurosurg 78:859–863, 1993.
76. Squires LA, Constantini S, Epstein F: Diffuse infiltrating astrocytoma of the cervicomedullary region: Clinicopathological entity. Pediatr Neurosurg 27:153–159, 1997.

# Approaches to Lateral and Third Ventricular Tumors

■ JOHN STRUGAR and JOSEPH PIEPMEIER

Tumors of the lateral and third ventricles tend to grow slowly and are often benign; thus, by the time that they present to the surgeon, most have reached a significant size. There are multiple surgical approaches to these tumors, but all attempt to utilize the pathways around the brain that least disturb and minimally displace normal anatomy. Before embarking on an approach, the surgeon should be familiar with both the ventricular anatomy and also the types and behavior of the lesions of the lateral and third ventricles. Some lesions, such as subependymal giant cell astrocytomas or nonobstructive colloid cysts, can be managed by close observation; others, such as sarcoid and germinomas, can be treated nonsurgically after a biopsy. Others, like teratomas and meningiomas, are best managed by complete resection. In this chapter we present an overview of the lateral and third ventricular anatomy, the radiologic appearance of the lesions presenting in these spaces, and the surgical approaches to these lesions.

## GENERAL ANATOMY

The lateral and third ventricles are divided into specific areas that help define both the pathology as well as the surgical approaches. Specific types of tumors tend to occur regularly in specific anatomic areas of the third and lateral ventricles, and an understanding of basic epidemiology will assist with the differential diagnosis.

### Lateral Ventricular Anatomy

The lateral ventricles are C-shaped cerebrospinal fluid (CSF)–filled cavities that can be divided into five areas: (1) the frontal horns, (2) the bodies, (3) the atriums, (4) the occipital horns, and (5) the temporal horns. The *frontal horns* are triangular extensions of the lateral ventricles anterior to the foramen of Monro and are bounded laterally by the head of the caudate, anteriorly and superiorly by the corpus callosum, and medially by the septum pellucidum. Posteromedially, the foramen of Monro marks the posterior extent of the frontal horns, and the boundary consists of

the forniceal columns that run just anterior to the foramen of Monro as they bend inferiorly to start their descent toward the mamillary bodies. The floor consists of the rostrum of the corpus callosum as it curves underneath the frontal horn. The frontal horn contains no choroid plexus but has on its wall surface two important veins that help with the surgical orientation. On its inferomedial border, the anteroseptal vein leads into the medial foramen of Monro, where it enters the velum interpositum in the roof of the third ventricle to join the internal cerebral vein (ICV). Laterally, the anterior caudate vein runs medioinferiorly to join the thalamostriate vein near the foramen of Monro.

*The body* of the lateral ventricles begins at the posterior edge of the foramen of Monro and extends posteriorly to the anterior border of the splenium of the corpus callosum, an area where the septum pellucidum tapers off. The body of the ventricle is covered superiorly by the corpus callosum, whereas the lateral wall consists of the body of the caudate. At the level of the foramen of Monro, just inferior to the caudate eminence in the lateral wall of the ventricle, the genu of the internal capsule can be found. There are two sets of veins that travel on the lateral wall of the body: the more anterior thalamocaudate (the size of which is inversely proportional to the thalamostriate vein) and the posterior caudate vein, which drains into the thalamostriate. Inferiorly, the junction of the lateral wall and floor of the body of the ventricle is demarcated by the striothalamic sulcus, which separates the caudate from the thalamus. In this sulcus one finds the thalamostriate vein coursing anteriorly to the foramen of Monro. The vein generally curves around the foramen of Monro to drain into the ICVs. The curve of this vein can often be seen on cerebral angiography and is called the venous angle. One should note that occasionally this vein drains more posteriorly through the choroidal fissure directly into the ICV without going through the foramen of Monro. Medial to this vein, the thalamus protrudes to make up the ventricular floor. Medial to the thalamus, separating the thalamus from the body of the fornix, lies the choroidal fissure. This fissure is obscured by the choroid plexus, in which the superior choroidal vein, which starts posteriorly in the atrium and may anastomose with the inferior choroidal vein, flows toward the foramen of Monro. The medial posterior choroidal artery, which enters the ventricular system just lateral to the pineal and travels anteriorly in the roof of the third ventricle in the velum interpositum, can be seen in the lateral ventricle as it ascends through the foramen of Monro and bends posteriorly to run in the direction of the choroid plexus. Coming from the atrial side of the ventricle, the lateral posterior choroidal artery courses anteriorly toward the foramen of Monro and may anastomose with the medial posterior choroidal artery. Medially, the two leaves of the septum pellucidum separate the two ventricles. On their surface one can see the posterior septal veins, which run inferiorly, pierce the choroid fissure, and drain into the ICVs.

The *trigone* or *atrium* of the lateral ventricles is a confluence of the body, temporal and occipital horns. The atrium begins as a continuation of the body at the posterior edge of the thalamus and ends further posteriorly as the bulb of the corpus callosum blends into the occipital lobe. The splenium (superiorly) and the tapetum of the corpus callosum (more posteriorly) make up the roof of the atrium. Because the roof bends into the lateral wall posteriorly, the tapetum covers this lateral wall segment. More anteriorly, the caudate tail covers the lateral wall as it curves downward, on its way toward the temporal lobe. On the surface of the lateral wall, just below the ependyma, the lateral atrial veins can be seen running inferiorly and medially toward the choroid fissure. This vein starts posteriorly in the occipital horn and empties, once through the choroidal fissure, in the basal vein, ICV, or great vein of Galen. The anterior boundary of the atrium starts just medial to the caudate tail with the pulvinar eminence. Medial to the pulvinar, covered by choroid, is the crus of the fornix. At the atrial level of the choroid plexus, two choroidal arteries can often be seen, one curving with the choroid medially, the anterior choroidal artery, which can course into the body of the ventricle. More laterally, the lateral posterior choroidal artery, which may have several branches, runs to supply the atrium and body of the choroid. The choroid plexus itself forms a triangular enlargement at the trigone called the glomus of the choroid plexus. The medial wall of the atrium has two prominences. The upper prominence consists of the forceps major fibers and is called the bulb of the corpus callosum. The lower prominence is called the calcar avis and is simply the ventricular protrusion of the calcarine sulcus. The floor similarly consists of the upward protrusion of the collateral sulcus forming the collateral trigone. On the surface of the medial wall, the medial atrial vein can be seen coursing toward the choroid fissure to pierce it and drain into the great vein of Galen, basal vein, or ICV.

The *occipital horn* is a posterior extension of the atrium and can vary in size. Medially, the wall consists of the same structures that make up the atrial medial wall, namely, the forceps major superior, and inferiorly, the calcar avis. Likewise, the collateral trigone forms the floor of the occipital horn. The roof and lateral wall blend into one and are both covered by the tapetum. There is no choroid in the occipital horn. The veins of the occipital horn are the posterior extension of the lateral and medial atrial veins.

The *temporal horn* is an extension of the lateral ventricles into the medial temporal lobe. The floor displays two prominences: (1) laterally the collateral eminence formed by the underlying deep collateral sulcus, and (2) medial to that, the hippocampus, which protrudes prominently into the floor. Seen running longitudinally over the hippocampal surface are a set of veins called the transverse hippocampal veins. These veins penetrate through the space between the fimbria and hippocampus into the ambient cistern, where they drain into the anterior and posterior hippocampal veins. The latter drain into the basal vein. The lateral wall, which angles into the roof of the temporal horn, is lined by the tapetum. In the medial part of the roof, the tail of the caudate projects anteriorly toward the amygdaloid nucleus. In this area, on the ventricular surface, the inferior ventricular vein runs in an anteromedial direction to exit through the choroid fissure at the level of the so-called "inferior choroidal point" and drain into the basal vein near the lateral geniculate body. Medial to the caudate tail, forming the medial wall of the temporal horn, is the thalamus, and inferior to it, the fimbria of the fornix. The choroid fissure separates the thalamus from the fornix. The choroid plexus is attached as it continues anteriorly to end just posterior to the amygdaloid nucleus at the "inferior choroidal point." The anterior choroidal artery enters the choroidal fissure at about this point and courses posteriorly in the plexus. More posteriorly, the lateral posterior choroidal artery enters the fissure and is seen more laterally in the choroid plexus. Starting at about the level of the atrium and draining anteriorly toward the "inferior choroidal point," the inferior choroidal vein is seen on the surface of the choroidal fissure. It drains into the basal vein. The temporal horn ends blindly anteriorly in the amygdaloid nucleus, on the surface of which can be seen the amygdalar vein, which drains into the inferior ventricular vein.[1–4]

## Third Ventricular Anatomy

The third ventricle communicates with the lateral ventricles via the foramen of Monro and drains posteriorly into the aqueduct of Sylvius. About one third of the third ventricle is located anterior to the foramen of Monro and extends inferiorly to the optic chiasm. The anterior wall consists mainly of the lamina terminalis, which is a thin sheet of pia and gray matter that runs between the optic chiasm inferiorly to the rostrum of the corpus callosum superiorly. The columns of the fornix are found at the superior lateral margins, and the anterior commissure crosses the anterior wall at its upper end. The lateral wall of the third ventricle is formed inferiorly by the hypothalamus and superiorly and posteriorly by the thalamus. The separation between these two structures can sometimes be noted on the lateral wall by the hypothalamic sulcus, which runs between the foramen of Monro and the aqueduct of Sylvius. At the upper and posterior end of the third ventricle, a thalamic projection, the massa intermedia often connects (in 75% of cases) with its counterpart on the other side. The floor of the third ventricle starts anteriorly and inferiorly at the optic chiasm; progressing posteriorly, the floor dips into the infundibular recess. The floor slants superiorly and posteriorly over the tuber cinereum then the two mamillary bodies and posterior perforated substance, which is located anterior to the cerebral peduncles. Posterior to the level of the peduncles is the aqueduct, which is surrounded by the tegmentum of the midbrain. The roof of the third ventricle starts anteriorly at the foramen of Monro and ends posteriorly in the suprapineal recess. The roof is separated from the lateral wall by the choroidal fissure, which runs in the cleft between the upper part of the thalamus and the fornix. Over the anterior part of the roof, the fornices run in parallel and are often attached into the body of the fornix, whereas over the posterior roof, the fornices separate into the forniceal crura, and the roof is draped by interforniceal-connecting white matter called the hippocampal commissure. However, the fornices and hippocampal commissure in the roof of the third ventricle are covered by a loose trabecular pial tissue that forms a double layer called the tela choroidea. In between these two layers of tela choroidea is a space, the velum interpositum, through which the ICVs and the medioposterior choroidal arteries course. The internal cerebral veins start at the posterior edge of the foramen of Monro and run posteriorly to exit the velum interpositum just above the pineal body. The third ventricular choroid plexus is attached to the roof by the tela choroidea, which communicates through the choroidal fissure with the lateral ventricular tela choroidea. The posterior wall of the third ventricle begins at the aqueduct of Sylvius anteriorly and inferiorly. Proceeding in a posterior and superior direction, the posterior wall of the third ventricle contains the posterior commissure, the pineal body, the habenular commissure, and the suprapineal recess above.[5–7]

## CLINICAL PRESENTATION

### Lateral Ventricular Tumors

Tumors of the lateral ventricles tend to present with similar symptoms. The clinical presentation depends more on location and less on individual pathology. Eighty-five percent of lateral ventricular tumors grow slowly; as a result, most symptoms present insidiously and are of long-term duration. Most of these patients present with hydrocephalus, which is often obstructive and unilateral. Headaches (which can be unilateral), gait disturbance, and cognitive changes are the hallmarks of hydrocephalus. The cognitive changes are related to the side of the obstruction; however, generally, in classic hydrocephalus, there is a split in the verbal intelligence quotient (IQ) compared with the performance IQ, with a comparative drop in the performance IQ when compared with the verbal IQ. Infiltrative lesions, such as astrocytomas, can cause more pronounced symptoms related to the site of invasion of surrounding brain. Frontal horn lesions tend to present with headaches and changes in personality. Lesions arising from the thalamus tend to present with hemiparesis and, paradoxically to a much lesser extent, sensory deficits. Lesions in the atrium and occipital horn are susceptible to visual deficits.[8–11]

### Third Ventricular Tumors

Symptoms tend to depend on whether the tumor presents in the anterior or posterior part of the third ventricle. Most of the lesions within the third ventricle grow slowly, and thus symptoms tend to be insidious. Almost all lesions tend to present with hydrocephalus; the posterior third ventricular lesions tend to present earlier in their course. Tumors exerting pressure on the posterior third ventricle, either by tumor itself or secondary to the hydrocephalus, can present with upgaze paralysis, mydriasis, and retraction nystagmus on attempted upgaze (Parinaud's syndrome). Lesions of the anterior third ventricle can present with endocrine abnormalities, particularly diabetes insipidus, and a decrease in growth hormone levels, although these hormonal manifestations present late in the disease. In children, hypothalamic gliomas have presented with a syndrome of emaciation combined with hyperalertness, which has been called the *diencephalic syndrome*. Visual symptoms are not a hallmark of anterior third ventricular tumors; when present, these symptoms indicate the presence of an optic pathway tumor. Behavioral changes are, however, commonly seen in tumors affecting this area and can include apathy and loss of recent memory.[12–16]

## PATHOLOGY AND RADIOLOGY

### Pathology of Lateral Ventricular Tumors

The tumors found in the lateral ventricles are varied in their pathology and arise from cellular elements found within and around the ventricular walls. There is an age- and location-dependent presentation of most tumor types which, in conjunction with adequate radiologic studies, help in the preoperative differential diagnosis. For instance, meningiomas can occur generally in adults and in the trigone of the ventricle, whereas primitive neuroectodermal tumors (PNETs) tend to present in children and in the frontal horns.

Most (85%) lateral ventricular tumors are low-grade, slow-growing tumors. These include low-grade gliomas, which make up 50% of lateral ventricular tumors, and choroid plexus papillomas and meningiomas, which together account for an additional 35%. Neurocytomas, congenital tumors (teratomas and ependymomas), and metastases each account for about 5% of lateral ventricular tumors. Recent use of immunohistochemistry has helped to identify neurocytomas that exhibit positive staining with synaptophysin. It is likely that neurocytomas are more common than was previously recognized. The location of tumor presentation helps to define the pathology. Most of the tumors arise in the trigone; an estimated 50% of all lateral ventricular tumors arise here. The most common tumors of the trigone in adults are meningiomas, followed by choroid plexus papillomas; however, all the pathologic types can be seen in this location (Fig. 59–1). The second most common site in lateral ventricular tumors is found in the body of the lateral ventricle, accounting for 35% of all ventricular tumors. The gliomas and neurocytomas are more common, but meningiomas are occasionally found in this location. The frontal horns account for 10% of ventricular tumors, and here the gliomas predominate. The temporal horn is the least common lateral ventricular site; only

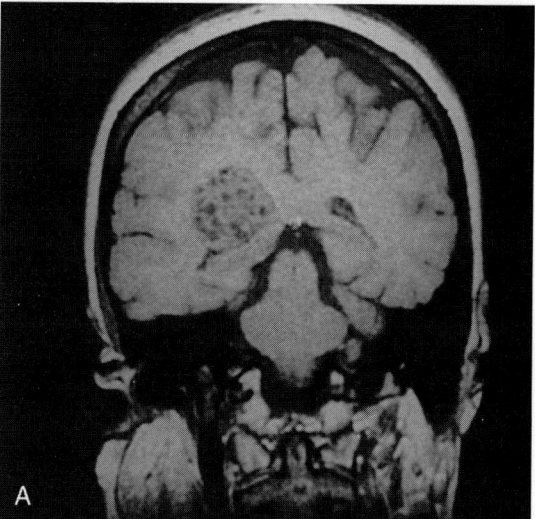

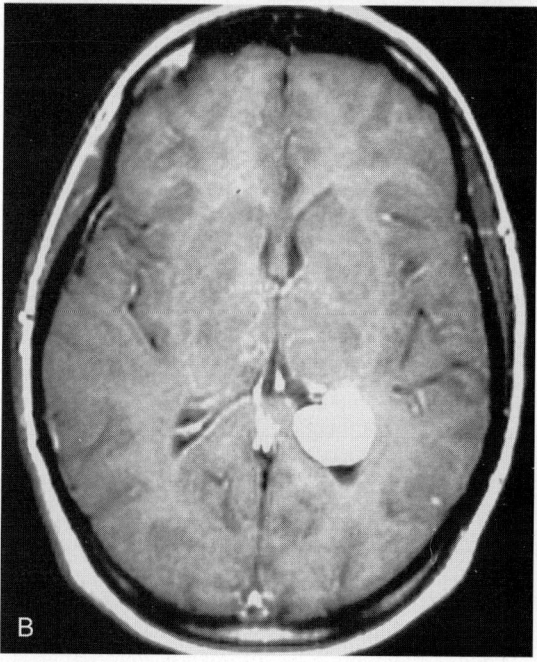

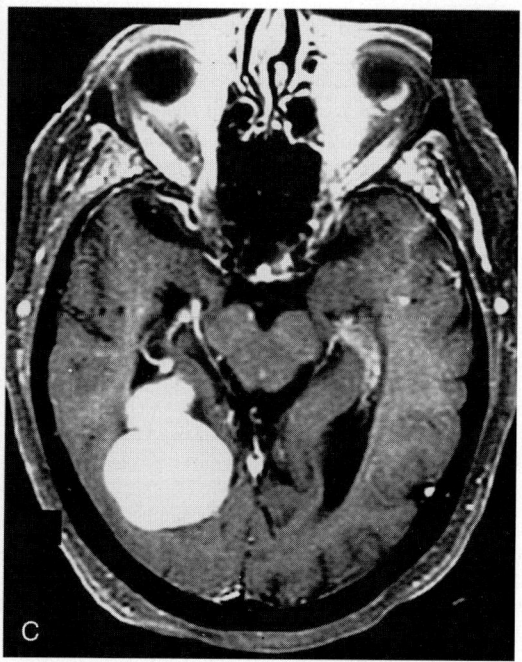

**FIGURE 59–1** ■ Meningiomas presenting in the trigone of the lateral ventricle. Intraventricular meningiomas are found most commonly at this site. *A,* A coronal $T_1$-weighted image reveals an isointense well-demarcated mass with areas of calcifications. Most meningiomas (60%) are isointense on $T_1$-weighted images, whereas a hypointense signal is seen in most of the rest. *B,* After injection of gadolinium contrast, the tumor exhibits intense enhancement. Note the absence of hydrocephalus, the symptoms of which usually bring patients with ventricular tumors to medical attention. This patient presented incidentally. *C,* A $T_1$-weighted contrast-enhancing trigone meningioma extends into the temporal horn in a patient who exhibits hydrocephalus.

5% of the tumors arise at this site. Meningiomas and ependymomas predominate in the temporal horn.[17, 18]

*Gliomas* as a group comprise 50% of lateral ventricular tumors. These lesions arise from surrounding ependymal and subependymal tissues and expand into the low-resistance ventricle. Astrocytomas can arise anywhere along the ventricular wall; tumors that originate from thalamic tissue tend to expand mainly within the ventricle. These tumors appear on a computed tomography (CT) scan as large well-circumscribed lesions of lower density with variable contrast enhancement. There can be minimal surrounding edema and for the size of the tumors, minimal parenchymal displacement. A magnetic resonance imaging (MRI) scan is beneficial to establish the diagnosis. Low-grade astrocytomas have low signal intensity on $T_1$ images, whereas on $T_2$-weighted images, these tumors have a high signal. The less common higher-grade astrocytomas will exhibit areas of both increased and decreased signal intensity within the tumors, and in the case of glioblastomas, areas of necrosis,

pronounced enhancement, and peritumoral edema. The treatment for these tumors is biopsy, followed by radiation therapy for the high-grade lesions (Fig. 59–2).[8, 17, 18]

*The subependymal giant cell astrocytoma* is a variant of astrocytomas found in patients with tuberous sclerosis. These tumors are low grade and slow growing and can be found anywhere along the ventricular system, although they tend to prefer the area around the foramen of Monro. The diagnosis is made along with the other stigmata of this phakomatosis. On a CT scan, these lesions appear hyperintense with areas of calcification. They also enhance more briskly than the standard low-grade astrocytomas. These tumors can be followed with serial scans, and unless there is evidence of malignant transformation (a rare occurrence) or obstructive hydrocephalus, they are left alone.[19]

*Ependymomas* may arise anywhere in the ventricular system but are usually found in the area of the trigone. They are less common than the low-grade astrocytomas; however, like them, they tend to grow slowly and often

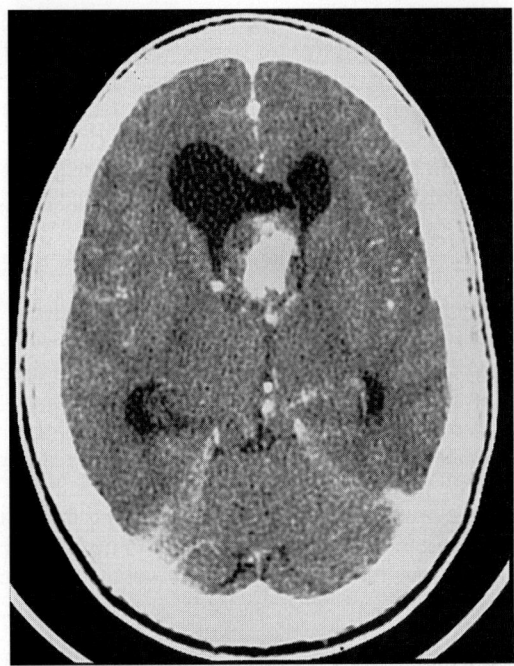

FIGURE 59–2 ■ Mixed glioma arising in the area of the foramen of Monro and extending into both lateral ventricles. Gliomas comprise half of the lateral ventricular masses, most of which are astrocytomas. This contrast computed tomography (CT) scan image shows an isodense tumor with a small amount of enhancement and a large calcified central area. Most astrocytomas are isodense on a CT scan with variable enhancement pattern, but calcifications are rare.

include a large intraventricular component. On a CT scan, they are isodense to the surrounding brain and enhance more prominently than the low-grade astrocytomas. Calcification can be seen in 50%. On an MRI scan, the $T_1$-weighted images are heterogeneous and either isodense or hypodense to surrounding brain, whereas the $T_2$-weighted images are hyperintense. Surgical resection is the treatment of choice. Intraventricular seeding and local regrowth is common with these lesions.[12, 20]

*Subependymomas* are rare tumors with a nodular appearance that arise anywhere within the ventricular system but seem to favor the frontal horns and body of the lateral ventricles. On a CT scan, other than their nodular appearance, they are hypodense compared with surrounding tissues; they are not generally calcified; and they have homogeneous minimal enhancement. MRI $T_1$-weighted images exhibit hypointense or isointense characteristics. The $T_2$-weighted images show a hypointense signal that may be heterogeneous. These tumors grow slowly, and surgical resection for these tumors is rarely needed unless they exhibit significant growth or an obstruction to CSF flow (Fig. 59–3).[21]

*Oligodendrogliomas* often present as mixed astrocytic tumors; they are generally low grade; and they include a parenchymal component in addition to their intraventricular extension. Their preferred site appears to be within the body of the ventricle. On a CT scan, these tumors are hypointense, with occasional calcifications and heterogeneous enhancement. An MRI scan reveals $T_1$-weighted images that are hypointense, whereas the $T_2$-weighted images tend to be heterogeneously hyperintense. These le-

sions are treated with resection, with a long-term prognosis favored by good resection, assuming that the pathology exhibits few astrocytic components and no anaplasia.[22–24]

*Neurocytomas* are rare tumors of neuronal origin that tend to be found at the inferior septum pellucidum near the foramen of Monro. Previously, they were often mistaken for oligodendrogliomas, but in the last two decades these tumors have been better identified by the use of immunohistochemistry. They tend to occur in the second to fourth decade of life; they are slow growing and benign and appear to be well demarcated within the ventricle. On a CT scan, as well as $T_1$- and $T_2$-weighted MRI scans, the tumor is heterogeneously isointense or slightly hyperintense with a lobulated appearance and possible cysts. Calcification can be present, and enhancement is heterogeneous. The treatment for these tumors is surgical excision. It appears that regrowth is slow in subtotal resections (Fig. 59–4).[25, 26]

*Choroid plexus papillomas* are the most common lateral ventricular tumors in children and are infrequent in adults. Their preferred site is the atrium. Most are benign, although a few can undergo carcinomatous changes. On a CT scan, these tumors appear frond-like and isodense to the brain with areas of calcification. On MRI $T_1$-weighted images, the density is isointense with the brain but enhances dramatically with contrast. The treatment is surgical. Rarely, choroid plexus carcinomas are malignant; they disseminate through the CSF spaces and invade the surrounding parenchyma. In these cases, neuraxis radiation is recommended.[27–29]

*Meningiomas* comprise 15% of all lateral ventricular tumors and tend to present in the atrium in the fourth to fifth decade of life. A CT scan shows an isodense well-circumscribed tumor, which may be calcified and enhances brightly. An MRI scan is isointense on $T_1$- and $T_2$-weighted images. These tumors are treated surgically, and complete resection is the goal.[30–32]

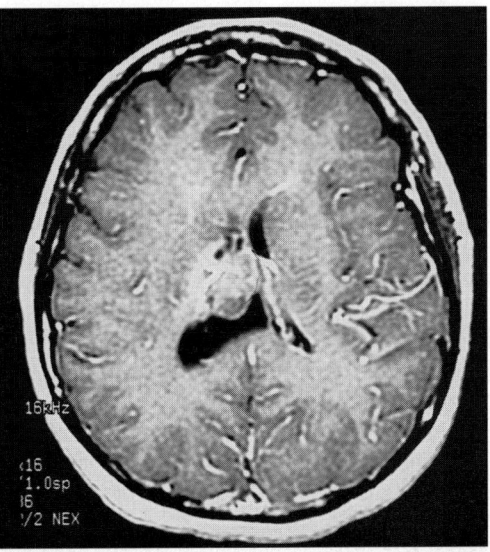

FIGURE 59–3 ■ Subependymoma presenting in the lateral ventricle with unilateral obstruction of cerebrospinal fluid pathways. On this $T_1$-weighted contrast image, the tumor appears as a lobulated, fairly well-demarcated isointense mass with moderate enhancement, which is fairly typical for this type of tumor.

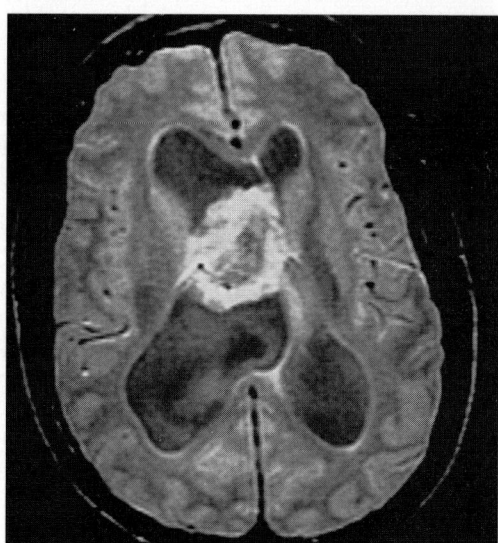

**FIGURE 59–4** ■ Neurocytoma of the lateral ventricle with obstructive hydrocephalus. This magnetic resonance imaging (MRI) scan exhibits fairly classic characteristics for this tumor. The lesion presents in the body of the lateral ventricle, with attachment to the lateral wall and bowing of the septum pellucidum contralaterally, hydrocephalus, and a small area of calcification. Heterogeneous signal intensity is caused by areas of calcification and cystic changes in the tumor. Note the vascular flow voids, another characteristic seen in these tumors.

## Third Ventricular Tumors

Tumors involving the third ventricle can arise primarily within the ventricle or outside with extension into the third ventricle, such as suprasellar tumors and pineal neoplasms. This division can be somewhat artificial, because some tumors that originate outside the third ventricle can be largely intraventricular on presentation. Like the lateral ventricular tumors, most of these lesions are low grade.

The most common primary intraventricular tumor in adults is the *colloid cyst*, which constitutes 20% of intraventricular lesions. These cysts present in mid-adulthood with obstructive hydrocephalus. Colloid cysts are believed to be congenital. They are located in the anterior roof of the third ventricle at the level of the foramen of Monro; they are filled with a dense hyaline substance; and they expand slowly. On a CT scan, the cyst appears as a round homogeneous hyperdense mass at the level of the foramen of Monro, without enhancement. An MRI scan reveals a hyperintense $T_1$-weighted image, with a variable (hypointense or hyperintense) signal on the $T_2$-weighted images. The variability depends on whether the cyst contains high-protein (hyperintense $T_2$) or high-cholesterol (hypointense $T_2$) content. Once symptomatic, these lesions are resected (Fig. 59–5).[33–36]

*Astrocytomas* are the next most common tumors to present inside the third ventricle, and their original site of origin is important in predicting the behavior of the tumor and the prognosis. In the anterior third ventricle, the most common type of astrocytoma is the juvenile pilocytic variant, which generally arises from the anterior floor or optic pathways. These tumors grow slowly; they present in childhood with hydrocephalus and behavioral changes; at a late stage in the disease, visual and endocrine abnormalities occur. Chiasmatic astrocytomas are generally low grade. In one third of cases, they are associated with neurofibromatosis type I. Astrocytomas must be differentiated from optic nerve gliomas, which tend to be more aggressive. Astrocytomas account for 25% of all posterior third ventricular tumors, and they are seen more frequently in the adult population. On a CT scan, these tumors appear hypodense or isodense and variably enhance. An MRI scan shows a $T_1$-weighted isointense or hypointense signal, whereas $T_2$-weighted images tend to be hyperintense. These tumors, although mainly benign, are not resectable, and debulking has to be outweighed against possible morbidity of surgery. A more aggressive surgical role is generally employed for the posterior third ventricular astrocytomas than for the anterior third ventricular astrocytomas. A variant, the subependymal giant cell astrocytomas, is seen in patients with tuberous sclerosis and is again, benign. These tumors have a predilection for the area around the foramen of Monro, and they occasionally grow into the third ventricle and obstruct the CSF pathway, necessitating surgery. Otherwise these giant cell astrocytomas are followed with serial scans and neuropsychological testing.[37–42]

*Germinomas* are rare tumors comprising about 1% of all intracranial tumors; however, they tend to be found in one of two places: pineal (80%) and suprasellar (20%) regions. These tumors present in childhood and have a 9:1 male:female predilection. The presenting symptoms depend on the site of growth and can include Parinaud's syndrome and precocious puberty. Subarachnoid and spinal seeding of the tumor is possible. On a CT scan, these lesions appear hyperdense, with homogeneous enhancement. MRI scans show isodense intensity on both $T_1$- and $T_2$-weighted images. These tumors are very radiosensitive, and complete surgical resection is not necessary if doing so increases morbidity. Total neuraxis radiation therapy is generally recommended in the postoperative management of germinomas.[43–47]

*Teratomas* are rare tumors that generally present in the posterior part of the third ventricle; they are usually well differentiated and do not infiltrate into surrounding tissues. The pineal region is the most common site of presentation of teratomas. Patients are boys or young men; they present with obstructive hydrocephalus or Perinaud's syndrome. A CT scan shows a heterogeneous mass with areas of fat, bone, and other soft tissue. There are various areas of enhancement. An MRI scan similarly exhibits a mixed signal on both $T_1$- and $T_2$-weighted images, reflecting the presence of tissue from all three germinal layers. In benign teratomas, surgery is the treatment of choice, because resection can be curative, whereas radiation therapy is generally not effective.[45, 48, 49]

Other *germ cell tumors* are rare and include choriocarcinoma, endodermal sinus tumor, embryonal cell carcinoma, and teratocarcinoma. These tumors exhibit markers in the CSF, and these markers can help with the diagnosis. Choriocarcinoma produces β-human chorionic gonadotropin (β-hCG); embryonal cell carcinoma produces α-fetoprotein and β-hCG; whereas an endodermal sinus tumor produces α-fetoprotein alone. These tumors occur in the first two decades of life and affect males. On MRI and CT scans, these tumors exhibit heterogeneous signals, as does the pattern of enhancement. Unlike most of the other third

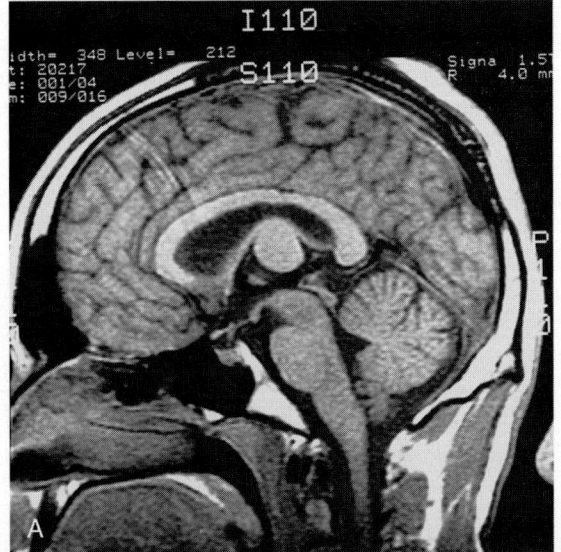

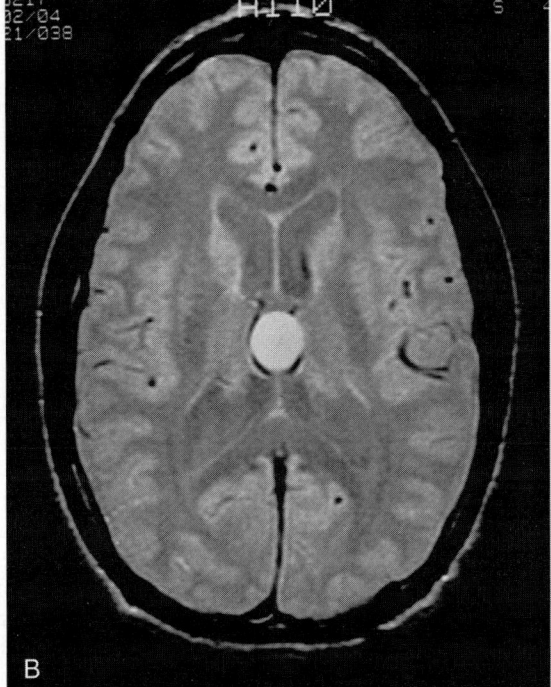

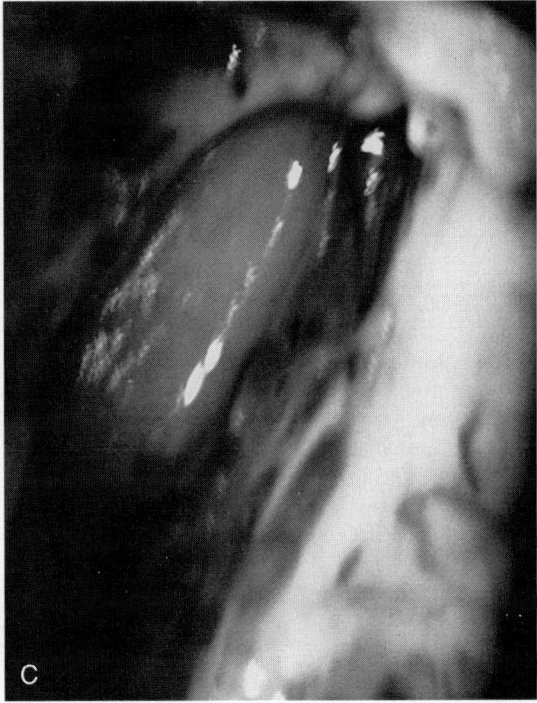

**FIGURE 59–5** ■ Third ventricular colloid (neuroepithelial) cyst. The colloid cysts make up 20% of all intraventricular tumors and are the most common type of third ventricular tumor. These lesions are most frequently found in the roof of the third ventricle near the foramen of Monro. *A*, Sagittal $T_1$-weighted image reveals the location of the tumor and its attachment to the third ventricular roof. These lesions are hyperintense on $T_1$-weighted image, smooth, round, and homogeneous. On $T_2$-weighted images, the signal is variable and depends on the colloid content. Hyperintensity on $T_2$ implies a high protein content, whereas hypointensity correlates with high cholesterol content. *B*, The same tumor on axial cuts shows splaying of the internal cerebral veins around the superior pole of the tumor. *C*, This tumor required a transchoroidal approach. Note that the tumor, by projecting into the field displacing the two internal cerebral veins, facilitates access to the tumor.

ventricular tumors, these tumors tend to be malignant and can metastasize through the CSF spaces. The treatment includes surgery, radiation, and chemotherapy; however, despite all that, the prognosis is poor.[45, 48, 49]

*Pineoblastomas and pineocytomas* are rare tumors of the pineal gland proper, pineoblastomas being five to six times as common as pineocytomas. The pineoblastomas are PNETs; they are infiltrative and can spread through CSF pathways. The pineocytomas often have portions that appear like pineoblastomas but tend to be less infiltrative and grow slowly. Both tumors present with hydrocephalus, whereas the pineoblastomas have an association with bilateral retinoblastomas. On a CT scan, the pineocytomas appear well circumscribed; they are isodense to hyperdense with homogeneous enhancement and occasional calcifications. Pineoblastomas appear similarly except for the inva-

sive nature of the tumor into the thalamus and midbrain. An MRI scan shows a low signal on $T_1$-weighted images and isointense or hyperintense on $T_2$-weighted images. The presence of invasion into adjacent tissues is more evident on an MRI scan and helps with the diagnosis. The treatment is surgery, followed by radiation; for pineoblastomas, the treatment is total neuraxis radiation.[44, 45, 50, 51]

*Epidermoids and dermoids* are uncommon third ventricular tumors that grow by displacing surrounding tissue rather than invading it. On a CT scan, these tumors are hypodense and do not enhance. The dermoids have fat and can be calcified, whereas the epidermoids do not. An MRI scan exhibits a homogeneous hypodense $T_1$-weighted image and a hyperdense $T_2$-weighted image. The treatment is surgery.

*Ependymomas* of the third ventricle are rare; they account for only 15% of ependymomas. They present with symptoms of hydrocephalus, and on presentation these tumors can be quite large. On a CT scan, the tumor shows hyperdensity, and there is quite a variable response to contrast. Approximately 50% show calcification, and this may be seen on a CT scan, as may intratumoral cysts. An MRI scan shows heterogeneous signals on both $T_1$- and $T_2$-weighted images with heterogeneous enhancement. Although complete removal is difficult to accomplish, surgery is recommended for these lesions, followed by radiation.

Craniopharyngiomas are tumors that commonly arise in the pituitary stalk. These tumors can expand superiorly into the anterior third ventricle. There are two peaks of incidence—the first, in the first two decades, the second in the fifth and sixth decades of life. Overall, craniopharyngiomas constitute 3% to 5% of all intracranial neoplasms, although only 20% present with only a suprasellar component. There are two types of craniopharyngiomas. The first, the so-called adamantinomatous type, is seen in the pediatric population and is often cystic, calcified, and more aggressive. The second type, which is more common in adults, is a papillary tumor and is seldom either calcified or cystic. Most of the third ventricular craniopharyngiomas appear to be papillary. Clinical presentation may present with diabetes insipidus, growth abnormalities in children, visual changes, and in large tumors, hydrocephalus. A CT scan shows an often cystic (in 90%), multilobulated mass with frequent calcifications. Enhancement is present in the solid portions and cyst wall. On an MRI scan, the signal intensity depends on the cystic contents and thus can vary. A high-protein content elicits a high signal on $T_1$- and $T_2$-weighted images. Intraventricular lesions tend to be papillary craniopharyngiomas, and generally they do not have cysts or calcification. The treatment approach is a surgical one with the intention being to remove the tumor completely, although the infiltrative nature of these tumors at their brain interface makes that goal difficult to attain.[52–55]

*Metastases* to the third ventricle are not only rare, they seldom occur in the absence of other intracerebral lesions. They have been reported in the anterior part of the third ventricle and can present with surrounding edema. On a CT scan, they are generally hyperdense with marked enhancement. Surgical resection depends on the overall life expectancy and the presence of other cerebral tumors.

There are several non-neoplastic entities that can present in the third ventricle and these need to be considered as part of the differential diagnosis. *Sarcoidosis* presents rarely in the CNS; however, when it does, it has a predilection for the hypothalamus and the floor of the third ventricle. On a CT scan, it exhibits a hyperdense signal that enhances homogeneously. When presenting in a patient with known sarcoid, the diagnosis is made without biopsy, and treatment is with steroids. *Histiocytosis* with CNS manifestations affects children more commonly, and this entity also has a predilection for the floor of the third ventricle. There is a male preponderance, and clinically patients present with pituitary dysfunction and bony skeletal lesions. Surgery, when performed, is for biopsy, because these lesions are radiosensitive. Cysticercosis is an infectious entity caused by the intestinal tapeworm *Taenia solium*. It is more common in some Third World endemic areas, but ventricular involvement has been seen occasionally in the

United States yet is nevertheless a rare entity. When the cysticercosis parasite develops in the ventricles, it can spread via the CSF pathways. The CT scan may have difficulty in picking up the cyst, and a ventriculogram may be necessary to visualize its outline. An MRI scan can pick out, on $T_1$-weighted images, both the cyst wall and the scolex. A diffuse ependymal inflammatory enhancement may be evident in some cases. On $T_2$-weighted images, the contents of the cyst generally appear higher in density than CSF. The treatment is surgical resection followed by praziquantel.[56, 57]

## APPROACHES TO THE LATERAL VENTRICLES

### Selection of Approach

There are several approaches to the ventricular system, and the choice of the best route is largely dictated by the location of the tumor. The goal is to have the shortest possible route to the tumor, while minimally disturbing the intracranial anatomy. Thus, sulci and fissures are used to their maximal extent, as is any pre-existing ventriculomegaly. Particular attention should be directed toward the vasculature, including the cortical draining veins, and, whenever possible, their drainage patterns should be evaluated preoperatively. If an angiogram is obtained preoperatively, in addition to the cortical draining veins, the deep venous system should be visualized well, especially for third ventricular lesions.

### Anterior Transcallosal Approaches to the Lateral Ventricle

This approach is commonly used to access the lateral and third ventricles. This route is useful for lesions affecting the body of the lateral ventricle as well as for access to the third ventricle. A preoperative cerebral angiogram or a magnetic resonance angiogram (MRA) is important in the preoperative planning. Cortical veins draining into the sagittal sinus can be a significant obstacle to interhemispheric access. Furthermore, the ventricular venous and arterial structures can be distorted by the tumor and should be noted preoperatively. The patient is placed in a supine position, with the head slightly flexed. A bicoronal incision is made just posteriorly to the coronal suture. The craniotomy, which measures about 4 to 6 cm in length and 4 cm lateral to the midline, is located two thirds in front of the coronal suture, one third behind. Access is optimized if the superior sagittal sinus (SSS) is exposed. The dura is opened with its base medially. Often, cortical draining veins enter the dura before reaching the midline and the superior sagittal sinus, and these veins may either be separated away from the overlaying dura, or the dura must be cut around the veins. Large veins should be preserved. If exuberant arachnoid granulations are encountered, they can be divided with sharp dissection and bipolar cautery. Once the midline is reached, the falx is followed to its depth. At the inferior edge of the falx, small cingulate gyrus veins may be encountered as they drain into the inferior sagittal sinus.

These veins may be sacrificed. The arachnoid below the falx may be adherent, and this arachnoid must be divided carefully in order not to injure the cingulate gyrus on either side. After placing protective patties over the brain surface, the frontal lobe is retracted no more than 2 cm laterally. Once the corpus callosum is reached, the two pericallosal arteries are visualized (Fig. 59–6). The best route to take is between the two arteries. At this point, the corpus callosotomy can be started just posterior to the genu and developed 3 cm posteriorly to gain access to the lateral ventricle. Occasionally, the opposite lateral ventricle is entered, and orientation is achieved by locating the foramen of Monro. At this point, the lateral ventricular tumor should be evident. Tumor resection proceeds by first doing internal debulking, then isolating tumor capsule away from surrounding ventricular structures.[1, 58–61]

## Anterior Transcortical, Transfrontal Approach

The transfrontal, transcortical approach is used occasionally for lesions found specifically in the anterior part of the lateral and third ventricular system, especially when associated with hydrocephalus. In addition, large, dominant draining cortical veins favor this approach over the transcallosal route, because it is lateral to the interhemispheric fissure. The craniotomy is similar to the one used for the transcallosal approach and utilizes a bicoronal incision, a preferably right-sided craniotomy, lateral to the midline, measuring 4 to 6 cm in length. The superior and middle frontal gyri need to be exposed, but almost always the middle frontal gyrus is accessed. A ventricular catheter may be initially passed from the cortical entry point into the ventricle to confirm the path. Once confirmed, a 2- to 3-cm gyral incision is made and developed down into the ventricle. Retraction allows visualization of lateral ventricular structures. Access into the third ventricle, if necessary, can be achieved by further developing this approach and

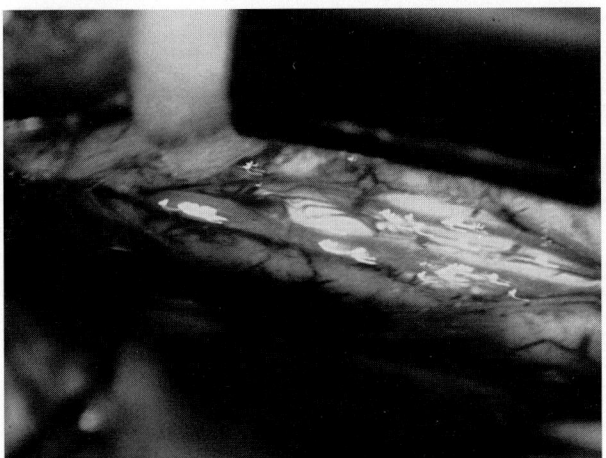

FIGURE 59–6 ■ A view of the corpus callosum through a standard anterior transcallosal approach. The brain is retracted no more than 2 cm, whereas another retractor is placed on the falcine side, without compressing the superior sagittal sinus. The arachnoid connecting the cingulate gyri is dissected, and the corpus callosum is visualized. The two pericallosal arteries are seen and help guide the surgeon toward the midline.

combining it with the subchoroidal dissection into the third ventricle (described later).[1, 34, 62, 63]

## Posterior Transcallosal Approach

The posterior transcallosal approach gains access to the roof and medial part of the atrium of the lateral ventricles. This is achieved, however, at the expense of splitting the splenium of the corpus callosum. The floor and lateral part of the atrium are not well visualized by this route. Preoperatively, as in the anterior approaches, an MRA or cerebral angiogram help to guide the placement of the craniotomy by visualizing the dominant cortical draining vessels. The patient is positioned in the three-quarter prone position, with the parietal area of the operated side uppermost in the field. The anterior extent of the craniotomy is at the posterior edge of the post central gyrus, and depending on the venous anatomy, the posterior edge is about 4 cm posterior to that. The craniotomy exposes the superior sagittal sinus and extends laterally 3 to 4 cm. The dura is reflected medially, and care is taken to maintain the large draining veins. The parietal lobe is gently retracted (about 2 cm) away from the falx. Once arachnoid adhesions are opened, the distal pericallosal arteries and the splenium are identified. Below the splenium, the ICVs join the vein of Galen, and these can be seen once the splenium is cut. The splenium is incised with a bipolar cautery, and this incision must be made lateral to the midline, because the atrium of the lateral ventricle deviates laterally. Access into the atrium is now achieved; however, tumors not found in the medial part of the atrium will be hard to resect by this route, and the surgeon should consider the posterior transcortical route for lateral atrial tumors.[1, 10, 64]

## Posterior Transcortical Approach

The posterior transcortical approach is the preferred route to the atrium of the lateral ventricle and allows access to both medial and lateral segments of the atrium (Fig. 59–7). The patient is positioned in the three-quarter prone position with the parietal area of interest at the highest point in the field. The craniotomy extends, as in the posterior transcallosal approach, from the posterior margin of the post central gyrus, posteriorly about 4 cm. Preoperative MRA or angiogram is helpful when determining the position of major draining veins. The craniotomy does not have to cross midline. Once the cortex is exposed, the cortical incision is made along the superior parietal gyrus. If the ventricular system is enlarged, prior to the cortical incision, it is useful to access the ventricle with a ventriculostomy. The atrium is more lateral at this location, and the direction of the dissection should reflect that. Once inside the atrium, should the tumor allow, the surgeon can visualize the pulvinar anteriorly, the choroid plexus more medially, and the crus of the fornix. The optic radiations course lateral to the atrium, and one should avoid dissecting into that area. The tumor should be debulked piecemeal before separating it from surrounding structures. Care should be taken to avoid blood pooling in the ventricles, which can lead to postoperative obstructive hydrocephalus. The vascular

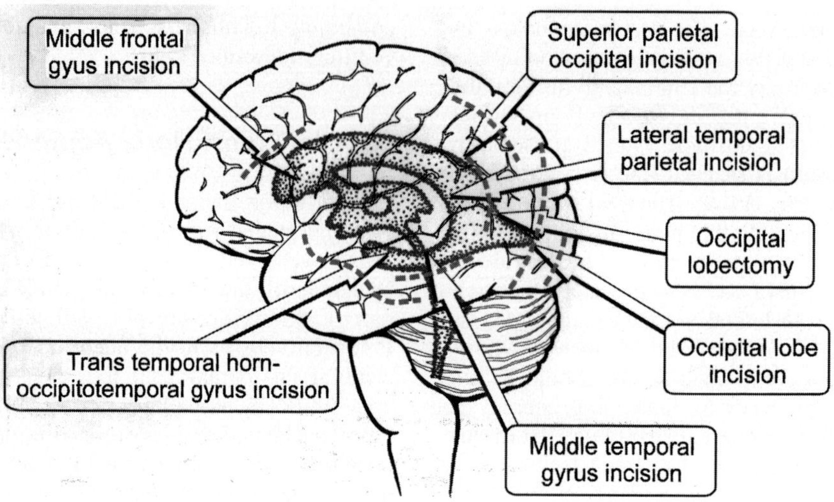

**FIGURE 59–7** ■ Lateral view of the brain showing the major transcortical routes to the lateral and third ventricular system. The *middle frontal gyrus incision* is utilized in the anterior transcortical approach to the anterior part of the lateral ventricle and for the transforaminal and subchoroidal approaches to the third ventricle. This route is facilitated in cases of ventricular enlargement. The *superior parietal occipital incision* and the *lateral temporal parietal incision* are utilized for the posterior transcortical approaches to posterior ventricular body and atrial lesions. The superior parietal approach avoids the visual pathways and reduces the risk for a postoperative field cut. The lateral temporal approach on the dominant hemisphere risks damage to speech and should be used on the nondominant side. The *occipital* approaches access the occipital horns and ventricular atria in patients with an established homonymous hemianopsia. The *middle temporal gyrus incision* and the *occipitotemporal gyrus incision* are utilized to access the temporal horn. The occipitotemporal approach is preferred on the dominant side through a subtemporal exposure.

pedicle of the tumor should be identified and coagulated at the earliest possible time to avoid excessive bleeding.[1, 65]

## Posterior Frontotemporal Approach

This approach is used to gain access to temporal horn lesions. The patient is placed supine, with the head tilted away by 45 degrees and extended. A reverse question mark incision is made starting at the level of the zygoma just anterior to the ear, then curving posteriorly over the ear and anteriorly toward the forehead. The temporalis muscle is mobilized anteriorly, and the craniotomy is extended inferiorly to the level of the zygoma. The dura is opened with its base anteriorly. Access to the ventricle is achieved either by first performing an anterolateral temporal lobectomy to include no more than the anterior 5 cm of the temporal lobe from the tip or by making a cortical incision in the middle or inferior temporal gyrus. Debulking of the tumor is followed by dissection away from surrounding tissues.[1]

## Transtemporal/Subtemporal Approach

The transtemporal approach to the atrium or lateral horn is a transcortical route for lesions that are located laterally in the atrium or within the temporal horn (see Fig. 59–7). The patient is positioned either supine with the head tilted at least 60 degrees away from the craniotomy side or the patient is placed in the lateral position. The reverse question mark incision runs about 5 cm posteriorly over the ear and behind it. The temporal craniotomy is performed across the base, just above the plane with the transverse sinus posteriorly. Extreme care should be taken not to injure the dura at this level, because the vein of Labbé travels under-

neath to drain at the junction of the transverse and sigmoid sinus. Once the dura is exposed, on the nondominant side, an incision into the posterior middle or inferior temporal gyrus will gain access to the atrium. The incision should be along the axis of the gyrus. Once the ventricle is accessed, the tumor is removed piecemeal, then separated away from surrounding tissues. On the dominant side, the approach can be varied to avoid impairment in language abilities. The inferior temporal bone and mastoid air cells can be drilled or rongeured to gain access to the subtemporal area. The cortical incision is then made in the occipitotemporal gyrus. Although this avoids more of the optic radiations and is further removed from the speech cortex, this route requires more temporal lobe retraction. Care should be taken to avoid stretching or kinking the vein of Labbé. Furthermore, on closure of the subtemporal craniotomy, the mastoid air cells must be waxed, and closure must be watertight to avoid postoperative CSF leakage.

## APPROACHES TO THE THIRD VENTRICLE

### Anterior Transcallosal Approaches: Transforaminal, Transchoroidal, Subchoroidal, and Interforniceal

The transcallosal approaches to the third ventricle are a continuation of the approaches described earlier for access into the lateral ventricles. The anterior transcallosal approach is the most commonly used for access to the third ventricle and affords an excellent, low morbidity pathway to the level of the lateral ventricle. There are several paths of dissection that the surgeon may undertake. The structures that are most at risk of injury during these approaches are the fornices and the vessels within the velum interpositum (the ICVs and the medial posterior choroidal arteries). These approaches are adequate for lesions from the foramen of Monro posteriorly. Lesions that are very anterior and inferior in the third ventricle may not be as readily accessible by this route.

Access to the anterior part of the third ventricle via the transcallosal route can be accomplished through an enlarged foramen of Monro. This transforaminal approach is particularly useful in situations in which the foramen of Monro is enlarged by a tumor. Colloid cysts can be removed in this fashion with minimal manipulation of the foramen and the encircling fornix. The use of angled view ventriculoscopes has allowed visualization of third ventricular structures. However, access to the third ventricle is limited by the size of the foramen of Monro, and when this limitation prohibits further removal of the tumor, one of four approaches to the third ventricle can be developed from this vantage point. The first method is enlargement of the foramen of Monro by unilateral transection of the fornix. This allows anterior access into the third ventricle. This approach, however, has been associated with potential significant morbidity in memory impairment. Thus, it is not a recommended route.[66–70]

A second approach is the interforniceal route to the third ventricle, which gains access by splitting the fornices in the sagittal plane, along the direction of their fibers. In this approach, the septum pellucidum is opened widely and used as a guide to the midline. The great advantage of this approach is that posterior dissection can be carried out to expose the entire third ventricle. The ICVs have no reported branches between them and must be separated. The disadvantage of this method is the potential bilateral damage to the fornices, which are closely adherent over the body of the fornix.[71–73]

The transchoroidal and subchoroidal routes are two related approaches that seek to gain access to the midline and posterior third ventricle without disturbing the forniceal body or columns. In the subchoroidal approach, the lateral ventricular choroid is separated from the thalamus. The tenia choroidea is cut, and the choroid plexus is reflected medially. The thalamostriate vein at the foramen of Monro is the anterior extent of the dissection, whereas posteriorly the exposure can be developed as far as the atrium. Once the tenia choroidea is cut, the velum interpositum and the ICVs are visualized. The velum is cut lateral to the ICVs, and both veins are displaced medially. The limitation in exposure with this maneuver can be the ipsilateral thalamic veins, which, if sacrificed, may lead to hemorrhagic thalamic infarcts. The advantage of this approach is the relative distance kept away from the body of the fornix and less manipulation of the ICVs.

In the transchoroidal route, the choroidal dissection is performed medial to the lateral ventricular choroid, through the tenia fornicis, separating the choroid from the body of the fornix. The choroid plexus is reflected laterally. This minimizes contact with the posterior choroidal artery and the superficial thalamic veins. Once the choroid is reflected laterally, the velum interpositum, the ICVs, and the medial posterior cerebral arteries are visualized. At this point the ICVs are separated, and a plane is developed between them. There are no reported bridging veins between these vessels; nevertheless, because they run closely together,

they require manipulation and intermittent compression to gain access to the third ventricle. The last layer in this approach to be split is the third ventricular choroid plexus, which must also be separated in the midline. Finally, one should keep in mind that the anatomy is often distorted; in this case, the preoperative radiologic studies are particularly useful.[3, 6, 74, 75]

## Subfrontal Approach

This approach is useful for midline suprasellar and anterior third ventricular lesions. The exposure can be unilateral or bilateral, with olfaction being at risk. The patient is positioned supine, and a bicoronal incision in utilized. The unilateral craniotomy starts laterally at the pterion, runs just above the orbital ridge, and goes past the midline. For bilateral subfrontal approaches, the craniotomy extends from pterion to pterion. The flap is developed 4 to 5 cm above the orbital ridge. The brain is relaxed with mannitol and CSF drainage, while the frontal lobe is retracted gently. To reduce retraction and increase the upward angle of vision, the orbital ridges can be removed. For unilateral approaches, the ipsilateral olfactory nerve is sacrificed. Care should be taken to coagulate small draining veins, because they may rupture during retraction. Past the planum sphenoidale, the optic nerves, the chiasm, and both internal carotids are visualized. The tumor is generally evident at this stage. The A1 branches must be identified bilaterally to the level of the anterior communicating artery. If the tumor has a cystic component, such as in craniopharyngiomas, it is useful to decompress the cyst at this point. Care should be taken not to allow cystic contents to escape into the ventricle or subarachnoid space, because it can cause aseptic meningitis. If the tumor does not contain a cystic component, then internal decompression is highly beneficial in reducing tension on surrounding structures during dissection of the capsule. The resection can be performed through the prechiasmatic space, the opticocarotid triangle, or the retrocarotid space. The latter two routes are the reasons for a wide craniotomy extending to the pterion. In patients with a pre-fixed chiasm, resection is particularly difficult to accomplish, and opening of the lamina terminalis must be performed. The lamina is opened above the chiasm and below the anterior cerebral vessels. In suprasellar tumors that extend upward into the anterior third ventricle, the anterior floor of the third ventricle is pushed upward. Thus, upon opening the lamina, the tumor is covered by a thin third ventricular floor, which every effort should be made to save. Occasionally, the tumor can be accessed and delivered through either the prechiasmatic space or the opticocarotid triangle.[76–79]

## Interhemispheric Approach

This approach is closely related to the subfrontal approach and allows access to suprasellar and anterior third ventricular lesions. The head position and incision are similar to those used in the the subfrontal approach. A bifrontal craniotomy is performed, with the inferior margin as close to the anterior fossa floor base as possible. The dural incision cuts across midline; thus, the anterior inferior segment of the superior sagittal sinus is sacrificed, as is the falx at this level. The olfactory nerves can be saved in most cases by dissecting the tracts away from the retracting frontal lobes. This approach affords good visualization of both optic nerves and carotid arteries as well as optimizes the access to the prechiasmatic space. However, this approach does put the frontal venous drainage system at risk.[80–82]

## Pterional Approach

This approach is a common one to suprasellar tumors that extend into the anterior third ventricle. The weakness of this approach is the poor visualization of the ipsilateral third ventricular extension and contralateral opticocarotid and retrocarotid space. The positioning is supine, with the head tilted about 45 degrees to the left and in about 20 degrees of extension. The incision follows a hairline curve from the zygoma anterior to the ear to the frontal region. It is important to stay flush with the pterional base; alternatively, an orbital osteotomy maximizes the upward angle. The sylvian fissure may need to be opened. Once CSF is released and brain relaxation is achieved, gentle retraction is applied to the frontal lobe. The tumor is accessed through the retrocarotid space, the opticocarotid triangle, and the prechiasmatic space. In addition, the lamina terminalis can be accessed and opened.[83]

## Approaches to the Posterior Third Ventricle

Lesions in and around the posterior third ventricle, especially those of the pineal region, are accessed via several approaches that aim to maintain the integrity of the ICVs and the vein of Galen and avoid injury to the midbrain. Most of these patients present with hydrocephalus, which must be relieved at the time of surgery, either with shunting or ventriculostomy. Spinal drainage in cases of obstructive hydrocephalus is not indicated, because compartmentalization of CSF may lead to herniation.

## Infratentorial Supracerebellar Approach

This approach is well suited for midline tumors in the pineal region and avoids retraction or manipulation of the supratentorial brain. The approach is not adequately suited if the tumor infiltrates laterally or superiorly above the tentorium. The patient can be placed in the sitting position, the three-quarter prone position, or the prone position. The sitting position is optimal for brain relaxation; the cerebellum falls away, while venous drainage is optimized. If this position is chosen, armrests are crucial in order for the surgeon to avoid rapid fatigue. Furthermore, the patient is susceptible to air embolism in this position, thus a central line, carbon dioxide monitor, and compression stockings are advised. The incision is midline, and the wide suboccipital craniotomy is performed bilaterally to the level of the mastoids, thus exposing the transverse sinus and torculum. Inferiorly, the craniotomy is developed to a distance of

about 1 cm from the foramen magnum. The dura is opened with its base superiorly. Retraction may be applied superiorly to the underside of the tentorium in the midline, while gentle inferior retraction can be placed on the vermis. Care should be taken to coagulate and divide cerebellar bridging veins, because they drain superiorly into the tentorium. The arachnoid is thick and should be divided before the parapineal vessels and the tumor are visualized. The precentral cerebellar vein connects the vermis to the vein of Galen. This vein can be sacrificed to gain access to the pineal. Resection of the tumor proceeds inferior to the vein of Galen, ICVs, and basal vein of Rosenthal. The quadrigeminal plate should be well visualized inferiorly. After resection, a postoperative shunt or ventriculostomy must be left to avoid immediate postoperative obstructive hydrocephalus.[84, 85]

## Occipital Transtentorial Approach

This approach is used for pineal and posterior third ventricular lesions with either supratentorial or infratentorial components, because it allows for a wide exposure. The patient can be placed in either the sitting or semiprone position, with the right side lower. However, whereas the sitting position helps in the infratentorial approach by allowing the cerebellum to fall away, the three-quarter prone position helps the occipital lobe to fall away, thus reducing need for retraction. The trapdoor incision is made with its base inferiorly and across the midline. The occipital craniotomy must extend across the midline and below the transverse sinus; it measures about 5 cm above the transverse sinus and lateral to the midline. The dura is opened with its base on the sinuses. Minimal retraction on the occipital lobe is necessary with adequate CSF drainage and brain relaxation. When retracting, the inferior tentorial surface should be retracted rather than the falx in order to avoid injuring the calcarine fissure. There are no significant draining veins from the medial occipital lobe into the tentorium, although there is a dominant cortical vein draining into the transverse sinus—the inferior cerebral vein, which should be lateral to the working area. The transection of the tentorium proceeds in a posterior to anterior direction by first making an incision proximally and then proceeding in a line about 1 cm off midline toward the tentorial edge. The tentorium is well vascularized, and hemostasis may require a bipolar cautery and clips. The thick arachnoid should be separated at the edge of the tentorium to avoid undue bleeding of small vessels. Once the tentorium is cut, it is gently retracted laterally with a suture. The deep veins around the pineal are surrounded in a thick arachnoid, which once cut reveal the anatomy. If necessary, the precentral cerebellar vein should be sacrificed to increase the working space. Tumor resection can proceed between the ICVs and the basal vein of Rosenthal. A variation on this approach, the *retrocallosal approach*, can be developed if further exposure is necessary. The falx can be cut about 1 cm in anterior to the insertion of the vein of Galen into the sinus, after coagulating or clipping the inferior sagittal sinus. Retraction on the falx allows further exposure. The splenium does not have to be cut but can be gently retracted upward to allow for extra exposure. Once the tumor is resected or debulked, the tentorium is simply returned to its position but does not need to be sutured.[86-88]

## Posterior Transcallosal Approach

This approach is suited for lesions in the mid to posterior third ventricle. The patient is placed in the lateral decubitus position; the side of approach (usually the right) is allowed to fall away. The craniotomy is centered more superiorly toward the area of the lambdoid suture, and the superior sagittal sinus is exposed. Generally, in the posterior third of the superior sagittal sinus, there are few noteworthy draining veins; however, an angiogram might be helpful in this position. The craniotomy is about 8 cm in the sagittal plane and extends laterally about 4 to 5 cm in a triangular fashion. The dura is opened with its base midline, and the hemisphere is separated away from the falx. The exposure of the corpus callosum must be made between the two pericallosal arteries from the splenium anteriorly for a distance of about 6 cm. A 3-cm corpus callosotomy is performed in the midline, leaving 2 to 3 cm of splenium intact posteriorly. The fornices should be just lateral to the midline, and care should be taken not to injure them. After the corpus callosum is cut, the tela choroidea is encountered, and the ICVs should be visible. A plane between the two can be developed widely to allow lateral displacement of the two vessels. Internal tumor debulking is performed before separating the tumor capsule away from the ventricular walls.[2, 89-91]

## COMPLICATIONS

Approaches to the lateral and third ventricles are difficult and potentially dangerous procedures and have a significant morbidity and mortality. Because of the numerous types of approaches, and the varied pathology involved, it is difficult to make wide generalizations regarding morbidity. The complications are very specific to the type of tumor and its location.

### Mortality

Surgery of the lateral and third ventricle has carried an extremely high mortality rate in the past (as high as 75%). With advances in microsurgery and improved understanding of anatomic pathways, the 30-day postoperative mortality at present is 5% to 12%. Among the immediate causes of the mortality were cerebral hemorrhage, infarction, brain swelling, and pulmonary embolus.

### Cognitive Deficits

Many patients undergoing lateral and third ventricular surgery exhibit immediate postoperative impairment of cognitive functions. Some of these symptoms are related to the corpus callosum disconnection and include disturbed consciousness, a transient state of mutism, memory impair-

ment and apathy, contralateral leg weakness, incontinence, and disinhibition. These symptoms can be seen in up to 75% of patients but tend to resolve spontaneously within 3 weeks. Permanent changes in cognition are reported in 5% to 10%. Neuropsychological testing is useful in these cases. Persistent focal neurologic deficits such impairment of motor function or a visual field cut are reported in 8% to 30% of cases.

### Seizures

Postoperative seizures are more common in patients who undergo transcortical procedures, and past reports have indicated that about one third of patients have seizures in the postoperative period. In patients undergoing transcallosal procedures, the incidence is unknown, although it is presumed to be lower. Although the majority of approaches avoid transversing cortical tissue, retraction injuries to brain may account for postoperative seizures.

### Hydrocephalus

Most of the lateral and third ventricular tumors present with hydrocephalus. Yet often, despite good resection of the tumor, hydrocephalus persists in up to 33% of patients. These patients require shunting. Furthermore, these shunts often (in >20%) malfunction, likely because of the higher protein content in the CSF of these postoperative patients, and there is an increased risk of shunt infection. Overshunting can add to the problem of postoperative subdural hematoma collections, which are found in about 40% of patients. Only one quarter of these require surgery for drainage of the subdural collection; nevertheless; this implies that approximately 10% of patients who undergo ventricular surgery will require drainage of a subdural collection later on. The more pronounced the preoperative ventriculomegaly, the higher is the risk of this complication.[92-97]

Multiple factors influence the successful outcome of surgery of the lateral and third ventricle. The approaches described have been developed to allow access to the ventricular system while minimizing manipulation of the surrounding brain. Among the numerous factors that are involved in choosing a particular surgical approach to these tumors are: the location in the ventricles, the size, vascularity, feeding the blood supply, the presumptive pathology, and the surgeon's comfort level with a particular approach. Although treatment of these lesions can be complex and often difficult, a good surgical outcome, which maximizes the patient's quality of life, can now be anticipated in most cases.

## REFERENCES

1. Tymurkaynak E, Rhoton AL Jr, Barry M: Microsurgical anatomy and operative approaches to the lateral ventricles. Neurosurgery 19:685–723, 1986.
2. Ono M, Rhoton AL Jr, Peace D, et al: Microsurgical anatomy of the deep venous system of the brain. Neurosurgery 15:621–657, 1984.
3. Nagata S, Rhoton AL Jr, Barry M: Microsurgical anatomy of the choroidal fissure. Surg Neurol 30:3–59, 1988.
4. Fuji K, Lenkey C, Rhoton AL Jr: Microsurgical anatomy of the

choroidal arteries: Lateral and third ventricle. J Neurosurg 52:165–188, 1980.

5. Yamamoto I, Rhoton AL Jr, Peace D: Microsurgery of the third ventricle: Microsurgical anatomy. Neurosurgery 8:334–356, 1981.

6. Wen WT, Rhoton AL Jr, deOliveira E: Transchoroidal approach to the third ventricle: An anatomic study of the choroidal fissure and its clinical application. Neurosurgery 42:1205–1219, 1998.

7. Rhoton AL Jr: Microsurgical anatomy of the third ventricular region. In Apuzzo MLJ (ed): Surgery of the Third Ventricle, 2nd ed. Baltimore: Williams & Wilkins, 1998, pp 89–158.

8. Piepmeier JM, Sass KJ: Surgical management of lateral ventricular tumors. In Paoletti P, Takakura K, Walker M, et al (eds): Neuro-oncology. Kluver: Dordrecht, 1991, p 333.

9. Fornari M, Savoiardo M, Morello G, Solero C: Meningiomas of the lateral ventricles. J Neurosurg 54:64, 1981.

10. Piepmeier J, Spencer D, Sass K, George T: Lateral ventricular masses. In Apuzzo MLJ (ed): Brain Surgery: Complications Avoidance and Management. New York: Churchill Livingstone, 1993, pp 581–600.

11. Collmann H, Kazner E, Sprung C: Supratentorial intraventricular tumors in children. Acta Neurochir Suppl 35:75–79, 1985.

12. Oppenheim JS, Strauss RC, Mormino J, et al: Ependymomas of the third ventricle. Neurosurgery 34:350–353, 1994.

13. Maeder PP, Holtas SL, Basibuyuk LN, et al: Colloid cyst of the third ventricle: Correlation of MR and CT findings with histology and chemical analysis. Am J Neuroradiol 11:575–581, 1990.

14. Bruce JN, Stein BM: Pineal tumors. Neurosurg Clin North Am 1:123–138, 1990.

15. Baumgartner JE, Edwards MS: Pineal tumors. Neurosurg Clin N Am 3:853–862, 1992.

16. Carmel PW: Tumors of the third ventricle. Acta Neurochir (Wien) 75:136–146, 1985.

17. Piepmeier JM: Tumors and approaches to the lateral ventricles. J Neurooncol 30:267–274, 1996.

18. Jelinek J, Smirnitopolous JG, Parisi JE, et al: Lateral ventricular neoplasms of the brain: Differential diagnosis based on clinical, CT and MR findings. Am J Neuroradiol 11:567–574, 1990.

19. Chow CW, Klug GL, Lewis EA. Subependymal giant-cell astrocytoma in children: An unusual discrepancy between histological and clinical features. J Neurosurg 68:880–883, 1988.

20. Swartz JD, Zimmerman RA, Bilaniuk LT: Computer tomography of intracranial ependymomas. Radiology 143:97–101, 1982.

21. Lobato RD, Cabello A, Carmena JJ, et al: Subependymomas of the lateral ventricles. Surg Neurol 15:144–147, 1981.

22. Morrison G, Sobel DF, Kelley WM, et al: Intraventricular mass lesions. Radiology 153:435–442, 1984.

23. Markwalder TM, Huber P, Markwalder RV, et al: Primary intraventricular oligodendroglioma. Surg Neurol 11:25–28, 1979.

24. Kikuchi K, Kowada M, Mineura K, et al: Primary oligodendroglioma of the lateral ventricle with computer tomographic and positron emission tomographic evaluations. Surg Neurol 23:483–488, 1985.

25. Chang KH, Han MH, Kim DG, et al: MR appearance of central neurocytoma. Acta Radiol 34:520–526, 1993.

26. Yasargil MG, von Ammon K, von Deimling A, et al: Central neurocytoma: Histopathologic variants and therapeutic approaches. J Neurosurg 76:32–37, 1992.

27. Raimondi AJ, Gutierrez FA: Diagnosis and surgical treatment of choroid plexus papillomas. Childs Brain 1:81–85, 1975.

28. Turcotte JF, Copty M, Bedard F, et al: Lateral ventricle choroid plexus papilloma and communicating hydrocephalus. Surg Neurol 13:143–146, 1980.

29. Boyd MC, Steinbok P: Choroid plexus tumors: Problems in diagnosis and management. J Neurosurg 66:800–805, 1987.

30. Gassel MM, Davies H: Meningiomas of the lateral ventricles. Brain 84:605, 1961.

31. Fornari M, Savorardo M, Morello G, et al: Meningiomas of the lateral ventricles: Neuroradiological and surgical considerations in 18 cases. J Neurosurg 54:64–74, 1981.

32. Wang AM, Power TC, Rumbaugh CL: Lateral ventricular meningioma. Comput Radiol 9:355–358, 1985.

33. Nitta M, Symon L: Colloid cyst of the third ventricle: A review of 36 cases. Acta Neurochir 76:99–104, 1985.

34. Little JR, MacCarty CS: Colloid cysts of the third ventricle. J Neurosurg 40:230–235, 1974.

35. Lach B, Scheitgauer BW, Gregor A, et al: Colloid cyst of the third ventricle: A comparative immunohistochemical study of neuraxis cysts and choroid plexus epithelium. J Neurosurg 78:101–111, 1993.

36. Wilms G, Marchal G, Van Hecke P, et al: Colloid cysts of the third ventricles: MR findings. J Comput Assist Tomogr 14:527–531, 1992.

37. Haugh RM, Markesbery WR: Hypothalamic gliomas and disturbances of behavior and endocrine and autonomic function. Arch Neurol 40:560–563, 1983.

38. Lee Y, Van Tassel P, Bruner JM, et al: Juvenile pilocytic astrocytomas: CT and MR characteristics. AJNR Am J Neuroradiol 10:363–370, 1989.

39. Forsyth PA, Shaw EG, Scheithauer BW, et al: Supratentorial pilocytic astrocytomas: a clinicopathologic, prognostic, and flow cytometric study of 51 patients. Cancer 27:1335–1342, 1993.

40. Imes RK, Hoyt WY: Childhood chiasmal gliomas: Update of the facts of patients in the 1969 San Francisco study. Br J Ophthalmol 70:179–182, 1986.

41. Fletcher WA, Imes RK, Hoyt WF: Chiasmal gliomas: Appearance and long term changes demonstrated by computer tomography. J Neurosurg 65:154–159, 1986.

42. Brown EW, Riccardi VM, Mawad M, et al: MR imaging of optic pathways in patients with neurofibromatosis. AJNR Am J Neuroradiol 8:1031–1036, 1987.

43. Jellinger K: Primary intrasellar germ cell tumors. Acta Neuropathol 25:291–306, 1973.

44. Chang T, Teng, Guo W, et al: CT of pineal tumors and intracranial germ cell tumors. AJNR Am J Neuroradiol 10:1039–1044, 1989.

45. Zee CS, Segall H, Apuzzo MLJ, et al: MR imaging of pineal region neoplasms. J Comput Assist Tomogr 15:56–63, 1991.

46. Hoffman HJ, Otsuba H, Hendrick EB, et al: Intracranial germ cell tumors in children. J Neurosurg 74:545–551, 1991.

47. Wara WM, Fellows CF, Sheline GE, et al: Radiation therapy for pineal tumors and suprasellar germinomas. Radiology 124:221–223, 1977.

48. Scheithauer BW: Neuropathology of pineal region tumors. Clin Neurosurg 32:351–383, 1985.

49. Nashold JR, Oakes WJ, Friedman HS, et al: Management of pineal non-germinoma germ cell tumor with residual teratoma and normal alpha-fetoprotein. Med Pediatr Oncol 22:137–139, 1994.

50. Futrell NN, Osborn DR, Burger PC, et al: Pineal region tumors: Computer tomographic-pathologic spectrum. Am J Radiol 137:951–956, 1981.

51. Mena H, Rushing EJ, Ribas JL, et al: Tumors of pineal parenchymal cells: A correlation of histological features, including nucleolar organizer regions, with survival in 35 cases. Hum Pathol 26:20–30, 1995.

52. Hoffman HJ, de Silva M, Humphries RP, et al: Aggressive surgical management of craniopharyngiomas in children. J Neurosurg 76:47–52, 1992.

53. Goldstein SJ, Wilson DD, Young AB, et al: Craniopharyngioma intrinsic to the third ventricle. Surg Neurol 20:249–253, 1983.

54. Crotty TB, Scheithauer BW, Young WF Jr, et al: Papillary craniopharyngioma: A clinicopathologic study of 48 cases. J Neurosurg 83:206–214, 1995.

55. Ahmadi J, Destian S, Apuzzo MLJ, et al: Cystic fluid in craniopharyngiomas: MR imaging and quantitative analysis. Radiology 182:783–785, 1992.

56. Zee CS, Segall HD, Apuzzo MLJ, et al: Intraventricular cysticercal cysts: Further neuroradiologic observations and neurosurgical implications. Am J Neuroradiol 5:727–730, 1984.

57. Zee CS, Segall HD, Destian S, et al: MRI of intraventricular cysticercosis: Surgical implications. J Comput Assist Tomogr 17:932–939, 1993.

58. Sugita K, Kobayashi S, Yokoo A: Preservation of large bridging veins during brain retraction. J Neurosurg 57:856–860, 1982.

59. Shucart WA, Stein BM: Transcallosal approach to the anterior ventricular system. Neurosurgery 3:339–343, 1978.

60. Geffen G, Walsh A Simppson D, Jeeves M: Comparison of the effects of transcortical removal of intraventricular tumors. Brain 103:773–788, 1980.

61. Sass K, Novelly R, Spencer D, Spencer S: Mnestic and attention impairments following corpus callosotomy section for epilepsy. J Epilepsy 1:61–66, 1988.

62. Viale GL, Turtas S: The subchoroidal approach to the third ventricle. Surg Neurol 14:71–76, 1980.

63. Shucart W: The anterior transcallosal and transcortical approaches. In Apuzzo MLJ (ed): Surgery of the Third Ventricle, 2nd ed. Baltimore: Williams & Wilkins, 1998, pp 369–389.

64. Dandy WE: Operative experience in cases of pineal tumor. Arch Surg 33:19–46, 1936.

65. Rhoton AL Jr, Yamamoto I, Pease DA: Microsurgery of the third ventricle. Part 2: Operative approaches. Neurosurgery 8:357–373, 1981.
66. Ehni G, Ehni BL: Considerations in transforaminal entry. In Apuzzo MLJ (ed): Surgery of the Third Ventricle, 2nd ed. Baltimore: Williams & Wilkins, 1998, pp 391–419.
67. Garcia-Bengochea F, Friedman WA: Persistent memory loss following section of the anterior fornix in humans: A historical review. Surg Neurol 27:361–364, 1987.
68. Sweet WH, Talland GA, Ervin FR: Loss of recent memory following section of fornix. Trans Am Neurol Assoc 84:76–82, 1959.
69. Tucker DM, Roeltgen DP, Tully R, et al: Memory dysfunction following unilateral transection of the fornix: A hippocampal disconnection syndrome. Cortex 23:465–472, 1988.
70. Ture U, Yasargil MG, Al-Mefty O: The transcallosal-transforaminal approach to the third ventricle with regard to the venous variations in this region. J Neurosurg 87:706–715, 1997.
71. Apuzzo MLJ, Chikovani OK, Gott PS, et al: Transcallosal interforniceal approaches for lesions affecting the third ventricle: Surgical considerations and consequences. Neurosurgery 10:547–554, 1982.
72. Hodges JR, Carpenter K: Anterograde amnesia with fornix damage following removal of the third ventricle colloid cyst. J Neurol Neurosurg Psychiatry 54:633–638, 1991.
73. Woiciechowsky C, Vogel S, Lehmann R: Transcallosal removal of lesions affecting the third ventricle: An anatomic and clinical study. Neurosurgery 36:117–122, 1995.
74. Lavyne MH, Patterson RH Jr: Sub-choroidal trans-velum interpositum approach to mid third ventricular tumors. Neurosurgery 12:86–94, 1983.
75. Petrucci RJ, Bucheit WA, Woodruff GC, et al: Transcallosal paraforniceal approach for third ventricle tumors: Neurophysiological consequences. Neurosurgery 20:457–464, 1987.
76. Patterson RH Jr: The subfrontal transsphenoidal and trans-lamina terminalis approaches. In Apuzzo MLJ (ed): Surgery of the Third Ventricle, 2nd ed. Baltimore: Williams & Wilkins, 1998, pp 471–487.
77. Choux M, Lena G, Genitori L: Craniopharyngioma in children. Neurochirurgie 37:1–174, 1991.
78. Tomita T, McLone D: Radical resection of childhood meningiomas. Pediatr Neurosurg 19:6–14, 1993.
79. King TT: Removal of intraventricular craniopharyngiomas through the lamina terminalis. Acta Neurochir (Wien) 45:277–286, 1979.
80. Susuki J, Katakura R, Mori T: Interhemispheric approach through the lamina terminalis to tumors of the anterior part of the third ventricle. Surg Neurol 22:157–163, 1984.
81. Kasama A, Kano T: A pitfall in the interhemispheric translamina terminalis approach for the removal of craniopharyngioma: Significance of preserving draining veins. Surg Neurol 32:116–120, 1989.
82. Yasui N, Nathal E, Fujiwara H, et al: The basal interhemispheric approach for acute anterior communicating aneurysms. Acta Neurochir 118:91–97, 1992.
83. Yasargil MG, Curcic M, Kis M, et al: Total removal of craniopharyngiomas: Approaches and long term results in 144 patients. J Neurosurg 73:3–11, 1990.
84. Stein BM: The infratentorial supracerebellar approach to pineal lesions. J Neurosurg 35:197–202, 1971.
85. Bruce JN, Stein BM: Surgical management of pineal region tumors. Acta Neurochir (Wien) 134:130–135, 1995.
86. Poppen JL: The right occipital approach to a pinealoma. J Neurosurg 25:706–710, 1966.
87. Reid WS, Clark WK: Comparison of the infratentorial and transtentorial approaches to the pineal region. Neurosurgery 3:1–8, 1978.
88. Clark WK, Batjer HH: The occipital transtentorial approach. In Apuzzo MLJ (ed): Surgery of the Third Ventricle, 2nd ed. Baltimore: Williams & Wilkins, 1998, pp 721–741.
89. Dandy WE: An operation for removing pineal tumors. Surg Gynecol Obstet 33:113–119, 1921.
90. Ono M, Rhoton AL Jr, Barry M: Microsurgical anatomy of the region of the tentorial incisura. J Neurosurg 60:365–399, 1984.
91. Westerveld M, Sass K, Spencer S, Spencer D: Neuropsychological function following corpus callosotomy for epilepsy. In Devinsky T (ed): Epilepsy and Behavior. New York: Alan Liss, 1991, pp 203–212.
92. Bruce DA: Complications of third ventricular surgery. Pediatr Neurosurg 17:325–330, 1991.
93. Alesh F, Kitz K, Koos WT, et al: Diagnostic potential of stereotactic biopsy of midline lesions. Acta Neurochir (Wien) Suppl 53:33–36, 1991.
94. Stein BM, Bruce JN: Surgical management of pineal region tumors. Clin Neurosurg 39:509–532, 1992.
95. Camacho A, Abernathey CD, Kelly PJ, Laws ER Jr: Colloid cysts: Experience with the management of 84 cases since the introduction of computer tomography. Neurosurgery 24:693–700, 1989.
96. Bellotti C, Pappada G, Sani R, et al: The transcallosal approach for lesions affecting the lateral and third ventricles: Surgical considerations and results in a series of 42 cases. Acta Neurochir (Wien) 111:103–113, 1991.

# Transcallosal Approach to the Third Ventricle

■ ARUN PAUL AMAR and MICHAEL L. J. APUZZO

Despite the highly refined nature of contemporary microneurosurgery, operations in and around the third ventricle continue to pose significant technical challenges. Optimal outcomes from such surgery require careful preoperative evaluation and planning, proper intraoperative technique, and vigilant postoperative management. The intricacies of such treatment constitute the subject matter of entire volumes.[1]

Before operative management of lesions within the third ventricle is undertaken, planning should consist of adequate multiplanar magnetic resonance imaging and angiography. This preparation provides the surgeon with necessary information about the pathologic nature of the third ventricular mass as well as definition of the anatomic substrate peculiar to the particular patient and identification of the major structures at risk from surgery. In addition, thorough neuropsychologic assessment establishes baseline functional data for each patient, allowing for selection of the best management strategy in individualized circumstances.

Complication avoidance also requires exquisite knowledge of the pertinent anatomic structures that demarcate the operative corridor, including the coronal suture, sagittal sinus and parasagittal draining veins, falx cerebri, cingulate gyrus, pericallosal arteries, corpus callosum, septum pellucidum, fornix, thalamostriate veins, foramina of Monro, tela choroidea, medial posterior choroidal arteries, and internal cerebral veins. Consideration of the consequences of injury to each neural or vascular component is essential as a stepwise progression evolves through the corridor of exposure. Appropriate instrumentation and technique are also essential. Postoperative management should include observation for memory deficits, hydrocephalus, and intraventricular hemorrhage. In this chapter, we discuss general issues related to surgical planning and technique in the treatment of third ventricular lesions, with an emphasis on transcallosal routes to the anterior third ventricle. The details of specific approaches can be found elsewhere.[1]

## SPECTRUM OF PATHOLOGY INVOLVING THE THIRD VENTRICLE

Pathologic lesions affecting the third ventricle encompass a wide range of neoplastic and inflammatory processes.[2]

Colloid cysts are the most common lesions intrinsic to the third ventricle itself. These lesions typically originate from the anterior roof of the ventricle and project inferiorly. They possess an inner epithelium composed of cuboidal cells, which secrete a mucinous substance that accumulates under pressure. Symptoms may result from persistent or intermittent obstruction of the foramina of Monro.[3]

Most other lesions encroach on the third ventricle from the surrounding parenchyma. Many of these are neoplastic, with astrocytic tumors representing the most common third ventricular neuroepithelial tumors. Central neurocytomas have been described, and many neoplasms that had previously been considered to be oligodendrogliomas were probably, in fact, neurocytomas.[4, 5]

Craniopharyngiomas may arise from the parasellar region and extend upward into the third ventricle, resulting in hydrocephalus and visual loss.[6] Rarely, these tumors may arise from the median eminence and be contained entirely within the ventricle. Other, less common, lesions include ependymomas and subependymomas, teratomas, germ cell tumors, cysticercosis, vascular malformations, histiocytosis X, pituitary adenomas, and sarcoidosis.[2]

## TRANSCALLOSAL APPROACH TO THE THIRD VENTRICLE

Based on the works of Dandy,[7] exposure of the third ventricle has historically been achieved via the transcortical route. This approach permits access to the lateral ventricle and is well suited to lesions that arise from or extend into this chamber, especially when accompanied by lateral ventricular dilatation. The studies of Bogen and Sperry[8–11] confirmed the relative safety of callosal sectioning when the splenium is spared. As a result, the past 20 years have witnessed an increased interest in transcallosal approaches to the third ventricle.[12–20] These latter routes have been applied to access the anterior third ventricle[12–15] as well as the region of the pineal body.[16, 17]

### Indications

The choice of surgical approach to lesions of the anterior third ventricle is predicated on the size and location of the mass, size of the lateral ventricles, and goals of the operation. Generally, if there is no associated hydrocephalus, a transcallosal approach to the lateral ventricle should be used.[12–15, 18–20] The surgeon can then gain passage into the third ventricular chamber by a number of secondary maneuvers that involve some manipulation of forniceal structure, by traversing the foramen of Monro (which may be expanded by the lesion or by the operative procedure), by the transchoroidal trans–velum interpositum approach, or by the interforniceal corridor.[14–15]

If the lesion is confined to the third ventricle, the transcallosal approach provides superior visualization of the entire ventricle. If, however, an extra-axial lesion arises inferiorly and extends upward into the caudal third ventricle, cranial base approaches may be more appropriate because the greatest volume of the mass may be accessed in this manner. Such approaches include the pterional, subfrontal, subtemporal, and transnasal-transsphenoidal routes. The orbitozygomatic craniotomy has been popularized as an approach to skull base lesions that secondarily invade the floor of the third ventricle.[21, 22] Originally developed to gain improved access to basilar territory aneurysms, this technique combines previously described zygomatic and temporopolar modifications of the classic pterional and subtemporal craniotomies. Removal of the zygomatic process allows the microscope to be maneuvered into a basal-to-vertex trajectory, enhancing exposure to areas of extension above the dorsum sellae. Likewise, removal of the orbital rim permits retraction of the globe and exposure of the interpeduncular fossa along the anterior-posterior axis. The enhanced operative corridor afforded by this approach may permit a greater extent of resection than is possible with conventional routes.

Establishment of a tissue diagnosis and reconstitution of cerebrospinal fluid pathways are the primary goals of transcallosal surgery for third ventricular lesions. Depending on the pathologic nature of the lesion (e.g., colloid cyst, cysticercosis), surgical extirpation may also be a reasonable goal. Otherwise, cytoreduction is a realistic objective.

Compared with transcortical routes, the major advantages afforded by the transcallosal approach include the following: (1) a short trajectory to the third ventricle; (2) flexibility to explore the entire third ventricular chamber, including the basal and posterior components[19]; (3) the absence of cortical transgression and diminished probability of seizures[23]; (4) bilateral exposure of the foramina of Monro; and (5) no requirement of ventriculomegaly.

## Operative Technique

High-potency glucocorticoids, anticonvulsants, and perioperative antibiotic prophylaxis are used for each patient.[13–15] After the induction of general anesthesia, the patient is positioned supine. The head is placed in neutral pin fixation and flexed to 15 degrees. Other options, such as the lateral decubitus position, offer some potential advantages[16, 17] but may distort the midline structures because of the effects of gravity, risking loss of orientation for the inexperienced surgeon. Various scalp flaps may be used, although we generally employ a two-limbed curvilinear incision that affords visualization of the coronal suture and at least 6 cm of the sagittal suture (Fig. 60–1).

For anterior third ventricular lesions, we use a 5 × 4 × 3 cm trapezoidal bone flap with complete sagittal sinus exposure, principally based on the right. To reduce the potential for venous infarction, placement of the bone flap in the anterior-posterior dimension should be based on assessment of the venous anatomy as determined by preoperative imaging. Review of 100 angiograms with particular attention to the distribution of the parasagittal venous complex disclosed that 42 studies had evidence of significant venous tributaries draining within 2 cm of the coronal suture, with most (70%) entering the sagittal sinus behind the suture and the remainder (30%) entering in front of it.[12] Whenever possible, the flap should be placed two thirds anterior and one third posterior to the coronal suture. Placement of the bone flap as far anteriorly as possible also provides an optimal angle of view to the foramina of Monro. Although some authors[24] suggest making the bony opening large enough so that the surgical strategy could be converted to a transcortical approach if a large parasagittal vein were encountered that would require sacrifice to proceed with the transcallosal route, this maneuver should not be necessary if adequate definition of venous tributaries and paramedian venous anatomy has been undertaken preoperatively. We have relied on magnetic resonance venography[25] or computed tomographic venography[26] for such planning, with both modalities revealing an average of 4.3 cortical veins draining into either side of the superior sagittal sinus.

After the application of dural tenting stitches, the Budde Halo self-retaining retractor system is secured in place. We then make a trapezoidal dural incision, with the broad base placed medially toward the sinus. This flap may be secured to the halo by several sutures, providing absolute midline exposure of the falx. As this flap is reflected, the bridging veins must be identified and preserved. Although we have sacrificed bridging veins that reside anterior to the coronal suture without untoward effects, every effort should be made to preserve them.

The falx-cortical interface is identified, and the plane is developed by placement of a large cottonoid patty into the space, followed by application of a 19-mm retractor blade from the right side of the field. This process is repeated in a serial fashion as the exposure is deepened. The surgeon should pause for 2 to 3 minutes between each advancement of the retractor blade to allow the brain to relax in the face of the pressure exerted by the retractor. This interhemispheric corridor should not exceed 5 cm in length and 1.5 cm in width, so as to minimize retraction injury. After identification of the inferior sagittal sinus, further dissection is accomplished with the aid of the operating microscope using either a 275-mm or 300-mm lens. Separation of the cingulate gyri often requires blunt dissection with microinstrumentation. Inexperienced surgeons commonly mistake the cingulate gyrus for the corpus callosum, but these structures can be distinguished by the fact that the former has the typical tan-gray color of the cortical-pial surface, whereas the latter is strikingly white.

Eventually the white callosal carpet is identified, with its associated pericallosal arteries. Once the corpus callosum is exposed, cotton balls or patties may be placed into the

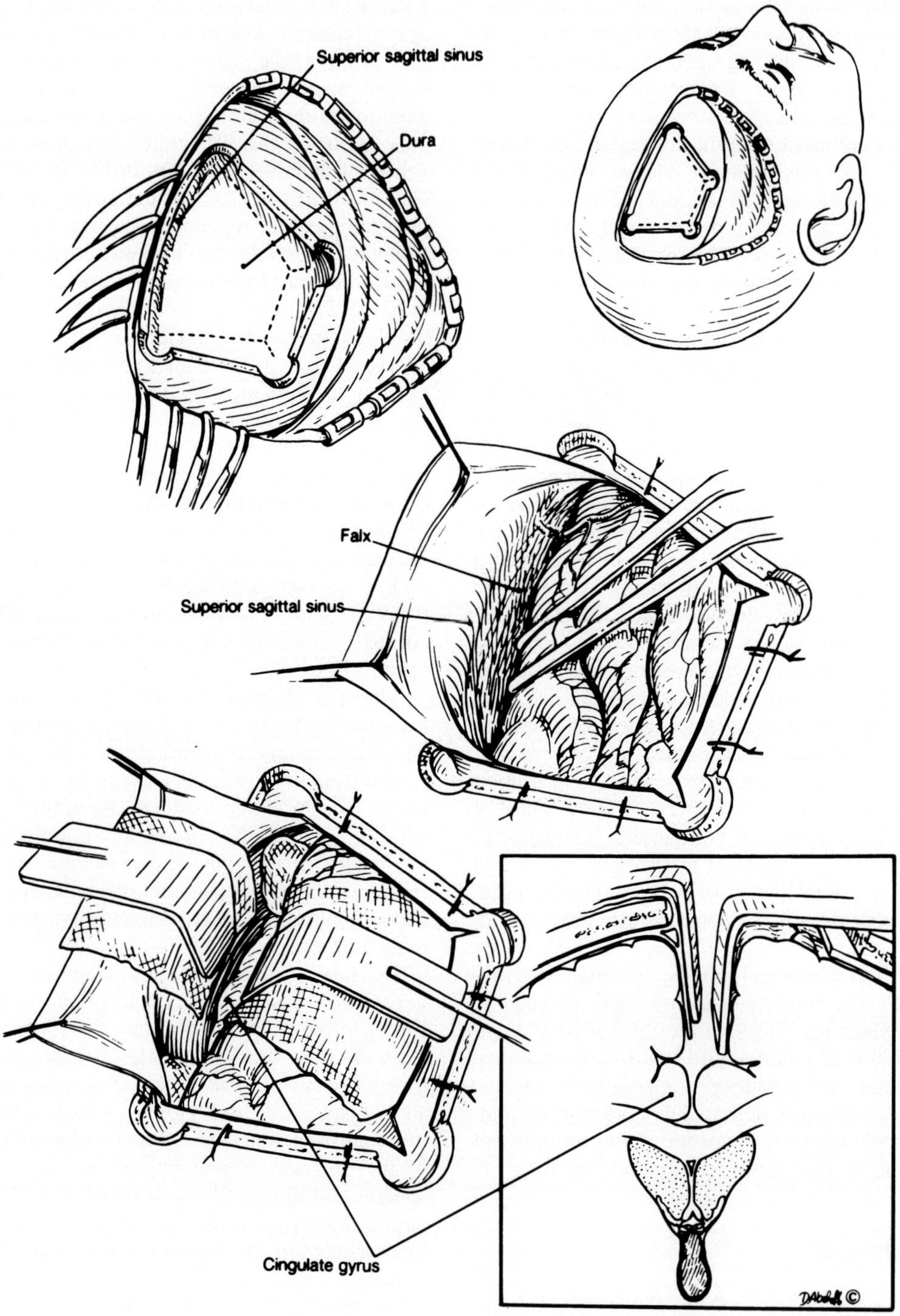

**FIGURE 60–1** ■ An L-shaped incision has been developed in a subperiosteal plane on the nondominant side. Subsequently, a trapezoidal free bone flap and dural incision are fashioned. The interhemispheric plane is then developed, exposing the corpus callosum. (From Apuzzo MLJ, Amar AP: Transcallosal interforniceal approach. In Apuzzo MLJ [ed]: Surgery of the Third Ventricle, 2nd ed. Baltimore: Williams & Wilkins, 1998, pp 421–452).

depths of the exposure at the anterior and posterior poles to aid in the maintenance of the hemispheric retraction. The size of the callosal exposure should be 1 × 3 cm. The falx is maintained as the midline reference point, with the original position of the pericallosal arteries serving as a secondary landmark.

After the corpus callosum and the pericallosal arteries are identified, ventricular entry is undertaken (Fig. 60–2). The site of the callosal incision depends on the position of the pericallosal arteries and may be either between the arteries or lateral to them. This entry is generally oval shaped and 2 to 2.5 cm long, depending on variables related to the angle of entry and the size of the lesion. Although some authors[27] recommend sectioning the thinnest part of the trunk to minimize postoperative neuropsychologic deficits, others[28, 29] argue that it is more important to plan the incision according to the most appropriate trajectory, which is usually anterior to the midportion of the corpus callosum. This region of the trunk may be approximated by the intersection of the corpus callosum with an imaginary line defined by the coronal suture in the midsagittal plane and the external auditory meatus; if continued inferiorly, this line would pass through the foramen of Monro.[19] With No. 5 French suction and bipolar coagulation, the corpus callosum is incised. The thickness of the trunk varies greatly and can range from a thin layer in the presence of hydrocephalus to more than 1 cm. Absolute control of ependymal bleeding must be obtained before proceeding because failure to do so may result in postoperative intraventricular hemorrhage. Once the ventri-cles are entered, the blade is advanced to retract the corpus callosum and the ipsilateral hemisphere.

Depending on the location of the callosal incision and its relation to the anterior-to-posterior and medial-to-lateral planes, the right or left lateral ventricle, forniceal body, or cavum septum pellucidum may be entered. Establishing proper orientation is critical before proceeding. If a cavum has been entered, the septum should be widely fenestrated. Otherwise, this maneuver should be performed after identification of ventricular landmarks, such as the choroidal fissure and foramen of Monro. Fenestration or excision of the septum provides potential bilateral midline exposure and alternate pathways for cerebrospinal fluid flow. Fenestration should not be less than 1 cm.[2]

Once the foramen and choroid plexus are identified, one of the following three routes may be used for entry into the third ventricular chamber: (1) transforaminal, (2) transchoroidal trans–velum interpositum, or (3) interforniceal (Fig. 60–3). Lesion character (size, vascularity, texture, location), foramen caliber, view lines, and personal skills and experience all guide the surgeon in selecting the most appropriate route. All strategies should be directed toward avoiding midline manipulation and minimizing the transmission of pressure gradients to paraventricular structures.

## Transforaminal Corridor

Inspection of the foramen of Monro often reveals the presence of the lesion (see Fig. 60–3, part 1). Initially an attempt to decompress the mass should be made via a

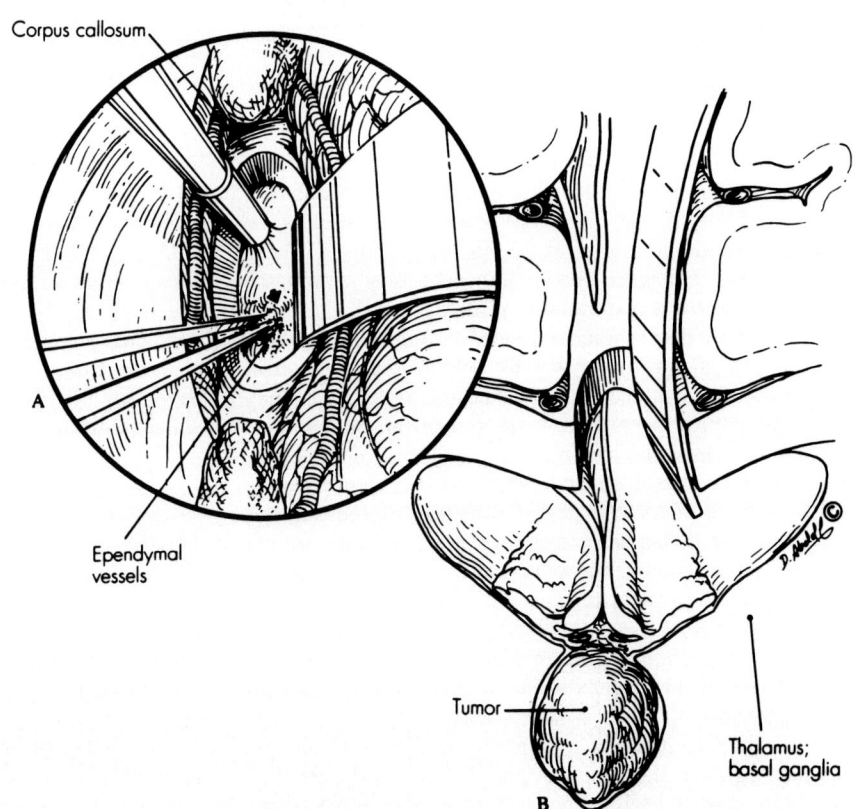

FIGURE 60–2 ■ After identification and preservation of the pericallosal arteries, the corpus callosum is traversed using bipolar cautery and suction. Care is taken to coagulate all visible ependymal vessels. (From Apuzzo MLJ, Litofsky NS: Surgery in and around the third ventricle. In Apuzzo MLJ [ed]: Brain Surgery: Complication Avoidance and Management. New York: Churchill Livingstone, 1992, pp 541–579.)

Corpus callosum

Ependymal vessels

Tumor

Thalamus; basal ganglia

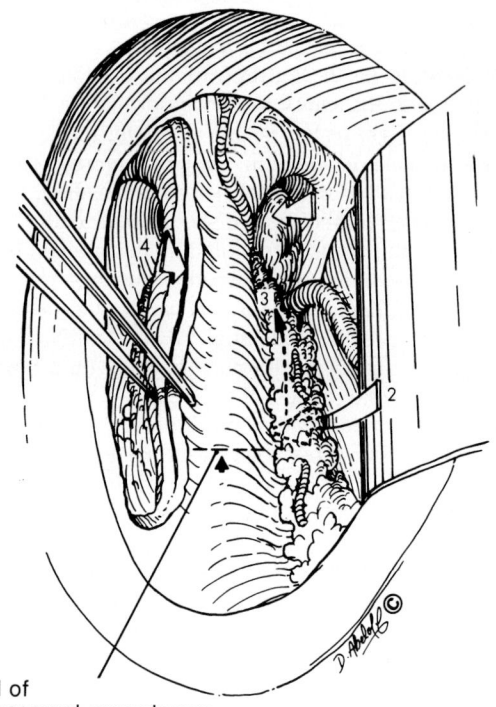

Level of
hippocampal commissure

**FIGURE 60–3** ■ Three routes of entry into the third ventricle from within the lateral ventricle. (1) The transforaminal corridor generally may be attempted initially, unless the lesion is so large and has such a consistency that it cannot be delivered through the foramen. (2) The transchoroidal transvelum interpositum corridor may be developed in order to gain a wider exposure of the ventricle. The thalamostriate vein (3) may be sectioned to enhance this exposure if the subchoroidal route is taken. (4) The interforniceal plane should be reserved for lesions that bulge upward, distending the fornices. (From Apuzzo MLJ, Litofsky NS: Surgery in and around the third ventricle. In Apuzzo MLJ [ed]: Brain Surgery: Complication Avoidance and Management. New York: Churchill Livingstone, 1992, pp 541–579).

transforaminal corridor,[30] especially if it is distended by presence of the mass itself or by attendant hydrocephalus. Cystic, soft, or easily resectable lesions may usually be removed via the foramen of Monro (Fig. 60–4). These lesions must be located far enough anteriorly within the ventricle to allow transforaminal visualization.[30]

When attempting to remove lesions through the foramen, the surgeon should never try to deliver the mass if it exceeds the size of the foramen because this action may injure the paraforniceal region. Moreover, all attachments to the third ventricular roof must be freed to avoid bleeding from the tela choroidea and injury to the fornix. Some surgeons have advocated partial resection of the anterior nucleus of the thalamus or section of the forniceal column to enlarge the foramen, but we do not endorse these maneuvers because the former risks uncontrollable bleeding from the internal cerebral vein,[3] whereas the latter may cause severe neuropsychologic impairment, especially if the contralateral fornix has already been compromised by the third ventricular lesion.

In the management of colloid cysts, the cyst may be aspirated through the foramen, and, subsequently, its wall may be coagulated with bipolar forceps (Fig. 60–5). This may be a definitive treatment if the cyst remnant does not appear to present a significant residual mass or obstruct cerebrospinal fluid flow.

## Transchoroidal Corridor

If transforaminal dissection fails to provide a safe route for access to the lesion, a transchoroidal trans–velum interpositum approach may be used to enter the third ventricle.[31–34] Similar to the interforniceal approach, it is especially well suited for lesions occupying the superior half of the third ventricle posterior to the foramen of Monro (Fig. 60–6). It may be technically more feasible than the interforniceal approach when the two internal cerebral veins are not clearly separate structures.[30]

Wen and colleagues[35] clarified two possible routes through the choroidal fissure that separates the thalamus inferiorly from the body of the fornix superiorly. In the classic subchoroidal approach, an incision is made along the taenia choroidea, the ependymal reflection between the dorsal surface of the thalamus and the inferolateral surface of the choroid plexus in the body of the lateral ventricle. Alternatively, access to the velum interpositum in the roof of the third ventricle can be gained along the taenia fornicis, the reflection of ependyma off the forniceal body onto the superomedial aspect of the choroid plexus. Although either taenia may be incised, Wen and colleagues[35] contend that the suprachoroidal approach between the dorsal aspect of the choroid plexus and the fornix is safer because superficial thalamic and caudate veins risk injury when the taenia choroidea is manipulated. In the subchoroidal approach, for instance, sacrifice of one thalamostriate vein is often necessary in lieu of sectioning or excessive local manipulation of the fornix.[33, 34] Although this maneuver may generally be accomplished without neurologic sequelae, complications such as hemiplegia, mutism, and drowsiness have been reported.[14, 32]

Once lateral ventricular entry is accomplished, the choroidal fissure is readily appreciated by the presence of the overlying choroid plexus. This structure serves as a guide to the foramen of Monro. In the subchoroidal route, the choroid plexus is elevated or coagulated, exposing the thalamus. As the choroid plexus is mobilized medially, the attachments of the velum interpositum must be divided (see Fig. 60–3). Subsequently, the third ventricular roof is dissected medially, opening the ventricle. Eventually the thalamostriate vein is encountered at the foramen. This vein may then be divided, completing the opening into the third ventricle.

## Interforniceal Corridor

Busch[36] initially described the interforniceal approach to a third ventricular lesion in 1944. Using this route, he was able to decompress a malignant glioma. This method is best suited for large lesions that distend the roof of the third ventricle and cannot be removed via the foramen of Monro (Fig. 60–7).[13] The method results in a wide exposure of the entire third ventricle, and it allows for simultaneous bilateral transforaminal and interforniceal manipulation of the mass, increasing the technical maneuvers available for tumor resection.

*Text continued on page 860*

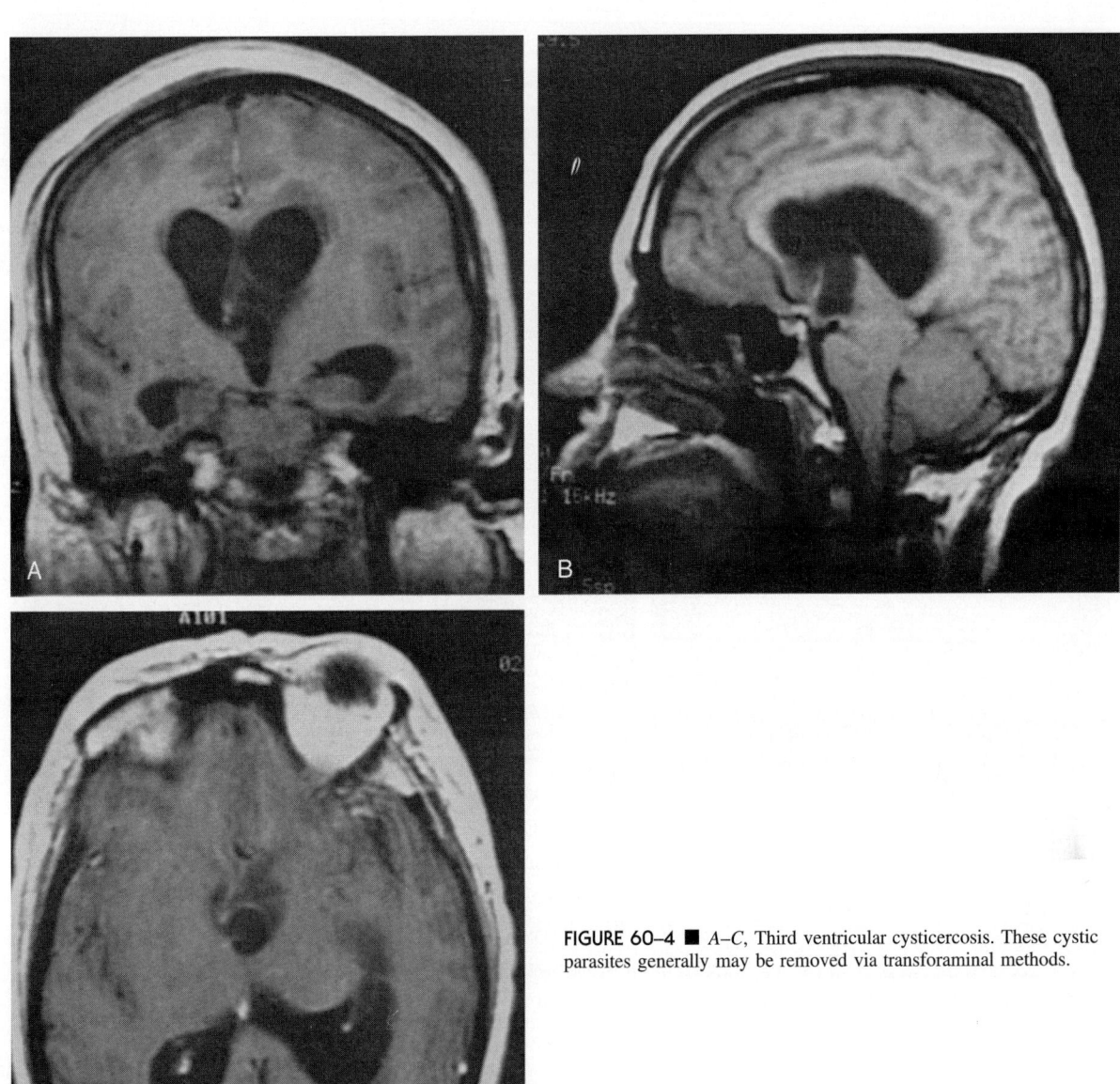

**FIGURE 60–4** ■ *A–C*, Third ventricular cysticercosis. These cystic parasites generally may be removed via transforaminal methods.

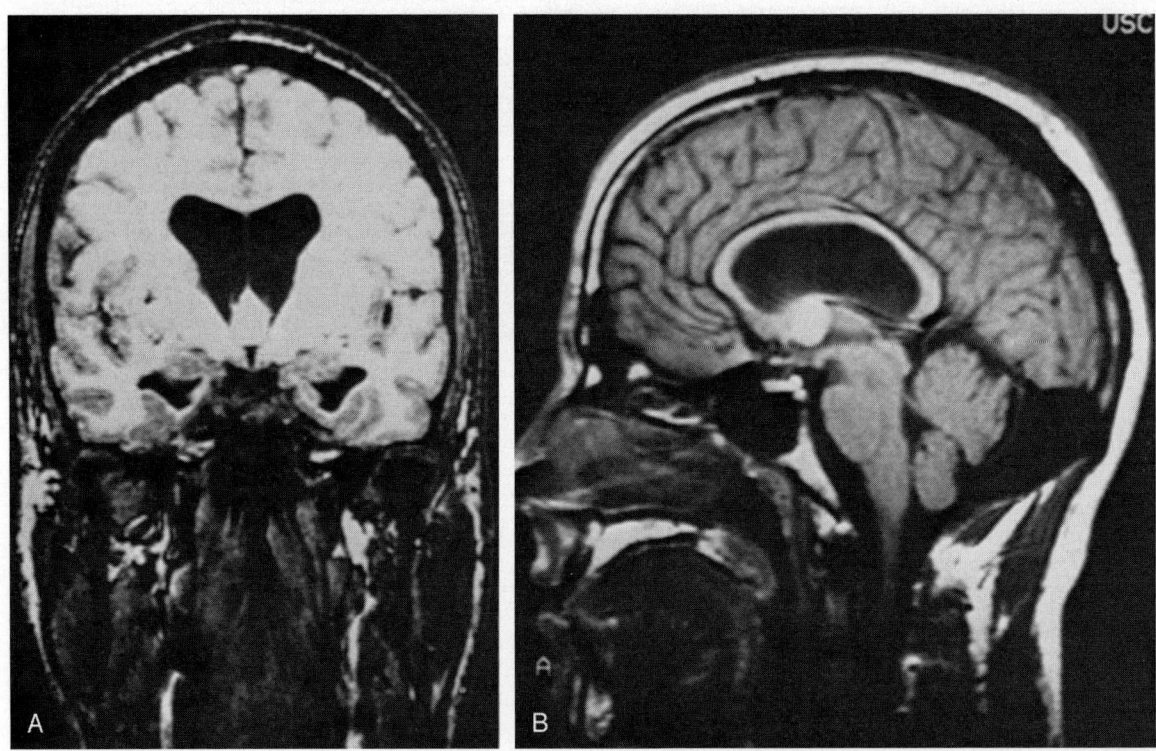

**FIGURE 60–5** ■ *A–B*, Colloid cyst. When these lesions are less than 1 cm, they may be aspirated through the foramen of Monro.

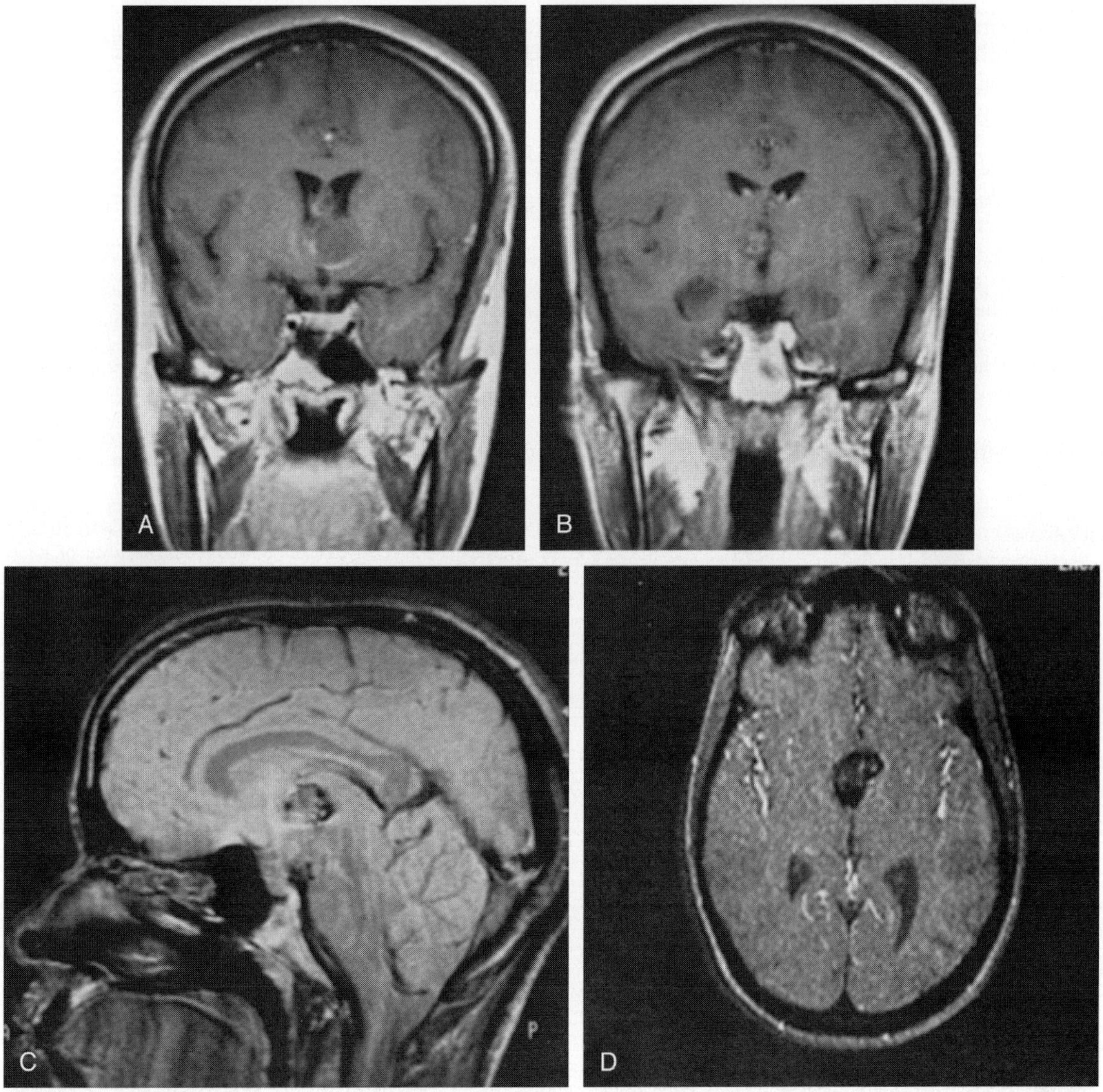

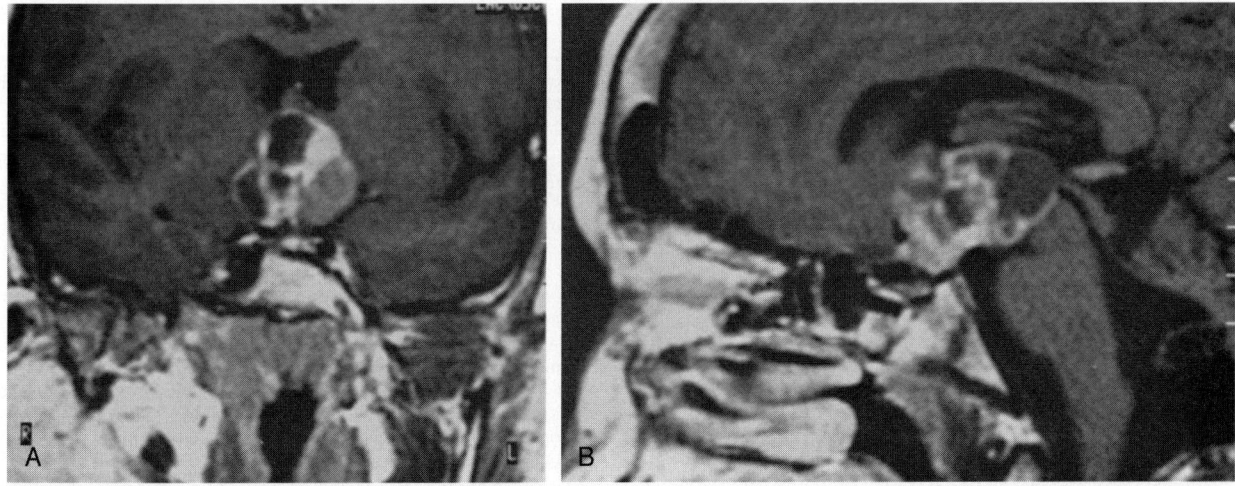

**FIGURE 60–6** ■ *A–D,* Cavernous angioma of the third ventricle. This lesion was resected through a subchoroidal transvelum interpositum approach.

**FIGURE 60–7** ■ *A* and *B,* Third ventricular craniopharyngioma. If such lesions are relatively confined to the third ventricle, a transcallosal approach may be used.

Once the septum pellucidum is fenestrated, the midline forniceal raphe in the roof of the third ventricle may be identified. This natural cleavage plane is developed with the use of a Sheehy canal knife, beginning at the foramen of Monro and extending posteriorly for 1 to 2 cm (see Fig. 60–3, part 4). The posterior dissection is limited by the presence of the hippocampal commissure, which, along with the internal cerebral veins and medial posterior choroidal arteries, must be preserved.[37] Secondary retraction at the level of the fornix is often not necessary; however, a 5-mm retractor blade tapered to 2 mm at the tip may be used to maintain exposure.

Large lesions tend to present themselves under pressure, facilitating their dissection. Once exposure is accomplished, the lesion is internally decompressed, then dissected from the surrounding structures.

## Complications

Discussions of the physiologic cost of manipulating critical brain structures encountered along the transcallosal corridor are beyond the scope of this chapter but have been reviewed in detail elsewhere.[13] Endocrinopathy, visual loss, and other features of diencephalic injury are possible complications, as well as hemiparesis, mutism, and memory disturbance. Additional untoward events include aseptic or infectious meningitis, seizures, hydrocephalus, intraventricular hemorrhage, and nonspecific postoperative complications.

Section of the corpus callosum (with sparing of the splenium) generally does not result in appreciable neurologic sequelae.[8–13, 38] Interhemispheric dissection may result in injury to the bridging veins. Although we have sacrificed tributaries anterior to the coronal suture without adverse effects, we always attempt to preserve them whenever possible. With care during midline entry in relation to cortical venous anatomy and minimization of midline retraction, the incidence of permanent paresis approaches zero, and incidence of transient paresis is less than 10%.[13]

Entry into the third ventricle is always associated with some degree of manipulation of the fornix. As a result, approximately one third of patients experience transient short-term memory difficulties, which typically resolve in less than 1 week. We believe that this effect is more related to the texture of the offending lesion than to its size, with firm masses creating a greater need for local manipulation. Additional complications include confabulation, aphasia, and astereognosis.[13, 14] In our experience, incision of the forniceal raphe and retraction of the body has not resulted in persistent amnestic syndromes, with mentation evaluated not only by standard bedside examination, but also by formal psychometric assessment.[12, 13]

## SUMMARY

Transcallosal approaches to the third ventricle provide avenues for the establishment of tissue diagnoses, reconstitution of cerebrospinal fluid pathways, and, occasionally, surgical cure of selected lesions. Proper understanding of the spectrum of third ventricular pathology and appropriate anatomic substrate optimizes patient selection and surgical outcomes.

## REFERENCES

1. Apuzzo MLJ (ed): Surgery of the Third Ventricle, 2nd ed. Baltimore: Williams & Wilkins, 1998.
2. Aldape KD, Davis RL: Pathological lesions of the third ventricle and adjacent structures. In Apuzzo MLJ (ed): Surgery of the Third Ventricle, 2nd ed. Baltimore: Wilkins & Wilkins, 1998, pp 289–306.
3. Little JR, MacCarty CS: Colloid cysts of the third ventricle. J Neurosurg 39:230–235, 1974.
4. Kim DG, Chi JG, Park SH, et al: Intraventricular neurocytoma: Clinicopathological analysis of seven cases. J Neurosurg 76:759–765, 1992.
5. Yasargil MG, von Ammon K, von Deimling A, et al: Central neurocytoma: Histopathological variants and therapeutic approaches. J Neurosurg 76:32–37, 1991.
6. Long DM, Chou SN: Transcallosal removal of craniopharyngiomas within the third ventricle. J Neurosurg 24:687–691, 1973.
7. Dandy WE: Diagnosis, localization, and removal of tumors of the third ventricle. Bull Johns Hopkins Hosp 33:188–189, 1922.
8. Bogen JE, Fisher D, Vogel PJ: Cerebral commissurotomy: A second case report. JAMA 194:1328–1329, 1965.
9. Bogen JE, Gazzaniga MS: Cerebral commiussurotomy in man: Minor hemisphere dominance for certain visual functions. J Neurosurg 23:394–399, 1965.
10. Bogen JE, Vogel PJ: Cerebral commissurotomy in man. Bull Los Angeles Neurol Soc 27:169–172, 1962.
11. Sperry RW, Gazzaniga MS, Bogen JE: Interhemispheric relationships: The neocortical commissures: Syndromes of hemisphere disconnection. Handbook Clin Neurol 4:273–290, 1969.
12. Apuzzo MJL, Chikovani O, Gott P, et al: Transcallosal interforniceal approaches for lesions affecting the third ventricle: Surgical considerations and consequences. Neurosurgery 10:547–554, 1982.
13. Apuzzo MLJ, Amar AP: Transcallosal interforniceal approach. In Apuzzo MLJ (ed): Surgery of the Third Ventricle, 2nd ed. Baltimore: Wilkins & Wilkins, 1998, pp 421–452.
14. Apuzzo MLJ, Litofsky NS: Surgery in and around the third ventricle. In Apuzzo MLJ (ed): Brain Surgery: Complication Avoidance and Management. New York: Churchill Livingstone, 1992, pp 541–579.
15. Apuzzo MLJ, Zee CS, Breeze RB, Day JD: Anterior and mid-third ventricular lesions: A surgical overview. In Apuzzo MLJ (ed): Surgery of the Third Ventricle, 2nd ed. Baltimore: Wilkins & Wilkins, 1998, pp 635–680.
16. McComb JG, Levy ML, Apuzzo MLJ: The posterior interhemispheric retrocallosal and transcallosal approaches to the third ventricle region. In Apuzzo MLJ (ed): Surgery of the Third Ventricle, 2nd ed. Baltimore: Williams & Wilkins, 1998, pp 743–778.
17. McComb JG, Apuzzo MLJ: Operative management of malformations of the vein of Galen. In Apuzzo MLJ (ed): Surgery of the Third Ventricle, 2nd ed. Baltimore: Williams & Wilkins, 1998, pp 779–786.
18. Winston KR, Cavazzuti V, Arkins T: Absence of neurological and behavioral abnormalities after anterior transcallosal operation for third ventricular lesions. Neurosurgery 4:386–393, 1979.
19. Shucart W: Anterior transcallosal and transcortical approaches. In Apuzzo MLJ (ed): Surgery of the Third Ventricle, 2nd ed. Baltimore: Williams & Wilkins, 1998, pp 369–390.
20. Shucart W, Stein BM: Transcallosal approach to the anterior ventricular system. Neurosurgery 3:339–343, 1978.
21. Levy ML, Khoo LT, Day JD, et al: Optimization of the operative corridor for the resection of craniopharyngiomas in children: The combined frontoorbitozygomatic temporopolar approach. Neurosurg Focus 3:1–10, 1997.
22. Zabramski JM, Kiris T, Sankhla SK, et al: Orbitozygomatic craniotomy: Technical note. J Neurosurg 89:336–341, 1998.
23. Bellotti C, Pappada G, Sani R, et al: The transcallosal approach for lesions affecting the lateral and third ventricles: Surgical considerations and results in a series of 42 cases. Acta Neurochir 111:103–107, 1991.
24. Garrido E, Fahs GR: Cerebral venous and sagittal sinus thrombosis after transcallosal removal of a colloid cyst of the third ventricle: Case report. Neurosurgery 26:540–542, 1990.

25. Mattle HP, Wentz KU, Edelman RR, et al: Cerebral venography with MR. Radiology 178:453–458, 1991.

26. Casey SO, Alberico RA, Patel M, et al: Cerebral CT venography. Radiology 198:163–170, 1996.

27. Woiciechowsky C, Vogel S, Lehmann R, Staudt J: Transcallosal removal of lesions affecting the third ventricle: An anatomic and clinical study. Neurosurgery 36:117–122, 1995.

28. Stein B: Comment on paper by Woiciechowsky et al. Neurosurgery 36:122–123, 1995.

29. Benes V: Advantages and disadvantages of the transcallosal approach to the IIIrd ventricle. Childs Nerv Syst 6:437–439, 1990.

30. Ehni G, Ehni BL: Considerations in transforaminal entry. In Apuzzo MLJ (ed): Surgery of the Third Ventricle, 2nd ed. Baltimore: Williams & Wilkins, 1998, pp 391–420.

31. Hirsch JF, Zouasui B, Reiner D, et al: A new surgical approach to the third ventricle with interruption of the striothalamic vein. Acta Neurochir (Wien) 47:135–147, 1979.

32. Lavyne MH, Patterson RH: Subchoroidal trans-velum interpositum approach. In Apuzzo MLJ (ed): Surgery of the Third Ventricle, 2nd ed. Baltimore: Williams & Wilkins, 1998, pp 453–470.

33. Lavyne MH, Patterson RH: Subchoroidal trans-velum interpositum approach to mid-third ventricular tumors. Neurosurgery 12:86–94, 1983.

34. Viale GL, Turtas S: The subchoroidal approach to the third ventricle. Surg Neurol 14:71–76, 1980.

35. Wen HT, Rhoton AL, de Oliveira E: Transchoroidal approach to the third ventricle: An anatomic study of the choroidal fissure and its clinical application. Neurosurgery 42:1205–1217, 1998.

36. Busch E: A new approach for the removal of tumors of the third ventricle. Acta Psychiatr Scand 19:57–60, 1944.

37. Heilman KM, Sypert GW: Korsakoff's syndrome resulting from bilateral fornix lesions. Neurology 27:490–493, 1977.

38. Jeeves MA, Simpson DA, Geffen G: Functional consequences of the transcallosal removal of intraventricular tumours. J Neurol Neurosurg Psychiatry 42:134–142, 1970.

CHAPTER 61

# Transcallosal Approach to Tumors of the Third Ventricle

■ ROBERTO M. VILLANI and GIUSTINO TOMEI

Tumors of the third ventricle include a wide variety of pathologic entities that can arise either within the ventricular cavity or from the neural structures that form the ventricle. According to anatomic site, tumors of the third ventricle are classified as primarily intraventricular (e.g., colloid cyst, ependymoma, craniopharyngioma) when their attachment to the ventricular wall is minimal and well circumscribed and secondarily intraventricular when they arise from the wall of the ventricle and secondarily occupy the cavity (e.g., glioma, craniopharyngioma, lymphoma).[1]

Tumors that originate within the neural elements of the different structures of the third ventricle (e.g., glial tumors affecting the thalamus and the hypothalamus; tumors growing from the intraventricular ependyma; germinomas; medulloblastomas) are classified as intra-axial. Extra-axial ventricular lesions are histologically benign tumors with a limited area of implantation to the ventricular wall. They include lesions of developmental, neoplastic, vascular, and infectious origin (e.g., colloid cyst, dermoids and epidermoids, arteriovenous malformations, cysticercosis, lymphocytic hypophysitis).[1]

Although these tumors are relatively rare, it is important to diagnose them before surgery and to distinguish, on the basis of neuroradiologic investigation, intra-axial from extra-axial neoplasms. Tumors arising from the base and invading and compressing from outside the third ventricular chamber (meningiomas, craniopharyngiomas, epidermoids, gliomas) (Fig. 61–1) should not be considered as tumors properly of the third ventricle.

The surgical approach to the region of the third ventricle should be tailored first according to the location of the tumor and, second, to the surgeon's experience and preference. In our experience, tumors arising from the anterior base and secondarily invading the third ventricle are better approached through a pterional or subfrontal route. When the tumor cannot be entirely removed with this approach, the anterior subfrontal approach can be combined with a superior approach (i.e., transcallosal or transcortical). Tumors of the pineal region, compressing the posterior part of the third ventricle, are better exposed through an infratentorial supracerebellar or suboccipital transtentorial entry.[2, 3]

Lesions located in the anterior or middle third ventricular chamber as well as those tumors that occupy the entire cavity of the third ventricle are approached with an anterior transcallosal route.[1, 4–11]

As for all central nervous system tumors, the first aim of surgery for masses in the third ventricle remains the improvement of neurologic signs and symptoms through as complete an excision as possible of the tumor. Second, because of the large variety of neoplasms encountered in this area, a precise histologic diagnosis for optimal completion of therapy is required. The third goal is the reopening of cerebrospinal fluid (CSF) pathways, because in more than 50% of cases the tumor occludes the foramen of Monro and can produce an acute or chronic hydrocephalus.[6]

Because the cavity of the third ventricle can be reached only by incision of neural structures, the complications of

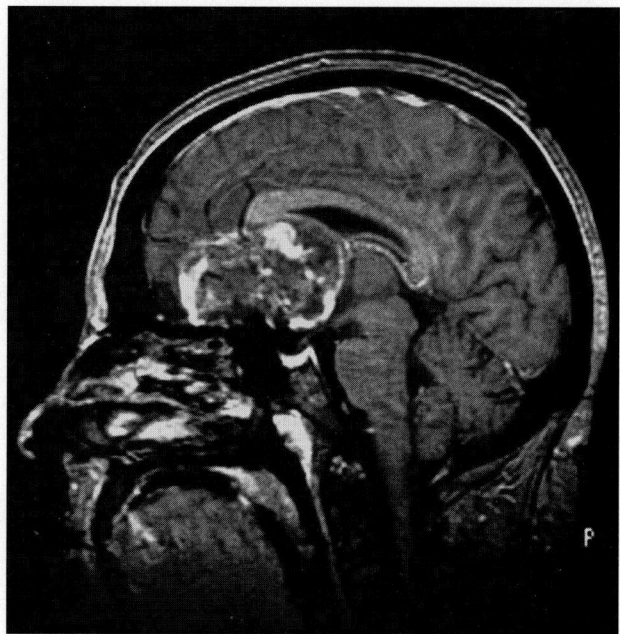

FIGURE 61–1 ■ Sagittal $T_1$-weighted magnetic resonance image of a large tumor arising from the anterior skull base and secondarily invading the third ventricle.

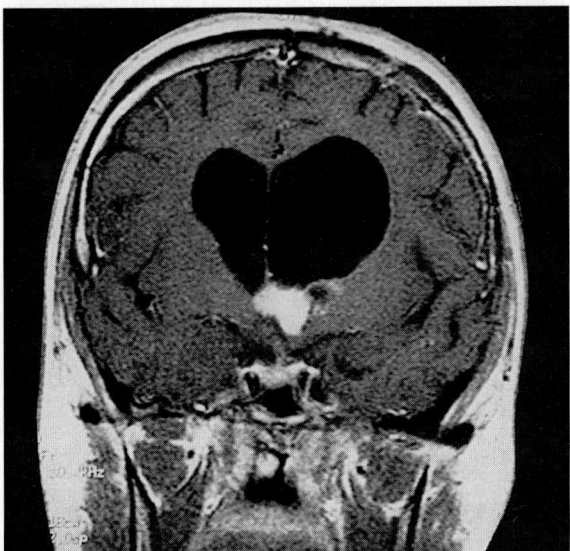

FIGURE 61-2 ■ Coronal T$_1$-weighted magnetic resonance image of a pilocytic astrocytoma of the third ventricle involving the foramen of Monro.

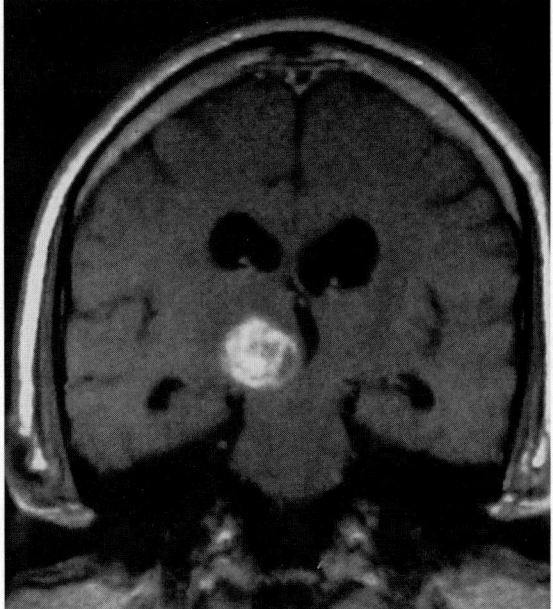

FIGURE 61-4 ■ Coronal T$_1$-weighted magnetic resonance of a thalamic tumor elevating and obliterating the unilateral foramen of Monro.

surgery of these tumors are the result of manipulation and alteration of a number of neural structures that form the third ventricular chamber and the brain areas surrounding it.[7, 8]

The appropriate corridor to reach tumors of the third ventricle should be chosen on the basis of precise neuroradiologic assessment: particular attention must be paid to the location of the mass and its relationship with the ventricular cavity, particularly with the fornix, the foramen of Monro, and the infundibulum. The size of the lateral and third ventricles, the thickness of the corpus callosum, and the anatomic characteristics of the septum have to be clearly borne in mind. Other important findings to be considered are the size of the mass and its relationship with the foramen of Monro (Figs. 61–1 to 61–4), the site of implant, the presence or absence of a CSF layer surrounding the mass, and the relationship of the mass with

the vascular structures—in particular, the internal cerebral vein.

The anterior approach to the third ventricle can be performed using either the transcortical or transcallosal route.[1, 4–6, 8–15] The transfrontal transcortical approach to the lateral and then the third ventricle requires an incision of the brain parenchyma. This procedure, along with many other disadvantages,[5] is followed by postoperative epilepsy in more than 20% of cases.[6]

The anterior transcallosal approach to the third ventricle does not seem, per se, to be responsible for significant postoperative deficits[1, 4–6, 9, 12]: this approach has been the method of choice for treating tumors of the third ventricle in our institution since the late 1980s.

The transcallosal approach is the most straightforward,

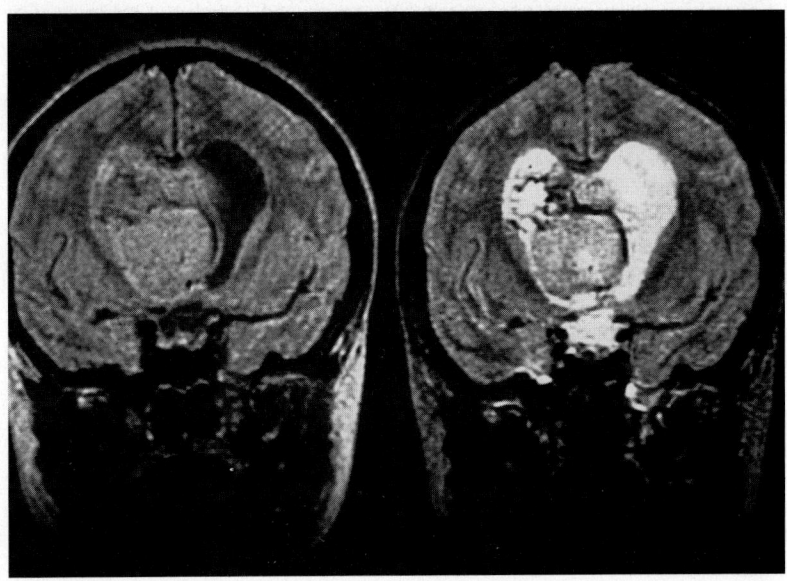

FIGURE 61-3 ■ Coronal T$_1$- and T$_2$-weighted magnetic resonance images of a tumor involving the entire cavity of the third ventricle.

shortest corridor to the third ventricle. The corpus callosum can be reached by simple retraction of the right hemisphere through a corridor between the bridging veins; cortical incision is not required. Incision of the anterior portion of the corpus callosum for a limited length (2 cm) allows entry into either or both lateral ventricles, providing exposure of the two foramens of Monro. The surgeon is then presented with different entry options for direct access to deep-seated lesions in the third ventricle, providing greater flexibility in the anteroposterior exposure of the ventricular cavity. Last, the transcallosal approach can be used even in the presence of a normal, not enlarged, lateral ventricle.

Because surgery of the diencephalic region still represents a major technical challenge in the surgical treatment of tumors of this area, the surgeon, in evaluating the operative approach to tumors of the third ventricle, should take into consideration the appropriateness of the tumor exposure through the chosen entry route, the risks associated with that particular corridor, and the transient or permanent postoperative deficits likely to follow. The region of the third ventricle remains difficult to explore and the operative field is often extremely limited. The most challenging problems are bleeding in the tumor bed and the dissection and separation of the external layer of the neoplasm from the surrounding neural structures. Surgery of the third ventricle requires a detailed knowledge of the anatomic landmarks and the intrinsic characteristics of the different tumors that involve this structure.

Results using the transcallosal approach to these tumors are satisfying; most of them can be completely removed, and long-term follow-up reveals good outcomes.[6]

## SURGICAL ANATOMY

The third ventricle is a narrow midline cavity of the brain located between the two thalami and under the body of the lateral ventricles[11, 16, 17] (Fig. 61–5). The cavity of the third ventricle communicates anterosuperiorly with the lateral ventricles through each foramen of Monro and posteriorly with the fourth ventricle through the aqueduct of Sylvius.

The third ventricular cavity can be approached and its inner structure exposed using different surgical options.

The upper part of the third ventricle comprises the fornix. The septum pellucidum connects the inner surface of the corpus callosum to the upper surface of the body of the fornix. The septum is tallest anteriorly and shortest posteriorly, disappearing near the junction of the body and the posterior columns of the fornix. At the posterior end of the septum pellucidum, the crura and the hippocampal commissure fuse with the lower surface of the corpus callosum.

The fornix consists of a body, two anterior limbs (the columns), and two posterior columns. The two anterior columns, viewed superiorly, form the foramens of Monro that open between the fornix and the thalamus into the lateral ventricles on each side and extend inferiorly into the third ventricle.

At the level of the opening of each foramen of Monro, the two anterior columns split away and terminate in the mamillary bodies. The anterior commissure fills the gap

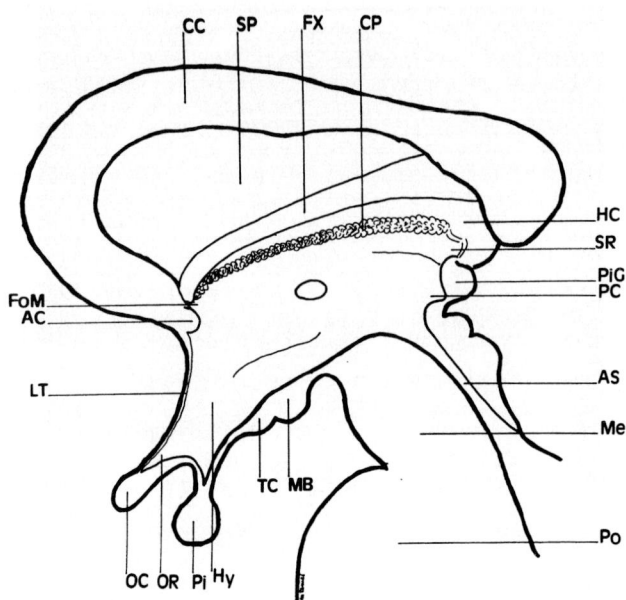

FIGURE 61–5 ■ Schematic drawing of the midsagittal section of the third ventricle. (CC, corpus callosum; SP, septum pellucidum; FX, fornix; CP, choroid plexus; HC, hippocampal commissure; SR, suprapineal recess; PiG, pineal gland; PC, posterior commissure; AS, aqueduct of Sylvius; Me, mesencephalon; Po, pons; MB, mamillary body; TC, tuber cinereus; Hy, hypothalamus; Pi, pituitary gland; OR, optic recess; OC, optic chiasm; LT, lamina terminalis; AC, anterior commissure; FoM, foramen of Monro.)

between the two anterior columns, below the foramens of Monro. The anterior commissure is connected to the optic chiasm by the lamina terminalis. The anterior wall of the third ventricle runs from the foramens of Monro to the optic chiasm.

The posterior limbs (crura) of the fornix are interconnected by the hippocampal commissure, which is fused with the lower surface of the corpus callosum.

Beneath the fornix is the tela choroidea, which is formed by two thin leptomeningeal membranes (the superior and inferior membranes) that contain a space called the velum interpositum, in which the vascular layer of the third ventricle runs.[11, 16] Beneath the velum interpositum is the choroid plexus of the third ventricle. The tela choroidea, through the choroidal fissure, forms a continuum with the choroid plexus of the lateral ventricle. The choroidal fissure is an incisura between the lateral edge of the fornix and the superomedial surface of the thalamus, and the choroid plexus of the lateral ventricle is attached to it. The attachment of the choroid plexus of the lateral ventricle to the fornix and to the thalamus is made by ependyma that, from the wall of the lateral ventricle, also covers the choroid plexus. The medial portion of the ependymal layer that attaches the plexus of the lateral ventricle to the fornix is called the taenia fornicis, and the lateral portion that attaches to the thalamus is called the taenia choroidea.[16]

The posterior aspect of the third ventricular cavity is covered by the tela choroidea beneath the hippocampal commissure. Viewed from the inner cavity of the ventricle, starting from above to below, the following structures are evident: the suprapineal recess extending from the posterior layer of the tela choroidea to the pineal gland; the pineal gland, which protrudes into the cavity; the pineal recess extending posteriorly toward the quadrigeminal cistern; and the two commissures of the posterior part of the third ventricle (the abenula and the posterior commissure), which cross the midline and the orifice of the aqueduct of Sylvius.

The oval medial surface of the thalamus (superiorly) and the hypothalamus (inferiorly), delineated from each other by the hypothalamic sulcus, form the lateral wall of the ventricle. The superomedial border of the thalamus is marked by the eminence of the striae medullaris thalami, close to the attachment of the tela choroidea. On the oval surface of the thalamus, almost in its mid-position, the massa intermedia often interconnects the two opposite thalami.

The floor of the third ventricle is formed by the hypothalamus anteriorly and by the mesencephalon posteriorly. The anteroinferior margin of the cavity of the third ventricle is formed by a prominence due to the optic chiasm. Behind this prominence, the infundibular recess extends into the infundibulum and, more posteriorly, the inner surface of the floor of the third ventricle is indented by the prominences of the mamillary bodies. The portion of the floor between the mamillary bodies and the aqueduct of Sylvius corresponds to the posterior perforated substance and the medial part of the cerebral peduncle.

Different vascular structures run within and around the third ventricle.[11, 16, 17] Between the two sheets of the tela choroidea (the superior and inferior membranes) lies the vascular layer of the roof of the third ventricle, in which the medial posterior choroidal arteries and the internal cerebral veins are located. The space in which the vascular layer of the third ventricle is located is known as the velum interpositum.

The medial posterior choroidal artery arises proximally from the posterior cerebral artery, which, in its course toward the quadrigeminal cistern and at the level of the pineal gland, gives rise to the medial branch for supply of the choroid plexus of the third ventricle.

The internal cerebral vein originates at the level of the foramen of Monro from the confluence of multiple veins. The internal cerebral veins course from anterior to posterior in the midline between the two layers of the tela choroidea. At the level of the superolateral surface of the pineal gland, the two internal cerebral veins diverge from the midline and, more posteriorly, converge together to form the vein of Galen.

On each side, the internal cerebral vein receives subependymal tributary veins that run in the wall of the lateral ventricle and collect blood from periventricular white and gray matter and converge into the internal cerebral vein at the level of the foramen of Monro. Three main groups of tributary veins are recognized: the medial group, the lateral group, and the direct lateral and medial veins. The septal vein is the principal medial vein; it crosses the septum pellucidum and the fornix. The lateral group includes the caudate veins, which cross the caudate nucleus and the thalamus from posterolateral to anteromedial, and the thalamostriate vein, which collects blood from the caudate veins. The thalamostriate vein courses from the posterolateral to the anteromedial aspect of the ependymal layer of the frontal horn between the caudate nucleus and the thala-

mus. At the level of the foramen of Monro, it curves medially and joins the internal cerebral vein.

The direct lateral vein runs across the caudate nucleus and the thalamus more posteriorly than the thalamostriate vein; the direct medial vein crosses the posterior part of the septum pellucidum, passes the fornix, and enters posteriorly to the internal cerebral vein.

Below the floor of the third ventricle, the tip of the basilar artery and the posterior part of the circle of Willis are located. Branches of the posterior communicating and posterior cerebral arteries (thalamogeniculate and thalamoperforating arteries) reach the thalamus, the hypothalamus, and the internal capsule. The internal capsule and the posteroinferior aspect of the thalamus also receive branches from the anterior choroidal artery.

The anterior and anterior communicating arteries are intimately related to the lamina terminalis of the anterior wall of the third ventricle; they give rise to perforating branches for the hypothalamus, fornix, septum pellucidum, and striatum.

The anterior cerebral artery, along its course around the corpus callosum, sends tributaries to the corpus callosum, septum pellucidum, and fornix.

## FUNCTIONAL ANATOMY

Compromised memory function is one of the more frequent postoperative deficits reported in surgery of the third ventricle. Although clinicopathologic studies have never clearly defined the precise anatomic substrates of memory, many structures around and within the third ventricle have been reported to be involved in memory disturbances.

### Corpus Callosum

The corpus callosum is a midline structure that interconnects the two hemispheres. Although the limbic system is responsible for temporary storage of short-term memory (see later), the rostral tract of the corpus callosum is implicated in memory retrieval, which depends on interhemispheric interaction and association.

It is well documented in the literature that section of the entire corpus callosum is followed by the disconnection syndrome (i.e., akinetic mutism, motor apraxia, tactile agnosia, auditory suppression, hemialexia, hemianopia).[12, 18–21]

Section of the corpus callosum that spares the splenium does not produce disconnection syndrome: mutism is rare and transient and so are the language, auditory, and somesthesic effects. Section of the splenium of the corpus callosum commonly causes left hemialexia with and without agraphia. Section of the anterior two thirds of the corpus callosum does not produce the disconnection syndrome; memory deficits are of a lesser degree compared with those in patients undergoing complete commissurotomy.

Limited section (2.5 cm) of the anterior portion of the corpus callosum does not produce measurable memory deficits.[1, 6, 12]

## Hippocampus, Fornix, Septum, Thalamus, and Gyrus Cinguli: The Limbic System

Alteration of the limbic system is almost always reported in many pathologic conditions (e.g., trauma, tumor, infarction, encephalitis, Alzheimer's disease, and Korsakoff's syndrome) that produce memory deficits.[21] Manipulation or significant lesions of the dorsal, lateral, and ventral aspects of the third ventricle can disrupt the major connections between the components of the limbic system, which, besides being manipulated during surgery, can be invaded by or can be the site of origin of tumors of the third ventricle.

The limbic system is composed of complex neural pathways that interconnect the various components to each other and includes the hippocampus, fornix, septum, thalamus, hypothalamus, and cingulate gyrus.[21–24]

The limbic system is the main system for the temporary storage of short-term memory traces, from which long-term memory is eventually consolidated at the cortical level. Moreover, the limbic system is responsible for spatial orientation of recent memory and, because it projects to endocrine and autonomic centers, also affects vegetative functions.

Lesions of the different neural components of the limbic system, as well as disconnection of each center from the others, have been reported to be responsible for memory deficits, spatial disorientation, inability to interact with the environment, and alteration of behavior.

Involvement of the hippocampal formation, mainly when bilateral, is followed by severe impairment of learning ability and loss of recent memory.

Although the role of the fornix and the consequences of its dissection in determining memory disturbances are still under debate, there is both clinical and experimental evidence that sectioning of the anterior columns of the fornix produces memory disturbances.[4, 6, 23–25]

Experimental lesions of the septum have led to a reduced ability to interact and pay attention to the environment, and produce hyperemotional responses. The medial and lateral nuclei of the septum are located in its anterior portion, in front of the anterior commissure. Fenestration of the septum to access the contralateral ventricle therefore must be performed in its highest portion, posterior to the foramen of Monro.

The thalamus and the dorsomedial thalamic nuclei seem to be more important in the process of recent memory storage than the hippocampus. Thalamic lesions result in severe memory disturbances and reduced initiative.

Other structures crucial to recent memory are the anterior commissure, the superior thalamic peduncle, and the thalamostriate pathway.

## Hypothalamus

The hypothalamus forms the floor of the third ventricle below the foramens of Monro and extends from the preoptic area to the mamillary bodies.[26] It contains a complex group of nuclei that play an important role in the regulation of anterior and posterior pituitary functions.

The tuberoinfundibular neurons are contained in the tuber cinereum, which, along with the median eminence of the infundibulum, gives rise to the pituitary stalk. The projection of these areas to the brain stem and forebrain is the anatomic basis for coordination of autonomic and behavioral responses to pituitary secretion.

The hypothalamic-hypophysial system plays a leading role in the regulation of homeostasis, endocrinologic patterns, and behavioral state. Alteration of this system results in dysregulation of water balance and body temperature; alterations in level of alertness and consciousness and the sleep-wake cycle; modification of pituitary functions (i.e., panhypopituitarism or hypopituitarism, hypogonadism, obesity, hypothyroidism, compromised adrenal function, hypotension), and changes in behavioral state.

## OPERATIVE APPROACH

### Preparation

Appropriate diagnosis and treatment of air embolism should be planned and a central venous catheter along with Doppler ultrasound and end-tidal $P_{CO_2}$ monitoring must be placed.

If tumor characteristics permit, a spinal needle for CSF drainage may be placed and mannitol used to relax the brain and obtain a wider exposure, necessitating less reflection of the brain.

The patient is positioned in the supine position with the back raised and the head flexed (35 degrees) and fixed by a pin-type headholder (Fig. 61–6). Care must be taken to prevent any change in head position during surgery. The position of the head has to be secured and the angle of the head has to be memorized by the surgeon to allow correct entry into the desired ventricle, neither too rostral nor too caudal to the foramen of Monro.

Tumors of the third ventricle are removed using standard microsurgical techniques.

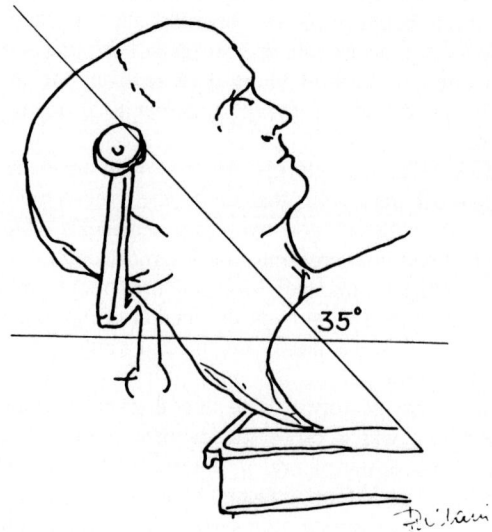

**FIGURE 61–6** ■ Positioning of the patient: the head is fixed and flexed 35 degrees from the longitudinal axis.

## Bone Flap

The corpus callosum is approached surgically through a frontal bone flap on the right side. The skin incision can be either linear or S-shaped or shaped like a question mark, with a tract parallel to the midline from anterior to posterior and then curving caudally toward the zygoma (Fig. 61–7).

The free bone flap can be either quadrangular (four holes) or triangular (three holes; our preferred method), with each margin not greater than 5 cm in length. The medial margin of the bone flap can be placed either 1 cm left of the midline or exactly along the midline, overlapping and exposing the sagittal sinus. The medial margin of the bone flap is cut in an oblique way. The inner table and the spongiosa covering the midline is then removed, providing good visualization of the superior sagittal sinus. With the outer table left intact, a good repositioning of the bone flap can be obtained (see Fig. 61–7).

The two bur holes along the midline are placed so that the medial anteroposterior margin of the bone flap will be anterior to the coronal suture for two thirds of its length and posterior for one third. Placing the posterior bur hole more than 2 cm posterior to the coronal suture can lead to positioning of the retractor just at the level of the supplementary motor area, thus increasing the chance of postoperative hemiparesis.

A U-shaped incision of the dura is made with its base along the sagittal sinus (see Fig. 61–7). The dural incision should reach the edges of the sagittal sinus and the flaps reflected and secured on the opposite side, thus permitting good visualization of the medial part of the frontal lobe and the falx. Dural flaps should not be so tight as to close the superior sagittal sinus.

## Approaching the Corpus Callosum

The medial aspect of the right frontal lobe should be retracted after the medial margin of the hemisphere is freed from Pacchioni granulations and cortical veins entering the sagittal sinus. These veins should be dissected and displaced from the sinus, without sacrificing them if possible, making an entry corridor through the bridging veins. Preoperative angiography can give useful information regarding the number and dimension of the cortical veins, and their relationship with the superior sagittal sinus. The bone flap can then be tailored according to the distribution of the veins, coagulation of which should be avoided because it can result in cerebral infarction, sometimes favored by the cerebral edema that follows positioning of the retractor over the hemisphere. Edema and infarction can be responsible for postoperative hemiparesis.

Displacement of the medial aspect of the hemisphere should not exceed 3 cm in length (the width of the retractor). If the tension on the brain is considered excessive, CSF drainage through the spinal needle or infusion of mannitol usually results in improved brain relaxation and eases the positioning of the retractors.

Entering the interhemispheric space, care must be taken in maintaining cortical pial layer integrity and identifying the cingulate gyri. The two cingulate gyri are often attached to each other and can be misidentified and confused with the corpus callosum. Entering the gyrus cinguli, besides making the approach to the corpus callosum more difficult, would result in direct injury to this structure. The cingulate gyrus is more vascularized than the callosum and contains gray matter. When the two cingulate gyri are displaced, one medially and one laterally, the main trunks of anterior cerebral arteries are visualized. Pericallosal arteries are

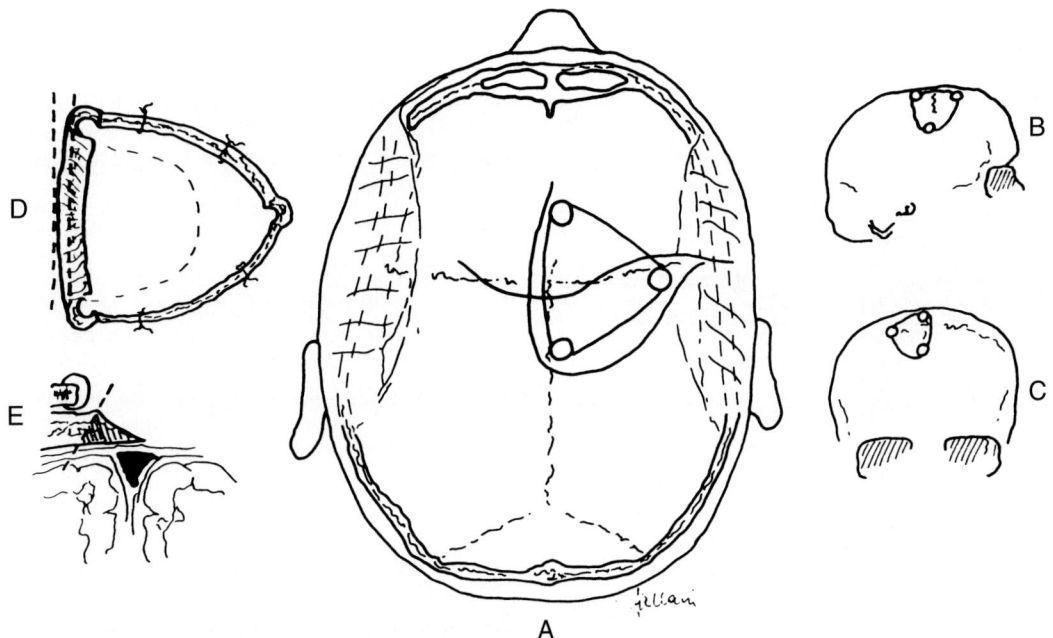

A

**FIGURE 61–7** ■ *A,* Different options of skin incision in relationship with the bur holes of the bone flap and the coronal suture. *B* and *C,* Lateral and anteroposterior views of the triangular bone flap for the access to the anterior portion of the corpus callosum. *D,* Line of incision for the dura opening. *E,* Coronal view of the medial margin of the bone flap cut obliquely. The inner table and the spongiosa *(hatched tract)* is removed over the midline, allowing a good visualization of the superior sagittal sinus. Leaving the outer table intact, the bone flap can be well repositioned.

easily displaced either to the left or to the right, or one to the right and one to the left. Dissection from the cingulate gyri sometimes requires the sacrifice of small tributaries from the pericallosal arteries.

At this point, the cortex must be protected with cottonoids, and a self-retaining retractor with a 2-cm blade can be positioned. A second retractor over the falx can also be set out, so that the falx is pushed toward the left and the view is enlarged (Fig. 61–8). The superficial layer of the corpus callosum appears whiter than the surrounding cortical structure, bright, and almost avascular, apart from some small running veins.[27]

After accurate cauterization of the pial layer of the corpus callosum, a vertical incision 2 cm long is made. The landmarks for a correct incision of the corpus callosum are the coronal suture for exact orientation of the angulation of the foramen of Monro, and the caudal border of the falx for the midline, thus avoiding incorrect entry into the left or right lateral ventricle. The incision of the corpus callosum can be placed over the midline or just to its left

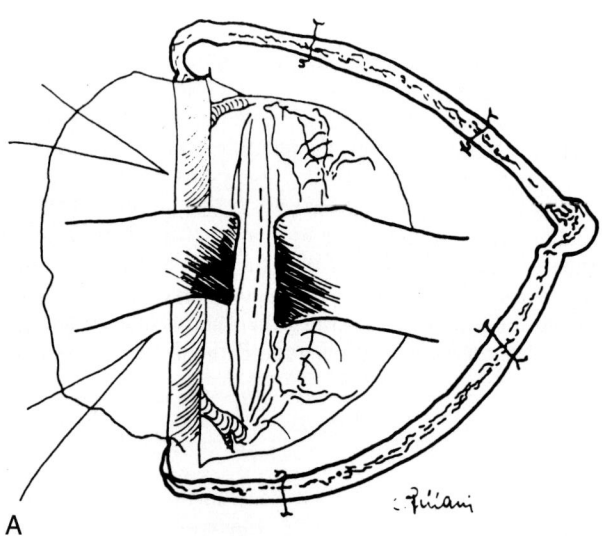

A

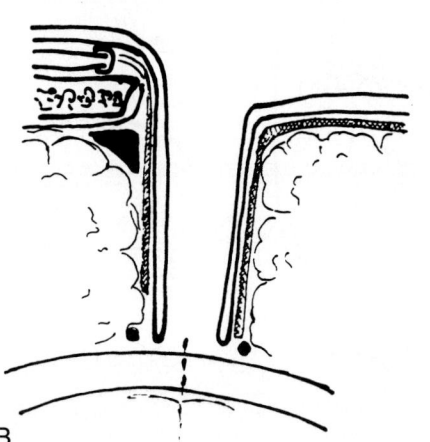

B

FIGURE 61–8 ■ Positioning of the retractors (over the hemisphere and the falx) to expose the corpus callosum after pericallosal and callosomarginal arteries have been divaricated. A, Superior view. B, Coronal view.

or right, according to what entry route into the third ventricle is desired, or which lateral ventricle the surgeon wants to reach.

The corpus callosum is penetrated by blunt dissection and suctioning. Its thickness can be calculated from sagittal magnetic resonance images (MRI); it varies greatly according to the degree of ventricular dilatation. The ependymal layer of the lateral ventricle is then easily recognized because the color and consistency of the tissue change. Opening the ependyma is followed by CSF leakage and visualization of the lateral ventricular cavity.

## Entering the Lateral Ventricle

At this point, it may be difficult for the surgeon to recognize whether the entry has been made into the left or right lateral ventricle. Precise landmarks are the choroid plexus, which runs from the lateral to the medial aspect of the lateral ventricle and terminates at the level of the foramen of Monro, and the thalamostriate and septal veins. However, in some circumstances, because of decompression of the entered ventricle, the septum pellucidum can be bent inward and obscure the view of the medial structures of the ventricle. The septum can be moved medially or can be widely fenestrated in its posterior part, allowing a complete exposure of both lateral ventricles.

When the desired lateral ventricle is exposed, the retractors are deeply advanced and the lateral and medial borders of the corpus callosum retracted.

## Corridors to the Third Ventricle

Two main corridors provide access to the third ventricular cavity: the transforaminal and the interfornicial entry[1, 4–6, 8, 12, 13, 25] (Fig. 61–9). The choice of appropriate entry largely depends on the position, size, and anatomic characteristics of the tumor (e.g., vascularization, consistency, adherence to surrounding structures) and its relationship to the foramen of Monro. The entry should be carefully evaluated and planned by the surgeon in light of detailed MRI in different planes.

### Transforaminal Entry

Lesions in the third ventricle can alter the foramen of Monro: it can be enlarged because of coexistent hydrocephalus, or it can be slit-like. Moreover, some tumors arising from the thalamus can elevate the floor of the lateral ventricle and obliterate the foramen (see Fig. 61–4).

Only tumors visible by direct microsurgical inspection of the foramen and that enlarge the foramen or come out from it (see Fig. 61–2) can be treated by a transforaminal entry (Fig. 61–10): we do not recommend the section of one or both fornices to enlarge the exposure anteriorly, or removal of tissue from the posteroinferior aspect of the foramen to gain a better posterior view, because severe postoperative deficits can arise.[25] To gain a better view of the posterior aspects of the foramen of Monro, we prefer alternative routes (see later). However, as reported by Ture and colleagues,[13] the foramen of Monro can be posteriorly

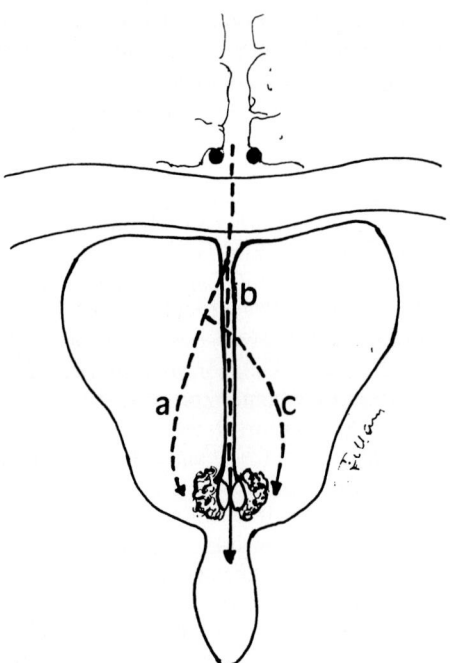

**FIGURE 61–9** ■ Diagram showing the two main options to enter the third ventricle cavity through the transcallosal approach: transforaminal (a) and interforniceal (b). Opening the septum allows the visualization of the contralateral foramen of Monro (c).

enlarged without tissue damage if the location of the junction between the anterior septal and internal cerebral veins is posterior.

The foramen provides access to the tumor, and space is gained by sharp dissection, gentle retraction, and intracap-

sular suction of the mass, getting the surface free from the surrounding cerebral structures by a progressive shrinking of the capsule itself. Any traction to the mass must be avoided because it can facilitate bleeding, mainly from the posterior portion of the tumor mass.

Anterosuperior detachment of the tumor could lead to some damage to the fornix from the manipulation of this structure; on the other hand, injury to the tela choroidea and internal cerebral veins remains the main risk during both the posterior enlargement of the foramen of Monro and the detachment of the posterior part of the tumor.

Difficulty in separating the tumor capsule from the choroid plexus, tela choroidea, and internal cerebral veins can lead to bleeding from the roof of the third ventricle, and sometimes the bleeding cannot be appreciated until the entire ventricle is filled with blood. Hemorrhage from a blind surface of the ventricle can be managed only with great difficulty; repeated rinsing and positioning of a piece of sponge and gently pushing, using a curved dissector as counterforce, can be very helpful.

After completion of tumor removal, care must be taken to determine the presence of tumor remnants or clots that can produce acute obstruction of the foramens of Monro or aqueduct of Sylvius. We recommend an accurate rinse and direct visualization of the third ventricular cavity using a mirror or an endoscope.

## Interforniceal Entry

The interforniceal approach must be planned before surgery using accurate neuroradiologic assessment. MRI in different planes and cerebral angiography or MR angiography can afford important information about vascular anatomy and, particularly, the anatomy of the corpus callosum, sep-

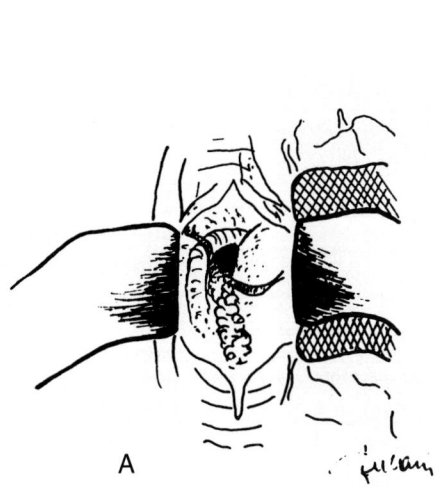

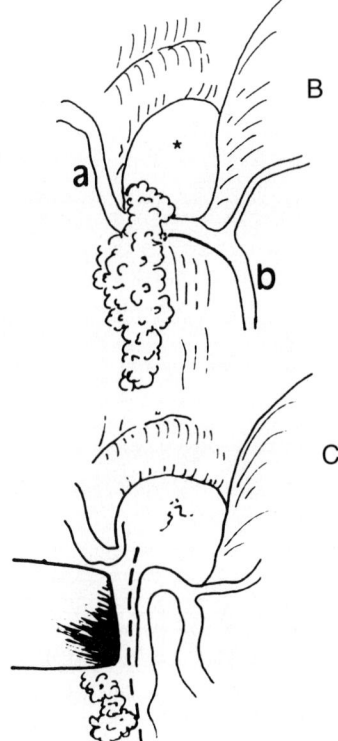

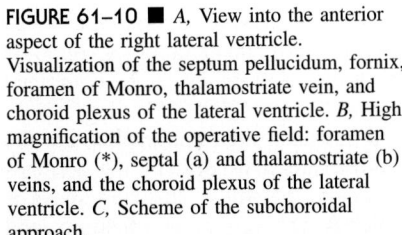

**FIGURE 61–10** ■ *A,* View into the anterior aspect of the right lateral ventricle. Visualization of the septum pellucidum, fornix, foramen of Monro, thalamostriate vein, and choroid plexus of the lateral ventricle. *B,* High magnification of the operative field: foramen of Monro (*), septal (a) and thalamostriate (b) veins, and the choroid plexus of the lateral ventricle. *C,* Scheme of the subchoroidal approach.

tum pellucidum, and fornices and their relationship with the mass in the ventricular cavity. Interforniceal entry is the corridor of choice for tumors located in the mid-third portion of the third ventricular chamber, or for tumors that occupy the entire cavity of the third ventricle (see Fig. 61–3).

After dissection of the corpus callosum, the surgeon has two options: identification and separation of the leaves of the septum before entering the lateral ventricle, or entering the lateral ventricle and sectioning the septum pellucidum.

After completion of the corpus callosum dissection and appreciation of the ependymal layer and underlying lateral ventricle, the line of attachment of the septum can sometimes be recognized.[4, 5] The two leaves of the septum can then be split away (this maneuver can be easily performed if a cavum Vergae is present), after which the median raphe of the fornices can be reached. However, in the presence of large masses that completely fill the cavity of the third ventricle, the roof of the third ventricle can be raised up by the tumor. In this case, the septum is no longer evident and the fornices are in direct contact with the corpus callosum, and sometimes spread apart; thus, once the dissection of the corpus callosum is completed, the surgeon can continue the dissection over the midline, obtaining entry to the third ventricle between the two fornices (Fig. 61–11; see also Fig. 61–3).

When the leaves of the septum are not identifiable from the ependymal layer of the lateral ventricle before entering it, the surgeon can enter the lateral ventricle and then, after identification of the different structures, can fenestrate the septum just posterior to the foramen of Monro and the septal vein, thus opening the contralateral ventricle.[4, 5] Because the septum is attached to the dorsomedial aspect of the fornices, it serves as a landmark for the midline, allowing a precise midline entry between the two fornices. These have to be bluntly and gently dissected for approximately 2 cm of posterior extension, starting just posterior to the foramen of Monro.

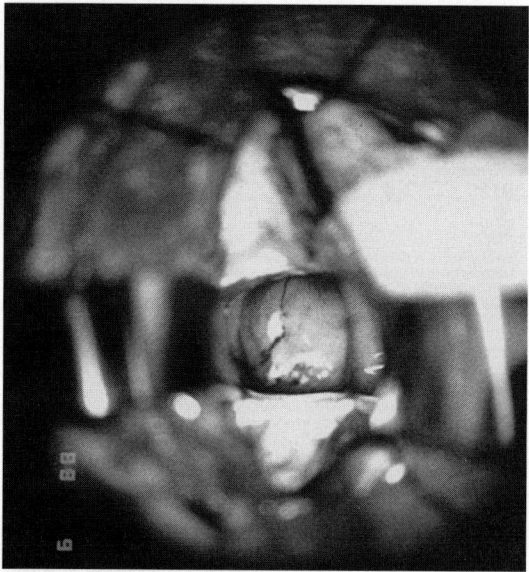

FIGURE 61–11 ■ Operative field of the transcallosal interforniceal approach: the tumor mass becomes apparent as soon as the fornices are divaricated.

The anterior and posterior boundaries of the interforniceal incision are represented by the anterior commissure and hippocampal commissure, respectively, which must be preserved because any lesion of these structures can lead to permanent memory deficits.

Once the interforniceal space is opened, the cavity of the third ventricle is apparent and the tumor is recognized. Entering the roof of the third ventricle through the interforniceal corridor, the surgeon must bear clearly in mind the anatomy of different vascular and nervous structures: tumors located in the middle portion of the third ventricle can displace the vascular layer, mainly the internal cerebral veins and medial posterior choroidal arteries, and modify their normal anatomy. Should these vessels be immediately recognized once dissection of the fornices is completed, the veins and arteries can be gently dissected and lateralized from the tela choroidea.

Standard microsurgical techniques are required to remove the tumor; when visible and distinguishable from surrounding normal tissue, the superficial layer of the mass can be coagulated and then incised, and the inner content progressively aspirated with an ultrasound aspirator. Difficulties in the total removal of intraventricular masses arise with tumors whose boundaries are not clearly separate and distinct from normal tissue. Particular attention must be paid to the lateral and anteroposterior boundaries of the tumor during its separation from the vascular structures of the roof (internal cerebral veins and posterior choroidal arteries), the lateral walls of the third ventricle (thalamus), and the anteroinferior portion of the floor of the third ventricle (hypothalamus). Removal of the more posterior portion of the tumor, sometimes not visible through the direct transcallosal interforniceal route, can be achieved by modifying the microscope's angulation or altering the patient's head positioning.

As soon as the inferior part of the tumor is completely removed, basal structures may be visualized progressively: from the posterior to anterior aspects, the surgeon can appreciate the prepontine cistern, basilar circulation vessels (basilar tip, posterior cerebral, and anterosuperior cerebellar arteries), clivus, posterior clinoids, anterior circulation vessels (anterior cerebral and communicating arteries), and dorsum sellae.

## Alternative and Combined Routes

When the surgeon is planning alternative routes to the third ventricle other than the aforementioned entries, detailed preoperative neuroradiologic evaluation of the anatomic relationships of the tumor is required. Tumors that are entirely confined in the third ventricle, located in its posteroinferior third, and do not alter either the foramen of Monro or the fornix and septum pellucidum, can be approached through a subchoroidal or transchoroidal route.[16, 28–30] In addition, if a transforaminal or interforniceal entry has been chosen and these corridors do not enable complete removal of the tumor, these alternative entry routes can be combined with that initially chosen.

The subchoroidal and transchoroidal approaches use the corridor between the inferolateral aspects of the fornices and the medial aspects of the thalamus. This thin space is filled by the choroid plexus, the velum interpositum, and the venous and arterial system of the diencephalon. There are two main options in relation to the thalamostriate vein, the anterior (subchoroidal) and the posterior (transchoroidal) approaches.

## SUBCHOROIDAL TRANS-VELUM INTERPOSITUM APPROACH

As soon as the right lateral ventricle is entered and all the structures well recognized, the choroid plexus of the lateral ventricle is anteriorly moved and elevated so that the dorsomedial aspect of the thalamus is exposed.[29]

To gain and enlarge the view, the plexus can be coagulated and shrunk and the leptomeninges of the velum interpositum gently cut (see Fig. 61–10). This procedure allows the surgeon to visualize the confluence of the septal and thalamostriate veins into the internal cerebral vein and the group of subependymal thalamic veins (mainly the anterior and posterior groups) that run on the anterior and superior aspects of the thalamus and drain to the thalamostriate and internal cerebral veins, respectively. The thalamostriate vein (sometimes with the septal vein) can be coagulated and cut: advancing the retractors along the medial wall of the thalamus and the inferior border of the fornix, a good access to the cavity of the third ventricle is gained. In this access, a corridor is created beneath the choroidal plexus of the lateral ventricle and the internal cerebral vein and above the superomedial aspect of the thalamus.

### TRANSCHOROIDAL APPROACH

Transchoroidal approaches enter the third ventricle through the velum interpositum behind the thalamostriate vein, and do not require its cutting.[28–30]

The corridor may be created either by dividing the attachment of the choroid plexus of the lateral ventricle from the fornix in its superior portion at the level of the choroidal fissure, or by separating the inferior aspect of the choroid plexus from the internal cerebral vein, the leptomeninges of the tela choroidea, and the superomedial aspect of the thalamus. Both these corridors enter the cavity of the third ventricle posterior to the thalamostriate vein and the foramen of Monro.

In the transchoroidal superior approach, the taenia fornicis can be easily identified because it is formed by the ependymal layer that covers the lateral ventricle and the plexus and is located between the inferolateral portion of the fornix and the superomedial aspect of the plexus of the lateral ventricle.[16] Once the taenia fornicis is opened, the superior membrane of the tela choroidea becomes apparent. The tela has to be opened so that the internal cerebral vein and the medial posterior choroidal artery can be exposed, separated, and gently moved laterally. Beneath these vessels are the inferior membrane of the tela choroidea and the plexus of the third ventricle: their dissection should start medial to the internal cerebral vein, from the posterior aspect of the third ventricle cavity toward the foramen of Monro. When dissection of the different layers of the tela choroidea is completed, the entire cavity of the third ventricle can be visualized. However, the presence of a mass in the third ventricle can grossly alter the anatomy of the various layers of the third ventricular roof: it may not be possible to distinguish the two membranes from each other,

and the vein and the artery can be displaced upward, inward, or laterally.

In the transchoroidal inferior approach, the taenia choroidea is opened. In this approach, manipulation of the upper thalamic surface and the veins than run in its superficial layer could increase the risk of their damage.[16]

The major risks in both transchoroidal entries are possible damage to the internal cerebral and thalamic veins as well as to the fornix, which sometimes must be elevated, and to the thalamus, which has to be displaced laterally to allow the entry to the third ventricular cavity.

Based on our experience, the different options for trans-velum interpositum access should be tailored during surgery. Sectioning the thalamostriate vein and the septal vein could lead to infarction of the thalamic and septal structures. This complication can increase the risk of postoperative hemiparesis and severe memory disturbances. Thus, thalamostriate and septal veins should be spared as often as possible and the approach to the posterior portion of the third ventricle should be gained first through a posterior enlargement of the foramen of Monro, with an anterior opening of the velum interpositum in there is a posterior location and junction between the anterior septal and internal cerebral veins,[16] or through a superior transchoroidal approach that initially spares the thalamostriate vein.

## Closure

When the tumor has been removed as completely as possible and meticulous hemostasis of the operative field obtained, an intraventricular catheter is placed into the cavity of the third ventricle, which is then filled with saline.

The retractors are gently removed under direct vision and the borders of the line of incision of the corpus callosum along with the medial aspect of the hemisphere are carefully inspected for bleeding. The closure of the dura, resecuring of the bone flap, positioning of drainage, and closure of the galea and skin are performed using standard surgical procedures.

The intraventricular catheter can then be connected to an external transducer for continuous intracranial pressure monitoring.

## COMPLICATIONS

Most of the complications of third ventricular surgery are related to the location of the lesion rather than to the approach.

Intraventricular and other intracranial hemorrhages (epidural and intracerebral) are rarely observed but require immediate reoperation to detect the source of bleeding. Massive intraventricular hemorrhage from the ependyma layer, choroid plexuses, and tumor remnants can be prevented by meticulous coagulation of any source of bleeding, continuous irrigation of the ventricular cavity, and adequate cauterization of tumor remnants when complete excision of the tumor is thought to be contraindicated. Indirect (using a mirror or an endoscopic device) or direct microscopic visualization of the ventricular cavity is highly recommended at the end of the operation. This allows the surgeon to visualize the possible presence of a blind site of bleeding, or occlusion of the aqueduct of Sylvius or the foramen of Monro. We routinely perform an immediate postoperative computed tomography (CT) scan to evaluate the presence of intracranial hemorrhages. Positioning of an intraventricular catheter, besides continuously measuring the intracranial pressure over the postoperative course, allows immediate drainage when a sudden increase of intracranial pressure is detected.

Postoperative pneumocephalus is often observed after third ventricular surgery and does not represent a major complication.

Persistent CSF subdural collection is often observed in the transcortical transventricular approach to the third ventricle, but is rare in the transcallosal approach, and has never been observed in our series.

Bacterial meningitis and ventriculitis are rare: the use of prophylactic antibiotics is questionable in preventing infectious complications. Serial CSF cell count and culture and identification of the infectious agent seem the best procedures for choosing a correct antibiotic regimen. Broad-spectrum antibiotic therapy should be started if there is an increase in CSF cells and proteins. Although the diagnosis is sometimes difficult, aseptic meningitis must be presumed when CSF cultures are persistently negative and CSF cell count and chemistry do not suggest infection. Aseptic meningitis can be observed after the removal of a colloid cyst or in the case of partial removal of an intra-axial tumor, and requires corticosteroid treatment.

Despite total removal of tumor masses in the third ventricle, the reopening of the foramens of Monro, and the avoidance of intraventricular bleeding, re-establishment of CSF pathways is not always obtained. Ventricular dilatation is present in more than 50% of patients with third ventricular tumors, and one third of these require a permanent CSF shunt.[6]

Early postoperative seizures are rarely observed after the transcallosal approach and are controlled with anticonvulsant therapy. Late epilepsy, observed in more than 20% of patients operated through a transcortical transventricular route, has never been observed in our series of patients operated with a transcallosal approach.[6]

Large or confined areas of brain edema or infarction, due to either direct venous drainage compromise or arterial occlusion or indirect occlusion by the retractor, are the main factors responsible for postoperative hemiparesis.[5, 8, 12] Hemiparesis is usually transient[5, 6] unless large portions of the hemispheres are involved.[14] Although vascular manipulation is a significant factor in this complication, postoperative hemiparesis may also be directly related to the tumor masses themselves, which may have required prolonged manipulation of the walls of the third ventricle to be removed.[7, 8] Accordingly, surgery of large intra-axial tumors that invade and distend the walls of the ventricle as well as extra-axial neoplasms that are strictly adherent to the ventricular walls could result in secondary injury to the thalamus, internal capsule, and deep diencephalic structures.

In our experience, diencephalohypothalamic involvement remains a major complication of third ventricular surgery because it produces severe metabolic derangement, gastrointestinal bleeding, diabetes insipidus, alterations of alertness and consciousness, and an akinetic mutism–like status.

Akinetic mutism is reported with variable incidence in the literature[5, 6, 10, 12, 15, 18–20] and is the result of involvement of the inferior frontal lobes and cingulate gyri outside the third ventricular region.[6, 12, 15, 21]

Memory disturbances have been reported frequently in patients submitted to transcallosal or transcortical approaches to third ventricular tumors; they usually involve short-term memory and in general are transient.[4–8, 12, 21–25, 31–34] Incision of the anterior part of the corpus callosum for the limited length necessary to provide access to the third ventricle (Fig. 61–12) does not seem, in itself, to produce permanent and measurable memory deficits.[5, 6, 12, 29] Psychological and memory disturbances are often observed as presenting symptoms in patients with third ventricular tumors, and in many instances they disappear after surgery.[6] Permanent memory losses are mainly related to the maneuvers necessary for removal of the tumor, rather than to the approach itself.[7, 8] In our experience, permanent memory loss was observed in a patient with postoperative alteration of the septal and forniceal areas.[6, 22–25, 31]

A disconnection syndrome or impairment of the frontal functions (i.e., attention, intelligence, and verbal fluency) usually is not observed at long-term neuropsychological evaluation of patients submitted to the transcallosal approach.[6]

## PERSONAL SERIES

Between 1984 and 1997, 193 patients with tumors located in and around the third ventricle were observed at our institution: 86 were operated on through different surgical approaches (transcortical transventricular, 21; transcallosal transventricular, 39; translamina terminalis, 4; pterional, 16; suboccipital transtentorial, 5; and suboccipital supracer-

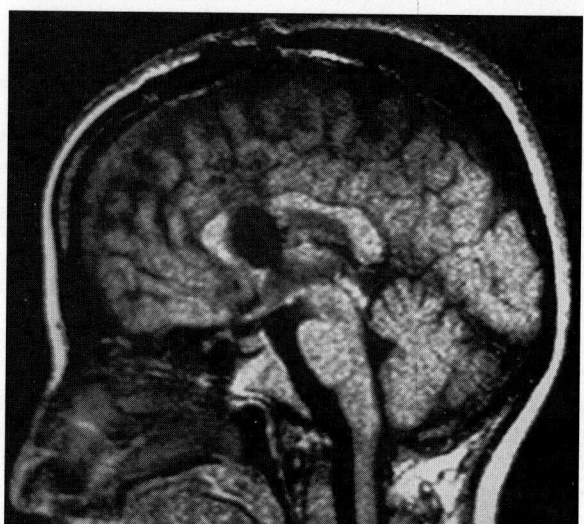

**FIGURE 61–12** ■ Postoperative sagittal T$_1$-weighted magnetic resonance image of a third ventricle tumor completely removed. The incision of the corpus callosum is evident.

ebellar, 1). Of 39 patients operated through a transcallosal route, 15 were male and 24 female. Age ranged from 4 to 65 years.

Headache was the most common initial complaint, usually referred to the frontal or retro-orbital area (33 cases; 84%); in four patients headache was paroxysmal or intermittent and positional (10%). Obesity, impotence, dysmenorrhea, diabetes insipidus, and sleep-wake cycle alterations were evident in nine patients (23%). Four patients (10%) had temporary loss of vision or diplopia. An epileptic seizure was the first symptom in one patient (2.5%).

Signs of increased intracranial pressure (papilledema with and without decreased visual acuity) were evident in 20 patients (51%). Hypothalamohypophysial dysfunction (partial or panhypopituitarism) was demonstrated in 23% of cases (nine patients). Gait disturbances and pyramidal tract signs were evident in five patients (13%). Decreased visual acuity or visual field defects were seen in five patients (13%). An organic mental syndrome (confusion, memory loss, and urinary incontinence) was reported in seven cases (18%); in addition, one patient was lethargic and one was comatose.

Lesions distending the foramen of Monro were approached by a transforaminal entry (20 cases; 51%; see Fig. 61–2). Fourteen patients harboring large masses distending and occupying the entire cavity of the third ventricle were approached by an interforniceal route (36%; see Fig. 61–3). An interseptal or trans-septal route provided complete exposure of the ventricular cavity, and the midline basal structures were largely exposed. Tumor masses located posterior to the foramen of Monro that were not visualized through a transforaminal route were approached by a transchoroidal or subchoroidal entry (five cases; 13%; see Fig. 61–4).

Four patients (10%) underwent a second operation: two were aged 10 and 6 years and had incomplete removal of tumor (one pilocytic and one low-grade glioma) demonstrated on postoperative MRI. They underwent a second procedure 3 and 5 months, respectively, after the first procedure, and the tumors were completely removed.

The remaining two patients were reoperated on 17 months and 5 years, respectively, after the first procedure for a regrowth of the tumor (one astrocytoma and one oligodendroglioma).

Complete resection of the mass, documented on postoperative CT or MRI, was achieved in all 15 patients with extra-axial tumors. In patients with intra-axial tumors (24 cases), total removal was achieved in 66% (16 patients) with the first procedure and in 75% after the second approach.

Histologic assessment of the third ventricular tumors of our series revealed that 61.5% of the tumors (24 patients) were intra-axial and 38.5% extra-axial (15 cases; Table 61–1). Among the former, low-grade gliomas (fibrillary and protoplasmatic variants of astrocytoma and giant cell astrocytoma) and pilocytic astrocytomas were more frequently observed. Rare tumors included ependymoma, ependymoblastoma, neurocytoma, and glioblastoma. Colloid cysts (nine cases) were the most common variant among the extra-axial tumors, whereas craniopharyngiomas (two cases) were less frequently observed. Rare tumors

### TABLE 61–1 ■ HISTOLOGY OF THIRD VENTRICULAR TUMORS: 39 CASES APPROACHED THROUGH THE TRANSCALLOSAL ROUTE

| Intra-axial (24) | |
|---|---|
| Pilocytic astrocytoma | 4 |
| Low-grade glioma* | 11 |
| Giant cell astrocytoma | 2 |
| Subependymoma | 3 |
| Ependymoma | 2 |
| Neurocytoma | 1 |
| Glioblastoma | 1 |
| **Extra-axial (15)** | |
| Colloid cyst | 9 |
| Craniopharyngioma | 3 |
| Pituitary adenoma† | 1 |
| Lymphocytic hypophysitis | 1 |
| Metastasis | 1 |

*Fibrillary and protoplasmatic variants.
†Ectopic.

included metastasis, ectopic pituitary adenoma, and lymphocytic hypophysitis.

As a result of the first surgical procedure, two patients died (5%). In one case, the patient with a lymphocytic hypophisitis, the postoperative course was characterized by an akinetic mutism–like status and a diencephalic syndrome (diabetes insipidus, electrolyte imbalance, hyperthermia), and the patient died 72 days after surgery. The second patient, with an ependymoma, died of postoperative hematoma 3 days after surgery.

Major postoperative complications were hemiparesis (five patients; 13%) and diabetes insipidus (six patients; 15%). Hemiparesis was moderate and had resolved in four patients by the 6-month follow-up. Persistent diabetes insipidus was present in one patient. Four of the seven patients with preoperative psychic disturbances experienced a normalization of mental performance. Epileptic seizures never appeared in the postoperative course of these patients.

Patients who underwent a second procedure had no mortality or significant morbidity.

In spite of an anatomically opened foramen of Monro after the surgical procedure, 10 of 21 patients with preoperative hydrocephalus had persistent ventricular enlargement; in 9 patients, a permanent CSF shunt was implanted.

## CONCLUSIONS

Reaching the third ventricular cavity obliges the surgeon to choose a route that invariably requires an incision of the brain parenchyma. Therefore, the method of choice is that which causes the least amount of clinically relevant brain damage. In the transcallosal approach, microsurgical techniques limit the damage because a 2-cm opening of the corpus callosum allows visualization and treatment of intraventricular lesions with sufficient safety.

Anatomically, the transcallosal approach has various advantages. The vascularization of the corpus callosum is modest and thus an incision does not cause great vessels sacrifice. Moreover, both ventricles can be reached through the same incision, and the dimension of the ventricles does not represent a contraindication to this approach. Last, dissection of the corpus callosum carries little or no incidence of postoperative epilepsy. Clinical and neuropsychological evaluations have documented that section of the corpus callosum limited to its anterior third does not, in itself, cause significant deficits in personality or behavior.

Evaluation of damage by partial dissection of the corpus callosum should be compared with those observed after the transcortical-transventricular approach to third ventricular tumors. However, none of the series reported in the literature allow for this because there is always a lesion involving the third ventricle, the removal of which necessarily implicates those structures of the third ventricle that are decisively involved in mnestic and neuropsychic functions.

However, with our data and clinical experience, we believe that the transcallosal approach is the route of first choice to approach tumors of the third ventricle because of its limited mortality and late postoperative morbidity. Although this decision also implies some technical and surgical considerations, the restricted access and the spatial limitations of the transcallosal route, along with the necessary attention to the manipulation of several structures (i.e., the bridging veins, the cortex of the medial aspect of the right hemisphere, the superior sagittal sinus, the pericallosal arteries, and the veins of the corpus callosum), have never prevented the treatment of these neoplasms.

Cases of subtotal or partial removal of tumor are always caused by the difficulty or impossibility of recognizing clear anatomic landmarks, and are never due to the limited corridor of access. Even lesions with heavy bleeding have not caused insurmountable problems of hemostasis, first because spontaneous hemorrhage usually ceases after tumor removal is completed, and second because the operative field is sufficiently exposed to allow direct hemostasis with traditional methods.

Surgical indications for the transcallosal route are confined to tumors that occupy the anterior and middle portion of the third ventricle, as well as those that completely fill the cavity of the third ventricle. The transcallosal route can be combined with subfrontal or interhemispheric approaches when the latter do not enable the surgeon completely to remove tumors arising from the base and secondarily invading the third ventricle.

Tumors of the posterior part of the third ventricle that primarily or secondarily invade the ventricle are better approached through transtentorial suboccipital or infratentorial supracerebellar routes, the discussion of which is beyond the scope of this chapter.

# REFERENCES

1. Apuzzo MLJ, Zee CS, Breeze RE, Day JD: Anterior and mid-third ventricular lesions: A surgical overview. In Apuzzo MLJ (ed): Surgery of the Third Ventricle, 2nd ed. Baltimore: Williams & Wilkins, 1998, pp 635–680.
2. Sano K: Pineal masses: General considerations. In Apuzzo MLJ (ed): Brain Surgery: Complication Avoidance and Management, Vol 1. Edinburgh: Churchill Livingstone, 1993, pp 463–473.
3. Takakura K, Matsumani M: Pineal region masses: Selection of an operative approach. In Apuzzo MLJ (ed): Brain Surgery: Complica-
tion Avoidance and Management, Vol 1. Edinburgh: Churchill Livingstone, 1993, pp 473–485.
4. Apuzzo MLJ, Chikovani O, Gott P et al: Transcallosal interforniceal approaches for lesions affecting the third ventricle: Surgical considerations and consequences. Neurosurgery 10:547–554, 1982.
5. Apuzzo LJ, Amar AP: Transcallosal interforniceal approach. In Apuzzo MLJ (ed): Surgery of the Third Ventricle, 2nd ed. Baltimore: Williams & Wilkins, 1998, pp 421–452.
6. Villani R, Papagno C, Tomei G, et al: Transcallosal approach to tumors of the third ventricle: Surgical results and neuropsychological evaluation. J Neurosurg Sci 41:41–50, 1997.
7. Woiciechowsky C, Vogel S, Lehmann R, et al: Transcallosal removal of lesions affecting the third ventricle: An anatomic and clinical study. Neurosurgery 36:117–123, 1995.
8. Woiciechowsky C, Vogel S, Meyer BU, et al: Neuropsychological and neurophysiological consequences of partial callosotomy. J Neurosurg Sci 41:75–80, 1997.
9. Hutter BO, Spetzger U, Bertalanffy H, et al: Cognition and quality of life in patients after transcallosal microsurgery for midline tumors. J Neurosurg Sci 41:123–129, 1997.
10. Bellotti C, Pappada G, Sani R, et al: The transcallosal approach for lesions affecting the lateral and third ventricle: Surgical considerations and results in a series of 42 cases. Acta Neurochir (Wien) 111:103–107, 1984.
11. Rhoton AL, Yamamoto I, Peace DA: Microsurgery of the third ventricle. Part 2: Operative approaches. Neurosurgery 8:357–373, 1981.
12. Ehni G, Ehni B: Considerations in transforaminal entry. In Apuzzo MLJ (ed): Surgery of the Third Ventricle, 2nd ed. Baltimore: Williams & Wilkins, 1998, pp 391–419.
13. Ture U, Yasargil MG, Al-Mephty O: The transcallosal-transforaminal approach to the third ventricle with regard to the venous variations in this region. J Neurosurg 87:706–715, 1997.
14. Shucart W: The anterior transcallosal and transcortical approach. In Apuzzo MLJ (ed): Surgery of the Third Ventricle, 2nd ed. Baltimore: Williams & Wilkins, 1998, pp 369–389.
15. Nakasu Y, Isozumi T, Nioka H, et al: Mechanism of mutism following the transcallosal approach to the ventricles. Acta Neurochir (Wien) 110:146–153, 1991.
16. When HT, Rhoton AL Jr., de Olivera E: Transchoroidal approach to the third ventricle: An anatomic study of the choroidal fissure and its clinical application. Neurosurgery 42:1205–1219, 1998.
17. Yamamoto I, Rhoton AL, Peace DA: Microsurgery of the third ventricle. Part 1: Microsurgical anatomy. Neurosurgery 8:334–356, 1981.
18. Bogen JE: Physiological consequences of complete or partial commissural section. In Apuzzo MLJ (ed): Surgery of the Third Ventricle, 2nd ed. Baltimore: Williams & Wilkins, 1998, pp 167–186.
19. Habib M: Syndromes de deconnexion calleuse et organization fonctionelle du corps calleux chez l'adulte. Neurochirurgie 44 (Suppl 1):102–109, 1998.
20. Sauerwein HC, Lassonde M: Neuropsychological alterations after split-brain surgery. J Neurosurg Sci 41:59–66, 1997.
21. Damasio AR, Van Hoesen GW, Tranel D: Pathological correlates of amnesia and the anatomical basis of memory. In Apuzzo MLJ (ed): Surgery of the Third Ventricle, 2nd ed. Baltimore: Williams & Wilkins, 1998, pp 187–204.
22. Garretson HD: Memory in man: A neurosurgeon's perspective. In Apuzzo MLJ (ed): Surgery of the Third Ventricle, 2nd ed. Baltimore: Williams & Wilkins, 1998, pp 211–214.
23. Gaffan D: Recognition impaired and association intact in the memory of monkeys after transection of the fornix. J Comp Physiol Psychol 86:1100–1109, 1974.
24. Gaffan D, Gaffan EA: Amnesia in man following transection of the fornix: A review. Brain 114:2611–2618, 1991.
25. McMackin D, Cockburn J, Ansow P, et al: Correlation of fornix damage with memory impairment in six cases of colloid cyst removal. Acta Neurochir (Wien) 135:12–18, 1995.
26. Page RB: Functional anatomy of the human hypothalamus. In Apuzzo MLJ (ed): Surgery of the Third Ventricle, 2nd ed. Baltimore: Williams & Wilkins, 1998, pp 233–251.
27. Kakou M, Velut S, Destrieux C: Vascularisation arterielle et veineuse du corp calleux. Neurochirurgie 44 (Suppl 1):31–37, 1998.
28. Nagata S, Rhoton AL, Barry M: Microsurgical anatomy of the choroidal fissure. Surg Neurol 30:3–59, 1988.
29. Lavyne MH, Patterson RH: The subchoroidal trans-velum interpos-

itum approach. In Apuzzo MLJ (ed): Surgery of the Third Ventricle, 2nd ed. Baltimore: Williams & Wilkins, 1998, pp 453–469.

30. Viale GL, Turtas S: The subchoroidal approach to the third ventricle. Surg Neurol 14:71–76, 1980.

31. Von Cramon DY, Markowitsch HJ, Schuri U: The possible contribution of the septal region to memory. Neuropsychologia 31:1158–1180, 1993.

32. Diamond SJ, Scammel RH, Brouwers EYM, et al: Functions of the centre section (trunk) of the corpus callosum in man. Brain 100:543–562, 1977.

33. Gordon HW: Neuropsychological sequelae of partial commissurotomy. In Boller F, Grafman J (eds): Handbook of Neuropsychology. New York: Elsevier, 1990, pp 85–87.

34. Petrucci RJ, Buchleit WA, Woodruff GC, et al: Transcallosal parafornicial approach for third ventricle tumors: Neuropsychological consequences. Neurosurgery 20:457–464, 1987.

# CHAPTER 62

# Neuroendoscopic Approach to Intraventricular Tumors

■ MICHAEL R. GAAB and HENRY W. S. SCHROEDER

With the development of endoscopic systems properly adapted to neurosurgical demands, endoscopic techniques have been used increasingly in the treatment of various neurosurgical conditions since the late 1980s. Initially, noncommunicating hydrocephalus was the main indication for an intracranial neuroendoscopic procedure. However, with increasing experience and technical advances in endoscopic instrumentation, cystic as well as solid lesions have been treated endoscopically.[1–18]

Intraventricular tumors are ideal lesions for the application of an endoscope. Located in a cerebrospinal fluid (CSF)–filled preformed cavity, which allows a clear view, they can be very well visualized. Intraventricular tumors often cause CSF pathway obstruction and ventricular enlargement, which gives sufficient space for maneuvering with endoscopes and instruments. However, ventricular dilatation is not a prerequisite for an endoscopic approach. With the aid of computerized neuronavigation, endoscopes can be inserted even into very small ventricles with high accuracy. Thanks to further improvements in endoscopic hemostasis, including the development of bipolar diathermy probes and suitable laser devices, selected highly vascularized tumors can also be completely resected.

Treatment of tumors arising in the ventricular system, however, remains a difficult neurosurgical challenge. These tumors must be approached over a considerable distance through normal brain tissue. In general, intraventricular lesions are treated by microsurgical resection.[19] Advantages of the endoscopic approach are that dissection and brain retraction can be reduced to a minimum. Craniotomies can be avoided because endoscopes are inserted through simple bur holes. Working through an operative sheath protects the surrounding structures such as fornix, hypothalamus, and vessels. To a certain extent, the procedure is comparable to Kelly's microsurgical stereotactic tube approach,[20, 21] but the endoscope sheath is much smaller (6.5 vs. 20 mm) and therefore less invasive. Along with tumor resection, CSF pathways can be simultaneously restored using the same endoscopic approach by performing ventriculostomies, septostomies, or stent implantations.[16]

## ENDOSCOPIC EQUIPMENT

For the endoscopic treatment of intraventricular tumors, a sophisticated and complex neuroendoscopic system is necessary. It should include various rigid and flexible endoscopes, effective instruments, bright cold light sources, a high-resolution video camera system, and an irrigation device. Combination with a guidance system is desirable. We use the universal GAAB neuroendoscopic system developed by the senior author and manufactured by Karl Storz GmbH & Co. (Tuttlingen, Germany).

## Endoscopes

The endoscopes are inserted through an operating sheath (outer diameter 6.5 mm; GAAB I system) that is initially introduced with the aid of a trocar (Fig. 62–1). This allows for intraoperative change of endoscopes without the need to reinsert the endoscopes through brain tissue, thus eliminating unnecessary damage to the surrounding brain. We prefer to use rigid rod-lens endoscopes (Hopkins II; 4-mm outer diameter) because of their brilliant optical quality, extreme wide-angle view, and ease of orientation and guidance. These endoscopes give an excellent overview of the intraventricular anatomy. Accurate assessment of tumor vascularization and the relation of the lesion to major vessels or other important structures is easily obtained. Even in the case of minor bleeding, which might blur the view, the surgeon can stay oriented, which is extremely difficult with the poor optics of a fiberscope. There are rigid endoscopes with four different angles of view available (0, 30, 70, and 120 degrees; Fig. 62–2). The 0- and 30-degree endoscopes are used for inspection and manipulation, and the 70- and 120-degree endoscopes for inspection only ("looking around a corner"). The main difference compared with other neuroendoscopic systems is the operating endoscope (wide-angle, straight-forward endoscope with angled eyepiece), which has no separate working channel but allows use of the whole inner diameter (approximately 6 mm) of the endoscopic sheath. This enables effective tissue removal. For removal of larger pieces of tumor, the forceps are withdrawn simultaneously with the endoscope after grasping tumor tissue. If manipulations "around a corner" are needed, we use steerable fiberscopes of two different diameters (2.5 and 3.5 mm; Fig. 62–3). An instrument channel of 1.2 mm is integrated. The high mobility of the tips (170 and 180 degrees upward, and 120 and 100

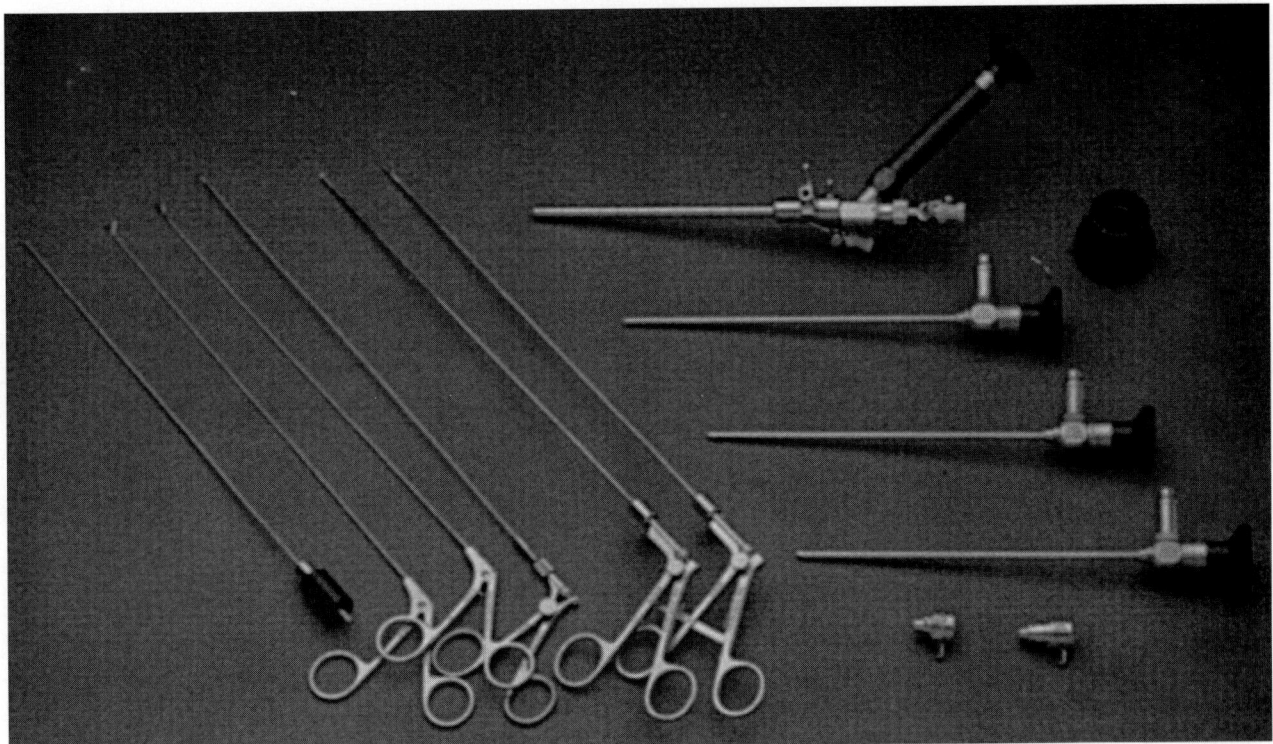

FIGURE 62–1 ■ The GAAB I universal neuroendoscopic system.

degrees downward movement) and wide angle of view (65 and 110 degrees) facilitates easy navigation through the ventricular spaces. These endoscopes are especially useful for inspecting the fourth ventricle through the aqueduct. In addition, a miniature endoscope (4-mm operating sheath outer diameter) for pediatric purposes has been developed (Fig. 62–4). This endoscope (GAAB II system) is based on semirigid minifiber optics (10,000 fibers/mm²) and incorporates an instrument channel as well as two separate channels for irrigation inflow and outflow. Using rigid 1.3-mm instruments, third ventriculostomies, aqueductoplasties, cystostomies, and tumor biopsies can be done.

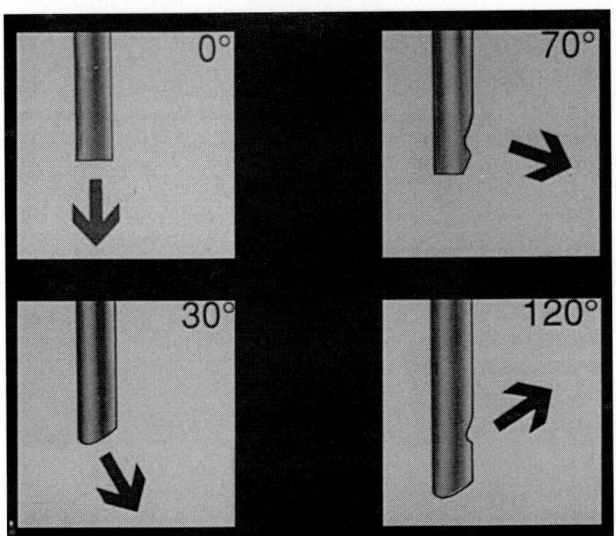

FIGURE 62–2 ■ Diagnostic scopes with different angles of view.

## Instruments

Various mechanical instruments of different sizes (1.7- and 2.7-mm outer diameter), including scissors, hooks, puncture needles, and biopsy and grasping forceps, are used for dissection and tissue removal (Fig. 62–5). The operating endoscope with the angled eyepiece as well as the miniature endoscope allow manipulations with rigid instruments in a straight line. This makes good tactile feedback from the tissue and easy guidance of the tools possible. For hemostasis and dissection, bipolar as well as monopolar diathermy probes and a laser guide that enables bending of the laser fiber tip are available (Fig. 62–6). We use a neodymium:yttrium-aluminum-garnet (Nd:YAG) laser (Opmilas YAG-M, 1.064 μm; Carl Zeiss, Oberkochen, Germany). Balloon catheters are applied for enlarging ventriculostomies or other fenestrations.

## Irrigation

In intraventricular endoscopy, the Malis CMS-II Irrigation Module (Codman & Shurtleff, Inc., Randolph, MA) is used. The flow of irrigation fluid is controlled with a foot switch. We use lactated Ringer's solution at 36°C to 37°C because postoperative increases in body temperature, often seen after abundant irrigation with saline, are rarely encountered. It is of utmost importance to make sure that the outflow channel is open to prevent dangerous increases in intracranial pressure. An irrigation-suction device combined with monopolar diathermy is used in transnasal-transsphenoidal tube-guided surgery. This helps considerably in hemostasis and maintaining a clear view.

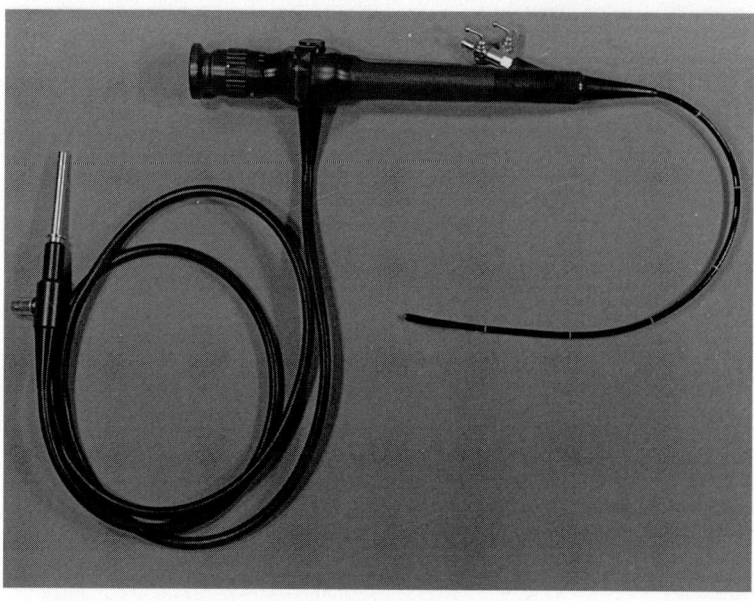

**FIGURE 62-3** ■ Steerable neurofiberscope.

## Light Sources, Cameras, and Video System

Xenon light sources provide the best illumination because the color temperature of xenon light resembles that of sunlight (6000 K). The light is transmitted by glass fiber or fluid (better light transmission, but more susceptible to kinking) cables from the light source to the endoscope. Although this system is called *cold light fountain*, the endoscope tip may become extremely hot.

Digital one-chip (horizontal resolution >450 lines) or three-chip (horizontal resolution >750 lines, separate processing of the three primary colors) mini-video cameras are attached by a sterile optical bridge to the endoscope.

Camera and bridge are draped with a sterile covering. This allows sterile intraoperative exchange of endoscopes using the same camera. Several functions of the digital video cameras, such as adjusting contrast, white balance, selection of different filters (e.g., anti-Moiré filter for fiberscopes to minimize the pixel appearance of the image), can be controlled directly by the surgeon pressing buttons on the camera. Of course, high-resolution video monitor screens are necessary to display the endoscopic picture obtained by the video cameras without loss of image quality. We use a Sony Trinitron monitor (horizontal resolution 800 lines, nonflickering, 100 Hz). Each endoscopic procedure is taped with an S-VHS recorder (a digital DVC system

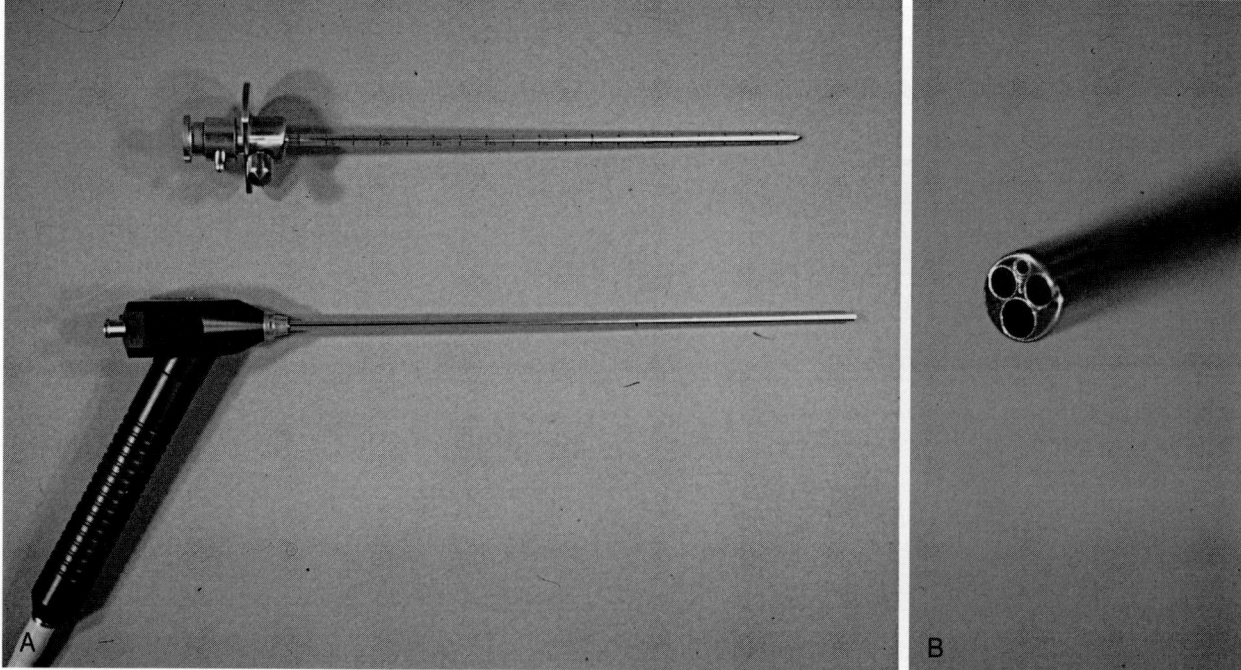

**FIGURE 62-4** ■ *A,* GAAB II miniature semirigid fiberscope. *B,* Tip of endoscope (0.8-mm optics, one working channel, two irrigation channels: inflow and outflow).

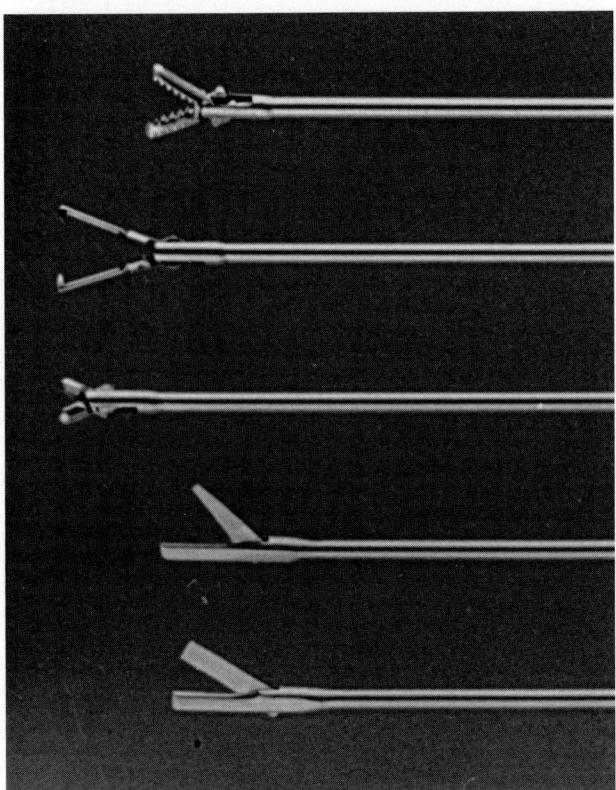

FIGURE 62–5 ■ Endoscopic scissors and biopsy and grasping forceps.

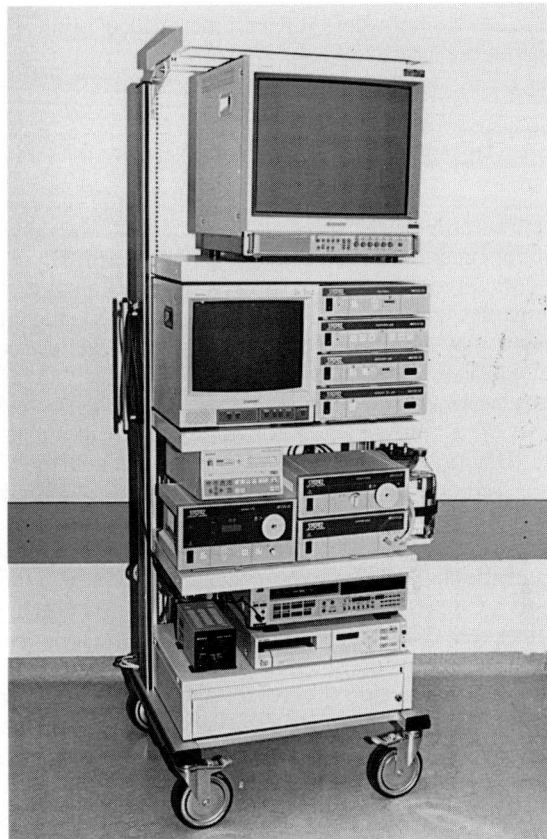

FIGURE 62–7 ■ Endoscopic equipment on a mobile videocart.

will be introduced in the near future). In addition, a digital still recorder (Sony) is used for documentation. The saved pictures can be modified on a computer and incorporated into slides or illustrations. Analogue video recordings can be processed with a digital processing unit (Digivideo) to enhance contrast as required. A video printer completes the documentation equipment.

For certain endoscopic procedures, the simultaneous use of two endoscopes is desirable. The images from both endoscopes can be displayed on one video monitor with the aid of a digital picture-in-picture device (Twinvideo), allowing the surgeon to obtain the input of both endoscopes by looking at one screen.

For convenience and ease of use, all the aforementioned video equipment can be placed on a mobile cart. Figure 62–7 shows our videocart, containing two monitors, two light sources, two endoscopic cameras, Twinvideo, Digi-

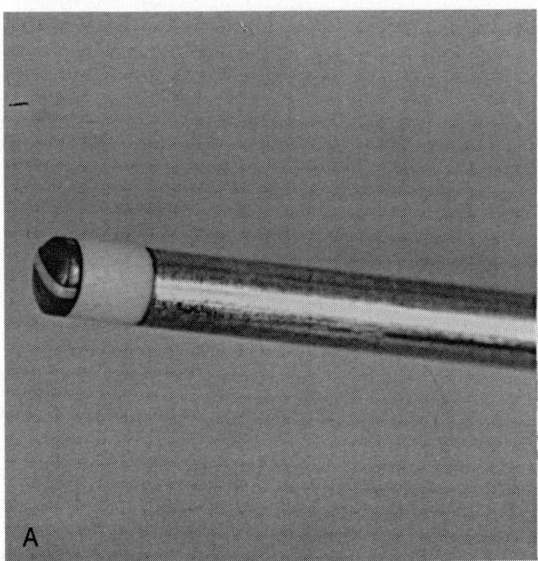
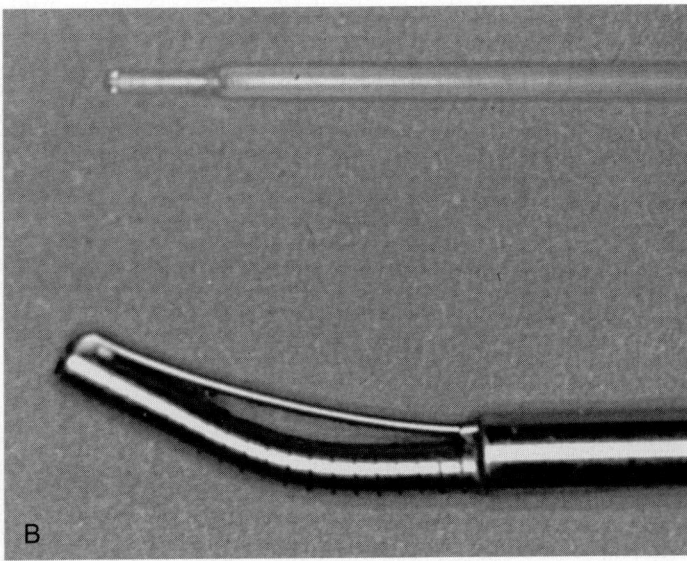

FIGURE 62–6 ■ *A,* Tip of a bipolar diathermy probe. *B,* Tip of a movable laser guide and a laser fiber tip.

video, S-VHS recorder, still recorder, video printer, and irrigation device.

## INDICATIONS FOR ENDOSCOPIC SURGERY

All intraventricular lesions that do not exceed a certain size limit are candidates for an endoscopic approach. However, it is difficult to determine the exact size limit of a tumor for an effective endoscopic resection. Endoscopic piecemeal removal may become time consuming and ineffective if the tumor is too large. The benefits of a minimally invasive approach are then outweighed by the length of the operation. A solid tumor should not exceed 2 cm in diameter; cystic lesions may be effectively treated even if they are larger. Tumor consistency and vasculature are additional considerations. Extirpation of soft lesions is easier and more rapid than removal of firm ones. The ideal indication for an endoscopic treatment is a small and avascular tumor located in the lateral or third ventricle, especially if the lesion causes CSF pathway obstruction resulting in enlargement of the ventricles. Ventricular dilatation gives sufficient space for manipulation of the endoscopes and instruments. However, using a computerized navigation system or ultrasound guidance, even very narrow ventricles can be approached accurately with an endoscope. With the aid of Nd:YAG laser and bipolar diathermy, even highly vascularized tumors such as cavernomas and hemangiomas can be removed. Large tumors with accompanying hydrocephalus, in which an endoscopic resection is not feasible, are indications for ventriculostomy or aqueductal stenting to restore CSF circulation. Tumor tissue sampling can be carried out on any tumor visible at the ventricular surface. The use of a second working portal enabling the insertion of larger instruments and thus accelerating tumor removal has been advocated.[5, 22] We do not routinely recommend two portals because it makes the approach more invasive and manipulations more difficult. If endoscopic tumor removal turns out to be ineffective, we do not hesitate to change in midprocedure to an open microsurgical operation. With a small keyhole approach and endoscope-assisted microsurgical techniques, an effective and minimally invasive tumor removal without extensive brain dissection, as proposed by Perneczky and colleagues,[23, 24] is feasible. We then simply switch our Leyla retractors from holding the endoscope sheath to holding small retractors for microsurgery. To date, in our series and using our system with one large working space, a second port has never been necessary.

## GENERAL OPERATIVE TECHNIQUE

Once general anesthesia is induced, the patient is commonly placed supine with the head in three-pin fixation and slight anteflexion. If infrared-based computer neuronavigation is to be used, a camera bar and dynamic reference frame are mounted. After patient registration and verification of accuracy (landmark test), the operating field is prepared and draped, allowing immediate change to

microsurgical intervention in case of ineffective tumor removal or complications. The operating microscope and microsurgical instruments are prepared for use. Just before starting the operation, the patient receives a bolus of 40 mg dexamethasone intravenously if no contraindications exist. Eight milligrams of dexamethasone are given every 6 hours for 2 days after surgery. Antibiotics are not administered routinely.

The entry point usually is selected according to information obtained by preoperative assessment of computed tomography (CT) scan or magnetic resonance imaging (MRI).[25] For lesions occupying the posterior part of the third ventricle or in ventricles that are very narrow, computerized neuronavigation has replaced the previously used frame-based stereotaxy to determine the ideal access route to the target. In cooperation with Carl Zeiss and Karl Storz, we developed a universal guiding system for endoscopic purposes. A light-emitting diode bar is attached to the optical bridge and can be used with different endoscopes or trocars (Fig. 62–8). With the aid of an infrared-based computerized navigation system (Surgical Tool Navigator; Carl Zeiss), the endoscopic sheath can be inserted precisely into the ventricles even if they are very small. Furthermore, this technique enables accurate planning of the approach—for example, in a straight line through the foramen of Monro to the aqueduct without injuring the fornix. Frameless computer navigation allows free-hand movement of the endoscope with real-time control of the endoscope tip's position and of the approach trajectory. The degree of accuracy is between 2 and 3 mm, which is sufficient for endoscopic purposes. After reaching the target point with neuronavigational guidance, minor position corrections can be made under endoscopic view.

If the ventricles or foramens of Monro are asymmetric in size, the approach should be made through the larger ventricle or foramen. If feasible, the entry point should be located opposite the dominant hemisphere. Once a 3-cm straight scalp incision has been made, a 10-mm bur hole is placed. After opening the dura, the operating sheath containing the trocar is introduced free-hand with or without navigational guidance into the lateral ventricle and fixed with two Leyla retractor arms (Fig. 62–9). The trocar is then removed and the rigid diagnostic endoscope inserted after white-balancing the camera. After inspection of the ventricle and identification of the main landmarks (i.e., choroid plexus, fornix, and veins), the tumor with its feeding arteries is visualized. Once the tumor has been explored, the diagnostic endoscope is replaced by the operating endoscope (Fig. 62–10). Capsule vessels are coagulated with the aid of a bipolar diathermy probe or a Nd:YAG laser in noncontact mode. Tumor specimens are taken for histologic investigation. Depending on the size of the lesion, tumor resection usually begins with intracapsular debulking or dissection in the plane between tumor and brain tissue. Feeding arteries should be identified early and cauterized before bleeding blurs the view. The Nd:YAG laser is especially useful for removal of highly vascularized lesions.[26] Initially, a chisel laser fiber is used in noncontact mode for tumor debulking and vessel coagulation. Tumor dissection is then performed with the chisel fiber or a conical fiber in contact mode for cutting. Laser-assisted resection requires vigorous irrigation to avoid thermal in-

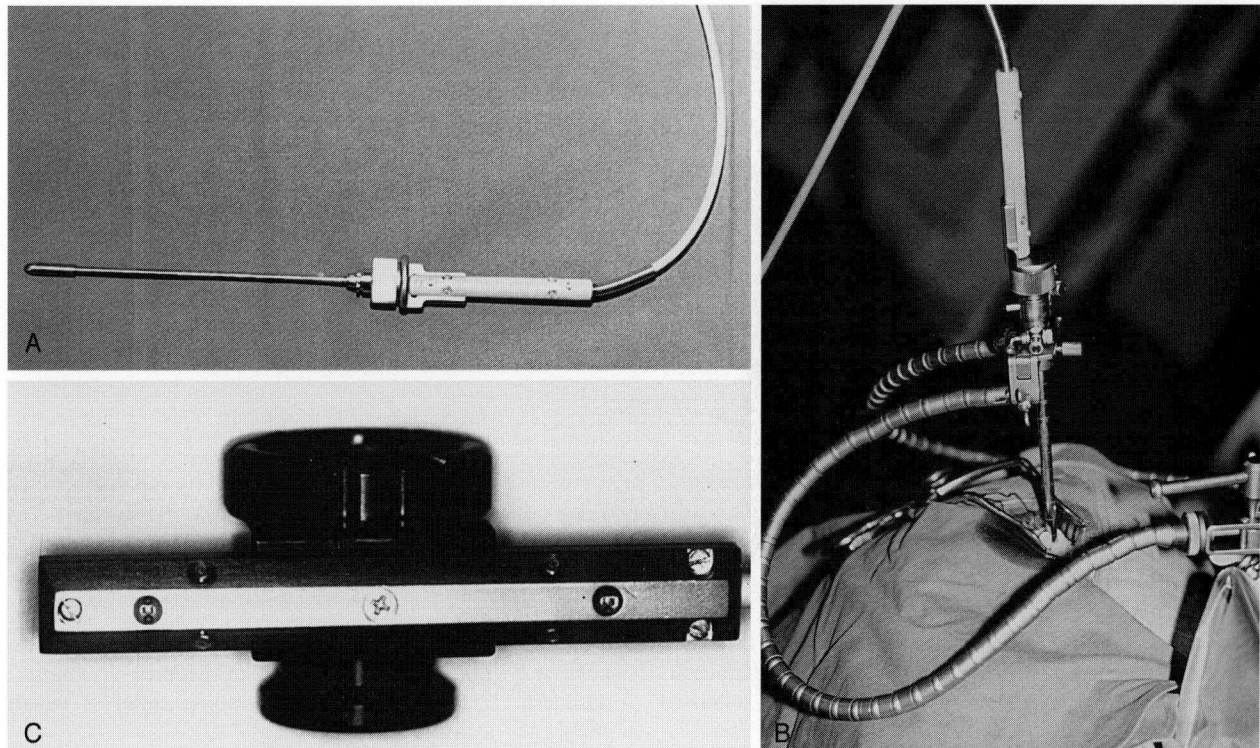

**FIGURE 62-8** ■ *A,* A trocar with a LED bar for computerized neuronavigation. *B,* An operating sheath inserted with the aid of navigational guidance. *C,* An optical bridge with a LED bar allowing navigation of the trocar and different scopes.

jury to the adjacent brain tissue.[27] After dissection of the tumor from the surrounding brain, the lesion is removed in piecemeal fashion with the aid of various grasping and biopsy forceps. The large operating sheath of our instrument enables removal of solid tumor pieces 6 mm in diameter, and even larger pieces of soft tumors. Details regarding the entry points for the different tumor locations are given later and in Table 62–1.

All endoscopic tumor operations are performed under continuous irrigation because each tumor resection causes some bleeding. A separate irrigation tube is used to focus the irrigation on the source of bleeding. For forced irrigating, a 20-ml syringe is helpful. Small hemorrhages usually cease spontaneously after a few minutes of irrigation. Rarely, irrigation for 20 minutes is necessary to stop a larger venous hemorrhage and to clear the view. It is ill-advised to remove the endoscope in case of bleeding; rather, stay in place, rinse, and wait. Larger vessels that are at risk of injury during tumor dissection should be cauterized with the bipolar diathermy probe before bleeding occurs. In rare cases of severe hemorrhage, aspiration of CSF is needed to obtain a dry field. With this "dry

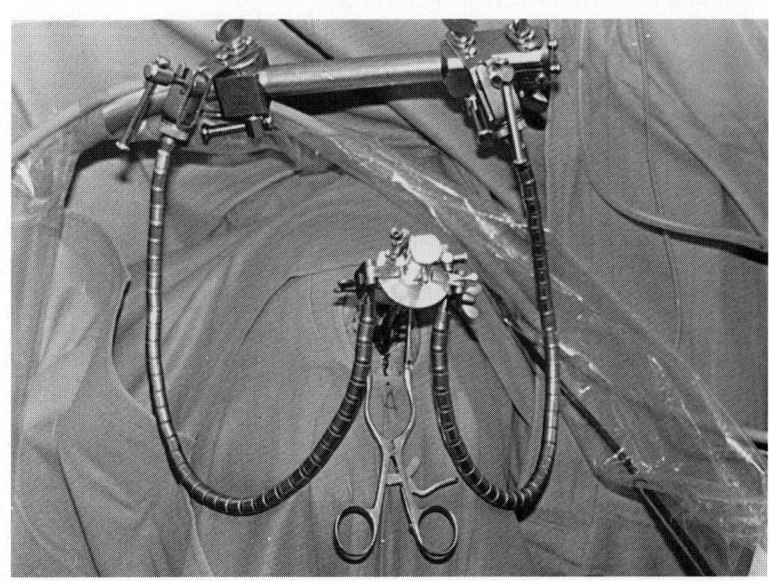

**FIGURE 62-9** ■ An endoscopic sheath fixed with standard microsurgical self-retaining retractors.

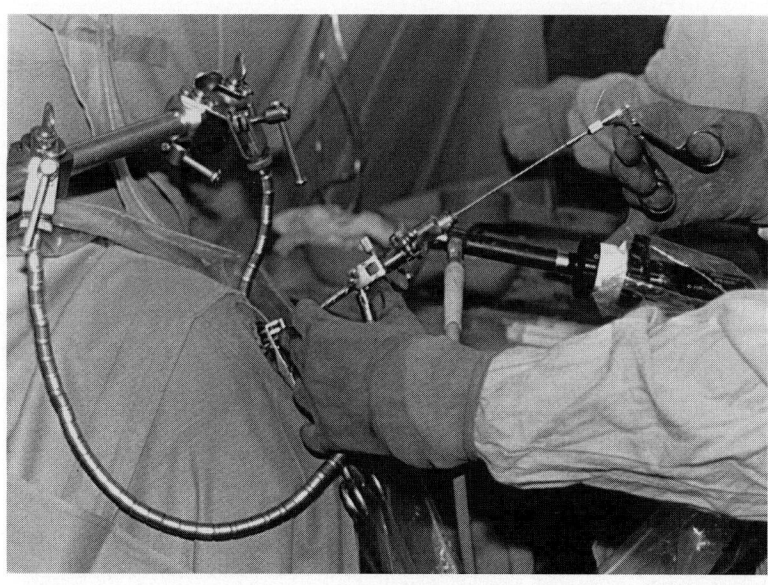

**FIGURE 62–10** ■ An operating endoscope guided with the left hand and an instrument used in a straight line with the right hand.

field" technique, bleeding vessels are more easily identified and hemostasis is quickly achieved. To avoid a dangerous increase in intracranial pressure, care must be taken to maintain sufficient outflow of irrigation fluid.

After tumor removal, the resection site is inspected with the diagnostic endoscope to check that there is no active bleeding. The ventricles are vigorously irrigated to remove any clots. The operating sheath is then withdrawn simultaneously with the endoscope to look for potential bleeding at the foramen of Monro or in the cortical puncture channel. In general, no external ventricular drainage is placed. We pack the bur hole with a gelatin sponge and tightly suture the galea to prevent subgaleal CSF accumulation and fistula formation. The skin is closed with running atraumatic sutures. CSF accumulation in spite of these measures indicates increased intracranial pressure mostly due to obstructed CSF flow. The patient usually is observed overnight in the intensive care unit.

## TUMORS OF THE LATERAL VENTRICLE

Tumors of the lateral ventricle are mostly benign or low-grade lesions such as gliomas, meningiomas, plexus papil-

**TABLE 62–1** ■ **ENDOSCOPIC APPROACHES FOR DIFFERENT TUMOR LOCATIONS**

| Tumor Location | Entry Point |
| --- | --- |
| Lateral ventricle—frontal horn | 2–3 cm parasagittal, coronal to 2 cm precoronal |
| Lateral ventricle—cella media | 2–3 cm parasagittal, coronal to 2 cm precoronal |
| Lateral ventricle—trigone | 2–3 cm parasagittal, 4–6 cm precoronal |
| Foramen of Monro | 3–5 cm parasagittal, 2–4 cm precoronal |
| Third ventricle—anterior part | 1–2 cm parasagittal, coronal |
| Third ventricle—posterior part | 1–2 cm parasagittal, 4–6 cm precoronal |

lomas, and hemangiomas.[28] Lesions located in the frontal horn may obstruct the foramen of Monro, resulting in unilateral hydrocephalus. The choroidal arteries usually supply the lesions.[29]

The patient is positioned supine with the head tilted slightly forward. For lesions of the frontal horn and ventricular body, a standard precoronal (3-cm paramedian) bur hole is placed. Tumors of the trigone are approached through a bur hole located more anteriorly to reach the target in a straight line through the ventricular body. A posterior approach is advisable only if marked ventricular dilatation provides enough space for manipulation with endoscope and instruments. In general, the CSF-filled working space in front of the tumor is very limited, which makes the inspection of the lesion, orientation, and dissection more difficult or even impossible. To date, we have had no experience with tumors arising in the temporal or occipital horn.

We prefer a transcortical insertion of the endoscope into the lateral ventricle. In a few patients, the endoscope was introduced using a transcallosal approach; this resulted in permanent memory loss in one patient, probably related to forniceal damage. We abandoned this approach for inserting the endoscope because it requires a small craniotomy and microsurgical dissection for exposing the corpus callosum (instead of a simple bur hole) and makes initial orientation more difficult. The transcortical bur hole approach has proved fast, easy, and safe owing to well-known landmarks. A higher seizure rate has been reported after the transcortical approach,[30, 31] although we have seen no seizures after the transcortical insertion of an endoscope in more than 180 cases.

Once the endoscopic sheath has been inserted into the lateral ventricle, the tumor is visualized. The relation of the tumor to the choroid plexus should be ascertained before starting tumor dissection. Because tearing of the choroid plexus may lead to bleeding at a distance from the operating field,[32] the choroid attachment of the lesion should be coagulated first with the aid of the Nd:YAG laser or bipolar probe (Fig. 62–11). Care must be taken to avoid injury to the thalamus, caudate nucleus, and fornices.

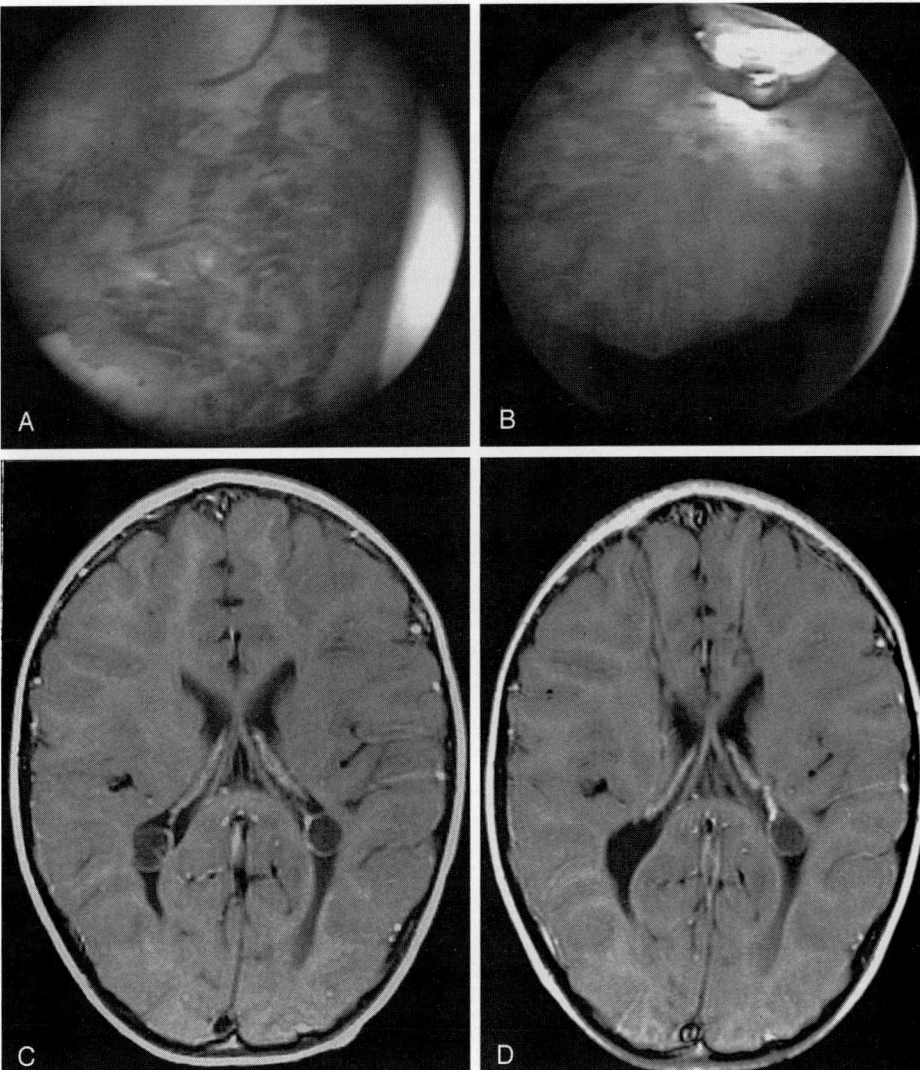

FIGURE 62–11 ■ A choroid plexus cystic lesion in the trigone of the lateral ventricle. *A,* Endoscopic view. *B,* Removal of a tumor using a neodymium:yttrium aluminum garnet laser. *C,* Axial $T_1$-weighted enhanced magnetic resonance (MR) image showing bilateral choroid plexus cysts in the trigone. *D,* An axial $T_1$-weighted enhanced postoperative MR image showing complete removal of the right lesion.

Patency of the foramen of Monro usually is achieved after tumor resection. If the foramen is still occluded, CSF circulation can be restored by performing a septostomy through the septum pellucidum. The septostomy can be made with the aid of laser, diathermy, scissors, and balloon catheters. The size of this fenestration should be approximately 10 mm². When the ventricles are very small or ventricular collapse occurs after ventricular puncture, there might be not enough working space for instrument manipulations. The endoscopic procedure must then be abandoned and the tumor removed microsurgically.

## TUMORS OF THE THIRD VENTRICLE

Tumors located in the third ventricle are among the most difficult lesions to expose and remove. A variety of approaches have been advocated in the literature, including the transsphenoidal, anterior and posterior transventricular, anterior and posterior transcallosal, subfrontal, frontotemporal, occipital transtentorial, and infratentorial supracerebellar approaches.[33–38] Division of the anterior column of the fornix,[33] division of the thalamostriate vein,[39] interforniceal midline division of the ventricular roof,[37, 40] and a subchoroid approach[41, 42] have been recommended for entering the third ventricle. The choice of approach depends on the surgeon and the tumor location. When working in the third ventricle, brain retraction should be minimized to avoid injury to important structures such as thalamus, fornix, veins, and hypothalamus. With endoscopic techniques, there is little need for retraction.[43] Frameless computerized neuronavigation aids in determining the exact entry point and the approach trajectory along which the endoscope is passed in a straight line through the foramen of Monro to the target without injuring the surrounding brain tissue. Neuronavigation has proven especially helpful for lesions in the posterior third ventricle.

Tumors originating in the third ventricle include astrocytomas (Fig. 62–12), ependymomas, epidermoids, colloid cysts (Fig. 62–13), craniopharyngiomas, pituitary adenomas, medulloblastomas, and gliosis (Fig. 62–14). In the pineal region, germinomas, nongerminomatous germ cell tumors, pineocytomas, pineoblastomas, and pineal cysts occur.[35]

The patient is placed in the supine position with the head slightly flexed. Tumors of the third ventricle are

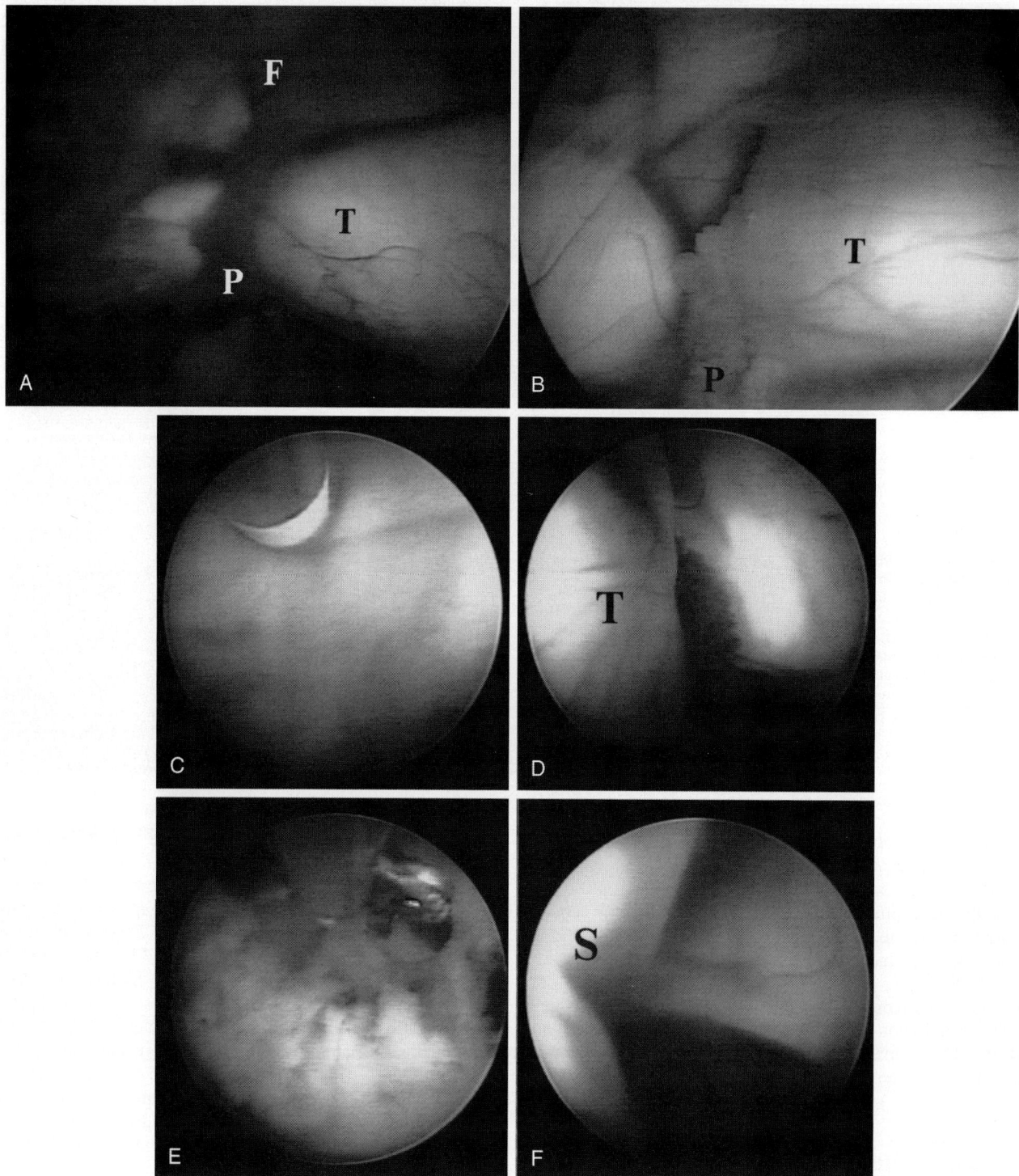

**FIGURE 62–12** ■ Benign astrocytoma within the foramen of Monro. *A,* View into the left lateral ventricle showing a tumor (T) medial from the choroid plexus (P) with an obstructed foramen of Monro (F). *B,* Closer view with an occluded foramen of Monro with a tumor (T) and choroid plexus (P). *C,* Septostomy in the septum pellucidum with a bipolar probe. *D,* View through the septostomy showing a tumor (T) bulging into the right lateral ventricle. *E,* Tumor resection using biopsy forceps. *F,* A stent (S) is inserted into the foramen of Monro.

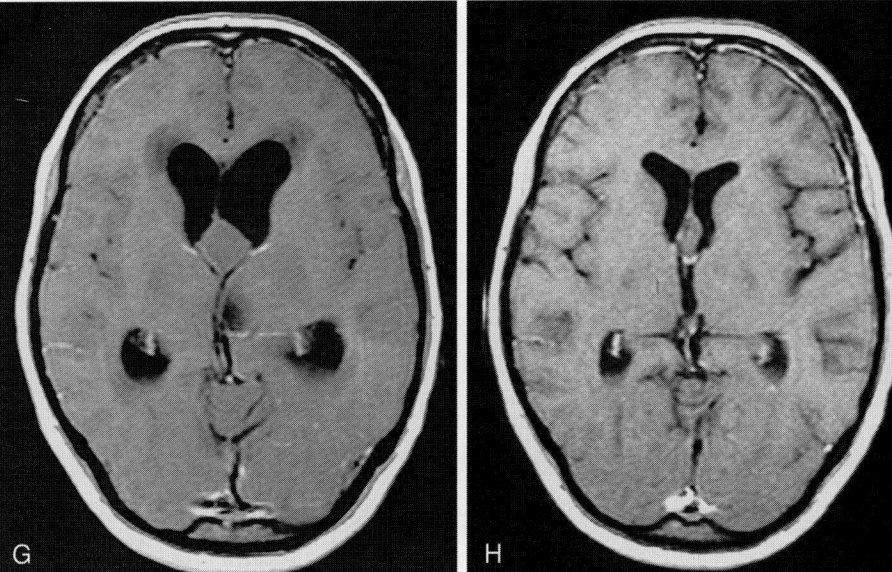

**FIGURE 62–12 ■** *Continued.*
*G,* Axial T₁-weighted enhanced magnetic resonance (MR) image showing a tumor with bilateral obstruction of the foramen of Monro and hydrocephalus. *H,* Axial T₁-weighted enhanced MR image obtained 10 months after surgery showing partial tumor resection (the fornices are spared!) and relief of hydrocephalus.

approached by a transcortical, transventricular, transforaminal route, regardless of anterior or posterior location. This is the standard approach in ventriculoscopy with clear landmarks. If the tumor is located in the anterior part of the ventricle, the entry point is at the coronal suture. If the tumor arises in the posterior part, the bur hole is made more anteriorly to pass the foramen of Monro in a straight line. For endoscopic procedures, we do not use the infratentorial supracerebellar approach,[36] which we prefer for microsurgical operations in the pineal region. Because a simple bur hole is not sufficient to identify the transverse sinus, a small craniotomy must be made. Thick arachnoid membranes often cover the pineal region and hinder accurate orientation. These membranes are more easily and safely divided microsurgically than endoscopically. Finally, the superior cerebellar bridging veins and deep incisural veins are at risk when introducing an endoscope.[44] These veins must be cauterized and divided. Hence, a strictly endoscopic infratentorial supracerebellar approach is inconvenient and possess a considerable risk. A better alternative is an endoscope-assisted microsurgical approach, as recommended by Perneczky.[45]

Tumors of the third ventricle are removed according to the guidelines described previously. When advancing the operating sheath through the foramen of Monro, care should be taken to avoid the fornix and the adjacent veins. Tilting the endoscopic sheath in the foramen of Monro can be done only with great caution, especially when the foramen is small. Cystic lesions are first punctured and the contents aspirated. Cyst collapse facilitates dissection from the adjacent brain. Capsule vessels are coagulated. Residual parts of the capsule firmly attached to the roof of the ventricle should be coagulated rather than vigorously removed because pulling may cause severe venous bleeding. After tumor removal, patency of CSF pathways should be verified. First, the entry of the aqueduct must be inspected to ensure there is no blockade by tumor debris. If the tumor resection is incomplete and residual tumor tissue may progress and occlude the CSF pathways in the future, a stent should be inserted. In tumors of the posterior part of the

third ventricle, such as in the pineal region, a short stent between fourth and third ventricles is sufficient to maintain CSF circulation. However, if the tumor occupies the entire third ventricle and blocks the foramen of Monro as well as the aqueduct, the stent should extend from the lateral to the fourth ventricle. Unilateral obstruction of the foramen of Monro may be managed by fenestration in the septum pellucidum (septostomy). Sometimes both stenting and septostomy are necessary to preserve CSF circulation.

Frame-based stereotactic MRI or CT-guided tumor biopsy is a well-established and safe option to obtain tumor tissue specimens. However, stereotactic puncture of tumors near the foramen of Monro has the potential for forniceal and venous injury.[46] Stereotactic biopsy of pineal lesions places the great vein and the internal veins at risk. Endoscopic biopsy offers some advantages over stereotactic biopsy. First, the lesions can be inspected. Changes in coordinates (e.g., after cyst aspiration) can be recognized early. Second, the procedure can be performed under direct vision and therefore be better controlled. Bleeding can be seen and hemostasis quickly achieved. For pineal lesions in particular, we consider the endoscopic approach the preferred method for obtaining a biopsy. Despite reports on large series of stereotactic biopsies of pineal lesions[47, 48] describing this technique as safe and reliable, we are concerned about the "blind" sampling of tissue in this area. We favor neuroendoscopic exploration and biopsy under direct view. Through the same bur hole, occluded CSF pathways can easily be restored by stenting of the aqueduct or third ventriculostomy. Thus, endoscopy offers simultaneous histologic verification and permanent restoration of blocked CSF pathways. After reaching an accurate histologic diagnosis, further treatment, such as microsurgical operation, irradiation, chemotherapy, or radiosurgery, is initiated.

## TUMORS OF THE FOURTH VENTRICLE

In our experience, tumors of the fourth ventricle are rarely suitable for an endoscopic resection because the ventricular

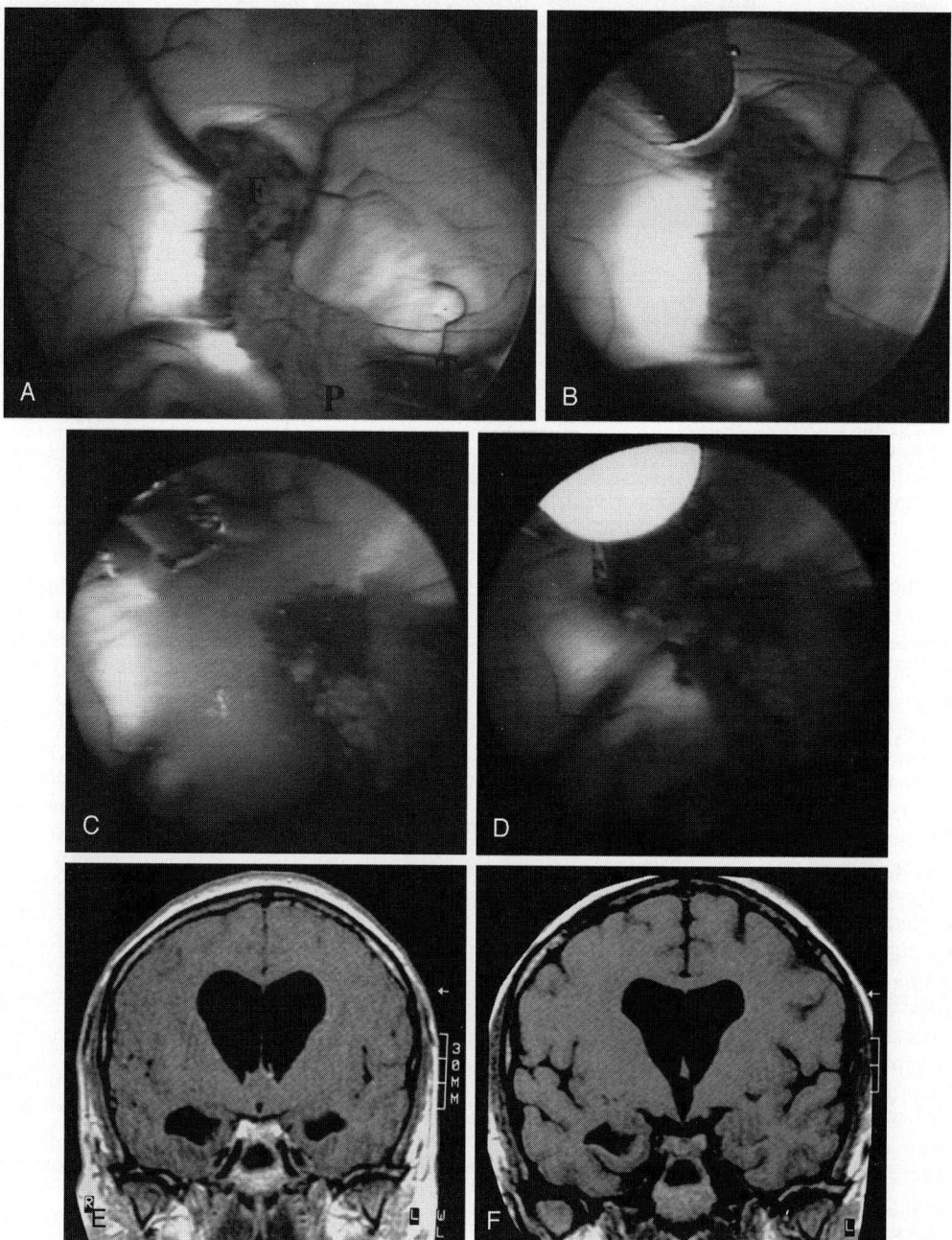

**FIGURE 62–13** ■ A colloid cyst in the third ventricle. *A,* A colloid cyst obstructing the foramen of Monro (F) covered by choroid plexus (P). Note the large thalamostriate vein (T) underneath the choroid plexus. *B,* Coagulation of capsule vessels and the choroid plexus with a bipolar probe. *C,* After opening the cyst, the yellow colloid contents bulge out of the cyst. *D,* Coagulation of the ependymal vein with a bipolar electrode. *E,* Coronal T$_1$-weighted enhanced magnetic resonance (MR) image showing a colloid cyst obstructing the foramen of Monro and ventricular dilatation. *F,* A postoperative coronal T$_1$-weighted enhanced MR image showing the complete removal of the cyst and a decrease in ventricular size.

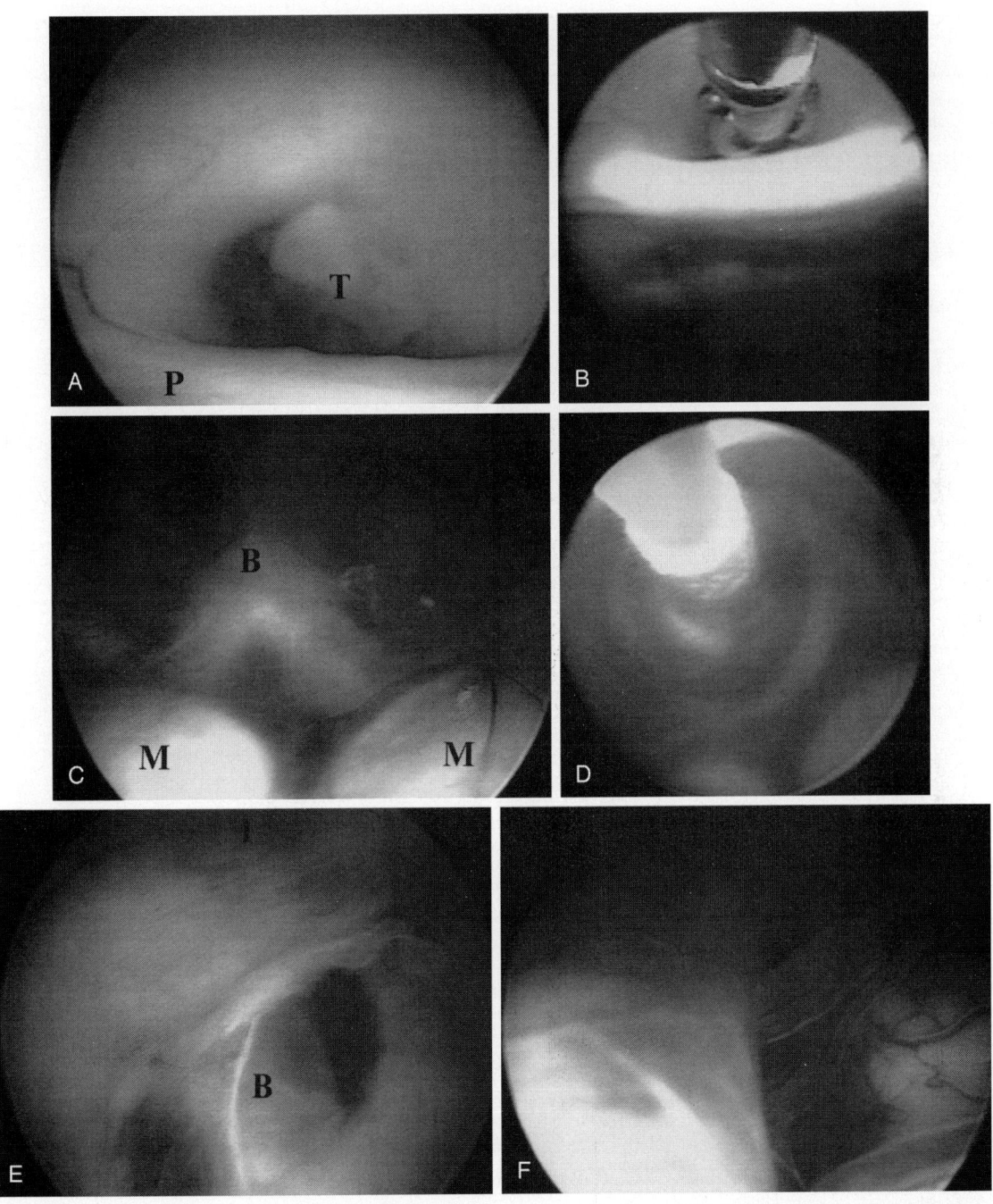

**FIGURE 62–14** ■ Aqueductal gliosis. *A,* Entry into the aqueduct above the posterior commissure (P) occluded by gliotic tissue (T). *B,* Biopsy with forceps. *C,* Translucent floor of the third ventricle with mamillary bodies (M) and a clearly visible basilar artery *(B). D,* Ventriculostomy with a Fogarty balloon catheter. *E,* Ventriculostomy behind the infundibular recess (I); basilar artery (B). *F,* View through a ventriculostomy into the interpeduncular cistern showing the basilar artery with pontine branches.

*Illustration continued on following page*

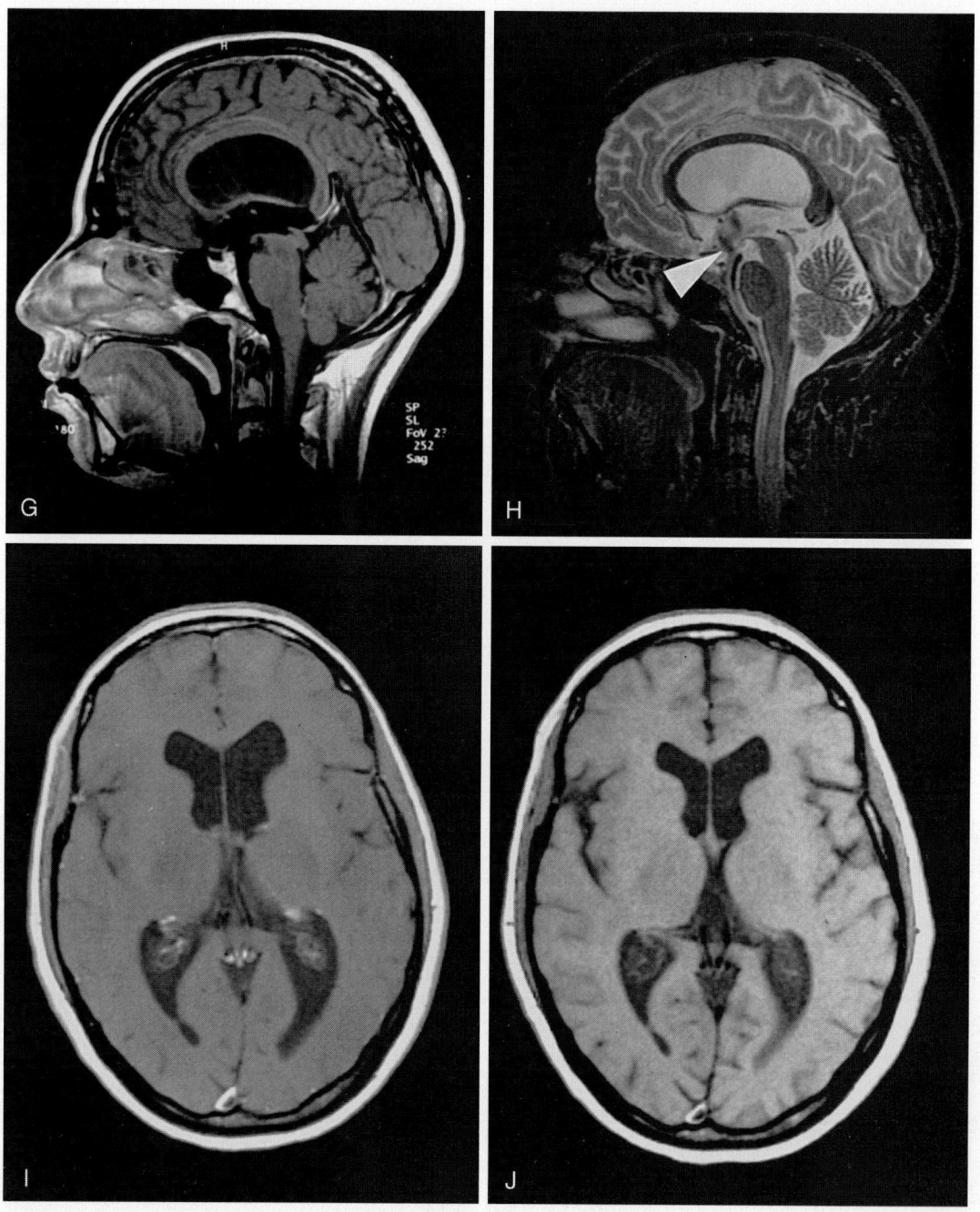

**FIGURE 62–14** ■ *Continued. G,* Sagittal T$_1$-weighted enhanced magnetic resonance (MR) image revealing a nonenhancing lesion within the aqueduct. *H,* Sagittal T$_2$-weighted MR image obtained 6 months postoperatively revealing a patent third ventriculostomy with a flow void sign *(arrow). I,* Axial T$_1$-weighted enhanced MR image showing ventricular enlargement. *J,* An axial T$_1$-weighted enhanced MR image obtained 6 months postoperatively showing a decrease in size of the ventricle.

space is very limited. However, because these lesions often become initially symptomatic with signs of increased intracranial pressure caused by obstructive hydrocephalus, a third ventriculostomy is indicated. In selected cases, biopsies are taken through the enlarged aqueduct.

## RESULTS

Forty-two patients harboring an intraventricular lesion underwent endoscopic treatment at our department between February 1993 and September 1998. Histologic examination revealed 11 colloid cysts, 7 astrocytomas, 3 subependymomas, 2 ependymomas, 2 germinomas, 2 craniopharyngiomas, 2 glioses, 1 pineocytoma/pineoblastoma (intermediate type), 1 pineoblastoma, 1 medulloblastoma, 1 arteriovenous hemangioma, 1 cavernoma, 1 plexus papilloma, 1 lymphoma, 1 pituitary adenoma, 1 neuroblastoma, 1 melanoma, 1 choroid plexus cyst, and 1 pineal cyst. In one specimen, no tumor tissue was detected. The mean follow-up period is 15 months.

None of the endoscopic procedures had to be stopped because of significant bleeding or poor orientation. Because of very firm tissue consistency, the endoscopic resection of two subependymomas larger than 2 cm in diameter was ineffective; the endoscopic procedure was discontinued and the tumors microsurgically removed. These two operations lasted 135 and 210 minutes, respectively. The mean surgical time for the strictly endoscopic procedures was 85 minutes, ranging from 30 to 170 minutes. One very small colloid cyst could not be detected endoscopically. Because the foramen of Monro was not narrowed, no further measures were undertaken. All other cystic lesions were completely evacuated and the membranes widely resected. In two colloid cysts, capsule remnants firmly attached to the roof of the third ventricle were not removed. However, MRI has not shown colloid cyst recurrence in any of the patients (follow-up periods of 15 to 60 months). Astrocytomas were partially resected. Patients with malignant tumors were referred for stereotactic precision irradiation or radiosurgery, and benign tumors were controlled with repeated MRI. Total endoscopic tumor removal was performed on the cavernoma, plexus papilloma, medulloblastoma metastasis, and arteriovenous angioma, and on one subependymoma. Follow-up MRIs have demonstrated no tumor recurrences. One craniopharyngioma, initially histologically classified as an epidermoid, recurred after 12 months. However, small ventricles indicated a patent septostomy and stent. Fourteen third ventriculostomies and four septostomies were performed. Six stents were inserted. In 13 patients, a tumor biopsy was taken. The hydrocephalus-related symptoms of increased intracranial pressure were relieved in all patients.

## COMPLICATIONS

There was no mortality related to the endoscopic procedure. Five patients died from progression of the tumor. Two patients died after microsurgical extirpation of the tumor (giant pituitary adenoma and craniopharyngioma) because of diencephalic dysfunction. Significant bleeding blurred the view in two cases. These hemorrhages were controlled endoscopically using the dry field technique. The postoperative course was uneventful in both cases. Memory loss attributed to forniceal damage was observed in two cases, and in one it remained permanent. Meningitis occurred in one patient and was treated with antibiotics. Because an external ventricular drainage was inserted 2 days before the endoscopic procedure, the meningitis was probably related to the external ventricular drainage rather than to the endoscopy. In one patient, a transient mutism occurred. We observed one transient trochlear palsy after biopsy of an aqueductal tumor, and one patient experienced transient confusion after biopsy of a suprasellar germinoma.

## CONCLUSION

In our preliminary experience, the endoscopic management of intraventricular tumors has proven to be effective and safe. The symptoms of obstructive hydrocephalus were relieved in all patients. All third ventriculostomies have remained patent. All stents have remained patent, and no dislocation has been observed. Shunting was completely avoided. The endoscopic procedure had to be abandoned and continued microsurgically in only two patients, and a histologic diagnosis was obtained in all tumors but one thalamic tumor.

With the application of neuroendoscopic techniques, the invasiveness of microsurgical procedures can be further reduced with similar or even better results. In selected cases, cystic and solid intraventricular tumors can be removed completely using endoscopic techniques. Craniotomies can be avoided and brain retraction minimized. A further advantage of the endoscopic approach is the rapid and straightforward access to the lesion. The combination of endoscopes with frameless computerized neuronavigation has improved the accuracy of the approach. The endoscopic procedures have usually been shorter than the analogous microsurgical procedure. The surgeon should be aware of potential complications, however, and all preparations should be made for immediate microsurgical intervention in case of complications or ineffectiveness of the endoscopic approach.

In our opinion, endoscopic techniques should be applied in the treatment of selected intraventricular lesions. In the future, endoscopic techniques will probably also be used for the treatment of paraventricular and intraparenchymal lesions. The combination of real-time computer-aided neuronavigation and intraoperative ultrasound (image fusion) will increase the accuracy of the approach and help control the extent of tumor removal.

## REFERENCES

1. Caemaert J, Abdullah J, Calliauw L, et al: Endoscopic treatment of suprasellar arachnoid cysts. Acta Neurochir (Wien) 119:68–73, 1992.
2. Gaab MR, Schroeder HWS: Neuroendoscopic approach to intraventricular lesions. J Neurosurg 88:496–505, 1998.

3. Schroeder HWS, Gaab MR, Niendorf W-R: Neuroendoscopic approach to arachnoid cysts. J Neurosurg 85:293–298, 1996.
4. Bauer BL, Hellwig D: Minimally invasive endoscopic neurosurgery: A survey. Acta Neurochir Suppl (Wien) 61:1–12, 1994.
5. Cohen AR: Endoscopic ventricular surgery. Pediatr Neurosurg 19:127–134, 1993.
6. Auer LM, Holzer P, Ascher PW, et al: Endoscopic neurosurgery. Acta Neurochir (Wien) 90:1–14, 1988.
7. Eiras Ajuria J, Alberdi Vinas J: Traitement endoscopique des lésions intracranienne: A propos de 8 cas. Neurochirurgie 37:278–283, 1991.
8. Hor F, Desgeorges M, Rosseau GL: Tumour resection by stereotactic laser endoscopy. Acta Neurochir Suppl (Wien) 54:77–82, 1992.
9. Merienne L, Leriche B, Roux FX, et al: Utilisation du laser Nd-YAG en endoscopie intracranienne: expérience préliminaire en stéréotaxie. Neurochirurgie 38:245–247, 1992.
10. Decq P, Yepes C, Anno Y, et al: L'Endoscopie neurochirurgicale: Indications diagnostiques et thérapeutiques. Neurochirurgie 40:313–321, 1994.
11. Fukushima T, Ishijima B, Hirakawa K, et al: Ventriculofiberscope: A new technique for endoscopic diagnosis and operation. J Neurosurg 38:251–256, 1973.
12. Fukushima T: Endoscopic biopsy of intraventricular tumors with the use of a ventriculofiberscope. Neurosurgery 2:110–113, 1978.
13. Griffith HB: Endoneurosurgery: Endoscopic intracranial surgery. Adv Tech Stand Neurosurg 14:2–24, 1986.
14. Grunert P, Perneczky A, Resch K: Endoscopic procedures through the foramen interventriculare of Monro under stereotactical conditions. Minim Invasive Neurosurg 37:2–8, 1994.
15. Abdullah J, Caemaert J: Endoscopic management of craniopharyngiomas: A review of 3 cases. Minim Invasive Neurosurg 38:79–84, 1995.
16. Oka K, Yamamoto M, Nagasaka S, et al: Endoneurosurgical treatment for hydrocephalus caused by intraventricular tumors. Childs Nerv Syst 10:162–166, 1994.
17. Jho H-D, Carrau RL: Endoscopic endonasal transsphenoidal surgery: Experience with 50 patients. J Neurosurg 87:44–51, 1997.
18. Caemaert J, Abdullah J: Endoscopic management of colloid cysts. Tech Neurosurg 1:185–200, 1996.
19. Collmann H, Kazner E, Sprung C: Supratentorial intraventricular tumors in childhood. Acta Neurochir Suppl (Wien) 35:75–79, 1985.
20. Kelly PJ, Kall BA, Goerss S, et al: Computer-assisted stereotaxic laser resection of intra-axial brain neoplasms. J Neurosurg 64:427–439, 1986.
21. Kelly PJ: Volumetric stereotactic surgical resection of intra-axial brain mass lesions. Mayo Clin Proc 63:1186–1198, 1988.
22. Jallo GI, Morota N, Abbott R: Introduction of a second working portal for neuroendoscopy: A technical note. Pediatr Neurosurg 24:56–60, 1996.
23. Perneczky A, Fries G: Endoscope-assisted brain surgery. Part I: Evolution, basic concept, and current technique. Neurosurgery 42:219–225, 1998.
24. Fries G, Perneczky A: Endoscope-assisted brain surgery. Part 2: Analysis of 380 procedures. Neurosurgery 42:226–232, 1998.
25. Gaab MR, Schroeder HWS: Endoscopic approach to lesions of the foramen of Monro (Abstract). Zentralbl Neurochir 56 (Suppl):42, 1995.
26. Schroeder HWS, Gaab MR, Niendorf W-R, et al: Neuroendoscopy in the treatment of brain tumors (Abstract). Zentralbl Neurochir (Suppl):50, 1996.
27. Goebel KR: Fundamentals of laser science. Acta Neurochir Suppl (Wien) 61:20–33, 1994.
28. Lapras C, Deruty R, Bret P: Tumors of the lateral ventricles. Adv Tech Stand Neurosurg 11:103–167, 1984.
29. Kempe LG, Blaylock R: Lateral-trigonal intraventricular tumors: A new operative approach. Acta Neurochir (Wien) 35:233–242, 1976.
30. McKissock W: The surgical treatment of colloid cyst of the third ventricle. Brain 74:1–9, 1951.
31. Little JR, MacCarty CS: Colloid cysts of the third ventricle. J Neurosurg 39:230–235, 1974.
32. Piepmeier JM, Westerveld M, Spencer DD, et al: Surgical management of intraventricular tumors of the lateral ventricles. In Schmidek HH, Sweet WH (eds): Operative Neurosurgical Techniques, 3rd ed. Philadelphia: WB Saunders, 1995, pp 725–738.
33. Rhoton AL, Jr., Yamamoto I, Peace DA: Microsurgery of the third ventricle. Part 2: Operative approaches. Neurosurgery 8:357–373, 1981.
34. Carmel PW: Tumours of the third ventricle. Acta Neurochir (Wien) 75:136–146, 1985.
35. Sawaya R, Hawley DK, Tobler WD, et al: Pineal and third ventricle tumors. In Youmans JR (ed): Neurological Surgery, 3rd ed. Philadelphia: WB Saunders, 1990, pp 3171–3203.
36. Stein BM: The infratentorial supracerebellar approach to pineal lesions. J Neurosurg 35:197–202, 1971.
37. Apuzzo MLJ, Chikovani OK, Gott PS, et al: Transcallosal, interforniccial approaches for lesions affecting the third ventricle: Surgical considerations and consequences. Neurosurgery 10:547–554, 1982.
38. Camins MB, Schlesinger EB: Treatment of tumours of the posterior part of the third ventricle and the pineal region: A long-term follow-up. Acta Neurochir (Wien) 40:131–143, 1978.
39. Hirsch JF, Zouaoui A, Renier D, et al: A new surgical approach to the third ventricle with interruption of the striothalamic vein. Acta Neurochir (Wien) 47:135–147, 1979.
40. Busch E: A new approach for the removal of tumours of the third ventricle. Acta Psychiatr Scand 19:57–60, 1944.
41. Viale GL, Turtas S: The subchoroid approach to the third ventricle. Surg Neurol 14:71–76, 1980.
42. Cossu M, Lubinu F, Orunesu G, et al: Subchoroidal approach to the third ventricle: Microsurgical anatomy. Surg Neurol 21:325–331, 1984.
43. Otsuki T, Jokura H, Yoshimoto T: Stereotactic guiding tube for open-system endoscopy: A new approach for the stereotactic endoscopic resection of intra-axial brain tumors. Neurosurgery 27:326–330, 1990.
44. Cohen AR: Comment on Ruge JR, Johnson RF, Bauer J: Bur hole neuroendoscopic fenestration of quadrigeminal arachnoid cyst: Technical case report. Neurosurgery 38:837, 1996.
45. Perneczky A: Comment on Ruge JR, Johnson RF, Bauer J: Bur hole neuroendoscopic fenestration of quadrigeminal cistern arachnoid cyst: Technical case report. Neurosurgery 38:837, 1996.
46. Lewis AI, Crone KR, Taha J, et al: Surgical resection of third ventricle colloid cysts: Preliminary results comparing transcallosal microsurgery with endoscopy. J Neurosurg 81:174–178, 1994.
47. Regis J, Bouillot P, Rouby-Volot F, et al: Pineal region tumors and the role of stereotactic biopsy: Review of the mortality, morbidity, and diagnostic rates in 370 cases. Neurosurgery 39:907–914, 1996.
48. Kreth FW, Schätz CR, Pagenstecher A, et al: Stereotactic management of lesions of the pineal region. Neurosurgery 39:280–291, 1996.

# Management of Pineal Region Neoplasms

■ HENRY H. SCHMIDEK

## SIGNS AND SYMPTOMS OF PINEAL NEOPLASMS

Pineal region neoplasms always present significant management issues. The decision-making process requires an appreciation of the biology of the lesions that occur at this location, then tailoring of the therapeutic approach to the specifics of a particular case. This chapter provides the information to be used in a therapeutic algorithm.

Pineal tumors are a heterogeneous group of mass lesions originating in, or located adjacent to, the pineal gland. Neoplasms in this region cause symptoms when they compress or invade local structures or are disseminated beyond the confines of the tumor. When these tumors occlude the cerebral aqueduct, obstructive hydrocephalus with intracranial hypertension occurs. If the superior colliculus and pretectal areas are involved, characteristic eye signs develop, which may include impairment of upward gaze and abnormalities of the pupil, paralysis or spasm of convergence, and nystagmus retractorius. This sylvian aqueduct syndrome is indicative of a periaqueductal lesion. Parinaud's syndrome, the paralysis of upward gaze alone, is often incorrectly used as a synonym for sylvian aqueduct syndrome. The anatomic substrate underlying these functions is located just anterior to the aqueduct and below the posterior part of the third ventricle. Downward gaze, which can also be impaired in these patients, is localized caudad to that of upward gaze in the brain stem. Raised intracranial pressure and Parinaud's syndrome are the commonest findings among patients with pineal region tumors. Compression or invasion of the cerebellum results in dysmetria, hypotonia, and intention tremor. Altered consciousness may occur as a result of intracranial hypertension or direct invasion of the brain stem by tumor. Some of these tumors metastasize to the spinal cord or cauda equina or to structures outside the nervous system. These metastases may pass through shunts inserted to treat intracranial hypertension. Less common symptoms, occurring in fewer than 10% of male patients with pineal tumors, are precocious puberty or delayed onset of sexual maturation. Even less common is the occurrence of pineal apoplexy, in which a patient undergoes sudden neurologic deterioration secondary to intratumoral hemorrhage and sudden expansion in the size of the posterior third ventricular tumor.

When there is suprasellar involvement by the anterior extension of a posterior third ventricular tumor, diabetes insipidus is the commonest sign. The diabetes insipidus may precede other findings by years. For example, in a case reported by Tarng and Huang,[14] a 13-year-old boy presented with diabetes insipidus. One year later, the patient's neurologic examination, computed tomography (CT) scan, and tumor markers were all normal. Three years later, the patient had signs of raised intracranial pressure, high levels of serum human β-chorionic gonadotropin, and a positive magnetic resonance imaging (MRI) scan for a pineal tumor.

Abnormalities of the visual system are the other common symptom complex with suprasellar tumor involvement. These abnormalities include reduction in visual acuity, often in conjunction with optic atrophy. There are also isolated reports of extraocular paralysis or severe exophthalmos caused by infiltration of tumor into the optic chiasm, nerves, and orbit. Papilledema may not be evident even in the presence of marked raised intracranial pressure resulting from an associated optic atrophy. Visual field studies may demonstrate bitemporal inferior scotomas indicating a lesion on the dorsum of the chiasm. Macular fiber involvement by tumor growing into the posterior and superior part of the chiasm associated with a bitemporal inferior scotomatous defect is particularly characteristic of this tumor.

Hypopituitarism is the third most common finding and often associated with growth arrest when the tumor occurs before puberty or with hypogonadism and amenorrhea when it occurs in older patients. Pathologic obesity, neurogenic hypernatremia, hyperphagia, abnormalities in temperature regulation, and excessive somnolence are other uncommon manifestations of these lesions. Suprasellar germinomas without pineal region tumor can also metastasize throughout the neuraxis.

Tinnitus with hearing loss is seen in about 18% of patients with pineal region tumors. This tinnitus is the result of involvement of the inferior colliculi and interference with the acoustic relay pathways in this region of the brain stem.

## SUPRASELLAR GERMINOMAS

Suprasellar germinomas are tumors that are histologically identical to pineal germinomas but arise in or beneath the anterior part of the third ventricle. Many suprasellar germinomas represent an anterior extension of a pineal germinoma; however, suprasellar germinomas have been shown to exist free of pineal involvement. When these tumors present as synchronous lesions in the pineal and the suprasellar region, the initial symptoms are usually attributable to the suprasellar lesion. In one report that includes 14 patients with proven germ cell tumors with suprasellar lesions, 5 were found to have intrasellar extension, and the normal pituitary was displaced anteriorly. Ten patients (45%) had multiple lesions. Kageyama and Belsky[2] categorized suprasellar germ cell tumors. Type 1 suprasellar germinomas are metastatic tumors from the pineal that invade the floor of the third ventricle, hypophysis, and optic pathways. The symptoms of type I suprasellar germinomas are the same as those of pineal tumor and of hypothalamic and chiasmatic involvement. An admixture of these signs and symptoms is common, indicating involvement of anterior and posterior third ventricular structures. Type II germinomas arise within the third ventricle and produce an obstructive hydrocephalus early in the disease; later findings are indicative of invasion of the hypothalamus, pituitary, and optic pathways. Type III germinomas originate in the optic chiasmal region, grow outside the ventricular system, and only late in the disease invade the third ventricle and hypothalamus.[1]

## CLASSIFICATION OF PINEAL TUMORS

The lesions in the posterior third ventricle represent a spectrum of neoplasia ranging from benign to extremely malignant tumors. Approximately 10% of pineal region lesions are truly benign and include the following:

Pineal cysts
Lipomas
Arteriovenous malformations and aneurysms
Pineocytomas
Meningiomas
Hemangiomas
Mature teratomas

Another 10% of tumors are relatively benign, such as low-grade gliomas including ganglioglioma and dermoid cysts. The remaining 80% of pineal region neoplasms are highly malignant lesions and include the following:

Germinoma (atypical teratoma) (40% of malignant tumors)
Teratocarcinoma
Choriocarcinoma
Endodermal sinus tumor
Pineoblastoma and mixed pineocytoma/blastoma
Glioblastoma
Sarcomas
Immature and malignant teratomas
Trilateral retinoblastomas
Metastatic tumors

## PREOPERATIVE EVALUATION

MRI with and without gadolinium enhancement of the head indicates the size and position of the pineal lesion; whether there is a calcific, cystic, or hemorrhagic component; the degree of hydrocephalus; and suprasellar, intraparenchymal, subependymal, and lateral ventricular involvement. Extension into the orbit and expansion of the optic nerves or chiasm may occur as a result of tumor infiltration. MRI is sensitive in the detection of pineal region tumors and provides superb anatomic detail of the lesion and regional anatomy, cerebrospinal fluid pathways, and subependymal tumor extension. MRI signal characteristics are often suggestive of the diagnosis, but there is always a lingering uncertainty until a tissue diagnosis is made. Magnetic resonance spectroscopy attempting to bridge the divide between anatomic and histopathologic data remains in its infancy at present. MRI examination of the spinal axis in patients with a posterior third ventricular neoplasm of undefined character is mandatory to identify asymptomatic spinal metastases and, if positive, as a baseline to assess the subsequent response to therapy.

*Magnetic resonance angiography* identifies aneurysms of the posterior cerebral artery, arteriovenous malformations, abnormalities of the vein of Galen, and meningiomas. Once identified, these lesions can be treated appropriately. Selective cerebral angiography provides information about the relationships of the internal cerebral veins, the vein of Galen, the basal veins of Rosenthal, and the straight sinus to the lesion—all of which are important in the surgical planning. In appropriate cases, angiography can be combined with embolization as another preoperative measure.

*Cytologic examination of cerebrospinal fluid* is important; the presence of malignant cells in the cerebrospinal fluid establishes the diagnosis and the extent of nervous system involvement. Seeding of the cerebrospinal fluid is a characteristic feature of germinomas but has been reported to occur with ependymomas, pineoblastomas, and glioblastomas.

The patient with a posterior third ventricular tumor requires careful *endocrine assessment*. Diabetes insipidus is the most common endocrine abnormality associated with pineal tumors; when present, it is often caused by anterior third ventricular extension of the neoplasm. Such patients are often overlooked. The appropriate provocative tests are performed to determine whether this condition is present. Tests of anterior pituitary function are performed to exclude corticotropin-releasing hormone deficiency and secondary, possibly life-threatening, insufficiency. Abnormalities of sexual maturation require that the levels of luteinizing hormone, follicle-stimulating hormone, testosterone, prolactin, and growth hormone as well as the melatonin-forming activity of the cerebrospinal fluid and serum be surveyed.

*Neuro-ophthalmologic examination* is mandatory to search for defects seen in conjunction with these lesions and to provide evidence of the extent of tumor involvement, which may not be apparent from the other studies.

*Immunoassay of the blood and cerebrospinal fluid* is performed to determine the presence of α-fetoprotein, human β-chorionic gonadotropin, and placental alkaline phosphatase. Endodermal sinus tumors, in particular, are identified with an elevation of α-fetoprotein levels; chorio-carcinomas, with an elevation of human β-chorionic gonad-otropin levels; and malignant teratomas or undifferentiated germ cell tumors, with an elevation of both of these mark-ers. The plasma level of these tumor markers correlates with tumor growth and regression and may be used to assess the patient's response to therapy.[5]

## SURGICAL OPTIONS AND GOALS

The surgical management of pineal region neoplasms in-volves identification of their probable nature from the ex-tensive preoperative investigation and tailoring of the fur-ther care to the specifics of the case. Even though it is feasible for an experienced surgeon to operate on pineal tumors at an acceptable risk, patients in whom the cerebro-spinal fluid shows malignant cells, patients with spinal or extraneural metastases that can be biopsied, and patients in whom one of the tumor markers is abnormal are harboring a germinoma or other malignant germ cell tumor and may require only relief of hydrocephalus before irradiation and chemotherapy.

Several different, preferably image-guided, craniotomy approaches exist that allow satisfactory exposure in the pineal region. A strong indication exists for such *interven-tion* in patients with a symptomatic cyst, meningioma, lipoma, or aneurysm. Another selected group of patients that should undergo direct surgical intervention are those patients who at some point were treated with shunt and radiation, without a tissue diagnosis, who subsequently develop progressive neurologic problems. These patients have often survived for years, and benign tumors are partic-ularly common among them.

Frame-based and frameless stereotaxis are techniques for the aspiration of cysts, biopsy of tumors, and insertion of interstitial isotopes for brachytherapy. There is significant experience with each of these approaches, and each has been successfully applied to patients with pineal region tumors. If doubt exists as to the nature of a pineal lesion, biopsy is mandatory, and these techniques allow this to be performed with relative safety. Among 370 stereotactic biopsy specimens of pineal region tumors collected at 15 French neurosurgical centers, the mortality rate was 1.3% (5 of 370 patients), and 3 patients suffered severe neuro-logic complications. Another center, using CT-guided ste-reotaxis for pineal tumor biopsy in 106 patients, was able to establish the histologic diagnosis in 103 of the 106 patients. These investigators also used this approach in some of these cases for cyst aspiration and brachytherapy. In this series, two patients died, and nine patients had perioperative morbidity.

Using a flexible, steerable neuroendoscope, a minimally invasive procedure can be performed through a bur hole, and cerebrospinal fluid can be obtained for cytologic exam-ination and for tumor markers, obstructive hydrocephalus can be relieved with a third ventriculostomy (ameliorating the need for a shunt), and the lesion can be biopsied under direct vision. This is a particularly attractive approach to posterior third ventricular tumors that is increasingly being used in the neurosurgical community.

The exquisite responsiveness of germinomas to radiation means that the surgical objective in these cases is relief of hydrocephalus and biopsy to establish a tissue diagnosis. There is no advantage to undertaking extensive surgical resection once one has the diagnosis of germinoma. Under these circumstances, further therapy involves some form of radiation therapy and subsequent chemotherapy. Gamma knife radiosurgery is well suited for the management of discrete posterior third ventricular masses. Alternately, ei-ther interstitial brachytherapy or conventional radiation therapy is effective. Dearnaley and colleagues[5] reported on the protocol and results obtained with radiation therapy of germ cell tumors treated at the Royal Marsden Hospital from 1962 to 1987. At that institution, patients with germ cell tumors are treated with radiation therapy to the neu-raxis with 50 Gy given to the tumor and 30 Gy to the remaining brain and spinal cord. This regimen is analogous to another report, in which the median dose of 54 Gy is delivered to the tumor bed, 36 Gy to the whole brain, and 24 Gy to the spinal axis. Craniospinal irradiation was associated with low morbidity in patients in whom spinal growth was complete. Craniospinal irradiation is also used in patients with disease involving more than one intracran-ial site, meningeal seeding, or positive cerebrospinal fluid cytology.

The absence of the blood-brain barrier in the pineal gland suggests that lesions located there may have an increased vulnerability to *systemic chemotherapy*. Objec-tive remission has been reported in a pineal tumor with pulmonary metastases treated with chlorambucil, metho-trexate, and dactinomycin. Testicular germinomas, which are histologically identical to pineal germinomas, have shown an 82% remission rate when treated with bleomycin, vinblastine, and cisplatin.[8] Although chemotherapy has been reserved for patients with systemic, extraneural metas-tases or for those with recurrent disease within the neuraxis after full courses of radiation therapy, in whom further radiation is not an option, this view concerning the role of chemotherapy in the management of pineal region malig-nant neoplasms is undergoing modification. Evidence exists that primary intracranial germ cell tumors can be induced to undergo remission with alternate courses of chemother-apy consisting of etoposide (VP-16) with cisplatin alternat-ing with vincristine, methotrexate, and bleomycin, without radiation therapy,[17] although the commoner approach is cisplatin-based chemotherapy in conjunction with radiation therapy to induce tumor remissions.[18, 19]

A heroic approach that has been used in relapsed or refractory germ cell tumors has been treatment with high-dose chemotherapy and marrow transplantation. Although the experience with pineal germ cell tumors is limited, this option might be considered for salvage therapy in otherwise untreatable cases.

## REFERENCES

1. Sugiyama K, Uozumi T, Kiya K, Mukada T: Intracranial germ-cell tumor with synchronous lesions in the pineal and suprasellar regions: Report of six cases and review of the literature. Surg Neurol 38:114–120, 1992.

2. Kageyama N, Belsky R: Ectopic pinealoma in the chiasma region. Neurology 11:318, 1961.
3. Schmidek HH (ed): Pineal Tumors. New York, Masson, 1977.
4. Linggood RM, Chapman PH: Pineal tumors. J Neurooncol 12:85–91, 1992.
5. Dearnaley DP, A'Hern RP, Whittaker S, Bloom HJ: Pineal and CNS germ-cell tumors: Royal Marsden Hospital experience 1962–1987. Int J Radiat Oncol Biol Phys 18:773–781, 1990.
6. Castaneda VL, Parmley RT, Geiser CF, Saldivar VA: Postoperative chemotherapy for primary intracranial germ cell tumor. Med Pediatr Oncol 18:299–303, 1990.
7. Patel SR, Buckner JC, Smithson WA, et al: Cisplatin-based chemotherapy in primary nervous system germ cell tumors. J Neurooncol 12:4752, 1992.
8. Itoyama Y, Kochi M, Yamamoto H, Kuratsu J: Clinical study of intracranial non-germinomatous germ cell tumors producing alpha-fetoprotein. Neurosurgery 27:454–460, 1990.
9. Haase J, Nielsen K: Value of tumor markers in the treatment of endodermal sinus tumors and choriocarcinomas in the pineal region. Neurosurgery 5:484, 1979.
10. Dempsey PK, Lunsford LD: Stereotactic radiosurgery for pineal region tumors. Neurosurg Clin North Am 3:245–253, 1992.
11. Nazzaro JM, Shults WT, Neuwelt EA: Neuro-ophthalmological function of patients with pineal tumors approached transtentorially in the semisitting position. J Neurosurg 5:746–751, 1992.
12. Nakagawa K, Aoki Y, Akanuma A, Sakata K: Radiation therapy of intracranial germ cell tumors with radiosensitivity assessment. Radiat Med 10:55–61, 1992.
13. Missoori P, Delfini R, Cantore G: Tinnitus and hearing loss in pineal region tumors. Acta Neurochir 135:154–158, 1995.
14. Tarng DC, Huang TP: Diabetes insipidus as an early sign of pineal tumor. Am J Nephrol 15:161–164, 1995.
15. Ziyal IM, Sekhar LN, Salas E, Olan WJ: Combined supra/infratentorial transsinus approach to large pineal region tumors. J Neurosurg 88:1050–1057, 1998.
16. Sawamura Y, de Tribolet N, Ishii N, Abe H: Management of primary intracranial germinomas: Diagnostic surgery or radical resection? J Neurosurg 87:262–266, 1997.
17. Regis J, Bouillot P, Rouby-Volot F, et al: Pineal region tumors and the role of stereotactic biopsy: Review of the mortality, morbidity, and diagnostic rates in 370 cases. Neurosurgery 39:907–912, 1996.
18. Kreth FW, Schatz CR, Pagenstecher A, et al: Stereotactic management of lesions of the pineal region. Neurosurgery 39:280–289, 1996.
19. Ferrer E, Santamarta D, Garcia-Fructuoso G, et al: Neuroendoscopic management of pineal region tumors. Acta Neurochir (Wien) 139:12–20, 1997.
20. Chasan CB, Goetsch S, Ott K: Radiosurgery for pineal tumors: Is biopsy indicated? Stereotact Funct Neurosurg 66 (Suppl 1):157–163, 1996.
21. Matsumoto K, Higashi H, Tomita S, Ohmoto T: Pineal region tumors treated with interstitial brachytherapy with low activity sources (192-iridium). Acta Neurochir (Wien) 136:21–28, 1995.
22. Huh SJ, Shin KH, Kim IH, et al: Radiotherapy of intracranial germinomas. Radiother Oncol 38:19–23, 1996.
23. Mandanas RA, Saez RA, Epstein RB, et al: Long-term results of autologous marrow transplantation for relapsed or refractory male and female germ cell tumors. Bone Marrow Transplant 21:569–576, 1998.

# Alternate Surgical Approaches to Pineal Region Neoplasms

■ KEIJI SANO

Because the pineal body is located in the center of the cranial cavity, Descartes (1596–1650), the greatest philosopher of 17th century France, thought that the pineal body might be the seat of the soul. This concept is wrong. The pineal body is, however, the seat of various kinds of neoplasms. Because of the central location of the pineal body, the distance between it and the surface of any portion of the scalp is almost the same, regardless of the surgical approach taken to the pineal region (Fig. 64–1). The surgical approach to this region should be chosen according to the size and extension of the neoplasm so that removal of the neoplasm is most extensive or complete, and damage to the normal brain is minimal. Neoplasms in the pineal region constitute 3.5% of all primary intracranial neoplasms in Japan (996 of 28,424 cases).[1] These neoplasms are mostly germinomas, or tumors of the two-cell pattern type, which form 2.3% of all primary Japanese intracranial neoplasms.[1] In the same statistics, pineocytoma constitutes 0.1%; pineoblastoma, 0.2%; teratoma, including malignant teratoma, 0.8%; and choriocarcinoma, 0.1% of all primary intracranial neoplasms. In the pineal region, germ cell tumors and tumors of pineal parenchymal origin are predominantly found.

This chapter discusses the surgery and management of germinoma, germinoma with syncytiotrophoblastic giant cells, embryonal carcinoma, endodermal sinus tumor (yolk sac tumor), choriocarcinoma, mature teratoma, immature teratoma, teratoma with malignant transformation, so-called mixed germ cell tumors, and pineocytoma with lymphocytic infiltration. I believe that only germinoma derives from primordial germ cells and is the true germ cell tumor.[2, 3] Among neoplasms of the two-cell pattern type in the pineal region, germinoma (true germ cell tumor) and pineocytoma with lymphocytic infiltration may be differentiated on the basis of the difference of the tumor cell–stroma relationship and placental alkaline phosphatase stain (positive in germinoma and negative in pineocytoma with lymphocytic infiltration).[2, 4] Both neoplasms are radiosensitive, however, and their biologic behaviors are similar.

## THERAPEUTIC PRINCIPLES

Diagnosis of a medium-sized or large tumor arising in the pineal region and the posterior third ventricle is not difficult because of the presence of increased intracranial pressure, paralysis of conjugate upward gaze (Parinaud's sign), and pseudo–Argyll Robertson pupil (reacting to accommodation but not to light). In the later stages, ataxia, choreic movements, or spastic weakness of the limbs may appear. Cerebral angiography is useful in the detection of the extent and vascularization of the tumor. Calcification in plain craniograms may sometimes be pathognomonic, especially in patients younger than 10 years of age. The most powerful noninvasive diagnostic tools are computed tomography (CT) and magnetic resonance imaging (MRI).

Levels of α-fetoprotein (AFP), human chorionic gonadotropin (hCG), and carcinoembryonic antigen should be determined in the serum or the cerebrospinal fluid in all cases. The first two tumor markers (AFP and hCG) are especially informative about the nature of tumors in this region. If hCG is present, the tumor must be a choriocarcinoma, a mixed germ cell tumor with choriocarcinomatous elements, or a germinoma with syncytiotrophoblastic giant cells. The last tumor type is not as malignant as choriocarcinoma and mixed tumors with choriocarcinomatous elements. The levels of serum hCG in choriocarcinoma cases are more than 2000 mIU/ml, whereas those in cases of germinoma with syncytiotrophoblastic giant cells are less than 1000 mIU/ml.[5] If AFP is present, the tumor must be an endodermal sinus tumor (yolk sac tumor) or a mixed germ cell tumor with endodermal sinus tumor elements. Prognosis of choriocarcinoma or endodermal sinus tumor, especially the former, is poor, even after surgical removal of the tumor and postoperative radiotherapy of the whole neuraxis.[2, 3, 5] Chemotherapeutic agents, such as dactinomycin (actinomycin D), cisplatin, vinblastine, bleomycin, etoposide, or their combinations, are reported to be useful.[5]

If AFP and hCG are not present, the tumor may be a germinoma, embryonal carcinoma, mature teratoma, immature teratoma, teratoma with malignant transformation mixed germ cell tumor with a combination of these tumor elements, or a pineal parenchymal tumor (pineocytoma, pineoblastoma, or pineocytoma with lymphocytic infiltration[2]). AFP and hCG are not present in pure embryonal carcinoma, which is rare. This tumor, however, is more frequently found as a mixed tumor with endodermal sinus tumor or choriocarcinoma. In these cases, AFP or hCG is present.

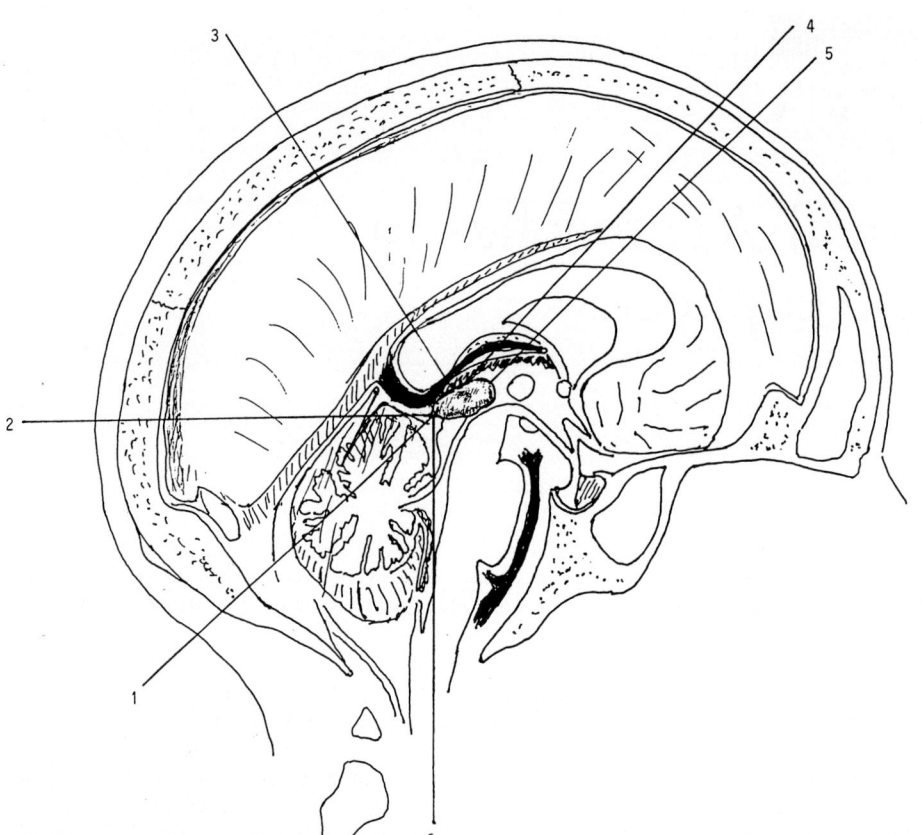

**FIGURE 64–1 ■** Various approaches to tumors in the pineal region and the posterior third ventricle: (1) infratentorial supracerebellar, (2) occipital transtentorial, (3) posterior transcallosal or posterior transventricular, (4) anterior transcallosal transventricular transvelum interpositum, (5) transcallosal interfornicial, (6) lateral-paramedian infratentorial.

If 20 Gy of local radiation effectively abolishes the tumor, as confirmed by CT scan or MRI, the tumor may be a germinoma or a two-cell pattern type of tumor of pineal parenchymal origin, which I call *pineocytoma with lymphocytic infiltration* or which used to be called *pinealoma,* in honor of Krabbe.[6] In this case, radiation should be continued to 50 Gy. If the tumor diameter is more than 2 cm (or sometimes > 1.5 cm), direct surgery and removal of the tumor followed by radiation is recommended. (For germinoma and pineocytoma with lymphocytic infiltration, local radiation is usually sufficient treatment.) Mature teratoma and immature teratoma can be cured only by removal of the tumor, and the prognosis is good after this treatment. Embryonal carcinoma and teratoma with malignant transformation usually show poor prognosis, even after surgical removal and postoperative radiotherapy of the whole neuraxis.[5] The chemotherapeutic agents mentioned earlier are also recommended in these patients. A flow chart of therapies for various tumors is presented in Figure 64–2.

Stereotactic biopsy of tumors of this region has been gaining in popularity. I am not particularly enthusiastic about this procedure, however, because different parts of the same tumor of this region may show different histology; a biopsy specimen of a small piece of the tumor may mislead the clinician as to the true nature of the tumor. I prefer exploration and debulking (unless removal is possible) of the tumor. Cytologic examination of the cerebrospinal fluid is important for diagnosis. If malignant neoplastic cells are identified cytologically, the patient may develop disseminated metastases in the cerebrospinal fluid space. For diagnostic purposes, I recommend millipore filter-cell culture[7] of the cerebrospinal fluid. This method is more sensitive than conventional cytologic studies. A positive culture result does not necessarily mean that the probability of disseminated metastases is high. During follow-up, repeated examinations of the tumor markers are useful to detect recurrence of the tumor that is producing these markers at the earliest possible stage.

## ANATOMIC CONSIDERATIONS

The artery supplying the pineal body is the medial posterior choroidal artery (ramus choroideus posterior medialis). This artery arises from the posterior cerebral artery lateral to its junction with the posterior communicating artery (pars postcommunicalis); runs in the ambient cistern, parallel to the posterior cerebral artery; supplies the pineal body and superior and inferior colliculi; and runs forward in the tela choroidea of the third ventricle. It then turns backward at the foramen of Monro, runs in the choroid plexus of the lateral ventricle, and anastomoses with the lateral posterior choroidal arteries, sending branches to the anterior thalamic nucleus, the medial geniculate body, and the pulvinar. This artery is usually single (69%) but is sometimes double (23.9%), triple (6.2%), or quadruple (0.9%).[8]

There are usually two lateral posterior choroidal arteries (rami choroidei posteriores laterales) (but they range from one to four). They arise from the posterior cerebral artery (pars postcommunicalis), run in the ambient cistern, go through the choroidal fissure, run into the choroid plexus

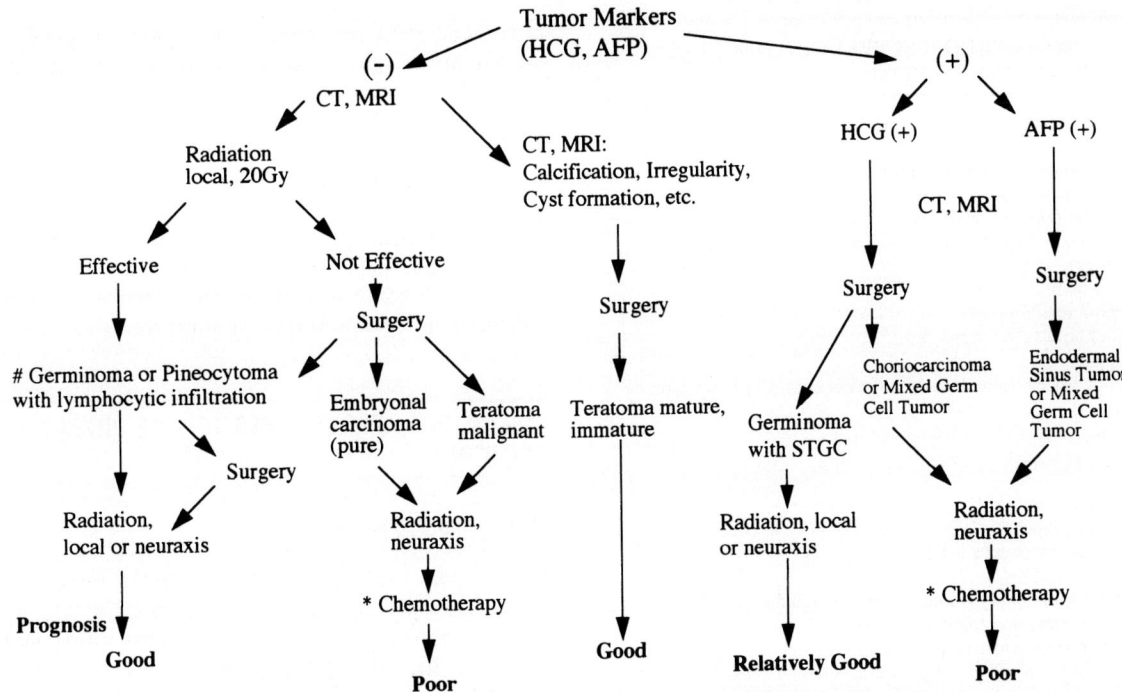

FIGURE 64–2 ■ Pineal tumors: flowchart of treatments. Pineocytoma or pineoblastoma may be treated in the same way as pineocytoma with lymphocytic infiltration.

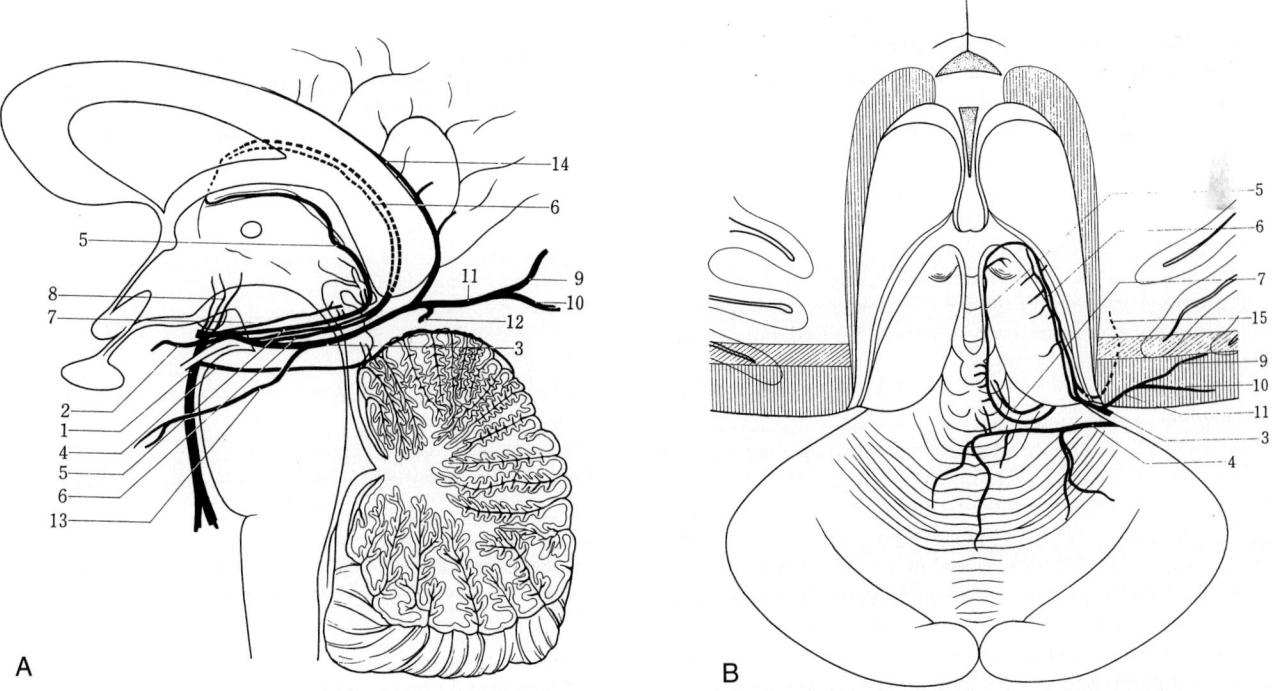

FIGURE 64–3 ■ *A,* Lateral view. *B,* View from above. Arteries supplying the pineal region and its neighborhood. (1) A. basilaris (basilar artery); (2) A. communicans posterior (posterior communicating artery); (3) A. cerebri posterior (posterior cerebral artery); (4) A. cerebelli superior (superior cerebellar artery); (5) ramus choroideus posterior medialis (medial posterior choroidal artery); (6) rami choroidei posteriores laterales (lateral posterior choroidal arteries); (7) A. laminae tecti, sive A. quadrigemina (quadrigeminal artery); (8) thalamoperforating arteries; (9) ramus parieto-occipitalis (parieto-occipital artery); (10) ramus calcarinus (calcarine artery); (11) A. occipitalis medialis; (12) A. temporalis posterior (posterior temporal artery); (13) A. temporalis anterior (anterior temporal artery); (14) A. pericallosa posterior (posterior pericallosal artery); (15) A. choroidea anterior. (From Sano K: Surgery of pineal tumors—anatomical consideration of various approaches. Neurol Surg [Tokyo] 12:1119–1129, 1984.)

## TABLE 64–1 ■ ARTERIES SUPPLYING THE PINEAL AND NEIGHBORING REGIONS

From the posterior cerebral artery (arteria cerebri posterior)
   From the pars precommunicalis
      Arteria laminae tecti (arteria quadrigemina)
         Colliculus superior
   From the pars postcommunicalis
      Medial posterior choroidal artery (ramus choroideus posterior
        medialis)
        Pineal body
        Corpora quadrigemina
        Tela choroidea ventriculi tertii
        Thalamus
      Lateral posterior choroidal arteries (rami choroidei posteriores
        laterales)
        Choroid plexus of the lateral ventricle
        Lateral geniculate body
        Thalamus
   From the peripheral trunk
      Arteria occipitalis medialis
      Calcarine artery (ramus calcarinus)
        Sulcus calcarinus
      Parieto-occipital artery (ramus parieto-occipitalis)
        Sulcus parieto-occipitalis and its area
      Posterior pericallosal artery
From the superior cerebellar artery (arteria cerebelli superior)
      Colliculus inferior

of the lateral ventricle, and anastomose with the medial posterior choroidal artery and the anterior choroidal artery, sending branches to the lateral geniculate body and parts of the thalamus. The arteria laminae tecti (arteria quadrigemina)[8] arises from the posterior cerebral artery medial to its junction with the posterior communicating artery (pars precommunicalis), runs in the ambient cistern, and supplies the superior colliculus. A branch of the superior cerebellar artery supplies the inferior colliculus. From the peripheral trunk of the posterior cerebral artery, the arteria occipitalis medialis arises and sends the calcarine artery (ramus calcarinus) to the calcarine sulcus and the parieto-occipital artery (ramus parieto-occipitalis) to the parieto-occipital sulcus and its area. These arteries are listed in Table 64–1 and are diagrammed in Figure 64–3. The arteries supplying various portions of the brain stem and the thalamus should always be preserved at surgery.

The draining veins from the pineal body and the habenular trigone were named the *superior* and *inferior pineal veins* by Tamaki and colleagues[9] and flow into the vein of Galen or the internal cerebral veins. The veins from the superior and inferior colliculi, the superior and inferior quadrigeminal veins (per Tamaki and colleagues[9]), or the tectal veins (per Matsushima and associates[10]) flow into the vein of Galen or the superior vermian vein. The basal veins of Rosenthal flow directly into the vein of Galen (28%[8]), into the internal cerebral veins (34%), into the confluence of the bilateral internal cerebral veins (28%), or directly into the straight sinus (about 9%). Many veins draining the frontal base, the lateral ventricle, and the hippocampus flow into the basal veins.

The anterior septal vein, the anterior caudate vein, the choroidal vein of the choroid plexus, and the thalamostriate (terminal) vein flow into the internal cerebral vein at the posterior rim of the foramen of Monro. In addition, the internal cerebral vein receives the posterior septal vein, the medial atrial vein (trigonal vein), and the direct lateral veins. The internal cerebral veins flow into the vein of Galen, which is 0.5 to 1.5 cm long and flows into the straight sinus (sinus rectus). The precentral cerebellar vein (one present in 46%, two in 54%) and the superior vermian veins (one present in 70%, two in 30%) flow into the vein of Galen or directly into the straight sinus. These veins are listed in Table 64–2 and are diagrammed in Figure 64–4. The veins draining portions of the brain stem and thalamus should always be preserved at surgery.

## OPERATIVE APPROACHES TO THE PINEAL REGION

### Historical Perspectives

Horsley was probably the first to try to remove a pineal tumor. He used the infratentorial supracerebellar approach but with poor results. He recommended supratentorial approaches. In 1913, Krause successfully removed a huge tumor in the region of the quadrigeminal plate from a 10-year-old boy by the infratentorial supracerebellar approach, which he reported on with Oppenheim, who diagnosed the case.[11] The tumor was reported to be a fibrosarcoma or an encapsulated mixed cell sarcoma but seems to have been a teratoma or meningioma, according to modern pathologic designation. The boy was reported to have been well at least until the first World War. In 1926, Krause[12] added two

## TABLE 64–2 ■ VEINS DRAINING THE PINEAL AND NEIGHBORING REGIONS

Great cerebral vein of Galen (vena cerebri magna)
   Pineal veins (superior and inferior)
      Pineal body
      Trigonum habenulae
   Quadrigeminal veins (superior and inferior) (tectal veins)
      Corporal quadrigemina
   Superior vermian vein
      Superior vermis
   Precentral cerebellar vein
      Cerebellum
      Superior cerebellar peduncle
   Posterior pericallosal vein
   Internal occipital vein
Internal cerebral veins (venae cerebri internae)
   Septal veins (anterior and posterior)
      Septum pellucidum
   Anterior caudate vein
      Caput nuclei caudata
   Thalamostriate vein (vena thalamostriata, terminal vein)
   Choroidal vein (vena choroidea)
      Choroid plexus of the lateral ventricle
   Medial atrial vein (trigonal vein)
      Trigonum of the lateral ventricle
   Direct lateral veins
Basal veins of Rosenthal (venae basales)
   Vena cerebri media profunda
   Venae centrales (striatae) inferiores
   Vena cerebri anterior
   Vena apicis cornus temporalis (hippocampal vein)
   Vena atrii lateralis (lateral atrial vein)
   Vena cornus temporalis (atriotemporal vein)

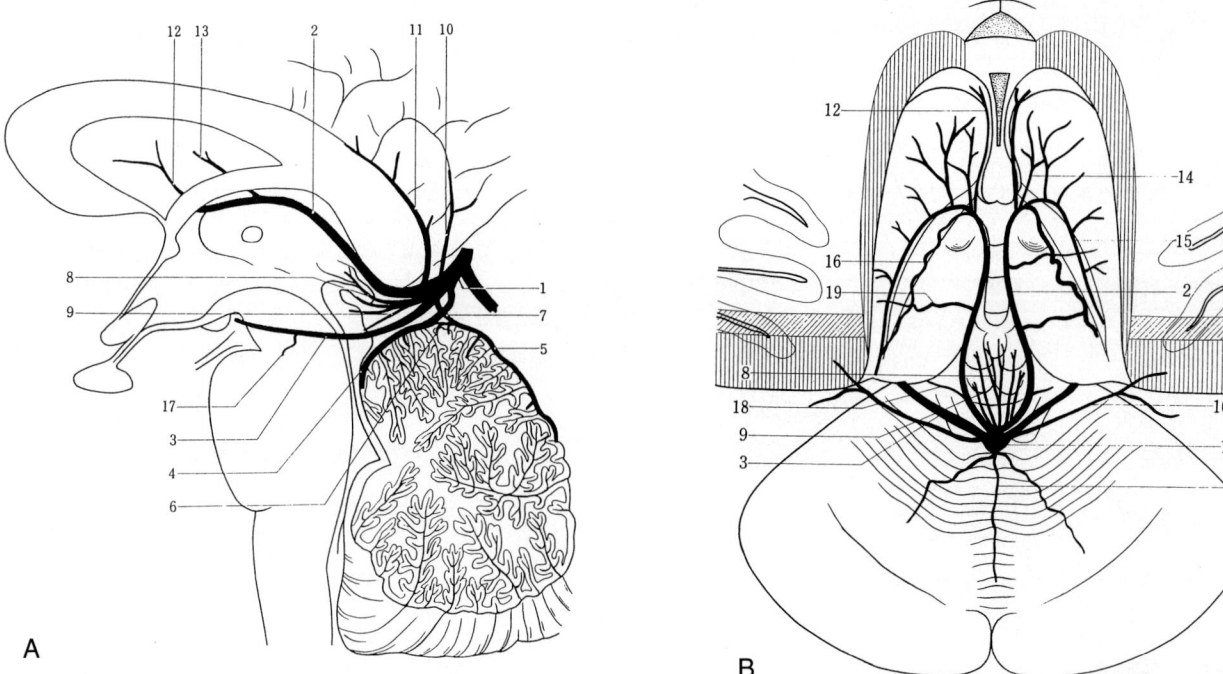

**FIGURE 64–4** ■ *A,* Lateral view. *B,* View from above. Veins draining from the pineal region and its neighborhood: (1) v. cerebri magna (great cerebral vein of Galen); (2) v. cerebri interna (internal cerebral vein); (3) v. basalis (basal vein of Rosenthal); (4) precentral cerebellar vein; (5) supraculminate vein; (6) pre- and intraculminate veins; (7) superior vermian vein; (8) superior and inferior pineal veins[9]; (9) superior and inferior quadrigeminal (tectal) veins; (10) internal occipital vein; (11) posterior pericallosal vein; (12) anterior septal vein; (13) posterior septal vein; (14) anterior caudate vein; (15) v. thalamostriata (thalamostriate vein, terminal vein); (16) choroidal vein (V. choroidea); (17) lateral mesencephalic vein; (18) medial atrial vein (trigonal vein); (19) direct lateral vein. (From Sano K: Surgery of pineal tumors: Anatomical consideration of various approaches. Neurol Surg 12:1119–1129, 1984.)

more patients, who were operated on by the same approach; in these two, however, he could not remove the tumors. In 1956, Zapletal[13] reported using practically the same approach. He reported on four cases: a malignant astrocytoma in the quadrigeminal region, a medulloblastoma of the upper vermis, an epidermoid, and a pineal tumor. The last one was successfully removed. In 1971, using microsurgical techniques, Stein[14] revived and elaborated this infratentorial supracerebellar approach, which has been widely used since then.

The parietal transcallosal approach was performed by Dandy[15] in 1921, then by Kunicki[16] and others. In 1931, Van Wagenen[17] proposed the posterior transventricular approach. This approach, however, has been used only rarely.

The occipital or parieto-occipital approach along the falx with or without splitting the tentorium and with or without splitting the splenium of the corpus callosum has been done by Heppner,[18] Poppen and Marino,[19] Glasauer,[20] Jamieson,[21] Lazar and Clark,[22] and many others. Special credit should be given to Jamieson, who established the occipital transtentorial approach. For huge tumors in the pineal region or the posterior third ventricle, Sano[4, 23–26] proposed the anterior transcallosal transventricular trans–velum interpositum approach. In 1990, Van den Bergh[27] proposed the lateral-paramedian infratentorial approach, which is a modification of the infratentorial supracerebellar approach. The unilateral cerebellopontine angle is explored, and from there, the tentorial notch is reached over the unilateral cerebellar hemisphere so that the tumor can be dissected between the

internal cerebral vein and the basal vein of Rosenthal. Other approaches, such as the subchoroidal approach[28, 29] and the transcallosal interfornicial approach,[30] are primarily used for lesions in the middle or anterior third ventricle. These may be used for tumors in the pineal-posterior third ventricular region.

Among various operative approaches to neoplasms in this region, I prefer the occipital transtentorial approach proposed by Poppen and Marino,[19] Jamieson,[21] and others; the infratentorial supracerebellar approach proposed by Krause and Oppenheim,[11, 12] Zapletal,[13] and Stein[14]; or the lateral-paramedian infratentorial approach proposed by Van den Bergh,[27] if the neoplasm is medium sized or small. If, however, the neoplasm is large enough to reach anterior to the adhesio interthalamica, the anterior transcallosal transventricular trans–velum interpositum approach, originally described as the frontal transcallosal approach by Sano,[4, 23–26] is recommended.

The infratentorial supracerebellar approach is described in another chapter. The parietal transcallosal approach[15] inevitably requires splitting of the splenium to cause disconnection syndrome. In the subchoroidal approach, the thalamostriate vein must be sacrificed; this process may damage the thalamus. The transcallosal interfornicial approach provides a narrow operative field, and there is a danger of a lesion of both fornices. In this chapter, only the occipital transtentorial, the lateral-paramedian infratentorial, and the anterior transcallosal transventricular trans–velum interpositum approaches are described.

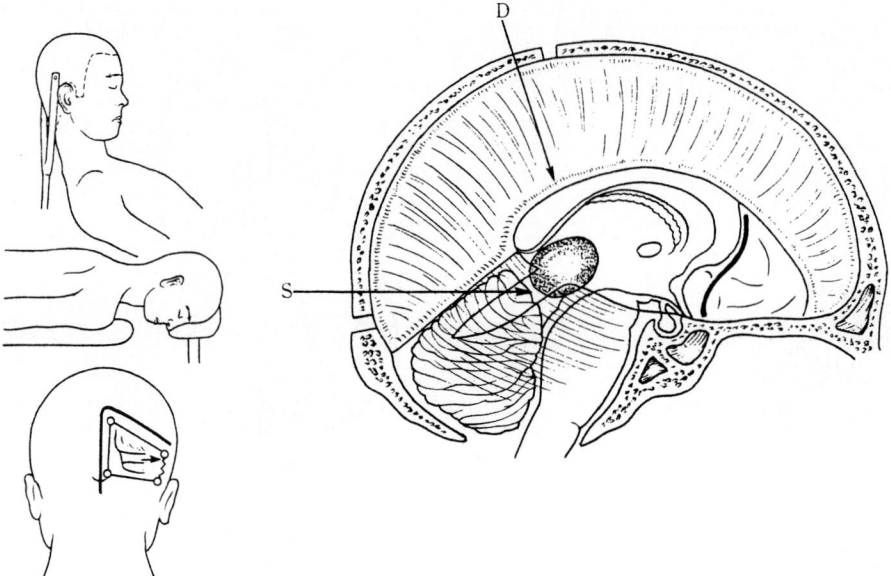

FIGURE 64–5 ■ Occipital transtentorial approach (S) and parietal transcallosal approach (D). (From Sano K: Pineal region tumors: Problems in pathology and treatment. Clin Neurosurg 30:59–91, 1983.)

## Occipital Transtentorial Approach

For the occipital transtentorial approach to a pineal neoplasm, I use the incision (usually on the nondominant side, i.e., on the right side) illustrated in Figures 64–5 and 64–6. The midline portion of the incision can be elongated to the suboccipital region if opening the posterior fossa for supracerebellar approach is necessary to add. Ziyal and coworkers[31] published a combined supratentorial and infratentorial trans-sinus approach. Sectioning the transverse sinus is not necessary in my opinion, however.

Craniotomy is close to the superior sagittal and the transverse sinuses. If necessary, the bone edge over the sinus is rongeured off. The patient is either in the prone position (the operating table should be slightly tilted to the side of craniotomy, i.e., the right side, so that the right occipital lobe sinks laterally and falls off the falx) or in the lounging position (see Fig. 64–5). The posterior horn is punctured through the dura mater, and a silicone rubber tube is inserted into the posterior portion of the lateral ventricle and secured to the dura (Fig. 64–7). The tube drains cerebrospinal fluid during the operation and makes

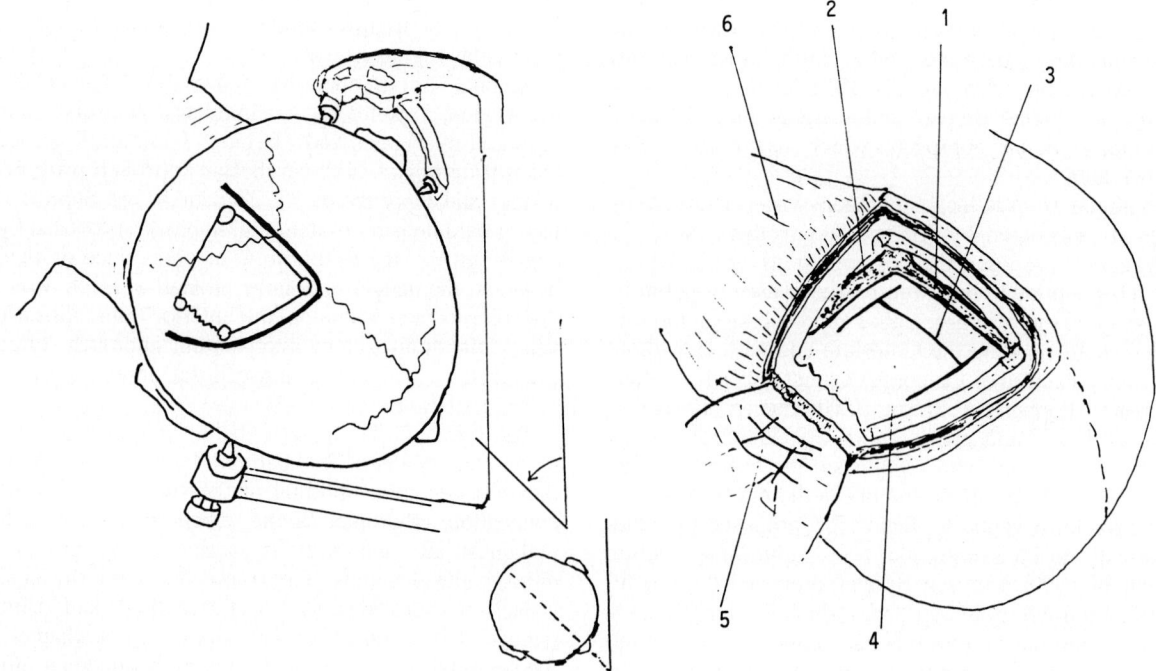

FIGURE 64–6 ■ Occipital transtentorial approach. The prone position is used, with the patient's head tilted toward the right side. (1) Superior sagittal sinus; (2) transverse sinus; (3) dural incision; (4) dura; (5) bone flap; (6) skin flap.

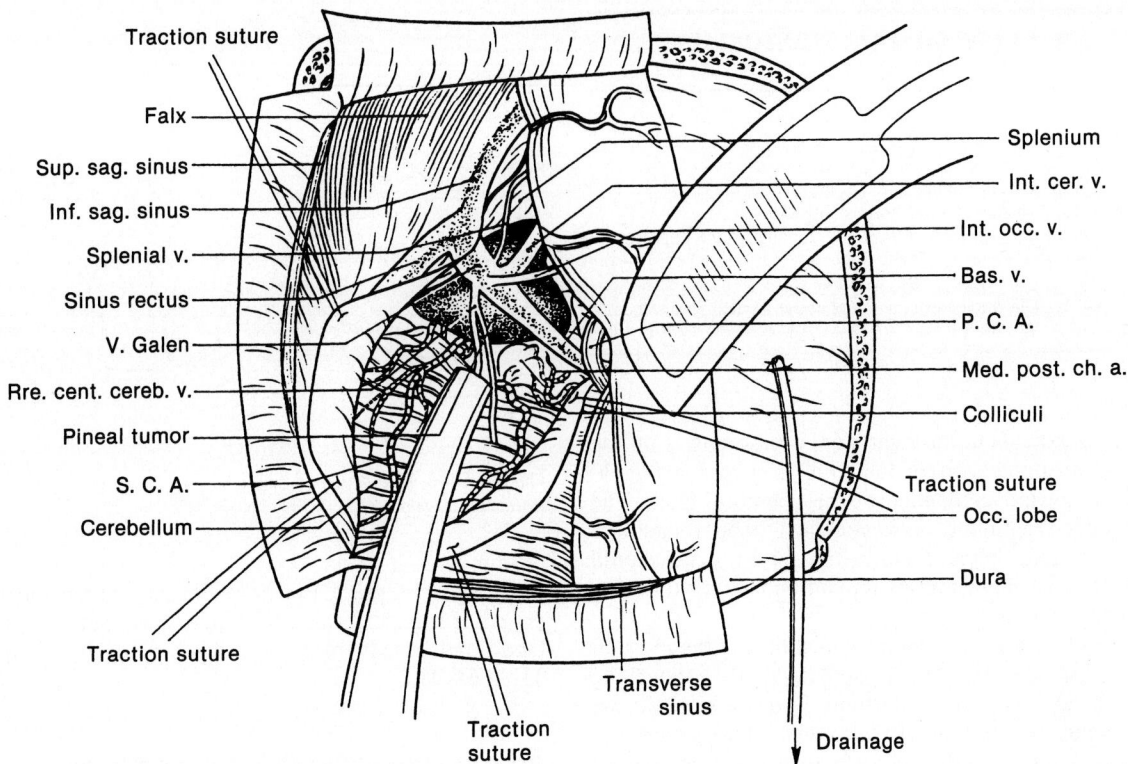

**FIGURE 64–7** ■ Occipital transtentorial approach (detailed view). Tumor (*dotted black*) is visible in front of the vein of Galen and the vein of Rosenthal. Sup. sag. sinus, superior sagittal sinus; Inf. sag. sinus, inferior sagittal sinus; Splenial v., splenial vein or posterior pericallosal vein; V. Galen, vein of Galen; Pre. Cent. Cereb. v., precentral cerebellar vein; S.C.A., superior cerebellar artery; Int. occ. v., internal occipital vein; Int. cer. v., internal cerebral vein; Bas. v., basal vein of Rosenthal; P.C.A., posterior cerebral artery; Med. post. ch. a.; medial posterior choroidal artery; Occ. lobe, occipital lobe. (From Sano K: Surgery of pineal tumors: Anatomical consideration of various approaches. Neurol Surg 12:1119–1129, 1984.)

lateral retraction of the occipital lobe unnecessary or easier. The dura is opened by an H-shaped incision close to the superior sagittal sinus.

The operating microscope is used from this stage. The tentorium is split close to the straight sinus, and the superior surface of the cerebellum is exposed. The arachnoid over the deep veins, which is tough and opaque, is sharply dissected. A pineal tumor is often visible rostral to the vermis, underneath the vein of Galen (see Fig. 64–7). If the tumor is located further rostrally, the splenium of the corpus callosum is split by suction to expose the tela choroidea of the third ventricle. If the tumor is large, it is often already breaking through the tela choroidea; if not, the tela is incised along the midline or close to the nondominant occipital lobe after cauterization with a bipolar coagulator. This approach enables the operator to use the low (parieto) occipital approach (as proposed by Poppen and Marino[19] and Jamieson[21]) and, if necessary, the high parieto-occipital approach (as proposed by Dandy[15] and others) or the additional infratentorial supracerebellar approach.

If the tumor is a pineocytoma with lymphocytic infiltration or a germinoma (germinomas are usually slightly tougher in consistency than the former), the tumor is removed piecemeal with or without the use of an ultrasonic aspirator. If the tumor is a teratoma, removal en bloc is sometimes feasible. After tumor removal, the other end of the silicone rubber tube (which has been inserted into the lateral ventricle) is brought into the lateral cistern or the pontine cistern to ensure an unobstructed cerebrospinal fluid pathway. This step is performed because the rostral portion of the aqueduct is often compressed by the tumor, and even after removal of the tumor, the effect of the compression may remain for a period of time. Care should always be taken not to disseminate tumor debris in the subarachnoid space or the ventricular system in any approach used.

This approach provides an excellent view above and below the tentorial notch. Reaching the part of a large tumor extending to the opposite side may be difficult, however. Rarely a danger of damaging the occipital lobe exists, as does a danger of damaging the splenium of the corpus callosum, resulting in disconnection syndrome. The approach is indicated in surgery of tumors that straddle the tentorial notch or are located above the notch. The advantages and disadvantages of this approach are listed in Table 64–3.

### Lateral-Paramedian Infratentorial Approach

The infratentorial supracerebellar approach is difficult when the tentorium is steep, and if the patient is in the sitting position, an air embolism may occur despite various precautionary measures, such as Doppler probe, central venous catheter, and modest pressure ventilation. In 1990, Van den Bergh[27] proposed a new infratentorial approach. The patient is positioned on the side, usually the right side;

## TABLE 64–3 ■ OCCIPITAL TRANSTENTORIAL APPROACH

Advantage
  Provides an excellent view above and below the tentorial notch
Disadvantages
  May damage the occipital lobe
  May damage the splenium of the corpus callosum
  May be difficult to reach parts of lesions extending to the opposite side
Indication
  Tumors that straddle the tentorial notch or those located above the notch

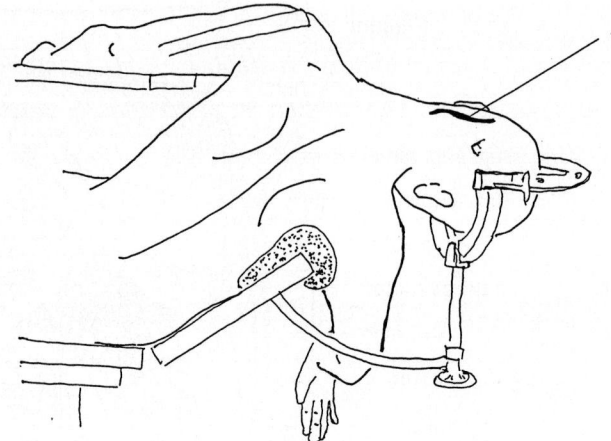

**FIGURE 64–8** ■ Position of the patient for lateral-paramedian infratentorial approach. (1, Skin incision.)

if the tumor extends to the right side, positioning is on the left side. The upper part of the trunk is raised about 30 degrees by upward inclination of the operating table. The head is flexed with the neck stretched, then rotated 45 degrees in a face-down fashion (Fig. 64–8). Care should be taken that the jugular veins remain unobstructed during flexion and rotation.

A flat, S-shaped incision is made just behind the mastoid process. The muscles are stripped away to expose the occipital bone. An oval craniectomy is made close to the sigmoid sinus laterally, to the transverse sinus superiorly, and caudally close to the foramen magnum (Fig. 64–9). The dura is opened in a cruciate fashion.

The superior surface of the cerebellar hemisphere is eased gently down. Bridging veins between it and the tentorium or the transverse sinus are electrocoagulated and severed. The petrosal vein and the precentral cerebellar vein are preserved. The tentorial incisura is easily reached. The arachnoid of the ambient cistern and the upper edge of the cerebellum are sharply dissected, permitting the cerebellum to descend further without retraction. The pineal tumor usually appears between the internal cerebral veins and the basal veins of Rosenthal (Fig. 64–10). The superior cerebellar artery appears at the rostral edge of the cerebellar hemisphere and gives branches to the cerebellar hemisphere and the vermis. This artery should be preserved. Elevating the straight sinus and the transverse sinus is unnecessary. The lateral-paramedian infratentorial ap-

proach may replace the infratentorial supracerebellar approach if it is performed by experienced hands. The advantages and disadvantages of this approach are listed in Table 64–4.

## Anterior Transcallosal Transventricular Trans–velum Interpositum Approach

The patient is positioned supine, with the head elevated 20 degrees in pin fixation. A coronal or horseshoe-shaped skin incision is made on the right (nondominant) side, in the frontal region. A quadrangular bone flap extending to the midline and anterior to the coronal suture is elevated (Fig. 64–11A, B). The dura is hinged toward the midline. The right frontal lobe is retracted away from the falx to expose the corpus callosum and the anterior cerebral arteries. The anterior part of the corpus callosum is split between these arteries, 3 to 4 cm in length, and the surgeon proceeds posteriorly to open the pars centralis of the right lateral ventricle (Fig. 64–12A, B). The velum interpositum (tela choroidea of the choroidal fissure) is cut just lateral to the tenia fornicis and medial to the choroid plexus of the lateral

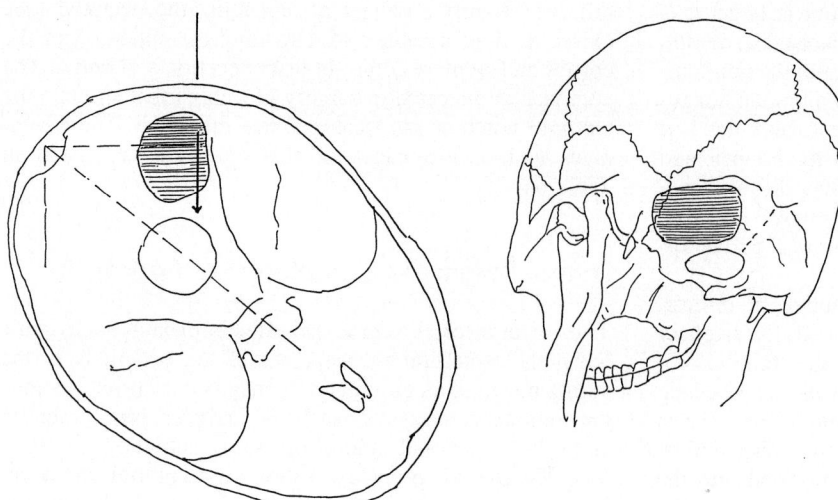

**FIGURE 64–9** ■ Lateral-paramedian infratentorial approach. Site of a craniectomy. (From Van den Bergh R: Lateral-paramedian infratentorial approach in lateral decubitus for pineal tumours. Clin Neurol Neurosurg 92:311–316, 1990.)

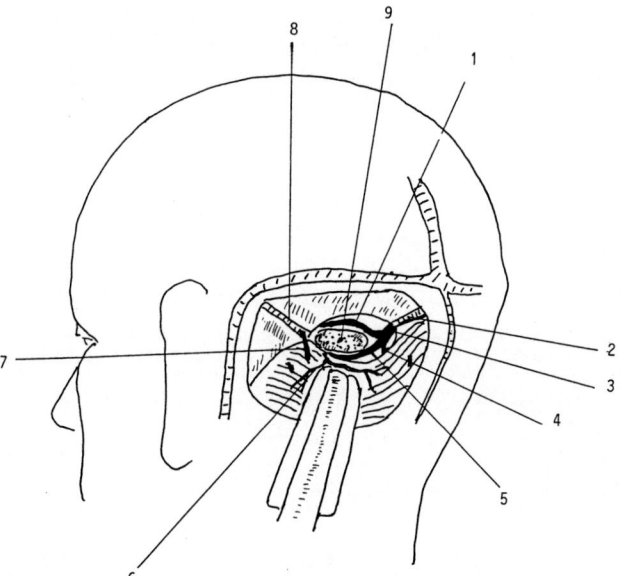

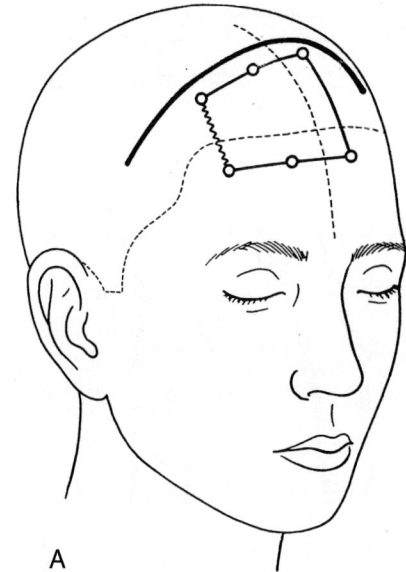

**FIGURE 64–10** ■ Lateral-paramedian infratentorial approach. (1) Internal cerebral vein; (2) straight sinus; (3) vein of Galen; (4) precentral cerebellar vein; (5) basal vein of Rosenthal; (6) superior cerebellar artery; (7) petrosal vein; (8) superior petrosal sinus; (9) tumor. (From Van den Bergh R: Lateral-paramedian infratentorial approach in lateral decubitus for pineal tumours. Clin Neurol Neurosurg 92:311–316, 1990.)

ventricle (Fig. 64–13A, B), as seen under the microscope. The velum tissue between the internal cerebral vein and the choroid plexus of the lateral ventricle is thin and easily cut (Fig. 64–14). The bilateral fornices and the internal cerebral veins are retracted to the medial side to explore the tumor between these structures and the right thalamus (Fig. 64–15). Section of the choroid plexus or the thalamostriate vein is not necessary. The tumor and the surrounding structures are viewed from above and from the front. Microsurgical manipulation of the tumor is easy because of the ample space provided. This approach provides an excellent view of tumors in the third ventricle and allows the surgeon to manage parts of tumors extending to the lateral ventricle. Damage, however, to the anterior portion of the corpus callosum occurs and may also occur to the fornix on the right side by retraction. This approach is indicated in cases of huge tumors in the pineal region or the posterior third ventricle that extend anterior to the adhesio interthalamica. The advantages and disadvantages of this approach are listed in Table 64–5. After this approach and its ana-

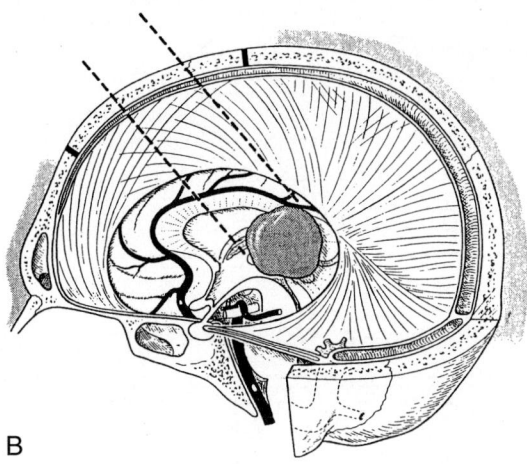

**FIGURE 64–11** ■ Anterior transcallosal transventricular trans-velum interpositum approach. A, Skin incision and craniotomy. B, The Approach to a tumor. (From Sano K: Surgery of pineal tumors: Anatomical consideration of various approaches. Neurol Surg 12:1119–1129, 1984.)

**TABLE 64–4 ■ LATERAL-PARAMEDIAN INFRATENTORIAL APPROACH**

Advantage
  Minimal damage to neural tissues
Disadvantages
  Narrow space
  Difficult to reach portions of tumor extending to the inferoposterior part of third ventricle
Indications
  Small tumors in the pineal region and the quadrigeminal area
  Biopsy

**TABLE 64–5 ■ ANTERIOR TRANSCALLOSAL TRANSVENTRICULAR TRANS–VELUM INTERPOSITUM APPROACH**

Advantages
  Provides an excellent view of lesions in the (posterior) third ventricle
  Allows the surgeon to manage parts of lesions extending to the lateral ventricle
Disadvantages
  Damage to the anterior portion of the corpus callosum
  Possible damage to the fornix
Indications
  Huge tumors in the pineal region or in the posterior third ventricle
  Tumors extending anterior to the level of the adhesio interthalamica

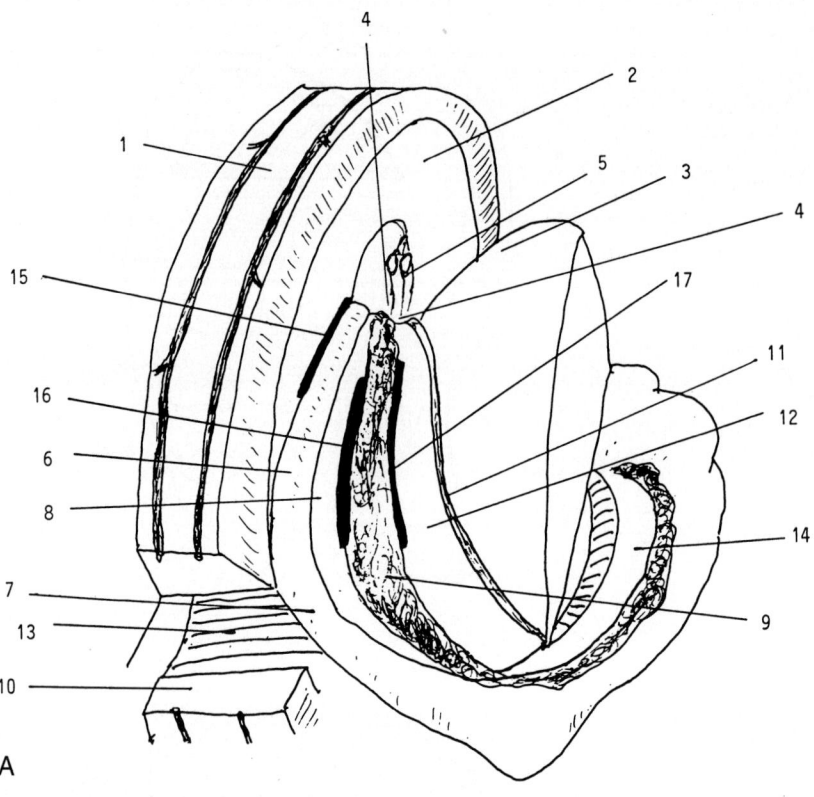

A

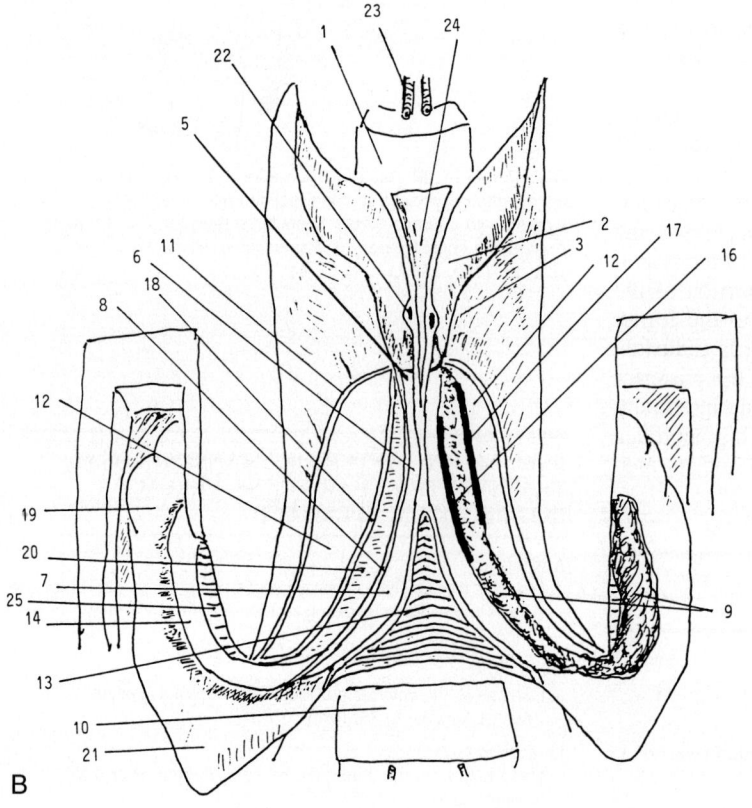

B

**FIGURE 64–12** ■ Approaches to the third ventricle. *A,* Right lateral ventricle opened; *B,* Corpus callosum stripped off. (1) Corpus callosum; (2) septum pellucidum; (3) head of the caudate nucleus; (4) foramen of Monro; (5) columna fornicis; (6) corpus fornicis; (7) crus fornicis; (8) tenia fornicis; (9) choroid plexus of the lateral ventricle; (10) splenium of the corpus callosum, (11) vena thalamostriata; (12) lamina affixa; (13) commissura fornicis (hippocampal commissure); (14) fimbria hippocampi; (15) development of the interfornicial plane; (16) transvelum interpositum approach; (17) development of the subchoroidal plane; (18) tenia choroidea; (19) hippocampus; (20) surface of the thalamus with the tela choroidea stripped off; (21) calcar avis; (22) anterior septal vein; (23) anterior cerebral artery; (24) cavum septi pellucidi; (25) gyrus dentatus. (Modified from Apuzzo MLJ, Chkovani OK, Gott PS, et al: Transcallosal interfornicial approaches for lesions affecting the third ventricle: Surgical considerations and consequences. Neurosurgery 10:547–554, 1982.)

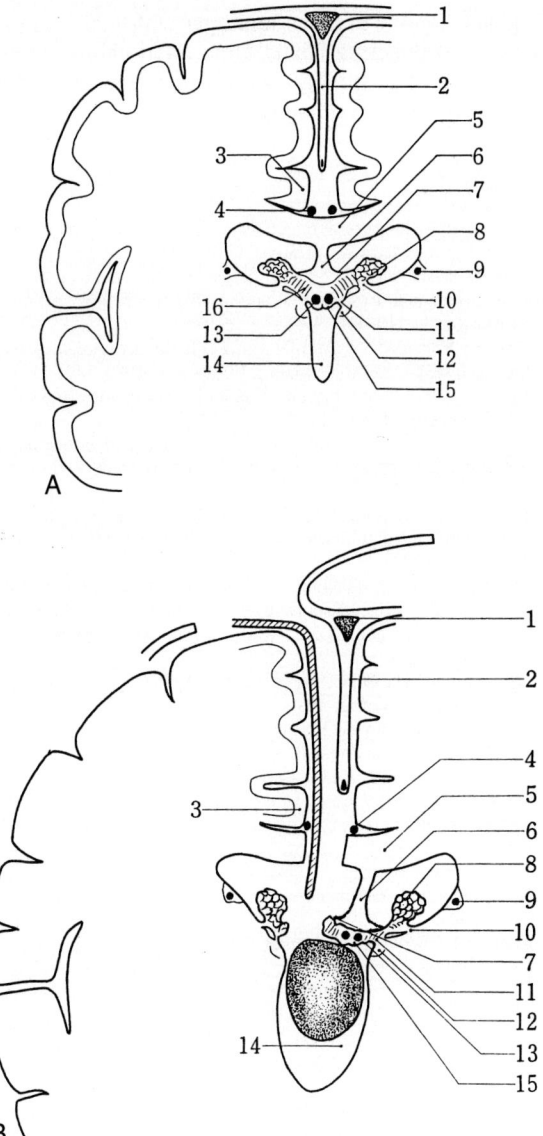

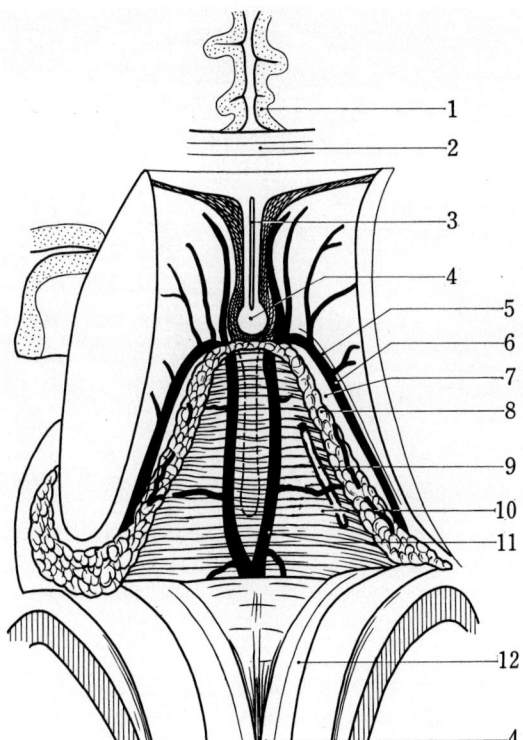

FIGURE 64–14 ■ The velum interpositum exposed with the fornix stripped away. Incision of the velum interpositum just lateral to the tenia fornicis on the right side. (1) Gyrus cinguli; (2) corpus callosum; (3) septum pellucidum; (4) fornix; (5) stria terminalis; (6) vena thalamostriata; (7) lamina affixa; (8) plexus choroideus ventriculi lateralis; (9) section of the velum interpositum; (10) velum interpositum; (11) vena cerebri interna; (12) tenia fornicis. (From Sano K: Surgery of pineal tumors. Anatomical consideration of various approaches. Neurol Surg 12:1119–1129, 1984.)

FIGURE 64–13 ■ *A,* Anatomy of the velum interpositum. *B,* Trans-velum interpositum approach and a tumor in the third ventricle. (1) Sinus sagittalis superior; (2) falx; (3) gyrus cinguli; (4) arteria cerebri anterior; (5) corpus callosum; (6) fornix; (7) tenia fornicis, (8) plexus choroideus ventriculi lateralis; (9) vena thalamostriata, stria terminalis, and lamina affixa; (10) tenia choroidea; (11) tenia thalami; (12) stria medullaris thalami; (13) vena cerebri interna; (14) ventriculus tertius; (15) plexus choroideus ventriculi tertii; (16) tela choroidea ventriculi tertii (8 + 16 + 15: velum interpositum). (From Sano K: Surgery of pineal tumors: Anatomical consideration of various approaches. Neurol Surg 12:1119–1129, 1984.)

tomic considerations were described,[23–26] Wen and colleagues[32] published and proposed a similar transchoroidal approach.

In all patients, steroids are administered before, during, and after the operation. Postoperative irradiation is indicated in cases of germinoma or pineocytoma with lymphocytic infiltration and usually consists of $^{60}$Co or LINAC (linear accelerator), the total dose being 50 to 60 Gy (the daily dose, 1 to 2 Gy). The field of irradiation is 6 × 6 cm to 8 × 8 cm, centering on the pineal region. In malignant neoplasms, whole-brain irradiation and spinal

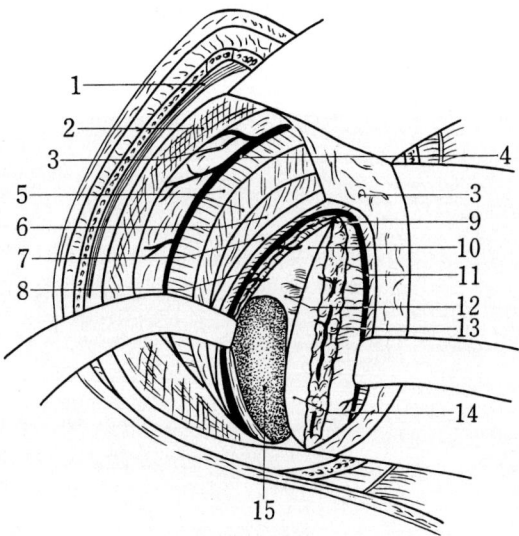

FIGURE 64–15 ■ Anterior transcallosal transventricular trans-velum interpositum approach. Actual operative view. (1) Sinus sagittalis superior; (2) falx; (3) gyrus cinguli; (4) arteria cerebri anterior sinistra; (5) corpus callosum; (6) septum pellucidum; (7) fornix; (8) vena cerebri interna dextra; (9) foramen of Monro; (10) ventriculus tertius; (11) vena thalamostriata dextra and lamina affixa; (12) adhesio interthalamica; (13) plexus choroideus ventriculi lateralis dexter; (14) thalamus dexter; (15) tumor. (From Sano K: Surgery of pineal tumors: Anatomical consideration of various approaches. Neurol Surg 12:1119–1129, 1984.)

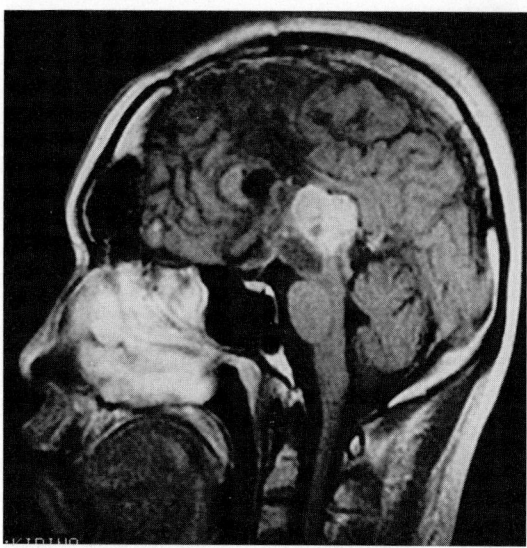

**FIGURE 64–16 ■** Recurrent endodermal sinus tumor. Gadolinium diethylenetriamine–penta-acetic acid enhancement of a 21-year-old man.

cord irradiation are added, but even in these cases, the total dose does not exceed 50 to 60 Gy. Chemotherapy may also be used before or after radiation therapy.[5] Figure 64–16 is a gadolinium-DTPA-enhanced MRI scan of a 21-year-old man with a recurrent endodermal sinus tumor with teratomatous tissue. His tumor was totally removed 5 years before this scan by anterior transcallosal transventricular trans–velum interpositum approach. He was treated by radiotherapy and chemotherapy consisting of cisplatin, vinblastine, and bleomycin. The radiotherapy and chemotherapy did not reduce the bulk of the tumor. The tumor was totally removed 7 months later by occipital transtentorial approach. Figure 64–17 is an MRI scan taken 6 years after the second operation. No tumor recurrence is observed, although the veins are enhanced by gadolinium-DTPA.

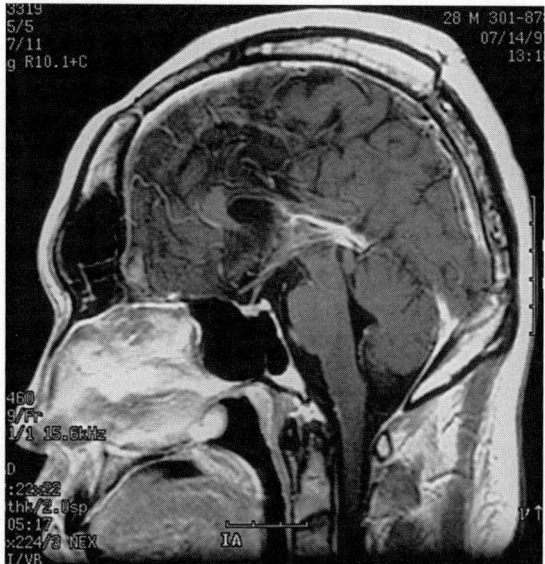

**FIGURE 64–17 ■** The same patient is shown 6 years after the tumor was totally removed. The veins are enhanced by gadolinium-diethylenetriamine–penta-acetic acid.

Malignant tumors, such as teratoma with malignant transformation, endodermal sinus tumor, and choriocarcinoma, often recur despite surgery, radiotherapy, and chemotherapy and may require second surgery.

## REFERENCES

1. Committee of brain tumor registry of Japan: Brain tumor registry of Japan. Neurol Med Chir (Tokyo) 32:395–438, 1992.
2. Sano K, Matsutani M, Seto T: So-called intracranial germ cell tumours: Personal experiences and a theory of their pathogenesis. Neurol Res 11:118–126, 1989.
3. Sano K: So-called intracranial germ cell tumors: Are they really of germ cell origin? Br J Neurosurg 9:391–401, 1995.
4. Sano K: Pineal region tumors: Problems in pathology and treatment. Clin Neurosurg 30:59–91, 1983.
5. Matsutani M, Sano K, Takakura K, et al: Primary intracranial germ cell tumors: A clinical analysis of 153 histologically verified cases. J Neurosurg 86:446–455, 1997.
6. Krabbe KH: The pineal gland, especially in relation to the problem of its supposed significance in sexual development. Endocrinology 7:379–414, 1923.
7. Sano K, Nagai M, Tsuchida T, Hoshino T: New diagnostic method of brain tumors by cell culture of the cerebrospinal fluid–millipore filter–cell culture method. Neurol Med Chir (Tokyo) 8:17–27, 1966.
8. Lang J: Praktische Anatomie. Kopf Teil B Gehirn- und Augenschädel. Berlin: Springer-Verlag, 1979.
9. Tamaki N, Fujiwara K, Matsumoto S, Takeda H: Veins draining the pineal body: An anatomical and neuroradiological study of "pineal veins." J Neurosurg 39:448–454, 1973.
10. Matsushima T, Rhoton AL Jr, de Oliveira E, Peace D: Microsurgical anatomy of the veins of the posterior fossa. J Neurosurg 59:63–105, 1983.
11. Oppenheim H, Krause F: Operative Erfolge bei Geschwülsten der Sehh ügel- und Vierhügelgegend. Berl Klin Wochenschr 50:2316–2322, 1913.
12. Krause F: Operative Freilegung der Vierhügel nebst Beobachtungen über Hirndruck und Dekompression. Zentralbl Chir 53:2812–2819, 1926.
13. Zapletal B: Ein neuer operativer Zugang zum Gebiet der Incisura Tentorii. Zentralbl Neurochir 16:64–69, 1956.
14. Stein BM: The infratentorial supracerebellar approach to pineal lesions. J Neurosurg 35:197–202, 1971.
15. Dandy W: An operation for the removal of pineal tumors. Surg Gynecol Obstet 33:113–119, 1921.
16. Kunicki A: Operative experience in 8 cases of pineal tumor. J Neurosurg 17:815–823, 1960.
17. Van Wagenen WP: A surgical approach for the removal of certain pineal tumors: Report of a case. Surg Gynecol Obstet 53:216–220, 1931.
18. Heppner F: Zur Operationstechnik bei Pinealomen. Zentralbl Neurochir 19:219–224, 1959.
19. Poppen JL, Marino R Jr: Pinealomas and tumors of the posterior portion of the third ventricle. J Neurosurg 28:357–364, 1968.
20. Glasauer FE: An operative approach to pineal tumors. Acta Neurochir (Wien) 22:177–180, 1970.
21. Jamieson KG: Excision of pineal tumors. J Neurosurg 35:550–553, 1971.
22. Lazar ML, Clark K: Direct surgical management of masses in the region of the vein of Galen. Surg Neurol 2:17–21, 1974.
23. Sano K: Surgery of pineal tumors: Anatomical consideration of various approaches. Neurol Surg (Tokyo) 12:1119–1129, 1984.
24. Sano K: Treatment of tumors in the pineal and posterior third ventricular region. In Samii M (ed): Surgery in and Around the Brain Stem and the Third Ventricle. Berlin, Heidelberg: Springer-Verlag, 1986, pp 309–317.
25. Sano K: Pineal region and posterior third ventricular tumors: A surgical overview. In Apuzzo MLJ (ed): Surgery of the Third Ventricle, 2nd ed. Baltimore: Williams & Wilkins, 1998, pp 801–819.
26. Sano K: Alternate surgical approaches to pineal region neoplasms. In Shimidek HH, Sweet WH (eds): Operative Neurosurgical Techniques, 3rd ed. Philadelphia: WB Saunders, 1995, pp 743–754.

27. Van den Bergh R: Lateral-paramedian infratentorial approach in lateral decubitus for pineal tumours. Clin Neurol Neurosurg 92:311–316, 1990.
28. Layne MH, Patterson RH: Subchoroidal trans-velum interpositum approach to mid-third ventricular tumors. Neurosurgery 12:86–94, 1983.
29. Viale GL, Turtas S: The subchoroidal approach to the third ventricle. Surg Neurol 14:71–76, 1980.
30. Apuzzo MLJ, Chikovani OK, Gott PS, et al: Transcallosal interfornical approaches for lesions affecting the third ventricle: Surgical considerations and consequences. Neurosurgery 10:547–554, 1982.
31. Ziyal IM, Sekhar LN, Salas E, et al: Combined supra/infratentorial transsinus approach to large pineal region tumors. J Neurosurg 88:1050–1057, 1998.
32. Wen HT, Rhoton AL Jr, de Oliveira E: Transchoroidal approach to the third ventricle: An anatomic study of the choroidal fissure and its clinical application. Neurosurgery 42:1205–1219, 1998.

# Supracerebellar Approach to Pineal Region Neoplasms

■ JEFFREY N. BRUCE and BENNETT M. STEIN

Pineal region tumors encompass a diverse group of tumors that can arise from pineal parenchymal cells, supporting cells of the pineal gland, or glial cells from the midbrain and medial walls of the thalamus.[1, 2] These tumors occupy a central position that is equidistant from various cranial points traditionally used as routes of exposure. The deep central location places these tumors in intimate contact with important components of the deep venous system that lie dorsally, including the vein of Galen, the precentral cerebellar vein, and the internal cerebral veins.[3] In some instances, there may be a dense attachment to these structures and the tela choroidea. The tumor is often fed by small-caliber branches of the posterior choroidal arteries and branches of the quadrigeminal arteries. These vessels usually do not supply any areas of the brain outside of the tumor.

Although pineal region tumors affect a relatively small number of patients, a comparatively large volume of literature has been generated about these neoplasms because of their variable histology and the difficult surgical challenge they present. This difficulty is underscored by Cushing's statement, "Personally, I have never succeeded in exposing a pineal tumor sufficiently well to justify an attempt to remove it."[4] Several other surgeons have emphasized the high mortality rate after pineal tumor surgery.[5–7] Despite this high rate of operative mortality, Dandy[8] continued to advocate their surgical exposure and removal. Suzuki and Iwabuchi[9] later reported a large series of pineal tumors that they successfully removed without incurring an overwhelming rate of morbidity or mortality. Over the decades, the historical perspective on surgical treatment of pineal tumors continued to evolve. Initially, the aggressive approach of surgery led to unacceptable mortality and morbidity rates. Based on these early disasters, a more conservative approach was adopted consisting of control of the hydrocephalus and irradiation of the tumor without benefit of a histologic diagnosis (blind radiation). Later, the advent of the operating microscope, a better understanding of pineal region anatomy, and improvement of sophisticated surgical techniques led to a rediscovery of microsurgical approaches to these lesions.[9–13] With experience, the mortality and morbidity rates from the various surgical approaches dropped steadily and led to the current manage-

ment philosophy for pineal tumors, which relies on an aggressive surgical approach for the removal of benign tumors and decompression and accurate histologic diagnosis of malignant tumors.[14]

## CLASSIC SURGICAL TECHNIQUES

Over the years, a variety of supratentorial and infratentorial approaches have been developed by several prominent neurosurgeons. Among the earliest was Dandy,[8] who was a master at approaching deep-seated brain tumors and cultivated a particular interest in pineal region tumors. He advocated an interhemispheric approach, with section of the posterior portion of the corpus callosum to reach the pineal region. This approach required sacrificing a number of parietal cortical veins and retracting a large portion of the parietal hemisphere (usually the right). Difficulties were encountered in dissecting around the deep venous systems adjacent to the gland, and many fatalities probably resulted from uncontrolled deep venous thrombosis and edema of the diencephalic region. Van Wagenen,[15] taking advantage of the hydrocephalus that usually accompanies these tumors, advocated an approach through the dilated right lateral ventricle. Tumor exposure still involved dissection of the deep venous system because the approach was primarily dorsal to the tumor. Because of the additional disadvantages of a transcortical incision and possible hemispheric collapse from the opening of the ventricle, this approach was seldom used. Poppen[16] advocated an approach under the occipital lobe, in which bridging veins were sacrificed, a large portion of the hemisphere was retracted, and the free edge of the tentorium was sectioned to expose the deep venous plexus in a more favorable position relative to the underlying tumor. Reid and Clark[10] have reviewed the merits of this approach. In 1926, Krause[17] reported three cases, each a different variety of tumor in the pineal or quadrigeminal region, which he approached through the posterior fossa, over the cerebellar hemispheres, and under the tentorium.

As Krause recognized, because most of these tumors are centrally located, the posterior fossa approach with the patient in the sitting position provides a natural advantage by providing a midline central exposure.[18] Furthermore, because most tumors lie primarily beneath the deep venous system, this exposure reduces the risk of venous injury. Overall, it provides exposure commensurate to supratentorial approaches and avoids injury to the parietal or occipital lobes and subsequent deficits in sensation or peripheral vision. However, when the tumor extends dorsally above the incisura or extends laterally to the trigone of the lateral ventricle, the posterior fossa approach is not recommended (Fig. 65–1). The tentorium may be cut, but it is still difficult to reach the periphery of the tumor. Overall, this approach provides excellent access and was used in 90% of the patients in our series.[14, 19]

## CLINICAL FEATURES

### Classification

Pineal tumors can be classified into four main categories (Table 65–1)[20]:

1. Germ cell tumors, which include malignant and benign varieties. This group comprises germinomas, embryonal cell carcinomas, choriocarcinomas, endodermal sinus tumors, benign teratomas, and dermoid and epidermoid cysts. Mixed germ cell tumors may occur that contain both malignant and benign elements or several different malignant elements.
2. Pineal cell tumors, which include benign and malignant varieties. Tumors in this group are pineocytomas, which are benign and malignant, and pineoblastomas, which are always malignant. Occasionally, mixed cell types can occur containing both pineocytoma and pineoblastoma or pineal cell and glial cell elements.
3. Glial cell tumors, which include astrocytomas,

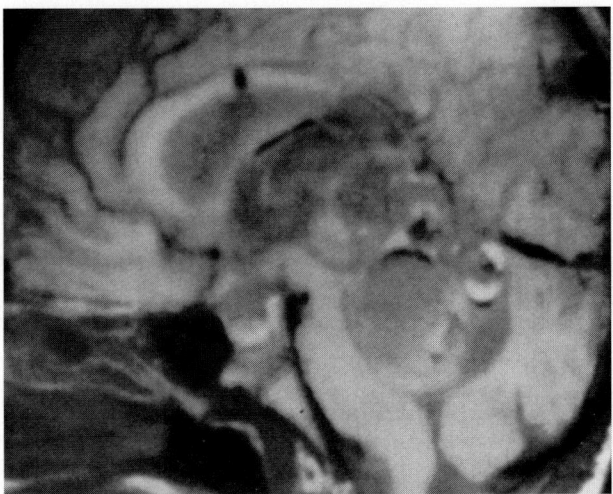

**FIGURE 65–1** ■ A sagittal magnetic resonance imaging scan showing a large teratoma extending well above the level of the incisura. A supratentorial approach is recommended for this tumor.

**TABLE 65–1** ■ **SUMMARY OF PATHOLOGIC FINDINGS IN 191 PATIENTS UNDERGOING SURGERY FOR PINEAL REGION TUMORS AT THE NEW YORK NEUROLOGICAL INSTITUTE**

| Tumor Pathologic Type | No. |
| --- | --- |
| **Germ Cell** | **62 (32%)** |
| Germinoma | 30 |
| Teratoma | 9 |
| Lipoma | 2 |
| Epidermoid | 1 |
| Mixed malignant germ cell | 16 |
| Immature teratoma | 2 |
| Embryonal cell carcinoma | 2 |
| **Pineal Cell** | **48 (25%)** |
| Pineocytoma | 27 |
| Pineoblastoma | 11 |
| Mixed pineal cell | 10 |
| **Glial Cell** | **52 (27%)** |
| Astrocytoma | 27 |
| Anaplastic astrocytoma | 3 |
| Glioblastoma | 4 |
| Ependymoma | 14 |
| Oligodendroglioma | 2 |
| Choroid plexus neoplasm | 2 |
| **Miscellaneous** | **29 (15%)** |
| Pineal cysts | 9 |
| Meningioma | 10 |
| Other malignant | 5 |
| Other benign | 4 |
| **Total** | **191** |

ependymomas, malignant astrocytomas, and, occasionally, oligodendrogliomas.
4. Miscellaneous tumors, which include meningiomas, hemangioblastomas, metastatic tumors, and lymphomas, among others.

In addition to these tumors, non-neoplastic vascular lesions such as arteriovenous malformations, aneurysms, vein of Galen malformations, and cavernous malformations can also be found.

Benign cysts of the pineal gland deserve special mention[21] (Fig. 65–2). The presence of these cysts has been detected with greater frequency as the use of computed tomography (CT) and magnetic resonance imaging (MRI) to evaluate minor neurologic complaints has increased. Histologically, these cysts are normal variants of the pineal gland consisting of a cystic structure surrounded by normal pineal parenchymal tissue. They are usually asymptomatic and do not require any intervention unless growth occurs or hydrocephalus develops. The natural history of these cysts usually defines them as static anatomic variants that need not be treated.

### Presenting Symptoms

Patients with pineal tumors commonly present with headache caused by raised intracranial pressure from obstruction of third ventricle outflow at the aqueduct of Sylvius. Impaired upward gaze and convergence, and other varia-

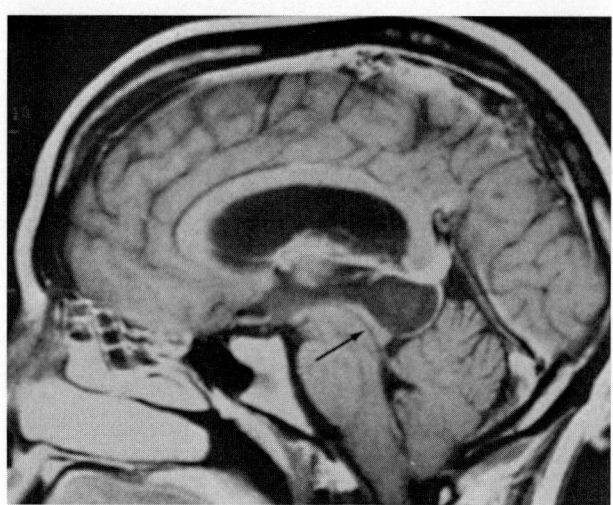

FIGURE 65-2 ■ A sagittal magnetic resonance imaging scan showing a benign pineal cyst and a patent sylvian aqueduct *(arrow)*. It is not uncommon to see enhancement of a portion of the cyst wall. Pineal cysts are normal anatomic variants and do not require treatment, except in rare cases when they become symptomatic.

tions of Parinaud's syndrome, often occur. Ataxia can result from compression of the superior cerebellar peduncle in the midbrain. Precocious puberty is a rare occurrence but can occasionally affect young boys.[22] The mechanism of this syndrome is thought to be ectopic secretion of human chorionic gonadotropin by a malignant germ cell tumor. Diabetes insipidus is another rare condition, and it is usually associated with tumor seeding of the hypothalamic region.

With the prevalent use of CT and MRI after head injuries or to evaluate patients with headaches, many asymptomatic pineal tumors are discovered. It is apparent that tumors can reach a significant size without producing symptoms.

## PREOPERATIVE EVALUATION

High-resolution MRI with gadolinium contrast is mandatory in the evaluation of all pineal region tumors (Fig. 65-3). Despite advances in radiographic imaging, histologic subtypes cannot be predicted consistently based on radiographic characteristics.[23-25] MRI can precisely define the size of the tumor, its vascularity, and its relationship with surrounding structures. Planning the operative approach depends on knowing the tumor's position within the third ventricle, its lateral and supratentorial extension, the degree of brain stem involvement, and the position relative to the deep venous system. Tumor invasiveness can sometimes be inferred by the degree of margination and irregularity on MRI; however, the true degree of encapsulation can be determined only at surgery. CT scans can provide details of calcification, blood-brain barrier breakdown, and degree of vascularity, as well as the presence of hydrocephalus. MRI, however, nearly always allows better visualization of the tumor than CT. Angiography is unnecessary unless a vascular anomaly is suspected.

Markers for malignant germ cell elements such as α-

fetoprotein and human chorionic gonadotropin should be measured in the cerebrospinal fluid (CSF) and blood as part of the routine preoperative work-up.[20, 26, 27] In addition to aiding in arriving at the correct diagnosis, the presence of these markers can be helpful in monitoring the patient's response to therapy and detecting early tumor recurrence. By definition, patients with elevated germ cell markers have malignant germ cell tumors and do not require a histologic diagnosis before commencing with chemotherapy or radiation therapy.[26]

## SURGICAL CONSIDERATIONS

Surgical intervention to obtain diagnostic tumor tissue is mandatory because of the wide variety of tumor subtypes that occur in the pineal region, each having implications for prognosis and selection of clinical management options.[20] Selection of a surgical approach for an individual patient depends on clinical features and radiographic findings. For most pineal tumors, the infratentorial supracerebellar approach performed in the sitting position is the method of choice. It offers the advantage of approaching the tumor from a midline trajectory while avoiding the inconvenience of working around the deep venous vessels that usually lie dorsal to the mass. With this approach, gravity is helpful in assisting with the tumor dissection. When the tumor is eccentric or grows laterally to the region of the trigone or superiorly to the corpus callosum, the posterior parietal-interhemispheric approach is recommended. Using this approach, a portion of the posterior corpus callosum is sectioned to reach the tumor. With the supratentorial approach, however, tumor extension to the contralateral side or into the posterior fossa can be difficult to visualize. The tentorium on the ipsilateral side can be sectioned to increase exposure of the posterior fossa component.

Stereotactic biopsy can be useful in addition to diagnostic biopsy in patients with disseminated tumor or those in whom extensive medical problems pose excessive surgical risks.[20, 28] Certain tumors that appear to invade the brain

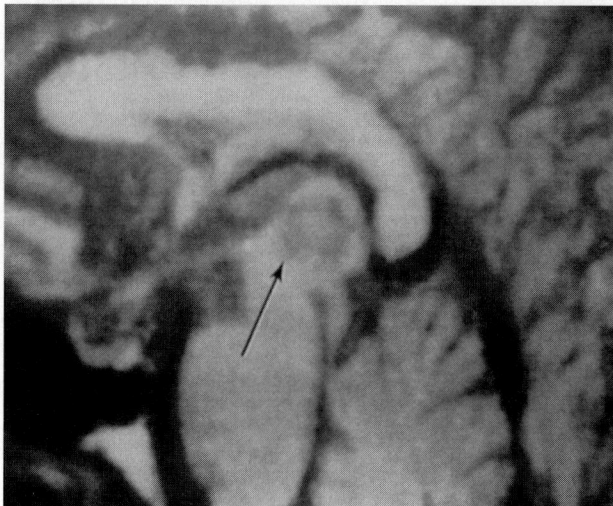

FIGURE 65-3 ■ A sagittal magnetic resonance imaging scan showing a large, variegated tumor compressing the aqueductal region *(arrow)*.

stem or thalamus likewise may benefit from stereotactic biopsy. Overall, however, the routine use of stereotactic biopsy is prohibited by problems of sampling error and the difficulties of making an accurate diagnosis through the study of small specimens.[29, 30] Furthermore, it ignores the advantages that open operation can provide in resecting benign tumors and debulking malignant tumors. Small tumors in particular are prone to risks of hemorrhage from damage to the deep venous system, whereas extremely vascular tumors, such as pineal cell tumors, are vulnerable to hemorrhage as well.

## OPERATIVE TECHNIQUE: SUPRACEREBELLAR APPROACH

Most patients with pineal tumors have raised intracranial pressure and hydrocephalus resulting from obstruction or compromise of the aqueduct. Hydrocephalus must be relieved before attempting any direct approach to the tumor. Stereotactic-guided third ventriculostomy is preferred over shunting procedures because it avoids the need for hardware, reduces the risk of ventricular collapse, and minimizes tumor seeding.[31] Treating hydrocephalus a week or two before surgical tumor removal allows the ventricular system sufficient time gradually to decompress. In situations of mild hydrocephalus where the tumor is likely to be resected, a ventricular drain can be placed at the time of craniotomy and then converted to a shunt on the second or third postoperative day if the hydrocephalus persists.

There are several positions that can be used for the infratentorial supracerebellar approach. Unless the patient is younger than 2 years of age and has a severe degree of hydrocephalus, the sitting position is preferred.[19] The three-quarter prone and lateral decubitus position and the Concorde position are possible alternatives; however, they do not allow gravity to work in the surgeon's favor.[32, 33]

The sitting position is accomplished by raising the back of the table to its maximal position. The patient's head, neck, and shoulders are brought forward by a pin-vise head fixation device such as the Mayfield headholder. The head must be strongly flexed so that optimal exposure of the tentorial notch can be achieved with the greatest comfort to the surgeon. The patient is tilted somewhat forward after being positioned on the operating table so that the surgeon actually works over the back of the patient's shoulders to the posterior fossa (Fig. 65–4). A Doppler probe, central venous catheter, end-tidal $PCO_2$ evaluation, and modest positive-pressure ventilation are used to recognize and avoid air embolism, which can occur during the bony opening or when large venous sinuses are exposed.

A self-retaining retractor, such as the Greenberg Universal retractor, is fixed by a bar to the operating table on the left side. The bars are then arranged in a rectangular configuration framing the operative field. The most important retractor is in the inferior position to depress the cerebellum. Occasionally, a superiorly placed retractor is desirable to elevate the tentorium a few millimeters. A cottonoid tray is fixed to the self-retaining retractor system and held by one of the retractor's arms.

A long midline incision is used, extending approximately

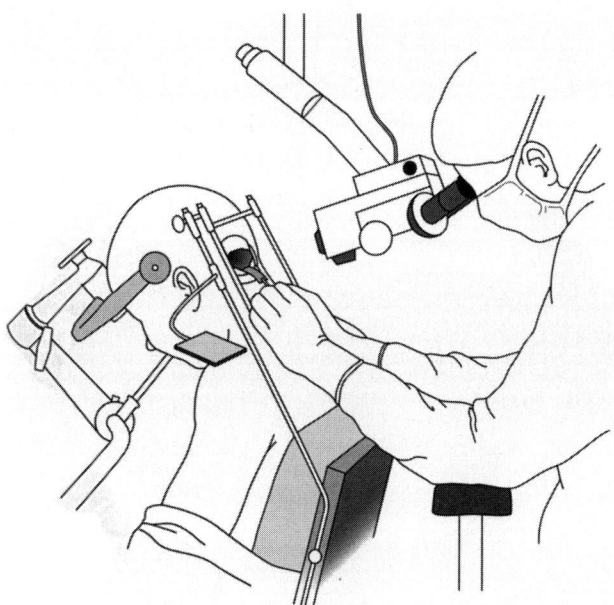

**FIGURE 65–4** ■ Diagram of the patient's position and operative setup for the supracerebellar approach.

from the spinous process of the third vertebral body up into the occipital region, so that the pericranium and muscle attachments can be elevated on either side without disrupting their continuity. Freeing up the muscle layer facilitates closure later on. A wide craniotomy is performed to include the lateral sinuses and torcular but without extending to the foramen magnum. We prefer to use a high-speed air drill to perform a suboccipital craniotomy so that the bone flap may be replaced at the end of the procedure. A craniotome is used to turn the flap after first exposing each of the dural sinuses to avoid tears. Brain relaxation and cerebellar retraction can be facilitated by mannitol, ventricular drainage, or removal of CSF from the cisterna magna. It is preferable to open the dura on either side of the midline so that the cerebellar falx and accompanying cerebellar sinus can be ligated and divided. The dural opening should extend bilaterally up to the lateral sinus (Fig. 65–5).

Once the dura is opened, all bridging veins over the dorsal surface of the cerebellum, including the hemispheres and vermis, can be sacrificed to free the cerebellum from the tentorium. The weight of cottonoids and a copper retractor, along with gravitational forces that are exerted in the sitting position, allow sufficient depression of the cerebellum to establish an unobstructed corridor to the pineal region under the tentorium (Fig. 65–6).

At this point, the operating microscope should be brought to the operating table. A microscope capable of varying the objective length from 275 to 400 mm is desireable because the operating distance for the surgeon changes throughout the operation, which extends from the dorsal surface of the cerebellum to the center of the third ventricle. The use of a free-standing armrest is also helpful in minimizing fatigue.

The arachnoid in the quadrigeminal region and around the incisura is usually thickened and opaque in the presence of tumors and must be opened by microdissection tech-

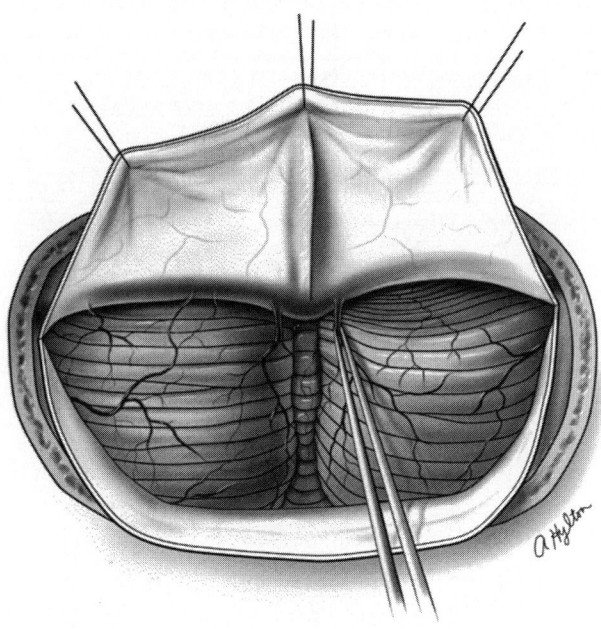

**FIGURE 65–5** ■ Drawing showing the dural opening and sacrifice of bridging veins.

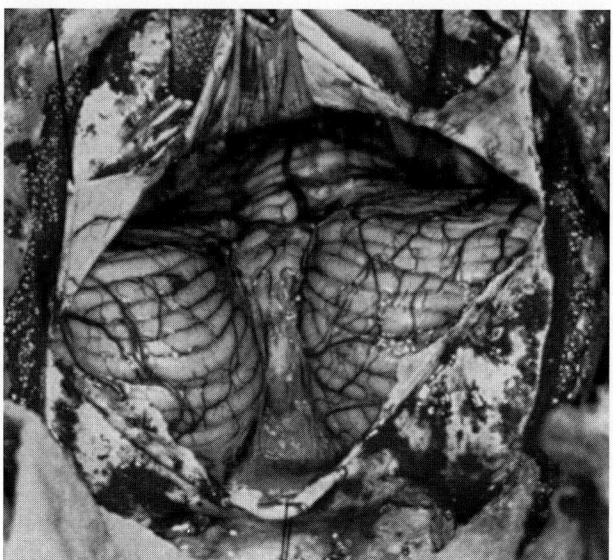

**FIGURE 65–6** ■ Full dural opening and the cerebellum, which is sagging because of gravity after the bridging veins have been divided.

niques to exposure the surface of the tumor. The precentral cerebellar vein, which can be seen extending from the edge of the vermis to the vein of Galen, should be cauterized and divided. The great vein of Galen and the internal cerebral veins are well above the tumor and are not encountered in these initial maneuvers.[3] Laterally, the medial aspect of the temporal lobe and the veins of Rosenthal can be seen as they course upward toward the confluence of veins in these regions. The thickened arachnoid should be opened widely to appreciate the underlying anatomy. Using sharp dissection, the arachnoidal opening must be kept close to the anterior surface of the vermis and cerebellar hemisphere to avoid injuring the deep venous system, keeping in mind that the initial trajectory is toward the vein of Galen. The anterior portion of the cerebellum is retracted by the inferior self-retaining retractor to expose the posterior surface of the tumor (Fig. 65–7). The tumor may be invested and supplied by branches of the choroidal arteries. The tumor capsule is then cauterized and opened by sharp dissection. Depending on its consistency, the tumor is removed with tumor forceps, small curets, suction, or cautery.

A portion of the tumor should be sent for frozen-tissue diagnosis early in the dissection. Although it may be helpful for intraoperative management, the frequent inaccuracy of frozen-section diagnosis for these tumors should be kept in mind when making intraoperative decisions.

Because many of these tumors extend well into the third ventricle, even to the region of the foramen of Monro, long instruments are required to reach the anterior margins of the tumor (Fig. 65–8). With tumors of firm consistency, a Cavitron with a long, curved tip can be helpful for debulking. The instrument is large and can be difficult to maneuver into the operative field, especially if an objective lens of less than 275 mm is used in the microscope.

In general terms, the trajectory of the operation is toward the velum interpositum (Fig. 65–9). This must be considered when attempting to remove segments of the tumor in the inferior portion of the third ventricle or directly over the quadrigeminal plate in relation to the anterior lobe of the cerebellum. The most difficult dissection involves the inferior portion of the tumor, where it is adherent to the collicular region of the dorsal midbrain. Small dental mirrors and angled instruments may be required to remove this portion of the tumor. Similarly, these techniques may

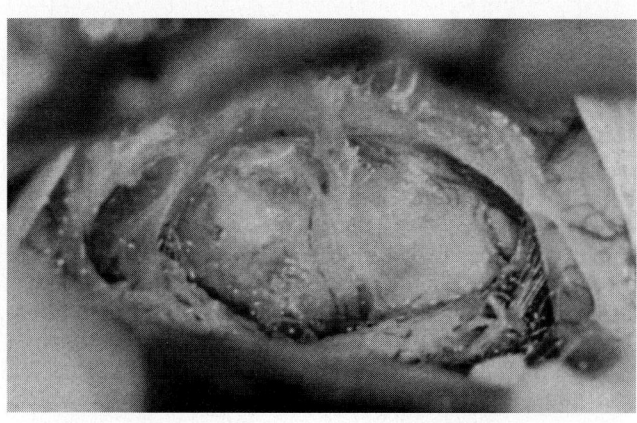

**FIGURE 65–7** ■ Operative view showing exposure of the posterior surface of a large meningioma, without dural attachment, in the pineal region.

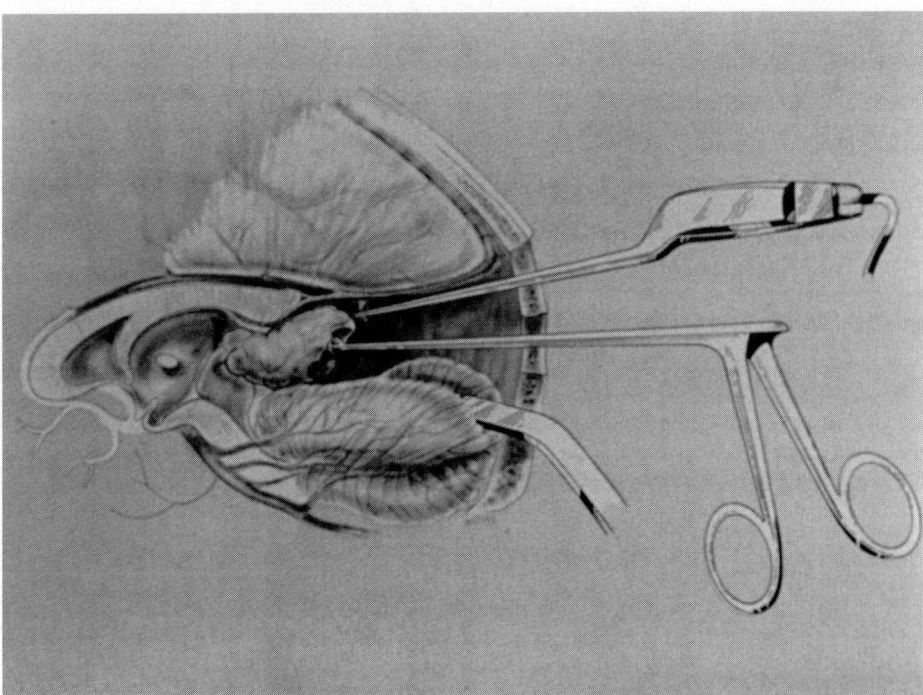

**FIGURE 65–8** ■ Drawing of the sagittal view showing the position of the pineal tumor and the extra-long instruments used in the posterior fossa approach.

be helpful for supratentorial tumor extensions. Further exposure can be gained by incising the tentorium if necessary.

Even with unresectable tumors, considerable benefit can be gained from internal decompression of the tumor or from sufficient tumor resection to expose the posterior third ventricle. Tumors that are benign or encapsulated can usually be removed completely. For most malignant tumors, an aggressive resection is desirable to improve the efficacy of adjuvant therapy, and complete resection is sometimes possible. One exception may be for germinomas, where the exquisite radiosensitivity of these tumors leaves surgical resection with little impact on long-term outcome.[34] With tumors that are incompletely resected, particularly vascular ones such as pineal cell tumors, meticulous hemostasis is crucial. Surgicel is the preferred hemostatic agent, and it should be placed carefully so that it does not float and obstruct the aqueduct when the third ventricle fills with CSF.

At the conclusion of the operation, after decompression of the tumor and the ventricular system, the dura can be closed to support the cerebellum. When a craniotomy has been performed, the bone flap is secured back in place with wires or miniplates. A greater degree of dural and bony closure seems to lower the incidence of postoperative aseptic meningitis.

## OPERATIVE COMPLICATIONS

Impairment of extraocular movements, particularly limitation of upward gaze and convergence, can be expected whenever the tumor is dissected from the quadrigeminal region.[14, 35] Other deficits, including pupillary abnormalities and difficulty focusing or accommodating, may also occur. These deficits usually are transient, but in some instances they may last for several months. The incidence of ataxia has been minimal and usually transient. Manipulation of the brain in the adjacent third ventricle or in the periaqueductal region of an infiltrating tumor can cause altered consciousness, which in severe instances can take the form of akinetic mutism. The incidence and severity of postoperative deficits are increased when significant symptoms are present after surgery, if prior radiation therapy has been given, and with tumors having highly malignant and invasive characteristics.

The most serious complication of pineal tumor surgery is postoperative hemorrhage, which can occur with a delay of up to several postoperative days.[35] It is seen most often with subtotally resected pineal cell tumors, which tend to

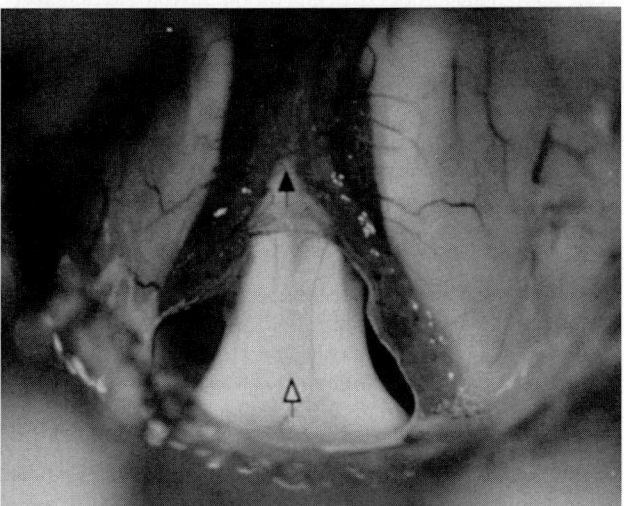

**FIGURE 65–9** ■ View of the interior of the third ventricle showing the columns of the fornix *(open arrow)* and the tela choroidea *(closed arrow)* after removal of a large pineal region tumor.

be soft and highly vascular. Hemorrhage has also been associated with stereotactic biopsy and has been known to occur before surgery as so-called *pineal apoplexy*.[36, 37]

Other complications related to the supracerebellar infratentorial approach in the sitting position include collapse of the ventricular system and entry of air into the ventricular system and subdural space.[35] These conditions usually improve with time and rarely is anything done to correct them. The incidence of air embolism causing complications is very low. Shunt malfunction can occur in up to 20% of patients after surgery. This problem can be minimized by leaving a catheter from the third ventricle into the cisterna magna at the time of surgery.

## POSTOPERATIVE MANAGEMENT

Malignant pineal cell tumors, germ cell tumors, and ependymomas have a propensity to seed along CSF pathways (Fig. 65–10). Patients with these tumors should be screened with an MRI scan of the complete spine to look for metastases. CSF cytology is also performed but is usually not particularly helpful in guiding management decisions. Spinal radiation is not given prophylactically but is reserved for patients who have radiographic documentation of spread of the tumor to the spine.[29, 38, 39]

All patients with malignant pineal tumors should be treated with a radiation dose of 4000 cGy to the whole brain and an additional 1500 cGy to the pineal region. The only exceptions to this include occasional ependymomas or low-grade pineal cell tumors that have been completely resected and have a benign histologic appearance. In this situation, a decision may be made to withhold radiation in lieu of close follow-up with serial MRI scans.

Nongerminomatous malignant germ cell tumors are the only pineal tumors that derive a significant benefit from

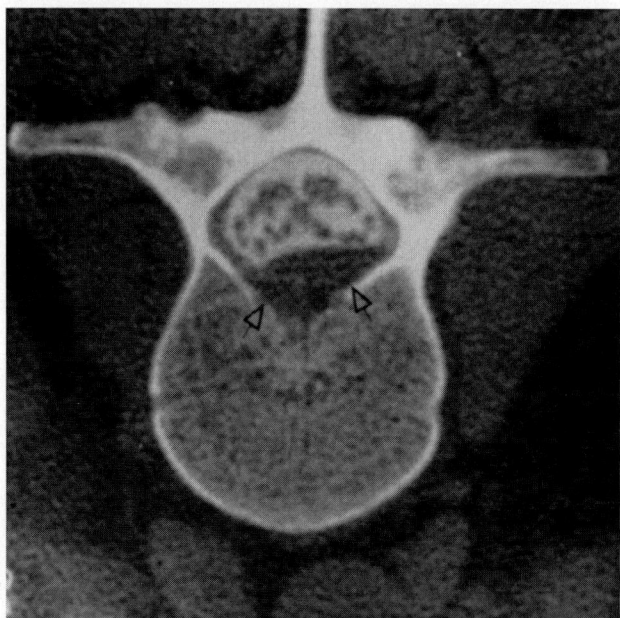

FIGURE 65–10 ■ A metrizamide-enhanced computed tomography myelogram showing subarachnoid metastases *(arrows)* from a pineocytoma.

chemotherapy.[20, 26] Chemotherapy usually is given before radiation therapy in patients with these tumors. Some preliminary results have suggested that chemotherapy may be useful in the treatment of pineal cell tumors and as an adjunct in the treatment of germinomas to reduce the amount of radiation therapy administered.

Studies of radiosurgery may ultimately prove it to be useful as an adjunct for recurrent tumors or to reduce the amount of conventional fractionated radiation necessary for other types of malignant tumors.[28, 40] The long-term effects of radiosurgery on the pineal region, however, are unknown.

## RESULTS

We have performed 196 operations for pineal region tumors at the New York Neurological Institute (Table 65–2). Surgery resulted in an excellent outcome in over 90% of patients, and a histologic diagnosis was made in all patients. For nearly all of the benign tumors, surgery alone was curative. Among all tumors, benign and malignant, a gross total resection was possible in 45% of cases.

Seven operative-related deaths occurred, all but one of which were associated with complications of postoperative hemorrhage. Delayed hemorrhage sometimes occurred several days after the surgery while the patient was making an otherwise satisfactory postoperative recovery. Permanent major morbidity occurred in 3% of patients and was most commonly associated with malignant tumors, prior radiation therapy, and the presence of significant preoperative neurologic impairment. Most patients had temporary disturbances in extraocular movements that gradually improved over time.

Overall, long-term results have been uniformly excellent for all tumors that were benign, which comprised one third of all pineal tumors. The long-term prognosis for patients with malignant tumors depends on the histologic diagnosis. Patients with pineal cell tumors have a 5-year survival rate in the range of 55%, and they also have the highest incidence of perioperative mortality and morbidity. Patients with germinomas have a 75% 5-year survival rate after undergoing surgery and radiation. Anecdotally, we have observed improved long-term survival in those patients with germinomas in whom a gross total resection was possible. Malignant germ cell tumors of a nongerminomatous variety, by contrast, have the poorest prognosis, with a 45% 2-year survival rate diminishing to 0% by 5 years despite aggressive treatment. With newer chemotherapy regimens, these results have been steadily improving and, at this writing we are following several patients in whom 5-year survival will likely be attainable.

Astrocytomas can vary depending on certain specific tumor characteristics. Cystic astrocytomas tend to be much more benign and completely resectable, with 100% 5-year survival rates. Noncystic astrocytomas clinically behave more like brain stem gliomas, and patients with these tumors have a 67% 5-year survival rate with surgery and radiation.

**TABLE 65–2 ■ SURGICAL RESULTS IN 196 OPERATIONS (191 PATIENTS) OF PINEAL REGION TUMORS AT THE NEW YORK NEUROLOGICAL INSTITUTE**

| Histology | Biopsy | Subtotal Resection | Total Resection | Transient/Minor/ No Morbidity | Permanent/ Major Morbidity | Death | Total |
|---|---|---|---|---|---|---|---|
| Benign | 0 | 6 | 58 | 63 | 0 | 1 | 64 |
| Malignant | 9 | 92 | 31 | 119 | 7 | 6 | 132 |
| Total | 9 | 98 | 89 | 182 | 7 | 7 | 196 |

## SUMMARY

Optimal management decisions in patients with pineal region tumors depend on making an accurate histologic diagnosis. Therefore, surgical exploration is mandated in all patients. The benefits of surgery extend beyond diagnostic purposes because one third of pineal tumors are benign and treatable with surgery alone. Malignant tumors may benefit from surgical debulking to reduce tumor burden before adjuvant therapy, and gross total resection is often possible.

The supracerebellar infratentorial approach offers several advantages over supratentorial techniques. By providing a midline trajectory beneath the deep venous system and taking advantage of the effects of gravity in the sitting position, the supracerebellar approach reduces the risk of complications and facilitates tumor removal. Improvements in microsurgical technique and neuroanesthesia have resulted in excellent outcomes after pineal surgery.

## REFERENCES

1. Neuwelt EA: The challenge of pineal region tumors. In Neuwelt EA (ed): The Diagnosis and Treatment of Pineal Region Tumors. Baltimore: Williams & Wilkins, 1984.
2. Schmidek HH: Pineal Tumors. New York: Masson, 1977.
3. Quest DQ, Kleriga E: Microsurgical anatomy of the pineal region. Neurosurgery 6:385–390, 1980.
4. Cushing H: Intracranial Tumors: Notes Upon a Series of Two-Thousand Verified Cases with Surgical Mortality Pertaining Thereto. Springfield, IL: Charles C Thomas, 1932.
5. Camins MB, Schlesinger EB: Treatment of tumors of the posterior part of the third ventricle and the pineal region: A long-term follow-up. Acta Neurochir Wien 40:131–143, 1978.
6. Cummins FM, Taveras JM, Schlesinger EB: Treatment of gliomas of the third ventricle and pinealomas: With special reference to the value of radiotherapy. Neurology 10:1031–1036, 1960.
7. Horrax G, Daniels JT: The conservative treatment of pineal tumors. Surg Clin North Am 22:649–659, 1942.
8. Dandy WE: Operative experience of cases of pineal tumor. Arch Surg 33:19–46, 1936.
9. Suzuki J, Iwabuchi T: Surgical removal of pineal tumors (pinealomas and teratomas). J Neurosurg 23:565–571, 1965.
10. Reid WS, Clark K: Comparison of the infratentorial and transtentorial approaches to the pineal region. Neurosurgery 3:1–8, 1978.
11. Sano K: Pineal region tumors: Problems in pathology and treatment. Clin Neurosurg 30:59–91, 1984.
12. Page LK: The infratentorial-supracerebellar exposure of tumors in the pineal area. Neurosurgery 1:36–40, 1977.
13. Stein BM: The infratentorial supracerebellar approach to pineal lesions. J Neurosurg 35:197–202, 1971.
14. Bruce JN, Stein BM: Surgical management of pineal region tumors. Acta Neurochir (Wien) 134:130–135, 1995.
15. Van Wagenen WP: A surgical approach for the removal of certain pineal tumors: Report of a case. Surg Gynecol Obstet 53:216–220, 1931.
16. Poppen JL: The right occipital approach to a pinealoma. J Neurosurg 25:706–710, 1966.
17. Krause F: Operative Frielegung der Vierhugel, nebst Beobachtungen uber Hirndruck und Dekompression. Zentralbl Chir 53:2812–2819, 1926.
18. Stein BM, Bruce JN, Fetell MR: Surgical approaches to pineal tumors. In Wilkins RH, Rengachary SS (eds): Neurosurgery Update 1: Diagnosis, Operative Technique, and Neuro-oncology. New York: McGraw-Hill, 1990, pp 389–398.
19. Bruce JN, Stein BM: Infratentorial approach to pineal tumors. In Wilson CB (ed): Neurosurgical Procedures: Personal Approaches to Classic Operations. Baltimore: Williams & Wilkins, 1992, pp 63–76.
20. Bruce JN: Management of pineal region tumors. Neurosurg Q 3:103–119, 1993.
21. Fetell MR, Bruce JN, Burke AM, et al: Non-neoplastic pineal cysts. Neurology 41:1034–1040, 1991.
22. Fetell MR, Stein BM: Neuroendocrine aspects of pineal tumors. Neurol Clin 4:877–905, 1986.
23. Ganti SR, Hilal SK, Stein BM, et al: CT of pineal region tumors. AJR Am J Roentgenol 7:97–104, 1986.
24. Muller-Forell W, Schroth G, Egan PJ: MR imaging in tumors of the pineal region. Neuroradiology 30:224–231, 1988.
25. Tien RD, Barkovich AJ, Edwards MSB: MR imaging of pineal tumors. AJNR Am J Neuroradiol 11:557–565, 1990.
26. Bruce JN, Fetell MR, Balmaceda CM, Stein BM: Tumors of the pineal region. In Black PM, Loeffler JS (eds): Cancer of the Nervous System. Malden, MA: Blackwell Science, 1996, pp 576–592.
27. Bjornsson J, Scheithauer BW, Okazaki H, Leech RW: Intracranial germ cell tumors: Pathobiological and immunohistological aspects of 70 cases. J Neuropathol Exp Neurol 44:32–46, 1985.
28. Kreth F, Schatz C, Pagenstecher A, et al: Stereotactic management of lesions of the pineal region. Neurosurgery 39:280–291, 1996.
29. Edwards MSB, Hudgins RJ, Wilson CB, et al: Pineal region tumors in children. J Neurosurg 68:689–697, 1988.
30. Kraichoke S, Cosgrove M, Chandrasoma PT: Granulomatous inflammation in pineal germinoma. Am J Surg Pathol 12:655–660, 1988.
31. Goodman R: Magnetic resonance imaging–directed stereotactic endoscopic third ventriculostomy. Neurosurgery 32:1043–1047, 1993.
32. Kobayashi S, Sugita K, Tanaka Y, Kyoshima K: Infratentorial approach to the pineal region in the prone position: Concorde position. J Neurosurg 58:141–143, 1983.
33. Ausman JI, Malik GM, Dujovny M, Mann R: Three-quarter prone approach to the pineal-tentorial region. Surg Neurol 29:298–306, 1988.
34. Sawamura Y, de Tribolet N, Ishii N, Abe H: Management of primary intracranial germinomas: Diagnostic surgery or radical resection? J Neurosurg 87:262–266, 1997.
35. Bruce JN, Stein BM: Supracerebellar approaches in the pineal region. In Apuzzo MLJ (ed): Brain Surgery: Complication Avoidance and Management. New York: Churchill-Livingstone, 1993, pp 511–536.
36. Peragut JC, Dupard T, Graciani N, Sedan R: De la prevention des risques de la biopsie stereotaxique de certaines tumeurs de la region pineale. Neurochirurgie 33:23–27, 1987.
37. Burres KP, Hamilton RD: Pineal apoplexy. Neurosurgery 4:264–268, 1979.
38. Bruce JN, Fetell MR, Stein BM: Incidence of spinal metastases in patients with malignant pineal region tumors: Avoidance of prophylactic spinal irradiation. J Neurosurg 72:354A, 1990.
39. Linstadt D, Wara WM, Edwards MS, et al: Radiotherapy of primary intracranial germinomas: The case against routine craniospinal irradiation. Int J Radiat Oncol Biol Phys 15:291–297, 1988.
40. Casentini L, Colombo F, Pozza F, Benedetti A: Combined radiosurgery and external radiotherapy of intracranial germinomas. Surg Neurol 34:79–86, 1990.

# Tumors of the Middle Cranial Fossa and Clivus

# CHAPTER 66

# Surgical Management of Lesions of the Clivus

■ GIULIO MAIRA

The clivus is a particular region of the skull characterized anatomically by the central and deep location
at the skull base and surgically by the difficulty in
reaching this structure.

Tumors that arise purely from the clivus are infrequent,
but the region can be involved with numerous processes
extending from the structures near the clivus, mainly from
the petrous-clival line. Tumors may be limited to a part of
the clivus, or they may involve the entire clivus. They may
also extend superiorly to the suprasellar region; inferiorly
to the foramen magnum and cervical spine; and, laterally,
to the cavernous sinus, subtemporal region, or pontocerebellar angle.

Different pathologic lesions can develop in this region.[1]
They can be benign (e.g., meningiomas, epidermoid cyst,
cholesterol granuloma, glomus jugulare tumors with major
petroclival involvement), of a low-grade malignancy (e.g.,
chordomas and chondrosarcomas), or of a high-grade malignancy (e.g., squamous cell cancer, adenocarcinoma,
basal cell carcinoma, osteogenic sarcoma). Some of these
tumors have an intradural location, whereas others are
extradural.

The lesions that most frequently involve this region are
meningiomas (commonly intradural) followed (much less
frequently) by chordomas, which are often extradural. The
former grows from the dura that covers the clivus or the
passage from the clivus and the petrous bone (petroclivus
fold),[2] whereas the latter originates directly from embryonic residues enclosed in the bone of the clivus.[3–6]

Tumors in the region of the clivus may involve the
lowest seven cranial nerves. Cranial nerve VI can be within
the tumor itself, while it runs through Dorello's canal
situated in the lateral region of the clivus. The brain stem
can be displaced posteriorly or laterally. The basilar artery
is usually displaced contralaterally; however, occasionally,
it is shifted posteriorly or encased by the tumor.

Major advances in imaging modalities over the last 2
decades have permitted a more precise delineation of the
anatomic extension of these tumors. In most cases, the
nature of the lesion can be suspected in advance.

Tumors in the region of the clivus are difficult to treat
using conventional neurosurgical approaches. Up until a
few decades ago, owing to the relative inaccessibility of

the clivus and its close proximity to the brain stem and
surrounding neurovascular structures, the results of surgical
treatment were so dismal that these tumors were often
considered to be incurable.[1]

Advances in microsurgery of the skull base have resulted
in the development and refinement of approaches to petroclival and clival lesions,[7–28] better methods for tumor
removal, and innovative techniques[29] to minimize injury to
neural and vascular structures during tumor removal. These
factors enable the surgeon to treat these tumors more effectively, aiming at a radical excision with an acceptable
morbidity and mortality.

In some cases, the combined effort of the neurosurgeon
with other disciplines interested in skull base surgery (otolaryngology or maxillofacial surgery) constitutes real progress in the realization of special approaches that aim at
improving the exposure of the tumor and reducing trauma
to the brain during surgery.

## SURGICAL ANATOMY

The clivus is located at the midline, which is the deeper
part of the skull base. It constitutes the inclined anteroinferior surface of the posterior cranial fossa and extends from
the dorsum sellae to the foramen magnum (Fig. 66–1A). It
is formed by a sphenoidal part (corresponding to the superior third) that extends from the dorsum sellae to the
spheno-occipital synchondrosis and by an occipital part
(corresponding to the inferior two thirds), which reaches
the anterior intraoccipital synchondroses.[3, 30]

Surgical access to the clivus is complicated by the presence of osseous barriers corresponding to the sphenoid and
facial bones, anteriorly and inferiorly, and to the petrous
bones, laterally. Posteriorly and laterally, there are critical
structures—the basilar artery, brain stem, cavernous sinus,
petrous carotid arteries, temporal lobes, and cranial nerves.

Owing to the complexity of the clivus and surrounding
structures, the knowledge of their anatomy is essential to
plan a correct surgical approach for patients who have a
tumor in this region.

The clivus is usually divided into the upper, middle, and

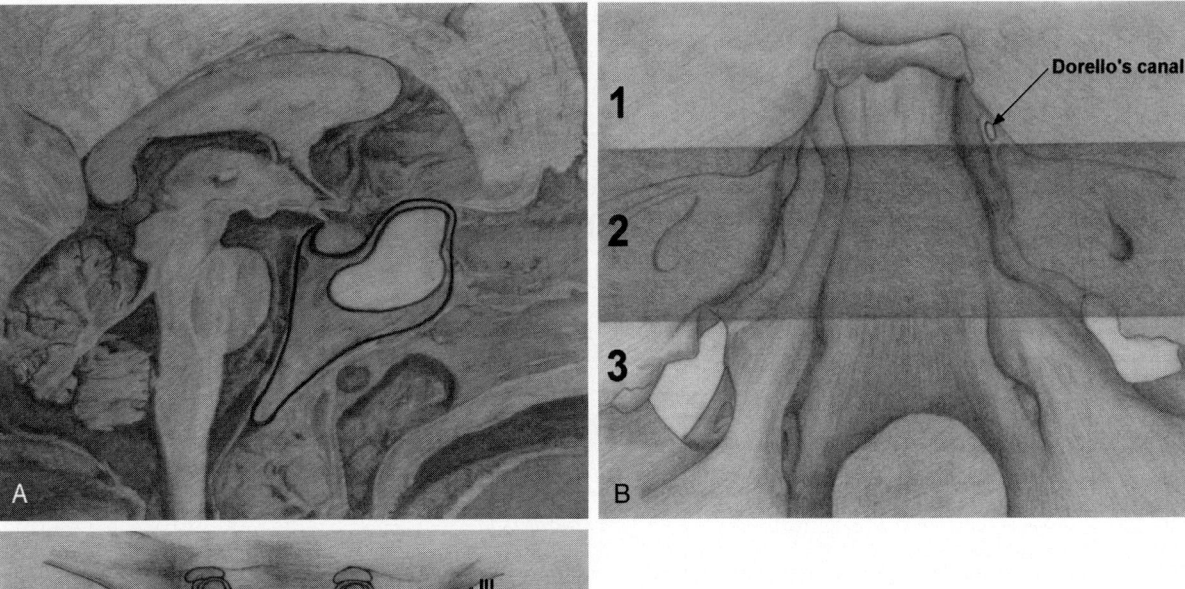

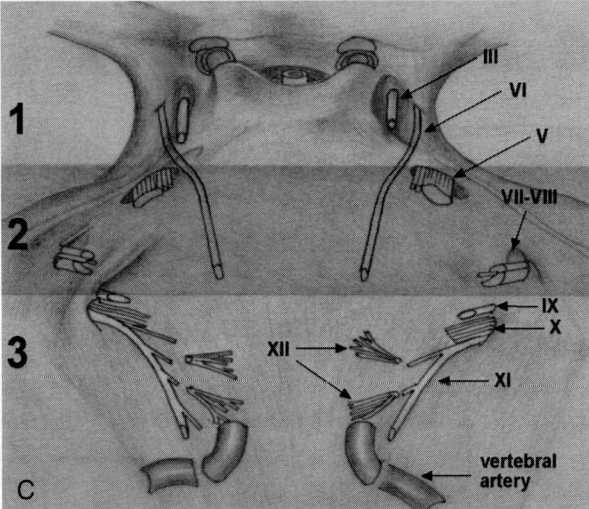

FIGURE 66–1 ■ *A*, Anatomy of the clivus and adjacent structures. *B*, Anatomic division of the clivus in upper (1), middle (2), and lower (3) regions. *C*, The clivus and cranial nerves III, V to XII.

lower clivus[25] (see Fig. 66–1*B, C*) or into superior and inferior halves of the clivus.[31]

- *The upper clivus* is the part above the crossing of the trigeminal and the abducens nerves from the posterior to the middle cranial fossa and includes the dorsum sellae and the posterior clinoid processes. This area is bounded anteriorly by the sella turcica and sphenoid sinus; posteriorly by the basilar artery and the midbrain; laterally by the cavernous sinus, the temporal lobes, and (from superior to inferior) cranial nerves III through VI.
- *The middle clivus* is the part between the exits of the trigeminal and the glossopharyngeal nerves. It is bounded anteriorly by the upper nasopharynx and retropharyngeal tissues, posteriorly by the basilar artery and by the pons, and laterally by the petrous apices and by cranial nerves VII and VIII.
- *The lower clivus* is the part from the glossopharyngeal nerve to the foramen magnum. It is bounded anteriorly by the lower nasopharynx and retropharyngeal tissues; posteriorly by the vertebral artery and the medulla; and laterally by the sigmoid sinus, jugular bulb, cranial nerves IX to XII.
- *The superior or inferior halves of the clivus* extend, respectively, above the internal auditory canal or below it.

The topographic anatomy of the clivus makes several surgical approaches feasible.[1, 11, 32, 33] The choice of an approach to remove a tumor from this region must take into account the nature of the lesion—whether the lesion is intradural or extradural, its position in respect to the clivus, and its lateral expansion.

The surgical approaches to the clivus are divided into three general groups: (1) anterior, (2) anterolateral, and (3) posterolateral:

- *Anterior approaches* are mainly used for extradural lesions that primarily involve the clivus and can extend extracranially, like chordoma and chondrosarcoma. For these tumors, the anterior approaches are usually extradural and include transnasal-transsphenoidal, transethmoidal, transoral-transpalatal, transmaxillary, and transcervical. A subfrontal transbasal extraintradural anterior approach can also be indicated for huge tumors with maximal involvement of the clival area and surrounding structures (e.g., chordoma, pituitary tumors, craniopharyngiomas).
- *Anterolateral approaches* are mainly utilized for intradural tumors involving the upper and middle clivus and extending into the surrounding regions. The *frontotemporal approach* exposes lesions of the upper clivus with

extension in the suprasellar region. The *subtemporal transtentorial approach* exposes lesions of the upper and midclival region, with extension in the middle fossa and tentorial edge (a zygomatic osteotomy and anterior petrosectomy increase the exposure inferiorly and toward the clivus).

• *Posterolateral approaches* are mainly utilized for tumors involving the medial and lower part of the clivus with extension to the petrous bone, cerebellopontine angle, foramen magnum, or upper cervical region. These approaches include the combined subtemporal suboccipital presigmoid with posterior petrosectomy (retrolabyrinthine, translabyrinthine, transcochlear, and total petrosectomy), the retrosigmoid, and the extreme lateral transjugular transcondylar approach.

## EXTRADURAL LESIONS: CHORDOMAS

Chordomas are the most frequent extradural tumors of the clivus. They arise from remnants of the embryonic notochord and are located in all places where the notochord existed: namely, the entire clivus, sella turcica, foramen magnum, C1, and nasopharynx.[3, 5] From there, they may spread to the upper cervical region, petrous bone, posterior fossa, cavernous sinus, middle fossa, nasopharynx, and sphenoid sinus.[3, 5]

Chordomas grow slowly but may present the characteristics of a malignant tumor in being locally aggressive with a tendency for regrowth.[34] Ten percent of chordomas show histologic signs of malignancy,[5] even if it is considered difficult to identify histologic features indicative of aggressiveness.[35, 36] Metastases are relatively rare.[36]

Chordomas infiltrate the bone and spread into the epidural space, seeding the dura with microscopic deposits well beyond the limits of the tumor bulk.[5, 37] For this reason, they may invade the dura and infiltrate the pia mater. The tumor is often gelatinous and soft, with a jelly-like consistency, but it can become very firm like cartilage.

Chordomas are usually classified according to the portion of clivus involved by the tumor and to the extension to surrounding structures: upper clivus, middle clivus, lower clivus, and craniocervical junction tumors, with or without invasion of sphenoid, cavernous sinus, and petrous bone.[1, 3]

A computed tomography (CT) scan and magnetic resonance imaging (MRI) are the most important radiologic tools for diagnosis. The CT scan reveals the destruction of bone, whereas the MRI shows the extension of the tumor, which appears isodense with the brain and with a variable contrast enhancement after gadolinium.[4]

The most commonly involved cranial nerve is the sixth, and diplopia is the most common presenting symptom, particularly in the midclivus chordomas. Other symptoms include headache, pituitary dysfunction, visual field defects, cerebellar syndrome, torticollis, and brain stem syndrome.[38]

### Surgical Treatment

The deep position (at the central base of the skull) and the tendency to infiltrate the bone make a total removal of the

clivus chordomas difficult. However, over the last decade, owing to the development of innovative and complex approaches to the clival area[39–43] or to the extensive application to this area of standard procedures,[12, 13, 16, 38, 44–48] many possibilities are at the disposal of the surgeon to attempt radical removal of these tumors.

As chordomas are basically extradural and midline tumors, they displace the neuraxis dorsally or dorsolaterally. Anterior midline extradural approaches are generally preferred (Fig. 66–2).[20, 37, 44, 49–52] These approaches allow a midline exposure of the clivus, with a short working distance, avoiding any retraction of the brain.

The choice of surgical approach depends on the location and extension of the tumor. Even when only anterior extracranial approaches are considered, many options exist. These include: the transbasal,[13] extended frontal,[52] transseptal transsphenoidal,[16,38,45,46] transsphenoethmoidal,[44] transmaxillary transnasal,[53] transfacial,[62] facial translocation,[54] transmaxillary,[55, 56] midfacial degloving,[51] transoral,[12] mandible-splitting transoral,[46] transcervical transclival,[57] anterior cervical[58] approaches, Le Fort I osteotomy,[59] unilateral Le Fort I osteotomy,[60] total rhinotomy, or pedicled rhinotomy.[61]

All these approaches are devoted to remove all clival lesions localized on the midline, without important lateral extent. In case of massive lateral expansion, so that a midline approach is insufficient for the removal of all the tumor, more complex lateral approaches can be utilized as a primary or secondary procedure[1, 5]: for lesions of the upper clivus, the subtemporal, transcavernous, and transpetrous apex approach; for lesions of the midclivus, a subtemporal and infratemporal approach; for lesions of lower

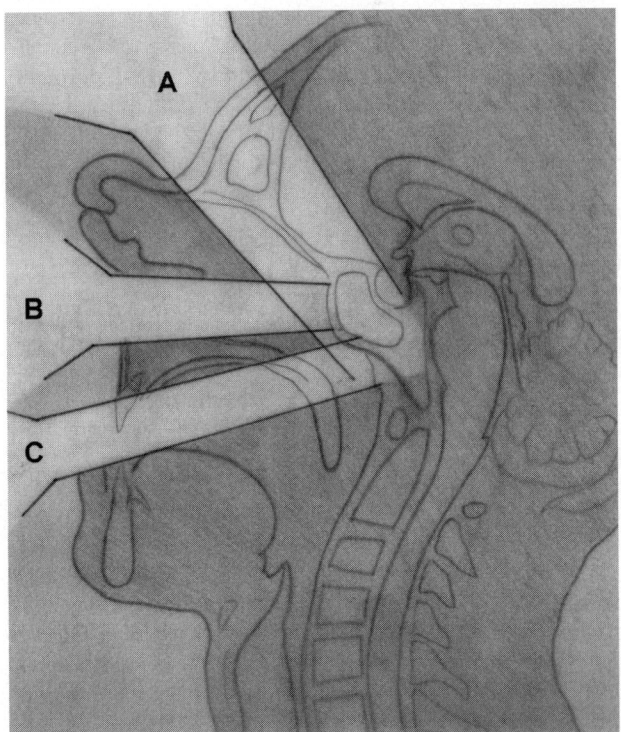

FIGURE 66–2 ■ Anterior approaches to the clivus: Subfrontal transbasal approach (A); transsphenoidal approach (B); and transoral approach (C).

clivus with lateral extension to the occipital condyle, jugular foramen, and cervical area, the extreme lateral transcondylar approach.[26]

According to the level of the clival lesion, the approaches that we more often utilize are the following:

- For chordomas located in the *upper and middle clivus*, we favor the *transsphenoidal approach.*
- For lesions of the *lower clivus* that involve the foramen magnum, C1, and C2, we prefer the *transoral approach*, with or without splitting the palate.
- For tumors located in the lower clivus, foramen magnum, and first cervical spinal bodies, with important lateral expansion, the approach used can be the *Le Fort I osteotomy with a midline incision of the hard and soft palate* and lateral swinging of the two flaps of the hard palate.
- For huge tumors involving all the clival area, the sphenoid, and the sellar region and extending anteriorly to the optic nerves, we utilize the *transbasal or frontal extended route.*
- For lesions that involve the lower clivus and the upper cervical region and that extend laterally into the occipital condyle and the jugular bulb on one side, *the extreme lateral, transcondyle approach* is particularly well suited.

Further anterior approaches can be utilized:

The *transsphenoethmoidal approach*[44] provides access to the entire sphenoid sinus, prepontine space, and superior clivus; a limited medial maxillectomy improves the access to the inferior clivus.

The *transfacial approach*[62] is indicated for extradural tumors confined on the midline and extending from the level of the sellar floor to the foramen magnum. This approach offers direct access to the clivus along its rostrocaudal extent up to the anterior arch of C1; with depression of the palate, the odontoid can also be visualized. The main advantage is to add, by this single facial route, the possibilities of the transsphenoidal and transoral routes, avoiding any injury to the hard and soft palate. The disadvantages are a facial scar and osteotomy of the facial skeleton.

## Transsphenoidal Approach

The transsphenoidal approach provides excellent exposure to chordomas of the sphenoid sinus, sella turcica, and upper and middle clivus (see Fig. 66–2), minimizing the morbidity of more complex surgical approaches[13, 16, 38, 48] with a route that, when necessary, can easily be repeated. The technique utilized for the sublabial, transseptal transsphenoidal procedure has been already described.[63] Extensive experience obtained with pituitary tumors[64, 65] and craniopharyngiomas[66] has made this route safe and effective, even for other pathologies (Figs. 66–3 to 66–5). Some papers have been published about the results obtained regarding chordomas.[38, 46, 47] These reports clearly indicate that gross total removal of the tumor can be achieved in up to the 70% of cases, with excellent long-term survival and no evidence of disease in all patients at a mean of 38.6 months after surgery.[38]

Its main disadvantages are represented by the limited lateral exposure and the deep and narrow field. Nevertheless, the correct use of long and angled curets can allow a skillful surgeon to remove even large tumors (>4 cm) that are not strictly confined to the midline. Application of endoscopy to the transsphenoidal route may increase the approach and allows even very extended tumors to be removed.

When the tumor is found to be located extraintradurally, an opening of the dura mater can be realized to remove the intradural tumor. Afterward, an accurate reconstruction must be realized. We usually use a dural patch and glue or fat tissue graft and human fibrin.

## Transoral Approach

The indication for the transoral route is for extradural lesions of the inferior clivus confined to the midline, protruding into the posterior pharyngeal region, and extended to C1 to C2 (see Fig. 66–2). The approach provides a good exposure with limited surgical trauma.[32, 67] This route has been used for many years for epidural tumors of the cervical spine.[68] Many reports have described the utilization of this surgical route to treat clivus chordomas.[69–71]

A modified transoral version has been described for these lesions.[56, 59] It combines the Le Fort I osteotomy with a midline incision of the hard and soft palate and allows lateral swinging of the two flaps of the hard palate based on their own palatine artery and nerves. The advantage is extensive exposure of the region, inferiorly and laterally (Fig. 66–6); the wound must be closed well in order to effect good occlusion and proper functioning of the palate. A unilateral Le Fort I osteotomy can be realized in laterally developed tumors.[60]

## Subfrontal Transbasal Approach or Extended Frontal Approach

This route can be utilized for chordomas with both intradural and extradural extension, with extensive involvement of the clivus and surrounding structures.[5] The approach is a modification of the "transbasal approach" of Derome.[13, 72] After a bifrontal craniotomy (including the orbital roof and nasal bones), the anterior skull base is exposed extradurally on both sides (Fig. 66–7; see also Fig. 66–2). The planum sphenoidale and part of the anterior wall of the sella are removed. The clivus is reached anterior to the sella and exposed up to the rim of the foramen magnum (see Fig. 66–2). If the lesion presents an intradural expansion, the frontal dura is opened. It also allows for the removal of tumors that extend near to the clivus— namely, the frontal suprasellar region, orbits, paranasal sinuses, and temporal fossa. This approach has been also used for different tumors, such as craniopharyngiomas (Fig. 66–8), meningiomas, or pituitary tumors.

## Extreme Lateral Transcondylar Approach

The approach is useful for the management of both intradural and extradural lesions that involve the lower clival and foramen magnum regions (Fig. 66–9), with extension into the occipital condyles and the jugular bulb on one side and the upper cervical spine.[15, 26, 73, 74] The technical steps of the approach are well described by many authors.[8, 26, 33]

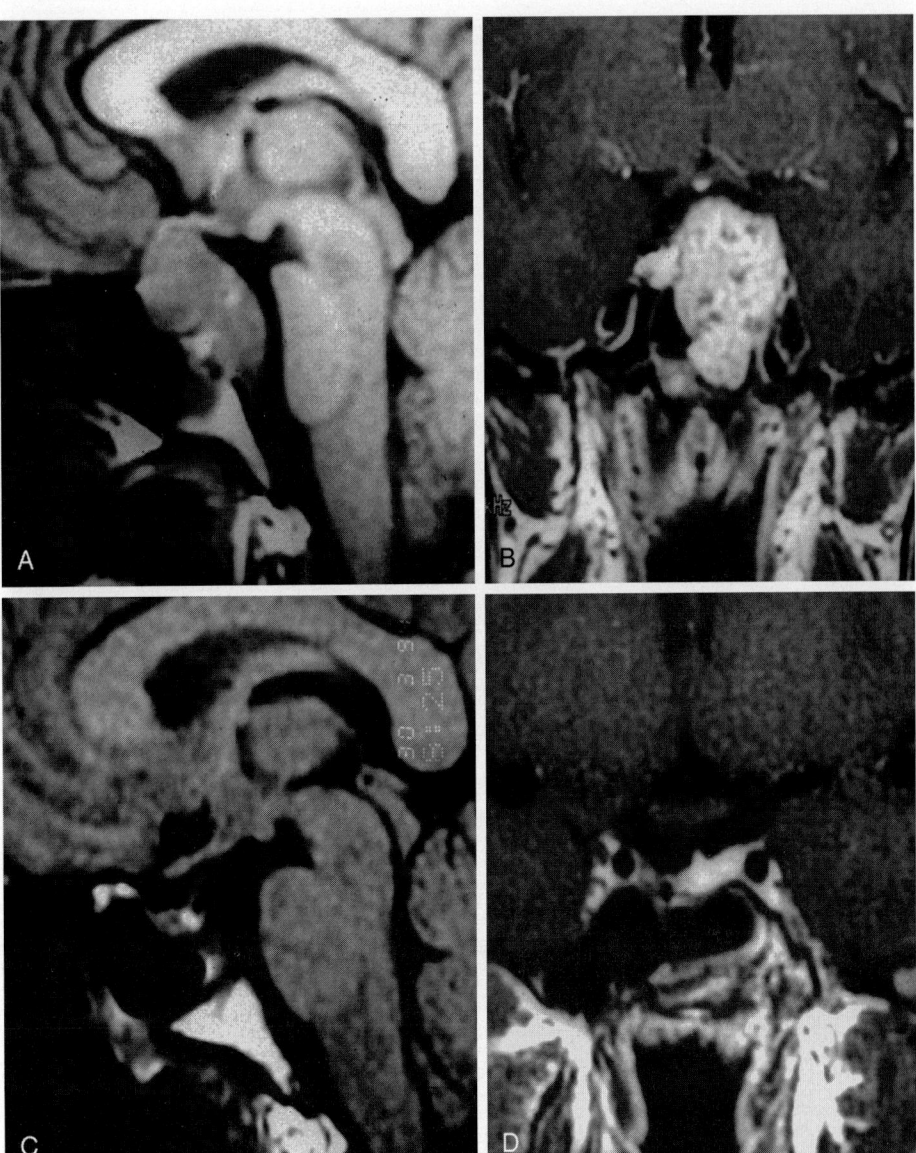

**FIGURE 66–3** ■ The transsphenoidal approach. An upper and middle clivus chordoma with retroclival diffusion and pontine compression. Contrast-enhanced magnetic resonance imaging is used. *A,* Preoperative sagittal image. *B,* Preoperative coronal image. *C,* Postoperative sagittal image. *D,* Postoperative coronal image.

The main advantage of this route is the direct view that it offers to the ventral aspect of the foramen magnum without requiring brain stem retraction.

The patient is placed in a full lateral decubitus position, with the head rotated downward. After a skin incision, the muscle mass is freed from along the nuchalis line. The paraspinous muscles are split until the spinous processes of C1 and C2 are exposed. The lateral mass of C1 and the vertebral artery from C1 to its dural entry are exposed. A C1 laminotomy is performed. A suboccipital craniotomy is performed. The occipital condyle and the lateral mass of C1 are removed. The vertebral artery is transposed during the dural opening.

## Postoperative Adjunctive Radiotherapy

Although the definitive modality of treatment for clival chordomas is surgical resection, an adjunctive treatment can be considered in selected cases. A correlation between radiation dose and length of the disease-free interval has been indicated,[75] but the prevailing opinion is somewhat skeptical as to the actual efficacy of postoperative radiotherapy in the management of chordomas.[76–78] Conventional external beam radiotherapy, after partial or subtotal removal, does not seem to affect the regrowth of the tumor.[79] Nevertheless, a better prognosis for small remnants is achieved with proton beam therapy.[80]

## INTRADURAL LESIONS: MENINGIOMAS

Meningiomas of the clivus and apical petrous bone are the most common intradural neoplasms of this region. Their natural history is characterized by a slow but progressive growth that eventually enables these tumors to achieve an enormous size before manifesting neurologic symptoms related to distortion of the brain stem or cranial nerves III to XII.

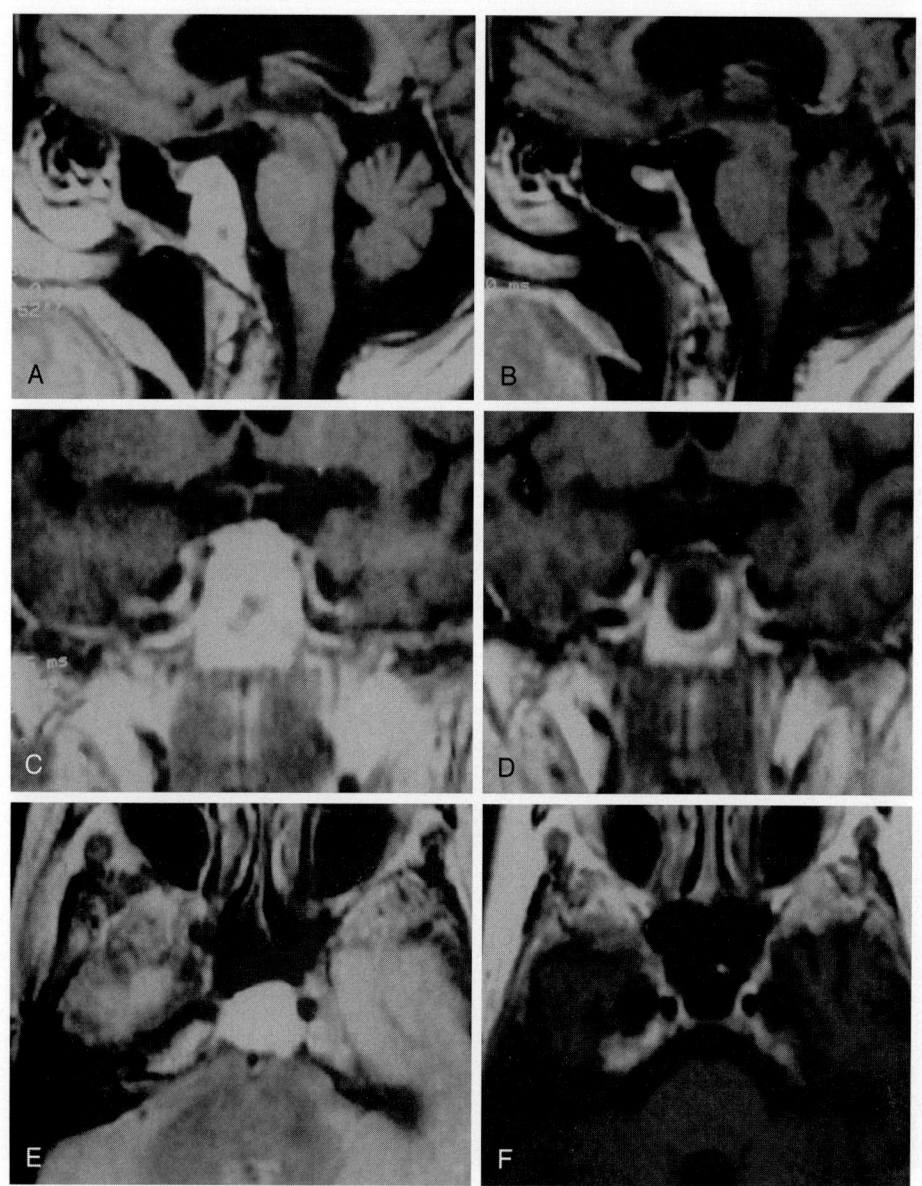

**FIGURE 66–4** ■ The transsphenoidal approach. An upper and middle clivus chordoma with a retroclival intradural diffusion *(E)*. Contrast-enhanced magnetic resonance imaging is used.
*A,* Preoperative sagittal image.
*B,* Postoperative sagittal image.
*C,* Preoperative coronal image.
*D,* Postoperative coronal image.
*E,* Preoperative axial image.
*F,* Postoperative axial image.

According to Yasargil and associates,[2] these meningiomas may be attached "at any of the lateral sites along the petroclival borderline, where the sphenoidal, petrous and clival bones meet." These authors suggested that such basal tumors could be divided into clival, petroclival, and sphenopetroclival, according to their point of insertion and extent.

*Clival meningiomas* originate from the clival dura. They are rare and frequently encase the basilar artery and its branches. *Petroclival meningiomas* are tumors that originate in the upper two thirds of the clivus at the petroclival junction, medial to the entry of the trigeminal root in Meckel's cave.[2, 81, 82] These meningiomas often displace the basilar artery and the brain stem on the opposite side; however, in up to 25%, there is encasement of the artery.[83] *Sphenopetroclival meningiomas* are the most extensive of these lesions. The clivus and the petrous apex are involved. They invade the posterior cavernous sinus and the sphenoid sinus, and they grow into the middle and posterior fossae.[82]

Classification of meningiomas of this area can also be based on the anatomic location of the tumor with reference to the clivus (upper, middle, and lower) and on the size and volume of the tumor (medium: up to 2.5 cm in average diameter; large: 2.5 to 4.5 cm; and giant: more than 4.5 cm).[84]

Structures that are in close proximity to the clivus may often be involved because of the growth of the tumor. Meningiomas of the upper clivus may involve the cavernous sinus, sella turcica, Meckel's cave, and tentorial notch; meningiomas of the middle clivus may involve the cerebellopontine angle; meningiomas of the lower clivus may involve the jugular bulb, hypoglossal foramina, and upper cervical region.

The location and volume of the tumor, its consistency and vascularity, the presence or absence of a subarachnoid plane between meningioma and the brain stem, arterial and nervous displacement or encasement, and correct choice of the surgical approach are the factors that, ultimately, decide

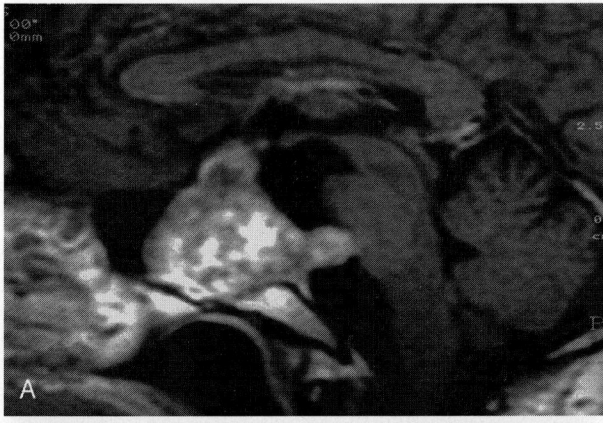

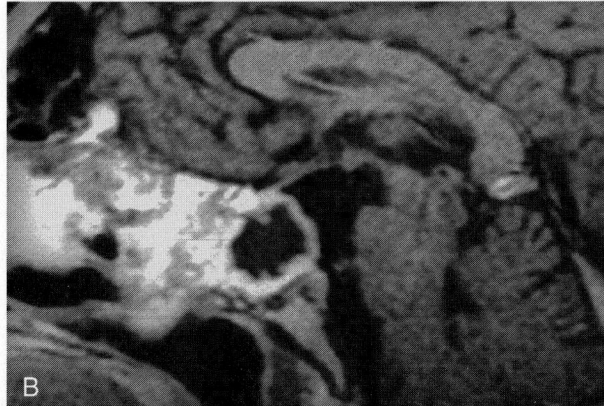

FIGURE 66–5 ■ The transsphenoidal approach. An upper and middle clivus chordoma with an intradural retroclival nodule compressing the brain stem. Contrast-enhanced magnetic resonance imaging is used. *A,* Preoperative sagittal image. *B,* Early postoperative sagittal image (1 month after surgery).

the extent of the surgical resection and the quality of the results.

## Surgical Treatment

For safe excision of these deep tumors, an adequate exposure (with a low or basal approach to limit or avoid brain retraction) is necessary. The combined supratentorial and infratentorial approach, which Malis called the petrosal approach,[9, 20, 85] was the first progress in the surgical exposure of the petroclival region. Thereafter, several surgical approaches have been proposed to reach tumors in this region.[33, 84, 86-88] In these approaches, the petrous part of the temporal bone is often removed to reduce retraction of the temporal lobe and cerebellum and provide better exposure of the clivus and ventral surface of the brain stem.

Surgical removal of the petrous bone was first used by King in 1970.[89] Limited anterior resection (anterior transpetrosal approach), with preservation of hearing, was reported by Kawase in 1985.[90] Since then, the transpetrosal approach has received many modifications and has become a relevant part of the surgical approaches to the clivus and brain stem.[14, 18, 22, 23, 42, 91-94] As suggested by Miller and associates, in 1993,[95] all described transpetrosal approaches can be divided basically into two types: (1) *anterior petrosectomy,* for lesions of the petrous apex and superior half

of the clivus, and (2) *posterior petrosectomy,* for lesions of the petroclival area and cerebellopontine angle.

Meningiomas of the petroclival region are reached through several routes, passing through the middle or posterior fossa (Fig. 66–10 and Table 66–1):

- **Anterolateral route**: *frontotemporal transsylvian approach* (usually combined with an orbitozygomatic osteotomy) for tumors of the upper clivus and tentorial notch
- **Lateral route**: *anterior subtemporal approach* with zygomatic osteotomy and anterior petrosectomy, for tumors of the petrous apex and upper half of the clivus
- **Posterolateral route**:
  - *Posterior subtemporal suboccipital presigmoid approach* with posterior petrosectomy for centrolateral midclival and petrous apex lesions. (In case of extensive meningiomas, this route can be combined with the anterior subtemporal approach.)
  - *Retrosigmoid approach* for lateral, small, and medium-sized tumors of the midclivus (which are eventually combined with the previous approach)
  - *Extreme lateral transcondylar approach* for tumors of the lower clivus, foramen magnum, and cervical spine

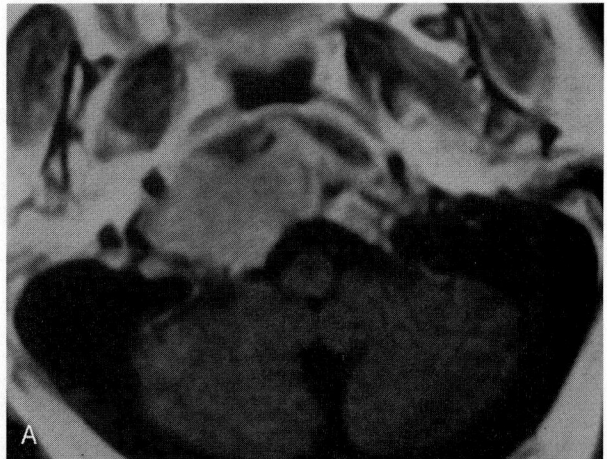

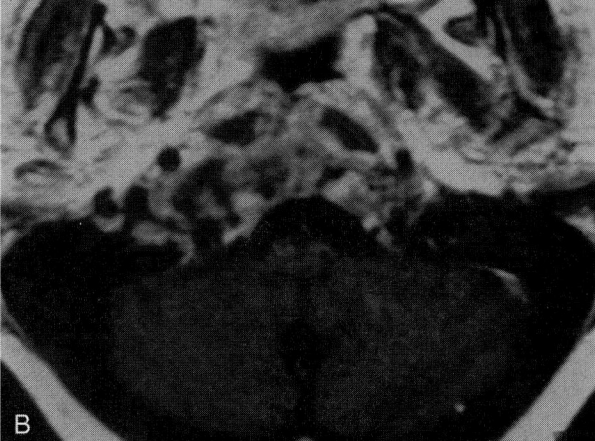

FIGURE 66–6 ■ A modified transoral approach. Le Fort I osteotomy with a midline incision of the hard and soft palate. The middle and lower clivus chordoma are shown with left lateral expansion. Contrast-enhanced magnetic resonance imaging is used. *A,* Preoperative axial image. *B,* Postoperative axial image.

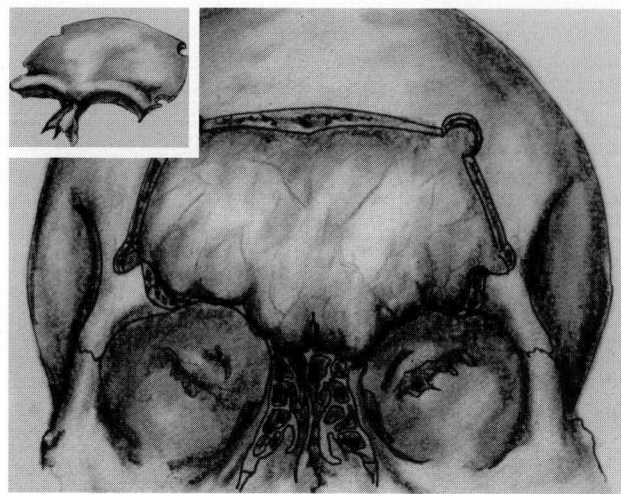

**FIGURE 66–7** ■ A subfrontal transbasal approach using a bifrontal craniotomy, including the orbital roof and nasal bones.

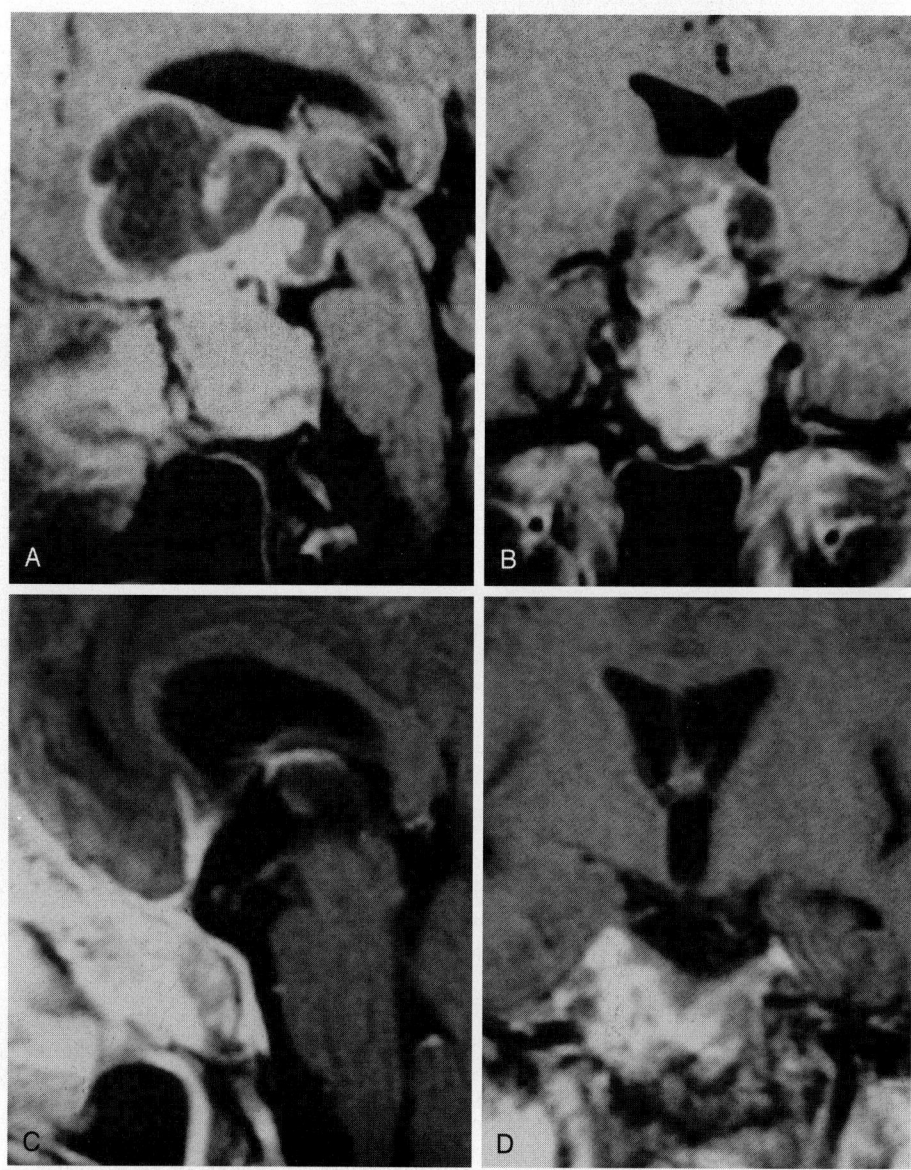

**FIGURE 66–8** ■ A subfrontal transbasal approach. An intraextradural craniopharyngioma with sellar, suprasellar, and retroclival extension is shown. Contrast-enhanced magnetic resonance imaging is used.
*A*, Preoperative sagittal image.
*B*, Preoperative coronal image.
*C*, Postoperative sagittal image.
*D*, Postoperative coronal image.

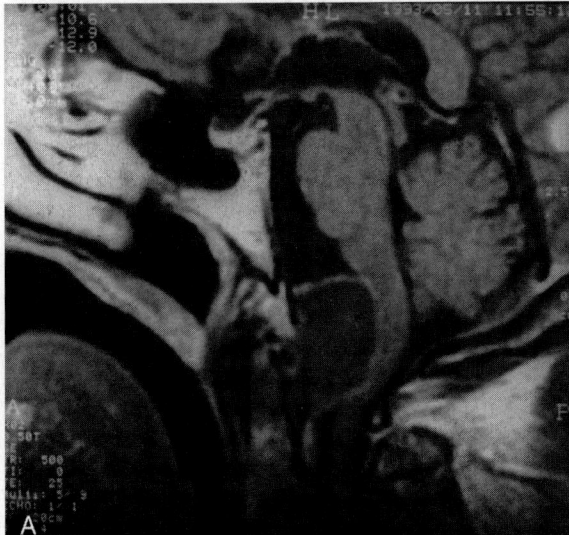

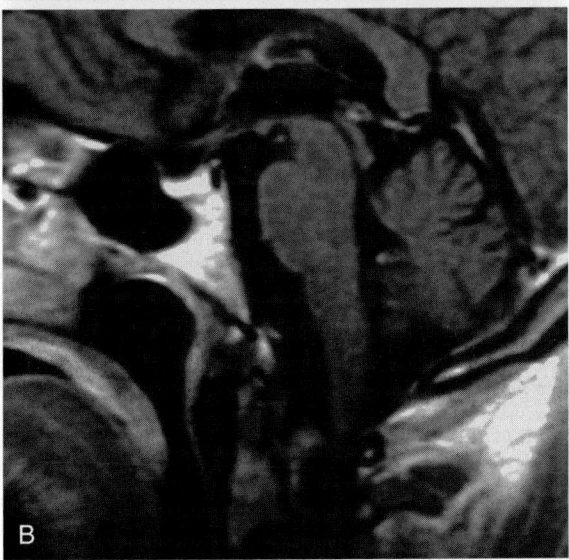

**FIGURE 66–9** ■ An extreme lateral transcondylar approach. Lower clivus and upper cervical chordoma. Contrast-enhanced magnetic resonance imaging is used. *A*, Preoperative sagittal image. *B*, Postoperative sagittal image.

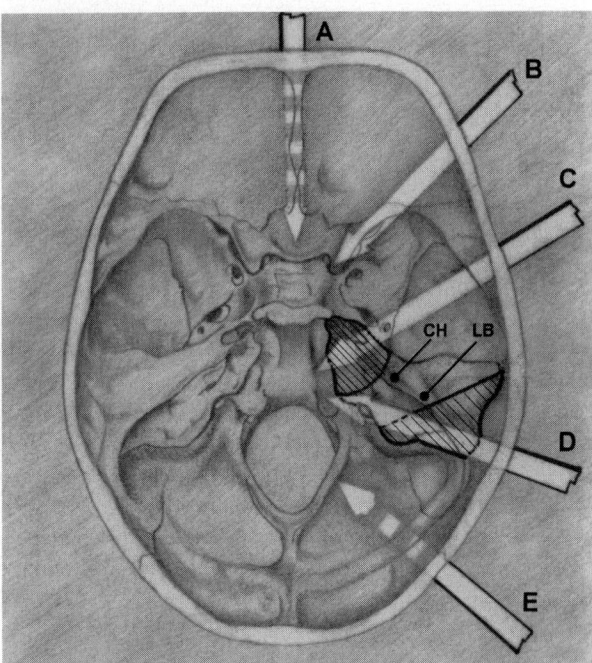

**FIGURE 66–10** ■ Approaches to the clivus: Anterior approaches (A); frontotemporal approach (B); anterior subtemporal approach with an anterior petrosectomy (C); presigmoid retrolabyrinthine approach with a posterior petrosectomy (D); extreme lateral transcondylar approach (E). (CH, cochlea; LB, labyrinth.)

## Frontotemporal Trans-sylvian Approach

This approach provides good exposure for removal of small tumors in the upper clivus and tentorial notch. If necessary, exposure of the floor of the middle fossa can be also obtained by performing a zygomatic or orbitozygomatic osteotomy with inferior displacement of the temporalis muscle.[17, 96, 97]

## Anterior Subtemporal Approach with Anterior Petrosectomy

The approach is indicated for lesions of the tip of the petrous bone or for those involving the middle upper clival area, which do not extend behind the internal auditory canal.[19] This approach is also indicated when the great part of the tumor is in the middle fossa, involving the cavernous sinus.[25, 84]

An anterior temporal craniotomy is performed, followed by an orbitozygomatic osteotomy to extend anteriorly or inferiorly the exposure of the conventional craniotomy. The superior orbital fissure, the foramen rotundum, and the foramen ovale are exposed. To expand the exposure at the petrous apex and midclivus, a part of the petrous bone is removed. Kawase[19] described a triangle in the petrous bone (lateral to the trigeminal nerve and medial to the internal auditory meatus) that can be drilled, thus providing a route toward the lesions located in the region of the midclivus (see Fig. 66–10). Anteroinferiorly to this area is the hori-

**TABLE 66–1** ■ **CHOICE OF SURGICAL APPROACH IN RELATION TO THE LOCATION OF THE TUMOR**

| Location of Lesion | Surgical Approach |
| --- | --- |
| Upper clivus | 1. Frontotemporal approach with orbitozygomatic osteotomy<br>2. Subtemporal approach with a zygomatic osteotomy and an anterior petrosectomy |
| Upper and middle third of the clivus | 1. Subtemporal craniotomy with an anterior petrosectomy<br>2. Subtemporal-suboccipital craniotomy with a posterior petrosectomy |
| Lower third of the clivus | Extreme lateral transcondylar approach |
| Middle and lower third of the clivus | Combined posterior petrosectomy with an extreme lateral approach |
| Entire clivus through the level of the foramen magnum | Far lateral/combined supratentorial and infratentorial approach (including posterior petrosectomy or total petrosectomy) |

zontal segment of the petrous carotid artery. The petrous apex can be drilled at the Glasscock triangle (demarcated laterally by a line from the foramen spinosum toward the arcuate eminence ending at the facial hiatus; medially by the greater petrosal nerve; and at the base, by the third trigeminal nerve division.[95] The exposure can be further increased by anterior displacement of the carotid artery or by drilling the region of the cochlea and thus sacrificing hearing. During this procedure, care should be taken not to damage the abducens nerve that runs through Dorello's canal just medial to this area.

The approach to the clivus can be obtained by the simple fenestration of the petrous bone and attached tentorium[19] or with an intradural transtentorial approach.[31, 93] In the last case, an intradural and extradural subtemporal approach is combined with division of the tentorium and intradural removal of the petrous bone from its apex to the cochlea.

In 1997, Taniguchi and Perneczky[94] suggested during the surgery of petroclival lesions, the application of the keyhole concept, which involves the reduction of the conventional approach to its essential parts.

## Subtemporo-Suboccipital Presigmoid Approach with a Posterior Petrosectomy

In 1992, Spetzler and associates[27] summarized neurosurgical approaches that required a posterior petrosectomy into three groups:

Group 1: approach that preserves hearing
Group 2: approaches involving sacrifice of hearing
Group 3: approaches involving mobilization of the facial nerve.

### APPROACH THAT PRESERVES HEARING

The presigmoid, retrolabyrinthine, transmastoid approach is most suitable for tumors of the clivus with extension in the middle and posterior fossa. This approach provides excellent exposure of the region ventral to the midbrain and pons. Described by Hakuba and associates[98] in 1977 and refined by Al-Mefty and associates in 1988, the approach requires a low posterior temporal craniotomy and a lateral retrosigmoid craniotomy.[91] A mastoidectomy is performed to expose the sigmoid sinus, the dura mater of the posterior cranial fossa situated anteriorly to the sinus, and the labyrinth. The sinus must be skeletonized along its entire course to provide adequate length for mobilization, and the labyrinthine complex must be freed completely from mastoid cells in order to gain as much space as possible (Fig. 66–11). A labyrinthectomy minimally improves access to the posterior fossa. Its use should be avoided unless hearing has been irreversibly lost. Some authors[99] have suggested the use of a partial labyrinthectomy to widen the exposure from the presigmoid route without affecting the hearing.

The dura mater of the posterior cranial fossa is incised anteriorly to the sigmoid sinus, and this incision is joined to that of the dura mater of the middle cranial fossa, thus preserving the sigmoid sinus as described by Al-Mefty and associates.[91] The superior petrosal sinus is then resected, and the tentorium is incised (see Fig. 66–11). The fourth

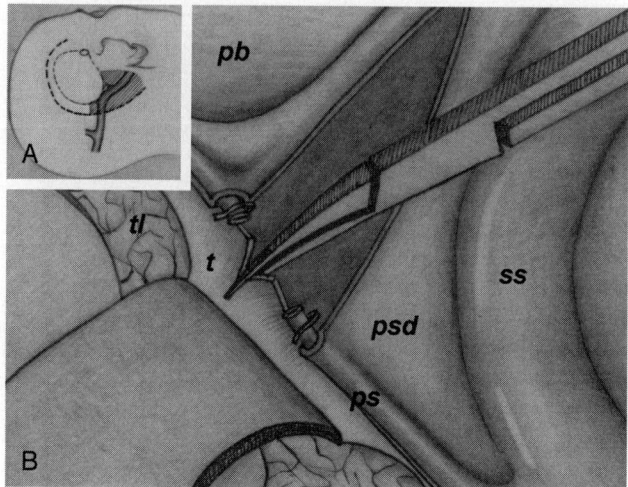

FIGURE 66–11 ■ Presigmoid retrolabyrinthine approach. *A*, Temporal craniotomy and retrolabyrinthine craniectomy and petrosectomy. *B*, Incision of tentorium after opening of the presigmoid and temporal dura. (tl, temporal lobe; t, tentorium; pb, petrous bone; ps, petrous sinus; psd, presigmoid dura; ss, sigmoid sinus.)

nerve is identified by moving the edge of the tentorium. A crucial step in the petrosal approach is the identification and preservation of the venous drainage of the posterior temporal lobe, namely the vein of Labbé and other basal veins. The transverse sinus may be divided to obtain improved exposure of structures below the auditory canal. This can be performed for patients who have good patency of the contralateral venous sinuses.

The advantages of this approach include minimal cerebellar and temporal lobe retraction and shortening of the operative distance to the tumor by 3 cm when compared with the retrosigmoid approach. The surgeon has surgical access more anterior and closer to the clivus, the latter factor being very important for the removal of lesions with a central location anterior to the brain stem (Figs. 66–12 and 66–13). Disadvantages are temporal lobe retraction and the possibility of injury to the vein of Labbé. Furthermore, paralysis of the lower cranial nerves constitutes one of the major sources of morbidity. Exposure of the lower clivus is limited by the jugular bulb, especially when it is high.

Access to the foramen magnum and inferior clivus can be improved by adding a retrosigmoid dural opening with anterolateral retraction of the sinus. If the lesion extends forward, one has to consider combining this approach with an anterior subtemporal zygomatic approach.

### APPROACHES INVOLVING SACRIFICE OF HEARING

The presigmoid translabyrinthine approach is an anterior extension of the presigmoid retrolabyrinthine approach. The approach involves the removal of the semicircular canals, thus enhancing the exposure. The transcochlear approach[100] involves the anterior extension of the translabyrinthine approach.

A combination of the transcochlear approach with more extensive bone removal and anterior mobilization of the petrous internal carotid artery is called a total petrosectomy approach.[33]

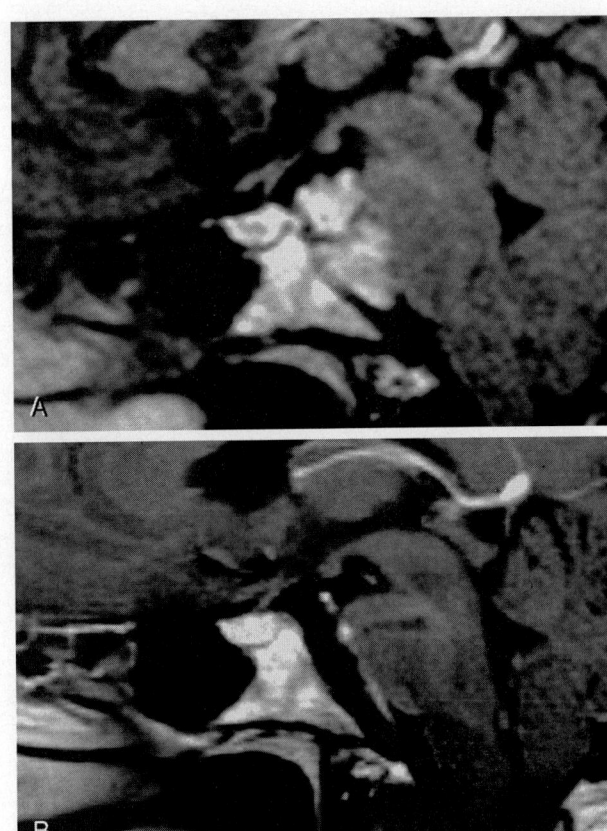

**FIGURE 66–12** ■ A presigmoid retrolabyrinthine approach. Central meningioma of the upper and middle clivus. Contrast-enhanced magnetic resonance imaging is used. *A*, Preoperative sagittal image. *B*, Postoperative sagittal image.

## APPROACHES INVOLVING MOBILIZATION OF THE FACIAL NERVE

Various elaborated transpetrous approaches have been described, some of which involve mobilization of the facial nerve. A total petrosectomy approach has been described by Sekhar and associates.[84, 93] The approach requires unroofing of the entire facial nerve and its posterior mobilization and anterior displacement of the petrous carotid artery.

## Retrosigmoid Approach

A retrosigmoid approach is indicated for lateral, small, and medium-sized tumors of the midclivus. The approach is easy, but it needs to work between the cranial nerves and blood vessels in the cerebellopontine angle[101] and does not provide adequate exposure of more medial or contralateral expansion of the lesions.

## Extreme Lateral Transcondylar Approach

This approach has already been described among the approaches for extradural lesions.

## Far Lateral/Combined Approach

This approach combines the far lateral approach with subtemporal and transpetrosal exposures in order to gain an extensive view of the entire petroclival region in case of tumors involving the entire clivus and also extending to the craniocervical region.[102, 103] The model incorporates a subtemporal craniotomy and posterior petrous bone resection into the far lateral approach in order to obtain an unobstructed view of the entire clivus and ventral brain stem.

## Surgical Adjuvants

1. Vascular embolization: Preoperative embolization of the external carotid artery feeders can be helpful for reducing intraoperative bleeding.
2. Intraoperative lumbar drainage of cerebrospinal fluid (CSF): Drainage of CSF is an important adjuvant to help relaxation of the brain.
3. Intraoperative monitoring of the brain and cranial nerve functions: It includes somatosensory evoked potential, auditory brain stem evoked potential, and monitoring of cranial nerves III, IV, VI, VII, X, XI, and XII.
4. Frameless stereotactic navigation: It improves the exposure and reduces the risks.
5. Contact neodymium:yttrium-aluminum-garnet laser: It increases the achievement of total removal, which can be realized faster and with less bleeding.[29]
6. Arterial bypass: When the tumor encases the petrous or cavernous carotid artery, if the patient fails the balloon occlusion test and vascular ligation is necessary, a vascular reconstruction is mandatory using a saphenous vein graft bypass or using an extracranial-intracranial arterial bypass.[104]
7. Adequate reconstruction of the skull base, in order to

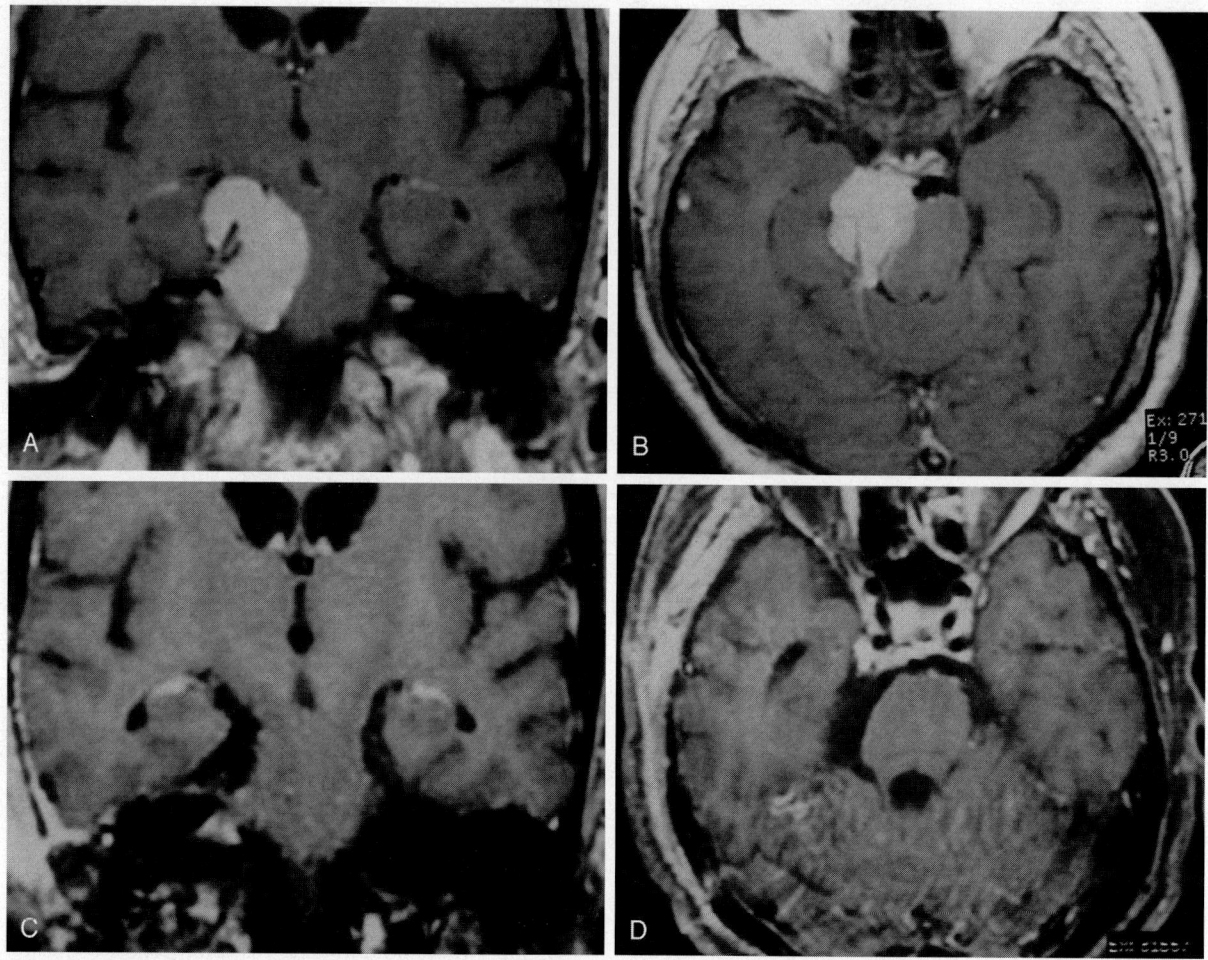

**FIGURE 66–13** ■ A presigmoid retrolabyrinthine approach. Petroclival meningiomas. Contrast-enhanced magnetic resonance imaging is used. *A*, Preoperative coronal image. *B*, Preoperative axial image. *C*, Postoperative coronal image. *D*, Postoperative axial image.

prevent CSF leakage: This is done by placing a pericranial flap or autologous fat and biologic glue.
8. Radiosurgery can be helpful for treating small remnants in critical areas.

## REFERENCES

1. Sekhar LN, Goel A, Sen CN: Extradural clival tumors. In Apuzzo MLJ (ed): Brain Surgery: Complication Avoidance and Management. New York: Churchill Livingstone, 1993, pp 2221–2244.
2. Yasargil MG, Mortara RW, Curcic M: Meningiomas of the posterior cranial fossa. In Krayenbuhl H (ed): Advances and Technical Standards in Neurosurgery, Vol 7. New York: Springer-Verlag, 1980, pp 4–115.
3. Lang J: Anatomy of clivus. In Samii M, Draf W (eds): Surgery of the Skull Base. Berlin: Springer-Verlag, 1989, pp 90–101.
4. Meyers SP, Hirsch WL, Curtin HD, et al: Chondrosarcomas of the skull base: MR imaging features. Radiology 184:103–108, 1992.
5. Gay E, Sekhar LN, Wright DC: Chordomas and chondrosarcomas of the cranial base. In Kaye AH, Laws ER Jr (eds): Brain Tumors. Edinburgh: Churchill Livingstone, 1995, pp 777–794.
6. Goel A: Chordomas and chondrosarcomas: Relationship to the internal carotid artery. Acta Neurochir (Wien) 133:30–35, 1995.
7. Al-Mefty O, Fox JL, Smith RR: Petrosal approach for petroclival meningiomas. Neurosurgery 22:510–517, 1988.
8. Bertalanffy H, Seeger W: The dorsolateral, suboccipital, transcondylar approach to the lower clivus and anterior portion of the craniocervical junction. Neurosurgery 129:815–821, 1991.
9. Bonnal J, Louis R, Combalbert A: L'abord temporal transtentoriel de l'angle ponto-cerebelleux et du clivus. Neurochirurgie 10:3–12, 1964.
10. Bricolo A, Turazzi S, Cristofori L, et al: Microsurgical removal of petroclival meningiomas: A report of 33 patients. Neurosurgery 31:813–828, 1992.
11. Cantore GP, Ciappetta P, Delfini R: Choice of neurosurgical approach in the treatment of cranial base lesions. Neurosurg Rev 17:109–125, 1994.
12. Crockard HA, Sen CN: The transoral approach for the management of intradural lesions at the craniovertebral junction: Review of 7 cases. Neurosurgery 28:88–98, 1991.
13. Derome PJ, Guiot G: Surgical approaches to the sphenoidal and clival area. In Krayenbuhl H (ed): Advances and Technical Standards in Neurosurgery, Vol 6. New York: Springer-Verlag, 1979, pp 101–136.
14. Fisch U, Kumar A: Infratemporal surgery of the skull base. In Rand RW (ed): Microneurosurgery, 3rd ed. St. Louis: CV Mosby, 1985, pp 421–454.
15. George B, Dematons C, Copignon J: Lateral approach to the anterior portion of the foramen magnum: Application to surgical removal of 14 benign tumors: Technical note. Surg Neurol 29:484–490, 1988.
16. Hardy J: L'abord transsphenoidal des tumeurs du clivus. Neurochirurgie 23:287–297, 1977.
17. Hakuba A, Liu S, Nishimura S: The orbitozygomatic infratemporal approach: A new surgical technique. Surg Neurol 26:271–176, 1986.
18. Hakuba A, Nishimura S, Jang BJ: A combined retroauricular and preauricular transpetrosal-transtentorial approach to clivus meningiomas. Surg Neurol 30:108–116, 1988.
19. Kawase T, Shiobara R, Toya S: Anterior transpetrosal-transtentorial approach for sphenopetroclival meningiomas: Surgical method and results in 10 patients. Neurosurgery 28:869–876, 1991.

20. Malis LI: Surgical resection of tumors of the skull base. In Wilkins RH, Rengashary SS (eds): Neurosurgery, Vol 1. New York: McGraw Hill, 1985, pp 1011–1021.

21. Malis L: The petrosal approach. Clin Neurosurg 37:528–540, 1990.

22. Samii M, Ammirati M: The combined supratentorial presigmoid sinus avenue to the petroclival region: Surgical technique and clinical applications. Acta Neurochir (Wien) 95:6–12, 1988.

23. Samii M, Ammirati M, Maharan A, et al: Surgery of petroclival meningiomas: Report of 24 cases. Neurosurgery 24:12–17, 1989.

24. Sekhar LN, Jannetta PJ, Burkhart LE, et al: Meningiomas involving the clivus: A six year experience with 41 patients. Neurosurgery 27:764–781, 1990.

25. Sekhar LN, Sen CN, Snyderman CH, et al: Anterior, anterolateral and lateral approaches to extradural petroclival tumors. In Sekhar LN, Janecka IP (eds): Surgery of Cranial Base Tumors. New York: Raven Press, 1993, pp 157–223.

26. Sen CN, Sekhar LN: An extreme lateral approach to intradural lesions of the cervical spine and foramen magnum. Neurosurgery 27:197–204, 1990.

27. Spetzler RF, Daspit CP, Pappas CTE: The combined supra and infratentorial approach for lesions of the petrous and clival regions: Experience with 46 cases. J Neurosurg 76:588–599, 1992.

28. Symon L: Surgical approaches to the tentorial hiatus. Advances and Technical Standards in Neurosurgery 9:69–112, 1982.

29. Maira G, Anile C, Vignati A, et al: Advances in treatment of supratentorial meningiomas of the skull base by microsurgical and laser techniques. In Samii M (ed): Skull Base Surgery. Basel: Karger, 1994, pp 190–193.

30. Lang J: Skull Base and Related Structures: Atlas of Clinical Anatomy. New York: Schattauer, 1995.

31. Harsh GR, Sekhar LN: The subtemporal, transcavernous, anterior transpetrosal approach to the upper brain stem and clivus. J Neurosurg 77:709–717, 1992.

32. Day JD, Koos WT, Matula C, et al: Color Atlas of Microneurosurgical Approaches. New York: Thieme, 1997.

33. Sekhar LN, Goel A: Intradural clival lesion. In Apuzzo MLJ (ed): Brain Surgery: Complication Avoidance and Management. New York: Churchill Livingstone, 1993, pp 2245–2264.

34. Saeger W, Ludecke DK, Muller S, et al: Chordome des clivus: Histologie, Ultrastruktur und Klinik. Tumor Diagnostik Therapie 4:74–79, 1983.

35. Goel A, Kobayashi S: Chordomas: A clinical review. In Kobayashi S, Goel A, Hongo K (eds): Neurosurgery of Complex Tumors and Vascular Lesions. New York: Churchill Livingstone, 1997, pp 293–306.

36. Chambers PW, Schwinn CP: A clinicopathologic study of metastasis. Am J Clin Pathol 72:765–776, 1979.

37. Crumley RL, Gutin PH: Surgical access for clivus chordoma: The University of California, San Francisco, experience. Arch Otolaryngol Head Neck Surg 115:295–300, 1989.

38. Maira G, Pallini R, Anile C, et al: Surgical treatment of clival chordomas: The transsphenoidal approach revisited. J Neurosurg 85:784–792, 1996.

39. Al-Mefty O, Fox JL, Rifai A, et al: A combined infratemporal and posterior fossa approach for the removal of giant glomus tumors and chondrosarcomas. Surg Neurol 28:423–431, 1987.

40. Canalis RF, Black K, Martin N, et al: Extended retrolabyrinthine transtentorial approach to petroclival lesions. Laryngoscope 101:6–13, 1991.

41. Gay E, Sekhar LN, Rubinstein E, et al: Chordomas and chondrosarcomas of the cranial base: results and follow-up of 60 patients. Neurosurgery 36:887–897, 1995.

42. Goel A: Extended middle fossa approach for petroclival lesions. Acta Neurochir (Wien) 135:78–83, 1995.

43. Sen CN, Sekhar LN, Schramm VL, et al: Chordoma and chondrosarcoma of the cranial base: an 8-year experience. Neurosurgery 25:931–941, 1989.

44. Lalwani AK, Kaplan MJ, Gutin PH: The transsphenoethmoid approach to the sphenoid sinus and clivus. Neurosurgery 31:1008–1014, 1992.

45. Laws ER Jr: Transsphenoidal surgery for tumors of the clivus. Otolaryngol Head Neck Surg 92:100–101, 1984.

46. Laws ER Jr: Clivus chordomas. In Sekhar LN, Janecka IP (eds): Surgery of Cranial Base Tumors. New York: Raven Press, 1993, pp 679–685.

47. Raffel C, Wright DC, Gutin PH, et al: Cranial chordomas: Clinical presentation and results of operative and radiation therapy in twenty-six patients. Neurosurgery 17:703–710, 1985.

48. Rougerie J, Guiot G, Bouche J, et al: Les voies d'abord du chordome du clivus. Neurochirurgie 13:559–570, 1967.

49. Harris JP, Godin MS, Krekorian TD, et al: The transoropalatal approach to the atlantoaxial-clival region: Considerations for the head and neck surgeon. Laryngoscope 99:467–474, 1989.

50. Menezes AH, VanGilder JC: Transoral-transpharyngeal approach to the anterior craniocervical junction: Ten-year experience with 72 patients. J Neurosurg 69:895–903, 1988.

51. Price JC: The midfacial degloving approach to the central skull base. Ear Nose Throat J 65:174–180, 1986.

52. Sekhar LN, Nanda A, Sen CN, et al: The extended frontal approach to tumors of the anterior, middle, and posterior skull base. J Neurosurg 76:198–206, 1992.

53. Rabadan A, Conesa H: Transmaxillary-transnasal approach to the anterior clivus: A microsurgical anatomical model. Neurosurgery 30:473–481, 1992.

54. Janecka IP, Sen CN, Sekhar LN, et al: Facial translocation: A new approach to the cranial base. Otolaryngol Head Neck Surg 103:413–419, 1990.

55. James D, Crockard HA: Surgical access to the base of the skull and upper cervical spine by exterior maxillotomy. Neurosurgery 29:411–416, 1991.

56. Anand VK, Harkey HL, Al-Mefty O: Open-door maxillotomy approach for lesions of the clivus. Skull Base Surg 1:217–225, 1991.

57. Stevenson GC, Stoney RJ, Perkins RK, et al: A transcervical transclival approach to the ventral surface of the brain stem for removal of a clivus chordoma. J Neurosurg 24:544–551, 1996.

58. George B, Lot G, Velut S, et al: Pathologie tumoral du foramen magnum. Neurochirurgie 39 (Suppl 1):1–89, 1993.

59. Sasaki CT, Lowlicht RA, Astrachan DI, et al: Le Fort I osteotomy approach for skull base tumors. Laryngoscope 100:1073–1076, 1990.

60. Bowles AP, Al-Mefty O: The transmaxillary approach to clival chordomas. In Al-Mefty O, Origitano TC, Harkey HL (eds): Controversies in Neurosurgery. New York: Thieme, 1996, pp 115–121.

61. Joseph M: Pedicled rhinotomy for exposure of the clivus. In Schmidek HH, Sweet WH (eds): Operative Neurosurgical Techniques. Philadelphia: WB Saunders, 1995, pp 469–475.

62. Swearingen B, Joseph M, Cheney M, et al: A modified transfacial approach to the clivus. Neurosurgery 36:101–105, 1995.

63. Hardy J: Transsphenoidal microsurgery of the normal and pathological pituitary. Clin Neurosurg 16:185–217, 1969.

64. Hardy J: Transsphenoidal microsurgery of prolactinomas: Report on 355 cases. In Tolis G, Stefanis C, Mountokalakis T, et al (eds): Prolactin and Prolactinomas. New York: Raven Press, 1983, pp 431–440.

65. Maira G, Anile C, De Marinis L, et al: Prolactin-secreting adenomas: Surgical results and long-term follow-up. Neurosurgery 24:736–743, 1989.

66. Maira G, Anile C, Rossi GF, et al: Surgical treatment of craniopharyngiomas: An evaluation of the transsphenoidal and pterional approaches. Neurosurgery 36:715–724, 1995.

67. Miller E, Crockard HA: Transoral transclival removal of anteriorly placed meningiomas at the foramen magnum. Neurosurgery 20:966–968, 1987.

68. Mullan S, Naunton R, Hekmat-panach J, et al: The use of an anterior approach to ventrally placed tumours in the foramen magnum and vertebral column. J Neurosurg 24:536–543, 1966.

69. Delgado TE, Garrido E, Harwick R: Labiomandibular, transoral approach to chordomas in the clivus and upper spine. Neurosurgery 8:675–679, 1981.

70. Gutkelch AN, Williams RG: Anterior approach to recurrent chordomas of the clivus. Neurosurgery 36:670–672, 1972.

71. Krayenbuhl H, Yasargil MG: Chondromas. Progr Neurol Surg 6:435–463, 1975.

72. Derome P, Visot A, Monteil JP, et al: Management of cranial chordomas. In Sekhar LN, Schramm VL (eds): Tumors of the Cranial Base. Mount Kisco: Futura, 1987, pp 607–622.

73. Perneczky A: The posterolateral approach to the foramen magnum. In Samii (ed): Surgery In and Around the Brain Stem and Third Ventricle. New York: Springer-Verlag, 1986, pp 460–466.

74. Spetzler RF, Graham TW: The far lateral approach to the inferior

clivus and upper cervical region: Technical note. BNI Q 6:35–38, 1990.

75. Heffelfinger MJ, Dahlin DC, MacCarty CS, et al: Chordomas and cartilaginous tumors at the skull base. Cancer 32:410–420, 1973.

76. Kondziolka D, Lunsford LD, Flickinger JC: The role of radiosurgery in the management of chordoma and chondrosarcoma of the cranial base. Neurosurgery 29:38–46, 1991.

77. Samii M: Comments. In Gay E, Sekhar LN, Rubinstein E, et al: Chordomas and chondrosarcomas of the cranial base: Results and follow-up of 60 cases. Neurosurgery 36:896–897, 1995.

78. Suit HD, Goitein M, Munzenrider J, et al: Definitive radiation therapy for chordoma and chondrosarcoma of base of skull and cervical spine. J Neurosurg 56:377–385, 1982.

79. Keisch ME, Garcia DM, Shibuya RB: Retrospective long-term follow-up analysis in 21 patients with chordoma of various sites treated at a single institution. J Neurosurg 75:374–377, 1991.

80. Austin-Seymour M, Muzenrider J, Goitein M, Verhey L, et al: Fractionated proton radiation therapy of chordoma and low-grade chondrosarcoma of the base of the skull. J Neurosurg 70:13–17, 1989.

81. Goel A, Nitta J, Kobayashi S: Surgical approaches to clival lesions. In Kobayashi S, Goel A, Hongo K (eds): Neurosurgery of Complex Tumors and Vascular Lesions. New York: Churchill Livingstone, 1997, pp 181–210.

82. Al-Mefty O: Operative Atlas of Meningiomas. Philadelphia: Lippincott Raven, 1998.

83. Long DM: Surgical approaches to tumors of skull base: An overview. In Wilkins RH, Rengachary SS (eds): Neurosurgery Update. I: Diagnosis, Operative Technique and Neuro-oncology. New York: McGraw-Hill, 1990, pp 266–276.

84. Sekhar LN, Javed T, Jannetta PJ. Petroclival meningiomas. In Sekhar LN, Janecka IP (eds): Surgery of Cranial Base Tumors. New York: Raven Press, 1993, pp 605–659.

85. Luyendijk W: Operative approaches to the posterior fossa. In Krayenbuhl H (ed): Advances and Technical Standards in Neurosurgery, Vol 3. New York: Springer-Verlag, 1976, pp 81–101.

86. Mayberg MR, Symon L: Meningiomas of the clivus and apical petrous bone: Report of 35 cases. J Neurosurg 65:160–167, 1986.

87. Samii M, Draf W: Surgery of the skull base. Berlin: Springer-Verlag, 1989.

88. Cantore GP, Delfini R, Ciappetta P: Surgical treatment of petroclival meningiomas: Experience with 16 cases. Surg Neurol 42:105–111, 1994.

89. King TT: Combined translabyrinthine-transtentorial approach to acoustic nerve tumors. Proc R Soc Med 63:780–782, 1970.

90. Kawase T, Toya S, Shiobara R, et al: Transpetrosal approach for aneurysms of the lower basilar artery. J Neurosurg 63:857–861, 1985.

91. Al-Mefty O: Surgery of the Cranial Base. Boston: Kluver, 1988.

92. Sen CN, Sekhar LN: The subtemporal and preauricular infratemporal approach to intradural structures ventral to the brain stem. J Neurosurg 73:345–354, 1990.

93. Sekhar LN, Pomeranz S, Janecka IP, et al: Temporal bone neoplasms: A report on 20 surgically treated cases. J Neurosurg 76:578–587, 1992.

94. Taniguchi M, Perneczky A: Subtemporal keyhole approach to the suprasellar and petroclival region: Microanatomic considerations and clinical applications. Neurosurgery 41:592–601, 1997.

95. Miller CG, van Loveren HR, Keller JT, et al: Transpetrosal approach: Surgical anatomy and technique. Neurosurgery 33:461–469, 1993.

96. Pellerin P, Lesoin F, Dhellemmes P, et al: Usefulness of the orbito-frontomalar approach associated with bone reconstruction for fronto-temporosphenoid meningiomas. Neurosurgery 15:715–718, 1984.

97. Zabramski JM, Kiris T, Sankhla SK, et al: Orbitozygomatic craniotomy: Technical note. J Neurosurg 89:336–341, 1998.

98. Hakuba A, Nishimura A, Tanaka K, et al: Clivus meningiomas: Six cases of total removal. Neurol Med Chir (Tokyo) 17:63–77, 1977.

99. Hirsch BE, Cass SP, Sekhar LN, et al: Translabyrinthine approach to skull base tumors with hearing preservation. Am J Otol 14:533–543, 1993.

100. House WF, Hitselberger WE: The transcochlear approach to the skull base. Arch Otolaryngol 102:334, 1976.

101. Lang J Jr, Samii M: Retrosigmoidal approach to the posterior cranial fossa: An anatomical study. Acta Neurochir (Wien) 111:147–153, 1991.

102. Baldwin HZ, Miller CG, van Loveren HR, et al: The far lateral-combined supra- and infratentorial approach: A human cadaveric prosection model for routes of access to the petroclival region and ventral brain stem. J Neurosurg 81:60–68, 1994.

103. Baldwin HZ, Spetzler RF, Wascher TM, et al: The far lateral-combined supra- and infratentorial approach: Clinical experience. Acta Neurochir (Wien) 134:155–158, 1995.

104. Linskey ME, Sekhar LN, Sen C: Cerebral revascularization in cranial base surgery. In Sekhar LN, Janecka IP (eds): Surgery of Cranial Base Tumors. New York: Raven Press, 1993, pp 45–68.

# Petroclival Meningiomas

■ ALBINO BRICOLO and SERGIO TURAZZI

Of the meningeal tumors of the basal posterior cranial fossa, petroclival meningiomas offer the greatest technical challenge to the neurosurgeon. Because of their rarity, their critical location in the center of the posterior skull base, and their proximity to the brain stem, cranial nerves III to XII, and arteries of the posterior circulation, the petroclival remains the most formidable of all meningiomas.[1-17]

Petroclival meningiomas arise in the area of the spheno-occipital synchondrosis, and in addition to the clivus and petrous apex, these tumors may involve the medial tentorium, Meckel's cave, the middle cranial fossa, the parasellar area, the petrosal and cavernous sinuses, and the transmission foramens of cranial nerves III to XII. Such tumors, often wedged in the brain stem, may encase cranial nerves and basilar and carotid arteries and their roots, perforate the dura, and invade the underlying bone.

Much was written in the 1990s about these tumors, particularly by skull base surgeons who have developed numerous complex approaches such that there is no aspect of the cranial base and underlying brain that may not be exposed if required by the circumstance.[18] Unfortunately, these advances in "access surgery" have not obtained the results anticipated by initial enthusiasts, and thus the intimidating reputation of these lesions has been reduced but not eliminated.

Advances in neuroimaging, microsurgery, and approaches to the skull base have provided better preoperative definition of these tumors while making their removal easier and less conducive to iatrogenic damage. Developments and improvements of microsurgical techniques, tools, and associated skull base approaches have also enabled total resection of these tumors with modest rates of morbidity and, specifically, mortality, because until the time of Olivercrona mortality was at an unacceptable level based on the general acceptance that tumors of the clivus were inoperable. Surgical morbidity remains consistent in all contemporary published series, although in clinical reality, at least in the authors' experience, a number of patients operated on for this lesion are not satisfied with the outcome and the surgeon's performance.

These slow-growing tumors tend to produce worrisome symptoms only after reaching considerable size and extension. Two aspects of petroclival meningiomas continue to plague the neurosurgeon: (1) the tumor is histologically benign and causes relatively mild neurologic impairment with which the patient can learn to live; and (2) major surgery is required for removal, with some risk that the patient will be neurologically worse after surgery (Fig. 67–1).

In this chapter, the surgical management of petroclival meningiomas is discussed based on the authors' experience. Current and relevant literature is also reviewed.

## PATHOLOGIC ANATOMY AND CLASSIFICATION

Petroclival meningiomas are considered rare tumors, accounting for approximately 3% to 10% of all posterior fossa meningiomas. However, the actual incidence of these lesions is difficult to establish because they are difficult tumors and are typically treated only by a few leading neurosurgical centers specializing in skull base surgery. In addition, incidence data are unreliable because of the lack of precise definition. Thus it is opportune first to discuss the criteria used to define petroclival meningiomas among the broad group of posterior skull base meningiomas, emphasizing that until a general consensus is established regarding this crucial problem, published series' will continue to remain poorly comparable.

Since the historical contribution of Cushing and Eisenhardt in 1938,[19] meningiomas have been classically grouped according to the dural site at origin, and with this broad grouping, some petroclival meningiomas were perhaps included in the gasseropetrosal group. With regard to posterior fossa meningiomas, the landmark classification adopted for many years was proposed in 1953 by Castellano and Ruggiero[20] based on Olivercrona's material. This classification, which was rigorously based on the site of dural attachment, also benefited from the often readily available postmortem material. In this classification, posterior fossa meningiomas were categorized as: (1) cerebellar convexity, (2) tentorium, (3) posterior surface of the petrosal bone, (4) clival, and (5) foramen magnum.

The advent of modern diagnostic imaging techniques and the introduction of surgical microscopes enabled surgeons to operate on numerous meningiomas as well as identify other criteria for subgrouping. As a consequence, in 1980, Yasargil and colleagues[17] proposed a new classification of posterior base meningiomas based on their extensive surgical experience: (1) clival, (2) petroclival, (3)

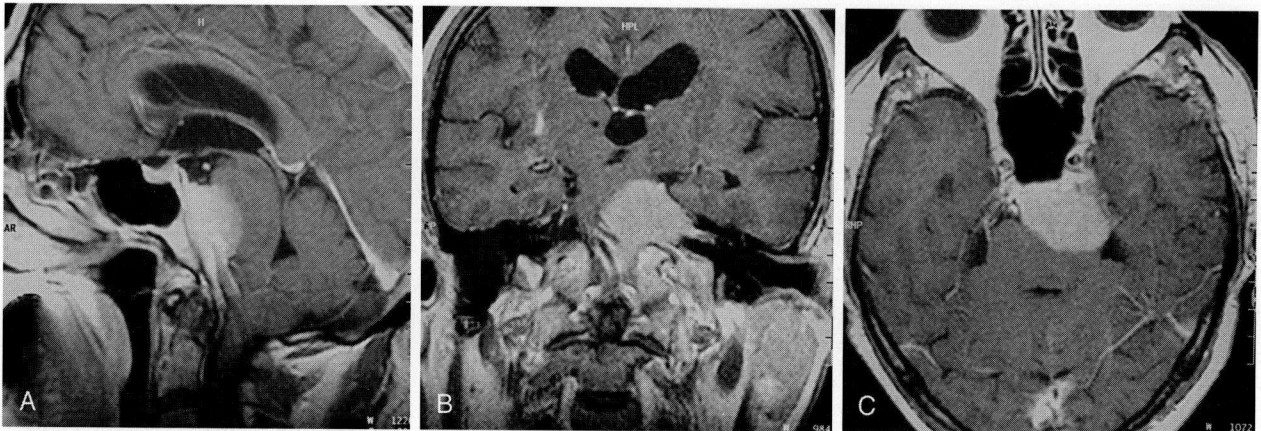

**FIGURE 67–1** ■ Sagittal *(A)*, coronal *(B)*, and axial *(C)* postcontrast $T_1$-weighted magnetic resonance imaging scan demonstrating a medium-sized petroclival meningioma with extensive adhesion to the clivus and involving the basilar artery. The patient complained only of transient diplopia and facial numbness. This case is typical not only for the characteristics of the tumor but also for the management decision. The encasement of the abducens, the trigeminal nerve, and the basilar artery are most likely; thus, surgery should be carefully evaluated.

sphenopetroclival, (4) foramen magnum, and (5) cerebello-pontine angle (CPA). This new classification was fundamental because Yasargil and colleagues were the first to deny the existence of a pure midline clivus meningioma, and they introduced the term *petroclival*, adding that "our impression is that these tumors arise along the petro-clival line . . . (lateral clivus)." These authors, capturing the difficulties inherent in precisely grouping meningiomas of the basal posterior fossa, pointed out that the separation of basal meningiomas into precise topographic areas is artificial because there are always transitional cases.

Today, however, there is still a problem with the so-called "petroclivals," a term that became relatively popular in the 1990s. The boundaries of this group of tumors lack precise definition, and as a result many authors prefer to describe such tumors as "meningiomas involving the clivus." Couldwell and associates[6] define "petroclivals" as those meningiomas with basal attachment at or medial to the skull base foramens of cranial nerves V through IX, X, and XI. Al-Mefty and Smith[3] emphasized that only those meningiomas arising medial to the trigeminal nerve should

be included in the petroclival group to differentiate them from those arising more laterally; the latter may be included in the broad family of CPA meningiomas, which are easily removed.

Identification of the origin of the dural attachment is not always possible on magnetic resonance imaging (MRI) or even during surgery, although it has been demonstrated that the difficulty of surgical removal increases with a progressively deeper and more centrally situated tumor origin. Reasons for this include: (1) the more medial the tumor, the greater the conflict with the brain stem; (2) more cranial nerves are involved; and (3) there is a closer relationship with the basilar artery and its branches. These factors also determine the degree of surgical difficulty and the approach; thus, issues of naming and classification cannot be regarded as merely a semantic dispute.

The authors' working hypothesis is that meningiomas at the posterior cranial base must be grouped not only according to the dural attachment, but with respect to the manner in which the cranial nerves are displaced by the tumor. Because the cranial nerves have a constant entry

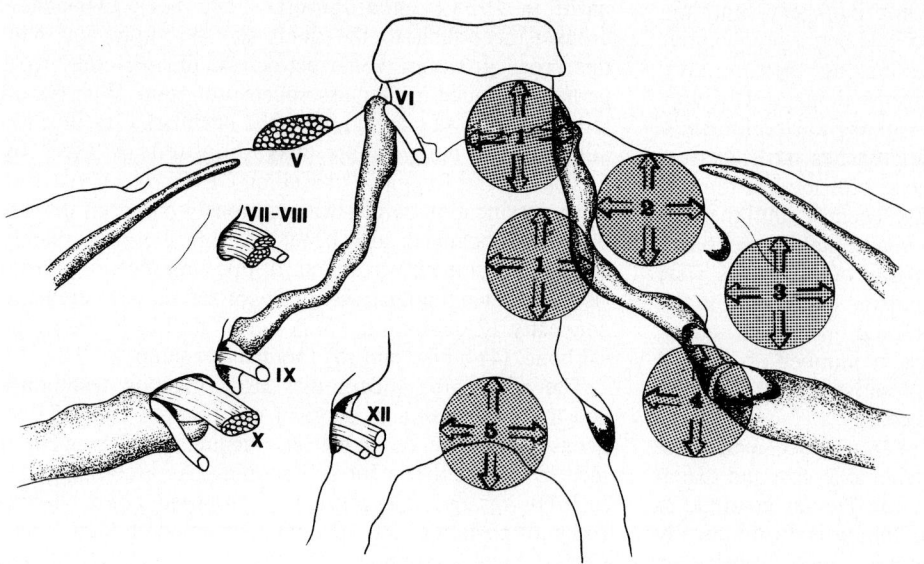

**FIGURE 67–2** ■ The site of the dural origin of the five groups of posterior skull base meningiomas: petroclival (1), anterior petrous (2), posterior petrous (3), jugular foramen (4), and foramen magnum (5).

**TABLE 67–1 ■ POSITION OF THE CRANIAL NERVES IN POSTERIOR SKULL BASE MENINGIOMAS**

| Meningioma | Cranial Nerves | | | | | | |
|---|---|---|---|---|---|---|---|
| | *III* | *IV* | *V* | *VI* | *VII, VIII* | *IX, X, XI* | *XII* |
| Petroclival | Superior Medial | Superior Lateral | Posterior Superior | Medial Anterior | Posterior | Inferior Posterior | Inferior |
| Anterior petrous | Medial Superior | Superior Medial | Anterior Medial | Medial Anterior | Posterior Inferior | Inferior | — |
| Posterior petrous | — | — | Anterior | Anterior | Anterior | Anterior Inferior | — |
| Jugular foramen | — | — | — | Medial | Superior | Posterior Lateral | Inferior |
| Foramen magnum | — | — | — | Posterior | Superior Posterior | Posterior Superior | Posterior |

and exit zone at the brain stem and the basal foramens, they are the most reliable "witnesses" of the growth pattern of the meningioma.

The authors have reconstructed the pathologic microsurgical anatomy of the last 150 posterior basal meningiomas they operated on by reviewing neuroimaging and intraoperative data. In the small area comprising the clivus and the petrous pyramid, crowded by cranial nerves and arteries, five homogeneous subgroups of meningiomas, differing in topography as well as in displacement or encasement of neurovascular structures, may be identified: (1) petroclival, (2) anterior petrous, (3) posterior petrous, (4) jugular foramen, and (5) foramen magnum meningiomas (Fig. 67–2). The cranial nerves and arteries have a relatively constant relationship to each of these subgroups of meningiomas, as shown in Tables 67–1 and 67–2.

When the tumor is exposed through the classic suboccipital retrosigmoid approach with the patient in a semisitting position, the relationship of the tumor to the cranial nerves gives an immediate understanding of the site of dural origin, and consequently the related difficulties in its removal (Fig. 67–3). The position of cranial nerves VII and VIII is a fundamental landmark for dividing these meningiomas into two main groups: those originating anterior to the acoustic meatus, which displace the cranial nerves VII and VIII complex posteriorly; and those growing from the dura posterior to the meatus, which displace cranial nerves VII and VIII anteriorly.

Both the petroclival and the anterior petrous displace cranial nerves VII and VIII posteriorly, and the lower cranial nerves posteriorly and inferiorly. What differentiates the two groups is the position of the trigeminal nerve: in petroclival meningiomas, its position is posterior-superior, whereas in the anterior petrous group, it is anterior-superior. In addition, simple visual examination of cranial nerve V, if the nerve is visible over the posterior surface of the tumor, ensures that its dural origin is in the clival area. Thus, it is more than reasonable that the term *petroclival* meningioma be limited to this particular type of tumor—although some anterior petrous meningiomas may be included in this group because of their extensive dural insertion around the petroclival line and the trigeminal encasement (Figs. 67–4 and 67–5).

In contrast to acoustic neuromas, which displace adjacent nerves and vessels, posterior skull base meningiomas often engulf or encase arteries and cranial nerves encountered during their growth. This propensity to envelope functionally important neurovascular structures is the major cause of the significant morbidity commonly reported after surgical excision. Therefore, based on the surgical and pathologic anatomy, it is reasonable to group these tumors into five groups, which are homogeneous in more ways than one: (1) by their dural origin; (2) by their spatial relationship to adjacent nerves and arteries; and (3) by the frequency with which they encase specific cranial nerves and arteries (Tables 67–3 and 67–4).

The authors reclassified their previous 150 cases of posterior cranial base meningiomas according to the aforemen-

**TABLE 67–2 ■ POSITION OF THE ARTERIES IN POSTERIOR SKULL BASE MENINGIOMAS**

| Meningioma | Posterior Cerebral Artery | Superior Cerebellar Artery | Basilar Artery | AICA | PICA | Vertebral Artery |
|---|---|---|---|---|---|---|
| Petroclival | Superior Medial | Superior Medial | Posterior Medial | Posterior Medial | Posterior Inferior | Posterior Inferior |
| Anterior petrous | Superior Medial | Medial | Medial | Anterior Medial | Inferior Medial | Medial |
| Posterior petrous | — | — | Anterior Medial | Anterior | Anterior | Anterior Medial |
| Jugular foramen | — | — | Medial | Superior | Inferior | Medial Inferior |
| Foramen magnum | — | — | — | Superior | Posterior | Posterior Lateral |

AICA, anterior inferior cerebellar artery; PICA, posterior inferior cerebellar artery.

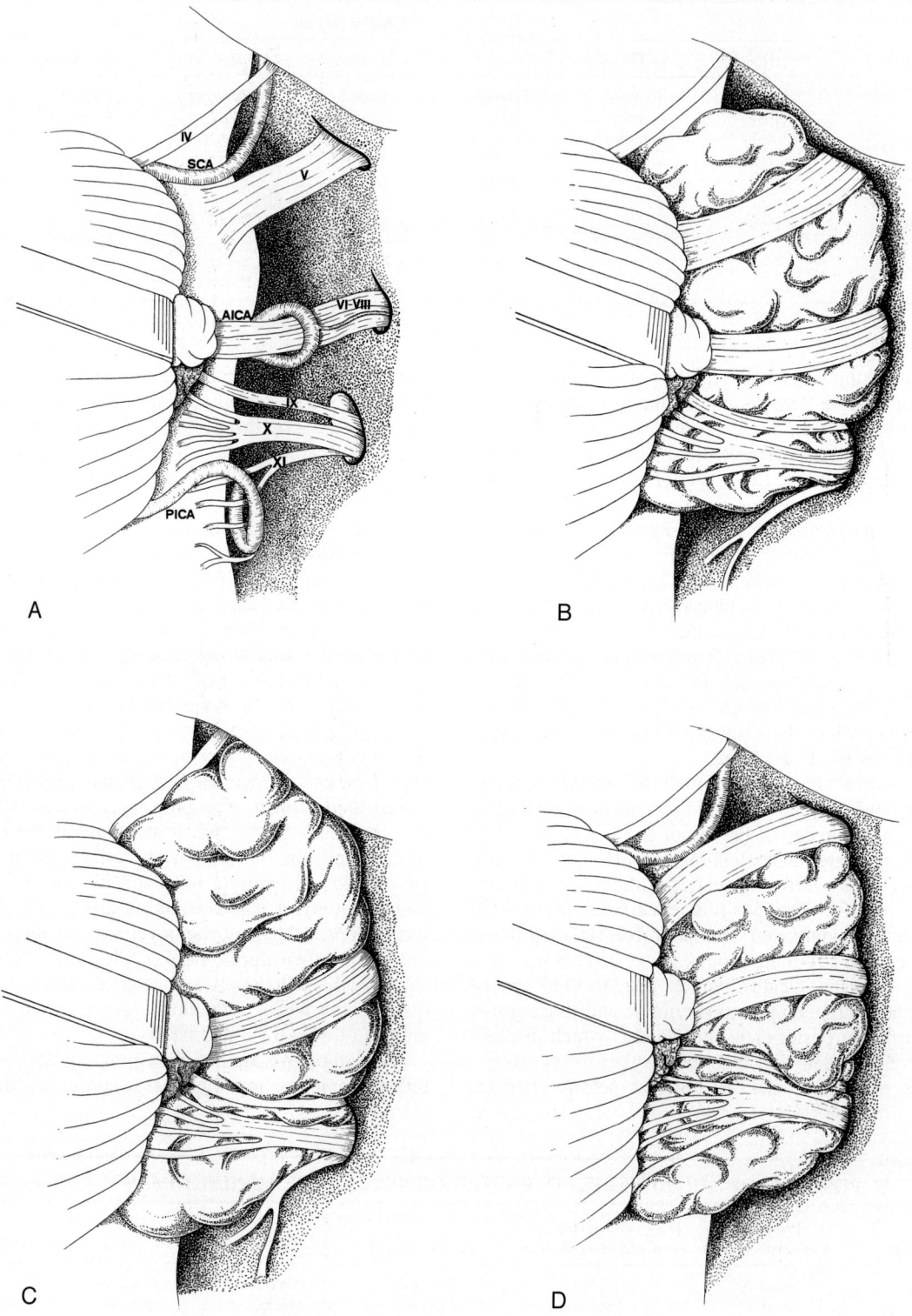

**FIGURE 67-3 ■** Schematic illustration of the cerebellopontine angle *(A)*. The cerebellum has been retracted to show (from top to bottom): the trochlear nerve (IV), the superior cerebellar artery (SCA), the trigeminal (V), facial and vestibulocochlear (VII-VIII) with the anteroinferior cerebellar artery (AICA), the glossopharyngeal (IX), vagus (X), and spinal accessory (XI) nerves with the posteroinferior cerebellar artery (PICA). Petroclival meningiomas *(B)* displace posteriorly the trigeminal, the VII and VIII and IX and X cranial nerves while in anteropetrous meningiomas *(C)*, the trigeminal nerve is displaced anteriorly and thus remains hidden by the tumor. The distinction between the two types of tumors is not always clear because the trigeminal nerve may assume an intermediate position *(D)* or may be encased by the tumor.

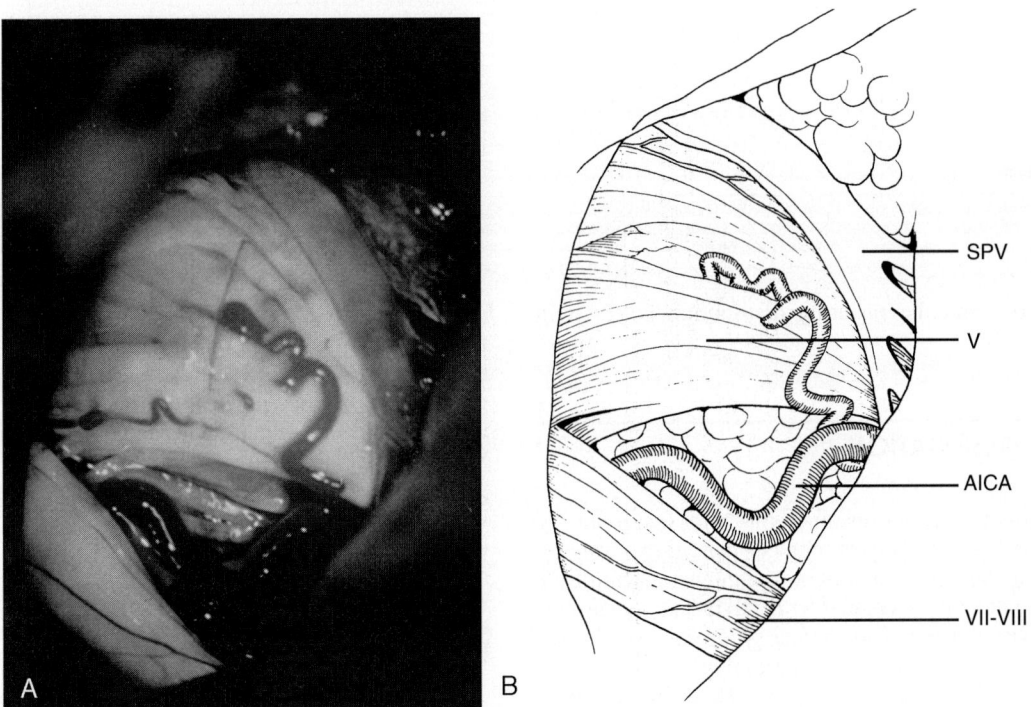

FIGURE 67–4 ■ *A* and *B,* Intraoperative microphotograph of a typical petroclival meningioma exposed using a left suboccipital lateral retrosigmoid approach with the patient in a semisitting position. The tumor originating from the clival area remains anterior to the trigeminal and faciovestibulocochlear nerves, which are shown to be stretched over the tumor.

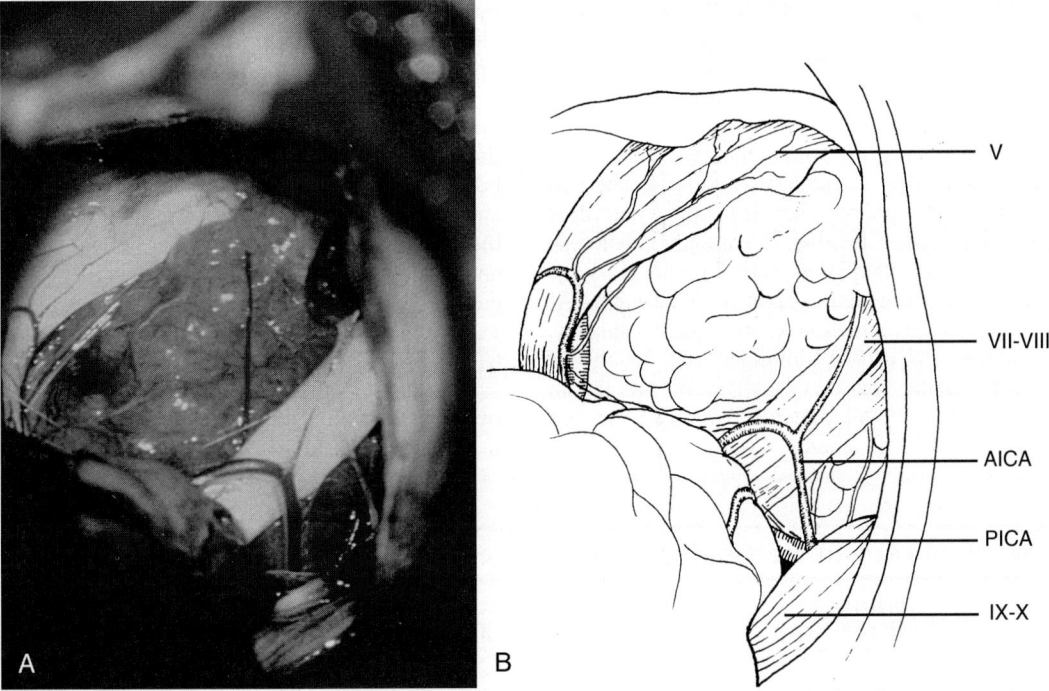

FIGURE 67–5 ■ *A* and *B,* Intraoperative microphotograph of a meningioma exposed using a right retrosigmoid approach. In this case, the trigeminal nerve is displaced upward and thus may still be considered as a petroclival meningioma.

**TABLE 67–3 ■ FREQUENCY OF CRANIAL NERVE ENCASEMENT IN POSTERIOR SKULL BASE MENINGIOMAS**

| Meningioma | Cranial Nerves | | | | | | |
|---|---|---|---|---|---|---|---|
| | *III* | *IV* | *V* | *VI* | *VII, VIII* | *IX, X, XI* | *XII* |
| Petroclival | + | + | + + | + + + | + + | + | — |
| Anterior petrous | — | + | + + + | + + | + + | — | — |
| Posterior petrous | — | — | — | — | + | — | — |
| Jugular foramen | — | — | — | — | + | + + + | + |
| Foramen magnum | — | — | — | — | — | + + | + + |

tioned criteria, and the resulting distribution is given in Table 67–5.

## CLINICAL PRESENTATION

Patients with petroclival meningiomas are first seen by neurosurgeons in a variety of clinical conditions, ranging from isolated trigeminal neuralgia or numbness to multiple cranial nerve deficits associated with ataxia and somatomotor and sensory deficits. The clinical syndrome is of insidious onset, often mimicking other pathologic processes; in elderly patients, the presenting symptoms are often attributed to vertebrobasilar insufficiency.

Headache, gait ataxia, facial dysesthesia, vertigo, and reduced hearing are the more frequent presenting symptoms, with the trigeminal nerve as the single structure most often involved from onset. Later symptoms (those appearing more recently and leading to diagnostic suspicion), in addition to gait ataxia, include double vision, swallowing difficulty, and somatomotor deficits of various types. Papilledema and changes in mental status are rare.

In the authors' first series of 33 petroclival meningiomas published in 1992,[4] the onset of symptoms usually occurred later on in the disease, varying from 7 months to 17 years (on average, 35 months for combined symptoms). The two most frequent early complaints were trigeminal neuralgia (43 months) and impaired hearing (35 months), whereas the two more common complaints nearer diagnosis were diplopia (4 months) and facial weakness (3 months). At the time of objective examination shortly before surgery, the clinical picture was usually dominated by deficits of the intermediate cranial nerves, which were present in various degrees in nearly all patients, with concomitant cerebellar signs in 60% of patients. Cranial nerve V was affected both earlier and more often (67% of patients), followed by cranial nerves IX, X, and XI (45%). The typical sign of a petroclival meningioma is a relatively fair preservation of hearing, in contrast to severe trigeminal involvement and impairment of the cranial nerves below VIII, with accompanying cerebellar signs. The preoperative performance status, as expressed by the Karnofsky scale, was higher than 70 in 23 patients (70%) and lower than 70 in 10 (30%).

## IMAGING EVALUATION

Computed tomography (CT), angiography, and MRI each play an important role in the preoperative evaluation of petroclival meningiomas, and none of these diagnostic methods has been able adequately to replace the other (Fig. 67–6). The general imaging characteristics of petroclival meningiomas do not differ from those of other meningiomas. Regarding skull base meningiomas and those of the clivus, it is particularly useful to apply or assemble all the information derived from the three investigative methods.

The most important information the surgeon needs to know before surgery includes the site and extension of dural attachment; tumor size, consistency, and vascularity; bone involvement; tumor–brain stem interface; the position and eventual encasement of the arteries; and extension of the tumor outside the proper petroclival area, particularly any involvement of the cavernous sinus. MRI, the latest entrant in the arsenal of diagnostic tools, is the single examination that answers many of these questions (Figs. 67–7 to 67–10).

The inability to define an arachnoid cleavage plane between extra-axial tumors and the brain stem is one of the most troubling situations confronting the surgeon, and is

**TABLE 67–4 ■ FREQUENCY OF ARTERIAL ENCASEMENT IN POSTERIOR SKULL BASE MENINGIOMAS**

| Meningioma | Posterior Cerebral Artery | Superior Cerebellar Artery | Basilar | AICA | PICA | Vertebral |
|---|---|---|---|---|---|---|
| Petroclival | + | + + + | + + + | + + + | + | + |
| Anterior petrous | + | + + | + + | + + | — | — |
| Posterior petrous | — | — | — | — | — | — |
| Jugular foramen | — | — | — | + | + + + | + |
| Foramen magnum | — | — | — | — | + + + | + + |

AICA, anterior inferior cerebellar artery; PICA, posterior inferior cerebellar artery.

TABLE 67–5 ■ **GROUPING THE POSTERIOR SKULL BASE MENINGIOMAS***

| Group | N (%) |
|---|---|
| Petroclival | 84 (56%) |
| Anterior petrous | 16 (11%) |
| Posterior petrous | 27 (18%) |
| Jugular foramen | 5 (3%) |
| Foramen magnum | 18 (12%) |

*In the authors' series of the last 150 posterior skull base meningiomas treated.

one of the primary reasons for abandoning a radical procedure, as well as being the major cause of postoperative complications.[13–15, 17, 21–23] Sekhar and colleagues[15] pointed out that some of these meningiomas have poor planes of dissection because of microvascular invasion of the brain stem pial layer. They concluded that this situation, which prohibits complete removal, may be predicted by the presence of brain stem edema on preoperative MRI, demonstrated by high signal intensity on $T_2$-weighted images, together with the lack of evidence of an arachnoid plane.

Sekhar and colleagues[15] also found a good correlation between radiologic and operative findings when signs of vascular encasement and tumoral blood supply from the basilar artery were seen in angiographic studies.

When MRI is not available, CT can be most useful; using high-resolution CT scanning, preoperative differentiation of petroclival meningiomas from other pathologic processes of the region is possible. CT scanning also permits the construction and display of three-dimensional images, which may allow better judgment of the relationship of the meningioma with the tentorium and other structures (Fig. 67–11).

Cerebral angiography is considered by many[24] to be mandatory for the preoperative work-up of tumors of this type, whereas some surgeons consider it necessary only for those cases with expected encasement of the basilar artery and its branches or direct vascularization of the tumor from the basilar artery.[4, 6, 15]

Angiography gives indirect evidence of the tumor mass in terms of dislocation of the basilar artery and its branches (posterior cerebral and superior, anterior, and posterior inferior cerebellar arteries); in addition, it reveals any "choking" of the basilar and carotid arteries by the tumor and provides some information about tumoral blood supply, although the extent of tumor vascularization is not always easy to determine. The tumors are supplied in various degrees by the meningohypophysial trunk of the internal carotid artery, the posterior branch of the middle meningeal artery, the meningeal branch of the vertebral artery, the clivus artery originating from the carotid siphon, the petrosal branches of the meningeal arteries, and the ascending pharyngeal branches of the external carotid artery. In 30% of patients in the authors' first series,[4] definite tumor staining was visible in the capillary and venous phases of angiography (Figs. 67–12 and 67–13).

## PATIENT SELECTION AND MANAGEMENT

Treatment strategies for difficult tumors such as the petroclival meningioma are complex issues because the patient may have a large tumor and minimal symptoms, the natural history is far from homogeneous, and total removal is difficult to achieve. Although the remarkable evolution of surgical techniques and facilities has led most authors to consider the results of this surgery acceptable, some express a more critical attitude.[6, 15, 23, 25–27] Although data on the natural history of unoperated patients are unavailable, follow-up in postoperative patients confirms progressive growth of the tumor at variable rates[11, 20]; it is well known, however, that some tumors may remain dormant for many years (Fig. 67–14).

As stated by Sekhar and colleagues,[14] "when and whether to operate a newly discovered tumor in patients with minimal symptoms can be a difficult decision." Important preoperative factors affecting patient outcomes include tumor size, degree of neurologic involvement, and patient age. Because tumor size is the most important factor affecting postoperative outcome in nonelderly, sympto-

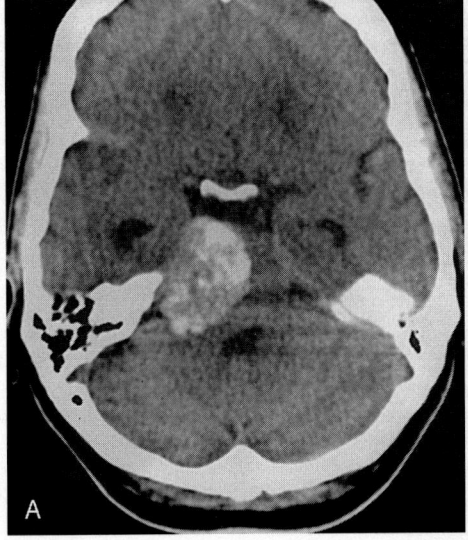
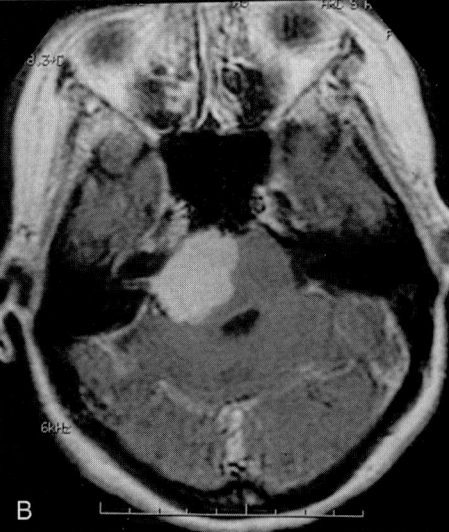

FIGURE 67–6 ■ A plain computed tomography scan *(A)* may show an extensive and dense calcification in a petroclival meningioma, which is not demonstrated by magnetic resonance imaging *(B)*.

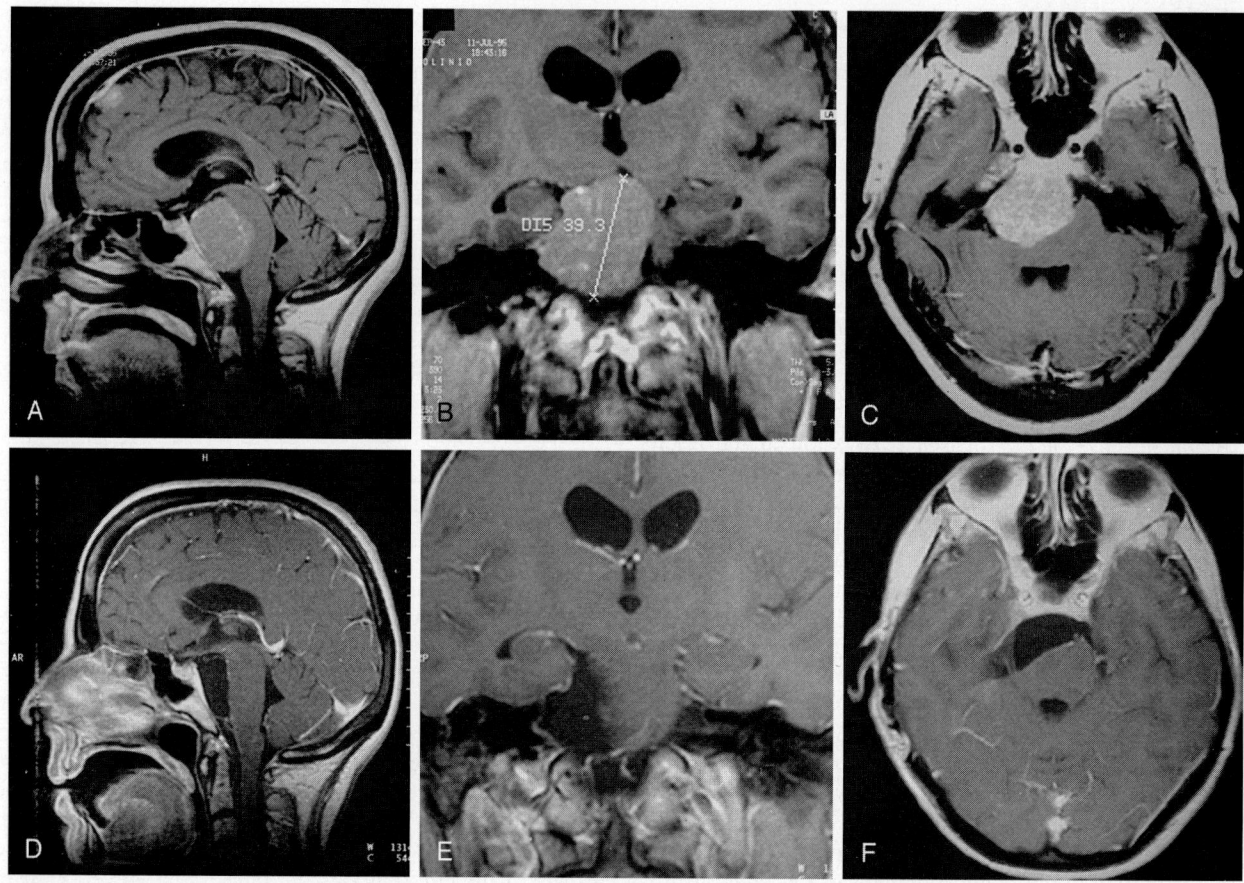

**FIGURE 67–7** ■ Preoperative sagittal *(A)*, coronal *(B)*, and axial *(C)* postcontrast T$_1$-weighted magnetic resonance imaging scan of a petroclival meningioma radically removed *(D–F)* through a lateral suboccipital retrosigmoid approach. The tumor–brain stem interface at surgery was well delineated by a good arachnoid plane. The patient, who was neurologically intact before surgery, remained asymptomatic after surgery.

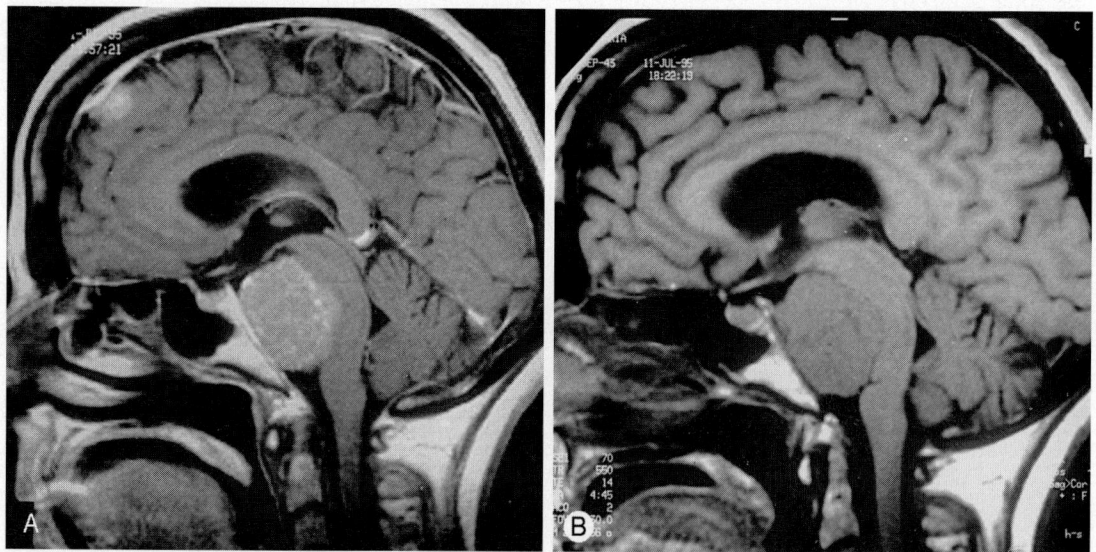

**FIGURE 67–8** ■ Sagittal contrast-enhanced *(A)* and plain *(B)* T$_1$-weighted magnetic resonance imaging (MRI) scans of the same patient as in Figure 67–7. Notice how contrast administration may sometimes hide the natural tumor–brain stem interface. The possibility that contrast-enhanced images may be misleading, suggesting brain stem edema or invasion, must be taken into consideration.

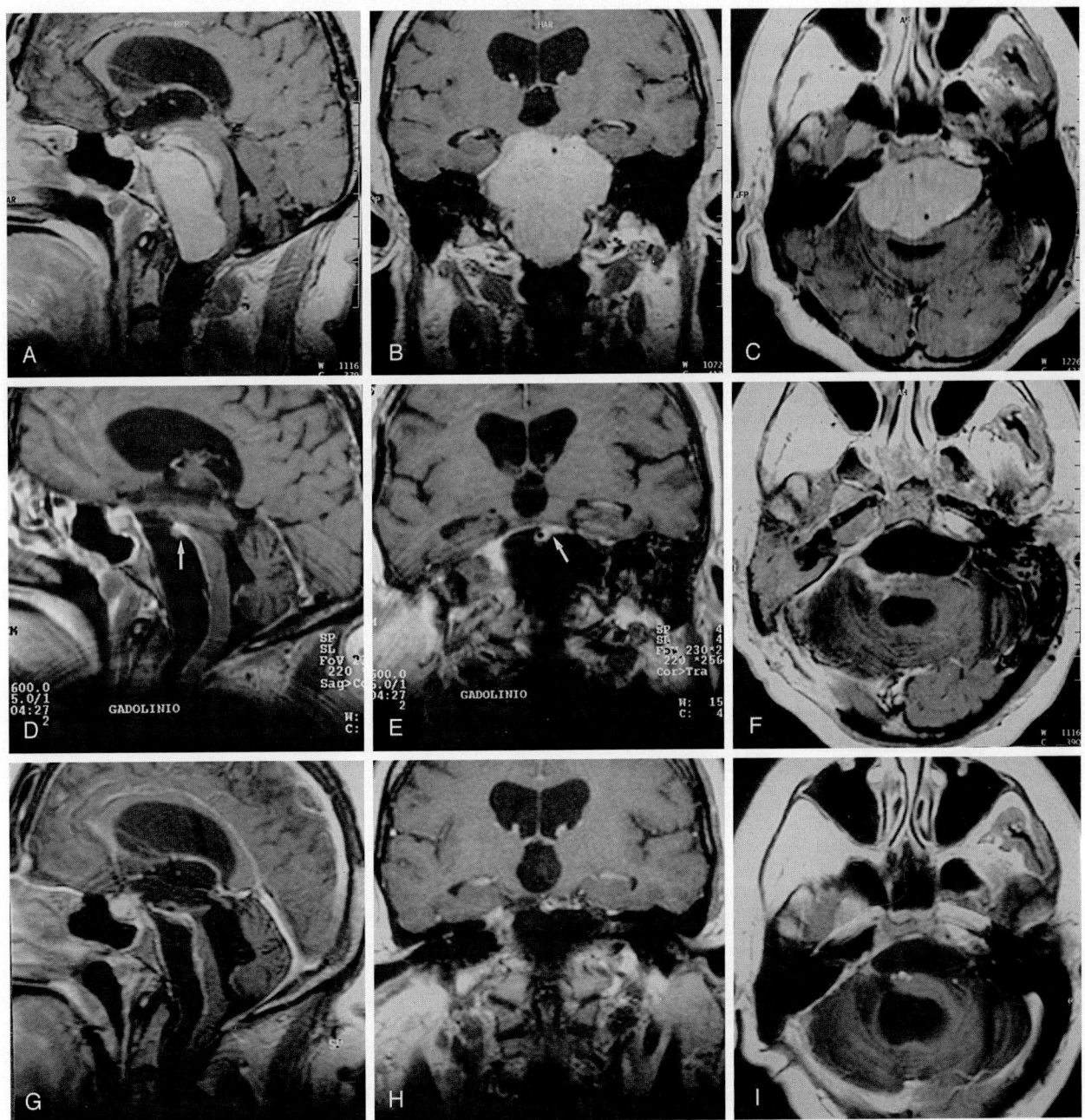

**FIGURE 67–9** ■ Preoperative sagittal *(A)*, coronal *(B)*, and axial *(C)* postcontrast T$_1$-weighted magnetic resonance imaging (MRI) scan of a giant panclival meningioma removed through a right suboccipital retrosigmoid dorsolateral approach. The signal voids represent the vertebral basilar arteries and its branches encased by the tumor, thus careful microdissection is required to avoid vessel injury. In this patient, the right vertebral artery, which was completely engulfed by the tumor, was dissected and freed while the top of the basilar artery and both anteroinferior cerebellar arteries (AICAs) were encased in a solid, calcified piece of tumor that was left in place. Comparable 4-week postoperative MRI scans *(E–G)* demonstrate removal of the tumor with a small remnant *(arrows)*. The patient, who was severely disabled before surgery, recovered well after a difficult perioperative course. Today, 4 years after surgery, the patient is almost self-sufficient and able to care for a large family. Notice the signs of brain stem atrophy on an MRI scan performed at a 4-year follow-up *(H–J)*, which contrast with the capability to perform daily functions.

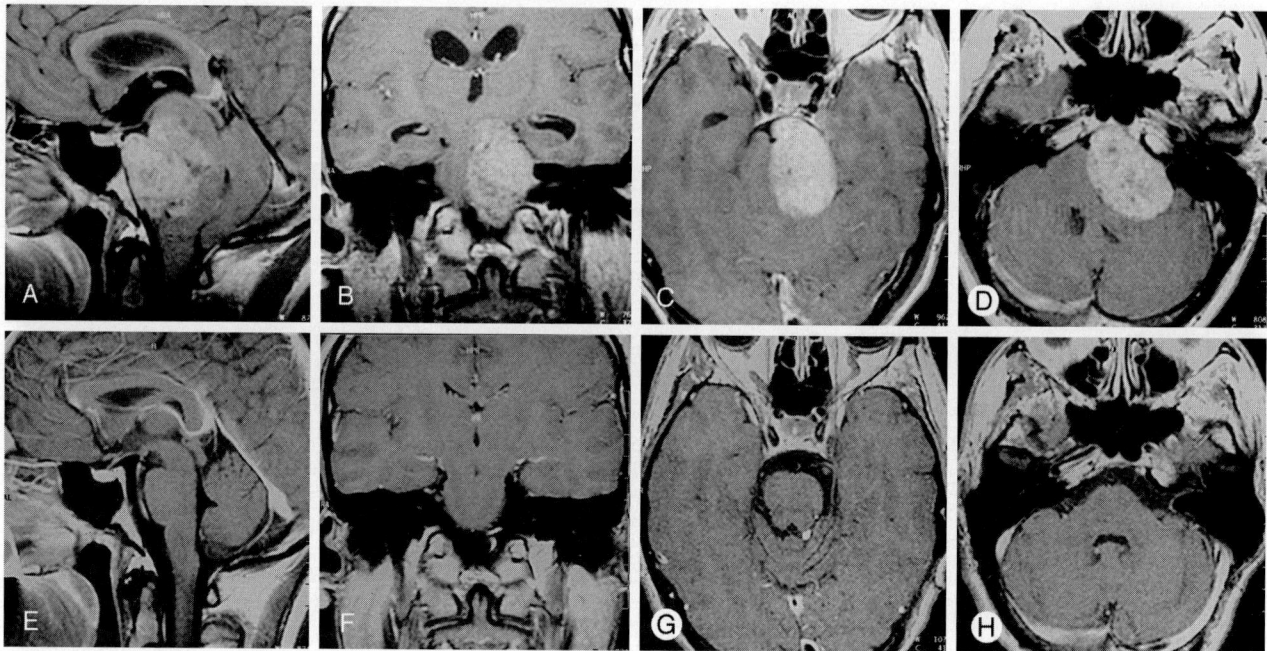

FIGURE 67–10 ■ Preoperative sagittal *(A)*, coronal *(B)*, and axials *(C and D)* postcontrast $T_1$-weighted magnetic resonance imaging scans of a petroclival meningioma that was totally *(E–H)* and easily removed through a lateral suboccipital retrosigmoid approach. The tumor's soft consistency and its weak adherence to the brain stem, cranial nerves, and arteries were favorable for radical removal with no morbidity.

matic patients with small or medium-sized tumors, surgery should be recommended even when symptoms are minimal. In this group of patients, total excision can be achieved with minimal morbidity and a low risk of moderate neurologic dysfunction. However, the surgeon should be cautious in considering the small tumor as "easy and without risk of morbidity" because these small tumors have not created a sufficient space to reach and remove them.

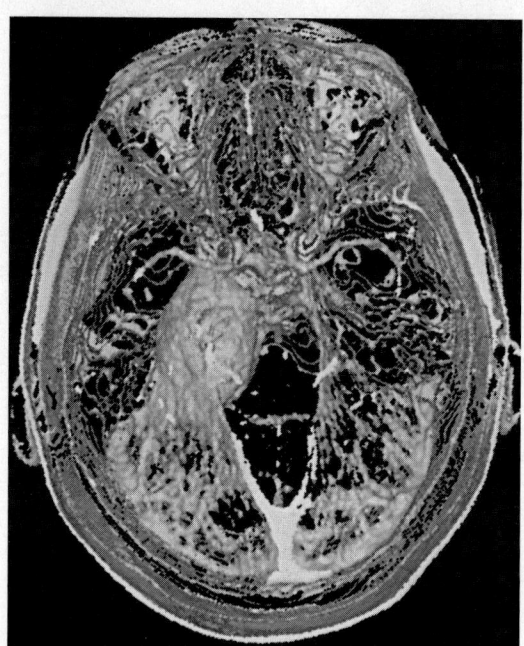

FIGURE 67–11 ■ A three-dimensional contrast-enhanced computed tomography reconstructed scan demonstrating the relationship of a petroclival meningioma with the tentorium, the clivus, and the basilar artery.

Patients with large, recurrent, or previously irradiated tumors have higher operative risks and the likelihood of worsened postoperative neurologic status, along with a reduced chance of obtaining total or satisfactory tumor removal.

Another issue in preoperative patient evaluation is the selection of approach based on tumor extension and site, and any neurologic dysfunction such as deafness.[16] Although objective criteria should be weighed and kept in mind, the operative choice is determined based on the surgeon's personal experience and preference.

The main issue in this difficult surgery is to determine at what point and at what price radical removal may be achieved. This problem, perhaps more of a management issue than of a technical nature, is also decided based on the surgeon's experience and personal philosophy.[28] Brain stem invasion by the tumor with an obscured arachnoid layer, vascular encasement (primarily the basilar artery and perforators), and cavernous sinus invasion are obstacles to radical removal that require intraoperative judgment and technique. When the tumor cannot be easily dissected, a subtotal removal is recommended with the residual monitored or treated by radiosurgery. Theoretical considerations and preoperative planning must be confronted by intraoperative practicability.

## SURGICAL MANAGEMENT

The removal of petroclival meningiomas continues to be regarded as a formidable challenge because the morbidity rates of published series remain high and mortality rates, although lower in the 1990s, are not zero. Furthermore, despite demanding and time-consuming surgery, radical

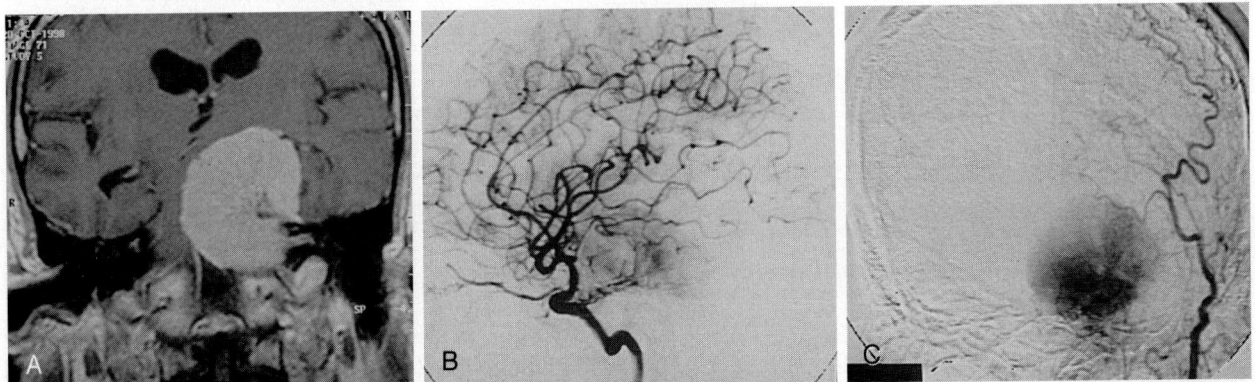

**FIGURE 67–12** ■ Coronal *(A)* T$_1$-weighted post-gadolinium magnetic resonance imaging scan showing a huge petroclival meningioma. Left internal carotid angiography *(B)* illustrates the early filling vessels (Bernasconi and Cassinari' arteries), and left external carotid angiography *(C)* shows the abundant amount of blood brought to the tumor by the ascending pharyngeal artery, which may be embolized.

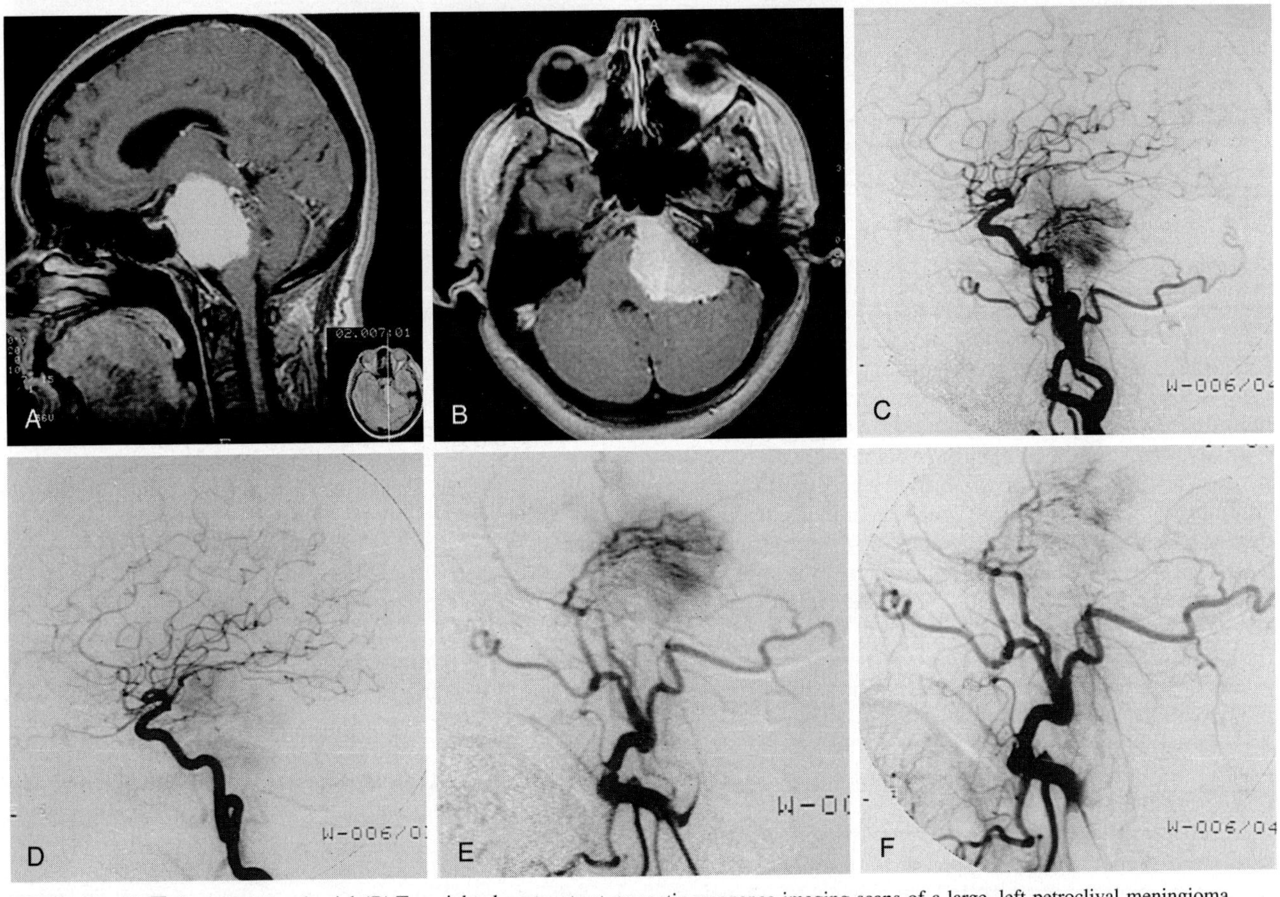

**FIGURE 67–13** ■ Sagittal *(A)* and axial *(B)* T$_1$-weighted postcontrast magnetic resonance imaging scans of a large, left petroclival meningioma suggesting the presence of rich vasculature at the tumor–brain stem interface with possible violation of the arachnoid and pial sheaths. Left common *(C)* and internal *(D)* carotid angiography illustrates the early filling vessels in a corkscrew configuration. Left external carotid angiography before *(E)* and after *(F)* embolization.

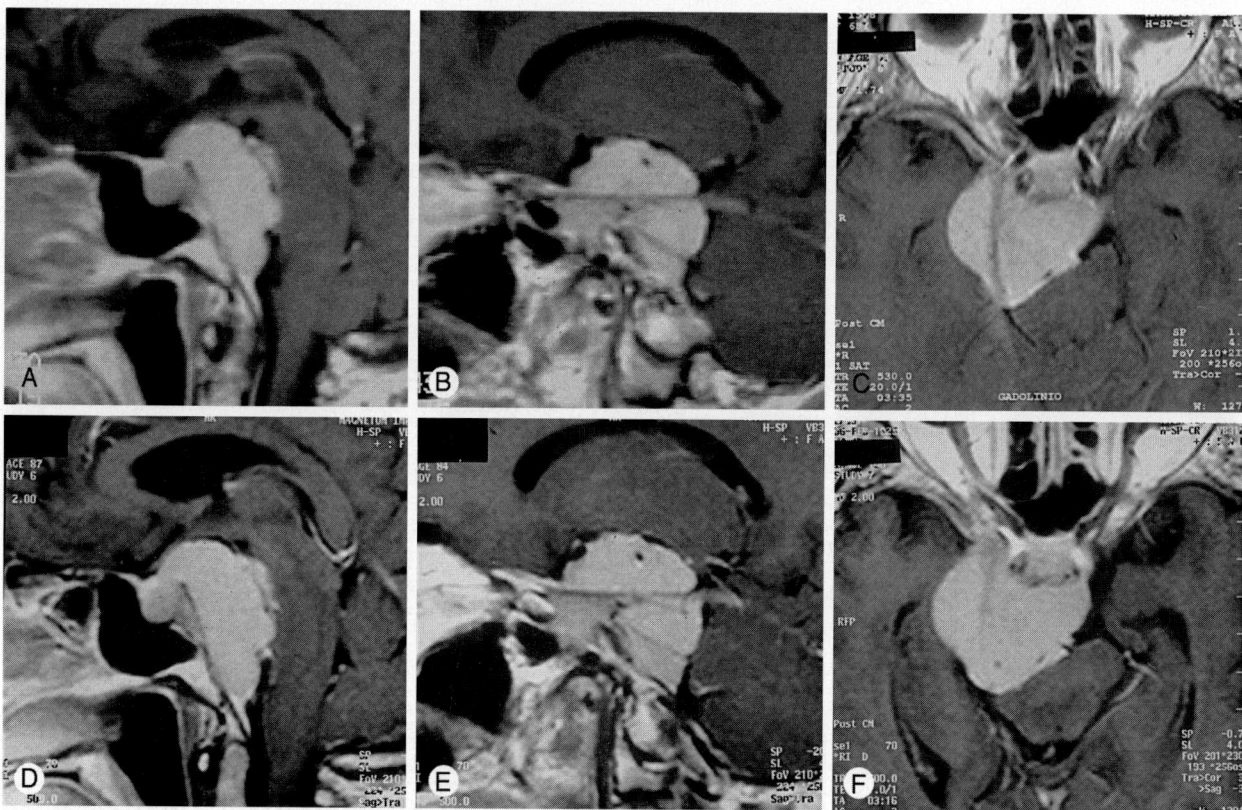

**FIGURE 67–14** ■ Sagittal *(A,* parasagittal *(B))* and axial *(C)* T₁-weighted postcontrast magnetic resonance imaging (MRI) scan performed in March 1992 in a 67-year-old woman who was neurologically intact and who complained only of a transient headache. The patient refused surgery and preferred periodically for follow-up. This large petroclival cavernous meningioma remained asymptomatic and practically unchanged in volume as demonstrated in the last MRI scan *(D–F),* which was performed in October 1998. The patient is still neurologically intact and leads a normal active life.

removal of these lesions is reported only in approximately 60% of cases, and occasional recurrence of disease indicates that radicality was only apparent; knowledge of the natural history of basal meningiomas and longer follow-up periods are therefore required.

In an attempt to attain the primary goal of surgery, which is radical removal with low morbidity and mortality, new, complex approaches and surgical techniques have been developed without regard to specialty-imposed surgical boundaries (mixing the competence of neurosurgeons and ear, nose, and throat surgeons). General surgical aggressiveness, which characterizes skull base surgery, enhanced by interdisciplinary work and innovation, have produced a myriad of new approaches and variations; however, such methods have only slightly reduced the intrinsic difficulty of removing a tumor that infiltrates the cranial nerves, encases the arteries and veins, and has a poor arachnoid plane with the brain stem.

Controversy has developed over the use of new, complex skull base approaches as opposed to more rational and modern adaptations of older and simpler neurosurgical approaches discredited because they belong to the premicrosurgical era. Only recently has a more analytical and critical evaluation of the most advantageous approaches emerged. The numerous published approaches for posterior skull base meningiomas may be categorized into three groups: middle fossa, lateral suboccipital, and combined supratentorial-infratentorial.

## Middle Fossa Approach

This approach is suitable for tumors involving the cavernous sinus, the upper clival area, and some of the middle clival area (sphenopetroclival meningiomas). The extradural approach to cavernous sinus lesions, proposed by Dolenc,[29, 30] was later extended by the same author for middle and upper clivus meningiomas by drilling the petrous apex and dividing the tentorium. The anterior middle fossa approach was described in 1991 by Kawase and associates[31] as the "anterior transpetrosal transtentorial approach" for sphenopetroclival meningiomas.

The area of pyramid resection in Kawase's procedure is bounded by the trigeminal nerve inferiorly and anteriorly, the eminentia arcuata posteriorly, the major petrosal groove laterally, and the carotid and internal auditory canal inferiorly. However, because this approach still resulted in a fairly restricted access to the clival area, in 1994 Kawase and associates[32] proposed its extension with a petrosectomy.

Sekhar and colleagues[14] termed this approach the *frontotemporal transcavernous* and sometimes combined it with orbitozygomatic osteotomy to minimize brain retraction. When the tumor has been removed from the cavernous sinus, the clival area is reached by removing the dorsum sellae, the posterior clinoid process, and the petrous apex, the lowest limit of exposure being the horizontal segment of the internal caroid artery (ICA). The tumor is removed by working between the supraclinoidal ICA and cranial nerve V. The advantage of this approach is that it allows the surgeon to work in the upper clival area without retraction of the posterior temporal lobe, and the tumor may be devascularized early.

The middle fossa approach may also be extended posteriorly to the subtemporal and the preauricular infratemporal approach, which requires resection of the mandibular condyle and exposure of the petrous ICA.[14, 33, 34]

## Retrosigmoid Approach

The lateral suboccipital approach has been a common method of access to tumors of the CPA since Dandy[35] proposed it in 1925. Today, using this access, we are able to remove pathologic processes radically and atraumatically in the deeper petroclival region, and it remains a preferred choice in our practice because it offers the simplest access to the CPA and lateral clivus.[36] The main disadvantage of this route is the difficulty of removing dural and extradural structures invaded by the tumor when approached from such a confined surgical field surrounded by cranial nerves and the already distorted brain stem.[17, 31]

As a rule, we place the patient in a semisitting position with the head flexed and rotated toward the side of the lesion (Fig. 67–15A). Particular care must be taken to extend bone drilling upward and laterally to unroof the lateral and sigmoid sinuses all the way to the jugular bulb (see Fig. 67–15B). With that done, the incised dura is drawn upward and sideways with retraction sutures arranged to pull the sinuses out of the surgeon's hands (see Fig. 67–15C). This creates a very lateral access to the CPA parallel to the posterior aspect of the fossa petrosa and to the insertion angle of the tentorium of the petrosal ridge, making it possible to initiate tumor exeresis by devascularization through coagulation of the dural attachment, first on the posterior surface of the petrous bone, then on the clivus. We then proceed to debulk the tumor with the ultrasonic aspirator throughout the fissure of the tentorium and cranial nerves V, VII and VIII, and IX and X (see Fig. 67–15D). The tumor is thus detached in succession from the cranial nerves and the brain stem; last, its insertion or site of attachment is demolished on the petrous apex, tentorium, and upper clivus.

The greatest possible care is taken to identify and preserve the arachnoid layers next to the cranial nerves, the brain stem, and the arteries (Fig. 67–16). At this stage of the procedure, coagulation is mostly abandoned and replaced by continuous irrigation with saline solution. When the CPA is completely freed of the tumor, an open space remains between the brain stem and the free margin of the tentorium through which the supratentorial space can be accessed. By this exposure, the surgeon can reach and remove even the more rostral projection of the tumor into the middle cranial fossa and parasellar area by dissecting it away from cranial nerves IV and III and from the arteries of the circle of Willis.

Supratentorial subtemporal and parasellar tumor expansion does not in itself disqualify or contradict this simple, well tested approach that has rewarded surgeons with excellent results. Access to this area is prepared by the tumor itself, located as it is in the tentorial hiatus, which can be enlarged by resecting the tentorial flap. Thus, the upper pole of the tumor, if not attached to the parasellar dura, can be dislocated downward and removed by separating it from the arachnoid of the interpeduncular, carotid, and chiasmatic cisterns, even though in some cases the excessive slope of the tentorium could direct the surgeon away from the floor of the middle cranial fossa, leaving the tumor lodgment out of view.

The working field is divided into narrow routes or corridors by cranial nerves crossing the CPA to their emerging foramens. The larger portion of the tumor is removed by dissecting between the inferior aspect of the tentorium and the vestibulocochlear nerves and trigeminal nerve. The middle clivus may be approached between cranial nerves VII and VIII and the caudal cranial nerves, and the lower clivus is reached by dissection below the caudal nerves.

The tumor enlarges the narrow space between the brain stem and the posterior surface of the pyramid laterally and the tentorium superiorly, making it possible to gain access to the clival area without intolerable retraction of the cerebellum and the already distorted brain stem. The elevation of the tentorium produced by the tumor creates a sizable space used for access to the tentorial incisure. The gap of the lateral suboccipital approach may be further enlarged upward by incising the tentorium laterally along the tentorial edge and downward, combining a transcondylar/C1 laminectomy approach.[14, 37–39] In tumors that involve the lower clivus and foramen magnum, after retrosigmoid craniectomy, the medial two thirds of the mastoid process and the posterior half of the occipital condyle are removed. The sigmoid sinus is then completely exposed and the C1 lamina is removed to the foramen transversarium. This approach provides sufficient lateral exposure of the tumor lying anterior to the brain stem without retraction of neural structures, and fusion procedures are not required because stability is not affected (Fig. 67–17).

## Combined Supratentorial and Infratentorial Approach

Meningiomas arising from the petroclival area occasionally extend above the tentorium to the cavernous sinus, and at the same time below to the foramen magnum. These tumors cannot be resected totally using a subtemporal or infratentorial approach alone; a combined supratentorial and infratentorial operation, as pioneered by Malis,[9] should be adopted.

Lateral approaches based on varying degrees of petrous bone resection combined with lateral suboccipital and subtemporal craniotomies have been termed the posterior subtemporal and the pure sigmoid transpetrosal approaches,[12, 14] the petrosal approach,[1, 40] the combined retroauricular and preauricular transpetrosal-transtentorial approach,[7] the combined supratentorial and infratentorial approach,[16] and the combined supraparapetrosal and infraparapetrosal approach.[41]

Bone removal ranges from the simpler retrolabyrinthine, presigmoid drilling to a total petrosectomy with transposition of the facial nerve. Simple bone destructive approaches, sometimes in two-stage operations, may be tai-

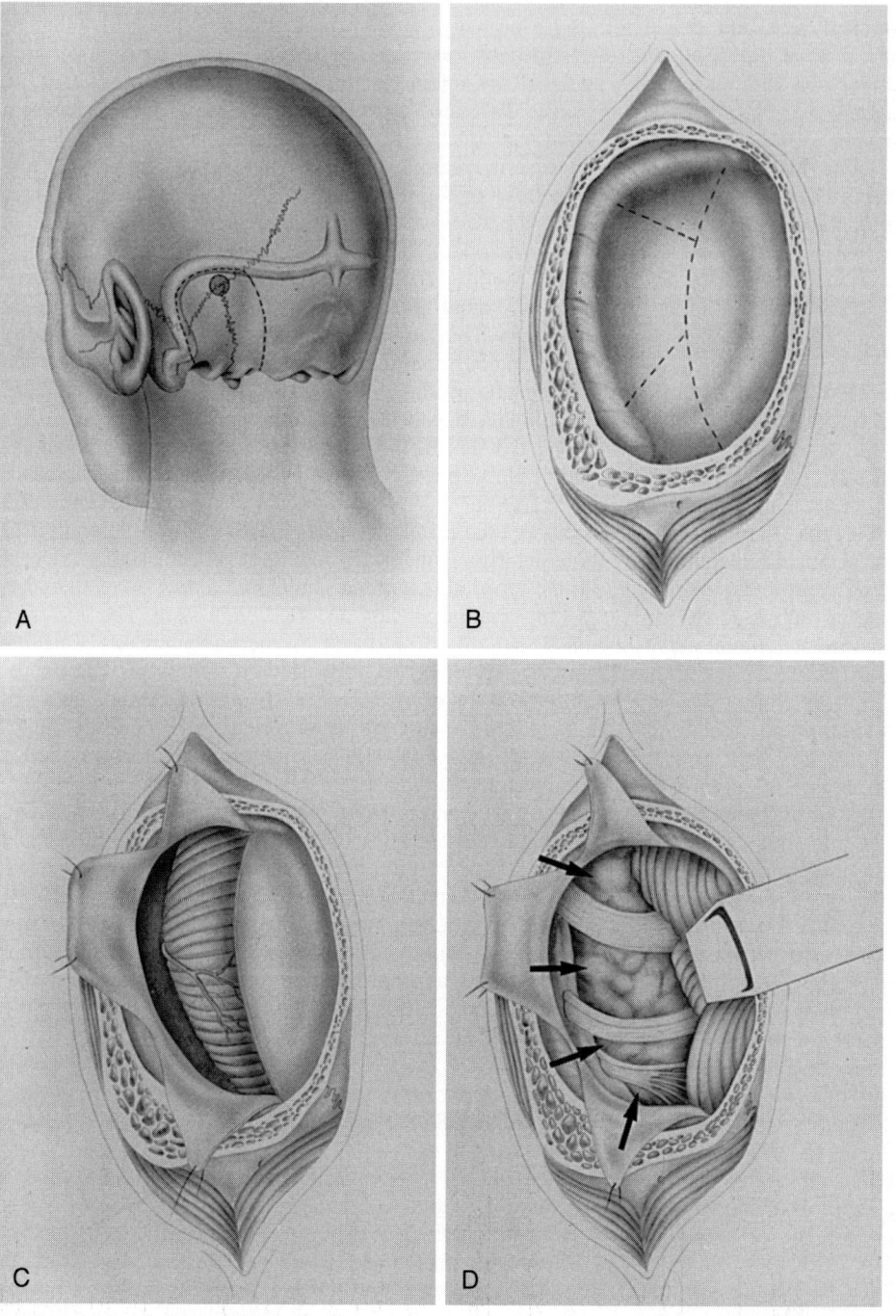

**FIGURE 67–15** ■ The simplest surgical approach to the petroclival area is the lateral suboccipital retrosigmoid route, preferably with the patient in a semisitting position. A retromastoid craniotomy (A) extended to unroof the lateral and sigmoid sinuses is performed (B), and a three-flap duratomy is retracted outside the surgical corridor (C) in order to improve the exposure and reduce the need for cerebellar retraction (D). The tumor is devascularized at its dural attachment and removed working through different routes (arrows) between the tentorium, cranial nerve V, cranial nerves VII and VIII and cranial nerves IX and X.

lored to the extension of the tumor and the presumed goal of surgery.

In the simpler and more rapid form described by Samii and colleagues,[12] a posterior subtemporal craniotomy is extended by lateral suboccipital craniotomy of the posterior cranial fossa; this provides the advantages of both approaches, and additional space at the petrous bone can be obtained through an extralabyrinthine presigmoidal mastoidectomy (Fig. 67–18).

The skin incision is basically an extended retromastoid incision that curves upward and forward into the temporal area. The temporal part of the craniotomy is performed first and must be extended to the floor of the middle fossa

and below the transverse sinus, which has been carefully unroofed by its groove. Next, a suboccipital craniotomy is done with a large cutting drill.

The last bony structures over the sigmoid sinus are removed with a cutting bur, exposing the presigmoid dura and the sinodural angle. Drilling is continued along the pyramid toward its apex. The dura is then opened in such a way that the temporal lobe with Labbé's vein may be elevated and the sigmoid sinus and cerebellum displaced posteriorly.

Next, the superior petrosal sinus is interrupted and the tentorium is incised along the petrous ridge close to its line of attachment. In this area, the large temporolateral Labbé's

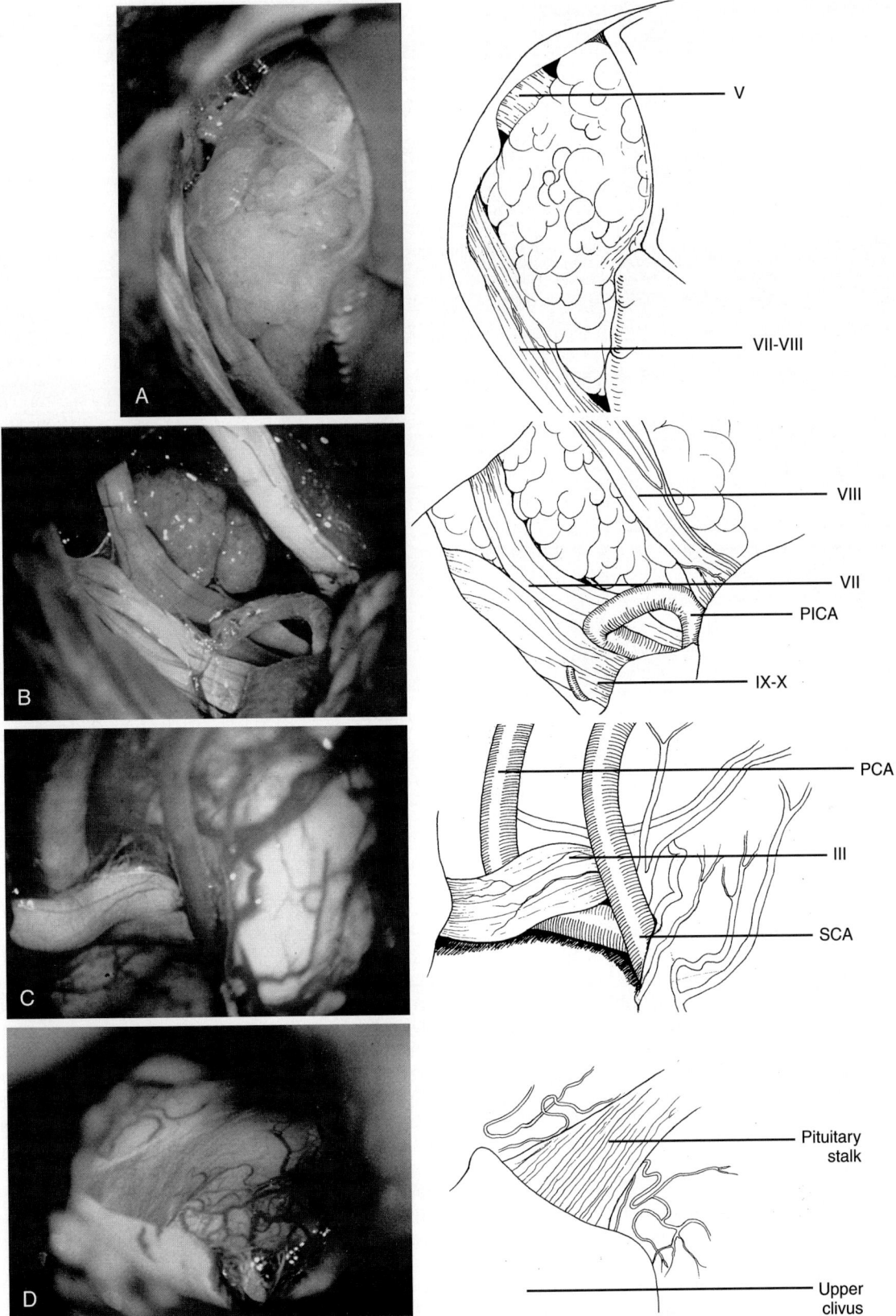

**FIGURE 67–16** ■ Intraoperative microphotographs of an anterior petrous meningioma exposed via a left retrosigmoid approach. The trigeminal nerve is displaced anteriorly and cranial nerves VII and VIII posteriorly and inferiorly *(A)*. The faciovestibulocochlear, glossopharyngeal, and vagus nerves and the PICA are dissected over the caudal extension of the tumor *(B)*. After the tumor is removed, the oculomotor nerve is seen emerging from the mesencephalon between the posterior cerebral artery and the superior cerebellar artery *(C)*. The pituitary stalk entering the sella is viewed from above *(D)*.

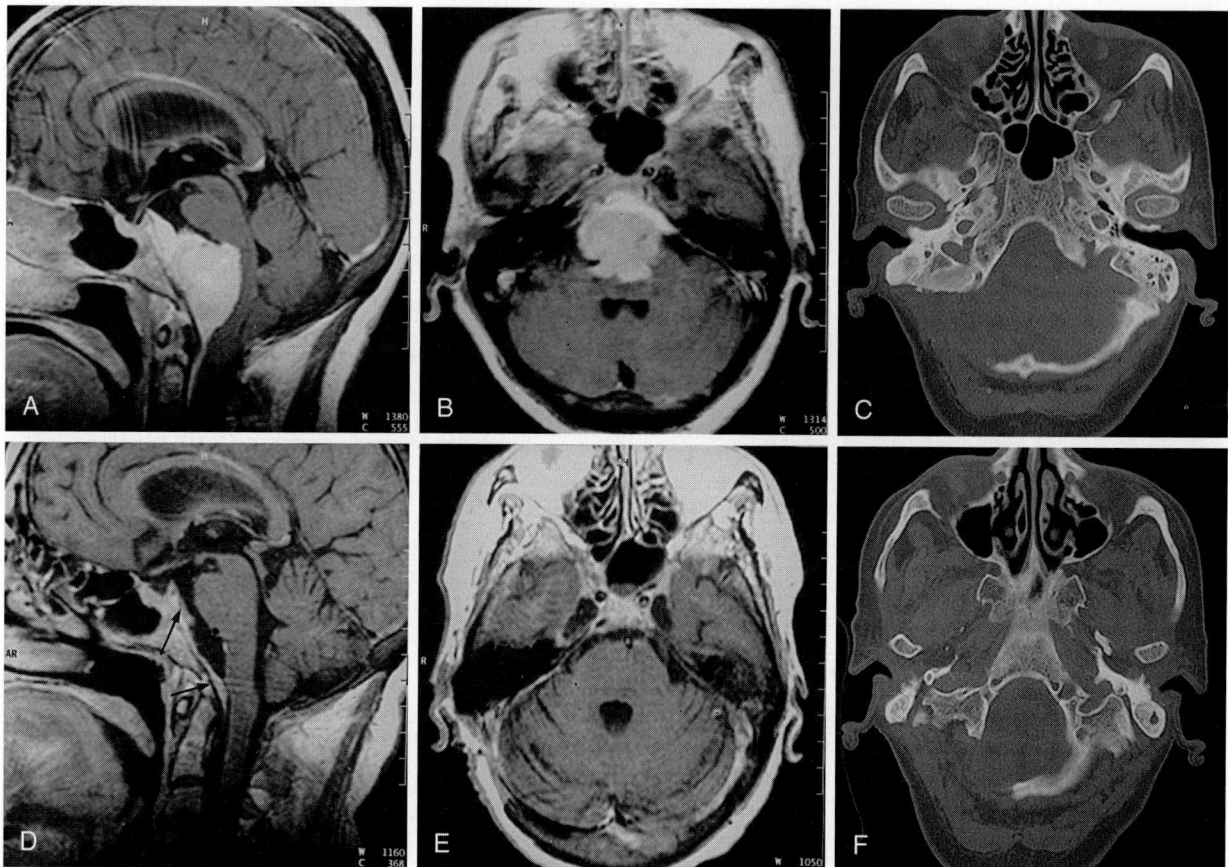

**FIGURE 67–17** ■ Preoperative sagittal *(A)* and axial *(B)* T₁-weighted contrast-enhanced magnetic resonance imaging scans of a large middle-lower clival meningioma approached and removed via a right retrosigmoid dorsolateral approach. Comparable 2-month postoperative images *(D and E)* demonstrate the gross total removal. *Arrows* indicate a possible tumoral residual infiltration. The postoperative computed tomography scans *(C and F)* show the extent of bone removal.

vein flows into the sinus system, and the surgeon must take great care not to injure it and to preserve its discharge into the sinus. The dural incision is then prolonged downward along the anterior margin of the sigmoid sinus, crossing the superior petrosal sinus, which can be divided without any associated risk. The posterior portion of the temporal lobe is then gently lifted with a self-retractor, taking particular care to maintain discharge of Labbé's vein into the sinus. The tentorium is then transected from lateral to medial in a line parallel to the petrous ridge as much as necessary to open the tentorial notch. Care should be taken to identify and preserve the trochlear nerve, which penetrates into the free edge of the tentorium. The tentorial division produces a good exposure of the upper clivus as well as of the anterior and lateral aspect of the brain stem, the basilar artery and its highest branches, and cranial nerves III, IV, and V. At this point, a second retractor is placed anterior to the sigmoid sinus to keep both the posterior edge of the transected tentorium and the cerebellum posterior and medial. Cerebellar retraction can be very slight because after transecting the tentorium, the cerebellum spontaneously withdraws from the posterior surface of the pyramid. Through this opening, the surgeon gains a good view of cranial nerves V to IX and of the medium and lower clivus. Neurosurgeons are particularly indebted to Al-Mefty and colleagues[1] and Samii and co-workers[12] for conceiving, carrying out, and clearly describ-

ing this elegant, tissue-preserving, and ample avenue to the skull base using a unilateral temporal suboccipital craniectomy and drilling of the petrosal bone to gain access to the tumor through the presigmoid (retrolabyrinthine) and subtemporal transtentorial approach (Fig. 67–19). This approach allows the surgeon to work approximately 2 cm closer to the tumor than would be possible through the retrosigmoid approach, and to remain in front of the brain stem (Fig. 67–20). Division of the tentorium reduces the need for retraction of the cerebellum and temporal lobe, preserves drainage of Labbé's vein, and creates an excellent exposure, opening a vista from the lowest cranial nerves to the sella. The combined posterior-subtemporal-suboccipital-presigmoid-transpetrous (retrolabyrinthine) approach without sinus division has proved to be the most elegant and least dangerous way to reach and possibly remove clival tumors that involve a large portion of the skull base from the lower clivus to the parasellar area (Fig. 67–21).

This access can be further enlarged by ligation and division of the transverse sinus laterally to the entrance of Labbé's vein.[7, 10–12, 14, 17] This is the simplest approach for centrolateral clival meningiomas. The advantage of this approach is that the surgeon may start working on the tumor in a reasonably short time, and mild cerebellar and tentorial retraction is well tolerated.

The translabyrinthine and total petrosectomy approach provides a wide exposure of the petroclival area but results

*Text continued on page 953*

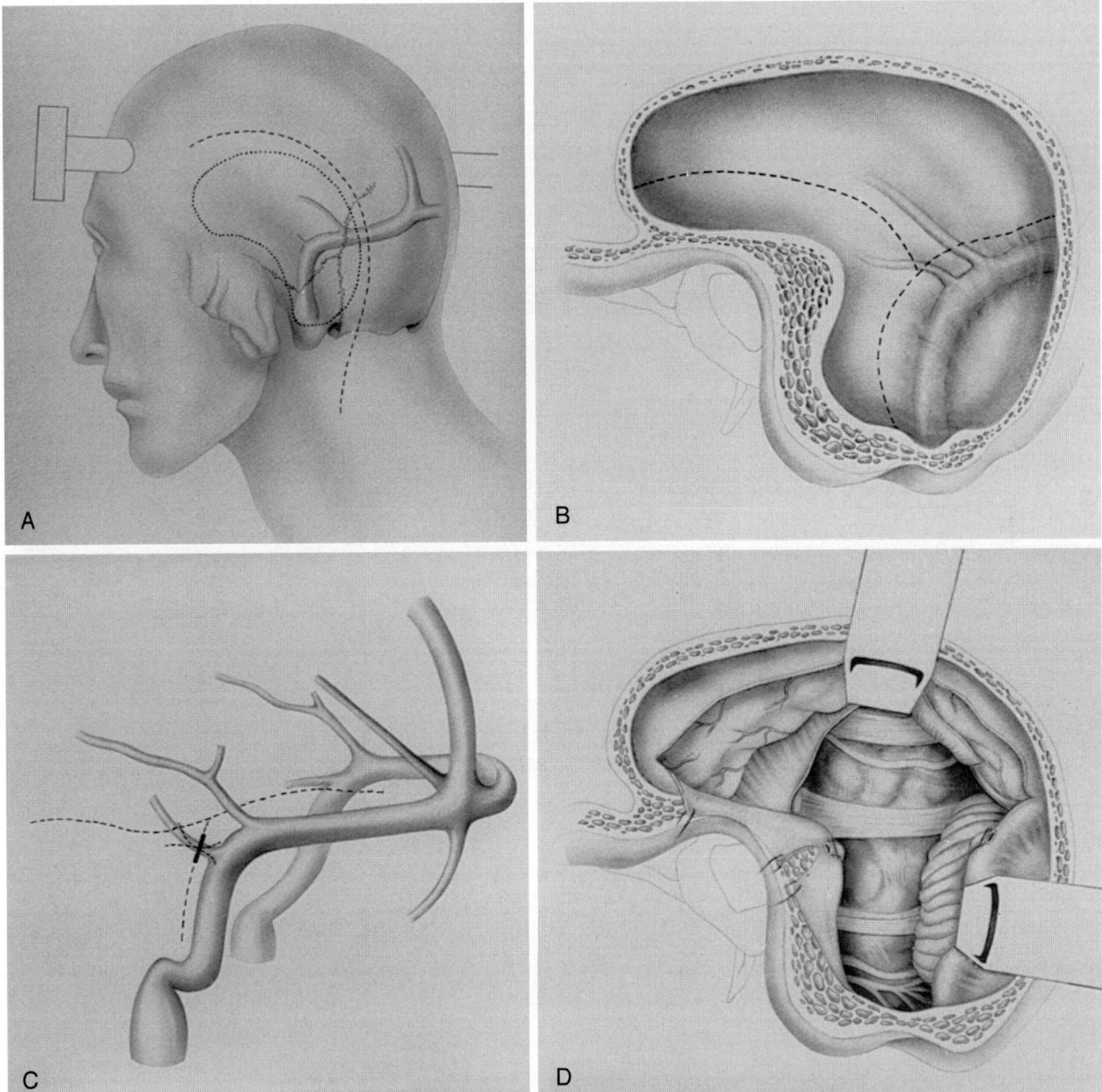

**FIGURE 67-18** ■ An artist's representation of the combined suprainfratentorial petrosal approach. *A,* The head position, the skin incision *(dashed lines),* and the extent of the craniotomy *(dotted line)* are shown. *B,* A temporal suboccipital bone flap is elevated exposing the transverse and sigmoid sinuses, and a mastoidectomy is performed exposing the sigmoid sinus until the jugular bulb and the dura anterior to the sigmoid sinus. The drilling of the petrous pyramid is done to expose the sinus dural angle and the superior petrosal sinus, barely stripping the labyrinth and staying out of the fallopian canal to avoid deafness and injury to the facial nerve. If the hearing is absent, a total labyrinthectomy is performed, which allows an increase of the anterolateral exposure of the tumor. *C,* The dura is opened along the floor of the temporal fossa using great care to preserve and protect the vein of Labbé and then along the anterior border of the sigmoid sinus. *D,* The superior petrous sinus is divided, and the tentorium is completely transected. One retractor is placed under the posterior flap of the tentorium in order to maintain suspended the temporal lobe, and the second is placed anteriorly to the sigmoid sinus to assist the spontaneous falling back of the cerebellum. Cranial nerves III to IX and X are exposed over the lateral aspect of the tumor.

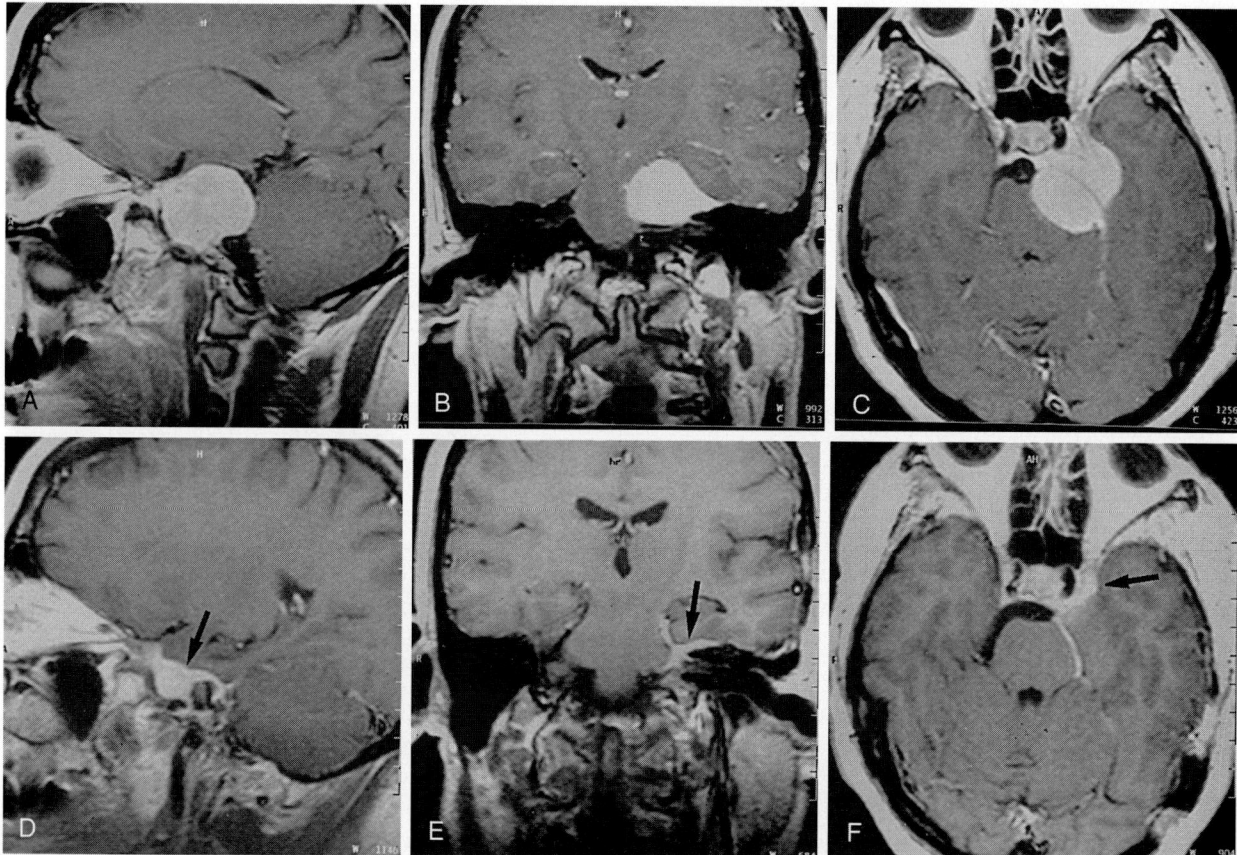

**FIGURE 67–19** ■ Parasagittal *(A)*, coronal *(B)*, and axial *(C)* postcontrast T₁-weighted magnetic resonance imaging scans demonstrate a medium-sized petroclival-cavernous meningioma. The tumor was approached and removed *(D–F)* through a combined temporal-suboccipital presigmoid petrosal route leaving a remnant in the cavernous sinus *(arrows)*. The patient had an uneventful postoperative course with the exception of transient trigeminal herpes. The residual tumor was treated by Gamma knife radiosurgery without waiting for signs of regrowth.

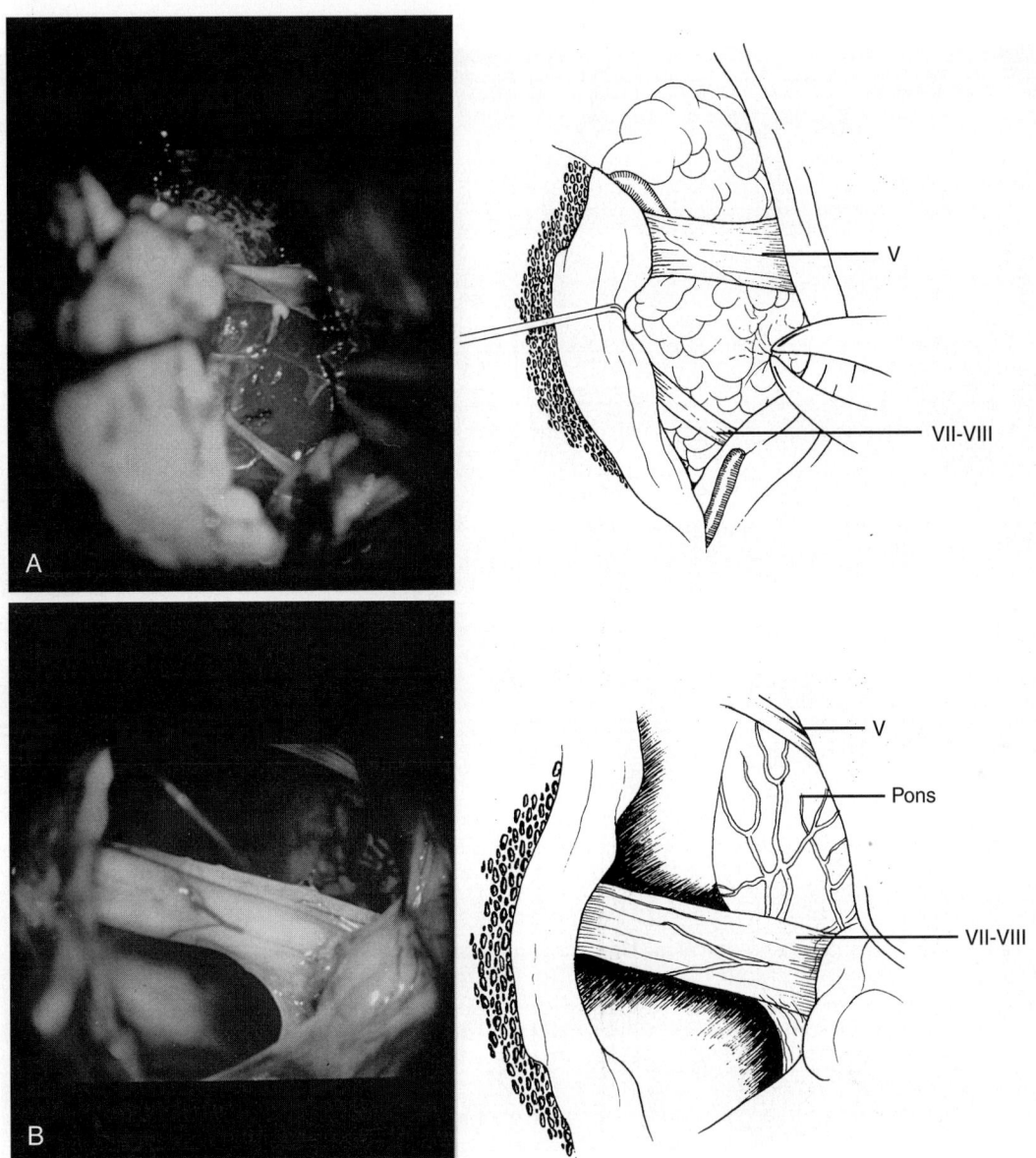

**FIGURE 67–20** ■ Intraoperative microphotographs of the lateral aspect of the petroclival meningioma in Figure 67–19 exposed using the combined subtemporal-presigmoid petrosal approach. The trigeminal nerve is displaced posteriorly and laterally and the faciovestibulocochlear complex, partially engulfed by the tumor, posteriorly and inferiorly *(A)*. After tumor removal, the faciovestibulocochlear appears reanimated *(B)*.

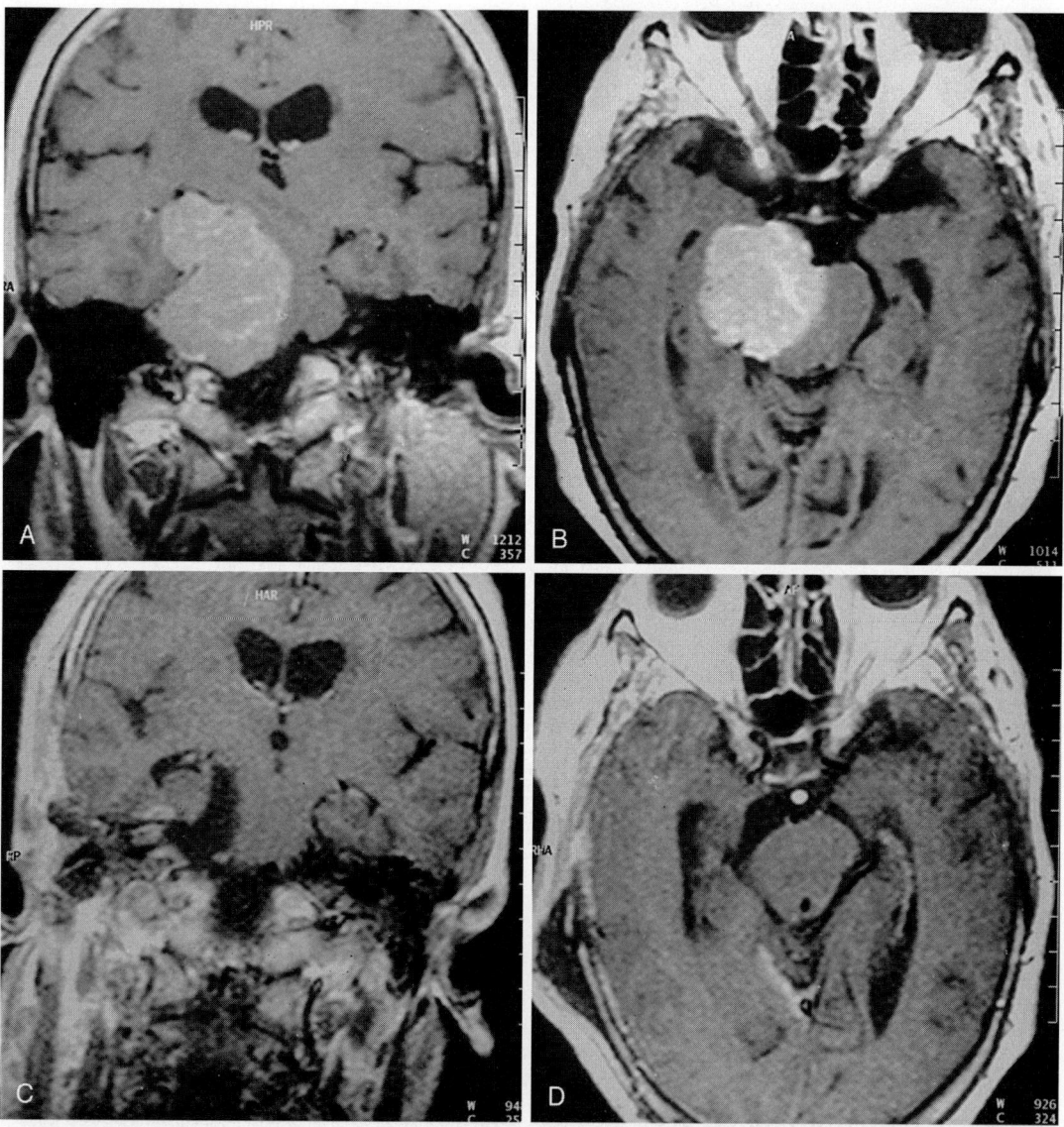

**FIGURE 67–21** ■ Preoperative coronal *(A)* and axial *(B)* postcontrast T$_1$-weighted magnetic resonance imaging scans of a large petroclival meningioma that was totally removed by a combined temporal-suboccipital presigmoid petrosal approach. Early postoperative comparable imaging *(C and D)* verify radicality.

in loss of hearing and varying degrees of facial palsy, and requires highly skilled bone work and reconstructive technique on the surgeon's part.

## RESULTS

A review of the major operative series in the microsurgical era indicates that the percentage of patients with petroclival meningiomas obtaining complete removal varies from 25% to 100% (Table 67–6). Based on these data, it may be estimated that so-called gross-total excision is obtained in approximately 60% of all reported cases.

Reported mortality rates in the series range from 17% to 0%. This low rate of mortality demonstrates the progress achieved in the surgical technique of tumor removal. Illustrating this progress, a review by Hakuba and colleagues[8] of 31 reported patients operated on before 1977 showed a mortality rate as high as 68%.

Operative morbidity tends to be high, exceeding 50% in most contemporary series. The actual morbidity rate is difficult to evaluate because most authors report transient and permanent complications in a different manner. However, it may be estimated that permanent morbidity of various degrees is present in roughly half of the cases operated on, and the incidence of severe disability is not negligible (15% to 20% of cases).

Major complications of surgery for petroclival meningiomas include (in order of frequency) cranial nerve dysfunction, long-tract deficits, cerebrospinal fluid leakage, stupor and coma, and sinus thrombosis.[2–4, 14, 15, 45] In almost all cases, the patient is in worse clinical and neurologic condition after surgery than before, and needs constant, meticulous assistance. What contributes more than anything else to postoperative neurologic deterioration is the onset of new cranial nerve deficits or the aggravation of pre-existing deficits. Only 8 (24%) of 33 patients in the authors' first series emerged from surgery without any change in cranial nerve function; all others showed the onset of at least one new cranial nerve deficit, and 12 showed definite aggravation of pre-existing deficits. Fortunately, many patients with either kind of deterioration showed some evidence of improvement within the first month after surgery, such that morbidity of this type was materially reduced at 4 weeks. The most dangerous type of impairment is palsy of cranial nerves IX and X, causing severe dysphagia and requiring utmost care to prevent aspiration pneumonia. A lesser but still significant contribution to overall neurologic deterioration is caused by the onset or aggravation of somatomotor deficits. In the authors' series, hemiparesis developed in four patients, abating in two within a few weeks. Altered states of consciousness, deregulation of brain stem functions, and functional impairment of the lowest cranial nerves were causes of respiratory problems, requiring mechanical ventilation beyond the second postoperative day in six patients and necessitating tracheostomy in two.

Cerebrospinal fluid leakage facilitated by the opening of the mastoid air cells is usually successfully treated by lumbar drainage for 1 week or more. Thrombosis of the transverse or sigmoid sinus is a life-threatening complication that must be immediately recognized and treated with intravenous heparin.[13]

## RECURRENCES

Unfortunately, surgical results of petroclival meningiomas are negatively affected by tumor remants. *Tumor recurrence* means that some remaining tumor tissue was capable of regrowing into a tumor mass. In approximately 30% of patients in reported series with subtotal tumor removal, recurrence was due either to incomplete excision or to regrowth after seemingly total removal. The broad dural

## TABLE 67–6 ■ REPORTED SERIES OF PETROCLIVAL MENINGIOMAS

| Authors | Year | No. of Patients | Total Removal (%) | Operative Morbidity* (%) | Mortality† (%) |
|---|---|---|---|---|---|
| Hakuba et al[8] | 1977 | 6 | 100 | — | 17 |
| Yasargil et al[17] | 1980 | 20 | 35 | 50 | 15 |
| Mayberg and Symon[11] | 1986 | 35 | 26 | 54 | 9 |
| Al-Mefty et al[1] | 1988 | 13 | 85 | 31 | 0 |
| Nishimura et al[42] | 1989 | 24 | — | 91 | 8 |
| Samii et al[12] | 1989 | 24 | 71 | 46 | 0 |
| Sekhar et al[14] | 1990 | 41 | 78 | 22 | 2 |
| Al-Mefty and Smith[3] | 1991 | 18 | 83 | — | 0 |
| Bricolo et al[4] | 1992 | 33 | 79 | 76 | 9 |
| Samii and Tatagiba[13] | 1992 | 36 | 75 | 42 | — |
| Spetzler et al[16] | 1992 | 46 | 91 | 56 | 0 |
| Sekhar et al[15] | 1994 | 75 | 60 | 60 | 0 |
| Cantore et al[43] | 1994 | 16 | 80 | 38 | 0 |
| Couldwell et al[6] | 1996 | 109 | 69 | 51 | 4 |
| Thomas and King[44] | 1996 | 16 | 44 | — | 0 |
| Zentner et al | 1997 | 19 | 68 | 58 | 5 |
| Bricolo and Turazzi[48] | 1999 | 110 | 66 | 47 | 4 |

*Operative morbidity is reported differently according to author. This table attempts to report the average occurrence of early postoperative dysfunction. A percentage of these are transient.

†A number of patients who died after surgery because of postoperative complications may not have been included.

**TABLE 67–7 ■ COMBINED FACTORS OPPOSING TOTAL REMOVAL IN 37 OF THE LAST 110 PETROCLIVAL AND ANTERIOR PETROUS MENINGIOMAS IN THE AUTHORS' SERIES**

| Factors | N |
|---|---|
| Tumor extension | 16 |
| Arterial encasement | 18 |
| Cranial nerve | 24 |
| Absent arachnoid plane | 12 |
| Dural invasion | 8 |
| Intraoperative failure | 2 |

base of most petroclival meningiomas and their tendency to grow en plaque with extensive bone and dural infiltration account for the high recurrence rate.

Although the goal of surgery should be complete removal of the lesion, these tumors also may be well controlled for a long period after a large and efficacious subtotal removal. In the series reported by Sekhar and associates,[15] only one of the five patients (20%) with residual tumor required reoperation. In the series of Mayberg and Symon,[11] 4 of 26 patients (15%) with subtotal removal had clinical progression and eventually died. In 1994, Kawase and associates[32] reported a rapid regrowth in 3 (7%) of 42 patients between 1 and 4 years after surgery, and stable residual tumor in 7 patients (17%).

Treatment of residual tumor depends on many factors: a small residual left because of neural or vascular structural encasement may be observed or treated by radiosurgery; the same can be done in elderly patients when a small amount of tumor remains after surgery. For larger residuals, Sekhar and colleagues[14] propose an early second operation before development of scar tissue. This aggressive surgical treatment seems justified because of unsatisfactory results and side effects of radiation therapy, which, however, still maintains a role in the treatment of large and fast-growing recurrences.

Prevention of recurrences may interfere with surgical wound closure. Ear, nose, and throat surgeons[46] who have resolved the problem of repairing large dural defects in the skull base by placing large pieces of autologous fat, claim the necessity of "as large as possible" dural removal to obtain true radicality and proper treatment of skull base meningiomas.

## FINAL REMARKS AND CONCLUSION

Evaluation of the authors' experience in the surgical management of more than 100 petroclival meningiomas and

review of major contemporary series demonstrate that it is not easy nor the rule to attain good clinical results after removal of such tumors. Surgical technical advancements associated with improved neuroanesthesia, postoperative intensive care, and rehabilitation make it possible to obtain much better results than in the past, and today surgical mortality rates approach 0%. However, morbidity, primarily from cranial nerve neuropathies, remains significant and unacceptable for more than a few patients.

The primary factors limiting total removal (Table 67–7) and reduction of operative morbidity are basically the same ones faced by many skull base surgeons who tend to use more extensive approaches.[47] It is the authors' belief that the real limitation in obtaining radical and safe removal is not inadequate exposure but rather the anatomicopathologic characteristics of the tumor.

Meningiomas of the clivus and petrous apex continue to pose surgical challenge and the optimal surgical management remains controversial. In a retrospective study, we reviewed all our experience in this field (Table 67–8).[48] In approximately 19 years (1981 to July 1999), 110 meningiomas of the petroclival region were treated. Separating the data into two groups by decades, one may note in the latter decade the following: (1) a slight increase in the use of a complex approach; (2) a reduction of the rate of total resection; and (3) a significant reduction in operative morbidity. Thus one may deduce that the "learning curve" has taught neurosurgeons to be less aggressive in tumor removal in an effort to avoid injury to the involved neurovascular structures. This attitude, also shared by others,[49] guarantees better clinical outcome based on the current technical capability.

A number of issues related to surgical management of petroclival meningiomas are still unresolved. The authors believe that preservation of function should take priority, and this remains the most important factor governing the procedure. Radical tumor removal at all costs, at the risk of adding permanent dysfunction to a pre-existing picture of brain stem distress, does not seem to be the appropriate strategy. If safe radical excision of a tumor is not feasible owing to its invasive nature, little room is left for complete removal, and severe brain stem indentation and arterial and cranial nerve encasement represent unresolved technical difficulties.

Although total eradication certainly remains the prime objective of surgery, the surgeon must also consider that a number of subtotally removed petroclival meningiomas remain stationary, often for long periods, and radiosurgery can control eventual regrowth.

## ACKNOWLEDGMENTS

*The authors thank Ms. Marina Longani for the illustrations, Ms. Cristina Bertolin for her preparation of*

**TABLE 67–8 ■ AUTHORS' SERIES OF 110 CONSECUTIVE PETROCLIVAL MENINGIOMAS**

| Period | No. of Patients | Retrosigmoid Approach | Skull Base Approach | Total Removal | Operative Morbidity | Mortality |
|---|---|---|---|---|---|---|
| 1981–1990 | 33 | 23 (70%) | 10 (30%) | 26 (79%) | 25 (72%) | 3 (9%) |
| 1991–1999 | 77 | 49 (64%) | 28 (36%) | 47 (61%) | 29 (37%) | 2 (3%) |
| Total | 110 | 72 (65%) | 38 (35%) | 73 (66%) | 54 (47%) | 5 (4%) |

*the photographic material, and Ms. Victoria Praino for editing.*

## REFERENCES

1. Al-Mefty O, Fox JL, Smith RR: Petrosal approach for petroclival meningiomas. Neurosurgery 22:510–517, 1988.
2. Al-Mefty O, Ayoubi S, Smith RR: The petrosal approach: Indications, technique, and results. Acta Neurochir Suppl (Wien) 53:166–170, 1991.
3. Al-Mefty O, Smith RR: Clival and petroclival meningiomas. In Al-Mefty O (ed): Meningiomas. New York: Raven Press, 1991, pp 517–537.
4. Bricolo A, Turazzi S, Cristofori L, et al: Microsurgical removal of petroclival meningiomas: A report of 33 patients. Neurosurgery 31:813–828, 1992.
5. Bricolo A: Radical surgical removal of clival meningiomas. In Al-Mefty O (ed): Controversies in Neurosurgery. New York: Thieme, 1996, pp 110–114.
6. Couldwell WT, Fukushima T, Giannotta S, et al: Petroclival meningiomas: Surgical experience in 109 cases. J Neurosurg 84:20–28, 1996.
7. Hakuba A, Nishimura S, Tanaka K et al: Clivus meningioma: Six cases of total removal. Neurol Med Chir (Tokyo) 17:63–77, 1977.
8. Hakuba A, Nishimura S, Jang BJ: A combined retroauricular and preauricular transpetrosal-transtentorial approach to clivus meningiomas. Surg Neurol 30:108–116, 1988.
9. Malis LI: The petrosal approach. Clin Neurosurg 37:528–540, 1991.
10. Malis LI: Suboccipital subtemporal approach to petroclival tumors. In Wilson CB (ed): Neurosurgical Procedures: Personal Approaches to Classic Operations. Baltimore: Williams & Wilkins, 1992, pp 41–51.
11. Mayberg M, Symon L: Meningiomas of the clivus and apical petrous bone: Report of 35 cases. J Neurosurg 65:160–167, 1986.
12. Samii M, Ammirati M, Mahran A, et al: Surgery of petroclival meningiomas: Report of 24 cases. Neurosurgery 24:12–17, 1989.
13. Samii M, Tatagiba M: Experience with 36 surgical cases of petroclival meningiomas. Acta Neurochir (Wien) 118:27–32, 1992.
14. Sekhar LN, Jannetta PJ, Burkhart LE, et al: Meningiomas involving the clivus: A six-year experience with 41 patients. Neurosurgery 27:764–781, 1990.
15. Sekhar L, Swamy NKS, Jaiswal V, et al: Surgical excision of meningiomas involving the clivus: Preoperative and intraoperative features as predictors of postoperative functional deterioration. J Neurosurg 81:860–868, 1994.
16. Spetzler RF, Daspit CP, Pappas CTE: The combined supra- and infratentorial approach for lesions of the petrous and clival regions: Experience with 46 cases. J Neurosurg 76:588–599, 1992.
17. Yasargil MG, Mortara RW, Curcic M: Meningiomas of basal posterior cranial fossa. Adv Tech Stand Neurosurg 7:3–115, 1980.
18. Uttley D: Skull base surgery. Br J Neurosurg 9:437–439, 1995.
19. Cushing HW, Eisenhardt L: Meningiomas: Their Classification, Regional Behavior, Life History and Surgical End Results. Springfield, IL: Charles C Thomas, 1938, pp 3–387.
20. Castellano F, Ruggiero G: Meningiomas of the posterior fossa. Acta Radiol (Suppl) 104:3–157, 1953.
21. Spetzler RF, Daspit CP, Pappas CTE: Combined approach for lesions involving the clivus and cerebellopontine angle: Experience with 23 cases. Presented at the International Symposium on Processes of the Cranial Midline, Vienna, May 21–25, 1990.
22. Couldwell WT, Weiss MH: Surgical approaches to petroclival meningiomas. I: Upper and midclival approaches. Contemp Neurosurg 16:1–6, 1994.
23. Zentner J, Meyer B, Vieweg U, et al: Petroclival meningiomas: Is radical resection always the best option? J Neurol Neurosurg Psychiatry 62:341–345, 1997.
24. McDermott MW, Wilson CB: Meningiomas. In Youmans J (ed): Neurological Surgery. Philadelphia: WB Saunders, 1997, pp 2782–2825.
25. Ojemann RG: Skull base surgery: A perspective. J Neurosurg 76:569–570, 1992.
26. Pomeranz S, Umansky F, Elidan J, et al: Giant cranial base tumors. Acta Neurochir (Wien) 129:121–126, 1994.
27. Holmes B. Sekhar L, Sofaer S, et al: Outcome analysis in cranial base surgery: Preliminary results. Acta Neurochir (Wien) 134:136–138, 1995.
28. Samii M, Tatagiba M: Petroclival approach. In Donald (ed): Surgery of the Skull Base. Philadelphia: Lippincott–Raven, 1998, pp 423–442.
29. Dolenc VV: Direct microsurgical repair of intracavernous vascular lesions. J Neurosurg 58:826–831, 1983.
30. Dolenc VN: Anatomy and Surgery of the Cavernous Sinus. New York: Springer-Verlag, 1989.
31. Kawase T, Shiobara R, Toya S: Anterior transpetrosal-transtentorial approach for sphenopetroclival meningiomas: Surgical method and results in 10 meningiomas. Neurosurgery 28:869–875, 1991.
32. Kawase T, Shiobara R, Ohira T: Middle fossa transpetrosal-transtentorial approaches for petroclival meningiomas: Selective pyramid resection and radicality. Acta Neurochir (Wien) 129:113–120, 1994.
33. Al-Mefty O, Anand VK: Zygomatic approach to skull-base lesions. J Neurosurg 73:668–673, 1990.
34. Sen CN, Sekhar LN: The subtemporal and preauricular infratemporal approach to intradural structures ventral to the brain stem. J Neurosurg 73:345–354, 1990.
35. Dandy W: An operation for the total removal of cerebellopontine (acoustic) tumors. Surg Gynecol Obstet 41:129–148, 1925.
36. Bricolo A, Turazzi A, Talacchi A, et al: Simple neurosurgical approaches to the clivus. In Samii M (ed): Skull Base Surgery. First International Skull Base Congress, Hannover 1992. Basel: Karger, 1994, pp 1055–1064.
37. Bertalanffy H, Gilsbach J, Seeger W, et al: Surgical anatomy and clinical application of the transcondylar approach to the lower clivus. In Samii M (ed): Skull Base Surgery. First International Skull Base Congress, Hannover, 1992. Basel: Karger, 1994, pp 1045–1048.
38. Sen CN, Sekhar LN: An extreme lateral approach to intradural lesions of the cervical spine and foramen magnum. Neurosurgery 27:197–204, 1990.
39. Al-Mefty O, Borba LAB, Aoki N, et al: The transcondylar approach to extradural nonneoplastic lesions of the craniovertebral junction. J Neurosurg 84:1–6, 1996.
40. King AK, Black KL, Martin NA, et al: The petrosal approach with hearing preservation. J Neurosurg 79:508–514, 1993.
41. Fukushima T: Combined supra- and infra-parapetrosal approach for petroclival lesions. In Sekhar LN, Janecka IP (eds): Surgery of Cranial Base Tumors. New York: Raven Press, 1992, pp 661–670.
42. Nishimura S, Hakuba A, Jang B, et al: Clivus and apicopetroclivus meningiomas: Report of 24 cases. Neurol Med Chir 29:1004–1011, 1989.
43. Cantore G, Delfini R, Ciappetta P: Surgical treatment of petroclival meningiomas: Experience with 16 cases. Surg Neurol 42:105–111, 1994.
44. Thomas NWM, King TT: Meningiomas of the cerebellopontine angle: A report of 41 cases. Br J Neurosurg 10:59–68, 1996.
45. Bricolo A, Turazzi S, Cristofori L, et al: Surgical treatment of meningiomas in the petroclival area: Experience in 28 cases (Abstract). Presented at the 1st Asian-Oceanic International Congress on Skull Base Surgery, Tokyo, June 18–20, 1991.
46. Sanna M, Mazzoni A, Saleh EA, et al: Lateral approaches to the median skull base through the petrous bone: The system of the modified transcochlear approach. J Laryngol Otol 108:1036–1044, 1994.
47. Lang DA, Neil-Dwyer G, Garfield J: Outcome after complex neurosurgery: The caregiver's burden is forgotten. J Neurosurg 91:359–363, 1999.
48. Bricolo A, Turazzi S: Surgical management of petroclival meningiomas: Experience on 110 cases (Abstract), presented at XLVIII Congress of the Italian Neurosurgical Society, Catanzaro, Sept. 12–15, 1999.
49. David CA, Spetzler RF: Petroclival meningiomas. BNI 15:5–14, 1999.

# CHAPTER 68

# Transtemporal Approaches to the Posterior Cranial Fossa*

■ FRANK D. VRIONIS, GALE GARDNER, JON H. ROBERTSON, and JASON A. BRODKEY

Traditional approaches to the posterior cranial fossa do not permit direct access to complex lesions of the lateral skull base, cerebellopontine angle (CPA), or clivus. To circumvent brain retraction and allow for complete resection, approaches have been developed that position the dissection both lateral and anterior to the brainstem and cerebellum. All of these skull base approaches are combinations and variations of transtemporal bone routes (Table 68–1 and Fig. 68–1). Unlike craniotomies performed elsewhere, entry to the posterior fossa through the temporal bone imposes special problems for the surgeon if the internal carotid artery (ICA), sigmoid sinus (SS), cranial nerves VII and VIII, and the specialized structures for hearing and balance are to be preserved. Despite the widely varied nomenclature, often only subtle differences exist between these approaches. It is imperative that the location, type, and extent of the lesion dictate the type of the approach. Tailored approaches to the lesion instead of standard ones are recommended for minimal disruption of normal structures. In this respect, transtemporal approaches represent an anatomic continuum of temporal bone dissection, with frequent overlaps and minor discrepancies or differences between the various approaches. The complicated nomenclature stems from the fact that skull base tumors tend to extend into different anatomic compartments, often necessitating combined approaches. Because of the overlap of neurosurgery and otology in this area, collaboration of neurosurgeons and otologists is mandatory.

This chapter is divided into three sections: Anterior Transpetrosal Approaches, describing anterior approaches within the temporal bone through the middle cranial fossa; Posterior Transpetrosal Approaches, for those that are situated more posteriorly through the mastoid process; and Combined Approaches. We define the external auditory canal (EAC) as the dividing structure between the anterior and posterior approaches. We divide each approach into sections, giving a brief historical perspective, indications, surgical technique, and complications/disadvantages.

---

*Portions of this chapter have been taken from Robertson JT, Robertson JH, Coakham H (eds): Cranial Bone Surgery. New York: Churchill Livingstone (in press).

---

TABLE 68–1 ■ **TEMPORAL BONE APPROACHES**

**Anterior Approaches**
Middle cranial fossa
Extended middle cranial fossa
Middle cranial fossa transtentorial

**Posterior Approaches**
Retrolabyrinthine—presigmoid
Retrolabyrinthine—retrosigmoid
Retrolabyrinthine—transsigmoid
Transotic
Translabyrinthine
Infralabyrinthine
Transcochlear
Transcanal-infracochlear

**Combined Approaches**
Petrosal
Infratemporal fossa

## ANTERIOR TRANSPETROSAL APPROACHES

Anterior transpetrosal approaches are based on a standard subtemporal extradural middle fossa approach. We divide the anterior approaches into three types: (1) middle fossa approach, (2) extended middle fossa approach (anterior petrosectomy), and (3) middle fossa transtentorial approach. The middle fossa approach provides a subtemporal extradural exposure of the middle fossa floor designed for removing acoustic neuromas situated laterally within the internal auditory canal (IAC). For more extensive tumors, the extended middle fossa approach provides additional exposure of the petrous apex and supraclival region. With the addition of division of the tentorium, the middle fossa transtentorial approach provides access to the midclival region and posterior fossa as well as the posterior cavernous sinus.

### Middle Fossa Approach

House developed the middle fossa access to the IAC and adjacent structures in 1961 in an effort to remove foci of

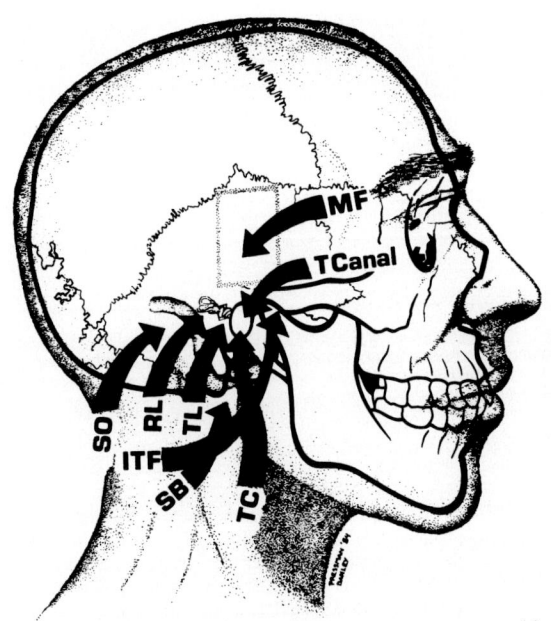

**FIGURE 68–1** ■ Multiple approach routes through the temporal bone to the posterior fossa. (SO, suboccipital; RL, retrolabyrinthine; TL, translabyrinthine; SB, skull base; TC, transcochlear; ITF, infratemporal fossa; MF, middle fossa; T Canal, transcanal.)

labyrinthine otosclerosis.[1–3] Although he used this approach briefly for the removal of acoustic tumors, he soon directed his efforts to a translabyrinthine approach. Fisch has further refined the middle fossa approach.[4]

Several techniques for localization of the IAC have been described. House's technique identifies the greater superficial petrosal nerve (GSPN), follows it to the geniculate ganglion (GG), and then proceeds along the labyrinthine segment of the facial nerve to the IAC.[2] Another popular method described by Fisch uses the superior semicircular canal (SSC) as the primary landmark.[66] Using this method, once the SSC is identified, the meatal plane overlying the IAC is located in a 60-degree plane centered over the SSC ampulla. Garcia-Ibanez and Garcia-Ibanez[5] advocate a technique beginning at the bisection of the angle between the GSPN and the arcuate eminence. The medial "safe" part of the IAC is first identified and is followed laterally. Because of the wide variations in anatomy[4, 5] and small working space, no single technique can ensure avoidance of injury to important structures. Careful dissection and a detailed understanding of the regional anatomy are important for success. Image-guided navigation through the temporal bone has been introduced as an accurate alternative method to localize the IAC without the need to expose the GG or the SSC.[6, 7]

## Indications

The middle fossa approach is best suited for lesions situated lateral within the IAC that have limited extension into the CPA (<1 cm) and where hearing preservation is the goal.[2, 8] It is especially useful when preoperative computed tomography (CT) of the temporal bone demonstrates close proximity of the posterior semicircular canal (PSC), common crus, or vestibule to the posterior lip of the IAC.

In those circumstances, retrosigmoid approaches are less preferable and the middle fossa approach becomes the hearing-preservation approach of choice. Tumors that are medial in position and do not extend to the fundus of the IAC are best approached by posterior approaches (e.g., retrosigmoid approach).

The middle fossa approach provides access to the labyrinthine segment of the facial nerve without sacrificing hearing. Thus, decompression of the facial nerve in trauma or Bell's palsy, or resection of facial nerve tumors can be accomplished. This approach also permits selective sectioning of the vestibular nerve fibers for Ménière's disease. In theory, it could also be used to expose the horizontal portion of the ICA, eustachian tube, and temporomandibular joint (TMJ). Other indications include advanced otosclerosis, nerve section for tinnitus, facial nerve repair and facial nerve neuroma, repair of middle fossa encephaloceles, and cerebrospinal fluid (CSF) leaks through the tegmen.[2]

## Surgical Approach

The patient is positioned supine on the operating table with the head turned opposite the side of the tumor.[2, 4, 5, 8, 9] Facial and auditory nerve monitoring is used. An incision is planned that begins at the level of the zygoma just anterior to the tragus and extends superiorly to approximately the superior temporal line. We prefer an S-shaped incision curving first anteriorly then posteriorly to allow for greater spreading of the soft tissues.

The temporalis muscle is divided and reflected anteriorly. A 4 × 5 cm bone flap is planned approximately two thirds anterior to the EAC and one third posterior. The inferior margin should be placed as close to the middle fossa floor as possible. A subtemporal craniectomy is performed. The dura is then elevated from the middle fossa floor from a posterior to anterior direction. This direction of dissection helps avoid inadvertent elevation of the GSPN and subsequent traction injury to the GG and facial nerve. Injury to the GSPN can produce a dry eye secondary to loss of lacrimal gland innervation. In approximately 16% of cases the GG is not covered by bone and inadvertent injury can occur.[4] To maintain a visible plane of dissection, a self-retaining brain retractor is used. Some retractors are limited to only 4 to 5 cm of spread, and thus too wide a craniotomy can impair the capability of the retractor to elevate the dura adequately.

Several landmarks need to be identified before bone removal can begin over the IAC: (1) the middle meningeal artery, (2) the arcuate eminence, (3) the GSPN, and (4) the facial hiatus (Fig. 68–2). The first landmark is typically the middle meningeal artery at the foramen spinosum. This can be obliterated and divided if necessary. The foramen may be rarely duplicated or absent. It marks the anterior limit of the dural elevation. As dural elevation continues, the arcuate eminence, a rounded elevation of the petrous bone, can be identified. It is usually produced by the underlying SSC. Lateral to the arcuate eminence is the tegmen tympani, a thin lamina of bone that forms the roof of the tympanic cavity. The GSPN originates from the GG, exits through the petrous bone at the facial hiatus, and runs extradurally in an anteromedial direction toward the tri-

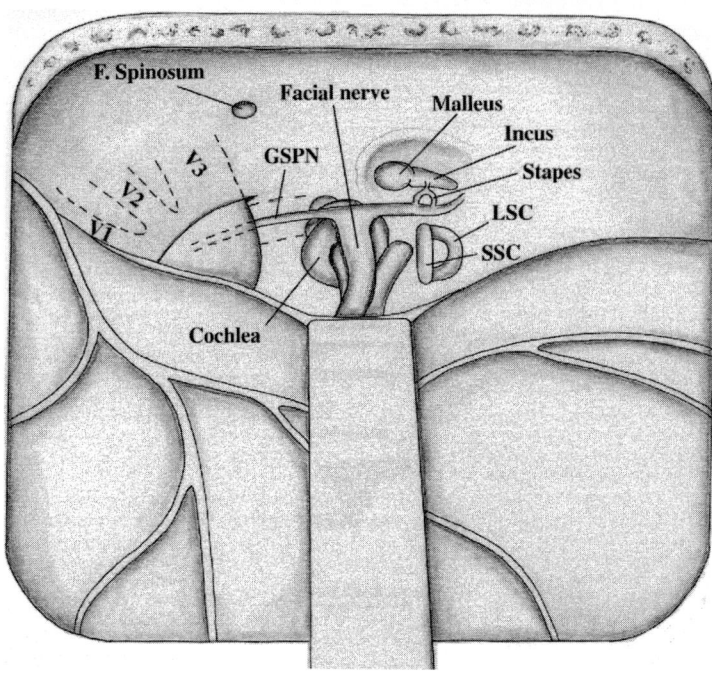

**FIGURE 68–2** ■ Middle fossa approach to the internal auditory canal (IAC). The illustration depicts the facial nerve, geniculate ganglion, and greater superficial petrosal nerve (GSPN). The petrous carotid artery is shown as a *dotted structure* under the GSPN. The tegmen is opened, and the head of the malleus, the incus, and the stapes are seen. Anteriorly, the branches of the trigeminal nerve (V1, V2, V3) are depicted.

geminal ganglion. The GSPN serves as a landmark for the lateral margin of the horizontal segment of the petrous carotid artery. Care should be taken at this stage not to apply force to the floor of the middle fossa because the bone over the carotid artery and the area of the tegmen can be quite thin and even dehiscent in up to 20% of cases.[4] The arcuate eminence is drilled until the dense bone of the SSC is encountered. The SSC is visualized with a bluish hue through the bone, the so-called "blue line." In approximately 15% of cases, however, the arcuate eminence is absent, and in 50% of cases where it is present it is rotated in relationship to the SSC.[10]

Once the key landmarks are identified, localization of the IAC can be accomplished using two key angles. Traditionally, the GSPN-SSC angle (120 degrees)[5] and the SSC-IAC angle (60 degrees)[11] have been used. Unfortunately, these angles have been shown to be quite variable,[9] and in one study the GSPN-SSC angle ranged from 90 to 135 degrees and the SSC-IAC angle from 34 to 75 degrees.[4] Thus, simply relying on angles may lead to inadvertent injury to the SSC and hence loss of hearing. House's technique places the facial nerve at risk because it is this structure that is first identified and followed to the IAC.[2] Fisch's technique places the SSC at risk. Orientation can be aided by removal of the tegmen and identification of the head of the malleus. This can help predict the location of the GG and IAC because these structures are usually colinear, at the expense of risking a CSF leak through the middle ear.[2] None of these techniques is fail-safe, and the best method of localizing the IAC is what the surgeon finds most comfortable in his or her own experience.

Once the IAC is identified, exposure proceeds from lateral to medial until the entire IAC is exposed along its superior surface. A safer technique is to begin medially, exposing first the porus acousticus and then working laterally, taking advantage of the larger margin for error in the region of the porus.[8, 9] At the fundus of the IAC, the vertical crest (Bill's bar), a bone spicule that separates the superior vestibular nerve from the facial nerve, is identified. Finally, the dura over the IAC is opened, first posteriorly over the superior vestibular nerve to avoid facial nerve injury.

In the case of vestibular schwannomas, the tumor can be removed by separating the superior vestibular nerve and tumor away from the facial nerve. The tumor is usually delivered posteriorly away from the facial nerve. Small hooks are necessary to palpate the limits of the IAC and gently free the tumor, particularly its inferolateral portion where the view is especially obscured. The approach carries a higher risk to the facial and cochlear nerves when the tumor less commonly arises from the inferior vestibular nerve. Closure of the IAC defect is accomplished with a small free graft of temporalis muscle.

## Complications and Disadvantages

The middle fossa approach requires retraction of the temporal lobe, and therefore potential injury can occur (e.g., aphasia, hemiparesis, seizure). There is potential for CSF leak through unwaxed air cells or through the middle ear, if the tegmen is opened. Careful hemostasis and tenting sutures can lessen the risk of postoperative hematoma (e.g., epidural hematoma).

As with any temporal bone approach, high-speed drilling can potentially cause injury to the underlying neurovascular structures owing to the vibration and heat from the drill. Using a diamond bur with continuous-suction irrigation lessens this risk.

Specific to the middle fossa approach, during drilling of bone over the facial nerve, there is a small margin for error, and inadvertent injury to the nerve, which is in the most superficial plane of the surgical field, can occur. The SSC, cochlea, and petrous portion of the carotid artery are obvious structures at risk with this approach. Also, the working zone is quite restricted, making this a somewhat technically demanding approach. If major bleeding occurs in the posterior fossa, control may necessitate conversion to a middle fossa transtentorial or to a translabyrinthine approach.

## Extended Middle Fossa Approach—Anterior Petrosectomy

The traditional middle fossa approach works well for lesions in the IAC[2, 3]; however, the exposure is limited. For that reason, extensions of the middle fossa approach have been developed to permit wider access to the petrous apex, clivus, and posterior fossa. The extended middle fossa approach involves a petrous apex resection in addition to the temporal craniotomy described for the middle fossa approach.[12] The horizontal segment of the carotid artery and the cochlea limit the inferior exposure to the level of the inferior petrosal sinus. The TMJ, ossicles, and petrous carotid artery laterally, the trigeminal ganglion anteriorly, and the SSC and vestibule posteriorly represent the limits of the extended middle fossa approach.

### Indications

The anterior petrosectomy provides access to the petrous apex and superior clival region. It provides access to the posterior fossa past the carotid artery and trigeminal and facial nerves. Although the extended middle fossa approach is considered a hearing-preservation approach, it can provide additional exposure in the posterior fossa by sacrificing the SSC and labyrinth, and thus hearing.[12, 13] Sacrifice of the cochlea improves visualization of the lateral extreme of the IAC, medial wall of the tympanic cavity, and the jugular foramen if needed.

This approach permits resection of vestibular schwannomas that extend more medially in the CPA. Meningiomas and chordomas of the anterior CPA and clivus can be resected through this approach, as well as lesions of the petrous apex (i.e., cholesterol granulomas, cholesteatomas, petrositis). Lesions of the petrous carotid artery, posterior cavernous sinus, basilar artery, and anterior brain stem can also be approached.

### Surgical Approach

A temporal craniotomy is performed, similar to the middle fossa approach. Occasionally, a zygomatic osteotomy is added for exposure of the middle fossa floor. The middle meningeal artery, foramen ovale, GSPN, and arcuate eminence are identified. The petrous carotid artery can be exposed at this point by drilling bone along the course of the GSPN (see Fig. 68–2). This area is also known as the posterolateral or Glasscock's triangle.[14] The boundaries of Glasscock's triangle are, laterally, a line extending from the foramen spinosum to the arcuate eminence; medially, the GSPN; and at the base, the third division of the trigeminal nerve (V3). Medial to this triangle is Kawase's or the posteromedial triangle, which consists of the bone in the area of the petrous apex. Drilling this bone provides access to the clivus and the infratentorial compartment.[15] Kawase's

triangle is defined laterally by the GSPN, medially by the petrous ridge, and at the base, by the arcuate eminence. The cochlea represents the posterolateral limit of exposure within Kawase's triangle.

The IAC is identified by one of the means described in the previous section. Once the IAC is identified, bone is removed, exposing the canal widely and the dura of the posterior fossa. The otic capsule bone is particularly dense and lighter in color than the remaining bone of the petrous apex. To identify the cochlea, Miller and colleagues[16] advocate drilling bone along an imaginary line extending from the tip of the vertical crest to the junction of the petrous carotid artery and cranial nerve V3 until the cochlea is identified. With this exposure, the dura along the medial temporal lobe and infratentorially to the level of the inferior petrosal sinus can be exposed. The superior petrosal sinus (SPS) can be clipped and divided. A dural incision can be extended across the SPS and then inferiorly into the posterior fossa. Occasionally, the dura over Meckel's cave is divided to mobilize the trigeminal nerve anteriorly and increase exposure of the petroclival region.

### Complications and Disadvantages

Complications are similar to those with the standard middle fossa approach. Because of the additional bone removal at the petrous apex, potential injury to the carotid artery and trigeminal nerve are possible. The disadvantage of this approach is the rather limited exposure of the posterior fossa. The main advantage of this approach compared with posteriorly based approaches (e.g., translabyrinthine, transcochlear), when used to remove petrous apex lesions, is hearing preservation.

## Middle Fossa Transtentorial Approach

This approach was first reported by Kawase and colleagues[15] in 1985 for approaching aneurysms of the midbasilar artery through the petrous pyramid. In 1991, Kawase and colleagues[17] applied this approach for resection of petroclival meningiomas that extended into the parasellar region (sphenopetroclival meningiomas). This approach uses a combination of the extended middle fossa approach with the addition of intradural resection of the tentorium to allow wider posterior fossa exposure. It is in many ways similar to the subtemporal transtentorial approach, with the added advantage of drilling the anterior petrous ridge.

### Indications

The middle fossa transtentorial exposure can be accomplished with an anterior or posterior petrosectomy or a combined petrosal approach.[12, 17–19] It is suitable for meningiomas extending along the superior and middle clivus or along the posterior wall of the petrous ridge, which can have long dural attachments. Hearing is preserved with this approach, as with all middle fossa approaches. It also permits resection of tumors that extend to the parasellar region and posterior cavernous sinus. It is particularly attractive for small tumors in the petroclival region, laterally located pontine lesions (cavernous malformations, gliomas), or basilar trunk aneurysms. Compared with the extended middle fossa approach, it provides wider posterior fossa exposure because of sectioning of the tentorium.

## Surgical Approach

The extent of petrous pyramid resection is similar to that obtained by the extended middle fossa approach. The dura is opened above and below the SPS. Cranial nerves IV and V are identified. The SPS is clipped between cranial nerves V and VII with care taken to avoid sacrificing the petrosal vein. The tentorium is cut until the tentorial notch is seen. The tentorium can then be tented open with retention sutures, exposing the petroclival region from cranial nerves III through VII.[18] The inferomedial triangle of the cavernous sinus can be visualized, mobilization of the trigeminal nerve can be accomplished by opening Meckel's cave, and Dorello's canal is seen through this exposure.

## Complications and Disadvantages

This approach carries the additional risk of injury to cranial nerve IV as a result of the tentorial incision. Furthermore, the degree of retraction and therefore the risk of possible injury to the temporal lobe may be slightly higher than in the middle fossa or extended middle fossa approaches.

## POSTERIOR TRANSPETROSAL APPROACHES

Most of these approaches involve a certain degree of mastoid resection, positioning the surgical corridor inferior to the middle fossa approaches. There are wide variations among these approaches, although often portions of approaches are used in combination to create more extensive exposure (e.g., presigmoid approach as part of the petrosal approach).

## Retrolabyrinthine Approaches

## Presigmoid Approach

The retrolabyrinthine presigmoid approach was first described by Hitselberger and Pulec[20] in 1972, and was popularized by Silverstein and Norrell[21] in 1977 and by House and associates[22] in 1984. It is performed through the mastoid air cells, with elevation of a dural flap between the labyrinth and the SS. The concept of this procedure is based on its allowing entry into the CPA anterior to the SS, thus lessening the need for cerebellar retraction. It was originally described as being useful for partial sectioning of the fibers of the sensory roots of cranial nerve V for trigeminal neuralgia. It has been used for selective sectioning of the vestibular division of cranial nerve VIII for treatment of vertigo and for endolymphatic duct surgery. It can be used, on occasion, to remove small acoustic tumors in cases in which preservation of hearing is desirable. The major advantage of this approach is that it provides direct access to the CPA without sacrificing hearing and without extensive cerebellar retraction. Its major disadvantage is

the limited exposure, which can be compromised even further by a large dominant SS or when the mastoid air space is contracted ("crowded mastoid").

## Transsigmoid Approach

This approach can be used as part of any posterior transpetrosal approach. Exposure is increased by ligating the SS, usually between the superior and inferior petrosal sinuses or between Labbé's vein and the SPS. Thus, Labbé's vein drains retrograde into the transverse sinus and into the opposite jugular system. A preoperative angiogram or magnetic resonance venogram is essential to ensure patency of the torcular. In general, a nondominant sinus in the presence of a patent torcular can be sacrificed in selected cases. Temporary clipping across the SS is recommended to assess for the presence of temporal lobe or cerebellar swelling. The SS can be opened and packed with Surgicel and its lumen sutured, or it can be ligated and clipped. Cadaver and angiographic studies show that the incidence of unilateral transverse sinus is rather infrequent (2.5%), and absence of any communicatin at the torcular is even rarer.[23, 24] Despite this, given the catastrophic results of ligating a unilateral SS, a preoperative arteriogram or magnetic resonance venogram is recommended.

## Retrosigmoid (Suboccipital) Approach

The retrosigmoid approach, also known as the lateral suboccipital approach, is not a true transtemporal approach. This approach is most familiar to neurosurgeons and has been the traditional exposure used for resection of tumors of the CPA.[25, 26] This approach provides wide entry into the posterior fossa with maximal exposure for tumors such as vestibular schwannomas. Using this approach, the neurovascular structures of the temporal bone are avoided at the expense of cerebellar retraction. The development of monitoring techniques using evoked response methods has greatly increased the practicality of this approach.

### INDICATIONS

Most tumors in the CPA can be approached through a suboccipital craniotomy (i.e., vestibular schwannomas, meningiomas, epidermoids). Cranial nerves V to XI can be visualized with this exposure. Tumors with extension into the petroclival region or with significant spread anterior to the brain stem are not optimally treated with this exposure because of the need for increased cerebellar retraction and a long surgical corridor. This exposure can be combined with other transpetrosal approaches to provide maximal supratentorial and infratentorial exposure for extensive lesions of the CPA.

### SURGICAL APPROACH

This approach can be done with the patient sitting, lateral, or three-fourths prone. An incision is made approximately 2 cm posterior to the mastoid tip, extending cephalad to slightly above the transverse sinus and caudally into the suboccipital musculature. The asterion is a useful landmark for the junction of the transverse and sigmoid sinuses. It represents the crossing of the lambdoid, parietomastoid, and occipitomastoid sutures and it can be palpated as a depression in the bone. A bur hole is placed immediately medial to the asterion, and a craniectomy or "silver-dollar" craniotomy can be performed such that the edges of the transverse and sigmoid sinuses and their junction are clearly identified. In difficult reoperative cases, a line drawn from the root of the zygoma to the inion can reliably locate the course of the transverse sinus.[27] Bone removal can include the posterior lip of the foramen magnum as well as the upper cervical lamina. The arachnoid at the foramen magnum should be opened first to permit CSF egress and facilitate cerebellar retraction.

In the case of vestibular schwannoma resection, the tumor is immediately visualized. The facial nerve usually lies anterior to the tumor. For tumors that extend into the IAC, the porus is drilled until the dura over the IAC is seen. In a cadaver study, the amount of posterior IAC canal that can be safely unroofed averaged 5.9 mm (range, 4 to 8 mm). The best available way to avoid critical labyrinthine structures during the suboccipital approach is to use preoperative high-resolution CT. A line is drawn on axial CT images from the medial aspect of the SS to the fundus of the IAC. If this line crosses any labyrinthine structures, the risk of injury and hearing loss during drilling of the IAC significantly increases.[28]

### COMPLICATIONS AND DISADVANTAGES

This exposure requires a certain amount of cerebellar retraction, and thus cerebellar edema or hematoma can occur. This is especially true for large tumors requiring lengthy surgery. If the surgeon maintains gentle retraction (1 to 2 cm), these types of complications can usually be avoided. Other complications include CSF leak and postoperative incisional pain attributed to adherence of the suboccipital muscles to the dura. The incisional pain can be lessened by either replacing the bone flap in the case of a craniotomy, or performing a cranioplasty to fill the bone defect. The incidence of CSF leak may be lessened by identifying and waxing small air cells in the IAC with the use of an endoscope. In 9% of cases, a high jugular bulb may make drilling of the meatus through the retrosigmoid approach impossible and is associated with increased risk of bleeding and air embolism.[29] As previously mentioned, loss of hearing can occur during drilling of the posterior aspect of the IAC.

## Translabyrinthine Approach

The first report of a translabyrinthine approach was in 1904 by Panse,[30] who advocated this approach for its shortest distance to the CPA. In 1961, William House[3] described the middle fossa approach for resection of vestibular schwannomas located laterally in the IAC with minimal CPA extension. Because of limited exposure, incidence of facial paresis, need for temporal lobe retraction, and limited control of vascular structures, House[31] introduced the translabyrinthine approach for resection of vestibular schwannomas. This was a more lateral approach and gave direct control of the facial nerve by drilling through the labyrinth.

He emphasized the vertical crest (Bill's bar) at the lateral end of the IAC as a landmark. Differentiation between the superior and inferior vestibular nerves was more readily apparent with this approach.

Variations of the translabyrinthine approach have been described for more extensive exposure of the SS with mobilization of the jugular bulb as well as drilling out of the infralabyrinthine air cells to increase access for large tumors.[32] Furthermore, there is evidence that in rare cases hearing preservation may be possible with the "translabyrinthine" approach, such that in one case ablation of all three semicircular canals with preservation of the cochlea and saccule left the patient with useful, although decreased hearing.[33] Another variation of the translabyrinthine approach is the addition of a suboccipital approach with a partial labyrinthectomy, such that only those elements that are required for visualization of Bill's bar and the lateral IAC are removed.[34]

One advantage of the translabyrinthine compared with the middle fossa approach is that after drilling the labyrinth, the tumor is encountered together with the superior and inferior vestibular nerves. Thus, the facial nerve, being anterior, is well protected. This is in contrast to the middle fossa approach, where the facial nerve is immediately beneath the dura. The advantage of the translabyrinthine approach over the suboccipital approach is the lack of cerebellar retraction. Thus, for large tumors when surgery is expected to be long, this approach minimizes the chance of postoperative cerebellar edema, hematoma, or infarction. Its main disadvantage is the added surgical time for the labyrinthectomy and the need for sacrificing hearing.

## Indications

The objective of the translabyrinthine approach is to expose the IAC and CPA through the labyrinth without entering the middle ear. Larger tumors occupying the IAC and CPA can be approached. Hearing and vestibular function are sacrificed by definition. Therefore, it is indicated only in those vestibular schwannomas with nonserviceable hearing (i.e., speech reception threshold >50 db and speech discrimination score <50%). It is an ideal approach for vestibular neurectomy for intractable vertigo when hearing is lost. For patients with normal hearing, this approach is contraindicated.

## Surgical Approach

The patient is positioned supine with the head turned opposite to the side of the tumor. A retroauricular C-shaped skin incision is made and an anteriorly based periosteal flap is elevated and preserved.[35]

A simple mastoidectomy is first accomplished by removing the mastoid cortex from the mastoid tip inferiorly, to the supramastoid crest superiorly, and to the posterior wall of the EAC anteriorly. The SS is visualized and skeletonized to the level of the jugular bulb. The angle between the middle fossa dura above, the posterior fossa dura below, and the SS is called the *sinodural angle*. After exposure of the sinodural angle, the SS and the transverse and superior petrosal sinuses are identified.

The mastoid antrum is then entered and the short process

of the incus in the fossa incudis is identified. This provides a useful landmark for the lateral semicircular canal (LSC), which is found immediately below. The solid angle is located medial to the mastoid antrum and houses the three semicircular canals (Fig. 68–3). The air cells are then removed inferiorly to the level of the digastric groove. The air cells posterior to the LSC are removed and the posterior semicircular canal, located between the LSC and the posterior fossa plate, is exposed. The vertical segment of the facial nerve is then located within the fallopian canal by removing the remaining inferior mastoid and retrofacial air cells. The facial nerve passes from the external genu at the inferior surface of the LSC to the stylomastoid foramen, located just anterior to the digastric ridge. The facial nerve is skeletonized only to facilitate exposure of the jugular bulb and foramen, and it is otherwise left within the dense bone of the fallopian canal. The SSC is identified by following the sinodural angle through the supralabyrinthine air cells. The final area of posterior exposure is removal of the middle, posterior, and sigmoid plates, completing the subtotal petrosectomy. The roughly triangular area of bone bounded by the SS, SPS, and bony labyrinth (i.e., solid angle) is known as *Trautmann's triangle*. This bone is drilled to expose the presigmoid posterior fossa dura.

After the retrofacial air cells, the jugular bulb is exposed next. At this point in the exposure, the tympanic and mastoid segments of the facial nerve mark the anterior limit, the jugular bulb the inferior limit, the SS the inferior limit, and the middle cranial fossa the superior limit of the dissection.

The lateral, posterior, and superior semicircular canals are removed as well as the bone over the posterior fossa,

revealing the endolymphatic sac. Next, the vestibule is opened and completely exposed beneath the facial nerve. Bone is removed over the medial and posterior vestibule until the nerves to the superior, lateral, and inferior ampullas are exposed. These nerves define the superior and inferior limits of the IAC. Bone removal continues over the IAC until a transparent shell remains. The transverse crest separating the superior and inferior division of the vestibular nerves can be seen through the thinned bone.

Identification of the facial nerve is then accomplished by palpation of the vertical crest (Bill's bar). Care should be taken when removing bone from the superior wall of the IAC because the facial nerve is superficial under the dura and can be injured. Once the facial nerve has been skeletonized, the remaining bone over the IAC is removed. The dura over the IAC can then be opened for tumor removal or vestibular neurectomy.

The wound is closed by placing a free muscle graft over the malleus, incus, and attic. To gain access to the middle ear, the facial recess is sometimes opened. The facial recess is a triangular area defined superiorly by the fossa incudis, medially by the facial nerve, and inferiorly by the chorda tympani (see Fig. 68–3). In this situation, a muscle plug is placed to close the opening of the eustachian tube. The cavity is filled with fat graft and the periosteal flap is closed. The skin is closed tightly and a pressure dressing is applied.

## Complications and Disadvantages

The main disadvantage of the translabyrinthine approach is the inadequate exposure of the tentorium, petroclival area,

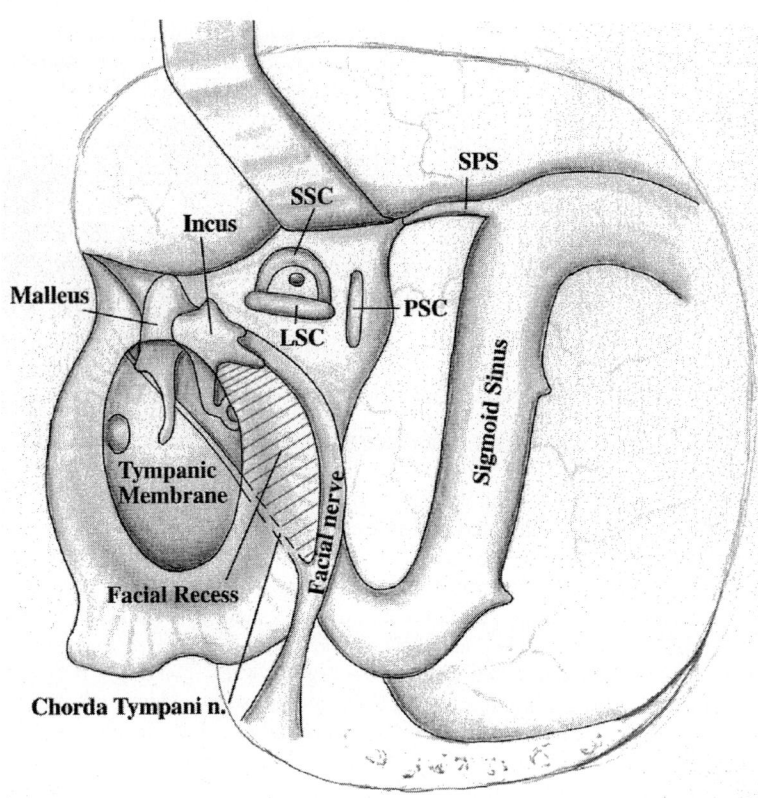

FIGURE 68–3 ■ Basic drawing depicting critical structures of the temporal bone as seen by posterior transmastoid approaches. The solid angle, housing the three semicircular canals, is shown. The facial recess anterior to the facial nerve (hatched area) is illustrated. Opening the facial recess provides access to the middle ear structures, ossicles, and round and oval windows.

and foramen magnum. Thus, for large posterior fossa tumors, especially meningiomas with broad-based tentorial attachment, the translabyrinthine approach by itself is inadequate. Also, it may be difficult to control vascular structures (e.g., anterior inferior cerebellar artery) if inadvertent injury occurs.

The main complication with this approach seems to be a high incidence of CSF leak (up to 30% in some series, usually in the 10% to 20% range).[36] Access to the eustachian tube through the middle ear (facial recess) or the epitympanum can lessen the risk of CSF leak but involves additional exposure and drilling. By placing a free muscle graft over the attic, filling the operative cavity with fat graft, and closing with a periosteal graft, the chance of CSF leak decreases.

In a series from the House Ear Clinic of 166 large (>4 cm) vestibular schwannomas resected using the translabyrinthine approach, complete resection was achieved in 95% of cases with acceptable facial nerve function at 2 years in 75% and good function in 42%.[37] Vascular complications, which included infarct or hematoma, occurred in 4.8%, CSF leak in 9.6%, and meningitis in 8.3%. There were no deaths. Most incidents of meningitis were aseptic and due to blood products or emulsified fat in the posterior fossa from the fat graft.

## Transotic Approach

The transotic approach was developed by Fisch[36] in response to the limitations of the translabyrinthine approach. Unlike the posteriorly directed translabyrinthine approach, the transotic approach permits more extensive temporal bone resection, and positions the dissection both anterior and posterior to the facial nerve, giving excellent visualization of the anterior CPA and petrous apex. The early description included transposition of the facial nerve and had similarities with the transcochlear approach of House and Hitselberger.[38] Unfortunately, the rate of facial nerve paralysis was unacceptable and modifications followed such that the facial nerve is not transposed but left in situ in the fallopian canal.[39, 40]

### Indications

The indication for this approach is essentially identical to that for the translabyrinthine approach. It was designed for vestibular schwannomas up to 2.5 cm in size,[37, 40] although it can certainly be used for larger schwannomas and other lesions, such as meningiomas, hemangiomas, arachnoid cysts, and mucosal cysts, involving the IAC.[41] In contrast to the translabyrinthine approach, the transotic approach circumvents the problem of a high jugular bulb because of the anterior exposure obtained.

This approach may be useful for large vestibular schwannomas because it provides an additional corridor anterior to the facial nerve compared with the translabyrinthine approach. Less extensive petrosectomies (e.g., translabyrinthine) are probably adequate for most vestibular schwannomas. Its other main advantage is the obliteration of the eustachian tube, resulting in a decreased chance for CSF leak.

## Surgical Approach

The surgical approach is similar to the transcochlear approach, with the important difference that the facial nerve is not mobilized (Fig. 68–4). It involves blind sac closure of the EAC, exenteration of the otic capsule including the cochlea, and exposure of the jugular bulb and petrous carotid artery. The additional exposure is obtained by drilling the bone anterior to the tympanic and mastoid segments of the facial nerve. The facial nerve from its entrance into the IAC to its exit at the stylomastoid foramen is exposed, yet remains within bone, thus reducing the potential risk for injury.[40, 41]

## Complications and Disadvantages

The original transotic approach was associated with a high incidence of facial nerve paralysis secondary to transposition of the facial nerve.[37] The modification of leaving the facial nerve within the fallopian canal reduced this risk.[39] In Fisch and Mattox's[40] series of 73 patients, for tumors less than 1.4 cm, all patients had normal facial nerve function at 2 years after surgery. For tumors measuring 1.5 to 2.5 cm, facial nerve function was normal in 61% at 2 years. CSF leak was contained subcutaneously in 4% and was transient in 3%, and no patient required revision. Removal of all of the middle ear mucosa and pneumatic air cells related to the middle ear space, and obliteration of the eustachian tube orifice combined with dural closure and filling of the defect with fat, lessen the chances for CSF leak.[41] In their series, meningitis occurred in 1%, and death in 1%. A disadvantage of this approach is that it adds operative time compared with other procedures (e.g., translabyrinthine approach).

## Transcochlear Approach

In 1976, House and Hitselberger[38] described the transcochlear approach. This approach is a forward extension of the translabyrinthine approach in which the facial nerve is mobilized and the cochlea removed. This exposure essentially removes the entire petrous bone, giving maximal transpetrous exposure.

The operative field given by the transcochlear approach is limited by the EAC canal wall and middle ear, and although more anterior than the translabyrinthine approach, still remains posteriorly directed. The modified transcochlear approach was developed to give additional anterior exposure by removing the EAC and the tympanic membrane.[37] It also offered more extensive exposure and circumferential control of the petrous ICA.[42–46] Some authors also include resection of the glenoid fossa, joint capsule, and meniscus, and partial resection of the posterior aspect of the zygomatic arch.[45] Others combine it with a neck dissection,[47] and some describe extended exposures including tentorial section for supratentorial exposure.[48]

### Indications

This approach was designed for large tumors in the CPA extending anterior to the IAC along the superior two thirds

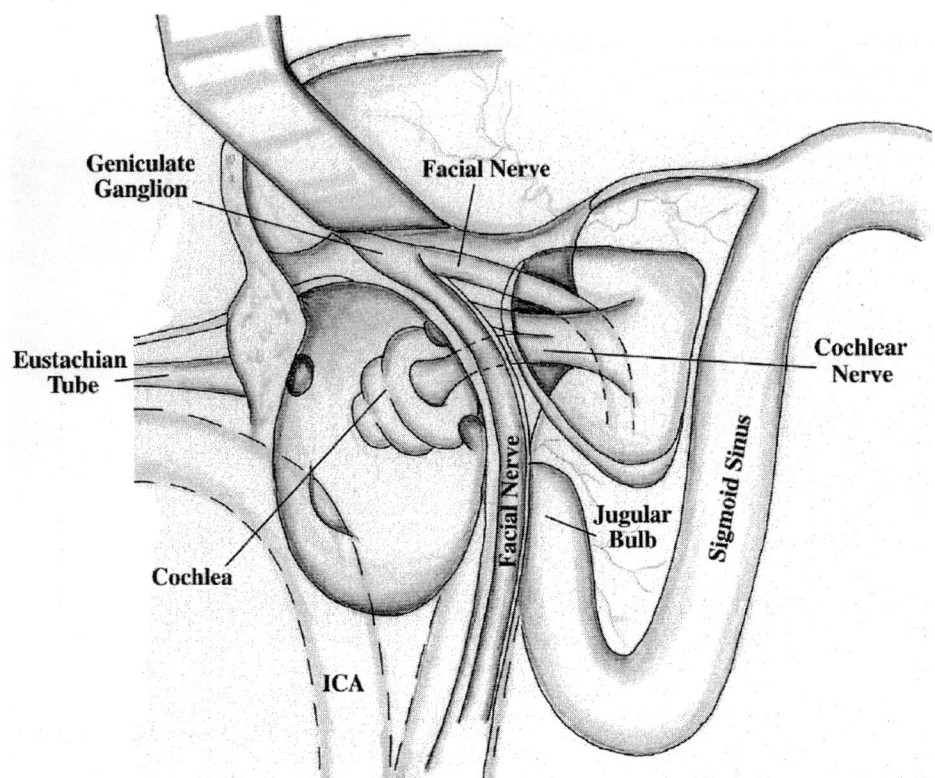

**FIGURE 68–4** ■ Exposure of the temporal bone as seen during a transcochlear approach. The cochlea is shown. The carotid artery is shown anterior and inferior to the cochlea. The facial nerve lies in its canal (not transposed).

of the clivus, as well as for aneurysms of the middle and lower basilar artery. Its main advantage is the broadness of the exposure, giving the surgeon a parallel triangular view of the mid-clivus. The addition of the modified transcochlear approach gives the surgeon a more direct and most laterally directed approach to the CPA, and circumferential exposure of the petrous ICA. This is important for selected cases in which a carotid bypass is required. It can be combined with resection of the mandibular condyle, closure of the EAC, zygomatic osteotomy, and drilling of the floor of the middle cranial fossa for tumors extending into the infratemporal fossa and nasopharynx.

## Surgical Approach

The initial exposure for this approach is similar to that for the translabyrinthine approach. A curvilinear C-shaped retroauricular skin incision is made and the skin of the cartilaginous EAC is everted and sewn shut (see Fig. 68–4). A musculoperiosteal flap from the mastoid process is used medially as a second layer of closure.[45] The skin of the bony EAC and tympanic membrane were initially left in place, but removal of this bone improves access to the midline without increasing morbidity. The entire osseous EAC can be removed without affecting the function of the mandibular condyle in the glenoid fossa.

A mastoidectomy is performed exposing the canal wall inferiorly. The middle and posterior fossa plates along with the SS are then skeletonized. The facial nerve is skeletonized from its entrance into the IAC to its exit from the stylomastoid foramen. The facial recess is opened. The middle ear space and epitympanum are entered and the ossicles can then be removed. In the original description,

the middle ear was not removed.[38] The chorda tympani is then sectioned inferiorly at its origin from the descending portion of the facial nerve. Drilling is continued into the retrofacial air cells. The GSPN is then divided just anterior to its origin at the GG. The facial nerve can then be mobilized from its bony canal and transposed posteriorly. This invariably results is facial nerve paralysis because it disrupts the blood supply to the GG. Obviously, it is best to leave the facial nerve within the canal, if possible. If transposition is necessary, then anterior transposition by mobilizing the mastoid segment and the nerve exiting at the stylomastoid foramen is safer.

Next, the cochlea is removed, including the bony septum between the basal turn and the ICA (see Fig. 68–6). The jugular bulb is also exposed completely. Care should be taken not to injure the underlying neurovascular structures, namely, cranial nerves IX through XI near the jugular bulb and foramen, as well as the facial nerve in the dura of the IAC.

The complete petrosectomy gives exposure from the SPS superiorly to Meckel's cave, and to the inferior petrosal sinus and jugular bulb inferiorly. The osseous removal extends anteriorly to the petrous carotid artery and TMJ, and medially to the clivus. The dura is opened in a triangular manner parallel to the SPS, inferior petrosal sinus, and SS, to the IAC. It can also be opened on both sides of the IAC. This exposes the CPA widely.

## Complications and Disadvantage

The main disadvantage of this approach is that hearing is sacrificed. The extensive mobilization of the facial nerve places it at risk, and most patients have a significant facial nerve paralysis. Although it usually improves after surgery, facial nerve function infrequently exceeds grade III on the House/Brackmann grading scale, and the nerve often is permanently impaired. Section of the GSPN can result in an ipsilateral dry eye. There is also a risk of CSF leak and meningitis. Resection of the mandibular condyle can result in TMJ dysfunction.

## Infralabyrinthine Approach

### Indications

In 1985, Gherini and coworkers[49] advocated the infralabyrinthine approach for the surgical management of cholesterol granulomas of the petrous apex and CPA. The purpose of this approach is to permit access to that portion of the petrous apex that is inferior to the labyrinth. As such, it is valuable in decompression of a cholesterol granuloma of the petrous apex. It can also be useful in conjunction with the suboccipital approach for resection of meningiomas of the petrous ridge with extension into the temporal bone, but without involvement of the labyrinth; hearing is therefore preserved.[47, 49]

### Surgical Approach

In this approach, a simple mastoidectomy is first performed. The middle and posterior fossa plates along with the SS are then skeletonized. At this point, the posterior and horizontal semicircular canals can be identified and protected. The facial nerve is identified and skeletonized along its mastoid segment and left in its bony canal. A communication between the labyrinth superiorly and the jugular bulb inferiorly is then developed until the petrous apex is entered. The bulb may be skeletonized and its superior portion carefully dissected to free it of its adjacent bony covering. It is then packed inferiorly with bone wax so that additional exposure is obtained. In the case of a cholesterol granuloma, on opening the cavity, drainage of dark, thick fluid, sometimes under pressure, occurs. Cultures are obtained and the opening into the cavity is widened to approximately 0.5 to 1 cm to provide permanent drainage.

### Complications and Disadvantages

If the jugular bulb is high in position, access below the labyrinth and above the bulb can be limited. A careful preoperative evaluation using high-resolution CT is useful.[28, 29] Measuring the distance between the labyrinth and jugular bulb on coronal images can be particularly useful; a distance of less than 1 cm was found to be inadequate for satisfactory drainage of cholesterol granulomas.[50] In those instances, another approach is recommended (e.g., transcanal-infracochlear; see later).

Other complications include injury to the facial nerve, carotid artery, jugular bulb, and labyrinth. Obviously, the opening made for drainage of the cholesterol granuloma may scar and the granuloma may recur.

## Transcanal-Infracochlear Approach

The transcanal part of the approach was first described by Farrior[52] in 1984.

### Indications

This approach is used for access to the petrous apex in cases where hearing preservation is a goal and the jugular bulb is positioned high, limiting exposure through an infralabyrinthine approach. Because this approach is directed cephalad, it provides dependent drainage for cholesterol granulomas of the petrous apex. In addition, the drainage is to a well aerated region near the eustachian tube.

### Surgical Approach

The transcanal-infracochlear approach uses a C-shaped retroauricular skin incision similar to that used for the translabyrinthine and infralabyrinthine approaches. The soft tissues are reflected forward and the ear canal is transected just medial to the bony cartilaginous junction. The anterior, inferior, and posterior portions of the ear canal skin are lifted superiorly to the level of the umbo. Bone is removed from over the anterior, inferior, and posterior portions of the bony canal wall, effectively achieving near-total removal of the tympanic bone and enlargement of the canal. The thin bone over the TMJ is preserved. The carotid artery is then skeletonized anterior and inferior to the eustachian tube orifice. Bone is then removed from between the ICA and internal jugular vein without actually exposing the jugular bulb. The region of the facial nerve is identified using continuous electrical monitoring, but the nerve is not exposed. Inferiorly, the cholesterol granuloma sac is identified, opened for drainage, and irrigated.

### Complications and Disadvantages

The complications are similar to those with the translabyrinthine approach except that injury to the cochlea, carotid artery, and jugular bulb is possible. This approach provides only limited exposure of the petrous apex, and therefore is useful only in the specific indications of drainage of a cholesterol granuloma or petrous apicitis.

# COMBINED APPROACHES

## Petrosal Approach

The petrosal approach is also referred to as the *combined suprainfratentorial approach* because it combines both supratentorial and infratentorial exposures to give wide anterior access to the CPA and ventral brain stem. The first reported transtentorial exposure was in 1896 by Stieglitz and colleagues,[53] in which a CPA tumor was approached through a supramastoid-suboccipital exposure. Several authors followed with modifications of the occipital flap with a suboccipital craniectomy, including ligation of the SS for wider exposure,[54] combined occipitotemporal craniotomy with or without ligation of the lateral sinus[55] and reapproximation of the lateral sinus,[56] and other approaches,[57, 58] including the addition of a mastoidectomy.[59, 60]

The petrosal approach was popularized by Malis,[60] who described ligation of the SS between its junction with the vein of Labbé and the SPS for increased exposure. Spetzler and colleagues[61] operated on 83 patients with the petrosal approach and sacrificed the SS in 50% of cases. Al-Mefty and colleagues[62] described the petrosal approach in detail, emphasizing an extensive petrous resection and directing the approach more laterally, thus lessening the operative distance to the clivus. They also stressed the importance of preserving the venous sinuses.

## Indications

The petrosal approach includes a combined temporal craniotomy with a posterior fossa craniectomy/craniotomy for supratentorial and infratentorial exposure. Crucial to this approach is sectioning of the tentorium. With the addition of an extensive petrous resection, the anterior surface of the brain stem can be approached to the level of the inferior one third of the clivus. The lowest portion of the clivus is often obscured by the jugular tubercle. The petrosal approach provides access to lesions in the CPA and petroclival junction (upper two thirds of the clivus) such as meningiomas, trigeminal schwannomas, epidermoids, or chondrosarcomas. For lesions of the lower one third of the clivus and the foramen magnum, the far lateral transcondylar approach provides better access.

## Surgical Approach

The patient is placed in a lateral position. The incision begins approximately 1 cm anterior to the ear and is directed posteriorly in a gentle curve to the postauricular area approximately 2 cm posterior to the mastoid process. The temporalis fascia and muscle are elevated and reflected anteriorly on a pedicle.

A mastoidectomy is first accomplished with preservation of the labyrinth and exposure of the mastoid segment of the facial nerve. A combined temporo-occipital bone flap is then raised (Fig. 68–5). The transverse and sigmoid sinuses have been previously identified during the mastoidectomy. This gives exposure along the middle fossa floor, transverse and sigmoid sinuses, and suboccipital dura. The dura can then be opened on the inferior aspect of the temporal lobe, and anterior or posterior to the SS. After opening the dura over the temporal lobe and the presigmoid dura, the SPS is clipped and divided. The tentorium can be divided in three different directions (Fig. 68–6). The first cut is done posteriorly along the transverse sinus to allow for retraction of the transverse-sigmoid sinus junction posteriorly, thus increasing the presigmoid corridor. The second cut is aimed medially toward the free edge to identify and protect the trochlear nerve. The third cut is parallel to the petrous pyramid and the SPS. This allows resection of the lateral tentorial leaflet and view of the supratentorial and infratentorial compartments. Ipsilateral cranial nerves IV through X are well visualized (Fig. 68–7). A retractor can be placed to retract the temporal lobe superiorly and another one to retract the transverse and sigmoid sinuses

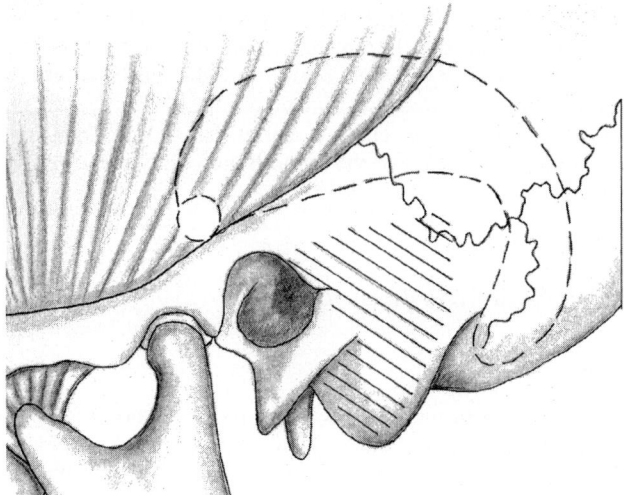

**FIGURE 68–5** ■ The petrosal approach. Outline of the craniotomy *(interrupted line)* and mastoidectomy *(hatched area).* The asterion and external auditory canal are shown.

posteriorly. If the surgeon decides to work through the retrosigmoid corridor, a cerebellar retractor can be placed. Care must be taken to avoid injury to the vein of Labbé. In certain cases, the presigmoid avenue is limited and ligation and division of the SS can provide maximum anterior exposure of the CPA.

Wound closure begins with reapproximation of the dura. A dural defect usually remains after suturing. Any opened air cells are waxed. The mastoid antrum is sealed with fascia or muscle and an autologous fat graft is used to fill the petrosectomy defect. Alternatively or additionally, the posterior temporalis vascularized flap can be used to cover the petrosectomy defect to prevent CSF leak. The inner table from the craniotomy can be shaped and anchored with miniplates for a more cosmetic mastoid appearance. Spinal drainage can be used for several days after surgery depending on preference.

## Complications and Disadvantages

Typical complications as described previously for any intracranial approach may be encountered. In addition, there is potential for injury to the sinuses and for significant blood loss and air embolism, if that occurs. Specific to this approach is the potential for injury to the vein of Labbé, which provides significant venous drainage to the temporal lobe. Hence, edema and venous infarction are a possibility. During drilling of the petrous apex, injury to the semicircular canals (especially the posterior one) and facial nerve may occur.

## Infratemporal Fossa Approach

The infratemporal fossa approach, developed by Fisch[63] in 1977, is a craniotemporocervical approach for exposure of the lateral inferior skull base. This approach is divided into three exposures, types A, B, or C, depending on the amount of anterior exposure required. The type A approach is similar to the combined lateral skull base approach reported

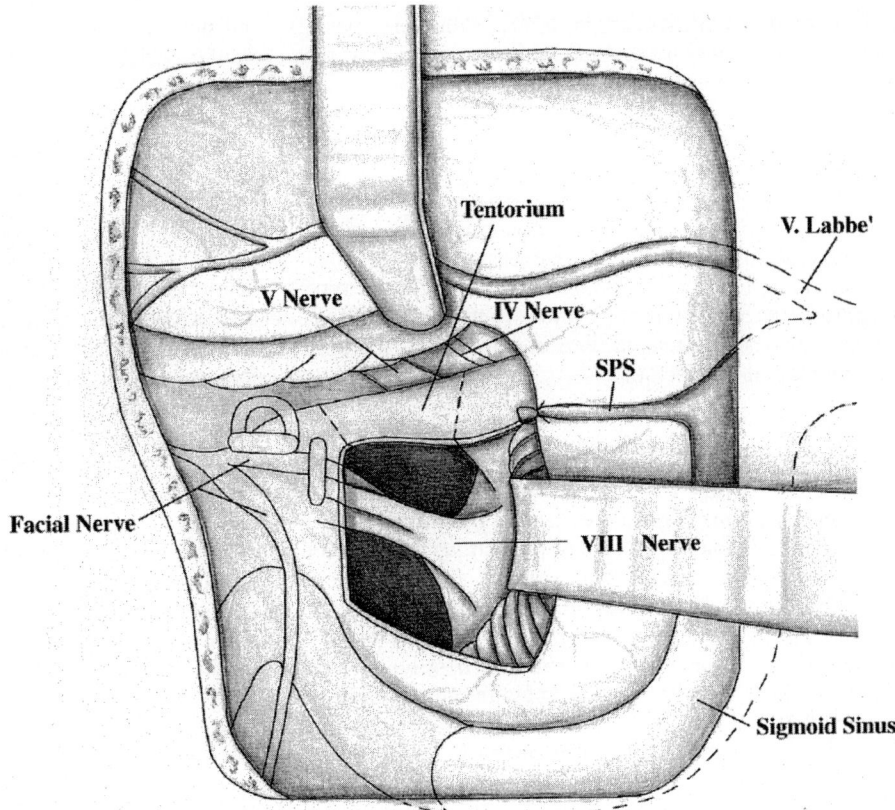

**FIGURE 68–6** ■ An artist's drawing of the exposure obtained by the petrosal approach. Two retractors (one superiorly and another posteriorly) elevate the temporal lobe and the cerebellum, respectively. The superior petrosal sinus is ligated. The vestibulocochlear nerve bundle as well as the facial nerve are shown as they course toward the internal auditory nerve. The semicircular canals are also shown. The tentorium is cut in three directions—one anterior parallel to the petrous pyramid; another medially toward the free edge (cranial nerves IV and V are shown medially); and one posteriorly along the transverse sinus (not shown here).

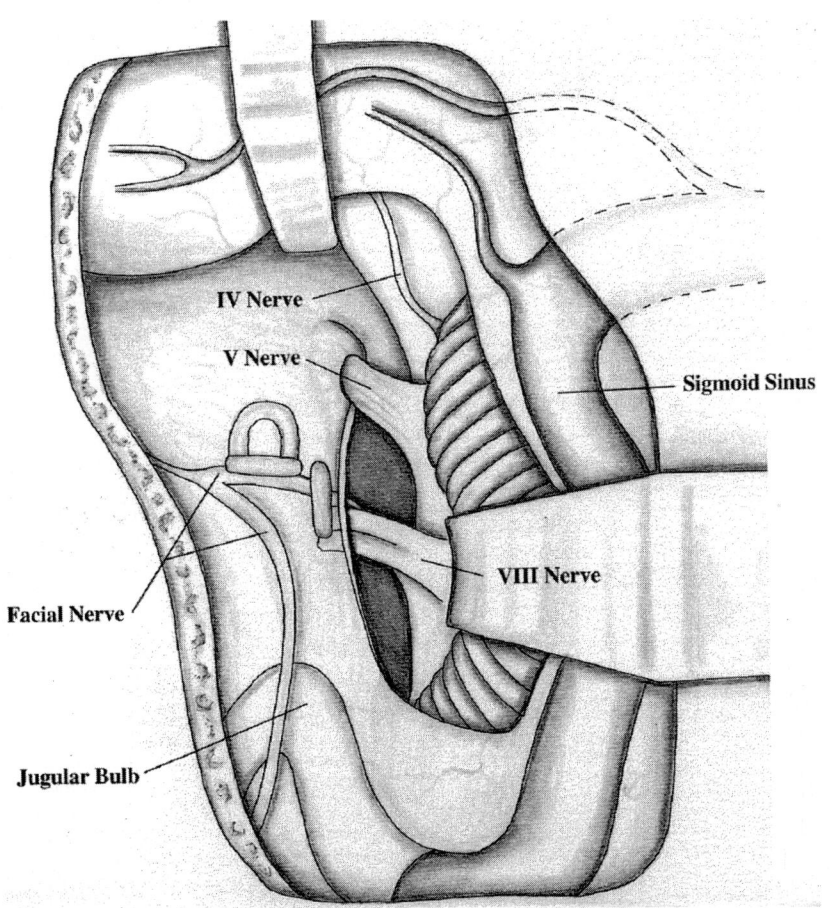

**FIGURE 68–7** ■ The petrosal approach. The presigmoid retrolabyrinthine corridor is shown. Exposure is obtained after sectioning the tentorium. The trochlear, trigeminal, facial, and vestibulocochlear nerves are seen.

by Gardner and colleagues[64] in 1977. With the type A exposure, a subtotal petrosectomy with transposition of the facial nerve is accomplished for exposure of the apical and infralabyrinthine temporal bone as well as the mandibular fossa and posterior infratemporal fossa. The type B exposure gives additional exposure of the clivus and horizontal segment of the ICA. The type C approach is an anterior extension of the type B approach, giving exposure of the infratemporal fossa, pterygopalatine fossa, parasellar region, and nasopharynx. With most indications for the type C approach, the surgeon can use a more anterior, preauricular pterional type of incision with a zygomatic osteotomy and subtemporal craniectomy.[65]

## Indications

According to Fisch,[63] the type A approach is useful for lesions involving the jugular foramen (e.g., class C and D glomus jugulare tumors), lesions of the petrous apex, lower cranial nerve schwannomas, high cervical and petrous carotid artery lesions, and certain infratemporal fossa lesions. The type B approach is indicated for lesions of the petrous apex and clivus. The type C approach is best for lesions such as juvenile nasopharyngeal angiofibroma and nasopharyngeal carcinoma, or those involving the pterygopalatine fossa, cavernous sinus, and nasopharynx.

## Surgical Approach

The details of these approaches have been elegantly described by Fisch[66] and are summarized here. The skin incision is an extension of the standard C-shaped retroauricular incision. The skin and periosteal flap is reflected anteriorly with transection and closure of the EAC. Next the great vessels (carotid artery, jugular vein) and nerves of the neck (glossopharyngeal, vagus, spinal accessory, and hypoglossal) are exposed (Fig. 68–8). The posterior belly of the digastric muscle is divided near its insertion at the mastoid process. The external carotid artery and its branches are ligated and transected above the lingual artery. The ICA is followed to the carotid foramen. Next, a subtotal petrosectomy is done by exposing the temporal bone and reflecting the sternocleidomastoid muscle away from the mastoid tip. The operation proceeds with removal of the EAC, mastoidectomy with complete mobilization of the facial nerve for anterior transposition, exposure, and possible ligation of the SS, removal of the styloid process for exposure of the ICA, obliteration of the eustachian tube, and exposure of the infratemporal fossa. This includes anterior translocation of the mandible. The exposure obtained with this approach spans from the middle ear, mastoid, and upper neck, exposing the posterior portion of the infratemporal fossa.

The type B approach includes exposure of the ICA from the neck to the cavernous sinus. To expose the horizontal segment of the ICA, the middle meningeal artery is divided and the eustachian tube is sacrificed. By sacrificing the eustachian tube at this point and preserving the middle ear cleft, hearing can be preserved. The approach to the clivus requires division of cranial nerve V3 and complete removal of the bony eustachian tube.

The type C approach adds anterior exposure to the type

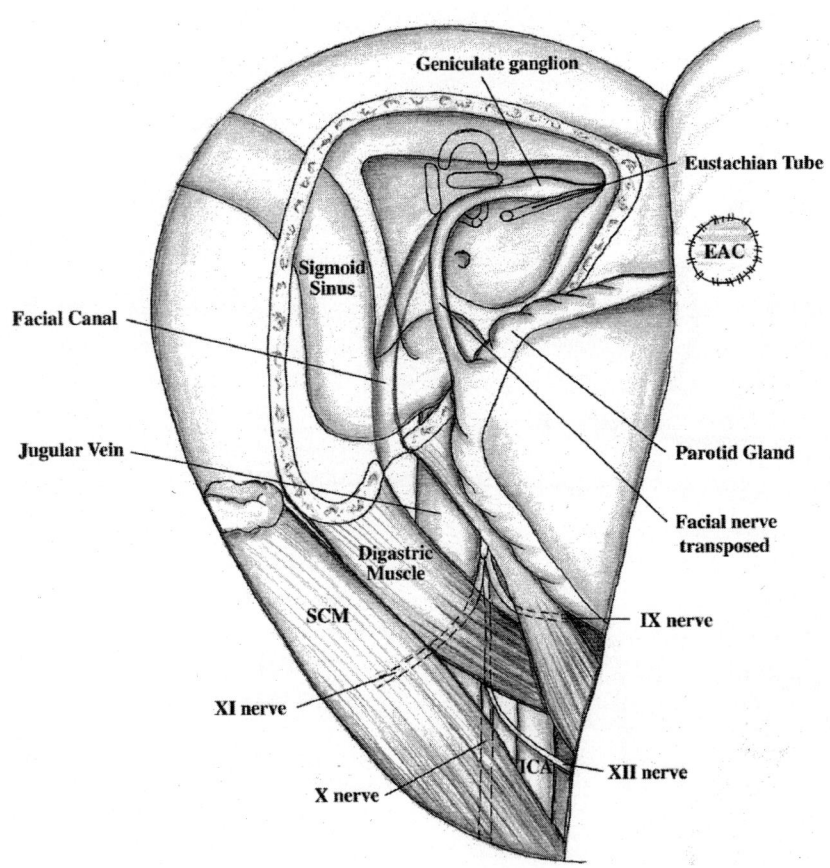

FIGURE 68–8 ■ Exposure is obtained by an infratemporal fossa approach type A. The sternocleidomastoid muscle (SCM) and posterior belly of the digastric muscle are shown. Cranial nerves IX, X, XI, and XII are shown in the neck. The external auditory canal, malleus, and incus have been removed. The facial nerve has been transposed anteriorly.

B approach. The nasopharynx can be entered by removing the lateral pharyngeal wall behind the medial pterygoid process. Exposure here gives visualization of the vomer, opposite inferior turbinate, and pharyngeal end of the opposite eustachian tube. The pterygopalatine fossa is exposed by removing the pterygoid process. To expose the parasellar region, the zygoma and basal portion of the sphenoid are removed. The ipsilateral sphenoid and maxillary sinus are opened. For complete exposure of the cavernous sinus, the maxillary nerve is divided and the bone at the floor of the middle fossa is removed for extradural elevation of the temporal lobe.

We have used a combination of middle fossa and infratemporal fossa approaches for treating en plaque meningiomas of the temporal bone (Fig. 68–9). This particular combination of approaches is a logical extension of either individual approach when both areas are involved pathologically. This approach could be of value in providing wider access to the petrous carotid artery.

## Complications and Disadvantages

According to Fisch and Mattox,[66] transposition of the facial nerve always results in some paresis, but the average recovery of function (to House/Brackmann grade II) was 80%. A conductive hearing loss is common in all infratemporal fossa approaches because of removal of the tympanic membrane and ossicles. Tachycardia can occur after removal of glomus jugulare tumors. Preoperative laboratory evaluation of suspected glomus tumors should include blood vanillylmandelic acid levels and possible use of α-adrenergic blockers. With the additional exposure of the eustachian

tube, ascending infection can occur even with subsequent primary closure of the eustachian tube. CSF leaks and meningitis can obviously occur. Fisch and Mattox[66] recommend obliteration of the wound with muscle rather than free fat graft to aid in closure of the eustachian tube. For the type C approach, the major risks include hearing loss, which occurs in most, and loss of mandibular function as a result of translocation of the mandibular condyle and resection of the articular disk and glenoid fossa during exposure. Initially there may be limitation in jaw opening, but this eventually resolves. Resection of cranial nerves V2 and V3 usually results in facial and tongue anesthesia; this generally improves over 9 months.[66]

## SUMMARY

The ability to approach the posterior cranial fossa in a variety of ways is advantageous because it allows the neurosurgeon more options to reach and treat tumors in this area. The ability to drill away selected segments of the temporal bone, without major sacrifice of function, to achieve access for surgical procedures presents a continuing and exciting challenge to both neurosurgeons and their otologic colleagues.

## ACKNOWLEDGMENT

*Portions of this chapter are reproduced with permission from Brodkey J, Vrionis FD: Surgical approaches through the temporal bone. In Robertson JT, Coakham H,*

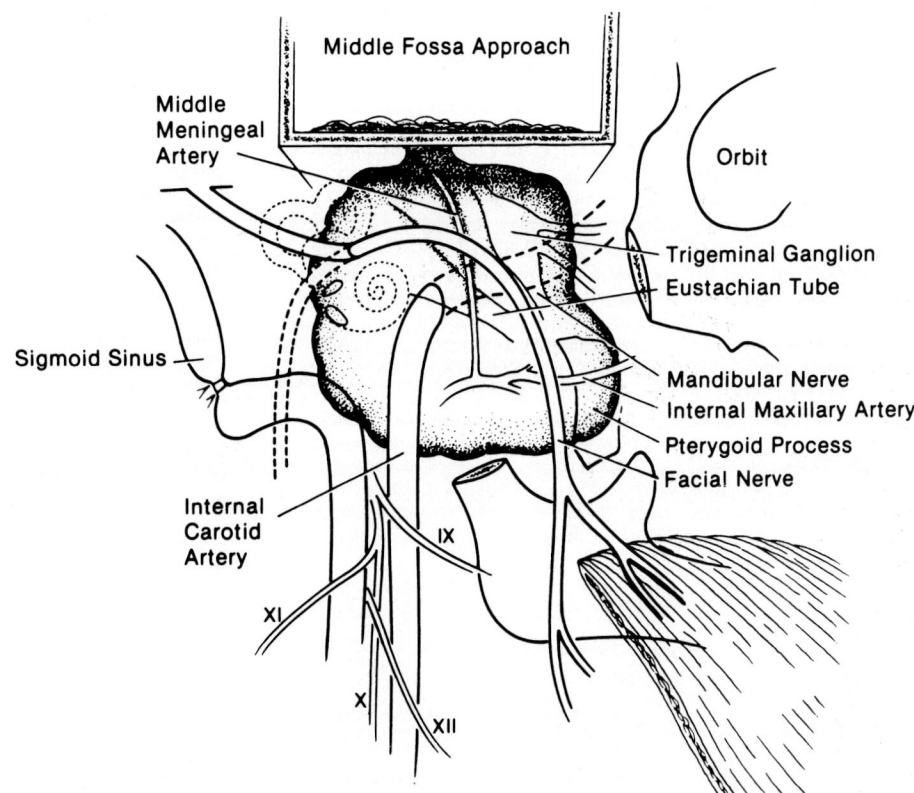

FIGURE 68–9 ■ Combined middle fossa–infratemporal fossa approach. Adjacent structures are shown. The facial nerve is displaced, and the internal carotid artery is exposed. (From Gardner G, et al: Transtemporal approaches to the posterior cranial fossa. Am J Otol [Suppl]:118, 1985.)

*Robertson JH (eds): Cranial Base Surgery: Management, Complications and Outcome. Edinburgh: Churchill Livingstone, in press.*

## REFERENCES

1. Parry RH: A case of tinnitus and vertigo treated by division of the auditory nerve. Laryngology 19:402–406, 1904.
2. House WF: Middle cranial fossa approach to the petrous pyramid: A report of 50 cases. Arch Otolaryngol 78:406–469, 1963.
3. House WF: Surgical exposure of the internal auditory canal and its contents through the middle cranial fossa. Laryngoscope 71:1363–1385, 1961.
4. Aristegui M, Cokkeser Y, Saleh E, et al: Surgical anatomy of the extended middle fossa approach. Skull Base Surg 4:181–188, 1994.
5. Garcia-Ibanez E, Garcia-Ibanez JL: Middle fossa vestibular neurectomy: A report of 373 cases. Otolaryngol Head Neck Surg 88:486–490, 1980.
6. Vrionis FD, Robertson JH, Foley KT, et al: Image-interactive orientation in the middle cranial fossa approach to the internal auditory canal: An experimental study. Comput Aided Surg 2:34–41, 1997.
7. Vrionis FD, Foley KT, Robertson JH, et al: Use of cranial surface anatomic fiducials for interactive image-guided navigation in the temporal bone: A cadaveric study. Neurosurgery 40:755–764, 1997.
8. Brackmann DE: Middle fossa approach for acoustic tumor removal. Clin Neurosurg 38:603–618, 1990.
9. Parisier SC: The middle cranial fossa approach to the internal auditory canal: An anatomic study stressing critical distances between surgical landmarks. Laryngoscope 87 (Suppl):1–19, 1977.
10. Kartush JM, Kemink JL, Graham MD: The arcuate eminence, topographic orientation in middle cranial fossa surgery. Ann Otol Rhinol Laryngol 94:25–28, 1985.
11. Fisch U, Mattox D: Transtemporal supralabyrinthine approach. In Fisch U, Mattox D (eds): Microsurgery of the Skull Base. New York: Thieme, 1988, pp 418–454.
12. Shiobara R, Ohira T, Kanzaki J, et al: A modified extended middle cranial fossa approach for acoustic tumors: Results of 125 operations. J Neurosurg 68:358–365, 1988.
13. King TI: Combined translabyrinthine-transtentorial approach to acoustic nerve tumors. Proc R Soc Med 63:780–782, 1970.
14. Glasscock ME: Middle fossa approach to the temporal bone. Arch Otolaryngol 90:41–53, 1969.
15. Kawase T, Toya S, Shiobara S, et al: Transpetrosal approach for aneurysms of the lower basilar artery. J Neurosurg 63:857–861, 1985.
16. Miller CG, van-Loveren HR, Keller JT, et al: Tranpetrosal approach: Surgical anatomy and technique. Neurosurgery 33:461–469, 1993.
17. Kawase T, Shiobara R, Toya S: Anterior tranpetrosal-transtentorial approach for sphenopetroclival meningiomas: Surgical method and results in 10 patients. Neurosurgery 28:869–876, 1991.
18. Kawase T, Shiobara R, Toya S: Middle fossa transpetrosal-transtentorial approaches for petroclival meningiomas: Selective pyramid resection and radicality. Acta Neurochir (Wien) 129:113–120, 1994.
19. Megerian CA, Chiocca EA, McKenna MJ, et al: The subtemporal-transpetrous approach for excision of petroclival tumors. Am J Otol 17:773–779, 1996.
20. Hitselberger WE, Pulec JL: Trigeminal nerve (posterior root) retrolabyrinthine selective section: Operative procedure for intractable pain. Arch Otolaryngol 96:412, 1972.
21. Silverstein H, Norrell H: Retrolabyrinthine surgery: A direct approach to the cerebellopontine angle. In Silverstein H, Norrell H (eds): Neurological Surgery of the Ear. Birmingham, AL: Aesculapius, 1977, pp 318–340.
22. House JW, Hitselberger WE, McElveen J, et al: Retrolabyrinthine section of the vestibular nerve. Otolaryngol Head Neck Surg 92:212–215, 1984.
23. Vrionis FD, Robertson JH, Heilman CB, et al: Asterion meningiomas. Skull Base Surg 8:153–161, 1998.
24. Durgun B, Ilglt ET, Cizmeli MO, et al: Evaluation by angiography of the lateral dominance of the drainage of the dural venous sinuses. Surg Radiol Anat 15:125–130, 1993.
25. Cushing H: Tumors of the Nervus Acousticus and the Syndrome of the Cerebellopontine Angle. New York: Hafner, 1917, pp 296–306.
26. Dandy WE: Operation for total extirpation of tumors in the cerebellopontine angle. Bull Johns Hopkins Hosp 33:344–355, 1922.
27. Day JD, Kellog JX, Tschabitscher M, et al: Surface and superficial surgical anatomy of the posterolateral cranial base: Significance for surgical planning and approach. Neurosurgery 38:1079–1084, 1996.
28. Yokoyama T, Uemura K, Ryu H, et al: Surgical approach to the internal auditory meatus in acoustic neuroma surgery: Significance of preoperative high-resolution computed tomography. Neurosurgery 39:965–970, 1996.
29. Shao KN, Tatagiba M, Samii M: Surgical management of high jugular bulb in acoustic neurinoma via retrosigmoid approach. Neurosurgery 32:32–37, 1993.
30. Panse R: Ein Gliom des Akustikus. Arch Ohrenheilkd 61:251–255, 1904.
31. House WF: Transtemporal bone microsurgical removal of acoustic neuromas. Arch Otolaryngol 80:599–756, 1964.
32. Naguib MB, Saleh E, Cokkeser Y, et al: The enlarged translabyrinthine approach for removal of large vestibular schwannomas. J Laryngol Otol 108:545–550, 1994.
33. McElveen JT, Wilkins RH, Erwin AC, et al: Modifying the translabyrinthine approach to preserve hearing during acoustic tumour surgery. J Laryngol Otol 105:34–37, 1991.
34. Feghali JG, Kantrowitz AB: Transcranial translabyrinthine approach to vestibular schwannomas. J Laryngol Otol 107:111–114, 1993.
35. Fisch U, Mattox D: Tranlabyrinthine approach. In Fisch U, Mattox D (eds): Microsurgery of the Skull Base. New York: Thieme, 1988, pp 546–576.
36. Fisch U, Mattox D: Transotic approach to the cerebellopontine angle. In Fisch U, Mattox D (eds): Microsurgery of the Skull Base. New York: Thieme, 1988, pp 75–98.
37. Briggs RJS, Luxford WM, Atkins JS, Hitselberger WE: Translabyrinthine removal of large acoustic neuromas. Neurosurg 34:785–792, 1994.
38. House WF, Hitselberger WE: The transcochlear approach to the skull base. Arch Otolaryngol 102:334–342, 1976.
39. Gantz BJ, Fisch U: Modified transotic approach to the cerebellopontine angle. Arch Otolaryngol 109:252–256, 1983.
40. Fisch U, Mattox D: Transotic approach to the cerebellopontine angle. In Fisch U, Mattox D (eds): Microsurgery of the Skull Base. New York: Thieme, 1988, pp 74–127.
41. Browne JD, Fisch U: Transotic approach to the cerebellopontine angle. Otol Clin North Am 25:331–346, 1992.
42. Sanna M, Mazzoni A, Saleh EA, et al: Lateral approaches to the median skull base through the petrous bone: The system of the modified transcochlear approach. J Laryngol Otol 108:1036–1044, 1994.
43. De La Cruz A: The transcochlear approach to meningiomas and cholesteatomas of the cerebellopontine angle. In Brackmann DE (ed): Neurological Surgery of the Ear and Skull Base. New York: Raven Press, 1982, pp 353–360.
44. Sekhar LN, Estonillo R: Transtemporal approach to the skull base: An anatomical study. Neurosurgery 19:799–808, 1986.
45. Horn KL, Hankinson HL, Erasmus MD, et al: The modified transcochlear approach to the cerebellopontine angle. Otolaryngol Head Neck Surg 104:37–41, 1991.
46. Sanna M, Mazzoni A, Gamoletti R: The system of the modified transcochlear approaches to the petroclival area and the prepontine cistern. Skull Base Surg 6:237–248, 1996.
47. Gardner G, Robertson JH, Clark C: Transtemporal approaches to the cranial cavity. Am J Otol vol 6(Suppl):114–120, 1985.
48. Thedinger BA, Glasscock ME, Cueva RA: Transcochlear transtentorial approach for removal of large cerebellopontine angle meningiomas. Am J Otol 13:408–415, 1992.
49. Gherini SG, Brackmann DE, Lo WWM, et al: Cholesterol granuloma of the petrous apex. Laryngoscope 95:659–664, 1985.
50. Brodkey JA, Robertson JH, Shea JJ, et al: Cholesterol granulomas of the petrous apex: Combined neurosurgical and otological management. J Neurosurg 85:625–633, 1996.
51. Giddings NA, Brackmann DE, Kwartler JA: Transcanal infracochlear approach to the petrous apex. Otolaryngol Head Neck Surg 104:29–41, 1991.
52. Farrior JB: Anterior hypotympanic approach for glomus tumor of the infratemporal fossa. Laryngoscope 94:1016–1020, 1984.
53. Stieglitz L, Gerster AG, Lilienthal H: A study of three cases of tumor of the brain in which operation was performed: One recovery, two deaths. Am J Med Sci 111:509–531, 1896.

54. Naffziger HC. Brain surgery with special reference to exposure of the brainstem and posterior fossa: The principle of intracranial decompression, and the relief of impactions in the posterior fossa. Surg Gynecol Obstet 46:241–248, 1928.
55. Fay T: The management of tumors of the posterior fossa by a transtentorial approach. Surg Clin North Am 10:1427–1459, 1930.
56. Bailey P: Concerning the technique of operation for acoustic neurinoma. Zentralbl Neurochir 4:1–5, 1939.
57. Samii M, Ammirati M, Mahran A, et al: Surgery of petroclival meningiomas: Report of 24 cases. Neurosurgery 24:12–17, 1989.
58. Tarlov E. Surgical management of tumors of the tentorium and clivus. In Schmidek HH, Sweet WH (eds): Operative Neurosurgical Techniques: Indications, Methods, and Results, Vol 1. New York: Grune & Stratton, 1977, pp 381–388.
59. Malis LI: Surgical resection of tumors of the skull base. Neurosurgery 1:1011–1021, 1985.
60. Malis LI: The petrosal approach. Clin Neurosurg 37:528–540, 1991.
61. Spetzler RF, Hamilton MG, Daspit CP: Petroclival lesions. Clin Neurosurg 41:62–82, 1994.
62. Al-Mefty O, Fox JL, Smith RR: Petrosal approach for petroclival meningiomas. Neurosurgery 22:510–517, 1988.
63. Fisch U: Infratemporal fossa approach to tumors of the temporal bone and base of the skull. J Laryngol Otol 92:949–967, 1978.
64. Gardner G, Cocke EW, Robertson JT, et al: Combined approach surgery for removal of glomus jugulare tumors. Laryngoscope 87:665–688, 1977.
65. Vrionis FD, Cano W, Heilman CB: Microsurgical anatomy of the infratemporal fossa as viewed laterally and superiorly. Neurosurgery 39:777–786, 1996.
66. Fisch U, Mattox D: In Fisch U, Mattox D (eds): Microsurgery of the Skull Base. New York: Thieme, 1988, pp 136–388.

# Posterior Fossa Tumors

# Surgical Management of Cerebellar Infarction and Cerebellar Hemorrhage

■ ANTONINO RACO

The management of patients with cerebellar infarction or cerebellar hemorrhage remains controversial.[1–59] Before the introduction of computed tomography (CT), the differential diagnosis between the two entities, on clinical grounds alone, was prohibitively difficult.[60–66] Because the coexistence or preponderance of signs and symptoms of brain stem compression further complicate the clinical presentation, diagnosis was frequently possible only at post mortem examination.

The treatment of vascular cerebellar syndromes, particularly hemorrhage, is not a new topic.[67–71] Yet only recently, thanks to the advent of CT and subsequently magnetic resonance imaging (MRI), have neurosurgeons recognized that not only cerebellar hemorrhage but also cerebellar infarction is sometimes a surgical emergency.[72–81]

## SURGICAL ANATOMY

The brain stem and the cerebellum are supplied by three pairs of arteries: (1) the posterior inferior cerebellar artery (PICA), (2) the anterior inferior cerebellar artery (AICA), and (3) the superior cerebellar artery (SCA). The three vessels in their arcuate course give branches that supply the brain stem. These arteries anastomose not only with the contralateral arteries, by means of their distal branches, but also with the ipsilateral contiguous arteries. Their terminal branches run along the folia and penetrate into the cerebellar fissures, spreading out into specific areas.[82]

### Posterior Inferior Cerebellar Artery

The PICA normally originates from the vertebral artery (82%) 1 to 3 cm caudally from the point where the two vertebral arteries unite in the basilar trunk. In a few cases it may originate from the basilar artery (10%), from a trunk in common with the AICA (6%) or from the AICA itself (2%).[83]

From its origin, the PICA runs transversally and back-wards around the bulbus; it then turns upward, continuing along the sulcus, which separates the dorsal part of the bulbus from the cerebellar tonsil. Between the cranial part of the tonsil and the inferior medullary veil, it takes a brusque turn backwards and downward, thus forming the tonsillar, choroidal, and bulbar branches.[83] In this way, it reaches the inferior surface of the cerebellum between the vermis and the tonsils, where it divides into two branches—a medial branch and a lateral branch. The medial branch, which is generally smaller, supplies a triangular area with a dorsal base and a ventral apex facing toward the fourth ventricle. This area includes the inferior vermis, nodulus, uvula, pyramis, tuber, and sometimes clivus and the internal part of the inferior semilunar lobe, gracile lobule, and the tonsil.[84]

When the medial branch of the PICA also supplies all or part of the lateral medullary territory,[85] its occlusion leads to Wallenberg's syndrome, although this is an uncommon occurrence (13%).[86] In some cases, anatomic variations may be observed in the territory of distribution: the medial ramus may be the only branch to supply the dorsolateral bulbar region and sometimes the retro-olivar area.[87, 88]

The lateral branch of the PICA is larger than the medial branch and supplies the inferior surface of the cerebellar hemisphere and tonsil.[83] Because this branch never supplies the bulbus, its occlusion may go unnoticed.[84]

The hemispheric branches of the PICA always form anastomoses with the hemispheric branches of the AICA and the SCA.

### Anterior Inferior Cerebellar Artery

The AICA normally originates from the inferior third of the basilar artery (75% of cases), sometimes from the middle third. However, it may originate from the vertebral artery or the basilar artery by means of a trunk in common with the PICA.[89] Sometimes, it is double (26%).[89] According to Lazorthes,[90] it is absent in 4% of the population.

From its origin, it runs along the caudal part of the pons,

supplying it with branches, and then crosses the abducens nerve; it then reaches the cerebellopontine angle, where it meets the acoustic-facial bundle. At the point where it crosses the acoustic-facial bundle (after giving rise to the labyrinthine artery), it divides into two branches. One branch runs laterally low down toward the anterior inferior portion of the cerebellar hemisphere. The other branch runs laterally and horizontally, forming a loop around the acoustic-facial bundle, to reach the flocculus, the middle cerebellar peduncle, and the middle part of the cerebellar hemisphere, thus forming vessels that supply these structures and the adjacent portion of the pons.

The AICA, therefore, feeds two distinct brain stem territories: (1) the proximal trunk supplies the lateral part of the pons, and (2) the lateral branches supply both the middle cerebellar peduncle and the tegmental part of the inferior two thirds of the pons.[89]

The cerebellar structures supplied include the flocculus. This is the only area of the brain stem to be supplied exclusively by the AICA, except in 3% to 5% of cases.[89] In 40% of the population, the AICA terminates in this zone; in the remainder, following the sulcus separating the semilunar lobe and the anterior lobe, it gives rise to terminal branches that supply the nearby lobes: anterior, simplex, superior and inferior semilunaris, gracilis, and biventer.[90, 91]

The AICA may substitute a hypoplastic PICA, supplying its entire distribution territory.[87, 91] The terminal branches of the AICA also anastomose with branches of the SCA and PICA.

## Superior Cerebellar Artery

Of the three arteries supplying the cerebellum, the SCA is the most constant in caliber and in distribution territory. In most cases, it is single (86%) and less frequently double (14%).[83] It originates from the basilar artery shortly before its bifurcation or, in a few cases (4%),[83] from the posterior cerebral artery.

From its origin it proceeds dorsally into the perimesencephalic cistern, running along the anterior edge of the pontomesencephalic sulcus, or within it, surrounding the cerebral peduncle. At this point, it gives rise to most of the collateral branches. Its initial segment is separated from the posterior cerebral artery by the common oculomotor nerve. It then divides into two principal branches, a medial and a lateral branch, which run parallel to the trochlear nerve.[82]

The medial branch, which runs between the inferior colliculus and the medial portion of the rostral edge of the cerebellum, divides into the vermian and paravermian arteries and occasionally into the intermediate arteries. The vermian arteries supply the ipsilateral rostral half of the vermis. The paravermian branches supply the medial part of the tentorial surface of the cerebellar hemisphere.

The lateral trunk runs around the lateral portion of the rostral edge of the cerebellum. It gives rise to between one and four lateral hemispheric branches and supplies the lateral portion of the tentorial surface of the cerebellum. In general, the SCA supplies most of the tentorial surface of the cerebellum, including the superior vermis, the dentate nucleus, and the superior cerebellar peduncle.[83]

The SCA connects with the AICA and PICA through anastomotic branches. Those between the PICA are particularly long. The anastomoses formed by these posterior cranial fossa vessels explain why clinically evident cerebellar infarction is comparatively less common than hemorrhage.

## HISTORICAL BACKGROUND

Spontaneous cerebellar hemorrhage has only recently been identified as a distinct nosologic entity.[68, 92] Morgagni and Lieutard were probably the first to recognize a spontaneous cerebellar hemorrhage, which was reported by Sédillot in 1813.[93] The first detailed descriptions of the disease date back to the 18th century. One paper, published in the *Lancet* in 1861, was written by Brown-Sequard[94]; another study was done by Hillairet.[95]

In 1906, Ballance was the first person to describe the successful removal of a cerebellar hemorrhage.[96] More recently, Mitchell and Angrist[92] reviewed a Queen Square series of 115 cases of intracerebral hemorrhage and reported on 15 patients with cerebellar hematoma.

The modern era of treatment for spontaneous cerebellar hemorrhage began with McKissock's report in 1960,[68] which was an update of the Queen Square experience based on 34 patients, followed by Fisher's report in 1965.[63] However, at that time, the choice of treatment still depended on clinical criteria that were much less reliable than the imaging methods available today. The advent of CT brought about a great improvement in the surgical results and overall management of these patients. As Little stated in 1978,[97] "the findings of CT investigations proved very helpful in defining appropriate therapy." They allowed the operating surgeon to distinguish patients with pure cerebellar hematomas amenable to surgical treatment from those with primitive brain stem hemorrhage and secondary ventricular involvement. Despite their poor quality compared with modern imaging, the first-generation CT images always permitted a differential diagnosis by exclusion with cerebellar infarction. In this context, the article written by Norris[61] (1969) is interesting for its historical value. One of the paper's subheadings, "Problems in differential diagnosis," gives an idea of the difficulties that our neurosurgical colleagues encountered about 30 years ago.

Other recent contributions, no longer regarding the diagnosis but the treatment of cerebellar hemorrhage, came from Weisberg[98] in 1986 and Taneda and coworkers[74] in 1987. Weisberg was the first to apply the concept of the "tight posterior fossa" to clinical practice.[98] After reviewing the case records of 20 consecutive patients with CT evidence of cerebellar hemorrhage, he selected 14 patients who had CT features of "tight posterior fossa," which was defined as effacement of the basal cisterns in the posterior fossa and ventricular enlargement consistent with obstructive hydrocephalus. All patients who harbored a tight posterior fossa suffered rapid neurologic deterioration, whereas none of the six patients who did not have a tight posterior fossa deteriorated; all recovered without surgery. One year later, in a large series of 75 patients with cerebellar hemorrhage diagnosed by CT scanning, Taneda assessed the relationship between the outcome and the CT appearance of the quadrigeminal cistern.[74] He concluded that "the CT grade of quadrigeminal cistern obliteration is an accurate indicator of outcome and is highly useful in selecting appropriate treatment for patients with cerebellar hemorrhage."

Previously in 1984, Laun and coworkers[58] had already reviewed their personal experience in seven patients with infarction of the PICA and showed how obliteration of the cisterns of the quadrigeminal plate and the vein of Galen was the determining factor when assessing the indications for suboccipital decompressive craniotomy.

During the last decade or so many investigators have proposed guidelines for the surgical treatment of cerebellar hemorrhage, among them Auer,[12] Van der Hoop,[51] Gilliard,[24] Van Loon,[52] Kobayashi,[31] and Luparello and associates.[35] Yet none have managed to set the gold standard, namely to select with absolute certainty the criteria valid for opting between surgical or conservative treatment in these patients.

Compared with hemorrhage in this site, cerebellar infarction attracted neurosurgical interest much more recently. The first to acknowledge cerebellar infarction as a neurosurgical emergency were probably Fairburn and Oliver[99] and Lindgren[100] in 1956. Among the several papers dealing with this subject since then, those published in 1975 by Duncan and coworkers[101] and Sypert and Alvord[102] deserve mention. In a clinicopathologic (two cases) and clinicosurgical description (one case), the former describes the most common type of cerebellar infarction—that of the PICA. Duncan emphasizes the difficulties in the clinical diagnosis between pure cerebellar infarction and symptoms attributable to concomitant involvement of the brain stem.[101] Interestingly, the clinical diagnosis made in two of the three cases was a benign labyrinthine disorder. Sypert and Alvord's paper considering 28 patients with acute, massive cerebellar infarction provided a detailed clinicopathologic correlation, which is up-to-date even today. Evidence of the difficult clinical diagnosis is that the studies published before the advent of CT scan came mainly from large autopsy series.[102] Indeed, Sypert and Alvord emphasized the similarities between the clinical pictures of cerebellar infarction and acute cerebellar hemorrhage, subdural or epidural hematoma, rapidly growing cerebellar tumor, or abscess in the posterior cranial fossa.

During the same period, a French journal published a detailed review of the literature based on 79 cases, including 11 personal ones; the salient feature was the low number of cases operated upon (only 17).[3] The papers published in the ensuing years show how the introduction of CT scanning and MRI into clinical practice allowed an early differential diagnosis and hence suitable treatment. It thus represented a turning point in the management of patients with cerebellar infarction. These diagnostic methods have also led to classification of cerebellar infarctions based on anatomic-radiologic criteria and correlations.

In 1995, Mathew and coworkers[36] published a surgical series of patients with cerebellar infarction predominantly treated conservatively or by external ventricular drainage.

Chen and coworkers surgically treated 11 patients with massive cerebellar infarction, by suboccipital decompressive craniectomy and ventricular drainage.[57] In recent years, Amarenco's papers on cerebellar infarction deserve credit for their new perspective and their contribution to knowledge about the angio-architecture of the posterior cranial fossa, as well as for their extremely interesting anatomic clinical correlations, supported by MRI findings.[89, 103–107] These studies have shed light on the physiopathologic mechanisms underlying territorial and nonterritorial infarction (i.e., a cerebellar infarct <2 cm).[108, 109]

In cerebellar hemorrhage, debate concerns mainly the identification and correlation of the criteria indicating surgical or conservative treatment: the neurologic status of the patient, the size of the hematoma, and the presence of a tight posterior fossa. Conversely, fewer reports address the surgical management of cerebellar infarction, and this remains controversial. Whereas some investigators believe that most cases respond satisfactorily to external ventricular drainage,[18, 36] others advocate treating cerebellar infarcts as space-occupying lesions.[57, 110]

## PATHOLOGY

Patients with cerebellar hemorrhage are generally hypertense; some have Charcot-Bouchard microaneurysms of the posterior circulation.[111] Cole and Yates demonstrated these lesions on the larger cerebellar cortical vessels that run along the folia and penetrate deeply within the cerebellar fissures.[112] Most lesions were multiple aneurysms located at the point where the perforating arteries branch in the region of the dentate nucleus.

Using a technique for serial sectioning of the surgical specimen, Wakai and Nagai,[113] in 14 patients with lobar intracerebral hemorrhage or cerebellar hemorrhage without vascular abnormalities on angiograms, detected definite microaneurysms in five patients and probable ones in two others. Histopathologic studies may disclose small angiomas known as "cryptic vascular malformations," which are no longer identifiable after massive hemorrhage.[114]

The cerebellar hemorrhage typical of microaneurysm is generally located deep in the region of the dentate nucleus. The vessels most frequently involved are the SCA and the AICA artery. Most patients are elderly and frequently present concomitant systemic diseases, such as diabetes, liver disease, and hematologic disorders.

Conversely, patients with cerebellar infarction mainly have embolic disease. The finding of atrial flutter and cardiac ischemia in these patients witnesses the cardiac origin of this disease.[1] In his study of 88 cases, Amarenco found that 43% of infarcts were cardioembolic and 35% were atherosclerotic.[104]

Symptomatic cerebellar infarction mainly affects the vertebral artery, usually unilaterally but in rare cases bilaterally, at the origin of the PICA. The PICA is, therefore, the most frequently affected vessel.

Reports have evaluated the concept of territorial infarcts involving the full territory of a cerebellar artery or its branches, as opposed to border-zone or nonterritorial infarcts.[108, 109] Territorial infarction has a thromboembolic mechanism, frequently due to cardioembolism. Nonterritorial infarcts may be caused by small emboli, usually in a clinical setting of hypercoagulation; sometimes, the mechanism is hemodynamic. Amarenco and Caplan affirmed that most SCA infarcts are embolic.[108] AICA infarcts arise equally from embolic and atherosclerotic occlusions, whereas PICA infarcts are predominantly atherosclerotic.

Nonterritorial infarcts rarely present a surgical indication. Of all territorial infarcts, those of the PICA most frequently require surgical treatment not only because they are the most common but also for anatomic reasons.

As Sypert emphasized in his detailed anatomicopathologic study, more than 40% of patients with cerebellar infarction suffer from hypertension. In his series of 88 cases, Amarenco noted that as many as 64% were hypertense.[104]

## PREOPERATIVE AND POSTOPERATIVE DIAGNOSTIC PROTOCOL

On admission to our hospital, patients with cerebellar hemorrhage are evaluated neurologically by means of standard neurologic tests as well as by other grading systems such as the Glasgow Coma Scale (GCS).[115, 116] A scrupulous general clinical examination, together with a complete battery of laboratory tests, completes the initial evaluation.

The preoperative diagnostic imaging work-up includes a CT study of the brain as well as an MRI, if necessary and feasible. In doubtful cases, MRI angiography or traditional angiography completes the diagnostic protocol. CT or MRI allows assessment of a series of variables that we believe to be important for prognostic evaluation and therapeutic purposes. These are essentially as follows:

- Location of the hemorrhage (vermian, hemispheric, or both)
- Size of the hemorrhage (the two major diameters in millimeters)
- Presence of blood in the ventricles (particularly the fourth ventricle)
- Invasion of blood into the brain stem
- Presence of hydrocephalus
- Signs of brain stem impairment
- Presence and extent of perilesional edema
- Evidence of tight posterior fossa (TPF), according to the criteria established by Weisberg[98]

Weisberg defined the anatomic and radiologic features of TPF as obliteration of the basal cisterns in the posterior cranial fossa; enlargement of the third ventricle and lateral ventricles, including the temporal horns; and effacement of the fourth ventricle (inconstant).

In addition to the imaging criteria, we also assess the presence of pre-existing or concomitant medical problems, including diabetes, arterial hypertension, hematologic disorders, and liver disease. We base our clinical assessment not only on the evolution of disease but also on a serial study using the same criteria used for the initial evaluation (general clinical and neurologic evaluation, GCS, and laboratory tests).

In the Department of Neurology and Neurosurgery, we also see patients with suspected cerebellar infarction. However, unlike patients with hemorrhage, who undergo priority transferral to the neurosurgical department, those with suspected infarcts are admitted to a neurologic ward or neurologic stroke unit, depending on their initial status. After admission, detailed background information is obtained on pre-existing or concomitant medical conditions and family history. We then evaluate on CT and MRI the following parameters that are essential for prognosis and therapy:

- Location of the infarct
- Size of the infarct
- Involvement of one or more arterial districts
- Secondary hemorrhagic infarction of the ischemic area
- Presence of hydrocephalus
- Presence and amount of perilesional edema
- Signs of brain stem compression

During the ensuing days, the initial assessment is repeated (preferably using the GCS).[115, 116]

## PERSONAL EXPERIENCE

During the past 8 years in our department, we have treated 50 patients with cerebellar hemorrhage (30 men and 20 women, with a mean age of 61 years) and 29 patients with cerebellar infarction (14 men and 15 women, with a mean age of 57 years). Patients with cerebellar hemorrhage showed a slight male preponderance and an older age than the group with infarction (Table 69–1).

Our patients with cerebellar hemorrhage typically presented with a clinical picture of rapid onset. Their symptoms began on average 13 hours before admission. On admission, most patients showed rapidly deteriorating neurologic status: 60% of the patients were in coma, and 22% had unmistakable signs of intracranial hypertension. In patients with cerebellar infarction, the initial symptoms had a less sudden onset. Between the onset of the clinical picture and the patient's admission to the hospital, an average of 48 hours had elapsed. Our patients with cerebellar infarction typically presented clinically with symptoms of dizziness, nausea, vomiting, and sometimes headache, whereas those with cerebellar hemorrhage first had a headache, which was described as a piercing and continuous pain centered in the neck and typically irradiating toward the posterior cervical region (Table 69–2). Cerebellar symptoms were predictably common in both diseases.

TABLE 69–1 ■ **CLINICAL CHARACTERISTICS OF THE 79 PATIENTS WITH CEREBELLAR HEMORRHAGE AND INFARCTION IN OUR SERIES**

| Cerebellar Hemorrhage | Cerebellar Infarction |
|---|---|
| 50 Cases | 29 Cases |
| Male 30 (60%) | Male 14 (48%) |
| Female 20 (40%) | Female 15 (52%) |
| Median age: 61 years | Median age: 57 years |
| Median presentation: 13 hours | Median presentation: 48 hours |

**TABLE 69–2 ■ PRESENTING SYMPTOMS AND GLASGOW COMA SCALE SCORE IN 79 PATIENTS**

| Cerebellar Hemorrhage (50 Patients) | Symptoms | Cerebellar Infarction (29 Patients) |
|---|---|---|
| 40  (80%) | Headache | 12  (41%) |
| 31  (62%) | Nausea, vomiting | 14  (48%) |
| 10  (20%) | Vertigo | 13  (44%) |
| GCS  =  3    4  (8%) | | GCS  =  3    2  (6%) |
| GCS  >9   26  (52%) | | GCS    >9    6  (20%) |
| GCS  >12  11  (22%) | | GCS  >12   15  (54%) |
| GCS  = 14   9  (18%) | | GCS  = 14    6  (20%) |

GCS, Glasgow Coma Scale.

Most of our patients with cerebellar hematomas were hypertensive; some had diabetes, hematologic disorders, or liver disease. Conversely, patients with cerebellar infarction sometimes had potentially embolic disease, such as atrial flutter or recent cardiac infarctions, endocarditis with vegetations, or a patent foramen ovale. Again, some of these patients (38%) were hypertensive. Spontaneous cerebellar hemorrhages occurred more frequently at a vermian site than at a hemispheric site. Later blood invasion into the fourth ventricle or into the lateral ventricles was common. About half of these patients had coexisting hypertensive hydrocephalus. In 38% of cases, these abnormalities led to the diagnosis of a TPF (Table 69–3).

The criteria for establishing the surgical indications for cerebellar hemorrhage in our department are extremely strict. For this reason, in this series, patients with hemispheric hematomas that exceeded a maximum diameter of 40 mm and a minimum diameter of 30 mm, or vermian hematomas more than 35 mm and less than 25 mm, and had a GCS of less than 13 underwent surgery. The identification of a TPF reduced by 10 mm the diameters indicating surgery. The remaining patients received conservative treatment with mannitol and corticosteroids. Surgery consisted of removal of the hematoma. A lobectomy was undertaken only for hematomas that occupied more than 80% of the total lobar volume. Patients who had been in deep coma for several hours before admission to the hospital did not undergo surgery. Of the 20 patients treated by craniectomy and placement of external drainage, six patients subsequently needed placement of a permanent ventriculoperitoneal shunt. Many patients needed postoperative mechanical ventilation, which was continued on average for 48 hours.

Preoperative and postoperative antibiotic prophylaxis practically eliminated the risks of local surgical sepsis but had no effect on the risk of bronchopulmonary infection, which is a frequent postoperative complication in our series. Hypertensive hydrocephalus, which is always treated promptly, did not influence the prognosis. Vermian hematomas had no less favorable an outcome than did hemispheric hematomas, possibly because we used distinct criteria for establishing the surgical indications for the two sites. Age did not unfavorably affect the course of the illness. Conversely, the presence of two or more general risk factors significantly influenced both mortality and the subsequent quality of life, despite preoperative attempts to restore normal function (e.g., by infusion of plasma and platelet supplements in patients with blood or coagulation disorders) before undertaking surgical treatment.

More than half of our patients with cerebellar hemorrhage had a good postoperative functional recovery (Table 69–4). The overall mortality rate was 24% (Table 69–5).

The surgical indications for cerebellar infarction, unlike those for hemorrhage, depend almost entirely on the patient's clinical conditions. In this series, we resorted to surgery much less frequently in patients with cerebellar infarction than in patients with hematoma. Most patients received conservative treatment with dexamethasone and mannitol. Patients whose clinical condition required surgery underwent placement of temporary ventricular drainage. Only 3 of 29 patients in this series underwent suboccipital craniectomy and removal of necrotic tissue.

Two thirds of our patients with cerebellar infarction had a good postoperative recovery. The overall mortality rate was 14%.

**TABLE 69–3 ■ ASSOCIATED HYDROCEPHALUS, SITE OF THE HEMATOMA AND ARTERY INVOLVED IN THE INFARCTION IN 79 PATIENTS**

| Cerebellar Hemorrhage | | | | Cerebellar Infarction | | | |
|---|---|---|---|---|---|---|---|
| Hydrocephalus | | 20 | (40%) | Hydrocephalus | | 6 | (20%) |
| Hemorrhage | Vermian | 16 | (32%) | *Infarction | PICA | 16 | (55%) |
| | Hemispheric | 30 | (60%) | | AICA | 3 | (10%) |
| | Both | 6 | ( 8%) | | SCA | 1 | ( 3%) |
| | | | | | Massive | 6 | (20%) |
| Tight posterior fossa | | 19 | (38%) | | | | |

*3 Cases (10%). The artery responsible for the infarction could not be detected with certainty.
PICA, posterior inferior cerebellar artery; AICA, anterior inferior cerebellar artery; SCA, superior cerebellar artery.

TABLE 69–4 ■ **MANAGEMENT OF THE 79 PATIENTS WITH CEREBELLAR HEMORRHAGE AND INFARCTION**

| Cerebellar Hemorrhage (50 Patients) | Cerebellar Infarction (29 Patients) |
|---|---|
| 18 Treated conservatively | 21 Treated conservatively |
| 4 Not treated due to coma depassé | 2 Not treated due to coma depassé |
| 28 Treated surgically | 6 Treated surgically |
| 20 Suboccipital craniectomy + external drainage | 2 Suboccipital craniectomy + external drainage |
| 8 Suboccipital craniectomy only | 1 Suboccipital craniectomy only |
| | 3 External drainage |

# CASE REPORTS

## Case Report 1

This 71-year-old man, with a history of untreated hypertension, presented with the sudden onset of a piercing occipital headache. This man, who was initially admitted to another hospital, had a brain CT scan that detected a hematoma 40 × 30 mm in the right cerebellar hemisphere with effacement of cisterns, slight ventricular dilatation, and secondary intraventricular hemorrhage (Fig. 69–1A–C). While undergoing the scan, the patient presented progressive impairment of consciousness, and he was therefore transferred on an emergency basis to our department for treatment. Because the patient was stuporous on admission and unable to obey commands, cerebellar function could not be tested: the Babinski sign was detectable bilaterally, breathing was arrhythmic.

The size of the hematoma, the effacement of cisterns in the posterior fossa, and the evolving clinical picture called for an immediate emergency surgical procedure. The patient underwent a right suboccipital craniectomy; the hematoma was removed; and a drainage system was inserted through the occipital horn in the right lateral ventricle and left in situ. After surgery, the patient's clinical status immediately improved. The patient was discharged 9 days later; he was mildly ataxic and had right cerebellar incoordination (see Fig. 69–1D, E).

## Case Report 2

This 29-year-old white woman with a history of diabetes presented to our emergency department after falling off her bicycle because of the onset of dizziness, severe nausea, and vomiting. On admission to the hospital, a neurologic examination showed severe impairment of consciousness, bilateral cerebellar incoordination, and cerebellar dysarthria.

The CT scan showed a large cerebellar hematoma that measured 5.5 × 3.8 cm with extensive intraventricular spread of blood above and below the tentorium. It also showed marked ventricular dilatation with a blood clot within the lateral ventricles and the third ventricle (Fig. 69–2A, B). In the meantime, the patient's overall neurologic status deteriorated and decerebrate posture developed.

The patient underwent an emergency removal of the hematoma and insertion of a ventricular drainage system through the right frontal horn (see Fig. 69–2C, D). Mechanical ventilation was maintained for 48 hours. About 72 hours after surgery, the patient's neurologic conditions improved, and a permanent ventriculoperitoneal shunt was placed. Nine days later, the patient was able to walk again. Two years later, she lives a normal life without neurologic sequelae.

## Case Report 3

A young boy, aged 9, was admitted to our pediatric department for investigation of a progressive syndrome characterized by vertigo, nausea, and vomiting. The boy had an acute headache. His body temperature was slightly raised (37.6°C). He had previously been diagnosed as having polymyositis. The other interesting finding was a family history of cerebral stroke. Three years earlier, the patient's father had suffered an MRI-documented left middle cerebral artery stroke, which left him with right hemiparesis. The patient's chest radiographs, electrocardiogram (ECG), and blood tests were unremarkable. The neurologic examination revealed mild ataxia and cerebellar incoordination.

An MRI obtained on the third day showed a cerebellar infarction in the right PICA territory, whereas MRI angiography showed the absence of PICA filling on the right side (Fig. 69–3A–C).

Conservative therapy was begun with 60 ml of 18% mannitol solution every 6 hours and 1.5 mg of dexamethasone every 8 hours plus gastric protection with cimetidine. Bed rest was continued for another week, and the patient's symptoms slowly subsided. Residual symptoms consisted of mild ataxia and right dysmetria.

## Case Report 4

A 64-year-old diabetic woman experienced the sudden onset of nausea and vomiting, followed by ver-

TABLE 69–5 ■ **MANAGEMENT AND MORTALITY IN THE 79 PATIENTS WITH CEREBELLAR HEMORRHAGE AND INFARCTION**

| Cerebellar Hemorrhage | | | Cerebellar Infarction | | |
|---|---|---|---|---|---|
| Overall mortality | 12 | (24%) | Overall mortality | 4 | (14%) |
| Operated cases | 8 | (16%) | Operated cases | 1 | ( 3%) |
| Treated conservatively | 0 | ( 0%) | Treated conservatively | 1 | ( 3%) |
| Not treated (coma depassé) | 4 | ( 8%) | Not treated (coma depassé) | 2 | ( 6%) |

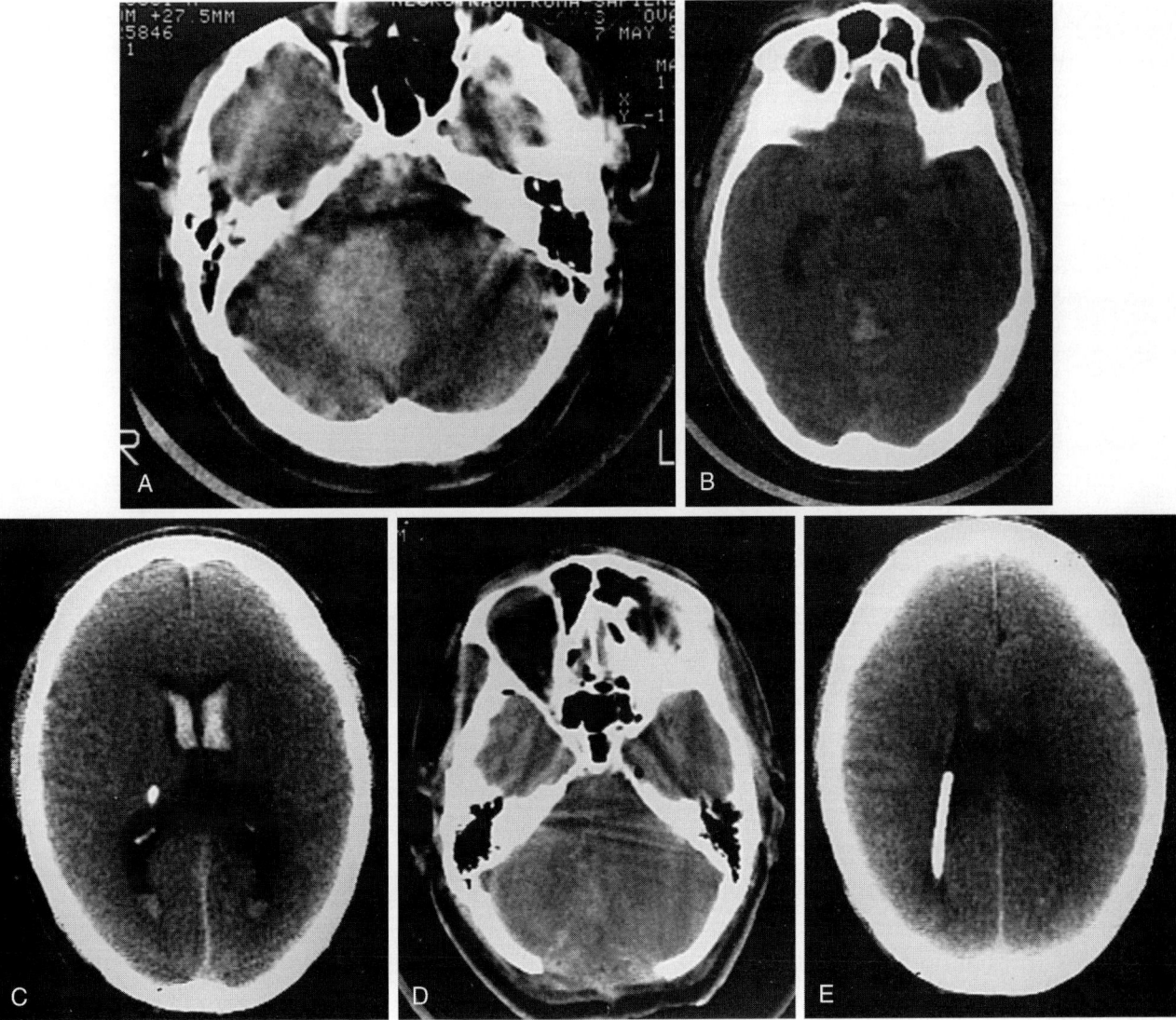

**FIGURE 69-1** ■ *A,* Case 1: A computed tomography (CT) scan showing a large acute right hemispheric cerebellar hematoma. *B,* Case 1: A CT scan showing effacement of the perimesencephalic cistern and initial dilatation of the temporal horns of the lateral ventricle. *C,* Case 1: A CT scan depicting supratentorial intraventricular hemorrhage in the same patient. *D,* Case 1: A postoperative CT scan showing evacuation of the hematoma. *E,* Case 1: A postoperative CT scan showing ventricular drainage, which is inserted through the right occipital horn and left in place, partially resolving obstructive hydrocephalus.

tigo. She was admitted to the emergency department of our hospital, where neurologic examination revealed gait ataxia and right-sided pyramidal tract signs. She complained of a persistent occipital headache. An ECG showed an atrial flutter, whereas the echocardiogram disclosed nothing remarkable. The result of the CT scan was negative. Nevertheless, therapy was begun with 4 mg of dexamethasone every 8 hours. Within 2 days, the symptoms had abated except for the headache. Another CT scan (Fig. 69–4A) detected a hypodense lesion in the medial left cerebellar hemisphere that was compatible with occlusion of the left PICA. For the next 3 days, 100 ml of 18% mannitol every 6 hours was added to the patient's therapy. An MRI scan (see Fig. 69–4B) confirmed the CT findings. The patient did not undergo MRI angiography. She had a complete functional recovery and was discharged 5 days later.

## DISCUSSION

For its definition as a distinct nosologic entity, cerebellar hemorrhage had to await the coming of the CT era. The diagnostic and semeiologic means available before the advent of CT scanning made cerebellar hemorrhage extremely difficult to recognize. Hence the surgical indications, relying as they did on indirect signs of the lesion alone, were also extremely imprecise. This shortcoming explains the considerable discrepancy between the various mortality rates reported in the literature throughout the years—from 73.5% reported by McKissock[68] in 1960 to 20% reported by Luparello[35] in 1995.

Spontaneous cerebellar hemorrhages occur predominantly in the older age groups—from the sixth to the eighth decades[9, 12, 14, 20, 31, 36, 38, 39, 51, 52, 73, 74]—both in our experience and in published series. However, this preference for el-

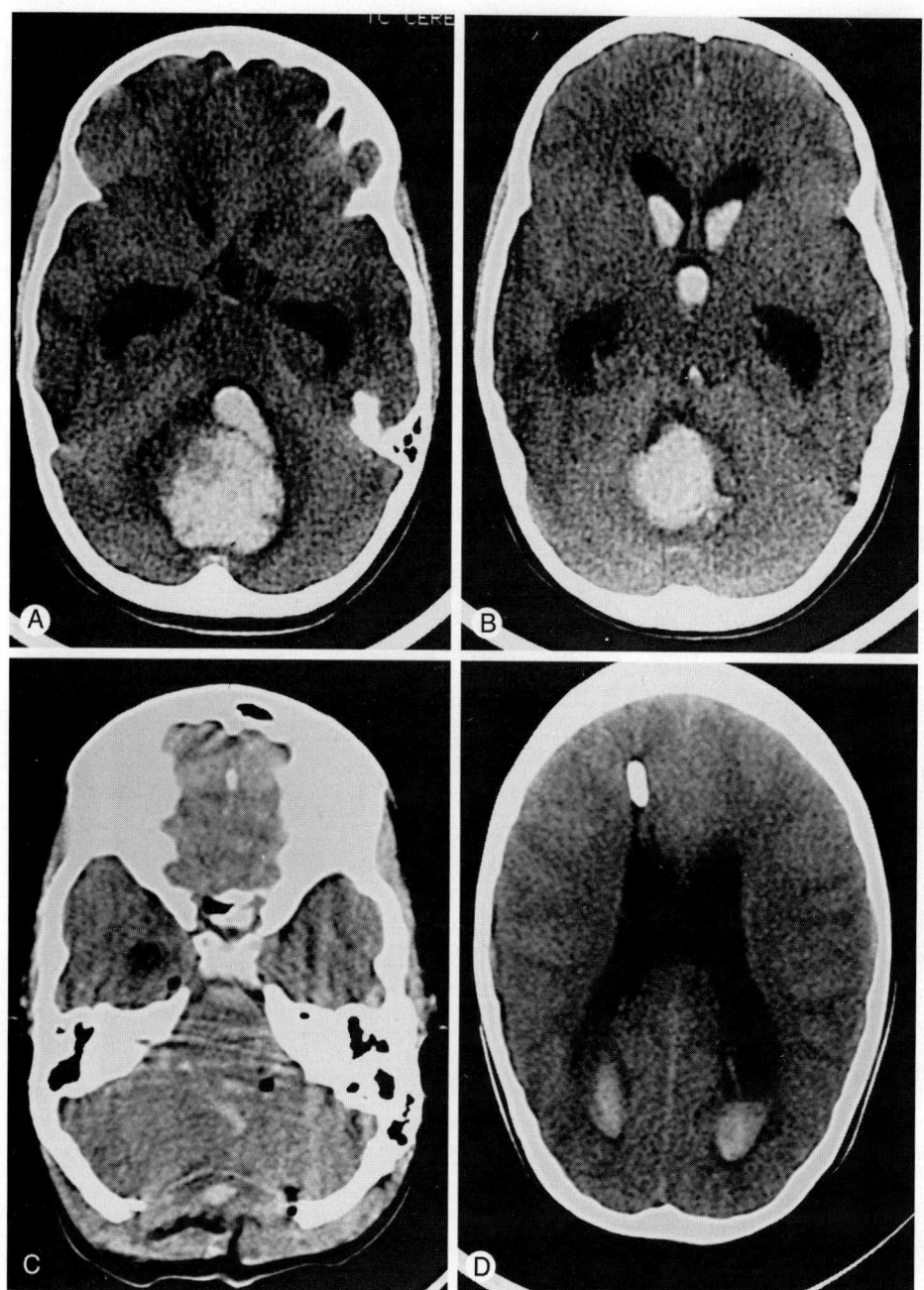

FIGURE 69–2 ■ *A*, Case 2: A computed tomography (CT) scan showing a large acute vermian hematoma with marked dilatation of the temporal horn of the lateral ventricles. *B*, Case 2: A CT scan showing the disappearance of the perimesencephalic cistern and an intraventricular blood clot. *C*, Case 2: A CT scan showing the evacuation of the hematoma. *D*, Case 2: The CT scan depicts a ventricular catheter inserted through the right frontal horn.

derly patients does not necessarily correspond with a less favorable prognosis, either in terms of mortality or quality of life. Neither does the patient's clinical status on admission influence operative mortality as long as surgery is done immediately.

In our experience, the location of the hematoma in the vermis rather than the cerebellar hemispheres did not seem to influence the prognosis, compared with other recent reports.[31, 35] Neither did hypertensive hydrocephalus seem to affect the prognosis unfavorably, as long as the condition was diagnosed and treated without delay. The presence of general risk factors (e.g., diabetes, arterial hypertension, hematologic disorders, and liver disease), if considered singly, had no significant influence on survival. However,

a combination of two or more risk factors statistically worsened the prognosis, as did the invasion of blood into the brain stem.

Neuroradiologic diagnosis plays an essential role in the staging of patients with hemorrhage.[9, 10, 12, 13, 18, 20, 22, 24, 26, 29, 31–33, 37–43, 48, 78, 53, 55, 73, 74, 76, 97] For early recognition of the disease, because MRI yields no better results than CT scanning, its higher costs hardly justify its use as an emergency procedure. Blood invasion into the brain stem, the presence of hypertensive hydrocephalus, blood in the ventricular system, and the size of the hematoma can be easily evaluated on unenhanced CT scans. For characterizing the bleeding in doubtful cases, MRI gives more detailed information on small vessel malformations and is ideal for

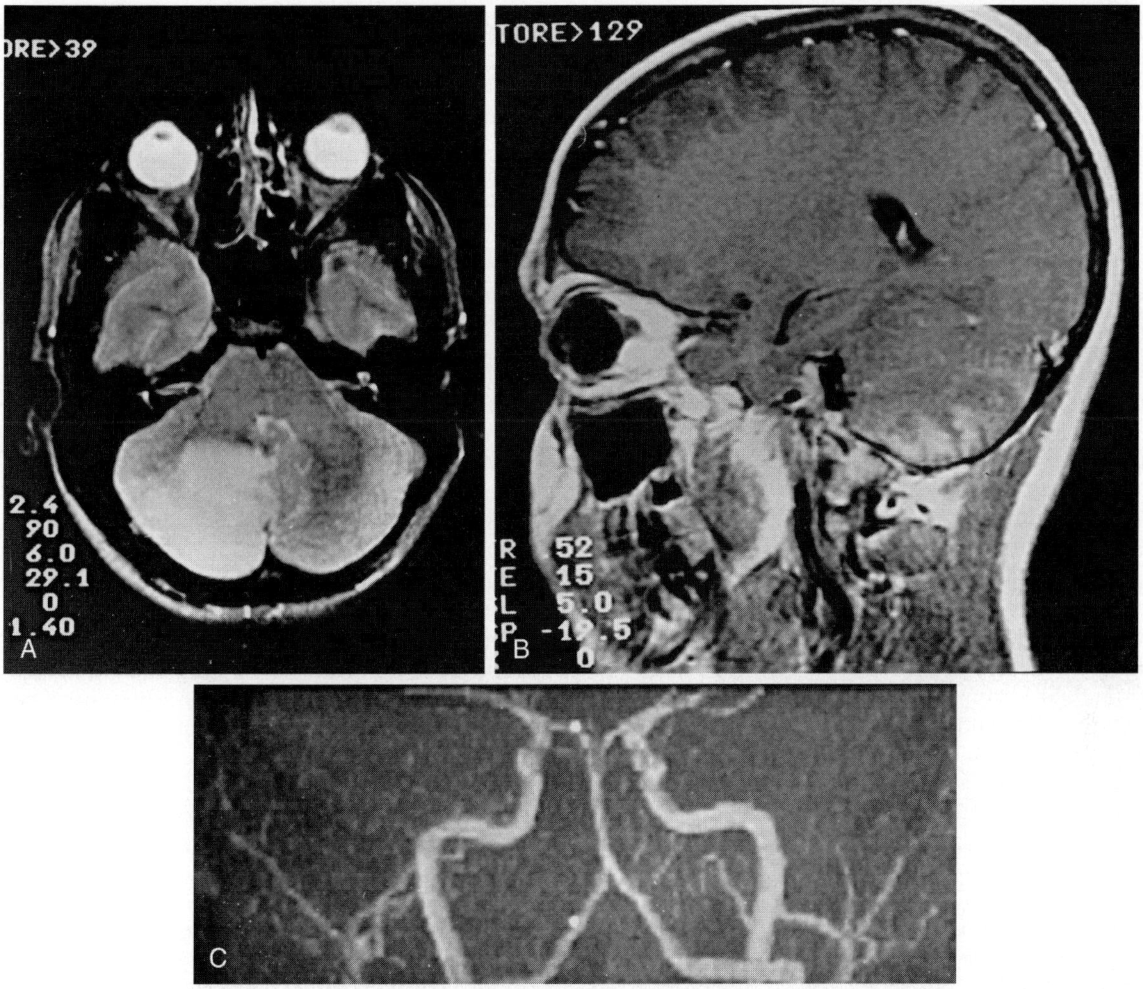

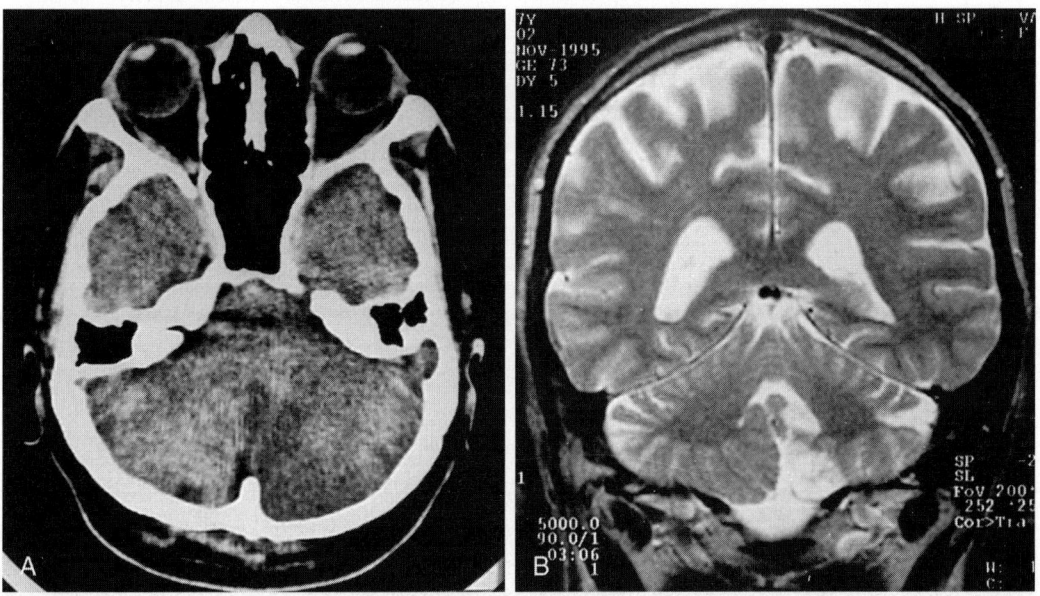

FIGURE 69–3 ■ *A,* Case 3: Magnetic resonance imaging (MRI) axial $T_2$-weighted images of an acute ischemic cerebellar infarction in the territory of the right posteroinferior cerebellar artery (PICA). *B,* Case 3: Sagittal $T_1$-weighted images with gadolinium enhancement in the same patient. *C,* Case 3: Angio-magnetic resonance imaging in a coronal section showing the absence of filling of the right PICA.

FIGURE 69–4 ■ *A,* Case 4: A computed tomography (CT) scan performed 48 hours after the onset of symptoms of acute cerebellar infarction in the left posteroinferior cerebellar artery (PICA) territory. *B,* Case 4: Coronal $T_2$-weighted magnetic resonance images of the same patient showing occlusion of the left medial branch of the PICA.

studying the brain stem. MRI angiography also allows noninvasive evaluation of eventual vascular abnormalities in this region.

As opposed to expansive lesions in the posterior cranial fossa, the role of perilesional edema is unimportant. It also has little practical value, because it is overshadowed by the role played by the compressive and destructive phenomena triggered by the hematoma.

Much controversy surrounds the indications for surgical treatment, especially the choice of criteria for the surgical indications.[1, 12–14, 18, 20, 22, 23, 29, 31, 35–37, 46, 49, 63, 73, 74, 97, 98] Obviously, the more prognostic factors assessed the more reliable they are for predicting the outcome. On the other hand, unduly strict adherence to these criteria may cause the surgeon's personal judgment acquired by experience to go unheeded.

Our experience suggests that a vermian hematoma larger than 35 × 25 mm, or a hemispheric hematoma bigger than 40 × 30 mm, represents an indication for surgery, because hematomas that are this size invariably lead to altered consciousness. The rationale for the distinction in size between vermian and hemispheric hematomas is that vermian hematomas lie closer to the brain stem and cerebrospinal fluid (CSF) pathways. Whether patients who belong in one of the two aforementioned categories but have a GCS of 13 or more should undergo surgery remains debatable, as reported also by Kobayashi.[31] Although we have not personally dealt with a similar clinical-radiologic presentation, we would implement a "watchful, armed wait-and-see" strategy. This type of management seems to be justified by the scarce clinical and neuroimaging progression observed in almost all of our patients who were not operated on and whose initial clinical conditions were satisfactory.

In our series, we had no cases of "spontaneous" cerebellar hemorrhage after supratentorial craniotomy, which was first described by Koenig and coworkers[119] and then by Van Loon and coworkers[52] in 2 of 49 cases of their series. In the series described by Toczek,[120] this event accounted for almost 5% of complications after temporal lobectomy.

One concept that requires careful evaluation is the presence of a TPF.[98] Obliteration of the cisterns does not depend only on the size of the hematoma. Hematomas of similar size may exert widely differing amounts of compression on the cisterns. The amount of compression probably depends also on various factors, including the patient's age, the amount of cerebellar atrophy, and the anatomy of the posterior cranial fossa. Therefore, identification of a TPF justifies changing the aforementioned surgical criteria, reducing by 10 mm the diameters indicating surgical treatment.

Although we have no experience with CT-guided stereotactic fibrinolysis techniques for removal of the hematoma, published data imply that this procedure is effective for hematomas that are considered borderline—namely those on the borderline between conservative and surgical treatment.[42, 117, 118]

The duration of hospitalization of these patients depends on how delicate and functionally important the surrounding brain is. The role of mechanical ventilation, when necessary, is predictably important for improving the prognosis for these patients. On the other hand, prophylactic postop-

erative mechanical ventilation seems to be unnecessary if blood gas analysis values and assessment of autonomous ventilation immediately after operation come within even the lowest values of the normal range.

Our strategy in managing comatose patients with cerebellar hemorrhage differs from that of others.[1, 56, 70, 72] Patients who are admitted in deep coma or with flaccid paralysis or loss of brain stem reflexes that lasts for more than 2 hours do not undergo surgery.

Of the simple, standardized methods for assessing the outcome of patients with cerebellar hemorrhage on admission, the one most commonly used is the GCS.[115, 116, 121] Even though the use of such a scale renders clinical evaluation less precise and less descriptive, it helps greatly with comparison of results. Despite these advantages, use of the GCS for the preoperative evaluation of patients with cerebellar hemorrhage is open to criticism. The GCS was conceived for patients with "head injuries," many of whom present neurologic deterioration "due to a supratentorial pathology and consequent transtentorial herniation."[115] This scale focuses on the level of consciousness and motor responsiveness of the patient. Heros[110] emphasized how "unresponsiveness and posturing" have different prognostic implications when the cause is a posterior fossa mass rather than herniation from a supratentorial mass.[67]

Particularly gratifying, considering their poor conditions on admittance, was the return of our patients to social activities. Most of the elderly patients almost reverted to their prepathologic level of activity.

Acknowledgment of direct surgical treatment of cerebellar infarct as a lifesaving maneuver is even more recent than treatment of cerebellar hemorrhage. In most cases, conservative treatment was preferred, particularly in the past, and the first surgically treated cases date back only as far as the middle 1950s.[99, 100] The true incidence of infarction of a cerebellar hemisphere is unknown and difficult to assess.[103] Contrary to previous beliefs, cerebellar infarction seems to be much more frequent than cerebellar hemorrhage, at least in post mortem series[102] and in CT studies.[18] In Amarenco's paper,[104] of 190 cases of cerebellar stroke, 85% were infarcts and 15% were hemorrhages. One explanation is the high incidence of asymptomatic (nonterritorial) cerebellar infarcts in diagnostic and post mortem series. Alternatively, some symptomatic cerebellar infarcts may be misdiagnosed.

In surgical series, similar numbers of patients with hemorrhage and with infarction undergo operation. Of 60 cases reported by Turgut and coworkers,[38] 39 were spontaneous cerebellar hemorrhages and 21 were infarcts; of the 89 cases reported by Mathew and associates,[36] 50 were infarcts and 39 were cerebellar hemorrhages. This finding implies that, despite autopsy observations and a wealth of CT and MRI studies, cerebellar infarcts still receive less attention than they deserve. In cases of infarction, MRI shows an area of increased signal on $T_2$-weighted images, whereas CT scans depict an area of hypodensity that is not usually detected in the first hours. Because of the limited CT scan resolution owing to the bony artifacts in the posterior cranial fossa, many cerebellar infarcts are overlooked initially.

Cerebellar infarcts may be due not only to atherosclerosis or acute vertebral artery occlusion of cardioembolic origin but also to various pathogenic causes, including cervical manipulation,[122] trauma,[4, 123] use of drugs such as cocaine,[124] and intra-extracranial dissection of vertebral arteries.[125–127] They may also represent the presenting symptom of polycythemia[128] or the result of the prolonged, though reversible, vasospasm that is sometimes associated with certain migraine syndromes or linked to congenital odontoid aplasia.[129–131]

Our series highlighted several differences between patients with cerebellar hemorrhage and infarction. First, patients with cerebellar infarction had a slightly lower average age than did patients with spontaneous cerebellar hemorrhage. In addition, patients with hemorrhage had a worse neurologic status evaluated according to the GCS.[103] Signs of brain stem compression also appear later in infarction than in hemorrhage. Cerebellar dysfunction is more frequent, because the neurosurgeon has longer to evaluate the course of the illness in patients with infarction, who tend to go into coma later and less frequently than patients with hemorrhage.

In the past few years, many published papers have addressed the clinical topographic correlations supplied by CT and above all by MRI.[77, 103, 132, 133] For this reason, we now know exactly which clinical pictures correspond with occlusion of the various arteries that supply the cerebellum.[81, 107, 134–137] In SCA infarcts, the clinical presentation is characterized by gait and limb ataxia, which is often accompanied by nystagmus.[137] In patients whose infarcts involve the lateral branch of the SCA, dysmetria, dysarthria, and axial lateropulsion predominate.[106] Vertigo and headache are much less common.

AICA infarcts are characterized by a pure vestibular syndrome or otherwise by dysmetria, Horner's syndrome, vestibular signs, contralateral pain and temperature sensory loss in the limbs, and facial sensory impairment.[89, 107]

Lastly, patients with PICA infarcts present with vertigo, headache, and gait imbalance. Nystagmus is a predominant sign and is sometimes associated with Wallenberg's syndrome with ipsilateral limb ataxia.[137] A comparison between the results of our series and other published data shows that cerebellar infarction requires open surgery less frequently than does hemorrhage, because in some cases medical treatment[69] or external ventricular drainage will suffice.[18, 138] In cerebellar hemorrhage, hydrocephalus is generally due to secondary blood extravasion into the fourth ventricle, whereas in cerebellar infarction, it arises from necrotic tissue obstructing the CSF pathways. This could explain why in our series cerebellar hemorrhages more often required a permanent ventriculoperitoneal shunt. None of our patients with cerebellar infarcts treated by an external shunt required a permanent ventriculoperitoneal shunt. Because none of them had intraventricular blood, once medical treatment or external drainage had resolved the acute edematous phase, CSF circulation returned to normal. Conversely, six of our patients with cerebellar hemorrhage needed a permanent ventriculoperitoneal shunt.

The choice of the most appropriate surgical treatment in patients with cerebellar infarction is still controversial. Many neurosurgeons have emphasized the success of surgical resection of the necrotic tissue in the infarcted territory.[59, 61, 69, 72, 79, 99–101, 110, 139] Others have reported good results with ventricular drainage and conservative management.[7, 18.]

Other noteworthy publication on the surgical management of cerebellar infarction include two studies[140, 141] by the same authors. The first,[140] a pilot study conducted retrospectively, compares the results in a group of patients in deep coma—stuporous or with posturing or cardiovascular instability and pinpoint pupils—with cerebellar infarcts treated by ventriculostomy. The results were significantly worse than those observed in a clinically matched group of patients who were treated prospectively with decompressive craniotomy.[140] The second,[141] conducted as a prospective observational multicenter trial, supports the notion that the level of consciousness is the most powerful predictor of outcome, superior to any other clinical sign and treatment assignment. These investigators, nevertheless, favor a gradual therapeutic approach that consists of medical therapy for awake patients, ventriculostomy for patients with hydrocephalus, and decompressive craniotomy for patients with signs and symptoms of brain stem compression.[140] We also opted for "specific" and "gradual" therapy. It depended specifically on clinical evaluation of the patients' neurologic conditions to detect signs of endocranial hypertension or brain stem compression. Therapy also included CT scanning or an MRI to detect hydrocephalus or brain stem compression. Patients who, despite conservative therapy, fail to show neurologic improvement or display radiologic signs of brain stem compression should undergo decompressive craniectomy and removal of the necrotic tissue.

In "awake" patients without symptoms of endocranial hypertension or signs of compression of the brain stem and ventricles, therapy to reduce edema is indicated, accompanied by frequent clinical and radiologic monitoring.[5, 7, 58, 140, 142] We disagree with those who warn that in cerebellar infarction positioning an external ventricular drainage system carries a real risk of upward transtentorial herniation.[6, 72] This undesirable complication can be virtually avoided by regulating CSF flow while simultaneously monitoring the patient's neurologic conditions.

External drainage may also be criticized, because it fails to decompress the brain stem. However, the good results obtained in our series (as in others) demonstrate that, in most cases, deterioration of the patient's neurologic status and level of consciousness coincided with the rise of intracranial pressure caused by obstructive hydrocephalus.[18, 138]

In cerebellar hemorrhage, on the other hand, the risks of an upward transtentorial herniation invariably contraindicate external ventricular drainage without a preceding decompressive craniectomy. In the series described by Van Loon and coworkers,[52] 2 of 26 patients treated by immediate ventricular drainage suffered upward herniation, and one of these patients died. In McKissock's series,[68] all nine patients who were treated by ventricular drainage alone died; in some of these patients, sudden deterioration occurred after ventricular tapping. Transtentorial upward herniation, therefore, remains a possible event in patients with cerebellar hemorrhage treated solely by ventricular drainage.

Although we cannot provide any statistics, we think that it is interesting that in their study[104] considering an autopsy series of 88 cerebellar infarcts in 56 patients, in 49 of 88 infarcts Amarenco and associates found an abnormal arterial arrangement. This observation merits attention even in the absence of an age- and sex-matched series of patients.

## Surgical Technique

The surgical treatment of cerebellar hemorrhage and infarction is generally a straightforward, standardized technique. In our department, we do not routinely use anesthetic gases or vapors. Anesthesia is induced with the aid of barbiturates such as sodium thiopental or propofol and maintained with the use of an analgesic (fentanyl) and a neuroleptic. Muscle relaxation is obtained and maintained with pancuronium bromide and vecuronium.

After being intubated by the oral or nasotracheal route, the patient is placed supine on the operating table. We prefer nasotracheal intubation whenever we consider that the patient's conditions could benefit from postoperative mechanical ventilation.

Monitoring includes a series of variables, including cardiac activity, blood gases, arterial pressure, urinary output, and rectal temperature.

The head is completely shaved and immobilized using the three-point headrest. For a predominantly vermian hematoma that only partially involves the cerebellar hemisphere, a median incision is made 2 cm above the inion as far as the spinous process of the fourth cervical vertebra. A Y-shaped incision is made in the deep fascia; the V-shaped portion of the incision of the fascia is lifted up and retracted posteriorly with silk sutures; and, using the electric scalpel, the median raphe is identified and cut to expose the spinous process of C2. The muscles with insertion on the occipital squama are partly incised, again with a Y-shaped incision, and superiorly retracted with the fascia: they are then partly detached laterally and maintained in situ with a self-retaining retractor. Once the occipital squama has been exposed, several bur holes are made, and a bone forceps is used to complete the craniectomy. Our experience suggests a wide craniectomy.

A Y-shaped incision of the dura mater is made, retracting the V-shaped flap superiorly and posteriorly with 3–0 silk sutures; the fixed flaps are retracted and suspended with 3–0 silk sutures. If the hematoma principally involves the cerebellar hemisphere, we prefer a paramedian incision; subsequently, the technique is similar to that used for exposing a neurinoma of the eighth cranial nerve. Although the craniectomy need not be extended as far as the transverse sinus and sigmoid sinus,[143] it should be wide enough to allow for treatment of an unsuspected pathologic condition, such as a hemorrhagic tumor or a vascular malformation.

Once the cerebellar surface has been exposed, a cortical incision is made that provides the most direct access yet the least injury to the cerebellar parenchyma and vessels. The hematoma is evacuated using a suction and irrigation technique. When most of the hematoma has been removed, the surgical microscope is brought into the operating field and the remaining clots are removed using forceps; thus, possible sources of bleeding are identified and coagulated. In our experience, bleeding rarely arises from a single source such as a single artery; it originates most often from the cavity walls and can be controlled using a hemostatic gelatin sponge or fibrillar collagen that is left in situ.

Hemostasis should be meticulous. To identify any persistent bleeding site, we usually raise the patient's blood pressure approximately 20 mm Hg over the monitored preoperative pressure. As a further check for eventual residual bleeding, the cavity is irrigated several times with a saline solution before closure. The dura mater is then closed with a continuous suture. Several dural suspension stitches are placed along the border of the craniectomy, and the watertightness of the dura mater is checked. The trapezius muscle, the muscles attached to the occipital protuberance, and the paraspinous muscles are sutured in two layers, and the skin is sutured using resorbable 3–0 silk thread.

The surgical techniques for cerebellar hemorrhage and cerebellar infarction use similar opening and closure stages. The cerebellar tissue at the site of the infarct is removed using low-suction aspiration and bipolar coagulation. The site of infarction is easy to recognize owing to its soft, fluffy consistency.

The amount of bleeding is usually moderate, and the infarcted or shifted cerebellar tonsil or tonsils are generally removed to favor proper restoration of CSF circulation. In patients with cerebellar infarcts and those with hemorrhage who have preoperative ventricular dilatation, an external ventricular shunt is usually placed using the standard technique and left in situ for 48 to 72 hours.

## Postoperative Care

Our patients go to the intensive care unit for the first 24 hours after surgery. Patients who are in satisfactory preoperative neurologic condition are extubated immediately after surgery, and their arterial pressure, pulse, ECG, water and electrolyte balance, and blood gases are closely monitored. The most important single aim is to avoid peaks of arterial hypertension. Patients in critical neurologic condition remain under mechanical ventilation and receive full doses of corticosteroids and mannitol; they undergo a CT scan within the first 24 hours. As soon as their neurologic condition has improved, patients are transferred to the neurosurgical ward until they are discharged from the hospital. During this time, they undergo serial CT scans.

## CONCLUSIONS

Vascular cerebellar syndromes occur predominantly in the elderly. The most frequent cause of cerebellar hemorrhage is arterial hypertension; the most frequent cause of infarction is cardioembolic disease. In our experience, hemorrhages require surgical treatment more frequently than do infarcts, mainly on an emergency basis. Cerebellar infarcts are diagnosed more frequently today than in the past. Most of them involve the territory of the PICA. The majority respond well to conservative management or external ventricular drainage for 48 to 72 hours. Comparatively few need a decompressive suboccipital craniectomy.

The choice of surgical option is based on neurologic

evaluation of consciousness. The essential criteria for the surgical assessment of intracerebellar hemorrhages are the diameter of the hematoma ($40 \times 30$ mm in hemispheric lesions and $35 \times 25$ mm in vermian lesions), the presence of a TPF (reducing the aforementioned diameters by 10 mm) and a GCS score of less than 13.

Blood invasion of the brain stem and the presence of two or more general risk factors considerably worsen survival. The presence of hypertensive hydrocephalus, if diagnosed and treated promptly, does not adversely influence the prognosis. Patients who are in a deep coma should be treated conservatively. Despite an often dramatic clinical onset, not all patients have an unfavorable course. Even patients with low preoperative GCS scores sometimes make a surprisingly good functional recovery.

## REFERENCES

1. Heros RC: Cerebellar hemorrhage and infarction. Stroke 13:106–109, 1982.
2. Tomaszek DE, Rosner MJ: Cerebellar infarction: Analysis of twenty-one cases. Surg Neurol 24:223–226, 1985.
3. George B, Cophignon J, George C, et al: Surgical aspects of cerebellar infarction: Based upon a series of 79 cases. Neurochirurgie 24:83–88, 1978.
4. Heros RC: Cerebellar infarction resulting from traumatic occlusion of a vertebral artery: Case report. J Neurosurg 51:111–113, 1979.
5. Chin D, Carney P: Acute cerebellar haemorrhage with brain stem compression in contrast with benign cerebellar haemorrhage. Surg Neurol 19:406–409, 1983.
6. Macdonnel RAL, Kalanis RM, Donnan GA: Cerebellar infarction: Natural history, prognosis and pathology. Stroke 18:849–855, 1987.
7. Cioffi FA, Bernini FP, Punzo A, et al: Surgical management of acute cerebellar infarction. Acta Neurochir (Wien) 74:105–112, 1985.
8. Kiwak KJ, Heros RC: Cerebellar hemorrhage and infarction: An update. Contemp Neurosurg 8:1–6, 1986.
9. Acampora S, Guarnieri L, Troisi F: Spontaneous intracerebellar hematoma: Report of ten cases. Acta Neurochir (Wien) 66:83–86, 1982.
10. Amacher AL: Spontaneous cerebellar hemorrhage: Evolution of an entity. Crit Rev Neurosurg 6:73–77, 1996.
11. Aoki N, Mizuguchi K: Expanding intracerebellar hematoma: A possible clinicopathological entity. Neurosurgery 18:94–96, 1986.
12. Auer LM, Auer T, Sayama I: Indications for surgical treatment of cerebellar hemorrhage and infarction. Acta Neurochir (Wien) 79:74–79, 1986.
13. Bogousslavsky J, Regli F, Jeanrenaud X: Benign outcome in unoperated large cerebellar haemorrhage: Report of two cases. Acta Neurochir (Wien) 73:59–65, 1984.
14. Brennan RW, Bergland RM: Acute cerebellar hemorrhage: Analysis and clinical findings and outcome in 12 cases. Neurology 27:527–532, 1977.
15. Brillman J: Acute hydrocephalus and death one month after nonsurgical treatment for acute cerebellar hemorrhage: Case report. J Neurosurg 50:374–376, 1979.
16. Chadduck WM: Cerebellar hemorrhage complicating cervical laminectomy. Neurosurgery 9:185–189, 1981.
17. Chadduck WM, Duong DH, Kast JM, et al: Pediatric cerebellar hemorrhages. Child's Nerv Syst 11:579–583, 1995.
18. Shenkin HA, Zavala M: Cerebellar strokes mortality, surgical indications and result of ventricular drainage. Lancet 2:429–432, 1982.
19. Cuny E, Loiseau H, Rivel J, et al: Amyloid angiopathy-related cerebellar hemorrhage. Surg Neurol 46:235–239, 1996.
20. Da Pian R, Bazzan A, Pasqualin A: Surgical versus medical treatment of spontaneous posterior fossa haematomas: A cooperative study on 205 cases. Neurol Res 6:145–151, 1984.
21. De Freixo MF, Garcia MJ, Alcelay LGO: Cerebellar hemorrhage: Nonsurgical forms (Letter). Ann Neurol 6:84, 1979.
22. Dunne JW, Chakera T, Kermode S: Cerebellar haemorrhage: Diagnosis and treatment: A study of 75 cases. Q J Med 64:739–754, 1987.
23. Freeman RE, Onofrio BM, Okazaki H, et al: Spontaneous intracerebellar hemorrhage: Diagnosis and surgical treatment. Neurology 23:84–90, 1973.
24. Gilliard C, Mathurin P, Passagia JG, et al: L'hématome spontanée du cervelet. Neurochirurgie 36:347–353, 1990.
25. Greenberg J, Shubick D, Shenkin H: Acute hydrocephalus in cerebellar infarct and hemorrhage. Neurology 29:409–413, 1979.
26. Guillermain P, Lena G, Reynier Y, et al: Hématomes intracérébelleux spontanées de l'adulte; 44 cas. Rev Neurol (Paris) 146:478–483, 1990.
27. Heiman TD, Satya-Murti S: Benign cerebellar hemorrhages. Ann Neurol 3:366–368, 1978.
28. Heros RC: Cerebellar hemorrhage and infarction. Stroke 12:17–22, 1981.
29. Kase CS: Cerebellar hemorrhage. In Kase CS, Caplan LR (eds): Intracerebral Hemorrhage. Boston: Butterworth-Heinemann, 1994, pp 425–443.
30. Kawasaki N, Uchida T, Yamada M, et al: Conservative management of cerebellar hemorrhage in pregnancy. Int J Gynecol Obstet 31:365–369, 1990.
31. Kobayashi S, Sato A, Kageyama Y, et al: A treatment of hypertensive cerebellar hemorrhage: Surgical or conservative management. Neurosurgery 34:246–251, 1994.
32. Kubo T, Sakata Y, Sakai SI, et al: clinical observations in the acute phase of cerebellar hemorrhage and infarction. Acta Otolaryngol (Stockh) 447:81–88, 1988.
33. Labauge R, Boukobza M, Zinszner J, et al: Hématomes spontanées du cervelet. Vingt huit observations personnelles. Rev Neurol (Paris) 139:193–204, 1983.
34. Lui T, Fairholm DJ, Shu T, et al: Surgical treatment of spontaneous cerebellar hemorrhage. Surg Neurol 23:555–558, 1985.
35. Luparello V, Canavero S: Treatment of hypertensive cerebellar hemorrhage—surgical or conservative management? Neurosurgery 37:552–553, 1995.
36. Mathew P, Teasdale G, Bannan A, et al: Neurosurgical management of cerebellar hematoma and infarct. J Neurol Neurosurg Psychiatr 59:287–292, 1995.
37. Matsumoto K, Shichijo F: A proposal of clinical grading for hypertensive cerebellar hemorrhage. No To Shinkei 34:55–62, 1982.
38. Turgut M, Ozcan OE, Erturk O, et al: Spontaneous cerebellar strokes: Clinical observations in 60 patients. Angiology 47:841–848, 1996.
39. Medrazzi JJM, Otero JM, Ottino CA: Management of 50 spontaneous cerebellar hemorrhages: Importance of obstructive hydrocephalus. Acta Neurochir (Wien) 122:39–44, 1993.
40. Melamed N, Satya-Murti S: Cerebellar hemorrhage: A review and reappraisal of benign cases. Arch Neurol 41:425–428, 1984.
41. Mitsuyama F, Katada K, Shinomiya Y, et al: Clinical investigation of the acute cerebrovascular disease. Part 4: Questions to the surgical indication of hypertensive intracerebral hemorrhage. Jpn J Stroke 4:25–29, 1982.
42. Neubauer U, Schwenk B: Therapy and prognosis in spontaneous cerebellar hematomas. Adv Neurosurg 21:57–60, 1993.
43. Noguki M, Nagashima T, Kwak S: Hypertensive cerebellar hemorrhage: Its symptoms and management. Neurol Med Chir (Tokyo) 21:751–755, 1981.
44. Patterson RH: Comment on treatment of hypertensive cerebellar hemorrhage: Surgical or conservative management. Neurosurgery 34:250, 1994.
45. Rosenthal D, Marquardt G, Sievert T: Spontaneous cerebellar hemorrhage: Acute management and prognosis. Adv Neurosurg 21:61–68, 1993.
46. Rousseaux M, Lesoin F, Combelle G, et al: Intéêt et limites de la dérivation ventriculaire isolée dans les hématomes cérébelleux non traumatiques. Neurochirurgie 30:41–44, 1984.
47. Seelig JM, Selhorst JS, Young HF, et al: Ventriculostomy for hydrocephalus in cerebellar hemorrhage. Neurology 31:1537–1540, 1981.
48. Suzuki A, Yasui N: Surgical indication of hypertensive cerebellar hematoma. Neurol Med Chir (Tokyo) 27:505–510, 1987.
49. Theodore WH, Striar J, Burger A: Nonsurgical treatment of cerebellar hematomas. Mt Sinai J Med 46:328–332, 1979.
50. Van Calenbergh F, Van Havenbergh T, Goffin J, et al: Les hématomes spontanées du cervelet au-delà de 60 ans. Neurochirurgie 42:162–168, 1996.
51. Van Der Hoop RG, Vermeullen M, Van Gijn J: Cerebellar hemorrhage: Diagnosis and treatment. Surg Neurol 29:6–10, 1988.

52. Van Loon J, Van Calenbergh F, Goffin J, et al: Controversies in the management of spontaneous cerebellar hemorrhage: A consecutive series of 49 cases and review of the literature. Acta Neurochir (Wien) 122:187–193, 1993.

53. Yoshida N, Kagawa M, Takeshita M, et al: Grading and operative indication for hypertensive cerebellar hemorrhage. Neurol Surg 14:725–731, 1986.

54. Yoshida S, Kobayashi S, Saito I, et al: Diagnosis and treatment of cerebellar hemorrhage: Comparison of hypertensive hemorrhage with hemorrhage caused by small angiomas, and CT findings. No To Shinkei 31:687–693, 1979.

55. Yoshida S, Sasaki M, Oka H, et al: Acute hypertensive cerebellar hemorrhage with signs of lower brain stem compression. Surg Neurol 10:79–83, 1978.

56. Waidhauser E, Hamburger C, Marguth F: Neurosurgical management of cerebellar hemorrhage. Neurosurg Rev 13:211–217, 1990.

57. Chen HJ, Lee TC, Wei CP: Treatment of cerebellar infarction by decompressive suboccipital craniectomy. Stroke 23:7, 1992.

58. Laun A, Busse O, Calatayud V, et al: Cerebellar infarcts in the area of the supply of the pica and their surgical treatment. Acta Neurochir 71:295–306, 1984.

59. Rousseaux M, Devos P, Lesoin F, et al: "Pseudotumoral" cystic cerebellar infarction with slow evolution. Neurosurgery 16:1, 1985.

60. Marshall J: Cerebellar vascular syndromes. In JF Toole (ed): Handbook of Clinical Neurology, Vol 11. III: Vascular Disease. New York: Elsevier Science, 1989, pp 89–94.

61. Norris JW, Eisen AA, Branch CL: Problems in cerebellar hemorrhage and infarction. Neurology 19:1043–1050, 1969.

62. Dinsdale Rb: Spontaneous hemorrhage in the posterior fossa. Arch Neurol 10:200–217, 1964.

63. Fisher CM, Picard EH, Polak A, et al: Acute hypertensive cerebellar hemorrhage. J Nerv Ment Dis 140:38–57, 1965.

64. Rey-Bellet J: Cerebellar hemorrhage: A clinico-pathological study. Neurology 10:217–222, 1960.

65. Rosenberg GA, Kaufmann DM: Cerebellar hemorrhage: Reliability of clinical evaluation. Stroke 7:332–336, 1976.

66. Sypert GW: Cerebellar hemorrhage and infarction. Comp Ther 3:42–47, 1977.

67. Abud-Ortega AF, Rajput A, Rozdilsky B: Observations in five cases of spontaneous cerebellar hemorrhage. Can Med Assoc J 106:40, 1972.

68. McKissock W, Richardson A, Walsh L: Spontaneous cerebellar hemorrhage: A study of 34 cases treated surgically. Brain 38:1–9, 1960.

69. Lehrich JR, Winkler GF, Ojemann RG: Cerebellar infarction and brain stem compression: Diagnosis and surgical treatment. Arch Neurol (Chicago) 22:490–498, 1970.

70. Ott KH, Kase CS, Ojemann RG, et al: Cerebellar hemorrhage: Diagnosis and treatment: A review of 56 cases. Arch Neurol 31:160–167, 1974.

71. Richardson AE: Spontaneous cerebellar hemorrhage. In Vinken PJ, Bruyn GJ (eds): Handbook of Clinical Neurology, Vol 12. New York: Elsevier Science, 1972, pp 54–67.

72. Hinshaw DB, Thompson JR, Hasso AN, et al: Infarctions of the brain stem and cerebellum: A correlation of computed tomography and angiography. Neuroradiology 137:105–112, 1980.

73. Salazar J, Vaquero J, Martinez P, et al: Clinical and CT scan assessment of benign versus fatal spontaneous cerebellar hematomas. Acta Neurochir 79:80–86, 1986.

74. Taneda M, Hayakawa T, Mogami H: Primary cerebellar hemorrhage: Quadrigeminal cistern obliteration on CT scans as a predictor of outcome. J Neurosurg 67:545–552, 1987.

75. Wizer B, Wall M, Weisberg L: The clinical and computed tomographic features of cerebellar peduncular hemorrhage. Neurology 38:1485–1487, 1988.

76. Zieger A, Vonofakos D, Steudel WI: Nontraumatic intracerebellar hematomas: Prognostic value of volumetric evaluation by computed tomography. Surg Neurol 22:491–494, 1984.

77. Barth A, Bogousslavsky J, Regli F: The clinical and topographic spectrum of cerebellar infarcts: A clinical magnetic resonance imaging correlation study. Ann Neurol 33:5, 1993.

78. Brusa L, Iannilli M, Bruno G, et al: Bilateral simultaneous cerebellar infarction in the medial branches of the posterior inferior cerebellar artery territories. Ital J Neurol Sci 17:433–436, 1996.

79. Ho SU, Kim KS, Berenberg RA, et al: Cerebellar infarction: A clinical and CT study. Surg Neurol 16:5, 1981.

80. Scotti G, Spinnler H, Sterzi R, et al: Cerebellar softening. Ann Neurol 8:2, 1980.

81. Thogi H, Takahashi S, Chiba K, et al: Cerebellar infarction: Clinical and neuroimaging analysis in 293 patients. Stroke 24:11, 1993.

82. Sobotta J, Becher H: Atlas der anatomie des Menschen. Munich: Urban & Schwarzenberg, 1988.

83. Marinkovic S, et al: The anatomical basis for the cerebellar infarcts. Surg Neurol 44:450–461, 1995.

84. Amarenco P, Roullet E, Hommel M, et al: Infarction in the territory of the medial branch of the posterior inferior cerebellar artery. J Neurol Neurosurg Psychiatry 53:730–735, 1990.

85. Fisher CM, Karnes WE, Kubik CS: Lateral medullary infarction: The pattern of vascular occlusion. J Neuropathol Exp Neurol 29:323–379, 1961.

86. Amarenco P, Hauw JJ, Henin D, et al: Les infarctus du territoire de l'artère cérébelleuse postero-inférieure: Etude clinico-pathologique de 28 cas. Rev Neurol (Paris) 145:277–286, 1989.

87. Duvernoy HM: Human Brain Stem Vessels. Berlin: Springer-Verlag, 1978.

88. Goodhart SP, Davison C: Syndrome of the posterior-inferior cerebellar arteries and of anterior-inferior cerebellar arteries and their branches. Arch Neurol Psychiatry 35:501–524, 1936.

89. Amarenco P, Hauw JJ: Cerebellar infarction in the territory of the anterior and inferior cerebellar artery. Brain 113:139–155, 1990.

90. Lazorthes G: Vascularisation et circulation cérébrales. Paris: Masson, 1961.

91. Takahashi M: The anterior inferior cerebellar artery. In Newton TH, Potts DG: Radiology of the Skull and Brain, Vol 2, Book 2. St. Louis: CV Mosby, pp 1796–1808.

92. Mitchell N, Angrist A: Spontaneous cerebellar hemorrhage: Report of fifteen cases. Am J Pathol 18:935–946, 1942.

93. Sedillot J: Epanchement de sang dans le lobe droit du cervelet suivi de la mort. J Gen Med Chir Pharm 47:375–379, 1813.

94. Brown-Sequard CE: Diagnosis of hemorrhage in the cerebellum. Lancet 2:391, 1861.

95. Hillairet JB: De L'haemorrhagie cerebelleuse. Arch Gen Med 1:149–169, 324–340, 411–432, 549–568, 1858.

96. Ballance H: A case of a traumatic hemorrhage into the left lateral lobe of the cerebellum, treated by operation with recovery. Surg Gynecol Obstet 3:223–225, 1906.

97. Little JR, Tubman DE, Ethier R: Cerebellar hemorrhage in adults. J Neurosurg 48:574–578, 1978.

98. Weisberg LA: Acute cerebellar hemorrhage and CT evidence of tight posterior fossa. Neurology 36:858–860, 1986.

99. Fairburn B, Oliver LC: Cerebellar softening: A surgical emergency. BMJ 1:1335–1336, 1956.

100. Lindgren SO: Infarctions simulating brain tumors in the posterior fossa. J Neurosurg 13:575–581, 1956.

101. Duncan GW, Parker SW, Fisher CM: Acute cerebellar infarction in the pica territory. Arch Neurol (Chicago) 32:364–368, 1975.

102. Sypert GW, Alvord EC Jr: Cerebellar infarction: A clinico-pathological study. Arch Neurol (Chicago) 32:357–363, 1975.

103. Amarenco P: The Spectrum of cerebellar infarctions. Neurology 41:973–979, 1991.

104. Amarenco P, Hauw JJ, Gautier JC: Arterial pathology in cerebellar infarction. Stroke 21:1299–1305, 1990.

105. Amarenco P, Hauw JJ: Cerebellar infarction in the territory of the superior cerebellar artery: A clinicopathologic study of 33 cases. Neurology 40:1383–1390, 1990.

106. Amarenco P, Roullet E, Goujon C, et al: Infarction in the anterior rostral cerebellum (the territory of the lateral branch of the superior cerebellar artery). Neurology 41:253–258, 1991.

107. Amarenco P, Rosengart A, Dewitt D, et al: Anterior inferior cerebellar artery territory infarcts: Mechanism and clinical features. Arch Neurol 50:154–161, 1993.

108. Amarenco P, Caplan L: Vertebrobasilar occlusive disease: Review of selected aspects. Cerebrovasc Dis 3:66–73, 1993.

109. Amarenco P, Levy C, Cohen A, et al: Causes and mechanism of territorial and nonterritorial cerebellar infarcts in 115 consecutive patients. Stroke 25:105–112, 1994.

110. Heros RC: Surgical treatment of cerebellar infarction (Editorial). Stroke 23:7, 1992.

111. Russel RWR: Observation on intracranial aneurysm. Brain 86:425–442, 1963.

112. Cole FM, Yates IO: The occurrence and significance of intracerebral micro-aneurysms. J Pathol Bact 2–93:393–411, 1967.

113. Wakai S, Nagai M: Histological verification of microaneurysms as a cause of cerebral hemorrhage in surgical specimen. J Neurol Neurosurg Psychiatry 52:595–599, 1989.
114. McCormick WF, Nafzinger JD: Criptic vascular malformations of the central nervous system. J Neurosurg 5:892–894, 1966.
115. Teasdale G, Jennet B: Assessment and prognosis of coma after head injury. Acta Neurochir (Wien) 34:45–55, 1976.
116. Teasdale G, Jennett B: Assessment of coma and impaired consciousness. A practical scale. Lancet ii:81–84, 1974.
117. Mohadjer M, Eggert R, May J, et al: CT-guided stereotactic fibrinolysis of spontaneous and hypertensive cerebellar hemorrhage: Long-term results. J Neurosurg 73:217–222, 1990.
118. Niizuma H, Suzuki J: Computed tomography-guided stereotactic aspiration of posterior fossa hematomas: A supine lateral retromastoid approach. Neurosurgery 21:422–427, 1987.
119. Koenig A, Laas R, Hermann HD: Cerebellar hemorrhage as a complication after supratentorial craniotomy. Acta Neurochir Wien 88:104–108, 1997.
120. Toczek MT, Morrell J, Silverberg GA, et al: Cerebellar hemorrhage complicating temporal lobectomy: Report of four cases. J Neurosurg 85:718–722, 1996.
121. Jennett B, Bond M: Assessment of outcome after severe brain damage: A practical scale. Lancet i:480–485, 1975.
122. Easton JD, Sherman DG: Cervical manipulation and stroke. Stroke 8:594–597, 1977.
123. Tyagi AK, Kirollos RW, Marks PV: Posttraumatic cerebellar infarction. Br J Neurosurg 9:683–686, 1995.
124. Aggarwal S, Byrne BD: Massive ischemic cerebellar infarction due to cocaine use. Neuroradiology 33:449–450, 1992.
125. Caplan LR, Baquis MD, Pessin MS, et al: Dissection of the intracranial vertebral artery. Neurology 38:868–877, 1988.
126. Mas JL, Bousser MG, Hasboun D, et al: Extracranial vertebral artery dissections: A review of 13 cases. Stroke 18:1037–1047, 1987.
127. Levine SR, Welch KMA: Superior cerebellar artery infarction and vertebral artery dissection. Stroke 19:1431–1434, 1988.
128. Hilzenrat N, Zilberman D, Sikuler E: Isolated cerebellar infarction as a presenting symptom of polycythemia vera. Acta Haematol 88:204–206, 1992.
129. Gomez CR, Gomez SM, Puricelli MS, et al: Transcranial Doppler in reversible migrainous vasospasm causing cerebellar infarction: Report of a case. Angiology 2:152–156, 1991.
130. Meco G, Bozzao L, Formisano R, et al: Complicated migraine: Case report. Ital J Neurol Sci 9:291–294, 1988.
131. Philips PC, Lorentsen KJ, Shropshire LC, et al: Congenital odontoid aplasia and posterior circulation stroke in childhood. Ann Neurol 23:410–413, 1988.
132. Chaves CJ, Caplan LR, Chung CS, et al: Cerebellar infarcts in the New England Medical Center Posterior Circulation Stroke Registry. Neurology 44:1385–1390, 1994.
133. Kase CS, White JL, Joslyn JN, et al: Cerebellar infarction in the superior cerebellar artery distribution. Neurology 35:943–948, 1985.
134. Tada Y, Mizutani T, Nishimura T, et al: Acute bilateral infarction in the territory of the medial branches of the posterior inferior cerebellar arteries. Stroke 25:3, 1994.
135. Matsushita K, Naritomi H, Kazui S, et al: Infarction in the anterior inferior cerebellar artery territory: Magnetic resonance imaging and auditory brain stem responses. Cerebrovasc Dis 3:206–212, 1993.
136. Terao S, Sobue G, Izumi M, et al: Infarction of superior cerebellar artery presenting as cerebellar symptoms. Stroke 27:1679–1681, 1996.
137. Kase CS, Norrvig B, Levine S, et al: Cerebellar infarction: Clinical and anatomic observations in 66 cases. Stroke 24:1, 1993.
138. Antonello RM, Pasqua M, Bosco A, et al: Massive cerebellar infarct complicated by hydrocephalus. Ital J Neurol Sci 13:695–698, 1992.
139. Feely MP: Cerebellar infarction. Neurosurgery 4:1, 1979.
140. Rieke K, Krieger D, Adams HP, et al: Therapeutic strategies in space-occupying cerebellar infarction based on clinical, neuroradiological and neurophysiological data. Cerebrovasc Dis 3:45–55, 1993.
141. Jauss M, Krieger D, Horning C, et al: Surgical and medical management of patients with massive cerebellar infarctions: Results of the German-Austrian cerebellar infarction studies. J Neurol 246:257–264, 1999.
142. Hornig CR, Rust DS, Busse O, et al: Space-occupying cerebellar infarction: Clinical course and prognosis. Stroke 25:2, 1994.
143. Kempe LG: Posterior Fossa: Spinal Cord and Peripheral Nerve Disease. Vol 2: Operative Neurosurgery. Berlin: Springer-Verlag, 1970, pp 34–35.

# C H A P T E R  7 0

# Surgical Management of Cerebellar Tumors in Adults

■ HENRY H. SCHMIDEK

In adults, the nature of cerebellar masses depends on the patient's age, clinical situation, and magnetic resonance imaging (MRI) characteristics of the lesion; however, 55% to 70% of cerebellar masses in adults are metastatic in origin, and the figure is higher if the patient is older than 40 years of age. Among the tumors that commonly involve midline structures of the cerebellum are the medulloblastoma, ependymoma, dermoid, and arachnoid cyst, whereas the cerebellar astrocytoma and hemangioblastoma are often found predominantly in the cerebellar hemispheres. Tumors anywhere in the posterior fossa can present with obstructive hydrocephalus, but this finding is seen most commonly in midline lesions. Midline cerebellar masses produce truncal and gait ataxia with a broad-based, unsteady gait and imperfect tandem walking, whereas hemispheric lesions give rise to limb ataxias manifested as dysmetria, abnormalities of rapid alternating movements, nystagmus, hypotonia, and hyporeflexia. Dysfunction of extraocular motility may be the result of the direct effect of the tumor on the brain stem and cerebellum, or the nonspecific result of raised intracranial pressure.[3] Horizontal gaze paretic nystagmus is seen with lesions around the fourth ventricle, and upbeat nystagmus is seen in patients with posterior fossa tumors and evidence of direct brain stem involvement. Vertigo is associated with laterally positioned tumors and may be disabling. Compression or invasion of brain stem structures produces numerous disturbances involving the cranial nerve nuclei and the motor and sensory pathways of the brain stem.

## PREOPERATIVE DIAGNOSTIC AND THERAPEUTIC MEASURES

Adults suspected of having a posterior fossa tumor require a chest radiograph to exclude a lung tumor and an MRI scan of the head. The radiographic appearance may suggest the tumor's histologic type. A metastatic tumor is usually situated at the gray-white interface of the cerebellar cortex and appears as a ring-like, enhancing mass with prominent peritumoral edema. The presence of more than one lesion suggests metastases or hemangioblastomas. Low-density,

cystic, extra-axial lesions without an enhancing mural nodule suggest an epidermoid tumor or an arachnoid cyst.[9] Cerebellar hemorrhages are high-density lesions with edema that produce a shift of midline structures and may occur in pre-existing tumors, producing a disproportionate shift of the intracranial contents. Cerebellar astrocytomas are characterized by a large cystic component, the walls of which consist of tumor tissue or an enhancing mural nodule of tumor. In adults, cystic lesions with mural nodules are likely to be cerebellar hemangioblastomas.[6] Medulloblastomas and ependymomas are usually centered in the fourth ventricle. Medulloblastomas have a heterogeneous density with variable contrast enhancement, and calcify in dense clumps, whereas ependymomas calcify in small, punctate aggregates. Typically, both low- and high-grade brain stem gliomas are low-density masses, with computed tomography (CT) images enhanced only slightly with contrast; gliomas enlarge the brain stem and displace the fourth ventricle.[5]

Magnetic resonance imaging is superior to CT in its sensitivity for detecting a posterior fossa lesion, defining the displacement of normal structures, and demonstrating the extent of the pathologic process (e.g., by scanning the spinal contents for evidence of tumor seeding). In one such study comparing these two modalities, a correct preoperative diagnosis was made in 83% of cerebellar tumors examined by MRI compared with 48% correctly diagnosed by CT. In addition, other MR systems allow noninvasive definition of the tumor's vascularity and blood supply, and proton MR spectroscopy can, in many cases, differentiate ependymomas, low-grade astrocytomas, and primitive neuroectodermal tumors (PNETs).[11]

## SURGICAL MANAGEMENT

The surgical management of masses in the posterior fossa depends on the patient's general condition and the presumed nature of the pathologic process.

The need for preoperative cerebrospinal fluid (CSF) shunting or ventricular drainage with an obstructive hydrocephalus secondary to a posterior fossa mass is a matter of surgical judgment. In my mind, the treatment of such hydrocephalus involves surgery, removal of as much tumor as is technically feasible and safe, and the reopening of the CSF pathways. The exception is the extremely ill patient in whom ventricular drainage is performed as a life-saving measure until definitive surgery can be performed.

Patients with posterior fossa mass lesions are operated on using the Radionics frameless stereotactic system with fiduciary markers placed before surgery on a patient who then undergoes a contrast-enhanced MRI scan of the head. The information provided by this system is used during surgery to fashion a craniotomy flap. The system allows the surgical exposure to be accurately centered on the lesion and ensures that it extends to the margins of the lesion. This planning allows exposures to be smaller and more accurately centered. The same technology, with its known limitations regarding brain shift, is also used intraoperatively to define the margins of the lesion.

Patients are begun on preoperative dexamethasone and antibiotics. Intubation is accomplished with particular care in the presence of raised intracranial pressure. Surgery is performed under controlled mechanical ventilation, which allows precise control of arterial $P_{CO_2}$ levels, reduces venous bleeding, and may decrease the incidence of air embolism. In the rare instances in which spontaneous ventilation is the preferable technique, it is accomplished with a shorter-acting inhalation agent, and the rate of respiration is increased by altering the concentration of the carbon dioxide inhaled. This technique is sometimes useful during surgery in or on the brain stem.

Operations in the posterior fossa can be performed with the patient in the full prone position, the lateral recumbent position, the supine position with the head turned away from the side of the lesion, or, nowadays, rarely, the sitting position.

The prone positions—fully prone, three-fourths prone, and lateral recumbent—also may be used for surgery in the posterior fossa. In the fully prone position, the patient is placed on a bolster to allow free abdominal excursion and avoid compression of the inferior vena cava. Pin fixation of the head is used in adult patients and older children. The surgeon must be careful repeatedly to ensure that the eyes have no pressure placed on them by the headrest during positioning, when the patient has reached the final position, and during the operation. Special care must also be taken to secure the endotracheal tube.

For operations in the prone position, the patient is placed in a minus Trendelenburg position of approximately 15 degrees to promote venous drainage.[15] The operative exposure chosen depends on the location and extent of the mass lesion. A midline posterior fossa craniectomy is suited for lesions situated on or close to the midline in the vermis, or for surgery on the cerebellar tonsils or in the region of the foramen magnum. This approach, modified to extend to one side, is also often used in managing large, space-occupying cerebellar lesions. A unilateral posterior fossa craniectomy is used in lesions restricted to one cerebellar hemisphere. A combined supratentorial and infratentorial approach can be used for large tumors involving these compartments.

## Midline Posterior Fossa Craniectomy

Lesions in the fourth ventricle, cerebellar vermis, and medial cerebellar hemispheres are best approached through a bilateral midline exposure. This exposure allows exploration from the superior aspect of the cerebellum, the cerebellar peduncles, and the midline structures to the foramen magnum.

A midline skin incision is made that extends from the inion to the cervical region. Hemostasis of the superficial layers is accomplished with Raney clips. The operation then proceeds in the midline to the avascular median raphe. The occipital muscles are separated and cut with the cautery 1 inch from their insertion. The periosteum is cleared, thereby exposing the occipital bone. Venous bleeding from muscle and bone should be controlled promptly; air emboli can occur with the patient in either the sitting or the prone position. If an air embolism is detected, the operative field is flooded with saline and packed with wet gauze sponges. When the patient's condition is stable, a diligent search is made for the site of air entry. Often, this source is not identified. Positive end-expiratory pressure increases the venous bleeding and aids in the identification of the source of the air embolization. It also reduces further air entry into the circulation. With the frameless stereotactic system, it is possible accurately to localize the tumor mass, and the exposure is tailored to the specifics of the case. The removal of bone is accomplished by thinning the occipital squama with a Midas Rex drill and then gently peeling away the shell of bone with a Kerrison rongeur. I usually do not use a craniotomy flap, nor do I attempt to replace bone into the skull defect at the end of intracranial surgery. The craniectomy may be enlarged to the foramen magnum. Dural attachments to the foramen magnum may be tenacious and require sharp dissection from the overlying bone. In a patient with tonsillar herniation, the arch of C1 and the yellow ligament between C1 and C2 are removed, allowing adequate decompression of the medulla and upper cervical spinal cord.

The dura is divided in a Y-shaped configuration. This opening crosses the occipital sinus and circular sinuses, which are cauterized and cut. The dura is reflected laterally and a small arachnoid opening is made to permit the gradual release of CSF. A midline craniectomy exposes the foramen of Magendie at the caudal end of the vermis. Lesions in or adjacent to the fourth ventricle (medulloblastoma, ependymoma) often protrude from this foramen, and their exposure requires coagulating the vermis and splitting it to gain adequate exposure of the tumor and the floor of the fourth ventricle.

## Management of Predominantly Midline Cerebellar Tumors

### Medulloblastoma

Medulloblastomas are reddish-gray, friable masses that frequently distend the vermis and protrude from the foramen of Magendie. Some of these tumors are located in the cerebellopontine angle or at the tentorium. In contrast to children, less than one half of medulloblastomas in adults are associated with hydrocephalus. In presumed cases of medulloblastoma, preoperative contrast-enhanced cranial and spinal MRIs are performed to identify the presence of tumor dissemination. Tumor dissemination is associated with a marked reduction in 5-year survival rates to approximately 25%.

These tumors are easily aspirated. Removing a tumor from between the cerebellar tonsils to identify the fourth ventricular outlet and floor is usually necessary. Once the foramen of Magendie is identified, the vermis is split to identify the upper margin of the tumor. Tumor removal can be accomplished by coagulation with the bipolar cautery followed by aspiration with the ultrasonic device. Tumor removal is continued so that the lateral recesses of the fourth ventricle and the aqueduct of Sylvius are visualized. Removing tumor adherent to the floor of the fourth ventricle may not be possible.

A radical approach to tumor removal followed by craniospinal irradiation has resulted in improved 5-year survival rates of 50% to 60%, compared with a 30% rate for cases managed by subtotal surgical removal. In general, survival is probably better in women. Medulloblastoma tends to recur in the posterior fossa, although subarachnoid and systemic metastases often cause further morbidity and mortality, and the occurrence of frontal lobe masses is not uncommon. Ventricular shunting has been implicated in the spread of these neoplastic cells beyond the neuraxis, and some authors therefore recommend the use of a millipore-type filter interposed in the shunt system. Survival after recurrence is poor in spite of additional radiation and chemotherapy.[12, 17]

## Ependymoma of the Fourth Ventricle

Ependymomas often arise at the obex and protrude into the upper cervical spinal canal, requiring a posterior fossa craniectomy and an upper cervical laminectomy for their exposure. Ependymomas characteristically conform to the shape and surfaces of the space into which they grow. Because most ependymomas of the fourth ventricle arise in the region of the hypoglossal and vagal trigone and are intimately adherent to underlying neural tissue, complete removal of these tumors may not be possible. Prognosis in these tumors is influenced by the preoperative Karnofsky performance grade (>70), extent of surgical removal, histologic grade, and evidence of spinal seeding. The 5-year survival rate for ependymomas of the fourth ventricle in adults is 60%, with the 10-year survival rate being 45%. Postoperative irradiation has markedly improved the 5-year survival rate. In these cases, postoperative irradiation is limited to the structures of the posterior fossa. Subarachnoid metastases occur in approximately 5% to 10% of patients and are associated with the more malignant forms of this tumor. These cases are treated with craniospinal irradiation, as are the histologically high-grade tumors.[1, 6]

## Posterior Fossa Cysts

Various midline cystic masses may be encountered in the posterior fossa, including extra-axial arachnoid cysts, the cysts associated with the Dandy-Walker syndrome. These lesions are symptomatic because of brain stem and cerebellar compression or obstructive hydrocephalus. Cyst fluid that is xanthochromic or has a protein content of greater than 20 mg/dl is unlikely to be associated with an arachnoid or Dandy-Walker cyst. In this case, the lesion is fully exposed, the cyst wall is carefully examined, and multiple biopsy specimens are obtained from the walls. Arachnoid cysts and Dandy-Walker cysts can usually be treated either by marsupialization or by cyst-peritoneal shunting. The supratentorial hydrocephalus occasionally associated with these lesions persists in spite of satisfactory shunting and may require either a separate ventriculoperitoneal shunt or a ventricular catheter joined through a Y-connector to the cyst-peritoneal shunt.

## Dermoid Tumors

Dermoid tumors in the posterior fossa typically arise near the midline, although they may be located in the cerebellopontine angle or at the skull base. These lesions may not be symptomatic until adult life, growing slowly into a cyst as sebaceous material and desquamated epithelium are discharged. Patients may have recurrent bouts of meningitis as a result of entrance of bacteria through a sinus tract or chemical inflammation from cholesterol leakage into the CSF. With aggressive surgery, these tumors are often completely removable and do not recur, whereas with subtotal removal there is a 30% recurrence rate within 8 years.[7]

## Unilateral Posterior Fossa Surgery for Cerebellar Mass Lesions

A unilateral exposure is usually adequate when the lesion involves one cerebellar hemisphere. Using the frameless stereotactic system during the planning phase of the operation, the surgeon can limit the size of the exposure and extent of soft tissue dissection. The surgery is centered on the lesion, and the rostrocaudal extent depends on the lesion's size. Often this surgery is performed through a skin incision located halfway between the mastoid process and the midline. The bone is thinned with a high-speed drill and removed with rongeurs. Before the dura is opened, a large cyst can be cannulated directly through an opening made in the posterior fossa dura to relieve the intracranial pressure.

## Cerebellar Astrocytoma

The cerebellar astrocytoma is the prototypical primary tumor of the cerebellar hemisphere. These tumors may be solid, cystic, or microcystic, and their location makes total excision the treatment of choice. After the dura is opened, the mass is exposed through a cerebellar corticectomy. If the tumor is solid, dissection is carried around its perimeter, or the tumor can first be debulked with the ultrasonic aspirator. For a cystic tumor with a mural nodule, a total excision of the mural nodule should be carried out. Removal of the wall of the cyst is not necessary. The 5-year survival rate for patients with benign cerebellar astrocytomas is approximately 85%. Some pathologic characteristics of cerebellar astrocytomas are of prognostic significance: patients with microcysts, leptomeningeal deposits, Rosenthal's fibers, and oligodendroglial elements (Winston's type A) have a 94% 10-year survival rate. Solid cerebellar astrocytomas and cerebellar astrocytomas located in the midline have a significantly higher incidence of recurrence. Every attempt should be made to effect total tumor removal with the first operation.[15]

Malignant astrocytoma of the cerebellum and cerebellar glioblastomas have a prognosis like that of malignant supratentorial gliomas and recur within 4 to 32 months regardless of the extent of removal or postoperative irradiation. These tumors often have a median location and extend into the fourth ventricle, cervical region, or outside the cranium. After surgery, patients with type A tumors undergo enhanced MRI studies biannually. Closer follow-up should be maintained for patients with solid or type B tumors. The optimal treatment of recurrent malignant cerebellar astrocytomas is unsettled.[2, 16]

## Metastatic Tumors of the Cerebellum

The course of patients with carcinomas of the breast, kidney, lung, or ovary is frequently complicated by solitary cerebellar metastases. These metastases are more life threatening than metastases in other locations, and considerably better results are obtained with their removal than if they are treated nonsurgically.

A cerebellar mass is considered for removal if survival of 3 to 6 months can be expected.[36] The procedures for surgical removal of metastatic masses from the cerebellum are the same as those for treating the cystic or solid cerebellar astrocytomas described earlier. The 1-year survival rate after surgery and radiation is 32% to 45% for patients with metastatic lung carcinomas, 45% to 63% for those with metastatic breast carcinomas, 30% to 52% for those with metastatic melanomas, and 30% to 31% overall for those with metastatic lesions to the brain.[36] Occasionally, a patient with contiguous posterior fossa metastatic lesions can have more than one lesion removed surgically with a useful prolongation of life.[14]

## Cerebellar Hemangioblastoma

Cerebellar hemangioblastomas are histologically benign vascular tumors often located in a cerebellar hemisphere. In approximately 75% of cases, the mass consists of a cystic tumor with a mural nodule. Complete removal of the tumor nodule is curative. Ten percent of patients harbor more than one tumor mass in the posterior fossa, especially in association with von Hippel-Lindau disease. Preoperative MR angiography is particularly important in these patients to assess the vascularity of the lesion and define the location and size of each tumor nodule. The arterial feeders known on the basis of angiographic studies to be supplying the mass should be interrupted before an attempt is made to remove the tumor, either before surgery by embolization or during surgery by a careful "search-and-destroy mission" to eliminate the blood supply to the tumor before removal of the mass. Even then, the surgeon should try to remove these tumors by going around the lesion rather than attempting a piecemeal resection because of the potential for serious intraoperative bleeding. Approximately one fourth of hemangioblastomas are solid tumors,[40] which are particularly difficult to remove and prone to invade the brain stem, making total excision impossible.[41]

In cystic lesions, a cortical incision is made into the cyst cavity after exposure of the cerebellum. Self-retaining retractors are used to hold the walls of the cyst apart, and a search is made for the mural nodule. This tumor often appears as a mulberry-sized mass. The area surrounding the tumor is cauterized with bipolar forceps, the tumor drawn into the cyst cavity, and its base cauterized. These tumors do not have a true capsule to assist in the dissection. If the surgeon encounters an obvious mural nodule, he or she must look for areas of discoloration or induration. The appearance of these lesions can be quite variable and requires careful correlation with the angiogram to identify the nidus of the tumor.

In the case of a large, solid hemangioblastoma that cannot be removed as a solitary mass, the surgeon should attempt to interrupt the tumor's arterial supply before trying to remove the lesion. Because the tumor's blood supply often arises from arterial branches passing through the tentorium, a combined supratentorial and infratentorial (occipitotranstentorial) approach may be necessary to interrupt the tumor's vascularity before the mass is removed. Tumor recurrence from undetected multiple or residual tumor is common, and reoperative surgery in these cases has a significantly higher mortality and morbidity rate; therefore, every attempt should be made at primary total tumor removal. Patients with evidence of postoperative residual hemangioblastomas should receive radiation to the posterior fossa, and follow-up MRI scanning should be performed every 6 months, so that if the mass enlarges or symptoms develop, its operative removal can again be attempted.

## Lhermitte-Duclos Disease (Dysplastic Gangliocytoma of the Cerebellum)

This lesion is a tumor-like mass of tissue resulting from the growth of dysplastic cortical neurons and thickening of the molecular layer, resulting in enlarged cerebellar folia and expansion of the cerebellar hemisphere. The MRI shows a parallel "tiger-striped" appearance of the cerebellum that is characteristic and indicative of the atrophic folia. Treatment recommendations are open biopsy or total excision with evidence of clinical progression.

## Combined Supratentorial and Infratentorial Approach to Posterior Fossa Tumors

Masses in the anterior and superior part of the cerebellum, high in the cerebellopontine angle, or involving the tentorial hiatus are difficult to expose. Some tumors extend from the posterior fossa through the tentorial notch. In these cases, a combined laterally situated supratentorial and infratentorial approach may be needed. Because this approach may require ligation of one lateral sinus, the preoperative contrast studies that provide information on the venous phase help to delineate the anatomy of the dural venous sinuses and to determine whether the ligation of the sinus ipsilateral to the side of the tumor is permissible. The combined supratentorial and infratentorial approach is performed after exposure of the occipital bone through a lateral skin incision. The incision is carried superiorly and is curved into a standard craniotomy incision. An occipital craniotomy is then performed above the transverse sinus, after which the bone over the transverse sinus is thinned with a high-speed drill and removed. If the main reason for exposing the tentorium is to obliterate the tumor's blood supply, ligating the transverse sinus may not be necessary. In this case, the dural incisions are made above and below the sinus, and the superior dural flap is situated lateral to Labbé's vein. This method leaves a bridge of dura containing the transverse sinus. Superomedial retraction of the occipital lobe exposes the superior surface of the tentorium. Bridging veins from the cerebellar surface to the dura are cauterized and divided, thereby exposing the inferior surface of the tentorium. Assessing the characteristics of the tumor mass and interrupting its arterial feeders should then be possible. The tumor mass below the tentorium is often debulked first. If additional exposure is needed, the tentorium is split, avoiding the deep veins, posterior cerebral artery, and cranial nerves III, IV, and VI at the incisura. Even greater exposure is provided by ligation and splitting of the transverse sinus.[8, 13, 14, 18]

After tumor surgery the posterior fossa dura is closed. Small rents in the dura may require interposition of pericranial fascia taken from a site adjacent to the operative field, and large defects are closed with an allograft. The subarachnoid space is filled with saline after the dural repair to ensure a watertight closure and replace CSF, thereby displacing intracranial air. Failure to close the dura of the posterior fossa after surgery is associated with an increased incidence of aseptic meningitis. The epidural space is drained with a Jackson-Pratt drain, and the muscle and skin layers are meticulously approximated.

Postoperative patient management is in the intensive care unit. Respiratory status must be carefully monitored, and the endotracheal tube is left in situ until the patient is awake, following commands, and able to exchange air and secretions adequately. External ventricular drainage is not used routinely unless there is an obstructive hydrocephalus that remains unrelieved.

Aside from the usual postoperative complications after posterior fossa surgery, an unusual complication not described elsewhere in this book is the so-called "posterior fossa syndrome," consisting of a transient loss of speech (cerebellar mutism) followed by dysarthria. Characteristically this is seen in children, but it is a complication occasionally seen in adults after the removal of vermian or paravermian tumors. The symptoms begin from 1 to 6 days after surgery and usually last for weeks to months. The mechanism is thought to be due to postsurgical edema of the pontine tegmentum interfering with afferent and efferent connections of the cerebellum involved in initiating speech and other complex motor and behavioral activities.[3, 4, 5, 9, 10]

## REFERENCES

1. McLaughlin MP, Marcus RB Jr, Buatti JM, McCollough WM: Ependymoma: Results, prognostic factors and treatment recommendations. Int J Radiat Oncol Biol Phys 40:845–850, 1998.
2. Djalilian HR, Hall WA: Malignant gliomas of the cerebellum: An analytic review. J Neurooncol 36:247–257, 1998.
3. Bhatoe HS: Mutism, oropharyngeal apraxia and dysarthria after posterior fossa tumor excision. Br J Neurosurg 11:341–343, 1997.
4. Pollack IF: Posterior fossa syndrome. Int Rev Neurobiol 41:411–432, 1997.
5. Kai Y, Kuratsu J, Suginohara K, et al: Cerebellar mutism after posterior fossa surgery: Two case reports. Neurol Med Chir (Tokyo) 37:929–33, 1997.
6. Ferrante L, Mastronardi L, Schettini G, et al: Fourth ventricle ependymomas: A study of 20 cases with survival analysis. Acta Neurochir (Wien) 131:67–74, 1994.
7. Talacchi A, Sala F, Alessandrini F, et al: Assesssment and surgical management of posterior fossa epidermoid tumors: Report of 28 cases. Neurosurgery 42:242–251, 1998.
8. Bartels RH, de Vries J, Van Overbeeke JJ, Grotenhuis JA: Occipitotranstentorial approach for lesions of the superior cerebellar hemisphere: Technical report. Neurosurgery 41:1127–1129, 1997.
9. Ersahin Y, Mutluer S, Cagli S, Dumman Y: Cerebellar mutism: Report of seven cases and review of the literature. Neurosurgery 38:60–65, 1996.
10. Wang Z, Sutton LN, Cnaan A, et al: Proton MR spectroscopy of pediatric cerebellar tumors. AJNR Am J Neuroradiol 16:1821–1833, 1995.
11. Colosimo C, Celi G, Settecasi C, et al: Magnetic resonance and computerized tomography of posterior cranial fossa tumors in childhood: Differential diagnosis and assessment of lesion extent (Abstract). Radiol Med (Torino) 90:386–395, 1995.
12. Becker RL, Becker AD, Sobel DF: Adult medulloblastoma: Review of 13 cases with emphasis on MRI. Neuroradiology 37:104–108, 1995.
13. Ogata N, Yonekawa Y: Paramedian supracerebellar approach to the upper brainstem and peduncular lesions. Neurosurgery 40:101–104, 1997.
14. Ampil FL, Nanda A, Willis BK, et al: Metastatic disease in the cerebellum: The LSU experience in 1981–1993. Am J Clin Oncol 19:509–511, 1996.
15. Hassounah M, Siqueira EB, Haider A, Gray A: Cerebellar astrocytoma: Report of 13 cases aged over 20 years and review of the literature. Br J Neurosurg 10:365–371, 1996.
16. Morreale VM, Ebersold MJ, Quast LM, Parisi JE: Cerebellar astrocytoma: Experience with 54 cases surgically treated at the Mayo Clinic, Rochester, Minnesota, from 1978 to 1990. J Neurosurg 87:257–261, 1997.
17. Le QT, Weil MD, Wara WM, et al: Adult medulloblastoma: An analysis of survival and prognostic factors. Cancer J Sci Am 3:238–245, 1997.
18. Kapp JP, Schmidek HH: The Cerebral Venous System and Its Disorders. Orlando: Grune & Stratton, 1984, pp 581–623.
19. Sato O: Transoccipital transtentorial approach for removal of cerebellar haemangioblastoma. Acta Neurochir (Wien) 59:195–208, 1981.

# CHAPTER 71

# Posterior Fossa Meningiomas*

■ DARREN S. LOVICK and ROBERT E. MAXWELL

Fewer than 9% of intracranial meningiomas occur in the posterior fossa.[1, 2] In Olivecrona's series of 4185 brain tumors, Castellano and Ruggiero reported a review of 803 intracranial meningiomas, of which 68 occurred in the posterior fossa, including 20 from the tentorium cerebelli.[3] Because of the complicated neurovascular anatomy of the posterior fossa and nature of tumor growth, meningiomas can be difficult to excise totally. The clinical presentation varies with the size and location of the tumor and depends primarily on the degree of involvement of the lower cranial nerves, cerebellum, brain stem, and fourth ventricle. Tumors of the posterior fossa are classified according to their site of attachment: the cerebellopontine angle (CPA), the posterior surface of the petrous ridge, the tentorium cerebelli, the clivus, the foramen magnum, the fourth ventricle, and the occipital squama over the cerebellar hemispheres.

Although the posterior fossa is a relatively small intracranial compartment, meningiomas within different locations may have vastly different presentations. Midline tumors arising along the basilic groove displace the brain stem and stretch the cranial nerves. The symptoms and signs are associated with dysfunction of the long motor tract and the lower six cranial nerves. The extremely rare tumors arising from the tela choroidea in the fourth ventricle produce obstructive hydrocephalus. Meningiomas arising from the posterolateral petrous ridge, from the occipital squama over the posterior cerebellar convexity, and from the tentorium cerebelli produce symptoms of cerebellar dysfunction. Because of their slow growth, these tumors often are well tolerated by the patient until signs and symptoms of increased intracranial pressure associated with hydrocephalus develop.

This chapter discusses the treatment of hydrocephalus due to posterior fossa meningiomas and describes the common clinical presentation, radiographic appearance, and surgical management of tentorial, CPA, and foramen magnum meningiomas.

## VENTRICULAR DRAINAGE FOR OBSTRUCTIVE HYDROCEPHALUS

Control of increased intracranial pressure and hydrocephalus is urgent. Lumbar puncture and drainage is contraindi-

cated because of the risk of transtentorial or foramen magnum herniation. If any delay in posterior fossa surgery is elected or necessary, the increased intracranial pressure associated with hydrocephalus is relieved by lateral ventriculostomy and ventricular drainage. Care should be taken to ensure that the cerebrospinal fluid (CSF) pressure is controlled and gradually reduced because upward transtentorial herniation or subdural hematoma can be induced by sudden changes in pressure. The sterile ventricular drainage system is kept open, but the height of the tubing is adjusted so that drainage occurs only at pressures exceeding 100 mm of water (7 to 8 mm Hg). The CSF pulsations or pressure waves are continually observed to ensure that the drainage system is not obstructed. The patient's vital signs and neurologic status are closely monitored for evidence of brain stem compression or ischemia associated with transtentorial herniation. Ventricular drainage is preferred to ventricular shunting because the system is better monitored and a foreign body is not permanently left in place. If a prolonged delay in definitive surgery is anticipated, however, a ventriculoperitoneal or ventriculoatrial shunt is preferred to lessen the risk of ventriculitis and to ease nursing care.

A preoperative ventriculostomy performed through a frontal twist drill or bur hole is preferred to one in the occipital or posterior parietal region. This method lessens the potential for contamination of the posterior fossa craniectomy wound. The right frontal site is chosen for primary shunting or ventriculostomy drainage. If ventriculostomy is necessary but subsequent shunting is a possibility, consideration should be given to placing the frontal ventriculostomy on the left side. If immediate posterior fossa surgery is carried out, an occipital bur hole is placed 7 cm above the inion and 3 cm to the right of the midline for lateral ventriculostomy (Fig. 71–1).

## MENINGIOMAS OF THE TENTORIUM CEREBELLI AND POSTERIOR PETROUS RIDGE

### Clinical Presentation

Meningiomas arising from the tentorium cerebelli account for 2% to 7% of all meningiomas and 18% of posterior fossa meningiomas.[4-7] As with meningiomas in other loca-

*This chapter has been adapted from Schmidek H: Meningiomas and their Surgical Management. Philadelphia: WB Saunders, 1991.

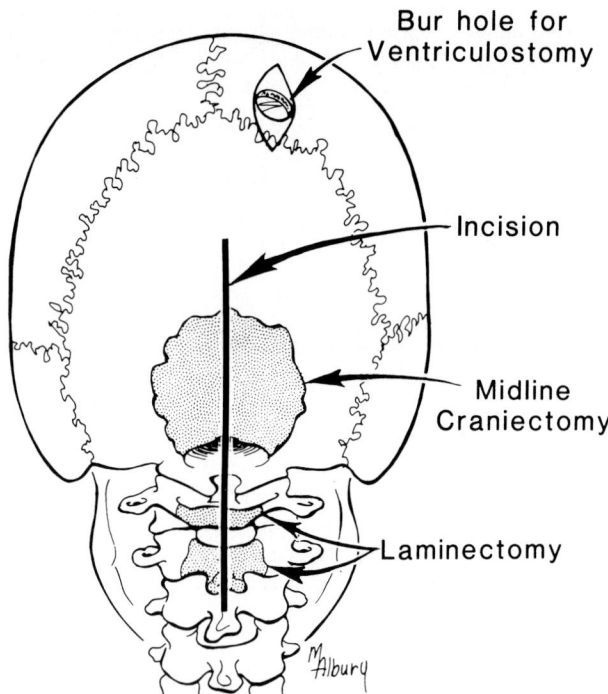

Bur hole for
Ventriculostomy

Incision

Midline
Craniectomy

Laminectomy

FIGURE 71–1 ■ A bur hole is placed 7 cm above the inion and 3 cm to the right of the midline for a lateral ventriculostomy when posterior fossa surgery is performed without previous ventricular drainage. Tumors in the region of the foramen magnum, the fourth ventricle, or the occipital squama overlying the medial posterior cerebellar hemisphere are approached by a midline suboccipital craniectomy. (From Maxwell RF, Chou SN: Posterior fossa meningiomas. In Schmidek HH, Sweet WH [eds]: Operative Neurosurgical Techniques: Indications, Methods, and Results, Vol 1, 2nd ed. Philadelphia: WB Saunders, 1988, p 572.)

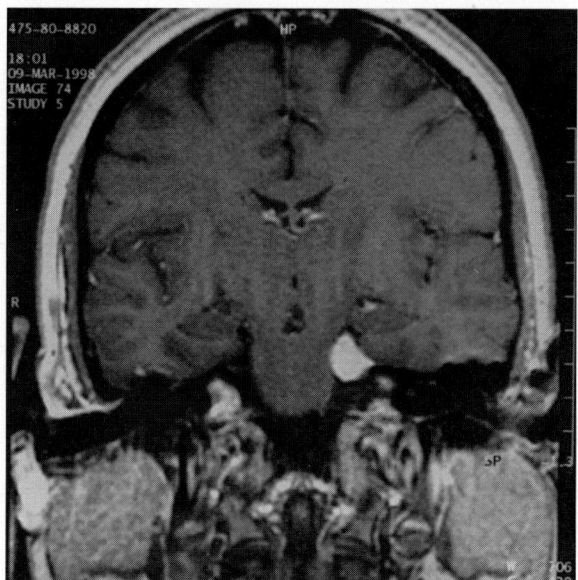

FIGURE 71–2 ■ Coronal gadolinium-enhanced magnetic resonance imaging scan demonstrating a meningioma with its origin at the tentorial incisura.

tions, women slightly outnumber men and the mean age at presentation is between the fourth and sixth decades of life. The clinical manifestations are dependent on the location along the tentorium and primary direction of growth. Large lesions that expand inferiorly over the cerebellar hemisphere may produce disturbances of gait with ataxia. Patients with anteroinferiorly directed meningiomas present with a progressive history of facial numbness or pain, weakness, or eighth nerve dysfunction. Trochlear palsy, although of significant localizing value, occurs infrequently or is seldom identified in history or examination. Headaches are the most common symptom and are frequently due to obstructive hydrocephalus and increased intracranial pressure.[8–10]

## Radiologic Appearance

Computed tomography (CT) with and without contrast detects 95% and 85% of meningiomas, respectively.[11] Hence, CT is a rapid, inexpensive screening study. One-millimeter serial axial CT images with coronal reconstructions aid in defining the bony anatomy and extent of invasion or hyperostosis. A knowledge of the peritumoral osseous anatomy aids in planning skull base approaches. CT is sensitive for identifying calcification and hemorrhage, which speak for and against the diagnosis of meningioma, respectively.

Meningiomas imaged with magnetic resonance imaging (MRI) demonstrate a relatively stereotypic appearance. Nearly all meningiomas demonstrate intense, rapid, and homogeneous enhancement with gadolinium[12] (Figs. 71–2 and 71–3). Ten to 15% of meningiomas may demonstrate cysts or rim-like enhancement.[13] Hemorrhage is uncommon.[14] Prominant dural enhancement, called the "dural tail" of the meningioma, may be present; however, its pathologic significance is controversial. Tokumaru and associates found neoplastic cells at 1 mm from the dura-tumor interface,[15] whereas Nakau and colleagues found meningioma cells at a distance of 4.5 mm in nearly half of patients with dural enhancement.[16] A trigeminal schwannoma shares many imaging characteristics with

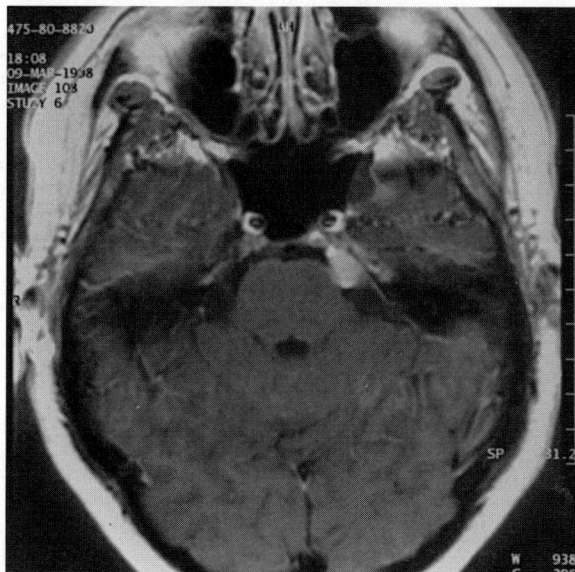

FIGURE 71–3 ■ Axial gadolinium-enhanced magnetic resonance imaging scan demonstrating an incisural tentorial meningioma.

meningioma but rarely demonstrates calcification and is more likely to undergo cystic change.

Multiplanar MRI with gadolinium enhancement delineates regional neurovascular anatomy. Patent vessels demonstrate a flow void, and the cranial nerves and brain stem can be visualized relative to the meningioma. The multiplanar images allow one to gauge the extent of tumor spread and plan a combined approach, if necessary, to access all the tumor. Magnetic resonance angiography and magnetic resonance venography can supplement MRI to define the vascular anatomy, but digital subtraction angiography (DSA) is preferred to determine the patency of sinuses and provide dynamic information regarding blood supply and presence of venous collaterals.

Angiography of the vertebral and internal and external carotid arteries is important when tentorial meningioma is a possible diagnosis. The blood supply is mainly from meningeal branches off the internal carotid artery.[17–19] The most prominent of these branches was described by Bernasconi and Cassinari[20] and has been called the "artery of the free margin of the tentorium."[18] This artery normally is small and may not be visible on routine angiograms, but as the artery enlarges it may become prominent in the presence of a tentorial meningioma. Meningiomas may also derive blood from other dural vessels—namely, the middle meningeal, occipital, and ascending pharyngeal arteries— or parasitize from intracranial pial vessels such as the terminal branches of the basilar.

Two studies from the 1980s suggest that sinus involvement with meningioma is underestimated with angiography.[9, 10] Dural sinus venography provides a more accurate assessment of sinus involvement and an opportunity for test occlusion.[21] Nonetheless, in most cases, DSA provides adequate information regarding venous sinus patency, dominance, and the extent of collateral development to determine whether the transverse sinus can be safely divided for a transtentorial resection.

## Choosing an Approach

Tentorial meningiomas present diagnostic and operative difficulties that in previously reported series resulted in an operative mortality rate between 16% and 34% and a case mortality rate, partly due to recurrences, as high as 54%.[5] With improved microsurgical techniques, more recent series describe a mortality rate of less than 10% and a morbidity rate of less than 30%, with the majority transient.[22, 23] Castellano and Ruggiero analyzed Olivecrona's patient material in 1953 and concluded that tentorial meningiomas are best removed from above, regardless of whether they are on the superior or inferior surface of the tentorium.[3] The following is a review of the current strategies for resection (dependent on location) and a description of a combined subtemporal-retrosigmoid approach.

The anatomy of the tentorial notch and a management strategy for incisural tentorial meningiomas have been described in detail by Samii and coworkers.[23] The approach for incisural meningiomas depends on the site of origin, lateral or posteromedial, and on the major extension, supratentorial or infratentorial. Lateral tumors with primarily infratentorial extension can be approached with a lateral

suboccipital retrosigmoid approach described for CPA meningiomas. A combined subtemporal-presigmoid approach is advantageous for lateral incisural meningiomas with supratentorial spread. Posteromedial meningiomas with an infratentorial component can be resected with an infratentorial-supracerebellar approach. A suboccipital transtentorial exposure is necessary for posteromedial incisural meningiomas with supratentorial extension.[23]

Malis,[24] Sugita and Suzuki,[25] and Guidetti and colleagues[10] each classified tentorial meningiomas using different terms and described a preferred operative approach. In general, the surgery is dictated by the tumor size, location along the tentorium, and pattern of growth above or below the tentorium. The approach to nonincisural tentorial meningiomas is discussed in terms of the following subgroups: lateral, falcotentorial, and torcular.

Meningiomas located at the lateral tentorium, tentorial leaf, or near the transverse sinus are managed with a craniotomy over the lesion and exposure of the transverse sinus. The necessity for a combined approach depends on the primary direction of spread. Angiography is important to determine the patency and size of each transverse sinus. An occluded sinus can be safely sacrificed. Usually, a nondominant transverse sinus can be divided,[26] although preoperative balloon test occlusion or intraoperative temporary occlusion is necessary prior to sacrifice.[7]

Falcotentorial meningiomas are approached via an occipital craniotomy with interhemispheric exposure and transtentorial resection. Again, the extent of the exposure depends on the configuration of the meningioma and patency of the venous sinuses. If the straight sinus is occluded, it may be resected to the vein of Galen.[27] Care must be taken to not interrupt important venous collaterals from the hemispheres into the superior sagittal sinus, convexity meningeal venous sinuses, or tentorial sinuses.[28] Tanaka and associates discuss meningiomas involving the straight sinus.[29]

Torcular meningiomas may involve the falx, tentorium cerebelli, and one to five venous sinuses (Figs. 71–4 and 71–5). The size and location of the craniotomy depend on the quadrant involved but must be generous enough to maintain venous control. Harsh and Wilson provide a management strategy and operative approach to torcular meningiomas.[30]

## Combined Supratentorial-Infratentorial Approach

The patient is placed in a three-quarters prone position with the ipsilateral shoulder elevated to avoid unnecessary twisting of the neck and obstruction of venous return. The head is slightly flexed and canted toward the opposite shoulder. The ipsilateral shoulder is pulled downward to provide better access to the suboccipital region, with care taken to pad the shoulder and avoid compression of the cervical or brachial plexus.

A slightly curved or hockey stick–shaped incision is started 6 cm above the ear and is extended in a posteromedial direction, passing midway between the inion and the mastoid process (Fig. 71–6). The neck in the suboccipital region is prepared and draped so that the incision can be

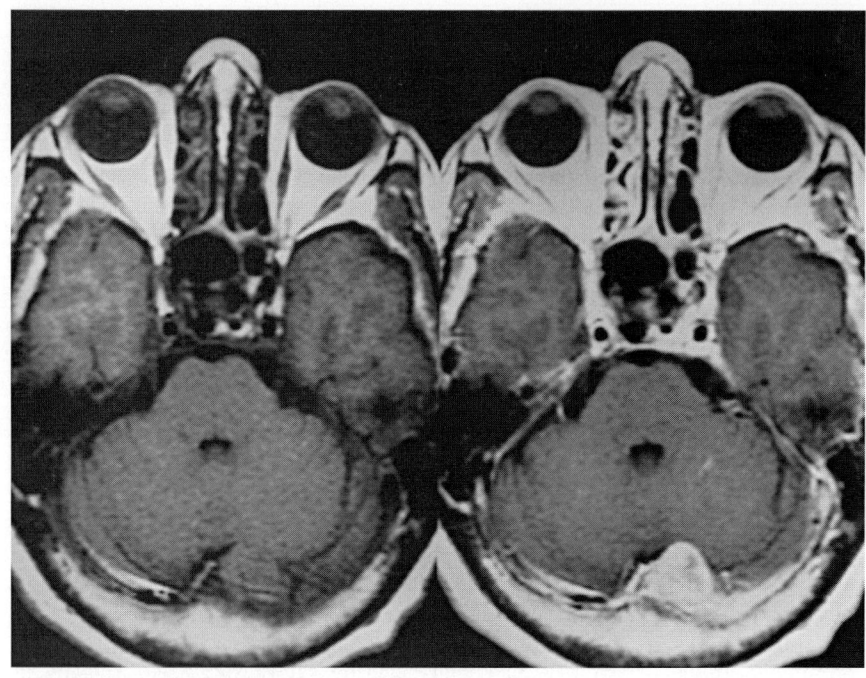

FIGURE 71–4 ■ Axial unenhanced and gadolinium-enhanced magnetic resonance imaging scan demonstrating a torcular meningioma involving the left transverse sinus.

extended as far as necessary to expose large tumors displacing the ipsilateral cerebellar hemisphere. The incision is carried down to the skull so that subperiosteal dissection with periosteal elevators and the scalpel permits adequate exposure.

After self-retaining retractors are inserted to maintain exposure, bur holes are placed in the temporal squama above the lateral sinus and in the posterior fossa below the lateral sinus and medially in relation to the mastoid air cells. A small temporo-occipital free bone flap is elevated. If extensive posterior fossa involvement by the tumor is

evident, proceeding immediately with a unilateral suboccipital craniectomy below and across the lateral sinus before opening the dura mater is probably best (see Fig. 71–6). Thus, the posterior temporal and occipital lobes of the brain are protected by dura while bone is being cut with a rongeur.

The dura mater is opened over the occipital lobe with the base of the dural flap at the lateral sinus (Fig. 71–7). This action promotes dural drainage and lessens the risk of tearing bridging cortical veins that pass toward the sinus before they are well exposed. The occipital lobe is gently

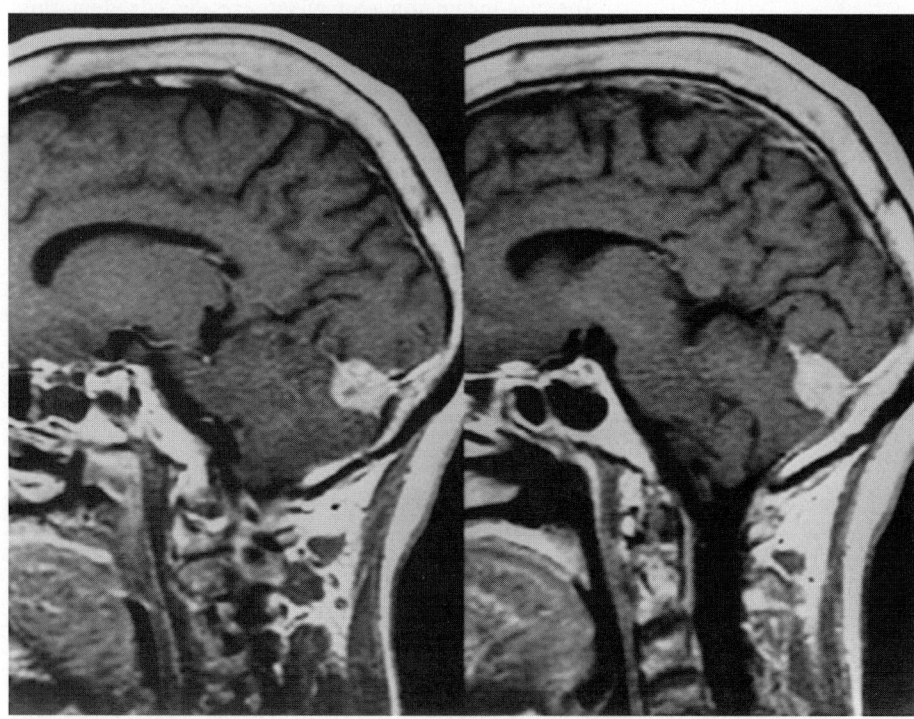

FIGURE 71–5 ■ Sagittal unenhanced and gadolinium-enhanced magnetic resonance imaging scan of a torcular meningioma involving the straight sinus.

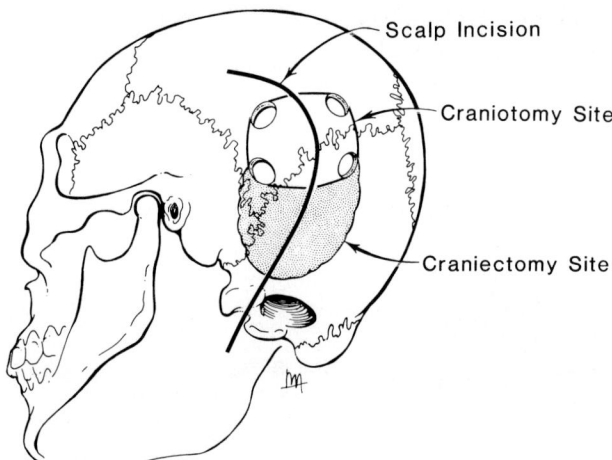

**FIGURE 71–6** ■ A combined supratentorial craniotomy and an infratentorial craniectomy is used to expose meningiomas above and below the tentorium cerebelli or large cerebellopontine angle tumors extending upward through the incisura. (From Maxwell RF, Chou SN: Posterior fossa meningiomas. In Schmidek HH, Sweet WH [eds]: Operative Neurosurgical Techniques: Indications, Methods, and Results, Vol 1, 2nd ed. Philadelphia: WB Saunders, 1988, p 575.)

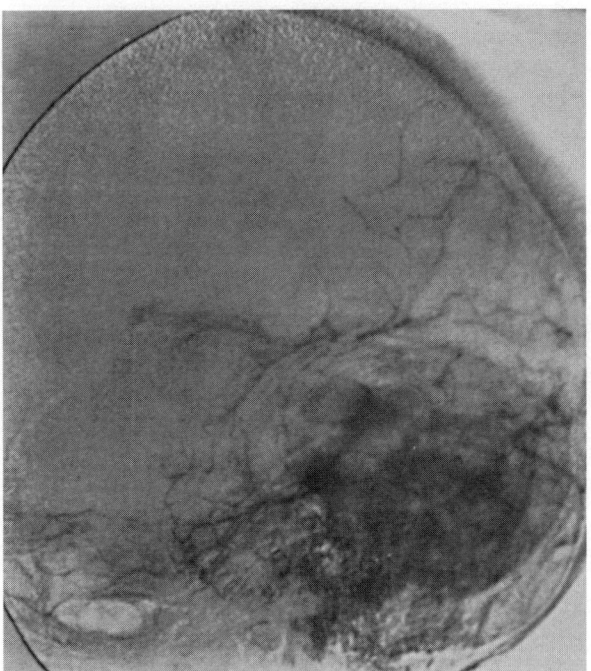

**FIGURE 71–8** ■ An angiogram showing a highly vascular tumor arising from the posterior petrous ridge, which proved to be an angioblastic meningioma. (From Maxwell RF, Chou SN: Posterior fossa meningiomas. In Schmidek HH, Sweet WH [eds]: Operative Neurosurgical Techniques: Indications, Methods, and Results, Vol 1, 2nd ed. Philadelphia: WB Saunders, 1988, p 577.)

retracted to expose the superior surface of the tentorium. Occipital bridging veins can be coagulated electively under direct vision at this time, but care should be taken to cut the veins well away from the dura mater and lateral sinus. The superior surface of the tentorium cerebelli is inspected for tumor, and the incisura is inspected for tumor growing upward along the brain stem.

The tentorium is elevated with a sharp hook and incised

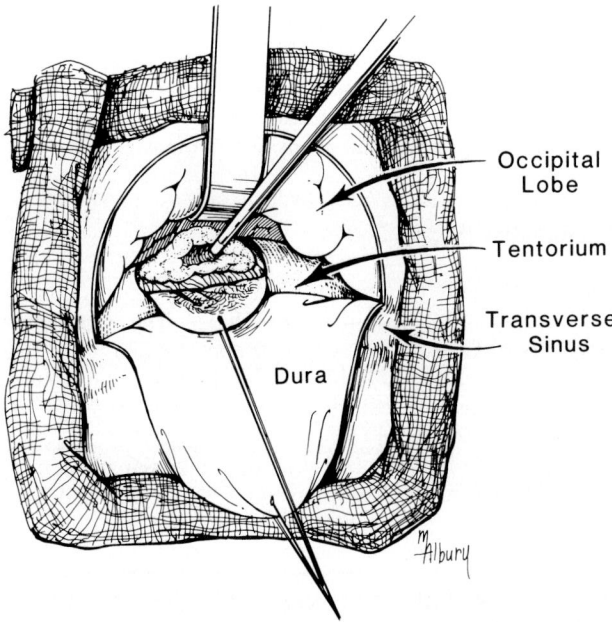

**FIGURE 71–7** ■ The temporo-occipital dura is opened and reflected toward the transverse sinus. Small tumors growing downward into the posterior fossa from the tentorium cerebelli are approached by a subtemporal-occipital approach with tentorial splitting. (From Maxwell RF, Chou SN: Posterior fossa meningiomas. In Schmidek HH, Sweet WH [eds]: Operative Neurosurgical Techniques: Indications, Methods, and Results, Vol 1, 2nd ed. Philadelphia: WB Saunders, 1988, p 576.)

posteriorly but well away from tumor attachment and the lateral sinus. The incision is carried toward the incisura, with care taken to identify and preserve the trochlear nerve adjacent to the tentorial edge. When possible, bipolar coagulation, rather than metallic clips, is used to control bleeding from the cut edge of the tentorium. Metallic clips cause refractive distortion on future CT and MRI images, hindering follow-up examinations for tumor recurrence.

Opening the tentorium back to the transverse sinus exposes the region of the CPA from above, provided that the tumor is not large. Although some tumors arise primarily from the underside of the tentorium, many tumors in this region arise from the posterior surface of the petrous ridge. These often grow to be large and may be quite vascular, with angioblastic features of the hemangiopericytic type (Fig. 71–8). In this situation, the best course is to elevate and incise the dura mater below the lateral sinus. Usually, a thin rim of cerebellum is stretched over the tumor. This rim of nonfunctional tissue is best excised, rather than retracted and undermined, which leaves devascularized, necrotic, swollen tissue behind.

If the tumor is huge and vascular, as meningiomas in this area tend to be, a useful technique involves temporary cross-clamping of the ipsilateral transverse sinus and observation of the brain and cortical veins for 5 minutes. If no swelling of the brain or venous engorgement is present, the transverse sinus can be safely ligated and divided because sufficient collateral venous drainage is available. This maneuver improves the exposure and obviates the need to work on the tumor resection alternately from above and below the lateral sinus (Fig. 71–9).

The large, firm, vascular tumor arising from the posterior

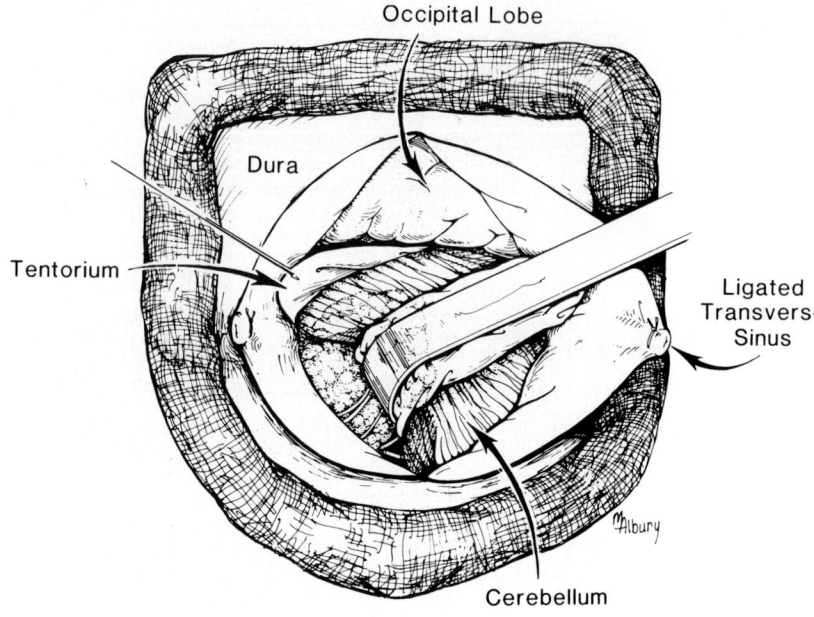

Occipital Lobe

Dura

Tentorium

Ligated
Transverse
Sinus

Cerebellum

FIGURE 71–9 ■ The dura mater was opened above and below the transverse sinus. The transverse sinus was subsequently ligated and divided after cross-clamping for 5 minutes produced no swelling of the brain or venous engorgement. (From Maxwell RF, Chou SN: Posterior fossa meningiomas. In Schmidek HH, Sweet WH [eds]: Operative Neurosurgical Techniques: Indications, Methods, and Results, Vol 1, 2nd ed. Philadelphia: WB Saunders, 1988, p 577.)

surface of the petrous ridge is technically challenging. Extracapsular dissection before enucleation of the tumor for the purpose of interrupting feeding vessels and devascularizing the tumor is precluded by the sensitivity of the brain stem and cranial nerves to compression or traction during tumor manipulation. Intracapsular removal of the bulk of the tumor is tedious if aspiration of the tumor is difficult. Troublesome bleeding is encountered when the cautery wire loop is used on highly vascular tumors. Heat spread to the brain stem and cranial nerves is also a concern. The ultrasonic aspirator, the carbon dioxide laser, or both may expedite this phase of the procedure.

After tumor removal, CSF flows freely through the tentorial incisura and the cranial nerves and carotid artery are well visualized. After meticulous hemostasis is achieved, a watertight dural closure is attempted and attention is given to obliterating any exposed mastoid air cells with bone wax or muscle. This action may prevent the occurrence of a CSF fistula in the immediate postoperative period before a dural neomembrane has a chance to form. The bone flap is plated into place; the temporalis fascia and galea are closed with nonabsorbable, inverted, interrupted sutures; and the skin closed with either staples or sutures.

## CEREBELLOPONTINE ANGLE MENINGIOMAS

The most common location for posterior fossa meningiomas is in the region of the CPA. Only 6% to 15% of CPA tumors are meningiomas, however.[31–33] Meningiomas originate from arachnoid cap cells in the vicinity of the CPA, specifically along the inferior border of the superior petrosal sinus, lateral border of the inferior petrosal sinus, or posterior temporal bone near the internal auditory canal.[34] This is in contrast with acoustic neuromas that arise from Schwann cells (peripheral myelin) on the vestibular divisions of cranial nerve VIII. Understanding this difference in origin aids in distinguishing the two neoplasms on

neuroimaging studies. Patients with acoustic neuromas and meningiomas present most commonly in their fourth and fifth decades of life. Meningiomas are more common in women.[32]

The clinical presentation depends on the site of origin and direction of growth. Meningiomas originating above the internal auditory canal frequently present with trigeminal neuralgia.[34] Meningiomas adjacent to the porus acousticus in the CPA cause symptoms similar to those associated with acoustic neuromas and cannot be distinguished with assurance on the basis of clinical findings alone. Meningiomas tend to involve cranial nerves V and VII more frequently than acoustic neuromas do, and additional involvement of any of the lower four cranial nerves suggests a meningioma, metastatic tumor, or epidermoid. Meningiomas tend to produce less auditory and vestibular nerve dysfunction than do acoustic neuromas.[35]

## Radiologic Appearance

Imaging features denoting a CPA mass versus an intraaxial lesion are listed in Table 71–1.[36] The differential diagnosis of CPA masses and their approximate respective frequency are listed in Table 71–2.[37] The three most common neoplasms are acoustic neuroma (75%), meningioma (10%), and epidermoid (5%).

Several radiologic findings can help distinguish acoustic neuromas from meningiomas on CT. Moller and col-

TABLE 71–1 ■ **MRI FEATURES DENOTING AN EXTRA-AXIAL MASS IN THE CEREBELLOPONTINE ANGLE (CPA)**

Enlarged ipsilateral CPA cistern
Cerebrospinal fluid density between mass and neural structures
Brain stem rotated
Gray-white junction distorted in adjacent neural structures

TABLE 71–2 ■ **MASSES OF THE CEREBELLOPONTINE ANGLE AND THEIR APPROXIMATE FREQUENCY**

| Mass | Percentage |
|---|---|
| Acoustic neroma | 75 |
| Meningioma | 10 |
| Epidermoid | 5 |
| Vascular (e.g., aneurysm) | 2 |
| Schwannoma (other than cranial nerve VIII) | 2 |
| Metastasis | 1 |
| Paraganglioma | 1 |
| Ependymoma | <1 |
| Choriod plexus papilloma | <1 |

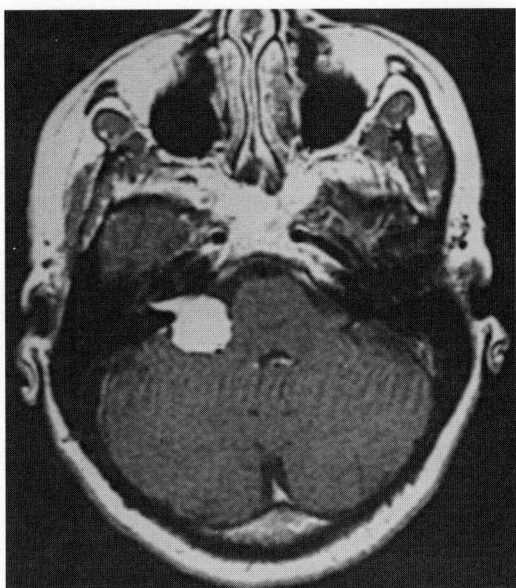

**FIGURE 71–10** ■ Axial gadolinium-enhanced magnetic resonance imaging scan demonstrating the "ice cream cone" appearance of an acoustic neuroma. The "cone" is formed from the shape of the expanded internal auditory canal (IAC) and the "ice cream" protrudes into the cerebellopontine angle.

leagues[38] analyzed CPA tumors with CT and found that CPA meningiomas were often calcified, the center of an acoustic neuroma rarely is anterior to the porus acousticus, and acoustic neuromas rarely extend as high as the dorsum sellae, a condition that may occur with CPA meningiomas. Meningiomas of the CPA may also protrude into the suprasellar cistern. Expansion of the internal auditory canal, which occurs with acoustic neuromas, is rare with CPA meningiomas. Meningiomas characteristically show a broad-based mass aligned with the petrous ridge rather than one centered over the internal auditory canal.[38]

Valavanis and associates carried out a detailed analysis of the CT findings in 16 surgically verified cases of meningioma of the posterior surface of the petrous bone.[39] They concluded that a correct preoperative diagnosis was possible in almost every case. Frequently occurring CT findings specific for meningioma of the posterior surface of the petrous bone include a hyperdense, homogeneously enhancing, extra-axial CPA mass; an inverse relationship between precontrast attenuation values and degree of contrast enhancement of the tumor; an oval shape; an obtuse angle between the lateral tumor border and the posterior surface of the petrous bone; and evidence of transcisternal, supratentorial tumor extension. Infrequently occurring specific CT findings include tumor calcification, hyperostosis or exostosis of the posterior surface of the petrous bone, a comma-shaped tumor configuration in cases with transcisternal tumor extension, and evidence of transtentorial tumor extension.

Both acoustic neuromas and meningiomas demonstrate enhancement on MRI with gadolinium. Acoustic neuromas typically have an "ice cream cone" appearance with the "cone" in the meatus and the "ice cream" representing the extracanalicular portion protruding into the CPA[37] (Fig. 71–10). Meningiomas typically do not involve the meatus but rather demonstrate a large broad attachment to the petrous temporal bone (Fig. 71–11). Calcification is common in meningiomas and rare in acoustic neuromas. Cystic change is more common in acoustic neuromas than in meningiomas.[32] The CN VII–VIII complex may be visualized with a meningioma, but such tumors are inseparable from acoustic neuromas.[32] Angiographically, meningiomas demonstrate a prolonged blush not seen with acoustic neuromas.[32]

## Choosing an Approach

Meningiomas and acoustic neuromas displace the regional anatomy differently. Acoustic neuromas have a consistent site of origin and thus impede on and displace the neurovascular structures in a predictable pattern. The CN VII–VIII complex is displaced anteriorly, vessels are stretched over the tumor capsule, and frequently an arachnoid plane is present to aid in the dissection. Conversely, meningiomas may displace CN VII and VIII posteriorly, the vessels may become incorporated into the tumor, and the arachnoid

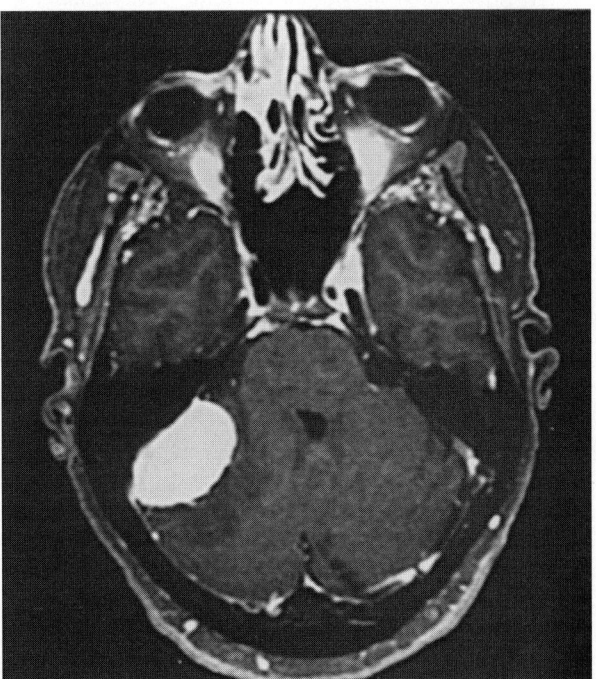

**FIGURE 71–11** ■ Axial gadolinium-enhanced magnetic resonance imaging scan demonstrating the broad sessile attachment of a cerebellopontine angle meningioma to the petrous bone.

plane is lost. Meningiomas may also spread upward significantly through the tentorium, medially involving the clivus, or inferiorly toward the jugular foramen.[32]

Hearing loss is less common with meningiomas; consequently, a hearing preservation approach is typically chosen and modified as necessary to gain access to tumor spread outside the CPA. The retrosigmoid approach is preferred for patients with serviceable hearing and a meningioma confined to the CPA, especially with an attachment lateral to the internal acoustic meatus. The retrosigmoid approach is combined with a subtemporal transtentorial approach when the meningioma extends above the tentorium. Giannotta and coworkers reported removal of two meningiomas over 4 cm in diameter via the translabrynthine approach with no deficit except hearing loss.[40]

## Retrosigmoid Approach

Meningiomas in the CPA can be approached through a paramedian incision and suboccipital craniectomy if the tumor is relatively small and confined to the posterior fossa (Fig. 71–12). The face is turned 45 degrees toward the side of the tumor, and the neck is flexed. The head is held in three-point skeletal fixation. A separate paramedian incision is made 7 cm above and 3 cm laterally in relation to the inion, and a bur hole is placed for ventriculostomy in case CSF decompression is necessary during or after surgery. The foot plate for the self-retaining retractor can be inserted at this site, which is well out of the main operative field.

Subperiosteal dissection is performed, and one or more bur holes are placed in the occipital squama. The craniectomy is enlarged with the use of instruments such as Leksell's double-action rongeur and large Kerrison's bone punches. The limits of the exposure, at least initially, are the transverse sinus superiorly, the mastoid air cell laterally, and the foramen magnum inferiorly. Sufficient bone is

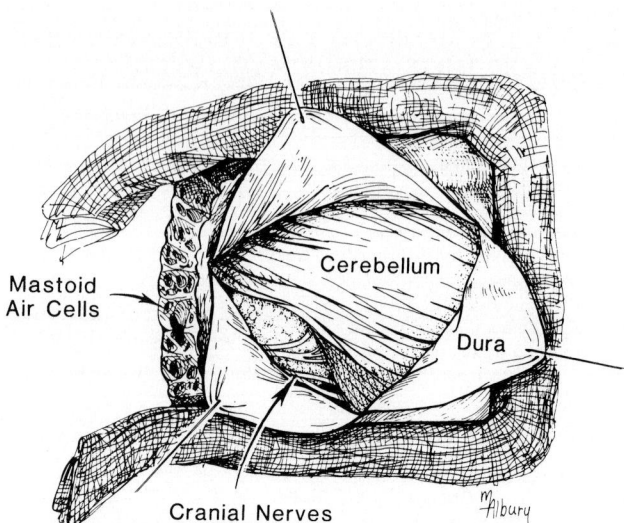

FIGURE 71–13 ■ A unilateral posterior fossa craniectomy is enlarged until the mastoid air cells are seen. The dura is opened in a triradiate (Y) fashion, and dural retention sutures are applied. The cerebellopontine angle meningioma displaces the lower cranial nerves. (From Maxwell RF, Chou SN: Posterior fossa meningiomas. In Schmidek HH, Sweet WH [eds]: Operative Neurosurgical Techniques: Indications, Methods, and Results, Vol 1, 2nd ed. Philadelphia: WB Saunders, 1988, p 579.)

removed medially to obtain good visualization of the tumor.

The dura mater is opened in a triradiate (Y) fashion, and dural retention sutures are applied (Fig. 71–13). The cerebellum is gently retracted to expose the tumor, and a self-retaining retractor with the blade placed on cotton padding maintains exposure with minimal tissue trauma. The operating microscope and microinstrumentation are important adjuncts for dissecting the capsule away from cranial nerves, vessels, and the brain stem. An en plaque meningioma may be unresectable and surgery limited to tissue biopsy. A globoid tumor may be multilobulated, but usually it has a limited area of dural attachment and is accessible for operative excision.

After the lower cranial nerves are identified and carefully dissected off the capsule wall, they are protected with moist cotton strips. The tumor capsule is incised, and the intracapsular removal of the tumor bulk is carried out via the techniques used for tissue removal and hemostasis discussed previously for meningiomas in other locations. When only a thin, pliable capsule remains, the capsular wall is carefully involuted while contiguous structures are dissected off the capsule.

CPA meningiomas tend to extend further up the clivus toward the dorsum sellae than do acoustic neuromas. They also are multilobulated, and important structures such as the anteroinferior cerebellar artery (AICA) and the facial nerve may be bound within the interstices of these lobules and surrounded by tumor, although technically they are still extracapsular. CN VII may be displaced in almost any direction or completely concealed by the tumor. The nerve may be displaced anteriorly by the capsular wall, but this finding varies far more than with acoustic neurinomas. Even with the aid of electrical nerve stimulation, the surgeon may not be able to identify and save the nerve and

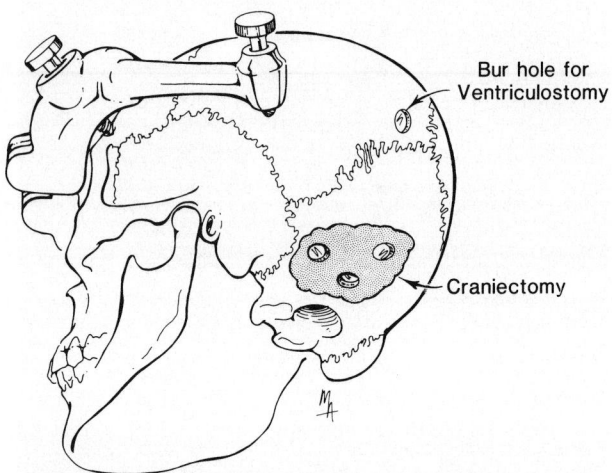

FIGURE 71–12 ■ Small meningiomas in the cerebellopontine angle (CPA) are exposed by a unilateral craniectomy. The head is rotated toward the side of the lesion, and the chin is flexed toward the ipsilateral shoulder. (From Maxwell RF, Chou SN: Posterior fossa meningiomas. In Schmidek HH, Sweet WH [eds]: Operative Neurosurgical Techniques: Indications, Methods, and Results, Vol 1, 2nd ed. Philadelphia: WB Saunders, 1988, p 574.)

still accomplish complete tumor removal. Palsy of CN VII is an even more profound problem if the trigeminal nerve root or descending tract also is compromised by tumor or damaged during surgery. Tarsorrhaphy or gold weights may be necessary to prevent corneal exposure keratitis, ulceration, and possible loss of ipsilateral vision. The corneal reflex and the ability to close the eye and blink should be checked as soon as the patient is awake in the recovery room. An eye ointment, artificial tears, and an eye patch may be indicated in the immediate postoperative period. If the lower cranial nerves are damaged and the gag reflex and ability to handle secretions are lost, a feeding gastrostomy and tracheostomy may prove necessary until function improves.

The surgeon's technical judgment is sorely taxed by large meningiomas in this region. The patient and the patient's family must be told in advance of the problems the surgeon may confront. Their understanding and philosophy regarding total or subtotal excision and possible functional loss complement the surgeon's judgment, which is based on the patient's age and condition and on the surgeon's previous experience with similar tumors.

Once the nerve root of CN V and CN VII are successfully identified, their dissection off the capsule is usually possible. The tumor is gently delivered from above into the space created by the intracapsular removal of tumor tissue. Arterial feeders from the AICA, the internal carotid artery, and the ascending pharyngeal artery are visualized, coagulated with the bipolar cautery, and divided. Bridging veins passing from the tumor to the superior petrosal sinus are similarly coagulated and are divided close to the tumor rather than to the sinus.

Tumor attached to the brain stem or involving the basilar artery, its perforating branches, or the AICA is better left behind. The AICA can loop out to the region of the porus acousticus, give off an internal auditory branch, and then return to supply the brain stem (Fig. 71–14). This vessel must be spared even when it appears to be well away from the brain stem in the vicinity of the porus acousticus.

An alternative method useful for resecting highly vascular meningiomas is to furrow quickly across the interior of the tumor near the pole attached to the petrous ridge (Fig. 71–15). Fibrillary collagen (Avitene), followed by light pressure with dry cotton pledgets, is applied to stem brisk bleeding. This action allows selective invagination of the capsule wall along the petrous ridge and coagulation and interruption of the main feeding vessels from the middle meningeal and ascending pharyngeal arteries through the dura mater at this site. Once this detachment is accomplished, the tumor is less vascular and its bulk can be removed much more quickly and with far less bleeding. The capsule is never placed under forceful traction. Extracapsular dissection is performed with magnification and microinstrumentation to spare the cranial nerves, important blood vessels such as the perforating arteries to the brain stem coming off the basilar artery, and the brain stem tissue itself.

On occasion, one encounters a huge, vascular posterior fossa meningioma arising from the posterior petrous ridge and extending up along the clivus in front of the brain stem and through the incisura alongside the brain stem. If tumor removal is tedious, the blood loss substantial, and

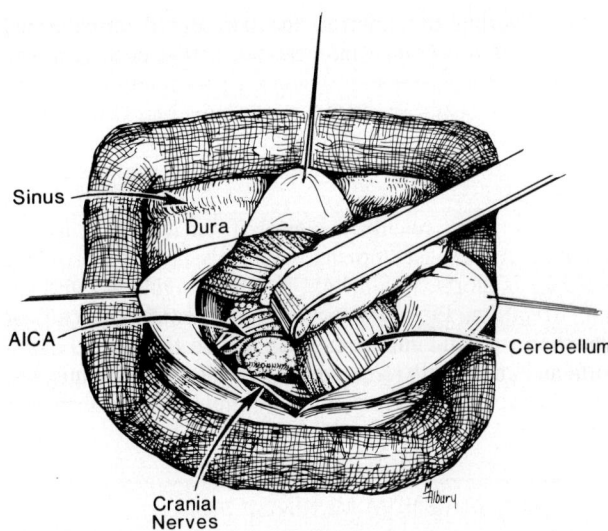

FIGURE 71–14 ■ The meningioma capsule is exposed, and the anteroinferior cerebellar artery (AICA) gives off an internal auditory branch before looping back to supply the brain stem. In this situation, leaving a small amount of tumor attached to the artery is preferable to risking sacrifice of the AICA. (From Maxwell RF, Chou SN: Posterior fossa meningiomas. In Schmidek HH, Sweet WH [eds]: Operative Neurosurgical Techniques: Indications, Methods, and Results, Vol 1, 2nd ed. Philadelphia: WB Saunders, 1988, p 580.)

brain stem function precarious as heralded by transient bradycardia and extrasystole, a staged procedure is considered. The dura is left open, the bone flap is freeze-preserved and stored in a saline-antibiotic solution, and the scalp is meticulously closed by careful approximation of the galea and dermis. Within 10 to 14 days, the second stage is carried out and the tumor is excised much more expedi-

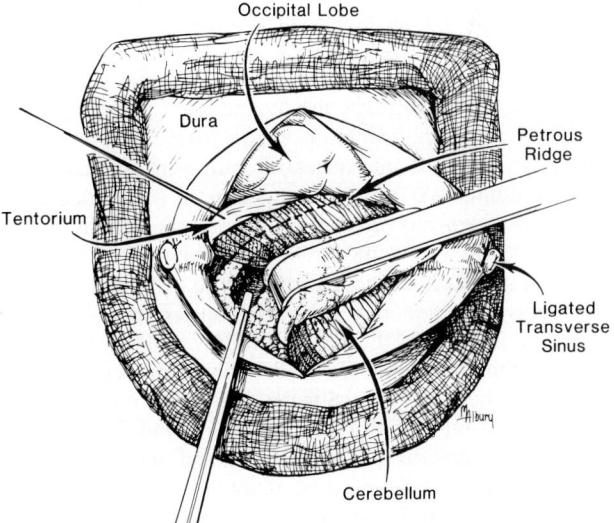

FIGURE 71–15 ■ A large, firm, vascular posterior petrous ridge meningioma is resected first by furrowing that is parallel to the ridge. The attachment to the dura and large feeding vessels from the middle meningeal artery can be coagulated. The bulk of the remaining tumor is then removed with less bleeding, and the thinned capsule adjacent to the brain stem is excised. (From Maxwell RF, Chou SN: Posterior fossa meningiomas. In Schmidek HH, Sweet WH [eds]: Operative Neurosurgical Techniques: Indications, Methods, and Results, Vol 1, 2nd ed. Philadelphia: WB Saunders, 1988, p 578.)

tiously. During the interim, the partially devascularized tumor tends to herniate into the site of the decompressed craniotomy (or craniectomy) and away from the brain stem, clivus, and incisura. Further tumor removal is accompanied by less blood loss, and the tumor capsule is more easily dissected off the brain stem without evidence of medullary dysfunction.

Hemostasis is readily achieved if the tumor is totally removed. Otherwise, oozing tumor tissue remains. This bleeding is stopped with light bipolar coagulation and saline irrigation. Fibrillary collagen, oxidized cellulose, or absorbable gelatin sponge is applied directly to the oozing surface if necessary. Closure of the dura mater, muscles, galea aponeurotica, and skin are as previously described.

## FORAMEN MAGNUM MENINGIOMAS

### Classification

By definition, foramen magnum meningiomas involve the lower third of the clivus (below the glossopharyngeal nerve) and the atlantoaxial region. Petroclival meningiomas occur between the internal acoustic meatus and in the upper two thirds of the clivus. This classification is helpful in terms of discussion, although meningiomas can involve several regions via contiguous spread. The following discussion pertains to meningiomas involving the lower clivus, atlas, and axis.

### Clinical Presentation

Foramen magnum meningiomas account for about 3% of brain and spinal cord meningiomas.[41] Meningiomas occur more frequently than either schwannomas or neurofibromas, constituting approximately two thirds of the tumors occurring at the foramen magnum.[41, 42] Kempe stated that the foramen magnum was the second most common location for meningiomas in the posterior fossa.[43] Most meningiomas are oriented anterolaterally with respect to the foramen magnum.[44] As with meningiomas in other locations, patients are typically in their fourth or fifth decade of life at presentation and women outnumber men 2 to 1.[45]

Cushing and colleagues classified foramen magnum meningiomas into "craniospinal" and "spinocranial" groups according to whether the site of origin was above or below the foramen magnum.[1] Cerebellar signs, increased intracranial pressure, and cranial nerve deficits are more characteristic of craniospinal meningiomas. Foramen magnum meningiomas tend to go unrecognized and undiagnosed for long periods because of their ubiquitous symptoms and lack of good localizing signs. Foramen magnum meningiomas were missed prior to MRI because incomplete myelographic studies fail to adequately define the anatomy around the foramen magnum. The diagnostic pitfalls associated with these tumors are emphasized in numerous reports.[42, 46, 47]

In the early stages of tumor growth, the clinical picture may be mistaken for cervical spondylosis with secondary radiculopathy. In advanced stages, an intramedullary, rather than extramedullary, lesion may be suspected. Elsberg and Strauss emphasized that the size of the upper spinal canal and foramen magnum permits tumors in this region to attain a large size and manifest radicular symptoms without myelopathy.[48, 49]

The most frequent initial symptom of foramen magnum tumors is suboccipital or neck pain (49%) and dysesthesia in the extremities (37%).[8] By the time patients undergo surgery, which is often many months after their initial symptoms develop, 95% have dysesthesia in their hands and fingers and 75% have posterior cervical or suboccipital pain. About 50% of these patients have weakness in the upper extremities or gait disturbance, and one third complain of bladder disturbance. Almost one half of patients with foramen magnum tumors have normal neurologic findings when first evaluated for their initial complaint. Hypalgesia in the C2 dermatomal distribution and spinal accessory nerve palsy are reliable localizing signs. Stereoanesthesia of the hands also occurs with foramen magnum tumors that compress or interfere with the blood supply to the posterior columns or their nuclei.[50, 51]

### Radiologic Appearance

Prior to MRI, complete cervical myelography with contrast medium carried through the foramen magnum was the imaging test of choice.[52–54] Multiplanar MRI with gadolinium enhancement demonstrates the meningioma in relation to the neurovascular structures, specifically the lower cranial nerves, vertebral arteries and its branches, and position of the medulla. Thin-slice CT with reconstructions delineates the bone involvement and assists in choosing a skull base approach.

The dura mater anterior to the foramen magnum is supplied by meningeal vessels from the carotid siphon, the ascending pharyngeal artery, and the middle meningeal artery. The dura mater posterior to the foramen magnum is supplied primarily by the occipital artery and by the posterior meningeal branch of the vertebral artery.[55] Selective angiography of the internal carotid, the external carotid, and the vertebral arteries is necessary to identify the blood supply to the meningioma. The position of the vertebral artery with reference to the meningioma is necessary for planning the subsequent approach.[45] For vascular tumors, one may consider preoperative embolization because it decreases blood loss, decreases the need for transfusion, and reduces bleeding-related intraoperative complications.[56]

### Choosing an Approach

George and associates[58] reviewed their approach to 40 meningiomas of the foramen magnum. Thirty-nine meningiomas were located along either the anterior or the lateral rim of the foramen magnum. In relation to the vertebral artery, 4 were above, 16 were below, and 20 were on both sides. Thirty-four meningiomas were intradural, two were solely extradural, and four were both intradural and extradural. Intradural anterior and lateral meningiomas were resected via the posterolateral approach with drilling of the occipital condyle or lateral mass of the axis depending on the position of the vertebral artery relative to the meningioma. Meningiomas with an extradural component were resected with an anterolateral approach with or without a posterior midline approach depending on tumor configuration. These approaches[57, 58] and others[59] are described in detail elsewhere. Access to the anterior foramen via a medullotomy is described by West.[60] An anterior, transoral approach has also been reported for exposing and resecting clival meningiomas.[61]

## Posterior and Posterolateral Approach

Posteriorly positioned foramen magnum meningiomas are removed through the posterior approach by a suboccipital craniectomy and upper cervical laminectomy (see Fig. 71–1). With the patient seated, the legs flexed and elevated, and vulnerable areas padded, the neck is flexed and the head is stabilized by three-point skeletal fixation. Hyperflexion of the neck is avoided by placing three fingers between the patient's chin and the sternum before tightening the headrest. A posterior midline incision extending from above the inion to the level of the spinous process of C5 is used. The head and neck are draped so that this incision can be extended, if necessary, to improve exposure. A separate vertical incision is made, and an occipital bur hole is placed 7 cm above the inion and 3 cm laterally in relation to the midline in case intraoperative or postoperative ventriculostomy for CSF decompression is required (see Fig. 71–1).

Subperiosteal dissection is carried out bilaterally over the occipital squama. The spinous processes and laminae of at least the upper three cervical vertebrae are exposed by sharp dissection. Care should be taken to avoid injuring the vertebral arteries where they pass over the posterior arch of the atlas in the lateral recess. Emissary veins opened during subperiosteal dissection should be waxed immediately. The condylar veins in the vicinity of the foramen magnum may require bipolar coagulation if troublesome bleeding occurs. Should the Doppler, electrocardiogram, or vital signs suggest air embolism, positive end-expiratory pressure (PEEP) is increased, the wound is filled with saline and covered with saline-soaked cotton sponges, and the patient is immediately lowered into the left lateral decubitus position. Air is aspirated through the catheter that was placed preoperatively in the right atrium. Meticulous attention to venous hemostasis with prompt bone waxing of open emissary veins lessens the risk of this complication, but veins and sinuses may be open without bleeding despite PEEP.

Bur holes are drilled bilaterally in the occipital squama, and care is taken to stay well off the midline so that a persistent occipital sinus is not perforated. The bur holes are placed well below the nuchal line and transverse sinus. The craniectomy is then enlarged by connecting the bur holes with Leksell's double-action rongeur and Kerrison's bone punches. The dura is carefully stripped away from the inner table of the skull with a dural separator. The craniectomy is enlarged until the edge of the transverse sinus is visible and the posterior rim of the foramen magnum is removed. Initially, the craniectomy may not have

to be enlarged so far laterally that the mastoid air cells are opened. Once entered, the mastoid air cells are sealed with bone wax. The posterior arch of the atlas is removed, and if pronounced tonsillar herniation or a significant intraspinal component to the tumor is evident preoperatively, the lamina and spinous process of C2 are also removed at this time.

The dura mater is always inspected and gently palpated before it is opened widely in the posterior fossa or upper cervical spinal canal. If the dura mater is unexpectedly tight or is not pulsating, a cannula is passed into the atrium of the right lateral ventricle through the occipital bur hole that was drilled earlier in the procedure for this purpose. Sudden intraventricular decompression, however, is avoided to prevent subdural or intraventricular bleeding.

The dura mater is opened with a Y-shaped incision. The cephalic leaf of dura is reflected cephalad and tacked up with dural sutures over a strip of cotton or absorbable gelatin sponge to protect the transverse sinus. The inferior tail of the Y incision extends below the level of the C1 arch and is tacked laterally with dural sutures over cotton strips or absorbable sponge pledgets. A persistent occipital sinus may be encountered at the junction of the Y limbs (Fig. 71–16). Bleeding from the sinus is controlled with metallic surgical clips or bipolar coagulation. The dura is kept moist throughout the procedure, and only bipolar coagulation is used on the dura. This method reduces shrinkage and permits a tight dural closure without necessitating a dural substitute graft.

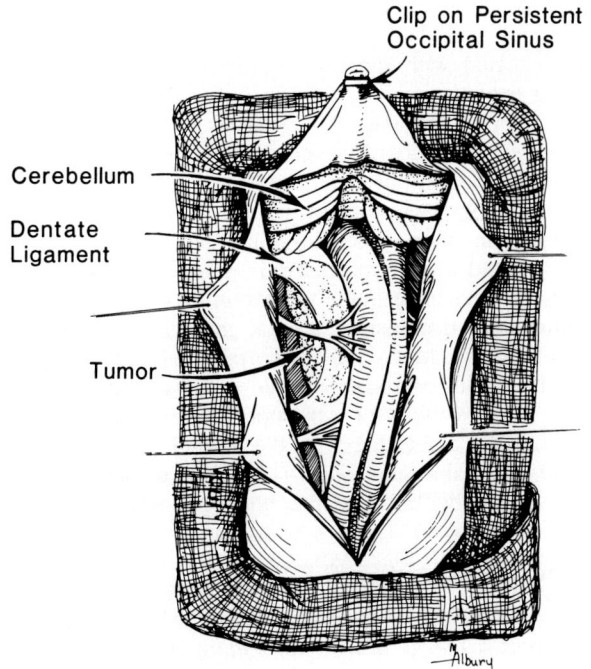

**FIGURE 71–16** ■ The dura mater is opened by a Y incision, and a persistent occipital sinus is clipped. The foramen magnum meningioma is located more on the left side and is ventrolateral to the spinomedullary junction. The dorsal root of C2 is stretched over the tumor and must be sectioned. The upper dentate ligament serves as a landmark of the site at which the displaced vertebral artery enters the intrathecal space. (From Maxwell RF, Chou SN: Posterior fossa meningiomas. In Schmidek HH, Sweet WH [eds]: Operative Neurosurgical Techniques: Indications, Methods, and Results, Vol 1, 2nd ed. Philadelphia: WB Saunders, 1988, p 581.)

This limited posterior exposure is not adequate for large tumors extending anterolaterally along the clivus. These tumors are exposed by an incision starting above the helix of the external ear and then angling across the occipital squama and down the posterior midline of the neck. This method then adds the exposure for posterior petrous ridge and CPA meningiomas with the region of the foramen magnum. The occipital condyle or lateral mass of the atlas is drilled to provide adequate exposure anteriorly.

The upper cervical spinal cord is displaced dorsally and is rotated away from the side on which the main tumor mass is located. The dorsal root of C2 may be stretched over the posterior surface of the tumor (see Fig. 71–16). The surgeon may need to section this nerve root and accept some ipsilateral scalp numbness. To the extent possible, the relationship of the tumor to the vertebral artery must be ascertained before surgery and at this stage of the operative exposure. If the artery is not seen, a helpful landmark is the highest dentate ligament that normally marks the level at which the vertebral artery enters the intrathecal space. The dentate ligament is sectioned where it is stretched over the tumor capsule (see Fig. 71–16). The spinal accessory nerve is identified, preserved, and protected with cotton strips. Dissection of the nerve off the tumor capsule may be necessary. Before the tumor capsule is opened for internal removal, the tumor is isolated from the intrathecal space with cotton strips to lessen the incidence and degree of postoperative aseptic meningitis associated with subarachnoid blood. The tumor then is enucleated via the techniques discussed previously.

As the capsule is collapsed inward, adhesions to the pia arachnoid over the cerebellum, spinal cord, and medulla are dissected with the use of microinstrumentation and bipolar coagulation. The capsule is dissected off the vertebral artery, if feasible. The site of dural attachment is cauterized with bipolar coagulation if the dura cannot be readily excised in this area.

After hemostasis is obtained, the cotton strips protecting the spinomedullary junction, spinal accessory nerve, and subarachnoid space are removed. A watertight closure of the dura mater is desirable to prevent an occipital pseudomeningocele. If necessary, a dural graft is used to achieve a tight closure. Meticulous hemostasis and a multilayered muscle closure with interrupted nonabsorbable sutures lessen the possibility of a postoperative seroma causing a complication associated with the wound. Inverted, interrupted absorbable sutures are used subcutaneously, and the skin is closed with interrupted, nonabsorbable sutures.

## ACKNOWLEDGMENTS

*We appreciate the assistance of Edward Michel, M.D., and Charles Truwit, M.D., in providing and interpreting the radiographs provided in this chapter.*

## REFERENCES

1. Cushing H, Eisenhardt L: Meningiomas: Their Classification, Regional Behavior, Life History, and Surgical End Results. Springfield, IL: Charles C Thomas, 1938.
2. Morley LP: Tumors of the cranial meninges. In Youmans JR (ed): Neurological Surgery, Vol 3, 3rd ed. Philadelphia: WB Saunders, 1990.
3. Castellano F, Ruggiero G: Meningiomas of the posterior fossa. Acta Radiol (Suppl) 104:1, 1953.
4. Frowein RA: Meningiomas of the tentorium. Acta Neurochir (Wien) 31:283, 1975.
5. Rostomily R, Eskridge J, Winn H: Tentorial meningiomas. Neurosurg Clin North Am 5(2):331–348, 1994.
6. Cantore G, Ciappettal P: Tentorial meningiomas. In Schmidek HH (ed): Meningiomas and Their Surgical Management. Philadelphia: WB Saunders, 1991, pp 390–403.
7. Maxwell R, Chou S: Posterior fossa meningiomas. In Schmidek HH (ed): Meningiomas and Their Surgical Management. Philadelphia: WB Saunders, 1991, pp 377–389.
8. Barrows HS, Harter DH: Tentorial meningiomas. J Neurol Neurosurg Psychiatry 25:40, 1962.
9. Sekhar L, Jannetta P, Maroon J: Tentorial meningiomas: Surgical management and results. Neurosurgery 145:268–275, 1984.
10. Guidetti B, Ciappettal P, Domenicucci M: Tentorial meningiomas: Surgical experience with 61 cases and long-term results. J Neurosurg 69:183–187, 1988.
11. New P, Aronow S, Hesselink J: National Cancer Institutes study; evaluation of computed tomography: The diagnosis of intracranial neoplasms IV meningiomas. Radiology 136:665–675, 1980.
12. Fujii K, Fujita N, Hirabuki N, et al: Neuromas and meningiomas: Evaluation of early enhancement with dynamic MR imaging. AJNR Am J Neuroradiol 13:1215–1220, 1992.
13. Fujii K, Fujita N, Hirabuki N, et al: Neuromas and meningiomas: Evaluation of early enhancement with dynamic MR imaging. AJNR Am J Neuroradiol 13:1215–1220, 1992.
14. Onesti S, Zahos P, Ashkenazi E: Spontaneous hemorrhage into a convexity meningioma. Acta Neurochir (Wien) 138:1250–1251, 1996.
15. Tokumaru A, Oguchi T, Ehuche T: Prominent meningeal enhancement adjacent to meningiomas on Gd-DTPA-enhanced MR images: Histopathologic correlation. Radiology 175:431–433, 1990.
16. Nakau H, Miyazawa T, Tamai S, et al: Pathological significance of meningeal enhancement (Flare sign) on meningiomas in MRI. Surg Neurol 48:584–591, 1997.
17. Berkmen YM: Angiographic demonstration of blood supply to the tentorium: Case report and review of the literature. J Neurosurg 25:90, 1966.
18. Papo I, Salvolini V: Meningiomas of the free margin of the tentorium developing in the pineal region. Neuroradiology 7:237, 1974.
19. Schechter MM, Zingesser LH, Rosenbaum A: Tentorial meningiomas. AJR Am J Radiol 104:123, 1968.
20. Bernasconi V, Cassinari V: Un segno carotidografico zipico di meningioma del tentorio. Chirurgia 11:586, 1956.
21. Halbach V, Higashida R, Heishima G: Venography and venous pressure monitoring in dural sinus meningiomas. AJNR Am J Neuroradiol 10:1209–1213, 1989.
22. Ciric I, Landau B: Tentorial and posterior cranial fossa meningiomas: Operative results and long-term follow-up: Experience with 26 cases. Surg Neurol 39:530–537, 1993.
23. Samii M, Carvalho G, Tatagiba M, et al: Meningiomas of the tentorial notch: Surgical anatomy and management. J Neurosurg 84:375–381, 1996.
24. Malis L: Surgical approaches to tentorial meningiomas. In Wilkins RH, Rengachary SS (eds): Neurosurgery Update I: Diagnosis, Operative Technique, and Neuro-Oncology. New York: McGraw-Hill, 1990, pp 399–408.
25. Sugita K, Suzuki Y: Tentorial meningiomas. In Al-Mefty O (ed): Meningiomas. New York: Raven Press, 1991, pp 357–361.
26. Vrionis D, Robertson J, Heilman C, Rustamzedah E: Asterion meningiomas. Skull Base Surg 8(3):153–161, 1998.
27. Odake G: Meningioma of the falcotentorial region: Report of two cases and literature review of occlusion of the galenic system. Neurosurgery 30(5):788–793, 1992.
28. Muthukumar N, Palaniappan P: Tentorial venous sinuses: An anotomic study. Neurosurgery 42(2):363–371, 1998.
29. Tanaka Y, Sugita K, Kogayashi S, Hongo K: Straight sinus meningioma. Surg Neurol 24:550–554, 1985.
30. Harsh G, Wilson C: Peritorcular meningiomas. In Wilkins RH, Rengachary SS (eds): Neurosurgery Update I: Diagnosis, Operative Technique, and Neuro-Oncology. New York: McGraw-Hill, 1990, pp 369–388.
31. Laird F, Harner S, Laws E Jr, et al: Meningiomas of the cerebellopontine angle. Otolaryngol Head Neck Surg 93:161, 1985.

32. Tator C, Duncan E, Charles D: Comparison of the clinical and radiologic features and surgical management of posterior fossa meningiomas and acoustic neuromas. Can J Neurol Sci 17:170–176, 1990.
33. Thomas N, King T: Meningiomas of the cerebellopontine angle: A report of 41 cases. Br J Neurosurg 10(1):59–68, 1996.
34. Rhoton A: Meningiomas of the cerebellopontine angle and foramen magnum. Neurosurg Clin North Am 5(2):349–377, 1994.
35. Katinsky SE, Toglis JV: Audiologic and vestibular manifestations of meningiomas of the cerebellopontine angle. J Speech Hear Disord 33:351, 1968.
36. Curnes J: MR imaging of peripheral intracranial neoplasms: Extraaxial versus intraaxial masses. J Comput Assist Tomogr 11:932–937, 1987.
37. Osborne A: Brain tumors and tumorlike masses: Classification and differential diagnosis. In Diagnostic Neuroradiology. St. Louis: CV Mosby, 1996, pp 401–528.
38. Moller A, Hatam A, Olivecrona H: The differential diagnosis of pontine angle meningioma and acoustic neuroma with computed topography. Neuroradiology 17:21, 1978.
39. Valavanis A, Schubiger O, Hayik J, et al: CT of meningiomas on the posterior surface of the petrous bone. Neuroradiology 22:111, 1981.
40. Giannotta S, Pulec J, Goodkin R: Translabyrinthine removal of cerebellopontine angle meningiomas. Neurosurgery 17:620–625, 1985.
41. Yasuoka S, Okazaki H, Daube J, et al: Foramen magnum tumors: Analysis of 57 cases of benign extramedullary tumors. J Neurosurg 49:828, 1978.
42. Dodge HW Jr, Love JG, Gottlieb CM: Benign tumors of the foramen magnum: Surgical considerations. J Neurosurg 13:603, 1956.
43. Kempe LG: Posterior fossa, spinal cord and peripheral nerve disease. In Kempe L (ed): Operative Neurosurgery, Vol 2. New York: Springer-Verlag, 1970, p 269.
44. Scott E, Rhoton A: Foramen magnum meningiomas. In Al-Mefty O (ed): Meningiomas. New York: Raven Press, 1991, pp 543–567.
45. Sekhar L, Wright D, Richardson R, Monacci W: Petroclival and foramen magnum meningiomas: Surgical approaches and pitfalls. J Neuro Oncol 29:249–259, 1996.
46. Howe JR, Taren JA: Foramen magnum tumors: Pitfall in diagnosis. JAMA 225:1061, 1973.
47. Krayenbühl H: Special clinical features of tumors of the foramen magnum. Schweiz Arch Neurol Neurochir Psychiatry 112:205, 1973.
48. Symonds CP, Meadows SP: Compression of the spinal cord in the neighborhood of the foramen magnum. Brain 60:52, 1937.
49. Elsberg CA, Strauss I: Tumors of the spinal cord which project into the posterior cranial fossal: Report of a case in which a growth was removed from the ventral and lateral aspects of the medulla oblongata and upper cervical cord. Arch Neurol Psychiatry 21:261, 1929.
50. Boshes B, Padberg F: Studies on the cervical spinal cord of man: Sensory pattern after interruption of the posterior columns. Neurology 3:90, 1953.
51. Rubenstein JE: Astereognosis associated with tumors in the region of the foramen magnum. Arch Neurol Psychiatry 39:1016, 1938.
52. Bakes HL Jr: Myelographic examination of the posterior fossa with positive contrast medium. Radiology 81:791, 1963.
53. Malis LI: The myelographic examination of the foramen magnum. Radiology 70:196, 1958.
54. Margolis MI: A simple myelographic maneuver for the detection of mass lesions at the foramen magnum. Radiology 119:482, 1976.
55. Salamon GM, Combalbert A, Raybaud C, et al: An angiographic study of meningiomas of the posterior fossa. 35:731, 1971.
56. Macpherson P: The value of preoperative embolization of meningiomas estimated objectively and subjectively. Neuroradiology 33(4):334–337, 1991.
57. George B, Lot G, Boissonnet H: Meningioma of the foramen magnum: A series of 40 cases. Surg Neurol 47:371–379, 1997.
58. George B, Dematons C, Cophigons J: Lateral approach to the anterior portion of the foramen magnum: Application to surgical removal of 14 benign tumors: Technical note. Surg Neurol 29:484–490, 1988.
59. Sen C, Sekhar L: An extreme lateral approach to intradural lesions of the cervical spine and foramen magnum. Neurosurgery 27:197–204, 1990.
60. West C: Access to anteriorly placed tumours in the posterior fossa by medullotomy. Br J Neurosurg 5:179–182, 1991.
61. Mullan S, Naunton R, Hekmatpanah J, et al: The use of an anterior approach to ventrally placed tumors in the foramen magnum and vertebral column. J Neurosurg 24:536, 1966.

# CHAPTER 72

# Suboccipital Transmeatal Approach to Vestibular Schwannoma

■ ROBERT G. OJEMANN

## OVERALL MANAGEMENT PLAN

Three management options are considered when a patient with a vestibular schwannoma is evaluated: (1) surgery, (2) radiosurgery or fractionated radiation therapy, and (3) observation. To decide on the best management plan for each patient, the physician must obtain the patient's history to have a clear idea of the patient's course and of how the symptoms are affecting the patient's life, make an objective assessment of any neurologic deficit, review carefully the radiographic studies to ensure they are adequate, and decide if any additional studies are needed. The management options are then evaluated. The physician must have up-to-date knowledge about these alternatives. What will be the impact of the proposed treatment on the patient's daily life? Will the treatment improve or arrest the progression of symptoms? Can further growth or recurrence of the tumor be prevented? What are the risks of the treatment? Do the short-term and long-term benefits justify these risks? The physician and patient should discuss the patient's hopes and expectations about the treatment. The informational brochures from the Acoustic Neuroma Association have been a great help to many patients and their families as they consider these questions.

In some patients, little doubt exists as to the treatment course. In other patients, the decision may be difficult because the symptoms are minimal or nonprogressive, the growth rate is unpredictable, no treatment plan is free of risk, and the long-term results of the radiosurgery and radiation therapy options are unknown. Vestibular schwannomas usually enlarge slowly. It has been well documented that some tumors stop growing, a few grow rapidly, and spontaneous regression rarely occurs.[1-3]

The indications for considering operation are as follows:

1. Recent or worsening symptoms except in some elderly patients with a tumor having 2 cm or less intracranial extension
2. Enlargement of the tumor in a patient who is being observed except in some elderly patients with a tumor having 2 cm or less intracranial extension
3. Enlargement of a tumor after radiosurgery once the initial swelling reaction has subsided

4. The patient's decision after discussion of the treatment options

The indications for considering radiation therapy (usually stereotactic radiosurgery unless hearing preservation is an issue, in which case, fractionated radiation therapy is considered) are as follows:

1. An elderly patient with an enlarging tumor or recent symptoms and 2 cm or less intracranial extension
2. Hearing loss or enlarging tumor in the only-hearing ear
3. Residual tumor or regrowth after subtotal removal
4. Major medical illness that significantly increases the risk of operation
5. The patient's decision after discussion of the treatment options

The indications for considering observation are as follows:

1. A long history of auditory symptoms in a patient of any age and with any sized tumor
2. An elderly patient with mild symptoms
3. An incidental finding of the tumor on a scan performed for some other reason
4. The patient's decision after discussion of the treatment options

## SURGICAL MANAGEMENT

### Overview

The microsurgical removal of a vestibular schwannoma can be performed by a suboccipital, translabyrinthine, or middle fossa approach. Good results after the removal of vestibular schwannomas have been reported with all three approaches by experienced groups of surgeons.[4] A thorough understanding of the anatomy of the cerebellopontine angle and petrous bone and the relationship of anatomic structures to the tumor is essential.[4-7] I prefer the suboccipital approach for most patients because of the wide visualization it allows, the ability to save hearing, and the good results that I[4, 8-19] and others[6, 20-29] have reported. I have used the middle fossa approach for some intracanalicular tumors that extend to the lateral end of the internal auditory canal when an attempt is being made to save hearing. The translabyrinthine approach is used for small tumors when there is no useful hearing. In a few patients, I have used a combined suboccipital-translabryinthine-transtemporal approach for large tumors growing far anteriorly. A similar approach has been described by Haddad and Al-Mefty,[30] in which a petrosal exposure can be combined with a translabyrinthine and transcochlear approach. Gormley and colleagues[26] also use a transpetrosal-retrosigmoid approach in some patients with large tumors.

Other modifications of the suboccipital approach have been described. Shelton and associates[31] combine a suboccipital approach with a mastoidectomy in some patients when they are attempting to save hearing. Poe and coworkers[32] have used a translabyrinthine drill-out from the suboccipital approach to combine the advantages of both exposures. Darrouzet and colleagues[25] describe a widened retrolabyrinthine approach exposing the temporal dura, sigmoid sinus, and retrosigmoid dura with removal of a portion of the mastoid bone. With some large tumors, Comey and associates[33] have suggested that a staged operation may be of benefit.

My operative approach and techniques for the suboccipital transmeatal approach have been described and illustrated in detail in previous publications.[4, 16–19] The operation is performed in collaboration with an otologic surgeon, who exposes the internal auditory canal and dissects the tumor in that area. This approach has also been described by several other groups.[5, 7, 21, 22, 34, 35]

## Preoperative Evaluation

In most patients, the diagnosis of vestibular schwannomas is established with magnetic resonance imaging (MRI) after gadolinium enhancement. Usually, MRI is the only imaging study needed. It has been suggested that computed tomography (CT) images with bone windows may be valuable in planning a hearing-saving operation, but this remains to be proven.[36, 37] Pure-tone audiometry and speech discrimination testing are usually performed as part of the patient's initial evaluation.[38] The information from these tests is used to help determine the probability of saving useful hearing and to evaluate hearing in the opposite ear.

## Management of Preoperative Hydrocephalus

Occasionally, patients with vestibular schwannomas have enlarged ventricles and no symptoms of hydrocephalus. No special treatment is needed for these patients.

High-pressure hydrocephalus is now uncommon in a patient with a vestibular schwannoma, but if it is present, the symptoms usually improve with steroid therapy. A ventricular drain may be needed at operation and for a few days postoperatively. Rarely does a patient need a ventriculoperitoneal shunt.

Occasionally an elderly patient is seen with a large tumor and large ventricles who has symptoms suggesting normal-pressure hydrocephalus. If the only symptom is hearing

loss, a ventriculoperitoneal shunt may be the only treatment needed. If symptoms of increasing cranial nerve or brain stem compression are also present, treatment consists of placement of a ventriculoperitoneal shunt and subtotal removal of the tumor, usually in the same operation. These patients generally have a good long-term result.

## Monitoring

Continuous electrophysiologic monitoring of facial nerve function during the operation has become an established procedure.[4, 39–41] The benefits of this monitoring have been documented.[42] Several different anesthetic techniques have been used to allow this monitoring. In one, a continuous drip of a muscle relaxant is carefully administered so that facial nerve function can be assessed. The dosage is monitored by following the twitches elicited with ulnar nerve stimulation. Another technique is to use continuous administration of a low dose of propofol. Facial nerve function is monitored by continuous recording of electromyographic activity with two recording electrodes, one in the orbicularis oculi and the other in the orbicularis oris muscles (Fig. 72–1). The muscle contractions, which can occur from stimulation of the facial nerve during coagulation when the electrodes are inactive, are recorded from a motion sensor placed on the cheek. Monopolar stimulation is used to locate the seventh nerve. Fifth nerve function is monitored with an electrode placed in the masseter muscle.

Monitoring of auditory function can be done using electrocochleography, brain stem auditory evoked potential recording, direct cochlear nerve recording, or a combination of these techniques. I use a system developed by Levine.[43–45] A transtympanic electrode is placed for electrocochleography, scalp electrodes are inserted for brain stem auditory evoked potential monitoring, and a microphone system is placed in the external ear canal to provide the sound stimulus (see Fig. 72–1).

## Perioperative Medical Therapy

Steroids are usually started before the induction of anesthesia. A high steroid dose is continued every 6 hours during the operation, then is gradually tapered over 5 to 10 days depending on the size of the tumor and neurologic and facial nerve function. The blood glucose level is monitored. An antibiotic is given intravenously starting just before surgery and is continued for 24 hours after surgery. To prevent deep venous thrombosis, alternating compression thigh-high air boots are placed.

After anesthesia is induced, an indwelling Foley catheter is inserted, and 10 to 20 mg of furosemide is administered intravenously. During preparation and exposure of the dura, a 20% solution of mannitol is given intravenously in a dose of 1 to 1.5 g/kg over 20 to 30 minutes.

## Patient Position

The semisitting, prone, supine-oblique, lateral or park bench, and lateral-oblique positions have been used for suboccipital removal of vestibular schwannomas.[4] My ex-

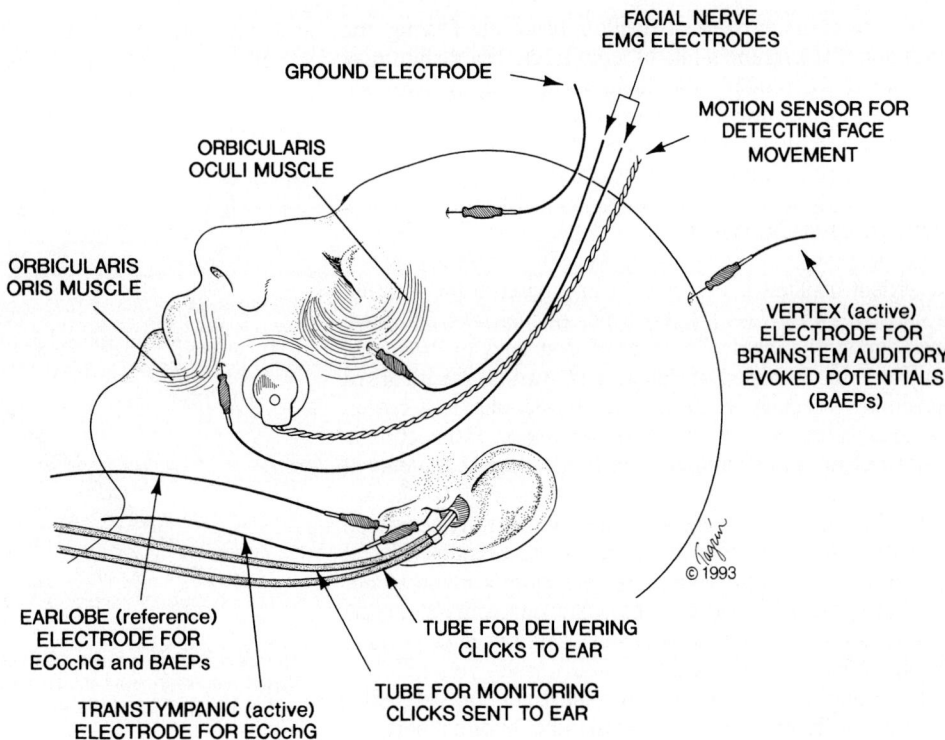

FIGURE 72–1 ■ Monitoring of facial and cochlear nerve function during operation. (Copyright © 1993, Edith Tagrin.)

perience with the semisitting position has been described previously.[11–12] No major permanent morbidity is related to this position, but occasional problems with air embolus and hypotension are encountered. Because of the risk of hypotension in older patients, a supine-oblique position is used. In addition to preventing hypotension, other advantages of this position are excellent visualization of the cerebellopontine angle, ease of tumor removal, no concern about air embolus, and comfort of the surgeon. This position is now used for removal of most cerebellopontine

angle tumors. If severe cervical spondylosis or limitation of neck motion exists from a previous injury, a lateral position is used. The intermittent pulsation of cerebrospinal fluid (CSF) into the operative area is not a problem and, in fact, keeps the neural and vascular structures from drying.

The operating table is turned so that the surgeon can sit behind the patient's head with his or her feet under the table. The patient lies supine with the shoulder that is ipsilateral to the tumor slightly elevated (Fig. 72–2). The head is turned parallel to the floor, elevated, and held

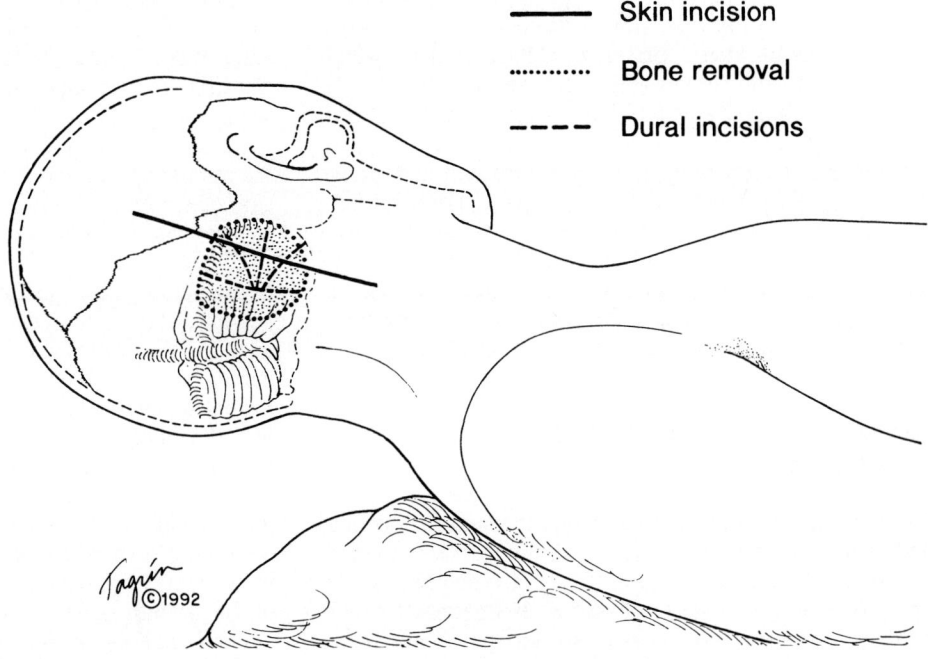

——— Skin incision

············ Bone removal

– – – Dural incisions

FIGURE 72–2 ■ Position, skin incision, craniotomy opening, and dural incisions. (Copyright © 1992, Edith Tagrin.)

with a three-point skeletal-fixation headrest. During the operation, the surgeon's line of sight to the brain stem may be altered by rotating the table from side to side. An armrest is placed for the surgeon's arm nearest the vertex. The other arm rests on the patient.

## Incision and Exposure

A vertical incision is centered 1 cm medial to the mastoid process (see Fig. 72–2). Other types of incisions that have been reported include an inverted J-shaped or L-shaped incision, an S-shaped incision, and various semicurved incisions.[4] A graft of pericranial tissue about 4 cm in diameter is taken from the occipital region. This graft is used in closing the cerebellar convexity dura at the end of the operation. The suboccipital muscles and fascia are incised in line with the incision and are carefully separated from their attachments to the bone by use of subperiosteal dissection and electrocautery. Special care is taken to occlude the arterial vessels as they are encountered in the muscle. An emissary vein is usually exposed in the region of the medial mastoid area.

The bone over the lateral two thirds of the cerebellar hemisphere is exposed. Visualizing the midline bone or rim of the foramen magnum is usually not necessary. A bur hole is placed, the dura is carefully separated from the overlying bone, and a free bone flap is cut (see Fig. 72–2). Care is taken not to take this initial opening too far laterally so as to avoid venous bleeding from the emissary veins or sigmoid sinus. The initial opening often exposes the edge of the transverse sinus. Further bone is removed as needed to expose the edge of the transverse sinus, the proximal sigmoid sinus, and the edge of the petrous bone laterally. This exposure allows the edge of the sinus to be retracted when the sutures are placed to hold the dural flaps, and it gives a direct line of sight down the posterior surface of the petrous bone. The mastoid air cells are usually entered and are occluded with bone wax.

The dura is opened vertically a few millimeters from the medial edge of the craniotomy. Stellate dural incisions provide superior, lateral, and inferior flaps of dura, which are held back with sutures (Fig. 72–3; see also Fig. 72–2).

The cerebellum is gently elevated, the arachnoid opened, and CSF allowed to drain (see Fig. 72–3). This process usually relieves any bulging of the cerebellum and allows exposure of the cerebellopontine angle with minimal retraction. The tip of a small catheter (No. 10 Bardic) is placed in the cistern and sutured to the inferior medial corner of the dural opening to drain CSF continuously during the operation. After placement of the self-retaining Greenberg retractors, the operating microscope is positioned.

## Removal of Small Tumors and Hearing Preservation

Under the microscope, arachnoid over the tumor is opened, and, if needed, the petrosal vein is coagulated and divided. The retractors are repositioned. It may also be necessary to open the arachnoid over the lower cranial nerves to facilitate the exposure. With small tumors, the eighth nerve

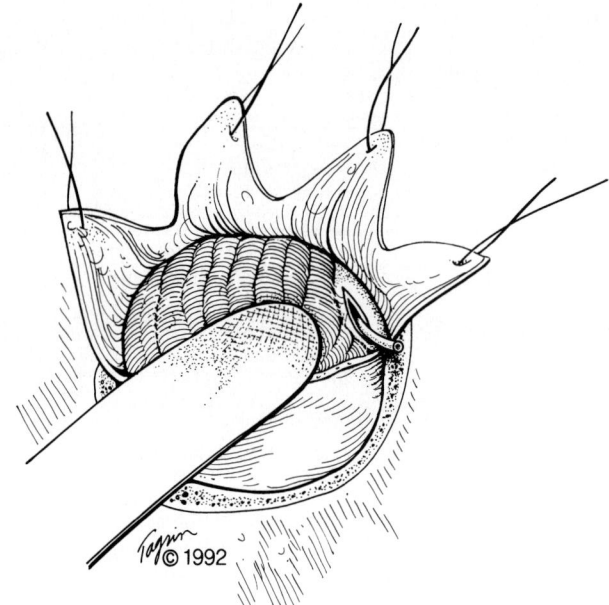

FIGURE 72–3 ■ Retraction of the dural flaps, elevation of the cerebellum, opening of the arachnoid, drainage of cerebrospinal fluid, and insertion of a catheter in the cistern. (Copyright © 1992, Edith Tagrin.)

complex is seen coming into the inferomedial side of the tumor. The facial nerve is usually on the anterior surface of the tumor. The capsule is stimulated to determine if there is an unusual course for the facial nerve. If there is a significant intracranial extension of the tumor, an internal decompression is done using sharp dissection.

The next step is exposure of the tumor in the internal auditory canal. Gelatin sponge (Gelfoam) is placed in the subarachnoid spaces to prevent dissemination of bone dust. Dura is removed over the region of the internal auditory canal, and bone is carefully removed by use of an air drill with constant suction-irrigation for cooling. The surgeon needs to remember that occasionally a high jugular bulb is exposed during the bone removal. Care is taken not to enter the labyrinth because this usually causes loss of hearing. If a semicircular canal is entered, it should be immediately closed with wax because hearing may still be preserved.[46] Once the internal auditory canal is exposed, the dura is opened over the tumor. An internal decompression of the tumor is done using sharp dissection so that the capsule can be mobilized with minimal pressure.

Dissection depends on an assessment of the relationship of the tumor to the vestibular and cochlear nerves. In most patients, the vestibular nerve fibers entering the medial edge of the tumor are divided, the cochlear and facial nerves are identified, and the dissection proceeds from medial to lateral. In a few patients, defining the cochlear nerve medially may be difficult. The tumor is then carefully rotated near the lateral end of the canal, while the surgeon looks for the seventh nerve anteriorly and superiorly and the cochlear nerve anteriorly and inferiorly (Fig. 72–4). Stretching or putting tension on the cochlear nerve must be avoided to prevent avulsion of the fibers. The position of the seventh nerve is confirmed with stimulation.

Dissection along the facial and cochlear nerves is per-

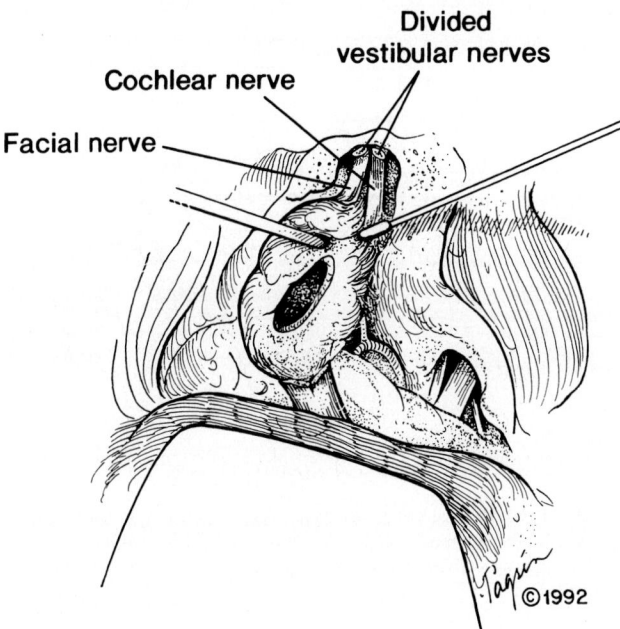

**FIGURE 72–4** ■ Exposure of a tumor and the seventh and eighth cranial nerves in the internal auditory canal. (Copyright © 1992, Edith Tagrin.)

formed with fine straight or curved microdissectors or canal knives and sharp dissection with microscissors. The tumor capsule is elevated laterally and superiorly. Dissection is alternated from different directions, depending on what direction provides the best exposure, the easiest plane of dissection, and the least traction on the nerves. When the cochlear and facial nerves have been clearly defined, the vestibular nerves coming into the tumor are divided on the lateral aspect of the tumor. In some patients, the lateral end of the tumor may not be exposed because of the limitation in bone removal. In these patients, the tumor is transected near the end of the canal, and the lateral extent of the tumor is removed with a small ring curet. To overcome the problem of inadequate visualization of the lateral end of the internal auditory canal, endoscopy has been used to ensure that all tumor has been removed and to visualize air cells that need to be occluded.[47–49] I have used this procedure and agree that excellent visualization can be achieved.

During the dissection, intermittent bleeding may occur along the nerves. A fine suction and irrigation keeps the field clean and does not damage the nerves. Most of the bleeding stops spontaneously. When hearing is to be saved, the surgeon should attempt to preserve any significant arterial vessel entering the internal auditory meatus.

## Removal of Medium-Sized and Large Tumors

Arachnoid between the posterior capsule of the tumor and cerebellum and over the lower cranial nerves is opened. A separate cystic collection of CSF containing xanthochromic fluid and surrounded by thickened arachnoid may occasionally be loculated in relation to the tumor capsule. The petrosal vein or one of its branches, which usually comes

off the cerebellum or middle cerebellar peduncle to the petrosal sinus just above the tumor, is coagulated and divided as needed. To complete the initial exposure of most of the posterior capsule, self-retaining retractors are repositioned. On occasion, it is necessary to shrink the cerebellar tissue next to the tumor with bipolar coagulation.

The posterior capsule is stimulated to locate the facial nerve. The facial nerve is usually on the anterior surface of the tumor, and no response occurs to this first stimulation. In some patients, the nerve is displaced superiorly, particularly in its lateral course. In this situation, a response may be seen on the initial stimulation over the superior capsule. Anteromedial displacement of the facial nerve along the brain stem and over the anterosuperior aspect of the tumor may also occur, and the facial nerve may be displaced against the fifth nerve. Rarely the nerve is inferior or across the posterior surface. The facial nerve was displaced posteriorly in only 1 patient in my series of 461 patients.[17]

The 9th, 10th, and 11th cranial nerves are identified, and arachnoid is carefully dissected to aid exposure of the inferomedial capsule. With larger tumors, the 9th and 10th nerves are carefully reflected off the tumor capsule. A small rubber dam is placed over these nerves for protection during the rest of the operation.

The next step is internal decompression of the tumor, which is performed intermittently as needed. This process allows all the pressure to be placed on the tumor capsule while separating it from the cranial nerves and brain stem. Ultrasonic aspiration, bipolar coagulation, and sharp dissection are used for internal decompression.

Dissection begins inferiorly and medially. In medium-sized tumors, the eighth nerve complex can usually be defined with moderate dissection (Fig. 72–5). These nerves are rarely seen initially in larger tumors. After carefully reflecting the capsule laterally and superiorly into the area of decompression, the surgeon looks for the eighth nerve complex along the inferomedial capsule. Being a right-handed surgeon, I use a fine suction in the left hand to retract the tumor and to keep the area of dissection clean. Care is taken to locate the facial nerve, which can be just under the eighth nerve complex or may be several

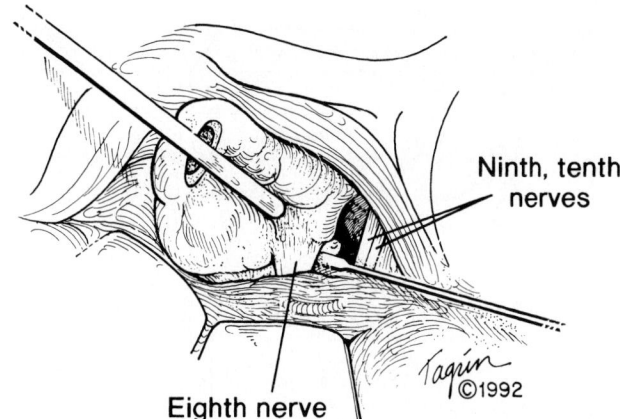

**FIGURE 72–5** ■ Visualization of the eighth cranial nerve on the inferior medial capsule after internal decompression of the tumor. (Copyright © 1992, Edith Tagrin.)

millimeters away. It can usually be recognized by its white or gray color, which is different from the adjacent brain stem. In many patients, the facial nerve is seen by elevating the eighth nerve complex, but when the seventh nerve is pushed against the brain stem and displaced anteriorly and medially, it is found by looking above the eighth nerve. If the seventh nerve has not been localized, intermittent stimulation is used. The vestibular and cochlear nerve fibers entering the tumor are divided using bipolar coagulation and sharp dissection. The surgeon must look carefully for a branch of the anterior-inferior cerebellar artery, which may loop just behind these nerves.

If the facial nerve is not seen anterior to the divided eighth nerve complex, it is usually located by reflecting the inferior and medial tumor capsule further laterally and superiorly (Fig. 72–6). Spontaneous electromyographic activity may indicate when the surgeon is near that nerve. Usually the facial nerve forms a solid band on the tumor capsule, but laterally it may be spread out over a wide area and occasionally is surrounded by the tumor.

As the dissection of the capsule progresses, not only is further internal decompression performed as indicated, but also sections of the tumor capsule are removed to allow room to reflect the capsule laterally. Arterial vessels adjacent to the tumor are preserved by division of only the branches entering the tumor (Fig. 72–7). Alternating dissection of the inferomedial capsule with dissection superiorly and medially to define the fifth nerve and brain stem attachments may be advantageous (Fig. 72–8). Vascular attachments are often in the region of the fifth nerve root entry zone. Small rubber dams may be placed on the brain stem for protection as the dissection progresses.

Dissection extends along the seventh nerve toward the internal auditory meatus (Fig. 72–9). When the point is reached where the bone over the internal auditory canal is impeding further dissection or the dissection is difficult, attention is directed to the tumor in the internal auditory canal. The exposure is the same as that described for small tumors except that the bone is removed to expose the lateral end of the canal entering the labyrinth if necessary.

After separation of the tumor from the facial nerve in

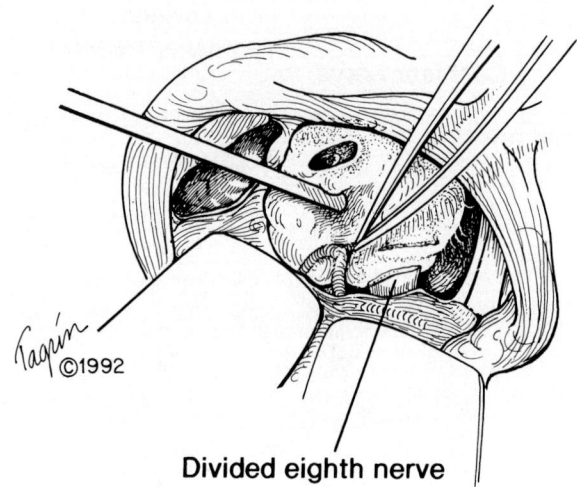

**Divided eighth nerve**

**FIGURE 72–7** ■ Division of the eighth cranial nerve and coagulation of a small arterial branch entering the tumor with preservation of the anterior inferior cerebellar artery branch. (Copyright © 1992, Edith Tagrin.)

the internal auditory canal, the attachments along the edge of the internal auditory meatus are divided. The facial nerve starts to turn anteriorly or anterosuperiorly as the posterior fossa is entered. The surgeon can then decide how best to proceed. The dissection may be continued medially along the brain stem and cerebellar peduncle, and the arachnoid and vascular attachments are divided as they are encountered, gradually freeing the facial nerve. Occasionally a large branch of the anterior-inferior cerebellar artery is embedded in the tumor capsule, but it can usually be dissected free by division of the small branches directly supplying the tumor. In large tumors, the trochlear nerve and superior cerebellar artery may be adherent superiorly, the 6th nerve adherent anteriorly, and the 9th and 10th nerves adherent inferiorly. The objective is to reduce the bulk and attachments of the tumor so that the surgeon is dealing only with dissection from the facial nerve and brain

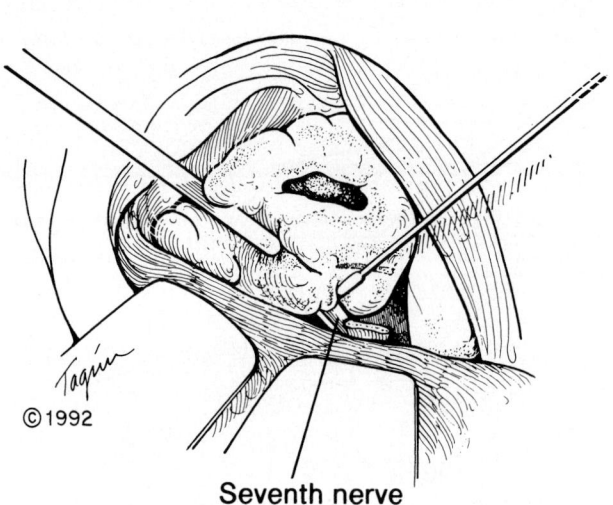

**Seventh nerve**

**FIGURE 72–6** ■ Identification of the seventh cranial nerve anterior to the divided eighth cranial nerve. (Copyright © 1992, Edith Tagrin.)

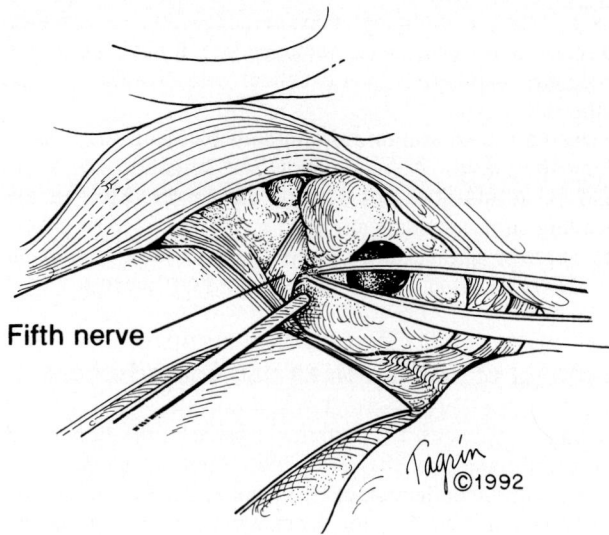

**Fifth nerve**

**FIGURE 72–8** ■ Exposure of the proximal segment of the fifth nerve. (Copyright © 1992, Edith Tagrin.)

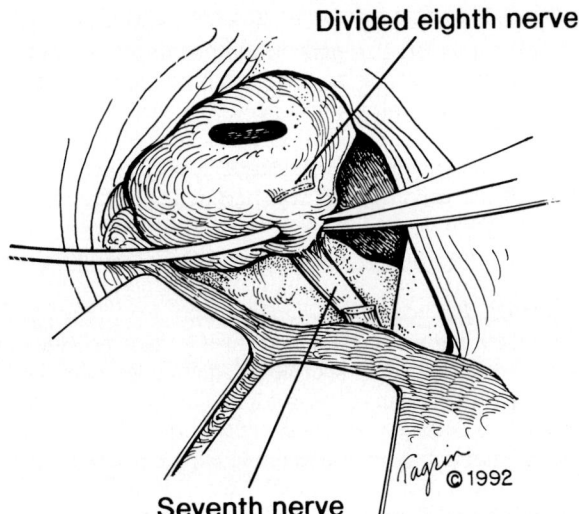

**Divided eighth nerve**

**Seventh nerve**

©1992

**FIGURE 72–9** ■ Dissection along the seventh cranial nerve. (Copyright © 1992, Edith Tagrin.)

stem. The facial nerve is usually most adherent to the tumor capsule in the posterior fossa near the internal auditory meatus, where the nerve may be splayed over the anterior-superior capsule, or it may occasionally be surrounded by tumor. Dissection in this area is often complicated by vascular and fibrous attachments. The surgeon must adapt to the characteristics of the tumor, and working alternately from various angles may be necessary.

If the tumor is large, the capsule may be so intimately adherent to the brain stem and cranial nerves that a plane cannot be developed. In such cases, a thin layer of tumor capsule is left (radical subtotal removal).[17]

## Closure

Once the tumor is removed, hemostasis is checked. The area of bone removal over the internal auditory meatus is carefully waxed to occlude air cells. An adipose tissue graft taken from a superficial incision on the lower abdomen is carefully placed in the area where bone has been removed. Surgicel is used to hold this graft in place and is also used to cover the area of resected or retracted cerebellum.

I close the dura in a watertight fashion by use of the graft of pericranial tissue taken at the beginning of the operation. The dura is covered with absorbable gelatin sponge (Gelfoam). The bone flap is replaced and held with stainless steel wire, which does not interfere with future imaging, and a dural tenting suture. An acrylic cranioplasty is done to occlude all of the bone defects and to place a thin layer over the bone flap. The wound is thoroughly irrigated with an antibiotic solution before closure.

## MANAGEMENT OF POSTOPERATIVE COMPLICATIONS

### Hematoma and Cerebellar Infarction

During the initial exposure, particular attention is paid to occlusion of the arterial vessels in the muscles as they are

encountered. During closure, the muscles are again carefully checked for bleeding. Postoperatively, blood pressure is controlled, beginning in the operating room with an intravenous antihypertensive medication, and is monitored continuously for as long as necessary.

If the cerebellum is unusually full at the end of the operation and good CSF drainage has occurred, cerebellar infarction or hematoma should be ruled out. In this situation, the lateral 1 to 2 cm of cerebellum may need to be resected. If there is doubt about the situation, the incision should be closed, and the patient should be kept intubated and taken immediately for a CT scan.

If the patient does not recover promptly from anesthesia, or if an unexpected significant neurologic deficit or a delayed neurologic deterioration occurs, a CT scan is performed immediately to look for cerebellar hematoma or infarction. Prompt removal of a significant hematoma or area of infarction can lead to a dramatic recovery.

### Cerebrospinal Fluid Leak

If a CSF leak develops, a lumbar drain is placed for 72 hours, and this often resolves the problem. When the leak persists, a transmastoid repair using an adipose tissue graft is performed.

### Hydrocephalus

In the postoperative period, the patient may develop neurologic symptoms that suggest hydrocephalus, or a tense subgaleal fluid collection may be present. Ventricular size is observed by CT scan. Persistent hydrocephalus is a rare complication. Most patients recover spontaneously, a few require a temporary lumbar drain, and only occasionally do patients require a ventriculoperitoneal shunt.

### Meningitis

When postoperative fever with headache or stiffness in the neck occurs, the possibility of either bacterial or aseptic meningitis must be considered. CT with contrast enhancement is performed to look for local infection. A lumbar puncture is performed, and broad-spectrum antibiotics are started. Subsequent treatment is guided by the results of the CSF examination and cultures. If the findings suggest an aseptic meningitis, steroids are administered.

### Wound Infection

When the infection is superficial and the organism is sensitive to antibiotics, removing the bone flap may not be necessary. If the infection is extensive, débridement of the wound and removal of the bone flap need to be done.

### Neurologic Disability

If any significant postoperative disability occurs, the patient is seen by physical and occupational therapists. Some patients note mild unsteadiness that clears over several days to several weeks. More severe impairment in walking and difficulties with coordination and dysarthria take longer to reverse, and permanent disability may result. If transient difficulty in focusing the eyes or diplopia occurs, it usually clears over days to a few weeks. Dizziness and vertigo are frequent complaints in the initial postoperative period, but these symptoms usually resolve quite rapidly.

Increased loss of facial sensation is usually not a problem except in the few patients who also have a facial paralysis (see Facial Nerve Function). Recovery from the facial numbness is variable.

Difficulty swallowing because of impaired function in the 9th and 10th nerves should be carefully evaluated with a modified barium swallow and followed by a specialist in swallowing disorders. Often the patient can be given instructions that facilitate his or her swallowing and prevent aspiration. If there is severe impairment in swallowing, a gastrostomy may need to be performed.

## Medical Complications

To prevent deep venous thrombosis, I use alternating-compression, thigh-high air boots, which are continued until the patient is ambulatory. Electrocardiographic changes and any cardiopulmonary symptoms are immediately evaluated by a cardiologist.

## Headache

Persistent headache remains a significant problem in a small percentage of patients. MRI rarely shows a structural abnormality, such as hydrocephalus. Harner and coworkers[50] found the incidence of significant headache was 23% at 3 months and 9% at 2 years after operation. Possible causes of headache that have been suggested include aggravation of pre-existing vascular headache, degenerative disease in the cervical spine, occipital nerve neuroma, myofascial scar, scar between the neck muscle and dura, and subarachnoid bone dust. A reduced incidence of headache with the use of methyl methacrylate cranioplasty has been reported,[50] and this has also been my experience. Catalano and associates[51] found that preventing the free circulation of bone dust by keeping the arachnoid relatively intact and using pieces of Gelfoam to block off the subarachnoid space during intradural drilling caused the most dramatic reduction in headache. Their patients also had a cranioplasty. Headache usually improves with time and responds to a program of physical therapy and medication.

## RESULTS FOR UNILATERAL VESTIBULAR SCHWANNOMA SURGICAL REMOVAL

### Overall Function

Good results using the suboccipital (posterior fossa) approach for removal of unilateral vestibular schwannomas have been reported by my group[4, 8–19] as well as others.[6, 20–29] My series of 461 patients with unilateral vestibular schwannomas operated by a suboccipital approach in conjunction with an otologist has been reviewed.[17] The size of the tumor has been recorded as intracanalicular or by size of the extension into the posterior fossa. The functional results of the operation are reported as good, fair, or poor. The term *good* is used for patients who were free of major neurologic deficit and returned to their pre-illness level of activity. Seventh and eighth nerve function was not considered. *Fair* described patients who were functionally independent but were unable to return to their previous full activity because of a neurologic deficit or who had a significant preoperative neurologic deficit that, although improved, continued to cause disability. Many of these patients returned to work and are leading normal lives. The term *poor* described patients who were dependent because of a major new or preoperative neurologic disability. In my overall series, 99% were independent in their activities. All patients with intracanalicular tumors or tumors extending 1 cm into the posterior fossa had a good result, as did 96% in the 1- to 1.9-cm group and 93% in the 2- to 2.9-cm group. Even patients with large tumors had an 80% chance of having a good outcome. The most common reasons for the fair results were impaired balance, gait, or coordination. Dysarthria or diplopia occurred in a few patients. In 6 of the 43 *fair* patients, a significant preoperative deficit improved but still limited the patient's activity. In a small percentage of patients, a significant headache problem lasted longer than expected, and it prevented full recovery, placing them into the fair result category.

In my series, there were two poor results (0.5%) and two deaths occurred (operative mortality, 0.5%). The operative mortality in most large series is close to 1%, and a high percentage of the patients return to normal activities.

## Extent of Tumor Removal and Recurrence

The goal of the operation is total removal of the tumor. This goal must be tempered, however, by surgical judgment, which considers the need to preserve and improve function as well as the long-term results. My experience indicates that a place exists for subtotal and radical subtotal removal of vestibular schwannomas because the recurrence rate has been low, and in larger tumors, the incidence of postoperative neurologic problems has been low, especially in elderly patients.

The term *radical subtotal removal* describes a procedure in which a small fragment of tumor is left, usually because it is densely adherent to the facial nerve or brain stem.[17] The term *subtotal removal* describes extensive removal of tumor in which a portion of the rim of the capsule is left attached to the brain stem and cranial nerves.

The reasons for performing a radical subtotal or subtotal removal include adherence of the tumor to the facial nerve or brain stem, age (≥70 years), treatment of a tumor affecting an only-hearing ear, and the patient's request. After carefully considering all the treatment options, some patients now request a less-than-total removal to reduce the risk to the facial nerve and the risk of neurologic disability.

The recurrence rate after radical subtotal and subtotal removal needs careful evaluation. Over the 15 years of the series I reported, none of the 43 patients with radical subtotal removals had a recurrence that required treatment.[17] These patients were followed for 1 to 14 years (average, 5.4 years). In seven patients, their tumors could not be seen on follow-up scans. Nine of 56 patients (16%) with subtotal removal had recurrence that required treatment (average follow-up, 5.2 years). Treatment options include further surgery and, in the past few years, radiosurgery and fractionated radiation therapy.

Wazen and coworkers[52] found that in 9 of 13 patients who had subtotal removal (aged 66 to 81 years), no growth occurred in the residual tumors in follow-up periods ranging from 6 months to 15 years. Klemink and associates[53] reported on 20 patients who had incomplete removal of the tumor to reduce operative risks. Two groups were defined: a subtotal group (resection of <95% of the tumor) and a near-total group (resection of ≥95% of the tumor). The subtotal group included mostly elderly patents (mean age, 68.5 years) with large tumors, and the near-total group consisted of young patients (mean age, 45.8 years). The mean length of follow-up was 5 years, and only one patient showed regrowth during this period. Lownie and Drake[54] reported that 9 of 11 patients followed for 10 to 22 years after radical intracapsular removal had recurrence. The two recurrences were at 2 and 3 years postoperatively. The low incidence of recurrence and the ability to treat recurrence effectively when it does occur suggests that a radical subtotal or subtotal removal should be considered in some patients with large tumors, particularly in the elderly.

Recurrence can also occur after apparent total removal of the tumor. The known recurrence rate in my series was 0.8% (3 of 360).[17] Samii and Matthies[28] reported a recurrence rate of 0.7% (6 of 880).

## Facial Nerve Function

With the development of microsurgical techniques and intraoperative monitoring of facial nerve function, preservation of facial nerve function has been possible in a high percentage of patients. Sampath and associates[41] have summarized the results of several large series. The House-Brackmann facial nerve grading system is used to record facial nerve function (Table 72–1).[55] In my series, evaluation of facial nerve function approximately 1 year after operation or the last time the patient was seen before 1

TABLE 72–1 ■ HOUSE-BRACKMANN FACIAL NERVE GRADING SYSTEM*

| Grade | Description |
| --- | --- |
| 1 | Normal |
| 2 | Mild: slight weakness only on close inspection |
| 3 | Moderate: obvious but not disfiguring difference |
| 4 | Moderately severe: obvious weakness |
| 5 | Severe: barely perceptible motion |
| 6 | Complete paralysis |

*Data from House JW, Brackmann DE: Facial nerve grading system. Otolaryngol Head Neck Surg 93:184–193, 1985.

year postoperatively revealed good function (grade I or II) as follows: intracanalicular, 26 patients (96%); up to 0.9 cm intracranial extension, 37 patients (100%); 1.0 to 1.9 cm intracranial extension, 122 patients (96%); 2 to 2.9 cm intracranial extension, 96 patients (77%); 3 to 3.9 cm intracranial extension, 102 patients (60%); and greater than 4 cm intracranial extension, 71 patients (58%).[17]

The facial nerve is so involved with tumor in some patients that it cannot be saved. A decision has to be made about whether to leave a small piece of tumor capsule with the nerve (radical subtotal removal), to divide the nerve and approximate the ends, or to perform a nerve graft with the sural nerve. Recovery after graft or anastomosis usually returned the face to at best a grade III, which is defined as a moderate weakness with an obvious but not disfiguring difference in the two sides of the face. Samii and Matthies[40] have reported on a large series of facial nerve reconstructions. I have left tumor in patients who, in the preoperative discussion, requested this to reduce the risk of facial paralysis, although they knew that they might need further surgery in the future. The results of long-term follow-up on these patients are encouraging.

Delayed onset of facial weakness can occur from a few hours to 2 weeks after removal of a vestibular schwannoma.[17, 56, 57] Most patients make an excellent recovery, often within a few weeks, and usually there is a full recovery by 6 months.

When the patient awakens from anesthesia with a facial paralysis or develops a delayed complete facial paralysis, the cornea must be protected. Initially the eyelids may almost close, but as muscle tone is lost, the opening becomes wider. Beginning immediately after surgery, the eyelids are approximated with tape. Artificial tears are used regularly during the day, and an ophthalmic ointment is used at night. The use of a tarsorrhaphy, a gold weight in the upper eyelid, or both is essential to the maintenance of a healthy cornea and prevention of visual loss and incapacitating pain. Which oculoplastic procedure is best suited for a particular patient depends on the patient's age, skin laxity, and presence or absence of corneal anesthesia. These procedures have the advantage of being reversible. When loss of corneal sensation occurs, the cornea is at great risk, and a medial and lateral tarsorrhaphy may be necessary for protection. When facial paralysis does not recover, improved function may result from use of a modification of the classic hypoglossal-facial anastomosis with partial division of the hypoglossal nerve and anastomosis of half of the nerve to the lower branch of the facial nerve. This procedure can be combined with one of the eye procedures and a temporalis transposition flap.[58]

## Cochlear Nerve Function

Preservation of useful hearing depends on the size of the tumor, the level of preoperative hearing, and the involvement of the internal auditory artery branches with the tumor. In 1984, my group published the results of a series of 22 patients in whom an attempt was made to save hearing.[14] Subsequent publications have updated this series.[4, 8, 9, 15, 17, 59] In 1988, Gardner and Robertson[60] reviewed the reports on hearing preservation published in the English literature from 1954 to 1986. Several publications have subsequently discussed hearing preservation with the suboccipital transmeatal approach.[22–24, 27, 29, 30, 61–70]

The question of what constitutes useful serviceable hearing has been discussed by several authors. The commonest criteria are a speech reception threshold of less than 50 db with a speech discrimination score of 50% or more.[71] Whittaker and Luetje[72] support the definition of speech discrimination score of 70% or better for serviceable hearing, whereas I have used a speech discrimination score of 35% or better because for some patients this level of hearing has been useful.

In patients with intracanalicular tumors, the rate of saving useful hearing in a series of reasonable size has ranged from 33% to greater than 90%.[17, 27, 29, 67] As the tumor grows into the posterior fossa and enlarges, this rate drops. Patients with tumors that are 2 cm or larger have a low probability of hearing preservation even if preoperative hearing is excellent.

In an attempt to help preserve hearing during removal of a vestibular schwannoma, I have investigated the monitoring of auditory evoked responses using a system developed by Levine.[14, 17, 43–45] Electrocochleography monitors the status of the cochlea and the auditory nerve peripheral to the tumor, and brain stem auditory evoked potential recording measures the neural activity central to the tumor. The goal of monitoring is to give an indication of early hearing compromise that is reversible and allows the surgeon to alter the dissection.[4, 15, 17, 73] This reversible hearing compromise has likely been the case in some patients in whom a change in the evoked response occurred that recovered when the dissection was stopped or altered. In some patients, no change occurs in the evoked responses. Monitoring has not made a difference in the outcome when abrupt loss of function has occurred without warning, presumably as a result of interruption of vascular supply.

Slavit and colleagues[69] compared two matched series of patients with and without auditory monitoring and concluded that there is a benefit from intraoperative monitoring. In an attempt to improve the use of monitoring in preserving cochlear nerve function, several techniques have been tried. Direct recording from the eighth nerve has been used, but this technique can be used only in patients with small tumors, and movement of the electrode remains a problem.[73] Matthies and Samii[74] using auditory brain stem response (ABR) waves I, III, and V reported that "useful recognition of significant waveform changes is possible and enables changes of microsurgical maneuvers to favor (ABR) recovery." Compton and colleagues,[62] Rowed and Nedzelski,[27] and Koos and associates[29] found monitoring to be of little help, however, and Post and coworkers[75] were not sure if there was help from the monitoring.

The long-term results of hearing preservation have been evaluated.[59, 66] McKenna and coworkers,[59] reporting on our series of 18 patients with follow-up periods ranging from 3.4 to 10.4 years (mean, 5.4 years), found four patients (22%) with a significant decline in hearing. Changes did not correlate with tumor size, preoperative hearing, intraoperative changes in hearing, interval between initial symptoms and surgery, sex, or age.

Concern about recurrence after removal of an acoustic neuroma with preservation of the cochlear nerve has been discussed in the literature. Thedinger and colleagues[76] emphasize that inadequate exposure of the lateral end of the internal auditory canal may be associated with leaving a remnant of tumor. Neely[64] reported that in patients in whom all of the tumor appeared to have been removed, residual tumor was found in the cochlear nerve, and he concluded that "histologic data suggests that complete tumor removal in attempts to preserve hearing may be beyond our surgical capabilities." Samii and Matthies,[67] however, reported a recurrence rate of 1.4% in 260 patients who had removal of vestibular schwannomas with hearing preservation. Post and associates[75] had a 4% recurrence rate in 56 patients. Our results show a 2% incidence of recurrence in this group of patients. A few patients have an area of gadolinium enhancement in the internal auditory canal on postoperative MRI. Whether this manifestation represents residual tumor or postoperative scar is unknown, but follow-up scans have usually remained unchanged, and the report of Weisman and colleagues[77] suggests that this finding is usually not due to tumor.

Tinnitus may persist after removal of an acoustic neuroma. There does not seem to be any difference in the incidence of tinnitus between patients who had the cochlear nerve preserved to save hearing and those in whom the cochlear nerve was divided for tumor removal.[78]

## REFERENCES

1. Bederson JB, yon Ammon K, Wichmann WW, et al: Conservative treatment of patients with acoustic neuroma. Neurosurgery 28:646–651, 1991.
2. Nedzelski JM, Canter RJ, Kassel EE, et al: Is no treatment good treatment in the management of acoustic neuromas in the elderly? Laryngoscope 96:825–829, 1986.
3. Valvassori GE, Shannon M: Natural history of acoustic neuroma. Skull Base Surg 1:165–167, 1991.
4. Ojemann RG, Martuza RL: Acoustic neuroma. In Youmans JR (ed): Neurological Surgery, 3rd ed. Philadelphia: WB Saunders, 1990, pp 3316–3350.
5. Camins MB, Oppenhiem JS: Anatomy and surgical techniques in the suboccipital transmeatal approach to acoustic neuromas. Clin Neurosurg 38:567–588, 1992.
6. Rhoton AL Jr: Microsurgical anatomy of the brain stem surface facing an acoustic neuroma. Surg Neurol 25:326–339, 1986.
7. Rhoton AL Jr: Microsurgical anatomy of the cerebellopontine angle. In Wilkins RH, Rengachary SS (eds): Neurosurgery. New York: McGraw-Hill, 1996, pp 1063–1084.
8. Nadol JB Jr, Levine RA, Ojemann RG, et al: Preservation of hearing in surgical removal of acoustic neuromas of the internal auditory canal and cerebellar pontine angle. Laryngoscope 97:1287–1294, 1987.
9. Nadol JB Jr, Chiong CM, Ojemann RG, et al: Preservation of hearing and facial nerve function in resection of acoustic neuroma. Laryngoscope 102:1153–1158, 1992.
10. Ojemann RG, Montgomery WW, Weiss AD: Evaluation and surgical treatment of acoustic neuroma. N Engl J Med 287:895–899, 1972.
11. Ojemann RG: Microsurgical suboccipital approach to cerebellopontine angle tumors. Clin Neurosurg 25:461–479, 1978.
12. Ojemann RG, Crowell RM: Acoustic neuromas treated by microsurgical suboccipital operations. Prog Neurol Surg 9:334–373, 1978.
13. Ojemann RG: Comments on Fischer G, Costantini JL, Mercier P: Improvement of hearing after microsurgical removal of acoustic neuroma. Neurosurgery 7:158–159, 1980.
14. Ojemann RG, Levine RA, Montgomery WM: Use of intraoperative auditory evoked potentials to preserve hearing in unilateral acoustic neuroma removal. J Neurosurg 61:938–948, 1984.
15. Ojemann RG: Strategies to preserve hearing during resection of acoustic neuroma. In Wilkins RH, Rengachary SS (eds): Neurosurgery Update I. New York: McGraw-Hill, 1990, pp 424–427.

16. Ojemann RG: Suboccipital approach to acoustic neuromas. In Wilson CB (ed): Neurosurgical Procedures: Personal Approaches to Classic Techniques. Baltimore: Williams & Wilkins, 1992, pp 78–87.
17. Ojemann RG: Management of acoustic neuroma (vestibular schwannoma). Clin Neurosurg 40:498–535, 1993.
18. Ojemann RG: Acoustic neurinoma (vestibular schwannoma)—the suboccipital approach. In Kaye AH, Laws ER Jr (eds): Brain Tumors. Edinburgh: Churchill Livingstone, 1995, pp 623–641.
19. Ojemann RG: Acoustic neuroma (vestibular schwannomas). In Youmans JR (ed): Neurological Surgery, 4th ed. Philadelphia: WB Saunders, 1996, pp 2841–2867.
20. Symon L, Bordi LT, Comptor JJ, et al: Acoustic neurinoma: A review of 392 cases. Br J Neurosurg 3:343–347, 1989.
21. Baldwin DL, King TT, Morrison AW: Hearing conservation in acoustic neuroma surgery via the posterior fossa. Laryngol Otol 104:463–467, 1990.
22. Ebersold MJ, Harner SG, Beatty CW, et al: Current results of retrosigmoid approach to acoustic neurinoma. J Neurosurg 76:901–909, 1992.
23. Klemink JL, LaRouare MJ, Kileny PR, et al: Hearing preservation following suboccipital removal of acoustic neuromas. Laryngoscope 100:597–601, 1990.
24. Fisher G, Fisher C, Remond J: Hearing preservation in acoustic neuroma surgery. J Neurosurg 76:910–917, 1992.
25. Darrouzet V, Guerin J, Aouad N, et al: The widened retrolabyrinthine approach: A new concept in acoustic neuroma surgery. J Neurosurg 86:812–821, 1997.
26. Gormley WB, Sekkhar LN, Wright DC, et al: Acoustic neuromas: Results of current surgical management. Neurosurgery 41:50–60, 1997.
27. Rowed DW, Nedzelski JM: Hearing preservation in removal of intracanicular acoustic neuroma via the retrosigmoid approach. J Neurosurg 86:456–461, 1997.
28. Samii M, Matthies C: Management of 1000 vestibular schwannomas (acoustic neuromas): Surgical management and results with an emphasis on complications and how to avoid them. Neurosurgery 40:11–23, 1997.
29. Koos WT, Day JD, Matula C, et al: Neurotopographic considerations in microsurgical treatment of small acoustic neuromas. J Neurosurg 88:506–512, 1998.
30. Haddad GF, Al-Mefty O: The road less traveled: Transtemporal access to the CPA. Clin Neurosurg 41:150–167, 1994.
31. Shelton C, Alavi S, Li JC, et al: Modified retrosigmoid approach: Use for selected acoustic tumor removal. Am J Otol 16:672–678, 1994.
32. Poe DS, Tarlov EC, Gadre AK: Translabyrinthine drillout from suboccipital approach to acoustic neuroma. Am J Otol 14:215–219, 1993.
33. Comey CH, Janetta PJ, Sheptak PE, et al: Staged removal of acoustic tumors: Technique and lessons learned from a series of 83 patients. Neurosurgery 37:915–921, 1995.
34. Eisenberg MB, Catalano PJ, Post KD: Management of acoustic schwannomas. In Tindall GT, Cooper PR, Barrow DL (eds): The Practice of Neurosurgery. Baltimore: Williams & Wilkins, 1996, pp 995–1004.
35. Buchheit WA, Getch CC: Tumors of the cerebellopontine angle: Clinical features and surgical management via retrosigmoid approach. In Wilkins RH, Rengachary SS (eds): Neurosurgery. New York: McGraw-Hill, 1996, pp 1085–1094.
36. Matthies C, Samii M, Krebs S: Management of vestibular schwannomas (acoustic neuromas): Radiological features in 202 cases—their value for diagnosis and their predictive importance. Neurosurgery 40:469–482, 1997.
37. Yokoyama T, Venura K, Ryu H, et al: Surgical approach to the internal auditory meatus in acoustic neuroma surgery: Significance of preoperative high resolution computed tomography. Neurosurgery 39:965–970, 1996.
38. Martuza RL, Parker SW, Nadol JB Jr, et al: Diagnosis of cerebellopontine angle tumors. Clin Neurosurg 32:177–213, 1985.
39. Eldridge R, Parry D: Summary: Vestibular Schwannoma (Acoustic Neuroma) Consensus Development Conference. Neurosurgery 30:962–964, 1992.
40. Samii M, Matthies C: Management of 1000 vestibular schwannomas (acoustic neuromas): The facial nerve—preservation and restitution of function. Neurosurgery 40:684–695, 1997.
41. Sampath P, Holliday MJ, Brem H, et al: Facial nerve injury in acoustic neuroma (vestibular schwannoma) surgery: Etiology and prevention. J Neurosurg 87:60–66, 1997.
42. Jellinek DA, Tan LC, Symon L: The import of continuous electrophysiological monitoring on preservation of the facial nerve during acoustic neuroma surgery. Br J Neurosurg 5:19–24, 1991.
43. Levine RA, Ojemann RG, Montgomery WM: Monitoring auditory evoked potentials during acoustic neuroma surgery: Insights into the mechanism of the hearing loss. Ann Otol Rhinol Laryngol 93:116–123, 1984.
44. Levine RA: Surgical monitoring applications of the brainstem auditory evoked response and electrocochleography. In Owen J, Donohoe C (eds): Clinical Atlas of Auditory Evoked Potentials. New York: Grune & Stratton, 1988, pp 103–106.
45. Levine RA: Monitoring auditory evoked potentials during cerebellopontine angle tumor surgery: Relative value of electrocochleography, brain-stem auditory evoked potentials, and cerebellopontine angle recordings. In Schramm J, Moelle AN (eds): Intraoperative Neurophysiologic Monitoring. Berlin: Springer-Verlag, 1991, pp 193–204.
46. Tatagiba M, Samii M, Matthies C, et al: The significance for postoperative hearing of preserving the labyrinth in acoustic neurinoma surgery. J Neurosurg 77:677–684, 1992.
47. McKennan KX: Endoscopy of the internal auditory canal during hearing conservation in acoustic neuroma surgery. Am J Otol 14:259, 1993.
48. Tatagita M, Matthies C, Samii M: Microendoscopy of the internal auditory canal in vestibular schwannoma surgery. Neurosurgery 38:737–740, 1996.
49. Valtonen JH, Poe DS, Heilman CD, et al: Endoscopically assisted prevention of cerebrospinal fluid leak in suboccipital acoustic neuroma surgery. Am J Otol 18:381–383, 1997.
50. Harner SG, Beatty CW, Ebersold MJ: Impact of cranioplasty on headache after acoustic neuroma removal. Neurosurgery 36:1097–1100, 1995.
51. Catalano PJ, Jacobowitz O, Post KD: Prevention of headache after retrosigmoid removal of acoustic tumors. Am J Otol 17:904–908, 1996.
52. Wazen J, Silverstein H, Norroll H, et al: Preoperative and postoperative growth rate in acoustic neuromas documented with CT scanning. Otolaryngol Head Neck Surg 93:151–155, 1985.
53. Klemink JL, Langman AW, Niparko JK, et al: Operative management of acoustic neuromas: The priority of neurologic function over complete resection. Otolaryngol Head Neck Surg 104:96–99, 1991.
54. Lownie SP, Drake CG: Radical intracapsular removal of acoustic neuroma: Long term follow-up review of 11 patients. J Neurosurg 74:422–425, 1991.
55. House JW, Brackmann DE: Facial nerve grading system. Otolaryngol Head Neck Surg 93:184–193, 1985.
56. Lalwani AK, Butt FY, Jackler RK, et al: Delayed onset of facial nerve dysfunction following acoustic neuroma surgery. Am J Otol 16:758–764, 1995.
57. Megerian CA, McKenna MJ, Ojemann RG: Delayed facial paralysis after acoustic neuroma surgery: Factors influencing recovery. Am J Otol 17:630–633, 1996.
58. Cheney ML, McKenna MJ, Megerian CA: Early temporalis muscle transposition for the management of facial paralysis. Laryngoscope 105:993–1000, 1995.
59. McKenna MJ, Halpin C, Ojemann RG, et al: Long-term hearing results in patients after surgical removal of acoustic tumors with hearing preservation. Am J Otol 13:134–136, 1992.
60. Gardner G, Robertson JH: Hearing preservation in unilateral acoustic neuroma surgery. Ann Otol Rhinol Laryngol 97:55–66, 1988.
61. Cohen NL: Retrosigmoid approach for acoustic tumor removal. Otolaryngol Clin North Am 25:295–310, 1992.
62. Compton JS, Bordi LT, Chesseman AD, et al: The small acoustic neuroma: A chance to preserve hearing. Acta Neurochir (Wien) 98:115–117, 1989.
63. Glasscock ME III, Hays JW, Monor LB, et al: Preservation of hearing in surgery for acoustic neuromas. J Neurosurg 78:872–870, 1993.
64. Neely JG: Is it possible to totally resect an acoustic tumor and conserve hearing? Otolaryngol Head Neck Surg 92:162–167, 1984.
65. Pensak ML, Tew JM Jr, Keith RW, et al: Management of the acoustic neuroma in an only hearing ear. Skull Base Surg 1:93–96, 1991.
66. Rosenberg RA, Cohen NL, Ransohoff J: Long term hearing preservation after acoustic neuroma surgery. Otolaryngol Head Neck Surg 97:270–274, 1987.
67. Samii M, Matthies C: Management of 1000 vestibular schwannomas (acoustic neuromas): Hearing function in 1000 tumor resections. Neurosurgery 40:248–262, 1997.

68. Shelton C, Hitselberger WE, House WF, et al: Hearing preservation after acoustic tumor removal: Long term results. Laryngoscope 100:115–119, 1990.

69. Slavit DH, Hamer SC, Harper CM Jr, et al: Auditory monitoring during acoustic neuroma removal. Arch Otolaryngol Head Neck Surg 117:1153–1157, 1991.

70. Umezu H, Aiba T, Tsuchida S, et al: Early and late postoperative hearing preservation in patients with acoustic neuromas. Neurosurgery 39:267–272, 1996.

71. Silverstein H, McDaniel A, Norrell H, Haber Kamp T: Hearing preservation after acoustic neuroma surgery with intraoperative direct eighth cranial nerve monitoring: A classification of results. Otolaryngol Head Neck Surg 95:285–291, 1986.

72. Whittaker CK, Luetje CM: Vestibular schwannomas. J Neurosurg 76:897–900, 1992.

73. Matthies C, Samii M: Direct brainstem recording of auditory evoked potentials during vestibular schwannomas resection: Nuclear BAEO recording. J Neurosurg 86:1057–1062, 1997.

74. Matthies C, Samii M: Management of vestibular schwannomas (acoustic neuromas): The value of neurophysiology for intraoperative monitoring of auditory function in 200 cases. Neurosurgery 40:459–468, 1997.

75. Post KD, Eisenberg MB, Catalano PS: Hearing preservation in vestibular schwannoma surgery: What factors influence outcome? J Neurosurg 83:191–196, 1994.

76. Thedinger BS, Whittaker CK, Luetje CM: Recurrent acoustic tumor after a suboccipital removal. Neurosurgery 29:681–687, 1991.

77. Weisman JL, Hirsch BE, Fukai MB, et al: The evolving MR appearance of structure in the internal auditory canal after removal of acoustic neuroma. AJNR Am J Neuroradiol 18:313–323, 1997.

78. Goel A, Sekhar LN, Langheinrich W, et al: Late course of preserved hearing and tinnitus after acoustic neurilemoma surgery. J Neurosurg 77:685–689, 1992.

# Translabyrinthine Approach to Vestibular Schwannomas

■ LARS POULSGAARD and SVEND ERIK BØRGESEN

V estibular schwannomas can be surgically accessed via a subtemporal, a translabyrinthine, or a suboccipital and retrosigmoid approach.[1, 2] The number of centers that has mastered all approaches has increased. The translabyrinthine approach was reintroduced about 35 years ago[3] and is successfully used by several otologic specialist centers.[4–6] Following developments in skull base surgery, neurosurgeons have become aware of the advantages of the translabyrinthine approach for vestibular schwannomas and for other skull base lesions.

## ADVANTAGES OF THE TRANSLABYRINTHINE APPROACH

The most obvious advantages of the translabyrinthine route are the direct approach it offers to the cerebellopontine angle and the fact that the cerebellum requires a minimum of retraction. The tumor is lifted away from the brain stem, avoiding pressure on the brain stem and cerebellum.

It has been stated that the usefulness of the translabyrinthine approach is limited to small tumors. In fact, no tumor is too large to be approached by the translabyrinthine route.[7–9] In large and giant tumors, it is a significant advantage to be able to go directly to the center of the tumor; after debulking the center of the tumor, the neoplasm collapses and is displaced toward the opening by the surrounding brain structure.

The procedure offers excellent exposure of the lateral end of the internal auditory meatus and allows identification of the facial nerve as it enters the fallopian canal. This identification ensures complete tumor removal from that area and the best chance to preserve the facial nerve.

We find it convenient that two surgeons may help each other in the removal of the tumor. As pointed out later, this approach offers two surgeons comfortable placement during a lengthy procedure.

## DISADVANTAGES OF THE TRANSLABYRINTHINE APPROACH

The procedure destroys the labyrinth and, as a consequence, hearing. This approach is not used if preservation of hearing is attempted. Only a limited number of patients with vestibular schwannomas have hearing worth preserving, however. If the tumor exceeds 2 cm in size, the chances of preserving hearing are known to be poor.[10]

If the patient has had active otitis media in the past, the approach involves crossing a potentially infected field, and alternative exposure should be considered. In the case of a mastoid cavity, a total obliteration with blind sac closure of the external auditory canal should be performed and healed before the translabyrinthine approach can be done. Finally, the procedure is generally more time-consuming than the suboccipital or middle fossa approach—a fact that must be considered if a limited duration of the operation is desirable.

## SURGICAL ANATOMY

The bone opening for the translabyrinthine approach is done in the mastoid part of the temporal bone (Fig. 73–1). The mastoid is filled with air cells, and the air cells are connected to the middle ear through the tympanic antrum. In the translabyrinthine approach, the bone is removed between the sigmoid sinus and the external ear canal. The sigmoid sinus is located in the sigmoid sulcus in the temporal bone. From the posterior aspect of the sigmoid sinus, emissary veins run through the mastoid foramen to subgaleal veins.[11–13]

Removing the air cells creates a space that is bounded posteriorly by the wall of the sigmoid sulcus, superiorly by the tegmen tympani, and anteriorly by the prominence of the lateral semicircular canal. Above the prominence of the lateral semicircular canal, the antrum communicates with the tympanic cavity. The facial canal runs close to the mastoid wall of the tympanic cavity. The genu of the facial canal is just inferior to the lateral semicircular canal, and it continues inferiorly to emerge below the skull base at the stylomastoid foramen (Fig. 73–2). The sigmoid sulcus meets the roof of the cavity at a sharp sinodural angle from which the superior petrosal sulcus runs anteriorly. When removing the bone in the sinodural angle, the superior petrosal sinus is exposed in a dural duplex.

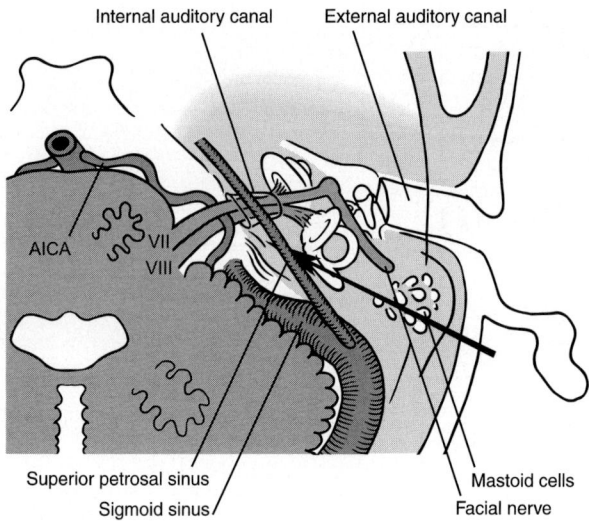

FIGURE 73–1 ■ Illustration of the approach to the cerebellopontine angle through the mastoid and labyrinth. The *arrow* indicates the surgical view after an extended mastoidectomy.

The lateral semicircular canal is an important landmark to the location of the entire labyrinth. After removing all three semicircular canals, the vestibule is open. The vestibule is the bone cavity that harbors the soft tissue part of the labyrinth-utricle and saccula. Through the aperture of the vestibular aqueduct runs the endolymphatic duct that connects the utricle to the endolymphatic sac. The internal auditory canal contains four separate nerves—two vestibular nerves, the facial nerve, and the cochlear nerve. Located laterally is the superior and inferior vestibular nerves separated at the fundus by a bony crest—the transverse crest. Anterior to the superior vestibular nerve, the facial nerve enters the fallopian canal. Laterally the facial nerve is separated from the superior vestibular nerve by a small vertical septum—the vertical crest, or *Bill's bar* (Fig. 73–3).

Most vestibular schwannomas arise from one of the vestibular nerves in the internal auditory canal. The facial nerve is often displaced in the internal auditory canal, and its location may vary. The nerve can always be identified laterally in the internal auditory canal.

After maximal translabyrinthine bone removal and opening of the dura, the cerebellopontine angle with its nerves and vessels is seen. Superiorly the exit of the fifth cranial nerve is seen on the pontine surface near the cerebellum. The exits of cranial nerves VI, VII, and VIII are located on a vertical line on the medulla oblongata near the crossing to the pons. The exit of the eighth nerve is just anterior and superior to the flocculus. The entry zone for the abducens nerve is anteriorly on the medulla oblongata. It runs in a superior direction anteriorly on the pons to enter the Dorello canal.

The blood vessels in the cerebellopontine angle display greater variability than do the nerves. The posterior-inferior cerebellar artery emerges from the vertebral artery. Loop formations of this artery are often seen to extend cranially to the level of the ninth and eighth nerves, and in these cases it may be seen using the translabyrinthine approach. The anterior-inferior cerebellar artery extends from the basilar artery, and in most cases it forms a loop that protrudes against or into the internal auditory canal. From the loop of the anterior-inferior cerebellar artery, the labyrinthine and the subarcuate artery extends.

## PREPARATION FOR SURGERY

A cephalosporin is given intravenously just before surgery and repeated every 3 hours. The patient is placed in a supine position on the operating table. The patient's head is turned toward the opposite side and maintained in position with a Sugita headframe. Excessive rotation of the

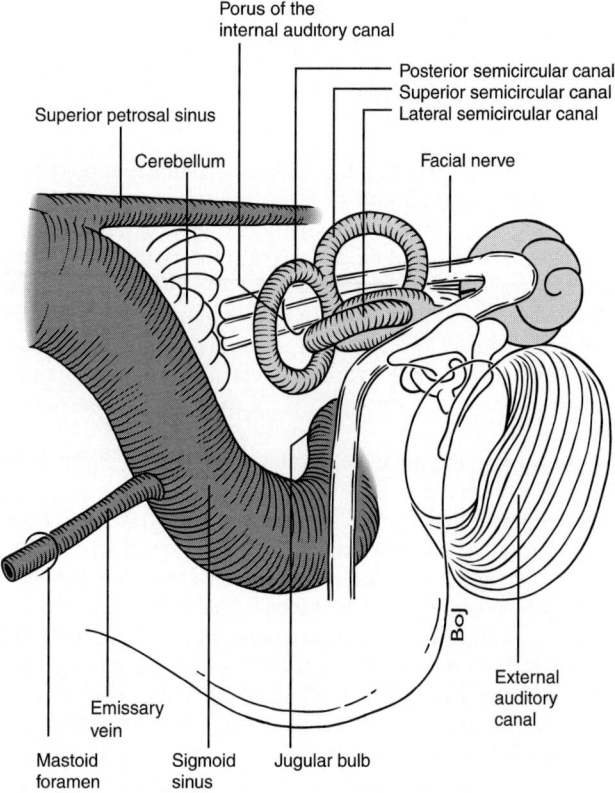

FIGURE 73–2 ■ The relationship between the labyrinth, the internal acoustic canal, the facial nerve, and the sigmoid sinus.

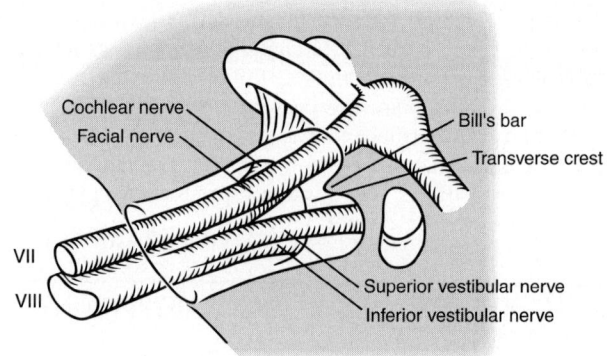

FIGURE 73–3 ■ The contents of the internal acoustic canal, which shows the relation of the facial nerve to "Bill's bar."

essary because even in large tumors, it is easy to access the cistern magna beneath the tumor, open the arachnoid, and allow cerebrospinal fluid (CSF) to drain. The incision is made using the cutting cautery to decrease the amount of bleeding from the skin. The incision starts at the upper edge of the helix, superior to the linea temporalis; it continues 4 to 5 cm posteriorly and turns inferiorly and ends near the tip of the mastoid process (Fig. 73–5).

The incision is made first only through the skin, and a large piece of muscle fascia and pericranium is harvested. The skin is elevated and turned anteriorly over the auricle, where it is covered with a piece of moist gauze and fixed with hooks attached to the Sugita headframe. The muscle fascia and pericranium are cut anteriorly just behind the external auditory canal up to the edge of the skin incision, which is then followed down to the mastoid process. The fascia and pericranium are used at the end of the operation for closure of the dural opening. Because of the size of the skin incision, it is not necessary to retract the skin at the superior, posterior, or inferior margin.

## Mastoidectomy

An extended mastoidectomy is performed with removal of bone over the sigmoid sinus and the middle cranial fossa (see Fig. 73–5). In cases with an anteriorly placed sigmoid sinus or in cases with large tumors, we also remove bone over the posterior cranial fossa behind the sigmoid sinus.[17, 18] The extended bone removal ensures good visualization of the entire surgical field. The power drill, driven by either an electric motor or an air turbine, is an essential tool in the translabyrinthine procedure. The cortical bone covering the mastoid region is removed by a large cutting drill. In cases with pronounced pneumatization, a large hole can be made quickly and safely. The anterior margin for cortical bone removal is just behind the external ear canal. The

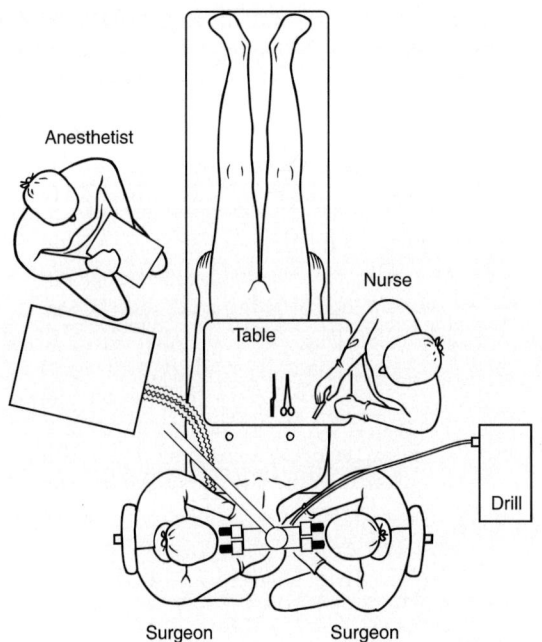

FIGURE 73–4 ■ Room arrangement for the translabyrinthine approach. Note the position of the two surgeons. Both have comfortable access to the microscope.

head should be avoided because it may cause venous obstruction in the neck. Decreased mobility of the neck in elderly patients may make sufficient rotation of the head difficult to achieve. This problem may be solved by lifting the ipsilateral shoulder with a pillow and by rotating the whole table.

Continuous electrophysiologic monitoring of facial nerve function is performed during the operation.[14–16] This monitoring has become an established procedure and is mandatory in our operations. To accomplish this, electrodes are placed in the frontal and in the oral orbicular muscles.

We use a ceiling-mounted operating microscope with the two surgeons sitting opposite each other on each side of the patient's head. This setup enables both surgeons a comfortable sitting position and a direct view in the microscope. The lead surgeon sits on the same side as the tumor. In left-sided tumors, the drill is placed between the two surgeons, and in right-sided tumors, the drill is placed between the scrub nurse and the surgeon on the right side (Fig. 73–4). The anesthesiologist is placed at the lower left side of the table at the level of the hip of the patient.

The surgical view of the cerebellopontine angle occurs along the posterior fossa dura. Posteriorly, it is limited by the sigmoid sinus and anteriorly by the horizontal part of the facial nerve. The operating microscope can be moved in all directions, and the table can be tilted in all directions. This capability ensures visualization of all surgical planes.

## SURGICAL PROCEDURE

Although some surgeons advocate routine cannulation of the lateral ventricle to relieve hydrocephalus or prevent surgically induced hydrocephalus, we do not find this nec-

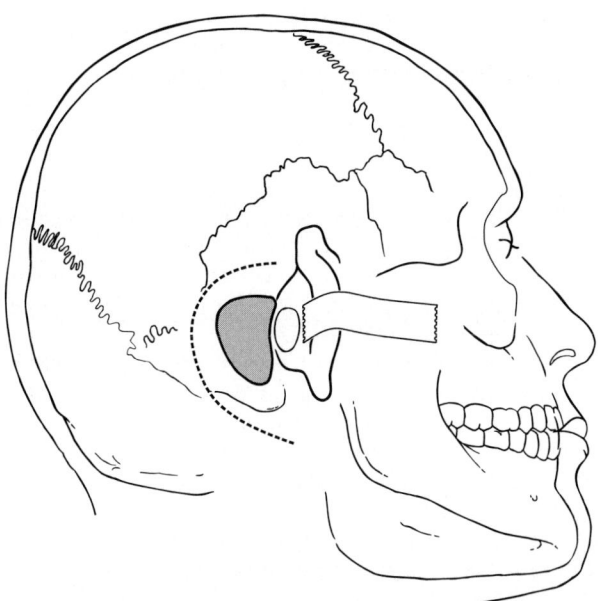

FIGURE 73–5 ■ Skin incision behind the right ear. The area planned for a mastoidectomy is indicated.

opening is gradually widened backward to the sigmoid sinus and upward to the dura in the middle cranial fossa. Removal of bone over the sigmoid sinus must be done carefully. If the cutting drill tears the sigmoid sinus, profuse bleeding ensues, requiring packing with Surgicel. Large emissary veins often drain into the posterior aspect of the sigmoid sinus. They can be identified through the bone as it is removed. The emissary veins must be controlled with bipolar coagulation and are filled with bone wax. As soon as the mastoid cortical bone has been removed and the sigmoid sinus and the middle fossa dura have been outlined, the operating microscope is used. With a diamond drill, the sigmoid sinus is skeletonized.

There are several methods to skeletonize the sigmoid sinus, including the eggshell method, total bone removal, and creation of *Bill's island of bone*. The aim of the eggshell method is to make the sigmoid sinus wall compressible without removing all bone. By continuous drilling with a large diamond drill and successive pressing of the bone with a dissector, the bony sinus wall becomes compressible because of the many microfractures in the *eggshell* bone. The preserved periosteum covering the sinus helps to avoid lesions in the sinus.

Total bone removal is initiated by carefully drilling away all the bone covering a small part of the sinus. Through this hole, the adjacent sinus wall can be depressed with a dissector, and the edge of the bone can safely be removed with the drill or a rongeur without touching the sinus wall. This method ensures an easily compressible sinus wall.

The method recommended by House and Hitselberger[19] is to leave a small island of bone (*Bill's island*) over the sigmoid sinus to protect the surface from the trauma of retraction. With a diamond drill, the bone around the outlined island is removed leaving a part of the sinus wall with an oval piece of bone. The sinus wall and the bony island can then be depressed, and the sinus wall that corresponds to the bony island is protected. We rarely use this method because of the risk of lesions in the sinus wall that may be produced by the sharp edge of the bony island. With blunt dissection, the adjacent dura in the middle and posterior cranial fossa is loosened, and the remaining bone may be removed by either rongeurs or drill.

## Labyrinthectomy

The facial nerve is an important landmark, and its position must be established early in the surgical dissection. After skeletonizing the middle fossa dura, the antrum is opened, and the compact bone of the labyrinth is visualized. We do not routinely remove the incus.

It is essential to open the antrum and to identify the lateral semicircular canal (Fig. 73–6). This canal is a main landmark, and once the position of this canal and antrum is known, the three-dimensional anatomy of the facial nerve is known. After identification of the facial nerve, the labyrinthectomy is performed. The bone in the sinodural angle is removed followed by opening along the superior petrosal sinus until the labyrinthine bone is encountered. The lateral semicircular canal is drilled away until the ampulla is reached anteriorly. Then the posterior and superior canals are identified and removed to their entrance in

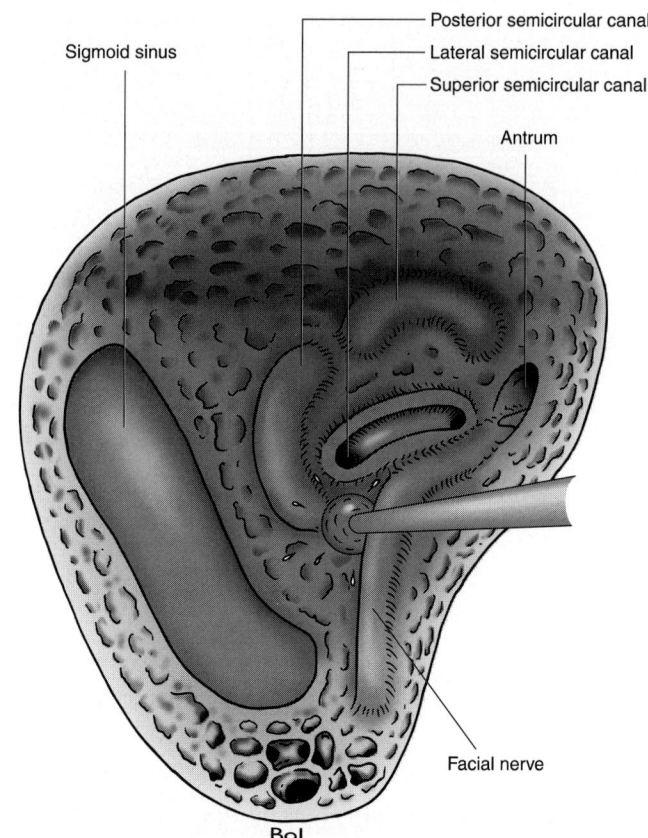

**FIGURE 73–6** ■ The facial nerve and the sigmoid sinus have been skeletonized. The lateral semicircular canal is opened.

the vestibule. After opening of the vestibule, the facial nerve is skeletonized from the genu inferiorly to near the stylomastoid foramen. It is not necessary to remove all the bone around the nerve. We always make a small window into the facial nerve canal near the second genu to ensure the position of the nerve and to ensure correct function of the facial nerve monitoring device. To avoid injury to the facial nerve, a thin, eggshell bone is left on the nerve. Only posteriorly, where access is needed to approach the cerebellopontine angle, is the nerve exposed.

After removal of all semicircular canals, the labyrinthectomy is completed, and the vestibule is opened. The endolymphatic duct must be excised from the endolymphatic sac on the posterior fossa dura. The vestibule is removed, and the cribriform area in the saccula marks the most lateral extent of the internal auditory meatus. In the center of the labyrinth, the subarcuate artery is located, and it is usually bleeding when it is opened by the drill.

## Internal Auditory Canal Dissection

The dura of the internal auditory canal is identified posteriorly, where it continues as dura of the posterior cranial fossa. The dura at the opening of the canal can be loosened from the bone with slightly bent sharp dissectors. The bone around the canal is gently removed with a diamond drill. A more than 180-degree arc of bone around the canal is removed. At this point, it is important to remove as much bone as possible on both sides below and above the meatus because this helps in accessing the superior and inferior borders of the tumor. Care is taken not to open the dura covering the nerves and tumor in the canal. If the dura is accidentally damaged, the facial nerve should be identified by stimulation.

All bone between the internal meatus and the jugular bulb is removed. The location of the jugular bulb varies extremely. When it is positioned low, all bone removal necessary for tumor removal can be performed without seeing the jugular bulb. In other cases, it is positioned high and occurs as a bluish spot in the bone after removing the ampulla of the posterior semicircular canal. The surgeon should always be aware of the blue color of the jugular bulb when drilling medial to the facial nerve and inferior to the posterior semicircular canal. All bone covering the jugular bulb must be removed in cases with a high-positioned jugular bulb, in which the bulb is an obstacle to proper bone removal from the inferior aspect of the internal acoustic meatus.

The technique of bone removal from the jugular bulb is the same as described for the sigmoid sinus. With the eggshell method, the bone can be thinned so much that the jugular bulb can be compressed and allow further removal of bone from the inferior part of the porus. Bone is removed until the cochlear aqueduct is identified. The cochlear aqueduct enters the posterior fossa directly inferior to the midportion of the internal auditory canal above the jugular bulb. It is an important landmark because it identifies the location of the cranial nerves IX, X, and XI in the neural compartment of the jugular foramen. Bone dissection should be confined to the area superior to the cochlear aqueduct to avoid injury to these nerves. After removal of bone on the inferior part of the internal auditory canal, the dissection is carried out on the superior and anterior parts.

The facial nerve often underlies the dura along the anterior-superior aspect of the internal auditory canal, and extreme care must be taken not to allow the bur to slip into the canal. The facial nerve is especially vulnerable at this point. The lateral end of the internal auditory canal is divided by the transverse crest in an inferior and a superior compartment (Fig. 73–7). The bone around the inferior compartment can be drilled away to the most lateral extent of the canal without risk of facial nerve injury. In the superior compartment, bone removal allows identification of a bar of bone (Bill's bar), which separates the superior vestibular nerve from the facial nerve. The bone is removed at the porus and the medial part of the internal auditory canal first, and the more difficult lateral part is left until last when most of the bone removal has been completed.

All bone between the middle fossa dura and the internal auditory canal must be removed. With the visualization of the most lateral end of the internal auditory canal, the bone work is completed. Until this point, all of the dissection has been extradural and the morbidity of the approach consequently low.

## Dural Opening

The dural incision is started superiorly in the sinodural angle near the sigmoid sinus continuing down to the porus

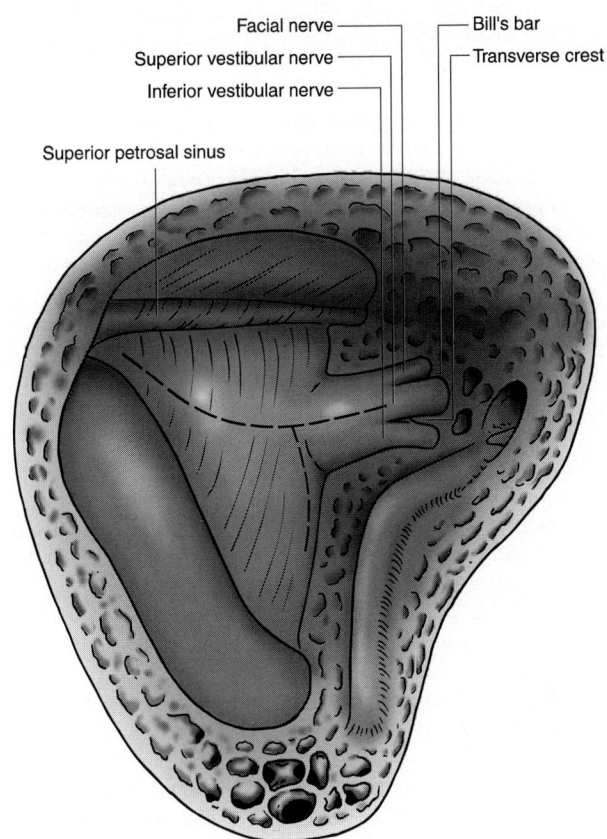

FIGURE 73–7 ■ The mastoidectomy has been completed. The internal auditory canal is opened and allows the facial nerve to be identified. The *broken lines* indicate the dural incisions.

(see Fig. 73–7). Care is taken to avoid vessels on the surface of the tumor. Posteriorly the petrosal vein lies just beneath the dura. This vein originates in the cerebellum and drains into the superior petrosal sinus near the level of the internal auditory canal. If the dura is pulled laterally with a small hook, the space between the cerebellum and the dura is enlarged, and injury to the vessels may be avoided. At the porus, a small incision is made on both sides of the porus. Around the porus, the dura often forms a distinct constriction ring that usually adheres to the surface of the tumor, and there are small vessels going from the dura to the tumor. The dural ring must be divided, and a further incision is made over the dura in the meatus. In the meatus, the dura is often extremely thin, and sometimes it is opened while removing the bone around the meatus. The small vessels in the thickened dura at the porus can be coagulated with bipolar coagulation. Hitching stitches are placed on the dural flap as it is retracted posteriorly. Cottonoids are advanced into the plane between the tumor and cerebellum. It is important to develop this plane accurately because doing so separates the major vessels of the cerebellopontine angle from the tumor. In cases in which the sigmoid sinus is prominent and blocking the view of the dural opening or the border between the tumor and the cerebellum, a retractor, attached to the Sugita frame, may be applied on the sinus.

## Tumor Removal

After opening the dura, the posterior part of the tumor is exposed. Rarely the facial nerve may lie on the posterior surface of the tumor and this surface must be carefully inspected for nerve bundles. In large tumors, it is essential to begin tumor removal with intracapsular debulking to reduce tumor size and subsequently develop the extracapsular dissection planes. In small tumors, the surgeon can identify readily the inferior and superior extracapsular dissection planes of the tumor. An ultrasonic aspirator is useful for debulking and removing intracapsular tumor.

### Identification of the Facial Nerve in the Fundus of the Internal Auditory Canal

In about 15% of vestibular schwannomas, the fundus of the internal auditory canal is empty, and all four nerves are visible and easy recognizable. In these cases, bone work in the internal auditory canal does not need to be as extensive as described. The identification of the vertical crest (Bill's bar) is not necessary. Exact determination of the facial nerve is done with stimulation.

In the remaining cases, the fundus of the internal auditory canal is filled up with tumor, and identification of the facial nerve is more difficult. During bone removal, the medial part of the fallopian canal is opened, which uncovers a labyrinthine segment of the facial nerve. Bill's bar separates the facial nerve anteriorly from the superior vestibular nerve. A fine hook is inserted lateral to Bill's bar and gently placed beneath the superior vestibular nerve and Bill's bar. The superior vestibular nerve can then be pulled out from its canal. Likewise the two nerves inferior to the transverse crest (the inferior vestibular nerve and the cochlear nerve) are pulled out from their canals along with the tumor (Fig. 73–8). Positive identification of the facial nerve at the lateral end of the internal auditory canal is one of the principal advantages of the translabyrinthine approach.

### Freeing the Tumor from the Facial Nerve in the Internal Canal

Arachnoid sheath completely surrounds the tumor, nerves, and vessels in the meatus, and the arachnoid strands that attach the facial nerve to the tumor must be divided. The meatal part of the tumor is gently retracted backward. Small hooks or fine microscissors are used to free the facial nerve from the arachnoid fibers that bind the nerve to the tumor. Because cutting of the arachnoid occurs along the facial nerve, it is important to have identified the inferior and the superior edges of the nerve accurately. Usually, it is relatively easy to develop the dissection plane between the facial nerve and the tumor in the internal auditory canal, but difficulties often arise at the porus. Around the entire circumference of the porus, dural adhesions to the tumor make dissection of the facial nerve from the tumor difficult. The exact position of the facial nerve in the porus must be established before the adhesions between dura and the tumor are removed. Inferiorly, freeing of the tumor from the porus is simpler because damage to the cochlear nerve is insignificant. Superiorly the facial nerve may be

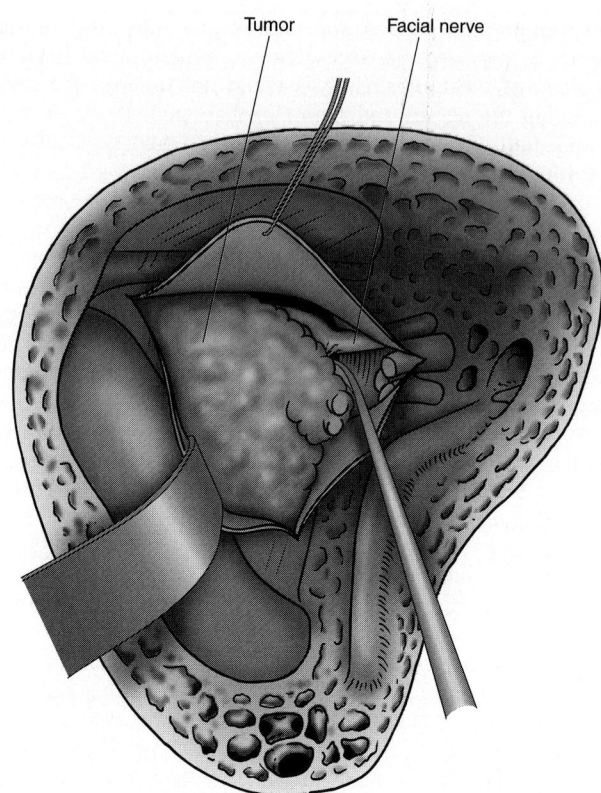

**FIGURE 73–8** ■ After dural opening, the tumor can be separated from the facial nerve in the internal auditory canal. The vestibular nerves and the cochlear nerve are divided lateral in the internal auditory canal.

at risk. At times, it is difficult to isolate the facial nerve at the porus. In these cases, it is wise to carry out a partial tumor removal, then identify the facial nerve medially and follow the nerve laterally until the porus is reached. During this work, the surgeon must be careful not to push the tumor forward or medially because stretching the facial nerve, especially at the porus level, can damage the nerve. Early mobilization of the tumor from the internal auditory canal has the advantage that the landmarks are well defined and are not obscured with blood, as tends to happen later in the surgical dissection.

### Reducing Tumor Size

In large tumors, there is inadequate space in the cerebellopontine angle to mobilize the tumor in the superior, inferior, and lateral directions, which is necessary to identify and free the facial nerve. In these cases, the posterior surface of the tumor capsule is incised in a superior-inferior direction, and an intracapsular removal is gently performed with the ultrasonic aspirator.

### Isolation of the Tumor

With tumors of all sizes, it is important to work in the proper cleavage plane between the tumor and the arachnoid. Tumor growth pushes the arachnoid membrane of the pontocerebellar cistern and causes it to double in the distal part of the internal auditory canal and in the cerebellopontine angle. In large tumors, there is duplication of the cerebellar cistern and the cerebellomedullary cistern, causing formation of the third and fourth arachnoid layers. Through these layers, the cranial nerves IX, X, and XI run at the inferior aspect of the tumor. The petrosal veins run through the layers of cisterna cerebelli at the superior-posterior aspect of the tumor.

## Tumor Removal

The principle for removal of large tumors is intracapsular gutting to reduce tumor bulk followed by mobilization and removal of the adjacent capsule segment. The point of attack must be changed progressively, and as the limits of mobilization are reached at one point, the surgeon moves to another. Packing the space between the tumor and the brain with cottonoids, then leaving them while the dissection is extended to another part is unwise because cottonoids may become stuck with fibrin to the brain, and redeveloping the plane is difficult. Once the interior part of the tumor has been extensively removed, the capsule is displaced into the tumor space. Opening of the arachnoid layers and dissecting within these layers facilitates the isolation of the tumor. Semisharp dissectors and sometimes small cottonoids are used in the proper dissection plane to separate the tumor from the surrounding structures. The dissection is made from four directions: inferior, superior, medial, and lateral.

### INFERIOR DISSECTION

Dissection at the inferior aspect of the tumor usually leads into the large cerebellomedullary cistern, which allows CSF to escape. This step improves the operative condition, and if any difficulties are encountered because of lack of room in the posterior fossa, draining the cerebellomedullary cistern as soon as possible is valuable.

On the inferior aspect of the tumor, it is possible to localize the cranial nerves IX and X, which are best identified near the jugular foramen medial to the jugular bulb. These nerves must be freed from the tumor and isolated. Sometimes, they are not well seen because they tend to lie around the corner of the opening. During manipulation of cranial nerves IX and X, changes in the pulse rate may occur. Stopping the manipulation restores the pulse rate.

The posterior-inferior cerebellar artery is at the inferior aspect of the tumor and must be carefully separated from the tumor capsule and preserved. The labyrinthine artery supplies branches to the facial nerve and should be preserved. Dissection inferior to the tumor continues until the brain stem is reached and is completed with removal of that portion of the capsule.

### SUPERIOR DISSECTION

The facial nerve is normally located anteriorly to the tumor, but it is not unusual to find the facial nerve over the top of the tumor. If the precise location of the facial nerve is unknown, when starting the dissection at the superior aspect of the tumor, it is imperative to inspect the tumor surface carefully and to use the nerve stimulator to identify the nerve and avoid injury.

The petrosal vein and cranial nerve V are located in the superior aspect of the tumor. These structures must be identified and carefully separated from the tumor. The trigeminal nerve is a broad white structure running in the inferior-posterior direction. Near the brain, the nerve lies in close contact to the tumor capsule but is usually easy to separate from the tumor. Handling the nerve must be avoided if recovery of sensory loss in the face is to be achieved. The petrosal vein and vein branches are stretched over the tumor and enter the superior petrosal sinus. To stay in the proper cleavage, it is better to separate the vein from the tumor rather than coagulate the vessels. The coagulation seals the layers together and makes later separation difficult. The superior dissection is continued until the pons is reached and the attachment of the trigeminal nerve to the brain stem is visualized.

### MEDIAL DISSECTION

The medial dissection is the most difficult part of the tumor removal because of the risk of damaging the facial nerve or the pons. After the posterior part of the tumor is debulked, a small portion of tumor capsule is left attached to the cerebellum and the pons. The tumor capsule is lifted, and the proper cleavage plane is identified. In large tumors, the posterior pole may protrude far under the cerebellum and deep into the brain stem. This protrusion requires maximal rotation of the operating table toward the surgeon to visualize the dissection plane. The vessels are dissected away, and the branches that extend into the capsule are coagulated and divided. The capsule and tumor remnant are pushed anteriorly, and arachnoid and veins are dissected from the capsule. When the brain stem has been reached from all directions and tumor gradually has been removed, the remaining small portion of tumor covers a part of the brain stem, facial nerve, and cochlear nerve.

### ANTERIOR DISSECTION AND FINAL TUMOR REMOVAL

In small tumors, the main approach is from the anterior aspect. In these cases, the facial nerve can easily be located at the brain stem, and the precise position of the nerve is easy to ascertain early. Separating the tumor from the facial nerve is done from the porus and against the brain stem.

In large tumors, the dissection of the facial nerve is done in an anterior and posterior direction. The small portion of tumor that covers the facial nerve from the brain stem to the porus is the most difficult to remove (Fig. 73–9). The anterior part of the tumor capsule usually contains a number of small vessels from arteries and vein, and dissection can easily provoke bleeding. Veins are often present around the facial nerve's entry zone from the brain stem. Coagulation of the bleeding vessels is dangerous and must be precise to avoid facial nerve injury.

For several reasons, the dissection on the anterior aspect of the tumor is troublesome and time-consuming:

1. The facial nerve is often stretched and spread out over the largest prominence of the tumor, which sometimes makes the nerve nearly invisible.
2. The facial nerve is not protected by an epineurium and is vulnerable to injury.

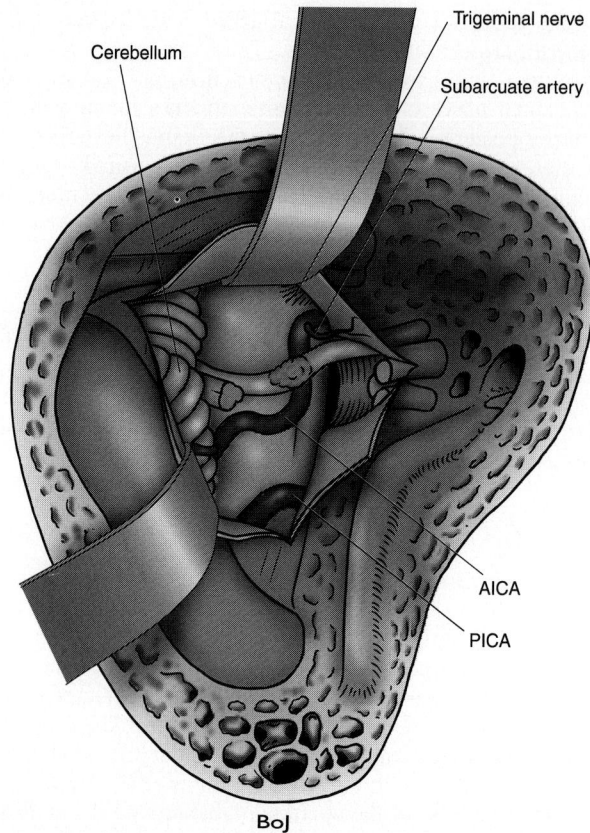

Cerebellum
Trigeminal nerve
Subarcuate artery
AICA
PICA
BoJ

**FIGURE 73–9** ■ The tumor has been removed. A small tumor remnant is left on the facial nerve.

3. At the porus, the facial nerve is often embedded in the tumor capsule, causing problems when loosening the tumor.

Care must be taken not to leave fragments of tumor on the nerve because the dissection continues inside the tumor and obscures the location of the nerve, which may be lost.

Once the facial nerve has been separated, the last bit of tumor is removed from the brain stem. The adhesions between the tumor and the brain stem are not usually dense, but if they are, clearing the brain stem of tumor demands particularly careful dissection. Once the tumor has been removed, the field is inspected, and the facial nerve is examined with the stimulator. If a signal can be obtained by stimulating the nerve at the brain stem, it is likely that the patient will have normal facial nerve function. The wound is then irrigated with saline, and all bleeding points are controlled. Absolute hemostasis is required and may take some time.

## Facial Nerve Repair

If the nerve has been divided during operation, one may get an acceptable level of function by anastomosing the nerve ends, provided that the central stump can be found and isolated. If the nerve ends can reach each other, they are anastomosed end-to-end and fixed with a suture and Tisseel.[20–22] If a gap exists, a great auricular nerve or sural nerve graft is used to bridge the gap between the nerve ends.

## Closure

An essential part of the wound closure involves preventing rhinorrhea. CSF may escape through the middle ear and the eustachian tube. The middle ear is packed with a small piece of muscle and Tisseel. The facial layer, harvested at the beginning of the operation, is packed to cover the opening into the tympanic cavity anteriorly and the dural opening posteriorly. The fascia is fixed with Tisseel. The mastoid cavity is filled with a large piece of adipose tissue taken from the abdomen. The postauricular skin incision is closed in two layers with absorbable subcutaneous suture and nylon suture in the skin. We do not use a subgaleal drain but make a solid compression of the wound by gauze supported by a solid elastic bandage.

## POSTOPERATIVE MANAGEMENT AND COMPLICATIONS

Surgery on large tumors in posterior fossa is not without risks.[23–25] Large tumors sometimes adhere strongly to the surface of the cerebellum and the brain stem. Dissection of the tumor from the surroundings may elicit cerebellar edema and infarction. Veins can often be coagulated, but sometimes packing is necessary, especially of the bulb of the sigmoid sinus and the petrosal vein. Hematomas or reactive edema of the cerebellum may necessitate immediate response. Close observation of the patient is necessary in the initial postoperative phase by trained nurses in the intensive care unit. Acute hydrocephalus resulting from obstruction of CSF drainage from the ventricles may occur because of edema or hematoma at the level of the fourth ventricle.

## Hematoma

Postoperative hematoma after a translabyrinthine approach is a rarity. Even when excellent hemostasis appears to have been achieved, however, postoperative hemorrhage may still occur[26] and seems most likely among elderly patients and patients with large tumors. The hematoma is most likely to occur shortly after the operation but may be seen 1 week after surgery.

The clinical course is often insidious. If the patient does not regain consciousness after surgery or if the patient after a period with normal sensorium develops decreasing consciousness, a hematoma must be suspected. If the symptoms develop quickly, it may be necessary to open the wound immediately. If the symptoms develop more slowly, a CT scan can confirm the diagnosis. Smaller hematomas that just fill up the tumor cavity and do not compress the brain stem further may be left for gradual resorption.

## Cerebellar Edema

Rarely, cerebellar edema may develop during surgery, unprovoked and early in the procedure. This complication may hinder further attempts of tumor removal. In such cases, it is necessary to keep the patient on moderate hyperventilation and only slowly take the patient off the respirator. Also, patients who do not wake up or who deteriorate after surgery in whom CT excludes significant hematoma may benefit from moderate hyperventilation.

## Acute Hydrocephalus

An acute dilatation of the cerebral ventricles may be observed either immediately postoperatively or in the following days. Failure to wake up or decreasing consciousness should rouse the suspicion, and a CT scan should be obtained. If the complication is diagnosed soon after surgery, ventricular drainage is undertaken. If the complication arises slowly and later after surgery, a permanent CSF shunt may be considered.

## Facial Paralysis

Facial paralysis is often difficult to detect immediately postoperatively, when full wakefulness and cooperation are absent and—for unknown reason—eye closure may be present. If the face is paralyzed, eye care is of great importance. In the first days after surgery, the eye is covered with a protective shield and viscous eye drops are used. Shortly thereafter, a tarsorrhaphy is performed. The patient is warned to protect the eye and to wear protective spectacles. An ophthalmologist should be consulted.

Even though the nerve seems anatomically intact at the end of the operation, some patients exhibit postoperative facial paralysis. These patients still have a good chance for some function of the facial nerve. At least 6 months of observation should be allowed before any further remedy is considered. If permanent facial paralysis exists, a faciohypoglossal anastomosis is carried out with a delay of about 1 year.[27]

## Cerebrospinal Fluid Leakage

CSF leakage is the most common complication after vestibular schwannoma surgery,[28] and it is seen in 5% to 15% of the cases. The leakage may occur either through the skin at the wound site or via the nose. Rhinorrhea is much more common than leakage through the wound. The diagnosis of postoperative CSF rhinorrhea is often obvious within a few days of operation, but its recognition may be delayed. Some patients report only a sensation of postnasal dripping or a salty taste in the mouth. In these cases, the diagnosis may be subtle. The patient should be tested in a head-down position for watery escape from the nose before discharge.

When rhinorrhea is diagnosed, a lumbar drain is inserted for 3 to 5 days; however, the success with CSF drainage is not as high as in the wound leakage, probably because the defect is located in the bone, which is not as easily overgrown as a defect in soft tissue. If the lumbar drainage fails to close the defect, reoperation and resealing the communication to the middle ear with muscle graft or bone wax in the communicating air cells is necessary.

CSF escape through the postauricular wound may be prevented by meticulous closure of the wound followed by a tight head bandage. If wound leakage occurs, spinal drainage is often sufficient to solve the problem, and reoperation is rarely necessary.

## Meningitis

Because the translabyrinthine approach is time-consuming and involves opening of an air-filled cavity, meningitis is among the more common complications, occurring in 5% to 10% of cases. The peak incidence is seen from the third to the fifth postoperative day. Delayed meningitis is often caused by a nondiagnosed otorhinorrhea. Early recognition of meningitis with demonstration of high polymorphonuclear cell count in CSF usually ensures rapid resolution.

A high or persistent fever combined with severe headache or signs of altered mental status is likely to be caused by meningitis. Because postoperative fever and headache are common after the translabyrinthine procedure, the clinician should have a low threshold for performing a lumbar puncture when suspicion of meningitis arises.

A large proportion of postoperative meningitis after vestibular schwannoma surgery is aseptic in nature.[29] It is not always clear from the CSF findings whether or not an infection is present. If there is any doubt, the patient should be treated with intravenous antibiotics.

## CONCLUSIONS

The results from translabyrinthine and retrosigmoid approaches are comparable, with less than 2% mortality, 97% total removal, anatomic preservation of facial nerve in 90% to 95%, and a functioning facial nerve in greater than 70% 1 year after surgery.[4, 30–32] Except for hearing preservation, the published results do not favor one method over the other, and preference of one method should be based mostly on personal experience.

No comparison exists regarding the clinical outcome of the two approaches in vestibular schwannomas larger than 3.5 cm. In such cases, hearing preservation is seldom an issue. The standard retrosigmoid approach, as used in most neurosurgical departments for other pathologies in the cerebellopontine angle, does not, in our opinion, offer the same control of the tumor surfaces, especially the relation to the brain stem, as that achieved by a large, translabyrinthine exposure.

### ACKNOWLEDGMENT

*We are indebted to Bo Jespersen, M.D., who provided all illustrations for this chapter.*

# REFERENCES

1. Helms J: Indications for the suboccipital, translabyrinthine, and transtemporal approaches in acoustic neuroma surgery. In Tos M, Thomsen J (eds): Proceedings of the First International Conference on Acoustic Neuroma. Amsterdam: Kugler, 1992, pp 501–502.
2. Jackler RK, Pitts LH: Selection of surgical approach to acoustic neuroma. Otolaryngol Clin North Am 25:361–387, 1992.
3. House WF (ed): Monograph. Transtemporal Microsurgical Removal of Acoustic Neuromas. Arch Otolaryngol Head Neck Surg 80:597–756, 1964.
4. Sterkers JM, Corlieu C, Sterkers O: Acoustic neuroma surgery (1300 cases), the translabyrinthine method. In Tos M, Thomsen J (eds): Acoustic Neuroma. Amsterdam: Kugler, 1992, pp 377–378.
5. Tos M, Thomsen J, Harmsen A: Results of translabyrinthine removal of 300 acoustic neuromas related to tumour size. Acta Otolaryngol Suppl (Stockh) 452:38–51, 1988.
6. King TT, Morrison AW: Translabyrinthine and transtentorial removal of acoustic tumours: Results of 150 cases. J Neurosurg 52:210–216, 1980.
7. Tos M, Thomsen J: The translabyrinthine approach for the removal of large acoustic neuromas. Arch Otorhinolaryngol 246:292–296, 1989.
8. Giannotta SL: Translabyrinthine approach for removal of medium and large tumors of the cerebellopontine angle. Clin Neurosurg 38:589–602, 1982.
9. Briggs RJ, Luxford WM, Atkins JS Jr, Hitselberger WE: Translabyrinthine removal of large acoustic neuromas. Neurosurgery 34:785–790, 1994.
10. Sanna M, Zini C, Gamoletti R, et al: Hearing preservation: A critical review of the literature. In Tos M, Thomsen J (eds): Proceedings of the First International Conference on Acoustic Neuroma. Amsterdam: Kugler, 1992, pp 631–638.
11. Rhoton AL Jr: Microsurgical anatomy of the brainstem surface facing an acoustic neuroma. Surg Neurol 25:326–339, 1986.
12. Rhoton AL Jr, Tedeschi H: Microsurgical anatomy of acoustic neuroma. Otolaryngol Clin North Am 25:257–294, 1992.
13. Anson BJ, Donaldson JA: Surgical Anatomy of the Temporal Bone and Ear, 2nd ed. Philadelphia: WB Saunders, 1973.
14. Hammerschlag PE, Cohen NL: Intraoperative monitoring of the facial nerve in acoustic cerebellopontine angle surgery. Otolaryngol Head Neck Surg 103:681–684, 1990.
15. Syms CA 3rd, House JR 3rd, Luxford WM, Brackmann DE: Preoperative electroneuronography and facial nerve outcome in acoustic neuroma surgery. Am J Otol 18:401–403, 1997.
16. Harner SG, Daube JR, Beatty CW, Ebersold MJ: Intraoperative monitoring of the facial nerve. Laryngoscope 98:209–212, 1988.
17. Brackmann DE, Green JD: Translabyrinthine approach for acoustic tumor removal. Otolaryngol Clin North Am 25:311–329, 1992.
18. Tos M, Thomsen J (eds): Translabyrinthine Acoustic Neuroma Surgery: A Surgical Manual. Stuttgart: Georg Thieme, 1991.
19. House WF, Hitselberger WE: Translabyrinthine approach. In House WF, Leutje CM (eds): Acoustic Tumors. Baltimore: University Park Press, 1979, pp 43–87.
20. Barrs DM, Brackmann DE, Hitzelberger WE: Facial nerve anastomosis in the cerebellopontine angle: A review of 24 cases. Am J Otol 5:269–272, 1984.
21. Fisch U, Dobie RA, Gmür A, Felix H: Intracranial facial nerve anastomosis. Am J Otol 8:23–29, 1987.
22. Luetje CM, Whittaker CK: The benefits of VII-XII neuroanastomosis in acoustic tumor surgery. Laryngoscope 101:1273–1275, 1991.
23. Benecke JE: Complications of acoustic tumor surgery and their management. Semin Hearing 10:341–345, 1989.
24. Sterkers JM: Life-threatening complications and severe neurologic sequelae in surgery of acoustic neurinoma. Ann Otolaryngol Chir Cervicofac 106:245–250, 1989.
25. Dawes JDK, Welch AR: Complications of acoustic neuroma surgery. Adv Otorhinolaryngol 34:156–159, 1984.
26. House WF, Hitselberger WE: Fatalities in acoustic tumor surgery. In House WF, Leutje CM (eds): Acoustic Tumors. Baltimore: University Park Press, 1979, pp 235–264.
27. Ebersold MJ, Quast LM: Long-term results of spinal accessory nerve–facial nerve anatomosis. J Neurosurg 77:51–54, 1992.
28. Hardy DG, Moffat DA: The management of cerebrospinal fluid leakage following acoustic neuroma surgery. In Tos M, Thomsen J (eds): Proceedings of the First International Conference on Acoustic Neuroma. Amsterdam: Kugler, 1992, pp 735–738.
29. Ross D, Rosegay H, Pons V: Differentiation of aseptic and bacterial meningitis in postoperative neurosurgical patients. J Neurosurg 69:669–674, 1988.
30. Ebersold MJ, Harner SG, Beatty CW, et al: Current results of the retrosigmoid approach to acoustic neurinoma. J Neurosurg 76:901–909, 1992.
31. Samii M, Matthies C: Management of 1000 vestibular schwannomas (acoustic neuromas): Surgical management and results with an emphasis on complications and how to avoid them. Neurosurgery 40:11–21, 1997.
32. Thomsen J, Tos M, Børgesen SE, Møller H: Surgical results after removal of 504 acoustic neuromas. In Tos M, Thomsen J (eds): Proceedings of the First International Conference on Acoustic Neuroma. Amsterdam: Kugler, 1992, pp 331–335.

# Vestibular Nerve Section in the Management of Intractable Vertigo

■ SETH I. ROSENBERG and HERBERT SILVERSTEIN

When medical management of a patient with Ménière's disease fails to control episodic vertigo and hearing is better than 80 db pure tone average and 20% speech discrimination, posterior fossa vestibular neurectomy has been the authors' procedure of choice since 1978.[1] Complications have been minor, and facial paralysis, meningitis, or death has not occurred in series by the authors.[1–7] In numerous studies, it has been demonstrated that vertiginous attacks have been cured or improved in greater than 90% of the authors' patients with preservation of hearing in most cases.[1–7] A review of the literature suggests that increasing emphasis is being placed on hearing preservation in surgery for vertigo and that more neuro-otologic surgeons are using the vestibular nerve section through the posterior fossa as their procedure of choice to cure vertigo caused by inner ear disease.[8] A survey of the American Otologic Society and the American Neurotologic Society in 1990 indicated that almost 3000 vestibular nerve sections had been performed in the United States, and 95% of these were done through the posterior fossa by retrolabyrinthine, retrosigmoid, or combined approaches.[5] In this series, representing the experience of 59 surgeons, the cure rate for vertigo exceeded 90%, as did the reported patient satisfaction rate.[5]

The modern trend toward interdisciplinary surgical approaches frequently combines the talents of both neurosurgeon and neuro-otologist during cranial nerve operations. The neurosurgeon's role in vestibular neurectomy may vary from primary surgeon to operative assistant, but in either event, the neurosurgeon must have a clear understanding of the disease process involving the vestibular system as well as of treatment options and surgical technique. The surgical anatomy and techniques involved in vestibular nerve section are also applicable to most posterior skull base operations.

## HISTORICAL PERSPECTIVE

Frazier[9] was the first to perform an eighth cranial nerve section through the posterior fossa to relieve the symptoms of *aural vertigo* in a patient with Ménière's disease in 1904. After 1924, when Dandy[10, 11] began his surgical series, the eighth nerve section received more widespread attention. Anatomic dissections of the eighth nerve by McKenzie[12, 13] in 1930 permitted him to be the first to section the vestibular nerve selectively, preserving the cochlear nerve in 117 patients. In 1932, Dandy began to perform the selective vestibular nerve section for a variety of balance disorders. His personal series of 624 procedures is still the largest in the world literature.[14] These procedures were performed without the benefit of microsurgical techniques and instrumentation. One half of Dandy's patients underwent a total eighth nerve section, and approximately 10% experienced a permanent facial paralysis. Although the procedure boasted excellent control of vertigo, it was not widely accepted because of the magnitude of these complications.

After Dandy's death in 1946, the vestibular nerve section fell into disuse until 1961, when House described a neurosurgical extradural approach to the internal auditory canal through the middle fossa.[15] Via this approach, the superior vestibular nerve could be exposed and sectioned. Because of the poor control of vertigo with this procedure, Fisch[16, 17] and Glasscock[18, 19] modified it to include sectioning of the inferior vestibular nerve and excision of Scarpa's ganglion. This modification yielded excellent control of vertigo with preservation of hearing in many cases. Although the middle fossa vestibular nerve section was performed frequently by Fisch[16, 17] and Garcia-Ibanez,[20] it never achieved widespread popularity in Europe or the United States. For many otologists, the middle fossa vestibular nerve section was formidable, and anatomic landmarks were difficult to determine reliably. The exposure was difficult and fraught with complications, including injury to the facial nerve, the cochlea, or the labyrinth. Generally, patients older than 60 years of age were not candidates because of the difficulty in elevating the thin dura from the skull and the risk of postoperative hematoma.

In 1972, Hitselberger and Pulec[21] described the retrolabyrinthine approach for section of the trigeminal nerve in the posterior fossa. The procedure was further modified by Brackmann and Hitselberger[22] in 1978 to allow for various posterior fossa operations. In 1978, during the removal of a glossopharyngeal neurilemmoma through the posterior fossa, the senior author (H.S.) noted the close proximity of the eighth nerve complex to the dural opening.[1] More importantly, he noted a well-delineated cleavage plane between the vestibular and cochlear constituents of the nerve. Gross anatomic and microscopic laboratory studies have confirmed that the vestibular nerve section can be performed routinely through the posterior fossa. The retrolabyrinthine exposure offered excellent exposure to the cerebellopontine angle with minimal cerebellar retraction, permitting vestibular nerve section within the posterior fossa. Since its introduction, posterior fossa vestibular nerve section, including the retrolabyrinthine approach and its subsequent modifications, the retrosigmoid–internal auditory canal approach and the combined retrolabyrinthine-retrosigmoid approach, has become the most popular means of selective vestibular nerve section.[5] Today, this exposure is widely used for vestibular nerve section as well as for the removal of acoustic neuromas in which hearing preservation is the goal. Many skilled otologists and neurosurgeons continue to perform retrolabyrinthine or middle fossa vestibular nerve sections with results quite similar to those achieved by the combined approach.[5] As endoscopic techniques and equipment improve, the possibility of endoscopic posterior fossa vestibular nerve section is a possibility. In contrast to the anecdotal results reported in earlier days of vestibular nerve sections, results today are objectively documented and established so that careful postoperative evaluation and comparisons are possible.[24, 25]

## DIFFERENTIAL DIAGNOSIS OF VESTIBULAR DISORDERS

Rarely is the neurosurgeon the initial consultant for the patient experiencing dizziness, but it is important for the neurosurgeon to be able to establish a correct diagnosis and have an understanding of vestibular disorders. The cause of the vertigo must be determined before any treatment is undertaken. The differentiation between peripheral and central vertigo is the first step in arriving at a diagnosis. Peripheral vertigo arises from the inner ear or vestibular nerve, whereas the origin of central vertigo is the brain stem or cerebellum. History and physical examination, combined with audiovestibular testing and diagnostic imaging, results in an accurate diagnosis.

Peripheral vertigo is characterized by an intense subjective sensation of spinning, accompanied by nystagmus. The vertigo is frequently induced by positional changes, and the vertigo and nystagmus rarely persist for 30 seconds, even when position is maintained. If the provocative moves are repeated, the signs and symptoms progressively lessen with each trial (fatigability). In contrast, central positional vertigo may occur with head movements in the recumbent patient, but the patient does not have the intense vertigo experienced with peripheral disorders. The vertigo persists as long as the position is maintained and lacks latency of onset and fatigability. Peripheral vertigo can be relieved by vestibular nerve section, whereas central vertigo cannot.

Ménière's disease classically affects middle-aged adults, producing a triad of symptoms. Early symptoms include fluctuating unilateral hearing loss and tinnitus; later in

the course of the disease, vertiginous attacks appear. The vertiginous attacks last from minutes to hours, disabling the victim, who prefers to lie immobilized in a dark, quiet place. Frequently the individual vertiginous attack is preceded by a sensation of increasing pressure or fullness in the involved ear. Vertigo attacks may undergo remissions and exacerbations and finally disappear as the disease *burns out*, whereas hearing and vestibular functions progressively deteriorate. Occasionally, vestibular symptoms may predominate from the start, with minimal hearing loss, a condition that leads to a diagnosis of vestibular Ménière's disease. Rarely, drop attacks, with or without vertigo, may occur as a manifestation of Ménière's disease.[18] Patients experiencing such attacks describe the sensation as a feeling of being pushed or shoved to the ground without loss of consciousness.

Otologic testing in patients with Ménière's disease reveals a hearing loss in the low frequencies early in the course of disease. Electronystagmography demonstrates a reduced caloric response in the affected ear, but imaging studies reveal no abnormalities. Profound hearing loss in all frequencies may occur, producing loss of serviceable hearing in the involved ear. In 15% to 40% of patients, the disease may involve both ears.

Most investigators agree that Ménière's disease results from endolymphatic hydrops or distention of the endolymphatic spaces, ultimately resulting in fibrosis of the labyrinth. The vertiginous episodes occur with the rupture of the endolymphatic membranes, allowing potassium-rich endolymph to mix with the potassium-poor perilymph. The potassium influx produces depolarization of the vestibular nerve endings, producing vertigo and nystagmus. As repair proceeds, symptoms resolve, and hearing may improve to near-normal, although each attack results in progressive degenerative changes in the cochlear and vestibular nerve endings.

The clinician must differentiate between Ménière's disease and other episodic peripheral vertigo disorders; the results of vestibular nerve section for Ménière's disease exceed the relief afforded for other conditions. Other important causes of acute vertiginous disorders include vestibular neuronitis and chronic labyrinthitis. Vestibular neuronitis occurs as a single or recurrent vertiginous episode without hearing loss. The cause appears to be an inflammatory process, possibly viral, involving the vestibular ganglia. Chronic labyrinthitis follows middle ear inflammatory disease or trauma to the labyrinth. Chronic labyrinthitis may result in recurrent episodes of vertigo but may also be associated with chronic dysequilibrium.

Benign positional vertigo must not be confused with Ménière's disease or other chronic vestibular disorders. In patients with benign positional vertigo, rapid changes in position result in brief vertiginous episodes. In the provocative test for this disorder, the patient quickly assumes the lateral supine position (Hallpike's maneuver). Symptoms occur only when the ear containing the diseased labyrinth is on the down side. Vertigo occurs and rotatory nystagmus appears. The nystagmus is fatigable on repeated provocative testing, and the disease is frequently self-limited. Disabling or persistent symptoms may require section of the nerve to the ampulla of the posterior semicircular canal.

The role of vascular cross-compression involving the

vestibular nerve deserves mention. Dandy,[11] in discussing Ménière's disease in 1937, stated, "In about 20 percent of the cases, a large artery (one of the branches of the superior-inferior cerebellar artery) lies against the nerve and, I think, is the cause of deafness and dizziness in this disease." Jannetta and associates[26] championed the cross-compression theory as the cause of vertigo that does not fit any other diagnostic profile. Typical symptoms consist of a constant positional vertigo or a dysequilibrium so severe that patients are disabled or constantly nauseated. Patients characteristically have motion intolerance, particularly when riding in an automobile or while pushing a shopping cart and gazing along the shelves. No demonstrable loss of auditory or vestibular function occurs. In the opinion of Jannetta and associates,[26] vascular compression of the vestibular nerve at the brain stem is responsible for this disorder. Vessels further distal along the course of the vestibular nerve are common and are not a source of the problem.

Disorders of the central nervous system, including multiple sclerosis or brain stem tumor, may produce acute central vertigo. Additional symptoms, signs, and imaging study results differentiate these disorders. Vertebral artery insufficiency rarely produces vertiginous attacks in the absence of other neurologic signs or symptoms. Acute occlusion of the labyrinthine artery may produce sudden hearing loss and vertigo, but the vertigo is self-limited once central accommodation occurs. Hearing loss is usually permanent.

## TREATMENT OF PERIPHERAL VESTIBULAR DISORDERS

Nonsurgical treatment forms the cornerstone of therapy for Ménière's disease and other peripheral labyrinthine disorders. Neurologists, internists, and otolaryngologists depend on vestibular depressant drugs, salt restriction, and diuretics to control symptoms. Time alone may produce a complete remission of symptoms. The unpredictability and the profound discomfort as well as the interruption of lifestyle that accompanies the episodic vertigo attacks compel the patient to seek surgical treatment. When the vertiginous attacks begin to interfere with everyday function, surgery is considered.

### Indications and Contraindications

Dandy reportedly performed a vestibular neurectomy on patients with a wide variety of dizzy disorders, some within 1 week of the onset of the vertigo.[14] Indications for surgery today are continued intractable vertigo attacks that have not responded to multiple trials of medical treatment. Approximately 20% of patients with Ménière's disease become surgical candidates. The selection of the initial procedure largely depends on the otologist's evaluation of the patient's hearing. With good hearing (≥80 dB pure tone average or <20% discrimination), preservation of auditory function is an additional goal of surgery; selective vestibular nerve section is the procedure of choice. Because preservation of any hearing in the involved ear is important, even in patients with poor hearing, vestibular nerve section is usually the initial procedure chosen. Occasionally, in a patient with poor hearing, some surgeons choose labyrinthectomy or eighth nerve section as the initial procedure.

Although the most common inner ear disorder treated by vestibular nerve section is classic Ménière's disease, the procedure is also useful in selected cases of recurrent vestibular neuronitis, traumatic labyrinthitis, and vestibular Ménière's disease. In deciding when to operate, the patient's perception of his or her disability is an important consideration. Some patients may have infrequent severe episodes of vertigo that do not affect their lifestyles sufficiently to warrant a major surgical procedure. Others, even those who have only a few attacks per year, may be so severely affected that they live in constant apprehension of the next attack. For some patients, attacks of vertigo may pose an occupational hazard that may jeopardize themselves, their coworkers, or the public. Often a patient decides to have surgery when he or she no longer has an aura preceding the onset of the vertigo.

Before surgery can be considered, objective evidence of unilateral inner ear disease should be documented with audiometry, electronystagmography, or electrocochleography. Early in the course of classic Ménière's disease, there is an ipsilateral low-frequency sensorineural hearing loss with good discrimination. As the disease progresses, the audiogram may flatten out or become downsloping, and the discrimination may deteriorate. During quiescence, electronystagmography may show normal or reduced caloric function in the involved ear. In the rare case in which an acute attack may be observed, spontaneous nystagmus toward the affected side and ipsilateral vestibular hyperfunction may be observed during the irritative phase. This activity is followed by a longer paralytic phase, characterized by spontaneous nystagmus away from the affected side and reduced vestibular response to caloric testing. Electrocochleography classically shows an elevated ratio of the summation potential to compound action potential, thought to be indicative of endolymphatic hydrops with distention of the basilar membrane.

The surgical candidate should be in good health and between vertigo attacks should have balance adequate to perform a tandem gait reasonably well. Elderly patients with good balance function are surgical candidates. Usually, however, they require more postoperative time and vestibular rehabilitation to regain good equilibrium than do younger patients. Vestibular nerve section has been performed on patients in their late 70s with excellent results and no additional morbidity.

Contraindications to vestibular nerve section include physiologic old age, poor general health, ataxia, unsteadiness, multisensory syndrome, and other evidence of central nervous system involvement. Patients with ataxia or dysequilibrium of central nervous system origin or a multisensory syndrome accommodate poorly after vestibular nerve section. Patients with these conditions may benefit from vestibular rehabilitation therapy. Those with severe disability are referred for a specialized rehabilitation program, but most respond well to home exercise regimens and are encouraged to maintain as active a lifestyle as possible. Poor hearing in the ear opposite to the one producing vertigo is a strong contraindication to vestibular neurectomy; the chance of hearing loss as a result of surgery must be considered. Bilateral Ménière's disease is another contraindication to vestibular neurectomy. Previous transmastoid surgery of the endolymphatic sac is not a contraindication to surgery.

The surgical candidate must be well educated in postoperative expectations. Several preoperative sessions with a surgeon are necessary to answer all the patient's questions. The patient must understand that the major purpose of the surgery is to relieve vertiginous attacks; tinnitus will likely be unaffected, and hearing loss may continue to progress, following the natural course of Ménière's disease. The greatest fear most patients profess is facial paralysis; this consequence must be discussed frankly and openly. Unless the possibility of cerebrospinal fluid (CSF) rhinorrhea and its treatment has been introduced before surgery, the uninformed patient assumes this to be a catastrophic complication if it occurs. The acute vertigo and the more subacute dysequilibrium experienced after vestibular nerve section, both of which subside spontaneously, must be carefully explained. The nurses caring for the patient after surgery must also be well versed in the postoperative course. Anxiety from an inexperienced nurse can rapidly be transferred to the patient.

## Surgical Anatomy

Multiple superbly illustrated microdissections of the cranial nerves in humans were published in 1865 by Bischoff.[27] Figure 74–1 reproduces some of their illustrations of the seventh and eighth cranial nerves and the nervus intermedius. McKenzie's[13] dissections led to the first practical localization of the vestibular portion of the eighth nerve in the cerebellopontine angle. Using McKenzie's[12] 1936 illustrations as an anatomic guide, a surgeon today could perform a differential section of the vestibular nerve in the cerebellopontine angle successfully. It is best to understand the changing anatomic relationships between the cochlear, vestibular, and facial nerves and the nervus intermedius throughout their course from the brain stem to their bony exits in the depths of the internal auditory canal. Throughout most of their course, minor individual anatomic variations occur; however, all nerves are constant in their position at the distal end of the internal auditory canal. Near the terminal end of the canal, which during surgery can be seen only by drilling away the bone that forms the posterior wall of the internal auditory canal, the superior and inferior vestibular nerves lie caudal (posterior), closest to the surgeon, obscuring the facial and cochlear nerves from view (Fig. 74–2). Terminally the vestibular nerves are separated by the transverse (falciform) crest. Anterior to and in front of the superior vestibular nerve lies the facial nerve. Below the facial nerve, the cochlear nerve lies in front of the inferior vestibular nerve. As the facial nerve enters its bony canal, it is separated from the superior vestibular nerve by the vertical crest, or *Bill's bar* (named in honor of William House).

The inferior vestibular nerve is formed by the fusion of the saccular and posterior ampullary nerves in the depths of the internal auditory canal. The saccule (innervated by the saccular nerve) has no apparent significant physiologic function in humans, which has important implications when

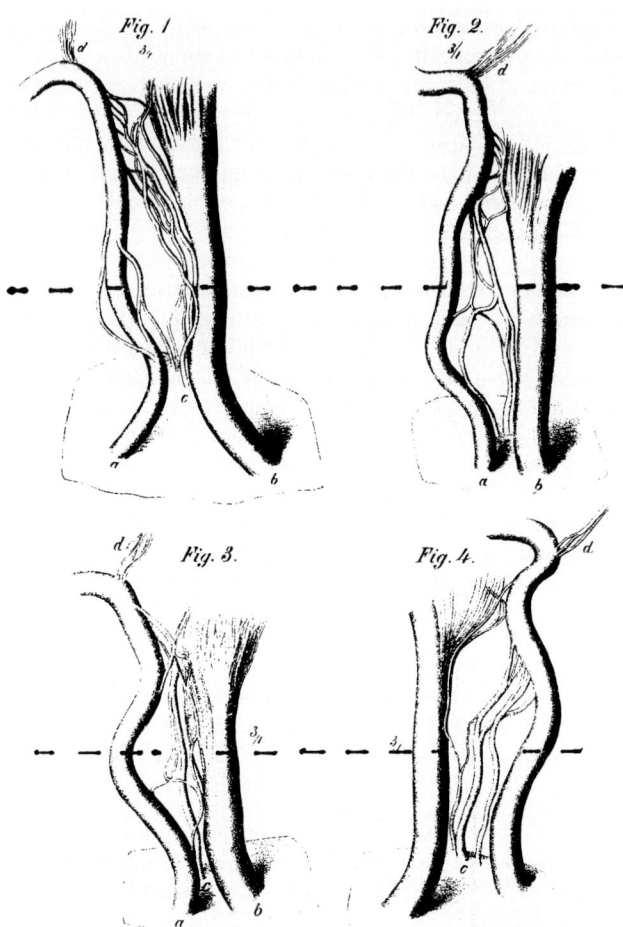

**FIGURE 74–1** ■ Dissection of nerves VII, VIII, and intermedius beginning at their emergence from the brain stem at a, b, and c, respectively, extending to their terminations within the petrous bone for nerves VIII and intermedius and to the knee of nerve VII at the point where it branches off the greater superficial petrosal nerve. Branches of the intermedius nerve unite about as often with nerve VIII as with nerve VII. Infrequently, this union occurs in the cerebellopontine cistern. The *dashed line* (- - -) through each drawing marks the approximate level of the opening into the internal auditory canal. (Courtesy of Bischoff EPE: Mikrospichen Analyse der Anastomosen der Kopfnerven. München: J.J. Leniner 1865, Tab. XLIII, p 52.)

section of the inferior vestibular nerve is considered. After innervating the saccule, the saccular nerve enters the terminal end of the internal auditory canal through its fenestrated posterior-inferior quadrant. Within 1 to 2 mm proximal to the terminal bony fenestrations, the saccular nerve is joined by the posterior ampullary nerve, which enters the posterior wall of the internal auditory canal through a small bony opening, the singular foramen (Fig. 74–3). The posterior ampullary nerve (singular nerve) innervates only the ampulla of the posterior semicircular canal. Almost immediately after the inferior vestibular nerve is formed, it begins to fuse with the cochlear nerve just medial to the falciform crest. Because of this early fusion, attempts to section the entire inferior vestibular nerve, even within the depths of the internal auditory canal, carry a significant risk of injury to the cochlear nerve. By the midportion of the internal auditory canal, the inferior vestibular nerve–cochlear nerve complex and superior vestibular nerve frequently fuse into a single bundle, the eighth nerve.

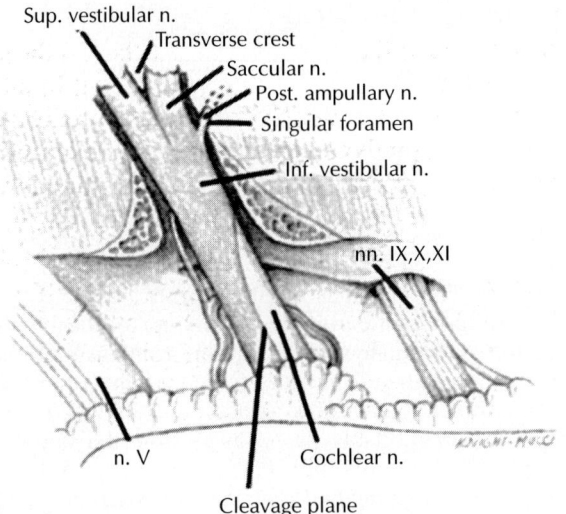

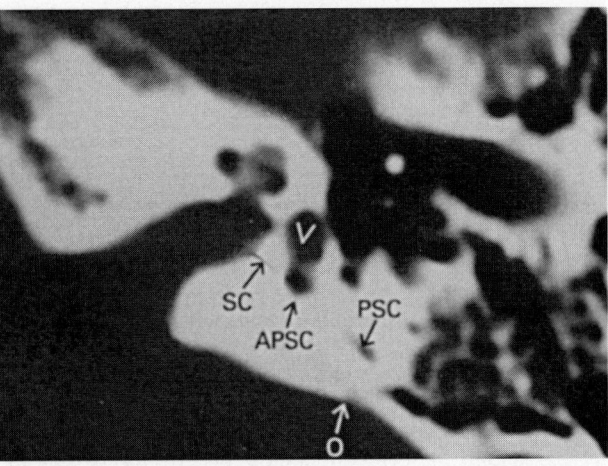

FIGURE 74–2 ■ Within the right internal auditory canal, the superior vestibular nerve obscures the facial nerve, while the inferior vestibular nerve hides the cochlear nerve. The distance from the singular foramen to the transverse crest is 2 ± 0.7 mm; the transverse crest would not be exposed during surgery.

FIGURE 74–3 ■ A computer-generated axial tomogram of the temporal bone demonstrates the singular canal (SC), the posterior semicircular posterior canal (PSC) and its ampulla (APSC), the vestibule (V), and the operculum (O) covering the endolymphatic duct.

As the nerves course through the internal auditory canal and the cerebellopontine cistern, rotation occurs. By the midportion of the internal auditory canal, the cochlear nerve has rotated more caudally (posteriorly) and dorsally to emerge from the porus acousticus closest to the surgeon, and the combined vestibular portions of the nerve have rotated rostrally away from the surgeon. Rotation continues so that when the nerves reach the midportion of the cerebel-

lopontine cistern, the cochlear nerve has rotated a full 90 degrees and is within full view of the surgeon (Fig. 74–4). As the eighth nerve emerges into the cerebellopontine cistern, a fine cleavage plane usually exists between the cochlear and vestibular nerves. Subtle color difference also assists the surgeon in identifying the separate components of the eighth nerve. The vestibular portion of the nerve, rostral and closest to the trigeminal nerve, appears grayer than the inferior white cochlear component that is closest to the ninth nerve. Maintaining its rostral position, the vestibular portion of the nerve enters the brain stem rostral

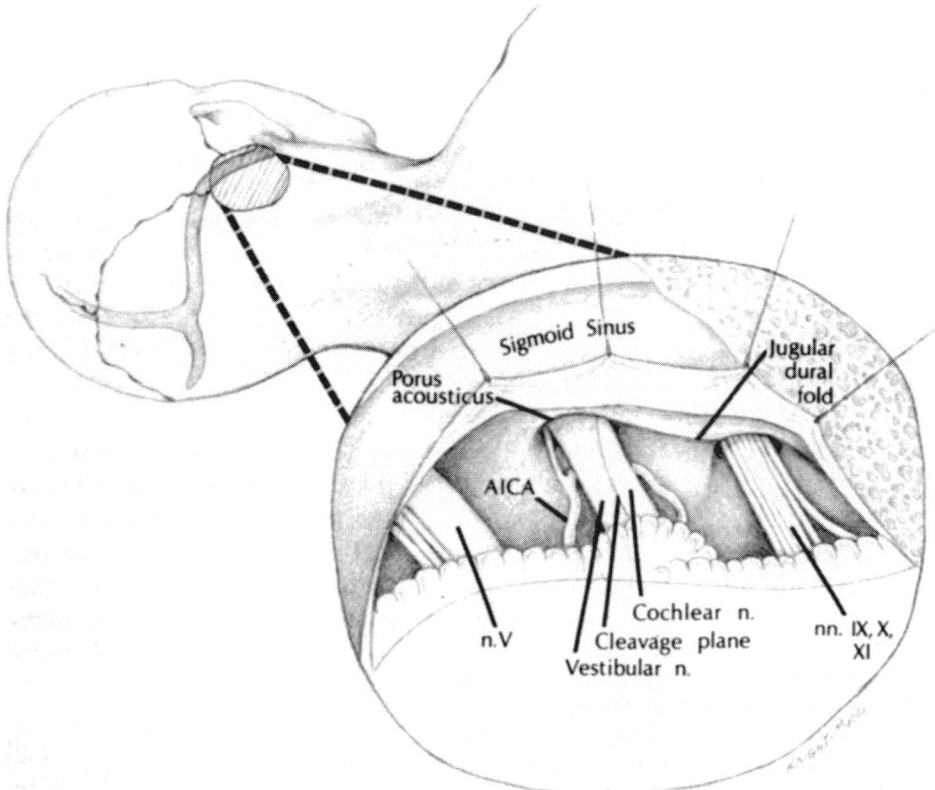

FIGURE 74–4 ■ Nerves of the right lateral posterior cranial fossa demonstrating the cochleovestibular cleavage plane. The facial nerve is hidden beneath the eighth nerve.

to the auditory portion through the middle cerebellar peduncle, and the auditory portion of the nerve enters the brain stem caudal and slightly more dorsally, where the restiform body disappears under the middle peduncle.

The facial nerve also participates in the rotation from the brain stem to its bony canal. The facial nerve emerges from the brain stem ventral and usually caudal to the eighth nerve; it is usually obscured from the surgeon's view by the eighth nerve throughout its course from the brain stem to the porus acousticus. Within the internal auditory canal, the seventh nerve rotates from caudal to rostral and from ventral to dorsal in its relationship to the cochlear portion of the eighth nerve before entering the bony facial canal. The nervus intermedius commonly originates as several twigs from the brain stem between the seventh and eighth nerves. Within the cerebellopontine cistern, the nervus intermedius fibers are intimately associated with the eighth nerve, usually attached to the ventral cleavage plane between the auditory and vestibular divisions of the nerve. In the midportion of the internal auditory canal, the nervus intermedius departs from the eighth nerve, joining the seventh nerve as it enters the facial canal.

A clear understanding of the rotation and changing relationship between the vestibular and cochlear portions of the eighth nerve is essential for surgeons performing surgery in the cerebellopontine angle. Before McKenzie's work, the changing position of the eighth nerve components was described but lacked practical value.[28] After the vestibular nerve section lost its popularity in the 1940s, the anatomy became less important, and more recent anatomic descriptions were misleading because they failed to note the rotation of the seventh and eighth nerves.[29] The resurrection of vestibular neurectomy and the possibility of hearing preservation during the removal of an acoustic neurinoma refocused attention on the importance of the eighth nerve rotation.[30, 31]

Rasmussen[32] was among the first to describe the histologic morphology of the eighth cranial nerve. He demonstrated the occasional complete separation between the cochlear and vestibular portions in the eighth nerve and the total intermingling of fibers within a single trunk in other specimens. The histologic difference between the two components of the nerve accounts for the surgical color difference. The cochlear fibers are uniform in size and more compact, appearing white under surgical magnification, whereas the loose fibers of the vestibular nerve produce a grayer color. Current histologic descriptions of the cleavage plane between the cochlear and vestibular nerves vary. Silverstein and colleagues[30] described an identifiable cleavage plane in 75% of specimens, realizing that in some cases vestibular fibers might still be contained within the cochlear portion of the nerve. Natout and coworkers[33] described an overlapping zone between the two divisions, in which the vestibular fibers were interspersed between the adjacent cochlear fibers. Schefter and Harner[34] studied the eighth nerve in 10 cadavers; they found no separation between the cochlear and vestibular fibers within the cerebellopontine angle in five specimens, and in the remaining cases, the eighth nerve was divided into many fascicles. No cochleovestibular cleavage plane was found in their study. Surgical outcome studies tend to favor at least some separation in most patients.

## Operating Room Setup

Before surgery, a thin-section computed tomography (CT) scan of the temporal bones is performed in addition to auditory and vestibular testing. This scan provides useful anatomic information about the labyrinths, venous sinuses, singular canals, and internal auditory canals.

Retrolabyrinthine and combined retrolabyrinthine-retrosigmoid operations for relief of peripheral vertigo are generally performed by teams of neurosurgeons and neuro-otologists. The positions of the patient, the surgeon, and the anesthesiologist during the surgery are identical to those used for the retrolabyrinthine and the combined retrolabyrinthine-retrosigmoid operations. The patient rests supine on an electrically controlled operating table, with the head turned and comfortably flexed away from the side of the surgery. Occasionally, pin-fixation head immobilization must be used, particularly in patients with thick, short necks. The patient need not be positioned in the "park-bench" position or prone, provided that an electric operating table is available to enable rotation. The surgeon sits directly behind the patient's head, with the anesthesiologist further down on the same side of the operating table. The surgical nurse is positioned directly opposite the surgeon, and the surgical microscope base is positioned at the head of the operating table. Electronic equipment is stacked at the foot of the operating table.

Intraoperative facial nerve monitoring is performed using the Silverstein Facial Nerve Monitor/Stimulator Model S8 (WR Medical Electronics, Stillwater, MN) and the Brackmann EMG Monitor (WR Medical Electronics, Stillwater, MN). The Silverstein monitor relies on an ultrasensitive piezoelectric strain gauge placed in the ipsilateral oral commissure that responds to facial movement. The electromyographic monitor senses facial myoelectric activity through bipolar electrodes placed in the facial musculature; the electrodes are typically placed in the ipsilateral orbicularis oris and orbicularis oculi muscles. The operation of these monitors has been described elsewhere. Intraoperative facial nerve stimulation is performed with the Silverstein Stimulator Probe (WR Medical Electronics, Stillwater, MN) and the Silverstein microinsulated neuro-otologic instruments (Storz Instruments, St. Louis, MO) using constant-current square wave pulse stimulation. Brain stem auditory evoked responses and direct eighth nerve potentials can be recorded during the operation. Cochlear nerve recordings are not considered to be an essential element in vestibular nerve section, but the use of this technique in these cases gives the surgeon a comfortable familiarity that is essential for acoustic neuroma surgery in which hearing preservation is the goal.

All patients receive perioperative intravenous antibiotics, starting immediately before incision and continuing for 24 hours. Intracranial pressure is lowered by the administration of mannitol (1.5 g/kg), and hypocarbia is produced by controlled hyperventilation. The mannitol is administered when the drilling begins. A urinary catheter is placed, and the urine output is monitored.

## Surgical Procedure

Adipose tissue is harvested from the left lower quadrant, and a suction drain is used to prevent hematoma formation.

This tissue is used to obliterate the postauricular surgical defect in the retrolabyrinthine and combined retrolabyrinthine-retrosigmoid vestibular nerve section procedures.

The retrolabyrinthine and the combined retrolabyrinthine-retrosigmoid operations begin with elevation of an anteriorly based, 4 × 5 cm U-shaped postauricular skin muscle flap. The flap, including the mastoid-occipital periosteum, is elevated in one layer. Anteriorly the spine of Henle should be visible. The mastoid emissary vein is frequently divided in the exposure, and bone wax is usually necessary to control the bleeding from the mastoid. Bleeding from the occipital artery should be controlled by suture ligation to avoid further intraoperative bleeding and postoperative hematoma formation.

## Retrolabyrinthine Vestibular Nerve Section

A complete mastoidectomy is performed, and the lateral venous sinus is skeletonized. The dura in front of and 1 cm behind the lateral venous sinus is exposed (Fig. 74–5). Bleeding from the lateral venous sinus is controlled by placing compressed Avitene and Gelfoam sponge over the bleeding site and holding it in place with a neurosurgical cottonoid sponge. Bleeding from a large emissary vein is controlled with bipolar cautery or an Avitene-Gelfoam pack. The endolymphatic sac is completely exposed, and the posterior semicircular canal is identified. The vertical segment of the facial nerve is delineated, and the retrofacial cells are opened. The dura over the posterior fossa is exposed from the middle fossa to the jugular bulb and from the lateral venous sinus to the posterior semicircular canal. The sigmoid sinus is compressed and retracted with the Silverstein lateral venous sinus retractor (Storz Instruments, St. Louis, MO), and the dura is incised around the endolymphatic sac anterior to the sigmoid sinus, forming a

C-shaped flap based on the labyrinth. The use of mannitol helps reduce the size of the cerebellum, allowing a wider exposure of the cerebellopontine angle.

A Penrose drain is placed over the cerebellum, which is then gently retracted with a Penfield elevator until the arachnoid is opened with an arachnoid knife (Storz Instruments, St. Louis, MO) to allow CSF to escape. As the cerebellopontine cistern is drained, the cerebellum falls away from the temporal bone to allow good exposure of the cerebellopontine angle and cranial nerves V, VII, VIII, IX, X, and XI without cerebellar retraction. Care must be taken not to traumatize the petrosal veins located above the fifth nerve and near the tentorium. Because of brain shrinkage from mannitol, these veins are stretched and can rupture easily. Bleeding is controlled with Avitene or bipolar cautery.

In 75% of cases, a good cochleovestibular cleavage plane exists between the cochlear and vestibular fibers of the eighth nerve in the cerebellopontine angle; the cochlear fibers constitute the caudal portion of the nerve and the vestibular fibers the cephalad portion. The orientation is important; the 5th cranial nerve is identified cephalad, and the 9th, 10th, and 11th nerves are identified caudally. The facial nerve should be identified. Occasionally the facial nerve is adherent to the vestibular nerve and must be separated from the vestibular nerve with a round knife. After the cleavage plane is identified under high magnification, an incision is made in the cleavage plane, the cochlear and vestibular fibers are separated, and the vestibular nerve is transected. The vestibular and cochlear nerves are separated longitudinally with an electrified sickle knife and nerve separator (Storz Instruments, St. Louis, MO), and the vestibular nerve is transected with microscissors and sickle knife. Transecting 75% of the vestibular nerve with microscissors and completing the transection with the

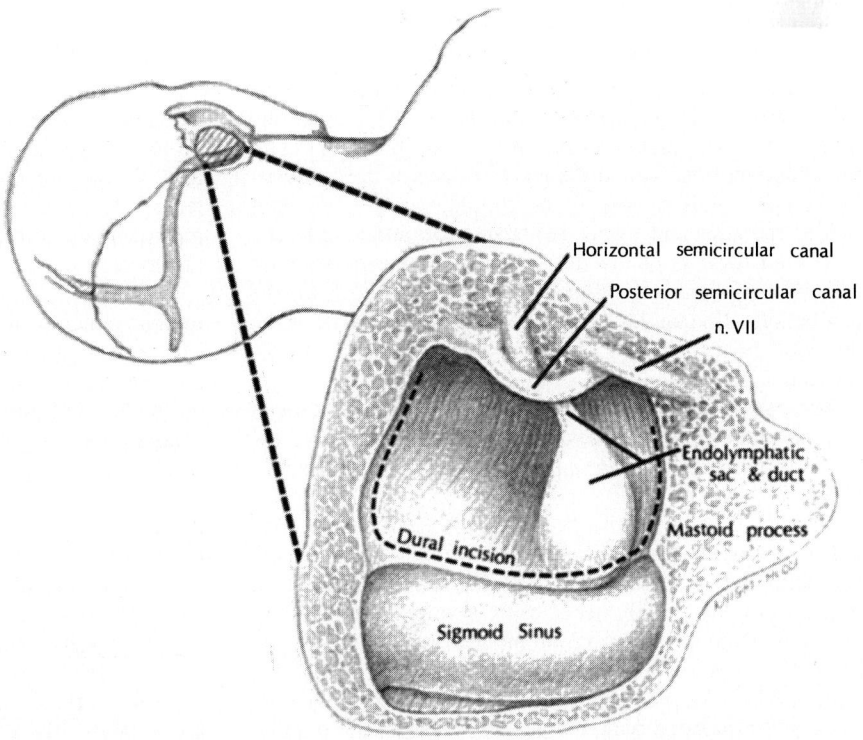

**FIGURE 74–5** ■ Removal of the right retrolabyrinthine bone exposes the sigmoid sinus and presigmoid sinus dura of the posterior fossa.

sickle knife helps avoid injury to the facial nerve and the internal auditory artery. The cephalad half of the eighth nerve is transected when a cleavage plane cannot be readily identified. When this technique is used, most vestibular fibers are transected, and most cochlear fibers are spared. The dural incision is completely closed with 4–0 silk sutures. Temporalis fascia is placed over the dural incision using fibrin glue, and the mastoid cavity is obliterated with abdominal adipose tissue and fibrin glue. The skin is closed with skin staples.

## Retrosigmoid–Internal Auditory Canal Vestibular Nerve Section

A U-shaped postauricular incision or a traditional neurosurgical straight suboccipital incision may be used. A round posterior fossa craniotomy 3 cm in diameter is made posterior to the lateral sinus. After the dura is opened with a posteriorly based U-shaped incision, the cerebellum is gently retracted with a self-retaining retractor blade to give exposure to the seventh and eighth cranial nerves and the internal auditory canal. The dura is closed in a watertight fashion, and the skin incision is closed. No fat graft is placed.

## Combined Retrolabyrinthine-Retrosigmoid Vestibular Nerve Section

A limited mastoidectomy is performed to expose 3 cm of the lateral venous sinus from the transverse sinus inferiorly. The lateral venous sinus is skeletonized, and the posterior fossa dura is exposed for 1.5 cm posterior to the lateral sinus (see Fig. 74–5). A dural incision is made 3 mm behind and parallel to the lateral sinus for 3 cm, and the lateral sinus is retracted anteriorly by means of stay sutures placed in the dural margin. A Penrose drain is placed against the cerebellum, and the cerebellum is gently retracted with a Penfield elevator. The landmark to the arachnoid over the cerebellopontine cistern is a white fold of dura, the jugular dural fold, attached to the temporal bone just lateral to the jugular foramen above the exit of the ninth nerve. The jugular dural fold is identified anterior to the endolymphatic sac on the inner surface of the temporal bone. The eighth nerve is found approximately 1 cm anterior to the cephalad extent of the jugular dural fold. The arachnoid layer is gently dissected, and the cerebellopontine cistern is entered. After the CSF is released from the cerebellopontine angle, the cerebellum falls away from the temporal bone, allowing good exposure of the cerebellopontine angle without cerebellar retraction.

The eighth nerve is examined, and the cleavage plane is sought between the cochlear and vestibular fibers. If the cochleovestibular cleavage plane is identified, the vestibular nerve section is performed as in the retrolabyrinthine approach. Sometimes the flocculus of the cerebellum is adherent to and hides much of the eighth nerve in the cerebellopontine angle. The flocculus must be dissected away from the eighth nerve with a round knife. If no cleavage plane is identified, an anteriorly based, U-shaped dural flap is elevated from the posterior surface of the temporal bone between the operculum and the porus acousticus. With diamond burs, the posterior wall of the internal

auditory canal is removed to the singular canal, exposing the branches of the vestibular nerve. Usually, 7 to 8 mm of bone is removed. This length is determined from the preoperative CT scan. The superior vestibular nerve and the posterior ampullary nerve are divided. The inferior vestibular nerve fibers that innervate the saccule are spared because of their close association with cochlear fibers. Because the saccule has no known vestibular function in humans, sparing these fibers does not result in postoperative vertigo attacks. The dura is closed in a watertight fashion, any exposed mastoid air cells are filled with bone wax, and the defect is filled with abdominal adipose tissue. The skin is closed with skin staples.

## Postoperative Care

Immediately after surgery, patients experience acute vertigo, nausea, and vomiting similar to a Ménière's attack. As the central nervous system vestibular compensation occurs, however, vertigo resolves rapidly over 3 to 4 days; the frequent complaint of dysequilibrium improves more slowly. Patients with near-normal preoperative vestibular function experience the greatest immediate postoperative vertigo and nausea after labyrinthine denervation. Early ambulation appears to hasten vestibular compensation, although immediately after surgery, patients usually have a wide-based gait and tend to fall to the operated side. One year after surgery, some patients may experience mild transient unsteadiness after abrupt head movement. Third-degree horizontal nystagmus beating away from the operated ear is seen early and diminishes quickly. It is not unusual, however, for a patient to have first-degree nystagmus for several days. Diplopia occurs in a small number of patients. It is difficult to document and clears rapidly. It appears to be due to ocular dysmetria or a skew deviation.

## Complications

Early postoperative bleeding in the posterior fossa requires prompt assessment by a neurosurgeon. The wound may have to be opened immediately. Meningismus with mild temperature elevation occurring soon after surgery usually represents a chemical meningitis caused by small amounts of blood in the CSF.

Spiking fever with nuchal rigidity and headache requires lumbar puncture for a CSF culture and sensitivity testing. The patient should then be treated empirically for meningitis, and the antibiotic coverage should be narrowed later on the basis of culture results. As yet, the authors have not encountered this complication.

Wound infection secondary to serum collected beneath the postauricular skin flap is treated with incision, drainage, culture, and appropriate antibiotics. This complication has been reduced by keeping the skin muscle flap in one layer during its elevation. Perioperative antibiotic administration has reduced wound infections to less than 1% of cases.

Postoperative CSF leak occurs in less than 5% of all cases.[3, 4] It was the most common early complication of retrolabyrinthine vestibular nerve section, occurring in approximately 10% of cases, and was seen occurring through the wound or as persistent rhinorrhea. When a leak is detected, lumbar drainage is immediately instituted and maintained for 3 to 5 days, avoiding re-exploration of the wound in most cases. Because the dura cannot be closed in a watertight fashion in the retrolabyrinthine approach, no way has been found to eliminate CSF leaks; however, the use of cryoprecipitate autologous fibrin glue appears to have reduced their incidence. The retrosigmoid–internal auditory canal and combined retrolabyrinthine-retrosigmoid approaches allow a watertight dural closure, and CSF leakage is rarely encountered.

Facial paralysis and transient facial weakness have been reported and are rare. The authors have not experienced either complication in their series.

## RESULTS

The retrolabyrinthine vestibular nerve section was developed in 1978 to replace the middle fossa vestibular nerve section. Results of this procedure have been good. In a review of 67 patients, 88% were completely cured of their vertigo, and 7% were substantially improved. Hearing has been maintained within 20 db of the preoperative level in 70%. Some patients experienced mild conductive loss in the low frequencies, which is presumed to be caused by bone dust or fat herniating into the attic and impeding ossicular motion. CSF leak occurred in 10% of patients and responded to lumbar drainage. Wound infection occurred in 3%. There were no cases of meningitis, facial paralysis, or death.

In 1985, the retrosigmoid–internal auditory canal vestibular nerve section was developed in an effort to improve results.[4] Because the cleavage plane between the cochlear and vestibular fibers is more completely developed within the internal auditory canal, a more complete and selective vestibular nerve section can be performed there. This approach resulted in a 92% cure rate for vertigo in 14 patients and hearing results similar to those with the retrolabyrinthine approach. Fifty percent of patients, however, experienced prolonged severe headaches that were difficult to control with non-narcotic analgesics. Two years after surgery, 25% of patients still experienced headaches requiring medication. The authors have speculated that removal of the dura from the bone at the porus and bone dust produced by drilling the internal auditory canal may have resulted in a prolonged arachnoiditis. Owing to the unacceptably high incidence of severe postoperative headaches, the authors abandoned the retrosigmoid–internal auditory canal approach in 1987. Only 15 procedures were performed.

The combined retrolabyrinthine-retrosigmoid vestibular neurectomy was developed in 1987.[3] This procedure incorporates the advantages of both of its predecessors. Depending on the presence of a good cochleovestibular cleavage plane in the cerebellopontine angle, the vestibular nerve section may be performed there, or the internal auditory canal may be opened and the superior vestibular and posterior ampullary nerves sectioned. Less bone removal is required, and surgical time is shortened. Also, a watertight dural closure may be accomplished. In the authors' series, vertigo has been cured in 90% of patients,

and hearing has been preserved to within 20 dB of preoperative levels in 84%. When the internal auditory canal was not opened, only 1% of patients developed headaches. Since October 1988, the internal auditory canal has not been drilled. Three of five patients requiring internal auditory canal exposure developed moderate headaches. There have been no cases of CSF leak, meningitis, facial paralysis, or death.

After vestibular nerve section in patients with vertigo attacks from labyrinthitis or vestibular neuronitis, the surgical results are slightly less impressive than in patients with Ménière's disease. Nguyen and colleagues[35] and Kemink[36] reported only a 70% improvement or complete resolution of symptoms in the non-Ménière's group of patients with chronic vertigo. There is a lack of correlation between surgical outcome and the surgeon's assessment of either the completeness of the vestibular neurectomy or the clarity of the cleavage plane.

Beyond relief of vertigo, some patients report relief of chronic unsteadiness, aural pressure, and tinnitus. The possibility of relief of any one of these symptoms, no matter how troublesome, in the absence of vertigo attacks, does not justify the performance of vestibular neurectomy.

Failure of surgery to relieve vertigo attacks requires re-evaluation of vestibular function. Approximately 3% of patients require additional surgery. If a patient continues to have vertigo attacks arising from the side of the original surgery, a decision must be made regarding further surgery. Labyrinthectomy, transcanal eighth nerve section, or middle fossa or posterior fossa total eighth nerve section should be performed. All of these procedures result in hearing ablation, but the results of vertigo relief are quite good.

## OUTCOMES STUDY

An important outcome measurement in any treatment modality is whether or not the patient feels better and considers himself or herself cured. In an effort to ascertain whether the patient's perception of the surgical outcome agrees with the surgeon's criteria of success, a comprehensive outcomes questionnaire was developed.[37] The questionnaire, which addresses patient lifestyle and incidence of vertigo, balance function, hearing, tinnitus, aural fullness, and incidence of failures or complications, was sent to all patients who underwent posterior fossa vestibular neurectomy. Of the patients that responded, 88% believed that the vertigo caused by their Ménière's disease was cured after surgery, and 78% believed that their hearing was maintained. After surgery, 95% believed that their balance function "rarely" or "never" prevented them from doing their normal daily activities. Overall, patient perception of outcome after posterior fossa vestibular neurectomy was similar to the surgeon's and to what has been previously reported.

## SUMMARY

In the nearly 90 years since Frazier first performed an eighth cranial nerve section through the posterior fossa for the treatment of Ménière's disease, the surgical management of Ménière's disease has come full circle. With refinements in surgical technique and advancements in instrumentation, optics, illumination, and neuromonitoring, a procedure that was once resoundingly condemned by the otologic community is now regarded as the procedure of choice in patients with serviceable hearing. The vestibular nerve section has experienced a renaissance. The posterior fossa vestibular nerve section has undergone an evolution, and the combined retrolabyrinthine-retrosigmoid vestibular nerve section represents the highest form. It is a significant improvement over its predecessors and the authors' procedure of choice in properly selected patients.

# REFERENCES

1. Silverstein H, Norrell H: Retrolabyrinthine surgery: A direct approach to the cerebellopontine angle. Otolaryngol Head Neck Surg 88:462–469, 1980.
2. Silverstein H, Norrell H, Smouha E: Retrosigmoid-internal auditory canal approach vs. retrolabyrinthine approach for vestibular neurectomy. Otolaryngol Head Neck Surg 97:300–307, 1987.
3. Silverstein H, Norrell H, Smouha E, et al: Combined retrolabyrinthine-retrosigmoid approach for vestibular neurectomy. Am J Otol 10:166–169, 1989.
4. Silverstein H, Norrell H, Rosenberg S: The resurrection of vestibular neurectomy: A 10-year experience with 115 cases. J Neurosurg 72:533–539, 1990.
5. Silverstein H, Wanamaker H, Flanzer J, Rosenberg S: Vestibular neurectomy in the USA 1990. Am J Otol 13:23–30, 1992.
6. Rosenberg S, Silverstein H, Norrell H, et al: Hearing results after posterior fossa vestibular neurectomy. Otolaryngol Head Neck Surg 114:32–37, 1996.
7. Silverstein H, Arruda J, Rosenberg S: Vestibular neurectomy. In Harris JP (ed): Ménière's Disease. Amsterdam: Kugler, 1998, pp 263–273.
8. Roland PS, Meyerhoff WL: Should the membranous labyrinth be destroyed because of vertigo? Otolaryngol Head Neck Surg 95:550–553, 1986.
9. Frazier CH: Intracranial division of the auditory nerve for persistent aural vertigo. Surg Gynecol Obstet 15:52–59, 1912.
10. Dandy WE: Ménière's disease: Its diagnosis and method of treatment. Arch Surg 16:1127–1152, 1928.
11. Dandy WE: Treatment of Ménière's disease by section of only the vestibular portion of the acoustic nerve. Bull Johns Hopkins Hosp 53:52–55, 1933.
12. McKenzie KG: Intracranial division of the vestibular portion of the auditory nerve for Ménière's disease. Can Med Assoc J 34:369–391, 1936.
13. McKenzie KG: Ménière's syndrome: A follow-up study. Clin Neurosurg 2:44–49, 1955.
14. Green RE: Surgical treatment of vertigo, with follow-up on Walter Dandy's cases. Clin Neurosurg 6:141–152, 1958.
15. House WE: Surgical exposure of the internal auditory canal and its contents through the middle cranial fossa. Laryngoscope 71:1363–1385, 1961.
16. Fisch U: Vestibular and cochlear neurectomy. Trans Am Acad Ophthalmol Otolaryngol 78:252–254, 1977.
17. Fisch U: Vestibular nerve section for Ménière's disease. Am J Otol 5:543–545, 1984.
18. Glasscock ME: Vestibular nerve section. Arch Otolaryngol 97:112–114, 1973.
19. Glasscock ME, Kveton JF, Christiansen SG: Middle fossa neurectomy: An update. Otolaryngol Head Neck Surg 92:216–220, 1984.
20. Garcia-Ibanez E, Garcia-Ibanez IL: Middle fossa vestibular neurectomy: A report of 373 cases. Otolaryngol Head Neck Surg 88:486–490, 1988.
21. Hitselberger WE, Pulec JL: Trigeminal nerve (anterior root) retrolabyrinthine selective section. Arch Otolaryngol 96:412–415, 1972.
22. Brackmann DE, Hitselberger WE: Retrolabyrinthine approach: Technique and newer applications. Laryngoscope 88:286–297, 1978.
23. Rosenberg SI, Silverstein H, Willcox TO, Gordon MA: Endoscopy in otology and neurotology. Am J Otol 15:168–172, 1994.
24. Pearson BW, Brackmann DE: Committee on hearing and equilibrium guidelines for reporting treatment results in Ménière's disease. Otolaryngol Head Neck Surg 93:579–581, 1985.
25. Monsell EM, Balkany TA, Gates GA, et al: Committee on hearing and equilibrium guidelines for the diagnosis and evaluation of therapy in Ménière's disease. Otolaryngol Head Neck Surg 113:181–185, 1995.
26. Jannetta PJ, Moller MB, Moller AR: Disabling positional vertigo. N Engl J Med 310:1700–1705, 1984.
27. Bischoff EPE: Mikrospichen Analyse der Anastomosen der Kopfnerven. Munchen: JJ Leniner, 1865.
28. Courville CB: Applied anatomy of the VIIIth nerve and its environs, the cerebellopontine angle.
29. Rhoton A: Neurosurgery of the internal auditory meatus. Surg Neurol 2:311–318, 1974.
30. Silverstein H, Norrell H, Haberkamp T, McDaniel AB: The unrecognized rotation of the vestibular and cochlear nerves from the labyrinth to the brain stem: Its implications to surgery of the eighth cranial nerve. Otolaryngol Head Neck Surg 95:543–549, 1986.
31. Malkasian DR, Rand RW: Microsurgical neuroanatomy. In Rand RW (ed): Microneurosurgery, 2nd ed. St. Louis, CV Mosby, 1978, pp 37–70.
32. Rasmussen AT: Studies of the VIIIth cranial nerve of man. Laryngoscope 50:67–83, 1949.
33. Natout MAY, Terr LI, Linthicum FH Jr, House WF: Topography of the vestibulocochlear nerve fibers in the posterior cranial fossa. Laryngoscope 97:954–958, 1987.
34. Schefter RP, Harner SG: Histologic study of the vestibulocochlear nerve. Ann Otolaryngol 95:146–150, 1986.
35. Nguyen CD, Brackmann DE, Crane RT, et al: Retrolabyrinthine vestibular nerve section: Evaluation of technical modification in 143 cases. Am J Otol 13:328–332, 1992.
36. Kemink IL: Retrolabyrinthine vestibular nerve section: A preliminary report. Am J Otol 5:549–551, 1984.
37. Rosenberg SI, Silverstein H, Hester TO, Deems D: Outcomes research after posterior fossa vestibular neurectomy—a 20 year experience. Am J Otol (in press).

# CHAPTER 75

# Surgical Management of Glomus Jugulare Tumors

■ CARL B. HEILMAN, JON H. ROBERTSON, GALE GARDNER, and NIKOLAS BLEVINS

The optimal management of a glomus jugulare tumor remains a challenge. This chapter presents a comprehensive review of this formidable lesion while emphasizing the relevant surgical anatomy and the importance of developing an individualized treatment plan for a particular lesion.

Glomus jugulare tumors are believed to arise from glomus bodies in the region of the jugular bulb. The first description of glomus tissue is credited to Valentin, who in 1840 noted a small cellular formation near the origin of the tympanic nerve that he thought was a ganglion.[4] In 1878, Krause[36] further described glomus tissue as being microscopic, indistinguishable from the carotid body, and occurring along the tympanic branch of the glossopharyngeal nerve in the inferior tympanic canaliculus. Valentin and Krause's work received little attention. It was not until 1941 that glomus tissue was rediscovered by Guild.[26] Guild coined the term *glomus jugularis*, or jugular body, to describe the paraganglionic tissue composed largely of capillary or precapillary vessels interspersed with numerous epithelioid cells that is found along the jugular bulb in human temporal bone sections. The relationship between the "glomus jugularis" described by Guild and the "carotid body like" tumor in the temporal bone was first recognized by Rosenwasser[50] in 1945. In 1953, after serially sectioning 88 human temporal bones, Guild[27] noted that approximately 50% of jugular bodies were situated in the adventitia of the jugular bulb dome. The remainder occurred with equal frequency along the course of the tympanic branch of the glossopharyngeal nerve (Jacobson's nerve) or the auricular branch of the vagus nerve (Arnold's nerve). This explained the observation that "glomus tumors" occur in the middle ear (*glomus tympanicum tumors*) as well as in the region of the jugular bulb (*glomus jugulare tumors*).

Rockley and Hawke[49] in 1990 published a systematic study of the exact anatomic distribution of glomus bodies in the temporal bone (Fig. 75–1). They noted that glomus bodies, which measured up to 1 mm in diameter, were found only along the course of parasympathetic nerves of the ear (Arnold's or Jacobson's nerve) or their identifiable branches. Histologically, the glomus bodies appeared as nests of epithelioid cells surrounded by a connective tissue capsule. On the surface of the capsule were tortuous arterioles, whereas thin-walled venous sinusoids coursed through the substance of the glomus body. Rockley and Hawke[49] concluded that dividing glomus tumors into two groups (glomus tympanicum and glomus jugulare tumors) was an artificial distinction based on observed clinical presentation rather than on actual anatomic distribution of glomus bodies. Tumors arising distally on Jacobson's nerve or on the promontory would manifest clinically as glomus tympanicum tumors. Tumors arising more proximally on Jacobson's nerve in the inferior tympanic canaliculus or adjacent to the jugular bulb would expand into the jugular bulb and manifest as glomus jugulare tumors. The discovery by Rockley and Hawke[49] of glomus bodies located along the course of Arnold's nerve adjacent to the facial nerve could account for the occasional clinical presentation of a glomus tumor in the descending facial canal.

The exact physiologic function of the glomus body remains unknown. Its histologic similarity to carotid and aortic bodies has suggested a chemoreceptor role responding to hypoxia, hypercarbia, or acidosis. Other possibilities are a role in regulating microcirculatory blood flow or the homeostasis of gas composition and pressure in the middle ear. On the basis of their anatomic study, Rockley and Hawke[49] suggested that temporal glomus bodies regulate the blood flow to the promontory with a secondary effect on gas pressure in the middle ear.

## EPIDEMIOLOGY

Although glomus jugulare tumors are second to vestibular schwannomas as the most common tumor involving the temporal bone, they are still uncommonly seen in neurosurgical practice. The age of presentation ranges from the second to the ninth decade, although most tumors manifest in middle age, with the disease affecting women more often than men.[9, 38, 66] In one study of 231 cases, glomus jugulare tumors were six times more common in women than in men.[9]

Most glomus jugulare tumors are benign, slow-growing neoplasms that are highly vascular and locally invasive.

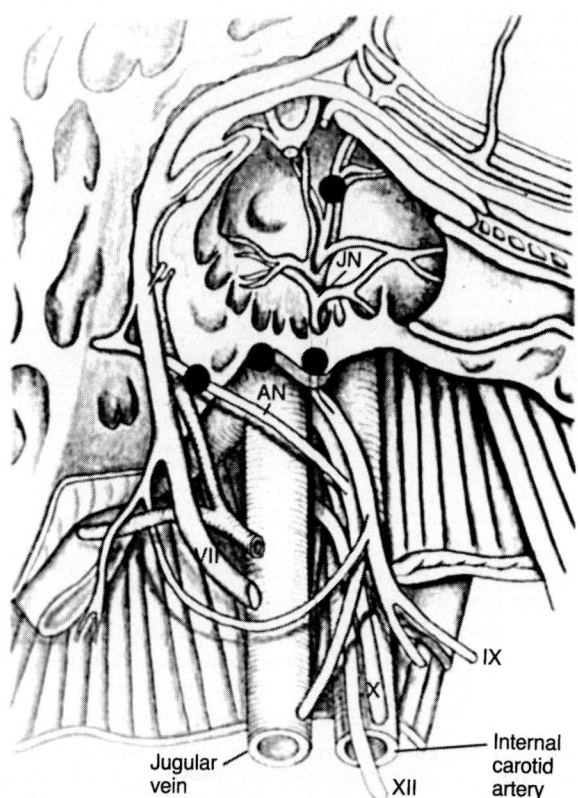

**FIGURE 75–1** ■ Lateral view of the temporal bone through the region of the jugular bulb demonstrating the anatomic location of the glomus bodies *(black dots).*

Symptoms may exist from months to decades before the diagnosis.[4, 38, 42, 65] In 1992, van der Mey and colleagues[65] reported a series of 52 patients with glomus jugulotympanicum tumors, of whom 20 underwent subtotal tumor removal and 13 patients were followed without treatment. All of these patients, except three who were lost to follow-up, were alive and without serious complaints with an average follow-up of 13.5 years (range, 1 to 32 years). Clinically, their disease was not progressive, with the exception of one case that required further surgery 5 years after incomplete surgical removal. Occasionally, however, the tumor is aggressive and grows rapidly; in rare cases (1% to 3%), it can metastasize to regional lymph nodes or distant sites.[3, 6, 9, 11, 13, 14, 35, 60, 70]

Glomus jugulare tumors may be bilateral or associated with other chemodectomas[2, 59, 61] (Fig. 75–2). In most series, familial glomus jugulare tumors comprise a minority; however, in a report by van der Mey and colleagues[65] from the Netherlands, familial cases of all glomus tumors (including carotid body tumors) made up approximately 50% of the entire series.

Catecholamine biosynthesis and secretion has been reported in approximately 4% of patients with glomus jugulare tumors.[1, 5, 15, 37, 41, 44, 51] Excess catecholamines may be responsible for hypertension preoperatively or for wide fluctuations in blood pressure during surgical manipulation. Preoperative 24-hour urinary studies to screen for vanillylmandelic acid, metanephrine, free catecholamine, and 5-hydroxyindole acetic acid (5-HIAA) may help predict which patients will have blood pressure fluctuations during tumor removal.

## PRESENTATION

The locally invasive and highly vascular nature of glomus jugulare tumors accounts for their clinical presentation. They usually present with progressive unilateral hearing loss from invasion of the mesotympanum and pulsatile tinnitus secondary to the tumor's rich vascularity. Other symptoms depend on the direction of tumor growth. Invasion of the cochlea or labyrinth produces sensorineural hearing loss or vertigo, respectively. Lower cranial nerve dysfunction, manifested as hoarseness or dysphagia, occurs more commonly with larger tumors but is generally well tolerated owing to its gradual onset and simultaneous compensation. In a series of 102 patients reported by Makek and associates,[40] cranial nerve VII was affected at presentation in 33% of patients. This cranial nerve was the most often affected on presentation in their series followed by cranial nerves X, IX, XII, and XI. In a series of 59 patients reported by Jackson and associates[32] in 1990, however, preoperative facial weakness was present in only 8%. Interestingly, the lack of preoperative nerve dysfunction does not preclude finding neural invasion at the time of surgery.[40] A complete jugular foramen syndrome is unusual unless advanced disease is present. Large glomus jugulare tumors may grow anteriorly and encase the carotid artery, producing Horner's syndrome, or extend medially and superiorly up into the cavernous sinus. Intracranial extension, either through the jugular foramen or via expansion in the epidural space along the posterior aspect of the petrous bone, may cause fifth and sixth cranial nerve dysfunction, brain stem compression, and hydrocephalus. Extracranial extension into and along the jugular vein may produce a mass visible in the oropharynx or palpable in the neck. Rarely, patients can present with palpitations and flushing from secretion of catecholamines.[62]

## SURGICAL ANATOMY

The jugular foramen in the posterolateral skull base is bounded anterolaterally by the petrous portion of the temporal bone and posteromedially by the occipital bone. The two jugular foramina are asymmetric, with the right side being larger in more than two thirds of cases.[12, 48] This is believed to be secondary to the asymmetry in the size of the transverse and sigmoid sinuses. The foramen is subdivided into two compartments by a fibrous or, less likely, bony septum that connects the jugular spine of the petrous bone with the jugular process of the occipital bone. In a systematic study of 129 dry skulls, Di Chiro and colleagues[12] noted a bony septum unilaterally in 13.2% and bilaterally in 4.7%. The posterolateral compartment, called the pars venosa, is larger and contains the jugular bulb, cranial nerves X and XI, and the posterior meningeal artery. The smaller anteromedial compartment, called the pars

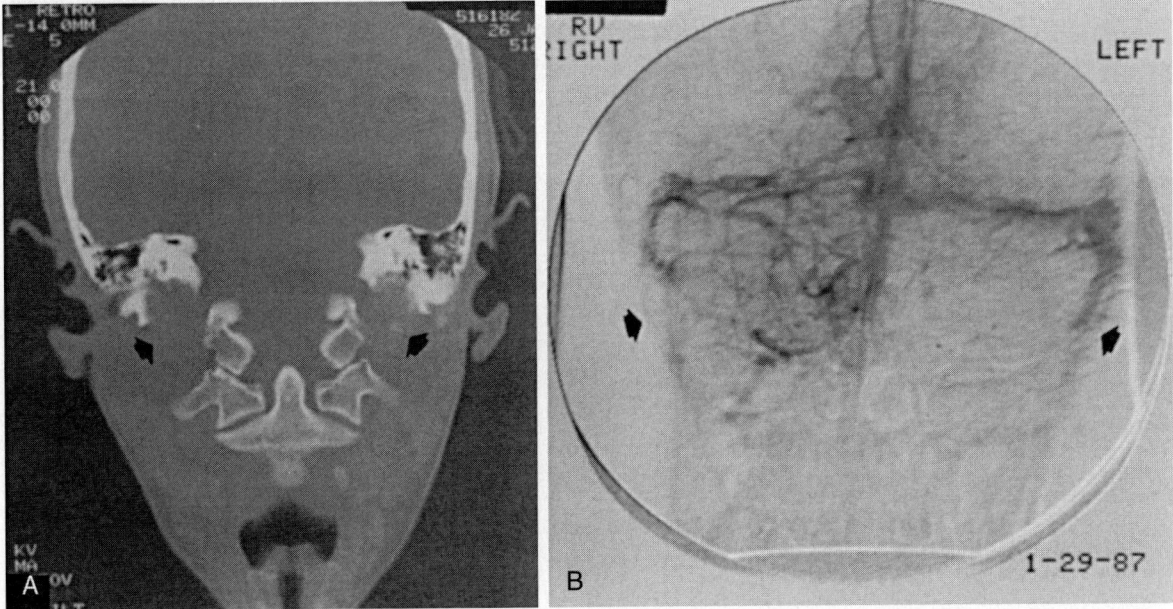

**FIGURE 75–2** ■ *A,* Coronal computed tomography scan of the skull base demonstrating bilateral glomus jugulare tumors. Note the irregular bone edges of the jugular foramina, which is typical for this locally invasive tumor *(arrows). B,* An anteroposterior venogram of the head in the same patient, demonstrating bilateral jugular bulb occlusion *(arrows).*

nervosa, contains cranial nerve IX and the venous channels of the inferior petrosal sinus (Fig. 75–3).[31]

The exact anatomic location of cranial nerves IX, X, and XI as they traverse the jugular foramen is variable, but in essentially every case, they are medial to the jugular bulb. The ninth cranial nerve travels alone, medial and slightly superior to cranial nerves X and XI, which are intimately associated with each other. In rare cases (6%), the glossopharyngeal nerve leaves the skull through a separate bony canal rather than through the pars nervosa.[48]

The venous anatomy of the jugular foramen is formed by the continuation of the horizontal limb of the sigmoid sinus into the jugular bulb. The jugular bulb then rises above the horizontal segment of the sigmoid sinus. Surrounding the dome of the jugular bulb in the temporal bone are numerous anatomic structures, including the posterior semicircular canal, the middle ear, the medial aspect of the external auditory canal, and cranial nerve VII. In 1975, Graham[24] reported that in some cases, the jugular bulb rose 0.75 inch above the horizontal limb of the sigmoid sinus, whereas in other cases, it rose not more than 0.25 inch. The jugular bulb lies inferior to the middle ear and, when small, is separated from the middle ear by bone. The bone separating a large jugular bulb from the middle ear may be thin or dehiscent with the venous wall of the bulb occasionally reaching the round window.[24] The facial nerve descends in the fallopian canal on the lateral aspect of the jugular bulb, often as close as 1 mm.

An understanding of the anatomy of the inferior petrosal sinus is critical during removal of glomus jugulare tumors. The inferior petrosal sinus is usually the largest vessel to empty into the jugular bulb, with the exception of the sigmoid sinus. The inferior petrosal sinus opens into the anterior medial aspect of the jugular bulb usually by multiple channels coursing through the fibrous septum separating the pars nervosa and pars venosa. Occasionally, the

vein of the cochlear aqueduct or a branch from the occipital sinus empties into the jugular bulb as well.[24] These multiple channels are a source of bleeding that must be controlled during the final stages of tumor excision without causing injury to the underlying cranial nerves.

As the contents of the jugular foramen leave the skull base, they are surrounded by vital structures, including the internal carotid artery, the facial nerve, and the hypoglossal nerve. Several relatively constant anatomic relationships are essential to successful dissection in this region. The stylomastoid foramen containing the facial nerve is located just lateral and posterior to the base of the styloid process. The glossopharyngeal nerve exits the medial and superior aspect of the jugular foramen and then passes lateral to the internal carotid artery. The spinal accessory nerve leaves the jugular foramen medial to the jugular vein. This nerve usually passes anterior to the jugular vein extracranially before passing under the sternocleidomastoid muscle. The hypoglossal nerve leaves the hypoglossal canal and passes around behind the vagus nerve before coursing anteriorly over the internal carotid artery toward the tongue. In summary, the nerves exiting the jugular foramen all travel medial to the jugular bulb, and all cranial nerves seen with this dissection (VII, IX, X, XI, and XII) pass lateral to the internal carotid artery.

## MANAGEMENT OF GLOMUS JUGULARE TUMORS

Patients presenting with a mass consistent with a glomus jugulare tumor should be evaluated by audiometry to determine the function of the middle and inner ear. In older patients with a large tumor, in whom blood pressure fluctuations would increase the risk of surgery, a 24-hour urinary catecholamine screen should be performed to rule

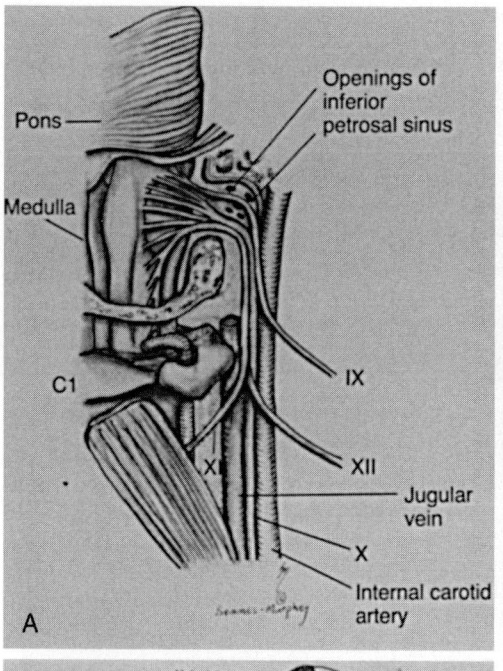

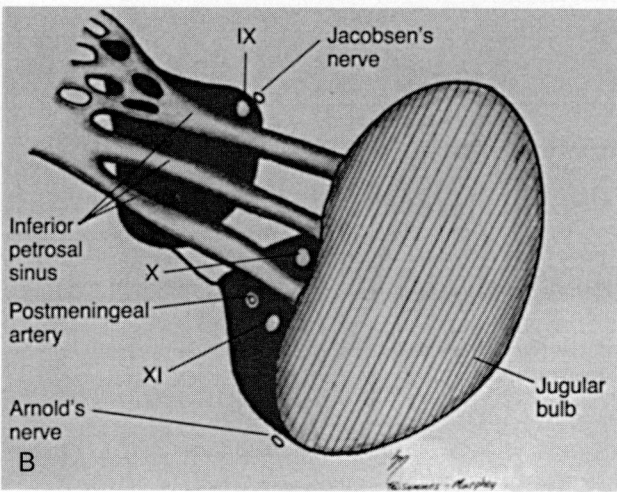

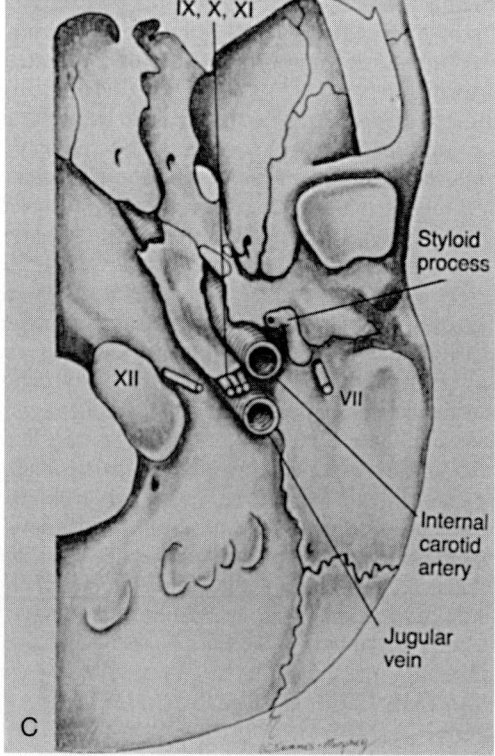

**FIGURE 75–3 ■** *A,* Lateral view of the jugular foramen with the jugular vein and bulb removed. *B,* Cross-section of the jugular foramen. *C,* Basal view of the skull base focusing on the region of the jugular foramen. (Copyright © Semmes-Murphey Clinic.)

out a catecholamine-secreting tumor. If elevated levels of catecholamines are detected, preoperative treatment with an α-blocker and β-blockade therapy during surgery are recommended. Magnetic resonance imaging (MRI), with and without gadolinium enhancement, provides excellent definition of the tumor and its relationship to both neural and vascular structures, particularly if there is intracranial extension. However, enhancement in the jugular foramen on MRI scans can occur with relatively static blood flow through a large jugular bulb in the absence of a tumor.[67] This enhancement can be erroneously interpreted as a glo-

mus jugulare tumor if MRI alone is used for diagnosis. Thin-section computed tomography (CT) is the preferred method for determining the extent of bony involvement.

Cerebral arteriography is useful for evaluating the tumor's blood supply, involvement of the internal carotid artery, and demonstration of the venous anatomy. It is important to know whether the sigmoid sinus and jugular bulb are occluded by the tumor, whether the opposite sigmoid sinus is patent, and whether there is communication across the torcular. Arteriography can also demonstrate an associated glomus vagale or carotid body tumor that is not seen on the CT or MRI scan. If sacrifice of the internal carotid artery is a possibility, arteriography combined with balloon test occlusion with cerebral blood flow studies can further evaluate collateral blood flow. In addition, the vascularity of the tumor and the potential for embolization can be assessed.

## Embolization

The use of preoperative embolization has been a major advance in the successful surgical management of glomus jugulare tumors.[18, 64, 68] Embolization has been shown to reduce operative blood loss, decrease the need for blood transfusion and shorten operating time.[30, 43, 56, 69] Preoperative embolization may increase the likelihood of complete tumor excision. In addition, embolization possibly decreases the incidence of postoperative cranial nerve palsy by improving visibility of the lower cranial nerves and by decreasing the need for bipolar coagulation in the region of the jugular foramen during tumor removal.

The main blood supply of glomus jugulare tumors is from the inferior tympanic branch of the ascending pharyngeal artery and the stylomastoid artery. The stylomastoid artery arises from the occipital artery in 60% of patients and from the posterior auricular artery in 40%.[29, 69] Occlusion of tumor vessels through these arteries is often the main goal of embolization. Large tumors may parasitize branches from either the internal carotid artery or the vertebral artery. Embolization of these vessels is advisable only in rare circumstances because of their small size and the risk of intracranial embolization. We have found that venous embolization of the inferior petrosal sinus and sigmoid sinus just upstream from the tumor can be performed in selective cases and may decrease venous bleeding during surgery.

## Surgery

The surgical management of glomus jugulare tumors has evolved gradually over the past 4 decades. Surgeons have been challenged by the tumor's rich vascularity, the complex regional anatomy, and the potential for injury to the carotid artery or lower cranial nerves. In the 1950s, radiation therapy alone or in combination with limited surgery became the preferred treatment because of the morbidity and mortality associated with radical surgery. Advances in neuroimaging in the 1960s led to better understanding of the tumor's size and anatomic location, which led to a renewed interest in surgical resection.

In 1964, Shapiro and Neues[53] established the general strategy for resecting a glomus jugulare tumor by combining a mastoidectomy with lateral skull base exposure through the neck. By rerouting the facial nerve, they were able to remove a tumor with minimal blood loss and no significant neurologic deficit. In the 1970s, the operating microscope, neuroanesthesia, and a better understanding of the surgical anatomy contributed to improved surgical results. Further refinements in technique led to the development of combined lateral skull base approaches[20, 22] and the infratemporal fossa approach,[17] both of which emphasized

exposure and control of the internal carotid artery. These approaches, with minor improvements, are the mainstays of surgical treatment today.

Although some authors continue to recommend radiation therapy as the initial treatment for all glomus jugulare tumors, we believe that in the young and middle-aged patients, the current definitive therapy is surgical. In elderly patients or those with major medical problems, we recommend radiosurgery or a "wait and see" policy.

In general, patients who present with complete ninth and tenth nerve palsy have compensated for this deficit because of its gradual onset. In our experience, these patients tolerate surgery extremely well. The patient with a large tumor and normal lower cranial nerve function, however, is more likely to have postoperative difficulty with swallowing and aspiration because of the acute onset of vagus nerve dysfunction.

## Surgical Approaches

The choice of surgical approach is based on the anatomic extent of the tumor and, to some extent, the patient's preoperative hearing function. A glomus tympanicum or glomus hypotympanicum tumor may be approached through the ear canal or mastoid, respectively. Glomus jugulare tumors require more extensive exposure and cannot be adequately approached through the mastoid alone.

### LATERAL SKULL-BASE APPROACH

The lateral skull-base approach is used for medium glomus jugulare tumors that extend up to the petrous portion of the internal carotid artery. After the induction of general anesthesia, with the patient supine, the head is turned away from the operative side. A retroauricular C-shaped incision is made that extends into the neck along the anterior border of the sternocleidomastoid muscle (Fig. 75–4). The greater auricular nerve is identified, divided, and tagged for reanastomosis or potential later use as a nerve graft. The ear canal is transected at the bony-cartilaginous junction. The ear canal skin is dissected off the ear canal cartilage and pulled out through the ear canal. It is then closed from the outside in an everted fashion with a running absorbable suture. A portion of the canal cartilage is removed from the membranous ear canal. Mastoid periosteum is then rotated over the opening of the ear canal and sutured down to complete a two-layer closure. An incision is then made in the periosteum of the skull, parallel and just inferior to the lower border of the temporalis muscle. A periosteal flap is then elevated inferiorly and kept in continuity with the sternocleidomastoid muscle as it is dissected off its attachment to the mastoid bone. This mastoid periosteal flap will be sewn to the inferior border of the temporalis muscle at the time of closure.

Attention is then turned to the neck. The internal carotid artery and adjacent cranial nerves are exposed medial to the sternocleidomastoid muscle. The facial vein must often be divided. The carotid bifurcation, external carotid artery, internal carotid artery, jugular vein, hypoglossal nerve, ansa hypoglossi, spinal accessory nerve, and vagus nerve are identified. The posterior belly of the digastric muscle is released from the digastric groove of the mastoid bone. If

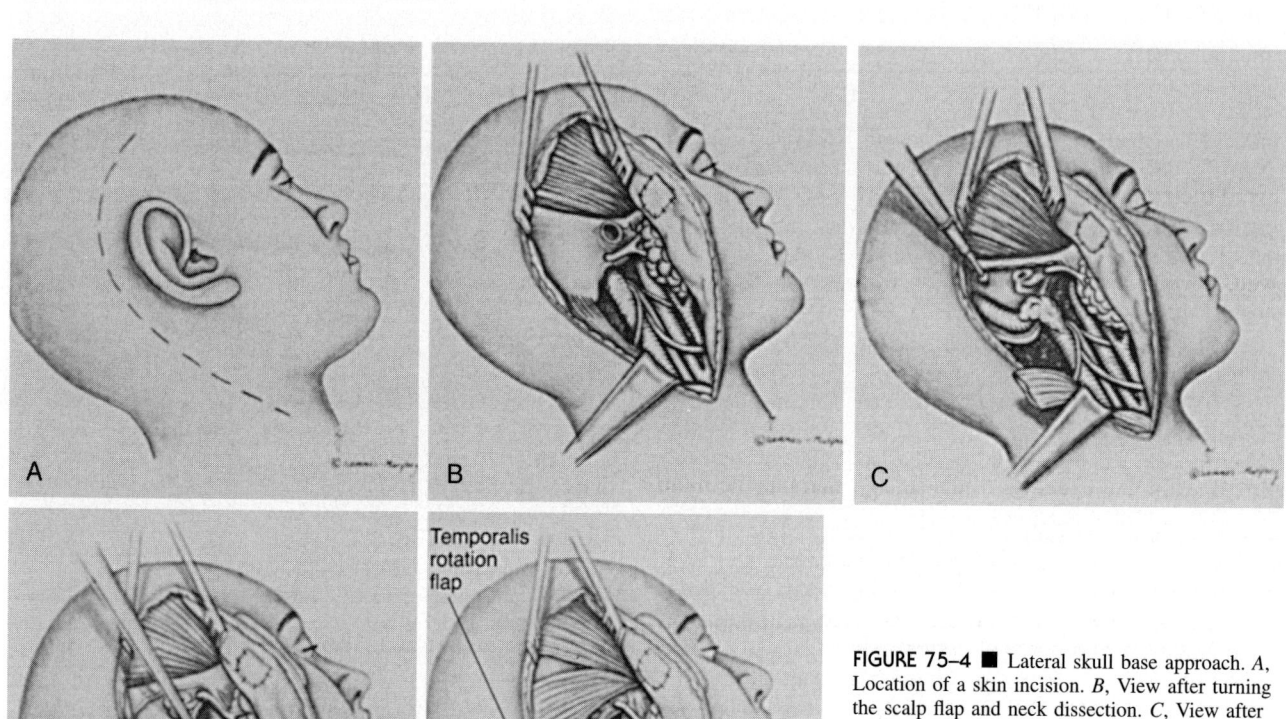

FIGURE 75–4 ■ Lateral skull base approach. *A,* Location of a skin incision. *B,* View after turning the scalp flap and neck dissection. *C,* View after the temporal bone dissection. *D,* Ligation of the sigmoid sinus and jugular vein with removal of the tumor. *E,* Reconstruction of the wound with fat packing and rotation of the temporalis muscle. (Copyright, © Semmes-Murphey Clinic.)

possible, the posterior belly of the digastric muscle and adjacent soft tissue are left attached to the soft tissue surrounding the facial nerve as it exits the stylomastoid foramen. This helps to preserve the facial nerve's blood supply and decreases the incidence of postoperative facial nerve paralysis. However, with large tumors, this muscle and attached soft tissue obstructs exposure and can be removed if necessary. The occipital artery is divided. The internal carotid artery and the jugular vein are dissected free of soft tissue and isolated. The distal styloid process and attached tendons are removed with a rongeur, and care is taken to protect the underlying internal carotid artery and ninth cranial nerve. The base of the styloid process is left in place at this point as a landmark. The glossopharyngeal nerve is identified. The transverse process of C1 lateral to the foramen transversaria can be removed to improve exposure if necessary. The soft tissue between the base of the skull and the transverse process of C1 is removed carefully in order to protect the underlying vertebral artery. The base of the styloid process is removed along with the soft tissue at the lateral edge of the jugular foramen.

A simple mastoidectomy is then performed with a high-speed drill and suction irrigation. Care is taken to avoid entering the semicircular canals or the cochlea unless sensorineural function has previously been destroyed by the tumor. The bone of the posterior aspect of the external auditory canal is removed. The tympanic membrane, malleus, and incus are removed after disarticulation of the

incostapedial joint. The mastoid and tympanic segments of the facial nerve are skeletonized. If possible, the facial nerve is left in a thin fallopian bridge.[46] Alternatively, the facial nerve can be drilled free of its bony canal from the geniculate ganglion to the stylomastoid foramen and transposed anterior and superior to the middle ear. This maneuver provides an unobstructed view of the tumor but essentially guarantees at least a temporary postoperative facial nerve paralysis. If the facial nerve was weak before surgery and is infiltrated by tumor, the involved portion of the nerve can be resected and grafted. If the facial nerve is transposed, it is placed proximally into a bony groove drilled into the epitympanum and distally into a groove in the substance of the parotid gland, as described by Fisch.[17]

The sigmoid sinus is then skeletonized, and the dura anterior and posterior to it is exposed. The bone of the lateral skull base between the digastric groove and the jugular foramen is removed.

The bony wall of the tympanum and hypotympanum is drilled away, exposing the petrous segment of the internal carotid artery. The eustachian tube is sealed with bone wax, fascia, and fibrin glue. The internal carotid artery is exposed from the neck to the horizontal segment in the petrous bone. The tumor is coagulated and mobilized inferiorly away from the carotid artery down toward the hypotympanum. Care is taken to avoid traumatizing the stapes.

The sigmoid sinus is then occluded in its descending portion above the tumor mass. This can be performed by packing Surgicel between the bone and the sigmoid sinus until the sigmoid sinus is occluded. Alternatively, the sigmoid sinus can be ligated with a 2–0 silk suture. Suture ligation, however, often violates the arachnoid and might increase the likelihood of CSF leak. The jugular vein is then ligated in the neck beyond the tumor extension. The lateral wall of the sigmoid sinus is then incised, and the inside of the sigmoid is packed with Surgicel down toward the jugular bulb. The lateral wall of the sigmoid is removed from the point of sinus occlusion down to the tumor. Typically, there is a preserved plane of dissection between the tumor and the medial wall of the jugular bulb. Bleeding from the inferior petrosal sinus or occipital sinus is controlled by packing with Surgicel. Care should be taken to avoid bipolar coagulation and excessive pressure on the Surgicel, because this force will be transmitted to the underlying cranial nerves. The tumor is then removed by working circumferentially in the plane between the tumor and the lower cranial nerves. The tumor cavity is inspected, and any remaining tumor remnants are removed. The dura of the posterior cranial fossa must be removed if it is in contact with tumor. The dural defect is closed with a graft of pericranium or temporalis fascia.

All remaining remnants of mastoid mucosa are drilled away, and the mastoid cavity is packed with fat and covered by downward rotation of the posterior temporalis muscle and upward mobilization of the previously prepared sternocleidomastoid-periosteal flap. The skin edges are closed in layers, and a Hemovac drain is placed if the dura was not violated. A spinal drain is placed at the end of the procedure if a dural graft was required.

### MODIFIED LATERAL SKULL-BASE APPROACH

In selected patients with relatively small tumors and good preoperative hearing, an attempt at preservation of middle ear function is reasonable.[23] The skin incision and cervical dissection proceeds as described for the lateral skull base approach. A mastoidectomy is performed, but in this case the posterior bony canal wall, tympanic membrane, and ossicles are preserved (Fig. 75–5). The tympanic segment of the facial nerve is left in place, and only the mastoid segment is mobilized. Alternatively, the facial nerve can be preserved in a thin canal of bone known as the fallopian bridge technique as described by Pensak and Jackler.[46] The facial nerve is not transposed but may be moved 1 cm forward and back during tumor removal. The tumor is mobilized out of the middle ear mainly through the facial recess. Tumor removal then proceeds as described for the lateral skull-base approach.

### INFRATEMPORAL FOSSA APPROACH

The development of the infratemporal fossa approach by Fisch has been a significant advance in the resection of large tumors.[17, 18] This approach is similar to the lateral skull-base approach, but the exposure is carried further in front of the ear canal into the infratemporal fossa. With this exposure, the bone over the glenoid fossa is removed, and the internal carotid artery is exposed from its extracranial portion up to the cavernous sinus (Fig. 75–6). The base of the skull can be removed anteriorly up to the

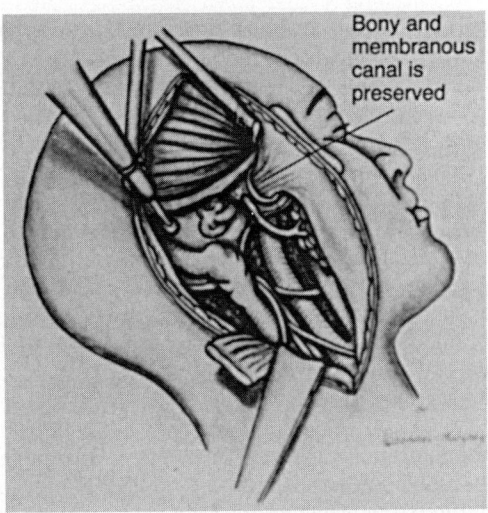

**FIGURE 75–5 ■** Surgical exposure with maintenance of the external auditory canal—the so-called canal wall-up approach. The facial nerve is only partially mobilized in its mastoid segment. (Copyright © Semmes-Murphey Clinic.)

foramen ovale or, with sectioning of this nerve, up to the foramen rotundum.

### INTRACRANIAL EXTENSION

Intracranial extension can be removed from a retrosigmoid, presigmoid retrolabyrinthine, translabyrinthine, or transcochlear approach, depending on the size and location of the tumor.

## Radiation

The role of radiation therapy in the management of glomus jugulare tumors remains controversial. No prospective controlled trial comparing radiation therapy with surgery has

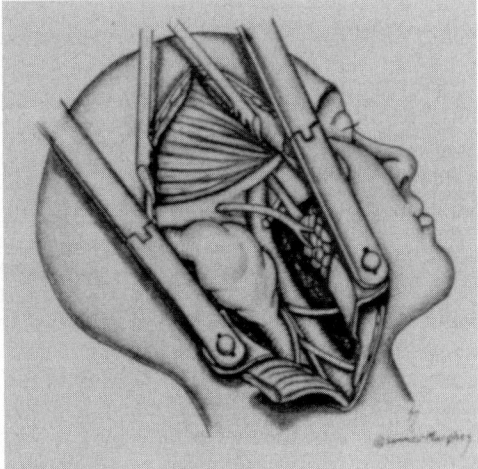

**FIGURE 75–6 ■** Infratemporal fossa approach with removal of the glenoid fossa, the floor of the middle cranial fossa, and complete release of the internal carotid artery from the petrous bone. The eustachian tube and the third division of the trigeminal nerve are visible. (Copyright © Semmes-Murphey Clinic.)

been performed to date. Long-term tumor control has been reported by many authors,[7, 10, 16, 38, 58, 66] although recurrence after radiation therapy is not rare.[21, 54, 55, 57] We use radiation therapy as the primary treatment modality in elderly patients with symptomatic tumors and in middle-aged patients with medical problems that substantially increase the risk of surgery. We have also employed postoperative radiation therapy for the rare case of subtotal tumor removal.

The argument against radiation therapy is primarily that the patient is not cured of the disease, and if the tumor recurs years or decades later, the morbidity of surgery in an irradiated field is thought to be increased. Radiation-induced osteonecrosis of the temporal bone has been reported rarely after conventional radiation[47] but probably will not be seen with radiosurgery. The development of new radiation induced neoplasms is often mentioned as a risk of radiation but is probably rare. Glomus jugulare tumors rarely decrease in size following radiation therapy and lack of growth is considered to indicate successful treatment.[38, 58, 66]

In 1997, Foote and colleagues reported on the use of stereotactic radiosurgery for nine patients with glomus tumors with an average of 20 months of follow-up.[19] In eight of the nine patients, the tumor remained stable in size. In one of the nine patients, the tumor decreased in size. However, none of the tumors enlarged with follow-up ranging from 7 to 65 months. In addition, seven of the nine patients reported a subjective decrease in symptoms, and there was no acute or chronic toxicity. In 1998, Liscak and associates reported on the use of Leksell Gamma knife radiosurgery for 14 patients with glomus jugulare and tympanicum tumors.[39] Eleven patients were available for follow-up ranging between 6 and 42 months, with an average of 20.5 months. Four of the 11 patients showed a decrease in tumor volume, but seven patients showed no change. Five of the 11 patients reported a decrease in symptoms. However, three patients had a further impairment in hearing, and two patients required a second radiosurgery treatment for infrabasal spread of tumor that was not delineated on the preoperative CT scan. Radiosurgery planning with MRI might eliminate this problem. The effectiveness of radiosurgery for the symptom of pulsatile tinnitus is not well known. In the series of Liscak and colleagues,[39] angiography was performed on follow up in three patients. One patient showed no pathologic vascularity at 1 year after radiosurgery. The other two patients had either a partial decrease or no effect on pathologic tumor vascularity at 12 months and 22 months, respectively. Tumor embolization followed by radiosurgery may prove to be effective for controlling pulsatile tinnitus.

Histologic studies of previously irradiated glomus tumors have concluded that the tumor cells appear unaffected by the irradiation. The primary effect of radiation is thought to be vascular injury.[8, 28] In addition, catecholamine secretion has not been shown to be affected by radiation therapy.[51] The primary argument against surgery is the risk of lower cranial nerve palsy with dysphagia and subsequent aspiration. In general, radiation therapy has not been shown to induce lower cranial nerve injury.

## COMPLICATIONS OF SURGERY

Complications after surgery for glomus jugulare tumors are mainly a function of the tumor's size, vascularity, and anatomic location, combined with the patient's preoperative condition, the surgeon's skill, and the choice of surgical approach. Complications can be minimized by proper patient selection, excellent surgical technique and knowledge of regional anatomy. Preoperative embolization can decrease intraoperative blood loss. This both aids in visualization of vital neurovascular structures and decreases the need for electrocautery around the lower cranial nerves as they pass through the jugular foramen. The major complications following surgery for glomus jugulare tumors are as follows:

- Cranial nerve injury
- Wound healing or CSF leak
- Bleeding or vascular injury
- Infection or meningitis

Other complications are catecholamine secretion, eustachian tube dysfunction, trismus, deep vein thrombosis with or without pulmonary embolism, and associated medical problems.

### Cranial Nerve Injury

Cranial nerve preservation after surgery is directly related to surgical technique, unless the tumor has invaded a specific cranial nerve. One would expect that a benign tumor would merely compress cranial nerves, but in a retrospective review of 83 patients with glomus temporale tumors, Makek and colleagues[40] detected neural infiltration in 30 of the tumors reviewed. They concluded that as tumor size increased, cranial nerve invasion increased as well. In addition, normal nerve function before surgery did not rule out the possibility of finding neural invasion at surgery.

The cranial nerves most commonly affected by the growth of glomus jugulare tumors are the facial nerve and the lower cranial nerves (IX, X, XI, and XII). If the facial nerve is normal preoperatively, good function can be expected if tumor removal can be accomplished without transposition of the facial nerve. In moderate to large tumors, however, transposition of the facial nerve often results in a temporary paralysis, probably owing to interruption of the nerve's blood supply in the tympanic and mastoid segments. In 1994, Green and associates reported good recovery of facial nerve function (House grades I to VI or II to VI) in 95% of patients in a series of 52 patients with previously untreated patients with glomus jugulare tumors.[25]

If neural invasion of the facial nerve is evident, resection of the involved segment is necessary, with reconstruction by end-to-end anastomosis of the remaining facial nerve or use of an interposition nerve graft. If the proximal stump of the facial nerve is lost at surgery, which might occur with a large intracranial extension, then an early hypoglossal to facial anastomosis should be considered if the hypoglossal nerve has functional integrity.

Postoperative facial nerve palsy should be managed aggressively with eye lubricants, an eye patch, and consideration of gold weight insertion in the upper lid or lateral canthoplasty. In most cases, satisfactory recovery of the facial nerve occurs if continuity of the facial nerve was maintained at surgery.

Lower cranial nerve palsies are potentially the most

serious complication after surgery for glomus jugulare tumors. A complete injury to the vagus nerve near the skull base is probably the least well tolerated. In a review of the subject, Tucker[63] pointed out that an acute vagal palsy at the skull base results in dysfunction of the entire upper aerodigestive tract, including airway control, swallowing, and phonation. Paralysis of the palate combined with some loss of pharyngeal sensation causes incoordination of swallowing, because the pharyngeal muscles fail to contract properly in combination with relaxation of the cricopharyngeus muscles. This may result in repeated aspiration with subsequent pneumonia and can be fatal if not promptly recognized and treated effectively. The aggregate loss of function of multiple lower cranial nerves may compound the risk of aspiration and, even if incomplete, may result in considerable short-term morbidity.

Injury to the lower cranial nerves can be minimized by not using cautery around the nerves as they pass medial to the tumor in the jugular foramen. In addition, Surgicel packing of the orifices of the inferior petrosal sinus must be performed carefully to avoid injury to the underlying cranial nerves. We think that preoperative embolization decreases intraoperative blood loss, improves visualization, and minimizes the need for electrocautery around the lower cranial nerves.

A patient with an acute postoperative vagal palsy should be evaluated by swallowing studies. If aspiration is present, early placement of a percutaneous endoscopic gastrostomy (PEG) tube should be considered. The patient should have hand-held suctioning devices available to assist in the control of saliva. Swelling of the vocal cords in the immediate postoperative period due to the endotracheal tube may sometimes mask an underlying vocal cord paralysis. As the swelling of the vocal cord resolves, the patient develops problems with hoarse voice and aspiration. Tracheostomy may be required in some patients, but because it further impairs swallowing function by limiting the upward movement of the larynx, we often try to avoid it. If the vagus nerve was preserved at surgery and recovery is expected in time, Gelfoam may be injected into the vocal cord to temporarily improve the patient's voice and cough. If unilateral vagus nerve function is permanently lost, a more permanent medialization of the vocal cord may be accomplished by either injecting Teflon or by performing a laryngoplasty.[45]

Most patients compensate for unilateral lower cranial nerve injury in 1 to 4 months. Persistent nasal regurgitation of food may be corrected with a palatoplasty, in which the paralyzed segment of the soft palate is unilaterally sutured to the posterior pharyngeal wall. Persistent dysphagia with recurrent aspiration despite vocal cord augmentation may on rare occasions require a cricopharyngeal myotomy.

Refinements in surgical technique and the successful management of lower cranial nerve palsies has decreased the morbidity associated with the surgical treatment of glomus jugulare tumors. In 1991, Jackson and colleagues[33] reported long-term follow-up on cranial nerve preservation in 100 patients with lesions of the jugular foramen, including 59 patients with glomus jugulare tumors. In their report, patients with small tumors had excellent cranial nerve preservation, and excellent long-term functional recovery was reported in cases in which cranial nerve sacrifice was

needed for tumor removal. On the basis of these data, Jackson and colleagues[33] concluded that the morbidity of cranial nerve loss associated with lateral skull-base surgery does not support the use of radiation therapy as the primary treatment of lesions of the jugular fossa, particularly small tumors.

In 1996, Jackson and colleagues reported on the success of attempts to preserve hearing during surgery for glomus jugulare tumors.[34] In a series of 122 patients with glomus jugulare tumors treated for 24 years, hearing conservation was attempted in 41 patients. Hearing preservation was successful in 38 patients (93%). In six cases (14.6%), hearing actually improved.

## Wound Healing and Cerebrospinal Fluid Leakage

Impaired wound healing after surgery for a glomus jugulare tumor may occur as the result of poor surgical technique, malnutrition, multiple medical problems, prolonged use of steroids, or previous radiation therapy. If a patient is malnourished preoperatively, surgery should be delayed until the nutritional status is normal. In all patients, nutrition should be resumed within several days of surgery. Patients with lower cranial nerve dysfunction and dysphagia often require tube feedings to maintain their nutritional status.

The prevention of cerebrospinal fluid (CSF) leakage depends on closure and healing of the surgical wound together with maintenance of normal intracranial CSF pressure. Small glomus jugulare tumors can often be removed with the dura intact. Adequate removal of large tumors often results in a large dural defect, which at the level of the jugular foramen can be difficult to close. Obliteration of the mastoid cavity with adipose tissue or by rotating the temporalis muscle downward is essential. In addition, careful closure of the external auditory ear canal along with sealing off of the eustachian tube is mandatory. CSF leakage may occur directly through the incision, through the external auditory canal, or down the eustachian tube into the oropharynx. A postoperative CSF leak may be detected by the Dandy maneuver, in which the patient is examined in the sitting position with the head held forward below the waistline for several minutes; CSF should drip out the nostril if a leak is present.

The intracranial CSF dynamics are often altered in the postoperative period by contamination with blood, bone dust, and the ensuing inflammatory reaction. This impairment in reabsorption of CSF in the early postoperative period may result in elevated CSF pressures and a secondary CSF leak. The use of continuous lumbar CSF drainage for several days after surgery allows for the CSF to clear and maintains a normal CSF pressure during the early stages of wound healing.

## Bleeding and Vascular Injury

The excessive bleeding encountered by earlier surgeons in their attempts to remove glomus jugulare tumors was one of the major factors that led to either limited surgery combined with radiation therapy or radiation therapy alone as the primary treatment of these lesions. The major blood supply of small to medium-sized glomus jugulare tumors is the tympanic branch of the ascending pharyngeal artery. Large tumors, however, may receive a large blood supply from other branches of the external carotid artery, the vertebrobasilar system, or the vasa vasorum of the internal carotid artery. Embolization has decreased the blood loss associated with operative excision, shortened operating time and we believe decreased the incidence of cranial nerve deficits. Small tumors whose blood supply is derived solely from the external carotid artery can be almost completely devascularized by embolization. Large tumors with blood supply from the vasa vasorum of the petrous segment of the internal carotid artery or from the vertebrobasilar system cannot be fully devascularized, because these vessels are often too small to catheterize and embolization carries an unacceptable risk of stroke.

Injury to the internal carotid artery may be life threatening if not managed appropriately. Proximal and distal control of the internal carotid artery must be secured before the tumor is dissected off the internal carotid artery. Patients with large tumors that encase the internal carotid artery should be evaluated with a preoperative internal carotid artery balloon occlusion test and either SPECT scanning or Xenon cerebral blood flow testing. If an adequate collateral cerebral circulation is present, there is some assurance (although not definitive) that carotid sacrifice will be tolerated. If balloon occlusion test is not tolerated; however, the surgeon must be prepared to perform interposition saphenous vein grafting or an extracranial-intracranial (EC-IC) bypass to the middle cerebral artery.

## Infection and Meningitis

Infections occurring with glomus jugulare tumor surgery are rare despite the extensive dissection, long duration of surgery, and potential for CSF leak. The presence of CSF leak, fever, elevated white blood cell count, changes in mentation, or signs of meningeal irritation should alert the surgeon to the possibility of meningitis. If meningitis is suspected, CSF should be obtained for the appropriate studies, and broad-spectrum CSF penetrating antibiotics should be started.

## Miscellaneous Complications

A few glomus jugulare tumors may produce and secrete catecholamines. Surgical manipulation of these tumors may produce surges in blood pressure as catecholamines are released. This may be prevented by preoperatively screening for excess catecholamine production and by treating patients found to have catecholamine secretion with α- and β-blockers preoperatively, as stated earlier in this chapter.

A history of previous bleeding problems should be thoroughly investigated because of the highly vascular nature of this neoplasm. In addition, medications with antiplatelet activity (e.g., aspirin) should be avoided during the week before surgery. The risk of lower extremity deep venous thrombosis can be minimized by the use of venous com-

### TABLE 75–1 ■ TREATMENT OF GLOMUS JUGULARE TUMORS AT UNIVERSITY OF TENNESSEE, MEMPHIS (1970–1998)

| Treatment | Glomus Jugulare | Glomus Tympanicum | Glomus Vagale | Total |
|---|---|---|---|---|
| Surgery alone | 31 | 30 | 4 | 65 |
| Surgery + preoperative radiation therapy | 7 | 0 | 0 | 7 |
| Surgery + postoperative radiation therapy | 4 | 0 | 0 | 4 |
| Radiation therapy only | 15 | 1 | 0 | 16 |
| No treatment | 5 | 5 | 1 | 11 |
| *Total* | 62 | 36 | 5 | 103 |

pression devices and early postoperative mobilization. Subcutaneous heparin is initiated on the first postoperative day. Catheterization of the veins of the neck or the contralateral subclavian vein is avoided because of the risk of thrombosis together with the fact that one jugular vein will be ligated during surgery.

Eustachian tube dysfunction may occur in patients with small tumors in whom the middle ear is preserved. This may result in serous otitis media, which can be managed with decongestants and antibiotics if needed. On occasion, a ventilation tube is required for definitive treatment if there is no evidence of CSF behind the tympanic membrane.

In patients with large glomus jugulare tumors encasing the internal carotid artery or extending up to the foramen lacerum, exposure of the infratemporal fossa is necessary. This can be accomplished by anteriorly dislocating the mandible. Early assessment by an oral surgeon to determine proper dental occlusion and an aggressive exercise program to increase range of motion is mandatory.

## UNIVERSITY OF TENNESSEE EXPERIENCE

Table 75–1 summarizes the cases of glomus tumors treated at University of Tennessee, Memphis, from 1970 to 1998.

## CASE REPORTS

### Case Report 1

***Typical Glomus Jugulare Tumor in a Young Patient***
A 24-year-old man developed right-sided pulsatile tinnitus and hearing loss. Physical findings were normal other than a red mass visible behind the right tympanic membrane. An MRI scan of the head with contrast showed a 3-cm enhancing mass enlarging the right jugular foramen and extending into the middle ear, consistent with a glomus jugulare tumor (Fig. 75-7). A cerebral arteriogram confirmed the typical vascular pattern of a glomus jugulare tumor and was followed by embolization.

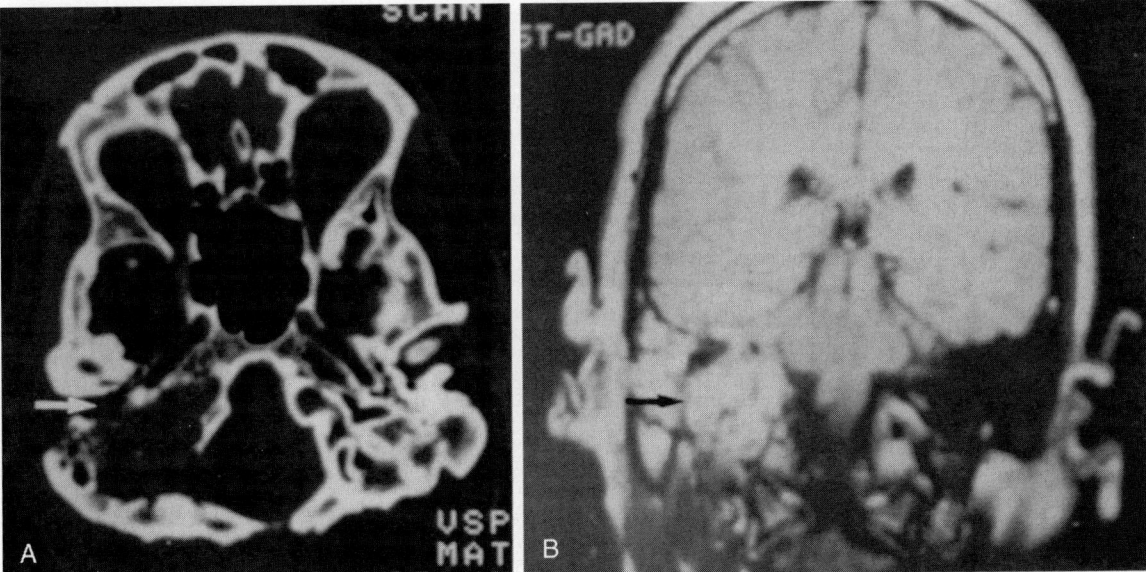

**FIGURE 75–7** ■ *A,* An axial computed tomography scan showing extensive bone destruction in the bone surrounding the jugular foramen in Patient 1 *(arrow). B,* A coronal-enhanced $T_1$-weighted magnetic resonance imaging scan of the head in the same patient, demonstrating a glomus jugulare tumor extending out from the jugular foramen *(arrow).*

Two days after the embolization, the patient was taken to surgery for a combined lateral skull-base approach and excision of the tumor. The mastoid segment of the facial nerve was found to be infiltrated by tumor over a 1-cm length. This segment of the facial nerve was resected, and through mobilization of the facial nerve from the geniculate ganglion to the soft tissue beyond the stylomastoid foramen, a primary facial nerve end-to-end anastomosis was performed. The tumor was found adjacent to, but not encasing, the petrous internal carotid artery and was carefully removed. Nonadherent, intraluminal tumor extension was found in the right transverse sinus as well as in the superior and inferior petrosal sinus. Resection of tumor after ligation of the upper sigmoid sinus and rostral jugular vein was accomplished with preservation of all lower cranial nerves.

The patient was neurologically intact after surgery, except for an immediate complete right facial palsy. A gold weight was placed in the right eyelid to assist in eye closure. The patient was discharged home on postoperative day 10. During the year after surgery, he returned to active employment in a lumber mill. Right facial nerve function returned but he had facial asymmetry and synkinesis when he smiled.

## Case Report 2

### Glomus Jugulare Tumor in a 64-Year-Old Patient

A 64-year-old woman presented with several months of left hearing loss, a hoarse voice, tinnitus, mild swallowing difficulty, and posterior occipital neck pain. On physical examination, she had left sensorineural hearing loss and a left vocal cord paralysis. An MRI scan showed a 2.5 × 3 cm left jugular foramen mass (Fig. 75–8). An arteriogram showed a vascular tumor in the left jugular foramen with occlusion of the left jugular bulb consistent with a left glomus

jugulare tumor. She was treated with Gamma knife radiosurgery. A follow-up MRI scan 2 years after radiosurgery treatment showed that the tumor was stable in size. Her headache and neck pain resolved. She denied tinnitus, and her voice was slightly less hoarse.

## Case Report 3

### Patient with a Hormone-Secreting Glomus Jugulare Tumor

A 35-year-old woman presented with a 3-month history of left-sided hearing loss and chronic hoarseness. She denied difficulty with swallowing. On physical examination, a red mass was visible behind the left tympanic membrane. She had a complete left 10th, 11th, and 12th cranial nerve palsy. A CT scan of the head showed a large mass in the region of the left jugular foramen with extension into the posterior fossa (Fig. 75–9). A biopsy performed through the ear canal confirmed the diagnosis of a glomus jugulare tumor. Each manipulation of the tumor during the biopsy resulted in a brief but marked rise in the systolic blood pressure. Measurements of 24-hour urinary catecholamines were elevated both before and 1 week after the biopsy. The patient was treated with 4500 Gy of preoperative radiation therapy in an attempt to decrease the tumor's vascularity. (This patient was treated prior to the availability of embolization.)

Four months after the radiation treatment, the patient was admitted and received 3 days of phentolamine and a long-acting β-blocker therapy. The large left glomus jugulare tumor was removed via the lateral skull-base approach combined with a tracheostomy and a tarsorrhaphy. Tumor manipulation did not produce significant changes in blood pressure. Although surgery was well tolerated, a CSF leak developed

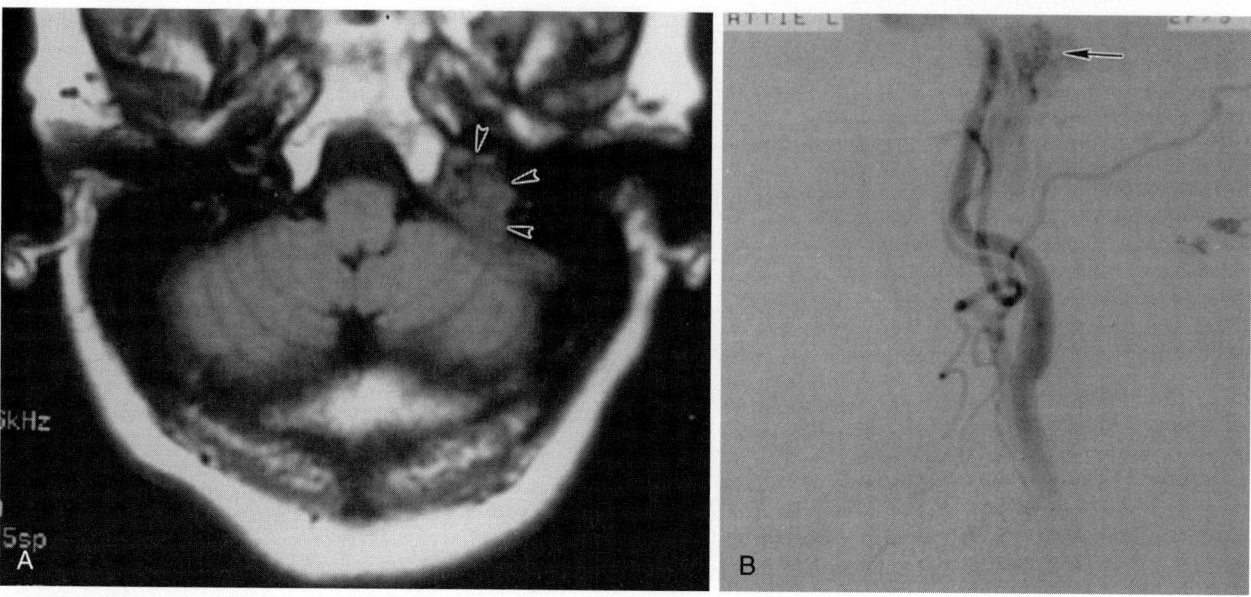

FIGURE 75–8 ■ *A*, Axial T$_1$-weighted magnetic resonance imaging scan in Patient 2, showing a left glomus jugulare tumor *(arrowheads)*. *B*, Lateral view of a left common carotid arteriogram showing the tumor blush in the jugular foramen *(arrow)*.

3 weeks postoperatively through an area of necrosis along the postauricular portion of the incision. This was treated successfully with débridement and primary closure.

Teflon injection of the left vocal cord was performed 1 month after tumor resection to help prevent aspiration and improve voice quality. The tracheostomy was removed. The patient returned to normal physical activities and has done well over the past 10 years, with mild facial asymmetry, left-sided hearing loss, and compensated left lower cranial nerve loss. Because of the complication associated with radiation therapy and the development of embolization techniques,

preoperative radiation therapy was abandoned after this case.

## Case Report 4

### Patient with Multiple Glomus Tumors

A 26-year-old woman presented with complaints of left-sided hearing loss, tinnitus, headache, intermittent dizziness, and an enlarging left anterior cervical mass. Three of her six siblings have had glomus tumors. An MRI scan and cerebral angiography showed bilateral carotid body, glomus vagale, and glomus jugulare tumors (Fig. 75–10). The tumors involving the left neck and jugular fossa were larger

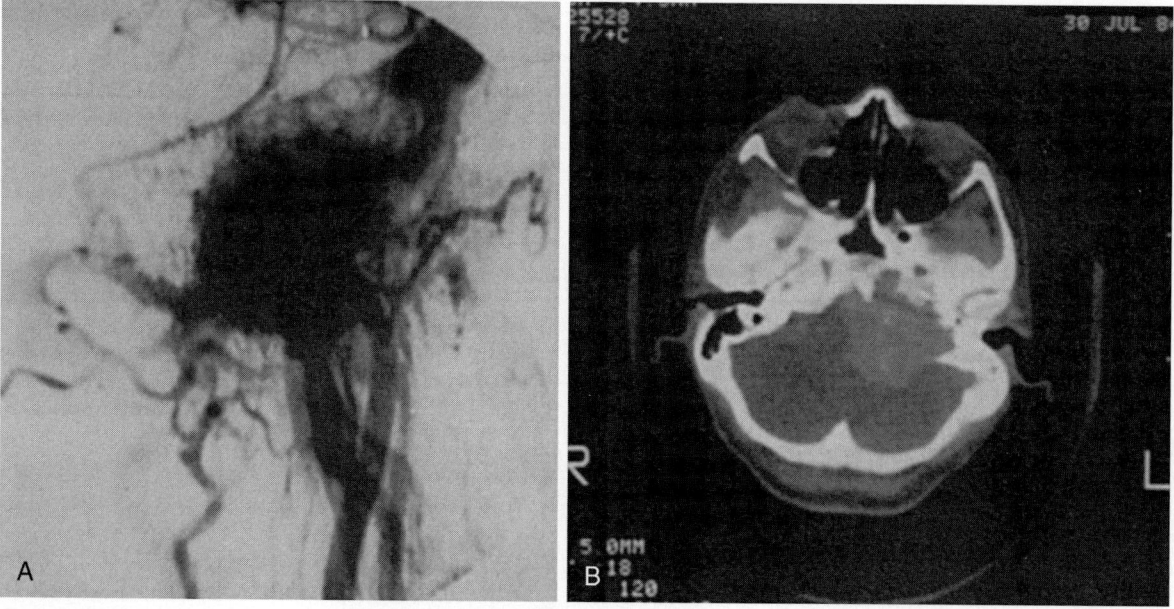

FIGURE 75–9 ■ A carotid angiogram and an axial computed tomography scan showing a large left glomus jugulare tumor with posterior fossa extension.

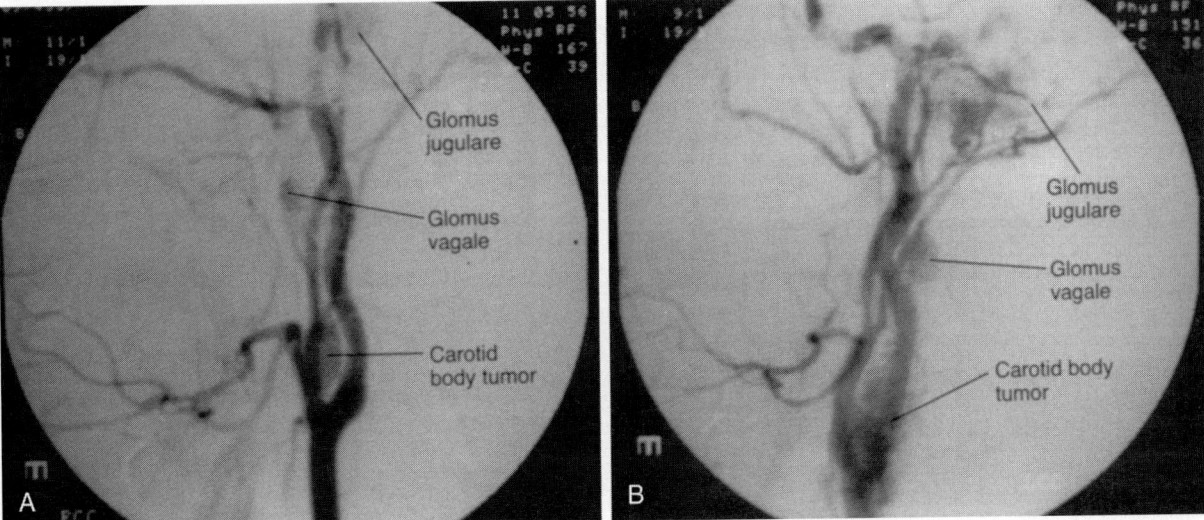

**FIGURE 75–10** ■ Right *(A)* and left *(B)* common carotid arteriograms in Patient 4 demonstrating bilateral carotid body tumors, glomus vagale tumors, and glomus jugulare tumors.

than those on the right. General physical examination showed a mobile, nontender mass of 3 to 4 cm in the left midcervical region anterior to the sternocleido-mastoid muscle. Neurologic examination was remarkable for mild left facial weakness and left-sided hearing loss. Embolization of the tumors on the left side was performed, followed by operative excision of all three of the left-sided glomus tumors. The mastoid segment of the facial nerve was encased by tumor, requiring excision of a 3-cm segment of the nerve; this was repaired by an interposition nerve graft using the greater occipital nerve. The lower cranial nerves were all anatomically preserved. Postoperatively, the patient had a complete left facial palsy and a partial left vagal palsy. A gold weight was implanted in the left eyelid to augment closure. The patient was able to tolerate oral feedings by postoperative day 7 without aspiration and was discharged home on postoperative day 10.

Ten months later, the patient had partial return of facial nerve function but an incomplete left vagus nerve palsy and left hearing loss remained. Surgical excision of the remaining three glomus tumors was considered, and cerebral arteriography with embolization was performed. Arteriography showed patency of the right sigmoid-jugular vein system, which was providing the major venous outflow of the brain. Because of the risk of bilateral vagal nerve dysfunction and the fear of complications related to taking the dominant right sigmoid-jugular venous drainage, it was elected to resect only the right carotid body tumor and to treat the smaller right glomus vagale and right glomus jugulare tumors with radiation therapy. Two years after initiating treatment, the patient remains independent in all activities and is employed. Clinically, she has mild facial asymmetry, left hearing loss, and compensated vagal nerve function.

This patient may have benefitted from a sigmoid sinus to jugular vein bypass on the left at the time of her first surgery. This technique has been reported by Sekhar.[52]

## SUMMARY

Glomus jugulare tumors are uncommon, slow growing, and locally invasive. The tumor is thought to arise from glomus tissue in the region of the jugular bulb. The most common presenting symptom is hearing loss with pulsatile tinnitus. In a few patients, the disease may be familial or multiple. In rare cases, the tumor can metastasize. The relevant surgical anatomy is compact and complex. Preoperative embolization decreases the difficulty of surgical excision. In healthy patients, the primary treatment should be surgical excision, although patients who are elderly or have major medical problems may benefit from radiation therapy or a "wait and see" policy.

## REFERENCES

1. Azzarelli B, Felten S, Muller J, et al: Dopamine in paragangliomas of the glomus jugulare. Laryngoscope 98:573–578, 1988.
2. Balatsouras DG, Eliopoulos PN, Economou CN: Multiple glomus tumors. J Laryngol Otol 106:538–543, 1992.
3. Bhansali SA, Bojrab DI, Zarbo RJ: Malignant paragangliomas of the head and neck: Clinical and immunohistochemical characterization. Otolaryngol Head Neck Surg 104:132, 1991.
4. Bickerstaff ER, Howell JS: The neurological importance of tumors of the glomus jugulare. Brain 76:576–592, 1953.
5. Blumenfeld JD, Cohen N, Laragh JH, Ruggiero DA: Hypertension and catecholamine biosynthesis associated with a glomus jugulare tumor (Letter). N Engl J Med 327:894, 1992.
6. Bojrab DI, Bhansali SA, Glasscock ME: Metastatic glomus jugulare: Long-term followup. Otolaryngol Head Neck Surg 104:261–264, 1991.
7. Boyle JO, Shimm DS, Coulthard SW: Radiation therapy for paragangliomas of the temporal bone. Laryngoscope 100:896–901, 1990.
8. Brackmann DE, House WF, Terry R, et al: Glomus jugulare tumors: Effect of radiation. Trans Am Acad Ophthalmol Otolaryngol 76:1423–1431, 1972.

9. Brown JS: Glomus jugulare tumors revisited: A ten year statistical follow-up of 231 cases. Laryngoscope 95:284–288, 1985.
10. Cole JM, Beiler D: Long-term results of treatment of glomus jugulare and glomus vagale tumors with radiotherapy. Laryngoscope 104:1461–1465, 1994.
11. Davis JM, Davis KR, Hesselink JR, et al: Malignant glomus jugulare tumor: A case with two unusual radiographic features. J Comput Assist Tomogr 4:415–417, 1980.
12. Di Chiro G, Fisher RL, Nelson KB: The jugular foramen. J Neurosurg 21:447–460, 1964.
13. Dinges S, Budach V, Stuschke M, et al: Malignant paragangliomas: The results of radiotherapy in 6 patients. Strahlenther Onkol 169:114–120, 1993.
14. El Finky FM, Paparella MM: A metastatic glomus jugulare tumor: A temporal bone report. Am J Otol 5:197–200, 1984.
15. Farrior J: Surgical management of glomus tumors: Endocrine-active tumors of the skull base. South Med J 81:1121–1126, 1988.
16. Ferrara P, Cimino A, Tortorici M: Role of radiation therapy in glomus tumor. Am J Otol 8:390–395, 1987.
17. Fisch U: Infratemporal fossa approach for extensive tumors of the temporal bone and base of the skull. In Silverstein H, Norrell H (eds): Neurological Surgery of the Ear. Birmingham, AL: Aesculapius, 1977, pp 34–53.
18. Fisch U, Mattox D (eds): Microsurgery of the Skull Base. Stuttgart: Thieme Medical Publishers, 1988.
19. Foote RL, Coffey RJ, Gorman DA, et al: Stereotactic radiosurgery for glomus jugulare tumors: A preliminary report. Int J Radiat Oncol Biol Phys 38:491–495, 1997.
20. Gardner G, Cocke EW, Robertson JT, et al: Combined approach to surgery for removal of glomus jugulare tumors. Laryngoscope 87:665–688, 1977.
21. Gibbins KP, Henk JM: Glomus jugulare tumors in South Wales: A twenty year review. Clin Radiol 29:607–609, 1978.
22. Glasscock ME, Harris PF: Glomus tumors: Diagnosis, classification, and management of large lesions. Arch Otolaryngol 108:401–410, 1982.
23. Glasscock ME, Harris PF, Newsome G: Glomus tumors: Diagnosis and treatment. Laryngoscope 84:2006–2032, 1974.
24. Graham MD: The jugular bulb: Its anatomic and clinical considerations in contemporary otology. Arch Otolaryngol 101:560–564, 1975.
25. Green JD, Brackman DE, Nguyen CD, et al: Surgical management of previously untreated glomus jugulare tumors. Laryngoscope 104:917–921, 1994.
26. Guild SR: A hitherto unrecognized structure: The glomus jugularis in man. Anat Rec 79 (Suppl 2):28–107, 1941.
27. Guild SR: Glomus jugulare in man. Ann Otol Rhinol Laryngol 62:1045–1071, 1953.
28. Hawthorne MR, Makek MS, Harris JP, Fisch U: The histopathological and clinical features of irradiated and nonirradiated temporal paragangliomas. Laryngoscope 98:325–331, 1988.
29. Hekster REM, Luyendijk W, Matricali B: Transfemoral catheter embolization: A method of treatment of glomus jugulare tumors. Neuroradiology 5:208–214, 1973.
30. Hilal SK, Michelsen JW: Therapeutic percutaneous embolization for extra-axial vascular lesions of the head, neck, and spine. J Neurosurg 43:275–287, 1975.
31. Hovelaque A: Osteologie, Vol 2. Paris: G Doin, 1934, pp 155–156.
32. Jackson CG, Cueva RA, Thedinger BA, Glasscock ME: Conservation surgery for glomus jugulare tumors: The value of early diagnosis. Laryngoscope 100:1031–1036, 1990.
33. Jackson CG, Cueva RA, Thedinger BA, Glasscock ME: Cranial nerve preservation in lesions of the jugular fossa. Otolaryngol Head Neck Surg 105:687–693, 1991.
34. Jackson CG, Haynes DS, Walker PA, et al: Hearing conservation in surgery for glomus jugulare tumors. Am J Otol 17:425–437, 1996.
35. Johnston F, Symon L: Malignant paraganglioma of the glomus jugulare: A case report. Br J Neurosurg 6:255–259, 1992.
36. Krause W: Die glandula tympanica des menschen. Zentralbl Med Wiss 16:737–739, 1878.
37. Kremer R, Michel RP, Posner B, et al: Case report: Catecholamine-secreting paraganglioma of glomus jugulare region. Am J Med Sci 297:46–48, 1989.
38. Larner JM, Hahn SS, Spaulding CA, Constable WC: Glomus jugulare tumors: Long-term control by radiation therapy. Cancer 69:1813–1817, 1992.
39. Liscak R, Vladyka V, Simonova G, et al: Leksell gamma knife radiosurgery of the tumor glomus jugulare and tympanicum. Stereotact Funct Neurosurg 70(Suppl 1):152–160, 1998.
40. Makek M, Franklin DJ, Zhao JC, Fisch U: Neural infiltration of glomus temporale tumors. Am J Otol 11:1–5, 1990.
41. Matishak MZ, Symon L, Cheeseman A, Pamphlett R: Catecholamine-secreting paragangliomas of the base of the skull. J Neurosurg 66:604–608, 1987.
42. McCabe BF, Fletcher M: Selection of therapy of glomus jugulare tumors. Arch Otolaryngol 89:182–185, 1969.
43. Murphy TP, Brackmann DE: Effects of preoperative embolization on glomus jugulare tumors. Laryngoscope 99:1244–1247, 1989.
44. Nelson MD, Kendall BE: Intracranial catecholamine secreting paragangliomas. Neuroradiology 29:277–282, 1987.
45. Netterville JL, Aly A, Ossoff RH: Evaluation and treatment of complications of thyroid and parathyroid surgery. Otolaryngol Clin North Am 23:529–552, 1990.
46. Pensak ML, Jackler RK: Removal of jugular foramen tumors: the fallopian bridge technique. Otolaryngol Head Neck Surg 117:586–591, 1997.
47. Pluta RM, Ram Z, Patronas NJ, Keiser H: Long-term effects of radiation therapy for a catecholamine-producing glomus jugulare tumor: Case report. J Neurosurg 80:1091–1094, 1994.
48. Rhoton AL, Buza R: Microsurgical anatomy of the jugular foramen. J Neurosurg 42:541–550, 1975.
49. Rockley TJ, Hawke M: Glomus bodies in the temporal bone. J Otolaryngol 19:51–56, 1990.
50. Rosenwasser H: Carotid body tumor of the middle ear and mastoid. Arch Otolaryngol 41:64–67, 1945.
51. Schwaber MK, Glasscock ME, Nissen AJ, et al: Diagnosis and management of catecholamine secreting glomus tumors. Laryngoscope 94:1008–1015, 1984.
52. Sekhar LN, Tzortzidis FN, Bejjani GK, Schessel DA: Saphenous vein graft bypass of the sigmoid sinus and jugular bulb during the removal of glomus jugulare tumors: Report of two cases. J Neurosurg 86:1036–1041, 1997.
53. Shapiro MJ, Neues DK: Technique for removal of glomus jugulare tumors. Arch Otolaryngol 79:219–224, 1964.
54. Sharma PD, Johnson AP, Whitton AC: Radiotherapy of jugulotympanic paragangliomas. J Laryngol Otol 98:621–629, 1984.
55. Simko TG, Griffen TW, Gerdes AJ, et al: The role of radiation therapy in the treatment of glomus jugulare tumors. Cancer 42:104–106, 1978.
56. Simpson GT, Konrad HR, Takahashi M, et al: Immediate postembolization excision of glomus jugulare tumors. Arch Otolaryngol 105:639–643, 1979.
57. Spector GJ, Fierstein J, Ogura JH: A comparison of therapeutic modalities of glomus tumors in the temporal bone. Laryngoscope 86:690–696, 1976.
58. Springate SC, Weichselbaum RR: Radiation or surgery for chemodectoma of the temporal bone: A review of local control and complications. Head Neck 12:303–307, 1990.
59. Tali ET, Sener RN, Ibis E, et al: Familial bilateral glomus jugulare tumors. Neuroradiology 33:171–172, 1991.
60. Taylor DM, Alford BR, Greenberg SD: Metastases of glomus jugulare tumors. Arch Otolaryngol 82:5–13, 1965.
61. Thompson JW, Cohen SR: Management of bilateral carotid body tumors and a glomus jugulare tumor in a child. Int J Pediatr Otorhinolaryngol 17:75–87, 1989.
62. Troughton RW, Fry D, Allison RS, Nicholls MG: Depression, palpitations and unilateral pulsatile tinnitus due to a dopamine-secreting glomus jugulare tumor. Am J Med 104:310–311, 1998.
63. Tucker HM: Rehabilitation of patients with postoperative deficits cranial nerves VIII through XII. Otolaryngol Head Neck Surg 88:576–580, 1980.
64. Valavanis A: Preoperative embolization of the head and neck: Indications, patient selection, goals, and precautions. AJNR Am J Neuroradiol 7:943–952, 1986.
65. van der Mey AGL, Fruns JHM, Cornelisse CJ, et al: Does intervention improve the natural course of glomus tumors? A series of 108 patients seen in a 32-year period. Ann Otol Rhinol Laryngol 101:635–642, 1992.
66. Wang ML, Hussey DH, Doornbos JF, et al: A comparison of surgical

and radiotherapeutic results. Int J Radiat Oncol Biol Phys 14:643–648, 1988.

67. Widick MH, Haynes DS, Jackson CG, et al: Slow-flow phenomena in magnetic resonance imaging of the jugular bulb masquerading as skull base neoplasms. Am J Otol 17:648–652, 1996.

68. Wiet RJ, Harvey SA, O'Connor CA: Recent advances in surgery of the temporal bone and skull base. South Med J 86:5–12, 1993.

69. Young NM, Wiet RJ, Russell EJ, Monsell EM: Superselective embolization of glomus jugulare tumors. Ann Otol Rhinol Laryngol 97:613–620, 1988.

70. Zak FG, Lawson W: Glomus jugulare tumors. In The Paraganglionic Chemoreceptor System. New York: Springer-Verlag, 1982, pp 339–391.

# CHAPTER 76

# Surgical Management of Nonglomus Tumors of the Jugular Foramen

■ CHUNG-CHENG WANG, ALI LIU, and CHUN-JIANG YU

Nonglomus tumors of the jugular foramen are rarely encountered, and account for only 0.3% of intracranial tumors (57 of 18,922) operated on at the Beijing Neurosurgical Institute between 1975 and 1997. Our series includes 37 schwannomas, 7 meningiomas, 5 chemodectomas, 3 chordomas, 2 myxomas, 2 chondrosarcomas, and 1 epidermoid cyst. Other kinds of neoplasm, such as neurenteric cysts,[1] petrous bone carcinomas,[2, 3] chondromyxoid fibromas,[4] hemangiopericytoma,[5] plasmacytoma,[6] metastatic melanoma,[7] and amyloidomas,[8] also have been reported in the literature. In the published materials, chemodectoma is the most common tumor, comprising 25% to 77% of jugular foramen tumors,[3, 9–11] with schwannoma the second most common.

## SCHWANNOMAS

The term *schwannoma* denotes a solitary nerve sheath tumor arising from perineural Schwann cells of the involved nerve. It is also called *neurinoma*, *neurilemmoma*, and *neurolemma*. It is different from neurofibroma, which originates from the axon-encasing Schwann cell and therefore contains trapped axons. The neurofibroma usually surrounds nerve fibers, making resection of tumor without nerve sacrifice impossible, whereas most schwannomas can be resected without nerve injury.[12, 13]

### Incidence

Intracranial schwannomas constitute approximately 8% of all primary brain tumors.[14] Schwannomas arising from cranial nerves IX, X, and XI comprise 2.9% of all intracranial schwannomas.[15] Schwannomas involving the jugular foramen are rare, with approximately 140 cases reported in the world literature. The jugular foramen neurilemmoma is an unusual tumor,[2, 15–22] and only a few centers have relatively large series. In 1984, Kaye and associates[23] reported 13 cases, Tan and colleagues[24] (1990) reported 14 cases, Sa-

saki and colleagues[25] (1991) reported 12 cases, Samii and coworkers[26] (1995) reported 16 cases, and in 1997, Mazzoni and colleagues[27] reported 19 cases.

From 1975 to 1997, the Beijing Neurosurgical Institute accumulated 1807 operated cases of intracranial schwannomas. Of these cases, only 37 (2%) arose in the region of the jugular foramen. The group consists of 13 men and 24 women, ranging in age from 16 to 70 years, with a mean age of 36 years. The preadmission duration of disease ranges from 1 month to 16 years.

## Anatomy

Cranial nerves IX, X, and XI emerge in a line from the medulla oblongata and then run laterally to the jugular foramen, leaving the posterior fossa. The jugular foramen is actually a canal. Tumors arising in the middle region tend to expand primarily into bone. The jugular foramen is bounded by the occipital bone medially and the temporal bone laterally and is divided by a fibrous or bony septum into an anteromedial (pars nervosa) compartment, containing the petrosal sinus and glossopharyngeal nerve, and a posterolateral (pars vasculara) compartment, containing the vagus and accessory nerves with the jugular vein.

Cranial nerves IX, X, and XI emerge from the anterior portion of the jugular foramen. Cranial nerve IX emerges between the internal carotid artery and the internal jugular vein, courses laterally to the internal jugular vein, and enters the sternocleidomastoid 1.5 to 2 inches (3.5 to 5 cm) below the mastoid tip. At the angle of the mandible, the cranial nerve XII parallels nerve X and is lateral to it. Nerves IX, X, and XI are anteroposterior, lateral to the internal carotid artery, and pass medially and then anterolaterally to the internal jugular vein, respectively. As the internal jugular vein comes to lie lateral to the internal carotid artery, the cranial nerve X lies behind and between the two vessels.

The parapharyngeal space is bounded medially by the vertebral column and the superior constrictor muscle, and superiorly by the ramus of the mandible and the internal

TABLE 76–1 ■ INITIAL SYMPTOMS OF JUGULAR FORAMEN SCHWANNOMA

| Initial Symptoms | No. | (%) |
|---|---|---|
| Swallowing difficulty | 14 | (38) |
| Glossal atrophy | 7 | (19) |
| Tinnitus | 8 | (22) |
| Hearing loss | 11 | (30) |
| Facial weakness | 2 | (5) |
| Headache | 13 | (35) |
| Vertigo | 5 | (14) |
| Cerebellar dysfunction | 20 | (54) |
| Facial paresthesias | 1 | (3) |
| Shoulder weakness | 2 | (5) |

pterygoid muscle. It is a potential anatomic space, and consists of the regions including the internal jugular vein, the carotid artery, four cranial nerves (IX, X, XI, and XII), and the cervical sympathetic chain. All of the nerves are encased by Schwann cells, which may give rise to a schwannoma.

## Disturbance of Cranial Nerves at Admission

The patient usually presents with a unilateral lesion of cranial nerves IX, X, or XI, or some combination of the three nerves. Occasionally, the patient presents with a retrocochlear lesion similar to a cerebellopontine angle tumor, such as an acoustic neuroma. In our series, 27 patients had initial symptoms involving cranial nerves IX to XI, and 10 had symptoms involving cranial nerves V to VIII (Table 76–1). All of the initially involved nerves are summarized in Table 76–2. In addition, 20 (54%) patients had cerebellar signs: 4 contralateral hemiparalysis, 12 papilledema, 8 suboccipital pain without intracranial hypertension, and 1 pharyngeal mass.

## Growth Patterns and Associated Symptomatology

The growth characteristics and associated symptomatology of these tumors are variable and can be grouped into

TABLE 76–2 ■ CRANIAL NERVE DISTURBANCE AT ADMISSION

| Cranial Nerve Involved | No. of Cases |
|---|---|
| V | 1 |
| V, VII | 1 |
| XI, XII | 1 |
| IX–XI | 2 |
| VIII–X, XII | 3 |
| VIII–XII | 3 |
| V, VII–XII | 2 |
| VIII | 7 |
| IX–X | 1 |
| VIII–X | 3 |
| IX–XII | 5 |
| V, VII–X | 5 |
| VII–XII | 1 |
| V–XI | 2 |
| Total | 37 |

three main categories. The first group is a jugular foramen syndrome with paralysis of the lower cranial nerves. The second common clinical picture is a cerebellopontine angle lesion with ipsilateral hearing loss, tinnitus, and vertigo, thus simulating acoustic neuroma. Less frequently, patients present with pulsatile tinnitus and a hypotympanic mass.

At least two classification systems have been developed for jugular foramen schwannomas, depending on the site and extent of the tumor. Franklin[28] classified the tumor into three groups: class A, tumor confined to the soft tissues of the neck; class B, tumor primary involvement of the neck with extension up to the jugular foramen; class C, tumor fills the jugular foramen with resultant bone expansion. Kaye and associates[23] classified the tumor as follows: type A tumors are primarily intracranial, with minimal extension into the bone foramen; type B tumors are primarily within the bone foramen, with or without an intracranial extension; and type C tumors are primarily extracranial, with only minor extension into the bone foramen or the posterior fossa. Samii and colleagues[26] and Pellet and coworkers[29] added another type, type D, comprising dumbbell-shaped tumors with both intracranial and extracranial extension.

### Type A: Primarily Intracranial Tumors

Twenty-six (70%) of the cases in our series are type A tumors. The tumors arise from the proximal nerve complex of cranial nerves IX, X, and XI, of which XI was involved the least. Patients had two types of symptoms; approximately half presented with a history of vertigo, tinnitus, or sensorineural hearing loss mimicking that of acoustic neuroma, and half had disturbances of cranial nerves IX to XI, such as hoarseness, weakness, or atrophy of the trapezius and sternocleidomastoid muscles.

Fifteen patients had jugular foramen enlargement, but none had an enlarged internal auditory meatus. All of the tumors were confirmed by surgery. Four patients had huge tumors, accompanied by hypoesthesia in the trigeminal distribution and hypodynamia of the facial nerve.

### Type B: Intraosseous Tumors

There are 6 (16%) cases with type B tumors in our series. Because the tumors grow in the jugular foramen, Vernet's syndrome provides the classic clinical signs. Motor and sensory disturbance of the soft palate, itching in the external auditory meatus, and tingling in the throat indicate a lesion of cranial nerve IX. Hoarseness results from vocal cord dysfunction due to a palsy of cranial nerve X, whereas weakness and atrophy of the sternocleidomastoid and trapezius indicate an accessory nerve lesion. The tumor tends to expand primarily into bone, with patients often exhibiting tinnitus, deafness, a middle ear mass, or involvement of the hypoglossal nerve.[23, 28, 30] The tumor in one case extended to the external auditory canal.

### Type C: Primarily Extracranial Tumors

These tumors grow in the segments of cranial nerves IX to XI that lie in the lateral pharyngeal wall, and can even reach the bifurcation of the carotid artery. They are primarily extracranial, or have only a minor extension into the bone, and usually manifest with single nerve palsy and a mass in the neck or lateral pharyngeal wall.[28] There are no cases of such tumors in our series.

## Type D: Dumbbell-Shaped Tumors With Intracranial and Extracranial Extension

There are five cases (13%) with type D tumor in our series. This type includes two or three types mentioned earlier (Fig. 76–1). Clinically speaking, the three other types cannot be distinctly divided, and they are classified artificially according to their different growing periods and the main location of the tumor. If treatment is not administered in a timely fashion, the tumor grows into a dumbbell-like shape and extends upward and downward from the jugular foramen. In one case, a mass was seen in the lateral pharyngeal wall. All of the previously mentioned symptoms and signs can be noted in clinical examination.

## Diagnosis

A jugular foramen tumor is highly likely to present in any adult who has initial symptoms of long duration originating from cranial nerves IX to XI and an enlarged jugular foramen. Most of them are glomus tumors, followed by schwannomas. The differential diagnosis of these tumors includes chemodectoma, acoustic neurinoma, and meningioma of the jugular fossa. Other tumors that involve the cerebellopontine angle, such as choroid plexus papillomas and exophytic pontine gliomas, should be considered.[6] The

preoperative diagnosis of jugular foramen schwannoma, based only on neurologic signs, is difficult because the initial symptoms sometimes are hearing disturbances, indicating involvement of the acoustic nerve. Awareness of a mass in the throat or neck is the most common complaint for parapharyngeal neurinomas. Complete neurologic evaluation is imperative for a correct diagnosis. Plain radiographic films should be obtained in each suspected case of jugular foramen syndrome. These images should include axial, Stenver's, and a special view of the jugular foramen. Tomography best demonstrates changes of the jugular foramen and should be obtained in the frontal, lateral, and basal projections. Thirteen of the 37 cases in our series underwent plain radiographic examination. All patients with tumors in the jugular foramen had radiographic abnormalities, whereas four patients with intracranial tumors did not have enlargement of the jugular foramen. Pneumoencephalographic examination and iophendylate cisternography were used in the past.[15, 31] Computed tomographic (CT) scanning and magnetic resonance imaging (MRI) outline the complete extent of these lesions. Angiography is helpful in determining the vascularity of the lesion and displacement of adjacent blood vessels, as well as the status of blood flow in the jugular bulb and the internal carotid artery. Angiography shows characteristic rapid filling and intense tumor blush in glomus tumors, but such a finding usually is absent in schwannomas.

## Computed Tomographic Scanning

High-resolution CT scanning has a decisive diagnostic value. CT scanning was available for use with 30 of the patients in our series. It was of considerable help in showing the extent of the tumors, not only intracranially but throughout the bone and extracranially. Smooth widening of the jugular foramen with discrete margins and no signs of bone infiltration was the most characteristic manifestation of jugular foramen schwannoma, which differentiated it from an acoustic neuroma (Fig. 76–2). CT scanning of the osseous skull base is extremely important. The simple enlargement or destruction of the foramen and adjoining area have a decisive differential diagnostic value. Contrast-enhanced CT scanning showed involvement of the base of the skull as well as extension into the posterior fossa. However, using only conventional CT scanning, differentiation of an extra-axial tumor from an intra-axial one is difficult. CT cisternography is required for demonstrating small intracranial extra-axial masses and for differentiating an extra-axial mass from an intra-axial one.[31–33]

The intracranial components of jugular foramen schwannomas showed as mixed low-density and isodense extra-axial masses, with ring-like enhancement in the cerebellopontine angle; such lesions were easily misdiagnosed as acoustic neurinomas (Fig. 76–3).

## Magnetic Resonance Imaging

Thirty-one cases were examined by MRI, and all were correctly diagnosed. MRI gives better information than CT. With the availability of different sequences, the absence of bone artifacts, and the ease of imaging in multiple planes, MRI showed jugular foramen schwannomas clearly as ex-

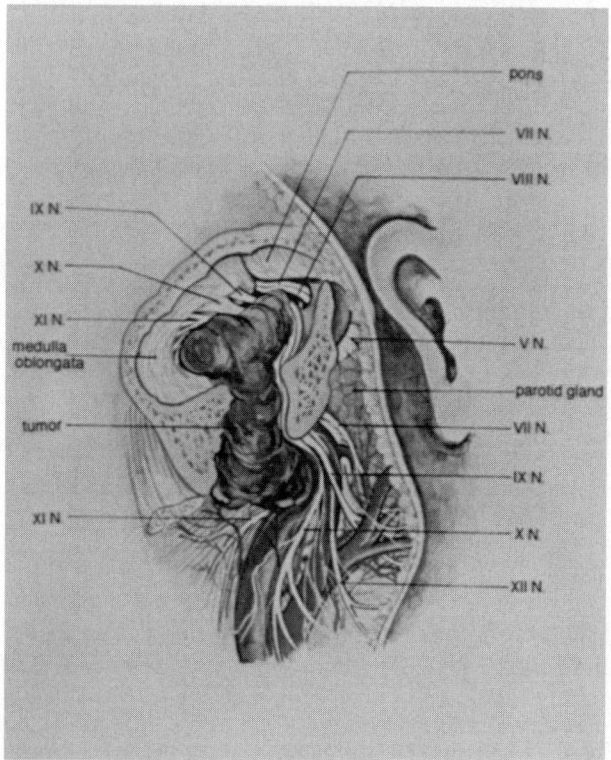

FIGURE 76–1 ■ Diagram of a tumor in the jugular foramen (type D, dumbbell-shaped tumor).

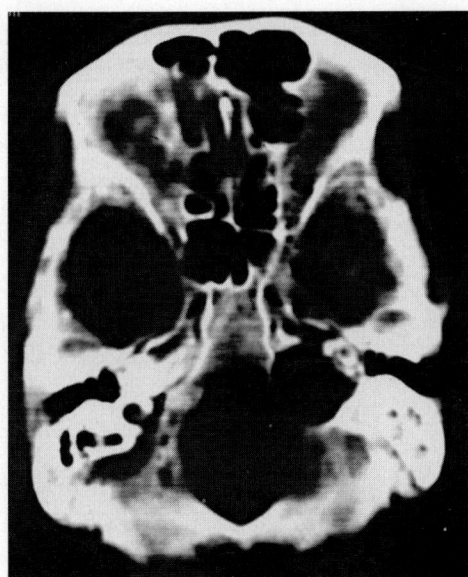

FIGURE 76-2 ■ A computed tomography scan shows enlargement of the left jugular foramen.

tra-axial posterior fossa masses with or without extracranial extension, and demonstrated the relationship of the tumor with the internal carotid artery. The coronal view clearly demonstrated the superior and inferior margins of the tumor, and the shape and nature of the tumor could be easily recognized (Fig. 76–4).

The intensities of jugular foramen schwannomas on $T_1$- and $T_2$-weighted images are similar to those of acoustic schwannomas, namely, long or isodense $T_1$ and long $T_2$ signals. Because MRI can reveal the facial and acoustic nerves, it is helpful in differentiating jugular foramen schwannomas from acoustic schwannomas. In addition, jugular foramen schwannomas mainly press on the medulla oblongata, whereas acoustic schwannomas tend to press on the pons. MRI is useful not only for preoperative diagnosis but for planning the surgical approaches and postoperative follow-up.

## Angiography

Carotid and vertebral angiography is helpful in determining the vascularity of the lesion and displacement of adjacent blood vessels, as well as the status of blood flow in the jugular bulb and the internal carotid artery. During the later phase of the angiogram, when the dural sinuses are opacified, obstruction of the jugular bulb or sigmoid sinus by a tumor mass projecting into the vein may be seen. Retrograde jugular venography is valuable in determining the extent of obstruction of the internal jugular vein and the presence or absence of tumor in the lumen of the jugular vein. Schwannomas tend to occlude the vein by external compression, whereas glomus tumors often grow intraluminally.[15]

Angiographic studies were done in 15 patients in our series; 2 were normal, 5 had tumor blush (Fig. 76–5), and most had tumors noted only as displacements of adjacent blood vessels. Jugular foramen tumors are supplied by the ascending pharyngeal artery originating from the external carotid artery. In the cases with tumor blush, the diameter of the artery increased greatly. The tumor can also be supplied by the occipital artery.[16] Angiography may help to differentiate a schwannoma from a glomus tumor because the glomus tumor is highly vascular, whereas the schwannoma has variable, often slight, vascularity. Preoperative arterial embolization during angiography may decrease operative blood loss and cause less injury to the four lower cranial nerves and other vital tissues during surgical manipulations.

Vessel displacements consist mainly of the anterior inferior cerebellar artery being pushed upward and backward, and the posterior inferior cerebellar artery being pushed downward and backward. Large intracranial tumors can displace the proximal superior cerebellar artery superiorly and medially and can even affect the proximal end of the posterior cerebral artery. However, the latter effect is less significant than with proximal superior cerebellopontine angle tumors. Slight displacement of the basilar artery and vertebral artery can be recorded. Large tumors in the jugular foramen can compress the internal carotid artery, leading to its stenosis or even complete occlusion.

## Surgery

Because jugular foramen schwannomas are benign, the purpose of surgical treatment is to achieve complete resec-

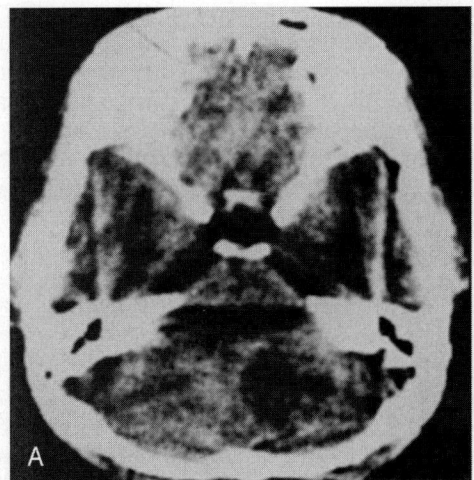
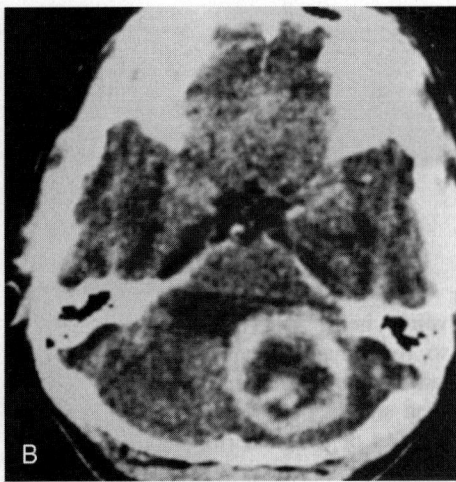

FIGURE 76-3 ■ A, Unenhanced computed tomography (CT) scan shows a mixed low-dense mass in the left cerebellopontine angle. B, An enhanced CT scan shows a ring-like enhancement.

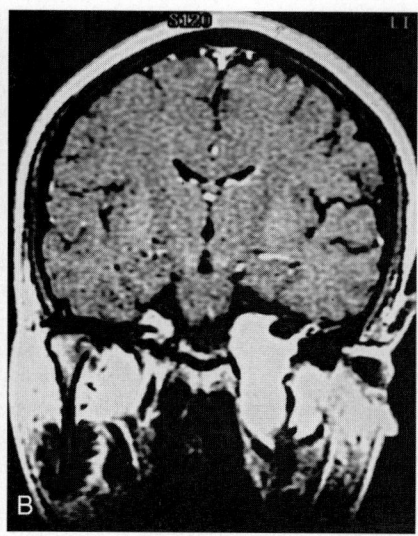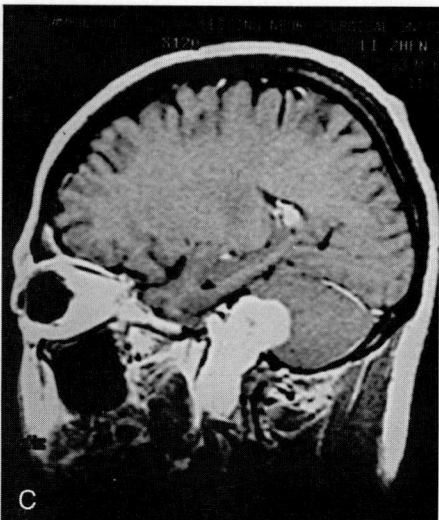

FIGURE 76–4 ■ A preoperative enhanced magnetic resonance imaging shows a type D schwannoma at the left jugular foramen. *A,* Axial view. *B,* Coronal view. *C,* Sagittal view.

tion at one procedure. Incomplete removal involves inevitable recurrence, and scarring from previous surgery adds greatly to the difficulties in preserving functional cranial nerves during a second procedure. Constantly evolving surgical approaches to the skull base, a better understanding of jugular foramen anatomy, improved electrophysiologic monitoring during operation, and improved microsurgical techniques have made the total removal of these tumors possible without causing major morbidity or mortality.

Accurate information about the size, location, and extent of the tumors and determination of involvement of the internal carotid artery and the internal jugular vein are very important in selecting an adequate surgical approach. Preoperative arterial embolization during angiography may decrease operative blood loss[34] and cause less damage to the lower cranial nerves. DasGupta and coworkers[35] indicated that benign schwannomas could be removed without resection of the involved nerves and the presumed nerve

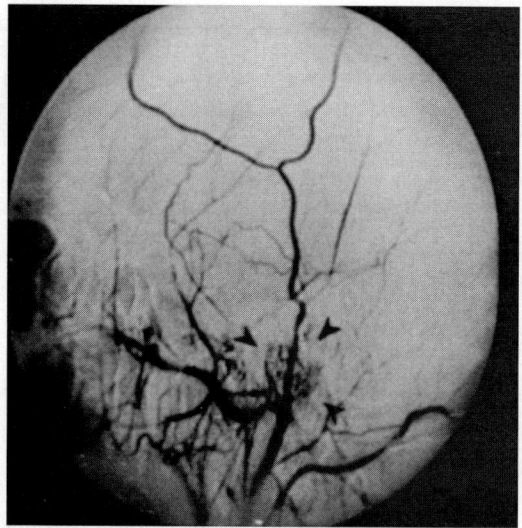

FIGURE 76–5 ■ A right external carotid angiogram that shows the tumor blush *(arrowheads)* supplied by ascending pharyngeal artery.

origin. In some of our cases, it seemed very easy to strip the tumor off its involved cranial nerves.

## Operative Technique

Because of their deep position and the complex surrounding neurovascular structures, surgical removal of jugular foramen tumors remains a difficult process. With the aid of recent microsurgical techniques, a variety of approaches to the jugular foramen have been devised. Arenberg and McCreary[15] and Neely[36] used the suboccipital approach on all of their patients. A transmastoid approach with subtotal removal was advocated by Gacek.[17] Crumley and Wilson[34] and Kinney[37] advocated a two-stage combined otologic and neurosurgical approach. These authors used an infratemporal approach, followed by a suboccipital craniectomy for intracranial extension. Horn and colleagues[30] used a single-stage procedure, including transmastoid, translabyrinthine, and infratemporal approaches, and Kamitani and associates[38] used a combined extradural-posterior petrous and suboccipital approach. More recently, Mazzoni and colleagues[27] used the petro-occipital transsigmoid approach.

The jugular foramen is located under the middle ear, the labyrinth, and the internal auditory canal, behind the vertical part of the petrosal segment of the internal carotid artery and lateral to the hypoglossal foramen. The infratemporal approach exposes the superior and anterior aspect of the jugular foramen by drilling part of the petrous bone. This approach requires a thorough knowledge of petrous bone anatomy, and exposes the patient to postoperative complications such as auditory loss, facial nerve palsy, and cerebrospinal fluid (CSF) leak.[39–42] George and colleagues[43] used the juxtacondylar approach to expose the posterior and inferior aspects of the jugular foramen. Exposing the inferior wall of the jugular foramen requires drilling a small part of the lateral aspect of the condyle and the bone above the condyle. This approach greatly reduces the risk of the complications.

The choice of surgical approach was determined by the

type of tumor extension. Samii and coworkers[26] use a lateral suboccipital approach for type A tumors, and a cervical-transmastoid approach for type B, C, and D tumors, which has the following advantages: (1) the facial nerve is left in its bone canal, and (2) drilling of the petrous bone inferior to the labyrinth and cochlea allows preservation of hearing and vestibular function.[26]

Our jugular foramen schwannomas were mainly in the posterior fossa, with only 11 cases with tumors confined to the jugular foramen and bone. For these cases, we used a lateral suboccipital approach (Fig. 76–6). The tumors are usually large and occupy the space between the jugular bulb and cranial nerves VII and VIII, which splay over the tumor surface (Fig. 76–7). The petrosal vein is identified, coagulated, and cut near the dura, and the tumor is coagulated, gutted, and collapsed. Under a microscope, the tumor capsule is carefully dissected from its surrounding tissue, including the brain stem and cranial nerves IX to XI (Fig. 76–8). We used the cervical-transmastoid approach in five patients with type D tumors. The incision extended into the neck along the anterior border of the sternocleidomastoid muscle to the level of the hyoid bone. The mastoid is exposed after mobilization of both the sternocleidomastoid muscle and the posterior belly of the digastric muscle (Fig. 76–9). The caudal cranial nerves are identified in the neck along with the internal jugular vein and followed cranially to the skull base. A part of the occipital squama is removed lateral to the occipitomastoid suture. The mastoid is removed, and to extend the exposure further, the posterior part of the occipital condyle may be removed, thus opening the jugular foramen dorsolaterally[26] (Fig. 76–10). Sometimes, successful total removal of skull base lesions requires complete control of the carotid artery and the inter-

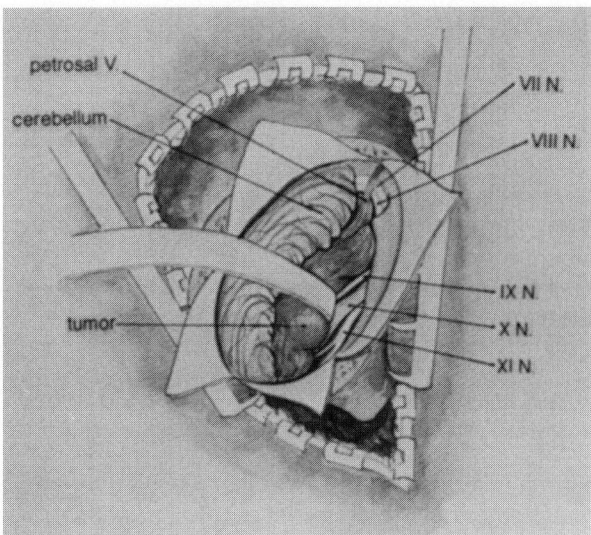

FIGURE 76–7 ■ Exposure of a huge schwannoma and lower cranial nerves.

nal jugular vein, so that the tumor may be removed from the vessels[40] (Fig. 76–11).

Cerebrospinal fluid leak must be prevented when the tumor extends from the posterior fossa into the bone or outside of it. CSF leaks can be averted by a layered compressive closure and use of a free fat graft to fill the extradural defect, as well as meticulous dural closure with a temporalis musculofascial graft, if necessary.

Preservation of adjacent cranial nerves in cases of schwannoma of the parapharyngeal space is usually possible at surgery, but those in the jugular foramen are extremely difficult to remove without damage to adjacent cranial nerves. If the vagus nerve is injured during tumor resection, microscopic reanastomosis or nerve grafting (greater auricular nerve) should be performed because near-normal return of function has been reported with these techniques.[44] Total excision of the tumor was achieved in

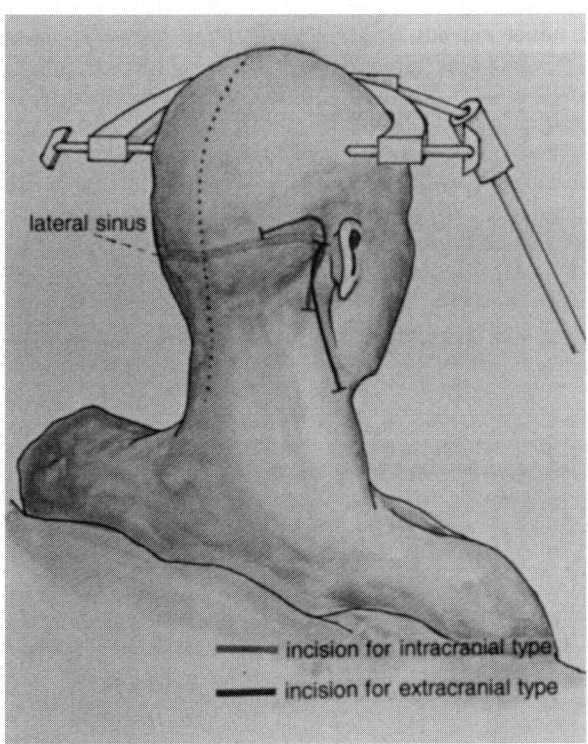

FIGURE 76–6 ■ Position of the patient for removal of a tumor involving the jugular foramen.

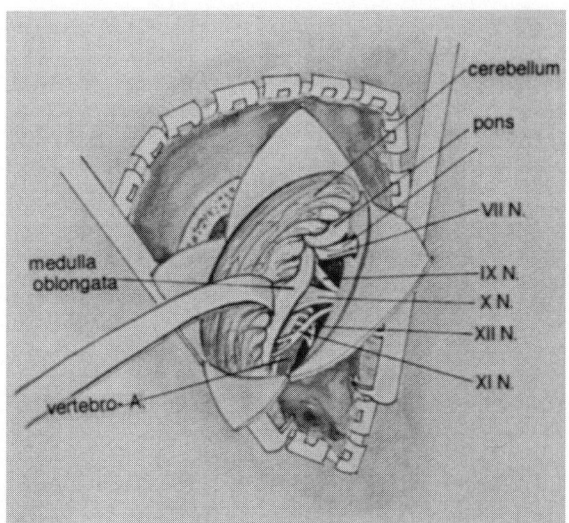

FIGURE 76–8 ■ After removal of a schwannoma, the brain stem and cranial nerves VII to XII are exposed.

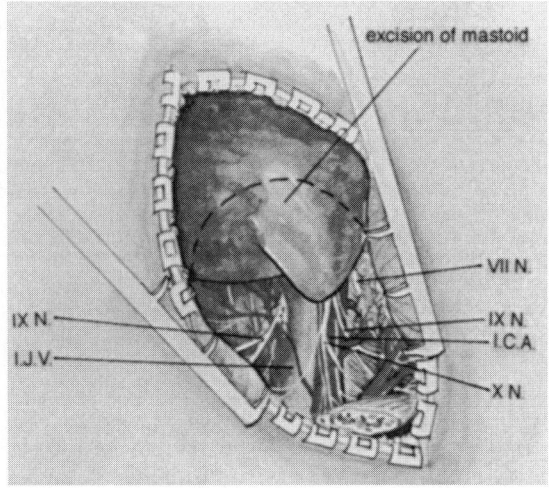

**FIGURE 76-9** ■ Diagram showing the excision of the mastoid.

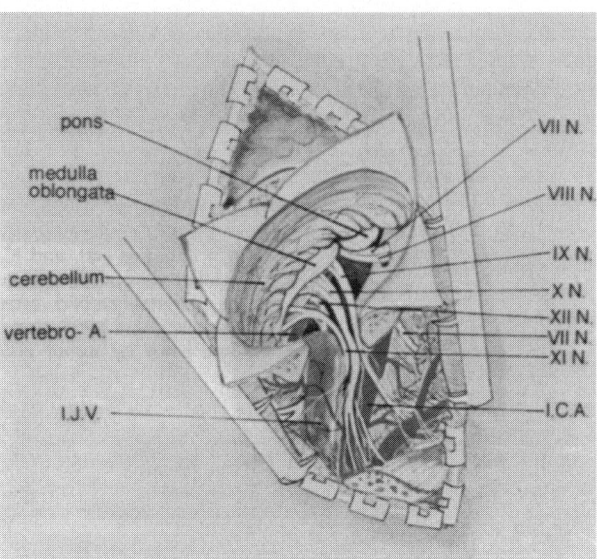

**FIGURE 76-11** ■ After the tumor has been removed.

our series in 27 patients, subtotal in 8, and partial in 2 patients. There was no operative mortality.

All patients presenting with lower cranial nerve dysfunction had the same or greater postoperative cranial nerve dysfunction. The long-term compensation for this deficit was good. Some patients had dramatic recovery from sensorineural hearing loss after total surgical removal of large intracranial jugular foramen schwannomas.[36]

## MENINGIOMAS

There were seven patients with a meningioma at the jugular foramen in our series. Such tumors arise from arachnoid villi associated with the jugular bulb, envelop the adjacent cranial nerves, and spread into the temporal bone, neck,

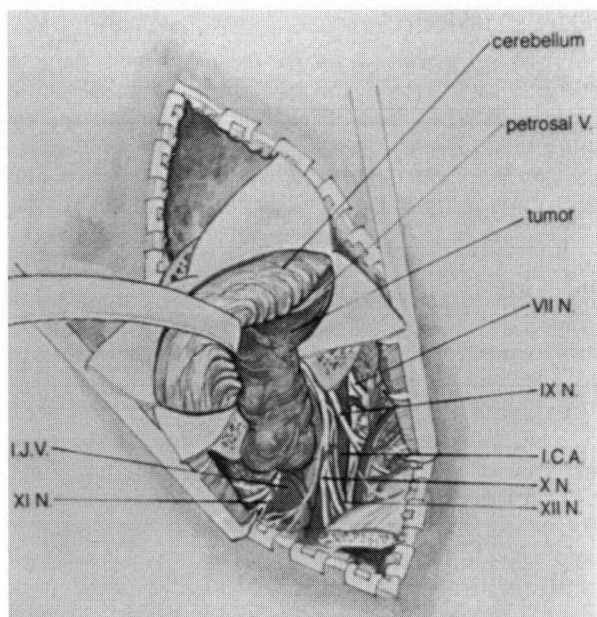

**FIGURE 76-10** ■ Exposure of the tumor involving the neck and related cranial nerves and vessels.

and posterior fossa.[45] The clinical manifestation of meningiomas is similar to that of neurinomas and glomus tumors. Meningiomas grow slowly but have a greater tendency to recur than do glomus tumors, even after "complete" extirpation.

Imaging studies are helpful in the differential diagnosis. On CT scanning, characteristic radiographic signs of sclerosis with little bone erosion at the edges of the tumor suggest a meningioma. Often, meningiomas show hyperostosis with loss of surrounding bony definition. Meningiomas are often hyperdense on noncontrast CT. MRI does not show a "salt-and-pepper" appearance or serpentine flow voids attributed to large vessels within the glomus tumor. Meningiomas strongly enhance with gadolinium, which indicates tumor size and involvement of adjacent soft tissue.[1] Angiography shows no tumor blush or less than that seen with glomus tumors. No early venous drainage can be seen, and differentiating a meningioma from a neurinoma of this area is not easy. If the lesion is rich with blood, embolization reduces blood loss during surgical procedures.

## EPIDERMOID CYSTS

Surgeons at our institute operated on 330 patients with cerebellopontine angle epidermoid. Approximately half of these tumors involved the jugular foramen, but only one primary epidermoid was at the jugular foramen, and the patient had initial symptoms involving cranial nerves IX to XI, and the patient's jugular foramen was extremely enlarged with smooth margin.

Computed tomography usually shows a hypodense, irregular or lobulated, nonenhancing mass, and MRI reveals an irregular, cauliflower-like surface. The most common signal pattern parallels that of CSF but may occasionally be hyperintense on $T_1$-weighted images if the solid cholesterin component is dominant.[46]

Surgical removal is the only treatment that provides a

cure. Preoperative CT scan and MRI can indicate the size and extent of the tumor, and the approach should be designed accordingly. A combined supratentorial and infratentorial incision is sometimes required for huge tumors. Removal of the whole capsule of a huge tumor is not usually necessary, lest it damage the cranial nerves, brain stem, and important vessels. However, the contents of tumor should be thoroughly cleared. Because a huge tumor of this kind cannot be completely exposed into the direct visual field, repeated physiologic saline irrigation should be applied after supposedly complete clearance of the contents, and the neurosurgeon should wait for new contents to flow out. This procedure must be performed several times until no new contents flow out. If clearance is not complete, tumor contents may flow into the subarachnoid space and cause arachnoid adhesion and intracranial hypertension.

The surgery achieves excellent results if the contents are completely cleared. The residue of the tumor capsule develops very slowly and takes a very long time to grow and give rise to recurrent symptoms. Some investigators advocate daubing the inner surface of the tumor capsule with formalin or alcohol to delay tumor development.

## CHORDOMAS

Chordomas are rare tumors arising from remnants of the embryologic notochord. Although chordomas are typically midline in site, we have encountered three cases of intracranial chordoma arising unilaterally in the petrous bone. All presented with Vernet's syndrome and bone erosion around the jugular foramen. The intraosseous portion of the internal carotid artery was displaced forward. CT demonstrated an extra-axial soft tissue mass associated with foci of calcification accompanied by bone destruction. MRI showed heterogeneous hypodensity. Calcified or ossified portions of the chordomas showed as moderate hypodensity on MRI.

The cranial nervous disturbance remained as it was before the operation. One patient died of other disease 2

years later, and the other is still alive and can take care of himself 10 years after the operation.

## MYXOMAS

Intracranial primary myxomas are rare. Most of the reported cases were either embolic or metastatic cardiac myxomas.[47–49] We had two female patients with primary myxomas, one with a 3-year and the other with a 13-year history of illness. Both had Vernet's syndrome as the initial set of symptoms. The patient with a shorter history had an intracranial tumor, and the other had a mixed tumor of the intracranium and extracranium. This patient's tumor extended upward, involving cranial nerve V, and downward into the neck through the jugular foramen.

Differentiating the tumor from a neurinoma in neuroradiologic examination is difficult. CT scan shows a hypodense image that can be enhanced. MRI can show abnormal signals in long $T_1$- and $T_2$-weighted images of the clear margin of the jugular foramen. No tumor blush was seen on angiograms in either of these cases except for some displacement of adjacent blood vessels. One tumor in our series extended into the neck, pressing the internal carotid artery to occlusion at the C2 level (Fig. 76–12). Surgical removal is the best treatment for myxomas. Myxomas have a capsule with a jelly-like content that is easy to clear away.

Primary myxomas are benign tumors arising from mesenchymal tissues and composed of stellate and spindle-shaped cells set in a loose, mucoid stroma containing hyaluronic acid.[50] They may occur at any age, and no sex predominates.[51]

## CHONDROSARCOMAS

Chondrosarcomas are malignant cartilage tumors arising from bone or pre-existing exostosis. They usually occur in the long bone of the limbs with some calcification.[52] Chondrosarcoma of the skull base is rare. Two cases in our

**FIGURE 76–12** ■ *A,* A left internal carotid artery (ICA) occluded at C2 vertebra, appearing beak-like by external compression. The ascending pharyngeal artery is enlarged, and the ICA siphon is filled via the collateral circulation from the external carotid artery (ECA). *B,* The venous phase with occlusion of the left transverse sinus by tumor compression.

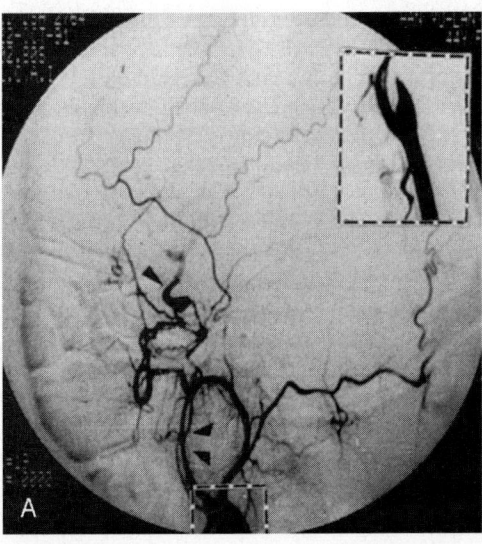
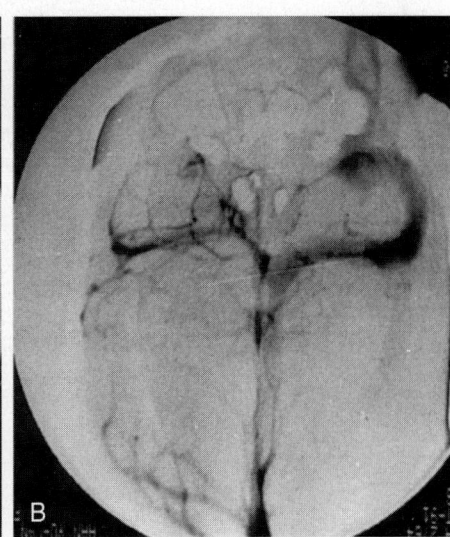

series presented with unilateral disturbance of cranial nerves IX to XII. CT showed a mixed hypodense lesion in the posterior fossa with the tumor extended into the foramen. MRI indicated a sharply delineated ovoid mass at the jugular foramen, with mixed low density on $T_1$-weighted images and low density with a high-signal rim on $T_2$-weighted images. Its clinical manifestations and radiologic appearance were similar to those of chordoma. The tumor was tough in consistency, with a violet-red surface and yellowish substantial content, and could not be easily suctioned to obtain a total excision. Postoperative radiation therapy can improve the survival rate.[47]

## REFERENCES

1. Harris CP, Dias MS, Brockmeyer DL, et al: Neurenteric cysts of the posterior fossa: Recognition, management and embryogenesis. Neurosurgery 29:893, 1991.
2. Maniglia AJ, Chandler JR, Goodwin WJ, et al: Schwannomas of the parapharyngeal space and jugular foramen. Laryngoscope 89:1405, 1979.
3. Takahashi M, Kamito T, Hatayama N, et al: Clinical analysis of eight cases treated with lateral skull base surgery. Nippon Jibiinkoka Gakkai Kaiho 94:1683, 1991.
4. Kitamura K, Niba K, Asai M, et al: Chondromyxoid fibroma of the mastoid invading the occipital bone. Arch Otolaryngol Head Neck Surg 115:384, 1989.
5. Megerian CA, Mckenna MJ, Nadol JB Jr: Non-paraganglioma jugular foramen lesions masquerading as glomus jugulare tumors. Am J Otol 16:94, 1995.
6. Comacchio F, Deredita R, Poletto E, et al: Hemangiopericytoma of skull base and Collet-Sicard syndrome: A case report. Ear Nose Throat J 74:845, 1995.
7. Schweinfurth JM, Johnson JT, Weissman J: Jugular foramen syndrome as a complication of metastatic melanoma. An J Otolaryngol 14:168, 1993.
8. Matsumoto T, Tani E, Maeda Y, et al: Amyloidomia in the cerebellopontine angle and jugular foramen. J Neurosurg 62:592, 1985.
9. Azm MEI, Samii M, Sepehrnia S, et al: Surgery of jugular foramen tumors. In First International Skull Base Congress. Hanover, Germany, June 14–20, 1992.
10. Jackson CG, Cueva RA, Thedinger BA, et al: Cranial nerve preservation in lesions of the jugular fossa. Otolaryngol Head Neck Surg 105:687, 1991.
11. Ramina R, Manigha JJ, Barrionuevo CE, et al: Surgical treatment of jugular foramen lesions. In First International Skull Base Congress. Hanover, Germany, June 14–20, 1992.
12. Conley JJ: Neurogenous tumors in the neck. Arch Otolaryngol Head Neck Surg 61:167, 1955.
13. Harkin JC, Read RJ: Tumors of the Peripheral Nervous System. Washington, DC: Armed Forces Institute of Pathology, 1969.
14. Russell DS, Rubinstein L: Pathology of Tumors of the Nervous System, 5th ed. Baltimore: Williams & Wilkins, 1989, p 537.
15. Arenberg IK, McCreary HS: Neurilemmoma of the jugular foramen. Laryngoscope 81:544, 1971.
16. Call WH, Pulec L: Neurilemmoma of the jugular foramen, transmastoid removal. Ann Otol Rhinol Laryngol 87:313, 1978.
17. Gacek RR: Schwannoma of the jugular foramen. Ann Otol Rhinol Laryngol 85:215, 1976.
18. Maniglia AJ: Intra and extracranial meningiomas involving the temporal bone. Laryngoscope 88 (Suppl 12):1, 1978.
19. Ito K, Suzuki M, Ottomo M, Suzuk S: Two cases of jugular foramen neurinoma: Review of 48 cases in the literature. Rinsho Shinkeigaku 17:499, 1977.
20. Bordi L, Compton J, Symon L: Trigeminal neuroma. Surg Neurol 31:272, 1989.
21. Hiscott P, Symon L: An unusual presentation of neurofibroma of the oculomotor nerve. J Neurosurg 56:854, 1982.
22. Columella F, Delzanno GB, Nicola GC: Les neurinomes des quatres demiers neuf craniens. Neurochirurgie 5:280, 1959.
23. Kaye AH, Hahn JF, Kinney SE, et al: Jugular foramen schwannoma. J Neurosurg 60:1045, 1984.
24. Tan LC, Bordi LL, Symon L, et al: Jugular foramen neuromas: A review of 14 cases. Surg Neurol 34:205, 1990.
25. Sasaki T, Takakara K: Twelve cases of jugular foramen neurinoma. Skull Base Surg 1:152, 1991.
26. Samii M, Babu RP, Tatagiba M, et al: Surgical treatment of jugular foramen schwannomas. J Neurosurg 82:924–932, 1995.
27. Mazzoni A, Sanna M, Saleh E, et al: Lower cranial nerve schwannomas involving the jugular foramen. Ann Otol Rhinol Laryngol 106:370, 1997.
28. Franklin DJ, Moore GF, Fisch U, et al: Jugular foramen peripheral nerve sheath tumors. Laryngoscope 99:1081, 1989.
29. Pellet W, Cannoni M, Pech A: The widened transcochlear approach to jugular foramen schwannomas. J Neurosurg 69:887, 1988.
30. Horn KL, House WF, Hitselberger WE: Schwannomas of the jugular foramen. Laryngoscope 95:761, 1985.
31. Baker HL Jr: Myelographic examination of the posterior fossa with positive contrast medium. Radiology 81:791, 1963.
32. Steele JR, Hoffman JC: Brainstem evaluation with CT cisternography. AJR Am J Roentgenol 136:287, 1984.
33. Uchino A, Hasuo K, Fukui M, et al: Computed tomography of jugular foramen neurinomas. Neurol Med Chir (Tokyo) 27:628, 1987.
34. Crumley RL, Wilson C: Schwannomas of the jugular foramen. Laryngoscope 94:772, 1984.
35. DasGupta TK, Brasfield RD, Strong WE, et al: Benign solitary schwannomas (neurilemmomas). Cancer 23:355, 1969.
36. Neely JG: Reversible compression neuropathy of the eighth cranial nerve from a large jugular foramen schwannoma. Arch Otolaryngol Head Neck Surg 105:555, 1979.
37. Kinney SE, Dohn DF, Hahn JF, et al: Neuromas of the jugular foramen. In Brackmann DE (ed): Neurological Surgery of the Ear and Skull Base. New York, Raven Press, 1982, p 361.
38. Kamitani H, Masnzawa H, Kanazawa I, et al: A combined extradural-posterior petrous and suboccipital approach to the jugular foramen tumors. Acta Neurochir (Wien) 126:179, 1994.
39. Al-mefty O, Fox JL, Rifar A, et al: A combined infratemporal and posterior fossa approach for the removal of giant glomus tumors and chondrosarcomas. Surg Neurol 28:423, 1987.
40. Fisch U, Pillsburg HC: Infratemporal fossa approach to lesion in the temporal bone and base of the skull. Arch Otolargyngol 125(2):99–107, 1979.
41. Hakuba A, Hashi K, Fujitani K, et al: Jugular foramen neurinomas. Surg Neurol 11:83, 1979.
42. Patel SJ, Sekhar LN, Cass SP, et al: Combined approaches for resection of extensive glomus jugular tumors. J Neurosurg 80:1026, 1994.
43. George B, Lot G, TraBahuy P, et al: The juxtacondylar approach to the jugular foramen (without petrous drilling). Surg Neurol 44:279, 1995.
44. Reddick LP, Myers RT: Neurilemmoma of the cervical portion of the vagus nerve. Am J Surg 125:744, 1972.
45. Molony TB, Brackmann DE, Lo WW: Meningiomas of the jugular foramen. Otolaryngol Head Neck Surg 106:128, 1992.
46. Osborn AG: Intracranial lesions: Cerebellopontine angle and internal auditory canals. In Osborn AG (ed): Handbook of Neuroradiology. St. Louis, Mosby-Year Book, 1991, p 347.
47. Branch CL Jr, Laster DW, Kelly DL Jr: Left atrial myxoma with cerebral emboli. Neurosurgery 16:675, 1985.
48. Budzilovich G, Aleksic S, Greco A, et al: Malignant cardiac myxoma with cerebral metastasis. Surg Neurol 11:461, 1979.
49. Jungreis CA, Sekhar LM, Martinez AJ, et al: Cardiac myxoma metastatic to the temporal bone. Radiology 170:244, 1989.
50. Stout AP: Myxoma, the tumor of primitive mesenchyme. Ann Surg 127:706, 1984.
51. Canalis RF, Smith GA, Konrad HR: Myxomas of the head and neck. Arch Otolaryngol 102:300, 1976.
52. Seidman MD, Nichols RD, Raju UB, et al: Extracranial skull base chondrosarcoma. Ear Nose Throat J 68:626, 1989.

# Vascular Disorders of the Nervous System

# CHAPTER 77

# Surgical Management of Extracranial Carotid Artery Disease

■ JOHN H. HONEYCUTT, JR. and CHRISTOPHER M. LOFTUS

Since the first description of a carotid endarterectomy for the prevention of stroke,[12] the operation has been widely debated and often criticized; yet the numbers of endarterectomy procedures performed annually have steadily increased. Early studies suggested that medical management was superior to surgical intervention.[20, 47] This is clearly no longer the case. Gratifying and unimpeachable results from multicenter trials have advocated surgical therapy over medical management in specific cases[14, 38, 40] of both asymptomatic and symptomatic carotid stenosis. The North American Symptomatic Carotid Endarterectomy Trial (NASCET) data indicate that carotid endarterectomy has benefit in all symptomatic patients with lesions of greater than 70% linear stenosis and for specific subgroups of symptomatic patients with greater than 50% stenosis.[40] The Asymptomatic Carotid Atherosclerosis Study (ACAS) results indicate that asymptomatic patients with greater than 60% stenosis have a better outcome with carotid endarterectomy than with medical management.[14]

In this chapter, we describe our standard technique for carotid endarterectomy, as well as discussing the various surgical options and different variations of the procedure. Although there are numerous ways to perform carotid endarterectomy, the surgeon must adhere to several basic principles of carotid reconstruction. The surgeon must have complete preoperative knowledge of the patient's vascular anatomy, must maintain complete vascular control at all times, must have sufficient working anatomic knowledge to prevent harm to adjacent structures, and must ensure the patient a widely patent repair free of technical errors.

## SURGICAL TECHNIQUE

### Surgical Magnification

We perform the operation with $3.5\times$ loupe-magnified technique. Microscopic repair of the internal carotid artery (ICA), which we have also tried, allows a primary repair that is unquestionably finer and superior to loupe-magnified technique[2, 20, 48, 49] but that in our experience did not alter the overall patient outcome or incidence of restenosis or acute occlusion. In the ongoing effort to reduce morbidity, we have adopted instead universal patch grafting with collagen impregnated Dacron (Hemashield graft), which has essentially eliminated the problem of acute postoperative thrombosis or rapid restenosis. In our opinion, the graft procedure is more easily and expeditiously accomplished with $3.5\times$ magnification rather than the microscope. There is no doubt that the suture lines are not as fine with this method, but the added lumen diameter with patch angioplasty renders this unnecessary.

## Anesthetic Technique

General anesthesia and local anesthesia are both in common use for carotid endarterectomy. We routinely use general anesthesia with full-channel electroencephalographic (EEG) monitoring. Proponents of local anesthesia tout the advantages of patient response to questioning as a superior method of assessing the need for intraoperative shunting while minimizing anesthetic risks, reducing postoperative morbidity, and shortening length of stay. The patient has local anesthesia with light sedation, which allows him or her to perform a simple task with the contralateral hand during cross-clamping. The disadvantages include risk of contamination and patient movement during the procedure, along with the increased psychological stress of remaining awake. A review comparing our technique and that of an institutional vascular surgeon using local anesthesia showed decreased incidence of EEG changes and intraoperative shunting with local anesthesia. However, there was no difference in stroke rate, complication, length of stay, or overall outcome.[56] We prefer general anesthesia for a number of reasons, not the least of which is the controlled environment. In addition, all commonly used inhalational anesthetic agents and intravenous barbiturates significantly reduce the cerebral metabolic rate of oxygen,[23] giving a theoretical advantage with regard to cerebral ischemia. We keep our patients normocapneic. Although there has been much interest in arterial levels of carbon dioxide, nonphysiologic hypercapnia and hypocapnia provide no cerebral protection.[4, 8, 22, 43] Gross and colleagues[28] found that there was a 40% decrease in EEG changes with cross-clamping in those patients receiving either one or two units of 6% hetastarch (500 to 1000 ml). They had acceptable outcomes with a postoperative stroke and mortality rate of 1.3%.[28] This warrants further research with a controlled, prospective study. Finally, blood pressure is maintained at normotensive levels with a tolerance of up to 20% increase in systolic pressure.[23] Although some surgeons prefer to induce hypertension at cross-clamping if there are EEG changes and then shunt if no improvement is seen in the EEG recordings, we shunt immediately if EEG changes are evident.

## Monitoring Techniques

Monitoring techniques can be divided into two categories: (1) tests of vascular integrity, such as stump pressure measurements, xenon regional cerebral blood flow studies, transcranial Doppler, and, to a lesser extent, intraoperative oculoplethysmography, Doppler/duplex scanning, and angiography; and (2) tests of cerebral function, such as EEG, EEG derivatives, or somatosensory evoked potential monitoring. The newly described near-infrared spectroscopy technique bridges both categories. We use a full-channel EEG interpreted by a neurologist on-line. After completion of arteriotomy closure, an intraoperative Doppler examination is performed of the common carotid artery, the ICA, and the external carotid artery.

## Intraoperative Shunting

There are three schools of thought about intraoperative shunting: carotid surgeons shunt in every case; shunt when indicated by some form of intraoperative monitoring; or never place a shunt. In our institution, we perform monitor-dependent shunting based on EEG criteria. We use a custom commercial shunt of our own design (Loftus Carotid Endarterectomy Shunt; Heyer-Schulte Neurocare, Pleasant Prairie, WI). In our experience, we shunt approximately 15% of carotid endarterectomies. This increases to approximately 25% if the contralateral carotid is occluded. After the shunt is placed, the monitoring parameters should return to baseline. If this does not occur, the shunt must be inspected for possible kinking, thrombosis, or misplacement. We always auscultate the shunt with a Doppler probe that confirms patency and shunt flow.

Proponents of universal shunting tout the benefits of a maximum degree of cerebral protection in every case while eliminating dependence on specialized intraoperative monitoring techniques. They assert that shunt placement is benign and allows extra time to ensure meticulous intimal dissection and arteriotomy repair.[5, 25, 31, 41, 46, 53]

Proponents of nonshunting believe that shunt placement is not benign. In one series, there was a higher stroke rate with shunting compared with nonshunting,[44] indicating that embolization from shunt placement, especially by surgeons inexperienced in the procedure, is a real risk. Another documented concern is distal intimal damage leading to embolization or carotid artery dissection.[35]

Many surgeons, in part because of the aforementioned concerns, choose not to shunt. There have been multiple

series that have had good surgical results with no shunts being used.[1, 3, 7, 15–19] These authors do not deny the existence of postoperative stroke, but they strongly believe that neurologic deficits from carotid artery surgery are invariably embolic rather than hemodynamic in nature and that intraoperative monitoring or shunt placement will not further reduce the already low morbidity rate in their series.[18]

As discussed previously, we prefer to shunt when there are changes in the EEG with cross-clamping. This policy has been well supported by several reports with large series of patients.[36, 52] There are also several authors who normally practice selective shunting but who advocate shunting all patients who have had recent strokes or reversible neurologic events (based on their belief that intraoperative monitoring is unreliable in the face of recent ischemic events).[37, 45] Although we understand their concerns, this has not been our practice.

## Patch Graft Angioplasty

Almost all carotid surgeons perform patch angioplasty for recurrent carotid stenosis. Many also use selective patching in cases where the internal carotid is small, where plaque and arteriotomy has extended far up the ICA, or in any similar case where compromise of the lumen and a high risk for thrombosis is anticipated. We have taken this policy one step further, and for 4 years have used a Hemashield patch graft in all of our patients. We have not encountered any restenosis or acute occlusions since using the patch universally. If patching is used, several synthetic grafts are available, in addition to autologous saphenous vein graft. There is the concern of central patch rupture in autologous vein grafts, especially in women and diabetic patients, but the risk can be reduced by harvesting the graft from a high femoral site rather than at the ankle.

## Heparinization

A single dose of intravenous heparin is given to the patient at some point before cross-clamping. This dose is between 2500 and 10,000 units of heparin, depending on the surgeon's preference; there are no studies to support one dose versus another. Some surgeons reverse the heparinization with protamine after the operation[17, 18]; we have not found any benefit in this. For those patients who come to the operating room on a continuous heparin drip, we continue the infusion until the arteriotomy closure is finished. With meticulous technique, bleeding in these cases has not been a problem.

## Tacking Sutures

Tandem sutures to secure the distal intima in the ICA after plaque removal are considered a great advance by some[25] and deemed unnecessary by others.[17, 18, 31] The concern with tacking sutures is that they may narrow the lumen, but to us this risk seems small compared with that of intimal dissection from an unsecured intimal flap. Several authors[17, 18, 41] state that if the arteriotomy is carried far enough to see normal intima distal to the plaque, then the tacking sutures are unnecessary. We strongly agree with an arteriotomy that extends past the plaque, but we are not always satisfied with how the intimal plaque tapers. Because of negative experiences with plaques that do not feather cleanly when they are pulled down from the distal ICA, we have begun to use fine scissors to "trim" the plaque cleanly in the ICA as it is removed. When this is done, tacking sutures are rarely necessary. We estimate that we selectively place tacking sutures in the distal ICA in approximately 10% of cases.

## SURGERY

We think that the meticulous anatomic dissection and identification of vital cervical structures needed to minimize postoperative complications can be achieved only with a bloodless field. Accordingly, we do not consider elapsed time to be a factor in the performance of carotid artery surgery. In our institution, carotid endarterectomy requires from 2 to 2.5 hours of operating time, and the average cross-clamp time is between 30 and 40 minutes. No untoward effects from the length of the procedure have been observed in any patient, and we are convinced that the risk of cervical nerve injury or postoperative complications related to hurried closure of the suture line is significantly reduced by meticulous attention to detail.

Two surgeons trained in the procedure are always present during carotid surgery. Both surgeons may stand on the operative side, the primary surgeon facing cephalad and the assistant facing the patient's feet, or the surgeons may stand on either side of the table. The operative nurse may stand either behind or across the table from the primary surgeon. The patient is positioned supine on the operating room table with the head extended and turned away from the side of operation. Several folded pillowcases are placed between the shoulder blades to facilitate extension of the neck, and the degree of rotation of the head is determined by the relationship of the external and internal carotid arteries on preoperative angiography or magnetic resonance angiography. The carotid vessels are customarily superimposed in the anteroposterior plane, and moderate rotation of the head swings the internal carotid laterally into a more surgically accessible position. In those patients in whom the ICA can be seen angiographically to be laterally placed, the head rotation need not be as great. On the other hand, occasional patients demonstrate an ICA that is rotated medially under the external carotid, and in such cases no degree of head rotation yields a satisfactory exposure. In these cases, the surgeon must be prepared to mobilize the external carotid more extensively and swing it medially to expose the underlying ICA (even tacking it up to medial soft tissues if necessary).

The position of the carotid bifurcation is likewise determined before surgery from the angiogram, and the skin incision is planned accordingly. We always use a linear incision along the anterior portion of the sternocleidomastoid muscles (Fig. 77–1). This may go as low as the suprasternal notch and as high as the retroaural region, depending on the level of the bifurcation. The skin and

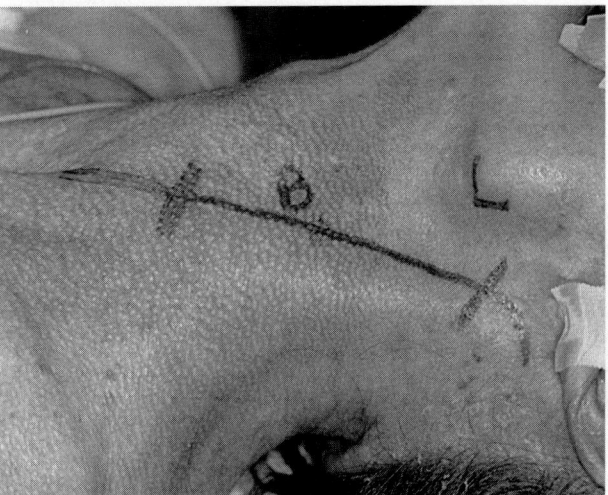

FIGURE 77–1 ■ Photograph showing positioning and surgical incision planning in a left carotid endarterectomy. The incision parallels the anterior border of the sternomastoid muscle. The "B" indicates the palpable position of the carotid bulb. The "L"-shaped mark indicates the angle of the mandible.

subcutaneous tissues are divided sharply to the level of the platysma, which is always identified and divided sharply as well. Hemostasis often requires generous use of bipolar electrocautery. If careful attention is paid to all bleeding points during the opening, there will be little or no bleeding when heparin is administered and the closure will be much simpler.

Self-retaining retractors are next placed and the underlying fat is dissected to identify the anterior edge of the sternocleidomastoid muscle. Retractors are left superficial at all times on the medial side to prevent retraction injury to the laryngeal nerves, but laterally retractors may be more deeply placed. Dissection proceeds in the mid-portion of the wound down the sternocleidomastoid muscle until the jugular vein is identified. Care must be taken under the sternocleidomastoid muscle, however, to prevent injury to the spinal accessory nerve, which can be inadvertently transected or stretched.

The jugular vein is the key landmark in this exposure and complete dissection of the medial jugular border should always be carried out before proceeding to the deeper structures. In some obese patients, the vein is not readily apparent and a layer of fat between it and the sternocleidomastoid must be entered to locate the jugular itself. If this is not done, it is possible to fall into an incorrect plane lateral and deep to the jugular vein. As soon as the jugular is identified, dissection is shifted to come along the medial jugular border and the vein is held back with blunt retractors. The importance of the blunt retractor in preventing vascular injury at this point cannot be overemphasized. In this process, several small veins and one large common facial vein are customarily crossing the field and need to be doubly ligated and divided (Fig. 77–2). The underlying carotid artery is soon identified once the jugular is retracted. Most often, we come on the common carotid artery first, and at the point of first visualization, the anesthesiologist is instructed to give 5000 units of intravenous heparin, which, as discussed previously, is never reversed. Dissec-

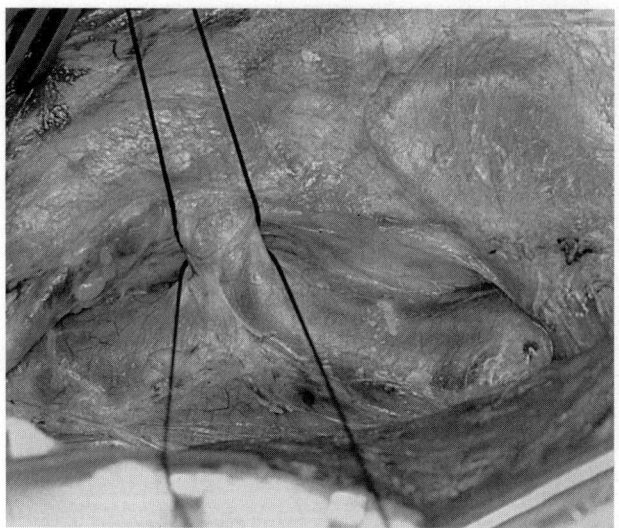

FIGURE 77–2 ■ Intraoperative photograph showing the left jugular vein with 2–0 silk sutures around the left common facial vein. The carotid cannot be visualized yet.

tion of the carotid complex is then straightforward, and the common, external, and internal carotid arteries are isolated with the gentlest possible dissection and encircled with 0–0 silk ties (or vessel loops if preferred) passed with a right-angle clamp. We no longer routinely inject the carotid sinus; however, the anesthesiologist is notified when the bifurcation is being dissected, and if any changes in vital signs ensue, the sinus can be injected with 2 to 3 ml of 1% plain lidocaine through a short 25-gauge needle (this has not been necessary for several years). Although the carotid complex is completely exposed, the common and external carotids are not dissected free from their underlying beds to prevent postoperative kinking and coiling of these vessels. These arteries are dissected circumferentially only in those areas where silk ties or clamps are placed around them. Posterior dissection is more extensive in the region of the ICA, where posterior tacking sutures occasionally may be placed later and tied.

The common carotid 0–0 silk is passed through a wire loop, which is then pulled through a rubber sleeve (Rummel tourniquet), thereby facilitating constriction of the vessel around an intraluminal shunt if this becomes necessary. The external and internal carotid ties or loops are merely secured with mosquito clamps. Particular attention is paid to the superior thyroid artery, which is dissected free and secured with a double-loop 0–0 silk ligature (some prefer an aneurysm clip for this). A hanging mosquito clamp keeps tension on this occlusive Pott's tie. Occasionally multiple branches of this artery are identified on the preoperative angiogram, and these must be individually dealt with so that no troublesome back-bleeding ensues during the procedure through ignorance of these vessels. It is also essential that the external carotid silk tie (and subsequent cross-clamp) be placed proximal to any major external branches, lest unacceptable back-bleeding occur during the arteriotomy and repair.

Proper placement of the retractors facilitates control of the carotid system. The hanging mosquitoes and silk ties are draped over these retractor handles to keep the field uncluttered. A blunt hinged retractor is invaluable in exposing the ICA when a far distal exposure is necessary. Dissection of the ICA must be complete and extend clearly beyond the distal extent of the plaque before cross-clamping is performed. A clear plane can be developed if the jugular vein is followed distally and dissection follows the plane between the lateral carotid wall and the medial jugular border. By following this plane, the hypoglossal nerve is readily identified as it swings down medial to the jugular and crosses toward the midline over the ICA. The nerve is mobilized along its lateral wall adjacent to the jugular vein, after which it can be isolated with a vessel loop and gently retracted from the field. Hypoglossal paresis is rare, and it seems to result in cases where the nerve is not visualized and is blindly retracted. On occasion, adequate mobilization of the hypoglossal nerve requires ligation of a small arterial branch of the external carotid to the sternocleidomastoid muscle, which loops over the nerve. We have never seen inadvertent transection of the hypoglossal nerve.

Several nerves can be injured during carotid exposure and endarterectomy. An important caveat in preventing nerve injury is the especially careful use of forceps once the carotid sheath is entered. From a long experience of working with trainees, it is apparent that less attention is paid to the forceps hand during dissection, and nerves can be "picked up" inadvertently and sustain a crush injury while the surgeon concentrates on the arterial dissection. The spinal accessory and hypoglossal nerves have already been discussed. The vagus nerve lies deep to the carotid in the carotid sheath and can be inadvertently cross-clamped if not identified. The marginal mandibular branch of the facial nerve can be stretched by medial retraction in the high exposure of the internal carotid, and the greater auricular nerve is at risk in a high incision, leaving the patient with a troublesome numb ear if it is transected. We have seen Horner's syndrome (always transient) from unrecognized injury to the pericarotid sympathetic chain. Cutaneous sensory nerves always are transected with the skin incision, and we advise patients that the anterior triangle of their neck will be numb for approximately 6 months after endarterectomy, after which sensation customarily reverts to normal.

It is vital to have adequate exposure of the ICA and control distal to the plaque before opening the vessel. The extent of the plaque can be readily palpated with some experience by a moistened finger. There is also a visual cue where the vessel becomes pinker (instead of hard and yellow) and more normal-appearing distal to the extent of the plaque. If high exposure is needed, the posterior belly of the digastric muscle can be cut with impunity, although this is necessary only in a small percentage of cases. When complete exposure is achieved, the final step in preparation for cross-clamping is to ensure that the shunt clamp can be fitted around the ICA to secure the shunt if one is used. We formerly used a Javid clamp for this purpose, but we have switched to a custom-designed, commercial spring-loaded pinch clamp (Loftus Carotid Shunt Clamp; Scanlan Instruments, St. Paul, MN), which is available in several angles and has a special head exactly sized to grasp the internal carotid and indwelling shunt without leakage. The Loftus shunt clamp is illustrated in Figure 77–3.

We also use a sterile marking pen to draw the proposed

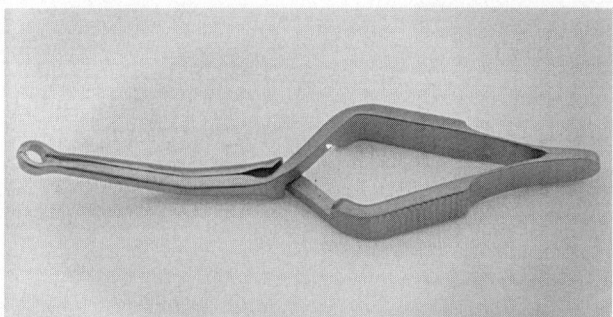

FIGURE 77–3 ■ The Loftus shunt clamp. This customized spring-loaded clamp is slightly angled with an encircling atraumatic end. This clamp is used to secure the indwelling shunt in the internal carotid artery.

arteriotomy line along the vessel, which is helpful in preventing a jagged or curving suture line (Fig. 77–4). The arteriotomy is made on the anterior surface of the internal carotid to facilitate the subsequent repair.

The monitoring system is then rechecked and the electroencephalographer is notified of impending cross-clamping. Once a suitable period of baseline EEG has been recorded, the common carotid is occluded with a large DeBakey vascular clamp, and small, straight bulldog clamps or Yasargil aneurysm clips are used to occlude the internal and external carotid arteries. We always occlude the ICA first in the belief that this approach has the lowest risk of embolization associated with clamping. A No. 11 blade is then used to begin the arteriotomy in the common carotid and, when the lumen is identified, a Pott's scissors is used to cut straight up along the marked line into the region of the bifurcation and then up into the ICA until normal ICA is entered (Fig. 77–5). In severely stenotic vessels with friable plaques, the lumen is not always easily discerned and false planes within the lesion are often encountered; one must take great care to ensure that the back wall of the carotid is not lacerated and that the true lumen is identified before attempting shunt insertion.

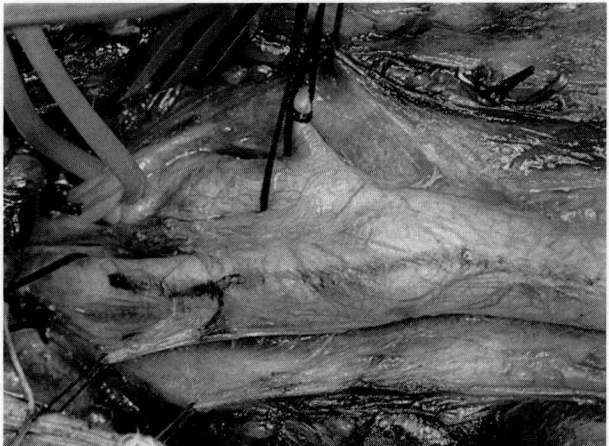

FIGURE 77–4 ■ The carotid system has been cleanly dissected, and the arteriotomy site has been marked with a black marking pen. In the left upper quadrant, the hypoglossal nerve has been dissected out and isolated with a vessel loop. The external carotid and superior thyroid artery have silk ties around them. In the left edge of the photograph, the internal carotid artery, which is free of plaque, has a silk tie around it.

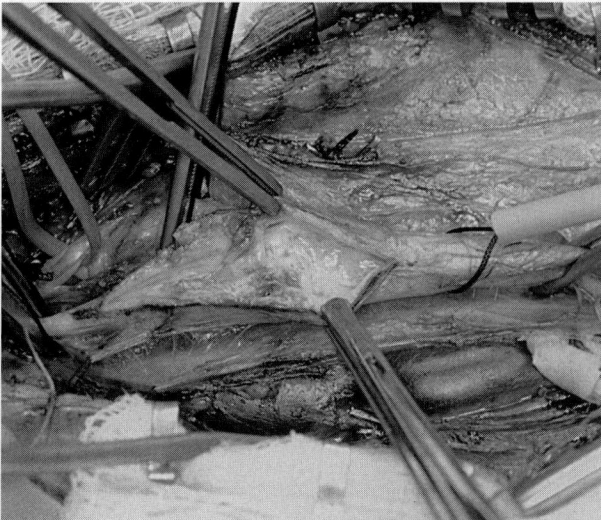

FIGURE 77–5 ■ After the vessel has been opened, the plaque can be best seen by gently everting the edges of the artery with vascular forceps.

Changes in the EEG mandate a rapid trial of induced hypertension. If there is no immediate reversal of these changes, an intraluminal shunt is used. The wisdom of shunt use is discussed elsewhere in the chapter. Numerous shunt types are available. We now use a customized indwelling shunt, the Loftus Carotid Endarterectomy Shunt (Fig. 77–6). This is a 15-cm, straight silicone tube, supplied in two diameters in the same kit, with tapered ends for easy insertion and a bulb at the proximal end to facilitate anchoring by the Rummel tourniquet. This shunt has a centrally placed black marker so that cephalad shunt migration can be readily discerned and corrected. The shunt is first inserted into the common carotid artery and secured by pulling up on the silk ties; a mosquito clamp then holds the rubber sleeve in place to snug the silk around both the vessel and the intraluminal shunt. The shunt tubing is held closed at its mid-portion with a heavy vascular forceps, then briefly opened to confirm blood flow and evacuate any debris in the shunt tubing. Suction is then used by the assistant to elucidate the lumen of the ICA, and the distal end of the shunt tubing is placed therein. After the shunt is again bled, flushing any debris from the ICA, the bulldog clamp is removed and the shunt is advanced up the ICA until the black dot lies in the center of the arteriotomy. The shunt, if properly placed, should slide easily into the ICA, and no undue force should be used to prevent intimal damage and possible dissection. The Loftus shunt clamp is then used to secure the shunt distally in the internal carotid. Visualization of the dot in the center of the arteriotomy confirms constant correct positioning of the shunt (Fig. 77–7). A hand-held Doppler probe can be applied to the shunt tubing to confirm flow audibly.

With or without the shunt, the plaque is next dissected from the arterial wall with a Freer elevator. A vascular pick-up is used to hold the wall, and the Freer is moved from side to side, developing a plane first in the lateral wall of the arteriotomy (Fig. 77–8). The plaque is usually readily separated in a primary case and we go approximately half way around the wall before proceeding to the

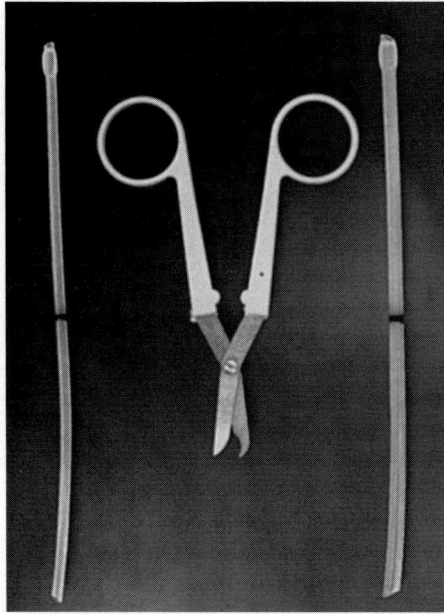
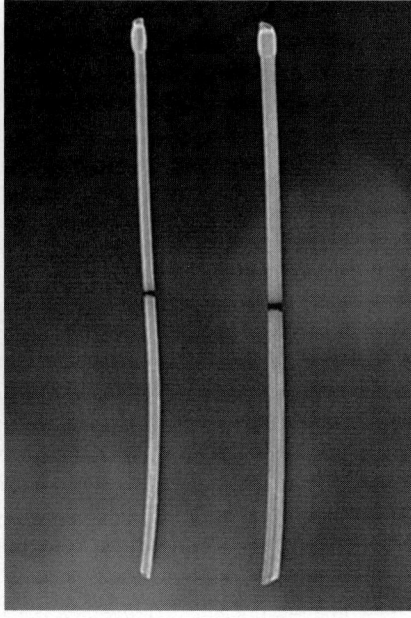

FIGURE 77–6 ■ The Loftus shunt set. The set contains two shunts of differing diameters, to allow for sizing preferences, as well as a special scissors (disposable) to hook and cut the shunt cleanly for removal without damaging the back wall of the carotid. The shunt is a straight silicone tube that is beveled and rounded at both ends for safe insertion. A built-up bulb is present on the proximal (CCA) end to anchor the shunt within the Rummel tourniquet.

other side. The plaque is then dissected on the medial side of the common carotid and transected proximally with a Pott's or Church scissors. A clean feathering away of the plaque is almost never possible in the common carotid and the goal here is to transect the plaque sharply, leaving a smooth transition zone. We like to pass a right-angle clamp between the plaque and the normal vessel and cut sharply along the clamp blade with the No. 15 knife (Fig. 77–9). Despite the direction of flow, the proximal end point can create a flap, and the surgeon should ensure that the common carotid end point is adherent. Attention is then directed to the ICA, where likewise the plaque is dissected

first laterally and then medially, after which an attempt is made to feather the plaque down smoothly from the ICA (Fig. 77–10). However, we find in some cases that no matter how far up the ICA we go, a shelf of normal intima remains and tacking sutures are required. Attention is finally directed to the final point of plaque attachment at the orifice of the external carotid. The vascular pick-up is used to grip across the entire plaque at the external carotid opening and, with some traction on the plaque, the external carotid can be everted such that the plaque can be dissected quite far up into that vessel (Fig. 77–11). The eversion of the external carotid and thus optimal plaque removal can be facilitated by "pushing" the distal external artery proximally with the clamp or forceps. The plaque is often tethered in the external carotid by the clamp, and as long as the lumen is held closed with the heavy forceps, this clamp can be removed without untoward bleeding, allowing avulsion of the distal plaque. The clamp must be

FIGURE 77–7 ■ The Loftus shunt in place. The shunt is secured at the common carotid end by a Rummel tourniquet, and in the internal carotid by the Loftus shunt clamp. The black band indicates the center of the shunt and helps to prevent unrecognized shunt migration (which should also be prevented by the fat bulb on the common carotid end anchored by the Rummel tourniquet).

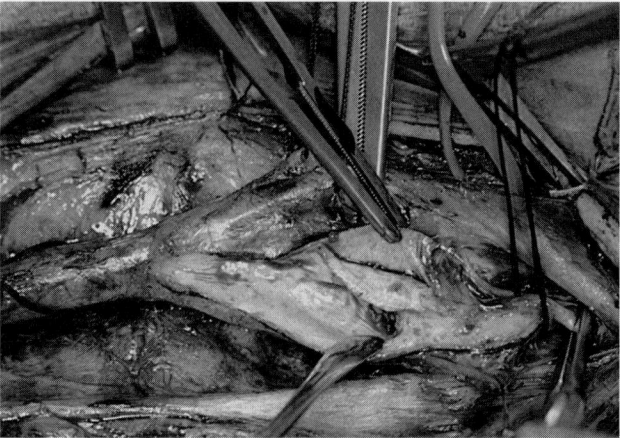

FIGURE 77–8 ■ Plaque dissection is started by using a Freer dissector to develop a plane at the lateral edge of the arteriotomy. In this left carotid endarterectomy, the medial edge has already developed a plane, while the surgeon starts on the lateral edge.

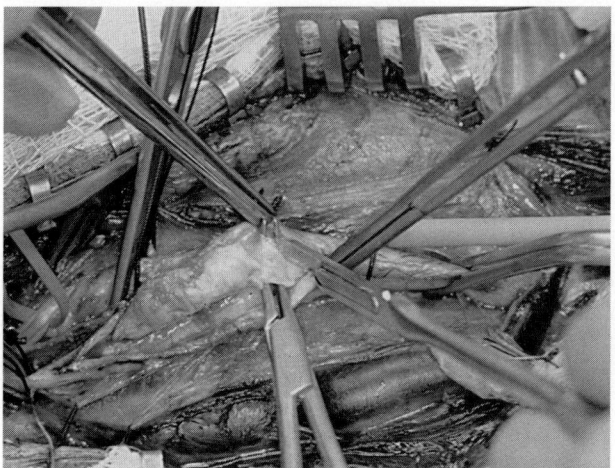

**FIGURE 77–9** ■ By using a right-angled clamp, the plaque can be incised in the common carotid artery by slipping the clamp under the plaque and then using a No. 15 knife to cut cleanly along the lower blade of the clamp.

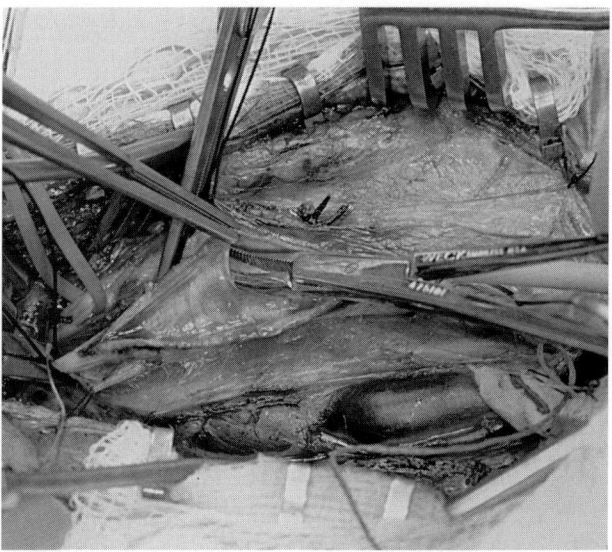

**FIGURE 77–11** ■ After the plaque has been removed from the internal and common carotid arteries, attention is then turned to the external carotid artery. The plaque is gently removed from the external artery with a fine hemostat and gentle traction.

quickly reapplied to stem back-bleeding that occurs when the plaque is removed from the external carotid. If plaque removal is inadequate in the external carotid artery, thrombosis may ensue that can occlude the entire carotid tree, with disastrous results. If there is any question of incomplete removal of the external plaque, we do not hesitate to extend the arteriotomy up the external carotid itself and close it using a separate suture line.

After gross plaque removal, a careful search is made for any remaining fragments adherent to the arterial wall (Fig. 77–12). Suspect areas are gently stroked with a peanut sponge and every attempt is made to remove all loose fragments in a circumferential fashion, elevating them the complete width of the vessel until they break free at the arteriotomy edge. Although it is important to remove all loose fragments, no attempt is made to elevate firmly attached fragments that pose no danger of elevating or breaking off.

Several special aspects of plaque removal need to be considered. The simplest plaques to remove are the soft,

friable ones with intraplaque hemorrhage and thrombus, which dissect quite readily and from which fragments are easily removed (Fig. 77–13). The more difficult are the severely stenotic, stony-hard plaques in which a plane of dissection at the lateral border of the carotid may not be readily apparent. This situation is analogous to the gross appearance in a case of recurrent carotid stenosis. In these instances, even the most gentle plaque removal results in areas of thinning where only an adventitial layer is left in the posterior wall of the carotid. These cases have been treated by primary plication with one or two double-armed interrupted stitches of 6–0 Prolene placed in the same fashion as the tacking sutures, and no untoward consequences have ensued. Likewise, we have occasionally encountered an intraluminal thrombus emanating from a congenital web or shelf in the lumen of the vessel, and this has been successfully plicated with a posteriorly placed

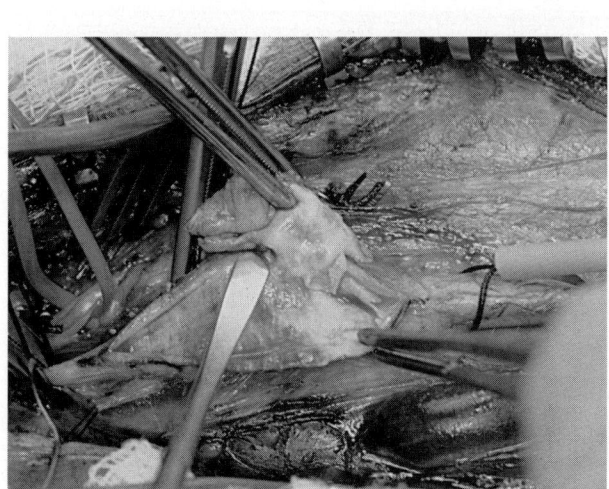

**FIGURE 77–10** ■ The dissection of the plaque is continued with the Freer elevator along the medial edge.

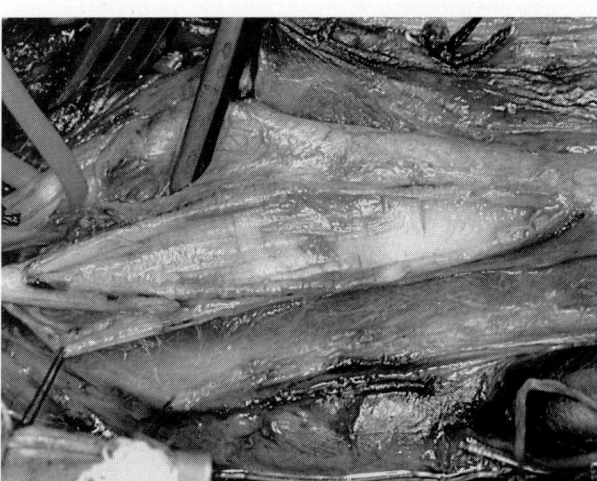

**FIGURE 77–12** ■ The lumen is then checked for any remaining fragments that might have adhered to the wall.

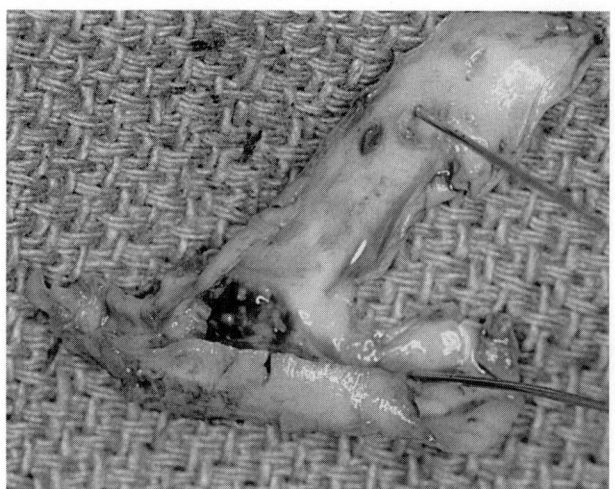

FIGURE 77–13 ■ A soft, friable plaque with a small thrombus is shown.

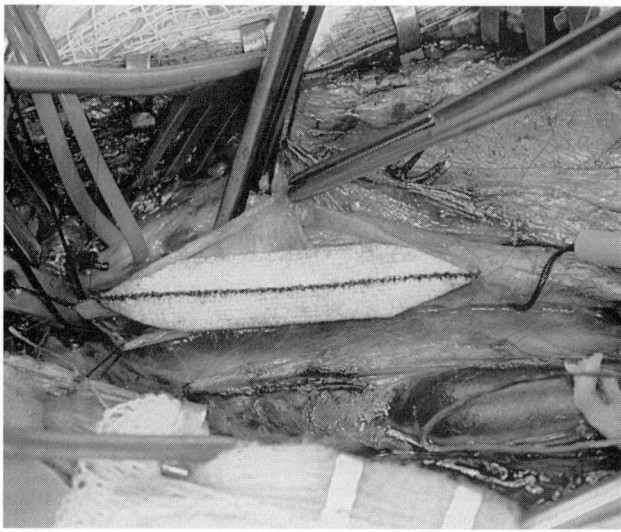

FIGURE 77–14 ■ The Hemashield patch is attached to both ends of the arteriotomy with a double-armed 6–0 Prolene stitch. The needles are left attached to allow closure of the patch graft. Notice that both ends of the patch are tapered.

stitch of double-armed 6–0 Prolene. In all cases, the goal is to leave as smooth an arteriotomy bed as possible with minimal areas of denudation or roughness available as sites for thrombus formation.

Attention is then directed to the arterial repair. If desired, the operating microscope can be brought into the field at this point, or in some cases sooner, to allow for removal of the small fragments under high magnification.[2, 21, 48, 49] Our preference is to continue with 3.5× loupe magnification. If tacking sutures are required, double-armed sutures of 6–0 Prolene are placed vertically from the inside of the vessel out, such that they traverse the intimal edge and are tied outside the adventitial layer. Most often, two such sutures are used, placed at the four and eight o'clock positions.

The patch, whatever material is used, is then fashioned if the surgeon has chosen this option. The patch material (Hemashield for the purposes of this description and illustrations) is placed over the arteriotomy and cut to the exact length of the opening. After removal from the field, the

ends are trimmed and tapered to a point with fine Metzenbaum scissors. Each end of the patch is then anchored to the arteriotomy with double-armed 6–0 Prolene sutures and the needles are left on and secured with rubber-shod clamps (Fig. 77–14). The medial wall suture line is closed first, and a running nonlocking stitch is brought from the ICA anchor to the common carotid anchor, where it is tied to a free end of the common carotid anchor Prolene (Fig. 77–15). The lateral wall is then closed (with the remaining limb of the ICA anchor stitch) from the ICA to just below the level of the carotid bulb. At this point, the second arm of the common carotid anchor stitch is used to run up the common carotid artery lateral wall to meet the ICA limb. Small bites are taken just at the arterial edge throughout (ensuring, however, that all layers are included) and sutures are placed relatively close together to prevent leaks. Care is also taken that no stray adventitial tags or suture ends are

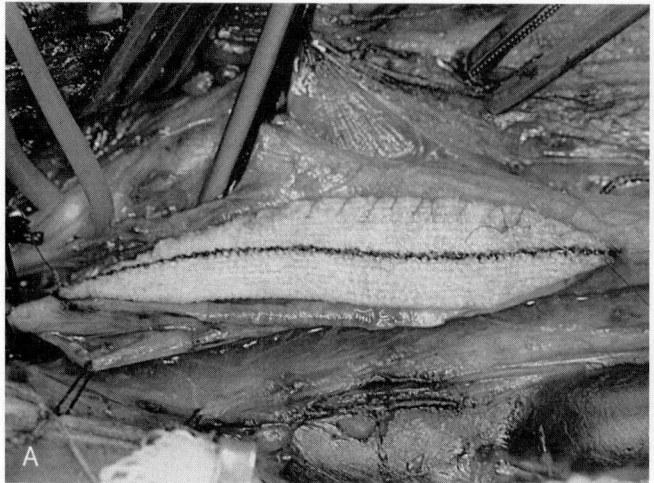

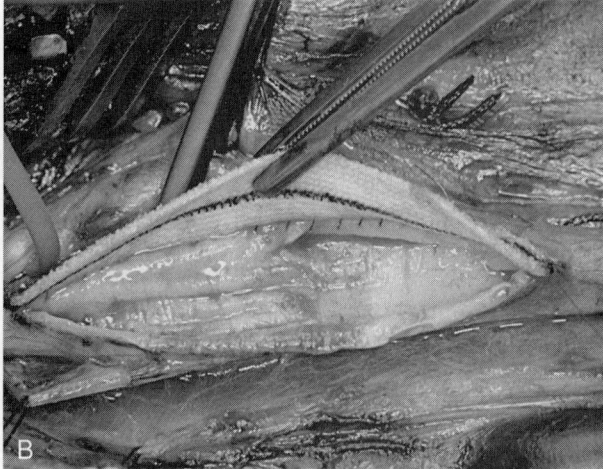

FIGURE 77–15 ■ A, The medial wall is closed first from the internal carotid artery to the common carotid artery. B, The patch is lifted to show the sutures from the luminal side.

sewn into the lumen, where they might induce thrombosis. Several millimeters of unsewn vessel are left on the lateral wall, ensuring room to remove the shunt if one has been used. After the electroencephalographer is again notified, the shunt is double-clamped with two parallel straight mosquitoes, then cut between them, and removed in two sections, one from each end. A common error at this point is to entangle the suture material in the shunt clamps and thereby hamper smooth shunt removal. With or without shunt, the arteriotomy is completely closed as follows: all three vessels are first opened and closed sequentially to ensure that back-bleeding is present from the internal, external, and common carotid arteries. The ICA is back-bled last to ensure that it is free of debris. The two stitches are then held taut by the surgeon while the assistant introduces a heparinized saline syringe with a blunt needle into the arterial lumen. The vessel is filled with heparinized saline and in this process all air is evacuated from the intraluminal space. As the stitches are drawn up and a surgeon's knot is thrown, the blunt needle is withdrawn, allowing no air to enter. Seven or eight further knots are then placed in this most crucial stitch (Fig. 77–16). The clamps are removed first from the external carotid, then from the common carotid, and finally, some 10 seconds later, from the ICA. In this fashion, all loose debris and remaining microbubbles of air are flushed into the external carotid circulation. Meticulous attention is paid to evacuation of all debris and air before opening the ICA in every case. However, in the rare case where there is a known external carotid occlusion (although most of these can be reopened at surgery with an external carotid endarterectomy), this technique is crucial because there is no external carotid safety valve and all intraluminal contents will be shunted directly into the intracranial circulation.

An alternative method for completing the repair involves removal of the ligature or clip from the superior thyroid artery or external carotid before final closure, allowing back-bleeding from that vessel to fill the lumen and eliminate the air and debris while the final stitches are placed and tied. We do not use this because we find the bleeding to be annoying.

When the clamps have been removed, the suture lines

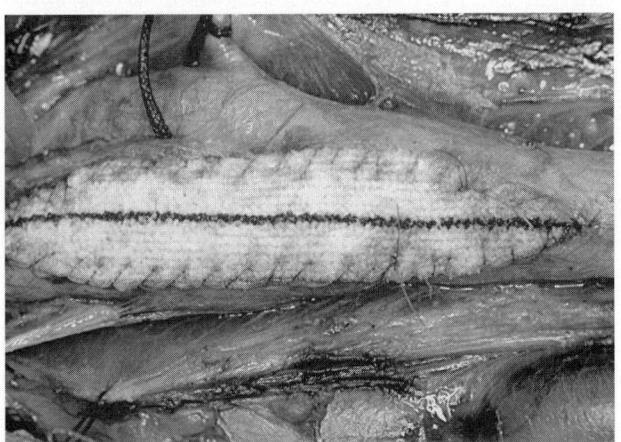

FIGURE 77–16 ■ The lateral wall is then closed half-way down the internal and then with the second stitch half-way up the common carotid artery.

are inspected for leaks, which are customarily controlled with pressure, patience, and Surgicel gauze. In occasional cases, a single throw of 6–0 Prolene is necessary to close a persistent arterial hemorrhage. Suture repairs of bleeding points are more likely if a patch graft has been placed. It is almost never necessary to reapply clamps to the artery if the repair has been properly performed. The repair is then lined with Surgicel and the three vessels are tested with a hand-held Doppler to ensure patency. Retractors are removed and hemostasis is confirmed both along the jugular vein and from the surrounding soft tissues. Persistent oozing is often encountered in these patients, who have often received large doses of antiplatelet agents is addition to their intraoperative heparin. A final Doppler check is made and the wound is closed in layers. The carotid sheath is closed first to provide a barrier against infection, and the platysma is then closed as a separate layer to ensure a good cosmetic result. Either running or interrupted subcuticular stitches may be used to close the skin edges. A Hemovac drain is left inside the carotid sheath; the drain is removed on the first postoperative day. Patients are continued on aspirin after surgery and are discharged in 1 to 2 days.

We manage any postoperative neurologic deficit, including transient ischemic attack (TIA) alone, with immediate assessment of the technical adequacy of repair. If high-quality color duplex ultrasonography is available, this may allow quick documentation of patency and identify any partially obstructing defects. Angiography is performed if ultrasonography is indeterminate or unavailable. Any postoperative occluded carotid is re-explored and repatched immediately, although since adopting the primary Hema-shield patch repair, the incidence of postoperative occlusion has been zero in our series.

## SPECIAL SITUATIONS

### Complete Occlusion

Surgery is usually indicated for cases of acute carotid occlusion if the patient is not so debilitated that recovery is unlikely. Surgery is essentially always indicated for known acute postoperative occlusion, reflecting technical error in most cases. Surgery is sometimes indicated for cases of subacute carotid occlusion, and in cases of chronic occlusion if the possibility of a "string sign" minimally patent vessel (which can usually be reopened) exists, justifying exploration. Our surgical technique for complete common carotid/ICA occlusion involves opening (or re-opening) the common carotid and ICA once the vessels have been controlled. The thrombus is usually seen at the carotid bulb and extending into the distal ICA; in our experience, the external carotid is usually patent. Removal of thrombus and associated ICA plaque may establish back-bleeding; if not, the ICA can be explored with a No. 8 feeding tube cut to a 15-cm length and attached to a 10-ml syringe. The tube is advanced into the ICA, and the syringe is drawn back to establish suction, which often pulls down the distal thrombus as the tubing is withdrawn. If this fails, Fogarty catheters are passed into the ICA, but the risk of establishing a carotid-cavernous fistula with these must be considered. If back-bleeding cannot be established, we cleanly ligate the distal and proximal ICA stumps and perform a common/external carotid endarterectomy and repair. If 6 hours or more have passed since occlusion, the likelihood of successful neurologic salvage is diminished, and the risk of intracerebral hemorrhage appears to increase.

## Stump Syndrome

The term *stump syndrome* describes the continuation of ipsilateral ischemic symptoms after internal carotid occlusion due to emboli from the ICA intraluminal thrombus that enters the intracranial circulation through the external carotid artery and its collateral blood flow. After strict criteria are met,[30] surgical correction is undertaken using a standard common to *external* carotid endarterectomy. After removal of the thrombus from the ICA stump, we attempt to reopen the ICA and establish back-bleeding. If this is not possible (it usually is not), the stump is obliterated with inside-out sutures or with external application of large Weck clips. We stress that the ICA lumen must be obliterated. A standard external carotid endarterectomy is then performed (we place a common to external patch graft) and the arteriotomy is closed in the usual fashion.

## Bilateral Carotid Endarterectomy

Bilateral carotid endarterectomy runs the risk of producing extreme swings in blood pressure from concurrent denervation of both carotid sinuses[54] and from risk of bilateral cranial nerve injury. For those patients who require bilateral endarterectomy, we recommend a staged procedure, with at least a 6-week window between the procedures. We customarily have the patient examined by an otolaryngologist to rule out an occult cranial nerve injury before the second procedure is undertaken. Unilateral nerve dysfunction in the cervical region is troublesome, but bilateral dysfunction can be disabling. We have sometimes deferred the second surgery because of an occult vocal cord paralysis. When this happens, the patient is maintained on medical management until cord function returns (as it usually does), after which the second-side carotid endarterectomy is performed.

## Plaque Morphology

The correlation of plaque ulceration with ischemic neurologic symptoms and the need for surgery is difficult for several reasons. First, studies have shown poor interobserver variability, either on ultrasound or arteriographic examinations, and poor correlation between pathologic specimens and radiographically demonstrated ulceration. Second, in symptomatic patients, deep ulceration is most commonly found with significant degrees of carotid stenosis, and it becomes difficult to separate clinical symptomatology between these two findings.[26, 55] The most recent data from NASCET[40] show that in medically treated patients with 50% to 99% stenosis (now proven to be un-

equivocal surgical candidates), the presence of plaque ulceration with stenosis significantly increases the risk of stroke.[13] The presence of ulceration in plaques of less than 50% linear stenosis requires surgical intervention remains an unanswered question that has not been addressed by cooperative trial data.

The significance of intraplaque hemorrhage as a predictor of ischemic symptoms is also unclear. In one study, heterogeneous plaque morphology on duplex scanning (consistent with intraplaque hemorrhage) was a significant risk factor for subsequent neurologic events if the underlying stenosis exceeded 50%.[51] Although one review also suggested that intraplaque hemorrhage was more common in patients with symptomatic carotid artery disease,[26] other studies suggest that there is a low correlation between ischemic symptoms and plaque hematoma in patients undergoing carotid endarterectomy.[34]

# CRITICAL STENOSIS/EMERGENCY SURGERY

## Intraluminal Thrombi

The problem of surgical timing in patients with angiographically demonstrated propagating intraluminal thrombus remains an open question among cerebrovascular experts.[6, 29] In patients who present with TIAs (which, in our experience, have always resolved with anticoagulation) and an intraluminal thrombus, we opt for delayed surgery (at 6 weeks after repeat angiography) in every case and have never seen a negative outcome from intercurrent embolization once heparin is instituted.

Likewise, there is a small subset of patients with postoperative neurologic events (most often a TIA) after carotid endarterectomy who are found to have a fresh thrombus adherent to the suture line (by angiography), partially occluding the artery, and which is presumably the source of embolic phenomena. If there is no other angiographic evidence of technical inadequacy, we manage these patients conservatively as well, with full anticoagulation and 6-week follow-up angiography. In every case the thrombus has resolved, and there have been no negative neurologic outcomes in our series with this plan of management. Despite the surgeon's natural inclination to fix a problem with bold action, we find that a measured, conservative approach yields good results in cases of fresh or propagating thrombus, and in our experience it is superior to undertaking a high-risk surgical procedure.

## Tandem Lesions of the Carotid Siphon

In the NASCET trial, symptomatic patients were excluded if the degree of siphon stenosis exceeded that at the carotid bifurcation.[40] The presence of stenotic disease at the carotid siphon has been proposed as a contraindication to carotid endarterectomy because of both the inability to pinpoint the symptomatic source and the reputed increased possibilities of postoperative occlusion from decreased carotid flow velocity. This has not been our experience, and we do not hesitate to operate on patients with tandem lesions if we are convinced that an active plaque at the carotid bifurcation is the source of their embolic phenomena.

## Concurrent Intracranial Aneurysm

There is always a concern that cervical carotid revascularization (for either symptomatic or asymptomatic carotid stenosis, especially high-grade stenosis) will lead to rupture of a known intracranial aneurysm when both lesions are present. Although this is no doubt a small risk, several articles have shown that it is safe to proceed with carotid endarterectomy with a silent intracranial aneurysm discovered on angiography.[33, 50] Obviously, the symptomatic lesion should be treated first. We do not hesitate to operate in the light of an asymptomatic intracranial aneurysm, but we do customarily recommend subsequent craniotomy and aneurysm clipping as well.

## Concurrent Coronary/Carotid Artery Disease

It is well established that patients with extracranial carotid artery disease have a higher-than-normal incidence of coronary artery disease as well as other peripheral vascular problems.[24, 39] Indeed, the risk of perioperative myocardial infarction exceeds the risk of perioperative stroke in many clinical series of carotid endarterectomy. Several major questions arise when planning treatment for concurrent coronary/carotid artery disease. First, what is the risk of coronary revascularization in a patient with a high-grade asymptomatic stenosis or bruit? Second, in patients with symptomatic carotid artery disease, what is the appropriate work-up of the coronary circulation? And third, if surgical degrees of both carotid artery and coronary artery disease are identified in the same patient, what is the appropriate surgical management (staged carotid and then coronary revascularization, combined procedure, or "reverse-staged" coronary revascularization and then delayed carotid endarterectomy)?

The first question regarding asymptomatic bruit in patients symptomatic with coronary artery disease is straightforward. ACAS has shown a surgical benefit for lesions with greater than 60% stenosis, and we recommend that these be staged before coronary revascularization whenever possible.

The second question regarding the appropriate work-up of coronary artery disease in patients with symptomatic carotid arteries is a more difficult one. In this situation, work-up is customarily guided by the history and symptomatology of the patient. It has been our practice to obtain cardiology consultation in any patient with a history of angina, known heart disease, or abnormal resting electrocardiogram. The work-up proceeds with a thallium stress test with exercise or dipyridamole, and, if there is any evidence of myocardial ischemia, coronary angiography is performed.[27, 32]

When the results of cardiac evaluation indicate the need for coronary revascularization, the question becomes one of timing of the surgical procedures. Our preference is to do staged procedures whenever possible. With careful hemodynamic monitoring and good anesthetic technique, we are able routinely to perform safe unilateral carotid endarterectomies before coronary revascularization. An occasional patient with severe unstable angina may require a combined procedure, but this entails a significantly higher surgical risk, and we attempt staged procedures whenever possible.[10, 27]

Most series dealing with reverse-staged coronary/carotid procedures (coronary artery revascularization first with delayed carotid endarterectomy) discuss them in the context of asymptomatic carotid disease. Although we previously believed that reverse-staged procedures in asymptomatic patients were not indicated, we now think that for unstable coronary disease with an unacceptable cardiac anesthetic risk, a reverse-staged procedure may be appropriate, because the ACAS data have validated surgery on silent carotid lesions.

It is our preference, then, to aggressively work up any patient with cardiac symptoms before carotid endarterectomy. If procedures in both circulations are indicated, staged procedures are preferable unless the coronary circulation disease makes anesthesia for carotid endarterectomy an untenable proposition. In such cases, a combined procedure may be acceptable. We see no indication for reverse-staged procedures in symptomatic patients and prefer to reconstruct an asymptomatic carotid stenosis exceeding 60% first, whenever possible.

## Recurrent Stenosis

There is a small but definite incidence of recurrent carotid stenosis after primary carotid endarterectomy. We have seen a decrease in our restenosis rate after adopting patching in all of our cases. Piepgras and colleagues[42] show a symptomatic restenosis rate of 1% and an asymptomatic restenosis rate of 4% to 5% at 2-year follow-up when a patch graft was used. Aside from technical inadequacies, it has been difficult to identify risk factors associated with recurrent carotid stenosis, although continuation of smoking habits after endarterectomy has proved to be a significant risk factor in several studies,[9, 11] whereas hypertension, diabetes mellitus, family history, lipid studies, aspirin use, and coronary disease may not be as important.

Reoperation for carotid stenosis is a technically difficult procedure. It is associated with significantly higher risks than primary endarterectomy. In our institution, the possibility of reoperation for carotid stenosis is entertained in patients who present with angiographically proved disease and classical neurologic symptoms referable to the appropriate artery, or with documented progression to severe stenosis while being followed with annual serial duplex examinations.

## CONCLUSIONS

Now that cooperative study data are available to support the clear superiority of surgery in the management of asymptomatic carotid stenoses greater than 60% and symptomatic stenoses exceeding 50%, carotid artery reconstruction will undergo continued technical refinements. Many of the basic neurovascular principles are standard, but conditions formerly thought to be unsuitable for carotid endarterectomy (e.g., contralateral occlusion, tandem stenosis, and fresh stroke) no longer prevent successful surgery in competent hands. In our opinion, this expanded acceptance of carotid surgery arises from more rigorous training and credentialing of surgeons, improved monitoring and anesthetic techniques, and the scientific application of cooperative trial methodology to the carotid problem.

The surgical methods presented here have produced acceptable postoperative results in a broad spectrum of patients with carotid disease. Minor technical details that may vary among surgeons are probably of little significance. On the other hand, subtleties of technique that may add operative time to the "routine" carotid procedure assume greater importance when difficult lesions or high exposures are encountered or when the patient is unstable. The importance of a good outcome under these more difficult circumstances leads us to approach all carotid surgery, no matter how simple it may seem, with the same technical strategy. Perhaps the most important factor in ensuring technically acceptable carotid surgery is the availability of a skilled cerebrovascular surgeon with a demonstrable morbidity and mortality rate below 3% and a proper understanding of both vascular principles and cerebral physiology.

## REFERENCES

1. Allen GS, Preziosi TJ: Carotid endarterectomy: A prospective study of its efficacy and safety. Medicine (Baltimore) 60:298–309, 1981.
2. Bailes J, Spetzler RF: Microsurgical Carotid Endarterectomy. New York: Lippincott–Raven, 1996.
3. Baker WH, Dorner DB, Barnes RW: Carotid endarterectomy: Is an indwelling shunt necessary? Surgery 82:321–326, 1977.
4. Baker WH, Rodman JA, Barnes RW, Hoyt JL: An evaluation of hypocarbia and hypercarbia during carotid endarterectomy. Stroke 7:451–454, 1976.
5. Benoit BG, Navavi NL: The "routine" use of intraluminal shunting in carotid endarterectomy. Can J Neurol Sci 5:339, 1978.
6. Biller J, Adams HP, Boarini D, et al: Intraluminal clot of the carotid artery. Surg Neurol 25:467–477, 1986.
7. Bland JE, Lazar ML: Carotid endarterectomy without shunt. Neurosurgery 8:153–157, 1981.
8. Boysen G, Ladegaard-Pedersen HG, Henriksen H, et al: The effect of $Pa_{CO_2}$ on regional cerebral blood flow and internal carotid arterial pressure during carotid clamping. Anesthesiology 35:286–300, 1971.
9. Clagett G, Rich N, McDonald P, et al: Etiologic factors for recurrent carotid artery stenosis. Surgery 2:313–318, 1983.
10. Cosgrove DM, Hertzer RN, Loop FD: Surgical management of synchronous carotid and coronary artery disease. J Vasc Surg 3:690–692, 1986.
11. Dempsey RJ, Moore R, Cordero S: Factors leading to early reoccurrence of carotid plaque after carotid endarterectomy. Surg Neurol 43:278–283, 1995.
12. Eastcott HHG, Pickering GW, Rob CG: Reconstruction of internal carotid artery in a patient with intermittent attacks of hemiplaegia. Lancet 2:994–996, 1954.
13. Eliasziw M, Streifler JW, Fox AJ, et al: Significance of plaque ulceration in symptomatic patients with high-grade carotid stenosis. Stroke 25:304–308, 1994.
14. Executive Committee for the Asymptomatic Carotid Atherosclerosis Study: Endarterectomy for asymptomatic carotid stenosis. JAMA 273:1421–1428, 1995.
15. Ferguson GG: Carotid endarterectomy: Indications and surgical technique. Int Anesthesiol Clin 22:113–121, 1984.
16. Ferguson GG: Carotid endarterectomy: To shunt or not to shunt? Arch Neurol 43:615–617, 1986.
17. Ferguson GG: Extracranial carotid artery surgery. Clin Neurosurg 29:543–574, 1982.
18. Ferguson GG: Intra-operative monitoring and internal shunt: Are they necessary in carotid endarterectomy? Stroke 13:287–289, 1982.
19. Ferguson GG: Shunt almost never. Int Anesthesiol Clin 22:147–152, 1984.
20. Fields WS, Maslenikov V, Meyer JS, et al: Joint study of extracranial arterial occlusion. V: Progress report of prognosis following surgery or nonsurgical treatment for transient cerebral ischemic attacks and cervical carotid artery lesions. JAMA 211:1993–2003, 1970.
21. Findlay JM: Carotid microendarterectomy. Neurosurgery 32:792–798, 1993.
22. Fourcade HE, Larson CP, Ehrenfeld WK, et al: The effects of $CO_2$ and systemic hypertension on cerebral perfusion pressure during carotid endarterectomy. Anesthesiology 33:383–390, 1970.
23. Gelb AW: Anesthetic considerations for carotid endarterectomy. Int Anesthesiol Clin 22:153–164, 1984.
24. Gerraty RP, Gates PC, Doyle JC: Carotid stenosis and perioperative stroke risk in symptomatic and asymptomatic patients undergoing vascular or coronary surgery. Stroke 24:1115–1118, 1993.
25. Gianotta SL, Dicks RE, Kindt GW: Carotid endarterectomy: Technical improvements. Neurosurgery 7:309–312, 1980.
26. Gomez CR: Carotid plaque morphology and risk for stroke. Stroke 21:148–151, 1990.
27. Graor RA, Hertzer NR: Management of coexistent carotid artery and coronary artery disease. Curr Concepts Cerebrovasc Dis Stroke 23:19–23, 1988.
28. Gross CE, Bednar MM, Lew SM, et al: Preoperative volume expansion improves tolerance to carotid artery cross-clamping during endarterectomy. Neurosurgery 43:222–228, 1998.
29. Heros RC: Carotid endarterectomy in patients with intraluminal thrombus. Stroke 19:667–668, 1990.
30. Honeycutt JH, Loftus CM: The carotid stump syndrome. In Loftus CM, Kresowik TF (eds): Textbook of Carotid Artery Surgery. New York: Thieme, 2000, pp 315–320.
31. Javid H, Julian OC, Dye WS, et al: Seventeen year experience with routine shunting in carotid artery surgery. World J Surg 3:167–177, 1979.
32. Jones RH, Loftus CM, Sheldon WC, et al: Concomitant carotid and coronary disease. Patient Care 15:49–66, 1992.
33. Ladowski JS, Webster MW, Yonas HO, Steed DL: Carotid endarterectomy in patients with asymptomatic intracranial aneurysms. Ann Surg 200:70–73, 1984.
34. Lennihan L, Kupsky WJ, Mohr JP, et al: Lack of association between carotid plaque hematoma and ischemic cerebral symptoms. Stroke 18:879–881, 1987.
35. Loftus CM, Dyste GN, Reinarz SJ, Hingtgen WL: Cervical carotid dissection following carotid endarterectomy: A complication of indwelling shunt? Neurosurgery 19:441–445, 1986.
36. Messick JM, Sharbrough F, Sundt T: Selective shunting on the basis of EEG and regional CBF monitoring during carotid endarterectomy. Int Anesthesiol Clin 22:137–145, 1984.
37. Moore WS, Yee JM, Hall AD: Collateral cerebral blood pressure: An index to tolerance to temporary carotid occlusion. Arch Surg 106:520–523, 1973.
38. MRC European Carotid Surgery Trial: Interim results for symptomatic patients with severe (70–99%) or with mild (0–29%) carotid stenosis. Lancet 337:1235–1243, 1991.
39. Newman DC, Hicks RG: Combined carotid and coronary artery surgery: A review of the literature. Ann Thorac Surg 45:574–581, 1988.
40. North American Symptomatic Carotid Endarterectomy Trial Collaborators: Beneficial effect of carotid endarterectomy in symptomatic patients with high grade stenosis. N Engl J Med 325:445–453, 1991.
41. Patterson RH: Technique of carotid endarterectomy. In Smith RR (ed): Stroke and the Extracranial Vessels. New York: Raven Press, 1984, pp 177–185.
42. Piepgras DG, Sundt TM, Marsh WR, et al: Recurrent carotid stenosis: Results and complications of 57 operations. In Sundt TM (ed): Occlusive Cerebrovascular Disease: Diagnosis and Surgical Management. Philadelphia: WB Saunders, 1987, pp 286–297.
43. Pistolese GR, Citone G, Faragilia V, et al: Effects of hypercapnia on cerebral blood flow during the clamping of the carotid arteries in surgical management of cerebrovascular insufficiency. Neurology 21:95–100, 1971.
44. Prioleau WH, Aiken AF, Hairston P: Carotid endarterectomy: Neurologic complications as related to surgical techniques. Ann Surg 185:678–683, 1977.

45. Rosenthal D, Stanton PE, Lamis PA: Carotid endarterectomy: The unreliability of intraoperative monitoring in patients having had a stroke or reversible ischemic neurological deficit. Arch Surg 116:1569–1575, 1981.
46. Schiro J, Mertz GH, Cannon JA, Cintora I: Routine use of a shunt for carotid endarterectomy. Am J Surg 142:735–738, 1981.
47. Shaw DA, Venables GS, Cartlidge NEF, et al: Carotid endarterectomy in patients with transient cerebral ischaemia. J Neurol Sci 64:45–53, 1984.
48. Spetzler RF, Martin N, Hadley MN, et al: Microsurgical endarterectomy under barbiturate protection: A prospective study. J Neurosurg 65:63–73, 1986.
49. Steiger HJ, Schaffler L, Liechti S: Results of microsurgical carotid endarterectomy. Acta Neurochir (Wien) 100:31–38, 1989.
50. Stern J, Whelan M, Brisman R, Correll JW: Management of extracranial carotid stenosis and intracranial aneurysms. J Neurosurg 51:147–150, 1979.
51. Sterpetti AV, Schultz RD, Feldhaus RJ, et al: Ultrasonographic features of carotid plaque and the risk of subsequent neurologic deficits. Surgery 104:652–660, 1988.
52. Sundt TM: The ischemic tolerance of neural tissue and the need for monitoring and selective shunting during carotid endarterectomy. Stroke 14:93–98, 1983.
53. Thompson JE: Protection of the brain during carotid endarterectomy. Int Anesthesiol Clin 22:123–128, 1984.
54. Wade JG, Larson CP, Hickey RF, et al: Effect of carotid endarterectomy on carotid chemoreceptor and baroreceptor function in man. N Engl J Med 282:823–829, 1970.
55. Wechsler LR: Ulceration and carotid artery disease. Stroke 19:650–653, 1998.
56. Wellman BJ, Loftus CM, Kresowik T, et al: The differences in electroencephalographic changes in awake versus anesthetized carotid endarterectomy patients. Neurosurgery 43:769–775, 1998.

# CHAPTER 78

# Surgical Exposure of the Distal Internal Carotid Artery

■ CALVIN B. ERNST and SONYA D. TUERFF

Since it was first successfully performed in the 1950s, the technique of carotid bifurcation endarterectomy has evolved so that the procedure has become standardized and safe. The approximately 108,000 carotid endarterectomies performed in the United States in 1996 are testimony to its widespread acceptance.[1] Less well standardized are exposure and reconstruction of the distal internal carotid artery, which is considered by some to be inaccessible. No doubt this is because of the infrequent need to correct such distal lesions, a requirement in only 3% of patients undergoing carotid endarterectomy.[2] In addition, such arteries are considered inaccessible because they are situated deep in the body or are obscured by bone, such as the mandible in the case of the internal carotid artery. However, seemingly inaccessible arteries often can be exposed surgically; when such exposure is not possible or prudent, reasonable therapeutic alternatives are usually available.

## LESIONS REQUIRING EXPOSURE OF THE DISTAL CAROTID ARTERY

Almost all carotid bifurcation lesions requiring surgical correction are atherosclerotic. Conversely, lesions requiring exposure and reconstruction of the distal carotid are rarely atherosclerotic and most commonly include traumatic lesions, aneurysms (true, false, or mycotic), recurrent (postoperative) stenoses, and fibromuscular dysplastic stenoses and kinks (Table 78–1). Occasionally, an atherosclerotic plaque originating at the carotid bifurcation may extend up to the skull base, beyond the limits of standard bifurcation endarterectomy, for which distal exposure is required (Fig. 78–1). The management of arterial complications of radiation therapy or the need for resection of benign or malignant neoplasms may require exposure of the distal carotid artery for reconstruction or ligation. Although rare, because a false aneurysm after a standard endarterectomy usually involves the accessible bifurcation, distal exposure may be required for repair, particularly if the pseudoaneurysm is large. The tendency of a thin-walled infected or mycotic aneurysm to rupture or for luminal contents to dislodge during dissection also mandates exposure of the distal carotid to manage such lesions successfully.

## ALTERNATIVES TO DISTAL EXPOSURE

For certain distal fibromuscular dysplastic lesions complicated by elongation and flow-reducing kinks or stenoses,

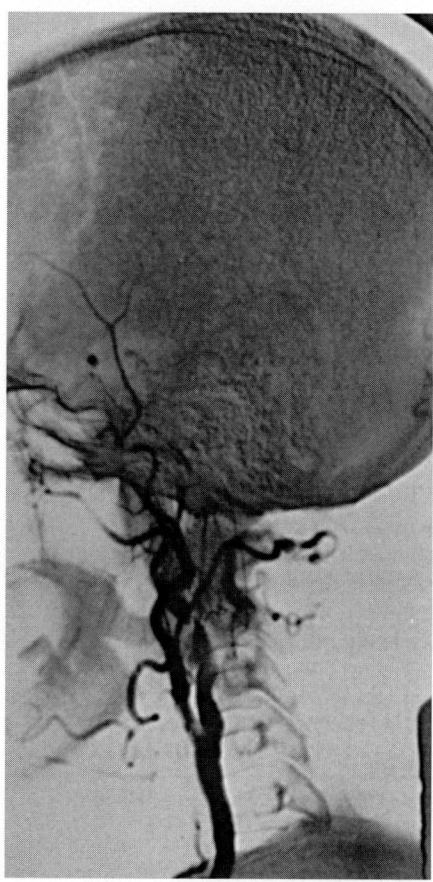

**FIGURE 78–1** ■ Selective carotid arteriogram demonstrating a preocclusive atherosclerotic lesion extending 4 to 5 cm into the internal carotid artery.

TABLE 78–1 ■ **LESIONS REQUIRING EXPOSURE OF THE DISTAL CAROTID ARTERY**

Distal extension of atherosclerotic bifurcation disease
Trauma
Fibromuscular dysplasia
Congenital loops or kinks
Aneurysm: true, false, or mycotic
Postirradiation arteriomalacia
Neoplastic involvement
Reoperation

an alternative to direct repair is proximal internal carotid resection, transluminal dilatation of the stenosis, and anastomosis to foreshorten and straighten the vessel (Figs. 78–2 and 78–3).

Certain extenuating circumstances may preclude carotid reconstruction, and one available alternative is distal ligation. Indications for ligation include radiation-induced arteriomalacia or necrosis, unreconstructable penetrating wounds, inaccessible aneurysms that act as a source of microemboli, friable, infected aneurysms, and unreconstructable carotid dissections. Under such circumstances, the benefits of ligation must be measured against the possible subsequent development of a stroke. Data suggest that a systolic carotid stump pressure of 70 mm Hg implies adequate intracranial circulation and is an index for safe ligation. Systolic stump pressures less than 70 mm Hg are associated with a 50% risk of stroke.[3] Alternatives to ligation of such lesions include external carotid–middle cerebral artery bypass[4]; cervical to petrous internal carotid artery vein bypass grafting[5]; and interventional radiologic

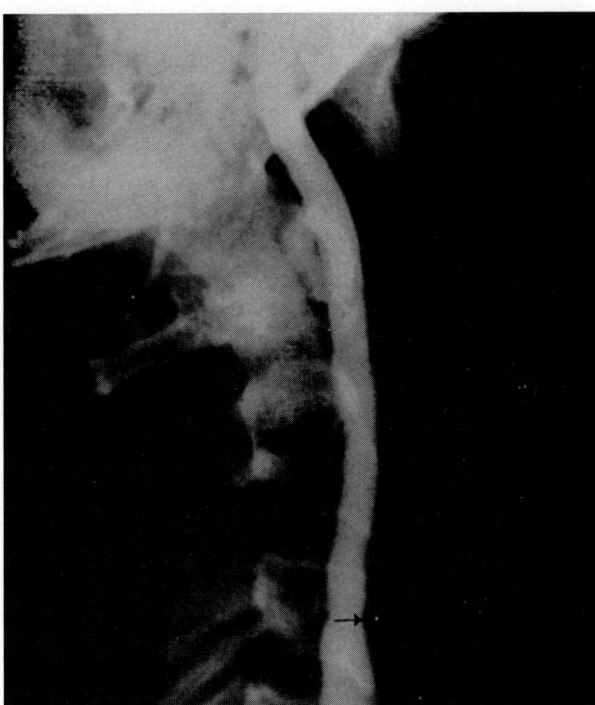

FIGURE 78–3 ■ Postoperative arteriogram of the patient in Figure 78–1 documenting satisfactory dilatation of the fibrodysplastic stenosis. A proximal end-to-end anastomosis *(arrow)* was performed after open transluminal dilatation and resection of a 1-cm segment of redundant carotid artery. (From Ernst CB: Exposure of inaccessible arteries. I: Carotid and arm exposure. Surg Rounds 8:21, 1985.)

techniques, including angioplasty and stent angioplasty, which are undergoing investigational trial.[6]

## TECHNIQUE OF EXPOSURE OF THE DISTAL CAROTID ARTERY

Various techniques have been suggested to facilitate distal internal carotid artery exposure.[2, 7–17] Some require resection of bone, and most are time consuming and complicated, and may be deforming or disabling. Temporary ipsilateral mandibular subluxation has been described as a simple and effective adjunct for exposing the distal internal carotid artery.[2, 7, 8]

### Anesthesia

Before anesthesia is induced, a cannula is inserted in the radial artery of the nondominant hand after an Allen's test is performed, to obtain blood samples for blood gas measurements and for continuous monitoring of systemic blood pressure. Nasotracheal intubation is performed in anticipation of the need for mandibular manipulation to facilitate exposure of the distal carotid. The depth of anesthesia must be closely modulated to ensure interpretable electroencephalographic monitoring, if this monitoring method is used during carotid occlusion. After adequate anesthesia is established, mandibular subluxation is performed.

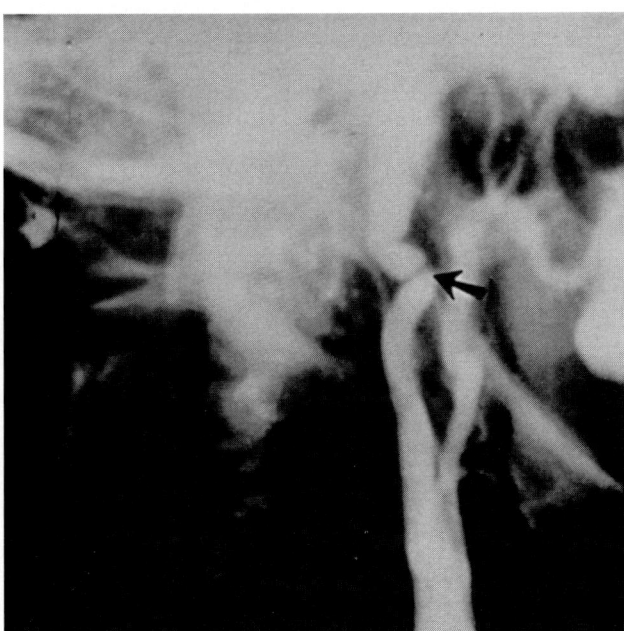

FIGURE 78–2 ■ An arteriogram demonstrating a preocclusive fibrodysplastic stenosis of the distal internal carotid artery *(arrow)*. Note the typical location of the lesion, several centimeters distal to the carotid bifurcation, close to the base of the skull. (From Ernst CB: Exposure of inaccessible arteries. I: Carotid and arm exposure. Surg Rounds 8:21, 1985.)

## Mandibular Subluxation

Ipsilateral mandibular subluxation is usually performed in cooperation with an oral surgeon. In dentate patients, the subluxation position is held by Ivy loop interdental diagonal wiring of an ipsilateral mandibular cuspid or bicuspid tooth using a 25-gauge stainless steel wire. In edentulous patients, 3/32-inch threaded Steinmann pins, which are inserted obliquely into the mandible and maxilla, are used. The Steinmann pins are placed into the contralateral maxillary alveolar process with a drill. The first pin should be placed 1 to 2 cm above the crest of the alveolar ridge and angled toward the angle of the mandible of the opposite side. The placement is stopped when the tip of the pin is felt protruding through the palatal mucosa. A second pin is inserted into the ipsilateral mandible 1 to 2 cm inferior to the alveolar crest and angled toward the angle of the mandible of the opposite side. The pins are cut so that 1 to 2 cm protrudes, and a loop of 25-gauge wire is used to secure the two pins after the temporomandibular joint is subluxed on the side of the carotid artery to be exposed. Gentle anterior pressure subluxes the mandible anteriorly from the temporomandibular fossa while the pins are secured by tightening the wire with a wire twister. Gentle, steady pressure is required to ensure that the distal and capsular ligaments are not overstretched or injured. Once maximum subluxation has been produced, the wire is twisted down tightly. Gauze coated with petroleum jelly is placed around the pins and the adjacent oral mucosa. When the carotid reconstruction has been completed, the pins are removed and the mandible restored to its anatomic position. Use of a rubber bite block or Molt Mouth Prop has also been described to stabilize the subluxed position.[7]

These mandibular subluxation methods convert the triangular operative field at the distal carotid artery into a rectangular one. The rectangular space provides an additional 2 cm of critical operating space for exposure of the distal carotid (Figs. 78–4 and 78–5).

Others have suggested osteotomies through the angle, body, or vertical or horizontal rami of the mandible.[9, 10, 12, 15–17] These procedures require exposing the mandible and incising and elevating the periosteum on its superficial and deep surfaces. After the carotid reconstructive procedure has been completed, the mandibular segments are reduced and wired together. Although these osteotomy techniques are helpful to know, they are rarely required; the less complex subluxation technique is preferred.

After ipsilateral subluxation is performed, the patient is positioned with the head turned to the opposite side and the neck slightly extended. The operating table is placed in a 15-degree reversed Trendelenburg position to minimize venous engorgement. The face, neck, and upper chest are prepared and draped. The ear should be included in the operative field in case the incision must be extended cephalad either anterior or posterior to the ear. If autogenous vein reconstruction is anticipated, either as a patch or as a replacement conduit, the groin must be prepared and draped for saphenous vein harvesting.

## Carotid Dissection and Exposure

Exposure of the distal internal carotid artery is best obtained through a longitudinal incision anterior to the sternocleidomastoid muscle. Preauricular or retroauricular extension of the incision may be required. The tip of the parotid

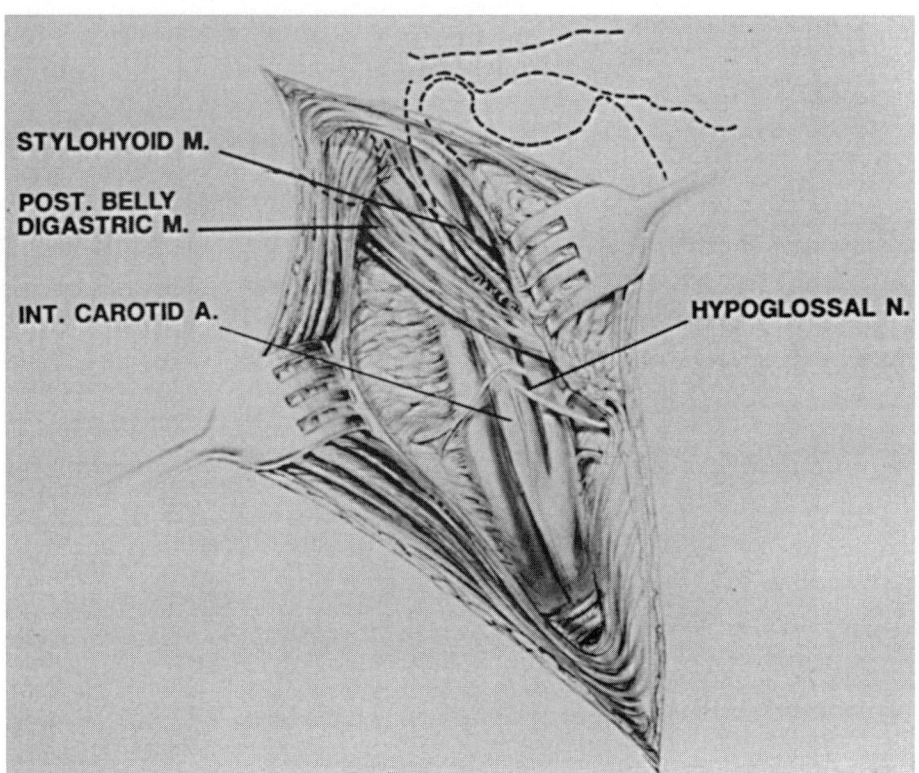

STYLOHYOID M.

POST. BELLY DIGASTRIC M.

INT. CAROTID A.

HYPOGLOSSAL N.

FIGURE 78–4 ■ The mandible in its anatomic position. Exposure of the carotid bifurcation through a standard cervical incision. Structures at the apex of the triangle obscure the distal internal carotid artery. Note the normal configuration of the temporomandibular joint (dotted line). (From Dossa C, Shepard AD, Wolford GD, et al: Distal internal carotid exposure: A simplified technique for temporary mandibular subluxation. J Vasc Surg 12:319–325, 1990.)

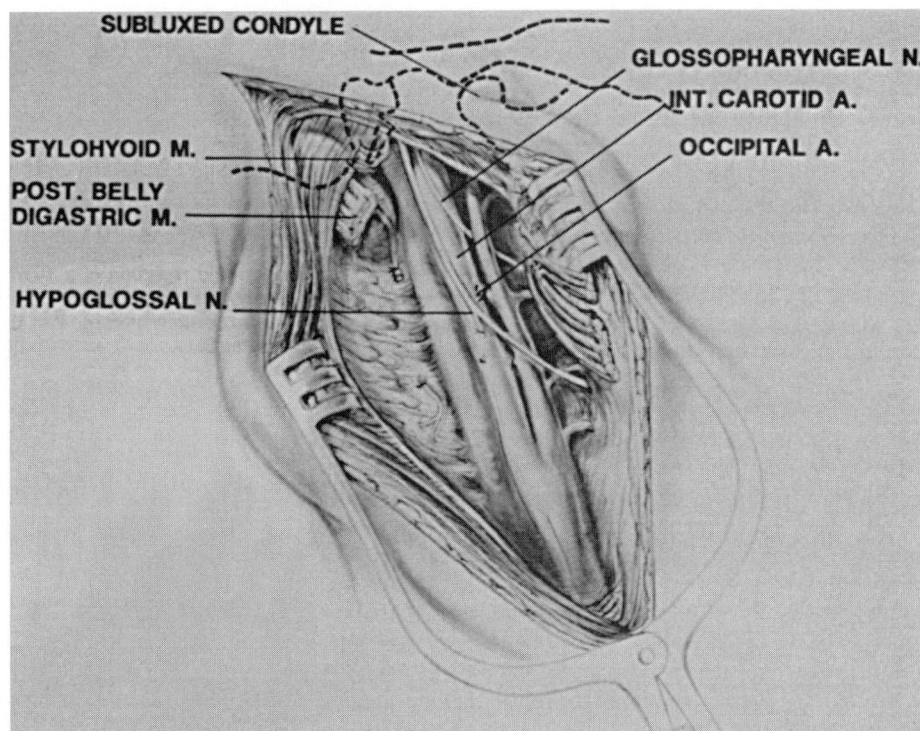

**FIGURE 78–5** ■ The mandible in a subluxed position *(dotted lines)* showing conversion of the triangular operative field into a rectangular one, thus gaining an additional 2 cm of exposure of the distal carotid. (From Dossa C, Shepard AD, Wolford GD, et al: Distal internal carotid exposure: A simplified technique for temporary mandibular subluxation. J Vasc Surg 12:319–325, 1990.)

gland can be mobilized anteriorly, or it can be divided if the tip is relatively small. After the sternocleidomastoid muscle is mobilized and retracted posteriorly, the carotid sheath is incised, and the carotid bifurcation is dissected, starting with the common carotid artery, which is encircled with a length of PE-90 polyethylene tubing that serves as a vessel loop to allow atraumatic traction. The external carotid artery is mobilized next, and the superior thyroid artery is ligated when necessary. The interval between the internal and external carotid artery is encircled with PE-90 tubing, which is threaded through an 8-cm segment of No. 18 French gauge Robinson catheter. This tubing later serves for external carotid snare occlusion. If hypotension or bradycardia occurs during carotid sinus manipulation, 1 to 2 ml of 1% lidocaine is injected into the adventitia of the carotid bifurcation to block the baroreceptor mechanism. The carotid sinus nerve is preserved. Traction on the polyethylene catheters allows gentle, atraumatic, "no-touch" dissection of the remainder of the carotid bifurcation while the internal carotid artery is mobilized.

After the vagus, hypoglossal, and glossopharyngeal (carotid sinus) nerves are identified, dissection proceeds toward the skull base. The ansa cervicalis branch of the hypoglossal nerve can serve as a marker to the hypoglossal nerve; this branch is usually divided 0.5 cm from the main trunk. Subluxation of the temporomandibular joint stretches the hypoglossal nerve and the digastric muscle; consequently, the hypoglossal nerve can be situated slightly cephalad to its usual anatomic location. Division of the posterior belly of the digastric muscle and the styloglossus, stylopharyngeus, and the stylohyoid muscles exposes the underlying internal carotid artery. If necessary, the styloid process can be excised after the mastoid insertion of the sternocleidomastoid muscle is divided. Styloid process excision is rarely required, but it can provide additional exposure if the process is a large structure. Care must be taken to protect the vagus, glossopharyngeal, and facial nerves during this dissection. Similarly, the spinal accessory nerve is vulnerable when the sternocleidomastoid muscle is mobilized and the styloid process is exposed.

During dissection of the distal internal carotid, many delicate veins must be carefully ligated. Avulsion or tearing of such vessels causes troublesome bleeding. Such bleeding obscures the nerves, which subsequently can be damaged in pursuit of hemostasis. In addition, the occipital artery overlies the internal carotid artery as it courses posteriorly and must be ligated and divided. Similarly, small branches from the external carotid artery to the sternocleidomastoid muscle must be ligated. The use of electrocautery is discouraged when the region of the hypoglossal nerve is being dissected. Mobilization, inferior traction, and displacement of the hypoglossal nerve, along with division of the muscles noted, particularly the digastric and the stylopharyngeus, provide ready access to the suprahypoglossal segment of the distal internal carotid artery.

After carotid reconstruction, the wound is closed without drainage. Deep structures are not reapproximated. Interrupted sutures are placed in the platysma layer, and staples are used on the skin. Once skin closure is complete, the mandibular retaining devices are removed and the mandible is replaced gently into its usual position.

## COMMENT

The dissection described here permits exposure of all but the distal 1 cm of the internal carotid artery before it enters the skull. Nonetheless, carotid reconstruction by graft interposition requires a distal segment adequate for application of the distal vascular clamp and sufficient remaining length for anastomosis. Additional space is available for distal suturing if the vessel is unencumbered by a distal vascular clamp, and a new clamp has been described to obviate this.[18] Another alternative for distal internal carotid occlusion is the placement of a No. 3 Fogarty intraluminal balloon catheter threaded into the distal artery and gently inflated. If electroencephalographic monitoring or stump pressure measurements suggest that an indwelling shunt is necessary, a balloon shunt has proved helpful. Balloon shunting or balloon occlusion is particularly useful if exposure of the distal carotid is required for trauma in cases in which expeditious hemostasis is of prime concern.

Complications of extended distal carotid exposure mainly relate to cranial nerve dysfunction, which can be avoided by clear knowledge of anatomy and meticulous dissection.[19] The most commonly injured nerves are XII, X, VII, and IX. Temporomandibular joint problems are rare after subluxation. Only 3 of 26 patients complained of transient discomfort over the temporomandibular joint, and a few noted gingival soreness that rapidly subsided.[2]

Occasionally, even with various bone resection or dislocation maneuvers, the distal internal carotid artery defies exposure, and alternatives to direct repair or even ligation are required. However, most distal internal carotid lesions can be treated definitively by meticulous, extended dissection and vigorous mandibular retraction facilitated by nasotracheal general anesthesia. Few lesions require mandibular subluxation or resection techniques, and fewer still require carotid ligation.

## REFERENCES

1. Hsia DC, Moscoe LM, Krushat WM: Epidemiology of carotid endarterectomy among Medicare beneficiaries: 1985–1995 update. Stroke 29:346–350, 1998.
2. Dossa C, Shepherd AD, Wolford DG, et al: Distal internal carotid exposure: A simplified technique for temporary mandibular subluxation. J Vasc Surg 1:727–733, 1984.
3. Ehrnefeld WK, Stoney RJ, Wylie EJ: Relation of carotid stump pressure to safety of carotid artery ligation. Surgery 93(2):299–305, 1983.
4. Numata T, Konno A, Takeuchi Y, et al: Contralateral external carotid-middle cerebral artery bypass for carotid artery resection. Laryngoscope 107:665–670, 1997.
5. Rostomily RC, Newell DW, Grady MS, et al: Gunshot wounds of the internal carotid artery at the skull base: Management with vein bypass grafts and a review of the literature. J Trauma 42:123–132, 1997.
6. Ernst CB: What's new in vascular surgery. J Am Coll Surg 182:191–200, 1996.
7. Coll DP, Ierdi, R, Mermet RW, et al: Exposure of the distal internal carotid artery: A simplified approach. J Am Coll Surg 186:92–95, 1998.
8. Frim DM, Padwa B, Buckley D, et al: Mandibular subluxation as an adjunct to exposure of the distal internal carotid artery in endarterectomy surgery. J Neurosurg 83:926–928, 1995.
9. Dew LA, Shelton C, Harnsberger HR, Thompson BG Jr: Surgical exposure of the petrous internal carotid artery: Practical application for skull base surgery. Laryngyscope 107:967–976, 1997.
10. Chang CY, O'Rourke DK, Cass SP: Update on skull base surgery. Otolaryngol Clin North Am 29:467–501, 1996.
11. Faggioli GL, Freyrie A, Stella A, et al: Extracranial internal carotid artery aneurysms: Results of a surgical series with long-term follow-up. J Vasc Surg 23:587–95, 1996.
12. Matsuyama T, Shimomomura T, Okumura Y, Sakaki T: Mobilization of the internal carotid artery for basilar artery aneurysm surgery. J Neurosurg 86:294–96, 1997.
13. Kuehne JP, Weaver FA, Papanicolaou G, Yellin AE: Penetrating trauma of the internal carotid artery. Arch Surg 131:942–48, 1996.
14. Alimi YS, Di Mauro P, Fiacre E, et al: Blunt injury to the internal carotid artery at the base of the skull: Six cases of venous graft restoration. J Vasc Surg 24:249–257, 1996.
15. Nelson SR, Schow SR, Stein SM, et al: Enhanced surgical exposure for the high extracranial internal carotid artery. Ann Vasc Surg 6:467–472, 1992.
16. Larsen PE, Smead WL: Vertical ramus osteotomy for improved exposure of the distal internal carotid artery: A new technique. J Vasc Surg 15:226–231, 1992.
17. Mock CN, Lilly MP, McRae RG, Carney WI Jr: Selection of the approach to the distal internal carotid artery from the second cervical vertebra to the base of the skull. J Vasc Surg 13:846–853, 1991.
18. Berkowitz HD: A new carotid clamp that facilitates distal internal carotid exposure. J Vasc Surg 24;2:301–2, 1990.
19. Hertzer NR, Feldman BJ, Beven EG, et al: A prospective study of the incidence of injury to the cranial nerves during carotid endarterectomy. Surg Gynecol Obstet 151:781, 1980.

# CHAPTER 79

# Management of Dissections of the Carotid and Vertebral Arteries

■ ROBERT J. SINGER and CHRISTOPHER S. OGILVY

Spontaneous or traumatic mural arterial dissections are produced by penetration of circulating blood into the wall of an artery and its subsequent extension for varying distances along the artery, often more distally than proximally.[12] Although a variety of systemic processes—Marfan's syndrome, fibromuscular dysplasia,[41] cystic medial necrosis, hypertension, atheromatous disease, and, questionably, smoking and contraceptive medications—have been implicated in the pathogenesis of spontaneous dissection, increasingly it is believed that minor traumatic events such as excessive head extension, flexion, and rotation may result in an intimal tear, precipitating a dissection.[3, 9, 10, 48] In other words, the so-called "spontaneous" dissection can be the result of an often unnoticed event. With advances in imaging techniques, our ability to define these lesions has increased immensely.[25, 30] Treatment protocols, although now aided somewhat by endovascular techniques, continue to be largely based on small clinical series and anecdotal experience.[2, 6, 8–10, 17, 24, 26, 27, 29, 44, 49, 51, 52] Surgical management is usually reserved for those clinical situations in which conservative management potentiates the risk of progressive neurologic deficit or potentially fatal outcome. This chapter reviews the basic anatomy of the cervicocephalic vasculature and describes surgical, endovascular, and conservative treatment strategies used in the management of these lesions.

The normal peripheral vasculature is composed of multiple layers of fibroelastic tissue with varying degrees of structural stability and compliance. Likewise, the extracranial neurovasculature is composed of the same basic layers—intima, internal elastic lamina, media, external elastic lamina, and adventitia—but has a proportionally thinner medial layer. With advancing age, changes in the vessel wall manifest primarily at the intima after reduplication or splitting of the internal elastic lamina. Subsequently, smooth muscle infiltrates from the media as well as collagen and glycosaminoglycans are deposited in the progressively thickening intimal layer. This process of diffuse intimal thickening, with progressive loss of vessel elasticity, begins at birth and progresses to adult life.[31–33] It is believed to be an early process in the development of atherosclerosis and possibly may be a predisposing factor to spontaneous dissection or that associated with minor trauma.[34]

Dissections of the extracranial neurovasculature most commonly involve the media, whereas those of the intracranial system are usually between the intima and media.[3, 8, 19, 22, 25, 49] False lumen formation and parent vessel stenosis can result in critical stenosis and subsequent hypoperfusion or thromboembolic complications. The plane of dissection may extend through the media, forming the so-called "true" aneurysm (with some remaining vessel wall components) or, in the setting of traumatic vessel wall disruption, form a false or "pseudoaneurysm," where the lateral wall of the vessel is formed by an organized thrombus (Fig. 79–1). The medial segment of the traumatic hematoma is cleared by parent artery flow and may generate emboli and neurologic sequelae.

## EXTRACRANIAL CAROTID DISSECTION

### Presentation

The extracranial carotid is the most common site of dissection.[3, 9, 12] The true incidence of such lesions is unknown, but an extracranial carotid artery dissection was documented angiographically in 11 (0.24%) of 4530 patients with acute cerebrovascular symptoms and 30 (2.5%) of 1200 consecutive patients with a first stroke.[42] Extracranial carotid dissection occurs most frequently in middle age. In most reported series, two thirds of the patients diagnosed with an extracranial carotid dissection are between the ages of 35 and 50 years. There is an increased incidence in men in most studies. Aneurysms occur in more than one third of cervical carotid dissections and most commonly involve the upper cervical segments.[42] Patients commonly present with a variety of combinations of headaches, focal ischemic attacks, stroke, oculosympathetic paresis, bruits, or cranial neuropathies.[3, 9, 12, 19, 21, 31, 32, 42]

The most common presenting complaint in an extracranial carotid dissection is ipsilateral neck or head pain.[42] The pain is usually described as throbbing and constant with varying intensity. Neck pain is usually over the region of the mastoid process or sternocleidomastoid muscle. Experimental stimulation of the perivascular plexus on the

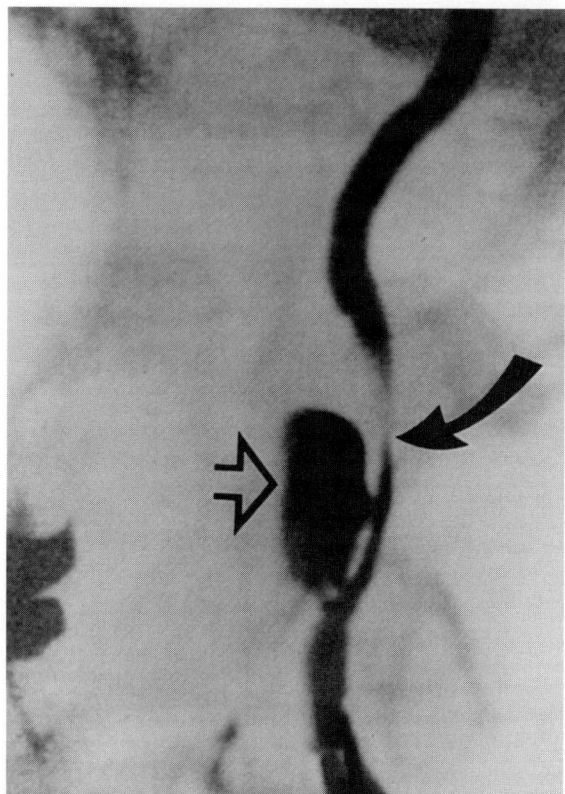

**FIGURE 79–1** ■ Digital subtraction angiogram demonstrating dissections of the cervical neurovasculature. The formation of a false lumen with resultant parent vessel stenosis *(curved arrow)* and extension of the plane of dissection through the media forming an aneurysm that may either be contained by the adventitia or, in the setting of vessel wall disruption, by organized thrombus forming the so-called "false aneurysm" *(open arrow)*. (Courtesy of Alexander M. Norbash, MD, Massachusetts General Hospital, Department of Interventional Neuroradiology.)

carotid artery has reproduced neck and hemicranial pain, lending some evidence to the notion that vessel damage may incite a painful stimulus.[3] Diffuse head and scalp pain has also been described.

The second most common presentation is focal neurologic symptoms. These may consist of transient ischemic attacks or overt stroke. These symptoms are often the result of either stenosis of the true lumen with hypoperfusion or thromboembolism, and tend to occur in the subacute period after dissection.

Oculosympathetic paresis is the third most commonly seen clinical manifestation of carotid dissection.[42] The paresis typically involves the oculomotor nerve while sparing those fibers traveling on the external carotid artery. Subsequently, patients have a classic third nerve lesion (involving the pupil) but have preserved facial sweating save for a small area in the frontosupraorbital region.[42] Pulsatile tinnitus has been noted in up to one third of patients and has been suggested to signify the onset of the dissection.[43]

In the setting of trauma, the diagnosis of carotid dissection is often made late.[3, 8, 9, 24, 26, 34, 44] Patients typically present with an altered level of consciousness, and symptoms such as head and neck pain are irrelevant. A head computed tomography (CT) scan and cervical spine films are almost universally acquired but are often negative. If a patient has an unexplained lateralizing deficit in this setting, assessment of the cervicocephalic vasculature is essential to rule of traumatic dissection.

## Diagnosis

Cervicocerebral angiography is the gold standard in establishing diagnosis.[42] Cervical internal carotid artery dissection typically occurs roughly 2 cm distal to the artery's origin and usually terminates proximal to its entry into the petrous bone.[3, 19, 34, 42] Extension into the petrous bone has been reported, however. Stenosis is the most common angiographic finding, but a wide variety of dissection patterns have been noted[19] (Fig. 79–2). Approximately 18% of cases are occluded at onset.[3] Aneurysms associated with dissection and stenosis are present in 35% to 40%. Aneurysms alone are seen in approximately 10%.[42] They are not likely to rupture but manifest clinically because of thromboembolic phenomena or by compressive cranial neuropathy.[3]

Other techniques for diagnosing and following dissections include magnetic resonance imaging (MRI) and CT. MRI offers an effective, noninvasive assessment of vessel dissection in the carotid and vertebral circulation (Fig. 79–3). Typically, axial images may demonstrate intramural clot and luminal stenosis. With serial images, blood degradation products change in signal intensity and may demonstrate clot resolution and vessel wall healing. CT angiography, with or without surface rendering techniques, is becoming more widely used in diagnosing and following dissection (Fig. 79–4) but requires contrast administration and a well-trained technologist for image acquisition.

## Treatment

### Nonsurgical

With the exception of penetrating injuries, anticoagulation is the most common initial mode of therapy for cervical

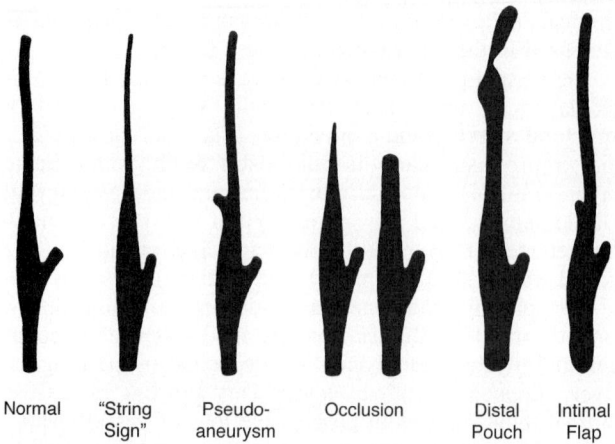

|     |     |     |     |     |     |
| --- | --- | --- | --- | --- | --- |
| Normal | "String Sign" | Pseudo-aneurysm | Occlusion | Distal Pouch | Intimal Flap |

**FIGURE 79–2** ■ Schematic rendering of various angiographic dissection patterns of the cervical internal carotid artery as originally described by Fisher CM, Ojemann RG, Robertson GH: Spontaneous dissection of the cervico-cerebral arteries. (Can J Neurol Sci 5:9–19, 1978.)

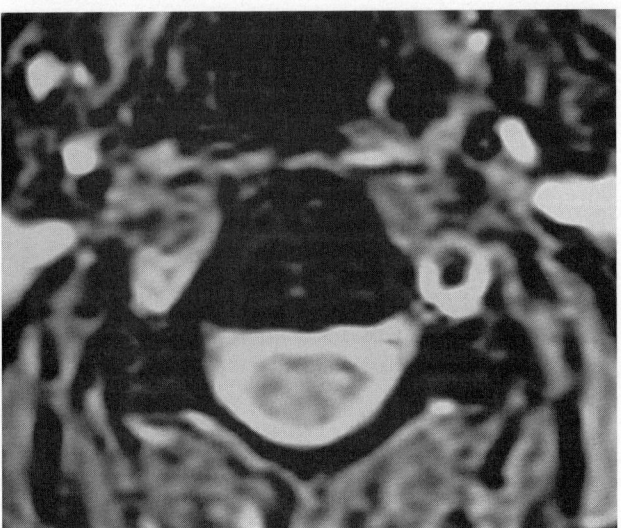

FIGURE 79–3 ■ Axial T₂-weighted image demonstrating an abnormal signal in the vertebral artery consistent with a subacute clot in the setting of post-traumatic vertebral artery dissection.

carotid dissection. Patients are anticoagulated acutely with heparin and then given oral anticoagulants (warfarin), usually for 3 months. Worsening with this therapy has been reported, with intracranial and visceral hemorrhages as a result of early anticoagulation.[40] Neurologic decline has been reported and speculatively associated with extension

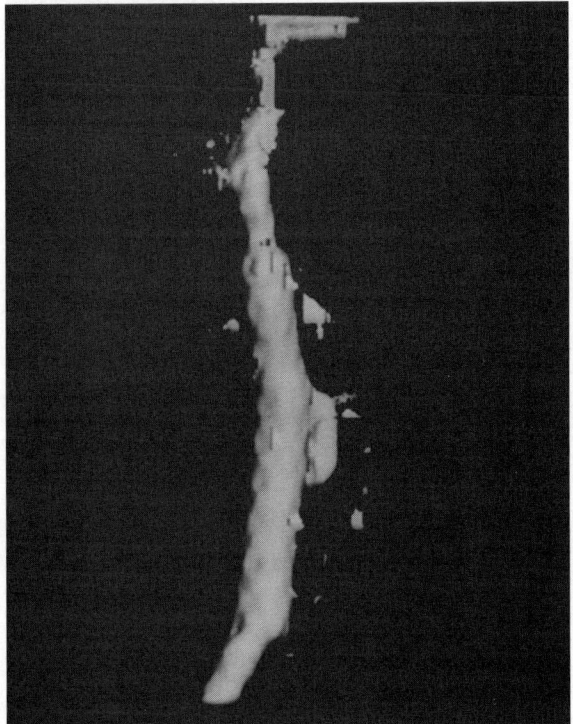

FIGURE 79–4 ■ Follow-up CTA image of a cervical internal carotid dissection treated with endovascular stenting. Persistent filling of the sidewall aneurysm is noted. (Courtesy of Alexander M. Norbash, MD, Massachusetts General Hospital, Department of Interventional Neuroradiology.)

of the intramural hemorrhage with resultant luminal stenosis and hypoperfusion.[9] The use of antiplatelet agents as an alternative to warfarin has also been reported and is suggested in the setting of warfarin allergy.[33] Follow-up imaging studies are usually obtained 3 months after initiation of treatment. Angiographically, improvement or resolution can be seen in 75% to 80% of cases.[42] Progression of stenosis or aneurysmal enlargement has been documented in 15% to 20%.[42] With evidence of residual dissection, a further period of anticoagulation is recommended because delayed resolution has been reported up to 16 months after initial diagnosis.[3, 12] Overall outcome with nonsurgical therapy is good in a reported 70% to 80% of patients.[42]

## Surgical/Interventional

Penetrating vessel wall injuries require prompt surgical exploration and repair.[2, 26, 32, 34] The prognosis for such lesions, which are frequently seen in the setting of trauma, is expectedly worse. The vessel should be repaired to preserve patency whenever possible. This may be achieved primarily or with patch or tube grafting, depending on extent of vessel damage. Parent vessel occlusion may be considered when backflow is lost, suggesting intracranial clot propagation, or when intraoperative monitoring (electroencephalography or stump pressures) suggests tolerance to ligation. Although studied in animals and mentioned in the literature,[2] acute external-internal carotid artery bypass procedures in this setting are rarely performed.[7, 8, 16, 28, 38, 50]

In nonpenetrating dissection,[14, 15, 18, 23] surgery or endovascular therapy is performed when anticoagulation has failed. Simple endarterectomy may be plausible if the involved segment can be adequately exposed and vessel integrity is sufficient. Unfortunately, these lesions often result in thin and friable vessel walls with the dissection extending to the skull base. Resection of the involved segment with saphenous vein or biopolymer grafting may be necessary in this setting.[28] An alternative to surgical management in this setting is stent placement, using either a covered or traditional stent construct depending on vessel architecture (Fig. 79–5). Stents have been shown to be effective in preserving antegrade flow and abating embolic phenomena.[44] When vessel patency cannot be restored, surgical or endovascular ligation may be required. Temporary balloon test occlusion should be considered if vessel ligation is possible. With this information, the need for extracranial-to-intracranial bypass can be addressed. Superficial temporal-to-middle cerebral anastomosis is most often used unless quantitative blood flow studies suggest the need for an early high-flow bypass, for which a saphenous vein graft may be more appropriate.[28]

## EXTRACRANIAL VERTEBRAL ARTERY DISSECTION

### Presentation

Vertebral artery dissection may occur spontaneously or as the result of trauma or cervical manipulation.[19, 21] It is less common than dissections of the extracranial carotid

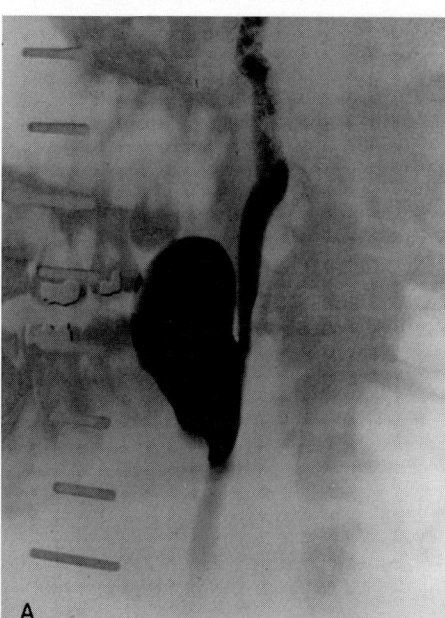
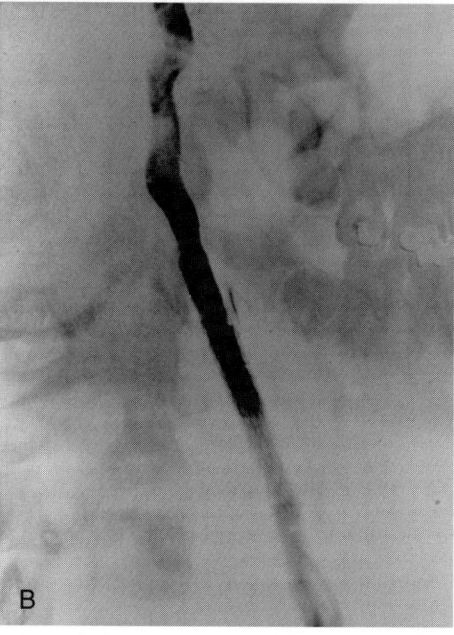

**FIGURE 79–5** ■ Right internal carotid artery dissection with pseudoaneurysm formation *(A)* treated with endovascular stenting and resultant preservation of parent vessel flows *(B)*. (Courtesy of Alexander M. Norbash, MD, Massachusetts General Hospital, Department of Interventional Neuroradiology.)

circulation. Traumatic lesions occur most frequently at the C1-C2 level, where the vessel exits the foramen transversarium and courses along the arch of C1.[3] Associated aneurysms are commonly seen along this horizontal segment and often have a broad neck. They may embolize but are not prone to rupture. The second most common location is at the portion of the vessel at the level of C2, which essentially is the portion traversing the foramen transversarium (Fig. 79–6). This section of the vessel is particularly vulnerable to injury from excessive motion, as often seen in the setting of trauma. As with carotid dissections, spontaneous lesions are seen in middle-aged patients complain-

ing of posterior cervical and occipital pain with an acute onset. The ictus of pain has been likened to subarachnoid hemorrhage (SAH), although this has not been known to occur in the setting of cervical vertebral dissection. Often, these lesions go unnoticed at ictus, only to be diagnosed as a result of an ischemic episode or infarction with or without radiographic confirmation. The usual manifestation of dissection is vertebrobasilar ischemia (80%), commonly lateral medullary syndrome from stenosis or emboli at the origin of the posterior inferior cerebellar artery. Other posterior vascular syndromes have also frequently been reported.[9, 12]

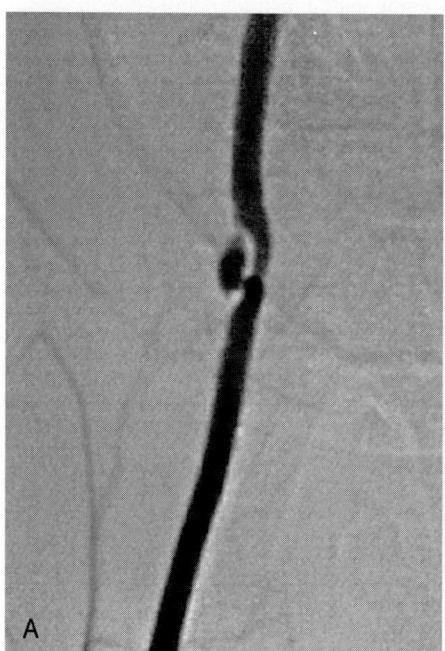
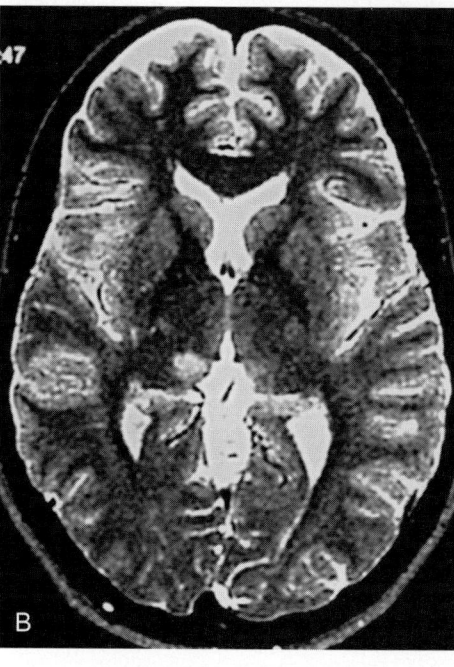

**FIGURE 79–6** ■ Digital subtraction angiogram *(A)* of a cervical vertebral dissection after minor trauma. The patient presented with vague left hemisensory changes and was found to have a small thalamic infarction *(B)*. She was anticoagulated, and she made an uneventful recovery.

## Treatment

As mentioned previously, anticoagulation is the primary mode of therapy, with surgery or endovascular therapy reserved for those patients with symptomatic or angiographic progression of disease. With anticoagulation, angiographic improvement has been documented in 26% to 33% of cases, normalization was seen in 61% to 63%, and progression to occlusion occurred in 6% to 11%. Angiographic improvement has been described by as early as 7 days. Healing is expected by 3 months. Overall, with anticoagulation alone, a good outcome has been in reported in 70% to 80% of patients.[42]

Surgical or intraluminal intervention is predicated on the angioarchitecture of the posterior circulation. A hypoplastic contralateral vertebral artery contraindicates proximal ligation or trapping unless a bypass or interposition graft is performed.[5, 40, 44] When necessary, a superficial temporal artery—saphenous vein—posterior cerebral artery bypass is preferred because it supplies a high-flow conduit with high patency rates and low risk.[28, 33, 35, 36]

## INTRACRANIAL ARTERIAL DISSECTION

Intracranial dissections are much less common than those involving the extracranial neurovasculature. They may or may not be related to a traumatic event, and usually manifest clinically as a result of embolism, occlusion, or SAH. As in the extracranial circulation, an association has been made with fibromuscular dysplasia, Marfan's syndrome, and cystic medial necrosis. In addition, syphilitic arteritis, polyarteritis nodosa, Takayasu's disease, homocystinuria, infection, medial degeneration, allergic arteritis, and, rarely, atherosclerosis have been mentioned as possible causative conditions in the setting of spontaneous dissection.[3, 9, 19] The pathogenesis remains unknown. Minor trauma in the setting of one of these conditions is often cited as a relatively frequent causative factor. Medial defects and fragmentation/disruption of the internal elastic lamina are commonly seen histologically. Intracranial dissections usually arise in the medial layer and can evolve to the subadventitia or intima with resultant aneurysm formation or thromboembolism/occlusion, respectively.[32] In contradistinction to extracranial dissections, which usually present subacutely, there is often a sudden onset of neurologic deficit secondary to ischemia, usually preceded by ipsilateral headache. Spontaneous intracranial dissection primarily occurs in the second to fourth decade of life, with the age peak between 20 and 30 years. The middle cerebral artery is the most frequently reported site (50%), followed by the internal carotid and basilar arteries.[49]

The major clinical findings of intracranial dissecting aneurysms are SAH[20] and ischemia or infarction due to stenosis, occlusion, or embolization. In a retrospective series of 147 patients, Yamaura[49] found that 57% of patients with intracranial dissections presented with SAH. SAH was more common in vertebrobasilar lesions (67%) than in carotid dissections (22%). Aoki and Sakai reviewed 60 cases of ruptured vertebral dissections and found that 18

(30%) were documented to have rebled, usually within several hours of the initial hemorrhage, justifying early treatment.[4] The rebleed rate for dissecting aneurysms in the carotid circulation was significantly lower. Patients without SAH present, in order of decreasing incidence, with headache, ischemia/infarction/vertigo, and seizures. Angiography is the diagnostic procedure of choice. Noninvasive techniques such as CT angiography, MRI, and MR angiography have played an increasingly effective role in demonstrating dissections for the purpose of initial diagnosis as well as follow-up assessment.

## Treatment

The optimal treatment for intracranial dissection has not been determined. Pozzati and colleagues[37] recommended angiographic monitoring in neurologically stable patients before intervention is planned. Dissections that result in a completed stroke are beyond treatment. Those with transient cerebral ischemia or stroke in evolution might be helped by treatment. Fatal intracranial hemorrhage has been reported in a case of heparinization after intracranial carotid dissection, and the use of anticoagulants in this setting is largely discouraged.[42]

Surgical and endovascular treatment options are varied and largely depend on the angioarchitecture and neurologic status of the patient. Clipping of an intracranial dissecting aneurysm is often not feasible given their morphometry. Encircling clips are available, however, which can be useful in securing a weakened segment when maintaining parent vessel patency is feasible. Proximal occlusion or trapping by endovascular or surgical means can be effective in abating thromboembolic phenomena and progression of a dissecting segment (Fig. 79–7). Revascularization may be necessary, and a variety of techniques for high-flow bypass using saphenous interposition grafts are available.[13, 28, 36, 39, 40, 45, 47, 50] Amin-Hanjani and coworkers[1] reported the use of flow reversal in the setting of a dissecting basilar aneurysm by clipping the basilar artery below the level of the anterior inferior cerebellar arteries. This eloquent procedure allows for retrograde flow through the posterior communicating arteries to provide continued basilar perfusion (Fig. 79–8).

## Outcome

In a review of the available literature, Yamaura,[49] using the Glasgow Outcome Scale, found a favorable outcome in 70% of patients with intracranial carotid or vertebral dissections. A poor outcome was seen in 5%, and 26% of the entire series died. The mortality rate was high in carotid lesions (49%), compared with 22% for lesions in the vertebrobasilar circulation. Patients with associated SAH had a mortality rate of 24%, compared with 29% in those without.

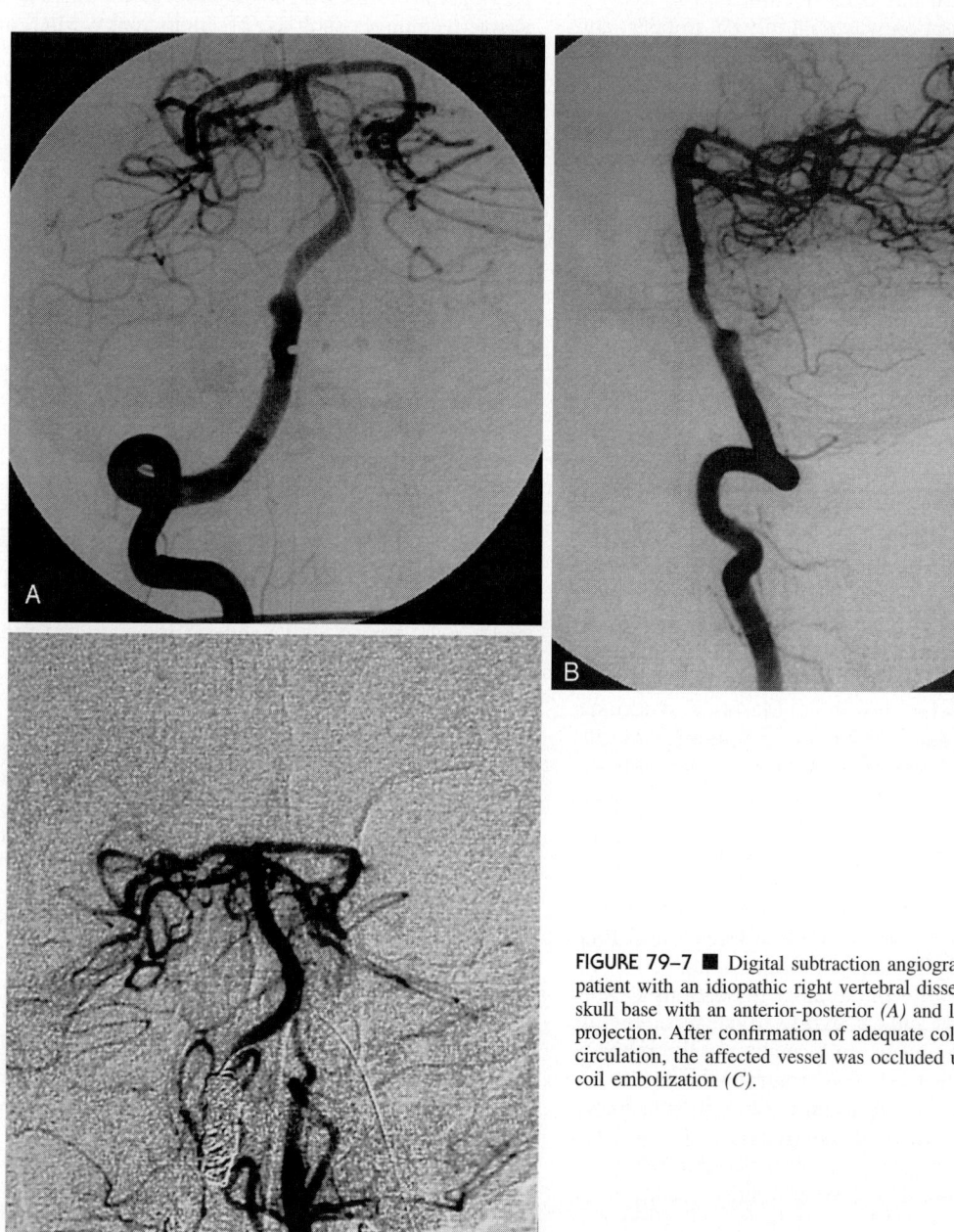

**FIGURE 79–7** ■ Digital subtraction angiography on a patient with an idiopathic right vertebral dissection at the skull base with an anterior-posterior *(A)* and lateral *(B)* projection. After confirmation of adequate collateral circulation, the affected vessel was occluded using detachable coil embolization *(C)*.

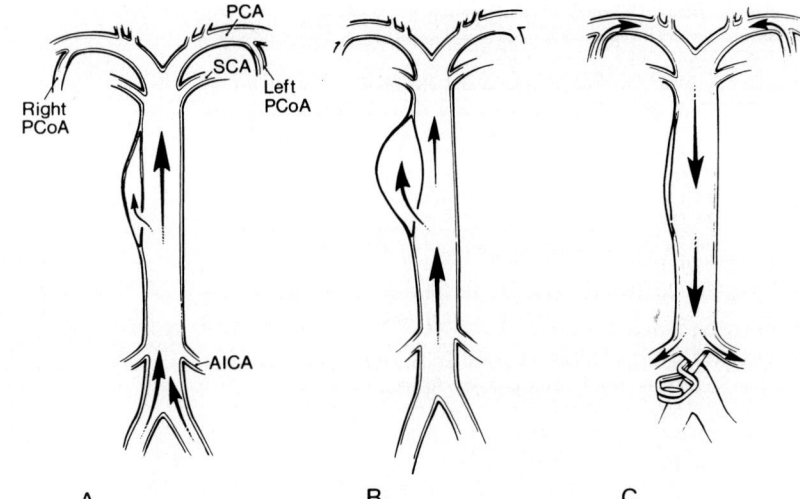

**FIGURE 79–8** ■ Schematic illustration of a dissecting basilar aneurysm before *(A, B)* and after *(C)* clip occlusion of the basilar artery. *Arrows* indicate the direction of blood flow. Reversal of blood flow prevents the progression of dissection and leads to obliteration of the pseudoaneurysm. (From Amin-Hanjani S, Ogilvy CS, Buonno FS, et al: Treatment of dissecting basilar artery aneurysm by flow reversal. Acta Neurochirurgica 139:44–51, 1997.)

A          B          C

## REFERENCES

1. Amin-Hanjani S, Ogilvy CS, Buonanno FS, et al: Treatment of dissecting basilar artery aneurysm by flow reversal. Acta Neurochir (Wien) 139:44–51, 1997.
2. Andrews BT: Treatment of acute traumatic internal carotid artery occlusion with extracranial-to-intracranial arterial bypass: Case report. Neurosurgery 25:90–92, 1989.
3. Anson J, Crowell RM. Cervicocranial arterial dissection. Neurosurgery 29:89–96, 1991.
4. Aoki N, Sakai T: Rebleeding from intracranial dissecting aneurysm in the vertebral artery. Stroke 21:1628–1631, 1990.
5. Ausman JI, Diaz FG, de los Reyes RA, et al: Extracranial-intracranial anastomoses in the posterior circulation. In Berguer R, Bauer BB, eds. Vertebrobasilar arterial occlusive disease. New York: Raven Press, 1984, pp 313–319.
6. Ausman JI, Diaz GF, de los Reyes RA, et al: Superficial temporal to proximal superior cerebellar artery anastomosis for basilar artery stenosis. Neurosurgery 9:56–59, 1981.
7. Bannister CM: Status of extracranial-intracranial anastomoses for cerebral ischemia two years after the International Bypass Study. Br J Neurosurg 2:139–141, 1988.
8. Batzdorf U, Bentson JR, Machleder HI: Blunt trauma to the high cervical carotid artery. Neurosurgery 5:195–201, 1979.
9. Biller J, Hingtgen WL, Adams HP, et al: Cervicocephalic arterial dissections: A ten year experience. Arch Neurol 43:1234–1238, 1986.
10. Bogousslavsky J, Despland PS-A, Regli F: Spontaneous carotid dissection with acute stroke. Arch Neurol 44:137–140, 1987.
11. Caplan LR, Baquis GD, Pessin MS, et al: Dissection of the intracranial vertebral artery. Neurology 38:868–877, 1988.
12. Caplan LR, Zarins CK, Hemmati M: Spontaneous dissection of the extracranial vertebral arteries. Stroke 16:1030–1038, 1985.
13. Chater N, Mani J, Tonnemacher K: Superficial temporal artery bypass for cerebrovascular occlusive disease. Cal Med 119:9–13, 1973.
14. Crowell RM, Olsson Y: Effect of extracranial-intracranial vascular bypass graft on experimental acute stroke in dogs. J Neurosurg 38:26–31, 1973.
15. Crowell RM, Ogilvy CS, Choi IS, Gress DR: Direct brain revascularization. In Schmidek H, Sweet WH (eds): Operative Neurosurgical Techniques. Philadelphia: WB Saunders, 1995, pp 909–928.
16. Crowell RM: Emergency STA-MCA bypass for acute focal cerebral ischemia. In Schmidek P, Gratzl O, Spetzler RF (eds): Microneurosurgical Anastomosis for Cerebral Ischemia. Berlin: Springer-Verlag, 1977.
17. DeBaets P, Delanote G, Jackers G, et al: Atherosclerotic dissection of the cervical internal carotid artery: A case report. Angiology 41:161–163, 1990.
18. Diaz FG, Ausman JL, Mehta B, et al: Acute cerebral revascularization. J Neurosurg 63:200–209, 1985.
19. Fisher CM, Ojemann RG, Robertson GH: Spontaneous dissection of the cervico-cerebral arteries. Can J Neurol Sci 5:9–19, 1978.

20. Friedman AH, Drake CG: Subarachnoid hemorrhage from intracranial dissecting aneurysm. J Neurosurg 60:325–334, 1984.
21. Greenberg MS: Cerebral arterial dissections. In Handbook of Neurosurgery, 3rd ed. Lakeland, FL: Greenberg Graphics, 1994, pp 786–790.
22. Hart RG. Vertebral artery dissection. Neurology 38:987–989, 1988.
23. Jaksche H, Scheffler P, Loew F, Papavero L: Indications for extra-intracranial bypass surgery: New orientation after the Toronto Bypass Study based on angiographic and non-invasive ultrasound flow measurements. Acta Neurochir (Wien) 95:34–39, 1988.
24. Krajewski LP, Hertzer NR: Blunt carotid artery trauma: Report of two cases and review of the literature. Ann Surg 191:341–346, 1980.
25. Lanzino G, Kaptain G, Kallmes DF: Intracranial dissecting aneurysm causing subarachnoid hemorrhage: The role of computerized tomographic angiography and magnetic resonance angiography. Surg Neurol 48:477–481, 1997.
26. LeBlanc KA, Benzel EC: Trauma to the high cervical carotid artery. J Trauma 24:992–996, 1984.
27. Leys D, Lesoin F, Pruvo JP, et al: Bilateral spontaneous dissection of the extracranial vertebral arteries. J Neurol 234:237–240, 1987.
28. Little JR, Furlan AJ, Bryerton B: Short vein grafts for cerebral revascularization. J Neurosurg 59:384–388, 1983.
29. Lomeo RM, Silver RM, Brothers M: Spontaneous dissection of the internal carotid artery in a patient with polyarteritis nodosa. Arthritis Rheum 32:1625–1626, 1989.
30. Mascalchi M, Bianchi MC, Mangiafico S, et al: MRI and MR angiography of vertebral artery dissection. Neuroradiology 39:329–340, 1997.
31. Mokri B, Houser OW, Sandok BA, et al: Spontaneous dissections of the vertebral arteries. Neurology 38:880–885, 1988.
32. Mokri B, Sundt TM Jr, Houser OW, et al: Spontaneous dissection of the cervical internal carotid artery. Ann Neurol 19:126–138, 1986.
33. Mokri B: Dissections of cervical and cephalic arteries. In Meyer FB (ed): Sundt's Occlusive Cerebrovascular Disease. Philadelphia: WB Saunders, 1994, pp 45–70.
34. O'Connell BK, Towfighi J, Brennan RW, et al: Dissecting aneurysms of the head and neck. Neurology 35:993–997, 1985.
35. Ojemann RG, Heros RC, Crowell RM: Surgical Management of Cerebrovascular Disease. Baltimore: Williams & Wilkins, 1987.
36. Onesti ST, Solomon RA, Quest DO: Cerebral revascularization: A review. Neurosurgery 25:618–628, 1989, discussion 628–629.
37. Pozzati E, Padovani R, Fabrizi A, et al: Benign arterial dissections of the posterior circulation. J Neurosurg 75:69–72, 1991.
38. Powers WJ, Grubb RL Jr, Raichle ME: Clinical results of extracranial-intracranial bypass surgery in patients with hemodynamic cerebrovascular disease (Comments). J Neurosurg 70:61–67, 1989.
39. Powers WJ, Martin WR, Herscovitch P, et al: Extracranial-intracranial bypass surgery: Hemodynamic and metabolic effects. Neurology 34:1168–1174, 1984.
40. Roski RA, Spetzler RF, Hopkins LN: Occipital artery to posterior inferior cerebellar artery bypass for vertebrobasilar ischemia. Neurosurgery 10:44–49, 1982.

41. Sato S, Hata J: Fibromuscular dysplasia: its occurrence with a dissecting aneurysm of the internal carotid artery. Arch Pathol Lab Med 106:332–335, 1982.

42. Sila CA, Awad IA: Arterial trauma and dissection. In Awad IA (ed): Cerebrovascular Occlusive Disease and Brain Ischemia. Parkridge, IL: American Association of Neurological Surgeons, 1992, pp 187–202.

43. Sila CA, Furlan AJ, Little JR: Pulsatile tinnitus. Stroke 18:252–256, 1987.

44. Singer RJ, Dake MD, Norbash AM, et al: Covered stent placement for neurovascular disease: a report of two cases. AJNR Am J Neuroradiol 18:507–509, 1997.

45. Sundt TM Jr, Piepgras DG: Bypass surgery for vertebral artery occlusive disease: Techniques and complications. Clin Neurosurg 26:346–352, 1979.

46. Sundt TM Jr, Piepgras DG: Occipital to posterior inferior cerebellar artery bypass surgery. J Neurosurg 48:916–928, 1978.

47. Sundt TM Jr, Whisnant JP, Piepgras DG, et al: Intracranial bypass grafts for vertebral-basilar ischemia. Mayo Clin Proc 53:12–18, 1978.

48. Tucci JM, Maitland CG, Pesolyar DW, et al: Carotid-cavernous fistula due to traumatic dissection of the extracranial internal carotid artery. AJNR Am J Neuroradiol 5:828–829, 1984.

49. Yamaura A: Nontraumatic intracranial arterial dissection: Natural history, diagnosis and treatment. Contemp Neurosurg 16:5, 1994.

50. Yasargil MG, Krayenbuhl HA, Jacobson JH. Microneurosurgical arterial reconstruction. Surgery 67:221–233, 1970.

51. Yonas H, Agamanolis D, Takaoka Y, et al: Dissecting intracranial aneurysms. Surg Neurol 8:407–415, 1977.

52. Young PH, Smith KR Jr, Crafts DC, et al: Traumatic occlusion in fibromuscular dysplasia of the carotid artery. Surg Neurol 16:432–437, 1981.

# CHAPTER 80

# Surgical Management of Unruptured Cerebral Aneurysms

■ OLAVI HEISKANEN and MATTI PORRAS

In the 1950s and 1960s, in patients with subarachnoid hemorrhage and multiple aneurysms, only the ruptured aneurysm was treated. Treatment of the responsible lesion alone was thought to give the best results,[1,2] although some neurosurgeons suggested that unruptured aneurysms carried a definite risk of bleeding and should be treated as well.[3-5] When more was learned about the risks of rupture of previously unruptured aneurysms in patients with multiple aneurysms, and once the operating microscope, microsurgical techniques, and new aneurysm clips were introduced, neurosurgeons started operating on the unruptured aneurysms of patients with multiple aneurysms. The advent of computed tomography (CT) and magnetic resonance imaging (MRI) also enabled physicians to detect more asymptomatic, incidental aneurysms. Although the natural history of incidental aneurysms was not well known, many neurosurgeons suggested that such aneurysms should also be treated.[6-9] In the 1990s, Guglielmi detachable coil (GDC) embolization has become an acceptable alternative to surgery in selected cases.

## MULTIPLE ANEURYSMS

### Incidence

The incidence of multiple aneurysms can be estimated based on autopsy series or on series of patients with four-vessel angiography. At autopsy, aneurysms must be specifically looked for, or some of them will be missed.[10,11] To find all aneurysms by angiography, a four-vessel study has to be performed (i.e., both carotid and both vertebral arteries must be investigated). An autopsy can also reveal very small aneurysms of 2 to 3 mm in diameter, whereas aneurysms of that size are difficult to see with angiography; in fact, many small aneurysms are found only during surgery.[12,13]

Varying incidences of multiple aneurysms have been reported in autopsy series of patients with intracranial arterial aneurysms. Chason and Hindman[14] found multiple aneurysms in 31.4% of 137 patients, Stehbens[11] in 20.6% of 252 patients, McCormick and Nofziger[10] in 25% of 153 patients, and Inagawa and Hirano[15] in 18% of 133 patients.

Varying incidences of multiple aneurysms have also been found in angiographic series. Björkesten and Halonen[16] performed four-vessel angiography in 113 patients with subarachnoid hemorrhage and found 84 patients with aneurysms and 25 (29.8%) with multiple aneurysms. Nehls and associates[17] detected multiple aneurysms in 33.5% of 206 patients with aneurysms, and a four-vessel study was performed in all except 2 patients. Wilson and colleagues[18] reported multiple aneurysms in 44.9% of 254 patients with ruptured aneurysms, and four-vessel angiography was performed in all but 21 of them. A much lower incidence of multiplicity in an ethnically homogeneous Norwegian population was reported by Nakstad and coworkers,[19] who found multiple aneurysms on four-vessel angiography in only 8.6% of 594 patients with subarachnoid hemorrhage and ruptured aneurysm. It may be assumed, however, that approximately 30% of patients with a ruptured aneurysm have one or more unruptured aneurysms.

## Age, Sex, and Hypertension

No correlation between multiple aneurysms and age was found by Inagawa[20] or Östergaard and Hog.[21] Andrews and Spiegel[22] maintain that increasing age correlates with an increasing number of aneurysms in women but not in men. Women account for most patients with multiple aneurysms. The percentage of women with multiple aneurysms has been reported by McKissock and colleagues[1] as 68%, by Paterson and Bond[2] as 70%, by Mizoi and associates[23] as 61%, by Fox[24] as 61%, by Wilson and colleagues[18] as 65.5%, and by Vajda and coworkers[25] as 72%. In a Finnish series,[26] the ratio between the sexes was more equal, with women comprising 53% of patients with multiple aneurysms. An exception is a series from Norway[19] that had only 45% women. Women also predominate in autopsy series.[10,11] Hypertensive patients have multiple aneurysms more often than normotensive patients.[21,22] Although hypertension is not significantly more prevalent in the patient population with aneurysm than in the general population, it does appear more often in women 18 to 54 years of age.[22]

## Number of Aneurysms

Most patients with multiple aneurysms have two aneurysms, although the number varies considerably in reports from different countries and populations. The proportion of patients with two aneurysms in the United States has been reported by Nehls and associates[17] as 50%, by Fox[24] as 71%, and by the Cooperative Study[27] as 74%. Other reported incidences are 78% in Japan,[23] 68% in Britain,[18] 77% in Finland,[26] and 78% in Hungary.[25] On the basis of these reports, approximately 70% of patients with multiple aneurysms may be expected to have two aneurysms. The proportion of patients with three aneurysms in the aforementioned studies ranges from 5% to 28%, and of those with four aneurysms, from 1.5% to 7.8%. The highest number of aneurysms the authors have seen and treated in the same patient is seven.

## Site of Aneurysms

It is generally accepted that all aneurysms that can be reached through the same approach should be clipped during the same session. Therefore, it is important to know how many aneurysms are situated on the same side so that they can be reached through the same approach. Marttila and Heiskanen[28] found that the aneurysms were situated on the same side in one third of the patients with two aneurysms. In patients with two aneurysms, the most frequent site combinations were as follows: symmetrically on opposite sides in 37% of patients; asymmetrically on opposite sides in 22%; and on the same side in 32%. A combination of aneurysms of the carotid and vertebrobasilar systems was seen in 9% of patients.

In the two series reported from Scandinavia[16, 19] in which the patients were studied with four-vessel angiography, the most common site for an aneurysm in patients with multiple aneurysms was the middle cerebral artery, followed by the anterior communicating and internal carotid arteries. In a series from the United States[17] and in one from Britain,[18] both incorporating four-vessel investigation, the most common site was the internal carotid artery (Table 80–1). The most frequent combinations in patients with two aneurysms were the bilateral internal carotid (Fig. 80–1), the bilateral middle cerebral (Fig. 80–2), and the middle cerebral and anterior communicating aneurysms. Vertebrobasilar aneurysms (Fig. 80–3) have been found in 10% to 14% of patients in the studies mentioned earlier,[16–18] but only in 4% in a Norwegian study[19] (see Table 80–1).

## Size of Aneurysms

The diameter of the aneurysm measured at autopsy does not provide information on its true size because aneurysms shrink after death.[29] The diameter measured from angiographic studies gives a better idea of the true size of the aneurysm.

In autopsy series, unruptured aneurysms are usually smaller than ruptured ones and are larger in only 4% of patients.[15] McCormick and Acosta-Rua[29] reported the average dimension of ruptured aneurysms to be 14.5 mm, in contrast with 4.8 mm for unruptured aneurysms. According to Crompton,[30] the critical size of an aneurysm once it becomes likely to rupture is between 2 and 5 mm. In contrast, Wiebers and coworkers[31] stated that aneurysms smaller than 10 mm in diameter have a very low probability of rupture. Kassel and Torner[32] disagreed with this statement and believed that aneurysms less than 10 mm in size cannot be considered innocuous. Juvela and associates[26] found that the median diameter of ruptured aneurysms was in the 10-mm range (4 to 28 mm), and that of unruptured aneurysms, 4 mm. This supports the contention that even very small aneurysms may bleed, as experience has indeed shown. The authors, too, disagree with Wiebers and colleagues[31] and believe that aneurysms less than 10 mm in diameter—and even less than 5 mm—are potentially dangerous and may hemorrhage.

## Identification of the Ruptured Aneurysm

In surgery of multiple aneurysms, the ruptured aneurysm should be identified first. If the aneurysms are situated so that they cannot be reached through the same approach, the ruptured aneurysm should be treated first.

Wood[33] reported that the ruptured aneurysm can be identified with the aid of total angiographic imaging in more than 95% of all cases. The largest aneurysm is usually the ruptured one. Evidence of intracranial hematoma is the most reliable indication of rupture. Vasospasm is less reliable because it may be widespread and distant from the ruptured aneurysm. Marttila and Heiskanen[28] found that the largest aneurysm had bled in 94% of cases. A secondary sac or local spasm was also a fairly reliable sign of rupture. Intracerebral hematoma was, of course, a sure sign of rupture. Almaani and Richardson[34] found that the ruptured aneurysm could be identified on the basis of angiographic signs in only 53% of cases. Sakamoto and colleagues[35] reported that the largest aneurysm had bled in 85% of the

TABLE 80–1 ■ SITES OF ANEURYSMS IN PATIENTS WITH MULTIPLE ANEURYSMS STUDIED WITH FOUR-VESSEL ANGIOGRAPHY

| Author | No. of Aneurysms | MCA (%) | ICA (%) | ACoA (%) | V-B (%) | Others (%) |
|---|---|---|---|---|---|---|
| Björkesten and Halonen, 1965[16] | 119 | 34 | 25 | 25 | 10 | 6 |
| Nehls et al., 1985[17] | 205 | 22 | 47 | 12 | 14 | 5 |
| Nakstad et al., 1988[19] | 103 | 52 | 19 | 21 | 4 | 4 |
| Wilson et al., 1989[18] | 414 | 24 | 43 | 19 | 10 | 4 |

MCA, middle cerebral artery; ICA, internal carotid artery; ACoA, anterior communicating artery; V-B, vertebral and basilar arteries.

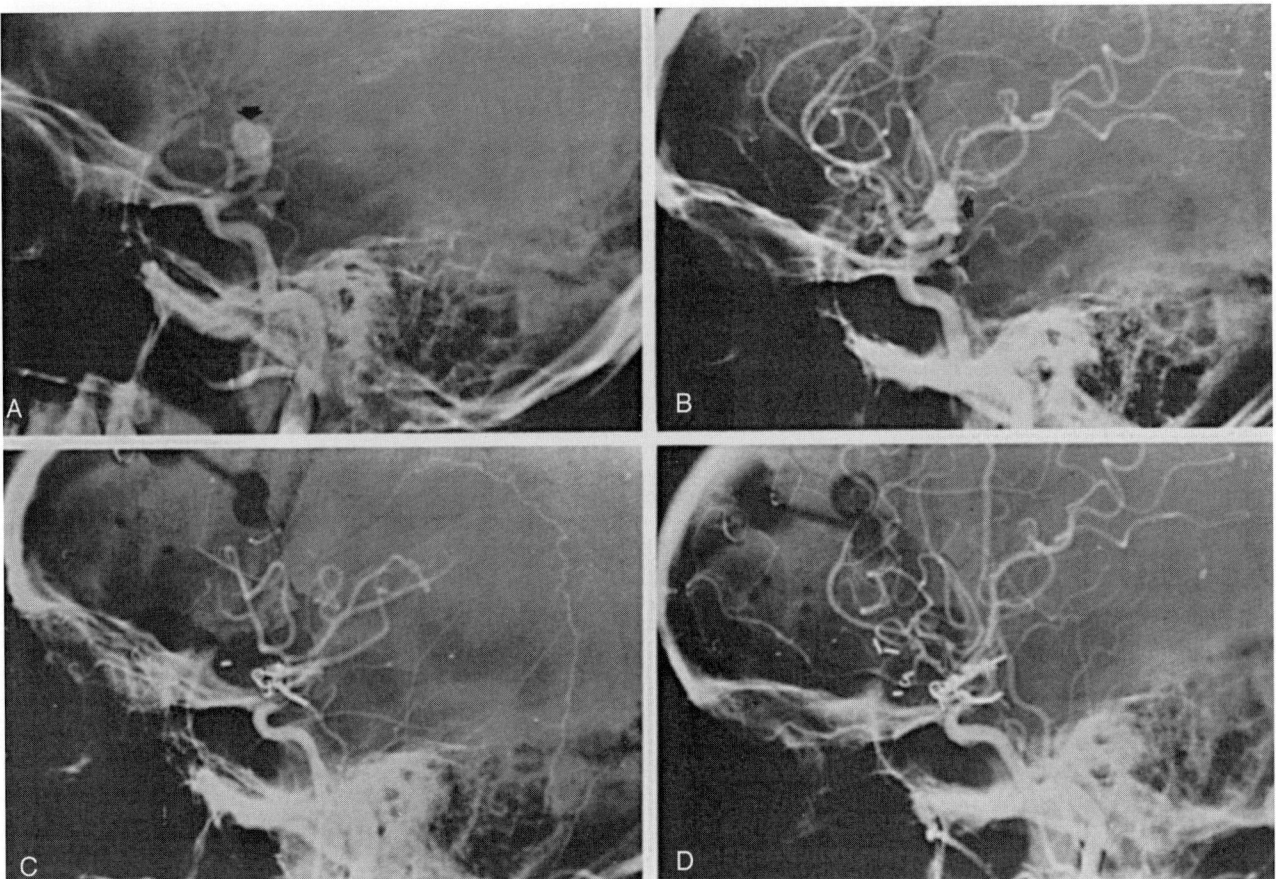

FIGURE 80–1 ■ *A*, Left carotid angiogram, lateral view. A large aneurysm of the carotid bifurcation *(large arrow)* and a small irregular aneurysm of the internal carotid artery are shown. The smaller aneurysm was the ruptured one. *B*, Right carotid angiogram, lateral view. A large aneurysm of the carotid bifurcation *(large arrow)* and a small aneurysm of the internal carotid artery *(small arrow)* are shown. Both are symmetric with the aneurysms on the left side. *C*, Left carotid angiogram, lateral view. Both aneurysms are clipped. *D*, Right carotid angiogram, lateral view. Both aneurysms are clipped.

cases studied. Nehls and coworkers[17] found the irregular outline of the aneurysm to be a more reliable indicator of rupture than its size. Whereas the largest aneurysm had bled in 83% of their cases, the irregularly outlined aneurysm had ruptured in 93%. Thus, when all the angiographic signs are combined, the ruptured aneurysm can be identified in 97% of cases.[17, 28] In combinations of anterior communicating aneurysm and aneurysm of any other site, it is usually the anterior communicating aneurysm that has bled.[17, 28, 33, 35]

## Risk of Rupture of an Unruptured Aneurysm

Only a few studies have assessed the risk of rupture of another aneurysm in patients with multiple aneurysms and one ruptured aneurysm. The risk has been assessed by following a series of patients with multiple aneurysms and subarachnoid hemorrhage in whom only the ruptured aneurysm was clipped.[36] The minimum follow-up time in this study was 10 years. The yearly risk of bleeding was 1.15% per year, and half of the hemorrhages were fatal. Winn and associates[37] monitored a similar group of patients for a mean follow-up time of 7 years and estimated the risk of bleeding as 1% per year. Juvela and coworkers[26]

followed yet another group of patients for a mean follow-up time of 14 years and calculated the risk of rupture to be 1.3% per year. The bleeding was fatal in 46% of their cases, and the cumulative rate of bleeding was 10% at 10 years, 25.6% at 20 years, and 32.4% at 30 years. The age of the patient seems to be the only significant factor predicting a rupture; younger patients have a higher risk of rupture than older patients.[26]

## Surgery for an Unruptured Aneurysm

The surgical risks of both mortality and morbidity for unruptured aneurysms in patients with multiple aneurysms are low. There are several studies on patients with multiple aneurysms that report no surgical mortality at all,[3, 4, 38] or very low mortality even in cases of posterior circulation aneurysms and in surgery performed on elderly patients.[20, 39, 40] The risk of permanent morbidity is also very low.[20, 38–40] Given the risk of bleeding, which is 10% over 10 years, with half of the hemorrhages being fatal, surgery seems to provide a clear margin of benefit. However, an unruptured aneurysm should be operated on only if the patient is basically a good candidate for surgery and has no other serious illness that would make the surgery exces-

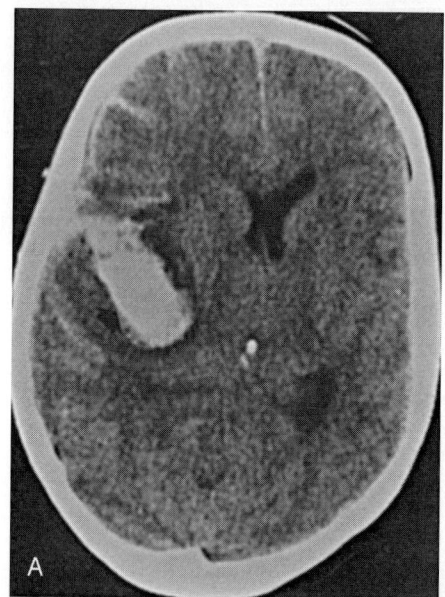

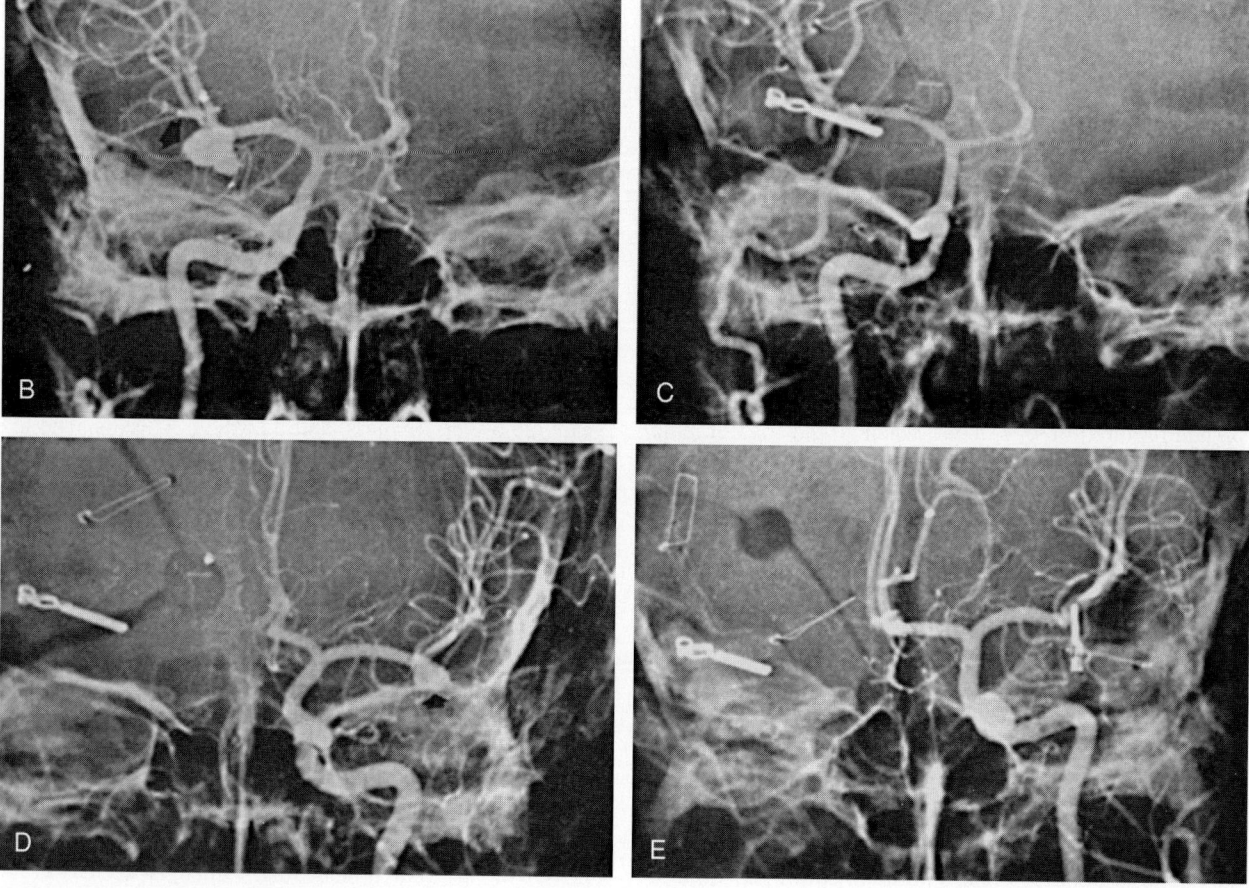

**FIGURE 80–2** ■ *A*, A computed tomography (CT) scan showing an intracerebral hematoma in the right temporal lobe. *B*, Right carotid angiogram, anteroposterior view. An aneurysm of the middle cerebral artery with a secondary sac *(arrow)*. This was the ruptured aneurysm. *C*, Right carotid angiogram, anteroposterior view. The middle cerebral artery aneurysm is clipped. *D*, Left carotid angiogram, anteroposterior view. This study was performed in connection with postoperative right carotid angiography. There is an aneurysm in the left middle cerebral artery *(arrow)*, which is symmetric with the middle cerebral aneurysm on the right side. *E*, Left carotid angiogram, anteroposterior view. The aneurysm is clipped.

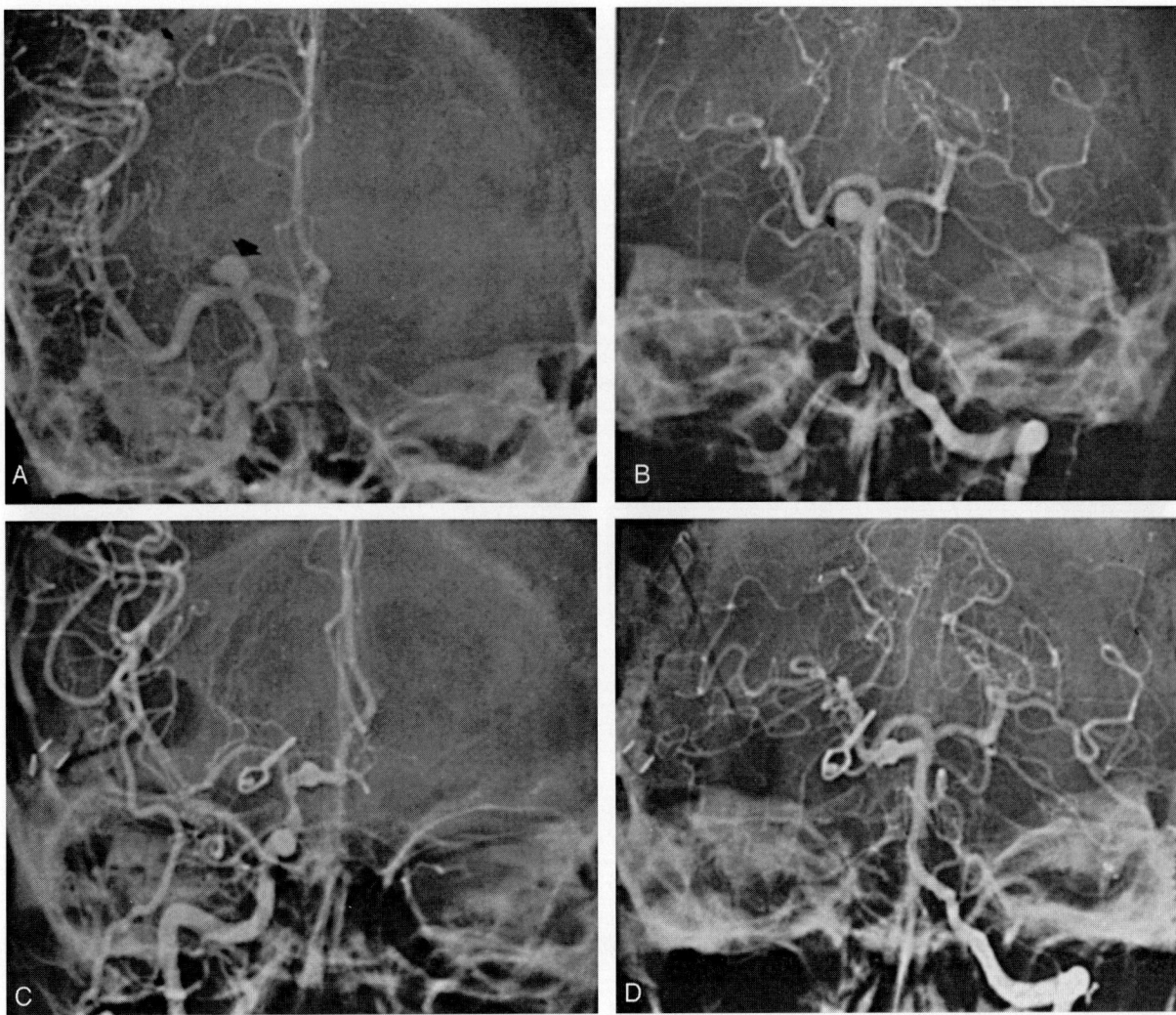

FIGURE 80–3 ■ *A*, Right carotid angiogram, anteroposterior view. An unruptured aneurysm of carotid bifurcation *(large arrow)*. There is also a small unruptured temporoparietal arteriovenous malformation *(small arrow)*. *B*, Vertebral angiogram anteroposterior view. An aneurysm of the basilar trunk on the right side between the posterior cerebral and superior cerebellar arteries *(arrow)*. This aneurysm was the one that had ruptured. *C*, Right carotid angiogram, anteroposterior view. The carotid bifurcation aneurysm is clipped. A moderate spasm of the carotid and middle cerebral arteries is shown. *D*, Vertebral angiogram, anteroposterior view. The basilar aneurysm is clipped.

sively risky. In general, all the aneurysms that can be reached through the same approach should be clipped at the same session. This is possible in aneurysms of the anterior circulation on the same side and in combinations of unilateral and midline aneurysms (i.e., aneurysms of the middle or internal carotid arteries and of the anterior communicating artery; aneurysms of the pericallosal artery and of the middle cerebral, internal carotid, or anterior communicating arteries; or aneurysms of the anterior circulation and of the basilar tip). The general neurosurgical techniques for operating on aneurysms of each particular site are the same as those described in the corresponding chapters of this book, and the authors refer the reader to them. In cases in which an aneurysm of the pericallosal artery occurs in combination with any other anterior circulation aneurysm, the authors prefer to make separate small parasagittal and pterional bone flaps, as recommended by Yasargil,[12] instead of one large bone flap. Two operations are usually necessary in symmetric aneurysms on opposite

sides. Some neurosurgeons clip unruptured aneurysms of the internal carotid arteries and even of the middle cerebral arteries from the contralateral side.[25, 41–43] This is technically possible, but should be undertaken by experienced neurosurgeons only.

If a second operation is necessary, the authors usually perform it approximately 3 to 4 weeks after the first operation. Some neurosurgeons suggest performing two separate operations in the same session to clip all the aneurysms.[20, 44] This method considerably lengthens the operating time and submits the patient to additional surgical stress. The authors prefer to give the patient time to recover between operations. The only situation in which the authors would operate on the other side immediately is when the wrong aneurysm has been identified as the ruptured one. If it can be determined that the aneurysm that has first been approached is not the ruptured one, the authors continue the operation on the opposite side in the same session. Otherwise, the patient runs a serious risk of rebleeding.

Mizoi and colleagues[23] use a bifrontal approach to clip all the anterior circulation aneurysms, but the authors have no personal experience with this approach.

Endovascular treatment of intracranial aneurysms, ruptured as well as unruptured, with the GDC system, first introduced in 1990, has become an accepted alternative to surgery. In this procedure, the aneurysm is packed with platinum microcoils using a microcatheter (Fig. 80–4). Embolization is not possible if the neck of the aneurysm is too wide to retain the coils or the proximal vessels are so tortuous that the aneurysm cannot be catheterized. The most common site of the aneurysm treated with GDC embolization is the basilar tip, but with nearly any aneurysm, embolization may be considered.[45, 46]

If the patient has a large intracerebral hematoma and a deteriorating level of consciousness, the hematoma must be evacuated in an emergency procedure and the ruptured aneurysm clipped.[47] These cases are urgent and, on admission, angiography should be performed only on the side of the hematoma. Angiography of the other side and eventually of the vertebrobasilar system should be performed in connection with postoperative angiography, and other unruptured aneurysms should be operated on later if the patient recovers reasonably well (see Fig. 80–2). The authors set no definite limit in millimeters on the size of aneurysm that should be operated on, as suggested by some neurosurgeons.[31, 48] Even very small (<5 mm) aneurysms may bleed.[26] Consequently, the authors treat all aneurysms that are large enough to be clipped. If, in the course of the operation, the authors find a very small aneurysm that has

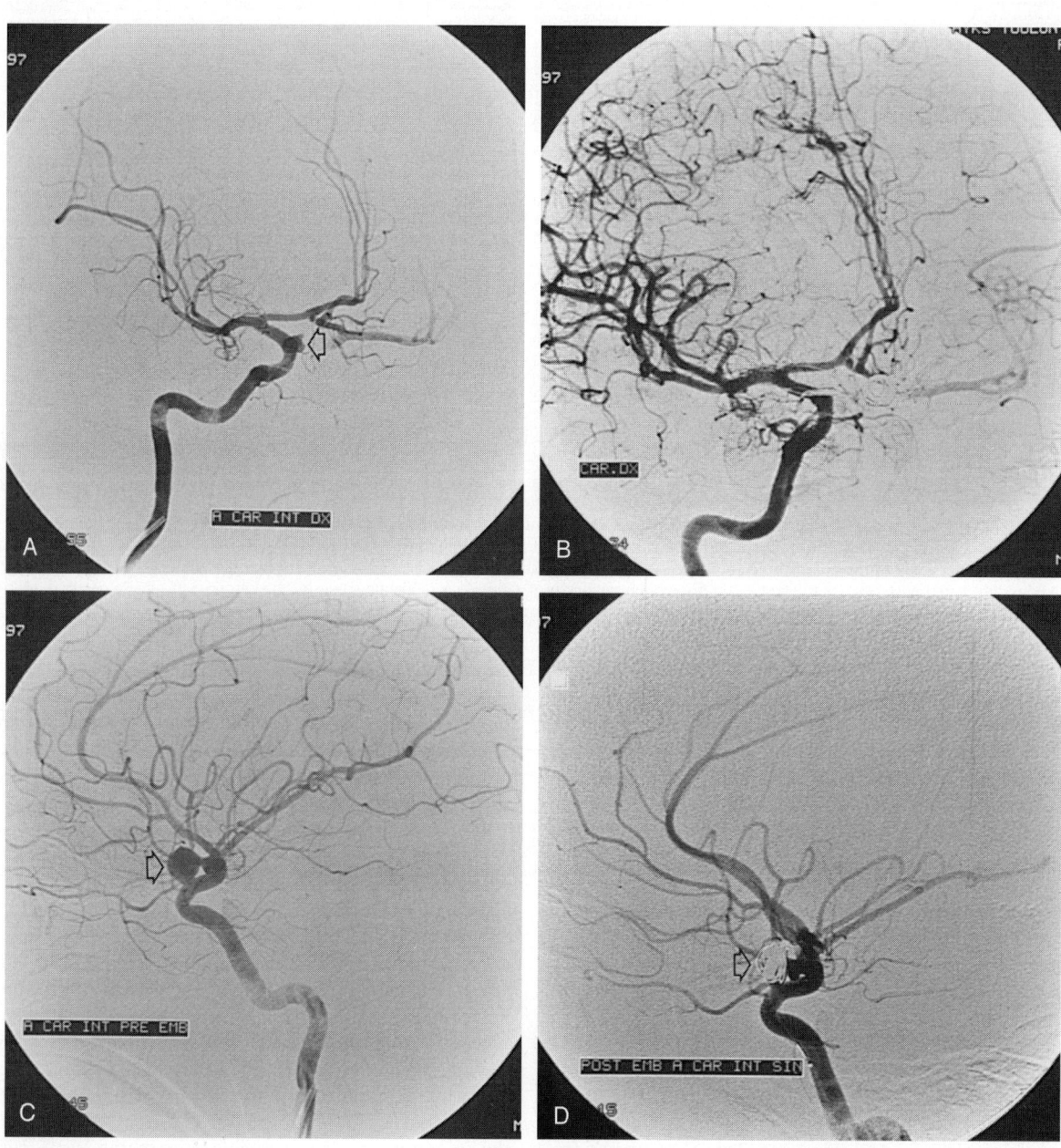

FIGURE 80–4 ■ *A,* Right carotid angiogram, oblique anteroposterior view. An incidental internal carotid aneurysm *(arrow). B,* The aneurysm is clipped. *C,* Left carotid angiogram, lateral view. A larger incidental internal carotid aneurysm with a narrow neck *(arrow). D,* The aneurysm embolized, and the aneurysmal sack is filled with coils *(arrow).*

not been detected in the angiogram and that is too small to clip, it is reinforced with fibrin sealant.

## Results of Surgery

According to several authors, the results of surgery on patients with multiple aneurysms do not differ from those of patients with single aneurysms, even if several aneurysms are clipped in the same session.[3, 4, 20, 23, 38] The surgical mortality rate is very low (0.6%), even in surgery on aneurysms of the posterior circulation in patients with multiple aneurysms.[40] Some authors, however, consider surgical treatment of multiple aneurysms a high-risk operation[49] or state that the outcome is poorer than for patients with single aneurysms.[50] The authors' experience has been that patients tolerate clipping of several aneurysms at the same session well, and the same is true for the second operation for an unruptured aneurysm. However, there seems to be a small risk of new aneurysm formation or de novo aneurysms. The risk is estimated as 1.6% per year, and it seems to be the same for patients with multiple and incidental aneurysms.[26] However, the risk of subarachnoid hemorrhage for these patients during the first 10 years is not higher than the incidence of subarachnoid bleeding in the general population.[26] With GDC embolization, complete occlusion of the aneurysm is achieved in 70% to 80%, and with repeated embolizations the percentage increases. In some cases, however, total occlusion is not possible, and in such cases regrowth of the aneurysm is possible. The rate of complications with permanent neurologic deficits with this procedure is approximately 4%.[51]

## INCIDENTAL ANEURYSMS

### Incidence, Age, and Sex

The prevalence of unruptured, incidental aneurysms in large autopsy series was reported to be 0.6% by Berry and associates[52] and 0.8% by Inagawa and Hirano.[53] It was higher in patients older than 60 years of age and highest, or 1.2%, in the seventh decade. The rate of female-to-male patients was 51:33. Atkinson and coworkers[54] reported the incidence of asymptomatic aneurysms as 1% in an angiographic study. These studies suggest that the incidence of asymptomatic aneurysms is very low overall. Iwata and associates[55] studied the incidence of aneurysms in 72 patients undergoing coronary angiography for angina pectoris by obtaining an intracranial digital subtraction angiogram and found the much higher incidence of 6.9%. Among asymptomatic members of families with familial intracranial aneurysms, the prevalence of incidental aneurysm is higher, approximately 10%.[56]

### Risk of Rupture of an Asymptomatic Aneurysm

The risk of rupture of an incidental aneurysm is not precisely known. It is assumed to be close to that of unruptured aneurysms in patients with multiple aneurysms,

which is 1.3% per year.[6, 26, 37] Furthermore, bleeding is eventually likely to be fatal in half of the patients. When surgical treatment of an incidental aneurysm is considered, the patient's age, other concurrent illnesses that possibly could increase the surgical risk, and the site and size of the aneurysm and its relationship to important arteries and structures should all be carefully weighed, as should the individual neurosurgeon's experience and skill in aneurysm surgery.[57]

## Risks of Surgery

Several studies have suggested that surgery of unruptured asymptomatic aneurysms is a very low-risk procedure. There has been no surgical mortality, and the rate of permanent morbidity has been very low (from 0% to 6.5%) in the published series.[6-8, 31, 58, 59] The authors' experience has been that it is technically easier to operate on unruptured, incidental aneurysm than on ruptured aneurysms. An unruptured aneurysm involves no adhesions; it is easily dissected free and tolerates much more manipulation without rupture. Giant aneurysms are naturally an exception because their size is always a technical problem and the surgical risks are higher. Basilar aneurysms may be another exception. They are technically difficult to manage and also entail higher surgical risks. For incidental aneurysms, GDC embolization is an acceptable alternative to surgery, as described previously for multiple aneurysms.

Therefore, an operation to clip an incidental, asymptomatic aneurysm or aneurysms should be suggested to patients who are otherwise well, free from a serious illness that might increase the surgical risk, and not too old. The authors would not suggest an operation for a patient older than 65 years of age. It should be made absolutely clear to the patient that the operation is intended only to prevent bleeding in the future and is unlikely to affect those symptoms for which the patient was initially examined, such as vertigo, headache, or seizures.[6] If the patient has more than one incidental aneurysm, all the aneurysms that can be reached through the same approach should be dealt with at the same session. If the other aneurysm or aneurysms can be clipped only through a separate approach, a second operation should be performed a few weeks after the first one. A recent report suggests, however, that in patients with unruptured aneurysm less than 10 mm in diameter and no subarachnoid hemorrhage from a different aneurysm the surgical risks may exceed the risks of rupture.[60] Van Crevel and colleagues[61] and Dell[62] have developed a special decision-making model for patients with incidental aneurysms.

## Summary

In patients with multiple aneurysms and subarachnoid hemorrhage, unruptured aneurysms should be clipped along with the ruptured aneurysm during the same operation if they are accessible through the same approach. However, the surgical priority should always be the ruptured aneurysm, which can be identified by angiographic signs in at least 97% of cases. If the unruptured aneurysm cannot be reached through the same approach as the ruptured aneurysm, it should be treated at a second operation a few weeks after the first operation, assuming that the patient is a good candidate for surgery and has no other serious illness that could increase the surgical risk.

Asymptomatic, incidental aneurysms should be treated surgically if the patient has no other serious illness that would increase the surgical risk unacceptably. On the whole, the surgical risks are very low for such patients, and the younger the patient, the stronger the indication for operation.

An alternative to surgery is GDC embolization. This procedure does not need general anesthesia and is thus suitable for patients with high anesthesia risks. The basilar tip is the most common site for aneurysms treated with embolization, but any aneurysm can be treated with GDC embolization if the neck of the aneurysm is not too wide and the aneurysm can be catheterized.

## REFERENCES

1. McKissock W, Richardson A, Walsh L, Owen E: Multiple intracranial aneurysms. Lancet 1:623–626, 1964.
2. Paterson A, Bond MR: Treatment of multiple intracranial arterial aneurysms. Lancet 1:1302–1304, 1973.
3. Mount LA, Brisman R: Treatment of multiple intracranial aneurysms. J Neurosurg 35:728–730, 1971.
4. Moyes PD: Surgical treatment of multiple aneurysms and of incidentally discovered unruptured aneurysms. J Neurosurg 35:291–295, 1971.
5. Poyanne H, Banayan A, Guerin J, Riemens V: Les anéurysmes sacculaires multiples du système carotidien supra clinoidie: Etude anatomo-clinique et thérapeutique. Neurochirurgie 19 (Suppl 1):1–96, 1973.
6. Heiskanen O, Poranen A: Surgery of incidental intracranial aneurysms. J Neurosurg 28:432–436, 1987.
7. Salazar JL: Surgical treatment of asymptomatic and incidental intracranial aneurysms. J Neurosurg 3:20–21, 1980.
8. Samson DS, Hodosh RM, Clark WK: Surgical management of unruptured asymptomatic aneurysms. J Neurosurg 6:731–734, 1977.
9. Wirth FP, Laws ER, Piepgras D, Scott MR: Surgical treatment of incidental intracranial aneurysms. Neurosurgery 12:507–511, 1983.
10. McCormick WF, Nofziger JD: Saccular intracranial aneurysms. J Neurosurg 22:155–159, 1965.
11. Stehbens WE: Aneurysms and anatomical variations of cerebral arteries. Arch Pathol 75:45–64, 1963.
12. Yasargil G: Microneurosurgery. II: Clinical consideration. In Surgery of the Intracranial Aneurysms and Results. Stuttgart: Georg Thieme, 1984, pp 305–328.
13. Inagawa T: Surgical treatment of multiple intracranial aneurysms. Acta Neurochir (Wien) 108:22–29, 1990.
14. Chason JL, Hindman WM: Berry aneurysms of the circle of Willis. Neurology 8:41–44, 1958.
15. Inagawa T, Hirano A: Ruptured intracranial aneurysms: An autopsy study of 133 patients. Surg Neurol 33:117–123, 1990.
16. Björkesten G, Halonen V: Incidence of intracranial lesions in patients with subarachnoid hemorrhage investigated by four-vessel angiography. J Neurosurg 23:29–32, 1965.
17. Nehls DG, Flom RA, Carter LP, Spetzler RF: Multiple intracranial aneurysms: Determining the site of rupture. J Neurosurg 63:342–348, 1985.
18. Wilson FMA, Jaspan T, Holland IM: Multiple cerebral aneurysms: Reappraisal. Neuroradiology 31:232–236, 1989.
19. Nakstad P, Nornes H, Hauge HN, Kjartansson O: Cerebral panangiography in spontaneous hemorrhage from intracranial aneurysms. Acta Radiol 29:633–636, 1988.
20. Inagawa T: Multiple intracranial aneurysms in elderly patients. Acta Neurochir (Wien) 106:119–126, 1990.
21. Östergaard JR, Hog E: Incidence of multiple intracranial aneurysms. J Neurosurg 63:45–55, 1985.
22. Andrews RJ, Spiegel PK: Intracranial aneurysms: Age, sex, blood pressure, and multiplicity in an unselected series of patients. J Neurosurg 51:27–32, 1979.
23. Mizoi K, Suzuki J, Yoshimoto T: Surgical treatment of multiple aneurysms. Acta Neurochir (Wien) 96:8–14, 1989.
24. Fox J: Intracranial Aneurysms. New York: Springer-Verlag, 1983, pp 36–37.
25. Vajda J, Juhasz J, Orosz E, et al: Surgical treatment of unruptured intracranial aneurysms. Acta Neurochir (Wien) 82:14–26, 1986.
26. Juvela S, Porras M, Heiskanen O: Natural history of unruptured intracranial aneurysms. J Neurosurg 79:161–173, 1993.
27. Locksley HB: Natural history of subarachnoid hemorrhage: Intracranial aneurysms and arteriovenous malformations. J Neurosurg 25:219–239, 1966.
28. Marttila I, Heiskanen O: Value of neurological and angiographic signs as indicators of the ruptured aneurysm in patients with multiple intracranial aneurysms. Acta Neurochir (Wien) 23:95–102, 1970.
29. McCormick WF, Acosta-Rua GJ: The size of intracranial saccular aneurysms: An autopsy study. J Neurosurg 33:422–427, 1970.
30. Crompton MR: Mechanism of growth and rupture in cerebral berry aneurysms. BMJ 1:1138–1142, 1966.
31. Wiebers NF, Whisnant JP, Sundt TM, O'Fallon N: The significance of unruptured intracranial saccular aneurysms. J Neurosurg 66:23–29, 1987.
32. Kassel NF, Torner JC: Size of intracranial aneurysms. Neurosurgery 12:291–297, 1983.
33. Wood EH: Angiographic identification of the ruptured lesion in patients with multiple cerebral aneurysms. J Neurosurg 21:182–198, 1964.
34. Almaani WS, Richardson AE: Multiple intracranial aneurysms: Identifying the ruptured lesion. Surg Neurol 9:303–305, 1978.
35. Sakamoto T, Kwak R, Mizoi K, et al: Angiographical study of ruptured aneurysm in the multiple aneurysms patients. No Shinkei Geka 6:549–553, 1978.
36. Heiskanen O: Risk of bleeding from unruptured aneurysm in cases with multiple intracranial aneurysms. J Neurosurg 55:524–526, 1981.
37. Winn HR, Almaani WS, Berga SL, et al: The long-term outcome in patients with multiple aneurysms. J Neurosurg 59:642–651, 1983.
38. Drake CG, Girvin JP: The surgical treatment of subarachnoid hemorrhage with multiple aneurysms. In Morley TP (ed): Current Controversies in Neurosurgery. Philadelphia: WB Saunders, 1976, pp 274–278.
39. Heiskanen O: Risks of surgery for unruptured intracranial aneurysms. J Neurosurg 4:51–453, 1986.
40. Rice BJ, Peerless SJ, Drake CG: Surgical treatment of unruptured aneurysm of the posterior circulation. J Neurosurg 73:165–173, 1990.
41. Milenkovicz Z, Gopic H, Antovic P, et al: Contralateral pterional approach to a carotid-ophthalmic aneurysm ruptured at surgery. J Neurosurg 57:823–825, 1982.
42. Nakao S, Kikuchi H, Takahashi N: Successful clipping of carotid-ophthalmic aneurysms through a contralateral pterional approach. J Neurosurg 54:532–536, 1981.
43. Yasargil MG, Gasser JC, Hodosh RM, Rankin TV: Carotid-ophthalmic aneurysms: Direct microsurgical approach. Surg Neurol 8:155–165, 1977.
44. Edner G, Kågström E, Wallstedt L: Total overall management and surgical outcome after aneurysmal subarachnoid hemorrhage in a defined population. Br J Neurosurg 6:409–420, 1992.
45. Fernandez ZA, Guglielmi G, Vinuela F, et al: Endovascular occlusion of intracranial aneurysms with electrically detachable coils: Correlation of aneurysms, neck size and treatment results. AJNR Am J Neuroradiol 15:815–820, 1994.
46. Standard S, Chavis T, Guterman L, et al: Endovascular occlusion of aneurysm. Neurosurg Q 4:201–219, 1994.
47. Heiskanen O, Poranen A, Kuurne T, et al: Acute surgery for intracerebral hematomas caused by rupture of an intracranial arterial aneurysm. Acta Neurochir (Wien) 90:81–83, 1988.
48. Piepgras DG: Management of incidental intracranial aneurysms. Clin Neurosurg 35:511–518, 1989.
49. Vajda J: Multiple intracranial aneurysms: A high risk condition. Acta Neurochir (Wien) 118:59–75, 1992.
50. Rinne J, Hernesniemi J, Niskanen M, Vapalahti M: Management outcome for multiple intracranial aneurysms. Neurosurgery 36:31–38, 1995.
51. Malisch TW, Guglielmi G, Vinuela F, et al: Intracranial aneurysms treated with the Guglielmi detachable coil: Midterm clinical results in a consecutive series of 100 patients. J Neurosurg 87:176–183, 1997.
52. Berry RC, Alpers BJ, White JC: The site, structure, and frequency of

intracranial aneurysms, angiomas and arteriovenous abnormalities. Res Publ Assoc Res Nerv Ment Dis 41:40–72, 1961.

53. Inagawa T, Hirano A: Autopsy study of unruptured incidental intracranial aneurysms. Surg Neurol 34:361–365, 1990.

54. Atkinson JLD, Sundt TM, Houser DW, Whisnant JP: Angiographic frequency of anterior circulation intracranial aneurysms. J Neurosurg 70:551–555, 1989.

55. Iwata K, Misus N, Terada K, et al: Screening for unruptured asymptomatic intracranial aneurysms in patients undergoing coronary angiography. J Neurosurg 75:52–55, 1991.

56. Ronkainen A, Hernesniemi J, Puranen M, et al: Familial intracranial aneurysms. Lancet 349(9049):380–384, 1997.

57. Weir B: Aneurysms Affecting the Nervous System. Baltimore: Williams & Wilkins, 1987, pp 48–53.

58. Pertuiset B, Mahdy M, Sichez JP, et al: Les anéurysmes arteriels sacculaires intracraniens nonrompus de l'adulte d'un diametre inférieur 20 mm. Rev Neurol (Paris) 147:111–120, 1991.

59. Wirth FP, Laws ER, Piepgras D, Scott RM: Surgical treatment of incidental intracranial aneurysms. Neurosurgery 12:507–511, 1983.

60. The International Study of Intracranial Aneurysm Investigators: Unruptured intracranial aneurysms—risk of rupture and risks of surgical intervention. N Engl J Med 339:1725–1733, 1998.

61. van Crevel H, Habbema JDF, Braakman R: Decision analysis of the management of incidental intracranial saccular aneurysms. Neurology 36:1335–1339, 1986.

62. Dell S: Asymptomatic cerebral aneurysm: Assessment of its risk of rupture. Neurosurgery 10:162–166, 1982.

# CHAPTER 81

# Perioperative Care After an Aneurysmal Subarachnoid Hemorrhage

■ NICHOLAS W. C. DORSCH, ANDREW KAM, and MICHAEL K. MORGAN

The definitive treatment for aneurysmal subarachnoid hemorrhage (SAH) is obliteration of the aneurysm through direct surgery and clipping of its neck or by interventional treatments such as detachable metal coils.[1] Of equal importance are other measures necessary to help the patient recover from the hemorrhage and from its complications. Although mostly nonsurgical in nature, these measures include ventricular shunting or angioplasty. The purposes of perioperative care after SAH are to keep the patient alive; to maximize the chances of surviving the surgery for the aneurysm; and to minimize the effect of complications, such as delayed hydrocephalus or vasospasm.

## BACKGROUND

Only in the last 2 to 3 decades has there been much active perioperative treatment for SAH. Until the 1970s, the perioperative treatment for SAH was strict bed rest, often with isolation in a quiet, darkened single room; sedation; and restriction of visitors and other stimuli for 10 to 14 days. Surgery was then carried out if the patient was fit enough. As with most patients with a serious intracranial problem, the tendency during this period was to keep the patient relatively dehydrated. This mode of management often resulted in significant systemic complications.[2] Although the overall management of SAH has become vastly more complicated, there has been an equivalent improvement in its effects on outcome.

## CAUSES OF SUBARACHNOID HEMORRHAGE

Cerebral aneurysm is only one of many possible causes of SAH, and the most common is head injury. Every patient with a fractured skull would, if submitted to a lumbar puncture, show blood staining of the cerebrospinal fluid (CSF). There has been considerable interest in traumatic

SAH, which has been shown to have a deleterious effect on the outcome of head injury,[3] and in the occurrence and treatment of post-traumatic vasospasm.[4] When restricted to spontaneous SAH, other causes apart from aneurysm include arteriovenous malformation, tumors, blood dyscrasias, anticoagulant drugs, systemic hypertension, and a significant proportion of cases in which no cause is ever found.[5] The hemorrhage in these cases is generally less severe, probably because less blood is spilled into the subarachnoid space, and it is at lower pressure. The risk of complications, such as cerebral vasospasm or hydrocephalus, is generally less, and there is less risk of early recurrent hemorrhage, so that definitive treatment is in general less urgent.

## CLINICAL PRESENTATION OF SUBARACHNOID HEMORRHAGE

### History

In most cases, the history of a SAH begins with the explosive onset of a headache of extreme severity. The headache is usually generalized but may be more posterior in location. Occasionally, it is mainly unilateral, and in such cases the aneurysm is usually located on the side of greater headache. Rarely the headache is less abrupt in onset or even absent. There is often a brief period of loss of consciousness, and there may be several such episodes. Nausea and vomiting are common. Focal symptoms are less common and may suggest an intracerebral hemorrhage, particularly if there is a persistent depression of consciousness.

### Symptoms and Signs

A conscious patient usually complains of severe headache. The clinical signs of SAH are also usually easily recognizable, being those of a chemical meningitis, and include

1102

photophobia, neck stiffness, and a positive Kernig sign. In some cases, a depressed conscious state or focal signs are seen. Fever and a peripheral leukocytosis may be present. The differentiation from infective meningitis may be impossible on examination alone, so that a knowledge of the history of onset may be vital to the diagnosis.

## Recognition and Misdiagnosis

A common problem in SAH is the failure of the first attending physician to diagnose the hemorrhage, particularly when it is less severe than in the classic case and is more in the nature of a *warning leak*.[6] Many misdiagnoses have been reported, and common among them are influenza, viral or other meningitis, migraine, tension headache, and cervical spine disorder.[7] A problem in this situation is that no symptom or sign (or diagnostic test) is completely accurate in diagnosing SAH, especially if negative.[8] It is essential for practicing neurosurgeons to take every possible opportunity to educate medical students, emergency department staff, and general practitioners to avoid misdiagnosing SAH because with a less severe hemorrhage, there is a perfect window of opportunity for successful definitive management if it is recognized in time.

## Unruptured Aneurysms

A small but increasing proportion of cerebral aneurysms are detected before rupture. Some are symptomatic and warrant treatment in any case. The best example is the sudden onset of a painful oculomotor nerve palsy as a result of expansion of an aneurysm at the origin from the internal carotid artery of the posterior communicating artery; such expansion may be a warning of imminent rupture and requires urgent treatment.

Many other intact aneurysms are detected when a computed tomography (CT) scan has been done for another indication, such as migraine or dizziness, or when relatives of a patient with an aneurysm are screened using one of the relatively noninvasive tests available today. These aneurysms are often operated on prophylactically, but the specific problems seen after SAH do not usually occur, so that management does not differ greatly from that which follows a craniotomy done for some other indication.

## DIAGNOSIS OF SUBARACHNOID HEMORRHAGE

### Computed Tomography Scan

The definitive diagnosis of SAH is usually made by CT scanning. This scanning shows the presence of blood in the basal cisterns and other subarachnoid spaces in nearly all cases if done early enough. When the scan is done in the first 12 hours after a hemorrhage, it is accurate in detecting about 98% of SAH.[9] The sensitivity of CT scanning drops rapidly, so that at the end of 1 week, only about 50% are detected.

CT scanning is useful in demonstrating other problems

associated with SAH, such as an intracerebral hematoma, intraventricular hemorrhage, hydrocephalus, or evidence of raised intracranial pressure (e.g., compression of basal cisterns or loss of gray-white differentiation). Subarachnoid blood or a hematoma may be concentrated in one part of the subarachnoid space, which can be a useful pointer to the location of the ruptured aneurysm. Occasionally, evidence pointing to the aneurysm itself may be seen.[10] When the SAH is due to another problem, such as an arteriovenous malformation or tumor, this is usually evident on a CT scan after contrast administration.

## Lumbar Puncture

Further testing, such as a lumbar puncture, is necessary only if the scan is negative and there is still a suspicion (no matter how slight this may be) that the patient has sustained a SAH. In some circumstances, such as the lack of availability of a CT scanner in a remote location, lumbar puncture may be justified as the first investigation. This approach is, however, safe only if the patient is conscious (with a Glasgow Coma Score[11] of ≥13), and if there is no clinical evidence of an intracranial mass or of raised intracranial pressure, such as hemiparesis, papilledema, or pupillary abnormalities.

Every effort must be made to avoid a traumatic lumbar puncture in this situation because such an occurrence makes the confirmation of SAH more difficult and uncertain. For this reason, the lumbar puncture should be done by a clinician who is expert at the procedure, rather than by a new intern or a student. The CSF specimen, even if it is apparently uniformly blood stained, must in any case be sent for pathologic examination for at least a cell count. Three separate tubes are collected, and the cell counts in all three are similar if there has been a SAH. A specimen must also be centrifuged and the supernatant examined for xanthochromia—this takes several hours to develop,[12] and the presence of xanthochromia may not be apparent in a specimen taken before 12 hours after the hemorrhage.

The CSF may apparently be clear if days or weeks have elapsed since the time of bleeding or at an early stage after a minor leak. Spectroscopic examination may be useful here for the demonstration of bilirubin[13] or oxyhemoglobin. The latter test may be too sensitive to be of great value, resulting in a number of false-positive findings.[13a]

## Magnetic Resonance Imaging

Magnetic resonance imaging (MRI) is not used routinely in the diagnosis of SAH, although it is, in fact, more sensitive than CT scanning in detecting small amounts of blood. The procedure is comparatively slow and cumbersome, and it is difficult to keep a confused patient or even someone with a severe headache still for long enough.

MRI is of more value in those with confirmed SAH and negative angiography in detecting other possible causes of hemorrhage. It can also be useful, particularly if some time has elapsed since the hemorrhage, in patients with more than one aneurysm. If more blood or hemosiderin is shown around one of the aneurysms, that one is more likely to have ruptured.

## DETERMINATION OF THE CAUSE OF SUBARACHNOID HEMORRHAGE

### Cerebral Angiography

Once the diagnosis of SAH has been confirmed, the next vital step is to determine the cause. This determination is done classically with selective pancerebral angiography, usually immediately after the CT scan before the patient leaves the radiology suite, if the clinical condition is stable. It is essential that both carotid and both vertebral arteries be studied thoroughly in case there are multiple aneurysms, which is the case in 10% or more of patients.[14] Often when one vertebral artery is injected, there is sufficient reflux down the other vertebral artery to show clearly the origin of the opposite posterior inferior cerebellar artery; if this is not the case, bilateral vertebral angiograms are necessary.

The standard projections include anteroposterior, lateral, and oblique views for the carotids and anteroposterior and lateral views for the vertebral injections. If necessary, further views, such as reverse oblique, lateral oblique, or submentovertical projections, may also be taken. On rare occasions, if an aneurysm is found that may need to be treated by proximal artery occlusion, cross-compression carotid studies or a vertebral angiogram with ipsilateral cervical carotid compression may be needed.

### Magnetic Resonance Angiography

For the reasons discussed earlier, magnetic resonance angiography is not generally used for aneurysm detection in the situation of acute SAH. It may be necessary if the patient has a contrast allergy, and it is also used later for confirmation if standard angiography has shown no cause for the hemorrhage, along with a standard MRI scan. Magnetic resonance angiography is not sensitive in detecting the smallest of aneurysms of 3 mm diameter or less.[15]

### Computed Tomography Angiography

CT angiography is a more recently developed technique that uses a helical CT scanner with 1-mm slices and reconstruction of the arteries, usually in a three-dimensional format, and has proved of great value in diagnosing cerebral aneurysms in general.[16] Because of the time needed for reconstruction, it is not always feasible in acute SAH, but it is being used instead of standard angiography in some centers.[17]

The main value of CT angiography in the acute situation is as a further test, done usually on the same or the next day, in patients with SAH in whom cerebral angiography was negative. Several small ruptured aneurysms, mostly less than 3 mm in diameter and not visible on angiograms even in retrospect, have been detected in this way in our experience. CT angiography has also been useful for providing more detail of large or giant aneurysms.[16]

## CLINICAL GRADING

### Relationship to Prognosis

The clinical state of a patient can and often does fluctuate widely over even a short period of time. Temporary loss of consciousness is common with even a less severe hemorrhage, and in the first few minutes the sufferer may appear moribund, then return quickly to full consciousness. Conversely, a patient may be reasonably well for several hours after the SAH, then deteriorate rapidly because of the development of cerebral edema or hydrocephalus. Nevertheless, numerous studies have shown that the clinical grade on admission to the hospital is correlated reasonably closely with prognosis. This correlation was well demonstrated in a review by Alvord and Thorn[18] as well as by Hunt and Hess[19] in the descriptions of their grading scale. Alvord and Thorn[18] have analyzed several large reported series of SAH patients and summarized the natural history of SAH in a single table of outcome according to grade.

Although there are imperfections in all the grading scales presently in use, they have enough accuracy to be of some use in outcome prediction for individual cases. In addition, a clinical assessment of this kind is essential when reporting large series of patients or when comparing the effect of different treatments (e.g., in drug trials) or the results from different centers.

### Grading Systems

Many grading systems, often not much different from each other, have been produced over the years. Only two are discussed in detail. An early grading method based on clinical state was introduced by Botterell and colleagues,[20] followed by the Hunt and Hess system,[19] which with slight modification from the original is probably the most widely used today (Table 81–1). This system consists of five

TABLE 81–1 ■ **HUNT AND HESS CLINICAL GRADING SCALE**

| Grade | State |
|---|---|
| 0 | Unruptured aneurysm |
| I | Asymptomatic, or minimal headache and slight nuchal rigidity |
| Ia | No acute meningeal or brain reaction but with fixed neurologic deficit |
| II | Moderate-to-severe headache, nuchal rigidity, no neurologic deficit other than cranial nerve palsy |
| III | Drowsiness, confusion, or mild focal deficit |
| IV | Stupor, moderate-to-severe hemiparesis, possibly early decerebrate rigidity, vegetative disturbances |
| V | Deep coma, decerebrate rigidity, moribund appearance |

From Hunt WE, Kosnik EJ: Timing and perioperative care in intracranial aneurysm surgery. Clin Neurosurg 21:79–89, 1974.

grades for SAH (a sixth, grade 0, was introduced later for unruptured aneurysms[21]). Grade I includes those least severely affected by the hemorrhage, with headache and neck stiffness but no other problems, and grade V patients are deeply unconscious or moribund or have decerebrate rigidity (see Table 81–1).

A committee of the World Federation of Neurosurgical Societies (WFNS), under the chairmanship of Drake,[22] devised a scale that is similar in principle but includes two major changes. The most important is the introduction into the grading of the Glasgow Coma Scale, which is now accepted almost everywhere as a simple, repeatable estimate of the conscious level and is more accurate than the rather descriptive estimates of conscious level used in the Hunt and Hess scale. In addition, neurologically normal patients are now all included in grade I, not in I or II depending on the severity of headache, which has little or no influence on prognosis. Decreased consciousness and focal deficits are given similar weight in the higher grades (Table 81–2).

## Grading by Computed Tomography Appearance

It was recognized in the late 1970s[23, 24] that the volume of subarachnoid blood visible on an early CT scan was closely related to the subsequent risk of developing cerebral vasospasm and bore some relationship to the ultimate prognosis. A quantitative measurement of the thickness of subarachnoid clot is given a rating of 1 to 4 in the Fisher scale,[23] and this has shown a strong correlation with the risk of later developing angiographic or symptomatic vasospasm (Table 81–3).

## Problems of Grading

There is no perfect grading system and in individual patients no way in which the outcome can reliably be predicted. It may be possible to state confidently that 60% of grade III patients eventually make a good recovery, but this can still differ widely in two apparently similar groups. Further, within any one group, it is essentially impossible to estimate which 60% of these clinically similar patients will be the good survivors.

TABLE 81–2 ■ **WORLD FEDERATION OF NEUROSURGICAL SOCIETIES (WFNS) GRADING SCALE**

| WFNS Grade | GCS Score | Focal Deficit* |
|---|---|---|
| I | 15 | Absent |
| II | 14–13 | Absent |
| III | 14–13 | Present |
| IV | 12–7 | Present or absent |
| V | 6–3 | Present or absent |

*Significant or major focal deficit: aphasia or hemiparesis or hemiplegia.
GCS, Glasgow Coma Scale.
From Drake CG: Report of World Federation of Neurological Surgeons Committee on a universal subarachnoid hemorrhage grading scale (Letter). J Neurosurg 68:985–986, 1988.

TABLE 81–3 ■ **DEVELOPMENT OF VASOSPASM ACCORDING TO FISHER COMPUTED TOMOGRAPHY SCALE**

| Fisher Grade | No. Patients | No. with Vasospasm* |
|---|---|---|
| 1—No visible blood | 11 | 4 |
| 2—Thin layer | 7 | 3 |
| 3—Clot or thick layer | 24 | 24 |
| 4—Intracerebral or ventricular | 5 | 2 |

*Angiographic vasospasm with (in 23 of 24 in group 3) or without clinical deterioration.
From Fisher CM, Kistler JP, Davis TM: Relation of cerebral vasospasm to subarachnoid hemorrhage visualized by computerized tomographic scanning. Neurosurgery 6:1–9, 1980.

The inclusion of a CT scale, such as that of Fisher and colleagues,[23] along with the clinical evaluation and grading helps to make outcome prediction a little more accurate. Many other factors contribute to the determination of prognosis, however, including the patient's age and general state of health, the presence of essential hypertension or other significant systemic disease, the state of the intracranial arteries, the size and location of the ruptured aneurysm, and any more direct complications of SAH that may develop, including recurrent hemorrhage, delayed vasospasm, and hydrocephalus.

Attempts have been made to analyze singly and in combination all of these determinants of outcome, in efforts to clarify rebleeding rates and long-term outcome in untreated patients[25] and in the short-term to develop a single, accurate means of prediction for use in individual cases. The latter especially have proved too complicated and not accurate enough for general use.

## DEFINITIVE TREATMENT

The most important aim of treatment is obliteration of the aneurysm that caused the SAH or its exclusion from the circulation, so that it is prevented from bleeding again in the future. Typically, this aim is best achieved by direct surgery to clip the aneurysm neck, but with developments in interventional neuroradiology techniques, particularly the use of Guglielmi detachable coils,[1] this situation is changing rapidly. When direct surgery is planned, one of the most important decisions to be made is the timing of the operation.

### Timing of Aneurysm Surgery

Until the late 1970s, the tendency in most centers was to delay direct surgery for the ruptured aneurysm until the state of the patient, especially the neurologic condition, was optimal. Early attempts at urgent operation, within hours or days of hemorrhage, had been hampered by the frequent finding of a red, swollen brain that could not be safely retracted,[26] and the results were generally poor.

A number of parallel advances have facilitated the resurgence of early operation. The most important has probably been the development of and rapid technologic advances in the binocular operating microscope, which provides an excellent stereoscopic view of the surgical field, with good illumination, good visualization of important small structures such as perforating arteries, and minimal need for brain retraction. Another vital factor is the greatly improved operating conditions; the move away from inhalational to more intravenous anesthetics, better control of parameters such as blood pressure and carbon dioxide levels, and more liberal use of techniques such as intraoperative mannitol or ventricular or lumbar drainage all contribute to a slack brain that can be retracted with little or no pressure. The situation has also been eased by improvements in monitoring (particularly when temporary occlusion of feeding arteries is necessary), so that evoked potential monitoring is now routine in many centers; by improved design of aneurysm clips and applicators; and by improvements in the associated microinstruments. Also important may be the move toward temporary clipping and away from induced systemic hypotension during difficult periods of dissection or when an aneurysm ruptures; the latter could make the whole brain ischemic, and the use instead of temporary vessel occlusion in these situations, with normal blood pressure and protective agents such as high-dose thiopental, is less disturbing to the whole brain.

## Early Operation

Several studies were reported showing reasonable outcomes after early operation,[27, 28] and in the 1980s, a large cooperative study was done on the timing of surgery.[29, 30] This was not, and there has not been, a randomized trial, which would be extremely difficult, if not impossible, to carry out. The results of the cooperative study showed no overall difference between outcomes according to the initially planned time of surgery, but there was a tendency toward worse outcomes when the time of surgery lay between 7 and 10 days.

## Advantages and Disadvantages

The most obvious benefit of early aneurysm operation is that it prevents any risk of further aneurysm rupture. In addition (and this is arguably an advantage over endovascular techniques), it provides the ability to remove cisternal blood and reduce the risk of delayed vasospasm, and if delayed ischemia does occur, it can be managed more effectively and safely with induced hypervolemia and hypertension. The average hospital stay is reduced, and the risks of prolonged immobilization are minimized.

The disadvantages of early surgery include the possibility, even with ventricular drainage as an adjunct and with perfect anesthetic techniques, of finding a red, swollen brain, to the extent occasionally of having to abandon the procedure altogether. The aneurysm can be more difficult to identify when surrounded by fresh clot, and there is more risk of damage to nearby vessels and other structures. Other problems are more logistical in nature—in all but the largest centers, it may be difficult at times to roster

anesthetic and operating room staff who are adequately familiar with cerebral aneurysm surgery. The state of tiredness of the operating surgeon and team also has to be considered. For these reasons, in many centers, a compromise is made by not operating late at night and leaving the procedure until early the next morning.

## Delayed Surgery

Delayed surgical treatment, in its classic form, involved delaying the surgery for at least 10 days to 2 weeks after hemorrhage, until the patient's neurologic condition had improved essentially to normal. During this time, the patient was kept at fairly strict bed rest in a quiet, darkened single room, with soft music, visits only from immediate family, diazepam for sedation, and a stool softener to prevent straining. Fluids were, in common with much of neurosurgical treatment of that period, restricted often severely (increasing the likelihood of delayed ischemia), and the whole regimen could adversely affect the patient's blood volume, red cell mass, bone calcium, muscle mass, and many other factors.[2] Hypostatic pneumonia and deep vein thrombosis or pulmonary embolism were more likely. The main advantage of the regimen was that patients who survived to operation had, by that time, usually recovered reasonably well from the neurologic point of view, so that the risks of surgery were considerably less. Because of this lessened risk, with late operation it was possible to obtain good surgical outcomes, although the overall management outcome was often comparatively poor.

## Advantages and Disadvantages

Late operation has the advantage that the brain is much less likely to be swollen and difficult to retract. Postoperative delayed ischemia as a result of vasospasm is less likely because in many cases the risk of vasospasm, which is maximal in the second week after SAH, has already passed.

The major risk of late surgery is that the patient, while waiting, has a recurrent hemorrhage, and this carries a death rate that may be two thirds or more.[25] The risk of further hemorrhage is highest soon after the first hemorrhage and decreases exponentially with time. Also, as noted earlier, metabolic and general effects can cause considerable problems with delayed operation.

## POOR-GRADE PATIENT

A proportion of patients are in a poor clinical state on admission, usually defined as being in grade IV or V (i.e., a Glasgow Coma Scale score of ≤12, with or without *major focal deficit*).[22] In most large series, depending, in part, on referral patterns and admission policy, the proportion is 20% to 40%.[31] This may be an understatement, especially in a series from a tertiary center, because patients who are initially admitted to a small district hospital are less likely to be transferred to a referral center if they are moribund or nearly so.

## Early Management

Patients whose conscious state is depressed as a result of SAH face the same risks as those with severe head injury. The brain has suffered a severe primary insult with the hemorrhage, and often there has been a period of reduced or absent cerebral perfusion,[32] possibly a mechanism for limiting the actual hemorrhage. Severe secondary damage can occur as a result of this period of partial or absolute ischemia, and, more importantly, additional insults can worsen these effects. As with head injury, it is vital in these patients to avoid hypotension or hypoxia.[3]

In grade IV or V patients, it is common for an early decision to be made to intubate and artificially ventilate, especially if there is any doubt about airway reflexes and if the patient is likely to vomit. These considerations apply even more in a district or peripheral hospital, if it is planned to transfer the patient to another institution. Great care has to be taken during intubation to avoid surges of blood pressure that may cause the aneurysm to bleed again, and intubation should always be done by a skilled operator.

Maintenance of the systemic blood pressure is equally as important. If blood pressure is allowed too high, there is a danger of rebleeding, and if it is too low, further ischemia may become a problem. In general, an upper limit for systolic pressure of about 160 mm Hg is reasonably safe, and it should not be allowed to fall to less than 110 mm Hg. Drug treatment may be needed to control blood pressure. The preferred agents vary considerably depending on local usage in different centers; for reducing blood pressure, nifedipine, hydralazine, or β-blockers are commonly used, whereas epinephrine, phenylephrine, or metaraminol is favored for raising blood pressure. Fluids, including crystalloids and colloid, but avoiding glucose because of the dangers of hyperglycemia if ischemia develops, are also important in maintaining a high blood pressure.

In many poor-grade patients, the cause of the poor condition is ischemia resulting from the initial hemorrhage. It is vital to ensure that no more reversible cause is present, however. Urgent CT scanning is necessary as soon as the airway and blood pressure have been stabilized, looking particularly for an intracerebral hematoma or early hydrocephalus. If a large hematoma is present, emergency evacuation is usually necessary, and often there is no time for a preliminary angiogram to localize exactly the aneurysm. Every effort should be made to find and treat the aneurysm after evacuating the clot because there is a real danger of further hemorrhage in the postoperative period if it is not clipped at this time. The approximate site of the aneurysm should be evident from the location of the hematoma, and sometimes the aneurysm is visible on the plain CT scan as a less dense area within the hematoma.

If hydrocephalus is present, an external ventricular drain should be inserted as soon as possible and *gentle* drainage started. Theoretically at least, and probably also in practice,[33] reduction of the intracranial pressure by draining CSF increases the risk of recurrent hemorrhage. If the patient's life is at risk from raised intracranial pressure as a result of hydrocephalus, however, reducing the pressure is essential. It should be done gradually, and it is reasonable in this situation to settle for a slightly high pressure of 20 mm Hg. Close observation of the patient is needed after this procedure, and if the clinical state shows signs of improving (even if it has not yet reached a better grade), consideration should be given to angiography and definitive surgery sooner rather than later.

Hydrocephalus does not develop instantaneously, and there may be problems with CSF absorption causing raised intracranial pressure even if an early CT scan shows apparently normal ventricles. For this reason, it is a common practice in poor-grade patients to insert a drain if the ventricles appear accessible, in the hope of obtaining some improvement as a result.

## Timing of Operation

Opinions differ widely on the optimal timing for definitive aneurysm surgery in grades IV or V. In some centers, the patient undergoes early operation once stabilized, regardless of grade. Good results can be obtained in some cases, but overall the death rate and morbidity are high in these patients. Probably a more common practice is as outlined previously, to resuscitate and maintain the patient, to drain some CSF to reduce the intracranial pressure if it is possible to insert a ventriculostomy, and to operate if the patient shows signs of improving clinically—this situation may have to be assessed periodically, usually once or twice daily, by reversing sedation or paralysis and assessing whether any improvement in responsiveness has taken place.

## General Care

*General care* is essentially the intensive management of the unconscious, intubated, ventilated patient, with a proviso on the importance of avoiding high or low extremes of blood pressure, as outlined earlier. Cardiac monitoring is important because cardiorespiratory problems, as a result of autonomic overactivity, include arrhythmias that may be life-threatening. Occasionally a genuine myocardial infarct, possibly resulting from coronary artery spasm, may occur. In addition, neurogenic pulmonary edema is more likely in this type of patient with a more severe SAH. In essence, these complications are treated symptomatically.

Pulmonary function, atelectasis, and chest infections have to be carefully checked in these patients. If respiratory complications develop or threaten, early treatment with intensive physical therapy may be necessary. Bladder care (usually with catheter drainage) is important. Parenteral or enteral feeding should be started as soon as possible. In the longer term, attention has to be paid to skin care, avoidance of contractures, and avoidance of thromboembolic complications.

An observation has arisen in the controlled trials in SAH of the 21-aminosteroid drug tirilazad mesylate. Overall, there was an improvement in outcome in male patients only[34]; the most marked improvement was seen in patients in grade IV or V on entry. In later studies in women with a higher dose, meta-analysis has again shown some improvement in poor-grade patients only. The possibility is raised that this may be the first treatment to influence the otherwise generally dismal course of these patients.

## POSTOPERATIVE TREATMENT

Once the ruptured aneurysm has been clipped, the postoperative management is largely as after any craniotomy. Close clinical observation is necessary for complications such as postoperative hematoma or cerebral edema. Some complications are more specific to aneurysms, including intraoperative arterial branch occlusions or incomplete aneurysm clipping and recurrent hemorrhage. In many centers, intraoperative angiography or Doppler measurements have been carried out to avoid these problems.

Observation for vasospasm is essential, with daily transcranial Doppler examination of the arterial flow velocity and often a postoperative angiogram. Fluid maintenance is vital, to avoid dehydration and maintain relative hypervolemia. Monitoring of at least the central venous pressure is routine, and in some centers, much more intensive monitoring, with Swan-Ganz catheterization and monitoring of pulmonary wedge pressure, is used in preference.[35] Serum electrolytes must be checked regularly, usually at least once daily. Early postoperative mobilization, with appropriate nursing care and physical therapy, helps to minimize complications from prolonged bed rest.

## COMPLICATIONS OF SUBARACHNOID HEMORRHAGE

### Recurrence of Hemorrhage

Despite the worldwide tendency toward early operation, rebleeding of the aneurysm remains probably the most common complication of SAH. In the first 24 hours, rebleeding affects 2% to 4% of patients and in the first 2 weeks, 20%.[36, 37] After that, the rebleeding rate falls gradually up to about 6 months, then remains static at about 3% annually.[25] There is a strong tendency for rebleeding to be more dangerous than the initial hemorrhage. The death rate after a first bleed is probably about 40%, but for recurrence, it is in many series two thirds or more.[25, 38] The reason for this worse outcome is presumably the cumulative effect of another severe cerebral insult, with a further period of ischemia, on top of the first.

The best way to prevent rebleeding is an early operation. Before this approach became feasible, the risk was minimized by the use of antifibrinolytic drugs, usually epsilon-aminocaproic acid or tranexamic acid, whose effect was to slow down dissolution of the clot that was plugging the tear in the aneurysm wall. A number of trials confirmed the efficacy of this treatment in reducing rebleeding.[39] In the long run, however, there was no improvement in the overall outcome of SAH patients because the cisternal clots persisted for longer, leading to a higher incidence of delayed vasospasm and ischemia. The ill effects of this complication balanced the improvement resulting from a reduction in rebleeding.[40]

## Cerebral Vasospasm

Delayed vasospasm is due to breakdown products of the blood in the subarachnoid space, most likely oxyhemoglobin.[41] It is logical that the risk of spasm should be greater if more blood is present. The Fisher scale described earlier,[23] rating the thickness of the subarachnoid deposits of blood on an early CT scan, is reasonably successful in quantifying this risk.

It is common for angiographic vasospasm to develop, and it may be that if it were possible to repeat the angiogram daily, spasm would be seen in nearly all patients.[42] Transcranial Doppler studies of middle cerebral artery flow velocities have shown that at least some increase in velocity occurs in most patients, starting between the 4th and 10th days posthemorrhage and peaking at 10 to 20 days.[43]

The incidence of delayed ischemic deficits or symptomatic vasospasm is much lower than that of angiographic spasm. There are several reasons for this. The diameter of a blood vessel needs to be considerably narrowed, usually by more than half, before the flow through it is reduced (Fig. 81-1).[44] This narrowing is reflected in an increase in the velocity of flow, as measured by transcranial Doppler. Even when the flow eventually begins to fall, the brain can compensate further to some extent, by increasing the extraction of oxygen from the blood; there is a decrease in the jugular venous oxygen tension and an increase in the oxygen extraction ratio. The cerebral blood flow may have to fall by half or more before there is any disturbance of function, and even when this has occurred, irreversible damage does not follow unless the reduction is profound or prolonged.

### Incidence and Effects of Vasospasm

The natural history of vasospasm has been studied extensively. In a review of the topic, angiographic vasospasm

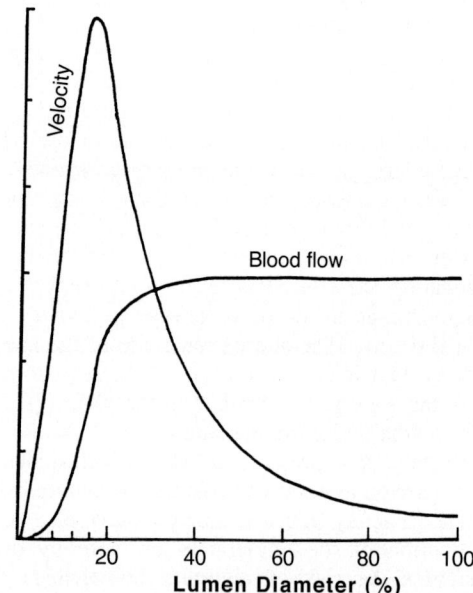

FIGURE 81-1 ■ A diagrammatic representation of the vessel diameter, volume flow, and flow velocity with increasing constriction. (Adapted from Spencer MP, Reid JM: Quantitation of carotid stenosis with continuous-wave (C-W) Doppler ultrasound. Stroke 10:326–330, 1979).

was found to occur overall in more than 40% of all patients. When angiography was carried out at the time of maximal risk, late in the first week and into the second week after hemorrhage, the incidence was approximately two thirds—1842 of 2738 patients, or 67.3%.[45] As noted earlier, the incidence of delayed ischemic deficits is much lower, and it affects about one third of patients (from 297 reports, 10,445 of 32,188 patients [32.5%]).

Delayed vasospasm undoubtedly affects the outcome of SAH adversely. From 25 publications, the death rate for all patients with aneurysmal SAH was 31% (1067 of 3482) in those who had vasospasm and 17% (1015 of 6098) in its absence ($P < .0001$; common odds ratio [COR], 3.3; 95% confidence interval [CI], 2.9 to 3.7). Good outcome was seen in 44% and 70% ($P < .0001$; COR, 3.1; 95% CI, 2.7 to 3.4). The actual outcome of established delayed ischemic deficits, analyzed in 3327 patients (106 reports), was that 30% died and 34% were left with permanent deficits.

## Diagnosis

The most certain diagnostic test to confirm the presence of vasospasm is the cerebral angiogram. This test may, however, miss spasm in small arteries that are not fully visualized on angiograms. Transcranial Doppler velocity measurement[43] is in common use; it detects changes in the velocity of flow in large arteries, and in skilled hands, the middle, anterior, and posterior cerebrals, internal carotid, and basilar arteries can be insonated. An increase in flow velocity may be due to vasospasm, with narrowing of the vessel, or to hyperemia, with an increased flow through an unchanged vessel. If facilities for measuring cerebral blood flow directly (e.g., xenon clearance CT) are available, the differentiation is simple.[46] Otherwise, measurement of flow velocity in the cervical internal carotid, with calculation of the middle cerebral to carotid ratio, is used.[47]

There is a classical clinical picture for the onset of symptomatic vasospasm. At around the end of the first week, the patient often complains of increased headache. Hours or days later, an ill-defined deterioration starts, with the onset of mild confusion. More definite focal signs, relevant to the involved area, tend to follow later, rather than being the first sign of ischemia. This picture is quite variable, and in some cases the clinical deterioration can be so rapid as to be mistaken for a recurrent hemorrhage.

## Prevention and Treatment

### CLEARANCE OF BLOOD

It seems logical that if subarachnoid blood and its products cause vasospasm, early removal of the blood would help to prevent it. There is evidence that this is the case; in one series, for example, surgery within 48 hours was more successful if radical attempts were made to remove all subarachnoid clot.[48] Mechanical removal of blood at operation is, however, not without its risks. In other series, reported elsewhere,[49] different maneuvers, such as lumbar drainage, ventriculocisternal perfusion, and instillation of streptokinase or urokinase, have been used with variable success.

Recombinant tissue plasminogen activator has been un-der trial—it is instilled into the subarachnoid space either directly at operation after aneurysm clipping or via a subarachnoid catheter postoperatively. As with the other techniques listed earlier, the intention is that it dissolves or removes subarachnoid clots much more rapidly than normally occurs and lessens the risk of spasm. Preliminary results suggest that recombinant tissue plasminogen activator is successful from that point of view, but improvements in outcome have not yet been convincingly shown.[50]

### HHH THERAPY

The use of induced hypertension was first reported in the late 1970s for the treatment of ischemic deficits resulting from established vasospasm.[51] Later, variations, including simply fluid loading or induced hypervolemia, then the induction of hemodilution, in some studies including venipuncture and blood removal, were used. This approach resulted in HHH or triple H therapy, including *h*ypervolemia, *h*ypertension, and *h*emodilution. As a result of increased awareness of the effects of prolonged dehydration and recumbency,[2, 52] variations of HHH therapy began to be used for the prevention as well as the treatment of delayed vasospasm.

In 31 publications in which the prophylactic use of variations of HHH treatment was specified, there were 443 cases of delayed ischemic deficits (18%) in 2516 patients.[49] This incidence is considerably lower than the 32.5% incidence recorded for the natural history; with the large numbers reported, the likelihood is that this treatment is effective in lessening the risk of vasospasm, even though it has not been submitted to formal trial.

When used for the treatment of established delayed ischemic deficits, HHH therapy is effective. From 72 reports of 2111 patients, the overall death rate was 17.5%, and there were permanent deficits in 28.5%.[49] The death rate, in particular, was lower than would be expected from the natural history figures. The results of a number of studies on HHH therapy have been summarized by Pritz and associates[53] in a meta-analysis.

### CALCIUM ANTAGONISTS

A number of calcium antagonists have been used in the management of vasospasm. The most experience has been gained with the *cerebral-selective* dihydropyridine analogue nimodipine, which has a more powerful vasodilating effect on cerebral arteries than on systemic vessels. It has been the subject of many controlled trials as well as in frequent general use in SAH. Several of the trials and two meta-analyses have confirmed that nimodipine is effective in reducing the proportion of fatal or otherwise bad outcomes after aneurysm rupture[54, 55] as well as lowering the incidence of delayed ischemia.[49]

Overall, the incidence of delayed ischemic deficits when nimodipine was used for prophylaxis, from 58 references that included 5826 patients, was 16%. It appears likely, although this has never been tested in a controlled trial, that the intravenous preparation is more effective, possibly because a more steady blood level can be maintained. With oral administration of nimodipine, the incidence of delayed ischemic deficits was 22%, and with the intravenous formulation it was 14%.[49]

When used for the treatment of established delayed ischemic deficits, nimodipine also appeared useful. When it was continued for therapy in patients who developed delayed ischemic deficits while on prophylactic nimodipine, the death rate was 18%, and permanent deficits occurred in 32%. By contrast, when the drug was given only after delayed ischemic deficits had developed, 13% died, and 20% remained disabled.[49]

Where intravenous nimodipine is available, the drug is given through a central line, starting at a low dose of 7.5 μg/kg/min (0.5 mg or 2.5 ml/hr). Provided that the blood pressure does not fall excessively (more likely in previously hypertensive patients), the dose is increased over 2 hours to the maintenance level of 10 ml/hr. This dose is continued for 1 to 2 weeks, then changed to oral treatment of 60 mg six times daily, which is continued until the end of the third week. The dose may be altered if clinical ischemia develops or if daily transcranial Doppler monitoring shows a significant increase in flow velocity, to a maximum of 15 ml/hr. Central venous pressure must be monitored and maintained at 6 mm Hg or more; fluid maintenance is important to minimize systemic hypotension. The use of nimodipine results in closer attention being paid to fluid balance, which is one of several possible mechanisms of action of calcium antagonists.[56] Experience has also been gained with other calcium antagonists, notably nifedipine, flunarizine,[57] and nicardipine.[58] Results have at times been impressive.

## TIRILAZAD MESYLATE

Tirilazad mesylate is one of the newly introduced group of 21-aminosteroid drugs, in which the steroid moiety has been altered to abolish any glucocorticoid or mineralocorticoid action and a large amine group added to the 21 carbon position. Tirilazad is a potent inhibitor of iron-dependent lipid peroxidation, which is one of the main processes involved in cell membrane disruption in vasospasm and ischemia.

Tirilazad has been the subject of several large controlled clinical trials in different countries.[34, 59] In one study in Europe and Australasia,[59] with intravenous nimodipine as background therapy, with the highest dose tested (6 mg/kg/day), there was a significant overall improvement in outcome at 3 months, and a strong trend toward a reduction in delayed ischemia. The improved outcome was seen essentially in male patients only. In a similar trial in North American centers,[34] in which oral nimodipine was included as background treatment, there was no significant improvement in overall outcome, but a strong effect was seen in male patients.

Two further studies have been done in women with aneurysmal SAH, with tirilazad mesylate 15 mg/kg/day compared with drug vehicle. In the first of these,[59a] a marked, significant reduction in the incidence of delayed ischemic deficits was seen, but overall outcome was not improved. There was a concomitant decrease in the need for therapeutic or *rescue* HHH therapy in the tirilazad-treated group, which it is believed has masked a possible

improvement in outcome resulting from the drug. Analysis of these trials is continuing.

## TRANSLUMINAL ANGIOPLASTY

Transluminal angioplasty was introduced by Zubkov and colleagues[60] in the mid-1980s. Initially, balloon angioplasty was used exclusively, and later intra-arterial drugs, usually papaverine or a calcium antagonist, were used also. The aim of angioplasty is to restore stenotic segments to normal caliber and normalize blood flow. This treatment forms the third major category of interventional options, after hemodynamic intervention with HHH therapy and *cerebral protection* by drugs such as calcium channel blockers, tirilazad, or barbiturates.

In a review of transluminal angioplasty treatment,[49] results were impressive, particularly when one considers that patients treated in that comparatively early stage in development of this therapy were mostly severely affected and that other vasospasm treatment had already failed. Of 242 reported patients at that time, most treated with balloon angioplasty and 43 with nicardipine or papaverine, 20% died, and 55% made a good recovery. In general, good results have been reported with balloon[61–64] and chemical angioplasty.[65–68] Each, however, has problems: Papaverine has a limited duration, may cause seizures or hemodynamic instability (probably related to the infusion rate), and may be relatively ineffective[67]; balloon angioplasty needs specialized equipment and expertise, is restricted to proximal vessels, may not be possible in the A1 segments, and has more risk of catastrophic complications.[69]

Given the growing evidence for early intervention,[68, 70] in some centers, treatment is started when there is significant angiographic vasospasm but no clinical deterioration.[70] Balloon angioplasty lasts longer (Fig. 81–2),[71] but the problems outlined previously make its uniform adoption impractical in its present state of development. Combining chemical and balloon angioplasty may be superior to either alone. Such a protocol has been used since 1992 at the North and West Cerebrovascular Unit of the University of Sydney (Table 81–4).[71a]

Of the first 200 SAH patients treated this way, 108 (54%) had on admission a decreased level of consciousness or a focal neurologic deficit. At 3 months, 131 were neurologically normal, 30 were abnormal but independent, 28 were dependent, and 11 were dead. Of the 92 who were neurologically normal on admission, 86 were normal at 3 months, and none had died. Vasospasm was diagnosed angiographically in 85 patients, of whom 84 received intra-arterial papaverine with or without balloon angioplasty (which was initially used sparingly). These patients averaged four separate angioplasties (range, 1 to 23). There was no significant difference in recovery to independence between those with and those without vasospasm. This strict regimen of perioperative management with fluids, drugs, and angioplasty appears to offer hope of reducing poor outcomes from aneurysmal SAH but is yet to be tested in a formal trial and awaits validation.

## Fluid and Electrolyte Disturbances

Disturbed fluid and electrolyte profiles have been reported in 30% to 50% of SAH patients.[72, 73] Diabetes insipidus,

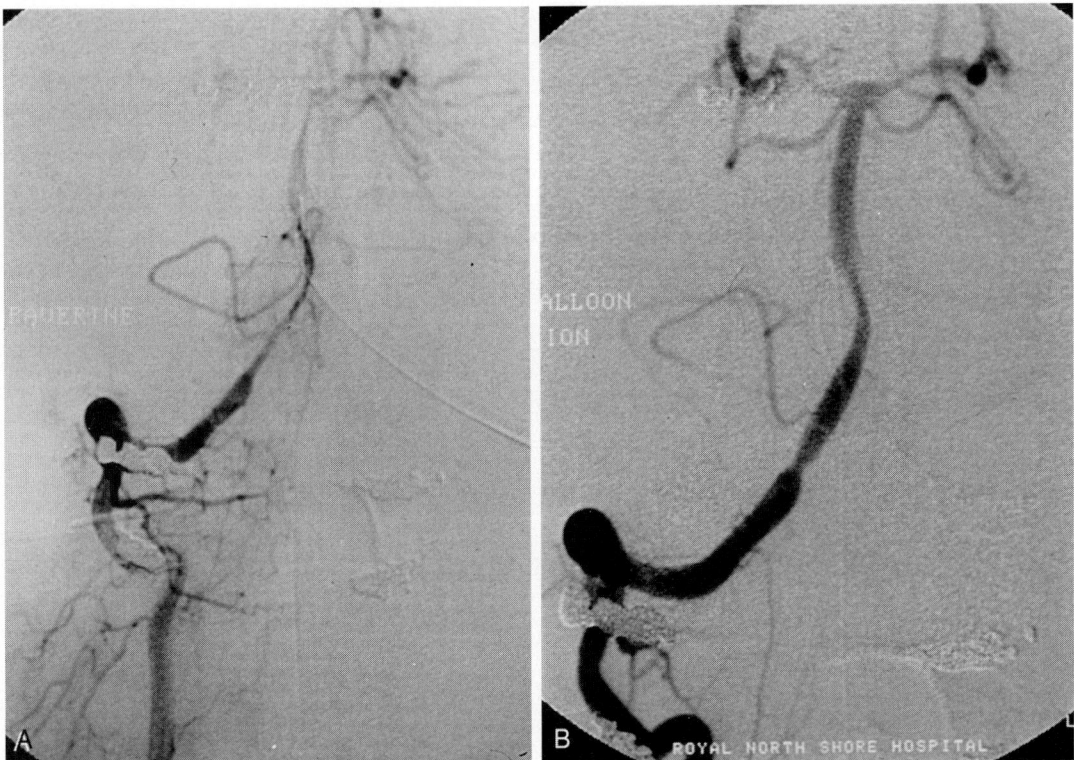

**FIGURE 81–2** ■ An example of vertebrobasilar vasospasm *(A)* treated successfully with balloon angioplasty *(B)* after unsuccessful papaverine angioplasty.

cerebral salt-wasting syndrome, and syndrome of inappropriate antidiuretic hormone secretion (SIADH) are examples. Hyponatremia is seen in SIADH and cerebral salt-wasting syndrome; it is vital to distinguish between them because the management is quite different. Fluid restriction to reduce cerebral edema and aggressive hypervolemia as part of HHH therapy to combat vasospasm can also result in electrolyte abnormalities. Other causes include local compression of the hypothalamic region by a large anterior

communicating aneurysm, and ischemia/infarction in the area secondary to vasospasm of or injury to perforating vessels.

## Regulation of Intravascular Volume and Electrolytes

A key role in the maintenance of intracellular solute concentration and volume is the $Na^+$, $K^+$-ATPase pump,

**TABLE 81–4 ■ INTENSIVE THERAPY PROTOCOL FOR PATIENTS WITH ANEURYSMAL SUBARACHNOID HEMORRHAGE AT THE NORTH AND WEST CEREBROVASCULAR UNIT OF THE UNIVERSITY OF SYDNEY**

| | |
|---|---|
| Admission Criteria | Aneurysmal SAH within 72 hr with GCS ≥5 (worse grade acceptable if due to intracerebral hemorrhage, hydrocephalus, pulmonary edema, or heart failure) |
| Angiography and Aneurysm Operation | Within 48 hr of admission |
| Fluid Regimen | 1.7 ml/kg/hr normal saline, adjusted for positive fluid balance (including postangiogram diuresis). Volume depletion corrected with blood if hemoglobin <10 g/dl and albumin if >10 g/dl |
| Body Temperature | Maintained <37.5°C |
| Oxygen Saturation | Maintained >95% |
| Blood Pressure | Maintained at 120–150 mm Hg systolic unless vasospasm present, in which case it is increased >150 mm Hg |
| Calcium Channel Blockade | Intravenous nimodipine 20–30 μg/kg/hr for 12 days followed by oral nimodipine for 21 days from SAH |
| Inotropic Support | Norepinephrine infusion as needed. In presence of cardiac failure or neurogenic pulmonary edema, dobutamine is also infused |
| Postoperative Initial Angiogram | Between day 5 and 7, or for a GCS decline by ≥2, or for a new focal neurologic deficit, or if hyponatremia develops |
| Presence of significant vasospasm on angiography | Papaverine infusion until spasm is reversed, or no further improvement is demonstrated at interval angiography, or 800 mg of papaverine has been infused into a single territory |
| Repeat angiography 24 hr after papaverine angiography | Papaverine infusion repeated if spasm again significant. If needed, consider balloon angioplasty for vertebrobasilar or carotid spasm |

SAH, subarachnoid hemorrhage; GCS, Glasgow Coma Scale.

which normally regulates cellular electrolytes in hyperosmolar or hypo-osmolar conditions. Cellular injury in SAH may disrupt these mechanisms, leading to cellular swelling and edema. The aim of sodium regulation is the maintenance of adequate blood pressure and intravascular volume. Physiologic systems to regulate this include the renin-aldosterone system; the sympathetic nervous system; and natriuretic factors, such as atrial natriuretic peptide or atrial natriuretic factor (ANF). A decrease in systemic blood pressure leads to the release of renin and eventually angiotensin II, with multiple effects that include aldosterone secretion from the adrenal cortex, direct vasoconstriction, and stimulation of the hypothalamic thirst mechanism. Reabsorption of sodium and the passive movement of water are promoted.

ANF is also produced and released from the atrium of the heart in response to increased atrial pressure.[74–76] ANF appears to counterbalance the effects of the antidiuretic hormone and renin-angiotensin-aldosterone system, regulating cerebral blood flow, blood-brain barrier function, and CSF production.[77] Natriuresis, diuresis, reduced thirst, and vasodilatation are some of the effects of ANF. The presence of intraventricular or cisternal blood may influence serum ANF,[78] and high serum ANF has also been shown by others.[79, 80]

## Syndrome of Inappropriate Antidiuretic Hormone Secretion

Antidiuretic hormone is an octapeptide released from the neurohypophysis in response to changes in serum osmolality and intravascular volume and increases renal reabsorption of water. In SIADH, excessive antidiuretic hormone is secreted as a result of ectopic production, pathologic pituitary oversecretion, or drug-induced pituitary oversecretion. This excessive secretion results in expansion of the extracellular fluid volume, with hypervolemia and a dilutional hyponatremia. Other causes of hyponatremia must be excluded (Tables 81–5 and 81–6). Criteria for SIADH include hyponatremia; low serum osmolality; high urinary sodium; urinary osmolality greater than serum osmolality; normal

### TABLE 81–5 ■ CONDITIONS THAT PRODUCE HYPONATREMIA

Water retention
  Hyperosmolar states (e.g., mannitol, alcohol, hyperlipidemia)
  Pain and stress
  CCF
  Hepatic cirrhosis
  Pregnancy
  Drugs
  SIADH
Sodium loss
  Diuretics
  Glucocorticoid/mineralocorticoid deficiency
  Hypothyroidism
  Salt-wasting nephropathies
  Cerebral salt wasting
  Elevated ANF

CCF, congestive cardiac failure; SIADH, syndrome of inappropriate antidiuretic hormone secretion; ANF, atrial natriuretic factor.

### TABLE 81–6 ■ DIFFERENCES BETWEEN DIABETES INSIPIDUS, INAPPROPRIATE ANTIDIURETIC HORMONE SECRETION, AND CEREBRAL SALT-WASTING SYNDROME

| | CSWS | SIADH | DI |
|---|---|---|---|
| Plasma volume | ↓ | ↑ | ↓ |
| Salt balance | Negative | Variable | ↓ |
| Symptoms and signs of dehydration | Present | Absent | Present |
| Weight | ↓ | ↑ or no change | ↓ |
| Pulmonary capillary wedge pressure | ↓ | ↑ or N | ↓ |
| Central venous pressure | ↓ | ↑ or N | ↓ |
| Hematocrit | ↑ | ↓ or no change | ↑ ↑ |
| Serum osmolality | ↑ or N | ↓ | ↑ ↑ |
| Urinary sodium concentration | ↑ ↑ | ↑ | ↓ |

CSWS, cerebral salt-wasting syndrome; SIADH, syndrome of inappropriate antidiuretic hormone secretion; DI, diabetes insipidus; ↓, decreased; ↑, increased; ↑ ↑, greatly increased; N, normal.
Modified from Harrigan MR: Cerebral salt wasting syndrome: A review. Neurosurgery 38:152–160, 1996.

thyroid, adrenal, and renal function; and no peripheral edema or dehydration.[81]

## Cerebral Salt-Wasting Syndrome

In some of the hyponatremic states seen in SAH, natriuresis and hypovolemia have been shown,[79–83] different from the profile of SIADH, in which there is hypervolemia. The natriuresis and hypovolemia of cerebral salt-wasting syndrome are associated with the presence of elevated natriuretic factors previously discussed, and fludrocortisone, a mineralocorticoid, has been shown to reduce the natriuresis.[73]

Primary treatment of these two syndromes differs. In SIADH, fluid restriction is needed, whereas in cerebral salt-wasting syndrome, there is usually already a depleted intravascular compartment. Cerebral salt-wasting syndrome needs fluid and salt replacement, and further fluid restriction can result in a critical hypovolemic state. In the setting of SAH and possible vasospasm, this state must be avoided.[84] The use of hypertonic saline has been tried, with encouraging results for intracranial pressure in the setting of hypovolemia after trauma.[85, 86] Hypertonic saline increases the intravascular fluid compartment by drawing in free water from the interstitial space, with maintenance of blood pressure and cardiac output and reduction of intracranial pressure.

Rapid correction of hyponatremia is not recommended because it has been associated with central pontine myelinolysis. Unless there is severe, symptomatic hyponatremia, it is recommended not to exceed a correction of serum sodium of 0.5 to 0.7 mEq/L/hr, for a maximum increase of 10 to 15 mEq/L/day.[87]

## Diabetes Insipidus

Diabetes insipidus is caused by a deficiency of antidiuretic hormone. Clinically, there is polyuria, with losses as high as 10 L a day. The diagnosis is confirmed by high outputs

(> 200 to 300 ml hourly) of dilute urine of low osmolality, with hypernatremia and a serum osmolality greater than 300 mOsm/kg. In a conscious patient, there is usually increased thirst. Although uncommon in SAH, diabetes insipidus has been reported related mainly to anterior communicating or cerebral aneurysms.[88–90] The pathogenesis may be related to ischemia involving the anterior hypothalamus, which receives blood from the anterior communicating complex.[79, 91] Hydrocephalus has also been suggested as a possible cause,[88, 92] with the dilated third ventricle exerting direct pressure on the hypothalamic region.[33]

The treatment of diabetes insipidus involves judicious fluid replacement, usually with 5% dextrose solution or other hypotonic solutions. When it is difficult to keep up with replacement, desmopressin (1-deamine-8-D-arginine vasopressin), a synthetic analogue of antidiuretic hormone, can be administered intravenously, intranasally, or subcutaneously to reduce diuresis, and this is usually effective.

Attention to fluid balance and electrolyte profile of the SAH patient is essential. Accurate diagnosis of diabetes insipidus, cerebral salt-wasting syndrome, or SIADH is important in ongoing management. The treatment of these clinical states, if misdiagnosed, can lead to serious consequences and a worse or even fatal outcome.

## Hydrocephalus

Hydrocephalus is common after SAH. It may present at the onset or develop over hours to weeks. The diagnosis is made on CT scan when the bicaudate index exceeds the 95th percentile for the age. The large variation in reports of the incidence (5% to 50%) of hydrocephalus is probably related to differences in diagnostic criteria.[93, 94]

Post-SAH hydrocephalus can be obstructive or communicating. The ventricular system may be obstructed by intraventricular blood at sites such as the foramen of Monro, aqueduct of Sylvius,[95] or the fourth ventricle cavity or outlets. Communicating hydrocephalus may result from the blood or blood products scarring the pial-subarachnoid space or the arachnoid granulations, or elsewhere.[96] In a review, Suarez-Rivera[97] reported an incidence of acute hydrocephalus after SAH of approximately 20%, two thirds clinically symptomatic. Spontaneous recovery was seen in half of these patients. Acute hydrocephalus is defined as ventriculomegaly in the first 2 weeks after SAH, with chronic hydrocephalus developing after this time. The presence of early hydrocephalus is a risk factor for long-term shunting. In one series of 835 SAH patients, 294 had early hydrocephalus, and 67 of these required long-term shunting (23%) versus 14 (2.6%) in the other 541.[98]

From the International Study on the Timing of Aneurysm Surgery and other studies, factors associated with clinical hydrocephalus included intraventricular hemorrhage, admission level of consciousness, pre-existing hypertension, increasing age, Fisher grade, and posterior circulation aneurysms.[99, 100] The location of the aneurysm may also have a role in the incidence of acute or chronic hydrocephalus, with a greater likelihood in posterior circulation aneurysm and less in middle cerebral aneurysms.[101, 102] In one report, a larger proportion of vertebrobasilar aneurysms required shunting (53%) than anterior communicating artery aneurysms (19%).[102] The ability at operation to open the lamina terminalis for a third ventriculostomy or the membrane of Liliequist may reduce the incidence of acute hydrocephalus and the need for shunting.[103]

In the acute setting, especially if there is an altered level of consciousness associated with hydrocephalus, external ventricular drainage can lead to improvement sufficient to allow definitive aneurysm surgery,[104] even though it may increase the risk of rebleeding.[33] The intracranial pressure should be monitored throughout, and care should be taken to have CSF draining against pressures of no less than 15 to 20 mm Hg.[97, 105] Despite the risk of increased rebleeding rates and ventriculitis, the benefits of ventricular drainage include improvements in neurologic state, the ability to monitor intracranial pressure in poor-grade patients, control of intracranial pressure by CSF release, and removal of some of the blood products that may contribute to vasospasm. To reduce the risk of infection, Khanna and associates[106] described the insertion of a drain via a long subcutaneous tunnel. Prophylactic antibiotics were used in the perioperative period only, and no infection was noted up to 16 days. The infection rate was fewer than 3 per 1000 ventricular drainage days. Daily CSF sampling for microscopy was recommended.

Another clinical syndrome has been described,[95] in which external hydrocephalus develops, with a subdural fluid collection in association with ventriculomegaly. This syndrome is the result of tears in the arachnoid membrane (and is seen after trauma also), allowing CSF to flow into the subdural space. Treatment usually requires ventricular shunting. This condition must be differentiated from subdural hygromas, in which the ventricular size is usually not enlarged; ventricular shunting in that situation could lead to worsening.

## REFERENCES

1. Malisch TW, Guglielmi G, Viñuela F, et al: Intracranial aneurysms treated with the Guglielmi detachable coil: Midterm clinical results in a consecutive series of 100 patients. J Neurosurg 87:176–183, 1997.
2. Maroon JC, Nelson PB: Hypovolemia in patients with subarachnoid hemorrhage: Therapeutic implications. Neurosurgery 4:223–226, 1979.
3. Eisenberg HM, Gary HE Jr, Aldrich EF, et al: Initial CT findings in 753 patients with severe head injury: A report from the NIH Traumatic Coma Data Bank. J Neurosurg 73:688–698, 1990.
4. Kakarieka A, Braakman R, Schakel EH: Subarachnoid haemorrhage after head injury. Cerebrovasc Dis 5:403–406, 1995.
5. Schwartz TH, Solomon RA: Perimesencephalic nonaneurysmal subarachnoid hemorrhage: Review of the literature. Neurosurgery 39:433–440, 1996.
6. Gillingham FJ: The management of ruptured intracranial aneurysms. Scot Med J 12:377–383, 1967.
7. Dorsch NWC: Cerebral aneurysms and the "missed haemorrhage." Aust N Z J Med 16:486–490, 1986.
8. Tobias E: Eli's pearls. Surg Neurol 49:661, 1988.
9. van der Wee N, Rinkel GJE, Hasan D, et al: Detection of subarachnoid haemorrhage on early CT: Is lumbar puncture still needed after a negative scan? J Neurol Neurosurg Psychiatry 58:357–359, 1995.
10. Noguchi K, Ogawa T, Fujita H, et al: Filling defect sign in CT diagnosis of ruptured aneurysm. Neuroradiology 39:480–482, 1997.
11. Teasdale G, Jennett B: Assessment of coma and impaired consciousness: A practical scale. Lancet 2:81–84, 1974.
12. Vermeulen M, Hasan D, Blijenberg BG, et al: Xanthochromia after subarachnoid haemorrhage needs no revisitation. J Neurol Neurosurg Psychiatry 52:826–828, 1989.

13. Page KB, Howell SJ, Smith CM, et al: Bilirubin, ferritin, D-dimers and erythrophages in the cerebrospinal fluid of patients with suspected subarachnoid haemorrhage but negative computed tomography scans. J Clin Pathol 47:986–989, 1994.

13a. Kam A, et al: Noise pollution in the anesthetic and intensive care environment. Anesthesia 49:982–986, 1994.

14. Mount LA, Brisman R: Treatment of multiple aneurysms—symptomatic and asymptomatic. Clin Neurosurg 21:166–170, 1974.

15. Horikoshi T, Fukamachi A, Nishi H, et al: Detection of intracranial aneurysms by three-dimensional time-of-flight magnetic resonance angiography. Neuroradiology 36:203–207, 1994.

16. Young N, Dorsch NWC, Kingston R, et al: Spiral CT scanning in the detection and evaluation of aneurysms of the circle of Willis. Surg Neurol 50:50–61, 1998.

17. Anderson GB, Findlay JM, Steinke DE, et al: Experience with computed tomographic angiography for the detection of intracranial aneurysms in the setting of acute subarachnoid hemorrhage. Neurosurgery 41:522–528, 1997.

18. Alvord EC Jr, Thorn RB: Natural history of subarachnoid hemorrhage: Early prognosis. Clin Neurosurg 24:167–175, 1977.

19. Hunt WE, Hess RM: Surgical risk as related to time of intervention in the repair of intracranial aneurysms. J Neurosurg 28:14–20, 1968.

20. Botterell EH, Lougheed WM, Scott JW, et al: Hypothermia and interruption of carotid, or carotid and vertebral circulation, in the management of intracranial aneurysms. J Neurosurg 13:1–42, 1956.

21. Hunt WE, Kosnik EJ: Timing and perioperative care in intracranial aneurysm surgery. Clin Neurosurg 21:79–89, 1974.

22. Drake CG: Report of World Federation of Neurological Surgeons Committee on a universal subarachnoid hemorrhage grading scale (Letter). J Neurosurg 68:985–986, 1988.

23. Fisher CM, Kistler JP, Davis TM: Relation of cerebral vasospasm to subarachnoid hemorrhage visualized by computerized tomographic scanning. Neurosurgery 6:1–9, 1980.

24. Yamamoto I, Hara M, Ogura K, et al: Early operation for ruptured intracranial aneurysms: Comparative study with computed tomography. Neurosurgery 12:169–174, 1983.

25. Jane JA, Winn HR, Richardson AE: The natural history of intracranial aneurysms: Rebleeding rates during the acute and long term period and implication for surgical management. Clin Neurosurg 24:176–184, 1977.

26. Kassell NF, Boarini DJ, Adams HP Jr, et al: Overall management of ruptured aneurysm: Comparison of early and late operation. Neurosurgery 9:120–128, 1981.

27. Hunt WE, Miller CA: The results of early operation for aneurysm. Clin Neurosurg 24:208–215, 1977.

28. Ljunggren B, Brandt L, Kägström E: Results of early operations for ruptured aneurysms. J Neurosurg 54:473–479, 1981.

29. Kassell NF, Torner JC, Haley EC Jr, et al: The international cooperative study on the timing of aneurysm surgery. Part 1: Overall management results. J Neurosurg 73:18–36, 1990.

30. Kassell NF, Torner JC, Jane JA, et al: The international cooperative study on the timing of aneurysm surgery. Part 2: Surgical results. J Neurosurg 73:37–47, 1990.

31. Säveland H, Brandt L: Which are the major determinants for outcome in aneurysmal subarachnoid hemorrhage? Acta Neurol Scand 90:245–250, 1994.

32. Nornes H: The role of intracranial pressure in the arrest of hemorrhage in patients with ruptured intracranial aneurysm. J Neurosurg 39:226–234, 1973.

33. Paré L, Delfino R, Leblanc R: The relationship of ventricular drainage to aneurysmal rebleeding. J Neurosurg 76:422–427, 1992.

34. Haley EC Jr, Kassell NF, Apperson-Hansen C, et al: A randomized, double-blind, vehicle-controlled trial of tirilazad mesylate in patients with aneurysmal subarachnoid hemorrhage: A cooperative study in North America. J Neurosurg 86:467–474, 1997.

35. Finn SS, Stephensen SA, Miller CA, et al: Observations on the perioperative management of aneurysmal subarachnoid hemorrhage. J Neurosurg 65:48–62, 1986.

36. Kassell NF, Torner JC: Aneurysmal rebleeding: A preliminary report from the cooperative aneurysm study. Neurosurgery 13:479–481, 1983.

37. Kassell NF, Torner JC, Adams HP Jr: Antifibrinolytic therapy in the acute period following aneurysmal subarachnoid hemorrhage: Preliminary observations from the cooperative aneurysm study. J Neurosurg 61:225–230, 1984.

38. Broderick JP, Brott TG, Duldner JE, et al: Initial and recurrent bleeding are the major causes of death following subarachnoid hemorrhage. Stroke 25:1342–1347, 1994.

39. Fodstad H, Forsell Å, Liliequist B, et al: Antifibrinolysis with tranexamic acid in aneurysmal subarachnoid hemorrhage: A consecutive controlled clinical trial. Neurosurgery 8:158–165, 1981.

40. Tsementzis SA, Hitchcock ER, Meyer CHA: Benefits and risks of antifibrinolytic therapy in the management of ruptured intracranial aneurysms: A double-blind placebo-controlled study. Acta Neurochir 102:1–10, 1990.

41. Macdonald RL, Weir BKA, Runzer TD, et al: Etiology of cerebral vasospasm in primates. J Neurosurg 75:415–424, 1991.

42. White RP: Vasospasm. II: Clinical considerations. In Fox JL (ed): Intracranial Aneurysms. New York: Springer-Verlag, 1983, pp 250–271.

43. Harders AG, Gilsbach JM: Time course of blood velocity changes related to vasospasm in the circle of Willis measured by transcranial Doppler ultrasound. J Neurosurg 66:718–728, 1987.

44. Spencer MP, Reid JM: Quantitation of carotid stenosis with continuous-wave (C-W) Doppler ultrasound. Stroke 10:326–330, 1979.

45. Dorsch NWC, King MT: A review of cerebral vasospasm in aneurysmal subarachnoid haemorrhage. I: Incidence and effects. J Clin Neurosci 1:19–26, 1994.

46. Clyde BL, Resnick DK, Yonas H, et al: The relationship of blood velocity as measured by transcranial Doppler ultrasonography to cerebral blood flow as determined by stable xenon computed tomographic studies after aneurysmal subarachnoid hemorrhage. Neurosurgery 38:896–905, 1996.

47. Lindegaard K-F, Nornes H, Bakke SJ, et al: Cerebral vasospasm diagnosis by means of angiography and blood velocity measurements. Acta Neurochir 100:12–24, 1989.

48. Taneda M: The significance of early operation in the management of ruptured intracranial aneurysms—an analysis of 251 cases hospitalized within 24 hours after subarachnoid haemorrhage. Acta Neurochir 63:201–208, 1982.

49. Dorsch NWC: A review of cerebral vasospasm in aneurysmal subarachnoid haemorrhage. II: Management. J Clin Neurosci 1:78–92, 1994.

50. Findlay JM, Kassell NF, Weir BKA, et al: A randomized trial of intraoperative, intracisternal tissue plasminogen activator for the prevention of vasospasm. Neurosurgery 37:168–178, 1995.

51. Kosnik EJ, Hunt WE: Postoperative hypertension in the management of patients with intracranial arterial aneurysms. J Neurosurg 45:148–154, 1976.

52. Kudo T, Suzuki S, Iwabuchi T: Importance of monitoring the circulating blood volume in patients with cerebral vasospasm after subarachnoid hemorrhage. Neurosurgery 9:514–520, 1981.

53. Pritz MB, Zhou X-H, Brizendine EJ: Hyperdynamic therapy for cerebral vasospasm: A meta-analysis of 14 studies. J Neurovasc Dis 1:6–9, 1996.

54. Tettenborn D, Dycka T: Prevention and treatment of delayed ischemic dysfunction in patients with aneurysmal subarachnoid hemorrhage. Stroke 21(Suppl IV):IV85–IV89, 1990.

55. Barker FG II, Ogilvy CS: Efficacy of prophylactic nimodipine for delayed ischemic deficit after subarachnoid hemorrhage: A meta-analysis. J Neurosurg 84:405–414, 1996.

56. Dorsch NWC: A review of cerebral vasospasm in aneurysmal subarachnoid haemorrhage. III: Mechanisms of action of calcium antagonists. J Clin Neurosci 1:151–160, 1994.

57. Fujita S, Kawaguchi T, Shose Y, et al: Flunarizine treatment in poor-grade aneurysm patients. Acta Neurochir 103:11–17, 1990.

58. Haley EC Jr, Kassell NF, Torner JC, et al: A randomized controlled trial of high-dose intravenous nicardipine in aneurysmal subarachnoid hemorrhage: A report of the cooperative aneurysm study. J Neurosurg 78:537–547, 1993.

59. Kassell NF, Haley EC Jr, Apperson-Hansen C, et al: Randomized, double-blind, vehicle-controlled trial of tirilazad mesylate in patients with aneurysmal subarachnoid hemorrhage: A cooperative study in Europe, Australia and New Zealand. J Neurosurg 84:221–228, 1996.

59a. Lanzino G, Kassell NF: Double-blind, randomized, vehicle-controlled study of high dose tirilazad mesylate in women with aneurysmal subarachnoid hemorrhage. Part II. A cooperative study in North America. J Neurosurg 90(6):1018–1024, 1999.

60. Zubkov YN, Nikiforov BM, Shustin VA: Balloon catheter technique for dilatation of constricted cerebral arteries after aneurysmal SAH. Acta Neurochir 70:65–79, 1984.

61. Bejjani GK, Bank WO, Olan WJ, et al: The efficacy and safety of angioplasty for cerebral vasospasm after subarachnoid hemorrhage. Neurosurgery 42:979–987, 1998.
62. Smith RR, Connors JJ, Yamamoto Y, et al: Balloon angioplasty for vasospasm: Theoretical and practical considerations. In Sano K, Takakura K, Kassell NF, Sasaki T (eds): Cerebral Vasospasm. Proceedings of the IVth International Conference on Cerebral Vasospasm, Tokyo, 1990. Tokyo: University of Tokyo Press, 1990, pp 415–420.
63. Takashita A, Yoshimoto H, Mizoi K, et al: Transcranial balloon angioplasty for vasospasm after subarachnoid hemorrhage. In Sano K, Takakura K, Kassell NF, et al (eds): Cerebral Vasospasm. Proceedings of the IVth International Conference on Cerebral Vasospasm, Tokyo, 1990. Tokyo: University of Tokyo Press, 1990, pp 429–432.
64. Brothers MF, Holgate RC: Intracranial angioplasty for the treatment of vasospasm after subarachnoid hemorrhage: Technique and modification to improve branch access. AJNR Am J Neuroradiol 11:239–247, 1990.
65. Yoshimura S, Tsukahara T, Hashimoto N, et al: Intra-arterial infusion of papaverine combined with intravenous administration of high-dose nicardipine for cerebral vasospasm. Acta Neurochir 135:186–190, 1995.
66. Clouston JE, Numaguchi Y, Zoarski GH, et al: Intraarterial papaverine infusion for cerebral vasospasm after subarachnoid hemorrhage. AJNR Am J Neuroradiol 16:27–38, 1995.
67. Polin RS, Hansen CA, German P, et al: Intra-arterially administered papaverine for the treatment of symptomatic cerebral vasospasm. Neurosurgery 42:1256–1267, 1998.
68. Morgan M, Halcrow S, Sorby W, et al: Outcome of aneurysmal subarachnoid haemorrhage following the introduction of papaverine angioplasty. J Clin Neurosci 3:139–142, 1996.
69. Linskey ME, Horton JA, Rao GR, et al: Fatal rupture of the intracranial carotid artery during transluminal angioplasty for vasospasm induced by subarachnoid hemorrhage: Case report. J Neurosurg 74:985–990, 1991.
70. Smith RR, Zubkov YN, Tarassoli Y: Cerebral Aneurysms. New York: Springer-Verlag, 1994, pp 46–51.
71. Morgan MK, Sekhon L, Halcrow S, et al: Effective management of cerebral vasospasm with balloon angioplasty after failed papaverine angioplasty: Case report. J Clin Neurosci 3:162–165, 1996.
71a. Morgan M, Jonker B, Finfer S, et al: Aggressive management of aneurysmal subarachnoid haemorrhage based on a papaverine angioplasty protocol. J Clin Neurosci (in press).
72. Fox JL, Falik JL, Shalour RJ: Neurosurgical hyponatremia: The role of inappropriate antidiuresis. J Neurosurg 34:506–514, 1971.
73. Woo MH, Kale-Pradhan PB: Fludrocortisone in the treatment of subarachnoid hemorrhage-induced hyponatremia. Ann Pharmacother 31:637–639, 1997.
74. de Bold AJ: Atrial natriuretic factor of the rat heart: Studies on isolation and properties. Proc Soc Exp Biol Med 170:133–138, 1982.
75. Keeler R, Azzarolo AM: Effects of atrial natriuretic factor on renal handling of water and electrolytes in rats. Can J Physiol Pharmacol 61:996–1002, 1983.
76. Sonnenberg H, Chong CK, Veress AT: Cardiac atrial factor—an endogenous diuretic? Can J Physiol Pharmacol 59:1278–1279, 1981.
77. Burnett JC Jr, Granger JP, Opgenorth TJ: Effects of synthetic atrial natriuretic factor on renal function and renin release. Am J Physiol 247:f863–f866, 1984.
78. Diringer MN, Lim JS, Kirsch JR, et al: Suprasellar and intraventricular blood predict elevated plasma atrial natriuretic factor in subarachnoid hemorrhage. Stroke 22:577–581, 1991.
79. Berendes E, Walter M, Cullen P, et al: Secretion of brain natriuretic peptide in patients with aneurysmal subarachnoid haemorrhage. Lancet 349:245–249, 1997.
80. Kurokawa Y, Uede T, Ishiguro M, et al: Pathogenesis of hyponatremia following subarachnoid hemorrhage due to ruptured cerebral aneurysm. Surg Neurol 46:500–508, 1996.
81. Doshi R, Neil-Dwyer G: A clinicopathological study of patients following a subarachnoid hemorrhage. J Neurosurg 52:295–301, 1980.
82. Isotani E, Suzuki R, Tomita K, et al: Alterations in plasma concentrations of natriuretic peptides and antidiuretic hormone after subarachnoid hemorrhage. Stroke 25:2198–2203, 1994.
83. Wijdicks EF, Van Dongen KJ, Van Gijn J, et al: Enlargement of the third ventricle and hyponatraemia in aneurysmal subarachnoid haemorrhage. J Neurol Neurosurg Psychiatry 51:516–520, 1988.
84. Wijdicks EF, Vermeulen M, Hijdra A, et al: Hyponatremia and cerebral infarction in patients with ruptured intracranial aneurysms: Is fluid restriction harmful? Ann Neurol 17:137–140, 1985.
85. Vassar MJ, Perry CA, Holcroft JW: Prehospital resuscitation of hypotensive trauma patients with 7.5% NaCl versus 7.5% NaCl with added dextran: A controlled trial. J Trauma 34:622–633, 1993.
86. Wisner DH, Schuster L, Quinn C: Hypertonic saline resuscitation of head injury: Effects on cerebral water content. J Trauma 30:75–78, 1990.
87. Gross P, Reimann D, Neidel J, et al: The treatment of severe hyponatremia. Kidney Int 64(Suppl):S6–11, 1998.
88. Correa AJ, Rodriquez M, Carey ME: SIADH after subarachnoid hemorrhage and craniotomy. South Med J 73:932–934, 1980.
89. Landolt AM, Yasargil MG, Krayenbuhl H: Disturbances of the serum electrolytes after surgery of intracranial arterial aneurysm. J Neurosurg 37:210–218, 1972.
90. McMahon AJ: Diabetes insipidus developing after subarachnoid haemorrhage from an anterior communicating artery aneurysm. Scot Med J 33:208–209, 1988.
91. Dawson BH: The blood vessels of the human optic chiasma and their relation to those of the hypophysis and hypothalamus. Brain 81:207–217, 1958.
92. Wise BL: Syndrome of inappropriate antidiuretic hormone secretion after spontaneous subarachnoid hemorrhage: A reversible cause of clinical deterioration. Neurosurgery 3:412–414, 1978.
93. Mehta V, Holness RO, Connolly K, et al: Acute hydrocephalus following aneurysmal subarachnoid hemorrhage. Can J Neurol Sci 23:40–45, 1996.
94. Milhorat TH: Acute hydrocephalus after aneurysmal subarachnoid hemorrhage. Neurosurgery 20:15–20, 1987.
95. Yoshimoto Y, Ochiai C, Kawamata K, et al: Aqueductal blood clot as a cause of acute hydrocephalus in subarachnoid hemorrhage. AJNR Am J Neuroradiol 17:1183–1186, 1996.
96. Rinkel GJ, Wijdicks EF, Vermeulen M, et al: Acute hydrocephalus in nonaneurysmal perimesencephalic hemorrhage: Evidence of CSF block at the tentorial hiatus. Neurology 42:1805–1807, 1992.
97. Suarez-Rivera O: Acute hydrocephalus after subarachnoid hemorrhage. Surg Neurol 49:563–565, 1998.
98. Tapaninaho A, Hernesniemi J, Vapalahti M, et al: Shunt-dependent hydrocephalus after subarachnoid haemorrhage and aneurysm surgery: Timing of surgery is not a risk factor. Acta Neurochir 123:118–124, 1993.
99. Graff-Radford NR, Torner J, Adams HP Jr, et al: Factors associated with hydrocephalus after subarachnoid hemorrhage: A report of the Cooperative Aneurysm Study. Arch Neurol 46:744–752, 1989.
100. Vale FL, Bradley EL, Fisher WS III: The relationship of subarachnoid hemorrhage and the need for postoperative shunting. J Neurosurg 86:462–466, 1997.
101. Kallmes DF, Lanzino G, Dix JE, et al: Patterns of hemorrhage with ruptured posterior inferior cerebellar artery aneurysms: CT findings in 44 cases. AJR Am J Roentgenol 169:1169–1171, 1997.
102. Pietila TA, Heimberger KC, Palleske H, et al: Influence of aneurysm location on the development of chronic hydrocephalus following SAH. Acta Neurochir 137:70–73, 1995.
103. Sindou M: Favourable influence of opening the lamina terminalis and Lilliequist's membrane on the outcome of ruptured intracranial aneurysms: A study of 197 consecutive cases. Acta Neurochir 127:15–16, 1994.
104. Rajshekhar V, Harbaugh RE: Results of routine ventriculostomy with external ventricular drainage for acute hydrocephalus following subarachnoid haemorrhage. Acta Neurochir 115:8–14, 1992.
105. McKhann GM II, LeRoux PD: Perioperative and intensive care unit care of patients with aneurysmal subarachnoid hemorrhage. Neurosurg Clin North Am 9:595–614, 1998.
106. Khanna RK, Rosenblum ML, Rock JP, et al: Prolonged external ventricular drainage with percutaneous long-tunnel ventriculostomies. J Neurosurg 83:791–794, 1995.

# CHAPTER 82

# Anesthetic Management of the Patient After an Aneurysmal Subarachnoid Hemorrhage

■ STEPHEN N. STEEN and VLADIMIR ZELMAN

Subarachnoid hemorrhage (SAH) is a multisystem illness that requires coordination of a wide variety of medical resources and practitioners. The anesthesiologist's role in the care of aneurysm patients may be wideranging and include preoperative and postoperative care as well as intraoperative management.[1] With this in mind and that "the anesthetic management . . . encompasses concerns about cerebral ischemia, blood loss, pharmacologic therapy for vasospasm, optimal timing for surgery, specific predictions of outcome, and, in the occasional patient, the problem of elevated 'intracranial pressure',"[2] some of these aspects are discussed in this chapter as well as in several other chapters of this book.

## PREOPERATIVE CONSIDERATIONS

Preoperative considerations are vasospasm, rebleeding, and timing of operation. In an attempt to assess the surgical risk and improve patient outcome, grading scales are used (Tables 82–1, 82–2, and 82–3). Patients are placed in the next less favorable category if serious systemic disease is present (e.g., diabetes, chronic pulmonary disease, severe atherosclerosis, hypertension, or serious vasospasm as seen on arteriography).

The Glasgow Coma Scale (GCS) (Table 82–4) is a clinical scale in which "these aspects of behaviour are independently measured—motor responsiveness, verbal performance, and eye opening" to assess "the depth and duration of impaired consciousness and coma."[7] A more recent grading scale based on the GCS was suggested by the World Federation of Neurologic Surgeons (see Table 82–3). The GCS scale should not be confused with the Glasgow Outcome Scale (Table 82–5), which assesses outcome after brain damage.[8] All patients who have a decreased level of consciousness should be treated as though they were scheduled for emergency surgery and receive nothing by mouth.

## Vasospasm

"Cerebral vasospasm following SAH is one of the most important causes of cerebral ischemia, and is the leading cause of death and disability after aneurysm rupture."[88] "The mere presence or absence of vasospasm is not as important clinically as the degree and distribution of such spasm and the adequacy of the patient's compensatory mechanisms."[10] Pathogenesis of cerebral vasospasm appears to be multifactorial, for which there is no satisfactory animal model of vasospasm. At this time, the cause of vasospasm is not known.

## Rebleeding

Rebleeding from a ruptured aneurysm is second only to vasospasm as a cause of morbidity and surpasses vasospasm as a cause of mortality among survivors of SAH. "Although aneurysm clipping removes the risk of aneurysmal rebleeding as a cause of neurologic deterioration after SAH, during the subsequent 2 to 3 weeks patients remain at risk for cerebral vasospasm, hydrocephalus, seizures, and other complications that pose a threat to neurologic and medical recovery."[1] "Intraoperative rupture of an intracranial aneurysm can . . . jeopardize the patient's chances for a favorable outcome."[11]

TABLE 82–1 ■ **CLINICAL GRADES ACCORDING TO BOTTERELL AND COWORKERS**

| Grade | Criteria |
|---|---|
| I | Conscious with or without meningeal signs |
| II | Drowsy without significant neurologic deficit |
| III | Drowsy with neurologic deficit and probable cerebral clot |
| IV | Major neurologic deficits present |
| V | Moribund with failing vital centers and extensor rigidity |

From Botterell EH, Lougheed WM, Scott JW, Vandewater SL: Hypothermia, and interruption of carotid, or carotid and vertebral circulation, in the surgical management of intracranial aneurysms. J Neurosurg 13:1–42, 1956.

## TABLE 82–2 ■ CLASSIFICATION OF SUBARACHNOID HEMORRHAGE PATIENTS ACCORDING TO SURGICAL RISK

| Grade | Criteria |
|---|---|
| 0 | Incidental aneurysm, no hemorrhage |
| I | Asymptomatic |
| I(A) | Fixed neurologic deficit, no meningeal reaction |
| II | Headache, nuchal rigidity |
| III | Drowsiness, confusion, mild focal deficit |
| IV | Stupor, major hemiparesis, early decerebrate rigidity, vegetative disturbances |
| V | Deep coma, deep cerebrate rigidity, moribund |
| X(s) | (s) denotes serious systemic illness or age >60 years |

Modified from Hunt WE, Hess RM: Surgical risk as related to time of intervention in the repair of intracranial aneurysms. J Neurosurg 281:14–19, 1968.

## Electrocardiography

In 1947 electrocardiogram changes (large, upright T waves; long QT intervals) were first noted in three patients with SAH.[12] In 1953, 67 factors affecting the T wave were listed, and further cases of abnormal electrocardiograms associated with intracranial aneurysm were noted.[13] Electrocardiogram findings suggestive of myocardial ischemia in a patient with SAH occurring after the induction of anesthesia present the anesthesiologist and the surgeon with a dilemma.[14] Delay of surgery may result in further neurologic deficit,[15] possibly caused by catecholamines, potentiated by corticosteroids and the associated potassium deficiency, which have been suggested as responsible for electrocardiogram abnormalities in patients with SAH.[16]

## MANAGEMENT OF SUBARACHNOID HEMORRHAGE

The principles of anesthetic management of patients with SAH are similar to those associated with other areas of anesthesia (i.e., intracerebral and cardiovascular homeostasis with optimization of surgical conditions).[27] Notwithstanding the introduction of new drugs, the anesthetic management depends to a great extent on the clinical preference and ability of the anesthesiologist. Premedication is unnecessary for patients with decreased levels of consciousness

## TABLE 82–3 ■ WORLD FEDERATION OF NEUROLOGICAL SURGEONS' GRADING SCALE

| WFNS Grade | GCS Score | Motor Deficit |
|---|---|---|
| I | 15 | Absent |
| II | 14–13 | Absent |
| III | 14–13 | Present |
| IV | 12–7 | Present or absent |
| V | 6–3 | Present or absent |

WFNS, World Federation of Neurological Surgeons; GCS, Glasgow Coma Scale.
From Drake CG: Report of World Federation of Neurological Surgeons Committee on a universal subarachnoid hemorrhage grading scale. J Neurosurg 68:985–986, 1988.

## TABLE 82–4 ■ GLASGOW COMA SCALE

| Response | Reaction | Score |
|---|---|---|
| Best motor response | Obeys | 6 |
| | Localizes | 5 |
| | Withdraws | 4 |
| | Abnormal flexion | 3 |
| | Extensor response | 2 |
| | Nil | 1 |
| Verbal response | Orientated | 5 |
| | Confused conversation | 4 |
| | Inappropriate words | 3 |
| | Incomprehensible sounds | 2 |
| | Nil | 1 |
| Eye opening | Spontaneous | 4 |
| | To speech | 3 |
| | To pain | 2 |
| | Nil | 1 |

Score 3–15

From Teasdale G, Jennett B: Assessment of coma and impaired consciousness. Lancet 1:81–84, 1974. © by The Lancet Ltd, 1974.

(grades III to V). After the preoperative visit, if anxiety is not reduced, a small dose of a benzodiazepine or other appropriate drugs may be administered to awake and otherwise alert patients.

## ANESTHETIC CONSIDERATIONS

### Preanesthetic Assessment

Some particular issues that should be considered during the preanesthetic assessment include a history of cocaine usage, because sudden transient increases of blood pressure may result in SAH.[31] The first report of SAH from cocaine snorting was in 1984.[33] The authors state that "it may prove prudent to prevent surges in blood pressure (BP) with appropriate prophylactic medications when cocaine is being used for topical anesthesia of mucous membranes," with which we concur.

### Pregnancy

Management of the pregnant patient with SAH is similar to that of the nonpregnant patient. In pregnant women,

## TABLE 82–5 ■ GLASGOW OUTCOME SCALE

| Grade | Neurologic Status |
|---|---|
| 1 | Good recovery; patient can lead a full and independent life with or without minimal neurologic deficit |
| 2 | Moderately disabled; patient has neurologic or intellectual impairment but is independent |
| 3 | Severely disabled; patient is conscious but totally dependent on others to get through daily activities |
| 4 | Vegetative survival |
| 5 | Dead |

From Jennett B, Bond M: Assessment of outcome after severe brain damage: A practical scale. Lancet 1:480–484, 1975. © by The Lancet, Ltd, 1975.

cerebral arteriovenous malformations cause 50% of symptomatic SAHs, and spontaneous SAH occurs in about 1 to 2 per 10,000 pregnancies with a mortality of approximately 10%. In the general population, cerebral arteriovenous malformations are present in about 1 per 10,000 population and are responsible for approximately 10% of SAHs. A careful history and neurologic examination with an early computed tomography (CT) brain scan (with lead shielding of the abdomen) and close fetal monitoring are warranted in all cases of suspected SAH.[34]

Since 1956, 48 cases of pregnant women with cerebral aneurysms have been reported; in many cases, rupture had occurred. Cesarean section or vaginal delivery was performed followed by clipping or resection of the aneurysm. Because the fetus is fully anesthetized after 1 hour of general anesthesia, it is ill advised to plan delivery after a long surgical procedure under general anesthesia.[35] The anesthetic management of these cases was diverse and included induced hypotension and hypothermia. Perinatal mortality has been low. Pregnant patients in the third trimester are treated as patients with a full stomach, and a rapid-sequence induction and tracheal intubation technique is currently employed.

Indirect evidence suggests that the risk of SAH is increased in pregnant patients compared with nonpregnant patients.[36] In a review of 118 patients with SAH, 92% occurred antepartum, and the surgical management was associated with lower maternal and fetal mortality.[37] As to the incidence of SAH during pregnancy, the best estimate is less than 0.01%. "The tendency to rupture may be related to hemodynamic, hormonal, and coagulation changes that occur during the third trimester, including the increase in blood volume."[28]

The differential diagnosis of postpartum headache is fraught with difficulty because it includes not only SAH, but also postdural puncture, migraine, hypertension, caffeine withdrawal, and myriad other possibilities. If a headache is suspicious in nature, a CT scan should be performed. If the result is negative, a lumbar puncture should be done.

## ANESTHETIC AGENTS

Anesthetic agents used for induction or maintenance are generally administered by intravenous (IV), inhalational, or intramuscular routes. The IV agents comprise the barbiturates (thiopental sodium [Hypnopento, Intraval, Farmotal, Nesdonal, Pentothal, Thiopentone, Trapanal], thiamylal sodium [Surital], and methohexital [Brevital, Brietal, Methohexitone, Sombrilex]) and the nonbarbiturates (opioids and nonopioids). More than 20 years ago, thiopental was reported to produce "no significant alteration in intracranial pressure, and the cerebral perfusion pressure remained above 85 mm Hg despite moderate reductions in arterial pressure"[40] when the drug was used for the induction of anesthesia in patients with normal pressures before thiopental, whether the intracranial pressure was elevated or not. These significant findings attest to the beneficial clinical effects observed by clinicians over the many years that thiopental has been used in neuroanesthesia. Doses may

reach 15 mg/kg[41] for induction alone, in which case volatile or narcotic agents should be reduced, particularly before the end of the procedure, so that awakening of the patient is not delayed. The elimination half-life of about 12 hours is doubled in patients with marked obesity and halved in pediatric patients.[42] Barbiturates may impart a limited degree of brain protection.[43–45]

## Opioids[46]

*Morphine* is metabolized primarily in the liver. In general, the metabolites are excreted within 24 hours after a single dose. It is metabolized to the 3β-glucuronide and the 6β-glucuronide; the latter form has greater analgesic activity than morphine and may constitute 15% of all of the metabolites and contribute to the long duration of action of morphine. The onset of respiratory depression occurs after the onset of analgesic effects, with peaks occurring at 30 to 60 minutes and 15 to 30 minutes. This difference between onsets and peaks may result in postoperative oversedation and potential respiratory obstruction leading to apnea and other complications.

*Meperidine* (Demerol, pethidine) has a shorter onset time and duration of analgesic effect than morphine (Table 82–6). One of the metabolites is normeperidine, a convulsant, with a half-life of 12 hours, which may result in significant accumulation.

*Fentanyl* (Phentanyl, Sublimaze) has a hepatic extraction similar to that of meperidine, which accounts for its poor effect when given orally. Because the drug (usually given intravenously in doses of 50 to 100 μg) has a long half-life (Table 82–7), cumulative effects are likely to occur after repeated administration. High blood levels are attained when the portal circulation is bypassed (i.e., buccal, intranasal, or transdermal routes).

*Sufentanil* (Sufenta), a derivative of fentanyl, is more potent than fentanyl and has been reported to raise intracranial pressure (as does fentanyl).

*Alfentanil* (Alfenta, Rapifen), a slightly less potent derivative of fentanyl, has a rapid onset of action, with peak analgesic and respiratory depressant effects occurring within a few minutes. The induction dose for adults varies from 0.5 to 5 mg, depending on the length of the procedure. The pharmacokinetics of alfentanil are such that it is less likely to produce cumulative effects after continuous infu-

TABLE 82–6 ■ **PROPERTIES OF COMMONLY USED OPIOID ANALGESICS**

| Agent | Equivalent Dose* | Duration† |
|---|---|---|
| Morphine | 1.00 | 3–4 |
| Meperidine | 10.00 | 2–3 |
| Fentanyl | 0.01 | 0.5–1.0 |
| Sufentanil | 0.001 | 0.5–1.0 |
| Alfentanil | 0.05 | 0.2–3.0 |

*Intravenously administered dose in milligrams.
†Hours after first single injection.
From Steen SN, Zelman V: Neuroanesthesia. Part V. Anesthesia and operative technique. In Youmans JR (ed): Neurological Surgery. A Comprehensive Reference Guide to the Diagnosis and Management of Neurosurgical Problems. Philadelphia: WB Saunders, 1996, pp 709–723.

## TABLE 82–7 ■ ELIMINATION HALF-LIFE OF COMMONLY USED ANESTHETIC AGENTS

| Agent | Half-Life (hr) |
|---|---|
| Midazolam | 2–2.5 |
| Diazepam | 20–40 |
| Flumazenil | 1 |
| Thiopental | 11.5 |
| Methohexital | 2.5–4.0 |
| Morphine | 2 |
| Meperidine | 3–4 |
| Fentanyl | 3–4 |
| Sufentanil | 2.5 |
| Alfentanil | 1.5 |
| Droperidol | 2 |
| Etomidate | 2–7 |
| Ketamine | 2.5 |

From Steen SN, Zelman V: Neuroanesthesia. Part V. Anesthesia and operative technique. In Youmans JR (ed): Neurological Surgery. A Comprehensive Reference Guide to the Diagnosis and Management of Neurosurgical Problems. Philadelphia: WB Saunders, 1996, pp 709–723.

sion or repeated doses. Careful titration of the alfentanil maintenance infusion to achieve the desired effect is required because of interpatient variability, in pharmacokinetic data and pharmacodynamic responses, to minimize the possibility of postoperative respiratory depression.[47–49] Alfentanil has been reported to raise intracranial pressure, and it has been suggested that the use of this drug in patients with intracranial pathology should be contraindicated.[50, 51] This suggestion was not confirmed in a study of patients with and without intracranial pathology.[52]

Hormonal changes from the intraoperative administration of the opioids are of relatively little clinical importance.[53] Small doses of opioids produce pupillary constriction, which may be reversed with opioid antagonists or ganglionic blockers (e.g., atropine). Pupillary constriction may be important in the subsequent neurologic evaluation of the patient.

Equianalgesic doses can be difficult to determine when opioids with different analgesic time-effect curves are being compared. Fentanyl is claimed to have about 100 times the potency of morphine, a number that measures analgesia over time (i.e., area under the curve); however, the peak effect after an intravenous bolus may be double this number.[54] Reversal of opioids should be undertaken with care because hemodynamic changes and pulmonary edema may occur, and death has been reported.[55–60]

*Naloxone* (Narcan), administered IV, is the only commercially available parenteral opioid antagonist.

## Nonopioids[61]

*Propofol* (Diprivan, disoprofol), di-isopropylphenol, is formulated as a 1% egg lecithin emulsion and can be given by bolus or continuous infusion as is or with normal saline; the larger the vein, the less likely is pain on administration. The drug is usually administered slowly (1 to 2 mg/kg IV), and it is advisable to label the milk-colored infusion line as propofol to differentiate it from any parenteral infusion fluids that are being administered. It has a rapid onset and recovery, with little nausea and emesis, benefits that

outweigh the potential for pain on injection. The cardiovascular depression that occurs does not appear to be clinically significant in healthy patients when cardiac filling pressures are maintained by IV fluid administration, and the responsiveness of cerebral blood flow to changes in arterial carbon dioxide is maintained during propofol–nitrous oxide analgesia.[62, 63] These effects may make propofol an appropriate drug for the high-risk patient and for sedation (e.g., in pediatric magnetic resonance imaging), but disinhibition occurs in some patients during conscious sedation, as does amnesia.[64–66] Tachyphylaxis for repeated procedures (50 occasions) has been reported despite a depth of anesthesia believed adequate. Propofol appears not to trigger malignant hyperthermia.[67] Anaphylactoid reactions to propofol have been reported.[68, 69]

*Droperidol* (Dehydrobenzperidol, Droleptan, Inapsine), a butyrophenone, is used more for its antiemetic effect (about 1.25 mg IV) than its sedative properties (2.5 to 5 mg IV) and appears to have little effect on the cerebrovascular system, although anxiety, restlessness, and extrapyramidal reactions have been reported postoperatively, even at the lower doses.[70] It reduces postoperative nausea and vomiting.[71] When 2.5 mg/ml of droperidol is combined with 50 µg/ml of fentanyl (Innovar) in amounts necessary for general anesthesia with nitrous oxide, the recurrence of respiratory depression during postanesthesia recovery may present a clinical risk. Two cases of anaphylaxis from droperidol have been reported.[72]

*Etomidate* (Amidate, Hypnomidate) appears to have less of a respiratory depressant effect than barbiturates and has been used as a sedative in the intensive care unit. It appears that when electroencephalogram burst suppression was achieved with the drug (128 ± 0.11 mg/kg, mean ± SE) in eight patients, there was a 50% decrease in intracranial pressure and minimal changes in cerebral perfusion pressure, which were maintained after laryngoscopy and endotracheal intubation.[73] The drug (1 mg/hr IV bolus followed by 10 µg/kg/min) has also been used for burst suppression because it produces significant depression of cerebral metabolism with minimal cardiotoxicity.[74] Because there does not appear to be any proven method for cerebral protection, maintenance of adequate perfusion pressure and the avoidance of hyperglycemia seem to be the most relevant factors to be controlled by the anesthesiologist.

*Ketamine* (Ketalar, Ketaject) produces marked increases in intracranial pressure in patients with normal or elevated levels, suggesting that it should not be used in the latter group (Table 82–8). Because the drug may increase arterial pressure (25%), it is contraindicated if a significant elevation of blood pressure could constitute a serious hazard (e.g., patients with aneurysm, cerebral trauma).

## Inhalational Agents (see Table 82–8)

The clinical potency of an inhaled anesthetic is the minimal alveolar concentration necessary to prevent movement in 50% of individuals subjected to a painful stimulus, usually an incision. Because minimal alveolar concentrations are additive, their total is the sum of the individual concentrations (contributed by more than one inhaled anesthetic or intravenous agents). The use of neuromuscular agents to

TABLE 82–8 ■ **EFFECTS OF INHALATIONAL AGENTS COMMONLY USED IN ANESTHESIA**

| Agent | Intracranial Pressure | Cerebral Blood Flow | Systemic Vascular Resistance | Heart Rate | Myocardial or Respiratory Depresion |
|---|---|---|---|---|---|
| Nitrous oxide | + | + | | (+) | + |
| Halothane | + | + + | 0 | 0 | + + |
| Isoflurane | + | + | − | + | + |
| Enflurane | + | + | + | (+) | + + |
| Desflurane | * | * | − | + | + |
| Sevoflurane | * | * | − | (+) | + |

+, increase; −, decrease; *, not known; 0, no change; (), possibly.

From Steen SN, Zelman V: Neuroanesthesia. Part V. Anesthesia and operative technique. In Youmans JR (ed): Neurological Surgery. A Comprehensive Reference Guide to the Diagnosis and Management of Neurosurgical Problems. Philadelphia: WB Saunders, 1996, pp 709–723.

prevent movement during light muscular anesthesia may result in awareness, recall, and litigation.

## Nitrous Oxide

Nitrous oxide is about 30 times more soluble than nitrogen in blood. The nitrogen is replaced rapidly by nitrous oxide, and in a closed cavity, such as the cranium, the increased volume may increase the pressure, a potentially adverse effect. Because nitrous oxide increased cerebral blood flow and reached a plateau at approximately 30% in 20 of 24 healthy male volunteers, it has been suggested that the use of nitrous oxide must be considered carefully for patients with cerebral pathology or if autoregulation is impaired.[75] The present belief is that it is not necessary to discontinue its use to avoid an increase in intracranial pressure or expansion of intracranial air, although some anesthesiologists discontinue the agent 20 to 30 minutes before the termination of surgery to minimize postoperative nausea and vomiting.[76]

A common practice is to administer 70% nitrous oxide in oxygen combined with a reduced concentration of other inhalational agents. The inhalational agents are liquids that may be volatilized by vaporizers or by direct injection of the liquid into the anesthetic circuit, where they vaporize because their boiling points are lower than conventional ambient temperatures. A graphical method for administering volatile agents is based on the classic technique formulated by Lowe and Ernst.[77, 78] Volatile anesthetics include the halogenated hydrocarbon halothane (Fluothane) and halogenated ethers enflurane (Alyrane, Ethrane), isoflurane (AErrane, Forane, Nederane), desflurane (Suprane), and sevoflurane (Ultane) (Table 82–9).

When more than two drugs are administered drug interactions are to be expected—in some desirable, others unwanted. Isoflurane at 1.0 MAC (minimal alveolar concentration) with hyperventilation was reported to provide adequate safety for 13 patients undergoing surgery for SAH[79] and is one of the current inhalational agents in use. The newer inhalational agents (sevoflurane, desflurane) may permit a faster induction and emergence but do not appear to impart any clear-cut advantage.[80]

Hypocapnia induced by hyperventilation usually eliminates the increase in intracranial pressure, most reliably during isoflurane anesthesia. Low-flow isoflurane–nitrous oxide anesthesia offers substantial economic advantages at one third to one half of the cost of high-flow and medium-flow techniques.[81] Patients with intracranial lesions should not receive halothane until measures to produce hyperventilation have been instituted. Enflurane should be used with care in these patients because it may produce seizures in cases of hypocapnia; convulsions are less likely if concentrations are maintained at less than 1.5% to 2%. Thiopental constricts cerebral vessels and is frequently used to attenuate the responses in intracranial pressure during the use of volatile agents. Because supplementation of IV narcotics often occurs intraoperatively with low concentrations of enflurane, there appears to be little justification for the preferential use of any one inhalational agent until sufficient data are available on a large number of such patients to confirm or deny the choice.[82]

## Intravenous Agents (see Table 82–9)

Thiopental is the most commonly used IV agent, and doses of 20 mg/kg have been used safely for controlled hypertension in 30 patients with SAH.[83] An obvious disadvantage is the prolonged recovery period. As to etomidate, although its successful clinical use has been reported, we are concerned about the potential for muscle rigidity, especially on induction. With respect to propofol and the occurrence of electroencephalogram abnormalities and convulsions, clinicians are undecided as to its clinical use when these occur. "The court is still out on the verdict." As regards ketamine, the prevailing opinion is that it is not indicated in patients with hypertension.

TABLE 82–9 ■ **EFFECTS OF SOME INTRAVENOUS AGENTS COMMONLY USED IN ANESTHESIA**

| Agent | Intracranial Pressure | Cerebral Blood Flow |
|---|---|---|
| Diazepam | − | − |
| Thiopental | − | − |
| Etomidate | − | − |
| Propofol | − | − |
| Ketamine | + | + |

+, increase; −, decrease.

From Steen SN, Zelman V: Neuroanesthesia. Part V. Anesthesia and operative technique. In Youmans JR (ed): Neurological Surgery. A Comprehensive Reference Guide to the Diagnosis and Management of Neurosurgical Problems. Philadelphia: WB Saunders, 1996, pp 709–723.

## Neuromuscular Blocking Agents (Table 82–10)

Neuromuscular blocking agents[84] are used for skeletal muscle relaxation to facilitate ventilation and endotracheal intubation, to relieve laryngospasm, and to decrease the depth of anesthesia when general anesthesia alone is used (but not to compensate for inadequate anesthesia). The blocking drugs may be divided into nondepolarizing blocking drugs (see Table 82–10), which compete with acetylcholine for cholinergic receptor sites, and the depolarizing drug succinylcholine dichloride (Anectine, Curaryl, Scoline, Sucostrin, Quelicin).

Reversal of the neuromuscular blocking effect, if desirable, may be undertaken if there is a muscle response of one or more twitches to peripheral nerve stimulation. If more than 50% fade on train-of-four twitches, a phase II block has occurred. After a plateau in recovery has been reached, reversal can be quantitated using a peripheral neuromuscular transmission monitor. The dosage requirements of all neuromuscular blocking drugs are decreased by about one third to one half (compared with nitrous oxide used alone) when inhalational agents are used. The duration of the neuromuscular block by these agents increases with many antibiotics.

## Depolarizing Drug (Succinylcholine Dichloride)

An advantage of succinylcholine is its short duration of action. It is rapidly metabolized to succinyl monocholine (which is about 5% as potent) in about 95% of patients; the remaining patients have prolonged blockade. Succinylcholine usually results in a slight increase (1 mEq/L) in serum potassium concentrations, which is of little consequence in the normal individual. Marked dysrhythmias (usually transient asystole and nodal rhythm) after a second injection of succinylcholine have been reported in adults after inhaled anesthetic induction with halothane and nitrous oxide.[85–87] Etomidate does not possess a protective effect against succinylcholine-induced dysrhythmias, as does thiopental.[85] Malignant hyperthermia, one of the greatest hazards in clinical anesthesia, may be triggered by succinylcholine in susceptible patients. Succinylcholine increases intracranial pressure and may increase cerebral blood flow. Its use in patients with increased intracranial pressure, whether pretreated or not with a neuromuscular blocking drug, is controversial; more important is avoidance of hypercapnia and light anesthesia. Mydriasis from ganglionic blockade may occur when continuous IV infusions are administered. This effect may hinder neurologic evaluation.

## TABLE 82–10 ■ NEUROMUSCULAR BLOCKING AGENTS

| Agent | Dose (mg/kg) |
| --- | --- |
| Rocuronium (Zemuron) | 0.6 |
| Atracurium (Tracrium) | 0.5 |
| Doxacurium (Nuromax) | 0.5 |
| D-Tubocurarine (Tubarine) | 0.3 |
| Cisatracurium (Nimbex) | 0.2 |
| Mivacurium (Mivacron) | 0.2 |
| Pancuronium (Pavulon) | 0.1 |
| Pipecuronium (Arducon) | 0.1 |
| Vecuronium (Norcuron) | 0.1 |

# ANESTHETIC MANAGEMENT

## Induction

Induction of anesthesia may be by the slow IV administration of thiopental (3 to 5 mg/kg), propofol (1.5 to 2.5 mg/kg), or etomidate (0.1 to 0.2 mg/kg). We do not advocate the use of etomidate because of its potential for muscle rigidity. It is essential to attenuate the responses to laryngoscopy and intubation and to avoid straining, coughing, or any induced movement during this phase because rebleeding[88] may occur.

Frequently, IV narcotics (e.g., sufentanil 0.5 to 1 μg/kg or fentanyl 5 to 10 μg/kg) are added to the induction sequence 3 to 5 minutes before laryngoscopy and intubation to blunt the hemodynamic responses that often result. Lidocaine, esmolol (Brevibloc) (0.5 mg/kg), or labetalol (10 to 20 mg) 1 to 2 minutes before laryngoscopy may be given in lieu of or in addition to the narcotics. When esmolol is used to block the cardiovascular response to intubation, the drug acts as a hypotensive agent before a hypertensive stimulus occurs and "not every patient will benefit from a 25% reduction in MAP [mean arterial pressure]."[89] IV lidocaine, 1.5 mg/kg, was preferred to laryngotracheal administration for blunting the increases in heart rate associated with laryngoscopy and endotracheal intubation, and it prevented (data indicated *less*) intracranial hypertension in patients who had brain tumors estimated to be larger than 3 cm in diameter by CT scan.[90] Light nitrous oxide barbiturate anesthesia was used during data collection on these patients, although more recent findings indicated that the administration of IV lidocaine at the extreme high dose of 5 mg/kg did not blunt the cardiovascular and catecholamine response to laryngoscopy and intubation in American Society of Anesthesiologists (ASA) I patients after rapid induction of general anesthesia.[91] Techniques for blunting this sympathetic response have been reported.[92, 93] There is little need to employ such drugs when a good topical anesthetic appropriately applied is safer.

## Maintenance

Maintenance of anesthesia after induction is usually with one of the volatile anesthetic agents and oxygen, with or without nitrous oxide. A narcotic and a nondepolarizing muscle relaxant are frequently added. A volatile inhalational agent with hyperventilation may also be used.

The maintenance of stable hemodynamics during induction and throughout the operative intervention (e.g., the anticipation of painful stimuli; from the insertion of skull pins of the headholder), is of prime importance. Local infiltration of an anesthetic at the sites of pin insertions before the application of a headholder is usually performed, and we recommend this procedure with dilute concentrations of a vasopressor if surgically required because hypertension may occur about 30 minutes thereafter with a concentrated solution.

Intraoperative fluid administration is based on blood loss, urinary output, and the maintenance requirements of the patient. Glucose, commonly administered IV during the intraoperative period, may have adverse effects that outweight the potential benefits; for example, when brain ischemia may occur intraoperatively, it has been recommended that the blood glucose level be maintained at less than 200 mg/dl.[94]

## Emergence and Recovery

At the end of the surgical procedure, neuromuscular blockade should be reversed (if indicated) and the anesthetic agents turned off (if indicated). In some situations, the surgeon may not want the patient to be awakened immediately. Untoward response (e.g., movement, increased blood pressure) during extubation, suctioning, and placement of the head dressing should be avoided. The use of a small dose of an opioid (e.g., IV fentanyl 0.5 to 1 mg/kg or IV lidocaine 1.5 mg/kg) has been suggested to attenuate these responses. We do not believe that these practices are particularly helpful, and we prefer to instill 2% lidocaine down the endotracheal tube or use a small IV dose of succinylcholine (20 to 40 mg) for suctioning and extubation, provided there is no previously known reason not to do so (e.g., intraoperative complications, such as aneurysmal rupture or cardiovascular instability; delayed recovery from succinylcholine based on patient history; or drug overdose by patient or anesthesiologist). If the patient is believed to have a full stomach, the dilemma for the anesthesiologist is whether to extubate under deep anesthesia or have the patient in a conscious state as soon as possible. We prefer the latter condition (if feasible) because it permits early neurologic evaluation. To control any undue rise in blood pressure at this time, antihypertensive drugs with or without a β-blocker of labetalol may be used.[28] "Patients who have intraoperative complications, such as rupture of the aneurysm or extensive surgical trauma, or grade IV patients, who had depression of consciousness before surgery" should retain their tracheal tube until their neurologic status is stable and an unobstructed airway can be assured.[2]

Transfer of the patient to the postanesthesia room should be with all appropriate monitors in place and functioning. All monitored parameters should be recorded at least every 15 minutes or more frequently if indicated.

## SPECIAL ANESTHETIC TECHNIQUES

### Deliberate Hypotension

Hypotension techniques,[98] when originally employed, permitted spontaneous respiration.[22] "When hypothermia... became fashionable, there was a disturbing incidence of cardiac arrythmias when (these) cooled patients were allowed to breath on their own, but matters improved when

ventilation was controlled."[99] Of special concern in the postanesthesia recovery period is hypotension with bradycardia and bradypnea, which may result from raised pressure in the posterior fossa. As the pressure rises, drowsiness (not apparent under general anesthesia), respiratory depression (evident with manually assisted or spontaneous ventilation), and fluctuations in heart rate occur with increased sensitivity to sedative medications and with impaired protective reflexes. Bradycardia may occur when the special receptors of the trachea are stimulated. Tracheal suctioning frequently produces bradycardia by producing hypoxia or by increasing vagal tone, which may be successfully treated with bupivacaine or other local anesthetics.[100]

In 1991, controlled hypotension was briefly reviewed and the statement made "that as neurosurgeons and neuroanesthetists gain more experience with regional vessel clipping, the use of controlled hypotension for cerebral aneurysm surgery will be of historical interest only."[101] Additional evidence was reported the same year for a retrospective study of 112 SAH patients who underwent early surgery. Of patients, 85 received hypotensive anesthesia (only to 80 to 90 mm Hg), and the remainder acted as controls; no differences in outcome were noted (with no reduction in the incidence of intraoperative rerupture).[102] "Evolving opinion of the neurosurgery-anesthesia community is that it is preferable to minimize blood pressure reduction and to reserve hypotension for the control of intraoperative rupture or perhaps for brief periods preceding clip application,"[103] as used at our medical center.

There has been much discussion about the safe limits of controlled hypotension. Adhering to the principle that physicians should not harm the patient, we defer to a conservative 40% decrease of mean arterial pressure (MAP), where $MAP = 1/3 (BP_{systolic} - BP_{diastolic}) + BP_{diastolic}$, so that an individual with a normal blood pressure of 120/80 mm Hg would have mean arterial pressure lowered to 56 mm Hg, and a hypertensive patient with a blood pressure of 200/110 mm Hg would be lowered to 84 mm Hg. The rapid induction of hypotension to a mean arterial pressure of 40 to 50 mm Hg or lower is questioned by the authors because the neurologic outcome was improved in patients who did not have hypotension during their cerebroaneurysmal surgery.[104] An adequate intravascular volume is necessary before any induced hypotensive technique is initiated.

### Hypothermia

Hypothermia has been used successfully,[105] but unless there is an indication mandating its use (e.g., cardiac bypass) and the facilities are available for the procedure, there appears to be little need to subject the patient to this more complex anesthetic technique.

## ANESTHETIC COMPLICATIONS

### Airway Obstruction and Aspiration

Although reinforced (e.g., wire spiral, armored) endotracheal tubes are commonly used in neurosurgery, the potential for obstruction exists. Aspiration pneumonitis, although uncommon (1.4 to 6 per 10,000 anesthetics), is a potentially preventable complication of anesthesia. A 0.05% incidence of aspiration was reported from a computer-aided study of 183,358 anesthetics; of the 83 cases of aspirations, the four patients who died were in poor physical condition preoperatively.[106] "A recent large retrospective study found 69% of all aspirations to have occurred in association with either laryngoscopy or extubation."[107] The incidence of aspiration in patients at risk (undergoing emergency surgery) was 0.11%.[108] "There appears to be no increased risk of aspiration with controlled versus spontaneous ventilation or in the pediatric population when the laryngeal mask airway (LMA) device is used for airway management."[109] "The true incidence of aspiration with the LMA (laryngeal mask airway) is unknown."[110] Pulmonary aspiration may occur as a result of laryngeal incompetence because of aging or drugs. "Anesthetic-related depression of the glottic reflex lasts at least 2 hours and sometimes as long as 8 hours after tracheal extubation, even in patients who appear alert."[111] Patients with clinically apparent aspiration who did not develop symptoms within 2 hours of aspiration on completion of the procedure were unlikely to have respiratory sequelae.[107] Pharmacologic prophylaxis is considered prudent in patients at increased risk, including patients undergoing emergency surgery, with delayed gastric emptying, with increased intra-abdominal pressure, or with impaired protective reflexes as well as in infants, the elderly, and obese patients. Prophylaxis consists of $H_2$ receptor antagonists (ranitidine [Zantac], cimetidine [Tagamet], or the new proton-pump inhibitor omeprazole [Prilosec]).

## Anaphylaxis

Intraoperative anaphylaxis is uncommon in anesthetic practice. Anaphylactoid reactions while under anesthesia occur in 1 of 5000 to 25,000 anesthetics, with a 3.4% mortality rate. Anaphylaxis in response to latex products has been reported outside and inside the operating room. Anaphylaxis may occur late, especially in at-risk patients. Because approximately 10% of such individuals require a second injection of epinephrine after apparent stabilization, all should be observed for 6 hours for late deterioration.[112, 113] Treatment for mild reactions usually consists of antihistamines and reassurance; for severe reactions, ventilation with or without endotracheal intubation, appropriate medications, and cardiopulmonary resuscitation may be necessary.

Anaphylaxis is well known for anesthetic agents and for neuromuscular blocking drugs. We believe that it behooves the anesthesiologist to be "constantly prepared to deal successfully with this rare but potentially catastrophic eventuality,"[114] because "all drugs may produce side effects (many adverse) and that includes placebo (which latter not infrequently produce beneficial effects)."[115]

The major complications of blood transfusions continue to be infection and alloimmunization (Table 82–11). Alloimmunization occurs when a recipient of a blood component produces antibodies that may be directed against antigens, leukocytes, and platelets, resulting in poor increments in blood component values after transfusions.

TABLE 82–11 ■ IMMUNE-MEDIATED ADVERSE EFFECT

| Adverse Effect | Estimated Frequency per Unit |
|---|---|
| Acute anaphylaxis | 1 : 20,000–50,000 |
| Allergic transfusion reaction | 1 : 333 |
| Acute hemolytic reaction | |
| Death | 1 : 100,000–800,000 |
| ABO incompatibility | 1 : 6000–33,000 |
| Delayed hemolytic reaction | |
| Hemolytic reaction | 1 : 4000 |
| Serologic reaction | 1 : 1500 |
| Febrile transfusion reaction (nonhemolytic) | 1 : 2000 |
| Transfusion-related acute lung injury | 1 : 5000 |

Data from I. Shulman. Personal communication, 1998.

The too-rapid correction of serum sodium in severely hyponatremic patients can be dangerous and has resulted in acute central pontine myelinolysis when chronic hyponatremia was corrected with sodium chloride. The treatment consists of diuresis with furosemide (Lasix) or mannitol and the administration of salt solutions, guided by repeated determinations of serum sodium values, which should not increase more rapidly than 1 to 2 mEq/L/hr.[116]

## Cardiac Arrest

Cardiac arrest frequently is preceded by bradycardia. Sudden arrest may be caused by a massive increase in the plasma potassium concentration. The differential diagnosis of sudden cardiopulmonary arrest during anesthesia includes administration error (e.g., potassium or other overdose), exsanguinating blood loss, primary ventricular fibrillation or asystole, myocardial infarction, and embolization to the pulmonary or coronary circulation. A protocol for circulatory arrest has been published in detail for patients with a cerebral aneurysm.[3]

## Miscellaneous Complications

Hypertensive emergencies require immediate blood pressure reduction (not necessarily to normal ranges) to prevent or limit target organ injury.[117] Examples include hypertensive encephalopathy and intracranial hemorrhage. Hypertension may result from the interaction of morphine and other opioids with monoamine oxidase inhibitors.

Muscle rigidity more often occurs during the induction of general anesthesia when a large IV bolus is administered than during the maintenance phase, although the response has been reported during emergence from anesthesia. Doses as low as 50 μg of fentanyl may produce this effect and, if pronounced, result in *lead pipe* rigidity, prohibiting ventilation of the patient. This severe complication may be treated successfully with a small dose of muscle relaxant, such as succinylcholine, if not contraindicated.

Embolism during the perioperative period is one of the catastrophes with which the anesthesiologist must be fully conversant,[116] as well as the diagnosis and treatment of malignant hyperthermia.[118] Nausea and vomiting are common effects of opioids and of large volumes of contrast media. A useful antiemetic appears to be ondansetron (Zofran) (serotonin receptor blocker), although other drugs, such as droperidol, metoclopramide (Reglan), prochlorperazine (Compazine), and domperidone (Motilium), are relatively effective and economical.

## MONITORING

Monitoring in neuroanesthetic procedures includes measurements of blood pressure, temperature, and respiratory rate; use of the electrocardiogram (three leads or more); and use of a pulse oximeter, capnograph, and stethoscope. In selected procedures, a peripheral nerve stimulator,[119] catheters (e.g., Foley, intra-arterial, pulmonary arterial, central venous), monitoring of electrolytes (i.e., potassium and sodium), electroencephalography, and monitoring of intracranial pressure may be of value.

The indications for pulmonary artery catheterization remain controversial 20 years after its introduction. We continuously monitor the arterial blood gases (because blood carbon dioxide can affect the cerebral flow and intracranial pressure), the cerebral oxygen saturation (noninvasively), and the cardiac output and data derived therefrom. Several methods should be considered for monitoring the adequacy of cerebral blood flow, including the level of consciousness, the electroencephalogram,[121] and evoked potential responses.[122]

*Electroencephalogram monitoring* has been advocated for the intraoperative detection of cerebral ischemia during deliberate hypotension and for the intraoperative or perioperative assessment of pharmacologic interventions. High concentrations of isoflurane or desflurane can cause periods of electrical silence interspersed with brief episodes of activity. Similar effects are seen by many IV sedative drugs, such as barbiturates. This pattern is termed *burst suppression*. At this time, we use propofol for burst suppression. "A total of 50% of the brain $O_2$ consumption has been attributed to the energy requirement for the generation of EEG activity,"[123] but the electroencephalogram is not a reliable indicator of reversible ischemia.

*Evoked potential responses* are small electrical signals generated after stimulation and are used to monitor the functional integrity of various neural pathways. Examples are brain stem auditory evoked responses, visual evoked responses, motor evoked potential responses, and somatosensory evoked potential responses. Routine use of evoked potential monitoring is not advocated at this time because of the high percentages of false-positive and false-negative results.[3] Of interest is a report that the effect of clonidine in reducing the requirements of anesthetics during general anesthesia is not seen in the cortical somatosensory evoked potential responses and does not influence isoflurane-induced burst suppression in the electroencephalogram.[124] Evoked potential responses are discussed in other chapters.

Years ago, the monitoring of human brain chemistry using microdialysis[125–127] was speculative. With new probes becoming available, the potential for future monitoring of, for example, neurotransmitters is unlimited.

## ACKNOWLEDGMENTS

*We are indebted to Steven L. Giannotta, MD, Department of Neurosurgery, Los Angeles County–University of Southern California Medical Center, to Ms. Kay Moon for secretarial services, the Norris Medical Library of the University of Southern California Medical Center, Rosemarie D. Murray (Library Assistant II/Photocopy Services), Rochelle Flowers-Pyle (Library Assistant II/ Interlibrary Borrowing Services), and Alice Witkowski (Librarian/Head of Access Services).*

## REFERENCES

1. McGrath BJ, Guy J, Borel CO, et al: Perioperative management of aneurysmal subarachnoid hemorrhage. Part 2: Postoperative management. Anesth Analg 81:1295–1302, 1995.
2. Manninen PH, Gelb AW: Anesthesia for cerebral aneurysms and arteriovenous malformations. In Porter SS (ed): Problems in Anesthesia. Philadelphia: JB Lippincott 1990, pp 81–93.
3. Eng CC, Lam AM: Cerebral aneurysms: Anesthetic considerations. In Cottrell JE, Smith DS (eds): Anesthesia and Neurosurgery. St Louis: Mosby, 1994, pp 376–405.
4. Botterell EH, Lougheed WM, Scott JW, Vandewater SL: Hypothermia, and interruption of carotid, or carotid and vertebral circulation, in the surgical management of intracranial aneurysms. J Neurosurg 13:1–42, 1956.
5. Hunt WE, Hess RM: Surgical risk as related to time of intervention in the repair of intracranial aneurysms. J Neurosurg 281:14–19, 1968.
6. Drake CG: Report of World Federation of Neurological Surgeons Committee on a universal subarachnoid hemorrhage grading scale. J Neurosurg 68:985–986, 1988.
7. Teasdale G, Jennett B: Assessment of coma and impaired consciousness. Lancet 2:81–84, 1974.
8. Jennett B, Bond M: Assessment of outcome after severe brain damage: A practical scale. Lancet 1:480–484, 1975.
9. Kassell NF, Sasaki T, Colohan ART, Nazar G: Cerebral vasospasm following aneurysmal subarachnoid hemorrhage. Stroke 16:562–572, 1985.
10. Fisher CM, Roberson GH, Ojemann RG: Cerebral vasospasm with ruptured saccular aneurysm: The clinical manifestations. Neurosurgery 1:345–348, 1977.
11. Batjer H, Samson D: Intraoperative aneurysmal rupture: Incidence, outcome, and suggestions for surgical management. Neurosurgery 18:701–707, 1986.
12. Byer E, Ashman R, Toth LA: Electrocardiograms with large, upright T waves and long Q-T intervals. Am Heart J 33:796–806, 1947.
13. Levine HD: Non-specificity of the electrocardiogram associated with coronary artery disease. Am J Med 15:344–355, 1953.
14. Samra SK, Kroll DA: Subarachnoid hemorrhage and intraoperative electrocardiographic changes simulating myocardial ischemia—anesthesiologist's dilemma. Anesth Analg 4:86–89, 1985.
15. White JC, Parker SD, Rogers MC: Preanesthetic evaluation of a patient with pathologic Q waves following subarachnoid hemorrhage. Anesthesiology 62:351–354, 1985.
16. Cruickshank JM, Neil-Dwyer G, Stott AW: Possible role of catecholamines, corticosteroids, and potassium in production of electrocardiographic abnormalities associated with subarachnoid haemorrhage. Br Heart J 36:697–706, 1974.
17. Barinaga M: Subarachnoid hemorrhage. Science 281:33–34, 1998.
18. Guy J, McGrath BJ, Borel CO, et al: Perioperative management of aneurysmal subarachnoid hemorrhage: Part 1. Operative management. Anesth Analg 81:1060–1072, 1995.
19. Zager EL: Surgical treatment of intracranial aneurysms. Neuroimaging Clin North Am 7:763–782, 1997.
20. Weir BK: Intracranial aneurisms and A-V malformations: Surgical considerations. In Albin MS (ed): Textbook of Neuroanesthesia with Neurosurgical and Neuroscience Perspectives. New York: McGraw-Hill, 1997, pp 845–859.
21. Nathanson M, Gajraj N: Anaesthesia for cerebral aneurysm surgery. Br J Hosp Med 54:405–408, 1995.
22. Sellery GR, Aitken RR, Drane CG: Anaesthesia for intracranial aneurysms with hypotension and spontaneous respiration. Can Anaesth Soc J 20:468–478, 1973.

23. Wallace CT: Anesthesia for intracranial aneurysms. South Med J 68:725–729, 1975.
24. Geevarghese KP: Anesthetic considerations in craniotomy for supratentorial lesions. Int Anesthesiol Clin 15:143–163, 1977.
25. Michenfelder JD: Foreword. In Varken GP (ed): Anesthetic Considerations in the Surgical Repair of Intracranial Aneurysms. Boston: Little, Brown, 1982, pp xii–xiv.
26. Frost EA: Anesthesia for intracranial vascular malformations. Bull N Y Acad Med 60:759–768, 1984.
27. Herrick IA, Gelb AW: Anesthesia for intracranial aneurysm surgery. J Clin Anesth 4:73–85, 1992.
28. Newfield P, Hamid RKA, Lam AM: Intracranial aneurisms and A-V malformations: Anesthetic management. In Albin MS (ed): Textbook of Neuroanesthesia with Neurosurgical and Neuroscience Perspectives. New York: McGraw-Hill, 1997, pp 871–900.
29. Marrubini MB: General anesthesia for intracranial surgery. Br J Anaesth 37:268–287, 1965.
30. Grundy BL, Pashayan AG, Mahla ME, Shah BD: Three balanced anesthetic techniques for neuroanesthesia: Infusion of thiopental sodium with sufentanil or fentanyl compared with inhalation of isoflurane. J Clin Anesth 4:372–377, 1992.
31. Roizen MF: Preoperative evaluation. In Miller RD (ed): Anesthesia, 4th ed. New York: Churchill Livingstone, 1994, pp 827–882.
32. Symon L: Smoking and subarachnoid haemorrhage. BMJ 1:577–578, 1979.
33. Lichtenfeld PJ, Rubin DB, Feldman RS: Subarachnoid hemorrhage precipitated by cocaine snorting. Arch Neurol 41:223–224, 1984.
34. Pritz MB, Giannotta L, Kindt GW, et al: Treatment of patients with neurological deficits associated with cerebral vasospasm by intravascular volume expansion. Neurosurgery 3:364–368, 1978.
35. Reichman OH, Karlman RL: Berry aneurysm. Surgery in the Pregnant Patient 75:115–121, 1995.
36. Wilterdink JL, Feldmann E: Cerebral hemorrhage. In Devinsky O, Feldmann E, Hamline B (eds): Neurological Complications of Pregnancy. New York: Raven Press, 1994, pp 13–23.
37. Dias MS, Sekhar LN: Intracranial hemorrhage from aneurysms and arteriovenous malformations during pregnancy and the puerperium. Neurosurgery 27:855–867, 1990.
38. Weeks SK: Postpartum headache. In Chestnut DH (ed): Obstetric Anesthesia. Part 8. Anesthetic Complications. St Louis: Mosby-Year Book, 1994, pp 606–620.
39. Drake CG: Management of cerebral aneurysms. Stroke 12:273–283, 1981.
40. Shapiro HM, Galindo A, Wyte SR, et al: Rapid intraoperative reduction of intracranial pressure with thiopentone. Br J Anaesth 45:1057–1062, 1973.
41. McDermott MW, Durity FA, Borozny M, Mountain MA: Temporary vessel occlusion and barbiturate protection in cerebral aneurysm surgery. Neurosurgery 25:34–61, 1989.
42. Department of Drugs, Division of Drugs and Toxicology: Drug Evaluations Annual 1993. Chicago: American Medical Association, 1993, pp 165–166.
43. Messick JM, Newberg Milde L: Brain protection. Adv Anesthesiol 4:47–88, 1987.
44. Drummond T: Do barbiturates really protect the brain? Anesthesiology 78:611–613, 1993.
45. Michenfelder JD: Heresy? Anesthesiology 78:613, 1993.
46. Bailey PL, Stanley TH: Intravenous opioid anesthetics. In Miller RD (ed): Anesthesia, 4th ed. New York: Churchill Livingstone, 1994, pp 291–387.
47. Jaffe RS, Coalon D: Recurrent respiratory depression after alfentanil administration. Anesthesiology 70:151–153, 1989.
48. Maitre PO, Vozeh S, Heykants J, et al: Population pharmacokinetics of alfentanil: The average dose-plasma concentration relationship and interindividual variability in patients. Anesthesiology 66:3–12, 1987.
49. Shafer S, Sung M-L, White PF: Pharmacokinetics and pharmacodynamics of alfentanil infusions during general anesthesia. Anesth Analg 65:1021–1028, 1986.
50. Huggins NJ: Alfentanil and intracranial pathology. Anesthesiology 48:453–454, 1993.
51. Moss E: Alfentanil increases intracranial pressure when intracranial compliance is low. Anaesthesia 47:134–136, 1992.
52. Mayberg TS, Lam AM, Eng CC, et al: The effect of alfentanil on cerebral blood flow velocity and intracranial pressure during isoflurane-nitrous oxide anesthesia in humans. Anesthesiology 78:288–294, 1993.
53. Sebel PS, Bovill JG, Schellekens APM, et al: Hormonal responses to high-dose fentanyl anaesthesia. Br J Anaesth 53:941–948, 1981.
54. Rosow C: Pharmacology of opioid analgetic agents. In Rogers MC, Tinker JH, Covino BG, et al (eds): Principles and Practice of Anesthesiology, Vol 2. St Louis: Mosby-Year Book, 1993, pp 1157, 1158.
55. Andree RA: Sudden death following naloxone administration. Anesth Analg 59:782–784, 1980.
56. Azar I, Turndorf H: Severe hypertension and multiple atrial premature contractions following naloxone administration. Anesth Analg 58:524–525, 1979.
57. Flacke JW, Flacke WE, Williams CE: Acute pulmonary edema following naloxone reversal of high-dose morphine anesthesia. Anesthesiology 47:376–378, 1977.
58. Michaelis LL, Hickey PR, Clark TA, Dixon WM: Ventricular irritability associated with the use of naloxone. Ann Thorac Surg 18:608–614, 1974.
59. Partridge BC, Ward CF: Pulmonary edema following low-dose naloxone administration. Anesthesiology 65:709–710, 1986.
60. Tanaka GY: Hypertensive reaction to naloxone. JAMA 228:25–26, 1974.
61. Reves JG, Glass PSA, Lubarsky DA: Nonbarbiturate intravenous anesthetics. In Miller RD (ed): Anesthesia, 4th ed. New York: Churchill Livingstone, 1994, pp 247–289.
62. Fox J, Gelb AW, Enns J, et al: The responsiveness of cerebral blood flow to changes in arterial carbon dioxide is maintained during propofol-nitrous oxide anesthesia in humans. Anesthesiology 77:453–459, 1992.
63. Illevich UM, Petricel W, Schramm W, et al: Electroencephalographic burst suppression by propofol infusion in humans: Hemodynamic consequences. Anesth Analg 77:155–160, 1993.
64. Crawford M, Pollock J, Anderson K, et al: Comparison of midazolam with propofol for sedation in outpatient bronchoscopy. Br J Anaesth 70:419–422, 1993.
65. Lefever EB, Potter PS, Seeley NR: Propofol sedation for pediatric MRI. Anesth Analg 76:919–920, 1993.
66. Moore-Jeffries E, Steen SN: Efficacy of propofol for conscious sedation under regional anesthesia. Rev Esp Anestesiol Reanim 39(Suppl 1):9, 1992.
67. Khan KJ, Cooper GM: Propofol and malignant hyperthermia: A case for day-case anesthesia? Anaesthesia 48:455–456, 1993.
68. Laxenaire MC, Gueant JL, Monerek-Vautrim DA, et al: Chocs anaphylactiques an propofol lors de la premiere utilisation. Ann Fr Anesth Reanim 9(Suppl):R125, 1990.
69. McHale S, Konieczko K: Anaphylactoid reaction to propofol. Anaesthesia 48:446, 1993.
70. Melnick B, Sawyer R, Karambelkar D, et al: Delayed side effects of droperidol after ambulatory general anesthesia. Anesth Analg 69:748–751, 1989.
71. Williams OA, Clark FL, Harris RW, et al: Addition of droperidol to patient-controlled analgesia: Effect on nausea and vomiting. Br J Anaesth 70:479P, 1993.
72. Occelli G, Saban Y, Pruneta RM, et al: Two cases of anaphylaxis from droperidol. Ann Fr Anesth Reanim 3:440–442, 1984.
73. Modica PA, Tempelhoff R: Intracranial pressure during induction of anaesthesia and tracheal intubation with etomidate-induced EEG burst suppression. Can J Anaesth 39:236–241, 1992.
74. Samson D, Batjer HH, Bowman G, et al: A clinical study of the parameters and effects of temporary arterial occlusion in the management of intracranial aneurysms. Neurosurgery 34:22–28, 1994.
75. Field LM, Dorrance DE, Krezeminska EK, Barsoum LZ: Effect of nitrous oxide on cerebral blood flow in normal humans. Br J Anaesth 70:154–159, 1993.
76. DeCiutiis V, Carter T, Steen S: PONV is no laughing matter (Abstract P75). Acta Anaesthesiol Scand 110(Suppl):181, 1997.
77. Lowe HJ, Ernst AE: The Quantitative Practice of Anesthesia: Use of Closed Circuit. Baltimore: Williams & Wilkins, 1981.
78. Pollock CG: A graphical method for administering volatile agents. Anaesthesia 48:450–451, 1993.
79. Gordon E, Lagerkranser EGM, Rudehill A, von Holst H: The effect of isoflurane on cerebrospinal fluid pressure in patients undergoing neurosurgery. Acta Anaesthesiol Scand 32:108–112, 1988.

80. Artru AA, Lam AM, Johnson JO, Sperry RJ: Intracranial pressure, middle cerebral artery flow velocity, and plasma inorganic fluoride concentrations in neurosurgical patients receiving sevoflurane or isoflurane. Anesth Analg 85:587–592, 1997.
81. Pederson J, Nielsen M, Guldager LH: Low-flow isoflurane-nitrous oxide anaesthesia offers substantial economic advantages over high- and medium-flow isoflurane-nitrous oxide. Acta Anaesthesiol Scand 37:509–512, 1993.
82. Steen SN, Zelman V: Neuroanesthesia. Part V. Anesthesia and operative technique. In Youmans JR (ed): Neurological Surgery: A Comprehensive Reference Guide to the Diagnosis and Management of Neurosurgical Problems. Philadelphia: WB Saunders, 1996, pp 709–723.
83. Bendtsen AO, Cold GE, Astrup J, Rosenorn J: Thiopental loading during controlled hypotension for intracranial aneurysm surgery. Acta Anaesthesiol Scand 28:473–477, 1984.
84. Savarese JJ, Miller RD, Lien CA, Caldwell JE: Pharmacology of muscle relaxants and their antagonists. In Miller RD (ed): Anesthesia, 4th ed. New York: Churchill Livingstone, 1994, pp 417–487.
85. Abdul-Rasool IH, Sears DH, Katz RL: The effect of a second dose of succinylcholine on cardiac rate and rhythm following induction of anesthesia with etomidate or midazolam. Anesthesiology 67:795–797, 1987.
86. Schoenstadt DA, Whitcher CE: Observations on the mechanisms of succinylcholine-induced cardiac arrhythmias. Anesthesiology 24:358–362, 1962.
87. Williams CH, Deutsch S, Linde HW, et al: Effects of intravenously administered sucinylcholine on cardiac rate, rhythm and arterial blood pressure in anestetized man. Anesthesiology 22:947–954, 1961.
88. Tsementzis SA, Hitchcock ER: Outcome from "rescue clipping" of ruptured intracranial aneurysms during induction anaesthesia and endotracheal intubation. J Neurol Neurosurg Psychiatry 48:160–163, 1985.
89. James RH: Does esmolol block the cardiovascular response to intubation? Anaesthesia 52:1119, 1997.
90. Hamill JF, Bedford RF, Weaver DC, Colohan AR: Lidocaine before endotracheal intubation: Intravenous or laryngotracheal? Anesthesiology 55:578–581, 1981.
91. Koveleskie JR, Stafford NC, Mok MS, Steen SN: Effect of 5.0 mg/kg intravenous lidocaine prior to intubation on the catecholamine and cardiovascular responses. J Anaesth Clin Pharmacol 12:175–179, 1996.
92. Kautto U-M: Attenuation of the circulatory response to laryngoscopy and intubation by fentanyl. Acta Anaesth Scand 26:217–221, 1982.
93. Payne KA, Murray WB, Oosthuizen JHC: Obtunding the sympathetic response to intubation. S Afr Med J 73:584–586, 1988.
94. Sieber FE, Smith DS, Traystman RJ, Wollman H: Glucose: A reevaluation of its intraoperative use. Anesthesiology 67:72–81, 1987.
95. Frost EAM: Postanesthetic care. In Frost EAM (ed): Clinical Anesthesia in Neurosurgery, 2nd ed. Boston: Butterworth-Heinemann, 1991, pp 501–513.
96. Frost EAM: Neurosurgical intensive care. In Frost EAM (ed): Clinical Anesthesia in Neurosurgery, 2nd ed. Boston: Butterworth-Heinemann, 1991, pp 515–532.
97. Petrozza PH, Prough DS: Postoperative and intensive care. In Cåthell JE, Smith DS (eds): Anesthesia and Neurosurgery. St Louis: CV Mosby, 1994, pp 625–659.
98. Cottrell JE, Hartung J: Induced hypotension. In Cåthell JE, Smith DS (eds): Anesthesia and Neurosurgery. St. Louis: Mosby, 1994, pp 425–434.
99. Aitken RR, Drake CG: A technique of anesthesia with induced hypotension for surgical correction of intracranial aneurysms. Clin Neurosurg 21:107–114, 1976.
100. Park GR, Stapak G: Bupivacaine protects against vagal bradycardias during tracheal suction. Anaesthesia 48:455, 1993.
101. Ruta TS, Mutch WAC: Controlled hypotension for cerebral aneurysm surgery: Are the risks worth the benefits. J Neurosurg Anesthesiol 3:153–156, 1991.
102. Inomata S, Mizuyama K, Sato S, et al: The effect of deliberate hypotension anesthesia on the prognosis of patients who underwent early surgeries for ruptured cerebral aneurysms. Jpn J Anesth 41:207–213, 1992.
103. Drummond JC: Deliberate hypotension for intracranial aneurysm surgery: Changing practices (Letter to Editor). Can J Anaesth 38:935–946, 1991.
104. Giannotta SL, Openheimer JH, Levy ML, Zelman V: Management of intraoperative rupture of aneurysm without hypotension. Neurosurgery 18:531–536, 1991.
105. Messick JM, Newberg LA, Nugent M, Faust RJ: Principles of neuroanesthesia for the neurosurgical patient with CNS pathophysiology. Anesth Analg 64:143–174, 1985.
106. Olsson GL, Hallen B, Hambraeus-Jonzon K: Aspiration during anesthesia: A computer-aided study of 185,358 anaesthetics. Acad Anesthesiol Scand 30:84–92, 1986.
107. Warner MA, Warner ME, Weber JG: Clinical significance of pulmonary aspiration during the perioperative period. Anesthesiology 78:56–62, 1993.
108. Brian AIJ: Historical aspects and future directions. In Ferson DZ, Brimacombe JR, Brian AIJ (eds): The Laryngeal Mask Airway. Philadelphia: Lippincott-Raven Publishers, 1998, pp 1–18.
109. Brimacombe JR, Berry AM, White PF: The laryngeal mask airway. Int Anesthesiol Clin 36:155–182, 1998.
110. Brimacomb JR, Dary H: The incidence of aspiration associated with the laryngeal mask airway: A meta-analysis of published literature. J Clin Anesth 7:297–305, 1995.
111. James CF: Pulmonary aspiration of gastric contents. In Gravenstein N, Kirby R (eds): Complications in Anesthesiology. Philadelphia: Lippincott-Raven Publishers, 1996, pp 175–190.
112. Fisher MM: Clinical observations on the pathophysiology and treatment of anaphylactic cardiovascular collapse. Anaesth Intensive Care 14:17–21, 1986.
113. Soreide EM, Buxrud T, Harboe S: Severe anaphylactic reactions outside hospital: Aetiology, symptoms and treatment. Acta Anaesthesiol Scand 32:339–342, 1988.
114. Fisher M, Baldo BA: Anaphylaxis during anesthesia: Current aspects of diagnosis and prevention. Eur J Anesth 11:263–284, 1994.
115. Steen SN, Canas M, Zelman V: Complications: Rare and unusual. Semin Anesth 15:238–249, 1996.
116. Gravenstein N (ed): Manual of Complications During Anesthesia. Philadelphia: JB Lippincott, 1991.
117. Joint National Committee on Detection, Evaluation, and Treatment of High Blood Pressure. NIH Publication No. 93-1088. Bethesda: National Institutes of Health, 1993.
118. Malignant hyperthermia. In Gravenstein N, Kirby RR (eds): Complications in Anesthesiology, 2nd ed. Philadelphia: Lippincott-Raven Publishers, 1996, pp 141–162.
119. Viby-Mogensen J: Neuromuscular monitoring. In Miller RD (ed): Anesthesia, 4th ed. New York: Churchill Livingstone, 1994, pp 1345–1361.
120. Naylor CD, Sibbald WJ, Sprung CL, et al: Pulmonary artery catheterization: Can there be an integrated strategy for guideline development and research promotion? JAMA 269:2407–2411, 1993.
121. Levy WJ: Neurophysiologic brain monitoring: Electroencephalography. In Cåthell JE, Smith DS (eds): Anesthesia and Neurosurgery. St Louis: CV Mosby, 1994, pp 240–245.
122. Sloan TB: Evoked potentials. In Albin MS (ed): Textbook of Neuroanesthesia with Neurosurgical and Neuroscience Perspectives. New York: McGraw-Hill, 1997, pp 221–226.
123. Vender JS, Gilbert HC: Monitoring the anesthetized patient. In Barash PG (ed): Clinical Anesthesia. Philadelphia: Lippincott-Raven Publishers, 1996, pp 621–641.
124. Porkkala T, Jantti V, Hakkinen V, Kaukinen S: Clonidine does not attenuate median nerve somatosensory evoked potentials during isoflurane anesthesia. J Clin Monit Comput 14:165–170, 1998.
125. Hamberger A, Runnerstam M, Nystrom B, et al: The neuronal microenvironment after subarachnoid hemorrhage: Correlation of amino acid and nucleoside levels with post-operative recovery. Neurol Res 17:97–105, 1995.
126. Såveland H, Nilsson OG, Boris-Moller F, et al: Intracerebral microdialysis of glutamate and aspartate in two vascular territories after aneurysmal subarachnoid hemorrhage. Neurosurgery 38:12–19, 1996.
127. Enblad R, Valtysson J, Andersson J, et al: Simultaneous intracerebral microdialysis and positron emission tomography performed in the detection of ischemia in patients with subarachnoid hemorrhage. J Cereb Blood Flow Metab 16:637–644, 1996.

# Aneurysms of the Carotid Circulation

# Surgical Management of Posterior Communicating, Anterior Choroidal, and Carotid Bifurcation Aneurysms

■ HENRY H. SCHMIDEK

Supraclinoid internal carotid artery (ICA) aneurysms are common and amenable to surgical treatment. In 1933, Norman Dott[1] became the first surgeon to operate on a cerebral aneurysm demonstrated by cerebral angiography. The patient, a 23-year-old woman, who experienced a severe headache and a left oculomotor nerve palsy, had a 7-mm aneurysm at the junction of the left internal carotid artery with its posterior communicating branch. This aneurysm was treated by cervical carotid ligation on March 24, 1933. The patient made an excellent general recovery and regained the oculomotor nerve function. In 1936, Walter Dandy[2] began to treat aneurysms of the internal carotid artery by a trapping procedure that involved ligation of the involved vessel proximal and distal to the aneurysm. He then introduced the direct intracranial clipping of a saccular aneurysm while preserving the parent artery. This procedure was first carried out in a 43-year-old alcoholic with an oculomotor nerve paralysis. Based on clinical findings, without angiographic studies, surgical exploration was performed. A pea-sized aneurysm was found projecting from the internal carotid artery adjacent to the posterior communicating artery. The aneurysm arose by a narrow neck, projected beneath the tentorial dura, and was attached to the oculomotor nerve. A silver clip was placed across the neck of the sac flush with the wall of the internal carotid artery and then the aneurysm was cauterized. Within 3 days the patient's ptosis and extraocular movements began to improve and were normal at 7 months.[2] In the 6 decades since these pioneering efforts, one of the major activities of the neurosurgical community has been directed toward understanding the natural history of cerebral aneurysms and improving their perioperative and intraoperative management. This chapter discusses one approach to the treatment of internal carotid artery aneurysms arising at the level of the posterior communicating artery, anterior choroidal artery, and the carotid bifurcation.

Internal carotid artery aneurysms occur in patients of any age, with the peak incidence between ages 35 and 65.

They have been operated on successfully within the first month of life. Although uncommon in children, cerebral aneurysms often exist in association with bacterial endocarditis, chronic lung infections, polycystic kidney disease, aortic coarctation, Marfan's syndrome, or Ehler-Danlos syndrome, and may appear in certain families. Familial aneurysms often occur in younger patients, who may harbor multiple aneurysms, suggesting a congenital arterial defect predisposing to early rupture. Although 10 times less common than arteriovenous malformations, cerebral aneurysms in children are more prone to rupture and account for approximately one third of the cases of spontaneous subarachnoid hemorrhage (SAH) in patients between the ages of 4 and 15 years. The clinical features are the same as those in adults. Fewer than 5 percent of the aneurysms in children produce a mass effect.

Most intracranial aneurysms are asymptomatic prior to rupture, but with aneurysmal expansion both adults and children may become symptomatic with headache, retro-orbital or facial pain, or visual complaints due to compression of the optic pathways. The highest incidence of warning signs before aneurysmal rupture exists among the aneurysms of the posterior communicating artery junction and aneurysms at the carotid bifurcation. A retrospective review reported that such warning signs have been described in 69.2% of the posterior communicating artery cases and in 60% of the carotid bifurcation aneurysms.[3]

Most of the aneurysms of the internal carotid artery distal to the ophthalmic artery are discovered after they rupture. In 40% of patients, an oculomotor palsy develops sometimes immediately or sometimes within a few days of the ictus. Before SAH occurs, ipsilateral retro-orbital and frontal head pain may exist for months or years before the aneurysm ruptures or produces an oculomotor palsy. In many cases, oculomotor palsy appears within 2 weeks of the onset of pain, and in these patients, oculomotor palsy is often the only sign of disease. The overall incidence of oculomotor palsy is approximately 38% in patients with posterior communicating artery aneurysms. When the oculomotor nerve is affected by an aneurysm, paresis is usually complete, with involvement of the levator, extraocular muscles, and the pupillary sphincter. Nontraumatic oculomotor palsy with pupillary involvement results from compression of the oculomotor nerve at the posterior end of the cavernous sinus and is, until proved otherwise, indicative of an intracranial aneurysm or tumor. Visual defects rarely occur in conjunction with these aneurysms and result from compression of the optic tract, thereby producing a contralateral homonymous hemianopia. Mental derangements may arise when the aneurysm compresses the mamillary bodies or the blood supply to the diencephalon, or pituitary insufficiency may occur when the aneurysm grows into the sella turcica.

Aneurysms that arise at the carotid bifurcation frequently present as an SAH in conjunction with an orbitofrontal or temporal intracerebral hematoma. They may grow without rupturing and mimic a suprasellar tumor. This type of growth can produce a bitemporal field defect, or if the aneurysm expands posteriorly and medially, it can compress an optic tract. If it expands posteriorly and inferiorly, it can compress the oculomotor nerve.

The patient presenting with an incidentally discovered intracranial aneurysm, often in the carotid circulation, noted on computed tomography (CT), magnetic resonance imaging (MRI), or cerebral angiography performed for some other purpose is an increasingly common phenomenon. The management requires consideration of the specifics of the patient's medical and psychological situation. In the context of an ICA aneurysm 4 to 5 mm or larger, in a suitable patient, the author's preference is for the elective clipping of these aneurysms.

## DIAGNOSTIC EVALUATION

The sudden onset of an excruciating or unusually severe headache (especially if following a history suspicious of SAH or of recent cocaine usage), or altered consciousness, in a patient who may be confused, drowsy, or amnestic for events, often in association with persistent headache and neck stiffness, requires an immediate CT scan of the head. Within the first 12 hours after SAH the CT scan is positive in over 95% of cases. After 12 hours the sensitivity of this study in detecting SAH remains over 90%. The CT scan also provides useful information about the intraparenchymal or subarachnoid distribution of the hemorrhage and the ventricular size, and often is suggestive of the site of the aneurysm that has bled. Should the CT scan be negative in a suspected case of SAH, and there is no major intracranial mass or coagulation defect, a lumbar puncture is performed. Blood in the cerebrospinal fluid (CSF) is diagnostic of an SAH unless there has been a traumatic spinal puncture.

Cerebral angiography is usually performed under sedation and local anesthesia. All four vessels are visualized and oblique, basal, magnification, and subtraction views are taken to assess the size, site, and configuration of the aneurym(s) and to examine cerebral blood vessels.

With a supraclinoid internal carotid aneurysm, the angio-

grams are specifically assessed to determine the exact relationships of the posterior communicating artery to the aneurysmal neck and whether the ipsilateral posterior communicating artery provides a major blood supply to the posterior cerebral artery. Anterior choroidal artery aneurysms usually arise from the inferior wall of the supraclinoid carotid artery and project downward. These aneurysms often present as a diffuse dilatation of the wall of the carotid artery and extend toward the carotid bifurcation, with the anterior choroidal artery incorporated in this dilatation; as a result, the aneurysm may not be amenable to clipping. Aneurysms arising at the carotid bifurcation can be difficult to delineate angiographically. Oblique and subtraction views are particularly important studies to find and characterize the aneurysm among the vessels present at the termination of the carotid artery.

In patients in whom the cerebral angiographic study is negative following SAH, a repeat four-vessel cerebral angiogram is performed 1 to 2 weeks after the first studies. In about 20% of SAH cases the initial four-vessel cerebral angiograms are negative. Repeat angiograms will demonstrate an aneurysm in an additional 5% of patients. These aneurysms are most commonly on the anterior cerebral–anterior communicating artery complex, followed in frequency by aneurysms of the middle cerebral and internal carotid arteries. The author has had one patient who underwent a third angiographic study after a second subarachnoid hemorrhage in whom an anterior communicating artery aneurysm was finally demonstrated. Another patient underwent a second angiographic study and an MRI angiogram, both of which were interpreted as showing an ICA–posterior communicating artery aneurysm. Surgical exploration did not demonstrate an aneurysm in this patient. The patient subsequently required a VP shunt for a post-SAH communicating hydrocephalus. After the shunt procedure, the patient made an excellent recovery during the last few years and has not suffered another hemorrhage.

## PREOPERATIVE MANAGEMENT

Following an SAH patients are managed in an intensive care (ICU) setting, which allows continuous monitoring. Triple-lumen central venous catheter and Foley catheters allow optimal fluid management. The preoperative management after aneurysmal SAH is designed to provide symptomatic relief, establish the diagnosis, reduce the tendency to rehemorrhage from aneurysms, and correct medical problems. The program involves bed rest, analgesics, anticonvulsants, control of blood pressure (systolic blood pressure is maintained at normotensive levels frequently with nitroprusside and the calcium-channel blocker nimodipine). Agitated, uncooperative patients are heavily sedated, often with propofol (Diprivan), following their intubation. This sedation may be reversed periodically to reassess the patient or may be continued until the surgery.

The lazaroids are 21-aminosteroids that inhibit lipid membrane peroxidation and act as oxygen-free radical scavengers. These agents were studied as potential cerebral protective agents following SAH, cerebral vasospasm, or focal cerebral ischemia. The initial encouraging results were not confirmed by a cooperative study of 900 cases of SAH reported in March, 1997. This study does not show improvement of outcome after SAH with the use of these agents.

The timing of surgical intervention depends on the clinical status of the patient. Ideally, all aneurysms should be surgically obliterated to eliminate the risk of rehemorrhage. In the Massachusetts General Hospital series of 108 patients admitted after SAH, 68 underwent craniotomy, 20 underwent endovascular mobilization, and 20 were managed nonsurgically owing to major medical contraindications to operation.

In an obtunded patient with significant angiographically demonstrated vasospasm present after SAH and prior to surgery, surgical intervention is deferred until repeat angiography no longer demonstrates the vasospasm. The patient is maintained on the medical regimen just described and is reassessed frequently; when appropriate, surgery is undertaken at a later date.

In patients whose problem is complicated by an intracerebral hemorrhage, those who have neurologic deterioration but are potentially salvageable and useful individuals undergo immediate surgery. At the time of surgery, the hemorrhage is removed and the aneurysm is dealt with definitively, if this is technically feasible.

## SURGICAL ANATOMY

The supraclinoid segment of the internal carotid artery (ICA) begins as the artery emerges from the cavernous sinus and passes medial to the anterior clinoid process. The ophthalmic, posterior communicating, and anterior choroidal arteries arise from this segment. The commonest site of ICA aneurysms is at the posterior communicating artery junction, and aneurysms arising at the ICA–anterior choroidal junction and the bifurcation of the ICA are uncommon. Aneurysms arising distally of the ICA are rare.

The posterior communicating artery arises from the posteromedial surface of the ICA and runs backward for 5 to 10 mm to anastomose with the posterior cerebral artery. The posterior communicating artery varies greatly in size from rudimentary to large. Occasionally this vessel is so large that the posterior cerebral artery appears to be arising from the internal carotid rather than from the basilar artery. The posterior communicating artery is frequently larger on the left side. If the posterior cerebral artery fills predominantly from the basilar artery, its occlusion is associated with little risk, whereas if the posterior cerebral artery fills primarily from the posterior communicating artery, its occlusion may result in a major infarction.

### Posterior Communicating Artery

The posterior communicating artery gives rise to 4 to 12 branches. These branches supply the genu and anterior third of the posterior limb of the internal capsule, the anterior third of the thalamus, and the walls of the third ventricle. This vessel gives off branches to the optic tract, the optic chiasm, the cerebral peduncle, and the tuber cinereum and terminates as the anterior thalamic perforating artery.

Aneurysms that arise at the junction of the internal carotid and posterior communicating arteries are globular, elongated, multilobular, or irregular in shape. They also vary greatly in size, although aneurysms greater than 2.5 cm in diameter are rare.

The most common type of aneurysm arising at the posterior communicating artery–ICA junction projects posterolaterally in 86% of cases and involves the oculomotor nerve in one third of cases. The aneurysm frequently overlies the origin of the posterior communicating artery. In the presence of multiple aneurysms, there is a 65% chance of one of the aneurysms being situated at this site. Because these aneurysms are the most likely to bleed into the basal cisterns, they are also the most likely to produce a communicating hydrocephalus, a complication encountered in approximately one third of patients after SAH resulting from an aneurysm in this location.

In a smaller group of patients, the aneurysm is directed posterolaterally and extends above the tentorial edge. This type is more difficult to approach because retraction of the temporal lobe may result in the aneurysm's intraoperative rupture. Temporal lobe hemorrhages may occur among this group of patients.

Medially situated aneurysms arising at the ICA–posterior communicating artery junction occur in 3.6% of the cases. These lesions tend to extend beneath the optic nerve and produce visual symptoms and subarachnoid hemorrhage. Aneurysms at this location are approached by mobilizing the frontal and temporal lobes, thereby gaining exposure of the ICA proximal and distal to the aneurysm.[5]

### Anterior Choroidal Artery

The anterior choroidal artery is an important source of blood supplying the internal capsule. This artery originates a few millimeters above the posterior communicating artery from the posterior surface of the ICA. This vessel arises either as two separate arteries or as a single trunk that divides a short way from its origin. It is often larger on the left side. This vessel takes a course along the optic tract, around the cerebral peduncle to the lateral geniculate body, to reach the choroid plexus of the lateral ventricle, and it anastomoses with branches of the posterior choroidal artery. It supplies branches that terminate in the lateral geniculate body, caudate nucleus, and the posterior limb, infralenticular, and retrolenticular portions of the internal capsule.

Although occlusion of this artery does not invariably lead to a profound neurologic deficit, its injury may result in contralateral hemiplegia, hemianesthesia, hemianopia, stupor, and death. This vessel is at risk during any surgical procedure performed near the supraclinoid internal carotid artery. Many aneurysms arising from the supraclinoid ICA involve this vessel in their wall, especially if the aneurysm is larger than 5 mm. Aneurysms also tend to coexist at this location, a situation that may not be appreciated preoperatively. Clinically, these aneurysms may be indistinguishable from the ICA–posterior communicating artery aneurysm, even with involvement of the oculomotor nerve. In addition, because the anterior choroidal artery can be attached to the fundus of a posterior communicating aneurysm, this artery must be identified before the aneurysm is clipped.

Anterior choroidal aneurysms usually project from the inferior aspect of the ICA, 3 to 6 mm proximal to the carotid bifurcation, and project laterally, whereas the anterior choroidal artery itself curves medially. The aneurysms often obscure the origin of the anterior choroidal artery; however, an angle of separation usually exists between the parent vessel and the aneurysm, which should allow a clip to be applied to the aneurysmal neck without injury to the anterior choroidal artery.

ICA bifurcation aneurysms represent about 5% of intracranial aneurysms and, following their rupture, often produce a frontal intracerebral hematoma. Because these aneurysms are often small they may be difficult to delineate angiographically and are hidden by other vessels. Morphologically, the aneurysms either represent a direct continuation of the ICA trunk, or they have a broad-based origin that incorporates the junction of the ICA and anterior cerebral arteries or the ICA–middle cerebral artery junction and include parts of the main trunk of the anterior or middle cerebral artery. Most of these lesions project superiorly or superiorly and ventrally beneath the orbitofrontal lobe in the region of the anterior perforated substance. Most of these aneurysms are 3 to 9 mm in size.

Giant aneurysms are unusual at this site. The dome of the aneurysm is usually covered by the frontal lobe or may be located in the sylvian fissure. Among aneurysms of the supraclinoid ICA, these giant aneurysms are the most likely to present with an intracerebral hematoma. Exposure of these lesions requires delineation of the vessels at the bifurcation, the lenticulostriate vessels, and the anterior choroidal artery, which is best accomplished by dissecting along the anterior and inferior margins of the major vessels while leaving the fundus, which is usually buried in the frontal lobe, alone.

## OPERATIVE PROCEDURE

Craniotomy is performed with the patient under general endotracheal anesthesia, with controlled ventilation, and continuous monitoring of cardiogram, blood gases, arterial pressure, and urinary output. The patient is brought to the operating room under sedation and with arterial and venous lines, is anesthetized, and is gently intubated without raising of the blood pressure. Neither spinal fluid drainage nor hypothermia is routinely used. The radial artery catheter must be calibrated to reflect the blood pressure at the level of the head. The patient is in a supine position, and the area of the surgery is shaved. The head is turned 15 degrees from the side of the aneurysm, and the head position is maintained in a three-point headrest. The arms and legs are protected with blankets, and a warming blanket is placed on the patient. The operating table is flexed. Intermittent compression boots are applied.

As the skin incision is made, the patient is receiving mannitol (1.5 g/kg), furosemide (20 to 40 mg IV), and antibiotics. On a separate Mayo stand there is a tray holding Yasargil, Scoville, Sugita, Drake, Mayfield, Heifitz,

and Sundt temporary and permanent aneurysm clips and appliers. This allows the surgeon a wide selection of clips in order to choose the right optimal configuration. Very often a gently curved Yasargil clip will work best. The preferred operating microscope is the Zeiss on the Contraves stand, which allows effortless changes in magnification and position.

The skin is cleansed with povidone-iodine (Betadine), and the area of surgery is infiltrated with 0.5% lidocaine (Xylocaine) with adrenalin for hemostasis. A small scalp flap is made, taking into account the position of the frontal branch of the facial nerve, which extends from the zygomatic process of the temporal bone and curves anteriorly to intersect the hairline at approximately the midpoint of the superior orbital ridge. Separate skin and muscle flaps can be reflected. A frontotemporal craniotomy is fashioned flush with the anterior cranial fossa, and the dura is then separated from the skull to allow removal of the lateral third of the greater wing of the sphenoid. Microfibrillar collagen is inserted beneath the bone edges, and tenting sutures are placed.

If an intracerebral hematoma is present, and if the brain is still tense after the administration of mannitol and furosemide, and with hyperventilation, the hematoma is cannulated, and about 5 ml of blood are removed. The extraction of this amount of blood often makes it possible to open the dura without brain herniation. Alternatively, the ventricle is cannulated before opening the dura if the brain remains tense and no intracerebral hemorrhage is present.

Under loupe magnification ×3 and headlight illumination the dura is opened to expose the lateral aspect of the frontal lobe and the anterior temporal lobe, and the dissection proceeds along the sphenoid ridge to the anterior clinoid process. By retraction of the frontal lobe with a ½- to 1-inch Silastic-coated brain retractor, dissection is carried down to the optic nerve. The optic nerve is exposed, and the arachnoid is opened adjacent to the carotid artery. CSF is removed to provide additional exposure. The retractor then is fixed in position; if necessary, a second narrow brain retractor can be introduced to retract the temporal tip and provide exposure to the tentorial notch. It is at this stage that the operating microscope is used until the aneurysm is clipped. Dissection is carried out at 6 to 16× magnification, depending on the structures to be examined. Unless it is a particularly difficult aneurysm, these lesions usually can be clipped without induced hypotension or application of temporary clips. Dissection is continued inferiorly along the internal carotid artery until the aneurysm is identified, and the upper and lower borders of the aneurysmal neck are separated from the arachnoid. The arachnoid around the carotid artery vessel and the aneurysmal neck is gently cut, and a passage, which is free of vessels, is developed on both sides of the neck. Often, the vessels adjacent to the aneurysm blend with the arachnoid covering the aneurysm, necessitating dissection beyond this arachnoidal layer while preserving the vessels in it. Before clipping the neck of the aneurysm, the surgeon must determine the locations of the anterior choroidal and posterior communicating arteries. The clip is applied across the neck of the aneurysm and, if necessary, reapplied to ensure preservation of these vessels. The aneurysm is occluded immediately adjacent to the parent vessel to prevent recurrence of the aneurysm proximal to the clip. Most aneurysms at this location can be obliterated with a single gently curved Yasargil or Sugita clip. Before applying a clip to the aneurysmal neck, the surgeon must test the clip and the clip applier to ensure that the clip can be easily and smoothly released from its holder.

If the aneurysm extends below the tentorium, additional exposure is achieved by coagulation and division of the veins of the temporal lobe tip and gradual retraction of the temporal lobe posteriorly to expose the tentorial edge and the proximal internal carotid artery and the aneurysm. If the aneurysmal sac projects above the tentorium and is buried in the temporal lobe, retraction is limited to the frontal lobe so as to expose the aneurysmal neck without disturbing the lesion further.

Carotid bifurcation aneurysms are frequently encased in dense adhesions between the aneurysm, the anterior and middle cerebral arteries, and vessels entering the anterior perforated substance. One or more vessels may be incorporated in the aneurysm, and clip occlusion may compromise major arterial trunks. Dissection is continued along the internal carotid artery up toward the bifurcation, staying along the anterior and inferior margin of the anterior and middle cerebral arteries while trying to identify the lenticulostriate vessels and anterior choroidal artery. When a carotid bifurcation aneurysm is not adequately visualized by a proximal-to-distal dissection along the internal carotid artery, the sylvian fissure is split and this approach usually provides excellent exposure and access to the aneurysm. If the aneurysm cannot be obliterated with clips, several alternatives are available, including wrapping the aneurysm and parent vessel with surgical gauze or wrapping the entire lesion in surgical or muslin gauze, or deferring to endovascular techniques to obliterate the lesion

Following clipping of the carotid aneurysm, the basal cisterns are irrigated of blood. If an intracerebral hemorrhage is present, enough of the clot is removed before the aneurysm is exposed to carry out the dissection; not until after the aneurysm has been clipped is the remainder of the clot removed. In patients with oculomotor nerve palsy, the aneurysm can be aspirated after clipping to reduce the pressure against this nerve, but no attempt is made to dissect the aneurysm from the nerve.

After the aneurysm is clipped, the patient's blood pressure is maintained at normotensive levels, and hemostasis is confirmed. The microscope may be removed. The cisterns are filled with saline and the brain retractors are removed. The dura is closed. If approximating the dural edges is difficult, a dural graft is interposed. A Jackson-Pratt drain (Heyerschulte, Worcester, MA) is placed subdurally to allow CSF drainage. Postoperative antibiotics are continued until the drain is removed. The bone flap is reinserted and fixed in position with a microplating system using self-tapping screws. The galea and skin are closed as separate layers. The incision and exit sites of the drain are covered with an antibiotic ointment, and a dressing is applied.

Postoperatively, the patient is maintained on sedation, analgesics, anticonvulsants, and nimodipine, and the central venous pressure is maintained at about 10 to 13 mm Hg with fluids and salt-poor albumen. Hypertension is induced if there is evidence of cerebral vasospasm. A baseline postoperative CT is done on day 1 after surgery. Other aspects of the postoperative management are the anticipation and immediate treatment of problems commonly encountered after SAH: bleeding at the surgical site, cerebral vasospasm, cerebral salt-wasting, hydrocephalus, seizures, and cardiopulmonary complications.

## RESULTS

Over the past 50 years, there has been a significant improvement in the outcome of aneurysm patients after they arrive in the hospital. In the 1950s only 15 of every 100 patients who had aneurysms made a useful recovery after reaching the hospital and undergoing angiography. The unfavorable outcomes seen at present result from hemorrhages in older patients and from the immediate effects of the SAH on the brain, compounded by the effects of rebleeding, and of secondary complications inside and outside the nervous system. Currently, most surgical series report that 65% of patients are able to continue their previous activities, 15% are moderately disabled, and there is a 10% mortality rate. The surgical mortality rate is about 5% and the management mortality rate is 4% for grades 1 and 2 patients, 20% for grade 3, and 45% for grades 4 and 5. In patients over age 65 the mortality rate is approximately 15%.

The overall quality of life after SAH remains a concern even as the mortality and morbidity rates drop. Even patients with good outcome may require months to years to fully recover cognitive and behavioral function. These areas must be addressed with patient and family so as to provide ongoing support.

## REFERENCES

1. Dott NM: Intracranial aneurysms: Cerebral arterio-radiography; surgical treatment. Med J (Edinb) 40:219, 1933.
2. Dandy WE: Intracranial aneurysm of the internal carotid artery cured by operation. Ann Surg 107:654, 1938.
3. Okawara SH: Warning signs prior to rupture of the intracranial aneurysm. J Neurosurg 38:575, 1973.
4. Mizukami M, Takemae T, Tazawa T, et al: Value of computerized tomography in the prediction of cerebral vasospasm after aneurysm rupture. Neurosurgery 7:583, 1980.
5. Fisher CM, Kistler JP, Davis JM: Relation of cerebral vasospasm to subarachnoid hemorrhage visualized by computerized tomographic scanning. Neurosurgery 6:1, 1980.
6. Adams HP Jr, Kassell NJ, Kongable GA, et al: Intracranial operation within seven days of aneurysmal subarachnoid hemorrhage: Results in 50 patients. Arch Neurol 45:1065–1069, 1988.
7. Saveland H, Hillman J, Brandt L, et al: Overall outcome in aneurysmal subarachnoid hemorrhage. A prospective study from neurosurgical units in Sweden during a 1-year period. J Neurosurg 79:729–734, 1992.
8. Kassell NF, Torner JC, Jane JA, et al: The International Cooperative Study on the Timing of Aneurysm Surgery. J Neurosurg 73:18–47, 1990.
9. Roos YB, Beenen LF, Groen RJ, et al: Timing of surgery in patients in aneurysmal subarachnoid haemorrhage: Rebleeding is still the major cause of poor outcome in neurosurgical units that aim at early surgery. J Neurol Neurosurg Psychiatry 63:490–493, 1997.
10. Hop JW, Rinkel GJ, Algra A, van Gijn J: Case fatality rates and functional outcome after subarachnoid hemorrhage: A systemic review. Stroke 28:660–664, 1997.
11. Findlay JM: Current management of aneursymal subarachnoid hemor-

rhage guidelines from the Canadian Neurosurgical Society. Can J Neurol Sci 24:161–170, 1997.

12. Le Roux PD, Elliott JP, Newell DW, et al: Predicting outcome in poor-grade patients with subarachnoid hemorrhage: A retrospective review of 159 aggressively managed cases. J Neurosurg 5:39–49, 1996.

13. LeRoux PD, Elliott JP, Downey L, et al: Improved outcome after rupture of anterior circulation aneurysms: A retrospective 10-year review of 224 good-grade patients. J Neurosurg 83:394–402, 1995.

14. Ogilvy CS, Carter BS: A proposed comprehensive grading system to predict outcome for surgical management of intracranial aneurysms. Neurosurgery 42:959–968, 1998.

15. Germano A, Tisano A, Raffaele M, et al: Is there a group of early aneurysmal SAH patients who can expect to achieve a complete long-term neuropsychological recovery? Acta Neurochirurg 139:507–514, 1997.

16. Ogden JA, Utley T, Mee EW: Neurological and psychosocial outcome 4 to 7 years after subarachnoid hemorrhage. Neurosurgery 41:25–34, 1997.

17. Enblad P, Perrsson L: Impact on clinical outcome of secondary brain insults during the neurointensive care of patients with subarachnoid hemorrhage: A pilot study. J Neurol Neurosurg Psychiatry 62:512–516, 1997.

# CHAPTER 84

# Surgical Management of Paraclinoid Aneurysms

■ KAZUHIKO KYOSHIMA, MASATO SHIBUYA, and SHIGEAKI KOBAYASHI

Paraclinoid aneurysms include aneurysms in the C2 and distal C3 portions (Fisher's classification) of the internal carotid artery (ICA).[1] Surgery of these aneurysms presents special difficulties because of their anatomic features as their proximity to complicated bony and dural structures. Some of these aneurysms were considered unclippable or associated with disastrous results when approached surgically, mainly because of the difficulty in securing the proximal parent artery. Furthermore, these aneurysms are often large and adhere tightly to the surrounding structures. Temporary carotid occlusion is often necessary during dissection and clip application, necessitating both preoperative complete circulation study including balloon test occlusion and protection of the brain from ischemic damage during occlusion.[2, 3] In addition to straight clips, special clips are often necessary; a combination of ring clips is essential for ventrally developed aneurysms.[4] With the recent refinement of microsurgical techniques and advancement of surgical anatomic study, their management has changed from conservative surgery to direct neck clipping. With the advent of intravascular surgery,[5] the treatment strategy is gradually changing, but direct clipping is currently the treatment of choice whenever feasible.[6–10]

## ANATOMIC CONSIDERATIONS

Characteristic anatomic features of these aneurysms in this area are their relation to the anterior clinoid process, cavernous sinus, optic nerve, and ophthalmic artery.

The ICA enters into the intracranial space through the carotid canal, which is covered with periosteum. The ICA courses in the space between the dura propria and the periosteum (cavernous sinus) at the middle skull base, where it occasionally produces a mild bony impression called the carotid groove. The ICA then turns posteriorly to form a curve at the bony sulcus at the foundation of the anterior clinoid process; this definite bony sulcus is called the infraclinoid carotid groove.[11] The ICA finally courses into the intradural space and penetrates the dura propria. This penetrating portion is the carotid dural ring (distal ring). The venous space around the ICA in the infraclinoid carotid groove is called the infraclinoid carotid groove sinus (infraclinoid sinus), which is surrounded by the periosteum at the bony side of the carotid groove and the dura propria at the other side and is a peripheral venous space of the cavernous sinus the same as the intercavernous or basilar venous sinus.[11] The entrance of the infraclinoid sinus is the proximal ring, and it is ended by the dural ring distally. The infraclinoid sinus, which is a peripheral venous space and is not a venous lake like the cavernous sinus, could be differentiated from the cavernous sinus. The ICA in this sinus is called the clinoid segment (infraclinoid carotid groove or infraclinoid segment).[11] On the medial side of the dural ring, in most of cases a dural pouch called the carotid cave is present.[12] It is an intradural space seated in the infraclinoid carotid groove with its apex pointing toward proximally. The connection of the dural ring with the ICA at this area is relatively loose. A few superior hypophyseal arteries often arise from the ICA in the carotid cave. The carotid cave may not always exist.

This anatomic relation is obtained by removing the anterior clinoid process and opening the optic canal. In the operating field via the pterional approach with the patient's head rotated to the opposite side about 45 degrees (Fig. 84–1), the carotid cave is located approximately in the ventral side of the ICA. After the anterior clinoid process is completely removed, the periosteal wall of the infraclinoid sinus is seen. By opening the periosteal wall, the infraclinoid segment is exposed. The ICA penetrates the dural ring obliquely, and the lateral side of the ICA at this level of the carotid cave, therefore, belongs to extradural area. The curved portion of the ICA, before it penetrates the dural ring, is called the surgical genu of the ICA. The genu is usually observed horizontally in the operating field, and the concave portion of the genu is called the axilla of the ICA.[12, 13]

The ophthalmic artery usually originates from the superior wall of the carotid artery (Table 84–1) immediately after the carotid artery penetrates the dura propria and it enters the optic canal penetrating the dura propria.[14–16] The ophthalmic artery originates occasionally from extradural portion of the ICA.[4, 16–18] The segment of the ICA between the branching points of the ophthalmic and posterior communicating arteries is the ophthalmic segment; its length

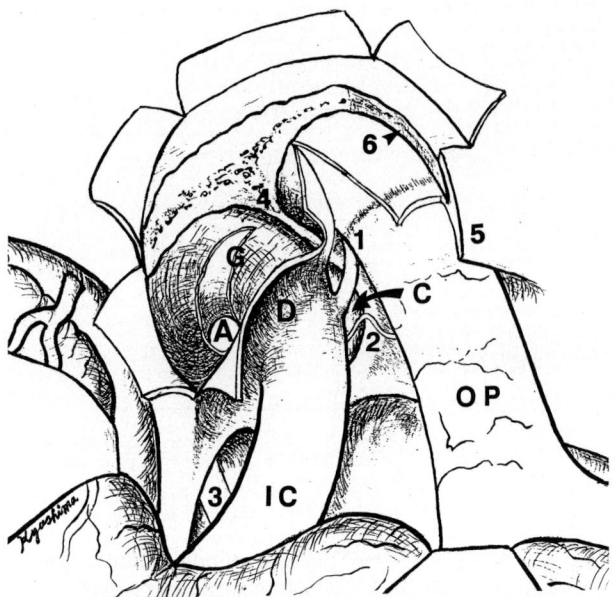

FIGURE 84–1 ■ Schematic drawing of surgical anatomy in the operating field after removal of the anterior clinoid process and optic roof via the left pterional approach with the patient's head rotated to the opposite side about 45 degrees.[11] Note that the internal carotid artery (ICA) penetrates the dural ring obliquely in the field, and the carotid cave is located ventrally where the superior hypophyseal artery originates from the ICA. The infraclinoid portion of the ICA is partially exposed by dissecting the periosteum. The ICA in this area runs horizontally, and the dural ring adheres to the ICA tightly in the dorsal to lateral side. (A, axilla of the ICA; C, carotid cave; D, dural ring; G, surgical genu of the ICA; OP, optic nerve; IC, internal carotid artery; 1, ophthalmic artery; 2, superior hypophyseal artery; 3, oculomotor nerve; 4, optic strut; 5, falciform fold; 6, optic roof.) (From Kyoshima K, Koike G, Hokama M, et al: A classification of juxtadural ring aneurysms with reference to surgical anatomy. J Clin Neurosci 2:61–64, 1996.)

varies from 6 to 15 mm (mean, 9.6 mm) because of anatomic variation of the branching point of the posterior communicating artery along the ICA.[14]

## TERMINOLOGY AND DEFINITION

With regard to surgical difficulty in clipping aneurysms arising from the C2 portion of the ICA, the anterior clinoid process has formerly been considered as an important landmark to describe the limitation of clippability of these aneurysms. Aneurysms in the supraclinoid portion are clippable because they are in the subarachnoid space, whereas those in the infraclinoid portion cannot be clipped

**TABLE 84–1 ■ ORIGIN OF THE OPHTHALMIC ARTERY FROM THE SUPERIOR WALL OF THE CAROTID ARTERY (%)**

|  | Medial Third | Central Third | Lateral Third |
| --- | --- | --- | --- |
| Renn[16] | 72 | 13 | 4 |
| Gibo[14] | 78 | 22 | 0 |
| Lang[15] | 55 | 25 | 20 |

because they are in the cavernous sinus. By the recent surgical and anatomic advancement, those aneurysms in the infraclinoid portion have become feasible for direct surgical treatment with removal of the anterior clinoid process, and the surgical attention is now focused more appropriately on the aneurysm's relationship to the dural ring, instead of the anterior clinoid process. Many aneurysms arising from the C2 and distal C3 portions, however, have no direct relationship to the branching arteries such as the ophthalmic or superior hypophyseal artery. As a result, these lesions are often described according to their relationship to adjacent anatomic landmarks or to the location of aneurysm neck on the ICA, hence such varying terms as para-, supra- and infraophthalmic; para- and supraclinoid; sub-, para- and suprachiasmal; and carotid cave aneurysms, or proximal ICA, global, ventral, and dorsal aneurysms.[19, 20]

We consider that paraclinoid aneurysms in distal C3 and C2 portions can then be classified into two categories as intradural aneurysms near the carotid dural ring. In the first category, aneurysms arising from the ICA within the ophthalmic segment, which is between the branching points of the ophthalmic and posterior communicating arteries and also includes the branching point of the ophthalmic artery, are defined as ophthalmic segment aneurysms abbreviated as ophthalmic aneurysms (Figs. 84–2 and 84–3; see also Figs. 84–7 and 84–8). In the ophthalmic aneurysms, those that have clear relation to the definite branching artery are described as carotid-ophthalmic artery aneurysms abbreviated as carotid-ophthalmic aneurysms if in relation to the ophthalmic artery (see Fig. 84–5), or superior hypophyseal (artery) aneurysms (see Fig. 84–6) if in relation to the superior hypophyseal artery.[19, 21] The ophthalmic segment aneurysms have been classically called "ophthalmic artery aneurysms." But the term of "ophthalmic artery aneurysm" should be used only for the aneurysm arising from the ophthalmic artery itself. Some ophthalmic aneurysms are located far distally from the anterior clinoid process, because of anatomic variations of the arterial branching points. In these cases, the proximal parent artery and aneurysm neck are easily exposed, such as in the ordinary carotid-posterior communicating artery aneurysms. These cases may not be included in paraclinoid aneurysms. In the second category, intradural aneurysms arising from the ICA proximal to the branching level of the ophthalmic artery (usually in the carotid cave) are carotid cave aneurysms (Fig. 84–4).[11, 12, 22] Most of these aneurysms could not be recognized by removal of the anterior clinoid process alone; additional opening of the dural ring enabled their exposure. They were traditionally considered as infraclinoid or cavernous sinus aneurysms and, therefore, were considered unclippable.

Aneurysms may arise at any locations around the cross-section of the ICA,[23] and the difficulties in clipping paraclinoid aneurysms depend not only on the existence of an arterial division or complicated anatomic features but also on their locations in the cross-section of the ICA in the operating field. Therefore, from the surgical point of view, these aneurysms may be categorized. In the operating field, these aneurysms are seen via the pterional approach with the patient's head rotated to the opposite side about 45 degrees, according to their location in relation to the cross-

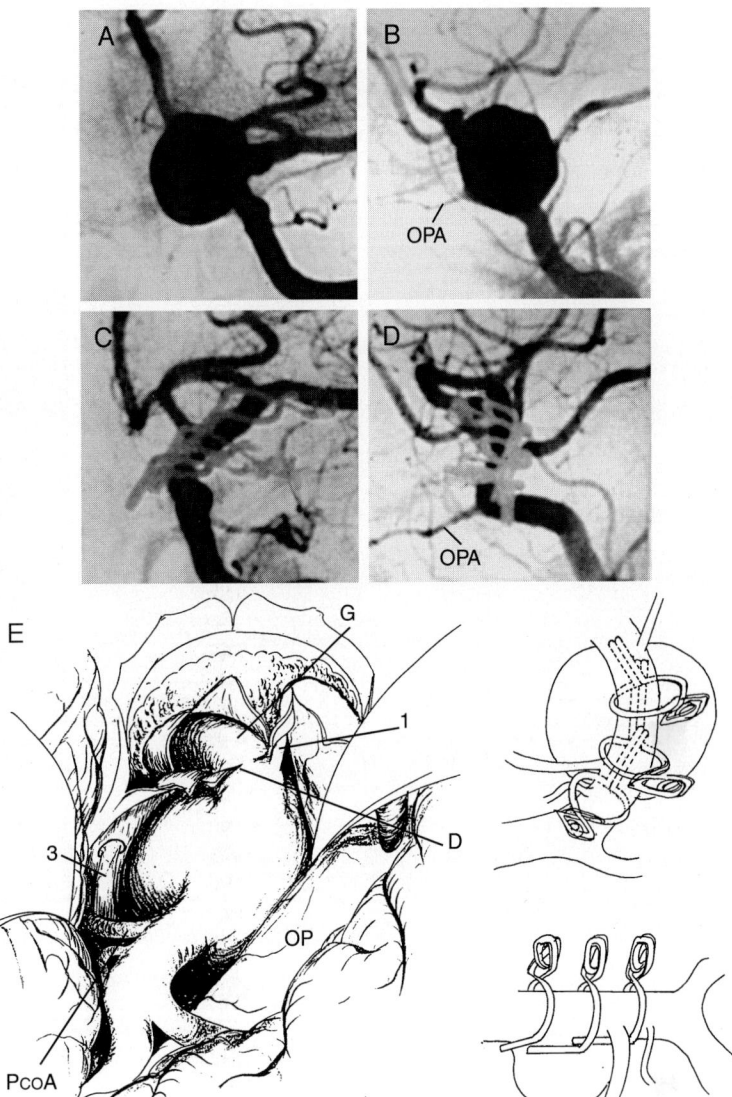

**FIGURE 84–2** ■ A 66-year-old woman with a left ruptured giant ophthalmic aneurysm (ventral type). *A* and *B*, Preoperative angiograms, anteroposterior and lateral views. Note that the aneurysm is directed medially on the anteroposterior view and inferiorly on the lateral view. *C* and *D*, Postoperative angiograms show that the aneurysm was clipped with multiple clips preserving the natural curvature of the internal carotid artery (ICA). (OPA, ophthalmic artery.) *E*, Intraoperative view. A giant aneurysm was seen projecting ventrally. After exposure of the cervical ICA, removal of the anterior clinoid process, unroofing of the ophthalmic artery, sectioning of the dural ring, mobilization of the ophthalmic artery, and exposure of the infraclinoid segment, multiple clipping with ring clips was placed in tandem fashion with direct puncture method under temporary occlusion of the cervical ICA, the ICA distal to the posterior communicating artery (PCoA), the ophthalmic artery, and the PCoA. Postoperatively the patient showed temporary right hemiparesis. In this earlier case, the dural ring was not dissected circumferentially. (D, dural ring; G, surgical genu of the ICA; OP, optic nerve; 1, ophthalmic artery; 3, oculomotor nerve.) (From Kyoshima K, Kobayashi K, Orz YI: Ophthalmic aneurysms. In Kaye AH, Black PM [eds]: Operative Neurosurgery. London, Churchill Livingstone, 1999.)

section of the ICA, as lateral, medial, ventral, or dorsal type.

Lateral-type ICA aneurysms are those that are directed laterally under the tentorium. Medial-type ICA aneurysms are directed medially toward or occasionally under the optic nerve. Ventral-type ICA aneurysms are located in the far side of the approaching route behind the ICA. Dorsal-type ICA aneurysms are located above the tentorium or the optic nerve projecting toward the approaching route in the operative field. A rare type of aneurysms also exists, called global-type aneurysms,[24] which involve the whole circumference of the carotid artery, and whose origins are not easy to identify.

Carotid-ophthalmic aneurysms are usually seen as a medial (Fig. 84–5) type protruding from the medial or dorsomedial wall of the ICA in the operating field. Ventral-type aneurysms may also arise from the medial side of the branching orifice on the ICA.

Carotid cave aneurysms are all of the ventral type depending on the anatomic location of the carotid cave (see Figure 84–4). They may grow out of the cave into the intradural subarachnoid space or the infraclinoid carotid groove sinus beyond the thin dura (propria). When a carotid cave aneurysm has grown distally, it may sometimes be difficult to differentiate from a carotid-ophthalmic aneurysm.

## INCIDENCE

The reported incidence of ophthalmic aneurysms, which may or may not include different types of aneurysms, varies from 0.5% to 5.4%.[23, 25–27]

We have operated on 129 patients with paraclinoid aneurysms, including 44 patients with large to giant aneurysms (34%) at Nagoya University Hospital, Shinshu University Hospital, and their affiliated hospitals. Clinical statistics of Nagoya University counted 41 patients with paraclinoid aneurysms: seven patients with carotid cave aneurysms and 34 patients with ophthalmic aneurysms, including 16 global aneurysms. Researchers at Shinshu University counted 88

*Text continued on page 1141*

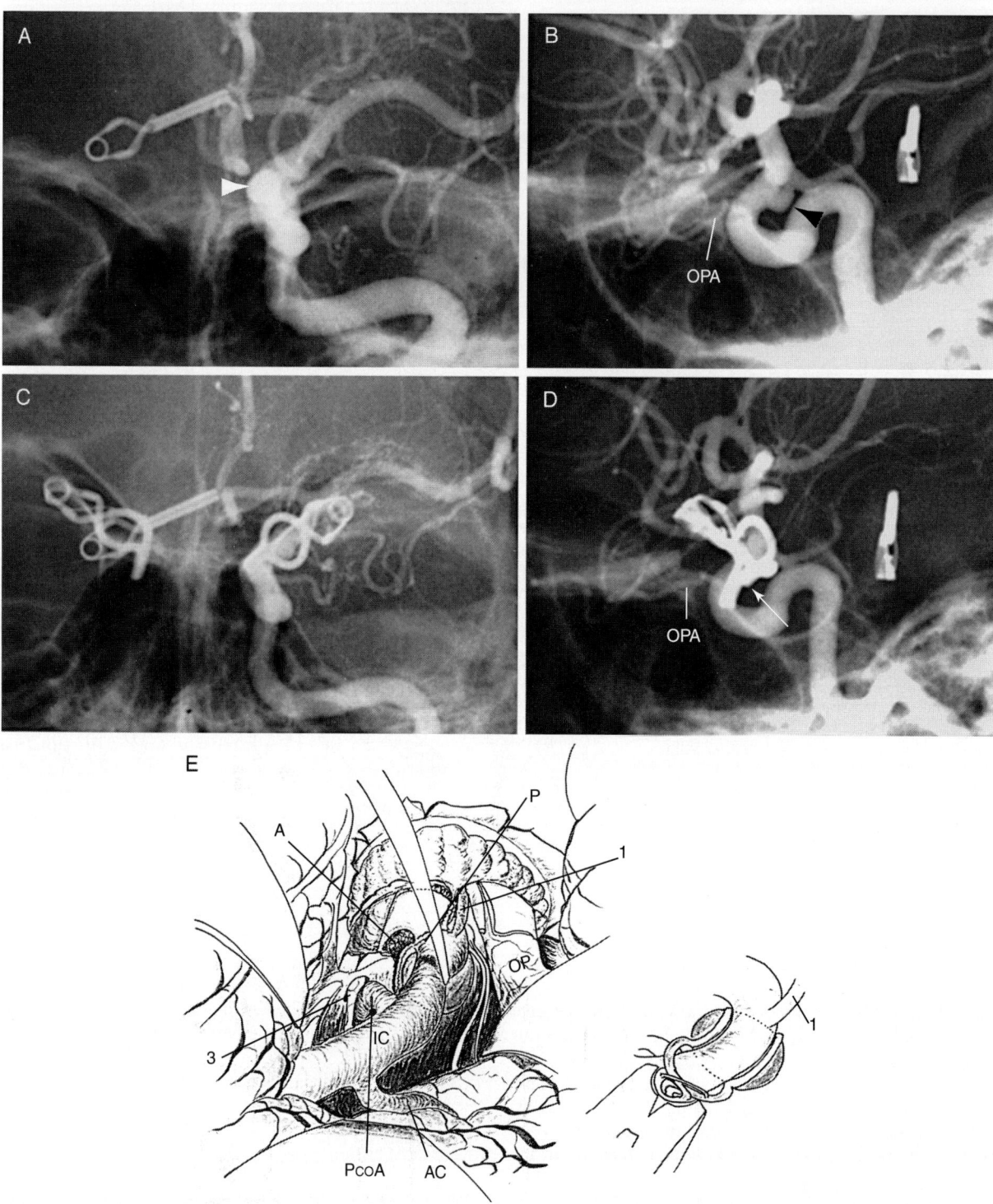

**FIGURE 84–3 ■** A 34-year-old woman with left ophthalmic aneurysms (ventral type), a right carotid cave aneurysm (ventral type), and a ruptured basilar aneurysm (which was clipped earlier). *A* and *B*, Preoperative left carotid angiograms with anteroposterior and lateral views. Note that the left ophthalmic aneurysm is located distally to the ophthalmic artery and directed just medially on the anteroposterior view and inferiorly on the lateral view. *C* and *D*, Postoperative angiograms are taken after clipping both internal carotid aneurysms. The arrowhead indicates the aneurysms. The *arrow* indicates a clip for the aneurysm. (OPA, ophthalmic artery.) *E*, This intraoperative view of the left ophthalmic aneurysm shows that the aneurysm is projecting ventrally. The aneurysm is located just distally to the branching level of the ophthalmic artery and was clipped with a curved-blade ring clip after the procedures of untethering exposure method. (A, axilla of the internal carotid artery; D, dural ring; AC, anterior cerebral artery; OP, optic nerve; PCoA, posterior communicating artery; *Arrow*, left ophthalmic aneurysm; 1, ophthalmic artery; 3, oculomotor nerve.) (From Kyoshima K, Kobayashi K, Orz YI: Ophthalmic aneurysms. In Kaye AH, Black PM [eds]: Operative Neurosurgery. London, Churchill Livingstone, 1999.)

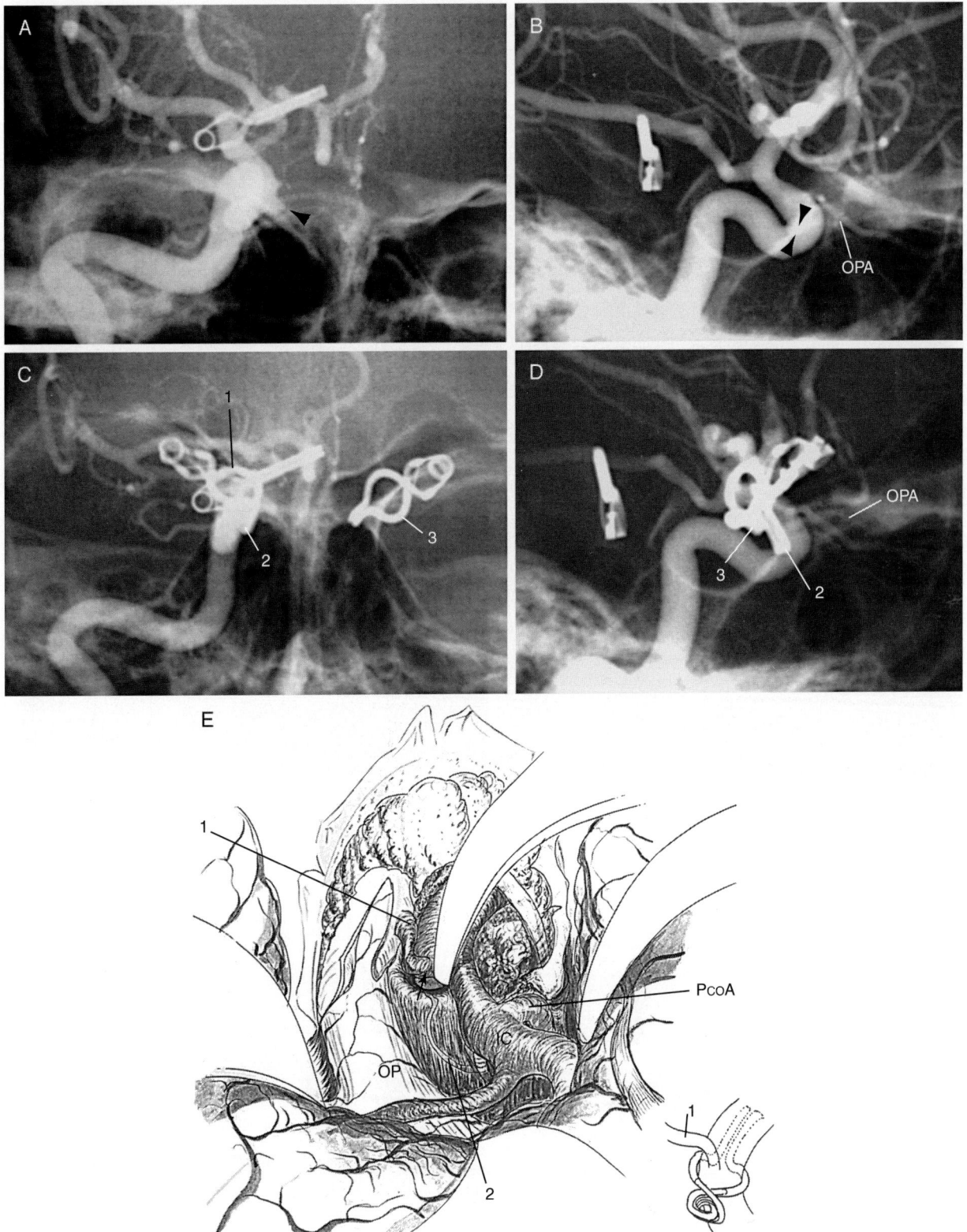

**FIGURE 84–4** ■ A right carotid cave aneurysm (ventral type) of the same case as found in Figure 84–3 (the basilar and left ophthalmic segment aneurysms were previously clipped). *A* and *B*, Preoperative right carotid angiograms with anteroposterior and lateral views. Note that the carotid cave aneurysm is directed medially on the anteroposterior view and located proximally to the ophthalmic artery, superimposing at the hairpin curve of the angiographic genu on the lateral view. *C* and *D*, Postoperative angiograms, which were taken after clipping both internal carotid aneurysms, show that the site of the aneurysm is precisely confirmed by the position of the clip blades. (1, clip for the basilar aneurysm; 2, clip for the carotid cave aneurysm; 3, clip for the opposite ophthalmic segment aneurysm; OPA, the ophthalmic artery.) The *arrowhead* indicates a carotid cave aneurysm. *E*, This intraoperative view shows that the aneurysm is ventrally located in the carotid cave and was clipped with a curved-blade ring clip after the untethering exposure method (see text) with prior exposure of the cervical internal carotid artery (ICA). The ophthalmic artery originated from the ICA extradurally in this case. (PCoA, posterior communicating artery.) The arrow indicates the aneurysm. (From Kyoshima K, Kobayashi K, Orz YI: Ophthalmic aneurysms. In Kaye AH, Black PM [eds]: Operative Neurosurgery. London, Churchill Livingstone, 1999.)

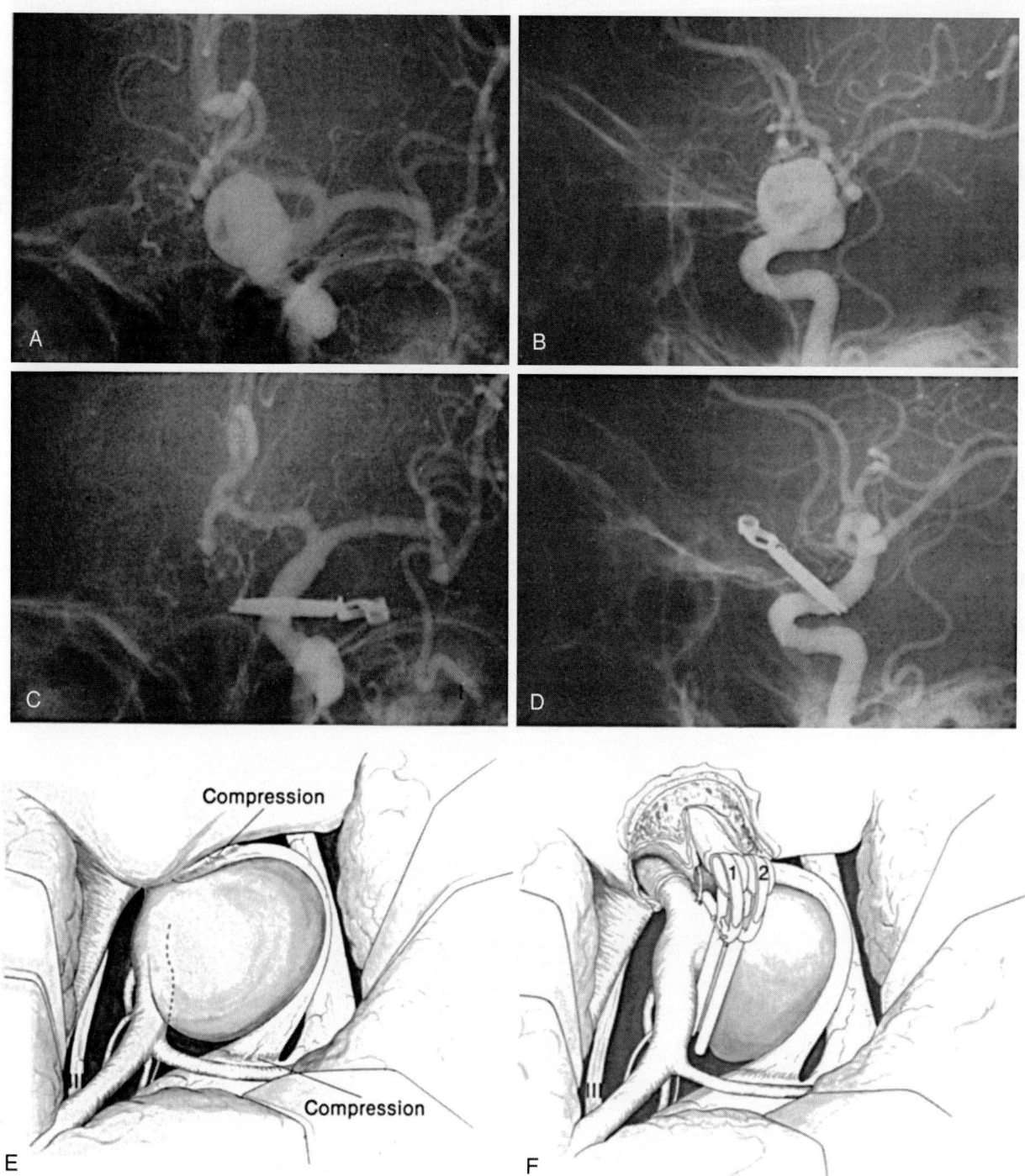

**FIGURE 84–5** ■ A carotid-ophthalmic aneurysm (medial type). *A* and *B*, Preoperative left carotid angiograms with anteroposterior and lateral views. *C* and *D*, Postoperative anteroposterior and lateral views. *E*, An intraoperative view before clipping shows that the left optic nerve was greatly displaced dorsomedially. The optic nerve was compressed anteriorly by the falciform process and posteriorly by the A1 segment of the anterior cerebral artery. *F*, Intraoperative view during clipping. Clip No. 1, which was applied perpendicularly, was not strong enough to close the aneurysm and opened with each pulsation. The larger clip No. 2 closed the aneurysm completely, and clip No. 1 was removed.

patients with 92 paraclinoid aneurysms—42 carotid cave aneurysms and 50 ophthalmic aneurysms.

Paraclinoid aneurysms have a female preponderance, a high incidence of multiple aneurysms, symmetric aneurysms, large size (75% are larger than 10 mm), and high incidence of visual disturbance as the initial symptom as well as subarachnoid hemorrhage (Table 84–2).[7, 23, 25, 27, 28] In carotid cave aneurysms, no patients showed preoperative visual symptoms.

## PREOPERATIVE EVALUATION

### Cerebral Angiography

Transfemoral four-vessel cerebral angiography is preferable to delineate the anatomic relationships among the aneurysm, the carotid, ophthalmic, posterior communicating and anterior choroidal arteries, the anterior clinoid process, and the optic canal. In addition to straight anteroposterior (AP) and lateral views, oblique and basal views are often helpful to identify the neck of an aneurysm. Cross-circulation through the anterior communicating artery and the posterior communicating artery must also be fully examined. Vertebral angiography with ipsilateral carotid compression often helps to determine the collateral flow through the posterior communicating artery and to identify the distal neck of the aneurysm. Balloon occlusion test is mandatory for most patients with paraclinoid aneurysms.

The anatomic relationship between large to giant paraclinoid aneurysms and the optic nerve is often difficult to predict from preoperative angiograms alone. Results of comparative studies of angiographic and intraoperative findings suggest that paraclinoid aneurysms with a closed carotid siphon, and aneurysms that grow inferiorly to the carotid artery stay beneath the optic nerve and compress the nerve from inferiorly (ventral type), although some ophthalmic aneurysms grow above the optic nerve (medial type) and displace it medially.[29] Compression by these aneurysms is usually much less than that by ventral-type aneurysms.

On angiograms, it is difficult to predict the location of the dural ring. But the ophthalmic artery, when visible, and the angiographic genu of the ICA will give approximate landmarks of the ring, which is usually proximal to the ophthalmic artery and located at the level of the angiographic genu. The medial side of the hairpin curve portion

of the angiographic genu corresponds to the level of the carotid cave, and its lateral side is the extradural portion. Because the ICA penetrates the dural ring obliquely (see Fig. 84–1), there is a discrepancy between the angiographic genu and the surgical genu as obtained by the pterional approach. The surgical genu is located more proximally than the angiographic genu.[11] The ophthalmic aneurysm is located at or distally to the branching point of the ophthalmic artery (see Figs. 84–2, 84–3, and 84–7), whereas the carotid cave aneurysm is located proximally (see Fig. 84–4).

In relation to the cross-section of the ICA, the direction of aneurysm projection seen in the operating field can roughly be estimated from the preoperative angiogram. In lateral-type aneurysms, they are directed laterally on the anteroposterior (AP) view and inferiorly on the lateral view. In medial-type aneurysms, they are directed medially on the AP view and superiorly on the lateral view. In ventral-type aneurysms, they are directed medially on the AP view and inferiorly on the lateral view (see Fig. 84–3). In dorsal-type aneurysms, they are directed laterally on the AP view and superiorly on the lateral view. When dorsal-type aneurysms are superimposed with the ICA on the AP view, many of them are adhered to the basal surface of the frontal lobe in the operative field, and when they are superimposed with the ICA on the lateral view, many of them are adhered to the medial surface of the temporal lobe.[30]

Carotid cave aneurysms are located medially on the AP view and posteriorly or laterally on the lateral view, and proximally to the origin of the ophthalmic artery. Then, they project ventrally in the operating field approached pterionally with the patient's head rotated about 45 degrees contralaterally. They are anatomically intradural aneurysms and are located angiographically at the angiographic genu or the anterior siphon knee (see Fig. 84–4).

### Computed Tomography and Magnetic Resonance Imaging

Computed tomography (CT) scan will reveal all giant aneurysms and most large aneurysms as an uniformly enhancing mass. Three-dimensional (3-D) CT scan is useful for planning surgical approach. Thin-slice CT scans are especially helpful in the surgical planning for large to giant paraclinoid aneurysms. Both plain and enhanced CT scans are needed. The former may reveal calcification of the carotid artery and aneurysmal wall,[23] which often disturbs clipping. The shape and size of the anterior clinoid process must also be examined carefully. Air cells in the anterior clinoid process may lead to postoperative cerebrospinal fluid (CSF) leakage. The anterior clinoid process may coalesce with the middle clinoid process to form a bony foramen around the carotid artery; drilling of the anterior clinoid process is extremely difficult in such cases.[31–33] Enhanced CT scans help to determine each relationship of the aneurysm, the carotid artery, and the anterior clinoid process, so that characteristics can be clearly kept in mind when the anterior clinoid process is drilled. Partial intramural thrombus may be revealed by CT scan as irregular enhancement, but magnetic resonance imaging (MRI) is superior for such purposes, as well as for 3-D display of anatomic relation-

TABLE 84–2 ■ DEMOGRAPHIC CHARACTERISTICS OF PATIENTS WITH PARACLINOID ANEURYSMS

| | Yasargil[23]* | Weir[27]* | Present Series |
|---|---|---|---|
| Total number of patients | 272 | 207 | 129 |
| Male/female (%) | 25/75 | 19/81 | 23/77 |
| Multiple aneurysms (%) | 18 | 49 | 40 |
| Symmetric aneurysms (%) | 21 | 11 | 12 |
| Initial symptoms: visual (%) | 11 | 30 | 20 |
| Subarachnoid hemorrhage (%) | 76 | 56 | 23 |

*Patients with "classic" ophthalmic artery aneurysms.

ships between the aneurysm and optic nerve and also surrounding structures. A 3-D CT scan would give better operative view of the aneurysm in relation to the parent artery than that provided by MRI; however, finer arteries like the superior hypophyseal artery are not shown.

## SURGICAL TREATMENT

All the information about the patient's condition, age, and the multiplicity and characteristics of the aneurysm as well as the collateral circulation must be carefully evaluated so that the most appropriate form of treatment is selected; that is, direct clipping, carotid occlusion with or without bypass surgery, or endovascular surgery. The results of balloon test occlusion of the carotid artery provide important information for making such a decision.[3]

### Positioning and Craniotomy

The ipsilateral pterional approach is usually taken for most paraclinoid aneurysms. Contralateral and interhemispheric approaches are limited to special cases of symmetric aneurysms or small, medially directed aneurysms.[34] The patient's head is elevated 25 to 45 degrees (depending on the estimation of intraoperative bleeding from the infraclinoid and cavernous sinus), then rotated 45 degrees to the contralateral side and fixed to the headholder with four pins. In the direct approach to paraclinoid aneurysms, more contralateral rotation of the head than in other cases of ICA aneurysms is required, because the optic nerve and ICA are overlapped at their proximal portions, and ophthalmic aneurysms have an intimate relation to the optic nerve, which covers and tends to hide their origin. By an extra head rotation, the optic nerve and the ICA can be seen more or less parallel, allowing less retraction of the ICA or optic nerve.

The ipsilateral neck must be cleaned and draped in the same operative field so that the carotid artery can be compressed manually in case of emergency. We usually expose the cervical carotid artery to allow temporary occlusion in difficult cases.

A semicoronal skin incision is made from just anterior to the tragus, crossing the midline behind the hairline to the contralateral side by about 4 cm. The frontal branch of the superficial temporal artery should always be preserved as a donor for anastomosis if needed.[35] A frontotemporal craniotomy is made with three bur holes. Medial enlargement of the craniotomy by 2 to 3 cm gives more freedom for clip application. After substantial removal of the sphenoid wing to the lateral corner of the superior orbital fissure, we usually open the dura and dissect the sylvian fissure to inspect the aneurysm and to secure the carotid artery distal to the aneurysm.

### Dissection of the Aneurysm

Wide splitting of the sylvian fissure may allow easier retraction of the brain. In large to giant aneurysms that

compress the optic nerve, sectioning the falciform ligament of the optic canal should be undertaken first before proceeding to the following procedures.

In acute-stage surgery performed when the brain is swollen, lumbar CSF drainage or ventricular drainage may be helpful for easy and safe brain retraction. We use a soft suction tube made of a ventricular tube from a ventriculoperitoneal shunt to keep the operating field clean and dry by constantly removing blood, CSF, or bone dust.

The important procedure in direct surgery of paraclinoid aneurysms is freeing the parent ICA by untethering it from the surrounding structures. Surgical procedures such as extensive removal of the anterior clinoid process, unroofing of the optic canal, mobilization of the ophthalmic artery, exposure of the infraclinoid segment by opening the infraclinoid sinus, and circumferential sectioning of the dural ring allow an excellent exposure and mobilization of the parent ICA (untethering exposure method), thus providing enough proximal exposure for temporary carotid clipping, if required, to facilitate clip application.

On removal of the anterior clinoid process, we prefer to observe it both extradurally and intradurally by cutting the dura mater vertically toward the anterior clinoid process as needed,[33] because premature rupture of the aneurysm during an exclusively epidural drilling can lead to an catastrophy.[36] Dural covering must be left to protect the aneurysm or parent ICA, and temporary cervical carotid occlusion may be helpful to decrease the tension and size of the aneurysm during critical drilling; however, this has to be done carefully and for a short time to avoid thromboembolism. Constant irrigation is mandatory to protect the optic nerve from heat injury. The optic canal should be completely opened anteriorly to the orbit, laterally to the floor by drilling the optic strut along with the anterior clinoid process with a high-speed diamond drill.[31, 32] The medial wall of the optic canal must be carefully drilled, and the surgeon should try not to open the sphenoid air sinus. Once opened, they should be packed with muscle, fibrin glue, or Biobond. Exenteration of the sinus is not recommended; rather, it should be covered by the mucosa to keep the sinus clean.

The ophthalmic artery is mobilized from the dura in the optic canal. In order to find the origin of the ophthalmic artery, direct retraction of the ICA laterally is helpful as the optic sheath is opened.

The infraclinoid segment of the ICA is exposed by opening the periosteum over the infraclinoid sinus. Bleeding from the infraclinoid sinus is easily controlled by elevation of the patient's head and packing with Oxycel cotton, Gelfoam, or Surgicel proximally along the wall of the ICA. However, excessive packing may compress the cranial nerves and disturb further dissection by forming a mass. The dural ring is finally cut circumferentially and thus substantial untethering of the ICA is obtained.

Although the extent of bone removal of the optic canal and the anterior clinoid process depends on the characteristics of each aneurysm, the untethering exposure method is necessary in cases of the paraclinoid aneurysm whose neck is located close to the dural ring or of large to giant aneurysms to secure the proximal parent artery and aneurysm neck. Without sectioning the dural ring, it may disturb the advancement of the clip blades and result in incomplete clipping.

Gentle retraction of the tip of the temporal lobe preserving bridging veins is required. Cutting the dura at medial side of the attachment of bridging veins and retraction of the temporal tip with the dura including the sphenoparietal sinus will facilitate further retraction of the temporal tip, if necessary.

Dissection of the aneurysm from the carotid artery and optic nerve is carried out with silver dissectors. Those with various shapes and sharpness of blades or bends of the tips should be prepared. The most difficult part of surgery for large to giant aneurysms in this location is dissection of the thin aneurysmal wall from thick fibrous adhesion to the basal dura. Unless over two thirds of the circumference of the aneurysmal wall is dissected free, clipping cannot be performed in a good shape without slipping. Sharp dissection with a knife or scissors and the use of a solid and less malleable dissector shorten the time to dissect tough and fibrous adhesions around the aneurysm.

Direct retraction of the ICA and optic nerve may facilitate the procedures. Careful retraction of the ICA laterally or the optic nerve medially brings the proximal portion of the internal carotid artery and the neck of the aneurysm into view. Retraction of the optic nerve should be undertaken as minimally as possible. However, if it is necessary, a normal optic nerve can be retracted as much as about 5 mm intermittently and during the procedures protection of the optic nerve with Silastic sheet is advisable.[37–39]

## Carotid Occlusion

Temporary or permanent occlusion of the carotid artery may be needed for surgical treatment of the paraclinoid aneurysms. Temporary occlusion is performed when a critical region is drilled or dissected or when the aneurysm is trapped and punctured. Permanent occlusion may be performed as the final treatment with or without bypass surgery.[40] Before the carotid artery is occluded, the brain should be protected from ischemic injury. We usually administer the following drugs: heparin sodium (3000 to 4000 IU),[41] thiamylal sodium (150 to 250 mg), methylprednisolone (250 mg), mannitol (20%, 100 ml), or low molecular weight dextran (10%, 40 ml/hr) and diphenylhydantoin (125 to 250 mg). Although the brain is monitored continuously by electroencephalography or by somatosensory evoked potential, temporary occlusion should be kept as short as possible. When longer trapping time is needed, it should be divided into several intermittent occlusions, and during periods of occlusion, the systemic blood pressure should be elevated above the preoperative level. Brain ischemia is usually more severe during surgery than at the time of preoperative balloon test occlusion because of the additional factor of brain retraction. If the patient cannot tolerate balloon test occlusion because of poor collateral circulation, an extracranial-intracranial bypass must be performed before the surgery to occlude the aneurysm.

## Decompression of Aneurysm

In large to giant aneurysms, it is important to collapse the aneurysm to achieve satisfactory clipping and also to decompress the optic apparatus in the case with visual signs.

Aneurysms do not collapse by the temporary trapping of the carotid artery alone; however, to make them collapse, blood must be withdrawn either by direct puncture of the aneurysmal dome,[42] from the internal carotid artery,[43] or from a branch of the external carotid artery in the neck.[44] We use a 21-gauge butterfly-type needle. Recently, we have used a specially designed puncture needle[45] to puncture the aneurysm after temporary trapping, with the needle held by a small hemostat, which is fixed to a self-retaining retractor. Fifty to 200 ml of blood is withdrawn from the tube connected to the butterfly needle. When an aneurysm is punctured, the needle must be inserted at a point as distal from the neck as possible so that the puncture site will not be involved in the clipping site. When multiple clips are applied, 1.5- to 2-mm width of aneurysmal wall is needed for each blade. Sometimes, this method of withdrawing blood is unsatisfactory, and the aneurysm does not collapse because blood comes through the ophthalmic artery when temporary trapping is made between the infraclinoid segment and the ICA proximal to the posterior communicating artery or through anastomoses between the internal and external carotid arteries when proximal trapping is made at the cervical ICA. Under these circumstances rapid suction is used; once the aneurysm is collapsed, its wall must be dissected from the surrounding tissues as quickly as possible to shorten the trapping time, whereby a special care should be taken not to traumatize the optic nerve.

## Clip Application

Clipping techniques vary depending on the anatomic situation and the size of the aneurysm. A large clip with a stronger closing force is often needed because of high intramural pressure and a thick aneurysmal wall. In these cases, a Sugita booster clip, by which 250 g can be added to the closing force, is useful.

For aneurysms free of the arterial division, perpendicular clipping (the clip blades are placed in a direction perpendicular to the axis of the ICA) may be applied, but parallel clipping (clip blades are placed parallel to the axis) is generally recommended. When an aneurysm is obliterated perpendicularly, the neck becomes tensive and tearing at the neck or kinking of the parent artery may occur. Neck tearing is more likely to occur because the ICA is larger and often harder than other major cerebral arteries. For small aneurysms located free of the arterial division, however, the parallel clipping is occasionally difficult as clip blades may slip off the small dome of the aneurysm.

For aneurysms related to the arterial division, perpendicular clipping is possible (see Fig. 84–5). As the clip blades close the aneurysm neck, a branching artery approximates to the side of the parent artery, and this will reduce the tension at the aneurysm neck by the decreased angle between the branching artery and the parent ICA. For aneurysms with a wide neck, however, parallel clipping or multiple clipping is required.

In lateral-type aneurysms, it is important to try to identify the posterior communicating artery during surgery, even though it is not seen on the preoperative angiogram. Medial-type aneurysms are often related to the ophthalmic artery, and most of them are carotid-ophthalmic aneurysms. Ventral-type aneurysms are located in the far side of the approaching route under the ICA and sometimes have a relation to the ophthalmic artery. It is usually very difficult to occlude them with conventional clips; however, with the introduction of ring clips, especially an angled ring clip with or without curbed-blades, their obliteration has become relatively easy.[4, 12, 46, 47] Using an angled ring clip, clip blades naturally become parallel to the axis of the ICA and the parent artery is reconstructed by the ring portion of the clip. All carotid cave aneurysms belong to this type. On clipping of carotid cave aneurysms, the untethering exposure method is essential. It is important to dissect the ICA from the dural ring completely and to place the tips of clip blades in the axilla for prevention of the parent artery stenosis or obstruction by clipping. Dorsal-type aneurysms include not only blister-like aneurysms but also usual saccular aneurysms.[30, 48–50] They are frequently adherent to the frontal or temporal lobe. Large to giant aneurysms are rare in this type.[51] Blister aneurysms are unlikely to grow large without rupture. They are usually small, fragile, and wide-based and at surgery intraoperative rupture occurs very frequently, requiring special techniques.[30, 50] Parallel clipping should be undertaken with an L-shaped or curved-blades clip, and a clip should be placed in such a way that the clip blades partially include the wall of the parent artery causing some stenosis. Reversed parallel clipping (a clip is applied from the proximal side of the ICA) is advisable to avoid tearing of the aneurysm neck caused by pressure on the clip head when brain retraction is released. Temporary occlusion of the parent artery at the time of clipping is necessary. The perpendicular clipping is contraindicated, because it may cause tearing of the fragile neck.

## Large to Giant Aneurysms

A large to giant aneurysm with a very broad neck presents a much greater problem. A single long clip may not completely close the aneurysm neck, owing to a high intraluminal pressure and thick, broad aneurysm neck, and is likely to kink or occlude the ICA because the clip is pushed down by a bulbous sac. A multiple clipping technique in various combinations[46–48, 52] is feasible to prevent the straightening of the ICA to conform to its natural curvature at the C2-C3 portion and to obtain a sufficient closing force to occlude the neck completely.

Most of the large to giant aneurysms are of the ventral type and are rarely of the dorsal type. Ventral-type aneurysms may grow very large because their wall is protected by the overlying internal carotid artery and underlying dura of the pituitary fossa.

In large to giant ventral-type aneurysms, it is easier to expose the aneurysm neck or to identify arteries around the neck than in smaller ones. In those aneurysms, the neck is spread almost in the same plane of the dorsal wall of the ICA, whereas, in small aneurysms with a diameter less than that of the ICA, the aneurysm neck is likely hidden by the ICA. For clipping of large to giant ventral-type aneurysms, ring clips are usually the first choice. Clips

must be applied along the course of the artery to keep the lumen of the artery adequately wide. For such purposes, use of multiple ring clips[4] with short blades is better than use of a single clip with long blades, and ring clips with curved blades that fit the C2-C3 curve are especially useful (see Figs. 84–3, 84–4, and 84–6). Clips are made specifically for such purposes for the right and left carotid arteries. A side-angled clip applier is also useful in this location, especially for medially directed aneurysms. Apertures of the Sugita ring clips are 3 or 5 mm in diameter, and the diameter of the carotid artery is usually a little less than 5 mm. To keep the lumen of the carotid artery as wide as possible, the clip must be inserted deep enough so that the near rim of the ring almost touches the dorsal wall of the carotid artery. When multiple ring clips are applied, the spring portion of the clips must be placed as parallel to each other as possible to keep a good alignment and to avoid cross-biting of the blades. Narrowing of the carotid artery caught in the ring almost always results from lack of dissection of adhesion of the aneurysm to the surrounding tissue, usually the dura mater. When the branching artery does not originate from the aneurysm, the aneurysm can be occluded with ring clips in tandem fashion (see Fig. 84–2). When the major branching artery originates from the neck or near the body of the aneurysm, the branching artery can be reconstructed with a straight ring clip (branching artery formation clipping).[4] It is often preferable to occlude the distal part of the aneurysm neck by a regular non-ring clip from the lateral or medial side of the ICA in order to preserve fine perforating arteries.[4] After the clips are applied and the patency of the carotid artery preserved, care must be taken not to constrict the posterior communicating, anterior choroidal arteries and their perforating branches when brain retraction is released, because the angled clips tend to rotate when the brain returns to its original place. Such rotation can be avoided by breaking the pia mater of the frontal lobe where the spring portion of the clip is hitting.

In lateral or medial type of large to giant aneurysms with a wide neck, clipping is often more difficult than for large to giant ventral aneurysms. Sometimes, in the case of a giant aneurysm it is impossible, because ring clips cannot be used as for ventral aneurysms, and the perpendicular clipping may cause tearing of the neck or kinking of the parent artery and placing clip blades parallel to the parent artery is technically difficult. In this situation, an attempt should be made to place the clip blades as parallel as possible with multiple clips. If the clip blades are placed perpendicularly, it is advisable to place them away from the aneurysm neck to the dome side.[4]

In some cases, kinking of the anterior or middle cerebral artery caused by elongation or displacement of the ICA by clipping a large aneurysm may occur and result in cerebral infarction. When the kinking is observed, alternative methods, which include relocation of the clip(s), replacement of the clip(s) to another clip(s) with shorter blades, or changing of the combination of clips may be tried.[52]

Partially thrombosed aneurysms are particularly difficult to clip. Clips applied to the neck of these aneurysms may not close completely but slide to or away from the parent artery unless the thrombus is removed. Intra-aneurysmal endarterectomy is often needed in such cases. Great care must be taken to prevent thrombi from migrating into the carotid stream; use of heparin and careful application of clips are important for this purpose. Ultrasonic Doppler flow meter (EME, Germany or VTI Surgical Doppler, USA) and intraoperative angiography help to check the clipping and to avoid kinking of the parent artery.

## Closure

The defected portion by opening the infraclinoid carotid groove is covered with a piece of temporalis muscle. If fibrin glue is applied, care should be taken to avoid direct contact of the glue to the optic or oculomotor nerve. Small titanium plates are useful to prevent a depression of the bone flap postoperatively.

## Bypass Surgery

The carotid artery may be occluded without causing neurologic deficits in patients with sufficient collateral flow. Balloon occlusion of the carotid artery is often the treatment of choice in elderly patients with difficult extradural aneurysms, but long-term results of such treatment in patients with paraclinoid aneurysm are not known. Furthermore, later development of hypertension or aneurysm in the remaining carotid artery[53] may have to be considered, especially in younger patients. Occlusion of the carotid artery in patients with poor collateral flow must be preceded by an intracranial-extracranial bypass, which can rescue patients with unclippable aneurysms, or those with hard calcification in the wall, fusiform aneurysm, or rupture of the aneurysm near the neck. Superficial temporal artery to middle cerebral artery anastomosis[35] may be performed if the superficial temporal artery is well developed, but flow through such a bypass is usually small and an insufficient substitute to that of the carotid artery. External carotid artery to middle cerebral artery bypass using either a saphenous vein,[41, 54] or a radial artery graft[55] are usually superior to superficial temporal artery to middle cerebral artery anastomosis. However, long-term follow-up of patients who have had these bypass surgeries must be accumulated to evaluate the most appropriate methods. Such bypass surgery may have to be performed even temporarily for patients with very poor collateral flow yet who need temporary carotid occlusion. After successful clipping of the aneurysm, with patency of the carotid artery preserved, the bypass may close spontaneously.

## Results

Of 129 patients with paraclinoid aneurysms, direct clipping was performed in 123 patients, wrapping in four, and trapping in two. Prophylactic superficial temporal artery to middle cerebral artery anastomosis was performed in one patient. External carotid artery to M2 bypass using saphenous vein graft was performed in three sides of two patients whose aneurysms were trapped together with the internal carotid artery. Patency was obtained in all anastomoses.

In small aneurysms, 80 of 85 patients obtained excellent results (94%) and resumed their full daily activities; 12 patients showed some postoperative visual deficits due to surgical manipulation. Wrapping was performed in two carotid cave aneurysms at early stage of this series. Three patients were poor; two patients did not improve from their poor preoperative condition due to rupture of the accompanied aneurysms, and another patient became disabled due to intraoperative thrombosis related to temporary occlusion of the ICA. Two patients died owing to worsening of preoperative poor condition; one was due to ICA occlusion, and another was due to subcortical hematoma.

In large to giant aneurysms, however, the results of these patients were not as good, with 33 of 44 patients obtaining excellent results (75%) and 4 of the 44 patients, with unruptured large or giant aneurysms, becoming moderately or severely disabled, probably because of complications of temporary carotid occlusion. Three patients had no improvement from their poor preoperative condition because of subarachnoid hemorrhage. Another patient (Hunt grade IV), who had bilateral ophthalmic aneurysms, did not improve after surgery. One patient in whom a giant basilar tip aneurysm and a large ophthalmic aneurysm were clipped on the same day became severely disabled because of intraoperative midbrain ischemia complicating the clipping of the basilar aneurysm. Two patients died; one patient with a giant global aneurysm died of progressive thrombosis because of narrowing of the internal carotid artery caused by a dislocated clip, and another patient with a giant nonruptured aneurysm died of postoperative rupture owing to slipping out of the clip.

Representative cases are described in the following case reports.

## C A S E   R E P O R T S

### Case Report 1 (see Fig. 84–5)

A carotid-ophthalmic aneurysm occurred in a 61-year-old woman with finger counting ability only in the left eye, a homonymous right lower quadrantanopia with a central scotoma in the left eye, and a mild left ptosis. A left carotid angiogram revealed a 16-mm aneurysm protruding superomedially from the C2 portion of the internal carotid artery. The angiogram also showed a defect due to an intramural thrombus (see Fig. 84–5A, B). The left carotid artery was secured in the neck. Intracranially, the left optic nerve was markedly pinched between the aneurysm and the falciform process anteriorly and between the aneurysm and the A1 posteriorly (see Fig. 84–5E). The optic canal was opened, and the anterior clinoid process was removed with a diamond bur. The aneurysm originated just distal to the ophthalmic artery and was protruding medially in the operating field (medial type). A No. 18 straight clip (No. 1 in Fig. 84–5F) was applied perpendicularly to the neck of the aneurysm, but this clip opened with each pulsation, which required the addition of a stronger, No. 19a clip (No. 2 in Fig. 84–5F) parallel to the first clip, which was then removed (see Fig. 84–5C, D). The oculomotor nerve was compressed by the carotid artery, which was displaced laterally by the aneurysm. The patient's visual acuity was unchanged after the surgery, but her ptosis disappeared.

*Comment.* Securing the carotid artery in the neck is safer for difficult ophthalmic aneurysms, or the neck should at least be draped along with the operative field so that the carotid artery can be compressed without a delay in an emergency. Carotid-ophthalmic aneurysms usually grow underneath the optic nerve, as seen in this case. Straight clips can be applied perpendicularly for most carotid-ophthalmic aneurysms, which arise at the branching point of the ophthalmic artery medially to the carotid artery in the operating field. A booster clip (or a larger clip) should be used when the closing force of a clip is insufficient. The extent of opening of the optic canal and removal of the anterior clinoid process should be decided after inspection of the anatomic relation of the aneurysm to the surrounding structures such as the optic nerve, the carotid artery, and the anterior clinoid process.

## Case Report 2 (Fig. 84–6)

A superior hypophyseal aneurysm occurred in a 51-year-old woman. This patient had a subarachnoid hemorrhage 6 weeks before surgery. A ventriculoperitoneal shunt had been inserted for the treatment of hydrocephalus in another hospital. At admission, the patient had no neurologic deficits. A right carotid angiogram showed a small aneurysm protruding medially from the C2 portion (see Fig. 84–6A, B). Intraoperatively, the aneurysm was hidden underneath the optic nerve and the anterior clinoid process (medial type) (see Fig. 84–6E). The proximal neck of the aneurysm was found when the well-pneumatized roof of the optic canal and the anterior clinoid process were removed. The superior hypophyseal artery originated from the proximal part of the aneurysm (Fig. 84–6F). A No. 73 ring clip with curved blades successfully obliterated the aneurysm, as confirmed by postoperative angiography (see Fig. 84–6C, D). It should be noted that the clip blades follow the natural curve of the carotid artery. The opened air cells in the roof of the optic canal and the anterior clinoid process were packed with muscle and fibrin glue. The patient was discharged without neurologic deficits.

*Comment.* Curved blades of the clip fit the natural curve of the carotid artery without causing kinking. Both bayonet and angled clips had been tried over the carotid artery, but their tips did not proceed deeply enough, and they hit a bone of the sella turcica. Consequently, they would have to be applied perpendicularly and not in parallel to the long axis of the carotid artery if such a clip as used in this patient was not available.

## Case Report 3 (Fig. 84–7)

A giant ventral-type (or global type) aneurysm occurred in a 60-year-old woman, who came to the hospital complaining of poor vision in the right eye (20/600) and had good vision in the left (20/25). Angiograms showed a 40-mm aneurysm projecting inferomedially from the C2 portion of the left carotid artery that occupied the suprasellar space (see Fig. 84–7A, B). Collateral flow through both the anterior communicating and the posterior communicating arteries was good, and the patient tolerated the balloon test occlusion for 20 minutes. During surgery, the aneurysm markedly elevated the bilateral optic nerves and chiasm, especially in the right optic nerve, which was severely pinched between the aneurysm and the right A1, and it was considered to be the cause of poor vision in the right eye (see Fig. 84–7E). After heparinization and brain protection, the aneurysm was trapped and collapsed by puncturing it with a butterfly needle held by a hemostat and a self-retaining retractor and connected to a syringe for suctioning blood. Severe adhesion of the aneurysmal wall to the basal dura was sharply dissected, and the aneurysm was occluded with three ring clips applied in tandem or vis-à-vis fashion (facing or crossing fashion[46]) (see Fig. 84–7F). Total trapping time of the carotid artery was 21 minutes. Postoperative angiograms showed obliteration of the aneurysm and patency of the carotid artery and its branches well preserved (see Fig. 84–7C, D). However, the patient suffered from moderate right hemiparesis due to infarction in the territory of the lenticulostriate arteries, which could not be detected by the intraoperative electroencephalographic monitoring.

*Comment.* Application of multiple ring clips is the treatment of choice for such a giant ventral carotid aneurysm. Multiple clips with shorter blades must be used rather than a single clip with longer blades so that the lumen of the carotid artery is kept open. Collapse of the aneurysm is essential for clipping. We prefer a direct aneurysmal puncture to withdrawal of blood than from the carotid artery in the neck. The aneurysm must be punctured at the dome, leaving enough distance away from the parent artery (longer than 6 mm when three clips are applied) so that the punctured hole is not involved under the clip blades.

## Case Report 4 (Fig. 84–8)

Bilateral ophthalmic aneurysms occurred in a 67-year-old woman, who suffered subarachnoid hemorrhage and was admitted in a semicomatose state. A CT scan revealed a severe subarachnoid hemorrhage in the basal cistern. Carotid angiograms showed a giant dorsal-type left and a large medial-type right ophthalmic aneurysm. The left A1 was hypoplastic, and bilateral anterior cerebral arteries were supplied by the right carotid artery (see Fig. 84–8A, B). Collateral flow through the posterior communicating artery was also not seen. Cerebral blood flow measured with Tc-hexamethylpropyleneamine oxime (HM-PAO) showed that the blood flow was severely decreased during compression of the carotid artery in the cervical region in the left side. Because of the lack of collateral circulation, bypass surgery was considered essential, even during temporary carotid occlusion. Although no preoperative evidence existed to determine which aneurysm had ruptured, the larger one on the left side was operated on first.

Two weeks after the hemorrhage, a left external

*Text continued on page 1150*

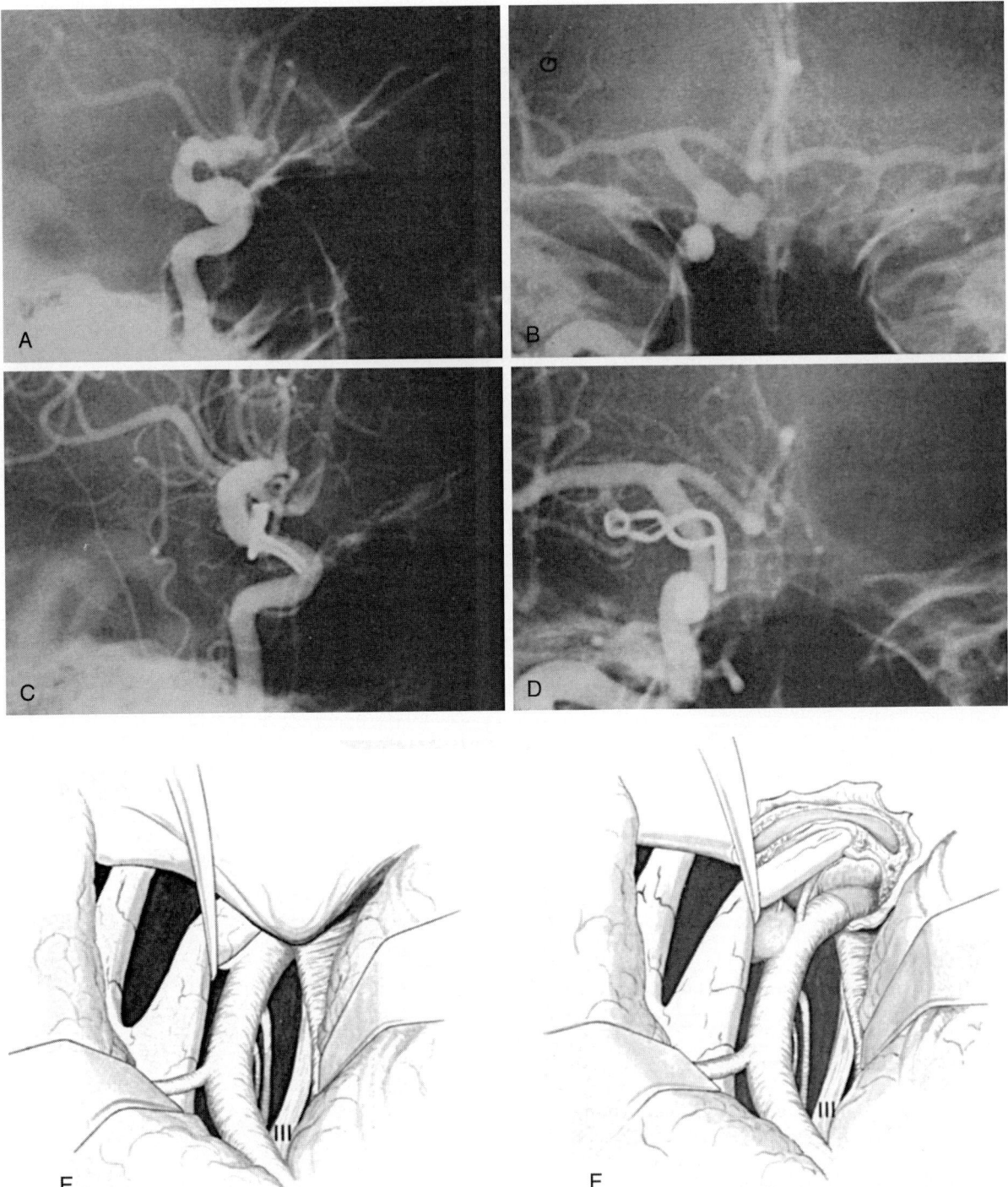

**FIGURE 84–6** ■ A superior hypophyseal aneurysm (medial type). *A* and *B*, Preoperative right carotid angiograms containing lateral and anteroposterior views with manual compression of the left carotid artery. *C* and *D*, Postoperative angiograms show that the fenestrated clip with curved blades fits the curve without causing narrowing of the carotid artery. *E* and *F*, Intraoperative views show that the aneurysm was hidden behind the optic nerve and the anterior clinoid process and was well visualized after opening the optic canal and removing the anterior clinoid process.

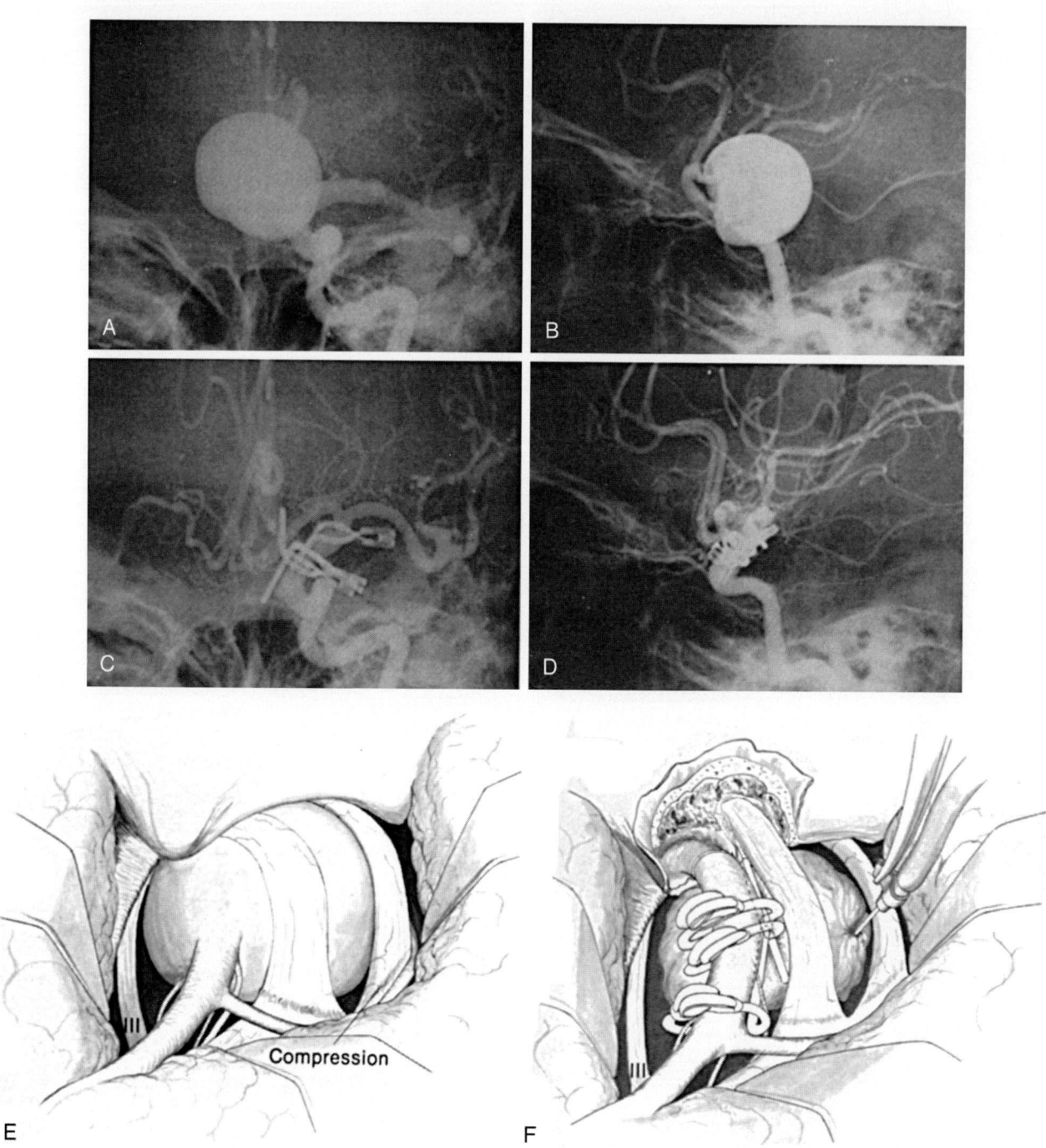

**FIGURE 84-7** ■ A giant ophthalmic aneurysm (ventral type). *A* and *B*, A preoperative left carotid angiogram with anteroposterior and lateral views. *C* and *D*, Postoperative angiograms show that the aneurysm has been excluded and the lumen of the internal carotid artery is well preserved. *E* and *F*, Intraoperative views show that the giant aneurysm developed ventral to the internal carotid artery, compressing both optic nerves from below. After the internal carotid artery was temporarily trapped, the aneurysm was punctured with a butterfly needle, which was held by a self-retaining retractor. The aneurysm was occluded with three fenestrated clips that were applied in tandem and vis-à-vis fashion.

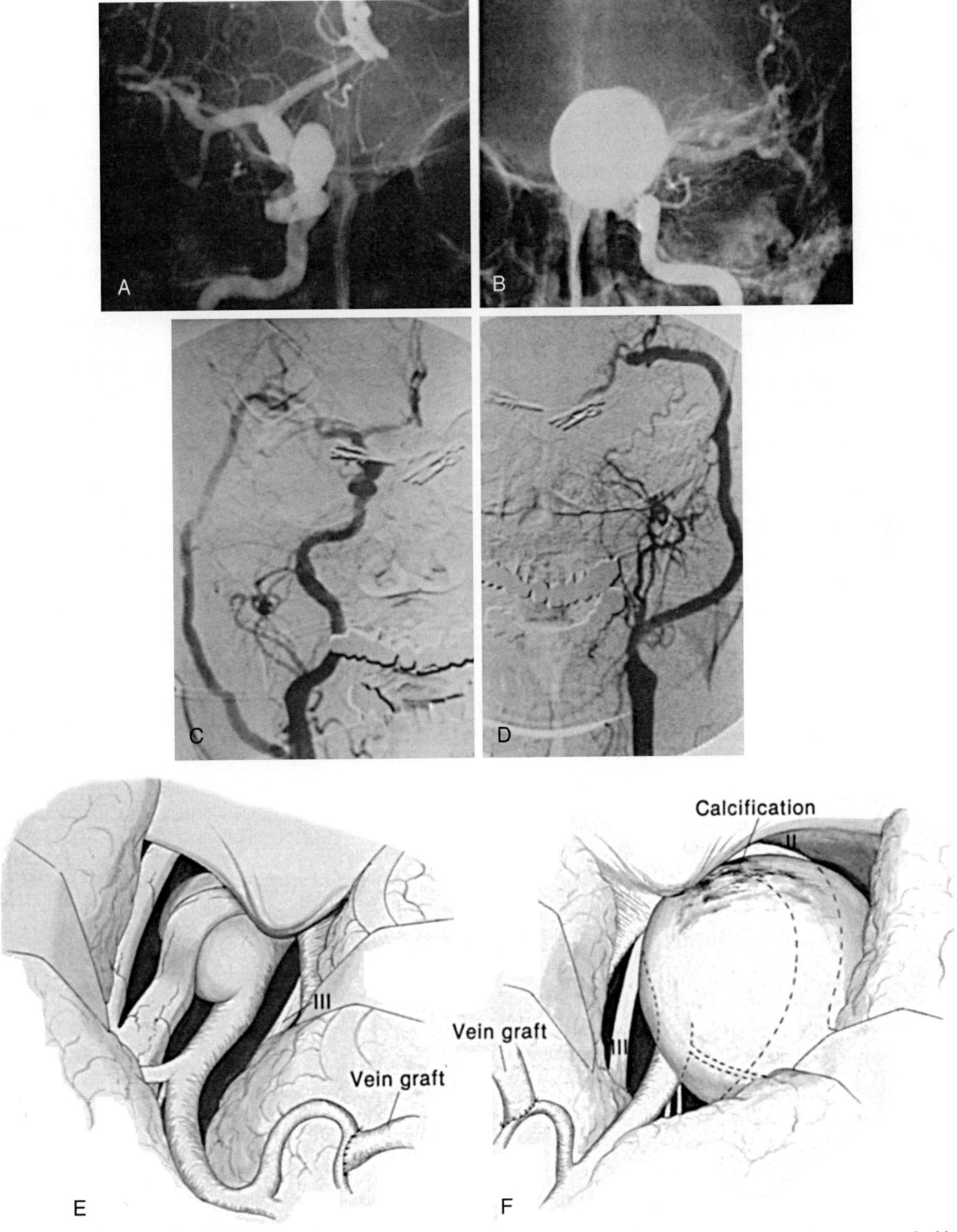

**FIGURE 84–8** ■ Right large medial-type *(A)* and left giant dorsal-type *(B)* ophthalmic aneurysms in the same patient, which were treated with clipping following a bilateral saphenous vein EC-IC bypass. Preoperative four-vessel angiography showed that blood flow through the A1 segment of the left anterior cerebral artery and both posterior communicating arteries was absent. The patient did not tolerate the balloon occlusion test. *C* and *D*, Postoperative carotid angiograms show exclusion of the aneurysms and patent external carotid-middle cerebral bypasses. *E* and *F*, Intraoperative views. The right large aneurysm required 35 minutes of intermittent carotid occlusion, but it was clipped successfully. The left giant aneurysm developed dorsally distal to the origin of the ophthalmic artery compressing the left optic nerve medially. Hard calcifications at the neck of the aneurysm made clipping impossible. The aneurysm was cut, and the carotid artery was trapped permanently.

carotid to M2 bypass with a saphenous vein graft was performed immediately before direct surgery via a frontotemporal craniotomy. The aneurysm was so large that dissection could not proceed without proximal occlusion of the internal carotid artery in the neck. The aneurysm displaced the optic nerve medially and grew above the left optic nerve (dorsal type) (see Fig. 84–8F). The optic canal was opened, and the anterior clinoid process was removed to dissect the C3 portion of the internal carotid artery. The anterior aneurysmal wall was calcified near the neck, as suggested by a preoperative CT scan, making neck clipping impossible. The posterior wall was so thin and tightly adhered to the dura that it prematurely ruptured near the neck during dissection, which made body clipping useless. Thus, the left internal carotid artery was permanently trapped between the common carotid bifurcation and the C2, just proximal to the posterior communicating artery. Patency of the bypass was confirmed by the postoperative carotid angiogram (see Fig. 84–8D).

One week after this surgery, the right ophthalmic aneurysm was operated on via a right frontotemporal craniotomy. Because of absent collateral flow, a prophylactic external carotid artery to M2 vein bypass was performed in a similar fashion. The aneurysm on this side was beneath the optic nerve (medial type) (see Fig. 84–8E). After removal of the roof of the optic canal and anterior clinoid process, the dural ring was cut to free the C3 portion. During dissection of the aneurysm from the surrounding tissues, the right internal carotid artery was occluded intermittently up to 35 minutes. The aneurysm was successfully obliterated perpendicularly with a No. 18 straight clip. During both surgeries, the patient was heparinized, and brain protection was instituted before carotid occlusion (using the drug regimen as described earlier in the text). Postoperative angiography 1 week after surgery showed that the aneurysm had been obliterated and that patency of both the bypass and the internal carotid artery were well preserved (see Fig. 84–8C). Postoperative CT scans showed no evidence of ischemia; however, the patient's condition remained unchanged from the preoperative, severely disabled state 1 month after the last surgery.

*Comment.* External carotid artery to M2 bypass surgery is preferred in these patients because direct surgery can be performed without the concern about blood flow when trapping of the internal carotid artery is needed, because abundant collateral flow can be expected through the bypass. Temporary external carotid artery to M2 bypass using synthetic material would be ideal for such conditions as existed in the right side of this patient because of the high possibility of successful neck clipping and preservation of the carotid flow in patients in whom the bypass is needed only during surgery.

## SUMMARY

Paraclinoid aneurysms are characterized by female preponderance, multiple or symmetric aneurysms, frequent visual symptoms, and surgical difficulty. The most appropriate form of treatment is determined by considering the patients' age, specific characteristics of the aneurysm, the collateral circulation, and whether direct clipping or carotid occlusion with bypass surgery is indicated.

We proposed classification of paraclinoid aneurysms according to the long axis and cross-section of the ICA from surgical points.

Although the extent of opening of the optic canal and removal of the anterior clinoid process depends on the location and size of the aneurysms, the untethering exposure method is basically necessary in cases of the paraclinoid aneurysm whose neck is located close to the dural ring or large to giant aneurysms. It allows an excellent exposure of the ICA freed from the surrounding structures, providing enough space for temporary carotid occlusion and enabling necessary mobilization of the ICA at clipping.

For difficult or complicated cases involving large to giant aneurysms, the carotid artery should be isolated in the neck initially. The patient should be heparinized, and the brain should be protected from ischemic injury during carotid occlusion. Clips should be applied after most of the aneurysm wall is dissected free from the surrounding structures; clips are usually placed with the carotid artery trapped and the aneurysm punctured and collapsed. Surgeons should be prepared to perform bypass surgery on patients with poor collateral circulation.

In lateral or medial type aneurysms, straight clips can usually be applied; in the case of a large to giant aneurysm, the clip blades should be tried to be placed as parallel as possible with multiple clips. If the clip blades are placed perpendicularly, it is advisable to place the clip blades away from the aneurysm neck to the dome side. In large to giant ventral type aneurysms, multiple clipping with ring clips, especially in tandem fashion, would be the treatment of choice.

In 129 patients, good results were obtained in almost all of the patients with small aneurysms (94%); 12 patients had postoperative visual impairment caused by surgical manipulation. Good results were accomplished in only 75% of patients with large to giant aneurysms. To improve these results, further refinement and advancement in operative techniques and management for ischemia are needed.

## ACKNOWLEDGMENT

*This chapter is dedicated by the authors to the memory of the late Professor Kenichi Sugita.*

## REFERENCES

1. Knosp E, Muller G, Perneczky A: The paraclinoid carotid artery: Anatomical aspects of a microneurosurgical approach. Neurosurgery 22:896–901, 1988.
2. Miller JD, Jawad K, Jennet B: Safety of carotid ligation and its role in the management of intracranial aneurysms. J Neurol Neurosurg Psychiatry 40:64–72, 1977.
3. Linskey ME, Sekhar LN, Horton JA, et al: Aneurysms of the intracavernous internal carotid artery: A multidisciplinary approach to treatment. J Neurosurg 75:525–534, 1991.
4. Sugita K, Kobayashi K, Kyoshima K, et al: Fenestrated clips for unusual aneurysms of the carotid artery. J Neurosurg 57:240–246, 1982.
5. Hieshima GB, Higashida RT, Halbach VV, et al: Intravascular balloon

embolization of a carotid-ophthalmic artery aneurysm with preservation of the parent artery. AJNR Am J Neuroradiol 7:916–918, 1986.

6. Almeida GM, Shibata MK, Bianco E: Carotid-ophthalmic aneurysms. Surg Neurol 5:41–45, 1976.

7. Drake CG, Vanderlinden RG, Amacher AL: Carotid-ophthalmic aneurysms. J Neurosurg 29:24–31, 1968.

8. Heros RC, Nelson PB, Ojemann RG, et al: Large and giant paraclinoid aneurysms: Surgical techniques, complications, and results. Neurosurgery 12:153–163, 1983.

9. Nutik SL: Ventral paraclinoid carotid aneurysms. J Neurosurg 69:340–344, 1988.

10. Yasargil MG, Gasser JC, Hodosch RM, Rankin TV: Carotid ophthalmic aneurysms: Direct microsurgical approach. Surg Neurol 8:155–165, 1977.

11. Kyoshima K, Koike G, Hokama M, et al: A classification of juxtadural ring aneurysms with reference to surgical anatomy. J Clin Neurosci 2:61–64, 1996.

12. Kobayashi S, Kyoshima K, Gibo H, et al: Carotid cave aneurysms of the internal carotid artery. J Neurosurg 70:216–221, 1989.

13. Kyoshima K, Kobayashi S: Carotid Cave Aneurysms of the Internal Carotid Artery: Intracranial Aneurysms and Arteriovenous Malformations. Nagoya: Nagoya University COOP Press, 1990, pp 197–207.

14. Gibo H, Lenkey C, Rhoton AL Jr: Microsurgical anatomy of the supraclinoid portion of the internal carotid artery. J Neurosurg 55:560–574, 1981.

15. Lang J: Clinical Anatomy of the Head, Neurocranium-Orbit-Craniocervical Regions. Translated by Wilson RR, Winstanley DP (eds). Berlin: Springer-Verlag, 1983.

16. Renn WH, Rhoton AL Jr: Microsurgical anatomy of the sellar region. J Neurosurg 43:288–298, 1975.

17. Engel A: Ursprungs- und Verlaufsvariationen der ersten Ophthalmica-Strecke. Wurzburg: Diss, 1975.

18. Hayreh SS: The ophthalmic artery. I: Normal gross anatomy. In Newton TH, Potts DG (eds): Radiology of the Skull and Brain; Angiography. St. Louis: CV Mosby, 1974, pp 1333–1410.

19. Day AL: Aneurysms of the ophthalmic segment: A clinical and anatomical analysis. J Neurosurg 72:677–691, 1990.

20. Kobayashi S, Koike G, Orz Y, et al: Juxta-dural ring aneurysms of the internal carotid artery. J Clin Neuroscience 2:345–349, 1995.

21. Gibo H, Kobayashi S, Kyoshima K, et al: Microsurgical anatomy of the arteries of the pituitary stalk and gland as viewed from above. Acta Neurochir 90:60–66, 1988.

22. Kobayashi S, Hongo K, Nitta J, et al: Carotid cave aneurysm of the internal carotid artery. In Kobayashi K, Goel A, Hongo K (eds): Neurosurgery of Complex Tumor and Vascular Lesions. London: Churchill Livingstone, 1997, pp 3–19.

23. Yasargil MG: Internal carotid artery aneurysms. In Yasargil MG (ed): Microneurosurgery II. Stuttgart; Georg Thieme Verlag, 1984, pp 33–123.

24. Thurel C, Rey A, Thiebaut JB, et al: Anevrysmes carotido-ophtalmiques. Neurochirurgie 20:25–39, 1974.

25. Locksley HB: Report on the cooperative study of intracranial aneurysms and subarachnoid hemorrhage. Section V, Part I: Natural history of subarachnoid hemorrhage, intracranial aneurysms and arteriovenous malformations: Based on 368 cases in the cooperative study. J Neurosurg 25:219–239, 1966.

26. Kodama N, Mineura K, Fujiwara S, Suzuki J: Surgical treatment of the carotid-ophthalmic aneurysms. In Suzuki J (ed): Cerebral Aneurysms. Tokyo: Neuron Publishing Company, 1979, p 269.

27. Weir B: Carotid ophthalmic aneurysm. In Weir B (ed): Aneurysms Affecting the Nervous System. Baltimore: Williams & Wilkins, 1987, p 447.

28. Ferguson GG, Drake CG: Carotid-ophthalmic aneurysms: Visual abnormalities in 32 patients and the results of treatment. Surg Neurol 16:1–8, 1981.

29. Kothandaram P, Dawson BH, Kruyt RC: Carotid ophthalmic aneurysms: A study of 19 patients. J Neurosurg 34:544–548, 1971.

30. Shigeta H, Kyoshima K, Nakagawa F, et al: Dorsal internal carotid artery aneurysms with special reference to angiographic presentation and surgical management. Acta Neurochir 119:42–48, 1992.

31. Dolenc VV: A combined epi- and subdural direct approach to carotid-ophthalmic artery aneurysm. J Neurosurg 62:667–672, 1985.

32. Nutik SL: Removal of the anterior clinoid process for exposure of the proximal intracranial carotid artery. J Neurosurg 69:529–534, 1988.

33. Perneczky A, Knosp E, Czech TH: Para- and infraclinoidal aneurysms. Anatomy, surgical technique and report on 22 cases. In Dolenc VV (ed): The Cavernous Sinus. Vienna: Springer-Verlag, 1987, p 253.

34. Nakao S, Kikuchi H, Takahashi N: Successful clipping of carotid-ophthalmic aneurysms through a contralateral pterional approach. J Neurosurg 54:532–536, 1981.

35. Gelber BR, Sundt Jr TM: Treatment of intracranial and giant carotid aneurysms by combined internal carotid ligation and extra- to intracranial bypass J Neurosurg 52:1–10, 1980.

36. Wada K, Nakagawara J, Sasaki T, et al: Angiographic selection of combined extra- and intradural direct approach as operative approach to internal carotid ophthalmic artery. Surg Cereb Stroke 19:99–102, 1991.

37. Hongo K, Kobayashi S, Yokoh A, et al: Monitoring retraction pressure on the brain: An experimental and clinical study. J Neurosurg 66:270–275, 1987.

38. Shibuya M, Sugita K, Kobayashi S: Intraoperative protection of cranial nerves and perforating arteries by silicone rubber sheet. J Neurosurg 74:677–679, 1991.

39. Tanaka Y, Kobayashi S, Hongo K, et al: Intraoperative protection of cranial nerves and arteries by split silicone tube. Neurosurgery 33:523–525, 1993.

40. Nishioka JH: Report on the cooperative study of intracranial aneurysms and subarachnoid hemorrhage: Section VIII, Part 1. Results of the treatment on intracranial aneurysms by occlusion of the carotid artery in the neck. J Neurosurg 25:660–682, 1966.

41. Diaz FG, Ausman JI, Pearce JE: Ischemic complications after combined internal carotid occlusion and extracranial-intracranial anastomosis. Neurosurgery 10:563–570, 1982.

42. Flamm ES: Suction decompression of aneurysms: Technical note. J Neurosurg 54:275–276, 1981.

43. Samson DS, Batjer HH: Aneurysms of the anterior carotid wall (ophthalmic). In Intracranial Aneurysm Surgery-Techniques. Mount Kisco, NY: Futura Publishing, 1990, p 41.

44. Tamaki N, Kim S, Ehara K, et al: Giant carotid-ophthalmic artery aneurysms: Direct clipping utilizing the "trapping-evacuation" technique. J Neurosurg 74:567–572, 1991.

45. Kyoshima K, Kobayashi S, Wakui K, et al: A newly designed puncture needle for suction decompression of giant aneurysms. J Neurosurg 76:880–882, 1992.

46. Kobayashi S, Tanaka Y: Aneurysm clip design, selection, and application. In Apuzo MLJ (ed): Brain Surgery. London: Churchill Livingstone, 1993, pp 825–846.

47. Kobayashi S, Hongo K, Goel A, et al: Giant aneurysms of the internal carotid artery. In Kobayashi K, Goel A, Hongo K (eds): Neurosurgery of Complex Tumor and Vascular Lesions. London: Churchill Livingstone, 1997, pp 21–36.

48. Diraz A, Kyoshima K, Kobayashi S: Dorsal internal carotid artery aneurysms: classification, pathogenesis, and surgical considerations. Neurosurg Rev 16:197–204, 1993.

49. Kobayashi S, Hongo K, Shigeta H, et al: Dorsal internal carotid artery aneurysms. In Kobayashi S, Goel A, Hongo K (eds): Neurosurgery of Complex Tumor and Vascular Lesions. London: Churchill Livingstone, 1997, pp 38–46.

50. Nakagawa F, Kobayashi S, Takemae T, et al: Aneurysms protruding from the dorsal wall of the internal carotid artery. J Neurosurg 66:303–308, 1986.

51. Diraz A, Kobayashi S, Okudera H, et al: Suprachiasmal carotid-ophthalmic artery aneurysm: Report of two cases. Neurol Med Chir 32:952–956, 1992.

52. Tanaka Y, Kobayashi S, Kyoshima K, et al: Multiple clipping technique for large to giant internal carotid artery aneurysms and complications: Angiographic analysis. J Neurosurg 80:635–642, 1994.

53. Keravel Y, Sindou M: Surgical occlusion of the carotid axis. In Keravel Y, Sindou M (eds): Giant Intracranial Aneurysms. Berlin: Springer-Verlag, 1984, pp 62–85.

54. Spetzler RF, Rhodes RS, Roski RA, Likavec MJ: Subclavian to middle cerebral artery saphenous vein bypass graft. J Neurosurg 53:465–469, 1980.

55. Ito Z: Long radial artery grafting. In Ito Z (ed): Microsurgery of Cerebral Aneurysms. Amsterdam: Niigata, Elsevier/Nishimura, 1985, pp 270–279.

56. Kyoshima K, Kobayashi K, Orz YI: Ophthalmic aneurysms. In Kaye AH, Black PM (eds): Operative Neurosurgery. London: Churchill Livingstone, 1999.

# Distal Anterior Cerebral Artery Aneurysms

■ WILLIAM A. SHUCART, CARL B. HEILMAN, and LYNDELL Y. WANG

## SURGICAL MANAGEMENT OF ANTERIOR CEREBRAL ARTERY ANEURYSMS DISTAL TO THE ANTERIOR COMMUNICATING ARTERY

Aneurysms arising from the anterior cerebral artery (ACA) distal to the anterior communicating artery (ACoA) are uncommon: the reported incidence is 2% to 9% of all intracranial aneurysms.[9, 10, 12, 13, 16, 24–26] Reviews emphasize that patients with distal anterior cerebral aneurysms have a high incidence of multiple aneurysms.[9, 16, 24, 26] Although often relatively small, these aneurysms are notoriously difficult to treat surgically.

Distal ACA aneurysms are similar to intracranial aneurysms found at other locations. They are saccular and are probably flow related, and they occur at arterial bifurcations. The commonest location for aneurysms of the distal ACA is where it branches into the pericallosal and callosal marginal arteries (Fig. 85–1).[21] Aneurysms also arise just distal to the ACoA where the orbitofrontal branch arises, at the origin of the frontopolar branch, and much less commonly at the callosal marginal branches. Mycotic aneurysms can occur in the distal ACA as the result of septic emboli, and traumatic aneurysms from both penetrating and closed head injuries have also been described.[3] In closed head injury, the aneurysm is presumed to form as the result of arterial wall injury occurring as the brain and ACA impact against the falx. Finally, aneurysms can form on vessels that feed arteriovenous malformations, and malignant aneurysms may occur in the distal ACA territory as the result of tumor emboli.[14, 15]

Most patients who have a distal ACA aneurysm come to medical attention because of subarachnoid hemorrhage. Imaging studies typically show a focal interhemispheric hemorrhage and sometimes a frontal lobe hematoma. Other patients may present with diffuse subarachnoid hemorrhage, intraventricular hemorrhage, corpus callosal hemorrhage, or interhemispheric subdural hematoma.[2, 5] With wider use of magnetic resonance imaging (MRI), an increasing number of patients have aneurysms that are found incidentally.

Some authors have stated that distal ACA aneurysms tend to bleed when relatively small, an effect that leads to

technical problems that differ from those associated with larger aneurysms (e.g., clip placement may compromise the lumen of the parent vessel, and these aneurysms commonly have a sessile base, which makes perfect clip placement more difficult). Some authors report that these aneurysms rupture infrequently intraoperatively, whereas others (ourselves included) have been impressed with how easily they can rupture intraoperatively. They rupture easily because the dome of the aneurysm is often embedded in a frontal lobe, and during retraction, the dome can be torn from the aneurysm.

The surgical mortality rate for distal ACA aneurysms remains at 8% to 10%, despite advances in surgical and anesthetic techniques; however, most series remain small, thus variation in one or two cases greatly affects the percentages. Reported complications of surgical treatment of these aneurysms include recent memory problems, hemiparesis (generally with the leg more severely involved than the arm), and decreased verbal output, which is usually temporary but may last for months.

Surgical intervention is often more difficult than would be suspected from either the size or the angiographic appearance of the aneurysm, particularly for aneurysms occurring from the ACoA to the top of the genu of the corpus callosum. The reasons for the difficulty are numerous; the space between the hemispheres is narrow, which limits exposure. The subarachnoid space between the hemispheres (the callosal cistern) is small; therefore, the release of cerebrospinal fluid does not provide the excellent exposure that it gives in other locations. The neck of the aneurysm is often atherosclerotic and broad; and dense adhesions often exist between the cingulate gyri. The approach is also difficult, partly because this area is not commonly dealt with.

## OPERATIVE PLANNING

We prefer to operate on patients early if they are in reasonably good condition. The usual preoperative routine of ensuring that the patient is in good cardiopulmonary status is followed. Anticonvulsants are started when the patient

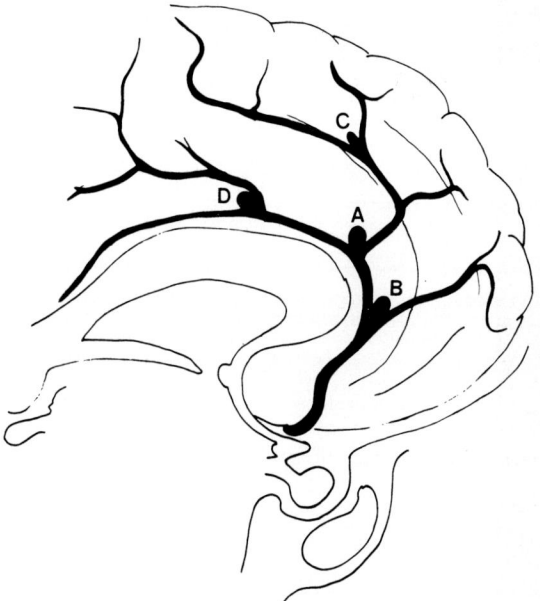

**FIGURE 85–1** ■ Anatomic location of pericallosal aneurysms. The junction of the pericallosal and callosal marginal arteries is shown (A). This is the most common location. The junction of the frontopolar and pericallosal arteries is indicated (B). This is probably the second most common location. The callosal marginal artery bifurcation is also shown (C). The pericallosal artery bifurcation (D) is a typical location for aneurysms that develop after a closed head injury.

is admitted to the hospital, and corticosteroids are started just before surgery. Lumbar spinal drainage is used in all patients to facilitate brain retraction. Mannitol is given when the bone flap is being elevated; the usual adult dose is 12.5 to 25 g administered intravenously. Systemic hypotension is seldom used during surgery for distal ACA aneurysms. With these aneurysms, we prefer to begin with known anatomy and proceed toward the abnormal site. Without the aid of intraoperative image-guided navigation systems, attempts to descend directly on the dome of the aneurysm are often confusing; the surgeon can have difficulty deciding whether the parent artery first identified is proximal or distal to the aneurysm or whether it is on the right or left side.

Currently available image-guided navigation systems can allow dissection directly to the aneurysm instead of localizing using a proximal-to-distal dissection. Origitano and Anderson[17] reported the use of computed tomography angiogram (CTA)-guided frameless stereotaxy to aid in the clipping of a distal posterior inferior cerebellar artery (PICA) aneurysm. Accuracy when locating distal ACA aneurysms would be greater than with PICA aneurysms owing to the constant location of the adjacent falx as a landmark. We have operated on one pericallosal aneurysm by incorporating magnetic resonance angiography (MRA) source images into the Radionics Optical Tracking System.

On or before the day of the surgery, the patient undergoes MR or CT angiography imaging with fiducial markers distributed over the head (usually six on the forehead and one anterior to each tragus are adequate). If the study is performed far in advance of surgery, the locations of the fiducials can be marked with indelible ink and the fiducials removed. At the time of surgery, the fiducials are replaced

in the premarked locations. An MRA or CTA is not sensitive enough to image aneurysms smaller than 3 mm.[19, 22] If the aneurysm is not visible on MRA or CTA, its location can be approximated by correlation with vessel patterns on conventional angiography.

The data obtained by the following CTA protocol was entered into a "Neurostation" frameless stereotactic system by Origitano and Anderson.[17] Contrast was administered at 3 to 5 ml/sec with a total dose of 90 ml after an 8- to 15-second delay and the images were presented on a 30-cm field of view. The slices were 1 to 2 mm thick without gantry tilt. This protocol requires only 1 to 2 minutes of scanning time. Schwartz and associates[19] described the following protocol for obtaining MRAs at their institution. They used a 1.5-Tesla MRI with either three-dimensional time-of-flight (54/4.4 repetition time msec/echo time msec) or three-dimensional phase-contrast (24/4.7, 20-degree flip angle, 60 cm/sec velocity encoding, 20-cm field of view, 256 × 128 matrix) technique. Reconstructions were obtained with a maximum intensity projection (MIP) algorithm. For the case done at our institution, we downloaded two-dimensional time-of-flight (TR 35/TE 7.3) MRA source images (Fig. 85–2).

Using the navigational wand, the trajectory is mapped out, and this becomes the center of the scalp incision and craniotomy for an interhemispheric approach. If the planned entry is in front of the hairline, a bicoronal incision is used to avoid a forehead scar. A craniotomy is planned with the medial edge just to the right of midline. Bur holes are placed as needed, and a craniotomy is done. The dura ipsilateral to the side of the aneurysm is opened in a horseshoe pattern with the flap hinged on the sagittal sinus. The falx adjacent to the aneurysm is located using the wand. The dissection is then directed toward the ACA approximately 1 cm proximal to the neck of the aneurysm. Once located, the aneurysm/artery complex is dissected free and secured as described in the following section on surgical approach.

Investigations into the accuracy of frameless navigational systems have shown target errors of less than 5 mm.[1, 6, 7, 23, 27] Maciumas and associates[11] have reported accuracy of less than 1 mm when implantable fiducial markers are used. Sipos and colleagues reported an accuracy of 2.51 mm using the fiducial-fit method of the "Viewing Wand" by Elekta and an accuracy of 3.03 mm using the surface-fit method. As Roberts and associates[18] observed, we found that the frameless navigational system was most accurate in the beginning of the case before the drainage of cerebrospinal fluid (CSF), administration of mannitol, or retraction of the intracranial structures. By the end of our case, the frontal cortex was visibly shifted by more than 1 cm owing to gravity and CSF drainage, making the image-guided system too inaccurate for further use.

CTA and MRA each has its own advantages and disadvantages, and the approach should be made individually for each case depending on the amount and age of blood surrounding the aneurysm. CTA allows visualization of slow turbulent flow as well as a thrombus in the aneurysm, which are not as well seen on an MRA. Although the thrombus may not be reconstructed into the three-dimensional CT scan owing to lack of contrast filling, the clot can easily be seen on the source images.[4] Scanning is faster

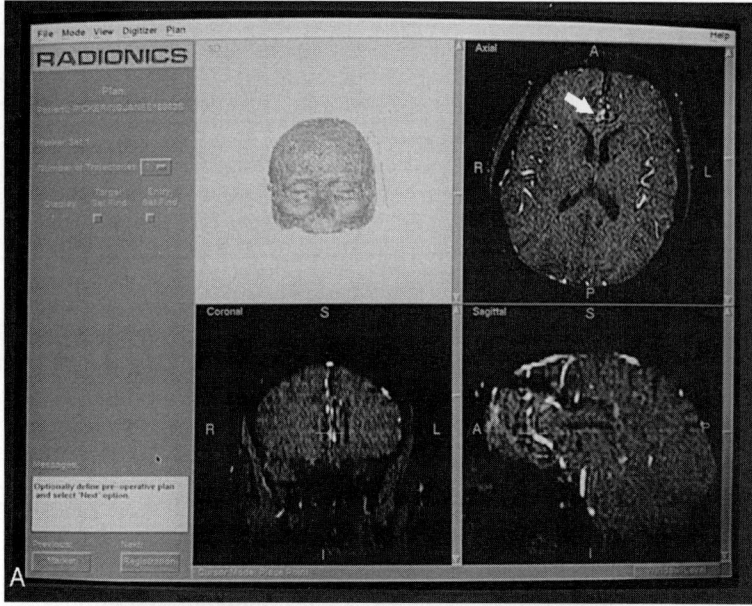

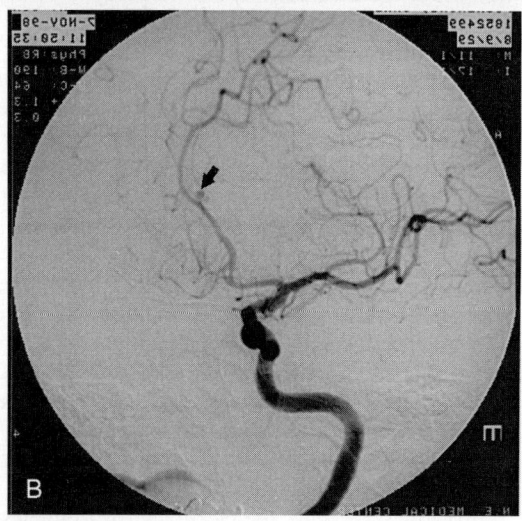

**FIGURE 85–2** ■ *A,* The monitor screen of the Radionics Optical Tracking System showing images of a patient with a ruptured right pericallosal anterior cerebral artery (ACA) aneurysm. Two-dimensional time of flight magnetic resonance angiogram source images were downloaded into the system for intraoperative localization. The *arrow* points to the pericallosal aneurysm. *B,* An oblique angiogram of the case shown in *A.* The *arrow* points to the pericallosal ACA aneurysm.

using CTA than MRA. Subarachnoid blood can obscure CT visualization of the aneurysms in certain cases. The $T_1$-weighted images on MR can present a similar problem if the aneurysm is surrounded by blood, depending on the age of the blood. MR has the advantage of differentiating arterial from venous flow, and gadolinium, if used, is safer than CT contrast. The three-dimensional CTA is approximately 30% of the cost of a conventional angiogram and 70% of the cost of an MRA. As far as size of aneurysm, both MRA and CTA are limited to imaging aneurysms greater than 3 mm.[19] Schwartz and associates[19] compared the use of helical CTA and MRA and concluded that they are comparable in demonstrating aneurysms. Dorsch and associates[4] found that spiral CT allowed visualization of the ACA past the ACom and usually past the bifurcation into the pericallosal and callosal marginal arteries. The same group also reports a case of a ruptured ACom aneurysm that was not visualized on conventional angiogram but was seen on the spiral CTA. Harbaugh and colleagues[8] state that they prefer three-dimensional CT over MRA for preoperative evaluation of cerebrovascular lesions, because it provides better detail.

In the future, the input of selected three-dimensional imaging information into the operative microscope may make localization even easier without the need for a navigational wand.

## SURGICAL APPROACH

We use three different approaches to the distal ACA aneurysms, depending on location. For those on the A2 segment just distal to the ACoA, a standard pterional craniotomy is used, and partial unilateral gyrus rectus resection is often needed. Aneurysms more than 1 cm beyond the ACoA to the top of the genu of the corpus callosum are approached differently from those located on the top of the body of the corpus callosum.

All distal ACA aneurysms are approached from the right unless specific reasons exist to do otherwise, such as when the dome of the aneurysm is large and embedded in the right hemisphere so that retraction would be hazardous. For aneurysms arising more than 1 cm distal to the ACoA up to the genu of the corpus callosum, a basal frontal interhemispheric approach is used (Fig. 85–3).[20] In this operation, the patient is placed in the supine position with the neck slightly extended. The head is kept straight or turned approximately 5 degrees to the left and is fixed in head pins. A bicoronal skin incision is made that extends slightly further toward the zygomatic process on the right side than on the left, and the scalp flap is reflected to the supraorbital ridge. A unilateral right frontal bone flap is made that extends from the supraorbital ridge to a point approximately 8 cm above the ridge in the midline. The bone flap must be long enough in the sagittal plane to provide room to operate around the draining veins without the need to sacrifice a vein of significant size. If the frontal sinus is small, the anteromedial bur hole is placed just above it with the medial edge just to the right of the midline. If the frontal sinus is large, the surgeon should go through it to facilitate exposure. If the sinus is entered, it is repaired in the usual fashion of stripping the mucosa, packing it with fat, and swinging down a pericranial flap to the dura to exclude the frontal sinus. As the bone flap is being removed, the patient is given 12.5 to 25 g of mannitol intravenously. The floor of the frontal fossa must be reached, and the lateral aspect of the sagittal sinus must be exposed. The surgeon does not need to go across the midline. A dural flap about the same size as the bone flap is then raised and hinged along the sagittal sinus. As the dura is elevated, care is taken not to avulse any of the underlying corticodural veins. One or two small draining veins to the sagittal sinus usually have to be cauterized and divided to allow hemispheric retraction.

Without an image-guided navigation system, we find it least confusing to approach the aneurysm from normal proximal arteries, a method that also provides proximal vascular control. The closer the aneurysm is to the ACoA, the more imperative it is to begin as inferiorly and proxi-

mally as possible. The right cerebral hemisphere is gently retracted to expose the falx, which is then followed to the crista galli. Care is taken to avoid injury to the olfactory tracts. Once the crista is identified, the right frontal lobe is gently retracted, and the adhesions between the frontal lobes are sharply divided. Retraction is carried back to expose the optic chiasm and the ACoA complex just above it. The two pericallosal arteries are then sharply dissected free in the subarachnoid space. The surgeon should know from the preoperative studies how far distally on the pericallosal artery dissection must be carried out, and, if MRI has been obtained, whether or not and where the dome is embedded in the brain.

The further distally toward the genu the aneurysm is located, the greater the surgeon's temptation to come directly down on it and not do the tedious dissection required when approaching from the ACoA. Unfortunately, without the aid of image-guided navigation systems, the surgeon often ends up exposing the pericallosal arteries distal to the aneurysm without realizing it, or the aneurysm may rupture secondary to retraction before the proximal or distal vascular anatomy is identified.

As dissection proceeds distally on the pericallosal arteries above the ACoA complex, the pericallosal arteries run more anteriorly, closer to the surgeon. When the proximal portion of the neck of the aneurysm is reached, careful retraction and dissection are used to identify the distal pericallosal arteries before the aneurysm neck is approached. Determining the exact anatomy of the origin of the aneurysm before surgery is not always possible, but this finding must be made at the time of surgery. The magnification on the microscope is progressively increased as the aneurysm is approached. Because the aneurysm neck is often broad, the clip is best applied along the long axis of the parent artery (Fig. 85–4). If the aneurysm neck is very atherosclerotic, care is taken to avoid fracturing it

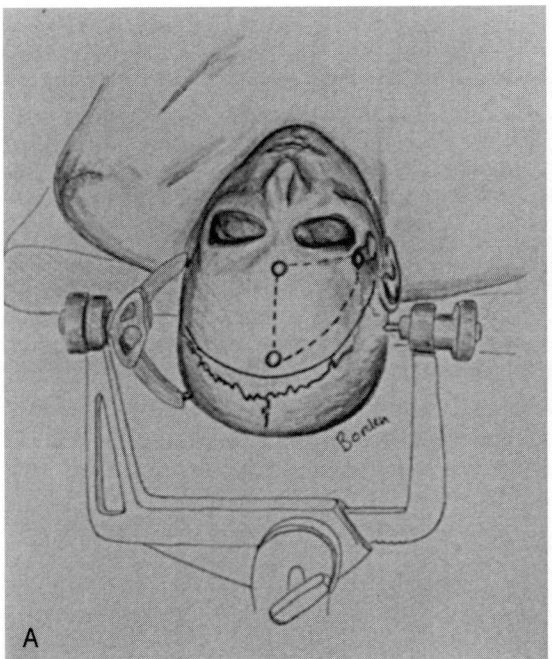
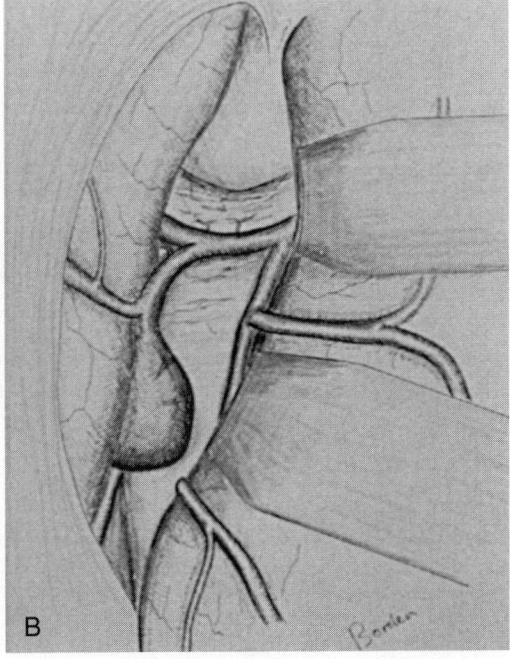

**FIGURE 85–3** ■ A basal frontal interhemispheric approach is shown. *A*, Patient positioning. *B*, Operative exposure.

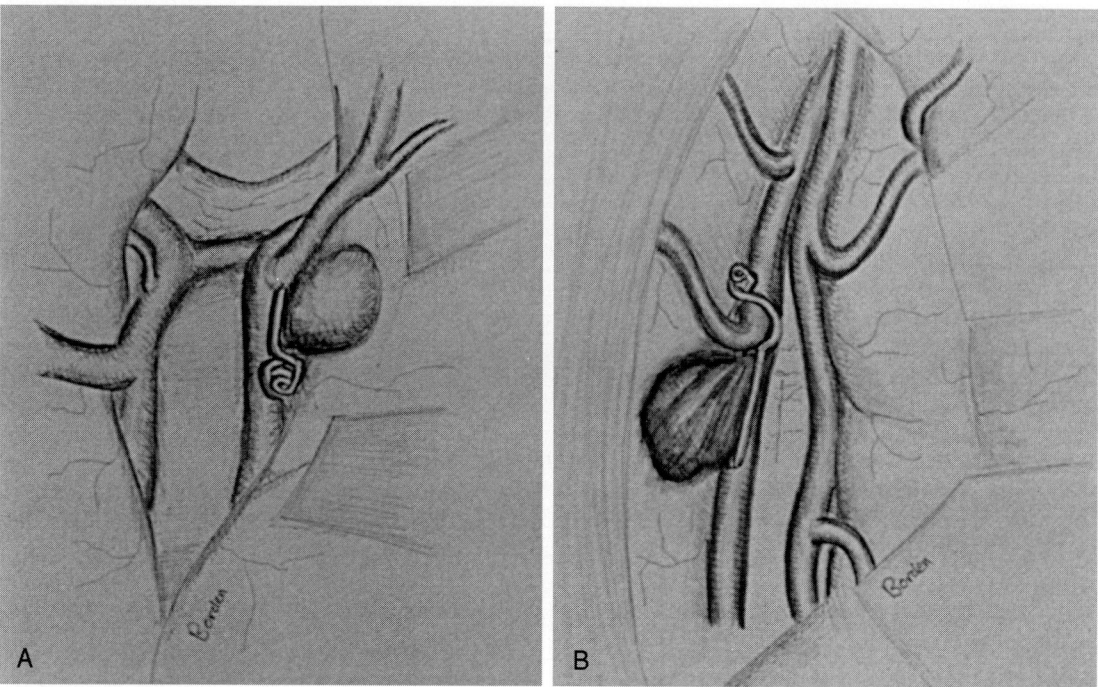

**FIGURE 85–4** ■ Optimal clip placement is often parallel to the pericallosal artery. *A,* A basal frontal interhemispheric approach. *B,* A direct interhemispheric approach.

during clip application. Occasionally, temporary clips proximal and distal to the aneurysm facilitate the dissection and the clipping by decreasing the turgor in the aneurysm. If temporary clipping is used, a cerebral protectant (either etomidate or thiopental) is given, and the blood pressure is elevated slightly. After the clip is applied, the dome of the aneurysm should be further shriveled, either by aspiration or with bipolar cautery, thus allowing complete inspection around the clip to ensure that the parent vessel is patent.

Aneurysms that are more distal on the corpus callosum are easier to deal with, but the surgeon should still obtain proximal control. We use a direct interhemispheric approach for these aneurysms (Fig. 85–5). A shorter coronal skin incision can be used that is guided by the location of the aneurysm. Even without image-guided navigational systems, MRI is helpful when planning the incision and bone flap. The coronal suture can often be identified on the sagittal MRI, and its location relative to the aneurysm

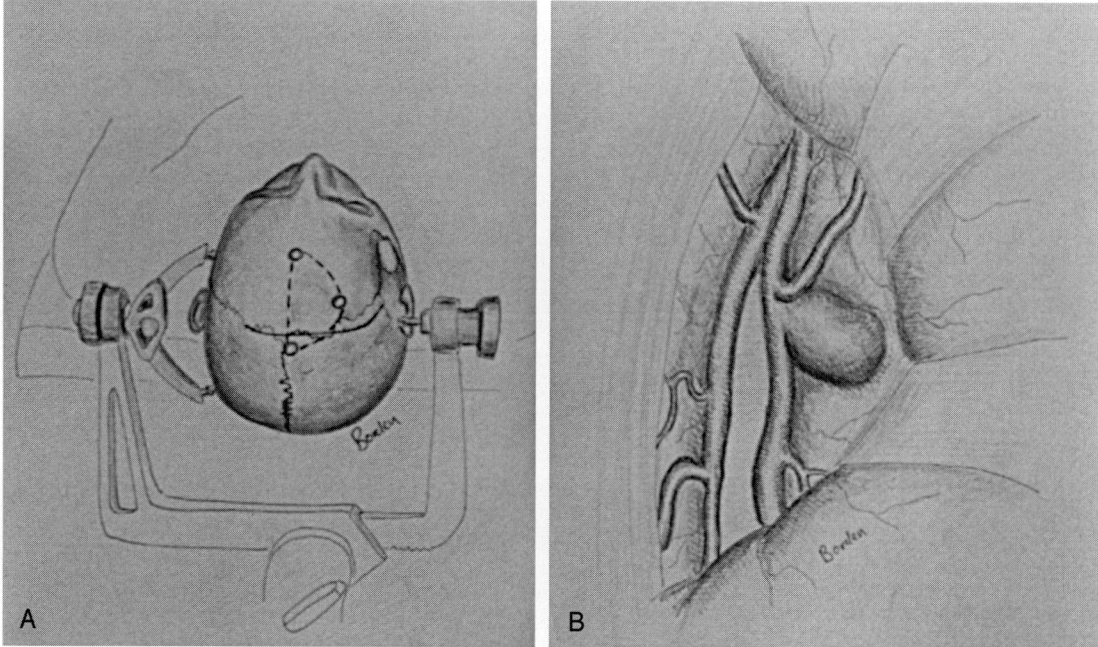

**FIGURE 85–5** ■ A direct interhemispheric approach. *A,* Patient positioning. *B,* Operative exposure.

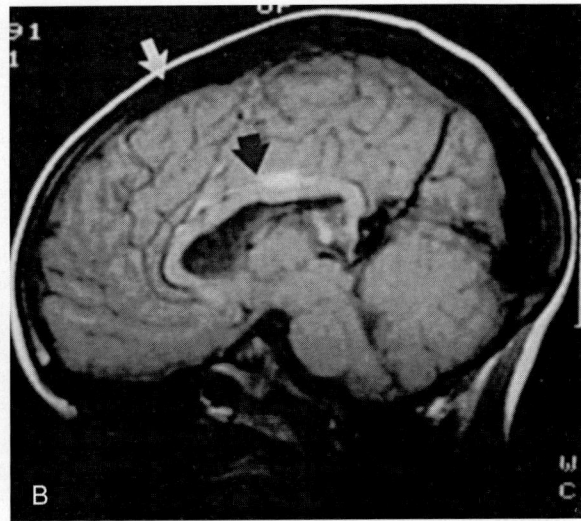

**FIGURE 85-6** ■ *A,* A lateral carotid arteriogram of a patient with a traumatic distal pericallosal artery aneurysm. *B,* A sagittal magnetic resonance imaging (MRI) scan of the same patient. The *small arrow* is on the coronal suture. The *large arrow* is on the aneurysm. Note that the relationship between the coronal suture on the surface of the skull and the location of the aneurysm can be determined from the MRI image. In addition, the distance from the skull to the aneurysm can be measured. This information can help when planning the bone flap once the skin incision has been made and the coronal suture has been identified.

dictates where the incision should be made relative to the coronal suture (Fig. 85–6). The same policy of careful, limited retraction of the hemisphere and preservation of the larger draining veins is followed. The exposure to reach the proximal portion of the pericallosal artery as it comes around the curve of the genu of the corpus callosum is the same as the approach to the corpus callosum itself. A self-retaining retractor is used to gently hold the frontal lobe away from the falx. In some patients, fenestrations are present in the falx where dense arachnoid adhesions must be divided sharply. The vertical depth of the falx varies, but it rarely extends deep enough to separate the cingulate gyri. Thus, once the edge of the falx is visualized, the dissection must still be performed to separate the cingulate gyri, which are often adherent to one another. The corpus callosum is identified by its very white color, and in the absence of hydrocephalus, the two pericallosal arteries are usually close together and must both be identified. If only one pericallosal artery is identified, it may not be the parent vessel. As before, both the proximal and distal portions of the ACA should be seen before the clip is applied. These aneurysms are rarely large enough to require aspiration of the aneurysm before the clip is placed. Because of the small size of the distal ACA, clip placement perpendicular to the parent vessel can compromise the vessel lumen; clip placement parallel to the pericallosal artery usually provides the best anatomic result.

Careful preoperative study of the arteriogram is essential for anatomic correlations. Preoperative MRIs are helpful to determine the true size and location of the dome of the aneurysm, particularly if the aneurysm contains thrombus or is buried in the medial surface of one hemisphere.

## COMPLICATIONS

Complications that arise with these aneurysms are much the same as those occurring with other aneurysms. Delayed ischemic deficits remain a significant problem and are treated the same as ischemic deficits occurring with aneurysms in other locations, primarily with hypervolemia and moderate hypertension. The interhemispheric exposure creates some of its own problems, especially if retraction is too aggressive and prolonged against the cingulate gyri. Such prolonged retraction can give rise to a syndrome similar to akinetic mutism that is usually transient. A similar picture can be seen with rupture of the aneurysm if significant hemorrhage has occurred in or around the cingulate gyri. Intentional sacrifice or accidental damage to the medial frontal draining veins can result in venous hemorrhagic infarction. This risk can be minimized by meticulous technique, limited retraction, and avoidance of deliberate sacrifice of medially draining veins, if possible. The small size of the pericallosal arteries and the fact that the neck is often atherosclerotic make compromise of the lumen of the parent vessel a hazard. The status of this anatomy can be difficult to evaluate at the time of surgery, and complications are best avoided by the surgeon's awareness of the possibility and the use of meticulous technique. Topical papaverine can be helpful for at least temporarily increasing the size of the pericallosal arteries to evaluate the adequacy of the clipping and the lack of compromise of the parent vessel. The small hematomas often associated with these aneurysms are usually best left alone, unless they are more than a few cubic centimeters in volume or they interfere with the dissection, or both.

## REFERENCES

1. Barnett GH, Kormos DW, Steiner CP, et al: Intraoperative localization using an armless, frameless stereotactic wand. J Neurosurg 78:510–514. 1993.
2. Batjer HH, Samson D: Distal anterior cerebral artery aneurysms. In Neurosurgical Operative Atlas, Vol 2. Baltimore: Williams & Wilkins, 1992, pp 119–132.
3. Becker D, Newton T: Distal anterior cerebral artery aneurysm. Neurosurgery 4:495–503, 1979.
4. Dorsch NWC, Young N, Kingston RJ, et al: Early experience with

spiral CT in the diagnosis of intracranial aneurysms. Neurosurgery 36:230–238, 1995.

5. Fein JM, Rovit RL: Interhemispheric subdural hematoma secondary to hemorrhage from a calloso-marginal artery aneurysm. Neuroradiology 1:183–186, 1970.

6. Golfinos JG, Fitzpatrick BC, Smith LR, et al: Clinical use of a frameless stereotactic arm: Results of 325 cases. J Neurosurg 83:197–205, 1995.

7. Guthrie BL: Graphic-interactive cranial surgery. Clin Neurosurg 41:489–516, 1994.

8. Harbaugh RE, Schlusselberg DS, Jeffery R, et al: Three-dimensional computed tomographic angiography in the preoperative evaluation of cerebrovascular lesions. Neurosurgery 36:320–327, 1995.

9. Hernesneimi J, Tapaninaho A, Vapalahti M, et al: Saccular aneurysms of the distal anterior cerebral artery and its branches. Neurosurgery 31:994–999, 1992.

10. Laitinen L, Snellman A: Aneurysms of the pericallosal artery. J Neurosurg 17:447–458, 1960.

11. Maciumas RJ, Fitzpatrick JM, Galloway RL Jr, et al: Extreme Levels of Application Accuracy Are Provided by Implantable Fiducial Markers for Interactive Image-Guided Neurosurgery: Interactive Image-Guided Neurosurgery. Park Ridge: American Association of Neurological Surgeons, 1993, pp 261–270.

12. Mann KS, Yue CP, Wong G: Aneurysms of the pericallosal-callosal marginal junction. Surg Neurol 21:261–266, 1984.

13. McKissock W, Paine KWE, Walsh LS: An analysis of the results of treatment of ruptured intracranial aneurysms. J Neurosurg 17:726–776, 1960.

14. Montaut J, Hepner H, Tridon P, et al: Aspects pseudo-vasculaires des métastases intracraniennes des chorio-épithéliomes. Neurochirurgie 17:119–128, 1971.

15. New PFJ, Price DL, Carter B: Cerebral angiography in cardiac myxoma: Correlation of angiographic and histopathological findings. Radiology 96:335–345, 1970.

16. Ohno K, Monma S, Suzuki R, et al: Saccular aneurysms of the distal anterior cerebral artery. Neurosurgery 27:907–913, 1990;

17. Origitano TC, Anderson DE: CT angiographic-guided frameless stereotactic-assisted clipping of a distal posterior inferior cerebellar artery aneurysm: Technical case report. Surg Neurol 46:450–454, 1996.

18. Roberts DW, Hartov A, Kennedy FE, et al: Intraoperative brain shift and deformation: A quantitative analysis of cortical displacement in 28 cases. Neurosurgery 43:749–760, 1998.

19. Schwartz RB, Tice HM, Hooten SM, et al: Evaluation of cerebral aneurysms with helical CT: Correlation with conventional angiography and MR angiography. Radiology 192:717–722, 1994.

20. Shucart WA: Distal anterior cerebral artery aneurysms. In Apuzzo MLJ (ed): Brain Surgery: Complication Avoidance and Management. New York: Churchill Livingstone, 1993, pp 1035–1040.

21. Sindou M, Pelissou-Guyotat I, Mertens P, et al: Pericallosal aneurysms. Surg Neurol 30:434–440, 1988.

22. Tampieri D, Leblanc R, Oleszek J, et al: Three-dimensional computed tomographic angiography of cerebral aneurysms. Neurosurgery 36:749–755, 1995.

23. Watanabe E, Mayanagi Y, Kosugi Y, et al: Open surgery assisted by the neuronavigator: A stereotactic, articulated, sensitive arm. Neurosurgery 28:792–800, 1991.

24. Wisoff JH, Flamm, ES: Aneurysms of the distal anterior cerebral artery and associated vascular anomalies. Neurosurgery 20:735–741, 1987.

25. Yasargil MG, Carter LP: Saccular aneurysms of the distal anterior cerebral artery. J Neurosurg 40:218–223, 1974.

26. Yoshimoto T, Uchida K, Suzuki J: Surgical treatment of distal anterior cerebral artery aneurysms. J Neurosurg 50:40–44, 1979.

27. Zinreich SJ, Tebo SA, Long DM, et al: Frameless stereotaxic integration of CT imaging data: Accuracy and initial applications. Radiology 188:735–742, 1993.

# Surgical Management of Aneurysms of the Middle Cerebral Artery

■ JAAKKO RINNE, HU SHEN, RIKU KIVISAARI, and JUHA A. HERNESNIEMI

Surprisingly few reports deal with such a common aneurysm site as the middle cerebral artery (MCA), and especially the overall management outcome of this specific group of patients.[1-12] MCA aneurysms (MCAAs) might be considered too common and routine, or perhaps the results of the treatment are too unfavorable to be reported. Because of the lack of sufficient collateral circulation, inadvertent occlusion of the MCA, or even of its branches, in most cases leads to calamitous infarction and death, especially in acute (1 day after subarachnoid hemorrhage [SAH]) and early surgery (2 to 3 days after SAH). In his pioneering work on surgery for intracranial aneurysms, Dandy[13] considered MCAAs hazardous for surgical management, even inoperable. Although currently only a few MCAAs are inoperable, they still present striking problems as compared with other aneurysms in the anterior circulation. Because MCAAs are less suitable for endovascular surgery, owing to anatomic reasons and frequent association with expanding hematomas, neurosurgeons should focus on the safe treatment of these lesions.[14-20]

Typically, Finnish patients—among other Arctic people—have a higher frequency of MCAAs than reported in other series.[17, 21-24] Consequently, we have had a unique opportunity to treat and scrutinize a large group of patients with these aneurysms (≥1000). This chapter is based on our scrutiny of 561 patients with a total of 690 MCAAs treated in our institution in Kuopio University Hospital from 1977 to 1992.[17] The baseline characteristics of these patients are shown in Table 86–1. One third of our patients with intracranial aneurysms harbor multiple lesions; among them, MCAAs are the most frequent.[17, 25, 26]

## DIAGNOSTIC WORK-UP

Most MCAAs are diagnosed as a cause of hemorrhagic stroke (i.e., SAH and intracerebral hematoma). Large or giant MCAAs can cause hemiparesis, seizures, or even ischemic symptoms as a result of embolic seeding. Unruptured, asymptomatic MCAAs are found in patients with

multiple lesions, incidentally, or by screening for possible familial aneurysms.[25, 27] Studies have shown that 10% of intracranial aneurysms have familial occurrence. In our series, the most frequent site for familial aneurysms is the MCA.[27-29]

The bedrock of the surgical management of MCAAs is proper imaging. Conventional angiography, with or without digital subtraction, is still the gold standard. Modern digital techniques and advances in catheters as well as in guide-wires have made this study safer with a 0.5% risk of permanent morbidity or mortality.[25, 30] The technique through femoral artery and selective internal carotid injection allows the use of significantly lower amounts of con-

## TABLE 86–1 ■ BASELINE CHARACTERISTICS OF 561 PATIENTS WITH MIDDLE CEREBRAL ARTERY ANEURYSMS

| Variable | Single MCAA | MIA with One MCAA | MIA with Multiple MCAAs |
|---|---|---|---|
| No. of patients | 340 | 110 | 111 |
| Mean age (yr) | | | |
| All | 47.7 | 51.0 | 50.3 |
| Females | 50.0 | 55.5 | 51.9 |
| Males | 45.5 | 47.5 | 49.0 |
| Females (%) | 48.2 | 43.6 | 45.0 |
| Size range of MCAAs (%) | | | |
| 2–7 mm | 27 | 63 | 51 |
| 8–14 mm | 45 | 27 | 32 |
| 15–24 mm | 19 | 6 | 13 |
| ≥25 mm | 9 | 4 | 4 |
| SAH (%) | 91.7 | 90.0 | 91.8 |
| MCAA rupture (% of patients) | 91.7 | 31.8 | 81.8 |
| Preoperative or admission grade in SAH, HH (mean) | 2.9 | 2.8 | 2.7 |
| ICH (%) in SAH | 43 | 45* | 33* |
| Familial (%) | 11 | 11 | 14 |
| Arterial hypertension (%) | 28 | 32 | 36 |

*With symptomatic MCAA.

MCAA, middle cerebral artery aneurysm; MIA, multiple intracranial aneurysms; SAH, subarachnoid hemorrhage; HH, preoperative or admission grade by Hunt and Hess; ICH, intracerebral hematoma.

TABLE 86–2 ■ **NUMBER OF ANEURYSMS AT DIFFERENT SITES IN 1314 PATIENTS WITH INTRACRANIAL ANEURYSMS**

| Site of Aneurysm | All (1314 patients) | MIA (302 patients) | MIA with One MCAA (110 patients) | MIA with Multiple MCAAs (111 patients) |
|---|---|---|---|---|
| ICA | 413 | 186 | 64 | 29 |
| MCA | 690 | 350 | 110 | 240 |
| ACoA | 433 | 115 | 60 | 16 |
| Peric | 96 | 53 | 25 | 9 |
| VBA | 119 | 34 | 9 | 2 |
| *Total* | 1751 | 738 | 268 | 296 |

MIA, multiple intracranial aneurysms; MCAA, middle cerebral artery aneurysm, ICA, internal carotid artery; MCA, middle cerebral artery; ACoA, anterior communicating artery; Peric, pericallosal artery; VBA, vertebrobasilar arteries.

trast material. The proper angiographic study has at least three projections: lateral, anteroposterior, and oblique. Sometimes more tailor-made views are mandatory to delineate the presence of the aneurysm or the neck, which is often, especially in larger MCAAs, broad and complex. Because of many vessel loops close to the MCA bifurcation or trifurcation, smaller aneurysms (one fifth of the ruptured aneurysms are <5 mm in diameter) can remain undetected without special views. We try to study all four vessels at the first session—except for highly urgent cases with large hematomas—because associated aneurysms can be treated in the same operation.

Magnetic resonance arteriography allows the imaging of intracranial vessels noninvasively, even without contrast material. The major limitation of this technique is the poorer resolution compared with digital subtraction angiography, leading to false-negative results in smaller lesions.[27, 31, 32] The longer study time and sensitivity to movement artifacts rules out this study from the basic work-up for patients with acute SAH, who are often uncooperative. Magnetic resonance angiography is the method of choice, however, when screening for unruptured aneurysms.[27, 28]

A plain computed tomography (CT) scan remains the cornerstone for the diagnosis of SAH, for the bleeding aneurysms in the case of multiple lesions, and for demonstration of intracerebral or intraventricular bleeding. Advances in CT have led to a possibility to detect any aneurysm greater than 3 mm in diameter on CT angiography, accounting for most aneurysms.[33–39] This technique is currently diagnostically equivalent at least with magnetic resonance angiography. The advantages of CT angiography are that it is truly three-dimensional, giving a possibility to view the aneurysm from all angles; it can take into account the bony background; it can show thrombosed aneurysms; and, most important, it can be used in emergent cases. CT angiography is a promising instrument in planning microsurgical procedures, especially in giant, thrombosed, or otherwise complicated aneurysms. In MCAAs, sometimes it might be difficult to visualize the anatomic relations of the neck of the aneurysm and the efferent branches of the vessel. To obtain good-quality CT angiography scans, fast spiral CT, capable of scanning slices thin enough, is needed. Also, the timing between contrast material injection and scanning is crucial to obtain acceptable images. The venous enhancement in acute SAH can lead

to a misdiagnosis (e.g., crossing veins can mimic small aneurysms, or cavernous sinus enhancement can be diagnosed as a paraclinoid aneurysm of the internal carotid artery).[35] In the most ultimate emergency situation with an unconscious patient harboring a large intraparenchymal hematoma, the diagnosis of MCAA can be based on a plain CT scan. The presence and more detailed anatomy of the ruptured aneurysm has to be studied under the operating microscope.[40]

## ANATOMIC FEATURES OF MIDDLE CEREBRAL ARTERY ANEURYSMS

### Site and Directions of Middle Cerebral Artery Aneurysms

Among our patients with intracranial aneurysms, MCAAs are most frequent (Table 86–2). Of 1314 patients with intracranial aneurysms,[17, 23, 26, 41] 43% had at least one MCAA (561 patients with 690 MCAAs), and of patients with multiple intracranial aneurysms, 73% had at least one MCAA. From the total number of 1751 intracranial aneurysms, 690 were MCAAs (39%). According to their site, MCAAs can be divided into three groups: proximal, bifurcation, and distal MCAAs (Table 86–3).

Proximal MCAAs constitute 16% of MCAAs, and their presence often indicates other associated aneurysms. Three fourths of patients with proximal MCAAs have other aneu-

TABLE 86–3 ■ **FREQUENCIES (%) OF MIDDLE CEREBRAL ARTERY ANEURYSMS AT DIFFERENT SITES**

| Site | Single MCAA (340 patients) | MIA with One MCAA (110 patients) | MIA with Multiple MCAAs (111 patients) |
|---|---|---|---|
| Proximal | 9 | 24 | 22 |
| Bifurcation | 89 | 74 | 72 |
| Distal | 2 | 2 | 6 |

MCAA, middle cerebral artery aneurysm; MIA, multiple intracranial aneurysms.

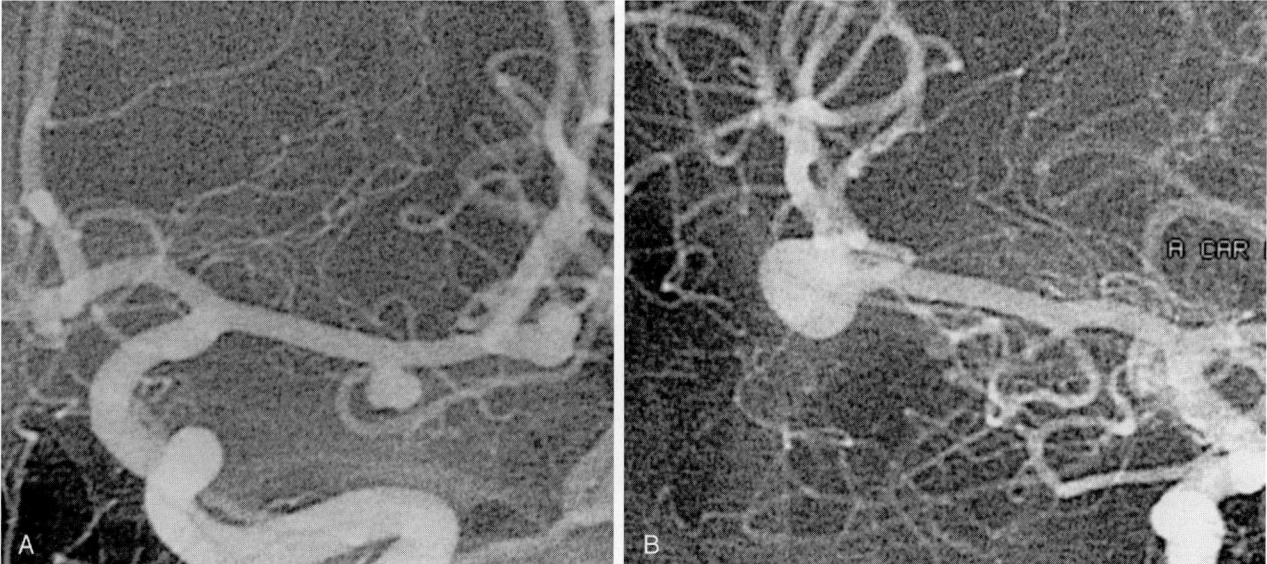

FIGURE 86-1 ■ *A* and *B*, A 64-year-old woman had three grade 2 aneurysms of the middle cerebral artery (MCA). The left bifurcation aneurysm had ruptured and was operated on 3 days after it bled once. The left proximal MCA aneurysm was also ligated. *A*, The patient had a good recovery. Four months later, the largest but unruptured MCA aneurysm on the contralateral side was operated. *B*, The patient had a good recovery.

rysms, making the surgical planning more demanding. Typically, proximal MCAAs are located at the origin of the anterior temporal artery (first branch of the main trunk) and are pointing downward, or are at the origin of lenticulostriatal perforators and are pointing upward (Fig. 86–1). A common feature among proximal MCAAs is that the neck is often wide and partially incorporates the small efferent vessels, making clipping and coiling of these more difficult.

Most of the MCAAs (80%) are located at the bifurcation or trifurcation (see Table 86–3), usually pointing laterally and inferiorly (Figs. 86–2 to 86–4). In anteroposterior angiograms, 45% of MCAAs pointed laterally; 38%, inferiorly; 15%, superiorly; and only 2%, medially (Fig. 86–5). The last-mentioned, however, carries the highest risk for perforator injury in surgery. In the lateral view, one third are projected inferiorly, and the rest are divided equally among the other three directions.

Distal MCAAs are less frequent (Fig. 86–6); in our series, 4% of MCAAs were located distally (see Table 86–3). Distal aneurysms may be fusiform or mycotic, but true saccular aneurysms are found in even the most distal parts of the MCA. Common to all types of distal aneurysms is that they are difficult to find during surgery, made easier today by more accurate neuronavigation systems.[6]

The frequency of multiple intracranial aneurysms in Finnish patients with cerebral aneurysms is at least 30%.[25] Because MCAAs are the most frequent aneurysms, most of these patients harbor multiple intracranial aneurysms. The MCA is the most frequent site to present mirror aneurysms (i.e., intracranial aneurysms at the same site but on different sides). Two thirds of our patients with multiple MCAAs had mirror aneurysms. Most of the proximal MCAAs (72%) were in patients with multiple intracranial aneurysms, and a patient with a proximal MCAA has an almost three times higher risk for associated aneurysms than patients with bifurcation or distal MCAAs.

## Size, Side, Shape, and Type

MCAAs are larger than symptomatic aneurysms at other sites, although 77% of the symptomatic bifurcation MCAAs and 92% of the symptomatic proximal MCAAs were 2 to 14 mm in size. More importantly, MCAAs often have broad necks, making their open and especially endovascular treatment more challenging. Nine percent of the single MCAAs were giant aneurysms, more than in any other aneurysmal site in our material.

Ruptured MCAAs were divided equally between both sides; for some reason, two thirds of the proximal ones were left-sided. Nearly all of the ruptured MCAAs are irregular by their shape. The shape of the dome depends more on whether the aneurysm has ruptured than on its site and is one of the most important signs to show the ruptured lesion in the absence of CT scan or when a delay in admission has occurred. In our series, the smaller MCAA often proved to be the ruptured one, even though statistically the larger ones are more commonly the ruptured ones. Fusiform, atherosclerotic, or mycotic MCAAs are rare (0.6%), and they remain one of the most difficult lesions to treat.[23, 26, 42–44]

## SPECIAL CLINICAL FEATURES OF MIDDLE CEREBRAL ARTERY ANEURYSMS

Once they rupture, MCAAs tend to do so more severely than intracranial aneurysms at other sites. The mean preoperative or admission Hunt and Hess grade[44a] among our patients with ruptured MCAAs was 2.9, as compared with 2.4 at other anterior circulation sites. Also, severe bleeding significantly more often causes death among patients with MCAAs than among patients with other aneurysms. This difference is partly explained by the high frequency of

*Text continued on page 1165*

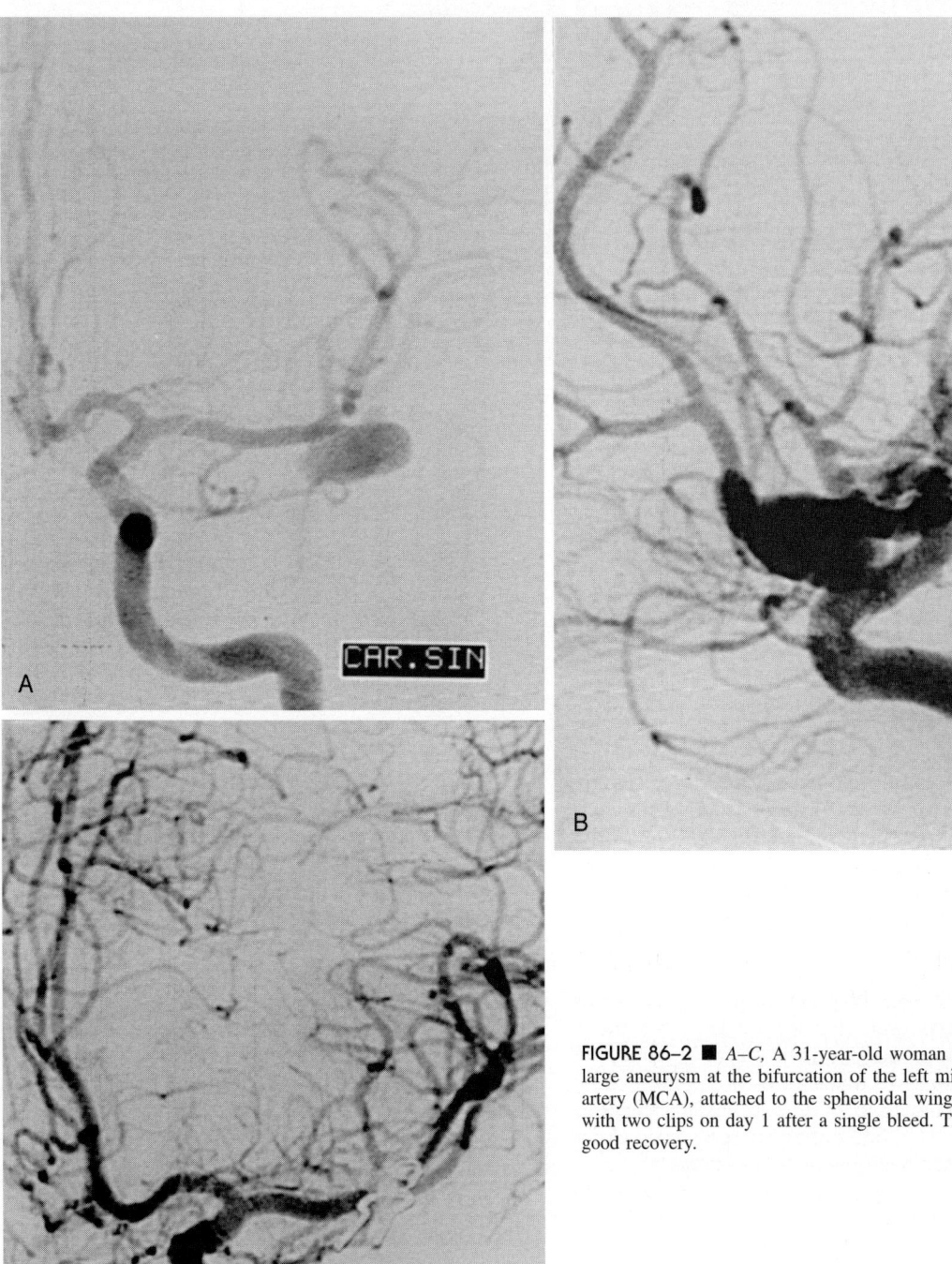

**FIGURE 86–2** ■ *A–C*, A 31-year-old woman had a grade 2, large aneurysm at the bifurcation of the left middle cerebral artery (MCA), attached to the sphenoidal wing. Clipping occurred with two clips on day 1 after a single bleed. The patient had a good recovery.

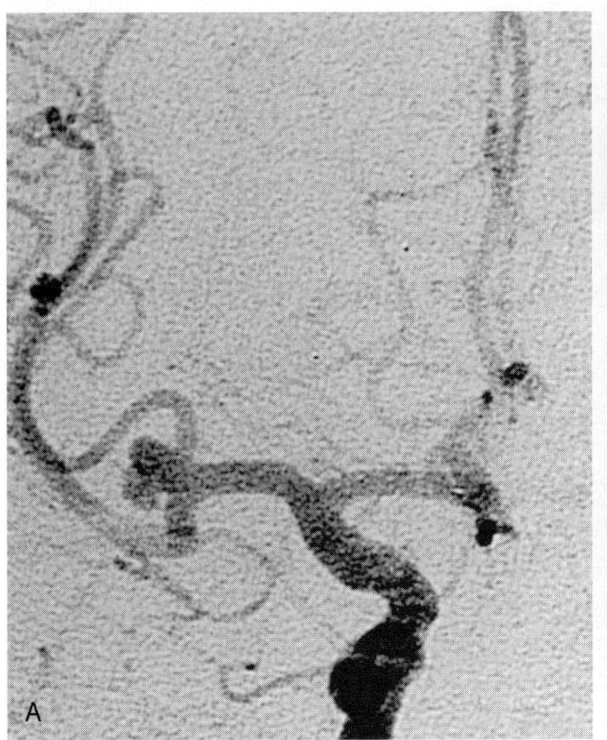

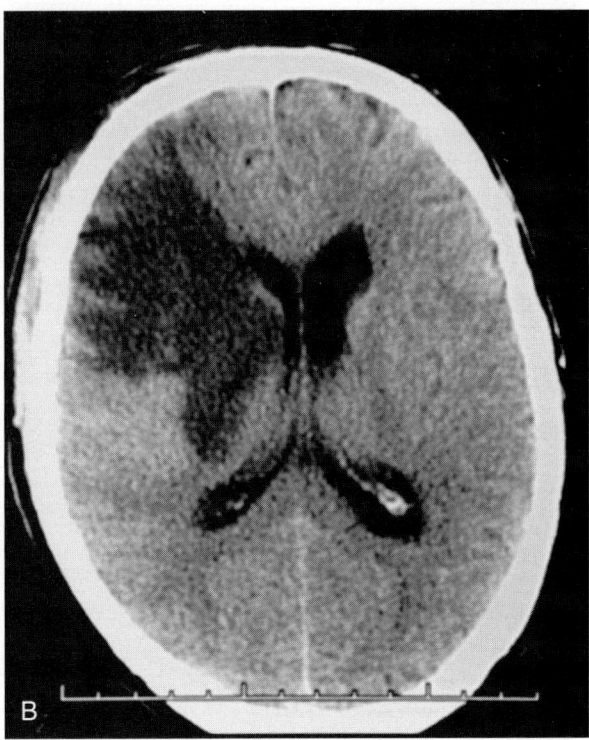

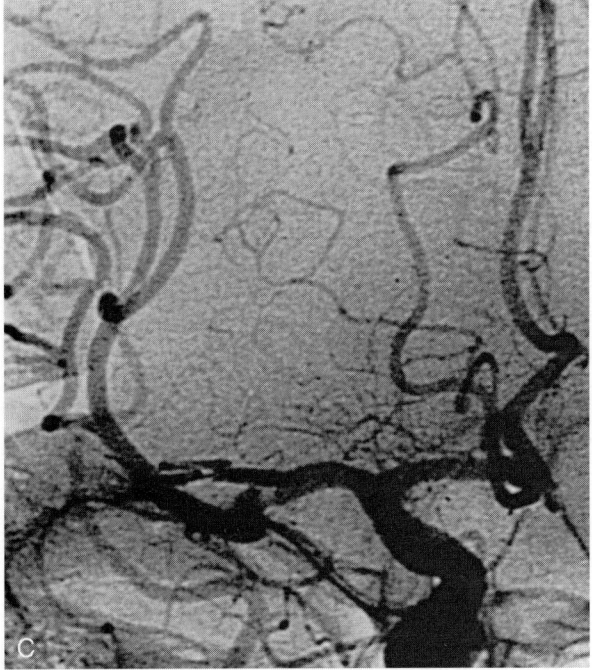

FIGURE 86–3 ■ *A–C,* A 49-year-old man had a grade 2, small ruptured bifurcation middle cerebral artery aneurysm, which was operated on day 1. *A,* A large infarction *(B)* caused by closure of the frontal bifurcation branch. *C,* No reoperation was necessary. Postoperatively, the patient had severe left hemiparesis. The patient recovered and lived independently, except with left hemiparesis.

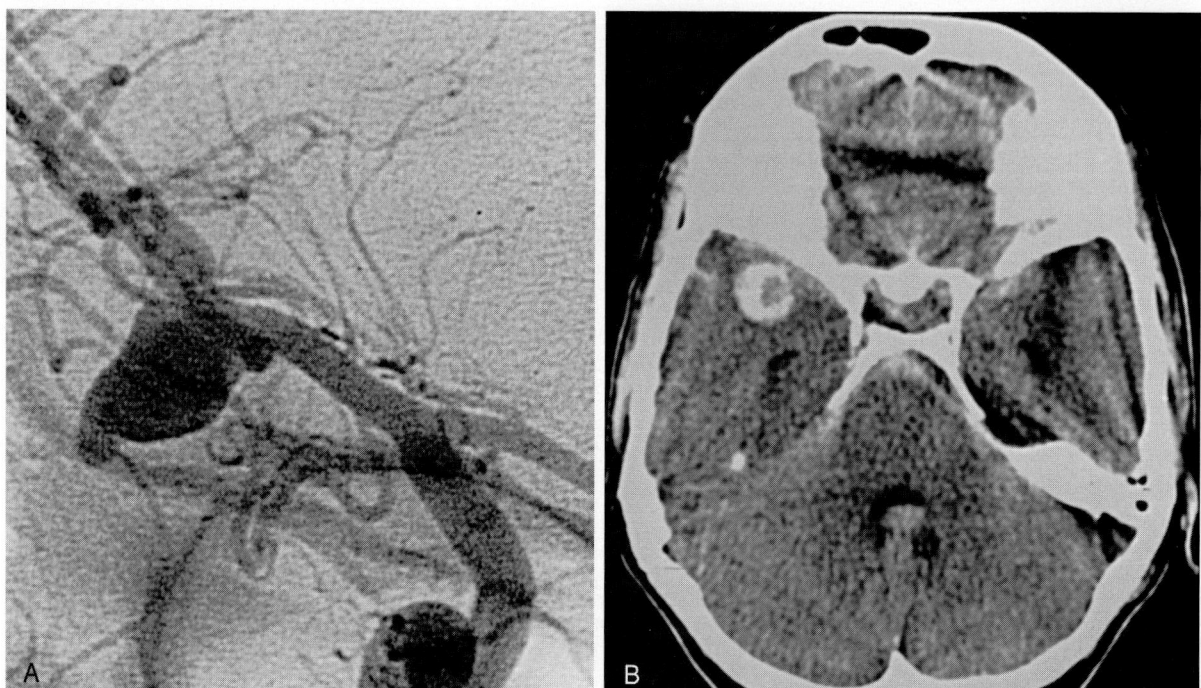

**FIGURE 86–4 ■** *A* and *B,* A 39-year-old woman had a grade 3, large partially calcified aneurysm at the middle cerebral artery (MCA) bifurcation *(A).* Calcification seen in a nonenhanced CT scan *(B).* The presence of calcification may predict difficult clipping. The patient had surgery on day 1. She recovered well.

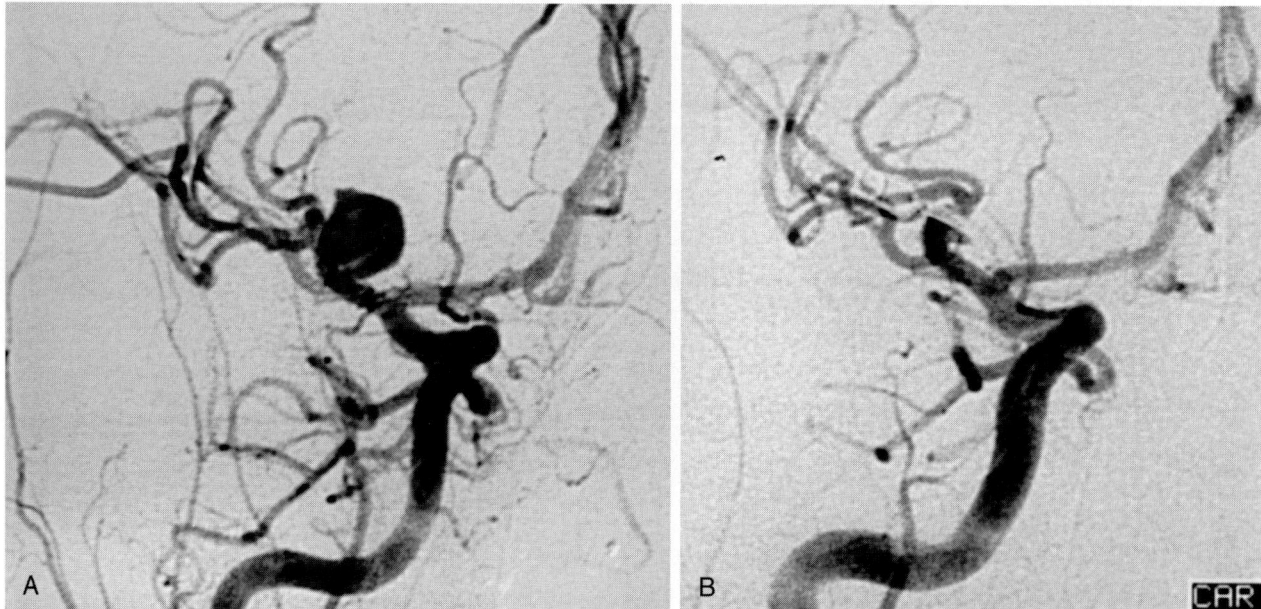

**FIGURE 86–5 ■** *A* and *B,* A 34-year-old man had a grade 3 tumor. The angiogram revealed a large superiorly and medially projecting bifurcation MCA aneurysm. *A,* A postoperative angiogram shows closure of the aneurysm. *B,* The patient had a good recovery.

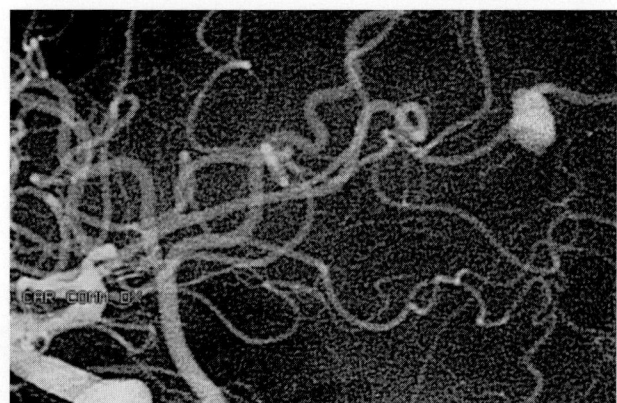

FIGURE 86–6 ■ A 39-year-old man had a grade 2, distal fusiform middle cerebral artery aneurysm. He was operated on day 1 after bleeding for a second time. A bypass from the superficial temporal artery to the MCA was performed before the resection of the aneurysm. After operation, the patient had slight left hemiparesis, which subsided rapidly, and the anastomosis was patent. He had a good recovery.

intracerebral hematomas (largest diameter ≥2.5 cm) associated with ruptured MCAAs (Fig. 86–7). The reported incidence of intracerebral hematoma in patients with aneurysmal SAH varies from 5% to 34%.[4, 16, 18, 19, 23, 45, 46] In our series, the frequency of intracerebral hematomas in patients with a single MCAA was significantly higher than in patients with any other single aneurysm (43% versus 11%),

making the goals of surgery two-fold: securing the aneurysm and evacuation of the hematoma. The risk for intracerebral hematoma increased as the site of the ruptured aneurysm became more distal, where it is more closely surrounded by the brain because the cistern is tighter. The frequency of intracerebral hematoma was 12% with an aneurysm at the carotid bifurcation (origin of MCA), 29%

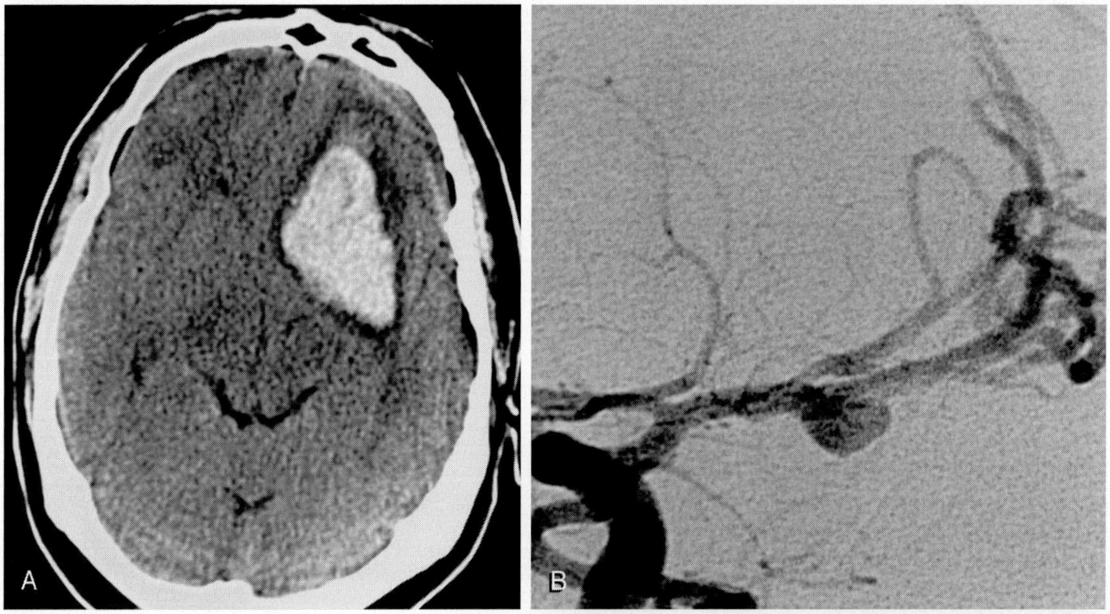

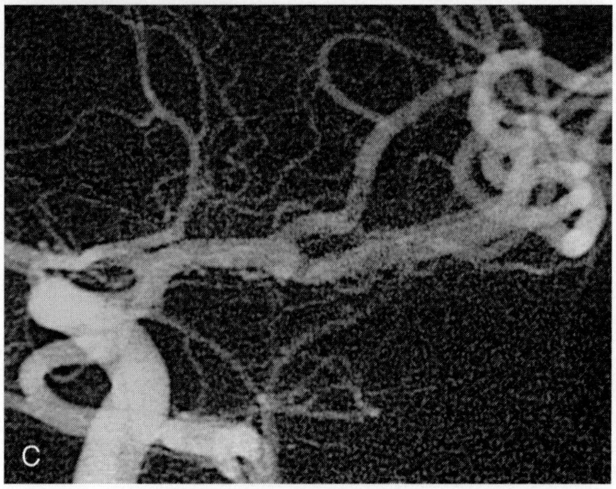

FIGURE 86–7 ■ A–C, A 38-year-old man had a grade 2, large medially located intracerebral hematoma without a subarachnoid hemorrhage (A). A bifurcation middle cerebral artery aneurysm is seen on angiography surprisingly projecting laterally, not medially as suspected from the site of an intracerebral hematoma (B). The hematoma was evacuated, and the aneurysm was clipped 3 days after the single bleed. The patient had a good recovery.

with a proximal MCAA, 43% with a bifurcation MCAA, and 44% with a distal MCAA. With MCAAs at the bifurcation, the frequency of intracerebral hematoma was highest for aneurysms directed laterally in anteroposterior angiograms, 58%. The sacks—and the bleeding sites—of these aneurysms point toward the temporal lobe, and the fundi are more parallel to the main trunk and so under a higher hemodynamic stress.

Moderate or severe intraventricular bleeding, one of the most important findings predicting poor outcome,[23, 41, 46] was observed in 24% of patients with ruptured bifurcation MCAAs, 19% of patients with proximal MCAAs, and 11% of patients with distal MCAAs. The frequencies for moderate or severe preoperative hydrocephalus were the same for each MCAA site as the frequencies for intraventricular hematoma. In a few cases with an acute hydrocephalus, an emergency ventricular drain can be life-saving; in these instances, we secure the aneurysm in the same session to prevent rebleeding.

## SURGICAL MANAGEMENT

In the case of ruptured MCAA, the timing of surgery plays a crucial role. In SAH, acute and early surgery (done in the first 72 hours) has a beneficial effect on outcome through two of the most important independent factors influencing outcome: It prevents rebleeding, and it allows the surgeon actively to prevent and to treat the vasospasm with intravenous nimodipine and HHH (hemodilution, hypervolemia, hypertension) therapy. In the extreme group of poor-grade (Hunt and Hess grade V) patients without a remarkable hematoma, the favorable effect of early surgery is less clear, and delaying surgery might be justified.[47] With our clinical experience, we operate on these patients if they improve or stabilize because as long as the bleeding site is not secured, the aggressive treatment of vasospasm (HHH therapy) may turn hazardous, as is waiting without obliterating the aneurysm. The incidence of surgical complications might be independent of the patient's grade.[48] In an unselected population and in a population without any referral bias such as ours, there are always patients presenting to the hospital with aneurysms that have bled so severely that the patients are beyond any treatment. Because these patients die in a few hours, they are not admitted to metropolitan centers, which consequently have better management or surgical results in their selected series. In our series, the reasons for nonsurgical treatment were initial poor grade (49), poor grade caused by rebleeding (7), old age (5), technical reasons (3), and patient refusal (1), comprising 11% of all patients with MCAAs. Early surgery (within 72 hours of SAH) was achieved in 60% of the ruptured MCAAs, but the number has increased in more recent years.

Especially in aneurysm surgery, the results are reflected by the quality of the team, by the skills and experience of the surgeon, and by referral biases.[49] Unless it is an emergency situation, it might be wise to delay an aneurysm operation from night to the next morning, when more experienced team and back-up is available. If the number of aneurysm operations in one institution is low, it is

impossible to gather enough experience, and the overall results remain too unfavorable.[50, 51] Large, giant, or otherwise complex aneurysms should be treated by experienced vascular neurosurgeons, capable of reconstructing or bypassing the vessels.[52]

## Positioning and Approach

All except rare distal MCAAs can be reached through a standard pterional approach, which is used exclusively in our institutions. A more subfrontal approach has also been used by creating only a small frontal flap with some removal of the sphenoid wing. For the surgery, the patient is positioned supine, with the head elevated clearly above the cardiac level to reduce the cranial venous pressure and the intra-aneurysmal arterial pressure. The head is fixed with three or four pins in the head frame (Mayfield or Sugita) and rotated 15 to 20 degrees toward the opposite side, tilted slightly downward (Fig. 86–8). The most common error is overrotating, which leads to covering of the sylvian fissure by the temporal lobe, which requires the surgeon to retract the temporal lobe more and predisposes to difficult dissection of the aneurysm. If the head is tilted downward too much, the basal orbital bony structures may obscure the operating field. A working channel parallel to the skull base is adequate, and removal of the superior orbital rim or the zygomatic arch to gain a more upward working direction is not necessary. The anesthesiologist is prepared

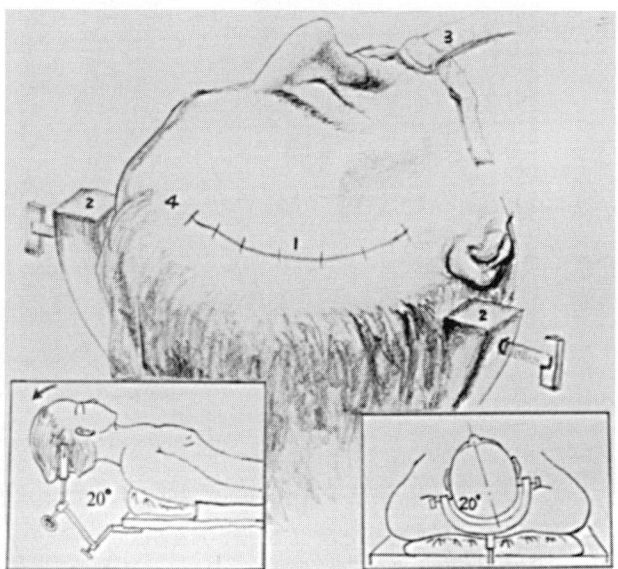

FIGURE 86–8 ■ For operation, the head is elevated clearly above the level of the heart to reduce the cranial venous pressure and even the intra-aneurysmal pressure. The head, which is fixed with three or four pins in the headframe (Mayfield or Sugita), is rotated approximately 20 degrees toward the opposite side and is tilted slightly downward. The most common error is overrotation, which leads to "covering" the sylvian fissure by the temporal lobe. If the head is tilted downward too much, the basal orbital bone structures may obscure the operating field. The working channel parallel to the skull base is adequate, and removal of the superior orbital rim or the zygomatic arch to gain a more upward-working direction is unnecessary. (1. Scalp incision; 2. Head frame; 3. Intubation tube; 4. Hair line.)

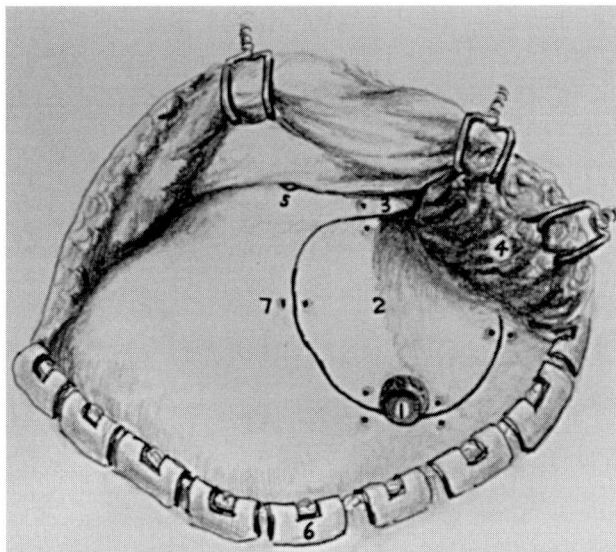

FIGURE 86–9 ■ The skin-galea-muscle flap is elevated after step-by-step detachement from the bone by diathermy in one layer, thus avoiding any injury to the branches of the facial nerve by spring hooks, until the superior orbital rim and the anterior zygomatic arch are exposed. The number of bur holes is determined by the size of the flap, the thickness of the bone, and adherence of the dura. Usually one or two bur holes are placed, one posteriorly just below the insertion line of the temporal muscle, and if necessary the other just over the pterion. The flap is detached mainly by a side-cutting craniotome, but the basal part is drilled off before lifting the flap. (1. Bur hole; 2. Temporal line; 3. Zygomatic process; 4. Temporal muscle; 5. Supraorbital foramen; 6. Scalp clip; 7. Bur holes for bone flap fixation.)

access may be done if needed to gain proximal control of the MCA. In the case of large hematomas and giant aneurysms, the skin flap is planned slightly more posteriorly to allow a better handling of the giant aneurysm or evacuation of the posteriorly, and many times deep centrally, projecting hematomas. The incision line is infiltrated abundantly with a mixture of lidocaine and epinephrine to prevent unnecessary oozing of the wound and rise of blood pressure of the patient during incision. The area of the skin flap is covered with self-adhesive transparent plastic.

The skin-galea-muscle flap is elevated after step-by-step detachment from the bone by diathermy in one layer, avoiding any injury of the branches of the facial nerve, by spring hooks until the superior orbital rim and the anterior zygomatic arch are exposed. The number of bur holes is determined by the size of the flap, thickness of the bone, and adherence of the dura. Usually one or two bur holes are placed, one posteriorly just below the insertion line of the temporal muscle and, if necessary, the other just over the pterion (Fig. 86–9). The flap is detached mostly by side-cutting craniotome, but the basal part is drilled off before lifting the flap. The operating microscope can be introduced at this point for high-speed drilling of the lateral sphenoid bone. The lateral sphenoid ridge and vertical bone on both sides is drilled off until the bony exposure is along the skull base, oozing from the cut bony surfaces, and the dura is controlled by bone wax and bipolar coagulation of the dural vessels (Fig. 86–10).

The dura is opened in a curvilinear incision pointing anterolaterally and elevated with stitches. The operating microscope is brought to place. We try to minimize the use of spatulas for brain retraction. The suction in the left hand can be used for intermittent brain retraction as well as the bipolar coagulating forceps or microscissors in the right hand. This technique necessitates frequent adjustment of the operating microscope to the proper position to keep the working channel minimum. We prefer a mouth-controlled and balanced microscope with magnetic brakes as designed by Yasargil. Besides the three extraordinary benefits of magnification, light microscopic view, and stereoscopic

for frequent adjustment of the position of the operating table.

Shaving should be minimal but allow a large enough oblique frontotemporal skin incision, behind the hairline if possible. In ordinary cases, we prefer a short incision placed slightly over the estimated location of the sylvian fissure and more frontally as the approach to the sylvian fissure is made from the frontal side. A more frontobasal

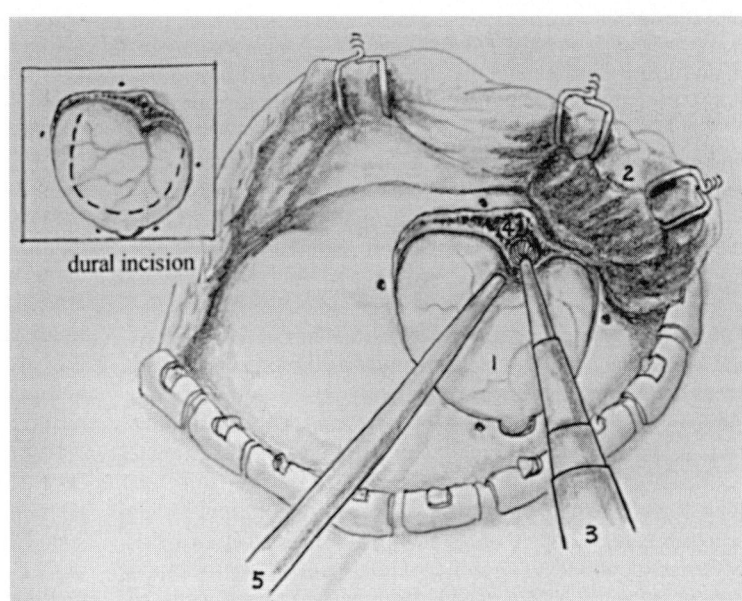

dural incision

FIGURE 86–10 ■ An operating microscope can be introduced for high-speed drilling of the lateral sphenoid bone. The lateral sphenoid ridge and vertical bone on both of its sides are drilled off until the bony exposure is along the skull base, oozing from the cut bone surfaces, and the dura is controlled by bone wax and bipolar coagulation of the dural vessels. The dura is opened in a curvilinear incision pointing anterolaterally and is elevated with stitches. (1. Dura; 2. Temporal muscle; 3. Drill; 4. Sphenoid; 5. Sucker.)

view, the modern microscope gives the surgeon free movements—especially with the use of a mouthpiece—giving an opportunity for as atraumatic exposure as possible. Elbow and arm support using a slim adjustable table lifted frequently according to the needs of proper working direction and height gives comfort and support. Microsurgery is a mixture of equipment, technique, knowledge of anatomy, and way of thinking.

## Strategy

The strategy for exposure basically depends on site, size, and especially direction of the aneurysm and existence of hematoma or associated aneurysms. It is wise to imagine three-dimensionally how the aneurysm is exactly located and projected when positioning the head of the patient in the skull clamp. With proximal MCAAs and with bifurcation MCAAs with a short MCA main trunk, the sylvian fissure may be opened medially. The opticocarotid cisterns are approached frontobasally and opened. Cerebrospinal fluid (CSF) is drained slowly giving more space. The frontal lobe is gently retracted. Especially when dealing with recently ruptured aneurysms, the direction of the aneurysm must be taken into account before any retraction. The carotid bifurcation is exposed by opening the cisterns widely. The dissection is then carried along the main trunk of the MCA opening the fissure mediolaterally, until the aneurysm is encountered. Any injury to the perforators at the bifurcation and at the medial wall of the MCA must be cautiously avoided. Proximal MCAAs are usually small, but their necks are wide. Also at the origin of the anterior temporal artery, the neck is often incorporated with that vessel, and careless clip placement can lead to kinking and closure of the vessel. Proximal MCAAs pointing upward or medially are involved with lenticulostriatal perforators. To secure these aneurysms properly and avoid calamitous infarcts, all small vessels must be meticulously separated from the neck before clipping. If the aneurysm is at the bifurcation, at the time of dissection, the part of the main trunk free of perforators is observed for possible temporary clip placement.

We usually approach nearly all MCAAs directly by opening the fissure laterally. Even in acute SAH, in most cases enough space can be obtained by patiently removing CSF after the fissure is first open. If the brain is edematous and swollen and the fissure tight, CSF can be first removed by opening the frontobasal cisterns or lamina terminalis or both. Gentle injection of fluid inside the sylvian fissure helps in its opening (water dissection). Spinal CSF drainage has not been used in MCAAs. Once enough room is achieved, the lateral dissection is carried deeper into the fissure, and one of the distal MCA branches is followed to the aneurysm. Many times, the sylvian fissure is opened straight over the aneurysm (Fig. 86–11). Usually, at this stage of dissection, the need for lobe retraction is minimal and is achieved with small cotton patties. If additional retraction is needed, it should be directed away from the lobe toward which the aneurysm dome is pointing. Once the bifurcation area is encountered, the main trunk of the MCA is identified to obtain proximal control or if temporary occlusion is to be applied. The main trunk can usually

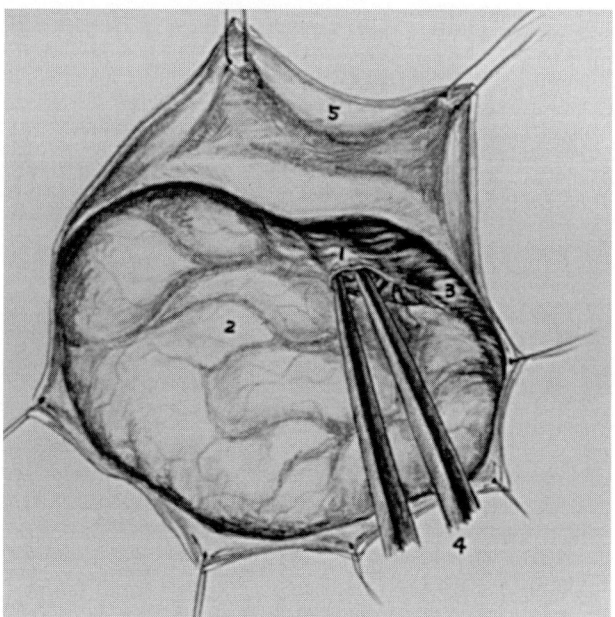

**FIGURE 86–11** ■ We usually approach almost all middle cerebral artery aneurysms (MCAAs) directly by opening the fissure laterally. Even in an acute subarachnoid hemorrhage, in most cases enough space can be obtained by patiently removing cerebrospinal fluid (CSF) after the fissure is first opened. If the brain is very edematic and swollen and the fissure is very tight, CSF can first be removed by opening the frontobasal cisterns, or the lamina terminalis, or both. Gentle injection of fluid inside the sylvian fissure helps to open it (via water dissection). CSF drainage from the spine has not been used in MCAAs. Once enough room is achieved, the lateral dissection is carried deeper into the fissure, and one of the distal MCA branches is followed to the aneurysm. Often, the sylvian fissure is opened straight over the aneurysm. (1. Arachnoid; 2. Frontal lobe; 3. Sylvian veins; 4. Bipolar forceps; 5. Dura.)

be found dissecting under or beside the bifurcation away from the aneurysm. Thereafter the dissection is concentrated in the neck, and all manipulation of the dome—and the bleeding site—must be avoided as long as possible (Fig. 86–12). All main branches must be identified and carefully dissected free. After a clip has been applied, the dome is dissected free, and the position of the blades is checked (Fig. 86–13).

If the clip is closing the neck, the sac is punctured and coagulated (Fig. 86–14). It must be ascertained that there is no obstruction in the main trunk or branches or that none of the medial perforators is trapped between the blades. Sometimes it is difficult to assess visually whether there is enough flow in M2 branches after clipping, especially under hypotension. Mini-Doppler ultrasound is a practical tool for this purpose: It is simple and easy to use, it gives an unmistakable sound if there is flow, and it is relatively cheap. In the most complicated aneurysms, intraoperative angiography is more helpful.[53, 54] This technique, however, demands special utilities and is more costly: It must be prepared preoperatively, and it requires decent fluoroscopy, a special headrest, a special operative table, and a neuroradiologist to do it. Mini-Doppler ultrasound has been proven to be cost-effective in cases with higher risk for technical troubleshooting.[53, 54] If used routinely, mini-Doppler ultrasound detects at least some unex-

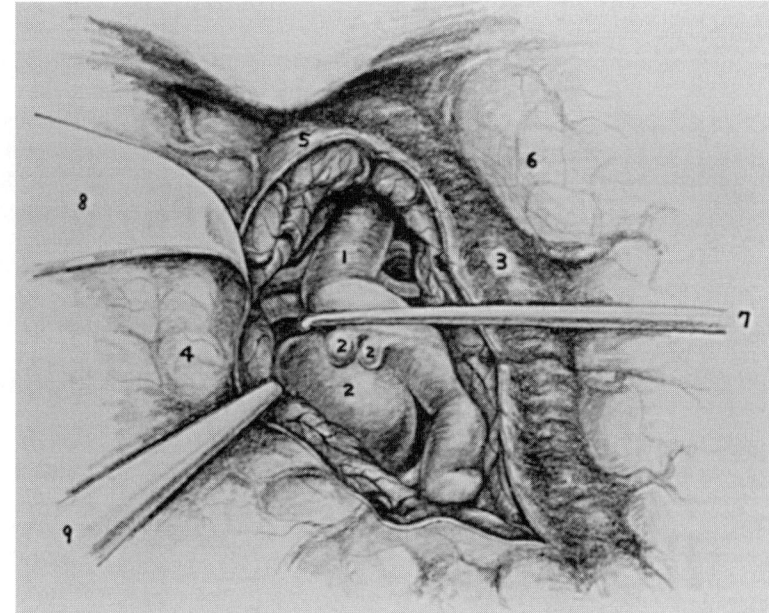

**FIGURE 86–12** ■ Once the bifurcation area is encountered, the main trunk of the middle cerebral artery may be identified to get proximal control. The main trunk can usually be found by dissecting under or beside the bifurcation away from the aneurysm—in this case M1 is below the bifurcation and its aneurysms. Thereafter, the dissection is concentrated in the neck, and all manipulation of the dome (and the bleeding site) must be avoided as long as possible. All the main branches must be identified and carefully dissected free. (1. M2; 2. Aneurysm; 3. Sylvian veins; 4. Frontal lobe; 5. Arachnoid; 6. Temporal lobe; 7. Hook; 8. Retractor; 9. Sucker.)

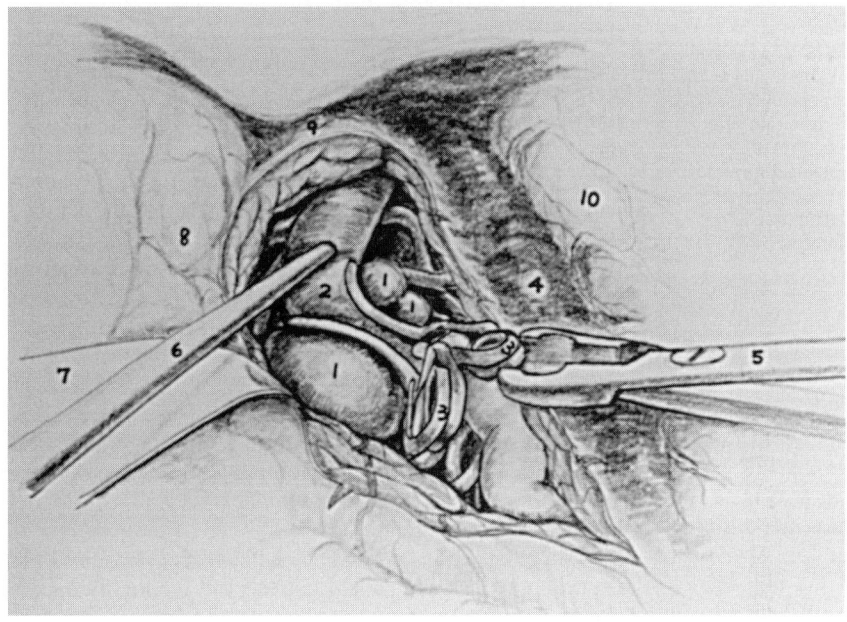

**FIGURE 86–13** ■ After a clip has been applied, the dome is dissected free and the position of the blades is checked. (1. Aneurysm; 2. M2; 3. Aneurysm clip; 4. Sylvian veins; 5. Clip applier; 6. Sucker; 7. Retractor; 8. Frontal lobe; 9. Arachnoid; 10. Temporal lobe.)

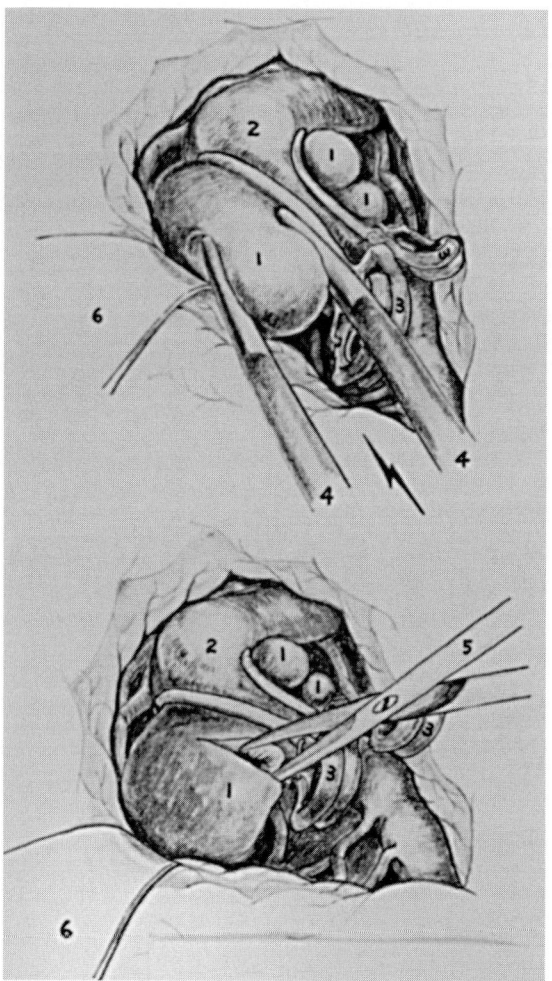

**FIGURE 86–14** ■ If the clip is closing the neck, the sac is punctured and coagulated. It must be secured so that there is not the slightest obstruction in the main trunk or branches and so that none of the medial perforators is trapped between the blades. Sometimes, it is hard to visually assess whether there is enough flow in M2 branches after clipping, especially under hypotension. Mini-Doppler ultrasound is a practical tool for this purpose: It is simple and easy to use; it gives an unmistakable sound effect if there is flow; and it is relatively cheap. (1. Aneurysm; 2. M2; 3. Aneurysm clip; 4. Bipolar forceps; 5. Microscissors; 6. Retractor.)

pected arterial occlusions, which otherwise would lead to clinically evident strokes, if not corrected.

In certain cases, one must consider leaving a small neck remnant—"dog ear"—rather than risking possible closure of a branch (Fig. 86–15). If the remnant is thin, it should be clipped with a miniclip. If the remaining part is strong walled, it should be left alone because a too-tight clipping may lead to occlusion of the branches (see Fig. 86–3). In larger aneurysms, the force in the tips of the clip blades might be insufficient for complete closure of the neck. In those cases, a booster clip must be applied above the first one, either parallel with it or crossing with the tips of the blades of the first one. The tricks of Drake[55] and Peerless with tandem and piggyback clips may also be used. Local administration of papaverine to prevent vasospasm has been used routinely. In a few cases, it has caused a frightening unilateral or bilateral mydriasis lasting a few hours.

## Intracerebral Hematoma Associated with Ruptured Middle Cerebral Artery Aneurysms

A significant intracerebral hematoma (>2.5 cm) is often associated with a ruptured MCAA. This situation often alters surgical strategy. The hematoma cavity can be used as a route to the aneurysm, but this route is unclear and dangerous. The aneurysm is pointing toward the cavity, and the first part of the aneurysm to be encountered is usually the bleeding site, raising the risk for intraoperative rupture. It is preferable to remove only a sufficient part of the hematoma to obtain enough space, then continue with the clear anatomy of the trans-sylvian approach. Once the aneurysm is secured, the rest of the hematoma can be removed. Commonly, the most superior and posterior parts of the hematoma remain unevacuated if three-dimensional anatomy of the hematoma is not appreciated. As a result, a second operation may be required to remove hematoma, edematous brain, and sometimes temporal lobe.

## Multiple Aneurysms

Our series consisted of 221 patients with multiple intracranial aneurysms and at least one MCAA. Surgical management of these patients should follow the guidelines for treatment of multiple intracranial aneurysms.[26, 50] The symptomatic aneurysm must be treated first. The associated aneurysms should be secured in the same session if possible because the overall outcome of these patients seems to be slightly better. The choice of one-stage or two-stage operation is strongly biased, however, and depends on the severity of SAH, brain swelling, sites of the aneurysms, and the experience of the surgeon and the team. In troublesome perioperative conditions, the pursuit of the intact sacs is abandoned. Our analysis also showed that in the cases of multiple intracranial aneurysms, only two thirds of all the aneurysms could be secured.

Of our patients with multiple MCAAs, 100 had bilateral and 11 unilateral MCAAs. Two thirds (63) of the patients with bilateral MCAAs had mirror aneurysms, and in half of these cases, they were the only aneurysms the patient had. Thirty-four percent of the associated bifurcation MCAAs were directed inferiorly in both angiogram projections, perhaps making them most suitable at this site for contralateral clipping. In 124 patients out of 221 with multiple intracranial aneurysms and at least one MCAA, all aneurysms were secured in 46 in a one-stage operation. In 18 patients, ipsilateral and contralateral aneurysms were clipped through the same craniotomy (Fig. 86–16). Contralateral aneurysms should not be clipped in the presence of red, swollen brain associated with recent severe SAH. Contralateral surgery should be reserved for highly experienced neurosurgeons.

## Giant Aneurysms

About 5% of all aneurysms are giant (diameter ≥2.5 cm by definition). Six percent of our MCAAs were giant aneurysms, and the MCA proved to be the most frequent site for these lesions (Fig. 86–17). The surgery for giant aneurysms

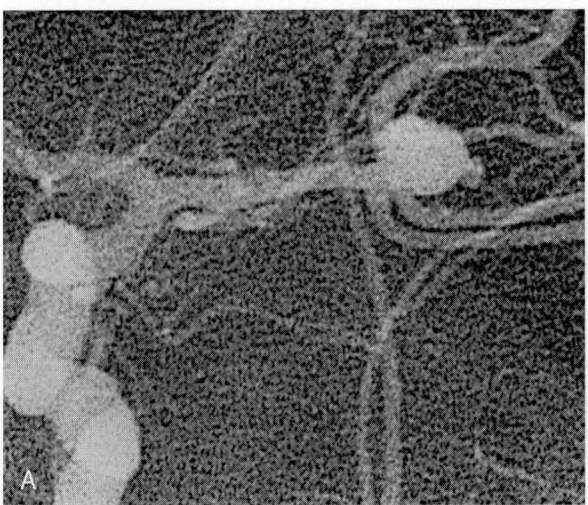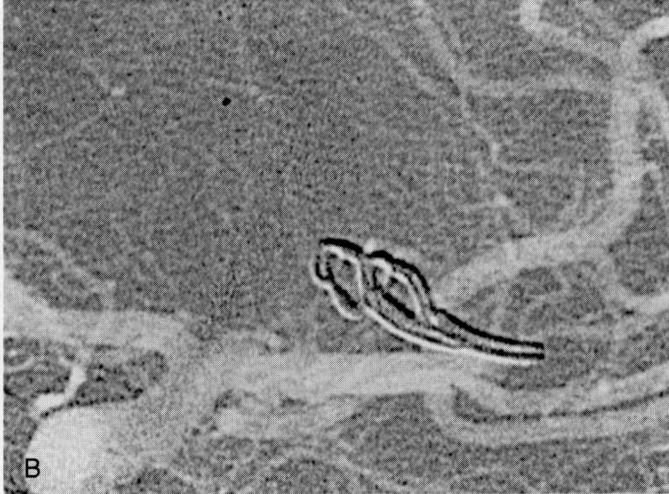

FIGURE 86–15 ■ *A* and *B*, A 48-year-old woman had a grade 2, left-sided middle cerebral artery (MCA) aneurysm, which was operated on the day of bleeding *(A)*. A small remnant of the neck is seen on the follow-up angiogram. *B*, The patient had a good recovery. An unruptured contralateral MCA aneurysm was operated on uneventfully 6 weeks later.

requires exceptionally careful imaging and planning, including preparation for bypass surgery or surgery with circulatory arrest under hypothermia.[52, 56–58] Direct clipping is reported to be possible in about two thirds of the cases (38% to 71%), and some reconstructive surgery is often needed (Figs. 86–18 to 86–21).[58] To soften the aneurysm dome, temporary occlusion is almost mandatory. Occlusion times are frequently remarkably longer than with smaller lesions. The risk for permanent iatrogenic ischemic lesion might be lowered by perioperative electroencephalogram monitoring.[59] The lateral asymmetry in wave patterns indicates hypoxia, which can turn to ischemia if the circulation remains restricted.

The thrombosed mass inside the aneurysm can be removed with an ultrasound aspirator. In some cases, the securing of the aneurysm leads to occlusion of the parent

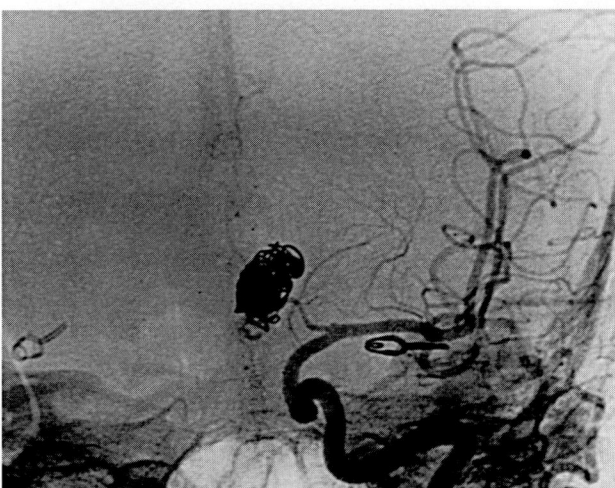

FIGURE 86–16 ■ A 53-year-old woman had a ruptured basilar aneurysm which was treated successfully with coils. Angiograms revealed bilateral unruptured middle cerebral artery (MCA) aneurysms that were treated through a single right-sided craniotomy. The patient had a good recovery.

artery. Sufficient circulation may be preserved by bypassing the MCA with superficial temporal artery or with external carotid artery using venous graft. Only in children can adequate oxygen content be provided by the collateral network. In most reported experience, indications for aneurysm clipping under circulatory arrest with hypothermia and barbiturate brain protection are giant or complicated posterior fossa lesions.

Ruptured giant aneurysms seem to carry practically the same risk for rebleeding as smaller ones. In a series from the Mayo Clinic, the risk for rebleeding was greater than 18% in the first 14 days after admission.[58, 60] This risk advocates early surgery, although real pros and cons remain controversial. In the same series, of patients surviving for surgery, 72% had a favorable outcome. This rate is higher than usually reported. The outcome figures are, however, affected more by the site of the aneurysm (anterior versus posterior) and clinical grade (Hunt and Hess grade I to II versus grade IV to V) than merely by early surgery itself. The experience of the whole team and referral pattern also have a strong impact on overall outcome.

## Temporary Arterial Occlusion

The indications for temporary arterial occlusion are premature aneurysm rupture during dissection and if the structure of the aneurysm (size, shape, location of the branches) requires manipulation of the sac to apply the clip properly. Sometimes the backflow from M2 branches is so brisk that temporary occlusion not only of the main trunk but also of the branches must be employed to decrease the sac sufficiently. The common practice to protect the brain during temporary occlusion is to raise blood pressure and administer a bolus of mannitol and barbiturates before occlusion.[59, 61, 62] The real influence of these factors to prevent iatrogenic infarction remains unproven. Moderate hypothermia (without cardiac arrest) may give some additional brain protection. It can be used in complicated large or giant MCAAs. High risk for an ischemic event during temporary occlusion

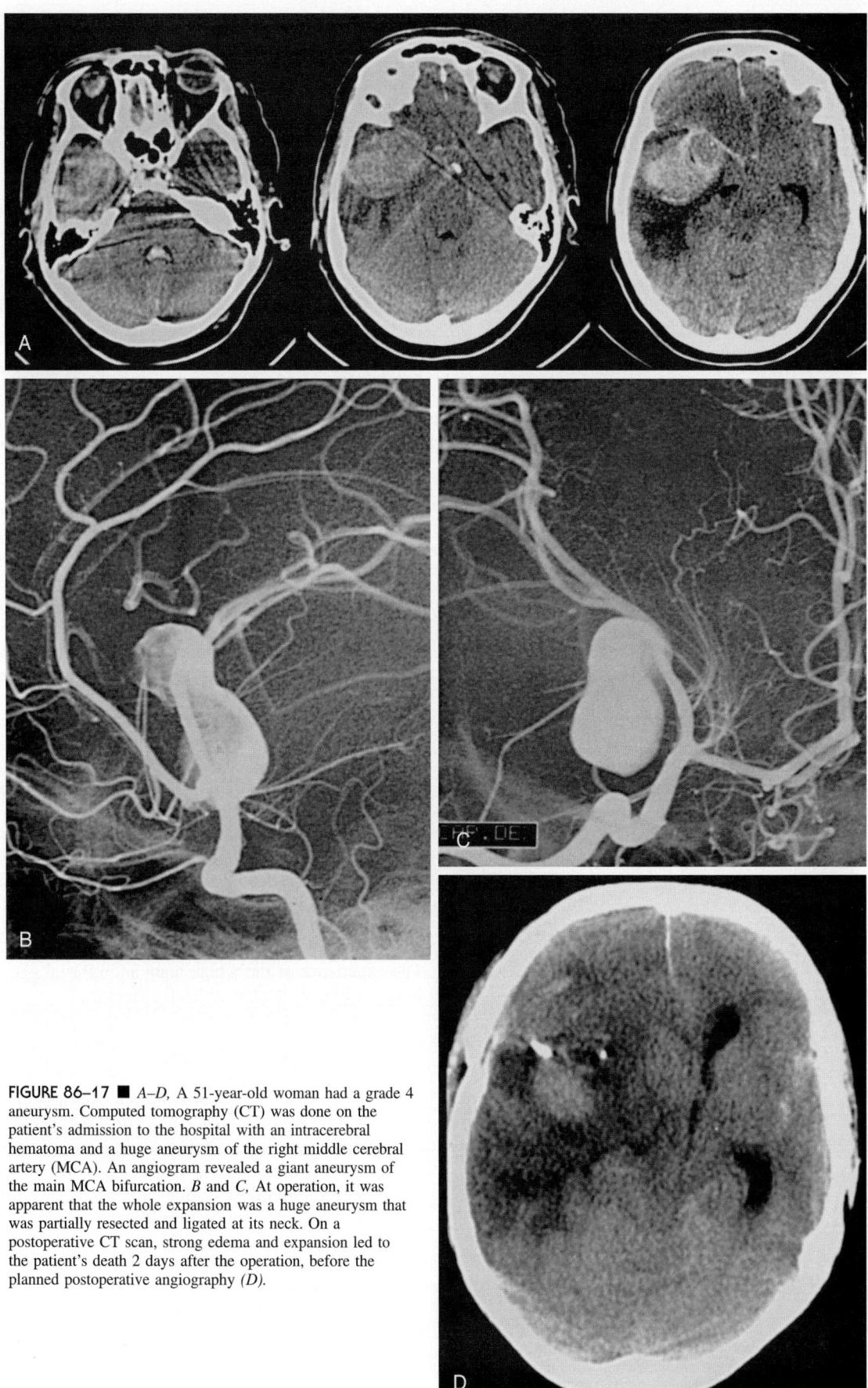

**FIGURE 86–17 ■** *A–D,* A 51-year-old woman had a grade 4 aneurysm. Computed tomography (CT) was done on the patient's admission to the hospital with an intracerebral hematoma and a huge aneurysm of the right middle cerebral artery (MCA). An angiogram revealed a giant aneurysm of the main MCA bifurcation. *B* and *C,* At operation, it was apparent that the whole expansion was a huge aneurysm that was partially resected and ligated at its neck. On a postoperative CT scan, strong edema and expansion led to the patient's death 2 days after the operation, before the planned postoperative angiography *(D).*

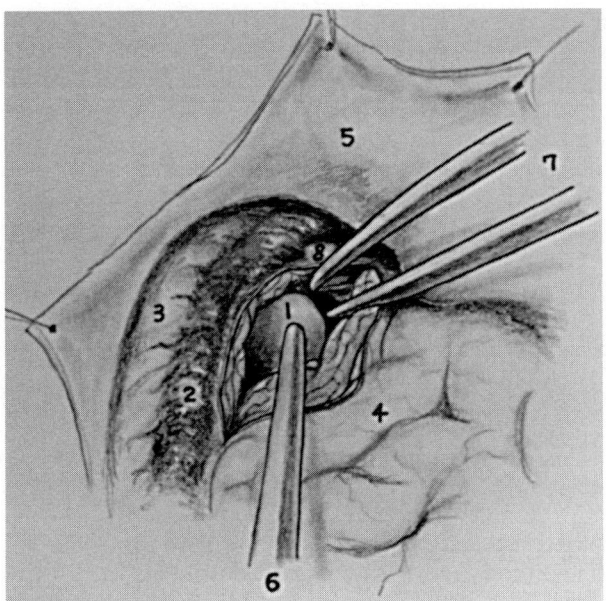

FIGURE 86–18 ■ A small part of the fundus of a left-sided giant middle cerebral artery aneurysm is seen after splitting of the sylvian fissure. (1. Aneurysm; 2. Sylvian veins; 3. Temporal lobe; 4. Frontal lobe; 5. Dura; 6. Sucker; 7. Bipolar forceps.)

endosaccular coils (i.e., coiling) has provided an optional and increasingly used method of treatment.[15, 63–66] With advances in microcatheters and guidewires, the site of the aneurysm is merely a factor in selecting patients for this treatment. The neck must be clearly visualized and be free from efferent branches, and the width of the neck should be preferably less than the diameter of the dome.

Because of the lack of adequate follow-up studies, the long-term effectiveness of this technique is unclear. It has been increasingly used in the treatment of unruptured and ruptured intracranial aneurysms, although more studies are needed to aid clinicians in selecting an optimal treatment modality in a specific clinical situation. MCAAs are the aneurysms least suitable for coiling.[15, 20, 63, 66] In giant aneurysms, the experience of coiling is even more limited, but in a few cases the outcome has been dismal. The traditional endovascular parent vessel occlusion is not a real option in giant MCAAs.[65] Theoretically, coiling could be used as a first-stage treatment to secure the lesion from rebleeding, providing a possibility for more delayed surgery or aggressive vasospasm management. According to our experience, later surgery for previously coiled aneurysms might be more complicated than thought because of the adhesions and lower mobility of the sac. Many times the sac must be

is clearly related to occlusion time (if >30 minutes), placement of the clip (if also occluding perforators), and operative conditions (emergency situation versus elective occlusion).[62]

Temporary occlusion is safe when used for fewer than 5 minutes except for a few local technical complications. There is no safe upper limit, but caution should be used with times more than 15 minutes. One single temporary occlusion is preferred. Temporary occlusion should be used with normotensive or hypertensive levels of blood pressure. Temporary occlusion should be used in aged patients and those in poor grades before surgery cautiously, and associated aneurysms should be left for a second craniotomy when using temporary occlusion. Temporary occlusion should be preserved only for cases that absolutely cannot be managed without it.

The role of the somatosensory evoked potential response or electroencephalogram monitorings in helping to protect the brain from ischemic lesions during temporary occlusion is controversial.[61] There is evidence that somatosensory evoked potential responses deteriorate in about 10 minutes after the closure of the MCA, but the brain tissue recovers completely without any new sequelae if the recirculation is obtained in another 10 minutes. Asymmetric slowing of waves on an electroencephalogram indicates hypoxia early enough to be reversible. These techniques have their limitations: There are false-negative results; they require educated staff and special hardware; and they work out best in elective surgery, not in cases done in the middle of the night.

## Endovascular Treatment

Since the introduction of Guglielmi detachable coils, the endovascular embolization of intracranial aneurysms with

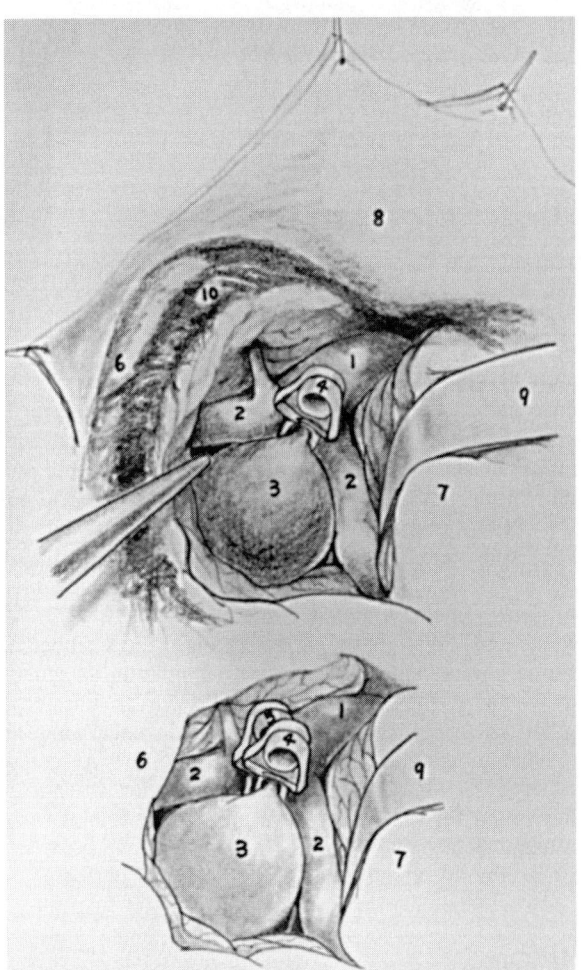

FIGURE 86–19 ■ The first clip is applied on the sclerotic, thick neck. Even with two clips, the aneurysm is still pulsating. (1. M1; 2. M2; 3. Aneurysm; 4. Aneurysm clip; 5. Aneurysm clip; 6. Temporal lobe; 7. Frontal lobe; 8. Dura; 9. Retractor; 10. Sylvian veins.)

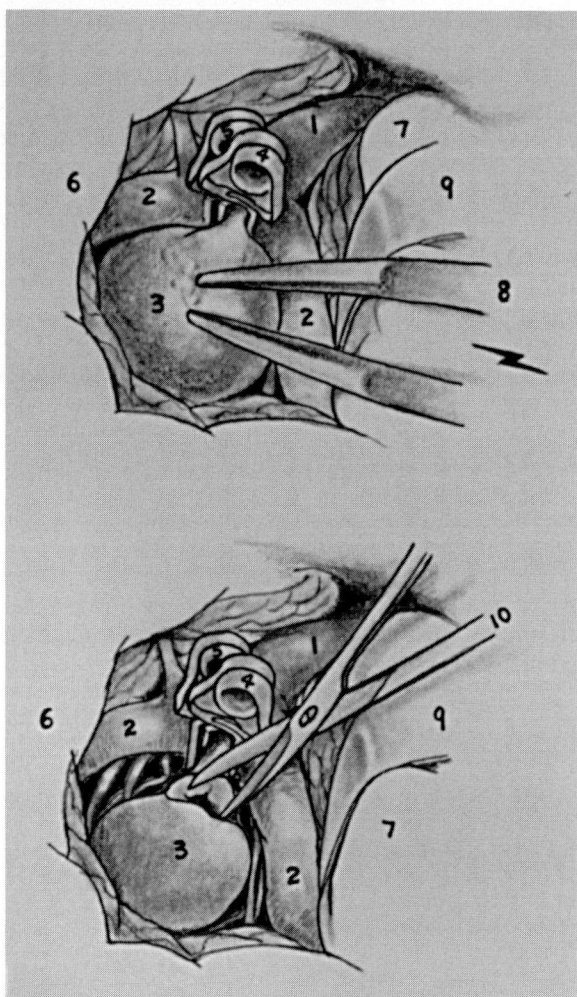

FIGURE 86–20 ■ The giant aneurysm is coagulated and opened. (1. M1; 2. M2; 3. Aneurysm; 4. Aneurysm clip; 5. Aneurysm clip; 6. Temporal lobe; 7. Frontal lobe; 8. Bipolar forceps; 9. Retractor; 10. Scissors.)

opened and the coils removed before the neck clipping is possible. Also the relief of other symptoms (i.e., cases with epilepsy, mass symptoms) may be more questionable with Guglielmi detachable coils treatment, even though the pulsatile effect might be diminished. Hypothetically the risk for vasospasm might be higher in ruptured aneurysms with Guglielmi detachable coils because the clot in the subarachnoid space remains untouched.

A randomized study in our institution of the treatment of ruptured intracranial aneurysms with Guglielmi detachable coils versus early surgery showed that in an unselected population, one third of the symptomatic aneurysms are not suitable for Guglielmi detachable coils.[20] At certain sites (e.g., the MCA), the aneurysms are often structurally better suited for surgery or have more complications with Guglielmi detachable coils. A modern neurovascular unit must be able to offer both of these treatment options.

## OUTCOME

Our patients with MCAAs fared poorly overall, despite the good surgical results in good-grade patients: a greater than

86% frequency for good outcome in grade 0 to grade II patients (Table 86–4). These results were equal to other patients with another symptomatic anterior circulation aneurysm. The immediate postoperative results were the same in all patients with symptomatic MCAAs as in patients with aneurysms at other sites, but 30% of the patients with a single MCAA had a poor outcome, being severely disabled or having died by 12 months' follow-up, compared with a 23% frequency for unfavorable outcome in patients with a single intracranial aneurysm at other sites in the anterior circulation. This significant difference is explained by the higher frequency of severe persistent deficits—dysphasia, severe hemiparesis, visual field deficits, and late epilepsy—associated with symptomatic MCAAs. In patients with multiple intracranial aneurysms and one MCAA, the frequency for poor outcome was 38%, and in patients with multiple MCAAs, it was 35%. These figures are worse than those generally seen in our patients with multiple intracranial aneurysms. Table 86–5 shows the outcome of ruptured MCAAs related to their site and clinical grade.

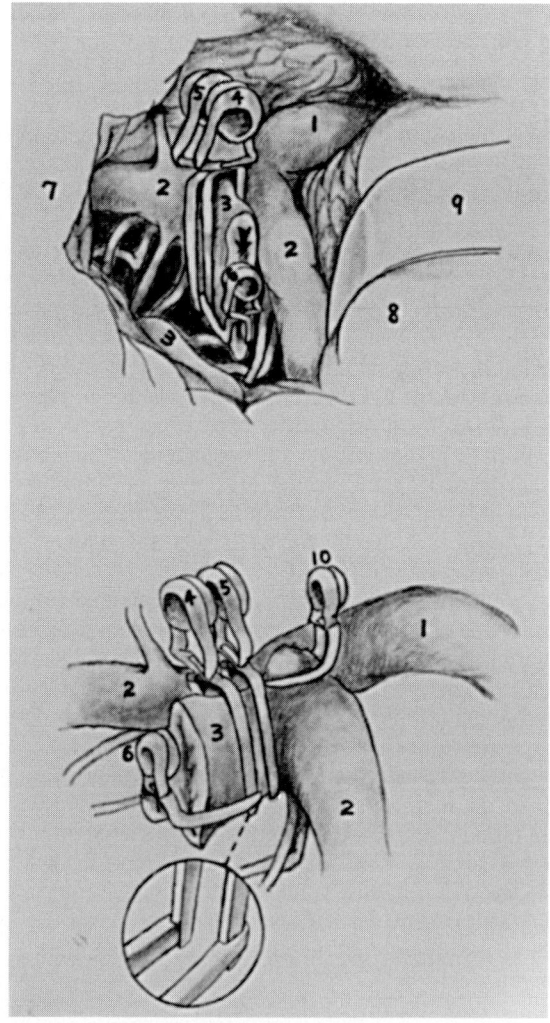

FIGURE 86–21 ■ Finally, after the resection of the aneurysm, a booster clip is applied. A small additional aneurysm is ligated with a miniclip. (1. M1; 2. M2; 3. Aneurysm remnant; 4. Aneurysm clip; 5. Aneurysm clip; 6. Booster clip; 7. Temporal lobe; 8. Frontal lobe; 9. Retractor; 10. Miniclip.)

| Grade† (no. patients) | Good Recovery | Moderate Disability | Severe Disability | Dead |
|---|---|---|---|---|
| 0 (33) | 88 | 12 | — | — |
| I (46) | 87 | 9 | — | 4 |
| II (171) | 85 | 6 | 4 | 5 |
| III (124) | 47 | 27 | 13 | 13 |
| IV (59) | 15 | 25 | 24 | 36 |
| V (24) | 8 | 17 | 29 | 46 |
| Total | 62 | 15 | 10 | 13 |

*No patient in a vegetative state at 12 months.
†Preoperative or admission grade according to Hunt and Hess.
GOS, Glasgow Outcome Scale.

In other published series of MCAAs, similar frequencies for surgical outcome can be seen.[7] In the series of Suzuki and colleagues[10] of 413 patients, 94% were in good or excellent condition 6 months after treatment. Half of these patients were operated late, their aneurysms were unruptured, or they had good grades (0 to I). In a Hungarian series of 289 patients with MCAAs, only 18% had poor outcome after surgery in a long-term follow-up.[8] Yasargil[12] reported unfavorable results only in 6% of his 231 patients with MCAAs. Excellent results were published by Sundt and coworkers,[44] with a 14% frequency for poor results after surgery for MCAAs. All these are surgical series and may reflect not only excellent surgical skills, but also selection and referral bias.

The overall management outcome was almost equal for all MCAA sites: 34% poor outcome in patients with ruptured proximal MCAAs, 32% with ruptured bifurcation MCAAs, and 30% for ruptured distal MCAAs. The frequency for poor outcome in good-grade patients was highest among patients with a proximal MCAA. This result is explained by a high frequency of anatomic variation, in which the neck of the aneurysm is partly incorporated with the smaller efferent vessel, leading easily to its inadvertent occlusion by the clip. Poor results were most common in patients who had a bifurcation MCAA directed laterally in the anteroposterior angiogram because these patients had

| Grade* | Proximal MCAA (41 patients) | Bifurcation MCAA (376 patients) | Distal MCAA (9 patients) |
|---|---|---|---|
| I | 12 | 3 | — |
| II | 18 | 11 | 20 |
| III | 40 | 25 | 100 |
| IV | 67 | 62 | — |
| V | 100 | 89 | 100 |

*Preoperative or admission grade according to Hunt and Hess. GOS, Glasgow Outcome Scale; MCAA, middle cerebral artery aneurysm.

significantly more temporal intracerebral hematomas. The best results were achieved in patients with a bifurcation MCAA pointing inferiorly in both projections: a 9% frequency of poor outcome. This outcome reflects a lower number of intracerebral hematomas and the fewest technical problems in the surgery of these aneurysms.

The larger the size of ruptured MCAA, the poorer the long-term outcome: 29% of patients with very small MCAAs (2 to 7 mm), 33% with small MCAAs (8 to 14 mm), 31 with large MCAAs (15 to 24 mm), and 43% with giant MCAAs had poor outcome (Figs. 86–22 and 86–23). Patients with large and giant MCAAs had significantly more intracerebral hematomas (59%) than those with smaller MCAAs (34%). An irregular or multilobular shape of the MCAA correlated with a more unfavorable outcome—33% compared with 7% in patients with a smooth-walled MCAA. This correlation was not caused by more frequent intraoperative ruptures but mainly by the significantly more severe (classified by CT according to Fisher) bleedings seen with these aneurysms—60% and 23%. We also studied the factors influencing outcome by multivariate analysis in selected patients with SAH (MCAA ruptured) confirmed by early CT. The following four variables had the most significant independent contributions to outcome: grade, vasospasm, postoperative hematoma, and age. Temporal intracerebral hematomas together with vasospasm and inadvertent occlusion of main vessels or thalamostriate perforators explain the specific late disabilities, described in detail subsequently, seen in patients with MCAAs.

## SPECIFIC LATE DISABILITIES

### Epilepsy

The incidence of late epilepsy after SAH varies from 7% to 25% in different studies.[67–72] The risk factors have shown to be the site (MCA) of the symptomatic intracranial aneurysms, temporal intracerebral hematoma, brain ischemia, and hypertension. Multiplicity of intracranial aneurysms increases the risk for late epilepsy. In our series, late epilepsy occurred in 18% of the long-term survivors with a single MCAA. The frequencies were even higher in patients with multiple intracranial aneurysms and one MCAA (20%) and with multiple MCAAs (27%). This frequency is significantly higher than with any other symptomatic aneurysms. Whether the symptomatic MCAA was proximal, bifurcation, or distal, the frequencies for late epilepsy were not significantly different—22%, 24%, and 30%. Of the patients with a bifurcation MCAA and late epilepsy, 52% had a temporal intracerebral hematoma, whereas only 23% of those who were seizure-free had a temporal intracerebral hematoma. Half of the long-term survivors with symptomatic MCAAs and late epilepsy had had intracerebral hematoma.

### Hemiparesis

As a result of feeding areas and the scarcity of the collateral circulation as well as the high number of intracerebral

*Text continued on page 1178*

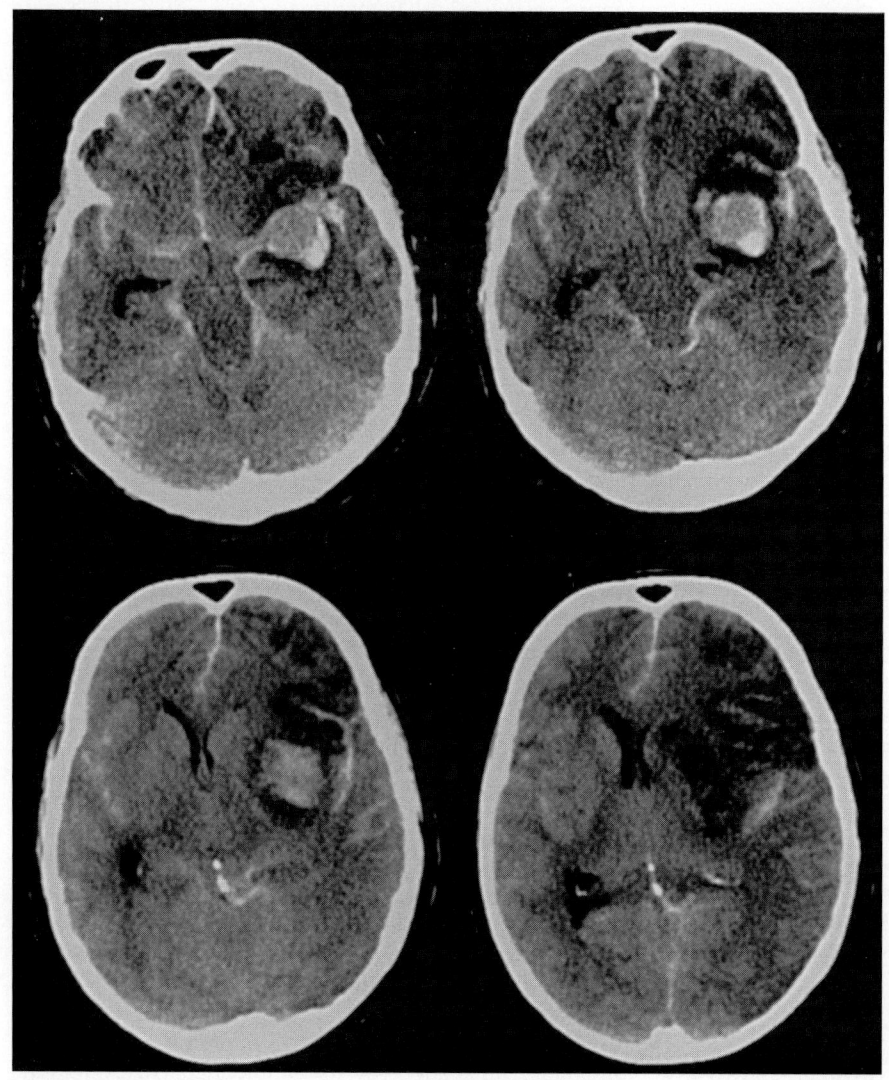

**FIGURE 86–22** ■ A 58-year-old woman was found unconscious at her home. This nonenhanced computed tomography (CT) scan shows a subarachnoid hemorrhage and a large middle cerebral artery aneurysm surrounded with blood. The patient had a large infarction and edema. The patient died 2 days after hospitalization. No operation was performed.

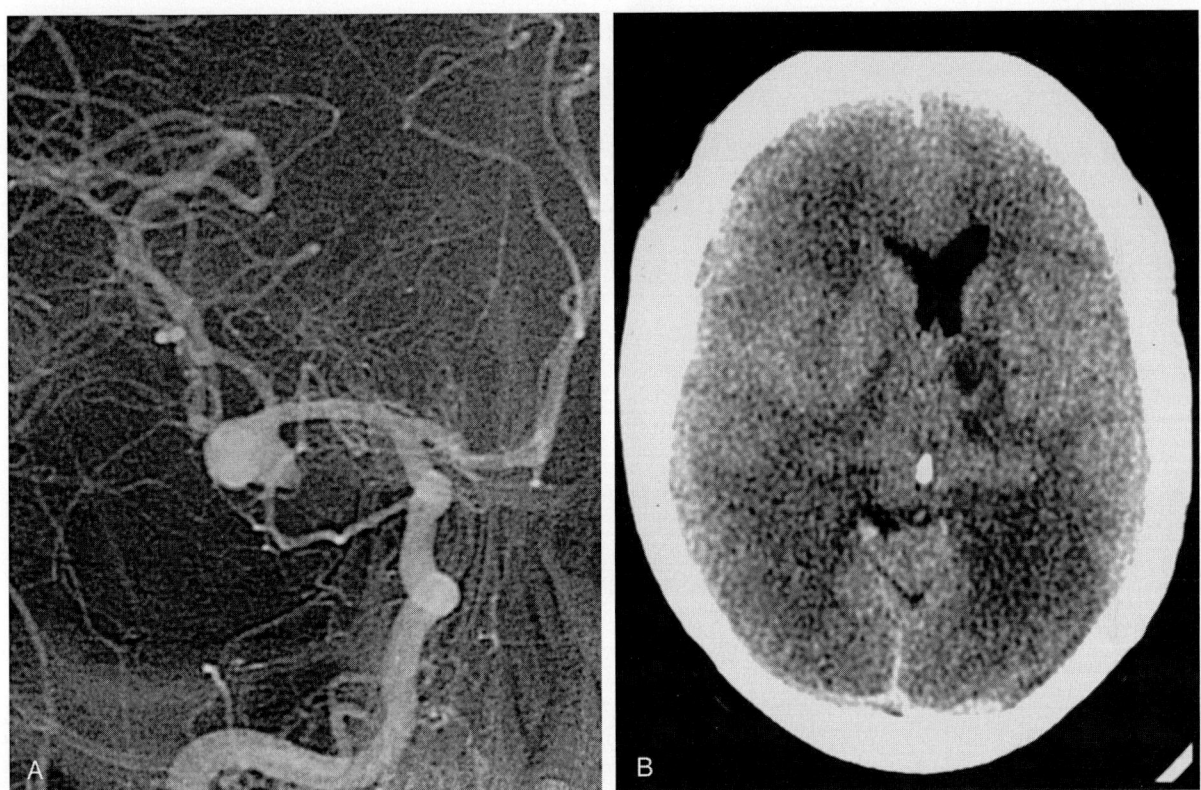

**FIGURE 86–23** ■ *A* and *B*, A 37-year-old woman had a grade 4 aneurysm after a second bleed of a middle cerebral artery bifurcation aneurysm *(A)*. She was operated on day 1 after the second bleed. Two weeks postoperatively, large diffuse ischemic lesions were seen on the computed tomography scan *(B)*. The patient remained in poor condition.

hematomas related to MCAAs, lesions—and spasm—of an MCA frequently cause hemiparesis, dysphasia, or both. There were significantly more cases of severe hemiparesis among long-time survivors with symptomatic MCAAs than among those with symptomatic aneurysms at other sites. The frequency of severe hemiparesis was significantly higher in patients with proximal than bifurcation MCAA—27% versus 12%. This difference may be ex-

plained by technical difficulties associated with proper clipping of proximal MCAAs, leading to occlusion or kinking of the anterior temporal artery or to occlusion of the thalamostriate perforator in a superiorly directed aneurysm by the clip (Fig. 86–24). The frequencies for hemiparesis were equal whether the patient had a single MCAA, multiple intracranial aneurysms with one MCAA, or multiple MCAAs.

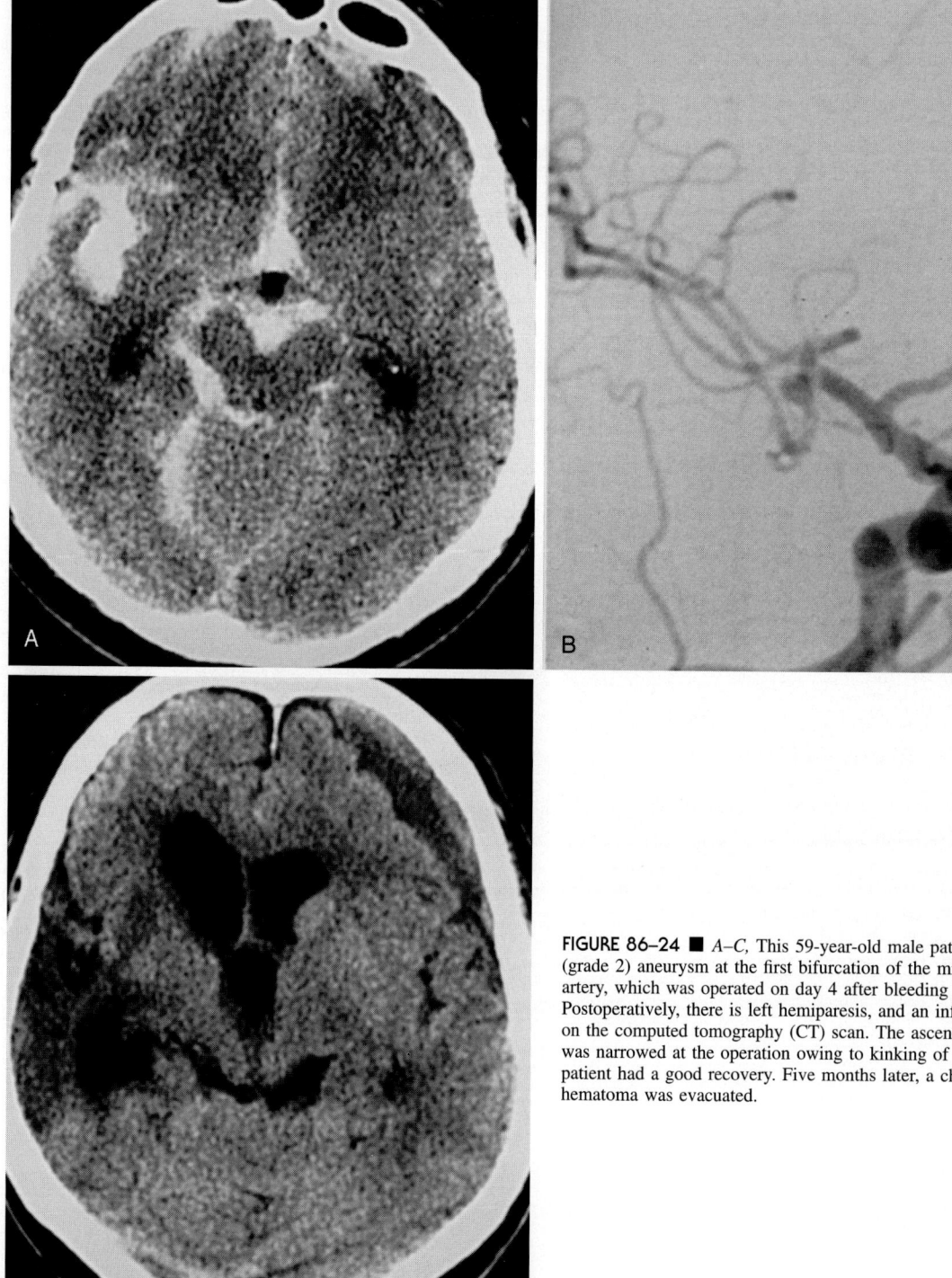

FIGURE 86–24 ■ A–C, This 59-year-old male patient had a small (grade 2) aneurysm at the first bifurcation of the middle cerebral artery, which was operated on day 4 after bleeding had started. Postoperatively, there is left hemiparesis, and an infarction is seen on the computed tomography (CT) scan. The ascending branch was narrowed at the operation owing to kinking of the clip. The patient had a good recovery. Five months later, a chronic subdural hematoma was evacuated.

## Visual Field Deficits

Visual field deficits were significantly more common in patients with MCAAs than in patients with any other aneurysms—20% versus 11%. There were no differences in the frequencies among different MCAA sites. Also, visual impairment was equally common in patients with a single MCAA, with multiple intracranial aneurysms and one MCAA, or with multiple MCAAs. In two thirds (69%) of the cases, visual field deficits were at least partly caused by the close anatomic relationship between the course of the optic tract and temporal intracerebral hematoma.

## REFERENCES

1. Aydin IH, Takci E, Kadioglu HH, et al: The variations of lenticulostriate arteries in the middle cerebral artery aneurysms. Acta Neurochir (Wien) 138:555–559, 1996.
2. Fox J: Technique of aneurysm surgery: IV. Middle cerebral artery aneurysms. In Fox J (ed): Intracranial Aneurysms, Vol 2. New York: Springer-Verlag, 1983, pp 1012–1023.
3. Heros R: Middle cerebral artery aneurysms. In Wilkins RH, Rengachary SS (eds) Neurosurgery, Vol 2. New York: McGraw-Hill, 1985, pp 1376–1382.
4. Heros R: Aneurysms in the middle cerebral artery. In Symon L, Thomas DGT, Clarke K (eds): Rob and Smith's Operative Surgery: Neurosurgery. New York: Chapman & Hall, 1994, pp 171–179.
5. Hosoda K, Fujita S, Kawaguchi T, et al: Saccular aneurysms of the proximal (M1) segment of the middle cerebral artery. Neurosurgery 36:441–446, 1995.
6. Malik JM, Kamiryo T, Goble J, et al: Stereotactic laser-guided approach to distal middle cerebral artery aneurysms. Acta Neurochir (Wien) 1–3:138–144, 1995.
7. Ogilvy CS, Crowell RM, Heros RC: Surgical management of middle cerebral artery aneurysms: Experience with transsylvian and superior temporal gyrus approaches. Surg Neurol 43:15–24, 1995.
8. Pasztor E, Vajda J, Juhasz J, et al: The surgery of middle cerebral artery aneurysms. Acta Neurochir (Wien) 82:92–101, 1986.
9. Peerless SJ: The surgical approach to middle cerebral and posterior communicating aneurysms. Clin Neurosurg 21:151–165, 1974.
10. Suzuki J, Yoshimoto T, Kayama T: Surgical treatment of middle cerebral artery aneurysms. J Neurosurg 61:17–23, 1984.
11. Weir BK, Findlay JM, Disney L: Middle cerebral artery aneurysms. In Apuzzo MLJ (ed): Brain Surgery, Vol 1. New York: Churchill Livingstone, 1993, pp 983–1008.
12. Yasargil MG: Middle cerebral artery aneurysms. In Yasargil MG (ed): Microneurosurgery, Vol 2. Stuttgart: Thieme Verlag, 1984, pp 124–164.
13. Dandy WE: Surgical treatment of aneurysms of the middle cerebral artery. In Dandy WE: Intracranial Artery Aneurysms. Ithaca, NY: Comstock Publishing Company, 1945, p 129.
14. Heiskanen O, Poranen A, Kuurne T, et al: Acute surgery for intracerebral haematomas caused by rupture of an intracranial aneurysms: A prospective randomized study. Acta Neurochir (Wien) 90:81–83, 1988.
15. Kuether TA, Nesbit GM, Barnwell SL: Clinical and angiographic outcomes, with treatment data, for patients with cerebral aneurysms treated with Guglielmi detachable coils: A single-center experience. Neurosurgery 43:1016–1025, 1998.
16. Papo I, Bodosi M, Doczi T: Intracerebral hematomas from aneurysm rupture: Their clinical significance. Acta Neurochir (Wien) 89:100–105, 1987.
17. Rinne J, Hernesniemi J, Niskanen M, et al: Analysis of 561 patients with middle cerebral artery aneurysms: Anatomic and clinical features as correlated to management outcome. Neurosurgery 38:2–11, 1996.
18. Tapaninaho A, Hernesniemi J, Vapalahti M: Emergency treatment of cerebral aneurysms with large haematomas. Acta Neurochir (Wien) 91:21–24, 1988.
19. Tokuda Y, Inagawa T, Katoh Y, et al: Intracerebral hematoma in patients with ruptured cerebral aneurysms. Surg Neurol 3:272–277, 1995.
20. Vanninen R, Koivisto T, Saari T, et al: Acute endovascular treatment of ruptured intracranial aneurysms with electrically detachable coils: A prospective randomized study. Radiology 211:325–366, 1999.
21. Bjorkesten G, Halonen V: Incidence of intracranial vascular lesions in patients with subarachnoid hemorrhage investigated by four-vessel angiography. J Neurosurg 23:29–32, 1965.
22. Fogelholm R: Subarachnoid hemorrhage in Middle-Finland: Incidence, early prognosis and indications for neurosurgical treatment. Stroke 3:296–301, 1981.
23. Hernesniemi J, Vapalahti M, Niskanen M, et al: One-year outcome in early aneurysm surgery: A 14-year experience. Acta Neurochir (Wien) 122:1–10, 1993.
24. Sarti C, Tuomilehto J, Narva E, et al: Epidemiology of subarachnoid hemorrhage in Finland during years 1982–85. Stroke 22:848–853, 1991.
25. Rinne J, Hernesniemi J, Puranen M, et al: Multiple intracranial aneurysms in a defined population: Prospective angiographic and clinical study. Neurosurgery 35:803–808, 1994.
26. Rinne J, Hernesniemi J, Niskanen M, et al: Management outcome for multiple intracranial aneurysms. Neurosurgery 36:31–38, 1995.
27. Ronkainen A, Puranen M, Hernesniemi JA, et al: Intracranial aneurysms: MR angiographic screening in 400 asymptomatic individuals with increased familial risk. Radiology 195:35–40, 1995.
28. Ronkainen A, Hernesniemi J, Puranen M, et al: Familial intracranial aneurysms. Lancet 349:380–384, 1997.
29. Ronkainen A, Miettinen H, Karkola K, et al: Risk of harboring an unruptured intracranial aneurysm. Stroke 29:359–362, 1998.
30. Kallmes DF, Kallmes MH, Lanzino G, et al: Routine angiography after surgery for ruptured intracranial aneurysms: A cost versus benefit analysis. Neurosurgery 41:629–641, 1997.
31. Horikoshi T, Fukamachi A, Nishi H: Detection of intracranial aneurysms by three-dimensional time-of-flight magnetic resonance angiography. Neuroradiology 36:203–207, 1994.
32. Nagasawa S, Ohta T, Tsuda E: Magnetic resonance angiographic source images for depicting topography and surgical planning for middle cerebral artery aneurysms: Technique application. Surg Neurol 50:62–64, 1998.
33. Dillon EH, van Leeuwen MS, Fernandez MA, et al: Spiral CT angiography. Am J Radiol 160:1273–1278, 1993.
34. Harbaugh RE, Schlusselberg DS, Jeffrey R, et al: Three-dimensional computerized tomography angiography in the diagnosis of cerebrovascular disease. J Neurosurg 76:408–414, 1992.
35. Nakajima Y, Yoshimine T, Yoshida H, et al: Computerized tomography angiography of ruptured cerebral aneurysms: Factors affecting time to maximum contrast concentration. J Neurosurg 88:663–669, 1998.
36. Ogawa T, Noguchi K, et al: Cerebral aneurysms: Evaluation with three-dimensional CT angiography. AJNR Am J Neuroradiol 3:447–454, 1996.
37. Tampieri D, Leblanc R, Oleszek J, et al: Three-dimensional computed tomography angiography of cerebral aneurysms. Neurosurgery 4:749–754, 1995.
38. Vieco PT, Shuman WP, Alsofrom GF, et al: Detection of circle of Willis aneurysms in patients with acute subarachnoid hemorrhage: A comparison of CT angiography and digital subtraction angiography. AJR Am J Roentgenol 165:425–430, 1995.
39. Young N, Dorsch NWC, Kingston RJ, et al: Spiral CT scanning in the detection and evaluation of aneurysms of the circle of Willis. Surg Neurol 50:50–61, 1998.
40. Le Roux PD, Dailey AT, Newell DW, et al: Emergent aneurysm clipping without angiography in the moribund patient with intracerebral hemorrhage: The use of infusion computed tomography scans. Neurosurgery 33:189–197, 1993.
41. Niskanen M, Hernesniemi J, Vapalahti M, et al: One-year outcome in early aneurysm surgery: Prediction of outcome. Acta Neurochir (Wien) 123:25–32, 1993.
42. Anson JA, Lawton MT, Spetzler RF: Characteristics and surgical treatment of dolichoectatic and fusiform aneurysms. J Neurosurg 84:185–193, 1996.
43. Hacein-Bey L, Connolly ES Jr, Mayer SA, et al: Complex intracranial aneurysms: Combined operative and endovascular approaches. Neurosurgery 43:1304–1313, 1998.
44. Sundt TM, Kobayashi S, Fode NC, et al: Results and complications of surgical management of 809 intracranial aneurysms in 722 cases: Related and unrelated to grade of patient, type of aneurysm, and timing of surgery. J Neurosurg 56:753–765, 1982.

44a. Hunt WE, Hess RM: Surgical risk as related to time of intervention in the repair of intracranial aneurysms. J Neurosurg 28:14–20, 1968.
45. Findlay JM: Current management of aneurysmal subarachnoid hemorrhage guidelines from the Canadian Neurosurgical Society. Can J Neurol Sci 24:161–170, 1997.
46. Säveland H, Hillman J, Brandt L, et al: Overall outcome in aneurysmal subarachnoid hemorrhage: A prospective study from neurosurgical units in Sweden during a 1-year period. J Neurosurg 76:729–734, 1992.
47. Fogelholm R, Hernesniemi J, Vapalahti M: Impact of early surgery on outcome after aneurysmal subarachnoid hemorrhage: A population-based study. Stroke 24:1649–1654, 1993.
48. Le Roux PD, Elliott JP, Newell DW, et al: The incidence of surgical complications is similar in good and poor grade patients undergoing repair of ruptured anterior circulation aneurysms: A retrospective review of 355 patients. Neurosurgery 38:887–894, 1996.
49. Whisnant JP, Sacco SE, O'Fallon WM, et al: Referral bias in aneurysmal subarachnoid hemorrhage. J Neurosurg 78:726–732, 1993.
50. Mayberg M, Batjer HH, Dacey R, et al: Guidelines for the management of aneurysmal subarachnoid hemorrhage. A statement for healthcare professionals from a Special Writing Group of the Stroke Council, American Heart Association. Stroke 25:2315–2328, 1994.
51. Solomon RA, Mayer SA, Tarmey JJ: Relationship between the volume of craniotomies for cerebral aneurysm performed at New York state hospitals and in-hospital mortality. Stroke 27:13–17, 1996.
52. Lawton MT, Raudzens PA, Zabramski JM, et al: Hypothermic circulatory arrest in neurovascular surgery: Evolving indications and predictors of patient outcome. Neurosurgery 43:10–21, 1998.
53. Kallmes DF, Kallmess MH: Cost-effectiveness of angiography perfomed during surgery for ruptured intracranial aneurysms. AJNR Am J Neuroradiol 18:1453–1462, 1997.
54. Payner TD, Horner TG, Leipzig TJ, et al: Role of intraoperative angiography in the surgical treatment of cerebral aneurysms. J Neurosurg 3:441–448, 1998.
55. Drake CG: Giant intracranial aneurysms: Experience with surgical treatment in 174 patients. Clin Neurosurg 26:12–95, 1979.
56. Gewirtz RJ, Awad IA: Giant aneurysms of the anterior circle of Willis: Management outcome of open microsurgical treatment. Surg Neurol 5:409–420, 1996.
57. Lawton MT, Spetzler RF: Surgical management of giant intracranial aneurysms: Experience with 171 patients. Clin Neurosurg 42:245–266, 1995.
58. Piepgras DG, Khurana VG, Whisnant JP: Ruptured giant intracranial aneurysms: Part II. A retrospective analysis of timing and outcome of surgical treatment. J Neurosurg 3:430–435, 1998.
59. Samson DS, Batjer HH, Bowmann G, et al: A clinical study of the parameters and effects of temporary arterial occlusion in the management of intracranial aneurysms. Neurosurgery 34:22–29, 1994.
60. Khurana VG, Piepgras DG, Whisnant JP: Ruptured giant intracranial aneurysms: Part I. A study of rebleeding. J Neurosurg 3:425–429, 1998.
61. Mizoi K, Yoshimoto T: Permissible temporary occlusion time in aneurysm surgery as evaluated by evoked potential monitoring. Neurosurgery 33:434–440, 1993.
62. Ogilvy CS, Carter BS, Kaplan S, et al: Temporary vessel occlusion for aneurysm surgery: Risk factors for stroke in patients protected by induced hypothermia and hypertension and intravenous mannitol administration. J Neurosurg 84:785–791, 1996.
63. Debrun GM, Aletich VA, Kehrli P, et al: Selection of cerebral aneurysms for treatment using Guglilemi detachable coils: The preliminary University of Illinois experience. Neurosurgery 43:1281–1297, 1998.
64. Eskridge JM, Song JK, et al: Endovascular embolization of 150 basilar tip aneurysms with Guglielmi detachable coils: Results of the Food and Drug Administration multicenter clinical trial. J Neurosurg 89:81–86, 1998.
65. Standard SC, Guterman LR, Chavis TD, et al: Endovascular management of giant intracranial aneurysms. Clin Neurosurg 42:267–293, 1995.
66. Vinuela F, Duckwiler G, Mawad M: Guglielmi detachable coil embolization of acute intracranial aneurysm: Perioperative anatomical and clinical outcome in 403 patients. J Neurosurg 86:475–482, 1997.
67. Baker CJ, Prestigiacomo CJ, Solomon RA: Short-term perioperative anticonvulsant prophylaxis for the surgical treatment of low-risk patients with intracranial aneurysms. Neurosurgery 5:863–870, 1995.
68. Cabral RJ, King TT, Scott DF: Epilepsy after two different neurosurgical approaches to the treatment of ruptured intracranial aneurysm. J Neurol Neurosurg Psychiatry 39:1052–1056, 1976.
69. Fabinyi GCA, Artiola-Fortuny L: Epilepsy after craniotomy for intracranial aneurysms. Lancet 1:1299–1300, 1980.
70. Keränen T, Tapaninaho A, Hernesniemi J, et al: Late epilepsy after aneurysm operation. Neurosurgery 17:897–900, 1985.
71. Kotila M, Waltimo O: Epilepsy after stroke. Epilepsia 33:495–498, 1992.
72. Ukkola V, Heikkinen E: Epilepsy after operative treatment of ruptured cerebral aneurysms. Acta Neurochir (Wien) 106:115–118, 1990.

# Surgical Management of Anterior Cerebral and Anterior Communicating Artery Aneurysms

■ R. P. SENGUPTA

The anterior communicating artery region is the most common site of intracranial aneurysms. About 35% of all intracranial aneurysms arise in this region, yet the surgical obliteration of these is considered the most difficult of all aneurysms in the anterior circulation.[1] Lying buried in between the frontal lobes, in close proximity to the hypothalamus and optic chiasm, they are often enclosed and obscured by the parent vessels and pose a considerable hazard at surgery.[2] Even in patients in good clinical condition, most postoperative complications result from injury to vessels or the brain during surgery. With recent advances in endovascular therapy, some aneurysms can be obliterated with Guglielmi detachable coils, particularly in patients in poorer clinical condition. This technique is still unproven, and surgical obliteration remains the ideal treatment.[3, 4]

## NATURAL HISTORY

The natural history of intracranial aneurysms has been well elucidated for the past 50 years. The fact that an aneurysm at each location has its own natural history,[1] however, is not appreciated. Embryologically the anterior communicating artery region is the weakest part in the circle of Willis, and a vascular anomaly in this region is common and is the most frequent site for the development of an aneurysm. Although aneurysms usually become symptomatic when patients are between the ages of 40 and 60 years, most aneurysms in patients younger than 30 years can be seen at this location. Although intracranial aneurysms occur twice as frequently in women as in men, anterior communicating artery aneurysms have a slight preponderance in men. Anterior communicating artery aneurysms are rarely associated with other aneurysms, and when they are, they are frequently the source of hemorrhage. Although an anterior communicating artery aneurysm can grow to a giant size, it is the least common site for a giant aneurysm because anterior communicating artery aneurysms often bleed while small. This situation is confirmed by the small incidence of unruptured anterior communicating artery an-

eurysms in the International Study of Unruptured Intracranial Aneurysms (ISUIA) finding. As a result of the congregation of many vessels in this region, small aneurysms are difficult to visualize on angiograms, and despite a definite subarachnoid hemorrhage (SAH), such aneurysms can remain undiagnosed. Computed tomography (CT) and magnetic resonance angiography may disclose some of these aneurysms.

## PATHOPHYSIOLOGIC CHANGES AFTER SUBARACHNOID HEMORRHAGE

Until the advent of CT scanning, pathologic changes produced within the brain were studied from postmortem specimens. Such information available to the neurosurgeon came only from fatal cases of either SAH or surgical failure. The ongoing pathologic changes in the living brain occurring after SAH can now be ascertained with the help of CT, which is extremely valuable in the management of SAH and is an essential prerequisite for the improvement of management outcome as well as surgical planning.

Pathologic changes produced within the brain after rupture of an anterior communicating artery aneurysm depend on the severity of the bleed, the morphology of the aneurysm itself, and the interval between the study and the ictus. In a catastrophic bleed, the brain is devastated by the massive hemorrhage, often within the ventricle, with massive rise in intracranial pressure (ICP), which leads to death. With a major nonfatal hemorrhage, subarachnoid blood exists in varying degrees. A rise in blood pressure occurs with the initial rise in ICP, conforming to Cushing's reflex. When the ICP decreases, the blood pressure returns to normal. Reducing the blood pressure with medication is harmful because when ICP is raised, perfusion pressure drops. Because they are close to the third ventricle, blood clots within the anterior part of the third ventricle can cause acute ventricular obstruction, which, if detected with CT scanning, can be easily treated with a ventricular drain. An aneurysm projecting upward can cause a hematoma in the interhemispheric fissure or in the frontal lobe. An aneurysm projecting backward and laterally can cause damage to the internal capsule and basal ganglia. One of the most significant problems created by a posteriorly directed aneurysm is damage to the hypothalamus, with disturbance of the limbic system, and the autonomic and biochemical control centers that is not detected on CT scan. Such a disturbance creates intracellular and interstitial edema, leading to an edematous brain.

Blood clots surround the neighboring vessels, and a continuing rise in ICP can lead to vasospasm and cerebral ischemia. Perforating vessels supplying the hypothalamus become obliterated, leading to necrosis of the vital centers. In patients with an intact circle of Willis, the effect of vasospasm on major vessels is not too severe, but in those with an anomalous circle, it may be profound (see later). Depending on the projection of the aneurysm, significant blood clots can spread along the parasellar cistern to the sylvian fissure, leading to spasm of the internal carotid artery or middle cerebral artery (see Fig. 87–17). Even after a modest SAH, the subarachnoid space may become incompetent for free flow and absorption of cerebrospinal fluid (CSF), causing delayed communicating hydrocephalus.

## CLINICAL PRESENTATION

Of patients with anterior communicating artery aneurysms, 99% present with rupture, and the remaining 1% present with a compressive mass lesion from an intact aneurysm. Because of the protective effect of the surrounding brain, as in middle cerebral artery aneurysms, a minor leak from these aneurysms may remain unnoticed and create an atypical presentation. Clinical presentation of rupture depends on the severity of the bleed and its specific projection. At least 10% of patients with aneurysms present with a catastrophic hemorrhage, and the patient succumbs to the bleed within 24 hours. In some of these patients, a history suggesting prior warning leak is obtained. A significant but nonfatal hemorrhage is the commonly encountered presentation.

Headache is the commonest initial symptom (80%), followed by loss of consciousness (44%) and seizures (6%).[1] Bleeding into the third ventricle with blockage of the foramen of Monro can present as acute hydrocephalus, causing profound restlessness, coma, and acute papilledema. Damage to the hypothalamic region may be associated with memory disturbance, autonomic instability, disturbance of biochemical control centers, and other features of diencephalic syndrome. Depending on the projection of the aneurysm, a mass effect of a frontal lobe hematoma and disturbance of the internal capsule or basal arteries, causing hemiparesis, may be seen.

The clinical presentation may be atypical in many patients with a ruptured anterior communicating artery aneurysm. The author has encountered various initial diagnoses in these patients, including head injury, neck injury, backache with sciatica, migraine, hysteria, depression, and symptoms of communicating hydrocephalus.[1] A correct diagnosis in any of these presentations is possible from an accurate and comprehensive history, and a correct diagnosis is extremely valuable because the surgical outcome is good. On rare occasions, when accompanied by other aneurysms, a leak from an anterior communicating artery aneurysm can be confirmed from prodromal symptoms of lower limb weakness at the time of ictus, if no other clue from CT scan or angiogram is available. A giant unruptured anterior communicating artery aneurysm can produce symptoms of compression of optic pathways, hydrocephalus from blockage of the foramen of Monro, or diencephalic symptoms resulting from compression of the hypothalamus.

## INITIAL MANAGEMENT AND PATIENT SELECTION

With careful evaluation of a patient after rupture of an anterior communicating artery aneurysm of any severity, not only can some patients in poor condition be saved and have an improved management outcome, but also a suitable time for definitive surgery for each aneurysm can be selected for improved surgical outcome. Early surgery prevents rebleeding and can preempt the development of ischemia from vasospasm. Some patients undeniably fair better from delay in definitive surgery, but even in these patients, partial coiling can prevent early rebleeding.

Although patients with aneurysmal SAH are grouped into various grades that define their clinical status, clinical evaluation alone is not sufficient to determine the pathologic status within the brain. For example, a patient in grade III may harbor a swollen brain or hydrocephalus. Surgery in the former situation is detrimental, whereas in the latter, it is beneficial. Furthermore, clinical grading immediately after SAH is erroneous: For example, a patient presenting with seizure or coma may be categorized as grade V, whereas in a short period of time, he or she may be recategorized as grade I or grade II. CT scan when performed within the first few days may provide a variety of information, including mild or modest SAH without effect on the brain, massive SAH, massive ventricular hemorrhage, hematoma with midline shift, dilated ventricles resulting from blockage of CSF pathways, and swollen brain with slit ventricles. This author's plan for initial management is given in Figure 87–1.

More neurosurgeons are now turning to early surgery for aneurysms in patients in good clinical condition. Although the author is a strong advocate of early surgery, in his view, each aneurysm becomes ready for its safe obliteration at a specific time. Based on experience and retrospective analysis of earlier cases, the author assesses specific risk factors to determine the timing of surgery, including the clinical status of the patient, the presence of angiographic vasospasm and anomaly of the circle of Willis, the morphology of the aneurysm that may present technical difficulties, the age of the patient, and the patient's associated medical condition. Together, all these factors constitute a hypothetical 100% risk. Computer analysis of each factor has yielded guidelines of how much risk each factor poses. The following list gives the proportion of each risk factor:

| | |
|---|---|
| Clinical status | 60% |
| Angiographic vasospasm | 10% |

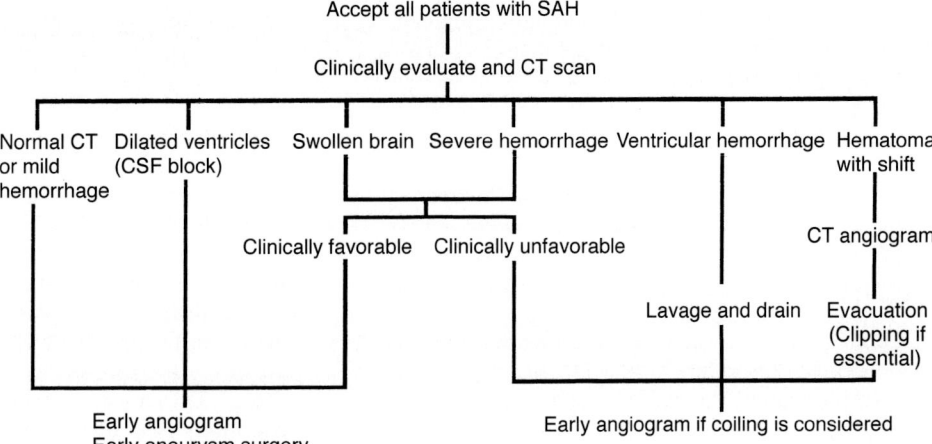

FIGURE 87–1 ■ Initial management policy for an aneurysmal subarachnoid hemorrhage at the neurosurgical center. (SAH, subarachnoid hemorrhage.)

| | |
|---|---|
| Anomaly of the circle of Willis | 10% |
| Technical hazard | 10% |
| Age of patient | 5% |
| Associated medical condition | 5% |

Clinical status is the most important factor in the selection of the timing of surgery. If a patient is alert and has a Hunt and Hess grade of I or II and a Glasgow Coma Scale of 15, surgery at the earliest possible moment poses no risk. Conversely, if the patient is obtunded without hydrocephalus and has a Hunt and Hess grade of III and Glasgow Coma Scale of less than 15, surgery poses a considerable risk. If the patient is improving, the risk score is 20, but if the patient is unstable, it increases to 30. When the patient's clinical condition is extremely poor and he or she has a Hunt and Hess grade of IV or V and a Glasgow Coma Scale of less than 12, there is no point in operating on the aneurysm until the condition improves with initial management and medical therapy. Clinical status may change, as may the risk score.

Angiographic vasospasm without clinical effect has only a small risk score of 10. Good clinical condition despite vasospasm suggests that the territory of the spastic artery has a good collateral circulation and does not depend entirely on the supply from the spastic vessel. If, however, the vasospasm is associated with clinical effect, the risk score is the combination of both of these factors. The anomaly of the circle of Willis is an underrated risk factor. The anomaly at the anterior part of the circle, particularly at the anterior communicating region, is frequently associated with an aneurysm, as is further discussed in Surgical Anatomy. When one of the proximal anterior cerebral arteries (ACAs) is hypoplastic, collateral circulation through the hypoplastic vessel is deficient. If the dominant vessel is injured or in spasm, its territory cannot receive blood from the opposite side. If the internal carotid artery with fetal posterior cerebral artery goes into spasm, the effect is worse. When no anomaly exists, the risk from this factor is nil, but in the worst scenario, the risk is maximum. Some anterior communicating artery aneurysms, particularly those of a giant size, can pose technical difficulties requiring considerable manipulation of the brain and its blood vessels, posing a risk. In the elderly, the cardiopulmonary system is not as efficient as in the young. Although

surgery in these patients can be safe, an element of surgical and anesthetic risk exists. Similarly, patients with SAH may have an underlying medical condition, such as hypertension, diabetes, chronic bronchitis, and ischemic heart disease. These conditions can pose some risk for anesthesia and surgery.

Taking all these factors into account, the author adds up the risk score and chooses the timing of surgery as follows:

| Risk Score | Timing of Surgery |
|---|---|
| 0–10 | Immediately or as soon as possible |
| ≤20 | Any time in the first week but not immediately |
| ≥25 | Second week or later |
| 60 | No surgery |

A patient with a risk score of 10 or less can be operated on immediately. Patients with a risk score up to 20 should be observed for a day or so. When the risk score is 25 or higher, the patient should be observed until the clinical status becomes stable or is improving. If the risk score remains at 60, which is the worst clinical status, no benefit is to be gained from elective aneurysm surgery.

## MEDICAL THERAPY

Every neurosurgeon with a large experience in aneurysm surgery has his or her own method of preoperative management. In this section, the author's personal preference is given. All patients with SAH, regardless of its severity, are given standard medical treatment, including the following:

1. Absolute bed rest in a quiet and darkened room to relieve headache and photophobia. The head should be moderately elevated to promote venous drainage and to reduce cerebral edema.
2. Elastic stockings to prevent venous thrombosis in the calves.
3. Laxative, such as lactulose, 30 mg at bedtime to avoid straining at stool.
4. Codeine phosphate, 60 mg every 4 hours as required for headache.

5. Anticonvulsants, such as phenytoin, 300 mg/day.

6. Treatment of hypertension. If a patient is a known hypertensive, his or her usual medication should be maintained. For reflex hypertension as a result of raised ICP, reducing blood pressure with drugs is counterproductive. If the ICP can be lowered by sedation, by analgesics, or by repeated lumbar puncture, when no space-occupying hematoma is present, blood pressure returns to normal. If blood pressure remains consistently raised, nimodipine is used intravenously.

7. Nimodipine. The value of this calcium antagonist is doubtful in the author's view, despite its various well-received claims.[5] Given intravenously, it often lowers blood pressure, which is undesirable, and in cases of proven vasospasm, release of spasm has not been demonstrated. Its protective value on brain metabolism has yet to be proved. Although the author believes the effect is marginal, nimodipine 60 mg orally every 4 hours is used or, in patients with poor enteral absorption, nimodipine infusion 200 μg/ml starting at a rate of 5 ml/hr, increasing after 2 hours to 10 ml/hr.

8. Fluids. In a brain affected by SAH, the fluid and electrolyte regulatory centers in the hypothalamus are affected, causing fluid retention.[6, 7] The author has found that a maximum of 1500 ml of fluid in 24 hours in the first few days is beneficial, although a much larger fluid volume is currently used by many.[5] The type of fluid should be guided by electrolyte values.

9. Blood transfusion. Red cells tend to break down in patients with SAH. A low hemoglobin level may merit preoperative blood transfusion.

10. Treatment for progressive neurologic deterioration resulting from vasospasm. Hypertensive therapy ("hypertensive hypervolemic") with colloid and inotropes (dopamine) is the initial therapy of choice. If deterioration is not reversed quickly, intra-arterial papaverine therapy is used (see Postoperative Complications).

## SURGICAL ANATOMY

The surgical approach to aneurysms in the anterior communicating artery region largely depends on the anatomy of the artery and its variations. The ACA arises from the internal carotid at its bifurcation at the medial end of the sylvian fissure. It then passes anteromedially above the optic chiasm or optic nerve beneath the anterior perforated substance to reach the midline and enters the interhemispheric fissure. Both ACAs are joined by the anterior communicating artery near the entrance into the interhemispheric fissure, then ascend in front of the lamina terminalis. Above the lamina terminalis, each artery smoothly curves around the genu of the corpus callosum, passing backward over the corpus callosum in the pericallosal cistern and continuing as the pericallosal artery.

The proximal part of the ACA (A1) gives rise to the perforating arteries in groups of two or three and turns laterally to supply the genu and posterior limb of the internal capsule and rostral thalamus. One group supplies the anterior limb of the internal capsule, hypothalamus, and basal ganglia. Another group, close to the anterior communicating artery, sends branches to the optic chiasm, adjacent hypothalamus, and anterior commissure. The recurrent artery of Heubner also arises from the distal part of A1 in 14% of cases.[8] It runs laterally beneath A1 to the anterior perforated substance and supplies much of the striatum and internal capsule.

The distal part of the ACA (A2) has a few central branches, but the Heubner artery arises from this segment close to the anterior communicating artery in 78% of cases.[8] This artery, however, turns sharply away laterally and rarely is in contact with the aneurysm in the region of the anterior communicating artery. The cortical branches arising from the A2 segment include a branch to the olfactory tract, the orbitofrontal artery, the frontopolar artery, and the callosomarginal artery. Other than the Heubner artery, these perforating arteries supply various portions of the frontal lobe.

The average length of the anterior communicating artery is 4 mm, but sometimes two arteries are fused. The artery gives rise to a maximum of three central branches, which supply the fornix, the corpus callosum, the septal region, and the anterior cingulum.

## ANOMALIES

Even in the normal brain, anatomic variations of ACAs and anterior communicating arteries are considerable and are commoner in patients harboring an aneurysm.[9–12] Hypoplasia of A1 can be seen in 28% of cases and aplasia in 3%. A fenestrated A1 has been reported in 1% of cases. Hypoplasia is distinguished from arterial spasm by the presence of a smooth continuation of the middle cerebral artery from the internal carotid artery, the opposite A1 being unusually large.

Anomaly in the anterior communicating artery region includes absence of the artery when both ACAs are fused at the point of contact. The anterior communicating artery can be duplicated or triplicated or be a net of small channels. Anomaly in the A2 segment includes fusion of both ACAs to form a common trunk (azygous ACA) or more than two ACAs. Anomaly of other components of the circle of Willis, such as fetal origin of the posterior cerebral artery or the persistence of a trigeminal artery, should be recognized. From these anatomic studies, several observations of profound surgical significance can be made.

*First*, the A1 segment, particularly its most proximal end, gives rise to most of the vital central perforating branches. Damage to these branches by surgical manipulation or vasospasm could produce severe neurologic deficit.

*Second*, the anterior communicating artery itself contributes little vascular supply because its main function is as a conduit.[1] If the artery is occluded, these vessels can still be nourished from the opposite ACA.

*Third*, as the A1 segment runs forward and medially from its origin, the region of the anterior communicating artery lies anterior to the carotid bifurcation. Entering deep and then dissecting superficially to explore the anterior communicating artery region is unnecessary because retraction and manipulation, necessary to reach the bifurcation point and adjacent A1 segment, may be harmful.

*Fourth*, because of the variations of the ACA and other vascular anomalies, the circulation through the anterior part of the circle is variable. This variability has important bearing on various surgical procedures and the effect of vasospasm because the available collateral circulation differs. The author has noted four types of circulation through the anterior part of the circle of Willis.[13]

## Type I (Fig. 87–2)

Type I, or ipsilateral, anomalies occur in 66% of cases. During angiography, the injection of contrast material into one carotid artery fills the aneurysm and ipsilateral or both A2 segments. Injection of contrast material in the contralateral carotid fills the A2 segment on the same side. In this type of circulation, surgical obliteration of the anterior communicating artery, if necessary, is not harmful. More significantly, if vasospasm of the parent A1 occurs, its territory can be nourished with blood from the opposite

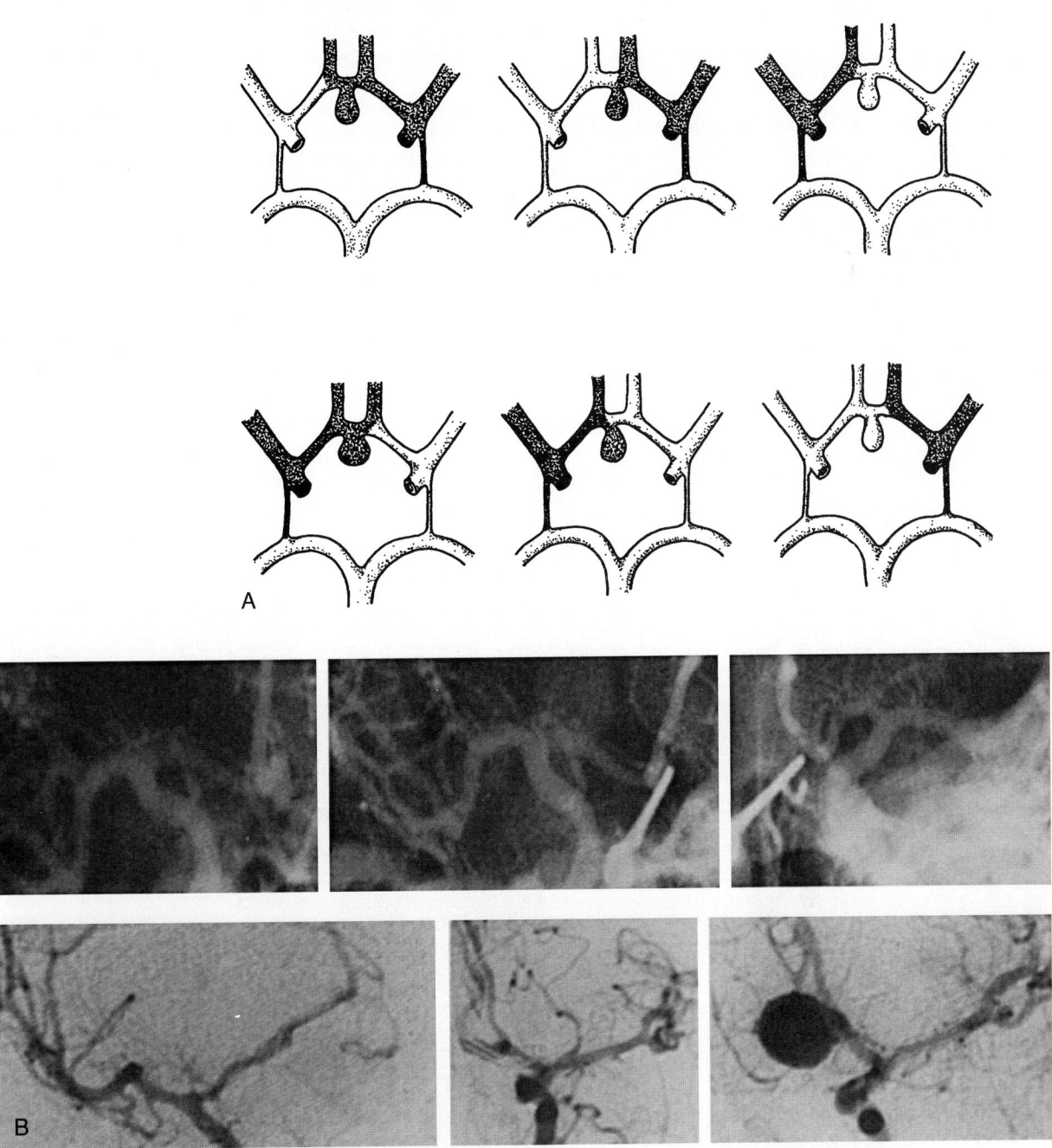

TYPE I IPSILATERAL

A

B

**FIGURE 87–2** ■ *A,* Type I circulation (ipsilateral) (see text). *B,* Example of type I circulation. *Upper Row,* Right anterior cerebral–anterior communicating aneurysm. *Lower Row,* Left anterior cerebral–anterior communicating aneurysm.

hemisphere and from the posterior circulation through the posterior communicating artery.

## Type II (Fig. 87–3)

Type II, or bilateral, anomalies occur in 14% of cases. In this type, the aneurysm and both A2 segments fill with contrast material from either carotid injection. Because of the extremely good collateral flow, the effect of vasospasm is minimal. This pattern of circulation is often associated with a rudimentary or nonexisting anterior communicating artery. In fact, the two ACAs may be fused before continuing as two separate A2 segments. In such situations, the application of a clip may lead to kinking of both ACAs.

## Type III (Figs. 87–4 and 87–5)

Type III, or dominant ACA, anomalies occur in 12% of cases. In this type, the contrast material fills the aneurysm, which arises from the bifurcation of the hypertrophic A1 segment into two A2 segments. Injection into the opposite carotid shows the middle cerebral artery to be a direct continuation of the internal carotid artery without filling of the ACA. Because there is no cross-flow from the opposite carotid system, the effect of vasospasm is considerable.

## Type IV (see Figs. 87–4 and 87–5)

Type IV anomaly, or dominant ACA with fetal posterior cerebral artery, occurs in 8% of cases. In this type, the contrast material fills as in type III. The posterior cerebral artery appears to arise from one or both internal carotid arteries. Vertebral injection in such situations demonstrates that the P1 segment from the basilar bifurcation is hypoplastic. Here the effect of vasospasm is worst because the area supplied by the spastic vessel has suffered from lack of collateral circulation, not only from the opposite hemisphere, but also from the posterior circulation.

## MORPHOLOGY OF THE ANEURYSM

Preoperative knowledge of the location of the neck of the aneurysm, configuration of its sac, and its relation to major vessels as well as projection of the fundus is crucial in surgical planning and dissection. All this information can be obtained from a good-quality angiogram performed with subtraction technique. In addition to routine views, oblique views through the orbit with and without cross-compression display the region well. Oblique orbital views correspond to the anatomy as seen at operation through the pterional approach. The angiographic evidence may occasionally be misleading, however.

### Location of the Aneurysm Neck

Most aneurysms arise from the crouch of the anterior communicating artery and one of the distal A2 segments. An aneurysm can arise from any of the following locations (Fig. 87–6):

1. The junction of the anterior communicating artery and the right A2

**TYPE II BILATERAL**

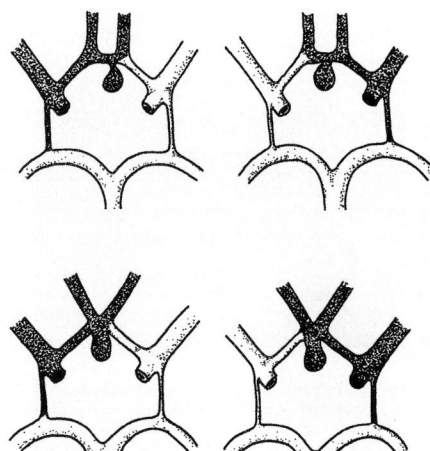

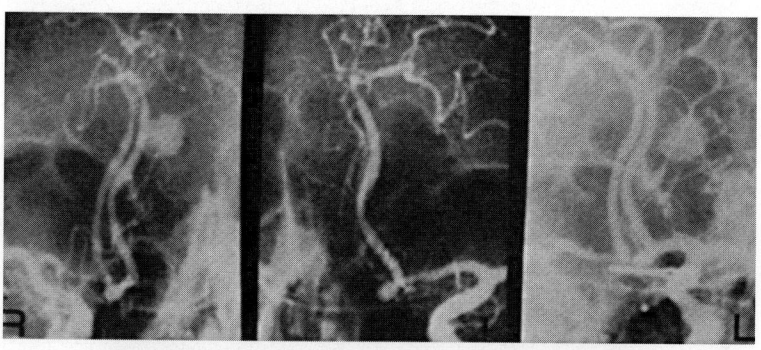

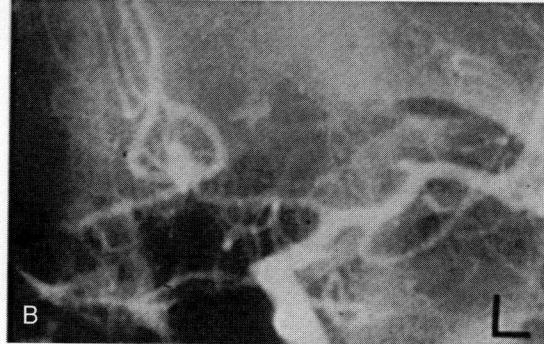

**FIGURE 87–3** ■ *A,* Type II circulation (bilateral) (see text). *B,* Angiogram in type II circulation. *Upper,* Prominent anterior communicating artery. *Lower,* Rudimentary anterior communicating artery.

TYPE III DOMINANT A.C.A.

TYPE IV DOMINANT A.C.A.
with fetal P.C.A.

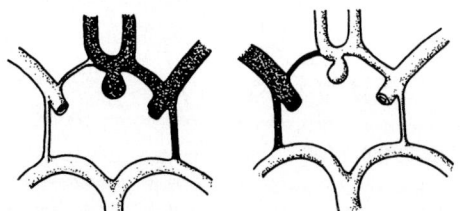

a) Dominant R a.c.a.

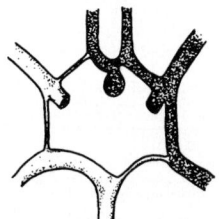

a) Ipsilat. fetal P.c.a.

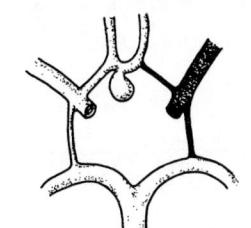

b) Dominant L a.c.a.

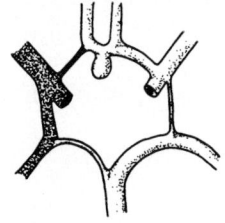

b) Contralat. fetal P.c.a.

**FIGURE 87-4** ■ *Left,* Type III circulation (dominant). *Right,* Type IV circulation (see text).

2. The junction of the anterior communicating artery and the left A2
3. The junction of the anterior communicating artery and the right A1
4. The junction of the anterior communicating artery and the left A1
5. The junction of both A2 segments with a dominant A1
6. The anterior communicating artery only

Most of the aneurysms have a neck of origin other than the anterior communicating artery blowing itself out. In a giant aneurysm, which is rare at this location, the configu-

ration of the neck is wide, irregular, and bulbous. Rarely are the neck and parent vessels atherosclerotic.

## Relationship of the Aneurysmal Sac to Adjacent Vessels

To avoid injury to adjacent vessels and to keep postoperative spasm to a minimum, the author relies on minimal dissection confined to the adherent vessels to isolate the neck. Precise knowledge of the vessels that need to be

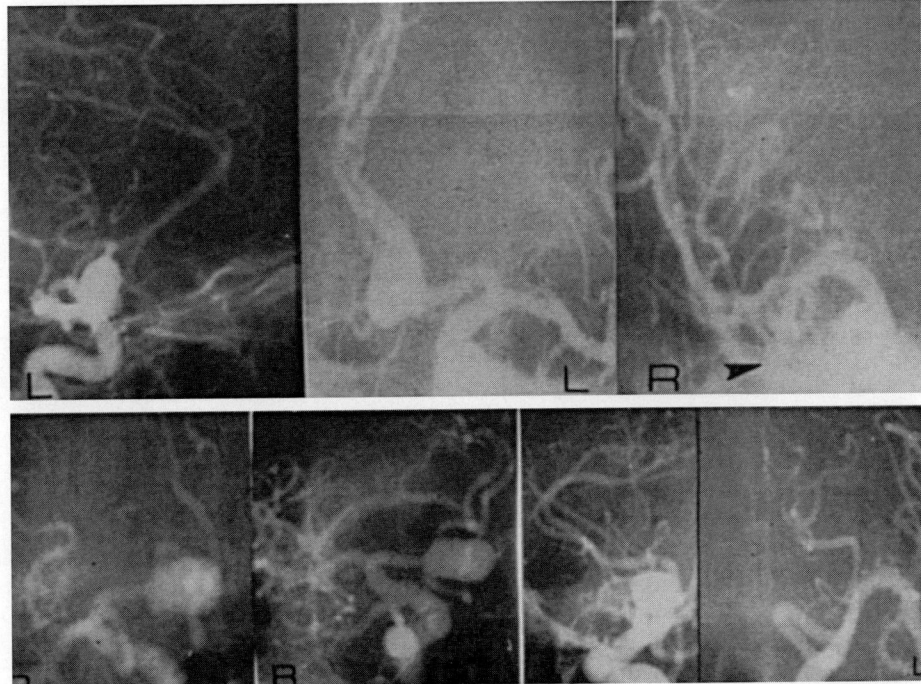

**FIGURE 87-5** ■ *Upper Row,* Angiogram in type III circulation. *Lower Row,* Angiogram in type IV circulation.

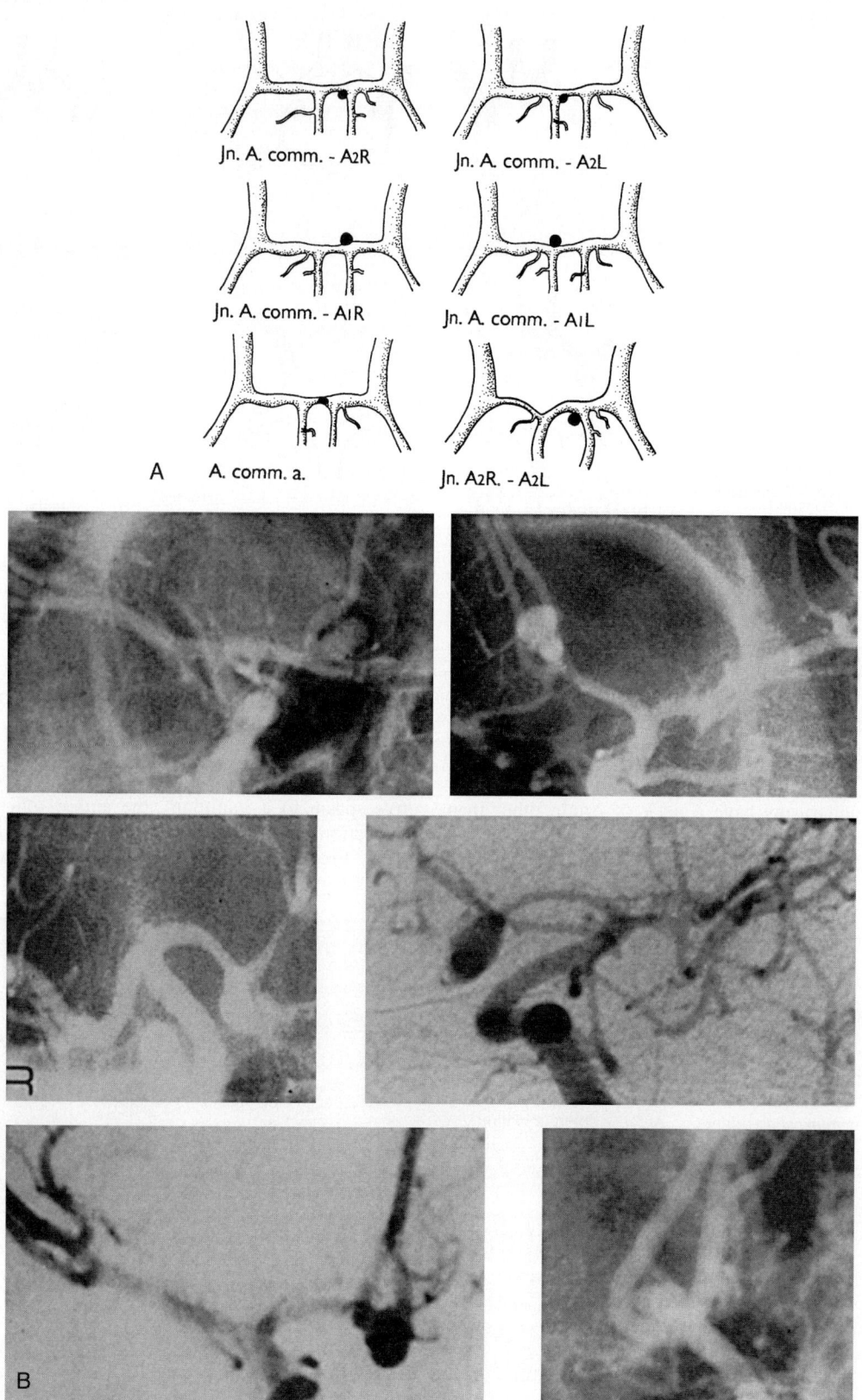

**FIGURE 87–6** ■ *A,* Diagrams of the location of the necks of anterior communicating artery aneurysms (see text). *B,* Angiograms showing various locations of the necks of aneurysms as in *A.*

dissected from the sac is helpful. Such knowledge also clarifies from which side the aneurysm is best approached. The intimate relationship of the sac to the neighboring vessels depends on the projection of the aneurysm. Those projecting anteriorly and inferiorly are free from both A2 segments. Conversely, those projecting superiorly and posteriorly along the course of A2 are closely related to these vessels. In most cases, the aneurysm projects to one or the other side with one major vessel in close contact. The following relationships of the sac to the major vessel may be seen on scrutiny of various views of the angiogram (Fig. 87–7):

1. No relationship to any major vessel
2. Anterior communicating artery alone
3. Anterior communicating artery and the right A2
4. Anterior communicating artery and the left A2
5. Anterior communicating artery and both A2 segments
6. Right A2 alone
7. Left A2 alone

The recurrent artery of Heubner is usually not adherent to the aneurysm, in contrast to the fronto-orbital artery, which may, however, be sacrificed if it is difficult to separate from the sac. The perforating arteries to the hypothalamus are adherent only when the aneurysm is large.

## PROJECTION OF THE ANEURYSM

Projection of the aneurysm (Fig. 87–8), or the direction in which the fundus points, is an important consideration

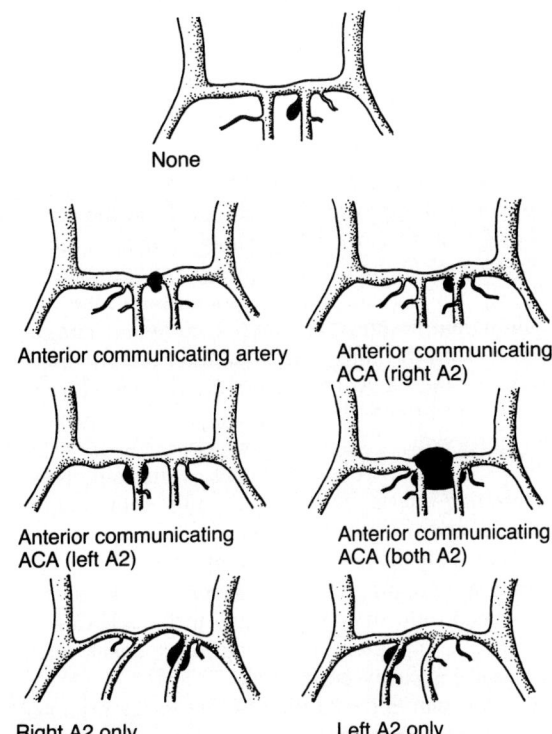

FIGURE 87–7 ■ Diagrams showing various relationships of the aneurysmal sac to major vessels.

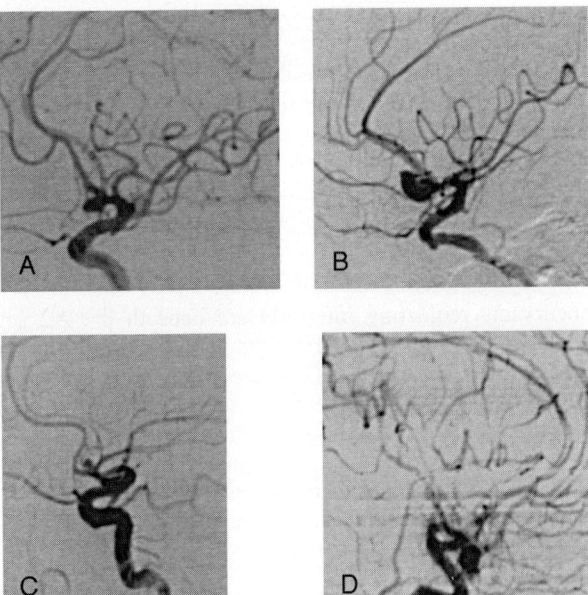

FIGURE 87–8 ■ Some examples of primary directions of aneurysm projection. A, Forward and slightly downward. B, Forward and slightly upward. C, Upward. D, Downward.

while planning surgical approach and dissection. Most information about the projection can be gathered from the relationship of the sac to the major vessels. Further information is helpful to appreciate the relationship of the aneurysm to other surrounding structures. Because aneurysms bleed most frequently from the fundus, its avoidance during dissection can reduce the incidence of intraoperative rupture. An aneurysm of the anterior communicating region can project in any direction. It is useful to classify the possibilities into four basic groups, although in reality various combinations arise.

### Anterior Projection

The aneurysm lies in close relationship to the optic nerves or pituitary stalk. It can obscure the contralateral A1 in the pterional approach but is rarely adherent to any significant vessels. It is not necessary and even harmful to dissect any of the related structures for clipping. Anteriorly projecting aneurysms are technically the easiest of all anterior communicating aneurysms.

### Superior Projection

Aneurysms projecting upward usually follow the course of the ipsilateral A2 and are pointing toward the gyrus rectus. These aneurysms are usually responsible for frontal lobe hematomas. Ipsilateral fronto-orbital and frontopolar arteries are closely adherent to the aneurysm and can also obscure visualization of the opposite A2. Selecting the appropriate side of approach to avoid the fundus can prevent premature rupture while retracting the frontal lobe.

## Posterior Projection

Aneurysms projecting posteriorly lie between the two A2 segments and often overlap the opposite A2 and its branches. Because the fundus lies underneath the gyrus rectus, its resection during the early part of dissection may cause intraoperative rupture.

## Inferior Projection

Aneurysms projecting inferiorly are beneath the A2 segments and closely related to the lamina terminalis and hypothalamic structures. They are often adherent to the perforators supplying these vital areas. They are the most difficult aneurysms from the technical viewpoint and tend to produce the maximal impairment of higher cerebral functions. For these aneurysms, an interhemispheric approach may protect many of the surrounding vessels from surgical trauma.

## SURGICAL APPROACHES

With the appalling natural history of aneurysms at the anterior communicating artery complex, obliteration of these common aneurysms by ligature or by clip became a neurosurgeon's task shortly after Dott[14] illustrated an aneurysm by angiography in 1931. Tonnis[15] was the first to operate directly on an anterior communicating artery aneurysm in 1936. Because of the technical difficulty of exposure, better understanding of the surgical anatomy of the anterior communicating artery complex and the morphology of the aneurysm, appreciation of the pathologic changes within the brain that occur after SAH, and a desire to obliterate the aneurysms as early as possible, surgical approaches to these aneurysms have undergone a continual change. The evolution of surgical approaches has been described by Fox and Sengupta[16] and Sengupta and McAllister.[1] No doubt other approaches to these aneurysms will be introduced in the future.

The purpose of the evolution of all these approaches was to ensure: (1) minimal brain retraction, (2) the prevention of premature bleed, (3) the avoidance of injury to vessels, and (4) a reduction in the incidence of postoperative vasospasm and ischemia. Three principal approaches can be used to treat these aneurysms, as follows:

1. Pterional trans-sylvian approach with exposure of the ACA from its origin to the region of the anterior communicating artery complex. A right-sided craniotomy is almost always performed.
2. Pterional subfrontal gyrus rectus approach without exposing the carotid bifurcation. The side for craniotomy is determined by the morphology of the aneurysm (Fig. 87–9).
3. Interhemispheric approach through a bifrontal craniotomy.

## Pterional Approaches

In the approach, advocated by Yasargil,[17] the pterional trans-sylvian approach, the anatomy of the anterior commu-

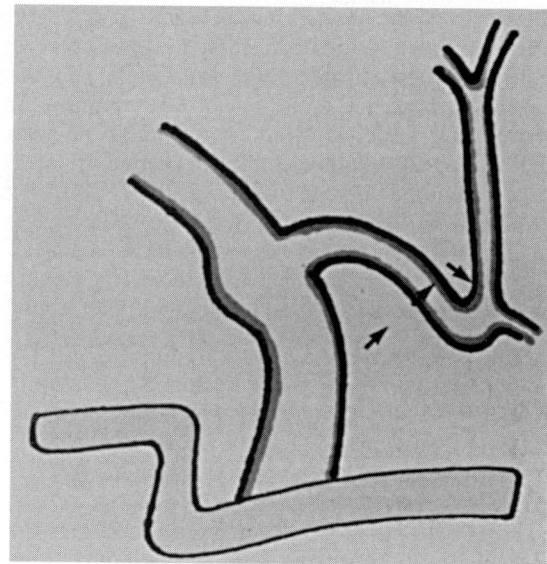

**FIGURE 87–9 ■** The direction of aneurysmal dissection in the subfrontal gyrus rectus approach.

nicating artery complex is well displayed by microsurgical dissection, and all the vessels surrounding the aneurysm are accounted for before the clip is applied. Rarely a small part of the gyrus rectus is removed. The difficulty with this approach is that A1 is the source of most of the vital central vessels. Dissection of these vessels in patients with recent SAH may lead to spasm and obliteration of some of the perforators. The carotid bifurcation is the deepest part of the circle, and opening the anterior part of the sylvian fissure, which is difficult because it has been obliterated by recent SAH, is necessary to avoid undue retraction. Considerable skill in microtechniques is required for dissection and protection of all the vessels.

The pterional subfrontal gyrus rectus approach has been adopted and modified by the author for the following reasons:

1. The course of the ACA, as seen at operation through the pterional approach, is such that from the point of its origin at the carotid bifurcation, which is the deepest part of the circle, it passes forward and slightly upward until it meets its fellow in the longitudinal fissure. The anterior communicating artery region is much more superficial than the proximal course of the ACA, and dissecting deeply with more retraction to the brain is unnecessary for exposure of this aneurysm.
2. The proximal ACA is the source of the important perforating arteries to the basal ganglia, the internal capsule, and the hypothalamus. In this approach, dissection of this artery can be avoided.
3. Temporary clipping of A1, if necessary, can be performed immediately proximal to the anterior communicating artery. Exposing the opposite A1, if necessary, is easily performed.
4. This approach allows a direct route to the origin of the neck of the aneurysm and the vessel that needs to be dissected free from the sac.
5. The distal ACA (A2) gives rise to few central

branches, other than the Heubner artery, which is always away from the aneurysm. Dissection of A2 close to the anterior communicating artery is less hazardous. Resection of part of the gyrus rectus prevents any torque on the aneurysm complex.

The disadvantages of this approach are as follows:

1. Part of the gyrus rectus is invariably resected, and this area is highly epileptogenic.
2. Precise knowledge of the location of the neck, fundus, and surrounding vessels from the angiogram is essential to avoid premature rupture and vessel injury.
3. In this approach, because the surrounding vessels are not well displayed and the application of the clip depends on the angiographic assessment of the location of these vessels, the possibility of vascular occlusion remains. This consequence is unlikely when the procedure is performed by an experienced surgeon.
4. When a left-sided approach is used, the dominant hemisphere is exposed.
5. For inexperienced right-handed surgeons, dissection on the left side may prove difficult.

Despite these possible disadvantages, the author has found the surgical outcome in these aneurysms to be most gratifying.

## Interhemispheric Approach

In the interhemispheric approach, used by Suzuki and colleagues[18] for hundreds of anterior communicating artery aneurysms, brain retraction is modest; no brain resection is necessary; and for anteriorly and inferiorly projecting aneurysms, the neck and parent vessels are exposed before the sac. Because the patient is placed supine with the head in the midline, the anatomic course of the vessels is in synchrony with the operative exposure, allowing safer dissection, and some surgeons find that orientation and identification of anatomic structures to be easier. The interhemispheric approach should be considered in the following situations: (1) The aneurysm is projecting anteriorly or inferiorly. (2) There is an associated aneurysm of the pericallosal artery. (3) Attempted clipping by the pterional approach has been unsuccessful.

There are some major disadvantages, which is why the interhemispheric approach is not universally adopted. The longitudinal fissure is often obliterated after recent SAH, and separation of the two embracing frontal lobes is not easy. In superiorly projecting aneurysms, the fundus is exposed first, risking premature bleeding. When both A1 segments are exposed for temporary clipping, the benefit of modest brain retraction is lost. The risk of bilateral olfactory nerve injury exists. Venous infarction after this approach in patients with acute SAH was reported.[19] There is also relatively late visualization and control of the A1 segments, and temporary clips can be difficult to apply.

## Summary

Each of the surgical approaches has its merits and works well for its advocates. The inherent disadvantages are not apparent in the literature, making it difficult for the inexperienced surgeon to adopt a particular approach. The author strongly believes that the only way to learn a particular technique is to spend time with an experienced surgeon who practices various approaches. The pterional trans-sylvian approach and the interhemispheric approach have been well described elsewhere.[16, 18] The author's own approach is described in detail in this chapter.

## TECHNICAL AIDS FOR INTRACRANIAL ANEURYSM SURGERY

The author employs the following technical aids for surgery:

1. Operating microscope. It is difficult for surgeons today to believe that a ruptured aneurysm can be successfully obliterated without the use of a microscope. Suzuki and colleagues,[18] however, reported 1500 cases of intracranial aneurysms that were treated surgically without a microscope, and the author operated on his first 300 patients without a microscope and achieved results no different from those achieved today. Nevertheless, the value of the microtechnique in aneurysm surgery is overwhelming. According to the availability of funds, various sophisticated microscopes can be used, but the basic model, which has magnification, illumination, and observation facilities for scrub nurses and others, is all that is required.
2. Microinstruments. Because most dissection is carried out with bipolar forceps, forceps of various shapes and sizes must be available during the procedure. The tips of the bipolar forceps should also be of various shapes and sizes.
3. Bipolar coagulation.
4. Self-retaining retractors. In the author's view, the introduction of self-retaining retractors in aneurysm surgery is as significant as that of the microscope.
5. Suction apparatus. At least two sets of suction apparatus must be available. The apparatus used during dissection should be of low pressure, not more than 4 lb/in$^2$, and controllable at the sucker tip.
6. Aneurysm clips. Various forms of nonferrous aneurysm clips are available. Although, theoretically and under laboratory conditions, these clips appear unaffected by strong magnetic fields, there remains at present an international moratorium on using magnetic resonance imaging in patients with any form of aneurysm clip in situ. Most widely used clips are designed by Yasargil and Sugita. Clips designed by Perneczky have the advantage of a smaller applicator tip that holds the clip from inside, allowing less obscuration of the target area during clipping. All these clips have their specific uses in a given situation.
7. Reinforcing agent. Muslin and glue (Histoacryl) are used by the author.
8. Spasmolytic agent. Papaverine 2.5% solution is used.
9. Lumbar drain. A lumbar drain is used unless a need exists for an external ventricular drain.

10. Urinary catheter. Because mannitol is always used in aneurysm surgery, the insertion of a urinary catheter is essential.

11. Endoscope. The introduction of this device to complement microsurgery allows the surgeon to visualize any obscured areas of the anatomy during and after clipping.

## ANESTHESIA

### Preoperative Preparation

The patient's neurologic status is assessed routinely, as are associated medical disorders that may affect the anesthesia. Sedative premedication is not routinely prescribed, but if it is specifically indicated, a 10- to 20-mg dose of temazepam is given orally.

### Induction

In the anesthetic room, the patient is attached to routine monitoring equipment before induction: electrocardiograph, noninvasive arterial pressure monitor, and pulse oximeter. A 22-gauge cannula is introduced, and glycopyrrolate 200 μg and fentanyl 100 to 200 μg are given. Oxygen is administered by face mask, and anesthesia is induced in a 15-degree head-up position by means of thiopentone 200 to 500 mg and vecuronium for muscle relaxation. Gentle hyperventilation with oxygen–nitrous oxide and isoflurane is employed until full relaxation is achieved. A second dose of thiopentone, 75 to 100 mg, may be used to obtund the reflex pressor response to laryngoscopy. Intubation is performed by use of an armored endotracheal tube, a pharyngeal pack is inserted, and the tube is firmly fixed in place with waterproof strapping. A 20-gauge cannula is inserted in the nondominant radial artery for invasive pressure monitoring, and a 12- or 14-gauge cannula is placed in a peripheral vein. A urinary catheter is also established. Central venous pressure is not routinely monitored. A lumbar drain is frequently placed at this stage to allow later withdrawal of CSF.

Positive-pressure ventilation that aims for an end-tidal carbon dioxide concentration of about 3.5% in a normal patient is employed. In those with suspected lung disease, arterial blood gases may be measured to determine serious discrepancies between end-tidal and arterial measurements. Continuous oximetry is routine.

### Maintenance

The patient is transferred to the operating room, is placed on the operating table in a slightly head-up position, and is infused with 0.75 to 1 g/kg of mannitol. Anesthesia is maintained with oxygen, nitrous oxide, and isoflurane, perhaps with an increment of 50 to 100 μg of fentanyl if there is a noticeable response to scalp incision. An infusion of vecuronium at about 4 mg/hr by use of nerve-stimulator control ensures continued muscle relaxation.

Arterial pressure may tend to sag in the postinduction phase before surgery begins. The combination of isoflurane-induced vasodilatation, lack of surgical stimulus, and perhaps covert fluid depletion often causes a degree of systemic hypotension and typically a marked respiratory swing on the arterial trace. Infusion of colloid in the form of modified gelatin is usually sufficient to counteract this effect. Occasionally, ephedrine, titrated in 3-mg increments, is required.

During craniotomy, arterial blood pressure is kept at or slightly below the preoperative level. After dural opening, the systolic pressure tends to fall to 90 to 100 mm Hg even without the use of specific hypotensive agents. This level is usually satisfactory for the surgeon, but a further gentle fall can usually be achieved by a modest increase in inspired isoflurane concentration. If greater levels of hypotension are called for than can be obtained in this way, and if the heart rate is high and the patient does not have obstructive pulmonary disease, labetalol may be given in 10-mg increments. Sodium nitroprusside may also be used. These measures may not be necessary if the patient is already receiving an infusion of nimodipine because arterial pressure may tend to fall. Induction of hypotension must be carried out in a normovolemic patient. Strict attention to fluid depletion or blood loss is essential.

After clipping of the aneurysm, blood pressure is allowed to return to preoperative levels to ensure hemostasis. The patient is extubated as tranquilly as possible and, after initial recovery in the operating room, is transferred to the intensive care unit for postoperative observation and care. Intra-arterial monitoring is continued in the recovery phase to allow early detection and correction of hypertension or hypotension.

## SURGICAL TECHNIQUE

### Side of Craniotomy

Aneurysms at the region of the anterior communicating artery are generally approached from the right, nondominant side except in the presence of a left frontal hematoma or a dominant left A1. The author plans his approach on the basis of the position of the neck of the aneurysm and the relationship of the sac to major vessel to procure the shortest route to the aneurysm and ease of separation of vessels from the sac. Information about the projection of the aneurysm suggests its likely relationship to major vessels and other structures. The presence of a large hematoma during elective surgery is unusual, but when present, the side of the exposure is determined by the hematoma. Dominance of A1 is a less important consideration because both A1 segments can be exposed from either side when required. A left-sided craniotomy is performed under the following circumstances (Fig. 87–10):

1. When the neck is located at the left A1 and the anterior communicating artery junction
2. When the sac is intermittently adherent to the left A2
3. In the presence of a large left frontal hematoma
4. When the left A1 is dominant and the right A2 is free from the aneurysm

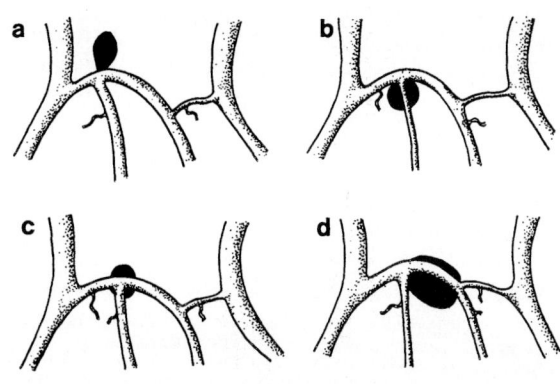

*a, b, c.* Left sided     *d,* Right sided (for dominant left ACA)

A

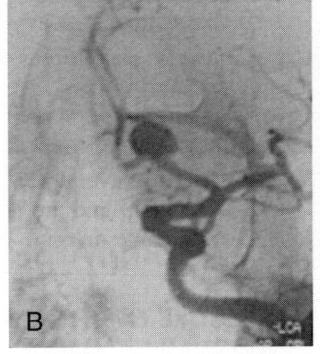 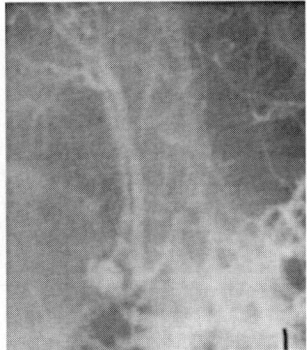 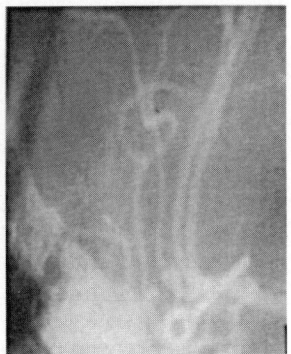

FIGURE 87–10 ■ *A,* Indications determining the side of a craniotomy. *B,* The aneurysm (left) was approached from the left side because it was intimately related to the left A2. Although the left A1 is dominant (center), the aneurysm was approached from the right because it was closely related to the right A2. Postoperative angiogram (right), as in the center.

If none of these circumstances is present, a right-sided craniotomy is performed. Although the author formerly approached large or giant aneurysms through a bilateral craniotomy, with experience, he has found a unilateral craniotomy to be adequate. Exposure of the dominant hemisphere has not been a problem, and there has been no difficulty in dissecting from the left for the right-handed surgeon in 30% of operations carried out from the left side.

## Position of Patient on the Operating Table
(Fig. 87–11)

Anterior communicating artery aneurysms are located deep in the midline on the floor of the anterior cranial fossa in the region of the tuberculum sella. To expose these lesions with minimal brain retraction, special care is required in positioning the patient.

The patient is placed supine on the operating table with its chest piece elevated 30 degrees and head piece lowered 15 degrees. During the early part of the operation, while the craniotomy is performed, the head piece can be kept elevated for convenience. The head is turned 45 degrees to the opposite side and placed on a ring, rather than fixed in a clamp, to allow change of angle during surgery, if necessary; however, the same effect can be achieved with various head clamps. The ipsilateral shoulder is raised on a sandbag to avoid venous congestion. The aim of this positioning is to allow the pterion to face directly upward. This position allows the frontal lobe to fall away from the floor when the arachnoid dissections are complete. A good position

for this approach is confirmed when the optic nerve can be seen with only little retraction before the microscope is brought into the operating field to begin arachnoidal dissection. The operative field is now prepared, and the line of incision for the scalp flap is marked and infiltrated with local anesthetic and epinephrine solution. The operation site is now isolated with drapes.

## Skin Incision and Scalp Flap (Fig. 87–12)

The goal of the scalp incision is to protect the superficial temporal artery, to allow the bone flap to reach the floor of

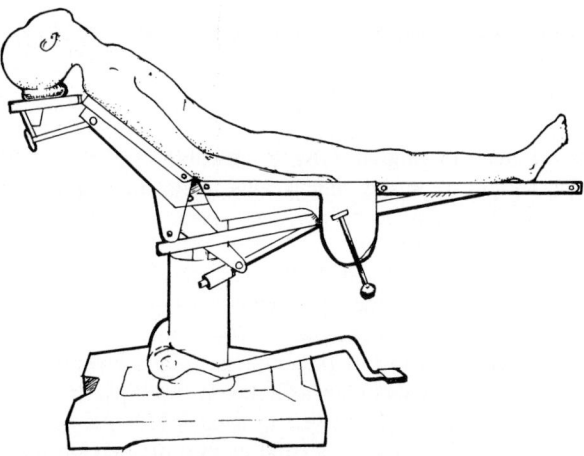

FIGURE 87–11 ■ The position of the patient on the table.

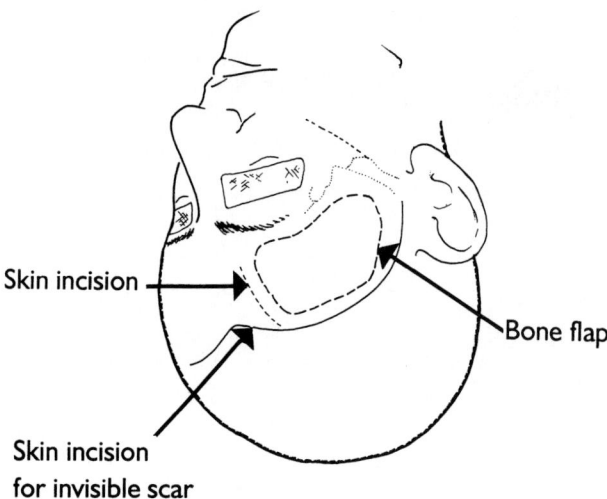

Skin incision

Bone flap

Skin incision
for invisible scar

**FIGURE 87-12** ■ Skin incision, scalp flap, and craniotomy (see text).

the anterior cranial fossa, and to provide a good cosmetic appearance. The skin is incised along a line, starting in front of the tragus, gently curving behind the hair line medially and anteriorly to the midline, then gently moving backward up to a point in the midpoint of the opposite pupil. If a cosmetic scar is not of paramount importance, a short incision curving forward to about 1.5 cm in front of the hairline at the level of ipsilateral pupil is quicker. While the scalp is incised, care is taken to avoid injury to the main stem of the superficial temporal artery and the temporalis muscle. Hemostasis in the scalp margin is achieved with Raney clips attached to the free border with curved hemostats over the attached margin. The scalp flap is reflected over the brow. While the scalp flap is elevated, the midline should be marked for orientation during placement of the bur holes. The supraorbital and supratrochlear nerves are carefully separated from the periosteum and are positioned with the scalp flap. The scalp is then held back with fish hooks. Location of the osteoplastic bone flap is now planned and prepared by division of the pericranium and temporalis muscle with cutting diathermy. The pericranium, which dries up with heat from the overhanging lights, must be kept moist at all times with gauze soaked in saline.

## Craniotomy and Bone Removal (see Fig. 87-12)

Placement of the craniotomy is crucial. The bone flap should be generous and should extend as close to the floor of the anterior cranial fossa as possible, and the medial limb should be in the plane of the ipsilateral pupil. If the frontal sinus cannot be avoided, special precautions are taken to seal up the sinus with bone chips and pericranium before the dura is opened. The crucial bur hole is in the pterion itself over the zygomatic process of the frontal bone, a position that should expose frontal and temporal fossas. Although use of the craniotome and power drill is now common, the author still favors multiple bur holes connected with the Gigli saw to avoid excessive vibration of the brain. Craniotomy should expose the sylvian fissure well. The lateral half of the sphenoidal wing must be

resected and the bone margin waxed. Before the bone flap is lifted, it is separated from the dura with a periosteal dissector and wide brain retractor. In the elderly, the dura is often intimately adherent to the bone, and great care is necessary to prevent laceration of the dura and, at times, the brain, which could result from tearing of the cortical veins. If the saw guide cannot be passed easily between the two bur holes, a small craniectomy with narrow, pointed rongeurs should be made to clear the path for the guide. After the bone flap is reflected, its margin is smoothed by the rongeur, and all the venous channels in the bone flap are carefully cauterized and waxed because, on a osteoplastic flap, slow oozing of blood may lead to extradural hematoma. The bone flap with attached temporalis muscle is now reflected laterally and is held in position with fish hooks. After the bone flap is elevated, the borders of the skull defect are also waxed and covered with a narrow strip of Surgicel, and the dura is hinged against the bone margin with the pericranium to prevent extradural bleeding.

## Assessment and Reduction of Brain Tension

Brain tension can be easily assessed by palpation of the exposed dura. If any tension exists, CSF is removed through a lumbar drain. If the ventricle is found to be enlarged on CT scan, which may occur in a significant number of patients with these aneurysms, the frontal horn of the lateral ventricle is cannulated, and a ventricular catheter is introduced to remove CSF and is later used as a continuous ventricular drain. Excessive removal of CSF at this stage makes subsequent arachnoidal dissection difficult owing to obliterations of the cisterns.

## Dural Opening

Once the dura is slack, a linear dural incision is made 1 cm above the anterior margin of the bony opening along its entire length. Several vertical cuts are then made in the anterior dural flap and are held up with sutures and hemostats against the bone margin.

## Exposure of the Optic Nerve and Internal Carotid Artery (Fig. 87-13)

After the dura is opened, the head piece of the table is lowered to allow maximal extension of the head, and care is taken to ensure that the head is resting comfortably on the ring and the endotracheal tube is not disturbed. A 1.5-cm-wide hand-held retractor is now used to retract the orbital surface of the frontal lobe. If the optic nerve can be visualized with minimal frontal lobe retraction, the position of the head is ideal. The retractor is now attached to the Leyla-Aesculap self-retaining retractor system, which is mounted on the left side of the operating table. The operating microscope, which has a 300-mm lens, is now brought into the operating field.

The paraoptic cisterns are opened with a sharp 22-gauge needle, bent 90 degrees at the tip, and mounted on a suitable handle. This device is the cheapest and finest arachnoidal knife available in any operating room. As the CSF starts to flow from the cistern, it is sucked up with the left sucker. If the scale of sucker pressure is used with a controllable sucker tube, the arachnoid membrane is kept open and divided with fine scissors. With fine division of the arachnoid from the prechiasmatic cistern medially to the lateral limit of exposure, the frontal lobe gradually falls further back. The arachnoid over the medial end of the sylvian fissure is thick. Careful division of this thick band causes the frontal lobe to fall further back without any tension on the temporal lobe. While the arachnoid medial to the optic nerve is dissected, care must be taken not to disturb the anteriorly projecting aneurysms or the blood clots in the prechiasmal cistern.

If an angiogram has suggested a difficult backward and inferiorly projecting aneurysm, the arachnoid over the opposite optic nerve and A1 is also divided for temporary proximal occlusion. During these early stages, the retractor over the frontal lobe should be kept over the lateral aspect of its orbital surface to avoid any tension on the aneurysm complex. Exposure of the sylvian fissure is not necessary. Once the proximal part of the internal carotid artery and the olfactory tract are exposed, this stage of the operation is complete because exposure of the carotid bifurcation or A1 is avoided in this approach. Occasionally the internal carotid artery is short, and the proximal part of the ACA comes into view with the anteriorly projecting aneurysms at its medial end. In this unlikely event, the aneurysm is approached, as is discussed later.

The brain retractor is now gently replaced over the medial aspect of the orbital surface of the frontal lobe, just above the olfactory tract, without any tension on the interhemispheric fissure. A site below the olfactory tract is now selected for corticectomy in the gyrus rectus (Fig. 87–14). A 1.5-cm incision over the cortex is made with bipolar coagulation. By use of a sucker, 1 cm³ of cortical tissue is removed in such a way that enables the interhemispheric fissure to be reached. The sucker pressure is critical during this step because arachnoid in the interhemispheric fissure or the aneurysm complex should not be disturbed at all. If the frontopolar or orbitofrontal artery creates a hazard for smooth dissection, these arteries should be sacrificed. After removal of the cortical tissue, a suitably

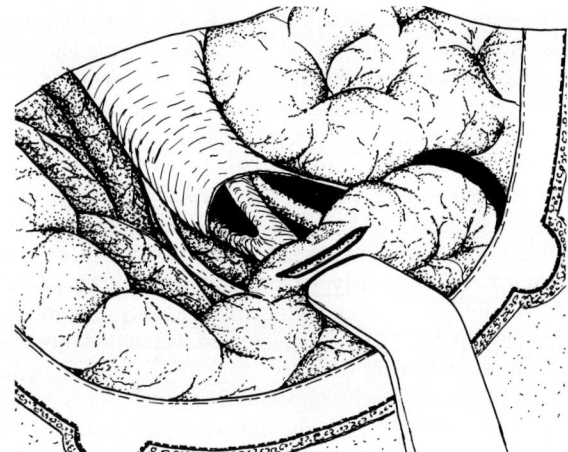

**FIGURE 87–14** ■ The location of a corticectomy.

sized retractor can be placed over the olfactory tract deep into the cavity created by corticectomy, and the frontal lobe can be further retracted without any tension on the aneurysm complex.

## Dissection in the Target Area

The surgeon is now in the "*tiger* territory." The risk of premature bleeding is highest at this stage, and every attempt should be made to minimize this hazard. The blood pressure should be allowed to fall gradually over a period of at least 4 minutes to prevent failure of autoregulation, to a level of 80 mm Hg systolic in a normotensive patient and to about 100 mm Hg in a hypertensive patient. Magnification is increased to a comfortable level. A second suction apparatus, with high suction pressure, is kept in readiness, and a temporary clip is kept mounted on its applicator.

Despite all preoperative planning, the anatomy of the aneurysm complex may appear confusing at the beginning of this stage. With the help of a suction tip set at a low pressure and fine-tipped bipolar forceps, however, the pia-arachnoid in the interhemispheric fissure is gently dissected. This process exposes the proximal part of A2 or the anterior communicating artery region or even the adjacent A1. Whichever part of the vascular anatomy is exposed, the dissection is kept on the outer side to avoid interference with the aneurysm and injury to the perforating vessels. Despite hypotension, if the aneurysm appears tense and intimately adherent to the vessel, proximal occlusion of A1 is useful. The distal part of the ipsilateral A1 is cleared of arachnoid, and a site free of perforators is chosen for a temporary clip. If a temporary clip proves necessary, elevating the blood pressure is not needed when the configuration of the circle is normal because enough blood flows through the communicating artery to nourish the area of the brain supplied by the occluded A1. If a temporary clip is applied to both A1 segments or to the dominant A1 segment, elevation of blood pressure to 100 mm Hg or greater is safe.

The vasculature ipsilateral to the aneurysm complex and the adjacent ACA is best seen with this approach, but the opposite side of the aneurysm and the opposite ACA re-

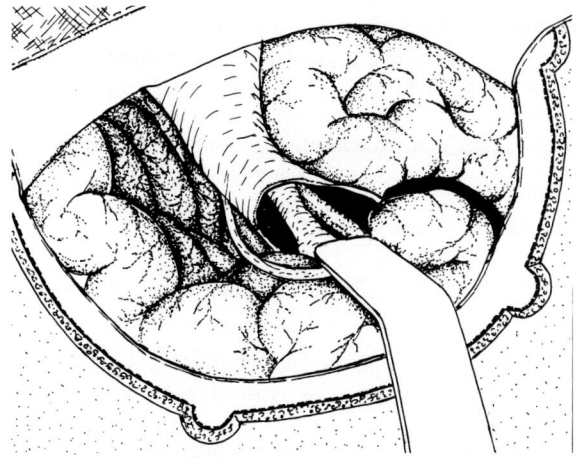

**FIGURE 87–13** ■ Initial exposure.

main obscured by the aneurysm itself. An attempt is made to pass a fine hook through the free border of the aneurysmal neck before the adherent side is dissected. If this attempt fails, coagulation of part of the sac with broad-tipped bipolar forceps shrinks the aneurysm sufficiently to discover or create a cleavage for passage of the clip. If one of the cortical vessels gets in the way at this stage, it is coagulated and divided but not separated from the sac. The Heubner artery is always distant from the sac, and it is not seen unless unnecessarily looked for. Perforating vessels from the anterior communicating artery are also not looked for because these become segregated when the neck is shrunken all around at the final stage of dissection. After the neck is cleared on the opposite side, attention is drawn to the ipsilateral side with the adherent A2 (Fig. 87–15). Again, gentle coagulation of the adjacent part of the sac, with the patient still under hypotension, exposes a potential space, which is further dissected free with microscissors. If the aneurysm is projecting laterally underneath A2, the vessel is separated with a temporary clip to A1. With the sac now slack, careful coagulation of the sac exposes the ipsilateral border of the neck. If the aneurysm leaks, gentle pressure on a cottonoid with the left sucker allows continued dissection or coagulation of the rent. If the aneurysm is a blowout of the communicating artery itself, no attempt is made to isolate this artery from the aneurysm.

## Temporary Vascular Occlusion

Temporary occlusion of the parent artery may permit safer dissection and reduce the size of the aneurysm and the pressure within it, facilitating neck clipping. This useful technique can be dangerous if not used judiciously. In addition to intimal injury, its prolonged use can cause irreversible cerebral ischemia. Maintenance of the blood pressure at its preoperative level in some situations during temporary clipping is essential to allow collateral circulation. Temporary clipping can be dangerous if the circle of Willis is incompetent. Somatosensory evoked potential responses from the posterior tibial nerves may predict poor perfusion in the anterior cerebral territory before irreversible ischemia sets in. Temporary clipping cannot be maintained for more than 15 to 20 minutes at a time without harm. Brain-protecting agents during temporary clipping include the following:

1. Mannitol, 1 g/kg body weight infused 1 hour before the temporary clipping.
2. Thiopental, 10 g/kg as a loading dose, then titrated until electroencephalogram burst suppression occurs.[20]
3. Etomidate, 0.3 mg/kg. This agent acts similar to a barbiturate but without cardiovascular depression. It has been used during temporary occlusion with good results.[21]

## Clipping of the Neck

Application of a clip to the neck is the goal of direct surgery. With bipolar coagulation, it is possible to render a broad neck clippable. The need to protect the anterior communicating artery has been exaggerated, however. In patients with a normal circulatory pattern, this artery can be occluded with the aneurysm, if necessary, without any harmful effect. Although the perforating vessels arising from the communicating artery should be protected whenever possible, excessive dissection to do this is counterproductive. As has been pointed out, the perforating vessels arising from the communicating artery are still nourished from the opposite A1 if the communicating artery is occluded on one side. The possible effect of clipping the anterior communicating artery in various circulatory patterns is shown in Figure 87–16, which demonstrates that although a clip on the neck is ideal, occlusion of the anterior communicating artery along with the neck is harmless in some patients and lethal in others.

Once the neck has been entirely isolated, the surgeon must decide which size and shape of clip is most appropriate to obliterate the aneurysm without compromising major vessels. By applying the clip in the correct direction, the vessels on the opposite side, even when not visualized, can be kept safe. If any doubt about their safety exists, the aneurysm is further reduced in size after the initial clip is applied so that the opposite A2 is safe. When the clip is advanced gradually, it should pass well beyond the neck of the aneurysm and be released gradually to avoid a tear in the neck. One of the problems with the Sugita clip applicator is engaging it when the clip needs to be repositioned. Adjusting the angle of vision of the microscope or using a multiangle applicator can overcome this problem. Although Drake clips, which have an aperture for a major artery, seem to be ideal, the appropriate size for a particular situation is difficult to determine.

## Steps After Clipping and Closure

The author takes the following steps after clipping and closure:

1. Pieces of muslin are placed around the clipped neck.
2. Papaverine solution 2.5% is instilled over the exposed vessels.
3. While the retractor is being removed, distortion of the clip by the overlying frontal lobe should be checked

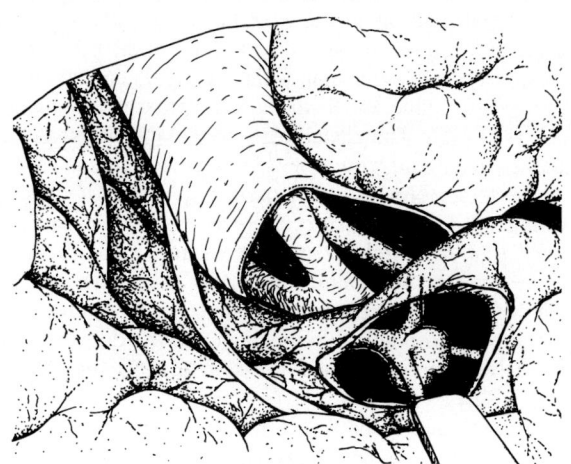

**FIGURE 87–15** ■ Exposure of the aneurysm.

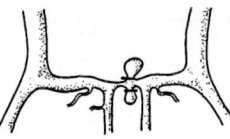

1. Clip on the neck *(ideal)*

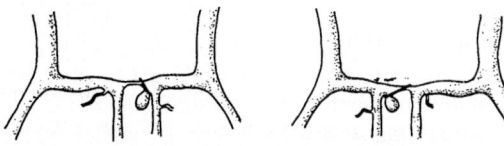

2. Clip on anterior communicating artery *(harmless)*

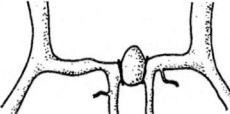

3. Clip on anterior communicating artery *(minimal risk)*

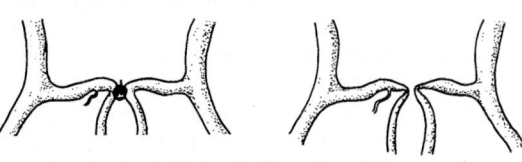

4. Clip on anterior communicating artery *(dangerous)*

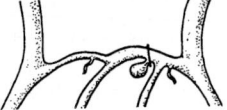
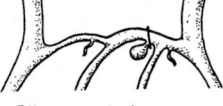

5. Clip on anterior communicating artery *(lethal)*

A

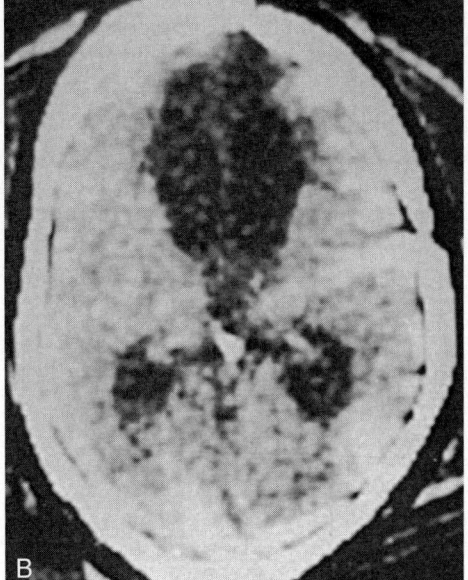

B

**FIGURE 87-16** ■ *A,* The effect of placement of a clip in various positions. *B,* A postoperative computed tomography (CT) scan showing an infarction of both frontal lobes due to kinking of both anterior communicating arteries in a patient with a rudimentary anterior communication artery.

to avoid kinking of the vessel or pressure on the optic nerve. Usually the head of the clip is accommodated by the space created by corticectomy. If not, space should be created to accommodate it in the frontal lobe.
4. The dura is left open in all cases of acute ruptured aneurysm. Alternatively the space can be enlarged by dural graft to provide a space for subsequent brain swelling.
5. Ventricular drainage is continued in cases of enlarged ventricles.
6. The bone flap is secured loosely to the pericranium and muscles.
7. A suction drain is placed underneath the scalp flap in such a way that the tip of the catheter cannot suck any CSF, as the dura is left open.
8. At the conclusion of the operation, the ipsilateral pupillary size is checked because papaverine can cause dilatation of the pupil, and unnecessary anxiety later regarding this sign can be avoided.
9. The patient is allowed to wake up and is nursed in the intensive care unit.
10. On rare occasions, if the patient does not wake up, a CT scan or angiography is performed to determine the presence of surgical complications. If none exists,

the patient receives elective ventilation for 24 hours in the intensive care unit, with ICP monitoring.

## POSTOPERATIVE MANAGEMENT

Successful obliteration of a ruptured aneurysm is only one facet of the patient's recovery. The ongoing pathologic changes in the brain that occur after SAH can be compounded by the additional assault of surgery. Complications in the postoperative period can arise abruptly and insidiously from many sources. Only strict monitoring in a unit equipped for this purpose, such as the intensive care unit, and, above all, the watchful eyes of trained nurses can prevent and detect these complications. The purpose of postoperative care includes the following:

1. To allow the brain to recover from the injury of the operation and SAH
2. To detect complications specific to craniotomy
3. To prevent and detect general complications that may arise from disturbance of consciousness
4. To detect and prevent early complications specific to the aneurysm, in the region of the anterior communicating artery

The postoperative care regimen includes the following areas.

**Clinical Assessment.** A baseline assessment is necessary to compare with any subsequent deterioration.

**Intensive Nursing Care.** The value of continuous observation by skilled nurses cannot be overemphasized. The watchful eyes of nurses who are trained in the observation and assessment of this type of patient are much more reliable than are the monitoring systems. Blood pressure, respiratory rate, temperature, fluid intake and output, and drug administration are routinely recorded, and neurologic records are kept according to the Glasgow Coma Scale.

**Routine Laboratory Tests.** Profound changes in the cellular and plasma component of blood occur secondary to SAH, craniotomy, and the administration of various drugs. Careful monitoring of complete blood count, serum electrolyte, blood urea nitrogen, creatinine levels, and osmolality can detect these changes. Arterial blood gases, particularly $Po_2$ and $Pco_2$, are assessed by bedside gas analyzers.

**Continuous Monitoring Program.** In the intensive care unit, patients are attached to various monitoring devices, but relying entirely on these is not safe. The following devices are routine:

Cardiograph—to record cardiac rhythm and pulse rate.
Pulse oximeter—to record oxygen saturation.
Arterial transducer—to record blood pressure continuously. The blood pressure is maintained at the preoperative level with a volume expander and medication, if required.
ICP—used only when patients are receiving ventilation.
Atrial pressure—monitored when a large amount of fluid intake is necessary, such as during the use of dopamine.
Transcranial Doppler—to assess flow velocity in intracranial vessels to detect early vasospasm.

**Medication.** All medication used in the preoperative regimen is continued.

**Venous Stasis Prophylaxis.** Elastic stocking or pneumatic compression boots and passive leg exercise are employed to prevent venous stasis.

**Fluid Intake.** The total fluid intake during the first postoperative days is limited to 1500 ml/day and consists of colloid and dextrose in saline. The surgeon and the anesthetist tend to underestimate blood loss during surgery. If the hemoglobin level is less than 12 g/dl in the postoperative period, 2 units of blood is routinely given.

**Angiography.** The author favors postoperative angiography for the following reasons: (1) A part of the aneurysm may remain unoccluded. (2) A clip may be misplaced or may have slipped off a large aneurysm. (3) If limited angiography has been performed, four-vessel angiography is mandatory to detect any other aneurysm. (4) Before operating on an incidental aneurysm, it is essential to know that satisfactory occlusion of the aneurysm, with preservation of the neighboring vessels, has been achieved. (5) Reassurance for the patient and the surgeon is desirable.

# RESULTS

Between 1970 and 1997, the author personally operated on 1246 patients with intracranial aneurysms. This number does not include patients operated on abroad because there are insufficient records for these patients. It is significant that from 1993 only 131 patients have been added to the surgical list. Among other reasons for this, introduction of endovascular therapy has diminished the enthusiasm of primary physicians for referring patients with SAH to neurosurgery. This change has produced a detrimental effect on the management outcome, in the author's opinion. Because the detailed records of cases after 1992 are incomplete and their long-term outcome not known, the results of surgery on the 1115 patients before 1993 are given here.

Of 1115 patients, 274 patients (146 men and 128 women) had aneurysms at the anterior communicating artery complex. Another 21 patients with anterior communicating artery aneurysms, who were devastated by recurrent hemorrhage or ischemia on admission, did not have surgery. Of the 274 patients, only 1, in whom the offending aneurysm was an initially undiagnosed posteroinferior cerebellar artery aneurysm, had an incidental anterior communicating artery aneurysm. Only two giant aneurysms occurred, one of which also presented as an SAH. Thirty-eight patients were younger than 30 years; 192, between 30 and 59 years; and 44, between 60 and 79 years.

At the time of admission, 193 patients had grades I and II aneurysms, and 81 patients had lower grades. At the time of elective surgery of the aneurysm, the total number in grades I and II was 206; in grade III, 59; in grade IV, 8; and in grade V, 1. The only patient in grade V in whom the aneurysm was clipped presented with a massive hematoma in the frontal lobe. While the hematoma was being removed, the aneurysm gave way and had to be clipped. Between the time of admission and surgery, the clinical status fluctuated considerably. All patients whose aneurysms were categorized in the poorer grade were treated according to the regimen suggested earlier, and the optimal time for aneurysm surgery was chosen. Twenty-seven patients were operated on between days 0 and 4 from ictus; 54, between days 5 and 7; 77, between days 8 and 11; 41, between days 12 and 14; 21, between days 15 and 18; 20, between days 19 and 21; and 34, beyond 21 days. The number of patients undergoing early surgery was small because of delay in the referral pattern.

All of the aneurysms were operated on personally by the author, who used the modified pterional subfrontal gyrus rectus approach. Sixty-nine patients were operated on electively from the left side. Earlier in this series, total obliteration of aneurysm was not achieved in 10 patients, whereas in another 9, after sac obliteration, the aneurysm complex was wrapped with muslin. In one patient, A1 was permanently occluded. With increasing experience, clipping all the aneurysms has been possible. The surgical outcome in relation to clinical grade is presented in Table 87–1.

Of 206 grade I and II patients, 174 (84%) had either excellent or good (with minor symptoms) outcome, 25 patients were independent but not working because of residual neurologic symptoms, 6 patients were severely disabled, and 1 patient died. In most cases, poor outcome

TABLE 87–1 ■ **SURGICAL OUTCOME BY GRADE AT OPERATION**

| Grade* | Good† | Fair† | Poor† | Dead | Total |
|---|---|---|---|---|---|
| I–II | 174 | 25 | 6 | 1 | 206 |
| III–V | 28 | 27 | 4 | 9 | 68 |
| Total | 202 (74%) | 52 (19%) | 10 (3.5%) | 10 (3.5%) | 274 |

*Hunt and Hess.
†Good = no deficit; fair = major defect but independent; poor = totally disabled.

in a good-grade patient resulted from postoperative cerebral ischemia from vasospasm.

Results in poor-grade patients were mostly affected by the SAH. Forty-one percent of poor-grade patients had a good outcome, and mortality was 13%. The outcome in relation to the timing of surgery is given in Table 87–2.

Eighty-one patients were operated on within the first week after SAH, with only one dead and 79% doing well. Most of the patients operated on after 3 weeks were categorized as poor grade with various complications of SAH and were treated initially with life-saving therapy. The reasons for poor outcome, particularly in grade I and II patients, are discussed later. Although some of the complications, such as hydrocephalus and seizures, were well controlled with therapy, ischemic complication was the predominant factor in preventing a good outcome.

## POSTOPERATIVE COMPLICATIONS

Postoperative complications after surgical treatment of anterior communicating artery aneurysms may arise from one or more of four sources: (1) craniotomy, (2) complications specific to aneurysm surgery, (3) disturbance in the anterior communicating artery region, and (4) ongoing pathologic process of SAH in general. Rational postoperative care can prevent many of these problems, but when they arise, management requires a clear appreciation of how problems arise, how to prevent them, and how to treat them. In addition to the preoperative factors previously discussed, various anesthetic drugs, the skill and experience of the anesthetist and the surgeon, and the patient's anxiety can inflict additional assault on the brain, even in a patient in good clinical condition. Furthermore, SAH is an ongoing

TABLE 87–2 ■ **SURGICAL OUTCOME BY TIMING OF SURGERY**

| | Days from Ictus | | | | | |
|---|---|---|---|---|---|---|
| Outcome | 0–4 | 5–7 | 8–11 | 12–21 | >21 | Total |
| Good | 19 | 45 | 56 | 59 | 23 | 202 |
| Fair | 6 | 8 | 15 | 14 | 9 | 52 |
| Poor | 1 | 1 | 2 | 5 | 1 | 10 |
| Dead | 1 | 0 | 4 | 4 | 1 | 10 |
| Total | 27 | 54 | 77 | 82 | 34 | 274 |

pathologic process that can manifest its complications in the postoperative period.

Non-neurologic complications, such as deep venous thrombosis and pulmonary embolism, infection, and stress bleeding, can occur in any surgical patient. In the author's series, no patient suffered permanent damage from any of these complications.

Progressive neurologic deterioration is one of the most worrisome complications of aneurysm surgery. The earlier the condition is detected, the better the chances are of complete recovery. The causes of progressive neurologic deterioration include the following:

1. Cerebral ischemia from brain swelling
2. Cerebral ischemia from vasospasm
3. Cerebral ischemia from vessel injury
4. Hydrocephalus
5. Seizures
6. Biochemical disturbances
7. Disturbances of blood gases
8. Intracranial hematoma
9. Rebleeding from a treated aneurysm or from another aneurysm.

### Brain Swelling

Brain swelling, without concurrent vasospasm, can cause ischemia. Because it is a constituent of traumatic inflammation, brain swelling or edema always occurs after craniotomy. Swelling of the brain within a rigid cranium after recent SAH, when the cerebral autoregulation is vulnerable, can produce a rise of ICP and can compromise perfusion pressure. With brain swelling, the ventricles become small, and this can be detected on CT scan, making a ventricular drain ineffective. Fluid restriction is often all the treatment that is necessary. Diuretics, such as furosemide or mannitol, may be required in some cases, and in extreme circumstances, removal of the bone flap may be necessary.

### Vasospasm

Vasospasm is the most dreaded cause of ischemic complication after SAH and may occur even after a successful operation on a grade I or II patient. Its cause is unknown, and its treatment remains elusive. Vasospasm is difficult to detect early, although it is extremely important to do so because the result of treatment after established cerebral ischemia is poor. With the help of Doppler ultrasound, CT scan, and CT angiography, a tentative diagnosis can be made as soon as clinical suspicion is aroused. Of 274 patients with anterior communicating artery aneurysm, 33 patients (12.2%) had postoperative vasospasm.

There are two ways the author treats vasospasm: First, one needs to prevent or reverse the effect of diminished perfusion to the involved territory. The various measures designed to achieve the first goal are empirical and largely futile. The calcium antagonist nimodipine has not achieved these aims. The treatment of cerebral ischemia before infarction has occurred can be achieved by increasing the perfusion pressure. Therapy is as follows:

Stage I
1. Control of ICP
   a. Reduction of fluid intake, depending on the biochemical parameters
   b. Mannitol (20%), 100 ml every 6 hours.
   c. Ventricular drainage if ventricles are dilated
2. Raising of blood pressure
   a. Blood or colloid
   b. Dopamine, if necessary
3. If no effect has been achieved within 2 hours, proceed to stage II.

Stage II
Angiography, with a view to angioplasty with or without infusion of papaverine. The results are far from satisfactory.

## Hydrocephalus

Hydrocephalus after SAH or after direct surgical treatment of an aneurysm occurs more frequently than is appreciated. Postoperative hydrocephalus is usually communicating in type with gradual onset because of blockage of the subarachnoid cisterns with blood, producing impairment of the absorptive mechanism of the arachnoidal villi and postoperative adhesions. Obstructive hydrocephalus can also occur as a result of blood clot acutely blocking the ventricle.

The insidious onset of impaired mentation and memory disturbance associated with gait disturbance and loss of sphincter control are classic features of communicating hydrocephalus. In acute ventricular obstruction, a sudden loss of consciousness occurs that mimics a rebleed or an unobserved seizure. A CT scan establishes the diagnosis of hydrocephalus. Most patients with communicating hydrocephalus recover after a few lumbar punctures. Definitive shunt insertion was required in 5.8% of cases in the author's series. In acute ventricular obstruction, an emergency ventricular drain is life-saving. The following case report is illustrative.

### Case Report 1

A 40-year-old man was admitted with grade IV clinical status with massive coma-producing SAH. CT scan showed scattered blood in the subarachnoid space and ventricle. Sixteen days later, his condition improved to a stable grade III, and repeat CT scan showed only mild ventricular dilatation (Fig. 87–17A). Angiography showed a large anterior communicating artery aneurysm that had obviously bled and a small, incidental posterior communicating artery aneurysm on the left side (see Fig. 87–17B). During operation, the clip had to be readjusted a few times because needling the aneurysm showed that it had not been totally occluded. The patient woke up from anesthesia without any additional neurologic deficit. Two hours after the operation, he suddenly became apneic and suffered bradycardia and dilated and fixed pupils. After 1 or 2 minutes, breathing returned spontaneously, the pupil became small, but his eyes deviated to the right, and he had involuntary movement of the right arm.

The immediate question was whether he had a seizure or a rebleed from the treated aneurysm or the untreated posterior communicating artery aneurysm. A CT scan showed massive dilatation of the ventricle and blood in the lateral third and fourth ventricles but no hematoma at the site of the operation (see Fig. 87–17C).

An immediate external ventricular drain was installed, followed a few days later by a ventriculoperitoneal shunt. Angiography showed complete obliteration of the aneurysm (see Fig. 87–17D). It became apparent that when the aneurysm was punctured during operation, a brief, brisk bleeding had occurred, and blood had entered into the ventricular system. It took 2 hours to produce the dramatic clinical picture that could have been avoided with an external ventricular drain after clipping of the aneurysm.

## Biochemical Abnormalities

Various biochemical abnormalities occurring after SAH, and particularly after surgery on an anterior communicating artery aneurysm, are more common than is recognized. These abnormalities include neurogenic hypernatremia as a result of disturbance of the thirst-controlling center; hyponatremia, often resulting from excessive fluid intake; diabetes insipidus and inappropriate secretion of antidiuretic hormone resulting from disturbance in the diencephalon; elevation of blood glucose, a reflection of the extent of acute brain damage; and, rarely, other endocrine disturbances, such as hypopituitarism and myxedema resulting from disturbance of the pituitary hypothalamic axis. The author has seen most of these problems, but with appropriate action, no permanent damage was noted.[1, 22]

## Seizures

Despite the routine use of anticonvulsant therapy, one or more seizures occurred in 5% of cases in this series. The seizures were quickly aborted with an intravenous injection of diazepam 5 to 10 mg in addition to regular anticonvulsant medication. For continued seizures, diazepam or clonazepam through an intravenous drip was given, and a careful watch was kept on blood pressure and breathing. Occasionally the patient needed to be paralyzed and given ventilation. Seizure in the immediate postoperative period is one of the most unpleasant factors that produces a poor outcome.

## Rebleeding

Rebleeding is a rare but serious complication specific to aneurysm surgery. Rebleeding can occur under some of the circumstances that have previously been described. If the wrong aneurysm is obliterated, however, leaving behind the offending aneurysm in cases of multiple aneurysms, the risk of rebleeding from the ruptured aneurysm is high. The following case is illustrative.

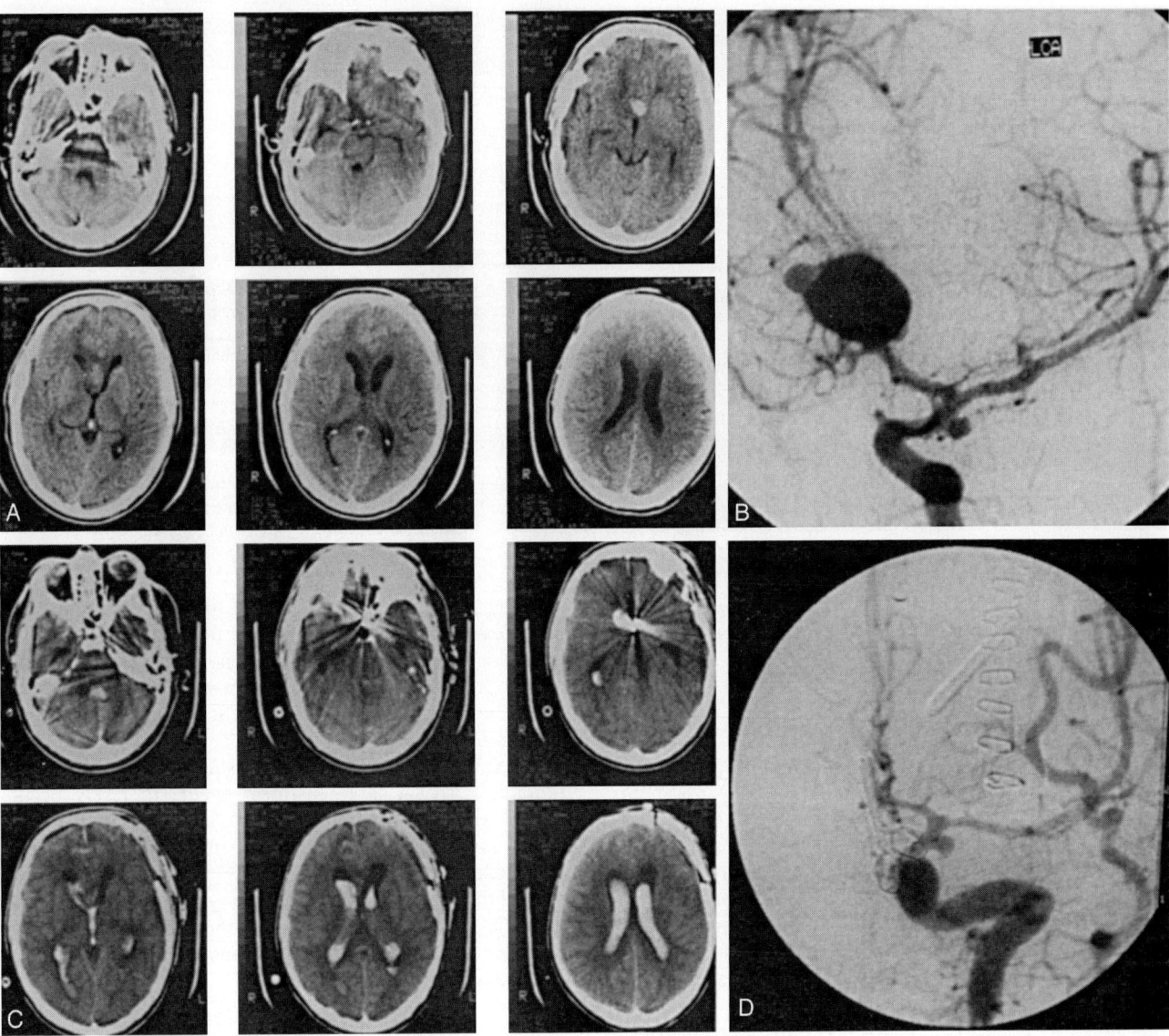

**FIGURE 87-17 ■** *A,* Case report 1: A computed tomography (CT) scan 16 days after a massive subarachnoid and intraventricular hemorrhage, which disappeared after an external ventricular drain and which now only shows mild ventricular dilatation. *B,* A left carotid angiogram (oblique view) showing a large anterior communicating artery aneurysm and a small incidental posterior communicating artery aneurysm. *C,* A postoperative CT scan showing massive ventricular blood. Note that apart from a clip artefact, there is no blood at the site of the aneurysm. *D,* A postoperative left carotid angiogram (Towne's view) showing total obliteration of the aneurysm. The unoccluded posterior communicating aneurysm was treated later.

## Case Report 2

A 63-year-old woman was admitted in grade III clinical condition. CT scanning showed modest ventricular dilatation and blood in the sylvian fissure (Fig. 87–18). Angiography revealed a middle cerebral aneurysm and a small anterior communicating aneurysm. On the basis of the CT scan, the middle cerebral aneurysm was considered to be the offending lesion and was occluded. At operation, because of blood in the sylvian fissure, the diagnosis was not in doubt. During the immediate postoperative period, however, the patient suddenly became comatose, with acute ventricular dilatation and fresh blood in the interhemispheric fissure (see Fig. 87–18). With an external ventricular drain, her condition improved,

and the anterior communicating artery aneurysm was clipped successfully.

## Psychiatric Disturbance

Psychiatric disturbance, both temporary and permanent, in patients with an anterior communicating artery aneurysm is more frequent than in any other aneurysm.[23–25] Severe Korsakoff's syndrome, commonly consisting of hallucinations, confusion, amnesia, and confabulation, is often a reflection of severe disturbance of the limbic system from SAH but can also occur from vessel injury. Loss of initiative, personality change, emotional lability, memory impairment, and intellectual impairment are detected in increasing numbers of formal psychometric studies. With

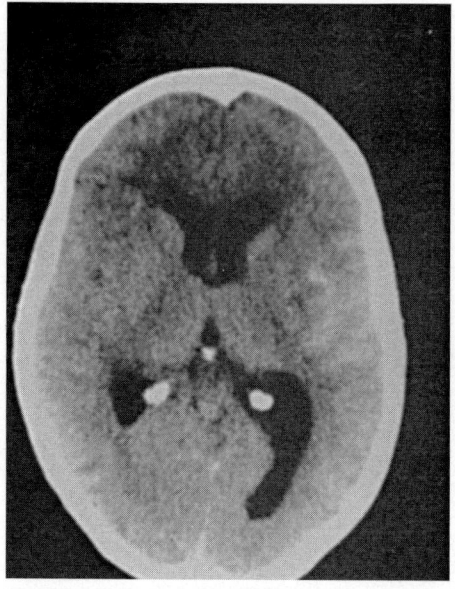
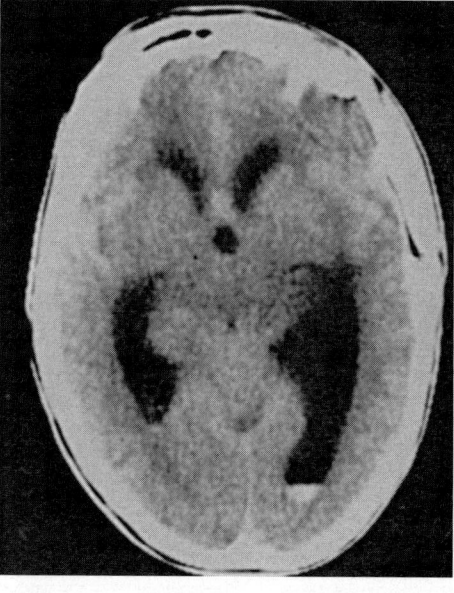

FIGURE 87–18 ■ Case report 2: A computed tomography (CT) scan (left) on admission showing modest ventricular dilatation with blood in the left sylvian fissure. CT scan (right) shortly after operation on the middle cerebral artery aneurysm showing acute ventricular dilatation and blood in the interhemispheric fissure from rupture of an associated anterior communicating artery aneurysm.

improved surgical technique in patients with grade I or II aneurysms, the quality of survival can be improved.[26–28]

## ANEURYSMS OF THE PROXIMAL ANTERIOR CEREBRAL ARTERY

Aneurysms of the proximal (A1) segment of the ACA usually arise at its posterior border from the origin of one of the perforating arteries and, less frequently, from the proximity of the carotid bifurcation or anterior communicating artery.[29] Occasionally an aneurysm may also arise from an anomalous vessel, such as a fenestrated A1.[30] Although several authors[29, 31–34] have reported an incidence of 1% to 2% of intracranial aneurysm at this location, in the author's series of 703 patients, only four aneurysms were found at the proximal anterior cerebral artery, an incidence of 0.6%. Some of the aneurysms at the carotid bifurcation of the anterior communicating artery region may have been included in the reported series. Because of their rarity, however, some of the aneurysms are often not

seen on angiography because CT findings of rupture are no different from those of rupture of an aneurysm at two other locations (Fig. 87–19). Even at operation, because of the small size and frequent association with vascular anomalies, these aneurysms are difficult to find unless they are carefully looked for.

These aneurysms are usually small and saccular and produce SAH. A large fusiform aneurysm rarely occurs at this site that presents with visual symptoms.[35] These aneurysms are more common in men and are often associated with multiple aneurysms.[29, 31, 33] When they are associated with an anterior communicating artery aneurysm, the latter is usually the source of the hemorrhage, but the presence and rupture of an A1 aneurysm should not be overlooked.

These aneurysms are approached through an ipsilateral pterional trans-sylvian route, as described by Fox and Sengupta.[16] The position of the patient on the table, the skin incision, the craniotomy and bone removal, the dural opening, and the initial exposure are similar to those used for the pterional gyrus rectus approach for anterior communicating artery aneurysms, described in this chapter. Because the

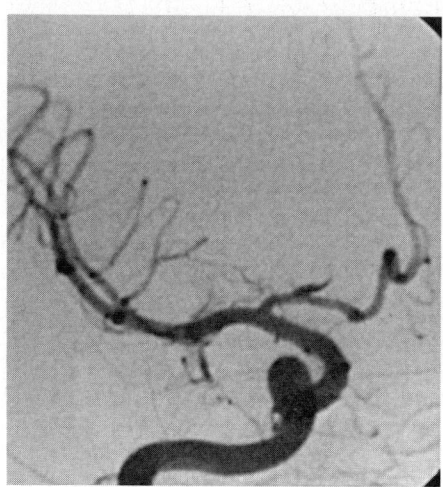
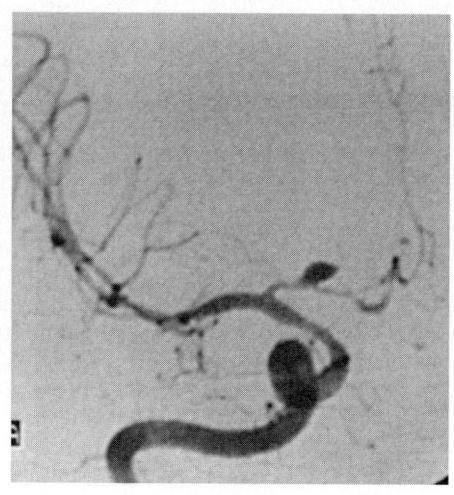

FIGURE 87–19 ■ Proximal A1 aneurysm. The aneurysm (left) was missed in the initial angiogram as a result of poor filling. A repeat angiogram (right) shows the aneurysm.

carotid bifurcation is deepest in the anterior part of the circle of Willis, the dissection must be deeper and more posterior. The medial part of the sylvian fissure is opened widely by dissection of the arachnoid medial to the sylvian veins. The dissection is continued until the carotid bifurcation and origin of the middle cerebral artery are reached. Once the frontal lobe is separated from the temporal lobe, further retraction of the frontal lobe exposes the A1 without excessive retraction. Placement of the retractor and brain retraction must be extremely gentle to avoid premature rupture of the aneurysm. The ACA is followed from the carotid bifurcation until the aneurysm is found (Fig. 87–20). The ACA can be safely dissected along its anterior border, and the presence of an anomalous vessel should be borne in mind. The aneurysm is often invested with perforating arteries, resembling a candelabra. Separation of these tiny vessels from the neck of the aneurysm is facilitated by increased magnification and proximal control with a temporary clip. Bipolar coagulation should be used judiciously to avoid injury to the tiny vessels. Aneurysms arising close to the anterior communicating artery are approached in the same way as those in the anterior communicating artery, and exposure of the carotid bifurcation is not necessary.

## CONCLUSION

The technique for surgical management of anterior communicating artery aneurysms the author describes has worked well for him. Other techniques are undoubtedly equally good, although each technique must conform to a set of ground rules. Any neurosurgeon with skill in microtechnique can obliterate an aneurysm and preserve the vessels. The surgeon's challenge is how to improve the management outcome by preventing the onset of vasospasm and early rebleeding. Improving management outcome is possible by operating at the earliest possible moment on the basis of the risk score.

Even in poor-grade patients, early rebleeding can be reduced by coiling the aneurysm, at least partially. The patient can then be treated more aggressively to recover from the effects of SAH.

Although endovascular therapy is attractive as a minimally invasive approach for treating intracranial aneurysms,[36] it is not without morbidity related to the procedure itself. The problem regarding long-term efficacy in preventing subsequent growth or rupture is still unsettled. More significantly, surgical treatment after coiling appears to be hazardous.[37]

## ACKNOWLEDGMENTS

*The author is grateful to Dr. Laurence Watkins and Dr. Giorgio Rubin for their help during revision of this chapter. I am also grateful to Olga Mapletoft for typing the manuscript with considerable patience and skill.*

## REFERENCES

1. Sengupta RP, McAllister VL: Subarachnoid Hemorrhage. Berlin: Springer-Verlag, 1986.
2. Paul RL, Arnold JC: Operative factors influencing mortality in intracranial aneurysm surgery: Analysis of 186 consecutive cases. J Neurosurg 32:289–294, 1970.
3. Hodes JE, Aymard A, Gobin YP, et al: Endovascular occlusion of intracranial vessels for curative treatment of unclippable aneurysms: Report of 16 cases. J Neurosurg 75:694–701, 1991.
4. Waro T, Nishi S, Yamashita K, et al: Selection and combination of various endovascular techniques in the treatment of giant aneurysms. J Neurosurg 77:37–42, 1992.
5. MacDonald RL, Weir B: Perioperative care of the patient following aneurysmal subarachnoid hemorrhage. In Schmidek HH, Sweet WH (eds): Operative Neurosurgical Techniques—Indications, Methods and Results, 3rd ed. Philadelphia: WB Saunders, 1994, pp 937–955.
6. Collins WF: Neurosurgical complications: Fluid and electrolytes imbalance. Clin Neurosurg 23:417–423, 1977.
7. Shenkin HA, Bezier HS, Bouzarth WF: Restricted fluid intake: Rational management of the neurosurgical patient. J Neurosurg 45:432–436, 1976.
8. Pearlmutter D, Rhoton AL: Microsurgical anatomy of the distal anterior cerebral artery. J Neurosurg 49:204–228, 1978.
9. Alpers BJ, Berry RG, Paddison RM: Anatomical studies of the circle of Willis in normal brain. Arch Neurol Psychiatry 81:409–418, 1959.
10. Baptista AG: Studies on the arteries of the brain: The anterior cerebral artery, some anatomical features and their clinical implications. Neurology 13:825–835, 1963.
11. Wilson G, Riggs HE, Rupp C: The pathological anatomy of ruptured cerebral aneurysms. J Neurosurg 11:128–134, 1954.
12. Pearlmutter D, Rhoton AL Jr: Microsurgical anatomy of the anterior cerebral-anterior communicating-recurrent artery complex. J Neurosurg 45:259–272, 1976.
13. Sengupta RP: Anterior Communicating Aneurysms and Their Management After Subarachnoid Hemorrhage. Thesis. Newcastle: University of Newcastle, 1977.
14. Dott MM: Intracranial aneurysms: Cerebral arterioradiography, surgical treatment. Edinb Med J 40:219–240, 1933.
15. Tonnis W: Erfolgreiche Behandlung eines Aneruysma der arteria communicans anterior cerebri. Zentralbl Neurochir 1:39–42, 1936.
16. Fox JL, Sengupta RP: Anterior communicating artery aneurysms. In Apuzzo MLJ (ed): Brain Surgery: Complication Avoidance and Management, Vol 1. New York: Churchill Livingstone, 1993, pp 1009–1010.
17. Yasargil MG: Microsurgery Applied to Neurosurgery. Stuttgart: Georg Thieme Verlag, 1969.
18. Suzuki J, Kodama N, Ebina T, et al: Surgical treatment of anterior communicating artery aneurysms. In Suzuki J (ed): Cerebral Aneurysms. Tokyo: Neuron Publishing Company, 1979, pp 238–249.

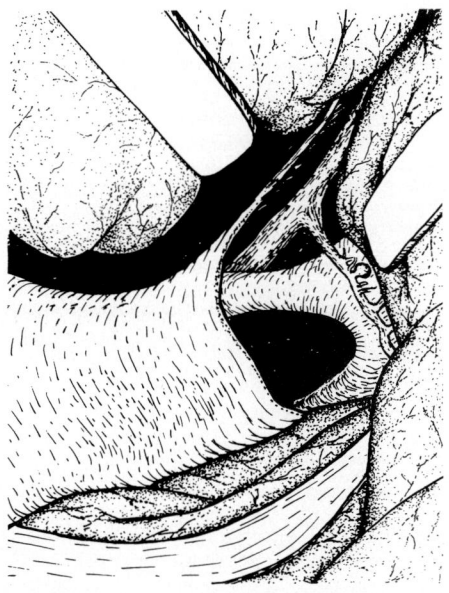

**FIGURE 87–20** ■ A pterional trans-sylvian approach for a proximal A1 aneurysm (see text).

19. Tsutsumi K, Shiokawa Y, Sakai T, et al: Venous infarction following the interhemispheric approach in patient with acute subarachnoid hemorrhage. J Neurosurg 74:715–719, 1991.
20. Taylor CL, Selman WR, Kiefer SP, Ratcheson RA: Temporary vessel occlusion/intracranial aneurysm repair. Neurosurgery 39:893–906, 1996.
21. Batjer HH, Franfurt AI, Purdy PD, et al: Use of etomidate, temporary arterial occlusion and intraoperative angiography in surgical treatment of large and giant cerebral aneurysms. J Neurosurg 68:234–240, 1988.
22. McIver B, Connacher A, Whittle I, et al: Adipsic hypothalamic diabetes insipidus after clipping of anterior communicating artery aneurysm. BMJ 303:1465–1467, 1991.
23. Logue V, Durward M, Pratt RTC, et al: The quality of survival after rupture of an anterior cerebral aneurysm. Br J Psychiatry 114:137–160, 1968.
24. Lindqvist G, Norlen G: Korsakoff's syndrome after operation on ruptured aneurysm of the anterior communicating artery. Acta Psychiatr Scand 42:24–34, 1966.
25. Stenhouse LM, Knight RG, Longmore BE, et al: Long-term cognitive deficits in patients after surgery on aneurysms of the anterior communicating artery. J Neurol Neurosurg Psychiatry 54:909–914, 1991.
26. Sengupta RP, Chiu JSP, Brierly H: Quality of survival following direct surgery for anterior communicating artery aneurysm. J Neurosurg 43:58–64, 1975.
27. Irle E, Wowra B, Kunert HJ, et al: Memory disturbances following anterior communicating artery rupture. Ann Neurol 31:473–480, 1992.
28. Hutter BO, Gilsbach JM: Cognitive deficits after rupture and early repair of anterior communicating artery aneurysms. Acta Neurochir (Wien) 116:6–13, 1992.
29. Suzuki M, Onuma T, Sakurai Y, et al: Aneurysms arising from the proximal (A1) segment of the anterior cerebral artery. J Neurosurg 76:455–458, 1992.
30. Minakawa T, Kawamata M, Hayano M, et al: Aneurysms associated with fenestrated anterior cerebral arteries: Report of four cases and review of the literature. Surg Neurol 24:284–288, 1985.
31. Handa J, Nakasu Y, Matsuda M, et al: Aneurysms of the proximal anterior cerebral artery. Surg Neurol 22:486–490, 1984.
32. Kassell NF, Torner JC: Size of intracranial aneurysms. Neurosurgery 12:291–297, 1983.
33. Wakabayashi T, Tamaki N, Yamashita H, et al: Angiographic classification of the horizontal segment of the anterior cerebral artery. Surg Neurol 24:31–35, 1985.
34. Yoshimoto T, Kayama T, Kodama N, et al: Distribution of intracranial aneurysm. In Suzuki J (ed): Cerebral Aneurysms. Tokyo, Neuron Publishing Company, 1979, pp 14–19.
35. Morota N, Kobayashi S, Sugita K, et al: Giant aneurysms of the horizontal segment of the anterior cerebral artery: Report of two cases. Neurosurgery 29:97–101, 1991.
36. Moret J, Pierot L, Boulin A, et al: Endovascular treatment of anterior communicating artery aneurysms using Guglielmi detachable coils. Neuroradiology 38:800–805, 1996.
37. Mizoi K, Yoshimoto T, Takashi A, Nagamine Y: A pitfall in the surgery of a recurrent aneurysm after coil embolization and its histological observation: Technical case report. Neurosurgery 39:165–169, 1996.

# CHAPTER 88

# Surgical Management of Giant Aneurysms of the Anterior Circulation*

■ ADAM I. LEWIS, DAVID SCALZO, JOHN M. TEW, Jr., and ROBERT R. SMITH

The treatment of giant intracranial aneurysms has continued to evolve during the past decade. The most notable advances have come in endovascular techniques and refinement of hypothermic circulatory arrest as an adjunct to surgical clipping.[1-4] These therapies have been developed because the anatomic characteristics of giant aneurysms often preclude simple surgical clipping. When aneurysms grow to giant proportions, the neck widens and may incorporate the branching arteries. Frequently there is intra-aneurysmal thrombus, and the wall is calcified. To overcome these difficulties, Charles Drake relied on collateral flow of the cerebrovasculature to obliterate giant aneurysms. In the 1970s, Drake used a tourniquet to gradually occlude the proximal parent artery.[5] However, 10% to 15% of the patients did not have sufficient collateral blood flow. In the 1980s, Thor Sundt championed aneurysm trapping and revascularization with bypass grafts to avoid cerebral ischemia.[6] In the 1990s, preoperative balloon test occlusion (BTO), intraoperative angiography, silicone detachable balloons, Guglielmi detachable coils (GDCs), and endovascular remodeling techniques were developed or came into widespread use.[4] For several years, intravascular stents have been used to open narrowed coronary arteries. These intravascular stents are now being adapted for use in the cerebrovasculature and will likely be the next innovation in the treatment of intracranial aneurysms.

Published in 1969, the Cooperative Aneurysm Study classified giant intracranial aneurysms as greater than 2.5 cm in diameter.[7] Thirty years later, the goals of obliterating the aneurysm, maintaining adequate cerebral blood flow, and relieving mass effect remain a technical challenge as evidenced by the variety and complexity of surgical strategies. Current treatment options include hunterian ligation of the parent artery or proximal endovascular occlusion, trapping the aneurysm with or without a bypass graft, intra-aneurysmal endovascular coil occlusion, and direct surgical repair with vessel reconstruction. Most cerebrovascular centers use a team approach that combines endovascular and surgical treatments in a complementary fashion.

Although surgical management of giant anterior circulation aneurysms is the focus of this chapter, the role of endovascular techniques is also presented because of its increasing importance. In fact, endovascular techniques are the primary mode of therapy for giant carotid cavernous aneurysms. The indications for treatment, preoperative planning, principles of aneurysm surgery, and surgical and endovascular techniques for obliterating giant aneurysms of the anterior circulation are presented in this chapter. The aneurysm types are categorized by the arterial branches of the anterior circulation. Traumatic aneurysms, dissecting aneurysms, fusiform aneurysms, and mycotic aneurysms have been excluded from the discussion because they generally do not reach giant dimensions and their management differs significantly from that of giant saccular aneurysms.

## INDICATIONS FOR TREATMENT

The decision to treat giant aneurysms is based on the clinical presentation, age of the patient, and location and type of aneurysm (saccular, fusiform, mycotic, or traumatic). Once symptomatic, patients with giant aneurysms have a poor prognosis and require prompt treatment.[8, 9] In a large series of giant aneurysms from the Mayo Clinic, the risk of rebleeding was 18% and the mortality rate was 33% in the first 2 weeks after aneurysm rupture; these percentages are similar to those for small aneurysms.[10] Patients with giant aneurysms had an overall management mortality rate of 21% compared with just 8.6% for surgically treated patients.[11] It is notable that patients with a giant aneurysm who do not suffer a subarachnoid hemorrhage (SAH) are more likely to survive with independent function (50%) than are those patients who do (18%).[12] Therefore, the authors recommend treatment for patients with hemorrhage, progressive headache, worsening of ex-

*This chapter is dedicated to the memory of Yuri Zubkov, who previously coauthored this chapter. He was found murdered outside his apartment in St. Petersburg, Russia, on February 7, 1997.

isting cranial nerve palsies, medically intractable seizures, and aneurysm enlargement.

The clinical presentation and natural history vary by aneurysm location. Giant carotid cavernous and paraclinoid aneurysms, which comprise almost 55% of all giant aneurysms,[13] usually cause symptoms related to mass effect. Giant aneurysms of the internal carotid artery (ICA) compress primarily the optic and oculomotor nerves, which leads to vision loss and ophthalmoparesis, respectively. In a review of nine series comprising 641 patients with giant aneurysms, Pia and Zierski found a 35% (range, 13% to 76%) incidence of SAH.[14] Subarachnoid hemorrhage is often the first presentation among patients with aneurysms of the anterior communicating artery, ICA bifurcation, and basilar artery apex. Half of all patients with middle cerebral artery (MCA) aneurysms suffer SAH and intracerebral hemorrhage.[15] Symptomatic MCA giant aneurysms usually cause temporal lobe seizures, hemiparesis, and hemianopsia. Posterior communicating artery giant aneurysms cause oculomotor palsies, facial pain, and SAH. Although more than 60% of giant aneurysms are partially thrombosed, cerebral infarction caused by distal thromboembolism occurs in less than 10%.[16] Fusiform and dolichoectatic aneurysms have a higher incidence of thromboembolic stroke compared with giant saccular aneurysms.

Before the advent of magnetic resonance imaging (MRI), many giant aneurysms resembled tumors on computed tomography (CT) images. MRI scans show flow void and multiple laminated layers of thrombus that differentiate giants aneurysms from tumors. Enlargement of giant aneurysms occurs from either slow progressive dilatation of the aneurysm lumen or from continued formation of thrombus within the sac. Twenty percent of giant aneurysms have a rim of calcification that can be visualized by CT and radiographs of the skull.[14] As the aneurysm enlarges, the arterial pulsations can erode the skull base (Fig. 88–1).[17] Giant aneurysms that erode into the sphenoid sinus should be obliterated because rupture can cause massive epistaxis.

## PREOPERATIVE PLANNING

Preoperative planning is complex and requires a cerebral arteriogram with multiple views of the aneurysm. When thrombus is present within the aneurysm, cerebral angiography shows only the filling portion of the aneurysm (Fig. 88–2). Therefore, MRI or CT is performed to visualize the thrombus and determine the true dimensions of the aneurysm. MRI is better than CT to define mass effect, parenchymal edema, and the relationship of the aneurysm to the surrounding structures (Fig. 88–3). CT is better than MRI to visualize hemorrhage, calcium within the neck and wall of the aneurysm, and erosion of the skull base.

Cerebral angiography produces two-dimensional (2-D) images but limited information on the true three-dimensional (3-D) anatomy, because the giant size frequently obscures the relationship of the aneurysm neck to the normal arteries. CT and magnetic resonance (MR) angiography can provide 3-D images but are hampered by lower resolution and difficulties detecting flowing blood through the vessels. Artifacts from surgical clips and coils make evaluation of neck remnants and parent artery compromise virtually impossible. Nevertheless, 3-D CT is useful in delineating the vascular anatomy and its relation to the cranial base structures.[18] Understanding the relationship of the aneurysm to the skull base is important in planning the operative approach.

New advances in angiography equipment and computer processing allow rapid-image intensity rotation and acquisi-

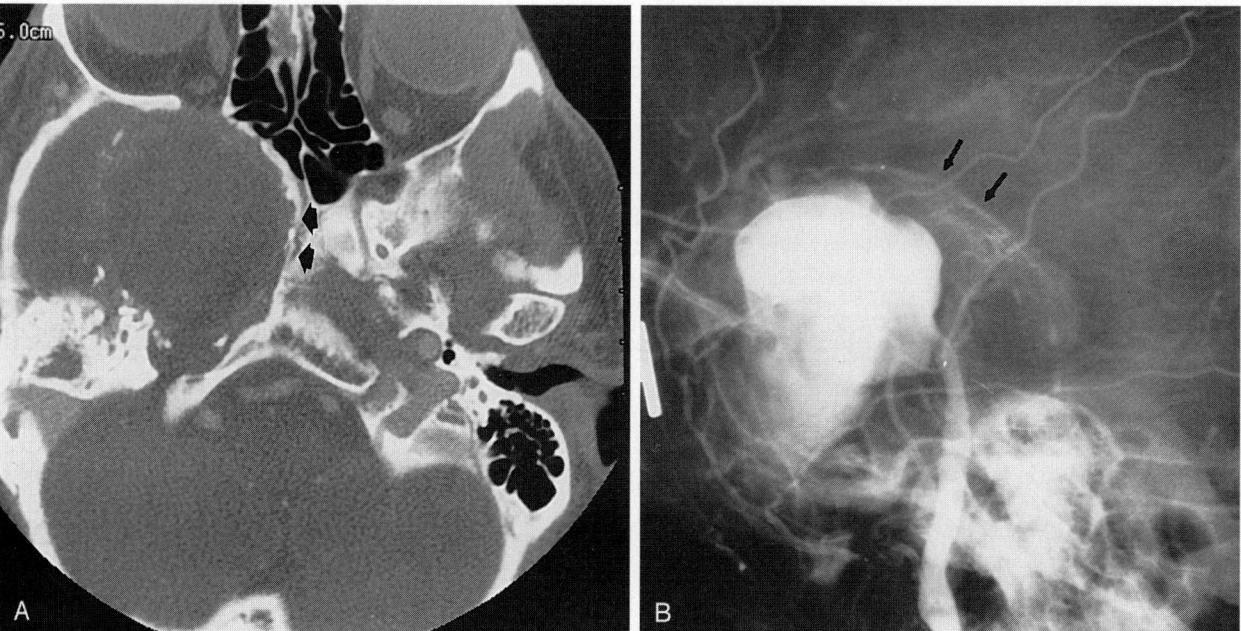

**FIGURE 88–1** ■ Giant aneurysms may erode the base of the skull. *A,* The computed tomography (CT) scan shows the giant internal carotid artery (ICA) aneurysm *(arrowheads)* has eroded the sphenoid wing and petrous apex causing proptosis of the right eye. *B,* The angiogram shows partial filling of the aneurysm with a rim of calcium *(arrows)* outlining the sac.

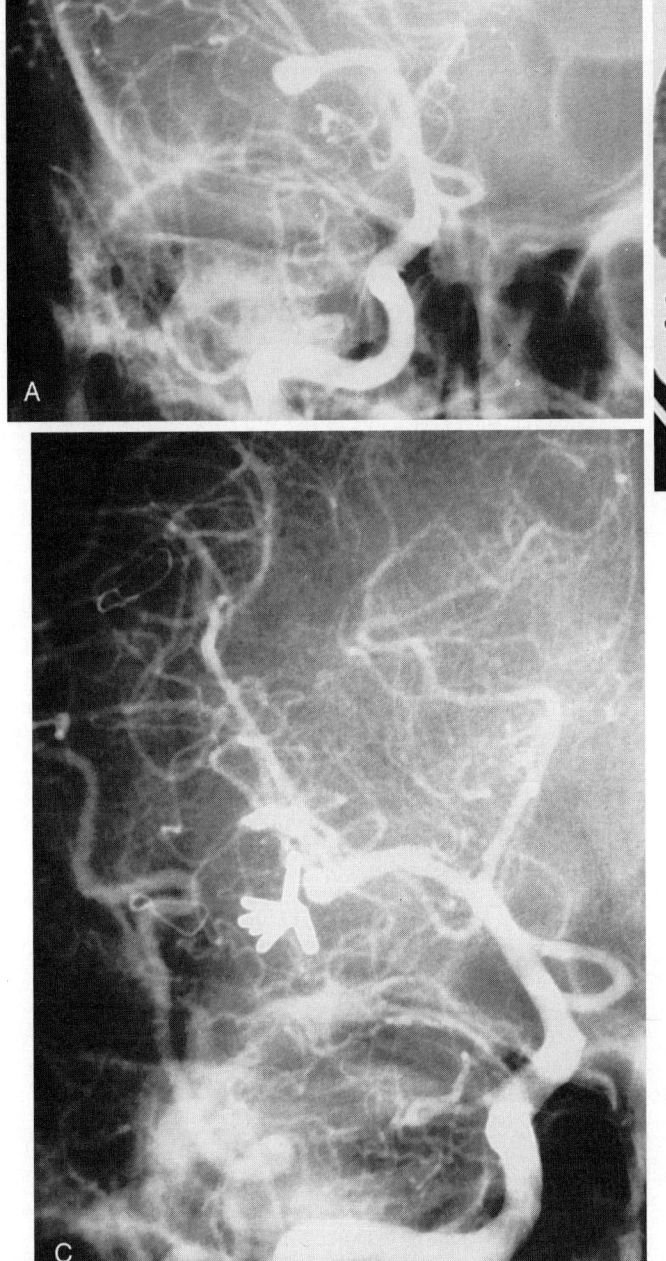

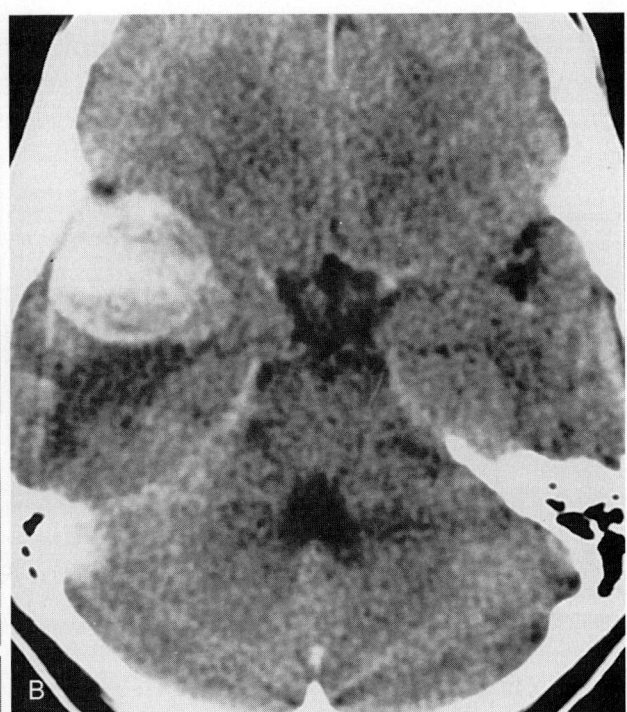

**FIGURE 88–2** ■ Cerebral angiography shows only the filling portion of the aneurysm. *A*, The cerebral angiogram shows a small middle cerebral artery (MCA) aneurysm. *B*, The computed tomography scan shows a giant aneurysm filled predominantly with thrombus. *C*, The postoperative angiogram shows reconstruction of the MCA branches with a small remnant of the aneurysm remaining to prevent parent artery occlusion.

tion of multiple-projection angiograms over a 210-degree arc with subsequent data reconstruction into 3-D surface-rendered images (General Electric, Milwaukee, WI); these images can be rotated about any angle. Virtual endoscopy can be performed within the vessels to provide important information on the dimensions of the aneurysms sac, neck, and parent artery. The 3-D angiograms show the extent of involvement of the parent artery and whether it can be reconstructed or must be sacrificed (Fig. 88–4). Finally, a

residual aneurysm neck after clipping or coiling is defined better by 3-D angiography than standard angiography.

Collateral circulation can be inferred on static images by the size and cross-flow of the posterior and anterior communicating arteries. The potential for collateral circulation must be assessed with carotid cross-compression and the Alcock test. Balloon test occlusion is combined with a cerebral blood flow study to quantitate the risk for cerebral ischemia (Fig. 88–5). Cerebral blood flow studies using

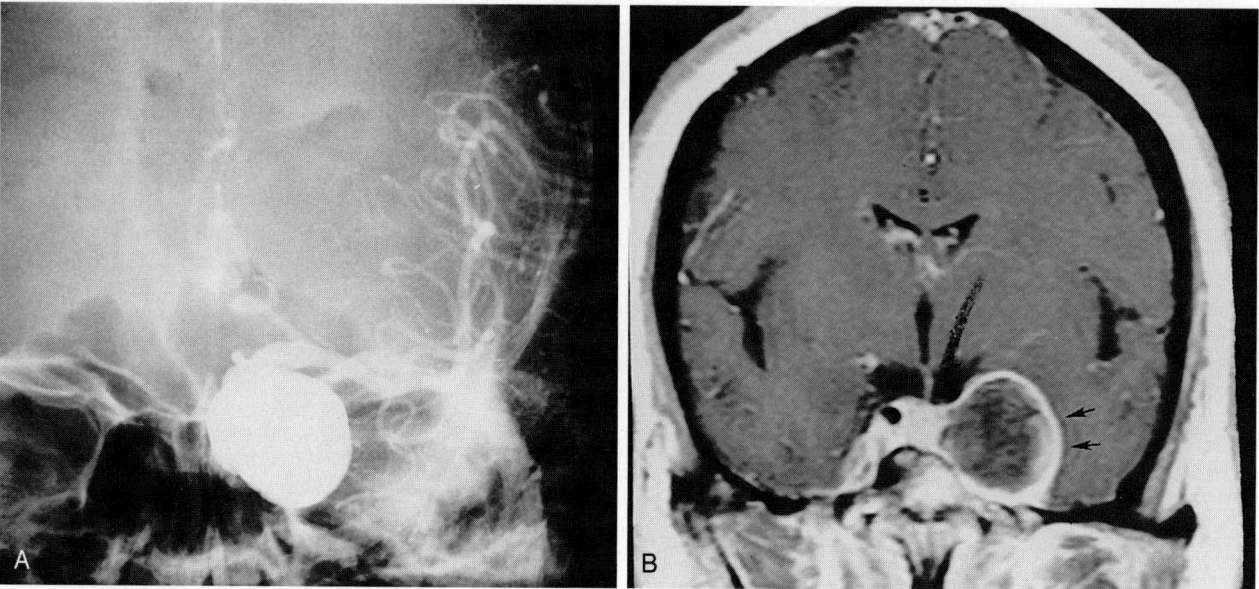

**FIGURE 88–3** ■ Magnetic resonance imaging (MRI) is useful to identify thrombus within the aneurysm and understand the relationship of the aneurysm to the surrounding stuctures. *A,* The cerebral angiogram shows a giant carotid cavernous aneurysm. *B,* The MRI shows that the same aneurysm is confined to the cavernous sinus *(arrows).*

xenon CT or single photon-emission computed tomography (SPECT) imaging follow the balloon test occlusion to identify borderline areas of cerebral ischemia.

## PRINCIPLES OF ANEURYSM SURGERY

Many principles of surgery for small aneurysms apply to large and giant aneurysms.[19] The surgical approach is chosen to maximize exposure of the surgical anatomy. Early surgery is preferred and performed as soon as the patient and the surgical team are prepared.

The most important determinant of surgical outcome is the experience of the surgeon and operating team. Because giant aneurysms comprise only 5% to 10% of all intracranial aneurysms, most are treated at a tertiary center that specializes in cerebrovascular surgery. A complete surgical team must be available. The details of the surgical plan must be communicated to all the members of the team, including neuroradiologists, neuroanesthesiologists, operating room nurses, and technicians.

Early surgery of the ruptured aneurysm poses an increased risk of intraoperative rupture. Even with unruptured aneurysms, removing the bone flap, draining cerebrospinal fluid (CSF), or retracting on the frontal and temporal lobes

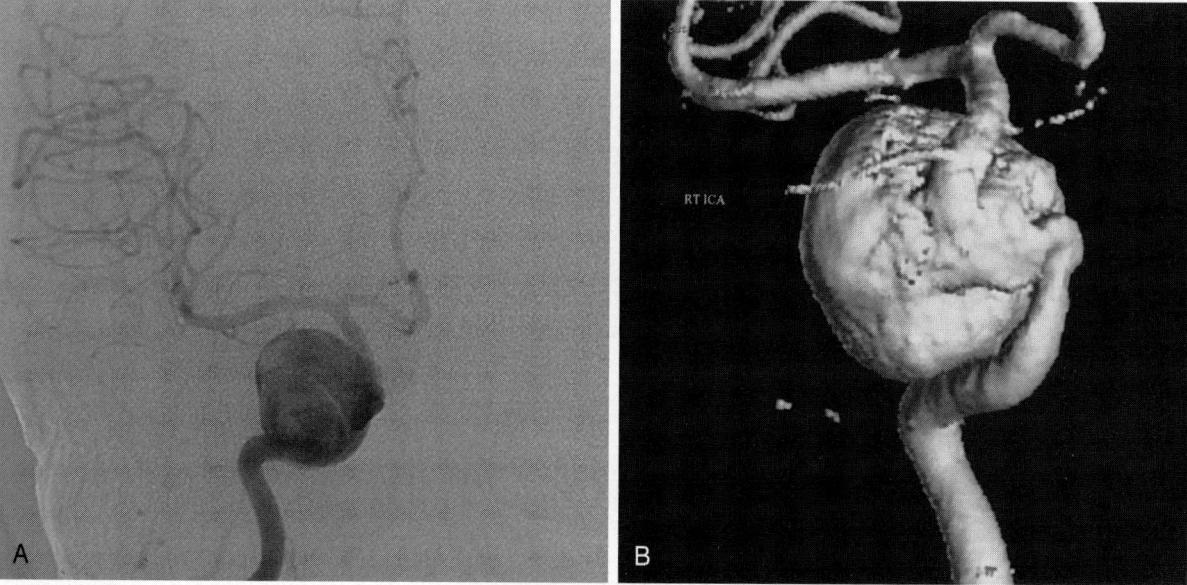

**FIGURE 88–4** ■ New advances in cerebral angiography include rotational angiography and three-dimensional reconstructed images. *A,* Digital subtraction angiogram shows a giant right carotid cavernous aneurysm. *B,* Three-dimensional reconstructed image identifies the exact origin and width of the aneurysm neck. The entire circumference of the internal carotid artery appears irregular, and the lumen could not be reconstructed.

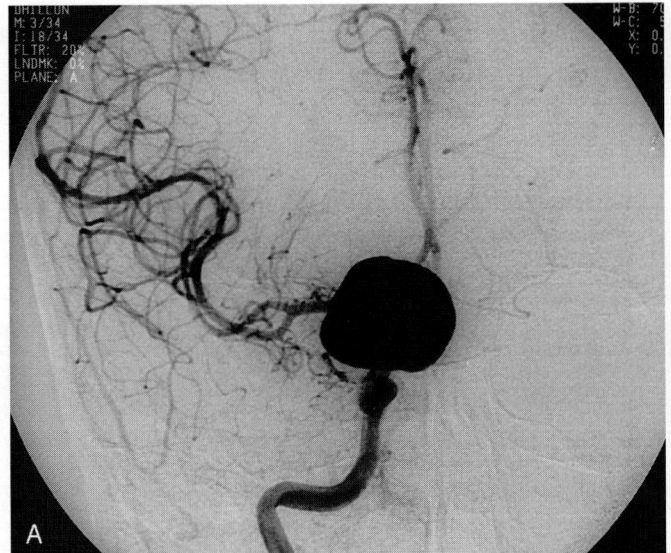

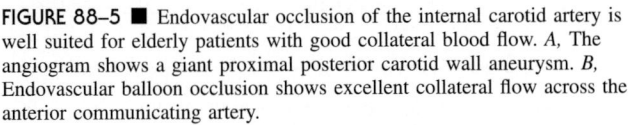

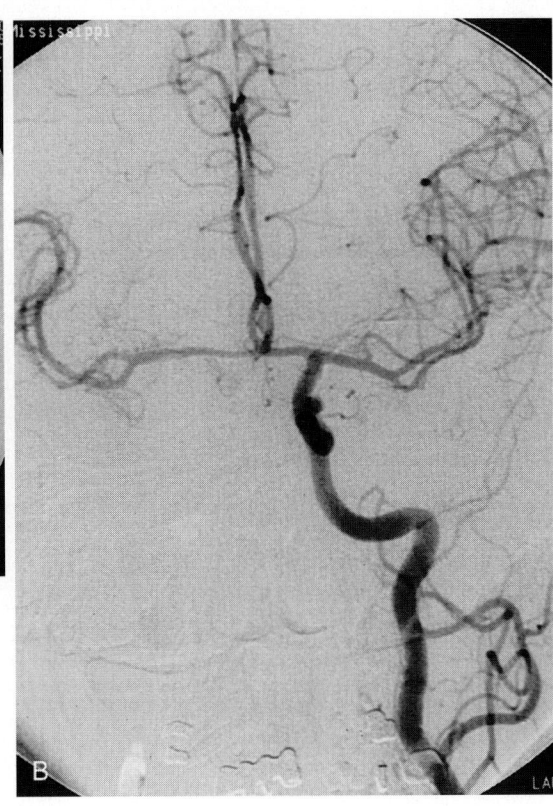

FIGURE 88–5 ■ Endovascular occlusion of the internal carotid artery is well suited for elderly patients with good collateral blood flow. *A,* The angiogram shows a giant proximal posterior carotid wall aneurysm. *B,* Endovascular balloon occlusion shows excellent collateral flow across the anterior communicating artery.

may precipitate rupture. Therefore, the microscope is draped at the beginning of the operation; the self-retaining brain retractor system is in place before opening the dura; and the aneurysm clips are loaded on the clip appliers before microdissection.

Brain relaxation is achieved by hyperventilation, osmotic diuresis with mannitol and Lasix, and removal of CSF through a lumbar drain, arachnoid cisterns, or direct intraoperative catheterization of the frontal horn of the lateral ventricle. Resection of noneloquent brain tissue (e.g., anterior temporal lobe, gyrus rectus) is preferable to excessive retraction of brain tissue. Administration of neuroprotective agents such as pentobarbital, etomidate, and propofol will also aid in brain relaxation. The surgeon must be prepared to delay or terminate the operation if brain relaxation is insufficient.

Proximal vascular control of the parent artery is the first objective. If proximal control cannot be achieved intracranially, then exposure of the cervical ICA or temporary intravascular balloon occlusion is required. The authors prefer isolation of the cervical ICA because heparinization is not required and the balloon catheter does not remain in the common carotid artery as a potential source for emboli. For giant aneurysms of the basilar artery, however, proximal control with temporary balloon occlusion may obviate the need for extensive bone removal of the skull base or circulatory arrest with cardiopulmonary bypass.

Giant aneurysms require greater operative exposure. For giant aneurysms of the anterior circulation, a wide splitting of the sylvian fissure is necessary. Removal of the skull base is required for paraclinoid aneurysms. In addition to the standard pterional craniotomy, the lesser sphenoid wing, anterior clinoid process, and the roof of the optic

canal are removed. Removal of the lateral superior rim of the orbit or an orbitozygomatic osteotomy increases exposure for giant anterior communicating artery aneurysms.

After bone removal and splitting of the sylvian fissure, sharp dissection is performed to identify the proximal parent artery, the distal branch arteries, and then the aneurysm neck. Sharp dissection is preferable to blunt dissection to avoid excessive manipulation of the aneurysm. Once the aneurysm neck is defined, critical perforating arteries adjacent to the neck are preserved and dissected away. In the case of giant aneurysms, frequently the aneurysm must be trapped and collapsed by removing the blood and thrombus to visualize the perforators and enable placement of a clip at the base of the aneurysm. Multiple clips in tandem or parallel are often required to obliterate the aneurysm.

Temporary clipping is almost always needed in giant aneurysm surgery to avoid intraoperative rupture and to facilitate clip application. During temporary clipping, raising the systemic blood pressure improves collateral circulation. Hypothermia and intravenous barbiturates are given for cerebral protection. After the temporary clips are applied, the aneurysm should be obliterated and flow reestablished in less than 20 minutes. If temporary clipping beyond 20 minutes is anticipated, then a cardiopulmonary bypass is performed to avoid cerebral infarction.

Aneurysms clips are applied along the long axis of the parent artery. Perpendicular clipping increases the risk of constricting or occluding the parent artery or tearing the aneurysm base. Application of multiple clips in tandem or in parallel is preferable to forcing a single clip onto a complex aneurysm. Once the primary clip is placed and temporary clips are removed, the aneurysm is punctured with a fine needle to check for residual filling. Residual

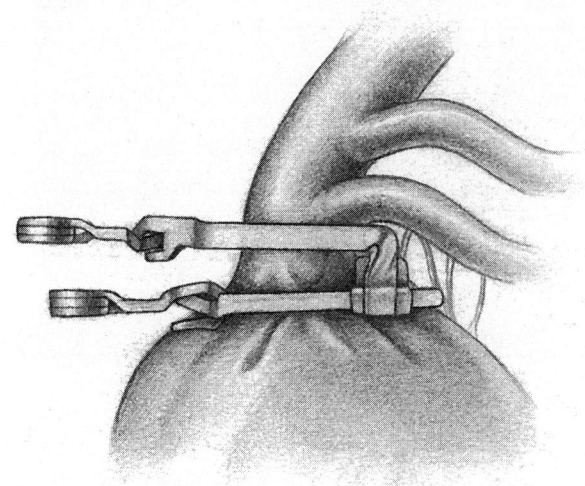

**FIGURE 88–6** ■ Booster or reinforcing clips may be required to increase the closing force on giant aneurysms with a wide neck. The booster clip is placed over the distal end of the primary clip blades. When booster, fenestrated, or encircling clips are applied, the neck is often obscured and intraoperative angiography is required to document that the aneurysm is completely obliterated and the distal branches are preserved. (From Tew JM Jr, van Loveren HR: Atlas of Operative Microneurosurgery, Vol 1. Philadelphia: WB Saunders, 1994.)

filling requires repositioning of the clip, the use of multiple clips, or a reinforcing clip to increase closing pressure (Fig. 88–6). The success of the clip closure is best determined when the patient's blood pressure is returned to normal.

After aspirating the aneurysm, the surgeon mobilizes the sac, inspects the aneurysm base, and repositions the clip if the parent artery or perforating vessels are in the clip. In large and giant aneurysms, the clip tends to slide down the neck onto the parent artery because of the thick wall or calcification at the base, high intra-aneurysmal pressure, or thrombus within the sac. Removal of the thrombus in the sac and calcium in the neck may be the only solution to achieve proper clip placement. In some cases, leaving a small aneurysm rest is required to avoid occluding the parent. Patency of the parent artery and elimination of flow in the aneurysm are assessed with intraoperative micro-Doppler and confirmed with intraoperative angiography.[20] When giant aneurysms have a wide neck or fusiform dilatation and clips cannot be applied to reconstruct the parent artery, then bypass grafting is required. There are various options to increase collateral flow. Saphenous vein bypass, superficial temporal artery to MCA bypass, radial artery interposition grafts, and reimplantation of branching vessels into the parent arteries may be used to avoid cerebral ischemia.[21]

## Aneurysms by Location

### Carotid Cavernous Aneurysms

Carotid cavernous aneurysms account for approximately 5% of all intracranial aneurysms and occur mainly in women during the fifth and sixth decades. Most aneurysms arise from the C3 segment or anterior genu (47%) followed by the C4 or horizontal segment (34%) and the C5 or posterior portion (19%).[22] Morphologically, 90% of spontaneous aneurysms are saccular and 10% are fusiform. Almost half (48%) are large (1.2 to 2.5 cm); 34% are small (<1 cm); and 16% are giant (>2.5 cm).[23] In the authors' experience with more than 100 carotid cavernous aneurysms, 7% were bilateral and 8% were multiple, including intradural aneurysms.

### INDICATIONS FOR TREATMENT

Most carotid cavernous aneurysms have a benign natural history. Thus, observation is appropriate if the aneurysm is asymptomatic and if it does not originate from or extend into the subarachnoid space.[24] Treatment should be initiated emergently for subarachnoid hemorrhage, epistaxis, progressive visual loss, or ocular paresis. Severe ipsilateral facial or retro-orbital pain and radiographic evidence of aneurysm enlargement should be treated promptly. Stable cranial nerve palsies may be managed conservatively, because they will improve spontaneously in 25% of patients.[23, 24]

### TREATMENT OPTIONS

Aneurysms of the cavernous portion of the ICA are difficult to treat by direct surgery because of the surrounding cavernous sinus. The goal of treatment is elimination of the aneurysm and mass effect. Historically, hunterian ligation of the ICA has been the primary treatment for giant ICA aneurysms.[25] Latex detachable balloons replaced hunterian ligation for giant unclippable ICA aneurysms.[26] Currently, silicone detachable balloons or GDCs are used to occlude the ICA. Small and large aneurysms may be treated with intra-aneurysmal GDC placement and preservation of the ICA.[27, 28] In most patients, ICA occlusion is well tolerated with minimal morbidity.[29] Perioperative antiplatelet agents have significantly reduced the risk of delayed cerebral ischemia after ICA occlusion.

Preoperative BTO of the ICA is performed to predict tolerance for occlusion. We combine test occlusion with $^{99m}$Tc-hexamethylpropyleneamineoxime (HMPAO)-photon emission CT and nipride-induced hypotension to identify patients with poor collateral circulation who are at risk for stroke. Our protocol begins with a 10-minute occlusion of the ICA followed by a 30% decrease in mean arterial pressure. We drop the blood pressure with nitroprusside to identify patients at risk for delayed stroke in case of a hypotensive episode during anesthesia induction, surgical blood loss, or other unforeseen situations. The HMPAO study is graded from 0 to 2 (none to minimal decrease in uptake) and 3 to 4 (moderate to severe decrease in uptake. Other assessments (quantitative stable xenon CT, transcranial Doppler sonography, electroencephalogram (EEG) monitoring, and measurement of arterial back pressures) of cerebral blood flow can be done during the BTO. Patients are grouped according to the results of the BTO and the HMPAO scan. In 80% of cases (group 1), the BTO is negative and the HMPAO scan is graded 0 to 2. In 8% of cases (group 2), the BTO is negative and the HMPAO scan is graded 3 to 4. In 12% of cases, group 3, the BTO is positive and the HMPAO scan is graded 3 to 4. Patients in groups 2 and 3 require a bypass graft before carotid sacri-

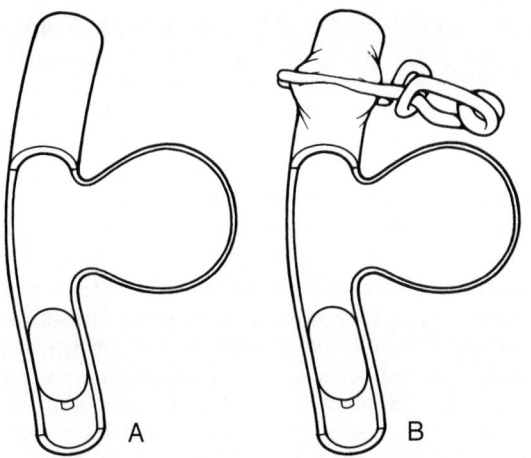

FIGURE 88–7 ■ Endovascular (A) proximal occlusion or trapping (B) remains a first-line approach for giant internal carotid artery aneurysms. Patients who fail the balloon test occlusion and cerebral blood flow study will require a bypass graft to augment collateral flow.

fice. For patients who do not tolerate ICA occlusion, we perform an extracranial to intracranial saphenous vein bypass. Alternative bypass procedures include superficial temporal artery to MCA and saphenous vein bypasses from the petrosal ICA to the supraclinoid ICA. For direct surgical approaches to cavernous sinus aneurysms, some authors advocate a petrosal to superclinoid ICA bypass graft because the saphenous vein is similar in size to the ICA; the bypass is performed through the same exposure; and the procedure takes only slightly longer than other bypass grafts.[30] Another advantage of the petrosal to supraclinoid ICA bypass graft is a relatively short bypass length, which reduces the risk for thrombosis and eliminates vascular dead space that might promote thrombus formation. The petrosal to supraclinoid ICA bypass is difficult to perform; therefore, addition of an orbitozygomatic osteotomy provides a shorter working distance and a wider exposure that reduces the technical difficulty.[31]

Most BTO results show that the ICA can be sacrificed safely. However, the authors prefer to preserve the ICA when possible because there is a small risk for delayed transient ischemic episodes, de novo aneurysm formation, and major hemispheric infarction after carotid occlusion. If the neck of the aneurysm is well defined and the risk for distal embolization is low, GDCs are placed in the aneurysm. When the aneurysm neck is wide or poorly defined, proximal occlusion or trapping of the ICA is performed (Fig. 88–7). Trapping eliminates retrograde flow from the ophthalmic artery and reduces the length of thrombus within the ICA. Stenting may provide another alternative for these sidewall and fusiform aneurysms and may preserve patency of the ICA. If the ICA is stenotic or tortuous and a catheter cannot be navigated through the cavernous segment of the ICA, then direct surgical exposure of the cavernous sinus and clipping of the aneurysm are performed.[32, 33]

## Paraclinoid Carotid Aneurysms

Paraclinoid aneurysms arise from the carotid artery segment immediately distal to the cavernous sinus. There are

three basic types: ophthalmic artery aneurysms, superior hypophyseal artery aneurysms, and proximal posterior carotid wall artery aneurysms.[34] All are partially obscured by the anterior clinoid process. The ophthalmic artery aneurysms arise at the branch point between the ICA and the ophthalmic artery, project superiomedially, and displace the optic nerve superiorly and medially. Superior hypophyseal giant aneurysms project primarily medially and posteromedially and elevate and laterally displace the ICA. The proximal posterior carotid wall aneurysms project laterally and posterolaterally, with the ICA elevated superiorly. The proximal posterior carotid wall aneurysms arise immediately distal to the proximal dural ring and proximal to the posterior communicating artery.

Similar to carotid cavernous aneurysms, paraclinoid aneurysms require a BTO and HMPAO-SPECT study to assess collateral flow. Proximal control of paraclinoid aneurysms requires either temporary balloon occlusion of the proximal ICA or exposure of the cervical ICA in the neck. Alternatively, the ICA can be isolated through a petrous carotid exposure.[35] We prefer to expose the ICA in the neck because the exposure is easy to perform and the ICA can be opened and closed rapidly. Exposure of the cervical ICA is performed through a transverse incision below the angle of the mandible medial to the anterior border of the sternocleidomastoid.

In addition to a standard pterional craniotomy, the lesser sphenoid wing, anterior clinoid process, and orbital roof are removed. An orbitozygomatic osteotomy is not required for removal of paraclinoid aneurysms. However, giant aneurysms require wide splitting of the sylvian fissure and removal of the entire anterior clinoid process and orbital roof. If the cavernous sinus is entered during drilling or dissection, bleeding is controlled by packing with Oxycel (Becton Dickinson, Franklin Lakes, NJ) or Surgicel (Johnson & Johnson, Arlington, TX). The falciform ligament and distal dural ring are opened with a No. 11 scalpel blade. Direct clipping of giant paraclinoid aneurysms rarely can be achieved without suction and decompression of the aneurysm sac.[36] This maneuver is performed by trapping the aneurysm with temporary clips and aspirating through direct puncture of the cervical ICA. The assistant evacuates the blood from the aneurysm while the surgeon defines the neck and applies the aneurysm clip. Occasionally, the giant aneurysm has a small neck and clipping is relatively straightforward with a standard clip. For most giant paraclinoid aneurysms, however, the ICA can only be reconstructed with a fenestrated aneurysm clip. Multiple aneurysm clips are often required and may be placed in tandem or in parallel. Intraoperative angiography is performed to ensure that there is no stenosis or occlusion of the ICA. Excessive change in the direction of the ICA is avoided because straightening the ICA may lead to kinking distally and delayed occlusion of the MCA.[37] When the aneurysm neck is wide and extends into the cavernous sinus, trapping is performed. If collateral flow is insufficient, a bypass graft is performed.

## Internal Carotid Artery Bifurcation Aneurysms

Giant aneurysms of the ICA bifurcation usually displace the A1 and M1 segment arteries away from one another so that no definable aneurysm neck exists. The aneurysm must be trapped and excised. A saphenous vein bypass graft is performed between the external carotid artery and the M2 segment. The A1 segment receives collateral blood supply from the anterior communicating artery and cortical collaterals. If there is poor collateral flow to the A1 segment, the aneurysm base can be reconstructed so that the ICA flows directly into the ipsilateral anterior cerebral artery.

It is important to avoid excessive manipulation of the sac when removing the thrombus, because the neck and parent arteries are atherosclerotic and can tear. If the parent artery is torn, then an intraposition graft, reimplantation, placement of an encircling clip, or suturing of the tear is required. The surgeon must be able to perform these maneuvers, recognize which option is best, and rapidly switch from one option to another.

## External Carotid-Internal Carotid Bypass Grafting

When a patient fails the BTO or has a borderline risk for cerebral ischemia from ICA occlusion, we perform a bypass graft before trapping the aneurysm (Fig. 88–8). Our preferred method is to place a saphenous vein graft between the cervical external carotid artery and the M2 temporal branch of the MCA. Most graft failures occur within 24 hours after surgery, and the failure rate is 14% at 1 year.[38] When grafts fail acutely, more than 70% are symptomatic; however, when the graft failure is delayed, only 20% develop new neurologic symptoms.

Patients are given 6000 U of intravenous heparin before undergoing the bypass. Approximately 15 mm of the M2 branch of the MCA is exposed to perform the distal anastomosis; small branches along this 15-mm segment are ligated with 9–0 nylon suture. A 2-cm segment of the external carotid artery between the superior thyroid and lingual arteries is exposed to perform the proximal anastomosis. The vein graft measures approximately 15 cm, and the

distal anastomosis to the M2 segment is performed first. The vein is passed in front of the ear down to the external carotid artery via a 26-gauge chest tube. The orifice of the vein graft is cut obliquely so that the length is 2½ times the diameter of the recipient artery. A microedged tapered or BV-100 needle with 9–0 or 10–0 monofilament suture is used to perform the distal anastomosis. The proximal end of the vein graft is anastomosed to the external carotid artery in the same fashion using 7–0 monofilament suture. This anastomosis is easier to perform because it is more superficial. The anastomosis is easier to perform by suturing from right to left and closing the back wall first. The needle holders and forceps are 7½ inches long and have a diamond edge finish (Scanlan Instruments, Minneapolis, MN). The needle holders have a gentle narrow tapered tip that prevents the suture from becoming hooked on the hinge. An angled needle holder is useful when suturing in the sylvian fissure. The foot pedal on the microscope is used to zoom into place the stitch and zoom out to retrieve and reposition the needle in the needle holder. The mouthpiece on the microscope helps maintain focus and keep the surgeon's hands free to perform the anastomoses. We prefer titanium instruments so that the needles do not become magnetized.

If there is good filling of the saphenous vein graft on intraoperative angiography and poor filling of the aneurysm, then ICA occlusion is performed in a delayed fashion. If the bypass graft and the aneurysm fill simultaneously, then the aneurysm is trapped to ensure that the graft will stay open. If there is concern for adequate collateral flow, then a repeat BTO study is performed postoperatively, and a Crutchfield or Silverstone clamp is used to gradually occlude the cervical ICA.

## Middle Cerebral Artery Aneurysms

The pterional craniotomy is modified with a half-and-half exposure of the frontal and temporal lobes. A radiolucent

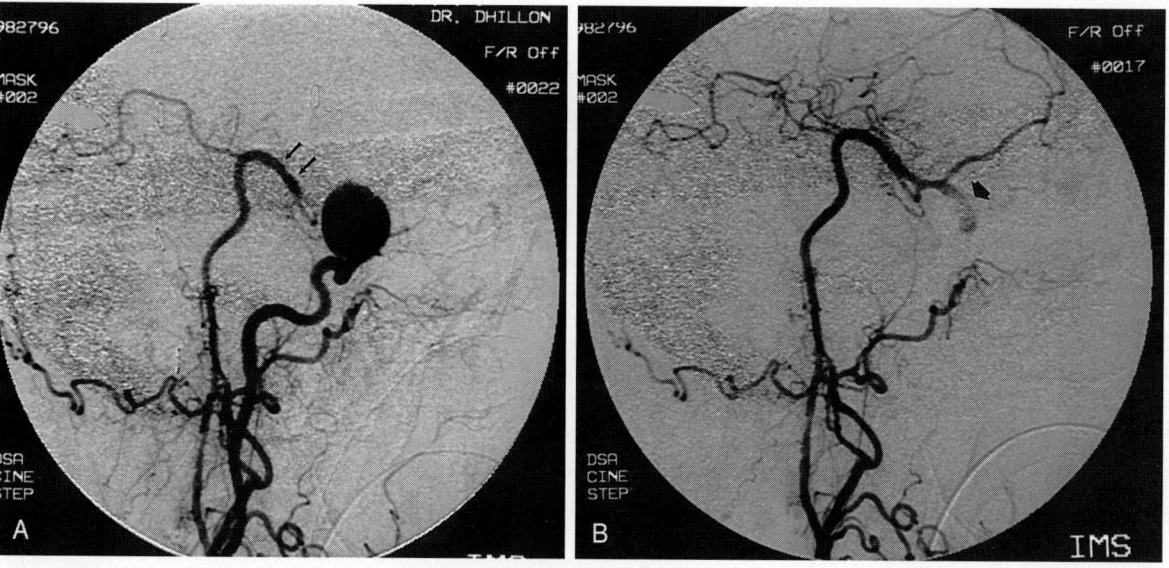

FIGURE 88–8 ■ A saphenous vein bypass from the external carotid artery to the M2 temporal branch is an excellent option to increase collateral flow. *A,* An intraoperative angiogram shows simultaneous filling of a giant ophthalmic artery aneurysm and the saphenous vein graft *(arrows). B,* Immediately after proximal occlusion, the vein graft fills the anterior and middle cerebral artery territories and there is a small amount of retrograde filling of the giant aneurysm *(arrowhead).*

head fixation device is used for intraoperative angiography (Ohio Medical Instruments, Cincinnati, OH). The sylvian fissure must be split widely to expose the M1 and M2 segments. Temporary clipping of the parent branches is required to decompress the aneurysm, remove the thrombus, and reconstruct the normal blood flow. Before trapping the MCA aneurysm, cerebral protection is administered by the anesthesiologist and the blood pressure is elevated to promote cortical collateral flow. When the aneurysm has no definable neck, then a high-flow vein graft from the cervical external carotid artery to the M2 segment or intraoperative reimplantation of the M2 arteries into the M1 segment is required (Fig. 88–9). During decompression of the aneurysm, the surrounding veins frequently bleed and obscure the operative field. Gelfoam (Upjohn, Kalamazoo, MI) and self-retaining retractors may be used to compress the veins and stop the bleeding.

There is generally less than 20 minutes of temporary clamp time to obliterate the aneurysm and reconstruct the middle cerebral arteries without causing a permanent ischemic deficit. Patients older than 60 years of age and those in poor neurologic condition do not tolerate temporary occlusion as well.[39] Likewise, if the clipping is performed between the 4th and 10th days after SAH, if multiple clipping episodes are required, or if intraoperative rupture occurs, then the risk of postoperative stroke is higher after temporary clipping.[40] Most postoperative ischemic deficits, however, are not related to temporary clipping. Overall, the stroke rate after temporary clipping ranges from 2% to 5%.[40, 41] The thrombus within the aneurysm is usually well organized and is best removed with an ultrasonic aspirator to avoid excessive manipulation of the parent arteries (Fig. 88–10). Once the sac is evacuated and the ostia are identified, the sac is amputated leaving a 1-cm cuff at the base of the aneurysm. The neck can then be reconstructed using aneurysm clips, suture, or vascular clips. The temporary clips are removed to test the security of the closure. Micro-Doppler records the patency of the M1 and M2 segment

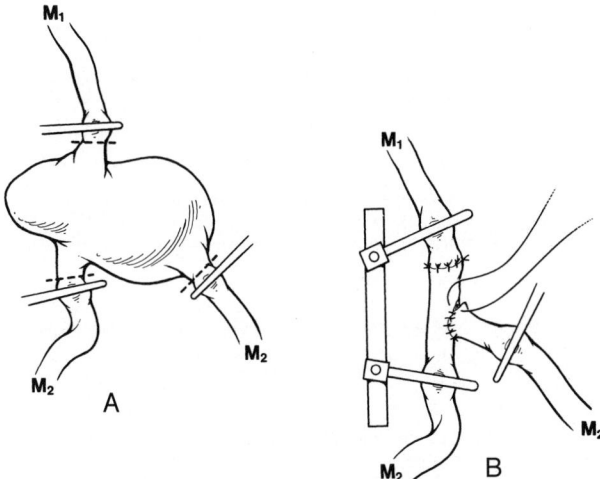

**FIGURE 88–9** ■ Giant aneurysms of the internal carotid artery bifurcation and middle cerebral artery (MCA) bifurcation often have displaced branching arteries that preclude surgical clipping. There is no neck and reimplantation techniques or bypass grafts must be performed. *A,* Trapping and excising a giant MCA aneurysm. *B,* Reimplantation of the M2 branches using a 10–0 monofilament suture.

arteries, and an intraoperative angiogram confirms the micro-Doppler findings.

## Anterior Communicating Artery Aneurysms

Giant aneurysms of the anterior communicating artery follow the same surgical principles of MCA aneurysms. Control of the A1 and A2 segments is essential. In general, cardiopulmonary circulatory arrest is reserved for posterior circulation giant aneurysms; however, calcified thrombosed giant aneurysms of the anterior communicating artery may also require circulatory arrest. In most cases, a unilateral pterional craniotomy with a generous frontal exposure is sufficient. A wide resection of the ipsilateral gyrus rectus will expose the ipsilateral A2 segment and the neck of the aneurysm. An orbitozygomatic osteotomy may provide a wide exposure, shorten the angle of approach,[42] and enhance exposure of the contralateral A2 segment. After temporary clipping of the A1 and A2 anterior cerebral arteries, the blood pressure is raised and pentobarbital is added to an infusion of lidocaine and propofol. The assistant performs suction decompression to shrink the aneurysm, and the surgeon identifies the neck and clips the aneurysm. Preservation of the anterior communicating segment and the perforators are attempted. The microdissection is primarily anterior to the sac to avoid injury to the posteriorly pointing hypothalamic perforators. After the temporary clips are removed, a micro-Doppler is used to establish patency of the A1 and A2 segment vessels. An intraoperative angiogram is performed to confirm obliteration of the aneurysm and preservation of the normal arteries.

### ENDOVASCULAR TECHNIQUES

Endovascular techniques play an increasing important role in the surgical management of patients with giant aneurysms, particularly preoperative BTO, intraoperative proximal vessel occlusion, and intraoperative angiography. When the operative exposure does not allow for a temporary clip proximal to the aneurysm, intraoperative endovascular balloon occlusion can be used instead to gain proximal vascular control.[43, 44] This is especially useful for paraclinoid and basilar artery aneurysms. Multiple clips, fenestrated clips, and booster clips frequently obscure the aneurysm neck and branching arteries. Intraoperative angiography confirms obliteration of the aneurysm and preservation of the parent artery and can assess patency of the bypass grafts.

Up until the early 1990s, placement of detachable latex and silicone balloons inside the aneurysm was used but was also associated with incomplete occlusion and balloon deflation.[45] The balloons caused a "water hammer" effect that led to aneurysm rupture (Fig. 88–11).[46] In addition, there was a high rate of ischemic complications caused by balloon migration and occlusion of the parent artery. The advent of GDCs (Target Therapeutics, Fremont, CA) in 1991 replaced detachable balloons because the coils conform better to the shape of the aneurysm, are retrievable, and provide a much more dense packing to reduce the risk of rupture.[47] When the safety issues regarding silicone breast implants were extended to silicone balloons, an

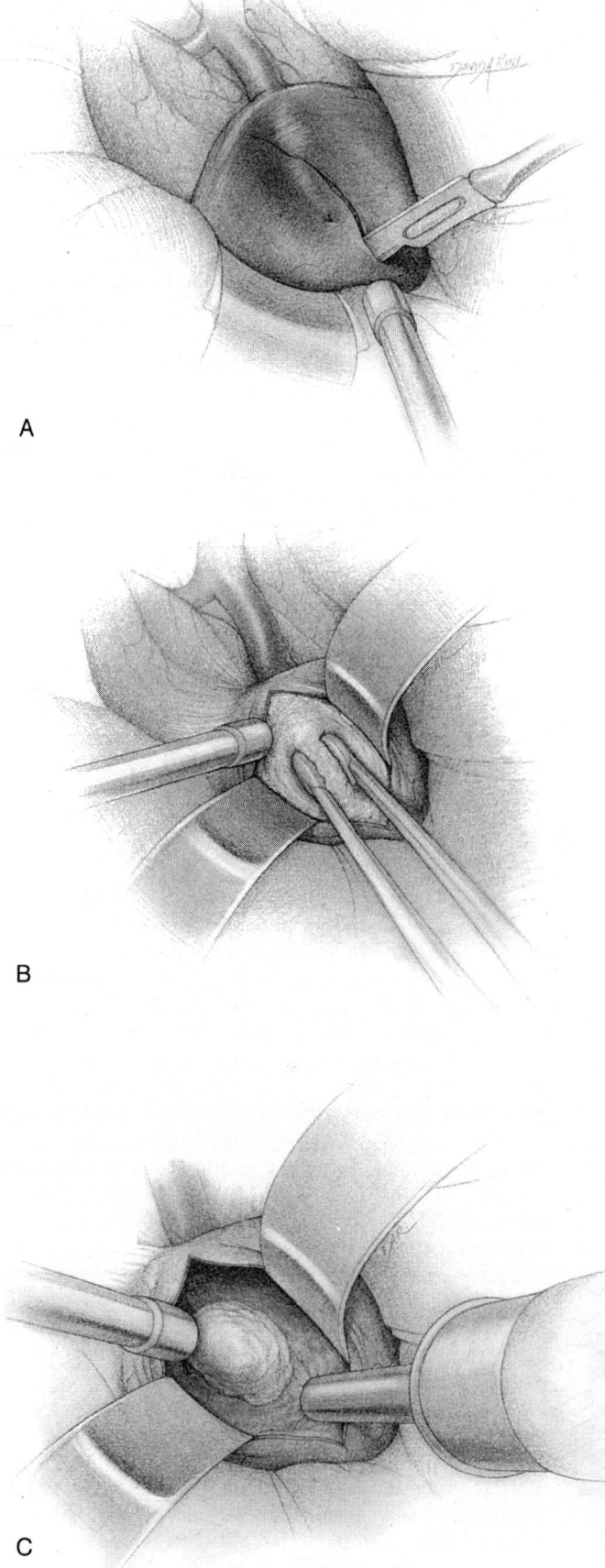

A

B

C

**FIGURE 88–10** ■ Giant aneurysms filled with thrombus require evacuation of the sac before clipping. *A,* The sac is opened widely with a scalpel. *B,* Retractors are placed inside the sac to enlarge the opening and the soft thrombus is removed with forceps. *C,* When the thrombus is well organized and calcified, it is removed with an ultrasonic aspirator. The soft red thrombus overlying the filling portion of the aneurysm is not evacuated until temporary clips are applied.

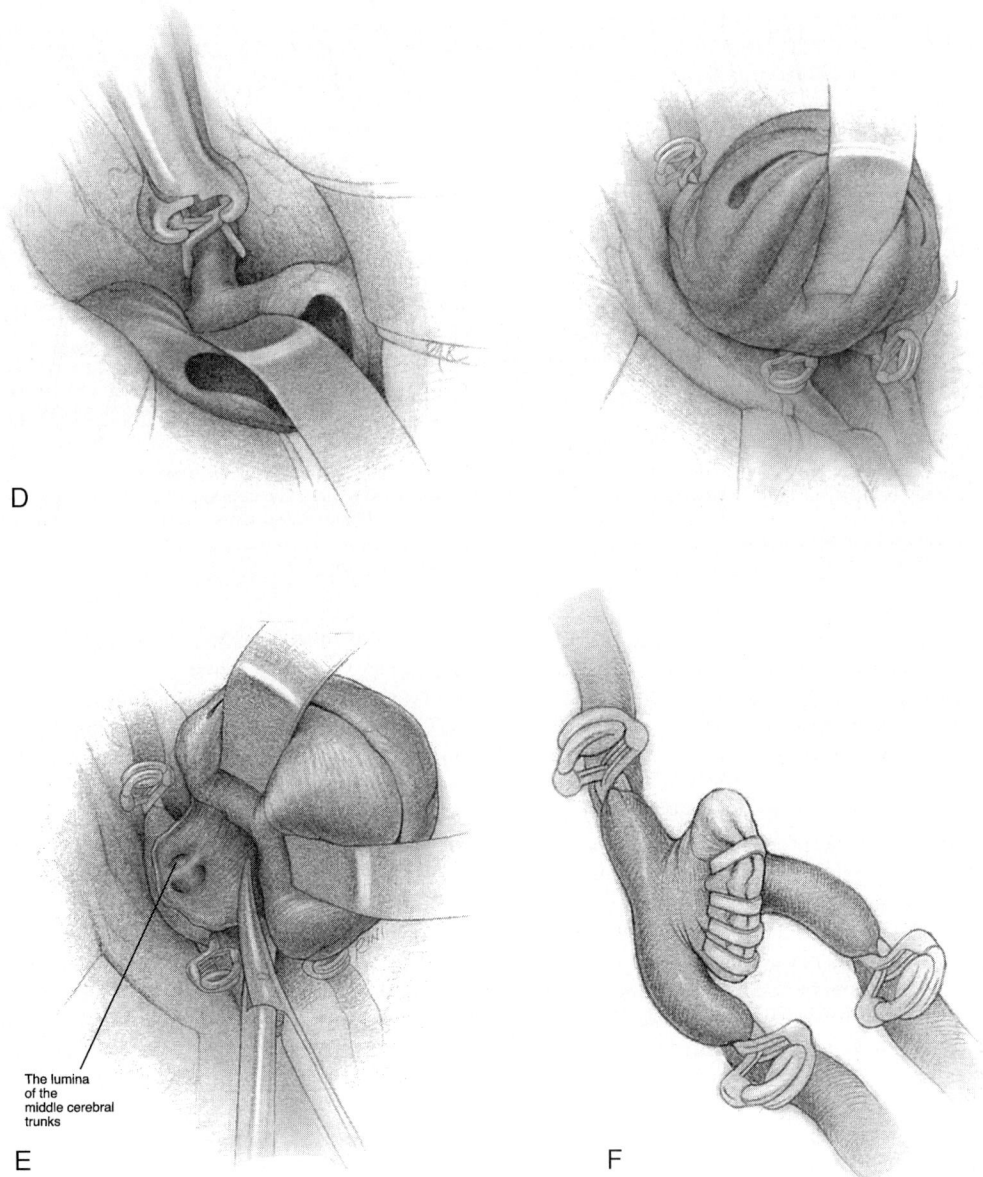

D

E

The lumina
of the
middle cerebral
trunks

F

**FIGURE 88–10** ■ *Continued. D,* The sac is collapsed and temporary clips are applied to the M1 and M2 branches to trap the aneurysm. *E,* The remaining soft thrombus is removed, and the sac is excised with a 1-cm cuff of the aneurysm left at the base. *F,* Multiple aneurysm clips, continuous monofilament suture, or hemostatic clips are used to reconstruct the M1 and M2 branches. (From Tew JM Jr, van Loveren HR: Atlas of Operative Microneurosurgery, Vol 1. Philadelphia: WB Saunders, 1994.)

investigator device exemption was required by the Food and Drug Administration in order to use the balloons. Not until November 1998 were detachable silicone balloons (Target Therapeutics, Fremont, CA) approved for commercial use.

Giant aneurysms are better suited for surgical clipping because of their anatomic characteristics (i.e., wide neck, thrombus formation, mass effect) (Fig. 88–12).[6, 27] In a large series of coiled aneurysms, complete thrombosis was achieved in 85% of small-necked aneurysms but only 15% of the wide-necked aneurysms.[48] Good results were achieved with GDC placement for aneurysms up to 18 mm; however, giant aneurysms had a high rate of rebleeding after GDC placement.[49] Partial coiling of the aneurysm offers some protection compared with the natural history,

but the long-term rates of aneurysm regrowth and hemorrhage are not well defined. A patient with an aneurysm remains at risk for SAH; additionally, aneurysm regrowth has been documented more than 2 years after GDC placement (Fig. 88–13).[50] Thrombosed aneurysms are not well suited for GDC placement because they tend to migrate into the thrombus, leading to a high rate of aneurysm regrowth (Fig. 88–14). In fact, more than 60% of giant aneurysms are partially thombosed.[15] Furthermore, a friable thrombus often poses an increased risk a of thromboembolism.

The GDCs have a circular memory so that coils tend to prolapse into the parent artery when the aneurysm has a wide neck. In general, dense packing of wide-necked aneurysms is more difficult to achieve than small-necked

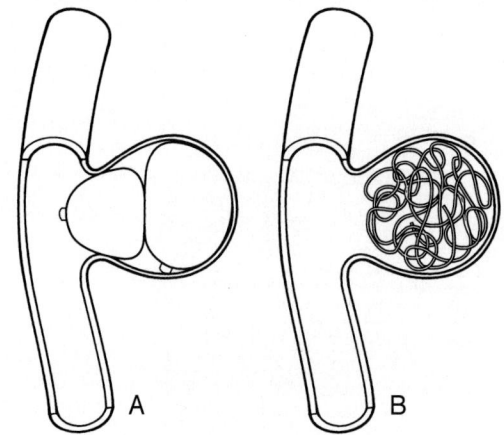

**FIGURE 88–11** ■ Endovascular balloon occlusion has been abandoned because there was a high rate of rupture and infarction due to balloon deflation and migration, respectively. In 1999, detachable platinum coils became the mainstay for endovascular treatment of aneurysms. *A,* Endovascular balloon occlusion. *B,* Endovascular coil occlusion.

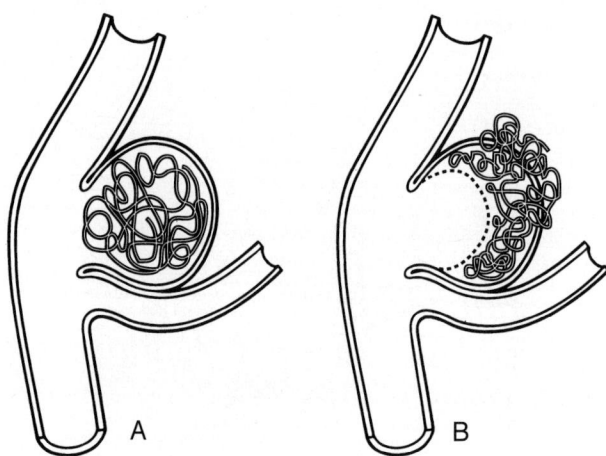

**FIGURE 88–13** ■ Once the aneurysm is coiled, it is difficult or impossible to remove the coil mass because it becomes impacted into the wall. *A,* Loose endovascular coiling of the aneurysm. *B,* Compaction and migration of the coils across the aneurysm wall.

aneurysms. Loose packing can lead to compaction of the coils, coil rotation and migration, and aneurysm regrowth. Remodeling of the parent artery with balloon angioplasty or stent-assisted GDC placement may allow wide-necked aneurysms to be treated more completely with denser packing and, theoretically, a reduced risk of aneurysm regrowth (Fig. 88–15).[51–54] If parent artery narrowing or distal thromboembolism occurs during the procedure, the coils can be withdrawn, and intra-arterial thrombolysis can be performed to lyse the embolus.

Dense GDC packing is essential to avoid aneurysm regrowth because the platinum coils are not very thrombogenic. However, dense packing creates mass effect that may exacerbate headaches, worsen cranial nerve palsies, and create additional pressure on the surrounding brain. Most cranial nerve palsies improve or remain the same but increased mass effect on the brain stem may have severe consequences. In a large series of aneurysms treated with GDCs, approximately 20% of patients had worsening of the cranial nerve palsies[55]; 32% showed complete resolution at

follow-up of the symptoms; 42% improved; 21% remained unchanged; and 5% worsened. In patients with smaller aneurysms, symptoms were more likely to improve following GDC treatment. The increased physical weight of the coil mass may also lead to compression or kinking of the parent artery branches and distal branch occlusion (Fig. 88–16). Development of GDCs impregnated with thrombogenic material may allow for loose packing while lessening mass effect to achieve aneurysm obliteration.

At leading endovascular centers the complication rate for GDC placement is approximately 9% major morbidity and 2% mortality. Aneurysm perforation, embolization, parent artery occlusion, coil migration, arterial vasospasm, and rebleeding account for most of the complications. These percentages will likely decline with inprovements in catheters and guidewires and increasing experience with the GDC. For example, general anesthesia is now favored over neuroleptic analgesia so that complications can be treated more effectively. High-quality fluoroscopy with roadmapping also provides more precision in GDC place-

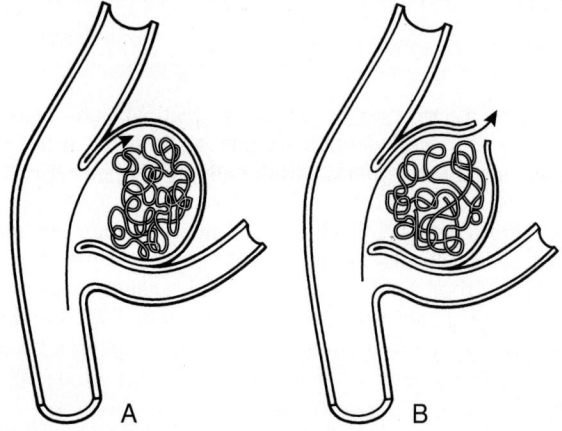

**FIGURE 88–12** ■ When previously coiled aneurysms regrow, there is a risk of rupture, especially on the inflow side of the aneurysm. *A,* Compaction of the coils allows blood to enter the sac. *B,* Rupture can occur between the coils and the aneurysm wall.

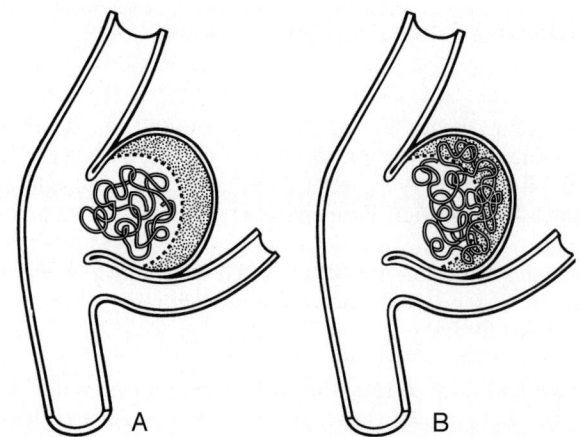

**FIGURE 88–14** ■ Coils are poorly suited for aneurysms filled with thrombus. *A,* Endovascular coiling of a partially thrombosed aneurysm. *B,* Compaction of the coils into the thrombus with regrowth of the aneurysm.

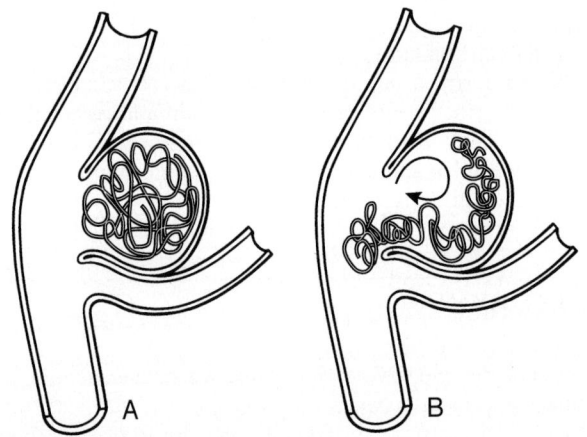

FIGURE 88–15 ■ It is difficult to achieve a dense and complete packing of coils in wide-necked aneurysms. Loose endovascular coiling of the aneurysm (A) results in blood flow into the aneurysm (B) causing rotation and migration of the coils into the parent artery.

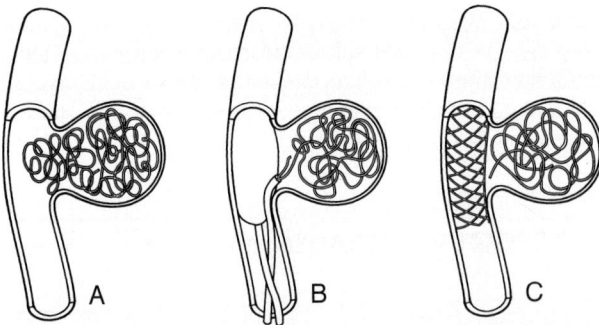

FIGURE 88–17 ■ It is difficult to achieve a complete coil packing of a wide-necked aneurysm because the coils may prolapse into the parent artery. Endovascular remodeling techniques reconstruct the parent artery. A, Endovascular coiling of the aneurysm with coils extending into the parent artery. B, Balloon-assisted technique with placement of coils into the sac. C, Stenting with coil placement to reconstruct the parent artery.

ment. Remodeling techniques are increasing the rate of aneurysm obliteration, and flexible intracranial stents and other aneurysm neck–blocking devices are being developed that may solve some of the problems with current GDC technology (Fig. 88–17).

Increasing operator experience is providing ingenious solutions to complications that occur during GDC placement. For example, intra-arterial thrombolysis and balloon angioplasty have become important adjuncts in the treatment of distal thromboembolism and parent artery narrowing, respectively. Most aneurysm perforations are caused by the coils, guidewire, or microcatheter.[56] However, the risk of aneurysm perforation during GDC placement is low (2%) and will continue to decline as the technology and experience with GDC improve.

Cost comparisons are difficult between surgical clipping and endovascular coiling because the effects of new technical innovations and the long-term results of GDC placement are unknown. Repacking of aneurysms with coils may add costs because of repeat procedures and additional imaging studies. Future improvements in endovascular techniques, including placement of 2-D and 3-D coils, remodeling techniques, and stenting, may expand the use

of GDC treatment for giant aneurysms. However, for giant aneurysms in locations other than the cavernous sinus, surgical treatment offers the best opportunity for cure and should be the primary method of treatment. Endovascular treatment should be reserved for patients with a major medical illness or a heavily calcified aneurysm neck.

## EXPERIENCE AND PERSPECTIVE

The poor prognosis of symptomatic giant aneurysms mandates an aggressive approach to treatment, which nonetheless can raise morbidity and mortality rates. The surgeon should have extensive experience with the repair of small and large intracranial aneurysms before operating on giant intracranial aneurysms. Likewise, the surgeon should be able to perform bypass and reimplantation vascular grafts. Because giant aneurysms are uncommon, performing bypass grafts in a microneurosurgery laboratory may be required to maintain proficiency.

Most giant aneurysms occur on the carotid cavernous segment and paraclinoid segment of the ICA in elderly patients and can usually be treated with parent artery occlusion. A patient in the sixth or seventh decade of life with good collateral flow should not be subjected to a bypass graft or a skull base procedure simply to preserve the ICA. Similarly, performing a bypass graft or an orbitozygomatic osteotomy and anterior clinoidectomy for "practice" or to achieve an ideal angiographic picture is not a valid reason to perform surgical clipping.

Skull base exposures including anterior and posterior petrosectomies, orbitozygomatic osteotomy, and far lateral craniotomies have been extremely useful for posterior circulation aneurysms. However, skull base approaches for anterior circulation aneurysms have limited value, except for paraclinoid aneurysms. In the case of paraclinoid aneurysms, the pterional craniotomy is expanded to include removal of the lateral wall of the superior orbital fissure, orbital roof, and anterior clinoid process. A large pterional craniotomy with wide splitting of the sylvian fissure suffices to expose most giant posterior communicating, anterior communicating, ICA bifurcation, and MCA aneurysms.

When a patient has bilateral aneurysms of the anterior

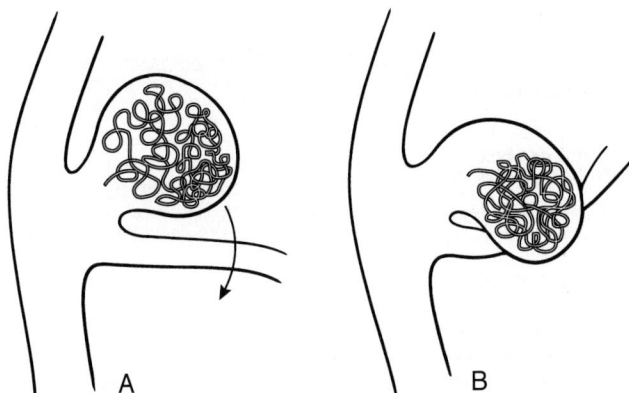

FIGURE 88–16 ■ Dense packing of giant aneurysms may lead to mass effect and prolapse of the sac. A, Endovascular coil occlusion of the aneurysm. B, Compression and occlusion of the branching artery.

circulation, treatment should be reserved for the symptomatic side. A contralateral saccular aneurysm is a relative contraindication to ICA occlusion, because a change in flow dynamics may precipitate aneurysm growth or rupture in the contralateral aneurysm.

## POSTOPERATIVE MANAGEMENT

The postoperative course depends on the patient's preoperative status, the method and complexity of the surgical operation, the type of operation performed, and the interval during which temporary occlusion of vessels was required. Vasospasm, hydrocephalus, and raised intracranial pressure may create additional postoperative morbidity. Patients who suffer subarachnoid hemorrhage receive the calcium channel blocker nimodipine and steroids to reduce the risk of cerebral ischemia. Patients are monitored daily with transcranial Doppler ultrasound. Prophylactic hypervolemia and allowing the blood pressure to rise (systolic range, 160 to 200 mm Hg) in hypertensive patients are measures to avoid cerebral ischemia in patients with borderline collateral flow or asymptomatic patients with elevated transcranial Doppler velocities. Those who show clinical deterioration due to vasospasm are treated with hypervolemic, hypertensive, and hemodilutional (triple H) therapy. If reversal of neurologic deficits does not occur within 2 hours from the initiation of triple H therapy, then intra-arterial papaverine is administered and transluminal angioplasty is performed to avoid a fixed neurologic deficit.

## COMPLICATIONS

Surgical morbidity in the treatment of giant aneurysms results primarily from cerebral ischemia. Intraoperative aneurysm rupture increases the rate of postoperative morbidity and mortality. Surgical clipping can result in cerebral infarction caused by prolonged temporary clipping, occlusion of the parent artery, or distal thromboembolism.

Although uncommon, BTO may produce a carotid dissection, stenosis, and occlusion. Despite systemic heparinization, thromboemboli from the balloon can cause a delayed stroke. The bypass graft is prone to pseudoaneurysm formation, thrombosis, or intimal dissection. Occlusion of the ICA may lead to propagation of a distant thrombus, de novo aneurysm formation, or accelerated atherosclerosis.

Impaired extraocular motility, which is the most frequent complication of surgery for giant carotid cavernous and paraclinoid aneurysms, is usually temporary and resolves within 3 months. Injury to the optic nerve, however, is usually permanent. Excessive retraction of the optic nerve, heating and vibration of the drill, or unroofing the optic canal with a Cloward punch instead of a drill can cause blindness. The falciform ligament binds the optic nerve laterally and compresses the optic nerve over the aneurysm. The most common visual loss is an inferior and lateral visual field defect. The falciform ligament must be opened to decompress the optic nerve and avoid blindness from excessive retraction. In a few cases, damage to the ophthalmic artery or clipping of the ophthalmic artery may lead to ipsilateral blindness.

CSF rhinorrhea may occur postoperatively after removing the anterior clinoid process if the ethmoid or sphenoid sinus was entered inadvertently. The rhinorrhea may stop spontaneously or require a temporary lumbar drain or re-exploration and closure of the leak.

## CONCLUSION

In this chapter, we have tried to present a balanced, complementary approach between endovascular and surgical techniques for the treatment of giant anterior circulation aneurysms. Complex intracranial aneurysms often require combined management strategies. For example, coils can be used to obliterate residual aneurysms after incomplete surgical clipping.[57] Placement of GDCs in the aneurysm remnant is more challenging because the residual aneurysm is not saccular and the aneurysm clip may obscure the true dimensions of the aneurysm neck. Conversely, incomplete endovascular GDC placement may be followed by surgical clipping.[58, 59] Here too, surgical clipping after coil placement is extremely hazardous because the aneurysm must be trapped and opened to remove the coils so that the neck will accept a clip. If the coils embed in the wall of the aneurysm, coil removal is impossible without tearing the neck and perforators. Removing the coils may also dislodge thrombus into the distal parent arteries. Close neurosurgical follow-up is important in patients who have undergone endovascular treatment, because 10% will require surgery to obliterate a remnant.[59] Bypass grafting followed by endovascular parent artery occlusion aneurysms has achieved good results in giant MCA aneurysms.[60] Other options include partial packing of the dome with GDCs followed by delayed surgical clipping and parent artery occlusion followed by decompression of the aneurysm sac to relieve mass effect.[61] When unexpected events occur during the course of treatment, the cerebrovascular team must be able to adapt and change. These innovative strategies listed earlier can expand the treatment options and improve the outcome.

## ACKNOWLEDGMENTS

*The authors thank Mary Kemper for editorial assistance and Michael Shank and David Rini for medical illustration.*

## REFERENCES

1. Ausman JI, Malik GM, Tomecek FJ, et al: Hypothermic circulatory arrest and the management of giant and large cerebral aneurysms. Surg Neurol 40:289–298, 1993.
2. Solomon RA: Principles of aneurysm surgery: Cerebral ischemic protection, hypothermia, and circulatory arrest. Clin Neurosurg 41:251–363, 1994.
3. Spetzler RF, Hadley MN, Rigamonti D, et al: Aneurysms of the basilar artery treated with circulatory arrest, hypothermia, and barbiturate cerebral protection. J Neurosurg 68:868–879, 1988.
4. Standard SC, Guterman LR, Chavis TD, et al: Endovascular management of giant intracranial aneurysms. Clin Neurosurg 42:267–293, 1995.

5. Drake CG: Giant intracranial aneurysms: Experience with surgical treatment in 174 patients. Clin Neurosurg 26:12–96, 1979.

6. Sundt TM Jr, Piepgras DG, Fode NC, et al: Giant intracranial aneurysms. Clin Neurosurg 37:116–154, 1991.

7. Sahs AL, Perret GE, Locksley HBO, et al: Intracranial Aneurysms and Subarachnoid Hemorrhage: A Cooperative Study. Philadelphia: JB Lippincott, 1969.

8. Barrow DL, Alleyne C: Natural history of giant intracranial aneurysms and indications for intervention. Clin Neurosurg 42:214–244, 1995.

9. Kodama N, Suzuki J: Surgical treatment of giant aneurysms. Neurosurg Rev 5:155–160, 1992.

10. Khurana VG, Piepgras DG, Whisnant JP: Ruptured giant intracranial aneurysms. I: A study of rebleeding. J Neurosurg 88:425–429, 1998.

11. Piepgras DG, Khurana VG, Whisnant JP: Ruptured giant intracranial aneurysms. II: A retrospective analysis of timing and outcome of surgical treatment. J Neurosurg 88:430–435, 1998.

12. Hamburger C, Schonberger J, Lange M: Management and prognosis of intracranial giant aneurysms: A report on 58 cases. Neurosurg Rev 5:97–103, 1992.

13. Fox JL: Intracranial Aneurysms, Vol 1. New York: Springer Verlag, 1983.

14. Pia HW, Zierski J: Giant cerebral aneurysms. Neurosurg Rev 5:117–148, 1982.

15. Weir B: Giant aneurysms. In Weir B (ed): Aneurysms Affecting the Nervous System. Baltimore: Williams & Wilkins, 1987, pp 187–206.

16. Lawton MT, Spetzler RF: Surgical management of giant intracranial aneurysms: Experience with 171 patients. Clin Neurosurg 42:245–266, 1995.

17. Fisher A, Som PM, Mosesson RE, et al: Giant intracranial aneurysms with skull base erosion and extracranial masses: CT and MR findings. J Comp Assist Tomogr 18:939–942, 1994.

18. Sekhar LN, Kalia KK, Yonas H, et al: Cranial base approaches to intracranial aneurysms in the subarachnoid space. Neurosurgery 35:472–483, 1994.

19. Tew JM, Jr, van Loveren HR: Atlas of Operative Microneurosurgery, Vol 1. Philadelphia: WB Saunders, 1994, pp 80–81.

20. Bailes JE, Tantuwaya LS, Fukushima T, et al: Intraoperative microvascular Doppler sonography in aneurysm surgery. Neurosurgery 40:965–970, 1997.

21. Lawton MT, Hamilton MG, Morcos JJ, et al: Revascularization and aneurysm surgery: Current techniques, indications, and outcome. Neurosurgery 38:83–92, 1996.

22. Linskey ME, Sekhar LN, Hirch WL Jr, et al: Aneurysms of the intracavernous carotid artery: Clinical presentation, radiographic features, and pathogenesis. Neurosurgery 26:71–79, 1990.

23. Linskey ME, Sekhar LN, Hirch WL Jr, et al: Aneurysms of the intracavernous carotid artery: Natural history and indications for treatment. Neurosurgery 26:933–938, 1990.

24. Kupersmith MJ, Hurst R, Berenstein A, et al: The benign natural course of cavernous carotid artery aneurysms. J Neurosurg 77:690–693, 1993.

25. Drake CG, Peerless SJ, Ferguson GG: Hunterian proximal arterial occlusion for giant aneurysms of the carotid circulation. J Neurosurg 81:656–665, 1994.

26. Debrun G, Fox, A, Drake C, et al: Giant unclippable aneurysms: Treatment with detachable balloons. AJNR Am J Neuroradiol 2:167–173, 1981.

27. Guglielmi G, Vinuela F, Dion J, et al: Electrothrombosis of saccular aneurysms via endovascular approach. II: Preliminary clinical experience. J Neurosurg 75:8–14, 1991.

28. Vinuela F, Duckwiler G, Mawad M: Guglielmi detachable coil embolization of acute intracranial aneurysm: Perioperative anatomical and clinical outcome in 403 patients. J Neurosurg 1997; 86:475–482.

29. Larson JJ, Tew JM Jr, Tomsick TA, et al: Treatment of aneurysms of the internal carotid artery by intravascular balloon occlusion: Long-term follow-up in 58 patients. Neurosurgery 36:26–30, 1995.

30. Spetzler RF, Fukushima T, Martin N, et al: Petrous carotid-to-intradural carotid saphenous vein graft for intracavernous giant aneurysm, tumor, and occlusive vascular disease. J Neurosurg 73:496–501, 1990.

31. Lawton MT, Spetzler RF: Surgical strategies for giant intracranial aneurysms. Neurosurg Clin North Am 4:725–742, 1998.

32. Dolenc VV: A combined epi- and subdural direct approach to carotid-ophthalmic artery aneurysms. J Neurosurg 62:667–672, 1985.

33. van Loveren HR, Keller JT, El-Kalliny M: The Dolenc technique for

34. Batjer HH, Kopitnik TA, Giller CA, et al: Surgery for paraclinoidal carotid artery aneurysms. J Neurosurg 80:650–658, 1994.

35. Kattner KA, Bailes J, Fukushima T: Direct surgical management of large bulbous and giant aneurysms involving the paraclinoid segment of the internal carotid artery: Report of 29 cases. Surg Neurol 49:471–480, 1998.

36. Batjer HH, Samson DS: Retrograde suction decompression of giant paraclinoidal aneurysms: Technical note. J Neurosurg 73:305–306, 1990.

37. Tanaka Y, Kobayashi S, Kyoshima K, et al: Multiple clipping technique for large and giant internal carotid artery aneurysms and complications: Angiographic analysis. J Neurosurg 40:635–642, 1994.

38. Regli L, Piepgras DG, Hansen KK: Late patency of long saphenous vein bypass grafts to the anterior and posterior cerebral circulation. J Neurosurg 83:806–811, 1995.

39. Samson D, Batjer HH, Bowman G, et al: A clinical study of the parameters and effects of temporary arterial occlusion in the management of intracranial aneurysms. Neurosurgery 34:22–28, 1994.

40. Ogilvy CS, Carter BS, Kaplan S, et al: Temporary vessel occlusion for aneurysm surgery: Risk factors for stroke in patients protected by induced hypothermia and hypertension and intravenous mannitol administration. J Neurosurg 84:785–791, 1996.

41. Charbel FT, Ausman JI, Diaz FG, et al: Temporary clipping in aneurysm surgery: Technique and results. Surg Neurol 36:83–90, 1991.

42. Smith RR, Al-Mefty O, Middleton TH: An orbitocranial approach to complex aneurysms of the anterior circulation. Neurosurgery 24:385–381, 1989.

43. Bailes JE, Deeb ZL, Wilson JA, et al: Intraoperative angiography and temporary balloon occlusion of the basilar artery as an adjunct to surgical clipping: Technical note. Neurosurgery 30:949–953, 1992.

44. Shucart WA, Kwan ES, Heilman CB: Temporary balloon occlusion of a proximal vessel as an aid to clipping aneurysms of the basilar and paraclinoid internal carotid arteries: Technical note. Neurosurgery 27:116–119. 1990.

45. Higashida RT, Halbach VV, Barnwell SL, et al: Treatment of intracranial aneurysms with preservation of the parent vessel: Results of percutaneous balloon embolization in 84 patients. AJNR Am J Neuroradiol 11:633–641, 1990.

46. Kwan ESK, Heilman CB, Shucart WA, et al: Enlargement of basilar artery aneurysms following balloon occlusion—"water hammer effect": Report of 2 cases. J Neurosurg 75:963, 1991.

47. Guglielmi G, Vinuela F, Sepetke I, et al: Electrothrombosis of saccular aneurysms via endovascular approach. I: Electrochemical basis, technique, and experimental results. J Neurosurg 75:1–7, 1991.

48. Fernandez-Zubillaga A, Guglielmi G, Vinuela F, et al: Endovascular occlusion of intracranial aneurysms with electrically detachable coils: Correlation of aneurysm neck size and treatment results. AJNR Am J Neuroradiol 15:815–820, 1994.

49. Malisch TW, Guglielmi G, Vinuela F, et al: Intracranial aneurysms treated with the Guglielmi detachable coil: Midterm clinical results in a consecutive series of 100 patients. J Neurosurg 87:176–183, 1997.

50. Mericle RA, Wakhloo AK, Lopes DK, et al: Delayed aneurysm regrowth and recanalization after Guglielmi detachable coil treatment: Case report. J Neurosurg 89:142–145, 1998.

51. Baxter BW, Rosso D, Lownie: Double microcatheter technique for detachable coil treatment of large, wide-necked intracranial aneurysms. AJNR Am J Neuroradiol 19:1176–1178, 1998.

52. Levy DI, Ku A: Balloon-assisted coil placement in wide-necked aneurysms: Technical note. J Neurosurg 86:724–727, 1997.

53. Mericle RA, Wakhloo AK, Rodriguez R, et al: Temporary balloon protection as an adjunct to endovascular coiling of wide-necked cerebral aneurysms: Technical note. Neurosurgery 41:975–978, 1997.

54. Moret J, Pierot L, Boulin A, et al: "Remodeling" of the arterial wall of the parent vessel in the endovascular treatment of intracranial aneurysms. Proceedings of the 20th Congress of the European Society of Neuroradiology (Abstract). Neuroradiology 36 (Suppl):S83, 1994.

55. Malisch TW, Guglielmi G, Vinuela F, et al: Unruptured aneurysms presenting with mass effect symptoms: Response to endosaccular treatment with Guglielmi detachable coils. I: Symptoms of cranial nerve dysfunction. J Neurosurg 89:956–961, 1998.

56. McDougall CG, Halbach VV, Dowd CF, et al: Causes and manage-

ment of aneurysmal hemorrhage occurring during embolization of Guglielmi detachable coils. J Neurosurg 89:87–92, 1998.

57. Thielen KR, Nichols DA, Fulgham JR, et al: Endovascular treatment of cerebral aneurysms following incomplete clipping. J Neurosurg 87:184–189, 1997.

58. Civit T, Auque J, Marchal JC, et al: Aneurysm clipping after endovascular treatment with coils: A report of eight patients. Neurosurgery 38:955–960, 1996.

59. Gurian JH, Martin NA, King WA, et al: Neurosurgical management of cerebral aneurysms following unsuccessful or incomplete endovascular embolization. J Neurosurg 83:843–853, 1995.

60. Weill A, Cognard C, Levy D, et al: Giant aneurysms of the middle cerebral artery trifurcation treated with extracranial-intracranial arterial bypass and endovascular occlusion: Report of two cases. J Neurosurg 89:474–478, 1998.

61. Hacein-Bey L, Connolly ES, Mayer SA, et al: Complex intracranial aneurysms: Combined operative and endovascular approaches. Neurosurgery 43:1304–1313, 1988.

# CHAPTER 89

# Intraoperative Endovascular Techniques in the Management of Intracranial Aneurysms

■ KAZUO MIZOI, HIROYUKI KINOUCHI, AKIRA TAKAHASHI, and TAKASHI YOSHIMOTO

With current advances in microsurgical techniques, the surgical treatment of cerebral aneurysms is approaching a satisfactory level. However, technical difficulties in aneurysm surgery are determined by two main factors, the size and the location of the aneurysms. Many problems remain with surgery of large aneurysms of the proximal internal carotid artery (ICA) and the vertebrobasilar artery. In surgery of these aneurysms, there is considerable difficulty in gaining both proximal arterial control and a sufficient operative field. Since 1986, with the introduction of digital subtraction angiography (DSA) in our operating room, we have attempted to operate on surgically difficult aneurysms with the aid of intravascular catheter techniques. Such techniques include using (1) a balloon catheter placed into the parent artery of the aneurysm to obtain temporary proximal occlusion; (2) a double-lumen balloon catheter for large aneurysms to aspirate blood and collapse the aneurysm; and (3) intraoperative DSA to evaluate the result of aneurysm clipping. In this chapter, we review our experiences with the combined use of intravascular and neurosurgical approaches in surgically difficult aneurysms.

## PATIENT SELECTION

From January 1986 to December 1996, 1067 patients with cerebral aneurysms underwent surgery at our institution. Among those patients, 71 (7%) were treated with the aid of intravascular catheter techniques. All 71 patients had complex aneurysms with difficulty in gaining proximal arterial control or risk of arterial narrowing after clip placement. A total of 75 aneurysms were treated surgically in 71 patients: 57 aneurysms of the ICA in 53 cases and 18 posterior circulation aneurysms in 18 cases. The ICA aneurysms included 22 large paraclinoid carotid aneurysms, 15 carotid cave aneurysms,[1] 15 broad-based posterior communicating artery (PcomA) aneurysms, one anterior choroidal artery aneurysm, and 4 unusual dorsal ICA aneurysms.

The paraclinoid aneurysms ranged from 15 to 30 mm in diameter, with an average size of 21 mm. Posterior circulation aneurysms included eight basilar tip aneurysms, seven basilar trunk aneurysms, one vertebral artery aneurysm, one distal anterior inferior cerebellar artery aneurysm, and one distal superior cerebellar artery aneurysm. The latter two distal aneurysms were associated with arteriovenous malformations (AVMs) located on their feeding arteries.

## INTRODUCTION OF BALLOON CATHETER

The patient is placed on a radiolucent operating table. After induction of anesthesia, the head is fixed in the desired position with a standard Mayfield head holder. A No. 7 or 5 French gauge heparinized angiographic catheter[2] (Anthron; Toray Industries, Inc., Tokyo, Japan) is introduced coaxially through the femoral sheath to the vessels of interest under fluoroscopic control. For patients who undergo surgery in the prone or the lateral "park bench" position, transfemoral catheterization is done before fixation of the patient's position. Preoperative DSA (Model DF 5000; General Electric, Milwaukee, WI) is performed routinely to confirm that the aneurysm not being obscured by the head holder or skull fixation pins. Although we use a standard Mayfield three-pin head holder, satisfactory images can be obtained simply by adjusting the angle of the C-arm fluoroscope. More recently, we have introduced a radiolucent carbon-head holder (Mizuho Medical Instrument Co., Tokyo, Japan; Fig. 89–1). The silicone balloon (0.7 to 1.5 mm in uninflated diameter) attached to a No. 1.5 French gauge polyethylene catheter (DowCorning Corporation, Tokyo, Japan) is advanced through the angiographic catheter to the desired location for temporary vascular occlusion. The balloon is inflated temporarily to assess the appropriate inflation volume for occlusion of the parent artery, after which the balloon catheter is withdrawn back into the angiographic catheter to prevent thrombus formation. Both the femoral sheath and the angiographic

1221

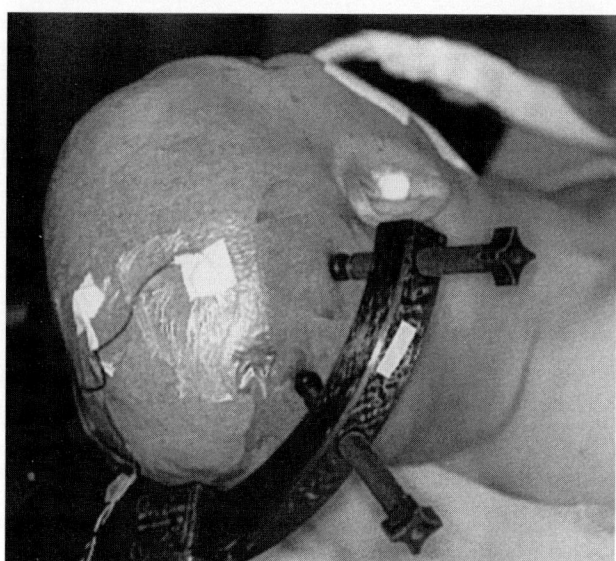

FIGURE 89-1 ■ The patient's head is fixed with a radiolucent carbon composite headholder. The electrodes for evoked potential monitoring were also placed.

catheter are flushed continually at 0.5 ml/min with heparinized saline (10 U/ml). In some patients operated on in a prone position, the balloon catheter is left in place throughout the surgery because catheter manipulations are often difficult during surgery. The femoral sheath can also be used intraoperatively as the arterial line for systemic blood pressure monitoring. The groin is sterilely draped and covered for the subsequent intraoperative catheterization procedures, and the craniotomy begun.

## SURGICAL PROCEDURES

Internal carotid artery aneurysms are ordinarily exposed through a standard pterional craniotomy; however, when

extensive removal of the anterior clinoid process is required for large paraclinoid ICA aneurysms or carotid cave aneurysms, we use Dolenc's combined epidural and intradural approach.[3] For posterior circulation aneurysms, various surgical approaches are used according to the location of the aneurysm: standard subtemporal approach, transzygomatic trans-sylvian approach, subtemporal transtentorial approach, transpetrosal approach, combined subtemporal and suboccipital approach, suboccipital retromastoid approach, and occipital transtentorial approach. In the case of aneurysms associated with AVMs, both lesions are treated in a single procedure.

The operation proceeds in a routine fashion until the stage of aneurysm dissection is reached, at which point the operation is temporarily interrupted. The operating microscope is moved, and the sterilely draped C-arm fluoroscope is positioned around the patient's head (Fig. 89-2). The balloon catheter is advanced again to the aimed location under fluoroscopic guidance. After confirming that the tip of the balloon catheter is placed in a suitable position for proximal vascular control, the C-arm is again moved and the operating microscope brought back for use. When these procedures are completed, the balloon is inflated for temporary vascular occlusion. This maneuver can be performed without fluoroscopic control because the appropriate inflation volume has been verified beforehand. For cerebral protection during temporary occlusion, we administer a solution of 500 ml of 20% mannitol with 500 mg of phenytoin and 500 mg of vitamin E.[4, 5] In surgery for posterior circulation aneurysms, the occluding balloon is placed in the basilar or vertebral artery approximately 1 cm proximal to the aneurysm. For PcomA or carotid cave aneurysms, the balloon is inflated at the horizontal cavernous segment of the ICA.

### Case Report 1

A 40-year-old man had a moderate subarachnoid hemorrhage 2 weeks before surgery. Preoperative angiography demonstrated a small basilar trunk aneu-

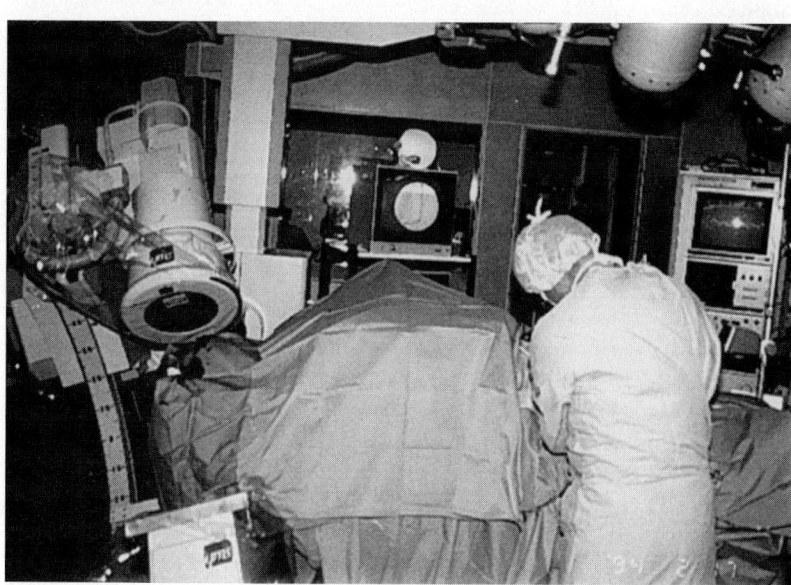

FIGURE 89-2 ■ The operating room setup during intraoperative angiography. The operating microscope was displaced, and the sterilely draped C-arm fluoroscope was positioned around the patient's head.

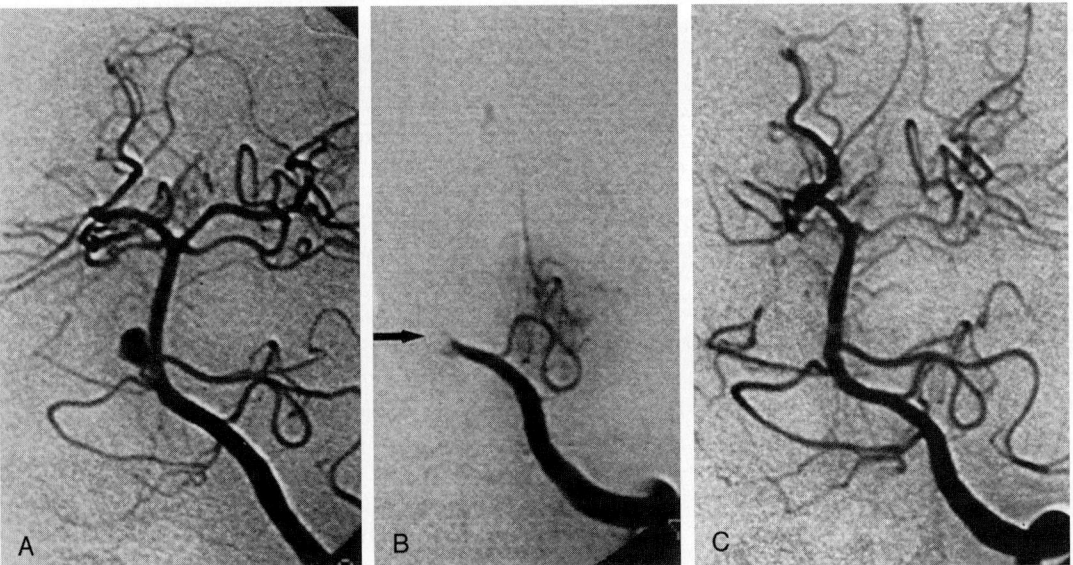

**FIGURE 89–3** ■ *Case 1. A,* Preoperative left vertebral angiogram, anteroposterior view, demonstrating a small basilar trunk aneurysm projecting laterally. This aneurysm was located 2.8 cm below from the posterior clinoid process. *B,* Intraoperative digital subtraction angiogram (DSA) demonstrating temporary balloon occlusion *(arrow)* of the basilar artery just proximal to the aneurysm. *C,* Intraoperative angiogram following clip placement showing the successful obliteration of an aneurysm.

rysm arising from the basilar artery at the distal crotch of the anterior inferior cerebellar artery origin (Fig. 89–3*A*). After induction of anesthesia, a balloon catheter was introduced into the basilar artery to approximately 1 cm proximal to the aneurysm. The balloon was temporarily inflated under DSA control to determine its suitable inflation volume (see Fig. 89–3*B*). Craniotomy was then begun with the balloon catheter left in place. Because the aneurysm was located relatively low (28 mm below the posterior clinoid process), it was approached through the right transpetrosal route. After the apex of the petrous bone was drilled off extradurally, the tentorium was widely opened. The aneurysm was identified below the eighth cranial nerve without retraction of the brain stem and cranial nerves. At this point, the balloon within the basilar artery was inflated. The aneurysm was then dissected and successfully clipped. The duration of basilar artery occlusion was 30 minutes. The initial intraoperative DSA after clip placement demonstrated a false-positive finding of basilar artery occlusion, but the final DSA after removal of the balloon catheter from the basilar artery showed successful clipping and vessel patency (see Fig. 89–3*C*). The patient did not have any postoperative neurologic deficits and returned to his previous work.

## RETROGRADE SUCTION DECOMPRESSION TECHNIQUE

For large or giant paraclinoid aneurysms, a retrograde suction decompression technique is used.[6, 7] A No. 5 or 7 French gauge double-lumen occlusion balloon catheter (Medi tech, Hanako, Inc., Tokyo, Japan) is introduced into the cervical ICA and the balloon is inflated. After tempo-

rary trapping of the aneurysm by balloon occlusion of the cervical ICA and clipping of the intracranial ICA distal to the aneurysm, retrograde aspiration of blood is initiated manually using a 20-ml heparinized syringe (Fig. 89–4). With this procedure, the aneurysm is completely deflated and its dissection greatly facilitated. It is often the case that in large paraclinoid aneurysms projecting inferiorly, the PcomA cannot be identified either in the preoperative angiograms or by intraoperative direct inspection. It is most important to preserve the patency of the anterior choroidal

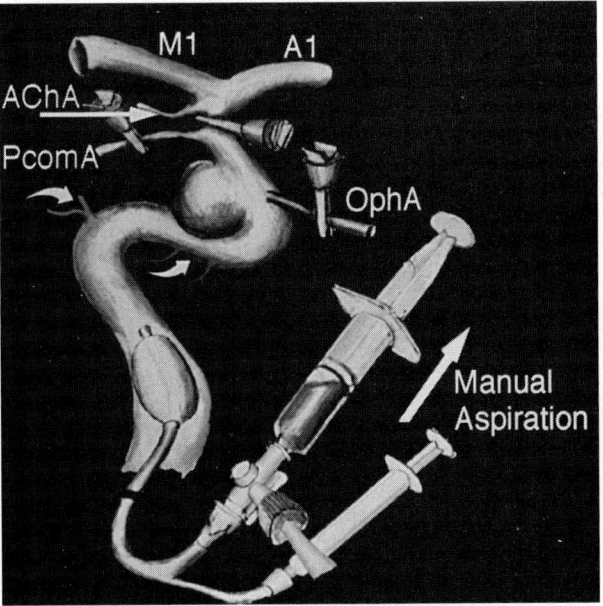

**FIGURE 89–4** ■ Schematic drawing showing the retrograde balloon suction decompression technique. (AChA, anterior choroidal artery; PcomA, posterior communicating artery; OphA, ophthalmic artery; A1, A1 segment of anterior cerebral artery; M1, M1 segment of middle cerebral artery.)

artery and clip the aneurysm while preserving sufficient lumen of the ICA.

In all of our cases, we confirm the results of clipping using intraoperative DSA, and if the results were unsatisfactory, the clip is readjusted. The catheter is removed after final examination of intraoperative DSA, but the femoral sheath is left in place until the end of the operation.

## Case Report 2

A 50-year-old woman presented with progressive loss of vision in the left eye. Computed tomography scan revealed a round mass lesion in the left suprasellar region and angiography demonstrated a 26-mm left paraclinoid ICA aneurysm (Fig. 89–5). Surgery was performed using the retrograde balloon suction decompression method. Under general anesthesia, the double-lumen balloon catheter was introduced into the left ICA by the transfemoral route. After confirming sufficient balloon inflation volume, the catheter was temporarily withdrawn back into the introducing catheter. A left pterional craniotomy was then performed. The anterior clinoid process was removed extradurally and the optic canal was unroofed. Because this large aneurysm had projected inferiorly and expanded close to the carotid dural ring, the proximal dome of the aneurysm was tightly adherent to the surrounding dura mater (Fig. 89–6A). At this point, the balloon catheter was again advanced into the cervical ICA and inflated to occlude the cervical ICA. The intracranial ICA (C1 segment) was also occluded, and retrograde suctioning begun. The aneurysm collapsed completely and was easily dissected (see Fig. 89–6B). The anterior choroidal artery was recognized

on the distal side of the aneurysm neck. Two Sugita fenestrated clips were applied in cross-wise fashion to reconstruct the lumen of the ICA (see Fig. 89–6C). The duration of temporary trapping of the ICA was 20 minutes. Approximately 200 ml of blood was aspirated during this procedure and simultaneously returned to the patient. The operation was completed after confirming the results of clip placement by DSA (Fig. 89–7). The patient awoke from anesthesia with no new neurologic deficits. Three months later, she had full recovery of vision in the left eye.

## RESULTS

### Intraoperative Digital Subtraction Angiography

In 20 of 75 aneurysms (27%), surgical alterations were required based on results obtained with intraoperative DSA. In nine paraclinoid or carotid cave aneurysms, narrowing of the parent artery was demonstrated by DSA and corrected by clip replacement. In 11 aneurysms, residual neck of the aneurysm was identified and corrected by clip repositioning or additional clip placement. However, of these 11 aneurysms, 2 were cases of giant posterior circulation aneurysm. In both cases, complete neck occlusion was impossible and surgery resulted in clipping the body of the aneurysms. Most of the early series of patients underwent postoperative conventional angiography. The findings of postoperative angiography were essentially identical to those obtained with intraoperative DSA. There were no false-negative results in the intraoperative DSA studies.

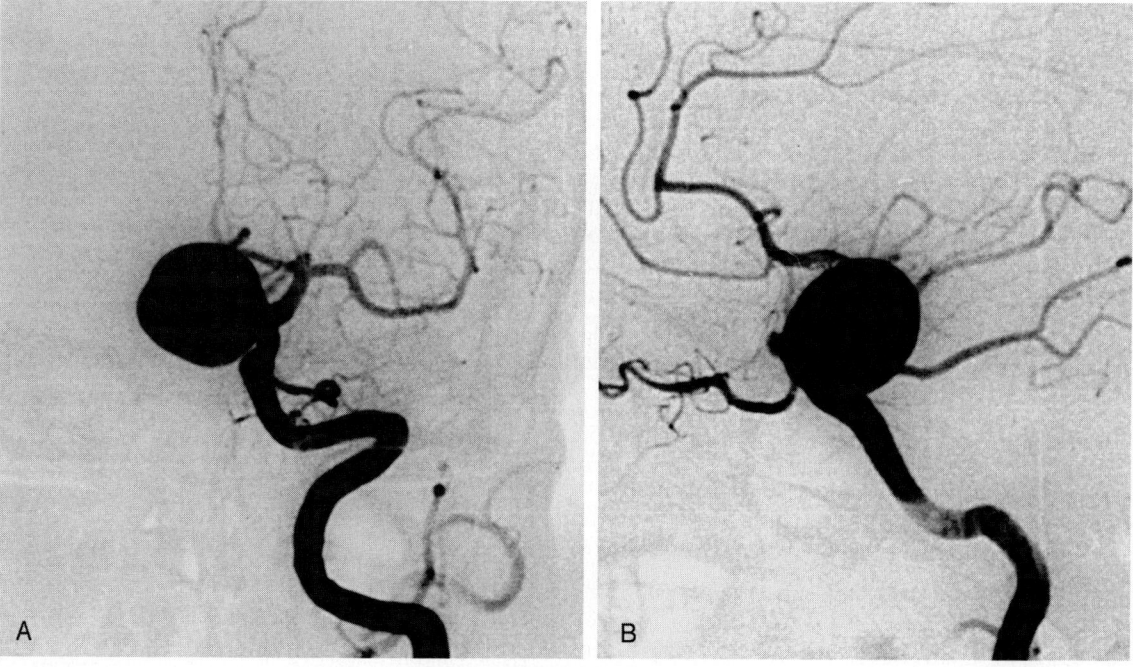

**FIGURE 89–5** ■ *Case 2.* Preoperative angiogram of the left internal carotid artery, demonstrating a giant paraclinoid aneurysm. *A*, Anteroposterior view. *B*, Lateral view.

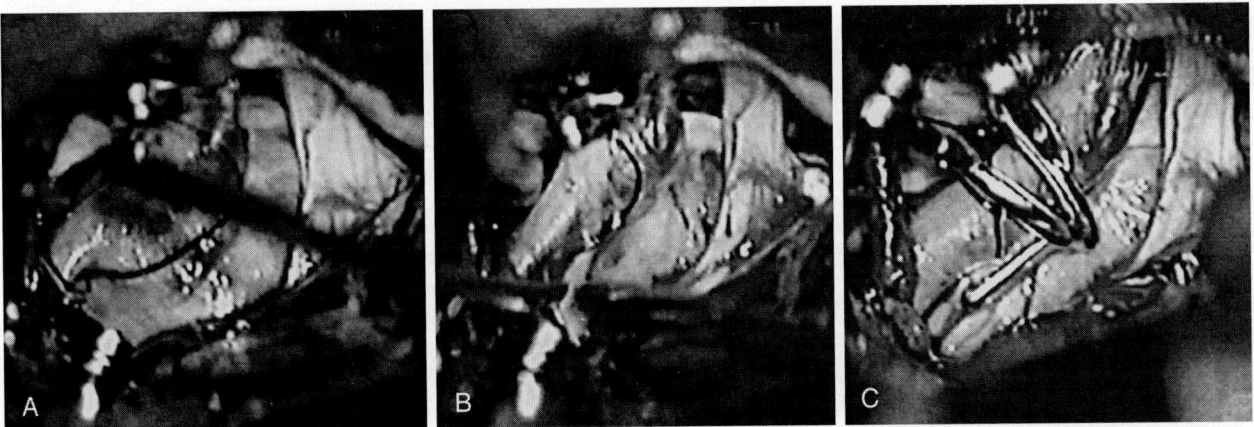

**FIGURE 89–6** ■ *Case 2. A*, Operative photographs of a giant paraclinoid aneurysm compressing the left optic nerve. *B*, The aneurysm was deflated and easily dissected with the aid of retrograde continuous blood aspiration. *C*, Two Sugita fenestrated clips were applied in cross-wise fashion to reconstruct the sufficient lumen of the internal carotid artery.

## Temporary Balloon Occlusion

In the operations for 48 aneurysms, the balloon catheter was placed in the vessels of interest, but temporary balloon occlusion was actually achieved in 37 aneurysms (78%). The remaining 11 aneurysms were treated without the use of temporary occlusion. The time required for the performance of preoperative vessel catheterization and intraoperative balloon technique was approximately 60 minutes. The duration of temporary occlusion among these 37 aneurysms ranged from 6 to 50 minutes, with a mean of 20.5 minutes. Intraoperative somatosensory evoked potential (SSEP) monitoring was also performed in most cases. Significant changes in SSEPs were not observed during occlusion in any case. There were no cases with postoperative sequelae attributable to ischemia caused by temporary balloon occlusion.

## Balloon Suction Decompression

We have used this method in 22 aneurysms in 21 patients. Carotid stump pressure was monitored through the distal lumen of the double-lumen balloon catheter placed in the cervical ICA. On inflating the balloon, the stump pressure fell to approximately 50%; however, contrary to expectations, after occlusion of the intracranial ICA above the aneurysm, the pressure increased to above the preocclusion level (Fig. 89–8). Operative findings also indicated that the aneurysm became more tense. However, on beginning retrograde aspiration, the aneurysm collapsed completely. The rate of blood aspiration was between 10 and 20 ml/min. When the syringe was exchanged and the aspiration temporarily interrupted, the aneurysm again inflated. The aspirated blood was returned to the patient intravenously. The total volume of aspirated blood differed among the patients, but was between 200 and 500 ml.

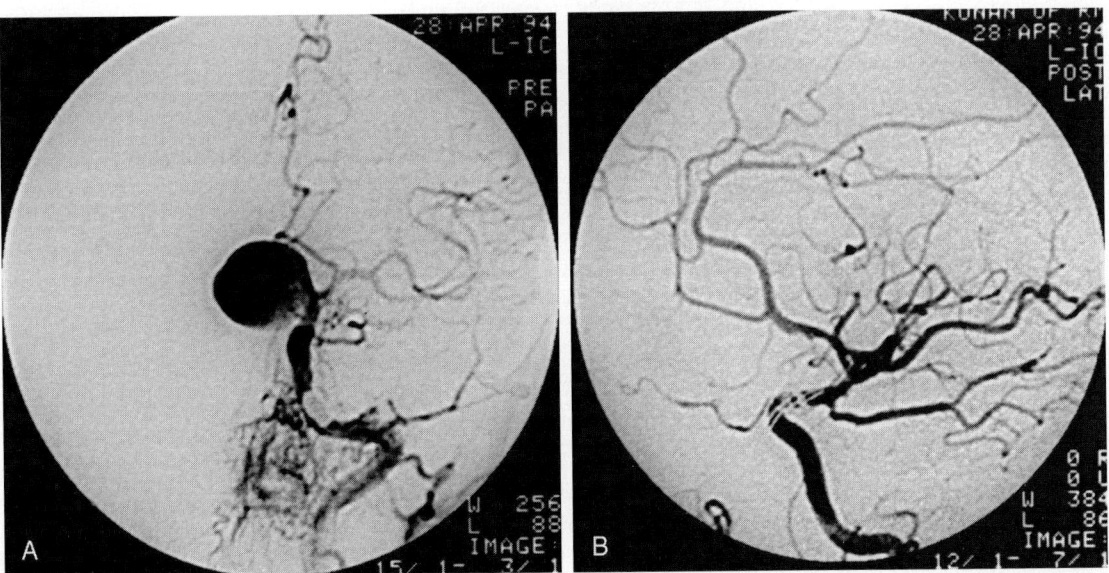

**FIGURE 89–7** ■ *Case 2. A*, Intraoperative angiogram before clip placement, demonstrating a large paraclinoid aneurysm. *B*, Intraoperative angiogram after aneurysmal clipping, showing a successful result.

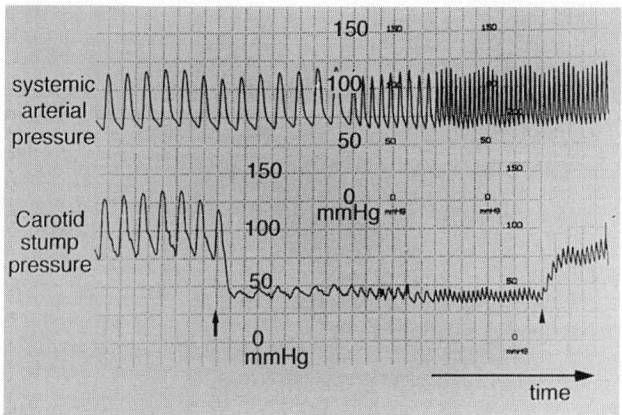

**FIGURE 89–8** ■ Continuous monitoring of the carotid stump pressure during the balloon suction decompression. On inflating the balloon within the cervical ICA *(arrow)*, the stump pressure decreased to approximately 30% of the preocclusion level; but subsequent occlusion of the ICA distal to the aneurysm *(arrowhead)* caused a paradoxical increase in stump pressure.

## Complications

Embolic complications attributable to the catheterization maneuver were seen in two cases. Both patients had large paraclinoid aneurysms treated using the retrograde suction decompression technique. In one patient, embolectomy was immediately carried out and no new neurologic deficits were observed after surgery. In another patient, the embolic complication was not detected during surgery and the patient had a postoperative persistent left hemiparesis.

## DISCUSSION

### Intraoperative Digital Subtraction Angiography

The need for intraoperative angiography in neurovascular surgery was recognized relatively early, and reports using such a technique in AVM surgery appeared by the late 1960s.[8–10] More recently, the development of portable DSA equipment has led to its use in many institutions.[11–16] Although it has been used in cases of cerebral aneurysm, AVM, bypass surgery, carotid endarterectomy, and spinal AVM, DSA is not always essential in such cases. Because intraoperative angiography is used primarily to detect inadequate surgical results before dural closure, its significance is not great in simple and uncomplicated operations. The experience and skill of the surgeon is the principal determinant of intraoperative angiography's usefulness.

Crucial for success in aneurysm surgery is complete closure of the aneurysm neck and preservation of patency of the parent artery and all adjacent arterial branches. Intraoperative DSA is used in complex aneurysms in which it may be difficult to accomplish these goals. From our experience, it is useful in surgery of large and broad-based aneurysms, as well as in surgery of aneurysms in deep locations where a wide operative field cannot be obtained, such as proximal ICA aneurysms and posterior circulation aneurysms. A wide operative field can usually be obtained

for middle cerebral artery aneurysms.[17] In complex anterior communicating artery aneurysms, a bifrontal interhemispheric approach allows for a sufficiently wide surgical field,[18] and intraoperative DSA rarely is needed.

Clip repositioning was required in 20 of 75 aneurysms. As Barrow and associates[15] have argued, if intraoperative DSA is available, the initial attempt at clipping is apt to be relatively easy and the results immediately examined. In all cases, an effort should be made to complete aneurysm clipping at the first attempt.

### Temporary Balloon Occlusion

Typically, proximal vascular control is difficult to obtain in large paraclinoid ICA and basilar trunk aneurysms. In such cases, temporary balloon occlusion can be used. Shucart and colleagues[19] and Bailes and coworkers[20] reported on a balloon occlusion method that we had developed independently in 1985.[21] Some surgeons may argue that the traditional method for exposing the cervical ICA provides sufficient proximal control for ICA aneurysms, but for lower basilar trunk aneurysms, there is no method for effective proximal control other than balloon occlusion.[22]

The most serious complication when using intraoperative occlusion technique is embolism. To prevent this complication, in most cases we keep the balloon catheter within the heparinized angiographic catheter during the surgery, proceed with the operation until balloon occlusion is required, and then advance the balloon catheter. This method has the disadvantage that the surgical procedure must be temporarily interrupted, but the interruption usually lasts only 15 to 20 minutes, during which the surgeon can relax and consider the plan for the subsequent operation. In all cases, a heparinized angiographic catheter is left in place throughout surgery. Systemic heparinization is not used, but embolic complications did not appear despite the catheter being kept in place for 4 to 8 hours. From our experiences with such cases, it seems that the heparinized catheter allows for prolonged intravascular placement without incurring embolic complications.[2]

We usually initiate vascular occlusion before dissection of the aneurysm itself. In the current series, the duration of balloon occlusion was relatively long (average, 21 minutes), but there were no ischemic symptoms caused by temporary occlusion. The administration of brain protective agents[4, 5] might achieve such good results. However, because there were no changes in SSEP monitoring during occlusion, these findings indicate that there was sufficient collateral flow in all cases.[23]

### Retrograde Balloon Suction Decompression

Flamm[24] was the first to report on a suction decompression method for giant aneurysms, in which the aneurysm was directly punctured using a No. 21 scalp vein needle. In puncturing the aneurysmal wall before treatment of the aneurysm, however, that technique may invite troublesome intraoperative bleeding. Subsequently, Batjer and Samson[25] and Tamaki and coworkers[26] reported retrograde suction methods in which the cervical ICA is exposed surgically and blood is aspirated from an angiocatheter inserted into the cervical ICA after clamping of both the cervical and intracranial ICA. Scott and colleagues[6] reported a less invasive modification of that method in which retrograde suction was done using a double-lumen balloon catheter. They also reported on their experience with the treatment of supraclinoid carotid aneurysms using balloon suction decompression in 12 patients, and described one complication of monocular blindness.[27] The balloon suction decompression technique is extremely effective for dissection of large paraclinoid aneurysms. However, even when the aneurysm is completely deflated, basic surgical procedures for the treatment of aneurysms in this location, such as extensive removal of the anterior clinoid process and sufficient exposure of the carotid dural ring, are still essential. Moreover, to make this method more certain and safer, further technologic improvements of the double-lumen balloon catheter are required. If the tip of the catheter makes contact with the inner surface of arterial wall, blood can no longer be aspirated. To avoid this problem, we have devised a new catheter with side holes, which is now being tested.

We noted an interesting phenomenon in our experience of this method.[7] While monitoring the carotid stump pressure by means of a double-lumen balloon catheter placed in the cervical ICA, inflation of the balloon (proximal occlusion) resulted in a sudden decrease in stump pressure to approximately 50% of the preocclusion level; subsequent occlusion of the intracranial ICA (distal occlusion), however, resulted in an increase in stump pressure to above the preocclusion level. This finding indicates that when an aneurysm is incompletely trapped, intra-aneurysmal pressure can be elevated by the retrograde flow through the remaining small branches. Even in cases where the ophthalmic artery, PcomA, and anterior choroidal artery have been occluded, similar increases in stump pressure are observed, suggesting the notable participation of retrograde flow from the cavernous ICA branches involving the meningohypophysial trunk. To our knowledge, this paradoxical phenomenon has not been previously reported. However, as Batjer and Samson[25] pointed out, many neurosurgeons may empirically be aware of this phenomenon through their experience that simple trapping of a large aneurysm by cervical ICA clamping and intracranial distal clipping does not adequately soften the lesion because of a brisk retrograde flow through the ophthalmic artery and cavernous branches. This phenomenon also implies that risk of aneurysmal rupture may increase after such a simple trapping as a result of the paradoxical rise in intra-aneurysmal pressure. There have been several case reports of patients who died from fatal rupture of a previously unruptured giant aneurysm after an extracranial-intracranial bypass with proximal carotid artery ligation.[28, 29] It is possible that the cause of rupture in those cases is a hemodynamic change similar to that seen in simple trapping.

We have used the suction decompression method only in cases of ICA aneurysms, but the indications for its use may expand with advances in technology to include giant posterior circulation aneurysms.

## REFERENCES

1. Kobayashi S, Kyoshima K, Gibo H, et al: Carotid cave aneurysms of the internal carotid artery. J Neurosurg 70:216–221, 1989.
2. Noishiki Y, Yamane Y, Takahashi M, et al: Prevention of thrombosis-related complications in cardiac catheterization and angiography using a heparinized catheter (Anthron). ASAIO Trans 33:359–365, 1987.
3. Dolenc VV: A combined epi- and subdural direct approach to carotid-ophthalmic artery aneurysms. J Neurosurg 62:667–672, 1985.
4. Suzuki J, Fujimoto S, Mizoi K, et al: The protective effect of combined administration of antioxidants and perfluorochemicals on cerebral ischemia. Stroke 15:672–679, 1984.
5. Suzuki J, Abiko H, Mizoi K, et al: Protective effect of phenytoin and its enhanced action by combined administration with mannitol and vitamin E in cerebral ischemia. Acta Neurochir (Wien) 88:56–64, 1987.
6. Scott JA, Horner TG, Leipzig TJ: Retrograde suction decompression of an ophthalmic artery aneurysm using balloon occlusion: Technical note. J Neurosurg 75:146–147, 1991.
7. Mizoi K, Takahashi A, Yoshimoto T, et al: Combined intravascular and neurosurgical approach for paraclinoid internal carotid artery aneurysms. Neurosurgery 33:986–992, 1993.
8. Loop JW, Foltz EL: Application of angiography during intracranial operation. Acta Radiol Diagn 5:363–367, 1966.
9. Bartal AD, Tirosh MS, Weinstein M: Angiographic control during total excision of a cerebral arteriovenous malformation: Technical note. J Neurosurg 29:211–213, 1968.
10. Peeters FLM, Walder HAD: Intraoperative vertebral angiography in arteriovenous malformations. Neuroradiology 6:169–173, 1973.
11. Foley KT, Cahan LD, Hieshima GB: Intraoperative angiography using a portable digital subtraction unit: Technical note. J Neurosurg 64:816–818, 1986.
12. Hieshima GB, Reicher MA, Higashida RT, et al: Intraoperative digital subtraction neuroangiography: A diagnostic and therapeutic tool. AJNR Am J Neuroradiol 8:759–767, 1987.
13. Batjer HH, Frankfurt AI, Purdy PD, et al: Use of etomidate, temporary arterial occlusion, and intraoperative angiography in surgical treatment of large and giant cerebral aneurysms. J Neurosurg 68:234–240, 1988.
14. Martin NA, Bentson J, Vinuela F, et al: Intraoperative digital subtraction angiography and the surgical treatment of intracranial aneurysms and vascular malformations. J Neurosurg 73:526–533, 1990.
15. Barrow DL, Boyer KL, Joseph GJ: Intraoperative angiography in the management of neurovascular disorders. Neurosurgery 30:153–159, 1992.
16. Mizoi K, Takahashi A, Yoshimoto T, et al: Surgical excision of giant cerebellar hemispheric arteriovenous malformations following preoperative embolization: Report of two cases. J Neurosurg 1992; 76: 1008–1011.
17. Suzuki J, Yoshimoto T, Kayama T: Surgical treatment of middle cerebral artery aneurysms. J Neurosurg 61:17–23, 1984.
18. Suzuki J, Mizoi K, Yoshimoto T: Bifrontal interhemispheric approach to aneurysms of the anterior communicating artery. J Neurosurg 64:183–190, 1986.
19. Shucart WA, Kwan ES, Heilman CB: Temporary balloon occlusion of a proximal vessel as an aid to clipping aneurysms of the basilar and paraclinoid internal carotid arteries: Technical note. Neurosurgery 27:116–119, 1990.
20. Bailes JE, Deeb ZL, Wilson JA et al: Intraoperative angiography and temporary balloon occlusion of the basilar artery as an adjunct to surgical clipping: Technical note. Neurosurgery 30:949–953, 1992.
21. Suzuki J, Takahashi A, Yoshimoto T, et al: Use of balloon occlusion and substances to protect ischemic brain during resection of posterior fossa AVM: Case report. J Neurosurg 63:626–629, 1985.
22. Mizoi K, Yoshimoto T, Takahashi A, et al: Direct clipping of basilar trunk aneurysms using balloon temporary occlusion. J Neurosurg 80:230–236, 1994.
23. Mizoi K, Yoshimoto T: Permissible temporary occlusion time in aneurysm surgery as evaluated by evoked potential monitoring. Neurosurgery 33:434–440, 1993.
24. Flamm ES: Suction decompression of aneurysms: Technical note. J Neurosurg 54:275–276, 1981.
25. Batjer HH, Samson DS: Retrograde suction decompression of giant paraclinoidal aneurysms: Technical note. J Neurosurg 73:305–306, 1990.
26. Tamaki N, Kim S, Ehara K, et al: Giant carotid-ophthalmic artery aneurysms: Direct clipping utilizing the "trapping-evacuation" technique. J Neurosurg 74:567–572, 1991.

27. Scott JA, Horner TG, Leipzig TJ: Retrograde suction decompression of an ophthalmic artery aneurysm using balloon occlusion: Technical note. J Neurosurg 75:146–147, 1991.

28. Matsuda M, Shiino A, Handa J: Rupture of previously unruptured giant carotid aneurysm after superficial temporal-middle cerebral artery bypass and internal carotid occlusion. Neurosurgery 16:177–184, 1985.

29. Scott RM, Liu HC, Yuan R, Adelman L: Rupture of a previously unruptured giant middle cerebral artery aneurysm after extracranial-intracranial bypass surgery. Neurosurgery 10:600–603, 1982.

# Index

Note: Page numbers in *italic* indicate illustrations; those followed by t refer to tables.